P9-AQX-656

YOUMANS
Neurological Surgery

VOLUME

1

Introduction to Neurological Surgery

Michel Kliot

Oncology

Henry Brem and Raymond Sawaya

VOLUME

2

Vascular

Robert F. Spetzler and Fredric B. Meyer

Epilepsy

Daniel L. Silbergeld

VOLUME

3

Functional Neurosurgery

Roy A. E. Bakay and Kim J. Burchiel

Pain

Kim J. Burchiel

Pediatric Neurosurgery

T. S. Park and R. Michael Scott

VOLUME

4

Peripheral Nerve

Michel Kliot

Radiation Therapy and Radiosurgery

L. Dade Lunsford and William A. Friedman

Spine

Volker K. H. Sonntag and Dennis G. Vollmer

Trauma

Lawrence F. Marshall and M. Sean Grady

Special Features

Marc R. Mayberg and Joel D. MacDonald

YOUMANS

Neurological Surgery

Fifth Edition

H. Richard Winn, MD
Professor of Neurological Surgery
and Neuroscience
Mount Sinai School of Medicine
New York, New York

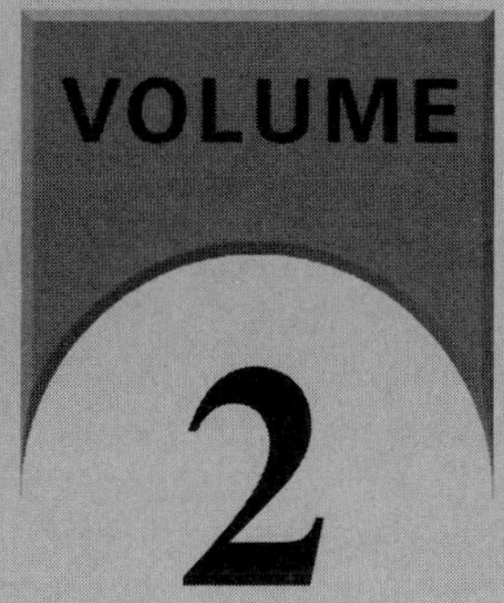

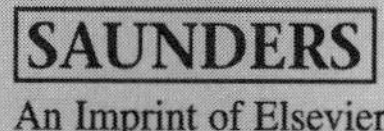

An Imprint of Elsevier

SAUNDERS
An Imprint of Elsevier

The Curtis Center
Independence Square West
Philadelphia, Pennsylvania 19106

YOUMANS NEUROLOGICAL SURGERY
Copyright 2004, Elsevier Inc. All rights reserved. ISBN 0-7216-8291-x.

No part of this publication may be reproduced, stored in a retrieval system, or transmitted in any form or by any means, electronic, mechanical, photocopying, recording, or otherwise, without prior permission of the publisher (Saunders, The Curtis Center, Independence Square West, Philadelphia, PA 19106-3399).

Notice

Neurosurgery is an ever-changing field. Standard safety precautions must be followed, but as new research and clinical experience broaden our knowledge, changes in treatment and drug therapy become necessary or appropriate. Readers are advised to check the product information currently provided by the manufacturer of each drug to be administered to verify the recommended dose, the method and duration of administration, and the contraindications. It is the responsibility of the treating physician, relying on experience and knowledge of the patient, to determine dosage and the best treatment for each individual patient. Neither the publisher nor the editor assumes any responsibility for any injury and/or damage to persons or property arising from this publication.

The Publisher

First Edition 1973. Second Edition 1982. Third Edition 1990. Fourth Edition 1996.

Library of Congress Cataloging-in-Publication Data

Youmans neurological surgery / [edited by] H. Richard Winn.—5th ed.

p. cm.

Rev. ed. of: Neurological surgery / editor-in-chief, Julian R. Youmans; associate editors, Donald P. Becker . . . [et al.]. 4th ed. c1996.

Includes bibliographical references and index.

ISBN 0–7216–8291–X

1. Nervous system—Surgery. I. Title: Neurological surgery. II. Winn, H. Richard. III. Youmans, Julian R., 1928–
[DNLM: 1. Neurosurgical Procedures. 2. Nervous System Diseases—surgery. 3. Neurosurgery—methods. WL 368 Y671 2003]

RE593 N4153 2003

617.4′8—dc21 2002017677

Vice President, Global Surgery: Richard Lampert

Developmental Editors: Anne Snyder, David Orzechowski

Project Manager: Jodi Kaye

Printed in the United States of America.

Last digit is the print number: 9 8 7 6 5 4 3 2 1

To my wife and family, and to my residents who have carried the message.

EDITOR-IN-CHIEF

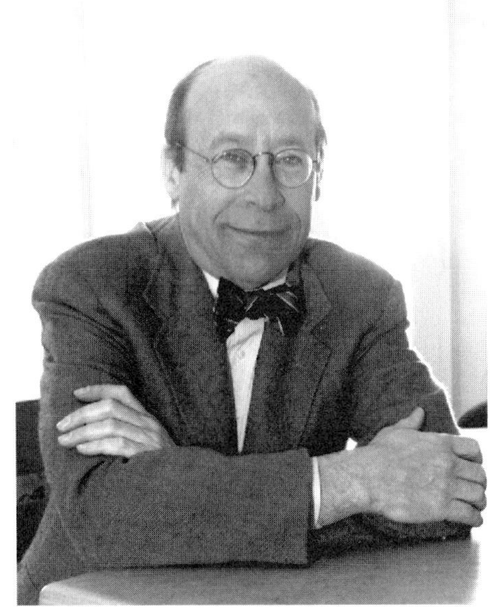

H. Richard Winn, MD
Professor of Neurological Surgery and Neuroscience
Mount Sinai School of Medicine
New York, New York

DEPUTY EDITOR-IN-CHIEF

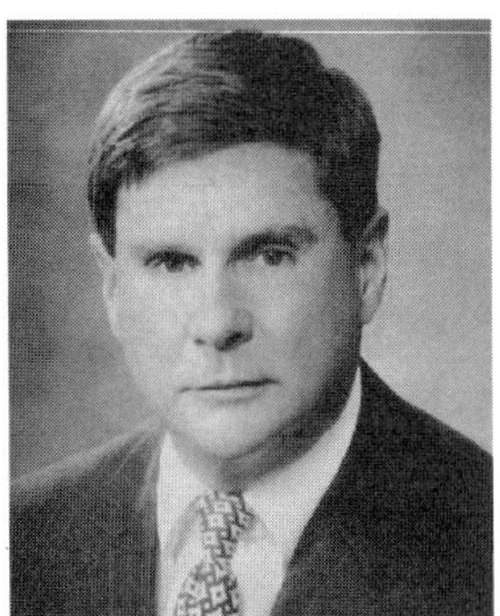

Ralph G. Dacey, Jr., MD
Henry G. and Edith R. Schwartz Professor and Chairman
Department of Neurological Surgery
Washington University School of Medicine
St. Louis, Missouri

SECTION EDITORS

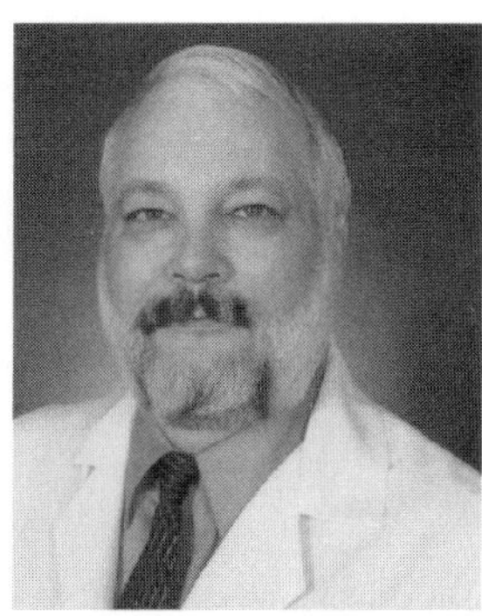

Roy A. E. Bakay, MD
Professor and Vice Chairman
Department of Neurosurgery
Rush Medical Center
Chicago, Illinois
Functional Neurosurgery, Volume 3

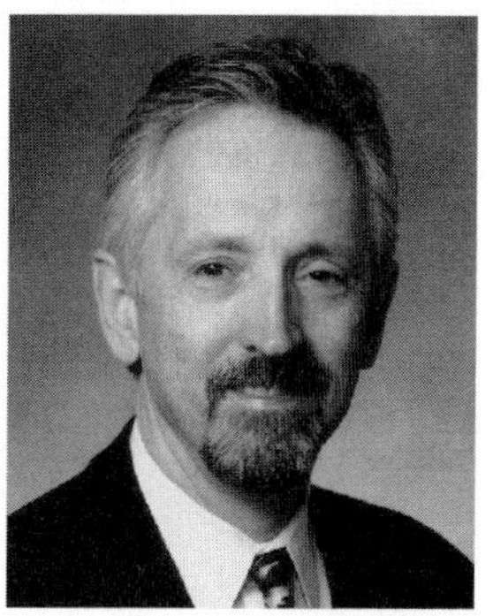

Kim J. Burchiel, MD
Professor and Chairman
Department of Neurological Surgery
Oregon Health & Science University
School of Medicine
Portland, Oregon
Functional Neurosurgery and Pain, Vol. 3

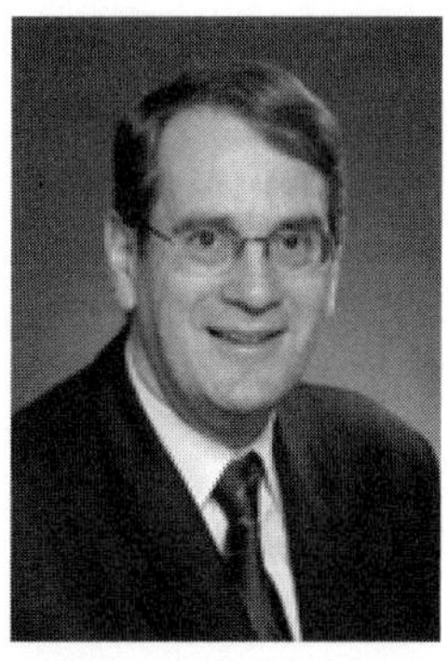

Henry Brem, MD
Harvey Cushing Professor of Neurosurgery,
Ophthalmology, and Oncology
Chairman, Department of Neurosurgery
Johns Hopkins University School of Medicine
Baltimore, Maryland
Oncology, Volume 1

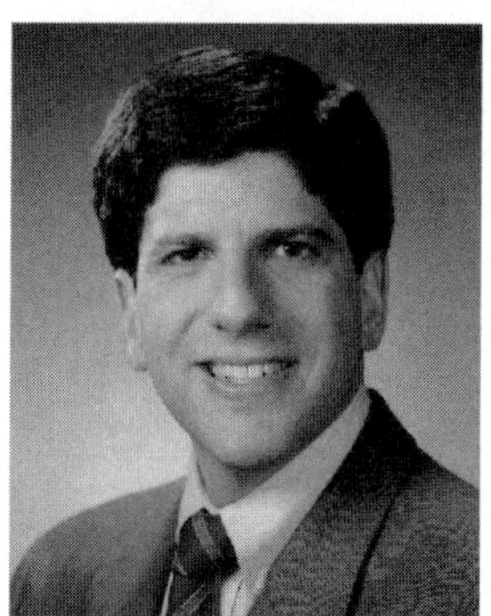

William A. Friedman, M.D.
Professor and Chair,
Department of Neurosurgery
University of Florida,
Gainesville, Florida
Radiation Therapy and Radiosurgery, Volume 4

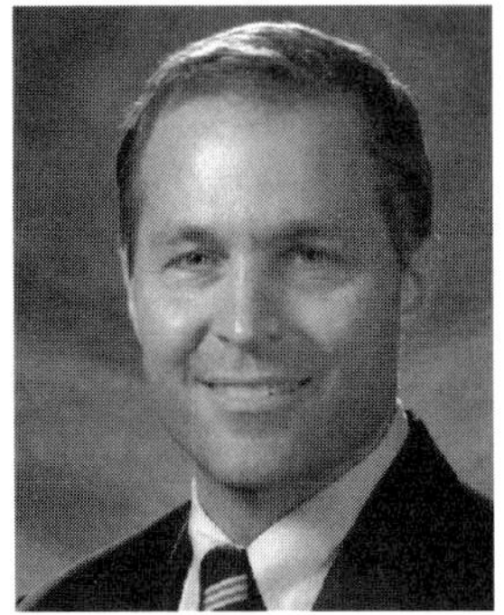

M. Sean Grady, MD
Charles Harrison Frazier Professor and Chair of the Department of Neurosurgery
University of Pennsylvania School of Medicine
Philadelphia, Pennsylvania

Trauma, Volume 4

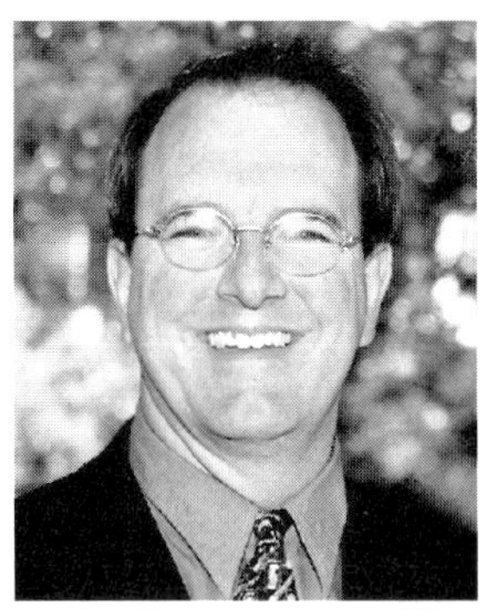

Joel D. MacDonald, MD
Assistant Professor of Neurosurgery
University of Utah Medical Center
Salt Lake City, Utah

Special Features

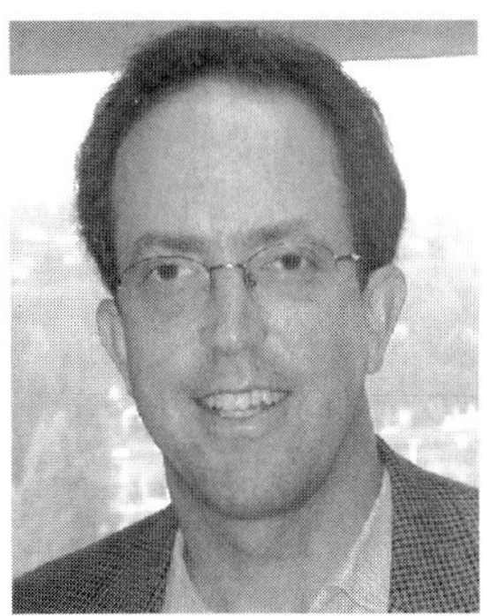

Michel Kliot, MD
Associate Professor of Neurosurgery
University of Washington School of Medicine
Seattle, Washington

Introduction to Neurological Surgery, Volume 1; Peripheral Nerve, Volume 4

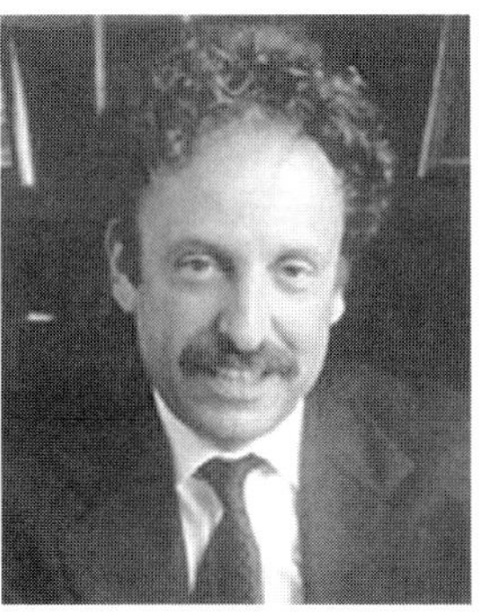

Lawrence F. Marshall, MD
Professor of Neurological Surgery
University of California, San Diego, School of Medicine
San Diego, California

Trauma, Volume 4

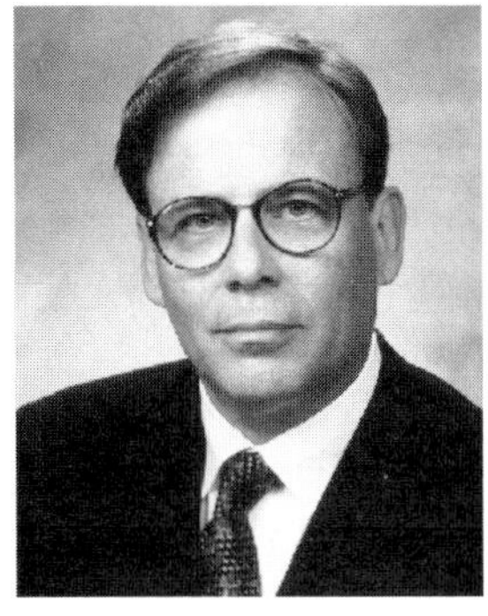

L. Dade Lunsford, MD
Lars Leksell Professor and Chairman of Neurological Surgery, Radiology, and Radiology Oncology
University of Pittsburgh School of Medicine
University of Pittsburgh Medical Center
Pittsburgh, Pennsylvania

Radiation Therapy and Radiosurgery, Volume 4

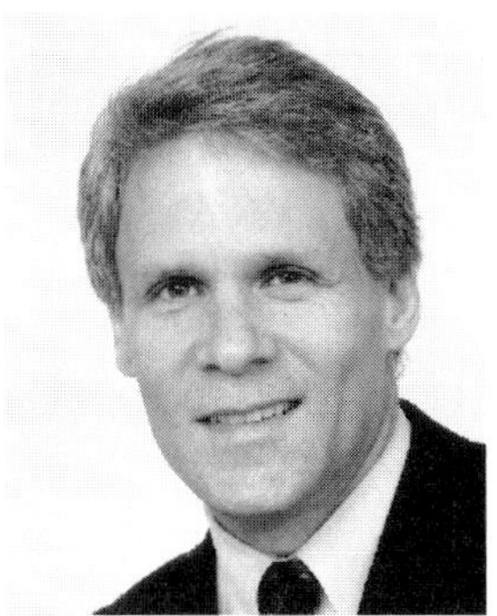

Marc R. Mayberg, MD
Chairman, Department of Neurosurgery
Cleveland Clinic Foundation
Cleveland, Ohio

Special Features

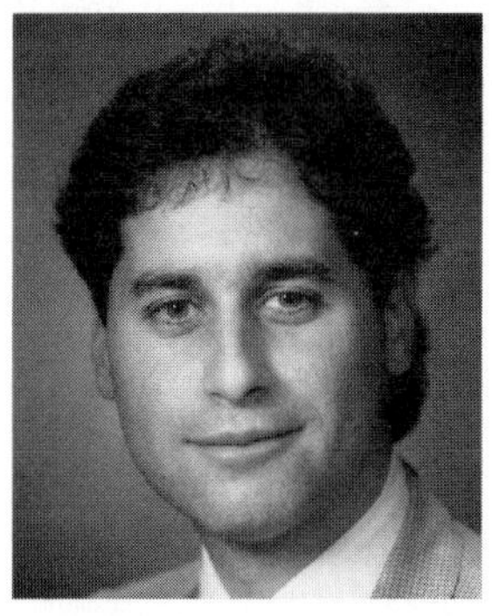

Fredric B. Meyer, MD
Professor of Neurosurgery
Mayo Medical School
Rochester, Minnesota
Vascular, Volume 2

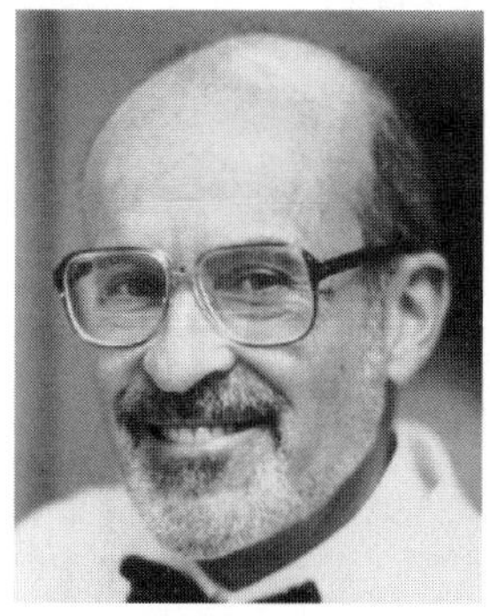

R. Michael Scott, MD
Professor of Neurological Surgery
Harvard Medical School
Boston, Massachusetts
Pediatric, Volume 3

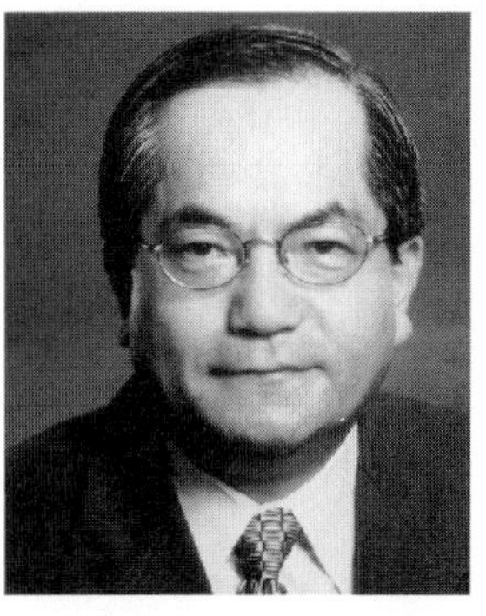

T. S. Park, MD
Shi H. Huang Professor of Neurosurgery and
Professor of Pediatrics and Anatomy and
Neurobiology
Washington University School of Medicine
St. Louis, Missouri
Pediatric, Volume 3

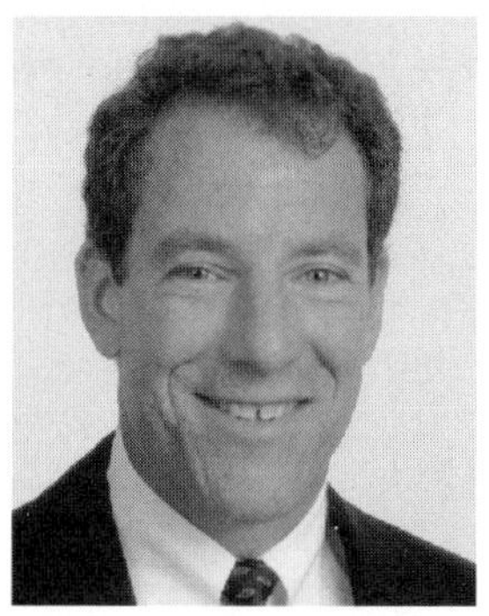

Daniel L. Silbergeld, MD
Associate Professor, Department of
Neurological Surgery
University of Washington School of Medicine
Seattle, Washington
Epilepsy, Volume 2

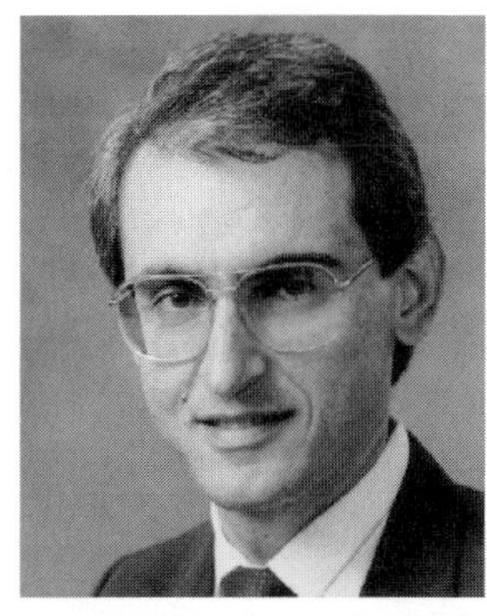

Raymond Sawaya, MD
Professor of Neurosurgery
University of Texas–Houston Medical School
Department of Neurosurgery
The University of Texas MD Anderson Cancer Center
Houston, Texas
Oncology, Volume 1

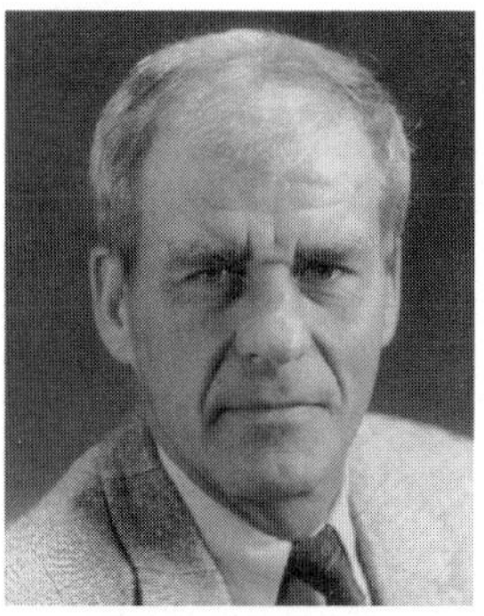

Volker K. H. Sonntag, MD
Clinical Professor of Neurosurgery
University of Arizona College of Medicine
Tucson, Arizona
Vice Chairman, Division of Neurological Surgery
Barrow Neurological Institute
Phoenix, Arizona
Spine, Volume 4

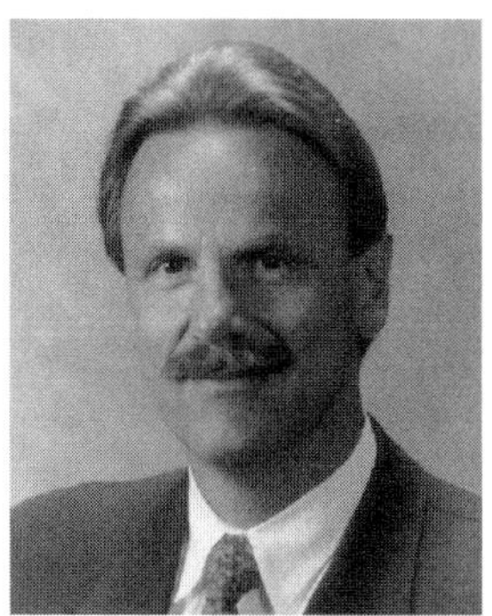

Robert F. Spetzler, MD
Professor, Department of Surgery,
Section of Neurosurgery
University of Arizona College of Medicine
Tucson, Arizona
Director and J. N. Harbor Chairman of
Neurological Surgery
Barrow Neurological Institute
Phoenix, Arizona
Vascular, Volume 2

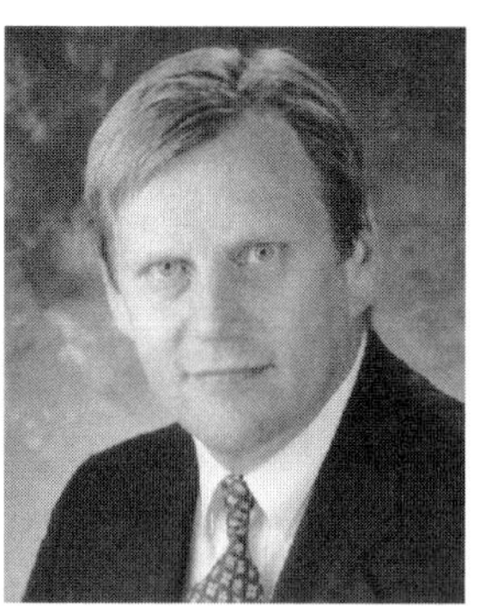

Dennis G. Vollmer, MD
Professor of Neurosurgery
University of Texas Health Science Center at Houston
Houston, Texas
Spine, Volume 4

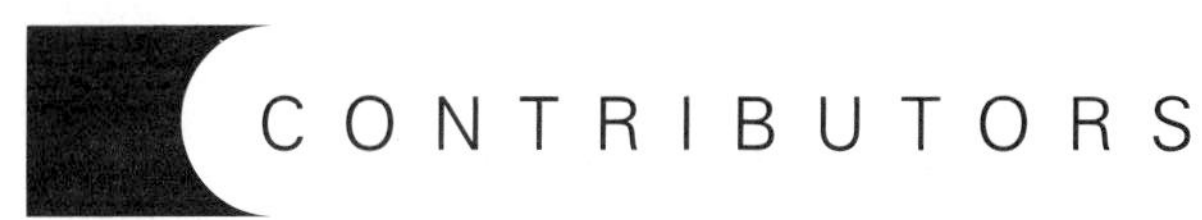

CONTRIBUTORS

Khaled M. Abdel Aziz, MD, PhD

Resident, Department of Neurosurgery, University of Cincinnati College of Medicine and University Hospital, Cincinnati, Ohio

Dorsal Rhizotomy and Dorsal Root Ganglionectomy

Muwaffak M. Abdulhak, MD

Clinical Instructor, Department of Neurosurgery, Medical College of Wisconsin, Milwaukee, Wisconsin

Bone Metabolism as It Relates to Spinal Disease and Treatment

Saleem I. Abdulrauf, MD

Assistant Professor, Neurological Surgery and Director, Cerebrovascular and Skull Base Surgery Program, Saint Louis University School of Medicine; Director, Cerebrovascular and Skull Base Surgery Program, Saint Louis University Hospital, St. Louis, Missouri

Meningiomas

Dima Abi-Said, MD

Attending, Department of Neurosurgery, The University of Texas M.D. Anderson Cancer Center, Houston, Texas

Metastatic Brain Tumors

John R. Adler, Jr., MD

Professor, Department of Neurosurgery, Stanford University School of Medicine, Stanford, California

General and Historical Considerations of Radiotherapy and Radiosurgery

Robin Albert, MD, MPH

Research Coordinator, Center for Endovascular Surgery, Institute for Neurology and Neurosurgery, Beth Israel Medical Center, New York, New York

Endovascular Management of Brain Arteriovenous Malformations

A. Leland Albright, MD

Professor of Neurosurgery, University of Pittsburgh School of Medicine; Chief, Pediatric Neurosurgery, Childrens Hospital of Pittsburgh, Pittsburgh, Pennsylvania

Patient Selection in Movement Disorder Surgery; Brainstem Gliomas

Felipe C. Albuquerque, MD

Staff Neurosurgeon and Assistant Director, Endovascular Neurosurgery, Barrow Neurological Institute, Phoenix, Arizona

Carotid Angioplasty and Stenting: Interventional Treatment of Occlusive Vascular Disease; Basilar Trunk Aneurysms

Kenneth Aldape, MD

Assistant Professor, Department of Pathology, Neuropathology Unit, University of California, San Francisco, School of Medicine, San Francisco, California

Low-Grade Gliomas: Astrocytoma, Oligodendroglioma, and Mixed Gliomas

Eben Alexander III, MD

Associate Professor of Surgery, Department of Surgery, Division of Neurosurgery, University of Massachusetts Medical School; Attending Neurosurgeon, University of Massachusetts-Memorial Hospitals, Worcester, Massachusetts

Linac Radiosurgery

Michael J. Alexander, MD

Assistant Professor, Department of Surgery, Divisions of Neurosurgery and Interventional Neuroradiology, Duke University School of Medicine, Durham, North Carolina

Nonatherosclerotic Carotid Lesions

Mir Jafar Ali, MD

Resident, Department of Neurosurgery, University of Michigan Hospital, Ann Arbor, Michigan

Basilar Apex and Posterior Cerebral Artery Aneurysms

Ahmed Alkhani, MD

Fellow in Functional Neurosurgery, University of Toronto Faculty of Medicine and Toronto Western Hospital, Toronto, Ontario, Canada

Pallidotomy for Parkinson's Disease

Cargill H. Alleyne, Jr., MD

Co-Director, Neurosurgery Residency Program, University of Rochester School of Medicine and Dentistry; Chief, Division of Stroke and Cerebrovascular Surgery, Department of Surgery, Rochester General Hospital, Rochester, New York

Carotid Angioplasty and Stenting: Interventional Treatment of Occlusive Vascular Disease; Traumatic Carotid Injury

Ossama Al-Mefty, MD
Professor and Chairman, Department of Neurosurgery, University of Arkansas for Medical Sciences, Little Rock, Arkansas
Meningiomas

Mahmoud Al-Yamany, MD
Department of Neurosurgery, Riyadh Medical Complex, King Saud University Affiliated Hospital, Riyadh, Saudi Arabia
Intracranial Internal Carotid Artery Aneurysms

Arun Paul Amar, MD
Clinical Instructor, Department of Neurosurgery, University of Southern California Keck School of Medicine; Staff, Children's Hospital of Los Angeles, Los Angeles, California
Ventricular Tumors; Vagus Nerve Stimulation for Intractable Epilepsy

Christopher Ames, MD
Assistant Professor, Department of Neurological Surgery, University of California, San Francisco, School of Medicine, San Francisco, California
Differential Diagnosis of Altered States of Consciousness

Sepideh Amin-Hanjani, MD
Instructor in Surgery, Harvard Medical School; Assistant Visiting Surgeon, Department of Neurosurgery, Massachusetts General Hospital, Boston, Massachusetts
Cerebral Lymphoma

Norberto Andaluz, MD
Clinical Fellow, Department of Neurosurgery, University of Cincinnati College of Medicine, Cincinnati, Ohio
Dorsal Rhizotomy and Dorsal Root Ganglionectomy

Peter Angevine, MD
Resident, Department of Neurological Surgery, Columbia-Presbyterian Medical Center, New York, New York
Anterior Lumbar Instrumentation

Ronald I. Apfelbaum, MD
Professor of Neurosurgery, University of Utah School of Medicine; Attending, University of Utah Hospital and Clinics, Salt Lake City, Utah
Treatment of Axis Fractures

Michael L. J. Apuzzo, MD
Edwin M. Todd/Treat M. Wells, Jr. Professor of Neurological Surgery and Professor of Radiation Oncology, Biology, and Physics, University of Southern California Keck School of Medicine; Staff, USC Care Medical Group, USC University Hospital, and USC/Norris Cancer Hospital, Los Angeles, California
Ventricular Tumors; Vagus Nerve Stimulation for Intractable Epilepsy

Claire Ardouin, MA
Psychologist, Hôpital Albert Michallon, Grenoble, France
Deep Brain Stimulation for Movement Disorders

E. Joy Arpin-Sypert, MD
Sypert Institute, Fort Myers, Florida
Evaluation and Management of the Failed Back Syndrome

James I. Ausman, MD
Professor of Neurosurgery, University of Illinois at Chicago, Chicago, Illinois; Editor, *Surgical Neurology*
Extracranial Vertebral Artery Disease

Issam A. Awad, MD, MSc
Ogsbury-Kindt Professor and Chairman, Department of Neurosurgery, and Professor of Neurosurgery, Neurology, and Pathology, University of Colorado School of Medicine, Denver, Colorado
Surgical Management of Supratentorial Cavernous Malformations

Julian E. Bailes, MD
Professor and Chairman, Department of Neurosurgery, West Virginia University School of Medicine, Morgantown, West Virginia
Carotid Endarterectomy

Roy A. E. Bakay, MD
Professor and Vice Chairman, Director of Movement Disorder Surgery, Rush-Presbyterian-St. Luke's Medical Center, Chicago Institute of Neurosurgery and Neuroresearch, Chicago, Illinois
History of Functional Neurosurgery; Cellular Transplantation in the Central Nervous System

Perry A. Ball, MD
Attending Neurosurgeon, Section of Neurosurgery, Dartmouth-Hitchcock Medical Center, Lebanon, New Hampshire
Treatment of Disk Disease of the Lumbar Spine

Gordon H. Baltuch, MD, PhD
Assistant Professor, Department of Neurosurgery, University of Pennsylvania School of Medicine; Attending Neurosurgeon, Hospital of the University of Pennsylvania, Pennsylvania Hospital, and Philadelphia Veterans Administration Medical Center, Philadelphia, Pennsylvania
Topectomy: Uses and Indications

Gene H. Barnett, MD
Professor of Surgery, Ohio State University College of Medicine and Public Health, Columbus; Chairman, Brain Tumor Institute, Cleveland Clinic Foundation, Cleveland, Ohio
Surgical Navigation for Brain Tumors

Stanley L. Barnwell, MD, PhD

Associate Professor of Neurological Surgery, Oregon Health & Science University School of Medicine; Staff, Dotter Interventional Institute, Portland, Oregon

Cerebral Venous and Sinus Thrombosis

Jean-Claude Baron, MD

Professor of Stroke Medicine, Department of Neurology, University of Cambridge Faculty of Medicine; Neurology Consultant, Addenbrooke's Hospital, Cambridge, England

Positron Emission Tomography in Cerebrovascular Disease

Daniel L. Barrow, MD

MBNA-Bowman Professor and Chairman, Department of Neurological Surgery, Emory University School of Medicine; Chief, Neurological Service, and Co-Director, Emory Stroke Center, Emory University Hospital, Atlanta, Georgia

Treatment of Lateral-Sigmoid and Sagittal Sinus Dural Arteriovenous Malformations

Juan Bartolomei, MD

Assistant Professor, Department of Neurosurgery, Yale University School of Medicine, New Haven, Connecticut

Anterior Approach including Cervical Corpectomy (Degenerative)

Jonathan J. Baskin, MD

Attending Neurosurgeon, Atlantic Neurosurgical Specialists, Chatham, New Jersey

Carotid Angioplasty and Stenting; Interventional Treatment of Occlusive Vascular Disease; Anterior Cervical Instrumentation; Occipitocervical Fusion

H. Hunt Batjer, MD

Professor and Chair, Department of Neurological Surgery, Northwestern University Feinberg School of Medicine; Chairman, Department of Neurological Surgery, Northwestern Memorial Hospital, Chicago, Illinois

Basilar Apex and Posterior Cerebral Artery Aneurysms

Thomas K. Baumann, PhD

Associate Professor, Department of Neurological Surgery and Department of Physiology and Pharmacology, Oregon Health and Science University School of Medicine, Portland, Oregon

Physiologic Anatomy of Pain

Andrew Beaumont, MD

Neurosurgical Fellow, Virginia Commonwealth University School of Medicine, Richmond, Virginia

Physiology of the Cerebrospinal Fluid and Intracranial Pressure

Joshua Bederson, MD

Professor, Department of Neurosurgery, Mount Sinai School of Medicine; Vice Chairman, Department of Neurosurgery, Mount Sinai Medical Center, New York, New York

Infectious Intracranial Aneurysms

Ghassan K. Bejjani, MD

Clinical Assistant Professor, Department of Neurosurgery, University of Pittsburgh School of Medicine; Neurosurgeon, Presbyterian University Hospital, Pittsburgh, Pennsylvania

Orbital Tumors

J. Brad Bellotte, MD

Resident, Department of Neurosurgery, Allegheny General Hospital, Pittsburgh, Pennsylvania

Brain Death; Diagnosis and Management of Seventh and Eighth Cranial Nerve Injuries due to Temporal Bone Fractures

Alim L. Benabid, MD, PhD

Professor of Biophysics, University Joseph Fourier Medical School; Head, Neurosurgery, and Director, INSERM U.318 Research Laboratory of Preclinical Neurosciences, Hôpital Albert Michallon, Grenoble, France

Deep Brain Stimulation for Movement Disorders

Eduardo E. Benarroch, MD

Professor of Neurology, Mayo Medical School; Consultant in Neurology, Mayo Clinic, Rochester, Minnesota

Cerebral Blood Flow and Metabolism

Abdelhamid Benazzouz, PhD

Research Fellow, University of Bordeaux School of Medicine; Director of Research, Neurophysiology Laboratory, University Victor Segalan, Bordeaux, France

Deep Brain Stimulation for Movement Disorders

Bernard R. Bendok, MD

Assistant Professor, Department of Neurological Surgery, Northwestern University Feinberg School of Medicine, Chicago, Illinois

Basilar Apex and Posterior Cerebral Artery Aneurysms

Gregory J. Bennett, MD

Clinical Assistant Professor of Neurosurgery, University of Buffalo; Clinical Director of Neurosurgery, Erie County Medical Center, Buffalo, New York

Spondylolysis and Spondylolisthesis

Alejandro Berenstein, MD

Professor of Radiology, Neurosurgery, and Neurology, Albert Einstein College of Medicine of Yeshiva University, Bronx; Director, Center for Endovascular Surgery, and Director, Institute for Neurology and Neurosurgery, Beth Israel Medical Center, New York, New York

Endovascular Management of Brain Arteriovenous Malformations

Mitchel S. Berger, MD

Professor and Chair, Department of Neurological Surgery, University of California, San Francisco, School of Medicine, San Francisco, California

Low-Grade Gliomas: Astrocytoma, Oligodendroglioma, and Mixed Gliomas; Hemangioblastomas of the Central Nervous System; Interstitial and Intracavitary Irradiation of Brian Tumors

Matt A. Bernstein, PhD

Assistant Professor of Radiologic Physics, Mayo Medical School; Senior Associate Consultant in Radiology, Mayo Clinic, Rochester, Minnesota

Magnetic Resonance Angiography

José Biller, MD

Professor and Chairman, Department of Neurology, Indiana University School of Medicine, Indianapolis, Indiana

Carotid Occlusive Disease: Natural History and Medical Management

Jeffrey R. Binder, MD

Professor, Department of Neurology, Medical College of Wisconsin, Milwaukee, Wisconsin

Functional Magnetic Resonance Imaging in Epilepsy Surgery

Barry D. Birch, MD

Attending, Department of Neurosurgery, Mayo Clinic Scottsdale, Scottsdale, Arizona

Anterior Thoracic Instrumentation

Rolfe Birch, MChir

Visiting Professor, University College and Imperial College, London University, London; Orthopaedic Surgeon, Peripheral Nerve Injury Unit, Royal National Orthopaedic Hospital, Stanmore, England

Management of Acute Peripheral Nerve Injuries

Peter M. Black, MD, PhD

Franc D. Ingraham Professor of Neurosurgery, Harvard Medical School; Neurosurgeon-in-Chief, Brigham and Women's Hospital and Children's Hospital, and Chief, Neurosurgical Oncology, Dana-Farber Cancer Institute, Boston, Massachusetts

Craniopharyngioma in the Adult

Miroslav P. Bobek, MD

Attending Surgeon, Providence Medford Medical Center, Medford, Oregon

Brain Edema and Tumor-Host Interactions

Anne Boulin, MD

Neuroradiologist, Hôpital Foch, Suresnes, France

Osseous Tumors

Blaise F. D. Bourgeois, MD

Director, Division of Epilepsy and Clinical Neurophysiology, Department of Neurology, Children's Hospital, Boston, Massachusetts

Antiepileptic Medications: Principles of Clinical Use

Guy Bouvier, MD

Professor of Neurosurgery, University of Montreal Faculty of Medicine, Montreal; Neurosurgeon, Hôpital Notredame, Montreal; Medical Advisor to the Vice President, Western Region, Workers' Compensation Board of Appeal, St. Lambert, Quebec, Canada

Selective Peripheral Denervation for Spasmodic Torticollis

Frank J. Bova, PhD

Professor of Neurosurgery, University of Florida College of Medicine; Staff, Shand's Hospital, Gainesville, Florida

Fractionated and Stereotactic Radiation, Extracranial Stereotactic Radiation, Intensity Modulation, and Multileaf Collimation

Robin Bowman, MD

Assistant Professor of Neurosurgery, Northwestern University Feinberg School of Medicine; Attending Neurosurgeon, Children's Memorial Hospital, Chicago, Illinois

Birth Head Trauma

Adam Brant, MD

Staff Neurosurgeon, St. Agnes Medical Center, Fresno, California

Traumatic Cerebrospinal Fluid Fistulas

Henry Brem, MD

Harvey Cushing Professor of Neurosurgery, Ophthalmology, and Oncology and Chairman, Department of Neurosurgery, Johns Hopkins University School of Medicine; Director, Hunterian Neurosurgical Laboratory, and Neurosurgeon-in-Chief, Johns Hopkins Hospital, Baltimore, Maryland

Brain Tumors: General Considerations; Basic Principles of Cranial Surgery for Brain Tumors

Steven Brem, MD

Professor and Chief, Neurosurgery Service/Director, Neuro-oncology Research Laboratory/NABTT; and Investigator/Program Leader, Neuro-oncology Program, H. Lee Moffitt Cancer Center and Research Institute, Tampa, Florida

Angiogenesis and Brain Tumors

Gavin W. Britz, MD

Assistant Professor, Department of Neurological Surgery, University of Washington School of Medicine; Attending Neurosurgeon, Harborview Medical Center, Seattle, Washington

The Natural History of Unruptured Saccular Cerebral Aneurysms; Traumatic Cerebral Aneurysms Secondary to Penetrating Intracranial Injuries; Endovascular Treatment of Spinal Cord Arteriovenous Malformations; Magnetic Resonance Imaging for Peripheral Nerve Disorders

Carolyn D. Brockington, MD

Attending, Department of Neurology, Herbert and Nell Singer Division, Beth Israel Medical Center, New York, New York

Acute Medical Management of Ischemic Disease and Stroke

Jason A. Brodkey, MD

Staff, Michigan Brain & Spine Institute, Michigan Orthopedic Center, Ypsilanti, Michigan

Glomus Jugulare Tumors

Richard A. Bronen, MD

Associate Professor of Diagnostic Radiology and Neurosurgery, Yale University School of Medicine, New Haven, Connecticut

Preoperative Evaluation for Epilepsy Surgery: Computed Tomography and Magnetic Resonance Imaging

David J. Brooks, MD, DSc

Hartnett Professor of Neurology, Imperial College Faculty of Medicine; Consultant Neurologist, Hammersmith Hospital, London, England

Positron Emission Tomography in Movement Disorders

Jeffrey A. Brown, MD

Professor, Department of Neurosurgery, Wayne State University School of Medicine, Detroit, Michigan

Percutaneous Techniques (Trigeminal Neuralgia)

Robert D. Brown, Jr., MD

Associate Professor of Neurology, Mayo Medical School and Mayo Graduate School of Medicine; Chair, Division of Cerebrovascular Diseases, and Consultant, Department of Neurology, Mayo Clinic, Rochester, Minnesota

Natural History of Intracranial Vascular Malformations

Jeffrey N. Bruce, MD

Associate Professor of Neurological Surgery, Colombia University College of Physicians and Surgeons; Associate Attending in Neurological Surgery, New York Presbyterian Hospital, New York, New York

Pineal Tumors

John M. Buatti, MD

Professor and Head, Department of Radiation Oncology, University of Iowa Roy J. and Lucille A. Carver College of Medicine; Attending, University of Iowa Hospitals and Clinics, Iowa City, Iowa

Radiobiology; Radiotherapy for Benign Skull Base Tumors; Fractionated and Stereotactic Radiation, Extracranial Stereotactic Radiation, Intensity Modulation, and Multileaf Collimation

Robert J. Buchanan, MD

Assistant Professor, Department of Psychiatry, University of California, San Diego, School of Medicine; Chief Resident, Division of Neurosurgery, UCSD Medical Center, San Diego, California

Traumatic Cerebrospinal Fluid Fistulas

Dennis E. Bullard, MD

Associate Clinical Professor, Department of Surgery, Division of Neurosurgery, University of North Carolina at Chapel Hill School of Medicine, Chapel Hill; Chief, Division of Neurosurgery, Rex Hospital, Raleigh, North Carolina

Caudalis Nucleus Dorsal Root Entry Zone Procedure for the Treatment of Intractable Facial Pain

M. Ross Bullock, MD, PhD

Virginia Commonwealth University School of Medicine, Richmond, Virginia

Surgical Management of Traumatic Brain Injury

Kim J. Burchiel, MD

Professor and Chairman, Department of Neurological Surgery, Oregon Health & Science University School of Medicine, Portland, Oregon

Pain: General Historical Considerations; Alternative Surgical Treatments for Trigeminal Neuralgia

Matthew V. Burry, MD

Resident in Neurosurgery, University of Florida College of Medicine, Gainesville, Florida

Vein of Galen Malformations

Richard W. Byrne, MD

Assistant Professor of Neurosurgery, Rush Medical College of Rush University; Attending Neurosurgeon, Rush-Presbyterian-St. Luke's Medical Center, Chicago, Illinois

Multiple Subpial Transection

Jeffrey W. Campbell, MD

Assistant Professor of Neurosurgery, University of South Carolina College of Medicine; Director, Pediatric Neurosurgery, MUSC Children's Hospital, Charleston, South Carolina

Cerebellar Astrocytomas in Children

Martin B. Camins, MD

Clinical Professor of Neurological Surgery, Mount Sinai School of Medicine; Attending Neurosurgeon, Mount Sinai Hospital, New York, New York

Tumors of the Vertebral Axis: Benign, Primary Malignant, and Metastatic Tumors

Michael E. Carey, MD, MS

Professor of Neurosurgery, Louisiana State University School of Medicine in New Orleans, New Orleans, Louisiana

Bullet Wounds to the Brain among Civilians

Carlos Carlotti, MD

Neurosurgeon, Da Universidade de São Paulo, São Paulo, Brazil

Encephaloceles

Thomas Carlstedt, MD, DM

Associate Professor, Karolinska Institute, Stockholm, Sweden; Visiting Professor, Imperial College, London University, London, England; Consultant Orthopaedic Surgeon, Royal National Orthopaedic Hospital, Peripheral Nerve Injury Unit, Stanmore, England

Management of Acute Peripheral Nerve Injuries

Peter Carmel, MD, DMedSci

Professor and Chairman Department of Neurological Surgery, University of Medicine and Dentistry of New Jersey—New Jersey Medical School; Attending, University Hospital, Newark, New Jersey

Craniopharyngiomas; Brain Tumors of Disordered Embryogenesis

Andrew L. Carney, MD

Clinical Associate Professor of Neurosurgery, Radiology, and Orthopedics, University of Illinois at Chicago College of Medicine, Chicago, Illinois

Extracranial Vertebral Artery Disease

Benjamin S. Carson, Sr., MD

Professor of Neurosurgery, Oncology, Plastic Surgery, and Pediatrics, Johns Hopkins University School of Medicine; Director, Pediatric Neurosurgery, Johns Hopkins Hospital, Baltimore, Maryland

Ependymoma; Achondroplasia and Other Dwarfism

L. Philip Carter, MD

Clinical Professor of Neurosurgery, University of Arizona School of Medicine; Private Practice, Western Neurosurgery, Ltd., Tucson, Arizona

Historical Considerations [Vascular]

Kenneth F. Casey, MD

Associate Professor of Neurosurgery, Drexel University School of Medicine, Philadelphia; Attending, Department of Neurosurgery, Allegheny Hospital, Pittsburgh, Pennsylvania

Ablative Surgery for Spasticity

Mauricio Castillo, MD

Professor of Radiology and Chief and Program Director of Neuroradiology, University of North Carolina School of Medicine, Chapel Hill, North Carolina

Webster K. Cavenee, PhD

Professor of Medicine, Cancer Genetics Program, University of California, San Diego, School of Medicine; Director, Ludwig Institute for Cancer Research, La Jolla, California

Molecular and Cytogenetic Techniques

C. Michael Cawley, MD

Assistant Professor, Department of Neurological Surgery, Emory University School of Medicine, Atlanta, Georgia

Treatment of Lateral-Sigmoid, and Sagittal Sinus Dural Anteriovenous Malformations

Stephan Chabardès, MD

Assistant Neurosurgeon, Hôpital Albert Michallon, Grenoble, France

Deep Brain Stimulation for Movement Disorders

Marc C. Chamberlain, MD

Professor of Neurology and Neurosurgery, University of Southern California Keck School of Medicine; Co-Director, Neuro-oncology Program, Norris Comprehensive Cancer Center and Hospital, Los Angeles, California

Neoplastic Meningitis: Diagnosis and Treatment

Amitabha Chanda, MD, MCh

Staff, AMRI-Apollo Hospitals, Kolkata, West Bengal

Chordoma and Chondrosarcoma

Chandrasekar Kalavakonda, MD

Anna Nagar, Chennai, India

Chordoma and Chondrosarcoma

Eric L. Chang, MD

Staff, Department of Radiation Oncology, The University of Texas M.D. Anderson Cancer Center, Houston, Texas

Metastatic Brain Tumors

Steven D. Chang, MD

Assistant Professor, Department of Neurosurgery, Stanford University School of Medicine, Stanford, California

Surgical and Radiosurgical Management of Giant Arteriovenous Malformations; General and Historical Considerations of Radiotherapy and Radiosurgery

Tailoi Chan-Ling, MOptom, PhD

Associate Professor and National Health and Medical Research Council, Senior Research Fellow, Department of Anatomy, University of Sydney Faculty of Medicine, Sydney, New South Wales, Australia

Astrocytes

Paul H. Chapman, MD

Professor of Surgery (Neurosurgery), Harvard Medical School; Neurosurgical Director, Proton Radiosurgery Group, Massachusetts General Hospital, Boston, Massachusetts

Proton Radiosurgery

Ali Charara, PhD

Post-Doctoral Fellow, Department of Neuroscience, University of Pittsburgh School of Medicine, Pittsburgh, Pennsylvania

Anatomy and Synaptic Connectivity of the Basal Ganglia

Fady T. Charbel, MD

Professor and Head, Department of Neurosurgery, University of Illinois at Chicago College of Medicine, Chicago, Illinois

Extracranial Vertebral Artery Disease

Thomas C. Chen, MD, PhD

Assistant Professor of Clinical Surgery, University of Southern California University Hospital, Los Angeles, California

Intradiskal and Percutaneous Treatment of Lumbar Disk Disease

Gopal Chopra, MD

Neurosurgeon, Department of Neurosurgery, St. John Regional Hospital, Saint John, New Brunswick, Canada

Surgical Approaches for Anterior Circulation Aneurysms

Cindy Christian, MD

Assistant Professor of Pediatrics, University of Pennsylvania School of Medicine; Chair, Child Abuse and Neglect Prevention and Director, Child Abuse Program, Children's Hospital of Philadelphia, Philadelphia, Pennsylvania

Child Abuse

Richard C. Clatterbuck, MD, PhD

Assistant Professor, Department of Neurosurgery, Johns Hopkins University School of Medicine; Attending, Johns Hopkins Hospital, Baltimore, Maryland

Surgical Positioning and Exposures for Cranial Procedures; Sarcoidosis, Tuberculosis, and Xanthogranuloma

Elizabeth B. Claus, PhD, MD

Associate Professor, Department of Epidemiology and Public Health, Yale University School of Medicine, New Haven, Connecticut

Scalp Tumors; Shunt Infection

Charles S. Cobbs, MD

Associate Professor of Neurological Surgery, Department of Surgery, University of Alabama School of Medicine; Attending, Kirklin Clinic, UAB Medical Center, Birmingham, Alabama

Meningeal Hemangiopericytoma

Kimberly Peele Cockerham, MD

Assistant Professor, Drexel University School of Medicine, Philadelphia; Director, Neuro-ophthalmology, Orbital Disease and Reconstruction, Allegheny General Hospital, Pittsburgh, Pennsylvania

Orbital Tumors

P. H. Cogen, MD

Chairman, Department of Neurosurgery, Children's National Medical Center, Washington, DC

Occult Spinal Dysraphism and the Tethered Spinal Cord

Alan R. Cohen, MD

Professor of Neurological Surgery and Pediatrics, Case Western Reserve University School of Medicine; Chief, Pediatric Neurosurgery, Rainbow Babies and Children's Hospital, Cleveland, Ohio

Myelomeningocele and Myelocystocele; Intervertebral Disk Disease in Children

Wendy A. Cohen, MD

Professor of Radiology and Neurosurgery, University of Washington School of Medicine; Chief, Neuroradiology, Harborview Medical Center, Seattle, Washington

Radiology of the Spine

Domingos Coiteiro, MD

Staff, Dobelle Institute, Lisboa, Portugal

Revascularization Techniques for Complex Aneurysms and Skull Base Tumors

Antony Colantonio, MD

Pain Fellow, Department of Anesthesiology, Oregon Health & Science University, Portland, Oregon

Management of Pain by Anesthetic Techniques

Andrew J. Cole, MD

Associate Professor of Neurology, Harvard Medical School; Associate Neurologist, Massachusetts General Hospital, Boston, Massachusetts

Identification of Candidates for Epilepsy Surgery

John J. Collins, MD

Assistant Professor of Neurosurgery, Loma Linda University School of Medicine; Chief, Pediatric Neurosurgery, Loma Linda University Children's Medical Center and Loma Linda University Medical Center, Loma Linda, California

Nonsyndromic Craniosynostosis and Abnormalities of Head Shape

Edward S. Connolly, MD

Attending, Ochsner Clinic Foundation, New Orleans, Louisiana

Metabolic and Other Nondegenerative Causes of Low Back Pain

E. Sander Connolly, Jr., MD

Irving Assistant Professor, Department of Neurological Surgery, Columbia University College of Physicians and Surgeons; New York, New York

Techniques for Deep Hypothermic Circulatory Arrest

Stephen W. Coons, MD

Staff, Division of Neuropathology, Barrow Neurological Institute, Phoenix, Arizona

Proliferation Markers in the Evaluation of Gliomas

James J. Corbett, MD

McCarty Professor and Chairman, Department of Neurology, and Professor of Ophthalmology, University of Mississippi School of Medicine, Jackson, Mississippi; Lecturer in Ophthalmology, Harvard Medical School, Boston, Massachusetts

Neuro-ophthalmology

Daniel M. Corcos, PhD

Professor, Department of Kinesiology, College of Associated Health Professions, University of Illinois at Chicago; Director, Clinical Motor Control Laboratory, Department of Neurological Sciences, Rush-Presbyterian-St. Luke's Medical Center, Chicago, Illinois

Management of Spasticity by Central Nervous System Infusion Techniques

G. Rees Cosgrove, MD

Associate Professor of Surgery, Harvard Medical School; Associate Visiting Neurosurgeon, Massachusetts General Hospital, Boston, Massachusetts

Identification of Candidates for Epilepsy Surgery; Neurosurgery of Psychiatric Disorders

Neil R. Crawford, PhD

Coordinator, Spinal Biomechanics, Barrow Neurological Institute, Phoenix; Adjunct Assistant Professor, Department of Bioengineering, Arizona State University, Tempe, Arizona

Basic Principles of Spinal Internal Fixation

Kerry R. Crone, MD

Associate Professor of Neurosurgery, Director of Graduate Education in Pediatric Neurosurgery, University of Cincinnati College of Medicine; Director, Department of Pediatric Neurosurgery, Cincinnati Children's Hospital Medical Center, Cincinnati, Ohio

Neuroendoscopy

Raimondo D'Ambrosio, PhD

Associate Professor of Neurosurgery, University of Washington; Seattle, Washington

Basic Science of Post-traumatic Epilepsy

Carlos A. David, MD

Director, Cerebrovascular and Skull Base Surgery, Lahey Clinic, Burlington, Massachusetts

Intracranial Occlusion Disease and Moyamoya

Arthur L. Day, MD

Professor of Neurosurgery, Program Director, and Associate Chairman, Department of Neurosurgery, Harvard Medical School; Director, Cerebrovascular Center, Brigham and Women's Hospital, Boston, Massachusetts

Surgical Treatment of Intracavernous and Paraclinoid Internal Carotid Artery Aneurysms

J. Diaz Day, MD

Associate Professor of Neurosurgery, Drexel University School of Medicine, Philadelphia; Director, Center for Cerebrovascular Surgery and Stroke, Allegheny General Hospital, Pittsburgh, Pennsylvania

Basilar Trunk Aneurysms; Cavernous Carotid Fistulas

A. Lee Dellon, MD

Professor of Plastic Surgery, Johns Hopkins University School of Medicine and University of Maryland School of Medicine, Baltimore, Maryland; Professor of Plastic Surgery and Neurosurgery, University of Arizona College of Medicine, Tucson, Arizona; Private Practice, Institute for Peripheral Nerve Surgery, Baltimore, Maryland, and Institute for Peripheral Nerve Surgery: Southwest, Tucson, Arizona

History of Peripheral Nerve Surgery

Mahlon R. Delong, MD

Professor and Chairman, Department of Neurology, Emory University School of Medicine, Atlanta, Georgia

Rationale for Surgical Interventions in Movement Disorders

Franco Demonte, MD

Associate Professor, Department of Neurosurgery, University of Texas–Houston Medical School; Clinical Associate Professor, Department of Neurosurgery, Baylor College of Medicine; Attending, The University of Texas M.D. Anderson Cancer Center, Houston, Texas

Neoplasms of the Paranasal Sinuses

Robert J. Dempsey, MD

Professor and Chair, Department of Neurosurgery, University of Wisconsin Medical School; Attending, University of Wisconsin Hospitals and Clinics, Madison, Wisconsin

Recurrent Carotid Stenosis

Milind Deogaonkar, MD

Department of Neurosurgery, University of Arizona Health Sciences Center, Tucson, Arizona

Historical Considerations [Vascular]

Antonio A. F. De Salles, MD, PhD

Professor, Division of Neurosurgery, Department of Surgery, David Geffen School of Medicine at UCLA; Co-Director, Epilepsy Surgery Program, West LA Veterans Administration Medical Center, Los Angeles, California

Molecular Imaging of the Brain with Positron Emission Tomography; Sympathectomy for Pain

Nicolas De Tribolet, MD

Professor, University of Geneva Faculty of Medicine; Attending, Department of Neurosurgery, University Hospital, Geneva, Switzerland

Aspects of Immunology Applicable to Brain Tumor Pathogenesis and Treatment

Paul W. Detwiler, MD, PhD

Staff, Tyler Neurosurgical Group, Tyler, Texas

Infratentorial Cavernous Malformations; Classification of Spinal Cord Vascular Lesions

Harel Deutch, MD

Instructor, Department of Neurosurgery, Emory University School of Medicine; Spinal Surgery Fellow, Department of Neurosurgery, Emory University Hospital, Atlanta, Georgia

Complication Avoidance in Neurosurgery

Paul T. Diamond, MD

Associate Professor, Department of Physical Medicine and Rehabilitation, University of Virginia School of Medicine, Charlottesville, Virginia

Rehabilitation and Prognosis after Traumatic Brain Injury

Mark S. Dias, MD

Staff, Department of Neurosurgery, Section of Neurosurgery, Milton Hershey Medical Center, Pittsburgh, Pennsylvania

Normal and Abnormal Embryology of the Spinal Cord and Spine

Curtis A. Dickman, MD

Associate Chief, Spine Section, and Director, Spinal Research, Division of Neurological Surgery, Barrow Neurological Institute, Phoenix, Arizona

Basic Principles of Spinal Internal Fixation; Anterior Cervical Instrumentation; Occipitocervical Fusion; Thoracoscopic Approaches to the Spine

Pierre-Yves Dietrich, MD

Associate Professor, University of Geneva Faculty of Medicine; Head, Laboratory of Tumor Immunology, Division of Oncology, University Hospital, Geneva, Switzerland

Aspects of Immunology Applicable to Brain Tumor Pathogenesis and Treatment

Francesco DiMeco, MD

Faculty Member, Department of Neurosurgery, Istituto Nazionale Neurologico, Milan, Italy

Brain Tumors during Pregnancy

Jacques E. Dion, MD

Professor of Neuroradiology and Neurosurgery, Department of Radiology, Emory University School of Medicine; Director, Interventional Neuroradiology, Emory University Hospital, Atlanta, Georgia

Treatment of Lateral-Sigmoid and Sagittal Sinus Dural Arteriovenous Malformations

Carl B. Dodrill, PhD

Professor, Departments of Neurology, Neurological Surgery, and Psychiatry and Behavioral Sciences, University of Washington School of Medicine; Associate Director, Regional Epilepsy Center, Harborview Medical Center, Seattle, Washington

Neuropsychological Assessment of the Neurosurgical Patient; The Intracarotid Amobarbital Procedure or Wada Test

Aclan Dogan, MD

Fellow, Division of Neurosurgery, Louisiana State University Health Sciences Center, Shreveport, Louisiana

Recurrent Carotid Stenosis

Vinko V. Dolenc, MD, PhD

Professor of Neurosurgery, Medical School at Ljubljana University; Head, Neurosurgical Department, University Hospital Center, Ljubljana, Slovenia

Skull and Skull Base Tumors

Egon M. R. Doppenberg, MD

Resident, Department of Neurosurgery, Medical College of Virginia Hospitals, Richmond, Virginia

Pediatric Head Injury

Zeena Dorai, MD

Resident, Department of Neurosurgery, University of Texas Southwestern Medical Center at Dallas, Dallas, Texas

Posterior Fossa Arteriovenous Malformations

Stephen E. Doran, MD

Clinical Assistant Professor of Neurosurgery, Department of Surgery, University of Nebraska College of Medicine; Neurosurgeon, University Medical Associates and Midwest Neurosurgery, Omaha, Nebraska

Brain Tumors: Population-Based Epidemiology, Environmental Risk Factors, and Genetic and Hereditary Syndromes

Catherine J. Doty, MD

Clinical Assistant Professor in Pediatrics, Washington University School of Medicine; Attending, St. Louis Children's Hospital, St. Louis, Missouri

Cerebral Palsy: An Overview

James M. Drake, MBBCh, MSc

Associate Professor, Division of Neurosurgery, University of Toronto Faculty of Medicine; Neurosurgeon, The Hospital for Sick Children, Toronto, Ontario, Canada

Physiology of Cerebrospinal Fluid Shunt Devices

Ann-Christine Duhaime, MD

Professor of Neurosurgery, Dartmouth Medical School; Director, Pediatric Neurosurgery, Dartmouth-Hitchock Medical Center, Lebanon, New Hampshire

Child Abuse

Christopher M. Duma, MD

Medical Director, Hoag Gamma Knife Program, Hoag Memorial Hospital Presbyterian, Newport Beach, California

Functional Radiosurgery

Charles Duncan, MD

Professor and Head, Section of Pediatric Neurosurgery, Department of Neurosurgery, Yale University School of Medicine; Chief, Pediatric Neurosurgery, Yale–New Haven Hospital, New Haven, Connecticut

Shunt Infection

Marc E. Eichler, MD

Clinical Instructor, Harvard Medical School; Associate Surgeon, Department of Neurosurgery, Brigham and Women's Hospital and Boston Children's Hospital, Boston, Massachusetts

Cervical Spine Trauma

F. J. Eismont, MD

Vice Chairman, Department of Orthopedics and Rehabilitation, University of Miami School of Medicine; Orthopedic Surgeon, Jackson Memorial Hospital, Miami, Florida

Diagnosis and Management of Thoracic Spine Fractures

Elizabeth A. Eldredge, MD

Instructor in Anesthesia, Harvard Medical School; Staff Anesthesiologist, Children's Hospital, Boston, Massachusetts

Neuroanesthesia in Children

Hikmat El-Kadi, MD, PhD

Clinical Associate Professor of Neurosurgery, University of Pittsburgh School of Medicine, Pittsburgh Pennsylvania

Brain Death

Richard G. Ellenbogen, MD

Associate Professor, Department of Neurological Surgery, University of Washington School of Medicine; Chief and Theodore S. Roberts Endowed Chair, Division of Pediatric Neurological Surgery, Children's Hospital and Regional Medical Center, Seattle, Washington

Diagnosis and Management of Juvenile Angiofibroma; Choroid Plexus Tumors; Craniofacial Trauma

J. Paul Elliott, MD

Assistant Professor, Department of Neurosurgery, University of Colorado School of Medicine; Chief, Neurosurgery, Denver Health Medical Center, Denver, Colorado

Traumatic Cerebrovascular Injury

Syed A. Enam, MD, PhD

Staff Physician, Department of Neurosurgery, Henry Ford Hospital, Detroit, Michigan

Invasion in Malignant Glioma

Fred J. Epstein, MD

Professor of Neurosurgery, Albert Einstein School of Medicine of Yeshiva University, Bronx; Attending Physician, Institute for Neurology and Neurosurgery, Beth Israel Medical Center, New York, New York

Intraspinal Tumors in Infants and Children

Nancy E. Epstein, MD

Clinical Professor of Neurological Surgery, Albert Einstein College of Medicine of Yeshiva University, Bronx; Adjunct Clinical Associate Professor of Surgery/Neurosurgery, Cornell University, Joan and Sanford I. Weill Medical College, New York; Attending Neurosurgeon, North Shore–Long Island Jewish Health System, Manhasset and New Hyde Park, and Winthrop University Hospital, Mineola, New York

Lumbar Spinal Stenosis

Joseph Eskridge, MD

Professor, Departments of Radiology and Neurosurgery, University of Washington School of Medicine, Seattle, Washington

Endovascular Treatment of Spinal Cord Arteriovenous Malformations

Matthew G. Ewend, MD

Assistant Professor of Neurosurgery and Section Chief of Neuro-oncology Clinical Research, University of North Carolina Lineberger Comprehensive Cancer Center, University of North Carolina, Chapel Hill, North Carolina

Meningeal Sarcoma

Gary G. Ferguson, MD, PhD

Professor of Neurosurgery, Department of Clinical Neurological Sciences (Neurosurgery), University of Western Ontario Faculty of Medicine; Attending Neurosurgeon, London Health Sciences Centre, London, Ontario, Canada

Distal Anterior Cerebral Artery Aneurysms

Richard G. Fessler, MD, PhD

Professor of Neurosurgery, Department of Surgery, University of Chicago, Division of the Biological Sciences, Pritzker School of Medicine; Chief, Section of Neurosurgery, University of Chicago Hospital and Clinics, Chicago, Illinois

Benign Extradural Lesions of the Dorsal Spine; Posterior Lumbar Instrumentation

Matthew E. Fewel, MD

Instructor, Department of Neurosurgery, University of Michigan Medical School, Ann Arbor, Michigan

Skull Tumors

Paul E. Fewings, MBBS

Consultant Neurosurgeon, Hull Royal Infirmary, Hull, England

Medical Management of Chronic Pain

J. Max Findlay, MD, PhD

Clinical Professor, Division of Neurosurgery, University of Alberta Faculty of Medicine; Neurosurgeon, University of Alberta Hospital, Edmonton, Alberta, Canada

Cerebral Vasospasm

Andrew D. Fine, MD

Staff, Neurological Associates, PA, Sarasota, Florida

Benign Extradural Lesions of the Dorsal Spine

Howard A. Fine, MD

Branch Chief, Neuro-Oncology, National Cancer Institute, National Institute of Health, Bethesda, Maryland

Principles of Chemotherapy

Jill B. Firszt, PhD

Assistant Professor and Director, Koss Cochlear Implant Program, Department of Otolaryngology and Communication Sciences, Medical College of Wisconsin; Attending, Froedtert & Medical College Hospital and Children's Hospital of Wisconsin, Milwaukee, Wisconsin

Neuro-otology

Michael T. Fitch, MD, PhD

Resident in Emergency Medicine, Carolina Medical Center, Charlotte, North Carolina

Cellular and Molecular Mechanisms Mediating Injury and Recovery in the Nervous System

James D. Fleck, MD

Clinical Assistant Professor, Department of Neurology, Indiana University School of Medicine, Indianapolis, Indiana

Carotid Occlusive Disease: Natural History and Medical Management

Ian G. Fleetwood, MD

Chief Resident, Department of Neurosurgery, Foothills Medical Centre, Calgary, Alberta, Canada

Hemorrhagic Disease: Arteriovascular Malformations

Kelly D. Flemming, MD

Assistant Professor, Mayo Graduate School of Medicine; Consultant in Neurology, Mayo Clinic, Rochester, Minnesota

Natural History of Intracranial Vascular Malformations

Susan Fletcher, MB

Acting Assistant Professor of Anesthesiology, University of Washington School of Medicine; Attending Anesthesiologist, Harborview Medical Center, Seattle, Washington

Anesthesia: Preoperative Evaluation

John C. Flickinger, MD

Professor of Radiation Oncology and Neurological Surgery, University of Pittsburgh School of Medicine, Pittsburgh, Pennsylvania

Fractionated Radiotherapy for Pituitary Tumors

Nancy Foldvary, DO

Staff Neurologist, Cleveland Clinic, Cleveland, Ohio

[Surgical Treatment of Epilepsy in Children] Recognition of Surgical Candidates and the Presurgical Evaluation

Kenneth A. Follett, MD, PhD

Professor, Department of Neurosurgery, University of Iowa College of Medicine, Iowa City, Iowa

Neurosurgical Management of Intractable Pain

Kelly D. Foote, MD

Assistant Professor, Department of Neurosurgery, University of Florida School of Medicine, Gainesville, Florida

Radiosurgery for Arteriovenous Malformations

Daryl R. Fourney, MD

Assistant Professor, Division of Neurosurgery, University of Saskatchewan Faculty of Medicine; Attending, Royal University Hospital, Saskatoon, Saskatchewan, Canada

Neoplasms of the Paranasal Sinuses

Valerie Fraix, MD, PhD

Assistant Neurologist, Hôpital Albert Michallon, Grenoble, France

Deep Brain Stimulation for Movement Disorders

Paul C. Francel, MD, PhD

Associate Professor, Department of Neurosurgery, University of Oklahoma College of Medicine, Oklahoma City, Oklahoma

Mild Brain Injury in Children, including Skull Fractures and Growing Fractures

Itzhak Fried, MD, PhD

Associate Professor of Neurosurgery and Psychiatry and Biobehavioral Sciences, David Geffen School of Medicine at UCLA, Los Angeles, California; Associate Professor of Neurosurgery, Sackler School of Medicine, Tel-Aviv University, Tel-Aviv, Israel; Director, of Epilepsy Surgery, and Co-Director, UCLA Seizure Disorder Center, UCLA Medical Center, Los Angeles, California; Director, Functional Neurosurgery Unit, Tel-Aviv Medical Center, Tel-Aviv, Israel

Surgery for Extratemporal Lobe Epilepsy

Jonathan A. Friedman, MD

Chief Resident, Department of Neurologic Surgery, Mayo Clinic, Rochester, Minnesota

Middle Cerebral Artery Aneurysms

William A. Friedman, MD

Professor and Chair, Department of Neurosurgery, University of Florida; Attending, Shand's Hospital, Gainesville, Florida

Radiobiology; Radiosurgery for Arteriovenous Malformations; Fractionated and Stereotactic Radiation, Extracranial Stereotactic Radiation, Intensity Modulation, and Multileaf Collimation

David M. Frim, MD, PhD

Assistant Professor of Surgery and Pediatrics, University of Chicago, Division of the Biological Sciences, Pritzker School of Medicine; Chief, Pediatric Neurosurgery, University of Chicago Children's Hospital, Chicago, Illinois

Benign Tumors of the Vertebral Column in Children

Michael J. Fritsch, MD

Fellow in Neurological Surgery, University of Miami School of Medicine, Miami, Florida

Surgical Management of Supratentorial Arteriovenous Malformation

Herbert E. Fuchs, MD, PhD

Associate Professor, Department of Surgery, Division of Neurosurgery, Duke University School of Medicine, Durham, North Carolina

Benign Tumors of the Skull, including Fibrous Dysplasia

Gregory N. Fuller, MD, PhD

Professor of Pathology, University of Texas–Houston Medical School; Chief, Section of Neuropathology, The University of Texas M.D. Anderson Cancer Center, Houston, Texas

Brain Tumors: An Overview of Histopathologic Classification

Aurelie Funkiewiez, MA

Staff, Department of Neurology, Centre Hospitalier Universitaire de Grenoble, Grenoble, France

Deep Brain Stimulation for Movement Disorders

Michael R. Gallagher, MD

Clinical Assistant Professor, Department of Surgery, University of Tennessee, Chattanooga, College of Medicine; Staff Neurosurgeon, Baroness Erlanger Hospital and Memorial Hospital, Chattanooga, Tennessee

Spondyloarthropathies, including Ankylosing Spondylitis

Ira M. Garonzik, MD

Neurosurgery Fellow, Department of Neurosurgery, Johns Hopkins Hospital, Baltimore, Maryland

Thalamotomy for Tremor

Hugh Garton, MD, MHSc

Assistant Professor, Department of Neurosurgery, University of Michigan Medical School, Ann Arbor, Michigan

Neurosurgical Epidemiology and Outcomes Assessment

Marilyn L. Gates, MD

Assistant Professor, Uniformed Services University of the Health Sciences, Medicine; Assistant Director, Complex Spine Surgery, National Naval Medical Center Hospital, Bethesda, Maryland

Bone Metabolism as It Relates to Spinal Disease and Treatment

Stephen S. Gebarski, MD

Professor, Department of Radiology, Division of Neuroradiology, University of Michigan Medical School, Ann Arbor, Michigan

Skull Tumors

Christopher C. Getch, MD

Assistant Professor, Department of Neurological Surgery, Northwestern University Feinberg School of Medicine, Chicago, Illinois

Basilar Apex and Posterior Cerebral Artery Aneurysms

Sanjay Ghosh, MD

Staff, Senta Clinic, Division of Skull Base Surgery, San Diego, California

Ventricular Tumors; Cavernous Carotid Fistulas

Steven L. Giannotta, MD

Professor of Neurological Surgery, University of Southern California Keck School of Medicine; Chief, Neurosurgery, and Medical Director, USC University Hospital, Los Angeles, California

Basilar Trunk Aneurysms

Philip L. Gildenberg, MD, PhD

Clinical Professor of Neurosurgery and Radiation Oncology, Baylor College of Medicine; Clinical Professor of Psychiatry, University of Texas–Houston Medical School, Houston, Texas

Brainstem Procedures for Management of Pain

Howard J. Ginsberg, MD

Senior Resident, University of Toronto, Division of Neurosurgery, Toronto, Ontario, Canada

Physiology of Cerebrospinal Fluid Shunt Devices

Ziya L. Gokaslan, MD

Clinical Assistant Professor, Department of Neurosurgery, University of Texas–Houston Medical School; Attending, The University of Texas M.D. Anderson Cancer Center, Houston, Texas

Treatment of Disk and Ligamentous Diseases of the Cervical Spine

Joel Goldwein, MD

Professor of Radiation Oncology, University of Pennsylvania School of Medicine; Chief, Pediatric Radiation Oncology, Children's Hospital of Philadelphia, Philadelphia, Pennsylvania

Intracranial Ependymomas

Robert Goodkin, MD

Associate Professor, Department of Neurological Surgery, University of Washington School of Medicine; Chief, Neurosurgical Section, Veterans Administration Puget Sound Health Care System, Seattle, Washington

Legal Issues; General Principles of Operative Positioning; Magnetic Resonance Imaging for Peripheral Nerve Disorders

James Tait Goodrich, MD, PhD

Professor of Clinical Neurological Surgery, Pediatrics, and Plastic and Reconstructive Surgery, Leo Davidoff Department of Neurological Surgery, Albert Einstein College of Medicine of Yeshiva University; Director, Division of Pediatric Neurosurgery, Montefiore Medical Center, Bronx, New York

Neurological Surgery in Childhood: General and Historical Considerations

John P. Gorecki, MD

Clinical Assistant Professor, The University of Kansas Medical School, Wichita, Kansas

Dorsal Root Entry Zone and Brainstem Ablative Procedures

M. Sean Grady, MD

Charles Harrison Frazier Professor and Chair of the Department of Neurosurgery, University of Pennsylvania School of Medicine, Philadelphia, Pennsylvania

Cellular Basis of Injury and Recovery from Trauma; Initial Resuscitation and Patient Evaluation; Modern Neurotraumatology: A Brief Historical Review

Sylvie Grand, MD, PhD

Assistant Professor of Biophysics and Radiology, University Joseph Fourier; Staff Neuroradiologist, Hôpital Albert Michallon, Grenoble, France

Deep Brain Stimulation for Movement Disorders

Gerald A. Grant, MD

Acting Instructor, Department of Neurological Surgery, University of Washington School of Medicine; Attending, Children's Hospital and Regional Medical Center, Seattle, Washington

The Blood-Brain Barrier; Diagnosis and Management of Juvenile Angiofibroma; General Principles in Evaluating and Treating Peripheral Nerve Injuries; Magnetic Resonance Imaging for Peripheral Nerve Disorders

B. A. Green, MD

Professor and Chairman, Department of Neurosurgical Surgery, University of Miami School of Medicine; Chief, Department of Neurosurgery, Jackson Memorial Medical Center, Miami, Florida

Diagnosis and Management of Thoracic Spine Fractures

Michael W. Groff, MD

Director, Spinal Surgery, Indiana University Hospital, Indianapolis, Indiana

Concepts and Mechanisms of Biomechanics

Andreas Gruber, MD

Professor, Department of Neurosurgery, University of Vienna Medical School, Vienna, Austria

Embolization of Arteriovenous Malformations as a Primary Treatment Modality

Joseph S Gruss, MBBCh

Professor, Department of Surgery; Adjunct Professor, Department of Neurosurgery; and Marlys C. Larson Professor and Endowed Chair in Pediatric Craniofacial Surgery, University of Washington School of Medicine; Chief, Division of Craniofacial, Plastic and Reconstructive Surgery, Children's Hospital and Regional Medical Center; Attending Surgeon, Harborview Medical Center, Seattle, Washington

Craniofacial Trauma

Michael Guarnieri, PhD, MPH

Research Associate, Johns Hopkins University School of Medicine, Baltimore, Maryland

Ependymoma

James D. Guest, MD, PhD

Assistant Professor of Neurological Surgery, University of Miami School of Medicine; Scientific Faculty, The Miami Project to Cure Paralysis; Attending Neurosurgeon, University of Miami Hospital and Clinics and Miami Veterans Administration Medical Center, Miami, Florida

Biologic Strategies for Central Nervous System Repair

Abhijit Guha, MSc, MD

Associate Professor, Division of Neurosurgery, University of Toronto Faculty of Medicine; Attending Neurosurgeon, University Health Network; Co-Director, Arthur and Sonia Labatts Brain Tumor Center, The Hospital for Sick Children, Toronto, Ontario, Canada

Management of Peripheral Nerve Tumors

Mary Kay Gumerlock, MD

Professor of Neurosurgery, University of Oklahoma, College of Medicine, Oklahoma City, Oklahoma

Epidermoid, Dermoid, and Neurenteric Cysts

Murat Gunel, MD

Assistant Professor of Neurosurgery, Yale University School of Medicine, New Haven, Connecticut

Surgical Management of Supratentorial Cavernous Malformations

Kern H. Guppy, MD, PhD

Assistant Professor of Neurosurgery, University of Illinois at Chicago College of Medicine, Chicago, Illinois

Extracranial Vertebral Artery Disease

Nalin Gupta, MD, PhD

Assistant Professor, Department of Neurosurgery, University of California, San Francisco, School of Medicine, San Francisco, California

Benign Tumors of the Vertebral Column in Children

Lee R. Guterman, MD, PhD

Assistant Professor, Department of Neurosurgery and Co-Director Toshiba Stroke Research Center, University at Buffalo; Neurosurgeon, Kaleida Health, Buffalo, New York

Endovascular Treatment of Aneurysms

Barton L. Guthrie, MD

Associate Professor of Neurological Surgery, Department of Surgery, University of Alabama School of Medicine; Co-Director, Health South/UAB Gamma Knife Program, Health South Medical Center, Birmingham, Alabama

Meningeal Hemangiopericytoma

P. W. Gutin, MD

Chief, Department of Neurosurgery, Memorial Sloan-Kettering Cancer Center, New York, New York

Interstitial and Intracavitary Irradiation of Brain Tumors

Eldad Hadar, MD

Assistant Professor, Department of Surgery, Division of Neurosurgery, University of North Carolina at Chapel Hill School of Medicine, Chapel Hill, North Carolina

General and Historical Considerations of Epilepsy Surgery

Georges F. Haddad, MD

Clinical Assistant Professor, Department of Neurosurgery, American University of Beirut, Beirut, Lebanon

Regis W. Haid, MD

Associate Professor, Department of Neurological Surgery, Emory University School of Medicine, Atlanta, Georgia

Spondyloarthropathies, including Ankylosing Spondylitis

Stephen J. Haines, MD

Professor and Chair, Department of Neurological Surgery, Medical University of South Carolina College of Medicine, Charleston, South Carolina

Neurosurgical Epidemiology and Outcomes Assessment

H. Bruce Hamilton, MD

Private Practice, Neurosurgery, Waco, Texas

Metabolic and Other Nondegenerative Causes of Low Back Pain

Mark G. Hamilton, MDCM

Associate Professor of Neurosurgery, Department of Clinical Neurosciences, University of Calgary Faculty of Medicine; Director, Pediatric Neurosciences, Alberta Children's Hospital, Foothills Medical Centre, Calgary, Alberta, Canada

Hemorrhagic Disease: Arteriovascular Malformations

Thomas A. Hammeke, PhD

Professor, Department of Neurology (Neuropsychology), Medical College of Wisconsin, Milwaukee, Wisconsin

Functional Magnetic Resonance Imaging in Epilepsy Surgery

Patrick P. Han, MD

Chief Resident, Division of Neurological Surgery, Barrow Neurological Institute, Phoenix, Arizona

Epidemiology and Natural History of Cavernous Malformations

Russell W. Hardy, Jr., MD
Professor of Neurological Surgery, Department of Surgery, Case Western Reserve University School of Medicine; Co-Director, University Hospitals Spine Center, Cleveland, Ohio
Treatment of Disk Disease of the Lumbar Spine

Raymond I. Haroun, MD
Instructor, Department of Neurosurgery, Johns Hopkins University School of Medicine, Baltimore, Maryland
Anterior Communicating Artery and Anterior Cerebral Artery Aneurysms; Achondroplasia and Other Dwarfism

Mark R. Harrigan, MD
Lecturer, Department of Neurosurgery, University of Michigan Medical School, Ann Arbor, Michigan
Pregnancy and Treatment of Vascular Disease

Griffith R. Harsh IV, MD
Professor, of Neurosurgery, Stanford University School of Medicine; Director, Stanford Brain Tumor Center, Stanford, California
Cerebral Lymphoma

Jaimie M. Henderson, MD
Associate Staff, Department of Neurosurgery, Cleveland Clinic, Cleveland, Ohio
Medical Management of Chronic Pain

Jeffrey S. Henn, MD
Assistant Professor, Department of Neurological Surgery, University of Florida College of Medicine, Gainesville, Florida
Giant Aneurysms

Roberto C. Heros, MD
Professor, Department of Neurological Surgery, University of Miami School of Medicine; Attending Neurosurgeon, Jackson Memorial Hospital, Miami, Florida
Surgical Management of Supratentorial Arteriovenous Malformation

Karl Herrup, PhD
Professor of Neurosciences and Neurology, Case Western Reserve University School of Medicine; Director, University Memory and Aging Center, University Hospitals of Cleveland, Cleveland, Ohio
Neurons and Neuroglia

Jason Heth, MD
Chief Resident, Department of Neurosurgery, University of Iowa Hospitals and Clinics, Iowa City, Iowa
Tumors of the Craniovertebral Junction

Julian T. Hoff, MD
Professor and Chair, Department of Neurosurgery, University of Michigan Medical School, Ann Arbor, Michigan
Brain Edema and Tumor-Host Interactions; Skull Tumors; Treatment of Intractable Vertigo

Dominique Hoffmann, MD
Staff Neurosurgeon, Hôpital Albert Michallon, Grenoble, France
Deep Brain Stimulation for Movement Disorders

Brian L. Hoh, MD
Clinical Fellow in Surgery, Harvard Medical School; Resident, Neurosurgical Service, Massachusetts General Hospital, Boston, Massachusetts
Vertebral Artery, Posterior Inferior Cerebellar Artery, and Vertebrobasilar Junction Aneurysms

Anna Depold Hohler, MD
Chief, Neurology Clinic, Madigan Army Medical Center, Tacoma, Washington
Approach to Movement Disorders

Eric C. Holland, MD, PhD
Staff, Departments of Surgery (Neurosurgery), Neurology, and Cell Biology, Memorial Sloan-Kettering Cancer Center, New York, New York
Molecular Genetics and the Development of Targets for Glioma Therapy

James P. Hollowell, MD
Associate Professor of Neurosurgery, Medical College of Wisconsin; Staff, Neuroscience Research Laboratory and Veterans Affairs Medical Center, Milwaukee, Wisconsin
Concepts and Mechanisms of Biomechanics; Bone Metabolism as It Relates to Spinal Disease and Treatment

Mark D. Holmes, MD
Associate Professor of Neurology, University of Washington School of Medicine; Director of EEG, Regional Epilepsy Center, Harborview Medical Center, Seattle, Washington
Approaches to the Diagnosis and Classification of Epilepsy

John Honeycutt, MD
Assistant Professor, Department of Neurosurgery, University of Oklahoma College of Medicine, Oklahoma City, Oklahoma
Mild Brain Injury in Children, including Skull Fractures and Growing Fractures

L. Nelson Hopkins, MD
Professor and Chairman, Department of Neurosurgery, and Professor of Radiology, School of Medicine and Biomedical Sciences, State University of New York at Buffalo, Buffalo, New York
Endovascular Treatment of Aneurysms

Frank P. K. Hsu, MD, PhD

Assistant Professor of Neurosurgery, Department of Surgery, Loma Linda University School of Medicine, Loma Linda, California

Cerebral Venous and Sinus Thrombosis

Sherwin E. Hua, MD, PhD

Resident and Fellow, Department of Neurosurgery, Johns Hopkins Hospital, Baltimore, Maryland

Sarcoidosis, Tuberculosis, and Xanthogranuloma; Thalamotomy for Tremor

Alan R. Hudson, MBChB

Professor, Department of Surgery, University of Toronto Faculty of Medicine, Toronto, Ontario, Canada

Management of Peripheral Nerve Tumors

Robin P. Humphreys, MD

Emeritus Professor, Department of Surgery, University of Toronto Faculty of Medicine, Division of Neurosurgery, The Hospital for Sick Children, Toronto, Ontario, Canada

Arteriovenous Malformations and Intracranial Aneurysms in Children

John Huston III, MD

Assistant Professor of Radiology, Mayo Medical School; Consultant in Neurologic Radiology, Mayo Clinic, Rochester, Minnesota

Magnetic Resonance Angiography

Mark Iantosca, MD

Assistant Clinical Professor, Department of Neurosurgery, University of Connecticut School of Medicine; Director, Pediatric Neurosurgery, Connecticut Children's Medical Center, Farmington, Connecticut

Encephaloceles

Koji IIhara, MD

Attending, Department of Neurosurgery, Toronto Western Hospital, University Health Network, Toronto, Ontario, Canada

Surgical Approaches for Anterior Circulation Aneurysms

Robert J. Jackson, MD

Department of Neurosurgery, Baylor College of Medicine; Attending, The University of Texas M.D. Anderson Cancer Center, Houston, Texas; Surgeon, Massoudi and Jackson Neurosurgical Medical Associates, Laguna Hills, California

Treatment of Disk and Ligamentous Diseases of the Cervical Spine

Deane B. Jacques, MD

Medical Director, The California Neuroscience Institute, Oxnard, California

Functional Radiosurgery

George I. Jallo, MD

Assistant Professor, Departments of Neurosurgery and Pediatrics, Albert Einstein School of Medicine of Yeshiva University, Bronx; Attending Physician, Institute for Neurology and Neurosurgery, Beth Israel Medical Center, New York, New York

Intraspinal Tumors in Infants and Children

C. David James, PhD

Professor of Laboratory Medicine, Mayo Medical School, Rochester, Minnesota

Molecular and Cytogenetic Techniques

John A. Jane, Sr., MD, PhD

Chairman, Department of Neurosurgery, University of Virginia School of Medicine, Charlottesville, Virginia

Esthesioneuroblastoma

Damir Janigro, PhD

Director, Cerebrovascular Center, Department of Neurosurgery, Cleveland Clinic, Cleveland, Ohio

The Blood-Brain Barrier; Electrophysiologic Properties of the Mammalian Nervous System

Peter J. Jannetta, MD

Professor of Neurosurgery, Drexel University College of Medicine, Philadelphia; Vice Chairman, Department of Neurosurgery, Allegheny General Hospital, Pittsburgh, Pennsylvania

Trigeminal Neuralgia: Microvascular Decompression of the Trigeminal Nerve for Tic Douloureux

Abel D. Jarell, MD

CPD Medical Corps, Department of the Army, Washington, DC

Growth Factors and Brain Tumors

Jeffrey G. Jarvik, MD, MPH

Associate Professor, Departments of Radiology and Neurosurgery, University of Washington School of Medicine; Adjunct Associate Professor, Department of Health Services, University of Washington School of Public Health; Director, Neuroradiology Fellowship, University of Washington Medical Center, Seattle, Washington

Radiology of the Spine; Magnetic Resonance Imaging for Peripheral Nerve Disorders

Kurt A. Jellinger, MD

Professor, University of Vienna Medical School, and Director, Ludwig Boltzmann Institute of Clinical Neurobiology, Vienna, Austria

Neuropathology of Movement Disorders

Arthur L. Jenkins III, MD, BA

Assistant Professor, Department of Neurosurgery, Mount Sinai School of Medicine, New York, New York

Complication Avoidance in Neurosurgery; Tumors of the Vertebral Axis: Benign, Primary Malignant, and Metastatic Tumors; Cervical Spine Trauma

Eric W. Johnson, MD

Chief, Molecular Genetics–Neurogenetics, Division of Neurology/Division of Neurosurgery, Barrow Neurological Institute, Phoenix, Arizona

The Genetics of Cerebral Cavernous Malformations

John Patrick Johnson, MD

Director, Cedars-Sinai Institute for Spinal Disorders, Los Angeles, California

Sympathectomy for Pain

Wayel Kaakaji, MD

Staff Neurosurgeon, Michigan Brain and Spinal Surgery Institute, Detroit, Michigan

Alternative Surgical Treatments for Trigeminal Neuralgia

Michael G. Kaiser, MD

Assistant Professor, Department of Neurological Surgery, Columbia University College of Physicians and Surgeons; Attending Neurosurgeon, New York Presbyterian Hospital, New York, New York

Anterior Thoracic Instrumentation; Anterior Lumbar Instrumentation

Iain H. Kalfas, MD

Head, Section of Spinal Surgery, Department of Neurosurgery, Cleveland Clinic, Cleveland, Ohio

Image-Guided Spinal Navigation

Paul M. Kanev, MD

Attending Neurosurgeon, Department of Surgery, Milton Hershey Medical Center, Hershey, Pennsylvania

Arachnoid Cysts

Yücel Kanpolat, MD

Professor and Chairman, Department of Neurosurgery, University of Ankara Faculty of Medicine; Ankara, Turkey

Cordotomy for Pain

Stuart S. Kaplan, MD

Assistant Professor of Neurosurgery, University of Cincinnati College of Medicine; Attending Neurosurgeon, Cincinnati Children's Hospital Medical Center, Cincinnati, Ohio

Birth Brachial Plexus Injury

Michael G. Kaplitt, MD, PhD

Assistant Professor, Department of Neurosurgery, Director, Center for Stereotactic and Functional Neurosurgery, Director, Laboratory of Molecular Neurosurgery, Cornell University Joan and Sanford I. Weill Medical College, New York, New York

Deep Brain Stimulation for Chronic Pain

Zvonimir S. Katusic, MD, PhD

Professor of Pharmacology, Mayo Medical School, Rochester, Minnesota

Cerebral Blood Flow and Metabolism

Bruce A. Kaufman, MD

Professor of Neurosurgery, Medical College of Wisconsin; Chief, Division of Pediatric Neurosurgery, Children's Hospital of Wisconsin, Milwaukee, Wisconsin

Medulloblastoma

Howard H. Kaufman, MD

Department of Neurosurgery, West Virginia University School of Medicine, Morgantown, West Virginia

Brain Death

Robert F. Keating

Associate Professor, Department of Neurosurgery, George Washington University School of Medicine; Chief, Children's National Medical Center, Washington; DC

Occult Spinal Dysraphism and the Tethered Spinal Cord

G. Evren Keles, MD

Assistant Professor, Department of Neurosurgery, University of California, San Francisco, School of Medicine; San Francisco, California

Low-Grade Gliomas: Astrocytoma, Oligodendroglioma, and Mixed Gliomas

John S. Kennerdell, MD

Professor of Ophthalmology, Drexel University Medical School, Philadelphia, and Adjunct Professor of Ophthalmology, University of Pittsburgh School of Medicine; Chairman, Department of Ophthalmology, Allegheny General Hospital, Pittsburgh, Pennsylvania

Orbital Tumors

Lawrence T. Khoo, MD

Department of Neurosurgery, University of Southern California Keck School of Medicine, Los Angeles, California

Intradiskal and Percutaneous Treatment of Lumbar Disk Disease

Vini G. Khurana, MD, PhD

Sundt Fellow, Departments of Neurologic Surgery and Molecular Pharmacology and Experimental Therapeutics, Mayo Clinic, Rochester, Minnesota

Cerebral Blood Flow and Metabolism

Monika Killer, MD
Attending, Christian Doppler Medical Center, Salzburg, Austria
Embolization of Arteriovenous Malformations as a Primary Treatment Modality

Jung Kim, MD
Professor, Department of Pathology, Yale University School of Medicine, New Haven, Connecticut
Unusual Gliomas

Thomas A. Kim, MD
Assistant Professor, Department of Radiology, University of Washington School of Medicine; Staff Neuroradiologist, Harborview Medical Center, University of Washington Medical Center, and Veterans Administration Puget Sound Medical Center, Seattle, Washington
Magnetic Resonance Imaging of Brain

Wesley A. King, MD
Associate Professor, Department of Neurosurgery, Mount Sinai School of Medicine; Attending Neurosurgeon, Mount Sinai Hospital, New York, New York
Neuro-otology

Gregory A. Kinney, PhD
Assistant Professor, University of Washington School of Medicine; Associate Director, Surgical Neuromonitoring University of Washington Medical Center and Harborview Medical Center, Seattle, Washington
Physiology of the Peripheral Nerve

Paul Klimo, MD
Resident, Department of Neurosurgery, University Hospital, Salt Lake City, Utah
Treatment of Axis Fractures

David G. Kline, MD
Boyd Professor and Chairman, Department of Neurosurgery, Louisiana State University School of Medicine at New Orleans; Visiting Staff, Medical Center of Louisiana at Charity Hospital and University Hospital; Academic Staff, Ochsner Foundation Hospital; Senior Staff, Touro Infirmary, S. Baptist and Mercy Hospitals; Consultant, Veterans Administration Hospital, New Orleans, Louisiana; and Keeslor AFB Hospital, Biloxi, Mississippi
Management of Peripheral Nerve Tumors

Michel Kliot, MD
Associate Professor of Neurosurgery, University of Washington School of Medicine; Attending Neurosurgeon, University of Washington Medical Center and Veterans Administration Puget Sound Health Care System, Seattle, Washington
Cellular and Molecular Mechanisms Mediating Injury and Recovery in the Nervous System; General Principles in Evaluating and Treating Peripheral Nerve Injuries; Magnetic Resonance Imaging for Peripheral Nerve Injuries; Carpal Tunnel Syndrome; Entrapment Syndromes of Peripheral Nerve Injuries

Douglas Kondziolka, MD, MSc
Professor of Neurological Surgery and Radiation Oncology, University of Pittsburgh School of Medicine, Pittsburgh, Pennsylvania
Patient Selection in Movement Disorder Surgery; Fractionated Radiotherapy for Pituitary Tumors; Gamma Knife Radiosurgery

Thomas A. Kopitnik, MD
Professor of Neurosurgery, University of Texas Southwestern Medical School; Director of Cerebrovascular Surgery, University of Texas Southwestern Medical Center at Dallas, Dallas, Texas
Posterior Fossa Arteriovenous Malformations

Oleg Kopyov, MD, PhD
Research Director, The California Neuroscience Institute, Oxnard, California
Functional Radiosurgery

Karl F. Kothbauer, MD
Assistant Professor, Department of Neurological Surgery, Albert Einstein College of Medicine of Yeshiva University, Bronx; Attending, Beth Israel Medical Center, New York, New York
Intraspinal Tumors in Infants and Children

Adnah Koudsié, MD
Staff Neurosurgeon, Hôpital Albert Michallon, Grenoble, France
Deep Brain Stimulation for Movement Disorders

Paul Krack, MD
Professor of Neurology, University Joseph Fourier Medical School; Staff Neurologist, Hôpital Albert Michallion, Grenoble, France
Deep Brain Stimulation for Movement Disorders

Michael A. Kraut, MD, PhD
Associate Professor of Radiology, Johns Hopkins University School of Medicine; Chief of Neuro–MRI, Johns Hopkins Hospital, Baltimore, Maryland
Radiologic Features of Central Nervous System Tumors

Lynda Kulawiak, RN
Research Associate, Department of Anesthesiology and Perioperative Medicine, Oregon Health & Science University, Portland, Oregon
Management of Pain by Anesthetic Techniques

V. G. R. Kumar, MBBS
Consultant Neurosurgeon, West Bank Hospital, Calcutta, West Bengal, India
Cervical Spondylotic Myelopathy

Lara J. Kunschner, MD

Assistant Professor, Department of Neurology, Drexel University College of Medicine, Philadelphia; Attending, Allegheny General Hospital, Allegheny Neurological Associates, Pittsburgh, Pennsylvania

Medulloblastoma

Charles Kuntz IV, MD

Assistant Professor of Neurosurgery, University of Cincinnati School of Medicine; Associate Director, Spine and Peripheral Nerve Surgery, The Maxfield Clinic and Spine Institute, and Director, Spine and Peripheral Nerve Research, Department of Neurological Surgery, The Neuroscience Institute, Cincinnati, Ohio

Approach to the Patient and Medical Management of Spinal Disorders

Inam Kureshi, MD

Department of Neurovascular Surgery, Hartford Hospital Stroke Center, Hartford, Connecticut

Revascularization Techniques for Complex Aneurysms and Skull Base Tumors

Arthur M. Lam, MD

Professor of Anesthesiology and Neurological Surgery, University of Washington School of Medicine; Head, Division of Neuroanesthesia, Harborview Medical Center, Seattle, Washington

Anesthesia: Preoperative Evaluation; Transcranial Doppler Ultrasonography

Lois A. Lampson, PhD

Associate Professor of Neurosurgery, Brigham and Women's Hospital, Harvard Medical School, Boston, Massachusetts

Basic Principles of Central Nervous System Immunology

Frederick F. Lang, Jr., MD

Attending, Department of Neurosurgery, The University of Texas M.D. Anderson Cancer Center, Houston, Texas

Medulloblastoma; Metastatic Brain Tumors

Guiseppe Lanzino, MD

Associate Professor, Department of Neurosurgery, University of Illinois College of Medicine at Peoria; Chief, Section of Cerebrovascular Surgery, Illinois Neurological Institute, Peoria, Illinois

Endovascular Treatment of Aneurysms

Donald Larsen, MD

Associate Professor, Department of Neurological Surgery, University of Southern California Keck School of Medicine; Director of Neuro-interventional Section, USC University Hospital, Los Angeles, California

Cavernous Carotid Fistulas

Sean D. Lavine, MD

Assistant Professor of Neurosurgery and Radiology, Columbia University, College of Physicians and Surgeons; Clinical Director, Endovascular Neurosurgery and Interventional Neuroradiology, Columbia-Presbyterian Medical Center, New York, New York

Basilar Trunk Aneurysms

Michael T. Lawton, MD

Tong-Po Kan Assistant Professor of Neurological Surgery, University of California, San Francisco, School of Medicine; Chief of Cerebrovascular Surgery, University of California, San Francisco Medical Center, San Francisco, California

Surgical Approaches for Posterior Circulation Aneurysms

Edward R. Laws, MD

Professor, Department of Neurosurgery, University of Virginia, Charlottesville, Virginia

Daniel A. Lazar, MD

Resident, Department of Neurological Surgery, University of Washington Hospitals, Seattle, Washington

Cellular and Molecular Mechanisms Mediating Injury and Recovery in the Nervous System

Jean F. Le Bas, MD, PhD

Professor of Biophysics and Radiology, University Joseph Fourier Medical School; Head, Division of Neuroradiology and MRI, and Director, Institut Federatif de Recherche eu IRM, Hôpital Albert Michallon, Grenoble, France

Deep Brain Stimulation for Movement Disorders

Chong C. Lee, MD, PhD

Resident, Department of Neurological Surgery, University of Washington, Seattle, Washington

Carpal Tunnel Syndrome; Entrapment Syndromes of Peripheral Nerve Injuries

Jang-Chul Lee, MD, PhD

Associate Professor, Department of Neurosurgery, Keimyung University School of Medicine, Taegu, Korea

Diagnostic Biopsy of Peripheral Nerves and Muscle

Jung-Il Lee, MD

Associate Professor, Department of Neurosurgery, Samsung Medical Center, Sungkyun Kwan University School of Medicine, Seoul, Korea

Thalamotomy for Tremor

Sunghoon Lee, MD

Administrative Chief Resident, Yale Neurosurgery Program, Yale–New Haven Medical Center, New Haven, Connecticut

Unusual Gliomas; Intracranial Monitoring

Elizabeth A. Leedom, JD
Lecturer, University of Washington School of Law, Seattle, Washington
Legal Issues

James W. Leiphart, MD, PhD
Resident in Neurosurgery, UCLA Medical Center, Los Angeles, California
Surgery for Extratemporal Lobe Epilepsy

G. Michael Lemole, Jr., MD
Private Practice, Huntingdon Valley, Pennsylvania
Giant Aneurysms

Frederick A. Lenz, MD
Professor of Neurosurgery, Johns Hopkins University School of Medicine; Attending Neurosurgeon, Johns Hopkins Hospital, Baltimore, Maryland
Thalamotomy for Tremor

Phillipp M. Lenzlinger, MD
Division of Trauma Surgery, Department of Surgery, University Hospital, Zuroch, Switzerland
Cellular Basis of Injury and Recovery from Trauma

Jeffrey R. Leonard, MD
Assistant Professor, Department of Neurosurgery, Washington University School of Medicine; Attending Neurosurgeon, St. Louis Children's Hospital, St. Louis, Missouri
Dandy-Walker Syndrome

Peter D. Le Roux, MB, ChB, MD
Associate Professor of Neurosurgery, University of Pennsylvania School of Medicine, Philadelphia, Pennsylvania
Surgical Decision Making for the Treatment of Cerebral Aneurysms

Allan D. O. Levi, MD, PhD
Assistant Professor, University of Miami School of Medicine; Chief, Section of Neurospinal Services, Jackson Memorial Hospital, Miami, Florida
Spine Trauma: Approach to the Patient and Diagnostic Evaluation

Elad I. Levy, MD
Neurosurgical Chief Resident, University of Pittsburgh Medical Center System, Pittsburgh, Pennsylvania
Trigeminal Neuralgia: Microvascular Decompression of the Trigeminal Nerve for Tic Douloureux

Michael L. Levy, MD, PhD
Associate Professor, Department of Neurosurgery, University of Southern California Keck School of Medicine, Los Angeles, California
Vagus Nerve Stimulation for Intractable Epilepsy

David H. Lewis, MD
Associate Professor of Radiology, University of Washington School of Medicine; Director, Division of Nuclear Medicine, Harborview Medical Center, Seattle, Washington
Single-Photon Emission Computed Tomography and Positron Emission Tomography

Patricia Limousin, MD, PhD
Senior Lecturer, Institute of Neurology, and Honorary Consultant Neurologist, National Hospital for Neurology and Neurosurgery, Queen's Square, London, England
Deep Brain Stimulation for Movement Disorders

E. Paul Lindell, MD
Attending Radiologist, Department of Radiology, Mayo Clinic, Rochester, Minnesota
Magnetic Resonance Imaging of Brain

Lawrence S. Liu, MD
Attending, Department of Neurosurgery, Kaiser-Permanente Los Angeles Medical Center, Los Angeles, California
Technical Aspects of Bone Graft Harvest and Spinal Fusion

Jay S. Loeffler, MD
Andreas Soriano Professor of Radiation Oncology, Harvard Medical School; Chair, Department of Radiation Oncology, Massachusetts General Hospital, Boston, Massachusetts
Proton Radiosurgery

Christopher Loftus, MD
Professor and Chairman, Department of Neurosurgery, University of Oklahoma College of Medicine, Oklahoma City, Oklahoma
Carotid Occlusive Disease: Natural History and Medical Management

William J. Logan, MD
Professor of Pediatrics and Medicine, University of Toronto Faculty of Medicine; Attending, Division of Neurology, The Hospital for Sick Children, Toronto, Ontario, Canada
Neurological Examination in Infancy and Childhood

Donlin M. Long, MD, PhD
Distinguished Service Professor of Neurosurgery, Johns Hopkins University School of Medicine; Active Staff, Johns Hopkins Hospital; Principal Staff, Applied Physics Laboratory, Johns Hopkins University, Baltimore, Maryland
Acoustic Neuroma

Luca Longhi, MD
Terapia Intensiva Neuroscienze, Padiglione Beretta Neuro II piano (Rianimazione), Ospedale Maggiore Policlinico IRCCS, Milano, Italy
Cellular Basis of Injury and Recovery from Trauma

James B. Lowe III, MD, MBA
Instructor in Surgery, Division of Plastic and Reconstructive Surgery, Washington University School of Medicine, St. Louis, Missouri
Ulnar Nerve Entrapment at the Elbow

Andres M. Lozano, MD, PhD
Professor of Neurosurgery and R. R. Tasker Chair in Functional Neurosurgery, University of Toronto Faculty of Medicine; Attending, Toronto Western Hospital, Toronto, Ontario, Canada
Pallidotomy for Parkinson's Disease; Deep Brain Stimulation for Chronic Pain

Mark Luciano, MD, PhD
Chief, Pediatric and Congenital Neurosurgery Section, and Director, Cleveland Clinic Hydrocephalus Project, Cleveland Clinic, Cleveland, Ohio
Infantile Posthemorrhagic Hydrocephalus

Jürgen Lüders, MD, PhD
Chairman, Department of Neurology, Cleveland Clinic Foundation, Cleveland, Ohio
General and Historical Considerations of Epilepsy Surgery

David Lundin, MD
Resident, Department of Neurological Surgery, University of Washington, Seattle, Washington
Spondylolisthesis

L. Dade Lunsford, MD
Lars Leksell Professor of Neurological Surgery, Radiology, and Radiology Oncology and Chairman, Department of Neurological Surgery, University of Pittsburgh School of Medicine; Director, Center for Image-Guided Neurosurgery, University of Pittsburgh Medical Center, Pittsburgh, Pennsylvania
Patient Selection in Movement Disorder Surgery; Radiosurgery of Tumors

W. David Lust, PhD
Professor of Neurological Surgery, Case Western Reserve University School of Medicine; Attending, Department of Neurological Surgery, and The Research Institute of University Hospitals of Cleveland, Cleveland, Ohio
Intraoperative Cerebral Protection

R. Loch MacDonald, MD, PhD
Professor, Department of Surgery, Division of the Biological Sciences, Pritzker School of Medicine University of Chicago; Attending Neurosurgeon, University of Chicago Medical Center, Chicago, Illinois
Perioperative Management of Subarachnoid Hemorrhage

Susan E. Mackinnon, MD
Shornberg Professor and Chief, Division of Plastic and Reconstructive Surgery, Department of Surgery, Washington University School of Medicine, St. Louis, Missouri
Ulnar Nerve Entrapment at the Elbow

Roger M. Macklis, MD
Professor of Radiology, Ohio State University College of Medicine and Public Health; Chairman, Department of Radiation Oncology, Cleveland Clinic, Cleveland, Ohio
Principles of Radiotherapy

Christopher Madden, MD
Clinical Assistant Professor, Ohio State University, Columbus, Ohio
Cervical Spondylotic Myelopathy

Parley W. Madsen III, MD, PhD
Staff, Department of Neurological Surgery, Conemaugh Memorial Medical Center, Johnstown, Pennsylvania
Diagnosis and Management of Thoracic Spine Fractures

Dennis J. Maiman, MD, PhD
Professor, Department of Neurosurgery, and Director, Spine Surgery Fellowship, Medical College of Wisconsin; Physical Medicine and Rehabilitation, Froedtert Hospital; Attending Neurosurgeon, Veterans Affairs Medical Center, Milwaukee, Wisconsin
Concepts and Mechanisms of Biomechanics

Allen Maniker, MD
Assistant Professor, Department of Neurological Surgery, University of Medicine and Dentistry of New Jersey, Newark; Attending Neurosurgeon, University Hospital, Newark, and Hackensack University Hospital, Hackensack, New Jersey
Peripheral Nerves

Scott C. Manning, MD
Professor, Department of Otolaryngology, University of Washington School of Medicine; Chief, Division of Pediatric Otolaryngology, Children's Hospital and Regional Medical Center, Seattle, Washington
Diagnosis and Management of Juvenile Angiofibroma

Timothy B. Mapstone, MD
Professor and Vice-Chairman, Department of Neurological Surgery, Emory University School of Medicine; Director, Pediatric Neurosurgery, Children's Health Care of Atlanta, Atlanta, Georgia
Intracranial Germ Cell Tumors

Kenneth Maravilla, MD

Professor of Radiology and Director of Neuroradiology, Department of Neurological Surgery, University of Washington School of Medicine; Research Affiliate, Center on Human Development and Disability, Seattle, Washington

Magnetic Resonance Imaging for Peripheral Nerve Disorders

Douglas A. Marchuk, PhD

Associate Professor, Department of Genetics, Duke University School of Medicine, Durham, North Carolina

The Genetics of Cerebral Cavernous Malformations

Paul J. Marcotte, MD

Associate Professor of Neurosurgery, University of Pennsylvania School of Medicine; Attending, Department of Neurosurgery, Hospital of the University of Pennsylvania, Philadelphia, Pennsylvania

Technical Aspects of Bone Graft Harvest and Spinal Fusion

Anthony Marmarou, PhD

Professor and Vice Chairman, Director of Research, Division of Neurosurgery, Virginia Commonwealth University School of Medicine, Richmond, Virginia

Physiology of the Cerebrospinal Fluid and Intracranial Pressure

Joseph C. Maroon, MD

Clinical Professor and Heindl Scholar, Department of Neurosurgery, University of Pittsburgh School of Medicine; Vice Chairman, Department of Neurosurgery, UPMC-Presbyterian Hospital, Pittsburgh, Pennsylvania

Orbital Tumors

Lawrence F. Marshall, MD

Professor of Neurological Surgery, University of California, San Diego, School of Medicine; Chief, Division of Neurosurgery, UCSD Medical Center, San Diego, California

Differential Diagnosis of Altered States of Consciousness; Modern Neurotraumatology: A Brief Historical Review; Traumatic Cerebrospinal Fluid Fistulas

Sharon B. Marshall

Director of Clinical Research, Department of Neurosurgery, University of California, San Diego, San Diego, California

Modern Neurotraumatology: A Brief Historical Review

Neil A. Martin, MD

Professor and Chair, Department of Neurosurgery, David Geffen School of Medicine at University of California, Los Angeles, Los Angeles, California

Revascularization Techniques for Complex Aneurysms and Skull Base Tumors

Timothy J. Martin, MD

Associate Professor of Surgical Sciences/ Ophthalmology, Department of Ophthalmology, Wake Forest University School of Medicine; Attending, Baptist Medical Center and Wake Forest University Eye Center, Winston-Salem, North Carolina

Neuro-ophthalmology

Robert E. Maxwell, MD, PhD

Professor and Chair, Department of Neurosurgery, University of Minnesota Medical School; Neurosurgery Clinical Service Chief, Fairview University Medical Center, Minneapolis, Minnesota

Standard Temporal Lobectomy and Transsylvian Amygdalohippocampectomy

Nina A. Mayr, MD

Professor and Director, Radiation Oncology, Oklahoma University Health Sciences Center, Oklahoma City, Oklahoma

Radiobiology

Kevin McCarthy, MD

Assistant Professor and Director, Department of Medicine, Nuclear Medicine Division, Louisiana State University School of Medicine in New Orleans, New Orleans, Louisiana

Intracranial Monitoring

Paul C. McCormick, MD, MPH

Professor of Clinical Neurosurgery, Department of Neurological Surgery, Columbia University College of Physicians and Surgeons; Attending Neurosurgeon, New York Presbyterian Hospital, New York, New York

Anterior Thoracic Instrumentation; Anterior Lumbar Instrumentation; Spinal Cord Tumors in Adults

M. W. McDermott, MD

Assistant Professor, Department of Neurological Surgery, University of California, San Francisco, School of Medicine, San Francisco, California

Interstitial and Intracavitary Irradiation of Brain Tumors

Cameron G. McDougall, MD, FRCS(C)

Director, Division of Endovascular Neurosurgery, Barrow Neurological Institute, Phoenix, Arizona

Carotid Angioplasty and Stenting: Interventional Treatment of Occlusive Vascular Disease

Tracy K. McIntosh, PhD

Professor of Neurosurgery, Pharmacology, and Bioengineering, Vice-Chair for Research and Director, University of Pennsylvania Head Injury Center, University of Pennsylvania, Philadelphia, Pennsylvania

Cellular Basis of Injury and Recovery from Trauma

Guy M. McKhann II, MD

Assistant Professor, Department of Neurological Surgery, Columbia University College of Physicians and Surgeons; Staff, The Neurological Institute, and Attending, New York Presbyterian Hospital, New York, New York

Electrophysiologic Properties of the Mammalian Central Nervous System

David G. McLone, MD, PhD

Staff, Department of Pediatric Neurosurgery, Children's Memorial Hospital, Chicago, Illinois

Normal and Abnormal Embryology of the Spinal Cord and Spine

Max B. Medary, MD

Director, Orlando Neurosurgical Foundation, Celebration, Florida

Carotid Endarterectomy

Sanford L. Meeks, PhD

Associate Professor of Radiology, University of Iowa Roy J. and Lucille A. Carver College of Medicine; Director of Medical Physics, Department of Radiation Oncology, University of Iowa Health Care, Iowa City, Iowa

Radiobiology; Radiotherapy for Benign Skull Base Tumors; Fractionated and Stereotactic Radiation, Extracranial Stereotactic Radiation, Intensity Modulation, and Multileaf Collimation

Minesh P. Mehta, MBChB

Associate Professor, Department of Human Oncology, University of Wisconsin—Madison Medical School, Madison, Wisconsin

Fractionated Radiation Therapy for Malignant Brain Tumors

Vivek Mehta, MD, MSc

Assistant Professor, Department of Neurosurgery, University of Alberta Faculty of Medicine; Attending, Walter MacKenzie Health Sciences Center, Edmonton, Alberta, Canada

Craniopharyngioma in the Adult

William P. Melega, PhD

Associate Professor, Department of Molecular and Medical Pharmacology, David Geffen School of Medicine at UCLA, Los Angeles, California

Molecular Imaging of the Brain with Positron Emission Tomography

Arnold H. Menezes, MD

Professor and Vice Chairman, Department of Neurosurgery, University of Iowa College of Medicine; Attending Neurosurgeon, University of Iowa Hospitals and Clinics, Iowa City, Iowa

Developmental Abnormalities of the Craniovertebral Junction; Acquired Abnormalities of the Craniocervical Junction; Tumors of the Craniovertebral Junction

Robert A. Mericle, MD

Assistant Professor, Department of Neurosurgery, University of Florida College of Medicine; Staff, McKnight Brain Institute, Gainesville, Florida

Vein of Galen Malformations

Glen S. Merry, MD

Professor of Neurosurgery, University of Queensland Faculty of Medicine; Consultant Neurosurgeon, Royal Brisbane Hospital, Brisbane Queensland, Australia

Mild Head Injury in Adults

Ali Mesiwala, MD

Resident, University of Washington Hospitals, Seattle, Washington

General Principles of Operative Positioning

Fredric B. Meyer, MD

Professor of Neurosurgery, Mayo Medical School; Staff, Departments of Diagnostic Radiology and Neurological Surgery, Mayo Clinic, Rochester, Minnesota

Cerebral Blood Flow and Metabolism; Multimodality Management of Complex Cerebrovascular Lesions

Jeff Michalski, MD

Associate Professor, Department of Radiation Oncology, Washington University School of Medicine; Clinical Director, Department of Radiation Oncology, Barnes-Jewish Hospital, St. Louis, Missouri

Radiotherapy of Tumors of the Spine

J. Parker Mickle, MD

Professor, Department of Neurosurgery, University of Florida College of Medicine; Staff, McKnight Brain Institute, Gainesville, Florida

Vein of Galen Malformations

Rajiv Midha, MD, MSc

Associate Professor, Department of Surgery, Division of Neurosurgery, University of Toronto Faculty of Medicine; Staff Neurosurgeon, Sunnybrook and Women's College Health Sciences Centre, Toronto, Ontario, Canada

Peripheral Nerve: Approach to the Patient

Tom Mikkelsen, MD

Co-Director, Hermelin Brain Tumor Center, and Attending, Henry Ford Hospital, Detroit, Michigan

Invasion in Malignant Glioma

Andrew N. Miles, MBBS

Consultant Neurosurgeon, Western Australian Comprehensive Epilepsy Service and Department of Neurosurgery, Royal Perth Hospital, Perth, Western Australia, Australia

Tailored Resections for Epilepsy

John W. Miller, MD, PhD

Professor of Neurology and Neurological Surgery, University of Washington School of Medicine; Director, Regional Epilepsy Center, University of Washington Medical Center, Seattle, Washington

Approaches to the Diagnosis and Classification of Epilepsy

Neil R. Miller, MD

Professor of Ophthalmology, Neurology, and Neurosurgery and Frank B. Walsh Professor of Neuro-Ophthalmology, Johns Hopkins University School of Medicine, Baltimore, Maryland

Pseudotumor Cerebri

Pedro Molina-Negro, MD, PhD

Professor of Surgery (Neurosurgery), University of Montreal Faculty of Medicine, Howick, Quebec, Canada

Selective Peripheral Denervation for Spasmodic Torticollis

Jacques J. Morcos, MD

Associate Professor, Department of Neurosurgery, University of Miami School of Medicine, Miami, Florida

Spontaneous Intracerebral Hemorrhage: Non–Arteriovenous Malformation, Nonaneurysm

Michael Kerin Morgan, MD

Professor of Neurosurgery, University of Sydney Faculty of Medicine, Sydney, New South Wales, Australia

Classification and Decision Making in Treatment and Perioperative Management, including Surgical and Radiosurgical Decision Making

Glenn Morrison, MD

Professor of Neurological Surgery, University of Miami School of Medicine; Chief, Division of Neurological Surgery, Miami Children's Hospital, Miami, Florida

Temporal and Extratemporal Lobe Resections for Childhood Intractable Epilepsy

Richard S. Morrison, PhD

Professor, Department of Neurological Surgery, University of Washington School of Medicine, Seattle, Washington

Growth Factors and Brain Tumors

Wade M. Mueller, MD

Associate Professor, Department of Neurosurgery, Medical College of Wisconsin, Milwaukee, Wisconsin

Functional Magnetic Resonance Imaging in Epilepsy Surgery

J. Paul Muizelaar, MD, PhD

Professor and Chair, Department of Neurological Surgery, University of California, Davis, School of Medicine, Davis; University of California, Davis, Medical Center, Sacramento, California

Clinical Pathophysiology of Traumatic Brain Injury

Jenny Multani, MD

Resident, Department of Neurosurgery, West Virginia University School of Medicine, Morgantown, West Virginia

Occult Spinal Dysraphism and the Tethered Spinal Cord

Karin M. Muraszko, MD

Associate Professor of Neurosurgery and Pediatric and Communicable Diseases, University of Michigan Medical School; Director, Pediatric Neurosurgery Program, C. S. Mott Children's Hospital, University of Michigan Hospital and Health Centers, Ann Arbor, Michigan

Primitive Neuroectodermal Tumors

Antonio C. M. Mussi, MD

Research Fellow, Department of Neurological Surgery, University of Florida College of Medicine, Gainesville, Florida

Surgical Anatomy of the Brain

Neal J. Naff, MD

Assistant Professor of Neurosurgery, Johns Hopkins University School of Medicine, Baltimore, and Uniformed Services University of Health Sciences, F. Edward Hébert School of Medicine, Bethesda; Chief of Neurosurgery, Sinai Hospital of Baltimore, Baltimore, Maryland

Endovascular Techniques for Brain Tumors

Blaine S. Nashold, MD

Professor Emeritus, Department of Surgery, Division of Neurosurgery, Duke University School of Medicine; Director, Neurosurgical Stereotactic Laboratory and Neuroprosthesis Laboratory, Duke University Medical Center, Durham, North Carolina

Caudalis Nucleus Dorsal Root Entry Zone Procedure for the Treatment of Intractable Facial Pain

Gary M. Nesbit, MD

Associate Professor, Department of Neurological Surgery, Diagnostic Radiology, and Neurology, Oregon Health & Science University School of Medicine and Dotter Interventional Institute; Chief, Neuroradiology and MRI, University Hospital, Portland, Oregon

Cerebral Venous and Sinus Thrombosis

David W. Newell, MD

Professor, Department of Neurological Surgery, University of Washington School of Medicine; Attending Neurosurgeon, Harborview Medical Center, University of Washington Medical Center, Children's Hospital Medical Center, and Veterans' Hospital Medical Center, Seattle, Washington

Transcranial Doppler Ultrasonography; Traumatic Cerebral Aneurysms Secondary to Penetrating Intracranial Injuries; Traumatic Cerebrovascular Injury

Douglas A. Nichols, MD

Associate Professor, Departments of Radiology and Neurosurgery, Mayo Medical School, Rochester, Minnesota

Multimodality Management of Complex Cerebrovascular Lesions

Ajay Niranjan, MBBS, MS, MCh

Assistant Professor, Department of Neurological Surgery, University of Pittsburgh School of Medicine; Director, Radiosurgery Research, University of Pittsburgh Medical Center System, Pittsburgh, Pennsylvania

Radiosurgery of Tumors

Russ P. Nockels, MD

Associate Professor and Vice Chair, Departments of Neurological Surgery and Orthopedic Surgery, Loyola University Stritch School of Medicine, Loyola University Medical Center, Maywood, Illinois

Diagnosis and Management of Thoracolumbar and Lumbar Spine Injuries

Michael J. Noetzel, MD

Professor of Neurology and Pediatrics, Washington University School of Medicine; Director, Clinical Services, Division of Pediatric Neurology, Washington University Medical Center; Medical Director, Clinical and Diagnostic Neuroscience Services, St. Louis Children's Hospital, St. Louis, Missouri

Acute Pediatric Neurorehabilitation

Patrick Noonen, MD

Department of Radiology, National Naval Medical Center, Bethesda, Maryland

Endovascular Techniques for Brain Tumors

Richard B. North, MD

Professor of Neurosurgery, Anesthesiology, and Critical Care Medicine, Johns Hopkins University School of Medicine, Baltimore, Maryland

Spinal Cord and Peripheral Nerve Stimulation for Chronic, Intractable Pain

Eric Nottmeier, MD

Chief Resident, Division of Neurosurgery, University of Missouri Hospitals and Clinics, Columbia, Missouri

Intracranial Occlusion Disease and Moyamoya

W. Jerry Oakes, MD

Professor of Neurosurgery and Pediatrics, University of Alabama School of Medicine; Chief, Pediatric Neurosurgery, University of Alabama Hospitals, Birmingham Alabama

Chiari Malformations

Maureen O'Donnell, MD, MSc

Assistant Professor and Head, Division of Developmental Pediatrics, Department of Pediatrics, University of British Columbia Faculty of Medicine; Medical Director, Child Development and Rehabilitation Program, Children's and Women's Health Centre of British Columbia, Vancouver, British Columbia, Canada

Intrathecal Baclofen Infusion

Christopher S. Ogilvy, MD

Associate Professor of Surgery, Harvard Medical School; Visiting Neurosurgeon, Massachusetts General Hospital, Boston, Massachusetts

Vertebral Artery, Posterior Inferior Cerebellar Artery, and Vertebrobasilar Junction Aneurysms

George A. Ojemann, MD

Professor of Neurological Surgery, University of Washington School of Medicine; Staff, University of Washington Regional Epilepsy Center, Seattle, Washington

Tailored Resections for Epilepsy

Jeffrey G. Ojemann, MD

Assistant Professor of Neurosurgery, Department of Neurological Surgery, and Assistant Professor of Pediatrics, Anatomy, Psychology, and Neurobiology, Washington University School of Medicine; Attending Neurosurgeon, St. Louis Children's Hospital, St. Louis, Missouri

Dandy-Walker Syndrome

Michael S. Okun, MD

Assistant Professor of Neurology, University of Florida College of Medicine; Co-Director, Movement Disorders Center, Department of Neurology, McKnight Brain Institute, Gainesville, Florida

Surgery for Dystonia

Edward H. Oldfield, MD

Chief, Surgical Neurology Branch, National Institute of Neurological Diseases and Stroke, National Institutes of Health, Bethesda, Maryland

Spinal Arteriovenous Malformations

Alessandro Olivi, MD

Professor of Neurosurgery, Johns Hopkins University School of Medicine, Baltimore, Maryland

Brain Tumors during Pregnancy

Stephen L. Ondra, MD

Assistant Professor of Neurosurgery, Northwestern University Feinberg School of Medicine, Chicago, Illinois

Adult Thoracolumbar Scoliosis

Michael Ostad, MD

Clinical Adjunct Assistant Professor of Urology, Cornell University, Joan and Sanford I. Weill College of Medicine; Attending Urologist, New York Presbyterian Hospital, New York, and North Shore University Hospital, Manhasset, New York

Neurourology

Renatta J. Osterdock, MD

Pediatric Neurosurgery Fellow, University of Tennessee, Memphis, College of Medicine and Semmes-Murphy Clinic, Memphis, Tennessee

Lipomyelomeningocele

Jeffrey H. Owen, PhD

President and Owner, Sentient Medical Systems, Cockeysville, Maryland

Intraoperative Electrophysiologic Monitoring of the Spinal Cord and Nerve Roots

Dachling Pang, MD

Professor of Clinical Neurosurgery, University of California, Davis, School of Medicine, Davis; Chief, Regional Center for Pediatric Neurosurgery, Kaiser Permanente Hospital, Oakland, California

Pediatric Vertebral Column and Spinal Cord Injuries

T. S. Park, MD

Shi H. Huang Professor of Neurosurgery and Professor of Pediatrics and Anatomy and Neurobiology, Washington University School of Medicine; Neurosurgeon-in-Chief, St. Louis Children's Hospital, St. Louis, Missouri

Birth Brachial Plexus Injury; Selective Dorsal Rhizotomy for Spastic Cerebral Palsy

Andrew T. Parsa, MD, PhD

Assistant Professor, Department of Neurological Surgery, University of California, San Francisco, School of Medicine, San Francisco, California

Anterior Thoracic Instrumentation; Anterior Lumbar Instrumentation

Michael Partington, MD

Neurosurgeon, Department of Pediatrics, Gillette Children's Specialty Healthcare, St. Paul, Minnesota

Normal and Abnormal Embryology of the Spinal Cord and Spine

Naresh P. Patel, MD

Assistant Professor of Neurosurgery, Mayo Medical School Scottsdale; Assistant Attending, Mayo Clinic Scottsdale, Scottsdale, Arizona

Complication Avoidance in Neurosurgery

Jogi V. Pattisapu, MD

Clinical Faculty, Department of Molecular Biology and Microbiology and Department of Nursing, College of Health Sciences, University of Central Florida; Medical Director, Pediatric Neurosurgery, Arnold Palmer Hospital for Women and Children, Florida Children's Hospital, Wade's Center for Hydrocephalus Research, HRI, Orlando, Florida

Infantile Posthemorrhagic Hydrocephalus

Richard D. Penn, MD

Professor of Neurosurgery, University of Chicago, Division of the Biological Sciences, Pritzker School of Medicine; Attending, Neuroscience Institute, Neurosurgery Division, Rush-Presbyterian-St. Luke's Medical Center, and University of Chicago Hospitals, Chicago, Illinois

Management of Spasticity by Central Nervous System Infusion Techniques; Intrathecal Drug Infusion for Pain

Noel I. Perin, MD

Clinical Associate Professor of Neurosurgery, Columbia University College of Physicians and Surgeons; Attending Physician, St. Luke's Roosevelt Beth-Israel Hospital, New-York, New York

Sacral Fractures

Richard G. Perrin, MD, MSc

Associate Professor of Neurological Surgery, Division of Neurosurgery, University of Toronto Faculty of Medicine; Staff, St. Michael's Hospital, Toronto, Ontario, Canada

Tumors of the Vertebral Axis: Benign, Primary Malignant, and Metastatic Tumors

Jonathan R. Perry, MD

Professor, Department of Radiology, University of Washington School of Medicine, Seattle, Washington

Radiology of the Spine

John A. Persing, MD

Professor, Department of Neurosurgery, Yale University School of Medicine; Chief, Section of Plastic Surgery, Yale–New Haven Hospital, New Haven, Connecticut

Scalp Tumors; Craniofacial Syndromes

Michael E. Phelps, PhD

Norton Simon Professor and Chair, Department of Molecular and Medical Pharmacology, David Geffen School of Medicine at UCLA; Director, Crump Institute for Molecular Imaging; Associate Director, Laboratory of Structural Biology and Molecular Medicine and Chief, Division of Nuclear Medicine, UCLA Medical Center, Los Angeles, California

Molecular Imaging of the Brain with Positron Emission Tomography

Loi K. Phuong, MD

Resident, Department of Neurology, Mayo Clinic, Rochester, Minnesota
Pediatric Cerebral Hemispheric Tumors

David G. Piepgras, MD

Professor of Neurologic Surgery, Mayo Medical School; Chairman, Department of Neurologic Surgery, Mayo Clinic, Rochester, Minnesota
Middle Cerebral Artery Aneurysms

Joseph Piepmeier, MD

Nixdorff-German Professor and Vice Chairman for Clinical Affairs, Department of Neurosurgery, Yale University School of Medicine; Director, Neuro-oncology Unit, Yale Comprehensive Cancer Center, New Haven, Connecticut
Unusual Gliomas

Webster H. Pilcher, MD, PhD

Professor and Chair, Department of Neurological Surgery, University of Rochester School of Medicine and Dentistry and School of Nursing; Staff, Eastman Dental Center and Strong Memorial Hospital, Rochester, New York
Epilepsy Surgery: Outcome and Complications

Frank A. Pintar, PhD

Professor, Department of Neurosurgery, Medical College of Wisconsin; Adjunct Professor of Biomedical Engineering, Marquette University; Director, Neuroscience Research Laboratories, and Principal Investigator/Biomedical Engineer, Veterans Administration Medical Center, Milwaukee, Wisconsin
Concepts and Mechanisms of Biomechanics

Joseph D. Pinter, MD

Assistant Professor of Neurology, University of California, Davis, School of Medicine, Davis; Attending, UC Davis Medical Center, Sacramento, California
Neuroembryology

Serge Pinto, PhD

Hôpital Albert Michallon, Service de Neurologie Grenoble and University Joseph Fourier, Grenoble, France
Deep Brain Stimulation for Movement Disorders

Farhad Pirouzmand, MD

Assistant Professor of Neurosurgery, University of Saskatchewan Faculty of Medicine; Program Director, Division of Neurosurgery, Royal University Hospital, Saskatoon, Saskatchewan, Canada
Arteriovenous Malformations and Intracranial Aneurysms in Children

Ian F. Pollack, MD

Professor of Neurosurgery, University of Pittsburgh School of Medicine; Co-Director, University of Pittsburgh Cancer Institute Brain Tumor Center, Children's Hospital of Pittsburgh, Pittsburgh, Pennsylvania
Brainstem Gliomas

Pierre Pollak, MD, PhD

Professor of Neurology, University Joseph Fourier Medical School; Head, Movement Disorders Unit, Hôpital Albert Michallon, Grenoble, France
Deep Brain Stimulation for Movement Disorders

Bruce E. Pollock, MD

Associate Professor, Department of Neurological Surgery, Mayo Medical School, Rochester, Minnesota
Multimodality Management of Complex Cerebrovascular Lesions

Randall W. Porter, MD

Chief, Interdisciplinary Skull Base Section, Barrow Neurological Institute, Phoenix, Arizona
Infratentorial Cavernous Malformations; Classification of Spinal Cord Vascular Lesions

Kalmon D. Post, MD

Professor and Chairman, Department of Neurosurgery, Mount Sinai School of Medicine; Chairman, Department of Neurosurgery, Mount Sinai Medical Center, New York, New York
Complication Avoidance in Neurosurgery; Trigeminal Schwannomas

Sujit S. Prabhu, MD

Director, Department of Neurosurgery, M.D. Anderson Cancer Center, Houston, Texas
Surgical Management of Traumatic Brain Injury

Charles J. Prestigiacomo, MD

Assistant Professor of Cerebrovascular/Endovascular Surgery, Departments of Neurological Surgery and Radiology, University of Medicine and Dentistry of New Jersey—New Jersey Medical School; Attending, Neurological Institute of New Jersey, University Hospital, Newark, New Jersey
Neurosonology

Robert Prost, PhD

Assistant Professor of Radiology, Medical College of Wisconsin; Attending, Froedtert & Memorial Lutheran Hospital, Milwaukee, Wisconsin
Magnetic Resonance Imaging of Brain

Chad J. Prusmack, MD

Resident, Department of Neurosurgery, University of Miami Hospital and Clinics, Miami, Florida
Spontaneous Intracerebral Hemorrhage: Non–Arteriovenous Malformation, Nonaneurysm

Donald O. Quest, MD

Professor, Department of Neurological Surgery, Columbia University College of Physicians and Surgeons; Attending, Department of Neurological Surgery, Neurological Institute of New York Presbyterian Hospital, and New York Presbyterian Medical Center, New York, New York

Neurosonology

Corey Raffel, MD, PhD

Professor of Neurosurgery, Mayo Medical School, Rochester, Minnesota

Pediatric Cerebral Hemispheric Tumors

Ramesh Raghupathi, PhD

Assistant Professor, Department of Neurobiology and Anatomy, Drexel University College of Medicine, Philadelphia, Pennsylvania

Cellular Basis of Injury and Recovery from Trauma

Frank A. Raila, MD

Professor Emeritus, Department of Radiology, University of Mississippi School of Medicine, Jackson, Mississippi

Radiology of the Skull

Zvi Ram, MD

Associate Professor of Surgery, Division of Neurosurgery, Tel Aviv University Sackler School of Medicine, Tel Aviv; Deputy Chairman, Department of Neurosurgery, Chaim Sheba Medical Center, Tel Hashomer, Israel

Principles of Gene Therapy

Bruce R. Ransom, MD, PhD

Professor and Chairman, Department of Neurology, University of Washington School of Medicine, Seattle, Washington

Astrocytes

Robert A. Ratcheson, MD

Professor of Neurological Surgery, Department of Neurological Surgery, Case Western Reserve University School of Medicine; Director, Department of Neurological Surgery, and the Research Institute, University Hospitals of Cleveland, Cleveland, Ohio

Intraoperative Cerebral Protection

Peter Raudzens, MD

Anesthesiologist, Department of Neuroanesthesia, Barrow Neurological Institute, Phoenix, Arizona

Anesthesia in Cerebrovascular Disease

Shlomo Raz, MD

Professor of Urology, Head of Reconstructive and Female Urology, David Geffen School of Medicine at UCLA, Los Angeles, California

Neurourology

Gary L. Rea, MD, PhD

Private Practice, University Orthopedic Physicians, Columbus, Ohio

Alyssa T. Reddy, MD

Assistant Professor of Pediatrics and Neurology, University of Alabama School of Medicine; Pediatric Neurologist, The Children's Hospital of Alabama, Birmingham, Alabama

Intracranial Germ Cell Tumors

Patrick M. Reilly, MD

Assistant Professor of Surgery, University of Pennsylvania School of Medicine, Philadelphia, Pennsylvania

Initial Resuscitation and Patient Evaluation

Harold L. Rekate, MD

Clinical Professor of Surgery, Division of Neurosurgery, University of Arizona College of Medicine, Tucson; Chairman, Section of Pediatric Neurosciences, and Director, Pediatric Neurosurgical Research Laboratory, Barrow Neurological Institute, Phoenix, Arizona

Hydrocephalus in Children

Ali R. Rezai, MD

Associate Professor and Head, Section for Stereotactic and Functional Neurosurgery, Department of Neurological Surgery, The Cleveland Clinic Foundation, Cleveland, Ohio

Deep Brain Stimulation for Chronic Pain

Laurence D. Rhines, MD

Assistant Professor of Neurosurgical Oncology, Department of Neurosurgery, University of Texas–Houston Medical School; Director, Spine Program, Department of Neurosurgery, The University of Texas M.D. Anderson Cancer Center, Houston, Texas

Brain Tumors during Pregnancy; Sarcoidosis, Tuberculosis, and Xanthogranuloma

Albert L. Rhoton, Jr., MD

R.D. Keene Family Professor, Chairman Emeritus, Department of Neurosurgery, University of Florida College of Medicine, Gainesville, Florida

Surgical Anatomy of the Brain

Teresa Ribalta, MD, PhD

Associate Professor of Pathology, University of Barcelona Medical School; Consultant, Department of Pathology, Hospital Clinic of Barcelona, Barcelona, Spain

Brain Tumors: An Overview of Histopathologic Classification

Bernd Richling, MD

Professor of Neurosurgery, Private Medical University of Salzburg, Salzburg Austria

Embolization of Arteriovenous Malformations as a Primary Treatment Modality

Charles J. Riedel, MD

Assistant Professor of Neurosurgery, Columbia University College of Physicians and Surgeons; Attending, Department of Neurological Surgery, Columbia-Presbyterian Medical Center, New York, New York

Surgical Exposures and Positioning for Spinal Surgery

Daniele Rigamonti, MD

Professor, Department of Neurosurgery, Johns Hopkins University School of Medicine; Director, Skeletal Dysplasias and Genetics, Johns Hopkins Hospital, Baltimore, Maryland

Anterior Communicating Artery and Anterior Cerebral Artery Aneurysms; Achondroplasia and Other Dwarfism

Howard A. Riina, MD

Assistant Professor of Neurological Surgery, Neurology, and Radiology, Cornell University Joan and Sanford I. Weill Medical College; Attending Neurosurgeon, New York Presbyterian Hospital, New York, New York

Giant Aneurysms; Classification of Spinal Cord Vascular Lesions

Michael E. C. Robbins, PhD

Professor, Department of Radiology, Wake Forest University School of Medicine; Head, Radiation Biology Section, Wake Forest Baptist Medical Center, Winston-Salem, North Carolina

Radiobiology

Claudia Robertson, MD

Professor, Department of Neurosurgery, Baylor College of Medicine; Medical Director, Neurosurgical Intensive Care Unit, Ben Taub General Hospital, Houston, Texas

Critical Care Management of Traumatic Brain Injury

Jon H. Robertson, MD

Chairman, Department of Neurosurgery, University of Tennessee, Memphis, College of Medicine, Memphis, Tennessee

Glomus Jugulare Tumors

Lawrence Robinson, MD

Professor and Chair, Department of Rehabilitation Medicine, University of Washington School of Medicine; Director, Electrodiagnostic Laboratory, Harborview Medical Center, Seattle, Washington

Electrodiagnostic Evaluation of Peripheral Nerves: Electromyography, Somatosensory Evoked Potentials, Nerve Action Potentials

Shenandoah Robinson, MD

Assistant Professor, Department of Neurological Surgery, Case Western Reserve University School of Medicine; Pediatric Neurosurgeon, Rainbow Babies and Children's Hospital, Cleveland, Ohio

Myelomeningocele and Myelocystocele; Intervertebral Disk Disease in Children

Mark A. Rockoff, MD

Professor of Anesthesia, Harvard Medical School; Vice-Chairman, Department of Anesthesia, Children's Hospital, Boston, Massachusetts

Neuroanesthesia in Children

Mark L. Rosenblum, MD

Chairman, Department of Neurosurgery, and Co-Director, Hermelin Brain Tumor Center, Henry Ford Hospital, Detroit, Michigan

Invasion in Malignant Glioma

Walter Royal III, MD

Associate Professor, Departments of Neurology, Morehouse School of Medicine, Atlanta, Georgia

Multiple Sclerosis

Ronald Ruff, PhD

Clinical Professor, Department of Psychiatry, University of California, San Francisco, School of Medicine, San Francisco, California

Sequelae of Traumatic Brain Injury

James T. Rutka, MD, PhD

Professor and Chairman, Division of Neurosurgery, University of Toranto Faculty of Medicine; Staff Neurosurgeon, The Hospital for Sick Children, Toronto, Ontario, Canada

Encephaloceles

Kathryn E. Saatman, MD

Associate Professor, Department of Neurosurgery, University of Pennsylvania School of Medicine, Philadelphia, Pennsylvania

Cellular Basis of Injury and Recovery from Trauma

Oren Sagher, MD

Associate Professor, Section of Neurosurgery, University of Michigan Medical College, Ann Arbor, Michigan

Diagnosis and Nonoperative Management [Trigeminal Neuralgia]

Sean A. Salehi, MD

Chief Resident, Department of Neurological Surgery, Northwestern Memorial Hospital, Chicago, Illinois

Adult Thoracolumbar Scoliosis

Ali Samii, MD

Assistant Professor of Neurology and Neurological Surgery, University of Washington School of Medicine, Seattle, Washington

Approach to Movement Disorders

Madjid Samii, MD

Professor and Chairman, Department of Neurosurgery, International Neuroscience Institute, Hanover, Germany

Basic Principles of Skull Base Surgery

Prakash Sampath, MD

Assistant Professor of Neurosurgery and Assistant Professor of Clinical Neurosciences, Brown University School of Medicine; Director, Neurosurgical Oncology, and Chief of Neurosurgery, Roger Williams Hospital, Providence, Rhode Island

Acoustic Neuroma; Sarcoidosis, Tuberculosis, and Xanthogranuloma

Duke Samson, MD

Professor and Chair, Department of Neurosurgery, University of Texas Southwestern Medical School, Dallas, Texas

Posterior Fossa Arteriovenous Malformations

Paul Santiago, MD

Resident, Department of Neurological Surgery, University of Washington Hospitals, Seattle, Washington

Malignant Gliomas: Anaplastic Astrocytoma, Glioblastoma Multiforme, Gliosarcoma, Malignant Oligodendroglioma; Benign Extradural Lesions of the Dorsal Spine

Harvey B. Sarnat, MD

Professor of Pediatrics (Neurology) and Pathology (Neuropathology), David Geffen School of Medicine at UCLA; Director, Division of Pediatric Neurology, and Neuropathologist, Cedars-Sinai Medical Center, Los Angeles, California

Neuroembryology

Raymond Sawaya, MD

Professor of Neurosurgery, University of Texas–Houston Medical School; Director, Brain Tumor Center, and Chairman, Department of Neurosurgery, The University of Texas M.D. Anderson Cancer Center, Houston, Texas

Brain Tumors: General Considerations; Metastatic Brain Tumors

Paul D. Sawin, MD

Private Practice, Orlando, Florida

Biology of Bone Grafting and Healing in Spinal Surgery; Posterior Cervical Stabilization and Fusion Techniques

Wouter I. Schievink, MD

Assistant Clinical Professor, Department of Neurological Surgery, University of California, Irvine, School of Medicine, Irvine; Attending Neurosurgeon, Cedars-Sinai Medical Center, and Co-Director, Neurovascular Surgery Program, Cedars-Sinai Neurosurgical Institute, Los Angeles, California

Genetics of Intracranial Aneurysms

Jay J. Schindler, MD, MS

Assistant Professor, Department of Neurologic Surgery, Mayo School of Medicine; Resident, Mayo Clinic, Rochester, Minnesota

Multimodality Management of Complex Cerebrovascular Lesions

James M. Schuster, MD, PhD

Assistant Professor of Neurosurgery, University of Pennsylvania School of Medicine; Attending, Department of Neurosurgery, Hospital of the University of Pennsylvania, Philadelphia, Pennsylvania

Growth Factors and Brain Tumors; Motor, Sensory, and Language Mapping and Monitoring for Cortical Resections; Posterior Thoracic Instrumentation

Theodore H. Schwartz, MD

Assistant Professor of Neurosurgery, Cornell University Joan and Sanford I. Weill Medical College; Assistant Attending in Neurosurgery, New York Presbyterian Hospital, New York, New York

Spinal Cord Tumors in Adults

R. Michael Scott, MD

Professor of Neurological Surgery, Harvard Medical School; Director, Clinical Pediatric Neurosurgery, The Children's Hospital and Medical Center, Boston, Massachusetts

Choroid Plexus Tumors; Cerebellar Astrocytomas in Children

Raymond Sekula, MD

Resident, Department of Neurosurgery, Allegheny General Hospital, Pittsburgh, Pennsylvania

Ablative Surgery for Spasticity

Laligam N. Sekhar, MD

Private Practice, Annandale, Virginia

Chordoma and Chondrosarcoma

Warren R. Selman, MD

Professor of Neurological Surgery, Department of Neurological Surgery, Case Western Reserve University School of Medicine; Vice Chairman, Department of Neurological Surgery, and The Research Institute, University Hospitals of Cleveland, Cleveland, Ohio

Intraoperative Cerebral Protection

Chandranath Sen, MD

Chairman, Department of Neurosurgery, and Co-Director, Center for Cranial Surgery, St. Luke's-Roosevelt Medical Center, New York, New York

Trigeminal Schwannomas

Joel L. Seres, MD

Clinical Professor, Department of Neurosurgery, Oregon Health Sciences University School of Medicine; Director, Northwest Occupational Medicine Center, Portland, Oregon

Approach to the Patient with Chronic Pain

Franco Servadei, MD

Professor of Neurotraumatology, Post-Graduate Medical School, University of Catania, Ancona; Director, WHO Neurotrauma Collaborating Center, Division of Neurosurgery, Hospital M. Bufalini, Cesena, Italy

Mild Head Injury in Adults

Avi Setton, MD

Attending, Center for Endovascular Surgery, Institute for Neurology and Neurosurgery, Beth Israel Medical Center, New York, New York

Endovascular Management of Brain Arteriovenous Malformations

Christopher I. Shaffrey, MD

Professor, Department of Neurological Surgery and Department of Orthopaedic Surgery, University of Virginia School of Medicine, Charlottesville, Virginia

Spondylolisthesis; Approach to the Patient and Medical Management of Spinal Disorders; Posterior Approach to Cervical Degenerative Disease

David Shafron, MD

Neurosurgeon, Phoenix Children's Hospital, Phoenix, Arizona

Benign Extradural Lesions of the Dorsal Spine

William R. Shapiro, MD

Professor of Neurology, University of Arizona College of Medicine, Tucson; Chief, Neuro-oncology, Division of Neurology, Barrow Neurological Institute, Phoenix, Arizona

Clinical Features: Neurology of Brain Tumor and Paraneoplastic Disorders

Michael Shea, MD

Attending, Department of Radiation Oncology, Hoag Memorial Hospital Presbyterian, Newport Beach, California

Functional Radiosurgery

Jonas M. Sheehan, MD

Chief, Division of Neuro-oncology and Cranial Base Surgery, Department of Neurosurgery, Pennsylvania State University Hospitals, Hershey, Pennsylvania

Esthesioneuroblastoma

Joseph H. Shin, MD

Assistant Professor of Surgery, Section of Plastic Surgery, Department of Surgery, Yale University School of Medicine; Director, Yale Craniofacial Center, Yale–New Haven Hospital, New Haven, Connecticut

Craniofacial Syndromes

Raj K. Shrivastava, MD

Chief Resident, Department of Neurosurgery, Mount Sinai Medical School,, New York, New York

Trigeminal Schwannomas

David Sibell, MD

Assistant Professor, Department of Anesthesiology and Perioperative Medicine, Oregon Health & Science University, Portland, Oregon

Management of Pain by Anesthetic Techniques

Bo K. Siesjö, Md, PhD

Professor, Center for the Study of Neurological Disease, The Queen's Neuroscience Institute, Honolulu, Hawaii

Cerebral Metabolism and the Pathophysiology of Ischemic Brain Damage

Peter Siesjö, MD, PhD

Assistant Professor, Department of Neurosurgery, University of Lund School of Medicine; Consultant, University Hospital, Lund, Sweden

Cerebral Metabolism and the Pathophysiology of Ischemic Brain Damage

Daniel L. Silbergeld, MD

Associate Professor, Department of Neurological Surgery, University of Washington School of Medicine, Seattle, Washington

Malignant Gliomas: Anaplastic Astrocytoma, Glioblastoma Multiforme, Gliosarcoma, Malignant Oligodendroglioma; Motor, Sensory, and Language Mapping and Monitoring for Cortical Resections

Jerry Silver, Ph.D.

Professor, Department of Neurosciences, Case Western Reserve University School of Medicine, Cleveland, Ohio

Cellular and Molecular Mechanisms Mediating Injury and Recovery in the Nervous System

Scott L. Simon, MD, MPH

Resident, Department of Neurosurgery, Hospital of the University of Pennsylvania, Philadelphia, Pennsylvania

Posterior Thoracic Instrumentation

Ran Vijai P. Singh, MBBS

Resident, Department of Neurosurgery, University of Miami Hospital and Clinics, Miami, Florida

Spontaneous Intracerebral Hemorrhage: Non–Arteriovenous Malformation, Nonaneurysm

Ash Singhal, MD

Senior Resident, Department of Neurosurgery, University of Toronto Faculty of Medicine, Toronto, Ontario, Canada

Tumors of the Vertebral Axis: Benign, Primary Malignant, and Metastatic Tumors

Grant Sinson, MD

Associate Professor of Neurosurgery, Medical College of Wisconsin, Milwaukee, Wisconsin

Initial Resuscitation and Patient Evaluation [Moderate and Severe Traumatic Brain Injury]

Stephen L. Skirboll, MD

Assistant Professor, Department of Neurosurgery, Stanford University; Staff, Palo Alto Veterans Affairs Medical Center, Palo Alto, California

Monitoring and Mapping of Vision in the Neurosurgical Patient

Jefferson Slimp, PhD

Associate Professor, Department of Rehabilitation Medicine, University of Washington School of Medicine; Director, Neurophysiological Monitoring, University of Washington Medical Center, Seattle, Washington

Electrodiagnostic Evaluation of Peripheral Nerves: Electromyography, Somatosensory Evoked Potentials, Nerve Action Potentials

Yoland Smith, PhD

Professor of Neurology, Emory University School of Medicine; Staff, Yerkes National Primate Research Center, Atlanta, Georgia

Anatomy and Synaptic Connectivity of the Basal Ganglia

P. K. Sneed, MD

Professor in Residence, Department of Radiation Oncology, University of California, San Francisco, San Francisco, California

Interstitial and Intracavitary Irradiation of Brain Tumors

Robert A. Solomon, MD

Byron Stookey Professor and Chairman, Department of Neurological Surgery, Columbia University College of Physicians and Surgeons, New York, New York

Techniques for Deep Hypothermic Circulatory Arrest

Volker K. H. Sonntag, MD

Clinical Professor of Surgery (Neurosurgery), University of Arizona College of Medicine, Tucson; Vice Chairman, Division of Neurological Surgery, Director, Residency Program, and Chairman, Spine Section, Barrow Neurological Institute, Phoenix, Arizona

Anterior Approach including Cervical Corpectomy; Anterior Cervical Instrumentation; Basic Principles of Spinal Internal Fixation; Occipitocervical Fusion; Overview and Historical Considerations [Spine];

Sulpicio G. Soriano, MD, MSEd

Associate Professor of Anesthesia, Harvard Medical School; Associate in Anesthesia, Children's Hospital, Boston, Massachussetts

Neuroanesthesia in Children

Dennis D. Spencer, MD

Professor, Department of Neurosurgery, Yale University School of Medicine, New Haven, Connecticut

Intracranial Monitoring

Robert F. Spetzler, MD

Professor, Department of Surgery, Section of Neurosurgery, University of Arizona College of Medicine, Tucson; Director and J. N. Harbor Chairman of Neurological Surgery, Barrow Neurological Institute, Phoenix, Arizona

Anesthesia in Cerebrovascular Disease; Traumatic Carotid Injury; Surgical Approaches for Posterior Circulation Aneurysms; Giant Aneurysms; Infratentorial Cavernous Malformations; Classification of Spinal Cord Vascular Lesions

Brett Stacey, MD

Associate Professor, Department of Anesthesiology and Perioperative Medicine, Oregon Health & Science University, Portland, Oregon

Management of Pain by Anesthetic Techniques

Gary K. Steinberg, MD, PhD

Lacroute-Hearst Professor and Chairman, Department of Neurosurgery, Stanford University School of Medicine, Stanford, California

Surgical and Radiosurgical Management of Giant Arteriovenous Malformations; General and Historical Considerations of Radiotherapy and Radiosurgery

Paul Steinbok, MBBS

Professor, Department of Surgery, University of British Columbia Faculty of Medicine; Head, Division of Pediatric Neurosurgery, Children's and Women's Health Centre, Vancouver, British Columbia, Canada

Intrathecal Baclofen Infusion

Barney J. Stern, MD

Professor and Executive Vice Chairman, Department of Neurology, Emory University School of Medicine, Atlanta, Georgia

Sarcoidosis, Tuberculosis, and Xanthogranuloma

David A. Steven, MD

Chief Resident, Department of Clinical Neurological Sciences (Neurosurgery), University of Western Ontario Faculty of Medicine, London, Ontario, Canada

Distal Anterior Cerebral Artery Aneurysms

Kimberly J. Stewart, PhD

Clinical Neuropsychologist, Hampton Roads Neuropsychology, Inc., Virginia Beach, Virginia
Rehabilitation and Prognosis after Traumatic Brain Injury

Charles B. Stillerman, MD

Clinical Professor, Department of Surgery, University of North Dakota School of Medicine, Grand Forks; Director, Department of Neurosurgery, Trinity Medical Center, Minot, North Dakota
Intradiskal and Percutaneous Treatment of Lumbar Disk Disease

John H. Suh, MD

Clinical Director, Department of Radiation Oncology, Cleveland Clinic, Cleveland, Ohio
Principles of Radiotherapy

Peter P. Sun, MD

Assistant Clinical Professor, Department of Neurological Surgery, University of California, San Francisco, School of Medicine, San Francisco; Chief, Division of Neurosurgery, Children's Hospital and Research Center at Oakland, Oakland, California
Pediatric Vertebral Column and Spinal Cord Injuries

Leslie N. Sutton, MD

Professor of Neurosurgery, University of Pennsylvania School of Medicine; Chief, Neurosurgery, Children's Hospital of Philadelphia, Philadelphia, Pennsylvania
Intracranial Ependymomas

Phillip D. Swanson, MD, PhD

Professor of Neurology, University of Washington School of Medicine, Seattle, Washington
History and Physical Examination [Introduction: Approach to the Patient]

Sara J. Swanson, PhD

Associate Professor, Department of Neurology, Medical College of Wisconsin, Milwaukee, Wisconsin
Functional Magnetic Resonance Imaging in Epilepsy Surgery

George W. Sypert, MD

Sypert Institute, Fort Myers, Florida
Evaluation and Management of the Failed Back Syndrome

Derek A. Taggard, MD

Chief Resident, Division of Neurosurgery, University of Iowa Hospitals and Clinics, Iowa City, Iowa
Treatment of Occipital C1 Injury

Jamal M. Taha, MD

Taha Neurosurgical Clinic Kettering; Ohio
Dorsal Rhizotomy and Dorsal Root Ganglionectomy

Rafael J. Tamargo, MD

Associate Professor, Department of Neurosurgery and Otolaryngology, Division of Head and Neck Surgery, Johns Hopkins University School of Medicine; Director, Division of Cerebrovascular Neurosurgery, Department of Neurosurgery, Johns Hopkins Hospital, Baltimore, Maryland
Surgical Positioning and Exposures for Cranial Procedures; Anterior Communicating Artery and Anterior Cerebral Artery Aneurysms

Nitin Tandon, MD

Chief Resident, Center for Neurosurgical Sciences, University of Texas Health Science Center; Chief Resident, University Hospital, Audie L Murphy VA Hospital, San Antonio, Texas
Infections of the Spine and Spinal Cord

Ronald Tasker, MD

Emeritus Professor, Division of Neurosurgery, Department of Surgery, University of Toronto Faculty of Medicine, Toronto, Ontario, Canada
Deep Brain Stimulation for Chronic Pain

Marcos Tatagiba, MD, PhD

Professor and Chairman, Department of Neurosurgery, University of Tuebingen, Tuebingen, Germany
Basic Principles of Skull Base Surgery

Christopher L. Taylor, MD

Resident, Department of Neurological Surgery, University Hospitals of Cleveland, Cleveland, Ohio
Intraoperative Cerebral Protection

Steven A. Telian, MD

John L. Kemink Professor of Neurotology, Department of Otolaryngology–Head and Neck Surgery, University of Michigan Medical School; Director, Division of Otology, Neurotology and Skull Base Surgery, and Medical Director, Cochlear Implant Program, University of Michigan Hospitals, Ann Arbor, Michigan
Treatment of Intractable Vertigo

Kamal Thapar, MD

Assistant Professor, Department of Neurosurgery, University of Toronto Faculty of Medicine, Toronto, Ontario, Canada

Nicholas Theodore, MD

Chief, Section of Neurosurgical Trauma, Division of Neurosurgery, Barrow Neurological Institute, Phoenix, Arizona
Anesthesia in Cerebrovascular Disease; Thoracoscopic Approaches to the Spine

Philip V. Theodosopoulos, MD

Assistant Professor, Department of Neurological Surgery, University of Cincinnati College of Medicine; Director, Skull Base Surgery, Mayfield Clinic, Cincinnati, Ohio

Ossification of the Posterior Longitudinal Ligament and Other Enthesopathies

B. Gregory Thompson, MD

Associate Professor, Department of Neurosurgery, University of Michigan Medical School; Director, Cerebrovascular and Skull Base Section, University of Michigan Hospitals, Ann Arbor, Michigan

Spinal Arteriovenous Malformations; Pregnancy and Treatment of Vascular Disease

Todd P. Thompson, MD

Chief of Neurosurgery, Straub Clinic and Hospital, Honolulu, Hawaii

Patient Selection in Movement Disorder Surgery

William E. Thorell, MD

Resident, Department of Neurosurgery, University of Nebraska Medical Center, Omaha, Nebraska

Brain Tumors: Population-Based Epidemiology, Environmental Risk Factors, and Genetic and Hereditary Syndromes

Robert Tiel, MD

Associate Professor, Department of Neurosurgery, Louisiana State University School of Medicine at New Orleans; Attending Neurosurgeon, Charity Hospital and Ochsner Hospital, New Orleans, Louisiana

Management of Peripheral Nerve Tumors

Suzie C. Tindall, MD

Professor, Department of Neurosurgery, Emory University School of Medicine, Atlanta, Georgia

Carpal Tunnel Syndrome; Entrapment Syndromes of Peripheral Nerve Injuries

Paul Tolentino, MD

Resident, Department of Neurosurgery, University of Florida College of Medicine, Gainesville, Florida

Posterior Lumbar Instrumentation

Tadanori Tomita, MD

Yeager Professor of Pediatric Neurosurgery, Northwestern University Feinberg Medical School; Chairman, Division of Neurosurgery, Children's Memorial Hospital, Chicago, Illinois

Birth Head Trauma

Steven A. Toms, MD, MPH

Assistant Professor, Department of Neurological Surgery, and Head, Section of Neurosurgical Oncology, Oregon Health & Science University School of Medicine; Chief, Section of Neurosurgery, Portland VA Medical Center, Portland, Oregon

Tumor Suppressor Genes and the Genesis of Brain Tumors

Kathleen R. Tozer, MD

Resident, Department of Neurosurgery, University of Washington, Seattle, Washington

Monitoring and Mapping of Vision in the Neurosurgical Patient

Bruce D. Trapp, PhD

Professor, Department of Neurosciences, Case Western Reserve University School of Medicine, Cleveland; Professor, Department of Cell Biology, Neurobiology, and Anatomy, Ohio State University, Cleveland; Professor Department of Chemistry, Cleveland State University, Cleveland; Professor Department of Cellular and Molecular Biology, Kent State University, Kent; Chairman, Department of Neurosciences, Lerner Research Institute, Cleveland Clinic Foundation, Cleveland, Ohio

Neurons and Neuroglia

Vincent C. Traynelis, MD

Professor of Neurosurgery, Department of Surgery, University of Iowa College of Medicine; Staff Neurosurgeon, University of Iowa Hospitals and Clinics, Iowa City, Iowa

Tumors of the Craniovertebral Junction; Treatment of Occipital C1 Injury

R. Shane Tubbs, MS, PA-C

Instructor in Anatomy, University of Alabama School of Medicine; Physician Assistant, Pediatric Neurosurgery Section, Children's Hospital, Birmingham, Alabama

Chiari Malformations

Ramachandra Tummala, MD

Resident, Department of Neurosurgery, University of Minnesota Medical School, Minneapolis, Minnesota

Standard Temporal Lobectomy and Transsylvian Amygdalohippocampectomy

Michael Tymianski, MD, PhD

Assistant Professor, Department of Surgery, University of Toronto Faculty of Medicine; Staff Neurosurgeon, Toronto Western Hospital, University Health Network, Toronto, Ontario, Canada

Surgical Approaches for Anterior Circulation Aneurysms

Atsushi Umemura, MD

Fellow in Stereotactic and Functional Neurosurgery, Department of Neurosurgery, University of Pennsylvania School of Medicine, Philadelphia, Pennsylvania

Topectomy: Uses and Indications

G. Edward Vates, MD, PhD

Staff, Department of Neurological Surgery, Brigham and Women's Hospital, Boston, Massachusetts

Hemangioblastomas of the Central Nervous System; Surgical Approaches for Posterior Circulation Aneurysms

A. Giancarlo Vishteh, MD

Co-Director, Neurotrauma, John C. Lincoln North Mountain Hospital, Phoenix, Arizona

Anesthesia in Cerebrovascular Disease; Traumatic Carotid Injury; Anterior Cervical Instrumentation;

André Visot, MD

Chief, Neurosurgical Service, Hôpital Foch, Suresnes, France

Osseous Tumors

Jerrold L. Vitek, MD, PhD

Professor, Department of Neurology, Emory University School of Medicine, Atlanta, Georgia

Surgery for Dystonia

Kenneth P. Vives, MD

Assistant Professor, Department of Neurosurgery, Yale University School of Medicine; Neurosurgeon, Yale Neurovascular Surgery Program, Neurovascular-Neuroscience Intensive Care Unit, Yale–New Haven Hospital, and Backus Hospital, New Haven, Connecticut

Unusual Gliomas; Surgical Management of Supratentorial Cavernous Malformations; Intracranial Monitoring

Dennis G. Vollmer, MD

Professor of Neurosurgery, University of Texas Health Science Center at Houston; Director, Comprehensive Center for Cerebrovascular Surgery, Memorial Hermann Hospital, Houston, Texas

Overview and Historical Considerations [Spine]; Infections of the Spine and Spinal Cord; Cervical Spine Trauma

Jennifer Vookles, MD

Assistant Professor, Department of Anesthesiology and Perioperative Medicine, Oregon Health & Science University, Portland, Oregon

Management of Pain by Anesthetic Techniques

Phillip A. Wackym, MD

John C. Koss Professor and Chairman, Department of Otolaryngology and Communication Sciences, Medical College of Wisconsin; Chief, Otolaryngology–Head and Neck Surgery, Froedtert & Medical College Hospital, and Children's Hospital of Wisconsin, Milwaukee, Wisconsin

Neuro-otology

Tom Wagner, PhD

Instructor, Department of Oncology, Mayo Graduate School of Medicine, Mayo Clinic; Therapeutic Radiological Physicist, St. Luke's Hospital, Jacksonville, Florida

Fractionated and Stereotactic Radiation, Extracranial Stereotactic Radiation, Intensity Modulation, and Multileaf Collimation

Gregory R. Wahle, MD

Clinical Associate Professor of Urology, Indiana University School of Medicine, Indianapolis, Indiana

Neurourology

Marion L. Walker, MD

Professor of Neurosurgery and Professor of Pediatrics, University of Utah School of Medicine; Chairman, Division of Pediatric Neurosurgery, Primary Children's Medical Center/University of Utah Medical Center, Salt Lake City, Utah

Nonsyndromic Craniosynostosis and Abnormalities of Head Shape

Paul R. Walker, PhD

Private Docent, University of Geneva, Faculty of Medicine; Biologist, University Hospital Geneva, Geneva, Switzerland

Aspects of Immunology Applicable to Brain Tumor Pathogenesis and Treatment

M. Christopher Wallace, MD

Chief, Division of Neurosurgery, University of Toronto Health Network, Toronto, Ontario, Canada

Intracranial Internal Carotid Artery Aneurysms

John W. Walsh, MD, PhD

Professor of Neurosurgery and Pediatrics, Tulane University Medical School; Chief, Section of Pediatric Neurosurgery, Tulane University Hospital and Clinic, New Orleans, Louisiana

Lipomyelomeningocele

Paul P. Wang, MD

Attending, Department of Neurological Surgery, Johns Hopkins Hospital, Baltimore, Maryland

Glomus Jugulare Tumors

John D. Ward, MD

Professor and Vice Chairman, Division of Neurosurgery , Department of Surgery, Virginia Commonwealth University School of Medicine, Richmond, Virginia

Pediatric Head Injury

Benjamin C. Warf, MD

Formerly Professor of Neurosurgery, University of Kentucky College of Medicine, Lexington, Kentucky

Tethered Spinal Cord

Ronald E. Warnick, MD
Professor of Neurosurgery, University of Cincinnati School of Medicine, Cincinnati, Ohio
Surgical Complications and Their Avoidance

Katherine E. Warren, MD
Tenure-Track Clinician, Pediatric Neuro-oncology, National Cancer Institute, National Institutes of Health, Bethesda, Maryland
Principles of Chemotherapy

W. Lee Warren, MD
Chief Resident, Department of Neurosurgery, Allegheny General Hospital, Pittsburgh, Pennsylvania
Diagnosis and Management of Seventh and Eighth Cranial Nerve Injuries due to Temporal Bone Fractures

Kyle D. Weaver, MD
Department of Neurosurgery, University of North Carolina at Chapel Hill School of Medicine, Chapel Hill, North Carolina

Jon Weingart, MD
Associate Professor of Neurosurgery and Oncology, Johns Hopkins University School of Medicine; Attending Neurosurgeon, Johns Hopkins Hospital, Baltimore, Maryland
Basic Principles of Cranial Surgery for Brain Tumors

Philip R. Weinstein, MD
Professor of Neurosurgery, University of California, San Francisco, School of Medicine, San Francisco, California
Ossification of the Posterior Longitudinal Ligament and Other Enthesopathies

Bryce Weir, MD
Interim Dean, Biological Sciences Division, University of Chicago Medical Center, Chicago, Illinois
Perioperative Management of Subarachnoid Hemorrhage

Hung Tzu Wen, MD
Courtesy Assistant Professor, Department of Neurological Surgery, University of Florida College of Medicine, Gainesville, Florida; Clinical Instructor, Division of Neurosurgery Hospital Das Clínicas—University of São Paulo; Clinical Associate, Hospital Samaritanod, São Paulo, Brazil
Surgical Anatomy of the Brain

G. Alexander West, PhD, MD
Associate Professor, Department of Neurological Surgery, Oregon Health & Science University Portland, Oregon
Traumatic Cerebral Aneurysms Secondary to Penetrating Intracranial Injuries

Michael F. Whelan, MD, DDS
Assistant Professor, Department of Surgery, Division of Craniofacial Plastic and Reconstructive Surgery, University of Washington School of Medicine; Attending Plastic and Craniofacial Surgeon, Children's Hospital and Regional Medical Center and Harborview Medical Center, Seattle, Washington
Craniofacial Trauma

Walter W. Whisler, MD
Professor and Chairman Emeritus, Department of Neurosurgery, Rush Medical College; Attending Neurosurgeon, Rush-Presbyterian-St. Luke's Medical Center, Chicago, Illinois
Multiple Subpial Transection

Jonathan White, MD
Assistant Professor of Neurosurgery, University of Texas Southwestern Medical School, Dallas, Texas
Posterior Fossa Arteriovenous Malformations

Thomas Wichmann, MD
Associate Professor of Neurology, Emory University School of Medicine, Atlanta, Georgia
Rationale for Surgical Interventions in Movement Disorders

Agadha Wickremesekera, MBChB (Ontario),
Consultant Neurosurgeon, Wakefield Hospital, Wellington, New Zealand
Infantile Posthemorrhagic Hydrocephalus

Gregory C. Wiggins, MD
Staff Neurosurgeon, David Grant Medical Center, Travis AFB, California
Posterior Approach to Cervical Degenerative Disease

James C. Wilberger, MD
Chair, Department of Neurosurgery, Allegheny General Hospital, Pittsburgh, Pennsylvania
Diagnosis and Management of Seventh and Eighth Cranial Nerve Injuries due to Temporal Bone Fractures

David M. Wildrick, PhD
Attending, Department of Neurosurgery, The University of Texas M.D. Anderson Cancer Center, Houston, Texas
Metastatic Brain Tumors

Lorna Sohn Williams, MD
Assistant Professor, Department of Radiology, University of Florida College of Medicine, Gainesville, Florida
Vein of Galen Malformations

H. Richard Winn, MD

Professor of Neurological Surgery and Neuroscience, Mount Sinai School of Medicine, New York, New York

The Natural History of Unruptured Saccular Cerebral Aneurysms; Surgical Decision Making for the Treatment of Cerebral Aneurysms; Traumatic Cerebral Aneurysms Secondary to Penetrating Intracranial Injuries; Monitoring and Mapping of Vision in the Neurosurgical Patient

Diana Barrett Wiseman, MD

Spine Fellow, Department of Neurological Surgery, University of Washington School of Medicine, Seattle, Washington

Spondylolisthesis

Jeffrey H. Wisoff, MD

Associate Professor of Neurosurgery and Pediatrics, New York University School of Medicine; Director, Division of Pediatric Neurosurgery, New York University Medical Center, New York, New York

Optic Pathway and Hypothalamic Gliomas in Children

Timothy F. Witham, MD

Department of Neurological Surgery, University of Pittsburgh School of Medicine, Pittsburgh, Pennsylvania

Gamma Knife Radiosurgery

W. Putnam Wolcott, MD

Department of Neurological Surgery, University of Virginia School of Medicine, Charlottesville, Virginia

Approach to the Patient and Medical Management, of Spinal Disorders

Donald C. Wright, MD

Surgeon, Washington Brain & Spine Institute, Bethesda, Maryland

Elaine Wyllie, MD

Head, Pediatric Epilepsy Program, Cleveland Clinic, Cleveland, Ohio

Recognition of Surgical Candidates and the Presurgical Evaluation

Kevin Yao, MD

Resident, Department of Neurosurgery, Mount Sinai Medical Center, New York, New York

Infectious Intracranial Aneurysms

Narayan Yoganandan, PhD

Professor and Chair, Department of Biomedical Engineering, and Professor, Department of Neurosurgery, Medical College of Wisconsin; Adjunct Professor of Biomedical Engineering, Marquette University, Milwaukee, Wisconsin

Concepts and Mechanisms of Biomechanics

Howard Yonas, MD

Peter J. Jannetta Professor of Neurological Surgery, University of Pittsburgh School of Medicine; Vice Chairman, Neurological Surgery, and Chief, Cerebrovascular Surgery, and Co-Director, University of Pittsburgh Medical Center Stroke Institute, University of Pittsburgh Medical Center-Presbyterian, Pittsburgh, Pennsylvania

Xenon Computed Tomography

Julie E. York, MD

Instructor, Department of Neurosurgery, Loyola University of Chicago Stritch School of Medicine, Maywood, Illinois

Treatment of Axis Fractures; Diagnosis and Management of Thoracolumbar and Lumbar Spine Injuries

Andrew S. Youkilis, MD

Chief Resident, Department of Neurosurgery, University Hospital, Ann Arbor, Michigan

Primitive Neuroectodermal Tumors; Diagnosis and Nonoperative Management [Trigeminal Neuralgia]

George P. H. Young, MD

Associate Professor of Clinical Urology, Cornell University Joan and Sanford I. Weill Medical College; Associate Attending Urologist and Director, Female Urology, Neurourology, Urodynamics, and Reconstructive Urology Unit, New York Presbyterian Hospital, New York, New York

Neurourology

David M. Yousem, MD

Professor of Radiology, Johns Hopkins University School of Medicine; Director, Division of Neuroradiology, Johns Hopkins Hospital, Baltimore, Maryland

Radiologic Features of Central Nervous System Tumors

Eric C. Yuen, MD

Associate Director of Clinical Research, Department of Clinical Neuroscience, Merck Research Laboratories, West Point, Pennsylvania

Peripheral Neuropathies; Electrodiagnostic Evaluation of Peripheral Nerves: Electromyography, Somatosensory Evoked Potentials, Nerve Action Potentials

Joseph M. Zabramski, MD

Chairman, Section of Cerebrovascular Surgery, Division of Neurological Surgery, Barrow Neurological Institute, Phoenix, Arizona

Epidemiology and Natural History of Cavernous Malformations; The Genetics of Cerebral Cavernous Malformations

Alois Zauner, MD

Clinical Instructor, Department of Radiology; University of California, Los Angeles, California

Surgical Management of Traumatic Brain Injury

Seth M. Zeidman, MD

Assistant Professor of Neurosurgery, University of Rochester School of Medicine and Dentistry; Chief, Division of Complex Neurological Surgery, Strong Memorial Hospital, and Attending Neurosurgeon, Highland Hospital, Park Ridge Hospital, and Rochester Memorial Hospital; Private Practice, Rochester Brain and Spine Neurosurgery, Rochester, New York

Hyperextension and Hyperflexion Injuries of the Cervical Spine

Gregory J. Zipfel, MD

Resident, Department of Neurological Surgery, University of Florida School of Medicine, Gainesville, Florida

Surgical Treatment of Intracavernous and Paraclinoid Internal Carotid Artery Aneurysms

Justin A. Zivin, MD, PhD

Professor of Neuroscience, University of California, San Diego, School of Medicine, La Jolla, California

Acute Medical Management of Ischemic Disease and Stroke

Geoffrey Zubay, MD

Chief Resident, Division of Neurological Surgery, Barrow Neurological Institute, Phoenix, Arizona

Basic Principles of Spinal Internal Fixation

Alexander Y. Zubkov, MD, PhD

Resident, Department of Neurology, University of Mississippi Medical Center, Jackson, Mississippi

Radiology of the Skull

Marike Zwienenberg-Lee, MD

Resident in Neurosurgery, Department of Neurological Surgery, University of California, Davis, Medical Center, Sacramento, California

Clinical Pathophysiology of Traumatic Brain Injury

PREFACE

Neurological surgery is a dynamic field, but one that is built on and sustained by the broad shoulders of earlier scientific discoveries and clinical experiences. The fifth edition of *Neurological Surgery* reflects this ever-changing discipline and combines what is "new" with that which is not only "old," but enduring. Thus, this latest volume continues the original intent of the first[1] and subsequent texts edited by Julian Youmans. Reflecting the breadth and complexity of neurosurgery at the beginning of the 21st century, this new volume has had a long gestation period.

This edition has been radically restructured to reflect the ever-changing nature of our discipline. The initial section is focused on the key basic science areas and associated clinical disciplines, the knowledge of which is a necessity for the rational practice of neurosurgery. Subsequent sections reflect the mixture of time-tested information and new advances in the areas of oncology, vascular system, epilepsy, functional, pain, pediatrics, peripheral nerve, radiation therapy and radiosurgery, spine, and trauma. Each section begins with a consideration of general features and historical background that allows the reader to place in context the advances within each section. There then follow chapters dealing with basic scientific information and advances relevant to each area, whereas the subsequent topics within each section deal with clinical advances and surgical techniques. Thus, in all sections, we have added a wealth of new horizontally and vertically integrated information.

The overall aim of each section reflects the unifying goal of the entire book: to provide comprehensive knowledge of disorders and surgery of the nervous system to the student, whether that "student" is a junior resident or an experienced practitioner. Moreover, I hope that future physicians dealing with surgery of the nervous system, whether they are mechanical or biological surgeons,[2] will value the information contained in this text.

It is self-evident that these volumes represent the diligent work of many individuals. I enthusiastically express my appreciation to each of the Section Editors who contributed many long hours to the success of this effort: Roy Bakay (Functional), Henry Brem (Oncology), Kim Burchiel (Functional and Pain), Bill Friedman (Radiation Therapy and Radiosurgery), Sean Grady (Trauma), Michel Kliot (Introduction and Peripheral Nerve), Dade Lunsford (Radiation Therapy and Radiosurgery), Joel MacDonald (Special Features), Larry Marshall (Trauma), Marc Mayberg (Special Features), Fred Meyer (Vascular), T. S. Park (Pediatric), Ray Sawaya (Oncology), Michael Scott (Pediatric), Dan Silbergeld (Epilepsy), Volker Sonntag (Spine), Robert Spetzler (Vascular), and Dennis Vollmer (Spine). A special acknowledgement and thanks go to my long-time colleague, Ralph Dacey, Deputy Editor-in-Chief.

To bring to fruition a work of this magnitude requires a highly professional and disciplined editorial effort and for this I thank the members of the Saunders/Elsevier team: Publishing Directors, Richard Lampert and Richard Zorab (formerly); Developmental Editors, Anne Snyder and David Orzechowski (formerly); and Project Manager, Jodi Kaye. Most importantly, Margaret Connelly, my Editorial Assistant throughout this entire project, should be recognized for her vital and superb contributions.

A personal note of gratitude goes to my wife Debbie, our daughter Allison and her husband Adam, and our son Randy and his wife Tamara for their sustaining support and encouragement.

Lastly, matching the stellar quality of the Deputy Editor-in-Chief, the Section Editors, and the editorial team at Saunders/Elsevier, are the authors of the 335 chapters. With much enthusiasm, I thank them one and all. Their contributions are truly the broad shoulders upon which future care and advances in Neurosurgery will stand.

H. Richard Winn, MD
Editor-in-Chief
Professor of Neurological Surgery and Neuroscience
Mount Sinai School of Medicine New York, New York

1. Youmans JR: Neurological Surgery. Philadelphia, WB Saunders, 1973, pp xvii–xviii.
2. Winn HR, Howard MA: The next 100 years of neurosurgery. Lancet 354(Suppl):36, 1999.

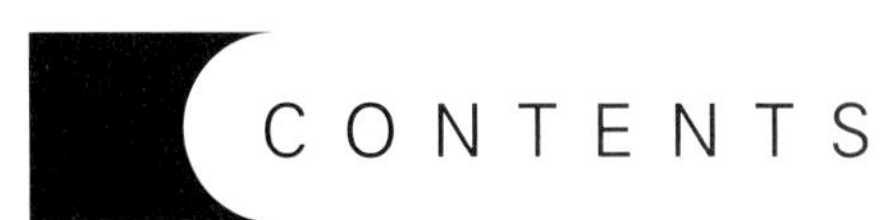

CONTENTS

VOLUME 1

SECTION I

Introduction to Neurological Surgery

PART 1

Basic Science for the Neurological Surgeon—Overview 3

1 *Surgical Anatomy of the Brain* 5
Hung Tzu Wen, Antonio C. M. Mussi, and Albert L. Rhoton, Jr.

2 *Neuroembryology* 45
Joseph D. Pinter and Harvey B. Sarnat

3 *Neurons and Neuroglia* 71
Bruce D. Trapp and Karl Herrup

4 *Astrocytes* 97
Bruce R. Ransom and Tailoi Chan-Ling

5 *Cerebral Metabolism and the Pathophysiology of Ischemic Brain Damage* 117
Peter Siesjö and Bo K. Siesjö

6 *The Blood-Brain Barrier* 153
Gerald A. Grant and Damir Janigro

7 *Physiology of the Cerebrospinal Fluid and Intracranial Pressure* 175
Anthony Marmarou and Andrew Beaumont

8 *Cellular and Molecular Mechanisms Mediating Injury and Recovery in the Nervous System* 195
Daniel A. Lazar, Michael T. Fitch, Jerry Silver, and Michel Kliot

9 *Electrophysiologic Properties of the Mammalian Central Nervous System* 215
Guy M. McKhann II and Damir Janigro

10 *Neurosurgical Epidemiology and Outcomes Assessment* 235
Hugh Garton and Stephen J. Haines

PART 2

Approach to the Patient 263

11 *History and Physical Examination* 263
Phillip D. Swanson

12 *Differential Diagnosis of Altered States of Consciousness* 277
Christopher Ames and Lawrence F. Marshall

13 *Neuro-ophthalmology* 301
Timothy J. Martin and James J. Corbett

14 *Neuro-otology* 327
Phillip A. Wackym, Jill B. Firszt, and Wesley A. King

15 *Neurourology* 357
Gregory R. Wahle, George P. H. Young, Shlomo Raz, and Michael Ostad

16 *Neuropsychological Assessment of the Neurosurgical Patient* 385
Carl B. Dodrill

17 *Brain Death* 393
Hikmat El-Kadi, Howard H. Kaufman, and J. Brad Bellotte

18 *Legal Issues* 407
Elizabeth A. Leedom and Robert Goodkin

PART 3

Fundamentals of Radiology 419

19 *Radiology of the Skull* 419
Frank A. Raila and Alexander Y. Zubkov

20 *Magnetic Resonance Imaging of Brain* 439
Thomas A. Kim, Robert Prost, and E. Paul LIndell

21 *Molecular Imaging of the Brain with Positron Emission Tomography* 477
William P. Melega, Antonio A. F. De Salles, and Michael E. Phelps

22 *Radiology of the Spine* 497
Jonathan R. Perry, Wendy A. Cohen, and Jeffrey G. Jarvik

PART 4

Perioperative Evaluation and Treatment 547

23 *Anesthesia: Preoperative Evaluation 547*
Susan Fletcher and Arthur M. Lam

24 *Complication Avoidance in Neurosurgery 561*
Arthur L. Jenkins III, Harel Deutch, Naresh P. Patel, and Kalmon D. Post

PART 5

Surgical Exposures and Positioning 595

25 *General Principles of Operative Positioning 595*
Robert Goodkin and Ali Mesiwala

26 *Surgical Positioning and Exposures for Cranial Procedures 623*
Richard C. Clatterbuck and Rafael J. Tamargo

27 *Surgical Exposures and Positioning for Spinal Surgery 631*
Charles J. Riedel

28 *Peripheral Nerves 647*
Allen Maniker

SECTION II

Oncology

PART 1

Overview 659

29 *Brain Tumors: General Considerations 659*
Henry Brem and Raymond Sawaya

PART 2

Basic Science of Neuro-oncology 661

30 *Brain Tumors: An Overview of Histopathologic Classification 661*
Teresa Ribalta and Gregory N. Fuller

31 *Basic Principles of Central Nervous System Immunology 673*
Lois A. Lampson

32 *Proliferation Markers in the Evaluation of Gliomas 689*
Stephen W. Coons

33 *Molecular Genetics and the Development of Targets for Glioma Therapy 711*
Eric C. Holland

34 *Growth Factors and Brain Tumors 725*
Richard S. Morrison, Abel D. Jarell, and James M. Schuster

35 *Tumor Suppressor Genes and the Genesis of Brain Tumors 739*
Steven A. Toms

36 *Molecular and Cytogenetic Techniques 747*
C. David James and Webster K. Cavenee

37 *Invasion in Malignant Glioma 757*
Tom Mikkelsen, Syed A. Enam, and Mark L. Rosenblum

38 *Angiogenesis and Brain Tumors 771*
Steven Brem

39 *Brain Edema and Tumor-Host Interactions 791*
Miroslav P. Bobek and Julian T. Hoff

40 *Brain Tumors: Population-Based Epidemiology, Environmental Risk Factors, and Genetic and Hereditary Syndromes 807*
Stephen E. Doran and William E. Thorell

41 *Principles of Gene Therapy 817*
Zvi Ram

PART 3

Approach to the Patient: Medical Considerations 825

42 *Clinical Features: Neurology of Brain Tumor and Paraneoplastic Disorders 825*
William R. Shapiro

43 *Radiologic Features of Central Nervous System Tumors 835*
David M. Yousem and Michael A. Kraut

44 *Endovascular Techniques for Brain Tumors 857*
Neal J. Naff and Patrick Noonan

45 *Brain Tumors during Pregnancy 867*
Alessandro Olivi, Laurence D. Rhines, and Francesco DiMeco

46 *Principles of Chemotherapy 877*
Katherine E. Warren and Howard A. Fine

47 *Aspects of Immunology Applicable to Brain Tumor Pathogenesis and Treatment 887*
Pierre-Yves Dietrich, Paul R. Walker, and Nicolas De Tribolet

PART 4

Surgical Considerations 899

48 *Basic Principles of Cranial Surgery for Brain Tumors 899*
Jon Weingart and Henry Brem

49 *Basic Principles of Skull Base Surgery 909*
Madjid Samii and Marcos Tatagiba

50 *Surgical Complications and Their Avoidance 931*
Ronald E. Warnick

51 *Surgical Navigation for Brain Tumors 941*
Gene H. Barnett

PART 5

Intrinsic Tumors 950

52 *Low-Grade Gliomas: Astrocytoma, Oligodendroglioma, and Mixed Gliomas 950*
G. Evren Keles, Kenneth Aldape, and Mitchel S. Berger

53 *Malignant Gliomas: Anaplastic Astrocytoma, Glioblastoma Multiforme, Gliosarcoma, Malignant Oligodendroglioma 969*
Paul Santiago and Daniel L. Silbergeld

54 *Unusual Gliomas 981*
Sunghoon Lee, Kenneth P. Vives, Jung Kim, and Joseph Piepmeier

55 *Primitive Neuroectodermal Tumors 997*
Karin M. Muraszko and Andrew S. Youkilis

56 *Pineal Tumors 1011*
Jeffrey N. Bruce

57 *Medulloblastoma 1031*
Lara J. Kunschner and Frederick F. Lang, Jr.

58 *Ependymoma 1043*
Benjamin S. Carson, Sr. and Michael Guarnieri

59 *Hemangioblastomas of the Central Nervous System 1053*
G. Edward Vates and Mitchel S. Berger

60 *Cerebral Lymphoma 1067*
Sepideh Amin-Hanjani and Griffith R. Harsh IV

61 *Metastatic Brain Tumors 1077*
Frederick F. Lang Jr., Eric L. Chang, Dima Abi-Said, David M. Wildrick, and Raymond Sawaya

PART 6

Extrinsic Tumors 1099

62 *Meningiomas 1099*
Georges F. Haddad, Ossama Al-Mefty, and Saleem I. Abdulrauf

63 *Meningeal Hemangiopericytoma 1133*
Barton L. Guthrie and Charles S. Cobbs

64 *Meningeal Sarcoma 1141*
Matthew G. Ewend, Mauricio Castillo, and Kyle D. Weaver

65 *Acoustic Neuroma 1147*
Prakash Sampath and Donlin M. Long

66 *Pituitary Tumors: Functioning and Nonfunctioning 1169*
Kamal Thapar and Edward R. Laws

67 *Craniopharyngioma in the Adult 1207*
Vivek Mehta and Peter M. Black

68 *Epidermoid, Dermoid, and Neurenteric Cysts 1223*
Mary Kay Gumerlock

69 *Neoplastic Meningitis: Diagnosis and Treatment 1231*
Marc C. Chamberlain

PART 7

Ventricular Tumors 1237

70 *Ventricular Tumors 1237*
Arun Paul Amar, Sanjay Ghosh, and Michael L. J. Apuzzo

PART 8

Skull and Skull Base Tumors 1265

71 *Skull and Skull Base Tumors 1265*
Vinko V. Dolenc

72 *Chordoma and Chondrosarcoma 1283*
Laligam N. Sekhar, Amitabha Chanda, Kalavakonda Chandrasekar, and Donald C. Wright

73 *Glomus Jugulare Tumors 1295*
Jon H. Robertson, Jason A. Brodkey, and Paul P. Wang

74 *Neoplasms of the Paranasal Sinuses 1311*
Daryl R. Fourney and Franco Demonte

75 *Esthesioneuroblastoma 1333*
Jonas M. Sheehan and John A. Jane, Sr.

76 *Trigeminal Schwannomas 1343*
Raj K. Shrivastava, Chandranath Sen, and Kalmon D. Post

77 *Diagnosis and Management of Juvenile Angiofibroma 1351*
Gerald A. Grant, Richard G. Ellenbogen, and Scott C. Manning

78 *Osseous Tumors 1361*
André Visot and Anne Boulin

79 *Orbital Tumors 1371*
Ghassan K. Bejjani, Kimberly Peele Cockerham, Joseph C. Maroon, and John S. Kennerdell

80 *Skull Tumors 1383*
Matthew E. Fewel, Stephen S. Gebarski, and Julian T. Hoff

81 *Scalp Tumors 1409*
Elizabeth B. Claus and John A. Persing

PART **9**

Non-Neoplastic Disorders Mimicking Brain Tumors 1419

82 *Pseudotumor Cerebri 1419*
Neil R. Miller

83 *Sarcoidosis, Tuberculosis, and Xanthogranuloma 1435*
Sherwin E. Hua, Richard E. Clatterbuck, Barney J. Stern, Prakash Sampath, and Laurence D. Rhines

84 *Multiple Sclerosis 1449*
Walter Royal III

VOLUME 2

SECTION **III**

Vascular

PART **1**

Overview 1461

85 *Historical Considerations 1461*
Milind Deogaonkar and L. Philip Carter

PART **2**

Basic Science 1467

86 *Cerebral Blood Flow and Metabolism 1467*
Vini G. Khurana, Eduardo E. Benarroch, Zvonimir S. Katusic, and Fredric B. Meyer

PART **3**

Approach to the Patient 1495

87 *Acute Medical Management of Ischemic Disease and Stroke 1495*
Carolyn D. Brockington and Justin A. Zivin

PART **4**

Anesthesia for Neurovascular Procedures 1503

88 *Anesthesia in Cerebrovascular Disease 1503*
A. Giancarlo Vishteh, Peter Raudzens, Robert F. Spetzler, and Nicholas Theodore

89 *Intraoperative Cerebral Protection 1515*
Warren R. Selman, Christopher L. Taylor, W. David Lust, and Robert A. Ratcheson

90 *Techniques for Deep Hypothermic Circulatory Arrest 1528*
E. Sander Connolly, Jr. and Robert A. Solomon

PART **5**

Vascular and Blood Flow Evaluations 1540

91 *Transcranial Doppler Ultrasonography 1540*
David W. Newell and Arthur M. Lam

92 *Neurosonology 1561*
Charles J. Prestigiacomo and Donald O. Quest

93 *Xenon Computed Tomography 1569*
Howard Yonas

94 *Magnetic Resonance Angiography 1575*
John Huston III and Matt A. Bernstein

95 *Positron Emission Tomography in Cerebrovascular Disease 1600*
Jean-Claude Baron

PART 6

Occlusive Vascular Disease 1613

96 *Carotid Occlusive Disease: Natural History and Medical Management 1613*
James D. Fleck, José Biller, and Christopher M. Loftus

97 *Carotid Endarterectomy 1621*
Julian E. Bailes and Max B. Medary

98 *Carotid Angioplasty and Stenting: Interventional Treatment of Occlusive Vascular Disease 1651*
Felipe C. Albuquerque, Cargill H. Alleyne, Jr., Jonathan J. Baskin, and Cameron G. McDougall

99 *Recurrent Carotid Stenosis 1661*
Robert J. Dempsey and Aclan Dogan

100 *Traumatic Carotid Injury 1669*
Cargill H. Alleyne, Jr., A. Giancarlo Vishteh, and Robert F. Spetzler

101 *Nonatherosclerotic Carotid Lesions 1677*
Michael J. Alexander

102 *Extracranial Vertebral Artery Disease 1691*
Fady T. Charbel, Kern H. Guppy, Andrew L. Carney, and James I. Ausman

103 *Intracranial Occlusion Disease and Moyamoya 1715*
Carlos A. David and Eric Nottmeier

104 *Cerebral Venous and Sinus Thrombosis 1723*
Frank P. K. Hsu, Gary M. Nesbit, and Stanley L. Barnwell

PART 7

Intracerebral Hemorrhage 1733

105 *Spontaneous Intracerebral Hemorrhage: Non–Arteriovenous Malformation, Nonaneurysm 1733*
Ran Vijai P. Singh, Chad J. Prusmack, and Jacques J. Morcos

PART 8

Hemorrhagic Vascular Disease: Aneurysms 1769

106A *Genetics of Intracranial Aneurysms 1769*
Wouter I. Schievink

106B *The Natural History of Unruptured Saccular Cerebral Aneurysms 1781*
Gavin W. Britz and H. Richard Winn

107 *Surgical Decision Making for the Treatment of Cerebral Aneurysms 1793*
Peter D. Le Roux and H. Richard Winn

108 *Perioperative Management of Subarachnoid Hemorrhage 1813*
R. Loch MacDonald and Bryce Weir

109 *Cerebral Vasospasm 1839*
J. Max Findlay

110 *Surgical Approaches for Anterior Circulation Aneurysms 1868*
Koji Ilhara, Gopal Chopra, and Michael Tymianski

111 *Surgical Treatment of Intracavernous and Paraclinoid Internal Carotid Artery Aneurysms 1895*
Gregory J. Zipfel and Arthur L. Day

112 *Intracranial Internal Carotid Artery Aneurysms 1915*
Mahmoud Al-Yamany and M. Christopher Wallace

113 *Anterior Communicating Artery and Anterior Cerebral Artery Aneurysms 1923*
Rafael J. Tamargo, Raymond I. Haroun, and Daniele Rigamonti

114 *Distal Anterior Cerebral Artery Aneurysms 1945*
David A. Steven and Gary G. Ferguson

115 *Middle Cerebral Artery Aneurysms 1959*
Jonathan A. Friedman and David G. Piepgras

116 *Surgical Approaches for Posterior Circulation Aneurysms 1971*
Michael T. Lawton, G. Edward Vates, and Robert F. Spetzler

117 *Vertebral Artery, Posterior Inferior Cerebellar Artery, and Vertebrobasilar Junction Aneurysms 2007*
Brian L. Hoh and Christopher S. Ogilvy

118 *Basilar Trunk Aneurysms 2025*
Sean D. Lavine, J. Diaz Day, Felipe C. Albuquerque, and Steven L. Giannotta

119 *Basilar Apex and Posterior Cerebral Artery Aneurysms 2041*
Bernard R. Bendok, Mir Jafar Ali, Christopher C. Getch, and H. Hunt Batjer

120 *Endovascular Treatment of Aneurysms 2057*
Guiseppe Lanzino, Lee R. Guterman, and L. Nelson Hopkins

121 *Giant Aneurysms 2079*
G. Michael Lemole, Jr., Jeffrey S. Henn, Robert F. Spetzler, and Howard A. Riina

122 *Infectious Intracranial Aneurysms 2101*
Kevin Yao and Joshua Bederson

123 *Revascularization Techniques for Complex Aneurysms and Skull Base Tumors 2107*
Neil A. Martin, Inam Kureshi, and Domingos Coiteiro

124 *Multimodality Management of Complex Cerebrovascular Lesions 2121*
Bruce E. Pollock, Jay J. Schindler, Douglas A. Nichols, and Frederic B. Meyer

125 *Traumatic Cerebral Aneurysms Secondary to Penetrating Intracranial Injuries 2131*
Gavin W. Britz, David W. Newell, G. Alexander West, and H. Richard Winn

PART 9

True Arteriovenous Malformations 2137

126 *Hemorrhagic Disease: Arteriovascular Malformations 2137*
Ian G. Fleetwood and Mark G. Hamilton

127 *Natural History of Intracranial Vascular Malformations 2159*
Kelly D. Flemming and Robert D. Brown, Jr.

128 *Classification and Decision Making in Treatment and Perioperative Management, Including Surgical and Radiosurgical Decision Making 2185*
Michael Kerin Morgan

129 *Endovascular Management of Brain Arteriovenous Malformations 2205*
Avi Setton, Alejandro Berenstein, and Robin Albert

130 *Embolization of Arteriovenous Malformations as a Primary Treatment Modality 2223*
Bernd Richling, Monika Killer, and Andreas Gruber

131 *Surgical Management of Supratentorial Arteriovenous Malformation 2231*
Michael J. Fritsch and Roberto C. Heros

132 *Posterior Fossa Arteriovenous Malformations 2251*
Thomas A. Kopitnik, Zeena Dorai, Jonathan White, and Duke Samson

133 *Surgical and Radiosurgical Management of Giant Arteriovenous Malformations 2267*
Steven D. Chang and Gary K. Steinberg

134 *Treatment of Lateral-Sigmoid and Sagittal Sinus Dural Arteriovenous Malformations 2283*
C. Michael Cawley, Daniel L. Barrow, and Jacques E. Dion

PART 10

Cavernous Malformations 2292

135 *Epidemiology and Natural History of Cavernous Malformations 2292*
Joseph M. Zabramski and Patrick P. Han

136 *The Genetics of Cerebral Cavernous Malformations 2299*
Eric W. Johnson, Douglas A. Marchuk, and Joseph M. Zabramski

137 *Surgical Management of Supratentorial Cavernous Malformations 2305*
Kenneth P. Vives, Murat Gunel, and Issam A. Awad

138 *Infratentorial Cavernous Malformations 2321*
Randall W. Porter, Paul W. Detwiler, and Robert F. Spetzler

139 *Cavernous Carotid Fistulas 2341*
Sanjay Ghosh, Donald Larsen, and J. Diaz Day

PART 11

Spinal Arteriovenous Malformations 2353

140 *Classification of Spinal Cord Vascular Lesions 2353*
Howard A. Riina, Paul W. Detwiler, Randall W. Porter, and Robert F. Spetzler

141 *Endovascular Treatment of Spinal Cord Arteriovenous Malformations 2363*
Gavin W. Britz and Joseph Eskridge

142 *Spinal Arteriovenous Malformations 2375*
B. Gregory Thompson and Edward H. Oldfield

PART **12**

Pregnancy and Treatment of Vascular Disease 2421

143 *Pregnancy and Treatment of Vascular Disease* 2421
Mark R. Harrigan and B. Gregory Thompson

SECTION **IV**

Epilepsy

PART **1**

Overview 2435

144 *General and Historical Considerations of Epilepsy Surgery* 2435
Eldad Hadar and Jürgen Lüders

145 *Basic Science of Post-traumatic Epilepsy* 2449
Raimondo D'Ambrosio

146 *Approaches to the Diagnosis and Classification of Epilepsy* 2461
Mark D. Holmes and John W. Miller

147 *Antiepileptic Medications: Principles of Clinical Use* 2469
Blaise F. D. Bourgeois

PART **2**

Preoperative Evaluation for Epilepsy 2475

148 *Single-Photon Emission Computed Tomography and Positron Emission Tomography* 2475
David H. Lewis

149 *Preoperative Evaluation for Epilepsy Surgery: Computed Tomography and Magnetic Resonance Imaging* 2483
Richard A. Bronen

150 *The Intracarotid Amobarbital Procedure or Wada Test* 2503
Carl B. Dodrill

151 *Functional Magnetic Resonance Imaging in Epilepsy Surgery* 2511
Thomas A. Hammeke, Wade M. Mueller, Sara J. Swanson, and Jeffrey R. Binder

152 *Identification of Candidates for Epilepsy Surgery* 2525
G. Rees Cosgrove and Andrew J. Cole

PART **3**

Intraoperative Mapping and Monitoring for Cortical Resections 2531

153 *Motor, Sensory, and Language Mapping and Monitoring for Cortical Resections* 2531
James M. Schuster and Daniel L. Silbergeld

154 *Monitoring and Mapping of Vision in the Neurosurgical Patient* 2541
Kathleen R. Tozer, Stephen L. Skirboll, and H. Richard Winn

PART **4**

Specific Operative Approaches 2551

155 *Intracranial Monitoring* 2551
Kenneth P. Vives, Sunghoon Lee, Kevin McCarthy, and Dennis D. Spencer

156 *Epilepsy Surgery: Outcome and Complications* 2565
Webster H. Pilcher

157 *Surgery for Extratemporal Lobe Epilepsy* 2587
James W. Leiphart and Itzhak Fried

158 *Standard Temporal Lobectomy and Transsylvian Amygdalohippocampectomy* 2605
Robert E. Maxwell and Ramachandra Tummala

159 *Tailored Resections for Epilepsy* 2615
Andrew N. Miles and George A. Ojemann

160 *Topectomy: Uses and Indications* 2629
Atsushi Umemura and Gordon H. Baltuch

161 *Multiple Subpial Transection* 2635
Richard W. Byrne and Walter W. Whisler

162 *Vagus Nerve Stimulation for Intractable Epilepsy* 2643
Arun Paul Amar, Michael L. Levy, and Michael L. J. Apuzzo

VOLUME 3

SECTION V

Functional Neurosurgery

PART 1

Overview 2653

163 *History of Functional Neurosurgery 2653*
Roy A. E. Bakay

PART 2

Movement Disorders: Basic Science 2671

164 *Rationale for Surgical Interventions in Movement Disorders 2671*
Thomas Wichmann and Mahlon R. Delong

165 *Anatomy and Synaptic Connectivity of the Basal Ganglia 2683*
Yoland Smith, Ali Charara

166 *Neuropathology of Movement Disorders 2699*
Kurt A. Jellinger

PART 3

Approach to the Patient and the Diagnosis 2729

167 *Approach to Movement Disorders 2729*
Anna Depold Hohler and Ali Samii

168 *Patient Selection in Movement Disorder Surgery 2745*
Todd P. Thompson, L. Dade Lunsford, Douglas Kondziolka, and A. Leland Albright

169 *Positron Emission Tomography in Movement Disorders 2755*
David J. Brooks

PART 4

Movement Disorders: Ablative Surgery of Movement Disorders 2769

170 *Thalamotomy for Tremor 2769*
Sherwin E. Hua, Ira M. Garonzik, Jung-Il Lee, and Frederick A. Lenz

171 *Pallidotomy for Parkinson's Disease 2785*
Andres M. Lozano and Ahmed Alkhani

172 *Surgery for Dystonia 2795*
Michael S. Okun and Jerrold L. Vitek

173 *Deep Brain Stimulation for Movement Disorders 2803*
Alim L. Benabid, Jean F. Le Bas, Sylvie Grand, Abdelhamid Benazzouz, Pierre Pollak, Paul Krack, Adnah Koudsié, Stephan Chabardès, Valerie Fraix, Patricia Limousin, Serge Pinto, Dominique Hoffmann, Claire Ardouin, and Aurelie Funkiewiez

174 *Cellular Transplantation in the Central Nervous System 2829*
Roy A. E. Bakay

175 *Neurosurgery of Psychiatric Disorders 2853*
G. Rees Cosgrove

PART 5

Spasticity 2863

176 *Ablative Surgery for Spasticity 2863*
Kenneth F. Casey and Raymond Sekula

177 *Management of Spasticity by Central Nervous System Infusion Techniques 2875*
Richard D. Penn and Daniel M. Corcos

178 *Selective Peripheral Denervation for Spasmodic Torticollis 2891*
Guy Bouvier and Pedro Molina-Negro

179 *Treatment of Intractable Vertigo 2901*
Steven A. Telian and Julian T. Hoff

SECTION VI

Pain

PART 1

Overview 2913

180 *Pain: General Historical Considerations 2913*
Kim J. Burchiel

PART 2

Basic Science 2917

181 *Physiologic Anatomy of Pain 2917*
Thomas K. Baumann

PART 3

Approach to the Patient 2937

182 *Approach to the Patient with Chronic Pain 2937*
Joel L. Seres

183 *Medical Management of Chronic Pain 2953*
Jaimie M. Henderson and Paul E. Fewings

184 *Management of Pain by Anesthetic Techniques 2970*
Brett Stacy, Antony Colantonio, Jennifer Vookles, David Sibell, and Lynda Kulawiak

PART 4

Trigeminal Neuralgia 2987

185 *Diagnosis and Nonoperative Management 2987*
Andrew S. Youkilis and Oren Sagher

186 *Percutaneous Techniques 2996*
Jeffrey A. Brown

187 *Trigeminal Neuralgia: Microvascular Decompression of the Trigeminal Nerve for Tic Douloureux 3005*
Peter J. Jannetta and Elad I. Levy

188 *Alternative Surgical Treatments for Trigeminal Neuralgia 3017*
Wayel Kaakaji and Kim J. Burchiel

PART 5

Surgical Treatment of Pain 3023

189 *Neurosurgical Management of Intractable Pain 3023*
Kenneth A. Follett

190 *Dorsal Rhizotomy and Dorsal Root Ganglionectomy 3033*
Jamal M. Taha, Khaled M. Abdel Aziz, and Norberto Andaluz

191 *Dorsal Root Entry Zone and Brainstem Ablative Procedures 3045*
John P. Gorecki

192 *Cordotomy for Pain 3059*
Yücel Kanpolat

193 *Brainstem Procedures for Management of Pain 3073*
Philip L. Gildenberg

194 *Caudalis Nucleus Dorsal Root Entry Zone Procedure for the Treatment of Intractable Facial Pain 3085*
Dennis E. Bullard and Blaine S. Nashold

195 *Sympathectomy for Pain 3093*
Antonio A. F. De Salles and John Patrick Johnson

196 *Spinal Cord and Peripheral Nerve Stimulation for Chronic, Intractable Pain 3107*
Richard B. North

197 *Deep Brain Stimulation for Chronic Pain 3119*
Michael G. Kaplitt, Ali R. Rezai, Andres M. Lozano, and Ronald Tasker

198 *Intrathecal Drug Infusion for Pain 3133*
Richard D. Penn

SECTION VII

Pediatric

PART 1

Overview 3145

199 *Neurological Surgery in Childhood: General and Historical Considerations 3145*
James Tait Goodrich

200 *Neurological Examination in Infancy and Childhood 3169*
William J. Logan

201 *Neuroanesthesia in Children 3187*
Sulpicio G. Soriano, Elizabeth A. Eldredge, and Mark A. Rockoff

PART 2

Developmental and Acquired Anomalies 3198

202 *Encephaloceles 3198*
James T. Rutka, Carlos Carlotti, and Mark Iantosca

203 *Myelomeningocele and Myelocystocele 3215*
Alan R. Cohen and Shenandoah Robinson

204 *Lipomyelomeningocele 3229*
John W. Walsh, Renatta J. Osterdock

205 *Tethered Spinal Cord 3245*
Benjamin C. Warf

206 *Occult Spinal Dysraphism and the Tethered Spinal Cord 3257*
R. F. Keating, J. Multani, and P. H. Cogen

207 *Dandy-Walker Syndrome 3285*
Jeffrey R. Leonard and Jeffrey G. Ojemann

208 *Arachnoid Cysts 3289*
Paul M. Kanev

PART **3**

Craniosynostosis, Chiari Malformation, and Achondroplasia 3300

209 *Nonsyndromic Craniosynostosis and Abnormalities of Head Shape 3300*
Marion L. Walker and John J. Collins

210 *Craniofacial Syndromes 3315*
Joseph H. Shin and John A. Persing

211 *Developmental Abnormalities of the Craniovertebral Junction 3331*
Arnold H. Menezes

212 *Chiari Malformations 3347*
W. Jerry Oakes and R. Shane Tubbs

213 *Achondroplasia and Other Dwarfism 3362*
Benjamin S. Carson, Sr., Daniele Rigamonti, and Raymond I. Haroun

PART **4**

Hydrocephalus 3374

214 *Physiology of Cerebrospinal Fluid Shunt Devices 3374*
Howard J. Ginsberg and James M. Drake

215 *Hydrocephalus in Children 3387*
Harold L. Rekate

216 *Infantile Posthemorrhagic Hydrocephalus 3405*
Mark Luciano, Jogi V. Pattisapu, and Agadha Wickremesekera

217 *Shunt Infection 3419*
Elizabeth B. Claus and Charles Duncan

218 *Neuroendoscopy 3427*
Kerry R. Crone

PART **5**

Vascular Disease 3433

219 *Vein of Galen Malformations 3433*
J. Parker Mickle, Robert A. Mericle, Matthew V. Burry, and Lorna Sohn Williams

220 *Arteriovenous Malformations and Intracranial Aneurysms in Children 3447*
Robin P. Humphreys and Farhad Pirouzmand

PART **6**

Head and Brain Trauma 3461

221 *Mild Brain Injury in Children, including Skull Fractures and Growing Fractures 3461*
Paul C. Francel and John Honeycutt

222 *Pediatric Head Injury 3473*
Egon M. R. Doppenberg and John D. Ward

PART **7**

Birth Trauma 3481

223 *Birth Head Trauma 3481*
Robin Bowman and Tadanori Tomita

224 *Birth Brachial Plexus Injury 3488*
T. S. Park and Stuart S. Kaplan

225 *Child Abuse 3499*
Ann-Christine Duhaime and Cindy Christian

226 *Pediatric Vertebral Column and Spinal Cord Injuries 3515*
Dachling Pang and Peter P. Sun

PART **8**

Benign Spine Lesions 3559

227 *Intervertebral Disk Disease in Children 3559*
Shenandoah Robinson and Alan R. Cohen

228 *Spondylolisthesis 3571*
Diana Barrett Wiseman, David Lundin, and Christopher I. Shaffrey

229 *Benign Tumors of the Vertebral Column in Children 3587*
Nalin Gupta and David M. Frim

PART 9

Tumors 3595

230 *Optic Pathway and Hypothalamic Gliomas in Children 3595*
Jeffrey H. Wisoff

231 *Intracranial Germ Cell Tumors 3603*
Alyssa T. Reddy and Timothy B. Mapstone

232 *Choroid Plexus Tumors 3612*
Richard G. Ellenbogen and R. Michael Scott

233 *Intracranial Ependymomas 3623*
Leslie N. Sutton and Joel Goldwein

234 *Medulloblastoma 3639*
Bruce A. Kaufman

235 *Cerebellar Astrocytomas in Children 3655*
Jeffrey W. Campbell and R. Michael Scott

236 *Brainstem Gliomas 3663*
A. Leland Albright and Ian F. Pollack

237 *Craniopharyngiomas 3671*
Peter Carmel

238 *Brain Tumors of Disordered Embryogenesis 3687*
Peter Carmel

239 *Pediatric Cerebral Hemispheric Tumors 3697*
Loi K. Phuong and Corey Raffel

240 *Intraspinal Tumors in Infants and Children 3707*
George I. Jallo, Karl F. Kothbauer, and Fred J. Epstein

241 *Benign Tumors of the Skull, including Fibrous Dysplasia 3717*
Herbert E. Fuchs

PART 10

Cerebral Palsy and Other Spastic Entities 3723

242 *Cerebral Palsy: An Overview 3723*
Catherine J. Doty

243 *Selective Dorsal Rhizotomy for Spastic Cerebral Palsy 3736*
T. S. Park

244 *Intrathecal Baclofen Infusion 3747*
Paul Steinbok and Maureen O'Donnell

PART 11

Surgical Treatment of Epilepsy in Children 3758

245 *Recognition of Surgical Candidates and the Presurgical Evaluation 3758*
Nancy Foldvary and Elaine Wyllie

246 *Temporal and Extratemporal Lobe Resections for Childhood Intractable Epilepsy 3769*
Glenn Morrison

PART 12

Rehabilitation 3783

247 *Acute Pediatric Neurorehabilitation 3783*
Michael J. Noetzel

VOLUME 4

SECTION VIII

Peripheral Nerve

PART 1

Overview 3794

248 *General Principles in Evaluating and Treating Peripheral Nerve Injuries 3795*
Gerald A. Grant and Michel Kliot

249 *History of Peripheral Nerve Surgery 3798*
A. Lee Dellon

PART 2

Basic Science 3809

250 *Physiology of the Peripheral Nerve 3809*
Gregory A. Kinney

PART 3

Approach to the Patient 3819

251 *Peripheral Nerve: Approach to the Patient 3819*
Rajiv Midha

252 *Peripheral Neuropathies 3831*
Eric C. Yuen

253 *Electrodiagnostic Evaluation of Peripheral Nerves: Electromyography, Somatosensory Evoked Potentials, Nerve Action Potentials 3851*
Eric C. Yuen, Lawrence Robinson, and Jefferson Slimp

254 *Magnetic Resonance Imaging for Peripheral Nerve Disorders 3873*
Gerald A. Grant, Gavin W. Britz, Robert Goodkin, Jeffrey G. Jarvik, Kenneth Maravilla, and Michel Kliot

PART **4**

Management of Peripheral Nerve Injuries 3889

255 *Carpal Tunnel Syndrome 3889*
Chong C. Lee, Suzie C. Tindall, and Michel Kliot

256 *Ulnar Nerve Entrapment at the Elbow 3897*
James B. Lowe III, Susan E. Mackinnon

257 *Entrapment Syndromes of Peripheral Nerve Injuries 3921*
Chong C. Lee, Suzie C. Tindall, and Michel Kliot

258 *Management of Peripheral Nerve Tumors 3941*
David G. Kline, Alan R. Hudson, Robert Tiel, and Abhijit Guha

259 *Diagnostic Biopsy of Peripheral Nerves and Muscle 3958*
Jang-Chul Lee

260 *Management of Acute Peripheral Nerve Injuries 3967*
Thomas Carlstedt and Rolfe Birch

SECTION **IX**

Radiation Therapy and Radiosurgery

PART **1**

Overview 3991

261 *General and Historical Considerations of Radiotherapy and Radiosurgery 3991*
Steven D. Chang, John R. Adler, Jr., and Gary K. Steinberg

PART **2**

Basic Science of Radiotherapy 3999

262 *Radiobiology 3999*
John M. Buatti, Sanford L. Meeks, Nina A. Mayr, Michael E. C. Robbins, William A. Friedman, and Frank J. Bova

263 *Principles of Radiotherapy 4005*
John H. Suh, Roger M. Macklis

PART **3**

Fractionated Radiation Therapy 4015

264 *Fractionated Radiation Therapy for Malignant Brain Tumors 4015*
Minesh P. Mehta

265 *Radiotherapy for Benign Skull Base Tumors 4027*
John M. Buatti and Sanford L. Meeks

266 *Fractionated Radiation Therapy for Pituitary Tumors 4033*
John C. Flickinger and Douglas Kondziolka

267 *Radiotherapy of Tumors of the Spine 4039*
Jeff Michalski

268 *Radiosurgery of Tumors 4053*
Ajay Niranjan and L. Dade Lunsford

269 *Radiosurgery for Arteriovenous Malformations 4073*
William A. Friedman and Kelly D. Foote

270 *Functional Radiosurgery 4087*
Christopher M. Duma, Michael Shea, Deane B. Jacques, and Oleg Kopyov

271 *Interstitial and Intracavitary Irradiation of Brain Tumors 4095*
M. W. McDermott, P. H. Gutin, Mitchel S. Berger, and P. K. Sneed

PART **4**

Techniques of Radiosurgery 4111

272 *Linac Radiosurgery 4111*
Eben Alexander III

273 *Gamma Knife Radiosurgery 4117*
Timothy F. Witham and Douglas Kondziolka

274 *Proton Radiosurgery 4123*
Paul H. Chapman and Jay S. Loeffler

275 *Fractionated and Stereotactic Radiation, Extracranial Stereotactic Radiation, Intensity Modulation, and Multileaf Collimation 4131*
Frank J. Bova, Sanford L. Meeks, Tom Wagner, William A. Friedman, and John M. Buatti

SECTION X

Spine

PART 1

Overview 4147

276 *Overview and Historical Considerations 4147*
Volker K. H. Sonntag and Dennis G. Vollmer

PART 2

Basic Science 4153

277 *Biologic Strategies for Central Nervous System Repair 4153*
James D. Guest

278 *Concepts and Mechanisms of Biomechanics 4181*
Dennis J. Maiman, Frank A. Pintar, Michael W. Groff, Narayan Yoganandan, and James P. Hollowell

279 *Intraoperative Electrophysiologic Monitoring of the Spinal Cord and Nerve Roots 4203*
Jeffrey H. Owen

280 *Bone Metabolism as It Relates to Spinal Disease and Treatment 4227*
Muwaffak M. Abdulhak, Marilyn L. Gates, and James P. Hollowell

281 *Normal and Abnormal Embryology of the Spinal Cord and Spine 4239*
Mark S. Dias, David G. McLone, and Michael Partington

PART 3

Approach to the Patient 4289

282 *Approach to the Patient and Medical Management of Spinal Disorders 4289*
Charles Kuntz IV, Christopher I. Shaffrey, and W. Putnam Wolcott

283 *Evaluation and Management of the Failed Back Syndrome 4327*
George W. Sypert and E. Joy Arpin-Sypert

284 *Metabolic and Other Nondegenerative Causes of Low Back Pain 4347*
Edward S. Connolly and H. Bruce Hamilton

PART 4

Infections 4363

285 *Infections of the Spine and Spinal Cord 4363*
Nitin Tandon and Dennis G. Vollmer

PART 5

Degenerative Disease 4395

286 *Treatment of Disk and Ligamentous Diseases of the Cervical Spine 4395*
Robert J. Jackson and Ziya L. Gokaslan

287 *Posterior Approach to Cervical Degenerative Disease 4409*
Gregory C. Wiggins and Christopher I. Shaffrey

288 *Anterior Approach including Cervical Corpectomy (Degenerative) 4431*
Juan Bartolomei and Volker K. H. Sonntag

289 *Cervical Spondylotic Myelopathy 4447*
V. G. R. Kumar, Christopher Madden, and Gary L. Rea

290 *Spondyloarthropathies, including Ankylosing Spondylitis 4459*
Michael R. Gallagher and Regis W. Haid

291 *Ossification of the Posterior Longitudinal Ligament and Other Enthesopathies 4475*
Philip V. Theodosopoulos and Philip R. Weinstein

292 *Benign Extradural Lesions of the Dorsal Spine 4491*
Paul Santiago, Andrew D. Fine, David Shafron, and Richard G. Fessler

293 *Treatment of Disk Disease of the Lumbar Spine 4507*
Russell W. Hardy, Jr. and Perry A. Ball

294 *Lumbar Spinal Stenosis 4521*
Nancy E. Epstein

295 *Spondylolysis and Spondylolisthesis 4541*
Gregory J. Bennett

296 *Adult Thoracolumbar Scoliosis 4557*
Sean A. Salehi and Stephen L. Ondra

PART **6**

Adult Congenital Abnormalities 4569

297 *Acquired Abnormalities of the Craniocervical Junction 4569*
Arnold H. Menezes

PART **7**

Techniques 4586

298 *Basic Principles of Spinal Internal Fixation 4586*
Goeffrey Zubay, Curtis A. Dickman, Volker K. H. Sonntag, and Neil R. Crawford

299 *Technical Aspects of Bone Graft Harvest and Spinal Fusion 4599*
Lawrence S. Liu and Paul J. Marcotte

300 *Biology of Bone Grafting and Healing in Spinal Surgery 4613*
Paul D. Sawin

PART **8**

Instrumentation 4621

301 *Anterior Cervical Instrumentation 4621*
Jonathan J. Baskin, A. Giancarlo Vishteh, Curtis A. Dickman, and Volker K. H. Sonntag

302 *Posterior Cervical Stabilization and Fusion Techniques 4639*
Paul D. Sawin

303 *Occipitocervical Fusion 4655*
Jonathan J. Baskin, Curtis A. Dickman, and Volker K. H. Sonntag

304 *Anterior Thoracic Instrumentation 4671*
Michael G. Kaiser, Andrew T. Parsa, Barry D. Birch, and Paul C. McCormick

305 *Posterior Thoracic Instrumentation 4693*
Scott L. Simon and James M. Schuster

306 *Anterior Lumbar Instrumentation 4701*
Michael G. Kaiser, Andrew T. Parsa, Peter Angevine, and Paul C. McCormick

307 *Posterior Lumbar Instrumentation 4731*
Paul Tolentino and Richard G. Fessler

308 *Image-Guided Spinal Navigation 4743*
Iain H. Kalfas

309 *Thoracoscopic Approaches to the Spine 4757*
Nicholas Theodore and Curtis A. Dickman

310 *Intradiskal and Percutaneous Treatment of Lumbar Disk Disease 4771*
Thomas C. Chen, Lawrence T. Khoo, and Charles B. Stillerman

PART **9**

Tumors of the Spine 4799

311 *Tumors of the Craniovertebral Junction 4799*
Arnold H. Menezes, Vincent C. Traynelis, and Jason Heth

312 *Spinal Cord Tumors in Adults 4817*
Theodore H. Schwartz and Paul C. McCormick

313 *Tumors of the Vertebral Axis: Benign, Primary Malignant, and Metastatic Tumors 4835*
Martin B. Camins, Arthur L. Jenkins III, Ash Singhal, and Richard G. Perrin

PART **10**

Spine Trauma 4869

314 *Spine Trauma: Approach to the Patient and Diagnostic Evaluation 4869*
Allan D. O. Levi

315 *Cervical Spine Trauma 4885*
Arthur L. Jenkins III, Dennis G. Vollmer, and Marc E. Eichler

316 *Hyperextension and Hyperflexion Injuries of the Cervical Spine 4915*
Seth M. Zeidman

317 *Treatment of Occipital C1 Injury 4925*
Derek A. Taggard and Vincent C. Traynelis

318 *Treatment of Axis Fractures 4939*
Julie E. York, Paul Klimo, and Ronald I. Apfelbaum

319 *Diagnosis and Management of Thoracic Spine Fractures 4951*
Parley W. Madsen III, F. J. Eismont, and B. A. Green

320 *Diagnosis and Management of Thoracolumbar and Lumbar Spine Injuries 4987*
Russ P. Nockels and Julie E. York

321 *Sacral Fractures* 5011
Noel I. Perin

SECTION **XI**

Trauma

PART **1**

Overview 5019

322 *Modern Neurotraumatology: A Brief Historical Review* 5019
Lawrence F. Marshall, Sharon B. Marshall, and M. Sean Grady

PART **2**

Basic Science (Biology of Brain Injury) 5025

323 *Cellular Basis of Injury and Recovery from Trauma* 5025
Luca Longhi, Kathryn E. Saatman, Ramesh Raghupathi, Phillipp M. Lenzlinger, M. Sean Grady, and Tracy K. McIntosh

324 *Clinical Pathophysiology of Traumatic Brain Injury* 5039
Marike Zwienenberg-Lee and J. Paul Muizelaar

PART **3**

Minor Head Injury 5065

325 *Mild Head Injury in Adults* 5065
Franco Servadei and Glen S. Merry

PART **4**

Moderate and Severe Traumatic Brain Injury 5083

326 *Initial Resuscitation and Patient Evaluation* 5083
Grant Sinson, Patrick M. Reilly, and M. Sean Grady

327 *Critical Care Management of Traumatic Brain Injury* 5103
Claudia Robertson

328 *Surgical Management of Traumatic Brain Injury* 5145
Sujit S. Prabhu, Alois Zauner, and M. Ross Bullock

329 *Sequelae of Traumatic Brain Injury* 5181
Ronald Ruff

330 *Traumatic Cerebrovascular Injury* 5203
J. Paul Elliott and David W. Newell

331 *Bullet Wounds to the Brain among Civilians* 5223
Michael E. Carey

332 *Craniofacial Trauma* 5243
Joseph S. Gruss, Richard G. Ellenbogen, and Michael F. Whelan

333 *Traumatic Cerebrospinal Fluid Fistulas* 5265
Robert J. Buchanan, Adam Brant, and Lawrence F. Marshall

334 *Diagnosis and Management of Seventh and Eighth Cranial Nerve Injuries due to Temporal Bone Fractures* 5273
W. Lee Warren, J. Brad Bellotte, and James E. Wilberger

PART **5**

Rehabilitation 5285

335 *Rehabilitation and Prognosis after Traumatic Brain Injury* 5285
Paul T. Diamond and Kimberly J. Stewart

Index i

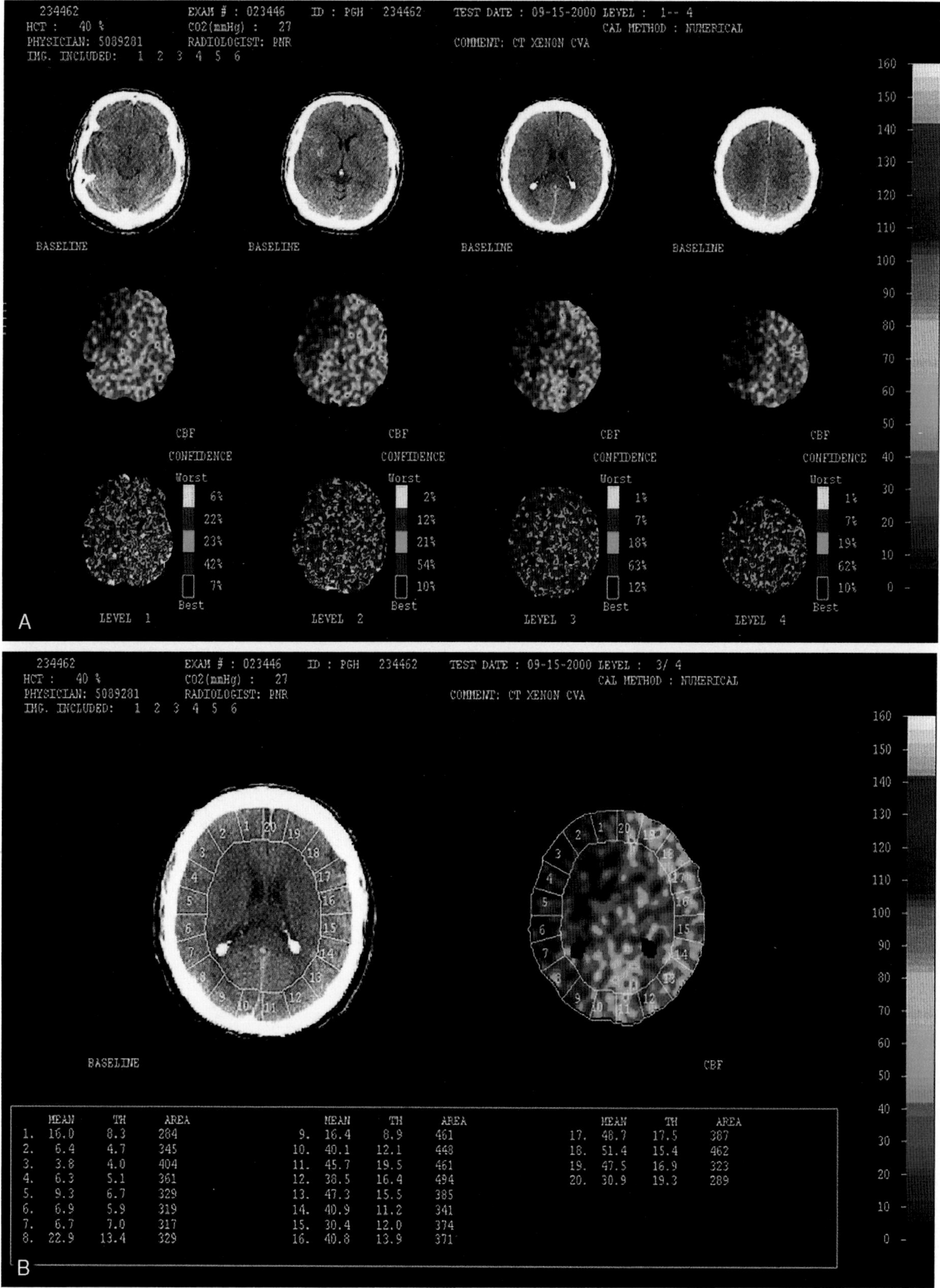

	MEAN	TH	AREA
1.	16.0	8.3	284
2.	6.4	4.7	345
3.	3.8	4.0	404
4.	6.3	5.1	361
5.	9.3	6.7	329
6.	6.9	5.9	319
7.	6.7	7.0	317
8.	22.9	13.4	329
9.	16.4	8.9	461
10.	40.1	12.1	448
11.	45.7	19.5	461
12.	38.5	16.4	494
13.	47.3	15.5	385
14.	40.9	11.2	341
15.	30.4	12.0	374
16.	40.8	13.9	371
17.	48.7	17.5	387
18.	51.4	15.4	462
19.	47.5	16.9	323
20.	30.9	19.3	289

FIGURE 93-1. *A,* Computed tomography (CT), cerebral blood flow (CBF), and confidence image for a four-level study. Each level is 10 mm thick and 5 mm apart. The color scale is fixed with direct reference to CBF measured in milliliters/100 g per minute. The uniform dark confidence image indicates a highly reliable quantitative study in a patient with right hemispheric ischemia due to middle cerebral artery occlusion. *B,* A standard cortical region of interest (ROI) placement shows both the CT image and the CBF image. The mean CBF for each ROI is displayed in the box below. The TH column indicates the standard deviation of the pixels within the ROI. The area column is the number of pixels within a ROI, each $1 \times 1 \times 10$ mm^3.

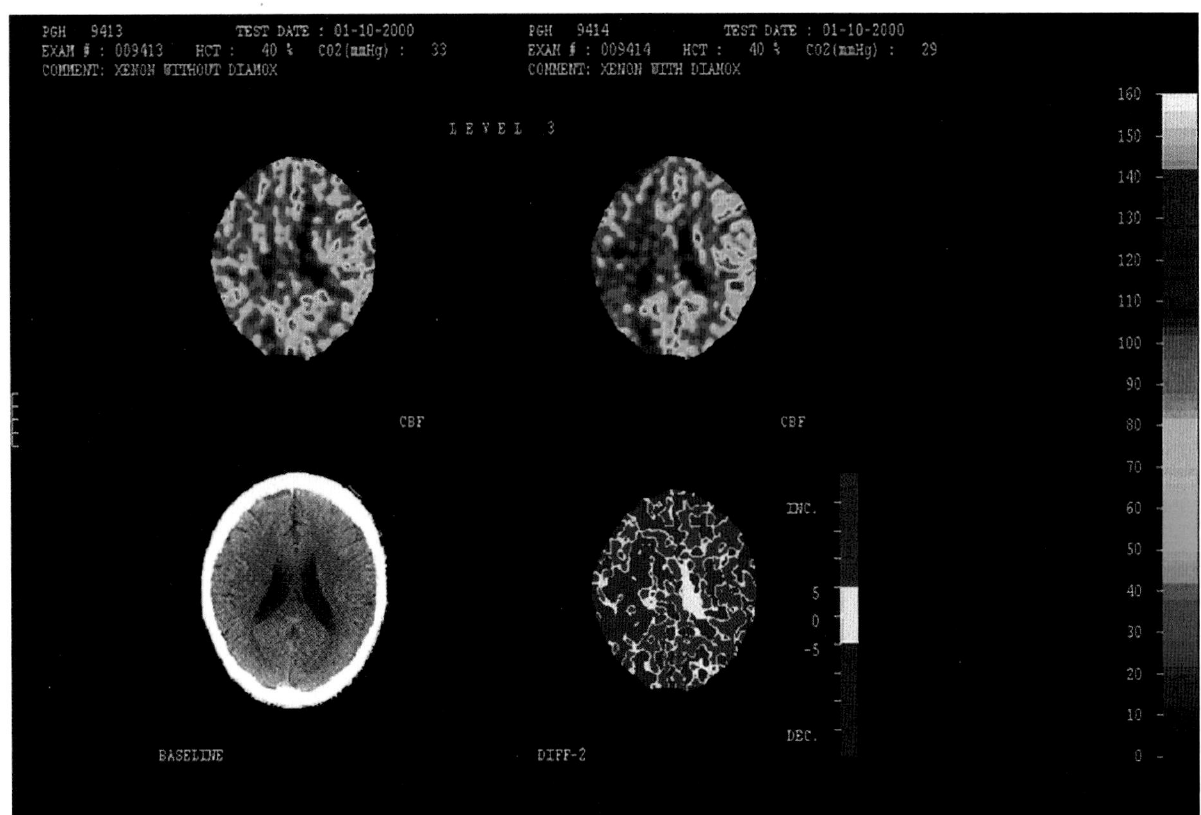

FIGURE 93-2. Acetazolamide (Diamox) challenge study with the baseline cerebral blood flow (CBF) image on the left and the corresponding image 20 minutes after acetazolamide administration. The computed tomographic image and the difference image are displayed below. This vasodilatory challenge normally increases CBF globally, and the difference image should be mostly red, indicating an increase in CBF of at least 5 mL/100 g per minute. The blue in the right hemisphere indicates a decrease in CBF by greater than 5 mL/100 g per minute ("steal phenomenon") in this patient with internal carotid artery occlusion, indicating increased stroke risk.

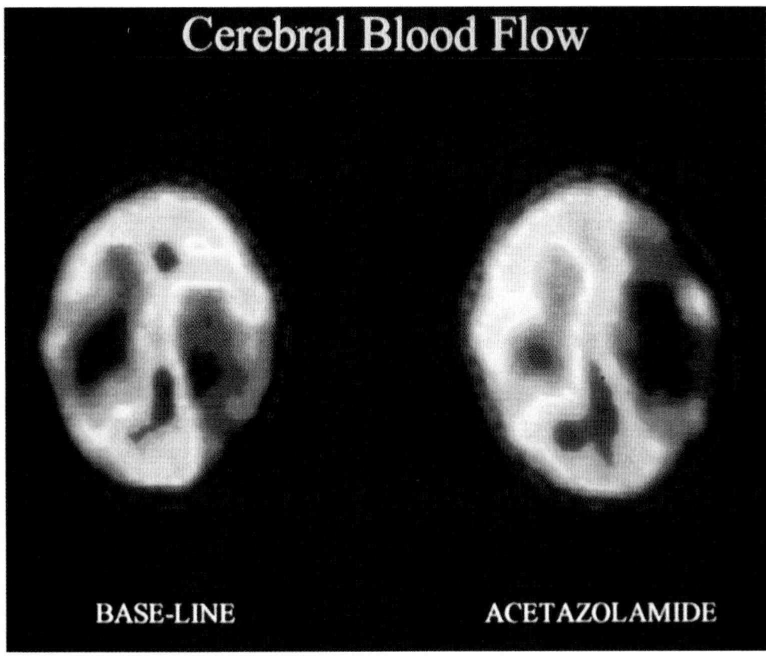

FIGURE 95-1. Impaired hemodynamic reserve. Resting and post-acetazolamide PET of cerebral blood flow (CBF) in a patient with repeated transient ischemic attacks owing to left internal carotid artery occlusion with revascularization through the ipsilateral ophthalmic artery and the contralateral internal carotid artery. Although the resting scan (*left*) showed little or no alteration in CBF in the affected hemisphere, the vasodilation challenge (*right*) induces a marked increase in CBF in the unoccluded side, but no increase in CBF on the occluded side with a decrease in the posterior and anterior parts of the left carotid territory, suggesting hemodynamic steal.

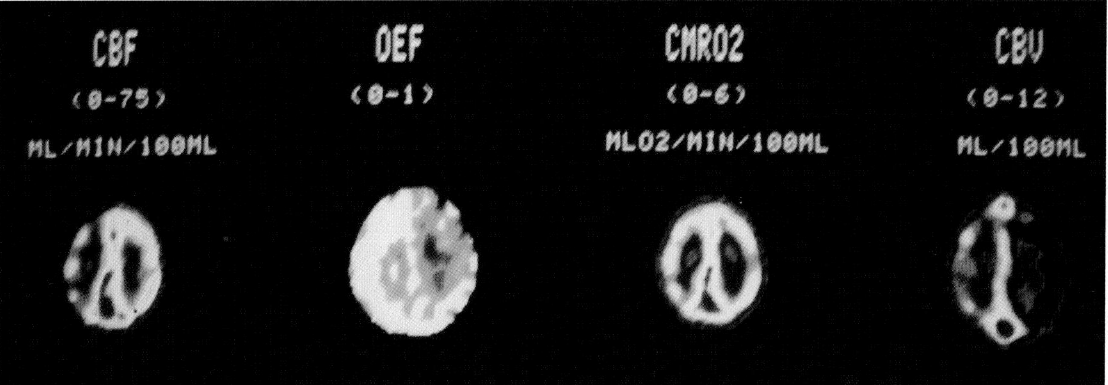

FIGURE 95-2. Misery perfusion: stage 2 of hemodynamic failure. Occlusion of the right internal carotid artery was diagnosed when the patient presented after an ipsilateral transient ischemic attack. Repeated transient ischemic attacks followed despite closely supervised antiplatelet and anticoagulant treatment. Some of the transient ischemic attacks were triggered on standing. PET performed several weeks later showed moderate hypoperfusion in the territory of the right carotid artery with a completely normal cerebral metabolic rate of oxygen. As a result, the oxygen extraction fraction was increased, causing *misery perfusion.* These data suggest inability of the collateral circulation to compensate fully for occlusion of the carotid artery and that the pressure of the blood supply to the brain downstream of the circle of Willis is insufficient to maintain cerebral blood flow (i.e., the local autoregulation mechanism has been overcome). This interpretation is supported by the observation of a marked increase in the cerebral blood volume on the side of the occlusion.

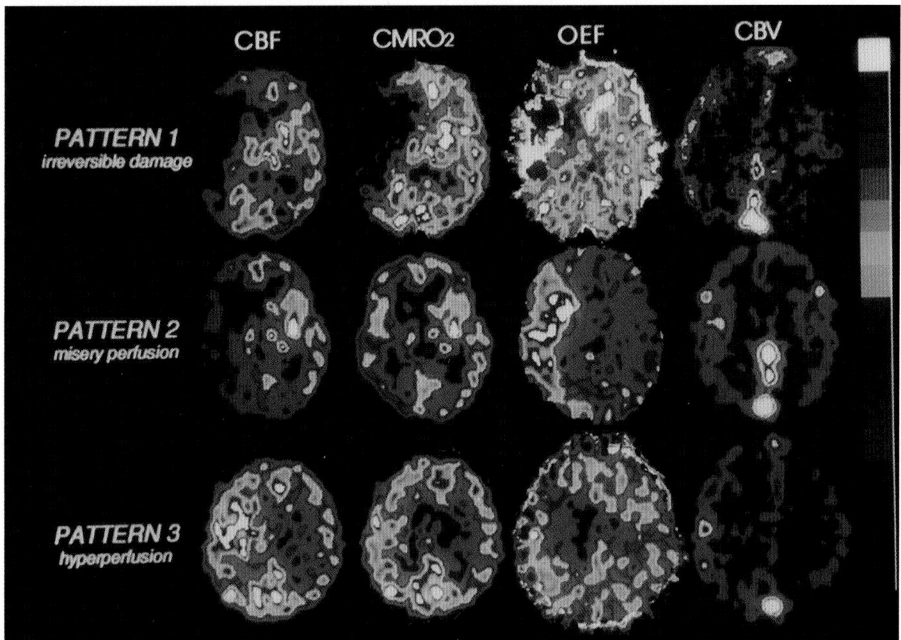

FIGURE 95-3. Illustrative PET patterns in acute middle cerebral artery (MCA) territory stroke. The three PET patterns of cerebral blood flow (CBF) and cerebral metabolic rate of oxygen ($CMRO_2$) changes observed within 18 hours of onset of MCA territory stroke. *Top row,* An example of *early extensive irreversible damage* in a patient with right-sided MCA territory stroke studied with PET 17 hours after symptom onset. There was a near-zero CBF and $CMRO_2$ in the whole right MCA territory (*pattern 1*), together with patchy oxygen extraction fraction (OEF) (black pixels represent unmeasurable OEF). The patient survived, but outcome was poor, and the whole MCA territory was infarcted at follow-up CT. *Middle row, Misery perfusion* in this patient with acute stage right MCA territory stroke; the PET study performed 12 hours after onset revealed a markedly reduced CBF in the whole right MCA territory, associated with relatively preserved $CMRO_2$ (except in the lenticulostriate area) and extremely elevated OEF. This example corresponds to a typical *pattern 2* of PET changes. This patient died 3 days after the PET study. *Bottom row,* An example of *early luxury perfusion (pattern 3)* in a patient studied with PET 13 hours after onset of right-sided MCA territory stroke. There is markedly increased CBF in the central right MCA territory, associated with normal or slightly increased $CMRO_2$ and decreased OEF. This patient made a full recovery, and the follow-up CT scan showed a small periventricular infarct.

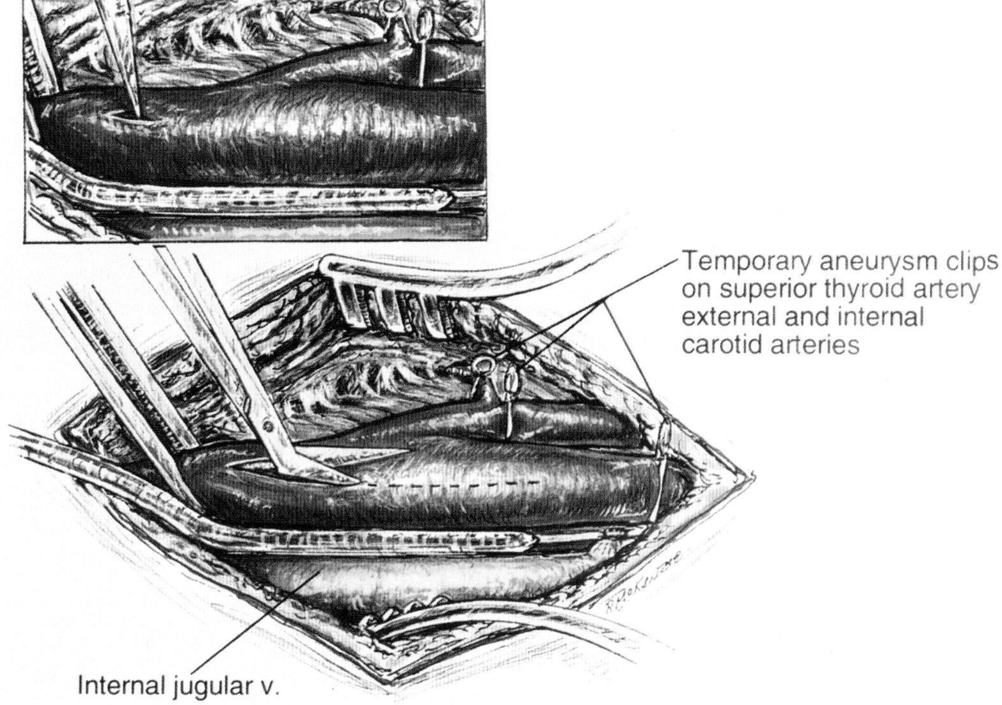

FIGURE 97-10. Once the common carotid artery is occluded with the vascular clamp and the superior thyroid and external and internal carotid arteries are occluded with temporary aneurysm clips, the arteriotomy is started by creating a 5-mm incision with a no. 11 scalpel blade. With an angled Pott's scissors, the arteriotomy is performed, beginning in the common carotid artery proximal to the atherosclerotic lesion and extending distally in the internal carotid artery to a point beyond the lesion. Care must be taken not to extend the arteriotomy too far medially, which will cause it to veer into the bifurcation or region of the origin of the external carotid artery. Likewise, making the arteriotomy too far laterally in the internal carotid artery will make subsequent closure difficult. (From Bailes JE, Spetzler RF [eds]: Microsurgical Carotid Endarterectomy. New York, Lippincott-Raven, 1996.)

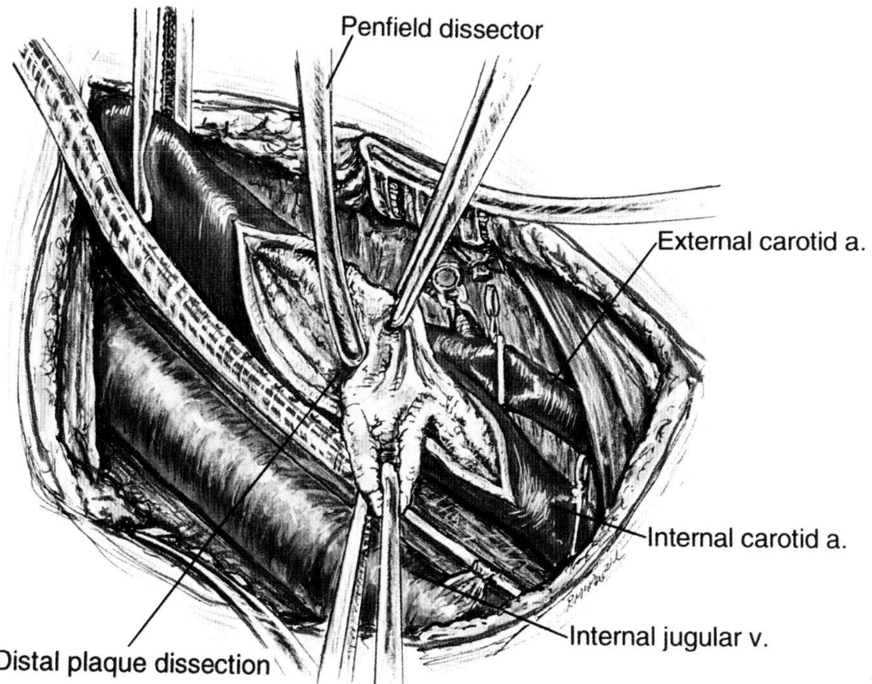

FIGURE 97-13. The plaque is everted and transected from its entrance into the superior thyroid and external carotid arteries. The remaining distal portion in the internal carotid artery is dissected free and removed with the intent of creating a smooth or feathering distal transition, avoiding the formation of an intimal flap. (From Bailes JE, Spetzler RF [eds]: Microsurgical Carotid Endarterectomy. New York, Lippincott-Raven, 1996.)

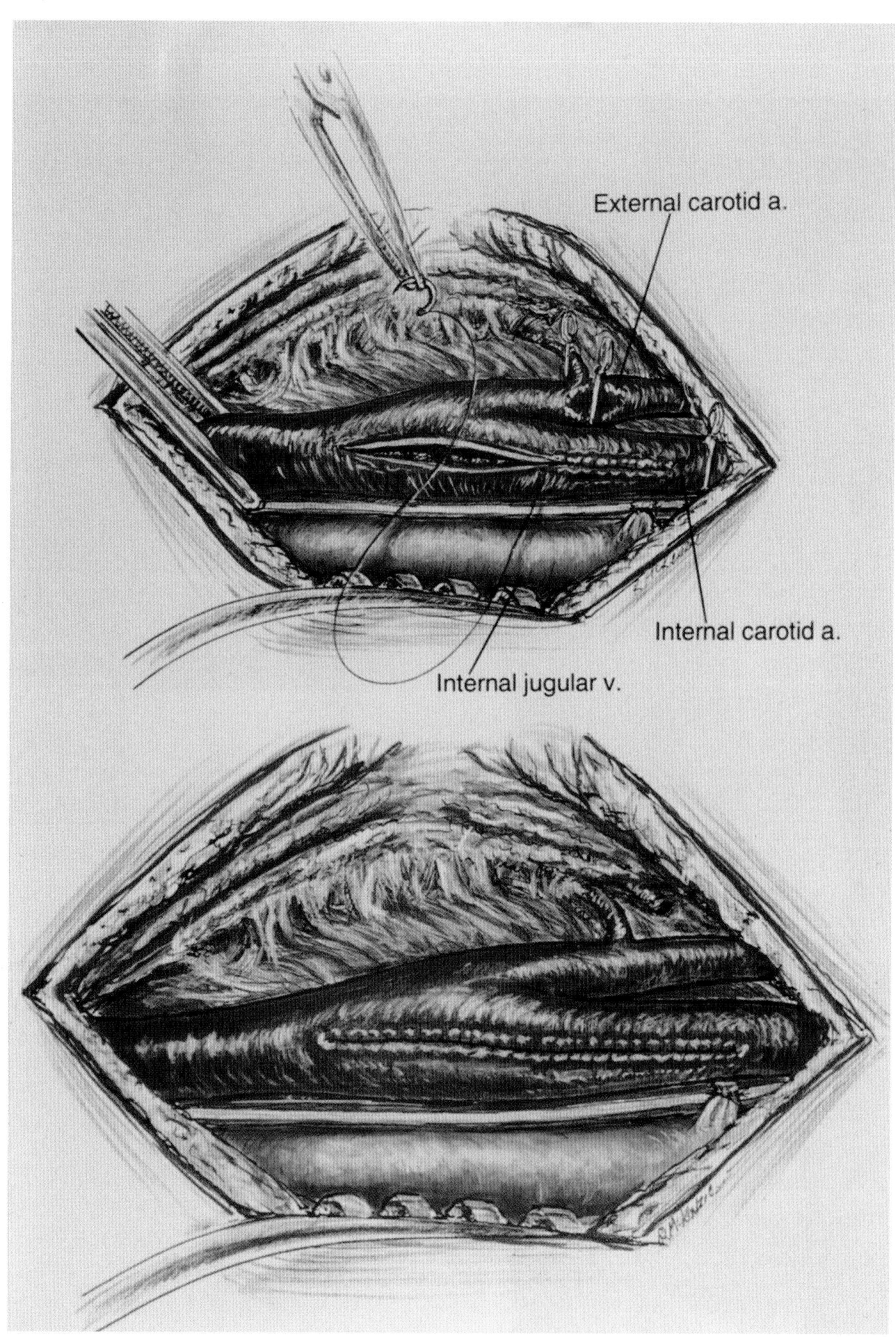

FIGURE 97-14. After the arteriotomy is closed, backbleeding and deocclusion are accomplished in the correct manner in an attempt to expel any air or debris out the lumen or into the distribution of the external (not internal) carotid artery. (From Bailes JE, Spetzler RF [eds]: Microsurgical Carotid Endarterectomy. New York, Lippincott-Raven, 1996.)

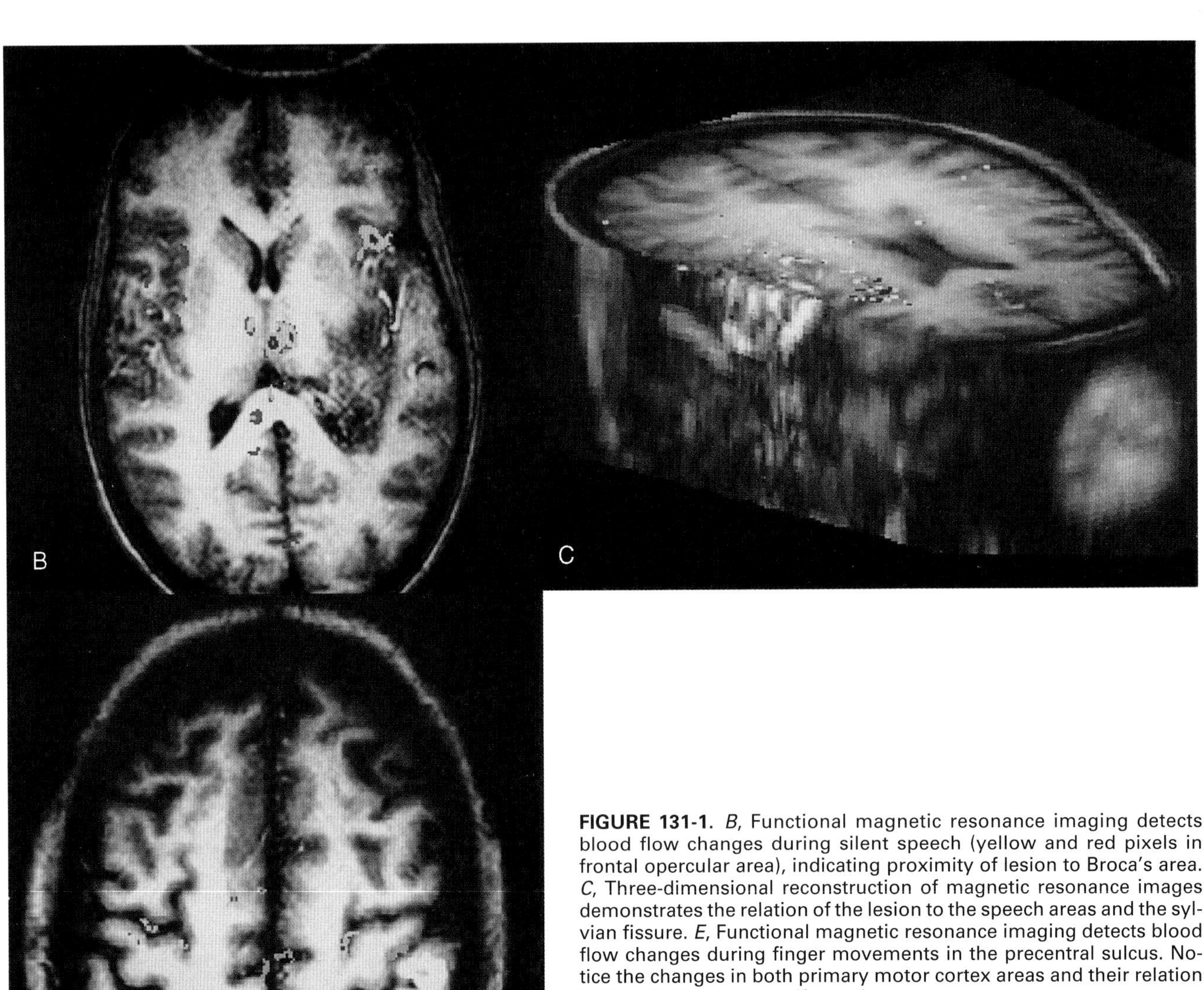

FIGURE 131-1. *B*, Functional magnetic resonance imaging detects blood flow changes during silent speech (yellow and red pixels in frontal opercular area), indicating proximity of lesion to Broca's area. *C*, Three-dimensional reconstruction of magnetic resonance images demonstrates the relation of the lesion to the speech areas and the sylvian fissure. *E*, Functional magnetic resonance imaging detects blood flow changes during finger movements in the precentral sulcus. Notice the changes in both primary motor cortex areas and their relation to the arteriovenous malformation.

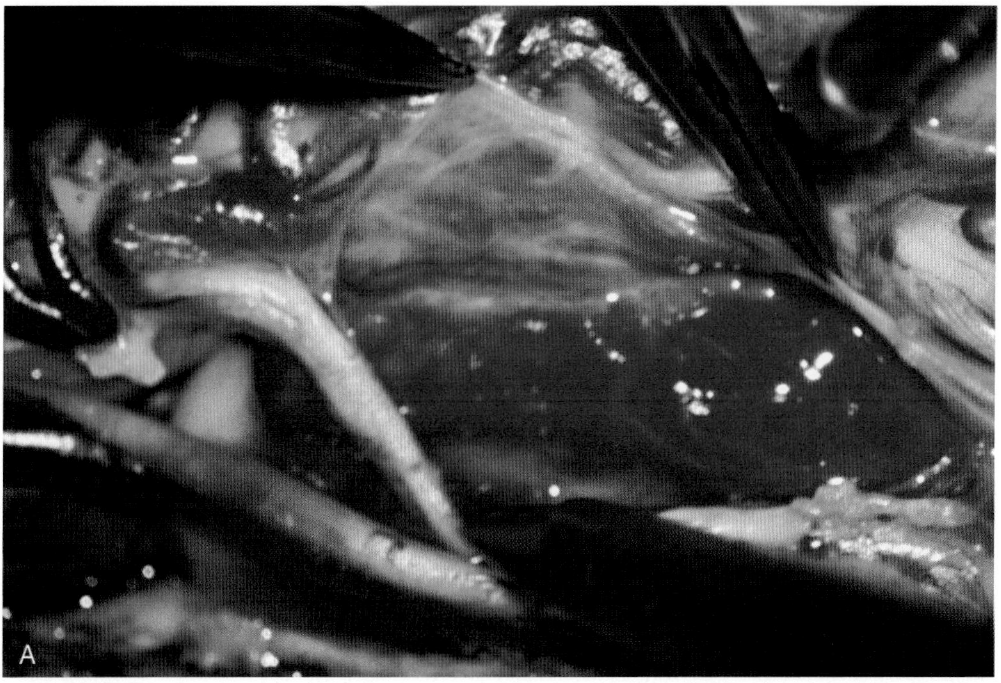

FIGURE 140-1. Intramedullary T9 hemangioblastoma situated arteriorly. The dentate ligamet is cut. *A*, Intraoperative photograph. (From Spetzler RF, Koos WT, Richling B, Lang J: Color Atlas of Microneurosurgery, vol 3, 2nd ed. Stuttgart, Germany, Georg Thieme Verlag, 1999.)

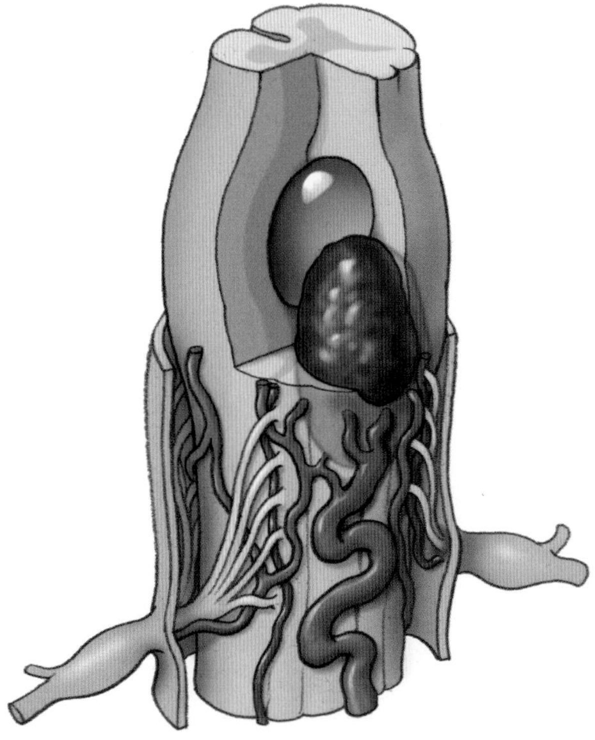

FIGURE 140-2. Cystic hemangioblastoma of the spinal cord. (Courtesy of Barrow Neurological Institute, Phoenix, AZ.)

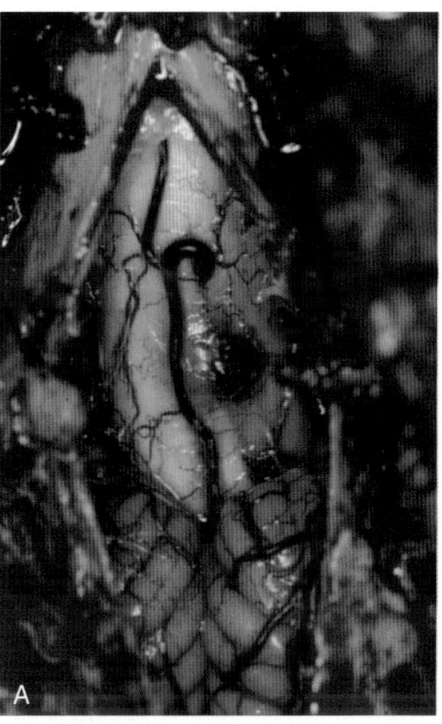

FIGURE 140-3. Intraoperative photograph *(A)* of a spinal cavernous malformation and associated venous anomaly. The cerebellum is at the bottom of the photograph. (From Spetzler RF, Koos WT, Richling B, Lang J: Color Atlas of Microneurosurgery, vol 3, 2nd ed. Stuttgart, Germany, Georg Thieme Verlag, 1999.)

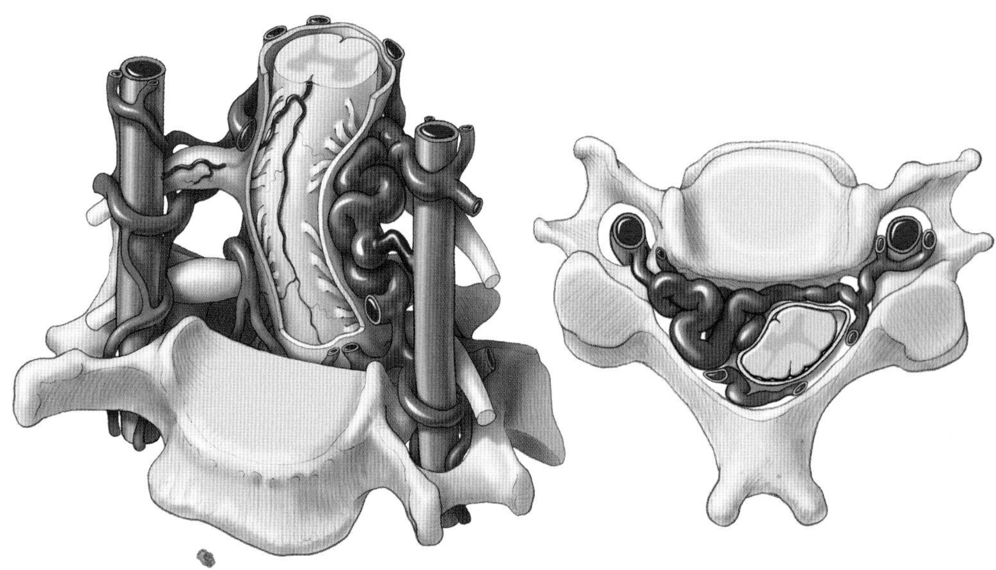

FIGURE 140-5. Extradural arteriovenous fistula. (From Spetzler RF, Detwiler PW, Riina HA, Porter RW: Modified classification of spinal cord vascular lesions. J Neurosurg [Spine 2] 96:145–156, 2002.)

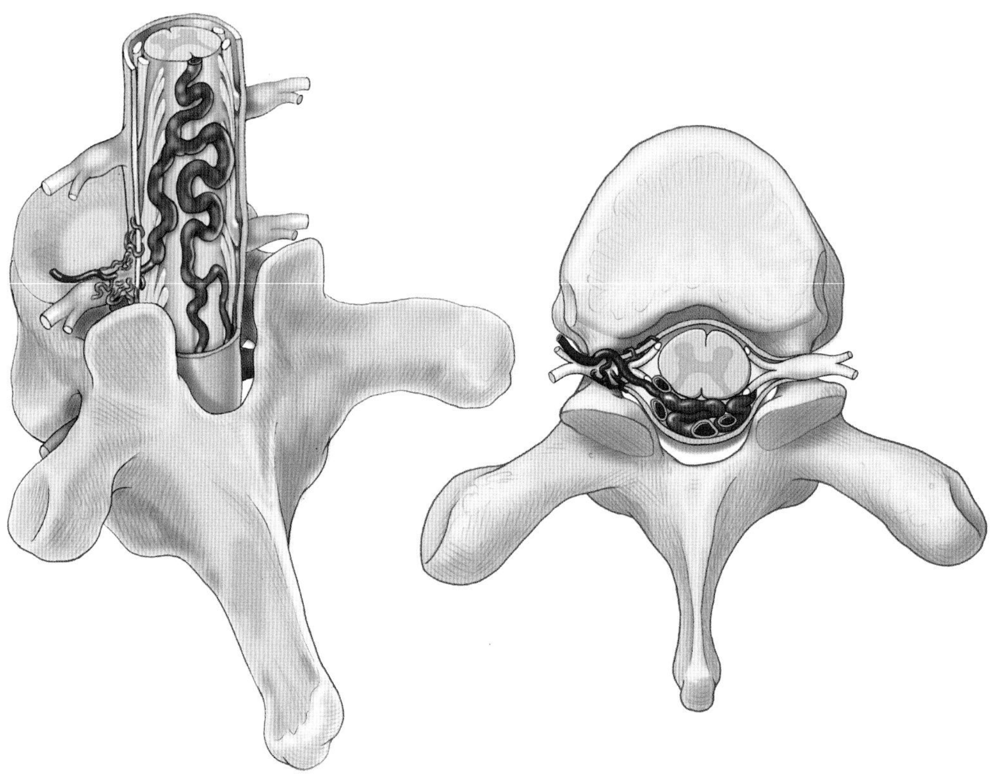

FIGURE 140-6. Dorsal intradural arteriovenous fistula. (From Spetzler RF, Detwiler PW, Riina HA, Porter RW: Modified classification of spinal cord vascular lesions. J Neurosurg [Spine 2] 96:145–156, 2002.)

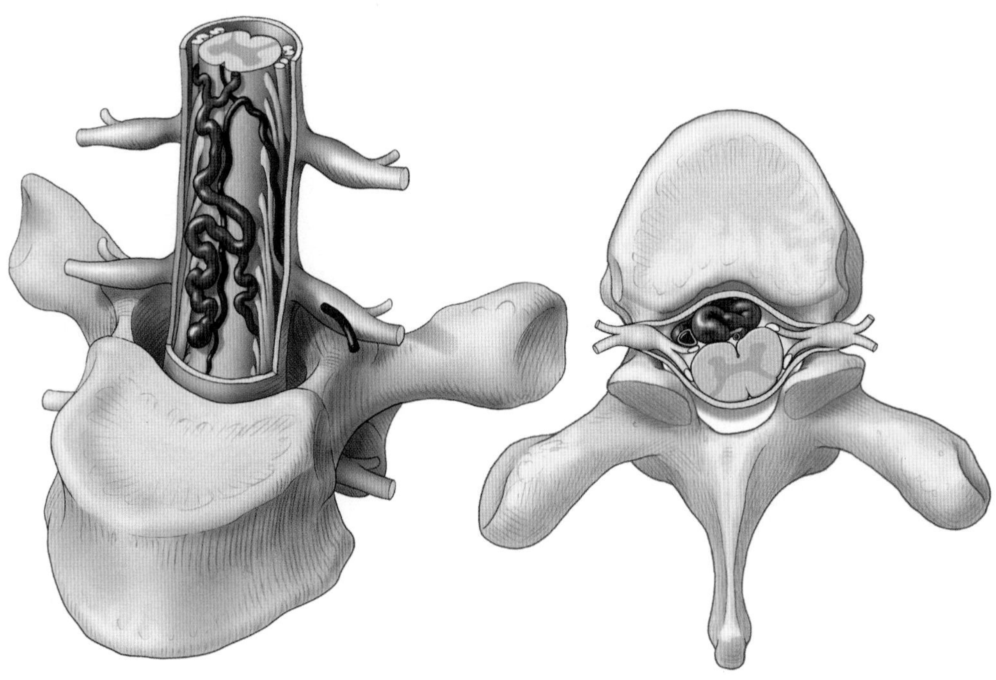

FIGURE 140-7. Ventral intradural arteriovenous fistula. (From Spetzler RF, Detwiler PW, Riina HA, Porter RW: Modified classification of spinal cord vascular lesions. J Neurosurg [Spine 2] 96:145–156, 2002.)

FIGURE 140-8. Ventral intradural arteriovenous fistula with connection to a dilated, engorged venous system. (Courtesy of Barrow Neurological Institute, Phoenix, AZ.)

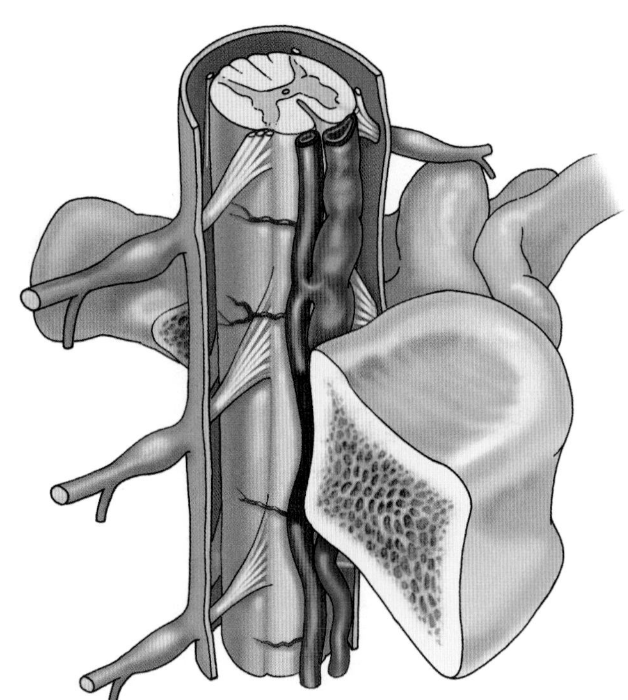

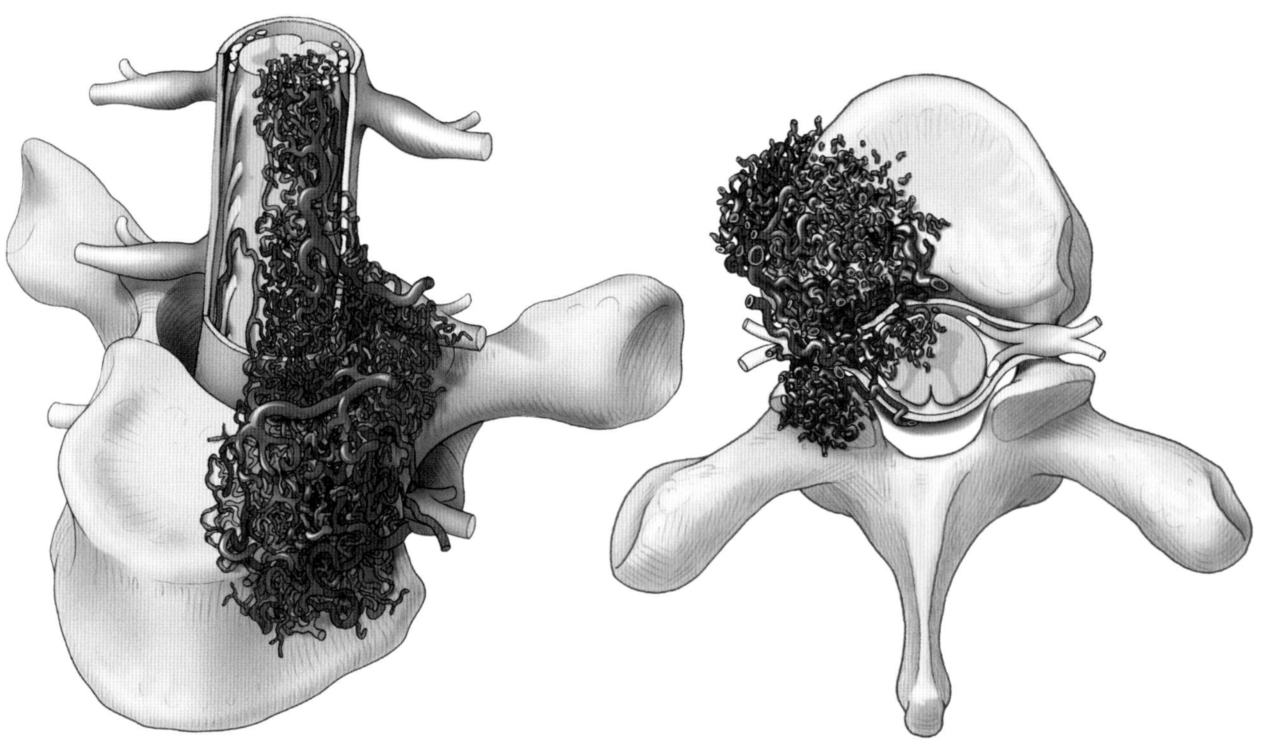

FIGURE 140-9. Complex extradural-intradural spinal arteriovenous malformation. (From Spetzler RF, Detwiler PW, Riina HA, Porter RW: Modified classification of spinal cord vascular lesions. J Neurosurg [Spine 2] 96:145–156, 2002.)

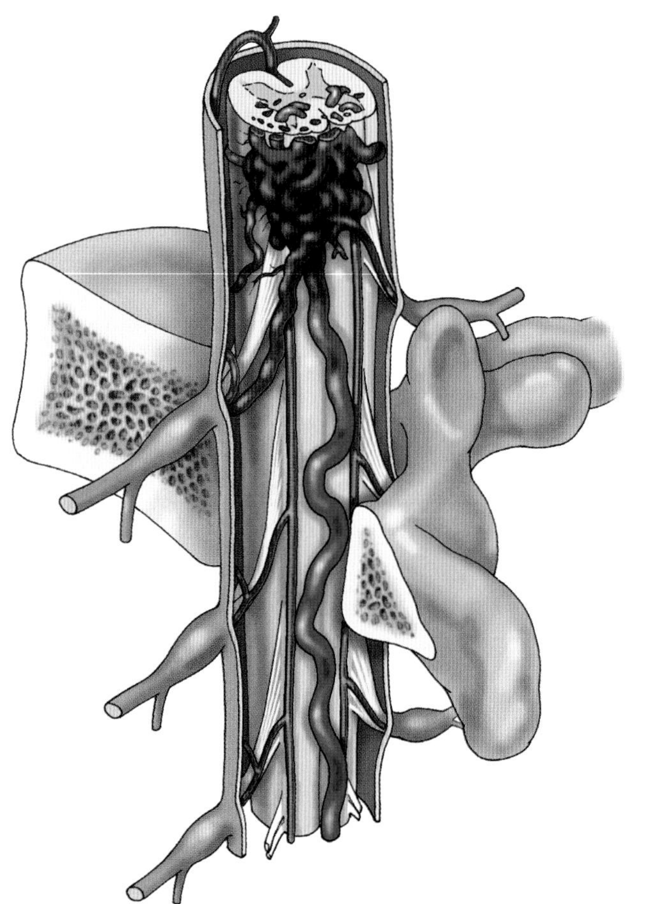

FIGURE 140-10. Intramedullary arteriovenous malformation. (Courtesy of Barrow Neurological Institute, Phoenix, AZ.)

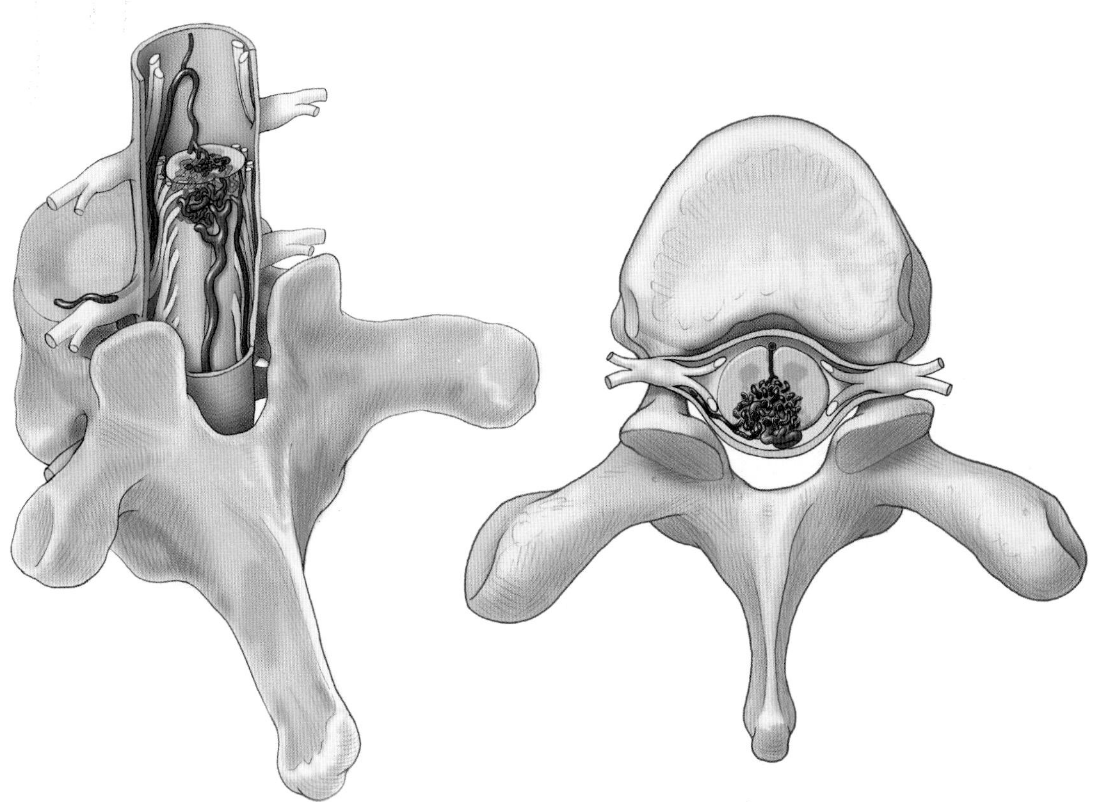

FIGURE 140-11. Intramedullary arteriovenous malformation with a compact nidus. (From Spetzler RF, Detwiler PW, Riina HA, Porter RW: Modified classification of spinal cord vascular lesions. J Neurosurg [Spine 2] 96:145–156, 2002.)

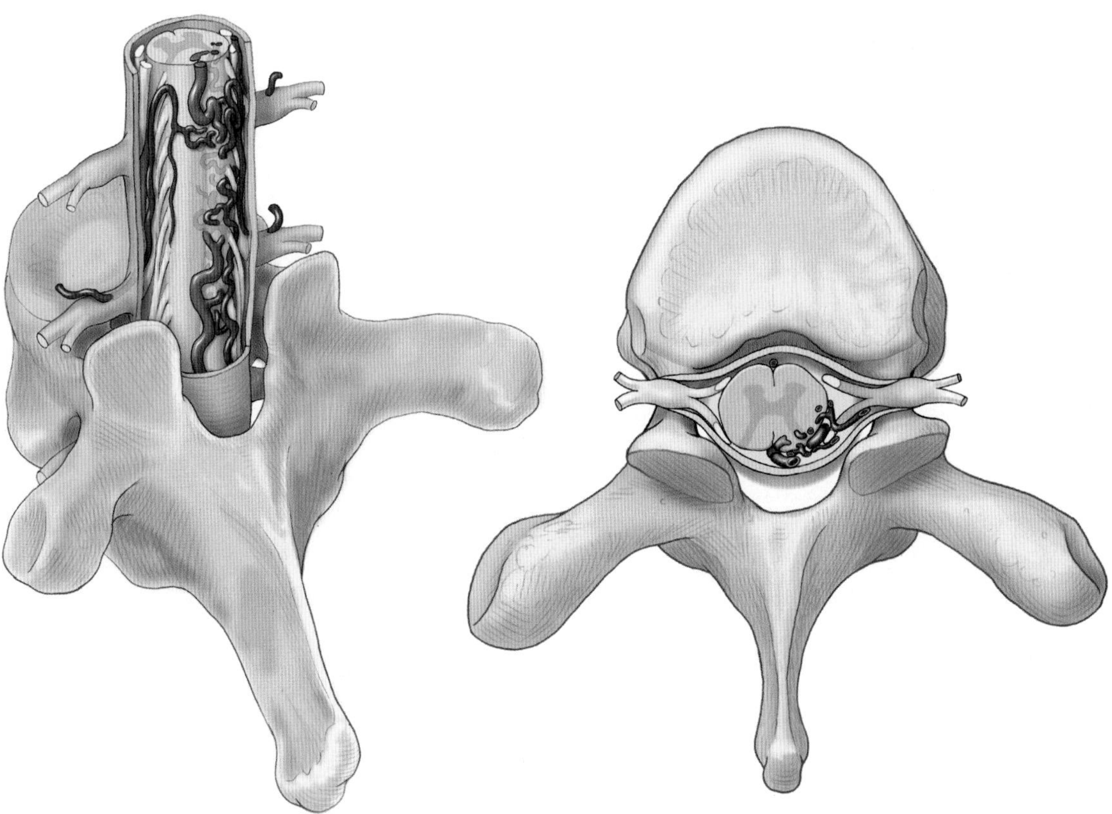

FIGURE 140-12. Intramedullary arteriovenous malformation with a diffuse nidus. (From Spetzler RF, Detwiler PW, Riina HA, Porter RW: Modified classification of spinal cord vascular lesions. J Neurosurg [Spine 2] 96:145–156, 2002.)

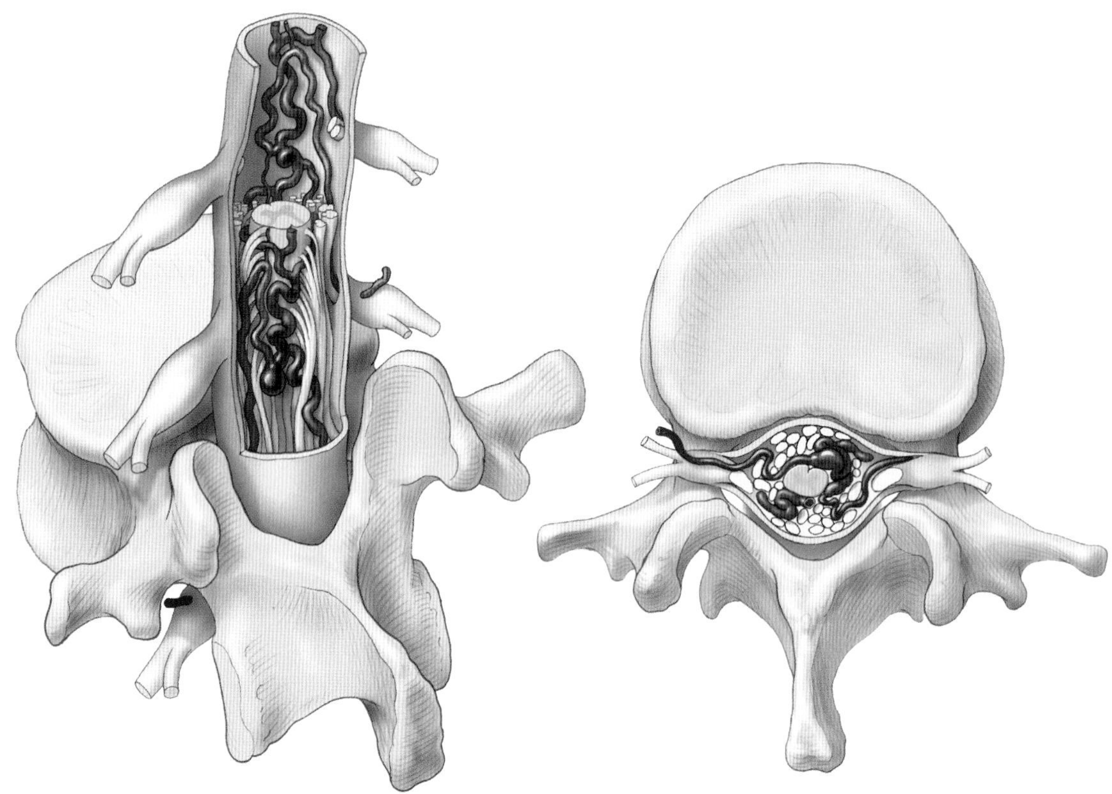

FIGURE 140-13. Conus arteriovenous malformation. (From Spetzler RF, Detwiler PW, Riina HA, Porter RW: Modified classification of spinal cord vascular lesions. J Neurosurg [Spine 2] 96:145–156, 2002.)

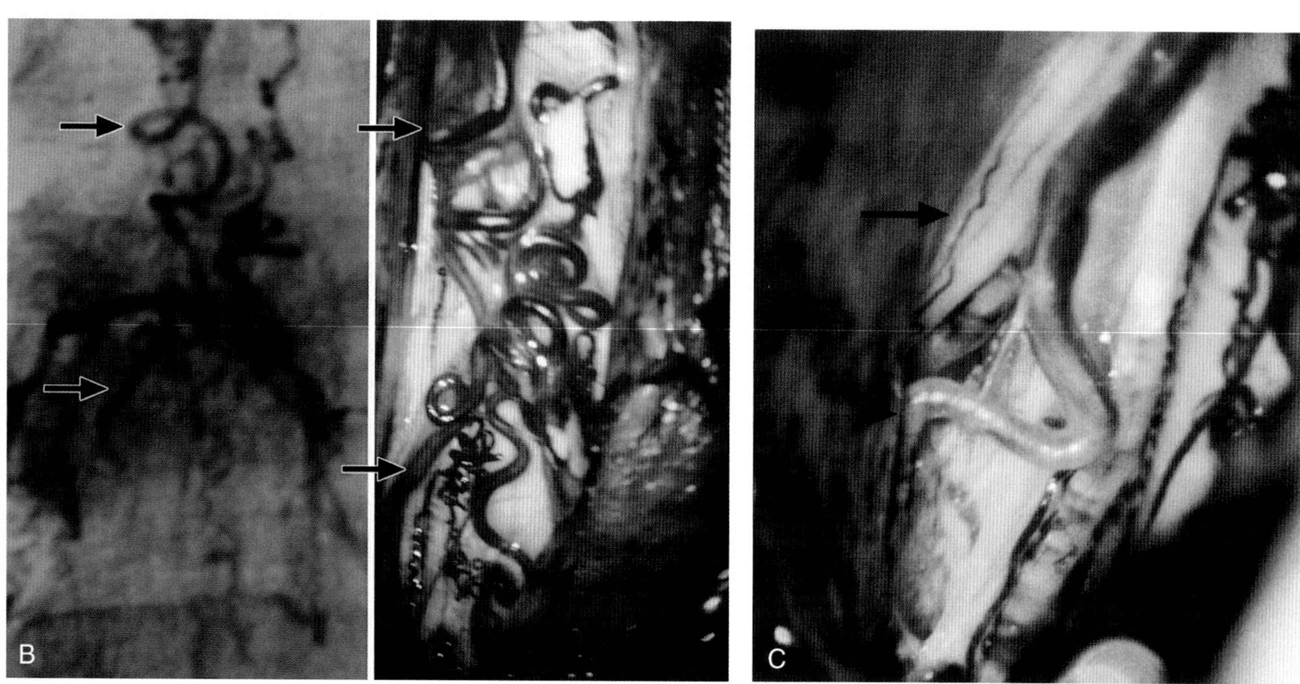

FIGURE 142-22. A 67-year-old woman with a 6-month history of progressive gait disturbance, lower extremity claudication, and bladder dysfunction. *B*, Preoperative arteriogram and intraoperative view. An anteroposterior spinal arteriogram (*left*; seen from the surgeon's view) demonstrates filling of the spinal dural arteriovenous fistula (AVF) and the pattern of the vessels of the coronal venous plexus. Note the congruency of the vascular pattern compared to an intraoperative view (*right*) of the dorsal surface of the spinal cord at the same level. By studying the vascular pattern of the arteriogram, correlation with the intradural vessels (*top arrows*) is possible, which allows ready identification of the intradural draining vein *(bottom arrows)*. *C*, Intradural draining vein (medullary vein). This magnified view demonstrates the relationship of the intradural draining vein of the AVF *(arrowhead)* to the dural penetration of the nerve root *(arrow)*. The fistula is effectively treated with coagulation and division of this vessel. (From Watson JC, Oldfield EH: The surgical management of spinal dural vascular malformations. Neurosurg Clin N Am 10:73–87, 1999.)

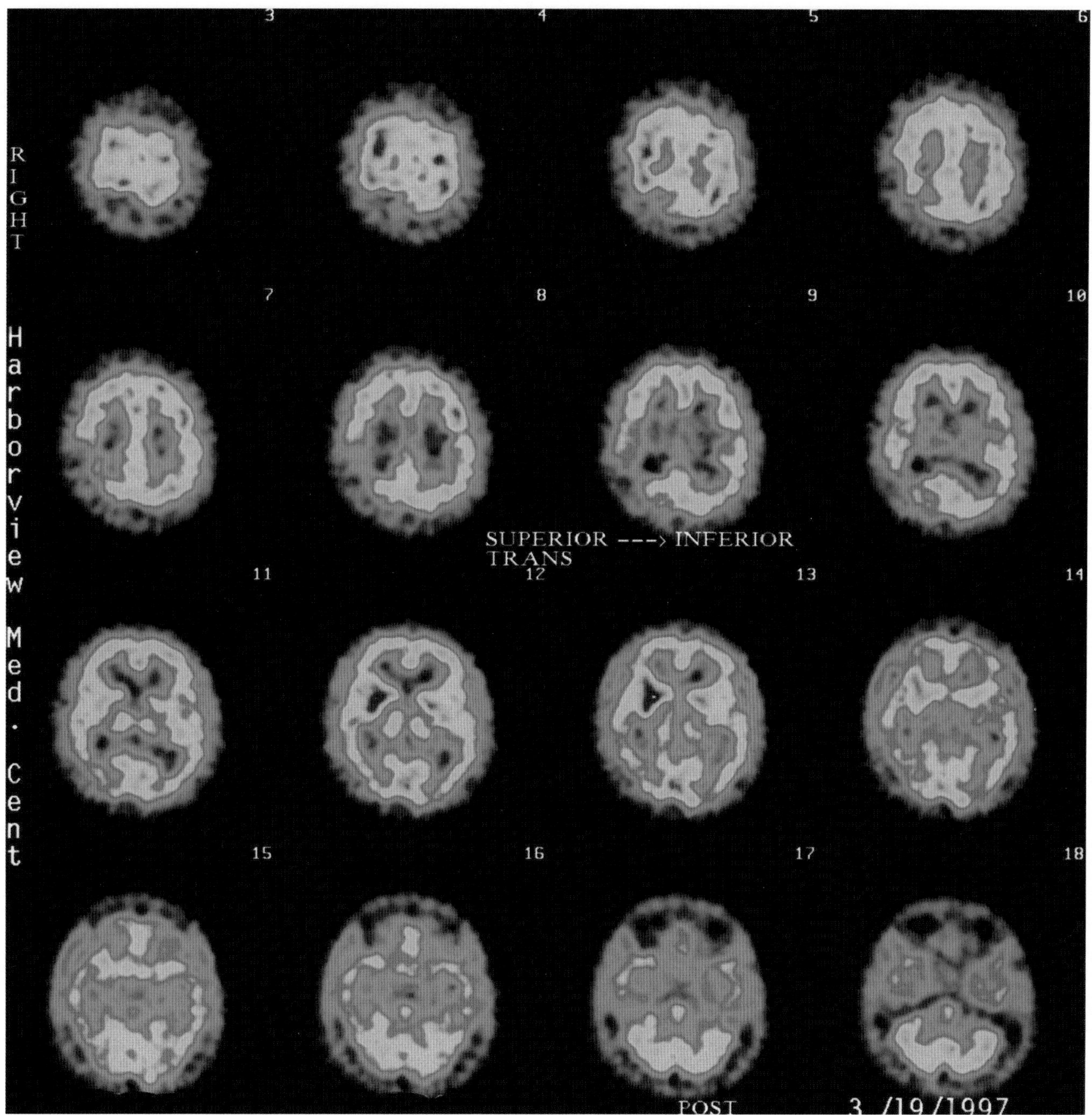

FIGURE 148-1. Transverse axial view of ictal injection of technetium-99m ethyl cysteinate dimer for regional cerebral perfusion in epilepsy. This patient had intractable epilepsy despite previous surgical resection in the right parietal cortex. Ictal image shows hyperperfusion (*red zone*) in the right insular cortex. After resection of this area, the patient was seizure-free.

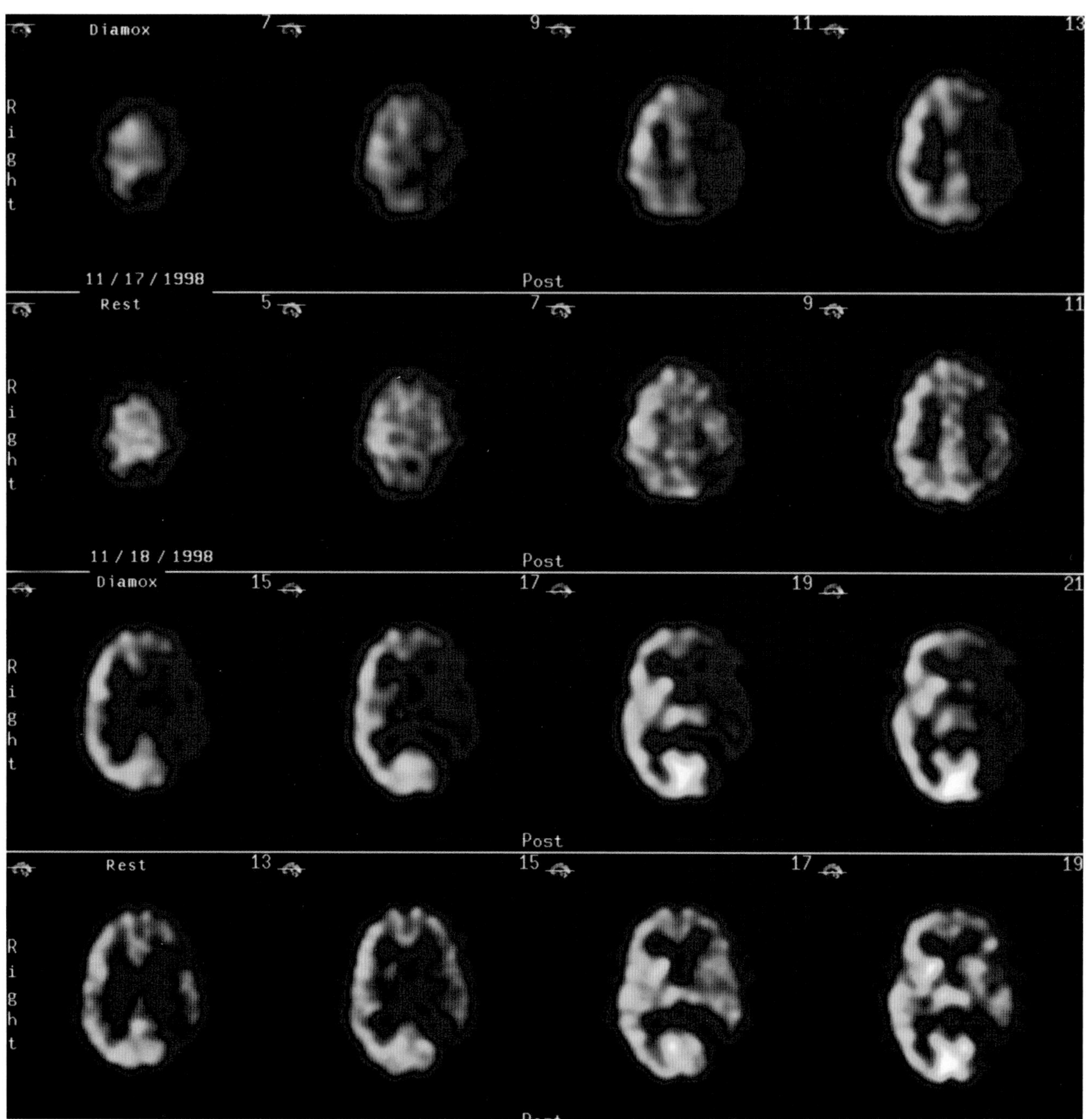

FIGURE 148-2. Transverse axial view of cerebral perfusion SPECT with technetium-99m ethyl cysteinate dimer with acetazolamide challenge (*rows 1 and 3*) and at rest. Images show severe lack of vasodilatory reserve in the left hemisphere with residual fixed defects in the watershed zones.

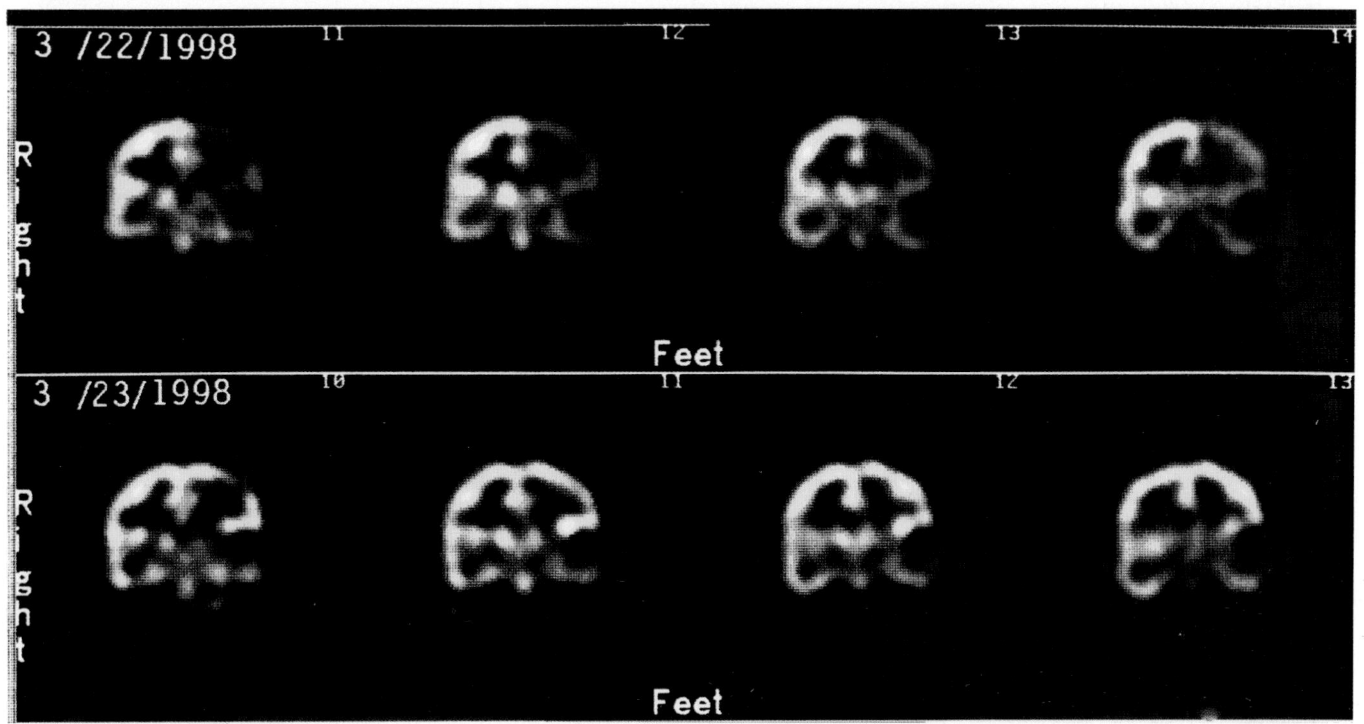

FIGURE 148-3. Coronal axial view of technetium-99m ethyl cysteinate dimer cerebral perfusion SPECT images before (*top*) and after (*bottom*) left middle cerebral artery balloon angioplasty for severe left middle cerebral artery vasospasm after subarachnoid hemorrhage. Images show significant improvement in perfusion to the left hemisphere.

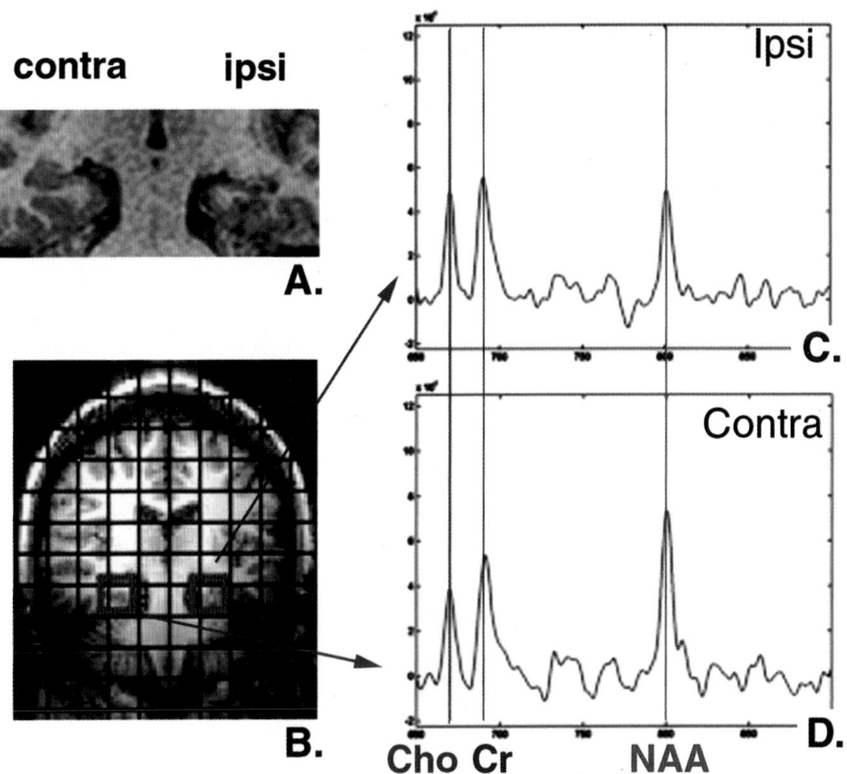

FIGURE 149-24. ^{1}H spectroscopy of temporal lobe epilepsy. *A*, Coronal T1-weighted image shows left hippocampal atrophy (ipsi) consistent with hippocampal sclerosis. *B*, Spectroscopic imaging yields spectra from multivoxels with spectra from ipsilateral abnormal hippocampus (ipsi) shown in *C* and the normal contralateral one (contra) in *D*. Compare the height of the peaks of NAA to Cr. The NAA/Cr ratio is decreased ipsilaterally. NAA, *N*-acetyl aspartate; Cr, creatine; Cho, choline. (Images courtesy of Hoby Hetherton and Edward Novotny.)

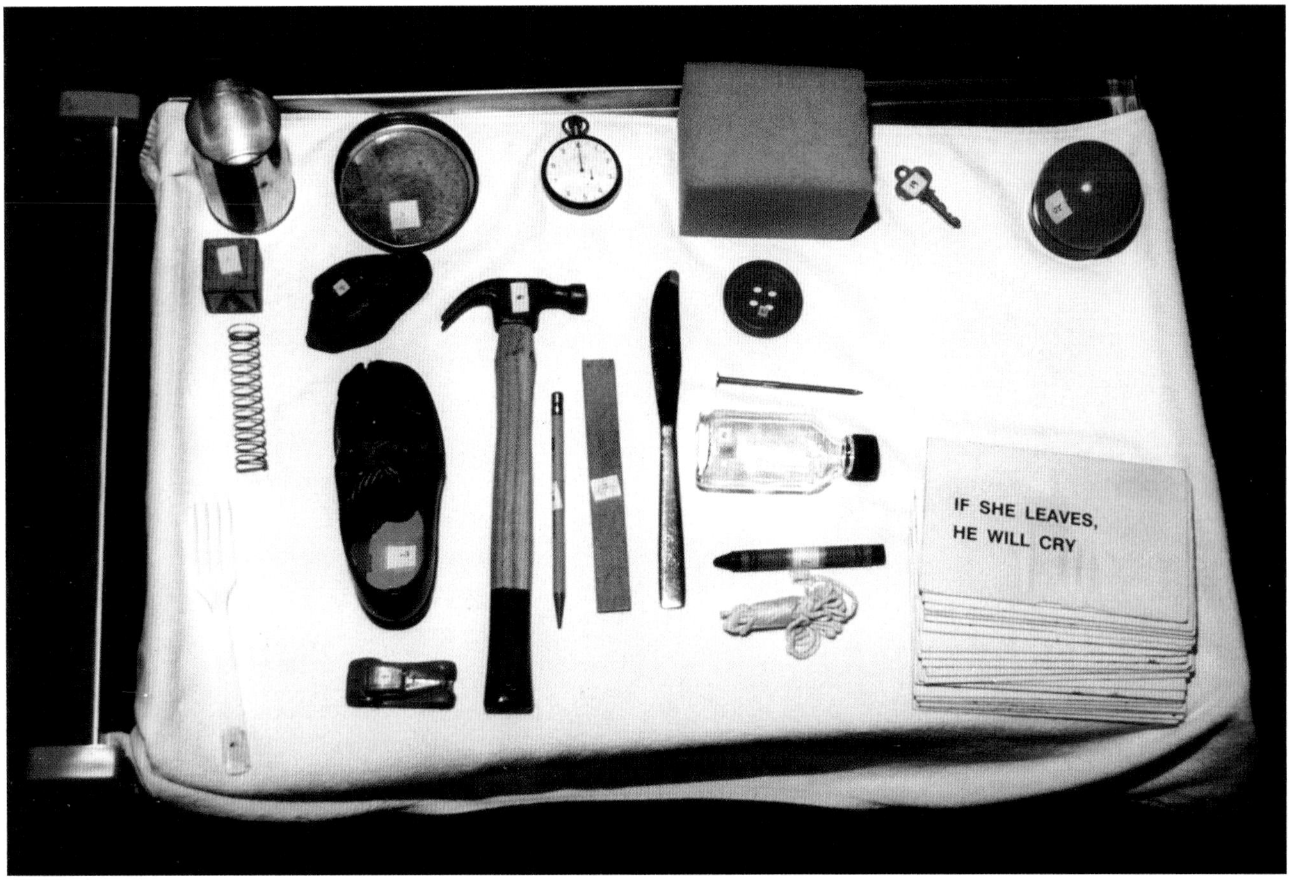

FIGURE 150-1. Psychological test materials used in the Seattle form of the intracarotid amobarbital procedure.

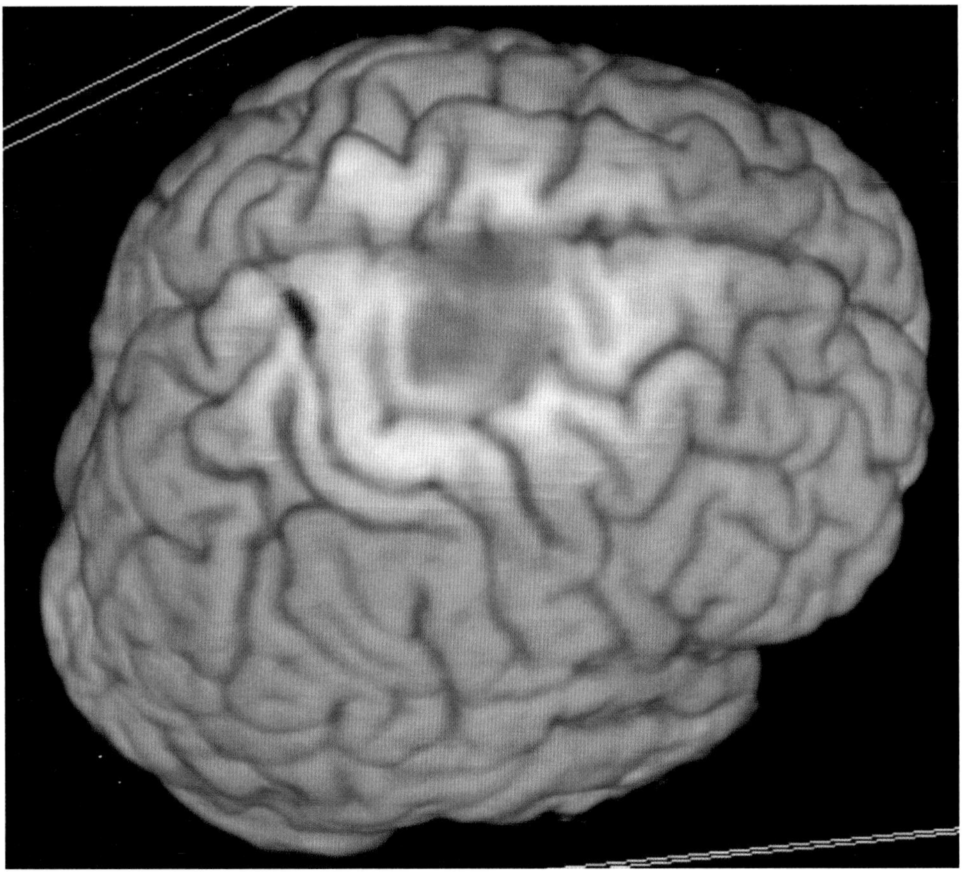

FIGURE 152-3. Functional magnetic resonance image superimposed on a three-dimensional surface rendering of a patient with focal motor seizures of the left hand. This image shows a low-grade glioma in the right superior frontal gyrus immediately anterior to the rolandic somatomotor area for hand function. Area of cortical activation during a left finger-tapping task is identified in red.

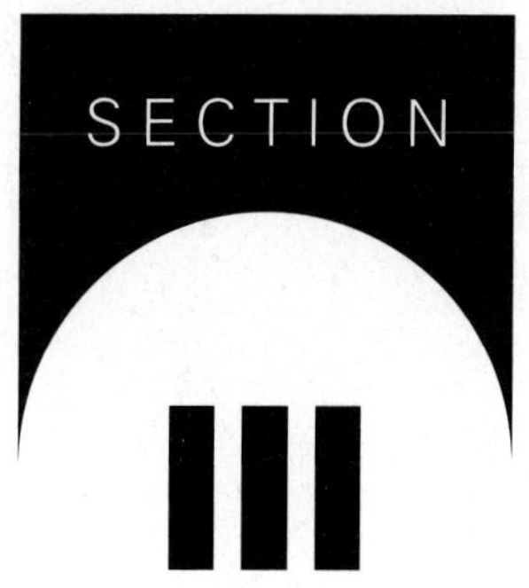

Vascular

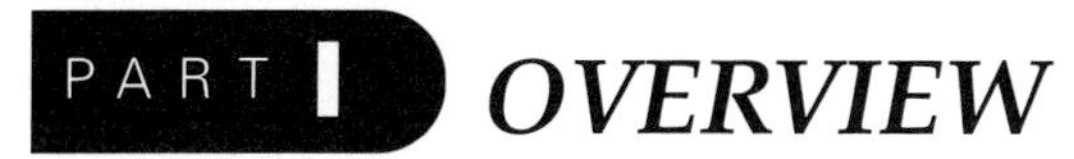

CHAPTER 85

Historical Considerations

MILIND DEOGAONKAR ■ L. PHILIP CARTER

What is past is prologue.

—William Shakespeare, 1611

In a numbingly complex and rapidly growing scientific discipline such as cerebrovascular diseases, it is imperative to consider the past to appreciate the progress. More than just an intellectual exercise, a historical perspective deepens our understanding of the present and clarifies the best path forward. The distance achieved since Galen[1] (130–200 AD) proposed that "the vital spirits, produced by the left ventricle of the heart, are carried towards the brain by the carotid arteries" is considerable. An Oxford-based English physician, Thomas Willis, provided the first scientific account of the architecture of cerebral circulation in 1664. His book *Cerebri Anatome*[2] remains a classic in the history of brain sciences.

INTRACRANIAL ANEURYSMS

Intracranial and subarachnoid hemorrhages have been recognized as a cause of death since Biblical times. Ancient Greek and Egyptian medical texts discussed the poor outcome associated with these hemorrhages. In 1761, Morgagni,[3] an anatomist from Padua, published the first description of an intracranial aneurysm. In 1765, Biumi[4] of Milan reported another cavernous sinus aneurysm, describing its postmortem appearance in detail. In 1813, Blackhall[5] published the first clinical account of a ruptured intracranial aneurysm. He demonstrated the presence of a basilar tip aneurysm and intraventricular blood in a young woman at autopsy.

In 1875, Hutchinson[6] first recognized an intracranial aneurysm based on neurological signs. He diagnosed the aneurysm 11 years before his patient died and proposed carotid ligation as treatment. After the patient's death from a pelvic abscess, an egg-sized aneurysm was found in the middle fossa at autopsy. In 1851, Brinton[7] published the first series of intracranial aneurysms with a systematic analysis of symptoms and location. He analyzed 52 cases of ruptured intracranial aneurysms collected from the literature. In 1859, Gull[8] published 62 cases of intracranial aneurysms. Although he believed that aneurysms could be recognized only at autopsy, he made the important observation that "young persons dying of apoplexy probably had an aneurysm." In 1868, Charcot and Bouchard[9] described microaneurysms. In 1872, Bartholow[10] reviewed the symptoms of 114 patients with aneurysms.

In 1887, Eppinger,[11] followed by Fearnsides in 1916,[12] proposed a congenital defect in the elastic properties of the arterial wall as the origin of aneurysms. In 1918, Turnbull[13] classified aneurysms based on their pathology: infective, congenital, and degenerative. About this time, the evolution of two diagnostic procedures changed the practical management of ruptured intracranial aneurysms. In 1891, Quincke[14] introduced the technique of lumbar puncture. In 1927, Egaz Moniz[15] introduced cerebral angiography, giving physicians a means to diagnose intracranial aneurysms. The first angiographic documentation of a cerebral aneurysm followed in 1931.[16]

In 1885, Sir Victor Horsley[17] attempted the first surgical treatment of an intracranial aneurysm. He successfully ligated carotid arteries to treat an aneurysm at the base of the brain. Early surgical attempts were confined to extracranial or intracranial carotid ligation. Horsley[17, 18] and many other surgeons performed such operations.

Carotid ligation appeared to be effective for aneurysms of the carotid artery, but there was a significant risk of hemiplegia and severe infarction. Because of this, gradual occlusion of the common or internal carotid artery became popular, and a series of carotid clamps were developed that were gradually tightened over several days to permit the progressive occlusion of the vessel. If the patient became obtunded or hemiplegic, the clamp could be opened. These instruments were designed by Dott, Selverstone, Poppen, and Crutchfield.[19] Proximal occlusion was popularized by

Valentine Logue[20] and was also carried intracranially, with occlusion of the feeding anterior cerebral artery for an anterior communicating artery aneurysm. Such proximal occlusive techniques were extended to the vertebral-basilar circulation by notable neurosurgeons such as Walter Dandy and Charles Drake. However, over the years, direct surgical attack on aneurysms gradually replaced the proximal occlusive techniques.

On April 22, 1931, Norman Dott[21] pioneered the direct surgical attack on aneurysms when he treated a carotid bifurcation aneurysm by wrapping it with muscle. Dandy[22] was also the first to clip the neck of an aneurysm successfully (Fig. 85–1). In 1938, soon after Dandy published his monograph on intracranial aneurysms, clipping the necks of aneurysms became the gold standard for their treatment.

The design of aneurysmal clips underwent numerous improvements after their introduction. As discussed by DeLong and Ray,[23] Schwartz and Mayfield developed the first spring clip in early 1950s. In 1966, Scoville[24] developed a lightweight, torsion-bar spring clip that could be applied temporarily or permanently. Since then, a variety of spring clips have been developed.[25]

Although exclusion of an aneurysm by clipping its neck is the most physiologically satisfactory treatment, it is not always possible because of anatomic complexities. Consequently, other treatments were developed to prevent rebleeding from an aneurysm. The aneurysmal sac has been reinforced with methyl methacrylate with acetone,[26] polyvinyl copolymer,[27] silicone,[28] and muslin gauze.[29]

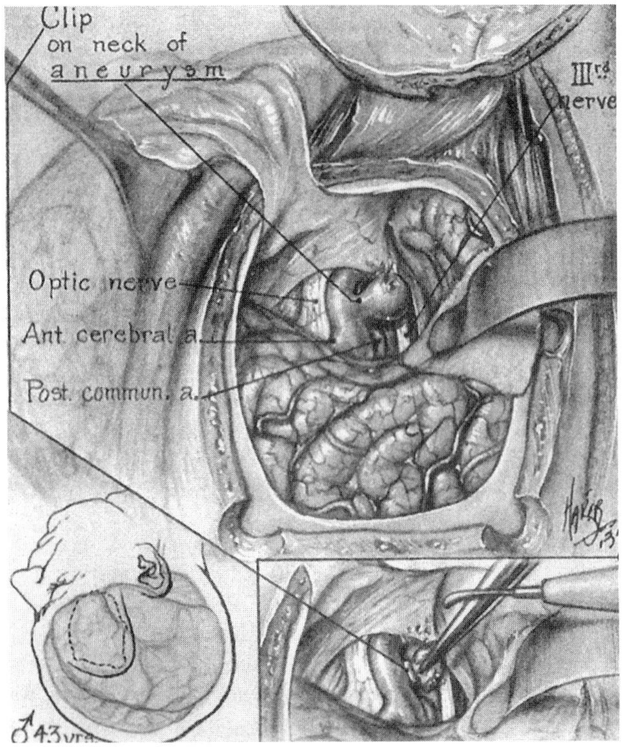

FIGURE 85–1. Dandy's operative planning in his first case of clipping the neck of an internal carotid aneurysm. (From Dandy WE: Intracranial aneurysms of the internal carotid artery. Ann Surg 107:656, 1938.)

Concomitant developments in anesthesia, operating techniques, and surgical instruments have helped to improve the safety of aneurysm surgery. Introduction of the operating microscope in 1962 by Jacobson and coworkers[30] improved appreciation of anatomic details. Yasargil, one of the pioneers of microneurosurgery, emphasized the importance of using the operating microscope during aneurysm surgery. In 1940, Greenwood[31] introduced bipolar diathermy, which has been immensely beneficial for working in the depths of tissue and around vital structures. As described by Lougheed and Marshall,[32] in 1953, White and Sweet introduced the use of hypothermia for cerebral protection during cerebrovascular procedures, thereby reducing postoperative morbidity. In 1962, Uihlein and coworkers[33] performed aneurysm surgery using hypothermia and circulatory arrest. In 1971, the practical management of aneurysms improved further when computed tomography (CT) became available, developed by a group that included Godfrey Hounsfield.[34] Newer imaging techniques such as digital subtraction angiography[35] and magnetic resonance imaging[36] have further contributed to the study and management of ruptured intracranial aneurysms. Charles Drake[37] modified the surgical treatment of posterior circulation aneurysms, demonstrating that they could be treated with an acceptable risk.

Classifications that correlated a patient's clinical condition with outcome provided a means of grading the clinical severity of a subarachnoid hemorrhage (SAH). The scale introduced by Hunt and Hess[38] and other such grading systems improved prognosis estimation and management of these patients. In 1951, Ecker and Riemenschneider[39] showed that cerebral vasospasm was a complication of SAH. Various multicenter studies, including a cooperative study[40] and the International Study of Unruptured Aneurysms,[41] have clarified the natural history and clinical behavior of intracranial aneurysms. Endovascular treatment of intracranial aneurysms is a recent milestone in the treatment of intracranial aneurysms.

CEREBROVASCULAR MALFORMATIONS

Cerebrovascular malformations are a diverse group of clinicopathologically distinct lesions. As discussed by Pool,[42] Luschka (1854) and Virchow (1863) made the first major attempts to classify lesions of this type. In 1895, Steinheil[43] first clinically diagnosed a cerebral arteriovenous malformation (AVM). In 1897, Giordano[44] exposed a cerebral AVM surgically. In 1908, Krause[45] attempted to treat a cerebral AVM by ligating its feeding arteries. In 1928, Cushing and Bailey[46] and Dandy[47] pioneered the systematic clinical study of these lesions. Cushing and Baily,[46] writing about the treatment of these lesions, admonished neurosurgeons: "The surgical history of most of the reported cases shows not only the futility of an operative attack upon one of these angiomas, but the extreme risk of serious cortical damage which is entailed. . . .The lesion, in short, when accidentally exposed by the surgeon, had better be left alone." In 1932, Olivecrona and Riives[48] excised the first cerebral AVM. As Pool and Potts[49] noted, Bergstrand reported the first angiographic diagnosis of AVMs in 1936. In 1948, Schwartz[50] first excised a cerebellar AVM.

Since the early days of contemporary neurosurgery, the philosophy of treating AVMs has changed tremendously. This change reflects advances in microsurgical techniques, diagnostic studies, endovascular therapy, and radiosurgery, as well as a better understanding of the natural history of these lesions. In 1966, McCormick[51] classified cerebral angiomas into five pathologic types: telangiectasia, varix, cavernous angioma, AVM, and venous angioma.

As the natural history of AVMs became clear, the need for an objective assessment to predict the technical difficulties and the risks associated with treatment was recognized. In 1928, Dandy[47] recommended considering certain key factors such as size, location, arterial and venous patterns, and blood flow through the AVM while planning treatment. The various grading schemes introduced since then have included some or all of these factors.[52, 53] Understanding phenomena such as normal perfusion pressure breakthrough has further improved the practical management of cerebral AVMs.[54] Use of microsurgery with adjuncts such as lasers and embolization has made the treatment of cerebral AVMs safer. Multimodality therapy, including surgery, embolization, and radiosurgery, is the currently accepted strategy.

CEREBROVASCULAR ACCIDENTS

The devastating consequences of cerebrovascular accidents (CVAs) were appreciated even before the Biblical era. In Hippocratic writings, the term *apoplexy* was often used to describe patients afflicted with major strokes. In 400 BC, Hippocrates[55] also observed minor transient ischemic attacks, which he described as episodes of tingling and numbness on the same side of the body that precede major stroke. He noticed that patients usually died on the third to fifth day of their illness and that those who stayed alive for 1 week after the stroke usually survived.

Donley[56] reported that Wepfer first mentioned the relationship between cerebral arteries and ischemic symptoms in his book *Treatise de Apoplexia,* published in 1658. As discussed by Clarke,[57] Hunt described the syndrome of contralateral hemiparesis and ipsilateral monocular blindness caused by occlusion of the carotid artery in 1914. Magladery[58] reported that Wilks differentiated traumatic from spontaneous intracerebral hematomas in 1859. Fazio[59] stated that, as early as 1834, Piorry had recommended trepanation for the treatment of intracerebral hemorrhage. In 1888, MacEwan[60] performed the first successful craniotomy for an intracerebral hematoma. Cushing's[61] interest in intracerebral hematoma was stimulated by his observations of intracranial hypertension.

Surgical treatments for brain ischemia varied from carotid endarterectomy to various revascularization procedures. The history of cerebral revascularization procedures merits a detailed review and is discussed later in this chapter. The surgical treatment of hemorrhagic strokes is quite controversial. In 1903, Cushing[61] reported removing an intracerebral hematoma. In 1932, Bagley[62] differentiated deep from superficial intracerebral hematomas and described their surgical significance. In 1933, Penfield[63] detailed the technique for removing intracerebral hematomas. In a landmark study in 1961, McKissock and coworkers[64] compared the medical and surgical treatments for intracerebral hematomas. Their randomized, prospective clinical study failed to find significant differences in the outcomes of surgically treated and medically treated groups. As discussed by Hamilton and Zabramski,[65] three other modern prospective studies (performed by Auer in 1983, Juvela in 1989, and Batjer in 1990) suggest that surgical therapy may benefit lobar hematomas but not deep-seated hematomas. Surgical evacuation of intracerebral hematomas has also been attempted using stereotactic aspiration,[66] neuroendoscopy,[67] and real-time CT-guided aspiration. Further multicenter, randomized, prospective trials are needed to determine the optimal treatment for the many different subgroups of patients with intracerebral hematomas.

ARTERIAL RECONSTRUCTION

C. Miller Fisher[68] demonstrated the close association of cerebral ischemia and extracranial occlusive disease. This soon led to development of carotid endarterectomy by Pickering and Robb[69] in 1953. Endarterectomy over the years has been shown to be a highly effective means of preventing further cerebral ischemic symptoms, and in the landmark clinical study funded by the National Institutes of Health and directed by Henry Barnett,[70] endarterectomy was found to be a highly effective treatment in preventing cerebral infarction.

The vertebrobasilar arterial tree has not been nearly as amenable to surgical repair. Most of these patients have been treated with anticoagulants. Although there have been multiple surgical procedures that have had some degree of success in relieving vertebrobasilar insufficiency, direct vertebral endarterectomy is a surgical challenge and has been successful on numerous occasions. Probably a more effective operation is vertebral-carotid transplantation, in which the vertebral artery is transplanted into the carotid artery.

CEREBRAL REVASCULARIZATION PROCEDURES

In 1942, Kredel[71] made the first surgical attempt to increase collateral circulation to the brain directly by applying a temporalis muscle flap over the convexity of the brain in five stroke patients. In 1950, Henschen[72] used bilateral temporalis muscle flaps in a patient with bilateral carotid occlusion. As described by Carter and coworkers,[73] Goldsmith, Yasargil, and Yonekawa used omental transposition to treat ischemic cortical tissue in dogs in separate experiments in 1970. In 1977, Karasawa and coworkers[74] transposed the temporalis muscle over ischemic cortex to treat moyamoya disease and demonstrated revascularization of cortical branches of the middle cerebral artery (MCA) with the arteries of the muscle flap. In 1980, Spetzler and coworkers[75] described a simple procedure that involved suturing adventitia of a mobilized segment of the superficial temporal artery (STA) to the underlying arachnoid. Soon, Matsushima and colleagues[76] described a similar technique and called it *encephaloduroarteriosynangiosis.* After this procedure, abundant collaterals were evident on angiography.

In 1963, Chou[77] performed the first successful embolectomy of the MCA without the aid of the microscope. In 1965, Pool[49] placed a plastic tube from the STA to the anterior cerebral artery (ACA) to avoid sacrificing the parent vessel while operating on an aneurysm of the ACA. In 1963, Woringer and Kunlin[78] placed a saphenous vein graft between the common carotid (CCA) and supraclinoid internal carotid artery (ICA). The microsurgical vascular anastomosis techniques introduced by Jacobsen and Suarez[79] in 1960 radically changed the approach to revascularization procedures. On June 7, 1967, Donaghy and Yasargil[80] simultaneously completed the first vascular anastomoses of the STA to the MCA in Vermont and Zurich, respectively.

From this point, various microvascular procedures aimed at diverting blood from the external circulation to ischemic brain evolved rapidly. In 1974, Spetzler and Chater[81] introduced anastomosis of the occipital artery to the MCA. In 1979, Nishikawa and coworkers[82] used the middle meningeal artery (MMA) for the same purpose. In 1975, Tew[83] used a saphenous vein graft to anastomose the CCA and supraclinoid ICA. In 1978, Story and associates[84] used a saphenous vein graft to anastomose a cortical branch of the MCA. In 1983, Little and coworkers[85] performed an STA-MCA bypass using a saphenous vein interposition graft. Pool and Potts[49] and Story and colleagues[84] also used synthetic grafts. In 1976, Ausman's group[86] and Khodadad[87] reported a technique for posterior circulation revascularization when they performed an occipital artery–to–posterior inferior cerebellar artery (PICA) bypass. In 1976, Ausman and associates[88] used a radial artery interposition graft in a distal vertebral artery–to–PICA bypass. In 1979, Ausman and colleagues[89] reported a STA–to–superior cerebellar artery (SCA) bypass. In 1982, Sundt and coworkers[90] used a saphenous vein graft in an external carotid artery (ECA)–to–proximal posterior cerebral artery (PCA) bypass.

In 1977, the International Cooperative Extracranial-Intracranial (EC-IC) Bypass Study[91] was initiated as a multicenter, prospective, randomized trial to test the efficacy of EC-IC bypass in preventing subsequent strokes in patients with symptomatic atherosclerotic lesions of the MCA or ICA. This study was organized and conducted by Barnett and colleagues in London, Ontario, and the results were published in 1985. Seventy-one centers randomized 1377 patients. The results of the study, which failed to show a benefit of EC-IC anastomosis in preventing cerebral ischemia, shocked the neurosurgical community. The conclusions of the study were as follows: "... fatal and nonfatal strokes were not prevented by anastomosis of STA to MCA. This negative result held for all patients and all individual subgroups."[91] As a result of this study, governmental and third-party agencies stopped reimbursing EC-IC bypass surgery.

When the results of the study were evaluated critically, however, major concerns about its methodology surfaced. Selective randomization with a large number of asymptomatic patients, poor sample size, differences among surgeons' expertise at different centers, and the lack of assessment of cerebrovascular reserve or collateral circulation before decision making were some of the major flaws of the study. EC-IC bypass procedures are slowly regaining their popularity. The subgroups of patients for whom EC-IC bypass is unequivocally effective include those with giant aneurysms, skull base tumors, moyamoya disease, posterior circulation disease, and special atherosclerotic occlusions with poor collateral blood flow and poor cerebrovascular reserve.

ENDOVASCULAR THERAPY

As techniques for excluding aneurysms from the circulation by direct surgery progressed, less invasive methods for treating these lesions were sought. In 1941, Werner and coworkers[92] used wires and electrothermic coagulation to treat a giant aneurysm of the right ICA. In 1963, Gallagher[93] used a special gun to inject hog hair into an aneurysm to initiate intraluminal thrombosis. In 1964, Mullan and coworkers[94] used electrodes and bioelectric phenomena to cause intraluminal thrombosis. In 1964, Luessenhop and Velasquez[95] used a Silastic sphere to produce intraluminal thrombosis by temporarily occluding the orifice. With a silk attached to it, this sphere was floated up to the neck of the aneurysm through the carotid artery.

In 1974, Mullan[96] published his work on inducing surgical thrombosis in aneurysms and caroticocavernous fistulae using copper and beryllium-copper alloy wires. Of 15 patients treated this way, 12 had satisfactory thrombosis. Alksne and coworkers[97] used iron coils held in place by a stereotactically placed magnet for embolization. In 1973, Serbinenko[98] used a detachable latex balloon to obliterate an aneurysm while maintaining patency of the parent artery. In 1976, Kerber[99] described a balloon microcatheter capable of injecting isobutyl cyanoacrylate. As described by Livingston and colleagues,[100] Debrun, Berenstein, and Fox proposed the endovascular treatment of giant inaccessible aneurysms by balloon occlusion of the parent artery in the 1980s. In 1988, Goto and associates[101] described silicone balloons that could be filled with 2-hydroxyethyl methacrylate (HEMA) and inflated permanently. In the same year, Hilal[102] first used platinum microcoils to occlude an aneurysm. In 1991, Guglielmi and coworkers.[103] introduced a detachable, thrombogenic coil for packing aneurysms.

Endovascular technology is still in its early stages. Large, multicenter, randomized, prospective trials are under way to evaluate the efficacy of endovascular technology for the long-term obliteration of aneurysms.

REFERENCES

1. Galen: Oeuvres anatomiques, physiologiques et medicales de Galien, vol 1. Translated by C Daremberg. Paris, JB Bailliere, 1854, pp 706–786.
2. Willis T: Cerebri Anatome, Cui Accessit Nervorum Descriptio et Usus. London, 1664.
3. Morgagni JB: De sebiuset causis morborumper anatomenin sagatis venetis et topog remondiama, book 1, letter 4. 2VXCVI: 298, 1761.
4. Biumi F: Observationes anatomicae observatio V. In Sandifort: Thesaurus Dissertationum. Lugd Bat, S & J Lightmans, 3:373–379, 1765.
5. Blackhall L: Observation on the Nature and Cure of Dropsies. London, Longman, 1813, p 126.
6. Hutchinson J: Aneurism of the internal carotid within the skull diagnosed eleven years before patient's death: Spontaneous cure. Trans Clin Soc Lond 8:127–131, 1875.
7. Brinton W: Report on cases of cerebral aneurysms. Trans Pathol Soc Lond 3:47–49, 1851.
8. Gull W: Cases of aneurysms of the cerebral vessels. Guy's Hosp Rep (3rd series) 5:281–304, 1859.
9. Charcot JM, Bouchard C: Nouvelles recherches sur la pathogenie de l'hemorrhagie cerebrale achives de physiologie normale et de pathologie. Arch Physiol (Paris) 1:110–127, 1868.
10. Bartholow R: Aneurisms of the arteries at the base of the brain: Their symptomatology, diagnosis and treatment. Am J Med Sci 64:373–386, 1872.
11. Eppinger H: Pathogenesis (histogenesis and hemologie) der Aneurysmen einschliesslich des Aneurysm equiverminosum. Arch Klin Chir 35(Suppl):1–563, 1887.
12. Fearnsides EG: Intracranial aneurysms. Brain 39:224–296, 1916.
13. Turnbull HM: Intracranial aneurysms. Brain 41:50–56, 1918.
14. Quincke H: Die Lumberpunction des Hydrocephalus. Klin Wochenschr 28:929–965, 1891.
15. Moniz E: L'encephalographie arterielle, son importance dans la localisation des tumeurs cerebrales. Rev Neurol 2:72–90, 1927.
16. Moniz E: Aneurisme intra-craien de la carotid interne droit rendu visible par l'arteriographie cerebrale. Rev Otoneuroophthalmol 11:746–748, 1933.
17. Horsley V: Discussion of paper by AH Bennett and RS Godlee. Case of cerebral tumor: The surgical treatment. Br Med J 2: 988–989, 1885.
18. Horsley V: Remarks on ten consecutive cases of operations upon the brain and cranial cavity to illustrate the details and safety of the method employed. Br Med J 1:863–865, 1887.
19. Crutchfield WG: Instruments for use in treatment of certain intracranial vascular lesions. J Neurosurg 16:471, 1959.
20. Logue V: Surgery in spontaneous subarachnoid hemorrhage: Operative treatment of aneurysms on anterior cerebral and anterior communicating artery. Br Med J 1:473, 1956.
21. Dott NM: Intracranial aneurysms. Cerebral arterioradiography: Surgical treatment. Trans Med Chir Soc Edinb 40:219–240, 1933.
22. Dandy WE: Intracranial aneurysms of the internal carotid artery. Ann Surg 107:654–659, 1938.
23. DeLong WB, Ray RL: Metallurgical analysis of aneurysm and microvascular clips. J Neurosurg 48:614–621, 1978.
24. Scoville WB: Miniature torsion bar spring aneurysm clip. J Neurosurg 25:97–104, 1966.
25. Rhoton AL Jr, Merz W: Spring clip for aneurysm surgery. Surg Neurol 19:14–16, 1993.
26. Dutton JEM: Intracranial aneurysms: A new method of surgical treatment. Br Med J 2:585–586, 1956.
27. Selverstone B, Ronis N: Coating and reinforcement of intracranial aneurysm with synthetic resin. Bull Tuffs N Engl Med Centre 4:8–12, 1958.
28. Todd EM, Shelden CH, Crue BL Jr, et al: Plastic jackets for certain intracranial aneurysms. JAMA 179:935–939, 1962.
29. Gillingham FJ: The management of ruptured intracranial aneurysms. Ann R Coll Surg Engl 23:89–117, 1958.
30. Jacobson JH 2nd, Wallman LJ, Schumacher GA, et al: Microsurgery as an aid to middle cerebral artery endarterectomy. J Neurosurg 19:108–115, 1962.
31. Greenwood J Jr: Two point coagulation: New principle and instrument for applying coagulation current in neurosurgery. Ann J Surg 50:267–270, 1940.
32. Lougheed WM, Marshall BM. The place of hypothermia in the treatment of intracranial aneurysms. Prog Neurol Surg 3: 115–148, 1969.
33. Uihlein A, Terry HR Jr, Payne WS, et al: Operation on intracranial aneurysm with induced hypothermia below 15 degrees C and total circulatory arrest. J Neurosurg 19:237–239, 1962.
34. Hounsfield GN: Computerized transverse axial scanning (tomography). 1. Description of system. Br J Radiol 46:1016–1022, 1973.
35. Crummy AB, Strother CM, Sackette JF, et al: Computerized fluoroscopy: Digital subtraction for intravenous angiocardiography and arteriography. AJR Am J Roentgenol 135:1131–1140, 1980.
36. Damadian R: Tumor detection by nuclear magnetic resonance. Science 171:1151–1153, 1971.
37. Drake CG: The treatment of aneurysms of posterior circulation. Clin Neurosurg 26:96–144, 1979.
38. Hunt WE, Hess RM: Surgical risk as related to the time of intervention in the repair of intracranial aneurysms. J Neurosurg 28:14–20, 1968.
39. Ecker A, Riemenschneider PA: Arteriographic demonstration of spasm of the intracranial arteries with special reference to saccular artery aneurysm. J Neurosurg 8:660–667, 1951.
40. Sahs AL, Perett GE, Locksley HB, et al: Intracranial Aneurysms and SAH: A Co-operative Study. Philadelphia, JB Lippincott, 1966.
41. The International Study of Unruptured Aneurysms Investigators: Unruptured intracranial aneurysms—risk of rupture and risks of surgical intervention. N Engl J Med 339:1725–1733, 1998.
42. Pool JL: Treatment of arteriovenous malformations of cerebral hemispheres. J Neurosurg 19:136–141, 1962.
43. Steinheil SO: Ueber einen fall von varix aneurysmaticus im Bereich der Gehirngefaesse. Wurzburg, F Fromme, 1895.
44. Giordano: Compendio di Chirurgia Operatoria Italiana. 2:100, 1897.
45. Krause F: Chirurgie Des Gehirns und Ruckenmarks nach eigenen Erfahrungen. Berlin, Urban & Schwarzenberg, 1908.
46. Cushing H, Bailey P: Tumors Arising From the Blood Vessels of the Brain: Angiomatous Malformations and Hemangioblastomas. Springfield, IL, Charles C Thomas, 1928.
47. Dandy WE: Arteriovenous aneurysm of the brain. Arch Surg 17:190–198, 1928.
48. Olivecrona H, Riives J: Arteriovenous aneurysms of the brain: Their diagnosis and treatment. Arch Neurol Psychiatry 59:567–602, 1948.
49. Pool JL, Potts DG: Aneurysms and Arteriovenous Malformations of the Brain: Diagnosis and Treatment. New York, Harper & Row, 1965, pp 326–373.
50. Schwartz HG: Arterial aneurysm of posterior fossa. J Neurosurg 5:312–317, 1948.
51. McCormick WF: The pathology of vascular ("arteriovenous") malformations. J Neurosurg 24:807–816, 1966.
52. Luessenhop AJ, Gennarelli TA: Anatomical grading of supratentorial arteriovenous malformations for determining operability. Neurosurgery 1:30–35, 1977.
53. Spetzler RF, Martin NA: A proposed grading system for arteriovenous malformations. J Neurosurg 65:476–483, 1986.
54. Spetzler RF, Wilson CB, Weinstein P, et al: Normal perfusion pressure breakthrough theory. Clin Neurosurg 25:651–672, 1978.
55. Hippocrates: The genuine works of Hippocrates. Adams F, trans. London, Sydenham Society 1849, pp 470–482.
56. Donley JE: John James Wepfer, a renaissance student of apoplexy. Bull Johns Hopkins Hosp 20:1–7, 1909.
57. Clarke E: Cerebrovascular system: Historical aspects. In Newton TH, Potts DG (eds): Radiology of Skull and Brain, vol 2, bk 1. Angiography. Great Neck, NY, Mosby, 1974, pp 875–889.

58. Magladery JW: Natural course of cerebrovascular haemorrhage. Clin Neurosurg, 9:106–116, 1963.
59. Fazio C: Clinical pathology of hypertensive intracerebral haemorrhage: Historical aspects. In Mizukami M, Kogure K, Kanaya H, et al (eds): Hypertensive Intracerebral Haemorrhage. New York, Raven Press, 1983, pp 105–113.
60. MacEwan W: An address on the surgery of the brain and the spinal cord. Br Med J 2:302–311, 1888.
61. Cushing H: The blood pressure reaction of acute cerebral compression, illustrated by cases of intracranial hemorrhage. Am J Med Sci 125:1017–1023, 1903.
62. Bagley C Jr: Spontaneous cerebral haemorrhage: Discussion of four types with surgical considerations. Arch Neurol Psychiatry 27:1133–1149, 1932.
63. Penfield W: The operative treatment of spontaneous intracerebral hemorrhage. Can Med Assoc J 28:369–374, 1933.
64. McKissock W, Richardson A, Taylor J: Primary intracerebral hemorrhage: A controlled trial of surgical and conservative treatment in 180 unselected cases. Lancet 2:221–232, 1961.
65. Hamilton MG, Zabramski JM: Intracerebral hematomas. In Carter LP, Spetzler RF, Hamilton MG (eds): Neurovascular Surgery. New York, McGraw-Hill, 1995, pp 477–496.
66. Nizuma H, Shimizu Y, Yonemitsu T, et al: Results of stereotactic aspiration in 175 cases of putaminal haemorrhage. Neurosurgery 24:814–819, 1989.
67. Auer LM, Deinsberger W, Niederkorn K, et al: Endoscopic surgery versus medical treatment for spontaneous intracerebral hematomas: A randomized study. J Neurosurg 70:530–535, 1989.
68. Fisher CM: Occlusion of the internal carotid artery. Arch Neurol Psychiatry 69:346, 1951.
69. Barnett, HJM, Stein BM, Mohr IP, Yatsu FM (eds): Stroke, vol 2. New York, Churchill Livingstone, 1986; p 1003.
70. North American Symptomatic Carotid Endarterectomy Trial Collaborators: Beneficial effect of carotid endarterectomy in symptomatic patients with high-grade carotid stenosis. N Engl J Med 325:445–453, 1991.
71. Kredel FE: Collateral cerebral circulation by muscle graft: Technique of operation with report of three cases. South Surg 11: 234–244, 1942.
72. Henschen C: Operative revascularization des zirkulatorisch geschadigten Gehirns durch Anlegen gestielter Muskellappen. Langenbecks Arch Chir 264:392–401, 1950.
73. Carter LP, Temeltas O, Guthkelch AN: Cerebral revascularization. In Carter LP, Spetzler RF, Hamilton MG (eds): Neurovascular Surgery. New York, McGraw-Hill, 1995, pp 441–456.
74. Karasawa J, Kikuchi H, Furuse S, et al: A surgical treatment of "Moyamoya" disease "encephalo-myosynangiosis." Neurol Med Chir (Tokyo) 17:29–37, 1977.
75. Spetzler RF, Roski RA, Kopaniky DR: Alternative superficial temporal artery to middle cerebral artery revascularization procedure. Neurosurgery 7:484–487, 1980.
76. Matsushima Y, Fukai N, Tanaka K, et al: A new surgical treatment for moya moya disease in children: A preliminary report. Surg Neurol 15:313–317, 1981.
77. Chou SN: Embolectomy of middle cerebral artery: Report of a case. J Neurosurg 20:161–163, 1963.
78. Woringer E, Kunlin J: Anastomosis between the common carotid and the intracranial carotid or the sylvian artery by a graft, using the suspended suture technic. Neurochirurgie 200:181–188, 1963.
79. Jacobsen JH, Suarez EL: Microsurgery in anastomosis of small vessels. Surg Forum 11:243–245, 1960.
80. Donaghy RPM, Yasargil MG: Extra-intracranial blood flow diversion. Paper presented at the meeting of the American Association of Neurological Surgeons, April 11, 1968, Chicago. Abstract 52.
81. Spetzler RF, Chater N: Occipital artery-middle cerebral artery anastomosis for cerebral artery occlusive disease. Surg Neurol 2:235–238, 1974.
82. Nishikawa M, Hashi K, Shiguma M: Middle meningeal–middle cerebral artery anastomosis for cerebral ischemia. Surg Neurol 12:205–208, 1979.
83. Tew JM Jr: Reconstructive intracranial vascular surgery for prevention of stroke. Clin Neurosurg 22:264–280, 1975.
84. Story JL, Brown WE Jr, Eidelberg E, et al: Cerebral revascularization: Common carotid to distal middle cerebral artery bypass. Neurosurgery 2:131–135, 1978.
85. Little JR, Furlan AJ, Bryerton B: Short vein grafts of cerebral revascularization. J Neurosurg 59:384–388, 1983.
86. Diaz FG, Umansky F, Ausman J, et al: Cerebral revascularization: A historical review. In Erickson DL (ed): Revascularization for the Ischemic Brain. Mount Kisco, NY, Futura Publishing, 1988, pp 5–11.
87. Khodadad G: Occipital artery–posterior inferior cerebellar artery anastomosis. Surg Neurol 5:225–227, 1976.
88. Ausman JI, Nicoloff DM, Chou SH: Posterior fossa revascularization: Anastomosis of vertebral artery to PICA with interposed radial artery graft. Surg Neurol 9:281–286, 1978.
89. Ausman JI, Lee MC, Chater N, et al: Superficial temporal artery to superior cerebellar artery anastomosis for distal basilar artery stenosis. Surg Neurol 12:277–282, 1979.
90. Sundt TM Jr, Piepgras DG, Houser OW, et al: Interposition saphenous vein grafts for advanced occlusive disease and large aneurysms in the posterior circulation. J Neurosurg 56:205–215, 1982.
91. International Cooperative Extracranial-Intracranial (EC/IC) Bypass Study Group: Failure of extracranial-intracranial arterial bypass to reduce the risk of ischemic strokes: Result of an international randomized trial. N Engl J Med 313:1191–1200, 1985.
92. Werner SC, Blakemore AH, King BC: Aneurysm of internal carotid artery within skull, wiring and electrothermic coagulation. JAMA 116:578–582, 1941.
93. Gallagher JP: Obliteration of intracranial aneurysm by pilojection. JAMA 183:231–236, 1963.
94. Mullan S, Beckman F, Vailati G, et al: An experimental approach to the problem of cerebral aneurysm. J Neurosurg 21:838–845, 1964.
95. Luessenhop AJ, Velasquez AC: Observations on the tolerance of intracranial arteries to catheterization. J Neurosurg 21:85–91, 1964.
96. Mullan S: Experiences with surgical thrombosis of intracranial berry aneurysms and carotid-cavernous fistulae. J Neurosurg 41:657–670, 1974.
97. Alksne JF, Fingerhut AG, Rand RW: Magnetically controlled focal thrombosis in dogs. J Neurosurg 25:516–525, 1966.
98. Serbinenko FA: Balloon catheterization and occlusion of major cerebral vessels. J Neurosurg 41:125–145, 1974.
99. Kerber C: Balloon catheter with a calibrated leak: A new system for superselective angiography and occlusive catheter therapy. Radiology 120:547–550, 1976.
100. Livingston K, Guterman LR, Gibbons KJ: Endovascular therapy of cerebral aneurysms. In Carter LP, Spetzler RF, Hamilton MG (eds): Neurovascular Surgery. New York, McGraw-Hill, 1995, pp 789–806.
101. Goto K, Halbach VV, Hardin CW, et al: Permanent inflation of detachable balloons with a low viscosity hydrophilic polymerising system. Radiology 169:787–790, 1988.
102. Hilal SK: Synthetic fibre coated platinum coils successfully used for the endovascular treatment of arteriovenous malformations, aneurysms and direct arteriovenous fistulae of the central nervous system [abstract]. Radiology 169(Suppl):28–29, 1988.
103. Guglielmi G, Vinuela F, Sepetka I, et al: Electrothrombosis of saccular aneurysms via endovascular approach. Part 1. Electrochemical basis, technique, and experimental results. J Neurosurg 75:1–7, 1991.

PART II BASIC SCIENCE

CHAPTER 86

Cerebral Blood Flow and Metabolism

VINI G. KHURANA ■ EDUARDO E. BENARROCH ■ ZVONIMIR S. KATUSIC ■ FREDRIC B. MEYER

The average rate of cerebral blood flow (CBF) is approximately 55 mL per 100 g of brain tissue per minute (expressed as 55 mL/100 g/min). Given that the average adult brain weighs between 1400 and 1600 g, representing 2% to 3% of total body weight, it is remarkable that at any one time, this organ receives about one fifth of the cardiac output and consumes a similar proportion of total body oxygen at rest. Even more remarkable is that, despite its enormous metabolic demand, the brain's utilization of energy amounts to a mere 20-watt output![1] Supporting this apparently modest utility, however, are complex biologic machineries responsible for preserving cerebral homeostasis by continually regulating blood flow in the brain while maintaining its tight coupling to cerebral metabolism. In this light, the present chapter is devoted to presenting a contemporary and integrative basic sciences review of CBF and metabolism and is divided into three sections. The first section details fundamental hemodynamic and rheologic concepts related to CBF, the physiology of blood flow regulation in the brain, and the techniques used to assess CBF and metabolism. The second section focuses on important metabolic pathways in the brain and the specific roles of neurons, astrocytes, and the blood-brain barrier (BBB) in cerebral metabolism. The final section describes the basis of flow-metabolism coupling. It should be noted at the outset that the material covered in this chapter serves to highlight the more salient aspects of each area from a neurosurgical perspective and, although comprehensive, is by no means exhaustive. The reader is therefore referred to several important texts and articles related to CBF[1–13] and metabolism[12–19] and to ongoing articles published in journals dedicated specifically to this field.

CEREBRAL BLOOD FLOW

Fundamental Concepts

HEMODYNAMICS

There are several equations that are extremely useful in understanding the principles of CBF. Recall that Ohm's law, pertaining to electrical conduction, defines the following relationship between current flow (I), applied voltage (ΔV; or "voltage difference"), and electrical resistance (R_e) in a system:

$$I = \Delta V/R_e \quad (1)$$

That is, current flow varies directly with the voltage difference but inversely with the system's electrical resistance. As applied to the vasculature, replacing in equation 1 current flow with blood flow (Q), voltage difference with pressure difference (ΔP; i.e., difference in pressure between blood inflow and outflow), and electrical resistance with vascular resistance (R_v), then the equation becomes:

$$Q = \Delta P/R_v \quad (2)$$

Empirically, this equation tells us that blood flow varies directly with blood pressure and inversely with vascular resistance. Analogously, in the brain, CBF varies directly with cerebral perfusion pressure (CPP) and inversely with cerebrovascular resistance (CVR):

$$CBF = CPP/CVR \quad (3)$$

There are several important features of this fundamental equation that are worth mentioning. First, CPP is defined as the difference between mean arterial pressure (MAP) and intracranial pressure (ICP):

$$CPP = MAP - ICP \quad (4)$$

For a given (constant) ICP, therefore, CPP varies directly with MAP. Second, MAP is not simply the average of the systolic (SP) and diastolic (DP) pressures but rather defined as follows:

$$MAP = [1/3 \times (SP - DP)] + DP \quad (5)$$

Third, the single most important site of resistance in

the cerebral vasculature is at the level of the penetrating precapillary arterioles, that is, those vessels derived from pial arteries that arise perpendicular to the conducting arteries on the brain's surface and enter the brain parenchyma. However, up to 50% of the total CVR arises from smaller pial arteries (150 to 200 μm diameter) and arteries of the circle of Willis.[20, 21] Fourth, Virchow's description of a triad of hemodynamic parameters for venous thrombosis, namely, rate of blood flow, status of the vessel wall, and blood coagulability,[22] suggests that there are many "other" factors that affect blood flow, some of which are represented in the Hagen-Poiseuille equation for general hemodynamics:

$$Q = (p \cdot r^4 \cdot \Delta P)/(8 \cdot \eta \cdot L) \quad (6)$$

Here, r refers to the vessel radius, η to blood viscosity, and L to vessel length, the last of which is generally regarded as invariable.[20] From this equation, it is apparent that blood flow varies proportionally with vessel radius and inversely with blood viscosity. Lastly, the situation in the brain is made even more complex by the presence of cerebrovascular autoregulation (discussed in detail later), any arterial stenosis, and the diameter and extent of arterial collaterals.[23] Whereas the main extracranial collateral channels are the carotid and vertebral arteries, the circle of Willis represents the main intracranial site of collateral blood flow. However, in situations where a major cerebral artery is occluded, the leptomeningeal arteries of the cortical surface become an important source of collateral supply.

RHEOLOGY

Unlike water, which is referred to as a newtonian fluid because of its relatively uniform flow through an even tube, blood traveling through a vessel demonstrates "laminar" (nonuniform) flow.[24] This property is imparted by both the presence of formed elements within blood (i.e., cells) and a variably adhesive endoluminal surface (i.e., the vascular endothelium). Together, these result in maximal flow velocity in the centermost axial portion of the stream with the slowest flow velocity in the outermost peripheral lamina directly adjacent to the vessel wall, the latter being subject to the greatest internal friction. For most purposes, the viscosity of blood refers to its consistency or "thickness," which is related to its cellular and protein composition and intravascular frictional drag. Shear *rate* refers to the velocity gradient between the axial and peripheral laminae, varying directly with the overall velocity of blood flow and inversely with the radius of the vessel,[25, 26] whereas shear *stress* can be taken as the mechanical effects of blood flow on the endothelium and also increases with any increment in flow velocity. Notably, viscosity and shear rate are themselves related, as evidenced in the Fahraeus-Lindqvist effect. Here, during high shear rates such as in the microcirculation composed of vessels less than 100 μm in diameter, there is an apparent fall in blood viscosity as aggregates of erythrocytes known as "rouleaux" disperse into individual cells. This property of blood, termed *thixotropy*, is dependent on erythrocyte cytoskeletal flexibility and aggregational tendency in addition to shear rate. Eventually, however, a critical radius is reached, where vessel diameter decreases to less than that of an erythrocyte (6 to 8 μm), resulting in a steep rise in blood viscosity and therefore an inversion phenomenon (i.e., reversal of the Fahraeus-Lindqvist effect).[27, 28] From these observations it is clear that the absolute number and flexibility of erythrocytes and other cells, in addition to their tendency to adhere and aggregate (increased in low velocity states for erythrocytes and proinflammatory conditions for platelets and leukocytes), are major determinants of blood viscosity and that the hematocrit only partially reflects these features. Furthermore, it is apparent that these properties (including hematocrit) are even more critical to blood flow in situations of poor perfusion. In a circulatory bed subject to poor perfusion, such as in focal ischemia, adverse effects of low blood velocity and shear rate are greatly compounded by the presence of high viscosity from raised hematocrit and plasma protein levels,[29] and knowledge of this concept underlies the clinical use of hemodilution techniques as a means of improving perfusion.

FLOW THRESHOLDS

Although the average rate of global CBF is 50 to 55 mL/100 g/min, regionally it is greater for gray than white matter (70 mL/100 g/min versus 20 mL/100 g/min, respectively), an observation that reflects the richer concentration of neuropils and synapses in the former. In general, the rate of global CBF is kept relatively constant through cerebral autoregulation (see later); however, it may vary in situations where the normal limits of autoregulation are breached, such as in profound acute hypotension or hypertension, or in conditions where autoregulation may be impaired, such as cerebral ischemia, traumatic brain injury, or after aneurysmal subarachnoid hemorrhage (SAH). On the other hand, rates of locoregional CBF may vary even under normal physiologic conditions, such as with increased neuronal activity during conscious mental effort or in rapid eye movement (REM) sleep, although they may also vary in pathologic conditions, such as focal epilepsy, migraine, focal ischemia, and with space-occupying lesions.

An important concept with regard to CBF is that of flow thresholds (Table 86–1). Remarkably, clinical evidence of a neurological deficit may not appear until average regional flow has fallen to 50% or below of normal levels (i.e., to 25 to 30 mL/100 g/min). At this threshold, global neurological impairment is noted; below this, the margin between reversible and irreversible ischemic damage becomes narrow.[30] Brain "electrical failure" begins at rates of 16 to 20 mL/100 g/min, whereas cytotoxic edema from failure of ionic pumps, particularly Na^+,K^+-ATPases, develops at 10 to 12 mL/100 g/min. Finally, metabolic failure with gross disturbance of cellular energy homeostasis occurs at rates of less than 10 mL/100 g/min.

TABLE 86–1 ■ **Cerebral Blood Flow (CBF) Thresholds**

ISCHEMIC THRESHOLD	RATE OF CBF (mL/100 g/min)	NEUROLOGIC MANIFESTATION
(Normal)	(50–60)	(No deficit)
First	25–30	Mild-moderate deficit from electrical impairment
Second	16–20	Severe deficit from electrical failure
Third	10–12	Profound deficit from pump failure and cytotoxic edema
Fourth	<10	Impending death from gross metabolic failure

THE MONRO-KELLIE DOCTRINE

In 1783, Alexander Monro proposed that the incompressibility of the cranial vault mandated a relatively constant intracranial blood volume at all times, a notion supported by George Kellie at the turn of the 19th century.[31] However, in the middle of the 19th century, this proposal was challenged by Sir George Burrows, who postulated that any variation in the volume of one of the three principal intracranial contents, namely, brain parenchyma (1200 to 1600 mL), blood (100 to 150 mL), and cerebrospinal fluid (CSF, 100 to 150 mL), was accompanied by a compensatory change in the volume of the other two.[31] In fact, this latter notion forms the basis of the relationship between ICP and cerebral blood volume (CBV).[20] This pressure-volume relationship implies that to maintain a constant ICP in the face of rising CSF volume, blood volume must fall and when this can no longer occur, the brain will herniate caudad. Importantly, as ICP rises there is a fall in CBF (see equations 3 and 4) in association with reduced CBV, most likely from structural compression of the vasculature.

Mechanisms

CEREBRAL BLOOD FLOW REGULATION

The regulation of CBF is a complex, integrated process involving all layers of the blood vessel wall (i.e., endothelium, smooth muscle, and adventitial nerve fibers), in addition to brain parenchymal neurons and glial cells, intracranial blood, CSF, and extracellular/interstitial fluid compartments. An adequate description of cerebrovascular regulation therefore must include endothelial, myogenic, neurogenic, and metabolic mechanisms. At present, there is no single hypothesis that decisively unifies and explains the biomechanics of CBF regulation. Compartmentalization of the cerebrovascular microenvironment[8] into vascular endothelium, smooth muscle cells, perivascular nerves, and extracellular and subarachnoid spaces aids in classifying vasoactive mediators according to their putative sites of action (Table 86–2) but does not shed any light on their mechanisms of action and interaction. Although it is beyond the scope of this chapter to discuss every mediator listed in Table 86–2 (see reviews elsewhere[4, 5, 8–10, 13]), it is of some benefit to consider those mediators of known or emerging primary importance. As measured by its pivotal vascular actions and extensive crosstalk with a variety of other vasoactive systems,[8, 32] it is clear that the nitric oxide (NO) signaling system is a major candidate in this arena, possibly part of a "final common pathway" of vascular modulation. Other important vasomodulators that will be considered are carbon monoxide (CO), eicosanoids (arachidonic acid metabolites), oxygen-derived free radicals, and endothelins. Myogenic, endothelial, and neurogenic aspects of CBF regulation are discussed under cerebral autoregulation, followed by a description of the vasomodulatory effects of arterial O_2 and CO_2. An important group of vasoactive "metabolic factors" associated with neuroglial activity is discussed in the

TABLE 86–2 ■ **Putative Vasoactive Mediators by Cerebrovascular Microcompartment***

Extracellular (Circulating/Humoral)

Adenosine and related compounds (adenosine diphosphate [ADP], adenosine triphosphate [ATP])
Aggregating platelets (releasing serotonin [5-HT], platelet activating factor [PAF], thromboxane [TXA_2])
Cations (Ca^{2+}, H^+, K^+, Mg^{2+})
CO_2 and O_2
Inflammatory cytokines (γ-interferon [IFN-γ], interleukin-1β [IL-1β], lipopolysaccharide [LPS], tumor necrosis factor-α [TNF-α])
Low density lipoprotein (LDL) cholesterol
Oxyhemoglobin
Peptides (angiotensin [AT], bradykinin [BK], natriuretic peptides, vasopressin [VP])
Vascular endothelial growth factor (VEGF)

Vascular Endothelium

Arachidonic acid metabolites (leukotrienes [LTs], prostaglandins [PGs, e.g., PGE_2, PGI_2, $PGF_{2\alpha}$], TXA_2)
Carbon monoxide (CO; from constitutive heme-oxygenase [HO-2])
Cation channels (ATP-sensitive K^+ [K_{ATP}] channels, nonspecific cation channels [NSCCs], voltage-gated Ca^{2+} channels [VGCCs])
Endothelin-1 (ET-1)
Endothelium-derived hyperpolarizing factor (EDHF)
Heat shock protein 90 (Hsp90)
Nitric oxide (NO; from constitutive/endothelial NO synthase [eNOS])
Oxygen-derived free radicals and related species (hydroxyl [OH•] and superoxide [O_2•] radicals, peroxide [H_2O_2], peroxynitrite [$ONOO^-$])

Vascular Smooth Muscle

ATP
Cation channels (K_{ATP} channels, stretch-activated cation channels [SACCs], VGCCs)
CO (from inducible HO [HO-1])
NO (from inducible NOS [iNOS])

Perivascular Nerves

Aminergic (acetylcholine [ACh], dopamine [DA], histamine [H], norepinephrine [NE], 5-HT)
Nitrergic (NO from constitutive/neuronal NOS [nNOS])
Peptidergic (calcitonin gene–related peptide [CGRP], neurokinin A [NKA], neuropeptide Y [NPY], substance P [SP], vasoactive intestinal peptide [VIP])

*Most important mediators in italics (see text for details).

third section of this chapter as part of flow-metabolism coupling.

Nitric Oxide

Endogenous production of oxides of nitrogen by mammals was first suggested by Mitchell and coworkers[33] in 1916. However, it was not until 1987 and 1988 that Furchgott and Zawadzki[34] presented evidence for an endothelium-derived substance required for relaxation of blood vessels. In 1987 and 1988, Furgchott[35] and Ignarro and associates[36] independently proposed that this substance, initially referred to as endothelium-derived relaxing factor (EDRF), was in fact the short-lived, highly diffusible gaseous molecule NO. Although some controversy still exists regarding the precise identity of EDRF, it is now widely accepted that NO or a derivative nitroso compound accounts for the biologic activity of EDRF.[35–43] The importance of the discovery and characterization of NO signaling was formally acknowledged in 1998 by awarding of the Nobel Prize for Medicine and Physiology to Robert Furchgott, Louis Ignarro, and Ferid Murad, the three widely recognized pioneers of NO research.

The NO signal transduction pathway is involved in a wide variety of physiologic functions and contributes to the pathogenesis of numerous diseases. The components of this pathway are detailed in Table 86–3.[2, 8, 44–50] Evidence for the presence of NO signaling in the cerebral vasculature has come from several lines of study. First, using antibodies raised against purified NO synthase (NOS), Bredt and colleagues[51] have shown that this enzyme is, among other sites in the rat brain, localized to the endothelial layer of large cerebral blood vessels and nerve fibers in their adventitia; other groups have detected NOS immunoreactivity in cerebral microvessels.[52, 53] The origin of perivascular "nitrergic" nerve fibers is the pterygopalatine ganglion, referred to as the sphenopalatine ganglion in animals.[54, 55] In vasospastic cerebral arteries, Pluta and associates[56] have observed a loss of nitrergic fibers as measured by a reduction in overall perivascular neuronal NOS (nNOS) immunoreactivity. Interestingly, treatment with endotoxin (bacterial lipopolysaccharide) or proinflammatory cytokines such as interleukin-1β and tumor necrosis factor-α has been shown to induce NOS expression in smooth muscle cells, includ-

TABLE 86–3 ■ **Features of the Nitric Oxide (NO) Signal Transduction Pathway***

COMPONENT	ROLE	MAJOR CHARACTERISTICS
L-Arginine (L-arg)	NOS substrate	Amino acid obtained from diet or endogenous biosynthesis; D-arginine is not a substrate.
Nitric oxide synthase (NOS)	NO biosynthesis	Uses L-arg and O_2 to form NO and L-citrulline; functions as a 260-KDa homodimer; needs many cofactors, including flavins, NADPH, BH_4, and calmodulin; three NOS isoforms exist: eNOS (endothelial), nNOS (neuronal), and iNOS (inducible); former two are Ca^{2+} dependent and synthesize NO transiently; the last is Ca^{2+} independent and produces NO in a sustained manner; NOS may be found constitutively in endothelial cells, neurons, and astrocytes, but its expression is induced (especially by proinflammatory cytokines) in vascular smooth muscle cells and in activated macrophages and neutrophils; endogenous regulation of NOS activity occurs by phosphorylation, fatty acylation, NO autoinhibition, L-arg analogues, heat-shock protein 90 (Hsp90), and transcriptional control by nuclear transcription factor NF-κB.
NO	Second messenger	Labile, diffusible substance; biosynthesis from endothelial cells stimulated by shear-stress/pulsatile flow or G protein–coupled receptor activation (e.g., by neurotransmitters such as ACh and 5-HT and peptides such as BK, ET-1, NK, SP, and VP); pivotal vasoregulatory actions include facilitation of vascular relaxation and prevention of smooth muscle proliferation, platelet and leukocyte adherence, and platelet aggregation; note that the actions of NO are generally cGMP dependent (see below); however, NO can also activate K^+ channels to cause hyperpolarization and relaxation in a cGMP-independent manner.
Guanylate cyclase (GC)	Target enzyme	Present in vascular smooth muscle cells; found in soluble (cytosolic; directly activated by NO) and particulate (membrane associated; activated through peptide receptors) forms; converts guanosine triphosphate (GTP) into cyclic guanosine monophosphate (cGMP).
Cyclic GMP (cGMP)	Second messenger	Synthesized by GC in vascular smooth muscle cells; facilitates vasorelaxation through protein kinase G (PKG)-mediated membrane hyperpolarization via activation of K^+ channels and/or closure of L-type VGCCs; note that PKG also facilitates vasorelaxation through phosphorylation and inactivation of myosin light-chain kinase (MLCK).

*See Table 86–2 and text for additional abbreviations.

ing those found in the cerebral vasculature.[55, 57] Second, several pharmacologic studies using inhibitors of NOS such as L-N^G-monomethyl arginine (L-NMMA) indicate that these agents elicit endothelium-dependent contractions in resting cerebral arteries.[57, 58] Endothelium-independent contractions to L-NMMA have also been observed in these vessels, indicating that the inhibition of nonendothelial sources of NOS (i.e., constitutive in perivascular nerve fibers or induced in vascular smooth muscle) may also be involved.[57, 58] Third, physiologic studies involving transmural electrical nerve stimulation of isolated cerebral arteries have also shown that vasorelaxation produced by this means is abolished by the presence of L-NMMA or hemoglobin and by extracellular Ca^{2+} depletion,[55, 59] findings consistent with the active presence of NOS here. Additionally, recent advances in molecular biology and genetics have facilitated a greater understanding of cerebrovascular NO signaling through the phenotypic study of targeted NOS isoform deletions in otherwise intact animals[56, 60] and the transgenic expression of NOS isoforms in hosts using genetically engineered viral vectors.[61–64] Murine NOS gene knockout models have demonstrated an association between endothelial NOS (eNOS) gene deletion and systemic hypertension and worsened cerebral ischemia; on the other hand, nNOS gene deletion is reported to be neuroprotective in the setting of ischemia, whereas deletion of the inducible isoform (iNOS) appears to be protective against hypotensive shock but impairs incisional wound healing.[2, 6, 56, 60] In vitro and in vivo studies involving recombinant NOS gene transfer to canine cerebral arteries using adenoviral vectors delivered periadventitially have demonstrated augmentation of NO-mediated vasodilatation in intact arteries, reversal of ET-1–induced constriction in endothelium-denuded arteries, and localization of recombinant eNOS in periadventitial fibroblasts.[61–64] Finally, NO-mediated signaling in human cerebral arteries has recently been characterized both structurally using eNOS immunohistochemistry and functionally via isometric force recording (Fig. 86–1).[65] Taken together, these findings unequivocally establish the presence of a NO-mediated signaling system in the cerebral vasculature. However, a key question in NO vascular biology is whether NO plays a role in the maintenance of resting vascular tone in vivo. The consensus is that direct application of NOS inhibitors onto cerebral arteries in vivo results in their constriction, an effect reversed by topical application of the NOS substrate L-arginine.[7, 66–68] In support of this, intravenous administration of NOS inhibitors has been found to reduce resting CBF, an effect not attributable to altered cerebral energy metabolism, because NOS inhibitors do not affect resting cerebral glucose utilization or cerebral oxygen consumption.[7] Furthermore, in vitro studies using isolated, perfused arteries have shown that shear stress facilitates the Ca^{2+}-dependent biosynthesis and release of NO from endothelial cells, a finding analogous to the presence of shear forces associated with pulsatile blood flow in vivo. It should be noted that despite much investigation, the relative contribution of endothelial versus neuronal NOS isoforms to basal NO release is not precisely known; however, more recent work[69] using NOS isoform knockout mice suggests that eNOS may be the predominant isoform involved here. It can therefore be concluded that a NO signaling path-

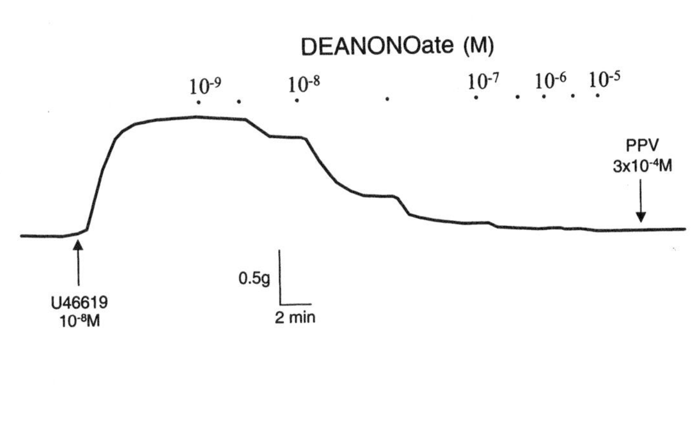

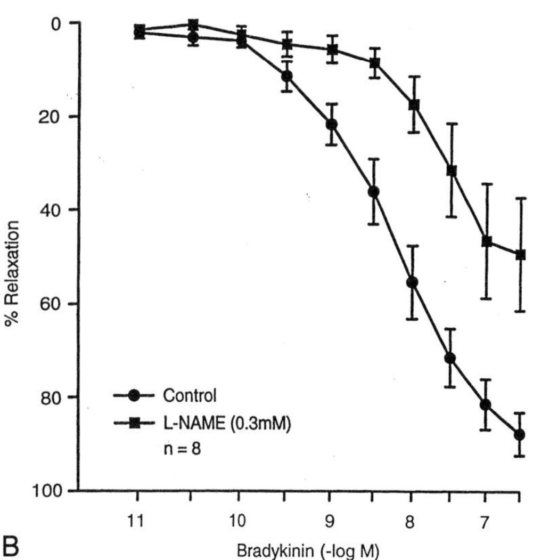

FIGURE 86–1. Functional evidence for human cerebroarterial nitric oxide (NO) signaling. Isometric force recording was carried out in isolated human pial arteries to demonstrate NO-mediated vasoreactivity. *A*, Actual recording from a human pial artery contracted *(upward deflection of trace)* from optimal resting tension with thromboxane analog U46619, and relaxed *(downward deflections of trace)* with progressively increasing concentrations of a NO donor diethylamine NONOate. Note almost complete relaxation compared with maximal relaxation induced by 3×10^{-4} M papaverine (PPV). *B*, Concentration-response curve showing relaxing effect of endogenous peptide bradykinin (control; *filled circles*) in human pial artery. Relaxations to bradykinin are mediated by NO, as evidenced by their significant inhibition in presence of a NO synthase inhibitor, L-nitroarginine methylester (L-NAME; n = 8 patients; $P < .05$; *filled squares*).[65]

way is present in the cerebral vasculature where it participates in the maintenance of basal vascular tone. The predominant isoform appears to be eNOS; however, the level of its contribution may vary between species and even between cerebrovascular territories.[7, 70]

Carbon Monoxide

CO is formed as an endogenous by-product of the metabolism of heme to free (ferric) iron and biliverdin by the enzyme heme oxygenase (HO).[71] Like NOS, HO also has inducible (HO-1) and constitutive (HO-2) isoforms, with expression of the former being inducible by heat shock (which accounts for its alternative name heat shock protein 32 [Hsp32])[3] and the presence of heavy metals, heme, proinflammatory cytokines, and prostanoids.[72] HO-1 is inducible in vascular smooth muscle and glial cells, whereas HO-2 is constitutively found in endothelial and nerve cells. In 1993, Verma and colleagues[73] reported a putative neuromodulatory role for CO after in situ hybridization studies of rat brain in which HO (particularly the constitutive isoform HO-2) was found in discrete neuronal populations throughout the brain. Furthermore, HO messenger RNA has been shown to be colocalized with that of the NO target enzyme guanylate cyclase, suggesting that a substantial portion of this enzyme may in fact serve as a target for CO.[51, 53, 73, 74] In fact, the similarities between NO and CO are striking.[3, 71–75] Both are short-lived, readily diffusible gases that bind to macromolecules containing the heme moiety such as guanylate cyclase and NOS (resulting in activation of the former and inhibition of the latter enzyme) and the blood's oxygen carrier hemoglobin (whereupon oxygen may be displaced, particularly by CO). The generating enzymes for NO and CO, namely, NOS and HO, respectively, have both been localized by immunohistochemistry to endothelial cells, vascular smooth muscle cells, and adventitial nerves of blood vessels. Both NO and CO are known to relax smooth muscle and inhibit platelet aggregation and have been implicated as neurotransmitter substances in the brain. NOS contains a cytochrome P450 reductase domain, and cytochrome P450 reductase is known to be an electron donor to HO.[76, 77] Expression of the inducible isoforms of these enzymes, iNOS and HO-1, is regulated by the nuclear transcription factor NF-κB, and HO may regulate the activity of NOS, not only via the competition between CO and NO for a binding site in their common target enzyme, guanylate cyclase, but also by the fact that NOS is a heme protein and HO is a metabolizer of heme.

The major implication of the aforementioned properties of CO is that this molecule may play an important role, perhaps no less important than NO, in the regulation of cerebral vasomotor tone and blood flow. In support of this is the finding by Zakhary and associates[75] that selective pharmacologic inhibition of HO-2 using tin protoporphyrin-9 (SnPP9) is associated with reversal of NOS inhibitor–insensitive relaxations in porcine pulmonary artery, suggesting that in this vascular bed at least, CO may play a role in the regulation of resting vascular tone. Furthermore, in a recent study by Suzuki and associates,[71] involving HO-1 mRNA quantification in an in vivo rat vasospasm model, a prominent induction of HO-1 mRNA production was found in vasospastic basilar arteries compared with controls. The authors also reported a significant correlation between the level of HO-1 mRNA induction and the lessened degree of vasospasm. These findings suggest that HO-1 plays a protective role in the setting of cerebral vasospasm after SAH. Undoubtedly, future HO knockout studies will help clarify the role of CO in the regulation of CBF under both resting and pathologic conditions.

Eicosanoids

The metabolic products of the membrane-bound fatty acid arachidonic acid are referred to as eicosanoids, and their individual biosynthetic pathways are shown in Figure 86–2. Arachidonic acid, which is not usually available for metabolism, is released from membrane phospholipids by the action of lipases, including phospholipases A_2, C, and D after membrane depolarization, receptor stimulation with second messenger system activation, and in the presence of oxyhemoglobin.[8, 78, 79] The vasomotor activity of cerebral arteries may be affected by arachidonic acid metabolites present locally in endothelial or vascular smooth muscle cells or in aggregating platelets or secreted from more distant cell types. This is an important consideration because endothelial cells tend to favor the release of vasodilatory eicosanoids under normal conditions, whereas aggregating platelets tend to favor release of vasoconstrictors.[78] This variability undoubtedly relates to the relative amounts and activities of arachidonic acid–metabolizing enzymes variably expressed in dif-

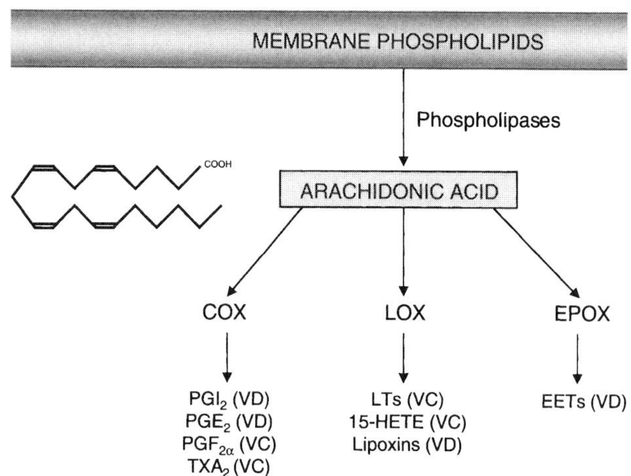

FIGURE 86–2. Metabolic cascades for arachidonic acid. Arachidonic acid is released from membrane phospholipids by the action of lipases and further metabolized by one or more of three enzyme systems, namely, cyclooxygenase (COX), lipoxygenase (LOX), and cytochrome P450 monoxygenases (such as epoxygenase, EPOX). The metabolic products of these cascades, known as eicosanoids, are important modulators of vasomotor reactivity (VC, vasoconstriction; VD, vasodilatation; see text and Table 86–2 for details and abbreviations).

ferent cell types depending on the prevailing cellular conditions.

There are three major enzyme systems that metabolize arachidonic acid, namely cyclooxygenase (COX), lipoxygenase (LOX), and epoxygenase (EPOX, a cytochrome P450 monooxygenase). These metabolic cascades result in the generation of a variety of vasoactive products, whose altering intracellular concentrations may affect the balance between vascular smooth muscle contraction versus relaxation. For example, the COX isoforms (i.e., constitutive COX-1 and inducible COX-2) produce potent vasoconstrictors such as prostaglandin $F_{2\alpha}$ ($PGF_{2\alpha}$) and thromboxane (TXA_2) and vasodilators such as prostaglandin I_2 (PGI_2, prostacyclin) and prostaglandin E_2 (PGE_2). Similarly, the LOX isoforms, 5-LOX and 15-LOX, produce vasoactive mediators such as leukotrienes (vasoconstrictors from 5-LOX), 15-hydroxyeicosatetraenoic acid (15-HETE, a vasoconstrictor from 15-LOX), and lipoxins (vasodilators from 15-LOX). EPOX and its related enzyme P450 ω-hydroxylase also produce a variety of vasoactive metabolites, namely epoxyeicosatrienoic acids (EETs, vasodilators derived from EPOX) and 20-HETE (a vasoconstrictor derived from P450 ω-hydroxylase), although their overall contribution to regulation of the cerebral circulation has not been elucidated.[78] It is likely that the products of arachidonic acid metabolism play a more important role in the regulation of CBF in pathologic rather than physiologic conditions. At present there are no data in support of a clear association between the use of selective COX and LOX inhibitors in vitro or in vivo and any major alteration in basal vasomotor reactivity or CBF, a sharp contrast to findings discussed earlier pertaining to the use of NOS inhibitors in this setting. On the other hand, both cerebral ischemia and aneurysmal SAH are associated with the increased release and metabolism of arachidonic acid and, particularly in aneurysmal SAH, the enhanced production of vasoconstrictive eicosanoids has been implicated in the pathogenesis of cerebral vasospasm.[8, 79, 80]

Oxygen-Derived Free Radicals

Oxygen-derived free radicals are molecular species formed during normal oxidative metabolism and characterized by the presence of an unpaired electron in an outer orbital. This feature renders them highly reactive from a biochemical point of view and, as such, free radicals are known to readily react with and damage cellular macromolecules, such as membrane lipids, nucleic acids, and structural, signaling, and enzymatic proteins. Three major types of free radicals produced in cells are superoxide ($O_2\cdot$), hydroxyl ($OH\cdot$), and NO (sometimes denoted as $NO\cdot$).[49, 72, 81] It should be noted that the endogenous species hydrogen peroxide (H_2O_2) and peroxynitrite ($ONOO^-$, formed from the chemical reaction between NO and $O_2\cdot$) are often referred to as free radicals but are in fact strong oxidants (they are not technically free radicals because neither contains an unpaired electron); they can, however, damage macromolecules by their own oxidizing properties or by decomposing into free radicals (as occurs with the formation of $OH\cdot$ from $ONOO^-$).[72, 81, 82] The major oxidative pathways associated with "physiologic" production of free radicals include normal mitochondrial respiration (see later section on cerebral metabolism), arachidonic acid metabolism by COX and LOX, and oxidative reactions carried out by xanthine oxidase (XO) and NOS (see later).[2, 6, 72] Endogenous free radical sequestration and inactivation are processes carried out by the enzymes superoxide dismutase (SOD), catalase, glutathione peroxidase (coupled to the antioxidant activity of glutathione), and HO (which is associated with the metabolism of the pro-oxidant, hemoglobin, and production of the antioxidant, bilirubin, from biliverdin) and vitamin scavengers such as vitamins C and E and β-carotene. The balance between intracellular production and sequestration/inactivation of free radicals is subject to tight regulation by the aforementioned enzymes under normal physiologic conditions, thereby limiting cellular "oxidative stress" from a relative overabundance of these reactive and potentially damaging species.

There is emerging interest in the role of NOS in the production of free radicals. It is now apparent that this enzyme contributes to the production of free radicals by one of two major mechanisms. The first is by producing NO itself, which has variable redox states, one of which is characteristic of a free radical, that is, associated with a reactive unpaired electron.[49] In this redox form (which happens to be its predominant state), NO may directly damage macromolecules in cells, particularly when it is produced in amounts that exceed endogenous radical scavenging capacity (e.g., via iNOS expressed in invading macrophages and neutrophils in inflammatory conditions or by nNOS in excitotoxic neurodegenerative diseases).[2, 49] Alternatively, NO may combine with other radical species, such as $O_2\cdot$, to form the highly damaging $ONOO^-$ anion.[72, 81, 82] The second mechanism whereby NOS contributes to free radical production is through its de novo synthesis of $O_2\cdot$ in certain settings.[6] In the absence of adequate amounts of its major substrate, L-arginine, or cofactors such as tetrahydrobiopterin (BH_4), NOS is known to act as a superoxide-generating enzyme due to the uncoupling of oxygen reduction and arginine oxidation.[6] The recent use of transgenic mouse models has been helpful in elucidating the role of free radicals in neuronal injury.[83] For example, overexpression of the human isoform of the free radical scavenger copper-zinc-SOD (CuZnSOD or SOD-1) is neuroprotective in the setting of cerebral ischemia,[84, 85] whereas SOD-1 or manganese-SOD (MnSOD or SOD-2) gene deletions in knockout mice have been found to increase the susceptibility of the brain to infarction compared with wild-type (i.e., genetically normal) or "control" mice.[83, 86] Interestingly, cerebral infarction is considerably reduced in nNOS knockout mice, suggesting that NO radicals produced by that isoform contribute to the pathogenesis of this condition.[2, 83] It is clear, therefore, that the relevance of free radical biology to CBF is via their link to NOS activity, which underlies cerebral vasomotor function, and via their role in the pathophysiology of conditions such as cerebral ischemia[87–90] and post-SAH vasospasm.[12, 80, 91–93]

Endothelins

Several groups have alluded to the concept of cerebrovascular tone being the product of a balance between endothelium-dependent relaxing and contracting factors.[94–97] In this context, it seems appropriate to consider the endothelins, a family of peptides that can regulate arterial tone and that have been shown to interact with NO signaling. Three endothelin (ET) isopeptides (ET-1 to ET-3) and two ET receptors (ET_A and ET_B) have been identified.[10, 94] ET_A receptors, found to predominate in vascular smooth muscle cells, are sensitive to ET-1 and ET-2 and mediate contraction, whereas ET_B receptors, which predominate in endothelial cells, are sensitive to all three isoforms and mediate smooth muscle relaxation.[4, 98] Of the three ET isoforms, ET-1 is perhaps the most important in vasoregulation. ET-1 can be produced in cerebral arteries from either circulating "big ET-1" (in humans, a 38–amino acid polypeptide precursor of ET-1, also known as "proendothelin"), which is cleaved to generate ET-1 by ET-converting enzyme (ECE) present in endothelial and vascular smooth muscle cells,[98] or by endogenous expression of ET-1 mRNA in cerebrovascular endothelial cells.[99] In vitro, ET-1 is known to have potent vasoconstrictive effects on human cerebral arteries[65] and a strong growth promoting action on cultured fibroblasts and vascular smooth muscle cells.[10, 100] In the presence of an intact endothelium, ET-1 acts on endothelial ET_B receptors and causes vasodilatation that has been shown to be mediated by NO.[4, 101, 102] However, when the endothelium is removed or disrupted, ET-1 produces profound and long-lasting vasoconstriction, most likely via a direct interaction with vascular smooth muscle ET_A, receptors leading to a phospholipase C–dependent elevation of intracellular Ca^{2+}.[94, 96, 100] In support of these findings, it has been shown that intracisternal injection of ET-1 produces strong constriction of cerebral arteries in vivo; however, cerebral intravascular injection may cause species- and territory-dependent vasoconstriction or vasodilatation.[98, 100]

There is increasing evidence for a functional link between the synthesis and activity of NO and ET-1. In human brain microvascular endothelial cells, ET-1 secretion has been shown to be stimulated by angiotensin II, bradykinin, calcium ionophore A23187, dopamine, norepinephrine, phorbol esters, serotonin, thrombin, and vasopressin.[98] Many of these agents are linked to NO-mediated relaxation, thereby providing circumstantial evidence for a balancing mechanism between ET-1–mediated vasoconstriction and NO-mediated vasodilatation. In an acute setting, endothelium-derived NO has been shown to inhibit the release of ET-1 in porcine aorta, whereas inhibition of NO production has been shown to potentiate the constrictive effect of this agent.[103] This manner of interaction between NO and ET-1 has been demonstrated in a variety of preparations, including human vascular tissue[104] and cultured rat vascular smooth muscle cells.[105] In a chronic setting, Redmond and associates[96] have shown that treatment of quiescent rat vascular smooth muscle cells with NO donors leads to an upregulation of (vasoconstrictive) ET_A receptor expression and an increase in the sensitivity of ET-1 for this receptor, effects mimicked by cyclic guanosine monophosphate but attenuated in the presence of the NOS inhibitor L-nitroarginine methylester (L-NAME). Together, these findings support the notion of physiologic antagonism between ET-1 and NO. Finally, it should be noted that, at present, it is not clear whether ET-1 plays a role in regulating resting cerebrovascular tone. Topical application of ET-1 to cerebral arteries in vivo causes significant vasoconstriction, an effect reversed in the presence of the selective ET_A receptor antagonist BQ-123.[98] However, topical application of ET receptor antagonists alone does not alter the diameter of cerebral vessels in vivo, suggesting that ET does not contribute to the maintenance of basal cerebrovascular tone.[4, 106, 107] Furthermore, because ET-mediated constriction is long lasting, it seems unlikely that ET contributes to the fine temporal regulation of CBF.[98] It is likely that the vasoconstrictive action of ET-1 is considerably augmented in pathologic conditions such as cerebral ischemia and vasospasm, where a defect in NO signaling is known to occur.

CEREBRAL AUTOREGULATION

From a functional perspective, the term *cerebral autoregulation,* first coined by Lassen in the 1950s,[108] refers to the ability of cerebral arteries to maintain CBF (and therefore brain perfusion) at a relatively constant level despite fluctuations in CPP. From a physical perspective, autoregulation involves relatively rapid changes in the caliber of cerebral resistance vessels, principally the precapillary arterioles, in response to changes in transmural pressure as CPP varies.[109] This phenomenon, first reported in feline pial vessels observed through a cranial window by Fog in the 1930s,[110, 111] has undoubtedly evolved to preserve cerebral homeostasis and protect against the development of cerebral ischemia and edema.[112] At the outset, it should be noted that there is often some confusion in use of the terms *cerebral autoregulation* versus *regulation of cerebral blood flow:* the former term refers to a vasomotor phenomenon that occurs *purely in response to changes in CPP* (i.e., akin to "pressure-associated regulation" or "pressure regulation") and may be mediated by a combination of myogenic, endothelial, and neurogenic but *not* metabolic factors; the latter term broadly encompasses a variety of vasomotor regulatory mechanisms of myogenic, endothelial, neurogenic, and metabolic causes and, unlike the former, is by no means limited to CPP-induced changes in vasomotor tone. Therefore, the former term may be thought of as a subset of the latter. In this chapter, the term *autoregulation* refers only to "pressure-regulation" and is described in terms of its myogenic, endothelial, and neurogenic causes. For a description of metabolic regulators of CBF see the later section on CBF-metabolism coupling.

Fundamental Principles

CBF is relatively independent of CPP between the physiologic limits of autoregulation, typically taken to be perfusion pressures of 50 to 60 mm Hg for the lower limit and 150 to 160 mm Hg for the upper (Fig. 86–3). In normal subjects, CPP varies directly with MAP (due to constant ICP), which in turn varies directly with systolic blood pressure. Across the autoregulatory range of approximately 100 mm Hg, to maintain a relatively constant CBF, cerebral arteries constrict as CPP rises and dilate as CPP falls.[113] As a result, CPP and CBV are inversely related by this phenomenon.[20] The limits of autoregulation are by no means invariable. For example, they may be shifted to the right in chronic hypertension (associated with increased sympathetic tone) and in states associated with increased renin release; on the other hand, left shift may be observed in sleep, in "physiologic hypotension" in athletes, in "pathologic hypotension" associated with hemorrhage, and in the presence of angiotensin-converting enzyme (ACE) inhibitors, prolonged hypoxemia, or hypercarbia.[114, 115] Furthermore, autoregulation of CBF may be disturbed in acute, severe hypotension or hypertension and profoundly impaired or even abolished in severe cerebral ischemia or brain injury and after aneurysmal SAH. Below the lower autoregulatory limit, a further decrease in CPP results in a relatively sharp fall in CBF and CBV, whereas above the upper limit, any increase in CPP results in a corresponding increase in these parameters (see Fig. 86–3).[20]

Mechanisms

The precise mechanism of cerebral autoregulation is not known. Proposed mechanisms include intrinsic changes in vascular smooth muscle tone (myogenic hypothesis) and the release of a variety of vasoactive substances from the endothelium (endothelial hypothesis) and periadventitial nerves (neurogenic hypothesis) in response to changes in transmural pressure. A "metabolic" or "humoral" hypothesis has also been proposed to aid in the explanation of cerebral autoregulation but for several reasons is better suited to a description of metabolic regulation of cerebral vasomotor function (see later section on CBF-metabolism coupling) rather than cerebral autoregulation. First, as measured by microdialysis, the extracellular and perivascular concentrations of H^+ and K^+, key mediators in metabolic vasoregulation, normally do not change in response to CPP alterations in the autoregulatory range.[5, 116] Second, as reported in studies measuring changes in cerebroarterial diameter or tone in response to variations in perfusion or transmural pressure, autoregulation begins within a few seconds of the pressure change and is typically complete within 15 to 30 seconds.[12, 116–118] Although not precluding their involvement in this process, this relatively rapid time course suggests that metabolic factors are less likely to be involved. Third, it has been reported that the brain's interstitial concentration of adenosine, another key mediator in the metabolic hypothesis, may be increased at the lower limit of autoregulation[12, 118, 119]; however, despite the possibility of adenosine contributing to autoregulation at this extreme, its concentrations are known not to vary across the bulk of the autoregulatory range. Fourth, the autoregulatory response has been observed in isolated, perfused vessels in vitro (i.e., not subject to alterations in neuroglial metabolism), providing further evidence against a metabolic hypothesis.[12, 120, 121] Taken together, these findings suggest that metabolic factors, despite being capable of strong regulation of cerebral vasomotor function, are unlikely to play a major role in autoregulation.

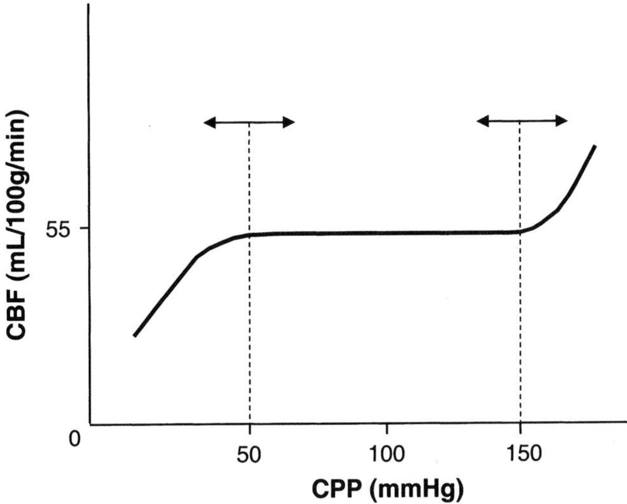

FIGURE 86–3. Classic cerebral autoregulation curve. Cerebral autoregulation maintains a relatively constant rate of cerebral blood flow (CBF) across a wide range of cerebral perfusion pressures (CPP) as shown *(plateau)*. The normal pressure limits of autoregulation *(vertical broken lines)* may be shifted to the left or right in certain conditions *(arrows)* and impaired or abolished in others (see text for details). Note the relatively steep rise and fall in CBF as CPP changes above and below, respectively, the normal limits of autoregulation.

In 1902, Bayliss[122] reported direct contraction and relaxation of canine hind limb arteries in response to increase and decrease, respectively, of intravascular pressure. This phenomenon, referred to as the "Bayliss effect," was attributed to intrinsic properties of vascular smooth muscle cells and formed the basis of the "myogenic hypothesis" of autoregulation. Importantly, contraction occurs in response to an increase in transmural pressure rather than intraluminal pressure alone and, as such, can be thought of as a vascular "stretch response." The single most important piece of evidence supporting the myogenic hypothesis is the presence of stretch-activated cation channels (SACCs) in myocytes. These channels have been shown to be present in a wide variety of cells, including all three types of muscle cells, in addition to epithelial and endothelial cells.[121] Experimentally, SACCs are studied by the patch clamp technique, their minute currents recorded via a cell-attached microelectrode following their gentle suction-induced activation.[123] The characteristic and reproducible pattern of ionic conductance through these channels precludes their currents from being attributable to passive "leak," instead suggesting that they are specific ionic responses to cell stretch. It has been postulated that suction may stress the cytoskeleton, thereby activating SACCs by a relatively rapid but yet undetermined mechanism.[124, 125] In smooth muscle cells, these channels are nonselective and readily permeable to monovalent cations such as Na^+ and K^+ and divalent cations such as Ca^{2+}.[123] SACC activation is associated with an influx of cations, leading to cell membrane depolarization. This, in turn, results in the opening of membrane voltage-gated calcium channels (VGCCs), and the heightened influx of Ca^{2+} into the smooth muscle cell facilitates "calcium-induced calcium release" from the sarcoplasmic reticulum; the end result is smooth muscle contraction. Davis and coworkers[126, 127] have recorded SACC activity in vascular smooth muscle cells and have shown that it is sufficient to cause contraction even in the presence of nifedipine, a dihydropyridine inhibitor of VGCCs, suggesting that the nonspecific Ca^{2+} influx through SACCs is adequate to trigger sarcoplasmic Ca^{2+} release. That the myogenic response is abolished in Ca^{2+}-free media to which Ca^{2+} buffer has been added provides further evidence for the pivotal role of Ca^{2+} in its mediation.[114, 128, 129] However, as suggested by the work of Nelson and colleagues,[130–134] it is likely that the extent of smooth muscle contraction is eventually limited by membrane hyperpolarization after Ca^{2+}-induced activation of Ca^{2+}-dependent K^+ (K_{Ca}) channels.

During the past decade, the role of the endothelium in the regulation of vasomotor function (first reported in 1980 by Furchgott and Zawadzki[34]) has been a relatively intense area of basic vascular research with strong clinical implications. It is clear that the endothelium is by no means a passive and inert barrier between the blood and vascular smooth muscle but rather a critical vasomodulatory "organ" that, in the brain, also serves as an enzymatic and molecular sieve that maintains the patency of the BBB (see later). Substances released by the endothelium include EDRFs, such as NO, PGI_2, and endothelium-derived hyperpolarizing factor (EDHF), and endothelium-derived contracting factors (EDCFs), such as ET-1 and TXA_2. In terms of an "endothelial hypothesis" for cerebral autoregulation, it has been suggested that the endothelium may act as a mechanoreceptor that senses and transduces variations in mechanical factors such as stretch (transmural pressure) and flow velocity (shear stress) into altered vascular tone.[112, 121] Increase in flow rate and shear stress without increase in transmural pressure can induce endothelial vasodilatation,[12] most likely through release of NO.[121] Rubanyi[135] and Katusic and colleagues[136] have shown a similar endothelial dependence of contractions to increased transmural pressure. This is considered to be due to depression of EDRF release and/or increase in EDCF release. Such work supports Harder's[120] observations that in feline middle cerebral arteries exposed in vitro to high transmural pressure, arterial contraction was associated with increased vascular smooth muscle membrane depolarization and action potential generation, effects abrogated by enzymatic de-endothelialization or "denudation." Importantly, patent vascular smooth muscle function was reported even after denudation, as indicated by preserved contractile responses to K^+ and serotonin.[120, 121] Finally, Rubanyi and associates[121] describe an ingenious set of bioassay experiments involving perfused arteries mounted in series where the perfused upstream artery is exposed to changes in transmural pressure and its perfusate subsequently used to perfuse the downstream artery to assess any alterations in the latter vessel's resting tone. The authors report that vasoconstriction in the downstream vessel in response to perfusion with the upstream vessel's perfusate is likely due to the effect of a humoral substance present in the perfusate and that such an effect involves an increase in some EDCF or a decrease in some EDRF. In addition, they note differences in such responses between species (e.g., a reduced release of NO [an EDRF] in canine carotid arteries and increased release of an unidentified EDCF in feline carotid artery).[121, 137]

It is widely accepted that cerebral arteries are subject to complex neurogenic regulation; and before considering the "neurogenic hypothesis" of cerebral autoregulation, it is appropriate to first consider the unique aspects of cerebrovascular innervation. First and foremost, it is important to appreciate that the "perivascular" nerve fibers arborizing throughout the adventitial layer of cerebral arteries have diverse origins and release a wide variety of neurotransmitter substances. The teleologic basis of this diversity may be to provide ultrafine-tuned neurochemical modulation, with the multiplicity and duplicity of neurovascular origins perhaps serving as a protective mechanism in the face of cerebral pathology such as ischemia-infarction, neurodegeneration, or trauma. The sources of cerebrovascular innervation may be either extrinsic (i.e., from remote neurons) or intrinsic (i.e., involving local neurons) and are detailed in Table 86–4. There is a wealth of morphologic and functional evidence supporting an active role for perivascular nerves in the regulation of vascular tone.[138] First, the dense innervation of cerebral arteries and the multitude of neurotransmitters contained in perivascular nerve fibers have been characterized by routine histologic and more advanced immuno/histochemical techniques.[12, 51, 58, 73, 114, 139] Second, the presence of specific receptors for neurochemical transmitters such as biogenic amines and peptides on vascular endothelial and smooth muscle cells has been widely established by both pharmacologic and immunochemical means.[114, 116, 140–142] Third, nerve stimulation studies have demonstrated the functional correlation between electrical stimulation of isolated arteries (even those subject to mechanical de-endothelialization) and altered vasomotor tone.[55, 59] Furthermore, during such studies, the inhibitory effects of specific receptor antagonists suggest that the vasomotor effects of nerve stimulation are mediated by neurotransmitter release from adventitial nerve fibers. Finally, isometric force recording of isolated cerebral arteries exposed to a variety of pharmacologic agents, such as acetylcholine, calcitonin gene-related peptide (CGRP), diethylamine NONOate (a NO donor), norepinephrine, serotonin, and substance P, have provided additional functional evidence for the importance of neurotransmitters in

TABLE 86–4 ■ **Origins of Neurovascular Innervation***

CLASSIFICATION	SUBDIVISION	SOURCE	NEUROTRANSMITTER	VASMOMOTOR EFFECT
"Extrinsic"				
Autonomic ganglionic	Sympathetic	Superior cervical ganglion	ATP	Vasoconstriction
			NPY	Vasoconstriction
			NE	Vasoconstriction (α)
	Parasympathetic	Pterygo/sphenopalatine and otic ganglia	ACh	Vasodilatation
			NO	Vasodilatation
			VIP	Vasodilatation
Nonautonomic ganglionic	Trigeminovascular peptidergic	Gasserian/trigeminal ganglion	CGRP	Vasodilatation
			NKA	Vasodilatation
			SP	Vasodilatation
Nuclear monaminergic	Catecholaminergic	Locus ceruleus, ventrolateral medulla	NE	Vasodilatation (β_2)
	Serotonergic	Raphe nuclei	5-HT	Vasodilatation or Vasoconstriction
"Intrinsic"	Local peptidergic	Adventitial local neurons	NPY	Vasoconstriction
			VIP	Vasodilatation

*See Table 86–2 for abbreviations.

regulating vasomotor function.[48, 58, 116, 140–142] These findings have been confirmed in a recent study of human cerebroarterial vasomotor reactivity.[65] Therefore, it is clear that cerebral arteries are endowed with a rich and active network of nerves that provides an important additional means of vascular regulation. In this light, the "neurogenic hypothesis" of cerebral autoregulation, which states that alterations in transmural pressure trigger changes in neurotransmitter release from perivascular nerve fibers, is likely to be true for the reasons just mentioned. Furthermore, the time course of neurotransmitter release, binding, and action is comparable to the relatively rapid time course of autoregulation. However, the precise signal triggering neurotransmitter release in the setting of increased transmural pressure remains to be determined. Although conjectural, the presence of nonspecific SACCs in perivascular nerve fibers, akin to those found in myocytes, could provide the local Na^+- and Ca^{2+}-mediated depolarization and Ca^{2+} entry required for transmitter release from perivascular nerve terminals. Lastly, a number of studies have reported the preservation of cerebral autoregulation in sympathetically and parasympathetically denervated animals[112, 143]; however, this does not preclude a neurogenic component of autoregulation, because multiple nonautonomic sources of neurochemical transmitters have been described and the network of fibers intrinsic to the vessel wall may contain local neurons still capable of independent neurosecretion.[12]

EFFECTS OF CO_2 AND O_2 ON CEREBRAL BLOOD FLOW

CO_2

The arterial partial pressure of CO_2 ($Paco_2$) exerts profound effects on CBF, particularly across the physiologic range (30 to 50 mm Hg; Fig. 86–4).[144] In mammals of all ages, hypercapnia (increased $Paco_2$) is found to cause cerebral vasodilatation whereas hypocapnia causes the reverse. In fact, inhalation of 5% to 7% CO_2 is associated with an almost exponential increase in CBF of 50% to 100%, rendering CO_2 one of the most potent vasodilatory influences on the cerebral circulation.[144, 145] Although several factors have been proposed to mediate hypercapnic vasodilatation, including H^+ (pH), prostanoids, and NO, it is most likely that the extracellular concentration of H^+ (and not molecular CO_2 itself) is the major determinant.[146, 147] Therefore, the "pH hypothesis" of hypercapnic vasodilatation states that the actions of CO_2 are mediated by the direct effects of H^+ on vascular smooth muscle.[144] The mechanism, however, is an indirect one, involving the chemical transformation of CO_2 to HCO_3^- and H^+ via carbonic anhydrase in astrocytes. When $Paco_2$ increases, molecular CO_2, but not HCO_3^- or H^+, diffuses across the BBB. The perivascular $Paco_2$ rises, and this is chemically coupled via astrocytic metabolism to an increase

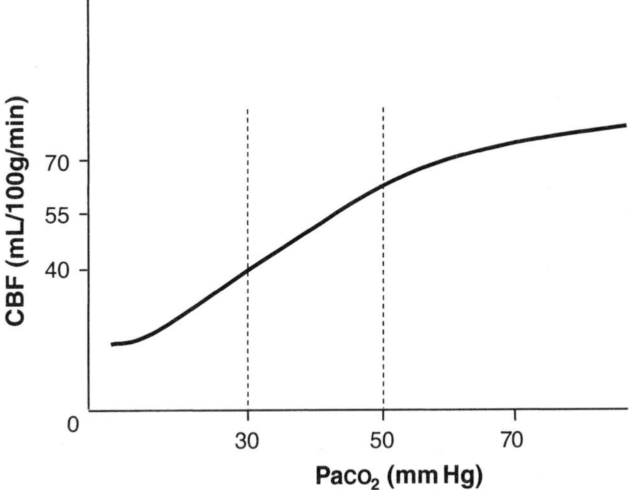

FIGURE 86–4. Effect of arterial partial pressure of CO_2 ($Paco_2$) on cerebral blood flow (CBF). Note that there is a linear relationship between CBF and $Paco_2$ across the physiologic range of $Paco_2$ as marked by the vertical broken lines.

in the extracellular or perivascular concentration of H^+; that is, there is a fall in local pH. This causes vasodilatation. The actual mechanism of vasodilatation may be via H^+-induced opening of adenosine triphosphate (ATP)-sensitive K^+ (K_{ATP}) channels in vascular smooth muscle cells or increased H^+-K^+ exchange favoring H^+ influx driven by an augmented H^+ chemical gradient.[148–152] Regardless, these events are associated with increased K^+ efflux and membrane hyperpolarization, resulting in the closure of VGCCs, reduced cytosolic Ca^{2+}, and facilitation of smooth muscle relaxation. Lastly, it should be noted that numerous experiments have shown attenuation of hypercapnic vasodilatation in the presence of NOS inhibitors, thereby implying a role for NO in mediating this phenomenon.[4, 7, 144, 153] However, this conclusion remains controversial; and, at best, it seems that NO may modulate rather than mediate hypercapnic vasodilatation under certain circumstances, such as moderate ($Paco_2$ of 50 to 60 mm Hg) but not severe ($Paco_2 > 100$ mm Hg) hypercapnia.[4, 7, 144, 154]

O_2

Unlike the situation for $Paco_2$, small fluctuations of Pao_2 above or below the normal physiologic range (60 to 100 mm Hg) do not affect CBF (Fig. 86–5).[115] However, moderately severe hypoxia ($Pao_2 < 50$ mm Hg) is associated with an exponential increase in CBF. This may reflect the vasodilatory effects of increased interstitial adenosine and/or extracellular acidosis and is likely to be related to an increased activity of K_{ATP} channels (see later section on CBF-metabolism coupling), whose opening is triggered by falling local Pao_2 and rising H^+ and adenosine levels, all of which are known to occur in moderate-to-severe hypoxia.[7, 115] Furthermore, it has been proposed that hypoxia-induced stimulation of oxygen-sensing neurons in the rostral ventrolateral medulla may increase CBF through neurogenic vasodilatation, although its precise mechanism remains to be elucidated.[115, 155] Lastly, there is an overall consensus that NO is probably not involved in mild-to-moderate hypoxic vasodilatation, because NOS inhibitors do not attenuate vasodilatation in this setting.[7, 156, 157] However, NO may be involved in severe hypoxia ($Pao_2 < 35$ mm Hg) because the NOS inhibitor L-NAME has been found to attenuate vasodilatation under these circumstances.[7]

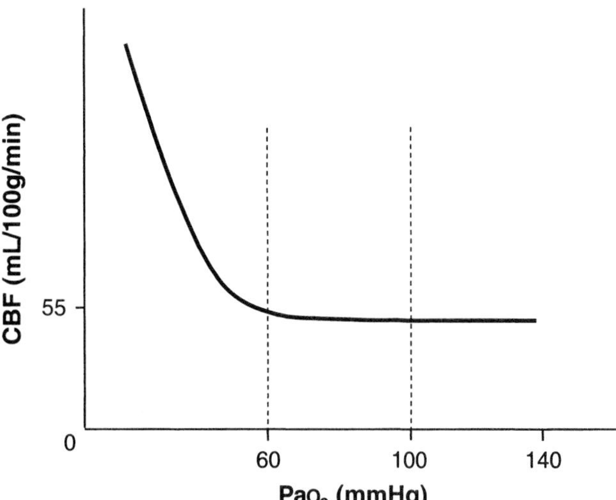

FIGURE 86–5. Effect of arterial partial pressure of O_2 (Pao_2) on cerebral blood flow (CBF). Note that there is a hyperbolic relationship between CBF and Pao_2. However, in the physiologic range of Pao_2 *(vertical broken lines)*, CBF remains relatively constant despite marked changes in Pao_2. Only when Pao_2 falls to levels indicative of marked hypoxia is there a compensatory (and relatively dramatic) increase in CBF.

Measurement

MODERN HISTORICAL DEVELOPMENTS

As applied to the cerebral circulation, the Fick principle states that the quantity of a tracer taken up by the brain per unit time is equal to the quantity entering the brain via arterial blood less the quantity leaving the brain via venous blood. The pioneering work of Kety and Schmidt,[158] which commenced in the 1940s, was founded on this principle and culminated in the first quantitative measurement of CBF in humans by means of jugular venous sampling of the inert, readily diffusible tracer gas nitrous oxide (N_2O).[1] Adding to this, Sokoloff and colleagues in the 1960s provided the first clear demonstration of increased CBF accompanying increased brain activity,[159] confirming the perceptive inference by Roy and Sherrington[160] in the previous century of the close coupling between functional activity, metabolic rate, and blood flow in the brain.[1] Around the same time, Lassen and colleagues, who were the first to apply the principles of capillary-tissue exchange of an inert gas, derived equations for measurement of regional CBF (rCBF) in humans using krypton 85 and later xenon 133.[161] Their techniques were soon adopted for the investigation of neuropsychiatric disorders and became the basis of early cognitive function studies.[1] The seed for the revolution in our understanding of the qualitative and quantitative aspects of rCBF and metabolism was sewn by Sokoloff and associates[162] in 1977 with the introduction of the 2-deoxyglucose (2-DG) technique based on the similar transport but subtly different metabolism of glucose and its competitive analog 2-DG. Here, measurement of radiolabeled 2-DG via standard autoradiographic techniques provided information regarding the brain's metabolism of glucose. Coupled with advances in imaging and computer technology, the considerable potential of this technique was fully exploited with the introduction of positron emission tomography (PET), which currently offers the most advanced and soundest approach to the noninvasive measurement of rCBF and metabolism in humans.[1] Interestingly, the equations developed for autoradiographic measurements of CBF and metabolism in animals[162, 163] provide the basis for PET studies in humans essentially unchanged.[1]

TECHNIQUES

It is clear that the measurement of CBF and metabolism in humans is invaluable for understanding brain function in normal and abnormal states, and in clinical practice it is exceedingly useful from both diagnostic and prognostic perspectives. Associated with a variety of underlying principles and unique sets of advantages, limitations, and clinical indications, there are numerous techniques currently available for the measurement of CBF metabolism, or both (Table 86–5).[1, 12, 23, 164–179] Conventional imaging techniques such as carotid ultrasonography, computed tomography (CT), magnetic resonance imaging/angiography (MRI/A), and cerebral angiography are not included in the table for the reason that in their basic forms these techniques provide useful structural, but no functional, data. Furthermore, some of techniques listed in the table such as autoradiography, bioassay, microspheres, and H_2, He, and thermal clearance are, for all intents and purposes, confined to a laboratory setting using animal models. Others such as optical intrinsic signal imaging and laser-Doppler flowmetry are currently in transit between experimental and clinical use, whereas techniques such as PET, single photon emission computed tomography (SPECT), xenon-enhanced CT (Xe-CT), and transcranial Doppler (TCD) ultrasonography are well established in clinical practice. At present, there is growing interest in the clinical applicability of the variants of MRI, namely, functional MRI (fMRI) and magnetic resonance spectroscopy (MRS), the latter of which may be usefully coupled to conventional MRI in MR spectroscopic imaging, whereas intracarotid xenon 133 and electroencephalography are used intraoperatively with great benefit in cerebrovascular surgery.

CEREBRAL METABOLISM

Fundamental Concepts

DEFINITIONS AND INDICES

Cerebral metabolism is a term used to denote the multitude of biochemical pathways in the brain collectively geared toward enzyme-mediated use of substrate to carry out cellular work. To function optimally, the brain is fueled by a continuous supply of glucose (the principal substrate) and oxygen from the circulation; and therefore, under normal conditions, cerebral metabolism is an aerobic process (i.e., carried out in the presence of oxygen). Aerobic metabolism of glucose enables the efficient execution of "cellular work," which includes the maintenance of ionic gradients; the formation, packaging, release, and uptake of neurotransmitter substances; facilitation of intracellular signaling cascades; and the biosynthesis, transport, and regulated turnover of cell macromolecules. There are several important indices one should bear in mind with regard to cerebral metabolism, all of which have been confirmed by PET and other functional imaging studies.[11, 179] In the adult brain, the global rate of glucose utilization, also known as the cerebral metabolic rate of glucose (CMRGlu), is 25 to 30 μmol/100 g/min, whereas that of oxygen ($CMRO_2$) is 150 to 160 μmol/100 g/min.[12] Notably, a CMRGlu in excess of the adult level is reached within the first few years of life, a finding attributable to relatively rapid brain growth and myelination, with a gradual return to normal adult levels by the end of the second decade.[180] At the average rate of global CBF (55 mL/100 g/min), the oxygen extraction fraction (i.e., the proportion of oxygen extracted by the brain relative to the amount delivered to it in arterial blood) is approximately 0.5 (or 50%), whereas the glucose extraction fraction is about 0.1 (10%).[12] Furthermore, under normal conditions, brain glucose levels vary directly with plasma concentrations, and the CSF/plasma-to-glucose ratio is approximately 2:3. These indices may alter dramatically in pathologic conditions such as ischemia and after SAH.[12, 80, 87–93]

ADENOSINE TRIPHOSPHATE

The critical link between the use of substrate and completion of "cellular work" is the generation of energy from a high-energy chemical intermediate; in the brain, this is ATP. This purine nucleotide is principally synthesized during the final stage of glucose metabolism, namely, oxidative phosphorylation (see later). Another high-energy phosphate, phosphocreatine (PCr), may play a similar role and can act as a potential short-term storage form of ATP through its ability to generate this molecule in a reaction involving adenosine diphosphate (ADP) and catalyzed by creatine kinase[15, 18]:

$$\text{PCr} + \text{ADP} + \text{H}^+ \leftrightarrow \text{ATP} + \text{Creatine} \qquad (7)$$

ATP represents the brain's energy currency, and its major function is to maintain the activity of a critical ionic pump, the ouabain-sensitive, ATP-dependent Na^+,K^+-ATPase. This pump, which maintains the membrane potential in neurons, establishes critical transmembrane fluxes for Na^+ and K^+ and continually utilizes a molecule of ATP each time it pumps (against their respective chemical gradients) two K^+ ions into and three Na^+ ions out of the cell. Cleavage of ATP into ADP by hydrolytic enzymes collectively referred to as ATP hydrolases (or "ATPases" for short) liberates its terminal orthophosphate (P_i) group. Similar hydrolytic degradations can occur for ADP and its metabolic product adenosine monophosphate (AMP). All of these reactions are exergonic (i.e., energy producing); the hydrolysis of ATP is associated with a free-energy ($\Delta G°'$) yield of -7.3 kcal/mol:

$$\text{ATP} + \text{H}_2\text{O} \rightarrow \text{ADP} + \text{P}_i + \text{H}^+ \,[+ \text{Energy}] \qquad (8)$$

The energy derived from this reaction drives the activity of Na^+,K^+-ATPase and other ATP-dependent pumps such as Ca^{2+}-ATPase and H^+-ATPase. Collectively, these pumps have a direct effect on cellular Na^+, K^+, Ca^{2+}, and H^+ fluxes. Indirectly, such gradients, particularly that for Na^+, may drive the activity and direction of other transporters, such as those involved in neurotransmitter reuptake and the Na^+-Ca^{2+} and Na^+-H^+ exchangers (which also contribute to cell Ca^{2+} levels and pH balance, respectively) and control the obligated flow of water, thereby participating in the

TABLE 86–5 ■ **Techniques of Measurement of Cerebral Blood Flow (CBF; l = local, r = regional; g = global) and Metabolism (M)**

TECHNIQUE	FORM	PRINCIPLES	DATA	ADVANTAGES	LIMITATIONS	USES	REFERENCES
Kety-Schmidt	CBF and M	Brain clearance of tracer (inhaled N_2O) estimated from its arteriovenous difference (Fick's principle)	gCBF, gCMRO$_2$, CMRGlu	Multiple measurements, quantitative, CBF and M both measured	No regional measurements, invasive (jugular puncture), anastomotic contamination	First technique used for animal and human CBF and M, laboratory technique only now	1, 164, 165
H_2 clearance	CBF only	Brain clearance of H_2 (generated locally electrochemically or inhaled to brain saturation) detected by probe	lCBF (rCBF if multiple probes used)	Inexpensive, reliable, serial, and quantifiable measurements	Brain penetration, complex analysis, inaccurate at high flows, point measurements	Lab only	164
He clearance	CBF only	Brain clearance of inhaled He detected by probe connected to a mass spectrometer	lCBF (rCBF if multiple probes used)	Multiple and quantifiable measurements, can measure tissue P_{CO_2} and P_{O_2}	Brain penetration, complex analysis, need mass spectrometer, point measurements	Lab only	164
Thermal clearance	CBF only	Thermistor probe measures temperature difference between heating element and brain via thermocouple	lCBF (rCBF if multiple probes used)	Can measure flow continously, inexpensive	Brain penetration, nonquantifiable, point measurements	Lab only	164
Microspheres	CBF only	Based on trapping of 10-μm spherical tracers (radiolabeled and injected into heart) in brain microcirculation	rCBF, gCBF	Quantitative, multiple measurements of CBF and flow in other organs	Invasive (cardiac catheter), poor resolution in smaller animals, mixing varies	Lab only	164
Autoradiography	CBF only	Brain tissue placed on x-ray film after accumulation of radioactive tracer ^{14}C iodoantipyrine injected IV	rCBF	High-resolution, quantifiable CBF measurements in multiple brain regions	Brain extraction required, measures flow at one instant only	Lab only	164, 166
Brain bioassay	M only	Direct biochemical measurement of tissue metabolites after brain extraction and fixation	ATP, PCr, glucose, lactate, etc.	Excellent for measurement of metabolite concentrations in $\geq$1 brain regions	Brain extraction required, autolytic changes may affect results	Lab only	12
Optical intrinsic signal (OIS) imaging	CBF only	Brain's transmission and reflectance of electromagnetic radiation correlate with its structure and chemical activity	rCBF, rCBV	Rapid, repeatable, no direct contact with brain, different tissue components detectable	Invasive (burr hole)	Spatial-functional cortical mapping, mainly lab use	167
Laser Doppler flowmetry	CBF only	Photons from probe laser hit blood cells and scatter, degree of scatter correlated with local perfusion	lCBF (rCBF if multiple probes used)	Easy to use, real-time, high resolution ($1 \times 1 \times 1$ mm^3), no brain penetration	Invasive (burr hole), nonquantifiable, point measurements, technical pitfalls	Can be used intraoperatively for point CBF in cerebrovascular surgery	164, 168

Intracarotid ^{133}Xe	CBF only	External radioactivity detectors used to measure brain washout of ^{133}Xe tracer injected into carotid	rCBF	Simultaneous measurement of CBF in multiple brain regions, quantitative	Invasive, slow, anastomotic artifacts, no or low-flow "look-through" phenomenon	Particularly useful in carotid endarterectomy	164, 169
Electroencephalography (EEG)	CBF only	Records cortical synaptic activity that can be regionally correlated to adequacy of cerebral perfusion	α, β, δ, τ waves	Continuous measurement, relatively sensitive and regionally specific	Nonquantifiable, artifacts from general anesthetic or preoperative EEG abnormalities	Intraoperative adjunct in cerebrovascular surgery	170, 171
Xenon-enhanced computed tomography (Xe-CT)	CBF only	Nonradioactive Xe gas (radiodense) is inhaled, diffuses into brain; CT detects distribution (i.e., perfusion)	rCBF	Rapid, repeatable, quantifiable, noninvasive high resolution ($1 \times 1 \times 5$ mm^3)	Significant radiation, mental status changes, and respiratory depression with Xe	Multiple applications plus measures cerebrovascular reserve (acetazolamide)	167, 172
Transcranial Doppler (TCD) ultrasonography	CBF only	Doppler effect; ultrasonographic measurement of direction and velocity of blood flow in large vessels	Flow velocity, change in CBF	Portable, inexpensive, real-time, noninvasive, bedside or intraoperatively	No quantitative measure of actual CBF, skull may reduce signal, large vessels only	Vasospasm, stenosis, embolism, arteriovenous malformation	23, 173
Functional magnetic resonance imaging (fMRI)	CBF only	Perfusion- or diffusion-weighted imaging modes for tracer (Gd-DTPA) or H_2O/proton tracking, respectively	rCBF, rCBV	Gd-DTPA biosafe, no radiation, diffusion mode is real-time, high resolution	Severe motion artifacts in diffusion-weighted fMRI; special hardware required	Subacute and chronic ischemia	167, 174, 175
Magnetic resonance spectroscopy (MRS)	CBF and M	Based on spectroscopic atomic profile of molecules in brain detected by MR unit using ^{31}P and ^{1}H tracers	ATP, PCr, P, pH, lactate, neuro-transmitters	Can fuse spectroscopic and MRI data sets into image, noninvasive, serial studies	Added scan time, movement artifacts, poor resolution of spectral data	May become imaging of choice for ischemia as technology develops	176
Positron emission tomography (PET)	CBF and M	Photons detected as positron (emitted from decaying radioisotope) collides with electron; many radioisotopes (IV or inhaled) used for measurements of various parameters	rCBF, rCBV, rOEF, $rCMRO_2$, rCMRGlu	Accurate, quantifiable, repeatable, excellent for detection of subtle occult abnormalities; numerous parameters measurable	Local cyclotron needed due to rapid tracer decay, course resolution ($5 \times 5 \times 5$ mm^3), radioactive markers needed, costs, expertise, space	Has provided wealth of information of CBF and M coupling; many uses, including measure of cerebrovascular reserve (acetazolamide)	167, 175, 177
Single photon emission computed tomography (SPECT)	CBF only	IV or inhaled radiopharmaceuticals emit single photon (g) radiation, detected by scanner; tracers include conjugates of ^{133}Xe, ^{123}I, or ^{99m}Tc	rCBF, rCBV	Long $T_{1/2}$ of tracers obviates need for cyclotron (more feasible than PET mainly for this reason)	Less quantifiable and lower resolution ($9 \times 9 \times 9$ mm^3) than PET, no metabolic measures because O, C, H, and N do not emit single photons	CBF and CBV in setting of ischemia or SAH; measures cerebrovascular reserve (acetazolamide)	167, 175, 178

CBF, cerebral blood flow; l, local; r, regional; g, global; M, metabolism; $CMRO_2$, cerebral metabolic rate of oxygen; CMRGlu, cerebral metabolic rate of glutamine; IV, intravenously; ATP, adenosine triphosphate; PCr, plasma creatinine; CBV, cerebral blood volume; Gd-DTPA, gadolinium–diethylenetriamine-penta-acetic acid; $T_{1/2}$, half-life; OEF, oxygen extraction fraction; SAH, subarachnoid hemorrhage; ^{133}Xe, xenon 133; ^{123}I, iodine 133; ^{99m}Tc, technetium 99m.

maintenance of overall cellular ionic and osmotic homeostasis. The overall importance of ATP and related adenine compounds in metabolism is reflected in the concept of "energy charge." Many metabolic reactions are governed by the energy status of the cell, and the energy charge represents one index of cellular energy status. It is represented by the following equation, and it ranges from 0 (all AMP) to 1 (all ATP):

$$\text{Energy charge} = ([\text{ATP}] + 0.5 \times [\text{ADP}])/([\text{ATP}] + [\text{ADP}] + [\text{AMP}]) \quad (9)$$

Normally, the cellular energy charge is 0.85 to 0.90, with higher energy charges usually stimulating ATP-utilizing pathways whereas inhibiting ATP-generating pathways.[18] Finally, it should be noted that the brain has minimal endogenous reserves of substrates such as free glucose and its associated polymer, glycogen, oxygen, and high-energy phosphates (ATP and PCr), with all of these moieties being subject to rapid depletion after interruption of CBF. In this light, it has been shown that brain ATP levels reduce to zero within 7 minutes of cessation of cerebral oxygen supply.[181]

Major Metabolic Pathways

GLUCOSE

Under normal conditions, brain glucose is derived principally from exogenous sources via the diet, albeit subject to hepatic regulation. Unlike oxygen, which passes from the blood to the brain by simple diffusion, plasma glucose is transported across the BBB via facilitated transport involving a single member of the family of glucose transporters (GLUT), namely, GLUT-1. In fact, of the several known GLUT isoforms, only GLUT-1 and GLUT-3 are found in the brain, the former localized to capillary endothelial cells and astrocytes, the latter to neurons.[182, 183] All GLUT isoforms are related structurally through the presence of 12 plasma membrane–spanning α-helical domains and functionally via their ATP independence, stereospecificity, and saturability. Furthermore, their absolute numbers in plasmalemmae are subject to upregulation or downregulation depending on the prevailing cellular conditions.[180] It is clear that astrocytes and neurons represent the two principal targets for glucose transported across the BBB. The former take up glucose via GLUT-1 present in their pericapillary foot processes and store it in the form of glycogen (see later), whereas the latter transport glucose via GLUT-3 and metabolize it principally via an elaborate metabolic pathway that commences with aerobic glycolysis.

Metabolism of Glucose

The complete pathway for the oxidative metabolism of glucose can be divided into four stages: glycolysis, synthesis of acetyl coenzyme A (acetyl CoA), Krebs cycle, and oxidative phosphorylation. At the outset, it should be noted that "glycolysis," "aerobic glycolysis," and "glycolytic pathway" are interchangeable terms used to denote the *first* stage of glucose metabolism, namely, its conversion to pyruvate under normal (aerobic) conditions. Furthermore, although all stages of glucose metabolism are necessarily dependent on the coordinated presence of each enzyme-catalyzed reaction, certain reactions are emphasized for their relative importance (Table 86–6 and Fig. 86–6). Three important aspects of glucose metabolism worthy of separate discussion relate to the concept of metabolic regulation, the net yield of ATP, and the major alternative pathways of glucose metabolism, namely, anerobic glycolysis and the pentose shunt.

The regulation of glucose metabolism represents an important mechanism of coupling energy supply and demand, and each of the four metabolic stages is characterized by the presence of enzymes whose activities are subject to feedback regulation by one or more ionic or molecular species. The occurrence of feedback regulation becomes even more important in pathologic conditions such as cerebral ischemia, where markedly abnormal levels of these species may interfere with the function of this and other metabolic pathways.[87–90] In the first stage of glucose metabolism (i.e., glycolysis; see Fig. 86–6*A*), the major site of regulation is at the level of phosphofructokinase (PFK), an enzyme that catalyzes the ATP-dependent addition of a phosphate group to fructose 6-phosphate early in the pathway. PFK activity can be inhibited by increases in ATP (the fundamental energy product of glucose metabolism), citrate (the first molecule generated in the Krebs cycle), and protons (which participate in numerous reactions in this pathway). Increases in the levels of these species indicate a relatively robust energy supply and therefore exert a negative feedback effect on PFK to dampen further glycolysis until their normal levels are restored. On the other hand, increases in adenosine monophosphate (AMP), cyclic AMP, ADP, K^+, NH_4^+, and P_i may indicate the reverse, thereby stimulating the activity of PFK. In the second stage of glucose metabolism (i.e., synthesis of acetyl CoA; see Fig. 86–6*B*), which is an irreversible process, the pyruvate dehydrogenase (PDH) complex is subject to regulation and is phosphorylated and deactivated by a specific kinase when the following ratios rise: $NADH/NAD^+$ (reduced nicotinamide adenine dinucleotide NADH, is formed in the first three stages of glucose metabolism); acetyl CoA: CoA (acetyl CoA is the entry point into the Krebs cycle); and ATP/ADP (ATP being the energy product of this metabolic pathway). Again, increases in these ratios indicate strong energy supply and exert negative feedback regulation. PDH is stimulated by increasing levels of its substrate pyruvate and by increases in intracellular Ca^{2+} (e.g., from G protein–coupled receptor activation by a variety of hormones). Its activity is also critically dependent on the presence of thiamine. The rate of the Krebs cycle, the third stage of glucose metabolism (see Fig. 86–6*C*), is also adjusted to meet the cell's need for ATP. For example, high ATP levels inhibit the activity of three enzymes in this cycle, namely, citrate synthase, isocitrate dehydrogenase, and α-ketoglutarate dehydrogenase. In oxidative phosphorylation, the fourth and final stage of glucose metabolism (see Fig. 86–6*D*), the most important factor regu-

TABLE 86–6 ■ **Features of Glucose Metabolism**

STAGE	LOCATION	ATP*	MAJOR CHARACTERISTICS
Aerobic glycolysis	Cytosol	2	A series of 10 enzymatic reactions. The substrate is glucose, and the end product is pyruvate; NADH is a by-product here. Regulation of aerobic glycolysis occurs at the early steps catalyzed by hexokinase and phosphofructokinase (PFK) and the late step catalyzed by pyruvate kinase. Of these, the PFK-catalyzed step is the most important regulatory site (see text).
Acetyl coenzyme A (acetyl CoA) synthesis	Mitochondrial matrix	0	A link stage between aerobic glycolysis and the Krebs cycle. Here, irreversible decarboxylation of pyruvate occurs, catalyzed by the pyruvate dehydrogenase (PDH) multienzyme complex. Like PFK, this trienzyme complex is subject to regulation (see text). The end product of PDH-mediated catalysis of pyruvate is acetyl CoA, with NADH formed as a by-product. Acetyl CoA represents the entry point into the Krebs cycle.
Krebs (tricarboxylic or citric acid) cycle	Mitochondrial matrix	2	A series of nine enzymatic reactions. The substrates are acetyl CoA (from stage 2) and oxaloacetate; the end product is also oxaloacetate (hence the term *cycle*) and the by-products are CO_2 and the electron donors NADH and $FADH_2$ (critical for stage 4). Note that the Krebs cycle is central to a number of biosynthetic pathways, providing molecular precursors for protein and lipid synthesis. It also represents the final common pathway for the oxidation of fuel molecules (amino acids, fatty acids, and carbohydrates).
Oxidative phosphorylation (Ox-phos)	Mitochondrial matrix and inner mitochondrial membrane	26	This stage is also known as the "electron transport" or "respiratory" chain. Here, electrons donated by NADH and $FADH_2$ (produced in stages 1–3) are transferred to O_2, producing H_2O, with the resultant release of energy used to drive the formation of ATP. Stage 4 involves four enzyme complexes (complexes I–IV), which are located in the inner mitochondrial membrane and act as electron carriers, and ends with ATP synthesis via ATP synthetase. The flow of electrons between the chain of carriers leads to the pumping of protons out of the mitochondrial matrix, thereby establishing a protonmotive force. This force (actually an electrochemical gradient) is used to drive ATP synthesis.
		Total = 30	

*Net yield of ATP molecules per glucose molecule entering each stage of the overall metabolic pathway for glucose.
ATP, adenosine triphosphate; NADH, reduced form of nicotinamide adenine dinucleotide; $FADH_2$, reduced form of flavin adenine dinucleotide.

lating its overall rate is the level of ADP. As ADP levels rise (reflecting higher consumption or inadequate production of ATP), oxidative phosphorylation is stimulated (i.e., the respiratory chain is activated by a need for ATP synthesis). Taken together, these complex and multiple regulatory mechanisms reflect precise control of glucose metabolism in response to the prevailing cellular conditions. It is likely that the evolution of such tight regulation is due to the need to accurately match energy supply and demand involving a variety of fuel molecules (all of which are oxidized in the Krebs cycle), including carbohydrates, amino acids, and fatty acids.

The net molecular yield of ATP from the aerobic metabolism of glucose is subject to debate.[12, 15, 18, 19, 180] Traditionally, it was thought that under aerobic conditions 36 molecules of ATP were generated from the complete oxidation of one molecule of glucose, and the overall equation was represented as follows:

$$C_6H_{12}O_6 + 6O_2 + 36ADP + 36P_i \rightarrow 6CO_2 + 42H_2O + 36ATP \quad (10)$$

However, owing to the somewhat variable transport processes and chemical reaction stoichiometries involved in the last stage of glucose metabolism (namely, oxidative phosphorylation), this estimate has been revised. Although most estimates for the ATP yield from the complete oxidation of one molecule of glucose range between 30 and 38 molecules of ATP, the revised number is 30 molecules (see Table 86–6).[18]

When the amount of oxygen is limiting (i.e., under cellular conditions associated with hypoxia or ischemia), there is a critical depletion of NAD^+ that is normally generated via reoxidation of its reduced form, NADH, during mitochondrial respiration. As a result, the reaction catalyzed by PDH (see Fig. 86–6*B*; equation 11), part of the second stage of glucose metabolism, can no longer occur effectively, thereby impairing the generation of ATP.

$$\text{Pyruvate} + NAD^+ + \text{CoA} \rightarrow \text{acetyl CoA} + CO_2 + \text{NADH} \quad (11)$$

Under these conditions, the metabolism of pyruvate is carried out by lactate dehydrogenase (LDH), which now produces some of the much needed NAD^+, but at the expense of also producing lactate:

$$\text{Pyruvate} + \text{NADH} + H^+ \leftrightarrow \text{Lactate} + NAD^+ \quad (12)$$

Thus, in anerobic glycolysis, lactate (not pyruvate) is the end product. The only purpose for the reduction of pyruvate to lactate is to regenerate NAD^+ so that

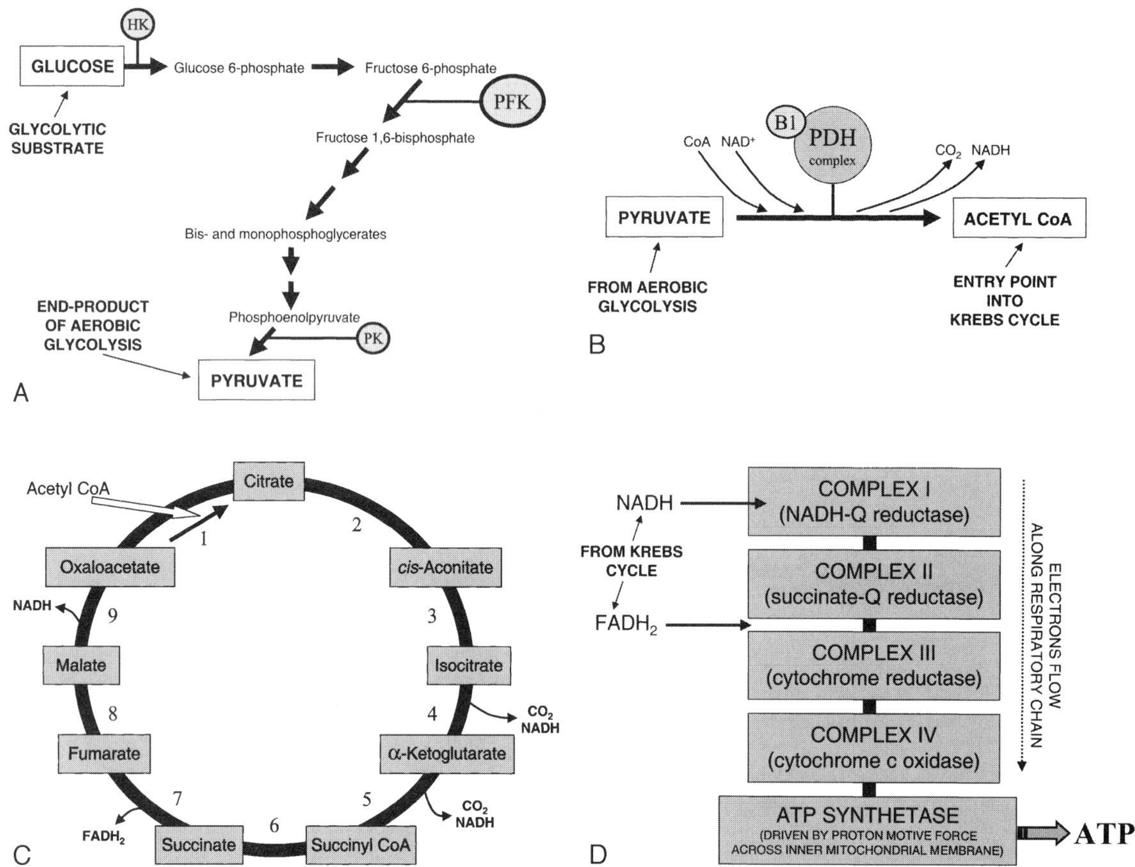

FIGURE 86–6. The four stages of glucose metabolism. *A,* Stage 1, aerobic glycolysis. The main glycolytic regulatory enzymes are hexokinase (HK), pyruvate kinase (PK), and especially phosphofructokinase (PFK). *B,* Stage 2, acetyl coenzyme A (acetyl CoA) synthesis via the thiamine (B_1)–dependent pyruvate dehydrogenase (PDH) multienzyme complex. *C,* Stage 3, Krebs cycle; *D,* Stage 4, oxidative phosphorylation (see text and Table 86–6 for details).

glycolysis can proceed. Lactate, however, is a dead-end metabolic product and is therefore reconverted by LDH (now acting in reverse) into pyruvate, which ultimately feeds into the Krebs cycle. Notably, ATP production from anerobic glycolysis is very inefficient compared with normal aerobic glycolysis, because only two molecules of ATP are generated per molecule of glucose (i.e., at least 15 times less than normal). Furthermore, there is an accumulation of lactate that is associated with potentially severe neurotoxicity from tissue lactic acidosis.[184] Of the total amount of glucose entering the glycolytic pathway under normal conditions, only about 85% actually enters the Krebs cycle for complete oxidative metabolism. Of the remaining 15%, 5% to 10% is converted to lactate as part of the *normal* occurrence of anerobic glycolysis (distinguished from the predominance of this pathway in pathologic conditions marked by true oxygen limitation) whereas a further 5% to 10% is metabolized by another important pathway of glucose metabolism known as the pentose (hexose monophosphate) shunt. Briefly, the main role of this shunt is to divert phosphorylated glucose (i.e., glucose 6-phosphate formed in the first step of glycolysis) into the production of ribose 5-phosphate and reduced nicotinamide adenine dinucleotide phosphate (NADPH):

$$\text{Glucose 6-phosphate} + 2NADP^+ + H_2O \rightarrow \text{ribose 5-phosphate} + 2NADPH + 2H^+ + CO_2 \quad (13)$$

Ribose 5-phosphate, a five-carbon (pentose) sugar, and its derivatives are incorporated into biomolecules such as ATP, CoA, NAD^+, flavin adenine dinucleotide (FAD), RNA, and DNA[18]; therefore, this metabolic shunt is critical for maintaining their synthesis. Furthermore, the production of NADPH is used both for the synthesis of the excitatory neurotransmitter glutamate (which is coupled to the synthesis of the neurotransmitters glutamine and γ-aminobutyric acid [GABA]) and the maintenance of the antioxidant glutathione in its reduced form, thereby preserving an important cellular defense mechanism against free radical-induced injury.

Metabolism of Glycogen

After its facilitated transport into astrocytes via their pericapillary foot processes, glucose is polymerized and stored as glycogen. This process, known as glycogenesis, is catalyzed by the actions of glycogen synthase and a branching enzyme on primed glucose subunits. In the adult brain, glycogen is stored exclusively in astrocytes; however, in neonatal brain, it is also found in neurons. Several important points can be made regarding glycogenolysis, the metabolic breakdown (catabolism) of glycogen. First, in adult brain, this process occurs only in astrocytes and is catalyzed by glycogen phosphorylase. Second, glycogenolysis is tightly and locally regulated (see later). Third, its end product is not glucose but rather lactate. Fourth, lactate must be transferred from astrocytes to neurons for use as an energy substrate. Fifth, although glycogen is an energy reserve even in steady-state conditions, alone it can maintain normal glycolytic flux for only a few minutes.[18, 19, 185–187] Lastly, in conditions of increased cerebral energy demand, glycogen is rapidly mobilized in astrocytes, with known stimulators of glycogenolysis including the neurotransmitters norepinephrine, vasoactive intestinal peptide, histamine, and serotonin and certain metabolic by-products of neuronal activity such as K^+ and adenosine.

Glycogenolysis is highly regulated by the actions of protein kinase (phosphorylation) and phosphatase (dephosphorylation) enzymes on glycogen phosphorylase and glycogen synthase. For example, the binding of the neurotransmitter norepinephrine to its adrenergic G protein–coupled receptor leads to the activation of adenylate cyclase, which increases the level of cyclic AMP. This second messenger activates a cyclic AMP–dependent protein kinase (protein kinase A [PKA]), which phosphorylates an enzyme called phosphorylase kinase. This enzyme, in turn, phosphorylates glycogen phosphorylase, thereby activating it to breakdown glycogen.[19, 185–187] Notably, PKA simultaneously phosphorylates glycogen synthase to *in*activate it; that is, PKA inhibits glycogenesis while facilitating glycogenolysis. Furthermore, phosphorylase kinase can also be activated by rising intracellular Ca^{2+} levels and is therefore subject to activation by hormones whose actions are coupled to Ca^{2+} modulation.

KETONE BODIES

Recall that pyruvate, the end product of aerobic glycolysis, is converted to acetyl CoA by the PDH complex and that acetyl CoA combines with oxaloacetate to form citrate in the first reaction of the Krebs cycle (see Fig. 86–6*A* to C). During prolonged hypoglycemia, the brain's ability to generate pyruvate becomes impaired from failure of glycolysis whereas peripheral sources of pyruvate and oxaloacetate are used by the liver for gluconeogenesis (this process occurs only minimally in the brain and typically involves the generation of glucose from noncarbohydrate precursors). Under these conditions, the body catabolizes adipose tissue, resulting in increased fatty acid oxidation and the generation of acetyl CoA. This is transported to the liver where it is metabolically diverted toward the generation of ketone bodies, principally acetoacetate and D-3-hydroxybutyrate.[18] After their release from the liver, these molecules are transported in the plasma and can cross the BBB. In the brain, they are metabolized to regenerate acetyl CoA, which can then enter the citric acid cycle for subsequent oxidative metabolism as described earlier. Interestingly, the rate of transport of ketone bodies across the BBB is the limiting step in terms of their cerebral metabolism. Under normal conditions, plasma ketone body levels are low and they contribute negligibly to brain metabolism. Within 24 hours of starvation, however, their plasma concentrations and contribution to cerebral metabolism have been shown to rapidly rise alongside their transport across the BBB.[18, 187, 188] Notably, the oxidation of ketone bodies in the brain represents one of the few energy-generating processes capable of replacing aerobic metabolism of glucose in a relatively effective manner.[189] In fact, during hypoglycemia, oxidation of ketone bodies may provide up to 75% of the total cerebral energy supply,[18, 190] although this metabolic pathway cannot maintain or restore optimal cerebral function in the absence of glucose.

GLUTAMATE AND RELATED COMPOUNDS

Glutamate is the major excitatory neurotransmitter and most abundant amino acid in the brain. Through its multiple biochemical interactions, it is involved in a variety of important functions in the brain (Fig. 86–7). Both astrocytes and neurons participate in the uptake of glutamate; however, it preferentially accumulates in the former.[191] Its synthesis can occur through several different pathways, including one catalyzed by glutamate dehydrogenase involving ammonia and α-ketoglutarate, a Krebs cycle intermediate, and by using NADPH as the reductant:

$$NH_4^+ + \alpha\text{-ketoglutarate} + \text{NADPH} + H^+ \leftrightarrow \text{Glutamate} + \text{NADP}^+ + H_2O \quad (14)$$

In a reaction driven by the hydrolysis of ATP, glutamate can be converted to the neurotransmitter glutamine by amidation catalyzed by glutamine synthetase, an enzyme found in astrocytes but not brain neurons:

$$\text{Glutamate} + NH_4^+ + \text{ATP} \rightarrow \text{Glutamine} + \text{ADP} + P_i + H^+ \quad (15)$$

Notably, glutamate can also be formed from glutamine through either the reductive amination of α-ketoglutarate by glutamate synthase or the hydrolysis of glutamine by glutaminase present in brain neurons. Furthermore, glutamate can be metabolized by glutamic acid decarboxylase to GABA, the major inhibitory neurotransmitter of the brain, and is both a precursor of several intermediaries of the Krebs cycle and a constituent of glutathione and an important enzymatic cofactor, folic acid. Additionally, cultured astrocytes have been shown to use glutamate as an energy substrate even in the presence of glucose.[192] Therefore, the metabolism of glutamate is associated with several important functions, including ammonia metabolism, protein and fatty acid biosynthesis, antioxidant-medi-

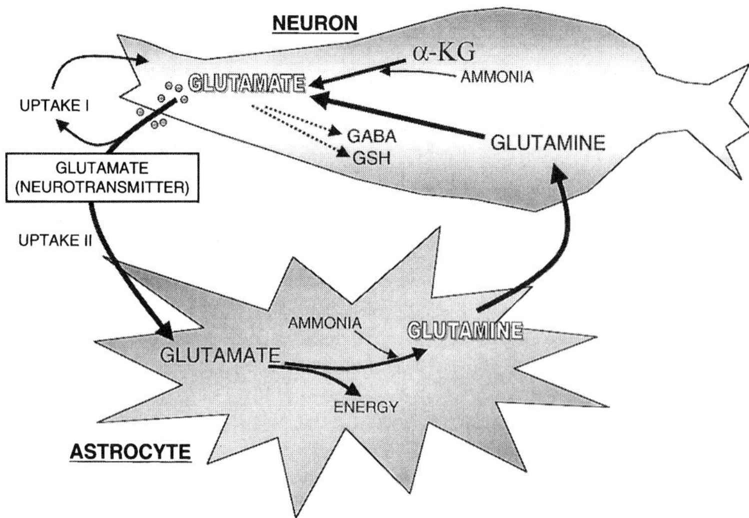

FIGURE 86–7. Functions of glutamate in the brain. Glutamate, synthesized from recycled astrocytic glutamine or neuronal α-ketoglutarate (α-KG), undergoes neuroglial uptake and participates in the glutamine/glutamate cycle between neurons and astrocytes. It is involved in normal excitatory neurotransmission (and therefore ionic homeostasis and the pathogenesis of excitotoxicity), ammonia metabolism, the biosynthesis of proteins, fatty acids, and glutathione (GSH, an antioxidant), astrocytic energy metabolism, and the synthesis and actions of neurotransmitters such as glutamine and γ-aminobutyric acid (GABA).

ated cytoprotection, astrocytic energy metabolism, and neurotransmitter biosynthesis and actions.

Metabolic Contributions of Brain Structural Elements

NEURONS

Neurons contribute to cerebral metabolism in three major ways. First, they are sites of energy (ATP) generation, including, under normal conditions, complete glucose oxidation and, during hypoglycemia, ketone body metabolism (see earlier). Second, they are major sources of ATP utilization principally for maintenance of the vast numbers of Na^+,K^+-ATPase pumps located in neuropil and axonal membranes. In addition to the pumping of ions, ATP is associated with numerous critical processes in neurons, including molecular motor-mediated axonal transport, protein chaperoning by means of heat shock proteins, macromolecule biosynthesis, purinergic (ATP- and adenosine-mediated) neurotransmission, and modulation of K_{ATP} channels (see later). Lastly, metabolic by-products from neurons are responsible for the tight coupling between brain metabolism and blood flow. Changes in local levels of ions such as H^+ and K^+ and molecules such as adenosine occur during neuronal activity, and the role of each of these in flow-metabolism coupling is elaborated later.

ASTROCYTES

Key to understanding the contribution of astrocytes to cerebral metabolism is the fact that astrocytes and neurons form two separate but highly interactive networks. This interaction occurs through the narrow extracellular space (ECS) and involves the flux of ionic and molecular metabolites and neurotransmitters between the two networks. Neuronal activity produces two important signals for astrocytes, namely, increase in extracellular K^+ concentration and release of neurotransmitters such as glutamate, which can act on astrocytic (in additional to neuronal) receptors. These signals depolarize astrocytic membranes and have three major consequences. First, K^+ accumulates and distributes within and between astrocytes. After its entry into astrocytes by both active and passive means, K^+ can flow across gap junctions, which are ion-permeable physical contacts linking the membranes of adjacent astrocytes. The phenomenon of K^+ flowing along a network of astrocytes is known as "K^+ spatial buffering" and is important to neurons because excessive accumulation of K^+ in the ECS after neuronal activity could potentially influence neuronal membrane polarity and neurotransmitter release, glucose metabolism, and CBF. Second, alkalinization of astrocytes occurs after the removal of H^+ from these cells. The extrusion of H^+, formed from metabolism of local CO_2 by astrocytic carbonic anhydrase, occurs through activation of an outward-directed lactate-H^+ cotransporter during astrocytic depolarization. This results in an "alkaline shift," corresponding to acidification of the ECS, and may be a negative feedback signal for neuronal activity because extracellular acidification is known to reduce the magnitude of depolarizing currents associated with activation of glutamate receptors.[193] Third, the influx of Ca^{2+} through astrocytic VGCCs activated by membrane depolarization is followed by its propagation as a "Ca^{2+} wave" across gap junctions. Again, Ca^{2+} is a pivotal intracellular signal and influences a host of cellular activities, including many related to metabolism. Taken together, it is clear that an increase in neuronal depolarization is coupled to an increase in astrocytic depolarization, which in turn influences local metabolic and electrical activity through K^+, H^+, and Ca^{2+} ions. However, there are three other major ways in which astrocytes influence neuronal function and energy metabolism: first, through the glutamate-glutamine cycle between neurons and astrocytes[194]; second, through lactate shuttling from astrocytes to neurons after astrocytic glycogenolysis[139]; and third, through regulating the development and maintenance of the BBB.[195]

Unlike neurons, astrocytes synthesize glutamine and related compounds such as glutathione from any neuronally derived glutamate that they sequester through "uptake II" (where "uptake I" refers to neuronal reuptake of secreted neurotransmitter). Glutamine, which is synthesized in astrocytes by glutamine synthetase (see equation 15), can subsequently be released by these cells into the ECS, where it is taken up by neurons and converted by a P_i-stimulated glutaminase to glutamate in the synaptic terminal. Interestingly, neuronal depolarization, through an increase in P_i derived from the hydrolysis of ATP, stimulates the glutaminase pathway, thereby making more glutamate available for release. It is clear that astrocytic uptake of glutamate is important for limiting the action of this excitatory neurotransmitter through decreasing its presence in the synaptic cleft, and the transfer of glutamine (rather than glutamate) across the ECS from astrocytes to neurons has the advantage of being an electrically "inert" (i.e., non-neuroexcitatory) process.[194] The occurrence of lactate shuttling highlights another important way in which metabolism in astrocytes differs from neurons. Glucose taken up into the astrocyte may have one of two primary fates: (1) it may be converted to lactate by means of astrocytic glycolysis, or (2) it may be converted by means of glycogenesis into the glucose storage polymer glycogen. In adult neurons, aerobic glycolysis results in the formation of pyruvate, not lactate, and glycogen metabolism and storage do not occur except in some large brainstem neurons. Lactate produced by astrocytes during glycogenolysis is secreted into the ECS through the H^+-lactate cotransporter and shuttles across to neurons where it is taken up and mainly converted to pyruvate via lactate dehydrogenase, with subsequent metabolism through the Krebs cycle and oxidative-phosphorylation. Notably, the use of lactate as a fuel under normal, aerobic conditions is only about half as effective in terms of energy production (i.e., the molecular yield of ATP) compared with aerobic glucose metabolism.[139] It should also be noted that glutamate stimulates the uptake of glucose by astrocytes in addition to their production and release of lactate.[139] Finally, the influence exerted by astrocytes on the BBB (which plays an important role in cerebral metabolism [see later]) is highlighted in two important ways: (1) contact of the astrocyte foot processes with endothelial cells of the BBB induces the formation of tight junctions in the latter, mainly by inducing the production of occludin, an integral protein of tight junctions, and (2) astrocytes also induce the expression of γ-glutamyltransferase (γ-GT) and GLUT-1 in, and regulate amino acid transport across, the BBB.[195, 196]

BLOOD-BRAIN BARRIER

The BBB facilitates cerebral homeostasis by isolating brain cells from variations in body fluid composition, thereby providing a stable environment for neural-neural and neural-glial interactions. It is in fact a "barrier" both structurally and functionally. Its structural component consists of an inner cellular layer formed by unfenestrated capillary endothelial cells connected by means of relatively impermeable tight junctions and an outer cellular layer formed by pericytes and the pericapillary foot processes of astrocytes. Its functional aspects represent its important contribution to cerebral metabolism, principally by two means. First, it acts as an ionic and molecular sieve through its involvement in ion and water exchange and selective transport of small molecules and certain proteins.[197] Second, it contains a battery of enzymes that act to protect the brain from circulating neurochemicals and toxins. Lipid-soluble substances such as CO_2, O_2, ethanol, nicotine, lipophilic pharmaceuticals, and volatile anesthetics, and very small polar molecules with a radius of less than 0.8 nm, diffuse readily across the BBB.[195] There is no specific transport mechanism for these substances, although their diffusion depends on their concentration gradients, any binding protein interactions, and the rate of CBF. Ions, on the other hand, are transported by active means.[197] For example, Na^+ exchange is known to occur through a primary active means, the Na^+,K^+-ATPase, as well as a secondary active means, the Na^+ transporter. Furthermore, the transport of ions (particularly Na^+) may be coupled to the obligatory flow of water via osmotic forces, and both the luminal Na^+ transporter and the antiluminal Na^+,K^+-ATPase are implicated in the secretion of extracellular fluid by brain capillaries. In general, larger polar molecules are excluded by the BBB, except for a select group of metabolically important molecules such as glucose, amino acids, monocarboxylic acids such as lactate and ketone bodies, and neurotransmitter precursors such as adenosine, arginine, and choline.[195] All of these molecules are critical to CBF and metabolism, and their entry into the brain is dependent on specific transport mechanisms.[197] For example, glucose and neutral amino acids are transferred by carriers such as GLUT-1 and the L–amino acid transporter, respectively. Interestingly, in conditions associated with hypoglycemia, the transport of lactate and ketone bodies into the brain is increased,[19, 180, 198, 199] demonstrating the ability of the BBB to be regulated through its adaptive response to an altering metabolic environment. Certain proteins such as insulin, transferrin, and insulin-like growth factor are taken up by a saturable receptor-mediated transcytosis mechanism involving vesicle formation at the luminal membrane, whereas others, particularly polycationic proteins, may cross the BBB through a nonspecific, non–receptor-mediated process referred to as absorptive transcytosis. It should be noted that capillary endothelial cells are also known to express the multidrug resistance transporter "P-glycoprotein," which actively pumps out toxic molecules or drugs that may have diffused into endothelial cells from the blood.[195] Finally, endothelial cells of the BBB are enriched with a battery of enzymes that also play a key role in preserving cerebral homeostasis. For example, amino acid decarboxylase, monoamine oxidase (MAO), pseudocholinesterase, GABA transaminase, aminopeptidases, alkaline phosphatase, and γ-GT are all present in brain capillaries.[12] Such enzymatic trapping mechanisms prevent the unrestricted entry of neurotransmitters, their precursors, and potential toxins into the brain.[195]

CEREBRAL BLOOD FLOW–METABOLISM COUPLING

Beginning with the early observations made by Roy and Sherrington over a century ago,[160] it is now well established through PET and other imaging techniques that increased cerebral functional activity is accompanied by rapid and regionally specific increases in oxygen utilization, glucose uptake and metabolism, and blood flow.[179, 200] In this light, there are two forms of coupling that must be recognized. The first is the coupling between neuronal activity and metabolism (which can be referred to as *excitation-metabolism* coupling), the critical mediator being Ca^{2+}. Briefly, during action potential generation and propagation, axonal membrane depolarization is associated with increased activity of Na^+,K^+-ATPase pumps, which act to remove excess intracellular Na^+ associated with the action potential. The massive influx of Na^+ into the cytoplasm during neuronal excitation reverses the direction of ion exchange carried out by the membrane Na^+-Ca^{2+} exchanger, whose activity and direction are dependent on ionic gradients such as that for Na^+. Under these circumstances, Na^+ is extruded in exchange for Ca^{2+} and the entering Ca^{2+} is the key signal for activation of intracellular metabolic pathways. This mechanism therefore provides a means of faithfully transducing the axon firing frequency into a proportional metabolic signal. The second form of coupling is that between neuronal metabolism and locoregional blood flow. This involves the tight matching of blood flow to oxygen and glucose demand in the brain and is referred to as *flow-metabolism* coupling. The mechanism underlying flow-metabolism coupling is complex; however, its principal mediators are metabolic, namely, chemical agents associated with electrical and biochemical activity of neurons. These chemical agents, which primarily include K^+, H^+ (related to local pH, lactate, and CO_2 levels), and adenosine, may affect vascular smooth muscle tone directly or indirectly through altered neurovascular transmission. The critical roles played by astrocytes, perivascular nerve fibers, NO, and K_{ATP} channels in CBF-metabolism coupling are discussed later, as is the involvement of Ca^{2+} (Table 86–7).

Chemical Mediators

POTASSIUM IONS

K^+ is released from neurons during physiologic neuronal activation and in large amounts during seizures, hypoxia, and ischemia.[201] Excessive extracellular K^+ accumulation is prevented by its uptake into local astrocytes (see K^+ spatial buffering, earlier), followed by its shunting toward their perivascular foot processes, where release into the ECS occurs.[12, 202] The vasomotor effects of astrocytic K^+ shunting and perivascular release have been shown by computer simulations of K^+ dynamics in the brain to be more rapid and effective than simple diffusion of K^+ through the ECS, particularly when the site of K^+ increase is remote from the vessel wall.[12, 202] In the range of 2 to 10 mM,[12] elevation of K^+ in the perivascular microenvironment leads to hyperpolarization of the vascular smooth muscle cell membrane via activation of the Na^+,K^+-ATPase and inwardly rectifying K^+ channels (which lead to K^+ efflux). This facilitates smooth muscle relaxation and vasodilatation through closure of VGCCs and decreased cytosolic Ca^{2+} levels. Above a perivascular concentration of 10 mM, K^+ is a vasoconstrictor, because excessive accumulation of this cation leads to

TABLE 86–7 ■ **Mediators of Cerebral Blood Flow–Metabolism Coupling**

MEDIATOR	ROLE
Cellular	
Neurons	Increased neuronal excitation and metabolism raises local CO_2 and extracellular K^+, H^+, and adenosine levels
Astrocytes	Buffer extracellular K^+, H^+, and Ca^{2+} levels; release vasoactive K^+ via perivascular foot processes
Perivascular nerves	May rapidly affect vascular tone via peptidergic, nitrergic, and/or aminergic neurotransmitter release in response to metabolic changes
Ionic	
K^+	From neuronal metabolism; extracellular [K^+] between 2 to 10 mM causes vasodilatation; >10 mM causes vasoconstriction
H^+ (pH)	From neuronal and astrocytic metabolism; decreasing extracellular pH (increasing H^+) leads to vasodilation
Ca^{2+}	Important intracellular signal secondarily associated with K^+ fluxes; decreasing extracellular or increasing intraendothelial Ca^{2+} causes vasodilatation; increasing cytosolic Ca^{2+} in vascular smooth muscle leads to vasoconstriction
Osmolarity	Increasing extracellular osmolarity causes vasodilatation; hypotonic cerebrospinal fluid facilitates vasoconstriction
Molecular	
Adenosine	From cellular metabolism; causes concentration-dependent vasodilatation
Adenosine triphosphate (ATP)	Critical cellular energy currency and neurotransmitter; increasing intracellular ATP leads to vasodilatation
K_{ATP} channels	K_{ATP} channels openers lead to vasodilatation (see text for details)
Nitric oxide (NO)	Vasodilator; may modulate K^+- and H^+-induced vasodilatation

K_{ATP}, adenosine triphosphate–sensitive K^+ channels.

depolarization of vascular smooth muscle from a massive chemical gradient not compensated for by cellular transport mechanisms.

HYDROGEN IONS

As described earlier, the well-known vasodilatory action of CO_2 is mediated mainly through the action of H^+ on cerebral arteries.[146] Active, healthy cells in addition to energetically compromised cells can lead to the production and extracellular accumulation of H^+. Acidification of the ECS, that is, lowering of extracellular pH from the local accumulation of H^+, leads to vasodilatation and reduced neuronal excitability. The origins of H^+ ions include local CO_2 production from oxidative metabolism of glucose in neurons (followed by CO_2 metabolism in and H^+ extrusion from astrocytes) and production of the metabolic intermediate, lactate. The precise mechanism of H^+-induced vasodilatation is not known but may involve K_{ATP} channel activation (see later) or facilitation of NO release, or both, because NOS inhibitors have been found to attenuate the vasodilatation elicited both by moderate hypercapnia and by topical application of acidic CSF.[4, 7, 50, 203]

ADENOSINE

Adenosine is a purine nucleoside whose physiologic activities in the brain include modulation of neuronal and synaptic activity and regulation of CBF.[204, 205] Based on microdialysis measurements in freely moving, unanesthetized animals, the best estimate of the free concentration of adenosine in the brain is 50 to 300 nM.[206] The level of adenosine increases sharply and relatively rapidly in the ECS during increased physiologic neuronal activity and with seizures, hypoxia, and ischemia. Intracellularly, the breakdown of AMP, a product derived from ATP and ADP hydrolysis during increased neuronal "work," and the metabolism of *S*-adenosyl homocysteine and other molecules lead to adenosine formation followed by its transport outside the cell by means of a nucleoside transporter.[204] Additionally, adenosine may be formed extracellularly from ectoenzyme-mediated catabolism of ATP acting as a neurotransmitter. Following its binding to *N*-methyl-D-aspartate (NMDA) receptors, the excitatory neurotransmitter glutamate can also elicit the release of adenosine. At cell surfaces, adenosine can act through two classes of P_1 (purinergic) receptors, A_1 and A_2.[204, 206] A_1 receptors are present on neurons and coupled to $G_{i/o}$ proteins, which reduce intracellular Ca^{2+} entry and accumulation and increase K^+ efflux through the effects of negative modulation of adenylate cyclase on Ca^{2+} and K^+ channel conductances. These receptors are therefore inhibitory, binding adenosine presynaptically (as negative feedback "autoreceptors") to decrease the release of glutamate and other neurotransmitters[207]; postsynaptically, A_1 receptors also lead to decreased neuronal excitability.[204] A_2 receptors, on the other hand, are present in both vascular smooth muscle and endothelial cells of cerebral blood vessels and are coupled to G_s proteins, which elicit cyclic AMP–mediated vasodilatation through stimulation of adenylate cyclase. Notably, the extracellular accumulation of adenosine reflects the level of neuronal functional and metabolic activity and can lead to local vasodilatation, and suppression of neurotransmitter release and neuronal excitability (equitable to a reduction of brain energy demand). The effects of adenosine-stimulated opening of K_{ATP} channels are described below. Together, these events are considered neuronally "protective," and therefore adenosine has been implicated not only as a mediator of flow-metabolism coupling but also as a neuroprotective agent in the setting of ischemia.[87–90, 148, 208]

Astrocytes and Perivascular Nerves

Astrocytes are particularly well suited to play an important role in CBF-metabolism coupling. Not only do they outnumber neurons by at least a factor of 2, but certain specialized processes from these cells also surround virtually all brain capillaries whereas others sheathe the neuronal synapses.[139] Their most important roles in coupling are manifest by their ability to spatially buffer K^+ levels (associated with K^+ shunting and release from perivascular foot processes) and metabolize locally produced CO_2, leading to acidification of the ECS. In general, these events occur in response to increased neuronal activity and under physiologic conditions lead to local vasodilatation. The rich endowment of blood vessels with plexuses of fibers that can rapidly and focally secrete aminergic, peptidergic, and nitrergic neurotransmitters suggests that perivascular nerves, too, may play an important role in coupling metabolism and flow; however, direct evidence is still lacking.[12, 139, 209]

K_{ATP} Channels and Calcium Fluxes

K_{ATP} channels are a subfamily of inward-rectifying K^+ channels found, among other sites, in vascular smooth muscle cells and neurons. They have been implicated in a wide variety of phenomena, including cardioprotection and neuroprotection, insulin secretion, modulation of vascular tone, neuronal excitability and neurotransmission, and mediation of excitation-metabolism and flow-metabolism coupling.[148–152] These channels are in fact 950-kd heterotetramers in which each of the four subunits is a sulfonylurea receptor bound to an inwardly rectifying K^+ channel (K_{IR}). The two most critical features of these channels from a coupling perspective are that their activity is modulated by a wide variety of metabolic signals and that their function directly impacts on VGCC activity (and therefore cytosolic Ca^{2+} levels). In terms of their modulation, K_{ATP} channels are closed by increasing intracellular levels of ATP (therefore termed *ATP-sensitive*) and in the presence of sulfonylurea drugs such as glibenclamide. Under normal physiologic conditions, where ATP is abundant, these channels are maintained in a closed state. However, they may be opened by nucleoside diphosphates such as ADP; G protein–coupled hormones such as adenosine, acetylcholine, CGRP, and catecholamines;

increasing intracellular levels of lactate and H^+; and drugs collectively known as "K^+ channel openers," such as pinacidil and aprikalim. When open, K^+ efflux occurs through these channels, a process that leads to membrane hyperpolarization and closure of VGCCs. For example, as intracellular ATP levels fall (such as during metabolic stress from starvation or hypoxia/ischemia), K_{ATP} channels open, leading to hyperpolarization and reduced cytosolic Ca^{2+}. It is clear that the functional consequences of their opening are decreased neuronal excitability and neurotransmitter release and increased vascular smooth muscle relaxation (and vasodilatation), events that are considered "neuroprotective." The activity of K_{ATP} channels has been shown to be associated with glibenclamide-sensitive relaxation of cerebral arteries in vitro and cerebrovascular dilatation in vivo,[210] although they do not appear to contribute to resting tone of cerebral blood vessels in vivo.[4]

Nitric Oxide

Although its role in flow-metabolism coupling remains controversial, NO has been implicated as a modulator of K^+ and Ca^{2+} conductances and as a mediator or modulator of the vasodilatory actions of increased extracellular H^+ and K^+, increased intraneuronal and intraendothelial Ca^{2+}, and moderate hypercapnia and severe hypoxia. NO is also known to be released from neurons after glutamate receptor activation and from perivascular nerve fibers after trigeminovascular nerve activation.[4, 7, 8, 50, 139, 211] NOS inhibitors such as 7-nitroindazole, which is selective for nNOS in vivo, have been shown in animal models to inhibit increases in CBF induced by neuronal activity and NMDA application, whereas studies in NOS knockout mice have provided evidence of a role for nNOS but not eNOS in flow-metabolism coupling.[4, 69, 212]

FUTURE DIRECTIONS

From a basic sciences perspective, the field of molecular biology currently holds the greatest promise for precisely elucidating the complex and integrated mechanisms underlying human biology, including blood flow and metabolism in the brain. In recent years, there has been prolific development and use of specific gene deletion (knockout) and insertion (recombinant transgenic) technologies that, along with the refinement of polymerase chain reaction and complementary DNA cloning techniques, have shed much needed light on the molecular basis of human physiology and pathophysiology. The field of NO signaling represents a prototype for the applicability and utility of molecular biological techniques, where NOS isoform cloning, specific gene deletions, and recombinant gene transfer have all been successfully carried out. Notably, such developments have been greatly complemented by advancements in histologic techniques, such as immunoelectron microscopy, ultrastructural protein analysis via x-ray crystallography, and biochemical methodologies such as tandem mass spectroscopy and its numerous variants. Further, the Human Genome Project is essentially complete, signifying the elucidation of the entire human genome. In this regard, the use of hand-held gene microarrays will undoubtedly become a standard means of rapid genetic screening while the possibility of correcting for genetic and other specific cellular defects through therapeutic recombinant gene transfer (or gene therapy) is progressively becoming a realistic treatment option. For neurosurgeons, therefore, a good working knowledge of the basic sciences is essential for both the continued advancement of neuroscience and the evolution of neurosurgical procedures and techniques.

REFERENCES

1. Kety SS: The circulation, metabolism, and functional activity of the human brain. Neurochem Res 16:1073–1078, 1991.
2. Hobbs AJ, Higgs A, Moncada S: Inhibition of nitric oxide synthase as a potential therapeutic agent. Annu Rev Pharmacol Toxicol 39:191–220, 1999.
3. Maines MD: The heme oxygenase system: A regulator of second messenger gases. Annu Rev Pharmacol Toxicol 37:517–554, 1997.
4. Brian JE Jr, Faraci FM, Heistad DD: Recent insights into the regulation of cerebral circulation. Clin Exp Pharmacol Physiol 23:449–457, 1996.
5. Wahl M, Schilling L: Regulation of cerebral blood flow—a brief review. Acta Neurochir 59:3–10, 1993.
6. Chen AFY, O'Brien T, Katusic ZS: Transfer and expression of recombinant nitric oxide synthase genes in the cardiovascular system. Trends Pharmacol Sci 19:276–286, 1998.
7. Iadecola C, Pelligrino DA, Moskowitz MA, Lassen NA: Nitric oxide synthase inhibition and cerebrovascular regulation. J Cereb Blood Flow Metab 14:175–192, 1994.
8. Khurana VG, Besser M: Pathophysiological basis of cerebral vasospasm following aneurysmal subarachnoid haemorrhage. J Clin Neurosci 4:122–131, 1997.
9. Shepherd JT, Katusic ZS: Endothelium-derived vasoactive factors: I. Endothelium-dependent relaxation. Hypertension 18: III76–III85, 1991.
10. Katusic ZS, Shepherd JT: Endothelium-derived vasoactive factors: II. Endothelium-dependent contraction. Hypertension 18: III86–III92, 1991.
11. Meyer FB (ed): Neurosurgery Clinics of North America: Cerebral Blood Flow, vol 7. Philadelphia, WB Saunders, 1996, pp 571–796.
12. Edvinsson L, Mackenzie ET, McCulloch J: Cerebral Blood Flow and Metabolism. New York, Raven Press, 1993, pp 1–683.
13. Welch KMA, Caplan LR, Reis DJ, et al (eds): Primer on Cerebrovascular Diseases. San Diego, Academic Press, 1997, pp 1–823.
14. Ginsberg MD: Local metabolic responses to cerebral ischemia. Cerebrovasc Brain Metab Rev 2:58–93, 1990.
15. Erecinska M, Silver IA: ATP and brain function. J Cereb Blood Flow Metab 9:2–19, 1989.
16. Siesjo BK, Bengtsson F: Calcium fluxes, calcium antagonists, and calcium-related pathology in brain ischemia, hypoglycemia, and spreading depression: A unifying hypothesis. J Cereb Blood Flow Metab 9:127–140, 1989.
17. Paschen W, Doutheil J: Disturbances of the functioning of endoplasmic reticulum: A key mechanism underlying neuronal cell injury. J Cereb Blood Flow Metab 19:1–18, 1999.
18. Stryer L: Biochemistry. New York, WH Freeman, 1995, pp 1–1064.
19. Siesjo BK: Brain Energy Metabolism. New York, John Wiley & Sons, 1978, pp 1–607.
20. Hurn PD, Traystman RJ: Overview of cerebrovascular hemodynamics. In Welch KMA, Caplan LR, Reis DJ, et al (eds): Primer on Cerebrovascular Diseases. San Diego, Academic Press, 1997, pp 42–44.
21. Tuor UI, Farrar JK: Contribution of the inflow arteries to alterations in total cerebrovascular resistance in the rabbit. Eur J Physiol 403:283–288, 1985.

22. Goldstone J: Veins and lymphatics. In Way LW (ed): Current Surgical Diagnosis and Treatment. Norwalk, CT, Appleton & Lange, 1994, pp 783–809.
23. Daffertshofer M, Hennerici M: Cerebrovascular regulation and vasoneural coupling. J Clin Ultrasound 23:125–138, 1995.
24. Owen CA Jr, Bowie EJW: Hematologic considerations in cerebrovascular surgery. In Fein JM, Flamm ES (eds): Cerebrovascular Surgery. New York, Springer-Verlag, 1985, pp 89–116.
25. Kee DB Jr, Wood JH: Influence of blood rheology on cerebral circulation. In Wood JH (ed): Cerebral Blood Flow: Physiologic and Clinical Aspects. New York, McGraw-Hill, 1987, pp 173–185.
26. Miller JD, Bell BA: Cerebral blood flow variations with perfusion pressure and metabolism. In Wood JH (ed): Cerebral Blood Flow: Physiologic and Clinical Aspects. New York, McGraw-Hill, 1987, pp 119–130.
27. Chien S: Shear dependence of effective cell volume as a determinant of blood viscosity. Science 168:977–978, 1970.
28. Davis AJ, Jafar JJ: Hemorheology of cerebral blood flow and ischemia. In Awad IA (ed): Cerebrovascular Occlusive Disease and Brain Ischemia. Park Ridge, IL, American Association of Neurological Surgeons, 1992, pp 25–58.
29. Wood JH, Kee DB: Clinical rheology of stroke and hemodilution. In Barnett HJM, Mohr JP, Stein BM, Yatsu FM (eds): Stroke: Pathophysiology, Diagnosis, and Management. New York, Churchill Livingstone, 1986, pp 97–108.
30. Naritomi H, Sasaki M, Kanashiro M, et al: Flow thresholds for cerebral energy disturbance and Na^+ pump failure as studied by in vivo ^{31}P and ^{23}Na nuclear magnetic resonance spectroscopy. J Cereb Blood Flow Metab 8:16–23, 1988.
31. Bell BA: Early study of cerebral circulation and measurement of cerebral blood flow. In Wood JH (ed): Cerebral Blood Flow: Physiologic and Clinical Aspects. New York, McGraw-Hill, 1987, pp 3–16.
32. Khurana G, Bennett MR: Nitric oxide and arachidonic acid modulation of calcium currents in postganglionic neurones of avian cultured ciliary ganglia. Br J Pharmacol 109:480–485, 1993.
33. Mitchell HH, Shonle HA, Grindley HS: The origin of nitrate in the urine. J Biol Chem 24:461, 1916.
34. Furchgott RF, Zawadzki JV: The obligatory role of endothelial cells in the relaxation of arterial smooth muscle by acetylcholine. Nature 288:373–376, 1980.
35. Furchgott RF: Studies on relaxation of rabbit aorta by sodium nitrite: The basis for the proposal that the acid-activatable inhibitory factor from retractor penis is organic nitrite and the endothelium-derived relaxing factor is nitric oxide. In Vanhoutte PM (ed): Vasodilatation: Vascular Smooth Muscle, Peptides and Endothelium. New York, Raven Press, 1988, pp 401–414.
36. Ignarro LJ, Buga GM, Wood KS, et al: Endothelium-derived relaxing factor produced and released from artery and vein is nitric oxide. Proc Natl Acad Sci U S A 84:9265–9269, 1987.
37. Palmer RMJ, Ferrige AG, Moncada S: Nitric oxide release accounts for the biological activity of endothelium-derived relaxing factor. Nature 327:524–526, 1987.
38. Marin J, Sanchez-Ferrer CF: Role of endothelium-formed nitric oxide on vascular responses. Gen Pharmacol 21:575–587, 1990.
39. Furchgott RF: The discovery of endothelium-derived relaxing factor and its importance in the identification of nitric oxide. JAMA 276:1186–1188, 1996.
40. Moncada S, Palmer RMJ, Higgs EA: Nitric oxide: Physiology, pathophysiology, and pharmacology. Pharmacol Rev 43:109–142, 1991.
41. Ignarro LJ, Lippton H, Edwards JC, et al: Mechanism of vascular smooth muscle relaxation by organic nitrates, nitrites, nitroprusside and nitric oxide: Evidence for the involvement of S-nitrosothiols as active intermediates. J Pharmacol Exp Ther 218:739–749, 1981.
42. Yamamoto S, Nishizawa S, Yokoyama T, et al: Subarachnoid hemorrhage impairs cerebral blood flow response to nitric oxide but not to cyclic GMP in large cerebral arteries. Brain Res 757:1–9, 1997.
43. Meyer B, Pfeiffer S, Schrammel A, et al: A new pathway of nitric oxide/cyclic GMP signaling involving S-nitrosoglutathione. J Biol Chem 273:3264–3270, 1998.
44. Szabo C: Physiological and pathophysiological roles of nitric oxide in the central nervous system. Brain Res Bull 41:131–141, 1996.
45. Garcia-Cardena G, Fan R, Shah V, et al: Dynamic activation of endothelial nitric oxide synthase by Hsp90. Nature 392:821–824, 1998.
46. Khurana VG, Shah V, Sessa WC, et al: Role of heat-shock protein 90 (Hsp90) in nitric oxide (NO)-mediated relaxation of cerebral arteries [abstract]. J Cereb Blood Flow Metab 19:S255, 1999.
47. Lincoln TM, Cornwell TL: Towards an understanding of the mechanism of action of cyclic AMP and cyclic GMP in smooth muscle relaxation. Blood Vessels 28:129–137, 1991.
48. Wong SKF, Garbers DL: Receptor guanylyl cyclases. J Clin Invest 90:299–305, 1992.
49. Watkins LD: Nitric oxide and cerebral blood flow: An update. Cerebrovasc Brain Metab Rev 7:324–337, 1995.
50. Persson PB: Modulation of cardiovascular control mechanisms and their interaction. Physiol Rev 76:193–244, 1996.
51. Bredt DS, Hwang PM, Snyder SH: Localization of nitric oxide synthase indicating a neural role for nitric oxide. Nature 347:768–770, 1990.
52. Iadecola C: Regulation of the cerebral microcirculation during neural activity: Is nitric oxide the missing link? Trends Neurosci 16:206–214, 1993.
53. Tomimoto H, Nishimura M, Suenaga T, et al: Distribution of nitric oxide synthase in the human cerebral blood vessels and brain tissues. J Cereb Blood Flow Metab 14:930–938, 1994.
54. Toda N, Ayajiki K, Yoshida K, et al: Impairment by damage of the pterygopalatine ganglion of nitroxidergic vasodilator nerve function in canine cerebral and retinal arteries. Circ Res 72:206–213, 1993.
55. Toda N, Okamura T: Nitroxidergic nerve: Regulation of vascular tone and blood flow in the brain. J Hypertens 14:423–434, 1996.
56. Pluta RM, Thompson BG, Dawson TM, et al: Loss of nitric oxide synthase immunoreactivity in cerebral vasospasm. J Neurosurg 84:648–654, 1996.
57. Faraci FM, Brian JE Jr: Nitric oxide and the cerebral circulation. Stroke 25:692–703, 1994.
58. Katusic ZS: Endothelium-independent contractions to N^G-monomethyl-L-arginine in canine basilar artery. Stroke 22:1399–1404, 1991.
59. Gonzalez C, Estrada C: Nitric oxide mediates the neurogenic vasodilation of bovine cerebral arteries. J Cereb Blood Flow Metab 11:366–370, 1991.
60. Huang PL, Fishman MC: Genetic analysis of nitric oxide synthase isoforms: Targeted mutation in mice. J Mol Med 74:415–421, 1996.
61. Chen AFY, O'Brien T, Tsutsui M, et al: Expression and function of recombinant endothelial nitric oxide synthase gene in canine basilar artery. Circ Res 80:327–335, 1997.
62. Tsutsui M, Chen AFY, O'Brien T, et al: Adventitial expression of recombinant eNOS gene restores NO production in arteries without endothelium. Arterioscler Thromb Vasc Biol 18:1231–1241, 1998.
63. Onoue H, Tsutsui M, Smith L, et al: Expression and function of recombinant endothelial nitric oxide synthase in canine basilar artery after experimental subarachnoid hemorrhage. Stroke 29:1959–1966, 1998.
64. Onoue H, Tsutsui M, Smith L, et al: Adventitial expression of recombinant endothelial nitric oxide synthase gene reverses vasoconstrictor effect of endothelin-1. J Cereb Blood Flow Metab 19:1029–1037, 1999.
65. Khurana VG, Smith LA, Weiler DA, et al: Adenovirus-mediated gene transfer to human cerebral arteries. J Cereb Blood Flow Metab 20:1360–1371, 2000.
66. Faraci FM: Role of nitric oxide in regulation of basilar artery tone in vivo. Am J Physiol 259:H1216–H1221, 1990.
67. Rosenblum WI, Nishimura H, Nelson GH: Endothelium-dependent L-Arg and L-NMMA-sensitive mechanisms regulate tone of brain microvessels. Am J Physiol 259:H1396–H1401, 1990.
68. Busija DW, Leffler CW, Wagerle LC: Mono-L-arginine-containing compounds dilate piglet pial arterioles via an endothelium-derived relaxing factor-like substance. Circ Res 67:1374–1380, 1990.
69. Dalkara T, Moskowitz MA: Nitric oxide and the cerebral circulation. In Welch KMA, Caplan LR, Reis DJ, et al (eds): Primer on

Cerebrovascular Diseases. San Diego, Academic Press, 1997, pp 96–98.
70. Faraci FM: Role of endothelium-derived relaxing factor in cerebral circulation: Large arteries vs. microcirculation. Am J Physiol 261:H1038–1042, 1991.
71. Suzuki H, Kenamaru K, Tsunoda H, et al: Heme oxygenase-1 gene induction as an intrinsic regulation against delayed cerebral vasospasm in rats. J Clin Invest 104:59–66, 1999.
72. Choi AMK, Alam J: Heme oxygenase-1: Function, regulation, and implication of a novel stress-inducible protein in oxidant-induced lung injury. Am J Respir Cell Mol Biol 15:9–19, 1996.
73. Verma A, Hirsch DJ, Glatt CE, et al: Carbon monoxide: A putative neural messenger. Science 259:381–384, 1993.
74. Bredt DS, Hwang PM, Glatt CE, et al: Cloned and expressed nitric oxide synthase structurally resembles cytochrome P-450 reductase. Nature 351:714–718, 1991.
75. Zakhary R, Gaine SP, Dinerman JL, et al: Heme oxygenase-2: Endothelial and neuronal localization and role in endothelium-dependent relaxation. Proc Natl Acad Sci U S A 93:795–798, 1996.
76. Wang M, Roberts DL, Paschke R, et al: Three-dimensional structure of NADPH-cytochrome P450 reductase: Prototype for FMN- and FAD-containing enzymes. Proc Natl Acad Sci U S A 94:8411–8416, 1997.
77. Masters BS, McMillan K, Sheta EA, et al: Neuronal nitric oxide synthase, a modular enzyme formed by convergent evolution: Structure studies of a cysteine thiolate-liganded heme protein that hydroxylates L-arginine to produce NO as a cellular signal. FASEB J 10:552–558, 1996.
78. Busija DW: Eicosanoids and cerebrovascular control. In Welch KMA, Caplan LR, Reis DJ, et al (eds): Primer on Cerebrovascular Diseases. San Diego, Academic Press, 1997, pp 93–96.
79. Takenaka K, Kassell NF, Foley PL, et al: Oxyhemoglobin-induced cytotoxicity and arachidonic acid release in cultured bovine endothelial cells. Stroke 24:839–845, 1993.
80. Wier B: The pathophysiology of cerebral vasospasm. Br J Neurosurg 9:375–390, 1995.
81. Beckman JS: Nitric oxide, superoxide, and peroxynitrite in CNS injury. In Welch KMA, Caplan LR, Reis DJ, et al (eds): Primer on Cerebrovascular Diseases. San Diego, Academic Press, 1997, pp 209–210.
82. Dalkara T, Moskowitz MA: The role of nitric oxide in cerebral ischemia. In Welch KMA, Caplan LR, Reis DJ, et al (eds): Primer on Cerebrovascular Diseases. San Diego, Academic Press, 1997, pp 207–208.
83. Chan PH: Transgenic mice. In Welch KMA, Caplan LR, Reis DJ, et al. (eds): Primer on Cerebrovascular Diseases. San Diego, Academic Press, 1997, pp 126–129.
84. Kinouichi H, Epstein CJ, Mizui T, et al: Attenuation of focal cerebral ischemic injury in transgenic mice overexpressing CuZn superoxide dismutase. Proc Natl Acad Sci U S A 88: 11158–11162, 1991.
85. Yang GY, Chan PH, Chen J, et al: Human copper-zinc superoxide dismutase transgenic mice are highly resistant to reperfusion injury after focal cerebral ischemia. Stroke 25:165–170, 1994.
86. Chan PH, Kamii H, Yang G, et al: Brain infarction is not reduced in SOD-1 transgenic mice after a permanent focal cerebral ischemia. Neuroreport 5:293–296, 1993.
87. Hertz L: Features of astrocytic function apparently involved in the response of central nervous tissue to ischemia-hypoxia. J Cereb Blood Flow Metab 1:143–153, 1981.
88. Crumrine RC, LaManna JC: Regional cerebral metabolites: Blood flow, plasma volume, and mean transit time in total cerebral ischemia in the rat. J Cereb Blood Flow Metab 11: 272–282, 1991.
89. Fiskum G, Murphy AN, Beal MF: Mitochondria in neurodegeneration: Acute ischemia and chronic neurodegenerative diseases. J Cereb Blood Flow Metab 19:351–369, 1999.
90. del Zoppo GJ: Microvascular changes during cerebral ischemia and reperfusion. Cerebrovasc Brain Metab Rev 6:47–96, 1994.
91. Sundt TM Jr, Whisnant JP: Subarachnoid hemorrhage from intracranial aneurysms: Surgical management and natural history of disease. N Engl J Med 299:116–122, 1978.
92. Khurana VG, Piepgras DG, Whisnant JP: Ruptured giant intracranial aneurysms: I. A study of rebleeding. J Neurosurg 88: 425–429, 1998.
93. Powers WJ, Grubb RL Jr: Hemodynamic and metabolic relationships in cerebral ischemia and subarachnoid hemorrhage. In Wood JH (ed): Cerebral Blood Flow: Physiologic and Clinical Aspects. New York, McGraw-Hill, 1987, pp 387–401.
94. Bakker ENTP, Van der Linden PJW, Sipkema P: Endothelin-1-induced constriction inhibits nitric-oxide–mediated dilation in isolated rat resistance arteries. J Vasc Res 34:418–424, 1997.
95. Zhu ZG, Li HH, Zhang BR: Expression of endothelin-1 and constitutional nitric oxide synthase messenger RNA in saphenous vein endothelial cells exposed to arterial flow shear stress. Ann Thorac Surg 64:1333–1338, 1997.
96. Redmond EM, Cahill PA, Hodges R, et al: Regulation of endothelin receptors by nitric oxide in cultured rat vascular smooth muscle cells. J Cell Physiol 166:469–479, 1996.
97. Noiri E, Hu Y, Bahou WF, et al: Permissive role of nitric oxide in endothelin-induced migration of endothelial cells. J Biol Chem 272:1747–1752, 1997.
98. Salom JB, Torregrosa G, Alborch E: Endothelins and the cerebral circulation. Cerebrovasc Brain Metab Rev 7:131–152, 1995.
99. Yoshimoto S, Ishizaki Y, Kurihara H, et al: Cerebral microvessel endothelium is producing endothelin. Brain Res 508:283–285, 1990.
100. Kobayashi H, Hayashi M, Kobayashi S, et al: Cerebral vasospasm and vasoconstriction caused by endothelin. Neurosurgery 28:673–679, 1991.
101. Namiki A, Hirata Y, Ishikawa M, et al: Endothelin-1- and endothelin-3-induced vasorelaxation via common generation of endothelium-derived nitric oxide. Life Sci 50:677–682, 1992.
102. Tsukahara H, Ende H, Magazine HI, et al: Molecular and functional characterization of the non-isopeptide-selective ET_B receptor in endothelial cells: Receptor coupling to nitric oxide synthase. J Biol Chem 269:21778–21785, 1994.
103. Boulanger C, Luscher TF: Release of endothelin from the porcine aorta: Inhibition by endothelium-derived nitric oxide. J Clin Invest 85:587–590, 1990.
104. Luscher TF, Yang Z, Tschudi M, et al: Interaction between endothelin-1 and endothelium-derived relaxing factor in human arteries and veins. Circ Res 66:1088–1094, 1990.
105. Okishio M, Ohkawa S, Ichimori Y, et al: Interaction between endothelium-derived relaxing factors, S-nitrosothiols and endothelin-1 on Ca^{2+} mobilization in rat vascular smooth muscle cells. Biochem Biophys Res Commun 183:849–855, 1992.
106. Kitazono T, Heistad DD, Faraci FM: Enhanced responses of the basilar artery to activation of endothelin B receptors in stroke-prone spontaneously hypertensive rats. Hypertension 25:490–494, 1995.
107. Foley PL, Caner HH, Kassell NF, et al: Reversal of subarachnoid hemorrhage-induced vasoconstriction with an endothelin receptor antagonist. Neurosurgery 34:108–113, 1994.
108. Lassen NA: Cerebral blood flow and oxygen consumption in man. Physiol Rev 39:183–238, 1959.
109. Heistad DD, Kontos HA: Cerebral circulation. In Shepherd JT, Abbourd FM (eds): Handbook of Physiology, vol 3. Bethesda, MD, American Physiological Society, 1983, pp 137–182.
110. Fog M: Cerebral circulation: The reaction of the pial arteries to a fall in blood pressure. Arch Neurol Psych 37:351–364, 1937.
111. Fog M: Cerebral circulation: II. Reaction of pial arteries to increase in blood pressure. Arch Neurol Psych 41:260–268, 1939.
112. Chillon JM, Baumbach GL: Autoregulation of cerebral blood flow. In Welch KMA, Caplan LR, Reis DJ, et al (eds): Primer on Cerebrovascular Diseases San Diego, Academic Press, 1997, pp 51–54.
113. Rosner MJ: Introduction to cerebral perfusion pressure measurement. Neurosurg Clin North Am 6:761–773, 1995.
114. Paulson OB, Strandgaard S, Edvinsson L: Cerebral autoregulation. Cerebrovasc Brain Metab Rev 2:161–192, 1990.
115. Golanov EV, Reis DJ: Oxygen and cerebral blood flow. In Welch KMA, Caplan LR, Reis DJ, et al (eds): Primer on Cerebrovascular Diseases. San Diego, Academic Press, 1997, pp 58–60.
116. Wahl M: Local chemical, neural, and humoral regulation of cerebrovascular resistance vessels. J Cardiovasc Pharmacol 7: S36–S46, 1985.
117. Paulson OB, Waldemar G, Schmidt JF, et al: Cerebral circulation under normal and pathologic conditions. Am J Cardiol 63: 2C–5C, 1989.

118. Strandgaard S, Paulson OB: Cerebral autoregulation. Stroke 15: 413–416, 1984.
119. Winn HR, Welsh JE, Rubio R, et al: Brain adenosine production in rat during sustained alteration in systemic blood pressure. Am J Physiol 239:H636–H641, 1980.
120. Harder DR: Pressure-induced myogenic activation of cat cerebral arteries is dependent on intact endothelium. Circ Res 60: 102–107, 1987.
121. Rubanyi GM, Freay AD, Kauser K, et al: Mechanoreception by the endothelium: Mediators and mechanisms of pressure- and flow-induced vascular responses. Blood Vessels 27:246–257, 1990.
122. Bayliss NM: On the local reactions of the arterial wall to changes of internal pressure. J Physiol 28:220–231, 1902.
123. Isenberg G: Nonselective cation channels in cardiac and smooth muscle cells. In Siemen D, Hescheler J (eds): Nonselective Cation Channels: Pharmacology, Physiology and Biophysics. Basel, Birkhauser Verlag, 1993, pp 247–260.
124. Sachs F: Biophysics of mechanoreception. Membr Biochem 6: 173–195, 1986.
125. Sachs F: Stretch-sensitive ion channels. Neuroscience 2:49–57, 1990.
126. Davis MJ, Donovitz JA, Hood JD: Stretch-activated single-channel and whole cell currents in vascular smooth muscle cells. Am J Physiol 262:C1083–C1088, 1992.
127. Davis MJ, Hester FK, Donovitz JA, et al: Whole-cell current and intracellular calcium changes elicited by longitudinal stretch of single vascular smooth muscle cells [abstract]. FASEB J 4: A844, 1990.
128. Halpern W, Mongeon SA, Root DT: Stress, tension, and myogenic aspects of small isolated extraparenchymal rat arteries. In Stephens NL (ed): Smooth Muscle Contraction. New York, Marcel Dekker, 1984, pp 427–455.
129. Osol G, Halpern W: Myogenic properties of cerebral blood vessels from normotensive and hypertensive rats. Am J Physiol 249:H914–H921, 1985.
130. Brayden JE, Nelson MT: Regulation of arterial tone by activation of calcium-dependent potassium channels. Science 256:532–535, 1992.
131. Nelson MT, Quayle JM: Physiological roles and properties of potassium channels in arterial smooth muscle. Am J Physiol 268:C799–C822, 1995.
132. Jaggar JH, Stevenson AS, Nelson MT: Voltage-dependence of Ca^{2+} sparks in intact cerebral arteries. Am J Physiol 274:C1755–C1761, 1998.
133. Knot HJ, Nelson MT: Regulation of arterial diameter and wall $[Ca^{2+}]$ in cerebral arteries of rat by membrane potential and intravascular pressure. J Physiol 508:199–209, 1998.
134. Knot HJ, Standen NB, Nelson MT: Ryanodine receptors regulate arterial diameter and wall $[Ca^{2+}]$ in cerebral arteries of rat via Ca^{2+}-dependent K^+ channels. J Physiol 508:211–221, 1998.
135. Rubanyi GM: Endothelium-derived vasoconstrictor factors. In Ryan US (ed): Endothelial Cell, vol 3. Cleveland, CRC Press, 1988, pp 61–74.
136. Katusic ZS, Shepherd JT, Vanhoutte PM: Endothelium-dependent contraction to stretch in canine basilar arteries. Am J Physiol 252:H671–H673, 1987.
137. Harder DR, Sanchez-Ferrer C, Kauser K, et al: Pressure releases a transferable endothelial contractile factor in cat cerebral arteries. Circ Res 65:193–198, 1989.
138. Branston NM: Neurogenic control of the cerebral circulation. Cerebrovasc Brain Metab Rev 7:338–349, 1995.
139. Magistretti PJ: Coupling of cerebral blood flow and metabolism. In Welch KMA, Caplan LR, Reis DJ, et al (eds): Primer on Cerebrovascular Diseases. San Diego, Academic Press, 1997, pp 70–75.
140. Linville DG, Hamel E: Acetylcholine and its receptors. In Welch KMA, Caplan LR, Reis DJ, et al (eds): Primer on Cerebrovascular Diseases. San Diego, Academic Press, 1997, pp 82–85.
141. McCulloch J: Neuropeptide transmitters and their receptors. In Welch KMA, Caplan LR, Reis DJ, et al (eds): Primer on Cerebrovascular Diseases. San Diego, Academic Press, 1997, pp 91–93.
142. Bonvento G, MacKenzie ET: Serotonin and its receptors. In Welch KMA, Caplan LR, Reis DJ, et al (eds): Primer on Cerebrovascular Diseases. San Diego, Academic Press, 1997, pp 80–82.
143. Busija DW, Heistad DD: Factors involved in the physiological regulation of the cerebral circulation. Rev Physiol Biochem Pharmacol 101:161–211, 1984.
144. Traystman RJ: Regulation of cerebral blood flow by carbon dioxide. In Welch KMA, Caplan LR, Reis DJ, et al (eds): Primer on Cerebrovascular Diseases. San Diego, Academic Press, 1997, pp 55–58.
145. Kety SS, Schmidt CF: The effects of altered arterial tensions of carbon dioxide and oxygen on cerebral blood flow and cerebral oxygen consumption of normal young men. J Clin Invest 27: 484–492, 1948.
146. Kontos HA, Raper AJ, Patterson JL: Analysis of vasoreactivity of local pH, P_{CO_2}, and bicarbonate on pial vessels. Stroke 8: 358–360, 1977.
147. Kontos HA, Wei EP, Raper AJ, et al: Local mechanisms of CO_2 action on cat pial arterioles. Stroke 8:226–229, 1977.
148. Bryan J, Agular-Bryan L: The ABCs of ATP-sensitive potassium channels: More pieces of the puzzle. Curr Opin Cell Biol 9: 553–559, 1997.
149. Quast U, Cook NS: Moving together: K^+ channel openers and ATP-sensitive K^+ channels. TiPS 10:431–435, 1989.
150. Terzic A, Jahangir A, Kurachi Y: Cardiac ATP-sensitive K^+ channels: Regulation by intracellular nucleotides and K^+ channel-opening drugs. Am J Physiol 269:C525–C545, 1995.
151. Jovanovic A, Jovanovic S, Lorenz E, et al: Recombinant cardiac ATP-sensitive K^+ channel subunits confer resistance to chemical hypoxia-reoxygenation injury. Circulation 98:1548–1555, 1998.
152. Alekseev AE, Kennedy ME, Navarro B, et al: Burst kinetics of co-expressed Kir6.2/SUR1 clones: Comparison of recombinant with native ATP-sensitive K^+ channel behavior. J Membrane Biol 159:161–168, 1997.
153. Niwa K, Lindauer U, Villringer A, et al: Blockade of nitric oxide synthesis in rats strongly attenuates the CBF response to extracellular acidosis. J Cereb Blood Flow Metab 13:535–539, 1993.
154. Iadecola C, Zhang F, Xu X: SIN-1 reverses attenuation of hypercapnic cerebrovasodilation by nitric oxide synthase inhibitors. Am J Physiol 267:R228–R235, 1994.
155. Golanov EV, Reis DJ: Oxygen-sensitive neurons of the rostral ventrolateral medulla contribute to hypoxic cerebral vasodilation. J Physiol 495:201–216, 1996.
156. McPherson RW, Koehler RC, Traystman RJ: Hypoxia, α_2-adrenergic and nitric oxide dependent interactions on canine cerebral blood flow. Am J Physiol 266:H476–H482, 1994.
157. Ichord RN, Helfaer MA, Kirsch JR, et al: Nitric oxide synthase inhibition attenuates hypoglycemic cerebral hyperemia in piglets. Am J Physiol 266:H1062–H1068, 1994.
158. Kety SS, Schmidt CF: The nitrous oxide method for the quantitative determination of cerebral blood flow in man: Theory, procedure, and normal values. J Clin Invest 27:475–483, 1948.
159. Sokoloff L: Local cerebral circulation at rest and during altered cerebral activity induced by anesthesia or visual stimulation. In Kety SS, Elkes J (eds): Regional Neurochemistry. Oxford, Pergamon Press, 1961, pp 107–117.
160. Roy CS, Sherrington CS: On the regulation of the blood supply of the brain. J Physiol 11:85–108, 1896.
161. Ingvar DH, Lassen NA: Quantitative determination of regional cerebral blood flow in man. Lancet ii:806–807, 1961.
162. Sokoloff L, Reivich M, Kennedy C, et al: The ^{14}C-deoxyglucose method for measurement of local cerebral glucose utilization: Theory, procedure, and normal values in the conscious and anesthetized albino rat. J Neurochem 28:897–916, 1977.
163. Kety SS: The theory and applications of the exchange of inert gas at the lungs and tissues. Pharmacol Rev 3:1–41, 1951.
164. Iadecola C: Principles and methods for measurement of cerebral blood flow: Experimental methods. In Welch KMA, Caplan LR, Reis DJ, et al (eds): Primer on Cerebrovascular Diseases. San Diego, Academic Press, 1997, pp 34–37.
165. Mayberg TS, Lam AM: Jugular bulb oximetry for the monitoring of cerebral blood flow and metabolism. Neurosurg Clin North Am 7:755–765, 1996.
166. Sakurada O, Kennedy C, Jehle J, et al: Measurement of local cerebral blood flow with iodo[^{14}C]antipyrine. Am J Physiol 234: H59–H66, 1978.
167. Mazziotta J, Cohen M, Toga A: The measurement of cerebral

blood flow and metabolism in humans. In Welch KMA, Caplan LR, Reis DJ, et al (eds): Primer on Cerebrovascular Diseases. San Diego, Academic Press, 1997, pp 38–41.
168. Arbit E, DiResta GR: Application of laser Doppler flowmetry in neurosurgery. Neurosurg Clin North Am 7:741–748, 1996.
169. Anderson RE: Cerebral blood flow xenon-133. Neurosurg Clin North Am 7:703–708, 1996.
170. McGrail KM: Intraoperative use of electroencephalography as an assessment of cerebral blood flow. Neurosurg Clin North Am 7:685–692, 1996.
171. Sundt TM Jr: Correlation of cerebral blood flow measurements and continuous electroencephalography during carotid endarterectomy and risk-benefit ratio of shunting. In Wood JH (ed): Cerebral Blood Flow: Physiologic and Clinical Aspects. New York, McGraw-Hill, 1987, pp 679–692.
172. Yonas H, Pindzola RR, Johnson DW: Xenon/computed tomography cerebral blood flow and its use in clinical management. Neurosurg Clin North Am 7:605–616, 1996.
173. Taormina MA, Nichols FT III: Use of transcranial Doppler sonography to evaluate patients with cerebrovascular disease. Neurosurg Clin North Am 7:589–603, 1996.
174. Lee CC, Jack CR Jr, Riederer SJ: Use of functional magnetic imaging. Neurosurg Clin North Am 7:665–683, 1996.
175. Knight RA, Chopp M: Imaging techniques for focal ischemic damage. In Welch KMA, Caplan LR, Reis DJ, et al (eds): Primer on Cerebrovascular Diseases. San Diego, Academic Press, 1997, pp 136–141.
176. Barker PB: Metabolism: Magnetic resonance spectroscopy and spectroscopic imaging. In Welch KMA, Caplan LR, Reis DJ, et al (eds): Primer on Cerebrovascular Diseases. San Diego, Academic Press, 1997, pp 650–660.
177. Derdeyn CP, Powers WJ: Metabolic studies using PET in stroke investigation. In Welch KMA, Caplan LR, Reis DJ, et al (eds): Primer on Cerebrovascular Diseases. San Diego, Academic Press, 1997, pp 644–650.
178. Mullan BP, O'Connor MK, Hung JC: Single photon emission computed tomography brain imaging. Neurosurg Clin North Am 7:617–651, 1996.
179. Villringer A, Dirnagl U: Coupling of brain activity and cerebral blood flow: Basis of functional neuroimaging. Cerebrovasc Brain Metab Rev 7:240–276, 1995.
180. Nehlig A: Cerebral energy metabolism, glucose transport and blood flow: Changes with maturation and adaptation to hypoglycemia. Diabetes Metab 23:18–29, 1997.
181. Siesjo BK: Cerebral circulation and metabolism. J Neurosurg 60: 883–908, 1984.
182. Pessin JE, Bell GI: Mammalian facilitative glucose transporter family: Structure and molecular regulation. Annu Rev Physiol 54:911–930, 1992.
183. Vannucci SJ: Developmental expression of GLUT1 and GLUT3 glucose transporters in rat brain. J Neurochem 62:240–246, 1994.
184. Hochachka PW, Mommsen TP: Protons and anaerobiosis. Science 219:1391–1397, 1983.
185. Gutman A: Regulation of glycogen metabolism. In Beitner R (ed): Regulation of Carbohydrate Metabolism, vol 2. Boca Raton, FL, CRC Press, 1985, pp 33–52.
186. Aghard CD, Chapman AG, Nilsson B, et al: Endogenous substrates utilized by rat brain in severe insulin-induced hypoglycemia. J Neurochem 36:490–500, 1981.
187. Ghajar JBG, Plum F, Duffy TE: Cerebral oxidative metabolism and blood flow during acute hypoglycemia and recovery in unanesthetized rats. J Neurochem 38:397–409, 1982.
188. De Feo P, Perriello G, De Cosmo S, et al: Comparison of glucose counterregulation during short-term and prolonged hypoglycemia in normal humans. Diabetes 35:563–569, 1986.
189. Sokoloff L: Circulation and energy metabolism of the brain. In Siegel GJ, Albers RW, Katzman R, et al (eds): Intermediary Metabolism in Basic Neurochemistry: Molecular, Cellular, and Medical Aspects. New York, Raven Press, 1989, pp 541–564.
190. Owen OE, Morgan AP, Kemp HG, et al: Brain metabolism during fasting. J Clin Invest 46:1589–1595, 1967.
191. Yu ACH, Hertz L: Uptake of glutamate, GABA, and glutamine into predominantly GABAergic and a predominantly glutamatergic nerve cell population in culture. J Neurosci Res 7: 23–35, 1982.
192. Yu ACH, Lee YL, Eng LF: Glutamate as an energy substrate for neuronal-astrocytic interactions. Prog Brain Res 94:251–259, 1992.
193. Trudeau LE, Parpura V, Haydon PG: Activation of neurotransmitter release in hippocampal nerve terminals during recovery from intracellular acidification. J Neurophysiol 81:2627–2635, 1999.
194. Yudkoff M, Pleasure D, Cregar L, et al: Glutathione turnover in cultured astrocytes: Studies with [^{15}N]glutamate. J Neurochem 55:137–145, 1990.
195. Stewart PA: Glial-vascular relations. In Welch KMA, Caplan LR, Reis DJ, et al (eds): Primer on Cerebrovascular Diseases. San Diego, Academic Press, 1997, pp 17–21.
196. Bradbury MWB: The structure and function of the blood-brain barrier. Fed Proc 43:186–190, 1984.
197. Pardridge WM: Blood-brain barrier transport mechanisms. In Welch KMA, Caplan LR, Reis DJ, et al (eds): Primer on Cerebrovascular Diseases. San Diego, Academic Press, 1997, pp 21–25.
198. Gjedde A, Crone C: Induction processes in blood-brain transfer of ketone bodies during starvation. Am J Physiol 229:1165–1169, 1975.
199. Pollay M, Stevens FA: Starvation-induced changes in transport of ketone bodies across the blood-brain barrier. J Neurosci 5: 153–172, 1980.
200. Silver IA: Cellular microenvironment in relation to local blood flow. In Elliott K, O'Connor K (eds): CIBA Foundation Symposium 56: Cerebral Vascular Smooth Muscle and Its Control. West Caldwell, NJ, CIBA-Geigy Publications, 1978, pp 49–61.
201. Dirnagl U, Dreier J: Regulation of cerebral blood flow by ions. In Welch KMA, Caplan LR, Reis DJ, et al (eds): Primer on Cerebrovascular Diseases. San Diego, Academic Press, 1997, pp 75–77.
202. Paulson OB, Newman EA: Does the release of potassium from astrocyte endfeet regulate cerebral blood flow? Science 237: 896–898, 1987.
203. Iadecola C: Does nitric oxide mediate the increases in cerebral blood flow elicited by hypercapnia? Proc Natl Acad Sci U S A 89:3913–3916, 1992.
204. Winn HR: Adenosine and its receptors: Influence on cerebral blood flow. In Welch KMA, Caplan LR, Reis DJ, et al (eds): Primer on Cerebrovascular Diseases. San Diego, Academic Press, 1997, pp 77–79.
205. Bennett MR, Kerr R, Khurana G: Adenosine modulation of calcium currents in postganglionic neurones of avian cultured ciliary ganglia. Br J Pharmacol 106:25–32, 1992.
206. Rudolphi KA, Schubert P, Parkinson FE, et al: Adenosine and brain function. Cerebrovasc Brain Metab Rev 4:346–369, 1992.
207. Corradetti R, Lo Conte G, Moroni F, et al: Adenosine decreases aspartate and glutamate release from rat hippocampal slices. Eur J Pharmacol 104:19–26, 1984.
208. von Lubitz DKJE, Dambrosia JM, Kempski O, et al: Cyclohexyladenosine protects against neuronal death following ischemia in the CA1 region of the hippocampus. Stroke 19:1133–1139, 1988.
209. Kuschinsky W: Coupling of function, metabolism, and blood flow in the brain. Neurosurg Rev 14:163–168, 1991.
210. Faraci FM, Heistad DD: Role of ATP-sensitive potassium channels in the basilar artery. Am J Physiol 264:H8–H13, 1993.
211. Dreier J, Korner K, Gorner A, et al: Nitric oxide mediates the CBF response to increased extracellular potassium. J Cereb Blood Flow Metab 15:914–919, 1995.
212. Faraci FM, Brian JE Jr: 7-Nitroindazole inhibits brain nitric oxide synthase and cerebral vasodilatation in response to NMDA. Stroke 26:2172–2176, 1995.

CHAPTER 87

Acute Medical Management of Ischemic Disease and Stroke

CAROLYN D. BROCKINGTON ■ JUSTIN A. ZIVIN

The administration of effective therapy in the setting of acute stroke is a race against time. The majority of acute ischemic strokes are caused by thromboembolic occlusion of an intracranial artery.[1] The clock begins to tick the moment cerebral blood flow (CBF) is diminished to a level too low to sustain tissue viability. The degree of ischemic injury is dependent on the specific neuronal vulnerability and the residual CBF through the collaterals.[2] After the reduction in CBF, a "window of opportunity" is available during which therapy must be instituted. Although reperfusion of the area can reduce the degree of ischemia, it can also produce neuronal injury.[3–5] This process has been referred to as *reperfusion injury.* Effective therapy for acute stroke must be able to reduce the degree of ischemic damage and minimize the effects of reperfusion injury.

Recombinant tissue plasminogen activator (rt-PA) is given to selected patients within 3 hours of stroke onset. Numerous other drugs have been studied in an attempt to provide further treatment options. Future stroke trials are likely to incorporate a combination of drugs to promote recanalization, block the effects of ischemia, and prevent reperfusion injury. This chapter provides information on the acute medical management of stroke.

PATHOPHYSIOLOGY OF STROKE AND MECHANISM OF THROMBOLYSIS

Most acute focal ischemic events in the brain are due to embolism or in situ thrombosis.[6] Thrombogenesis is dependent on a series of complex events that promote the formation of a stable clot. Platelet aggregation, endothelial injury, and fibrin formation are key components. Angiographic studies have revealed several preferential sites for atherothrombotic lesions. Lesions of the proximal internal carotid artery and common carotid artery bifurcation are found in 50% to 80% of ischemic stroke patients, and a cardioembolic source is suspected in approximately 15% to 20% of all ischemic strokes. Although any cardiac disease is a potential source for embolization, the clinical conditions most often associated are nonvalvular atrial fibrillation, prosthetic heart valves, acute myocardial infarction, rheumatic heart disease, and ventricular aneurysm. Hereditary or acquired hemostatic disorders associated with thrombotic conditions generally involve the venous rather than the arterial circulation and are frequently seen in young adult stroke patients (4% to 5%).

Cerebral infarction is the result of a series of pathophysiologic events. The disruption in blood flow causes a reduction in the supply of glucose and oxygen to the tissue. This event leads to the production of acidic end products and a reduction in intracellular pH. With the release of toxic substances, the glutamate channels and the Na^{+}-Ca^{2+} exchange pump are damaged. Pump failure allows the unrestricted entry of calcium into the cell, causing the malfunction of ion channels and membrane receptors. The simultaneous release of free radicals, breakdown of the blood-brain barrier, and inflammatory response may add to the magnitude of the injury produced.

Data obtained from animal studies and clinical observations suggest that the amount of time before ischemia produces irreversible injury is relatively brief. Irreversible focal damage begins within several minutes after a significant reduction in CBF and is complete within approximately 6 hours. Figure 87–1 depicts the relationship between the duration of ischemia and the severity of the resulting neurological deficit.[7] As the duration of ischemia is extended, there is a brief period during which neurological injury is completely reversible if blood flow is restored. This type of injury is termed a *transient ischemic attack.* In a short amount of time, however, an ischemic event can result in re-

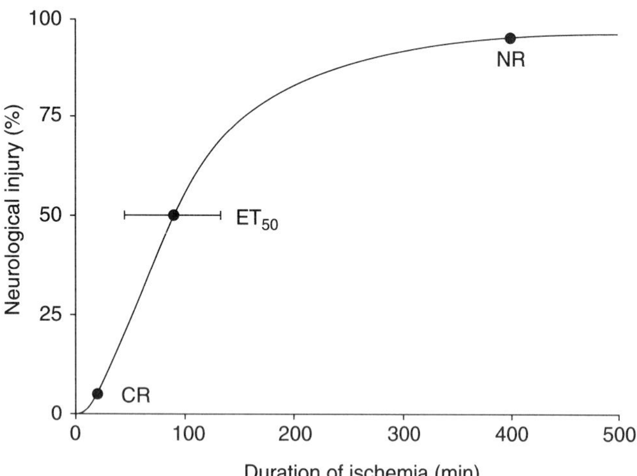

FIGURE 87–1. The degree of neurological injury as a function of the duration of ischemia. The neurological damage is the percentage of the monkeys exhibiting infarcts of any size. CR is the maximal duration of ischemia compatible with complete recovery. NR is the minimal time for no recovery. The ET_{50} represents the duration of ischemia that results in half-maximal damage. The error bar is the standard error at ET_{50}. (Data from Jones TH, Morawetz RB, Crowell RM, et al: Thresholds of focal cerebral ischemia in awake monkeys. J Neurosurg 54:773–782, 1981.)

versible injury, and as the ischemic period increases, the degree of the resulting neurological deficit increases. Ultimately, a point is reached where further ischemia cannot produce additional deficits. The injury produced is permanent, and no intervention will result in recovery of the tissue.

The site of the ischemic injury is an area in flux. If the center of the lesion is densely ischemic, it requires prompt restoration of blood flow to prevent irreversible damage. The area surrounding the core still receives some perfusion and is potentially salvageable if the cascade of cellular events resulting in neuronal death is blocked. This region has been referred to as the *ischemic penumbra*[8] and is the target of neuroprotective therapy. The size and duration of the penumbra are unknown for any individual patient.

Thrombolytic therapy is directed toward dissolution of the thrombus and subsequent restoration of blood flow. Thrombolytic agents act by promoting the conversion of plasminogen into plasmin, resulting in the degradation of fibrin and recanalization of the vessel. Spontaneous lysis can occur, but the rate of recanalization is not well established because it is impossible with current methods to continuously monitor clot dissolution in patients. The recanalization rate is dependent on a variety of factors, including the age, composition, and size of the thrombus, as well as the location of the occlusion.

Based on current evidence, acute stroke treatment must be initiated promptly if recovery is to be obtained. Without early intervention, the possibility of significant functional recovery is forfeited.

RECENT STROKE TRIALS

The safety and efficacy of thrombolytic therapy have been extensively studied in acute stroke. At present, t-PA is the only drug approved by the Food and Drug Administration for use in acute ischemic stroke. Data obtained from the National Institute of Neurological Disorders and Stroke (NINDS) trial showed that t-PA given within 3 hours of stroke onset improved the functional outcome at 3 months[9] (Table 87–1), and the benefit achieved with treatment was still present at 1 year.[10] The benefit of t-PA was seen across all ischemic stroke subtypes and was not affected by age, sex, or ethnicity. Although the symptomatic intracerebral hemorrhage (SICH) rate was greater in the group treated with t-PA (6.4% t-PA, 0.6% placebo), there was no significant difference in mortality at 3 months (17% t-PA, 21% placebo). Cost-benefit analyses have shown that thrombolysis not only reduces long-term disability but also saves the health care system money.[11]

The success of t-PA in acute ischemic stroke has led to the investigation of other thrombolytic agents. The Prolyse in Acute Cerebral Thromboembolism Trial II (PROACT II) evaluated the use of intra-arterial (IA) recombinant prourokinase (r-pro-UK) in patients with arteriogram-proven middle cerebral artery occlusions within 6 hours of stroke onset.[12] The results showed a significant difference favoring r-pro-UK over placebo (placebo 25%, pro-UK 40%) using the modified Rankin scale as a measure of global neurological function. Although patients who received r-pro-UK had a higher rate of SICH, the mortality rate at 90 days was similar for the two groups. The recanalization rate at 2 hours (complete plus partial patency; TIMI grades 2 and 3) was 66% for the r-pro-UK group, compared with 18% for the control group. The results demonstrated the efficacy and safety of r-pro-UK in selected individuals with middle cerebral artery occlusions of less than 6 hours' duration. Although IA thrombolytic agents such as r-pro-UK may be able to extend the therapeutic window longer than is possible with intravenous (IV) therapy, the availability of the required technology and the identification of appropriate patients may limit the clinical utility of this therapy.

The Emergency Management of Stroke (EMS) Bridging Trial investigated the efficacy and safety of combined IV and IA thrombolysis in acute ischemic stroke within 3 hours of symptom onset.[13] Thirty-five patients (17 assigned to the IV-IA group, 18 assigned to the placebo-IA group) were randomly assigned to receive either IV rt-PA or IV placebo, followed by immediate cerebral arteriography and local IA administration of rt-PA by microcatheter. Although the rate of recanalization was better with the combined IV-IA therapy, there was no difference in neurological outcome between the two groups. The rate of SICH was similar in the two groups, but the mortality rate was higher in the combined treatment arm. The baseline National Institutes of Health Stroke Scale (NIHSS) was found to have a direct correlation with the degree of clot burden on initial arteriography. This trial did not have sufficient power to detect the superiority of either form of treatment.

The Stroke Treatment with Ancrod Trial (STAT) investigated the safety and efficacy of a defibrinogenating agent in patients with acute ischemic stroke.[14] Low-

TABLE 87–1 ■ **Summary of Acute Stroke Trials**

TRIAL	RESULTS
NINDS Drug: Recombinant tissue plasminogen activator (rt-PA) (alteplase) Dose: 0.9 mg/kg (max 90 mg) Route: IV Time of administration: ≤3 hr Conclusions: Treatment with rt-PA within 3 hr of stroke onset improved functional outcome at 3 mo	Part 1 (at 24 hr): No significant difference between groups Part 2 (at 3 mo): Benefit was observed with rt-PA across all 4 outcome measurement scales Mortality: 21% (placebo) 17% (rt-PA) SICH: 0.6% (placebo) 6.4% (rt-PA)
PROACT II Drug: Recombinant prourokinase (r-pro-UK) Dose: 9 mg over 2 hr Route: IA Time of administration: <6 hr Conclusions: The results confirmed the efficacy and safety of r-pro-UK in selected patients with MCA occlusions of <6 hr duration	Primary end point (mRS ≤ 2 at day 90): 25% (control) 40% (r-pro-UK) Relative benefit: 60% Absolute benefit: 15% Mortality: 27% (control) 25% (r-pro-UK) SICH: 2% (control) 10% (r-pro-UK)
EMS Bridging Trial Drug: r-pro-UK Dose: 0.6 mg/kg (max 60 mg) Route: IV-IA compared with placebo-IA Time of administration: ≤3 hr Conclusions: The combined IV-IA therapy resulted in better recanalization, but there was no difference in clinical outcomes between the two groups	Primary end point (NIHSS of 0 or 1 at 7 days or ≥7-point improvement in score): 24% (IV-IA) 24% (placebo-IA) Mortality: 5 (29%) (IV-IA) 1 (5.5%) (placebo-IA) SICH: 11.8% (IV-IA) 5.5% (placebo-IA) at 72 hr
Ancrod Drug: Malaysian pit viper venom (serine protease) Dose: Starting dose based on body weight and initial fibrinogen level Route: IV Time of administration: ≤3 hr Conclusions: Ancrod was found to increase the functional independence of patients at 3 mo; the efficacy and safety appeared to be dependent on the level of defibrinogenation	Primary end point (BI at 90 days): 34.4% (placebo) 42.2% (ancrod) Mortality: 23% (placebo) 25.4% (ancrod) at 90 days SICH: 2.0% (placebo) 5.2% (ancrod)

BI, Barthel Index; EMS, Emergency Management of Stroke; IA, intra-arterial; IV, intravenous; mRS, modified Rankin Scale; NIHSS, National Institutes of Health Stroke Scale; NINDS, National Institute of Neurological Disorders and Stroke; PROACT, Prolyse in Acute Cerebral Thromboembolism; SICH, symptomatic intracerebral hemorrhage.

ering the fibrinogen level in the blood may increase spontaneous fibrinolysis and inhibit thrombus propagation. Ancrod is a serine protease that promotes rapid defibrinogenation by inducing the cleavage of the fibrinogen A-α chain. It is derived from Malaysian pit viper venom and has been used as a defibrinogenating agent in a variety of conditions, including deep vein thrombosis, peripheral vascular disease, and central retinal venous thrombosis.

Five hundred patients were randomized to receive either ancrod (n = 248) or placebo (n = 252) as a continuous 72-hour IV infusion with subsequent 1-hour infusions on days 4 and 5. All patients with ischemic strokes were eligible, and treatment was to be initiated within 3 hours of symptom onset. A functional assessment scale, the Barthel Index, was used to evaluate the patients' status. The primary efficacy end point was a favorable functional status, designated as a Barthel Index score of 95 or greater (indicating functional independence) or a score greater than or equal to the prestroke score at 90 days. The primary safety variables included mortality and SICH.

Treatment with ancrod was found to increase the functional independence of patients at 3 months, compared with placebo. The covariate-adjusted proportion of patients who achieved favorable functional status with ancrod was 42.2%, compared with 34.4% with placebo. The relative treatment effect was 22.7% (absolute 7.8%). Despite the greater risk of SICH with ancrod (5.2% ancrod, 2% placebo), the mortality rates of the two groups were the same. Further analysis revealed that the likelihood of SICH was greater when the mean fibrinogen maintenance level was below the target range at 9 to 72 hours. The highest risk of SICH (13.8%) was discovered in the subgroup in which the fibrinogen level was maintained below 40 mg/dL. The safety and efficacy of ancrod appeared to be dependent on the level of defibrinogenation achieved.

The efficacy of neuroprotection in acute stroke remains unclear. To date, several clinical trials have been unable to demonstrate a beneficial effect. The results of three recent large clinical trials were disappointing. The ECCO 2000 study compared citicoline with placebo.[15] It is believed that citicoline may reduce ischemic injury by stabilizing cell membranes and reducing free radical production. Although data from experimental models and previous studies suggested some possible benefit when citicoline was administered within 24 hours of the initial event, the results of the ECCO 2000 study were unimpressive. The trial involved 899 patients who were randomized to receive either oral citicoline (1000 mg twice daily) or placebo for 6 weeks. Inclusion criteria included treatment within 24 hours of ischemic stroke onset. No significant difference in outcome was found between patients given citicoline and those treated with placebo (52% citicoline, 51% placebo). The major side effect of citicoline was mild hypotension.

The Glycine Antagonist in Neuroprotection (GAIN) International Trial investigated the effectiveness of GV150526, a novel glycine site antagonist at the *N*-methyl-D-apartate receptor complex, in acute ischemic stroke.[16] Although the drug was found to be a potent neuroprotective agent in animal stroke models, the trial was unable to establish any benefit.

Some have postulated that the use of neuroprotective agents in combination with thrombolytic therapy might be effective in acute stroke treatment. One study investigated the use of IV t-PA with and without lubeluzole.[17] The patients were treated with t-PA according to the NINDS protocol and then randomly assigned to receive either IV lubeluzole (7.5 mg over 1 hour, followed by 10 mg/day) or placebo. The treatment was initiated before the end of the t-PA infusion and continued for a total of 5 days. The trial was terminated early ($N = 89$) because results of a concurrent trial investigating the efficacy of lubeluzole alone were negative. There was no significant difference in clinical outcome, mortality, or intracerebral hemorrhage between the two groups in the small combination study.

Despite the negative results, the evaluation of neuroprotection in acute ischemic stroke is still ongoing. It is likely that the time window for administration needs to be shortened in order to demonstrate a therapeutic benefit.

PATIENT EVALUATION

The initial evaluation of an acute stroke patient must be brief. The history obtained should include the time of symptom onset and any history of similar neurological events, including the existence of additional stroke risk factors (e.g., cardiac and vascular disease). Disease processes that can mimic stroke symptoms (e.g., migraine, hyperglycemia, postictal paralysis) should be excluded as causes if possible. In addition, the presence of serious coexisting illnesses and the recent use of oral anticoagulants should be determined for patient management.

To determine the degree of neurological deficit, the NIHSS can be used as a quick and efficient assessment.[18] The NIHSS is a graded examination that quantifies neurological deficits in 11 categories, including motor and sensory impairment, visual field deficits, language, and ataxia (Table 87–2). Use of the NIHSS is not obligatory.

During the evaluation process, a noncontrast computed tomographic scan should be performed to exclude the possibility of tumor, intracranial hemorrhage, and extensive early infarct signs. In the European Cooperative Acute Stroke Study (ECASS),[19] patients with early signs of ischemia in greater than 33% of the middle cerebral artery territory had an increased rate of mortality. If the infarct signs on computed tomography are obvious, the time of stroke onset should be reconfirmed.

To complete the evaluation, a series of laboratory tests, including chemistries, complete blood count with platelet count, and coagulation studies, must be obtained. Serial blood pressure measurements are imperative. A 12-lead electrocardiogram should be performed to evaluate for the possibility of a simultaneous myocardial infarction.

TISSUE PLASMINOGEN ACTIVATOR ADMINISTRATION

Inclusion criteria for IV t-PA administration include age 18 years or older, signs of a neurological deficit from an ischemic stroke on examination, and time of onset within 3 hours (Table 87–3). A reliable time of onset must be ascertained before administration of the drug. If the onset period cannot be established reliably, the time that the patient was last known to be normal (baseline) is used. This guideline includes stroke onset during sleep. Data from the ATLANTIS trial[20] has provided some information concerning the efficacy and safety of t-PA when administered beyond 3 hours. Five hundred fifty patients were randomized to receive either t-PA or placebo within 3 to 5 hours of stroke onset. Although the drug was not shown to be effective beyond the 3-hour window, the safety profile was similar to the results from the NINDS trial. This information provides physicians with some flexibility regarding administration of the drug within the 3-hour window.

There are several contraindications and warnings related to the administration of IV t-PA. Some of the exclusion criteria include evidence of intracranial hemorrhage on computed tomography, elevated blood pressure (systolic >185 mm Hg or diastolic >110 mm Hg) on repeated measurements despite antihypertensive administration, and known platelet diathesis and recent use of an anticoagulant with an elevated prothrombin time greater than 15 seconds (see Table 87–3). If the blood pressure can be successfully controlled with mild antihypertensive agents, t-PA may be given. The t-PA Stroke Study Group protocol guidelines sug-

TABLE 87–2 ■ **National Institutes of Health Stroke Scale**

1a. Level of Consciousness (LOC)
0 = alert
1 = lethargic, but arousable
2 = obtunded
3 = unresponsive or reflexive responses

1b. LOC Questions
0 = answers both questions correctly
1 = answers one question correctly
2 = answers neither question correctly

1c. LOC Commands
0 = performs both tasks correctly
1 = performs one task correctly
2 = performs neither task correctly

2. Best Gaze
0 = normal
1 = partial gaze palsy
2 = forced deviation or total gaze paresis

3. Visual
0 = no visual loss
1 = partial hemianopia
2 = complete hemianopia
3 = bilateral hemianopia

4. Facial Palsy
0 = normal symmetrical movement
1 = minor paralysis
2 = partial paralysis
3 = complete paralysis

5 and 6. Motor Arm and Leg*
0 = no drift
1 = drift
2 = some effort against gravity
3 = no effort against gravity
4 = no movement
9 = amputation, joint fusion

7. Limb Ataxia
0 = absent
1 = present in one limb
2 = present in two limbs

8. Sensory
0 = normal
1 = mild to moderate sensory loss
2 = severe to total sensory loss

9. Best Language
0 = normal
1 = mild to moderate aphasia
2 = severe aphasia
3 = mute or global aphasia

10. Dysarthria
0 = normal
1 = mild to moderate
2 = severe
9 = intubated or other physical barrier

11. Extinction and Inattention
0 = no abnormality
1 = inattention or extinction in one sensory modality
2 = profound hemi-inattention

* 5a, Left arm; 5b, right arm; 6a, left leg; 6b, right leg.

TABLE 87–3 ■ **Criteria for the Administration of Tissue Plasminogen Activator: 1997 Protocol Guidelines of the t-PA Stroke Study Group**

INCLUSION CRITERIA	EXCLUSION CRITERIA
Age 18 yr or older Signs of a measurable neurological deficit from an ischemic stroke on examination Time of onset of symptoms ≤3 hr	Evidence of intracerebral hemorrhage on pretreatment computed tomography Minor or rapidly improving symptoms Clinical presentation suggestive of subarachnoid hemorrhage Active internal bleeding Known platelet diathesis including but not limited to: Platelet count <100,000/mm^3 Heparin administration within 48 hr with elevated activated partial thromboplastin time Current or recent use of oral anticoagulants with an elevated prothrombin time >15 sec Major surgery or serious trauma in previous 14 days Any intracranial surgery, serious head trauma, or previous stroke within 3 mo History of gastrointestinal or urinary tract hemorrhage within 21 days Recent arterial puncture at noncompressible site or lumbar puncture Uncontrolled hypertension (systolic blood pressure >185 mm Hg or diastolic >110 mm Hg) on repeated measurements at time of treatment History of intracranial hemorrhage Abnormal blood glucose (<50 or >400 mg/dL) Post myocardial infarction Seizure at time of stroke onset Known arteriovenous malformation or aneurysm

TABLE 87–4 ■ Administration of Tissue Plasminogen Activator: 1997 Protocol Guidelines of the t-PA Stroke Study Group

Dose of t-PA = 0.9 mg/kg (max 90 mg). Ten percent of the total dose should be given as a bolus over 1 min. The remainder of the dose should be infused over 1 hr.
Monitor BP every 15 min during the antihypertensive therapy; observe for hypotension.
If an intracranial hemorrhage is suspected clinically, an emergent noncontrast computed tomographic scan should be obtained and the administration of t-PA discontinued.

PRETREATMENT	DURING AND AFTER TREATMENT
BP should be monitored every 15 min. The pressure should be <185/110. An elevated BP (>185/110) may be treated with nitroglycerin paste and/or one to two doses of IV labetalol 10–20 mg over 1 hr. If the treatment does not decrease the BP, the patient should not be treated with t-PA.	BP should be monitored for the first 24 hr after the start of treatment: every 15 min for 2 hr after the start of the infusion, then every 30 min for 6 hr, then every hour for 18 hr. If the diastolic BP is >140 mm Hg, start an IV infusion of sodium nitroprusside (0.5–10 μg/kg/min). If the systolic BP is >230 mm Hg or diastolic BP is 121–140 mm Hg, administer labetalol 20 mg IV over 1–2 min. The dose may be repeated and/or doubled every 10 min (max 150 mg). Alternatively, after the first bolus of labetalol, an IV infusion of 2–8 mg/min labetalol may be initiated and continued until the desired BP is achieved. If the desired response is not obtained, give some nitroprusside. If the systolic BP is 180–230 mm Hg or diastolic BP is 105–120 mm Hg on two readings 5–10 min apart, administer labetalol 10 mg IV over 1–2 min. The dose may be repeated or doubled every 10–20 min (max 150 mg). Alternatively, after the first bolus of labetalol, an IV infusion of 2–8 mg/min labetalol may be initiated and continued until the desired BP is reached.

BP, Blood pressure; IV, intravenous.

gest treatment with nitroglycerin paste, one to two doses of IV labetalol (10 to 20 mg) over 1 hour, or both (Table 87–4). The blood pressure should be monitored every 15 minutes before t-PA administration.

The dose of IV t-PA is 0.9 mg/kg (maximal dose 90 mg). Ten percent of the dose is administered as a bolus over 1 minute, followed by the remainder over 1 hour. Once the drug has been given, arrangements should be made to have the patient transferred to an appropriate monitored setting. The use of heparin, aspirin, or warfarin within the first 24 hours of symptom onset is not recommended.

Hemorrhagic complications are what most physicians fear when administering t-PA. The risk of intracranial and extracranial bleeding is increased with thrombolytic agents. In the NINDS trial, the percentage of patients with SICH was 6.4% with t-PA, compared with 0.6% with placebo.[9] Notably, the increased SICH did not alter mortality or morbidity between the two groups at 3 months, and the overall benefit favored the t-PA–treated group. Thus, despite an increased hemorrhage rate, t-PA treatment is licensed by the Food and Drug Administration and is recommended by the American Academy of Neurology and the American Heart Association.

If bleeding is suspected, several laboratory tests (hematocrit, hemoglobin, prothrombin time/INR, platelet count, partial thromboplastin time, and fibrinogen) should be ordered. Blood should be typed and crossmatched in preparation for possible transfusion. Infusion of thrombolytic therapy should be halted in the setting of any life-threatening intracranial or extracranial hemorrhage.

Suspicion of an intracranial hemorrhage warrants an emergent computed tomographic scan. Although the t-PA package insert recommends limiting treatment to facilities that can provide "appropriate evaluation and management of intracranial hemorrhage," the specific interventions that constitute appropriate treatment are unclear. No studies have demonstrated any benefit to surgical intervention or other therapies in this setting.

STROKE MANAGEMENT

After the administration of thrombolytic therapy, the patient should be transferred to a monitored setting for close observation. Appropriate management of the blood pressure is vital. Present guidelines suggest checking the blood pressure every 15 minutes for the first 2 hours, every 30 minutes for the next 6 hours, and then every hour for 18 hours.[21] The recommended goal is a blood pressure of less than 185/110. An elevated blood pressure is frequently noted in the acute period after stroke, followed by a gradual reduction to baseline over the ensuing days.

The management of blood pressure in an acute stroke patient is a balancing act. Aggressive blood pressure reduction might precipitate further ischemic injury, whereas sustained hypertension can lead to hemorrhagic transformation of the infarct, worsening cerebral edema, altered renal function, and cardiac ischemia. Some stroke experts advocate a conservative approach. Because many stroke patients suffer from altered cerebral autoregulation as a result of chronic hypertension, a rapid reduction in blood pressure to normotensive levels could result in a dramatic fall in CBF and worsening ischemia. A common approach is to discontinue the patient's regular antihypertensive therapy and treat the blood pressure as needed. Short-acting agents are recommended. Adequate glycemic control is also necessary to reduce the risk of further ischemic injury. Subcutaneous insulin administration is typically used to maintain appropriate levels.

The management of an acute stroke patient requires a multidisciplinary approach. Attention must be paid to a variety of issues, including airway and respiratory management, infection, cardiac status, deep vein thrombosis prophylaxis, and nutrition. Careful observation and a detailed care plan can significantly reduce the morbidity and mortality associated with acute cerebral infarction.

SURGICAL INTERVENTION

The prognosis for a patient who presents with a massive hemispheric stroke is poor. A malignant cerebral infarction can result from the occlusion of either the distal internal carotid artery or the trunk of the proximal middle cerebral artery and has been demonstrated in animal models[22, 23] and clinical studies.[24] The injury is typically associated with extensive brain edema and increased intracranial pressure, ultimately producing herniation and death. In light of the progressive clinical course and limited medical options, renewed interest has developed in decompressive craniectomies. The decompression can result in a significant decrease in intracranial pressure and may limit extension of the infarcted territory. The reduction in intracranial and mechanical pressure allows for an increase in cerebral perfusion pressure, leading to enhanced blood flow.

There is experimental evidence that the timing of the procedure is critical. Decompressive surgery performed 1 and 4 hours postictus in animal models of middle cerebral artery occlusion has resulted in improvement in neurological outcome and reduction in infarct volume.[22, 25] In clinical studies, surgery performed an average of 21 hours postictus resulted in a decreased mortality rate compared with surgery performed an average of 39 hours postictus.[26, 27] The influence of the patient's age on clinical outcome is still unknown, but there is some evidence that younger patients benefit more than older patients do.[28]

Most of the evidence in support of decompressive craniectomy for acute ischemic stroke has been limited to case series without controls. A recent study was conducted to investigate the clinical practice of hemicraniectomy using a case-control study of seven centers.[29] The results revealed that younger patients with massive strokes, early nausea, and fewer comorbid illnesses were more likely to undergo the surgery. Hemicraniectomy appeared to reduce the mortality rate associated with massive cerebral infarction compared with medical therapy alone (OR = 0.25, $P = 0.02$).

Decompressive surgery was compared with medical therapy in a prospective, nonrandomized, control study.[30] Thirty-two patients were selected for surgery, and 21 were treated medically. The control group consisted of 14 patients with extensive signs of left hemispheric infarction and global aphasia on presentation, 2 patients with severe medical complications, and 5 patients without informed consent. The mean age of the surgical group was 48.8 ± 12.4 years (range, 17 to 68), and the mean age of the control group was 58.4 + 7.7 years (range, 37 to 69). The Barthel Index measured the functional status. Six (18.8%) of the 32 surgical patients had a good outcome, compared with 0% in the medical arm; 15 surgical patients (46.9%) had moderate to severe disabilities, compared with 5 (23.8%) of the 21 medically treated patients. The mortality rate was dramatically reduced in the surgical group (34.4% surgery, 76.2% medical).

Although decompressive craniectomy in selected patients appears promising, many questions remain, including the timing of surgery and criteria for appropriate patient selection. At present, no form of surgery is a proven method of acute stroke management, but well-designed multicenter randomized clinical trials should provide some definitive answers.

CONCLUSION

Acute ischemic stroke needs to be approached as a medical emergency. Time is a critical factor, and patients need to be assessed and treated quickly. The approval of IV t-PA for acute ischemic stroke marked the start of a revolution in stroke therapy. Further investigation will provide alternative therapeutic options. Stroke is a difficult disease, and practicing physicians must stay abreast of the latest developments and practice guidelines.

REFERENCES

1. Fieschi C, et al: Clinical and instrumental evaluation of patients with ischemic stroke within the first six hours. J Neurol Sci 91: 311–321, 1989.
2. Ginsberg MD, Pulsinelli WA: The ischemic penumbra, injury thresholds, and the therapeutic window for acute stroke. Ann Neurol 36:553–554, 1994.
3. Halsey JH Jr, et al: The contribution of reoxygenation to ischemic brain damage. J Cereb Blood Flow Metab 11:994–1000, 1991.
4. Ito U, et al: Brain edema during ischemia and after restoration of blood flow: Measurement of water, sodium, potassium content and plasma protein permeability. Stroke 10:542–547, 1979.
5. Halsey JH, et al: The role of tissue acidosis in ischaemic tissue injury: The concept of the pH integral. Neurol Res 10:97–104, 1988.
6. Mohr JP, et al: The Harvard Cooperative Stroke Registry: A prospective registry. Neurology 28:754–762, 1978.
7. Zivin JA: Factors determining the therapeutic window for stroke. Neurology 50:599–603, 1998.
8. Astrup J, Siesjo BK, Symon L: Thresholds in cerebral ischemia — the ischemic penumbra. Stroke 12:723–725, 1981.
9. NINDS: Tissue plasminogen activator for acute ischemic stroke. The National Institute of Neurological Disorders and Stroke rt-PA Stroke Study Group. N Engl J Med 333:1581–1587, 1995.
10. Kwiatkowski TG, et al: Effects of tissue plasminogen activator for acute ischemic stroke at one year. National Institute of Neurological Disorders and Stroke Recombinant Tissue Plasminogen Activator Stroke Study Group. N Engl J Med 340:1781–1787, 1999.
11. Fagan SC, et al: Cost-effectiveness of tissue plasminogen activator

for acute ischemic stroke. NINDS rt-PA Stroke Study Group. Neurology 50:883–890, 1998.
12. Furlan A, et al: Intra-arterial prourokinase for acute ischemic stroke. The PROACT II study: A randomized controlled trial. Prolyse in Acute Cerebral Thromboembolism. JAMA 282:2003–2011, 1999.
13. Lewandowski CA, et al: Combined intravenous and intra-arterial r-TPA versus intra-arterial therapy of acute ischemic stroke: Emergency Management of Stroke (EMS) Bridging Trial. Stroke 30:2598–2605, 1999.
14. Sherman DG, et al: Intravenous ancrod for treatment of acute ischemic stroke. The STAT study: A randomized controlled trial. Stroke Treatment with Ancrod Trial. JAMA 283:2395–2403, 2000.
15. Gammans RE, Sherman DG, Investigators E: ECCO 2000 study of citicoline for treatment of acute ischemic stroke: Final results. Stroke 31:278A, 2000.
16. Lees KR, et al: Glycine antagonist (gavestinel) in neuroprotection (GAIN International) in patients with acute stroke: A randomized controlled trial. GAIN International Investigators. Lancet 355:1949–1954, 2000.
17. Grotta JC: Combination therapy stroke trial: rt-PA ± lubeluzole. Stroke 31:278A, 2000.
18. Lyden P, et al: Improved reliability of the NIH Stroke Scale using video training. NINDS TPA Stroke Study Group. Stroke 25:2220–2226, 1994.
19. Hacke W, et al: Intravenous thrombolysis with recombinant tissue plasminogen activator for acute hemispheric stroke. The European Cooperative Acute Stroke Study (ECASS). JAMA 274: 1017–1025, 1995.
20. Clark WM, et al: Recombinant tissue-type plasminogen activator (Alteplase) for ischemic stroke 3 to 5 hours after symptom onset. The ATLANTIS study: A randomized controlled trial. Alteplase Thrombolysis for Acute Noninterventional Therapy in Ischemic Stroke. JAMA 282:2019–2026, 1999.
21. NINDS and NINDS rt-PA Stroke Study Group: A systems approach to immediate evaluation and management of hyperacute stroke: Experience at eight centers and implications for community practice and patient care. The National Institute of Neurological Disorders and Stroke (NINDS) rt-PA Stroke Study Group. Stroke 28:1530–1540, 1997.
22. Doerfler A, et al: Decompressive craniectomy in a rat model of "malignant" cerebral hemispheric stroke: Experimental support for an aggressive therapeutic approach. J Neurosurg 85:853–859, 1996.
23. Engelhorn T, et al: Decompressive craniectomy, reperfusion, or a combination for early treatment of acute "malignant" cerebral hemispheric stroke in rats? Potential mechanisms studied by MRI. Stroke 30:1456–1463, 1999.
24. Hacke W, et al: "Malignant" middle cerebral artery territory infarction: Clinical course and prognostic signs. Arch Neurol 53: 309–315, 1996.
25. Forsting M, et al: Decompressive craniectomy for cerebral infarction: An experimental study in rats. Stroke 26:259–264, 1995.
26. Schwab S, et al: Hemicraniectomy in space-occupying hemispheric infarction: Useful intervention or desperate activism? Cerebrovasc Dis 6:325–329, 1996.
27. Schwab S, et al: Early hemicraniectomy in patients with complete middle cerebral artery infarction. Stroke 29:1888–1893, 1998.
28. Carter BS, et al: One-year outcome after decompressive surgery for massive nondominant hemispheric infarction. Neurosurgery 40:1168–1175; discussion 1175–1176, 1997.
29. Demchuk AM, et al: Multicenter evaluation of the clinical practice of hemicraniectomy in ischemic stroke. Stroke 32:295A, 2000.
30. Rieke K, et al: Decompressive surgery in space-occupying hemispheric infarction: Results of an open, prospective trial. Crit Care Med 23:1576–1587, 1995.

PART IV ANESTHESIA FOR NEUROVASCULAR PROCEDURES

CHAPTER 88

Anesthesia in Cerebrovascular Disease

A. GIANCARLO VISHTEH ■ PETER RAUDZENS ■ ROBERT F. SPETZLER ■ NICHOLAS THEODORE

Advances in the field of neuroanesthesiology in the last 10 years have paralleled the evolution of more sophisticated surgical management schemes for cerebrovascular pathologies. New approaches have been applied to old clinical problems, and new equipment has replaced existing diagnostic and surgical devices. For example, the operating microscope and use of temporary arterial clips have enabled greater precision and control during the dissection of cerebral aneurysms. In turn, the development of these techniques has prompted a trend toward early aneurysm surgery, which has led to two other important changes. First, antifibrinolytic agents (e.g., ϵ-aminocaproic acid), which were used widely to reduce the risk of rebleeding in patients being stabilized for "late" surgery, became unnecessary, thus avoiding serious side effects.[1,2] Second, the use of "controlled hypotension" to reduce the risk of hemorrhage from a ruptured aneurysm also decreased.[3–5] Pharmacologic agents and anesthetic strategies that have further revolutionized cerebrovascular surgery and improved outcomes include barbiturates[6–15] or hypothermia to provide cerebral protection, use of the calcium channel blocker nimodipine, and hypertensive-hypervolemic therapy.[16]

Another important aspect of anesthesia during cerebrovascular cases is neurophysiologic monitoring of the electrical activity of the central nervous system. Electroencephalography (EEG) and evoked potentials are used to assess, respectively, the functional states of the cortex and sensory systems of anesthetized (or comatose) patients.[17] Such monitoring permits the early detection of cerebral ischemia to prevent postoperative stroke.

Despite these advances, however, the goal of anesthesia remains the same: to provide an optimal surgical environment for the surgeon without compromising the patient's safety and comfort. Anesthetic techniques and agents continue to evolve. As a vital member of the neurovascular team, the anesthesiologist must incorporate the most recent advances in pharmacologic cerebral protection while monitoring intraoperative neurophysiologic factors and overseeing and maintaining the normal function of other organ systems (cardiovascular and renal). The anesthesiologist also oversees the preoperative medical clearance of patients who will undergo more involved procedures. As neurosurgery becomes compartmentalized into a host of subspecialties, neuroanesthesia must be tailored to individual procedures, especially within the realm of neurovascular surgery.

After reviewing the basics of cerebral metabolism and blood flow, this chapter details the specific anesthetic considerations for occlusive cerebrovascular disease, intracranial aneurysms, arteriovenous malformations (AVMs), cavernous malformations, and spinal vascular surgery. The neurophysiologic monitoring parameters used at the Barrow Neurological Institute are presented; a more detailed description of neurophysiology can be found elsewhere.[18–20]

CEREBRAL PHYSIOLOGY

Brain metabolism is a function of cerebral activity. It fluctuates with mental processes, time, and cell layers. About 60% of the required cerebral energy is used for synaptic activity, as reflected by EEG. The remaining 40% is used to maintain cellular integrity.[21,22] The brain has only minimal reserves of phosphorylase and glycogen and requires a continuous supply of oxygen and glucose to function normally (Table 88–1). As a result, the cerebral metabolic rate of oxygen ($CMRO_2$ = 3.5 mL O_2/min^{-1}/100 g^{-1} brain) is high, and blood flow in the brain is disproportionate compared with the rest of the body.[23]

TABLE 88–1 ■ **Normal Physiologic Parameters for the Brain**

PARAMETER	RATE
Global CBF	~50 mL/100 g^{-1}/min^{-1}
CBF (gray)	~80 mL/100 g^{-1}/min^{-1}
CBF (white)	~20 mL/100 g^{-1}/min^{-1}
CMR oxygen	~3.5 mL/100 g^{-1}/min^{-1}
CMR glucose	~4.5 mL/100 g^{-1}/min^{-1}
CBF/CMR oxygen	~15
Intracranial pressure	5–12 mm Hg
Venous Po_2	>35 mm Hg

CBF, cerebral blood flow; CMR, cerebral metabolic rate.

The brain constitutes only about 2% of body weight but receives about 15% of the cardiac output.[24] If this blood flow is interrupted, cerebral dysfunction is progressive. If cerebral blood flow (CBF) is less than 10 mL/100 g^{-1}/min^{-1} for 10 minutes, cellular activity fails irreparably.[25] If the ischemic thresholds of target tissues are recognized intraoperatively, safe periods of ischemia, such as during temporary clipping of arteries or hypothermic arrest, can be planned to achieve surgical repair without compromising neural function. This ischemic tolerance varies with age, temperature, $CMRO_2$, and collateral circulation.

Cerebral circulation is normally controlled by a number of metabolic, myogenic, and neurogenic factors. Neurological injury such as trauma, hypoxia, and seizures, and even diabetes and various pharmacologic agents such as anesthetics, can perturb this system.[26]

The cerebral arteries are sensitive to systemic arterial pressures between 50 and 150 mm Hg. Changes in cerebrovascular resistance maintain blood flow in this range.[27] Beyond these normal pressure limits, blood flow becomes pressure dependent. Symptoms of cerebral ischemia develop when systemic perfusion pressure is less than 40 mm Hg,[28] which probably represents the lowest safe limit of controlled hypotension. Systemic pressure above the autoregulation threshold can disrupt the blood-brain barrier and cause cerebral edema.

CBF is also coupled to metabolism by a variety of mechanisms. CBF is higher in metabolically active gray matter (80 mL/100 g^{-1}/min^{-1}) than in white matter (20 mL/100 g^{-1}/min^{-1}). As the $CMRO_2$ increases, there is a parallel increase in CBF.[29, 30]

Both oxygen (O_2) and carbon dioxide (CO_2) tensions can alter CBF by changing cerebrovascular resistance. When Pco_2 is between 20 and 80 mm Hg, CBF changes linearly at the rate of 1 mL/100 g^{-1} for every 1 mm Hg change in Pco_2. These acute changes can be buffered by restoring CBF to near normal within 6 to 8 hours. When Pco_2 is below 22 mm Hg, no further cerebral vasoconstriction occurs. Blood flow can be manipulated by hyperventilation and by reducing Pco_2. The goal of this change is to vasoconstrict normal cerebral vessels and redistribute blood to the maximally dilated vessels in an ischemic area of the brain. The benefits of this inverse steal (the so-called Robin Hood effect) are important for controlling intracranial pressure (ICP) but difficult to demonstrate for stroke prevention.[21]

Arterial Po_2 tension does not affect CBF until it falls below 50 mm Hg. Compensatory vasodilatation then occurs, and CBF subsequently increases.

Temperature is another important influence on CBF. As temperature decreases, CBF falls and viscosity increases. At extreme levels of hypothermia (<17°C), the $CMRO_2$ is reduced to 8% of normal, with a corresponding reduction in blood flow.[31, 32] This technique, together with barbiturate cerebral protection, is used to prolong a patient's tolerance for ischemia to 45 to 60 minutes during complicated cerebrovascular procedures.

The effects of adrenergic and cholinergic stimulation of the cerebral circulation are not well understood. Although sympathetic innervation of cerebral arteries is present, under normal circumstances other metabolic factors override neural influences.

INTRACRANIAL PRESSURE

The intracranial contents consist of cerebral blood volume (4%, or about 50 mL), brain tissue and interstitial fluid (84%, or 1100 mL), and cerebrospinal fluid (CSF; 12%, or 150 mL). The contents are contained within the rigid cranial vault, which is contiguous with the intraspinal neural contents.[33] In this closed system, a pressure-volume relationship can be plotted, and a patient's intracranial compliance can be measured by the pressure-volume index ($PVI = \Delta V/\log_{10} Pp/_{PO}$). To prevent ICP from increasing, a change in one compartment must be compensated for by a corresponding reduction in the other compartments. The pressure-volume index equals zero once the skull is opened.

Intracranial volume maintains a dynamic equilibrium. The volume of the circulating CSF is equal to the difference between CSF production in the choroid plexus and its absorption by the arachnoid villi. Blood volume can change abruptly and transiently. Cerebral interstitial fluid can also vary with injury, neoplasm, or infection.

The regulating mechanism driven by elevated ICP is cerebral perfusion pressure (CPP = mean arterial pressure − ICP). As ICP increases, the systemic perfusion pressure is driven up to maintain cerebral perfusion.

Typically, intracranial hypertension is defined as pressure sustained above 15 mm Hg, but it varies with the clinical situation. Although some patients are symptomatic at lower pressures, others tolerate significantly higher ICP (e.g., those with pseudotumor cerebri). Abnormally high ICP can lead to neural injury as a result of either cerebral ischemia or herniation of brain tissue around or through structures in the skull. Uncal herniation refers to the mesial temporal lobe protruding through the tentorial hiatus and compromising the cerebral peduncle and oculomotor nerve. The result is often occlusion of the posterior cerebral artery (P_2 segment). "Coning" refers to herniation of the cerebellar tonsils through the foramen magnum, with resultant compression of the medulla oblongata and dramatic and usually fatal respiratory failure and cardiovascular arrest. The degree and duration of elevated ICP determine the extent of injury.

Disorders of CSF outflow or resorption (e.g., congenital hydrocephalus, acquired congenital posterior fossa venous outflow obstruction), mass lesions (e.g., tumor, trauma, other intracranial hemorrhage), metabolic imbalance, infection, ischemia, numerous other disease states (e.g., respiratory disease, hypertension), and iatrogenic causes (e.g., anesthetics and fluid overload) can increase ICP. The management of such patients by an anesthetist requires an understanding of intracranial compliance and control of ICP.

A subarachnoid bolt, intraventricular catheter, intraparenchymal pressure monitor, or implanted epidural transducer can be used to measure ICP continuously and accurately. The technology most often used at our institution is the ventriculostomy catheter. The utility of this system for draining CSF and monitoring ICP is well established, and the risk of infection, if proper precautions are taken, is minuscule.[31, 32, 34, 35]

The treatment of increased ICP, especially in a surgical setting, usually combines operative and pharmacologic interventions: hyperventilation, head elevation, CSF drainage, surgical decompression, barbiturates, diuretics, and steroids. Initially, hyperventilation alone usually reduces ICP for 3 to 5 hours. ICP then increases to stabilize at a level lower than that of an untreated patient. In the case of patients with traumatic head injuries, cerebral perfusion pressure should be optimized, and excessive hyperventilation avoided. Technologies are being developed to determine which subsets of head-injured patients would potentially benefit from more profound hyperventilation.

During neurosurgical procedures, fluids are administered to maintain adequate cardiac filling pressure, as determined by either urinary output or pulmonary artery pressure. Volumes are maintained, and half the urine output is replaced, along with two to three times the estimated blood loss. Glucose-free isotonic crystalloid solutions are recommended to prevent shifts in cerebral fluids and to avoid exacerbating ischemic changes in tissue.[36, 37]

Two agents, which can be used independently or together, are frequently used to dehydrate the brain. Mannitol, an osmotic diuretic, is administered in doses of 0.25 to 1 g/kg^{-1}. Furosemide, a loop diuretic, is administered in doses of 0.5 to 1 mg/kg^{-1}. Mannitol rapidly reduces ICP for 2 to 4 hours but can transiently increase circulating volume. It should be used cautiously in patients with compromised cardiac reserve.[38] Electrolyte abnormalities can also be precipitated, and potassium may need to be replaced.[33, 39]

NEUROPHYSIOLOGIC MONITORING

Clinically useful evoked potentials for neurosurgical monitoring include somatosensory evoked potentials (SEPs) and brainstem auditory evoked potentials (BAEPs). BAEPs provide valuable information about the function of the brainstem auditory pathways during posterior fossa surgery. Cranial nerve electromyography can help identify the function of specific cranial nerves. The feasibility of monitoring motor evoked potentials to gauge the function of descending motor pathways is being investigated. This modality, which allows stimulation of the cortices via scalp electrodes, followed by evaluation of distal motor function, permits a more detailed and objective monitoring parameter for the cortical spinal pathways. Visual evoked potentials are seldom monitored because of the constraints imposed by the flash stimulus during surgery. This nonspecific, unfocused stimulus is mediated by extrageniculate pathways and, unlike patterned visual stimuli, does not correlate with visual activity. The utility of the test is limited to confirming continuity of the optic nerves only to the level of the optic chiasm. The efficacy of monitoring CBF by thermal diffusion flowmetry and Doppler flowmetry is also being evaluated.

The patient's own response to a stimulus, whether verbal, visual, or mechanical, is the most sensitive and predictive test of central nervous system function. Unfortunately, the range of responses in neurologically injured patients is often limited. The Glasgow Coma Scale was designed to stratify patient evaluation over time and institutions. Although initially designed strictly for neurotrauma patients, the Glasgow Coma Scale is a simple but reliable test that records the patient's best possible response to auditory or sensory stimuli as judged by eye opening, verbalization, and motor responses (Table 88–2). The scale ranges from a score of 15 for fully intact patients to a score of 3 (no eye opening, no verbalization, no motor response). The Glasgow Coma Scale, along with other neurological findings, can help clinicians make therapeutic decisions quickly.

In addition to their utility during neurosurgical pro-

TABLE 88–2 ■ **Glasgow Coma Scale**

BEHAVIOR	SCORE
Eyes Open	
Spontaneously	4
To verbal command	3
To pain	2
No response	1
Best Motor Response	
To verbal command	
Obeys	6
To painful stimulus	
Localizes pain	5
Flexion-withdrawal	4
Flexion-abnormal	3
Extension	2
No response	1
Best Verbal Response	
Oriented and converses	5
Disoriented and converses	4
Inappropriate words	3
Incomprehensible words	2
No response	1

cedures, multimodality monitoring that includes compressed spectral array (CSA), SEPs, and BAEPs is an effective substitute for more objective neurological testing in comatose patients or in those whose awakening after barbiturate cerebral protection is delayed.

Electroencephalography

One test of cerebral function in unresponsive or anesthetized patients is EEG. The time-varying waveform, recorded from the surface of the scalp, represents the spontaneous electrical discharge of pyramidal cells of the granular layer of the cerebral cortex.[40] Although these signals can be readily acquired and displayed as a graph of voltage change (y-axis) over time (x-axis), the ability to interpret their clinical relevance is limited.

The standard electroencephalogram is divided into four frequency bands: delta (0 to 3 Hz), theta (4 to 7 Hz), alpha (8 to 13 Hz), and beta (>13 Hz). These waves are recorded in 16 channels at a chart speed of 30 mm/sec. Interpreting 16 channels of complex waveforms requires an experienced observer.

To simplify both interpretation and record keeping, the frequency content of EEG can be reduced to just two or four channels and displayed in a compressed format for surgical applications.[41] One example of such "processed EEG" is power spectrum analysis, a frequency-time record of 2-second epochs of electroencephalographic output analyzed by a fast Fourier transform processor and displayed as a CSA (Fig. 88–1). Other techniques are zero-cross and aperiodic analysis.

EEG is sensitive to many stimuli but is not very specific for any one. Among the variables that can affect electroencephalographic activity are age, oxygen levels,[42] ischemia,[43] temperature,[44] electrolytic imbalance, hypocalcemia, endocrine disease, hypoglycemia, and anesthetic agents.[40] Older patients (78 ± 5 years), for example, are sensitive to barbiturates and display more electroencephalographic burst suppression than do younger patients (28 ± 3 years). Carbon dioxide levels higher than 100 mm Hg can either suppress the electroencephalographic waveforms or cause seizures. Calcium levels less than 5 mg/dL can also cause seizures. Hyperthyroidism can increase beta activity. Hypoxemia and reduction of CBF to less than 12 mL/100 g^{-1}/min^{-1} eliminate all spontaneous electroencephalographic activity. Temperatures below 20°C cause the progressive slowing and eventual cessation of all electroencephalographic output. Different anesthetic agents can suppress the electroencephalogram or occasionally cause seizure discharges.[45]

Electroencephalographic monitoring is most useful for detecting focal cerebral ischemia intraoperatively. Ischemia is easily identified on CSA as an asymmetrical loss of electroencephalographic frequency and power on the side of the ischemic hemisphere. It occurs in about 10% of patients after temporary occlusion of the common carotid artery during a carotid endarterectomy.[46] In many institutions, this change determines the need to place a shunt intraoperatively to restore perfusion. These changes can also occur during temporary clipping of major proximal cerebral arteries (e.g.,

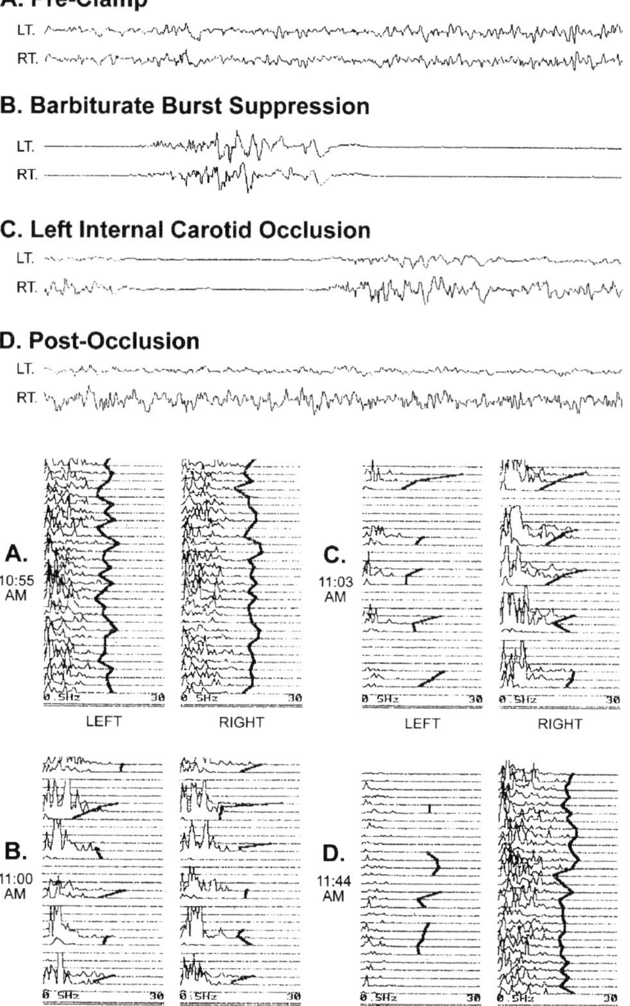

FIGURE 88–1. The electroencephalogram was recorded as a compressed spectral array (CSA) over the left and right hemispheres during left carotid endarterectomy for an 80% carotid stenosis. The top four traces show representative electroencephalographic segments corresponding to the four spectral array tracings below. Recordings were bipolar, F3-C3, F4, and C4, respectively. In the CSA, electroencephalographic epochs were 2 seconds long, displayed over a frequency range of 1 to 30 Hz. The thick line represents a 90% spectral edge. *A*, Barbiturates were infused at 10:55 AM. *B*, By 11:00 AM, a burst-suppression pattern was produced with good left-right symmetry. The typical period of electroencephalographic flattening was 4 to 10 seconds between bursts. *C*, At 11:03 AM, the left carotid artery was clamped, and the spectral pattern became asymmetrical, with a greater than 50% relative decrease in power over the left anterior hemisphere. *D*, Electroencephalographic asymmetry persisted after occlusion and after recovery from barbiturate-induced burst suppression. Postoperatively, the patient showed right hemiparesis and aphasia, which improved over time. The CSA program was written by Alexander Drachev and David Blum, M.D. (From Fisher RS, Raudzens P, Nunemacher M: Efficacy of intraoperative neurophysiological monitoring. J Clin Neurophysiol 12:97–109, 1995.)

during aneurysm or bypass surgery). If CBF falls below the patient's ischemic threshold, electroencephalographic activity is lost within 10 to 20 seconds and can be localized to the cortical "watershed" area. Typically, no neurological deficits occur if CBF is restored within 20 minutes. The longer it takes to recover electroencephalographic activity, the greater the incidence of postoperative stroke.

CSA-EEG can also be used to gauge the depth of pharmacologically induced burst suppression during high-risk cerebrovascular procedures that warrant some form of cerebral protection (e.g., administration of barbiturates). This form of monitoring facilitates cerebral protection by allowing pharmacologic agents to be titrated to their maximal effect (i.e., electroencephalographic burst suppression that corresponds to a 50% reduction in $CMRO_2$). Typically, this level of barbiturate suppression is tolerated without deleterious cardiovascular depression.[47]

Somatosensory Evoked Potentials

Unlike EEG, SEPs are sensory specific, and their amplitude (0.1 to 20 μV) is much smaller than an electroencephalographic signal (50 μV or more). SEPs are recorded from scalp electrodes placed over cortical sensory generators. The waveforms are generated after stimulation of a nerve, such as the median nerve of the upper extremity for a cortical procedure or a spinal procedure above C6, and the posterior tibial nerve of the lower extremity for lower spinal surgeries involving C6 to the lower thoracic levels. Other recording sites along the neuraxis, such as a lumbar potential, Erb's point, and a cervical potential, can be used.

The SEP signal is averaged from background electrical noise by presenting hundreds of stimuli to the patient and then filtering and amplifying the response. The process takes 3 to 5 minutes to generate individual response waveforms, which are then superimposed to demonstrate reproducibility. Finally, responses are obtained from the nonsurgical side to evaluate the possible effects of anesthetics, temperature, perfusion, and electrical artifact on response latency or amplitude. This time-consuming analysis is necessary to confirm that a recorded change in SEP is related temporally to a surgical event that may have interrupted sensory conduction in the tested pathway. Although SEPs take longer to generate than the spontaneous waveforms of the electroencephalogram, it enables sensory disturbances to be identified and corrected in time to prevent a possible postoperative neurological deficit.[17] Preservation of response morphology is consistent with functional integrity of the sensory pathway from stimulation site to sensory cortex.

SEPs are invaluable during patient positioning. The patient's head often must be rotated or positioned to optimize the exposure of a pathology. Patients with unsuspected cervical stenosis may not tolerate exaggerated positioning of the head. In such high-risk cases, we obtain baseline SEPs after the patient is intubated (sometimes before intubation) and again after the head is positioned. In a small number of patients, SEPs change markedly after head positioning, only to return to normal after the head is repositioned in the neutral position. This modality can therefore be invaluable in preventing iatrogenic and preventable causes of injury before surgery even begins.

Intraoperative SEPs are used to test spinal cord and cortical function during procedures involving spinal cord lesions, high aortic aneurysm repairs, and cerebrovascular surgery (Fig. 88–2). Although the cortical response is most altered by volatile anesthetics, the signal is more robust than the spontaneous electroencephalogram and can still be recorded at low levels of CBF (15 to 20 mL/100 g^{-1}/min^{-1}) and at low temperatures (20°C to 30°C) at which the electroencephalogram is suppressed. This feature is particularly useful in evaluating the adequacy of hemispheric perfusion after temporary clipping of cerebral vessels during aneurysm dissection.[48]

The effect of volatile anesthetics on SEPs is largely a dose-dependent increase in cortical latency and a decrease in cortical amplitude. For most volatile agents, the minimal alveolar concentration is greater than 1.5;

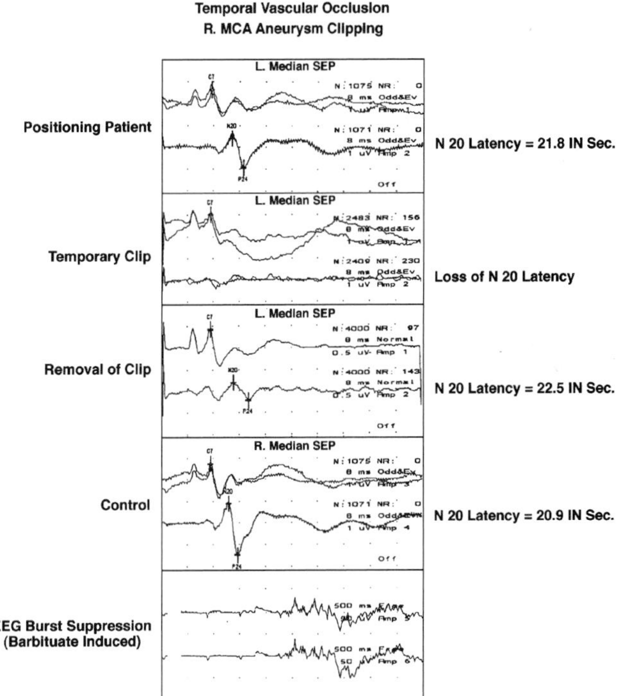

FIGURE 88–2. Neuromonitoring during cerebrovascular surgery. Both somatosensory evoked potentials (SEPs) and electroencephalography (EEG) were recorded during clipping of a right middle cerebral artery (R. MCA) aneurysm. In SEP recordings (*upper four frames*) the top tracing is from Erb's point, and the bottom is the cortical electrical potential. The Erb's point recording remains stable in all tracings and confirms the integrity of the electrophysiologic monitoring. During patient positioning, the N 20 latency of the right cortical potential tracing is robust. After temporary clipping of the right MCA, there is a loss of the N 20 cortical potential. After removal of the temporary clip, there is a return of the N 20 potential, and the patient awoke intact following surgery. The left cortical potential is used as a comparison and remains unchanged throughout the entire procedure. Simultaneous EEG recording (*last frame*) during the procedure demonstrates burst suppression.

at these values, the signal-to-noise ratio is reduced to less than 3:1, and the cortical response cannot be identified.[49–54] Even nitrous oxide in concentrations of 50% or more can degrade the SEP.[55, 56]

Intravenous anesthetics attenuate the SEP less than volatile anesthetics do and are the recommended agents for anesthetic maintenance when neurophysiologic monitoring is an important surgical adjunct.[57] In clinically effective doses, opioids have little effect on cerebral perfusion pressure. Curiously, two intravenous agents, etomidate and ketamine,[58] increase the amplitude of the SEP without changing its latency.

Temperature alters SEPs predictably. The lower the temperature, the longer the response latency, reflecting both reduced synaptic activity and delayed axonal conduction.[59, 60]

Brainstem Auditory Evoked Potentials

Intraoperatively, BAEPs are even more stable than SEPs. These short-latency responses from the auditory brainstem are recorded by far-field electrodes from the auditory relay nuclei in the medulla and pons. Like SEPs, they are pathway specific and provide information about the function of the eighth cranial nerve and some brainstem activity during exploration of lesions involving the seventh cranial nerve and posterior fossa. Because only a short extent of the brainstem is involved in generating the BAEP, the response is not sensitive to functional changes (e.g., during surgery involving the posterior circulation).[17]

ANESTHETIC AGENTS

Isoflurane is the preferred volatile anesthetic for neurological procedures. At a minimal alveolar concentration of 1.5, it causes less vasodilatation and less of an increase in CBF than do halothane (65%) and enflurane (35%).[61, 62] Isoflurane also reduces the $CMRO_2$ more than other agents do. Enflurane is undesirable because it induces hypocapnia and seizure discharges at 1.5 minimal alveolar concentration.[43] Sevoflurane, a newer volatile anesthetic, affects ICP much like isoflurane but also has demonstrated cerebral protective effects in the laboratory.[63, 64] In the future, it may be a better anesthetic choice. Another new volatile anesthetic, desflurane, increases ICP intraoperatively,[65] which may limit its usefulness. Nitrous oxide also increases CBF and ICP and should probably be avoided in patients with preexisting intracranial hypertension.

Intravenous anesthetics play an important role in neuroanesthesia. Barbiturates are used for cerebral protection because they can reduce $CMRO_2$ to 50% of normal.[66, 67] They also cause cerebral vasoconstriction,[68] a feature that can be used to reduce ICP before the dura is opened. These benefits must be weighed against the risk of cardiovascular depression at higher doses and delayed postoperative awakening.

Etomidate is a direct cerebral vasoconstrictor and reduces cerebral metabolism,[69, 70] but it exerts no clinically proven cerebral protective effect. It does not cause the same degree of hypotension that barbiturates induce, but adrenocortical suppression can occur with prolonged use.

Propofol is a new intravenous induction agent with properties that reduce $CMRO_2$ much like barbiturates do. Its cerebral protective properties have not yet been demonstrated. At higher doses, hypotension is a frequent complication.[71–73]

Benzodiazepines also reduce $CMRO_2$. The rapid-acting drug midazolam can be used as an effective anesthetic agent during the induction of neuroanesthesia.[74, 75] Its anxiolytic effect reduces undesirable sympathetic responses, and it can be combined with an opioid to prolong sympathetic suppression. Reversal with the benzodiazepine antagonist flumazenil is discouraged to prevent an increase in ICP.[76]

Opioids are used with good effect in neurosurgery. Sympathetic responses are blunted by morphine or fentanyl, which have little effect on CBF. Sufentanil has contradictory effects on ICP and CBF in different studies, but its potential to increase ICP could be overcome by hypocapnia.[77, 78]

The dissociative anesthetic ketamine[79, 80] is not used in neuroanesthesia because it increases cardiac output, $CMRO_2$, and CBF. These changes could increase the risk in a patient with preexisting intracranial hypertension.

Muscle relaxants are limited to nondepolarizing agents unless rapid-sequence intubation of the trachea is necessary. In that case, the depolarizing agent succinylcholine may be used, although hyperkalemia may develop in patients with paraplegia, closed head injury, and ruptured cerebral aneurysm.[81–83] Succinylcholine also increases ICP. Vasodilatation from nondepolarizing histamine release can cause hypotension. The histamine-releasing effect is the least with metocurine.[84] Atracurium can release laudanosine,[85] which has caused seizures in animals but is not a clinically significant problem in humans. Pancuronium is a long-acting muscle relaxant that has no effect on ICP, CBF, or $CMRO_2$.[85] Occasionally, its vagolytic properties are a problem. The most widely used agent for intubation and maintenance is vecuronium (0.10 to 0.40 mg/kg^{-1}). Good conditions for intubating can be achieved in 2 to 3 minutes without changing ICP, CBF, or hemodynamics.[86, 87]

NEUROANESTHETIC MANAGEMENT OF CEREBROVASCULAR DISORDERS

Occlusive Cerebrovascular Disease

In the management of occlusive cerebrovascular disease, it is vital for patients to undergo the appropriate preoperative evaluation of other potentially affected organ systems. Many patients who undergo surgery for occlusive extracranial vascular disease also have coexistent ischemic cardiovascular disease. Electrocardiography and, less commonly, echocardiography are indicated. A small subset of patients may need cardiac catheterization and angiography before carotid endarterectomy. In this high-risk subset of patients, cardiovascular function may be monitored intraoperatively via a Swan-Ganz catheter. We routinely monitor SEPs and CSA in patients undergoing surgery for occlusive cerebrovascular disease.

At our institution, all carotid endarterectomies are performed with patients under general inhalational anesthesia to diminish the demand for cerebral oxygen without increasing ICP. Although endarterectomies can be performed in awake patients with local anesthesia only, we believe that general inhalational anesthesia provides better patient comfort and a more relaxed surgical environment. During any portion of the procedure that involves temporary vessel occlusion, we administer barbiturates to obtain burst suppression on CSA. A bolus of heparin is also administered (3000 to 5000 U) during temporary occlusion. Artificial elevation of blood pressure above the baseline can also benefit patients during temporary occlusion by increasing systemic filling pressures and cross-circulation. Mild hypothermia may be helpful when more extended periods of temporary occlusion are anticipated. After carotid endarterectomy, a patient who develops an expanding neck mass may need emergent reintubation. Vascular shunts are used selectively as dictated by asymmetry on CSA.

In the surgical management of the rare symptomatic vertebral artery stenosis, BAEPs may also need to be monitored. Mild hypothermia is especially important during such procedures. Based on a patient's responsiveness, the amount of barbiturates used, and the function of the lower cranial nerves after a vertebral artery endarterectomy, we usually keep patients intubated overnight instead of extubating them immediately in the recovery room.

Intracranial Aneurysms

Practicing neuroanesthesiologists can expect to encounter aneurysms frequently. Although the incidence of intracranial aneurysms is about 1% based on autopsy studies, their incidence of rupture is much lower, about 1 in 8000.[88, 89] Aneurysmal rupture accounts for 80% to 90% of nontraumatic subarachnoid hemorrhage (SAH).[90, 91] SAH is reported to complicate 1 in 2000 to 10,000 pregnancies and is a leading cause of maternal death.[92, 93] The overall mortality rate associated with aneurysmal rupture is about 45% during the first year after hemorrhage. The risk of rebleeding is estimated at 3% annually. These dismal outcomes stipulate the need for therapeutic agents and techniques that offer more favorable management of aneurysms.[94]

Neurological function and symptoms are classified by Hunt and Hess grade (Table 88–3). A patient's Hunt and Hess grade at the time of initial treatment is the most important predictor of outcome. Typically, patients with a poor Hunt and Hess grade (4 or 5) at presentation have poor outcomes. Symptoms and signs associated with SAH include headache, photophobia, nausea, vomiting, systemic hypertension, and cardiac dysrhythmia. Electrocardiographic changes can be numerous and range from ST segmental abnormalities with the presence of Q and U waves to rhythmic disturbances such as bradycardia or tachycardia with associated ectopy.

The diagnostic gold standard for the evaluation of aneurysms is catheter cerebral angiography. Advances in computed tomographic angiography and magnetic resonance angiography, however, will probably lead to their replacing catheter angiography as the primary diagnostic modality in the near future.

Immediate management of ruptured aneurysms is directed at preventing further hemorrhage and controlling ICP. These patients are managed in the intensive care unit with invasive monitoring, including arterial lines, aggressive blood pressure control, and, when indicated, an intraventricular catheter. Preoperatively, patients are kept comfortable (with morphine sedatives). Tight control of blood pressure can be managed with labetalol or hydralazine hydrochloride. Nimodipine, approved by the Food and Drug Administration to help improve outcomes of patients with vasospasm, is also administered to patients with aneurysmal SAH.[16]

In preparation for surgery, patients are often sedated with 2 to 5 mg of midazolam as necessary, and blood pressure is strictly controlled. Hypertension during intubation is usually managed with a combination of sedation (Pentothal, midazolam), opioids (fentanyl, sufentanil), and beta-blockers (propranolol, labetalol, esmolol). After anesthesia has been induced, recording electrodes are applied to the patient for electroencepha-

TABLE 88–3 ■ **Hunt and Hess Neurological Grade and Surgical Risk**

GRADE	NEUROLOGICAL CRITERIA	PERIOPERATIVE MORTALITY (%)
0	Incidental aneurysm, no subarachnoid hemorrhage	0–2
1	Asymptomatic or mild headache or meningismus	0–5
2	Moderate to severe headache, nuchal rigidity, no deficit other than cranial nerve palsy	2–10
3	Drowsiness, confusion, mild focal deficit	10–15
4	Stupor, moderate to severe focal deficit, early decerebrate rigidity	60–70
5	Deep coma, decerebrate rigidity, moribund	70–100

Modified from Manninen PH, Gelb AW: Anesthesia for cerebral aneurysms and arteriovenous malformations. In Porter SS (ed): Problems in Anesthesia, vol 4. Philadelphia, Lippincott, 1990, pp 81–93.

lographic monitoring and SEP recording. Occasionally, sterile intraoperative recording leads are added. The electrophysiologic events are used to determine the levels of burst suppression and cerebral perfusion changes during surgery.

We operate early on patients with acute SAH from ruptured aneurysms. Therefore, the appropriate preoperative evaluation is of utmost importance. Many patients with acutely ruptured intracranial aneurysms develop severe pulmonary decompensation and respiratory failure (so-called neurogenic pulmonary edema). Some may also suffer myocardial infarctions or cardiovascular arrhythmias. Depending on the severity of the hemorrhage and the status of the other organ systems, the patient may also develop a coagulopathy. The appropriate coagulation parameters, including disseminated intravascular coagulation profiles, prothrombin time, partial thromboplastin time, and platelet count, must be evaluated.

During periods of temporary occlusion for aneurysm surgery, both hypothermia and pharmacologic hypertension are used with barbiturate-induced electroencephalographic burst suppression for cerebral protection. During the remainder of the procedure, however, patients may be kept mildly hypotensive or normotensive.

Intraoperatively, the surgeon is more likely to encounter elevated ICP in patients with acutely ruptured aneurysms than in those undergoing elective aneurysm surgery. In addition to mannitol and furosemide (where tolerated), barbiturates are extremely effective at providing cerebral protection and diminishing ICP. Because of their myocardial depressant effect, however, barbiturates may not be well tolerated by patients with cardiovascular compromise after SAH. ICP can also be reduced with hyperventilation and by placing a CSF diversion catheter in the ventricle or lumbar theca. In general, during aneurysm surgery, an attempt is made to keep systemic pressures at baseline levels or below, P_{CO_2} between 25 and 30 mm Hg, and fluid hydration at a minimum. Once the dura has been opened, the anesthetic requirements can be reduced because the hypertensive response to sympathetic stimulation does not occur. Anesthesia can usually be maintained with isoflurane and incremental doses of opioids or barbiturates if cerebral protection is planned. Patients must remain in burst suppression, and the mean arterial pressure must be elevated pharmacologically during periods of temporary occlusion. Any changes in the SEPs from baseline must be communicated to the surgeon. The time elapsed since the onset of temporary occlusion is also relayed to the surgeon at 2- to 5-minute intervals.

Once an aneurysm is clipped safely, an attempt is made to reduce the risk of postoperative vasospasm. Blood pressure is allowed to drift back to baseline levels or above by reducing anesthetic levels. P_{CO_2} is raised to normal capneic levels. The barbiturates are discontinued, and hydration is increased. Pulmonary capillary wedge pressure is raised to 15 to 18 mm Hg, and the hematocrit is diluted to 30% to 35% to improve perfusion.

The risks of deliberate hypotension induced with sodium nitroprusside, nitroglycerine, trimethaphan, and isoflurane are greater than the potential benefits. Instead, temporary arterial clipping should be used to control aneurysmal hemorrhage intraoperatively.[95, 96]

Moderate hypothermia (30°C to 32°C) may also be beneficial for these patients. The $CMRO_2$ decreases 7% to 13% for each degree the temperature decreases, which may provide some degree of cerebral protection.

At the end of surgery, every attempt is made to control systemic pressure and to avoid coughing or straining. Anesthesia should be maintained until the Mayfield head holder is removed and the only existing source of stimulation is the endotracheal tube. To avoid the serious complications of aspiration pneumonitis and subsequent hypercarbia, the patient should be extubated only when the appropriate response to verbal commands is observed. These procedures are often long, and drug clearance may be delayed, especially if barbiturate cerebral protection was used. Neurophysiologic monitoring is continued until a reliable neurological examination is possible.

As noted, hydrocephalus and elevated ICP are frequent complications of SAH.[97] Early surgery is usually delayed in patients with high ICP despite maximal medical therapy and ventricular CSF diversion. In our experience, patients with continuously and severely elevated ICP refractory to medical treatment do poorly after aneurysmal SAH.

The optimal timing of surgery for ruptured aneurysms is controversial. Early operation is recommended within 72 hours of the initial hemorrhage, but it should be timed to ensure that all appropriate angiographic and laboratory studies are complete and the surgical team is rested. These procedures are difficult and require an experienced, alert staff. Early surgery can potentially prevent rerupture and the need for antifibrinolytic agents such as aminocaproic acid (Amicar). The benefit of this drug in reducing the risk of early rebleeding is offset by the associated increase in ischemic complications.[2, 98]

Early clipping of aneurysms also permits aggressive treatment of vasospasm with pharmacologic hypertensive therapy. In the International Cooperative Study on the Timing of Aneurysm Surgery,[99] early surgery was not associated with a higher rate of surgical complications, and the ischemic injuries related to rebleeding were reduced, thereby improving outcomes. The mortality rate decreased to 20%, and 60% of patients had a favorable recovery. Aggressive treatment of vasospasm with calcium channel blockers and hypervolemic-hypertensive therapy lowered the mortality rate to 10%, and 75% of the patients made good recoveries. In good-grade patients (Hunt and Hess grades 1 to 3), the mortality rate was only 7%, and 81% of patients had good outcomes. Even in the high-risk, poor-grade patients, outcomes were better after early surgery than after late or nonoperative therapy.[100–103] Advocates of late surgery note that brain swelling is significantly reduced if surgery is delayed. The usual delay of 10 to 14 days, however, can be associated with about a 20%

risk of the aneurysm rerupturing.[99] The highest risk is in the 48 to 72 hours after initial rupture.

As more complex aneurysms have become amenable to surgery, a number of adjuncts have helped neurovascular surgeons obtain better outcomes. One such technique, hypothermic circulatory arrest, is used to manage giant posterior circulation aneurysms and occasionally anterior circulation aneurysms. Hypothermic circulatory arrest renders the giant aneurysm and its neck malleable by stopping intra-aneurysmal pulsatile blood flow and deflating the aneurysm. Giant calcified aneurysms should not be considered for hypothermic circulatory arrest because their hard casts do not respond to this procedure by deflating. Hypothermic circulatory arrest requires the assistance of a cardiovascular surgeon and involves cannulation of the femoral artery and vein via two large-bore catheters threaded into the right atrial appendage. Extracorporeal circulation, hypotension, and, ultimately, cardiac standstill follow. The femoral artery and vein catheters obviate the need for a thoracotomy.

Patients considered for hypothermic circulatory arrest must undergo a complete preoperative evaluation by a cardiologist and cardiovascular surgeon. Patients with preexisting cardiac conditions and peripheral vascular disease are not candidates for hypothermic circulatory arrest. Systemic heparin is administered, and extreme hypothermia to 15°C is used. Monitoring coagulation parameters is extremely important, especially during the rewarming period and during heparin reversal with protamine. Because of the prevalence of cardiac arrhythmias during rewarming, antiarrhythmic agents may be needed.

Because barbiturates are administered to patients undergoing hypothermic circulatory arrest, they are left intubated overnight in the intensive care unit. A brain computed tomographic scan is obtained that evening after surgery to rule out the presence of a postoperative surgical hematoma.

Cerebral aneurysms also can be controlled by endovascular techniques. Anesthesia for such endovascular procedures is similar to that used in general neurovascular procedures. However, because large amounts of angiographic dye are sometimes used during endovascular coiling procedures, more diligent attention must be directed to preoperative tests of renal function.

Arteriovenous Malformations

Cerebral AVMs are congenitally malformed blood vessels that shunt arterial blood directly into the venous system without the blood passing through a high-resistance capillary bed. The lesions can rupture and present as intraparenchymal hemorrhages or SAH. Mass effect or focal tissue irritation can lead to neurological deficits or seizures. Ischemia can also occur as the result of vascular steal. Men are affected twice as often as women. Like aneurysms, AVMs have a 2% to 3% annual risk of hemorrhage. The combined rate of morbidity and mortality with each hemorrhagic event is 30% to 35%. Treatment is based on the location, size, and accessibility of the lesion.

When surgical excision is planned, the anesthetic considerations are similar to those that apply to aneurysm surgery. Important concepts during AVM anesthesia include brain protection with barbiturates, mild hypothermia, and mild hypotension where indicated. The patient's hemodynamic status must be monitored during the entire procedure, because AVM ruptures cause extremely large volumes of blood to be lost in a brief period. Additional cardiovascular evaluation may be needed to supplement the routine preoperative blood work (i.e., hemoglobin, hematocrit, and coagulation profiles), electrocardiography, and chest radiography. Patients with a cardiovascular history need the appropriate medical clearance from a designated specialist. Preoperatively, a central venous line is placed, as is an arterial line. When indicated, a Swan-Ganz catheter is also placed. Because intraoperative angiography may be necessary, the anesthesiologist must be aware of the patient's renal function before surgery. Neurophysiologic monitoring for these cases includes CSA, SEPs, and cranial nerve monitoring where indicated (i.e., brainstem or cerebellar AVMs).

Owing to hemodynamic changes or previous hemorrhages, the surgeon may encounter cerebral swelling. Based on the patient's hemodynamic status, agents such as mannitol and furosemide may be administered in addition to barbiturates to help reduce ICP. In the absence of a mass lesion in the cranium, a preoperatively placed lumbar drain or ventriculostomy may also be used to help reduce ICP. We have found it helpful to have the anesthesiologist place a lumbar drain preoperatively, especially for patients with occipital lobe AVMs who will be positioned prone. Drainage of CSF from the lumbar drain prevents herniation of the occipital lobe through the craniotomy site after the dura has been opened.

Strict blood pressure control is of utmost importance during AVM surgery to prevent catastrophic surgical hemorrhage and cerebral edema. Once the resection has been completed, however, the surgeon may request artificial elevation of blood pressure to rule out potential bleeding from occult residual AVM. More recently, intraoperative angiography has been used to detect the presence of a residual AVM nidus.

The appropriate postoperative care of AVM patients is important. Meticulous blood pressure control is vital. Agents frequently used to control hypertension include labetalol, hydralazine, and enalapril (Vasotec). If the need arises, a nitroprusside drip may be used, despite the potential complications of increased ICP and cyanide and thiocyanate toxicity. In addition to the obvious risks of hemorrhage from residual AVM, brain swelling as the result of venous thrombosis is also a possibility and must be controlled by hyperventilation and antihypertensive agents. The control of postoperative hypertension is also important because of the danger of hemorrhage from surrounding tissue, or "normal perfusion pressure breakthrough."[104, 105] Normal perfusion pressure breakthrough refers to the sudden exposure of vessels surrounding an AVM to higher blood pressure after an AVM is resected. These vessels sometimes lose the ability to autoregulate to compensate for this pressure increase, and hemorrhages result. Ventriculostomy catheters can also help monitor ICP and drain CSF when indicated. Extubation of patients who have undergone AVM surgery largely depends on the complexity and size of the AVM, the amount of barbiturate used, and the location of the AVM itself. Patients who have undergone brainstem AVM surgery are kept intubated routinely for 24 hours while sedated. Patients can then be examined to rule out brainstem and lower cranial nerve deficits.

Preoperative treatment options for these complex pathologies include endovascular embolization. Embolization of deep arterial feeders in more complex, deep AVMs can facilitate surgical resection. The appropriate anesthetic care during such embolization sessions is also recommended. Preoperative stereotactic radiosurgery (e.g., gamma knife, linear accelerator) may help reduce large AVMs to more manageable sizes.

Cavernous Malformations

With the advent of magnetic resonance imaging, a large number of cerebrovascular pathologies previously designated "angiographically occult" vascular malformations are now diagnosed as cavernous malformations. If symptomatic, these lesions, for the most part, are amenable to resection based on location. Typically, patients with cerebral cavernous malformations are maintained in the euvolemic state. Barbiturates, however, are administered for cerebral protection, and CSA and SEPs are monitored. In the case of brainstem cavernous malformations, meticulous attention must be paid to brainstem functions. Therefore, the appropriate cranial nerves and BAEPs are also monitored.

Spinal Vascular Surgery

Various spinal vascular lesions are amenable to surgical or endovascular therapies: spinal AVM and fistula, spinal cavernous malformation, spinal hemangioblastoma (vascular tumor), and the rare spinal arterial aneurysm. These lesions are managed much like their cranial counterparts. Most spinal lesions are approached with the patient in a prone position. Therefore, particular attention must be paid during positioning to pad pressure points to avoid peripheral nerve palsies. A small subset of patients with spinal AVMs may need to undergo intraoperative angiography.[106]

Neurophysiologic monitoring plays a vital role during intramedullary spinal cord surgery. In addition to SEPs, we have also monitored motor evoked potential changes, which may indicate impending spinal cord injury to pyramidal pathways. While performing intramedullary spinal surgery, we have also administered the high-dose spinal cord methylprednisolone (Solu-Medrol) protocol (used for acute spinal cord injuries) to provide a measure of spinal cord protection. This strategy, however, is used on a case-by-case basis.

Most patients who undergo spinal cord surgery can be extubated at the end of the case. However, the respiratory functions of patients undergoing upper cervical or cervicomedullary surgery for vascular malformations must be monitored closely to avoid postoperative complications. Therefore, these patients may remain intubated during the early postoperative phase to ensure proper pulmonary function.

CONCLUSION

The field of neuroanesthesiology has grown tremendously, keeping pace with advances in the fields of neurosurgery and endovascular therapy. It can reasonably be expected that the surgical outcomes of patients with cerebrovascular disease will continue to improve in this new millennium. Many of the devastating postoperative neurological injuries related to cerebral ischemia can now be detected more accurately and treated more specifically with fewer complications. For example, motor evoked potentials, which detect conduction changes in descending pathways, could prevent intraoperative motor deficits. More continuous transcranial Doppler flow studies could identify early vasospasm. Newer calcium antagonists are being developed specifically to treat vasospasm. Short-acting beta-blockers are available for precise blood pressure control during the perioperative period.

Overall, the importance of preoperative optimization of patients in nonemergent cases, especially those with neurovascular pathologies, cannot be overemphasized. These factors, together with the myriad details of surgical intervention accumulated by the collective experience of skilled surgeons and anesthesiologists, are gradually improving the outcomes of patients with cerebrovascular disease.

REFERENCES

1. Fodstad H: Antifibrinolytic treatment in subarachnoid haemorrhage: Present state. Acta Neurochir (Wien) 63:233–244, 1982.
2. Kassell NF, Torner JC, Adams HP Jr: Antifibrinolytic therapy in the acute period following aneurysmal subarachnoid hemorrhage: Preliminary observations from the Cooperative Aneurysm Study. J Neurosurg 61:225–230, 1984.
3. Dernbach PD, Little JR, Jones SC, et al: Altered cerebral autoregulation and CO_2 reactivity after aneurysmal subarachnoid hemorrhage. Neurosurgery 22:822–826, 1988.
4. Ishii R: Regional cerebral blood flow in patients with ruptured intracranial aneurysms. J Neurosurg 50:587–594, 1979.
5. Voldby B, Enevoldsen EM, Jensen FT: Cerebrovascular reactivity in patients with ruptured intracranial aneurysms. J Neurosurg 62:59–67, 1985.
6. Branston NM, Hope DT, Symon L: Barbiturates in focal ischemia of primate cortex: Effects on blood flow distribution, evoked potential and extracellular potassium. Stroke 10:647–653, 1979.
7. Hoff JT, Pitts LH, Spetzler RF, et al: Barbiturates for protection from cerebral ischemia in aneurysm surgery. Acta Neurol Scand Suppl 64:158–159, 1977.
8. McDermott MW, Durity FA, Borozny M, et al: Temporary vessel occlusion and barbiturate protection in cerebral aneurysm surgery. Neurosurgery 25:54–62, 1989.
9. Nehls DG, Todd MM, Spetzler RF, et al: A comparison of the cerebral protective effects of isoflurane and barbiturates during temporary focal ischemia in primates. Anesthesiology 66:453–464, 1987.
10. Selman WR, Spetzler RF: Therapeutics for focal cerebral ischemia. Neurosurgery 6:446–452, 1980.
11. Selman WR, Spetzler RF, Anton AH, et al: Management of prolonged therapeutic barbiturate coma. Surg Neurol 15:9–10, 1981.

12. Selman WR, Spetzler RF, Roessmann UR, et al: Barbiturate-induced coma therapy for focal cerebral ischemia: Effect after temporary and permanent MCA occlusion. J Neurosurg 55: 220–226, 1981.
13. Selman WR, Spetzler RF, Roski RA, et al: Barbiturate coma in focal cerebral ischemia: Relationship of protection to timing of therapy. J Neurosurg 56:685–690, 1982.
14. Selman WR, Spetzler RF, Zabramski JM: Induced barbiturate coma. In Wilkins RH, Rengachary SS (eds): Neurosurgery. New York, McGraw-Hill, 1985, pp 343–349.
15. Silverberg GD, Reitz BA, Ream AK: Hypothermia and cardiac arrest in the treatment of giant aneurysms of the cerebral circulation and hemangioblastoma of the medulla. J Neurosurg 55: 337–346, 1981.
16. Pickard JD, Murray GD, Illingworth R, et al: Effect of oral nimodipine on cerebral infarction and outcome after subarachnoid haemorrhage: British aneurysm nimodipine trial. BMJ 298: 636–642, 1989.
17. Nuwer MR: Evoked Potential Monitoring in the Operating Room. New York, Raven Press, 1986.
18. Copper JR, Bloom FE, Roth RH: The Biochemical Basis of Neuropharmacology. New York, Oxford University Press, 1986.
19. Kandel ER, Schwartz JH: Principles of Neural Science. New York, Elsevier, 1985.
20. Siegel G, Agranoff B, Albers RW, et al: Basic Neurochemistry. New York, Raven Press, 1989.
21. Michenfelder JD: Anesthesia and the Brain. New York, Churchill Livingstone, 1988.
22. Michenfelder JD: Cerebral blood flow and metabolism. In Cucchiara RF, Michenfelder JD (eds): Clinical Neuroanesthesia. New York, Churchill Livingstone, 1990, p 1.
23. Lassen NA: Cerebral and spinal cord blood flow. In Cottrell JE, Turndorf H (eds): Anesthesia and Neurosurgery. St. Louis, CV Mosby, 1986, p 1.
24. Smith AL, Wollman H: Cerebral blood flow and metabolism: Effects of anesthetic drugs and techniques. Anesthesiology 36: 378–400, 1972.
25. Mihm FG, Cottrell JE, Hartung J, et al: Cerebral damage and pharmacological intervention. In Newfield P, Cottrell JE (eds): Neuroanesthesia: Handbook of Clinical and Physiologic Essentials. Boston, Little, Brown, 1991, p 59.
26. Siesjo BK: Cerebral circulation and metabolism. J Neurosurg 60: 883–908, 1984.
27. Strandgaard S, Olesen J, Skinhoj E, et al: Autoregulation of brain circulation in severe arterial hypertension. BMJ 1:507–510, 1973.
28. Hitchcock ER, Tsementzis SA, Dow AA: Short- and long-term prognosis of patients with a subarachnoid haemorrhage in relation to intra-operative period of hypotension. Acta Neurochir (Wien) 70:235–242, 1984.
29. Sokoloff L: Circulation and energy metabolism of the brain. In Sokoloff L (ed): Basic Neurochemistry. New York, Raven Press, 1989, p 565.
30. Lehninger AL: Principles of Biochemistry. New York, Worth, 1982.
31. Busto R, Globus MY, Dietrich WD, et al: Effect of mild hypothermia on ischemia-induced release of neurotransmitters and free fatty acids in rat brain. Stroke 20:904–910, 1989.
32. Hoffman WE, Werner C, Baughman VL, et al: Postischemic treatment with hypothermia improves outcome from incomplete cerebral ischemia in rats. J Neurosurg Anesthesiol 3:34–38, 1991.
33. Hochwald GM: Cerebrospinal fluid mechanisms. In Cottrell JE, Turndorf H (eds): Anesthesia and Neurosurgery. St. Louis, CV Mosby, 1986, p 33.
34. Bruce DA: Management of severe head injury. In Cottrell JE, Turndorf H (eds): Anesthesia and Neurosurgery. St. Louis, CV Mosby, 1986, p 150.
35. Uzzell BP, Obrist WD, Dolinskas CA, et al: Relationship of acute CBF and ICP findings to neuropsychological outcome in severe head injury. J Neurosurg 65:630–635, 1986.
36. Pulsinelli WA, Levy DE, Sigsbee B, et al: Increased damage after ischemic stroke in patients with hyperglycemia with or without established diabetes mellitus. Am J Med 74:540–544, 1983.
37. Welsh FA, Ginsberg MD, Rieder W, et al: Deleterious effect of glucose pretreatment on recovery from diffuse cerebral ischemia in the cat. II. Regional metabolite levels. Stroke 11:355–363, 1980.
38. Muizelaar JP, Lutz HA, Becker DP: Effect of mannitol on ICP and CBF and correlation with pressure autoregulation in severely head-injured patients. J Neurosurg 61:700–706, 1984.
39. Lundberg N: Monitoring of the intracranial pressure. In Critchley M, O'Leary JL, Jennett B (eds): Scientific Foundations of Neurology. Philadelphia, FA Davis, 1972, p 356.
40. Kiloh LG, McComas AJ, Osselton JW, et al: The neural basis of the EEG. In Kiloh LG, McComas AJ, Osselton JW (eds): Clinical Electroencephalography. London, Butterworth, 1981, p 24.
41. Levy WJ, Shapiro HM, Maruchak G, et al: Automated EEG processing for intraoperative monitoring: A comparison of techniques. Anesthesiology 53:223–236, 1980.
42. Woodbury DM, Rollins LT, Gardner MD, et al: Effects of carbon dioxide on brain excitability and electrolytes. Am J Physiol 192: 79, 1958.
43. Michenfelder JD, Cucchiara RF: Canine cerebral oxygen consumption during enflurane anesthesia and its modification during induced seizures. Anesthesiology 40:575–580, 1974.
44. Levy WJ: Quantitative analysis of EEG changes during hypothermia. Anesthesiology 60:291–297, 1984.
45. Spackman TN, Faust RJ, Cucchiari RF, et al: A comparison of aperiodic analysis of the EEG with standard EEG and cerebral blood flow for detection of ischemia. Anesthesiology 66:229–231, 1987.
46. Chiappa KH, Burke SR, Young RR: Results of electroencephalographic monitoring during 367 carotid endarterectomies: Use of a dedicated minicomputer. Stroke 10:381–388, 1979.
47. Spetzler RF, Hadley MN, Rigamonti D, et al: Aneurysms of the basilar artery treated with circulatory arrest, hypothermia, and barbiturate cerebral protection. J Neurosurg 68:868–879, 1988.
48. Symon L, Momma F, Murota T: Assessment of reversible cerebral ischaemia in man: Intraoperative monitoring of the somatosensory evoked response. Acta Neurochir Suppl (Wien) 42:3–7, 1988.
49. Peterson DO, Drummond JC, Todd MM: Effects of halothane, enflurane, isoflurane, and nitrous oxide on somatosensory evoked potentials in humans. Anesthesiology 65:35–40, 1986.
50. Pathak KS, Amaddio MD, Scoles PV, et al: Effects of halothane, enflurane, and isoflurane in nitrous oxide on multilevel somatosensory evoked potentials. Anesthesiology 70:207–212, 1989.
51. Domino EF, Corssen G, Sweet RB: Effects of various general anesthetics on the visually evoked response in man. Anesth Analg 42:735, 1963.
52. Uhl RR, Squires KC, Bruce DL, et al: Effect of halothane anesthesia on the human cortical visual evoked response. Anesthesiology 53:273–276, 1980.
53. Dubois MY, Sato S, Chassy J, et al: Effects of enflurane on brainstem auditory evoked responses in humans. Anesth Analg 61:898–902, 1982.
54. Manninen PH, Lam AM, Nicholas JF: The effects of isoflurane and isoflurane–nitrous oxide anesthesia on brainstem auditory evoked potentials in humans. Anesth Analg 64:43–47, 1985.
55. McPherson RW, Mahla M, Johnson R, et al: Effects of enflurane, isoflurane, and nitrous oxide on somatosensory evoked potentials during fentanyl anesthesia. Anesthesiology 62:626–633, 1985.
56. Sloan TB, Koht A: Depression of cortical somatosensory evoked potentials by nitrous oxide. Br J Anaesth 57:849–852, 1985.
57. McPherson RW, Sell B, Traystman RJ: Effects of thiopental, fentanyl, and etomidate on upper extremity somatosensory evoked potentials in humans. Anesthesiology 65:584–589, 1986.
58. Koht A, Schutz W, Schmidt G, et al: Effects of etomidate, midazolam, and thiopental on median nerve somatosensory evoked potentials and the additive effects of fentanyl and nitrous oxide. Anesth Analg 67:435–441, 1988.
59. Stockard JJ, Sharbrough FW, Tinker JA: Effects of hypothermia on the human brainstem auditory response. Ann Neurol 3: 368–370, 1978.
60. Dubois M, Coppola R, Buchsbaum MS, et al: Somatosensory evoked potentials during whole body hyperthermia in humans. Electroencephalogr Clin Neurophysiol 52:157–162, 1981.
61. Boarini DJ, Kassell NF, Coester HC, et al: Comparison of systemic and cerebrovascular effects of isoflurane and halothane. Neurosurgery 15:400–409, 1984.
62. Todd MM, Drummond JC: A comparison of the cerebrovascular

and metabolic effects of halothane and isoflurane in the cat. Anesthesiology 60:276–282, 1984.
63. Scheller MS, Tateishi A, Drummond JC, et al: The effects of sevoflurane on cerebral blood flow, cerebral metabolic rate for oxygen, intracranial pressure, and the electroencephalogram are similar to those of isoflurane in the rabbit. Anesthesiology 68: 548–551, 1988.
64. Werner C, Kochs E, Hoffman WE, et al: The effects of sevoflurane on neurological outcome from incomplete ischemia in rats. J Neurosurg Anesthesiol 3:237, 1991.
65. Lutz LJ, Milde JH, Milde LN: The cerebral functional, metabolic, and hemodynamic effects of desflurane in dogs. Anesthesiology 73:125–131, 1990.
66. Pierce EC, Lambersten CJ, Deutsch S, et al: Cerebral circulation and metabolism during thiopental anesthesia and hyperventilation in man. J Clin Invest 41:1664, 1964.
67. Michenfelder JD: The interdependency of cerebral functional and metabolic effects following massive doses of thiopental in the dog. Anesthesiology 41:231–236, 1974.
68. Shapiro HM, Galindo A, Wyte SR, et al: Rapid intraoperative reduction of intracranial pressure with thiopentone. Br J Anaesth 45:1057–1062, 1973.
69. Renou AM, Vernhiet J, Macrez P, et al: Cerebral blood flow and metabolism during etomidate anaesthesia in man. Br J Anaesth 50:1047–1051, 1978.
70. Milde LN, Milde JH, Michenfelder JD: Cerebral functional, metabolic, and hemodynamic effects of etomidate in dogs. Anesthesiology 63:371–377, 1985.
71. Dam M, Ori C, Pizzolato G, et al: The effects of propofol anesthesia on local cerebral glucose utilization in the rat. Anesthesiology 73:499–505, 1990.
72. Van Hemelrijck J, Fitch W, Mattheussen M, et al: Effect of propofol on cerebral circulation and autoregulation in the baboon. Anesth Analg 71:49–54, 1990.
73. Pinaud M, Lelausque JN, Chetanneau A, et al: Effects of propofol on cerebral hemodynamics and metabolism in patients with brain trauma. Anesthesiology 73:404–409, 1990.
74. Nugent M, Artru AA, Michenfelder JD: Cerebral metabolic, vascular and protective effects of midazolam maleate: Comparison to diazepam. Anesthesiology 56:172–176, 1982.
75. Forster A, Juge O, Morel D: Effects of midazolam on cerebral blood flow in human volunteers. Anesthesiology 56:453–455, 1982.
76. Fleischer JE, Milde JH, Moyer TP, et al: Cerebral effects of high-dose midazolam and subsequent reversal with Ro 15-1788 in dogs. Anesthesiology 68:234–242, 1988.
77. Milde LN, Milde JH, Gallagher WJ: Effects of sufentanil on cerebral circulation and metabolism in dogs. Anesth Analg 70: 138–146, 1990.
78. Marx W, Shah N, Long C, et al: Sufentanil, alfentanil, and fentanyl: Impact on cerebrospinal fluid pressure in patients with brain tumors. J Neurosurg Anesthesiol 1:3, 1989.
79. Davis DW, Mans AM, Biebuyck JF, et al: The influence of ketamine on regional brain glucose use. Anesthesiology 69: 199–205, 1988.
80. Takeshita H, Okuda Y, Sari A: The effects of ketamine on cerebral circulation and metabolism in man. Anesthesiology 36: 69–75, 1972.
81. Cooperman LH, Strobel GE Jr, Kennell EM: Massive hyperkalemia after administration of succinylcholine. Anesthesiology 32:161–164, 1970.
82. Stevenson PH, Birch AA: Succinylcholine-induced hyperkalemia in a patient with a closed head injury. Anesthesiology 51: 89–90, 1979.
83. Iwatsuki N, Kuroda N, Amaha K, et al: Succinylcholine-induced hyperkalemia in patients with ruptured cerebral aneurysms. Anesthesiology 53:64–67, 1980.
84. Vesely R, Hoffman WE, Gil KS, et al: The cerebrovascular effects of curare and histamine in the rat. Anesthesiology 66:519–523, 1987.
85. Lanier WL, Milde JH, Michenfelder JD: The cerebral effects of pancuronium and atracurium in halothane-anesthetized dogs. Anesthesiology 63:589–597, 1985.
86. Stirt JA, Maggio W, Haworth C, et al: Vecuronium: Effect on intracranial pressure and hemodynamics in neurosurgical patients. Anesthesiology 67:570–573, 1987.
87. Ginsberg B, Glass PS, Quill T, et al: Onset and duration of neuromuscular blockade following high-dose vecuronium administration. Anesthesiology 71:201–205, 1989.
88. Chason JL, Hindman WM: Berry aneurysms of the circle of Willis: Results of a planned autopsy study. Neurology (NY) 8: 41, 1958.
89. Cohen MM: Cerebrovascular accidents: Study of 201 cases. Arch Pathol 60:296, 1955.
90. Ingall TJ, Whisnant JP, Wiebers DO, et al: Has there been a decline in subarachnoid hemorrhage mortality? Stroke 20:718–724, 1989.
91. Suzuki S, Kayama T, Sakurai Y, et al: Subarachnoid hemorrhage of unknown cause. Neurosurgery 21:310–313, 1987.
92. Hunt HB, Schifrin BS, Suzuki K: Ruptured berry aneurysms and pregnancy. Obstet Gynecol 43:827–837, 1974.
93. Biller J, Adams HP Jr: Cerebrovascular disorders associated with pregnancy. Am Fam Physician 33:125–132, 1986.
94. Jane JA, Kassell NF, Torner JC, et al: The natural history of aneurysms and arteriovenous malformations. J Neurosurg 62: 321–323, 1985.
95. Ausman JI, Diaz FG, Malik GM, et al: Management of cerebral aneurysms: Further facts and additional myths. Surg Neurol 32: 21–35, 1989.
96. Jabre A, Symon L: Temporary vascular occlusion during aneurysm surgery. Surg Neurol 27:47–63, 1987.
97. Lobato RD, Rivas JJ, Portillo JM, et al: Prognostic value of the intracranial pressure levels during the acute phase of severe head injuries. Acta Neurochir Suppl (Wien) 28:70–73, 1979.
98. Vermeulen M, Lindsay KW, Murray GD, et al: Antifibrinolytic treatment in subarachnoid hemorrhage. N Engl J Med 311: 432–437, 1984.
99. Adams HP Jr, Kassell NF, Torner JC, et al: Predicting cerebral ischemia after aneurysmal subarachnoid hemorrhage: Influences of clinical condition, CT results, and antifibrinolytic therapy. A report of the Cooperative Aneurysm Study. Neurology 37:1586–1591, 1987.
100. Auer LM: Acute operation and preventive nimodipine improve outcome in patients with ruptured cerebral aneurysms. Neurosurgery 15:57–66, 1984.
101. Ljunggren B, Brandt L, Saveland H, et al: Outcome in 60 consecutive patients treated with early aneurysm operation and intravenous nimodipine. J Neurosurg 61:864–873, 1984.
102. Ljunggren B, Saveland H, Brandt L, et al: Early operation and overall outcome in aneurysmal subarachnoid hemorrhage. J Neurosurg 62:547–551, 1985.
103. Ohman J, Heiskanen O: Timing of operation for ruptured supratentorial aneurysms: A prospective randomized study. J Neurosurg 70:55–60, 1989.
104. Drake CG: Arteriovenous malformations of the brain: The options for management. N Engl J Med 309:308–310, 1983.
105. Graf CJ, Perret GE, Torner JC: Bleeding from cerebral arteriovenous malformations as part of their natural history. J Neurosurg 58:331–337, 1983.
106. Schievink WI, Vishteh AG, McDougall CG, et al: Intraoperative spinal angiography. J Neurosurg 90:48–51, 1999.

CHAPTER **89**

Intraoperative Cerebral Protection

WARREN R. SELMAN ■ CHRISTOPHER L. TAYLOR
W. DAVID LUST ■ ROBERT A. RATCHESON

Paradigms for understanding the pathophysiology of ischemic injury have become more complex as understanding of the mechanisms of cell death have expanded. The processes that occur between energy failure and cell death immediately after vessel occlusion now are being understood more clearly. Ischemia triggers many diverse biochemical and molecular biologic cascades, including active nuclear processes involving transcription and translation, which can injure the cell. Although necrosis is the predominant mode of cell death after prolonged focal ischemia, apoptosis can be observed after a transient interruption of blood flow. An understanding of the pathways leading to ischemic cell death is necessary to appreciate what measures can be taken to afford neural protection during cerebrovascular procedures.

PATHOPHYSIOLOGY OF ISCHEMIC INJURY

Cerebral Blood Flow Thresholds

In 1948, Kety and Schmidt[1] quantified normal cerebral blood flow (CBF) in "healthy young men" and found that it was 54 mL/100 g/minute. Sundt and others[2, 3] measured CBF during carotid endarterectomy and noted that CBF greater than 18 mL/100 g/minute was necessary to maintain a normal electroencephalogram (EEG). It is not until CBF is reduced to 6 to 12 mL/100 g/minute that the integrity of the cell membrane is inevitably lost,[4–8] as evidenced by a dramatic increase in the level of extracellular potassium (Fig. 89–1).

Ischemic Penumbra

In laboratory and clinical settings, occlusion of a large intracranial artery results in a spectrum of affected neurons. In the center of the affected territory, there is a *core* of irreversibly damaged cells surrounded by an area of electrically silent but physiologically viable cells. This area is known as the *ischemic penumbra*, analogous to the half-shaded zone around the center of a complete solar eclipse.[4, 9–11] The membranes of cells in the ischemic core rapidly lose their integrity and viability as evidenced by an elevated concentration of extracellular potassium. Cells in the penumbra receive sufficient blood flow to maintain the integrity of their membranes but cannot generate synaptic activity, as manifested by a loss of electroencephalographic or evoked potential activity.

If blood flow is reestablished within a brief time, these cells can recover their normal function. Not only the degree, however, but also the duration of ischemia determines whether the cells in the affected territory recover or are injured irreversibly (Fig. 89–2).[12] Although a time frame of hours of ischemic tolerance has been determined in experimental models, evidence suggests that the duration of safe occlusion may be in the range of minutes in a clinical setting.[13–16] *Cerebral protection* strategies have been used to extend the safe threshold of occlusion time. These protection schemes are intended to block primary or secondary events in the pathophysiologic alterations associated with ischemia.

Energy Failure

The most immediate biochemical change in neurons subjected to ischemia is the change from aerobic to anaerobic glycolysis. Cells that are unable to oxidize pyruvate further because sufficient oxygen is unavailable accumulate lactic acid from a reaction catalyzed by lactic dehydrogenase. Diminished blood flow also limits the removal of lactate. Lactic acidosis can impair cytoplasmic and mitochondrial enzyme activity. A decrease in pH less than 6.0 produces cerebral infarction when CBF and oxygen delivery are maintained at normal levels.[17]

Anaerobic glycolysis cannot generate the amount of adenosine triphosphate (ATP) that is obtained normally by oxidative phosphorylation. The energy failure that results from the decreased blood flow leads to impairment of the ability to maintain normal ionic gradients across the cell membrane. Neurons and glia ultimately depolarize as a result of the energy depletion, and somatodendritic and presynaptic voltage-dependent calcium channels become activated leading

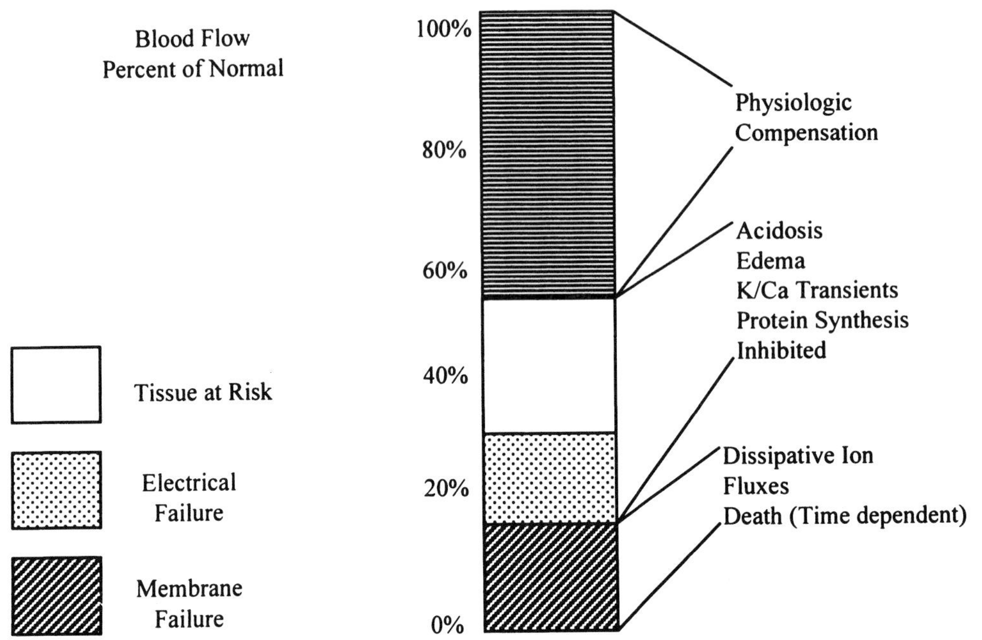

FIGURE 89-1. Cerebral blood thresholds for critical functions. (Adapted from Astrup J, Symon L, Branston NM, et al: Cortical evoked potential and extracellular K^+ and H^+ at critical levels of brain ischemia. Stroke 8:51–57, 1977.)

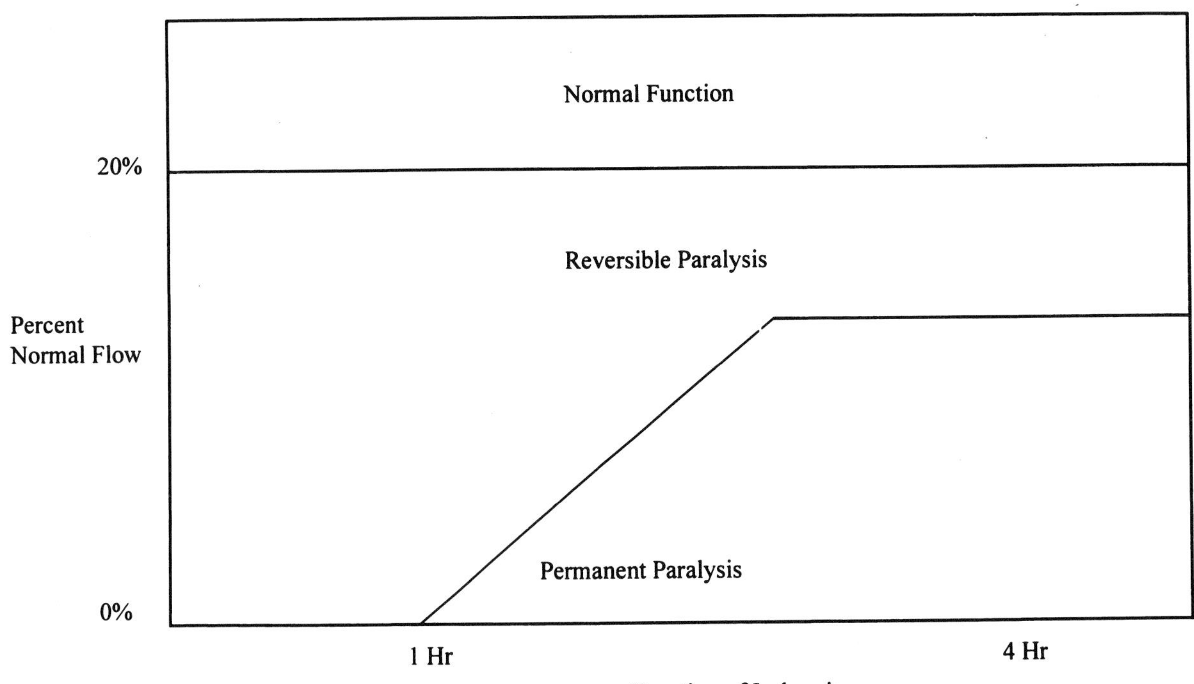

FIGURE 89-2. Relation between time of ischemia and reversibility of neurological deficit. (Adapted from Jones TH, Morawetz RB, Crowell RM, et al: Thresholds of focal cerebral ischemia in awake monkeys. J Neurosurg 54:773–782, 1981.)

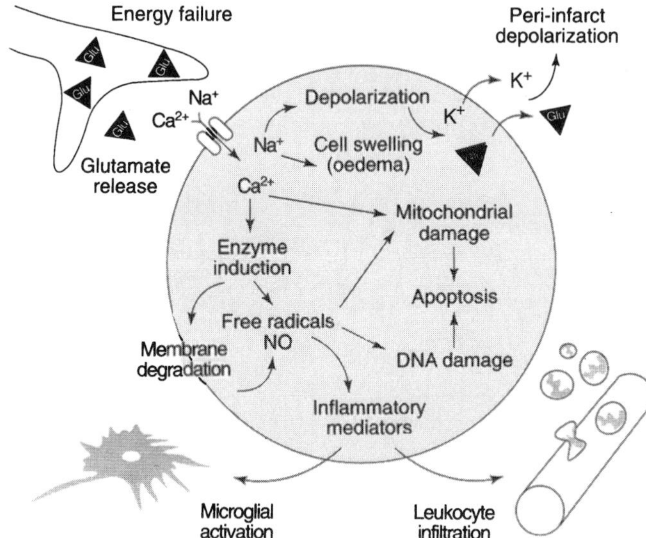

FIGURE 89-3. Simplified overview of pathophysiologic mechanisms in the focally ischemic brain. Energy failure leads to the depolarization of neurons. Activation of specific glutamate receptors dramatically increases intracellular levels of Ca^{2+}, Na^{+}, and Cl, whereas K^{+} is released into the extracellular space. Diffusion of glutamate (Glu) and K^{+} in the extracellular space can propagate a series of spreading waves of depolarization (peri-infarct depolarizations). Water shifts to the intracellular space via osmotic gradients, and cells swell (edema). The universal intracellular messenger Ca^{2+} overactivates numerous enzyme systems (e.g., proteases, lipases, endonucleases). Free radicals, which damage membranes (lipolysis), mitochondria, and DNA, are generated and in turn trigger caspase-mediated cell death (apoptosis). Free radicals also induce the formation of inflammatory mediators, which activate microglia and lead to the invasion of blood-borne inflammatory cells. (From Dirnagl U, Iadecola C, Moskowitz MA: Pathobiology of ischaemic stroke: An integrated view. Trends Neurosci 22:391–397, 1999. With permission from Elsevier Science.)

to the release of excitatory amino acids (Fig. 89–3). Activation of excitatory amino acid receptors contributes to intracellular overload of calcium. The ability to maintain the intracellular homeostasis of calcium is impaired if the amount of ATP is insufficient, and an altered concentration of intracellular calcium is central to many ischemia-related injury processes. The detrimental effects of abnormally elevated levels of intracellular calcium are due to the sustained release of excitatory amino acids *(excitotoxicity)*, overactivation of degradative enzymes, alterations in the activity of protein kinases, inhibition of mitochondrial oxidative phosphorylation, and secondary generation of reactive oxygen species.[18]

Altered Calcium Homeostasis

Depolarization mediated by energy failure leads to an initial influx of calcium through voltage-sensitive channels. Calcium-mediated activation of glutamate receptors results in further accumulation of intracellular calcium through agonist-sensitive channels (Fig. 89–4). The central role of calcium in mediating ischemic neuronal cell death initially was suggested in the 1980s and has been refined since.[18, 19] Energy failure leads to disturbances in homeostasis of the calcium ion and to an accumulation of intracellular calcium. These imbalances initiate a series of cytoplasmic and nuclear events: activation of proteolytic enzymes that degrade cytoskeletal proteins; activation of phospholipase A_2 and cyclooxygenase, which generate free radical species producing lipid peroxidation; and membrane damage.[20]

Excitotoxicity

In the presence of compromised energy stores, increased glutamate efflux and a failure of glutamate uptake can lead to a toxic elevation of extracellular glutamate. Glutamate neurotoxicity has been modeled as a three-stage process.[21–23] The calcium-mediated release of glutamate from depolarized neurons plays a major role in ischemic cell death.[21, 23, 24] In experimental models of ischemia, the levels of glutamate immediately and profoundly increase.[25] Glutamate binds to four classes of receptors: *N*-methyl-D-aspartate (NMDA) receptors that gate cation channels highly permeable to Ca^{2+}, two types of non-NMDA cation channels (α-amino-3-hydroxy-5-methylisoxazole-4-propionate [AMPA] and kainate) with variable permeability to Ca^{2+}, and metabotropic glutamate receptors that are coupled to G proteins. Under normal conditions, Mg^{2+} blocks the NMDA receptor, but this process is displaced in the setting of membrane deplorization and Ca^{2+} influx. The uptake of glutamate from the extracellular space is an energy-dependent process. It is believed that glial cells are primarily responsible for removing glutamate from the synaptic cleft.

In the penumbral region, cells can repolarize but at the expense of further energy consumption. In response to a continued increase in extracellular glutamate or potassium concentration, repetitive depolarizations, *peri-infarct depolarizations*, occur.[26] Such depolarizations have been recorded for 6 to 8 hours after an initial ischemic insult.[20] The depletion of energy stores for restoration of normal polarization is thought to contribute to the enlargement of an infarct.

Reactive Oxygen Species

Free radicals are highly reactive owing to the presence of an unpaired electron in their outer orbit. Free radicals target oxygen; transition metals; iron-sulfur clusters containing proteins; and heme-containing proteins that cause damage by inhibiting oxidative phosphorylation, glycolysis, and mitochondrial respiration and that directly damage deoxyribonucleic acid (DNA). Although free radicals can form during the period of ischemia, it is during the period of reperfusion, when oxygen returns to the ischemic regions, that most reactive oxygen species are formed. *Reperfusion injury* refers to the deleterious effects that result from the resumption of normal blood flow to a previously ischemic region.

One of the more widely studied free radicals is nitric oxide (NO). NO is synthesized from L-arginine and molecular oxygen by NO synthetase (NOS).[27] Three

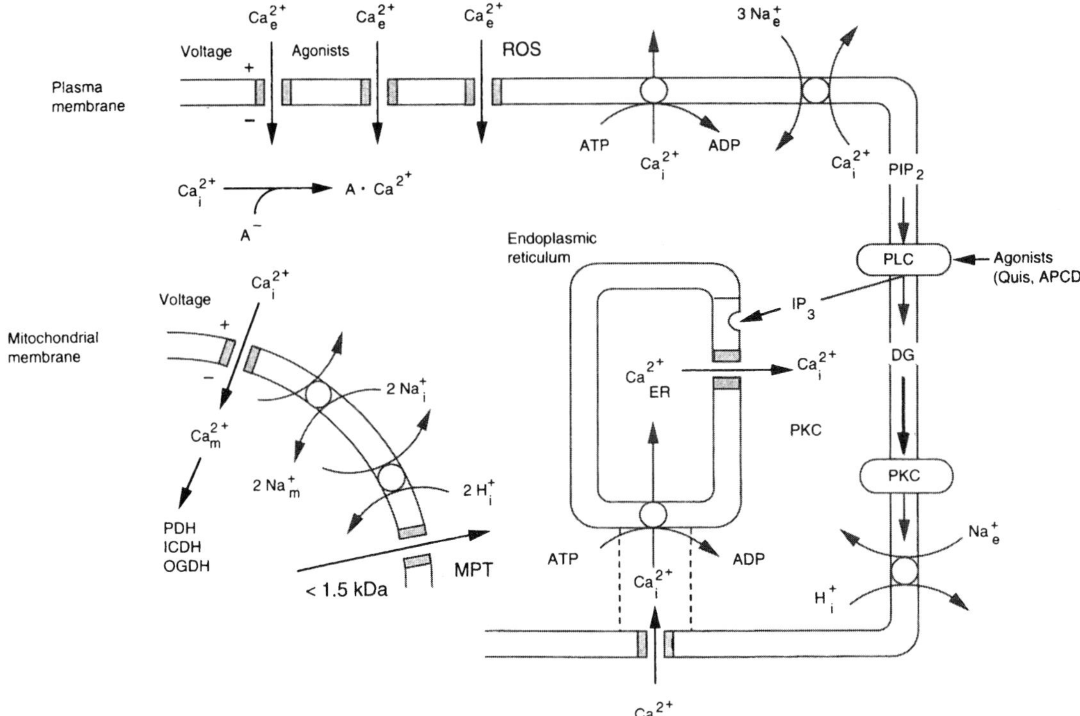

FIGURE 89-4. Calcium handling by cells. The calcium enters the cell through voltage-operated and agonist-operated channels and by more nonspecific channels, such as those opened by reactive oxygen species, whereas Ca^{2+} is extruded from the cell by an adenosine triphosphate (ATP)–driven pump or by Ca^{2+}-Na^+ exchange. Cystolic calcium (Ca_i^{2+}) is sequestered by mitochondria and endoplasmic reticulum (ER) at the expense of respiratory energy or ATP, and it is bound to calcium-binding molecules. Ca^{2+} is released from ER in response to agonist activation of receptors coupled to phospholipase C (PLC) and the formation of IP_3 from phosphatidyl inositol bisphosphate (PIP_2). A rise in (Ca_i^{2+} can cause translocation of protein kinase C (PKC) to membranes where the kinase may be activated by diglycerides (DG) formed during PIP_2 hydrolysis. Accumulation of Ca^{2+} in mitochondria can lead to the activation of an MPT (mitochondrial permeability transition) pore, leading to the release of Ca^{2+} and other molecules with molecular weights up to 1.5 kDa from intramitochondrial compartments. Quis, quisqualate; APCD, 1-aminocyclopentane-1S, 3R-dicarboxylic acid; PDH, pyruvate dehydrogenase; ICDH, isocitrate dehydrogenase; OGDH, oxoglutarate dehydrogenase ROS, reactive oxygen species. (From Kristian T, Siesjo BK: Calcium in ischemic cell death. Stroke 29: 707–718, 1998. With permission from Lippincott Williams & Wilkins.)

types of NOS have been described. Ca^{2+}-dependent neuronal NOS (nNOS) and endothelial NOS (eNOS) are constitutively expressed, whereas the Ca^{2+}-independent immunologic NOS (iNOS) is expressed in activated macrophages and other inflammatory cells.[28] Although NO may have a beneficial effect in ischemia at physiologic concentrations by acting as a vasodilator (previously identified as endothelium-derived relaxing factor),[29–31] deleterious effects resulting from direct neuronal toxicity can occur. NO is known to activate the nuclear enzyme poly (ADP-ribose) synthetase, leading to the depletion of cellular ATP.[32] Sustained production of NO by overstimulation of Ca^{2+}-mediated nNOS and induced iNOS during cerebral ischemia can cause neuronal death.[33–36]

Arachidonic Acid Metabolites

Cerebral ischemia and reperfusion lead to the accumulation of free fatty acids, in particular arachidonic acid. Arachidonic acid is released during ischemia by alteration of phosphatidylcholine synthesis from 1,2-diacylglycerol and the action of phospholipases. Metabotropic glutamate receptors and increases in intracellular calcium can activate phospholipase C and phospholipase A_2.[37] One possible link between excitotoxicity and peroxidative damage is that lipid peroxidation initiated by peroxynitrite, which is formed from the reaction of NO with the superoxide radical, releases arachidonic acid from cell membranes. Arachidonic acid is a substrate for the lipoxygenase and cyclooxygenase systems, which produce leukotriene C_4, prostaglandin E_2, and free radicals by oxidative metabolism. Leukotriene C_4, prostaglandin E_2, and arachidonic acid all are believed to be involved in producing neuronal death.[38]

Inflammatory Response

Reperfusion facilitates the arrival of inflammatory cells to the ischemic zone, and postischemic inflammation contributes to ischemic injury in several ways.[39] Inflammatory cells are responsible for the production of proteolytic enzymes and reactive oxygen species, which, as outlined previously, cause direct neuronal damage. The inflammatory process also contributes to ischemic injury by compromising blood flow in the microcirculation.[40–42] Postischemic inflammation is enhanced by chemoattractants, such as platelet-activating factor and interleukin-8, and is mediated by up-regulation of adhesion molecules, including selectins, integrins (CD11/CD18), and the immunoglobulin supergene family.[42] Tumor necrosis factor and interleukin-1 up-regulate selectins and intercellular adhesion molecule-1 (ICAM-1).

Apoptosis

As opposed to the unregulated and always pathologic process of cell necrosis, apoptosis is a highly regulated and selective homeostatic mechanism that eliminates cells that are beyond their useful life span. Apoptosis is a late manifestation of focal cerebral ischemia, although the events that trigger this process probably occur earlier. Synthesis of proteins from genes that promote apoptosis is required before programmed cell death occurs.[43]

Precisely how ischemia triggers apoptotic mechanisms is unknown. Genes involved in the regulation of programmed cell death may inhibit or promote this process. The gene product *Bcl-2* is thought to protect cells by suppressing lipid peroxidation, regulating an antioxidant pathway at sites in the mitochondria, endoplasmic reticula, and nuclear membranes where free radicals are generated.[44] Experimental studies reveal great variability in the expression of different gene families after ischemia, and the variability may be related to differences in the type, degree, and duration of ischemia (Fig. 89–5).[45] The increased production of destructive proteins may be activated by the increased activity of reactive oxygen species.[46]

Key destructive proteins in apoptosis are endonucleases and proteases. Endonucleases cleave DNA into oligonucleosomal fragments. The interleukin-1 beta-converting enzyme (ICE) family of proteases is the most highly conserved gene product involved in apoptosis. The calpain family of proteases is activated by calcium. Apoptosis may be differentiated from necrosis by the formation of DNA degradation products consisting of oligonucleosomal fragments in the former. These DNA fragments, indicating late neuronal death through apoptotic mechanisms, have been observed after focal ischemia by many investigators.[47–49] The relative contribution of apoptosis versus necrosis in the overall volume of cell death after cerebral ischemia is yet to be determined.

Integration of Injury Mechanisms

In the setting of focal ischemia, the biochemical changes discussed previously occur in a dynamic and highly interrelated fashion that may lead to a variety of end points. If adequate collateral circulation is available and the ischemia is sufficiently brief, temporary focal ischemia may be tolerated without any histologic or clinically evident sequelae. This situation can occur when perfusion through collateral channels maintains blood flow above that required for membrane integrity (approximately 10 mL/100 g/minute). As described previously, in the absence of sufficient collateral blood flow, cells in the ischemic core undergo necrosis-disorganized cell death. The prolonged survival of cells in the penumbral zone is not guaranteed by reperfusion,

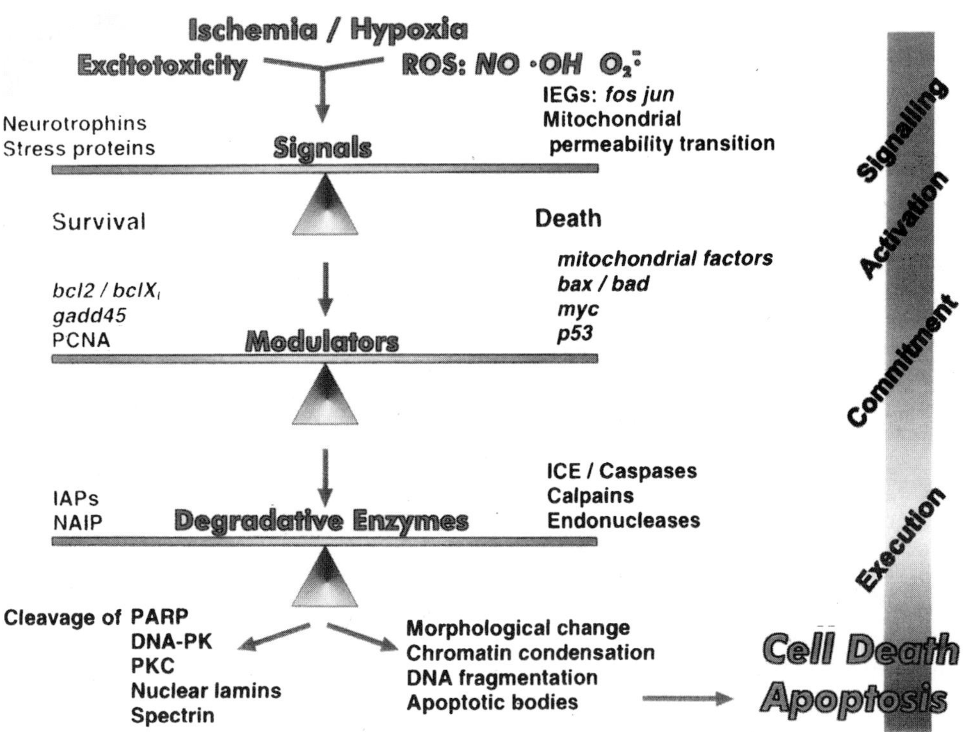

FIGURE 89-5. There are several steps between the initial hypoxic-ischemic insult and frank neuronal death. Within this cell death cascade, several molecules and proteins facilitate neuronal survival and compete with factors that contribute to the cell death cascade. Ultimately the balance between survival factors and death factors determines the fate of the cell. Pharmacologic approaches to stroke can be directed at facilitating the survival factors or inhibiting the cell death machinery, with the goal of preserving neurons until reperfusion and reoxygenation of the tissue can be established. (From MacManus JP, Linnik MD: Gene expression induced by cerebral ischemia: An apoptotic perspective. J Cereb Blood Flow Metab 17:815–832, 1997. With permission from Lippincott Williams & Wilkins.)

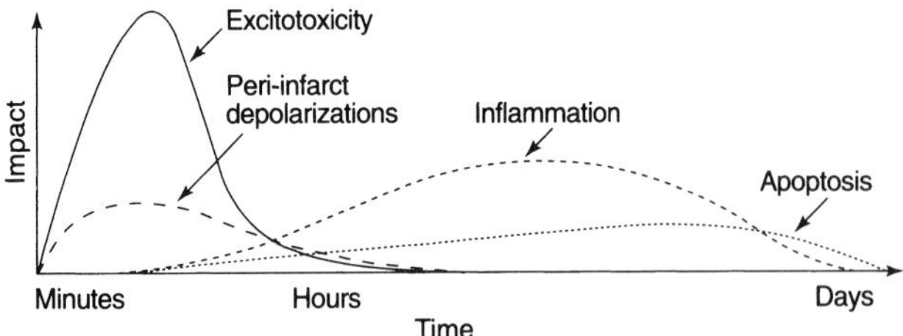

FIGURE 89-6. Putative cascade of damaging events in focal cerebral ischemia. Early after the onset of the focal perfusion deficit, excitotoxic mechanisms can damage neurons and glia lethally. Excitotoxicity triggers many events that can contribute further to the demise of the tissue. Such events include peri-infarct depolarizations and the more delayed mechanisms of inflammation and programmed cell death. The *x*-axis reflects the evolution of the cascade over time, whereas the *y*-axis illustrates the impact of each element of the cascade on final outcome. (From Dirnagl U, Iadecola C, Moskowitz MA: Pathobiology of ischaemic stroke: An integrated view. Trends Neurosci 22:391–397, 1999. With permission from Elsevier Science.)

however. These cells remain at risk because of the possibility of reperfusion injury and the occurrence in some instances of apoptosis or programmed cell death (Fig. 89–6).

CYTOPROTECTIVE STRATEGIES FOR FOCAL ISCHEMIA

Several strategies may be used in an attempt to provide cytoprotection during cerebrovascular procedures. Limiting the duration of ischemia is probably the most intuitive and direct method of reducing ischemic injury. Residual blood flow through collateral channels can be increased by induced hypertension. Decreasing the metabolic activity of tissue at risk can be achieved by lowering core temperature and by the use of certain anesthetic agents. A variety of pharmacologic agents have been tested in patients with ischemic stroke. Although not currently in routine use during surgery, cytoprotective agents with proven efficacy for treating ischemic stroke may benefit patients with temporary intraoperative ischemia.

Limiting Duration of Ischemia

The duration of focal ischemia that can be employed safely without clinically evident sequelae varies among individuals and different vascular territories.[50–54] Whether repetitive temporary occlusion for brief periods can provide increased safety as compared with a single episode of occlusion in intraoperative use remains unclear.

Reports of laboratory studies of multiple ischemic events in *focal* models have shown varying results.[54–58] Sakaki and coworkers[55] examined the response of cats to three 20-minute episodes of middle cerebral artery (MCA) occlusion compared with a single 1-hour period. The intermittent occlusion produced less damage than the single, longer occlusion. This report did not specify the length of reperfusion between the episodes of ischemia, so it is difficult to assess whether reperfusion injury could occur. Steinberg and colleagues[58] used a rabbit model of multiple intracranial vessel occlusion and showed a 59% decrease in the area of cortical ischemic neuronal damage. There were no differences in the extent of striatal ischemic damage with either intermittent occlusion or uninterrupted occlusion.

Goldman and colleagues[54] studied repetitive MCA occlusion in rats using a protocol designed to simulate intraoperative occlusion techniques. The total infarcted areas after 60, 90, and 120 minutes of uninterrupted occlusion were significantly greater than the infarcted areas after identical cumulative ischemic periods but with 5 minutes of reperfusion after every 10-minute ischemic period.

In an investigation of normotensive rats undergoing MCA occlusion by Selman and colleagues,[56] biochemical and pathologic evidence suggested that a single prolonged episode of reversible ischemia was more deleterious than multiple occlusions of a similar total duration. Statistical differences occurred only when total single occlusion time reached 2 hours.

To provide an infarct size that could be evaluated statistically among different treatments, experimental models required total occlusion times longer than those typically needed in clinical settings. The nature of these experimental paradigms and species differences must be recalled when attempting to generalize results and to apply them to clinical use.

Most reports on the use of temporary artery occlusion in humans have been retrospective analyses of case series in which the use (or absence) of temporary occlusion was based on the surgeon's experience and judgment.[13–15, 59–76] No randomized, prospective studies have been designed to compare the outcomes of cerebrovascular procedures with temporary occlusion with surgery without local circulatory arrest. No studies have compared the use of a single episode of temporary occlusion with intermittent reperfusion in the clinical setting.

In 1961, Pool[73] stated that bilateral anterior cerebral artery occlusion was safe for 20 minutes when associated with the protective effects of hypothermia. Suzuki's group[15] and Ljunggren's group[66] estimated the maximum periods of safe occlusion of the MCA to be 20 minutes under normothermia. More recently, most authors have recommended maintaining occlusion times less than 15 minutes when possible.[13, 61, 69, 70] Some authors have reported occlusions longer than 90 minutes without deficit, however.[67]

Samson and coworkers[13] reviewed 121 patients from a group of 234 consecutive aneurysm patients. A total of 100 patients who did not experience intraoperative complications were analyzed. These patients underwent elective temporary occlusion under a standard neuroanesthetic regimen, including etomidate-induced burst suppression, normotension, and normothermia. Infarctions were noted in specific arterial territories as follows: basilar, 41%; MCA, 26%; internal carotid, 7%; and anterior communicating, 16%. The authors identified the following factors as significant predictors of postoperative radiographic evidence of infarction: age

(≥61 years), poor preoperative grade (Hunt and Hess grades III to IV), protracted duration of temporary occlusion, and the use of incomplete circulatory arrest.[13] This series documents that temporary occlusion is not without risk; however, factors other than the length of temporary occlusion, such as aneurysm configuration and location of perforators, may be crucial in determining this risk.[77]

Ogilvy and colleagues[14] studied the results of 132 consecutive aneurysm clippings. Their report comprised a nonconcurrent, prospective analysis using temporary vascular occlusion in combination with mild hypothermia (33°C to 34°C), induced hypertension (systolic, 150 mm Hg), and the administration of mannitol (100 g). Multivariate analysis showed that intraoperative rupture and clipping longer than 20 minutes were associated independently with stroke outcome. The average clip application time in patients with radiographic evidence of stroke was approximately 42 minutes compared with 29 minutes for patients without radiographic evidence of stroke. In patients with a clinically significant stroke, the average time was 50 minutes.[14] The overall stroke rate of patients who were occluded less than 20 minutes (1 of 67 surgeries, 1.5%) was significantly less than that of patients who were occluded longer than 20 minutes (12 of 65 surgeries, 18%).[14]

Augmentation of Residual Blood Flow

Systemic arterial pressure can be manipulated readily in the setting of planned temporary ischemia. Symon and colleagues[78] showed that MCA occlusion in primates caused a loss of autoregulation in the ischemic region. Elevation of blood pressure should increase cerebral perfusion because of the passive nature of the vessels that have lost autoregulation in the ischemic territory. Other investigators have shown that the decrease in CBF with focal ischemia is less in animals with phenylephrine-induced hypertension than in controls.[79–81] The beneficial effect of induced hypertension may be limited to relatively brief episodes of ischemia. Smrcka et al[82] reported that hypertension reduced infarct size by 97% in rabbits subjected to 1 hour of arterial occlusion but achieved only a 45% reduction in animals with 2 hours of ischemia. In the clinical setting, the use of hypertension is limited by the patient's cardiac tolerance. Close monitoring of cardiac function and limiting blood pressure elevation to approximately 10% above baseline are advisable.

Reduction of Metabolic Activity

HYPOTHERMIA

In animal models of focal ischemia, hypothermia ameliorates primary and secondary mechanisms of ischemic injury, including metabolism, glutamate release, NO synthesis, and myeloperoxidase activity.[83–87] Mild (33°C to 34.5°C) and moderate (27.5°C to 30°C) hypothermia have been associated with a decrease in infarct size in experimental animals.[88–92] Cooling animals beyond 33°C does not appear to provide greater benefit.[93] Lo and Steinberg[94] found an equivalent benefit from mild and moderate hypothermia as measured by the recovery of evoked potentials and magnetic resonance imaging in rabbits that underwent permanent focal ischemia. Karibe and coworkers[95] reported that mild hypothermia was protective when delayed 30 minutes after the onset of ischemia, but hypothermia induced 60 minutes after the insult was not beneficial. These findings indicate that the initiation of hypothermia after unanticipated temporary vessel occlusion still may provide benefit.

BARBITURATES, ETOMIDATE, AND PROPOFOL

The beneficial effect of barbiturates in the treatment of experimental focal cerebral ischemia has been well documented.[67, 96–100] The systemic cardiovascular effects and prolonged depression of consciousness after barbiturate administration may complicate the use of high-dose barbiturates in clinical situations. Two groups of investigators have shown that rats anesthetized with barbiturate at doses that suppress the EEG mildly show an equivalent reduction of infarct volume as those with barbiturate dosed to maintain EEG burst suppression.[101, 102] The use of such lower doses in the clinical setting may permit the safer administration of barbiturates during cerebrovascular procedures.

Etomidate and propofol, short-acting anesthetics with EEG effects similar to barbiturates but without cardiovascular side effects, have been proposed for use in cerebrovascular procedures.[103–105] Studies on experimental animals using these agents have produced conflicting results with regard to neuroprotection.[106–109]

Lavine et al[16] retrospectively analyzed 49 patients who underwent surgery for MCA aneurysms. Thirty-eight patients received intravenous pentobarbital, etomidate, or propofol, and the remaining 11 patients received only inhaled isoflurane. Postoperative radiographic evidence of infarction was present in 45.5% of the patients receiving the inhalation agent compared with 15.8% of those who received intravenous anesthesia. The retrospective, nonrandomized, historical-control study design produces a definitive statement about the benefit of these agents or a comparison among them. It is the best evidence to date showing a protective effect with their use during temporary intracranial vessel occlusion.

SERUM GLUCOSE MODULATION

Hyperglycemia, resulting from lactic acidosis from increased anaerobic glycolysis immediately after ischemia, increases ischemic injury in the laboratory and clinical setting.[110] Consequently, it is prudent to limit the amount of glucose delivered in intravenous solutions during cerebrovascular procedures.

Cytoprotective Agents

Various pharmacologic agents that act at specific sites in the ischemic cascade have been developed. Drug development has been directed toward pharmaceuticals that protect patients with acute ischemic stroke. None of these agents have been tested systematically in the setting of iatrogenic focal ischemia. It seems intuitive, however, that if a drug can be shown to have benefit when given several hours after the onset of ischemic stroke, the same drug might be protective if given at or just before the onset of focal ischemia during cerebrovascular surgery. Several agents that have shown promise in clinical trials of stroke patients are discussed here.

Ca^{2+} CHANNEL BLOCKERS

In animal studies of focal cerebral ischemia, various Ca^{2+} channel antagonists have been associated with reduced infarct volume, decreased peri-infarct edema, improved CBF, and improved neurological outcome.[111–122] Nimodipine is a 1,4-dihydropyridine that is more lipophilic than nifedipine and dilates cerebral vessels at lower doses than those required for peripheral vasodilation.[123] Nimodipine given within 12 hours of ischemic stroke has been associated with reduced mortality rates and greater neurological improvement[124–127] but is not beneficial when given 48 hours after the ictus.[128–131] A trial of nimodipine administered within 6 hours of stroke is in progress.[132]

GLUTAMATE ANTAGONISTS

NMDA antagonists have shown beneficial effects in reducing the volume of infarction in a variety of experimental models.[133–140] NMDA antagonists with potential clinical efficacy include dextrorphan, dextromethorphan, licostinel, and magnesium.[137–144] The most promising of these agents for intraoperative use may be magnesium. Magnesium has reduced the extent of infarction in several experimental models and has a long history of safe use in humans.[145–151] Marinov and colleagues[148] reported that $MgSO_4$ given intra-arterially to rats before temporary MCA occlusion reduced the volume of infarction 19% to 28% depending on the duration of ischemia.

NITRIC OXIDE SYNTHASE INHIBITORS

NOS inhibitors and free radical scavengers have provided significant neuroprotection in experimental animals subjected to focal ischemia.[152–157] Tirilazad mesylate is a potent inhibitor of lipid peroxidation caused by suppression of inducible NOS.[158] Most studies have shown a significant reduction of infarct volume in focal ischemia models.[145, 159–164] Human studies for the treatment of ischemic stroke have produced conflicting results, however.[165, 166] A multicenter, randomized, placebo-controlled study of tirilazad in patients with acute ischemic stroke was halted prematurely because of a lack of benefit.[167]

LUBELUZOLE

Lubeluzole is a novel agent that may provide effective therapy for focal ischemia. This drug blocks the postischemic release of glutamate and taurine, blocks Ca^{2+} and sodium channels, and inhibits the glutamate-activated NOS pathway.[168–172] In focal ischemia models, lubeluzole reduces infarct volume by approximately 25%,[173, 174] and studies in humans have shown few side effects.[175–177] Three randomized, placebo-controlled studies of patients with acute ischemic stroke have reported encouraging results.[178–180] Improvement was measured by a different outcome in each study. Further clinical trials are needed to elucidate these disparate findings before routine use of lubeluzole can be recommended.

CITICOLINE

Citicoline (cytidine 5-diphosphocholine) supplies choline and cytidine, both of which are necessary substrates for the synthesis of phosphatidylcholine, a key membrane component. In animal models of focal ischemia, citicoline administration has been associated with reduced infarct volume.[181, 182] In a single multicenter, randomized, placebo-controlled, and blinded study of patients treated within 24 hours of ischemic stroke, citicoline was associated with improved neurological, cognitive, and functional outcomes.[183]

OTHER CYTOPROTECTIVE AGENTS

Several other classes of agents have shown promise in laboratory studies of focal ischemia but have had limited testing in the clinical setting, including antibodies designed to prevent leukocyte adhesion, growth factors, and caspase inhibitors. Antibodies to ICAM-1, CD11/CD18 integrin, and P-selectin have reduced infarct volume in focal models of ischemia.[184–186] An uncontrolled study of enlimomab (anti-ICAM-1 antibody) in patients with ischemic stroke showed minimal side effects,[187] but an increased mortality rate and poorer functional outcomes were reported from a placebo-controlled trial.[188]

SURGICAL PROTOCOL

Before aneurysm surgery or when an intracranial arterial bypass is planned, the concentrations of serum electrolytes and glucose are maintained in the normal range. Phenytoin is used routinely in supratentorial surgery for its anticonvulsant effect. Mannitol is used for decompression as needed but is not given specifically during occlusion. Core body temperature is gradually dropped (passively or actively) to about 33°C. Before arterial occlusion is instituted, mild hypertension to approximately 10% above the patient's baseline mean arterial pressure is induced with phenylephrine. A loading dose of thiopental (10 mg/kg) is given followed by a maintenance infusion titrated to maintain EEG burst suppression (about 3 to 5 mg/kg/hour). If possible, occlusion is performed in an intermittent fashion on the basis of time limitations or electrophysiologic evidence of altered function (Fig. 89–7). Barbitu-

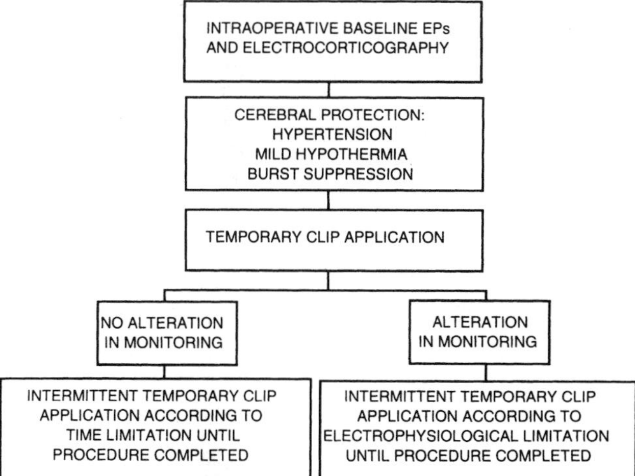

FIGURE 89-7. Paradigm for intraoperative evoked potentials (EPs) and electrocorticogram monitoring with temporary clip application. (From Taylor CL, Selman WR, Kiefer SP, et al: Temporary vessel occlusion during intracranial aneurysm repair. Neurosurgery 39:893–906, 1996. With permission from Lippincott Williams & Wilkins.)

rates are stopped and active rewarming is instituted as soon as blood flow is restored.

CONCLUSION

Whether iatrogenic or pathologic, temporary focal ischemia encompasses a complex cascade of events with a continuum of potential outcomes ranging from no measurable effect to devastating neurological injury. Studies that elucidate the biochemical mechanisms underlying ischemic injury provide potential sites for modulating these pathologic events. Although a wide variety of pharmacologic agents have shown beneficial effects in reducing infarct volume in laboratory animals, translating these successes to the clinical sphere has been complicated by toxic side effects and inconsistent results. It is hoped that as the mechanisms of ischemia-induced cell injury are understood better and clinical trials of various pharmacologic agents continue, specific cytoprotective agents will be developed that make cerebrovascular surgery safer.

REFERENCES

1. Kety SS, Schmidt CF: The nitrous oxide method for the quantitative determination of cerebral blood flow in man: Theory, procedure and normal values. J Clin Invest 27:476–483, 1948.
2. Sundt TM, Sharbrough FW, Anderson RE, et al: Cerebral blood flow measurements and electroencephalograms during carotid endarterectomy. J Neurosurg 41:310–320, 1974.
3. Waltz AG, Wanek AR, Anderson RE: Comparison of analytic methods for calculation of cerebral blood flow after intracarotid injection of 133 Xe. J Nucl Med 13:66–72, 1972.
4. Astrup J, Symon L, Branston NM, et al: Cortical evoked potential and extracellular K^+ and H^+ at critical levels of brain ischemia. Stroke 8:51–57, 1977.
5. Astrup J, Blennow G, Nilsson B: Effects of reduced cerebral blood flow upon EEG pattern, cerebral extracellular potassium, and energy metabolism in the rat cortex during bicuculline-induced seizures. Brain Res 177:115–126, 1979.
6. Branston NM, Strong AJ, Symon L: Extracellular potassium activity, evoked potential and tissue blood flow: Relationships during progressive ischaemia in baboon cerebral cortex. J Neurol Sci 32:305–321, 1977.
7. Meyer FB, Anderson RE, Sundt TM Jr, et al: Intracellular brain pH, indicator tissue perfusion, electroencephalography, and histology in severe and moderate focal cortical ischemia in the rabbit. J Cereb Blood Flow Metab 6:71–78, 1986.
8. Morawetz RB, Crowell RH, DeGirolami U, et al: Regional cerebral blood flow thresholds during cerebral ischemia. Fed Proc 38:2493–2494, 1979.
9. Astrup J, Siesjo BK, Symon L: Thresholds in cerebral ischemia—the ischemic penumbra. Stroke 12:723–725, 1981.
10. Symon L, Branston NM, Strong AJ, et al: The concept of thresholds of ischaemia in relation to brain structure and function. J Clin Pathol Suppl (R Coll Pathol) 11:149–154, 1977.
11. Heiss WD: Flow thresholds of functional and morphological damage of brain tissue. Stroke 14:329–331, 1983.
12. Jones TH, Morawetz RB, Crowell RM, et al: Thresholds of focal cerebral ischemia in awake monkeys. J Neurosurg 54:773–782, 1981.
13. Samson D, Batjer HH, Bowman G, et al: A clinical study of the parameters and effects of temporary arterial occlusion in the management of intracranial aneurysms. Neurosurgery 34:22–29, 1994.
14. Ogilvy CS, Carter BS, Kaplan S, et al: Temporary vessel occlusion for aneurysm surgery: Risk factors for stroke in patients protected by induced hypothermia and hypertension and intravenous mannitol administration. J Neurosurg 84:785–791, 1996.
15. Suzuki J, Kwak R, Okudaira Y: The safe time limit of temporary clamping of cerebral arteries in the direct surgical treatment of intracranial aneurysm under moderate hypothermia. Tohoku J Exp Med 127:1–7, 1979.
16. Lavine SD, Masri LS, Levy ML, et al: Temporary occlusion of the middle cerebral artery in intracranial aneurysm surgery: Time limitation and advantage of brain protection. J Neurosurg 87:817–824, 1997.
17. Kraig RP, Pulsinelli WA, Plum F: Hydrogen ion buffering during complete brain ischemia. Brain Res 342:281–290, 1985.
18. Kristian T, Siesjo BK: Calcium in ischemic cell death. Stroke 29:705–718, 1998.
19. Siesjo BK: Cell damage in the brain: A speculative synthesis. J Cereb Blood Flow Metab 1:155–185, 1981.
20. Dirnagl U, Iadecola C, Moskowitz MA: Pathobiology of ischaemic stroke: An integrated view. Trends Neurosci 22:391–397, 1999.
21. Rothman S: Synaptic release of excitatory amino acid neurotransmitter mediates anoxic neuronal death. J Neurosci 4:1884–1891, 1984.
22. Garthwaite G, Garthwaite J: Neurotoxicity of excitatory amino acid receptor agonists in rat cerebellar slices: Dependence on Ca^{2+} concentration. Neurosci Lett 66:193–198, 1986.
23. Choi DW, Rothman SM: The role of glutamate neurotoxicity in hypoxic-ischemic death. Ann Rev Neurosci 13:171–182, 1990.
24. Rothman SM, Olney JW: Glutamate and the pathophysiology of hypoxic-ischemic brain damage. Ann Neurol 19:105–111, 1986.
25. Benveniste H, Drejer J, Schousboe A, et al: Elevation of the extracellular concentrations of glutamate and aspartate in rat hippocampus during transient cerebral ischemia monitored by intracerebral microdialysis. J Neurochem 43:1369–1374, 1984.
26. Hossmann KA: Periinfarct depolarizations. Cerebrovasc Brain Metab Rev 8:195–208, 1996.
27. Marletta MA, Yoon PS, Iyengar R, et al: Macrophage oxidation of L-arginine to nitrite and nitrate: Nitric oxide is an intermediate. Biochemistry 27:8706–8711, 1988.
28. Samdani AF, Dawson TM, Dawson VL: Nitric oxide synthase in models of focal ischemia. Stroke 28:1283–1288, 1997.
29. Palmer RM, Ferrige AG, Moncada S: Nitric oxide release accounts for the biological activity of endothelium-derived relaxing factor. Nature 327:524–526, 1987.
30. Ignarro LJ, Buga GM, Wood KS, et al: Endothelium-derived relaxing factor produced and released from artery and vein is nitric oxide. Proc Natl Acad Sci U S A 84:9265–9269, 1987.
31. Moncada S, Higgs A: The L-arginine-nitric oxide pathway. N Engl J Med 329:2002–2012, 1993.

32. Zhang J, Dawson VL, Dawson TM, et al: Nitric oxide activation of poly(ADP-ribose) synthetase in neurotoxicity. Science 263: 687–689, 1994.
33. Huang PL, Dawson PM, Bredt DS, et al: Targeted disruption of the neuronal nitric oxide synthase gene. Cell 75:1273–1286, 1993.
34. Iadecola C, Xu X, Zhang F, et al: Marked induction of calcium-independent nitric oxide synthase activity after focal cerebral ischemia. J Cereb Blood Flow Metab 15:52–59, 1995.
35. Dawson VL, Kizushi VM, Huang PL, et al: Resistance to neurotoxicity in cortical cultures from neuronal nitric oxide synthase-deficient mice. J Neurosci 16:2479–2487, 1996.
36. Hewett SJ, Csernansky CA, Choi DW: Selective potentiation of NMDA-induced neuronal injury following induction of astrocytic iNOS. Neuron 13:487–494, 1994.
37. Choi DW: The excitotoxic concept. In Welch KMA, Caplan LR, Reis DJ, et al (eds): Primer on Cerebrovascular Disease. San Diego, CA, Academic Press, 1997, pp 187–190.
38. Kaufmann WE, Andreasson KL, Isakson PC, et al: Cyclooxygenases and the central nervous system. Prostaglandins 54:601–624, 1997.
39. Feuerstein GZ, Wang X, Barone FC: Inflammatory mediators and brain injury: The role of cytokines and chemokines in stroke and central nervous system disease. In Ginsberg M, Bogousslavsky J (eds): Cerebrovascular Disease: Pathophysiology, Diagnosis and Management. Philadelphia, Blackwell Science, 1998, pp 507–531.
40. Matsuo Y, Kihara T, Ikeda N, et al: Role of platelet-activating factor and thromboxane A2 in radical production during ischemia and reperfusion of the rat brain. Brain Res 709:296–302, 1995.
41. Nishigaya K, Yoshida Y, Sasuga M, et al: Effect of recirculation on exacerbation of ischemic vascular lesions in the rat brain. Stroke 22:635–642, 1991.
42. Jean WC, Spellman SR, Nussbaum ES, et al: Reperfusion injury after focal cerebral ischemia: The role of inflammation and the therapeutic horizon. Neurosurgery 43:1382–1397, 1998.
43. Shakikh AY, Uthayshanker RE, Liu PK, et al: Ischemic neuronal apoptosis: A view based on free radical-induced DNA damage and repair. Neuroscientist 2:88–95, 1998.
44. Park JR, Hockenbery DM: BCL-2, a novel regulator of apoptosis. J Cell Biochem 60:12–17, 1996.
45. Savitz SI, Rosenbaum DM: Gene expression after cerebral ischemia. Neuroscientist 5:238–253, 1999.
46. Greenlund LJ, Deckwerth TL, Johnson EM Jr: Superoxide dismutase delays neuronal apoptosis: A role for reactive oxygen species in programmed neuronal death. Neuron 14:303–315, 1995.
47. Linnik MD, Zobrist RH, Hatfield MD: Evidence supporting a role for programmed cell death in focal cerebral ischemia in rats. Stroke 24:2002–2009, 1993.
48. MacMannus JP, Hill IE, Huang Z-G, et al: DNA damage consistent with apoptosis in transient focal ischemic neocortex. Neuroreport 5:493–496, 1994.
49. Li Y, Chopp M, Jiang N, et al: Temporal profile of in situ DNA fragmentation after transient middle cerebral artery occlusion in the rat. J Cereb Blood Flow Metab 15:389–397, 1995.
50. Batjer H, Samson D: Intraoperative aneurysmal rupture: Incidence, outcome, and suggestions for surgical management. Neurosurgery 18:701–707, 1986.
51. Buchthal A, Belopavlovic M, Mooij JJ: Evoked potential monitoring and temporary clipping in cerebral aneurysm surgery. Acta Neurochir (Wien) 93:28–36, 1988.
52. Jabre A, Symon L: Temporary vascular occlusion during aneurysm surgery. Surg Neurol 27:47–63, 1987.
53. Symon L: Management of giant intracranial aneurysms. Clin Neurosurg 36:21–47, 1990.
54. Goldman MS, Anderson RE, Meyer FB: Effects of intermittent reperfusion during temporal focal ischemia. J Neurosurg 77: 911–916, 1992.
55. Sakaki T, Tsunoda S, Morimoto T, et al: Effects of repeated temporary clipping of the middle cerebral artery on pial arterial diameter, regional cerebral blood flow, and brain structure in cats. Neurosurgery 27:914–920, 1990.
56. Selman WR, Kiefer SP, Lust WD, et al: Metabolic evidence to support that single ischemic episodes are more devastating to the brain than are multiple insults of similar duration. J Cereb Blood Flow Metab 15:328, 1995.
57. Selman WR, Bhatti SU, Rosenstein CC, et al: Temporary vessel occlusion in spontaneously hypertensive and normotensive rats: Effect of single and multiple episodes on tissue metabolism and volume of infarction. J Neurosurg 80:1085–1090, 1994.
58. Steinberg GK, Panahian N, Sun GH, et al: Cerebral damage caused by interrupted, repeated arterial occlusion versus uninterrupted occlusion in a focal ischemic model. J Neurosurg 81: 554–559, 1994.
59. Batjer HH, Frankfurt AI, Purdy PD, et al: Use of etomidate, temporary arterial occlusion, and intraoperative angiography in surgical treatment of large and giant cerebral aneurysms. J Neurosurg 68:234–240, 1988.
60. Beck DW, Boarini DJ, Kassell NF: Surgical treatment of giant aneurysm of vertebral-basilar junction. Surg Neurol 12:283–285, 1979.
61. Charbel FT, Ausman JI, Diaz FG, et al: Temporary clipping in aneurysm surgery: Technique and results. Surg Neurol 36: 83–90, 1991.
62. Fox JL: Microsurgical treatment of ventral (paraclinoid) internal carotid artery aneurysms. Neurosurgery 22:32–39, 1988.
63. Heros RC, Nelson PB, Ojemann RG, et al: Large and giant paraclinoid aneurysms: Surgical techniques, complications, and results. Neurosurgery 12:153–163, 1983.
64. Hosobuchi Y: Direct surgical treatment of giant intracranial aneurysms. J Neurosurg 51:743–756, 1979.
65. Jabre A, Symon L: Temporary vascular occlusion during aneurysm surgery. Surg Neurol 27:47–63, 1987.
66. Ljunggren B, Saveland H, Brandt L, et al: Temporary clipping during early operation for ruptured aneurysm: Preliminary report. Neurosurgery 12:525–530, 1983.
67. McDermott MW, Durity FA, Borozny M, et al: Temporary vessel occlusion and barbiturate protection in cerebral aneurysm surgery. Neurosurgery 25:54–62, 1989.
68. Momma F, Wang AD, Symon L: Effects of temporary arterial occlusion on somatosensory evoked responses in aneurysm surgery. Surg Neurol 27:343–352, 1987.
69. Ogawa A, Sato H, Sakurai Y, et al: Limitation of temporary vascular occlusion during aneurysm surgery. Surg Neurol 36: 453–457, 1991.
70. Ohmoto T, Nagao S, Mino S, et al: Monitoring of cortical blood flow during temporary arterial occlusion in aneurysm surgery by the thermal diffusion method. Neurosurgery 28:49–55, 1991.
71. Peerless SJ, Drake CG: Treatment of giant cerebral aneurysms of the anterior circulation. Neurosurg Rev 5:149–154, 1982.
72. Pia HW, Zierski J: Giant cerebral aneurysms. Neurosurg Rev 5: 117–148, 1982.
73. Pool JL: Aneurysms of the anterior communicating artery: Bifrontal craniotomy and routine use of temporary clips. J Neurosurg 18:98–112, 1961.
74. Symon L, Vajda J: Surgical experiences with giant intracranial aneurysms. J Neurosurg 61:1009–1028, 1984.
75. White R, Yashon D, Olbin M: Temporary occlusion of afferent arteries in the treatment of arterial aneurysms [in Russian]. Vopr Neirokhir 1:3–7, 1975.
76. Yoshimoto T, Suzuki J: Intracranial definitive aneurysm surgery under normothermia and normotension—utilizing temporary occlusion of major cerebral arteries and preoperative mannitol administration [in Japanese]. No Shinkei Geka 4:775–783, 1976.
77. Solomon RA: Comment on Samson D, Batjer HH, Bowman G, et al: A clinical study of the parameters and effects of temporary arterial occlusion in the management of intracranial aneurysms. Neurosurgery 34:28–29, 1994.
78. Symon L, Branston NM, Strong AJ: Autoregulation in acute focal ischemia: An experimental study. Stroke 7:547–554, 1976.
79. Drummond JC, Oh YS, Cole DJ, et al: Phenylephrine-induced hypertension reduces ischemia following middle cerebral artery occlusion in rats. Stroke 20:1538–1544, 1989.
80. Chileuitt L, Leber K, McCalden T, et al: Induced hypertension during ischemia reduces infarct area after temporary middle cerebral artery occlusion in rats. Surg Neurol 46:229–234, 1996.
81. Cole DJ, Matsumura JS, Drummond JC, et al: Focal cerebral ischemia in rats: Effects of induced hypertension, during reperfusion, on CBF. J Cereb Blood Flow Metab 12:64–69, 1992.

82. Smrcka M, Ogilvy CS, Crow RJ, et al: Induced hypertension improves regional blood flow and protects against infarction during focal ischemia: Time course of changes in blood flow measured by laser Doppler imaging. Neurosurgery 42:617–625, 1998.
83. Baker CJ, Fiore AJ, Frazzini VI, et al: Intraischemic hypothermia decreases the release of glutamate in the cores of permanent focal cerebral infarcts. Neurosurgery 36:994–1002, 1995.
84. Toyoda T, Suzuki S, Kassell NF, et al: Intraischemic hypothermia attenuates neutrophil infiltration in the rat neocortex after focal ischemia-reperfusion injury. Neurosurgery 39:1200–1205, 1996.
85. Kader A, Frazzini VI, Baker CJ, et al: Effect of mild hypothermia on nitric oxide synthesis during focal cerebral ischemia. Neurosurgery 35:272–277, 1994.
86. Kaibara T, Sutherland GR, Colbourne F, et al: Hypothermia: Depression of tricarboxylic acid cycle flux and evidence for pentose phosphate shunt upregulation. J Neurosurg 90:339–347, 1999.
87. Winfree CJ, Baker CJ, Connolly ES Jr, et al: Mild hypothermia reduces penumbral glutamate levels in the rat permanent focal cerebral ischemia model. Neurosurgery 38:1216–1222, 1996.
88. Onesti ST, Baker CJ, Sun PP, et al: Transient hypothermia reduces focal ischemic brain injury in the rat. Neurosurgery 29: 369–373, 1991.
89. Chen H, Chopp M, Zhang ZG, et al: The effect of hypothermia on transient middle cerebral artery occlusion in the rat. J Cereb Blood Flow Metab 12:621–628, 1992.
90. Morikawa E, Ginsberg MD, Dietrich WD, et al: The significance of brain temperature in focal cerebral ischemia: Histopathological consequences of middle cerebral artery occlusion in the rat. J Cereb Blood Flow Metab 12:380–389, 1992.
91. Ridenour TR, Warner DS, Todd MM, et al: Mild hypothermia reduces infarct size resulting from temporary but not permanent focal ischemia in rats. Stroke 23:733–738, 1992.
92. Goto Y, Kassell NF, Hiramatsu K, et al: Effects of intraischemic hypothermia on cerebral damage in a model of reversible focal ischemia. Neurosurgery 32:980–984, 1993.
93. Kader A, Brisman MH, Maraire N, et al: The effect of mild hypothermia on permanent focal ischemia in the rat. Neurosurgery 31:1056–1061, 1992.
94. Lo EH, Steinberg GK: Effects of hypothermia on evoked potentials, magnetic resonance imaging, and blood flow in focal ischemia in rabbits. Stroke 23:889–893, 1992.
95. Karibe H, Chen J, Zarow GJ, et al: Delayed induction of mild hypothermia to reduce infarct volume after temporary middle cerebral artery occlusion in rats. J Neurosurg 80:112–119, 1994.
96. Smith AL, Hoff JT, Nielsen SL, et al: Barbiturate protection in acute focal cerebral ischemia. Stroke 5:1–7, 1974.
97. Black KL, Weidler DJ, Jallad NS, et al: Delayed pentobarbital therapy of acute focal cerebral ischemia. Stroke 9:245–249, 1978.
98. Selman WR, Spetzler RF, Anton AH, et al: Management of prolonged therapeutic barbiturate coma. Surg Neurol 15:9–10, 1981.
99. Selman WR, Spetzler RF, Roessmann UR, et al: Barbiturate-induced coma therapy for focal cerebral ischemia: Effect after temporary and permanent MCA occlusion. J Neurosurg 55: 220–226, 1981.
100. Selman WR, Spetzler RF, Roski RA, et al: Barbiturate coma in focal cerebral ischemia: Relationship of protection to timing of therapy. J Neurosurg 56:685–690, 1982.
101. Warner DS, Takaoka S, Wu B, et al: Electroencephalographic burst suppression is not required to elicit maximal neuroprotection from pentobarbital in a rat model of focal cerebral ischemia. Anesthesiology 84:1475–1484, 1996.
102. Schmid-Elsaesser R, Schroder M, Zausinger S, et al: EEG burst suppression is not necessary for maximum barbiturate protection in transient focal cerebral ischemia in the rat. J Neurol Sci 162:14–19, 1999.
103. Batjer HH: Cerebral protective effects of etomidate: Experimental and clinical aspects. Cerebrovasc Brain Metab Rev 5:17–32, 1993.
104. Batjer HH, Frankfurt AI, Purdy PD, et al: Use of etomidate, temporary arterial occlusion, and intraoperative angiography in surgical treatment of large and giant cerebral aneurysms. J Neurosurg 68:234–240, 1988.
105. Rosenwasser RH, Jimenez DF, Wending WW, et al: Routine use of etomidate and temporary vessel occlusion during aneurysm surgery. Neurol Res 13:224–228, 1991.
106. Drummond JC, Cole DJ, Patel PM, et al: Focal cerebral ischemia during anesthesia with etomidate, isoflurane, or thiopental: A comparison of the extent of cerebral injury. Neurosurgery 37: 742–749, 1995.
107. Guo J, White JA, Batjer HH: Limited protective effects of etomidate during brainstem ischemia in dogs. J Neurosurg 82:278–283, 1995.
108. Ridenour TR, Warner DS, Todd MM, et al: Comparative effects of propofol and halothane on outcome from temporary middle cerebral artery occlusion in the rat. Anesthesiology 76:807–812, 1992.
109. Pittman JE, Sheng H, Pearlstein R, et al: Comparison of the effects of propofol and pentobarbital on neurological outcome and cerebral infarct size after temporary focal ischemia in the rat. Anesthesiology 87:1139–1144, 1997.
110. Wass CT, Lanier WL: Glucose modulation of ischemic brain injury: Review and clinical recommendations. Mayo Clin Proc 71:801–812, 1996.
111. Benham CD, Brown TH, Cooper DG, et al: SB 201823-A, a neuronal Ca^{2+} antagonist is neuroprotective in two models of cerebral ischaemia. Neuropharmacology 32:1249–1257, 1993.
112. Harada K, Shiino A, Matsuda M, et al: Effects of a novel Ca^{2+} antagonist, KB-2796, on neurological outcome size of experimental cerebral infarction in rats. Surg Neurol 32:16–20, 1989.
113. Kittaka M, Giannotta SL, Zelman V, et al: Attenuation of brain injury and reduction of neuron-specific enolase by nicardipine in systemic circulation following focal ischemia and reperfusion in a rat model. J Neurosurg 87:731–737, 1997.
114. Kondoh Y, Mizusawa S, Murakami M, et al: Fasudil (HA1077), an intracellular calcium antagonist, improves neurological deficits and tissue potassium loss in focal cerebral ischemia in gerbils. Neurol Res 19:211–215, 1997.
115. Ohtaki M, Tranmer B: Pretreatment of transient focal cerebral ischemia in rats with the calcium antagonist AT877. Stroke 25: 1234–1239, 1994.
116. Perez-Pinzon MA, Yenari MA, Sun GH, et al: SNX-111, a novel, presynaptic N-type calcium channel antagonist, is neuroprotective against focal cerebral ischemia in rabbits. J Neurol Sci 153: 25–31, 1997.
117. Sakaki T, Tsujimoto S, Sasaoka Y, et al: The effect of a new calcium antagonist, TA3090 (clentiazem), on experimental transient focal cerebral ischemia in cats. Stroke 24:872–878, 1993.
118. Shiino A, Matsuda M, Susumu T, et al: Effects of the calcium antagonist nilvadipine on focal cerebral ischemia in spontaneously hypertensive rats. Surg Neurol 35:105–110, 1991.
119. Takizawa S, Matsushima K, Fujita H, et al: A selective N-type calcium channel antagonist reduces extracellular glutamate release and infarct volume in focal cerebral ischemia. J Cereb Blood Flow Metab 15:611–618, 1995.
120. Germano IM, Bartkowski HM, Cassel ME, et al: The therapeutic value of nimodipine in experimental focal cerebral ischemia: Neurological outcome and histopathological findings. J Neurosurg 67:81–87, 1987.
121. Meyer FB, Anderson RE, Yaksh TL, et al: Effect of nimodipine on intracellular brain pH, cortical blood flow, and EEG in experimental focal cerebral ischemia. J Neurosurg 64:617–626, 1986.
122. Uematsu D, Greenberg JH, Hickey WF, et al: Nimodipine attenuates both increase in cytosolic free calcium and histologic damage following focal cerebral ischemia and reperfusion in cats. Stroke 20:1531–1537, 1989.
123. Scriabine A, van den Kerckhoff W: Pharmacology of nimodipine: A review. Ann N Y Acad Sci 522:698–706, 1988.
124. Gelmers HJ, Gorter K, de Weerdt CJ, et al: A controlled trial of nimodipine in acute ischemic stroke. N Engl J Med 318: 203–207, 1988.
125. Paci A, Ottaviano P, Trenta A, et al: Nimodipine in acute ischemic stroke: A double-blind controlled study. Acta Neurol Scand 80:282–286, 1989.
126. Gelmers HJ, Hennerici M: Effect of nimodipine on acute ischemic stroke: Pooled results from five randomized trials. Stroke 21(12 suppl):IV81–84, 1990.
127. Mohr JP, Orgogozo JM, Harrison MJG, et al: Meta-analysis of

oral nimodipine trials in acute ischemic stroke. Cerebrovasc Dis 4:197–203, 1994.
128. Trust Study Group: Randomised, double-blind, placebo-controlled trial of nimodipine in acute stroke. Lancet 336:1205–1209, 1990.
129. American Nimodipine Study Group: Clinical trial of nimodipine in acute ischemic stroke. Stroke 23:3–8, 1992.
130. Kaste M, Fogelholm R, Erila T, et al: A randomized, double-blind, placebo-controlled trial of nimodipine in acute ischemic hemispheric stroke. Stroke 25:1348–1353, 1994.
131. Martinez-Vila E, Guillen F, Villanueva JA, et al: Placebo-controlled trial of nimodipine in the treatment of acute ischemic cerebral infarction. Stroke 21:1023–1028, 1990.
132. Fisher M, Bogousslavsky J: Further evolution toward effective therapy for acute ischemic stroke. JAMA 279:1298–1303, 1998.
133. Minematsu K, Fisher M, Li L, et al: Effects of a novel NMDA antagonist on experimental stroke rapidly and quantitatively assessed by diffusion-weighted MRI. Neurology 43:397–403, 1993.
134. Park CK, Nehls DG, Graham DI, et al: The glutamate antagonist MK-801 reduces focal ischemic brain damage in the rat. Ann Neurol 24:543–551, 1988.
135. Bertorelli R, Adami M, Di Santo E, et al: MK 801 and dexamethasone reduce both tumor necrosis factor levels and infarct volume after focal cerebral ischemia in the rat brain. Neurosci Lett 246:41–44, 1998.
136. Maier CM, Sun GH, Kunis DM, et al: Neuroprotection by the N-methyl-D-aspartate receptor antagonist CGP 40116: In vivo and in vitro studies. J Neurochem 65:652–659, 1995.
137. Steinberg GK, Panahian N, Perez-Pinzon MA, et al: Narrow temporal therapeutic window for NMDA antagonist protection against focal cerebral ischaemia. Neurobiol Dis 2:109–118, 1995.
138. Britton P, Lu XC, Laskosky MS, et al: Dextromethorphan protects against cerebral injury following transient, but not permanent, focal ischemia in rats. Life Sci 60:1729–1740, 1997.
139. Steinberg GK, Kunis D, DeLaPaz R, et al: Neuroprotection following focal cerebral ischemia with the NMDA antagonist dextromethorphan, has a favourable dose response profile. Neurol Res 15:174–180, 1993.
140. Takaoka S, Bart RD, Pearlstein R, et al: Neuroprotective effect of NMDA receptor glycine recognition site antagonism persists when brain temperature is controlled. J Cereb Blood Flow Metab 17:161–167, 1997.
141. Albers GW, Atkinson RP, Kelley RE, et al: Safety, tolerability, and pharmacokinetics of the *N*-methyl-D-aspartate antagonist dextrorphan in patients with acute stroke. Dextrophan Study Group. Stroke 26:254–258, 1995.
142. Albers GW, Saenz RE, Moses JA Jr: Tolerability of oral dextromethorphan in patients with a history of brain ischemia. Clin Neuropharmacol 15:509–514, 1992.
143. Albers GW, Saenz RE, Moses JA Jr, et al: Safety and tolerance of oral dextromethorphan in patients at risk for brain ischemia. Stroke 22:1075–1077, 1991.
144. Albers GW, Clark WM, Atkinson RP, et al: Dose escalation study of the NMDA glycine–site antagonist licostinel in acute ischemic stroke. Stroke 30:508–513, 1999.
145. Schmid-Elsaesser R, Zausinger S, Hungerhuber E, et al: Neuroprotective effects of combination therapy with tirilazad and magnesium in rats subjected to reversible focal cerebral ischemia. Neurosurgery 44:163–171, 1999.
146. Izumi Y, Roussel S, Pinard E, et al: Reduction of infarct volume by magnesium after middle cerebral artery occlusion in rats. J Cereb Blood Flow Metab 11:1025–1030, 1991.
147. Tsuda T, Kogure K, Nishioka K, et al: Mg^{2+} administered up to twenty-four hours following reperfusion prevents ischemic damage of the Ca1 neurons in the rat hippocampus. Neuroscience 44:335–341, 1991.
148. Marinov MB, Harbaugh KS, Hoopes PJ, et al: Neuroprotective effects of preischemia intraarterial magnesium sulfate in reversible focal cerebral ischemia. J Neurosurg 85:117–124, 1996.
149. Muir KW, Lees KR: Dose optimization of intravenous magnesium sulfate after acute stroke. Stroke 29:918–923, 1998.
150. Muir KW: New experimental and clinical data on the efficacy of pharmacological magnesium infusions in cerebral infarcts. Magnes Res 11:43–56, 1998.
151. Muir KW, Lees KR: Clinical experience with excitatory amino acid antagonist drugs. Stroke 26:503–513, 1995.
152. Coert BA, Anderson RE, Meyer FB: A comparative study of the effects of two nitric oxide synthase inhibitors and two nitric oxide donors on temporary focal cerebral ischemia in the Wistar rat. J Neurosurg 90:332–338, 1999.
153. Imaizumi S, Woolworth V, Fishman RA, et al: Liposome-entrapped superoxide dismutase reduces cerebral infarction in cerebral ischemia in rats. Stroke 21:1312–1317, 1990.
154. Liu TH, Beckman JS, Freeman BA, et al: Polyethylene glycol-conjugated superoxide dismutase and catalase reduce ischemic brain injury. Am J Physiol 256:H589–593, 1989.
155. Martz D, Rayos G, Schielke GP, et al: Allopurinol and dimethylthiourea reduce brain infarction following middle cerebral artery occlusion in rats. Stroke 20:488–494, 1989.
156. Spinnewyn B, Cornet S, Auguet M, et al: Synergistic protective effects of antioxidant and nitric oxide synthase inhibitor in transient focal ischemia. J Cereb Blood Flow Metab 19:139–143, 1999.
157. Trifiletti RR: Neuroprotective effects of NG-nitro-L-arginine in focal stroke in the 7-day old rat. Eur J Pharmacol 218:197–198, 1992.
158. del Pilar Fernandez M, Meizoso MJ, Lodeiro MJ, et al: Effect of desmethyl tirilazad, dizocilpine maleate and nimodipine on brain nitric oxide synthase activity and cyclic guanosine monophosphate during cerebral ischemia in rats. Pharmacology 57: 174–179, 1998.
159. Karki A, Westergren I, Widner H, et al: Tirilazad reduces brain edema after middle cerebral artery ligation in hypertensive rats. Acta Neurochir Suppl (Wien) 60:310–313, 1994.
160. Wilson JT, Bednar MM, McAuliffe TL, et al: The effect of the 21-aminosteroid U74006F in a rabbit model of thromboembolic stroke. Neurosurgery 31:929–933, 1992.
161. Young W, Wojak JC, DeCrescito V: 21-Aminosteroid reduces ion shifts and edema in the rat middle cerebral artery occlusion model of regional ischemia. Stroke 19:1013–1019, 1988.
162. Schmid-Elsaesser R, Zausinger S, Hungerhuber E, et al: Monotherapy with dextromethorphan or tirilazad—but not a combination of both—improves outcome after transient focal cerebral ischemia in rats. Exp Brain Res 122:121–127, 1998.
163. Clark WM, Hotan T, Lauten JD, et al: Therapeutic efficacy of tirilazad in experimental multiple cerebral emboli: A randomized, controlled trial. Crit Care Med 22:1161–1166, 1994.
164. Hellstrom HO, Wanhainen A, Valtysson J, et al: Effect of tirilazad mesylate given after permanent middle cerebral artery occlusion in rat. Acta Neurochir (Wien) 129:188–192, 1994.
165. Kassell NF, Haley EC Jr, Apperson-Hansen C, et al: Randomized, double-blind, vehicle-controlled trial of tirilazad mesylate in patients with aneurysmal subarachnoid hemorrhage: A cooperative study in Europe, Australia, and New Zealand. J Neurosurg 84:221–228, 1996.
166. Haley EC Jr, Kassell NF, Apperson-Hansen C, et al: A randomized, double-blind, vehicle-controlled trial of tirilazad mesylate in patients with aneurysmal subarachnoid hemorrhage: A cooperative study in North America. J Neurosurg 86:467–474, 1997.
167. RANTTAS Investigators: A randomized trial of tirilazad mesylate in patients with acute stroke (RANTTAS). Stroke 27:1453–1458, 1996.
168. Ashton D, Willems R, Wynants J, et al: Altered Na(+)-channel function as an in vitro model of the ischemic penumbra: Action of lubeluzole and other neuroprotective drugs. Brain Res 745: 210–221, 1997.
169. Lesage AS, Peeters L, Leysen JE: Lubeluzole, a novel long-term neuroprotectant, inhibits the glutamate-activated nitric oxide synthase pathway. J Pharmacol Exp Ther 279:759–766, 1996.
170. Maiese K, TenBroeke M, Kue I: Neuroprotection of lubeluzole is mediated through the signal transduction pathways of nitric oxide. J Neurochem 68:710–714, 1997.
171. Marrannes R, De Prins E, Clincke G: Influence of lubeluzole on voltage-sensitive Ca^{++} channels in isolated rat neurons. J Pharmacol Exp Ther 286:201–214, 1998.
172. Scheller DK, De Ryck M, Kolb J, et al: Lubeluzole blocks increases in extracellular glutamate and taurine in the peri-infarct zone in rats. Eur J Pharmacol 338:243–251, 1997.
173. Culmsee C, Junker V, Wolz P, et al: Lubeluzole protects hippo-

campal neurons from excitotoxicity in vitro and reduces brain damage caused by ischemia. Eur J Pharmacol 342:193–201, 1998.

174. De Ryck M, Keersmaekers R, Duytschaever H, et al: Lubeluzole protects sensorimotor function and reduces infarct size in a photochemical stroke model in rats. J Pharmacol Exp Ther 279: 748–758, 1996.

175. De Keyser J, Van de Velde V, Schellens RL, et al: Safety and pharmacokinetics of the neuroprotective drug lubeluzole in patients with ischemic stroke. Clin Ther 19:1340–1351, 1997.

176. Hacke W, Lees KR, Timmerhuis T, et al: Cardiovascular safety of lubeluzole (Prosynap) in patients with ischemic stroke. Cerebrovasc Dis 8:247–254, 1998.

177. Hantson L, Tritsmans L, Crabbe R, et al: The safety and tolerability of single intravenous doses of lubeluzole (Prosynap) in healthy volunteers. Int J Clin Pharmacol Ther 35:491–495, 1997.

178. Diener HC, Hacke W, Hennerici M, et al: Lubeluzole in acute ischemic stroke: A double-blind, placebo-controlled phase II trial. Lubeluzole International Study Group. Stroke 27:76–81, 1996.

179. Diener HC: Multinational randomised controlled trial of lubeluzole in acute ischaemic stroke. European and Australian Lubeluzole Ischaemic Stroke Study Group. Cerebrovasc Dis 8:172–181, 1998.

180. Grotta J: Lubeluzole treatment of acute ischemic stroke. The US and Canadian Lubeluzole Ischemic Stroke Study Group. Stroke 28:2338–2346, 1997.

181. Schabitz WR, Weber J, Takano K, et al: The effects of prolonged treatment with citicoline in temporary experimental focal ischemia. J Neurol Sci 138:21–25, 1996.

182. D'Orlando KJ, Sandage BW Jr: Citicoline (CDP-choline): Mechanisms of action and effects in ischemic brain injury. Neurol Res 17:281–284, 1995.

183. Clark WM, Warach SJ, Pettigrew LC, et al: A randomized dose-response trial of citicoline in acute ischemic stroke patients. Citicoline Stroke Study Group. Neurology 49:671–678, 1997.

184. Zhang RL, Chopp M, Li Y, et al: Anti-ICAM-1 antibody reduces ischemic cell damage after transient MCA occlusion in the rat. Neurology 44:1747–1751, 1994.

185. Goussev AV, Zhang Z, Anderson DC, et al: P-selectin antibody reduces hemorrhage and infarct volume resulting from MCA occlusion in the rat. J Neurol Sci 161:16–22, 1998.

186. Chen H, Chopp M, Zhang RL, et al: Anti-CD11b monoclonal antibody reduces ischemic cell damage after transient focal cerebral ischemia in rat. Ann Neurol 35:458–463, 1994.

187. Schneider D, Berrouschot J, Brandt T, et al: Safety, pharmacokinetics and biological activity of enlimomab (anti-ICAM-1 antibody): An open-label, dose escalation study in patients hospitalized for acute stroke. Eur Neurol 40:78–83, 1998.

188. Enlimolab Acute Stroke Trial Investigators: The enlimolab acute stroke trial: Final results [abstract]. Neurology 48:A270, 1997.

CHAPTER 90

Techniques for Deep Hypothermic Circulatory Arrest

E. SANDER CONNOLLY, JR ■ ROBERT A. SOLOMON

Advances in surgical technique have allowed for direct arterial reconstruction in most cases of intracranial aneurysms. Using modern clips, most cerebral aneurysms can be obliterated while fully arterialized. Many aneurysms present additional challenges, however. Large size, intimacy with crucial perforator branches, deep location, atherosclerotic walls, and the incorporation of afferent or efferent arteries in the dome represent factors that singly or in combination may hamper safe clipping while high-pressure circulation continues in the aneurysm. Circumferential dissection around the neck may be impossible without partial deflation of the dome. Dissecting adherent perforators may risk intraoperative rupture with thin-walled, tense sacs. Atherosclerotic aneurysms may have to be opened for thrombectomy and endarterectomy to close a clip on the aneurysm. Complex arterial reconstruction when the aneurysm involves a crucial branch point may be impossible without deflating the dome.

Three main strategies have been developed to address these situations by reducing pressure in an aneurysm dome: (1) systemic hypotension, (2) temporary clipping of major arterial branches, and (3) complete circulatory arrest. Systemic hypotension has fallen out of favor because of its negative effects on other organ systems and adjacent uninvolved areas of the brain. Focal circulatory arrest with one or more temporary clips has become the most common method for dealing with complex intracranial aneurysms. The length of time that temporary clips can be used before infarction develops poses limitations that, on occasion, can become a crucial issue. For these situations, complete circulatory arrest with the protection of deep hypothermia represents the ultimate approach to devascularize a complex intracranial aneurysm. Because this technique is a major undertaking and poses additional risks, it can be justified only in a few select cases.

This chapter discusses appropriate selection of cases with a special emphasis on the technique of circulatory arrest. Attention is given to the pathophysiology of cerebral ischemia as it relates to this specialized technique. Finally, the results achieved with this technique are discussed briefly.

HISTORY

Since the introduction of the temporary aneurysm clip in the early 1960s, several groups have experimented with its usefulness in facilitating dissection and reconstruction.[1–11] The result of that experience was the realization that all cerebral arteries can withstand short periods of temporary occlusion without cerebral infarction.[3] Nonetheless, ischemic tolerance varies dramatically among arterial distributions, with the proximal internal carotid artery perhaps allowing an hour or more, and the perforator-bearing segments of the middle cerebral artery or the basilar apex allowing only a few minutes.[6, 10] Although several agents can enhance cerebral tolerance (see later), these are of limited benefit in territories solely perfused by end arteries. If these end arteries are captured in a temporary clip, permanent endothelial damage may result, leading to intravascular thrombosis. When proximal occlusion is used without complete trapping, the low-pressure release of arterial blood through the hole in the aneurysm may lead to distal collateral steal, further minimizing the ischemic tolerance.

For these reasons, there continues to be a need for complete circulatory arrest. Using deep hypothermia to achieve this arrest safely is not a new concept. Pioneered nearly half a century ago, this technique lost favor because of complications related to anticoagulation and to primitive pump technology.[12, 13] In the 1970s, however, further elucidation of cerebral physiology during hypothermia combined with refinements in cardiac surgery techniques that accompanied the evolution of cardiac transplantation opened new possibilities for aneurysm surgery.[14, 15]

PROMINENT INDICATIONS

Anatomic Factors

ATHEROSCLEROTIC ANEURYSMS

Cessation of blood flow within giant aneurysms often is required for clipping. Heavily atherosclerotic necks

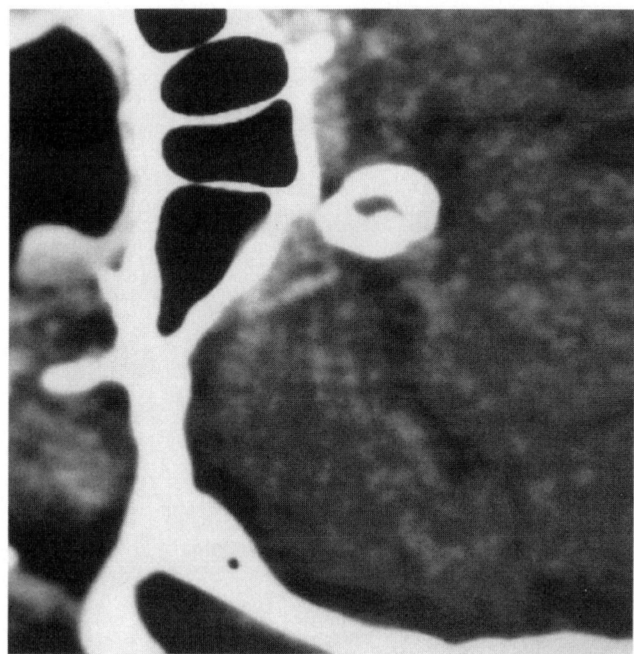

FIGURE 90–1. Coronal computed tomography scan shows extensive calcium in a paraclinoid aneurysm managed nonoperatively in an elderly woman. The appearance of such a finding in an aneurysm requiring treatment suggests the need for an endarterectomy of the neck region, which is facilitated greatly by the prolonged protection provided by arrest.

do not compress with standard clips. Consequently the dome of the aneurysm must be opened and the neck region endarterectomized to allow proper clipping. Axial imaging with three-dimensional reconstructed computed tomography is particularly useful in assessing lesions for this risk factor (Fig. 90–1).

PARTIALLY THROMBOSED ANEURYSMS

Frequently, giant aneurysms are filled with fresh or well-organized thrombotic debris. In either case, the solid mass of the aneurysm prevents safe clip application without first opening the dome and removing the contents of the aneurysm. Magnetic resonance imaging has been crucial in screening for this mass preoperatively (Fig. 90–2).

ANEURYSMS ADHERENT TO VITAL STRUCTURES

Often the dome of a giant aneurysm is adhered to vital structures, such as the visual apparatus, hypothalamus, or adjacent vascular structures. Clipping the aneurysm can cause the dome to tear away from these attachments, producing mechanical damage and hemorrhage. The best way to handle these problems is to cut off the dome of the aneurysm, leaving it attached to delicate structures, and create a separated neck region for clipping. Although total local circulatory arrest often can be achieved with temporary clips, this is not always safe or possible in certain anatomic situations.

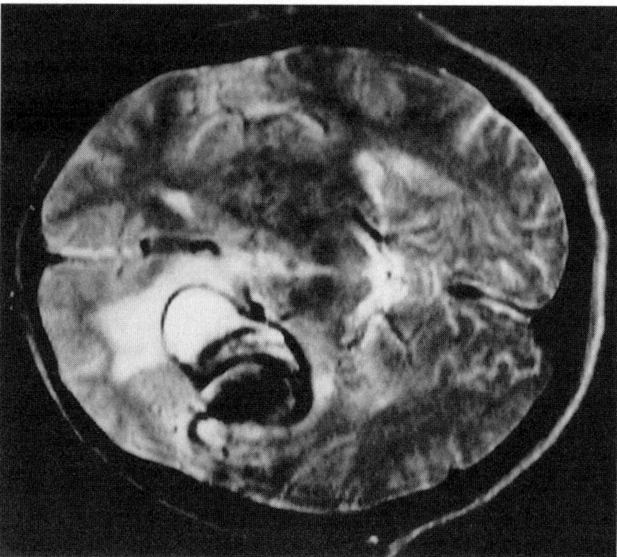

FIGURE 90–2. Partially thrombosed giant middle cerebral aneurysm as shown by magnetic resonance imaging. To ensure that clot does not compromise the inflow or outflow of such a lesion, the aneurysm may need to be opened and the clot removed with the cavitron. This requires prolonged flow arrest, which is possible only with profound hypothermia.

GIANT OPHTHALMIC AND PARACLINOID GIANT ANEURYSMS

With ophthalmic aneurysms (Fig. 90–3), the proximal carotid artery may reside well within the cavernous sinus and be impossible to clip safely. Occlusion of the cervical carotid still leaves intracavernous branches and the ophthalmic artery to supply the aneurysm, and endovascular balloon occlusion may produce suboptimal arrest. In addition, sacrifice of the carotid may lead to the development of flow-related aneurysms at other sites over time.

GIANT BASILAR ANEURYSMS

Basilar apex aneurysms (Fig. 90–4) can obscure the view of the contralateral posterior cerebral artery. Even if the apex can be totally trapped, there would be no supply to the perforators that emanate from the top of the basilar artery, usually located immediately behind the aneurysm dome. The territory supplied by these vessels cannot withstand more than a few minutes of loss of blood flow at normothermia. Although arrest usually is reserved for truly giant lesions in this location, smaller lesions may benefit from this technique when the aneurysm is oriented posteriorly into the interpeduncular cistern.

OTHER GIANT ANEURYSMS

With giant middle cerebral, anterior communicating (Fig. 90–5), and vertebral artery aneurysms, the mass of the aneurysm may obstruct the view of major efferent or afferent branches. When total local arrest must be achieved, the time required to incise the dome and

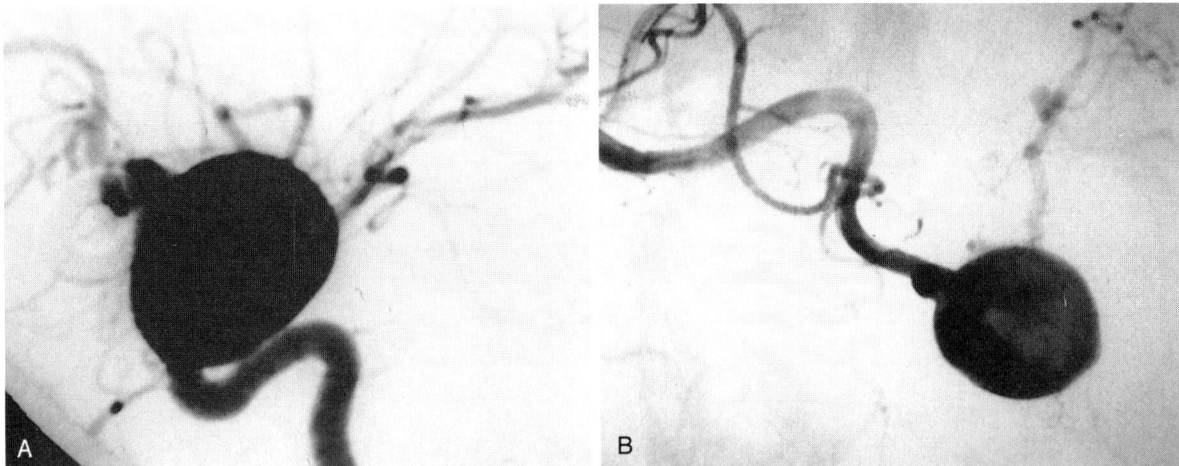

FIGURE 90–3. *A* and *B,* Giant carotid-ophthalmic aneurysm. Although these aneurysms may be approached with a focal arrest procedure using a neck dissection or intravascular balloon combined with distal trapping and suction decompression, not all patients can tolerate the ischemia time. In such cases, arrest may be appropriate.

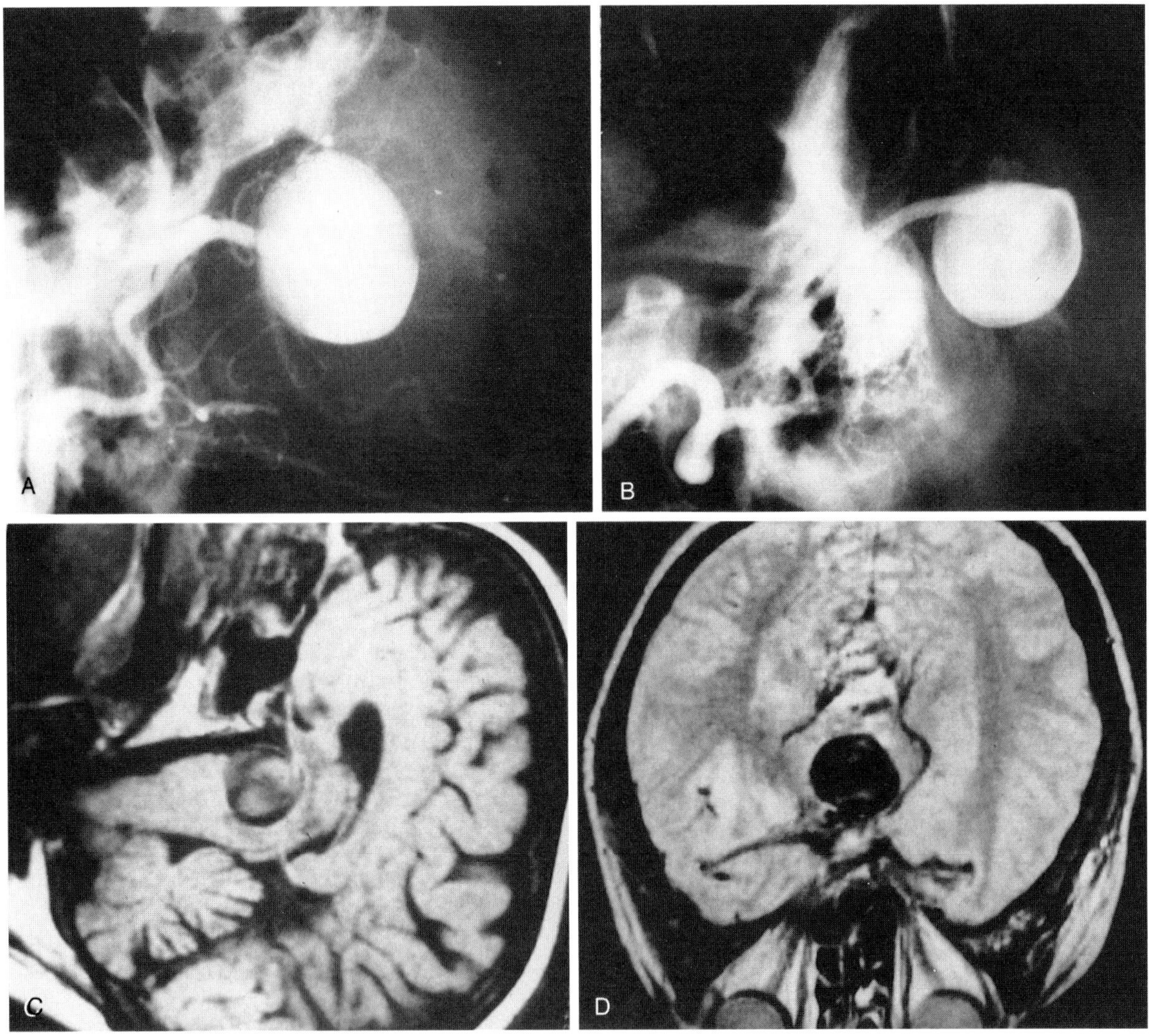

FIGURE 90–4. Giant basilar apex aneurysms such as this one *(A* and *B)* in general cannot be reconstructed satisfactorily without the use of arrest. Without arrest, the posterior wall cannot be freed successfully from the interpeduncular cistern *(C* and *D)*, and the perforators cannot be dissected safely. Although focal arrest of the basilar apex can soften the aneurysm, this can be accomplished only for a few minutes, and decompression is awkward and untenable in this location.

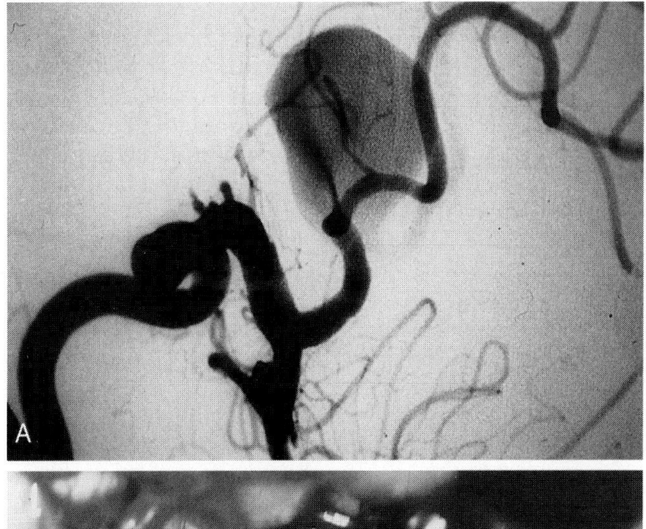

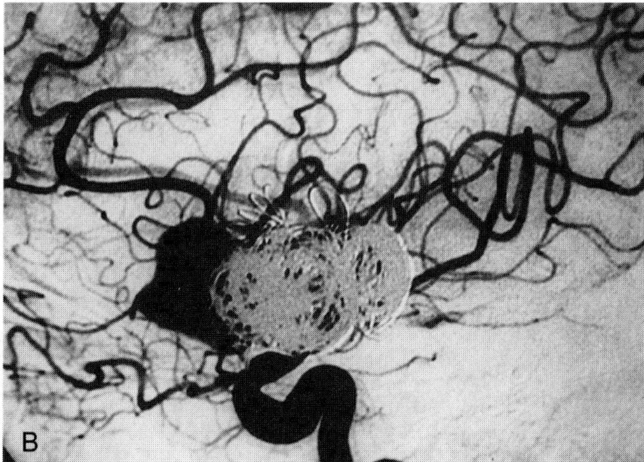

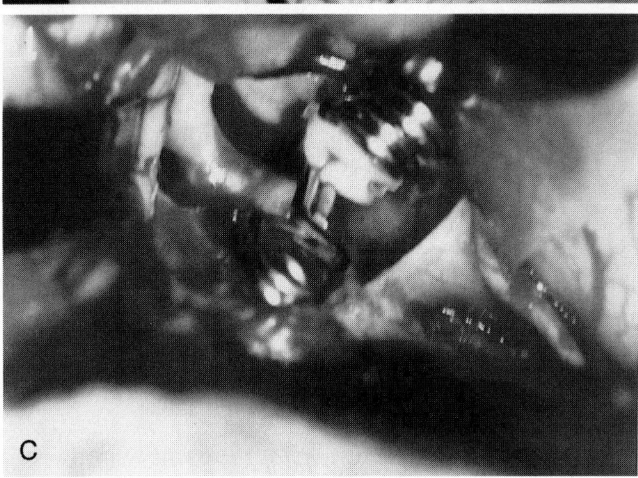

FIGURE 90–5. Giant anterior cerebral artery aneurysm. Although many of these lesions may be treated with parent vessel occlusion proximal to the discrete neck *(A)*, occasionally prior failed treatment efforts *(B)* necessitate arrest to mobilize the neck region for definitive clipping *(C)*.

perform the necessary maneuvers often exceeds the ischemic tolerance of the brain. It usually is not possible to predict accurately in advance the amount of time that temporary occlusion will be required.

Patient-Related Factors

Patients are selected for deep hypothermic circulatory arrest in one of two ways. Some patients are surgically explored and found to have aneurysms that are too difficult to clip with temporary clips alone. In these cases, surgery can be terminated, and a circulatory arrest procedure can be planned for the following week. Other candidates can be recognized from preliminary neuroradiologic studies. Giant basilar aneurysms of any configuration probably are handled best by circulatory arrest if clipping is to be pursued (Table 90–1). The safety of clipping aneurysms greater than 3 cm in diameter in most other locations usually is enhanced with deep hypothermic circulatory arrest.

In general, patients become candidates for hypothermic circulatory arrest based on the location, size, and anatomy of the vascular anomaly. Hunt and Hess grade, patient age, and time from subarachnoid hemorrhage may be important prognostically but do not represent contraindications to surgery. Preexisting disease, especially of the cardiopulmonary system, may contraindicate arrest surgery. A thorough preoperative medical examination is essential, and preoperative laboratory screening helps identify preexisting problems and provide the baseline values to be used in the postoperative period. Internal medicine consultation should be obtained if more specialized testing is required. An echocardiogram always is obtained to define cardiac

TABLE 90–1 ■ **Profound Hypothermic Circulatory Arrest: Indications**

	PRO	CON
Giant		
Posterior circulation	+ + +	
Proximal carotid	+	
MCA bifurcation	+ +	
Anterior communicating	+ +	
Atherosclerotic neck		
Basilar location	+ +	
Other	+	
Adherent structures		
Optic nerve	+	
Brainstem	+ +	
Patient		
>65 years old		+ +
Severe athero-occlusive disease		+ + +
Recent SAH (<10 day)		+
Aortic insufficiency		+

MCA, middle cerebral artery; SAH, subarachnoid hemorrhage.

function and valvular competency. Ultimately the decision to proceed is made after all areas of concern have been addressed, but young healthy patients usually derive great benefit with minimal additional risk.

PATHOPHYSIOLOGY OF CEREBRAL ISCHEMIA AND HYPOTHERMIC CEREBRAL PROTECTION

Occlusion of one of the major cerebral arteries to devascularize an aneurysm temporarily produces a zone of relatively ischemic tissue. This zone traditionally has been viewed as composed of two pathophysiologically distinct areas: (1) a central core of densely ischemic tissue and (2) the penumbra, where collateral circulation allows for prolonged viability. In the ischemic core, low flow leads to anaerobic glycolysis, acidosis, depletion of adenosine triphosphate (ATP) and, eventually, disrupted homeostasis. Sodium, chloride, and toxic calcium in turn enter the cell, resulting in intracellular acidosis, edema, and loss of structural integrity. Unless occlusion is reversed, the penumbra is recruited progressively into the core by several mechanisms. Although initially in possession of marginal yet adequate blood flow, the penumbra is exposed to increasing concentrations of toxic neurotransmitters, such as glutamate and nitric oxide, released from the actively infarcting ischemic core. These toxins cause further cellular depolarization and spreading neuronal death.[16, 17] Low blood flow in penumbral regions is associated with the expression of platelet and leukocyte adhesion molecules on the intact endothelium leading to progressive microvascular failure, which worsens flow further. Protection of the brain supplied by vessels destined for temporary ischemia requires strategies designed to halt this spreading death in anticipation of reperfusion.

Perhaps the most time-honored pharmacologic manipulation used is based on the fact that neurons expend energy/consume oxygen (CMRO) for two general purposes: (1) to maintain basic cellular structure and (2) to transmit electrical impulses. Interventions that decrease or eliminate the electrical activity of neurons reduce the CMRO of the brain and enhance membrane viability. Barbiturates are the best-studied agent for decreasing brain electrical activity and have been shown to reduce CMRO by 50%.[18] Barbiturates also redistribute blood flow to ischemic cortex, scavenge free radicals, and stabilize membranes. Because barbiturates have several adverse effects pertinent to hypothermic cardiac arrest, however, additional CMRO-reducing agents have been developed. These agents (etomidate, propofol, and isoflurane) are shorter acting and have fewer myocardial depressant effects than barbiturates.[19] Elimination of electrical activity reduces CMRO by only about 50%, however, and further use of any of these agents is ineffective in producing an additional lowering of CMRO. To extend tolerance beyond the limits of these agents requires the use of hypothermia.

Only hypothermia has been shown capable of slowing the energy expenditures of the cell required for maintenance of ionic gradients and structural homeostasis. Mild hypothermia down to 33°C has been shown to have demonstrable protective effects, but deep hypothermia to 18°C allows the brain to be totally deprived of blood flow for 1 hour without noticeable damage.[20] Ischemic tolerance induced by hypothermia is attributed primarily to ATP preservation.[18, 21] Hypothermic tolerance is related directly to the degree of temperature reduction and occurs in the presence of proportional reductions in cerebral blood flow.[22] In cell culture, oxygen consumption has been shown to decrease 50% for every 10°C drop in temperature. In vivo reductions in metabolism are greater (approximately 7% for each 1°C drop in temperature), probably owing to the combined effect of hypothermia on basal metabolic rate and electrical activity as well as excitatory neurotransmitter and inflammatory cytokine release.[6, 23–34] Despite the beneficial effects of hypothermia, and deep hypothermia in particular, humans cannot tolerate this condition for much more than 90 minutes, with intelligence quotient loss and neuropsychologic deficits being seen increasingly as membrane stability becomes threatened.[34–37] Many surgeons recommend temporary reperfusion for periods of arrest longer than 90 minutes.[38]

SIDE EFFECTS OF PROFOUND HYPOTHERMIA

If the use of cardiac arrest with profound hypothermia is considered for the treatment of giant and complex intracranial aneurysms, it is crucial for the surgeon to understand the effects that profound hypothermia has on the host as a whole and how these effects are best monitored (Table 90–2). Perhaps the least-recognized alteration that occurs with hypothermia is its ability to increase oxygen and carbon dioxide solubility. Although generally of little concern to the surgeon, these alterations have created an important controversy regarding the need for temperature correction of blood gases by adding carbon dioxide; this is unnecessary and may lead to unwanted cerebral swelling and intracranial pressure.[39–41] The second major physiologic effect of hypothermia that is of concern to neurovascular surgeons is its role in increasing blood viscosity. To avoid this increase, isovolemic hemodilution is pursued aggressively, with the final hematocrit titrated approximately to temperature (i.e., 18°C = hematocrit of 18).[42, 43] Profound hypothermia may exacerbate cerebral swelling by inducing a metabolic acidosis as noncardiac, non-neurological tissues become increasingly and relatively underperfused.[44, 45] Potentially cerebrotoxic hyperglycemia secondary to hypoinsulinemia occurs during profound hypothermia and requires close monitoring and avoidance of glucose-containing solutions. Adrenal corticosteroid release may be decreased after prolonged hypothermia, necessitating perioperative replacement as well as continued hypothalamic-adrenal axis surveillance for 1 year.[46] Profound hypothermia plays a potentially important role in

TABLE 90-2 ■ **Profound Hypothermic Circulatory Arrest: Side Effects**

	RESULT	SOLUTION
Direct effect of hypothermia		
Increased carbon dioxide solubility	Cerebral swelling	Avoid temperature correcting ABG
Metabolic acidosis	Cerebral swelling	Bicarbonate infusion
Increased blood viscosity	Reduced ischemic tolerance	Isovolemic hemodilution
Hyperglycemia	Reduced ischemic tolerance	Avoid D5W-containing fluids
Slowing of enzymatic coagulation	Coagulopathy	Rewarming
Platelet dysfunction	Coagulopathy	Rewarming
Decreased myocardial contractility	Impaired cardioversion	Propofol rather than barbiturate
Sinus bradycardia	Impaired cardioversion	Atropine/rewarming
Widening of the P-R interval	Impaired cardioversion	Digoxin/rewarming
Sensitization to cardiac medications	Arrhythmia	Adjust accordingly
Primary hepatic dysfunction	Dilantin toxicity	Adjust accordingly
Bypass circuit related		
Complement-mediated pneumonitis	Prolonged intubation	Nonpulsatile flow oxygenators
Hemolysis	ATN, anemia, platelet dysfunction	Heparinized circuitry
Blood product reaction	ATN	Osmotic alkalinization urine
Platelet dysfunction	Coagulopathy	Platelet transfusion
Visceral hypoperfusion	ATN	Generous fluid postoperatively

ABG, arterial blood gas; ATN, acute tubular necrosis; D5W, 5% dextrose in water.

pulmonary pathophysiology with the occasional development of a complement-mediated pneumonitis (i.e., pump-lung). Although increasingly rare as a result of improvements in the construction of oxygenators, flow rates, and the use of nonpulsatile flow, this pneumonitis can result in the need for prolonged postoperative intubation.[47, 48] Equally as rare, but important to recognize, especially in the elderly, is the rare occurrence of postoperative renal failure caused by transient decreases in glomerular filtration rate as well as hemolysis and blood product reactions.[45, 49–51] Osmotic alkalinization of the urine is particularly beneficial in the management of hemoglobinuria.[52, 53] Hypothermia can cause mild hepatic dysfunction that can result in overly high dilantin levels, but frank hepatic dysfunction is extraordinarily rare.

In contrast to these rare and essentially minor concerns is the common and frustrating problem of hypothermia-induced coagulopathy. This condition is due to platelet dysfunction and slowing of the enzymatic coagulation cascade.[54] Platelet dysfunction is mostly due to sequestration, which resolves within an hour of rewarming, and major clotting factors seem to be largely unaffected. Heparinization and extracorporeal circuitry account for the remainder of the coagulopathy, and although hypothermia may prolong the anticoagulant effects of the former, its half-life generally is less than 2 hours. As for the latter, removal of the circuits results in an immediate reduction in turbulence and shear-induced red blood cell and platelet destruction. Progressive hemoconcentration during warming also helps to correct the coagulopathy, and warming causes a decrease in plasmin-dependent fibrinolysis.[55–57]

Finally, hypothermia may have profound and lasting effects on myocardial contractility and conduction lasting well into the intensive care unit course. Systolic and diastolic dysfunction, sinus bradycardia, widening of the P-R interval, QRS changes, and sensitization to pharmacologic challenge all have been reported.[58]

Despite the protective effects of hypothermia, neurological sequelae still occur.[59–62] Prolonged hypothermia may contribute to neurological damage by a combination of macroembolization and microembolization as well as global hypoperfusion.[63] Age and preexisting cerebrovascular disease are the major risk factors for neurological complications, and despite increased experience, there is little evidence of these complications declining much further.[63, 64] Some improvement in neurological complication rates can be found with the use of barbiturate alternatives, which decrease cerebral metabolism more readily and with fewer cardiovascular effects.[55, 65–69]

CLINICAL TECHNIQUES

Technical Preparations

Before performing an institution's first arrest case, a multispecialty team needs to be assembled, with all members ideally having been trained in this technique at specialized centers. When this team is assembled, an operative protocol should be designed. Next, an appropriate operating suite should be identified. The size of this suite must accommodate two surgical teams and a significant amount of extra equipment (including neurophysiologic monitors, transesophageal ultrasound, heat-exchange pumps, perfusion pump and oxygenator, and cardiovascular surgery equipment trays). The electrical demands placed by this amount of equipment should not be underestimated, and coordination with hospital electricians is crucial.

Preoperative Medical Evaluation

When a patient is deemed an appropriate arrest candidate from a neurosurgical point of view, it is imperative that coronary or valvular heart disease, pulmonary disease, and systemic blood pressure abnormalities be addressed fully. In particular, aortic valve function should be evaluated carefully with transthoracic echocardiography. If insufficiency is detected, central cannulation and left ventricular venting through a median sternotomy may be required. The status of the patient's peripheral arterial disease should be assessed because it also might complicate peripheral cannulation. General medical examination with attention to renal and hepatic function as well as to the competence of the coagulation cascade is a prerequisite.

Choice of Cannulation Sites

Cannulation for cardiopulmonary bypass can be done peripherally through an inguinal incision (femoral-femoral) or centrally through a sternotomy (aortic–right atrial). With peripheral cannulation, the two surgical fields are comfortably separate, but neurosurgical instrumentation still must allow access to the sternal notch in the event central access suddenly becomes necessary. Cross-contamination, blood loss, and the risk of sternal osteomyelitis are reduced with this peripheral technique. In return, one accepts a 10% risk of more minor wound and vascular complications.

Advocates of central cannulation point out that direct exposure of the heart ensures rapid response to distention or fibrillation and claim that cooling and warming times are reduced. The authors prefer peripheral cannulation in the nonatherosclerotic patient, however, and have found that cooling and warming times are not significantly different from those obtainable with central cannulation. With aortic valve competence and continuous transesophageal echocardiography monitoring, ventricular fibrillation for lengthy periods is well tolerated in a decompressed, perfused heart, and parallel circuit venting systems replace a cardiotomy reservoir. Occasionally, if flow cannot be improved when bypass is begun, central cannulation may be required.

Patient Preparation

In addition to the usual equipment necessary for aneurysm surgery, cardiac arrest procedures require a Swan-Ganz catheter, a transesophageal echocardiography probe, scalp and cortical electroencephalography electrodes, a brain temperature needle probe, a cooling/warming blanket, and the placement of specialized grounding plates for defibrillation. These plates take some time to attach or insert, and a full day should be committed to this effort and an early start planned.

Neuroanesthetic Management

When these special monitoring devices have been arranged, the case may begin, and the neurosurgeon may concentrate on the superficial dissection as per routine. It is crucial that the neurosurgeon understands the routine to help solve problems. All patients are given perioperative antibiotics, steroids, and anticonvulsants. Steroids purportedly stabilize membranes, prevent vasogenic edema, and minimize complement generation.[70] Antibiotics are especially important because hypothermia increases the risk of infection (independently and in association with prolonged operative exposure). Anticonvulsants are employed only in the immediate perioperative period, and although their use has little scientific merit, dilantin especially may be mildly cerebroprotective. Anesthesia is induced with intravenous midazolam, fentanyl, and thiopental. Vecuronium, lidocaine, and esmolol are used immediately before intubation, and maintenance anesthesia consists of a balanced technique of narcotics, oxygen, and isoflurane. Ventilation is controlled to maintain a normal $Pa{CO_2}$, and the concentration of isoflurane is minimized (<0.75%) to facilitate electrophysiologic monitoring. In general aneurysm patients should have their fluids conservatively managed; however, hypothermic circulatory arrest often makes this difficult. The vasodilatory effects of warming, together with third space losses secondary to membrane dysfunction, often render the patient relatively hypovolemic. Euvolemic correction is guided by central pressures and urine output and maintained primarily with glucose-free isotonic crystalloids. Colloid as packed cells and albumin occasionally is necessary.

A crucial adjunct in optimizing fluids and by extension cardiopulmonary function is the use of a 5-MHz phased-array ultrasonic esophageal transducer, positioned so that left ventricular short-axis images can be obtained continuously at the level of the papillary muscles. Adjunctive intraoperative monitoring includes compressed spectral array electroencephalography analysis, which facilitates titration of anesthetics to burst suppression. In contrast to other groups, the authors have not found somatosensory evoked potentials or brainstem auditory evoked potentials to be useful adjuncts, and these modalities require an extra level of sophistication to interpret. Electroencephalogram burst suppression for cerebral protection is induced just before cardiopulmonary bypass with a loading dose of propofol followed by a constant infusion. Although considerably more literature exists regarding the use of barbiturates for this purpose, the authors have found the level of protection to be adequate with propofol, and emergence times are significantly shorter, leading to quicker extubations and potentially reducing pulmonary complications. Propofol appears to have less cardiosuppressive qualities than barbiturates, perhaps shortening overall bypass times. This propofol infusion is continued until the electroencephalogram becomes isoelectric secondary to cooling (around 25°C), at which time it is discontinued. Propofol is resumed at the same constant infusion rate on rewarming and continued until the patient is safely in the intensive care unit.

In contrast to routine aneurysm surgery in which mild hypothermia is induced with surface cooling blankets, deep hypothermic circulatory arrest requires the use of surface cooling and extracorporeal circulatory cooling. The latter requires the use of chilled intravenous solutions and a refrigerated water bath heat exchanger set at 8°C. Using these, cooling is more uniform than with a blanket alone and ensures better protection of all organ systems.[38] Despite this greater degree of protection, two caveats exist. First, cooling does not proceed in a uniform fashion, and second, the temperature should not be allowed to drift below 16°C.[42] To avoid problems, vasodilators are employed as are multiple temperature monitors to verify that equilibration has occurred. In the authors' center, esophageal, tympanic, pulmonary artery, and cortical brain temperature probes are used. Cortical brain temperature probes can be placed safely into the frontal lobe after cauterizing the pia; the authors find these less variable than epidural monitors and less bulky as well. Despite the suggestions of others that rectal temperature approximates brain temperature, the authors consistently observe brain cooling to lag behind esophageal cooling. Sole reliance on esophageal cooling could lead to premature initiation of arrest. In the authors' institution, surface cooling generally is employed preferentially from the beginning of the case, and during 1 to 2 hours, mild hypothermia to 33°C can be achieved. Only when the surgeon has finished the dissection and realizes that arrest is a certainty does final cooling begin. Surgeons should expect this cooling to take 30 to 45 minutes.

If circulatory arrest is determined to be necessary, operative times can be minimized by calling the cardiac surgeon 45 minutes before the need for arrest so that the cutdowns for cannula placement may be initiated. At this point, anticoagulation with heparin is titrated to an activated clotting time of 450 to 500 seconds. An initial bolus of 3000 IU/kg generally is adequate followed by an infusion. A 19F femoral artery cannula and a long 21F femoral venous right atrial cannula are used in conjunction with centrifugal bypass pumps and a membrane oxygenator. The pump is primed bloodlessly with saline or a colloid, such as mannitol. Although the appropriate flow rate and perfusion pressure are controversial, the authors have found that a rate of 2.5 L/min/m^2 works quite well. Ventricular fibrillation occurs during cooling (approximately 27°C), and potassium chloride can be given to induce diastolic arrest. Echocardiography monitoring is crucial to ensure that the heart does not distend at this point. When the brain temperature finally reaches 18°C, the circulation is arrested, and the patient is allowed to exsanguinate through the venous cannula until the neurovasculature is decompressed adequately. Too much exsanguination carries the risk of air embolism and a no-reflow phenomenon in small blood vessels, but arterial pressure is generally almost zero. Although others have used 72 minutes of circulatory arrest without adverse sequelae, the authors generally aim for no more than 45 to 60 minutes. If it appears that a longer time is needed, recirculation generally is performed for a period of 20 minutes or so, somewhere around the 40-minute mark.

When the neurosurgeon is satisfied with the clip placement, circulation is reestablished, and reperfusion is accompanied by rewarming. Because of the risk of hypoxia, acidosis, and air embolism, gradual rewarming is crucial. The perfusate temperature is increased gradually, never exceeding the venous temperature by more than 10°C (maximum of 40°C). At about 30°C, the heart may resume a sinus rhythm or develop ventricular fibrillation, which requires cardioversion (200 to 400 J). Mild ischemia and hypothermia may cause some myocardial depression requiring the temporary use of inotropic agents. With the abandonment of barbiturates, this situation has become rare. A final rewarming temperature of 37°C is targeted, allowing for some downward drift. Warming blankets, heated ventilation, and warmed intravenous solutions maintain the patient's temperature, and protamine is titrated carefully (1.3 mg protamine/mg heparin) to reverse the heparin-induced coagulopathy. Despite this, a mild ooze is noted well into rewarming as platelet damage and dilution of the clotting factors take some time to stabilize. In contrast to many groups who routinely infuse autologous whole blood, platelets, and fresh frozen plasma and occasionally use cryoprecipitate, the authors generally avoid these. Similarly the authors do not use desmopressin (improves platelet function) because complications have been reported. Instead the authors simply wait to leave the operative field until this ooze is entirely reversed and the patient is at least 34°C. This generally takes 1 to 2 hours. At the end of the procedure, the patient is taken to the intensive care unit with computed tomography monitoring, having removed the electrophysiologic monitors and the transesophageal echocardiography monitor. The patient is left intubated and is ventilated if necessary, and computed tomography scan helps confirm intracranial hemostasis.

Surgical Management

Craniotomy and initial dissection of the aneurysm are done in a standard fashion, with extra attention to hemostasis. A small ooze develops into a major one when heparin is given. At the point where further dissection seems unduly hazardous without aneurysm softening or decompression, the anesthesiologist places the patient in burst suppression with a propofol drip, and the cardiac surgeon institutes deep hypothermia. It is crucial that the cardiac team is immediately available because a delay lengthens the overall brain retraction time and may predispose to lobar hematoma formation. At this point, the operating surgeon generally takes a short break to review the films, while the assistant maintains close inspection of the field. With essentially no blood pressure and the brain at 18°C, aneurysm repair can proceed in an unencumbered environment. There is no mechanical intrusion of temporary clips, bleeding from opened arterial structures can be titrated to zero if required, and the ischemic tolerance of the brain shut off from blood flow does not begin to be an issue for at least 60 minutes after the initiation of complete circulatory arrest. A more perfect clipping generally can be achieved than with other techniques. Clip placement is checked by reinstituting pump circulation. Adjustments can be made by turning off the pump. When repair is deemed secure, full flows and normal pressures are restored. Special care needs to be taken to preserve all perforating vessels. During the arrest, these can appear to be bands of arachnoid rather than vessels. Once clipped or disrupted, the vessels may not refill, giving no signal to the surgeon that a major error has been committed. During heparinization, retractors should not be moved if possible to decrease the shear on small vessels; this also protects against lobar clot formation. All operative irrigation during the arrest period should be cooled so as to create no mismatch in brain temperature.

Complication Avoidance and Management

THROMBOPHLEBITIS

Deep venous thrombosis with pulmonary embolization is a potential complication of femoral cannulation.[12, 71, 72] Postoperative bed rest and the use of antifibrinolytic agents compound this problem. Some experts have suggested cannulation of the saphenous bulb with postoperative ligation as a potential solution, whereas others have advocated open-chest cannulation. The authors advocate the use of alternating compression stockings and early ambulation. In the authors' series, all of whom had femoral cannulation, no problems with thrombophlebitis were experienced.

DELAYED AWAKENING

The use of hypothermia, barbiturates, and narcotics contributes to a significant degree of postoperative somnolence. The degree of sedation varies among individuals, although the total dose of barbiturates is the major predictor of the length of postoperative sedation. Postoperative hepatic or renal dysfunction can delay elimination and recovery further.[73] The authors have nearly eliminated this problem by substituting propofol for barbiturate, and emergence times are now on the order of 3 hours.[74]

TEMPERATURE INSTABILITY

Temperature maintenance is mandatory in the early postoperative period to prevent cardiopulmonary instability and continued coagulopathy. Initially, core temperature is maintained by vasoconstrictive shunting, but as rewarming continues, vasodilation occurs, resulting in hypotension, tachycardia, and cardiac strain. Persistent hypothermia also increases sympathetic tone, shivering, and oxygen consumption.[75–77] Aggressive management is required. Vasodilators together with meperidine and prolonged muscle relaxation reduce shivering and provide for a smooth anesthetic emergence.[75, 76, 78]

COAGULOPATHIES

Although most problems with hemostasis are managed in the operating suite, continued bleeding diathesis can occur. The most common causes are further dilution, inadequate clotting factor replacement, and rebound heparinization. Less common causes include fibrinolysis, disseminated intravascular coagulopathy, and pharmacologic impairment of platelets by antibiotics, antihypertensive agents, and diuretics.[79, 80] Management requires close clinical and laboratory monitoring as well as appropriate fluid and temperature maintenance. Occasionally, clotting factor replacement is necessary to treat dilutional coagulopathies and disseminated intravascular coagulopathy.

INCREASED FLUID SHIFTS

Perioperatively, large volumes of fluids are required to maintain adequate circulating volume. This requirement, coupled with hypothermia-induced alterations of membrane permeability, leads to interstitial fluid sequestration.[81] Hypervolemic hemodilution for postoperative vasospasm compounds the situation. Most patients mobilize and eliminate these fluids, rarely requiring more than time and, occasionally, diuretics. Such patients are typically in a precarious position on the Starling curve, however, and the use of a pulmonary artery catheter can greatly simplify decision making.

CLINICAL RESULTS

From 1987 through 1999, the authors have performed 55 cardiac arrest procedures for giant or complex intracranial aneurysms at Columbia–Presbyterian Medical Center. All patients were placed on bypass via a femorofemoral technique. Beginning in 1991, propofol was substituted for barbiturates with no increase in complications and with a 73% reduction in the average time of emergence from 11 to 3 hours. Patient age ranged from 15 to 73 years (mean, 51 years). All but four patients operated had giant aneurysms, with 36% situated at the basilar bifurcation, 24% situated on the ophthalmic artery, and 42% situated elsewhere (19% midbasilar/vertebrobasilar junction, 8% middle cerebral artery, 8% anterior communicating artery). In approximately 25% of cases, the aneurysm was selected for arrest at least in part because of the presence of significant intraluminal atheroma or clot, which would necessitate complete aneurysm opening before clipping. Ten patients (20%) presented with subarachnoid hemorrhage; most came to medical attention for other reasons (46% nerve or brainstem compression, 16% headaches, 4% stroke, 4% hydrocephalus). Only one case was an incidental finding.

Functional outcomes at 3 months were good (Glasgow Outcome Scale I or II) in 74% of patients, 16% were dependent, and 10% were dead. Procedural complications occurred in 36% and can be divided into two broad categories: (1) complications related to the bypass procedure (14%) and (2) complications related to clip placement (22%). There were two cases of aortic root dissection in elderly patients resulting in death. There were six (12%) postoperative hematomas. One hematoma resulted in acute hydrocephalus and death; another resulted in a transient fluent aphasia and required anterior temporal lobectomy, but the patient ultimately did well. There were seven cases of perforator injury. There were three cranial nerve II injuries. Overall perioperative morbidity resulted in mild deficits that improved in 7 patients and permanently debilitating deficits in 11. Postoperative angiography was performed in only 22 cases. In 16 (73%) cases, the angiographic result was perfect; in 4 (18%), a vessel was obviously occluded; and in 1, a vessel was compromised but patent. In only one case was an aneurysm remnant seen (5%). Overall, length of stay averaged 21 days (range, 2 to 138 days). In uncomplicated cases, the average length of stay was 19 days (range, 4 to 52 days). Death resulted in shorter stays, and disability resulted in longer stays.

In the modern era (1980 to present), there have been several reports detailing the successes of deep hypothermic circulatory arrest in the management of complex intracranial aneurysms. Since Silverberg's report on the management of eight aneurysms with low morbidity and mortality, many neurosurgeons have begun using the technique with excellent results.[92] Since the 1980s, more than 100 cases have been reported in the searchable (Medline) literature.[71, 72, 82–95] These reports, usually a compilation of a few cases, illustrate several important points. The first is the prominent role of committed anesthesiologists in deep hypothermic circulatory arrest. The second is that subarachnoid hemorrhage, clinical grade, and acute presentation are not, in and of themselves, contraindications to arrest surgery.[94] The preponderance of cases either were operated in a delayed fashion or had presented with symptoms of mass effect. Third, even in centers with extremely heavy volumes of subarachnoid hemorrhage and where consultation for complex unruptured lesions is extremely common, arrest surgery is employed rarely (1% to 5% of all cases). This probably results from the fact that patients selected for this procedure are screened carefully. As a result, when significant complications do occur in these series, they rarely have been due to the bypass itself, but rather are due to factors that would have been more difficult to manage had the bypass not been chosen. Cumulatively the results achieved in these limited reports are laudable, with 82% experiencing excellent or good outcomes with only 10% dying.

CONCLUSIONS

Although deep hypothermic circulatory arrest represents an extremely useful adjunct for the treatment of complex aneurysms of the anterior and posterior circulations, results with this technique may not be generalizable to all institutions. Because of the need for an experienced team and the steep learning curve, cases best treated with arrest probably should be sent to regional centers. At such centers, the neurological protection afforded by this technique allows for the safe and lasting reconstruction of most giant posterior fossa lesions in young and middle-aged patients. Older patients with calcified, wide-necked aneurysms continue to represent a significant challenge. Open-chest techniques should be considered in these patients, as should other modalities, such as bypass and endovascular proximal vessel occlusion.

REFERENCES

1. Boecher-Schwarz HG, Ungersboeck K, Ulrich P, et al: Pre- and intraoperative methods of controlling cerebral circulation in giant aneurysm surgery. Neurosurg Rev 18:85–93, 1995.
2. Fujita S, Kawaguchi T: Monitoring of direct cortical responses during temporary arterial occlusion at aneurysm surgery. Acta Neurochir 101:23–28, 1989.
3. Mizoi K, Yoshimoto T: Permissible temporary occlusion time in aneurysm surgery as evaluated by evoked potential monitoring. Neurosurgery 33:434–440, 1993.
4. Momma F, Wang AD, Symon L: Effects of temporary arterial occlusion on somatosensory evoked responses in aneurysm surgery. Surg Neurol 27:343–352, 1987.
5. Mooij JJ, Buchthal A, Belopavlovic M: Somatosensory evoked potential monitoring of temporary middle cerebral artery occlusion during aneurysm operation. Neurosurgery 21:492–496, 1987.
6. Ogilvy CS, Carter BS, Kaplan S, et al: Temporary vessel occlusion for aneurysm surgery: Risk factors for stroke in patients protected by induced hypothermia and hypertension and intravenous mannitol administration. J Neurosurg 84:785–791, 1996.
7. Ohmoto T, Nagao S, Mino S, et al: Monitoring of cortical blood flow during temporary arterial occlusion in aneurysm surgery by the thermal diffusion method. Neurosurgery 28:49–54, 1991.
8. Pool JL: Aneurysms of the anterior communicating artery, bifrontal craniotomy, and routine use of temporary clips. J Neurosurg 18:98–103, 1961.
9. Sako K, Nakai H, Takizawa K, et al: Aneurysm surgery using temporary occlusion under SEP monitoring. No Shinkei Geka 23: 35–41, 1995.
10. Samson D, Batjer HH, Bowman G, et al: A clinical study of the parameters and effects of temporary arterial occlusion in the management of intracranial aneurysms. Neurosurgery 34:22–28, 1994.
11. Steinberg GK, Panahian N, Sun GH, et al: Cerebral damage caused by interrupted, repeated arterial occlusion versus uninterrupted occlusion in a focal ischemic model. J Neurosurg 81: 554–559, 1994.
12. Drake CG, Barr HWK, Coles JC, et al: The use of extracorporeal circulation and profound hypothermia in the treatment of ruptured aneurysms. J Neurosurg 21:575–580, 1964.
13. Patterson RH, Ray BS: Profound hypothermia for intracranial surgery: Laboratory and clinical experience with extracorporeal circulation by peripheral cannulation. Ann Surg 156:377–383, 1962.
14. McMurtry JG, Housepian EM, Bowman FO Jr, et al: Surgical treatment of basilar artery aneurysms: Elective circulatory arrest with thoracotomy in 12 cases. J Neurosurg 40:486–494, 1974.
15. Michenfelder JD, Gronert GA, Rehder K: Anesthesia for neurosurgical procedures. Clin Anesth 3:383–414, 1969.
16. Siesjo BK: Pathophysiology and treatment of focal cerebral ischemia: Part I. Pathophysiology. J Neurosurg 77:169–175, 1992.
17. Siesjo BK: Pathophysiology and treatment of focal cerebral ischemia: Part II. Mechanism of damage and treatment. J Neurosurg 77:337–349, 1992.
18. Smith AL, Wollman H: Cerebral blood flow and metabolism: Effects of anesthetic drugs and techniques. Anesthesiology 36: 378–389, 1972.
19. Ridenour TR, Warner DS, Todd MM, et al: Comparative effects of propofol and halothane on outcome from middle cerebral artery occlusion in the rat. Anesthesiology 83:1254–1265, 1995.
20. Solomon RA: Principles of aneurysm surgery: Cerebral ischemic protection, hypothermia, and circulatory arrest. Clin Neurosurg 41:351–363, 1994.
21. Fay T: Early experiences with local and generalized refrigeration of the human brain. J Neurosurg 16:239, 1959.
22. Schettini A, Stahurski B, Young HF: Osmotic and osmotic-loop diuresis in brain surgery. J Neurosurg 56:679, 1982.
23. Busto R, Dietrich WD, Globus MY: Small differences in intraischemic brain temperature critically determine the extent of ischemic neuronal injury. J Cereb Blood Flow Metab 7:729, 1987.

24. Busto R, Globus MY, Dietrich WD: Effects of mild hypothermia on ischemia-induced release of neurotransmitters and free fatty acids in rat brain. Stroke 20:904, 1989.
25. Conley RF, Sundt TM: Effect of dexamethasone on the edema of focal cerebral ischemia. Stroke 4:148, 1973.
26. Dempsey RJ, Combs DJ, Maley ME: Moderate hypothermia reduces postischemic edema development and leukotriene production. Neurosurgery 21:177, 1987.
27. Farrar JK, Gamache FW Jr, Ferguson GG: Effects of profound hypotension on cerebral blood flow during surgery for intracranial aneurysms. J Neurosurg 55:857, 1981.
28. Fox LS, Blackstone EH, Kirklin JW: Relationship of whole body oxygen consumption to perfusion flow rate during hypothermic cardiopulmonary bypass. J Thorac Cardiovasc Surg 83:239, 1982.
29. Gill R, Foster AC, Woodruff GN: Systemic administration of MK-801 protects against ischemia-induced hippocampal neurodegeneration in the gerbil. J Neurosci 7:3344, 1987.
30. Michenfelder JD, Milde JH: The effects of profound hypothermia (below 14 degrees C) on canine cerebral metabolism. J Cereb Blood Flow Metab 12:877, 1992.
31. Sheardown MJ, Nielsen EO, Hansen AJ: 2,3-dihydroxy-6-nitro-7-sulfamoyl-benzo (F) quinoxaline: A neuroprotectant for cerebral ischemia. Science 247:571, 1990.
32. Steen PA, Geesvold SE, Milde JH: Nimodipine improves outcome when given after complete cerebral ischemia in primates. Anesthesiology 62:406, 1985.
33. Steen PA, Newberg LA, Milde JH, Michenfelder JD: Hypothermia and barbiturates: Individual and combined effects on canine cerebral oxygen consumption. Anesthesiology 58:527, 1983.
34. Swan H: The importance of acid-base management for cardiac and cerebral preservation during open heart operations. Surg Gynecol Obstet 158:391, 1984.
35. Crawford ES, Saleh SA: Transverse aortic arch aneurysm: Improved results of treatment employing new modifications of aortic reconstruction and hypothermic cerebral circulatory arrest. Ann Surg 194:180, 1981.
36. Rittenhouse EA, Mohri H, Dillard DH, Merendino KA: Deep hypothermia in cardivascular surgery. Ann Thorac Surg 17:63, 1974.
37. Tharion J, Johnson DC, Celermajer JM: Profound hypothermia with circulatory arrest: Nine years' clinical experience. J Thorac Cardiovasc Surg 84:66, 1982.
38. Barret-Boyes BG, Simpson M, Nentz JM: Intracardiac surgery in neonates and infants using deep hypothermia with surface cooling and limited cardiopulmonary bypass. Circulation 43(suppl 1):125, 1971.
39. Henriksen L: Brain luxury perfusion during cardiopulmonary bypass in humans: A study of the cerebral blood flow response to changes in CO_2, O_2, and blood pressure. J Cereb Blood Flow Metab 6:366, 1986.
40. Murkin JM, Farrar JK, Tweed A: Cerebral autoregulation and flow/metabolism coupling during cardiopulmonary bypass: The influence of Pa_{CO_2}. Anesth Analg 66:825, 1987.
41. Stephan H, Sonntag H, Lange H, Rieke H: Cerebral effects of anesthesia and hypothermia. Anaesthesia 44:310, 1989.
42. Hedley-Whyte J, Burgess GE, Feely TW: Applied Physiology on Respiratory Care. Boston, Little, Brown, 1976.
43. Tommasino C, Moore S, Todd MM: Cerebral effects of isovolemic hemidilution with crystalloid or colloid solutions. Crit Care Med 16:862, 1988.
44. Delin NA, Kjartansson KB, Pollock L, et al: Redistribution of regional blood flow in hypothermia. J Thorac Cardiovasc Surg 49:511, 1965.
45. Zarins CK, Skinner DB: Circulation in profound hypothermia. J Surg Res 14:97, 1973.
46. Shedd S: Principles and techniques of hypothermia and cardiac arrest for neurovascular anomalies. In Carter LP, Spetzler RF, Hamilton MG (eds): Neurovascular Surgery. New York, McGraw-Hill, 1995, p 196.
47. Chenoweth DE, Cooper SW, Hugli TE: Complement activation during cardiopulmonary bypass: Evidence for generation of C3a and C5a anaphylatoxins. N Engl J Med 304:497, 1981.
48. Kirklin JK, Westaby S, Blackstone EH: Complement and the damaging effects of cardiopulmonary bypass. J Thorac Cardiovasc Surg 86:845, 1983.
49. Boylan JW, Hong SK: Regulation of renal function in hypothermia. Am J Physiol 211:1371, 1966.
50. Litwin MS, Walter CW, Jackson N: Experimental production of acute tubular necrosis. Ann Surg 152:1010, 1960.
51. Sears DA: Disposal of plasma heme in normal man and patients with intravascular hemolysis. J Clin Invest 49:5, 1970.
52. Finlayson DC, Kaplan JA: Cardiopulmonary bypass. In Kaplan JA (ed): Cardiac Anesthesia. New York, Grune & Stratton, 1979, pp 393-440.
53. Flores J, DiBona DR, Beck CH, Leaf A: The role of cell swelling in ischemic renal damage and the protective effect of hypertonic solute. J Clin Invest 51:118, 1972.
54. Patt A, McCroskey BL, Moore EE: Hypothermia-induced coagulopathies in trauma. Surg Clin North Am 68:775, 1988.
55. Cold GE, Eskesen V, Eriksen H: CBF and $CMRO_2$ during continuous etomidate infusion supplemented with N_2O and fentanyl in patients with supratentorial cerebral tumor: A dose-response study. Acta Anesthesiol Scand 29:490, 1985.
56. Patten BM, Mendell J, Brunn B: Double-blind study of the effects of dexamethasone in acute stroke. Neurology 22:377, 1972.
57. Spetzler RF, Martin N, Hadley MN: Microsurgical endarterectomy under barbiturate protection: A prospective study. J Neurosurg 65:63, 1986.
58. Okada M: The cardiac rhythm in accidental hypothermia. J Electrocardiol 17:123, 1984.
59. Aberg T, Ronquist G, Tyden H: Adverse effects on the brain in cardiac operations as assessed by biochemical, psychometric, and radiologic methods. J Thorac Cardiovasc Surg 87:99, 1984.
60. Messmer BJ, Schallberger U, Gattiker R, Senning A: Psychomotor and intellectual development after deep hypothermia and circulatory arrest in early infancy. J Thorac Cardiovasc Surg 72:495, 1976.
61. Settergren G, Ohqvist G, Lundberg S: Cerebral blood flow and cerebral metabolism in children following cardiac surgery with deep hypothermia and circulatory arrest: Clinical course and follow-up of psychomotor development. Scand J Thorac Cardiovasc Surg 16:209, 1982.
62. Treasure T, Naftel DC, Conger DA: The effect of hypothermic circulatory arrest time on cerebral function, morphology, and biochemistry. J Thorac Cardiovasc Surg 86:761, 1983.
63. Thomson IR: Neurological aspects of cardiopulmonary bypass. Problems in Anesthesia 3:394, 1987.
64. Slogoff S, Girgis KZ, Keats AS: Etiologic factors in neuropsychiatric complications associated with cardiopulmonary bypass. Anesth Analg 61:903, 1982.
65. Churchill-Davidson HC, McMillan IKR, Melrose DG, Lynn RB: Hypothermia: An experimental study of surface cooling. Lancet 2:1011, 1953.
66. Murkin JM, Farrar JK, Tweed WA: Cerebral blood flow, oxygen consumption, and EEG during isoflurane anesthesia. Anesth Analg 65:S107, 1986.
67. Newberg LA, Michenfelder JD: Cerebral protection by isoflurane during hypoxemia or ischemia. Anesthesiology 59:29, 1983.
68. Nugent M, Artru AA, Michenfelder JD: Cerebral, metabolic, vascular, and protective effects of midazolam maleate: Comparison to diazepam. Anesthesiology 56:172, 1982.
69. Woodstock TE, Murkin JM, Farrar JK: Isoflurane augments the hypothermia-induced reduction of cerebral metabolic rate during cardiopulmonary bypass. Can Anaesth Soc J 33:S82, 1986.
70. Anderson DC, Cranford RE: Corticosteroids in ischemic stroke. Stroke 10:68, 1979.
71. Baumgartner WA, Silverberg GD, Ream AK, et al: Reappraisal of cardiopulmonary bypass with deep hypothermia and circulatory arrest for complex neurosurgical operations. Surgery 94:242–249, 1983.
72. Silverberg GD, Reitz BA, Ream AK: Hypothermia and cardiac arrest in the treatment of giant aneurysms of the cerebral circulation and hemangioblastoma of the medulla. J Neurosurg 55: 337–346, 1981.
73. Heier T, Caldwell JE, Sessler DI, Miller RD: Mild intraoperative hypothermia increases duration of action and spontaneous recovery of vecuronium blockade during nitrous oxide-isoflurane anesthesia in humans. Anesthesiology 74:815, 1991.
74. Stone JG, Young WL, Marans ZS, et al: Consequences of electroencephalographic suppressive doses of propofol in conjunction

with deep hypothermic circulatory arrest. Anesthesiology 85: 497–501, 1996.
75. Casey WF, Smith CE, Katz JM: Intravenous meperidine for control of shivering during cesarian section under epidural anesthesia. Can J Anesthesiol 35:128, 1988.
76. Fassero JJ, Berend JZ, Sladen RN: Vecuronium infusion vs. meperidine in the treatment of shivering following cardiopulmonary bypass [abstract]. Anesthesiology 73:A1229, 1990.
77. Guffin A, Girard D, Kaplan JA: Shivering following cardiac surgery: Hemodynamic changes and reversal. J Cardiothorac Anesth 1:24, 1987.
78. Baker KZ, Young WL, Stone JG, et al: Deliberate mild intraoperative hypothermia for craniotomy. Anesthesiology 81:361–367, 1994.
79. Shedd S: Principles and techniques of hypothermia and cardiac arrest for neurovascular anomalies. In Carter LP, Spetzler RF, Hamilton MG (eds): Neurovascular Surgery. New York, McGraw-Hill, 1995, p 195.
80. Pifarre R, Babka R, Sullivan HJ: Management of postoperative heparin rebound following cardiopulmonary bypass. J Thorac Cardiovasc Surg 81:378, 1981.
81. Smith EEJ, Naftel DC, Blackstone EH, et al: Microvascular permeability after cardiopulmonary bypass. J Thorac Cardiovasc Surg 94:225, 1987.
82. Ausman JI, McCormick PW, Stewart M, et al: Cerebral oxygen metabolism during hypothermic circulatory arrest in humans. J Neurosurg 79:810–815, 1993.
83. Belopavlovic M, Buchthal A: Cardiac arrest during moderate hypothermia for cerebrovascular surgery. Anaesthesia 35:368–371, 1980.
84. Gonski A, Acedillo AT, Stacey RB: Profound hypothermia in the treatment of intracranial aneurysms. Aust N Z J Surg 56: 639–643, 1986.
85. Greene KA, Marciano FF, Hamilton MG, et al: Cardiopulmonary bypass, hypothermic circulatory arrest and barbiturate cerebral protection for the treatment of giant vertebrobasilar aneurysms in children. Pediatr Neurosurg 21:124–133, 1994.
86. Guegan Y, Scarabin JM, Le Guilcher C, et al: Extracorporeal circulation with deep hypothermia and circulatory arrest in the treatment of intracranial arterial aneurysms. Surg Neurol 24: 441–448, 1985.
87. Kato Y, Sano H, Zhou J, et al: Deep hypothermia cardiopulmonary bypass and direct surgery of two large aneurysms at the vertebro-basilar junction. Acta Neurochir 138:1057–1066, 1996.
88. Koch F, Thompson J, Chung RS: Giant cerebral aneurysm repair: Incorporating cardiopulmonary bypass and neurosurgery. AORN J 54:224–227, 1991.
89. Pacult A, Gratzick G, Voegele D, et al: Surgical clipping of difficult intracranial aneurysms using deep hypothermia and total circulatory arrest. South Med J 86:898–902, 1993.
90. Richards PG, Marath A, Edwards JM, et al: Management of difficult intracranial aneurysms by deep hypothermia and elective cardiac arrest using cardiopulmonary bypass. Br J Neurosurg 1:261–269, 1987.
91. Silverberg GD: Giant aneurysms: Surgical treatment. Neurol Res 6:57–63, 1984.
92. Silverberg GD, Reitz BA, Ream AK, et al: Operative treatment of a giant cerebral artery aneurysm with hypothermia and circulatory arrest: Report of a case. Neurosurgery 6:301–305, 1980.
93. Solomon RA, Smith CR, Raps EC, et al: Deep hypothermic circulatory arrest for the management of complex anterior and posterior circulation aneurysms. Neurosurgery 29:732–737, 1991.
94. Spetzler RF, Hadley MN, Rigamonti D, et al: Aneurysms of the basilar artery treated with circulatory arrest, hypothermia, and barbiturate cerebral protection. J Neurosurg 68:868–879, 1988.
95. Williams MD, Rainer WG, Fieger HG Jr, et al: Cardiopulmonary bypass, profound hypothermia, and circulatory arrest for neurosurgery. Ann Thorac Surg 52:1069–1074, 1991.

PART V VASCULAR AND BLOOD FLOW EVALUATIONS

CHAPTER 91

Transcranial Doppler Ultrasonography

DAVID W. NEWELL ■ ARTHUR M. LAM

BACKGROUND AND PRINCIPLES

History of Doppler Ultrasound

The origins of Doppler ultrasound can be traced back to the description of the Doppler effect by the Austrian physicist Christian Doppler. His work first was presented to the Royal Bohemian Society of Sciences in May 1842, entitled, "On the colored light of the double stars and certain other stars of the heavens." This presentation described the *Doppler effect* as it subsequently became known, which explains the shift in the frequency of a wave when neither the transmitter of the wave nor the receiver of the wave is moving with respect to the wave-propagating medium. This effect applies to sound, and sound emanating from or reflected by an object moving toward an observer is characterized by a higher frequency in proportion to the speed of the moving object. Conversely, if sound emanates from an object moving away from an observer, the sound has a lower frequency in proportion to the speed of the moving object. According to this principle, ultrasound can be used to measure the velocity of flowing blood. Ultrasound is generated by a small crystal and emitted from a probe, then reflected off the moving blood cells, and the reflected signal is received by the probe. The frequency shift between the emitted and the reflected ultrasound varies proportionally with the velocity of the flowing blood. Blood flowing toward the probe reflects the ultrasound at a higher frequency, producing a positive Doppler shift, and ultrasound reflected from blood flowing away from the probe is reduced in frequency or exhibits a negative Doppler shift. The signals are processed, and a spectral analyzer displays multiple spectral dots for the many reflections that are recorded.

The use of Doppler ultrasound to measure blood flow was reported initially by Satomora in 1959.[1] Satomora and Kaneko initially were interested in measuring cerebral blood flow; however, they concluded that the skull was an insurmountable barrier to the passage of ultrasound and focused on the extracranial carotid arteries in their initial investigations. After refinements in the equipment and advances in the technology, Doppler ultrasound was introduced as a clinical tool to examine blood flow velocity in the extracranial arteries. Doppler ultrasound then was used by vascular surgeons to examine the extracranial and peripheral arteries. Refinements in signal processing and the introduction of duplex followed by development of color flow ultrasound have continued to improve the diagnostic capabilities for peripheral vascular examinations.

Pulsed Doppler allows the examiner to reduce the sample volume to a small area and predetermine a location where the examining site is focused. Pulsed Doppler generates bursts of ultrasound at regular intervals, which is called the *pulse repetition frequency*. An electronic gate is used to sample the reflected pulses at certain intervals, which is usually the time taken for the ultrasound to travel to the preselected target and back, providing the method to determine a preselected recording depth. This feature is essential for transcranial Doppler (TCD) ultrasonography, allowing examination at specific recording sites. The sample volume or the size of the recording site can be varied by most equipment.

History of Transcranial Doppler

Aaslid and colleagues[2] first reported the ability to record blood flow velocity in the intracranial arteries using Doppler ultrasound in 1982, introducing TCD ultrasonography. TCD ultrasonography employed an optimized 2-MHz frequency with a pulsed Doppler range gated design. The lower 2-MHz frequency allowed penetration through the cranium in the thin portions of the bone. The introduction of TCD ultrasound allowed examination of the intracranial vasculature, which has improved the diagnosis of intracranial disease. TCD ultrasound initially was employed in the Department of Neurosurgery in Bern, Switzerland, for the diagnosis of vasospasm after subarachnoid hemorrhage.[3] Many subsequent uses have been described for this technology and are reviewed in this chapter.

Principles of Transcranial Doppler

EXAMINATION TECHNIQUES

A complete TCD examination normally includes examination through three transcranial windows: the transtemporal, transorbital, and transoccipital windows.[4] Through these three windows, most of the basal intracranial arteries can be examined (Fig. 91–1). The transtemporal window is used to examine the middle cerebral artery, (MCA), anterior cerebral artery, intracranial internal carotid artery (ICA), and proximal posterior cerebral artery. The transorbital window normally is used to examine the ophthalmic artery and intracavernous and supraclinoid ICA. The transoccipital window is used to examine the posterior circulation, specifically the two vertebral arteries and the basilar artery. The origin of the posterior inferior cerebellar arteries can be examined in many patients.

The original technique for examination was a handheld method, which uses manual manipulation of the probe with recordings of preselected depths and sample volumes to examine specific sites in the intracranial vasculature. Normally, as the distal intracranial arteries become vertically oriented in the sylvian fissure and in the intrahemisphere fissure, they are considered beyond the scope of the normal TCD examination.[5] Distal intracranial arteries occasionally can be examined in unusual circumstances, however, such as after craniotomy, when bone is removed and examination windows are created.

The Doppler signal reflected from the intracranial arteries measures ultrasound frequency shifts, which are converted into blood flow velocity in centimeters per second. To determine the actual blood flow in milliliters per minute, the total average velocity, vessel diameter, and angle of insonation need to be known precisely,[6, 7] and these parameters are not measured normally during routine TCD examinations. The angle of insonation (angle between the ultrasound beam and the vessel being recorded from) is important to consider when measuring TCD velocity. The true velocity and observed velocity are equal when the angle of insonation is equal to zero, as often happens when examining the MCA trunk. As the angle of insonation increases, there is a reduction in the observed frequency as a function of the cosine of the angle (Fig. 91–2). For example, if the angle between the ultrasound beam and the flow reflector is 30 degrees, 97% of the true velocity can be observed by the recording device. As the angle of insonation increases, the proportion of the true velocity observed decreases. If the angle of insonation is 60 degrees, 50% of the true velocity is observed by the recording equipment. TCD examination techniques incorporate this strategy to reduce the insonation angle to as low as possible when recording from different intracranial arteries. The introduction of color flow ultrasound adds the ability to determine the angle of insonation to some extent during the examination. Figure 91–3 illustrates a typical velocity recording from the MCA.

Since the introduction of TCD, the technology has undergone significant improvements secondary to technical improvements in equipment and signal processing allowing an increased capability to detect abnormalities in intracranial vascular structure and function. Table 91–1 lists milestones in the development of TCD, showing the progression to its current state. The performance of high-quality intracranial examination with TCD requires experienced examiners with a fundamen-

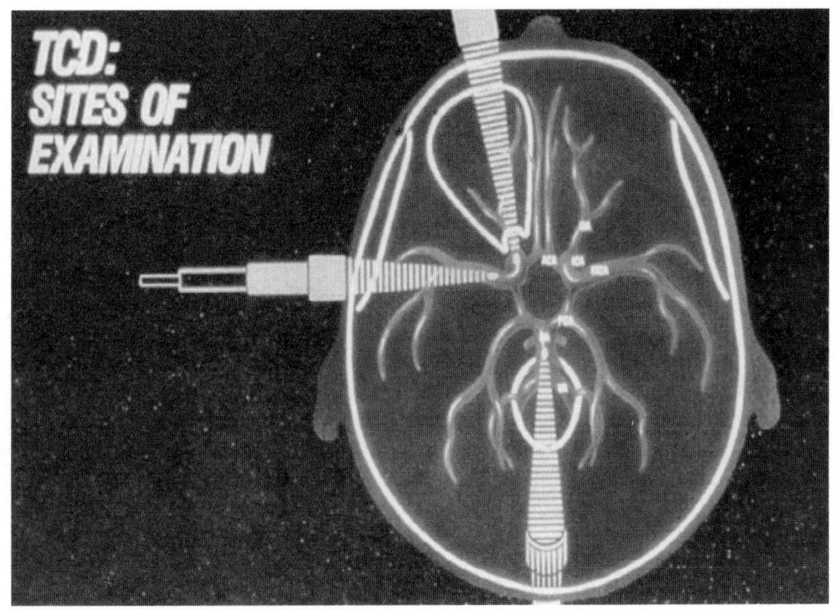

FIGURE 91–1. The three windows for transcranial Doppler examination of the basal cerebral vessels. Anteriorly the transorbital window is used to examine the carotid siphon as well as the ophthalmic artery. On the lateral portion of the skull is the transtemporal region used to examine the middle cerebral artery, proximal anterior cerebral artery, distal internal carotid artery, and proximal posterior cerebral artery. The third window is the transforaminal window, which can be used to examine the posterior circulation vessels. The two vertebral arteries and basilar artery are examined easily by this method. The posterior inferior cerebellar arteries sometimes can be examined.

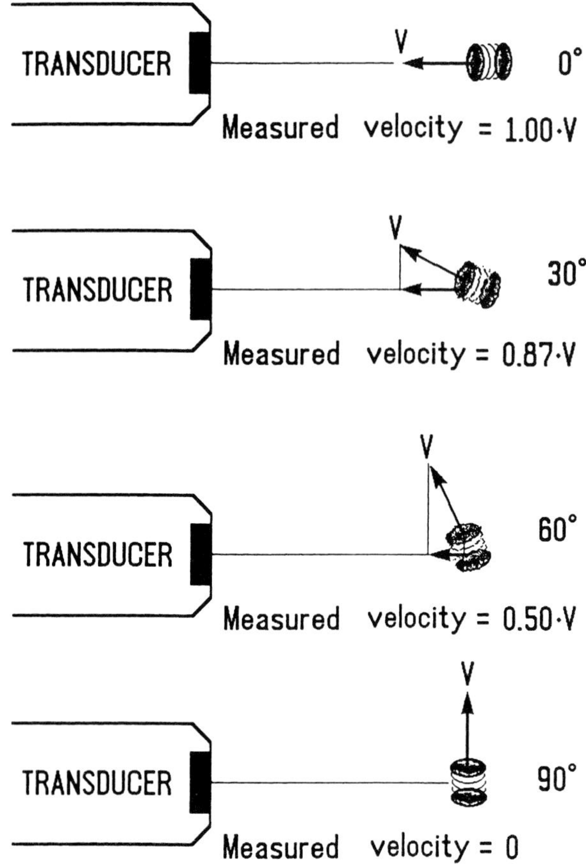

FIGURE 91–2. The effect of the insonation angle between the ultrasound beam and the artery on the velocity values. The percentage of the actual velocity measured changes as a function of the cosine of the insonation angle.

TABLE 91–1 ■ **Milestones in the Development of Transcranial Doppler**

First TCD range gated low-frequency ultrasound
Flow-mapping device for better vessel identification
Computerized recording devices to allow calculation in flow changes and events
Two-channel TCD allowing recording from multiple vessels
Emboli monitoring and automated emboli detection
Color flow and advances in transcranial B mode
Advances in probe holders and automatic adjustment
Multirange emboli detection
Reflected power recording and contrast agents
Miniaturization

TCD, transcranial Doppler.

tal knowledge of the intracranial anatomy and the relationships of the intracranial vessels to each other. To aid in vessel identification and complement the free-hand examination technique, Aaslid introduced a vessel mapping device that allowed computer-generated, three-dimensional maps of the vessel identification site, which was useful in documenting the recording sites from each of the intracranial vessels.[8] This device has largely been replaced by color flow and transcranial B-mode imaging.[9] Color flow Doppler has combined the advantages of color flow imaging with color-coded display of blood flow velocity and direction, with duplex scanning allowing simultaneous B-mode imaging to image the intracranial structures adjacent to the vasculature. Transcranial duplex scanning allows three-dimensional vessel maps to be constructed, and the recording site can be documented easily in most cases (Fig. 91–4). The advantages of this technology include an easier learning curve for beginning examiners as well as positive identification of abnormal vascular anatomy, which can be due to anatomic variations as well as pathologic changes from occlusions or displacement.

Middle Cerebral Artery

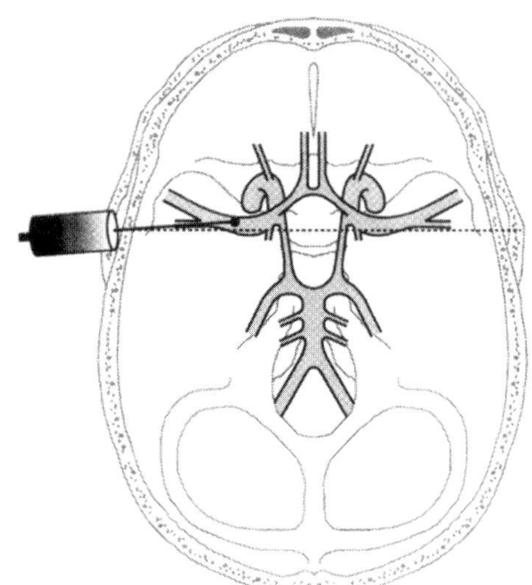

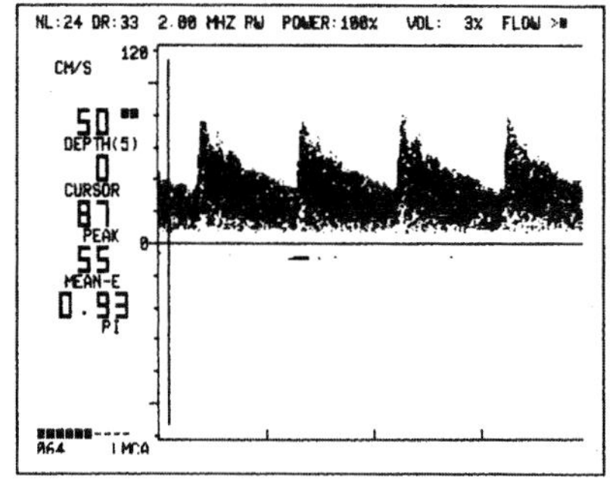

Depth:	30mm-60mm
Direction of Flow:	Toward
Spatial Orientation:	Same
Velocity[Mean]:	55 ± 12cm/sec
Response to Ipsilateral CCA Compressions:	Obliteration or Diminishment

FIGURE 91–3. Recordings from the middle cerebral artery through the transtemporal window. The spectral tracing is that of a low-resistance vascular bed, which is typical of the intracranial circulation. Normally the middle cerebral trunk is found at a depth of 30 to 60 mm from the scalp at the temporal window.

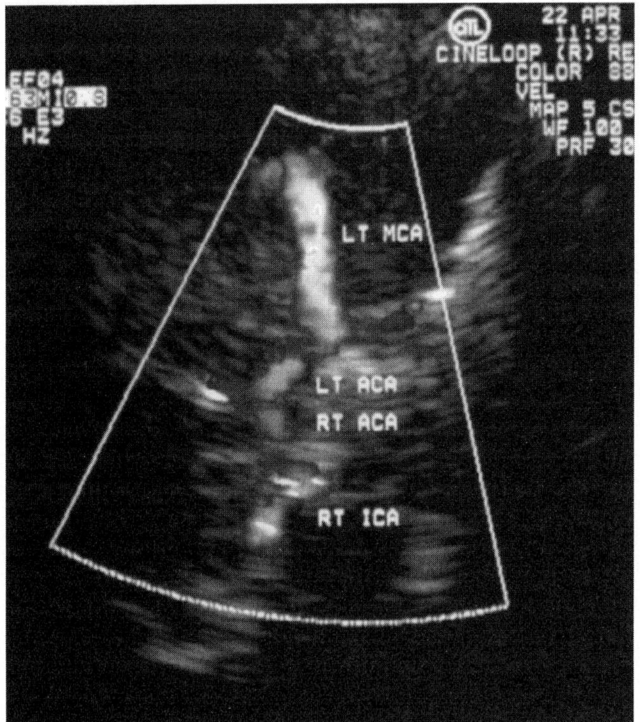

FIGURE 91–4. Sector scan from a color flow Doppler instrument. This black-and-white illustration shows images of the major components of the circle of Willis. The flow components directed toward the probe normally are coded in red and yellow. Flow directed away from the probe normally is coded in blue. When the scan is obtained, the examiner can place the Doppler sample volume on preidentified vessels to record the blood flow velocity. This method provides the examiner with increased confidence for and documentation of correct vessel identification. LT, left; RT, right; MCA, middle cerebral artery; ACA, anterior cerebral artery; ICA, internal carotid artery.

Advances in computerized recording devices and the miniaturization of computerized digital processing have allowed easier recording of Doppler signals for analyses. This development has allowed continuous recording of spectral outline and full spectral signals, permitting more detailed analyses of physiologic events.[10] Digital recording with the capability to display continuous data over time has allowed the calculation of changes in velocity secondary to blood flow changes evoked by physiologic stimuli and allowed the analyses of cerebrovascular control mechanisms, such as carbon dioxide (CO_2) autoregulation and evoked flow changes secondary to cortical activation (Fig. 91–5). Two-channel TCD ultrasound was introduced to resolve physiologic questions regarding the control of the cerebral circulation and to document simultaneous changes in venous and arterial flow.[6] Subsequently, multichannel TCD recording has been used to record signals simultaneously from both cerebral hemispheres recorded from both MCAs.[11] Multichannel recording has allowed emboli detection by recording from multiple sample volumes simultaneously.[12] Reflected power recordings have allowed calculation of relative flow volume, which can be used for scientific purposes to calculate changes in cerebral blood flow.[6] Power Doppler can be accomplished transcranially to provide further details in imaging intracranial vascular structures, such as aneurysms and arteriovenous malformations. Miniaturization has allowed TCD units to become more portable, and in the future battery-operated examination units may serve as a neurovascular stethoscope to allow rapid determination of vessel patency and flow characteristics.

PRINCIPLES OF DIAGNOSIS

TCD ultrasonography records blood flow velocity in the intracranial arteries, which can be altered in a variety of pathologic conditions. One of the common conditions to affect the intracranial circulation is intracranial stenosis resulting from a variety of causes. Intracranial stenosis can occur from atherosclerosis, cerebral vasospasm, moyamoya disease, sickle cell disease, vasculitis, recanalizing thrombi, inflammation, tumor-induced narrowing or stretching, among other causes.[13–19] Stenosis in the basal intracranial vessels produces accelera-

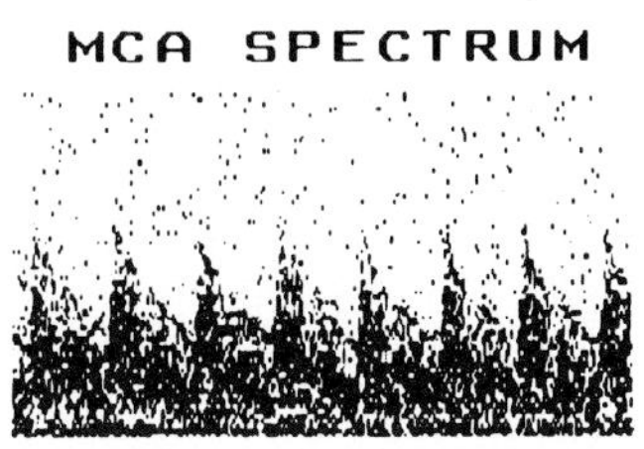

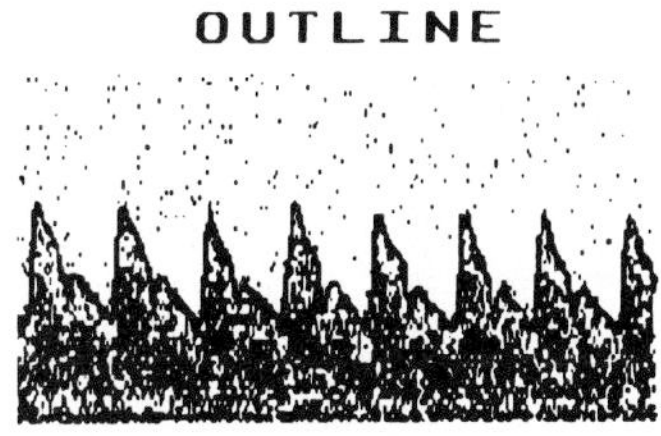

FIGURE 91–5. The derivation of the middle cerebral artery (MCA) outline or V_{max} (maximal velocity). The MCA spectrum is generated by a spectrum analyzer, then assigned an outline along the maximal spectral tracing. This maximal spectral outline is taken as an analogue signal and can be recorded continuously as a trend. The spectral outline or V_{max} corresponds to the flow velocity at the central portion of the artery during laminar flow.

tion in the velocity through the stenosis in proportion to the reduction in the cross-sectional area of the vessel if the blood flow remains constant. If the diameter of a vessel is reduced to half its original value, the velocity increases to 400% of the resting value. Accelerations in velocity can be indirect indicators of narrowing of the intracranial vessel from a variety of causes.

The following principles related to flow and velocity are crucial to obtaining diagnostic information using TCD. First, under conditions of constant flow and constant insonation angle, changes in velocity are inversely proportional to the changes in cross-sectional area of the vessel. Using this principle, TCD is able to detect stenosis resulting from either fixed lesions or reversible lesions of the intracranial arteries, such as vascular spasm. Second, under conditions in which the vessel diameter being recorded from is known to remain constant and the insonation angle does not change, changes in velocity are directly proportional to changes in volume flow through the vessel. This principle is the basis for continuous monitoring of blood flow velocity that can be used to detect *relative* changes in blood flow through the inflow artery (usually the MCA), which can be used to calculate vascular reactivity in the distal regulating arteries. Useful diagnostic information can be obtained from evaluation of waveform changes that can reflect progressive increases in resistance of the cerebral circulation, which in some cases can reflect high intracranial pressure.

Because velocity increases can occur with flow changes, interpretation of velocity changes must be done in the setting of each particular patient. Relative flow changes through the vessel can be calculated in the setting where intracranial vessel diameter does not change during a given interval and the probe is fixed for recording purposes.[20] For example, CO_2 reactivity and cerebral autoregulation as well as changes in evoked flow secondary to cortical activation can be calculated based on real-time recording of basal artery velocity in response to changes in blood pressure or in CO_2 concentration or activation of cerebral cortex in the vascular distribution of the vessel being recorded from.[21] By using this principle, valuable information can be obtained regarding control mechanisms of the cerebral circulation under normal and abnormal conditions (Fig. 91–6).

Another diagnostic capability of TCD ultrasound is the ability to examine the spectral signal for the detection of intracranial emboli. Substances that have different composition from the normal blood components flowing through arteries, such as formed element emboli or air bubbles, produce a sufficient interface between the surrounding blood and the embolic material that a distinct brief frequency change is noted,which can be heard audibly on the audio output of the equipment and can be observed in the spectral tracing.[22] There has been interest in the significance of intracranial emboli in conditions that predispose patients to stroke as well as during monitoring of neurovascular and other surgical procedures. There has been work on developing consensus opinions for the discrimination of intracranial emboli from artifacts and an attempt to determine the clinical significance of emboli.[23]

The use of contrast agents has increased the diagnostic capabilities of TCD by allowing signal enhancement in examination of intracranial arteries that may have weak or inadequate signals for diagnostic purposes under normal conditions.[24, 25] In elderly individuals and patients with hyperostotic bone, examination often cannot be completed or inadequate examination may result because of poor penetration and recording of ultrasound signals. Advances in fluorocarbon signal enhancement contrast agents have increased the duration of contrast remaining in the circulation during examination.[26]

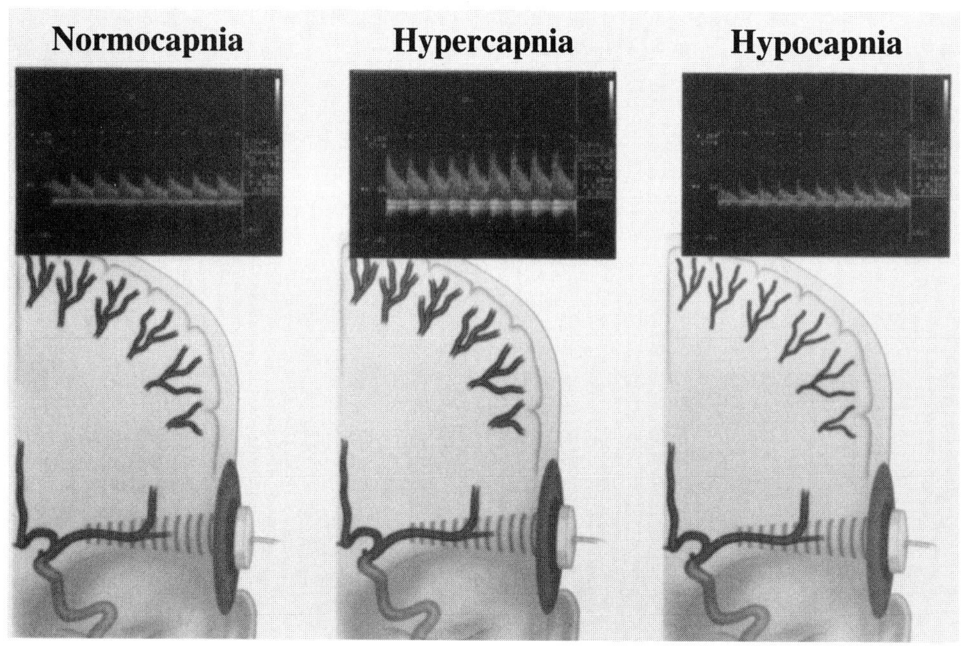

FIGURE 91–6. The tracings illustrating the principle of CO_2 reactivity. Continuous recordings are made from the middle cerebral arteries bilaterally at normocapnea, and the patient is instructed to inhale 6% CO_2. After this, the patient is instructed to hyperventilate. The percentage increase of flow velocity with CO_2 inhalation (hypercapnea) and percentage decrease with hyperventilation (hypocapnea) are used to indicate the cerebrovascular vasomotor reactivity. The changes in diameter of the distal regulating vessels at the different CO_2 levels affect the middle cerebral blood flow velocity. LMCA, left middle cerebral artery; RMCA, right middle cerebral artery.

APPLICATIONS OF TRANSCRANIAL DOPPLER IN NEUROSURGERY AND ANESTHESIA

One of the most common applications of TCD in the care of neurosurgical patients is for the detection of cerebral vasospasm after subarachnoid hemorrhage. TCD can be used to follow the onset, time course, and resolution of vasospasm, and it can be combined with other blood flow measurement techniques to offer useful information to clinicians managing patients with subarachnoid hemorrhage.[27]

Although the physiology of cerebral vasospasm is complex and not completely understood, the prompt diagnosis and institution of treatment for delayed ischemic neurological deficits (DINDs) secondary to vasospasm can be lifesaving and may prevent permanent ischemic brain damage after subarachnoid hemorrhage. It is useful to consider the physiology of large vessel spasm, which can produce transient or permanent DINDs. It is generally accepted that the risk for vasospasm is related closely to the degree of subarachnoid hemorrhage that occurs at the time of aneurysm rupture or is present after trauma, which can be assessed by the amount of blood clot in the basal cisterns on computed tomography (CT) scan obtained within several days of the bleeding episode.[28, 29] Most patients develop some degree of vessel narrowing after subarachnoid hemorrhage, and 70% of patients may develop angiographic vasospasm at some time during their hospital course; however, only approximately 30% of patients develop symptomatic vasospasm, characterized by DINDs.[30] Factors in addition to the degree of vessel narrowing may determine which patients develop DINDs from vasospasm; however, the degree and extent of basal vessel narrowing appears to play a major role in determining which patients eventually develop delayed ischemia. In addition, blood pressure response to medical treatment, hematocrit, and viscosity, which may influence oxygen delivery capacity, function of cerebral autoregulation, collateral circulation, intracranial pressure, and degree of overall brain dysfunction as well as other factors may influence the development of symptoms.[31] It is useful to think about large vessel spasm as progressing through stages that can affect the degree of narrowing in the basal cerebral vessels and the resulting cerebral blood flow. Table 91–2 outlines the various effects of the degree of vessel narrowing from vasospasm on TCD velocities, cerebral blood flow, and the occurrence of DINDs.

In the early stages of vasospasm, proximal vessel narrowing occurs, and the velocity values in the basal vessels increase on TCD examination often before there is any visible change angiographically. The next stage is characterized by further vessel narrowing with increased flow velocity through the narrow portion of the vessel but maintenance of blood flow (stage I). During the next stage, as the vessel narrows further, the degree of stenosis may be flow limiting; however, the cerebral autoregulation can compensate by lowering the distal vascular resistance, maintaining adequate cerebral blood flow (stage II). In some patients after subarachnoid hemorrhage, especially patients with poor initial grade, the autoregulatory mechanism may not be functioning to full capacity and may predispose patients to earlier critical reductions in cerebral blood flow. As further vessel narrowing occurs and the autoregulatory mechanism becomes exhausted, cerebral blood flow decreases in the given vascular distribution, and reduced cerebral blood flow may be detected on blood flow imaging studies, such as xenon-CT, single-photon emission computed tomography (SPECT), and positron emission tomography (PET), or other methods used to measure cerebral blood flow.[32, 33] As cerebral blood flow is reduced, increased oxygen extraction occurs, and cerebral metabolism and neuronal function are maintained (stage III). As further vessel narrowing occurs, blood flow drops to ischemic thresholds, synaptic transmission no longer functions, and neurological deficits ensue (stage IV). As the blood flow drops to lower levels or the time of ischemia is prolonged, permanent neuronal damage leading to infarction occurs.[34, 35] The characteristic findings during vessel narrowing from vasospasm in cerebral blood flow velocities, cerebral blood flow, and neurological condition are illustrated in Table 91–2. Figure 91–7 illustrates an example of velocity recordings and angiography in a patient with vasospasm after subarachnoid hemorrhage.

TABLE 91–2 ■ Stages of Vasospasm After Subarachnoid Hemorrhage: Relationship Between Diagnostic Findings and Clinical Symptoms

STAGE	ANGIOGRAPHIC VESSEL NARROWING	TCD VELOCITY	CBF	DIND
I	↑	↑	↔	No
II	↑ ↑	↑ ↑	↔	No
III	↑ ↑ ↑	↑ ↑ ↑	↓ ↓	No
IV	↑ ↑ ↑ ↑	↑ ↑ ↑ ↑ or ↑ ↑ ↑	↓ ↓ ↓	Yes

↑, mild; ↑ ↑, moderate; ↑ ↑ ↑, severe; ↑ ↑ ↑ ↑, very severe; ↔, no change; TCD, transcranial Doppler; CBF, cerebral blood flow; DIND, delayed ischemic neurological deficit.

When managing patients with subarachnoid hemorrhage who are at risk for cerebral vasospasm, it is helpful to keep in mind this framework that describes the stages of progression. TCD and cerebral blood flow measurements are useful to determine the state of contraction of the basal intracranial vessels as well as the response of cerebral blood flow.

Effect of Vessel Narrowing from Subarachnoid Hemorrhage on Blood Flow Velocity

Normal values for cerebral blood flow velocity have been published by multiple investigators. Under normal conditions, the average flow velocity in the MCA is 62 cm/second. Velocities greater than 120 cm/second

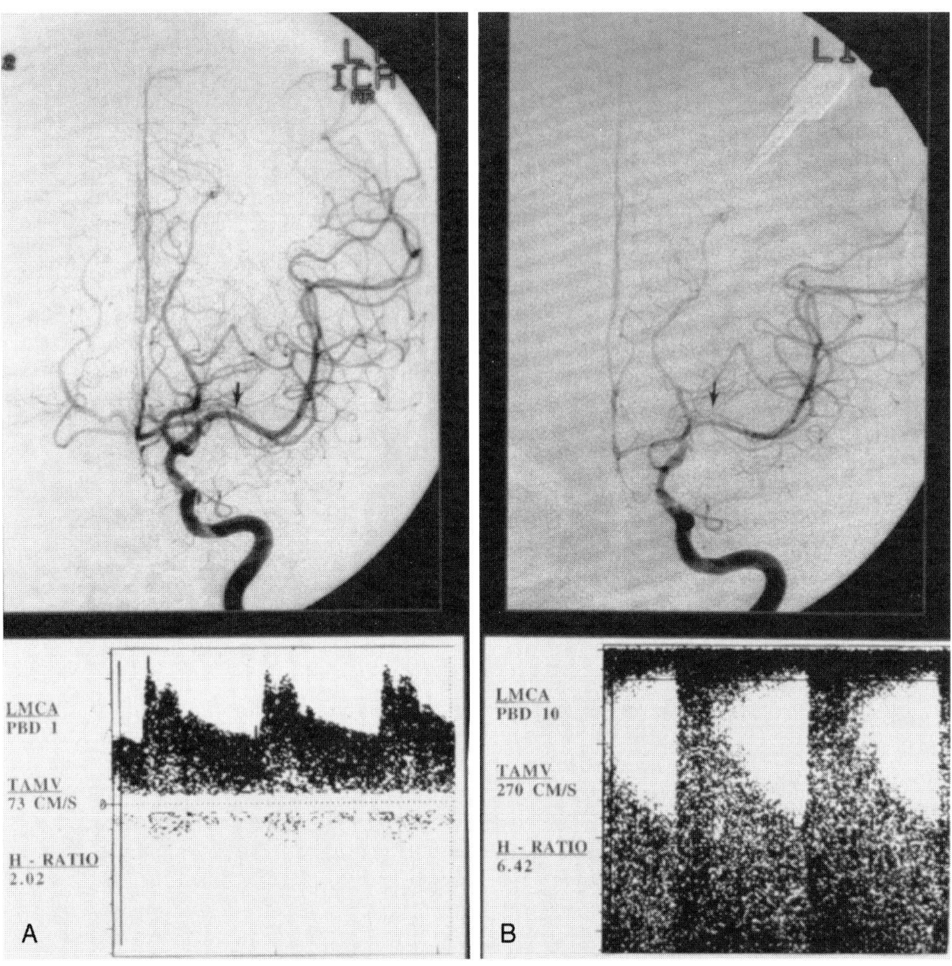

FIGURE 91–7. Transcranial Doppler recordings before and after the onset of vasospasm near the carotid termination in a patient with subarachnoid hemorrhage. *Arrow* indicates middle cerebral artery. Ratio indicates V_{MCA}/V_{ICA} (velocity in the middle cerebral artery divided by velocity in the extracranial internal carotid artery).

correlate with vasospasm, as evidenced by vessel narrowing on angiogram. Flow velocities greater than 200 cm/second often correlate with severe vasospasm seen angiographically and are associated with clinical episodes of ischemia and infarction.[13, 29, 36, 37]

Early studies performed by Aaslid and Seiler and their colleagues[13, 29, 37] in Bern, Switzerland, established the correlation between elevated velocities and cerebral infarction from vasospasm. Seiler and colleagues observed a group of 39 patients with subarachnoid hemorrhage followed with TCD ultrasonography. No patient developed cerebral infarct if blood flow velocities had not exceeded 140 cm/second. Blood flow velocities greater than 200 cm/second were associated with ischemic episodes and infarctions; however, some patients remained asymptomatic.[13, 29, 37] These observations are in keeping with previous angiographic studies of vasospasm indicating that there was not an absolute concordance between the degree of vessel narrowing and the development of delayed ischemia. Most patients who develop major episodes of delayed ischemia have significant vessel narrowing; however, other patients go on to severe vessel narrowing and preserve cerebral blood flow and do not develop DINDs. Occasionally, patients with subarachnoid clots located in the distal cerebral fissures may develop diffuse distal spasm, which is unaccompanied by proximal vessel spasm.[5] Often the careful examination of the CT scan for the presence of distally located blood clots can help to predict patients at risk for distal vessel vasospasm. Cerebral blood flow measurements and angiography are required to confirm the diagnosis.

Subsequent studies have correlated the degree of angiographic vasospasm with TCD velocities and found the best correlations in the MCA and distal ICA.[38, 39] Vasospasm in the distal anterior cerebral artery is not normally accessible by TCD, and the proximal anterior cerebral arteries sometimes can be problematic because of congenital atresia and other factors that lead to poor correlation between vessel diameter and increased velocity. Multiple physiologic factors have been shown to affect blood flow velocity in vasospasm, including intracranial pressure, hematocrit, blood pressure from induced hypertension, hyperdynamic therapy, and hyperemia, which can result from aggressive hemodynamic support.[40–42]

Aaslid and colleagues[13] initially described a mathematical ratio of flow velocities, which was analyzed further by Lindegaard and associates,[39] between the velocity in the MCA and the extracranial ICA (V_{MCA}/V_{ICA}) to correct for flow changes induced by vasospasm. Because velocity can change either from changes in flow or from changes in vessel diameter, the extracranial-to-intracranial ratio can be helpful in distinguishing hyperemia from elevated velocities caused by spasm. If vasospasm progresses to a severe degree whereby cerebral blood flow is reduced significantly, intracranial velocities may begin to decrease as the vessels become severely attenuated, leading to a decrease in blood flow velocity in the extracranial carotid artery as well, which decreases the intracranial velocity but results in a persistently elevated V_{MCA}/V_{ICA} ratio.

Predictive Value of Transcranial Doppler Ultrasound

The time course of vasospasm can vary according to the severity of the subarachnoid hemorrhage and the extent of the spasm. The peak incidence of vasospasm occurs in a delayed fashion after subarachnoid hemorrhage. Weir and coworkers[43] carefully measured angiograms from 293 patients with aneurysms. These investigators found that angiographic vasospasm initially occurred 3 days after subarachnoid hemorrhage and appeared to be maximal between days 6 and 8 and was much reduced by day 12. Subsequent studies using TCD confirmed the delayed onset and time course of vasospasm.[13, 29, 44] Multiple investigators have observed that patients who have early and more severe increases in flow velocities are at higher risk for the development of DINDs. The use of TCD has addressed several controversies in the past regarding the timing of vasospasm. Romner and associates[45] were unable to find significant vasospasm within 12 hours after subarachnoid hemorrhage in a group of patients harboring aneurysms. It previously was thought that an early and late phase of vasospasm existed leading to management decisions based on these preconceptions. These authors also showed that progression of vasospasm was more likely to occur in patients operated on 49 to 96 hours after aneurysmal rupture than in patients operated on within 48 hours of rupture, supporting the notion that early aneurysm surgery may be less likely to aggravate vasospasm than surgery during the time when vasospasm begins to occur to a significant extent.[46]

Grosset and colleagues[47] showed that rapid increases in velocity are predictive of patients who develop DINDs. These investigators examined 121 consecutive patients after acute subarachnoid hemorrhage with frequent repeated examinations for 14 days. The average highest velocity reached was greater in 47 patients who developed DINDs (186 cm/second) compared with the 74 patients who did not develop DINDs (149 cm/second). There was no significant difference, however, between symptomatic and asymptomatic patients when considering the velocities recorded before the onset of neurological deficit. The rate of increase in the TCD velocities was greater in patients who then developed DINDs, however. In these patients, there was a maximum velocity increase of 65 ± 5 cm/second per 24-hour period compared with increases of 47 ± 3 cm/second per 24-hour period in patients who did not develop DINDs. An increase greater than 50 cm/second per 24-hour period may help predict which patients go on to develop DINDs; information gathered from sequential recording may be useful in managing these patients.

Several treatments exist for cerebral vasospasm after subarachnoid hemorrhage, and it is useful to consider the effects of these treatments on vessel diameter and TCD values. Triple-H therapy (hypertension, hypervolemia, and hemodilution) may have unpredictable effects on basal vessel velocity recordings using TCD. Reports have indicated that in some cases increases in velocity after this treatment can be due to increases in blood flow and not further reduction of basal vessel diameter.[41, 48] The state of the cerebral autoregulation may play a role in determining the velocity changes after induction of triple-H therapy.[48] These reports underscore the need for combined assessment with cerebral blood flow measurements and the use of intracranial-to-extracranial ratios to correct for blood flow changes when using TCD to follow patients undergoing triple-H therapy for vasospasm.

Calcium channel blockers have been shown by several prospective randomized trials to be useful in the prevention of vasospasm and reduction in morbidity and mortality after subarachnoid hemorrhage.[49] It has been shown that cerebroselective calcium channel blockers cause reductions in subarachnoid hemorrhage–induced elevated intracranial blood flow velocities measured using TCD.[50]

Endovascular therapy has been useful in reversing vessel narrowing from vasospasm and improving cerebral blood flow. TCD ultrasonography and cerebral blood flow studies have shown improvements in blood flow and reduction in elevated blood flow velocities secondary to spasm after treatment.[51, 52] Interventional treatment with papaverine has been shown to decrease cerebral blood flow velocities and to improve cerebral blood flow, although the effect appears to be more transient. Figure 91–8 illustrates the reduction in velocities by transluminal angioplasty in a group of patients with vasospasm.

Arteriovenous Malformations

Hemodynamic changes in arteriovenous malformations have been well characterized by blood flow studies, direct pressure measurements, and TCD ultrasonography.[53] Classic arteriovenous malformations show high velocity in feeding arteries corresponding to elevated volume flow and show a low pulsatility index on TCD, which indicates a decreased vascular resistance. It has been shown by color flow Doppler that arteriovenous malformations can be imaged transcranially.[54] Their characteristic features on color flow imaging and the characteristic hemodynamic changes on TCD can lead to their diagnosis of arteriovenous malformation in patients examined for neurological symptoms such as headaches, seizures, or other focal findings that may lead to routine examination. For decision making regarding treatment planning, other imaging modalities, such as CT, magnetic resonance imaging, and angiography, are essential. Physiologic evaluations of arteriovenous malformations have been performed

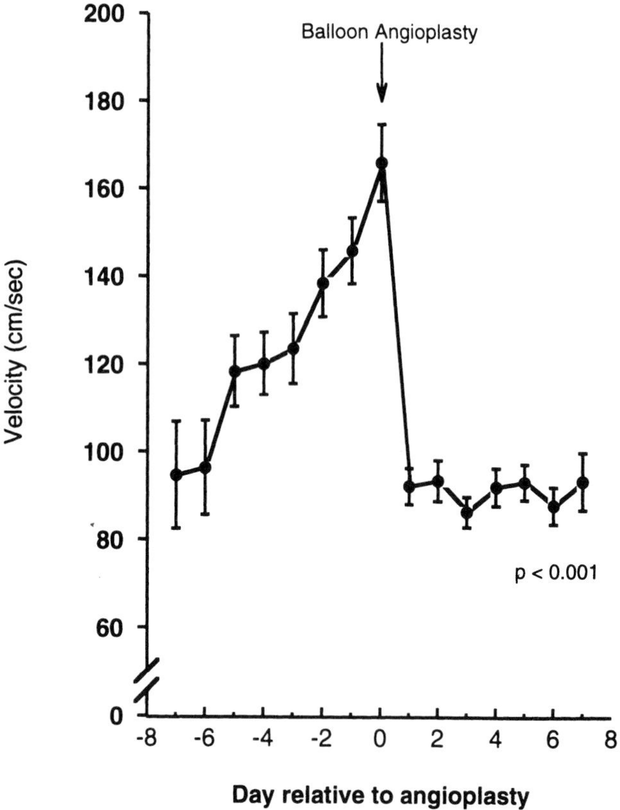

FIGURE 91–8. Graph shows the sequential changes in velocity values measured using transcranial Doppler before and after transluminal angioplasty in 101 distal internal carotid artery or proximal middle cerebral artery vessels in a group of 39 patients with subarachnoid hemorrhage and severe vasospasm indicating a sustained effect on the cerebral vessels.

using TCD, and feeding vessel mean velocity measured using TCD correlates with feeding artery mean arterial pressure.[55] It has been shown that these malformations do not react normally to physiologic stimulation, such as changes in CO_2 concentration. TCD can be useful in identifying arteriovenous malformations that previously were undiscovered in some patients and may be useful in evaluating physiologic aspects to monitor patients after embolization[56] or surgery. Intraoperative color flow imaging may have a role in defining residual arteriovenous malformation during surgery.

Detection of Intracranial Aneurysms

During standard TCD examination, characteristic multiphasic waveforms have been described occurring in intracranial aneurysms. Standard TCD generally has not been useful as a screening test to detect these aneurysms, however. With the introduction of color flow, two-dimensional transcranial color-coded sonography (TCCS) has shown increased sensitivity to detect aneurysms.[54, 57] The addition of intravascular contrast agents has been useful to improve the signal-to-noise ratio for examination. Klotzsch and colleagues[57] have reported the use of TCCS in 30 patients with known intracranial aneurysms. Twenty-nine angiographically proven aneurysms were detected by TCCS, with diameters ranging from 3 to 16 mm with a mean of 7.2 ± 3.6 mm. In another study, Baumgartner and associates[54] evaluated 29 patients with 30 radiographically proven cerebral aneurysms. Twenty-three of 27 (85%) nonthrombosed aneurysms with diameter 6 to 25 mm were identified. It appears that with improvements in contrast agents and signal processing, TCCS may be useful as a screening method in the future. Intraoperative color duplex Doppler imaging may be useful during aneurysm surgery to locate certain aneurysms and to ensure complete obliteration as well as preservation of proximal and distal vessels after clipping (Fig. 91–9).[58]

Monitoring During Carotid Endarterectomy

TCD monitoring during carotid endarterectomy (CEA) is being used increasingly in many institutions.[59] Monitoring probes can be placed unilaterally or bilaterally over the temporal windows for continuous recording of V_{MCA} without interfering with the surgical field. One distinct advantage of TCD over other types of monitoring is that TCD provides information relevant to all the major causes of perioperative cerebrovascular morbidity, including intraoperative and postoperative emboli, hypoperfusion during cross-clamping, intraoperative or postoperative thrombosis, and postoperative hyperperfusion syndrome.

MONITORING FOR CROSS-CLAMP HYPOPERFUSION

Controversy exists regarding the need for placement of an intraluminal shunt during CEA. Options include placement of a shunt in all cases, no shunt placement in any case, or selective shunting only in patients at high risk for cross-clamp hypoperfusion. Ideally, shunts should be placed only in the few patients who have critically reduced cerebral blood flow on carotid artery cross-clamping because they can cause vessel injury in some cases. The identification of patients who develop hypoperfusion has been inexact, however. Monitoring the V_{MCA} is useful in determining which patients may benefit from shunt placement. During the time of cross-clamping, in most cases there is a fall in V_{MCA} followed by a partial or full recovery during the next few seconds owing to autoregulatory vasodilation. The V_{MCA} then reaches a steady-state that usually is lower than it was before cross-clamping. The relative change in blood flow can be estimated by expressing the V_{MCA} 10 to 20 seconds after cross-clamping as a percentage of the V_{MCA} immediately before clamping.

Halsey[60] published results from a collaborative study of 1495 CEAs in an attempt to define the relationship between intraoperative measurements of V_{MCA} and the need for shunt placement. Patients were categorized according to the risk for ischemia (cross-clamp hypoperfusion) based on the reduction in V_{MCA} values during carotid artery clamping. The study indicated that patients with a high risk of ischemia (85% reduction in V_{MCA}) who were not shunted were at high risk

Basilar Artery Aneurysm Pre-Clipping

PCA

PCA

Basilar Artery Aneurysm

A

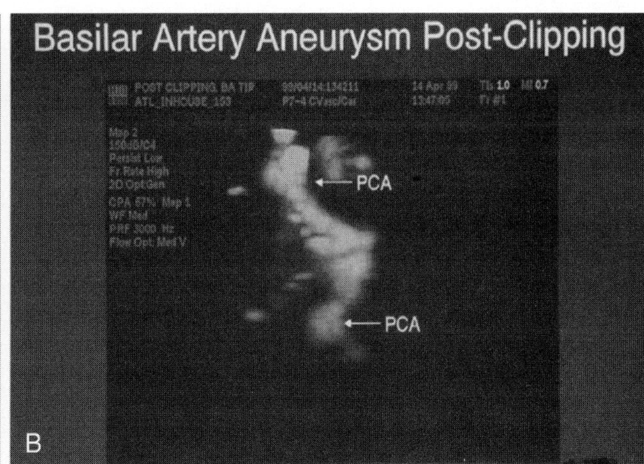

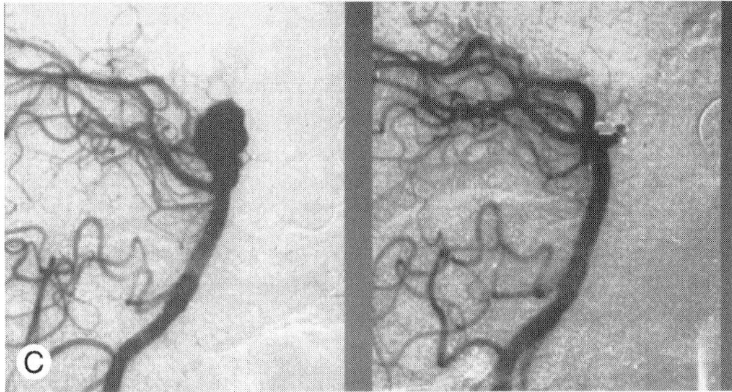

FIGURE 91–9. Transcranial color-coded power Doppler imaging of a basilar bifurcation aneurysm *(A)* before and *(B)* after surgical clipping, showing preservation of the parent and distal vessels and complete obliteration of the aneurysm. *C,* Angiogram of the same aneurysm before *(left)* and after *(right)* clipping.

of perioperative stroke. In more than 75% of patients with a low risk of ischemia (V_{MCA} fell by <60%), there was a better outcome in patients who were *not* shunted. In the group at intermediate risk for ischemia (V_{MCA} fall 60% to 85%), there was no difference in outcome between the shunted and nonshunted patients. Based on these data, if V_{MCA} stabilizes to at least 40% of the preclamp value, it is unlikely the patient would benefit from a shunt.

Comparison studies have been conducted between TCD and other methods of identifying patients at risk for cross-clamp ischemia who may benefit from an intraluminal shunt. There appears to be excellent correlation between TCD and electroencephalography (EEG) criteria of ischemia,[61, 62] although it is possible to have severe reduction in V_{MCA} and subsequent stroke without EEG evidence of ischemia.[63] Spencer and colleagues[64] reported a good correlation between V_{MCA} and stump pressure, but they found stump pressure to be sensitive to zeroing errors, and a small error in stump pressure estimation may represent a critical difference in cerebral perfusion.[64] Another method to monitor for cross-clamp hypoperfusion is to perform surgery on awake patients under local anesthesia. Cerebral symptoms in awake patients having CEA under local anesthesia may not always be accompanied by a significant fall in V_{MCA}; this is true in patients undergoing both types of monitoring.[65] It cannot be assumed, however, that all awake patients who develop ischemic symptoms would have suffered a stroke if they had been operated under general anesthesia without being shunted.

Some patients with severe ischemia on TCD criteria do not suffer stroke.[60] Sufficient residual flow may be preserved because of perfusion via cortical (leptomeningeal) collaterals that may be better developed in patients with severe carotid stenosis. False-positive values for diagnosis of critically reduced V_{MCA} can arise from technical problems, such as probe dislodgment or inadvertent monitoring of the distal ICA rather than the MCA.

Another advantage of TCD monitoring is the ability to give immediate feedback regarding adequacy of shunt function. When a shunt is used, TCD confirms restoration of MCA flow and provides a continuous monitor of shunt function. An obstructed shunt causes an immediate reduction in flow velocity that precedes any change in cerebral function or EEG. The major disadvantage of TCD monitoring is the failure to obtain adequate signals because of hyperostosis in some patients. It is useful to have an alternative form of monitoring available if this circumstance arises. The authors use a combination of intraoperative TCD and EEG to detect ischemia during cross-clamping and use selective shunting, which is employed if hypoperfusion is detected.

DETECTION OF EMBOLI

Postoperative thrombosis and cerebral emboli are the major cause of perioperative stroke from CEA.[66, 67] Microemboli detected by TCD are associated with stroke and ischemic events during and after CEA. Intra-arterial microemboli can be recognized easily using TCD monitoring by the characteristic *chirping, clicking,* or *whistling* sounds on the audio output and spectral display. The TCD features of particulate and gas emboli have been characterized and software has been developed for automatic emboli detection and counting.[68, 69] The prevalence and timing of perioperative cerebral emboli associated with CEA must be considered when using TCD monitoring. Some cerebral microemboli are noted during most CEAs (97% in one report[70]); however, most microemboli do not result in stroke. Most emboli are detected on restoration of ICA perfusion, but these are predominately air emboli, which are believed to be less harmful than particulate emboli and not associated with ischemic events. Emboli noted during dissection of the carotid artery[63] or frequent emboli detected immediately postoperatively are associated with postoperative stroke and ischemic events.[67, 71–73] Dextran or other antiplatelet drugs can be effective in reducing postoperative microemboli.[74, 75] Information gained from TCD monitoring may allow the surgeon to alter surgical technique or institute treatment postoperatively to reduce ischemic events.

POSTOPERATIVE HYPERPERFUSION

Postoperative hyperperfusion syndrome occurs in about 1% of patients after CEA, and when cerebral hemorrhage occurs, the prognosis is poor.[66, 76] The syndrome is thought to occur when abnormally high blood flow develops in vascular beds that have been habituated to a low perfusion pressure and are exposed suddenly to normal arterial pressure after restoration of normal perfusion pressure during CEA.[77, 78] Hyperperfusion can be associated with defective cerebral autoregulation at normal blood pressure[79] and can be diagnosed by TCD before clinical signs develop. Elevated ipsilateral V_{MCA} ranging from 30% to 230% is found in 10% to 20% of patients after CEA, only some of whom develop headaches or more serious sequelae.[80] Early diagnosis with TCD allows strict control of blood pressure to restore flow velocities to the normal range and perhaps to prevent serious complications.

POSTOPERATIVE OCCLUSION

Immediate postoperative cerebral ischemia may be due to technical problems at the site of endarterectomy, such as thrombosis or intimal flap, and may be affected by coagulability factors. Neurological deterioration in the recovery room should prompt immediate TCD evaluation for impending or completed postoperative occlusion, and if ipsilateral flow is poor, rapid re-exploration may be indicated to prevent stroke. Findings on TCD that suggest impending or completed carotid occlusion include frequent and increasing microemboli and decrease of V_{MCA} to postclamp values.[67]

Evaluation of Patients After Head Iinjury

Recording blood flow velocity from the basal cerebral arteries after closed head injury may be useful for the diagnosis of a variety of conditions that can occur and may contribute to delayed cerebral ischemia. Some of these conditions include impaired autoregulation, vasospasm, vessel injury and dissection, increased intracranial pressure (ICP), decreased cerebral perfusion pressure, and cerebral circulatory arrest. Continuous measurement of velocity changes in head-injured patients has added to understanding of the pathophysiology of disordered cerebrovascular control mechanisms and may provide information that may help with patient management and prognosis. Further advances in signal processing and analysis may allow the noninvasive estimation of ICP in patients with head injury.

BLOOD FLOW VELOCITY CHANGES FROM RELATIVE FLOW CHANGES

Monitoring of V_{MCA} waveforms can yield information that reflects relative changes in cerebral blood flow in response to a variety of circumstances in the neurosurgical intensive care unit. Blood flow changes in response to various waves in ICP can be assessed. Autoregulation can be evaluated by assessing the V_{MCA} change in response to an induced or spontaneous blood pressure change. Relative blood flow changes in response to changes in CO_2 concentration as well as in response to various medications can be assessed.

CARBON DIOXIDE REACTIVITY

Cerebrovascular reactivity to CO_2 reactivity can be impaired or abolished in head-injured patients, and this may have implications in their response to hyperventilation and barbiturate therapy as a treatment for ICP control.[81] Poor CO_2 reactivity after head injury is associated with a poor prognosis.[82] The use of TCD to measure CO_2 reactivity offers a noninvasive nonradioisotope method, with advantages over the previously used method of xenon blood flow devices.[10, 83]

EVALUATION OF CEREBRAL AUTOREGULATION

Autoregulation is the ability of the cerebral circulation to maintain constant blood flow under conditions of changing cerebral perfusion pressure and can be assessed using TCD. Autoregulation impairment has significant implications in head injury management. When autoregulation is abolished, the brain may be much more sensitive to hypotension, which can precipitate cerebral ischemia much more readily than in patients with normal cerebral autoregulation. Prevention of marked increases in arterial blood pressure is important in patients with poor autoregulation, to prevent cerebral swelling, edema, or secondary hemorrhages.[84] Autoregulation is important in mediating the responses of various therapies to control ICP. Muizelaar and colleagues[85] showed that mannitol can lower ICP more effectively in patients with intact autoregulation than in patients with impaired autoregulation.

Several different methods can be used to measure cerebral autoregulation using TCD. Response of the V_{MCA} to static changes in blood pressure or to rapidly induced dynamic changes in blood pressure has correlated well with changes in flow and can be used to indicate the effectiveness of the autoregulatory response.[20, 86] Other methods have been used to observe V_{MCA} in response to a transient reduction in cerebral perfusion pressure induced by carotid compression to evaluate the effectiveness of autoregulation[87] or to observe the relationships between spontaneous fluctuations in V_{MCA} and arterial blood pressure, ICP, or both.[88, 89]

The most commonly used method to calculate the autoregulatory response using TCD is observation of relative changes in the V_{MCA} in response to rapid or slow changes in arterial blood pressure. Rapid changes in blood pressure can be induced by releasing large thigh cuffs inflated to suprasystolic pressure for a period of 2 to 3 minutes. The release of the thigh cuffs produces a rapid moderate drop in blood pressure, which then triggers the dynamic autoregulatory response. A computerized model can be used to calculate the various responses based on the effectiveness of the autoregulatory response. This method of testing has been compared with the results of testing by more conventional methods using induced slower blood pressure changes (static or steady-state autoregulation) with phenylephrine infusion.[86, 90] In normal volunteers with intact autoregulation, then progressive impairment of autoregulation induced by the anesthetic agent isoflurane, both testing methods revealed similar results in detecting progressive impairment in autoregulation. There was a significant reduction in autoregulatory capacity after the administration of high-dose isoflurane, which could be shown using static ($P < .0001$) and dynamic ($P < .0001$) methods. Correlation between static or steady-state and dynamic autoregulation measurements by regression analysis was highly significant ($r = 0.93$, $P < .0001$) (Fig. 91–10).[86]

Clinical studies strongly indicate that the injured brain is more vulnerable to hypotensive insults, and this increased vulnerability is believed to be due to impaired cerebral autoregulation. The association between hypotension and poor outcome in head-injured patients has been well documented.[91–94] Information from the Traumatic Coma Data Bank indicates that lowered cerebral perfusion pressure as a result of hypotension or increased ICP is associated with a poor outcome after head injury.[91, 92] Pietropaoli and coworkers[93] found that intraoperative hypotension occurring in severely head-injured patients undergoing surgical procedures within 72 hours of admission to the hospital was associated with a significant increase in mortality and with a significant decrease in Glasgow Outcome Scale score compared with head-injured patients

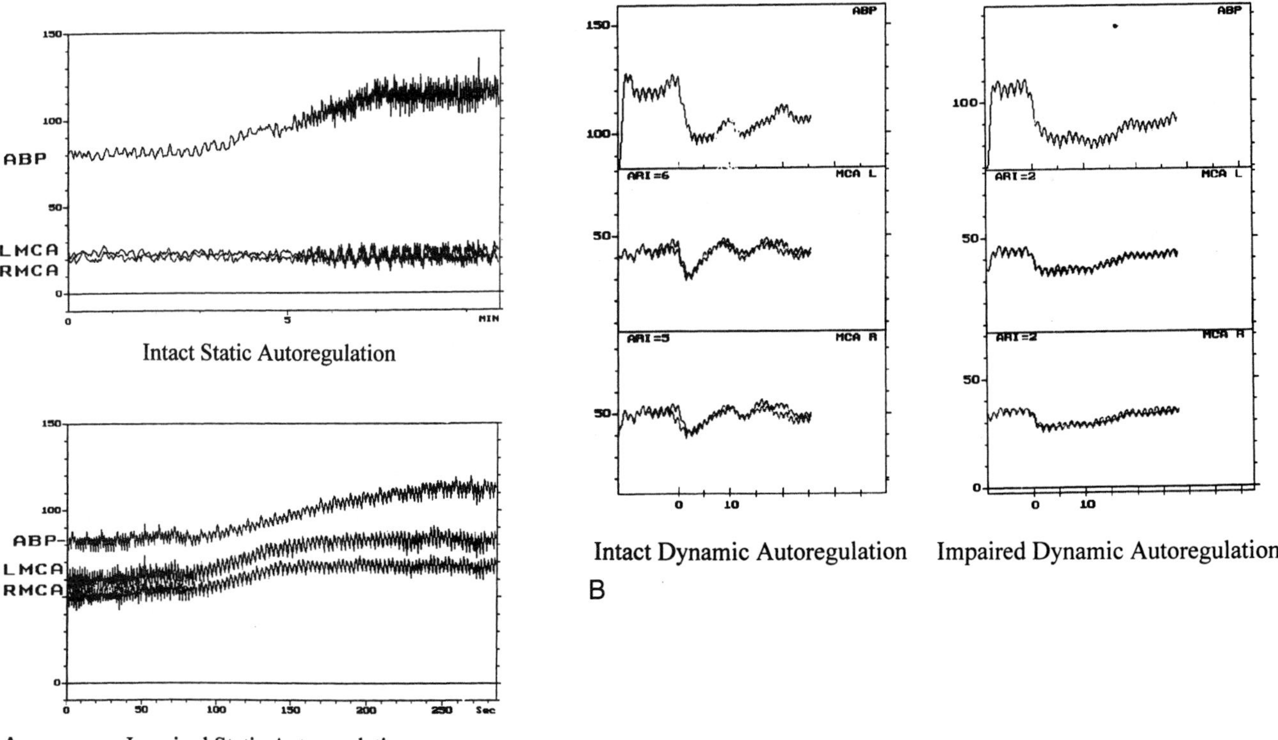

FIGURE 91–10. Autoregulation can be assessed with transcranial Doppler by using the middle cerebral artery velocity as an index of relative change in blood flow in response to a transient drop or a sustained change in blood pressure. *A*, Static autoregulation testing induced by increasing blood pressure with phenylephrine (Neo-Synephrine), with intact *(above)* and impaired *(below)* autoregulation testing. *B*, Intact and impaired dynamic autoregulation testing evaluates the relative blood flow change through the middle cerebral artery in response to a rapid change in blood pressure produced by deflating thigh blood pressure cuffs. LMCA, left middle cerebral artery; RMCA, right middle cerebral artery.

who did not become hypotensive during surgery. This same study found that intraoperative hypotension occurred frequently (32%) in this group of head-injured patients. Winchell and associates[94] showed that hypotension in the intensive care setting is associated with an adverse outcome after head injury, especially in patients with less severe injuries. The most marked effect of hypotension on outcome was in patients with less severe injuries (Glasgow Coma Scale score >8). Patients with absent or severely impaired autoregulation may be at high risk of ischemic brain damage if hypotension or increases in ICP occur. If patients without autoregulation undergo secondary surgical procedures for their injuries, moderate hypotension in the perioperative period could cause critical reductions in cerebral blood flow. The authors reported that a significant number (approximately 30%) of patients with minor head injury had absent or significantly impaired autoregulation within the first 2 days after head injury.[95] Measurement of cerebral autoregulation using TCD may be useful to identify head-injured patients at high risk for secondary ischemia from hypotension.

POST-TRAUMATIC VASOSPASM

Cerebral vasospasm can occur after head injury and is associated with traumatic subarachnoid hemorrhage. Post-traumatic vasospasm has been well documented and has been shown to be responsible for clinical deterioration and infarction in some patients with closed head injury.[27, 96–98] TCD is useful in monitoring head-injured patients for this complication. Initial investigations by Weber and colleagues[99] reported a 40% incidence of vasospasm, by TCD criterion, in a group of severely head-injured patients. Martin and coworkers[97] reported a 27% incidence of vasospasm using TCD in a group of head-injured patients. Detection of vasospasm in head-injured patients using TCD is made more difficult by the concurrent existence of cerebral hyperemia after head injury, which may result in false-positive values for vasospasm if the criteria for vasospasm in subarachnoid hemorrhage are used. Blood flow velocity recordings should be obtained from the most distal portion of the extracranial ICA in the neck, to allow the calculation of V_{MCA}/V_{ICA} ratios. V_{MCA}/V_{ICA} ratio should be used to correct for hyperemia when using TCD to detect post-traumatic vasospasm. Cerebral blood flow measurements using quantitative techniques are useful to identify patients at risk for cerebral ischemia.[96]

VASCULAR DISSECTION

Carotid artery dissection extracranially and at the skull base can be a complication after head injury, which sometimes can produce devastating delayed cerebral infarction. One of the diagnostic clues to extracranial dissection can be the presence of intracranial arterial emboli. The authors determined the incidence of intracranial emboli in the MCA on the side of ICA dissection in 10 patients with ICA dissection secondary to trauma and 7 with spontaneous ICA dissection.[100] The diagnosis was confirmed by carotid angiography and studied by TCD from the time of diagnosis through initiation of therapy.

Emboli were detected in the MCA distal to the dissection in 10 of 17 patients (59%). Patients with microemboli detected by TCD presented with a stroke (70%) much more frequently than patients without emboli (14%; $P = .0498$). It may be useful to employ TCD as an adjunctive tool to manage patients with suspected carotid dissection, and TCD may prove useful in evaluating the efficacy of treatment in reducing microemboli and subsequent stroke.

ISCHEMIA AND PROGNOSIS OF HEAD INJURY USING TRANSCRANIAL DOPPLER CRITERIA

Low velocities in the intracranial arteries after head injury can be due to low cerebral blood flow secondary to severely reduced cerebral metabolism or can be due to high ICP. Monitoring of V_{MCA} and jugular venous oxygen saturation has revealed that low jugular venous oxygen saturation concentrations, indicating cerebral ischemia, correlated well with increased MCA pulsatility index.[101] Increased pulsatility correlated with cerebral perfusion pressure in the lower range when it dropped to less than 70 mm Hg. The recording of low blood flow velocities on admission in head-injured patients can indicate a poor prognosis. Chan and associates[102] reported that low cerebral blood flow velocities of less than 28 cm/second in both MCAs predicted 80% of the early deaths in a series of head-injured patients.

Transcranial Doppler Findings with Increased Intracranial Pressure

Changes in V_{MCA} recordings have been described with increasing ICP. With early increases in ICP, the pulsatility index increases with progressive reduction of the diastolic velocity and initially no change in the mean velocity. With further increases in ICP, there is a simultaneous reduction in mean velocity and a further increase in pulsatility index.[103] It is likely that these changes occur as a result of progressive increases in the resistance of the cerebrovascular bed. At high ICPs that produce arrest of the cerebral circulation, the V_{MCA} waveform progresses through a predictable sequence. This sequence begins with a progressive reduction in diastolic velocity initially to zero, then the initiation of an alternating flow pattern with a reversed diastolic component (see Fig. 91–2). Further obstruction to flow causes progression to alternating flow, which is antegrade in systole and retrograde in diastole, of equal components. Further progression leads to small systolic peaks, then an absence of the waveform entirely. These characteristic TCD changes have correlated with previously described angiographic findings of nonfilling of the cerebral arterial tree in patients undergoing cerebral angiography.[103] It has been documented by cerebral angiography and radionucleide isotope scanning that an alternating flow pattern on TCD corresponds to arrest of the cerebral circulation (Fig. 91–11).[103, 104]

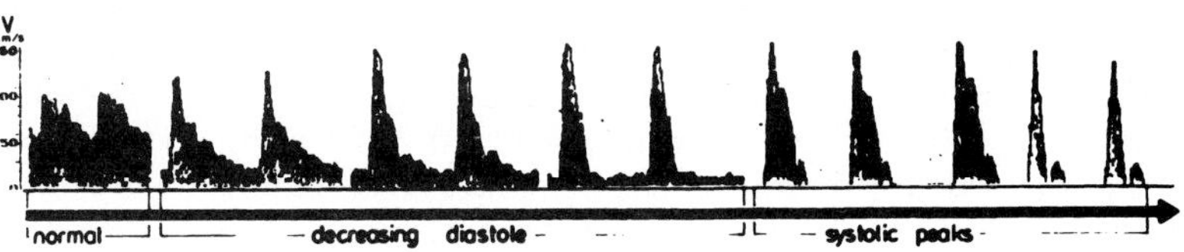

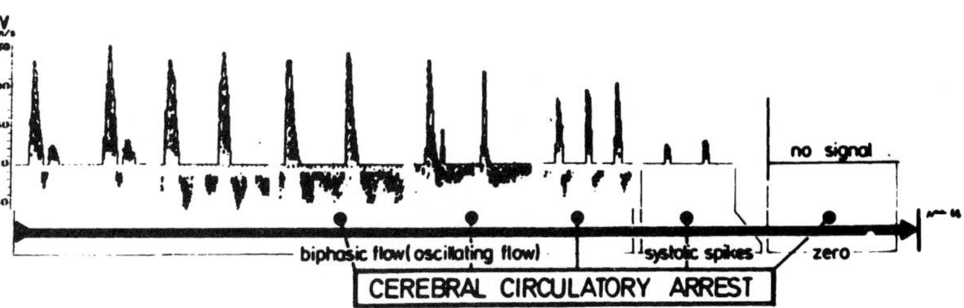

FIGURE 91–11. Tracing indicating progression of the velocity waveform from a normal pattern to one seen with cerebral circulatory arrest. With increased resistance to flow, there is a progressive decrease in the diastolic velocity, progressing to oscillating flow, and finally to small systolic peaks. (From Hassler W, Steinmetz H, Pirschel J: Transcranial Doppler study of intracranial circulatory arrest. J Neurosurg 71:195–201, 1989.)

Changes in pulsatility index and mean velocity alone are not specific for increased ICP. A high resistance in the cerebral vascular bed, producing increased pulsatility and decreased velocity, can be seen with intense vasoconstriction. Intense vasoconstriction can occur secondary to vigorous hyperventilation, low cerebral metabolism, and cerebral vasoconstricting drugs, such as barbiturates. For these reasons, the mean velocity and pulsatility index when taken in isolation cannot predict ICP reliably. Pulsatility index can be affected markedly by cardiac factors.[105] Progressive increases in the pulsatility index can indicate a progressive rise in ICP in patients who are observed carefully and are known not to have concomitant cardiac changes and changes in CO_2 or other factors that produce vasoconstriction.

The cerebrovascular tone pressure as well as the critical closing pressure of the cerebral circulation can be obtained by analysis of the V_{MCA} waveform and the arterial pressure waveform. It may be possible in the future to predict ICP more reliably from these parameters using TCD and arterial blood pressure recordings.[106, 107]

Transcranial Doppler as a Confirmatory Test for Brain Death

TCD sonography is useful as a confirmatory test in the diagnosis of brain death. Arrest of the intracranial circulation can be detected reliably with TCD, which is often but not always present when brain death occurs. The true diagnosis of brain death is a clinical diagnosis, and blood flow studies such as cerebral angiography, radioisotope scanning, and TCD are confirmatory tests. According to the President's Commission on guidelines for determination of brain death in the United States, confirmatory tests can be used to shorten the observation period in patients who fulfill the clinical criteria for brain death, before organ retrieval or discontinuation of mechanical ventilation can proceed.[104]

Many studies have examined the role of TCD in the determination of brain death, comparing clinical findings and the results of blood flow studies with sonographic waveforms in patients progressing to brain death.[104, 108–118] Most of the studies comparing TCD with clinical criteria for brain death have indicated sensitivities and specificities of the TCD technique approaching 100%.

Several caveats apply to TCD and any other cerebral blood flow method as confirmatory tests for brain death. False-negative and false-positive results can occur in rare circumstances. False-positive TCD recordings have been reported under several circumstances. Cerebral circulatory arrest can be transient, however, and reverse after a period of minutes in patients with subarachnoid hemorrhage who have a marked increase in ICP, resulting in temporary arrest of the cerebral circulation.[119, 120] For this reason, when using TCD to confirm arrest of the cerebral circulation, it should be repeated or be documented that cerebral circulatory arrest is present for a sufficient period of time (i.e., 30 minutes under normothermic conditions) to be incompatible with survival. Another possible cause of false-positive TCD findings can be in patients who have sustained cerebral circulatory arrest but have residual circulation to the brainstem, which may sustain respiratory effort or minimal cranial nerve function for a short time. False-positive TCD tracings showing alternating flow velocity patterns have been seen in unusual situations in which abnormally low diastolic pressure is present, such as in patients with intra-aortic balloon pumps.

False-negative TCD results (in which TCD indicates preserved flow and patients are clinically brain dead) have been reported in patients with clinical brain death. When massive destruction of the brainstem occurs as a result of destructive lesions or posterior fossa lesions, the brainstem function may be absent, and the patient fulfills the clinical criteria for brain death, with preserved supratentorial blood flow. EEG activity may persist, and TCD waveforms can indicate preserved blood flow.[117] These examples of false-positive and false-negative studies are not an indication of the failure of the TCD technique itself, but they emphasize why confirmatory tests do not always concur 100% with the clinical diagnosis of brain death. Despite these shortcomings, TCD can be especially useful in patients in whom the clinical diagnosis of brain death is made difficult owing to extensive trauma and cranial nerve damage and in patients after trauma who have been given paralytic agents, which make clinical evaluation difficult. A TCD examination may be helpful in avoiding unnecessary surgery in this situation.

APPLICATIONS OF TRANSCRANIAL DOPPLER IN STROKE AND CEREBROVASCULAR DISEASE

Intracranial Stenosis

TCD ultrasonography has extended the capability of Doppler ultrasound to diagnose intracranial arterial stenosis reliably, which may be caused by a variety of pathologic conditions other than vasospasm. A common cause of intracranial stenosis in patients presenting with symptoms related to cerebrovascular disease is atherosclerosis involving the basal intracranial vessels. Other conditions can cause intracranial arterial stenosis, including moyamoya disease, intracranial arterial dissection, vasculitis, preeclampsia, sickle cell disease, and arterial-to-arterial emboli undergoing various stages of recanalization.

Atherosclerotic disease of the intracranial vessels has received much less attention than similar lesions of the extracranial cerebral vessels.[121] Although intracranial arterial stenosis secondary to atherosclerosis is less common than extracranial stenosis in Western populations, intracranial atherosclerotic lesions can be a significant cause of stroke or transient ischemic attacks. Bogousslavsky and coworkers[122] analyzed the natural history of patients with MCA stenosis or occlusion entered into the extracranial-intracranial bypass study group. During a follow-up period of 42 months, 11.7% of the patients per year experienced recurrent cerebrovascular events (transient ischemic attack or stroke).

Several early studies reviewed the accuracy of TCD for the diagnosis of intracranial stenosis secondary to atherosclerosis.[14, 123, 124] Spencer and Whisler[123] compared carotid siphon stenosis assessed by angiography and TCD. In a group of 33 carotid siphons visualized angiographically, 11 showed stenosis ranging from 30% to 75%. Comparison of TCD with angiography revealed a sensitivity of 73% and specificity of 95%. Ley-Pozo and Ringelstein[124] compared intra-arterial digital subtraction angiography with TCD in detecting occlusive disease of the carotid siphon and MCA. Sixteen of 17 cases of carotid siphon stenosis were identified correctly using TCD. Rorick and colleagues[125] compared TCD with angiography for the diagnosis of intracranial stenosis. These investigators found that the presence of coexisting extracranial stenosis can be a confounding variable and affect the accuracy of TCD in detecting intracranial lesions. It has been useful to examine the intracranial arteries using TCD in patients with cerebrovascular symptoms who are not found to have significant pathology in the extracranial arteries.

Intracranial Hemodynamics

The evaluation of intracranial hemodynamics using TCD has allowed assessment of the vascular control of the cerebral circulation as well as identification of patients with cerebrovascular occlusive disease who are at higher risk for stroke. In patients with occlusive disease, the two most useful capabilities of TCD for hemodynamic parameters are the evaluation of collateral patterns and cross flow and direct assesment of hemodynamic changes in the distal vascular territories caused by proximal occlusive lesions.

The maintenance of adequate cerebral blood flow depends on sufficient cerebral perfusion pressure through the inflow vessels, from adequate blood pressure; intact anatomy of the extracranial and intracranial vasculature; and compensatory mechanisms when the vasculature or blood pressure becomes compromised. The normally configured circle of Willis functions as a manifold to normalize the perfusion pressure to the distal cerebral vessels if one or more extracranial vessels becomes occluded or becomes hemodynamically compromised secondary to stenosis. The circle of Willis normally allows nearly complete compensation in cases of carotid occlusion.[126]

Compensation for a carotid occlusion usually occurs through (1) crossover through the anterior communicating artery and reversed flow in the proximal anterior cerebral artery (A_1) ipsilateral to the occlusion, (2) forward flow in the posterior communicating artery ipsilateral to the occlusion, or (3) reversed flow in the ipsilateral ophthalmic artery.[127] Major differences in the functional capacity of the circle of Willis are found in the general population, however, and some patients cannot recruit sufficient flow to maintain an adequate cerebral perfusion pressure.

The use of TCD to evaluate vasomotor reserve is based on the principle that changes in velocity are proportional to changes in flow through a vessel if the vessel diameter is constant. Changes in blood flow velocity through the MCA can be used to reflect relative changes in blood flow in that artery owing to changes in CO_2 concentration or acetazolamide (vasomotor reserve) or moderate changes in arterial blood pressure (autoregulation). Using these principles, the functional capacity of the distal regulating vessels in the cerebral circulation can be assessed using TCD.

When cerebral perfusion pressure decreases as a result of proximal arterial stenosis or occlusion, the distal cerebral regulatory vessels become dilated maximally and exceed their functional capacity to autoregulate and to respond to CO_2. Acetazolamide has been used to effect distal cerebral vasodilation and probably works by a similar pH-dependent mechanism as CO_2 inhalation. Lack of responsiveness to CO_2 or to acetazolamide can be used to indicate indirectly reduced cerebral perfusion pressure in the MCAs resulting from the effects of proximal occlusive disease.

The total percentage change in velocity between normocapnea and hypercapnea added to the percent difference between normocapnea and hypocapnea has been termed *vasomotor reactivity* by Ringlestein and coworkers.[128] These investigators established normal values in a group of volunteers (age 20 to 75 years) for vasomotor reactivity in the MCA distribution. An average maximum increase in velocity of 52.5% with CO_2 inhalation (hypercapnea) and a decrease of 35.3% with hyperventilation (hypocapnea) were found, yielding an average vasomotor reactivity (VMR) of 87.8%. In a group of patients with carotid occlusions, VMR was reduced significantly in the ipsilateral MCA in 40 cases of unilateral occlusions. In 15 cases with bilateral occlusions, VMR was reduced severely bilaterally. All patients who were found to have low-flow infarctions on CT (n = 5), chronic ischemic ophthalmopathy (n = 2), or repeated hypostatic transient ischemic attacks (n = 2) had VMR measurements of less than 38%. The VMR value in patients with carotid occlusions depends highly on the configuration of the circle of Willis, and in a group of 64 patients with carotid occlusions, a significantly reduced VMR was found in patients with inadequate collateral vessels in the circle of Willis as compared with the subgroup with a normal circle.

Testing of VMR using TCD can provide valuable physiologic information regarding prognosis in patients with certain vascular lesions. Kleiser and Widder[126] reported the results of a natural history study of patients with unilateral carotid occlusions after VMR testing. In a group of 86 patients with unilateral carotid occlusion, 11 patients had exhausted VMR and had an increased ipsilateral stroke rate (17% per year during 3 years) compared with an ipsilateral stroke rate of 3% per year for the entire group (which is comparable to previously published series). Similar findings of an increased stroke risk in patients with carotid occlusion and impaired vascular reserve, measured using other methods including xenon-CT with acetazolamide challenge and PET, have been reported.[129, 130]

The prognosis of carotid stenosis may be influenced by the vasomotor reserve. Gur and associates[131] reported that patients with asymptomatic carotid stenosis with impaired VMR had a worse prognosis than those with intact VMR. Using VMR testing, it appears possible to identify patients with poor hemodynamic reserve with carotid stenosis or occlusion who have a high stroke risk and may benefit from medical or surgical therapy to improve cerebral perfusion.

Cerebral Autoregulation

Cerebral autoregulation is the ability of the brain to maintain constant cerebral blood flow despite changes in cerebral perfusion pressure. The methodology for determining cerebral autoregulation in the past was cumbersome and invasive, requiring radioisotopes for cerebral blood flow measurement and vasoactive medication to change the blood pressure. TCD can be used to determine autoregulation noninvasively in the MCA perfusion territories.[6, 20, 132] Preliminary clinical testing in patients with cerebrovascular occlusive disease indicates that cerebral autoregulation is absent in patients with severely impaired CO_2 reactivity.[133, 134] Noninvasive testing of the cerebral autoregulation using TCD may prove useful in the complete hemodynamic evaluation of patients with cerebrovascular occlusive disease.

Positional Vertebral Artery Obstruction

Cerebrovascular insufficiency sometimes can occur in the posterior circulation, secondary to positional obstruction of one or both vertebral arteries in the setting of impaired collateral pathways from the anterior circulation. Several reports have found TCD monitoring of the posterior cerebral arteries bilaterally during various head positions to be useful in detecting transient hemodynamic insufficiency in this condition.[135, 136] The most common cause of positional vertebral artery obstruction is cervical spondylosis, which can be treated surgically by anterolateral removal.[136] The essential diagnostic findings on TCD are a transient drop in posterior cerebral artery velocity signals with head turning and a rebound hyperemia on return to a neutral position. Examination with TCD is useful in differentiating true positional ischemia from positional vertigo and can identify patients who require angiography to define the location and nature of the obstruction.

Intracranial Emboli

Interest has developed in the ability of TCD to detect directly intracranial microemboli in the basal cerebral vessels and their relationship to stroke and ischemic symptoms in occlusive vascular disease. Doppler ultrasound previously was used clinically to detect intravascular air microemboli audibly during cardiac surgery[137] and during neurosurgical procedures in the sitting position.[138] The ability of TCD to detect intracranial microemboli first was recognized by monitoring the V_{MCA} during CEA and cardiac surgery.[22, 139]

Clinical evaluations of intracranial and extracranial microemboli detection have been described.[140] Intracranial microemboli have been detected in patients with atrial fibrillation, prosthetic heart valves,[141] carotid stenosis,[142, 143] fibromuscular dysplasia, arterial dissection,[100, 144] and intracranial stenosis as well as during invasive procedures, such as angiography,[145] angioplasty,[146] vascular and heart surgery,[147] and after aneurysm surgery.[148] Monitoring for intracranial air microemboli after venous injection has been useful in identifying patients with cardiac and pulmonary defects causing right-to-left circulation shunts.[149] Most microemboli do not cause overt symptoms; however, multiple microemboli have been associated with impaired neuropsychologic function after cardiac surgery.[150] The clinical utility of intracranial emboli monitoring still is being established; however, much has been learned about microembolism to the brain using TCD. Emboli monitoring using TCD has played a useful role in identifying the site of active embolization in the arterial system in patients with transient ischemic attacks or recent stroke, distinguishing embolic versus hemodynamic causes of stroke and transient ischemic attacks, identifying high-risk stages of neurovascular and surgical procedures, and identifying patients with vascular lesions at higher risk for ischemic events.

REFERENCES

1. Kaneko Z: First steps in the development of the Doppler flowmeter. Ultrasound Med Biol 12:1877–1895, 1986.
2. Aaslid R, Markwalder T-M, Nornes H: Noninvasive transcranial Doppler ultrasound recording of flow velocity in basal cerebral arteries. J Neurosurg 57:769, 1982.
3. Aaslid R, Huber P, Nornes H: Evaluation of cerebrovascular spasm with transcranial Doppler ultrasound. J Neurosurg 60: 37–41, 1984.
4. Fujioka KA, Douville CM: Anatomy and freehand examination techniques. In Newell DW, Aaslid R (eds): Transcranial Doppler. New York, Raven Press, 1996, pp 9–31.
5. Newell DW, Grady MS, Eskridge JM, Winn HR: Distribution of angiographic vasospasm after subarachnoid hemorrhage: Implications for diagnosis by transcranial Doppler ultrasonography. Neurosurgery 27:574–577, 1990.
6. Aaslid R, Newell DW, Stooss R, et al: Assessment of cerebral autoregulation dynamics from simultaneous arterial and venous transcranial Doppler recordings in humans. Stroke 22:1148–1154, 1991.
7. Giller CA, Hatab MR, Giller AM: Oscillations in cerebral blood flow detected with a transcranial Doppler index. J Cereb Blood Flow Metab 19:452–459, 1999.
8. Niederkorn K, Myers LG, Nunn CL, et al: Three-dimensional transcranial Doppler blood flow mapping in patients with cerebrovascular disorders. Stroke 19:1335–1344, 1988.
9. Baumgartner RW, Mattle HP, Aaslid R: Transcranial color-coded duplex sonography, magnetic resonance angiography, and computed tomography angiography: Methods, applications, advantages, and limitations. J Clin Ultrasound 23:89–111, 1995.
10. Newell DW, Aaslid R, Stooss R, et al: Evaluation of hemodynamic responses in head injury patients with transcranial Doppler monitoring. Acta Neurochir 139:804–817, 1997.
11. Newell DW, Aaslid R, Stooss R, Reulen HJ: The relationship of blood flow velocity fluctuations to intracranial pressure B waves. J Neurosurg 76:415–421, 1992.
12. Nabavi DG, Georgiadis D, Mumme T, et al: Detection of microembolic signals in patients with middle cerebral artery stenosis by means of a bigate probe: A pilot study. Stroke 27:1347–1349, 1996.
13. Aaslid R, Huber P, Nornes H: Evaluation of cerebrovascular spasm with transcranial Doppler ultrasound. J Neurosurg 60: 37, 1984.
14. Lindegaard KF, Bakke SJ, Aaslid R, Nornes H: Doppler diagnosis of intracranial artery occlusive disorders. J Neurol Neurosurg Psychiatry 49:510–518, 1986.
15. Alexandrov AV, Bladin CF, Norris JW: Intracranial blood flow velocities in acute ischemic stroke. Stroke 25:1378–1383, 1994.
16. Ries S, Schminke U, Fassbender K, et al: Cerebrovascular involvement in the acute phase of bacterial meningitis. J Neurol 244:51–55, 1997.
17. Qureshi AI, Frankel MR, Ottenlips JR, Stern BJ: Cerebral hemodynamics in preeclampsia and eclampsia. Arch Neurol 53:1226–1231, 1996.
18. Takase K, Kashihara M, Hashimoto T: Transcranial Doppler ultrasonography in patients with moyamoya disease. Clin Neurol Neurosurg 99(suppl 2):S101–S105, 1997.
19. Adams RJ, Nichols FT, Figueroa R, et al: Transcranial Doppler correlation with cerebral angiography in sickle cell disease. Stroke 23:1073–1077, 1992.
20. Newell DW, Aaslid R, Lam A, et al: Comparison of flow and velocity during dynamic autoregulation testing in humans. Stroke 25:793–797, 1994.
21. Newell DW, Aaslid R: Transcranial Doppler: Clinical and experimental uses. Cerebrovasc Brain Metab Rev 4:122–143, 1992.
22. Spencer MP, Thomas GI, Nicholls SC, Sauvage LR: Detection of middle cerebral artery emboli during carotid endarterectomy using transcranial Doppler ultrasonography. Stroke 21:415–423, 1990.
23. Ringelstein EB, Droste DW, Babikian VL, et al: Consensus on microembolus detection by TCD. International Consensus Group on Microembolus Detection. Stroke 29:725–729, 1998.
24. Ries F, Kaal K, Schultheiss R, et al: Air microbubbles as a contrast medium in transcranial Doppler sonography: A pilot study. J Neuroimaging 1:173–178, 1991.
25. Ries F: Clinical experience with echo-enhanced transcranial Doppler and duplex imaging. J Neuroimaging 7:S15–S21, 1997.
26. Main ML, Grayburn PA: Clinical applications of transpulmonary contrast echocardiography. Am Heart J 137:144–153, 1999.
27. Newell DW, Winn HR: Transcranial Doppler in cerebral vasospasm. Neurosurg Clin N Am 1:319–328, 1990.
28. Kistler JP, Crowell RM, Davis KR, et al: The relation of cerebral vasospasm to the extent and location of subarachnoid blood visualized by CT scan: A prospective study. Neurology 33: 424–436, 1983.
29. Seiler RW, Grolimund P, Aaslid R, et al: Cerebral vasospasm evaluated by transcranial ultrasound correlated with clinical grade and CT-visualized subarachnoid hemorrhage. J Neurosurg 64:594–600, 1986.
30. Heros RC, Zervas NT, Varsos V: Cerebral vasospasm after subarachnoid hemorrhage: An update. Ann Neurol 14:599–608, 1983.
31. Lodi CA, Ursino M: Hemodynamic effect of cerebral vasospasm in humans: A modeling study. Ann Biomed Eng 27:257–273, 1999.
32. Sekhar LN, Wechsler LR, Yonas H, et al: Value of transcranial Doppler examination in the diagnosis of cerebral vasospasm after subarachnoid hemorrhage. Neurosurgery 22:813–821, 1988.
33. Lewis DH, Newell DW, Winn HR: Delayed ischemia due to cerebral vasospasm occult to transcranial Doppler: An important role for cerebral perfusion SPECT. Clin Nucl Med 22: 238–240, 1997.
34. Powers WJ, Grubb RL Jr, Raichle ME: Physiological responses to focal cerebral ischemia in humans. Ann Neurol 16:546–552, 1984.
35. Powers WJ, Grubb RL Jr., Baker RP, et al: Regional cerebral blood flow and metabolism in reversible ischemia due to vasospasm: Determination by positron emission tomography. J Neurosurg 62:539–546, 1985.
36. Vora YY, Suarez-Almazor M, Steinke DE, et al: Role of transcranial Doppler monitoring in the diagnosis of cerebral vasospasm after subarachnoid hemorrhage. Neurosurgery 44:1237–1247, 1999.
37. Seiler R, Grolimund P, Huber P: Transcranial Doppler sonography: An alternative to angiography in the evaluation of vasospasm after subarachnoid hemorrhage. Acta Radiol Suppl Stockh 369:P99–102, 1986.
38. Sloan MA, Haley EC Jr, Kassell NF, et al: Sensitivity and specificity of transcranial Doppler ultrasonography in the diagnosis of vasospasm following subarachnoid hemorrhage. Neurology 39:1514–1518, 1989.
39. Lindegaard KF, Nornes H, Bakke SJ, et al: Cerebral vasospasm after subarachnoid haemorrhage investigated by means of transcranial Doppler ultrasound. Acta Neurochir Suppl Wien 42:P81–84, 1988.
40. Klingelhofer J, Dander D, Holzgraefe M, et al: Cerebral vasospasm evaluated by transcranial Doppler ultrasonography at different intracranial pressures. J Neurosurg 75:752–758, 1991.
41. Clyde BL, Resnick DK, Yonas H: The relationship of blood velocity as measured by transcranial Doppler ultrasonography to cerebral blood flow as determined by stable Xenon computed tomographic studies after aneurysmal subarachnoid hemorrhage. Neurosurgery 38:896, 1996.
42. Lindegaard KF: The role of transcranial Doppler in the management of patients with subarachnoid haemorrhage—a review. Acta Neurochir Suppl 72:59–71, 1999.
43. Weir B, Grace M, Hansen JEA: Time course of vasospasm in man. J Neurosurg 48:173, 1978.
44. Harders AG, Gilsbach JM: Time course of blood velocity changes related to vasospasm in the circle of Willis measured by transcranial Doppler ultrasound. J Neurosurg 66:718–728, 1987.
45. Romner B, Ljunggren B, Brandt L, Saveland H: Transcranial Doppler sonography within 12 hours after subarachnoid hemorrhage. J Neurosurg 70:732–736, 1989.
46. Romner B, Ljunggren B, Brandt L, Saveland H: Correlation of transcranial Doppler sonography findings with timing of aneurysm surgery. J Neurosurg 73:72–76, 1990.
47. Grosset DG, Straiton J, du Trevou M, Bullock R: Prediction of symptomatic vasospasm after subarachnoid hemorrhage by rapidly increasing transcranial Doppler velocity and cerebral blood flow changes. Stroke 23:674–679, 1992.

48. Manno EM, Gress DR, Schwamm LH, et al: Effects of induced hypertension on transcranial Doppler ultrasound velocities in patients after subarachnoid hemorrhage. Stroke 29:422–428, 1998.
49. Barker FG, Ogilvy CS: Efficacy of prophylactic nimodipine for delayed ischemic deficit after subarachnoid hemorrhage: A metaanalysis. J Neurosurg 84:405–414, 1996.
50. Harders A, Gilsbach J: Haemodynamic effectiveness of nimodipine on spastic brain vessels after subarachnoid haemorrhage evaluated by the transcranial Doppler method: A review of clinical studies. Acta Neurochir Suppl Wien 45:P21–28, 1988.
51. Elliott JP, Newell DW, Lam DJ, et al: Comparison of balloon angioplasty and papaverine infusion for the treatment of vasospasm following aneurysmal subarachnoid hemorrhage. J Neurosurg 88:277–284, 1998.
52. Lewis DH, Eskridge JM, Newell DW, et al: Brain SPECT and the effect of cerebral angioplasty in delayed ischemia due to vasospasm. J Nucl Med 33:1789–1796, 1992.
53. Harders A, Bien S, Eggert HR, et al: Haemodynamic changes in arteriovenous malformations induced by superselective embolization: Transcranial Doppler evaluation. Neurol Res 10:239–245, 1988.
54. Baumgartner RW, Mattle HP, Kothbauer K, Schroth G: Transcranial color-coded duplex sonography in cerebral aneurysms. Stroke 25:2429–2434, 1994.
55. Fleischer LH, Young WL, Pile-Spellman J, et al: Relationship of transcranial Doppler flow velocities and arteriovenous malformation feeding artery pressures. Stroke 24:1897–1902, 1993.
56. Duong H, Tampieri D, TerBrugge KG, et al: Transcranial Doppler ultrasonographic changes after embolization of cerebral arteriovenous malformations [published erratum appears in Can Assoc Radiol J 1995 Apr;46(2):130]. Can Assoc Radiol J 45: 447–451, 1994.
57. Klotzsch C, Nahser HC, Fischer B, et al: Visualisation of intracranial aneurysms by transcranial duplex sonography. Neuroradiology 38:555–559, 1996.
58. Woydt M, Greiner K, Perez J, et al: Intraoperative color duplex sonography of basal arteries during aneurysm surgery. J Neuroimaging 7:203–207, 1997.
59. Ackerstaff RG, van de Vlasakker CJ: Monitoring of brain function during carotid endarterectomy: An analysis of contemporary methods. J Cardiothorac Vasc Anesth 12:341–317, 1998.
60. Halsey JH Jr: Risks and benefits of shunting in carotid endarterectomy. The International Transcranial Doppler Collaborators. Stroke 23:1583–1587, 1992.
61. Fiori L, Parenti G, Marconi F: Combined transcranial Doppler and electrophysiologic monitoring for carotid endarterectomy. J Neurosurg Anesthesiol 9:11–16, 1997.
62. Jansen C, Vriens EM, Eikelboom BC, et al: Carotid endarterectomy with transcranial Doppler and electroencephalographic monitoring: A prospective study in 130 operations. Stroke 24: 665–669, 1993.
63. Jansen C, Ramos LM, van Heesewijk JP, et al: Impact of microembolism and hemodynamic changes in the brain during carotid endarterectomy. Stroke 25:992–997, 1994.
64. Spencer MP, Thomas GI, Moehring MA: Relation between middle cerebral artery blood flow velocity and stump pressure during carotid endarterectomy. Stroke 23:1439–1445, 1992.
65. Cao P, Giordano G, Zannetti S, et al: Transcranial Doppler monitoring during carotid endarterectomy: Is it appropriate for selecting patients in need of a shunt? J Vasc Surg 26:973–980, 1997.
66. Riles TS, Imparato AM, Jacobowitz GR, et al: The cause of perioperative stroke after carotid endarterectomy. J Vasc Surg 19:206–216, 1994.
67. Spencer MP: Transcranial Doppler monitoring and causes of stroke from carotid endarterectomy. Stroke 28:685–691, 1997.
68. Smith JL, Evans DH, Bell PR, Naylor AR: Time domain analysis of embolic signals can be used in place of high-resolution Wigner analysis when classifying gaseous and particulate emboli. Ultrasound Med Biol 24:989–993, 1998.
69. Droste DW, Hagedorn G, Notzold A, et al: Bigated transcranial Doppler for the detection of clinically silent circulating emboli in normal persons and patients with prosthetic cardiac valves. Stroke 28:588–592, 1997.
70. Smith JL, Evans DH, Gaunt ME, et al: Experience with transcranial Doppler monitoring reduces the incidence of particulate embolization during carotid endarterectomy. Br J Surg 85:56–59, 1998.
71. Gaunt M, Naylor AR, Lennard N, et al: Transcranial Doppler detected cerebral microembolism following carotid endarterectomy. Brain 121:389–390, 1998.
72. Levi CR, O'Malley HM, Fell G, et al:. Transcranial Doppler detected cerebral microembolism following carotid endarterectomy: High microembolic signal loads predict postoperative cerebral ischaemia. Brain 120:621–629, 1997.
73. Cantelmo NL, Babikian VL, Samaraweera RN, et al: Cerebral microembolism and ischemic changes associated with carotid endarterectomy. J Vasc Surg 27:1024–1031, 1998.
74. Hayes P, Lennard N, Smith J, et al: Vascular Surgical Society of Great Britain and Ireland: Transcranial Doppler-directed dextran therapy in the prevention of postoperative carotid thrombosis. Br J Surg 86:692, 1999.
75. Lennard N, Smith J, Dumville J, et al: Prevention of postoperative thrombotic stroke after carotid endarterectomy: The role of transcranial Doppler ultrasound. J Vasc Surg 26:579–584, 1997.
76. Jansen C, Sprengers AM, Moll FL, et al: Prediction of intracerebral haemorrhage after carotid endarterectomy by clinical criteria and intraoperative transcranial Doppler monitoring: Results of 233 operations. Eur J Vasc Surg 8:220–225, 1994.
77. Schroeder T, Sillesen H, Boesen J, et al: Intracerebral haemorrhage after carotid endarterectomy. Eur J Vasc Surg 1:51–60, 1987.
78. Schroeder T, Sillesen H, Sorensen O, Engell HC: Cerebral hyperperfusion following carotid endarterectomy. J Neurosurg 66: 824–829, 1987.
79. Jorgensen LG, Schroeder TV: Defective cerebrovascular autoregulation after carotid endarterectomy. Eur J Vasc Surg 7:370–379, 1993.
80. Jansen C, Sprengers AM, Moll FL, et al: Prediction of intracerebral haemorrhage after carotid endarterectomy by clinical criteria and intraoperative transcranial Doppler monitoring. Eur J Vasc Surg 8:303–308, 1994.
81. Cold GE: Measurements of CO2 reactivity and barbiturate reactivity in patients with severe head injury. Acta Neurochir 98: 153–163, 1989.
82. Cold GE, Jensen FT, Malmros R: The cerebrovascular CO2 reactivity during the acute phase of brain injury. Acta Anaesthesiol Scand 21:222–231, 1977.
83. Newell DW, Weber JP, Watson R, et al: Effect of transient moderate hyperventilation on dynamic cerebral autoregulation after severe head injury. Neurosurgery 39:35–44, 1996.
84. Simard JM, Bellefleur M: Systemic arterial hypertension in head trauma. Am J Cardiol 63:32C–35C, 1989.
85. Muizelaar JP, Lutz III HA, Becker DP: Effect of mannitol on ICP and CBF and correlation with pressure autoregulation in severely head-injured patients. J Neurosurg 61:700–706, 1984.
86. Tiecks FP, Lam AM, Aaslid R, Newell DW: Comparison of static and dynamic cerebral autoregulation measurements. Stroke 26: 1014–1019, 1995.
87. Giller CA: A bedside test for cerebral autoregulation using transcranial Doppler ultrasound. Acta Neurochir 108:7–14, 1991.
88. Czosnyka M, Guazzo E, Iyer V, et al: Testing of cerebral autoregulation in head injury by waveform analysis of blood flow velocity and cerebral perfusion pressure. Acta Neurochir Suppl Wien 60:P468–471, 1994.
89. Czosnyka M, Smielewski P, Kirkpatrick P, et al: Monitoring of cerebral autoregulation in head-injured patients. Stroke 27: 1829–1834, 1996.
90. Strebel S, Lam AM, Matta B, et al: Dynamic and static cerebral autoregulation during isoflurane, desflurane, and propofol anesthesia. Anesthesiology 83:66–76, 1995.
91. Marmarou A, Anderson RL, Ward JD, et al: Impact of ICP instability and hypotension on outcome in patients with severe head trauma. J Neurosurg 75:S59–S66, 1991.
92. Chesnut RM, Marshall SB, Piek J, et al: Early and late systemic hypotension as a frequent and fundamental source of cerebral

ischemia following severe brain injury in the Traumatic Coma Data Bank. Acta Neurochir Suppl (Wien) 59:121–125, 1993.
93. Pietropaoli JA, Rogers FB, Shackford SR, et al: The deleterious effects of intraoperative hypotension on outcome in patients with severe head injuries. J Trauma 33:403–407, 1992.
94. Winchell RJ, Simons RK, Hoyt DB: Transient systolic hypotension: A serious problem in the management of head injury. Arch Surg 131:533–539, 1996.
95. Junger EC, Newell DW, Grant GA, et al: Cerebral autoregulation following minor head injury. J Neurosurg 86:425–432, 1997.
96. Martin NA, Patwardhan RV, Alexander MJ, et al: Characterization of cerebral hemodynamic phases following severe head trauma: Hypoperfusion, hyperemia, and vasospasm. J Neurosurg 87:9–19, 1997.
97. Martin NA, Doberstein C, Zane C, et al: Posttraumatic cerebral arterial spasm: Transcranial Doppler ultrasound, cerebral blood flow, and angiographic findings. J Neurosurg 77:575–583, 1992.
98. Lee JH, Martin NA, Alsina G, et al: Hemodynamically significant cerebral vasospasm and outcome after head injury: A prospective study. J Neurosurg 87:221–233, 1997.
99. Weber M, Grolimund P, Seiler RW: Evaluation of posttraumatic cerebral blood flow velocities by transcranial Doppler ultrasonography. Neurosurgery 27:106–112, 1990.
100. Srinivasan J, Newell DW, Sturzenegger M, et al: Transcranial Doppler in the evaluation of internal carotid artery dissection. Stroke 27:1226–1230, 1996.
101. Chan KH, Miller JD, Dearden NM, et al: The effect of changes in cerebral perfusion pressure upon middle cerebral artery blood flow velocity and jugular bulb venous oxygen saturation after severe brain injury. J Neurosurg 77:55–61, 1992.
102. Chan KH, Miller JD, Dearden NM: Intracranial blood flow velocity after head injury: Relationship to severity of injury, time, neurological status and outcome. J Neurol Neurosurg Psychiatry 55:787–791, 1992.
103. Hassler W, Steinmetz H, Gawlowski J: Transcranial Doppler ultrasonography in raised intracranial pressure and in intracranial circulatory arrest. J Neurosurg 68:745–751, 1988.
104. Newell DW, Grady MS, Sirotta P, Winn HR: Evaluation of brain death using transcranial Doppler. Neurosurgery 24:509–513, 1989.
105. Newell DW: Transcranial Doppler ultrasonography. Neurosurg Clin N Am 5:619–631, 1994.
106. Aaslid R: Cerebral hemodynamics. In Newell DW, Aaslid R (eds): Transcranial Doppler. New York, Raven Press, 1992, pp 49–55.
107. Aaslid R, Newell DW: Pressure flow relationships in the cerebral circulation. J Cardiovasc Technol 9:90, 1990.
108. Bode H, Sauer M, Pringsheim W: Diagnosis of brain death by transcranial Doppler sonography. Arch Dis Child 63:1474–1478, 1988.
109. D'Avalos A, Rodriguez Rago A, Mate G, et al: [Value of the transcranial Doppler examination in the diagnosis of brain death]. Med Clin 100:249–252, 1993.
110. Ducrocq X, Pincemaille B, Braun M, et al: [Value of transcranial Doppler ultrasonography in patients with suspected brain death]. Ann Fr Anesth Reanim 11:415–423, 1992.
111. Ducrocq X, Hassler W, Moritake K, et al: Consensus opinion on diagnosis of cerebral circulatory arrest using Doppler-sonography: Task Force Group on cerebral death of the Neurosonology Research Group of the World Federation of Neurology. J Neurol Sci 159:145–150, 1998.
112. Hadani M, Bruk B, Ram Z, et al: Application of transcranial Doppler ultrasonography for the diagnosis of brain death. Intensive Care Med 25:822–828, 1999.
113. Kirkham FJ, Neville BG, Gosling RG: Diagnosis of brain death by transcranial Doppler sonography. Arch Dis Child 64:889–890, 1989.
114. Petty GW, Mohr JP, Pedley TA, et al: The role of transcranial Doppler in confirming brain death: Sensitivity, specificity, and suggestions for performance and interpretation. Neurology 40: 300–303, 1990.
115. Powers AD, Graeber MC, Smith RR: Transcranial Doppler ultrasonography in the determination of brain death. Neurosurgery 24:884–889, 1989.
116. Shiogai T, Takeuchi K: [Relationship between cerebral circulatory arrest and loss of brain functions—analysis of patients in a state of impending brain death]. Rinsho Shinkeigaku 33: 1328–1330, 1993.
117. Ropper AH, Kehne SM, Wechsler L: Transcranial Doppler in brain death. Neurology 37:1733–1735, 1987.
118. Zurynski Y, Dorsch N, Pearson I, Choong R: Transcranial Doppler ultrasound in brain death: Experience in 140 patients. Neurol Res 13:248–252, 1991.
119. Eng CC, Lam AM, Byrd S, Newell DW: The diagnosis and management of a perianesthetic cerebral aneurysmal rupture aided with transcranial Doppler ultrasonography. Anesthesiology 78:191–194, 1993.
120. Grote E, Hassler W: The critical first minutes after subarachnoid hemorrhage. Neurosurgery 22:654–661, 1988.
121. Toole JF: Middle cerebral artery stenosis—a neglected problem? Surg Neurol 27:44–46, 1987.
122. Bogousslavsky J, Barnett HJ, Fox AJ, et al: Atherosclerotic disease of the middle cerebral artery. Stroke 17:1112–1120, 1986.
123. Spencer MP, Whisler D: Transorbital Doppler diagnosis of intracranial arterial stenosis. Stroke 17:916–921, 1986.
124. Ley-Pozo J, Ringelstein EB: Noninvasive detection of occlusive disease of the carotid siphon and middle cerebral artery. Ann Neurol 28:640–647, 1990.
125. Rorick MB, Nichols FT, Adams RJ: Transcranial Doppler correlation with angiography in detection of intracranial stenosis. Stroke 25:1931–1934, 1994.
126. Kleiser B, Widder B: Course of carotid artery occlusions with impaired cerebrovascular reactivity. Stroke 23:171–174, 1992.
127. Wilterdink JL, Feldmann E, Furie KL, et al: Transcranial Doppler ultrasound battery reliably identifies severe internal carotid artery stenosis. Stroke 28:133–136, 1997.
128. Ringelstein EB, Sievers C, Ecker S, et al: Noninvasive assessment of CO2-induced cerebral vasomotor response in normal individuals and patients with internal carotid artery occlusions. Stroke 19:963-969, 1988.
129. Yonas H, Smith HA, Durham SR, et al: Increased stroke risk predicted by compromised cerebral blood flow reactivity. J Neurosurg 79:483-489, 1993.
130. Grubb RLJ, Derdeyn CP, Fritsch SM, et al: Importance of hemodynamic factors in the prognosis of symptomatic carotid occlusion. JAMA 280:1055–1060, 1998.
131. Gur AY, Bova I, Bornstein NM: Is impaired cerebral vasomotor reactivity a predictive factor of stroke in asymptomatic patients? Stroke 27:2188–2190, 1996.
132. Aaslid R, Lindegaard KF, Sorteberg W, Nornes H: Cerebral autoregulation dynamics in humans. Stroke 20:45–52, 1989.
133. Newell DW, Aaslid R, Douville CM, et al: Comparison of autoregulation and CO_2 reactivity in occlusive disease. Stroke 25: 748, 1994.
134. White RP, Markus HS: Impaired dynamic cerebral autoregulation in carotid artery stenosis. Stroke 28:1340–1344, 1997.
135. Fujioka KA, Ernsberger AM, Nicholls SC, Spencer MP: Transcranial Doppler assessment of mechanical compression of the vertebral arteries. J Vasc Surg 15:254–259, 1991.
136. Sturzenegger M, Newell DW, Douville C, et al: Dynamic transcranial Doppler assessment of positional vertebrobasilar ischemia. Stroke 25:1776–1783, 1994.
137. Spencer MP, Lawrence GH, Thomas GI, Sauvage LR: The use of ultrasonics in the determination of arterial aeroembolism during open-heart surgery. Ann Thorac Surg 8:489–497, 1969.
138. Maroon JC, Albin MS: Air embolism diagnosed by Doppler ultrasound. Anesth Analg 53:399–402, 1974.
139. Padayachee TS, Parsons S, Theobold R, et al: The detection of microemboli in the middle cerebral artery during cardiopulmonary bypass: A transcranial Doppler ultrasound investigation using membrane and bubble oxygenators. Ann Thorac Surg 44: 298–302, 1987.
140. Babikian VL, Hyde C, Pochay V, Winter MR: Clinical correlates of high-intensity transient signals detected on transcranial Doppler sonography in patients with cerebrovascular disease. Stroke 25:1570–1573, 1994.
141. Georgiadis D, Baumgartner RW, Karatschai R, et al: Further evidence of gaseous embolic material in patients with artificial heart valves. J Thorac Cardiovasc Surg 115:808–810, 1998.

142. Siebler M, Nachtmann A, Sitzer M, et al: Cerebral microembolism and the risk of ischemia in asymptomatic high-grade internal carotid artery stenosis. Stroke 26:2184–2186, 1995.
143. Siebler M, Sitzer M, Rose G, et al: Silent cerebral embolism caused by neurologically symptomatic high-grade carotid stenosis: Event rates before and after carotid endarterectomy. Brain 116:1005–1015, 1993.
144. Koennecke HC, Trocio SH Jr, Mast H, Mohr JP: Microemboli on transcranial Doppler in patients with spontaneous carotid artery dissection. J Neuroimaging 7:217–220, 1997.
145. Dagirmanjian A, Davis DA, Rothfus WE, et al: Silent cerebral microemboli occurring during carotid angiography: Frequency as determined with Doppler sonography. AJR Am J Roentgenol 161:1037–1040, 1993.
146. Markus HS, Clifton A, Buckenham T, Brown MM: Carotid angioplasty: Detection of embolic signals during and after the procedure. Stroke 25:2403–2406, 1994.
147. Markus H: Transcranial Doppler detection of circulating cerebral emboli: A review. Stroke 24:1246–1250, 1993.
148. Giller CA, Giller AM, Landreneau F: Detection of emboli after surgery for intracerebral aneurysms. Neurosurgery 42:490–494, 1998.
149. Di Tullio M, Sacco RL, Venketasubramanian N, et al: Comparison of diagnostic techniques for the detection of a patent foramen ovale in stroke patients. Stroke 24:1020–1024, 1993.
150. Stump DA, Rogers AT, Hammon JW, Newman SP: Cerebral emboli and cognitive outcome after cardiac surgery. J Cardiothorac Vasc Anesth 10:113–119, 1996.

CHAPTER **92**

Neurosonology

CHARLES J. PRESTIGIACOMO ■ DONALD O. QUEST

The use of ultrasonology in the evaluation and management of neurosurgical disease has undergone significant changes. The application of this technology has expanded over the years to serve not only as a means of intraoperative localization but also as a primary mode of assessment for cerebrovascular disease. In its current state, neurosonology is used for the real-time identification and localization of brain and spinal cord lesions, the safe and reproducible evaluation of carotid or vertebral artery disease, and the evaluation of intracranial flow dynamics. Although each of these uses involves the interpretation of reflected sound waves, their technologies and respective merits vary. This chapter reviews the basic physics of ultrasonology, the use of ultrasonography in the diagnosis of extracranial carotid disease in adults, and the role of intraoperative ultrasonography in neurological surgery.

THE PHYSICS OF ULTRASONOLOGY

General Principles

Modern ultrasound techniques have evolved through a greater understanding of the physics of sound and of its interactions with human tissue, as well as numerous technologic advances in data analysis. Any vibrating source placed in contact with a medium produces a sound wave of vibrating particles. In today's machines, a vibrating synthetic piezoelectric crystal generates a focused ultrasonographic pulse, which travels at a velocity of approximately 1540 m/sec through human tissue. As this pulse travels through the tissue in a well-defined direction, a portion of it is absorbed (known as attenuation) and a portion is transmitted through the tissue according to the tissue's unique acoustic properties. When the pulse reaches a point where tissues of different acoustic properties interface, a portion of the transmitted pulse is reflected (Fig. 92–1). This reflected signal returns to the transducer and mechanically distorts the same piezoelectric crystal, which induces a small voltage in the crystal. The amplitude and time of flight of the reflected signal is then recorded and analyzed by a computer. These echoes can subsequently be amplified and processed into several different formats for display.

The degree of sound attenuation is determined by the absorptive properties of the tissue and by the frequency of the ultrasonographic pulse. Most diagnostic ultrasonography is performed at frequencies from 1 to 15 megahertz (MHz). The higher the frequency of the pulse wave, the higher the attenuation and therefore the lower the tissue penetration. Thus, high-frequency ultrasonography produces a high-resolution image of a small amount of tissue.

B-Mode Ultrasonography

The basic principle underlying real-time brightness-mode (B-mode) imaging is the variable acoustic impedance that different body tissues naturally possess. When the technique was first developed, the intensity and time of flight for the reflected signal (echo) were represented as a unidimensional tracing, with the amplitude of the wave representing intensity and the dis-

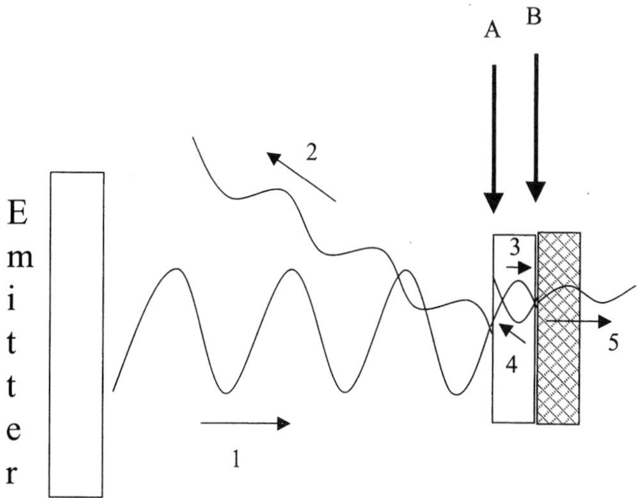

FIGURE 92–1. Properties of sound waves. An emitter sends a sound wave toward an object with a specific amplitude (wave height) and wavelength *(arrow 1)*. At the air-object (air-tissue) interface (A), some of the sound is reflected *(arrow 2)*, and some is transmitted *(arrow 3)*. As the sound strikes the interface of two objects (tissues) with different densities (B), again a portion of the sound is reflected *(arrow 4)* and the remainder is transmitted *(arrow 5)*.

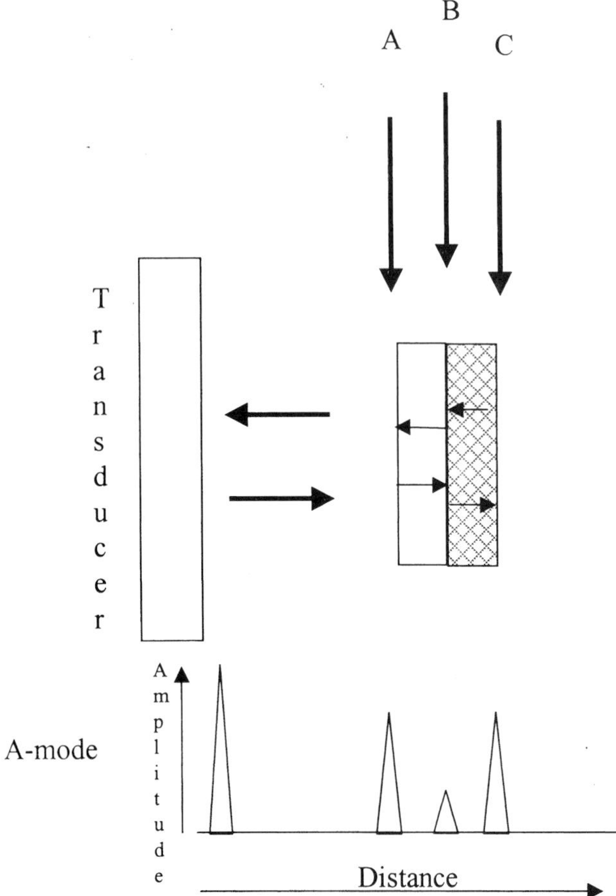

FIGURE 92–2. Schematic of A-mode ultrasonography. Sound is emitted and detected at the transducer. The time of flight and the amplitude of the reflected signal from the interfaces (A, B, C) are determined by the transducer and reflected in a tracing. The distance from the point of the sound's origin is a function of one-half the time of flight for that signal to return to the transducer. The height of the reflected signal depicts its relative amplitude.

tance along the x-axis representing the reflector depth or distance from the transducer (known as amplitude-modulation mode, or A-mode; Fig. 92–2). The standard display now allows for the visualization of tissue interfaces when sound waves are spatially represented by picture elements (pixels) on a video display, with the brightness of each pixel correlating to the amplitude or intensity of the echo signal (Fig. 92–3). Scanner screens use 256 shades of gray to represent the tissues' different ability to absorb or reflect sound.

When the piezoelectric crystal emits a pulse, this focused beam travels along a single plane. Any sound reflected back along this plane is recorded and presented on the display screen. By insonating adjacent segments of tissue with multiple crystals located within a sonographic head or with a rotating head, a two-dimensional representation of the object being insonated can be shown on the display screen. This B-mode display has become a standard mode of displaying the anatomy of insonated tissue (Fig. 92–4). The rapid processing and display of this data allow for "real-time" imaging in ultrasonography, such that pulsations of vessels and cerebrospinal fluid spaces can be identified.

Doppler Shift and Vascular Ultrasonography

In 1842, Doppler[1] first described the frequency shift of reflected or scattered signals that occurs whenever there is relative motion between the emitter and the object or interface reflecting the sound. Doppler quite elegantly demonstrated that the frequency of the reflected signal increases as a reflecting object moves toward the receiver and decreases as it moves away, such as is observed with the motion of stars or with the sound of a train whistle as it approaches and passes a stationary individual. Variables that affect the shift in frequency that accompanies insonation of a moving object, such as a red blood corpuscle in a stream of flowing blood, include the angle of insonation with respect to the vector of flow, the insonating frequency of the ultrasound beam, the velocity of the flow, and the speed of sound through the insonated tissue. By controlling the angle of insonation and the insonating frequency, and by knowing the speed of sound through insonated tissue, one can determine the velocity of flow by the degree of the Doppler frequency shift.

The first clinical applications of the Doppler principle involved the use of continuous-wave ultrasonography. This technology employs two crystals, with one acting as a continuous signal emitter and the other as a receiver. Lowering the frequency of the beam can increase penetration of the beam in tissue. Output data from these early devices consisted of either a complex audio signal or visual display denoting the average frequency shift of the Doppler beam. Because all reflectors within the insonated tissue contributed to the Doppler shift, the source of this reflected signal could not be precisely located. Limited by this inability to precisely locate the source of the reflected signal and the inability to extrapolate the precise frequency shift from a particular source given the complexity of the signal, researchers began to incorporate techniques such as beam focusing and spectral analysis into the field of ultrasonography. The technique of beam focusing allows the ultrasound instrument to "gate" the echo signals so that only the signal from a discrete portion along the beam's course is analyzed (known as range gating; Fig. 92–5). Despite the ability to focus the emitting beam, accurate localization of the origin of a particular frequency shift was not possible until the early 1970s with the advent of ultrasonic arteriography, which used a single piezoelectric crystal to emit and receive *pulsed* signals rather than a continuous beam.[2]

Spectral Analysis and Duplex Ultrasonography

Although the combination of beam focusing and pulsed Doppler arteriography improved the ability to localize the source of the reflected signal, Doppler spectral analysis of this signal, especially when it involved complicated blood velocity patterns, was still quite dif-

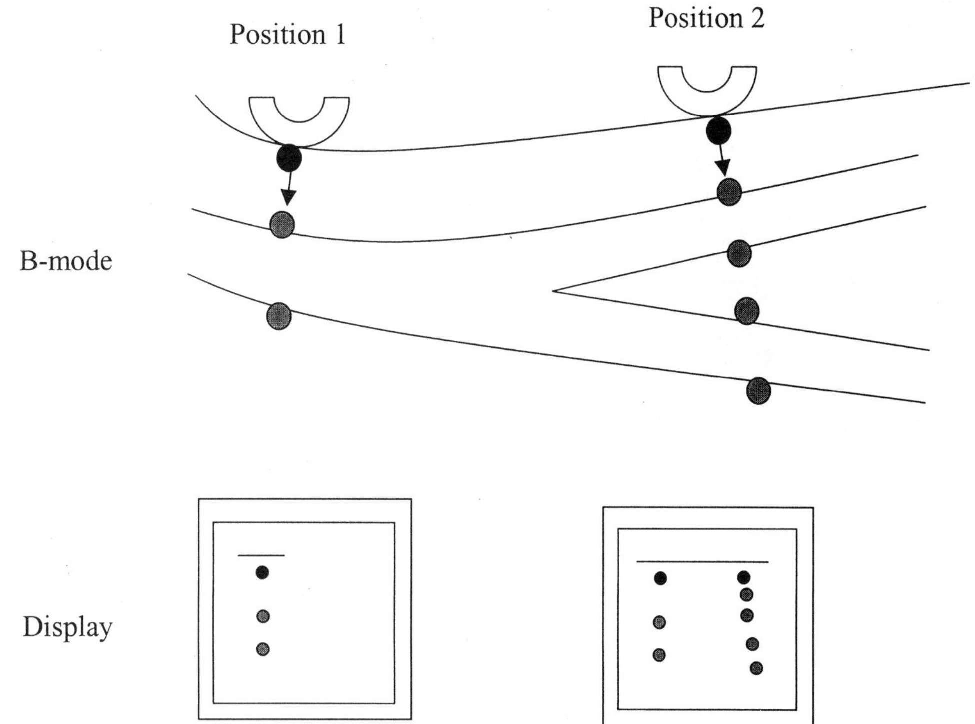

FIGURE 92–3. Schematic of B-mode ultrasonography. This modality allows the graphic display of reflected sound by plotting the reflected signal in the vertical direction and displaying the signal's amplitude by its relative brightness on a gray scale. With the transducer in position 1, insonation of a vessel through the skin results in reflection of sound at three distinct interfaces. These reflections are displayed on the screen. At position 2, sound is reflected by five distinct interfaces, which are also displayed on the screen.

ficult to interpret. Through the use of fast Fourier transformations, the complex reflected signal was separated into its numerous single-frequency components; the relative contribution of each single-frequency component to the original signal could then be visually displayed. This resultant "power spectrum" for the Doppler signal could be used to distinguish the various flow characteristics that exist in normal and diseased vessels (Fig. 92–6).

These technologies were later integrated with B-mode imaging, and duplex ultrasonography was born.[3]

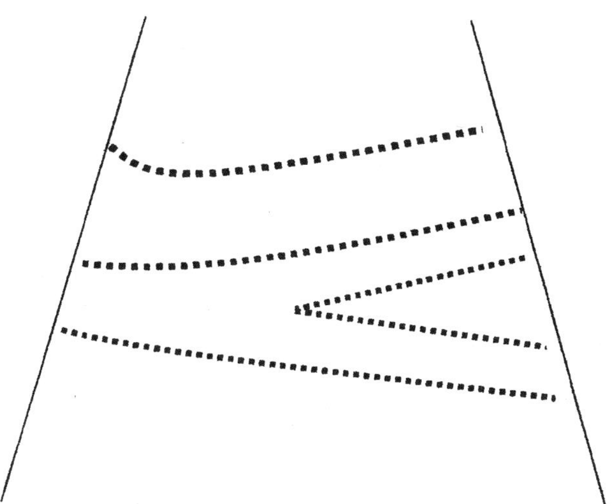

FIGURE 92–4. By combining the information in consecutive "slices" on one display, the resultant graphic representation depicts underlying tissue anatomy.

The advantage of the duplex scanner compared with existing technology was the ability to sample flow within the vessel while simultaneously displaying vessel wall anatomy. This allowed for reproducible acquisition of spectral waveform patterns from the pulsed Doppler crystals, which in turn allowed refinement of the criteria defining the varying degrees of vessel stenosis.

Modern duplex scanning uses one transducer (5 to 7 MHz) to produce simultaneous B-mode images and pulsed Doppler waveform analysis. The screen of the display module provides real-time anatomic B-mode data and a graphic representation of the Fourier-transformed pulsed spectral analysis (Fig. 92–7). The technologist also receives direct audio signals from the pulsed signal. The pitch of these audio signals is proportional to the velocity of the flowing blood, which is proportional to the frequency of the transformed spectral wave. In addition, the B-mode display contains a cursor (or Doppler gate) that allows one to focus the pulsed signal to a particular point along the beam's course and thus selectively insonate clearly identifiable vessels. This feature has allowed for greater standardization of frequency data for particular areas of the carotid system. Simultaneous gray-scale and spectral data have allowed for recognition of anatomic variants, such as vessel kinks and coils, and severe calcifications, as well as the evaluation of associated disease in accessible portions of the subclavian and vertebral arteries. An additional advantage of this diagnostic tool is that it has the ability to correct for variable angles of insonation, which, if not kept between 55 and 65 degrees, could significantly alter the recorded frequencies.

One of the major limitations of duplex scanning is

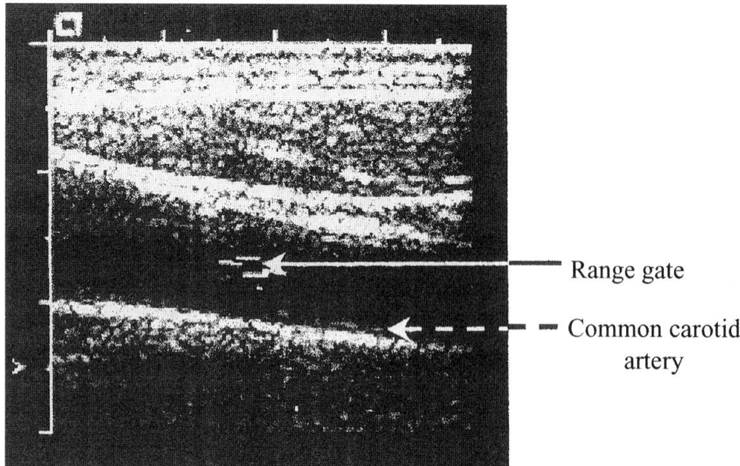

FIGURE 92–5. B-mode ultrasound image of the common carotid artery with the gating icon to demonstrate the region where flow analysis is being performed.

that only a small region of the artery can be studied at any one time. This technology is also only a two-dimensional representation of a three-dimensional dynamic process. Color-flow imaging, which combines real-time, B-mode gray-scale with color encoding of multigated Doppler flow information, begins to address these issues by sampling the mean Doppler frequency shift at various depths over the entire scan area. The color assigned to the frequency data depends on the magnitude and direction of flow, with hue (red versus blue) depicting the direction of flow, the hue's saturation denoting the magnitude of the frequency shift, and the brightness (luminance) demonstrating the variance in mean flow (i.e., the turbulence), which is superimposed on a gray-scale B-mode image depicting the surrounding anatomy. Color Doppler allows for more rapid identification of the component vessels than does duplex alone, and it also provides rapid identification of laminar flow patterns for placement of a single pulsed Doppler gate for acquisition of spectral waveform data. Today, the combined use of B-mode two-dimensional imaging and the real-time,

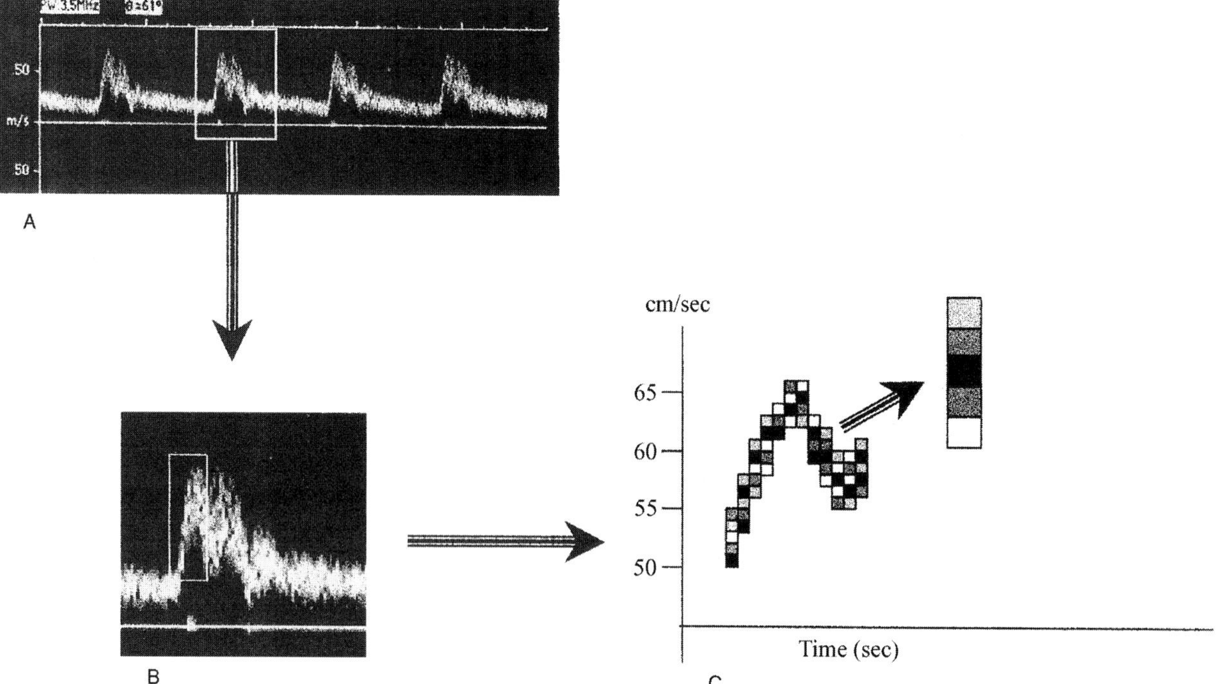

FIGURE 92–6. Doppler waveform during insonation of the common carotid artery. *A*, Spectral display demonstrates the pulse wave frequency (PW = 3.5 MHz) and the angle of insonation (θ = 61 degrees). Velocity is then plotted along the y-axis, and time along the x-axis. *B*, Magnified view of the spectral Doppler waveform demonstrating pixels of differing intensities. *C*, Schematic representation of the spectral waveform. Relative pixel intensity corresponds to the relative amount of flow at that particular velocity.

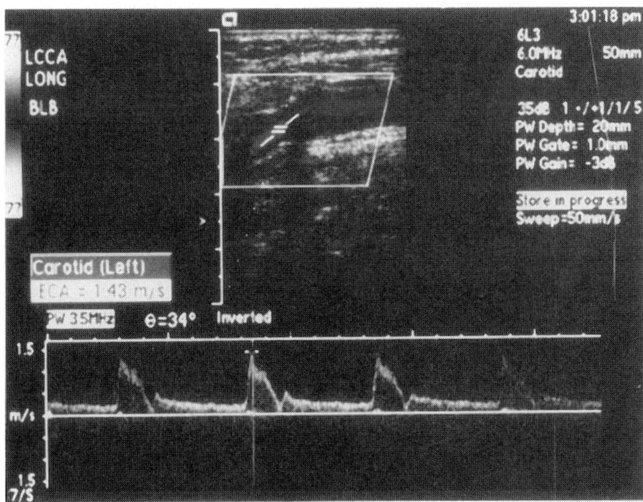

FIGURE 92–7. Duplex Doppler display with B-mode ultrasonogram at the top of the display, along with the Doppler spectral wave for the range-gated portion of the proximal external carotid artery below with normal flow pattern.

color-enhanced spectral analysis of pulsed-wave Doppler has enabled experienced operators to recognize carotid stenosis with sensitivities approaching 100%.

ULTRASONOGRAPHY FOR DIAGNOSIS

Diagnostic ultrasonography is an established, inexpensive, safe, noninvasive imaging tool in the diagnosis of fetal or neonatal intracranial pathology and adult cerebrovascular disease. The importance of fetal and neonatal ultrasonography is well documented elsewhere in this text and is not expounded on here.

Diseases of the Carotid Artery

Over the years, in efforts to reduce both the major and the minor risks of carotid endarterectomy, along with the associated risks of preoperative evaluation, several noninvasive methods of assessing carotid and intracranial blood flow have been used. Besides allowing clinicians to assess the degree of carotid stenosis with a sensitivity and specificity often greater than that of angiography, carotid duplex sonography has enabled clinicians to evaluate plaque morphology, which may have additional implications in the overall morbidity and mortality of carotid atherosclerosis. Further, in combination with other noninvasive imaging techniques, magnetic resonance angiography (MRA) in particular, carotid ultrasonography has essentially obviated the need for angiography in the evaluation and treatment of the vast majority of patients with carotid bifurcation disease.[4]

B-mode Doppler typically shows the carotid system as a pulsatile luminal structure with a thin echogenic line representing the intimal surface. High-resolution scanners have enabled technologists to visualize and characterize subintimal plaques using this technique. When Doppler shift analysis is employed, the normal internal carotid artery waveform possesses a sharp systolic upstroke and a broad peak due to the low-resistance cerebral vasculature. Normally, maximal systolic frequency is less than 4 kHz, and flow remains antegrade throughout diastole. The distribution of velocities insonated is narrow, because flow in the center of the vessel where the Doppler gate is focused is essentially laminar. The combination of these characteristics results in a clear window beneath the systolic peak. This is quite different from the signal produced by the external carotid artery, where the systolic upstroke is a sharp peak, followed by an abrupt downstroke and flow reversal early in diastole. The common carotid artery waveform has characteristics of both systems but resembles the internal more than the external, as 70% of the waveform is contributed by the former. Diastolic flow in the common carotid artery is consequently maintained above zero.

Of importance is the fact that some nonpathologic regions are associated with nonlaminar flow. This is the case at the carotid bulb, where the sudden dilatation of the vessel wall results in both turbulence and flow reversal. This phenomenon is termed *boundary separation,* and its absence can represent a pathologic state in which normal bulb dilatation is lost.

As the vessel narrows, which can be seen to some degree on the B-mode display, the velocity of flow increases, with consequent increases in pitch and frequency in the reflected Doppler signal. Despite this increase in frequency, arterial blood flow remains essentially laminar within the center of the lumen. The spectral analysis therefore continues to produce a waveform with a narrow band of frequencies. Progressive arterial narrowing secondary to disease, however, perturbs this "center-stream" laminar flow, resulting in "spectral broadening," especially in the turbulent area just distal to the stenosis. This spectral broadening is accompanied by an increase in the amplitude of the audio signal corresponding to an increase in blood flow. As the severity of stenosis increases, the resultant high-velocity jets encountered by Doppler result in increased peak systolic frequencies as well.

Certain characteristic waveforms have been recognized to correlate well with the degree of vascular obstruction.[5] Gentle spectral broadening, usually in the downslope of the systolic peak and in early diastole, is known to appear in mild stenosis (<50% reduction in diameter or <75% area reduction). With moderate (50% to 70%) and sometimes severe (80% to 99%) stenosis, increases in waveform frequencies are seen, and spectral broadening increases to such a degree that the window beneath the spectral waveform is filled (Fig. 92–8). In severe stenosis (greater than 90%), blood flow is limited, despite compensatory increases in velocity, resulting in a decrease in signal amplitude. If the internal carotid artery is completely occluded, no flow is visualized within the lumen, and the common carotid waveform begins to resemble the external carotid artery waveform. If the common carotid artery is occluded, the internal carotid artery may fill from the external carotid artery, and reversal of flow may be

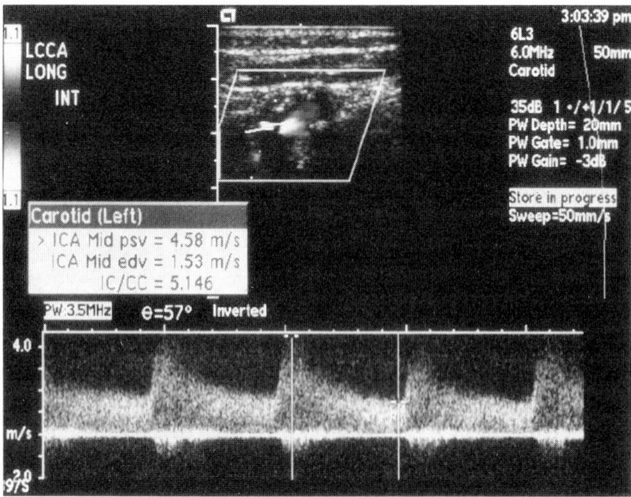

FIGURE 92–8. Doppler display of high-grade stenosis of the internal carotid artery, as demonstrated by broad spectral pattern.

evident in the external carotid artery throughout the cardiac cycle.

These waveform characteristics, although helpful in determining the severity of stenosis, are augmented by the following more rigorous parameters: (1) degree of stenosis by B-mode imaging; (2) peak systolic frequency (velocity); (3) peak diastolic frequency; (4) end-diastolic frequency; (5) ratio of systolic frequency between the internal and common carotid arteries; and (6) ratio of diastolic frequency between the internal and common carotid arteries. Although investigators disagree about which of these is most indicative of disease, peak systolic frequency, end-diastolic frequency, and systolic frequency ratio are considered the most important and the most predictive of stenosis.[6] Together, the aforementioned parameters raise the sensitivity and specificity of duplex sonography for the evaluation of carotid stenosis to 99% and 84%, respectively.[5] Moreover, correlation with angiography is excellent.[7] As will be discussed later, more recent studies suggest that although the sensitivity of angiography and duplex is roughly equivalent, the specificity of duplex sonography may actually be better.

The recognition of plaque irregularities has always been considered important in the evaluation of symptomatic patients. Although studies have demonstrated that there must be at least a 50% reduction in arterial diameter to cause flow-related ischemic neurological symptoms,[8] there have been numerous reports describing ischemic symptoms in patients with less than 50% stenosis.[9] It has thus been postulated that plaque irregularities and intraplaque hemorrhages are significant sources for embolic events.[10] Imparato and coworkers noted that the presence of intraplaque hemorrhage strongly correlated with the presence of ischemic symptoms.[11] Persson and colleagues noted that 85% of intraplaque hemorrhages communicated with the arterial lumen, implicating this as a possible mechanism for the acute thrombosis of the vessel.[12] Thus, although it is important to evaluate patients for the presence of stenosis, which can be accomplished by conventional or digital subtraction angiography, other, more subtle factors that may predispose individuals to cerebrovascular ischemia are not readily discernible with angiography.

B-mode sonography is capable of demonstrating intraplaque pathology based on the relative heterogeneity of these highly echogenic plaques. Although such information is not universally accepted, some investigators have shown that duplex scanning has a high degree of sensitivity and specificity (80% to 90%) in predicting findings at pathologic examination.[13] In addition to better evaluating plaque morphology, duplex scanning enables clinicians to noninvasively screen patients for hemodynamically significant stenosis when they present with evidence of neurovascular compromise (e.g., stroke, transient ischemic attack, evidence of coronary artery disease or carotid bruit on routine physical examination). When patients do not demonstrate hemodynamically significant lesions, duplex sonography allows clinicians to carefully follow them with repeat studies, thereby eliminating the excessive cost and risk of repeated angiography.

Despite the numerous advantages, duplex sonography has several limitations. It has been shown that calcifications within the arterial wall cast an "acoustic shadow," thus obscuring arterial anatomy. In addition, approximately 10% of patients presenting for duplex scanning cannot be successfully imaged because of anatomic limitations (e.g., high carotid bifurcations) or unusual vessel anatomy (e.g., coiled or redundant vessels). Differentiation between vessel occlusion and preocclusive critical stenosis may be difficult.[14, 15] Such a distinction is extremely important, because patients with carotid occlusion usually are not surgical candidates. Finally, duplex sonography is highly operator and interpreter dependent.

In recent years, some of the disadvantages associated with duplex sonography have been obviated by incorporating adjuvant modalities such as MRA in the evaluation of carotid stenosis. With the recent advances in MRA resolution, clinicians can now obtain the necessary anatomic data previously obtainable only by angiography, without the inherent risks of an invasive procedure.[14–16] The sensitivity of this technique has been compared with that of angiography on several occasions. For instance, Lustgarten and coworkers reported that duplex sonography used in conjunction with MRA (12-minute scan sequence) precluded the need for preoperative angiographic evaluation in 90% of patients presenting with carotid stenosis.[4] Those authors noted that the combined accuracy of the two procedures, when in concordance, was 100%, thus precluding the need for angiography in their patient population.

Angiography versus Carotid Duplex Ultrasonography

Carotid duplex ultrasonography is capable of detecting critical stenosis with nearly 100% sensitivity and specificity. By comparison, arteriography, which is the gold standard against which all noninvasive tests are compared, provides little physiologic information regarding flow and nearly no insight into the nature of the plaque (especially "low-grade" ulceration). When compared with surgical findings at endarterectomy, arteriography is also less sensitive than duplex ultrasonography in detecting anatomic stenosis (91% versus 99%).[17]

When the two modalities were compared in a blinded fashion with direct examination of the plaque, it was noted that duplex scanning not only was as sensitive as angiography in detecting greater than 50% luminal narrowing but also was associated with an overall 96% sensitivity and 100% specificity, compared with 92% sensitivity and 100% specificity for angiography.[17] In addition, duplex scanning was significantly more accurate in the detection of smaller plaque ulcerations and significantly more accurate in predicting vessel wall irregularities than was angiography. Finally, unlike angiography, duplex sonography (via its B-mode imaging) was able to denote plaque morphology as well as the presence of intraplaque hemorrhages.

Although some surgeons have discussed the use of duplex scanning in conjunction with conventional angiography for the preoperative evaluation of patients with carotid stenosis, angiography involves some risk in this patient population, as documented by several studies.[18] Although studies have demonstrated that contrast angiography carries a mortality rate of 0.5% and a major permanent neurological complication rate of 2% to 4%, these studies did not select for patients being evaluated for carotid stenosis.[18] Earnest and colleagues noted that in a prospective study of 1517 consecutive angiograms, 4.2% of patients undergoing angiography for the evaluation of cerebrovascular disease had a neurological complication.[19] Mortality was noted to be 0.06% in this group, with a fixed neurological deficit incidence of 0.6%. Thus, when evaluating the overall morbidity and mortality of carotid endarterectomy, in addition to the risk of major complication or death secondary to the surgery, one must consider the potential complications of angiography if the patient undergoes that procedure for the preoperative evaluation of carotid stenosis. Despite the risks, surgeons have stressed the need for angiography in cases of carotid stenosis because, unlike duplex ultrasonography, angiography can provide data concerning anatomic variations of the carotid system, as well as help document evidence of intracranial occlusive disease.[20] The advent of MRA and its use with duplex ultrasonognraphy has dramatically reduced the need for angiography to obtain such detailed anatomic information.

INTRAOPERATIVE ULTRASONOGRAPHY

The many advances in imaging and neuronavigation are a direct result of the need for precise localization and identification of lesions in the central nervous system. Image-guided frameless stereotactic devices that allow a coregistration of preoperative imaging with fixed topographic or artificial fiducial markers on the scalp fill today's neurosurgical operating rooms. Despite its precision, such technology has clearly been unable to compensate for the intraoperative displacement of the contents within the cranial vault, which may be secondary to the effects of gravity, loss of cerebrospinal fluid, or retraction. In certain situations, such displacement makes the lesion more difficult to find. Intraoperative ultrasonography provides the real-time imaging necessary for the precise localization of a lesion irrespective of the effects of gravity, retraction, or loss of cerebrospinal fluid. The craniotomy or laminectomy used for the surgery provides the acoustic window necessary to insonate the central nervous system tissue. Its portability, low cost, safety, and real-time evaluation make this technology an important adjunct in the treatment of neurosurgical disease. It has been shown to be useful in the management of intracranial and spinal tumors, abscesses, vascular malformations, and hematomas.

The size of the craniotomy or laminectomy determines the size of the transducer used. Subcortical lesions can be insonated at a frequency of 7 to 10 MHz, which provides a high-resolution image. Deeper lesions require a lower frequency transducer (perhaps 3 MHz), because attenuation is less for lower frequency sound. Once the craniotomy or laminectomy is complete, the transducer is placed in a sterile drape with sufficient coupling gel. Saline is used as a coupling medium at the surgical site. The tissue is scanned in the coronal and sagittal planes to delineate the lesion. The trajectory to the target is then determined by defining the shortest distance to the lesion.

For spinal lesions, intraoperative ultrasonography is helpful in determining the appropriate degree of exposure and in localizing the tumor. It can also evaluate the surgical bed for complete resection.[21, 22]

Several investigators have described the benefits of using intraoperative ultrasonography.[23, 24] In a study of 186 patients, Rubin and Dohrmann found intraoperative ultrasonography to be more useful for small, subcortical lesions.[25] The literature abounds with novel uses of intraoperative ultrasonography, which range from the more traditional localization of subcortical lesions to the localization of contusions in trauma[26] and the monitoring of ventricular catheter placement.[27] Although these anecdotal reports are helpful, formal studies to determine the efficacy of this technology as a possible standard of care have yet to be published.

The use of intraoperative micro-Doppler sonography has become invaluable to vascular neurosurgeons. With current technology, vessels less than 1 mm in diameter can be discretely insonated to assess for patency.[28] Though crude when compared with transcranial Doppler or duplex sonography, micro-Doppler can determine vessel patency, direction of flow, and presence of laminar versus turbulent flow. With this technology, anastomosis sites can be easily evaluated in bypass surgery, and the patency of parent vessels and their branches can be assessed during aneurysm clipping.

CONCLUSION

The use of ultrasonography in neurosurgery has undergone a significant resurgence. Concerns that this technology would become obsolete in this age of frameless magnetic resonance imaging and computed tomographic neuronavigation were once dominant, but new advances have significantly changed the role and future of neurosonology. Techniques such as endovascular ultrasonography provide innovative ways of evaluating vascular patency and anatomy. The potential for using ultrasonography as a therapeutic tool is still largely unexplored. Through its continued use and modification, this technology will remain a major tool in the armamentarium of the neuroscience community for the diagnosis and treatment of neurological disease.

REFERENCES

1. Doppler C: Uber das farbige lich der doppelsterne und eineger gestirne des himmels. Ges Wiss Prag 465–482, 1842.
2. Hockanson DE, Mozersky DJ, Summer DS, et al: Ultrasonic arteriography: A new approach to arterial visualization. Radiology 102:435–436, 1972.
3. Blackshear WM, Phillips DJ, Thiele BL, et al: Detection of carotid occlusive disease by ultrasonic imaging and pulsed Doppler spectrum analysis. Surgery 86:698–706, 1979.
4. Lustgarten JH, Solomon RA, Quest DO, et al: Carotid endarterectomy after noninvasive evaluation by duplex ultrasonography and magnetic resonance angiography. Neurosurgery 34:612–619, 1994.
5. Roederer GO, Langlois YE, Chan AT, et al: Ultrasound duplex scanning of the extracranial carotid arteries: Improved accuracy using new features from the common carotid artery. J Cardiovasc Ultrasonogr 1:373–380, 1982.
6. Zwiebel WJ: Doppler evaluation of carotid stenosis. In Zwiebel WJ (ed): Introduction Vascular Ultrasonography, 4th ed. Philadelphia, WB Saunders, 2000, pp 137–154.
7. Dawson DL, Zierler RE, Strandness DE, et al: The role of duplex scanning and arteriography before carotid endarterectomy: A propective study. J Vasc Surg 18:673–680, 1993.
8. Brice JG, Dowsett DJ, Lowe RD: Hemodynamic effects of carotid artery stenosis. BMJ 2:1363–1366, 1964.
9. Bartynski WS, Darbouze P, Nemir P: Significance of ulcerated plaque in transient cerebral ischemia. Am J Surg 141:353–357, 1981.
10. Executive Committee for the Asymptomatic Atherosclerosis Study: Endarterectomy for asymptomatic carotid artery stenosis. JAMA 273:1421–1429, 1993.
11. Imparato AM, Riles TS, Mintzer R, et al: The importance of hemorrhage in the relationship between gross morphologic characteristics and cerebral symptoms in 376 carotid artery plaques. Ann Surg 197:195–203, 1983.
12. Persson AV, Robichaux WT, Silverman M: The natural history of significant events in carotid plaque development. Arch Surg 118: 1048–1052, 1983.
13. Pan XM, Saloner D, Reilly LM, et al: Assessment of carotid artery stenosis by ultrasonography, conventional angiography, and magnetic resonance angiography: Correlation with ex vivo measurement of plaque stenosis. J Vasc Surg 21:82–88, 1995.
14. Litt AW, Eidelman EM, Pinto RS: Diagnosis of carotid stenosis: Comparison of 2DTF MR angiography with contrast angiography in 50 patients. AJNR Am J Neuroradiol 12:149–154, 1991.
15. Mattle HP, Kent C, Edelmann RR, et al: Evaluation of extracranial carotid arteries: Correlation of magnetic resonance angiography, duplex ultrasonography and conventional angiography. J Vasc Surg 13:838–845, 1991.
16. Huston J III, Lewis BD, Wiebers DO: Carotid artery: Prospective blinded comparison of two-dimensional time-of-light MR angiography with conventional angiography and duplex ultrasound. Radiology 186:339–344, 1993.
17. Rubin JR, Bondi JA, Rhodes RS: Duplex scanning versus conventional arteriography for the evaluation of carotid artery plaque morphology. Surgery 102:749–755, 1987.
18. Davies KN, Humphrey PR: Complications of cerebral angiography in patients with symptomatic carotid territory ischemia screened by carotid ultrasound. J Neurol Neurosurg Psychiatry 56:967–972, 1993.
19. Earnest F, Forbes G, Sandok B, et al: Complications of cerebral angiography: Prospective assessment of risk. AJR Am J Roentgenol 142:247–249, 1984.
20. Levien LJ, Voll CL, Lithgow-Jolly P, et al: The value of noninvasive investigation in the diagnosis of total occlusion of the internal carotid artery. Stroke 16:945–948, 1985.
21. Montalvo BM, Quencer RM: Intraoperative sonography in spinal surgery. Neuroradiology 28:551–590, 1986.
22. Rubin JM, Dohrmann GJ: The spine and spinal cord during neurosurgical operations: Real-time ultrasonography. Radiology 151:461–465, 1985.
23. Dohrmann GJ, Rubin JM: Use of ultrasound in neurosurgical operations: A preliminary report. Surg Neurol 16:362–366, 1981.
24. Dohrmann GJ, Rubin JM: Dynamic intraoperative imaging and instrumentation of brain and spinal cord using ultrasound. Neurol Clin 3:425–437, 1985.
25. Rubin JM, Dohrmann GJ: Efficacy of intraoperative ultrasound for evaluating intracranial masses. Radiology 157:509–511, 1985.
26. Andrews BT, Bederson JB, Pitts LH: The use of intraoperative ultrasonography to improve the diagnostic accuracy of exploratory burr holes in patients with traumatic tentorial herniation. Neurosurgery 24:345–347, 1989.
27. Rubin JM, Dohrmann GJ: Use of ultrasonically guided probes and catheters in neurosurgery. Surg Neurol 18:143–148, 1982.
28. Cathignol D, Chapelon JY, Jossinet J, et al: Detailed description of an implantable directional Doppler flowmeter. Biotelemetry 3: 117–128, 1976.

CHAPTER 93

Xenon Computed Tomography

HOWARD YONAS

The measurement of cerebral blood flow (CBF) began with the examination of tracers that had the capacity to move into the substance of the brain and thereby serve as a marker of CBF. The ability to measure the time course and extent of delivery of the tracer to the brain, as well as the time course and extent of return from the brain, allows the Fick principle to be applied and CBF calculated through solution of the Kety-Schmidt equation. Using xenon 133 as a CBF tracer, the fundamentals of CBF physiology were defined over the past 4 decades.

The measurement of CBF with the combination of computed tomography (CT) and stable xenon inhalation began with Winkler and Spira's observation that stable xenon gas is radiodense.[1] Xenon, although a noble (inert) gas, is next to iodine on the chart of molecular weights and therefore can be imaged in the same manner. Historically, xenon had been used as an anesthetic agent at a concentration of 80%, so it was known to be biologically safe and inert, although pharmacologically active. To measure CBF, the question became one of finding a dose level that was adequate for imaging but low enough to minimize the physiologic side effects. Another variable was the inhalation period, which needed to be limited to minimize side effects while providing enough data to characterize the movement of xenon within all tissue compartments. The hallmark paper by Gur and colleagues[2] in 1982 demonstrated that blood flow measurements could be achieved with stable xenon-enhanced CT CBF (xenon-CT CBF) for each of the 24,000 CT voxels per CT image, thereby providing a high-resolution map of CBF.

METHODOLOGY AND ASSUMPTIONS

The methodology and assumptions for xenon-CT CBF, as developed at the University of Pittsburgh in the early 1980s, have remained the same, despite the dramatic evolution of technologies on which this technique is based. Some of the assumptions were that (1) CBF measurement should be based on only arterial and tissue "wash-in" data, thereby minimizing the effects of flow activation due to xenon; (2) a single compartmental analysis of CBF should be made for each voxel, and that this unit of volume was small enough to adequately characterize either pure gray or white matter; (3) the partition coefficient should be solved for and integrated within the CBF calculation, providing greater accuracy in normal as well as diseased tissues; and (4) blood vessels should be deleted from the initial database so that only the movement of the tracer within brain substance would be displayed. All these assumptions have proved to be valid, providing a reliable, quantitative CBF map with high resolution as a result of a relatively brief (4.3 minutes) inhalation of a subanesthetic (33%) concentration of xenon.

CALCULATION OF CEREBRAL BLOOD FLOW

Like other methods that indirectly measure CBF, the stable xenon technique uses Kety's application of the Fick principle of indicator dilution, which relates the concentration of a freely diffusible, nonmetabolized indicator absorbed in the tissue per unit time as the difference between the arterial and venous concentrations of the indicator.[3] In the case of stable xenon gas, the gas's radiodensity allows its concentration in the brain to be determined directly by the CT scanner so that measurement of the venous concentration is unnecessary. Conceptually, the brain xenon concentration is related to the arterial concentration of xenon (which is itself time dependent), the brain blood flow, and the duration of exposure to xenon (because the equilibrium of xenon between brain and blood is not instantaneous). These factors determine the total amount of xenon presented to the brain. Uptake is also determined by the affinity of the brain for xenon, which is measured by the brain-blood partition coefficient, lambda (λ). This reflects the relative solubility of xenon gas in the brain and blood or, more simply, the xenon concentration in the brain and blood at equilibrium. These factors are related mathematically by the Kety-Schmidt equation modified for the xenon CT technique:

$$Cxe_{Br}(t) = \lambda k \int_{o}^{t} Cxe_{Art}(u)\, e^{-k(t-u)}\, du \qquad (1)$$

and

$$F = \lambda k \tag{2}$$

where Cxe_{Br} (t) is the time-dependent brain xenon concentration, λ is the brain-blood partition coefficient, k is the brain uptake flow rate constant, $Cxe_{Art}(u)$ is the time-dependent arterial xenon concentration, and F is CBF. The temporary variable μ stands for any selected subinterval between o and t.

Time-dependent arterial xenon buildup is described by:

$$Cxe_{Art}(u) = Cxe_{max}(1 - e^{-bu}) \tag{3}$$

where Cxe_{max} is the maximum arterial xenon concentration in milligrams per milliliter, u is the time, and b is the arterial uptake rate constant.

In practice, arterial xenon uptake is not measured directly but rather by assuming instantaneous equilibrium with end-tidal pulmonary xenon concentration. This assumption is valid in the absence of severe pulmonary disease or right-to-left intrapulmonary or intracardiac shunts. Maximum arterial xenon uptake in milligrams per milliliter is related to maximum percent arterial uptake by:

$$Cxe_{max} = C(\%)_{max}\,(5.15)\,(S_{Xe})\,(0.01) \tag{4}$$

where $C(\%)_{max}$ is the maximum percentage of xenon uptake, 5.15 is the density of xenon in milligrams per milliliter at 37°C and 1 atmosphere, and S_{Xe} is the Ostwald solubility of xenon in blood, related to hematocrit (Hct) by:

$$S_{Xe} = 0.1 + 0.0011\,(\%\ Hct) \tag{5}$$

Finally, the Hounsfield enhancement (HE) resulting from xenon in the brain is related to the concentration in milligrams per milliliter by:

$$HE = Cxe_{Br}/(u_p{}^{w}/u_p{}^{Xe}) \tag{6}$$

where $u_p{}^{w}$ and $u_p{}^{Xe}$ are the mass attenuation coefficients of water and xenon, respectively.

The measurement of xenon buildup in tissue is obtained in the following manner: Two baseline scans are obtained at four or more different 10-mm-thick levels before xenon inhalation. Six enhanced scans per level are then obtained during a 4.3-minute xenon inhalation. The baseline scan pair is averaged and then subtracted from each of the enhancement images to obtain $Cxe_{Br}(t)$ for each of the 15,000 to 30,000 voxels in each image. A thermoconductivity analyzer measures end-tidal xenon concentration. This inexpensive device approaches the accuracy of a mass spectrometer.[4]

With the relationships described previously, the brain uptake data are fitted to the Kety-Schmidt equation (equation 1) by using an iterative least-squares approach. The two unknown parameters, flow (F) and lambda (λ), are simultaneously derived from the resulting curves for each voxel at each level. Noise between voxels is minimized by pre- and postcalculation smoothing routines. Because head motion between images degrades the calculation, as many as two images can be deleted from the calculation without significantly altering the numeric results. If only three images (2.5 minutes of inhalation) are used, the stability of the flow calculation is diminished, and studies should be interpreted as qualitative rather than quantitative.

The image that results is a map of CBF values with a full width at half maximum resolution of about 4 mm. Depiction of the CBF map uses a color scale of 0 to 140 mL/100 g per minute. Flow values of 6 to 8 mL/100 g per minute have been displayed as violet in order to highlight this important threshold for irreversible ischemia. Numeric values of flow can be extracted by placing regions of interest (ROIs) of any shape or size on the CBF map to obtain mean and standard deviations of flow. When large cortical regions are measured, both gray and white matter are usually included in the ROI, and the flow measurement and standard deviation will reflect the averaging of these two compartments. The display also includes a "confidence image," which assesses the quality of the data. This image integrates a measurement of the degree of misregistration of images due to movement, the number of images used in the calculation, and the concentration of xenon. As a result, the presentation allows the reader to determine whether numeric information in one part or all of the flow image should be disregarded or interpreted as being qualitative rather than quantitative (Fig. 93–1; see color section in this volume).

A flow "phantom" has been created so that differences between scanners and x-ray tube instability over time can be compensated. A sequence of iodine-impregnated cylinders with prescribed densities (one baseline and six enhanced) is scanned, and flow is calculated by using a prescribed air curve designed to calculate 20, 40, and 80 mL/100 g per minute. Differences between the numbers calculated with any scanner and the phantom are then used to correct values with the introduction of a flow constant. Thus, the same flow values should be calculated by the current system with little or no dependence on operator judgment or individual scanner performance.

Owing to the inherent noise of the system, caution must be used in relying on numeric values from too small an ROI. Measurement accuracy rapidly improves as the number of included pixels increases, and it reaches an acceptable error of about 12% when the ROI is 1 cm^2 or larger, even in very low flow states. Thus, a value of 1.0 ± 1.0 mL/100 g per minute for the entire brain can be equated with flow at or very near zero with no statistically reasonable likelihood that there are flows compatible with tissue validity.

IMPACT OF COMPUTED TOMOGRAPHY, NETWORKING, AND COMPUTER TECHNOLOGIES

The dramatic advances that have occurred in the 1990s in the technologies on which xenon-CT CBF is directly dependent have had a favorable impact. A "best curve fit" approximation of the air curve was initially used,

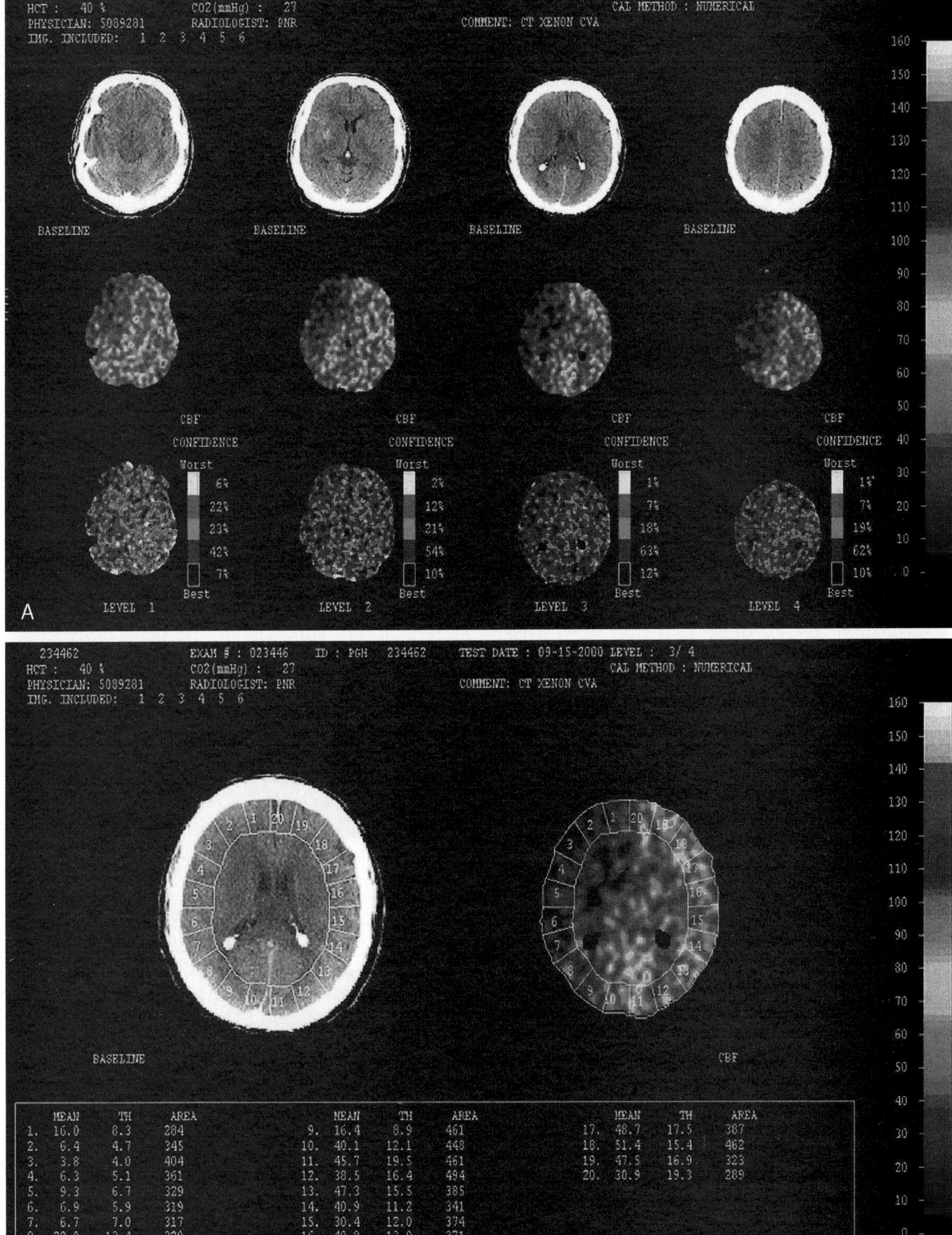

FIGURE 93–1. *A*, Computed tomography (CT), cerebral blood flow (CBF), and confidence image for a four-level study. Each level is 10 mm thick and 5 mm apart. The color scale is fixed with direct reference to CBF measured in milliliters/100 g per minute. The uniform dark confidence image indicates a highly reliable quantitative study in a patient with right hemispheric ischemia due to middle cerebral artery occlusion. *B*, A standard cortical region of interest (ROI) placement shows both the CT image and the CBF image. The mean CBF for each ROI is displayed in the box below. The TH column indicates the standard deviation of the pixels within the ROI. The area column is the number of pixels within a ROI, each 1 × 1 × 10 mm³ (see color section in this volume).

owing to the need for a short calculation time despite primitive computers. As computer speed increased, it became possible to use an analytic approach to the data, thereby using all data points, which has made the calculation more stable and reliable. The combination of modern scanners with very low noise levels, networking that allows rapid CT image movement, and faster computers has had a synergistic, positive effect. These factors have made it possible to perform studies at lower xenon concentrations (<28%) and at more levels of the brain and have resulted in user-friendly data presentation in a time frame (about 3 minutes) consistent with integration into prospective clinical decision making.

VALIDATION OF QUANTITATIVE NATURE OF MEASUREMENTS

Xenon-CT CBF has proved capable of reliable, quantitative CBF information both in the laboratory and clinically. Cross-correlation studies with microspheres,[5–7] iodoantipyrine,[8] and xenon 133[9] showed high degrees of correlation. Normative flow values obtained in a population of normal adults aged 20 to 80 years demonstrated the gentle decline of mixed cortical flow values from the high 50s to the mid-40s mL/100 g per minute, identical to that demonstrated with other quantitative technologies.[10] Although pure gray matter flow values fell dramatically over the decades, white matter flow values were very stable at 20 ± 2 mL/100 g per minute. Additional validation of the physiologic significance of xenon-CT CBF was obtained in a retrospective study of 160 patients undergoing balloon test occlusion.[11] From laboratory studies, we have learned that the onset of neurological deficits occurs when flow falls to less than 20 mL/100 g per minute. In this clinical study, patients who did not develop deficits despite internal carotid artery balloon test occlusion had middle cerebral artery flow values that did not fall below 20 mL/100 g per minute, even though 20% of patients had flow values that fell to between 20 and 30 mL/100 g per minute.

The accuracy of xenon-CT CBF measurements despite flow activation due to xenon inhalation has been explained by a series of simulation studies.[12–14] Because flow activation does not become significant until after 2.5 minutes of xenon inhalation and continues to rise well past 4 minutes, the three images obtained before 2.5 minutes characterize fast flow before flow activation occurs, thereby minimizing the impact of flow activation to less than 5%. Although some advocates of xenon-CT CBF have used an integrated "wash-in" and "wash-out" phase to improve the signal-to-noise ratio, integration of the "activated" wash-out flow values introduces a more significant error of measurement.[15]

The experimental studies include stroke modeling involving the lateral striate vessels as well as larger lateral cortical infarctions in subhuman primates. Following lateral striate occlusion, flow values less than 5 mL/100 g per minute were recorded within the caudate nucleus and remained stable for 6 hours. The same level of flow elevated to more than 120 mL/100 g per minute after 1 hour of occlusion followed by reperfusion. In both studies, all cells were defined as infarcted on electron microscopy.[16, 17] Twenty minutes of occlusion resulted in only a brief period of elevated flow values and a rapid return to normal, with only occasional nuclear changes on electron microscopy. Lateral cortical stroke models confirmed that persistent flow near 0 (<6) mL/100 g per minute was consistent with the acute (2 to 3 hours) development of visually apparent CT density changes (Nemoto, unpublished data).

In clinical studies, the fall of flow to below 20 mL/100 g per minute within the cortical mantle of the middle cerebral artery territory (about 50-50 gray and white matter) was correlated with the onset of neurological deficit and the increased likelihood of irreversible ischemic injury. Patients with hemispheric deficits due to embolic middle cerebral artery occlusion had a mean flow level of 15 mL/100 g per minute,[18] as did patients who developed delayed neurological hemispheric deficits following subarachnoid hemorrhage.[19] The timely return of flow values above the threshold of 20 mL/100 g per minute has been associated with a reversal of neurological deficits and the avoidance of infarction on follow-up CT.[20, 21] Conversely, following subarachnoid hemorrhage, the persistence of flow levels at or below 15 mL/100 g per minute was consistently followed by CT-defined infarction.[22] The volume of tissue with cortical middle cerebral artery flow values below 10 mL/100 g per minute following ischemic stroke was predictive of the volume of infarction on follow-up CT,[23] an increased risk of hemorrhagic complications,[19, 24] and the development of clinical herniation irrespective of intervention.[25] Near-zero flow values throughout the supra- and infratentorial compartments (except the lower pons and medulla, which are poorly imaged owing to CT artifact) have been used for brain-death criteria.[26, 27] Because flow values within the contralateral hemisphere as well as the cerebellum also fall with unilateral hemispheric stroke to a mean of about 34 mL/100 g per minute with a considerable and unpredictable variance,[20, 28, 29] the use of qualitative data to derive the preceding measurements is problematic.

Flow studies performed before and after a physiologic challenge have provided another validation of the stability of the data and the importance of quantitative measurements. The ability to isolate one variable—such as the flow response to a change of blood pressure—provides valuable information about the integrity of autoregulation. Following subarachnoid hemorrhage, the observation that both flow elevation and depression can be observed with blood pressure elevation provides an important insight into the potential benefit and harm that can come from the indiscriminate application of hypertensive "therapy."[30] Likewise, lowering of P_{CO_2} can reduce flow values to ischemic levels and be potentially harmful following head trauma, but it can also reduce hyperemic flow levels to normal and thereby improve the control of

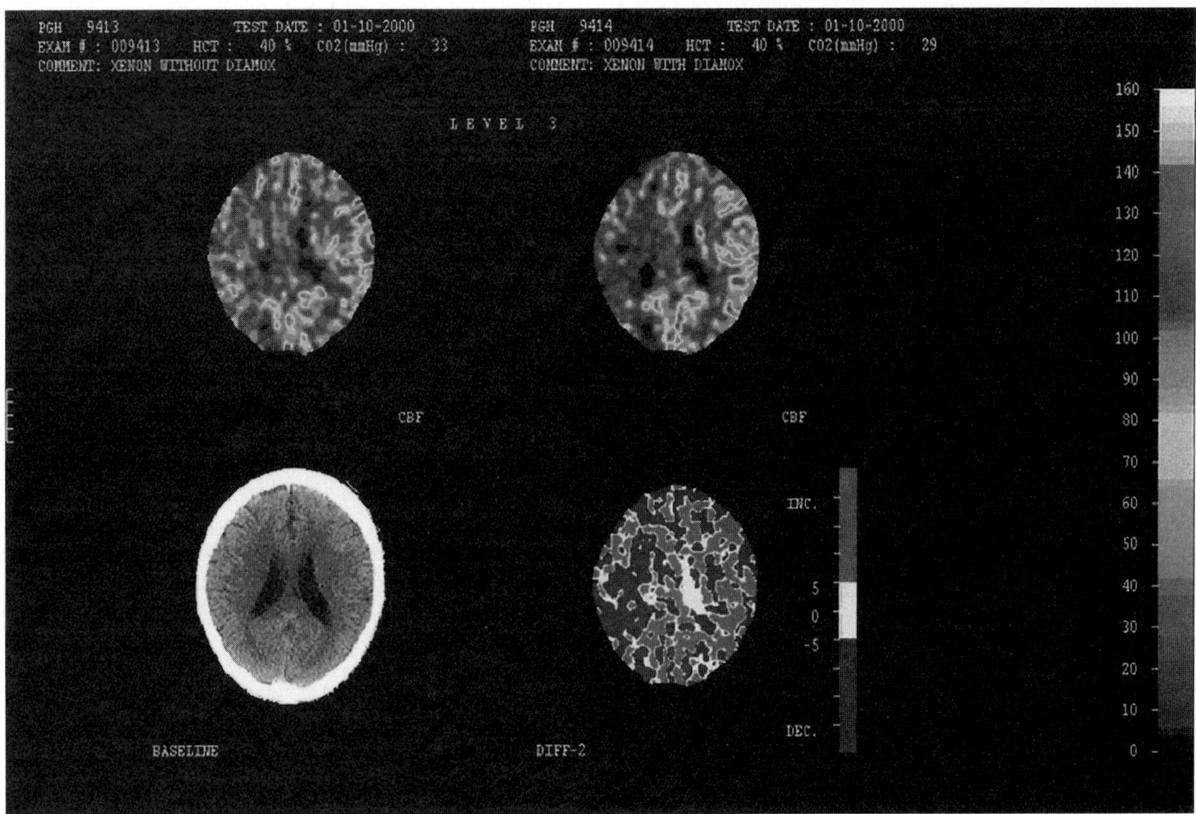

FIGURE 93–2. Acetazolamide (Diamox) challenge study with the baseline cerebral blood flow (CBF) image on the left and the corresponding image 20 minutes after acetazolamide administration. The computed tomographic image and the difference image are displayed below. This vasodilatory challenge normally increases CBF globally, and the difference image should be mostly red, indicating an increase in CBF of at least 5 mL/100 g per minute. The blue in the right hemisphere indicates a decrease in CBF by greater than 5 mL/100 g per minute ("steal phenomenon") in this patient with internal carotid artery occlusion, indicating increased stroke risk (see color section in this volume).

intracranial pressure.[31] The elevation of local tissue acidosis either by carbon dioxide retention or by the introduction of intravenous acetazolamide has provided an assessment of the cerebrovascular reserve, that is, the ability of the vasculature to increase CBF in response to a vasodilatory challenge (Fig. 93–2; see color section in this volume). This "challenge" study provides an indirect measure of the dependence of regional blood flow on secondary pial collaterals. The fall in CBF following acetazolamide ("steal" phenomenon) has been correlated with a dependence on pial collaterals[32] and has defined a group of patients at increased hemodynamic risk for stroke following spontaneous carotid occlusion.[33, 34] In this group of patients, the decrease of flow is most dramatic within the deep periventricular white matter, which is where infarction due to "low-flow" states tends to occur in association with symptoms of ischemic claudication.[35] Qualitative studies of CBF with the same physiologic challenge do not seem to have the ability to identify the same high-risk subgroups.[36, 37]

Xenon-CT CBF quantitative measurements have a broad range of clinical and experimental applications. As noted by Gur and coworkers[38] in 1989, this technology will only improve as the technologies on which it is based continue to evolve. The next evolutionary steps for xenon-CT CBF will involve the further lowering of xenon concentrations with maintenance of the signal-to-noise ratio, a movement correction for motion in any direction, and the ability to image nearly all of the brain.

REFERENCES

1. Winkler SS, Spira J: Radiopacity of xenon under hyperbaric conditions. AJR Am J Roentgenol 96:1035–1040, 1966.
2. Gur D, Good WF, Wolfson SK, et al: In vivo mapping of local cerebral blood flow by xenon-enhanced computed tomography. Science 215:1267–1268, 1982.
3. Kety SS: The theory and applications of the exchange of inert gas at the lungs and tissues. Pharmacol Rev 3:1–41, 1951.
4. Gur D, Herron JM, Molter BS, et al: Simultaneous mass spectrometry and thermoconductivity measurements of end-tidal xenon concentrations: A comparison. Med Phys 11:208–212, 1984.
5. Gur D, Yonas H, Jackson DL, et al: Measurements of cerebral blood flow during xenon inhalation as measured by the microspheres method. Stroke 16:871–874, 1985.
6. Fatouros PP, Wist AO, Kishore PR, et al: Xenon/computed tomography cerebral blood flow measurements: Methods and accuracy. Invest Radiol 22:705–712, 1987.
7. DeWitt DS, Fatouros PP, Wist AO, et al: Stable xenon versus radiolabeled microsphere cerebral blood flow measurements in baboons. Stroke 20:1716–1723, 1989.
8. Wolfson SK, Clark J, Greenberg JH, et al: Xenon-enhanced computed tomography compared with [^{14}C] iodoantipyrine for nor-

mal and low cerebral blood flow states in baboons. Stroke 21: 751–757, 1990.

9. Yonas H, Obrist W, Gur D, Good WF: Cross-correlation of CBF derived by ^{133}Xe and Xe/CT in normal volunteers. J Cereb Blood Flow Metab 9:S409, 1989.
10. Yonas H, Darby JM, Marks EC, et al: CBF measured by Xe-CT: Approach to analysis and normal values. J Cereb Blood Flow Metab 11:716–725, 1991.
11. Witt JP, Yonas H, Jungreis C: Cerebral blood flow response pattern during balloon test occlusion of the internal carotid artery. AJNR Am J Neuroradiol 15:847–857, 1994.
12. Marks EC, Yonas H, Sanders MH, et al: Physiologic implications of adding small amounts of carbon dioxide to the gas mixture during inhalation of xenon. Neuroradiology 34:297–300, 1992.
13. Witt JP, Holl K, Heissler HE, Dietz H: Stable xenon CT CBF: Effects of blood flow alterations on CBF calculations during inhalation of 33% stable xenon. AJNR Am J Neuroradiol 12: 973–975, 1991.
14. Obrist WD, Zhang Z, Yonas H: Effect of xenon-induced flow activation on xenon-enhanced computed tomography cerebral blood flow calculations. J Cereb Blood Flow Metab 18:1192–1195, 1998.
15. Good WF, Gur D: The effect of computed tomography noise and tissue heterogeneity on cerebral blood flow determination by xenon enhanced computed tomography. Med Phys 14:557–561, 1987.
16. Yonas H, Gur D, Claassen D, et al: Stable xenon enhanced computed tomography in the study of clinical and pathologic correlates of focal ischemia in baboons. Stroke 19:228–238, 1988.
17. Yonas H, Gur D, Claassen D, et al: Stable xenon-enhanced CT measurement of cerebral blood flow in reversible focal ischemia in baboons. J Neurosurg 73:266–273, 1990.
18. Firlik AD, Kaufmann AM, Wechsler LR, et al: Quantitative cerebral blood flow determinations in acute ischemic stroke. Stroke 28:2208–2213, 1997.
19. Goldstein S, Yonas H, Gebel JM, et al: Acute cerebral blood flow as a predictive physiologic marker for symptomatic hemorrhagic conversion and clinical herniation after thrombolytic therapy. Stroke 31:275, 2000.
20. Firlik AD, Rubin G, Yonas H, Wechsler LR: Relation between cerebral blood flow and neurologic deficit resolution in acute ischemic stroke. Neurology 51:177–182, 1998.
21. Firlik AD, Kaufmann AM, Jungreis CA, Yonas H: Effect of transluminal angioplasty on cerebral blood flow in the management of symptomatic vasospasm following aneurysmal subarachnoid hemorrhage. J Neurosurg 86:830–839, 1997.
22. Fukui MB, Johnson DW, Yonas H, et al: Xe/CT cerebral blood flow evaluation of delayed symptomatic ischemia after subarachnoid hemorrhage. AJNR Am J Neuroradiol 13:265–270, 1992.
23. Kaufmann AM, Firlik AD, Fukui MB, et al: Ischemic core and penumbra in human stroke. Stroke 30:93–99, 1999.
24. Rubin G, Firlik AD, Levy EI, et al: Xenon-enhanced computed tomography cerebral blood flow measurements in acute cerebral ischemia: Review of 56 cases. J Stroke Cerebrovasc Dis 8:404–411, 1999.
25. Firlik AD, Yonas H, Kaufmann AM, et al: Relationship between cerebral blood flow and the development of swelling and life-threatening herniation in acute ischemic stroke. J Neurosurg 89: 243–249, 1998.
26. Pistoia F, Johnson DW, Darby JM, et al: The role of xenon CT measurements of cerebral blood flow in the clinical determination of brain death. AJNR Am J Neuroradiol 12:97–103, 1991.
27. Ashwal S, Schneider S, Thompson J: Xenon computed tomography measuring cerebral blood flow in the determination of brain death in children. Ann Neurol 25:539–546, 1989.
28. Rubin G, Levy EI, Scarrow AM, et al: Remote effect of acute ischemic stroke: A xenon CT cerebral blood flow study. Cerebrovasc Dis 10:221–228, 2000.
29. Rubin G, Firlik AD, Levy EI, et al: Relationship between cerebral blood flow and clinical outcome in acute stroke. Cerebrovasc Dis 10:298–306, 2000.
30. Darby JM, Yonas H, Marks EC, et al: Acute cerebral blood flow response to dopamine-induced hypertension after subarachnoid hemorrhage. J Neurosurg 80:857–864, 1994.
31. Marion DW, Darby J, Yonas H: Acute regional cerebral blood flow changes caused by severe head injuries. J Neurosurg 74: 407–414, 1991.
32. Smith HA, Thompson-Dobkin J, Yonas H, Flint E: Correlation of xenon-enhanced computed tomography–defined cerebral blood flow reactivity and collateral flow patterns. Stroke 25:1784–1787, 1994.
33. Yonas H, Smith HA, Durham SR, et al: Increased stroke risk predicted by compromised cerebral blood flow reactivity. J Neurosurg 79:483–489, 1993.
34. Webster MW, Makaroun MS, Steed DL, et al: Compromised cerebral blood flow reactivity is a predictor of stroke in patients with symptomatic carotid artery occlusive disease. J Vasc Surg 21:338–345, 1995.
35. Firlik AD, Firlik KS, Yonas H: Physiological diagnosis and surgical treatment of recurrent limb shaking: Case report. Neurosurgery 39:607–611, 1996.
36. Yonas H, Pindzola RR, Meltzer CC, Sasser H: Qualitative versus quantitative assessment of cerebrovascular reserves. Neurosurgery 42:1005–1012, 1998.
37. Yokota C, Hasegawa Y, Minematsu K, Yamaguchi T: Effect of acetazolamide reactivity and long-term outcome in patients with major cerebral artery occlusive disease. Stroke 29:640–644, 1998.
38. Gur D, Yonas H, Good WF: Local cerebral blood flow by xenon-enhanced CT: Current status, potential improvements, and future directions. Cerebrovasc Brain Metab Rev 1:68–86, 1989.

CHAPTER **94**

Magnetic Resonance Angiography

JOHN HUSTON, III ■ MATT A. BERNSTEIN

FLOW EFFECTS IN MAGNETIC RESONANCE IMAGING

Flow effects are an important source of image contrast in magnetic resonance (MR) imaging. Flow effects can be used to enhance MR image quality because they enable angiographic methods, such as time of flight (TOF). They can degrade image quality, however, by introducing artifacts, such as ghosting and signal loss. Various techniques, such as gradient moment nulling (also known as *flow compensation*) and spatial presaturation (SAT), have been developed as countermeasures against this type of image degradation. This chapter briefly introduces some of the concepts underlying flow effects in MR imaging. Some of the most popular acquisition methods for MR angiography are described, and clinical applications are presented.

Amplitude Effects

Flow effects in MR imaging can be divided into two categories: *amplitude effects* and *phase effects*. Amplitude effects also are known as *magnitude* or *TOF effects.* Phase effects exploit the phase-sensitive nature of the MR data, and amplitude effects do not.

FLOW-RELATED ENHANCEMENT

Flow-related enhancement is the basic mechanism behind TOF angiographic methods.[1] To obtain an MR image, a selected slice (i.e., section) of magnetization is exposed to multiple radiofrequency (rf) excitations. Two such consecutive rf excitations are separated by the repetition time (TR). Incomplete T1 recovery between these repeated rf excitations reduces the signal intensity in the resulting image. This effect is called *T1 saturation*, or simply *saturation*.

Flow-related enhancement (FRE) is the mechanism by which spins flowing into the slice overcome the signal attenuation of T1 saturation. FRE also is known as the *wash-in* or *in-flow effect* and is illustrated in Figure 94–1. The signal intensity of stationary tissue within the slice is attenuated as a result of T1-saturation, but "fresh" unsaturated blood flows into the slice. The in-flowing blood has experienced fewer rf excitations and is less saturated so it appears brighter in the image.

In general, T1 saturation increases as the TR is reduced. T1 saturation is greater for tissues with higher values of T1. Additionally, T1 saturation increases as the flip angle of the rf excitation pulse increases. TOF angiography uses gradient-recalled echoes, and these acquisitions allow the operator to select the rf flip angle of the excitation pulse (typically 15 to 60 degrees).

A factor that affects the degree of FRE is the angle that the vessel makes with the imaging slice. Maximal FRE occurs when the vessel is perpendicular to the slice plane. FRE is not effective for in-plane flow, which explains signal loss in portions of the vertebral arteries in some axial two-dimensional (2D) TOF acquisitions (Fig. 94–2).

For gradient-recalled echoes, flow-related enhancement also increases with faster perpendicular flow velocity, until that component of velocity is approximately

$$v_{max} = \frac{\Delta z}{TR} \qquad (1)$$

where Δz is the slice thickness. Equation 1 can be interpreted as follows: When the perpendicular component of velocity exceeds v_{max}, the replacement blood entering the slice has experienced no rf excitations and is completely fresh or unsaturated. Further increases in velocity cannot increase the signal intensity. As an example of Equation 1, if TR = 50 msec, and Δz = 5 mm, then v_{max} = 10 cm/second. If the perpendicular component of velocity greatly exceeds v_{max}, and there is a nonuniform flow pattern (e.g., a laminar profile), the signal intensity may begin to decrease because of other mechanisms, such as intravoxel dephasing (described later).

For slow flow ($v < v_{max}$), FRE can be modeled mathematically as an effective T1 shortening of the blood. This model works because FRE and T1 shortening both increase signal intensity. FRE does not shorten the T1 of blood, however, as does the use of gadolinium-based contrast agents.

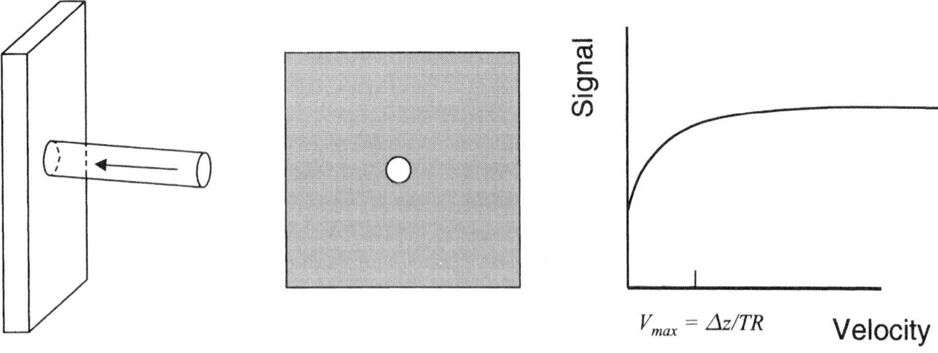

FIGURE 94–1. Flow-related enhancement. When flowing blood impinges on an imaging slice, increased signal intensity results. For gradient-recalled echo acquisitions, the signal increases until the perpendicular flow velocity approximately reaches the value V_{max}. See text.

ENTRY-SLICE EFFECT

Whenever multiple slices per pass are acquired, the exterior or *entry slice*s of each group of slices display greater FRE than the interior slices (Fig. 94–3). As the blood flows toward the interior slices, it becomes progressively more T1 saturated because of the repeated rf excitations that it experiences. The entry-slice effect becomes more pronounced the slower the flow and the higher the rf flip angle.

Sequential acquisitions, such as 2DTOF, acquire a single slice per pass—that is, all of the data for one slice are acquired before progressing to acquisition of data for the next slice. Every slice in a sequential acquisition is an entry slice. Most MR data collection strategies acquire more than a single slice per pass, however, because it is time-efficient to interleave the acquisition in this manner. There can be unequal FRE among the slices. In particular, three-dimensional (3D) acquisitions, such as 3DTOF, always acquire multiple slices per pass. With 3DTOF images, slower flowing blood often suffers signal loss beyond the entry slices. To counteract these image artifacts, techniques such as TONE (i.e., ramp) rf pulses and MOTSA have been developed. These techniques are described later.

SIGNAL LOSS WITH RADIOFREQUENCY SPIN ECHOES (BLACK BLOOD)

Spin-echo images can show FRE for slow velocities, but for moderate and rapid velocities the situation is

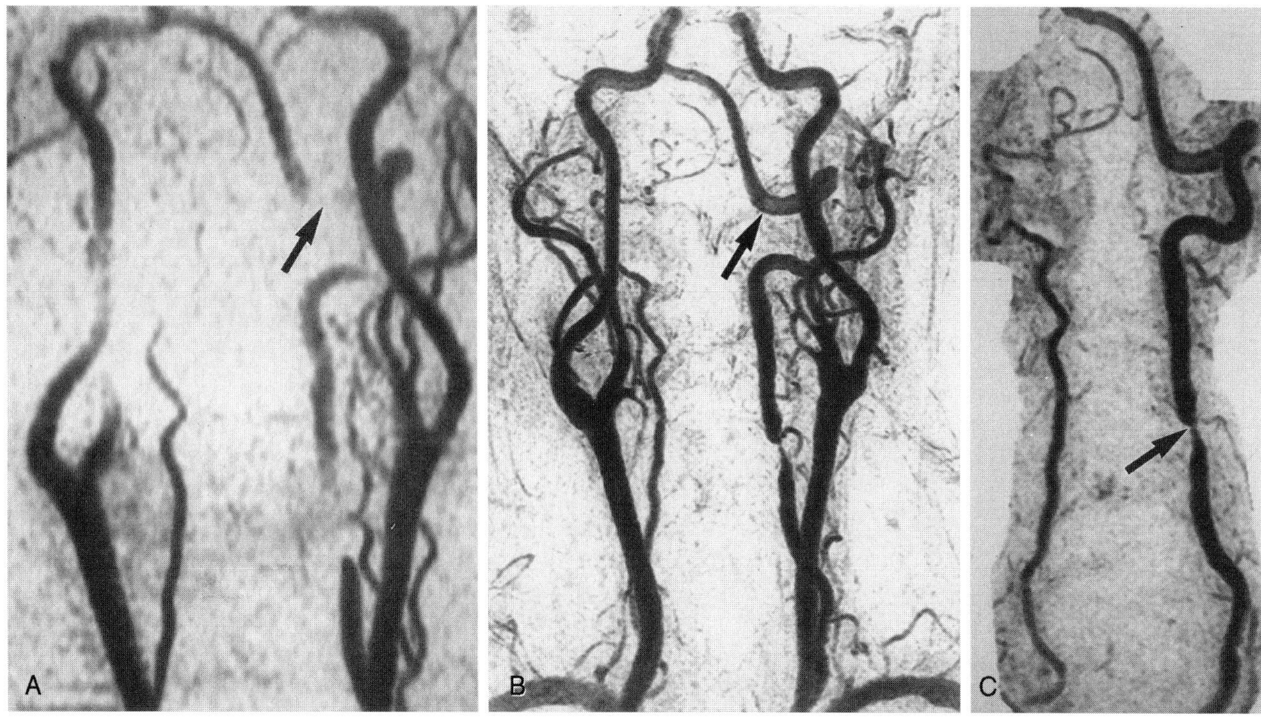

FIGURE 94–2. Patient with posterior transient ischemic attacks and normal intracranial imaging. *A*, Two-dimensional time-of-flight image signal loss in the horizontal portion of the left vertebral artery *(arrow)*. *B*, Bolus contrast-enhanced MR angiogram shows the horizontal portion of the left vertebral artery *(arrow)*. *C*, A subvolume of the bolus contrast-enhanced study including the posterior circulation shows that the small right vertebral artery ends in the posterior inferior communicating artery and that there is a high-grade stenosis in the midportion of the left vertebral artery *(arrow)*.

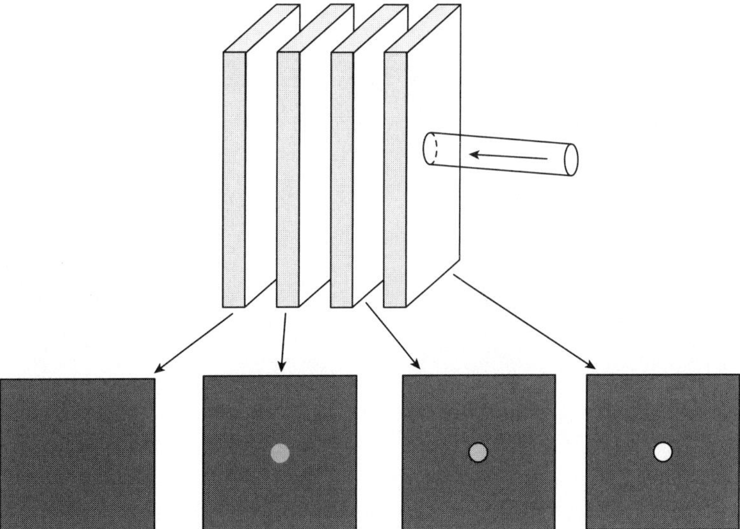

FIGURE 94–3. Entry slice effect. When multiple slices are acquired per pass, such as in the three-dimensional time-of-flight technique, the flow-related enhancement is strongest on the exterior entry slices.

different from images acquired with gradient-recalled echoes. If the flow has a perpendicular velocity on the order of, or faster than

$$v_{SE} = \frac{\Delta z}{\left(\frac{TE}{2}\right)} = \frac{2\Delta z}{TE} \qquad (2)$$

signal loss (i.e., *black blood*) results in the image. In Equation 2, TE/2 is the time between the 90-degree excitation pulse and the 180-degree refocusing pulse (i.e., one half the echo delay). The signal loss mechanism is illustrated in Figure 94–4: To produce an rf spin-echo signal, the magnetization must "see" both pulses. Rapidly moving blood can flow out of the selected slice before the 180-degree refocusing pulse is applied. The minimal velocity required to produce signal loss in spin-echo acquisitions is relatively slow, especially for T2-weighted scans, which have a longer

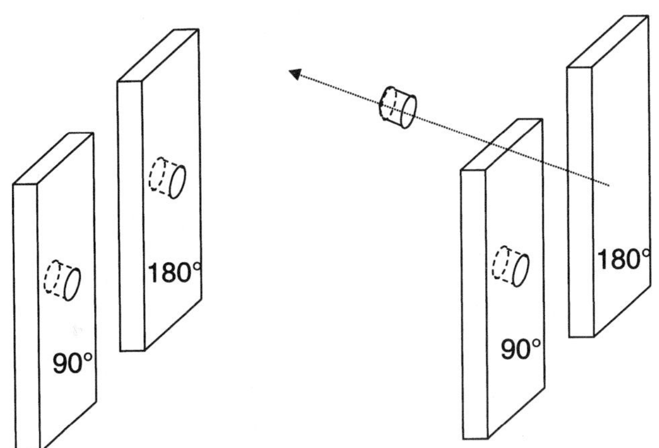

FIGURE 94–4. Signal loss in spin echo images. To produce a spin echo, the blood must *see* the 90-degree excitation and 180-degree refocusing pulse. If the blood flows out of the imaging slice before the refocusing pulse is applied, *black blood* results in the image.

echo time (TE). For example, if TE = 80 msec, and the slice thickness Δz = 4 mm, then the velocity in Equation 2, v_{SE}, is only 10 cm/second.

The signal loss in spin-echo imaging can be exploited to make *black blood* MR angiograms.[2] Normal T2-weighted spin-echo scans can serve as black blood angiograms (Fig. 94–5). Thin contiguous slices capable of being viewed from any plane with minimum intensity projections can be obtained with the 3D RARE (fast or turbo spin echo) technique.[3] A pitfall with the black blood technique is that slow or recirculating flow may not produce the desired hypointense signal. To suppress the blood signal further, black blood angiographic techniques often employ inversion recovery, SAT, or both.

SPATIAL PRESATURATION

SAT is a technique that eliminates MR signal from specified locations.[4] The SAT pulse usually consists of a spatially selective 90-degree rf pulse, followed by a gradient dephasing pulse. The gradient dephasing pulse eliminates the MR signal from the excited region. The region where the MR signal is eliminated is a thick slice, often called the *SAT band*. The thickness of the SAT band typically ranges from 10 to 80 mm.

SAT bands commonly are used to eliminate the signal from flowing blood. To eliminate venous signal from an axial slice of the carotid arteries, an axial SAT band is placed superior (i.e., cephalad) to the slice. SAT bands are employed routinely in the 2DTOF and 3DTOF multislab (MOTSA) techniques to eliminate venous signal. The distance in between the imaging slice and a parallel SAT band is called the *SAT gap*. Typically the SAT gap ranges from 5 to 30 mm.

DISPLACEMENT ARTIFACT

In MR imaging, spatial encoding for the three perpendicular axes (slice selection, phase encoding, and readout) does not occur simultaneously. In 2D pulse se-

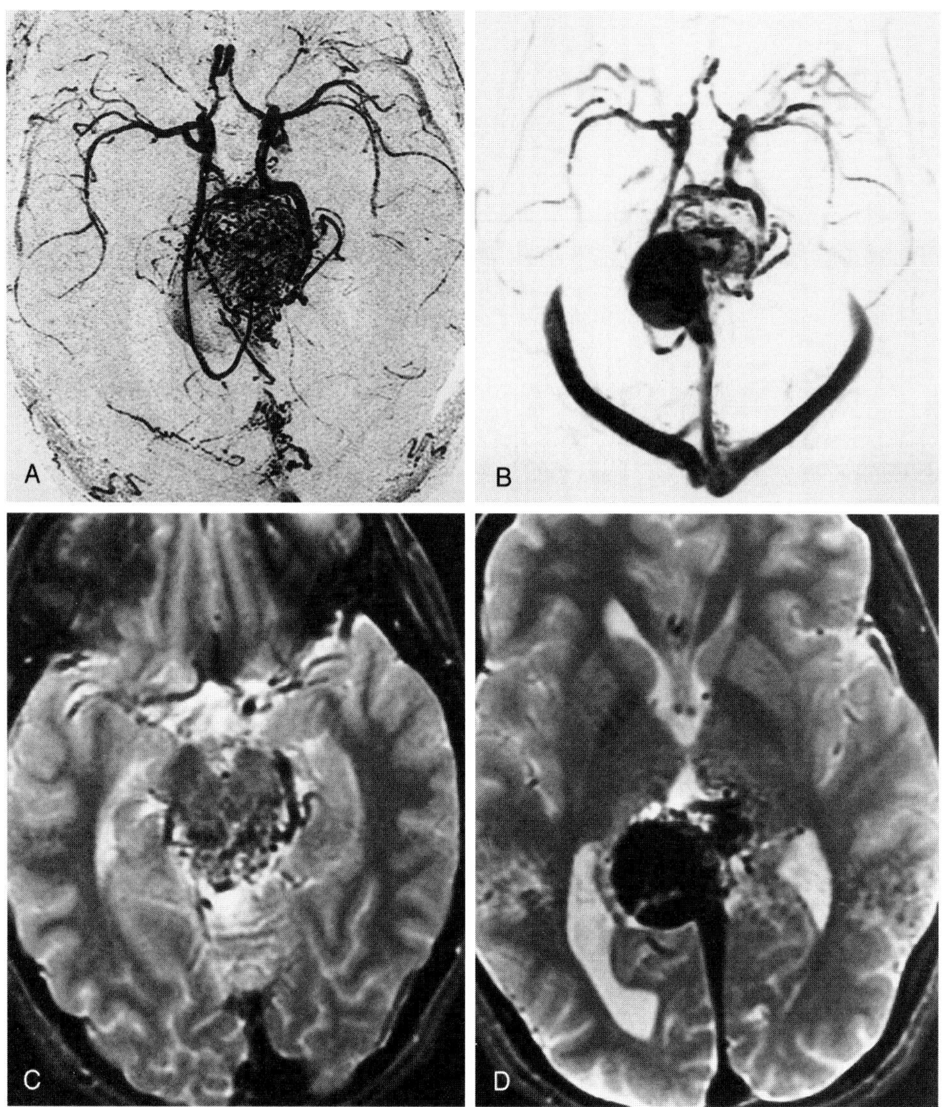

FIGURE 94–5. High-flow arteriovenous malformation (AVM) in the pineal region. *A*, Three-dimensional time of flight shows the feeding arteries and nidus of the AVM. *B*, A three-dimensional phase contrast acquisition shows better a slow flow varix associated with the AVM as well as the draining veins, including the dural sinuses. *C* and *D*, Standard T2-weighted images show the multiple signal voids within the nidus and the large area of decreased signal associated with the varix.

quences, slice selection occurs first, followed by phase encoding, and the readout is last. If there is a component of the flow velocity in more than one of these axes (i.e., oblique flow), there is misregistration between where the vessel appears in the image and its true location. This is called the *displacement artifact.*

Figure 94–6 illustrates an example of flow along an oblique readout-phase encode axis (i.e., an example of oblique flow). If the phase encoding gradient lobe is centered a time Δt before the center of the echo in the readout, the vessel displacement D is

$$D = v\,\Delta t \cos\theta \sin\theta = \frac{v\,\Delta t}{2}\sin(2\theta) \qquad (3)$$

where v is the velocity, and θ is the angle that the vessel makes with the readout (or phase encode) axis. The displacement artifact is maximal at $\theta = 45$ degrees, and it vanishes at $\theta = 0$ degrees and $\theta = 90$ degrees. There is no displacement artifact if the flow is purely along the readout or the phase encoded direction. For $v = 100$ cm/second, $\Delta t = 2$ msec, and oblique flow with $\theta = 45$ degrees, the displacement artifact $D = 1$ mm.

If a vessel contains blood that flows at a distribution of speeds (e.g., laminar flow), according to Equation 3, there also is a distribution of displacement values because D and v are directly proportional. At the edge of the vessel, where the flow velocity goes to zero, there is no displacement. In the center of the vessel, where the velocity is maximal, the displacement is also maximal. This can cause the signal apparently to *pile up* toward one edge of the vessel. Nishimura and colleagues[5] and Frank and associates[6] give a more complete description of the pile-up effect. If a vessel branches, oppositely directed pile-up artifacts from the two branches can overlap and cause a region of artifactual signal at the bifurcation point. This signal can mimic a basilar tip aneurysm (Fig. 94–7).

Several countermeasures have been developed to reduce the displacement artifact. A simple, effective method is to minimize the time Δt in Equation 3 (i.e., to apply the phase encoding gradient lobes as closely in time to the center of the echo as possible). (For 3D

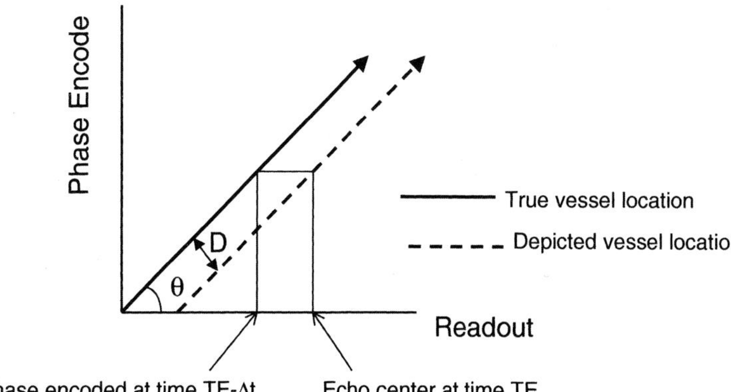

FIGURE 94–6. Displacement artifact. Because phase encoding occurs at a time Δt earlier than the peak of the echo, flow that is oriented obliquely between the readout and phase-encoded directions produces a displacement artifact. See text.

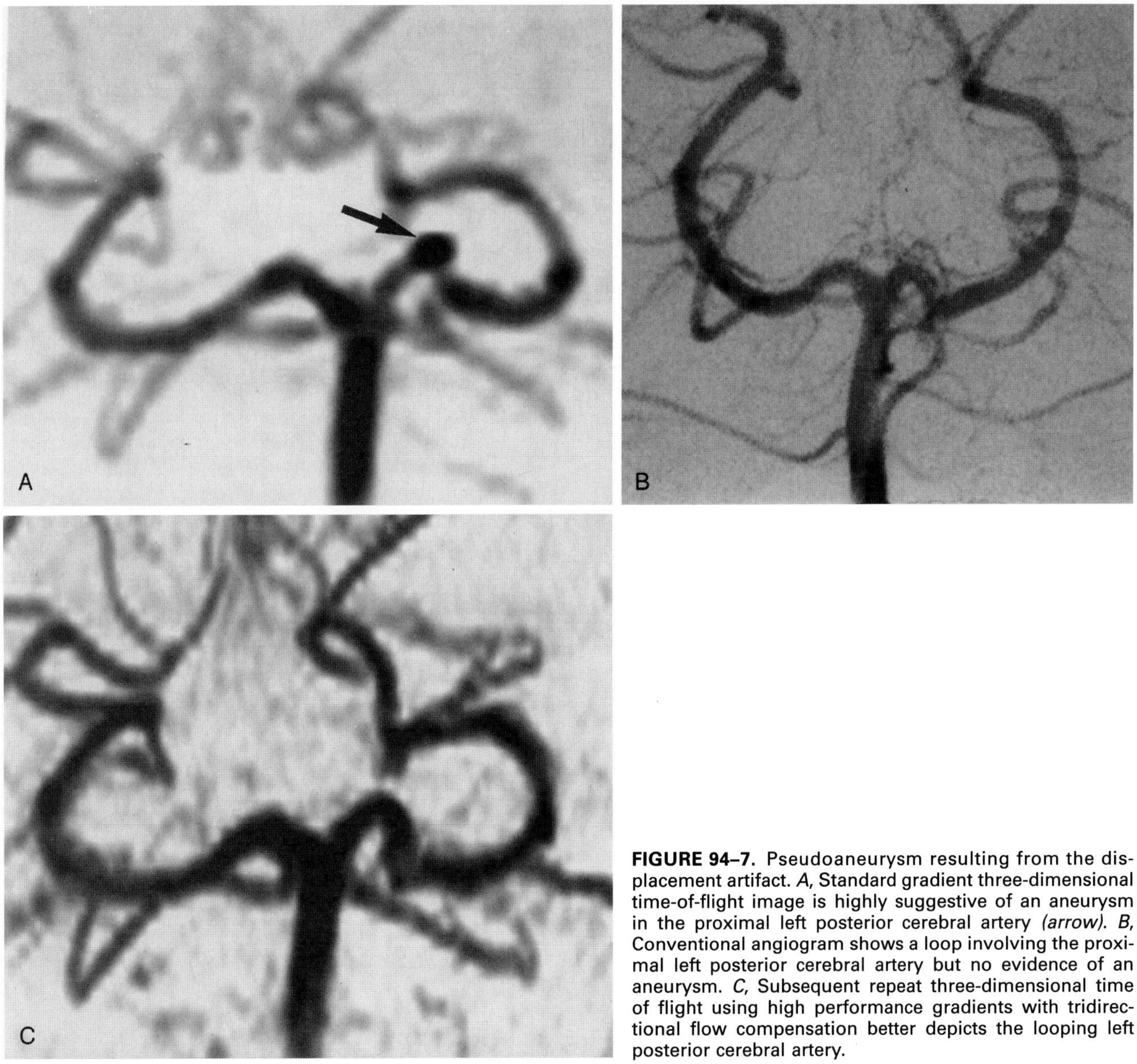

A

B

C

FIGURE 94–7. Pseudoaneurysm resulting from the displacement artifact. *A,* Standard gradient three-dimensional time-of-flight image is highly suggestive of an aneurysm in the proximal left posterior cerebral artery *(arrow). B,* Conventional angiogram shows a loop involving the proximal left posterior cerebral artery but no evidence of an aneurysm. *C,* Subsequent repeat three-dimensional time of flight using high performance gradients with tridirectional flow compensation better depicts the looping left posterior cerebral artery.

scans, the phase encoding gradient lobe on the slice axis also is applied as closely to the echo center as possible.) The advent of high-performance gradient subsystems has allowed pulse sequence designers to make more compact gradient lobes. Such systems typically have maximal gradient amplitudes in excess of 20 mT/m, and gradient slew rates in excess of 50 T/m/second. With these systems, it is often feasible to reduce Δt to submillisecond levels, at which the displacement artifact begins to be negligible.

An alternative countermeasure against the displacement artifact is to replace the standard unipolar phase encoding lobe with a bipolar phase encoding lobe that is gradient moment nulled (see later) for the time point at the center of the echo.[5] This method allows exact nulling of the displacement artifact. These bipolar phase encoding lobes require relatively large gradient amplitudes and durations so that the advent of high-performance gradients has made this method more feasible. A 3D pulse sequence with gradient moment nulling on its two phase encoded axes, in addition to its readout axis, sometimes is said to have *tridirectional flow compensation*. As shown in Figure 94–7*B*, the false basilar tip aneurysm apparent in Figure 94–7*A* is not apparent on an image acquired with tridirectional flow compensation and a high-performance gradient subsystem.

Phase Effects

In contrast to x-ray-based medical imaging modalities such as computed tomography, MR imaging is phase sensitive. The detected signal has a magnitude (i.e., strength) and a phase. The phase is the angle that the magnetization vector sweeps out as it precesses in the rotating frame (Fig. 94–8). The strength or magnitude of the signal is represented by the length of the arrow, and the phase is represented by the angle ϕ.

When an MR image is reconstructed with a Fourier transform, every pixel has magnitude and phase information. Normally the phase information is discarded during the reconstruction, and only a magnitude image is displayed. As described in this section, however, intrinsic phase effects in MR imaging can have a substantial effect on the magnitude image, even if the phase information is discarded.

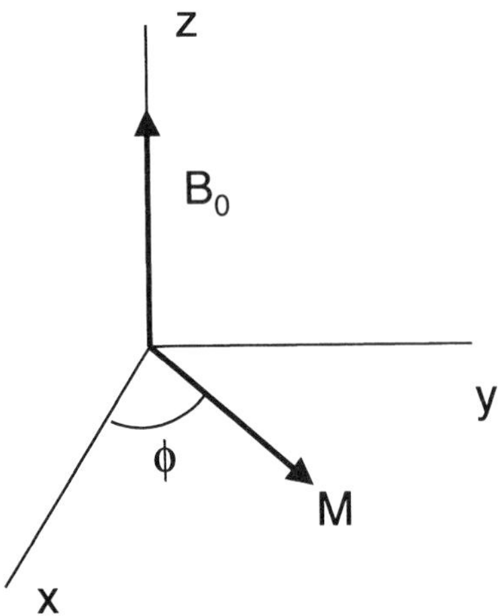

FIGURE 94–8. The magnetization *M* precesses about the main magnetic field B_0. The angle ϕ that a small element of magnetization sweeps out in the rotating frame provides the phase information for MR imaging.

INTRAVOXEL DEPHASING

When the phase information is discarded in the final reconstructed image, phase effects still can help determine the signal intensity, particularly within vessels. A mechanism for this is called *intravoxel dephasing*, or *intravoxel phase dispersion*.

The voxel is the basic 3D picture element in MR imaging. A voxel can be thought of as a rectangular box, in which the face of the box is a pixel (a 2D picture element), and the depth is the slice thickness. The total signal that is observed from a particular voxel is given by the phase-sensitive, or coherent, sum of all the isochromats within the voxel. This process is illustrated in Figure 94–9. An *isochromat* is magnetization from a microscopic section of the voxel where the phase is uniform.

The isochromats are denoted on diagrams such as Figure 94–9 by small arrows, where the orientation of the arrow represents its phase. All the isochromats in a phase-sensitive sum are added up by placing their arrows head-to-tail. The total magnitude signal from the voxel is given by the length of the arrow drawn from the tail of the first arrow to the head of the last one.

If all the arrows line up in the same direction (see Fig. 94–9*A*), the total signal (length of the bold arrow) is the simple sum of the signals from the subvoxels. That is the maximal possible value for the magnitude signal. The phase need not be zero, only the same constant value throughout the voxel. If the directions of the small arrows vary, however, as in Figure 94–9*B*, the length of the bold arrow is shorter, and the resulting magnitude signal for that voxel is reduced. Intravoxel dephasing is the loss of signal that results from the signal components within a voxel having nonuniform phase. It is possible for intravoxel dephasing to lead to complete signal loss. Intravoxel dephasing often occurs in vessels because blood flowing in the presence of the imaging gradients accumulates phase. Regions of complex flow, such as distal to stenoses, are particularly prone to signal loss from intravoxel dephasing.

Phase accumulation can occur from many other sources in MR imaging. In gradient echo imaging, lipid (fat) signal accumulates 180 degrees of phase relative to water at certain TE times (e.g., TE = 6.9 msec at the field strength of 1.5T). This phase accumulation is due to the chemical shift between fat and water. The resonant frequency of water is about 220 Hz higher than that of fat at 1.5T. Because of this 180-degree phase accumulation, the image intensity from voxels that contain fat and water is attenuated. This method of selecting the TE to attenuate the fat signal with intravoxel dephasing is known as placing fat and water *out of*

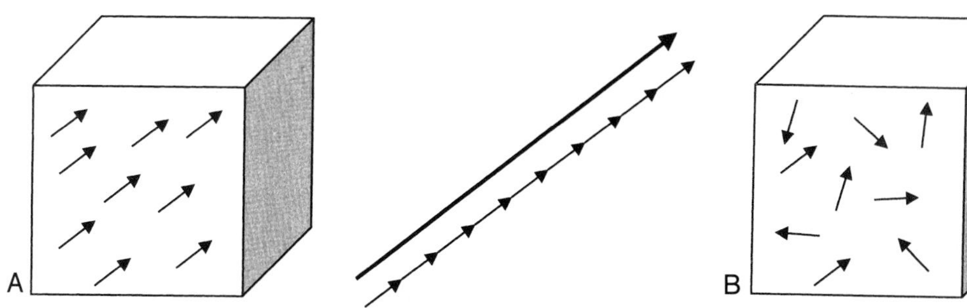

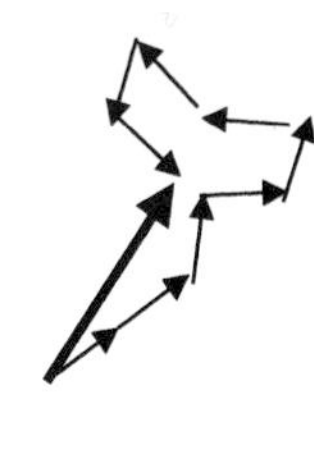

FIGURE 94–9. *A*, When all the isochromats within a voxel have a uniform phase, the magnitude signal is maximal. *B*, When the phase is inconsistent, intravoxel dephasing results, and the signal within that voxel is attenuated, even when a standard magnitude reconstruction is used.

phase and is used commonly in 3DTOF angiography. Intravoxel dephasing is a phase effect that can lead to signal loss in the standard magnitude image, even if the phase information is discarded from the reconstruction.

PULSATILE FLOW AND GHOSTING ARTIFACTS

Often arterial blood and cerebrospinal fluid flow is pulsatile (i.e., the flow velocity varies substantially with the phase of the cardiac cycle). MR image formation requires the collection of multiple (e.g., ≥128) views of data. Because the collection of subsequent views is separated by a time TR, pulsatile flow can lead to an *inconsistent* phase among the raw data views. This phase inconsistency, in turn, causes ghosting artifacts on MR images, in which the signal intensity from blood or cerebrospinal fluid is spread out in the phase-encoded direction (Fig. 94–10).

One method to reduce the pulsatile flow artifact is to trigger the acquisition of the views to a cardiac event, such as the detection of the QRS complex in an electrocardiogram waveform. In this way, all of the views have approximately consistent phases resulting from flow. For neurological MR imaging applications, often the exact relationship between the triggered acquisitions and the cardiac cycle is unimportant. To simplify the patient setup, peripheral triggering with a plethysmograph placed on a finger or toe can be used instead of electrocardiogram leads.

GRADIENT MOMENT NULLING (FLOW COMPENSATION)

Another method used to reduce the ghosting artifact is gradient moment nulling. Often the loss of signal intensity caused by intravoxel dephasing is undesirable. One method to avoid it is simply to make the voxels smaller. This method is seldom used, however, because the signal-to-noise (S/N) ratio is linearly proportional to the voxel volume. The increased imaging time required to retain the same S/N ratio with smaller voxels is usually impractical. A more practical countermeasure against the signal loss from intravoxel dephasing is called first-order *gradient moment nulling*, or *flow compensation*. This method typically introduces additional gradient lobes onto the readout and slice select gradient waveforms so that constant flow does not introduce any phase accumulation.

As mentioned previously, magnetization moving along a magnetic gradient accumulates phase. Consider a small element of flowing blood moving in the x-direction, so that its location is described by $x(t)$. Suppose also that an x-gradient $G_x(t)$ is applied. Then the accumulated phase for this isochromat of blood is given by

$$\phi = \gamma \sum_{t=0}^{TE} G_x(t)\, x(t) \qquad (4)$$

where γ is the gyromagnetic ratio. In Equation 4, $t = 0$ usually represents the peak of the rf excitation pulse. If the location, velocity, and acceleration of the blood are known at $t = 0$ (x_0, v_0, and a_0), its position $x(t)$ can be extrapolated at future times with the expansion

$$x(t) = x_0 + v_0\, t + \frac{1}{2} a_0\, t^2 + \ldots \qquad (5)$$

Substituting Equation 5 into Equation 4, we find that

$$\begin{aligned} \phi &= \gamma \sum_{t=0}^{TE} G_x(t) \left(x_0 + v_0\, t + \frac{1}{2} a_0\, t^2 + \ldots \right), \\ &= M_0 + v_0 M_1 + a_0 M_2 + \ldots \end{aligned} \qquad (6)$$

where

$$\begin{aligned} M_0 &= \gamma \sum_{t=0}^{TE} G_x(t); \quad M_1 = \gamma \sum_{t=0}^{TE} t\, G_x(t); \\ M_2 &= \frac{\gamma}{2} \sum_{t=0}^{TE} t^2\, G_x(t) \ldots \end{aligned} \qquad (7)$$

M_0 is simply the area under the gradient waveform, when its amplitude is plotted versus time. M_1 is called the *first moment*, which is the center of gravity of the gradient waveform.

According to Equation 6, if the gradient lobes are designed so that $M_1 = 0$, constant velocity does not contribute to the phase ϕ. This is flow compensation,

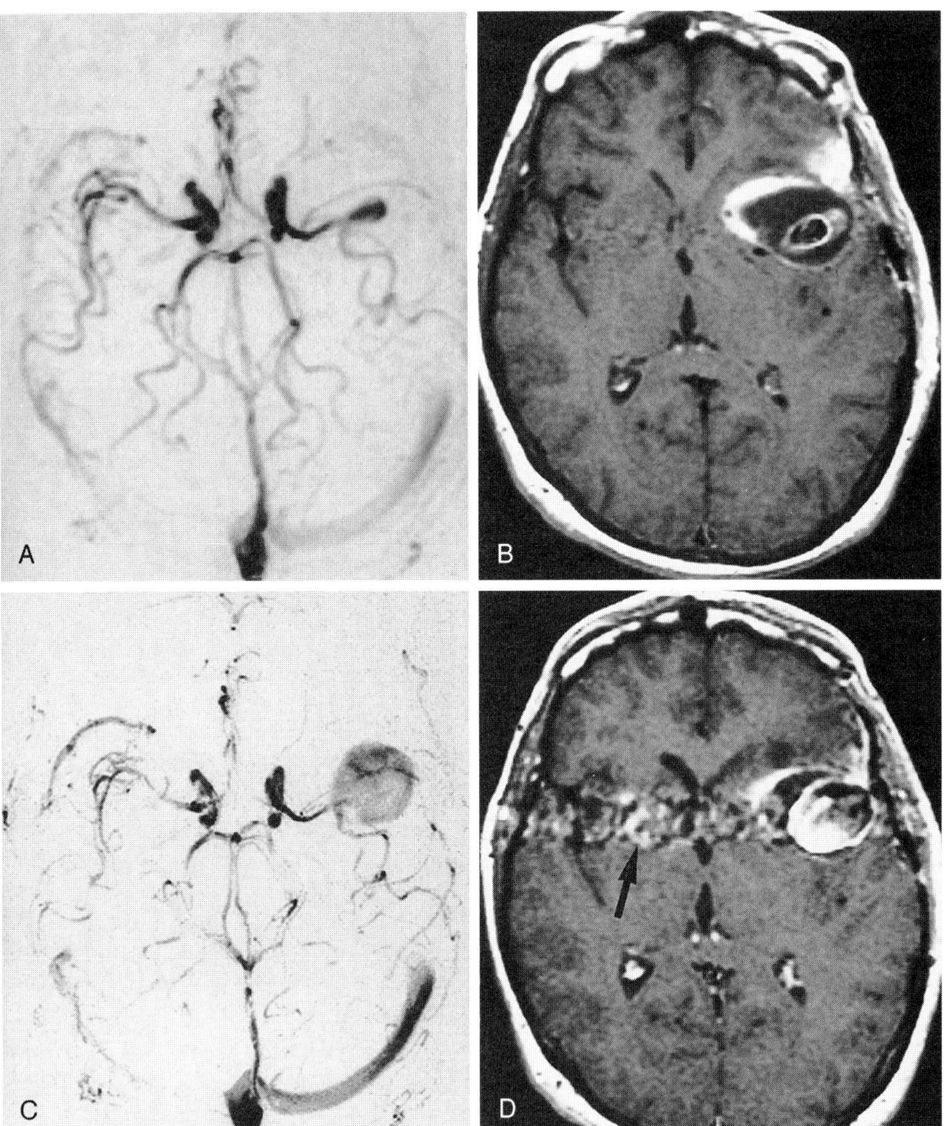

FIGURE 94–10. Follow-up MR angiogram shows aneurysm enlargement. *A*, A two-dimensional phase contrast sequence shows a left middle cerebral artery aneurysm. *B*, Axial T1-weighted image shows that the aneurysm is a giant aneurysm with considerable intraluminal thrombus. *C*, Follow-up two-dimensional phase contrast MR angiography shows considerable enlargement in the aneurysm lumen. *D*, Repeat T1-weighted image shows little overall change in the wall of the aneurysm; however, clot retraction has led to a considerable increase in the size of the patent lumen. Ghosting artifact in the phase encoding direction is seen as a result of the high flow through the aneurysm lumen (*arrow* in *D*).

and it can reduce intravoxel dephasing and ghosting artifacts.

Typically, flow compensation is not implemented on the phase encoding waveform because the strongest MR signals are acquired when the phase encoding gradient is stepped through amplitudes near zero (i.e., the center of k-space). According to Equation 7, the first moment is small when the gradient G is small so that M_1 often is negligible for these views anyway. It has been determined that, in practice, gradient moment nulling of the phase encoding waveform seldom is required. An exception is tridirectional flow compensation, which was discussed earlier as a method to combat the displacement artifact.

By definition, first-order gradient moment nulling zeroes M_1, second-order gradient moment nulling zeroes M_2, and so on. Equation 6 contains an infinite series and so is not practical to null all the moments. It is unusual to attempt to null any moments beyond M_1. Another strategy is to make these higher gradient moments as small as possible by designing the gradient to be compact in time, often by reducing TE. Partial echo readouts and asymmetric rf pulses[7] are helpful tools to accomplish this. High-performance gradient hardware, with their rapid rise and fall times, are useful for producing gradient waveforms that are compact in time.

MAGNETIC RESONANCE ANGIOGRAPHY TECHNIQUES

There are three main classes of MR angiography techniques in use today: TOF, phase contrast (PC), and contrast-enhanced MR angiography. Each has its own distinct advantages and its own applications.

Time-of-Flight Angiographic Techniques

TOF angiography is based on obtaining multiple slices that have a strong FRE effect. TOF angiograms use gradient-recalled echo acquisitions and can be obtained with either 2D or 3D techniques. Vessels are hyperintense on these angiograms so that TOF is a *white blood* technique. (Sometimes the images are viewed in inverse video so that the vessels appear black.) After the slices are reconstructed, they typically are postprocessed with a *maximum intensity projection* (MIP),[8] which enables the vessels to be viewed from any desired orientation.

TWO-DIMENSIONAL TIME OF FLIGHT

2DTOF angiograms are obtained by sequentially acquiring multiple thin (1 to 3 mm) slices that have a strong FRE.[9] The flip angle of the excitation pulse for the gradient echo acquisition is set relatively high (e.g., 50 to 70 degrees) to suppress the signal from the stationary tissue and maximize the FRE contrast.

A stack of axial slices typically is acquired to produce a 2DTOF angiogram. Sometimes an overlapping or overcontiguous acquisition is used (e.g., the slice thickness exceeds the center-to-center spacing of adjacent slices by 50%) to provide a smoother vessel appearance on the MIP.

Typically in a single MR angiogram, the clinician wishes to examine arteries or veins but seldom both. If one wants to image the carotid arteries with 2DTOF, it is important to suppress the signal from the jugular veins because it can be an overlapping structure. This is accomplished by placing an axial SAT band superior to each axial imaging slice. An SAT band that is moved with each slice so as to keep its SAT gap constant is said to be a *traveling* or *concatenated* SAT band. This method is used to ensure uniform venous suppression among the entire set of axial slices.

The venous flow suppression in 2DTOF is based solely on the direction of flow and not on any property of arterial or venous blood. If a carotid artery has a loop, instead of pure foot-to-head flow, the superior SAT band, which is designed to provide venous suppression, could provide inadvertent arterial suppression as well. This pitfall is illustrated in Figure 94–11.

It often is desirable to suppress the lipid signal in 2DTOF angiograms. A technique called *SLIP*[10] (spatially separated lipid presaturation) exploits the chemical shift of the SAT band. Suppose the rf bandwidth of the SAT pulse is 1000 Hz. At 1.5T, the 220-Hz chemical shift between fat and water translates to approximately one quarter of the thickness of the SAT band, or nearly 20 mm for an 80-mm-thick band. If the SAT gap is less than this value (e.g., 10 mm), effective lipid suppression can be obtained (Fig. 94–12). The pulse sequence can be designed so that chemical shift of the SAT band is always *toward* the imaging slice, regardless of factors such as the direction of patient entry (e.g., head first) or the direction of the main magnetic field within the bore.

THREE-DIMENSIONAL TIME OF FLIGHT

3DTOF angiograms are obtained with gradient-recalled echo volume acquisitions.[11] Similar to its 2D counterpart, 3DTOF relies on FRE to produce an intense signal from in-flowing blood. Because MR volume acquisitions employ a phase encoding gradient on the slice axis, 3DTOF has the ability to generate thin slices (approximately ≦1 mm) with much lower gradient strength than 2DTOF. As illustrated in Figure 94–13, 3DTOF can provide higher spatial resolution than 2DTOF without the high gradient moments that cause severe intravoxel dephasing. The main drawback of 3DTOF is the entry slice effect (i.e., signal from slow flow tends to be suppressed as the vessel penetrates further into the 3D volume). Several techniques designed to address this drawback are described next. In

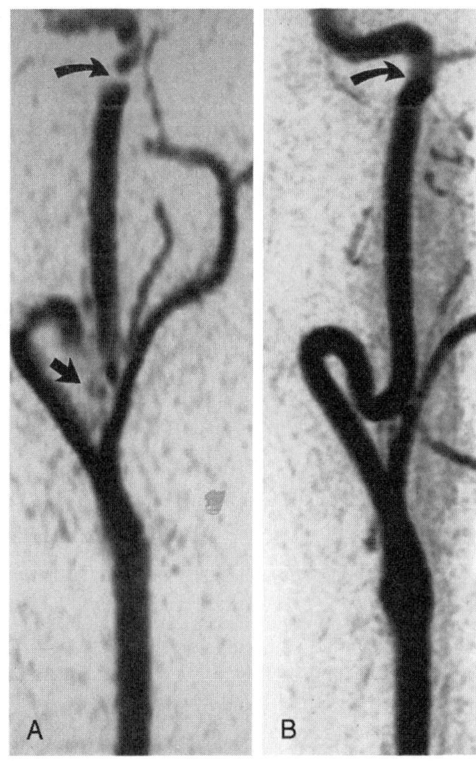

FIGURE 94–11. *A*, Two-dimensional time of flight shows loss of signal in a midcervical internal carotid loop *(arrow)* resulting from flow from the superior to inferior direction and resulting saturation. Also susceptibility artifact at the skull base *(curved arrow)* results in apparent high-grade stenosis. *B*, Contrast-enhanced technique depicts the looping midcervical internal carotid artery and is minimally degraded by susceptibility artifact at the skull base *(curved arrow)*.

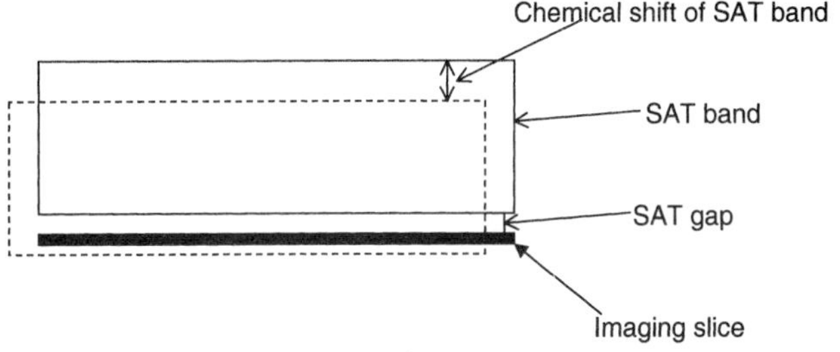

FIGURE 94–12. Lipid suppression in two-dimensional time-of-flight imaging. When the chemical shift of the spatial presaturation band exceeds the presaturation gap, lipid suppression results.

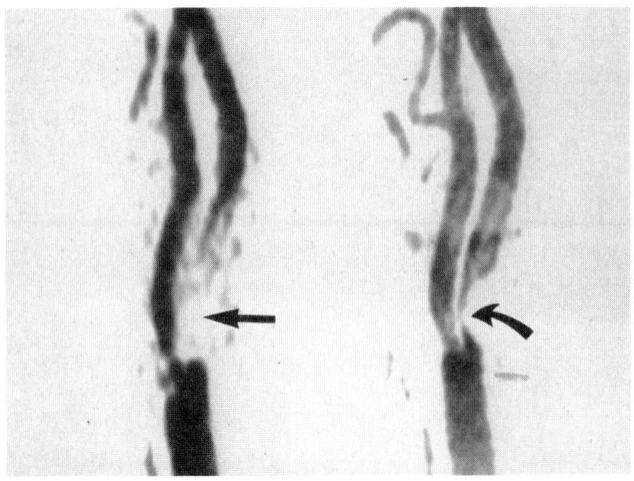

FIGURE 94–13. *Left,* Two-dimensional time of flight of the carotid artery shows a signal void caused by the presence of a high-grade stenosis *(arrow). Right,* Three-dimensional time of flight better depicts the high-grade stenosis *(curved arrow)* in part because submillimeter-thick slices can be obtained without producing large gradient moments. Three-dimensional time of flight is less sensitive to intravoxel dephasing distal to a stenosis than is two-dimensional time of flight.

addition, a general reconstruction method called *zero filling,* which is particularly useful for 3DTOF, is discussed.

3DTOF methods include MOTSA, ramp or TONE pulses, magnetization transfer, and zero filling. MOTSA (multiple overlapping thin slab acquisition) sequentially acquires multiple 3D volumes.[12] MOTSA offers improved visualization of slow flow compared with single thick slab 3DTOF because thin slabs provide improved FRE. A drawback to MOTSA is the *venetian blind* artifact that occurs at the slab boundaries. This artifact can be reduced by (1) overlapping the slabs so that some of the slices are acquired twice and (2) postprocessing the slices that are acquired twice with an MIP to form a single, resultant slice (Fig. 94–14). More advanced methods, such as *SLINKY,*[13] also have been proposed to reduce the venetian blind artifact further.

Another method that is useful for addressing the problem of signal loss from slow flow in 3DTOF is called the *TONE* or *ramp* rf pulse.[14] These excitation pulses do not attempt to produce a uniform flip angle across the 3D slab. Instead the entry slices receive a lower flip angle (e.g., 15 degrees), whereas the exit slices receive a larger flip angle (e.g., 40 degrees) (Fig. 94–15). Ramp pulses can be used with either single slab or MOTSA acquisitions.

Magnetization transfer (MT)[15] is used in 3DTOF as a method to improve small vessel detectability by reducing the stationary tissue signal. An MT rf pulse is applied at a frequency that is typically about 1000 Hz from the resonance frequency of water. The MT pulse has little or no direct effect on the MR signal of blood. Instead, it saturates *bound* protons in macromolecules that have a short T2 and, consequently, a broad spectrum. Although the bound protons themselves produce no signal in MR images, they are able to *transfer* their saturation to protons that do. The signal from tissue such as white matter is suppressed, increasing the conspicuity of small vessels.

Zero filling is an image reconstruction method that provides overlapped voxels.[16] It is particularly useful for 3DTOF acquisitions. If a 3DTOF volume contains 32 1-mm contiguous slices, zero filling the reconstruction in the slice direction provides 64 1-mm slices that are overlapped by 0.5 mm. In this case, zero filling provides 32 new interpolated slices (Fig. 94–16 illustrates this process with 8 slices). The location of each interpolated slice is midway between two adjacent original slices. The images from the original 32-slice location are not affected by the zero filling. Similarly, zero filling can be used to increase the in-plane matrix size (e.g., from 256 × 192 to 512 × 512). The zero-filled reconstruction provides a smoother MIP display of vessels because partial volume artifacts are reduced. Zero filling affects neither the acquisition time nor the S/N ratio of the images. Image reconstruction time is increased, however, when zero filling is used.

Phase Contrast Techniques

PC is an MR angiography technique that provides excellent stationary tissue suppression, can provide information about the flow direction, and has the ability to quantify flow velocity (cm/second) and volume rate (mL/minute).[17, 18] PC angiograms can be acquired in either 2D or 3D modes. Disadvantages of PC compared with TOF techniques are longer acquisition times and increased intravoxel dephasing. PC requires the operator to select an additional parameter, the *aliasing velocity,* or *VENC.* A brief introduction to PC techniques is given here.

The basic element of a PC pulse sequence is called the *bipolar gradient.* Two images are obtained—one with a bipolar gradient and the other with the bipolar gradient negated, or toggled (Fig. 94–17). The subtraction of

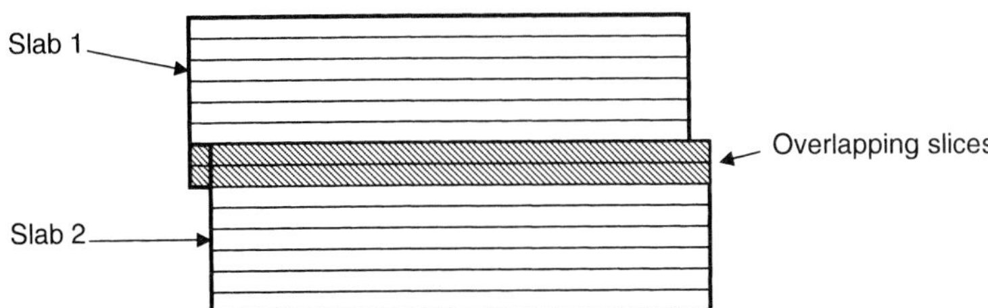

FIGURE 94–14. MOTSA. In this example, there are two slices that overlap slices in the adjacent slab. A maximum intensity projection is used to determine the resulting images in the overlap region.

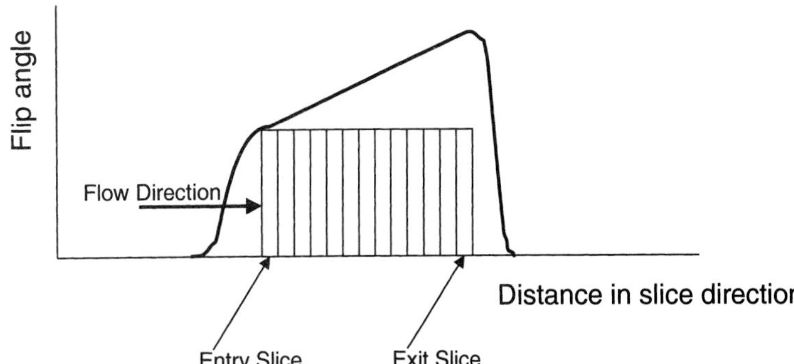

FIGURE 94–15. TONE radiofrequency pulse. The flip angle is ramped up from a small value at the entry slice to a larger value at the exit slice. This counteracts the entry slice effect and equalizes the signal intensity of flowing blood throughout the slab.

two images, each obtained with one of the settings of the bipolar gradient, is the source of vessel conspicuity. Each bipolar gradient introduces a phase into the MR image that is directly proportional to the velocity of the moving spins. The phase in the first image is given by

$$\phi_1 = \Phi + M_1 v \qquad (8)$$

where Φ is the phase in the image caused by effects besides the bipolar gradient (such as chemical shift, imperfect echo centering). M_1 is the first moment of the bipolar gradient waveform (Equation 7), and v is the component of the flow velocity along the direction of gradient. According to Equation 7, when one negates or toggles the bipolar gradient, its first moment reverses sign.

$$\phi_2 = \Phi - M_1 v \qquad (9)$$

The pair of phase images are subtracted on a pixel-by-pixel basis to form a *phase difference* image.

$$\textit{Phase difference} = \phi_1 - \phi_2 = \Delta\phi = 2\,M_1 v \qquad (10)$$

The purpose of forming the difference in Equation 10 is to eliminate the phase Φ, which is not due to flow, while accentuating the phase difference that arises entirely from flow.

The phase difference in Equation 10 is directly proportional to the velocity component, v, along the sensitizing gradient. Because one can calculate the value of M_1, one can extract *quantitative* information about the flow velocity in units of cm/second. One also can determine the flow *direction* because information about it is encoded in the *sign* of the phase difference.

If the phase difference is greater than 180 degrees (or < -180 degrees), flow-related aliasing occurs. A phase difference of 181 degrees is indistinguishable from a phase difference of -179 degrees. For a given value of M_1, the velocity that produces a phase difference of 180 degrees is known as *VENC*. Flow that is faster than VENC is disguised or *aliased* as slower flow. Because the signs of 181 degrees and -179 degrees are opposite, the flow direction also can be represented incorrectly when flow-related aliasing occurs.

The S/N ratio in PC images can be summarized[19] by the equation

$$(S/N)_{PC} \propto (S/N)_{MAG}\left(\frac{v}{VENC}\right), \quad |v| < VENC \qquad (11)$$

The first factor indicates that the S/N ratio in PC images is proportional to the S/N ratio that would be obtained if a standard magnitude image reconstruction were used instead. To optimize the vessel S/N ratio, attention to coil choice, sufficient voxel size, and maximizing FRE are required. A good PC imaging protocol begins with a good TOF protocol. The second factor indicates that S/N ratio in PC images is also proportional to the flow velocity and is *inversely* proportional to VENC.

Equation 11 presents a dilemma when developing a

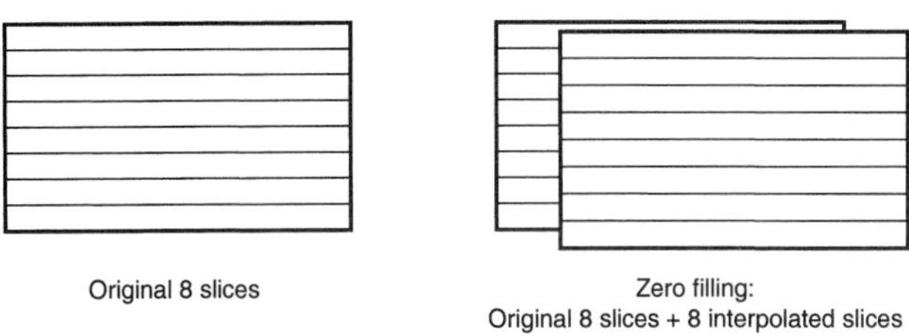

FIGURE 94–16. Zero filling. A normal three-dimensional reconstruction yields eight slices. By zero filling the raw data by a factor of 2, 8 additional interpolated slices are obtained, for a total of 16 slices.

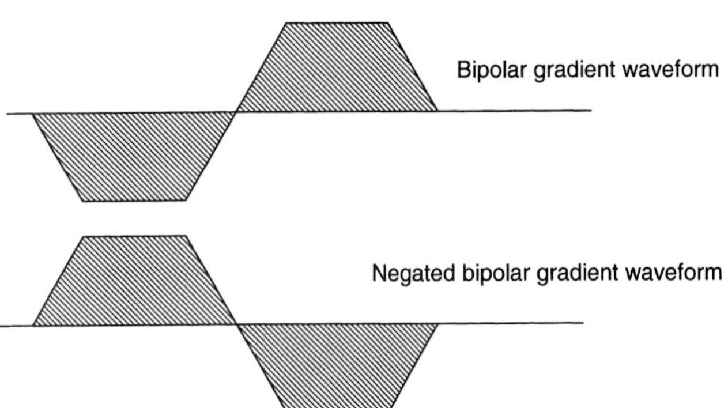

FIGURE 94–17. Bipolar gradient waveform. The toggled bipolar gradient waveform is the basis of phase contrast MR angiography. See text.

PC protocol: A large value for VENC should be selected to avoid flow-related aliasing, whereas a small value should be selected to maximize S/N ratio. In practice, often VENC is selected to be slightly larger than an estimated velocity in the vessel of interest.

A phase difference provides information about flow along a single direction. Often, clinicians wish to reconstruct angiograms that show flowing blood, regardless of its direction. This reconstruction can be accomplished by forming three separate phase differences (one for flow along x, one for flow along y, and one for flow along z), then forming the square root of the sum of the squares on a pixel-by-pixel basis. This provides an image whose intensity is proportional to the flow speed, regardless of flow direction. Directional flow information is not provided by this type of image. Because three phase differences are required to form a speed image, the data can be obtained with $2 \times 3 = 6$ acquisitions. This data acquisition can be accelerated by using a common phase reference image to perform the phase differences so that only $1 + 3 = 4$ acquisitions are required.[20] Often when only speed information is desired, the phase difference operation described by Equation 10 is replaced with a *complex difference* operation.[21] Often, more flow-related aliasing can be tolerated in speed images so that VENC can be lowered to improve the S/N ratio.

Because of the excellent background suppression available with PC, single thick-slice (e.g., 80 mm), or slab, acquisitions are feasible. These scans can provide an excellent scout view for the vessels of the head and neck. Figure 94–18 shows an example. The excellent suppression of stationary tissue with thick-slab PC also makes it an effective technique for postcontrast studies.

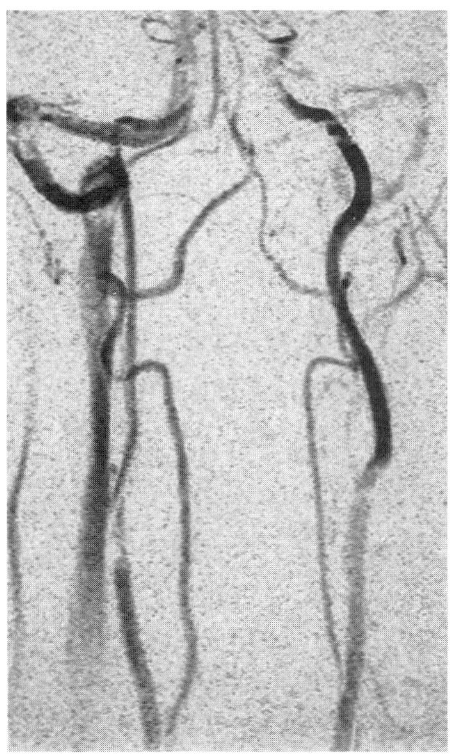

FIGURE 94–18. Two-dimensional phase contrast is a technique that offers large field of view with excellent background suppression and frequently is used as a scout sequence.

FLOW QUANTIFICATION

Equation 10 shows that one can determine quantitatively the flow velocity. Often, clinicians are interested instead in volume flow rate (in units of mL/minute) as a measure of blood or cerebrospinal fluid supplied to a particular organ.[18] Flow rate is the product of the perpendicular component of velocity v and the area A through which it flows. The volume flow rate can be determined by acquiring a PC image with the slice plane perpendicular to the vessel of interest. The volume flow rate can be calculated

$$\textit{Volume flow rate}\left(\frac{\text{mL}}{\text{min}}\right) = \frac{60\ \text{sec}}{\text{min}} A \sum_{i=1}^{N} v_i \qquad (12)$$

where A is the pixel area in cm^2, and v_i is the velocity in cm/second for the ith pixel. The sum is performed over all pixels that cover the vessel. Although Equation 12 can provide a good estimate of the flow rate, several systematic errors limit the accuracy of the measurement.[22, 23] Among the most serious is the precise definition of the vessel margin, leading to partial-volume errors. One fortunate property of the volume flow rate is that (to a first-order approximation) it is independent of the angle between the vessel and the slice. The decrease in the perpendicular component of the velocity is offset by an increase in the area of intersection between the vessel and the slice. This approximation breaks down rapidly as the slice thickness is increased or for values of θ far from the perpendicular.

Often, it is desirable to measure the volume flow rate as a function of time throughout the cardiac cycle. *Cine* phase contrast[24] and other rapid electrocardiogram-triggered techniques[25] can be used for this purpose.

Contrast-Enhanced Techniques

Contrast-enhanced MR angiography does not rely on FRE or phase effects to produce vessel contrast. Instead the T1 of blood is reduced by the injection of a contrast agent.[26] Typically, 10 to 40 mL of gadolinium chelates is injected intravenously as a bolus, preferably by a power injector. For neurological applications, gadolinium is injected at a relatively rapid rate (2 to 3 mL/second is typical). The gadolinium bolus injection often is followed by the injection of a saline flush. After transition through the pulmonary system, the gadolinium bolus remains partially intact and typically produces concentrations on the order of 1 to 10 mM in the arterial system. This reduces the T1 of blood by greater than an order of magnitude (e.g., to 50 msec), allowing short TR (e.g., TR <10 msec) 3D scanning with minimal signal loss from T1 saturation. It is important to synchronize the 3D acquisition to the arterial bolus arrival, either with a triggering or bolus timing method or by

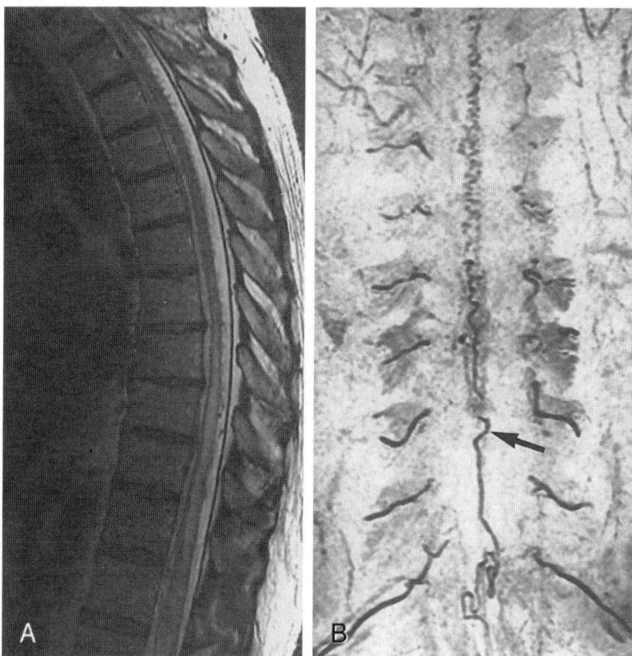

FIGURE 94–19. Spinal dural arteriovenous fistula. *A*, T2-weighted image of the thoracic spine shows an enlarged spinal cord with increased T2 signal and multiple signal voids in the subarachnoid space consistent with dilated veins. *B*, Bolus contrast-enhanced MR angiogram shows dilated veins within the thecal sac *(arrow)*. (Case provided by Jack Lane, MD.)

taking repeated 3D acquisitions. It is important to obtain images that solely show the arterial phase. In the cervical arteries, enhancement of the jugular vein typically occurs within 5 to 15 seconds of arterial enhancement.

TOF and PC techniques are analogous to ultrasound in that vessel signal depends on flow. Contrast-enhanced MR angiography is more analogous to conventional angiography, however, because its contrast depends on the lumen-filling properties of the contrast agent (Fig. 94–19).

The rapid acquisition speed and high S/N ratio of contrast-enhanced MR angiography has led to a rapid surge in its use. Contrast-enhanced MR angiography techniques have begun to displace some x-ray-based techniques in clinical practice.

SINGLE-PHASE METHODS WITH TIMING OR TRIGGERING; ELLIPTICAL CENTRIC VIEW ORDER

Sometimes a single 3D scan is acquired when the arterial concentration of gadolinium is high. The advantage of these single-phase acquisitions is that they allow for longer scan times, which in turn allow better coverage and spatial resolution. Many single-phase acquisitions employ the *elliptical centric* view order.[27] Elliptical centric view ordering is a method for acquiring 3D MR data. The center of k-space contains the views that govern the low spatial frequencies and the overall contrast in the image. In elliptical centric view ordering, the two standard nested loops used for 3D phase encoding are replaced by a single loop. The view ordering within this single loop is determined by the distance in k-space from that view to the center of k-space. Elliptical centric is a true centric k-space ordering for 3D acquisitions.

If a single 3D scan is acquired, it is crucial to synchronize it accurately to the bolus arrival in the artery of interest. One method to accomplish this is called *fluoroscopic triggering*.[27] In the time after the bolus injection, multiple 2D scans are acquired at the same slice location. The images are reconstructed and displayed in real-time. The frame rate is on the order of, or faster than, 1 image/second. When the bolus arrival is detected, the operator switches from the 2D to the 3D acquisition. An important performance parameter for fluoroscopic triggering is the latency time, which is the lag between the command to switch to the 3D acquisition and its actual start. Because of the rapid venous return, latency times of 1 second or less are desirable for carotid MR angiography studies. Fluoroscopic triggering requires a centric view ordering, preferably the elliptical centric method described previously.

Sometimes the switch from the bolus detection to the 3D scan is performed automatically by the computer system, as in the SmartPrep (General Electric Medical Systems, Milwaukee, Wis.) technique.[28] In the SmartPrep method, the operator places a small *tracker volume* on a vessel that is expected to enhance. A drawback of such techniques is they can fail to trigger properly if the patient moves during the injection, and the enhancing vessel moves out of the tracker volume; this can be particularly problematic when targeting smaller vessels such as the carotids.

The *test bolus timing* method[29] is an alternative to fluoroscopic triggering. In this timing method, a small test dose (e.g., 2 mL) of gadolinium is injected, followed by a saline flush. A series of rapid 2D images is acquired to display the arrival of the test dose at the artery of interest. This circulation time is estimated from the vessel enhancement, then it is recorded. Then the full gadolinium dose and saline flush are injected. If the elliptical centric view order is used, the 3D acquisition is initiated as soon as the recorded circulation time has elapsed. If a noncentric 3D acquisition is used, the 3D scan is initiated somewhat earlier so that the center of k-space is acquired concurrently with the maximal arterial enhancement.

Both the fluoroscopic triggering and test bolus timing methods have advantages. Fluoroscopic triggering allows the 3D angiogram to be acquired with a single injection, which can save time and reduce cost. Unwanted enhancement of veins and stationary tissue from the test bolus is avoided. The fluoroscopic triggering method is insensitive to variations in the patient's cardiac output, which could lead to possible changes in circulation time. The test bolus method requires less sophisticated hardware and does not require any real-time decision making. The uptake of gadolinium into late filling vessels and veins can be examined prospectively before the 3D acquisition so that the circulation time measurement can be fine-tuned accordingly. In the authors' experience, the fluoroscopic and the test bolus timing methods work well for carotid MR angiography when the elliptical centric view order is used.

MULTIPHASE METHODS

An alternative to fluoroscopic triggering or test bolus timing is to image the vessels of interest repeatedly with rapid 3D scans. If the same 3D volume is acquired repeatedly on the order of once every 10 seconds, it is virtually assured that one of these scans will display peak arterial enhancement, with minimal venous contamination. Such *multiphase* 3D acquisitions typically demand extremely short TRs (e.g., TR <5 msec). Even so, it is challenging to cover the entire carotid-vertebrobasilar system in the coronal plane with high spatial resolution (e.g., voxel size approximately 1 mm^3, before zero filling) with only a 10-second acquisition time. Multiphase methods can be particularly useful for examining late-filling structures.

Several techniques have been developed to alleviate the trade-offs between temporal and spatial resolution of multiphase methods. TRICKS[30] is a 3D technique that acquires the views in the center of k-space more frequently, then shares raw data among multiple phases. More recently, undersampled projection reconstruction methods have been developed[31] that may lead to greater improvements in spatial resolution.

CLINICAL APPLICATIONS

The techniques described in the previous section have important clinical applications. This section is divided into extracranial and intracranial applications of these techniques.

Extracranial Circulation

CAROTID ARTERY ATHEROSCLEROSIS

Interest in noninvasive carotid imaging has increased as extracranial atherosclerosis has become an increasingly important cause of cerebral ischemia. Ischemic stroke is now the third leading cause of death in the United States, with approximately 600,000 new cases each year, of which nearly 40% are fatal. Atherosclerotic disease involving the carotid bifurcation and the resulting thromboemboli account for a significant proportion of cerebral infarctions. Results of prospective randomized trials, including the North American Symptomatic Carotid Endarterectomy Trial

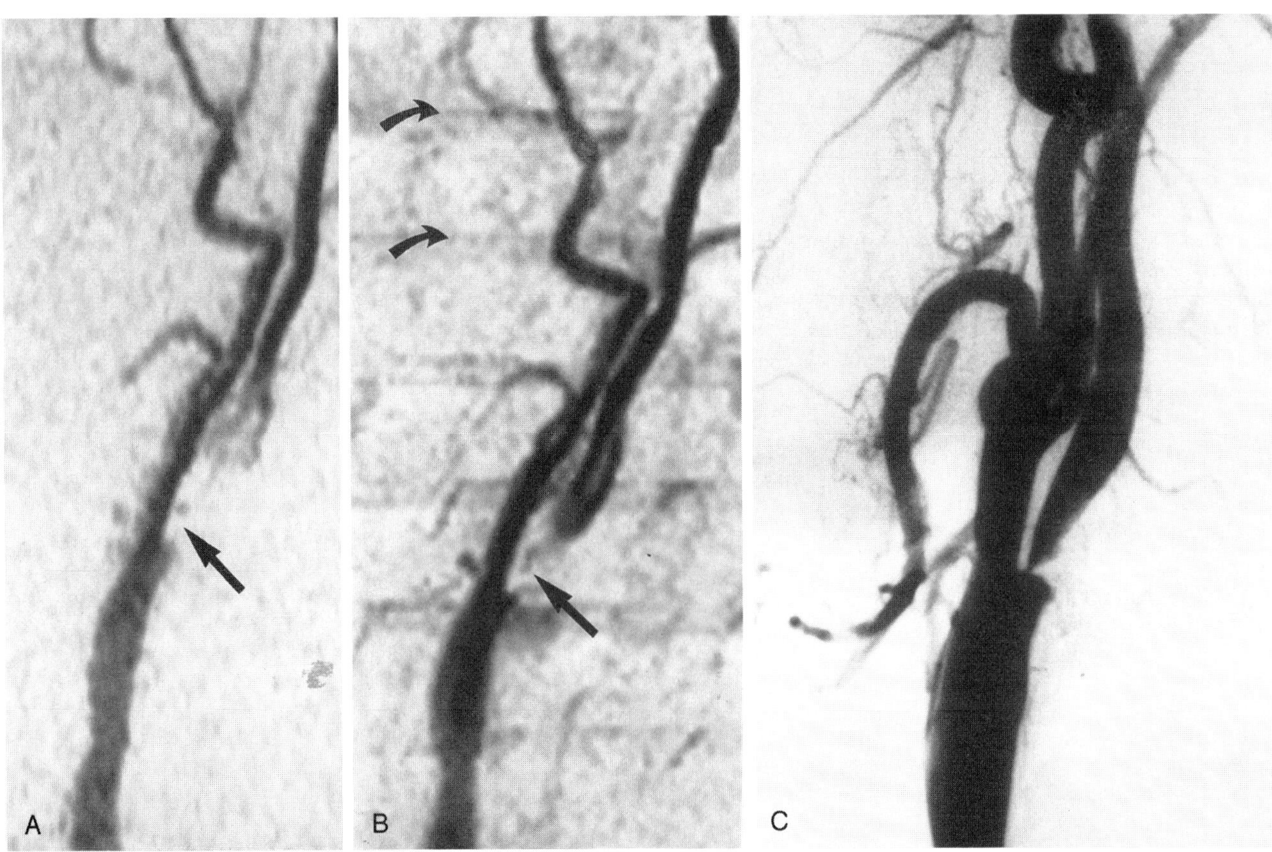

FIGURE 94–20. *A*, High-grade stenosis at the origin of the internal carotid artery is seen as a long segment signal void on two-dimensional time of flight *(arrow)*. *B*, MOTSA sequence better depicts the vascular anatomy and shows a signal void at the stenosis *(arrow)*. The slab interfaces are seen as subtle lines creating a venetian blind artifact on the MOTSA acquisition *(curved arrows)*. *C*, Conventional angiogram shows that the high-grade stenosis is at the origin of the internal carotid artery.

(NASCET),[32] have shown relative risk reductions ranging from 70% to 85% when an endarterectomy is performed in patients with an internal carotid artery diameter stenosis of 70% or greater. Final results of the NASCET have shown a surgical benefit for selected patients whose internal carotid artery stenosis is 50%. As criteria for identifying patients for carotid endarterectomy evolve from a single threshold to a more complex consideration of multiple factors, accurate grading of the degree of carotid stenosis increases in importance.

Interest in noninvasive techniques has grown as a method to control costs and to avoid the risk of conventional angiography. Comparison of the various techniques has been complicated by variation in study design and by the quality of reported studies. Since its introduction, MR angiography has shown progressive improvement in diagnostic accuracy. The introduction of contrast-enhanced 3D MR angiography techniques has allowed MR angiography to replace conventional angiography before an endarterectomy in most patients.

Early carotid artery MR angiography using 2DTOF techniques was introduced by Keller and associates[9] in 1989 as a reliable method to visualize the carotid arteries.[33] Advantages of the 2DTOF sequence were sensitivity to slow flow and excellent stationary tissue suppression. Carotid arteries uninvolved with disease were well depicted with the 2DTOF technique. The 2DTOF sequence had a tendency to overestimate the degree of stenosis and result in a signal void when a high-grade stenosis was present (Fig. 94–20).[34, 35] Consequently the 2DTOF sequence was shown to be sensitive to the presence of clinically significant stenosis. Because of the considerable overestimation, however, the technique had a low specificity.

MOTSA (described earlier) is technical advancement in MR angiography that combines 3D acquisitions with multiple thin slabs.[36] This hybrid technique offers the high spatial resolution of 3D imaging with resulting less intravoxel dephasing than 2DTOF (see Fig. 94-13). A deficiency of the flow-dependent 2DTOF and multislab 3DTOF techniques is insensitivity to stagnant flow, such as in carotid bulbs or ulcerations.[37]

The bolus contrast-enhanced MR angiography technique has shown the ability to generate high-quality images of the carotid bifurcation with lumen-filling characteristics physiologically analogous to conventional angiography (Figs. 94–21 through 94–23). Use of the bolus contrast-enhanced technique requires accurate initiation of the scan with the arrival of the contrast.[27] Typically a bolus of contrast material is injected

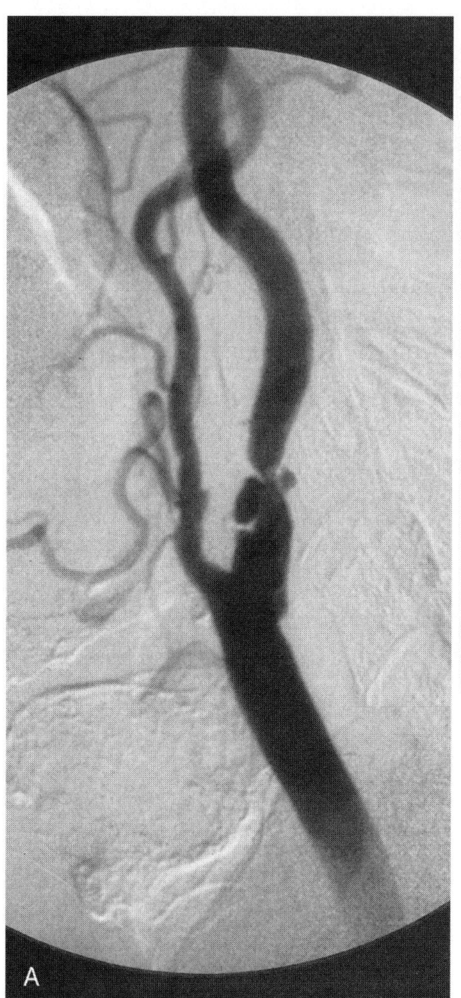

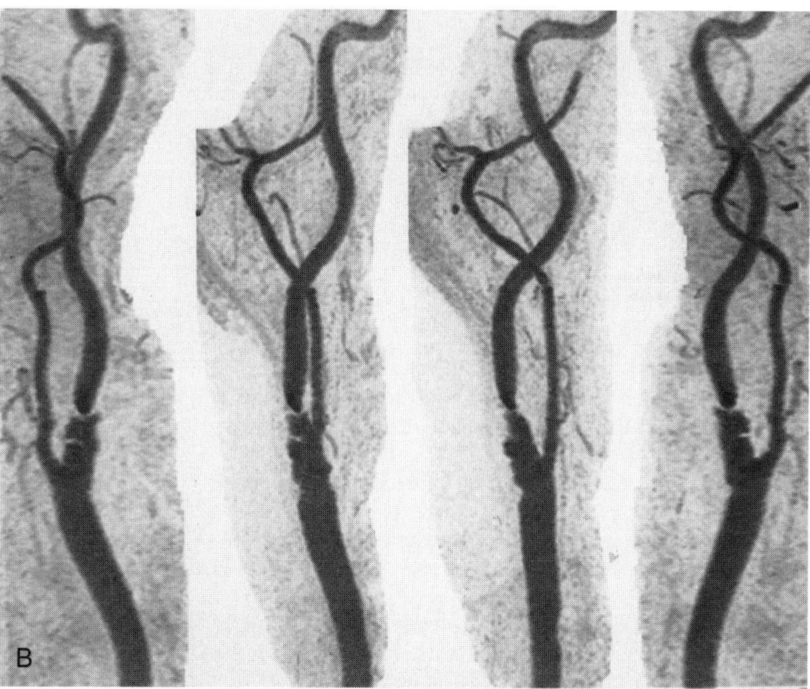

FIGURE 94–21. *A*, Conventional angiogram shows an ulcerated high-grade stenosis of the internal carotid artery. *B*, Bolus contrast-enhanced MR angiogram depicts well the complex ulcerated, highly stenotic atherosclerotic plaque. The three-dimensional nature of the bolus contrast-enhanced MR angiogram is illustrated by the multiple projections made possible with a single acquisition.

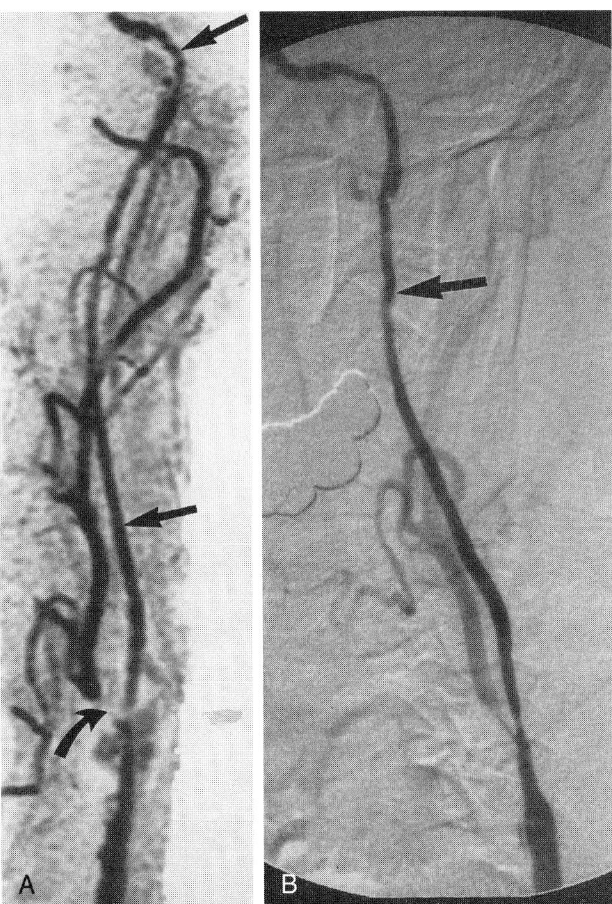

FIGURE 94–22. *A*, Bolus contrast-enhanced MR angiogram shows a near-occlusion of the internal carotid artery with a slim sign *(arrows)*. The high-grade stenosis at the origin of the external carotid artery is seen as a signal void *(curved arrow)*. *B*, Conventional angiogram confirms the presence of a nearly occluded internal carotid artery *(arrow)*. Faint filling of the external carotid branches is seen as a result of the high-grade stenosis at the external carotid origin.

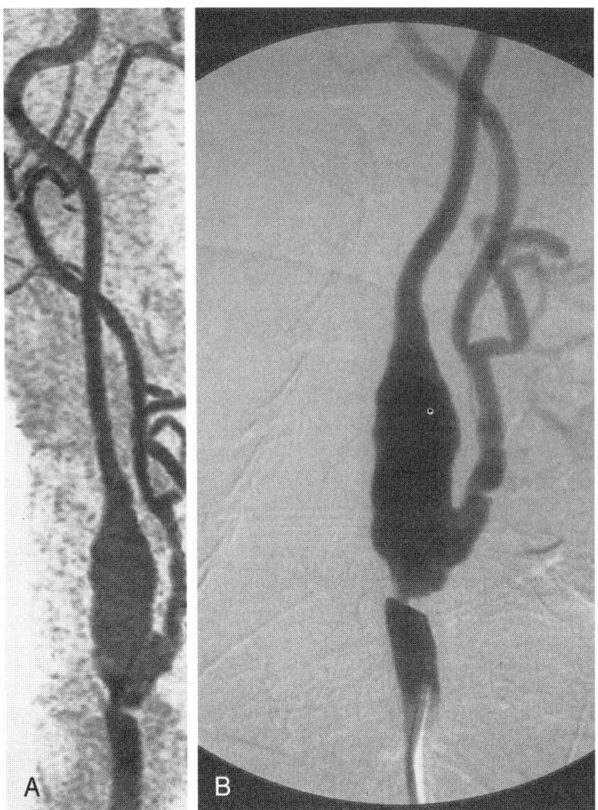

FIGURE 94–23. *A*, Bolus contrast-enhanced MR angiogram shows high-grade recurrent stenosis involving the distal common carotid artery with postoperative changes involving the bifurcation after an endarterectomy. *B*, Conventional angiogram confirms the recurrent stenosis and postoperative changes.

into an antecubital vein followed by a saline flush. The determination of the contrast material arrival in the carotid artery can be performed with MR fluoroscopy, use of a test injection, multiple short 3D acquisitions, or retrospective view sharing obtained during a continuous acquisition.

Bolus contrast-enhanced MR angiography is superior to previous MR angiography techniques.[38] The 2DTOF and multislab 3DTOF sequences are flow dependent and analogous to ultrasound. Signal loss occurs in these techniques as a result of slow flow, such as in the carotid bulb or in the presence of an ulcer. Signal loss can occur in a complex flow situation, such as high-grade stenosis. Because the bolus contrast-enhanced technique is physiologically more analogous to conventional angiography, its lumen-filling character results in visualization of slow or stagnant flow, including ulcerations.

VERTEBRAL ARTERY AND AORTIC ARCH ATHEROSCLEROSIS

Although flow-dependent TOF techniques have offered imaging of the carotid bifurcation and intracranial circulation, no reliable approach to the vertebral origins and aortic arch has been available. With the introduction of bolus contrast-enhanced MR angiography techniques, it now is possible to obtain a noninvasive evaluation of the entire cerebrovascular system from the aortic arch through the intracranial circulation.[39, 40] Although technical difficulties remain, this will be an important and expanding aspect of MR angiography in the future (Fig. 94–24; see also Fig. 94–2).

CAROTID ARTERY AND VERTEBRAL ARTERY DISSECTION

Carotid and vertebral dissections are acute disruptions of the arterial wall. An intramural hematoma splits the layers of the vessel, creating a false lumen that typically is surrounded by the external elastic lamina and adventitia. The hematoma within the media can cause compression and narrowing of the true lumen. Alternatively, it may expand outward, stretching the adventitia, and cause an enlargement of the lumen or a dissecting aneurysm.[41, 42] Dissections may be spontaneous or result from trauma that can be severe or minor, such as associated with coughing. Primary arterial diseases, such as fibromuscular dysplasia, have an association with dissections. Dissections predominantly involve middle-aged patients, with a higher incidence in

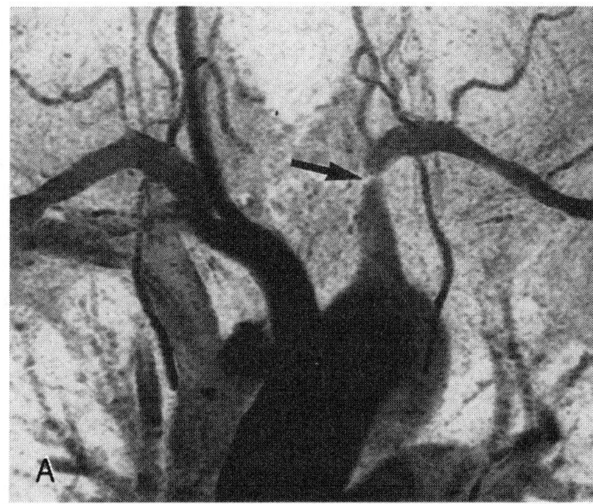
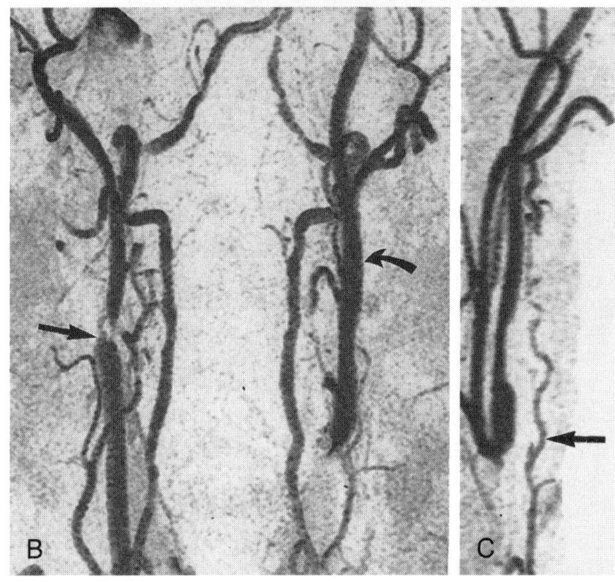

FIGURE 94–24. *A*, Bolus contrast-enhanced aortic arch MR angiogram shows occlusion of the left common carotid artery and a high-grade stenosis in the proximal left subclavian artery *(arrow)*. *B*, Bolus contrast-enhanced MR angiogram of the cervical, carotid, and vertebral arteries shows occlusion of the right internal carotid artery *(straight arrow)*, reconstitution of the left internal carotid artery through muscular collaterals *(curved arrow)* and a high-grade stenosis involving the distal left vertebral artery. *C*, Subvolume of the left carotid bifurcation better depicts the musculocollaterals *(arrow)*, contributing to reconstitution of the left internal carotid artery.

women. Headache frequently is associated with the occurrence of the dissection that is usually unilateral and often periorbital. Additional presenting manifestations include acute neurological ischemia and Horner's syndrome.

Angiographic findings in the setting of carotid or vertebral dissection include occlusion, stenosis, or aneurysmal dilation.[43] Tapering proximal to a stenotic segment is a typical finding, which can be helpful when attempting to differentiate a dissection from atherosclerotic stenosis. When a long segment stenosis is present, the lumen often is restored to the normal diameter as the artery enters the bone portion of the petrous canal. When present, the stenotic segment typically is elongated and irregular. Dissecting aneurysms occur in about one third of dissected vessels. Dissecting aneurysms can vary in size and are often ovoid or finger-like, typically paralleling the course of the native vessel. Occasionally, dissections can occur bilaterally.

Dissections have been noted on MR imaging with standard T1-weighted and T2-weighted imaging.[44–46] The typical appearance is a compromised lumen with crescent-shaped high signal on T1 and T2 surrounding the narrowed lumen. This signal change presumably is related to the presence of thrombosis within the vessel wall.

Noncontrast MR angiography techniques have allowed depiction of the luminal narrowing and dissecting aneurysm.[47] When correlated with the MR angiography source images, the degree of luminal narrowing and the dilation of the external diameter of the vessel can be evaluated. A useful application of MR angiography has been follow-up of known dissections. When a dissection has been documented on conventional angiography or MR angiography, the change in the lesion over time can be monitored noninvasively.

With the introduction of bolus contrast-enhanced MR angiography techniques, the usefulness of MR angiography has increased.[48] Noncontrast MR angiography often was degraded by a signal void in the setting of a high-grade stenosis. The loss of signal in the presence of slow flow, such as distal to a high-grade stenosis or within a pseudoaneurysm, resulted in nonvisualization of the flow. Bolus contrast-enhanced techniques allow better depiction of the stenotic segment and filling of the slow flow within the pseudoaneurysms (Fig. 94–25). Also with bolus contrast-enhanced MR angiography techniques, the entire vertebrobasilar system can be visualized. Noncontrast MR angiography has been unable to visualize the vertebral artery origins. With an appropriate choice of field of view, the vertebral artery origins as well as the basilar artery can be included within the field of view of the bolus contrast-enhanced MR angiography study.

Intracranial Circulation

ANEURYSMS

Saccular aneurysms are abnormal focal arterial dilations typically at bifurcations, but they may arise directly from the lateral wall of a nonbranching artery as well. The frequency of intracranial aneurysms is unknown, but it has been estimated to be approximately 5%.[49, 50] Although previously thought to result from a congenital defect in the arterial wall, it now generally is believed that hemodynamic stresses result in degeneration and weakness of the arterial wall, resulting in aneurysm development. Most saccular aneurysms are isolated lesions; however, there is an increased incidence in patients with a family history of subarachnoid hemorrhage, autosomal dominant polycystic kidney disease, fibromuscular dysplasia, and high-flow states such as arteriovenous malformations. Aneurysms are multiple in approximately 20% of patients. When multiple aneurysms arise, they are frequently in a mirrored location.

In the past, most aneurysms were discovered after

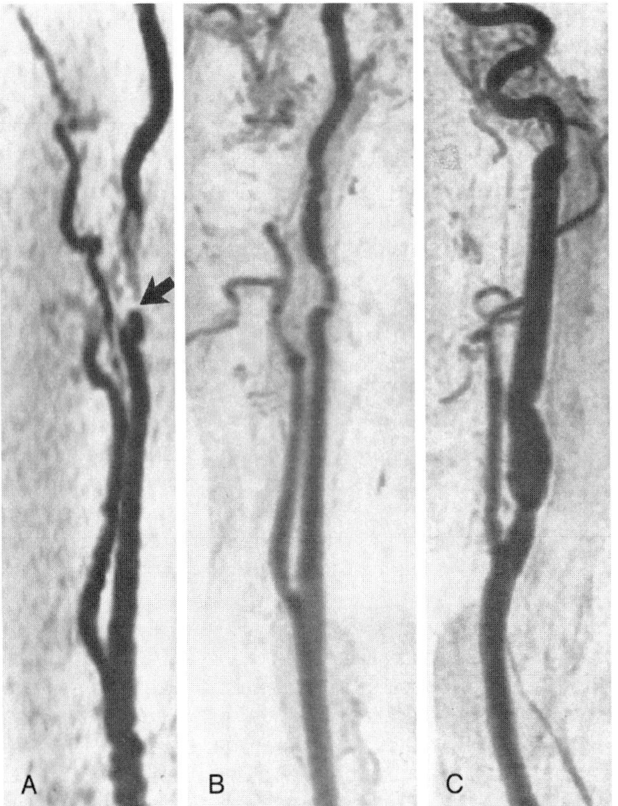

FIGURE 94–25. Bilateral carotid dissections. *A*, Two-dimensional time-of-flight MR angiogram of the right carotid artery shows a signal void *(arrow)* at the location of a high-grade stenosis secondary to a dissection. *B*, Bolus contrast-enhanced MR angiogram shows better the high-grade stenosis as well as vascular irregularity of the right internal carotid artery dissection. *C*, Bolus contrast-enhanced MR angiogram of the left internal carotid artery shows postoperative changes after an interposition vein graft for severe stenosis resulting from a previous dissection.

a subarachnoid hemorrhage. Rupture of intracranial aneurysms is the most common cause of nontraumatic subarachnoid hemorrhage. With the widespread use of cross-sectional imaging, including computed tomography and MR imaging, an increased number of incidental aneurysms are being identified (Fig. 94–26).

Greater than 90% of saccular aneurysms occur within the circle of Willis. The most frequent locations include the anterior communicating artery, posterior communicating artery, middle cerebral artery trifurcation, internal carotid artery including the cavernous portion, and the tip of basilar artery.[51] When MR angiography is used to search for aneurysms, the field of view typically is limited to increase the spatial resolution. Aneurysms are rare in the distal middle and anterior cerebral artery branches. These vascular territories often are not included within the imaging volume of the typical MR angiography study.

The role of MR angiography in the evaluation of patients with intracranial aneurysms is evolving. MR angiography has occupied a predominantly screening role. In some instances, a MR angiogram is the only diagnostic study before surgical clipping (Fig. 94–27). In general, patients presenting with subarachnoid hemorrhage still proceed to conventional angiography.

MR angiography techniques have been improving rapidly. Initial retrospective work suggested that MR angiography could detect aneurysms 3 mm or greater in size.[52, 53] Blinded prospective studies comparing PC with TOF techniques revealed that high-resolution TOF was superior to PC. When studied prospectively, however, 5 mm appeared to be a crucial diameter for the detection of aneurysms.[54] More recently, a combination of hardware and software improvements has led to the ability to identify routinely aneurysms 3 mm in diameter.[55] The morphology of aneurysms also often can be determined. One advantage of MR angiography over conventional angiography is the 3D nature of the data acquisition. Postprocessing allows virtually unlimited viewing angles to assess the morphologic

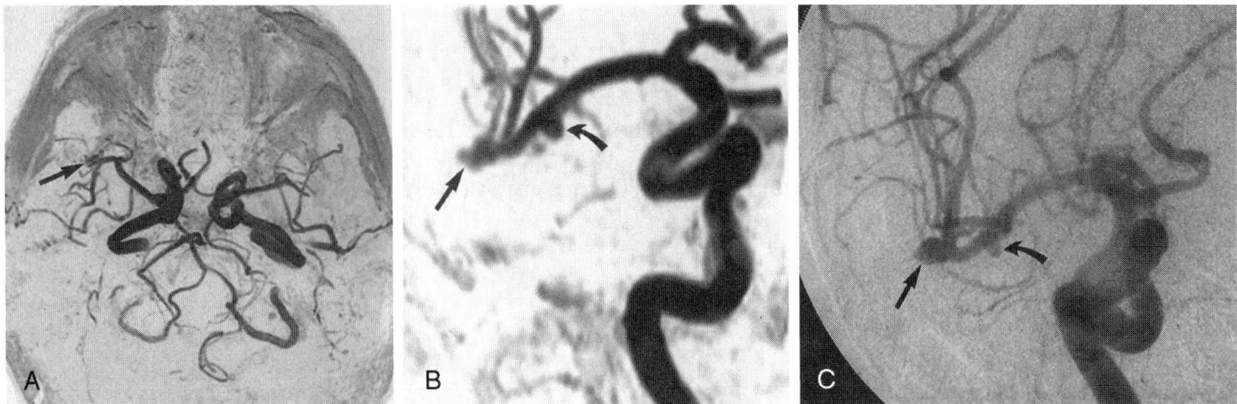

FIGURE 94–26. *A*, Three-dimensional time-of-flight MR angiography shows a laterally directed 3-mm middle cerebral artery trifurcation aneurysm *(arrow)*. *B*, MR angiography subvolume shows the laterally directed aneurysm is bilobed in nature *(straight arrow)* and the presence of a smaller, more proximal aneurysm *(curved arrow)*. *C*, Conventional angiogram confirms the presence of the two middle cerebral artery aneurysms *(straight arrow* and *curved arrow)*.

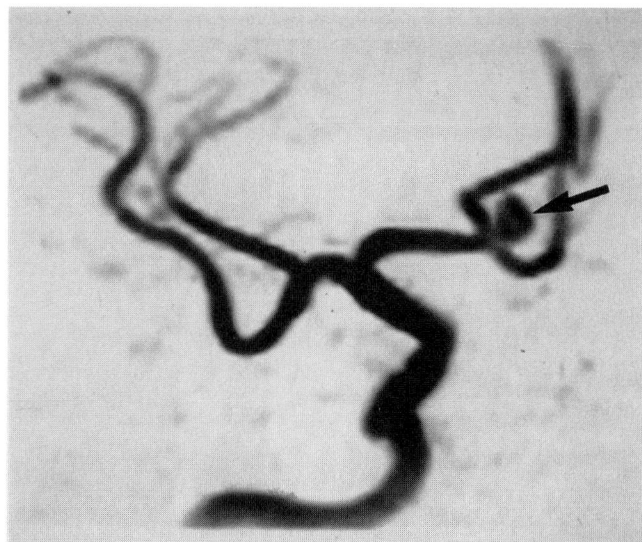

FIGURE 94–27. Three-dimensional time-of-flight MR angiography subvolume shows a 4-mm anterior communicating artery aneurysm *(arrow)* that was an incidental finding. The patient proceeded to surgical clipping without an conventional angiogram.

characteristics of the aneurysms, including the size of the aneurysm neck.

MR angiography occasionally can be used as a problem-solving technique when severe atherosclerotic disease increases the risk of an angiogram or an angiogram fails to identify an aneurysm in the setting of subarachnoid hemorrhage.[56]

An ideal use for MR angiography when an aneurysm has been identified is to monitor the aneurysm for change in size over time (see Fig. 94–10). The noninvasive nature of MR angiography reduces the risk of conventional angiography to a patient. This can have important implications for treatment considerations.

Fusiform aneurysms frequently are associated with thrombus and often involve the basilar artery (Fig. 94–28). The imaging characteristics of MR angiography techniques permit the detection of aneurysms between 3 and 15 mm equally well with PC and TOF. As aneurysm size increases beyond 15 mm, however, the 3D PC technique was progressively superior to 3DTOF. As a pragmatic consideration, aneurysms larger than 1.5 or 2 cm are depicted clearly with standard MR sequences. PC techniques reflect the patent lumen as depicted on conventional angiograms, whereas TOF techniques represent the patent lumen as well as subacute thrombus containing methemoglobin that has a short T1. A partially thrombosed fusiform aneurysm shows the aneurysmal thrombus to be of high T1 signal, which can simulate a patent lumen on a TOF sequence. The role of bolus contrast-enhanced MR angiography in the detection and characterization of intracranial aneurysms remains to be determined.[57]

VASCULAR MALFORMATIONS

Arteriovenous Malformations

Arteriovenous malformations are a congenital abnormality composed of a collection of abnormal vascular channels connecting arteries to veins without passing through a capillary bed. Typically, arteriovenous malformations are a mass of dilated vessels that have no intervening normal brain parenchyma (see Fig. 94–5). In the absence of a high-resistance capillary bed, there is rapid arteriovenous shunting through the malformations. Arteriovenous malformations can be associated with aneurysms involving the feeding arteries. With the use of microcatheters, there has been an increased appreciation of the high frequency of aneurysms within the nidus of the malformations. The high-volume, high-pressure flow through the venous system can result in dilation of draining veins as well as stenosis or occlusion; this occurs most frequently at the point where draining veins enter the dural sinuses. Arteriovenous malformations can occur throughout the brain but most frequently are located in the cerebral hemispheres. Approximately 20% of arteriovenous malformations become symptomatic before the patient turns 20 years old. Symptoms include hemorrhage, seizures, headaches, and progressive neurological deficits.

The risk associated with an arteriovenous malformation can be graded with imaging studies. Features that are associated with worse outcomes include a larger size, central venous drainage, deep location, involvement of eloquent cortex, and presence of aneurysms. MR imaging and MR angiography can help evaluate for all of these risk factors.

TOF and PC MR angiography techniques can have complementary roles in the evaluation of arteriovenous malformations.[58] TOF typically shows the nidus of the arteriovenous malformation and allows determination of the arterial supply. PC techniques are versatile owing to the ability to repeat the studies with multiple VENC values. With a slow velocity encoding, an image can show the internal slow flow within the nidus and the draining veins of an arteriovenous malformation. Using progressively higher velocity encoding, the arterial flow can be identified more clearly, and the slower flow within the nidus and veins is progressively less visible.

MR angiography techniques can reveal information about the flow dynamics of an arteriovenous malformation. Using cine-phase contrast MR angiography, it is possible to measure the blood flow to and from an arteriovenous malformation.[59] This measurement has been particularly useful when documenting a change in the flow after endovascular therapy. A particularly useful application of MR angiography with arteriovenous malformations is following treatment changes after radiosurgery (Fig. 94–29). Serial MR angiography examinations can document the decreasing size and flow through the lesion. When an absence of flow is shown, a single confirmatory conventional angiogram can be performed.

Dural Arteriovenous Fistulas

Dural arteriovenous fistulas consist of arterial-to-venous shunting without the nidus seen in an arteriovenous malformation. It is estimated that dural arteriove-

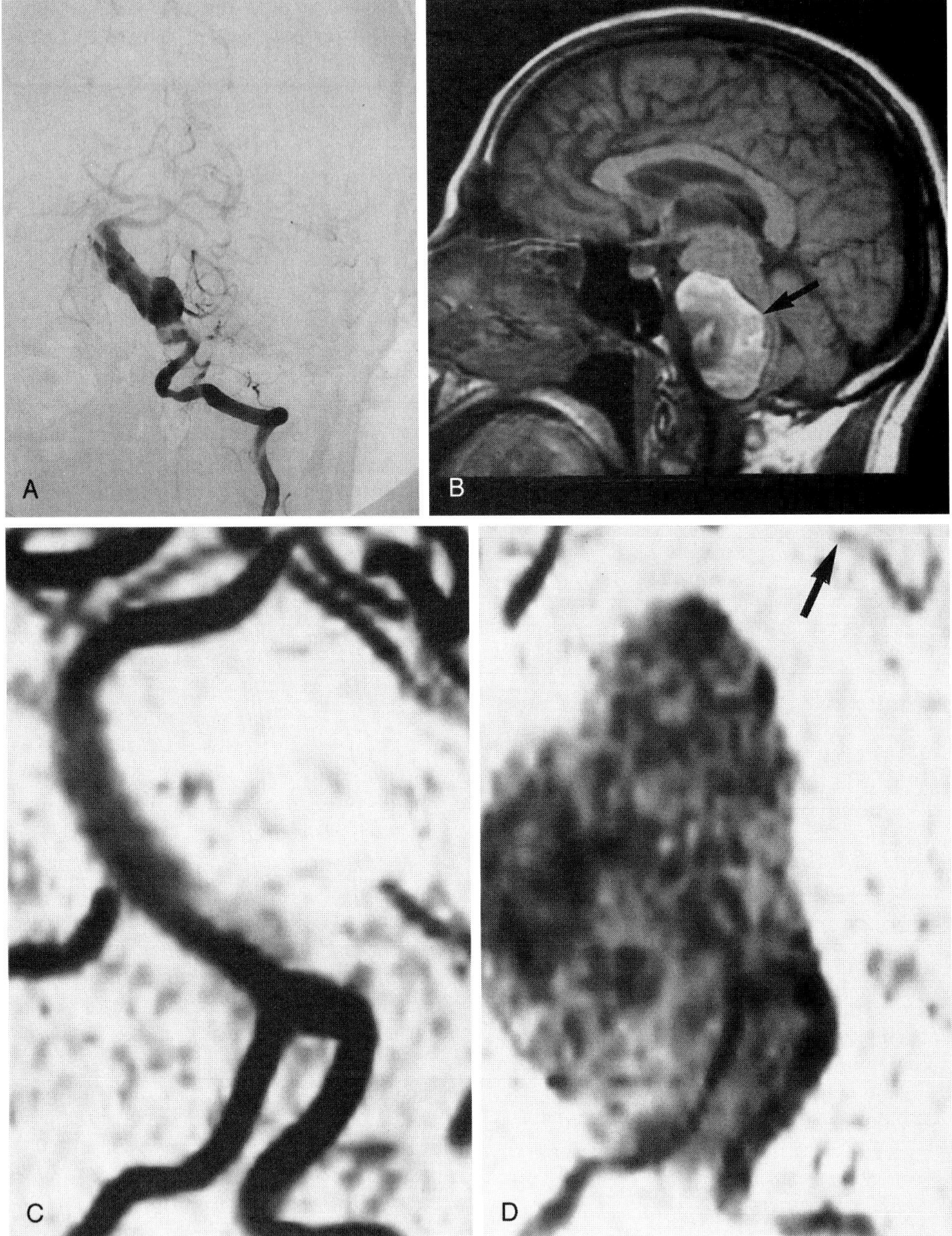

FIGURE 94–28. Partially thrombosed fusiform basilar artery aneurysm. *A*, Conventional angiogram shows the proximal aneurysmal lumen. *B*, Sagittal T1-weighted MR image shows a large amount of subacute thrombus containing methemoglobin extrinsic to the patent lumen *(arrow)*. *C*, Three-dimensional phase contrast (subvolume) is analogous to the conventional angiogram. *D*, Three-dimensional time-of-flight MR angiography does not allow a differentiation of the patent lumen from the subacute thrombus containing methemoglobin. Slow flow resulted in nonvisualization of the distal basilar artery owing to saturation effects. The left posterior cerebral artery *(arrow)* is visualized because of inflow of the unsaturated blood from the anterior circulation.

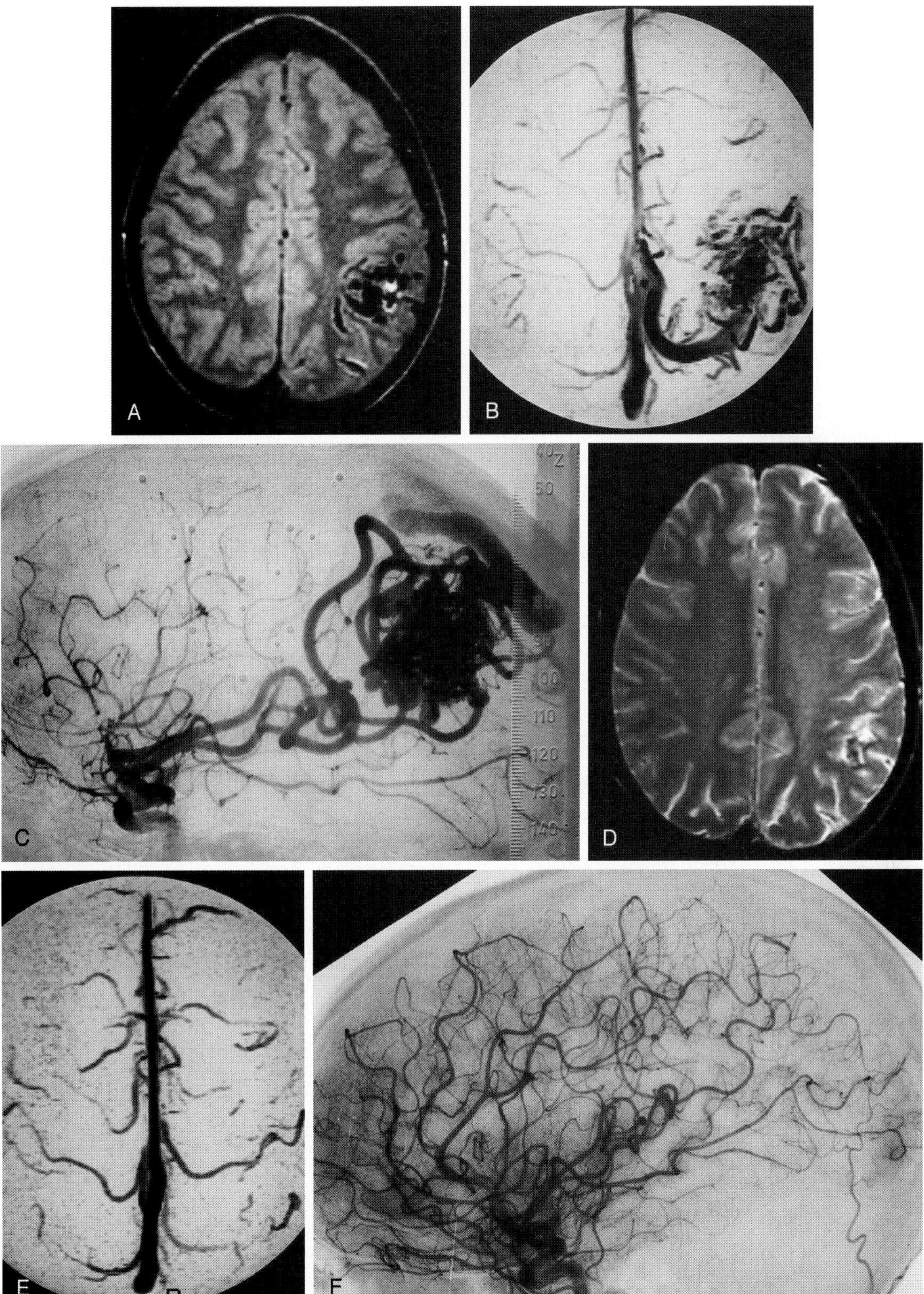

FIGURE 94–29. Left parietal arteriovenous malformation (AVM) treated with gamma-knife radiosurgery. *A,* T2-weighted image shows numerous signal voids corresponding to the AVM nidus. *B,* Two-dimensional phase contrast MR angiogram depicts well the AVM nidus and draining vein to the superior sagittal sinus. *C,* Conventional angiogram obtained during gamma-knife planning. *D,* Two years after therapy, the T2-weighted sequence shows areas of decreased T2 signal that may be confused with signal voids owing to residual AVM. These are areas of hemosiderin that frequently are seen after regression of the AVM after gamma-knife therapy. *E,* Two-dimensional phase contrast MR angiogram shows no evidence of a shunting lesion. *F,* Conventional angiogram confirms ablation of the AVM.

nous fistulas represent 10% of all intracranial vascular malformations. These fistulas are classified by their location and the pattern of venous drainage. In most cases dural arteriovenous fistulas involve the dural sinuses, including the cavernous, transverse, and sigmoid sinuses. The venous drainage can occur directly into the involved sinuses, into a combination of the sinus and cortical veins, or exclusively into the cortical veins. The clinical symptoms associated with dural arteriovenous fistulas often are a result of the route and type of venous drainage (Fig. 94–30).

Most dural arteriovenous fistulas are acquired lesions. One theory regarding the formation of dural arteriovenous fistulas is that after a sinus thrombosis or occlusion, subsequent recanalization results in direct artery-to-venous communications.[60]

MR angiography has a more limited role in the detection and characterization of dural arteriovenous fistulas.[61] MR angiography techniques can detect numerous dilated external carotid branches, occluded dural sinuses, or enlarged cortical veins. MR angiography frequently can miss symptomatic smaller lesions, especially involving the cavernous sinus.

Spinal dural arteriovenous fistulas have a typical clinical picture of an elderly man who presents with progressive weakness in the lower extremities during months to years. Loss of sensation in the low thoracic level frequently is present. Typically, MR imaging shows abnormal T2 signal within an enlarged cord, serpentine flow voids within the thecal sac, and possibly enhancement within the substance of the cord or of the dilated venous structures. Currently, MR angiography has a limited role in the characterization of spinal dural arteriovenous fistulas. Bolus contrast-enhanced techniques may be useful diagnostically in the future (see Fig. 94–19).

VENO-OCCLUSIVE DISEASE

The diagnosis of cerebral veno-occlusive disease is difficult because of the broad spectrum of nonspecific

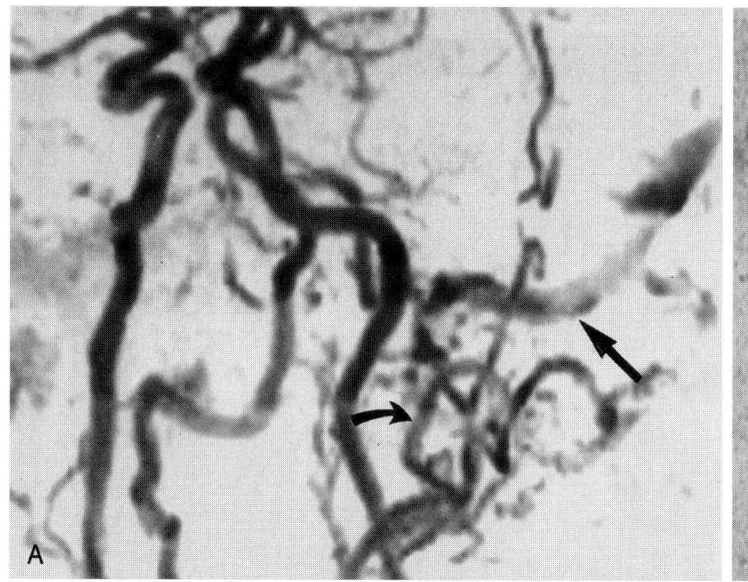

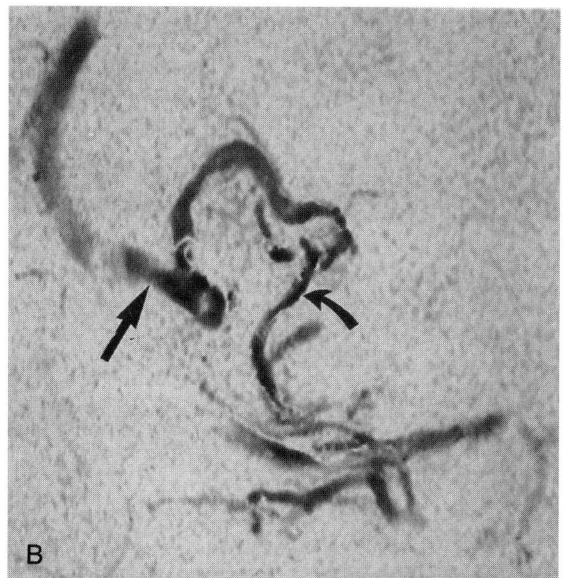

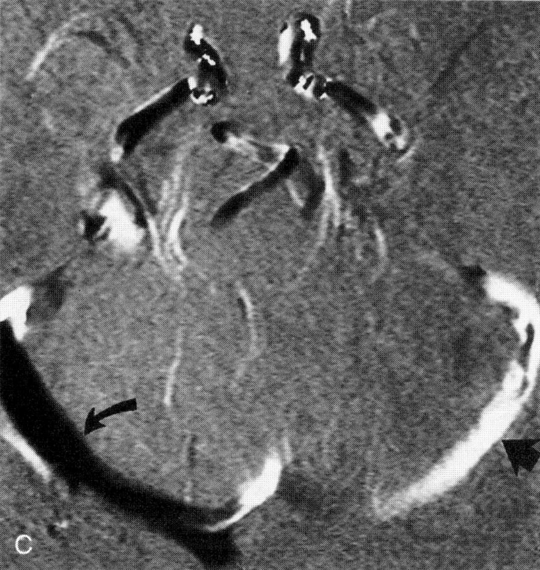

FIGURE 94–30. Dural arteriovenous fistula with retrograde flow in the transverse sinus. *A*, Three-dimensional time-of-flight MR angiogram shows enlarged left external carotid artery branches *(curved arrow)* and a prominent left sigmoid sinus *(straight arrow)*. *B*, Subvolume of the three-dimensional time-of-flight MR angiogram shows more clearly the feeding arteries *(curved arrow)* and sigmoid sinus *(straight arrow)* resulting from the arteriovenous fistula. *C*, Direction encoded two-dimensional phase contrast image shows normal posterior-to-anterior flow in the right transverse sinus *(curved arrow)* as black on a gray background, whereas there is retrograde flow in the left transverse sinus *(straight arrow)* shown as high signal on a gray background.

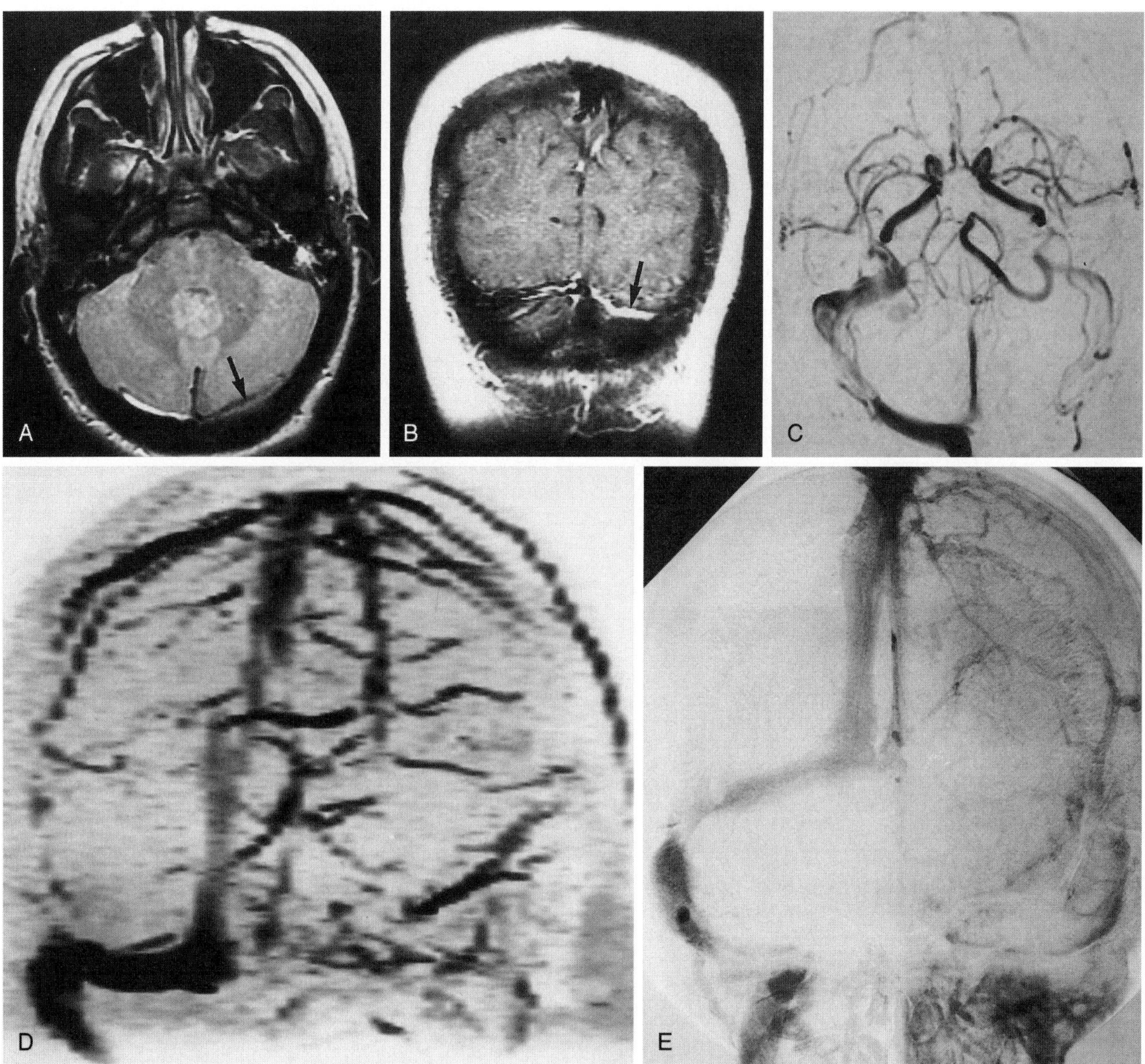

FIGURE 94–31. Thrombosis of the left transverse and sigmoid sinus. *A*, Proton density–weighted image shows equal size transverse sinuses with isointense signal on the left *(arrow)*. *B*, T1-weighted sequence after the administration of contrast material shows enhancement of the left transverse sinus *(arrow)*. Two-dimensional phase contrast *(C)* and two-dimensional time-of-flight *(D)*) images fail to show flow in the left transverse sinus. *E*, Conventional angiogram confirms occlusion of the left transverse and sigmoid sinuses.

symptoms. When interpreted in conjunction with standard imaging, MR angiography can identify thrombosis of the dural sinuses.[62, 63] MR venography can be performed with PC techniques with appropriate slow velocity encoding (e.g., VENC = 10 cm/second). MR venography often is used as a screening technique. Typically the most helpful technique for identifying dural sinus thrombosis is a coronally obtained 2DTOF sequence (Fig. 94–31). A potential pitfall is that thrombus with high T1 signal can mimic flow. The presence or absence of flow can be determined confidently, however, by review of source images and correlation with standard T1 imaging.

REFERENCES

1. Bradley WG Jr: Carmen lecture: Flow phenomena in MR imaging. AJR Am J Roentgenol 150:983–994, 1988.
2. Edelman RR, Mattle HP, Wallner B, et al: Extracranial carotid arteries: Evaluation with "black blood" MR angiography. Radiology 177:45–50, 1990.
3. Alexander AL, Buswell HR, Sun Y, et al: Intracranial black-blood MR angiography with high-resolution 3D fast spin echo. Magn Reson Med 40:298–310, 1998.
4. Felmlee JP, Ehman RL: Spatial presaturation: A method for suppressing flow artifacts and improving depiction of vascular anatomy in MR imaging. Radiology 164:559–564, 1987.
5. Nishimura DG, Jackson JI, Pauly JM: On the nature and reduction of the displacement artifact in flow images. Magn Reson Med 22:481–492, 1991.

6. Frank LR, Crawley AP, Buxton RB: Elimination of oblique flow artifacts in magnetic resonance imaging. Magn Reson Med 25: 299–307, 1992.
7. Schmalbrock P, Yuan C, Chakeres DW, et al: Volume MR angiography: Methods to achieve very short echo times. Radiology 175: 861–865, 1990.
8. Laub G: Displays for MR angiography. Magn Reson Med 14: 222–229, 1990.
9. Keller PJ, Drayer BP, Fram EK, et al: MR angiography with two-dimensional acquisition and three-dimensional display. Radiology 173:527–532, 1989.
10. Doyle M, Matsuda T, Pohost GM: SLIP, a lipid suppression technique to improve image contrast in inflow angiography. Magn Reson Med 21:71–81, 1991.
11. Ruggieri PM, Laub GA, Masaryk TJ, et al: Intracranial circulation: Pulse-sequence considerations in three-dimensional (volume) MR angiography. Radiology 171:785–791, 1989.
12. Parker DL, Yuan C, Blatter DD: MR angiography by multiple thin slab 3D acquisition. Magn Reson Med 17:434–451, 1991.
13. Liu K, Rutt BK: Sliding interleaved kY (SLINKY) acquisition: A novel 3D MRA technique with suppressed slab boundary artifact. J Magn Reson Imaging 8:903–911, 1998.
14. Atkinson D, Brant-Zawadzki M, Gillan G, et al: Improved MR angiography: Magnetization transfer suppression with variable flip angle excitation and increased resolution. Radiology 190: 890–894, 1994.
15. Wolff SD, Balaban RS: Magnetization transfer imaging: Practical aspects and clinical applications. Radiology 192:593–599, 1994.
16. Du YP, Parker DL, Davis WL, et al: Reduction of partial-volume artifacts with zero-filled interpolation in three-dimensional MR angiography. J Magn Reson Imaging 4:733–741, 1994.
17. Moran PR: A flow velocity zeugmatographic interlace for NMR imaging in humans. Magn Reson Imaging 1:197–203, 1982.
18. Pelc NJ, Sommer FG, Li KC, et al: Quantitative magnetic resonance flow imaging. Magn Reson Q 10:125–147, 1994.
19. Bernstein MA, Ikezaki Y: Comparison of phase-difference and complex-difference processing in phase-contrast MR angiography. J Magn Reson Imaging 1:725–729, 1991.
20. Pelc NJ, Bernstein MA, Shimakawa A, et al: Encoding strategies for three-direction phase-contrast MR imaging of flow. J Magn Reson Imaging 1:405–413, 1991.
21. Dumoulin CL, Souza SP, Walker MF, et al: Three-dimensional phase contrast angiography. Magn Reson Med 9:139–149, 1989.
22. Tang C, Blatter DD, Parker DL: Accuracy of phase-contrast flow measurements in the presence of partial-volume effects. J Magn Reson Imaging 3:377–385, 1993.
23. Wolf RL, Ehman RL, Riederer SJ, et al: Analysis of systematic and random error in MR volumetric flow measurements. Magn Reson Med 30:82–91, 1993.
24. Marks MP, Pelc NJ, Ross MR, et al: Determination of cerebral blood flow with a phase-contrast cine MR imaging technique: Evaluation of normal subjects and patients with arteriovenous malformations. Radiology 182:467–476, 1992.
25. Foo TK, Bernstein MA, Aisen AM, et al: Improved ejection fraction and flow velocity estimates with use of view sharing and uniform repetition time excitation with fast cardiac techniques. Radiology 195:471–478, 1995.
26. Prince MR: Gadolinium-enhanced MR aortography. Radiology 191:155–164, 1994.
27. Wilman AH, Riederer SJ, King BF, et al: Fluoroscopically triggered contrast-enhanced three-dimensional MR angiography with elliptical centric view order: Application to the renal arteries. Radiology 205:137–146, 1997.
28. Foo TK, Saranathan M, Prince MR, et al: Automated detection of bolus arrival and initiation of data acquisition in fast, three-dimensional, gadolinium-enhanced MR angiography. Radiology 203:275–280, 1997.
29. Kim JK, Farb RI, Wright GA: Test bolus examination in the carotid artery at dynamic gadolinium-enhanced MR angiography. Radiology 206:283–289, 1998.
30. Mistretta CA, Grist TM, Korosec FR, et al: 3D time-resolved contrast-enhanced MR DSA: Advantages and tradeoffs. Magn Reson Med 40:571–581, 1998.
31. Vigen KK, Peters DC, Grist TM, et al: Undersampled projection-reconstruction imaging for time-resolved contrast-enhanced imaging. Magn Reson Med 43:170–176, 2000.
32. North American Symptomatic Carotid Endarterectomy Trial Collaborators: Beneficial effect of carotid endarterectomy in symptomatic patients with high-grade carotid stenosis. N Engl J Med 325:445–453, 1991.
33. Heiserman JE, Drayer BP, Fram EK: Carotid artery stenosis: Clinical efficacy of two-dimensional time-of-flight MR angiography. Radiology 182:761–768, 1992.
34. Litt AW, Eidelman EM, Pinto RS, et al: Diagnosis of carotid artery stenosis: Comparison of 2DFT time-of-flight MR angiography with contrast angiography in 50 patients. AJNR Am J Neuroradiol 12:149–154, 1991.
35. Huston J III, Lewis BD, Wiebers DO, et al: Carotid artery: Prospective blinded comparison of two-dimensional time-of-flight MR angiography with conventional angiography and duplex US. Radiology 186:339–344, 1993.
36. Blatter DD, Bahr AL, Parker DL, et al: Cervical carotid MR angiography with multiple overlapping thin-slab acquisition: Comparison with conventional angiography. AJR Am J Roentgenol 161:1269–1277, 1993.
37. Huston J, Nichols DA, Luetmer PH, et al: MR angiographic and sonographic indications for endarterectomy. AJNR Am J Neuroradiol 19:309–315, 1998.
38. Huston J III, Fain SB, Riederer SJ, et al: Carotid arteries: Maximizing arterial to venous contrast in fluoroscopically triggered contrast-enhanced MR angiography with elliptical centric view ordering. Radiology 211:265–273, 1999.
39. Leclerc X, Martinat P, Godefroy O, et al: Contrast-enhanced three-dimensional fast imaging with steady-state precession (FISP) MR angiography of supraaortic vessels: Preliminary results. AJNR Am J Neuroradiol 19:1405–1413, 1998.
40. Krinsky G, Menahem M, Rofsky N, et al: Gadolinium-enhanced 3D MRA of the aortic arch vessels in the detection of atherosclerotic cerebrovascular occlusive disease. J Comput Assist Tomogr 22:167–178, 1998.
41. Mokri BN, Sundt TM Jr, Houser OW, et al: Spontaneous dissection of the cervical internal carotid artery. Ann Neurol 19:126–138, 1986.
42. Schievink WI, Mokri BN, Whisnant JP: Internal carotid artery dissection in a community: Rochester, Minnesota, 1987–1992. Stroke 24:1678–1680, 1993.
43. Houser OW, Mokri BN, Sundt TM Jr, et al: Spontaneous cervical cephalic arterial dissection and its residuum: Angiographic spectrum. AJNR Am J Neuroradiol 5:27–34, 1984.
44. Goldberg HI, Grossman RI, Gomori JM, et al: Cervical internal carotid artery dissecting hemorrhage: Diagnosis using MR[1]. Radiology 158:157–161, 1986.
45. Brugieres P, Castrec-Carpo A, Heran F, et al: Magnetic resonance imaging in the exploration of dissection of internal carotid artery. J Neuroradiol 16:1–15, 1989.
46. Bui LN, Brant-Zawadzki M, Verghese P, et al: Magnetic resonance angiography of cervicocranial dissection. Stroke 24:126–131, 1993.
47. Levy C, Laissy JP, Raveau V, et al: Carotid and vertebral artery dissections: Three-dimensional time-of-flight MR angiography and MR imaging versus conventional angiography. Radiology 190:97–103, 1994.
48. Leclerc X, Lucas C, Godefroy O, et al: Preliminary experience using contrast-enhanced MR angiography to assess vertebral artery structure for the follow-up of suspected dissection. AJNR Am J Neuroradiol 20:1482–1490, 1999.
49. Houspian EM, Pool JL: A systematic analysis of intracranial aneurysms from the autopsy file of Presbyterian Hospital, 1914–1956. J Neuropathol Exp Neurol 17:409–423, 1958.
50. Atkinson JLD, Sundt TM, Houser OW, et al: Angiographic frequency of anterior circulation intracranial aneurysms. J Neurosurg 70:551–555, 1989.
51. Wiebers DO, Whisnant JP, Sundt TM, et al: The significance of unruptured intracranial saccular aneurysms. J Neurosurg 66: 23–29, 1987.
52. Huston J III, Ehman RL: Comparison of time-of-flight and phase-contrast MR neuroangiographic techniques. Radiographics 13: 5–19, 1993.
53. Huston J III, Torres VE, Sullivan PP, et al: Value of magnetic resonance angiography for the detection of intracranial aneurysms in autosomal dominant polycystic kidney disease. J Am Soc Nephrol 3:1871–1877, 1993.

54. Huston J III, Nichols DA, Luetmer PH, et al: Blinded prospective evaluation of sensitivity of MR angiography to known intracranial aneurysms: Importance of aneurysm size. AJNR Am J Neuroradiol 15:1607–1614, 1994.
55. Chung TS, Joo JY, Lee SK, et al: Evaluation of cerebral aneurysms with high-resolution MR angiography using a section-interpolation technique: Correlation with digital subtraction angiography. AJNR Am J Neuroradiol 20:229–235, 1999.
56. Curnes JT, Shogry MEC, Clark DC, et al: MR angiographic demonstration of an intracranial aneurysm not seen on conventional angiography. AJNR Am J Neuroradiol 14:971–973, 1993.
57. Wiebers DO, and The International Study of Unruptured Intracranial Aneurysms Investigators: Unruptured intracranial aneurysms—risk of rupture and risks of surgical intervention. N Engl J Med 339:1725–1733, 1998.
58. Huston J III, Rufenacht DA, Ehman RL, et al: Intracranial aneurysms and vascular malformations: Comparison of time-of-flight and phase-contrast MR angiography. Radiology 181:721–730, 1991.
59. Marks MP, Pelc NJ, Ross MR, et al: Determination of cerebral blood flow with a phase-contrast cine MR imaging technique: Evaluation of normal subjects and patients with arteriovenous malformations. Radiology 182:467–476, 1992.
60. Houser OW, Campbell JK, Campbell RJ, et al: Arteriovenous malformation affecting the transverse dural venous sinus—an acquired lesion. Mayo Clin Proc 54:651–661, 1979.
61. Chen JC, Tsuruda JS, Halbach VV: Suspected dural arteriovenous fistula: Results with screening MR angiography in seven patients. Radiology 183:265–271, 1992.
62. Vogl TJ, Bergman C, Villringer A, et al: Dural sinus thrombosis: Value of venous MR angiography for diagnosis and follow-up. AJR Am J Roentgenol 162:1191–1198, 1994.
63. Wasenko JJ, Holsapple JW, Winfield JA: Cerebral venous thrombosis demonstration with magnetic resonance angiography. Clin Imaging 19:153–161, 1995.

CHAPTER 95

Positron Emission Tomography in Cerebrovascular Disease

JEAN-CLAUDE BARON

The advent of imaging of brain perfusion and metabolism by means of positron emission tomography (PET) in the late 1970s and early 1980s afforded new pathophysiologic insights into the understanding of acute cerebral ischemia, the hemodynamic and metabolic effects of carotid artery obstruction, and the neurobiologic mechanisms underlying the neurological expression of stroke and recovery. This new understanding has had major effects on patient management. It has become possible to test the concepts issued from PET in large patient samples thanks to widely available techniques such as single-photon emission tomography (SPECT) and diffusion-weighted and perfusion-weighted magnetic resonance (MR) imaging. This chapter discusses the major findings with PET in cerebrovascular disease with occasional reference to SPECT findings whenever they significantly contributed to present-day understanding.

VARIABLES AND TECHNIQUES

Variables

Table 95–1 lists the main physiologic variables assessable by functional imaging in humans and their commonly used abbreviations. The hemodynamic reserve expresses the vasodilatory capacity of the cerebrovascular bed and is assessed with vasodilation challenge, such as inhalation of 5% carbon dioxide (CO_2) or intravenous injection of acetazolamide (Fig. 95–1; see color section in this volume).

TABLE 95–1 ■ **Physiologic Variables**

PHYSIOLOGIC VARIABLE	ABBREVIATION
Cerebral blood flow	CBF
Cerebral blood volume	CBV
Mean transit time	MTT
Hemodynamic reserve	HR
CBF/CBV ratio	CBF/CBV
Local tissue hematocrit	tHt
Cerebral metabolic rate of oxygen	$CMRO_2$
Cerebral metabolic rate of glucose	CMRG
Tissular pH	pHt
Oxygen extraction fraction	OEF
Glucose extraction fraction	GEF
Tissue partial O_2 tension	PtO_2

Positron Emission Tomography Techniques

Using ^{15}O-labeled tracers such as water (H_2O), CO_2, carbon monoxide (CO), and oxygen (O_2), and the glucose analogue ^{18}F-fluoro-2-deoxy-D-glucose (FDG), PET allows the clinician to obtain quantitative tomographic

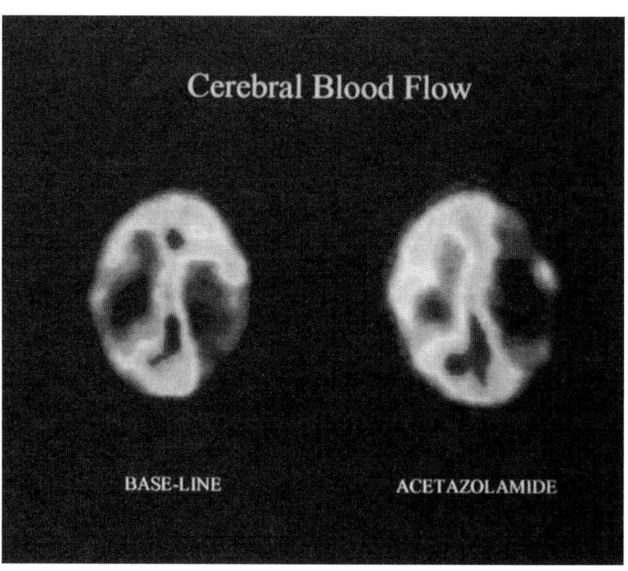

FIGURE 95–1. Impaired hemodynamic reserve. Resting and post-acetazolamide PET of cerebral blood flow (CBF) in a patient with repeated transient ischemic attacks owing to left internal carotid artery occlusion with revascularization through the ipsilateral ophthalmic artery and the contralateral internal carotid artery. Although the resting scan (*left*) showed little or no alteration in CBF in the affected hemisphere, the vasodilation challenge (*right*) induces a marked increase in CBF in the unoccluded side, but no increase in CBF on the occluded side with a decrease in the posterior and anterior parts of the left carotid territory, suggesting hemodynamic steal (see color section in this volume).

maps of cerebral blood flow (CBF), cerebral blood volume (CBV), cerebral metabolic rate of oxygen ($CMRO_2$), oxygen extraction fraction (OEF), and brain glucose utilization (CMRG) and as such is especially well suited for the investigation of ischemic stroke.[1] Access to CBF and CBV allows one to compute the CBV/CBF ratio, which represents the local circulatory mean transit time, and its corollary the CBF/CBV ratio, which reflects the local cerebral perfusion pressure (CPP).[2–4] Of interest for cerebrovascular disease are three specific markers: (1) ^{11}C-flumazenil, a radioligand specific for the neuronal benzodiazepine receptor[5]; (2) ^{11}C-PK 11-195, a radioligand of the peripheral benzodiazepine receptor, borne only by glial cells[5, 6]; and (3) ^{18}F-fluoro-misonidazole, a marker of tissue hypoxia presently under investigation as a potential marker of the ischemic penumbra.[7]

NORMAL PHYSIOLOGY AND BASIC PATHOPHYSIOLOGY

Normal Brain

In physiologic conditions, there exists a matching of local values of CBF, CMRG, $CMRO_2$, and CBV, according to linearly proportional relationships.[3, 8] This matching reflects the metabolic regulation of the cerebral circulation, such that in physiologic conditions the distribution of CBF is superimposable on that of $CMRO_2$ and CMRG. As shown subsequently, this coupling between perfusion, $CMRO_2$, and CMRG is preserved in areas exhibiting reduced metabolism owing to disconnection effects.

Autoregulation and Hemodynamic Failure

Table 95–2 shows the main hemodynamic and metabolic changes that occur in response to a fall in the CPP distal to an arterial obstruction, subdivided into four stages of increasing severity.[9–11] During the phase of *autoregulation*, when the CBF remains unchanged, there is a marked increase in CBV, which reflects the vasodilation of resistance vessels, tapping the hemodynamic reserve. This phase is identifiable as normal resting CBF with partial or complete loss of CBF reactivity to CO_2 inhalation or acetazolamide or even with a paradoxical CBF decrease (*hemodynamic steal*) (see Fig. 95–1). As soon as the CPP falls below the lower threshold of autoregulation, the CBF starts to decline, but the $CMRO_2$ at first remains unaltered, tapping the *perfusion reserve*. This flow-metabolism uncoupling translates as a focal increase in the OEF (up to the theoretical maximum of 1.00) and has been termed *misery* perfusion (Fig. 95–2; see color section in this volume).[12] In the moderate stage of misery perfusion, the brain is able to maintain $CMRO_2$ despite reduced CBF, at the expense of tissue hypoxia (see Fig. 95–2). This phase is designated as *oligemia*. If the CPP drops further, neuronal function becomes impaired, and the $CMRO_2$ falls despite maximally increased OEF, characterizing true ischemia, which initially is reversible (the *ischemic penumbra*) and thereafter becomes irreversible (i.e., *impending necrosis*) (Fig. 95–3; see color section in this volume). As shown in Table 95–2, PET studies in acute stroke have identified operational probabilistic voxel-based CBF and $CMRO_2$ thresholds for these stages (see more detailed discussion later).

Luxury Perfusion

Luxury perfusion is characterized by an oxygen supply in excess of demand,[13] and its hallmark is a focal reduction of the OEF.[9] It indicates full or partial reestablishment of perfusion within ischemic or already irreversibly damaged tissue (see Fig. 95–3). In luxury perfusion, the CBF may be increased (hyperperfusion), normal, or decreased (relative luxury perfusion), although by definition in excess of prevailing $CMRO_2$, which itself may be normal, increased, or reduced.

LONG-STANDING ARTERIAL OBSTRUCTION: MAPPING HEMODYNAMIC FAILURE

Hemodynamic Reserve and Misery Perfusion

Misery perfusion originally was described in a patient with internal carotid artery occlusion and continuing reversible ischemic attacks, some triggered by standing up.[12] PET and SPECT studies have documented repeatedly that *carotid artery disease* may have hemodynamic consequences on the distal cerebral vascular bed.[14–20]

TABLE 95–2 ■ **Four Stages of Brain Hemodynamic and Metabolic Impairment as a Function of Severity in Cerebral Perfusion Pressure Drop**

STAGE	CPP	CBV	CBF	OEF	$CMRO_2$
1—Autoregulation	60–100%	↑	N	N	N
2—Oligemia	40–60%	↑↑	17–50 mL/100 mL/min*	↑	N
3—Ischemic penumbra	20–40%	↑	7–17 mL/100 mL/min*	↑↑	>0.76 mL/100 mL/min†
4—Impending necrosis	<20%	↓	<8.4 mL/100 mL/min†	↑ to ↓	<0.76 mL/100 mL/min†

*Data from Furlan et al.[73]
†Data from Marchal et al.[67]
CPP, cerebral perfusion pressure; CBV, cerebral blood volume; CBF, cerebral blood flow; OEF, oxygen extraction fraction; $CMRO_2$, cerebral metabolic rate of oxygen.

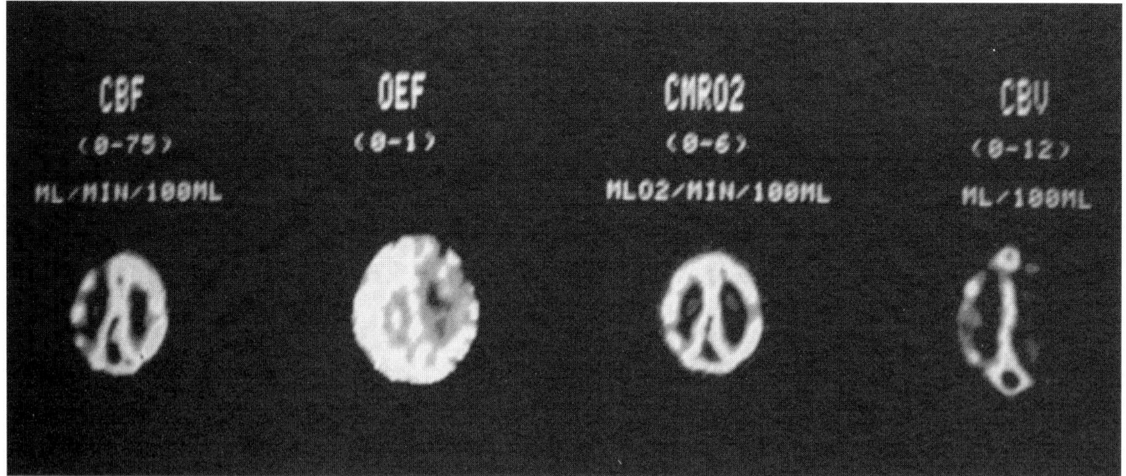

FIGURE 95–2. Misery perfusion: stage 2 of hemodynamic failure. Occlusion of the right internal carotid artery was diagnosed when the patient presented after an ipsilateral transient ischemic attack. Repeated transient ischemic attacks followed despite closely supervised antiplatelet and anticoagulant treatment. Some of the transient ischemic attacks were triggered on standing. PET performed several weeks later showed moderate hypoperfusion in the territory of the right carotid artery with a completely normal cerebral metabolic rate of oxygen. As a result, the oxygen extraction fraction was increased, causing *misery perfusion.* These data suggest inability of the collateral circulation to compensate fully for occlusion of the carotid artery and that the pressure of the blood supply to the brain downstream of the circle of Willis is insufficient to maintain cerebral blood flow (i.e., the local autoregulation mechanism has been overcome). This interpretation is supported by the observation of a marked increase in the cerebral blood volume on the side of the occlusion (see color section in this volume).

These studies also indicate that the severity of these hemodynamic disturbances is related to the degree of carotid artery obstruction (i.e., only >50% stenosis or occlusion appear to have measurable effects) as well as to the compensation afforded by the circle of Willis (with the most marked effects seen when compensation is essentially or exclusively through the ipsilateral ophthalmic artery). Other authors have found no relationship between the collateralization pattern and the OEF increase, however.[21] Similar effects have been reported in patients with long-standing middle cerebral artery (MCA) trunk stenosis or occlusion.[22, 23]

The hemodynamic effects observed, which reflect the extent to which the CPP is reduced, range from simply autoregulated (i.e., with normal resting CBF but increased CBV, reduced CBF/CBV ratio, and reduced vasodilatory capacity to CO_2 or acetazolamide stress) to true oligemia (i.e., reduced resting CBF, increased OEF, increased CBV, markedly reduced CBF/CBV ratio, and abolished vasodilatory capacity with occasional hemodynamic steal) (see Figs. 95–1 and 95–2).[2, 24–26] Whatever their severity, these changes often (but not always) predominate in watershed (border zone) territories.[14, 17, 27] Focal chronic misery perfusion has been documented as a forerunner of the development of watershed infarction in occasional patients with tight carotid artery stenosis or occlusion.[28, 29]

Regarding the specific case of moyamoya disease, the available PET data[30–33] indicate the presence of clear-cut hemodynamic insufficiency in the childhood-onset type (with transient ischemic attacks and ischemic strokes only as clinical manifestations) and in the adult-onset type (with transient ischemic attacks or brain hemorrhages or both). Impaired vasoreactivity to CO_2 inhalation or intravenous acetazolamide and reduced CBF/CBV ratio especially in the cerebral cortex have been reported, with misery perfusion observed in a fraction of the cases only and more frequently in children than in adults.

Few PET studies of *vertebrobasilar insufficiency* have been reported. This paucity of studies may be due at least in part to the lack of clear operational clinical criteria defining this entity and to the limitations of physiologic imaging in the posterior fossa. One study of eight patients reported significant reductions in CBF and increases in OEF with significant improvement after posterior fossa bypass surgery, but these changes were widespread to the whole brain, which was interpreted by the authors as reflecting chronic ischemia of autonomic brainstem centers[34]; the $PaCO_2$ was not reported. In a patient with symptoms of subclavian steal and multiple arterial obstructions resulting from Takayasu's arteritis, a PET study revealed hemodynamic effects of left arm exercise on CBF and OEF, but these effects were not confined to the posterior circulation.[35] Using SPECT, a clear-cut impaired vasodilatory response in the right cerebellum and occipital cortices, but not in the anterior circulation, was observed in a patient with bilateral vertebral artery disease and posterior circulation transient ischemic attacks; the patient went on to develop an infarct in the same areas depicted as abnormal by SPECT.[36] This seems to be the only example with clear-cut vertebrobasilar hemodynamic impairment reported so far.

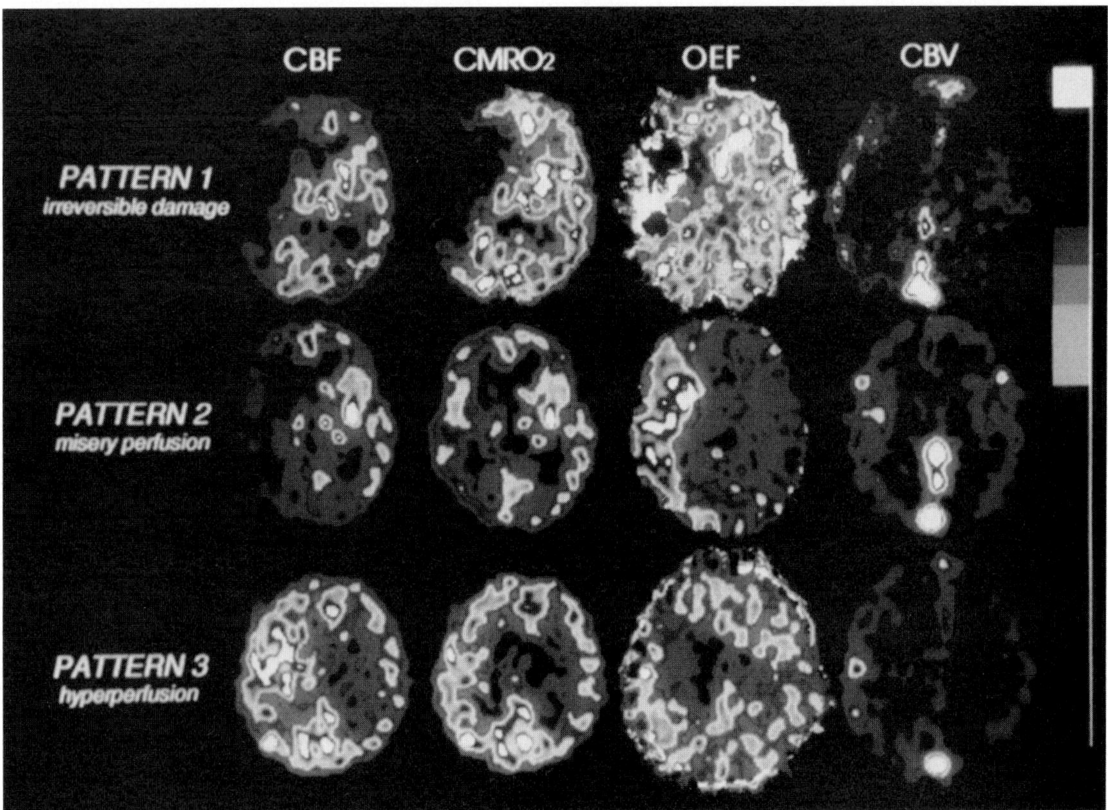

FIGURE 95–3. Illustrative PET patterns in acute middle cerebral artery (MCA) territory stroke. The three PET patterns of cerebral blood flow (CBF) and cerebral metabolic rate of oxygen ($CMRO_2$) changes observed within 18 hours of onset of MCA territory stroke. *Top row,* An example of *early extensive irreversible damage* in a patient with right-sided MCA territory stroke studied with PET 17 hours after symptom onset. There was a near-zero CBF and $CMRO_2$ in the whole right MCA territory (*pattern 1*), together with patchy oxygen extraction fraction (OEF) (black pixels represent unmeasurable OEF). The patient survived, but outcome was poor, and the whole MCA territory was infarcted at follow-up CT. *Middle row, Misery perfusion* in this patient with acute stage right MCA territory stroke. The PET study performed 12 hours after onset revealed a markedly reduced CBF in the whole right MCA territory, associated with relatively preserved $CMRO_2$ (except in the lenticulostriate area) and extremely elevated OEF. This example corresponds to a typical *pattern 2* of PET changes. This patient died 3 days after the PET study. *Bottom row,* An example of *early luxury perfusion* (*pattern 3*) in a patient studied with PET 13 hours after onset of right-sided MCA territory stroke. There is markedly increased CBF in the central right MCA territory, associated with normal or slightly increased $CMRO_2$ and decreased OEF. This patient made a full recovery, and the follow-up CT scan showed a small periventricular infarct (see color section in this volume).

Clinical Correlates and Implications for Therapy

The clinical correlates of these hemodynamic changes can be straightforward, as in the rare instances of orthostatic transient ischemic attacks.[12] In many instances, however, they are difficult to ascertain in the individual case because hemodynamic abnormalities can be found in asymptomatic subjects or in the asymptomatic hemisphere of symptomatic subjects. Nevertheless, a significant relationship exists between the presence of high OEF and that of ipsilateral ischemic symptoms.[37]

After the early report of Baron and colleagues,[12] many studies documented that successful cerebral revascularization, be it by means of carotid endarterectomy, superficial temporal artery–MCA (STA-MCA) bypass, or encephaloduroarteriosynangiosis, at least partially reverses the preoperatively observed hemodynamic compromise.[12, 14, 15, 38–43] This result also applies to moyamoya disease.[44, 45]

In the early 1980s, the documentation of a clear-cut compromise of brain circulation distal to internal carotid artery occlusion was advocated by some as the only rational basis for STA-MCA bypass in symptomatic patients.[12] This surgical procedure subsequently was shown to lack significant clinical benefit in a randomized study, which, however, was criticized for not having used physiologic imaging as an entry criterion.[46] Consistent with this, two retrospective nonrandomized studies from Powers' group[47, 48] suggested that the finding of hemodynamic compromise accurately predicted neither poor outcome if medical therapy was elected nor good outcome if STA-MCA bypass was performed. This view was disputed by several open studies, however, which concluded that severely impaired cerebrovascular reactivity carries a significantly increased risk of ipsilateral stroke despite best medical treatment.[15, 49–54] Formal confirmation was provided by the results of a prospective study of 81 patients with symptomatic internal carotid artery occlusion,[55] which showed in the subgroup with misery perfusion an increased risk of ipsilateral stroke at follow-up, with an odds ratio of 7.3 (P = .004). Based on this evidence, several authors now advocate the design of a new STA-MCA bypass study in which the selection of the patients would be based on the presence of clear hemodynamic compromise ascertained by imaging studies.[11, 56]

Patients with the most compromised cerebrovascular physiology also may be those most at risk of perioperative complications, such as low-pressure breakthrough of autoregulation with hyperperfusion, which results from long-term dysregulation of the cerebral circulation.[14, 15, 57] Also, in patients with carotid occlusion and no interval stroke in the follow-up, there is a tendency for the hemodynamic disturbances to resolve spontaneously, probably as a result of development of collaterals.[58] The results from functional imaging of each candidate for revascularization surgery need to be weighed carefully in relation to other clinical and instrumental data to assess the risk-to-benefit ratio of the surgical procedure under consideration.

Impaired brain hemodynamics in a patient with carotid artery disease should be considered in planning the medical management. For instance, systemic hypotension (as a result of drug therapy or any surgical procedure, especially cardiac) should be avoided carefully. Because embolic events may have more serious tissue consequences in a dysregulated vascular bed than they would in normal brain, medical measures to prevent embolism always should be considered.

ARTERIOVENOUS MALFORMATIONS

The use of PET in arteriovenous malformations (AVMs) is of theoretical interest because this technique in principle should allow identification of hemodynamic steal in brain areas surrounding the nidus in the form of reduced CBF/CBV ratio (or increased CBV/CBF ratio), exhausted hemodynamic reserve, and decrease in CBF during a vasodilation challenge or even in the form of misery perfusion. As reviewed elsewhere,[59] the hypothesis of hemodynamic steal as a mechanism for the occurrence of transient or fluctuating neurological deficits and postoperative *hyperperfusion syndrome* in AVMs has received some support from direct intraoperative measurements of the CPP and tissue perfusion. Studies of CBF alone performed in awake subjects outside the operating room have been inconclusive, however, or even paradoxical.[60] PET methods of perfusion and $CMRO_2$ measurement are not well suited for the assessment of AVMs for model reasons. All models make the assumption that the blood pool in the voxels is either negligible or small enough to be corrected accurately by means of the CBV scan.[1] In the case of AVMs, however, the large blood pools resulting from dilated draining veins may violate this assumption and cause errors in the calculated values not only of CBV, but also of CBF, the CBF/CBV ratio, the OEF, and the $CMRO_2$.[1] This problem presumably explains the nonphysiologic CBV values reported in some AVM PET studies. Although it should be possible to exclude from the analysis all the voxels above a given CBV value, this may lead to exclusion of large parts of the parenchyma, especially that surrounding the AVM itself.

With these caveats, all PET studies published so far tend to indicate the presence of hemodynamic disturbances in AVMs.[61–63] In one study, increased CBV/CBF ratio was observed in the hemisphere ipsilateral to the AVM in small lesions and in both hemispheres in large lesions.[61] In another study, a similar finding was observed in the tissue adjacent to the nidus, but the available data were interpreted as inconsistent with a steal mechanism.[63] Reduced CBF has been observed repeatedly, but unexpectedly accompanied by a normal or reduced OEF instead of the increased OEF that would be predicted by the steal hypothesis. Accordingly, reductions in $CMRO_2$ and especially of CMRG in the tissue around an AVM, in the whole affected hemisphere, and to a lesser extent in the opposite hemisphere have been reported. The interpretation given for this finding is that it may represent synapse or neuron loss resulting from long-standing reductions in CPP. Overall the available PET studies not only weakly support the steal hypothesis, but also have produced unclear findings that may be affected by methodologic artifacts. Clinical correlations have not been assessed completely, and the clinical relevance of these findings is unclear.

ACUTE ISCHEMIC STROKE: MAPPING THE CORE, PENUMBRA, AND REPERFUSED TISSUE

In this chapter, the acute stage of stroke is defined as the first 24 hours after onset of clinical symptoms because available evidence suggests this is the time window within which salvageable tissue might be expected to be present. Only a brief summary of the events that occur after this initial period is given here (see Baron[64, 65] for further details). Also, because MCA territory stroke is the most common and the prototype of acute ischemic stroke and has been the subject of all acute stroke PET studies so far, only this stroke subtype is dealt with here.

Three findings have been investigated in detail with respect to their time course and their prognostic value for tissue and clinical outcome: (1) the ischemic core (defined here as the *irreversibly damaged tissue* already present at time of imaging), (2) the *penumbral tissue* (defined as the tissue that could be saved from infarction by appropriate measures), and (3) the *hyperperfused tissue* (defined as the tissue with CBF higher than that in the contralateral homologous tissue).

Irreversibly Damaged Tissue

The ischemic core is characterized by a $CMRO_2$ value below a threshold of about 1.4 mL/100 mL/minute for gray matter regions,[8, 66] or about 0.9 mL/100 mL/minute for any voxel in brain tissue.[67] The corresponding values for CBF are approximately 12 and 8.5 mL/100 g/minute, although it is likely that these values depend on time since occlusion, as shown in the awake monkey.[68] In a large proportion of patients, irreversible damage affects the striatum early, associated in most instances with cortical misery perfusion.[69, 70] Presumably because of its end-artery system, and in contrast to the cerebral cortex, which has collaterals, the lenticulostriate territory constitutes the initial ischemic core and rapidly suffers irreversible damage. In a subset of patients, the area of irreversible damage affects extensive parts of the cortical territory only hours into stroke,[69–71] suggesting inadequate pial collaterals (see Fig. 95–3). These profoundly hypometabolic areas express variable CBF and in turn variable OEF. In most instances, however, the CBF also is reduced profoundly (see earlier), but partial reperfusion with variably reduced or nearly normal CBF occasionally is encountered, especially in small deep infarcts.[72]

Marchal and associates[67] found that the volume of severely hypometabolic or hypoperfused voxels (below the aforementioned thresholds) as assessed with PET 5 and 18 hours postonset, was highly linearly correlated to final infarct volume, as measured by computed tomography (CT) scanning about 1 month later. The former underestimated the latter by a factor of 2, however, because of subsequent metabolic deterioration of the penumbra (see later). Mapping the ischemic core in the acute stage of stroke provides an early assessment of already established damage and helps predict the volume of final infarction.

Penumbral Tissue

One major finding from PET has been the demonstration, hours into the episode, of wide zones of cortex with still critically ischemic tissue (see Fig. 95–3).[9, 69–71] This tissue is characterized by reduced CBF (below the penumbral threshold of approximately 20 mL/100 g/minute), massively increased OEF (often >0.80), and mildly to moderately reduced $CMRO_2$ (i.e., above the threshold for viability). These alterations are consistent with at-risk but still recuperable (i.e., penumbral) tissue. In their detailed voxel-based analysis of 11 patients studied within 5 to 18 hours after clinical onset of stroke, Furlan and coworkers[73] found that the range of CBF that characterized this tissue was 7 to 17 mL/100 g/minute, well within the classic ranges found in the monkeys.[68]

Extensive cortical penumbra has been reported in more than 50% of the patients studied within 9 hours of onset, in 25% of cases at 24 hours, and occasionally until 30 hours postonset, suggesting that the window for therapeutic opportunity may be protracted in at least a fraction of the cases. In one study, it was found that up to 16 hours after symptom onset, the fraction of the ultimately infarcted tissue still exhibiting physiologic characteristics compatible with penumbra could be as high as 52%, suggesting that delayed neuroprotection might have altered the functional outcome in such cases significantly.[71] Heiss and colleagues[75] reported different results, but scrutiny into their data suggests this discrepancy is more apparent than real. From a PET study of CBF alone (assessed in a semiquantitative way) performed in 10 patients within 3 hours of clinical onset, these authors concluded that the penumbral component was small, accounting for only 18% of the finally infarcted volume. These authors used an unconventional classification of tissue subtypes based on CBF only, however, and which comprises (1) a critically hypoperfused component, which inescapably undergoes necrosis if not rapidly reperfused; (2) a penumbral component, which may survive spontaneously and would be salvageable by neuroprotective agents; and (3) a sufficiently perfused component, which may suffer delayed neuronal death and be incorporated in the final infarct. According to the conventional definitions given earlier, the latter two tissue subtypes would be incorporated within the conventional penumbra because they are clearly at risk of infarction, whereas the former would include not only truly penumbral, but also already irreversibly damaged tissue. If one takes into account these differences, the data reported by Heiss and colleagues[74] are quite similar to those reported earlier by Marchal and associates[71] using a more conventional classification.

Fate of Penumbra

Transition of such penumbral areas toward infarction has been documented within hours to days and is signaled by a decline in $CMRO_2$ regardless of the local CBF, which may decline in parallel or remain stable.[69, 71, 75] With elapsing days, perfusion increases progressively in the necrotic tissue, representing neovascularization within necrotic tissue, before falling down again in the final cavity.[9, 76] This whole process is illustrated strikingly by the associated dramatic fall in the OEF, from initially high to massively low values (i.e., luxury perfusion), signaling the exhaustion of the tissue's oxygen needs.

Such a deleterious course of events does not always take place, however, and all or part of the penumbral tissue may escape infarction spontaneously.[73, 75] In this event, one hypothesis is that some favorable event (e.g., partial reperfusion, gradual dampening of glutamate release from the core) occurred after the PET study to save part or all of this tissue. PET studies of the MCA occlusion model in the baboon have documented that early reperfusion is capable of reversing the otherwise deleterious demise of the penumbra.[77, 78] Accordingly, Heiss and coworkers[79] reported in humans that large volumes of tissue with CBF less than 12 mL/100 g/minute (potentially penumbral) do not evolve to necrosis in patients successfully recanalized by intravenous thrombolysis within 3 hours from onset of stroke.

Early Spontaneous Hyperperfusion

Early hyperperfusion, which suggests recanalization of the occluded artery, has been observed in one third of cases studied between the 5th and the 18th hour after stroke onset (see Fig. 95–3).[70, 80] In most cases, hyperperfusion is not associated with reduced metabolism, but instead with a mildly increased $CMRO_2$, suggesting postischemic rebound of cellular energy-dependent processes.[72] The significantly reduced OEF and increased CBV indicate, however, luxury perfusion with abnormal vasodilation. In a sample of 10 patients, the hyperperfused areas consistently exhibited intact morphology at chronic stage CT,[72] suggesting that the spontaneous recanalization of the MCA that occurred at some undefined time point before the PET study resulted in efficient reperfusion of the previously ischemic and dysregulated, but still viable, tissue. At odds with the loose experimental concept according to which sudden tissue reoxygenation might exacerbate ischemic brain damage, these findings in humans suggest that postischemic hyperperfusion is not detrimental.[81] This suggestion is consistent in turn with the well-established notion that infarct size is reduced by early recanalization.[68]

Clinical Correlates

Marchal and associates[70, 80] conducted a prospective study that assessed the relationships between acute stage PET findings and clinical outcome. In their study of 30 patients with first-ever MCA territory stroke investigated with PET within 18 hours of symptom onset, each patient could be classified into one of three patterns of PET changes (see Fig. 95–3): *pattern 1*, characterized by a large subcorticocortical area of already extensive necrosis; *pattern 2*, characterized by the presence of presumably penumbral tissue without associated irreversible damage except possibly in the lenticulostriate area; and *pattern 3*, characterized by hyperperfusion without associated irreversible damage except possibly in a small area. There was a statistically highly significant relationship between PET patterns and subsequent neurological course. All patients classified as pattern 1 did poorly (early death from massive infarct or poor outcome), whereas all patients classified as pattern 3 did well (complete or nearly complete recovery in all). Patients classified as pattern 2 had a variable course, ranging from death to full recovery. These findings from functional imaging are consistent with evidence from clinical studies, which show that early recanalization is associated with rapid recovery, whereas persistence of MCA trunk occlusion is a risk factor for poor outcome and massive brain swelling. It was shown that the predictive value of these patterns for final outcome were independent of admission neurological scores (i.e., they significantly add to the value of clinical data alone).[80] Consistent findings regarding hyperperfusion have been reported by Heiss and associates,[82] who showed in a few cases studied before and after early intravenous thrombolysis that the early occurrence of hyperperfusion was associated with good clinical and tissue outcome, in contrast to severe and persisting hypoperfusion.

Likewise, SPECT investigations with technetium-99m (^{99m}Tc)–labeled HMPAO or ethyl-cysteinate dimer in acute ischemic stroke have reported similar patterns with similar (although slightly weaker) predictive value for clinical outcome and recovery as PET.[83–86] A normal SPECT scan (or with mild hyperfixation) is always predictive of good spontaneous outcome, whereas a profound and extensive hypofixation almost always predicts malignant infarction (or hemorrhagic transformation if subjected to thrombolysis[87]); patients with moderate ranges of hypoperfusion (in extent and in degree) have an uncertain prognosis. A different case with HMPAO SPECT is represented by well-demarcated areas of massively increased tracer uptake or *hot spots*, which appear to predict subsequent infarction,[88] although they may not represent true hyperperfusion, but rather abnormal tracer penetration in brain parenchyma owing to altered blood-brain barrier in already severely damaged tissue.

Alleviation of Penumbra: Its Role in Clinical Recovery

Alleviation of penumbra has long been hypothesized as one major mechanism underlying early recovery from ischemic stroke. Only more recently was this mechanism directly documented in a quantitative way.[74] In this study, the degree of neurological recovery during the succeeding 2 months was found to be correlated positively to the individual volume of acute stage penumbral tissue that escaped infarction, as assessed with chronic stage CT.[80] Unexpectedly the best correlation was observed with 2-month recovery scores, which suggests that survival of the penumbra influences not only early, but also late recovery. Survival of the penumbra not only allows for early return of function in the peri-infarct tissue, but also may provide an important opportunity for subsequent neural reorganization processes, in a synergistic rather than simply cumulative way. Survival of the penumbra would appear to be an important prerequisite for subsequent functional recovery. Confirmatory results were reported by Heiss and coworkers,[79] who found a significant positive relationship between the reduction in volume of critically hypoperfused tissue between prethrombolysis and post-thrombolysis PET and the change in neurological scores between admission and 3 weeks.

Implications for Therapy

IMPLICATIONS FOR GENERAL MANAGEMENT

Demonstration of high OEF in the setting of acute stroke implies that the autoregulation of CBF is overridden in the affected territory. This finding is especially important in view of the frequent occurrence of reactive hypertension in this clinical setting. Any lowering of systemic arterial pressure is likely to reduce the CPP further and, in turn, the CBF in the affected tissue, which may have potentially damaging effects. This situation may explain why reductions in systemic arterial pressure in acute stroke frequently have been associated with poorer outcome. Conversely, if low OEF with hyperperfusion is found, management of arterial hypertension may be warranted, particularly if early edema is shown by CT or MR imaging, because some experimental studies suggest that hyperperfusion in necrotic tissue may promote the development of malignant brain swelling.

IMPLICATIONS FOR SPECIFIC THERAPY AND TRIALS

Based on the data reviewed earlier, physiologic imaging would be helpful in depicting in each patient the pathophysiologic condition of the brain before aggressive therapy is considered. A theoretical framework would be as follows: (1) Pattern 3 suggests spontaneous recanalization already has occurred and is predictive of good spontaneous outcome so that patients with this profile would not be eligible. (2) Pattern 1 suggests poor outcome with considerable risk of massive brain swelling and early death so that patients with this profile also should be excluded from most trials apart from those directed against vasogenic edema, such as surgical brain decompression. (3) Pattern 2 patients have substantial penumbral tissue and would represent the best candidates for therapy. In practice, however, there is as yet no experience of PET or SPECT being used as a screening method for intravenous thrombolysis (i.e., within 3 hours from onset), and specific trials incorporating physiologic imaging should test whether this is a valuable addition (despite the added time required to perform the procedure). Likewise, although the aforementioned data suggest that pathophysiologically blind inclusion of acute stroke patients into trials may blur any beneficial effects of the agent being tested because of underlying pathophysiologic heterogeneity, whether adding physiologic imaging would result in improved sensitivity of therapeutic trials needs to be tested in its own right. A final point of potential importance is the observation of pattern 2 as late as 16 hours after stroke onset, suggesting that the individual therapeutic window needs to be considered in each case.[89] Beyond the 3-hour window, however, these patients would benefit from a trial of neuroprotection or intra-arterial thrombolysis rather than intravenous thrombolysis, but avoiding agents tend to reduce systemic arterial pressure.

REMOTE METABOLIC EFFECTS OF STROKE

Remote metabolic depression is characterized by coupled reductions in perfusion and metabolism in brain structures remote from, but connected with, the area damaged by the stroke. This effect widely is explained as depressed synaptic activity as a result of disconnection (either direct or transneural). Remote effects allow mapping of the disruption in distributed networks as a result of focal infarction. Although they often are referred to collectively as *diaschisis*,[90] this term conceals a variety of cellular derangements, from reversible hypofunction to evolving wallerian or transsynaptic degeneration, which all have the same PET expression. Some of these effects reflect purely functional, potentially recoverable synaptic derangement, which may participate in the acute clinical expression of stroke and its recovery.

Crossed Cerebellar Diaschisis

Crossed cerebellar diaschisis[9, 91] affects the cerebellar hemisphere contralateral to supratentorial stroke (Fig. 95-4). It occurs in about 50% of cortical or subcortical strokes but is more frequent and severe with large hemispheric or capsular strokes.[92] It generally results from damage to the glutamatergic corticopontocerebellar system (CPCS), inducing transneuronal functional depression, as further documented by observations of crossed cerebellar diaschisis after unilateral brainstem lesion at the level of the crus cerebri or basis pontis. Although it often is associated with hemiparesis,[92] this association is not systematic and presumably results from strokes encroaching the pyramidal and the CPCS fibers.

The fact that crossed cerebellar diaschisis may develop within the first hours of stroke and subsequently disappear[93] indicates that it can be a transient manifestation of deafferentation. Accordingly, crossed cerebellar diaschisis also can manifest transiently in instances of reversible functional depression of the cerebral cortex, such as transient ischemic attacks or balloon occlusion of the internal carotid artery.[94] In most stroke patients, however, it tends to persist,[77, 92] which suggests it might evolve into transneuronal degeneration in the long run. Even in long-standing crossed cerebellar diaschisis, atrophy rarely is shown by standard MR imaging, although ipsilateral atrophy of the cerebral peduncle is seen occasionally, consistent with CPCS damage.[95]

The lack of crossed cerebellar diaschisis in acute MCA territory stroke predicts good outcome, whereas its presence has little predictive value individually.[93] Although a relationship between crossed cerebellar diaschisis and ipsilateral ataxia has been reported anecdotally,[96] other studies indicate a lack of one-to-one association,[97] such that only ataxia caused by CPCS damage is translated into crossed cerebellar diaschisis. A relationship with ipsilateral flaccidity has been reported,[98] but this was not a one-to-one association.

Contralateral Cerebral Effects

Although contralateral cerebral effects have long been thought to underlie some symptoms such as agitation, confusion, and coma and exacerbate the focal deficit, they have been elusive because of confounding factors, such as the lack of adequate controls and the use of CBF, which has physiologic variability. No association between changes in contralateral hemisphere $CMRO_2$ and early changes in neurological deficits was re-

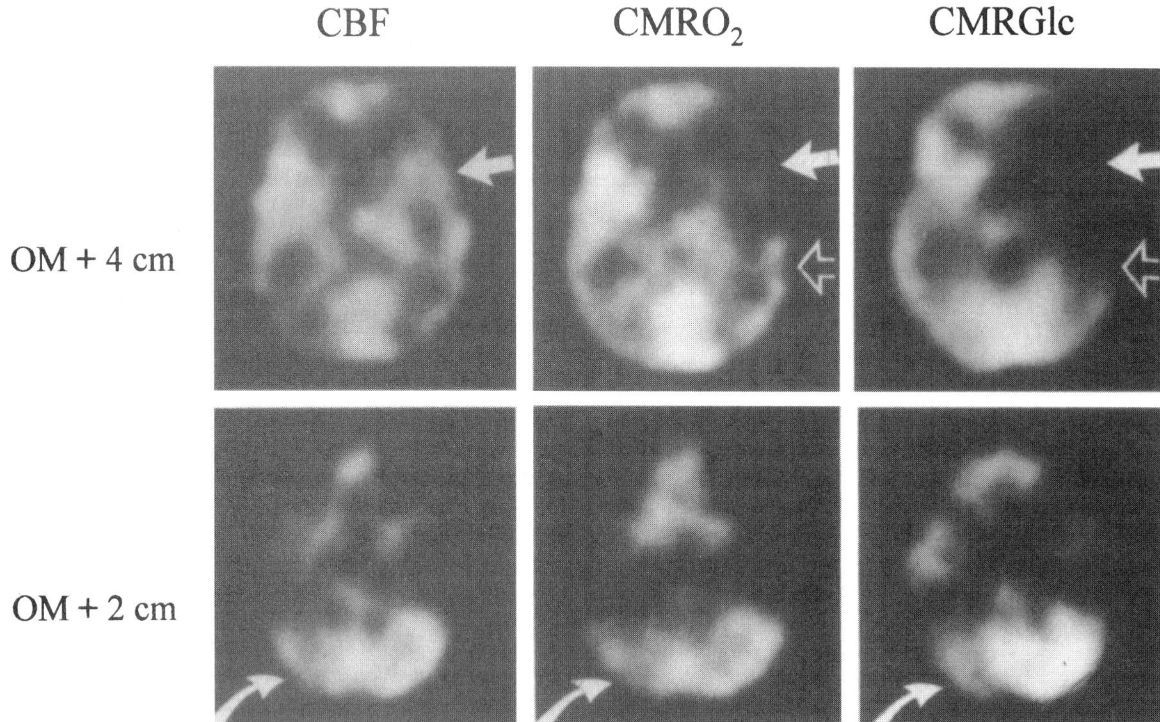

FIGURE 95–4. Crossed cerebellar diaschisis. Quantitative images of cerebral blood flow, cerebral metabolic rate of oxygen, and cerebral metabolic rate of glucose obtained at two brain levels in a 37-year-old patient 6 days after massive right middle cerebral artery infarction secondary to cardiac embolism. On these images, the right side of the brain is on the reader's right. The data show on level OM + 4 cm a profoundly reduced cerebral metabolic rate of oxygen and cerebral metabolic rate of glucose in the infarcted area associated with heterogeneous cerebral blood flow showing combined areas of markedly reduced, moderately reduced, and increased flow (luxury perfusion; *straight arrows*). On level OM + 2 cm, a proportional reduction in flow, oxygen consumption, and glucose utilization in the entire left cerebellar hemisphere (crossed cerebellar diaschisis), showing primary metabolic depression, is seen, a remote transneuronal effect of right middle cerebral artery infarction that damages the crossed corticopontocerebellar pathway.

ported.[99] Contralateral hemisphere hypometabolism develops in the subacute stage of MCA stroke, however, dissociated from the clinical recovery that takes place at this stage, presumably as a result of degeneration of severed transcallosal fibers.[99, 100] It may be that the slow recovery from contralateral hemisphere hypometabolism that appears to take place subsequently underlies late improvements in cognitive deficits.[100–102]

Subcorticocortical Effects

SUBCORTICAL APHASIA

Reduced cortical CMRG has been reported in small, deep, left-sided infarcts such as thalamic or thalamocapsular stroke with language impairment,[101, 103, 104] suggesting that subcortical aphasia could be related in part to this remote functional effect. This idea is supported by the finding of a positive correlation between the impairment in distinct aphasia items (oral and written comprehension, naming, and repetition) and the severity of left parietotemporal hypometabolism.[105, 106]

SUBCORTICAL NEGLECT

Marked ipsilateral cortical hypometabolism has been reported consistently after right-sided subcortical infarcts with left hemineglect.[101, 107, 108] Predominance of these effects over the frontal and parietal cortices suggests involvement of the subcorticocortical network for directed attention. Consistent with this interpretation, motor neglect is characterized by sparing of the primary motor circuit (striatum, cerebellum, and motor strip) but hypometabolism of the *supramotor* circuit (i.e., premotor, prefrontal, cingulate, and parietal cortices).[109, 110]

HEMIANOPIA

Damage to the optic radiations induces a significant reduction in glucose utilization in the disconnected part of the ipsilateral primary visual cortex,[111] sometimes spreading to the visual association areas and to the contralateral visual cortex.[112]

THALAMOCORTICAL DIASCHISIS

Infarcts in the anterior, medial, or lateral thalamus almost invariably induce a metabolic depression of the entire ipsilateral cortical mantle (maximal in the projection area of the affected nuclei), with lesser effects contralaterally,[101, 113, 114] presumably as a result of involvement of the excitatory thalamocortical projections. As noted earlier, there are significant relationships between the pattern of cortical hypometabolism and the aphasia profile or hemineglect after thalamic stroke.[101] A correlation between the degree of cognitive impairment after ventrolateral thalamotomy and the extent of thalamocortical diaschisis has been reported.[101] Thalamocortical diaschisis is absent in stroke involving the posterolateral thalamus, however.[115] Also, preferential frontal cortex hypometabolism has been associated with frontal-like syndromes and global amnesia after right-sided or left-sided thalamic infarction.[113, 114] In patients with severe permanent amnesia and apathy from bilateral paramedian thalamic infarction (*thalamic dementia* from *strategic infarcts*), marked neocortical hypometabolism has been reported.[116, 117]

Other Ipsilateral Effects

Striatal and thalamic hypometabolism is a frequent finding ipsilateral to corticosubcortical stroke.[9, 95, 103] Thalamic hypometabolism develops a few days after the stroke and presumably represents active retrograde degeneration of the damaged thalamocortical neurons, whereas striatal hypometabolism probably reflects loss of glutamatergic input from the cortex. Left caudate and thalamic hypometabolism are associated significantly with Broca's (i.e., nonfluent) aphasia, as compared with Wernicke's or conduction aphasia.[118] Thalamic hypometabolism has been associated with poor recovery of hand function after ischemic stroke.[119]

Role of Cortical Hypometabolism in Behavioral Recovery from Stroke

After subcortical stroke, the cortical metabolic depression tends to recover during the ensuing months, in parallel with cognitive recovery.[101, 120, 121] Some mechanism of synaptic reorganization must develop slowly after the early trans-synaptic effect, underlying cognitive recovery. The lesser the subacute stage defect in CMRG around Wernicke's and Broca's areas, the better outcome in terms of language comprehension and verbal fluency.[122] These observations that the peri-infarct area may be crucial for early recovery in aphasia are consistent with the aforementioned findings regarding the fate of the penumbra.[74] Although language recovery within the first year appears to be linked primarily to metabolic recovery in the dominant hemisphere,[102] long-term language improvements seem to be related to slow metabolic recovery in the contralateral hemisphere, specifically in the homotopic frontal and thalamic areas.[123] Taken together, the available evidence suggests that recovery of cortical metabolism, both ipsilateral and contralateral, partly predicts functional recovery after stroke and is one expression of neuronal reorganization after network damage.

RADIOLIGAND STUDIES IN CEREBROVASCULAR DISORDERS

Neuronal Marker

^{11}C-Flumazenil is an ideal potential in vivo marker of neuronal loss because the central benzodiazepine receptor is part of the γ-aminobutyric acid–A complex, which has widespread cortical distribution. In experimental and clinical stroke, loss of ^{11}C-flumazenil binding can be shown in the ischemic core within hours into arterial occlusion.[5, 124] In the chronic stage, decreases in cortical uptake of ^{11}C-flumazenil (or its SPECT analogue ^{123}I-iomazenil) have been reported, occasionally affecting areas not showing frank infarction on structural imaging.[125] This finding has been taken as evidence for selective neuronal loss, which might underlie neuropsychologic deficits after subcortical infarction. Benzodiazepine receptor imaging may facilitate differentiating cortical dysfunction induced by diaschisis from that caused by occult damage. Reduced tracer uptake in the hypometabolic cortex after striatocapsular infarction is not a universal finding,[126] however, and histopathologic confirmation of neuronal loss in areas with reduced in vivo binding has been lacking so far.

Glial Marker

^{11}C-PK 11195 is a ligand of the peripheral benzodiazepine receptor, which is borne by microglia and macrophages. As such, it may be an in vivo marker of glial proliferation after stroke. This possibility has been confirmed by studies in humans and nonhuman primates, showing progressively increasing ^{11}C-PK11195 uptake within the infarct, peaking at around 10 to 15 days.[5, 6]

Marker of Hypoxia

Read and colleagues[7] reported on the use of ^{18}F-fluoromisonidazole as a marker of tissue hypoxia in a series of 12 patients with acute MCA territory stroke. They reported widespread areas of increased tracer uptake in the affected cerebral hemisphere, found even later than 42 hours after clinical onset in some subjects. These findings would concur with earlier PET studies that suggested that the ischemic penumbra may persist for long intervals in a small subset of the cases (see earlier).

REFERENCES

1. Baron JC, Frackowiak RSJ, Herholz K, et al: Use of positron emission tomography in the investigation of cerebral hemodynamics and energy metabolism in cerebrovascular disease. J Cereb Blood Flow Metab 9:723–742, 1989.
2. Gibbs JM, Wise RJS, Leenders KL, et al: Evaluation of cerebral perfusion reserve in patients with carotid-artery occlusion. Lancet 1:310–314, 1984.
3. Sette G, Baron JC, Mazoyer B, et al: Local brain hemodynamics and oxygen metabolism in cerebro-vascular disease: Positron emission tomography. Brain 112:931–951, 1989.
4. Schumann P, Touzani O, Young AR, et al: Evaluation of the ratio of cerebral blood flow to cerebral blood volume as an

index of local cerebral perfusion pressure. Brain 121:1369–1379, 1998.
5. Sette G, Baron JC, Young AR, et al: In vivo mapping of brain benzodiazepine receptor changes by positron emission tomography after focal ischemia in the anesthetized baboon. Stroke 24:2046–2058, 1993.
6. Ramsay SC, Weiller C, Myers R, et al: Monitoring by PET of macrophage accumulation in brain after ischaemic stroke. Lancet 239:1054–1055, 1992.
7. Read SJ, Hirano T, Abbott DF, et al: Identifying hypoxic tissue after acute ischemic stroke using PET and 18F-fluoromisonidazole. Neurology 51:1617–1621, 1998.
8. Baron JC, Rougemont D, Soussaline F, et al: Local inter relationship of cerebral oxygen consumption and glucose utilization in normal subjects and in ischemic stroke patients: A positron tomography study. J Cereb Blood Flow Metab 4:140–149, 1984.
9. Baron JC, Bousser MG, Comar D, et al: Non invasive tomographic study of cerebral blood flow and oxygen metabolism in vivo: Potentials, limitations and clinical applications in cerebral ischemic disorders. Eur Neurol 20:273–284, 1981.
10. Frackowiak RSJ: The pathophysiology of human cerebral ischaemia: A new perspective obtained with positron tomography. QJM 223:713–727, 1985.
11. Derdeyn CP, Grubb RL, Powers WJ: Cerebral hemodynamic impairment: Method of measurement and association with stroke risk. Neurology 53:251–259, 1999.
12. Baron JC, Bousser MG, Rey A, et al: Reversal of focal "misery-perfusion syndrome" by extra-intracranial arterial bypass in hemodynamic cerebral ischemia: A case study with ^{15}O positron tomography. Stroke 12:454–459, 1981.
13. Lassen NA: The luxury perfusion syndrome and its possible relation to acute metabolic acidosis localised within the brain. Lancet 2:1113–1115, 1966.
14. Samson Y, Baron JC, Bousser MG, et al: Effects of extra-intracranial arterial bypass on cerebral blood flow and oxygen metabolism in humans. Stroke 16:609–616, 1985.
15. Derlon JM, Bouvard G, Viader F, et al: Impaired cerebral hemodynamics in internal carotid occlusion. Cerebrovasc Dis 2:72–81, 1992.
16. Herold S, Brown MM, Frackowiak RSJ, et al: Assessment of cerebral haemodynamic reserve: Correlation between PET parameters and CO_2 reactivity measured by the intravenous ^{133}xenon injection technique. J Neurol Neurosurg Psychiatry 51: 1045–1050, 1988.
17. Leblanc R, Yamamoto YL, Tyler JL, et al: Borderzone ischemia. Ann Neurol 22:707–713, 1987.
18. Levine RL, Dobkin JA, Rozental JM, et al: Blood flow reactivity to hypercapnia in strictly unilateral carotid disease: Preliminary results. J Neurol Neurosurg Psychiatry 54:204–209, 1991.
19. Powers WJ, Press GA, Grubb RL, et al: The effect of hemodynamically significant carotid artery disease on the hemodynamic status of the cerebral circulation. Ann Intern Med 106: 27–35, 1987.
20. Yamauchi H, Fukuyama H, Kimura J, et al: Hemodynamics in internal carotid artery occlusion examined by positron emission tomography. Stroke 21:1400–1406, 1990.
21. Derdeyn CP, Shaibani A, Moran CJ, et al: Lack of correlation between pattern of collateralization and misery perfusion in patients with carotid occlusion. Stroke 30:1025–1032, 1999.
22. Sgouropoulos P, Baron JC, Samson Y, et al: Sténoses et occlusions persistantes de l'artère cérébrale moyenne; conséquences hémodynamiques et métaboliques étudiées par tomographie à positons. Rev Neurol (Paris) 141:698–705, 1985.
23. Derdeyn CP, Powers WJ, Grubb RL: Hemodynamic effects of middle cerebral artery stenosis and occlusion. AJNR Am J Neuroradiol 19:1463–1469, 1998.
24. Vorstrup S, Engell HC, Lindewald H, et al: Hemodynamically significant stenosis of the internal carotid artery treated with endarterectomy. J Neurosurg 60:1070–1075, 1984.
25. Vorstrup S, Lassen NA, Henriksen L, et al: CBF before and after extracranial-intracranial bypass surgery in patients with ischemic cerebrovascular disease studied with ^{133}Xe-inhalation tomography. Stroke 16:616–626, 1985.
26. Vorstrup S, Brun B, Lassen NA: Evaluation of the cerebral vasodilatory capacity by the acetazolamide test before EC-IC bypass surgery in patients with occlusion of the internal carotid artery. Stroke 17:1291–1298, 1986.
27. Carpenter DA, Grubb RL, Powers WJ: Borderzone hemodynamics in cerebrovascular disease. Neurology 40:1587–1592, 1990.
28. Itoh M, Hatazawa J, Pozzilli C, et al: Positron CT imaging of an impending stroke. Neuroradiology 30:276–279, 1988.
29. Yamauchi H, Fukuyama H, Fujimoto N, et al: Significance of low perfusion with increased oxygen extraction fraction in a case of internal carotid artery stenosis. Stroke 23:431–432, 1992.
30. Kuwabara Y, Ichiya Y, Otsuka M, et al: Cerebral hemodynamic change in the child and the adult with moya-moya disease. Stroke 21:272–277, 1990.
31. Kuwabara Y, Ichiya Y, Sasaki M, et al: Response to hypercapnia in moya-moya disease. Stroke 28:701–707, 1997.
32. Taki W, Yonekawa Y, Kobayashi A, et al: Cerebral circulation and oxygen metabolism in Moyamoya disease of ischemic type in children. Childs Nerv Syst 4:259–262, 1988.
33. Taki W, Yonekawa Y, Kobayashi A, et al: Cerebral circulation and metabolism in adult's moya-moya disease: PET study. Acta Neurochir (Vienna) 100:150–154, 1989.
34. Ogawa A, Kameyama M, Muraishi K, et al: Cerebral blood flow and metabolism following superficial temporal artery to superior cerebellar artery bypass for vertebrobasilar occlusive disease. J Neurosurg 76:955–960, 1992.
35. Mase M, Yamada K, Matsumoto T, et al: Cerebral blood flow and metabolism of steal syndrome evaluated by PET. Neurology 52:1515–1516, 1999.
36. Delecluse F, Vooredecker P, Raftopoulos C: Vertebrobasilar insufficiency revealed by Xenon-133 inhalation SPECT. Stroke 20: 952–956, 1989.
37. Derdeyn CP, Yundt KD, Videen TO, et al: Increased oxygen extraction fraction is associated with prior ischemic events in patients with carotid occlusion. Stroke 29:754–758, 1998.
38. Gibbs JM, Wise RJS, Thomas DJ, et al. Cerebral haemodynamic changes after extracranial-intracranial bypass surgery. J Neurol Neurosurg Psychiatry 50:140–150, 1987.
39. Leblanc R, Tyler JL, Mohr G, et al: Hemodynamic and metabolic effects of cerebral revascularization. J Neurosurg 66:529–535, 1987.
40. Muraishi K, Kameyama M, Sato K, et al: Cerebral circulatory and metabolic changes following EC/IC bypass surgery in cerebral occlusive diseases. Neurol Res 15:97–103, 1993.
41. Powers WJ, Martin WRW, Herscovitch P, et al: Extracranial-intracranial bypass surgery: Hemodynamic and metabolic effects. Neurology 34:1168–1174, 1984.
42. Nariai T, Suzuki R, Matsushima Y, et al: Surgically induced angiogenesis to compensate for hemodynamic cerebral ischemia. Stroke 25:1014–1021, 1994.
43. Kuwabara Y, Ichiya Y, Sasaki M, et al: PET evaluation of cerebral hemodynamics in occlusive cerebrovascular disease pre- and postsurgery. J Nucl Med 39:760–765, 1998.
44. Ikezaki K, Matsushima T, Suzuki SO, et al: Cerebral circulation and oxygen metabolism in childhood Moyamoya disease: A perioperative positron emission tomography study. J Neurosurg 81:843–850, 1994.
45. Okada Y, Shima T, Nishida M, et al: Effectiveness of superficial temporal-artery-middle cerebral artery anastomosis in adult moya-moya disease. Stroke 29:625–630, 1998.
46. The EC/IC Bypass Study Group: Failure of extracranial-intracranial arterial bypass to reduce the risk of ischemic stroke. N Engl J Med 313:1191–1200, 1985.
47. Powers WJ, Grubb RL, Raichle M: Clinical results of extracranial-intracranial bypass surgery in patients with hemodynamic cerebrovascular disease. J Neurosurg 70:61–67, 1989.
48. Powers WJ, Templel LW, Grubb RL: Influence of cerebral hemodynamics on stroke risk: One-year follow-up of 30 medically treated patients. Ann Neurol 25:325–330, 1989.
49. Kleiser B, Widder B: Course of carotid artery occlusions with impaired cerebrovascular reactivity. Stroke 23:171–174, 1992.
50. Kuroda S, Kamiyama H, Abe H, et al: Acetazolamide test in detecting reduced cerebral perfusion reserve and predicting long-term prognosis in patients with internal carotid artery occlusion. Neurosurgery 32:912–919, 1993.
51. Webster MW, Makaroun MS, Steed DL, et al: Compromised cerebral blood flow reactivity is a predictor of stroke in patients

with symptomatic carotid artery occlusive disease. J Vasc Surg 21:338–345, 1995.

52. Yamauchi H, Fukuyama H, Nagahama Y, et al: Evidence of misery perfusion and risk for recurrent stroke in major cerebral arterial occlusive diseases from PET. J Neurol Neurosurg Psychiatry 61:18–25, 1996.
53. Yonas H, Smith HA, Durham SR, et al: Increased stroke risk predicted by compromised cerebral blood flow reactivity. J Neurosurg 79:483–489, 1993.
54. Gur AY, Bova I, Bornstein NM: Is impaired cerebral vasomotor reactivity a predictive factor of stroke in asymptomatic patients? Stroke 27:2188–2190, 1996.
55. Grubb RL, Derdeyn CP, Fritsch SM, et al: Importance of hemodynamic factors in the prognosis of symptomatic carotid occlusion. JAMA 280:1055–1060, 1998.
56. Klijn CJM, Kappelle LJ, Tulleken CAF, et al: Symptomatic carotid artery occlusion. Stroke 28:2084–2093, 1997.
57. Haisa T, Kondo T, Shimpo T, et al: Post-carotid endarterectomy cerebral hyperperfusion leading to intracerebral haemorrhage. J Neurol Neurosurg Psychiatry 67:546, 1999.
58. Derdeyn CP, Videen TO, Fritsch SM, et al: Compensatory mechanisms for chronic cerebral hypoperfusion in patients with carotid occlusion. Stroke 30:1019–1024, 1999.
59. Brown AP, Spetzler RF: Intracranial arteriovenous malformation: Cerebrovascular hemodynamics. In Hunt Batjer H (ed): Cerebrovascular Disease. Philadelphia, Lippincott-Raven, 1997, pp 833–842.
60. Batjer HH, Devous MD: The use of acetazolamide-enhanced regional cerebral blood flow measurement to predict risk to arteriovenous malformation patients. Neurosurgery 31:213–218, 1992.
61. Tyler JL, Leblanc R, Meyer E, et al: Hemodynamics and metabolic effects of cerebral arteriovenous malformations studied by positron emission tomography. Stroke 20:890–898, 1989.
62. De Reuck J, Van Aken J, Van Landegem W, et al: Positron emission tomography studies of changes in cerebral blood flow and oxygen metabolism in arteriovenous malformation of the brain. Eur Neurol 29:294–297, 1989.
63. Fink GR: Effects of cerebral angiomas on perifocal and remote tissue: A multivariate positron emission tomography study. Stroke 23:1099–1105, 1992.
64. Baron JC: Positron emission tomography. In Barnett HJM, Mohr JP, Stein BM, Yatsu FM (eds): Stroke: Pathophysiology, Diagnosis, and Management, 3rd ed. New York, Churchill Livingstone, 1998, pp 101–119.
65. Baron JC: Mapping the ischaemic penumbra with PET: Implications for acute stroke treatment. Cerebrovasc Dis 9:193–201, 1999.
66. Powers WJ, Grubb RL Jr, Darriet D, et al: Cerebral blood flow and cerebral metabolic rate of oxygen requirements for cerebral function and viability in humans. J Cereb Blood Flow Metab 5: 600–608, 1985.
67. Marchal G, Benali K, Iglesias S, et al: Voxel-based mapping of irreversible tissue damage by PET in the acute stage of ischemic stroke. Brain 122:2387–2400, 1999.
68. Jones TH, Morawetz RE, Crowell RM, et al: Thresholds of focal cerebral ischaemia in awake monkeys. J Neurosurg 54: 773–782, 1981.
69. Wise RJS, Bernardi S, Frackowiak RSJ, et al: Serial observations on the pathophysiology of acute stroke: The transition from ischaemia to infarction as reflected in regional oxygen extraction. Brain 106:197–222, 1983.
70. Marchal G, Serrati C, Rioux P, et al: PET imaging of cerebral perfusion and oxygen consumption in acute ischaemic stroke: Relation to outcome. Lancet 341:925–927, 1993.
71. Marchal G, Beaudouin V, Rioux P, et al: Prolonged persistence of substantial volumes of potentially viable brain tissue after stroke: A correlative PET-CT study with voxel-based data analysis. Stroke 27:599–606, 1996.
72. Marchal G, Furlan M, Beaudouin V, et al: Early spontaneous hyperperfusion after stroke: A marker of favorable tissue outcome. Brain 119:409–419, 1996.
73. Furlan M, Marchal G, Viader F, et al: Spontaneous neurological recovery after stroke and the fate of the ischemic penumbra. Ann Neurol 40:216–226, 1996.
74. Heiss W-D, Thiel A, Grond M, et al: Which targets are relevant for therapy of acute ischemic stroke? Stroke 30:1486–1489, 1999.
75. Heiss WD, Huber M, Fink GR, et al: Progressive derangement of periinfarct viable tissue in ischemic stroke. J Cereb Blood Flow Metab 12:193–203, 1992.
76. Lenzi GL, Frackowiak RSJ, Jones T: Cerebral oxygen metabolism and blood flow in human cerebral ischemic infarction. J Cereb Blood Flow Metab 2:231–235, 1982.
77. Touzani O, Young AR, Derlon JM, et al: Progressive impairment of brain oxidative metabolism reversed by reperfusion following middle cerebral artery occlusion in anaesthetized baboons. Brain Res 767:17–25, 1997.
78. Young AR, Sette G, Touzani O, et al: Relationships between high oxygen extraction fraction in the acute stage and final infarction in reversible middle cerebral artery occlusion: An investigation in anaesthetized baboons with positron emission tomography. J Cereb Blood Flow Metab 16:1176–1188, 1996
79. Heiss WD, Grond M, Thiel A, et al: Tissue at risk of infarction rescued by early reperfusion: A positron emission tomography study in systemic recombinant tissue plasminogen activator thrombolysis of acute stroke. J Cereb Blood Flow Metab 18: 1298–1307, 1998.
80. Marchal G, Rioux P, Serrati C, et al: Value of acute-stage PET in predicting neurological outcome after ischemic stroke: Further assessment. Stroke 26:524–525, 1995.
81. Marchal G, Young AR, Baron JC: Early post-ischaemic hyperperfusion: Pathophysiological insights from positron emission tomography. J Cereb Blood Flow Metab 19:467–482, 1999.
82. Heiss WD, Graf R, Löttgen J, et al: Repeat positron emission tomographic studies in transient middle cerebral artery occlusion in cats: Residual perfusion and efficacy of postischemic reperfusion. J Cereb Blood Flow Metab 17:388–400, 1997.
83. Giubilei F, Lenzi GL, Di Piero V, et al: Predictive value of brain perfusion single-photon emission computed tomography in acute ischemic stroke. Stroke 21:895–900, 1990.
84. Marchal G, Bouvard G, Iglesias S, et al: Predictive value of 99mTc-HMPAO for neurological outcome/recovery in the acute stage of stroke. Cerebrovasc Dis 10:8–17, 2000.
85. Berrouschot J, Barthel H, von Kummer R, et al: 99m technetium-ethyl-cysteinate-dimer single-photon emission CT can predict fatal ischemic brain edema. Stroke 12:2556–2562, 1998.
86. Berrouschot J, Barthel H, Hesse S, et al: Differentiation between transient ischemic attack and ischemic stroke within the first six hours after onset of symtoms by using 99mTc-ECD-SPECT. J Cereb Blood Flow Metab 18:921–929, 1998.
87. Ueda T, Hatakeyama T, Kumon Y, et al: Evaluation of risk of hemorrhagic transformation in local intra-arterial thrombolysis in acute ischemic stroke by initial SPECT. Stroke 25:298–303, 1994.
88. Shimosegawa E, Hatazawa J, Inugami A, et al: Cerebral infarction within six hours of onset: Prediction of completed infarction with technetium-99m-HMPAO SPECT. J Nucl Med 35: 1097–1103, 1994.
89. Baron JC, von Kummer R, Del Zoppo GJ: Treatment of acute ischemic stroke: Challenging the concept of a rigid and universal time window. Stroke 26:2219–2221, 1995.
90. Feeney D, Baron JC: Diaschisis. Stroke 17:817–830, 1986.
91. Baron JC, Bousser MG, Comar D, et al: "Crossed cerebellar diaschisis" in human supratentorial brain infarction. Trans Am Neurol Assoc 105:459–461, 1980.
92. Pantano P, Baron JC, Samson Y, et al: Crossed cerebellar diaschisis: Further studies. Brain 109:677–694, 1986.
93. Serrati C, Marchal G, Rioux P, et al: Contralateral cerebellar hypometabolism: A predictor for stroke outcome? J Neurol Neurosurg Psychiatry 57:174–179, 1994.
94. Brunberg JA, Frey KA, Horton JA, et al: (^{15}O)H_2O positron emission tomography determination of cerebral blood flow during balloon test occlusion of the internal carotid artery. AJNR Am J Neuroradiol 15:725–732, 1994.
95. Pappata S, Tran-Dinh S, Baron JC, et al: Remote metabolic effects of cerebrovascular lesions: Magnetic resonance and positron tomography imaging. Neuroradiology 29:1–6, 1987.
96. Tanaka M, Kondo S, Hirai S, et al: Crossed cerebellar diaschisis accompanied by hemiataxia: A PET study. J Neurol Neurosurg Psychiatry 55:121–125, 1992.

97. Pappata S, Mazoyer B, Tran-Dinh S, et al: Cortical and cerebellar hypometabolic effects of capsular, thalamo-capsular, and thalamic stroke: A positron tomography study. Stroke 21:519–524, 1990.
98. Pantano P, Formisano R, Ricci M, et al: Prolonged muscular flaccidity after stroke: Morphological and functional brain alterations. Brain 118:1329–1338, 1995.
99. Iglesias S, Marchal G, Rioux P, et al: Do changes in oxygen metabolism in the unaffected cerebral hemisphere underlie early neurological recovery after stroke? A positron emission tomography study. Stroke 27:1192–1199, 1996.
100. Heiss WD, Kessler J, Karbe H, et al: Cerebral glucose metabolism as a predictor of recovery from aphasia in ischemic stroke. Arch Neurol 50:958–964, 1993.
101. Baron JC, D'Antona R, Pantano P, et al: Effects of thalamic stroke on energy metabolism of the cerebral cortex. Brain 109: 1243–1259, 1986.
102. Mimura M, Kato M, Kato M, et al: Prospective and retrospective studies of recovery in aphasia: Changes in cerebral blood flow and language functions. Brain 121:2083–2094, 1998.
103. Kuhl DE, Phelps ME, Kowell AP, et al: Effects of stroke on local cerebral metabolism and perfusion: Mapping by emission computed tomography of ^{18}FDG and ^{13}NH3. Ann Neurol 8: 47–60, 1980.
104. Metter EJ, Wasterlain CG, Kuhl DE, et al: FDG positron emission computed tomography in a study of aphasia. Ann Neurol 10: 173–183, 1981.
105. Metter EJ, Riege WH, Hanson WR, et al: Subcortical structures in aphasia. Arch Neurol 45:1229–1234, 1988.
106. Karbe H, Szelies B, Herholz K, et al: Impairment of language is related to left parieto-temporal glucose metabolism in aphasic stroke patients. J Neurol 237:19–23, 1990.
107. Perani D, Vallar G, Cappa S, et al: Aphasia and neglect after subcortical stroke: A clinical/cerebral perfusion correlation study. Brain 110:1211–1229, 1987.
108. Bogousslavsky J, Miklossy J, Regli F, et al: Subcortical neglect: Neuropsychological, SPECT, and neuropathological correlations with anterior choroidal artery territory infarction. Ann Neurol 23:448–452, 1988.
109. Fiorelli M, Blin J, Bakchine S, et al: PET studies of cortical diaschisis in patients with motor hemi-neglect. J Neurol Sci 104: 135–142, 1991.
110. Von Giesen HJ, Schlaug G, Steinmetz H, et al: Cerebral network underlying unilateral motor neglect: Evidence from positron emission tomography. J Neurol Sci 125:29–38, 1994.
111. Bosley T, Rosenquist AC, Kushner M, et al: Ischemic lesions of the occipital cortex and optic radiations: Positron emission tomography. Neurology 35:470–484, 1985.
112. Kiyosawa M, Bosley TM, Kushner M, et al: Middle cerebral artery strokes causing homonymous hemianopia: Positron emission tomography. Ann Neurol 28:180–183, 1990.
113. Kuwert T, Hennerici M, Langen KL, et al: Regional cerebral glucose consumption measured by positron emission tomography in patients with unilateral thalamic infarction. Cerebrovasc Dis 1:327–336, 1991.
114. Szelies B, Herholz K, Pawlik G, et al: Widespread functional effects of discrete thalamic infarction. Arch Neurol 48:178–182, 1991.
115. Chabriat H, Levasseur M, Pappata S, et al: Cortical metabolism in postero-lateral thalamic stroke: A PET study. Acta Neurol Scand 86:285–290, 1992.
116. Levasseur M, Baron JC, Sette G, et al: Brain energy metabolism in bilateral paramedian thalamic infarcts: A positron emission tomography study. Brain 115:795–807, 1992.
117. Bogousslavsky J, Regli F, Delaloye G, et al: Loss of psychic self-activation with bithalamic infarction. Acta Neurol Scand 83: 309–316, 1991.
118. Metter EJ, Kempler D, Jackson C, et al: Cerebral glucose metabolism in Wernicke's, Broca's, and conduction aphasia. Arch Neurol 46:27–34, 1989.
119. Binkofski F, Seitz RJ, Arnold S, et al: Thalamic metabolism and corticospinal tract integrity determine motor recovery in stroke. Ann Neurol 39:460–470, 1996.
120. Baron JC, Levasseur M, Mazoyer B, et al: Thalamo-cortical diaschisis: PET study in humans. J Neurol Neurosurg Psychiatry 55:935–942, 1992.
121. Metter EJ, Jackson CA, Kempler D, et al: Temporoparietal cortex and the recovery of language comprehension in aphasia. Aphasiology 6:349–358, 1992.
122. Karbe H, Kessler J, Herholz K, et al: Long-term prognosis of poststroke aphasia studied with positron emission tomography. Arch Neurol 52:186–190, 1995.
123. Cappa SF, Perani D, Grassi F, et al: A PET follow-up study of recovery after stroke in acute aphasics. Brain Lang 56:55–67, 1997.
124. Heiss WD, Grond M, Thiel A, et al: Permanent cortical damage detected by flumazenil positron emission tomography in acute stroke. Stroke 29:454–446, 1998.
125. Nakagawara J, Sperling B, Lassen NA: Incomplete brain infarction of reperfused cortex may be quantitated with Iomazenil. Stroke 28:124–132, 1997.
126. Takahashi W, Ohnuki Y, Ohta T, et al: Mechanism of reduction of cortical blood flow in striatocapsular infarction: Studies using (123I)Iomazenil SPECT. Neuroimage 6:75–80, 1997.

CHAPTER 96

Carotid Occlusive Disease: Natural History and Medical Management

JAMES D. FLECK ■ JOSÉ BILLER ■ CHRISTOPHER M. LOFTUS

Stroke is a leading cause of death and disability. It is estimated that approximately 600,000 people suffer a new or recurrent stroke each year in the United States. Strokes killed an estimated 160,000 people in the United States in 1996 and rank behind only heart disease and cancer as the third leading cause of death.[1] Ischemic stroke accounts for approximately 80% to 85% of all strokes.[2] Although the causes of ischemic stroke may vary with the demographic characteristics of the patient population, the most common causes are large artery atherosclerotic disease and cardioembolic and small vessel or penetrating artery disease. Certainly, carotid artery occlusive disease or extracranial carotid disease is an important risk factor for and cause of stroke. This chapter focuses on the natural history and medical management of carotid atherosclerotic disease.

PATHOLOGIC MECHANISMS OF ATHEROSCLEROSIS

The word carotid, derived from the Greek word *karos*, means deep sleep. Hippocrates, around 400 BC, was one of the first to describe the symptoms of stroke.[3] Chiari is credited as being the first to propose that occlusive disease of the extracranial blood vessels could be responsible for neurological symptoms. In 1905, in a series of 400 autopsies, Chiari found seven patients who had thrombus superimposed on atherosclerosis near the carotid bifurcation. Four of these patients had suffered a cerebral embolism, and he presumed the source was the extracranial carotid artery.[4] In 1927 Egas Moniz described the first successful cerebral angiogram.[3] Initially, this technique was used predominantly to visualize the intracranial cerebral circulation; however, it represented an opportunity to visualize the carotid artery before direct visualization at surgery. Published in 1951, C. Miller Fisher's article, *Occlusion of the Internal Carotid Artery*, is unquestionably the landmark publication describing the relationship between carotid artery disease and transient ischemic attacks (TIAs) and stroke. Fisher described the clinical history, available premortem studies, and available postmortem examinations of the carotid arteries in eight patients with stroke.[5] Interestingly, the clinical descriptions of previous symptoms included several patients with transient monocular blindness ipsilateral to the diseased carotid artery. Fisher later reported the clinicopathologic results of 45 more patients with occlusion or near-occlusion of the carotid arteries.[6]

The pathology of the atherosclerotic plaque is quite complex. Essentially, however, it represents a disease of the arterial intima that, in subsequent stages, progresses to luminal narrowing. Over the years, various theories regarding the genesis and growth of atherosclerotic lesions have been promoted, usually concentrating on endothelial injury, smooth muscle cell proliferation, lipid accumulation, and more recently, inflammatory cells.[7, 8]

Infectious agents such as *Chlamydia pneumonia* and *Cytomegalovirus* have been associated with carotid atherosclerosis. Evidence of *Chlamydia pneumonia* organisms has been found in atherosclerotic plaques removed at the time of carotid endarterectomy by both reverse transcriptase polymerase chain reaction and immunohistochemical techniques.[9, 10] A population-based cohort study showed a graded relation between the odds of intimal-medial carotid artery thickening measured by carotid ultrasonography and the levels of *Cytomegalovirus* antibody titers in sera.[11] Whether these agents cause carotid atherosclerosis, contribute to its progression, or simply represent a superimposed infection remains to be studied.

A combination of these elements causes the development of significant plaque. Atherosclerosis is likely initiated by injury to or dysfunction of the endothelium.

The reactive endothelium allows the inward migration of mononuclear cells and lymphocytes, and stimulates medial smooth muscle cells to migrate and proliferate. Lipids are deposited or taken up by monocytes or macrophages through lipoproteins, most notably low-density lipoproteins (LDLs). Lipid-laden macrophages, or foam cells, continue to accumulate as do various connective tissue elements and smooth muscle cells.

Inflammatory cells also likely play a role in the progression of atherosclerotic plaque. Oxidative stress and free radical production also play a role in the pathogenesis of atherosclerosis. As the various elements accumulate, the lesion grows and the diameter of the vessel narrows. Eventually, a complicated lesion with a fibrous cap overlying a core of lipid and necrotic tissue is formed. Certainly, the atherosclerotic plaque is a complex environment of cells, connective tissue elements, lipids, cytokines, growth factors, and calcium. The plaque may fissure, ulcerate, or rupture, exposing thrombogenic nonendothelial cells and substances. The adherence of platelets and the formation of fibrin clot are precursors for further narrowing or occlusion of the artery and distal embolization.

Typically, the mechanism of ischemic stroke in atherosclerosis of the proximal internal carotid artery (ICA) is attributed to either "hemodynamically consequential" narrowing of the vessel lumen, proximal carotid artery-to-distal vessel embolus, or thrombosis of the proximal vessel leading to perhaps both hemodynamic compromise and potential artery-to-artery embolization. Blood flow in a larger artery like the ICA remains fairly constant until its internal diameter is reduced to approximately 70% of its normal diameter.[12] Further diminution in blood flow follows higher levels of stenosis. Some authors, however, argue that true cerebral hemodynamics cannot be assumed on the basis of the degree of carotid stenosis and that other factors, especially the adequacy of collateral circulation, play important roles.[13, 14]

Carotid atherosclerosis develops in regions of low wall shear stress. Symptomatic carotid artery plaque involves primarily the carotid artery bulb. Plaque morphology and, specifically, plaque ulceration may also play a role in the risk of stroke. Ulcerated, echolucent, and heterogenous plaque with a soft core may be unstable with a high risk of arterioarterial embolization.[15] Cranial computed tomography (CT) of patients with carotid artery plaque shows a six-fold increase in the frequency of cerebral infarction in patients with echolucent carotid artery plaque compared with patients with echogenic carotid artery lesions.[16] However, it is quite difficult to determine the exact risk associated with ulcerations given the various radiographic modalities used to image the carotid artery, the various definitions for the severity of ulcerations, and the various degrees of stenosis that accompany ulcerations.[17] In an analysis of patients with severe carotid stenosis (70% to 99%) in the North American Symptomatic Carotid Endarterectomy Trial (NASCET), the presence of angiographically defined ulceration for medically treated patients was associated with an increased risk of stroke.[18]

CLINICAL MANIFESTATIONS OF ATHEROSCLEROSIS

Recognition of the symptoms and signs of TIAs or strokes related to carotid artery atherosclerotic disease is important in evaluating patients (Table 96–1). Approximately 10% to 15% of those who experience a stroke have a history of preceding TIAs. Among patients with a TIA who survive 5 years, a third will experience a stroke. Estimates indicate that the risk of stroke after a TIA is approximately 5% during the first month after the event and 12% during the first year.[19] Patients with hemispheric TIAs have a greater risk of ipsilateral stroke than patients with retinal TIAs.[20] The ICA and its branches supply blood to the eye and the largest portions of the cerebral hemispheres. Therefore, it is almost impossible to describe one or a few sets of syndromes related to cerebral ischemia in its territory. The type and severity of symptoms depend on the location of the occlusion, the amount of brain or retinal tissue affected, and the availability of collateral circulation. The important clinical features of lesions of the carotid artery or its branches, including the ophthalmic artery, middle cerebral artery (MCA), anterior cerebral artery (ACA), anterior choroidal artery, and sometimes the posterior cerebral artery (PCA), are summarized.

The only feature that truly differentiates the ICA syndrome from the MCA syndrome is transient monocular blindness or amaurosis fugax. Patients describe the abrupt and painless onset of a visual disturbance in one eye, usually lasting 1 to 30 minutes. The classic description is one of a shade being pulled down over the eye, but it occurs only in a minority of patients. Blackout, graying, dimming of vision, or even a general constriction of the visual field in one eye can be described. Marginal perfusion causing diminished retinal blood flow or microemboli to the retinal circulation are the causes. Different types of microemboli may be seen on funduscopic evaluation of the retinal vessels, including bright plaques (Hollenhorst), so-called white plugs, or calcium. Hollenhorst plaques are composed of cholesterol crystals while "white plugs" typically consist of platelets and fibrin.[21]

The MCA is the most common site of ischemic stroke. The manifestations of an infarction in its territory can be extremely varied, depending on the site of occlusion. Contralateral weakness and sensory loss can occur. Often, the face and arm are more severely affected than the leg. Various types of aphasia are associ-

TABLE 96–1 ■ **Symptoms of Carotid Artery Territory Transient Ischemic Attacks**

- Ipsilateral monocular blindness (amaurosis fugax)
- Contralateral weakness, clumsiness, or paralysis
- Contralateral numbness, paresthesias, including loss of sensation
- Dysphasia
- Dysarthria
- Contralateral homonymous hemianopia
- Combinations of the above

ated with lesions in the dominant hemisphere; hemineglect and apractic syndromes are associated with damage to the nondominant hemisphere. Contralateral visual field deficits can occur, and paresis and apraxia of conjugate gaze to the opposite side are occasionally noted. Infarctions of the ACA typically lead to contralateral leg weakness more so than weakness of the arm. Various cognitive or psychiatric disturbances have also been associated with unilateral or bilateral medial frontal lobe infarctions.

Anterior choroidal artery infarctions typically result in contralateral hemiparesis caused by involvement of the posterior limb of the internal capsule, hemisensory loss caused by involvement of the posterolateral thalamus or its connections, and hemianopia related to involvement of the lateral geniculate body or its connections in the visual pathways. The classic deficit in PCA infarctions is contralateral visual field disturbances. Other symptoms and signs may occur, depending on site of occlusion and the extent of the cerebral hemisphere supplied by the PCA.

NATURAL HISTORY OF EXTRACRANIAL CAROTID DISEASE

As a prelude to discussing the medical management of extracranial carotid disease, knowledge of its prevalence, the importance of detecting carotid bruits, and its natural history can provide a helpful perspective. Some insight into the history of proposed treatments for extracranial carotid disease is necessary as a background to a discussion of the natural history. Armed with the thought that extracranial carotid artery disease might be a mechanism for stroke, surgeons began using carotid endarterectomy in the 1950s as a way to remove offending plaque, hoping to prevent strokes. In the 1970s, platelet antiaggregating agents such as aspirin were found to help prevent strokes. Several studies on the efficacy of aspirin in preventing stroke excluded patients who were to undergo surgical treatment such as carotid endarterectomy. Adequate prospective randomized controlled studies that compared carotid endarterectomy with "best medical care" did not appear until the 1990s. Also, initial observational studies did not control for the use of platelet antiaggregants or anticoagulants. Therefore, it is difficult to determine the actual natural history of carotid artery occlusive disease using data from these years.

Typically, patients with extracranial carotid disease reach a physician's attention in one of three ways. (1) An asymptomatic lesion is found on some type of noninvasive screening test, most often carotid ultrasonography. (2) A carotid bruit is auscultated on physical examination. (3) Extracranial carotid disease is found during the evaluation of a patient with a previous stroke or TIA symptoms. In unselected adult populations, the frequency of ICA stenosis of more than 50% on carotid duplex scanning was less than 5% but increased with age.[22, 23] The incidence is higher in patients with coronary artery disease, peripheral vascular disease, and high-risk factors for atherosclerosis.[24]

The prevalence of asymptomatic carotid artery bruits increases with age and has been assessed in two large population-based studies. In Evans County, Georgia, 4.4% of 1620 asymptomatic individuals at least 45 years of age had a carotid bruit.[25] In the Framingham study, 3.5% of asymptomatic people aged 44 to 54 years and 7% of those aged 65 to 79 years had a carotid bruit.[26] In both studies, the incidence of TIAs and strokes was higher in individuals with carotid bruits than in those without bruits, but the correlation between the location of the bruit and the location and proposed etiology of the cerebral ischemia was poor. In two studies that correlated cerebral angiographic findings and carotid bruits, the predictive value of carotid bruit for ipsilateral extracranial carotid atherosclerosis was approximately 75%[27] and the false-positive rate was 10%.[28] In the Asymptomatic Carotid Artery Study (ACAS), only about 10% of the randomized patients had an ipsilateral carotid bruit.[29] Auscultation of the carotid artery is useful and easy to accomplish at the bedside. Some patients, however, have no carotid bruit but have significant extracranial carotid disease, and not all patients with a carotid bruit have significant extracranial carotid disease.

The risk of stroke depends on the degree of carotid artery stenosis. Asymptomatic carotid artery stenosis of less than 75% carries an annual stroke risk of approximately 1%. When the stenosis is greater than 75%, the combined 1-year risk of TIA or stroke is about 10%. Most events are ipsilateral to the stenosed artery. The natural history of asymptomatic carotid artery occlusive disease was reported in studies from the 1980s. In a retrospective study of 640 neurologically asymptomatic patients with either pressure-significant ICA lesions determined by oculoplethysmography or carotid bruits without pressure-significant lesions, the annual stroke rate was 3.4% and 1.5%, respectively. However, only 56% of the strokes and TIAs occurred in a distribution ipsilateral to the oculoplethysmographic abnormality.[30] In a prospective study of 339 patients using serial Doppler examinations with a median follow-up of 29 months, the number of strokes varied with the degree of carotid stenosis. Two percent of those with 50% to 80% carotid stenosis, 8.3% of those with 80% to 99% stenosis, and 12.2% of those with a carotid occlusion had strokes.[31] Again, not all strokes occurred in the distribution of the abnormal carotid artery. Neither of these studies controlled for the use of platelet antiaggregants, and both excluded patients who had undergone carotid artery surgery.

Two large randomized prospective studies evaluated the effects of carotid endarterectomy in neurologically symptomatic patients, the European Carotid Surgery Trial (ECST) and the North American Symptomatic Carotid Endarterectomy Trial (NASCET). Both studies had patients with some degree of asymptomatic carotid stenosis contralateral to the symptomatic, randomized carotid, and the risk of stroke in the distribution of the asymptomatic artery has been published. ECST found that higher degrees of stenosis tended to have a higher risk of stroke; the 3-year risk of stroke was 1.8% in the 0% to 29% stenosis group, 2.1% in the 30% to 69%

stenosis group, and 5.7% in the 70% to 99% stenosis group.[32] In the NASCET trial, the risks of stroke over a 4-year period were 4.5%, 8.3%, and 14.5% for stenosis of less than 30%, 30% to 69%, and 70% to 99%, respectively.[33] These numbers should be compared carefully because the degree of carotid stenosis was measured differently in the two trials (50% NASCET stenosis = 75% ECST stenosis).

Patients with a TIA or minor nondisabling stroke in the distribution of a carotid stenosis appear to have a higher risk of subsequent ipsilateral stroke compared with patients with no neurological symptoms with known carotid stenosis. Data from the control or medically treated arms of NASCET and ECST provided stroke rates ipsilateral to the symptomatic carotid stenosis. In NASCET, the ipsilateral stroke rate was 26%, 22%, and 19% for 70% to 99%, 50% to 69%, and less than 50% stenosis, respectively. The major ipsilateral stroke rate was 13%, 7.2%, and 4.7% for 70% to 99%, 50% to 69%, and less than 50% stenosis, respectively.[34, 35] In ECST, the ipsilateral major stroke rate was 17.4%, 10.6%, and 6% for 70% to 99%, 50% to 69%, and less than 50% stenosis, respectively.[36] Again, interpretation must be cautious. Not only was the degree of carotid stenosis measured differently in ECST and NASCET, the duration of follow-up also varied. The mean follow-up was approximately 6 years in ECST, 2 years in the severe stenosis NASCET group, and 5 years in the mild and moderate stenosis NASCET group.

MEDICAL MANAGEMENT OF EXTRACRANIAL CAROTID DISEASE

This discussion of the medical management of carotid occlusive disease concentrates on secondary prevention rather than acute interventions. First, risk factors for stroke and carotid artery occlusive disease are considered, followed by various medical treatments that have been used to prevent complications of carotid artery occlusive disease (i.e., ischemic strokes). The risk factors for ischemic stroke are discussed in general and applied specifically to carotid artery occlusive disease when applicable. Most patients with significant cerebrovascular disease are likely to have other cardiovascular diseases or to be predisposed to develop them. Patients have no control over risk factors such as advancing age, gender, race, and previous TIA or stroke. Certain risk factors, however, are modifiable, and both patients and physicians must be aware of them: arterial hypertension, diabetes mellitus, tobacco smoking, heavy alcohol use, and hyperlipidemia, among others.

Risk Factors

Hypertension is the most prevalent and modifiable risk factor for stroke.[37] Its treatment substantially reduces the risk of stroke. Several prospective randomized controlled trials indicate that a 5 to 6 mm Hg decrease in diastolic blood pressure reduces the risk of stroke by 42%.[38] The treatment of isolated systolic hypertension in the elderly decreases the risk of stroke by 36%.[39] In this population of elderly patients, isolated systolic hypertension greater than 160 mm Hg strongly correlated with carotid stenosis, as measured by carotid ultrasonography.[40] In general, recommendations state that systolic blood pressure (BP) should be less than 140 mm Hg and diastolic BP should be less than 90 mm Hg. In patients with heart failure, renal insufficiency, diabetes, or other evidence of target organ damage or clinical cardiovascular disease (including stroke or TIA), drug therapy combined with lifestyle modifications should be considered when blood pressure is high-normal (systolic BP, 130 to 139 mm Hg or diastolic BP, 85 to 89 mm Hg).[41, 42]

Diabetes mellitus, a well-established risk factor for stroke, may increase the risk of stroke by several mechanisms: acceleration of large artery atherosclerosis, adverse effects on plasma lipoprotein levels, and promotion of plaque formation through hyperinsulinemia. Although it has been difficult to show conclusively that tight control of serum glucose levels reduces the risk of stroke, it does reduce some of the other microvascular complications of diabetes.[37, 43] Controlling elevated blood sugars, perhaps at less than 126 mg/dl,[41] is desirable.

Heavy alcohol consumption appears to be a risk factor for ischemic stroke.[44] However, light or moderate alcohol use may exert a protective effect.[45] This J-shaped curve also appears to hold true for early carotid atherogenesis. Light drinkers face a lower risk of incident carotid atherosclerosis detected by carotid ultrasonography than heavy drinkers or those abstaining from alcohol.[46]

Cigarette smoking is another ischemic stroke risk factor. Smokers have an approximate risk of 1.5.[47] The impact of cigarette smoking on the risk of stroke also applies to young adults (between 15 and 45 years old).[48] It also appears that smoking is an independent determinant of severe carotid artery stenosis in patients with previous strokes.[49] Therefore, all patients should be encouraged to quit smoking.

The relationship of hypercholesterolemia to stroke has been controversial, mainly because the outcomes of lipid-lowering regimens in preventing strokes have been inconsistent.[50] However, recent, large-scale, randomized, double-blind, placebo-controlled trials have shown that the hepatic hydroxymethyl glutaryl coenzyme A (HMG CoA) reductase inhibitors, or statins, can lower rates of myocardial infarction and fatal coronary events in patients with a history of coronary artery disease and various levels of total cholesterol and LDL cholesterol.[51–53] Two of these studies specified stroke as a secondary endpoint, and it appears that these medications lower the risk of stroke in these patients with coronary artery disease by 19% to 32%.[53, 54] Two meta-analyses of the data from reported clinical trials of the effectiveness of HMG CoA reductase inhibitors in patients with coronary artery disease also showed a 27% to 32% reduction in stroke rate.[55, 56] Several studies have shown that lovastatin or pravastatin reduce the development or progression of carotid atherosclerosis as measured by the thickness of the vessel initima-media complex on carotid ultrasonography.[57–61] We await the results of trials evaluating the effectiveness of these medications in lowering cholesterol and in preventing strokes in patients with primary cerebrovascular disease. At this time, we recommend following the guidelines on the detection, evaluation, and treatment of high blood cholesterol published by the National Cholesterol Education Program.[62]

Homocysteine (specifically, hyperhomocystinemia) is a risk factor for atherosclerosis and endothelial dysfunction, and therefore, likely for stroke as well. Proposed mechanisms for its proatherogenic effects are endothelial cell injury, increased platelet aggregation, enhancement of a prothrombotic environment, and smooth muscle cell proliferation.[63, 64] A case-control study in a group of British men aged 40 to 59 years showed that hyperhomocystinemia was a strong risk factor for stroke even after adjusting for multiple other risk factors.[65] A graded increase in the number of strokes was noted as homocysteine levels increased. Elderly subjects with an elevated homocysteine level also appear to be at higher risk of cardiovascular disease, including strokes.[66] Plasma homocysteine concentrations and extracranial carotid artery disease appear to be associated.[67, 68] In a cohort of patients from the Framingham Heart Study, the odds ratio of a carotid stenosis greater than or equal to 25% was 2.0 for subjects with the highest plasma homocysteine concentrations compared with those with the lowest concentrations.[67] Treatment with vitamins, specifically B_{12}, B_6, and folate, may lower plasma homocysteine concentrations, but their effectiveness in preventing stroke has not yet been determined. Ongoing trials of vitamins in preventing strokes are under way and should help answer that question.

Platelet Antiaggregant Therapy

This discussion of the medical management of carotid artery occlusive disease focuses on platelet antiaggregating drugs, which are mainstays in the prevention of stroke in arterial atherothromboembolic disease. Aspirin works by irreversibly inhibiting platelet cyclooxygenase, which prevents the formation of thromboxane A_2, a potent vasoconstrictor and inducer of platelet aggregation. In healthy individuals, a single aspirin results in a 98% inhibition of thromboxane A_2 production within 1 hour of ingestion. Several large, randomized and controlled clinical trials have found it to be beneficial in the secondary prevention of cardiovascular events and death.[69] An overview of randomized trials of platelet antiaggregant therapy in patients with a history of TIA or stroke showed about a 25% reduction in the risk of nonfatal stroke, nonfatal myocardial infarction, and death from vascular causes.[70] This risk reduction was independent of age, gender, and other risk factors.

Another advantage of aspirin is its effect on reducing cardiovascular deaths, a helpful feature for patients with carotid disease given their frequent combination of carotid and coronary atherosclerosis. Aspirin also helps reduce mortality rates after carotid endarterectomy.[71] In a retrospective analysis of the medically treated patients from the VA Cooperative Study on Asymptomatic Stenosis, patients not taking aspirin had a higher incidence of stroke and death than those taking aspirin. This finding provides some indirect evidence that aspirin may be useful in asymptomatic patients with significant carotid stenosis.[72] Higher doses of aspirin slowed the growth of carotid plaque in 27 patients, although this finding has not been duplicated in larger patient populations.[73]

The appropriate dose of aspirin in preventing stroke remains controversial. Studies showing its effectiveness in the secondary prevention of stroke have used doses ranging from 30 to 1500 mg/day. Some authors have advocated higher doses of aspirin, given that these doses may have useful effects unrelated to cyclooxygenase inhibition.[74] In the Aspirin in Carotid Endarterectomy Trial (ACE), 2804 patients who had a carotid endarterectomy were randomly assigned to compare the benefits of low-dose aspirin (81 to 325 mg/day) with high-dose aspirin (650 to 1300 mg/day). The primary endpoints in the ACE trial were stroke, myocardial infarction, or death. Three months after surgery, the risk of stroke, myocardial infarction, or death was 6.2% in the low-dose aspirin group compared with 8.4% in the high-dose aspirin group. The difference was less apparent when only stroke or death was evaluated as the endpoint.[75] Recently, the United States Food and Drug Administration recommended a dose of 50 to 325 mg/day of aspirin[76]

Ticlopidine is a platelet antiaggregant agent that works by inhibiting the adenosine phosphate pathway of platelet aggregation. Although it has not been studied specifically in patients with carotid atherosclerosis, it has been shown to reduce the risk of stroke, myocardial infarction, or vascular death in patients with recent noncardioembolic stroke.[77] Ticlopidine reduces the relative risk of death or nonfatal stroke by 12% compared with aspirin.[78] The recommended dose of ticlopidine is 250 mg twice daily. Ticlopidine has more side effects than aspirin, including diarrhea, nausea, dyspepsia, and rash. Its use, however, has been limited by significant hematologic side effects, including a reversible neutropenia and thrombotic thrombocytopenic purpura. The drug must be discontinued if the neutrophil count falls below 1200/mm^3.

Clopidogrel is also a platelet adenosine diphosphate receptor antagonist. In a study enrolling more than 19,185 patients with atherosclerotic vascular disease, which manifested as either recent ischemic stroke, recent myocardial infarction, or symptomatic peripheral arterial disease, clopidogrel (75 mg/day) was more effective than 325 mg of aspirin in reducing the combined risk of ischemic stroke, myocardial infarction, or vascular death.[79] After almost 2 years of follow-up, the absolute risk reduction was modest (annual risk of end points in clopidogrel-treated patients 5.32% versus 5.83% in aspirin-treated patients) although statistically significant. In the group of more than 6400 patients who entered the study with a stroke, there was a nonsignificant relative risk reduction of 7.3% in favor of clopidogrel. Most of these patients developed a recurrent stroke as their first outcome measure. The side effect profile of clopidogrel is relatively benign. There is no increased incidence of neutropenia, and the incidence of gastrointestinal hemorrhage and gastric or duodenal ulcers is lower compared with that of aspirin. Its use has not been tested specifically in patients who have carotid artery occlusive disease only.

Dipyridamole is a phosphodiesterase inhibitor that increases the levels of cyclic adenosine monophosphate (cAMP). Previous studies failed to demonstrate the benefit of adding dipyridamole to aspirin. A large, randomized, placebo-controlled, double-blind trial, however, was published in 1996. This European Stroke Prevention Study-2 (ESPS-2) randomized patients with prior TIA or stroke to treatment with aspirin alone (25 mg twice daily), modified-release dipyridamole (200 mg twice daily), the two agents in combination, or a placebo. The ESPS-2 investigators reported an additive effect of dipyridamole when it was coprescribed with aspirin. The stroke rate decreased in the combined treatment arm compared with either agent alone. Both low-dose aspirin and high-dose dipyridamole in a modified release form alone were associated with better outcomes than the placebo.[80] The main side effects of dipyridamole are gastrointestinal distress and headaches.

Platelet glycoprotein IIb–IIIa receptor inhibitors have been evaluated in cardiovascular disease, but their benefit in preventing ischemic stroke awaits randomized studies. Combinations of platelet antiaggregant therapy (aspirin + ticlopidine or aspirin + clopidogrel) are also used by clinicians, but no data have demonstrated their benefit over single agents alone in preventing ischemic stroke in general or carotid artery occlusive disease specifically.

Warfarin has also been used in the primary and secondary prevention of stroke in patients with nonvalvular atrial fibrillation. Warfarin is unequivocally effective in reducing the recurrence of stroke in patients with selective cardiac sources of emboli, especially nonvalvular atrial fibrillation. However, its relative efficacy compared with antiplatelet therapy in patients with atherothrombotic TIA or stroke has not been studied adequately. Many clinicians use warfarin to treat patients with high-grade intracranial stenosis and severe ICA stenosis, but randomized clinical data are not available to support its use. Trials comparing warfarin to aspirin in the secondary prevention of noncardioembolic stroke are ongoing. When available, these data, including subgroup analysis, may help define the usefulness of warfarin in treating carotid artery occlusive disease.

Surgical and catheter-based procedures such as angioplasty and stenting are also used to treat carotid artery occlusive disease. Numerous well-designed studies defining the effectiveness of carotid endarterectomy in preventing strokes in both neurologically symptomatic and asymptomatic patients have been published since 1990.[29, 34–36, 81] Trials of carotid angioplasty and stenting are getting started and are discussed elsewhere in this book. Further defining the appropriate treatment for patients with carotid occlusive disease, whether medical or surgical, will be the goal of ongoing and future research.

REFERENCES

1. Stroke facts: American Heart Association. http://www.americanheart.org/Heart_and_Stroke_ A_Z_Guide/strokes.html (Accessed 12/01/99.)
2. Mohr JP, Caplan LR, Melski JW, et al: The Harvard Cooperative Stroke Registry: A prospective registry. Neurology 28:754–762, 1978.
3. Fields WS, Lemak NA: A History of Stroke: Its Recognition and Treatment, New York, Oxford University Press, 1989.
4. Estol CJ: Dr C. Miller Fisher and the history of carotid artery disease. Stroke 27:559–566, 1996.
5. Fisher C: Occlusion of the internal carotid artery. Arch Neurol Psychiatry 65:346–377, 1951.
6. Fisher C: Occlusion of the carotid arteries: further experiences. Arch Neurol Psychiatry 72:187–204, 1954.
7. Ross R: The pathogenesis of atherosclerosis—an update. N Engl J Med 314:488–500, 1986.
8. Ross R: Atherosclerosis—an inflammatory disease. N Engl J Med 340(2):115–126, 1999.
9. Esposito G, Blasi F, Allegra L, et al: Demonstration of viable *Chlamydia pneumoniae* in atherosclerotic plaques of carotid arteries by reverse transcriptase polymerase chain reaction. Ann Vasc Surg 13:421–425, 1999.
10. Yamashita K, Ouchi K, Shirai M, et al: Distribution of *Chlamydia pneumoniae* infection in the atherosclerotic carotid artery. Stroke 29:773–778, 1998.
11. Nieto FJ, Adam E, Sorlie P, et al: Cohort study of *cytomegalovirus* infection as a risk factor for carotid intimal-medial thickening, a measure of subclinical atherosclerosis. Circulation 94:922–927, 1996.
12. Moore WS, Malone JM: Effect of flow rate and vessel calibre on critical arterial stenosis. J Surg Res 26:1–9, 1979.
13. Powers WJ, Press GA, Grubb RL Jr, et al: The effect of hemodynamically significant carotid artery disease on the hemodynamic status of the cerebral circulation. Ann Intern Med 106:27–34, 1987.
14. Powers WJ: Cerebral hemodynamics in ischemic cerebrovascular disease. Ann Neurol 29:231–240, 1991.
15. el-Barghouty N, Nicolaides A, Bahal V, et al: The identification of the high risk carotid plaque. Eur J Vas Endovasc Surg 11: 470–478, 1996.
16. Nicolaides A, Kalodiki E, Ramaswani G, et al: The significance of cerebral infarcts on CT scan in patients with transient ischemic attacks. In Bernstein EF, Callow A, Nicolaides A, Shifrin E (eds): Cerebral Revascularization, London, Med-Orion Publishing, 1993.
17. Wechsler LR: Ulceration and carotid artery disease. Stroke 19: 650–653, 1988.
18. Eliasziw M, Streifler JY, Fox AJ, et al: Significance of plaque ulceration in symptomatic patients with high-grade carotid stenosis. North American Symptomatic Carotid Endarterectomy Trial. Stroke 25:304–308, 1994.
19. Biller J, Saver JL: Transient ischemic attacks—populations and prognosis. Mayo Clin Proc 69:493–494, 1994.
20. Streifler JY, Eliasziw M, Benavente OR, et al: The risk of stroke in patients with first-ever retinal vs hemispheric transient ischemic attacks and high-grade carotid stenosis. North American Symptomatic Carotid Endarterectomy Trial. Arch Neurol 52:246–249, 1995.
21. Vascular Syndromes of the Cerebrum. In Brazis PW, Masdeu JC, Biller J (eds): Localization in Clinical Neurology, 3rd edition, Boston, Little, Brown and Co, 1996, pp 535–564.
22. Josse MO, Touboul PJ, Mas JL, et al: Prevalence of asymptomatic internal carotid artery stenosis. Neuroepidemiology 6:150–152, 1987.
23. Colgan MP, Strode GR, Sommer JD, et al: Prevalence of asymptomatic carotid disease: Results of duplex scanning in 348 unselected volunteers. J Vasc Surg 8:674–678, 1988.
24. Hennerici M, Aulich A, Sandmann W, et al: Incidence of asymptomatic extracranial arterial disease. Stroke 12:750–758, 1981.

25. Heyman A, Wilkinson WE, Heyden S, et al: Risk of stroke in asymptomatic persons with cervical arterial bruits: A population study in Evans County, Georgia. N Engl J Med 302:838–841, 1980.
26. Wolf PA, Kannel WB, Sorlie P, et al: Asymptomatic carotid bruit and risk of stroke. The Framingham study. JAMA 245:1442–1445, 1981.
27. Ingall TJ, Homer D, Whisnant JP, et al: Predictive value of carotid bruit for carotid atherosclerosis. Arch Neurol 46:418–422, 1989.
28. Ziegler DK, Zileli T, Dick A, et al: Correlation of bruits over the carotid artery with angiographically demonstrated lesions. Neurology 21:860–865, 1971.
29. Executive Committee for the Asymptomatic Carotid Atherosclerosis Study: Endarterectomy for asymptomatic carotid artery stenosis. JAMA 273:1421–1468, 1995.
30. Meissner I, Wiebers DO, Whisnant JP, et al: The natural history of asymptomatic carotid artery occlusive lesions. JAMA 258: 2704–2707, 1987.
31. Hennerici M, Hulsbomer HB, Hefter H, et al: Natural history of asymptomatic extracranial arterial disease. Results of a long-term prospective study. Brain 110(Pt 3):777–791, 1987.
32. The European Carotid Surgery Trialists Collaborative Group: Risk of stroke in the distribution of an asymptomatic carotid artery. Lancet 345(8944):209–212, 1995.
33. Chan R EB, Hachinski V, Barnett H: The risk of stroke in the territory of an asymptomatic stenosed extracranial internal carotid artery: Degree of stenosis, intermittent claudication and silent cerebral infarction as predictors of stroke. Stroke 27:194, 1996.
34. North American Symptomatic Carotid Endarterectomy Trial Collaborators: Beneficial effect of carotid endarterectomy in symptomatic patients with high-grade carotid stenosis. N Engl J Med 325:445–453, 1991.
35. Barnett HJ, Taylor DW, Eliasziw M, et al: Benefit of carotid endarterectomy in patients with symptomatic moderate or severe stenosis. North American Symptomatic Carotid Endarterectomy Trial Collaborators. N Engl J Med 339:1415–1425, 1998.
36. European Carotid Surgery Trialists Group: Randomised trial of endarterectomy for recently symptomatic carotid stenosis: Final results of the MRC European Carotid Surgery Trial (ECST). Lancet 351:1379–1387, 1998.
37. Gorelick PB, Sacco RL, Smith DB, et al: Prevention of a first stroke: A review of guidelines and a multidisciplinary consensus statement from the National Stroke Association. JAMA 281:1112–1120, 1999.
38. Collins R, Peto R, MacMahon S, et al: Blood pressure, stroke, and coronary heart disease. Part 2. Short-term reductions in blood pressure: Overview of randomised drug trials in their epidemiological context. Lancet 335:827–838, 1990.
39. SHEP Cooperative Research Group: Prevention of stroke by antihypertensive drug treatment in older persons with isolated systolic hypertension. Final results of the Systolic Hypertension in the Elderly Program (SHEP). JAMA 265:3255–3264, 1991.
40. Sutton-Tyrrell K, Alcorn HG, Wolfson SK, Jr, et al: Predictors of carotid stenosis in older adults with and without isolated systolic hypertension. Stroke 24:355–361, 1993.
41. Wolf PA, Clagett GP, Easton JD, et al: Preventing ischemic stroke in patients with prior stroke and transient ischemic attack: A statement for healthcare professionals from the stroke council of the American Heart Association. Stroke 30:1991–1994, 1999.
42. The Sixth Report of the Joint National Committee on prevention, detection, evaluation, and treatment of high blood pressure. Arch Intern Med 157:2413–2446, 1997.
43. Albers GW, Hart RG, Lutsep HL, et al: AHA Scientific Statement. Supplement to the guidelines for the management of transient ischemic attacks: A statement from the Ad Hoc Committee on Guidelines for the Management of Transient Ischemic Attacks, Stroke Council, American Heart Association. Stroke 30:2502–2511, 1999.
44. Gill JS, Zezulka AV, Shipley MJ, et al: Stroke and alcohol consumption. N Engl J Med 315:1041–1046, 1986.
45. Sacco RL, Elkind M, Boden-Albala B, et al: The protective effect of moderate alcohol consumption on ischemic stroke. JAMA 281: 53–60, 1999.
46. Kiechl S, Willeit J, Rungger G, et al: Alcohol consumption and atherosclerosis: What is the relation? Prospective results from the Bruneck Study. Stroke 29:900–907, 1998.
47. Shinton R, Beevers G: Meta-analysis of relation between cigarette smoking and stroke. BMJ 298:789–794, 1989.
48. Love BB, Biller J, Jones MP, et al: Cigarette smoking. A risk factor for cerebral infarction in young adults. Arch Neurol 47: 693–698, 1990.
49. Mast H, Thompson JL, Lin IF, et al: Cigarette smoking as a determinant of high-grade carotid artery stenosis in Hispanic, black, and white patients with stroke or transient ischemic attack. Stroke 29:908–912, 1998.
50. Atkins D, Psaty BM, Koepsell TD, et al: Cholesterol reduction and the risk for stroke in men. A meta-analysis of randomized, controlled trials. Ann Intern Med 119(2):136–145, 1993.
51. The Scandinavian Simvastatin Survival Study (4S): Randomised trial of cholesterol lowering in 4444 patients with coronary heart disease. Lancet 344:1383–1389, 1994.
52. Sacks FM, Pfeffer MA, Moye LA, et al: The effect of pravastatin on coronary events after myocardial infarction in patients with average cholesterol levels. Cholesterol and Recurrent Events Trial investigators. N Engl J Med 335:1001–1009, 1996.
53. The Long-Term Intervention with Pravastatin in Ischaemic Disease (LIPID) Study Group: Prevention of cardiovascular events and death with pravastatin in patients with coronary heart disease and a broad range of initial cholesterol levels. N Engl J Med 339:1349–1357, 1998.
54. Plehn JF, Davis BR, Sacks FM, et al: Reduction of stroke incidence after myocardial infarction with pravastatin: The Cholesterol and Recurrent Events (CARE) study. The Care Investigators. Circulation 99(2):216–223, 1999.
55. Blauw GJ, Lagaay AM, Smelt AH, et al: Stroke, statins, and cholesterol. A meta-analysis of randomized, placebo-controlled, double-blind trials with HMG-CoA reductase inhibitors. Stroke 28(5):946–950, 1997.
56. Crouse JR, 3rd, Byington RP, Hoen HM, et al: Reductase inhibitor monotherapy and stroke prevention. Arch Intern Med 157(12): 1305–1310, 1997.
57. MacMahon S, Sharpe N, Gamble G, et al: Effects of lowering average of below-average cholesterol levels on the progression of carotid atherosclerosis: Results of the LIPID Atherosclerosis Substudy. LIPID Trial Research Group. Circulation 97(18):1784–1790, 1998.
58. Hodis HN, Mack WJ, LaBree L, et al: Reduction in carotid arterial wall thickness using lovastatin and dietary therapy: A randomized controlled clinical trial. Ann Intern Med 124:548–556, 1996.
59. Furberg CD, Adams HP, Jr, Applegate WB, et al: Effect of lovastatin on early carotid atherosclerosis and cardiovascular events. Asymptomatic Carotid Artery Progression Study (ACAPS) Research Group. Circulation 90:1679–1687, 1994.
60. Salonen R, Nyyssonen K, Porkkala E, et al: Kuopio Atherosclerosis Prevention Study (KAPS). A population-based primary preventive trial of the effect of LDL lowering on atherosclerotic progression in carotid and femoral arteries. Circulation 92(7): 1758–1764, 1995.
61. Crouse JR, 3rd, Byington RP, Bond MG, et al: Pravastatin, Lipids, and atherosclerosis in the carotid arteries (PLAC-II). Am J Cardiol 75(7):455–459, 1995.
62. Adult Treatment Panel II: Summary of the second report of the National Cholesterol Education Program (NCEP) Expert Panel on Detection, Evaluation, and Treatment of High Blood Cholesterol in Adults. JAMA 269(23):3015–3023, 1993.
63. Welch GN, Loscalzo J: Homocysteine and atherothrombosis. N Engl J Med 338:1042–1050, 1998.
64. Stein JH, McBride PE: Hyperhomocysteinemia and atherosclerotic vascular disease: Pathophysiology, screening, and treatment. Arch Intern Med 158:1301–1306, 1998.
65. Perry IJ, Refsum H, Morris RW, et al: Prospective study of serum total homocysteine concentration and risk of stroke in middle-aged British men. Lancet 346:1395–1398, 1995.
66. Bots ML, Launer LJ, Lindemans J, et al: Homocysteine and short-term risk of myocardial infarction and stroke in the elderly: The Rotterdam Study. Arch Intern Med 159:38–44, 1999.
67. Selhub J, Jacques PF, Bostom AG, et al: Association between plasma homocysteine concentrations and extracranial carotid-artery stenosis. N Engl J Med 332:286–291, 1995.
68. McQuillan BM, Beilby JP, Nidorf M, et al: Hyperhomocysteinemia but not the C677T mutation of methylenetetrahydrofolate

reductase is an independent risk determinant of carotid wall thickening. The Perth Carotid Ultrasound Disease Assessment Study (CUDAS). Circulation 99:2383–2388, 1999.
69. Fuster V, Dyken ML, Vokonas PS, et al: Aspirin as a therapeutic agent in cardiovascular disease. Special Writing Group. Circulation 87:659–675, 1993.
70. Antiplatelet Trialists' Collaboration: Collaborative overview of randomised trials of antiplatelet therapy. I: Prevention of death, myocardial infarction, and stroke by prolonged antiplatelet therapy in various categories of patients. BMJ 308:81–106, 1994.
71. Kretschmer G, Pratschner T, Prager M, et al: Antiplatelet treatment prolongs survival after carotid bifurcation endarterectomy. Analysis of the clinical series followed by a controlled trial. Ann Surg 211:317–322, 1990.
72. Hobson RW 2d, Krupski WC, Weiss DG: Influence of aspirin in the management of asymptomatic carotid artery stenosis. VA Cooperative Study Group on Asymptomatic Carotid Stenosis. J Vasc Surg 17:257–265, 1993.
73. Ranke C, Hecker H, Creutzig A, et al: Dose-dependent effect of aspirin on carotid atherosclerosis. Circulation 87:1873–1879, 1993.
74. Dyken ML, Barnett HJ, Easton JD, et al: Low-dose aspirin and stroke. "It ain't necessarily so." Stroke 23:1395–1399, 1992.
75. Taylor DW, Barnett HJ, Haynes RB, et al: Low-dose and high-dose acetylsalicylic acid for patients undergoing carotid endarterectomy: A randomised controlled trial. ASA and Carotid Endarterectomy (ACE) Trial Collaborators. Lancet 353:2179–2184, 1999.
76. Food and Drug Administration: Internal analgesic, antipyretic, and antirheumatic drug products for over-the-counter human use: Final rule for professional labeling of aspirin, buffered aspirin, and aspirin in combination with antacid products. Fed Reg 63:56802–56819, 66015–66017, 1998.
77. Gent M, Blakely JA, Easton JD, et al: The Canadian American Ticlopidine Study (CATS) in thromboembolic stroke. Lancet 1: 1215–1220, 1989.
78. Hass WK, Easton JD, Adams HP, Jr, et al: A randomized trial comparing ticlopidine hydrochloride with aspirin for the prevention of stroke in high-risk patients. Ticlopidine Aspirin Stroke Study Group. N Engl J Med 321:501–507, 1989.
79. CAPRIE Steering Committee: A randomised, blinded, trial of clopidogrel versus aspirin in patients at risk of ischaemic events (CAPRIE). Lancet 348:1329–1339, 1996.
80. Diener HC, Cunha L, Forbes C, et al: European Stroke Prevention Study. 2. Dipyridamole and acetylsalicylic acid in the secondary prevention of stroke. J Neurol Sci 143:1–13, 1996.
81. European Carotid Surgery Trialists' Collaborative Group: MRC European Carotid Surgery Trial: Interim results for symptomatic patients with severe (70–99%) or with mild (0–29%) carotid stenosis. Lancet 337:1235–1243, 1991.

CHAPTER 97

Carotid Endarterectomy

JULIAN E. BAILES ■ MAX B. MEDARY

Few procedures in modern medicine have been as carefully scrutinized and highly debated as carotid endarterectomy (CEA). Spurred by the prevalence of stroke and the high medical and societal costs of caring for victims and survivors of stroke, the clinical considerations and techniques related to performing CEA have evolved. Although the efficacy of CEA in certain situations is still debated, this procedure has been deemed beneficial for many groups of patients.

CEA has often been considered merely a method of increasing ipsilateral cerebral blood flow and removing angiographically visualized stenoses. Our current knowledge has progressed to allow detailed analysis of the entire cerebrovascular supply, beginning at the aortic arch and continuing to the cerebral microcirculation. In conjunction with the neuroradiologic investigation, treatment can be individualized based on the clinical manifestations of each patient's embolic or hemodynamic phenomena. The past few years have seen tremendous advances in areas such as magnetic resonance angiography, transcranial Doppler (TCD) ultrasonography, cerebral blood flow, critical care medicine, cardiology, and anesthesiology, among others. These advances have greatly increased our ability to perform CEA successfully and improve outcomes compared with the natural history of the untreated disease.

The protocol described here, which is based on contemporary principles of neurological surgery such as use of the operating microscope, intraoperative monitoring of cerebral function, pharmacologic protection, and avoidance of the routine use of carotid shunts, has yielded favorable outcomes in patients undergoing endarterectomy.[1] This chapter describes the techniques of microsurgical CEA and thromboendarterectomy and focuses on the controversies surrounding the procedure. Major complications and their avoidance are also addressed.

HISTORICAL BACKGROUND

The development of carotid artery surgery has progressed stepwise, with several notable milestones, and reflects the disciplines of neurology, surgery, pathology, and radiology. In the 1940s, it was realized that ischemic symptoms related to the carotid distribution could be ascribed to narrowing or stenosis of the artery, distal embolization of clot or particulate matter, or complete occlusion. Patients suffering embolic ischemic phenomena were found to have no thrombus in any of the usual sources of systemic emboli, such as the left heart, ascending aorta, or pulmonary veins. Embolic strokes occurring in the territory of the middle cerebral artery (MCA) established the cervical carotid artery bifurcation as a common embolic source.[2] Carotid artery ligation for the repair of penetrating injuries and cervical carotid aneurysms was the earliest surgical procedure performed on this vessel. Ligation subsequently became standard treatment for many intracranial aneurysms. Cervical carotid excisional ligation and sympathectomy had been used in attempts to prevent thromboembolism and to abolish symptoms believed to cause vasospasm.[3] Fisher and coworkers[4] emphasized the role of carotid bifurcation atheroma and proposed the idea of bypassing carotid stenosis, causing surgical efforts to be directed toward restoring blood flow. Resection and reconstruction of carotid segments followed, performed by Carrea and colleagues in 1951 (as discussed in Fein[3]) and by Eastcott and coworkers in 1954.[5]

Originally, endarterectomy was developed for the lower extremities, but later it was adopted and modified for the carotid arteries, leading to the first published report of a successful CEA in 1953 by DeBakey (as discussed in Fein[3]). Although early studies demonstrated a benefit in certain patients, they also found that some of the best predictors of outcome were patient variables such as hypertension and cardiac disease. Consequently, surgical indications varied widely, and the number of procedures performed increased dramatically. In 1962, the first multicenter cooperative trial, the Joint Study of Extracranial Arterial Occlusion, began. This study enrolled 316 patients for 6 years, with a mean follow-up of 42 months.[6] It found that the number of asymptomatic survivors increased; however, it also highlighted a need to refine the surgical indications and improve the overall morbidity and mortality rates. Cardiac disease was the major cause of death in all groups studied. Further, the study documented that the surgical mortality rate decreased between the periods 1961 to 1965 and 1965 to 1969.[6]

Based on results that demonstrated an improved outcome, the use of CEA increased from 15,000 cases in 1971 to a peak of about 110,000 cases in 1985.[7, 8] By 1982, CEA had become the third most frequently performed surgery in the United States. However, serious doubts were raised about the procedure's risk-benefit ratio compared with that of medical therapy using aspirin.[6, 8–11] A second large cooperative study to evaluate the benefit of endarterectomy was begun by Shaw and associates[12] in 1965 but was not published until 1984. This study was discontinued after only 41 patients were enrolled because the rates of surgical morbidity and mortality were disproportionately high compared with those of patients in the medical control group. More recently, several large, multicenter, cooperative trials clearly demonstrated a benefit of CEA and better defined the appropriate indications for its use.[13–15] These studies also added to our knowledge of the disease and its ability to progress despite modern medical management. Nonetheless, controversies about diagnosis, surgical indications, techniques, and patient monitoring still remain.

CHARACTERISTICS AND PATHOPHYSIOLOGY OF CEREBROVASCULAR ACCIDENTS

Stroke is the third leading cause of death in the United States, accounting for 145,340 deaths in 1990, and it is the leading cause of morbidity.[16] Despite an encouraging decline in the number of strokes and in the number of fatalities from stroke in the past 20 years, the number of individuals disabled by stroke is increasing.[17–21] The American Heart Association estimates that 3,020,000 people have survived a stroke; many of them require long-term care and have significant disabilities.[16] Recent data indicate that as many as 750,000 people suffer stroke annually in the United States. The enormity of the human and economic impact of stroke is obvious and perhaps incalculable. Effective diagnostic methods and prophylactic treatments must be developed.

Infarction is the most common type of stroke, accounting for about 70% of all strokes in some studies.[16] The frequency of different causes of infarction has been examined in several noteworthy studies. The Framingham Study, which followed 5070 patients for 32 years, found that 50% of infarctions were the result of atherosclerotic and thrombotic vessel disease.[11] Cardioembolic strokes accounted for 17% to 22% of all strokes. Information from the Stroke Data Bank on 1273 patients showed that cardioembolic conditions caused 19% of strokes, whereas large vessel occlusion caused only 14%.[22] Of these 1273 strokes, 77% occurred in the territory of penetrating vessels, although the origin in 40% of cases was undetermined.[23]

Epidemiologic studies have examined and identified stroke risk factors. Age, female sex, hypertension, race, cholesterol level, tobacco use, diabetes, and degree of stenosis are the major predictors of the severity of the underlying disease.[15, 24–32] Several of the recent cooperative trials examined the importance of risk factors on outcome.[13–15] The North American Symptomatic Carotid Endarterectomy Trial (NASCET) found a significant and progressive increase in the risk of stroke among patients with an increasing number of risk factors,[15] but it did not identify the relative contribution of each factor. Several other multivariate analyses have found poor outcomes for patients with the risk factors of hypertension, diabetes, or smoking.[26, 33]

The development of carotid artery stenosis is analyzed by factoring multiple characteristics of systemic disease, plaque pathophysiology, effects on cerebral blood flow, and indicators of disease progression. The contribution of factors that may modify risk (such as hypertension, tobacco use, plaque ulceration, or degree of stenosis) must be studied.

Bruits

A cervical bruit is the most common physical manifestation of extracranial carotid artery disease. A bruit is an audible sign that can often be detected by auscultation during routine physical examination. The differential diagnosis of a carotid bruit is extensive.[10, 30, 34–43] A detailed history combined with a thorough physical examination can be used to reduce the list of possibilities.

Auscultation for the location, timing, and tone of a cervical bruit helps determine its cause. The characteristics of a neck bruit are difficult to correlate reliably with the underlying degree of carotid stenosis. Several clinical studies have evaluated the significance of bruits, but few have specified the proportion of bruits attributed to different causes. Rennie and coworkers[42] found that carotid atherosclerosis was the most common cause of a cervical bruit in young adults, hospital controls, and stroke patients. Cardiac causes, which ranked second, was responsible for 12% to 14% of bruits. Bruits related to carotid stenosis are audible vibrations of the carotid wall caused by turbulent blood flow distal to the stenosis. The degree of stenosis necessary to produce a bruit has been reported to be as low as 25%.[41] The presence of a bruit in a patient with carotid stenosis has been found to indicate a significant level (>50%) of stenosis on angiography in at least 70% of patients. False-positive rates of 10% to 40% and false-negative rates of 30% to 70% have been reported for cervical bruits. As many as half the patients with significant stenosis may not have cervical bruits.

Based on data from the Framingham and Evans County, Georgia, studies, an asymptomatic cervical bruit in the general population has been estimated to occur in 440 to 460 of 100,000 persons.[30, 40] These studies also demonstrated that the number of bruits increases markedly with age, hypertension, diabetes, and female sex.[30, 31, 40] Patients with bruits who were previously asymptomatic have an increased risk of neurological symptoms, but the true clinical significance of this finding has been the subject of much debate.[10, 31, 37, 38, 40, 44–48] The Framingham Study found that the risk of stroke and transient ischemic attacks (TIAs) in patients with bruits was two to three times the risk for patients without bruits.[31] Such patients were also 2.5 times more likely to have a myocardial infarction and 1.9 times more likely to die during the period of study. These results were similar to those found by Heyman and colleagues[49] in the Evans County, Georgia, study, which demonstrated more than a threefold increase in the risk of a new stroke for patients with bruits. However, the increased risk of ipsilateral neurological symptoms is substantially less than it appears to be from these impressive statistics. Bruits have been interpreted as general markers of atherosclerosis and thus warrant further investigation. They do not, however, necessarily predict the occurrence of a stroke.[50, 51]

Radiographic evaluation is necessary to discern the importance and extent of the atherosclerosis and to aid in selecting a treatment. Chambers and Norris[35] studied 500 patients with asymptomatic bruits who were followed for a mean of 23.2 months. They found a 6% annual rate of cerebral ischemia and an actual stroke rate of 1.7% at 12 months. However, only 42% of the strokes were ipsilateral to the carotid bruit. They also found a 7% annual rate of cardiac ischemic events and a 4% mortality rate for patients with bruits, primarily from a cardiac source.

Transient Ischemic Attacks

Carotid artery stenosis often presents with transient neurological symptoms. Patients may have symptoms caused by retinal ischemia, hemispheric ischemia, or both. In 1958, the Committee on Cerebrovascular Nomenclature defined a TIA as a temporary neurological deficit with an upper duration of 1 hour. As knowledge increased, this duration was revised to less than 30 minutes.[52] Then in 1990, TIA was redefined as a focal loss of brain function, including loss of vision, lasting less than 24 hours.[52, 53] The definition was based on clinical grounds, despite the ability of neuroimaging modalities such as magnetic resonance imaging and computed tomography to detect small areas of infarction associated with deficits that persist 24 hours.[52] Further, the decision to lump both hemispheric and retinal transient events together is unwarranted. The occurrence of stroke at 2 years increases more than twofold in patients with hemispheric TIAs compared with those who have retinal TIAs.[15]

The neurological symptoms characteristic of TIAs usually have a rapid onset and are maximal within 2 minutes, but sometimes they evolve over 5 minutes.[2, 49, 52, 54–57] Reports indicate that 75% of TIAs resolve within 5 minutes, and many last 1 minute or less.[49, 52, 58] TIAs rarely persist as long as the 24-hour limit. They completely resolve and are typically characterized by a symptom profile associated with the particular vascular distribution (e.g., carotid or vertebrobasilar) in which they occur. The variations in the definition of TIA and how it is distinguished from stroke have created confusion in interpreting studies on this topic. Thus, results across studies, especially those in different decades, must be compared cautiously.

The rate of occurrence of TIAs in the general population has received little attention during the past 3 decades. The prevalence of TIAs was examined in two large surveys published in the early 1970s. The Evans County, Georgia, survey studied 2455 people during the 1960s for evidence of stroke. This study contained 551 patients aged 65 years and older. The prevalence rate of TIAs in this age group was 18.1/1000.[40, 49] The Cook County survey, a similar study performed in an urban setting, consisted of 2772 patients between 65 and 74 years old. The prevalence rate of TIAs was 63/1000.[49, 55] Numerous explanations concerning the socioeconomic status of the two populations have been proposed to account for the differences between them, but none has ever been proved. Despite the population differences, both studies found that risk increased with age and was higher for women than for men.[40, 56] The incidence of TIAs in a defined population was examined in the Rochester, Minnesota, survey, which included 39,012 people, 9369 of whom were between 45 and 74 years old. The annual incidence in this age group was 93/100,000, and the overall incidence was 31/100,000.[49, 53] A similar figure of 110/100,000 was found in the Seal Beach, California, study, which included 10,500 people aged 52 years or older.[49, 59]

Studies of TIAs have also found a strong association with other vascular risk factors. In 1978, Toole and coworkers[57, 60] examined the association of risk factors in 225 patients with TIAs: 60% had ischemic cardiac disease, 30% had peripheral vascular disease, 30% had hypertension, and 20% had diabetes mellitus. The Framingham Study followed 171 patients for a mean of 4 years. Four patients (2.4%) had TIAs, and six (3.5%) experienced strokes. The incidence of myocardial infarction was doubled in patients who had bruits.[31] The mechanism underlying the occurrence of TIAs and stroke associated with carotid stenosis has been the subject of much speculation. The first mechanism proposed was a relative hypoperfusion state distal to a tight carotid stenosis. Another proposed mechanism was the occurrence of artery-to-artery thromboemboli. Other theories have included cardiac emboli, arrhythmic perfusion deficits, migraines, and a host of more obscure events.[52]

Cerebral hypoperfusion on a hemodynamic basis and thromboembolic-induced ischemia are explanations for TIAs. The embolic theory was confirmed by funduscopic observations made by Fisher[52] during an episode of amaurosis fugax in one of his patients (Fig. 97–1). Clinical research, such as that by Pessin and associates,[56] has offered angiographic support for the concept of thromboembolism in 66% of patients with TIAs or strokes. However, the remaining 34% of patients in this study had no evidence of a thromboembolic source. Instead, these patients had significant stenosis with hemodynamic compromise, thus providing support for the hemodynamic theory as well.[56] Angiographic assessments have shown structural lesions severe enough to account for strokes in patients with TIAs involving the carotid territory, but one in four lacked structural lesions, thus implicating emboli as the cause of their strokes.[61] Similarly, Fields and Lemak[62] reported identifiable lesions in only 73% of their patients. These findings strongly suggest the possibility

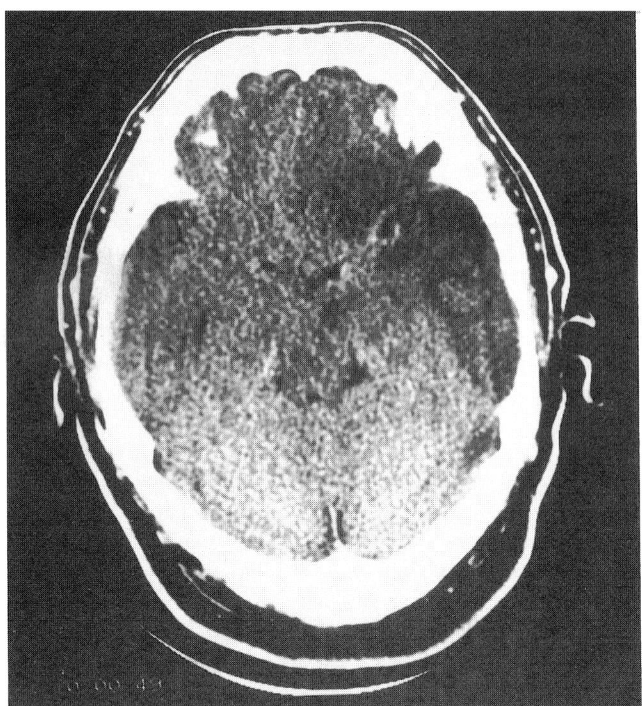

FIGURE 97–1. Computed tomographic scan obtained 24 hours after symptom onset showing embolism of the left middle cerebral artery. Subtle mass effect within the left hemisphere can be appreciated. (From Bailes JE, Spetzler RF [eds]: Microsurgical Carotid Endarterectomy. New York, Lippincott-Raven, 1996.)

of artery-to-artery emboli in patients who lack angiographic evidence of hemodynamically significant lesions to account for their symptoms.

These two mechanisms appear to cause TIAs, and often the difficulty is how to distinguish between them. Studies have revealed that TIAs presumed to be due to emboli (60% of emboli are not associated with TIAs) appear to persist for several hours; in contrast, hemodynamic TIAs tend to resolve in minutes.[49, 52, 54, 55] Fisher[52] found that when a patient had two or more TIAs or had a TIA and an episode of amaurosis on the same side, the most likely cause was significant carotid stenosis. In 88.5% of cases with multiple TIAs, the second TIA occurred within 7 days of the first event. When two TIAs occurred on the same day, occlusion was imminent. Additional support for the hemodynamic hypothesis came from Fisher's studies of carotid artery plaque.[52] He found a strong association between residual carotid lumina with a cross-sectional area of 1 mm or less and the occurrence of TIAs (98% of cases) and amaurosis (90%).

The correlation of TIAs with the risk of subsequent stroke has been studied extensively, and that risk ranges between 2% and 62% in TIA patients.[2, 16, 23, 44, 49, 54–56, 63–66] The consensus figure used by the American Heart Association is that 36% of patients who suffer one or more TIAs eventually experience a stroke; a large proportion of the remainder becomes asymptomatic. The data indicate that TIA patients are 9.5 times more likely than those without TIAs to experience a stroke.[16] Equally important is the percentage of patients who have a stroke without warning. In the Rochester, Minnesota, survey, Whisnant and colleagues[58] found that only 10% of patients reported TIA symptoms before their strokes. In contrast, Pessin and associates[67] in 1979 found that 54% of patients reported TIAs before stroke. Strokes of embolic origin, however, were preceded by TIAs in only 40% of patients. These findings emphasize the need to develop rational surgical guidelines for patients without neurological symptoms.

In summary, the occurrence of a TIA markedly increases the risk of stroke and the risk of death due to ischemic heart disease and thus merits an immediate and thorough diagnostic evaluation. Apparently, amaurosis fugax per se does not portend as serious a prognosis as hemispheric TIAs, but it should lead to a serious investigation.

Plaque Ulceration

Carotid plaque ulceration adversely affects a patient's risk.[68] Ulceration of the carotid artery has been described and categorized into three groups: small ulcers (type A), large ulcers (type B), and complex excavated ulcers (type C). Both experimental and clinical experience has shown a higher incidence of stroke as ulceration becomes more complex. The incidence of stroke associated with type C ulcers, for example, is seven times higher than that associated with type A ulcers (Fig. 97–2).

Apparently, the risk of stroke increases when plaque ulceration is present. Most studies, however, confirm that the risk factor of overwhelming importance remains the degree of stenosis of the ipsilateral vessel.[2] In the last 30 years, many studies have documented the progressive risk of ischemia as the level of stenosis increases. This relationship has also been illustrated in NASCET patients with symptomatic severe stenosis and ulceration. At 2 years, the risk of stroke associated

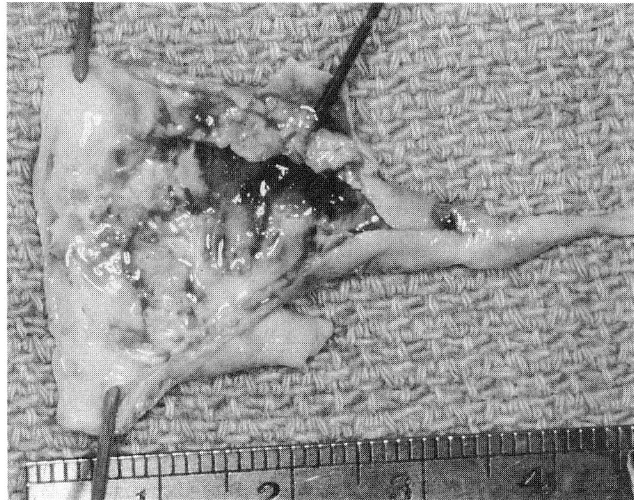

FIGURE 97–2. Typical complex atherosclerotic plaque occurring at the carotid artery bifurcation, with erosion through the plaque and platelet formation. (From Bailes JE, Spetzler RF [eds]: Microsurgical Carotid Endarterectomy. New York, Lippincott-Raven, 1996.)

with symptomatic 75% stenosis with ulceration was 26.3%, compared with a 73.2% risk in those with 95% stenosis.[15] Several fluid dynamic studies have modeled the mechanisms responsible for such changes. These data reveal that blood flow remains normal if the vessel diameter decreases by less than 60% (90% narrowing of cross-sectional area).[69] Blood flow decreases rapidly (by 40%) if the luminal diameter is diminished by 75%. If the luminal diameter is decreased by 84%, representing a 96% compromise of the cross-sectional area, blood flow decreases dramatically to 64% of normal.[70]

There is an even greater increase in the risk of stroke as stenosis increases and a contralateral carotid occlusion is present. An analysis of NASCET data reveals a marked increase in the ipsilateral 2-year stroke rate (56.3%) for patients with symptomatic severe stenosis and impressive but lower rates for the groups with minimal and moderate stenosis (22.5% and 22.4%, respectively).[15]

Although carotid atherosclerotic disease undoubtedly progresses, it is rarely asymptomatic. When the degree of stenosis is critical, it may lead to a recommendation for prophylactic CEA. Javid and colleagues[33] reported the only angiographic study on the evolution of carotid atherosclerosis. They studied 135 carotid artery bifurcations for 1 to 9 years. During this time, the carotid atherosclerotic lesion progressed in 62% of patients; in 30%, the lesions enlarged by more than 25% per year. This study suggested that moderate to severe atherosclerotic disease is particularly likely to progress to a critical degree of stenosis. In a carotid duplex scan study, a third of the carotid arteries progressively narrowed more than 50%.[66] Such progression remains a key indicator for performing CEA in asymptomatic individuals.

The following factors correlate with plaque progression: plaque size at the time of initial assessment, tobacco use, hypertension, and diabetes mellitus.[12, 19, 20, 24–26, 30, 32, 36, 60, 61, 66] Patients with known cervical carotid atherosclerotic disease should be followed closely, perhaps more frequently early in their course or if they have any other risk factors. Symptomatic patients typically proceed to surgical treatment. It is believed that control of vasculopathic risk factors may markedly slow the progression of the atherosclerotic process.

Cardiac Disease

The patient's cardiac status should also be evaluated thoroughly, because the occurrence of TIAs and surgical risk are strongly associated with ischemic cardiac disease.[16, 71] Indeed, the most frequent cause of death in many large studies of TIA patients has been myocardial infarction. For example, Fields and coworkers[72] and Toole and associates[57] reported mortality rates attributable to myocardial infarction of 58% and 57%, respectively. Since the 1960s, it has been firmly established that many patients have concurrent cerebral and coronary atherosclerosis. In fact, most patients who undergo CEA subsequently succumb to coronary disease.[73] Many patients have unknown or asymptomatic coronary disease. Because they are often unable to exercise, they may undergo thallium perfusion imaging or dobutamine stress echocardiography. A full preoperative cardiac evaluation is performed whenever indicated to reduce the risk of perioperative myocardial infarction to the lowest level achievable.

Clinical Studies

The indications, preoperative patient assessment, intraoperative technique, anesthetic management, and postoperative patient care associated with CEA have evolved. The NASCET study demonstrated a benefit from surgical intervention in 659 patients with greater than 70% symptomatic stenosis. Life-table estimates for the risk of ipsilateral stroke at 2 years were 26% in the medical group, compared with 9% in the surgical group. The absolute risk reduction for surgery compared with the best medical therapy was 17%, with a relative risk reduction of 65% for ipsilateral stroke and death from stroke.[74] Two additional contemporaneous trials, the European Carotid Surgery Trialists' Collaborative Group[13] and the Veterans Administration Asymptomatic Stenosis Trial,[14] corroborated the success of using endarterectomy to treat symptomatic stenosis.

The highly significant findings of NASCET, combined with these other two studies of symptomatic carotid stenosis patients, have withstood multivariate analyses and follow-up assessments to show a direct correlation between surgical benefit and extent of stenosis. Using the projections of these studies, six CEAs are necessary to prevent stroke in one patient, which is clinically and economically efficacious. NASCET analyzed 2226 randomized patients with moderate (50% to 69%) stenosis with a 5-year follow-up. In the surgical group, the ipsilateral stroke rate was 15.7%, compared with 22.2% in the medical management cohort—a statistically significant difference.[75]

Two major studies have shown the benefit of CEA for patients with asymptomatic carotid stenosis. The Veterans Administration Asymptomatic Stenosis Trial randomized 444 patients who had more than 50% stenosis and no ischemic symptoms. The rate of ipsilateral stroke tended to be lower in the surgical group than in the medical group, but the difference was not statistically significant.[76] The Asymptomatic Carotid Atherosclerosis Study randomized 1662 patients with stenosis greater than 60% to surgery or best medical management. The projected risk of stroke at 5 years was 5.1% for the surgical group and 11% for the medically managed patients. Overall, the risk of ipsilateral stroke was reduced 53%, which remained statistically significant at a 3-year follow-up.[77]

Although the results of these studies of asymptomatic patients with stenosis greater than 50% to 60% show a definitive benefit, we recommend careful selection within this subgroup. Patients with the following factors are considered likely candidates for elective CEA: complex or ulcerated lesions, documented progressive carotid stenosis on serial examinations, a reasonable life expectancy, lack of concurrent serious medical illness such as malignancy, a high number of atherosclerotic risk factors, and male sex. Careful selection of asymptomatic patients is paramount to improve their outcomes compared with the natural history of the condition, especially when additional information such as cerebral hemodynamic function is considered.

CONTROVERSIES IN CAROTID ENDARTERECTOMY

Notwithstanding the definition of populations that benefit from CEA, some areas remain controversial. Technical issues have centered around the avoidance of cerebral ischemia. Although the period of carotid cross-clamping was once considered paramount, experience has shown that it is usually well tolerated and that other technical factors may predominate in determining outcome. All aspects of the surgical protocol for CEA must be carefully considered and justified.

Tandem Carotid Lesions

Complete assessment of the cerebrovascular circulation begins with angiographic visualization of the aortic arch. It is important to visualize the origins of both the carotid and vertebral arteries.[78] Patients with cerebral ischemic symptoms may have atherosclerotic stenosis, ulcerative lesions, or occlusion of the origin of these great vessels. A full consideration of the cerebrovascular supply and an understanding of the patient's symptoms are impossible unless a comprehensive evaluation is performed. When tandem lesions exist, they usually involve the cervical carotid bifurcation, along with abnormalities in the cavernous portion of the internal carotid artery (ICA). However, carotid bifurcation lesions can also exist in tandem with stenosis of the origin of the common carotid artery.

Carotid siphon lesions do not seem to have the poor prognosis associated with high-grade stenosis of the cervical carotid bifurcation. However, the natural history has been reported to be an annual ipsilateral stroke rate of 8.1%, with 30% or greater stenosis of the siphon, concurrent with less extensive proximal carotid stenosis.[79] In patients with tandem lesions of the carotid bifurcation and carotid siphon, the former are usually responsible for cerebral ischemic symptoms. Cerebral infarction, which often occurs in the territory of the MCA, is more likely to have a thromboembolic than a hemodynamic origin. The characteristics of atheromatous plaques at the ICA origin are more likely to provide a substrate for atheromatous debris, thrombus, or platelet aggregate material for embolization than are plaques in the carotid siphon. Removing a lesion of the ICA origin should eliminate a symptomatic embolic source. In addition, studies using oculoplethysmography have shown that stenoses at the cervical carotid bifurcation and carotid siphon may have an additive hemodynamic effect.[80, 81] In terms of cerebral blood flow, lesions of the cervical carotid bifurcation have a greater detrimental impact than do lesions of the carotid siphon. Carotid siphon stenosis is a predictor of future coronary disease and indicates widespread systemic atherosclerotic changes.[82]

CEA can be performed successfully in patients with coexistent carotid siphon lesions without an apparent increased risk of morbidity and mortality. Severe preoperative carotid siphon stenosis may resolve after patients undergo CEA, emphasizing that tandem lesions are not a contraindication to CEA and that carotid siphon stenosis may be reversible.[83] Repeat angiography or magnetic resonance angiography may be beneficial to ascertain the status of a carotid siphon lesion. Carotid siphon tandem stenosis can be caused by embolization, reactive arterial spasm, anterograde flow disturbance, or a combination of factors. Alcock[83] demonstrated a similar phenomenon with occlusive lesions of the MCA. Little and coworkers[84] had a similar experience, which they termed pseudotandem stenosis, in two patients with resolving carotid siphon lesions. They postulated that laminar flow through the poststenotic carotid segment beyond the cervical bifurcation may produce the appearance of marked diminution in arterial caliber, either by reducing the amount of contrast medium or by the actual slow flow of contrast. Substantial collateral flow through either the anterior cerebral artery or posterior communicating artery likewise could displace or dilute a column of contrast medium.

It appears that most patients with tandem carotid lesions are probably symptomatic from the atheromatous plaque at the cervical bifurcation. It is believed that CEA can be performed safely in patients with tandem lesions without significantly increasing the incidence of cerebral ischemic symptoms or stroke.[85] CEA has been combined successfully with distal balloon angioplasty and is an example of providing surgical and endovascular therapy simultaneously.[86]

Cerebral Protection

Many technical facets of CEA focus on providing a good outcome by protecting cerebral tissue either directly or indirectly. Intraoperatively, the threshold for tolerating cerebral ischemia can be increased by a few select pharmacologic agents. Barbiturates have been used widely in cerebrovascular surgery, during both CEA and periods of temporary cerebral arterial occlusion, particularly in aneurysm surgery. The mechanism of action of barbiturates in providing cerebral protection is believed to be a reversible, dose-dependent depression of cerebral blood flow and, ultimately, of the cerebral metabolic rate.[87–90] When the electroencephalogram (EEG) reaches an isoelectric state, barbiturates have reduced cerebral blood flow and the cerebral metabolic rate of oxygen by about 50%. This protective effect is more prominent in nonischemic portions of the brain.[90] Vasoconstriction of normal portions of the brain occurs and is thought to improve cerebral blood flow to ischemic areas.[91] By reducing cerebral blood flow and cerebral blood volume, barbiturates decrease the rate of edema formation and intracranial pressure. Barbiturates may also serve as free radical scavengers and reduce the production of free fatty acids from damaged cells.[90, 92]

The exact mechanism of barbiturate cerebral protection in the setting of arterial occlusion is probably multifactorial and incompletely understood. Clearly, however, these agents modify or prevent cerebral damage related to focal ischemia.[90, 93, 94] Laboratory experience with a primate model has demonstrated that prior administration of barbiturates provides dramatic cerebral protection for as long as 6 hours of MCA occlusion.[87, 90, 95] This degree of cerebral protection far surpasses that provided by other general anesthetic agents. Barbiturates administered after the onset of cerebral ischemia are not believed to provide protection and, in fact, may be deleterious, especially in the presence of a permanent vascular occlusion.[96, 97]

The use of barbiturates has disadvantages, such as intraoperative hypotension, myocardial depression, and a prolonged postoperative wake-up period in some patients. The use of vasopressor agents and intravenous volume expansion prevents or corrects intraoperative hypotension. In patients with severe myocardial dysfunction, the anesthesiologist may be concerned that the cardiovascular effects of barbiturates could be detrimental or have a significantly adverse effect on function. In such cases, we have used etomidate with excellent results. Etomidate is a short-acting intravenous anesthetic agent that induces a reversible, dose-dependent reduction in the cerebral metabolic rate. The effects of etomidate on the EEG are similar to those of barbiturates: an isoelectric EEG pattern associated with about a 50% decease in the cerebral metabolic rate of oxygen. The cardiovascular depressive effects of etomidate are likely insignificant.[98] We have used this drug safely and efficaciously during CEA, and others have done so during temporary cerebral arterial occlusion.[99] The addition of barbiturate therapy for cerebral protection provides an opportunity for the surgeon to perform a precise and relaxed endarterectomy, including the time needed for complicated arterial reconstruction. In our series, the administration of barbiturates was both feasible and safe.[1]

Carotid Patch Graft

Carotid patch angioplasty has been performed using saphenous vein, Dacron, or polytetrafluoroethylene. Autogenous saphenous vein has been the preferred material because of its ease in handling; its relatively antithrombotic properties; and its size, tensile strength, and resistance to infection. Proponents of vein patch carotid angioplasty propose that this technique enlarges the endarterectomized segment and restores a normal contour to the carotid bulb. Disturbances to blood flow in the immediate postoperative period and later are thereby minimized. It is also thought to prevent or minimize intimal hyperplasia.[100, 101] The saphenous vein interposition graft contains viable endothelium that may reduce thrombogenicity compared with the otherwise denuded surface after conventional endarterectomy (Fig. 97–3).[102]

The routine use of saphenous vein patch grafts has been advocated during CEA to reduce the incidence of postoperative restenosis, which ranges from 1% to 49% in reported series.[73, 103–105] Sundt and coworkers[102, 105] regularly employed saphenous vein interposition grafts with excellent success. They believed that vein angioplasty enlarged the endarterectomized segment and improved blood flow in this region of the carotid bifurcation. It has been postulated that the saphenous vein interposition graft reorients the configuration of the bifurcation. Consequently, the ICA becomes the primary extension of the common carotid artery, improving the rheologic characteristics of the operative site.[102]

A saphenous vein interposition graft may be most beneficial in the immediate postoperative period, when the potential for thrombosis is highest. Little and associates[106] compared 70 cases of CEA and primary closure with 50 cases of CEA and saphenous vein interposition graft. Based on the early postoperative intravenous digital subtraction angiograms, the ICA was consistently larger and the incidence of thrombosis at the operative site was less in the patients who received saphenous vein interposition grafts. In the conventional CEA group, four patients had ICA occlusions; two patients had internal, external, and common carotid artery occlusions; and nine patients had various degrees of ICA stenosis. No patient with a saphenous vein interposition graft developed an occlusion postoperatively, and only two developed stenosis. In the conventional CEA patients with postoperative occlusions who underwent re-exploration, thrombosis was found in the angiographically nonvisualized arteries but could not be attributed to any obvious cause. Of the patients in the conventional CEA group, three had cerebral infarctions that were the main cause of postoperative morbidity. The difference between the two groups was statistically significant and led the authors to recommend the routine use of saphenous vein interposition grafts. In this study, the surgical microscope was not used, and heparinization was neutralized at the end of the procedure.

Others have reported similar encouraging benefits from the routine use of saphenous vein interposition grafts, which are thought to prevent early thrombosis and late recurrent stenosis.[102–104, 107] Rosenthal and colleagues,[108] however, retrospectively studied 1000 consecutive patients who underwent CEA. The patients were divided into four equal groups: 250 patients had a conventional endarterectomy closure, 250 patients had an expanded polytetrafluoroethylene patch, 250 had a Dacron patch, and 250 had a saphenous vein interposition graft. Postoperative patency was documented by B-mode ultrasonography. The difference in the incidence of early or late postoperative stroke and restenosis was not statistically significant among the groups. The authors recommended saphenous vein interposition graft angioplasty for patients with small arteries and for habitual smokers. Meyer and Windschitl[109] reported a prospective study of 290 consecutive CEAs in which a collagen-impregnated fabric graft was used for closure. The microvalve, knitted, double-Velour graft, which lessens the risk of suture

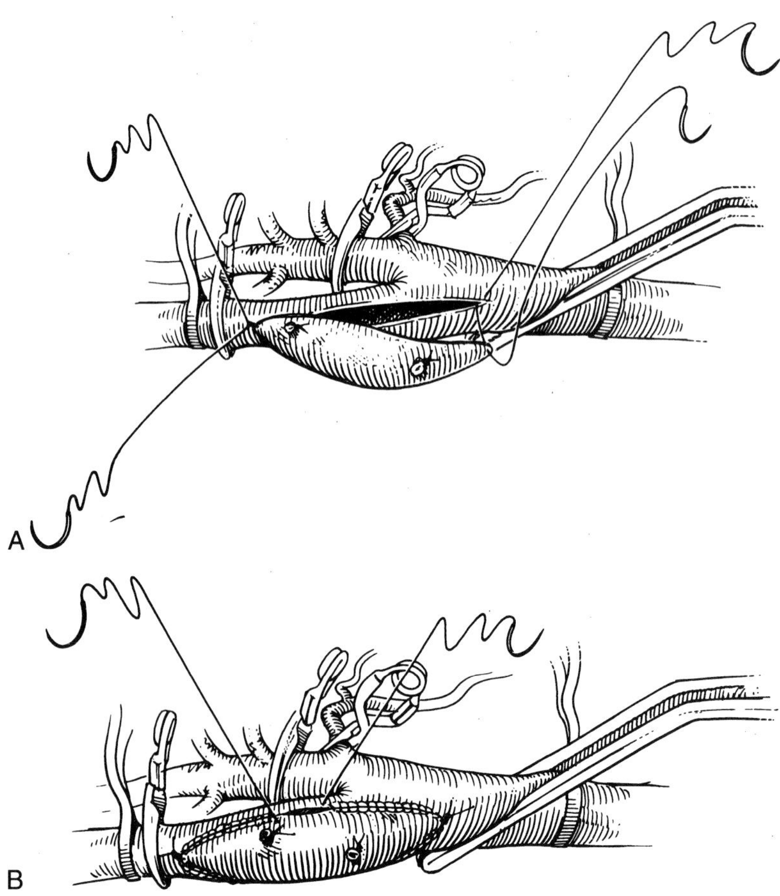

FIGURE 97–3. *A*, Placement and spacing of vein. *B*, Completion of vein patch closure. Saphenous vein patch grafts are occasionally necessary, usually when an endarterectomy must be redone. The customary method of inserting a vein patch graft is illustrated here. (Courtesy of Barrow Neurological Institute, Phoenix, AZ.)

line bleeding due to the added collagen, was a viable method of closure and reduced the higher risk of postoperative rupture associated with a saphenous vein patch graft. Their 30-day rate of major neurological morbidity and mortality was 1.7%. There were no postoperative occlusions or wound hematomas, and the early recurrent stenosis rate was less than 1%.

AbuRahma and coauthors[110] compared primary closure to patch closure (both saphenous vein and synthetic grafts) in 74 patients undergoing bilateral CEAs (mean follow-up, 29 months). In all categories evaluated, primary closure was associated with a higher rate of neurological complications (combined TIA and stroke rate: 12% for primary closure; 1% for patching), total ICA occlusion, and recurrent stenosis than was patch closure. With each patient serving as his or her own control, this study is one of the most compelling to date advocating patch closure. Nonetheless, the complication rate, which was higher than that reported in many studies, may contribute to the apparent major discrepancy between these two methods of closure.

In contrast, Hans[100] reported 90 patients undergoing CEA with a saphenous vein interposition graft. He performed arteriography at both intermediate (21 months) and late (55 months) follow-up examinations, documenting recurrent stenosis in three patients and carotid occlusion in five patients at the intermediate follow-up and recurrent stenosis in three additional patients at the late follow-up. He thus concluded that saphenous vein interposition grafts did not uniformly prevent either early or late postoperative carotid stenosis.

Both primary suture closure and saphenous vein interposition graft for CEA have received support. The consensus suggests that specific groups of patients may benefit most from saphenous vein interposition grafts: patients undergoing reoperation for postoperative recurrent carotid stenosis, patients with an unusually small ICA (primarily women), patients who have undergone cervical radiation treatments, patients who are habitual heavy smokers, and patients whose external arterial walls hold sutures poorly.

A saphenous vein interposition graft, however, does have disadvantages. It increases operative and carotid cross-clamping time because two suture lines are required. Postoperatively, the angioplasty segment can balloon, slowing blood flow or causing eddy currents. Such a pattern of blood flow can predispose patients to form mural thrombi and pseudoaneurysms. Vital lower extremity veins are often used and thus are unavailable if they are needed later for other arterial reconstruction (e.g., coronary artery bypass) procedures. The most dreaded complication of saphenous vein interposition graft angioplasty is rupture of the vein patch, which has been reported in 0.4% to 4% of patients. This catastrophic event most often occurs in the first few days after the procedure. Hypertension increases its incidence. The associated morbidity and mortality rates, which are high, follow hemorrhagic shock, cerebral ischemia, or airway compression.[101, 111]

Notwithstanding reports of the greater incidence of complications with primary closure, our experience suggests that the routine use of saphenous vein interposition grafts for microsurgical CEA is unnecessary.[1, 112] The microsurgical technique, with the gathering of only a minute portion of the arterial wall within the suture, helps explain the durability and excellent results obtained. Although not regularly performed in our patients, postoperative angiography has demonstrated a slight enlargement, not a narrowing, of the endarterectomized segment. Our low symptomatic early stroke rate of 1% suggests that postoperative patency rates can be excellent. It is doubtful that these rates could be improved by using a saphenous vein interposition graft or synthetic graft angioplasty.[1] We do, however, recommend using a saphenous vein interposition graft in operations for recurrent carotid stenosis and in extraordinary circumstances such as after cervical radiation for malignancy.

Intraoperative Carotid Shunt

There continues to be disagreement about the indications for placing a carotid artery shunt during carotid cross-clamping.[113, 114] Many surgeons believe that the cerebral ischemia induced during carotid cross-clamping is the primary reason for the complications associated with CEA. Others believe that embolic rather than hemodynamic events cause most cerebral ischemic episodes during CEA.[114, 115] Many surgeons, believing that hemodynamic intolerance to carotid cross-clamping is common, have reported excellent results with the use of intraluminal shunting.[116]

Various criteria have been used to determine the need for shunt placement during CEA. Sundt and colleagues[102] measured intraoperative regional cerebral blood flow using extracranial detection of intra-arterially injected xenon 133. Their protocol employed shunt insertion for all patients with an occlusion flow of less than 18 mL/100 g per minute. They concluded that with intraoperative carotid occlusion, the critical regional cerebral blood flow is approximately 15 mL/100 g per minute. Blood flow greater than 10 mL/100 g per minute during occlusion, which was seen in 8% of their patients, always produced rapid changes in the EEG pattern.[102] Intraoperative measurement of carotid stump pressures has also been used as an indication for shunting, with significant ischemia believed to occur with a mean blood pressure of less than 25 mm Hg.[117]

The use of intraoperative temporary carotid shunting is associated with its own risks.[116] Many believe that a shunt can produce more problems than benefits. An intraluminal shunt has several major drawbacks. First, the shunt may allow the embolization of atherosclerotic debris, thrombotic material, or air into the distal cerebral circulation. This phenomenon is often unrecognized by the surgeon until it is detected by changes in the EEG or by a signal change on TCD. At that point, sometimes little can be done to stop further embolization by this route or to reverse the damaging cerebral effects. Postoperatively, it can also occur without clinical detection. Second, when inserted, the shunt can injure the intimal surface of either the common carotid artery or the distal ICA. Such an injury can lead to postoperative thrombosis at the operative site. Finally, the presence of a shunt severely limits the surgeon's ability to expose and dissect the atheroma, especially the distal portion (Fig. 97–4). The creation of an intimal flap or the inability to recognize and repair the intima or to remove all the atherosclerotic debris can contribute to a poor technical outcome. This is true even when the surgical microscope, with its improved visualization, is used. Further, significant periods of ischemia can occur when the shunt is placed and after it is withdrawn, before the arteriotomy closure is completed and carotid cross-clamping is removed. Shunt occlusion and improper placement leading to potential upper extremity ischemia have also occurred.[8, 114, 116]

Ott and coauthors[118] prospectively studied 240 patients to determine the effectiveness of CEA performed without shunting. The incidence of perioperative stroke was 1.3%, and the mortality rate was 0.64%, the latter caused by myocardial infarction in two patients. The incidence of permanent neurological deficit compared favorably with that in other published series, regardless of whether shunting was used. Further, none of their 102 patients who had either partial or complete occlusion of the contralateral ICA experienced a postoperative stroke. Bland and Lazar[115] performed 280 consecutive CEAs without using EEG monitoring or an intraluminal shunt. A third of their patients had contralateral stenosis or ICA occlusion. Their carotid occlusion time, however, averaged only 10 minutes. They reported no operative mortality, no strokes in the immediate postoperative period, and only three strokes

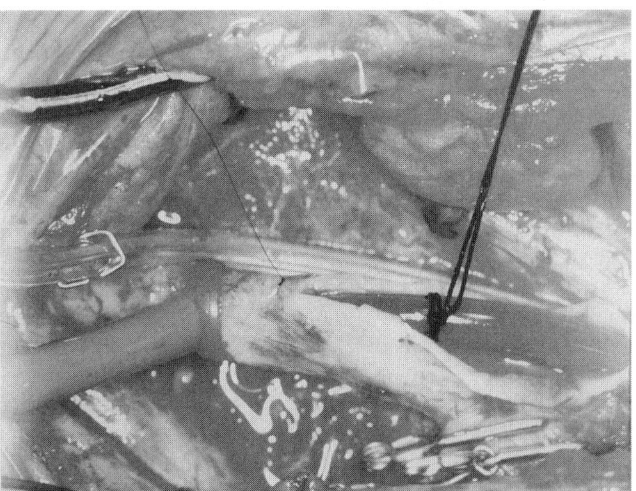

FIGURE 97–4. Although seldom used during our procedure, carotid artery shunting is vital to successful outcomes in cases identified by intraoperative encephalography, transcranial Doppler ultrasonography, or both. Either external (Javid) or internal (Sundt) shunts are used; the latter is pictured. (From Bailes JE, Spetzler RF [eds]: Microsurgical Carotid Endarterectomy. New York, Lippincott-Raven, 1996.)

(1.1%) during the first postoperative month. They concluded that intraluminal shunts and intraoperative monitoring such as EEG and carotid stump pressures are unnecessary, reinforcing the concept that most intraoperative strokes that occur during CEA are embolic. In 282 consecutive CEAs, Ferguson and coworkers[119] reported that intraoperative stroke occurred in four patients (1.4%), all of whom were in a small subgroup with major EEG changes and a mean carotid stump pressure of less than 25 mm Hg. They concluded that this subgroup of patients is at high risk for hemodynamic stroke and could benefit from shunting.

We prospectively studied 100 consecutive patients to determine the most reliable monitoring modality for CEA. The procedure was performed using microneurosurgical techniques. All patients were under general anesthesia and were monitored continuously with EEG and TCD. Pentobarbital or etomidate was administered to burst suppression throughout the period of carotid cross-clamping.

Eighty-two patients (82%) demonstrated competent collateral blood flow after carotid cross-clamping. In the MCA, the blood flow velocity fell a mean of 27% (range, 13% to 55%) after clamping. In nine patients (9%), collateral blood flow patterns were incompetent, and mean blood flow velocity decreased 75% from the preclamp baseline. The EEG evaluations remained normal despite the compromised blood flow as measured by TCD. Shunting was not performed because the EEGs were normal. In nine patients (9%), mean blood flow velocity decreased 98% (range, 90% to 100%) of the preclamp mean after ICA cross-clamping. Intraluminal shunting was performed in these nine patients who had both low blood flow and concomitant EEG changes. There was only one neurological complication in a patient who suffered permanent partial expressive aphasia caused by ICA thrombosis. In our experience, EEG monitoring remains the most reliable indicator for intraluminal shunting.

Halsey[116] reported a multicenter, retrospective study of 1495 CEA patients in which EEG, regional cerebral blood flow, and TCD were used to determine the ischemic threshold during carotid cross-clamping. The routine use of carotid shunting had no beneficial effect on neurological outcome, and he concluded that intraoperative monitoring could be used to determine the need for selective shunt placement (TCD <40% of baseline blood flow velocity).[116] Sandmann and colleagues[120] conducted a multicenter, randomized, prospective study in 503 patients to assess the need for or benefit of routine carotid shunting during CEA. Their overall stroke rate was 4%. The incidence of perioperative stroke did not differ significantly between patients who were routinely shunted (4.2%) and those whose endarterectomy was performed without a shunt (3.3%).

Carotid shunting is an answer to only one problem associated with CEA and cerebral hemodynamic insufficiency. Many other factors (e.g., technical, embolic, thrombotic, anesthetic, systemic, and experiential) play a major role, along with global cerebral blood flow.[115, 116, 120] In a small subpopulation of CEA patients, temporary carotid artery occlusion may cause hemispheric hypoperfusion that results in cerebral infarction, which is correctable by shunt placement. Many patients, however, respond to moderate induced hypertension, which increases collateral blood flow. We use a major change in EEG and, more recently, a change in TCD (mean ipsilateral MCA velocity reduced to less than a third of the preocclusion value) as indications for selective carotid intraluminal shunting if the patient fails to respond to induced hypertension.[121] A series by Jansen and associates[122] claimed that TCD may be more sensitive than EEG in detecting subcortical ischemia and embolic phenomena. Since instituting this criterion, 7% to 9% of our patients have required intraoperative shunts. None of these patients has experienced a permanent cerebrovascular accident postoperatively. EEG monitoring should be used. It predicts postoperative deficits[92, 105, 121] more accurately than TCD criteria alone, especially when cerebroprotective agents are circulated.

Operating Microscope

The operating microscope has revolutionized neurological surgery with its unparalleled lighting, visualization, and wide range of magnification, and it is the cornerstone of microsurgical CEA. The size of the operating field can be up to 12 times that of ordinary operating surgical loupes. The ability to zoom to higher magnifications to inspect fine details and to retreat to low degrees of magnification for portions of the procedure such as tying sutures makes this flexible instrument a mainstay in our surgical protocol. In addition, the operating microscope provides excellent illumination, even in the depths of a wound and in the intraluminal area of the carotid artery. The operating microscope is usually used once the gross portion of the atheromatous plaque and intraluminal thrombotic material has been removed. If ulcerated or indistinct plaques are present, the microscope can facilitate dissection in the correct plane. Remaining portions of the atheromatous material are best removed under higher magnification. The view is unequaled, and the luminal surface can be assessed in detail (Fig. 97–5).

Findlay and Lougheed[123] described their technique and results in 60 consecutive patients with symptomatic carotid stenosis who underwent microsurgical CEA. Only one patient (1.7%) suffered a perioperative stroke after common carotid artery occlusion, without an obvious cause. During a mean follow-up of 18 months, no patient experienced a postoperative hemorrhagic or ischemic stroke. These authors believed that using the surgical microscope helped minimize difficulties with the surgical technique. The benefits of using the surgical microscope when performing CEAs have also been emphasized by other neurosurgeons.[1, 92, 124, 125] A series from the Barrow Neurological Institute included 200 consecutive CEAs performed in 180 patients using a defined protocol of microsurgical endarterectomy. Barbiturate protection was used during carotid cross-clamping, the period of potential focal cerebral ischemia. The protocol also included preoperative antiplatelet therapy, barbiturate anesthesia, routine avoidance of an internal shunt, and strict postoperative

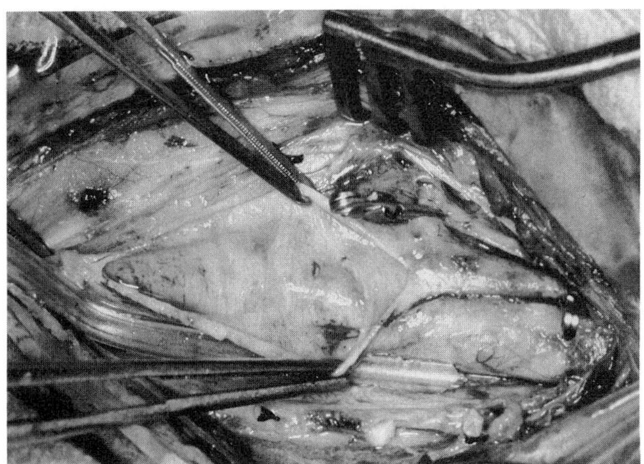

FIGURE 97–5. A view through the operating microscope shows the final stages after removal of the plaque and the excellent visualization of the luminal surface provided by the superior lighting and magnification of the operating microscope. (From Bailes JE, Spetzler RF [eds]: Microsurgical Carotid Endarterectomy. New York, Lippincott-Raven, 1996.)

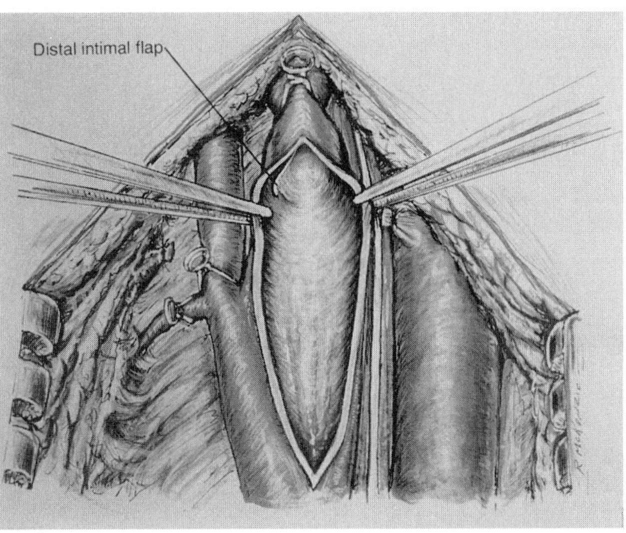

FIGURE 97–6. The superior lighting and magnification of the surgical microscope visualize the distal transition zone, where an intimal flap usually occurs. (From Bailes JE, Spetzler RF [eds]: Microsurgical Carotid Endarterectomy. New York, Lippincott-Raven, 1996.)

control of blood pressure. On the fifth postoperative day, one patient died from a hypertensive cerebral hemorrhage, and two patients suffered postoperative cerebrovascular accidents. The combined rate of permanent morbidity and mortality was 1.5%.[112] The results from our larger series have upheld our opinion that using the operative microscope greatly improves technical results and, ultimately, the clinical outcome of CEA.[1] The utility of the operating microscope and its ability to improve the manipulation of the diseased artery are highlighted when one realizes that embolic events and technical errors are probably the two leading causes of neurological morbidity associated with CEA.

In the series by Rosenthal and coworkers,[108] technical failures accounted for two thirds of the postoperative strokes. The causes were intimal flaps, lateral carotid tears, or carotid clamp injuries. The remaining strokes were caused by embolic occlusion of intracranial vessels. Moore and colleagues[126] described three patients who developed postoperative neurological deficits from thromboembolic propagation that originated from an intimal flap of the external carotid artery (ECA). Thrombotic material accumulated in the ECA and passed through the ICA into the cerebral distribution. This report emphasized the potential interaction between the external carotid circulation and the intracranial circulation. The importance of technical failures emphasizes the great benefit of an instrument such as the microscope that improves visualization and the performance of manual tasks (Fig. 97–6).

Magnification and illumination provided by the operating microscope improve the surgeon's ability to inspect the luminal surface of both the ECA and the ICA. Blaisdell and coauthors[127] reported that after routine use of intraoperative angiography, approximately 25% of the endarterectomized carotid arteries demonstrated a significant technical abnormality that would not have been noted without angiography. They believed that correcting these deficits at the time of angiography resulted in a 100% late patency rate in their endarterectomy series.

OPERATIVE ANATOMY AND TECHNIQUE FOR CAROTID ENDARTERECTOMY

For CEA, the patient is positioned supine with the head turned slightly to the contralateral side. A towel roll can be placed in the interscapular area to permit cervical extension and improve deep exposure. Care must be taken during surgical skin preparation to minimize the likelihood of mechanical dislodgment of atheromatous or thrombotic debris.

The surgical incision begins about two fingerbreadths above the clavicle and sternal notch, along the anterior border of the sternocleidomastoid muscle, and proceeds superiorly until it approaches the angle of the mandible. Further cephalad exposure is ordinarily attained by gently curving the incision posteriorly toward the mastoid tip. Directing the incision away from the side of the cheek improves cosmesis and avoids injury to the branches of the facial nerve (Fig. 97–7).

Operative planning is facilitated by reviewing the patient's angiogram to ascertain the location of the carotid bifurcation and the level and extent of the carotid lesion, which are noted in relation to the cervical vertebral bodies and mandibular angle. When the bifurcation is unusually high or low, the incision should be adjusted accordingly. A submandibular incision 1 cm below and parallel to the lower mandibular margin and a zigzag incision along the anterior border of the sternocleidomastoid muscle are alternatives that can

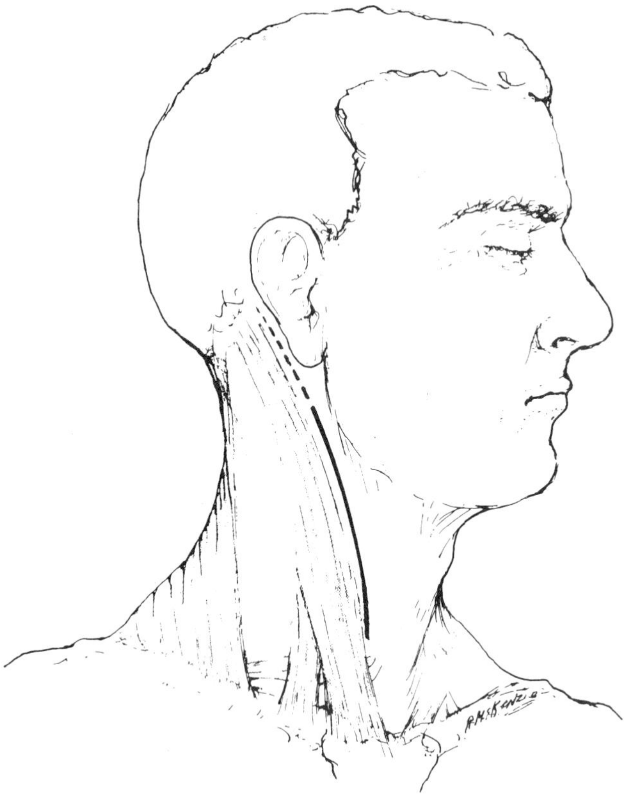

FIGURE 97–7. Exposure of the carotid artery is accomplished with an anterocervical longitudinal incision parallel to the medial border of the sternocleidomastoid muscle. For lesions that extend distally on the internal carotid artery, the incision is usually curved posteriorly behind the ear for cosmetic reasons and to avoid the facial nerve branches. (From Bailes JE, Spetzler RF [eds]: Microsurgical Carotid Endarterectomy. New York, Lippincott-Raven, 1996.)

also improve cosmesis. These incisions, however, require developing wide skin flaps and do not offer as good an exposure, particularly proximally on the common carotid artery. The incision along the anterior edge of the sternocleidomastoid is preferred and gives acceptable cosmetic results, especially with subcuticular suture closure.

The dissection next proceeds through the subcutaneous tissues and platysma along the medial border of the sternocleidomastoid. Hemostasis from the skin incision down to the carotid artery must be complete and meticulous, because heparinization is not reversed at the end of the procedure. The dermis often oozes after heparinization. The loose areolar tissue, which adheres the sternocleidomastoid to the strap muscles overlying the trachea, is dissected. A deep, self-retaining retractor or retaining sutures are placed to expose the carotid sheath. The pulse from the common carotid artery can serve as a guide to the proper dissection plane.

Several nerves are in the vicinity of the exposure, superficial to the sternocleidomastoid muscle. The great auricular nerve crosses obliquely over the sternocleidomastoid toward the posterior auricular region and mandibular angle. The lesser occipital nerve courses across the posterior sternocleidomastoid attachment to the occipital and mastoid regions. The spinal accessory nerve runs on the posterior aspect of the sternocleidomastoid across the posterior triangle to innervate the trapezius muscle. A cervical branch of the facial nerve runs deep to the platysma. By maintaining the dissection in the correct plane, these nerves are seldom encountered or injured during the endarterectomy. Often, however, the transverse cervical nerve, which crosses the midbelly of the sternocleidomastoid, is transected and causes transient numbness in the anterior neck. Typically, however, it regenerates, and the numbness disappears within 6 months. Because of the likelihood of injuring a nerve, it is important to avoid placing a self-retaining retractor medially in a deep plane.

As the dissection proceeds posteriorly, lymph nodes are often present. They are best handled by medial dissection and lateral deflection. In the upper end of the incision, the parotid gland may be recognized by its lobulated architecture and pale color compared with subcutaneous adipose tissue. The carotid sheath is opened with sharp dissection and careful bipolar coagulation of any small vessels within the fibrous sheath. The common carotid artery, located in the proximal region of the dissection posteromedial to the internal jugular vein, is exposed first. The vagus nerve usually is situated dorsal to the vessels within the carotid sheath. The internal jugular vein must be mobilized, which often requires dividing medial venous tributaries, the largest of which is usually the common facial vein located near the carotid bifurcation. Access to the carotid bifurcation and ICA is best facilitated by reflecting the internal jugular vein laterally.

The proximal extent of the exposure is usually the omohyoid muscle. This muscle may be divided partially or completely to attain adequate access to the common carotid artery; however, this maneuver is rarely necessary. Occasionally, as the dissection proceeds cephalad, the ansa cervicalis is encountered. It is composed of an inferior division, which originates from the ventral rami of the second and third cervical nerves, and a superior division, which descends from the hypoglossal nerve and connects with the inferior division after the latter courses over the internal jugular vein. Dividing the descending limb of the ansa cervicalis improves access to the carotid artery. This maneuver also shifts the hypoglossal nerve medially and slightly superiorly away from the carotid bifurcation, but it is not performed unless necessary. The carotid bifurcation is most often located at the level of the thyroid cartilage. In about 20% of cases, however, it bifurcates between the thyroid cartilage and the hyoid bone. Rarely, the bifurcation is below the thyroid cartilage or the common carotid artery is absent, and the ICA and ECA originate directly from the aortic arch or the innominate artery. These details are discernible on the preoperative angiogram and should be considered during preoperative planning.

The common carotid artery typically possesses no branches, although the superior thyroid artery may originate within 2 cm proximal to the carotid bifurcation. When the superior thyroid artery is dissected for temporary clipping, its posterior aspect—a location where the superior laryngeal nerve may be injured—should be avoided. The carotid body is ovoid, usually less than 5 mm, and situated immediately dorsal to the carotid bifurcation. Its chemoreceptor elements form a portion of the visceral afferent system innervated by the vagus nerve. The routine injection of local anesthetic into the carotid body to avoid reflexive bradycardia and hypotension is often advocated. However, experience has shown that carotid body injection does not significantly affect the patient's cardiovascular response. Consequently, this technique is seldom employed. If, however, the anesthesiologist notes hemodynamically significant changes during dissection or handling of this area, the physiologic effects may be blocked temporarily with an injection of 1% lidocaine.

The distal ICA must be dissected, usually 3 to 5 cm distal to the bifurcation, depending on the extent of the carotid plaque. This distal exposure is readily gained by dissecting laterally and superiorly to the hypoglossal nerve. Leaving the areolar connective tissue attached on the medial side tends to pull the hypoglossal nerve somewhat medially and superiorly, as desired. Occasionally, distal exposure is improved by careful placement of retraction sutures in the medial connective tissue or perineurium of the hypoglossal nerve, or by dividing or incising the digastric muscle. Often an external carotid branch to the sternocleidomastoid muscle, accompanied by a vein, is encountered and must be divided. Rarely, this structure, together with the hypoglossal nerve, has been the source of carotid compression, the so-called carotid sling. More complex maneuvers for distal exposure, such as osteotomy of the mandibular ramus, are seldom necessary. Careful and deliberate dissection along the distal ICA, working laterally to the hypoglossal nerve, typically provides adequate cephalad exposure. The adventitial layer, which must be included within the arteriotomy closures, should be avoided. Small venous tributaries of the internal jugular vein, which are often encountered in this area, can readily be handled by bipolar coagulation or suture ligation. The ECA is dissected about 2 cm beyond the bifurcation. Exposure is necessary only to guarantee vascular control and sufficient space for temporary clipping (Fig. 97–8).

Once the exposure is completed, the carotid artery is inspected to determine the extent of the plaque. The plaque is usually tinged yellow, in contrast to the gray walls of a healthy carotid artery. The step-off transition zone at the distal end of the lesion can be palpated gently with a moistened, gloved finger. This intraoperative judgment is combined with the preoperative angiographic data to confirm the location of the plaque, placement of the arteriotomy, and adequacy of proximal and distal dissection and thus vascular control.

Anticoagulation during periods of ICA occlusion is an important facet of this surgery. Heparin administration during vascular surgery is efficacious and helps prevent thrombosis in the period surrounding carotid cross-clamping. Heparin achieves this desired clinical effect in three main ways. Its primary action is to potentiate the action of antithrombin III by binding to it and producing a conformational change, which inactivates the intrinsic coagulation cascade (factors Xa, XIIa, XIa, and IXa and thrombin). Heparin also inactivates thrombin via heparin cofactor II and binds to and thus inhibits platelet function. Both activated partial prothrombin time and activated clotting time have been used to determine the patient's degree of anticoagulation. The latter method is often preferred, because it is considered more accurate and can be determined rapidly.[128] Generally, with both measures, levels twice normal are attained using standard heparin dosage regimens. There is, however, considerable individual variability in patients' responses to heparin administration. Heparin has proved safe and effective, but extreme values (e.g., more than 3 standard deviations above mean) may be associated with the forma-

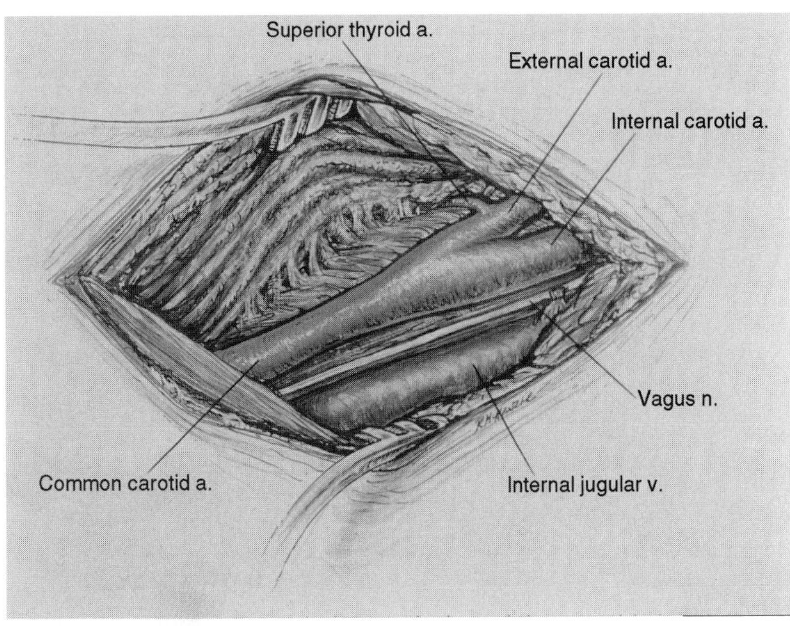

FIGURE 97–8. The dissection is carried posteriorly, and the carotid sheath is opened to isolate the common external and internal carotid arteries. This maneuver is best accomplished by retracting the internal jugular vein laterally. Crossing venous tributaries of the internal jugular are ligated and divided. (From Bailes JE, Spetzler RF [eds]: Microsurgical Carotid Endarterectomy. New York, Lippincott-Raven, 1996.)

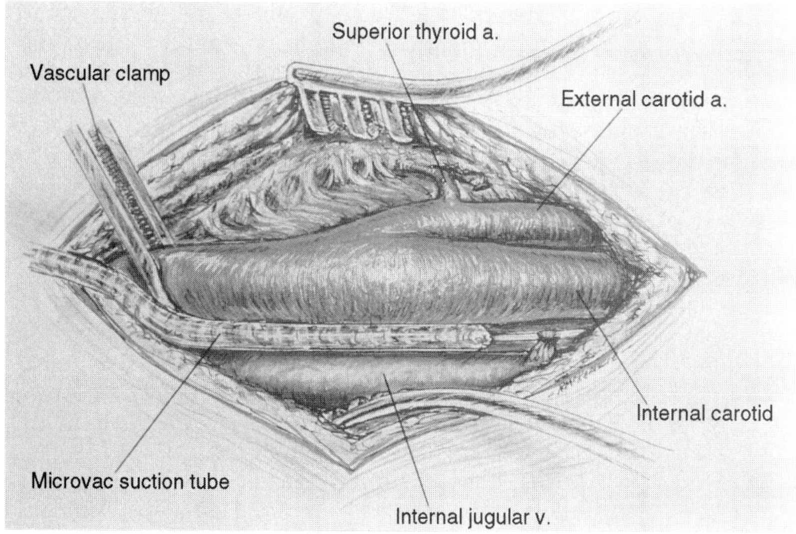

FIGURE 97–9. The vessels are prepared for temporary clipping, and an occlusive vascular clamp is positioned on the common carotid artery until needed. An indwelling suction tube is laid parallel with the carotid artery for constant evacuation of heparinized irrigant, obviating the need for an assistant to perform this task. (From Bailes JE, Spetzler RF [eds]: Microsurgical Carotid Endarterectomy. New York, Lippincott-Raven, 1996.)

tion of wound hematomas.[129] Poisik and coauthors[129] reported that a fixed dose of 5000 IU heparin achieves activated clotting times that are clinically comparable to those obtained with weight-based heparin administration. In addition, postoperative neurological and wound complications were not influenced by dosing methods.

At this juncture in the procedure, the patient undergoes full systemic heparinization when the anesthesiologist administers 85 IU/kg intravenously or, alternatively, a standard adult dose of 5000 IU. Cerebral protection is attained by placing the patient in 15- to 30-second EEG burst suppression, usually with bolus doses of thiopental (150 to 250 mg). Patients with considerable myocardial dysfunction receive an intravenous bolus loading dose of etomidate (0.4 to 0.5 mg/kg) and then 0.1 mg/kg to maintain burst suppression. During infusion of these agents—and particularly during carotid cross-clamping, when a moderate degree of hypertension is desired to optimize collateral cerebral blood flow—blood pressure must be controlled carefully. Infusion of phenylephrine or other appropriate agents may be required to maintain systemic blood pressure in the desired range.

When the blood pressure is stable and the EEG is in burst suppression, the distal ICA is occluded with a temporary aneurysm clip (Fig. 97–9). This initial maneuver prevents cerebral embolization of plaque or thrombotic material as the vessels are occluded. The proximal common carotid artery is immediately occluded with a 45-degree-angled DeBakey vascular clamp, tightened only enough to prevent hemorrhage. The ECA and superior thyroid artery are closed using temporary aneurysm clips. For ultimate proximal vascular control, a vascular loop with a rubber tubing occluder (Rummell tourniquet) can be placed proximal to the DeBakey clamp. When encircling tapes are placed for occlusion, the vessel should be dissected

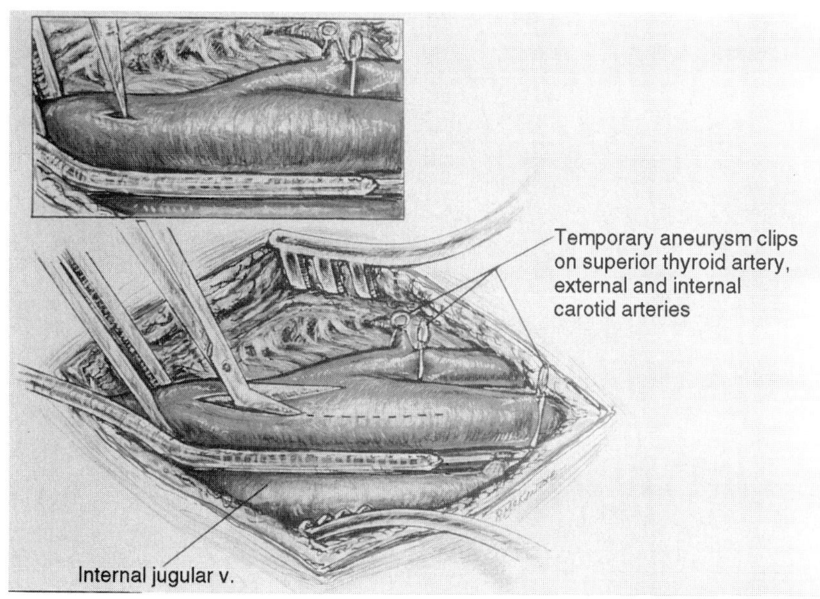

FIGURE 97–10. Once the common carotid artery is occluded with the vascular clamp and the superior thyroid and external and internal carotid arteries are occluded with temporary aneurysm clips, the arteriotomy is started by creating a 5-mm incision with a no. 11 scalpel blade. With an angled Pott's scissors, the arteriotomy is performed, beginning in the common carotid artery proximal to the atherosclerotic lesion and extending distally in the internal carotid artery to a point beyond the lesion. Care must be taken not to extend the arteriotomy too far medially, which will cause it to veer into the bifurcation or region of the origin of the external carotid artery. Likewise, making the arteriotomy too far laterally in the internal carotid artery will make subsequent closure difficult. (From Bailes JE, Spetzler RF [eds]: Microsurgical Carotid Endarterectomy. New York, Lippincott-Raven, 1996.)

from its underlying soft tissue only where the tape is to be passed. Otherwise, oozing from the relatively inaccessible back wall can be troublesome, especially after heparinization.

Using the angiographic data to judge the proximal extent of the lesion, the common carotid artery is incised, usually about 2 cm proximal to the carotid bifurcation (Fig. 97–10). The incision must penetrate through the plaque completely and proceed into the carotid lumen, extending about 5 mm in length. Otherwise, the muscularis layer may contract and, together with the adventitial layer, occlude the incision. An angled Pott's scissors is used to extend the arteriotomy cephalad into the ICA until the distal extent of the atherosclerotic plaque is passed. Care must be taken to extend the arteriotomy down the center axis of the ICA. The closure will be more difficult if the arteriotomy veers either medially into the region of the bifurcation or laterally on the vessel. Especially in tightly stenotic carotid arteries, it is important that the lower blade of the scissors seek and follow the remaining luminal channel. The surgeon should learn and appreciate a proprioceptive feel with the bottom blade of the Pott's scissors.

The endarterectomy is performed using two microsurgical dissectors to find the cleavage plane between the atherosclerotic plaque and the arterial wall (Fig. 97–11). However, the characteristics of these lesions vary. They usually begin in the distal common carotid artery, are thickest in the anterolateral position of the carotid sinus, and thin distally after considerable involvement at the ICA origin. Typically, the atherosclerotic plaque is first separated from the arterial wall in the common carotid artery using the dissectors to pass along the back or dorsal wall of the artery. The plaque is incised at its proximal end and lifted superiorly as the plaque-media interface is dissected in a distal direction into the ICA. The back wall must not be injured, nor should the media be dissected through the adventitial layer, which can be identified by its pinkish coloration (Fig. 97–12).

The plaque in the ECA is removed by an eversion technique that circumferentially dissects the plaque off the artery. Simultaneously, the ECA is grasped with

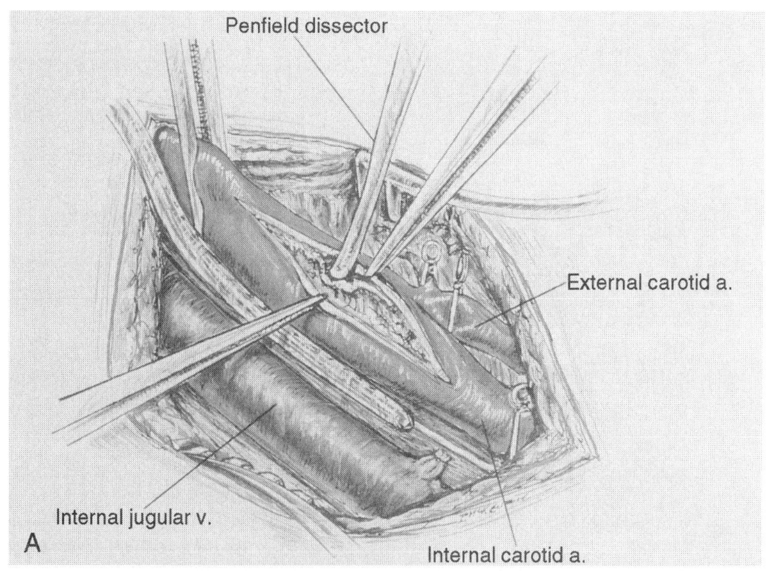

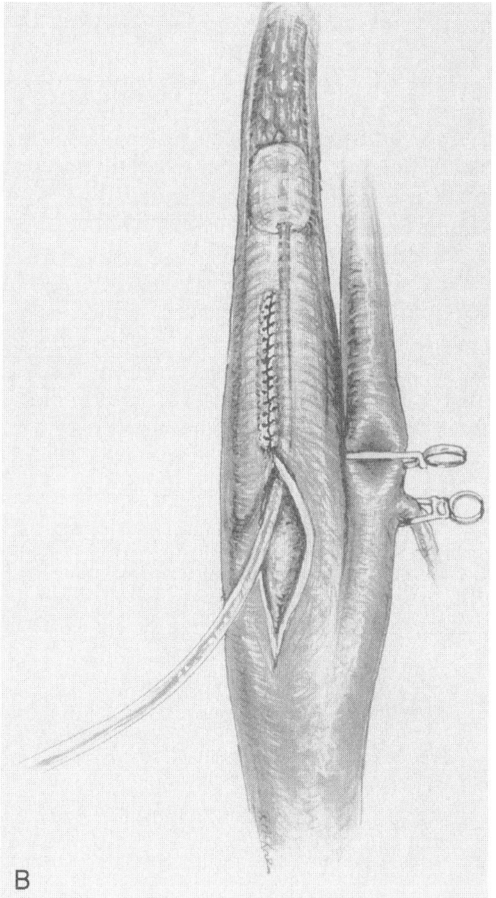

FIGURE 97–11. *A*, After the arteriotomy is completed and hemostasis is confirmed, the endarterectomy is begun by finding the correct plane between the arterial wall and the atherosclerotic plaque. This identification is best accomplished using microsurgical instruments and dissecting in a longitudinal direction and circumferentially. *B*, If distal internal carotid artery vascular control is lost or incomplete during the endarterectomy, hemostasis can be achieved with careful insertion of a balloon occlusive catheter. (From Bailes JE, Spetzler RF [eds]: Microsurgical Carotid Endarterectomy. New York, Lippincott-Raven, 1996.)

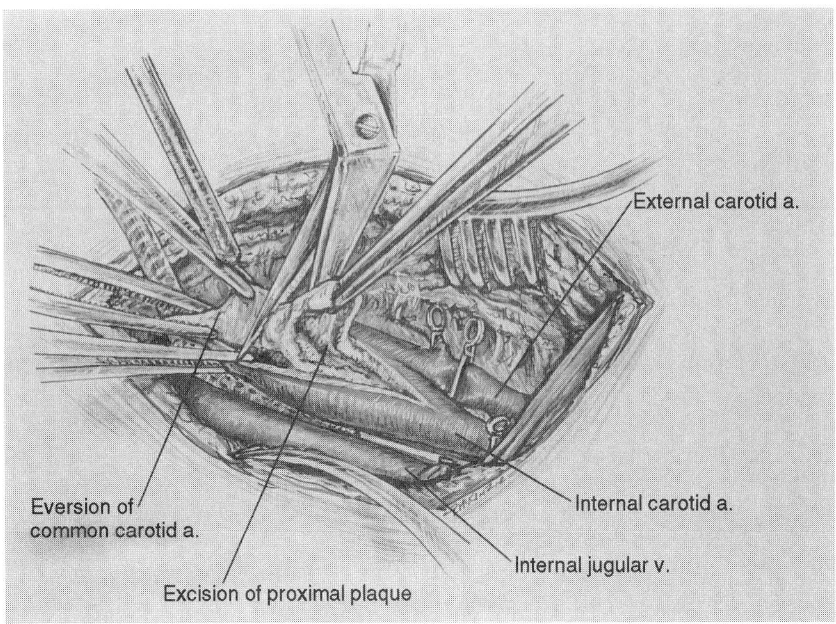

FIGURE 97–12. The proximal portion of the plaque is excised using Pott's scissors, allowing the lesion to be grasped and pulled superiorly with gentle traction so that further dissection in the correct plane is accomplished. (From Bailes JE, Spetzler RF [eds]: Microsurgical Carotid Endarterectomy. New York, Lippincott-Raven, 1996.)

forceps and pulled away from the atheroma. Removing this plaque can be assisted by opening the temporary clip briefly, allowing the tail of the lesion to be removed. This maneuver is often required when a calcified portion of the plaque involves the proximal ECA. If required to remove residual plaque or potential intimal plaque, a separate incision and endarterectomy of the ECA should be performed (Fig. 97–13; see color section in this volume).

The critical portion of plaque removal is that within the distal ICA. This plaque provides the leading edge of the plaque-vessel interface, which may lead to the formation of an intimal flap and postoperative thrombosis. Gentle elevation and traction of the plaque often cause it to break with an even contour or a feathering effect at the distal ICA transition zone. This maneuver not only removes the remainder of the hemodynamically offending lesion but also prevents an intimal flap from developing. Often, the final cleavage of the plaque can be optimized by combining traction and eversion of the plaque as the back wall of the vessel is pushed away. Transecting the plaque proximal to the end of the arteriotomy makes closure easier and avoids stenosis of the vessel. When the vessel wall is handled, the layers of the wall should not be separated. Rather, the walls should be held together only at the edges with slight pressure, using wide-grip vascular forceps. Fine sutures should not be picked up by or pinched between the jaws of the forceps, because doing so can crimp and weaken the sutures.

The operating microscope is now positioned to allow the surgeon and assistant unimpeded binocular

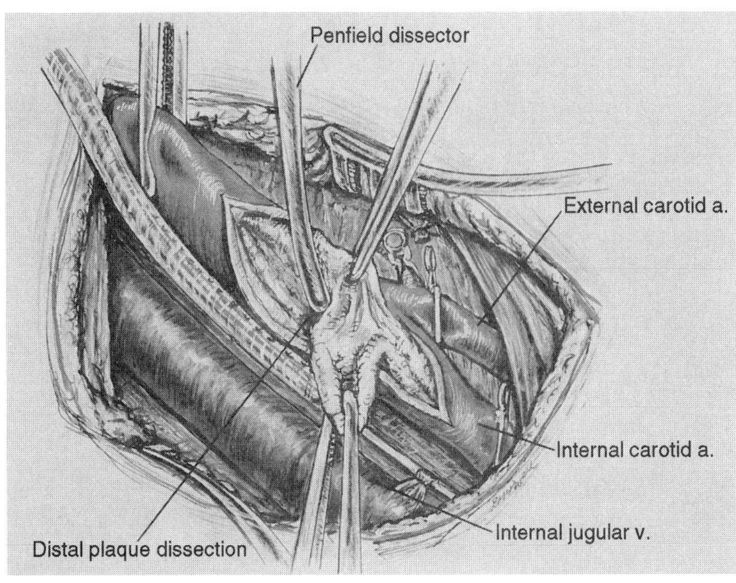

FIGURE 97–13. The plaque is everted and transected from its entrance into the superior thyroid and external carotid arteries. The remaining distal portion in the internal carotid artery is dissected free and removed with the intent of creating a smooth or feathering distal transition, avoiding the formation of an intimal flap (see color section in this volume). (From Bailes JE, Spetzler RF [eds]: Microsurgical Carotid Endarterectomy. New York, Lippincott-Raven, 1996.)

vision. The internal surface of the carotid artery is inspected carefully. Remaining atheromatous debris is removed, usually by stripping it circumferentially from the intimal surface. The luminal surface is irrigated continuously with heparinized saline (100 IU/L). Small fragments of plaque filaments are likewise removed. The arterial surface is inspected proximally and especially distally, where thrombosis-causing intimal flaps are usually located. More effective than tacking sutures is the use of microscissors to trim the intimal flap to where it becomes adherent to the wall. This maneuver often obviates the need for tacking sutures. If necessary, however, interrupted 8–0 monofilament (nylon) tacking sutures should be placed. The luminal surface is inspected in detail using the superior lighting and magnification afforded by the operating microscope. Shunting is not performed routinely and is reserved for patients who experience major EEG changes that cannot be reversed by inducing moderate hypertension. Both internal (e.g., Sundt) and external (e.g., Javid) shunts have been used successfully. Experience over the last several years indicates that only 7% to 9% of our patients require shunting, based on monitoring parameters.[1, 121]

Closure

Beginning distally, the arteriotomy is closed with a continuous 6–0 monofilament (Prolene) suture to below the bifurcation (Fig. 97–14; see color section in this

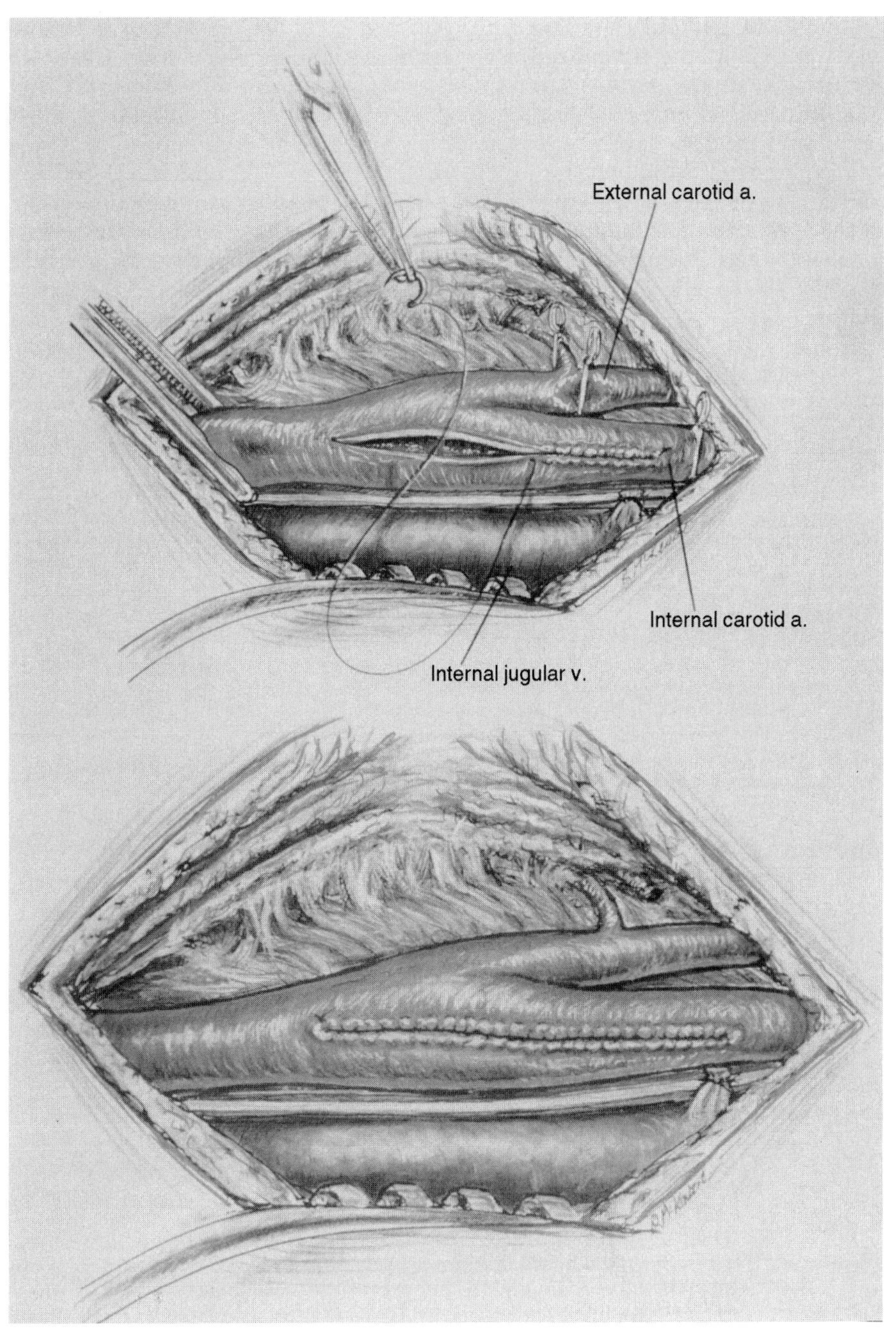

FIGURE 97–14. After the arteriotomy is closed, backbleeding and deocclusion are accomplished in the correct manner in an attempt to expel any air or debris out the lumen or into the distribution of the external (not internal) carotid artery (see color section in this volume). (From Bailes JE, Spetzler RF [eds]: Microsurgical Carotid Endarterectomy. New York, Lippincott-Raven, 1996.)

volume). Another 6–0 monofilament suture is used starting proximally on the common carotid artery, and the two are joined. Alternatively, a single 6–0 suture can be used to close distally to proximally, which is easier and the preferred method. When the arteriotomy is almost complete, but before the two sutures are tied, backbleeding of the ICA and ECA is accomplished by briefly opening the temporary aneurysm clips. The quality and extent of the backbleeding from the ICA are important. Poor or no blood flow often indicates thrombosis at or distal to the operative site. This requires immediate re-exploration and is usually caused by an unrecognized or insufficiently repaired intimal flap. Alternatively, a suture grabbing both the anterior and posterior walls of the artery may be responsible. The superior vision afforded by the operating microscope, however, has made this technical mistake exceedingly rare. In our experience, it occurs significantly less than 1% of the time. Failure to restore acceptable backflow once the sutures are removed implies distal ICA thrombosis and may necessitate balloon catheter or suction thrombectomy, intraoperative angiography, or intra-arterial thrombolysis.

The common carotid clamp is also opened momentarily to permit thrombotic or atheromatous material to be expelled through the open lumen. The superior thyroid artery clip is removed permanently. Consequently, the slow, continuous backbleeding pushes trapped air out through the arteriotomy opening or through the small spaces between the sutures. All microsutures must be handled delicately, and crimping must be avoided. Multiple throws are required to hold the knot of this suture. Including only 1 or 2 mm of the cut edge of the artery permits only small bites with each suture to avoid kinking of the vessel. Postoperative angiographic evaluation has shown consistently that no ICA stenosis is associated with the microsurgical closure (Fig. 97–15).

After arteriotomy closure, the vessels are opened in a specific order (Fig. 97–16). The ECA is opened first. The clamp of the common carotid artery is opened temporarily to permit atheromatous debris, thrombotic material, or air to wash up the distribution of the ECA and away from the hemispheric or retinal blood supply. Next, the ICA clip is released momentarily to allow any debris accumulated between the endarterectomy site and the distal ICA clip to travel by retrograde flow into the external carotid system. The first maneuver, opening both the external and common carotid arteries, is repeated. The common carotid clamp is then removed permanently, restoring anterograde flow through the ICA.

The arteriotomy suture line should be hemostatic except for slight oozing through the needle holes or between the sutures. Any source of pumping blood or an area that does not immediately stop bleeding is

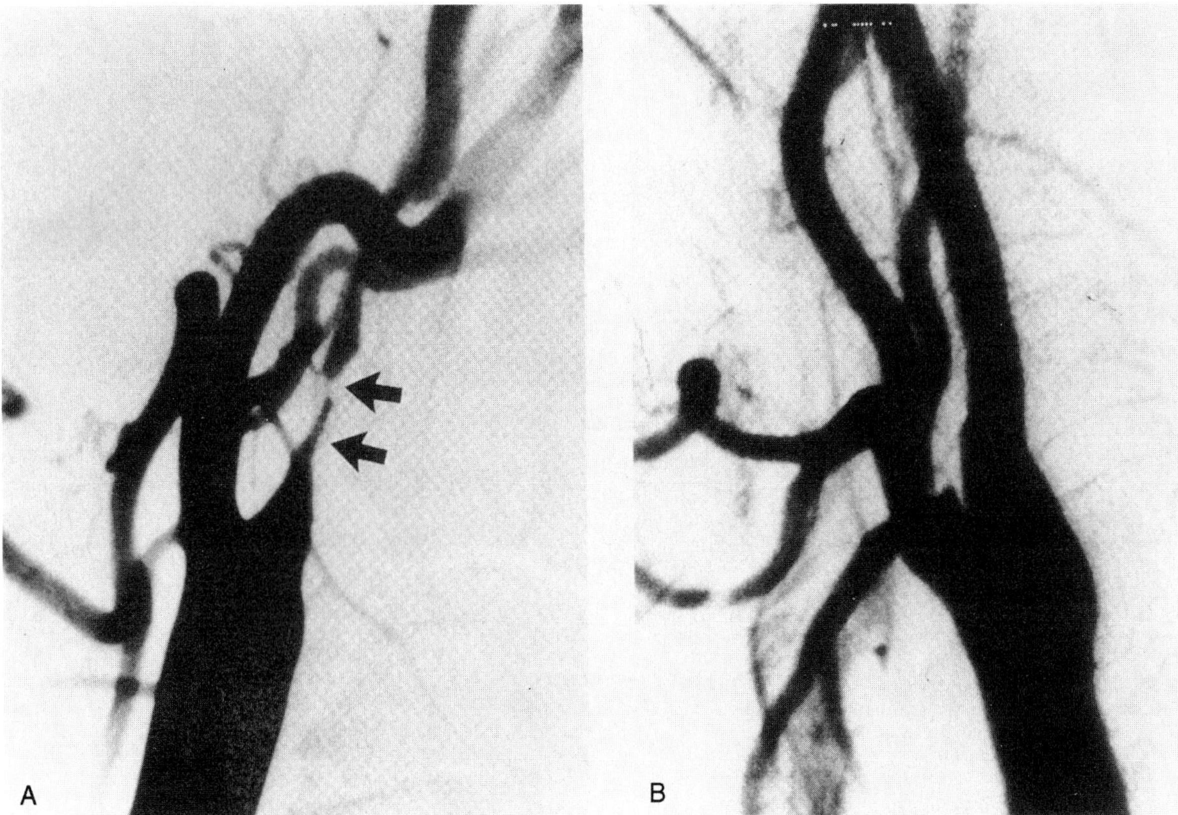

FIGURE 97–15. *A*, Preoperative angiogram showing a severe long-segment stenosis in the proximal internal carotid artery and distal common carotid artery *(arrows)*. *B*, After microendarterectomy, the postoperative angiogram shows excellent resolution of the lesion. (From Bailes JE, Spetzler RF [eds]: Microsurgical Carotid Endarterectomy. New York, Lippincott-Raven, 1996.)

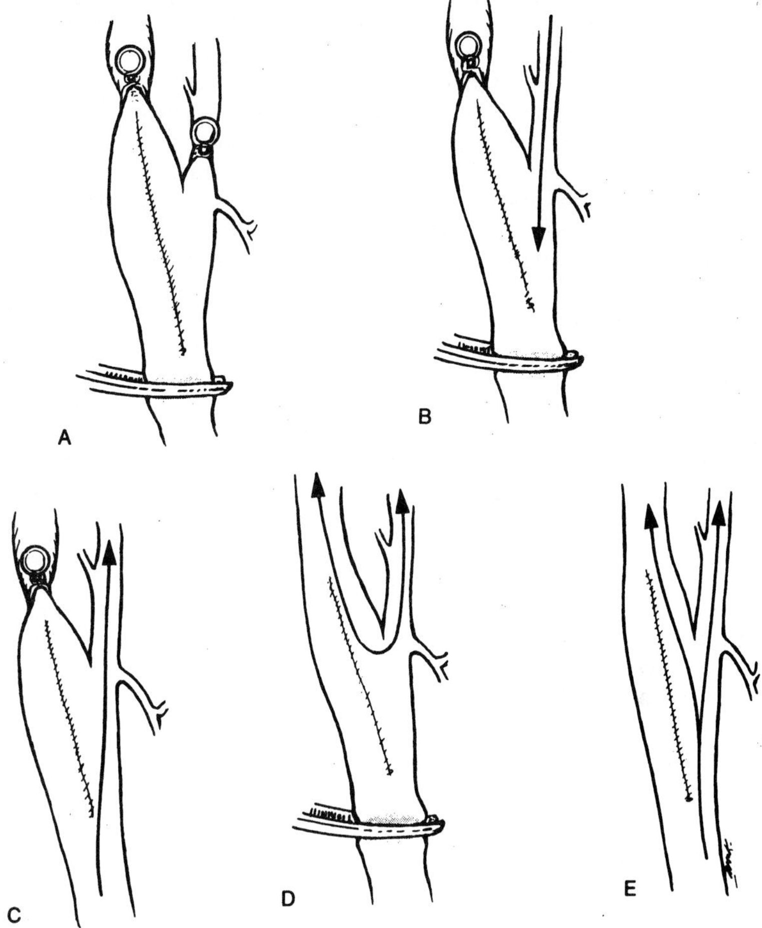

FIGURE 97–16. After the arteriotomy is completed, deocclusion is best accomplished by the following method. *A*, Careful attention is paid so that the suture line is not handled with forceps and so that bipolar coagulation of adventitial bleeding points does not occur near the sutures. The temporary aneurysm clip on the superior thyroid artery was removed previously, just before the arteriotomy was closed, which causes a constant, low-volume blood backflow through the arteriotomy site. This maneuver helps maintain a full column of fluid and expel air bubbles. *B*, The external carotid artery is opened to allow any trapped thrombotic or atherosclerotic debris, as well as air bubbles caused by retrograde flow, to be at least partially removed through the arteriotomy. In addition, this retrograde flow often reveals sources of significant leaks in the arteriotomy closure. *C*, With the internal carotid artery still occluded by a temporary aneurysm clip, the vascular clamp on the common carotid artery is opened for a few moments to allow blood and proximal debris to flow out through the external carotid system. *D*, With the proximal common carotid artery again temporarily occluded, the clip on the distal internal carotid artery is released, allowing any debris distal to the internal carotid clip to travel back into the external carotid artery by retrograde flow. The maneuver in *C* is then briefly repeated. *E*, All clips are removed, and the common carotid artery is opened, establishing anterograde flow in the internal carotid artery. In our experience, transcranial Doppler monitoring has shown that embolization into the cerebral circulation is markedly diminished or eliminated by using these maneuvers. (From Bailes JE, Spetzler RF [eds]: Microsurgical Carotid Endarterectomy. New York, Lippincott-Raven, 1996.)

closed with single, interrupted 6–0 monofilament sutures. Surgicel may be placed as a monolayer over the arteriotomy. Complete hemostasis is attained, and a topical hemostatic agent (Avitene, MecChem, Woburn, MA) can be applied to the wound after copious irrigation with a topical antibiotic solution. Blood pressure is brought to or very near normal to avoid hypertension-induced intracerebral hemorrhage in a dysautoregulated cerebral hemisphere. The systemic heparinization is not reversed. The wound is closed in two layers with absorbable sutures, and sterile strips are used for the skin.

In the recovery room and during the patient's first overnight stay, blood pressure must be strictly controlled to avoid hypertension. Hypertension can lead to intracerebral hemorrhage, especially after tightly stenotic lesions are reopened. In these patients, the autoregulation of the ipsilateral cerebral hemisphere is thought to be faulty. Conversely, hypotension can promote thrombosis at the operative site and should also be avoided. Aspirin (650 mg) is administered rectally in the recovery room and then orally each day for an indefinite period. Routine antibiotics are administered for 24 hours.

Invasive cardiac or other monitoring is performed postoperatively as indicated. Many patients who receive intraoperative barbiturates for cerebral protection may experience postoperative respiratory depression, neurological depression, or both. Usually these effects diminish rapidly. Even when patients are deeply obtunded pharmacologically, brainstem reflexes are intact, and meaningful movement or a withdrawal pattern to painful stimuli can be seen. Consequently, a basic examination typically detects focal or localizing findings even at this stage. In the occasional patient who is initially deeply sedated on arrival in the recovery room, EEG or TCD monitoring can be continued until a neurological examination is possible. Of all the methods of postoperative monitoring, TCD gives the earliest warning of impending carotid occlusion by showing a marked decline in ipsilateral blood flow velocities. Often, TCD findings significantly precede other methods of detection, even the clinical neurological examination, especially in a patient just emerging from general anesthesia.

Postoperative Care

The postoperative treatment of patients who have undergone CEA follows the guidelines for routine postoperative care, but several important aspects are given special consideration. Careful cardiac monitoring and assessment of the patient's cardiac clinical status are stressed in the immediate postoperative period.

In the past, patients were usually maintained in the intensive care unit for at least 24 hours after endarterectomy. Recent advances have shown that this may be unnecessary for many patients. Having patients maintain their oral medications, especially cardiac and hypertensive agents, the night before surgery and the morning of surgery (with a sip of water) seems to stabilize blood pressure postoperatively. Other maneuvers, such as optimizing medical conditions preoperatively and using regional anesthesia, appear to increase the number of patients who do not require intensive care postoperatively and reduce the overall length of hospitalization.[130, 131] Invasive monitoring (e.g., arterial blood pressure lines, Swan-Ganz catheters, central venous pressure catheters, saturation monitors) is used as indicated in selected patients. Patients who have received significant doses of intraoperative barbiturates (usually >1 g of thiopental) are subject to postoperative respiratory depression. This effect usually resolves in several hours. An occasional patient may require intubation and ventilation overnight and is often managed by consulting with specialists in intensive care medicine. Although prophylaxis for deep vein thrombosis (subcutaneous heparin) is considered safe in the postoperative period, we use it only in patients considered to be at high risk.

Patients are mobilized early in the postoperative period and allowed out of bed on the first postoperative day if their general and cardiac conditions permit. If patients are otherwise stable, they are transferred from the intensive care unit to a regular care bed on the first postoperative day. Postoperative antiplatelet therapy is continued indefinitely (650 mg aspirin daily), and patients are allowed a general diet and full ambulatory activity. During the next 2 days, blood pressure must be monitored closely, particularly as patients become fully ambulatory. Postoperative hypertension, even if mild, should be considered for aggressive treatment. Early postoperative hypertension, especially in patients with tight preoperative carotid stenotic lesions, may predispose to intracerebral hemorrhage. Symptoms such as severe ipsilateral headache, facial pain, or seizures may also herald a cerebral hyperperfusion syndrome and possible intracerebral hemorrhage. During these first postoperative days, the wound is inspected carefully for any evidence of hematoma or infection. If there are no complicating or extenuating events, patients are usually discharged on the second or third postoperative day and followed closely as outpatients.

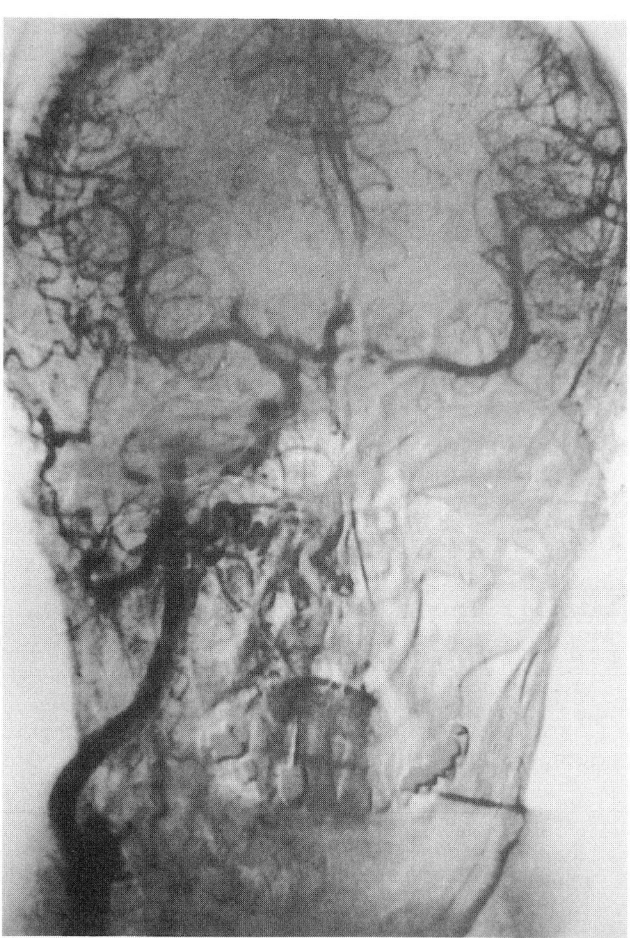

FIGURE 97–17. Approximately 95% of patients tolerate atherosclerotic occlusion of the internal carotid artery, which occurs slowly and is usually associated with adequate cross-filling from the contralateral carotid artery. (From Bailes JE, Spetzler RF [eds]: Microsurgical Carotid Endarterectomy. New York, Lippincott-Raven, 1996.)

CAROTID THROMBOENDARTERECTOMY

The clinical course and natural history of ICA occlusion are often considered uncertain. Although most occlusions of the ICA are discovered incidentally and are apparently asymptomatic, patients with associated signs and symptoms of stroke or TIAs may benefit from aggressive medical and surgical management (Fig. 97–17). Operative treatment is sometimes recommended for patients with acute blockages but no major neurological deficits. In such patients, ICA occlusion can potentially be opened successfully with minimal morbidity and mortality. Chronic ICA occlusion can cause symptoms resulting from embolization from the proximal segment (stump) of the ICA, and this phenomenon must be ruled out in these patients.[132]

The natural history of ICA occlusion is varied and was not clearly elucidated by some of the earlier literature. In several retrospective series, the incidence of subsequent stroke or TIAs after complete ICA occlusion varied between 0% and 23%.[133–135] Prospective series, which may be more sensitive indicators when minor syndromes are considered, found that the incidence of subsequent stroke was between 7% and 54% (mean, 23.6%).[48, 136, 137] The strokes occurred ipsilateral to the carotid occlusion in about two thirds of patients and were located in a contralateral distribution in one third. Fields and Lemak[137] followed 359 patients with ICA occlusion for a mean of 44 months. New strokes occurred in 25% of patients, and 64% of the strokes were ipsilateral to the occluded ICA. Furlan and colleagues[134] reported a 3% annual stroke rate after angiographically proven ICA occlusion; one third occurred on the contralateral side. The incidence of ischemia ipsilateral to an occluded ICA ranges from 5% to 10% annually for stroke and is approximately twice that for TIAs.[136, 138] Cardiac death is more likely to occur in the follow-up period[139] than is stroke.

Meyer and associates[140] described their experience with 34 patients with acute ICA occlusions who underwent carotid thromboendarterectomy. All the patients except one experienced changes in their level of consciousness and had major neurological deficits that began while they were hospitalized. Nine patients (26.5%) returned to normal, four patients (11.8%) were left hemiplegic, and seven patients (20.6%) died. Walters and coworkers[141] performed emergency thromboendarterectomies in 64 patients; 16 of these patients had presumed acute, complete occlusion, but in some, this later proved to be pseudo-occlusion. Blood flow through the ICA was reestablished in all cases. Postoperatively, 14 patients were unchanged or improved, 1 patient's neurological status deteriorated, and 1 patient died from cardiopulmonary arrest on the 24th postoperative day.

Results of surgical thromboendarterectomy in patients with ICA occlusions who presented early and without profound deficits have been reported. This category of patients was the one most likely to benefit from surgery. Hugenholtz and Elgie[142] excluded patients with drowsiness, major neurological deficits, and tandem lesions distal to the ICA occlusion. With these criteria, they reduced the surgical morbidity rate to 10% and the surgical mortality rate to 0% in a group of 35 patients. Using similar selection criteria in 47 patients, Hafner and Tew[139] reported surgical mortality and neurological morbidity rates of 0%. Kusunoki and colleagues[143] studied two groups of patients: those with and without neurological, medical, and angiographic risk factors (Fig. 97–18). There were no operative deaths in the latter group of 14 patients. Clearly, case series that excluded patients with severe neurological deficits demonstrated that restoring blood flow in the ICA is beneficial. Despite the identification of a subgroup of patients expected to benefit from restoring blood flow through the ICA and the publication of two clinical series showing favorable surgical morbidity and mortality rates in this group, a recent poll indicated that, according to expert opinion, ICA occlusion was a contraindication to ICA surgery. In fact, after reviewing 1000 CEAs, the responders categorized the 60 endarterectomies (6%) performed for complete ICA occlusion as inappropriate.[142]

The optimal treatment for carotid occlusion, especially surgical intervention, is thus controversial. The controversy partially reflects the difficulties in defining the population best suited for surgical intervention and in performing prospective studies to determine the outcomes of different treatment groups. However, there appears to be a subgroup of patients that fares well if they can be diagnosed and treated expeditiously before significant cerebral infarction occurs. As experience with intra-arterial thrombolytic therapy accrues, it is anticipated that some patients with acute ICA occlusion may benefit from such treatment. If restoration of anterograde blood flow is successful, carotid bifurcation and angioplasty of the ICA origin by balloon or stent techniques may be a temporizing or preferred treatment.[144] Protection against distal propagation of thrombotic material is of obvious importance. The significant advances made in endovascular therapy for arterial occlusion notwithstanding, the cerebrovascular surgeon should be aware of the natural history of, controversies surrounding, and technique of performing surgical thromboendarterectomy.

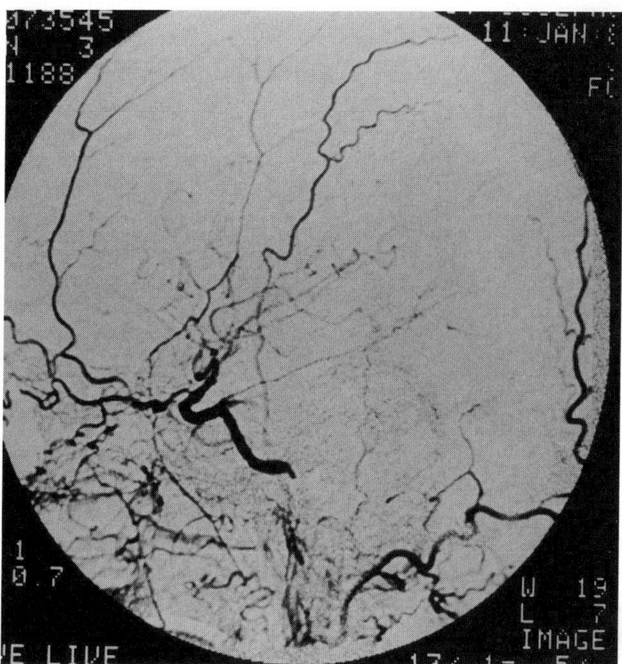

FIGURE 97–18. Lateral carotid angiogram showing reconstitution of the distal internal carotid artery (ICA) in a patient with occlusion of the ICA origin. With retrograde filling via ethmoidal branches and the ophthalmic artery, there is a good chance of reopening this vessel. (From Bailes JE, Spetzler RF [eds]: Microsurgical Carotid Endarterectomy. New York, Lippincott-Raven, 1996.)

Technique

In patients who are candidates for thromboendarterectomy, a standard CEA longitudinal incision is made along the medial border of the sternocleidomastoid muscle, through the platysma muscle and cervical fascia, to expose the carotid sheath. After the carotid artery is isolated above and below the level of the bifurcation, the vessel is inspected to determine its size and external appearance. If the ICA is small, thin, and fibrotic, no attempt is made to reopen it. Surgery is directed to performing a proximal remnant angioplasty (stumpectomy) if otherwise indicated. Before the common carotid artery is cross-clamped, thiopental sodium is administered intravenously to achieve 15- to 30-second EEG burst suppression.[112] Dissection is then completed to expose the common, internal, and external carotid arteries. Care is used to avoid manipulating the occluded ICA.

Next, a small arteriotomy is made on the lateral ICA beyond the obvious atheromatous disease. At this point, one of these phenomena occurs: (1) the clot spontaneously expresses itself with good backflow; (2) the clot does not exit spontaneously, and backflow is not observed; or (3) a small amount of clot exits and is followed by poor backflow. In the first instance, standard cross-clamping of the vessels is performed, followed by an endarterectomy. In the case of the latter two events, a 2F Fogarty catheter with a 0.2-mL balloon is passed up the ICA with very gentle pressure until it is near (a distance of 10 to 12 cm) the carotid siphon. The balloon is inflated with saline and gently withdrawn. In cases of acute or subacute thrombosis, especially where collateral blood flow has kept the distal ICA patent, it is often possible to remove the clot. Brisk bleeding from the distal ICA is then encountered immediately. After good retrograde flow is established, the distal ICA along with the common carotid artery should be occluded rapidly. The CEA is then completed in the standard fashion by extending the arteriotomy into the common carotid artery. Shunting is not recommended unless indicated by a major EEG change, as described in the standard CEA protocol. If the ICA cannot be reopened by passing the catheter approximately three times, it is safest to discontinue the effort.

When the ICA cannot be reopened or is atretic on inspection, a proximal remnant angioplasty and an external carotid endarterectomy, if indicated, are performed. Proximal remnant angioplasty is performed by closing the ICA flush at its origin with a large vascular clip, dissecting along the posterior wall of the ICA, and transecting it from the distal portion. These maneuvers avoid angulation as flowing blood passes into the ECA. This maneuver may reduce the propensity for stagnated blood, eddy currents, and embolic material to form in the area of the ICA origin.

In 1992, Barrow Neurological Institute reported its experience with 42 patients with symptomatic carotid occlusion.[145] Clinical presentations included focal TIAs in 68%, amaurosis fugax in 28%, new fixed deficits in 28%, and stroke in evolution in 9% of patients. Forty-six operations were performed on the 42 patients, including 24 (52%) successful ICA reopenings and 9 (20%) stumpectomies with concomitant external endarterectomies; 4 of the latter patients (9%) ultimately required extracranial-intracranial bypass for persistent ischemic symptoms. Three patients (7%) experienced transient surgical morbidity, and in one patient (2%), hemiparesis worsened with restoration of anterograde blood flow. There were no deaths.

Long-term arterial patency was assessed in 17 of the 24 patients undergoing ICA reopening (73%). Carotid Doppler ultrasound studies were performed a mean of 28 months after surgery. In 15 patients (88%), the ICA was widely patent. In the other two patients, one had more than 70% stenosis, and one had developed a reocclusion. Three patients were lost to follow-up, which, for the remaining 39 patients, was an average of 40 months after their last operation. Five patients (13%) died—two of cancer and three of myocardial infarction. Four patients (10%) experienced neurological events—TIAs in two and vertebrobasilar insufficiency in two. Six patients (15%) had new myocardial infarctions or new-onset angina. The outcome for patients with successful restoration of ICA flow was not significantly different from that of patients who were treated until asymptomatic with the alternative surgical strategies described. No patient had a subsequent stroke during the follow-up period, and the rates for neurological transient events (TIAs and vertebrobasilar insufficiency) for both groups were comparable with the expected natural history for completed stroke in nonsurgically treated patients.

These data strengthen the conclusion that the surgical morbidity and mortality rates will be low in a subgroup of patients chosen for restoration of ICA flow based primarily on the presenting neurological examination. The precise timing between ICA occlusion and attempted restoration of blood flow is known in few series. These series include postangiographic or postsurgical occlusions that represent a pathophysiology other than spontaneous occlusion associated with atherosclerotic disease. The impression of those reporting such series is that the earlier surgery is performed, the better patients fare.

The literature concerning thromboendarterectomy of spontaneously occluded symptomatic ICAs consistently demonstrates a subgroup of patients in whom blood flow is restored successfully and who have low morbidity and mortality rates. This subgroup is best defined as those without severe neurological deficits, a decreased level of consciousness, or intracerebral hemorrhage. Clinical experience with such patients at our institution and others shows that low surgical morbidity and mortality rates are associated with carefully performed thromboendarterectomy of the ICA. During long-term follow-up review, the vessels remained patent, and the patients had fewer strokes than would be anticipated from natural history data. Our patients followed a prospectively designed diagnostic, anesthetic, and surgical protocol. Their evaluation and treatment were interdisciplinary. The data, however, were collected retrospectively, and no simultaneous control group was available for comparison. This experience cannot definitively establish the efficacy of surgical management for ICA occlusion. Based on the available data, however, we currently recommend surgery for patients with acute symptomatic ICA occlusion who do not have a major neurological deficits or hemorrhage on computed tomography.

The natural history of carotid occlusion has been ill defined, and its treatment is controversial. Even when initially presenting in an asymptomatic fashion, probably as many as a fifth of patients suffer a cerebral infarction ipsilateral to the occluded carotid artery within 3 years. This likelihood suggests that occlusion of the ICA is of recent onset, and the diagnosis cannot always be made with certainty. It is often difficult to determine the optimal treatment for patients with documented symptomatic ICA occlusion. ICA occlusion can manifest with acute, transient, or evolving cerebral ischemic symptoms. In the past, emergency carotid thromboendarterectomy for patients with acute ICA occlusion was considered contraindicated by some specialists. This attitude reflects several perceptions. First, the incidence of neurological morbidity and mortality has been perceived as high. Second, it was thought that blood flow must be restored in the first few hours after the occlusion. Finally, lack of a definite benefit has also been perceived.

As microsurgical technique, anesthesia methods, and perioperative management have improved, however, the ability to reopen these occluded arteries with minimal neurological morbidity and no operative mortality has likewise improved. In recent years, we have also achieved a higher patency rate by developing our current protocol of operating on patients with acute, symptomatic carotid occlusions who have not experienced a decreased level of consciousness, hemiplegia, or aphasia. This approach is viable in appropriately selected patients. Current endovascular methods offer an alternative to surgical procedures for attempting to reopen an occluded carotid artery.[144] The indications and technology are continually evolving, and an individualized approach in every patient is warranted.[146–148] It nonetheless remains important for cerebrovascular surgeons to understand the concepts relating to the presentation and operative treatment of this patient population.

COMPLICATIONS OF CAROTID ENDARTERECTOMY

CEA is an efficacious treatment, but like any surgical procedure, it has inherent risks. Even if performed properly, intervention on the arterial vasculature carries low but definite risks. Despite traditional theory, the actual risk of temporary carotid occlusion (i.e., carotid cross-clamping) is now thought to be relatively low, especially when performed in the controlled environment of the operating theater and with the full complement of cerebral monitoring and the protective elements of general anesthesia and metabolic suppressive agents.

Embolization

The major risk of CEA is no longer attributed to temporary ischemia during the period of cross-clamping; rather, other phenomena account for the associated neurological morbidity. Embolization of thrombotic material, portions of atherosclerotic plaque material, or air particles has been reported. With TCD monitoring, emboli (usually gaseous) have been detected in one third of cases.

Intraoperative embolic events occur during three phases of CEA. The nurse preparing the surgical field with antiseptic solution should exercise care. The pressure transmitted transcutaneously during scrubbing can shear thrombotic material from fragile plaque lesions. During the operation, the dissection of vessels in preparation for endarterectomy can cause the embolization of particulate matter. This is the time of highest risk because of the necessary handling and manipulation of the carotid artery, the presence of the plaque, and the associated thrombotic material. Reopening the vessel after closure of the arteriotomy is another period of potential distal embolization, as confirmed by our experience with intraoperative TCD recording. Usually, however, the emboli are gaseous owing to incomplete evacuation of the intraluminal air and can be minimized or eliminated by meticulous attention to surgical technique. Surgeons must always attempt to establish a full column of fluid intraluminally before releasing the clamp. Backbleeding via an open superior thyroid artery or, in cases of inadequate backflow, filling the intraluminal carotid artery with heparinized saline solution helps establish this fluid-filled lumen.

Intraluminal carotid shunts have been controversial, and their use has been further complicated by a lack of agreement among scientific and surgical data. Although some advocate the routine use of intraluminal carotid shunts, there are several drawbacks, including a high incidence of cerebral embolization.

Carotid Artery Thrombosis

Thrombosis of the lumen can occur in the absence of technical errors and can cause ischemic complications. The thrombogenic nature of the fresh luminal surface after CEA makes it susceptible to mural thrombosis, subsequent embolization, or both. Removal of the atherosclerotic plaque exposes the underlying media and occasionally portions of the adventitial layer. When blood flow is restored, platelets actively adhere to the underlying collagen.[149] A pseudoendothelial monolayer of platelets, which is thought to be nonthrombogenic, forms.[118, 150, 151] The adhering platelets release vasoactive substances, including adenosine diphosphate and thromboxane A_2, both potent platelet aggregators. Factor XII is activated by the exposed collagen and initiates the hemostatic cascade that forms a fibrin clot. Platelet factor III, released by the activated platelets, dissipates when the intrinsic coagulation system is activated.[152–154] The combination of aggregated platelets, fibrin, and red blood cells constitutes a thrombus at the operative site. This thrombus can fragment with distal embolization, or the size of the clot can continue to increase locally until the vessel is occluded. The thrombus can also be propagated distally. Heparin is routinely administered before carotid cross-clamping to prevent intravascular thrombosis and thromboembolism of areas of stasis caused by the carotid occlusion.[155–157] Because the half-life of heparin is only 90 minutes, it appears that superior results are obtained if heparinization is not neutralized, because the platelet monolayer can form to protect the exposed elements in the media.[152] Some authors recommend the routine infusion of postoperative heparin. Such a regimen, however, has the potential to cause postoperative hematomas at the operative site and is probably unnecessary, except when there is unusual potential for postoperative vessel occlusion.

Aspirin affects normal platelet function by inhibiting the formation of thromboxane A_2 in adenosine diphosphate–induced platelet aggregation.[149] Findlay and associates[158] administered a combination of aspirin and dipyridamole or a placebo perioperatively to patients undergoing CEA. Autologous indium 3–labeled platelets were injected postoperatively, and platelet collection and deposition were measured at the endarterectomy site. The degree of platelet aggregation and accumulation in the treatment group was significantly reduced compared with the placebo group. Two patients in the control group had postoperative strokes. In one of these patients, a thick, white, mural thrombus, indicative of a platelet clot, was found on re-exploration. None of the patients had a postoperative wound hematoma. These authors recommended 300 mg of aspirin every 8 hours and 75 mg of dipyridamole every 8 hours. The cyclooxygenase system is inhibited by aspirin. Dipyridamole interferes with the platelet phosphodiesterase system, elevating the cyclic adenosine monophosphate levels in a synergistic fashion. We have used aspirin alone with excellent results. In canines, a single dose of aspirin (10 mg/kg) resulted in the formation of the platelet monolayer, which inhibited thrombus formation at the endarterectomy site. In contrast, doses in the range of 0.5 mg/kg were ineffective.[151]

The incidence of recurrent carotid artery stenosis after an endarterectomy may be decreased by antiplatelet treatment. Degranulated platelets release smooth muscle and fibroblast mitogens, which subsequently migrate to the underlying neointima. Exaggerated or exuberant growth of layers of this neointima may be the origin of recurrent stenosis. This growth is termed neointimal hyperplasia or fibromuscular hyperplasia.[47, 156, 159] One report suggested that aspirin plus dipyridamole was ineffective in reducing the incidence of carotid restenosis when evaluated at a 1-year follow-up.[160] Hansen and coworkers[161] likewise noted no difference in those treated with low doses of aspirin (75 mg daily) versus a placebo 1 year after CEA. Two months after surgery, 39% of patients had recurrent carotid artery stenosis of 30% or greater; stenosis recurred in 42% of patients 6 months after surgery. More than 50% stenosis was seen in 9% of patients, and 2% had an occlusion at the 6-month follow-up. Bischof and coauthors[162] compared antiplatelet therapy with anticoagulation in 328 patients who underwent CEA with a subgroup of patients treated without medication and found no statistically significant differences between the two groups. There was no difference in their cause of death or in the incidence of intracerebral hemorrhage. They concluded that long-term antiaggregant and anticoagulant therapy did not affect the rate of complications or survival after CEA. However, survival was increased in the treated group because the incidence of postoperative myocardial infarction was reduced. We advocate aspirin administered about a week before surgery and extended indefinitely in the postoperative period. As mentioned, aspirin is also administered to the patient rectally in the recovery room immediately after the procedure.

Intracerebral Hemorrhage

Intracerebral hemorrhage is an infrequent but potentially devastating complication of CEA.[163–166] Postoperative intracerebral hemorrhage, which usually occurs several days after the operation, has been the source of significant morbidity and mortality in series in which operative techniques have otherwise resulted in excellent outcomes. The incidence of postoperative intracerebral hemorrhage is thought to be less than 1%. In our series, intracerebral hematoma caused one postoperative complication and one death, which was the only neurologically related death in the series.[1] Bruetman and colleagues[164] reported that intracerebral hemorrhage complicated 6 of 900 (0.67%) endarterectomies.[164] In 1986, Spetzler and coworkers[112] reported a 0.5% incidence of postoperative intracerebral hematoma, which led to one death. Of 1930 CEAs, eight patients (0.41%) sustained a postoperative intracerebral hemorrhage.[167] Postoperative intracerebral hemorrhage was thought to occur only in patients with preexisting cerebrovascular accidents in which reperfusion of cerebral blood flow to that region could cause hemorrhage into or adjacent to the infarcted zone. In their 1978 review, Caplan and associates[165] described 17 patients, all of whom had preoperative stroke. Two of these patients had severe unilateral carotid stenosis and underwent CEA 4 and 5 weeks after cerebral infarction, respectively. However, most patients with postoperative intracerebral hemorrhage have had a recent antecedent brain infarct and preoperative hypertension. Postoperative intracerebral hemorrhage usually occurs in the first few days after surgery and is associated with systemic hypertension. In reported series, these hemorrhages occurred an average of 3 days after surgery and were ipsilateral to the CEA in more than 90% of cases.[99, 157, 165]

Hypertension often accompanies CEA and is especially critical in the immediate postoperative period. Lehv and coauthors[130] found that mean systolic blood pressure was elevated more than 15 mm Hg in 15 of 27 patients (55%) undergoing unilateral CEA. Seven of these patients developed neurological complications, and one died. In a third of these hypertensive patients, blood pressure was extremely elevated (systolic, 195 to 250 mm Hg; diastolic, 105 to 130 mm Hg). They believed that postoperative hypertension occurred after the normal carotid sinus reflex was interrupted and therefore was common after bilateral carotid procedures. In some patients, the absence of other systemic (e.g., retinal, renal, cardiac) signs of hypertension suggested that preoperative occult or asymptomatic hypertension did not exist and that a new onset of postoperative hypertension could cause capillary breakdown and hemorrhage.[165] Besides recent cerebral infarction and hypertension, TIAs and anticoagulation have been regarded as contributors to postoperative hemorrhage. Wong and coworkers[168] retrospectively studied 291 consecutive CEA patients and found that postoperative hypertension was significantly associated with stroke or death and was statistically correlated with heart complications. Postoperative hypotension and bradycardia did not correlate with outcome.

In addition to the risk caused by uncontrolled postoperative hypertension, Sundt and colleagues[105] documented that postoperative cerebral blood flow increased to the cerebral hemisphere ipsilateral to the CEA despite the absence of systemic hypertension. In certain patients, cerebral hyperperfusion may be symptomatic, causing severe headache, facial pain, orbital pain, and paroxysmal lateralizing epileptiform discharges.[155, 156, 169, 170] Brick and colleagues[171] reported a patient who developed acute confusion, agitation, and headaches 8 days after undergoing CEA. His evaluation disclosed that he had paroxysmal lateralizing epileptiform discharges and severe angiographic cerebral vasoconstriction. The symptoms subsided in 1 week, did not recur, and were thought to be related to impaired cerebral autoregulation. Both focal and generalized seizures have been described in patients with negative computed tomographic scans after CEA.[153] Akers and associates[172] found that somnolence, clinical depression, and psychiatric disturbances were present postoperatively in their CEA patients. These features were characteristic of patients who had high-grade stenoses corrected and were believed to be secondary to cerebral hyperperfusion syndrome. These phenomena tended to be self-limited and resolved within 8 weeks. TCD ultrasonography is an effective, accurate, and noninvasive method to document and follow patients with suspected hyperperfusion until it resolves.[163]

Solomon and colleagues[167] reported that six of eight patients with postoperative intracerebral hemorrhage after CEA had no evidence of previous cerebral infarction in the area of the subsequent hemorrhage. Most hemorrhages occurred within the first 5 days of surgery and were not associated with postoperative hypertension. It was believed that a cerebral hyperperfusion syndrome existed in these patients in areas where severe, chronic ICA stenosis had paralyzed autoregulation of cerebral blood flow. This state is reminiscent of and perhaps has an underlying mechanism similar to that of normal perfusion pressure breakthrough after resection of an arteriovenous malformation. In this circumstance, cerebral steal causes chronic ischemia in the area surrounding the malformation. The surrounding vessels are in a chronic state of maximal dilatation and have lost the capacity to autoregulate. When the arteriovenous malformation is removed, the surrounding cerebral tissue is unable to react to a normal perfusion pressure with normal vasoconstriction. In certain cases, cerebral hemorrhage or edema can result.

Myocardial Infarction

In series of microsurgical CEAs, myocardial infarction is one of the most common complications and certainly the greatest systemic complication associated with the procedure. In our series, it occurred in approximately 3% of patients and accounted for as many as 50% of late deaths.[1] Undoubtedly, its occurrence reflects the frequent concomitant presence of coronary and carotid artery atherosclerosis. In addition, the systemic or coronary operative stresses of CEA and general anesthesia are significant.

Despite thorough preoperative cardiac assessments, the reported general incidence of perioperative myocardial infarction with CEA remains at 2% to 3%. It is primarily due to the natural progression of the coronary atherosclerotic process. Various cardiac syndromes, including activation of previously stable angina, onset of unstable angina, and development of acute intraoperative or immediate postoperative myocardial infarction, occur. Myocardial oxygen demand, probably altered by increased catecholamine production, may exceed oxygen delivery. Intraoperative or postoperative hypertension, increased intravascular volume, and tachycardia can exacerbate this situation. In addition, if intraoperative barbiturates are used for cerebral protection, myocardial suppression may occur. Patients with aortic and mitral valve insufficiency seem especially vulnerable to this scenario and may suffer congestive failure with or without myocardial infarction.

Careful preoperative screening for critical coronary perfusion and myocardial function at rest and in response to stress is necessary to minimize complications. Strict attention to intraoperative hemodynamic parameters and their response to anesthetic manipulation is required. Immediate postoperative hemodynamic and cardiac monitoring helps minimize the possibility of perioperative cardiac morbidity.

CONCLUSION

Both the indications for and the techniques of CEA have evolved remarkably in recent years. Defined by the recent clinical trials for both symptomatic and asymptomatic populations, the procedure is now supported by firm data and more sophisticated methods. The cardiac, medical, and anesthetic management of these patients has also improved. Meticulous attention to technical details and the participation of qualified nursing and other support personnel contribute heavily to excellent outcomes. No other procedure in medicine so highlights the importance of minimizing operative morbidity and mortality if the natural history of the disease process is to be improved on. Current clinical research will continue to define the patient population most likely to benefit from this procedure and the ultimate role of future developments in endovascular techniques.

REFERENCES

1. Bailes JE, Spetzler RF (eds): Microsurgical Carotid Endarterectomy. New York, Lippincott-Raven, 1996.
2. Flamm ES, Demopoulos HB, Seligman ML, et al: Possible molecular mechanisms of barbiturate-mediated protection in regional cerebral ischemia. Acta Neurol Scand Suppl 64:150–151, 1977.
3. Fein JM: A history of cerebrovascular disease and its surgical management. In Smith R (ed): Stroke and the Extracranial Vessels. New York, Raven Press, 1984, pp 1–7.
4. Fisher CM, Gore I, Okabe N, et al: Atherosclerosis of the carotid and vertebral arteries—extracranial and intracranial. J Neuropathol Exp Neurol 24:455–476, 1965.

5. Eastcott HHG, Pickering GW, Rob CG: Reconstruction of internal carotid artery. Lancet 2:994–996, 1954.
6. Fields WS, Lemak NA, Franowski RF, et al: Controlled trial of aspirin in cerebral ischemic. Stroke 8:301–314, 1977.
7. Dyken ML, Pokras R: The performance of endarterectomy for disease of the extracranial arteries of the head. Stroke 15:948–950, 1984.
8. Winslow CM, Solomon DH, Chassin MR, et al: The appropriateness of carotid endarterectomy. N Engl J Med 318:721–727, 1988.
9. Barnett HJ, Plum F, Walton JN: Carotid endarterectomy—an expression of concern. Stroke 15:941–943, 1984.
10. Kuller LH, Sutton KC: Carotid artery bruit: Is it safe and effective to auscultate the neck? Stroke 15:944–947, 1984.
11. Weksler BB, Lewin M: Anticoagulation in cerebral ischemia. Stroke 14:658–663, 1983.
12. Shaw DA, Venables GS, Cartlidge NE, et al: Carotid endarterectomy in patients with transient cerebral ischemia. J Neurol Sci 64:45–53, 1984.
13. European Carotid Surgery Trialists' Collaborative Group: MRC European carotid surgery trial: Interim results for symptomatic patients with severe (70–99%) or with mild (0–29%) carotid stenosis. Lancet 337:1235–1243, 1991.
14. Mayberg MR, Wilson SE, Yatsu F, et al: Carotid endarterectomy and prevention of cerebral ischemia in symptomatic carotid stenosis. Veterans Affairs Cooperative Studies Program 309 Trialist Group. JAMA 266:3289–3294, 1991.
15. North American Symptomatic Carotid Endarterectomy Trial: Methods, patient characteristics, and progress. Stroke 22:711–720, 1991.
16. American Heart Association: Heart and Stroke Facts Statistics. January 1994.
17. Bonita R, Stewart A, Beaglehole R: International trends in stroke mortality: 1970–1985. Stroke 21:989–992, 1990.
18. Modan B, Wagener DK: Some epidemiological aspects of stroke: Mortality/morbidity trends, age, sex, race, socioeconomic status. Stroke 23:1230–1236, 1992.
19. Sarti C, Tuomilehto J, Sivenius J, et al: Stroke mortality and case-fatality rates in three geographic areas of Finland from 1983 to 1986. Stroke 24:1140–1147, 1993.
20. Wolf PA, O'Neill A, D'Agostino RB, et al: Declining mortality not declining incidence of stroke: The Framingham Study #101. Stroke 20:158, 1989.
21. Xue S, Burke GL, Sprafka M, et al: Trends in stroke mortality, morbidity, case-fatality and long-term survival from 1970–1985: The Minnesota Heart Survey. Paper presented at the 17th International Joint Conference on Stroke and Cerebral Circulation, 1992, Phoenix, AZ.
22. Mohr JP, Caplan LR, Melski JW, et al: The Harvard Cooperative Stroke Registry: A prospective registry. Neurology 28:754–762, 1978.
23. Chimowitz M: Clinical spectrum and natural history of cerebrovascular occlusive disease. In Awad IA (ed): Cerebrovascular Occlusive Disease and Brain Ischemia. Park Ridge, IL, AANS, 1992, pp 59–71.
24. Anderson RJ, Hobson RW 2nd, Padberg FT, et al: Carotid endarterectomy for asymptomatic carotid stenosis: A ten-year experience with 120 procedures in a fellowship training program. Ann Vasc Surg 5:111–115, 1991.
25. CASANOVA Study Group: Carotid surgery versus medical therapy in asymptomatic carotid stenosis. Stroke 22:1229–1235, 1991.
26. Collins R, Peto R, MacMahon S, et al: Blood pressure, stroke, and coronary heart disease. Part 2. Short-term reductions in blood pressure: Overview of randomised drug trials in their epidemiological context. Lancet 335:827–838, 1990.
27. Dyken M: Stroke risk factors. In Norris JW, Hachinski VC (eds): Prevention of Stroke. New York, Springer-Verlag, 1991, pp 83–101.
28. Kannel WB, Wolf PA, Verter J: Risk factors for stroke. In Smith RR (ed): Stroke and the Extracranial Vessels. New York, Raven Press, 1984, pp 47–58.
29. MacMahon S, Peto R, Cutler J: Blood pressure, stroke, and coronary heart disease. Part 1. Prolonged differences in blood pressure: Prospective observational studies corrected for the regression dilution bias. Lancet 335:765–774, 1990.
30. Wolf PA: An overview of the epidemiology of stroke. Stroke 21(Suppl II):II2–II6, 1990.
31. Wolf PA, Kannel WB, Sorlie P, et al: Asymptomatic carotid bruit and risk of stroke: The Framingham Study. JAMA 245: 1442–1445, 1981.
32. Wolf PA, Belanger AJ, D'Agostino RB: Management of risk factors. Neurol Clin 10:177–191, 1992.
33. Javid H, Ostermiller WE Jr, Hengesh JW, et al: Natural history of carotid bifurcation atheroma. Surgery 67:80–86, 1970.
34. Arkless HA: Cervical murmurs with normal hearts. QCIM 40: 114, 1946.
35. Chambers BR, Norris JW: Outcome in patients with asymptomatic neck bruits. N Engl J Med 315:860–865, 1986.
36. Gilroy J, Meyer JS: Auscultation of the neck in occlusive cerebrovascular disease. Circulation 25:300–310, 1962.
37. Hammond JH, Eisinger RP: Carotid bruits in 1000 normal subjects. Arch Intern Med 109:563–565, 1962.
38. Hennerici M, Hulsbomer HB, Hefter H, et al: Natural history of asymptomatic extracranial arterial disease: Results of a long-term prospective study. Brain 110:777–791, 1987.
39. Hertzer NR, Flannagan RA Jr, Bevens EG, et al: Surgical versus nonoperative treatment of symptomatic carotid stenosis: 290 patients documented by intravenous angiography. Ann Surg 204:163–171, 1986.
40. Heyman A, Wilkinson WE, Heyden S, et al: Risk of stroke in asymptomatic persons with cervical arterial bruits: A population study in Evans County, Georgia. N Engl J Med 302:838–841, 1980.
41. Ingall TJ, Homer D, Whisnant JP, et al: Predictive value of carotid bruit for carotid atherosclerosis. Arch Neurol 46:418–422, 1989.
42. Rennie L, Ejrup B, McDowell F: Arterial bruits in cerebrovascular disease. Neurology 14:751–756, 1964.
43. Welch LK, Crowley WJ: Bruits of the head and neck. Stroke 1: 245–247, 1970.
44. Busuttil RW, Baker JD, Davidson RK, et al: Carotid artery stenosis—hemodynamic significance and clinical course. JAMA 245:1438–1441, 1981.
45. Moore WS: Extracranial Cerebrovascular Disease—The Carotid Artery, 4th ed. New York, WB Saunders, 1993, pp 532–575.
46. Norris JW, Zhu CZ, Bornstein NM, et al: Vascular risks of symptomatic carotid stenosis. Stroke 22:1485–1490, 1991.
47. Thompson JE, Patman RD, Talkington CM: Asymptomatic carotid bruit: Long term outcome of patients having endarterectomy compared with unoperated controls. Ann Surg 188:308–316, 1978.
48. Wiebers DO, Whisnant JP, Sandok BA, et al: Prospective comparison of a cohort with asymptomatic carotid bruit and a population-based cohort without carotid bruit. Stroke 21:984–988, 1990.
49. Heyman A, Leviton A, Millikan CH, et al (Study Group on TIA Criteria and Detection): Transient focal cerebral ischemia: Epidemiological and clinical aspects. Stroke 5:277–287, 1974.
50. Caplan LR: Carotid artery disease. N Engl J Med 315:886–888, 1986.
51. Chambers BR, Norris JW: The case against surgery for asymptomatic carotid stenosis. Stroke 15:964–967, 1984.
52. Fisher CM: Guy Williams Jr Memorial Lecture, 1985: Concerning transient ischemic attacks. Clev Clin J Med 54:3–11, 1987.
53. Special report from the National Institute of Neurological Disorders and Stroke: Classifications of cerebrovascular diseases III. Stroke 21:637–676, 1990.
54. Adams HP, Putman SF Jr, Corbett JJ, et al: Amaurosis fugax: The results of arteriography in 59 patients. Stroke 14:742–744, 1983.
55. Ostfeld AM, Shekelle RB, Klawans HL: Transient ischemic attacks and risk of stroke in an elderly poor population. Stroke 4: 980–986, 1973.
56. Pessin MS, Duncan GW, Mohr JP, et al: Clinical and angiographic features of carotid transient ischemic attacks. N Engl J Med 296:358–362, 1977.
57. Toole JF, Yuson CP, Janeway R, et al: Transient ischemic attacks: A prospective study of 225 patients. Neurology 28:746–753, 1978.
58. Whisnant JP, Matsumoto N, Elveback LR: Transient cerebral ischemic attacks in a community, Rochester, Minnesota, 1955 through 1969. Mayo Clin Proc 48:194–198, 1973.

59. Friedman GD, Wilson WS, Mosier JM, et al: Transient ischemic attacks in a community. JAMA 210:1428–1434, 1969.
60. Toole JF: Cerebrovascular Disorders, 4th ed. New York, Raven Press, 1990.
61. Ueda K, Toole JF, McHenry LC Jr: Carotid and vertebrobasilar transient ischemic attacks: Clinical and angiographic correlation. Neurology 29:1094–1101, 1979.
62. Fields WS, Lemak NA: Joint study of extracranial arterial occlusion. IX. Transient ischemic attacks in the carotid territory. JAMA 235:2608–2610, 1976.
63. Gerraty RP, Gates PC, Doyle JC: Carotid stenosis and perioperative stroke risk in symptomatic and asymptomatic patients undergoing vascular or coronary surgery. Stroke 24:1115–1118, 1993.
64. Muuronen A: Outcome of surgical treatment of 110 patients with transient ischemic attack. Stroke 15:959–964, 1984.
65. Sorensen S, Marquardsen J, Pedersen H, et al: Long-term prognosis of reversible cerebral ischemic attacks. Paper presented at the 14th International Joint Conference on Stroke and Cerebral Circulation, 1989, San Antonio, TX.
66. Roederer GO, Langlois YE, Jager KA, et al: The natural history of carotid arterial disease in asymptomatic patients with cervical bruits. Stroke 15:605–613, 1984.
67. Pessin MS, Hinton RC, Davis KR, et al: Mechanisms of acute carotid stroke. Ann Neurol 6:245–252, 1979.
68. Hunter WJ, Sterpetti AV, Schultz RD, et al: Carotid plaque ulceration: Its significance in cerebral ischemia [abstract]. Stroke 20:158, 1989.
69. Norris JW, Zhu CZ: Stroke risk and critical carotid stenosis. J Neurol Neurosurg Psychiatry 53:235–237, 1990.
70. Mohr JP, Pessin MS: Extracranial carotid artery disease. In Burnett HJM, Mohr JP, Stein BM, et al (eds): Stroke. New York, Churchill Livingstone, 1986, pp 293–336.
71. Stallones RA: Epidemiology of stroke in relation to the cardiovascular disease complex. Adv Neurol 25:117–126, 1979.
72. Fields WS, Maslenikov V, Meyer JS, et al: Joint study of extracranial arterial occlusion. V. Progress report of prognosis following surgery or nonsurgical treatment for transient cerebral ischemic attacks and cervical carotid artery lesions. JAMA 211:1993–2003, 1970.
73. Thompson JE, Austin DJ, Patman RD: Carotid endarterectomy for cerebrovascular insufficiency: Long-term results in 592 patients followed up to thirteen years. Ann Surg 172:663–679, 1970.
74. North American Symptomatic Carotid Endarterectomy Trial Collaborators: Beneficial effect of carotid endarterectomy in symptomatic patients with high-grade carotid stenosis. N Engl J Med 325:445–453, 1991.
75. Barnett HG, Taylor DW, Eliasziw M, et al: Benefit of carotid endarterectomy in patients with symptomatic moderate or severe stenosis: North American Symptomatic Carotid Endarterectomy Trial. N Engl J Med 339:1415–1425, 1998.
76. Hobson RW 2nd, Weiss DG, Fields WS, et al: Efficacy of carotid endarterectomy for asymptomatic carotid stenosis: The Veterans Affairs Cooperative Study Group. N Engl J Med 328:221–227, 1993.
77. Executive Committee for the Asymptomatic Carotid Atherosclerosis Study: Endarterectomy for asymptomatic carotid artery stenosis. JAMA 273:1421–1428, 1995.
78. Fox JL: Cerebral arterial revascularization: The value of repeated angiography in selection of patients for operation. Neurosurgery 2:205–209, 1978.
79. Bogousslavsky J: Prognosis of carotid siphon stenosis [letter]. Stroke 18:537, 1987.
80. Keagy BA, Poole MA, Burnham SJ, et al: Frequency, severity, and physiologic importance of carotid siphon lesions. J Vasc Surg 3:511–515, 1986.
81. Thiele BL, Young JV, Chikos PM, et al: Correlation of arteriographic findings and symptoms in cerebrovascular disease. Neurology 30:1041–1046, 1980.
82. Craig DR, Meguro K, Watridge C, et al: Intracranial internal carotid artery stenosis. Stroke 13:825–828, 1982.
83. Alcock JM: Occlusion of the middle cerebral artery: Serial angiography as a guide to conservative therapy. J Neurosurg 27: 353–363, 1967.
84. Little JR, Sawhny B, Weinstein M: Pseudo-tandem stenosis of the internal carotid artery. Neurosurgery 7:574–577, 1980.
85. Pritz MB, Smolin MR: Treatment of tandem lesions of the extracranial carotid artery. Neurosurgery 15:233–236, 1984.
86. Widenka DC, Spuler A, Steiger HJ: Treatment of carotid tandem stenosis by combined carotid endarterectomy and balloon angioplasty: Technical case report. Neurosurgery 45:179–182, 1999.
87. Gross CE, Adams HP Jr, Sokoll MD, et al: Use of anticoagulants, electroencephalographic monitoring, and barbiturate cerebral protection in carotid endarterectomy. Neurosurgery 9:1–5, 1981.
88. Howe JR, Kindt GW: Cerebral protection during carotid endarterectomy. Stroke 5:340–343, 1974.
89. Imparato AM, Ramirez A, Riles T, et al: Cerebral protection in carotid surgery. Arch Surg 117:1073–1078, 1982.
90. Michenfelder JD, Milde JH, Sundt TM Jr: Cerebral protection by barbiturate anesthesia: Use after middle cerebral artery occlusion in Java monkeys. Arch Neurol 33:345–350, 1976.
91. Feustel PJ, Ingvar MC, Severinghaus JW: Cerebral oxygen availability and blood flow during middle cerebral artery occlusion: Effects of pentobarbital. Stroke 12:858–863, 1981.
92. Giannotta SL, Dicks RE 3rd, Kindt GW: Carotid endarterectomy: Technical improvements. Neurosurgery 7:309–312, 1980.
93. Sundt TM Jr, Anderson RE, Michenfelder JD: Intracellular redox states under halothane and barbiturate anesthesia in normal, ischemic, and anoxic monkey brain. Ann Neurol 5:575–579, 1979.
94. Moseley JI, Laurent JP, Molinari GF: Barbiturate attenuation of the clinical course and pathological lesions in primate stroke model. Neurology 25:870–874, 1975.
95. Nehls DG, Todd MM, Spetzler RF, et al: A comparison of the cerebral protective effects of isoflurane and barbiturates during temporary focal ischemia in primates. Anesthesiology 66:453–464, 1987.
96. Selman WR, Spetzler RF, Roski RA, et al: Barbiturate coma in focal cerebral ischemia: Relationship of protection to timing of therapy. J Neurosurg 56:685–690, 1982.
97. Corkill G, Chikovani OK, McLeish I, et al: Timing of pentobarbital administration for brain protection in experimental stroke. Surg Neurol 5:147–149, 1976.
98. Milde LN, Milde JH, Michenfelder JD: Cerebral functional, metabolic, and hemodynamic effects of etomidate in dogs. Anesthesiology 63:371–377, 1985.
99. Batjer HH, Frankfurt AI, Purdy PD, et al: Use of etomidate, temporary arterial occlusion, and intraoperative angiography in surgical treatment of large and giant cerebral aneurysms. J Neurosurg 68:234–240, 1988.
100. Hans SS: Late follow-up of carotid endarterectomy with venous patch angioplasty. Am J Surg 162:50–54, 1991.
101. Van Damme H, Grenade T, Creemers E, et al: Blowout of carotid venous patch angioplasty. Ann Vasc Surg 5:542–545, 1991.
102. Sundt TM Jr, Whisnant JP, Houser OW, et al: Prospective study of the effectiveness and durability of carotid endarterectomy. Mayo Clin Proc 65:625–635, 1990.
103. Deriu GP, Ballotta E, Bonavina L, et al: The rationale for patch-graft angioplasty after carotid endarterectomy: Early and long-term follow-up. Stroke 15:972–979, 1984.
104. Hertzer NR, Beven EG, O'Hara PJ, et al: A prospective study of vein patch angioplasty during carotid endarterectomy: Three-year results for 801 patients and 917 operations. Ann Surg 206: 628–635, 1987.
105. Sundt TM, Sandok BA, Whisnant JP: Carotid endarterectomy: Complications and preoperative assessment of risk. Mayo Clin Proc 50:301–306, 1975.
106. Little JR, Bryerton BS, Furlan AJ: Saphenous vein patch grafts in carotid endarterectomy. J Neurosurg 61:743–747, 1984.
107. Thomas M, Otis SM, Rush M, et al: Recurrent carotid artery stenosis following endarterectomy. Ann Surg 200:74–79, 1984.
108. Rosenthal D, Archie JP Jr, Garcia-Rinaldi R, et al: Carotid patch angioplasty: Immediate and long-term results. J Vasc Surg 12: 326–333, 1990.
109. Meyer FB, Windschitl WL: Repair of carotid endarterectomy with a collagen-impregnated fabric graft. J Neurosurg 88:647–649, 1998.
110. AbuRahma AF, Robinson PA, Saiedy S, et al: Prospective randomized trial of bilateral carotid endarterectomies: Primary closure versus patching. Stroke 30:1185–1189, 1999.

111. O'Hara PJ, Hertzer NR, Krajewski LP, et al: Saphenous vein patch rupture after carotid endarterectomy. J Vasc Surg 15: 504–509, 1992.
112. Spetzler RF, Martin N, Hadley MN, et al: Microsurgical endarterectomy under barbiturate protection: A prospective study. J Neurosurg 65:63–73, 1986.
113. Sundt TM Jr: The ischemic tolerance of neural tissue and the need for monitoring and selective shunting during carotid endarterectomy. Stroke 14:93–98, 1983.
114. Gumerlock MK, Neuwelt EA: Carotid endarterectomy: To shunt or not to shunt. Stroke 19:1485–1490, 1988.
115. Bland JE, Lazar ML: Carotid endarterectomy without shunt. Neurosurgery 8:153–157, 1981.
116. Halsey JH Jr: Risks and benefits of shunting in carotid endarterectomy: The International Transcranial Doppler Collaborators. Stroke 23:1583–1587, 1992.
117. Hunter GC, Sieffert G, Malone JM, et al: The accuracy of carotid back pressure as an index for shunt requirements: A reappraisal. Stroke 13:319–326, 1982.
118. Ott DA, Cooley DA, Chapa L, et al: Carotid endarterectomy without temporary intraluminal shunt: Study of 309 consecutive operations. Ann Surg 191:708–714, 1980.
119. Ferguson GG, Blume WT, Farras JK: Carotid endarterectomy: An evaluation of results in 282 consecutive cases in relationship to intraoperative monitoring [abstract 54]. Program presented at the annual meeting of the American Association of Neurologic Surgeons, Apr 23, 1985, Atlanta.
120. Sandmann W, Kolvenback R, Willeke F: Risks and benefits of shunting in carotid endarterectomy [letter]. Stroke 24:1098–1099, 1993.
121. Medary M, Bailes J, Teeple E, Davis D: Reliability of EEG as an indicator for intraluminal shunting during carotid endarterectomy. J Neurosurg 86:399A, 1997.
122. Jansen C, Vriens EM, Eikelboom BC, et al: Carotid endarterectomy with transcranial Doppler and electroencephalographic monitoring: A prospective study in 130 operations. Stroke 24: 665–669, 1993.
123. Findlay JM, Lougheed WM: Carotid microendarterectomy. Neurosurgery 32:792–798, 1993.
124. Barrow KL, Mizuno J: Carotid endarterectomy: Technical aspects and perioperative management. In Awad IA (ed): Cerebrovascular Occlusive Disease and Brain Ischemia. Chicago, American Association of Neurological Surgeons, 1992, pp 162–185.
125. Sundt TM Jr: Occlusive Cerebrovascular Disease: Diagnosis and Surgical Management. Philadelphia, WB Saunders, 1987.
126. Moore WS, Martello JY, Quinones-Baldrich WJ, et al: Etiologic importance of the intimal flap of the external carotid artery in the development of postcarotid endarterectomy stroke. Stroke 21:1497–1502, 1990.
127. Blaisdell FW, Lim R Jr, Hall AD: Technical result of carotid endarterectomy: Arteriographic assessment. Am J Surg 114:239–246, 1967.
128. Cipolle RJ, Uden DL, Gruber SA, et al: Evaluation of a rapid monitoring system to study heparin pharmacokinetics and pharmacodynamics. Pharmacotherapy 10:367–372, 1990.
129. Poisik A, Heyer EJ, Solomon RA, et al: Safety and efficacy of fixed-dose heparin in carotid endarterectomy. Neurosurgery 45: 434–442, 1999.
130. Lehv MS, Salzman EW, Silen W: Hypertension complicating carotid endarterectomy. Stroke 1:307–313, 1970.
131. Harbaugh KS, Harbaugh RE: Early discharge after carotid endarterectomy. Neurosurgery 37:219–225, 1995.
132. Bogousslavsky J, Regli F, Hungerbuhler JP, et al: Transient ischemic attacks and external carotid artery: A retrospective study of 23 patients with an occlusion of the internal carotid artery. Stroke 12:627–630, 1981.
133. Dyken ML, Klatte E, Kolar OJ, et al: Complete occlusion of common or internal carotid arteries: Clinical significance. Arch Neurol 30:343–346, 1974.
134. Furlan AJ, Whisnant JP, Baker HL Jr: Long-term prognosis after carotid artery occlusion. Neurology 30:986–988, 1980.
135. Gurdjian FS, Lindner DW, Hardy WG, et al: "Completed stroke" due to occlusive cerebrovascular disease: Analysis of 409 cases. Neurology 11:724–733, 1961.
136. Cote R, Barnett HJ, Taylor DW: Internal carotid occlusion: A prospective study. Stroke 14:898–902, 1983.
137. Fields WS, Lemak NA: Joint study of extracranial arterial occlusion. X. Internal carotid artery occlusion. JAMA 235:2734–2738, 1976.
138. Hennerici M, Hulsbomer HB, Rautenberg W, et al: Spontaneous history of asymptomatic internal carotid occlusion. Stroke 17: 718–722, 1986.
139. Hafner CD, Tew JM: Surgical management of the totally occluded internal carotid artery: A ten-year study. Surgery 89: 710–717, 1981.
140. Meyer FB, Sundt TM Jr, Piepgras DG, et al: Emergency carotid endarterectomy for patients with acute carotid occlusion and profound neurological deficits. Ann Surg 203:82–89, 1986.
141. Walters BB, Ojemann RG, Heros RC: Emergency carotid endarterectomy. J Neurosurg 66:817–823, 1987.
142. Hugenholtz H, Elgie RG: Carotid thromboendarterectomy: A reappraisal. Criteria for patient selection. J Neurosurg 53:776–783, 1980.
143. Kusunoki T, Rowed DW, Tator CH, et al: Thromboendarterectomy for total occlusion of the internal carotid artery: A reappraisal of risks, success rate and potential benefits. Stroke 9: 34–38, 1978.
144. Medary M, Bailes JE, Levy D: Management of complete carotid occlusion. In Loftus CM, Kresowik TF (eds): Carotid Artery Surgery. New York, Thieme, 2000, pp 291–301.
145. McCormick PW, Spetzler RF, Bailes JE, et al: Thromboendarterectomy of the symptomatic occluded internal carotid artery. J Neurosurg 76:752–758, 1992.
146. Sasaki O, Takeuchi S, Koike T, et al: Fibrinolytic therapy for acute embolic stroke: Intravenous, intracarotid, and intra-arterial local approaches. Neurosurgery 36:246–253, 1995.
147. Guterman LR, Budny JL, Gibbons KJ, et al: Thrombolysis of the cervical internal carotid artery before balloon angioplasty and stent placement: Report of two cases. Neurosurgery 38:620–624, 1996.
148. Diethrich EB, Ndjaye M, Reid DB: Stenting in the carotid artery: Initial experience in 110 patients. J Endovasc Surg 3:42–62, 1996.
149. Bailes JE, Quigley MR, Kwaan HC, et al: The effects of intravenous prostacyclin in a model of microsurgical thrombosis. Microsurgery 9:2–9, 1988.
150. Baumgartner HR, Haudenschild C: Adhesion of platelets to subendothelium. Ann N Y Acad Sci 201:22–36, 1972.
151. Ercius MS, Chandler WF, Ford JW, et al: Early versus delayed heparin reversal after carotid endarterectomy in the dog: A scanning electron microscopy study. J Neurosurg 58:708–713, 1983.
152. Dirrenberger RA, Sundt TM Jr: Carotid endarterectomy: Temporal profile of the healing process and effects of anticoagulation therapy. J Neurosurg 48:201–219, 1978.
153. Kieburtz K, Ricotta JJ, Moxley RT 3rd: Seizures following carotid endarterectomy. Arch Neurol 47:568–570, 1990.
154. Mustard JF, Jorgenson L, Hovig T, et al: Role of platelets in thrombosis. Thromb Diath Haemorrh Suppl 21:131–158, 1966.
155. Dolan JG, Mushlin AI: Hypertension, vascular headaches, and seizures after carotid endarterectomy: Case report and therapeutic considerations. Arch Intern Med 144:1489–1491, 1984.
156. Metke MP, Lie JT, Fuster V: Reduction of intimal thickening in canine coronary bypass vein grafts with dipyridamole and aspirin. Am J Cardiol 43:1144–1148, 1979.
157. Zierler RE, Bandyk DF, Thiele BL, et al: Carotid artery stenosis following endarterectomy. Arch Surg 117:1408–1415, 1982.
158. Findlay JM, Lougheed WM, Gentili F, et al: Effect of perioperative platelet inhibition on postcarotid endarterectomy mural thrombus formation: Results of a prospective randomized controlled trial using aspirin and dipyridamole in humans. J Neurosurg 63:693–698, 1985.
159. Waring PH, Kraftsow DA: Another complication of carotid artery shunting during endarterectomy [letter]. Anesthesiology 72:1099, 1990.
160. Harker LA, Bernstein EF, Dilley RB, et al: Failure of aspirin plus dipyridamole to prevent restenosis after carotid endarterectomy. Ann Intern Med 116:731–736, 1992.
161. Hansen F, Lindblad B, Persson NH, et al: Can recurrent stenosis after carotid endarterectomy be prevented by low-dose acetylsalicylic acid? A double-blind, randomized and placebo-controlled study. Eur J Vasc Surg 7:380–385, 1993.

162. Bischof G, Pratschner T, Kail M, et al: Anticoagulants, antiaggregants or nothing following carotid endarterectomy? Eur J Vasc Surg 7:364–369, 1993.
163. Bernstein M, Fleming JF, Deck JH: Cerebral hyperperfusion after carotid endarterectomy: A cause of cerebral hemorrhage. Neurosurgery 15:50–56, 1984.
164. Bruetman ME, Fields WS, Crawford ES, et al: Cerebral hemorrhage in carotid artery surgery. Arch Neurol 147:458–467, 1963.
165. Caplan LR, Skillman J, Ojemann R, et al: Intracerebral hemorrhage following carotid endarterectomy: A hypertensive complication? Stroke 9:457–460, 1978.
166. Templehoff R, Modica PA, Grubb RL Jr, et al: Selective shunting during carotid endarterectomy based on two-channel computerized electroencephalographic/compressed spectral array analysis. Neurosurgery 24:339–344, 1989.
167. Solomon RA, Loftus CM, Quest DO, et al: Incidence and etiology of intracerebral hemorrhage following carotid endarterectomy. J Neurosurg 64:29–34, 1986.
168. Wong JH, Findlay JM, Suarez-Almazor ME: Hemodynamic instability after carotid endarterectomy: Risk factors and associations with operative complications. Neurosurgery 41:35–43, 1997.
169. Leviton A, Caplan L, Salzman E: Severe headache after carotid endarterectomy. Headache 15:207–210, 1975.
170. Messert B, Black JA: Cluster headache, hemicrania, and other head pains: Morbidity of carotid endarterectomy. Stroke 9:559–562, 1978.
171. Brick JF, Dunker RO, Gutierrez AR: Cerebral vasoconstriction as a complication of carotid endarterectomy. J Neurosurg 73: 151–153, 1990.
172. Akers DL, Brinker MR, Engelhardt TC, et al: Postoperative somnolence in patients after carotid endarterectomy. Surgery 107:684–687, 1990.

CHAPTER **98**

Carotid Angioplasty and Stenting: Interventional Treatment of Occlusive Vascular Disease

FELIPE C. ALBUQUERQUE ■ CARGILL H. ALLEYNE, JR. ■
JONATHAN J. BASKIN ■ CAMERON G. MCDOUGALL

Each year, more than one-half million Americans suffer a cerebrovascular accident (CVA). Of these, 150,000 will die, rendering stroke the third leading cause of death in the United States and the most common and disabling neurological disorder among the elderly worldwide.[1–3] Ischemia accounts for approximately 85% of strokes, and the remaining are the sequelae of intracerebral hemorrhage.[3–6] In particular, atherosclerotic disease at the bifurcation of the common carotid artery (CCA) is associated with 20% to 30% of strokes.[1–3] Given these public health concerns, research in the latter half of the 20th century focused on the optimal treatment of carotid stenosis.

Prospective analyses such as the North American Symptomatic Carotid Endarterectomy Trial (NASCET), the Asymptomatic Carotid Atherosclerosis Study (ACAS), and the European Carotid Surgery Trial (ECST) demonstrated superior reduction in the incidence of stroke among symptomatic and a select group of asymptomatic patients undergoing carotid endarterectomy (CEA).[7–9] These studies established CEA as the therapeutic gold standard for carotid atherosclerosis.[7–11] Technical innovations in interventional radiology have renewed the debate about the optimal therapy.[12–17] Although retrospective analyses of angioplasty and stenting suggest that their clinical efficacy is comparable to that of endarterectomy, prospective evaluation is pending.

The concept of percutaneous transluminal angioplasty was first introduced by Dotter and Judkins in 1964.[18] Since then, the technique has been used extensively throughout the vascular system. In 1980, Kerber and colleagues[19] and Mullan and associates[20] first reported angioplasty in the carotid artery. The use of stents to maintain luminal patency after angioplasty evolved substantially with demonstrated successes in the coronary and distal arterial trees. The overall development of percutaneous angioplasty and stenting of the supra-aortic vessels, however, has proceeded at a more cautious rate than its use in the coronary and peripheral vessels. This caution reflects the risk of significant morbidity associated with embolic events in the cerebral arterial distribution.

Although the efficacy of percutaneous angioplasty and stenting in preventing stroke remains indeterminate, the technical ease of performing the procedure has reached almost 100%.[12, 21–30] The procedure is now commonly performed throughout the United States and Europe despite the lack of a prospective, randomized comparison with CEA. The Carotid Revascularization Endarterectomy versus Stent Trial (CREST) and the Carotid and Vertebral Artery Transluminal Angioplasty Study (CAVATAS) will attempt to address the efficacy of percutaneous angioplasty and stenting compared with CEA.[16, 31]

A number of retrospective studies of percutaneous angioplasty and stenting, however, have reported comparable results to those for CEA in terms of stroke and mortality rates.[12, 14, 21–30] These favorable results seem to support at least a limited role for percutaneous angioplasty and stenting in the management of specific subsets of patients with carotid stenosis. Typically, the procedure is reserved for patients deemed at highest risk of suffering complications after CEA.[22, 31, 32] Patients with lesions affecting the high cervical carotid artery and those suffering recurrent stenosis after CEA, radiation-induced stenosis, and carotid stenosis associated with contralateral occlusion are other groups that may benefit from endovascular treatment.[1, 2, 12, 14, 27, 33–36]

PATIENT SELECTION

A factor that must be considered when assessing the relative risks of CEA and percutaneous angioplasty with stenting is that the two procedures differ in terms of their applicability to specific patient populations and lesion types.[37] There is no consensus regarding the indications for angioplasty and stenting. In the absence of randomized, prospective, controlled data, there are

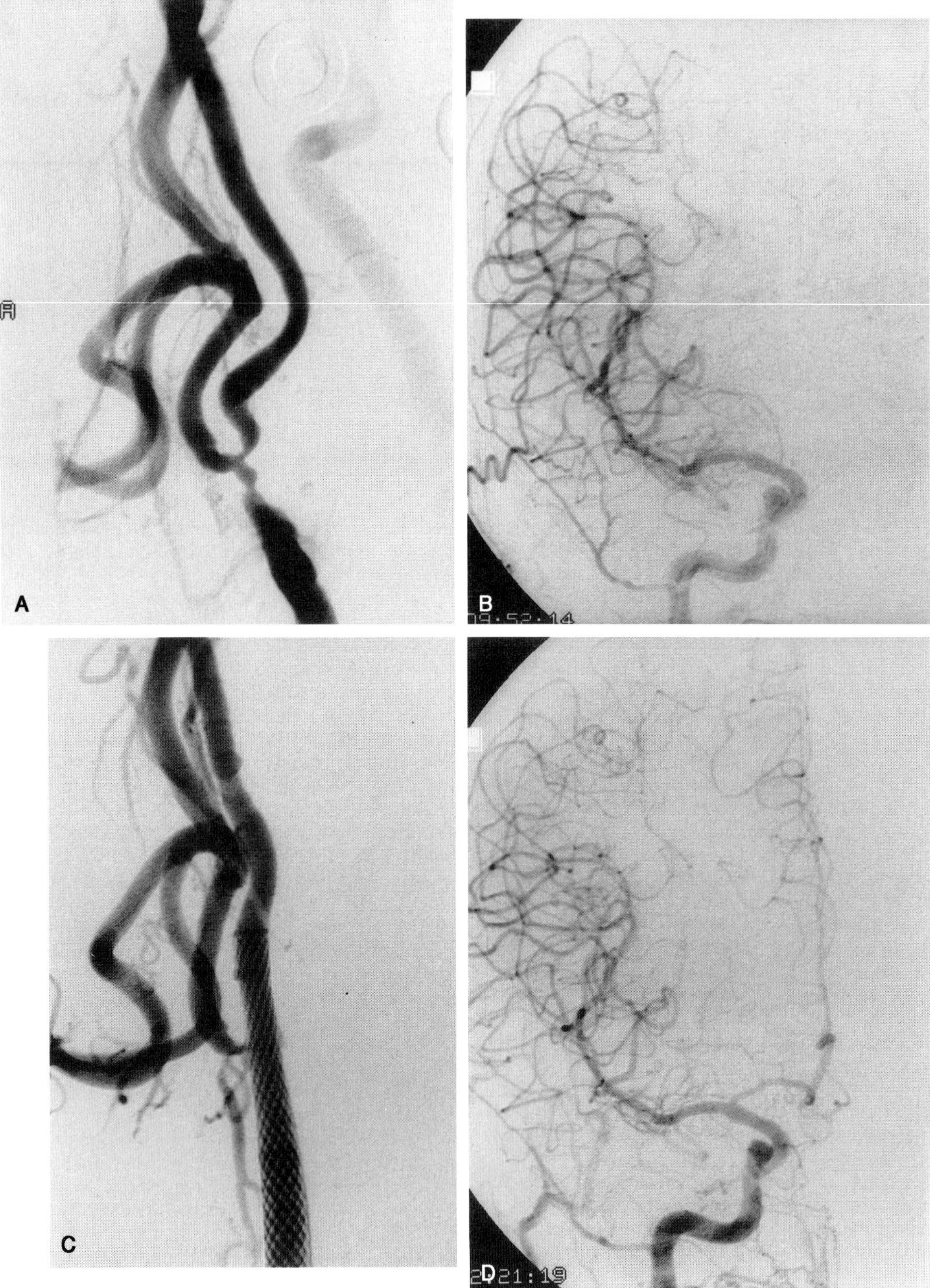

FIGURE 98–1. A 79-year-old woman presented for follow-up examination with high-grade restenosis of her right internal carotid artery (ICA) 7 months after endarterectomy. *A,* Angiography revealed high-grade restenosis of the common carotid artery (CCA) and the origins of the internal and external carotid arteries. *B,* The cerebral angiogram revealed poor filling of the ICA branches and almost no filling of the anterior cerebral artery. *C,* After angioplasty and stenting of the CCA and ICA, the patency of those vessels was almost normal. *D,* The cerebral angiogram confirmed markedly improved blood flow and renewed filling of the anterior cerebral artery and its distal branches.

several groups of patients for whom stent placement is particularly attractive as a treatment alternative. Common to each group is an increased risk of thromboembolic or ischemic stroke associated with the standard endarterectomy procedure.

The first group comprises patients with recurrent carotid stenosis (Figs. 98–1 and 98–2).[34, 35] Early restenosis (i.e., recurrence within 2 years) after CEA is largely related to fibroproliferation; late recurrences typically result from progressive atherosclerotic disease.[12, 35] The rate of restenosis after CEA ranges from 1.5% to 49% of cases and varies according to the criteria for defining restenosis and according to the method used to diagnose recurrent disease.[34, 38] Given the routine use of noninvasive screening methods such as Doppler ultrasonography and improvements in treating coexisting diseases in this patient population, the incidence of recurrent disease will likely increase.

Reports from the Mayo Clinic and Cleveland Clinic document a major complication rate between 4.6% and 10.9% for repeat CEA.[35, 39, 40] Reoperation is complicated by scar tissue that obscures and tethers the regional neurovascular structures and places them at increased risk of injury.[31] In 1983, Tievsky and coworkers[35, 41] first proposed that angioplasty was a safe alternative to a second CEA for the treatment of recurrent disease. Percutaneous angioplasty and stenting negate the effect of intracarotid and extracarotid scarring. They also permit treatment of lesions at the proximal and distal ends of the endarterectomy, sites that may be difficult to access surgically. Given the likelihood of higher recoil forces within highly fibrosed segments of a chronically diseased artery,[35] the rate of restenosis after percutaneous angioplasty and stenting for recurrent carotid disease may prove somewhat higher than that of primary percutaneous angioplasty and stenting.

The second patient group that lends itself to percutaneous angioplasty and stenting harbors lesions of the cervical internal carotid artery (ICA) that extend well beyond the bifurcation toward the skull base.[12, 37] Such lesions are easily accessed through an endovascular route but difficult to expose surgically. The increased

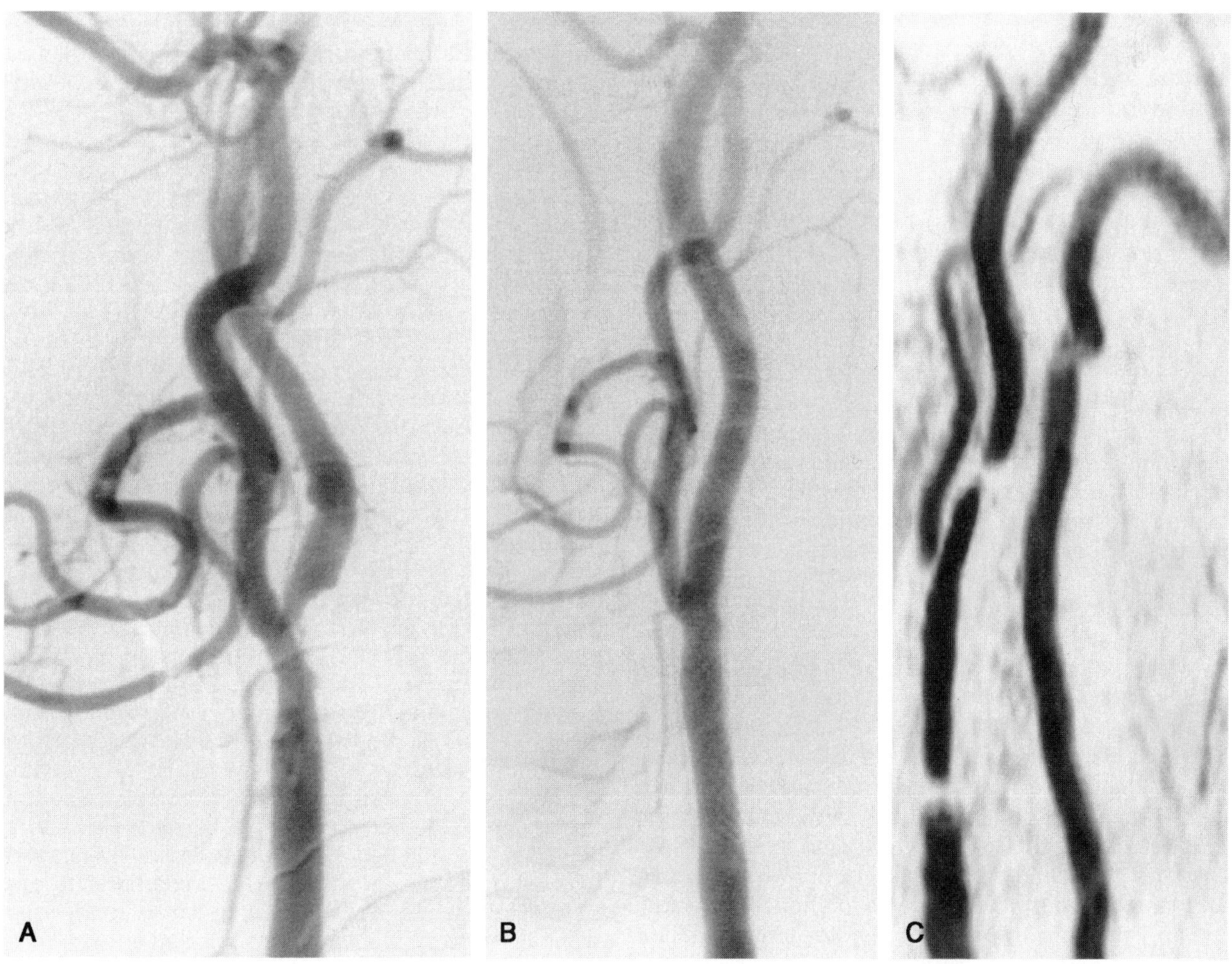

FIGURE 98–2. A 78-year-old woman with a history of coronary artery disease and atrial fibrillation had duplex ultrasonic evidence of carotid restenosis after endarterectomy. *A,* Angiography confirmed the presence of high-grade restenosis of the internal carotid artery at the bifurcation. *B,* After angioplasty and stenting across the site of stenosis, vessel patency improved significantly. *C,* Follow-up magnetic resonance angiogram revealed artifactual stenosis at the ends of the stent. The stented region, however, remained widely patent by angiography.

retraction and aggressive dissection required to expose such stenoses for endarterectomy predispose patients to a greater risk of cranial nerve injuries. The rate of cranial nerve injuries during CEA has ranged from 7.6% to 27% of cases.[9, 27]

Patients who have undergone prior extensive neck surgery or radiation therapy for malignant disease and those who suffer stenoses caused by diseases other than atherosclerosis (e.g., fibromuscular dysplasia) have adulterated anatomic planes and tissues with a poor capacity to heal.[12, 24, 37] Percutaneous stenting procedures through the femoral artery eliminate the problems associated with open surgery in this subgroup of patients and can be used to treat relatively long stenotic segments of the carotid artery.

Typically, radiation-induced stenosis occurs more than 2 years after treatment of a cervical malignancy but can develop as long as 50 years later.[42–44] In 1972, Glick first described the occurrence of symptomatic, radiation-induced narrowing of the carotid artery.[45] Commonly treated lesions include lymphomas and laryngeal carcinomas.[42–44] Patients who develop stenoses after radiation are also more likely to have undergone prior neck surgery, another factor that complicates CEA. A previous surgery increases the difficulty of the procedure and the likelihood of cranial nerve injury. Radiation-induced stenoses tend to be longer than atherosclerotic lesions, often extending from the origin of the ICA to the skull base. They are usually composed of atheromatous debris and sclerotic tissue.[42–44]

Patients with an occlusion of the contralateral ICA suffer more complications after CEA than those with unilateral disease.[9, 33] NASCET reported a 30-day risk of stroke and death of 14.3% for this patient group.[9, 33] The most likely precipitating factor for this higher-than-average complication rate after CEA is a long period of clamping the ICA (NASCET median, 32 minutes) in a patient with poor intracranial collateral circulation.[9] In this subpopulation, percutaneous angioplasty and stenting are advantageous because carotid occlusion during angioplasty is typically limited to 5 to 15 seconds per inflation of the angioplasty balloon.[33] Performing the procedure under sedative anesthesia permits repetitive neurological assessment during the treatment session.

Another potential application of percutaneous angioplasty and stenting is the treatment of spontaneous or traumatic carotid dissections.[46–54] With dissections, the intima of the vessel develops a tear, and a false lumen is created between the intimal and medial (or medial and adventitial) layers. The initial management of carotid dissection varies greatly among institutions and spans the range from expectant observation to treatment with antiplatelet agents or anticoagulation. Ischemic symptoms that persist despite anticoagulation (i.e., maximal medical therapy) or a progression of the radiographic defect usually indicate surgical intervention, including direct repair, embolectomy, proximal vessel ligation, and bypass procedures. Although there are no findings from randomized, controlled trials to guide the management of vascular dissections, stents can reapproximate an intimal flap against its parent vessel wall and maintain patency of the lumen.[55]

More definitive indications for angioplasty and stenting in the extracranial carotid circulation await the results of long-term follow-up and randomized, controlled trials that compare the stenting procedure with CEA. If the morbidity and mortality rates and long-term outcomes of stenting compare favorably with those of CEA, the indications for stenting will expand to include patients with primary carotid stenosis.

TECHNIQUE

Patients are routinely placed on oral antiplatelet agents 3 days before percutaneous angioplasty and stenting. Those undergoing the procedure emergently who cannot be pretreated are given an intravenous antiplatelet agent such as ReoPro (abciximab; Centocor B.V., Leiden, The Netherlands).

The patient is positioned supine on the table in the radiology suite. Light sedation is administered to enhance the patient's comfort while still permitting a neurological examination to be performed throughout the procedure. An anesthesiologist is present for the duration of the procedure to monitor the patient's comfort and hemodynamic fluctuations, which should be anticipated during angioplasty.

Familiarity with the various catheters and wires that compose the endovascular surgeon's armamentarium is elemental to performing stent-supported angioplasty optimally and safely. A formal description of these devices, along with their individual advantages and disadvantages, is outside the scope of this chapter and available in interventional radiology texts. The essential equipment should be checked carefully and arranged neatly on a sterile worktable. Typically, a 19-gauge, single-wall needle; 0.035-inch guide wire; 6-French sheath; 0.035-inch, stiff exchange wire; 0.018-inch exchange wire, two angioplasty balloon catheters; and an appropriate stent are needed. Real-time intravascular ultrasonography is optional but can be a useful adjunct.

The three types of stent most commonly used are the Palmaz (Johnson & Johnson Interventional Systems Company, Warren, NJ), the Wallstent (Snyder USA, Inc., Minneapolis, MN), and the Smart Stent (Cordis Corp., Miami, FL). The Palmaz stent is expanded to the selected diameter using an angioplasty balloon and offers the advantages of high radial strength, less metal, and accuracy of deployment. Its disadvantages include its rigidity and resistance to advancement and its tendency to deform when subjected to stress and bending. The metallic, self-expandable Wallstent has two components: an implantable metallic stent and a single-step delivery system. The stent is made from a superalloy monofilament wire braided into a tubular mesh configuration that imparts flexibility and compliance. The delivery system consists of inner and outer coaxial tubes. The Smart Stent, which is composed of nitinol, is also self-expanding and deployed with great accuracy. The U.S. Food and Drug Administration has yet to approve a stent for use in the carotid artery.

The percutaneous, retrograde femoral artery approach is most often used to deploy carotid stents although the direct carotid puncture technique has also been described.[28] Preventing a hematoma from forming by compressing the carotid artery after percutaneous angioplasty and stenting through a direct carotid puncture technique may compromise blood flow to the brain and through the newly stented segment. The direct puncture technique also subjects patients to a higher likelihood of sustaining injury to other critical structures of the neck.

The right femoral artery is used preferentially unless the right iliac artery is significantly stenotic or tortuous. The artery is located by palpation and cannulated with the 19-gauge, single-wall needle. The entry site is usually 3 fingerbreadths below the inguinal ligament, which is located deep to an imaginary line drawn from the anterosuperior iliac spine to the symphysis pubis. The entry site at the common femoral artery should be superficial to the medial aspect of the femoral head, against which the artery may be compressed at the end of the procedure. The fluoroscope can be used to localize the medial aspect of the femoral head. The needle is directed toward the umbilicus at a 45-degree angle.

After the artery has been punctured, the 0.035-inch guide wire is inserted and advanced to the abdominal aorta under fluoroscopic guidance. A 6-French sheath is placed into the common femoral artery over the wire, which is then removed. At this stage, heparin is infused intravenously to achieve an activated clotting time of 200 to 250 seconds. A suitable diagnostic catheter is placed over the guide wire, and the guide wire and catheter combination is advanced through the introducer sheath into the arterial system. The guide wire is then passed into the aortic arch, and the brachiocephalic trunk or left CCA is engaged selectively. The guide wire and catheter are advanced to the level of the distal CCA. The wire is withdrawn, and diagnostic images in multiple projections are obtained to confirm the stenosis and to permit measurements necessary for selecting the appropriately sized angioplasty balloons and stents. A marker of known size is used as a reference to determine the dimensions of the artery and the length of the stenosis (Fig. 98–3).

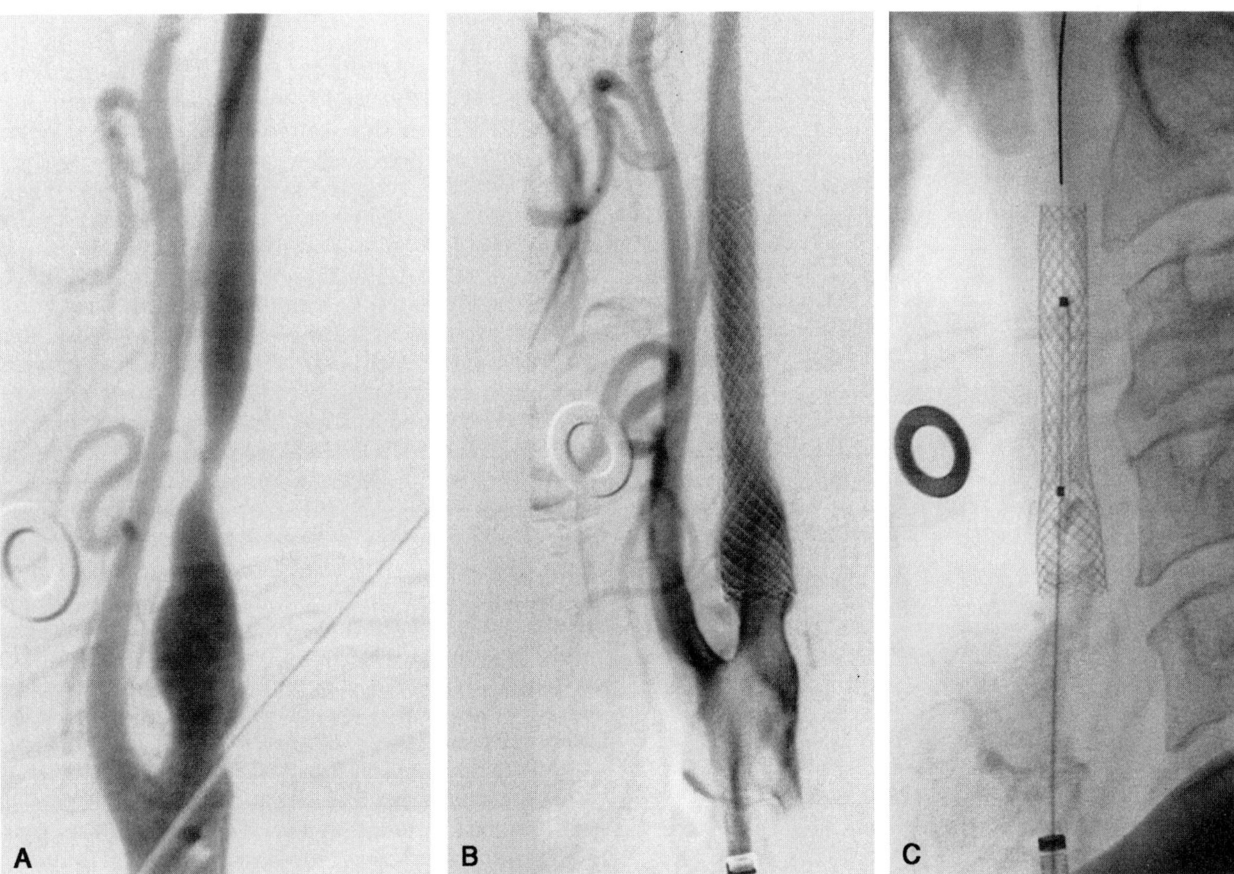

FIGURE 98–3. A 53-year-old man with a history of congestive heart failure and a previous stroke had duplex evidence of a high-grade stenosis of the left internal carotid artery. *A,* The lesion arose distal to the bifurcation and was confirmed angiographically. *B,* After angioplasty and stenting, the patency of the vessel was normal. *C,* The lateral radiograph showed the stent deployment device and exchange length guide wire across the site of stenosis. The metallic washer was used as a reference to measure the length of the stenosis and the diameter of the affected vessel.

Next, a roadmap image is obtained while a small amount of contrast medium is injected. The guide wire is directed into the external carotid artery (ECA), and the diagnostic catheter is advanced over it. The guide wire is removed, and the 0.035-inch-diameter, 260-cm-long, stiff exchange wire is passed through the diagnostic catheter and into the ECA. The initial placement of the catheter and guide wire system into the ECA leaves the diseased ICA undisturbed, reducing the risk of thromboembolic complications (Fig. 98–4).

The diagnostic catheter is removed. Along with the 6-French introducer sheath, a 90-cm-long, 7-French (inner diameter) guide sheath is advanced to the distal CCA. The stiff exchange wire is removed, and contrast medium is infused gently through the guide sheath to ensure satisfactory positioning. Another roadmap image is obtained through the new guide sheath. At this point, a 300-cm-long (exchange length), 0.018-inch-diameter wire is inserted into the ICA and passed across the lesion under roadmap guidance.

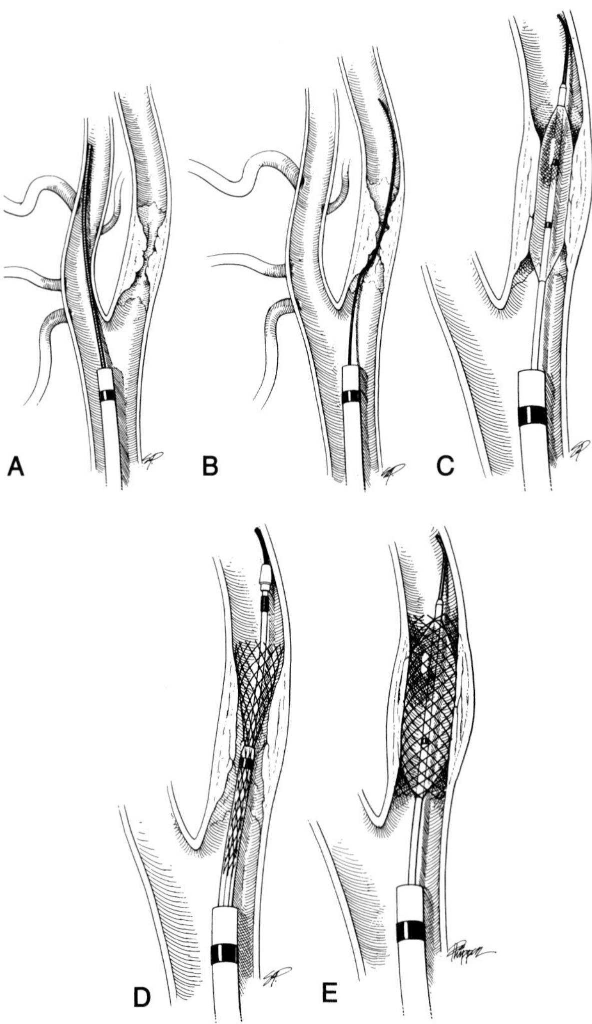

FIGURE 98–4. *A,* A 0.035-inch exchange wire is passed through the diagnostic catheter and into the external carotid artery. *B,* A 0.018-inch wire is inserted into the internal carotid artery and across the lesion. *C,* The predilation balloon is passed across the lesion and inflated for 10 to 15 seconds at 12 to 15 atm of pressure. *D,* The stent is deployed. *E,* The stent is further expanded by inflating a second, larger angioplasty balloon. (Courtesy of the Barrow Neurological Institute, Phoenix, AZ.)

An appropriately sized balloon is selected for predilation of the artery at the site of the lesion. Typical dimensions of the balloon are 3, 4, or 5 mm by 2 cm, with a 120-cm long shaft. An appropriate stent is also selected. The authors favor using the Wallstent or Smart Stent over the Palmaz stent because of the relative ease of deployment and low risk of permanent deformation if compressed.

As is the case with the manipulation of the carotid body during endarterectomy, angioplasty of the artery can precipitate arrhythmias, specifically bradycardia or asystole. A vagolytic agent such as atropine is administered before angioplasty is performed. External pacing leads are applied before the case is begun as a precaution should severe bradycardia or asystole occur. Central venous access is also secured.

The predilation balloon is passed across the lesion and inflated for 10 to 15 seconds at 12 to 15 atm of pressure. The balloon is deflated, and the effect of the angioplasty is assessed by injecting a small amount of contrast medium through the guide sheath. The stent is placed across the lesion, and its position is checked with an additional injection of contrast before the stent is deployed. After the stent has been deployed, it may be expanded further using a second, larger angioplasty balloon to achieve the desired size. If the stent extends from the ICA proximal to the bifurcation, a larger balloon may be necessary to implant the stent properly within the CCA. After further angiography confirms satisfactory angioplasty and stent placement, the exchange wire and guide catheter are withdrawn. If available, intravascular ultrasonography can be used to assess the apposition of the stent to the vessel wall. Obtaining serial activated clotting times during the procedure confirms appropriate heparinization.

After the procedure has been completed, the heparin is allowed to dissipate. Attention to groin hemostasis is critical after the sheath is removed, and patients are maintained supine for 6 hours thereafter. In lieu of manual compression, various hemostatic devices may be used to close the femoral puncture site and to permit the patient to be mobilized more rapidly. Postoperative assessment includes neurological examinations, groin checks for hematoma, and evaluation of distal limb perfusion. Typically, the patient is monitored in the intensive care unit overnight. Combined oral antiplatelet therapy is continued 3 weeks; thereafter, aspirin alone is used indefinitely.

As a means of preventing embolization into the distal cerebral circulation during the angioplasty phase, research has focused on the development of protection devices. Theron and colleagues[25] described the use of a triple coaxial catheter device that allows an occlusion balloon to be placed in the distal ICA during the angioplasty phase. A modification of this technique, using materials commercially available in the United States, employs a compliant silicone balloon to occlude the distal ICA during angioplasty.[25a] After angioplasty, debris is flushed into the ECA circulation if anastomoses with the intracranial circulation have been ruled out, or it is aspirated into the guiding catheter. The results of this technique and those of Theron and coworkers[25] suggest a significant decrease in the rate of morbidity associated with percutaneous angioplasty and stenting.[25a] The most salient drawback of these techniques is that they do not allow stent deployment during the protected phase. Future innovations in catheter technology will undoubtedly address this issue.

COMPLICATIONS AND OUTCOMES

Complications associated with percutaneous angioplasty and stenting of the carotid artery include arterial dissection with resulting cerebral infarction, embolic stroke, intracranial hemorrhage caused by reperfusion injury, acute bradycardia and asystole from carotid bulb compression during angioplasty, contrast-induced renal failure, and groin hematoma with associated dissection and pseudoaneurysm formation.[6, 12, 15, 21, 23–26, 36, 56–59] Restenosis is a common risk to CEA and percutaneous angioplasty and stenting. It occurs in the latter case at a frequency of 7% to 16%.[21–30, 56] Most patients who suffer restenosis after percutaneous angioplasty and stenting, however, are asymptomatic because their stented segments typically narrow through a process of neointimal hyperplasia.[12, 37] The proliferation of smooth muscle cells within the stented segments poses little risk of thromboembolism and produces symptoms only at its most severe extent when cerebral circulation is limited.

Given the nascency of endovascular techniques in the treatment of neurological diseases, it is reasonable to assume that technical advances will significantly reduce the number of associated complications. For example, the use of stents has reduced the risks associated with angioplasty on several levels. Carotid dissection from intimal fractures occurs during the angioplasty phase in as many as 25% of cases.[22] Stenting prevents acute occlusion after dissection by reapposing the intima to the vessel wall. It also decreases the rate of embolization by compressing friable regions of the diseased luminal wall. Stenting also has improved long-term patency by providing a rigid intra-arterial support structure that resists recoil from within fibrous segments of the diseased artery.

A practical advantage of percutaneous angioplasty and stenting compared with CEA is that, in most cases, the procedure is performed under local anesthesia.[35] A change in a patient's neurological status immediately alerts the endovascular neurosurgeon to the potential of thromboembolism.[35] Such occurrences can be addressed rapidly by administering intra-arterial thrombolytic agents or by using mechanical disrupting devices, such as microwires and balloon catheters. Asymptomatic branch occlusions also can be detected by angiography and addressed before symptoms begin.

A survey of major interventional centers worldwide prompted responses from 24 centers at which 2048 endovascular carotid artery stent procedures had been performed.[26] The overall rate of immediate technical success was 98.6% (defined as less than 30% residual stenosis in the treated region). The responding physicians reported that 66.4% of the patients had symptoms referable to the lesion. Minor strokes occurred in 63 patients (occurrence rate, 3.08%), and major strokes occurred in 27 patients (1.32%). All deaths occurring in a 30-day postoperative period (including those caused by myocardial infarction) were recorded. A combined major and minor stroke and death rate of 5.77% was obtained. Follow-up studies included Doppler ultrasonography 1 and 6 months after stent placement and angiography at 6 months as needed. The restenosis rate at 6 months was 4.8%.

In a review of 445 percutaneous angioplasty and stenting procedures performed in 404 patients, Vitek and associates[60] reported a combined 30-day morbidity and mortality rate of 8.4%. This rate included 8 deaths (1.9%), 3 major strokes (0.7%), and 26 minor strokes (5.8%), only 12 of which produced permanent symptoms. Their series included 40 patients with contralateral carotid occlusions and 70 cases of restenosis after CEA. The investigators further documented a progressive decrease in their incidence of minor strokes over time, reporting a rate of 7.2% during 1994 and 1995 and 2.2% during 1997 and 1998. Angiography or ultrasonography, performed in the follow-up evaluation of 80% of their patients, revealed a rate of significant restenosis of 5%. The physicians calculated that percutaneous angioplasty and stenting avoided neurological death or stroke in 92% ± 4% of their cases.

Theron and coworkers[25] reviewed their experience with angioplasty for carotid stenosis in 259 patients. Cerebral protection (i.e., inflation of a balloon distal to the lesion to prevent embolic showers and then aspiration and flushing through the ECA) was used in 136 cases. A stent was placed in 69 patients when imaging revealed a suboptimal angioplastic result. Among the 38 patients who underwent angioplasty without cerebral protection, 5% sustained a dissection and 8% experienced embolic phenomena. None of the 136 patients in whom cerebral protection was used developed embolic complications during angioplasty. Embolic complications occurred in 1% of patients during or after stent placement.

Yadav and colleagues[27] reported a 30-day risk of stroke and death of 7.9% after performing 126 percutaneous angioplasty and stenting procedures in a high-risk group of 107 patients. These complications included seven minor strokes, two major strokes, and one death. Of these patients, 77% would have failed the inclusion criteria in NASCET or ACAS because of severe coexisting disease. When only those strokes occurring ipsilateral to the treated artery are considered, the rate of complications fell to 1.6%. Restenoses were all asymptomatic and occurred in 3 of 61 patients undergoing angiography 6 months after percutaneous angioplasty and stenting.

After reviewing 271 percutaneous angioplasty and stenting procedures in 231 patients, Mathur and coworkers[36] determined that advanced age and the presence of long or multiple stenoses were independent factors predictive of procedurally related strokes. Seventeen patients (6.2%) had minor strokes, and two (0.7%) suffered a major CVA. When patients who would not have met criteria for NASCET were excluded, the rate of all strokes fell to 2.7%. Patients younger than 80 years of age demonstrated a 5.6% risk of periprocedural stroke, compared with 19.2% of patients 80 years of age or older.

In a report that reflects an early experience with percutaneous angioplasty and stenting, Diethrich and associates[29] reviewed their results in 110 nonconsecutive patients with more than 70% stenosis of the carotid artery as determined angiographically; 72% of patients were asymptomatic. Lesions were located in the ICA, middle CCA, distal CCA, proximal CCA, and ECA. Including all lesions, the mean stenosis rate was 86.5% ± 10.6%. The retrograde femoral technique and the direct carotid artery puncture technique were used.

A relatively high rate of major and minor complications in this series reflects the learning curve associated with percutaneous angioplasty and stenting. Vasospasm occurred in four patients (3.6%) and responded to treatment with intra-arterial papaverine. One (0.9%) flow-limiting dissection required deployment of a second stent. Four complications related to direct carotid puncture occurred: three hematomas and one arteriovenous fistula treated surgically. There were two complications related to the retrograde femoral artery approach. A pseudoaneurysm of the common femoral artery in one patient responded to compression, and a hematoma in a second patient required operative intervention. A stent could not be delivered by this approach in seven patients. A direct carotid artery puncture was performed in six of these patients, and CEA was the treatment in the seventh.

Major strokes occurred in two patients, one of whom died 6 weeks later. Minor strokes occurred in five patients, all of whom recovered in 1 month. Five patients had minor transient neurological symptoms. Two ICA stents occluded within 30 days of the procedure, and the clinical success rate was 89.1%. Over a mean follow-up period of 7.6 months, no patient developed new neurological symptoms. An 89% cumulative primary patency rate was found using life-table analysis.

Regarding the use of percutaneous angioplasty and stenting in the treatment of recurrent carotid stenosis after endarterectomy, Yadav and colleagues[61] reported no major strokes and only one minor stroke (4%) in 25 cases. Only eight patients, however, underwent follow-up angiography at 6 months. Of these, the mean stenosis was 19.4% ± 4.4%. None of these patients demonstrated restenosis greater than or equal to 50%, and none required retreatment. Lanzino and coworkers[35] reported no major periprocedural deficits or deaths in 25 procedures performed in 21 patients who developed restenosis after CEA. Of the five patients treated with angioplasty alone, however, three required retreatment. Of the 16 patients who were followed for at least 6 months, none developed neurological complications ipsilateral to the treated vessel. Only one patient manifested a significant restenosis (55%). This patient, however, was asymptomatic.

Mericle and associates[33] reported a 30-day complication rate of 0% after percutaneous angioplasty and stenting in a series of 26 angioplasty procedures performed in 23 patients with contralateral carotid occlusions. Most of these patients, moreover, were too high risk because of comorbid factors to have qualified for inclusion in NASCET. Complications included one death from respiratory arrest 2 months after percutaneous angioplasty and stenting, a second death from complications related to a prostate carcinoma 12 months after the procedure, and one minor stroke contralateral to the treated vessel 41 months after therapy. Although this study is limited by its small number of patients, the results suggest a role for percutaneous angioplasty and stenting in the treatment of this complex subgroup.

The efficacy of percutaneous angioplasty and stenting in the treatment of carotid dissection has yet to be determined. A number of case reports, including a review of 11 cases from our institution, reveal an acceptable rate of technical success and complications.[46–54] In most such cases, percutaneous angioplasty and stenting are performed only after a dedicated course of medical therapy and usually only in the presence of progressive, symptomatic disease. Associated pseudoaneurysms typically resolve with stenting of the dissected segment although coil embolization through the struts of the stent has also been described. Given that the surgical management of these lesions is difficult and may include vessel ligation and bypass, preserving affected vessels through percutaneous angioplasty and stenting is certainly an attractive treatment option.

CONCLUSIONS

Review of these studies indicates that the complication rates associated with stent placement are not dramatically different from those associated with CEA. As stent design and delivery systems are refined, techniques to prevent distal embolic phenomena improve, and experience increases, the long-term outcomes can be expected to improve and the procedural risks to decrease. Most equipment now used in carotid percutaneous angioplasty and stenting is designed for use in the coronary and peripheral arterial systems. Percutaneous angioplasty and stenting holds promise for the future and presents a viable alternative to CEA in the current management of select cases.

REFERENCES

1. Donnan GA, Davis SM, Chambers BR, et al: Surgery for prevention of stroke. Lancet 351:1372–1373, 1998.
2. Easton JD: Current advances in the management of stroke. Neurology 51:S1–S2,1998.
3. Kuller LH: Incidence rates of stroke in the eighties: The end of the decline in stroke? Stroke 20:841–843, 1989.
4. Kurtzke JF: Epidemiology of Cerebrovascular Disease. Berlin, Springer-Verlag, 1969.
5. Mohr JP, Caplan LR, Melski JW, et al: The Harvard Cooperative Stroke Registry: A prospective registry. Neurology 28:754–762, 1978.
6. Chaturvedi S: Medical, surgical, and interventional treatment for carotid artery disease. Clin Neuropharmacol 21:205–214, 1998.

7. European Carotid Surgery Trialists' Collaborative Group: MRC European Carotid Surgery Trial: Interim results for symptomatic patients with severe (70–99%) or with mild (0–29%) carotid stenosis. Lancet 337:1235–1243, 1991.
8. Executive Committee for the Asymptomatic Carotid Atherosclerosis Study: Endarterectomy for asymptomatic carotid artery stenosis. JAMA 273:1421–1428, 1995.
9. North American Symptomatic Carotid Endarterectomy Trial Collaborators: Beneficial effect of carotid endarterectomy in symptomatic patients with high-grade carotid stenosis. N Engl J Med 325:445–453, 1991.
10. Cebul RD, Snow RJ, Pine R, et al: Indications, outcomes, and provider volumes for carotid endarterectomy. JAMA 279:1282–1287, 1998.
11. Hertzer NR, O'Hara PJ, Mascha EJ, et al: Early outcome assessment for 2228 consecutive carotid endarterectomy procedures: The Cleveland Clinic experience from 1989 to 1995. J Vasc Surg 26:1–10, 1997.
12. Albuquerque FC, Giannotta SL, Teitelbaum G: The neurosurgical treatment of stroke. In Neurosurgery for the Neurologist: 4: 25–46, 1998.
13. Becker GJ: Should metallic vascular stents be used to treat cerebrovascular occlusive diseases? Radiology 191:309–312, 1994.
14. Bettmann MA, Katzen BT, Whisnant J, et al: Carotid stenting and angioplasty: A statement for healthcare professionals from the Councils on Cardiovascular Radiology, Stroke, Cardio-Thoracic and Vascular Surgery, Epidemiology, and Prevention, and Clinical Cardiology, American Heart Association. Stroke 29:336–338, 1998.
15. Dorros G: Stent-supported carotid angioplasty: Should it be done, and, if so, by whom? A 1998 perspective. Circulation 98: 927–930, 1998.
16. Hobson RW II, Brott T, Ferguson R, et al: Regarding "Statement regarding carotid angioplasty and stenting." J Vasc Surg 25: 1117,1997.
17. Wholey MH, Wholey M: Momentum growing for carotid stent placement. Diagn Imaging (San Franc) 20:65–75, 1998.
18. Dotter CT, Judkins MP: Transluminal treatment of arteriosclerotic obstruction. Description of a new technic and a preliminary report of its application. Circulation 30:654–670, 1964.
19. Kerber CW, Cromwell LD, Loehden OL: Catheter dilation of proximal carotid stenosis during distal bifurcation endarterectomy. AJNR Am J Neuroradiol 1:348–349, 1980.
20. Mullan S, Duda EE, Patronas NJ: Some examples of balloon technology in neurosurgery. J Neurosurg 52:321–329, 1980.
21. Brown MM, Crawley F, Clifton A, et al: Percutaneous transluminal angioplasty of the internal carotid artery. Br J Surg 84:729–730, 1997.
22. Gil-Peralta A, Mayol A, Marcos JR, et al: Percutaneous transluminal angioplasty of the symptomatic atherosclerotic carotid arteries: Results, complications, and follow-up. Stroke 27:2271–2273, 1996.
23. Roubin GS, Yadav S, Iyer SS, et al: Carotid stent-supported angioplasty: A neurovascular intervention to prevent stroke. Am J Cardiol 78:8–12, 1996.
24. Teitelbaum GP, Lefkowitz MA, Giannotta SL: Carotid angioplasty and stenting in high-risk patients. Surg Neurol 50:300–312, 1998.
25. Theron JG, Payelle GG, Coskun O, et al: Carotid artery stenosis: Treatment with protected balloon angioplasty and stent placement. Radiology 201:627–636, 1996.
25a. Albuquerque FC, Teitelbaum GP, Lavine SD, et al: Balloon-protected carotid angioplasty. Neurosurgery 46:918–921, discussion 922–923, 2000.
26. Wholey MH, Wholey M, Bergeron P, et al: Current global status of carotid artery stent placement. Cathet Cardiovasc Diagn 44: 1–6, 1998.
27. Yadav JS, Roubin GS, Iyer S, et al: Elective stenting of the extracranial carotid arteries. Circulation 95:376–381, 1997.
28. Diethrich EB, Marx P, Wrasper R, et al: Percutaneous techniques for endoluminal carotid interventions. J Endovasc Surg 3:182–202, 1996.
29. Diethrich EB, Ndiaye M, Reid DB: Stenting in the carotid artery: Initial experience in 110 patients. J Endovasc Surg 3:42–62, 1996.
30. Kachel R, Basche S, Heerklotz I, et al: Percutaneous transluminal angioplasty (PTA) of supra-aortic arteries especially the internal carotid artery. Neuroradiology 33:191–194, 1991.
31. Callow AD: Recurrent stenosis after carotid endarterectomy. Arch Surg 117:1082–1085, 1982.
32. Sundt TM, Sandok BA, Whisnant JP: Carotid endarterectomy: Complications and preoperative assessment of risk. Mayo Clin Proc 50:301–306, 1975.
33. Mericle RA, Kim SH, Lanzino G, et al: Carotid artery angioplasty and use of stents in high-risk patients with contralateral occlusions. J Neurosurg 90:1031–1036, 1999.
34. Hobson RW II, Goldstein JE, Jamil Z, et al: Carotid restenosis: Operative and endovascular management. J Vasc Surg 29:228–238, 1999.
35. Lanzino G, Mericle RA, Lopes DK, et al: Percutaneous transluminal angioplasty and stent placement for recurrent carotid artery stenosis. J Neurosurg 90:688–694, 1999.
36. Mathur A, Roubin GS, Iyer SS, et al: Predictors of stroke complicating carotid artery stenting. Circulation 97:1239–1245, 1998.
37. Albuquerque FC, Teitelbaum GP, Larsen DW, et al: Carotid endarterectomy compared with angioplasty and stenting: The status of the debate. Neurosurg Focus 5: Article 2, 1998.
38. Diethrich EB, Gordon MH, Lopez-Galarza LA, et al: Intraluminal Palmaz stent implantation for treatment of recurrent carotid artery occlusive disease: A plan for the future. J Interv Cardiol 8: 213–218, 1995.
39. Das MB, Hertzer NR, Ratliff NB, et al: Recurrent carotid stenosis. A five-year series of 65 reoperations. Ann Surg 202:28–35, 1985.
40. Rothwell PM, Slattery J, Warlow CP: A systematic review of the risks of stroke and death due to endarterectomy for symptomatic carotid stenosis. Stroke 27:260–265, 1996.
41. Tievsky AL, Druy EM, Mardiat JG: Transluminal angioplasty in postsurgical stenosis of the extracranial carotid artery. AJNR Am J Neuroradiol 4:800–802, 1983.
42. Mellière D, Becquemin JP, Berrahal D, et al: Management of radiation-induced occlusive arterial disease: A reassessment. J Cardiovasc Surg 38:261–269, 1997.
43. Rockman CB, Riles TS, Fisher FS, et al: The surgical management of carotid artery stenosis in patients with previous neck irradiation. Am J Surg 172:191–195, 1996.
44. Ahuja A, Blatt GL, Guterman LR, et al: Angioplasty for symptomatic radiation-induced extracranial carotid artery stenosis: Case report. Neurosurgery 36:399–403, 1995.
45. Glick B: Bilateral carotid occlusive disease. Following irradiation for carcinoma of the vocal cords. Arch Pathol 93:352–355, 1972.
46. Bejjani GK, Monsein LH, Laird JR, et al: Treatment of symptomatic cervical carotid dissections with endovascular stents. Neurosurgery 44:755–761, 1999.
47. Hong MK, Satler LF, Gallino R, et al: Intravascular stenting as a definitive treatment of spontaneous carotid artery dissection. Am J Cardiol 79:538,1997.
48. Coric D, Wilson JA, Regan JD, et al: Primary stenting of the extracranial internal carotid artery in a patient with multiple cervical dissections: Technical case report. Neurosurgery 43:956–959, 1998.
49. Crawley F, Brown MM, Clifton AG: Angioplasty and stenting in the carotid and vertebral arteries. Postgrad Med J 74:7–10, 1998.
50. Perez-Cruet MJ, Patwardhan RV, Mawad ME, et al: Treatment of dissecting pseudoaneurysm of the cervical internal carotid artery using a wall stent and detachable coils: Case report. Neurosurgery 40:622–626, 1997.
51. Griewing B, Brassel F, Schminke U, et al: Angioplasty and stenting in carotid artery dissection. Eur Neurol 40:175–176, 1998.
52. Hurst RW, Haskal ZJ, Zager E, et al: Endovascular stent treatment of cervical internal carotid artery aneurysms with parent vessel preservation. Surg Neurol 50:313–317, 1998.
53. Dorros G, Cohn JM, Palmer LE: Stent deployment resolves a petrous carotid artery angioplasty dissection. AJNR Am J Neuroradiol 19:392–394, 1998.
54. Horowitz MB, Miller G III, Meyer Y, et al: Use of intravascular stents in the treatment of internal carotid and extracranial vertebral artery pseudoaneurysms. AJNR Am J Neuroradiol 17:693–696, 1996.
55. Marks MP, Dake MD, Steinberg GK, et al: Stent placement for arterial and venous cerebrovascular disease: Preliminary experience. Radiology 191:441–446, 1994.
56. Crawley F, Clifton A, Taylor RS, et al: Symptomatic restenosis after carotid percutaneous transluminal angioplasty. Lancet 352: 708–709, 1998.

57. Eckert B, Thie A, Valdueza J, et al: Transcranial Doppler sonographic monitoring during percutaneous transluminal angioplasty of the internal carotid artery. Neuroradiology 39:229–234, 1997.
58. Heuser RR: Success with carotid stenting: A stroke of good luck or the wave of the future? Cathet Cardiovasc Diagn 44:7–8, 1998.
59. Markus HS, Clifton A, Buckenham T, et al: Carotid angioplasty. Detection of embolic signals during and after the procedure. Stroke 25:2403–2406, 1994.
60. Vitek J, Roubin G, Iyer S: Immediate and late outcome of carotid angioplasty with stenting [abstract]. In American Association of Neurological Surgeons, Cognitive Neuroscience Society, and American Society of Interventional Neuroradiology (eds): Program Book. Park Ridge, IL, American Association of Neurological Surgeons, 1999.
61. Yadav JS, Roubin GS, King P, et al: Angioplasty and stenting for restenosis after carotid endarterectomy. Initial experience. Stroke 27:2075–2079, 1996.

CHAPTER **99**

Recurrent Carotid Stenosis

ROBERT J. DEMPSEY ■ ACLAN DOGAN

OVERVIEW AND HISTORY

Carotid endarterectomy has been established to be a safe procedure with acceptable perioperative morbidity and mortality rates. A growing number of carotid endarterectomies have been performed in the world because several randomized trials have demonstrated the superiority of carotid endarterectomy over medical management for stroke prevention in both asymptomatic and symptomatic patients who have severe carotid artery stenosis.[1-4] Although the short-term benefits of surgery are well recognized, the long-term results of this operation are less well known. This is, in part, due to the presence of intercurrent cardiac disease in this population. In long-term survivors, however, the maintenance of luminal patency is required for durability of the procedure. Restenosis occurring months to years after the initial procedure may result in recurrent symptoms or vessel occlusion and late failure of this procedure. Restenosis of the carotid artery is any arterial narrowing at or near the site of an operative or interventional procedure for atherosclerosis[5] and was first described by Eastcott and colleagues[6] in 1954. The importance of restenosis is becoming increasingly recognized because of the growth in the number of carotid endarterectomies, improved survival from cardiac disease, and improved noninvasive diagnostic techniques used to evaluate postoperative carotid endarterectomy patients.

INCIDENCE

Long-term follow-up studies indicate that postoperative recurrent carotid stenosis and residual stenosis not repaired at the time of operation can occur in 1.2% to 49% of patients undergoing carotid endarterectomy, depending on the surveillance methods used and the presence of the residual lesions.[7-13]

By using oculopneumoplethysmography, which can detect only severe stenosis or occlusions, Kremen and associates[14] showed a total incidence of restenosis of 9.8%. Cantelmo and colleagues[15] reported an incidence of recurrent carotid stenosis of 12.1%. On the basis of angiograms, recurrent carotid stenosis that was sufficiently severe to warrant operation was identified in only 2.9% and 3.8% in two large series.[13, 16] The introduction of more reliable noninvasive serial assessment by duplex scanning has increased the discovery of patients with symptomless recurrent stenosis and the incidence of residual lesions after the initial surgery. This can vary greatly with the surgeon and surgical technique, including the use of a microscope. A patch or a shunt may effect these rates. The overall incidence of residual defects has been reported to be between 5.3% and 42.9%.[17-20] The actual clinically important incidence based on occurrence of neurological symptoms averages between 1% and 4%.[21, 22] In large surgical series, only about 5% of the total number of carotid endarterectomies requires a repeat operation.[23] This discrepancy may be explained by the asymptomatic nature of many restenoses and misinterpretation of the findings related to artifacts or normal features of postoperative arterial remodeling on noninvasive imaging.[16] In a compilation of series reported in the literature based on duplex scanning, the incidence of recurrent carotid stenosis (>50%) was 13% (Table 99–1).

ETIOLOGY

Many reports of recurrent carotid stenosis have tried to incriminate the usual systemic or local risk factors including hypertension, smoking, small internal carotid artery, hyperlipidemia, sex, age, diabetes mellitus, residual disease, and operative defects as being the primary causes for recurrence.[9, 24-34] None has clearly demonstrated that any of the recognized risk factors for atherosclerosis contribute to the process of restenosis. Although continued smoking probably has the greatest predictive value in the progression of the carotid atherosclerosis preoperatively[35-37] and postoperatively,[38, 39] not all reports have confirmed this relationship. Relatively younger age (<55 years) has been implicated in the higher incidence of both early postoperative carotid thrombosis and recurrent stenosis.[40] This may suggest that the factors leading to the need for the primary endarterectomy at such an early age are still active in the postoperative period. Although the relationship with female sex is not consistent, women, in general,

TABLE 99-1 ■ Incidence of Recurrent Stenosis (>50%) Based on Duplex Scanning in Published Series

REFERENCE	NUMBER OF OPERATIONS	RESTENOSIS (%)	SYMPTOMATIC (%)
Shanik et al.	80	13	1
Thomas et al.	257	8.9	1.2
Colgan et al.	80	13	1
Nicholls et al.	145	17–22	1.4
Zbornikova et al.	113	23.9	4.4
Curley et al.	72	14	3
Ouriel and Green	102	13.7	0
Sanders et al.	94	7	–
Bandyk et al.	250	12	0
Healy et al.	301	19–26	3.7
Clagett et al.	152	5.9	0.7
Sawchuk et al.	80	5	–
Sterpetti et al.	73	37	8
Bernstein et al.	484	8.5	–
Rosenthal et al.	717	3.3	0.5
Atnip et al.	184	6	1.6
Reilly et al.	131	18.1	–
Cook et al.	78	18	3
Nitzberg et al.	1043	–	1.8
Mattos et al.	544	12.7	2.8
Donaldson et al.	232	18.5	1.7
Powell et al.	107	16.8	2.8
Katz et al.	100	2	–
Lattimer et al.	482	17	2.3
Dempsey et al.*	500	1.5	0.4

*Unpublished data.
(Modified from Lattimer CR, Burnand KG: Recurrent carotid stenosis after carotid endarterectomy. Br J Surg 84:1206–1219, 1997.)

appear to be at higher risk for the development of early postoperative lesions resulting from myointimal hyperplasia.[41] Smaller vessel size and sex differences affecting smooth-muscle cell proliferation were thought to be potential causative factors for this female preponderance.[14, 42, 43] Hyperlipidemia may contribute to restenosis, but it is not consistently demonstrable in this population. Diabetes mellitus, the severity of the original stenosis, the presence of symptoms at the time of the original operation, bilateral disease, and hypertension have all been incriminated by individual reports but have not been confirmed by others.

Factors related to the surgery such as inadequate endarterectomy, difficult endpoints, clamp injuries, using of tacking sutures, and the presence of residual lesions including atheroma, myointimal flaps, intraluminal thrombi, and vein patch irregularities were thought to be associated with an increased incidence of late restenosis.[25, 32, 44–53] Unfortunately, it is not possible to form a consensus from the literature about the role of technical factors in recurrent carotid stenosis because each of the above-mentioned factors is variably reported as having and as not having a correlation with subsequent restenosis.[17, 22, 32, 47, 54–56] Although exact etiologic factors remain debated, technical perfection at the time of carotid endarterectomy appears to be of great import. This should include minimal dissection of the diseased portion of the artery to decrease the risk of embolization before clamping, the careful application of clamps with or without the insertion of shunts, and meticulous suture closure with magnification of vision.

The data from the literature suggest that patients with small internal carotid arteries, especially female patients, are at a greater risk of restenosis or occlusion. This has led some surgeons to suggest that patch angioplasty may decrease the risk and should be considered in these patients.[32, 57] Although the routine use of patching in all arteriotomy closures has been proposed as one means of preventing recurrent carotid stenosis by increasing the lumen size,[51] this has not been proved by randomized study. In fact, the use of too large a patch may predispose the patient to turbulence and increase the risk of recurrent disease. The use of autologous vein as a patch material may provide an unwelcome additional source of proliferating smooth muscle cells, but it may also provide the endarterectomized vessel with an additional source of endothelial cells.[58]

There is no consensus on the choice of vein or prosthetic material for the patch. The effectiveness of saphenous vein patch grafting in protecting the internal carotid artery and the distal site of the endarterectomy from recurrent carotid stenosis has been demonstrated by several authors.[53, 59] The very interesting question of the effects of introducing muscle or endothelial calls into the postoperative site remains to be studied.

Excellent results with primary closure are reported by experienced surgeons. This is the most common type of closure.[60–63] Generally, patches are applied when the vessel is less than 3 to 5 mm in diameter and shunt insertion is difficult or impossible. In experienced hands, with the routine use of the microscope for closure, it has been shown that primary closure of the endarterectomized vessel will still increase its diameter approximately threefold. On average, these vessels reach to 87% of the theoretical maximum lumen, as estimated by measure of the distal internal carotid artery remote from the stenotic area.[39]

PATHOGENESIS

It has been suggested that the pathogenesis of recurrent carotid stenosis is a dynamic process of arterial healing beginning at the time of the initial endarterectomy. Surgical manipulation, clamp injury, shunt trauma, endovascular angioplasty, and the placement of distal tacking sutures all produce various degrees of injury. There are a number of studies showing that thrombosis can occur at any time after carotid endarterectomy.[13, 19, 64] Immediately after blood flow is re-established, a layer of platelets, fibrin, red blood cells, and leukocytes can be seen to cover the endarterectomized surface. Mural thrombus caused by injury has been implicated in the production of growth factors, cytokines, and other molecules, including platelet-derived growth factor (PDGF), basic fibroblast growth factor (bFGF), interleukin-1 (IL-1), tumor necrosis factor-α (TNF-α), transforming growth factor-β (TGF-β), angiotensin II, oxygen free radicals, and thrombin. These elements have been shown to stimulate smooth muscle proliferation, and migration as well as matrix formation. As a potential balance to these mitogens several factors including heparin, IL-1, high concentrations of

TGF-β, and TNF-α can inhibit smooth muscle proliferation. Heparin may decrease the neointimal thickening by its antiaggregatory effects on platelets, as well as by direct inhibition of smooth muscle proliferation and migration. This effect of heparin is thought to be the result of altering the composition of the extracellular matrix and the sequestration of bFGF. Interferon-γ (IFN-γ) produced by T lymphocytes has also been shown to decrease the cross-sectional intimal area of lesions by 50% in experimental studies.

PDGF is a major chemoattractant for monocytes and neutrophils and mitogen in platelets. Neointimal formation after angioplasty has been reduced by inhibition of PDGF by approximately 40%.

bFGF is released by injured and dying cells. It is a potent smooth muscle cell mitogen and a stimulator of angiogenesis; it can also stimulate endothelial cell regrowth. The neutralization of bFGF by an antibody before balloon catheter de-endothelialization in rats has markedly reduced medial smooth muscle cell proliferation by 80%.[65]

Histopathology

The morphologic appearance of a recurrent stenosis depends on the mechanism and the time interval following endarterectomy. It has been generally accepted that residual carotid lesions due to technical defects at the time of operation are responsible for immediate fixed lesions. Acute thrombosis can be due to a hypercoagulable status in the absence of a structural defect because of the presence of the newly exposed collagen in the endarterectomized segment. Although it has been suggested that the two processes may represent different stages of a single lesion causing a recurrent stenosis,[66, 67] early-appearing recurrences that develop within the first 2 years are usually the result of myointimal hyperplasia, whereas late lesions (appearing after 2 years) more typically consist of atherosclerotic material. Whether they are early or late recurrences, it is clear that platelet deposition is necessary for the formation of these lesions.[68] Early stenosis had a greater cellular component with spindled shaped nucleated cells, small nests of lymphocytes, and polymorphs surrounded by dense accumulations of collagen and acid mucopolysaccharide (Fig. 99–1).[69] The lack of lipid accumulation and hemosiderin is noted.[22, 70] In the later lesions, the presence of macrophages, needle-shaped cholesterol clefts, foam cells lying immediately beneath the endothelium, abundant collagen, and calcium deposits are more apparent (Fig. 99–2). Abundant lipid may be seen as small intracellular globules and large extracellular lakes. Immunoreactivity for desmin and actin is found only in the early restenotic lesions whereas capillary ingrowth (neovascularization) is evident in both the early (44%) and late (75%) specimens. At the time of reoperation, a mother-of-pearl appearance is characteristic of myointimal hyperplasia with a smooth, firmly adherent localized thickening at the site of the previous endarterectomy. Conversely, atherosclerotic lesions tend to be irregular, friable, and more pronounced at

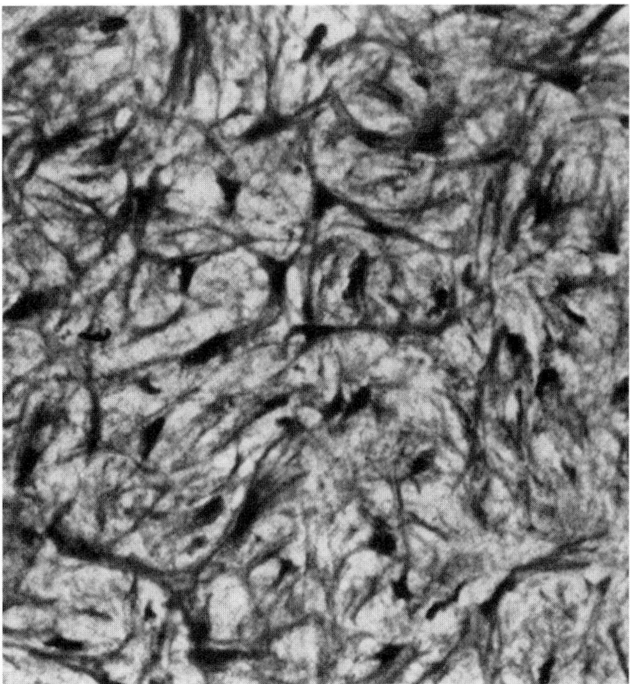

FIGURE 99–1. Early recurrent lesion characterized by myointimal hyperplasia with spindle-shaped and stellate cells. Hematoxylin-eosin stain; original magnification × 200. (From Schwarcz TH, Yates GN, Ghobrial M, et al: Pathologic characteristics of recurrent carotid artery stenosis. J Vasc Surg 5:280–288, 1987.)

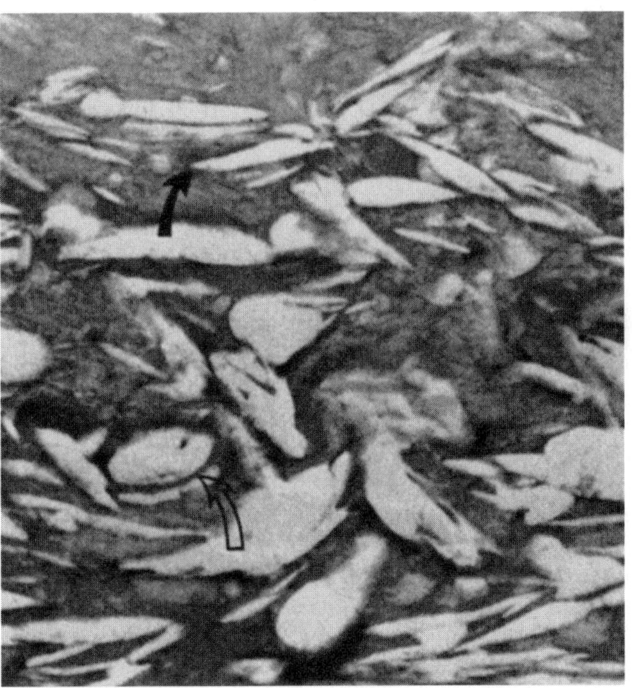

FIGURE 99–2. Late recurrent lesion with needle-shaped cholesterol clefts *(black arrow)* and circular defects consistent with extracellular fat *(open arrow)*. Hematoxylin-eosin stain; original magnification × 200. (From Schwarcz TH, Yates GN, Ghobrial M, et al: Pathologic characteristics of recurrent carotid artery stenosis. J Vasc Surg 5:280–288, 1987.)

the proximal and distal endpoints.[21] The presence at the old suture line and a step off in the common carotid artery are usually distinguishing features for recurrent atherosclerosis.

CLINICAL PRESENTATION AND NATURAL HISTORY

Although the incidence of recurrent carotid stenosis after endarterectomy has been reported in up to 49% of cases, only 1% to 4% of patients with recurrent carotid stenosis have neurological symptoms.[21, 22, 42, 71] Those with symptoms do not necessarily develop them in the same arterial territory as their initial symptoms.[31, 54, 72] This is often due to the systemic nature of atherosclerosis. Symptoms, when they do occur, are typically transient in nature and are more likely to appear once the lesion progresses to higher than 80% stenosis. The early stenotic lesions have been shown to lead to significantly fewer neurological symptoms than late restenosis.[73] Myointimal hyperplasia also has the potential to improve.[26, 42, 47, 61, 74, 75] However, there are no data about factors that are associated with regression. Two mechanisms have been postulated to account for regression. These are, first, an adaptive remodeling response of the arterial wall to new hemodynamic conditions which occur typically after the initial proliferative phase, and, second, a reduction of the intimal mass by the organization and resolution of mural thrombosis.

DIAGNOSIS

Intraoperative assessment of the carotid artery after endarterectomy is an important part of the operative procedure and has been done by many methods. The routine use of B-mode imaging in the diagnosis and postoperative follow-up of patients with carotid disease has provided useful information regarding the course of healing at the endarterectomy site and the progression of the disease.[9, 54, 75] In comparison to other methods such as oculopneumoplethysmography and intravenous digital angiography, duplex scanning is thought to have material advantages of high sensitivity and reproducibility, lack of known risks, and patient acceptance.[76–79] Caps and coworkers[80] have described a duplex ultrasound finding of two dense lines separated by an echolucent zone (double line) predictive of healing without restenosis after carotid endarterectomy. In addition, the development of platelet aggregation at the endarterectomy site and the abnormal hemodynamics associated with distal ICA kinking or angulation with arteriotomy closure can be reliably identified in several planes by Doppler flow analysis. The detection of these same conditions by angiography is difficult because of the unpredictable image resolution and vessel projection of intraoperative studies.[54] Angiographically, postoperative neointimal thickening can be seen as a concentric ringlike stenosis with a normal luminal diameter at the bifurcation or in the internal carotid artery. In patients in whom an extensive surgical procedure extending into the common carotid artery has been performed, a scalloped appearance may be present.[81] In contrast, recurrent atherosclerosis is characterized by marked irregularity of the lumen with focal areas of ulceration and stenosis.[82]

TREATMENT

The management of recurrent carotid artery stenosis depends on the type of recurrence and its related symptoms. Most carotid restenoses are asymptomatic or hemodynamically nonsignificant. Less than 4% of all patients undergoing carotid endarterectomy have symptomatic hemodynamically significant recurrent carotid stenosis.[12, 53, 83] Although there is a clear consensus that a hemodynamically significant recurrent carotid stenosis that produces hemispheric symptoms should be repaired, there is still controversy regarding the most appropriate management of asymptomatic recurrent carotid stenosis.

The possibility of a devastating stroke that might accompany disease progression to total occlusion has led several surgeons to operate on asymptomatic patients. O'Donnell and associates found a higher stroke rate in patients with asymptomatic recurrent carotid stenosis who did not undergo operation and suggested a more aggressive surgical approach.[84] On the other hand, a more conservative nonoperative approach has been advocated by others who found that recurrent carotid stenosis tends to run a benign course in their patients.[73, 85] Although symptoms occur less frequently in early recurrent carotid stenosis, these lesions are just as likely as those with recurrent atherosclerosis to have evidence of thrombus as a potential cause of symptoms. It would appear logical to recommend surgery for symptomatic patients with hemodynamicaly significant stenosis and follow the asymptomatic patients with noninvasive surveillance of the recurrent lesion unless the adequacy of the arterial lumen is significantly compromised.[28, 29]

Medical Management

The use of pharmacologic agents to prevent intimal thickening in recurrent carotid stenosis is based on the response-to-injury hypothesis of such thickening. This hypothesis relates endothelial injury, thrombosis, cytokine, and growth factor release to smooth muscle cell migration, proliferation, and secretion.[86] Treatment should be based on interrupting these processes.

Agents that inhibit platelet aggregation and release at the site of arterial injury have been extensively studied to prevent neointimal thickening. Aspirin, dipyridamol, coumadin, thromboxan inhibitors, heparin, fish oils, alpha adrenergic antagonists, nitric oxide agonists, nitric oxide donors, and prostacyclin analogs have all been shown to be effective in laboratory investigations. All of them remain unproven in humans. Prospective clinical studies have had limited success.[87, 88] Patient survival after carotid endarterectomy, however, seems to be prolonged with aspirin and heparin because of a reduction in the number of cardiac deaths and vascular events in general.

Several agents including heparin, angiotensin II inhibitors, antimetabolites, methotrexate, corticosteroids, and angiopeptin have also been shown to inhibit smooth muscle cell proliferation in in vitro models. As with antithrombotic agents, these drugs are yet to be proven in reducing recurrent carotid stenosis in clinical trials.[88–90] More recently, experimental methods have targeted gene therapy[91] to decrease smooth muscle cell replication. Other molecular therapies include those to express antithrombotic substances such as tissue plasminogen activator, and antibodies to platelets IIa and IIIb integrin, PDGF, and bFGF. Bioabsorbable stents may soon be available that maintain lumen caliber while releasing biologically active agents.

Antisense oligonucleotides may also act to prevent accumulation of neointimal mass by direct delivery to the arterial wall of agents which inhibit smooth muscle division. Photodynamic therapy has recently been shown to reduce induced intimal hyperplasia experimentally by targeting the action of various photosensitive agents to the site of catheter injury.

Surgical Management

The surgical approach to recurrent carotid stenosis may differ from primary endarterectomy. The following approaches have been used: endarterectomy alone; saphenous vein patch, polytetrafluoroethylene (PTFE) patch, or Dacron patch alone; endarterectomy with patching; excision of the segment with graft interposition using saphenous vein, basilic vein, Dacron, PTFE, bovine artery, hypogastric artery, or superficial femoral artery; carotid bifurcation advancement; and saphenous vein bypass.[92] The lack of consensus would suggest none of these procedures has been proven to be superior in all cases.

The operative strategy for recurrent carotid stenosis most commonly involves carotid endarterectomy with patch angioplasty (Fig. 99–3). Carotid patch angioplasty alone has been advocated by several authors, especially for myointimal hyperplasia in which an endarterectomy plane cannot be established or if the symptoms prompting reoperation are believed to be due to reduction in cerebral blood flow and are not likely to be embolic.[16, 57, 93, 94] However, in theory, carotid patch angioplasty alone may cause anatomic changes in the configuration of the artery, resulting in altered hemodynamics with laminated thrombus formation and ultimately secondary recurrent carotid stenosis. In addition, patch angioplasty may rarely cause late aneurysm formation and catastrophic patch ruptures.[17, 50, 51] In considering patch material, there is a preference in the literature for autogenous saphenous vein.[51] Nevertheless, some have chosen predominantly prosthetic patches (PTFE and woven Dacron).[16, 93–95]

Carotid resection with the placement of an interposition graft is another surgical option (Fig. 99–4). This option has been reserved for those patients in whom repeat carotid endarterectomy or patch angioplasty is not possible usually because the luminal surface is damaged extensively. Resection and bypass grafting eliminates the previously endarterectomized area but replaces the risk of thrombosis of the normal segment with the risk of thrombus within the graft. Treiman and associates[96] demonstrated that, in their hands, carotid resection with saphenous vein interposition graft placement was as safe and effective as repeat carotid endarterectomy with patch angioplasty. The use of a shunt may be strongly considered because a repeat procedure is usually more difficult and lengthy than a primary operation and by its nature the pathophysiology more

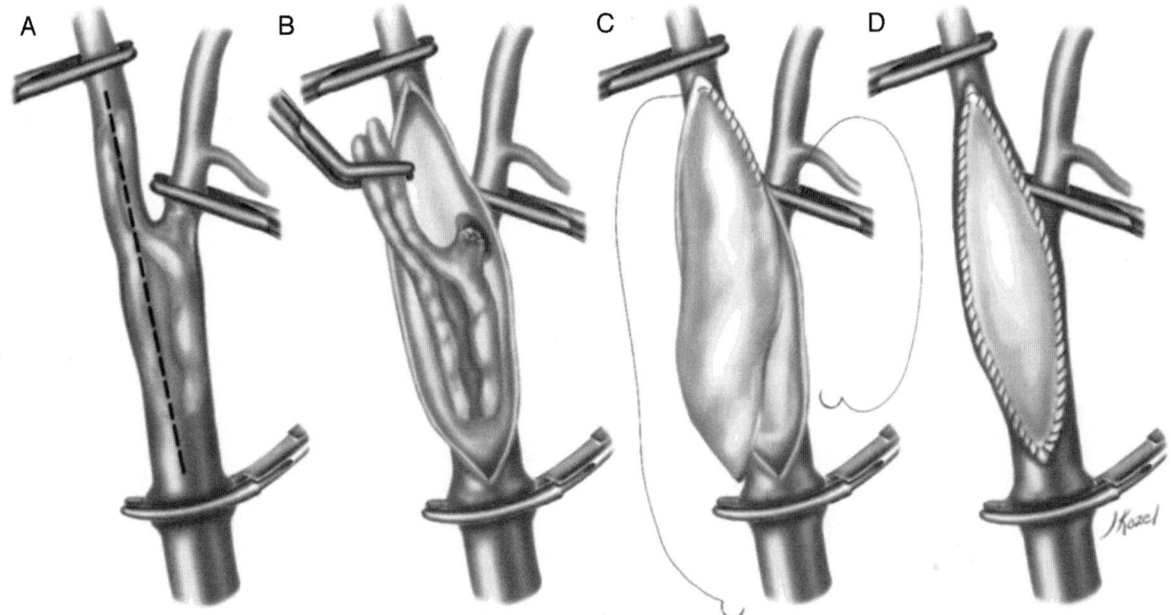

FIGURE 99–3. *A–D,* Patch angioplasty with endarterectomy.

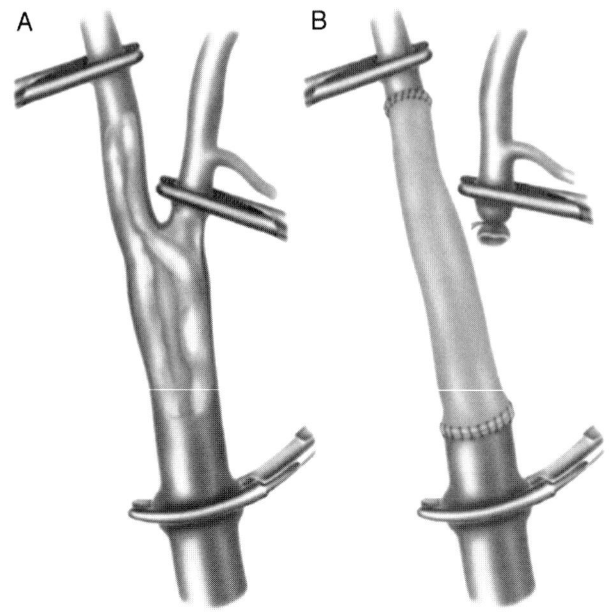

FIGURE 99–4. *A, B,* Interposition vein graft placement on the carotid artery.

commonly involves patients with flow-related symptoms than does primary atherosclerosis.

Although it is generally recognized that repeat carotid endarterectomy is associated with a higher risk than is surgery for primary disease, redo operations may have an acceptable perioperative stroke and mortality rate.[23] Given the technical challenges of a repeated operation, it is not surprising that the complication rate appears to be somewhat higher than that after primary carotid endarterectomy. The reported incidence of stroke following surgery for recurrent carotid stenosis ranges from 0% to 6.5% and death from 0% to 3.1%, with a combined incidence of stroke and death of 5.5%.[16, 30, 93–95] Of particular concern is the danger of cranial nerve deficits. Cranial nerve palsies occur in a range of 0% to 20% of patients and are usually temporary in the majority of cases.[16, 30, 93–95] The mandibular branch of the facial, vagus, glossophayngeal, and hypoglossal nerves are at risk.[16, 93] The increased operative morbidity rate is attributed to the greater manipulation required to dissect the carotid bifurcation out of scar tissue with an attendant increase in the risk of thromboembolic complications, dilated vessel, or patch rupture.[97] Wound hematomas has been reported to occur in about 4% of patients.[84]

ANGIOPLASTY

Percutaneous transluminal angioplasty has been proposed as a therapeutic alternative to surgery for recurrent carotid stenosis. Experience is limited, but initial reports suggest some utility of this method of treatment. It can be associated with serious complications such as cerebral embolization, carotid dissection, and carotid occlusion. Intraoperative angioplasty with the common carotid artery exposed under local anesthesia has been advocated as a safer alternative to percutaneous angioplasty in patients with recurrent stenosis. This approach allows backbleeding from the internal carotid artery to wash out potential debris following catheter withdrawal in an attempt to reduce the risk of embolization.

The risk of restenosis after ballon angioplasty is real. Drawing from the experience of balloon angioplasty in coronary arteries, stenting has also been considering for treatment of recurrent carotid stenosis. These stents are under development but the experience in the case of restenosis is very limited. The result of randomized studies of stenting for primary atherosclerosis may not be generalizable to the restenosis population as the pathophysiology is often different.

CONCLUSIONS

Carotid endarterectomy is an established and effective operation with a low incidence of symptomatic recurrent stenosis from 0.8% to 2%. Symptomless recurrence is, however, much more common (from 1.3% to 37%); it usually has a benign course, but the patient may regress. Early recurrent stenosis, occurring within 24 months after initial endarterectomy, is usually due to myointimal hyperplasia, whereas late recurrences, occurring 24 months or more after surgery is usually caused by an atherosclerotic lesion. Intraoperative assessment of carotid endarterectomy by completion angiography and duplex scanning demonstrates that recurrent stenosis may occur in arteries that have had excellent operations, although there is some evidence that a poor technical result may predispose to early and more severe narrowing. The use of a vein patch, shunt, or tacking sutures has not been shown to have a causative effect on restenosis. Similarly, there is no clear association with smoking, hypertension, diabetes, hyperlipidaemia, or male or female sex, although all such factors have been implicated by small or correlational studies.

Many operations have been advocated to treat recurrent stenosis, but there is limited experience at most centers and the nature of the evidence is anecdotal. A previously endarterectomized artery that is heavily infiltrated with atheroma, or an artery in which a sharp dissection plane is difficult to find because of severe myointimal hyperplasia, should be considered for patch angioplasty or replacement with an autologous interposition or prosthetic graft. Balloon angioplasty and stenting is under development for small lesions. Repeat endarterectomy with or without patch angioplasty is acceptable in circumstances with good surgical planes and an adequate resulting lumen. Symptomless carotid restenoses do not necessarily require surgery. Unlike the case of primary disease, we do not have a clinical trial demonstrating a clear benefit of surgery in terms of patient survival or stroke reduction for asymptomatic restenosis. We suggest that the indications for revision surgery on symptomatic recurrent carotid stenosis should be the same as those for the original operation, with the understanding by both surgeon and patient that the secondary operation is more difficult and the complications of stroke, transient neurological events, and cranial nerve palsies are increased. The decision for surgery would then result from a clear understanding of the risks and benefits for this procedure.

REFERENCES

1. Mayberg MR, Wilson SE, Yatsu F, et al: Carotid endarterectomy and prevention of cerebral ischemia in symptomatic carotid stenosis. Veterans Affairs Cooperative Studies Program 309 Trialist Group [see comments]. JAMA 266:3289–3294, 1991.
2. Endarterectomy for asymptomatic carotid artery stenosis. Executive Committee for the Asymptomatic Carotid Atherosclerosis Study [see comments]. JAMA 273:1421–1428, 1995.
3. Beneficial effect of carotid endarterectomy in symptomatic patients with high-grade carotid stenosis. North American Symptomatic Carotid Endarterectomy Trial Collaborators [see comments]. N Engl J Med 325:445–453, 1991.
4. MRC European Carotid Surgery Trial: Interim results for symptomatic patients with severe (70%–99%) or with mild (0–29%) carotid stenosis. European Carotid Surgery Trialists' Collaborative Group [see comments]. Lancet 337:1235–1243, 1991.
5. Lattimer CR, Burnand KG: Recurrent carotid stenosis after carotid endarterectomy. Br J Surg 84:1206–1219, 1997.
6. Eastcott HHG, Pickering GW, Rob CG: Reconstruction of internal carotid artery in a patient with intermittent attacks of hemiplegia. Lancet ii:994–996, 1954.
7. Carballo RE, Towne JB, Seabrook GR, et al: An outcome analysis of carotid endarterectomy: The incidence and natural history of recurrent stenosis. J Vasc Surg 23:749–753; discussion 753–775, 1996.
8. Gagne PJ, Riles TS, Jacobowitz GR, et al: Long-term follow-up of patients undergoing reoperation for recurrent carotid artery disease. J Vasc Surg 18:991–998; discussion 999–1001, 1993.
9. Barnes RW, Nix ML, Wingo JP, et al: Recurrent versus residual carotid stenosis. Incidence detected by Doppler ultrasound. Ann Surg 203:652–660, 1986.
10. DeGroote RD, Lynch TG, Jamil Z, et al: Carotid restenosis: long-term noninvasive follow-up after carotid endarterectomy. Stroke 18:1031–1036, 1987.
11. Civil ID, O'Hara PJ, Hertzer NR, et al: Late patency of the carotid artery after endarterectomy. Problems of definition, follow-up methodology, and data analysis. J Vasc Surg 8:79–85, 1988.
12. Healy DA, Zierler RE, Nicholls SC, et al: Long-term follow-up and clinical outcome of carotid restenosis. J Vasc Surg 10:662–668; discussion 668–669, 1989.
13. Piepgras DG, Sundt TM, Jr, Marsh WR, et al: Recurrent carotid stenosis. Results and complications of 57 operations. Ann Surg 203:205–213, 1986.
14. Kremen JE, Gee W, Kaupp HA, et al: Restenosis or occlusion after carotid endarterectomy: A survey with ocular pneumoplethysmography. Arch Surg 114:608–610, 1979.
15. Cantelmo NL, Cutler BS, Wheeler HB, et al: Noninvasive detection of carotid stenosis following endarterectomy. Arch Surg 116: 1005–1008, 1981.
16. Das MB, Hertzer NR, Ratliff NB, et al: Recurrent carotid stenosis. A five-year series of 65 reoperations. Ann Surg 202:28–35, 1985.
17. Curley S, Edwards WS, Jacob TP: Recurrent carotid stenosis after autologous tissue patching. J Vasc Surg 6:350–354, 1987.
18. Barnes RW, Garrett WV: Intraoperative assessment of arterial reconstruction by Doppler ultrasound. Surg Gynecol Obstet 146: 896–900, 1978.
19. Blaisdell FW, Lim R, Jr, Hall AD: Technical result of carotid endarterectomy. Arteriographic assessment. Am J Surg 114:239–246, 1967.
20. Rosental JJ, Gaspar MR, Movius HJ: Intraoperative arteriography in carotid thromboendarterectomy. Arch Surg 106:806–808, 1973.
21. Stoney RJ and String ST: Recurrent carotid stenosis. Surgery 80: 705–710, 1976.
22. Cossman D, Callow AD, Stein A, et al: Early restenosis after carotid endarterectomy. Arch Surg 113:275–278, 1978.
23. Mansour MA, Kang SS, Baker WH, et al: Carotid endarterectomy for recurrent stenosis. J Vasc Surg 25:877–883, 1997.
24. Reilly LM, Okuhn SP, Rapp JH, et al: Recurrent carotid stenosis: A consequence of local or systemic factors? The influence of unrepaired technical defects. J Vasc Surg 11:448–459; discussion 459–460, 1990.
25. Salvian A, Baker JD, Machleder HI, et al: Cause and noninvasive detection of restenosis after carotid endarterectomy. Am J Surg 146:29–34, 1983.
26. Thomas M, Otis SM, Rush M, et al: Recurrent carotid artery stenosis following endarterectomy. Ann Surg 200:74–79, 1984.
27. Mattos MA, Shamma AR, Rossi N, et al: Is duplex follow-up cost-effective in the first year after carotid endarterectomy? Am J Surg 156:91–95, 1988.
28. Ricotta JJ, O'Brien MS, DeWeese JA: Natural history of recurrent and residual stenosis after carotid endarterectomy: Implications for postoperative surveillance and surgical management. Surgery 112:656–661; discussion 662–663, 1992.
29. Avramovic JR, Fletcher JP: The incidence of recurrent carotid stenosis after carotid endarterectomy and its relationship to neurological events. J Cardiovasc Surg (Torino) 33:54–58, 1992.
30. Coyle KA, Smith RB 3rd, Gray BC, et al: Treatment of recurrent cerebrovascular disease. Review of a 10-year experience. Ann Surg 221:517–521; discussion 521–524, 1995.
31. Clagett GP, Rich NM, McDonald PT, et al: Etiologic factors for recurrent carotid artery stenosis. Surgery 93:313–318, 1983.
32. Ouriel K, Green RM: Clinical and technical factors influencing recurrent carotid stenosis and occlusion after endarterectomy. J Vasc Surg 5:702–706, 1987.
33. Rapp JH, Qvarfordt P, Krupski WC, et al: Hypercholesterolemia and early restenosis after carotid endarterectomy. Surgery 101: 277–282, 1987.
34. Cossman DV, Treiman RL, Foran RF, et al: Surgical approach to recurrent carotid stenosis. Am J Surg 140:209–211, 1980.
35. Dempsey RJ, Diana AL, Moore RW: Thickness of carotid artery atherosclerotic plaque and ischemic risk. Neurosurgery 27:343–348, 1990.
36. Dempsey RJ, Moore RW: Amount of smoking independently predicts carotid artery atherosclerosis severity. Stroke 23:693–696, 1992.
37. Tell GS, Howard G, McKinney WM, et al: Cigarette smoking cessation and extracranial carotid atherosclerosis. JAMA 261: 1178–1180, 1989.
38. Bodily KC, Zierler RE, Marinelli MR, et al: Flow disturbances following carotid endarterectomy. Surg Gynecol Obstet 151:77–80, 1980.
39. Dempsey RJ, Moore RW, Cordero S: Factors leading to early recurrence of carotid plaque after carotid endarterectomy. Surg Neurol 43:278–282; discussion 282–283, 1995.
40. Pedrini L, Pisano E, Sacca A, et al: Carotid endarterectomy in young adults. Int Angiol 10:220–223, 1991.
41. Ten Holter JB, Ackerstaff RG, Thoe Schwartzenberg GW, et al: The impact of vein patch angioplasty on long-term surgical outcome after carotid endarterectomy. A prospective follow-up study with serial duplex scanning. J Cardiovasc Surg (Torino) 31:58–65, 1990
42. Nicholls SC, Phillips DJ, Bergelin RO, et al: Carotid endarterectomy. Relationship of outcome to early restenosis. J Vasc Surg 2: 375–381, 1985.
43. Bernstein EF, Humber PB, Collins GM, et al: Life expectancy and late stroke following carotid endarterectomy. Ann Surg 198: 80–86, 1983.
44. Javid H, Ostermiller WE, Jr, Hengesh JW, et al: Natural history of carotid bifurcation atheroma. Surgery 67:80–86, 1970.
45. Julian OC, Javid H: Surgical management of cerebral arterial insufficiency. Curr Probl Surg Mar:1–42, 1971.
46. Edwards WS, Wilson TA, Bennett A: The long-term effectiveness of carotid endarterectomy in prevention of strokes. Ann Surg 168:765–770, 1968.
47. Aldoori MI, Baird RN: Prospective assessment of carotid endarterectomy by clinical and ultrasonic methods. Br J Surg 74:926–929, 1987.
48. Ackroyd N, Lane R, Appleberg M: Carotid endarterectomy. Long term follow-up with specific reference to recurrent stenosis, contralateral progression, mortality and recurrent neurological episodes. J Cardiovasc Surg (Torino) 27:418–425, 1986.

49. Sundt TM, Sandok BA, Whisnant JP: Carotid endarterectomy. Complications and preoperative assessment of risk. Mayo Clin Proc 50:301–306, 1975.
50. Katz MM, Jones GT, Degenhardt J, et al: The use of patch angioplasty to alter the incidence of carotid restenosis following thromboendarterectomy. J Cardiovasc Surg (Torino) 28:2–8, 1987.
51. Hertzer NR, Beven EG, O'Hara PJ, et al: A prospective study of vein patch angioplasty during carotid endarterectomy. Three-year results for 801 patients and 917 operations. Ann Surg 206: 628–35, 1987.
52. Archie JP Jr: Prevention of early restenosis and thrombosis-occlusion after carotid endarterectomy by saphenous vein patch angioplasty. Stroke 17:901–905, 1986.
53. Eikelboom BC, Ackerstaff RG, Hoeneveld H, et al: Benefits of carotid patching: A randomized study. J Vasc Surg 7:240–247, 1988.
54. Bandyk DF, Kaebnick HW, Adams MB, et al: Turbulence occurring after carotid bifurcation endarterectomy: A harbinger of residual and recurrent carotid stenosis. J Vasc Surg 7:261–274, 1988.
55. Colgan MP, Kingston V, Shanik G: Stenosis following carotid endarterectomy. Its implication in management of asymptomatic carotid stenosis. Arch Surg 119:1033–1035, 1984.
56. Stewart GW, Bandyk DF, Kaebnick HW, et al: Influence of vein-patch angioplasty on carotid endarterectomy healing. Arch Surg 122:364–371, 1987.
57. Rosenthal D, Archie JP Jr, Garcia-Rinaldi R, et al: Carotid patch angioplasty: immediate and long-term results [see comments]. J Vasc Surg 12:326–333, 1990.
58. Myers SI, Valentine RJ, Chervu A, et al: Saphenous vein patch versus primary closure for carotid endarterectomy: Long-term assessment of a randomized prospective study. J Vasc Surg 19: 15–22, 1994.
59. Sundt TM Jr, Houser OW, Fode NC, et al: Correlation of postoperative and two-year follow-up angiography with neurological function in 99 carotid endarterectomies in 86 consecutive patients. Ann Surg 203:90–100, 1986.
60. Ojemann RG, Crowell RM: Surgical Management of Cerebrovascular Disease. Baltimore, Williams & Wilkins, 1983.
61. Baker WH, Hayes AC, Mahler D, et al: Durability of carotid endarterectomy. Surgery 94:112–115, 1983.
62. Diaz FG, Patel S, Boulos R, et al: Early angiographic changes after carotid endarterectomy. Neurosurgery 10:151–161, 1982.
63. Hertzer NR, Beven EG, Modic MT, et al: Early patency of the carotid artery after endarterectomy: Digital subtraction angiography after two hundred sixty-two operations. Surgery 92:1049–1057, 1982.
64. Takolander R, Bergentz SE, Bergqvist D, et al: Management of early neurological deficits after carotid thrombendarterectomy. Eur J Vasc Surg 1:67–71, 1987.
65. Raines EW, Ross R: Smooth muscle cells and the pathogenesis of the lesions of atherosclerosis. Br Heart J 69:S30–S37, 1993.
66. Sterpetti AV, Schultz RD, Feldhaus RJ, et al: Natural history of recurrent carotid artery disease. Surg Gynecol Obstet 168: 217–223, 1989.
67. Imparato AM, Bracco A, Kim GE, et al: Intimal and neointimal fibrous proliferation causing failure of arterial reconstructions. Surgery 72:1007–1017, 1972.
68. Zucker MB: The functioning of blood platelets. Sci Am 242: 86–103, 1980.
69. Schwarcz TH, Yates GN, Ghobrial M, et al: Pathologic characteristics of recurrent carotid artery stenosis. J Vasc Surg 5:280–288, 1987.
70. Callow AD: Recurrent stenosis after carotid endarterectomy. Arch Surg 117:1082–1085, 1982.
71. Bandyk DF, Moldenhauer P, Lipchik E, et al: Accuracy of duplex scanning in the detection of stenosis after carotid endarterectomy. J Vasc Surg 8:696–702, 1988.
72. Hunter GC, Palmaz JC, Hayashi HH, et al: The etiology of symptoms in patients with recurrent carotid stenosis. Arch Surg 122:311–315, 1987.
73. Washburn WK, Mackey WC, Belkin M, et al: Late stroke after carotid endarterectomy: The role of recurrent stenosis. J Vasc Surg 15:1032–1036; discussion 1036–1037, 1992.
74. Sanders EA, Hoeneveld H, Eikelboom BC, et al: Residual lesions and early recurrent stenosis after carotid endarterectomy. A serial follow-up study with duplex scanning and intravenous digital subtraction angiography [see comments]. J Vasc Surg 5:731–737, 1987.
75. Zierler RE, Bandyk DF, Thiele BL, et al: Carotid artery stenosis following endarterectomy. Arch Surg 117:1408–1415, 1982.
76. Ricotta JJ, Bryan FA, Bond MG, et al: Multicenter validation study of real-time (B-mode) ultrasound, arteriography, and pathologic examination. J Vasc Surg 6:512–520, 1987.
77. Keagy BA, Edrington RD, Poole MA, et al: Incidence of recurrent or residual stenosis after carotid endarterectomy. Am J Surg 149: 722–725, 1985.
78. Chilcote WA, Modic MT, Pavlicek WA, et al: Digital subtraction angiography of the carotid arteries: A comparative study in 100 patients. Radiology 139:287–295, 1981.
79. Dempsey R: Neurosonology. In Youmans J (ed): Neurological Surgery. Philadelphia, WB Saunders, 1996, pp 214–222.
80. Caps MT, Hatsukami TS, Primozich JF, et al: A clinical marker for arterial wall healing: The double line. J Vasc Surg 23:87–93, discussion 93–94, 1996.
81. Palmaz JC, Hunter G, Carson SN, et al: Postoperative carotid restenosis due to neointimal fibromuscular hyperplasia. Clinical, angiographic, and pathological findings. Radiology 148:699–702, 1983.
82. Hunter GC: Edgar J. Poth Memorial/W.L. Gore and Associates, Inc. Lectureship. The clinical and pathological spectrum of recurrent carotid stenosis. Am J Surg 174:583–588, 1997.
83. Raithel D: Technique and results of carotid endarterectomy in patients with contralateral carotid occlusion. In Current Critical Problems in Vascular Surgery. St. Louis, Quality Medical Publishing, 1990, pp 407–413.
84. O'Donnell TF, Jr, Rodriguez AA, Fortunato JE, et al: Management of recurrent carotid stenosis: Should asymptomatic lesions be treated surgically? J Vasc Surg 24:207–212, 1996.
85. Cook JM, Thompson BW, Barnes RW: Is routine duplex examination after carotid endarterectomy justified? J Vasc Surg 12:334–340, 1990.
86. Ross R: The pathogenesis of atherosclerosis: A perspective for the 1990s. Nature 362:801–809, 1993.
87. Harker LA, Bernstein EF, Dilley RB, et al: Failure of aspirin plus dipyridamole to prevent restenosis after carotid endarterectomy. Ann Intern Med 116:731–736, 1992.
88. Dangas G, Fuster V: Management of restenosis after coronary intervention. Am Heart J 132:428–436, 1996.
89. Colburn MD, Moore WS, Gelabert HA, et al: Dose responsive suppression of myointimal hyperplasia by dexamethasone. J Vasc Surg 15:510–518, 1992.
90. Emanuelsson H, Beatt KJ, Bagger JP, et al: Long-term effects of angiopeptin treatment in coronary angioplasty. Reduction of clinical events but not angiographic restenosis. European Angiopeptin Study Group [see comments]. Circulation 91:1689–1696, 1995.
91. Ohno T, Gordon D, San H, et al: Gene therapy for vascular smooth muscle cell proliferation after arterial injury [see comments]. Science 265:781–784, 1994.
92. Rosenman J, Edwards WS, Robillard D, et al: Carotid arterial bifurcation advancement. Surg Gynecol Obstet 159:260–264, 1984.
93. Bartlett FF, Rapp JH, Goldstone J, et al: Recurrent carotid stenosis: Operative strategy and late results. J Vasc Surg 5:452–456, 1987.
94. Kazmers A, Zierler RE, Huang TW, et al: Reoperative carotid surgery. Am J Surg 156:346–352, 1988.
95. AbuRahma AF, Snodgrass KR, Robinson PA, et al: Safety and durability of redo carotid endarterectomy for recurrent carotid artery stenosis. Am J Surg 168:175–178, 1994.
96. Treiman GS, Jenkins JM, Edwards WH Sr, et al: The evolving surgical management of recurrent carotid stenosis. J Vasc Surg 16:354–362; discussion 362–363, 1992.
97. Meyer FB, Piepgras DG, Sundt TMJ, et al: Recurrent carotid stenosis. In Meyer FB (ed): Sundt's Occlusive Cerebrovascular Disease. Philadelphia, WB Saunders, 1994, pp 310–321.

CHAPTER **100**

Traumatic Carotid Injury

CARGILL H. ALLEYNE, JR. ■ A. GIANCARLO VISHTEH ■ ROBERT F. SPETZLER

The terms *pseudoaneurysms, dissecting aneurysms,* and *false aneurysms* have been applied to traumatic (and spontaneous) injury of the carotid artery. A mural arterial dissection or dissecting aneurysm occurs when blood penetrates the wall of the artery and enters along the wall a variable distance. A false lumen can be created in the media close to the intima (subintimal) or close to the adventitia (subadventitial). The false lumen can narrow or compress the true lumen or may expand toward the adventitia, causing a dissecting aneurysm. Pseudoaneurysms or false aneurysms are collections of blood that communicate with the blood vessel lumen but are not contained by elements of the blood vessel wall. The latter are usually caused by penetrating injury. Most carotid artery dissections occur at the cervical segment of the internal carotid artery (ICA). Dissections also occur along transition points between the cervical and petrous or petrous and cavernous segments. A ruptured traumatic dissecting aneurysm in the cavernous segment of the ICA can lead to the formation of a carotid-cavernous fistula. An ICA dissection causing a traumatic aneurysm to form is rare along the supraclinoid segment of the ICA. Because the ICA is tethered along its clinoidal segment by dural rings and its proximity to the bony skull base, traumatic acceleration or deceleration can cause such vascular injuries.

HISTORY

The earliest treatment of a carotid artery injury was reported in 1552 by Ambroise Paré, who stopped a hemorrhage from the lacerated right common carotid artery (CCA) of a duelist.[1] Although he did not report the event until 1804, in 1798, John Abernethy[1] ligated the CCA of a patient who was gored in the neck by a bull. Although the hemorrhage was controlled, the patient died 30 hours later from hypotensive blood loss. An ICA dissection from blunt, nonpenetrating injury was reported in 1872,[2] but the next case was not reported until 1942.[3]

PATHOGENESIS

Traumatic injury of the CCA and ICA may result from penetrating or blunt trauma. Iatrogenic causes of carotid injury (e.g., needle puncture, arterial catheterization) during angiography have been described.[4–6] Most series of carotid artery injuries have documented that injuries related to penetrating trauma are more common than those related to blunt trauma. Handguns cause most penetrating injuries to the carotid artery. For example, a review of 703 carotid artery injuries in the English literature revealed 244 gunshot wounds, 90 stab wounds, 133 other penetrating injuries, and 73 blunt injuries.[7]

Penetrating injury can completely or partially disrupt a vessel, pseudoaneurysm, arteriovenous fistula, or local hemorrhage. Blunt injury to the carotid artery usually is associated with motor vehicle accidents, but a variety of precipitating factors such as falls, boxing, altercations, direct trauma to the neck, diagnostic carotid compression, and chiropractic manipulation have been reported.[8]

Various mechanisms of blunt carotid injury have been postulated. Hyperextension and rotation to the contralateral side can stretch the cervical ICA against the transverse processes of the second and third vertebral bodies. Hyperextension and contralateral lateral flexion can produce the same effect.[9] Sudden hyperflexion can compress the ICA between the angle of the mandible and the upper cervical vertebrae.[10] Extreme head rotations can impinge the ICA against a prominent styloid process.[11]

CLINICAL MANIFESTATIONS AND INDICATIONS

A high index of suspicion for carotid artery injury needs to be maintained. About one half of all patients with a traumatic carotid artery injury do not manifest external signs of injury to the neck. Many patients manifest only minor external signs (i.e., bruises around the neck). Conversely, many patients with a penetrating neck injury may not have an arterial injury.[12] The physical examination, although invaluable in the assessment of patients with suspected carotid artery injury, cannot be relied on exclusively to make an accurate diagnosis. Traumatic extracranial carotid artery (ECA) injuries can manifest as exsanguination, as soft tissue hemorrhage with or without airway impairment, or as an aneurysm. The latter may become symptomatic in a delayed fashion and cause difficulty with breathing and swallowing, or cranial nerve deficits.

The diagnosis of a traumatic artery injury can be compounded by the presence of an accompanying head injury (e.g., patients involved in motor vehicle accidents). Diagnosis can be delayed or even missed. In a series of 51 patients with blunt carotid artery trauma reported before 1967, diagnosis was delayed in 94% of patients for as long as several days because symptoms occurred after a period of latency or resembled symptoms associated with a closed head injury. In a later report of 96 patients with blunt carotid artery trauma (which included the former series),[13] physical signs of trauma were absent in one half of the cases, and the onset of symptoms was more than 24 hours after presentation in 35% of the patients. The neurological manifestations of carotid artery injury include unilateral motor or sensory loss, amaurosis fugax, aphasia, decreased level of consciousness, Horner's syndrome, transient ischemic attacks, and dysgenesia.

As outlined by Mokri,[14] indications for carotid artery imaging include focal and neurological deficits with a normal head computed tomographic study or one that does not explain the deficits, progressive neurological deficits with computed tomography (CT) of the head that is normal or that does not explain the deficit, and delayed neurological deficits with CT that fails to explain the clinical findings. We also recommend an imaging study for patients who manifest fractures involving the carotid canal on head CT with a bone algorithm.

GENERAL EVALUATION OF MANAGEMENT OF PENETRATING NECK INJURIES

Historically, the neck has been divided into 3 zones. Zone I is below a horizontal line 1 cm above the clavicular-manubrial junction or inferior to the cricoid cartilage, zone II is between zone I and the angle of the mandible, and zone III is between the angle of the mandible and the base of the skull (Fig. 100–1).[15] This classification has been useful in describing the management of patients with penetrating neck injuries. The more aggressive approach of routinely exploring wounds that penetrate the platysma was espoused in the past. This resulted in a high percentage of negative explorations, and a more selective approach based on symptomatology, arteriography, esophageal studies, and location of the neck injury is generally done at most institutions. In general, patients with zone I injuries undergo angiography, esophagoscopy, and bronchoscopy unless they are unstable. If hemodynamically unstable, they should be taken directly to the operating room. Patients with zone II injuries who are unstable or who have evidence of airway compromise or hemorrhage should be explored promptly. Stable patients with zone II injuries should be locally explored. Wounds that do not penetrate the platysma should be closed. Most of the remainder of zone II injuries can be observed. Patients with zone III injuries require carotid and vertebral angiography if there is evidence of arterial bleeding.

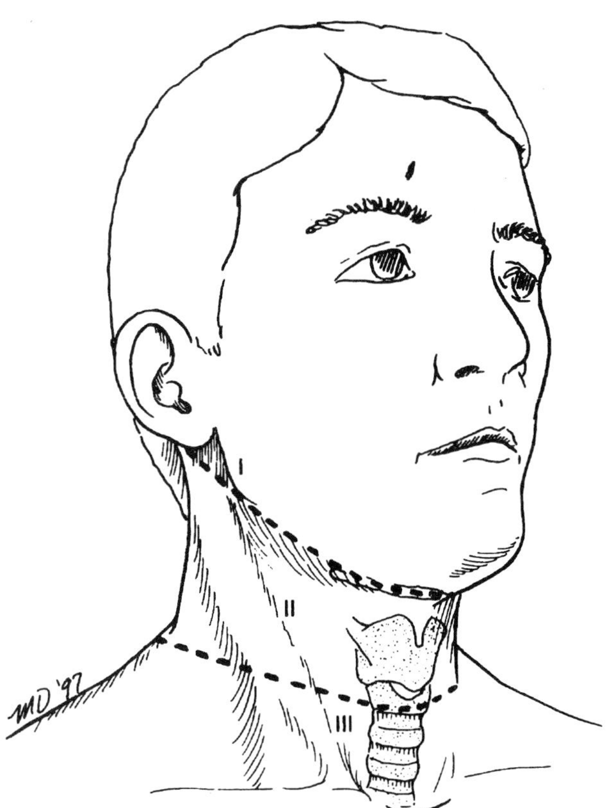

FIGURE 100–1. Diagram of Monson's zones of the neck. (From Schwartz SI [ed]: Principles of Surgery, 7th ed. New York, McGraw-Hill, 1999, p 166.)

Biffl and colleagues[16] reviewed their 18-year, prospective evaluation of a selective approach to the management of these injuries. Of 312 patients, 75% were stabbed, and 24% were shot. Zones I, II, and III were penetrated in 13%, 67%, and 20% of cases, respectively. In all, 105 (34%) were symptomatic and were explored (29% in zone I, 38% in zone II, and 22% in zone III). Eighty-eight patients (84%) had 111 injuries warranting exploration. There were 36 venous, 26 arterial, 19 digestive tract, 17 airway, and 13 miscellaneous injuries. Of the 207 (67%) patients observed, 1 (0.5%) required delayed exploration. The authors conclude that selective management of penetrating neck injuries is safe and does not mandate routine diagnostic testing for patients with injuries in zones II and III.

DIAGNOSTIC EVALUATION

Plain CT of the head is essential in the evaluation of patients with neurological deficits who are suspected of having a carotid dissection. The diagnosis should be further suspected if CT is negative or does not explain the clinical manifestations. Although evidence of ischemia typically appears 24 to 48 hours after the event, massive infarctions may be diagnosed earlier. The bone windows on the CT are helpful in diagnosing fractures in the carotid canal at the skull base. CT of the neck can arouse suspicion for carotid artery injury if a fracture through the lateral masses or subluxation is identified.

Arteriography remains the gold standard for the evaluation of arterial pathology. Arteriography reveals the site of injury, type of injury (i.e., dissection, intimal flap, stenosis, aneurysm, thrombosis, distal pouches, and distal branch occlusion, which are the hallmarks of cerebral emboli). Plain radiography may be helpful in the diagnosis of facial fractures and cervical fractures that may be associated with carotid artery injuries.

Duplex ultrasonography of the ICA may reveal indirect and direct signs of dissection.[17] The latter include tapering of the lateral carotid artery lumen more than 2 cm distal to the bulb, an irregular membrane crossing the ICA lumen, and demonstration of a true and false lumen. The use of this modality is limited in injuries involving the high cervical carotid artery. Magnetic resonance angiography is becoming increasingly popular as a noninvasive diagnostic tool that can diagnose arterial dissections, especially on axial, fat-suppressed images.

Patients who present with delayed ischemic symptoms or continued ischemic symptoms despite conservative therapy (i.e., anticoagulation) may be candidates for revascularization. Patients who cannot be placed on anticoagulation (i.e., coexistent systemic injuries) and who continue to have progressive ischemia may be candidates for revascularization. Preoperative xenon–computed tomographic study with or without a Diamox challenge may be useful in patients with delayed ischemic symptoms because this blood-flow study can reveal the presence and degree of vascular steal and the loss of vascular reserve. This information can help determine the need for a high-flow or low-flow bypass procedure.

TREATMENTS AND OUTCOMES

The natural history of traumatic ICA injury is somewhat worse than that of spontaneous ICA injury. Mokri and coworkers[8, 14, 18] retrospectively reviewed the records of 21 patients with traumatic extracranial ICA dissections and 70 patients with spontaneous ICA dissections. Aneurysms were more common in the traumatic group than in the spontaneous group. Likewise, significantly fewer aneurysms resolved or became smaller, fewer stenoses resolved or improved, and more stenoses progressed to occlusion in the traumatic group. Traumatic dissections were also more likely to result in persistent neurological deficits. A significantly higher percentage of patients with spontaneous dissections was asymptomatic at follow-up examinations compared with the traumatic group.

Medical Therapy

The optimal treatment of traumatic dissections has been controversial. Some physicians have proposed conservative medical management for patients[9, 13] with traumatic carotid artery dissections. Pathology is often located at the level of upper cervical vertebrae, where surgical accessibility is limited. The injury to the vessel often renders it fragile and precludes direct repair. The risk of postoperative parent vessel occlusion may also be high.

Stringer and Kelly[9] reported six cases of traumatic dissections of the ECA that were successfully treated conservatively. Five of the six patients received anticoagulation therapy. Batzdorf and coworkers[19] reported using supportive therapy or trapping the injured segment as an alternative to direct thromboendarterectomy, which has yielded dismal results in some studies.[20]

Most physicians favor anticoagulation as the initial therapy for patients with a carotid artery injury.[8, 10–14, 18, 21–23] After a brief period of heparinization, the patient is placed on warfarin. Follow-up studies, such as magnetic resonance angiography, are obtained periodically (e.g., every 3 months) to assess healing of the injury. If the injury has healed, the anticoagulation therapy can be stopped, and an antiplatelet agent can be added. No controlled studies have compared antiplatelet with anticoagulation therapy or compared surgical with medical therapy.

Surgical Therapy

The surgical options for the treatment of carotid artery injury include vessel reconstruction and direct repair, thromboendarterectomy, vessel ligation, surgical trapping, or revascularization procedures. Some surgeons have adopted a more surgically aggressive approach to carotid artery injury. In a review of 52 patients with carotid artery injury, 37% of those undergoing surgery and 65% of those undergoing nonoperative management had a stroke or died.[24] In another series of 96 patients, 32% of the surgically treated group were asymptomatic compared with 4% of the conservatively treated group. Fifty-three percent of the surgically treated group suffered a severe deficit or died, compared with a mortality rate of 86% for the conservatively treated group.[13]

Unger and associates[7] documented the outcome of 722 patients with carotid artery trauma. Of the patients undergoing arterial repair, 34% improved compared with 14% of patients undergoing carotid ligation or not undergoing surgical treatment. Stroke or coma was an independent predictor of that outcome. In patients with preoperative neurological deficits, there was no evidence to suggest that prompt arterial repair yielded better results than delayed repair.

In addition to thromboendarterectomy and trapping, revascularization procedures can also be considered in appropriate patients. The presence of systemic traumatic injury in patients with carotid artery injury may preclude heparinization. Patients who manifest recurrent ischemic symptoms or progressive ischemic deficits may also be considered for revascularization. Vishteh and colleagues[23] reported the results of 13 patients who underwent 16 revascularization procedures for symptomatic traumatic ICA dissection. The 13 patients made up 17% of a population of 76 patients diagnosed with traumatic ICA dissections during a 7-year period. Blunt trauma and penetrating trauma were the causes in 11 and 2 patients, respectively. Six patients underwent "early" revascularization after stabilization of other systemic injuries. Two of these patients continued to experience recurrent transient ischemic attacks despite anticoagulation therapy. Both patients had an ipsilateral ICA occlusion distal to the dissection. Two other patients had multiple visceral injuries that precluded systemic anticoagulation therapy. The two remaining patients developed cavernous ICA aneurysms that ruptured and carotid-cavernous fistulas associated with their dissections. Seven patients underwent delayed revascularization procedures after initially responding to medical therapy, but they eventually developed refractory cerebrovascular ischemia.

In this study, four different revascularization procedures were used. A cervical-to-petrous ICA bypass was performed in eight patients, a cervical ICA–to–middle cerebral artery (MCA) bypass in three patients, a petrous-to-supraclinoid ICA bypass in three patients, and

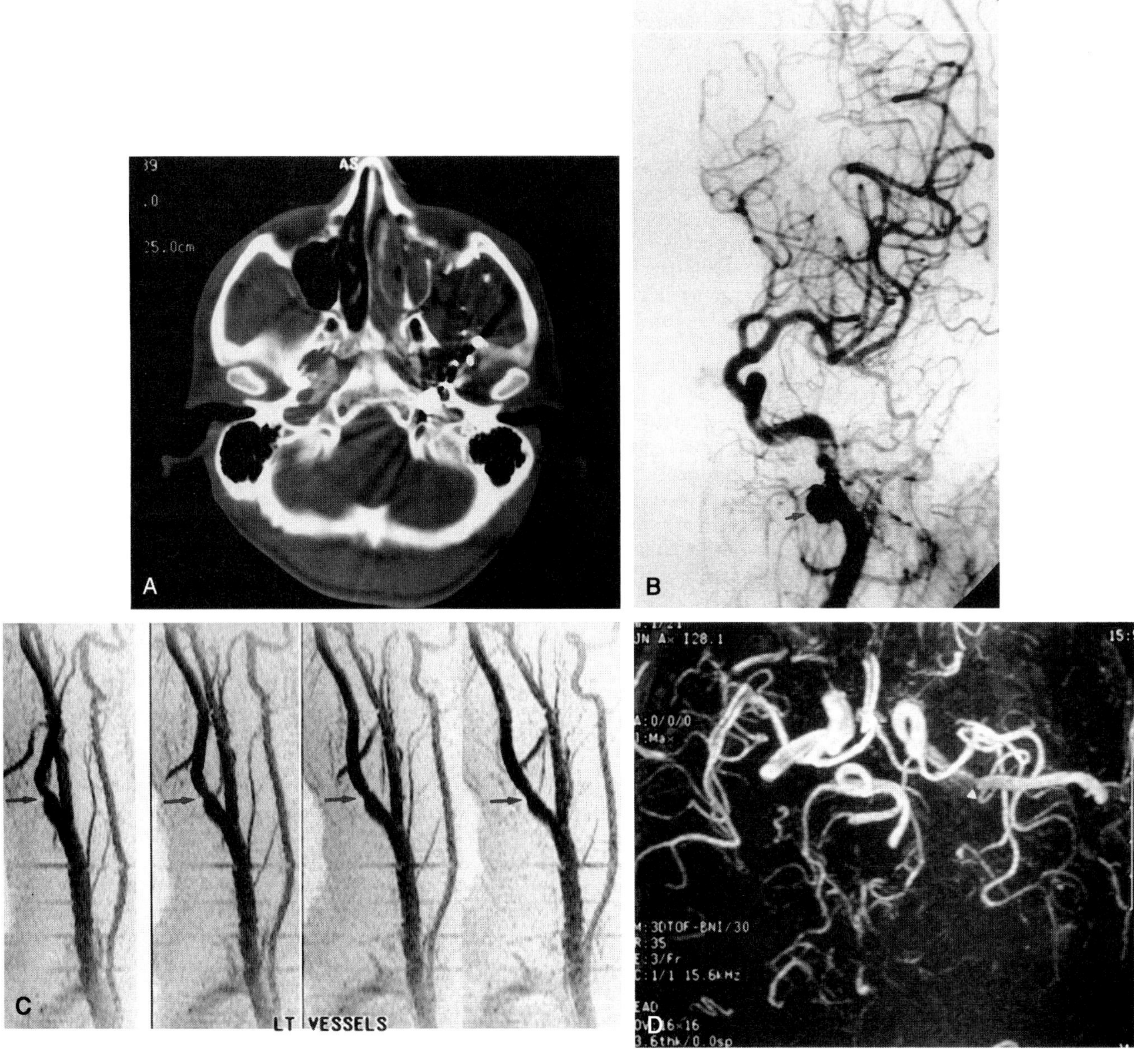

FIGURE 100–2. Cervical-to-petrous bypass for a traumatic dissecting internal carotid artery (ICA) aneurysm after penetrating (gunshot) trauma. *A,* Axial computed tomogram (bone algorithm) shows a bullet lodged near the left carotid canal. *B,* Lateral angiogram of the left common carotid artery shows dissection and the resulting aneurysm *(arrow)* at the cranial base. *C* and *D,* After cervical-to-petrous bypass surgery, the 1-year follow-up magnetic resonance angiograms show graft patency at the level of the left cervical ICA *(arrows)(C)* and petrous ICA *(white arrowhead) (D).* A minor amount of artifact from the petrous carotid clip is at the distal anastomosis site, but good flow signal distally can be seen. (From Vishteh AG, Marciano FF, David CA, et al: Long-term graft patency rates and clinical outcomes after revascularization for symptomatic traumatic internal carotid artery dissection. Neurosurgery 43:761–767, 1998.)

a superficial temporal artery (STA)–to–MCA bypass in two patients. All bypasses were performed under barbiturate-burst suppression after an intravenous bolus of heparin.

CERVICAL-TO-PETROUS INTERNAL CAROTID ARTERY BYPASS

For the high-flow bypasses, the saphenous vein was harvested as previously described.[25–27] The cervical ICA was exposed in the neck, and a pterional-subtemporal (half and half) craniotomy was performed to expose the petrous ICA and Glasscock's triangle.[28] The saphenous vein interposition graft was secured by performing an end-to-end anastomosis of the cervical ICA and an end-to-side anastomosis at the petrous ICA (Fig. 100–2).

CERVICAL INTERNAL CAROTID ARTERY–TO–MIDDLE CEREBRAL ARTERY BYPASS

The cervical ICA was exposed in the neck and the saphenous vein was harvested. A pterional craniotomy

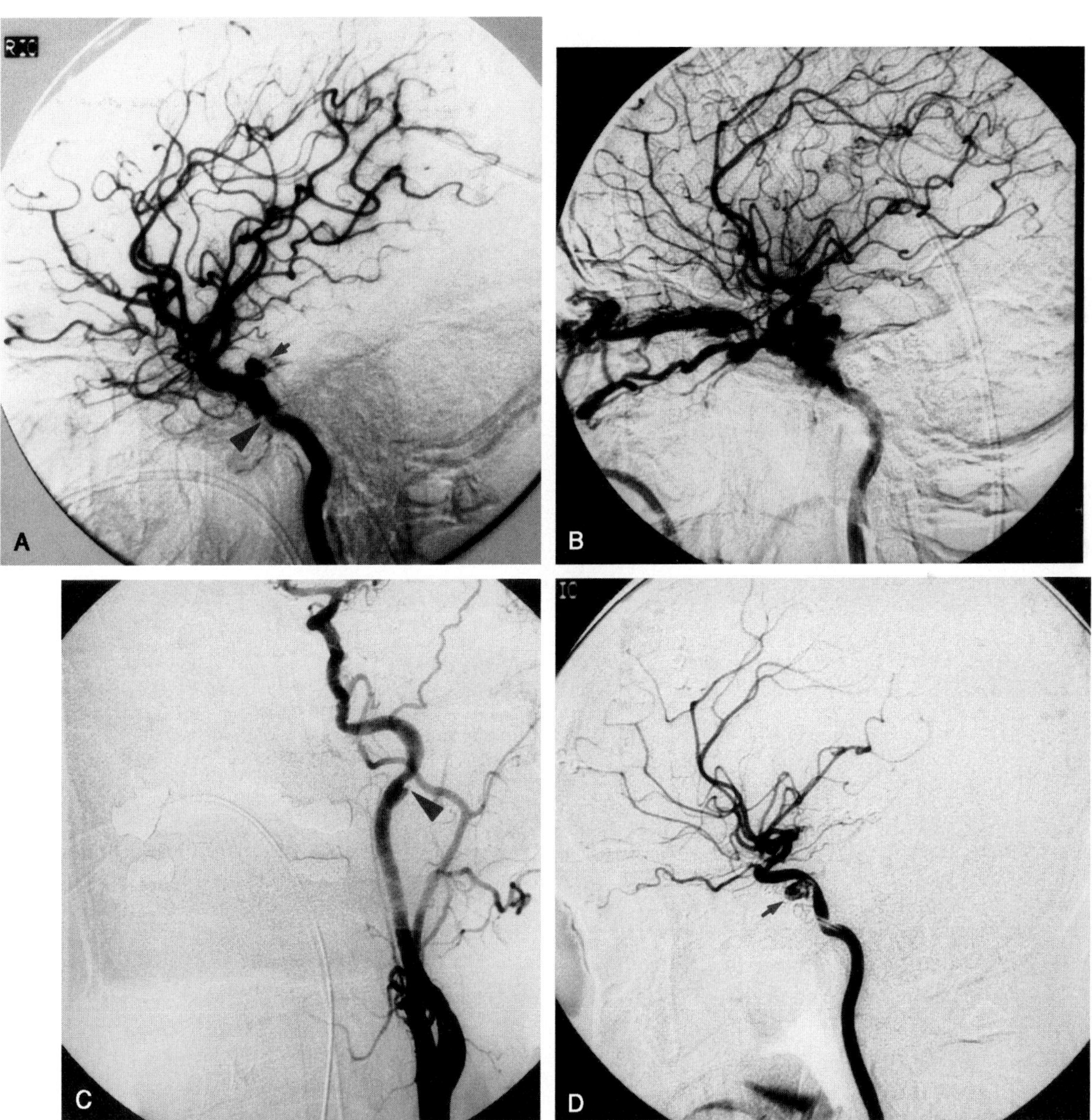

FIGURE 100–3. Bilateral petrous-to-supraclinoid bypasses for refractory cavernous-carotid fistulas after rupture of dissecting aneurysms (blunt trauma). *A,* Lateral view angiogram of the right internal carotid artery (ICA) shows dissection with a flap *(arrowhead)* and the resulting aneurysm *(arrow)*. *B,* Follow-up angiogram shows carotid-cavernous fistula (CCF) formation. *C,* Angiogram of the left common carotid artery shows the ICA dissection flap *(arrowhead)* (resolved at follow-up). *D,* Angiogram of the left ICA shows the left cavernous carotid aneurysm *(arrow)*. Digitally subtracted coils (from failed endovascular therapy) and a clip are superimposed from the contralateral side.

Illustration continues on following page.

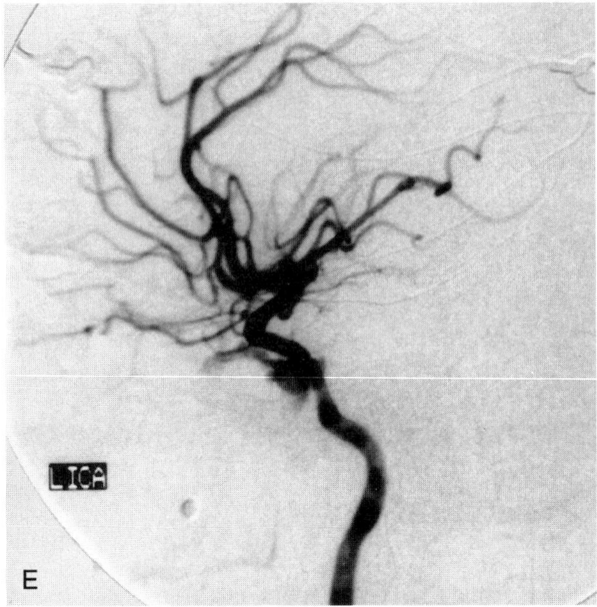

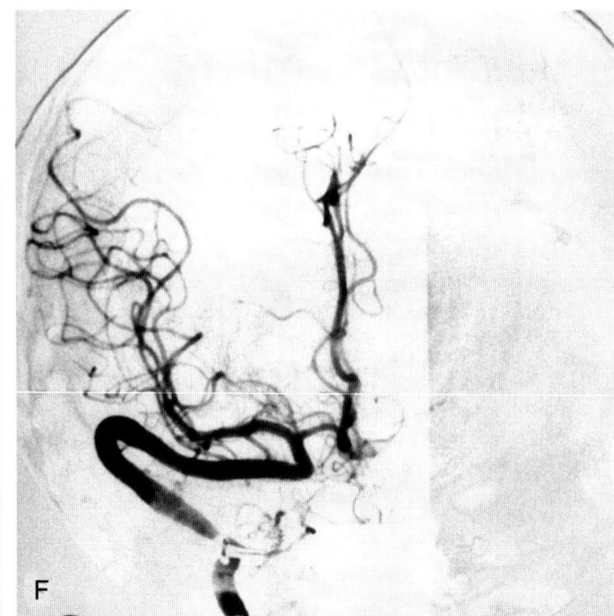

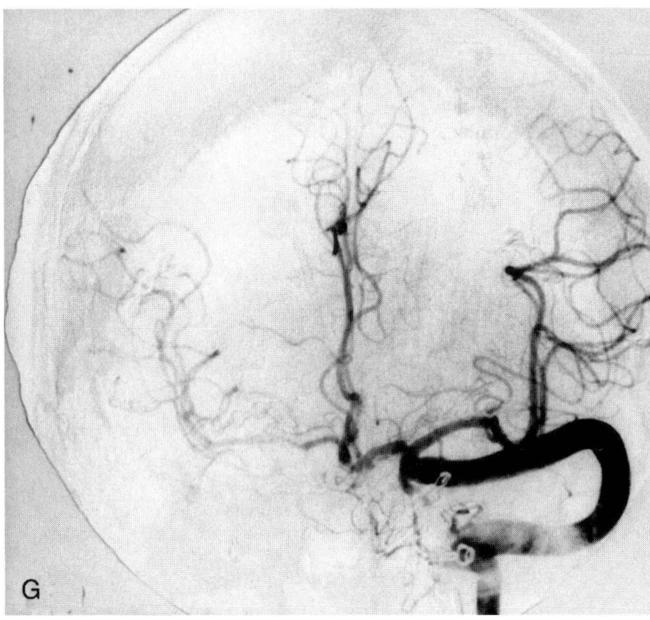

FIGURE 100–3. *Continued. E,* Follow-up angiogram of the left ICA shows the formation of a CCF. *F* and *G,* The 2-year follow-up angiograms, obtained after bilateral petrous-to-supraclinoid bypass surgery, show patency of right *(F)* and left *(G)* ICA grafts. (From Vishteh AG, Marciano FF, David CA, et al: Long-term graft patency rates and clinical outcomes after revascularization for symptomatic traumatic internal carotid artery dissection. Neurosurgery 43:761–767, 1998.)

was performed, and the sylvian fissure was widely dissected to expose the proximal MCA segments. An end-to-side anastomosis was performed at the M2 branch, and an end-to-end anastomosis was performed at the cervical ICA.

PETROUS-TO-SUPRACLINOID INTERNAL CAROTID ARTERY BYPASS

The petrous ICA was exposed in Glasscock's triangle.[28] The sylvian fissure was widely dissected and the supraclinoid ICA was exposed. The harvested saphenous vein graft was sewn end-to-side at the petrous ICA and the supraclinoid ICA (Fig. 100–3).

SUPERFICIAL TEMPORAL ARTERY–TO–MIDDLE CEREBRAL ARTERY BYPASS

The main trunk of the STA and its parietal branch were identified by using intraoperative Doppler ultrasonography. The STA was dissected, and a temporoparietal craniotomy was made over Chatter's point. The STA branch was then sewn end-to-side to a superficial MCA branch. Three patients underwent bilateral bypass procedures, and all received antiplatelet therapy after surgery.

OUTCOMES OF SURGERY

Immediately after surgery, graft patency was confirmed in 15 cases. The mean clinical follow-up of the 13 patients undergoing 16 revascularization procedures was 44.3 months. All patients had Glasgow Outcome Score (GOS) scores of 5 and Glasgow Coma Scale (GCS) scores of 15 at follow-up, and no patient was experiencing transient ischemic attacks.

One cervical-to-petrous ICA saphenous vein bypass occluded in the immediate postoperative period but was successfully reopened after thrombectomy. Subsequent angiography documented graft patency. At long-term follow-up (mean, 24 months), graft patency was confirmed by angiography in five patients, magnetic resonance angiography in four patients, and duplex ultrasonography in four patients. One patient developed a postoperative epidural hematoma that was evacuated. A cerebrospinal fluid leak in one patient with a cervical-to-petrous bypass responded to a short course of lumbar drainage.

One patient with bilateral ICA dissections died of a pulmonary embolus soon after her 12-month follow-up examination when her GCS score was 15 and her GOS score was 4. She had mild hemiparesis and patent grafts.

All patients with preoperative hemiparesis or dysphasia improved after surgery. Ophthalmoplegia resolved in one eye of a patient with bilateral ICA dissections, ruptured cavernous-carotid aneurysms, and carotid-cavernous fistulas, but he remained blind and ophthalmoplegic in the other eye. Another patient with an enlarging traumatic cavernous aneurysm experienced ophthalmoparesis that resolved after bypass surgery. Horner's syndrome resolved in one patient and was unchanged in the other after surgery.

Endovascular Therapy

Since the concept of percutaneous transluminal angioplasty was first introduced by Dotter and Judkins in 1964,[29] the technique has revolutionized the field of vascular medicine, especially the treatment of coronary disease. The technique of maintaining luminal patency with a stent after angioplasty has been refined considerably. The treatment of supra-aortic vessels, however, has lagged behind that of the coronary system, mainly because the risk of morbidity associated with distal embolization in this arterial distribution is significant.

Although the role of angioplasty and stenting procedures in traumatic carotid injury awaits further elucidation, stents have been used successfully to treat traumatic carotid dissections by reapproximating an intimal flap against the parent vessel and maintaining patency of the lumen, especially along the straight segments of the ICA.[30]

CONCLUSIONS

Traumatic carotid artery injury remains a significant cause of morbidity and mortality among the relatively young. The effects of injury to the carotid artery may not be obvious immediately after injury, and a high index of suspicion must be maintained for the diagnosis. When symptomatic, manifestations of carotid artery injury can be varied but range from the subtle (e.g., Horner's syndrome) to the profound (e.g., coma). Concomitant intracranial injury can confound the diagnosis. A variety of diagnostic tests, including angiography, magnetic resonance angiography, Doppler ultrasonography, and CT, can be used. The treatment of carotid artery injury remains somewhat controversial but includes expectant management, medical therapy (e.g., anticoagulation, antiplatelet therapy), and surgical intervention (e.g., direct repair, ligation, trapping, revascularization). Although not yet completely defined, early endovascular treatment of these injuries with stents is promising.[30] Endovascular therapy will probably become the mainstay of treatment in medically refractory cases of traumatic ICA dissection, especially for dissections involving straight segments or the petrous portion of the ICA. Revascularization can be reserved for medically refractory cases, involving segments deemed too risky for stent deployment. Overall, however, the decision regarding the appropriate management remains difficult and must be individualized by careful consideration of all available data.

REFERENCES

1. Abernethy J: Surgical Observations Containing a Classification of Tumours, with Cases to Illustrate the History of Each Species; an Account of Diseases which Strikingly Resemble the Veneral Disease; and Various Cases Illustrative of Various Surgical Subjects. London, England, Longman & Rees, 1804.
2. Verneil M: Contusions multiples, delire violent, hemiplegie adroite, signes de compression cerebrale. Bull Acad Natl Med (Paris) 1:46–56, 1872.
3. Cairns H: Vascular aspects of head injuries. Lisboa Med 19: 375–410, 1942.
4. Crawford T: The pathological effects of cerebral angiography. J Neurol Neurosurg Psychiatry 19:217–221, 1956.
5. Tangchai P, Pisitbutr M: Angiographic dissecting aneurysm of internal carotid artery: An autopsy case report. J Med Assoc Thai 54:598–601, 1971.
6. Davis JM, Zimmerman RA: Injury of the carotid and vertebral arteries. Neuroradiology 25:55–69, 1983.
7. Unger SW, Tucker WS Jr, Mrdeza MA, et al: Carotid arterial trauma. Surgery 87:477–487, 1980.
8. Mokri B, Piepgras DG, Houser OW: Traumatic dissections of the extracranial internal carotid artery. J Neurosurg 68:189–197, 1988.
9. Stringer WL, Kelly DL Jr: Traumatic dissection of the extracranial internal carotid artery. Neurosurgery 6:123–130, 1980.
10. Zelenock GB, Kazmers A, Whitehouse WM Jr, et al: Extracranial internal carotid artery dissections. Arch Surg 117:425–432, 1982.
11. Anson J, Crowell RM: Cervicocranial arterial dissection. Neurosurgery 29:89–96, 1991.
12. Fry RE, Fry WJ: Extracranial carotid artery injuries. Surgery 88: 581–587, 1980.
13. Krajewski LP, Hertzer NR: Blunt carotid artery trauma. Report of two cases and review of the literature. Ann Surg 191:341–346, 1980.
14. Mokri B: Dissections of cervical and cephalic arteries. In Meyer FB (ed): Sundt's Occlusive Cerebrovascular Disease, 2nd ed. Philadelphia, WB Saunders, 1994, pp 45–70.
15. Monson DO, Saletta JD, Freeark RJ: Carotid vertebral trauma. J Trauma 9:987–999, 1969.
16. Biffl WL, Moore EE, Rehse DH, et al: Selective management of penetrating neck trauma based on cervical level of injury. Am J Surg 174:678–682, 1997.
17. Sturzenegger M: Ultrasound findings in spontaneous carotid artery dissection: The value of duplex sonography. Arch Neurol 48:1057–1063, 1991.
18. Mokri B: Traumatic and spontaneous extracranial internal carotid artery dissections. J Neurol 237:356–361, 1990.
19. Batzdorf U, Bentson JR, Machleder HI: Blunt trauma to the high cervical carotid artery. Neurosurgery 5:195–201, 1979.
20. Little JM, May J, Vanderfield GK, et al: Traumatic thrombosis of the internal carotid artery. Lancet 2:926–930, 1969.
21. Rubio PA, Reul GJ Jr, Beall AC Jr, et al: Acute carotid artery injury: 25 years' experience. J Trauma 14:967–973, 1974.

22. Harris ME, Barrow DL: Arterial dissection. In Tindall GT, Cooper PR, Barrow DL (eds): The Practice of Neurosurgery. Baltimore, Williams & Wilkins, 1995, pp 1899–1906.
23. Vishteh AG, Marciano FF, David CA, et al: Long-term graft patency rates and clinical outcomes after revascularization for symptomatic traumatic internal carotid artery dissection. Neurosurgery 43:761–767, 1998.
24. Yamada S, Kindt GW, Youmans JR: Carotid artery occlusion due to nonpenetrating injury. J Trauma 7:333–342, 1967.
25. Towne JB: The autogenous vein. In Rutherford RB (ed): Vascular Surgery, 4th ed. Philadelphia, WB Saunders, 1995, pp 482–491.
26. Cooley DA: Techniques in Cardiac Surgery, 2nd ed. Philadelphia, WB Saunders, 1984.
27. Waga S, Morikawa A, Fujimoto K: Carotid-cavernous fistula associated with traumatic aneurysm of the internal carotid artery. Surg Neurol 9:367–369, 1978.
28. Glasscock MEI: Exposure of the intra-petrous portion of the carotid artery. In Hamberger C-A, Wersäll J (eds): Disorders of the Skull Base Region. Proceedings of the Tenth Nobel Symposium, Stockholm, August 1968. Stockholm, Almqvist & Wiksell, 1969, pp 135–143.
29. Dotter CT, Judkins MP: Transluminal treatment of arteriosclerotic obstruction. Description of a new technic and a preliminary report of its application. Circulation 30:654–670, 1964.
30. Prall JA, Brega KE, Coldwell DM, et al: Incidence of unsuspected blunt carotid artery injury. Neurosurgery 42:495–498, 1998.

CHAPTER **101**

Nonatherosclerotic Carotid Lesions

MICHAEL J. ALEXANDER

The origins of the pathologies involving the cervical carotid artery are highly variable, yet the principles of their treatment are similar. This chapter deals with the nonatherosclerotic causes of disease in the cervical carotid artery: tumor, primarily carotid body tumors; arteriopathy, as seen in fibromuscular dysplasia; aneurysms, from infections and various other causes; nontraumatic dissection; and iatrogenic pathology (i.e., radiation-induced stenosis). The principles of the management and treatment of these diseases are reviewed. First, the history and physical examination help establish the chronicity and extent of involvement of the disease. Second, an appropriate diagnostic evaluation is critical in planning the method of treatment. High-quality cervical and cerebral angiograms are key for determining collateral blood flow before treatment. Third, the modality of treatment, surgical or endovascular, should maximize efficacy and minimize risks to the patient. Finally, intraoperative monitoring, with neuronal protection during carotid occlusion, can help reduce complications. In each of these pathologies, preservation of the carotid artery is the primary goal of both surgical and endovascular treatment. If the carotid artery cannot be preserved, a patch graft or bypass may be necessary.

CAROTID BODY TUMORS

In 1743, von Haller[1] reported the anatomy of the carotid body. He described the carotid body as a nodule about the size of a kernel of wheat at the bifurcation of the common carotid artery (CCA). Anatomic dissection revealed that the structure was contained in a dense meshwork at the base of the carotid bifurcation.[2] Believing that the structure was nerve tissue, he called it the "intercarotid ganglion."

In 1862, Luschka, as discussed by Balfour and Wildner,[2] characterized the carotid body microscopically after examining hundreds of specimens. He described it as 5 to 7 mm long, 2.5 to 4 mm wide, and 1.5 mm thick and as having the primary histologic characteristics of a gland. Years later, Kohn defined the carotid body as chromaffin cells embedded in the sympathetic nerve fibers about the carotid artery and coined the term *paraganglion*.[3]

Lahey and Warren[4] reported that Marchand attempted the first surgical resection of a carotid body tumor in 1880. The report detailed an aggressive tumor resection with division of the carotid artery; jugular vein; and vagus, hypoglossal, and sympathetic nerves. The patient died 3 days after surgery. Lahey and Warren[4] also noted that in 1886 Maydl reported excising a carotid body tumor with division of the common, internal, and external carotid arteries. The patient developed aphasia and hemiplegia. These early attempts included ligation and resection of the carotid artery bifurcation but no attempts at reconstruction. It was not until 1889 that Albert first resected a carotid body tumor (the size of an apple) by dissecting the tumor, preserving the internal carotid artery (ICA), and ligating the external carotid artery (ECA). The tumor recurred at its original site within a year and required re-excision, as reported by Keen and Funke[5] and Paltauf.[6] In 1917, Lund[7] described the first successful resection of bilateral carotid body tumors.

By the 1960s and 1970s, several hundred cases of carotid body tumors had been reported, but the complication rates associated with surgical treatment were still high. The larger series reported mortality rates of 5% to 15% with surgical excision, cerebrovascular complications in 8% to 20% of patients, and postoperative cranial nerve injuries in 32% to 44% of patients.[8] These reports, however, preceded the widespread use of electroencephalograms (EEGs) and cerebral blood flow monitoring techniques to determine the usefulness of intraoperative shunting during carotid cross-clamping. Today, early diagnosis with gadolinium-enhanced magnetic resonance imaging of the neck, improved surgical and endovascular techniques, and radiotherapy adjuncts have considerably reduced the morbidity rates associated with treating these tumors.

Anatomy

The carotid body is a light brown structure within the adventitial layer of the dorsal aspect of the CCA bifurcation. The vascular supply is from the carotid bifurcation, and the primary innervation is the carotid sensory branch of the glossopharyngeal nerve. This branch is also known as the carotid sinus nerve or the nerve of Hering.[9] The carotid body is connected to the CCA bifurcation by a fibrovascular band called the ligament of Mayer. Embryologically, the carotid body may have constituents of both the third branchial arch mesoderm and neural elements of the neural crest ectoderm.[10]

Carotid bodies are part of a group of neuroepithelium-derived aggregates known as paraganglia. Tumors of these cells have also been known as paragangliomas, glomus tumors, and chemodectomas. Tumors of similar histology arise in several locations, including the ciliary body of the orbit, aortic-pulmonary paraganglia, carotid body (glomus caroticum), middle ear (glomus tympanicum), ganglion nodosum of the vagus nerve (glomus vagale), jugular body (glomus jugulare), and adrenal medulla (pheochromocytoma). Although most glomus tumors appear to be composed of nonchromaffin cells that are physiologically silent, some contain secretory granules that may secrete catecholamines similar to pheochromocytomas.[10]

Histology

Carotid body tumors consist of epithelioid cells grouped into cords or clusters, also known as *Zellballen*. Typically, the cells are polyhedral with granular cytoplasm (Fig. 101–1). The stroma is composed of a fine mesh of reticulin fibers.[11] Intertwined is a rich network of capillaries, giving the general appearance of a glomerulus. Several reports have detailed the chromaffin-positive nature of the secretory granules, indicating that the carotid body and tumors of it may be capable of secreting catecholamines such as norepinephrine and dopamine.[12–15]

Genetics

A genetic cause of carotid body tumors is highly suggested from examples of familial occurrence. In the sporadic form, the rate of bilateral tumor occurrence is 5%. An autosomal-dominant expression of bilateral tumors, however, occurs in 32% of patients with a familial occurrence.[16, 17] Comorbid cervical paragangliomas (glomus vagale, glomus jugulare) are relatively common in patients with carotid body tumors. Gardner and coworkers[18] reviewed 11 patients with carotid body tumors, 3 of whom had other head and neck paragangliomas.

Seminal genetic studies have indicated an increased expression of the oncogenes *c-myc*, *bcl-2*, and *c-jun* in most carotid body tumor specimens studied.[19] Wang and colleagues[20] suggested that the expression of the oncoprotein bcl-2 may deregulate apoptosis, thus suppressing programmed cell death, a critical step in the tumorigenesis of carotid body tumors.

Clinical Presentation

The most common manifestation of carotid body tumors is a palpable neck mass in the high cervical region. Less common initial presentations include cranial nerve deficits such as laryngeal dysfunction (hoarseness), difficulty swallowing, and unilateral tongue atrophy or weakness. These symptoms reflect the tumor's proximity to the vagus and hypoglossal nerves. There have also been reports of patients who became symptomatic with Horner's syndrome[21] or carotid sinus syndrome.[22]

There is no reported sex predominance in carotid body tumors. Typically, diagnosis is between 30 and 60 years of age. The youngest reported patient was 7 years old.[23–25]

Radiographic and Medical Evaluation

Cervical magnetic resonance imaging with and without gadolinium can help differentiate carotid body

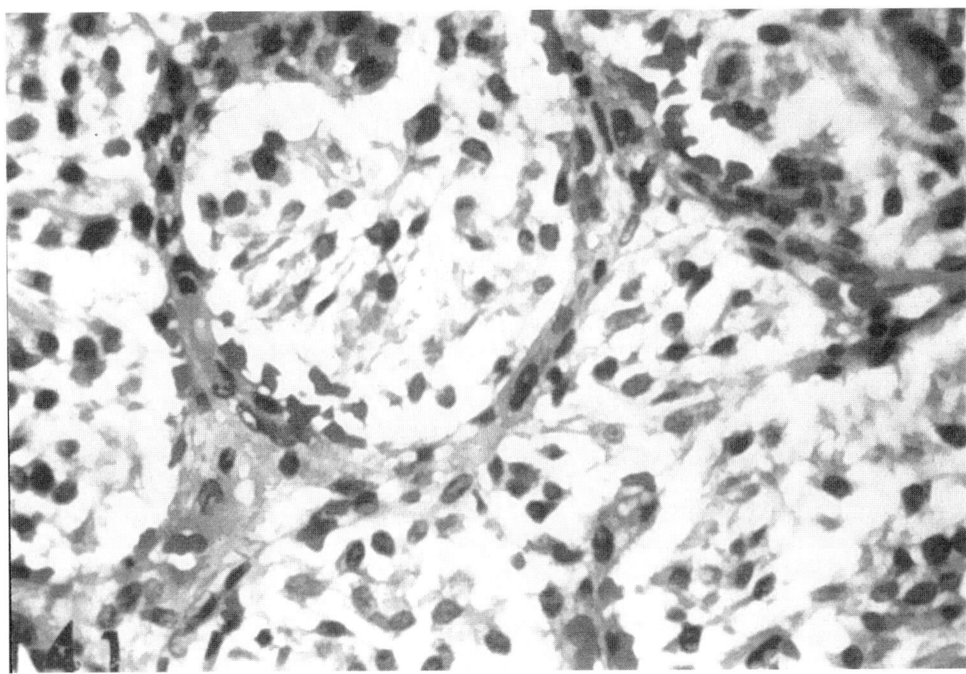

FIGURE 101–1. Photomicrograph of carotid body tumor showing the characteristic cluster of cells known as *Zellballen*, composed of octahedral cells in a glomerulus-like shape.

tumors from other lesions that arise in the same region—carcinomas, enlarged lymph nodes, branchial cleft cysts, and leiomyomas.[22, 26] Magnetic resonance imaging demonstrates a brightly enhancing, well-circumscribed mass at the cervical carotid bifurcation (Fig. 101–2). Magnetic resonance angiography can be useful by displaying the hypervascular nature of the tumor and the characteristic splaying of the ECA and ICA (Fig. 101–3).

Angiography can help confirm the diagnosis. These tumors are extraordinarily vascular (Fig. 101–4). The ascending pharyngeal artery often provides the majority of the vascular supply, and the superior thyroid artery almost always provides a minority contribution. The blood supply of the tumor can also be derived from the ICA, vertebral artery, and thyrocervical trunk. If angiography is planned, a concomitant session to embolize the tumor can be coordinated. Studies have shown that preoperative embolization significantly reduces blood loss during resection of a carotid body tumor.[27, 28]

An evaluation of the endocrine system may be warranted, particularly in patients who have elevated blood pressure or tachycardia. Clinicians must be aware of the potential comorbidity of a pheochromocytoma and that some carotid body tumors secrete catecholamines. In such patients, α-adrenergic blockade must be induced pharmacologically 2 weeks before surgery. Once this blockade is established, β-adrenergic blockade is recommended to control heart rate and cardiac arrhythmias.[22] Careful preoperative assessment of blood pressure may indicate the need for urine metanephrine analysis.

Characteristics of Tumor Growth

In an effort to assess the preoperative risks of tumor resection, Shamblin and associates[29] devised a classification scheme for carotid body tumors. Group I tumors are restricted to the space between the ICA and ECA. Generally, these tumors dissect easily from the surrounding structures. Neither the carotid vessels nor adjacent nerves travel through the tumor. Group II tumors partially involve the ECA and ICA but do not encase the arteries completely. Tumor involving the adventitia of the artery can still be dissected free. Finally, group III tumors totally encase the ICA and invade the adventitia into the muscularis. Dissecting group III tumors from the artery requires reconstruction or sacrifice of the ICA. In this challenging group,

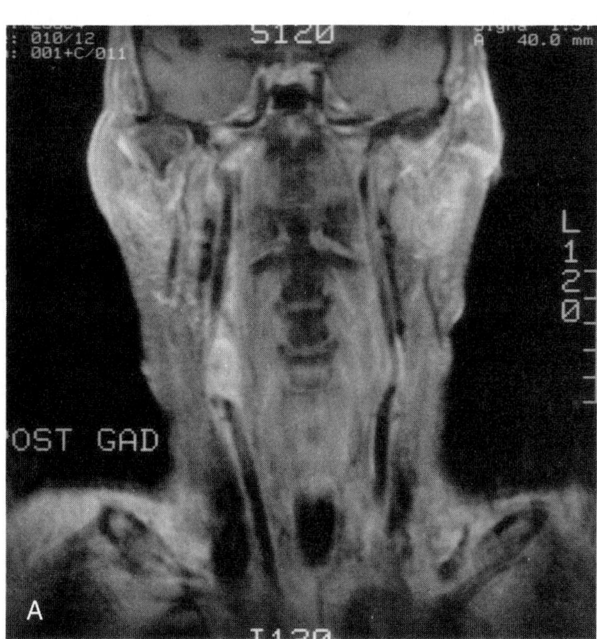

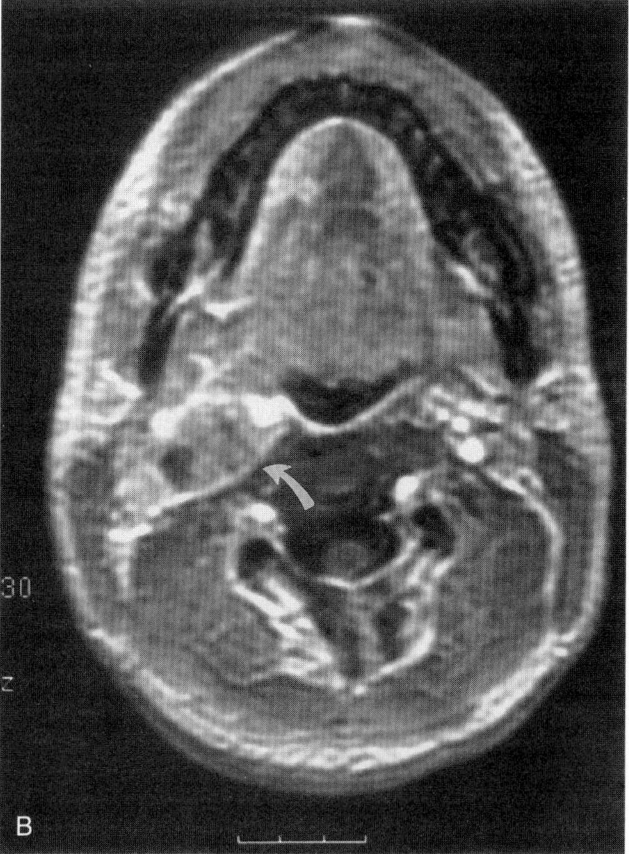

FIGURE 101–2. *A*, Coronal magnetic resonance imaging with gadolinium enhancement of carotid body tumors can help surgical planning by demonstrating the cervical level of the carotid bifurcation, as well as the superior and inferior extents of tumor. *B*, Axial magnetic resonance imaging with gadolinium enhancement can help determine the Shamblin[29] grade of the carotid body tumor *(arrow)* preoperatively.

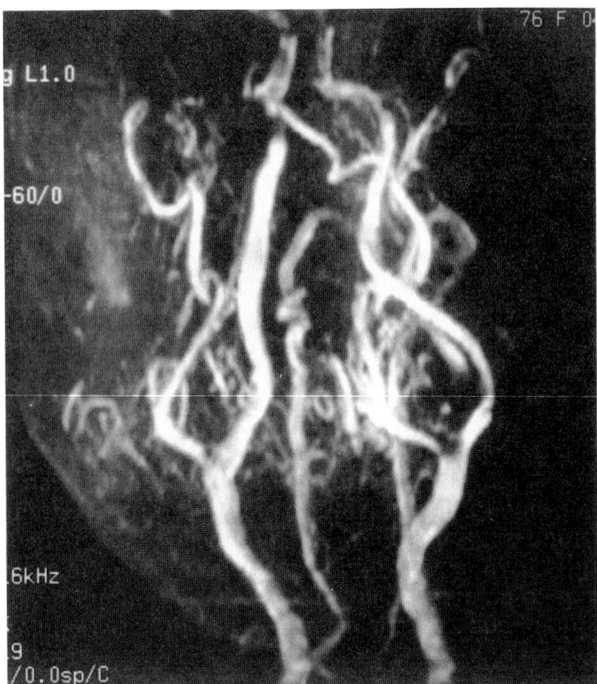

FIGURE 101–3. Preoperative magnetic resonance angiogram of the cervical vessels showing characteristic splaying of the external and internal carotid arteries near the carotid bifurcation in larger tumors. Splaying is shown on both sides in a patient with bilateral carotid body tumors.

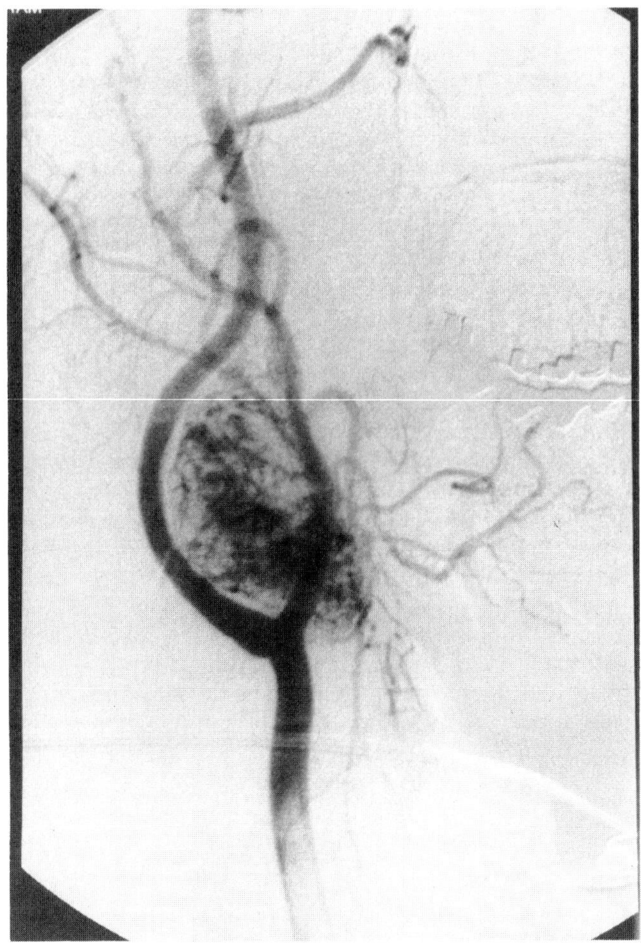

FIGURE 101–4. Digital subtraction angiography demonstrates a characteristic tumor blush at the carotid bifurcation. The carotid body tumor is typically fed by the ascending pharyngeal artery, with a smaller contribution from the superior thyroid artery.

the superior laryngeal and hypoglossal nerves may traverse the tumor.

Metastasis

Most carotid body tumors are benign. They are problematic only in their local invasion of vascular and nervous structures and, occasionally, the oropharynx. Staats and coworkers[24] reviewed 500 patients and found a 6.4% incidence of malignancy with local or distant metastases. Distant metastases have been reported in lymph nodes, bone, lung, liver, pancreas, thyroid, kidney, brain, and breast.[30–32]

Surgical Treatment

Preoperative planning is critical to reduce morbidity in patients with carotid body tumors. As mentioned, a thorough medical evaluation is necessary, particularly to rule out endocrine abnormalities. Preoperative embolization helps reduce blood loss during resection, but diagnostic cerebral angiography is equally important for assessing collateral blood flow. A temporary balloon test occlusion may be warranted, particularly in patients with group III tumors with apparent marginal collateral blood flow on angiography. In such cases, surgeons may anticipate intraoperative shunting to maintain adequate cerebral blood flow.

I routinely use compressed spectral array electroencephalograms (CSA-EEGs) to monitor the patient's cerebral function during resection. Therefore, intraoperative shunting is not routinely performed, even for large tumors; the need for shunting is based on changes in the CSA-EEG.

The initial incision primarily reflects the size and extent of the tumor. For example, a small group I tumor may be accessed through a transverse incision along a cervical skin crease, giving the best cosmetic result. Larger tumors with group II or III extension require a larger exposure to control the proximal and distal carotid artery for possible shunting. Here, an oblique incision along the medial border of the sternocleidomastoid muscle is indicated. As in a standard exposure for carotid endarterectomy, the common facial vein is ligated and cut to mobilize the jugular vein laterally. The hypoglossal and vagus nerves are identified. Frequently, the hypoglossal nerve may be displaced superiorly and posteriorly by the tumor[8]; consequently, care must be exerted during dissection of the superior aspect of the tumor to avoid damaging this nerve. In the more challenging group III tumors, nerves may actually traverse the tumor, making dissection difficult and tedious. In rare cases, the vagus nerve can be involved with tumor. Tumor invasion into the carotid arterial wall requires temporary occlusion, with or without shunting, to dissect the tumor and, if necessary, to patch the arterial wall defect with a graft.[8]

Perioperatively, the patient's blood pressure should be monitored closely, particularly immediately after surgery. Labile blood pressure, presumed to be secondary to baroreceptor failure from loss of carotid sinus function, has been reported after resection of a carotid body tumor.[33, 34] Netterville and coworkers[34] reviewed 30 patients with 46 carotid body tumors and found baroreceptor failure in 10 patients. Interestingly, first-bite pain occurred in 10 of 25 patients assessed postoperatively.

The role of radiotherapy in managing carotid body tumors remains unclear. Radiotherapy is not used as the sole primary treatment of carotid body tumors, but it is the preferred therapy in recurrent or residual tumor with intracranial extension.[8, 28, 35] Radiosurgery may be useful for a metastasis or intracranial extension, but no significant series of this relatively rare pathology has been reported.

FIBROMUSCULAR DYSPLASIA

Fibromuscular dysplasia (FMD) can be a unifocal or multifocal disease that manifests as arteriopathy of medium to large arteries. In 1938, Leadbetter and Burkland[36] reported the first clear description of FMD in the pathologic findings of a patient who had hypertension secondary to FMD of the renal artery. In fact, most cases of FMD in the literature involve the renal artery. In 1964, Palubinskas and Ripley[37] provided the first angiographic description of FMD of the extracranial ICA in an addendum to their report of FMD in extrarenal arteries. Several reports of cephalocervical FMD followed in the 1960s and 1970s, particularly of the extracranial ICA and vertebral artery.[38–43] Subsequently, cases of intracranial artery involvement with FMD expanded our understanding of the disease process.[44, 45] Two major institutional reviews of cerebral angiography—one reviewing 6100 angiograms, the other 13,955—found a 0.53% and 0.6% incidence of FMD, respectively.[46, 47]

Histologic studies indicate that the arterial dysplasias present as three primary pathologies: intimal fibroplasia, medial fibroplasia, and subadventitial hyperplasia.[48] In medial fibroplasia, also known as fibromuscular hyperplasia, the expression of the disease ranges from fibrodysplasia limited to the outer media to complete involvement of the entire media. Collagen and ground substance accumulate in the inner media in the milder form of the disease, separating the disorganized smooth muscle cells. In the severe form, the media is profoundly disorganized, with fibroblasts and collagen replacing the smooth muscle.[49]

Cause

The exact cause of FMD is becoming better defined as we begin to understand the multifactorial pathology, with a spectrum of phenotypic expressions. Its prevalence in women is much higher than that in men, with an approximate 9:1 ratio. Stanley and colleagues[49] suggested that progestin and estrogen play a role in the development of the disease, because 94% of the patients they reviewed were women. Mettinger's familial analysis of patients with FMD suggests that it is an inheritable dominant trait with limited penetrance in men.[50, 51]

Mechanical and anatomic factors have also been evaluated in the development of FMD. Stanley and colleagues[49] implied that mechanical stresses on the vessel walls play a role in the development of FMD. Likewise, the disease appears to involve primarily arteries with a paucity of vasa vasorum, indicating that arterial wall ischemia may contribute to disease progression. Long-term follow-up of some cases has indicated a definite progression of the disease in some patients with carotid FMD.[42]

Clinical Presentation

Patients with cervical carotid FMD typically present in their 50s to 60s. On physical examination, about two thirds of symptomatic patients have a cervical bruit that is audible on auscultation.[46] Symptoms of cerebral ischemia have been reported in 18% to 56% of patients.[52] In such cases, the sequential arrangement of the fibromuscular rings reduces blood flow while increasing turbulence within the vessel. In addition to ischemic symptoms, FMD has been associated with spontaneous carotid artery dissection,[53, 54] aneurysm formation,[55, 56] carotid-cavernous fistula,[57, 58] and thromboembolism.[46] In Mettinger's review of 284 patients with aortocranial FMD, a surprising 21% had associated intracranial aneurysms.[51]

Angiographic Findings

In 1977, Osborn and Anderson[48] described the angiographic appearance of carotid FMD variants in a summary report. The classic angiographic appearance, present in more than 80% of patients, is the "string of beads"—multiple, irregularly spaced arterial constrictions with normal or ectatic intervening segments. Angiographically, it is similar to stationary arterial waves or circular spastic contractions, although these show more regularly spaced constrictions with no associated dilated segments. The second variant is that of smooth, concentric tubular stenosis. Angiographically, this variant can be distinguished from Takayasu's arteritis, which affects the proximal segments of the aortic branches. In contrast, FMD typically spares the origins and proximal segments. The third variant, termed "atypical" FMD by Houser and Baker,[38] usually involves one wall of the affected segment, creating a smooth or corrugated outpouching of the vessel.

Treatment

The treatment of FMD should be tailored to the patient's symptoms. Incidentally diagnosed FMD should be followed radiographically by noninvasive studies such as magnetic resonance angiography or carotid duplex ultrasonography. No convincing evidence suggests that the disease progresses as a rule, although notable exceptions have been reported. Therefore, asymptomatic patients should not be treated unless their disease progresses. In patients with an embolic presentation, antiplatelet medication such as aspirin, ticlopidine, or clopidogrel is recommended. Intervention is warranted in patients whose symptoms persist despite antiplatelet therapy.

A report by DeBakey's group in 1968 described the surgical luminal dilatation of the ICA in 12 patients and of the vertebral artery in 1 patient.[59] This report is interesting from a historical perspective, but it also documents intraluminal pressures at the proximal and distal ends of the affected segments in two patients. Before dilatation, they found pressure gradients of 25 and 50 mm Hg; after surgical treatment, there were no discernible gradients. These findings demonstrated that multiple tandem rings, as seen in FMD, significantly reduce arterial pressure and blood flow, although individual stenotic rings do not narrow the carotid artery significantly.

Contemporary treatment has used the endovascular techniques of balloon angioplasty and stenting for medically refractory cervical FMD lesions (Fig. 101–5). In the early 1980s, several reports documented the successful treatment of FMD by percutaneous balloon angioplasty.[60–64] By the mid-1980s, the limitations of this technology were revealed in reports of complications of percutaneous transluminal angioplasty for FMD, including dissection[65] and aneurysm formation.[66] The transfemoral access route has significantly reduced the morbidity of endovascular procedures. Subsequently, endoluminal stenting, performed in coordination with angioplasty for cervical FMD, has become increasingly more prominent as the primary treatment method in medically refractory cases.

EXTRACRANIAL CAROTID ARTERY ANEURYSMS

Although aneurysms of the extracranial carotid artery were first described in 1687,[67] they are exceedingly

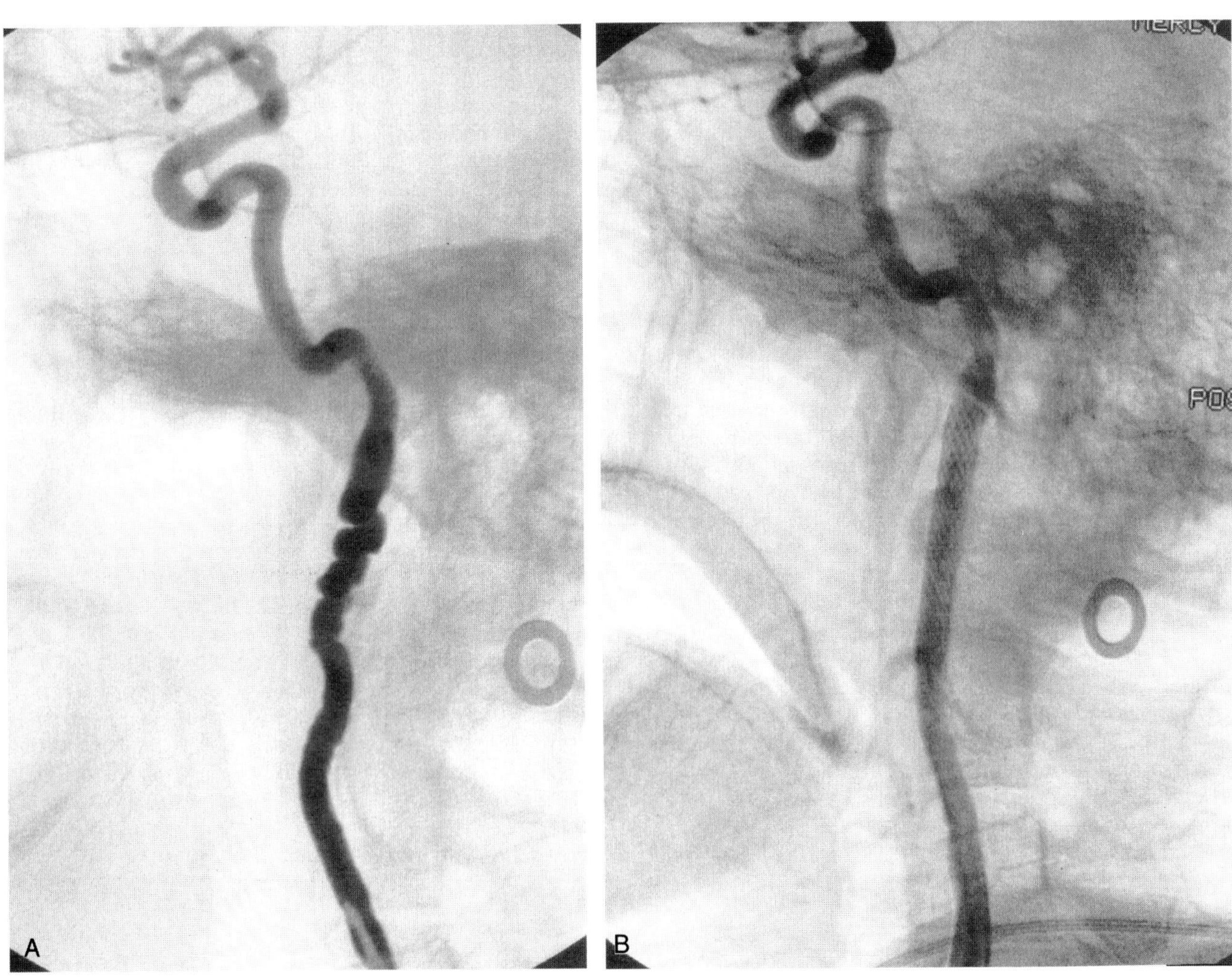

FIGURE 101–5. *A*, Lateral left internal carotid artery angiogram showing fibromuscular dysplasia in a 56-year-old woman who presented with left hemisphere transient ischemic attacks refractory to treatment with aspirin. *B*, Lateral angiogram after the deployment of a Palmaz stent (Johnson & Johnson Interventional Systems Company, Warren, NJ). (*A* and *B* courtesy of Barrow Neurological Institute, Phoenix, AZ.)

rare. Interestingly, successful surgical treatment of an extracranial carotid aneurysm was reported in 1836 by Cooper, who used hunterian ligation of the proximal CCA.[68]

Early treatment, which was effective to a degree, consisted of proximal ligation but no attempt at resecting the aneurysm, reestablishing circulation, or bypassing the diseased segment. However, Winslow's[69] 1926 review of a series of patients with extracranial ICA aneurysms stressed the importance of treatment. He reported a 71% mortality rate related to the aneurysm in untreated patients, compared with a 30% mortality rate in patients who underwent hunterian ligation.

Treatment of these aneurysms evolved to attempts to preserve the cerebral circulation and to avoid hunterian ligation. In 1952, Dimtza[70] first successfully excised an extracranial carotid aneurysm and reanastomosed the ICA to reestablish circulation. In the ensuing years, it became clear that the risk of operating on aneurysms in this location held just a slightly higher risk than a standard carotid endarterectomy when proper vascular techniques were used.[71]

Clinical Presentation

The clinical symptoms associated with extracranial carotid aneurysms vary according to their location and size. Larger aneurysms usually present as pulsatile cervical or parapharyngeal masses that may or may not be tender.[72] Rarely, patients become symptomatic with hemorrhage, which may result in a neck hematoma or epistaxis, depending on the location of the aneurysm. Some patients may present with transient ischemic attacks related to emboli produced by the turbulent blood flow associated with a larger, tortuous aneurysm.[73, 74]

These aneurysms may be caused by trauma, infection, or iatrogenic causes such as previous carotid surgery. Most true aneurysms of the cervical carotid artery, however, are caused by atherosclerotic disease of the artery.[75] There have been reports of extracranial or skull base carotid aneurysms in which the cause was related to genetic vascular diseases, such as Marfan syndrome or progeria, but these are the minority of cases.[76, 77]

Treatment

The treatment of extracranial carotid artery aneurysms depends on the size, shape, cause, and location of the aneurysm. The primary goals of treatment should be exclusion of the aneurysm and preservation of adequate cerebral blood flow. Therefore, the hunterian ligation employed by Cooper for this pathology is no longer applicable to most cases. The results of small, contemporary operative series involving preservation of the carotid artery have been good. Painter and coworkers[78] reviewed the literature on extracranial carotid aneurysms treated surgically over a 10-year period by methods other than ligation (e.g., segmental resection, aneurysmorrhaphy). Of the 61 operative

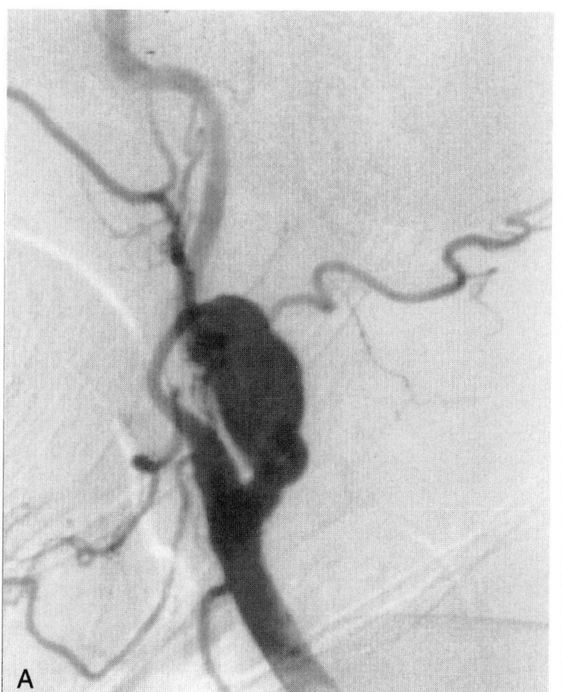

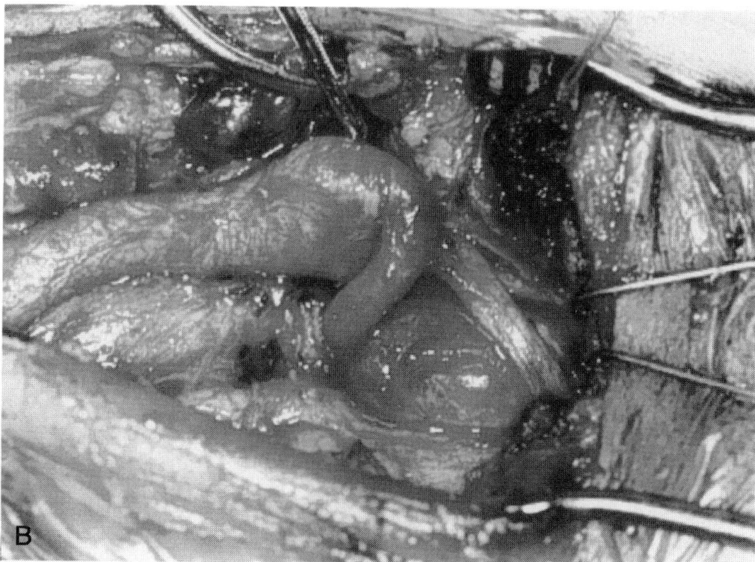

FIGURE 101–6. *A*, Cervical common carotid angiogram showing a large fusiform aneurysm of the internal carotid artery in a 58-year-old woman who presented with a pulsatile left cervical mass. *B*, Operative exposure for excision of the aneurysm and primary reanastomosis of the internal carotid artery. (*B*, Courtesy of George Thieme Verlag.)

cases they found, 3 patients (5%) had permanent neurological deficits from the surgery, and 1 died (1.6%).

If an aneurysm is in the low to midcervical region, it can be approached directly. Even fusiform aneurysms (Fig. 101–6) can be excised surgically, with primary reanastomosis of the proximal and distal artery. When primary reanastomosis is infeasible, a Dacron or saphenous vein patch graft can be used to reconstruct the carotid artery. Temporary clipping of the CCA or ICA is necessary during the procedure. Therefore, intraoperative EEG monitoring, pentobarbital burst suppression, and intravenous heparin are recommended. Should the EEG change during the procedure, intraoperative shunting may be necessary, as in a carotid endarterectomy procedure.

In aneurysms of the high cervical ICA, a direct approach is infeasible without extensive dissection of the skull base or upper neck. Coffin and associates[79] described 14 patients with high cervical carotid aneurysms resulting from spontaneous dissection, blunt trauma, FMD, or atheroma. With all aneurysms extending to C1 or higher, they were able to revascularize 12 arteries and ligate 3 (one after an extracranial-intracranial bypass). Overall, their results were good. Postoperatively, only one patient had a transient ischemic attack, and four patients had lower facial nerve palsies (from the extended cervical approach). In such cases, trapping the diseased segment and performing a high-flow vein bypass constitute the preferred treatment (Fig. 101–7). Aneurysms of the high cervical segment may be related to parapharyngeal infection or iatrogenic trauma. In such cases, the field is contaminated, and primary direct repair of the carotid artery is infeasible. Nor are endovascular stents indicated, because placing a foreign body in an infected region is inadvisable. Carotid occlusion is a reasonable alternative if the patient passes a balloon test occlusion. If the patient fails balloon test occlusion, bypass with carotid occlusion is the preferred long-term strategy.

If an infected site is not an issue, an endoluminal stent may be considered. One advantage of a stent is preservation of the ICA. It may be particularly useful in the high cervical region, which is difficult to access surgically. Likewise, if the contralateral carotid artery is diseased, preservation of the ipsilateral carotid artery is preferable to relying on bypass patency. Hurst and colleagues[80] reported a few cervical ICA aneurysms treated with stents alone; the aneurysms were thrombosed, and the parent artery was preserved.

SPONTANEOUS CAROTID ARTERY DISSECTION

The first case of spontaneous dissection of the ICA was reported by Jentzer[81] in 1954. Spontaneous carotid dissections have been reported in association with arteriopathies secondary to FMD, cystic medial necrosis, and Marfan syndrome, but the cause of most cases is

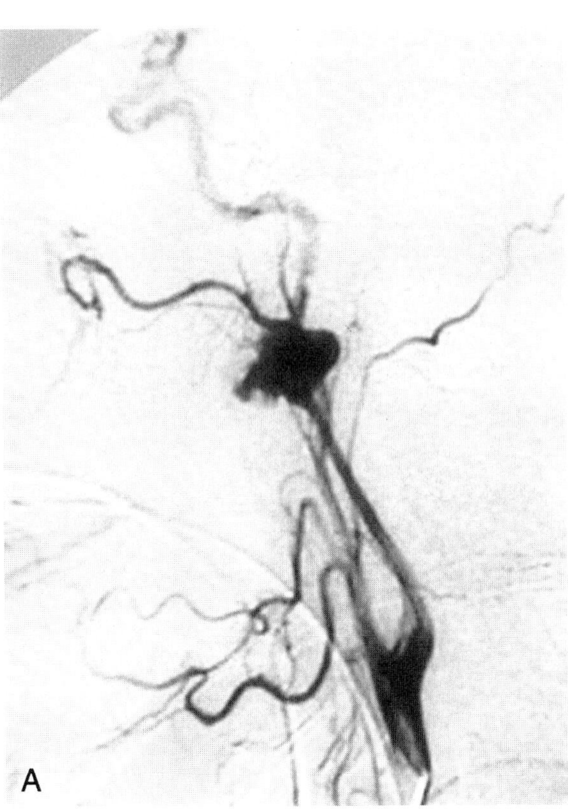

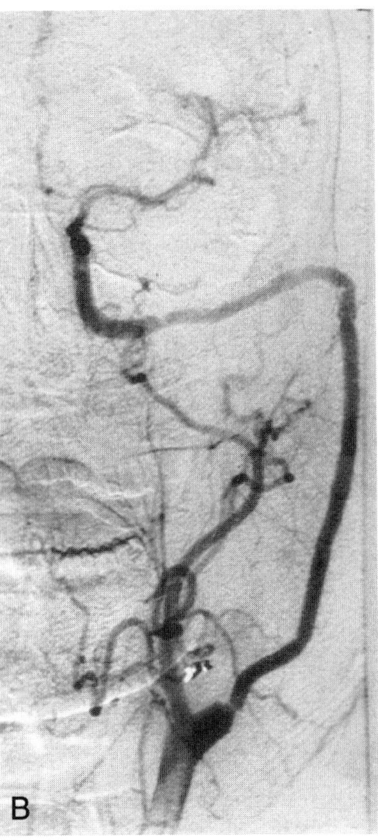

FIGURE 101–7. *A*, Lateral angiogram of a patient with a parapharyngeal abscess showing a pseudoaneurysm of the high cervical internal carotid artery. *B*, Owing to the high position of the aneurysm, a cervical–to–petrous carotid artery bypass was performed, with a saphenous vein interposition graft and trapping of the carotid artery pseudoaneurysm. (Courtesy of Barrow Neurological Institute, Phoenix, AZ.)

unknown. Likewise, a few familial cases have been reported, but they are rare.[82–84]

Dissections of the carotid artery are considered spontaneous in the absence of a history of trauma, even a seemingly minor trauma. In the dissected segment, blood traverses the arterial wall into the media. It forms a false channel or false lumen that may expand inward to narrow the true lumen or expand outward to develop a dissecting aneurysm. Some authors use the term *pseudoaneurysm* to describe the latter manifestation. Technically, it is a misnomer, because pseudoaneurysms have no arterial wall structures that compose the aneurysm wall, and the dissecting aneurysm has at a minimum an adventitial layer. A pseudoaneurysm may form when all layers of the arterial wall have been breached. The result is a hematoma that tamponades the artery. In this case, the pseudoaneurysm wall is merely the capsule of the hematoma.

Clinical Presentation

Typically, spontaneous dissection of the cervical carotid artery manifests with symptoms of headache and transient ischemic attacks or stroke. Meissner and Mokri[85] reviewed 80 patients with spontaneous ICA dissection. Headache was the most common symptom, occurring in 83% of patients. The headache manifested as frontal or periorbital pain in some and as periauricular pain in others. Strangely, neck pain was comparatively infrequent, occurring in 21% of patients. Focal cerebral ischemic symptoms, manifesting as transient ischemic attacks, strokes, or both, occurred in 60% of these patients, and an atypical Horner's syndrome was seen in half the patients.

There seems to be no overwhelming trend toward spontaneous carotid dissection in either gender. The age of onset is typically younger than 50 years, although younger individuals have been affected. In contrast, stroke tends to affect elderly patients more frequently.

Preliminary data suggest that a deficiency in type III collagen may predispose patients to spontaneous carotid dissection by compromising the integrity of the arterial wall. Van den Berg and colleagues[86] performed protein analysis of type I and type III collagen in 16 patients with spontaneous cervical arterial dissections and in 41 healthy controls. Although they found no type III collagen gene mutations by single-stranded conformation polymorphism–heteroduplex analysis in patients with dissections, a few patients had a low type III–type I collagen ratio.

The physical examination of patients with spontaneous carotid dissection should accurately assess neurological deficits from any presenting or evolving transient ischemic attack or stroke. Interestingly, the oculosympathetic palsy caused by an ICA dissection is not associated with the classic triad of Horner's syndrome (i.e., ptosis, miosis, and anhidrosis). Typically, these patients have only ptosis and miosis. Facial sweating is seldom affected, a pattern that reflects the anatomy of the sympathetic fibers. The sympathetic fibers leading to the eyes travel along the ICA and are affected in dissection. In contrast, the sympathetic fibers leading to the facial sweat glands travel with the ECA and are seldom affected.[84]

A thorough examination should assess for the presence of a carotid bruit, which was present in more than 40% of Meissner and Mokri's patients.[85] Patients rarely become symptomatic with lower cranial nerve palsies, although a complete cranial nerve examination is warranted before any treatment is instituted.

A few authors have recommended following patients with ICA dissection by measuring their retinal artery pressure with oculopneumoplethysmography.[84] Increasing retinal artery pressures and the resolution of the luminal stenosis related to arterial dissection are reliably correlated.

Angiographic Findings

The classic description of carotid arterial dissection is a long, tapered narrowing of the ICA just distal to the carotid bulb, also known as the "string sign."[87] Dissecting aneurysms also occur in the affected segment (Fig. 101–8). Of course, complete occlusion of the ICA is also possible with these lesions. In patients with complete occlusions from spontaneous dissections who were treated with anticoagulation therapy, the long-term recanalization rate was 47% in the report by Pozzati and coworkers[88, 89] and 43% in that by Bogousslavsky and associates.[90]

Treatment

The mainstay of treatment for patients with spontaneous carotid artery dissection is anticoagulant medical therapy. In patients with symptomatic ischemia from vessel narrowing due to dissection or embolic events despite anticoagulant therapy, surgical or endovascular intervention is indicated. Direct surgical repair of the dissection is seldom feasible, although surgical options include either a superficial temporal artery–to–middle cerebral artery bypass or a high-flow saphenous vein graft bypass, depending on the need for cerebral blood flow.

An endovascular option is available even in patients with high cervical dissections. Angioplasty and stenting remain viable options, even as primary treatment considerations. In complex cases or dissections resulting in a double lumen, the difficulty lies in identifying which is the true lumen and which is the false one. Provided the stent is well opposed to the lumen wall, small pseudoaneurysms or vessel irregularities outside the stent typically thrombose with time, even when patients are receiving antiplatelet medical therapy. Long-term follow-up in a large series of patients with carotid dissections treated with endoluminal stents has yet to be reported. Therefore, the durable efficacy of this treatment is still under evaluation.

RADIATION STENOSIS

Radiation is commonly used to treat many vascular pathologies, including arteriovenous malformations,

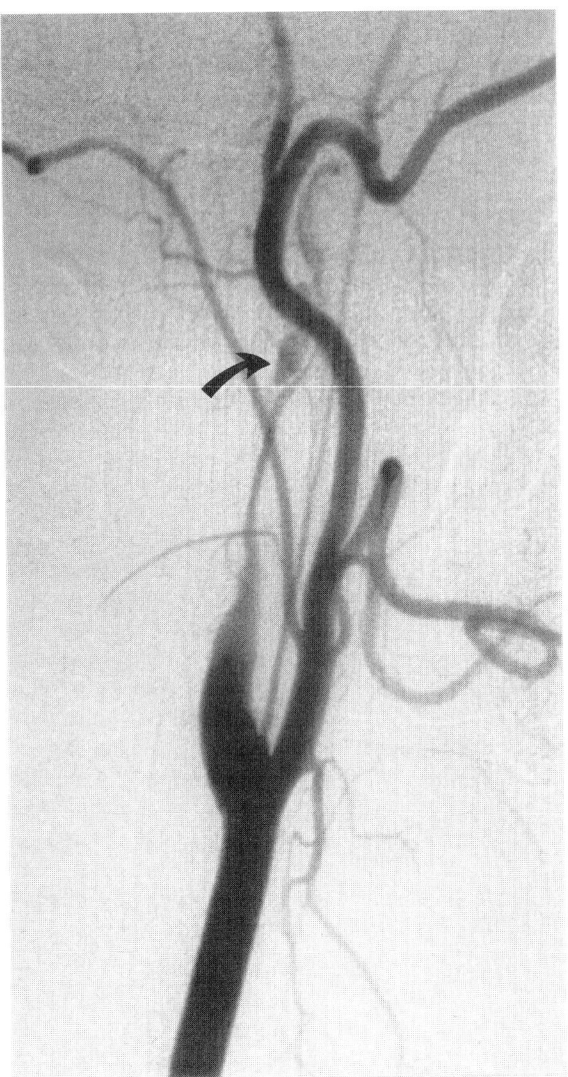

FIGURE 101–8. Cervical angiogram demonstrating a spontaneous dissecting aneurysm in the middle of the internal carotid artery *(arrow)*.

arteriovenous fistulas, cavernous malformations, and vascular tumors. In some cases, however, radiation to the normal artery can induce pathology.[91–94] Histologic studies have demonstrated that radiation has variable effects, depending on the arterial size and radiation dose.[95]

Not long after the discovery of x-rays by Roentgen, the adverse effects of radiation became known. In 1899, Gassman described histologically the small-vessel endothelial proliferation associated with radiodermatitis.[96] In 1909, Wolbach[97] noted that this endothelial proliferation also caused obliteration or thrombosis of the capillary lumina. In 1944, Sheehan[98] reported a more detailed study in which he described the development of plaquelike thickenings in the intima of small arteries secondary to the accumulation of foam cells, hyalin, and fibrin in the endothelial lining and internal elastic membrane. Working with a radiation injury model in the carotid artery of rabbits, Konings and coworkers[99] determined that endothelial cells damaged by irradiation do not function properly as a barrier to plasma lipoprotein infiltration in the arterial wall. This dysfunction leads to lysosomal activation and cellular proliferation within the vessel wall, resulting in intimal plaque formation.

With the expanded use of radiation in the treatment of neck and mediastinal malignancies, reports of radiation changes in larger arteries became more prevalent. In 1940, Cade[100] briefly mentioned a case of presumed radiation injury to the aorta of a patient treated for esophageal cancer. Thomas and Forbus,[101] however, are credited with the first clinical report of a patient with radiation injury in a large artery. In 1959, they detailed the course of a 19-year-old patient who underwent radiotherapy for mediastinal lymphoma.

Clinical Evaluation

Imaging studies are indicated for patients who develop symptoms of cerebral ischemia or emboli after radiotherapy to the head, neck, or mediastinum. Although radiation changes in large arteries look very similar to the atherosclerotic changes seen in the carotid bulb in atherosclerotic vaso-occlusive disease, the spectrum of radiation stenosis is more varied. First, the arterial changes associated with radiation stenosis can occur in regions typically unaffected by atherosclerosis, such as the CCA.[102] Second, the surrounding tissues in radia-

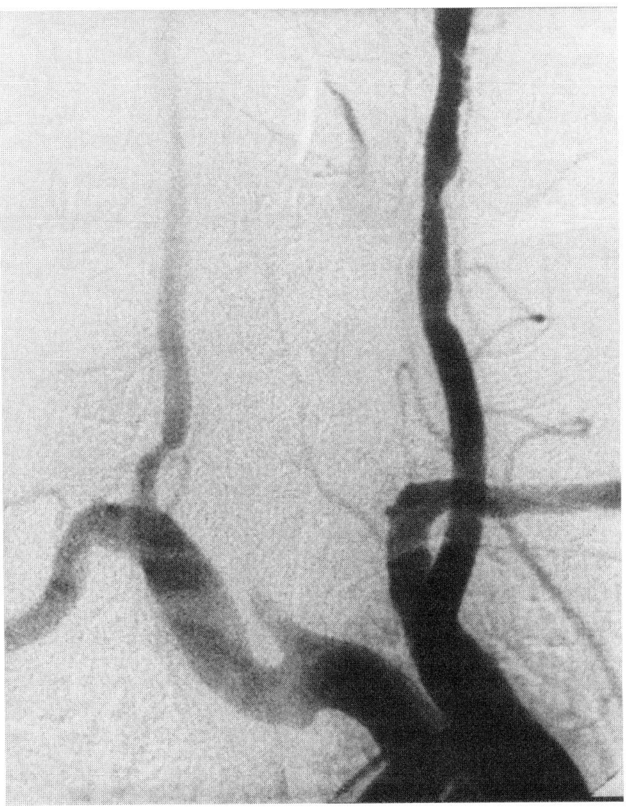

FIGURE 101–9. Aortic arch angiogram showing occlusion of the right common carotid artery and left vertebral artery and atheromatous disease over a diffuse segment of the left common carotid artery in a 46-year-old woman 2 years after mediastinal radiation.

tion stenosis can be severely affected, requiring myocutaneous flaps after surgical intervention. Third, some authors speculate that the carotid arterial wall is damaged, making carotid endarterectomy in these patients more dangerous than a standard carotid endarterectomy.[103] A carotid duplex scan should give sufficient information about most of the cervical carotid artery, but it is a poor choice for the evaluation of the proximal CCA and the distal cervical ICA. Magnetic resonance angiography of the arteries can give a more complete view of the arterial origins and high cervical segments[104] but may not be obtainable in some patients. Cervical and cerebral angiography remain the gold standards for evaluating potential radiation stenosis. Figure 101–9 shows an aortic arch angiogram of a 46-year-old woman with a history of radiation for lymphoma who presented with a right hemisphere stroke. The angiogram demonstrated an occlusion of the right CCA near the origin, in addition to an occlusion of the left vertebral artery. The figure shows the type of changes seen in radiation-associated atherosclerosis over a diffuse segment of the left CCA.

Treatment

Some authors have reported that it is more difficult to dissect plaques caused by radiation stenosis than to dissect atherosclerotic plaques, because the former are more adherent to the intima.[103] Patients with radiation-associated carotid atherosclerosis were previously thought to be unacceptable candidates for surgical carotid endarterectomy, but their surgical risks are actually comparable to those of patients undergoing standard carotid endarterectomy. In 1999, Kashyap and associates[105] reported 24 patients who received a mean dose of 6300 rad and who underwent 26 carotid artery operations. In this series, 58% of patients had cerebral or monocular transient ischemic attacks, 27% had asymptomatic high-grade stenosis, 12% had prior stroke, and 4% had tumor invasion in the carotid artery. Two thirds of the patients had severe scarring or fibrosis of the skin of the neck, and four patients had permanent tracheostomies. Yet complications were limited to two restenoses, two wound infections, and four cranial nerve palsies. Based on carotid artery backpressure or EEG monitoring, selective intraoperative shunting was performed in 31% of the cases. A patch graft arterial repair was necessary in 79% of the surgically treated patients.

Endovascular treatment is also a viable option in the treatment of radiation stenosis of the carotid arteries. Because of concerns associated with soft tissue fibrosis, operating through an area of a previous myocutaneous flap, and more proximal arterial involvement, endovascular angioplasty and stenting have emerged as the primary treatment for radiation stenosis. The long-term efficacy of stenting in this setting has yet to be analyzed, but the short-term results are promising.[106, 107]

REFERENCES

1. von Haller A: Elementa physiologia corporis humani, iv. 1743, p 1766.
2. Balfour DC, Wildner F: The intercarotid paraganglion and its tumors. Surg Gynecol Obstet 18:203–213, 1914.
3. Kohn A: Die paraganglien. Arch Mikr Anat 62:263–265, 1903.
4. Lahey FH, Warren KW: A long term appraisal of carotid body tumors with remarks on their removal. Surg Gynecol Obstet 85: 281–288, 1941.
5. Keen WW, Funke J: Tumors of the carotid gland. JAMA 47: 469–479, 1906.
6. Paltauf: Ziegler's Beitr z path Anat u alleg Path, vol xi. 1892.
7. Lund FB: Tumors of the carotid body. JAMA 69:348–352, 1917.
8. Meyer FB, Sundt TM Jr, Pearson BW: Carotid body tumors: A subject review and suggested surgical approach. J Neurosurg 64:377–385, 1986.
9. Williams PL, Warwick R, Dyson M, et al: Gray's Anatomy, 37th ed. London, Churchill Livingstone, 1989.
10. Pryse-Davies J, Dawson IM: Some morphologic, histochemical, and chemical observations on chemodectomas and the normal carotid body, including a study of the chromaffin reaction and possible ganglion cell elements. Cancer 17:185–202, 1964.
11. Byrne JJ: Carotid body and allied tumors. Am J Surg 95:371–384, 1958.
12. Rossi P, Russo F, Paganelli C, et al: Carotid chemodectoma: A clinical case report and review of the literature [Italian]. G Chir 15:21–28, 1994.
13. Ikejiri K, Muramori K, Takeo S, et al: Functional carotid body tumor: Report of a case and a review of the literature. Surgery 119:222–225, 1996.
14. Hirano S, Shoji K, Kojima H, et al: Dopamine-secreting carotid body tumor. Am J Otolaryngol 19:412–416, 1998.
15. Levit SA, Sheps SG, Espinosa RE, et al: Catecholamine-secreting paraganglioma of glomus-jugulare region resembling pheochromocytoma. N Engl J Med 281:805–811, 1969.
16. Grufferman S, Gillman MW, Pasternak LR, et al: Familial carotid body tumors: Case report and epidemiologic review. Cancer 46: 2116–2122, 1980.
17. Rush BF Jr: Familial bilateral carotid body tumors. Ann Surg 157:633–636, 1963.
18. Gardner P, Dalsing M, Weisberger E, et al: Carotid body tumors, inheritance, and a high incidence of associated cervical paragangliomas. Am J Surg 172:196–199, 1996.
19. Wang DG, Barros D'Sa AA, Johnston CF, et al: Oncogene expression in carotid body tumors. Cancer 77:2581–2587, 1996.
20. Wang DG, Johnston CF, Barros D'Sa AA, et al: Expression of apoptosis-suppressing gene bcl-2 in human carotid body tumours. J Pathol 183:218–221, 1997.
21. Sankar NM, Munene J, Arumugam SB, et al: Benign carotid body tumor presenting with Horner's syndrome: A case report. Tex Heart Inst J 23:180–182, 1996.
22. Sampson JH, Wilkins RH: Paragangliomas of the carotid body and temporal bone. In Wilkins RH, Rengachary SS (eds): Neurosurgery. New York, McGraw-Hill, 1996, pp 1559–1571.
23. Fletcher WE, Arnold JH: Carotid body tumor: A review of the literature and report of an unusual case. Am J Surg 87: 617–623, 1954.
24. Staats EF, Brown RL, Smith RR: Carotid body tumors, benign and malignant. Laryngoscope 76:907–916, 1966.
25. Harrington SW, Clagett OT, Dockerty MD: Tumors of the carotid body: Clinical and pathological considerations of twenty tumors affecting nineteen patients (one bilateral). Ann Surg 114:820–833, 1941.
26. Reiner SA, Medina J, Minn KW: Vascular leiomyoma of the carotid sheath simulating a carotid body tumor. Am J Otolaryngol 19:127–129, 1998.
27. Litle VR, Reilly LM, Ramos TK: Preoperative embolization of carotid body tumors: When is it appropriate? Ann Vasc Surg 10:464–468, 1996.
28. Liapis C, Gougoulakis A, Karydakis V, et al: Changing trends in management of carotid body tumors. Am Surg 61:989–993, 1995.
29. Shamblin WR, ReMine WH, Sheps SG, et al: Carotid body tumor (chemodectoma): Clinicopathologic analysis of ninety cases. Am J Surg 122:732–739, 1971.
30. Romanski R: Chemodectoma (non-chromaffinic paraganglioma) of the carotid body with distant metastases. Am J Pathol 30: 1–9, 1954.
31. Rangwala AF, Sylvia LC, Becker SM: Soft tissue metastasis of a chemodectoma: A case report and review of the literature. Cancer 42:2865–2869, 1978.

32. Kawai A, Healey JH, Wilson SC, et al: Carotid body paraganglioma metastatic to bone: Report of two cases. Skeletal Radiol 27: 103–107, 1998.
33. Boyle JR, London NJ, Tan SG, et al: Labile blood pressure after bilateral carotid body tumour surgery. Eur J Vasc Endovasc Surg 9:346–348, 1995.
34. Netterville JL, Reilly KM, Robertson D, et al: Carotid body tumors: A review of 30 patients with 46 tumors. Laryngoscope 105:115–126, 1995.
35. Leonetti JP, Donzelli JJ, Littooy FN, et al: Perioperative strategies in the management of carotid body tumors. Otolaryngol Head Neck Surg 117:111–115, 1997.
36. Leadbetter WF, Burkland CE: Hypertension in unilateral renal disease. J Urol 39:611–626, 1938.
37. Palubinskas AJ, Ripley HR: Fibromuscular hyperplasia in extrarenal arteries. Radiology 82:451–455, 1964.
38. Houser OW, Baker HL Jr: Fibromuscular dysplasia and other uncommon diseases of the cervical carotid artery: Angiographic aspects. Am J Roentgenol Radium Ther Nucl Med 104:201–212, 1968.
39. Bergan JJ, MacDonald JR: Recognition of cerebrovascular fibromuscular hyperplasia. Arch Surg 98:332–335, 1969.
40. Momose KJ, New PF: Non-atheromatous stenosis and occlusion of the internal carotid artery and its main branches. Am J Roentgenol Radium Ther Nucl Med 118:550–566, 1973.
41. Pollock M, Jackson BM: Fibromuscular dysplasia of the carotid arteries. Neurology 21:1226–1230, 1971.
42. Galligioni F, Iraci G, Marin G: Fibromuscular hyperplasia of the extracranial internal carotid artery. J Neurosurg 34:647–651, 1971.
43. Sandok BA, Houser OW, Baker WL Jr, et al: Fibromuscular dysplasia: Neurologic disorders associated with disease involving the great vessels in the neck. Arch Neurol 24:462–466, 1971.
44. Frens DB, Petajan JH, Anderson R, et al: Fibromuscular dysplasia of the posterior cerebral artery: Report of a case and review of the literature. Stroke 5:161–166, 1974.
45. Iosue A, Kier EL, Ostrow D: Fibromuscular dysplasia involving the intracranial vessels: Case report. J Neurosurg 37:749–752, 1972.
46. So EL, Toole JF, Moody DM, et al: Cerebral embolism from septal fibromuscular dysplasia of the common carotid artery. Ann Neurol 6:75–78, 1979.
47. Corrin LS, Sandok BA, Houser OW: Cerebral ischemic events in patients with carotid artery fibromuscular dysplasia. Arch Neurol 38:616–618, 1981.
48. Osborn AG, Anderson RE: Angiographic spectrum of cervical and intracranial fibromuscular dysplasia. Stroke 8:617–626, 1977.
49. Stanley JC, Gewertz BL, Bove EL, et al: Arterial fibrodysplasia: Histopathologic character and current etiologic concepts. Arch Surg 110:561–566, 1975.
50. Mettinger KL, Ericson K: Fibromuscular dysplasia and the brain. I. Observations on angiographic, clinical and genetic characteristics. Stroke 13:46–52, 1982.
51. Mettinger KL: Fibromuscular dysplasia and the brain. II. Current concept of the disease. Stroke 13:53–58, 1982.
52. Hopkins LN, Budny JL: Fibromuscular dysplasia. In Wilkins RH, Rengachary SS (eds): Neurosurgery. New York, McGraw-Hill, 1996, pp 2169–2172.
53. Andersen CA, Collins GJ Jr, Rich NM, et al: Spontaneous dissection of the internal carotid artery associated with fibromuscular dysplasia. Am Surg 46:263–266, 1980.
54. Ringel SP, Harrison SH, Norenberg MD, et al: Fibromuscular dysplasia: Multiple "spontaneous" dissecting aneurysms of the major cervical arteries. Ann Neurol 1:301–304, 1977.
55. Ehrenfeld WK, Wylie EJ: Fibromuscular hyperplasia of the internal carotid artery. Arch Surg 109:676–681, 1974.
56. Bergentz SE, Ericsson BF, Linell F, et al: Bilateral fibromuscular hyperplasia in the internal carotid arteries with aneurysm formation. Acta Chir Scand 142:501–504, 1976.
57. Zimmerman R, Leeds NE, Naidich TP: Carotid-cavernous fistula associated with intracranial fibromuscular dysplasia. Radiology 122:725–726, 1977.
58. Kaufman HH, Lind TA, Mullan S: Spontaneous carotid-cavernous fistula with fibromuscular dysplasia. Acta Neurochir (Wien) 40:123–129, 1978.
59. Morris GC Jr, Lechter A, DeBakey ME: Surgical treatment of fibromuscular disease of the carotid arteries. Arch Surg 96: 636–643, 1968.
60. Garrido E, Montoya J: Transluminal dilatation of internal carotid artery in fibromuscular dysplasia: A preliminary report. Surg Neurol 16:469–471, 1981.
61. Hasso AN, Bird CR, Zinke DE, et al: Fibromuscular dysplasia of the internal carotid artery: Percutaneous transluminal angioplasty. AJR Am J Roentgenol 136:955–960, 1981.
62. Dublin AB, Baltaxe HA, Cobb CA 3rd: Percutaneous transluminal carotid angioplasty in fibromuscular dysplasia: Case report. J Neurosurg 59:162–165, 1983.
63. Starr DS, Lawrie GM, Morris GC Jr: Fibromuscular disease of carotid arteries: Long term results of graduated internal dilatation. Stroke 12:196–199, 1981.
64. Wilms GE, Smits J, Baert AL, et al: Percutaneous transluminal angioplasty in fibromuscular dysplasia of the internal carotid artery: One year clinical and morphological follow-up. Cardiovasc Intervent Radiol 8:20–23, 1985.
65. Jooma R, Bradshaw JR, Griffith HB: Intimal dissection following percutaneous transluminal carotid angioplasty for fibromuscular dysplasia. Neuroradiology 27:181–182, 1985.
66. Lord RSA, Graham AR, Benn IV: Radiologic control of operative carotid dilatation: Aneurysm formation following balloon dilatation. J Cardiovasc Surg (Torino) 27:158–162, 1986.
67. Mokri B, Piepgras DG, Sundt TM Jr, et al: Extracranial internal carotid artery aneurysms. Mayo Clin Proc 57:310–321, 1982.
68. Cooper A: Account of the first successful operation performed on the common carotid artery for aneurysm. Guys Hosp Rep 1: 53–59, 1836.
69. Winslow N: Extracranial aneurysm of the internal carotid artery: History and analysis of the cases registered up to August 1, 1925. Arch Surg 13:689–729, 1926.
70. Dimtza A: Aneurysms of the carotid arteries: Report of two cases. Angiology 7:218–227, 1956.
71. Taylor SP, Langan EM 3rd, Snyder BA, et al: Nonendarterectomy procedures of the carotid artery: A five-year review. Am Surg 65:323–327, 1999.
72. Ekestrom S, Bergdahl L, Huttunen H: Extracranial carotid and vertebral artery aneurysms. Scand J Thorac Cardiovasc Surg 17: 135–139, 1983.
73. Petrovic P, Avramov S, Pfau J, et al: Surgical management of extracranial carotid artery aneurysms. Ann Vasc Surg 5:506–509, 1991.
74. McCollum CH, Wheeler WG, Noon GP, et al: Aneurysms of the extracranial carotid artery: Twenty-one years' experience. Am J Surg 137:196–200, 1979.
75. Kaupp HA, Haid SP, Jurayj MN, et al: Aneurysms of the extracranial carotid artery. Surgery 72:946–952, 1972.
76. Ohyama T, Ohara S, Momma F: Aneurysm of the cervical internal carotid artery associated with Marfan's syndrome—case report. Neurol Med Chir (Tokyo) 32:965–968, 1992.
77. Green LN: Progeria with carotid artery aneurysms: Report of a case. Arch Neurol 38:659–661, 1981.
78. Painter TS, Hertzer NR, Beven EG, et al: Extracranial carotid aneurysms: Report of six cases and review of the literature. J Vasc Surg 2:312–318, 1985.
79. Coffin O, Maiza D, Galateau-Salle F, et al: Results of surgical management of internal carotid artery aneurysm by the cervical approach. Ann Vasc Surg 11:482–490, 1997.
80. Hurst RW, Haskal ZJ, Zager E, et al: Endovascular stent treatment of cervical internal carotid artery aneurysms with parent vessel preservation. Surg Neurol 50:313–317, 1998.
81. Jentzer A: Dissecting aneurysm of the left internal carotid artery. Angiology 5:232, 1954.
82. Freidman A: Arterial dissections. In Wilkins RH, Rengachary SS (eds): Neurosurgery. New York, McGraw-Hill, 1996, pp 2173–2176.
83. Mokri B, Piepgras DG, Wiebers DO, et al: Familial occurrence of spontaneous dissection of the internal carotid artery. Stroke 18:246–251, 1987.
84. Mokri B, Sundt TM Jr, Houser OW, et al: Spontaneous dissection of the cervical internal carotid artery. Ann Neurol 19:126–138, 1986.
85. Meissner I, Mokri B: Vascular diseases of the cervical carotid artery. Cardiovasc Clin 22:161–188, 1992.

86. van den Berg JS, Limburg M, Kappelle LJ, et al: The role of type III collagen in spontaneous cervical arterial dissections. Ann Neurol 43:494–498, 1998.
87. Petro GR, Witwer GA, Cacayorin ED, et al: Spontaneous dissection of the cervical internal carotid artery: Correlation of arteriography, CT, and pathology. AJR Am J Roentgenol 148:393–398, 1987.
88. Pozzati E, Giuliani G, Acciarri N, et al: Long-term follow-up of occlusive cervical carotid dissection. Stroke 21:528–531, 1990.
89. Pozzati E, Gaist G, Poppi M: Resolution of occlusion in spontaneously dissected carotid arteries: Report of two cases. J Neurosurg 56:857–860, 1982.
90. Bogousslavsky J, Despland PA, Regli F: Spontaneous carotid dissection with acute stroke. Arch Neurol 44:137–140, 1987.
91. Nardelli E, Fiaschi A, Ferrari G: Delayed cerebrovascular consequences of radiation to the neck: A clinicopathologic study of a case. Arch Neurol 35:538–540, 1978.
92. Murros KE, Toole JF: The effect of radiation on carotid arteries: A review article. Arch Neurol 46:449–455, 1989.
93. Dubec JJ, Munk PL, Tsang V, et al: Carotid artery stenosis in patients who have undergone radiation therapy for head and neck malignancy. Br J Radiol 71:872–875, 1998.
94. Elerding SC, Fernandez RN, Grotta JC, et al: Carotid artery disease following external cervical irradiation. Ann Surg 194: 609–615, 1981.
95. Fonkalsrud EW, Sanchez M, Zerubavel R, et al: Serial changes in arterial structure following radiation therapy. Surg Gynecol Obstet 145:395–400, 1977.
96. Gassman A: Zur Histologie der Röntgenulcera. Fortschr Geb Roentgenstr 2:199–207, 1899.
97. Wolbach SB: The pathologic history of chromic x-ray dermatitis and early x-ray carcinoma. J Med Res 21:415–449, 1909.
98. Sheehan JF: Foam cell plaques in the intima of irradiated arteries. Arch Pathol 37:297–307, 1944.
99. Konings AW, Hardonk MJ, Wieringa RA, et al: Initial events in radiation-induced atheromatosis. I. Activation of lysosomal enzymes. Strahlentherapie 150:444–448, 1975.
100. Cade S: Malignant Disease and Its Treatment by Radium. Baltimore, Williams & Wilkins, 1940, p 248.
101. Thomas E, Forbus WD: Irradiation injury to the aorta and the lung. Arch Pathol 67:256–263, 1959.
102. Chung TS, Yousem DM, Lexa FJ, et al: MRI of carotid angioplasty after therapeutic radiation. J Comput Assist Tomogr 18: 533–538, 1994.
103. Silverberg GD, Britt RH, Goffinet DR: Radiation-induced carotid artery disease. Cancer 41:130–137, 1978.
104. Atkinson JL, Sundt TM Jr, Dale AJ, et al: Radiation-associated atheromatous disease of the cervical carotid artery: Report of seven cases and review of the literature. Neurosurgery 24:171–178, 1989.
105. Kashyap VS, Moore WS, Quinones-Baldrich WJ: Carotid artery repair for radiation-associated atherosclerosis is a safe and durable procedure. J Vasc Surg 29:90–99, 1999.
106. Melliere D, Becquemin JP, Berrahal D, et al: Management of radiation-induced occlusive arterial disease: A reassessment. J Cardiovasc Surg (Torino) 38:261–269, 1997.
107. Teitelbaum GP, Lefkowitz MA, Giannotta SL: Carotid angioplasty and stenting in high-risk patients. Surg Neurol 50:300–311, 1998.

CHAPTER 102

Extracranial Vertebral Artery Disease

FADY T. CHARBEL ■ KERN H. GUPPY ■ ANDREW L. CARNEY ■
JAMES I. AUSMAN

As early as 1844, Quain[1] described the anatomy and operative surgery of the extracranial vertebral artery in lithographic drawings. In 1893, Matas[2] described the contributions made in the early 1800s by other surgeons such as Dietrich, Velpeau, and Maisonneuve for the treatment of penetrating trauma to the vertebral artery. In 1831, Dietrich first proposed ligating the distal vertebral artery in the occipital-atloid region. In 1833, Velpeau ligated the vertebral artery at its proximal portion. Twenty years later, Maisonneuve successfully ligated the vertebral artery at the transverse foramen of the sixth cervical vertebra for a stab wound to the neck. The patient later died from a cerebral septic embolism.

As the discovery of extracranial vertebral artery disease became more extensive, new methods of treatment evolved. Pathologic injury to the vertebral artery, caused by erosion of its wall by a tuberculous abscess, was repaired by ligation by Smythe in New Orleans in 1864. Alexander[3] also used ligature of the vertebral arteries to treat epilepsy, sometimes ligating both arteries at the same time. Elective ligation of the vertebral artery was also used to treat aneurysms. In 1888, Matas[2] was the first surgeon who did not rely on ligation of the vertebral artery as treatment but fully excised an aneurysm between the occiput and the atlas through a posterior approach.

For the next 50 years, few advances were made in the medical treatment of extracranial vertebral disease until Moniz[4] performed the first vertebral angiogram in 1927 (Moniz won the Nobel Prize not for this discovery but for the prefrontal lobotomy). Radner[5] first reported selective angiography of the vertebral artery. This technique allowed researchers to correlate occlusive disease with symptoms. In 1946, Kubik and Adams[6] first described basilar artery insufficiency caused by thrombosis of the basilar artery. Ten years later at the Mayo Clinic, Millikan and Siekert[7] reported studies of cerebrovascular disease and the syndrome of intermittent insufficiency of the basilar arterial system. They introduced the use of anticoagulation drugs in the treatment of thrombosis of the basilar artery and noted a substantial reduction in the incidence of brainstem infarctions.[8]

With this revolution in the diagnosis of diseased arteries, more aggressive surgical techniques were developed. The cause of brain ischemia was assumed to be hypoperfusion, with the solution being revascularization. In 1958, Crawford and coworkers[9] presented their results of surgical treatment of brainstem ischemia by reconstructing the vertebral artery after removing atherosclerotic plaque. The next year, Cate and Scott[10] first described the technique of trans-subclavian endarterectomy of the subclavian-vertebral artery.

In 1961, angiography allowed Reivich and colleagues[11] to describe the process of reversed flow in the vertebral artery with proximal left subclavian stenosis in two patients with associated neurological dysfunction. This phenomenon was called *subclavian steal syndrome*. Angiography also allowed visualization of other causes of extracranial vertebral artery disease, including extrinsic compression of the vertebral artery by osteophytes,[12] constricting bands,[13] and rotational obstruction,[14] all of which were diagnosed and treated by surgical decompression.

Angiography also provided the first extensive cooperative study of the incidence of extracranial arterial stenosis caused by atherosclerotic lesions in patients with cerebrovascular insufficiency. In 1968, *stenosis* was defined as a compromised lumen of more than 50% by the Joint Study of Extracranial Arterial Occlusion.[15] Of 4748 patients, 80% had four-vessel angiograms that were categorized by location of the arterial stenosis. For the first time, this study provided a frequency distribution of surgically accessible sites with stenosis caused by atherosclerosis of the extracranial vertebral artery.[15]

As microsurgery evolved in the 1970s, various reconstructive techniques also developed. Wylie and Ehrenfeld[16] first treated pathology of the proximal vertebral artery by the transposition technique, with anastomosis between the vertebral artery and the common carotid artery (CCA). Berguer and associates[17] used vein grafts in this region of the vertebral artery to connect the subclavian artery to the proximal vertebral artery. In January 1977, Carney and Anderson[18] performed the first vein bypass from the CCA to the distal vertebral artery at the level of C1 and C2. Subsequently,

Carney used the supply from the subclavian artery, external carotid artery (ECA), internal carotid artery (ICA), and occipital artery to supply the distal vertebral artery.[19]

The treatment of penetrating vertebral artery injuries also changed significantly with the advent of the Vietnam War. Surgeons no longer relied solely on ligation of the artery as treatment; in many cases, they actually reconstructed the vertebral artery.[19] In the civilian population, vertebral artery injuries were less common; Perry and coworkers[20] reported no such injuries among 508 penetrating arterial injuries.

Angioplasty was first introduced by Dotter and Judkins[21] in 1964 using flexible dilators, but it was not until the 1980s that angioplasty was successfully performed in the subclavian and vertebral arteries. In 1980, Bachmann and Kim[22] first reported dilatation of the subclavian artery for the treatment of subclavian steal syndrome. In 1986, Higashida and colleagues[23] reported successful percutaneous transluminal angioplasty of the vertebral arteries.

Today, many of the medical, surgical, and endovascular techniques described so far are still in use. The most rapid developments have been made in endovascular techniques. As the evolution of neurovascular surgery in the 1960s was used to remedy occlusion of the carotid and vertebral arteries, it is not difficult to imagine that we may be witnessing a new evolution in the management and diagnosis of extracranial vertebral artery disease.

CLINICAL SIGNIFICANCE

The external vertebral arteries provide blood flow to a large distribution via the basilar artery and posterior cerebral arteries. Therefore, symptoms can arise from the occipital or temporal lobes, cerebellum, pons, and brainstem with its cranial nerves. The term *intermittent insufficiency of the basilar arterial system* was first used by Millikan and Siekert[7] when they observed clinical symptoms in patients with basilar artery occlusions. These symptoms occurred in 70% of the patients before occlusion. Today, this syndrome is known as *vertebrobasilar insufficiency* (VBI) and is characterized by intermittent episodes of multiple symptoms that can be sudden or severe. Eventually, the symptoms either resolve or become permanent. These symptoms are caused not only by embolic or thrombotic sources but also by other hemodynamic changes. Fields and Lemak[24] noted that in 168 patients with angiographically proven subclavian steal syndrome, changes in the blood flow of the vertebral artery accounted for symptoms of VBI. Fluctuations in vertebral artery blood flow have also been reproduced by head turning, as demonstrated by Toole and Tucker.[25]

After a critical review of the literature, Ausman and coworkers[26] concluded that the symptoms of VBI have multiple causes and that one can seldom localize pathologic lesions in the posterior circulation by clinical examination alone. Most physicians use the presence of any two of the common symptoms to define the syndrome (Table 102–1).

TABLE 102–1 ■ **Symptoms of Vertebrobasilar Insufficiency**

Motor or sensory symptoms, or both	Alternating paresthesias
Dysarthria	Homonymous hemianopsia
Imbalance	Diplopia
Dizziness or vertigo	Other cranial nerve palsies
Tinnitus	Dysphagia

The presence of at least two symptoms is required to diagnose vertebrobasilar insufficiency.

The most common symptom that physicians (including neurologists and neurosurgeons) have difficulty relating to VBI is vertigo or dizziness. First, this symptom is often associated with other diseases. In addition, many articles have ruled out the occurrence of vertigo or dizziness as evidence of transient ischemic attacks. The dogma that vertigo or dizziness alone is not a presenting symptom of VBI was thereby established.[27] These patients are often treated empirically or referred to an otolaryngologist for further evaluation.

Studies by Grad and Baloh[27] and Kumar and associates[28] raised significant questions about how extensive an evaluation is needed in patients with isolated symptoms of vertigo. Kumar's group found that vertigo, dizziness, and imbalance—individually or collectively—can be exclusive symptoms of VBI and that vestibular test results (decruitment and hyperactivity) show a clinically significant sensitivity for distinguishing labyrinthine or brainstem-cerebellum (posterior neuraxis) lesions. In general, the vagueness of the presenting symptoms of VBI requires a team approach to analyze these patients. Because the final determination of the cause of VBI requires invasive and expensive tests, a clear-cut approach to making the diagnosis is essential.

ANATOMY OF THE EXTRACRANIAL VERTEBRAL ARTERY

The vertebral artery varies in diameter from 0.5 to 5.5 mm and in length from 5 to 35 cm. It is a high-resistance artery, and both sides accommodate blood flow rates of about 120 mL/min. The left vertebral artery is larger than the right in about 75% of cases.[19]

The extracranial vertebral arteries can be divided into three regions: proximal, middle, and distal (Fig. 102–1). This division is helpful because the associated pathology appears to differ among the segments. In many cases, the surgical approaches are similarly divided by these anatomic regions.

Proximal Vertebral Artery. The proximal vertebral artery extends from the superior portion of the subclavian artery to enter the transverse foramen of C6. It

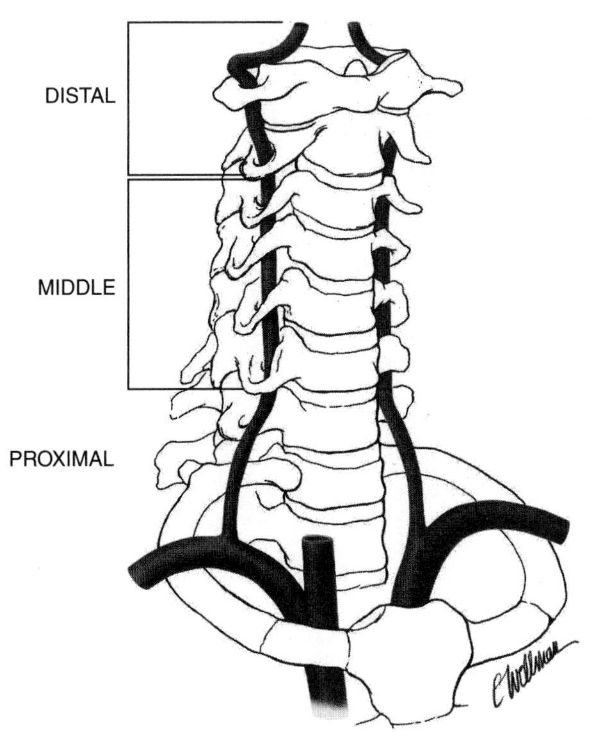

FIGURE 102–1. Segments of the vertebral artery. It is divided into the proximal vertebral artery, from the subclavian artery to the beginning of its entry to the transverse foramen of C6; the middle vertebral artery, between the exit of the artery from the transverse foramen of C6 to its entry to the transverse foramen of C2; and the distal vertebral artery, from the exit from the transverse foramen of C2 to its entry through the dura.

enters at levels other than C6 10% of the time (C5, 7%; C6, 90%; C7, 3%). Instead of arising from the superior portion of the left subclavian artery, the left vertebral artery can arise from the proximal subclavian trunk. In 5% of cases, it arises separately from the aortic arch. Typically, the right vertebral artery is the first branch of the right subclavian artery, but it can arise from various places: from the right CCA or the right ICA, from the aortic arch directly, or from the right subclavian artery distal to the thyrocervical trunk.[29]

Middle Vertebral Artery. The middle vertebral artery describes the region between the transverse foramen of C6 and where it exits the transverse processes of C2. As the vertebral artery enters the transverse foramen of C6, it ascends in a vertical path through the upper cervical foramen until it approaches C2. Then it deviates laterally as it ascends through the C2 transverse foramen (see Fig. 102–1).

Distal Vertebral Artery. The distal vertebral artery extends from where it exits the transverse foramen ofC1 to its entry through the atlanto-occipital membrane. From the C2 transverse foramen, it courses slightly anteriorly to pass through the transverse foramen of C1. As the artery exits the cervical spine, it enters the dura and foramen magnum by moving dorsally, resting on the posterior arch of C1. It turns superomedially before piercing the dura (see Fig. 102–1).

PATHOPHYSIOLOGY OF EXTRACRANIAL VERTEBRAL ARTERY DISEASE

The pathophysiology of extracranial vertebral artery disease is not as well understood as that of the carotid system. Vertebrobasilar symptoms arise from interruption of the blood supply to the brain and brainstem. The interruption can be the result of hypoperfusion caused by hemodynamic changes or by thromboembolic sources. Ischemia from hemodynamic mechanisms rarely causes infarction initially; rather, the symptoms are short-lived and repetitive. They are, however, still dangerous if the hypoperfusion persists. In contrast, emboli are more likely to cause dangerous infarctions and leave patients with permanent deficits. Most vertebrobasilar symptoms are likely caused by emboli, although exact percentages are lacking in the literature.

Hemodynamic Causes

Hemodynamic changes can result from either an interruption of the source of blood supply or blockage of the conduit that provides the blood flow. The former occurs in cardiac insufficiency or postural hypotension from systemic disease. The latter is related to obstruction of blood flow in the arterial system, but obstruction of blood flow in one vertebral artery may be insufficient to cause hemodynamic changes. Anatomic variations in the other artery—such as a hypoplastic vertebral artery, termination of one artery into the posterior inferior cerebellar artery, or complete occlusion of the contralateral vertebral artery—can also occur.[29] There also may be associated pathology in the carotid system or an incomplete circle of Willis.[19]

The mere presence of an obstruction or stenosis does not necessarily mean that blood flow in that particular artery will be significantly reduced. In 1938, Mann and colleagues[30] first demonstrated that a decrease in the flow rate of the carotid artery does not become significant until a critical narrowing occurs (called *critical stenosis*). May and coworkers[31] confirmed this finding in later studies and showed that critical stenosis depends on the baseline rate of blood flow. For example, if symptoms appear in a low-flow system when the rate of blood flow is reduced 25%, the critical stenosis is about 85%. For a high-flow system, however, the critical stenosis for the same percentage of change in the rate of blood flow may be as low as 35%. This fact is often not fully appreciated, especially when a similar criterion for critical stenosis is used for both the carotid and vertebral arteries, even though the flow rate in the CCA approaches 300 mL/min, compared with about 120 mL/min in the vertebral artery. Hence, the criterion for critical stenosis of the carotid artery cannot be applied to the vertebral artery.

Examples of diseases in the extracranial vertebral arteries that cause hemodynamic changes include atherosclerosis, compressive syndromes, traumatic or spontaneous dissections of these vessels, and subclavian steal syndrome. Atherosclerosis is the most common form of vertebral artery disease. Although it is a source of thromboembolic plaque, it can cause significant hypoperfusion by obstructing blood flow. Details of the incidence, clinical manifestations, and prognosis of hypoperfusion caused by this disease process are still lacking. One of the most extensive studies on the incidence of extracranial disease in symptomatic patients was presented by Hass and associates[15] from the Joint Study of Extracranial Arterial Occlusion. They found that the most common site of plaque formation in the vertebrobasilar arterial system was the origin of the proximal vertebral artery (right vertebral artery, 18.4%; left vertebral artery, 22.3%). The second most common site was the middle vertebral artery. In this region, it is believed that the blood flow rate is dampened as it passes through the foramen. Atherosclerosis occurs less frequently intracranially in the midbasilar artery and at the entry of the vertebral artery through the dura.

Spontaneous dissections are associated with systemic diseases affecting the arterial walls. In both the carotid and vertebral arteries, fibromuscular dysplasia is the most common cause of spontaneous dissection. It tends to affect areas where there is significant movement of the cervical spine and therefore occurs in the middle and distal segments of the vertebral artery. The formation of pseudoaneurysms is also quite common, although these lesions are often asymptomatic.[19]

Trauma is the third most common cause of vertebral artery disease. Both blunt and penetrating trauma can dissect the vertebral artery. Blunt injury occurs from cervical spine fractures and dislocations that may result in occlusion, pseudoaneurysm, or arteriovenous fistula (AVF) of the vertebral artery, especially in the middle portion. This type of injury can also be created iatrogenically from chiropractic manipulation. The most frequent site of thrombosis is at the level of C2 in the distal vertebral artery. This tendency may reflect the posterior placement of the vertebral foramina with respect to the vertebral body. The vertebral artery has an increased vulnerability for compression by subluxation of the cervical apophyseal joints. Blunt injury to the vertebral artery may be more common than has been quoted in the literature because these patients seldom undergo angiography unless they show symptoms of vertebral insufficiency. Penetrating trauma to the vertebral artery is less common than blunt trauma. In 1971, Perry and coworkers[20] examined 508 penetrating arterial injuries in the civilian population and found no involvement of the vertebral artery in any of the cases. Only during periods of war and with the advent of shrapnel on the battlefield did the incidence of these injuries increase.

Compression of the vertebral artery can cause VBI. The anterior scalene muscle has been found to compress the vertebral artery at the level of C6. Osteophytes and disk spurs, found between levels C6 and C2, can encroach on and compress the middle vertebral artery, causing vascular symptoms. Usually, rotation or extension of the neck triggers symptoms. Dynamic angiography has been recommended for patients who show vertebral artery symptoms on flexion, extension, or rotation of the neck.[19]

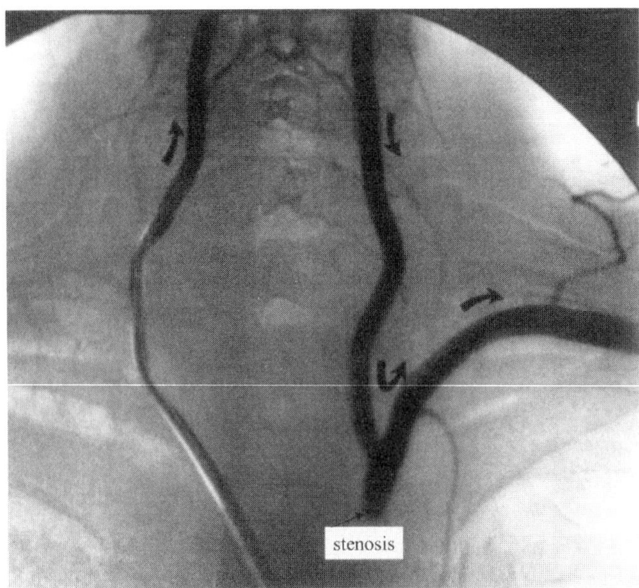

FIGURE 102–2. Angiogram showing blood flow in a patient with subclavian steal syndrome. As indicated, blood returns to the subclavian artery because of the proximal obstruction in it.

Subclavian steal syndrome was first described by Reivich and colleagues[11] in 1961 when they discovered reverse flow in the vertebral artery. It is caused by stenosis or occlusion in the subclavian or innominate artery proximal to the vertebral artery. If the pressure in the subclavian artery distal to the obstruction is low enough, it acts as a "sink" for the flow of blood from the vertebral artery and drains blood from the contralateral vertebral artery and even as far as the circle of Willis (Fig. 102–2). Hence, patients can experience vertebrobasilar symptoms and may also have cerebrum, cerebellum, and brainstem symptoms. Most of these symptoms are caused by use of the extremities when the demand for blood flow is increased and the pressure sink becomes more pronounced. In many cases, patients rarely experience symptoms at rest.

Embolic Causes

The pathology that causes hemodynamic changes and the sources of emboli often overlap. Embolism arising from within or outside the vertebral system seeks the terminal branches of the basilar artery or the posterior cerebral arteries. Consequently, symptoms can manifest as simple cranial nerve palsies or brainstem vascular syndromes (e.g., Wallenberg's syndrome, Weber's syndrome). Acute visual field defects or symptoms of occipital lobe infarction can also be presenting symptoms.

Emboli or thrombi may originate from the vertebral arteries themselves or from the subclavian or aortic arches. They also can come from pathologic heart valves, abnormal cardiac wall behavior, or arrhythmias. Atherosclerotic plaque is usually the source of emboli or thrombi from the aorta or subclavian or vertebral arteries. If not treated with anticoagulation, thrombi from the spontaneous rupture of vessels or after trauma to the extracranial vertebral arteries will obstruct the smaller branches of the vertebral arteries.

DIAGNOSTIC EVALUATION

The symptoms associated with disease of the extracranial vertebral artery are multiple and often vague. Distinguishing patients with true VBI is therefore a significant challenge. Once such patients have been diagnosed, the treatment must be individualized to best suit the specific patient. A statement by one of the senior authors of this chapter 20 years ago still holds true today: "The surgeon operating on the vertebral artery must address not only the surgical technique, but also the diagnostic approach, the hemodynamic documentation."[19]

The diagnostic approach to extracranial vertebral artery disease consists of ruling out patients who present with VBI-type symptoms caused by disorders other than vertebrobasilar artery insufficiency, identifying the cause and thus identifying patients with extracranial vertebral artery disease, and determining whether the cause is embolic or hemodynamic.

Many systemic and neurological diseases can cause VBI-type symptoms. Meniere's disease, infection or dysfunction of the vestibular and labyrinthine structures, demyelinating diseases, seizures, tumors of the cerebellopontine angle, spinal column dysfunction, and compression of structures in the posterior fossa from either masses (intra-axial cerebellum tumors) or bony encroachment (Chiari's malformation) can all manifest with VBI-type symptoms.

Reduced cardiac output can also cause symptoms of VBI. Cardiac disease such as dysrhythmias, cardiac insufficiency, and infarction can result in poor cardiac output. Thromboembolic causes from cardiac valvular disease, bacterial endocarditis, dysrhythmias, and hematologic diseases (thrombocytosis, bleeding disorders, sickle cell) can cause symptoms of VBI. Other systemic diseases such as diabetes can cause autonomic dysfunction that causes orthostatic hypotension. Severe cases of hypovolemia associated with poor autonomic function can manifest with symptoms of VBI. Therefore, a careful medical and diagnostic workup is necessary when evaluating these patients.

History and Physical Examination

The first process in any evaluation is to obtain a good history of the patient's presenting symptoms. The history must identify the onset of symptoms, their duration, and the predisposing conditions that elicit or relieve symptoms. VBI is a vascular phenomenon, and the onset of symptoms is sudden. Hypertension, smoking, and, in women, contraceptive medications can be contributing factors. The patient's work history and any family history of migraine headaches or cardiac or neurological diseases need to be known. Patients on medications, particularly antihypertensive medications, can present with low blood pressure and have symptoms of VBI.

A thorough physical examination is the second step in identifying the cause of VBI-type symptoms or true VBI. An abnormal neurological examination permits the symptoms to be isolated to a particular region of the central nervous system. However, many VBI patients present with no detectable neurological findings.

Routine Laboratory Evaluation

A routine metabolic and blood workup should be obtained. Patients on medications that require therapeutic levels should be monitored, because many VBI symptoms can be related to overmedication (e.g., antihypertensives). If the patient's work history indicates exposure to unusual chemicals known to be toxic, the appropriate level should be determined. A 12-lead electrocardiogram, a 24-hour Holter monitor and, if possible, an echocardiogram (if indicated) can be the first steps in evaluating the heart.

Audiometric and Vestibular Tests

In some cases, the presentation of vertigo or dizziness with no other findings requires consultation with an otolaryngologist to rule out labyrinthitis or vestibular causes. By the time patients are seen by a neurologist or neurosurgeon, most of them have already been treated with medications for labyrinthitis or Meniere's disease. Before more invasive procedures such as cerebral angiography are recommended, these patients should undergo audiometric and vestibular tests. Audiometric tests include a pure-tone audiogram and a speech discrimination test to indicate hearing loss. A vestibular test can indicate decruitment and hyperactivity, which can be strong indicators of a centrally located lesion (sensitivity of 92%).[28]

Brain Imaging Techniques

The brain and the posterior fossa must be imaged as part of the evaluation. Computed tomography is an excellent imaging technique for ruling out mass lesions or hemorrhages. Magnetic resonance imaging (MRI) is highly sensitive and can detect demyelinating disease, stroke, and mass lesions. MRI of the arterial system, or magnetic resonance angiography (MRA), is a good noninvasive screening technique for evaluating the intracranial and extracranial arteries. Its ability to accurately identify stenosis is limited, however. The use of contrast enhancement can increase the utility of magnetic resonance angiography.[32]

For patients with VBI, metabolic changes occur immediately. MRI and computed tomography cannot detect such changes acutely (<24 hours). Single photon emission computed tomography evaluates the metabolic function of the brainstem and cerebellum, as does xenon computed tomography. Both modalities, however, are of limited use in the posterior fossa because of imaging difficulties. Diffusion-weighted imaging and perfusion imaging, two new magnetic resonance technologies, are becoming increasingly available for the evaluation of acute ischemic stroke patients.[33] Diffusion-weighted imaging provides early information about the location of acute focal ischemic brain injury, and perfusion imaging can document the presence of disturbances in microcirculation perfusion.

Cerebral Angiography

Cerebral angiography is considered the gold standard for evaluating the intracranial and extracranial vessels of the brain. Unlike MRA, it is an invasive procedure and carries a low risk of stroke (1% overall incidence of neurological deficit, and 0.5% incidence of persistent deficit).[34]

In cases of extracranial vertebral artery disease, the aortic arch must be visualized, as well as the four major intracranial arteries. VBI symptoms are caused predominantly by intracranial disease, and good visualization of the intracranial vessels is essential. Similarly, subclavian steal syndrome manifests with VBI symptoms, although the pathology is located in the subclavian artery.

Compared with MRA, cerebral angiography is a dynamic study. As the contrast medium diffuses, a quantitative sense of the hemodynamics can be obtained. In the hands of an experienced neuroradiologist or neurosurgeon, the blood flow in the basilar artery can be determined as low or high. Similarly, retrograde flow, as occurs in subclavian steal syndrome, can be seen. Dynamic angiography can also be used to monitor vascular changes associated with head position. This feature is needed in patients with an occlusion or reduced blood flow in the vertebral artery from an obstruction caused by soft tissue (ligament or muscle), neuronal tissue, or bone.[19]

Hemodynamic Evaluation

Once an obstructive lesion has been identified, it is important to determine whether the VBI symptoms are from poor perfusion caused by the obstruction or by emboli. Cerebral angiography can give some sense of the cause, but it is far from reliable. Several methods have been used to evaluate the hemodynamics. Ultrasonography of the vertebral arteries has been used, but insonation is difficult, and its sensitivity is questionable. Interequipment, interinstitution, and technician variability make this method unsatisfactory.[35] Intracranial hemodynamic changes have also been monitored with transcranial Doppler ultrasonography, but this technique is also difficult to use in the posterior fossa.

Since the 1980s, flow quantification using phase-contrast MRI of the blood vessel has been studied.[36-42] Although static MRI or conventional angiography is useful for determining the anatomy of the vessel, phase-contrast MRI provides actual flow rates of blood in the vessel (in milliliters per minute). Both in vitro and in vivo flow studies have shown that velocities and volumetric flow rates can be estimated accurately for the carotid, vertebral, and major cerebral arteries.[41, 42] Normal values for flow rates in these vessels have been estimated.[41]

Therefore, phase-contrast MRI provides a noninvasive method for analyzing the cause of VBI symptoms. Rates of blood flow in both the vertebral and basilar arteries can be estimated using this technique. Based on knowledge of the normal range of flow rates in these vessels,[41] it can be determined whether obstructive lesions are significant enough to cause hypoperfusion of the vertebral artery. This knowledge is essential in planning treatment.

Other Evaluation Techniques

Once the diagnostic data are analyzed, one should have a clear indication of whether the cause of VBI is hemodynamic changes or emboli. If the treatment plan involves surgery or endovascular management that will change hemodynamics, further investigation is required. Several alternatives are available, but the optimal choice must provide reperfusion with the smallest risk to the patient. In the past, this decision was based solely on the surgeon's bias and training.

The use of mathematical models provides a unique method of testing alternative surgical strategies before they are implemented.[43, 44] Many models have been presented in the literature, but the most common difficulties are their lack of patient specificity and their inaccuracy.[44] We routinely use such models for planning surgery by simulating alternative procedures and evaluating the flow rate distribution after each one. The extracranial vertebral arteries are not isolated hemodynamically. Reconstruction of the vessels affects blood flow in the entire extracranial and intracranial system for both carotid and vertebral arteries. Therefore, careful planning is necessary.

By the time a treatment plan is chosen, the evaluation should indicate the cause of the VBI symptoms. In cases of hemodynamic compromise, removing the obstruction by surgery or endovascular angioplasty or bypassing the lesion may be indicated. For emboli, medical management is recommended initially in most cases. If the symptoms persist, surgical options can be used. Removing or bypassing the lesion with ligation of the offending vessel is often used.

MEDICAL MANAGEMENT

The use of medical management for vertebrobasilar ischemia dates to the 1950s,[8] with the use of heparin, and to the 1970s,[45] with the use of oral anticoagulation. This type of medical treatment for vertebrobasilar ischemia was associated with good outcomes. These early studies were flawed, however, because no angiographic studies were performed to identify the cause and significance of the extracranial disease. Without these data, the conclusions are anecdotal because the causes of extracranial vertebral artery disease are so variable.

Medical therapy of the extracranial vertebral arteries is used to prevent thrombus formation anywhere in the vertebral arteries or to prevent emboli from plaque. Vertebral artery dissections with the potential to form thrombi have been treated successfully with anticoagulation therapy. Once a thrombus has formed and caused hypoperfusion, however, it can be treated with angioplasty with anticoagulation or with local infusion of streptokinase or urokinase to dissolve the clot. The administration of tissue plasminogen activator has met with great success in dissolving clots.

Thrombi and emboli can also come from systemic sources. Typically, they migrate to the anterior circulation but can make their way to the posterior circulation. Medical therapy and, in particular, anticoagulants are used to prevent this thromboembolic formation from systemic sources. Medical therapy is also used to reduce the risk and complications of stroke, which include hypertension and high cholesterol levels.

Several antiplatelet trials have shown that aspirin reduces the relative risks of stroke, myocardial infarction, and vascular death by about 25%.[46] Ticlopidine is more effective than aspirin but has important side effects. Clopidogrel is as effective as ticlopidine, with fewer side effects. In 1996, the European Stroke Prevention Study showed that dipyridamole effectively prevents stroke and, when combined with aspirin, is equivalent to ticlopidine or clopidogrel.[47] These results can be applied to the medical treatment of extracranial vertebral artery disease.

Warfarin has also been used to prevent stroke and myocardial infarction. In 1995, the Warfarin-Aspirin Symptomatic Intracranial Disease Study showed a significant difference in stroke rates in patient with intracranial disease taking warfarin versus aspirin (stroke rate, 10.4/100 patient-years versus 3.6/100 patient-years). In many cases of extracranial vertebral artery disease, there is an associated intracranial component.[48] The use of warfarin is encouraged in these cases.

ENDOVASCULAR MANAGEMENT

Endovascular management of the external vertebral artery is in its infancy, and only selected procedures are performed. Vertebral AVFs have been treated by embolization with latex balloons. Beaujeux and colleagues[49] treated 46 AVFs that occurred between C1 and C2 in 21 patients, between C2 and C5 in 5 patients, and below C5 in 20 patients. More recently, electrical detachable coils were used to treat an AVF; the 5-month follow-up showed obliteration of the fistula.[50]

Although percutaneous transluminal angioplasty has been widely used to treat the ICA with or without the placement of stents, vertebral artery angioplasty is becoming more common. Its main application to the external vertebral artery is for the treatment of atherosclerotic plaque, which most often occurs at the origin of the vertebral artery. The plaque is often fibrous with a smooth surface (ulcerated in <4% of cases), making it ideal for percutaneous transluminal angioplasty.[51] Restenosis poses a major problem; in one series, it was reported in 3 of 34 arteries.[52, 53] The use of stents can alleviate this complication. Storey and associates[54] reported three patients who failed medical therapy and conventional angioplasty of the proximal vertebral artery and developed restenosis within 3 months. Stents were placed, and a 9-month follow-up showed no restenosis and no symptoms. This method is becoming the standard technique for treating stenosis of the proximal vertebral artery.

■ CASE HISTORY 1

A 53-year-old right-handed man was seen in the emergency room after complaining of the sudden onset of horizontal diplopia, dizziness, and ataxia. His medical history was significant for heart disease and hypertension, for which he was treated medically. The neurological examination was significant for nystagmus. The cranial nerves were intact, as were his sensation to pinprick and motor function. The cerebellar examination was significant for right-sided dysmetria. T1-weighted MRI showed hypodense areas in the right lateral medulla. The patient was placed on warfarin, but the dizziness continued intermittently for 3 months. After an extensive workup for other causes of his dizziness, the patient underwent four-vessel cerebral angiography, which showed 90% stenosis at the proximal vertebral artery (Fig. 102–3). The patient underwent angioplasty and stent placement. He was asymptomatic during a 3-month follow-up.

SURGICAL MANAGEMENT

Unlike those for the carotid artery, no clinical trials have shown the beneficial effect of surgery for high-grade stenosis of the vertebral artery.[55] If an extensive evaluation shows hypoperfusion or the patient is refractory to medical management, either endovascular or surgical management is indicated. The surgical approach to each anatomic segment of the extracranial vertebral artery is different. However, treatments intended for a given segment can sometimes be used for a preceding segment. The following discussion of the surgical management of extracranial vertebral artery disease is divided into the different surgical procedures that can be performed in each anatomic segment.

Surgery of the Proximal Vertebral Artery

Several operations have been devised to treat lesions of the proximal artery.[56–59] Transposition of the proximal vertebral artery onto the CCA is the most common procedure performed in this section of the artery. Bypasses using vein grafts are also performed from the adjacent subclavian artery or CCA to the proximal vertebral artery. Endarterectomy of the subclavian artery or the proximal vertebral artery can also be performed. Vertebral artery angioplasty with stent placement, however, is becoming the first choice of nonmedical management.

Approach to the Proximal Vertebral Artery. The standard approach to the proximal vertebral artery is a supraclavicular approach (Fig. 102–4*A*). The patient's head is placed in a headrest. Downward traction of the arm provides better exposure. We prefer to keep the head midline for this approach. A supraclavicular inci-

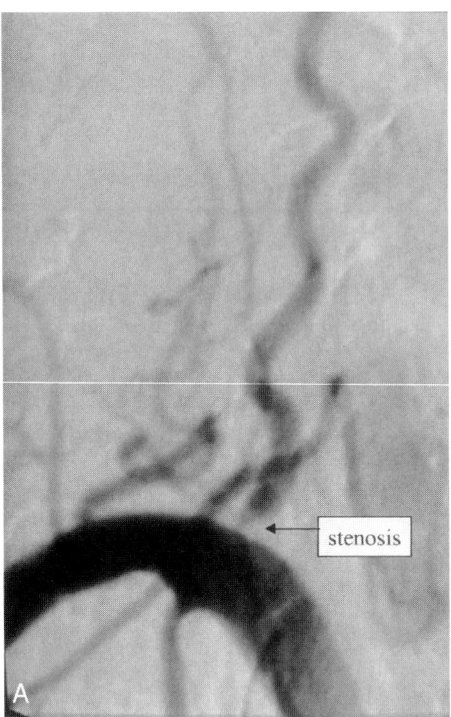

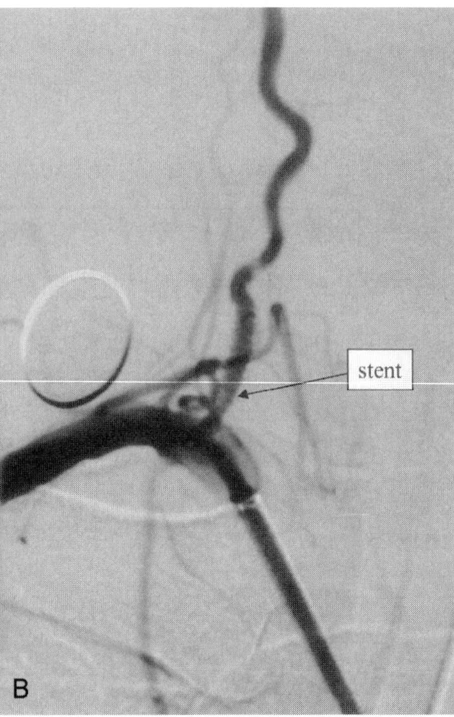

FIGURE 102–3. Angiograms of the right subclavian artery showing stenosis of the proximal vertebral artery *(A)* and after angioplasty with placement of a stent *(B)*.

sion is made about 2 cm above and parallel to the clavicle and extends from the suprasternal notch to 7 to 8 cm laterally. The skin is retracted superiorly and inferiorly, leaving the platysma intact. The platysma is divided horizontally. The superficial veins flank the edges of the sternocleidomastoid muscle as the external jugular vein comes from the lateral edge and crosses the muscle at the middle level (see Fig. 102–4*B*). The sternocleidomastoid muscle has two origins: the clavicular head from the superior surface of the medial third of the clavicle, and the sternal head from the anterior surface of the manubrium of the sternum.

The clavicular head is divided, leaving a cuff on the clavicle, and the muscle is retracted superiorly and laterally. The omohyoid muscle can also be divided (see Fig. 102–4C). The dissection is kept medial to expose the carotid sheath. The anterior scalene muscle lies laterally, with the phrenic nerve lying on top of it. This muscle is usually far lateral to the exposure and rarely requires division. The carotid sheath is separated from the overlying fascia and opened. Inside can be found the CCA, the internal jugular vein, and the vagus nerve. The jugular vein and vagus nerve are retracted laterally, and the CCA is retracted medially. From this point, dissection proceeds below the deep fascia layer caudally.

If the right side is exposed, several steps are needed. The lymphatic drainage on the right side of the neck is different from that on the left. Delicate lymphatic trunks empty into the right subclavian and jugular veins, which are usually smaller than the lymphatic ducts on the left. Because they do not coagulate completely, it is better to identify and ligate them. The right recurrent laryngeal nerve exits the vagus nerve and loops below the right subclavian artery as it approaches the trachea and larynx. Consequently, medial retraction of the trachea can cause ipsilateral paresis of the vocal cord.

If the left side is exposed, the thoracic duct is encountered as it arches from the side of the esophagus laterally to the angle between the internal jugular and subclavian veins. The proximal portion of this duct is ligated twice (see Fig. 102–4C), and smaller branches are also ligated. The left recurrent laryngeal nerve can be retracted with greater ease because it loops around the aortic arches and approaches the trachea much lower.

The vertebral artery can now be identified (see Fig. 102–4*D*). It is the first branch of the subclavian artery and exits from its posterosuperior surface. This feature distinguishes it from the thyrocervical trunk, which has multiple branches and exits from the anterosuperior surface. Alternatively, the vertebral artery can be located superiorly as it exits the transverse foramen of C6. The transverse process of C6 can be identified adjacent to its foramen. The artery arises from the apex of two muscles as they attach to the carotid tubercle: the anterior scalene muscle and the longus colli. The vertebral vein, which overlies the artery, can be divided or retracted. The vertebral vein is formed at the lower end of the canal of the transverse foramina from a venous plexus within the canal around the vertebral artery. The vein is anterior to the artery and often adheres to it.

It is important to identify and preserve the sympathetic chain. The vertebral artery is looped and dissected from C6 to the subclavian artery. Care is exerted to avoid destroying the sympathetic trunks and stellate or intermediate ganglia that lie on it. The anterior surface is freed.

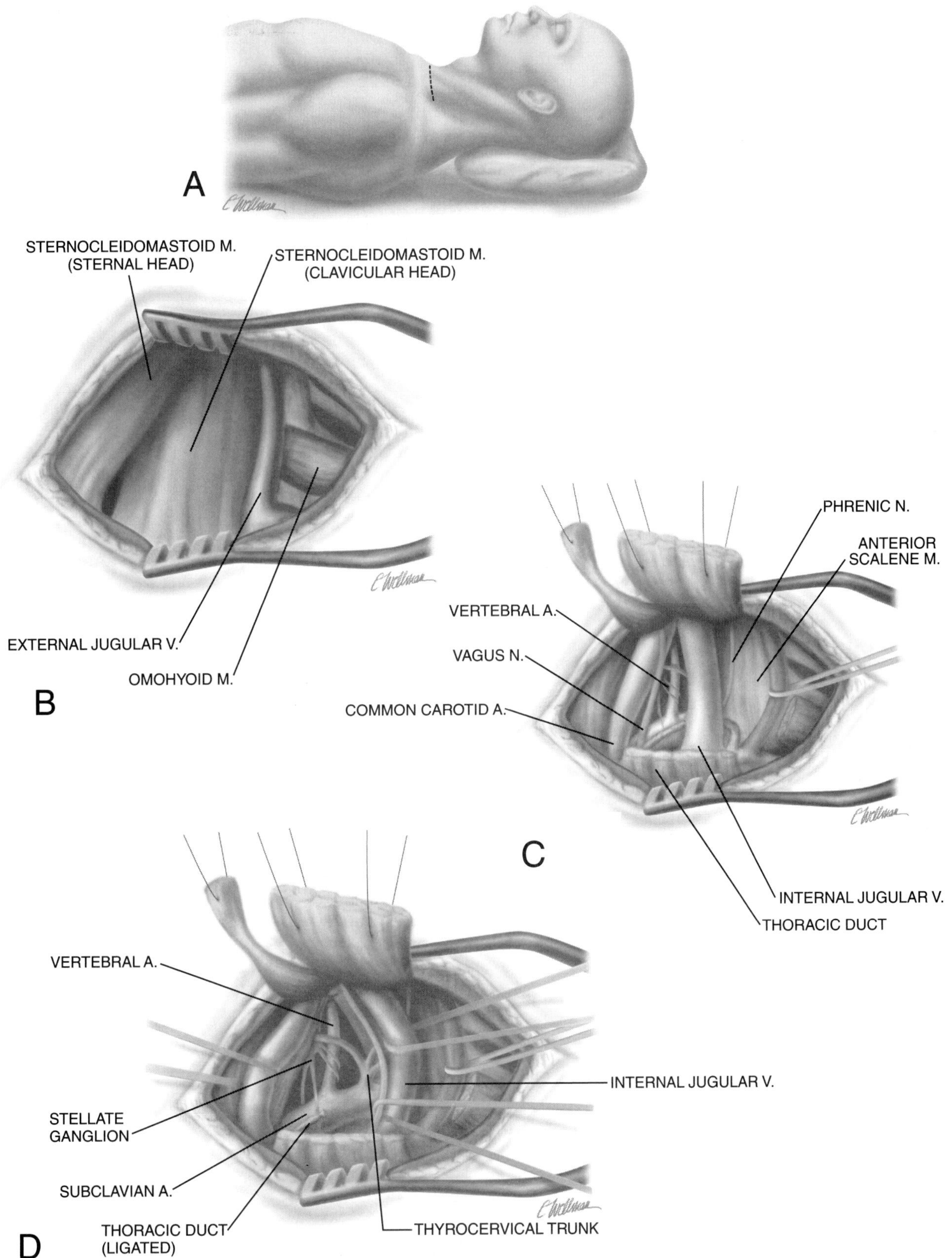

FIGURE 102–4. Supraclavicular approach to the proximal vertebral artery. *A*, The incision is placed 2 cm above and parallel to the clavicle. *B*, Exposure of the sternocleidomastoid muscle and the external jugular vein. *C*, The clavicular head is divided, leaving a cuff on the clavicle, and the muscle is retracted superiorly and laterally. The omohyoid muscle can also be divided to expose the vascular contents and thoracic duct. *D*, Exposure of the vertebral artery.

Transposition of Proximal Vertebral Artery to Common Carotid Artery. This procedure, first described by Wylie and Ehrenfeld[16] in 1970, is used because of the ease of exposure. Its limitation, however, is the requirement for simultaneous occlusion of both carotid and vertebral arteries (Fig. 102–5*A*). Using the standard approach described earlier for isolation of the proximal vertebral artery, the CCA is prepared for the vertebral artery. The CCA is already isolated during the dissection of the vertebral artery. Adventitia is cleared from the carotid artery. The patient is given a bolus of 3000 to 5000 U of heparin. Five minutes later, the vertebral artery is clamped at the level of C6 with a temporary clip. The proximal vertebral artery just above the stenosis is occluded with a hemoclip and cut above it. The artery is freed from the surrounding sympathetic trunk and moved medially toward the CCA. If the vertebral artery is not lax enough, it may be necessary to remove it from the C6 transverse process. A fish-mouth opening is made in the proximal end of the vertebral artery.

A partially occluding clip is placed on the carotid artery at the selected level and used to rotate the vessel medially. This maneuver allows the anastomosis to be performed on the posterolateral wall of the CCA in line with the trajectory of the vertebral artery. With 7–0 monofilament nylon suture, the superior and inferior ends of the fish-mouth opening are sutured to the corresponding ends of the hole in the carotid artery. One suture is used to form a running anastomosis on the back wall and is tied to the opposite end on completion. The front walls are then sutured. Before the last suture is tied, the lumina of both arteries are flushed with heparinized saline. First the vertebral artery and then the CCA are back-flushed. The final suture is tied, and all clamps are removed. If blood continues to ooze, gentle pressure is placed over the anastomosis with Gelfoam. After copious irrigation and when hemostasis is obtained, the neck opening is ready to be closed.

The sternocleidomastoid muscle is reapproximated. A suction drain is placed in the neck and should be removed in 24 hours.

Vein Graft Bypass from Subclavian Artery or Common Carotid Artery. When transposition is infeasible because of the length of the proximal vertebral artery or an endarterectomy cannot be done, a vein graft bypass is indicated.[17, 57] Berguer and Feldman[57] anastomosed a saphenous vein graft to the subclavian artery distal to the site of origin of the vertebral artery and then attached it by an end-to-side anastomosis to the subclavian artery (see Fig. 102–5*B*). Although this procedure does not interrupt carotid blood flow, it requires two anastomoses and is time consuming. The proximal vertebral artery can be bypassed from the subclavian artery to the thyrocervical trunk (see Fig. 102–5*C*) or CCA.

For any bypass to be successful, one of the three brachiocephalic arteries must be free of significant stenosis. Usually, the left carotid and innominate arteries are less likely to be stenotic. If the carotid artery is stenotic or otherwise compromised, the subclavian artery can be used. The desired segment of the subclavian artery is in the area of the anterior scalene muscle or more distally. The vein is usually autogenous saphenous, although prosthetic materials have been used. As described previously, this approach uses an end-to-side anastomosis.

Subclavian-Vertebral Endarterectomy. In 1959, Cate and Scott[10] described an endarterectomy of the origin of the vertebral artery through a subclavian approach (see Fig. 102–5*D*). They chose this approach because the vertebral artery is too fragile to accommodate vertical dissection. The dissection requires exposure of the proximal and distal subclavian artery. As described earlier, a more extensive approach is required distally. The anterior scalene muscle is divided, and care is exerted to preserve the phrenic nerve. The thyrocervical trunk and internal mammary artery need not be sacrificed but can be clamped with temporary aneurysm clips. Again, the thoracic duct must be ligated on the left, as described previously.

Heparin (5000 U) is given. Five minutes later, the proximal and distal portions of the subclavian artery are clamped. A horizontal incision is made in the subclavian artery below its junction with the vertebral artery. The plaque is removed from the subclavian artery and followed into the stoma of the vertebral artery. If intimal flaps remain at the margins, they are tacked up with 6–0 monofilament suture. In this region, the plaque is usually short and does not require this procedure. The incision in the subclavian wall is closed with 6–0 monofilament nylon after back-flushing from the vertebral artery and from the proximal and distal subclavian artery. Hemostasis is obtained, and the wound is closed.

An alternative approach is to apply a vein patch obtained from the saphenous or jugular vein to a vertical incision made in the vertebral artery that extends into the subclavian artery. After the plaque is removed, the vein patch is used to close the incision.

Although subclavian-vertebral endarterectomies have been used successfully since the 1960s, they are still associated with several technical problems. The endarterectomy is a difficult approach to use with a low-lying subclavian artery. Some have advocated the use of intrathoracic approaches. With other safer alternatives now available, the procedure is seldom used today.

Decompression of the Proximal Vertebral Artery. The proximal vertebral artery can be compressed by bands from the tendon of the anterior scalene or the longus colli muscle.[58, 59] The approach was described earlier. The vertebral artery is mobilized from its origin to the transverse foramen of C6. Ligaments, muscles, and bands overlying the artery are excised. In some cases, the sympathetic ganglia or nerve fibers can constrict the artery. If the ganglia are divided, a mild Horner's syndrome will develop.

Segmental resection and end-to-end anastomosis can be used when obstruction is caused by entrapment.[56] The vertebral artery must be long and its diameter adequate. If the ganglia must be excised to relieve the

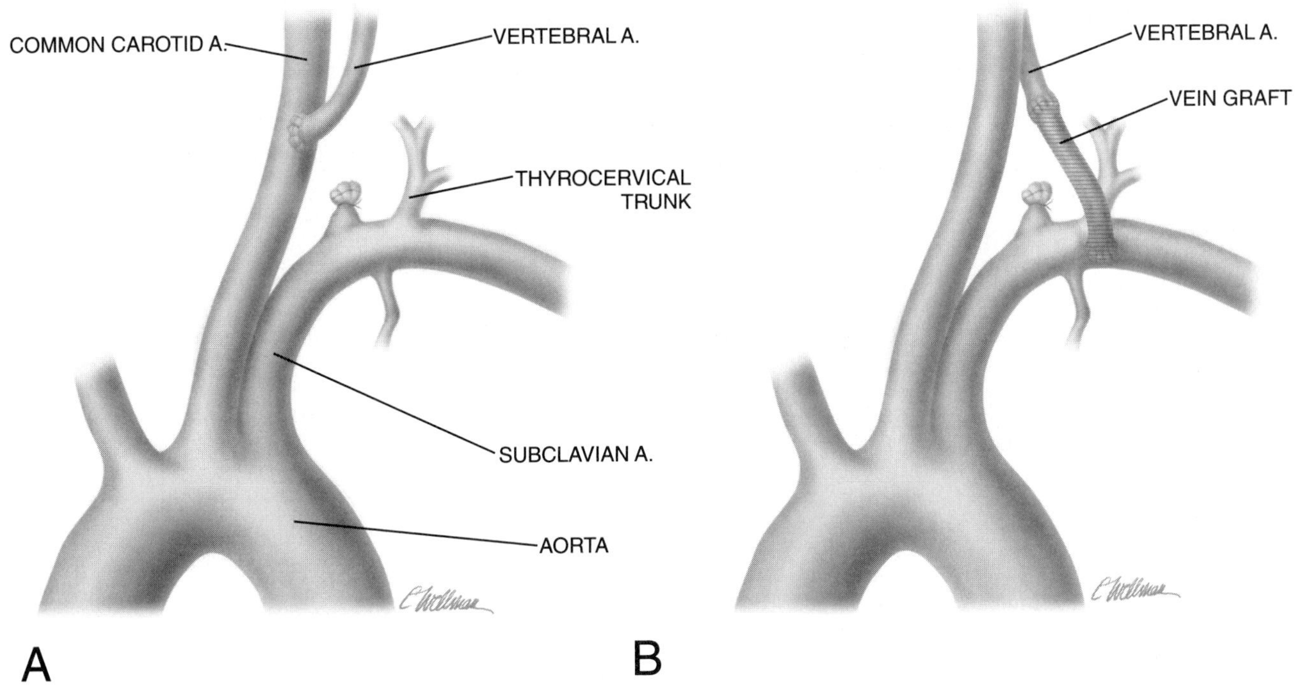

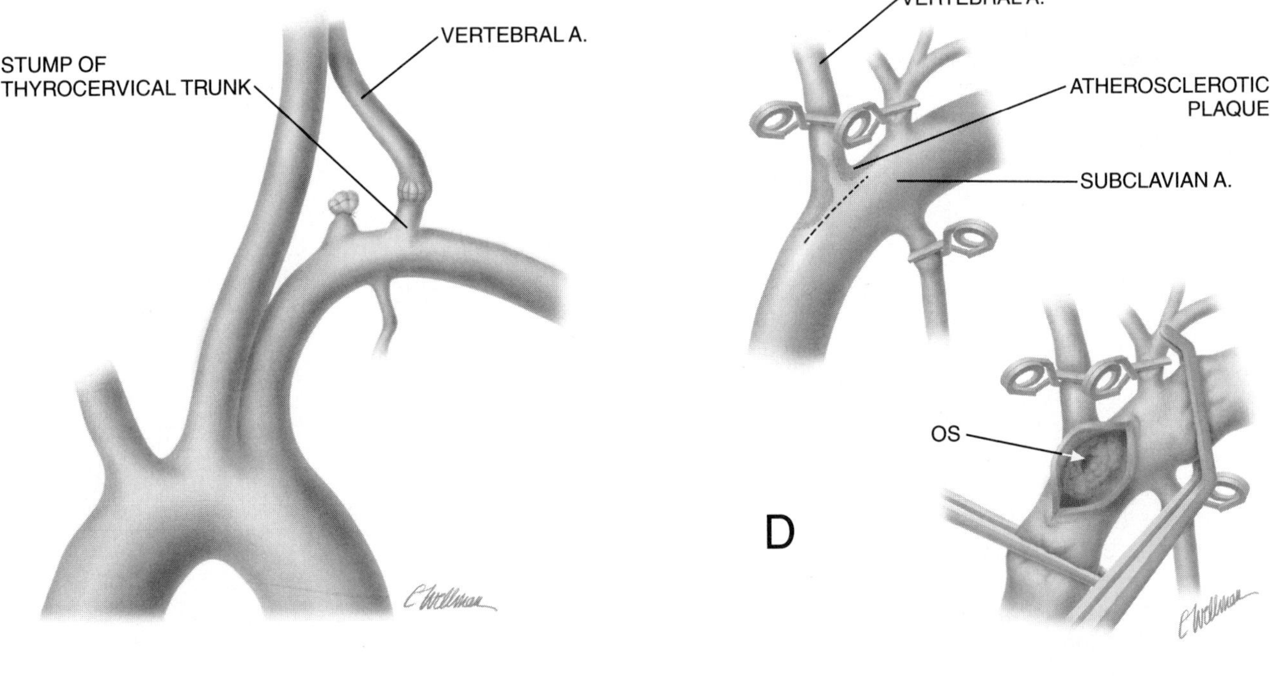

FIGURE 102–5. Different methods of proximal vertebral artery reconstruction. *A*, Vertebral-carotid transposition. *B*, Vertebral-subclavian vein bypass. *C*, Vertebral-thyrocervical trunk vein bypass. *D*, Vertebral artery endarterectomy.

compression, this technique can be used instead of removing the ganglia, which will worsen the Horner's syndrome.

Other Procedures. If high-grade stenosis of the proximal vertebral artery is present, the inferior thyroid artery can become well developed. Carney[59] proposed an end-to-end anastomosis of the inferior thyroid artery to the proximal vertebral artery.

■ CASE HISTORY 2

A 65-year-old right-handed man was referred to our institution for persistent vertigo and dizziness. The patient had undergone multiple neurovascular surgeries, including a left carotid endarterectomy 14 years earlier and a left carotid–to–subclavian artery bypass 12 years earlier. His medical history was significant for hypertension, severe hypercholesterolemia, benign prostate hypertrophy, gastroesophageal reflux, and a questionable myocardial infarction.

He was alert, oriented, pleasant, and in no acute distress. He had a carotid endarterectomy scar on the left. The rest of his physical examination was normal. Cranial nerves II through XII were intact. His pupils were equally round and reactive. His motor strength was 5/5 in all extremities, and his facial expressions were symmetrical. There was no evidence of decreased sensation. His reflexes were symmetrical, and no Babinski's reflex was present. His gait was steady, but he was unable to tandem walk. There was no dysmetria, but the Romberg test was positive.

The patient underwent an extensive evaluation by the ear, nose, and throat service to rule out a vestibular cause for the symptoms. The evaluation was negative and led to MRI and MRA. Angiograms showed occlusion of the left subclavian–to–carotid artery bypass and occlusion of the left origin of the subclavian artery. The origin of the right vertebral artery was 70% stenotic (Fig. 102–6*A*).

Based on these data, the patient's symptoms were attributed to stenosis of the right vertebral artery. The treatment of choice, angioplasty of the lesion and stent placement, was unsuccessful. The patient then underwent a right vertebral artery–to–carotid artery transposition in a similar manner as described previously. His hospital course was uneventful. His symptoms resolved, and 6-month follow-up studies showed the transposition to be patent (see Fig. 102–6*B*).

Surgery of the Middle Vertebral Artery

Surgical reconstruction of the middle vertebral artery is rarely undertaken, although it is possible to bypass diseased segments.[60, 61] Most surgeons use angioplasty

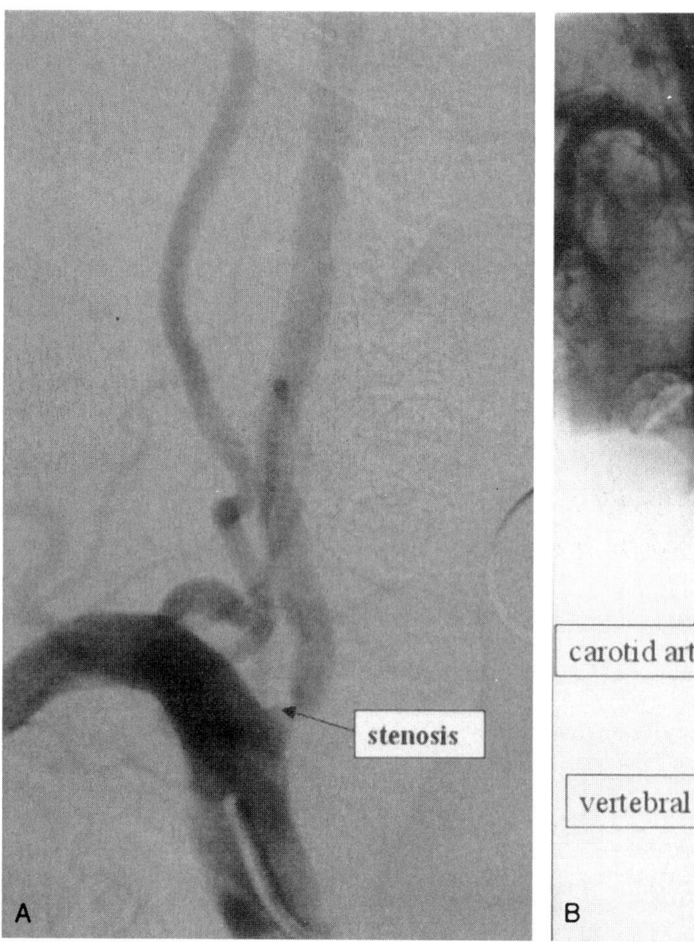

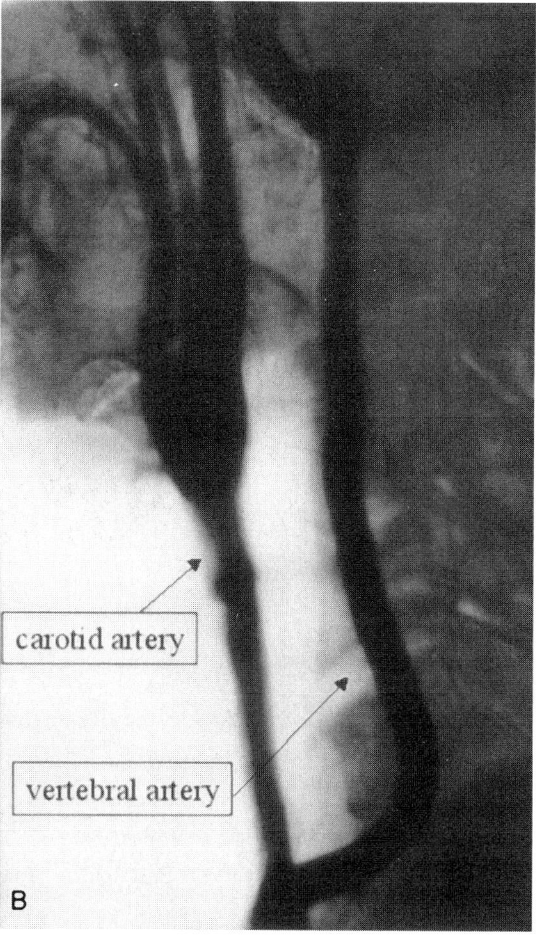

FIGURE 102–6. Angiograms of the right vertebral artery showing stenosis of the proximal vertebral artery *(A)* and after vertebral-carotid transposition *(B)*.

as the first choice of treatment or may bypass at the level of the distal vertebral artery. Single or minor extrinsic lesions can be removed to relieve compression on or kinking of the vertebral artery. In some cases of extensive proximal artery disease, it may be necessary to revascularize the middle vertebral artery. The proximal artery or a portion of the middle vertebral artery is ligated. After the vertebral artery is dissected, any of the previously described techniques can be used to attach the middle vertebral artery.

Approach to the Middle Vertebral Artery. The middle vertebral artery can be accessed from an anterior or anterolateral approach.[19] The incision can traverse a skin crease or be made longitudinally along the anterior border of the sternocleidomastoid muscle (Fig. 102–7*A*), depending on whether the pathology involves one or two levels. Initially, a cervical radiograph is used to define the level of interest and should be repeated intraoperatively before the transverse process is drilled. The skin is retracted, and the platysma is left intact until it is completely exposed. An incision is then made longitudinally along the anterior border of the sternocleidomastoid muscle (see Fig. 102–7*B*). By blunt dissection, a plane is developed between the strap muscles, trachea, and esophagus, which are retracted medially, and the sternocleidomastoid muscle and carotid sheath, which are retracted laterally. The longus colli muscle can be seen on the anterior vertebral body (see Fig. 102–7*C*). For a more lateral approach, the carotid sheath is opened. Care is taken to identify the vagus nerve, which lies posteriorly. An incision is made over the posterior carotid sheath to expose the prevertebral fascia over the transverse processes.

The sympathetic ganglia seen on the lateral aspect of the longus colli need to be preserved (see Fig. 102–7*C*). As noted, the vertebral artery can be located at the transverse foramen of C6 between the longus colli muscle medially and the anterior scalene laterally. Using a periosteal elevator, the dissection proceeds subperiosteally to remove the muscles from their attachment to the anterior surface of the transverse process. The muscles are reflected laterally with sutures. The transverse process is removed using a high-speed drill or curet (see Fig. 102–7*D*). Immediately below the transverse process, anterior to the vertebral artery, is the venous plexus, which is coagulated meticulously. Care is taken to preserve radiculomedullary arteries that exit from the vertebral artery between C1 and C5 and supply the spinal cord.

Decompression of the Middle Vertebral Artery. Several surgeons have operated in this segment of the vertebral artery to treat external compressive lesions (Fig. 102–8*A*).[14, 60–62] The anterior approach is used. Once the transverse process is reached, the level of the compression can be identified and decompressed. Plain anteroposterior cervical radiographs identify the level. Osteophytes are drilled off or removed with curets. The periosteum must be removed; otherwise, adhesions to the artery can persist. The artery is dissected circumferentially and displaced laterally. In some cases, degenerative changes of the zygapophyseal joint can result in protrusion and compression of the artery, and it must be removed. At the end of the procedure, the artery should be free of all restrictions.

Vein Grafts. Vein grafts can be used to connect the middle vertebral artery to the CCA (see Fig. 102–8*B*), subclavian artery, or ICA. In 1966, Clark and Perry[63] used a saphenous vein graft to connect the ECA to the vertebral artery at C2-3. The advantage of the ECA as the donor supply is that the proximal and distal anastomoses do not interfere with the cerebral circulation. A disadvantage occurs when the source of blood is from the ICA or CCA. Harvesting the vein and the potential for graft occlusions may pose a problem.

Synthetic grafts have also been used with similar donor sources. However, they have other disadvantages, including infection and pseudoaneurysm formation. Further, the use of grafts is limited over regions of constant movement because of rigidity and the corresponding wear caused by traction.

Pritz and associates[64] reported using the trunk of the ECA to connect to the middle vertebral artery after an aneurysm was found at C4. The vertebral artery was ligated distal to the aneurysm, and the trunk of the ECA was connected to the vertebral artery. In some cases, if the ECA is too short to reach the vertebral artery, use of the occipital artery can be considered.

Middle Vertebral Artery Endarterectomy. In the case of limited focal stenosis of the middle vertebral artery, a selective vertebral endarterectomy can be performed (see Fig. 102–8*C*). The artery is removed from the transverse foramen and incised vertically. The procedure is performed in the standard fashion with the artery clamped proximally and distally. The plaque is removed in its entirety. When the proximal artery is occluded into the middle segment of the vertebral artery, this approach is used to access the vertebral artery. A limited endarterectomy[60] is performed with a possible vein graft or transposition from the middle vertebral artery to the CCA.

Transposition of Middle Vertebral Artery to Common Carotid Artery. Transposition of the vertebral artery to the ICA, ECA, or CCA is feasible but can be surgically challenging. The main concern is to dissect enough of the vertebral artery to reach the donor site (see Fig. 102–8*D*). It is easier to use a vein graft or to go higher to the distal vertebral artery.

■ CASE HISTORY 3

A 53-year-old right-handed man suffered "black-out" episodes when he turned his neck to the right while driving. The patient had no significant medical history, except for a 30-year smoking history and neck pain during the past 5 years. His neurological examination was unremarkable.

Plain cervical radiographs showed degenerative disease of the spine with a large osteophyte at C6. After an extensive evaluation, the patient underwent aortic arch and dynamic four-vessel angiography. The right vertebral artery was occluded at the C6 foramen when the patient's head was turned to the right (Fig. 102–9).

The patient underwent an anterolateral approach. Cer-

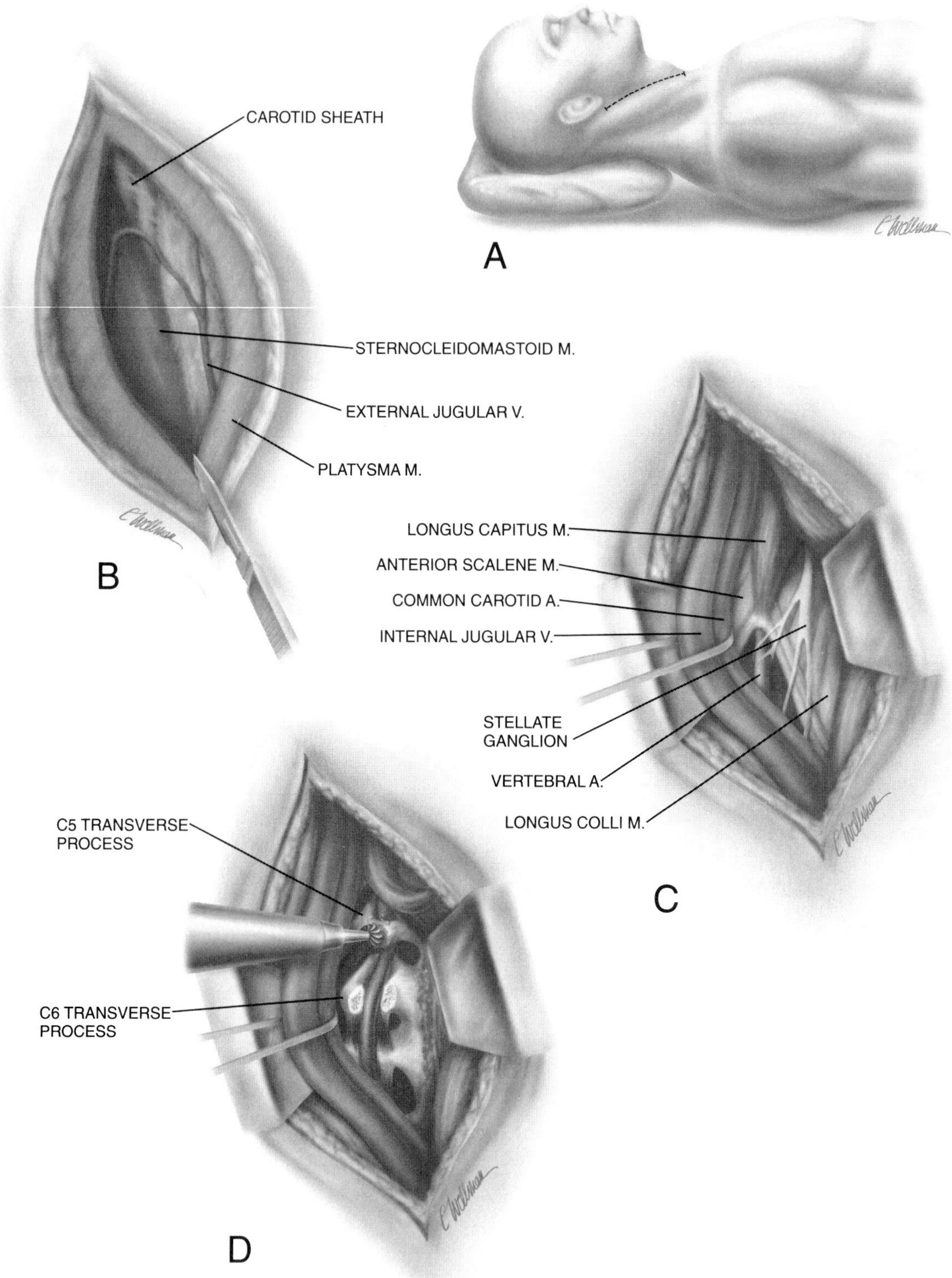

FIGURE 102–7. Anterior approach to the middle vertebral artery. *A*, The incision is placed along the medial border of the sternocleidomastoid muscle. *B*, The skin is retracted, and the platysma is left intact initially until it is completely exposed. Then an incision is made longitudinally along the anterior border of the sternocleidomastoid muscle. *C*, By blunt dissection, a plane is developed between the strap muscles, trachea, and esophagus, which are retracted medially, and the sternocleidomastoid muscle and carotid sheath, which are retracted laterally. The longus colli muscle can be seen on the anterior vertebral body. *D*, The vertebral artery is exposed by drilling away the bone surrounding the transverse foramen.

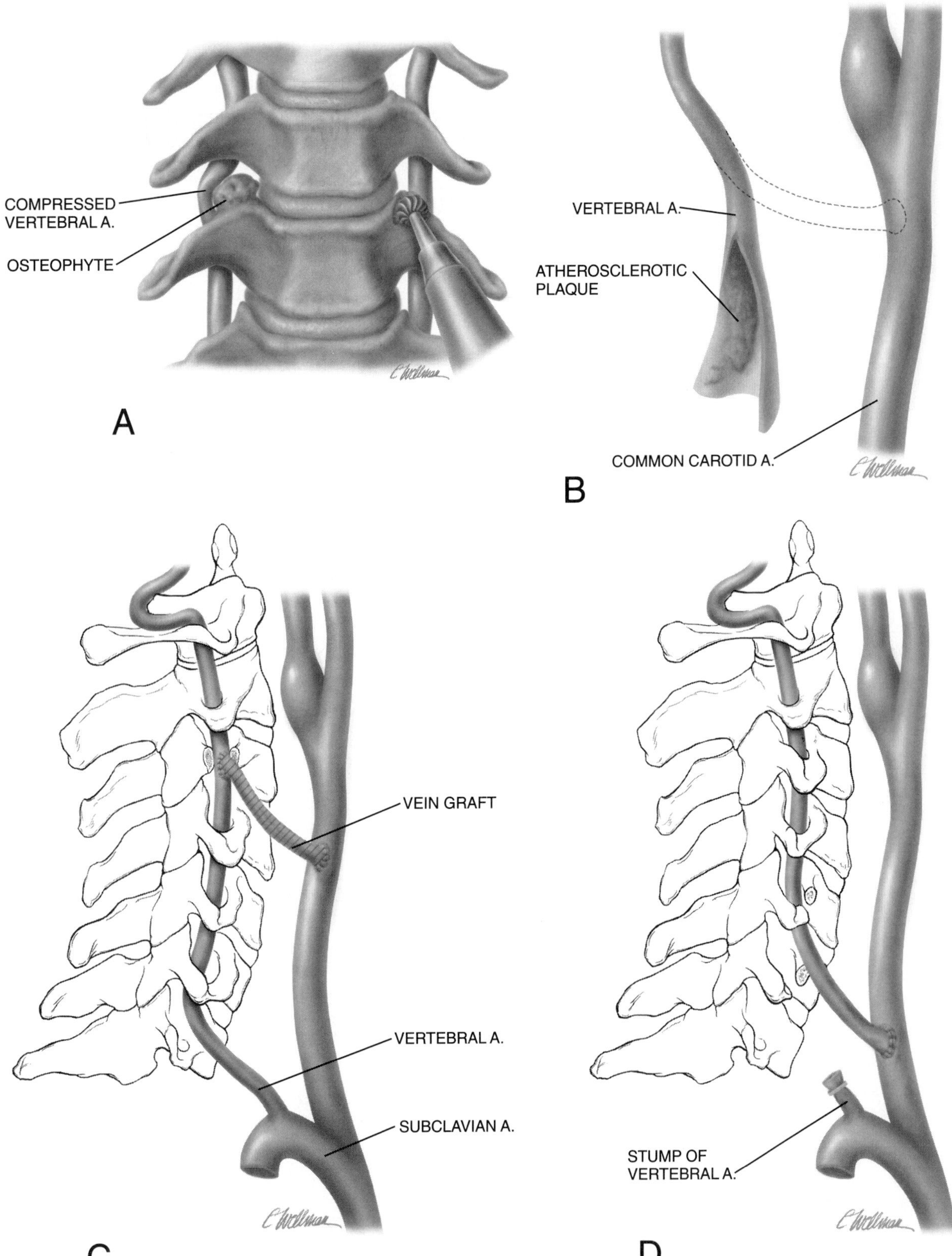

FIGURE 102–8. Different methods of middle vertebral artery reconstruction (right side). *A,* Decompression of osteophytic compression of the vertebral artery. *B,* Vertebral-carotid vein graft. *C,* Vertebral artery endarterectomy. *D,* Vertebral artery–to–common carotid artery transposition.

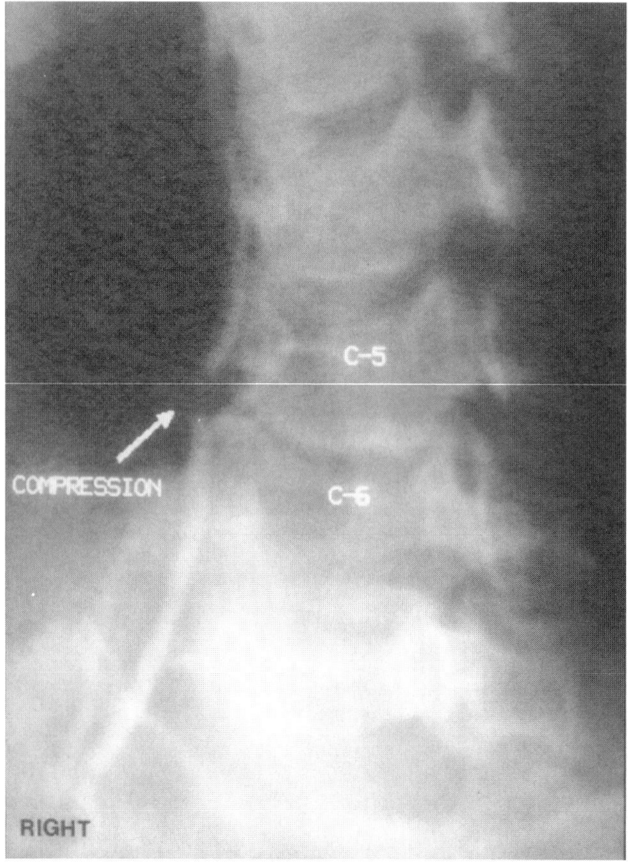

FIGURE 102–9. Angiogram showing osteophytic compression of the right vertebral artery at C5-6 when the patient's neck is turned to the right.

vical radiography was used to identify the center of the incision at C6. The osteophyte was drilled off and removed with curets. The artery was dissected circumferentially and displaced laterally. The patient did well postoperatively and had no symptoms immediately after surgery.

Surgery of the Distal Vertebral Artery

The distal vertebral artery is vulnerable to blunt trauma, and injury to the intima can result in thrombosis, embolization, and dissection.[19] This region has a high incidence of AVF formation and aneurysmal degeneration. Patency of the distal segment is often maintained through cervical collaterals. In many cases, if angiography reveals collaterals from the occipital artery, this artery is left intact.

Before planning any type of procedure, surgeons must consider the biomechanics of the spine at this level. Rotation occurs with the axis line posterior to the neck. Therefore, it is best to place grafts posteriorly to avoid undue torsion. An appropriate length must be used to avoid kinking or torsion.

Approach to the Distal Vertebral Artery. The approach to the distal vertebral artery depends on the revascularization technique used. The most common techniques are the anterolateral approach[65–67] and the posterior approach.[58] The former is used for an ECA–to–distal vertebral artery bypass or an occipital–to–distal vertebral artery bypass. These arteries can be anastomosed directly end to side or end to end, or an interposition graft from a vein or the radial artery can be used to connect the arteries. The latter approach is used to gain greater exposure of the vertebral artery for an occipital artery–to–distal vertebral artery bypass or to decompress an obstructed vertebral artery.

In the anterolateral approach, the exposure is made high in the anterior triangle. In some cases, disarticulation of the jaw provides additional exposure. The incision is made on the medial edge of the sternocleidomastoid muscle and extends in a curvilinear fashion over the mastoid bone (Fig. 102–10*A*). The incision is brought down to the platysma muscle, which is separated from the subcutaneous tissue. Along the medial border of the sternocleidomastoid muscle, the carotid sheath is entered, and the internal jugular vein is identified. The parotid gland is freed from the sternocleidomastoid muscle and reflected anteriorly. In the posterosuperior corner, the greater auricular nerve crossing the sternocleidomastoid muscle is sacrificed. A self-retaining retractor is placed to retract the internal jugular vein medially and the sternocleidomastoid muscle laterally (see Fig. 102–10*B*). Below the sternocleidomastoid muscle, the accessory nerve is visible. This nerve is protected by placing a loop around it and retracting it laterally. The belly of the digastric muscle is retracted superiorly, or it can be divided. Below the digastric muscle, the C1 tubercle is palpated. The fascia is cleared, and the fibers of the levator scapulae and splenius cervicis become visible (see Fig. 102–10*C*). These muscles are detached from the tubercle. If the anatomy does not appear correct, the C1 tubercle can be identified with the use of a clamp, and a lateral cervical radiograph can be obtained.

The C2 tubercle is also palpated, and the levator scapulae is cut to reveal the anterior ramus of the C2 nerve root, which passes laterally to the vertebral artery. Cutting this nerve exposes the vertebral artery (see Fig. 102–10*D*). Dissection of the overlying tissue reveals a venous plexus surrounding the vertebral artery. Careful coagulation or the use of Gelfoam prevents injury to the artery. Approximately 1 to 2 cm of vertebral artery is exposed. Further exposure can be obtained by removing the lateral wall of the transverse foramen of C1.

External Carotid Artery–to–Distal Vertebral Artery Bypass. This technique requires a carotid bifurcation free of disease and a long ECA trunk. The anterolateral approach is used to isolate both the vertebral artery and the ECA. The major drawback of this procedure is the need to mobilize the ECA to reach the vertebral artery. The ECA is skeletonized, and all its branches are divided and ligated before the appropriate length is selected (Fig. 102–11*A*). We sometimes leave the occipital branch intact, primarily because musculoskeletal branches from the occipital artery always feed the more distal vertebral artery. The ECA is mobilized laterally either below or above the ICA and connected to the distal segment of the vertebral artery by an end-to-end

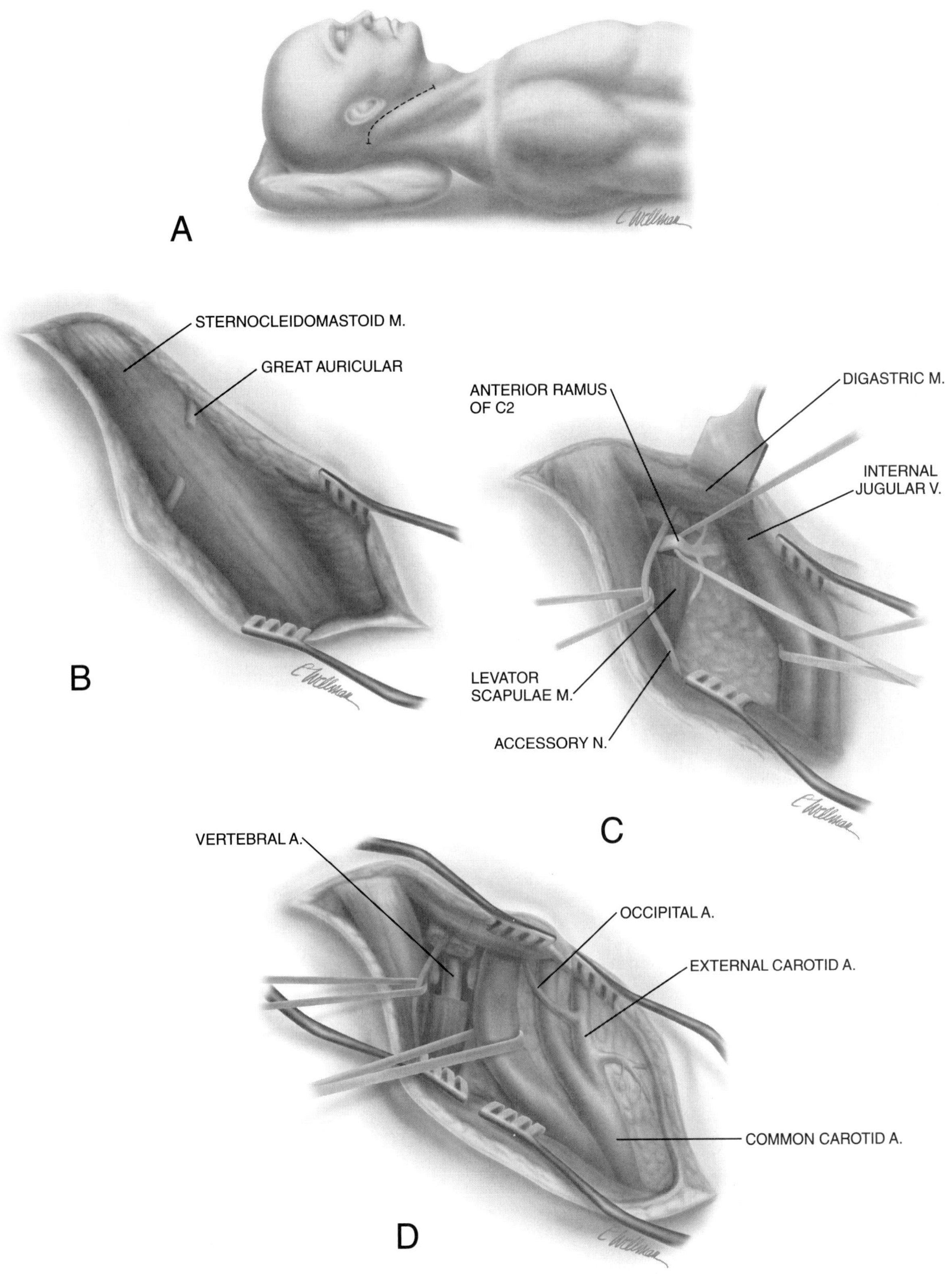

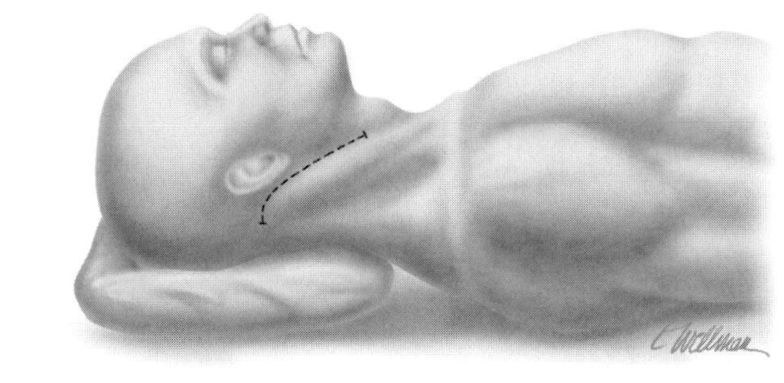

FIGURE 102–10. Anterolateral approach to the distal vertebral artery. *A*, The incision is placed along the medial border of the sternocleidomastoid muscle and extends posteriorly over the mastoid bone. *B*, The skin is retracted and the platysma is cut, exposing the sternocleidomastoid muscle with the great auricle nerve, which is also cut. The levator scapulae muscle, which covers the anterior ramus of C2, is visible. *C*, The levator scapulae muscle is cut to reveal the anterior ramus of C2. *D*, The vertebral artery is revealed. Medial exposure of the carotid sheath shows the common, internal, and external carotid arteries.

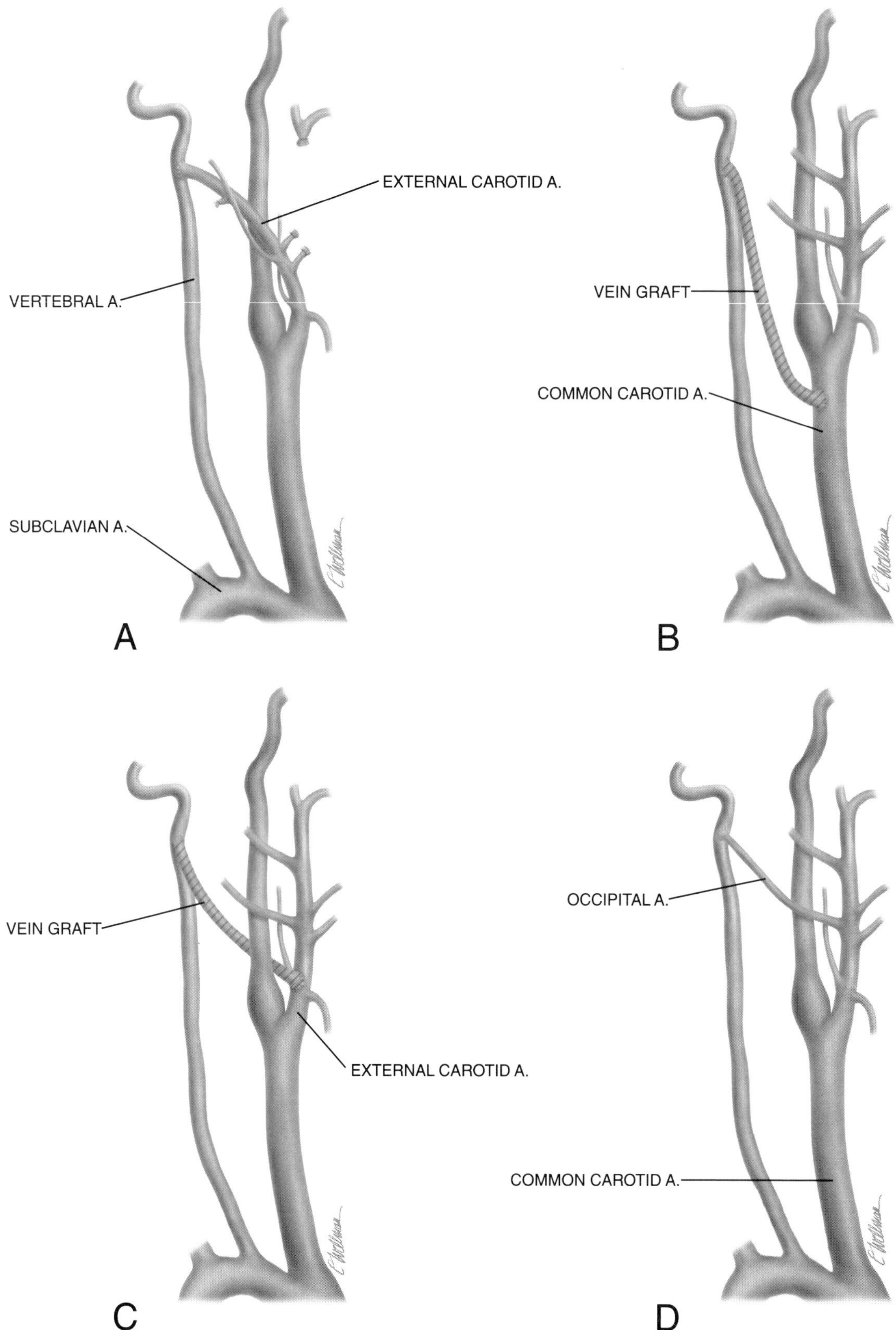

FIGURE 102–11. Different methods of distal vertebral artery reconstruction. *A*, External carotid artery–to–distal vertebral artery transposition leaves the occipital artery intact while other branches are sectioned. *B*, Common carotid artery–to–distal vertebral artery vein bypass. *C*, External carotid artery–to–distal vertebral artery vein bypass. *D*, Occipital artery–to–distal vertebral artery transposition.

anastomosis. The proximal vertebral artery is permanently occluded with a clip. Some authors have used an interposition graft, but it has a high likelihood of thrombosis with frequent head motion.

Vein Bypass from the Distal Vertebral Artery. Using the anterolateral approach, both the vertebral artery and the carotid artery are exposed. The donor site can be the CCA (see Fig. 102–11*B*), ICA, or ECA (see Fig. 102–11*C*).

A saphenous vein of selected length is removed from the leg. The vein is prepared, and its valves removed. The patient is given heparin (5000 U). After 5 minutes, the vertebral artery is gently pulled up with the loop to isolate a 2-cm section. Two Sugita clips are used to isolate the vertebral artery, and an incision is made equivalent to the fish-mouth end of the vein graft. The vein is connected to the vertebral artery with an end-to-side anastomosis using 8–0 polypropylene. If the artery is occluded in the proximal segment, the ECA and vertebral artery can be anastomosed end to end. The J-clamp is removed. If backflow through the graft is good, a temporary clip is used to occlude the vein.

The proximal end of the graft is passed below the CCA or ECA. The CCA (see Fig. 102–11*B*) is cleared of any surrounding tissue, and a cross-clamp is applied to its proximal and distal portions. Using an aortic punch, a 4- or 5-mm elliptical arteriostomy is made in the posterior wall of the CCA. With 6–0 polypropylene, the vein graft is anastomosed end to side. Again, backflow is allowed from the vein and distal CCA before the final suture is placed. The clamp on the proximal carotid artery is then removed.

The ECA can be anastomosed end to end to the proximal portion of the artery from the vein graft. The distal portion of the ECA is tied off permanently (see Fig. 102–11*C*).

We do not recommend the use of a vein graft for the ECA–to–distal vertebral artery bypass (see Fig. 102–11*C*), because rotation of the head often leads to thrombosis of the graft. This is especially true if the graft is passed below the carotid artery.

Occipital–to–Distal Vertebral Artery Bypass. As discussed, collateral blood flow to the distal vertebral artery comes from the occipital artery. In such cases, transposing the occipital artery directly to the distal vertebral artery has minimal effect. In cases of acute occlusion with inadequate collateral blood flow, a simple anastomosis between the occipital artery and the distal vertebral artery from the anterolateral approach can be used (see Fig. 102–11*D*).

The posterior approach for an occipital artery–to–distal vertebral artery bypass has been advocated by others.[58] This approach is more familiar to neurosurgeons because the patient is in a full prone or three-quarter prone position. The incision is made from the C3-4 spinous process to the inion in a hockey-stick fashion to the mastoid bone.[58, 67] Details of this approach can be found elsewhere.[58] All occipital approaches have the same disadvantages, with the added challenge that the occipital artery tends to be more tortuous as it emerges from the trapezius muscle, and large lengths of it can be difficult to isolate. However, the distal vertebral artery is easily accessed with a large exposure from the dura to C1 by removing the C1 foramen as inferiorly as the exit of C2.

Decompression of the Distal Vertebral Artery. An occasional patient may have severe local obstruction of the vertebral artery caused by compression from arterial branches or neighboring nerves. This can easily be treated by using the posterolateral approach with division of the obstruction.

Sometimes acute angulation or constriction can compromise blood flow. In such cases, the vertebral artery is removed as inferiorly as C3. The redundant section is cut, and an end-to-end anastomosis is reestablished. Constriction can also be caused by head rotation. In some reported cases, occlusion of the distal vertebral artery followed lateral head rotation. Traditionally, these patients were simply fused between the skull, C1, and C2. In younger patients, however, it is best to explore the anatomy and remove the pathology. If the artery is too short, an appropriate bypass should be used.

■ CASE HISTORY 4

A 77-year-old right-handed man was admitted to another hospital with pulmonary edema and right-sided weakness. In the emergency room he became hypotensive and unresponsive. He was hospitalized, and his neurological examination revealed double vision, nystagmus, dysphagia, and paresthesias of the hands and feet. MRI of the brain showed right medullary and cerebellar infarctions in the territory of the right posterior inferior cerebellar artery. MRA showed narrowing of the basilar artery with small vertebral arteries. His electrocardiogram was abnormal, and congestive heart failure developed. After medical management, he was transferred to a rehabilitation program.

The patient was transferred to our institution for further evaluation. Four-vessel cerebral angiography showed both carotid arteries to be normal, with good filling of posterior cerebral arteries via patent posterior communicating arteries. His left vertebral artery was narrow and terminated in the posterior inferior cerebellar artery. His right vertebral artery was 90% stenotic at its origin on the subclavian artery (Fig. 102–12) and fed the basilar artery by musculoskeletal branches from the occipital artery (Fig. 102–13). The basilar artery was poorly visualized, but segmental stenosis of this artery was possible. Phase-contrast MRI showed that blood flow in the basilar artery was 28 mL/minute. Blood flow in the right vertebral artery was 12 mL/minute. Both values were substantially low compared with normal.

Based on these findings, the patient's symptoms were attributed to hypoperfusion of the basilar artery. Although his vertebral artery filled, it was segmented. Therefore, it was not clear if the entire vertebral artery was patent. Angioplasty of the proximal vertebral artery stenosis was recommended. This procedure failed because the lesion could not be penetrated, and an ECA–to–distal vertebral artery bypass was recommended.

An anterolateral approach followed. Because the patient's occipital artery supplied musculoskeletal branches that fed the vertebral artery, the only branch from the

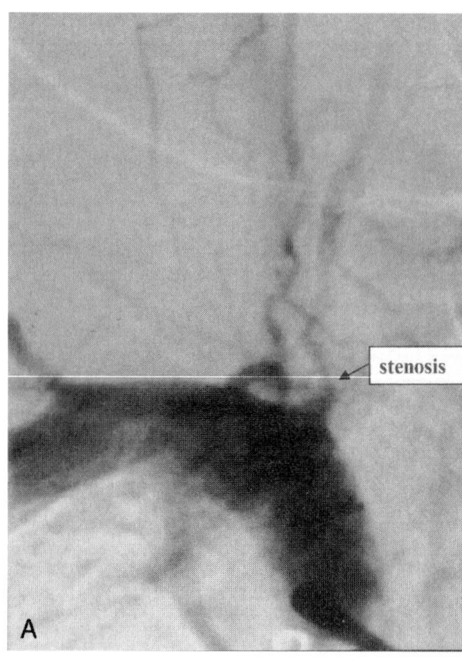

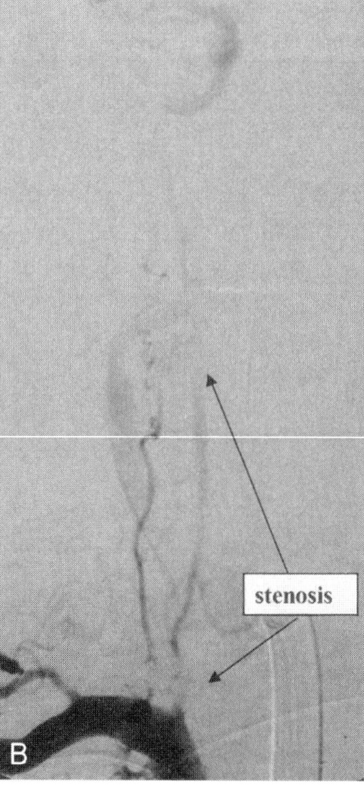

FIGURE 102–12. *A*, Anteroposterior angiographic view of proximal vertebral artery stenosis. *B*, Entire length of the vertebral artery showing segmental stenosis.

ECA that was not ligated was the occipital artery. An end-to-end anastomosis was completed between the ECA and the distal vertebral artery. Intraoperative flow measurements showed that when the ECA proximal to the occipital artery was temporarily occluded, there was no flow in the vertebral artery. The patient tolerated the procedure without difficulty. Phase-contrast MRI showed that the blood flow in the basilar artery was 50 mL/minute. He was returned to his rehabilitation program with no further symptoms.

Postoperative angiography showed patent distal vertebral artery–to–ECA anastomosis (Fig. 102–14). With better flow in the basilar artery, the segmental stenosis of the vertebral artery was more noticeable. The patient is now asymptomatic. If further symptoms are noted or if follow-up phase-contrast MRI shows a substantial decrease in

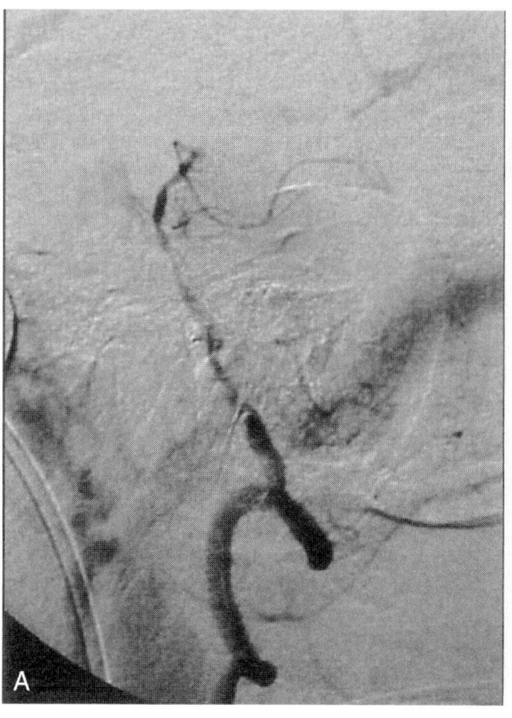

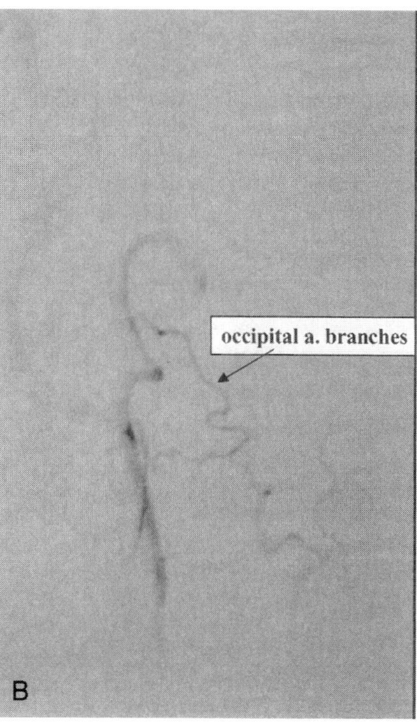

FIGURE 102–13. *A*, Lateral angiographic view of the basilar artery showing segmental stenosis. *B*, The distal vertebral artery with occipital artery branches to the distal vertebral artery.

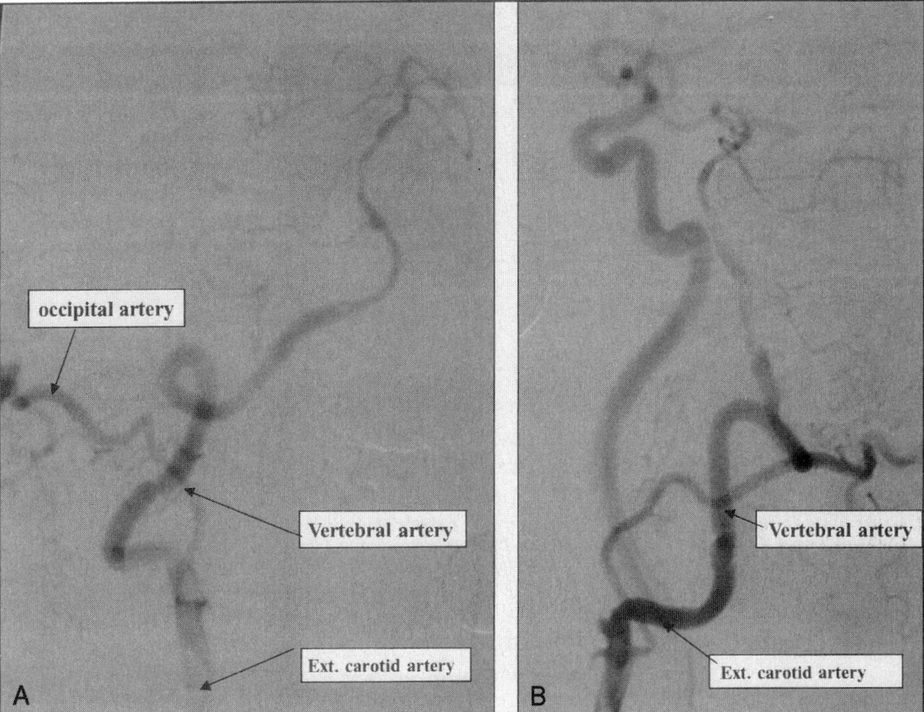

FIGURE 102–14. *A*, Postoperative anteroposterior angiographic view showing external carotid artery–to–distal vertebral artery transposition, with a view of the segmental stenosis of the basilar artery. *B*, Lateral angiographic view of the external carotid artery–to–distal vertebral artery transposition.

basilar artery flow, the patient will be considered for angioplasty of the basilar artery via his new anastomosis.

OUTCOMES AND COMPLICATIONS

Two studies have reported outcomes from medical therapy for extracranial vertebral artery disease. Millikan and colleagues[8] showed a decline in the mortality rate from 43% to 14% when heparin was used systemically to treat extracranial vertebral artery disease. Twenty years later in a 4-year follow-up, Whisnant and coworkers[45] reported that the incidence of brainstem stroke decreased from 35% to 15% when oral anticoagulants were used. In neither study were the patients chosen randomly, nor did most of the patients undergo angiography. A well-controlled, randomized, multicenter study is needed to address the efficacy of medical therapy for extracranial vertebral artery disease. Meanwhile, outcome studies on the use of antiplatelet medications and anticoagulants in the anterior circulation and the use of warfarin for intracranial disease are well documented. The findings can be applied to the extracranial vertebral arteries, but with caution.

There are few studies on the complications and outcomes associated with endovascular management of extracranial vertebral artery disease. During a 12-year period, Beaujeux and associates[49] treated 46 patients with AVF involving the extracranial vertebral arteries, 35 of which were treated by endovascular therapy. Thirty-two (91%) of these patients had complete occlusion, and three patients (9%) had partial occlusion. They reported no complications.

Few studies have reported long-term outcomes for percutaneous transluminal angioplasty of the extracranial vertebral arteries. Higashida and coworkers[52] performed percutaneous transluminal angioplasty for hemodynamically significant stenosis of the proximal vertebral artery in 34 cases and of the distal vertebral artery in 5 cases. For the former, three cases of postprocedural transient ischemic attacks occurred. Short-term follow-up showed restenosis in three patients, two of whom again underwent angioplasty. In 12 months, symptoms in all patients improved, except for one who died of an unrelated aneurysm. For the distal vertebral artery, two patients died from complications during the procedure. The other three were symptom free 12 months later.

In 1996, Storey and colleagues[54] observed restenosis within 3 months of angioplasty of the vertebral artery. Subsequently, they recommended the use of stents. In the next few years, the long-term outcome of angioplasty with and without stenting compared with medical therapy for vertebral artery stenosis will be available with the results of the Carotid and Vertebral Artery Transluminal Angioplasty Study.

The outcome of patients undergoing surgery of the external vertebral artery depends on the cause of the disease, the segment of the vertebral artery affected, and the type of treatment performed. In the hands of an experienced surgeon, surgery is associated with a very low mortality rate, and life expectancy is not substantially different from that of the general population with cerebrovascular disease. These individuals usually die within 10 years of cardiac disease.[68, 69]

Berguer[68] detailed the long-term outcome and experience with surgery of the proximal vertebral artery. Of 230 patients, 2 died. Complications included recurrent laryngeal nerve palsy in 2%, Horner's syndrome in 15%, lymphocele in 4%, chylothorax in 0.5%, and im-

TABLE 102–2 ■ **Common Surgical Approaches to the Vertebral Artery**

PROXIMAL VERTEBRAL ARTERY	MIDDLE VERTEBRAL ARTERY	DISTAL VERTEBRAL ARTERY
Subclavian artery–vertebral artery angioplasty	Decompression	Transposition of distal vertebral artery to external carotid artery
Transposition of proximal vertebral artery to common carotid artery	Vertebral angioplasty, if isolated lesion	Vein graft to external carotid artery, common carotid artery, or subclavian artery
Vein graft bypasses to subclavian artery or common carotid artery		Vertebral artery angioplasty, if isolated lesion

mediate thrombosis in 1%. Symptoms resolved substantially or were cured in 83% of the patients. Patency rates were 95% and 91% at 5 and 10 years, respectively.

For middle vertebral artery disease, decompression for osteoarthritic spurs was associated with excellent results in series by Hardin and colleagues[12] and Nagashima.[62] Diaz and coworkers[60] reported surgical treatment (vertebral endarterectomy and vertebral-to-carotid transposition) in 11 of 12 patients with middle vertebral artery disease. Patency was found in 11 of the 12 patients. One patient had an occluded graft and continued to have transient ischemic attacks. VBI, however, was relieved in all patients. Follow-up ranged from 4 to 34 months.

Berguer and colleagues[69] published the outcomes of 100 consecutive reconstructions of the distal vertebral artery over a 14-year period. They performed 72 distal vertebral artery–to–CCA, –ICA, or –ECA venous grafts. Twenty-three procedures were transposition of the distal vertebral artery to the ECA or occipital artery. In two patients, the ICA was used. Other methods were used in three patients. Of 16 graft abnormalities (16%) noted on postangiographic studies, 11 required revisions. Four patients died of perioperative stroke, and there was one nonfatal hemispheric stroke. Symptoms resolved in 87 patients, and the patency rate was 75% and 70% at 5 and 10 years, respectively.

Koskas and associates[70] also reported revascularization of the distal vertebral artery segment in 92 patients, 91 of whom underwent direct transposition of the vertebral artery to the ICA. They performed endarterectomy of the ICA during the same operation in 26.1% of the cases. There were no deaths or strokes. VBI symptoms were alleviated in 57.5%, 2.3% were unchanged, and the rest improved. Eight patients (8.7%) had thromboses of the vertebral artery. The patency rate was 89.1% at 5 years.

CONCLUSION

The literature reports many series using different approaches to the extracranial vertebral artery with great success. Table 102–2 summarizes the endovascular and surgical approaches to the extracranial vertebral artery that we believe should be initiated before more sophisticated techniques are used. We must emphasize, however, the need to analyze the clinical and laboratory data of each patient methodically and to define the cause of the symptoms. If surgical intervention is indicated, the choice of procedure must optimize blood flow while minimizing the treatment risk of death or morbidity to the patient.

There will always be unique cases that require special approaches to the three segments of the extracranial vertebral artery. In general, however, as more sophisticated endovascular techniques are developed, the use of angioplasty and stent placement to treat occlusive disease will likely become more common. Such a trend has already occurred with the proximal vertebral artery. For the distal vertebral artery, ECA–to–vertebral artery transpositions or vein graft surgeries are the most common procedures used to revascularize this region and will continue to be used. The middle vertebral artery will not be operated on as frequently as the other segments unless compressive lesions are easily accessible. Other cases of segmental occlusion in this region can be approached more distally.

REFERENCES

1. Quain R: The Anatomy of the Arteries of the Human Body and Its Application to Pathology and Operative Surgery, with a Series of Lithographic Drawings. London, Taylor & Walton, 1844.
2. Matas R: Aneurysms and wounds of the vertebral arteries. Ann Surg 18:477–516, 1893.
3. Alexander W: The treatment of epilepsy by ligature of the vertebral arteries. Brain 5:170–187, 1882.
4. Moniz E: L'encephalographie arterielle son importance dans la localisation des tumeurs cerebrales. Rev Neurol (Paris) 2:72–90, 1927.
5. Radner S: Intracranial angiography via the vertebral artery: Preliminary report of a new technique. Acta Radiol (Stockh) 28: 838–842, 1947.
6. Kubik CS, Adams RD: Occlusion of the basilar artery—a clinical and pathological study. Brain 69:73–121, 1946.
7. Millikan CH, Siekert RG: Studies in cerebrovascular disease. I. The syndrome of intermittent insufficiency of the basilar arterial system. Mayo Clin Proc 30:61–68, 1955.
8. Millikan CH, Siekert RG, Shick RM: Studies in cerebrovascular disease. III. The use of anticoagulant drugs in the treatment of insufficiency or thrombosis within the basilar arterial system. Mayo Clin Proc 30:116–126, 1955.
9. Crawford ES, De Bakey ME, Fields WS: Roentgenographic diagnosis and surgical treatment of basilar artery insufficiency. JAMA 168:509–514, 1958.
10. Cate WR Jr, Scott HW Jr: Cerebral ischemia of central origin: Relief by subclavian-vertebral artery thromboendarterectomy. Surgery 45:19–31, 1959.
11. Reivich M, Holling HE, Roberts B, et al: Reversal of blood flow through the vertebral artery and its effect on cerebral circulation. N Engl J Med 265:878–885, 1961.
12. Hardin CA, Williamson WP, Steegmann AT: Vertebral artery insufficiency produced by cervical osteoarthritic spurs. Neurology 10:855–858, 1960.
13. Husni EA, Bell HS, Storer J: Mechanical occlusion of the vertebral artery. JAMA 196:475–478, 1966.

14. Hardin CA, Poser CM: Rotational obstruction of the vertebral artery due to redundancy and extraluminal cervical fascial bands. Ann Surg 158:133–137, 1963.
15. Hass WK, Fields WS, North RR, et al: Joint study of extracranial arterial occlusion. II. Arteriography, techniques, sites and complications. JAMA 203:969–976, 1968.
16. Wylie EJ, Ehrenfeld WK: Extracranial Cerebrovascular Disease. Philadelphia, WB Saunders, 1970.
17. Berguer R, Andaya L, Bauer RB: Vertebral artery bypass. Ann Surg 111:976–979, 1976.
18. Carney AL, Anderson EM: Carotid distal vertebral bypass for carotid occlusion: Case report and technique. Clin Electroencephalogr 9:105–109, 1978.
19. Carney AL: Vertebral artery surgery: Historical development, basic concepts of brain hemodynamics, and clinical experience of 102 cases. Adv Neurol 30:249–279, 1981.
20. Perry MO, Thal ER, Shires GT: Management of arterial injuries. Ann Surg 173:403–408, 1971.
21. Dotter CT, Judkins MP: Transluminal treatment of arteriosclerotic obstruction: Description of a new technic and a preliminary report of its application. Circulation 30:654–670, 1964.
22. Bachman DM, Kim RM: Transluminal dilation for subclavian steal syndrome. AJR Am J Roentgenol 135:995–996, 1980.
23. Higashida RT, Hieshima GB, Tsai FY, et al: Percutaneous transluminal angioplasty of the subclavian and vertebral arteries. Acta Radiol Suppl (Stockh) 369:124–126, 1986.
24. Fields WS, Lemak NA: Joint study of extracranial arterial occlusion. VII. Subclavian steal—a review of 168 cases. JAMA 222: 1139–1143, 1972.
25. Toole JF, Tucker SH: Influence of head position upon cerebral circulation: Studies on blood flow in cadavers. Arch Neurol 1: 616–623, 1960.
26. Ausman JI, Shrontz CE, Pearce JE, et al: Vertebrobasilar insufficiency: A review. Arch Neurol 43:803–808, 1985.
27. Grad A, Baloh RW: Vertigo of vascular origin: Clinical and electronystagmographic features in 84 cases. Arch Neurol 4:281–284, 1989.
28. Kumar A, Mafee M, Dobben G, et al: Diagnosis of vertebrobasilar insufficiency: Time to rethink established dogma? Ear Nose Throat J 77:966–974, 1998.
29. Osborne AG: Diagnostic Cerebral Angiography, 2nd ed. New York, Lippincott Williams & Wilkins, 1999.
30. Mann FC, Herrick JF, Essex HE, et al: The effect on blood flow of decreasing the lumen of a blood vessel. Surgery 4:249–252, 1938.
31. May AG, DeWeese JA, Rob CG: Hemodynamic effects of arterial stenosis. Surgery 53:513–524, 1963.
32. Parker DL, Tsuruda JS, Goodrich KC, et al: Contrast-enhanced magnetic resonance angiography of cerebral arteries: A review. Invest Radiol 33:560–572, 1998.
33. Karonen JO, Vanninen RL, Liu Y, et al: Combined diffusion and perfusion MRI with correlation to single-photon emission CT in acute ischemic stroke: Ischemic penumbra predicts infarct growth. Stroke 30:1583–1590, 1999.
34. Heiserman JE, Dean BL, Hodak JA, et al: Neurologic complications of cerebral angiography. AJNR Am J Neuroradiol 15:1401–1411, 1994.
35. Srinivasan J, Mayberg MR, Weiss DG, et al: Duplex accuracy compared with angiography in the Veterans Affairs Cooperative Studies Trial for Symptomatic Carotid Stenosis. Neurosurgery 36:648–655, 1995.
36. Bryant DJ, Payne JA, Firmin DN, et al: Measurement of flow with NMR imaging using a gradient pulse and phase difference technique. J Comput Assist Tomogr 8:588–593, 1984.
37. Hofman MBM, Visser FC, van Rossum AC, et al: In vivo validation of magnetic resonance blood volume flow measurements with limited spatial resolution in small vessels. Magn Reson Med 33:778–784, 1995.
38. Zhao M, Charbel FT, Loth F, et al: Improving quantification of blood flow in intracranial vessels with 3D localization and vessel contouring algorithm. Paper presented at the 10th Annual International Workshop on Magnetic Resonance Angiography, Sept 29–Oct 3, 1998, Park City, Utah.
39. Charbel FT, Zhao M, Quek F, et al: Phase contrast MR flow measurement system using volumetric constrained image interpolation and color-coded image visualization. Paper presented at the 47th Annual Meeting of the Congress of Neurological Surgeons, 1997, New Orleans.
40. Meier D, Maier S, Bosiger P: Quantitative flow measurements on phantoms and on blood vessels with MR. Magn Reson Med 8: 25–34, 1988.
41. Enzman DR, Ross MR, Marks MP, et al: Blood flow in major cerebral arteries measured by phase-contrast cine MR. AJNR Am J Neuroradiol 15:123–129, 1994.
42. Mattle H, Edelman RR, Wentz KU, et al: Middle cerebral artery: Determination of flow velocities with MR angiography. Neuroradiology 181:527–530, 1991.
43. Charbel FT, Shi J, Quek F, et al: Neurovascular flow simulation review. Neurol Res 20:107–115, 1998.
44. Clark ME, Zhao M, Loth F, et al: A patient-specific computer model for prediction of clinical outcomes in the cerebral circulation using MR flow measurements. Proceedings of the 2nd International Conference of Medical Image Computing and Computer-Assisted Intervention, Sept 1999, Cambridge, England.
45. Whisnant JP, Cartlidge NE, Elveback LR: Carotid and vertebral-basilar transient ischemic attacks: Effect of anticoagulants, hypertension, and cardiac disorders on survival and stroke occurrence—a population study. Ann Neurol 3:107–115, 1978.
46. Weksler BB, Lewin M: Anticoagulation in cerebral ischemia. Stroke 14:658–663, 1983.
47. Easton JD: What have we learned from recent antiplatelet trials? Neurology 51(3 Suppl):S36–S38, 1998.
48. Chimowitz MI, Kokkinos J, Strong J, et al: The warfarin-aspirin symptomatic intracranial disease study. Neurology 45:1488–1493, 1995.
49. Beaujeux RL, Reizine DC, Casasco A, et al: Endovascular treatment of vertebral arteriovenous fistula. Radiology 183:361–367, 1992.
50. Miralbes S, Cattin F, Andrea I, et al: Vertebral arteriovenous fistula: Endovascular treatment with electrodetachable coils. Neuroradiology 40:761–762, 1998.
51. Mortarjeme A, Keifer JW, Zuska AJ: Percutaneous transluminal angioplasty of the brachiocephalic arteries. AJNR Am J Neuroradiol 3:457–462, 1982.
52. Higashida RT, Tsai FY, Halbach VV, et al: Transluminal angioplasty for atherosclerotic disease of the vertebral and basilar arteries. J Neurosurg 78:192–198, 1993.
53. McKenzie JD, Wallace RC, Dean BL, et al: Preliminary results of intracranial angioplasty for vascular stenosis caused by atherosclerosis and vasculitis. AJNR Am J Neuroradiol 17:263–268, 1996.
54. Storey GS, Marks MP, Dake M, et al: Vertebral artery stenting following percutaneous transluminal angioplasty. J Neurosurg 84:883–887, 1996.
55. North American Symptomatic Carotid Endarterectomy Trial Steering Investigators: Clinical alert: Benefit of carotid endarterectomy for patients with high-grade stenosis of the internal carotid artery: National Institute of Neurological Disorders and Stroke-Trauma Division. Stroke 22:816–817, 1991.
56. Diaz FG, Ausman JI, De Los Reyes RA, et al: Surgical reconstruction of the proximal vertebral artery. J Neurosurg 61:874–881, 1984.
57. Berguer R, Feldman AJ: Surgical reconstruction of the vertebral artery. Surgery 93:670–675, 1983.
58. Anson JA, Spetzler RF: Surgery for vertebral basilar insufficiency: Extracranial. In Carter LP, Spetzler RF, Hamilton MG (eds): Neurovascular Surgery. New York, McGraw-Hill, 1995, pp 383–403.
59. Carney AL: Vertebral artery surgery: Pathology, hemodynamics, and technique. In Robicsek F (ed): Extracranial Cerebrovascular Disease: Diagnosis and Management. New York, Macmillan, 1986, pp 395–424.
60. Diaz FG, Ausman JI, Shrontz C, et al: Surgical correction of lesions affecting the second portion of the vertebral artery. Neurosurgery 19:93–100, 1986.
61. Brink B: Approach to the second segment of the vertebral arteries. In Berguer R, Bauer RB (eds): Vertebrobasilar Arterial Occlusive Disease: Medical and Surgical Management. New York, Raven, 1984, pp 257–264.
62. Nagashima C: Surgical treatment of vertebral artery insufficiency caused by cervical spondylosis. J Neurosurg 32:512–521, 1970.

63. Clark K, Perry MO: Carotid vertebral anastomosis: An alternative technic for repair of the subclavian steal syndrome. Ann Surg 163:414–416, 1966.
64. Pritz MB, Chandler WF, Kindt GW: Vertebral artery disease: Radiological evaluation, medical management, and microsurgical treatment. Neurosurgery 9:524–530, 1981.
65. Henry AK: Extensile Exposures. Baltimore, Williams & Wilkins, 1957.
66. Verbiest H: Anterolateral operations for fractures and dislocations in the middle and lower parts of the cervical spine. J Bone Joint Surg Am 51:1489–1530, 1969.
67. Verbiest H: A lateral approach to the cervical spine: Techniques and indications. J Neurosurg 28:191–203, 1968.
68. Berguer R: Long-term results of vertebral artery reconstruction. In Yao JST, Pearce WH (eds): Long-Term Results in Vascular Surgery. Norwalk, Conn, Appleton & Lange, 1993, pp 69–80.
69. Berguer R, Morasch MD, Kline RA: A review of 100 consecutive reconstructions of the distal vertebral artery for embolic and hemodynamic disease. J Vasc Surg 27:852–859, 1998.
70. Koskas F, Kieffer E, Rancure G, et al: Direct transposition of the distal cervical artery into the internal carotid artery. Ann Vasc Surg 9:515–524, 1995.

CHAPTER **103**

Intracranial Occlusion Disease: Moyamoya

CARLOS A. DAVID ■ ERIC NOTTMEIER

Moyamoya, the Japanese word for puff of smoke, is a term first coined by Suzuki and Takaku[1] to describe the angiographic appearance of abnormal collateral vasculature involving the circle of Willis and proximal intracranial vessels. It has come to signify both a disease of unknown etiology and a syndrome or angiographic appearance associated with poor intracranial perfusion caused by a known disorder such as arteriosclerosis. The disease is characterized by chronic progressive stenosis of the arteries of the circle of Willis. The initial manifestation is often stenosis of the bilateral supraclinoid carotid arteries, with the associated development of abnormal collateral circulation at the base of the brain and basal ganglia. The disease can progress to involve the middle cerebral (MCA) and posterior cerebral arteries. These vascular changes can lead to ischemic strokes or spontaneous intracranial hemorrhages.

The first reported case is credited to Takeuchi and Shimizu[2] in 1957. In the ensuing years, Nishimoto and Takeuchi[3] reported 96 cases and outlined diagnostic criteria and definitions for the disease. The disease, also called spontaneous occlusion of the circle of Willis, is a specific disease entity most often encountered in Japan. Since 1977, moyamoya disease has been an area of intense study and effort sponsored by the Ministry of Health and Welfare of Japan. The pathogenesis, etiology, epidemiology, and treatment of the disease have been investigated systematically. Despite this intense study, the etiology and pathogenesis of the disease remain poorly understood. However, several successful surgical treatments have been developed and are described in this chapter.

EPIDEMIOLOGY

Although it was once believed to be endemic among the Japanese, moyamoya disease is now recognized to occur worldwide. Its prevalence, however, is highest in Japan, followed by China and Korea. In Japan, it is estimated that 100 new cases are identified each year.[4] It appears to involve both sexes, although the incidence is higher in women (1.7:1).[4] The age of onset is bimodal, as is the manner of presentation. The disease predominates in children younger than age 10 years and tends to manifest as an ischemic disorder in this group.[4] A second smaller peak occurs in the fourth decade and tends to manifest as hemorrhage. The isolated sporadic variety of the disease predominates, but a familial version has been identified. In a study of 474 families, the incidence of the familial subtype was estimated at 8.82%.[4]

PATHOGENESIS AND ETIOLOGY

The pathogenesis of moyamoya disease remains obscure. The basic manifestation of the disease is typically attributed to the deposition of smooth muscle and an associated chronic inflammatory response.[5] Aoyagi and coworkers[6] found evidence of this mechanism in deoxyribonucleic acid synthesis experiments involving smooth muscle cells obtained from moyamoya patients. Their work suggested a delayed repair mechanism for vascular walls in which a slow but long-term proliferation of smooth muscle during the repair process led to the progressive occlusion of intracranial vessels.

The role of angiogenic growth factors has also been investigated.[7] These substances, in particular b-fibroblast growth factor (b-FGF), have been proposed as possible mediators of the neovascular response in moyamoya disease.[8] The precise mechanisms, however, have yet to be elucidated. Genetic studies have suggested a multifactorial process. Recent studies in Japan have focused on the human leukocyte antigen (HLA) class 2 genes.

At present, it appears that moyamoya disease occurs in certain individuals with some predisposition, be it race, familial, genetic, some unknown factor, or a combination of factors. In the past, factors, such as childhood tonsillitis, conjunctivitis, otitis media, bronchitis, and other head and neck infections were proposed as causes, but more recent data appear to refute these associations.[9]

PATHOLOGY

The pathologic changes associated with moyamoya disease are well characterized and similar in both adults and children. The primary lesion occurs in the intimal layer of the cerebral vessel. Fibrous deposition with intimal thickening causes stenosis of the vessel. The internal elastic lamina becomes infolded, tortuous, and redundant. Minimal to no chronic inflammatory response is noted. The findings have been likened to the early stages of arteriosclerosis without the lipid deposition in macrophages.[5]

Owing to the resultant oligemic state induced by the primary lesion, a rich, fragile collateral circulation develops secondarily. This abnormal capillary and collateral network involves the base of the brain and leptomeningeal vessels on the surface of the brain. Dilated and tortuous collaterals at the base of the brain involve the basal ganglia and deep structures and form complex anastomoses with the distal intracranial vessels and leptomeningeal collaterals. The vessels are believed to be dilated lenticulostriate and thalamoperforating arteries. Pathologically, the dilated collaterals exhibit a disrupted internal elastic lamina, medial fibrosis, microaneurysms, and areas of rupture.[10] These changes are thought to underlie the hemorrhagic subtype of the disease.

CLINICAL PRESENTATION

The slow progressive stenosis and occlusion cause a rich, fragile collateral network to form. If the blood flow through the collateral network is insufficient, cerebral ischemia and infarction may occur. Hence, in the pediatric population, moyamoya disease tends to manifest as ischemic events. Transient ischemic attacks (TIAs) or completed strokes lead to various clinical symptoms. The TIAs are precipitated by crying, coughing, and straining and have also occurred in children playing wind instruments. Associated seizure activity is another common symptom in children. Some patients complain of headaches, visual disturbances, and sensory changes. Apart from the overt ischemic episodes, involuntary choreic-type movements have been described. Intellectual impairment and deterioration to retardation have occurred in both adults and children.

In adults, the most common symptoms of moyamoya disease are related to hemorrhage from the fragile collateral vessels. The hemorrhages most often occur in the basal ganglia and thalamus but can also manifest as intraventricular hemorrhage and subarachnoid hemorrhage. These hemorrhages are thought to be associated with the increasing hemodynamic stress associated with aging, which is imparted on the fragile collaterals.

The prognosis for adults and children is significantly different. Adults with a hemorrhagic presentation have a worse overall prognosis compared with children with ischemic manifestations. The ischemic manifestations tend to resolve, but cognitive deterioration continues over the ensuing decade.[11]

DIAGNOSTIC EVALUATION

The diagnosis of moyamoya disease is based primarily on radiologic features and clinical inclusion and exclusion criteria. Definitive diagnosis usually requires angiography. The following diagnostic guidelines have been proposed by the Ministry of Health and Welfare of Japan.[12]

1. Stenosis or occlusion at the terminal portion of the internal carotid artery or at the proximal portion of the anterior cerebral arteries or the MCAs
2. Abnormal vascular networks in the vicinity of the occlusive or stenotic lesions in the arterial phase
3. Bilateral findings
4. No other identifiable cause

The use of magnetic resonance imaging (MRI) has been suggested to avoid subjecting patients to the risks associated with angiography. Other tests include computed tomography (CT), cerebral blood flow (CBF) studies, and electroencephalography (EEG).

Angiography

The diagnosis of moyamoya disease is based primarily on angiographic findings (Fig. 103–1). Until recently, conventional angiography was mandatory to confirm a diagnosis of moyamoya disease. Based on angiographic observation, Suzuki and Takaku[1] proposed a series of six stages in the development and progression of the disease. Stage 1 is characterized by bilateral stenosis of the supraclinoid carotid arteries. Stage 2 reveals the development of the abnormal basal vascular network. In stage 3, the major trunks of the anterior circulation are severely stenotic, and the collaterals are more prominent. In stages 4 and 5, the collateral vessels progressively diminish in response to complete occlusion of the intracranial vessels, and abnormal extracranial-to-intracranial anastomoses develop. In Stage 6, the moyamoya collaterals and the intracranial vessels have completely disappeared. The cerebrum is perfused through the abnormal extracranial-to-intracranial anastomosis.

Magnetic Resonance Imaging

The use of MRI and magnetic resonance angiography (MRA) has been suggested for the evaluation of patients suspected of harboring moyamoya disease. The changes that suggest the diagnosis are multiple, dilated abnormal vessels and flow voids in the basal ganglia and thalamus, narrowing and occlusion of the circle of Willis, and parenchymal changes consistent with ischemia. These changes, particularly the collateral vessels, can be difficult to visualize on MRI scans. If conventional angiography is not used, high-quality MRI is paramount.

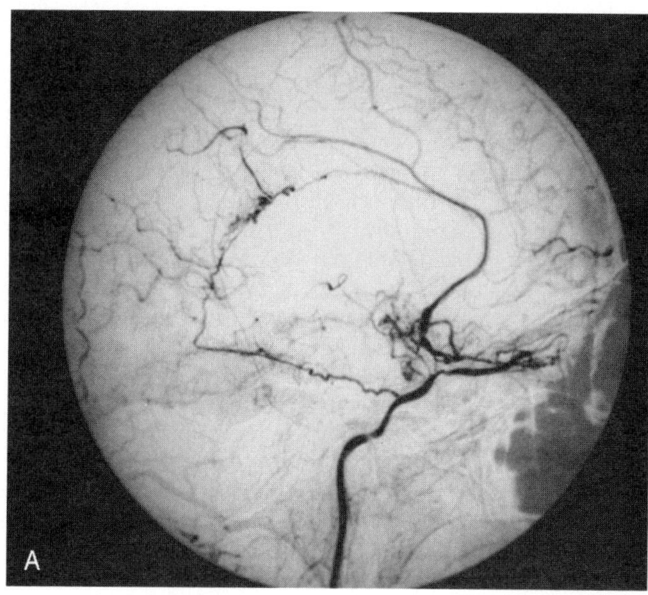

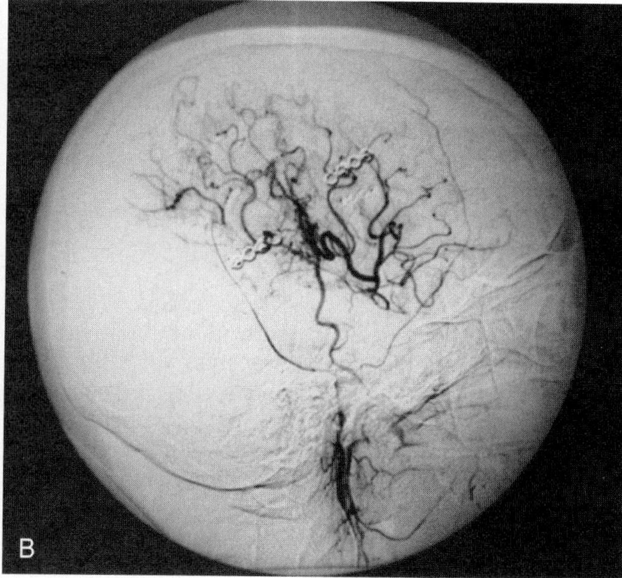

FIGURE 103–1. *A*, Preoperative internal carotid arteriogram revealing advanced moyamoya disease, with occlusion of the middle cerebral artery (MCA), the development of moyamoya collaterals, and a dural-to-anterior cerebral artery anastomosis via the tentorial artery. *B*, Postoperative arteriogram after pial synangiosis procedure. Note the marked filling of the previously unseen MCA territory.

Computed Tomography

In the early stages of the disease, CT studies are often normal. In the latter stages, CT may reveal multiple areas of hypodensity from previous infarction, particularly in the watershed regions (Fig. 103–2). Atrophy can be present in various degrees. Overall, MR imaging is considered superior to CT for demonstrating the changes associated with moyamoya disease.

Cerebral Blood Flow

CBF has been measured by xenon-enhanced CT, single photon-emission computer tomography, or positron-emission tomography. The findings reveal that CBF is significantly decreased in children, whereas CBF is relatively normal in adults.[13] In children, CBF was redistributed to the occipital lobes owing to the later involvement of the posterior circulation as the disease progressed. Furthermore, autoregulation in response to hypotension and hypercapnia was impaired.

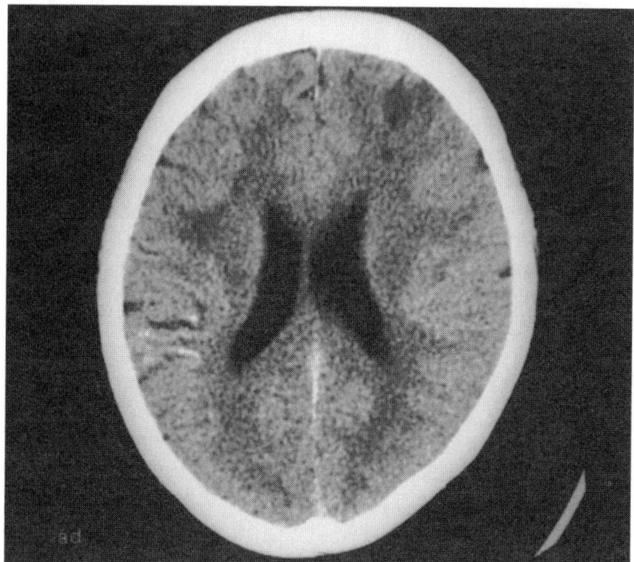

FIGURE 103–2. Computed tomographic scan of a moyamoya patient showing multiple areas of hypodensity and gyral enhancement.

Electroencephalography

The characteristic findings of moyamoya disease are slow waves involving the posterior hemispheres and centrotemporal regions. Sleep spindle depression and diffuse low-voltage waves have also been described. A pathognomonic finding in children is the re-buildup phenomenon in which a normal buildup induced by hyperventilation is followed immediately or concurrently with another buildup of slow, irregular, lower voltage waves. This peculiar EEG phenomenon, which occurs only in children, is attributed to a delayed response to carbon dioxide reactivity.[14]

Differential Diagnosis

Because the etiology of moyamoya disease is unknown, other diseases with a similar presentation and radiologic criteria must be excluded. These disorders include meningitis, in particular the tuberculous variety. Other disorders are arteriosclerosis, autoimmune diseases, vasculitis, Down syndrome, von Recklinghausen's disease, postradiation arteriopathy, and fibromuscular dysplasia.

Associated Conditions

Intracranial saccular aneurysms as opposed to the microaneurysms found on collateral vessels have been noted in patients with moyamoya disease. These aneurysms are similar to those in the general population; however, aneurysms in patients with moyamoya disease tend to occur in the posterior circulation. The basilar bifurcation seems to be the location most commonly involved. This predominance of aneurysms on the basilar bifurcation has been attributed to the added hemodynamic stress placed on the posterior circulation as the anterior circulation vessels succumb to stenosis and occlusion.[15]

Although extremely rare, arteriovenous malformations have been reported associated with moyamoya disease. An attempt to link these two conditions has been proposed, but the relationship between the two conditions remains unclear and may be coincidental.

Other conditions reported in association with moyamoya disease include primary pulmonary hypertension, fibromuscular dysplasia of the renal vessels, and Fanconi's syndrome.

TREATMENT

The treatment of moyamoya disease depends on the patient's clinical presentation and the stage of the disease. Treatment options include observation, medical therapy, surgical therapy, or various combinations thereof. At present, no definitive recommendations can be given, primarily because randomized or long-term follow-up studies are lacking.

Medical Management

Various medical treatments have been suggested, such as vasodilators, anticoagulant drugs, hemostatic agents, anticonvulsants, and steroids. Because no definitive medical treatment is available, these treatments are aimed at the symptoms and manifestations of the disease.

Surgical Management

The primary goals of surgical intervention are to provide effective revascularization and to prevent cerebral ischemia. The revascularization is thought to promote the regression of the fragile collateral moyamoya vessels and thereby decrease the risk of hemorrhage. No long-term studies, however, have supported this conclusion.

Revascularization for moyamoya disease can be accomplished by several means, from placing burr holes to creating direct bypasses. In general, revascularization procedures can be grouped as direct and indirect. The direct methods involve creating actual bypasses, typically a superficial temporal artery (STA)–MCA bypass. Indirect methods rely on the propensity of the ischemic brain to develop collateral vessels from any available source.[16] The most commonly used indirect methods are encephalo-duro-arterio-synangiosis (EDAS), encephalo-myo-synangiosis (EMS), and various combinations of the two. Other procedures involve dural inversion, galeal apposition, and omental transplants.

The direct method of STA-MCA bypass immediately augments the cerebral tissue with a significant amount of new blood flow. Theoretically, it would be the procedure of choice. In practice, however, creating an STA-MCA bypass in moyamoya patients can be a formidable challenge. Frequently, the caliber of the donor STA and recipient branches is unsuitable for a direct anastomosis, particularly in children. In addition, the already taxed cerebral circulation may not tolerate the time needed to occlude the MCA temporarily during the creation of the bypass. Given these difficulties, indirect methods have become the treatments of choice.

Indirect methods attempt to augment blood flow by inducing extradural collaterals to the ischemic brain. Several methods have been described, and each has its proponents. In 1977, Karawasa and colleagues[17] described EMS, in which the inner surface of the temporalis muscle is approximated to the cerebral surface. The procedure appeared to decrease the incidence of TIAs and major stroke. However, associated problems, such as the development of subdural hematomas and seizures, have tempered some of the enthusiasm for the procedure. In 1981, Matsushima and coworkers[18] proposed EDAS in the hope of avoiding some of these problems. In the EDAS procedure, the intact and continuous STA is approximated to the cerebral surface and sutured to the dural edges. A subsequent report by Matsushima and colleagues[19] analyzing their results in 65 patients revealed a gradual decrease in the incidence of TIAs and the maintenance of cognitive function. Other investigators have failed to reproduce these results, and many argue that EDAS alone fails to provide the degree of revascularization achieved with other procedures.

In 1993, Kinugasa and colleagues[20] proposed a combination of EDAS and EMS that achieved excellent revascularization. This combination procedure referred to as EDAMS (encephalo-duro-arterio-myo-synangiosis) approximates the STA and muscle flaps to the surface of the brain and sutures them to the dural edge.

The procedure preferred by the senior author involves a modification of the EDAS technique that has good and sometimes dramatic results (see Fig. 103–1). Some of the poor outcomes associated with EDAS may be due to the intact arachnoid membrane acting as a barrier to the development of new collaterals. Opening this arachnoid layer promotes more aggressive development of collaterals either through direct contact or the promotion of granulation and other inductive factors. This pial synangiosis, as termed by Adelson and Scott,[21] promotes significant collateral development and obviates some of the difficulties associated with other procedures. In severe cases, we have also used muscle in combination with the pial synangiosis; however, focal seizures have been encountered. The pial synangiosis alone is preferred.

Operative Technique

After general anesthesia has been induced and EEG electrodes have been placed for compressed spectral array monitoring, the patient is positioned supine with a shoulder roll. The head is turned laterally to the opposite shoulder and fixated in a standard three-point fixation clamp. Doppler ultrasonography with a small pencil probe is used to determine the course of the STA, which is marked with a marking pen. A curvilinear skin incision is planned over the course of the STA, and a small strip of hair is clipped over the area. To decrease the possibility of injuring the STA, no local anesthetic is infiltrated.

Under loop magnification or occasionally the microscope, the skin is incised over the STA. Using sharp technique, the subcutaneous layer is incised until the layer harboring the STA is encountered. Bleeding points from the skin edges are carefully coagulated using very fine jeweler bipolar forceps. Dissection proceeds along the entire course of the STA until the tissue is dissected free of the subcutaneous tissues. Small branches from the STA are coagulated and divided with fine bipolar forceps. A self-retaining retractor is used to retract the skin edges. The galea surrounding the STA is divided using a needle-tip Bovie cauterization device. A generous cuff of soft tissue is left (Fig. 103–3). When the STA is dissected free, it is retracted laterally and protected under a papaverine-soaked cottonoid.

The underlying temporalis muscle and fascia are divided with electrocauterization in line with the incision and reflected laterally with the self-retaining retractors. Two burr holes are placed at the inferior and superior limits of the planned craniotomy flap. An elliptical bone flap is fashioned and removed. Dural-tenting sutures are placed along the bone edges. At this point, the STA is centered over the craniotomy area (see Fig. 103–3). If undue tension on the STA is apparent, the vessel should be freed further by expanding the dissection proximally and distally. The goal is a redundant STA that can be placed over the desired area without tension or stretching.

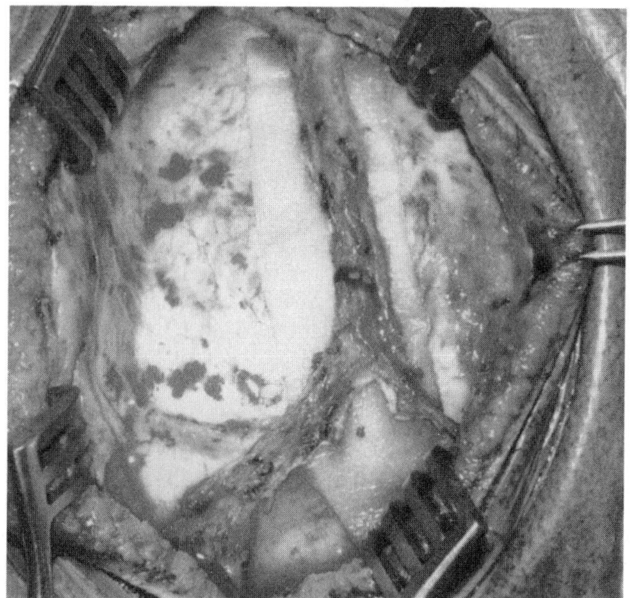

FIGURE 103–3. Intraoperative depiction of the dissected superficial temporal artery (STA) and craniotomy area. A generous cuff of galea remains on the STA.

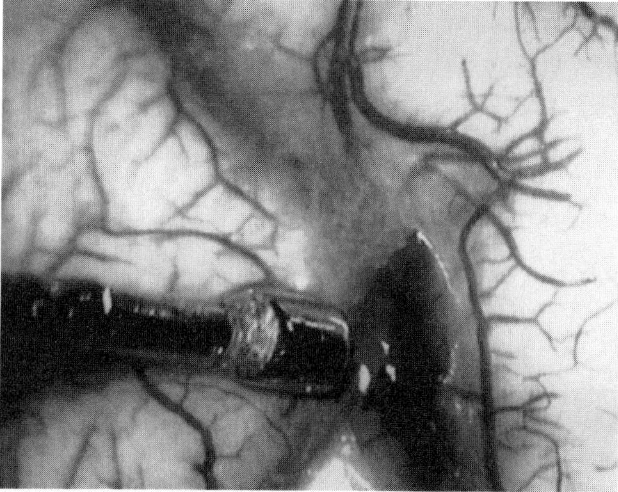

FIGURE 103–4. Intraoperative photograph depicting the opening of the pia-arachnoid membrane.

The dura is opened in a cruciate manner. Care is taken to avoid disturbing or injuring any naturally developed transdural collaterals. If the middle meningeal artery (MMA) is providing significant dural collaterals to the brain, the incision is modified to preserve it. Under the operating microscope and using microsurgical technique, the arachnoid over the gyral and sulcal areas is opened (Fig. 103–4). The MCA branches are inspected for their suitability for direct bypass.

The continuous STA is positioned over the open sulcal regions and anchored using interrupted 10-0 nylon sutures. The needle of the suture is passed through the galeal cuff and the adjacent pial area (Fig. 103–5). When this maneuver is completed, the dural edges are loosely approximated with 4-0 silk sutures. A layer of Gelfoam is placed over the dura, and the bone flap is replaced with miniplates and screws. The STA should pass through the burr holes without undue tension or kinking that could occlude and thrombose the vessel. The scalp is closed in two layers using 3-0 Vicryl and staples. The hair is washed, and sterile ointment is placed on the incision without dressing.

Anesthetic Considerations and Complications

The complications associated with the surgical treatment of moyamoya disease can be divided into anesthetic and surgical issues. The most significant complication is the development of perioperative ischemia and stroke. In children, the ischemic symptoms of moyamoya disease can be precipitated by hyperventilation. Hence, the use of hyperventilation during surgery must be avoided. End-tidal CO_2 and arterial CO_2 must be monitored carefully. Volume status and blood pressure should be maintained strictly. Hypotension during or after induction must be avoided. The use of

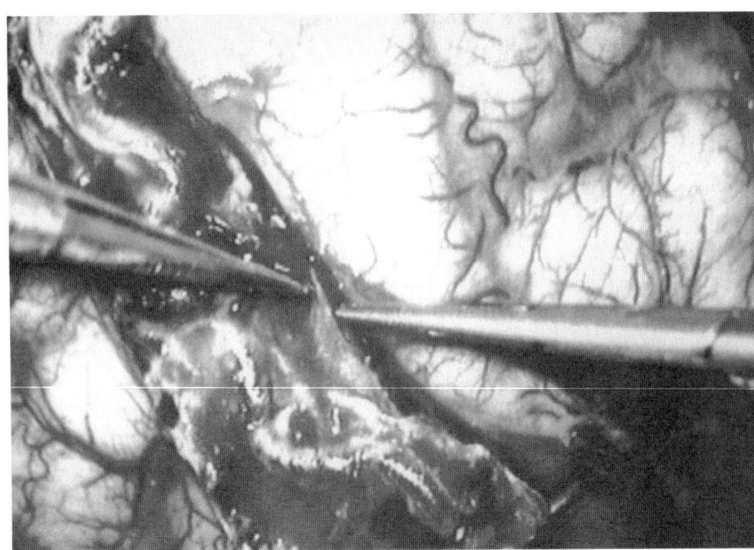

FIGURE 103–5. The superficial temporal artery sutured to the adjacent edge of the pia-arachnoid membrane.

relative hypercapnia during anesthetic management has been advocated to avoid the vasoconstrictive effects of hypocapnia. Sato and coworkers,[22] however, have suggested that the ischemic vascular territories and cerebral arteries may already be dilated maximally. If other vascular territories are induced to dilate with hypercapnia, steal to the already ischemic territories may ensue. Sato and associates[22] found that the use of inhalational anesthetics decreased regional CBF and suggested using total intravenous anesthesia instead.

Ischemic complications related to surgery are rare and are usually the result of disrupted transdural collateral vessels and temporary occlusion during direct bypass. The most common surgical complication is the development of acute and chronic subdural hematomas, particularly when muscle is involved in the procedure. During an EMS procedure, strict hemostasis must be maintained. Postoperative focal seizures are another complication of EMS, but most are easily controlled with anticonvulsant therapy. Fortunately, wound complications are rare. Meticulous attention to proper surgical technique during closure and tissue handling appears to eliminate these risks.

OUTCOMES

Although the surgical treatment of ischemic moyamoya disease has been accepted as successful, the indications for surgery and associated long-term outcomes compared to the natural history of the disease are controversial. Unfortunately, few well-controlled studies have critically investigated the natural history of moyamoya disease. It has been suggested that many patients will stabilize and experience no further symptoms after a period of time. Others have suggested that gradual deterioration will occur, particularly in young children in whom severe cognitive disabilities have been noted.

Several studies evaluating the different surgical procedures have suggested an improvement in symptoms and a decrease in the frequency of TIAs and stroke. However, a summary report of 628 patients over 5 years revealed no difference in the outcomes of surgical and medical treatments.[23] It appears that in as many as 80% of cases, the natural history is benign, with the disease burning itself out.

Given these conflicting data, the precise indications for surgical intervention in moyamoya disease remain undefined. Undoubtedly, further long-term follow-up studies will answer the question of ultimate prognosis after surgery.

MOYAMOYA DISEASE AND PREGNANCY

There have been few reports and no extensive studies on the effect of moyamoya disease on pregnancy. Because moyamoya disease is more common in women who tend to be of childbearing age, recommendations for the management of pregnancy and delivery are needed. Recently, Komiyama and colleagues[24] reviewed all cases in the literature to date. They found no evidence that pregnancy increases the risk of cerebrovascular accident or that bypass surgery decreases it. The causes underlying the few poor outcomes for mothers or newborns were related to hemorrhagic manifestations of the disease and not to cerebral ischemia. Either cesarean section or vaginal delivery could be accomplished without sequelae.

CONCLUSION

Moyamoya disease remains a chronic occlusive cerebrovascular disorder of unknown etiology. Seen most commonly in Asian populations, the disease affects both children and middle-aged adults. Characterized by progressive occlusion of the proximal intracranial vessels and the development of fragile collateral circulation, the disease manifests with ischemic symptoms, stroke, and hemorrhage.

The natural history of moyamoya disease remains poorly understood, but patients with progressive ischemic insults are thought to benefit from surgical management. Various procedures exist for augmenting CBF in moyamoya disease. Indirect procedures that take advantage of the propensity of the ischemic brain to develop extracranial-to-intracranial collaterals are used most often. These revascularization procedures are thought to improve the circulation and to prevent further ischemic injury and perhaps hemorrhage. However, the true long-term outcome of surgical treatment compared to the natural history of the disease is unknown. Precise criteria and indications for surgical intervention remain to be defined.

REFERENCES

1. Suzuki J, Takaku A: Cerebrovascular "moyamoya" disease. Disease showing abnormal net-like vessels in base of brain. Arch Neurol 20:288–299, 1969.
2. Takeuchi K, Shimizu K: Hypoplasia of the bilateral internal carotid arteries. Brain Nerve 9:37–43, 1957.
3. Nishimoto A, Takeuchi S: Abnormal cerebrovascular network related to the internal carotid arteries. J Neurosurg 29:255–260, 1968.
4. Fukui M: Current state of study on moyamoya disease in Japan. Surg Neurol 47:138–143, 1997.
5. Peerless SJ: Risk factors of moyamoya disease in Canada and the USA. Clin Neurol Neurosurg 99:S45–S48, 1997.
6. Aoyagi M, Fukai N, Sakamoto H, et al: Altered cellular responses to serum mitogens, including platelet-derived growth factor, in cultured smooth muscle cells derived from arteries of patients with moyamoya disease. J Cell Physiol 147:191–198, 1991.
7. Yoshimoto T, Houkin K, Takahashi A, et al: Angiogenic factors in moyamoya disease. Stroke 27:2160–2165, 1996.
8. Hojo M, Hoshimaru M, Miyamoto S, et al: Role of transforming growth factor-beta1 in the pathogenesis of moyamoya disease. J Neurosurg 89:623–629, 1998.
9. Yamaguchi T, Matsushima Y, Takada Y, et al: Case-control study of moyamoya disease. [article in Japanese.] No To Shinkei 41: 485–491, 1989.
10. Yamashita M, Oka K, Tanaka K: Histopathology of the brain vascular network in moyamoya disease. Stroke 14:50–58, 1983.
11. Ueki K, Meyer FB, Mellinger JF: Moyamoya disease: The disorder and surgical treatment. Mayo Clin Proc 69:749–757, 1994.
12. Fukui M: Guidelines for the diagnosis and treatment of spontaneous occlusion of the circle of Willis ('moyamoya disease'). Research Committee on Spontaneous Occlusion of the Circle of Willis (Moyamoya Disease) of the Ministry of Health and Welfare, Japan. Clin Neurol Neurosurg 99:S238–S240, 1997.
13. Ogawa A, Yoshimoto T, Suzuki J, et al: Cerebral blood flow in moyamoya disease. Part 1: Correlation with age and regional distribution. Acta Neurochir (Wien) 105:30–34, 1990.
14. Kodama N, Aoki Y, Hiraga H, et al: Electroencephalographic findings in children with moyamoya disease. Arch Neurol 36: 16–19, 1979.
15. Kwak R, Ito S, Yamamoto N, et al: Significance of intracranial aneurysms associated with moyamoya disease. (Part 1). Differences between intracranial aneurysms associated with moyamoya disease and usual saccular aneurysms—review of the literature (article in Japanese). Neurol Med Chir (Tokyo) 24:97–103, 1984.
16. Nariai T, Suzuki R, Matsushima Y, et al: Surgically induced angiogenesis to compensate for hemodynamic cerebral ischemia. Stroke 25:1014–1021, 1994.
17. Karasawa J, Kikuchi H, Furuse S, et al: A surgical treatment of "moyamoya" disease "encephalo-myo-synangiosis." Neurol Med Chir (Tokyo) 17:29–37, 1977.
18. Matsushima Y, Fukai N, Tanaka K, et al: A new surgical treatment of moyamoya disease in children: A preliminary report. Surg Neurol 15:313–320, 1981.
19. Matsushima Y, Aoyagi M, Koumo Y, et al: Effects of encephalo-duro-arterio-synangiosis on childhood moyamoya patients—swift disappearance of ischemic attacks and maintenance of mental capacity. Neurol Med Chir (Tokyo) 31:708–714, 1991.
20. Kinugasa K, Mandai S, Kamata I, et al: Surgical treatment of moyamoya disease: Operative technique for encephalo-duro-arterio-myo-synangiosis, its follow-up, clinical results, and angiograms. Neurosurgery 32:527–531, 1993.
21. Adelson P, Scott R: Pial synangiosis for moyamoya syndrome in children. Pediatr Neurosurg 23:26–33, 1995.
22. Sato K, Shirane R, Kato M, et al: Effect of inhalational anesthesia on cerebral circulation in Moyamoya disease. J Neurosurg Anesthesiol 11:25–30, 1999.
23. Yonekawa Y, Summary report of the research committee on spontaneous occlusion of the circle of Willis (moyamoya disease) (1988–1992). In Yonekawa Y (ed): 1992 Annual Report of the Research Committee on Spontaneous Occlusion of the Circle of Willis, Tokyo, Japanese Ministry of Health and Welfare, 1992, pp 1–11.
24. Komiyama M, Yasui T, Kitano S, et al: Moyamoya disease and pregnancy: Case report and review of the literature. Neurosurgery 43:360–369, 1998.

CHAPTER **104**

Cerebral Venous and Sinus Thrombosis

FRANK P. K. HSU ■ GARY M. NESBIT ■ STANLEY L. BARNWELL

HISTORY AND CLINICAL SIGNIFICANCE

Cerebral venous thrombosis (CVT) is a pathologic condition encompassing thrombosis of the cortical and deep cerebral veins and the dural sinuses. It was first described by Ribes in the early 19th century.[1] He reported a 45-year-old man with systemic malignancy harboring thrombosis of the superior sagittal sinus demonstrated at autopsy. CVT is thought to be a rare clinical problem, but the exact incidence is unknown. Because of the rarity of the disease and its nonspecific presentation, the diagnosis of CVT is difficult and frequently delayed.

PATHOGENESIS

When thrombosis occurs in the cerebral veins and the dural sinuses, the resulting venous hypertension causes hypoxia of the brain, similar to the syndrome of a carotid cavernous fistula, with resultant neuronal ischemia.[2] The spectrum ranges from cerebral edema of varying degrees to extreme progression to massive hemorrhage and often bilateral cerebral infarcts. The potential causes of and risk factors associated with CVT are numerous. The underlying mechanisms are related to alterations in the physical properties of the vasculature, the chemical properties of blood, or the hemodynamic properties of blood flow.

Vascular injury due to trauma causes local endothelial damage and altered hemodynamics. Trauma, neoplasms, and other mass lesions can cause vascular compression and altered hemodynamics as well. The association between dural arteriovenous fistulas and CVT has been recognized.[3] This link is also thought to be related to the altered hemodynamics induced by the dural arteriovenous fistula.

Hypercoagulable states are associated with numerous conditions. Factors involved in hypercoagulability include protein C, protein S, antithrombin III, and plasminogen. A disequilibrium or altered functionality of these factors can result in hypercoagulable states, contributing to CVT.

Protein C is a vitamin K–dependent, thrombin-activating regulatory protein. Activated protein C has been reported to have potent anticoagulation properties.[4] The activity of protein C increases 10,000-fold when bound to its vitamin K–dependent cofactor, protein S, on phospholipid surfaces.[5] Deficiency of proteins C and S is associated with hypercoagulability. Protein C–activated resistance can also cause a hypercoagulable state,[6] and it has been reported as a cause of CVT.[7–9] Further, factor V gene mutation (factor V Leiden)[8, 10] and prothrombin (factor II) gene mutation[11] have been determined to be risk factors for CVT. A hypercoagulable state may be present in patients with lupus anticoagulants, which are circulating autoantibodies directed primarily against phospholipids. Lupus anticoagulants have been reported to be associated with CVT.[12] Anticardiolipin antibodies may be a contributing factor in the pathogenesis of CVT.[13]

A number of coagulation system abnormalities that are rarely associated with CVT have been reported in Behçet's disease,[14–16] inflammatory bowel diseases (e.g., ulcerative colitis),[17–19] Wegener's granulomatosis,[20] and Cogan's syndrome.[21]

Infection is thought to cause CVT by altering the coagulation cascade, and hypercoagulable states have been described in those with infections. Infection used to be a major cause of CVT, but with contemporary antibiotic therapy, this has become less common. Ameri and Bousser reported that 8.2% of CVT cases are due to infection.[22] Cavernous and lateral sinus thrombosis is most frequently related to infections such as sinusitis, otitis, and mastoiditis. *Staphylococcus aureus* is the most frequently reported pathogen. In chronic forms, gram-negative rods and fungi such as *Aspergillus* species are more commonly isolated.[23, 24]

CVT is more common in young women than in other groups,[14, 22, 25–28] and CVT that develops during puerperium is still common in developing countries.[14, 29] Oral contraceptives may play a role in the pathogenesis of CVT in young women.[8, 14, 29] Ameri and Bousser reported that 8% of their cases of CVT were thought to be caused by the use of oral contraceptives.[22] Martinelli and colleagues reported an association between oral contraceptive use and the development of CVT.[8] The risk is much higher in women using oral contraceptives who also have the prothrombin gene mutation. A postmenopausal woman taking estrogen-progesterone therapy was reported to develop CVT.[30]

Despite a long list of possible causes for CVT, the inciting factors remain undetermined in some cases. Some investigators estimate that as many as 40% of cases are idiopathic.[31, 32]

In summary, CVT may be associated with numerous conditions. Most of these conditions involve alterations in the physical properties of the vasculature, the chemical properties of blood coagulation, or the hemodynamic properties of blood flow. An extensive workup is usually required to identify an underlying cause for CVT.

INCIDENCE

Although the exact incidence of CVT is unknown, it is agreed that this is a relatively rare disease.[22] Most of the estimates are derived from autopsy studies. Autopsy cases may introduce bias, however, because the most severe cases with the worst outcome are overrepresented. Ehler and Courville found 16 cases of superior sagittal sinus thrombosis in a series of 12,500 autopsies.[33] Over a 20-year period, Barnett and Hyland found only 39 cases of noninfective CVT that were proved by autopsy.[34] Later autopsy studies reported the incidence to be as low as 0.03%[35] and as high as 9% in 182 adult cases.[36] Scotti and coworkers observed CVT in approximately 4% of cerebral angiograms performed in 240 children.[37]

CVT affects all age groups and both sexes, but with a strong preponderance in women between 20 and 40 years old.[38] This may reflect the fact that women in that age group are more likely to use oral contraceptives[39] and undergo puerperium.

CLINICAL PRESENTATION

The clinical presentation of CVT varies widely.[22, 26, 27, 40–42] Headache is the most common and often the earliest symptom.[22] It is seen in nearly 80% of cases.[14] Nausea, vomiting, and visual changes are other symptoms experienced by patients. Increased intracranial pressure is thought to be the underlying cause for these symptoms. Papilledema is seen in about half of those afflicted, and confusion, agitation, and other mental status changes occur in about 25% of cases.[22] Focal neurological deficits are present in 50% to 75%, often caused by venous hypertension and cerebral infarction or hemorrhage.[14] Aphasia, hemianopia, or hemisensory deficits may also occur. Seizure is another common symptom,[43] with simple or generalized seizures complicating nearly 33% of cases.

The mode of onset is quite variable. Although an acute presentation can mimic acute ischemic stroke, subacute presentations are more common. In 70% of cases, the patients' complaints are present for days to weeks, and the symptoms can be fluctuating or progressive.

The clinical presentation also varies according to the site and extent of thrombosis. When thrombosis is limited to the superior sagittal sinus or lateral sinus, the most frequent pattern of presentation is isolated intracranial hypertension. If the thrombosis extends to cortical veins, focal deficits and seizures may occur. Bilateral deficits are typical as late signs of superior sagittal sinus thrombosis. Transverse sinus CVT may be associated with otalgia, otorrhea, cervical tenderness, and lymphadenopathy from an underlying infection such as mastoiditis or otitis media. In cavernous sinus CVT, symptoms often include eyelid edema, chemosis, retro-orbital pain, and exophthalmos. Paralysis of cranial nerves III, IV, V_1, V_2, and VI may occur, due to their involvement within the cavernous sinus. When the thrombosis involves the deep venous system, the patient can present with akinetic mutism, coma, or decerebration. Mild cases causing memory disturbances or minor confusion may occur. Cortical vein thrombosis without sinus involvement can present as stroke syndromes.[44] Cerebellar vein thrombosis is extremely rare and often lethal.[25]

DIAGNOSTIC EVALUATION

Because the clinical presentation is highly variable and the symptoms are usually nonspecific, the key to making the diagnosis of CVT is to have a high level of suspicion. Historically, CVT was first documented radiographically with a direct injection of the superior sagittal sinus.[22, 25] Diagnostic modalities currently used for the confirmation of CVT include computed tomography (CT), magnetic resonance imaging (MRI), and cerebral angiography.

CT is usually the initial diagnostic test performed on patients who are suspected of having CVT or who present with acute mental deterioration.[22, 25] The dense vein and cord sign may be seen in approximately 20% of cases with non–contrast-enhancing CT (Fig. 104–1).[31, 45, 46] The cord sign and the dense triangle sign correspond to spontaneously hyperdense cortical veins or sinuses, respectively. They can be seen during the first 1 to 2 weeks after thrombosis and may be falsely positive in neonates, dehydrated individuals, and those with elevated hemoglobin. Sometimes a dense triangle, also known as the delta sign, may be seen as the thrombus occupies the superior sagittal sinus (Fig. 104–2). On contrast-enhanced CT, the empty delta sign consists of peripheral dural leaf enhancement, along with a central nonopacified thrombus; it occurs in 10% to 30% of cases of superior sagittal sinus thrombosis.[47–50] Unfortunately, the false-negative rate for CT diagnosis of CVT is high, estimated at between 4% and 25%. CT can also show hemorrhagic infarctions as a result of poor drainage secondary to CVT (Fig. 104–3). The infarctions are usually bilateral.

MRI has recently become the chosen modality for detecting CVT.[42, 51–55] With magnetic resonance angiography (MRA) and magnetic resonance venography (MRV), the arterial and venous phases can be examined

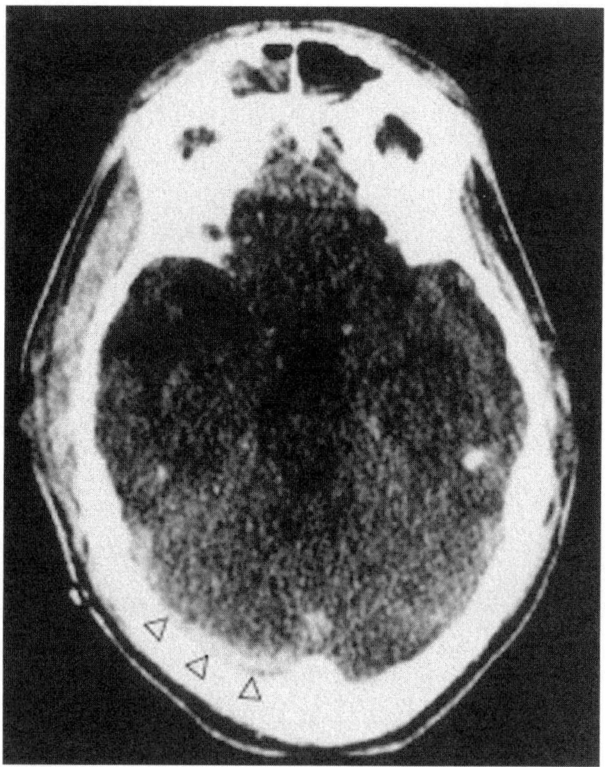

FIGURE 104–1. Nonenhanced computed tomographic scan demonstrating hyperdense signal signifying clot in the right transverse sinus as a result of thrombosis *(arrowheads).*

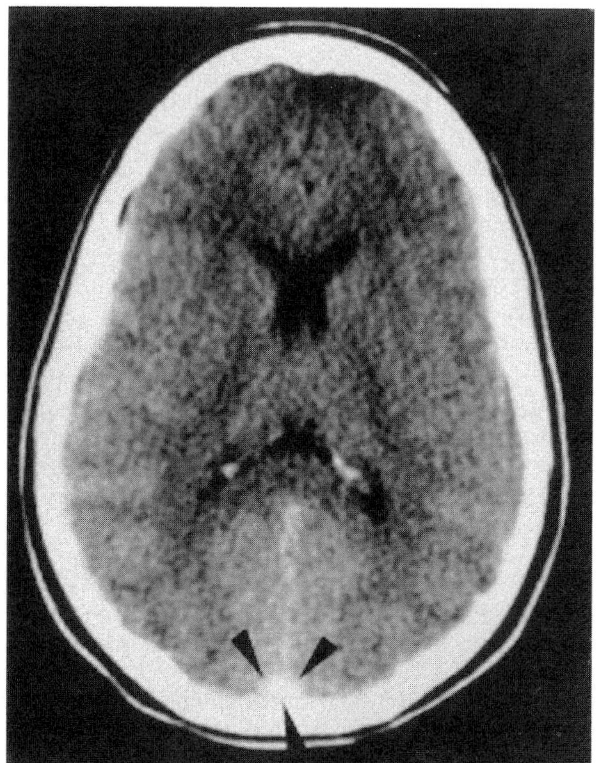

FIGURE 104–2. Nonenhanced computed tomographic scan demonstrating a delta sign—triangular hyperdensity signifying clot in the superior sagittal sinus *(arrowheads).*

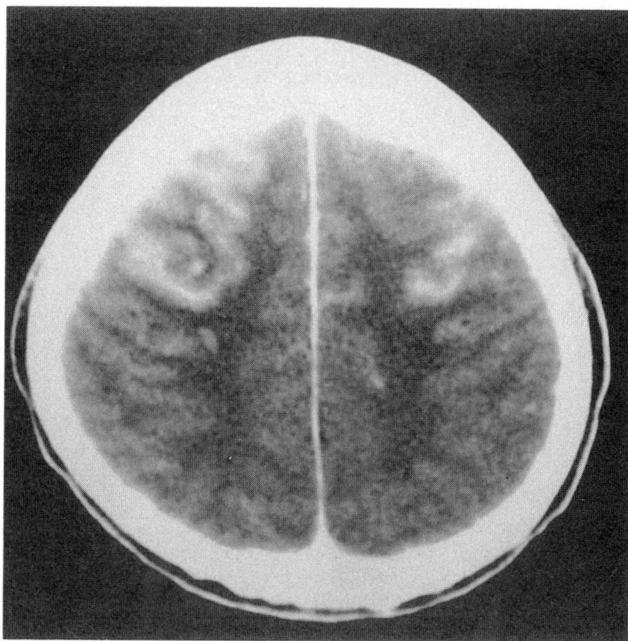

FIGURE 104–3. Nonenhanced computed tomographic scan demonstrating bilateral hemorrhagic infarctions as a result of superior sagittal sinus thrombosis.

concomitantly or separately. MRA-MRV is now the best method for detecting CVT (Figs. 104–4 and 104–5). MRI offers certain advantages: the thrombus can be directly visualized, and the cerebral lesions, such as edema and hemorrhagic infarct, can be detected. These MRI changes are best seen in superior sagittal sinus, lateral sinus, straight sinus, and vein of Galen thrombosis;

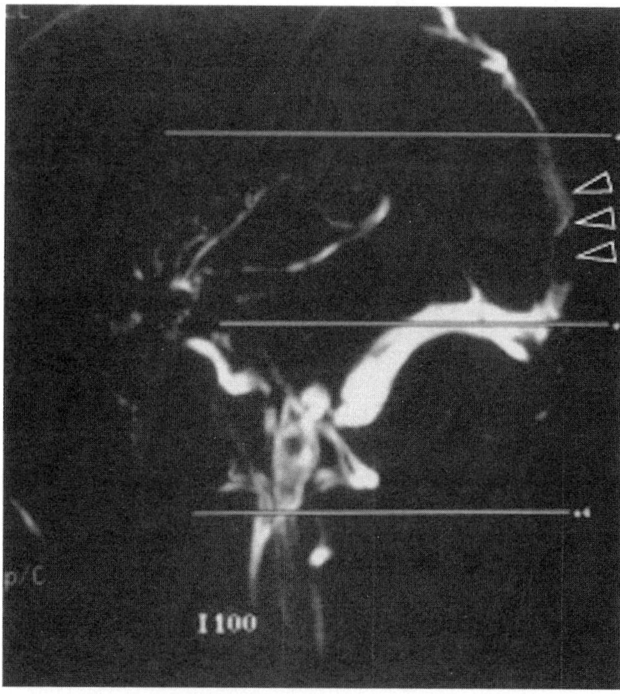

FIGURE 104–4. Magnetic resonance venography showing decreased blood flow in the superior sagittal sinus *(arrowheads).*

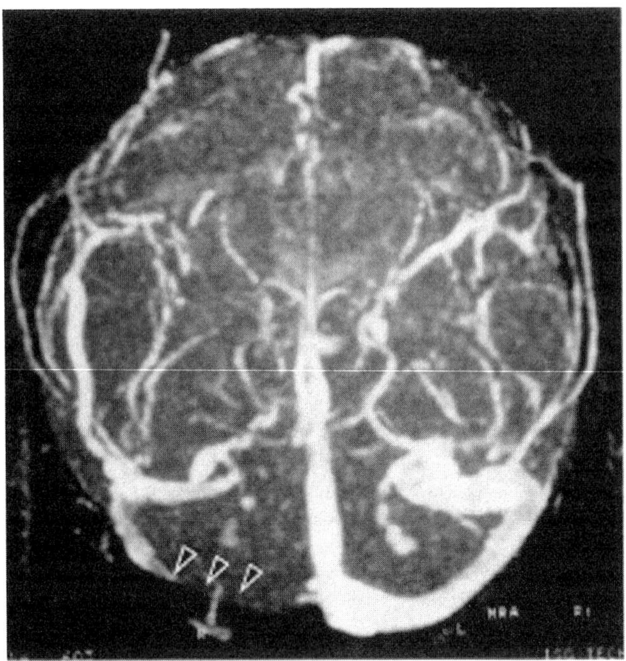

FIGURE 104–5. Magnetic resonance venography showing absence of blood flow in the right transverse sinus *(arrowheads)*.

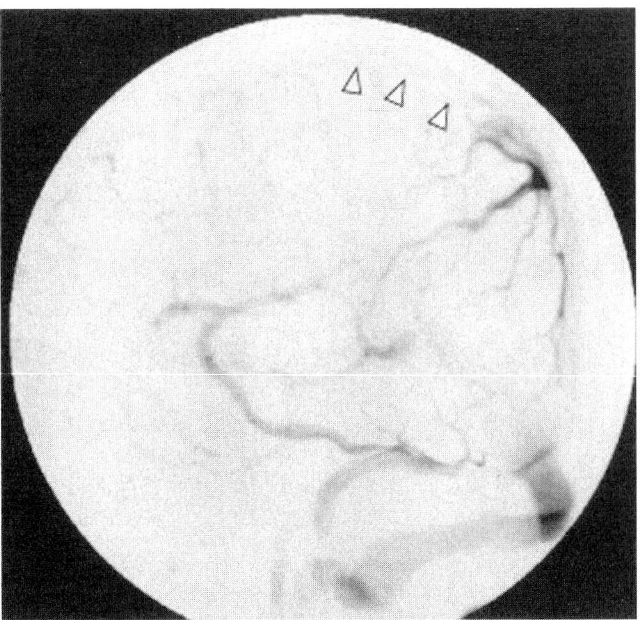

FIGURE 104–6. Lateral view of the venous phase of a cerebral arteriogram demonstrating thrombosis of the superior sagittal sinus *(arrowheads)*.

they are far less obvious in cavernous sinus and cortical vein thrombosis, which sometimes remains difficult to diagnose. Although MRA-MRV is the most sensitive modality for detecting CVT, it may give inaccurate results in some circumstances. False-positive identification may occur when sinuses are congenitally absent or hypoplastic. False-negative identification may occur when the signal of methemoglobin mimics that of flowing blood, or when loss of signal occurs secondary to magnetic susceptibility artifact.

Cerebral angiography used to be the standard in making the diagnosis of CVT.[56] It is now indicated only when MRI diagnosis is uncertain or neuroradiologic intervention is desired. The typical finding is nonvisualization of all or part of a sinus during the venous phase of an angiogram (Fig. 104–6). In cortical vein thrombosis, there is a sudden stop of the occluded vein, which may be surrounded by dilated collateral "corkscrew vessels."[22]

The value of conventional transcranial Doppler ultrasonography was examined by Canhão and colleagues.[57] It was suggested that using transcranial ultrasound to detect the velocity increase in the deep middle cerebral vein and basal vein of Rosenthal aided the diagnosis of superior sagittal sinus thrombosis.

TREATMENT

Therapy for patients with CVT should be directed at treating the underlying causative process, symptoms secondary to elevated intracranial pressure, and seizures or focal deficits caused by cerebral edema and infarction. If an underlying cause is found, it should be treated. If an infectious process is identified, broad-spectrum antibiotics or drainage of purulent collections should be part of the treatment.[22, 25] Patients presenting with CVT should initially be stabilized with appropriate airway and circulation management. Subsequent supportive measures should be instituted. Increased intracranial pressure can be treated with mannitol, temporary short-term hyperventilation, cerebrospinal fluid drainage through ventriculostomy or lumbar puncture, barbiturate coma, or surgical craniectomy.[22, 25, 58] Cerebral perfusion pressure should be kept at an adequate level to prevent secondary ischemic insults. Seizure is a frequent symptom and should be treated with anticonvulsant medications.

Antithrombotics

The natural course of CVT is variable, and the guidelines directing treatment are controversial. The use of heparin for the treatment of CVT was initially reported by Stansfield in 1942.[59] Since then, several other authors have reported the beneficial effects of heparin in those with CVT,[14, 15, 60] but there has been only one prospective, randomized, controlled study using heparin. Einhäupl and coworkers published the results of their series of 20 patients in 1991.[61] The efficacy of systemic heparin was compared with placebo in a double-blind, randomized study. The group of patients receiving heparin had a better outcome at 3 days, 8 days, and 3 months. Although the power of this study was reduced because the investigators did not meet all the criteria for a double-blind, randomized study, the advantage of heparin in treating CVT was strongly suggested.

Despite the risk for intracerebral hemorrhage, the benefit of using systemic heparin was examined in a large retrospective study by Ameri and Bousser.[22] Their

82 patients were treated with heparin for CVT, and no mortality or worsening of clinical status was found.

The current trend is to use heparin.[22, 26, 62] The goal for heparin anticoagulation is to maintain the activated partial thromboplastin time at 2 to 2.5 times normal. Once the patient's condition has stabilized, warfarin therapy is initiated. The therapeutic international normalized ratio is kept between 2 and 3 for 6 months. There are few scientific data or guidelines for the dosage and duration of heparin and warfarin therapy in the literature on CVT. The stated protocol is empirically determined.

Levine and associates[63] found that patients treated with anticoagulation and antibiotics for cavernous sinus thrombosis in the early stage (<7 days after initial onset) showed a significant reduction in morbidity compared with patients treated with antibiotics alone. However, if anticoagulant treatment began at a later stage of the disease, no beneficial effect was found.

Systemic Thrombolytics

Thrombolytic agents, such as streptokinase, urokinase, and tissue plasminogen activator, have been used systemically in small experimental series.[64] Unfortunately, only anecdotal reports are available on the clinical management of thrombolytic agents.[65–69]

The major risks of the systemic administration of thrombolytics are gastrointestinal or intracranial hemorrhage. Contraindications to thrombolytic therapy include recent childbirth, history of a bleeding diathesis, recent major surgery, recent major trauma, active gastrointestinal bleeding, or inflammatory bowel disease. It has been suggested that local infusion of thrombolytic agents via interventional neuroradiologic techniques can minimize the major complications from systemic thrombolysis.

Interventional Neuroradiology

Recent advances in endovascular techniques enable the local delivery of thrombolytic agents to selective venous channels where thrombosis occurs (Table 104–1 provides a summary of the reported cases of endovascular thrombolytic therapy in the English literature). The local infusion of thrombolytics offers advantages, including minimization of systemic effects and local clot lysis with higher concentration of thrombolytic agents. Historically, Scott and colleagues reported the first case of local fibrinolytic therapy.[70] A young patient with CVT and a rapidly deteriorating clinical course was treated with midline craniotomy and direct catheterization of the superior sagittal sinus. Urokinase was infused at 4000 U/minute for 3 hours and then 1000 U/minute for 8 hours. The patient progressed from being unresponsive initially to having just mild dysphasia at 4 weeks.

Higashida and associates proposed a more aggressive modality of therapy for CVT patients with clinical deterioration.[71] These investigators successfully performed direct puncture of the superior sagittal sinus in a neonate and infused urokinase, resulting in clot lysis over 12 hours. This was the first reported attempt at locally infused thrombolytic treatment for CVT without a craniotomy.

Barnwell and coworkers reported direct endovascu-

TABLE 104–1 ■ **Endovascular Urokinase Treatment of Cerebral Venous Thrombosis Reported in the Literature**

AUTHOR	YEAR	NO. OF PATIENTS	DOSES	SHORT-TERM OUTCOME
Scott et al[70]	1988	1	240,000 U/hr × 3 hr 60,000 U/hr × 8 hr	Mild dysphasia at 4 wk
Higashida et al[71]	1989	1	1000 U/hr × 12 hr in 3.7-kg infant	Normal development at 3 yr
Barnwell et al[72]	1991	3	58,000 U/hr × 5–10 days	2 of 3 clinically improved; follow-up 12–24 mo
Tsai et al[73]	1992	5	200,000–600,000 U; total duration n/a	4 of 5 totally recovered; follow-up time n/a
Smith et al[74]	1994	7	20,000–150,000 U/hr × 163 hr (88–244)	6 of 7 clinically improved; follow-up 8–37 mo
Horowitz et al[75]	1995	12	50,000–500,000 U bolus 73,600 U/hr × 50 hr (12–84)	8 of 12 with excellent outcome; 2 of 12 with good outcome; follow-up time n/a
Barnwell et al[63]	1995	6	100,000 U bolus 40,000–80,000 U/hr up to 48 hr	3 of 6 completely recovered; 1 of 6 blind, 2 of 6 died; follow-up time n/a
Spearman et al[76]	1997	2	200,000–283,300 U/hr × 3 hr	2 of 2 minor neurological deficits; follow-up time 6 mo
Holder et al[77]	1997	1	150,000 U bolus × 2 100,000 U/hr × 3 days	Complete recovery; follow-up time 6 mo
Rael et al[78]	1997	1	250,000 U bolus × 2 80,000 U/hr × 165 hr	No neurological deficit; follow-up time 30 d
Smith et al[79]	1997	2	1 million U; total duration n/a	2 of 2 complete recovery; follow-up time 18 mo
Dowd et al[80]	1999	1	3,000,000 U total over 2 days, AngioJet used	Minimal cognitive deficit; follow-up time 6 mo

n/a, not available.

lar thrombolytic therapy in three patients.[72] All three patients had dural arteriovenous fistulas, and all three were treated by direct transjugular infusion of urokinase. The period of continuous infusion for thrombolysis ranged from 4 to 10 days. In two patients, the clinical signs and symptoms improved, with angiographic evidence of clot lysis and dural sinus recanalization. Angiography indicated that one patient had partial resolution of a clot in the torcular Herophili and transverse sinus, but that patient showed no clinical improvement. These preliminary results were encouraging and suggested that transjugular local infusion of thrombolytic agents can be an effective treatment for symptomatic, thrombosed dural sinuses.

Tsai and colleagues reported five cases of successful direct transfemoral thrombolytic treatment.[73] Smith and associates reported on seven patients with symptomatic dural sinus thrombosis who had failed a trial of medical treatment and were treated with direct infusion of urokinase into the thrombosed sinus.[74] The patients received urokinase doses ranging from 20,000 to 150,000 U/hour, with a mean infusion time of 163 hours (range, 88 to 244 hours). Patency of the affected dural sinus was achieved with antegrade flow in all patients. Six patients either improved neurologically over their prethrombolysis state or were healthy after thrombolysis. The only complications were an infected femoral access site and transient hematuria.

Horowitz and coworkers added 12 more cases to the literature.[75] They reported that despite the presence of preinfusion infarct in five patients, four of whom were hemorrhagic, they incurred no major therapeutic morbidity. Functional sinus patency was achieved in 11 of 12 patients, with the only true failure occurring in an individual with symptoms of at least 2 months' duration. Good to excellent clinical outcomes were achieved in 10 of 11 patients.

Barnwell and colleagues reported an additional six cases of local thrombolytic therapy.[62] Three patients did well and made complete recoveries. Two of these patients had extensive thrombosis and presented with severe clinical pictures but made full functional recoveries. One patient, with extensive dural sinus thrombosis that had been observed but not treated for 3 weeks, had minimal improvement on the post-therapy angiogram and became blind from optic neuropathy, probably secondary to optic nerve damage from increased intracranial pressure. Two patients with extensive dural sinus thrombosis, bilateral parietal lobe infarcts, and coma had no improvement and died, both from intractable intracranial hypertension and stroke.

Spearman and associates reported two patients with CVT who were deteriorating rapidly.[76] Endovascular thrombolysis was performed, and both patients survived with minimal deficits. Holder's and Rael's groups each contributed one additional case to the literature.[77,78] Smith and colleagues reported two additional cases.[79]

Dowd and associates presented a novel application of a transvascular rheolytic thrombectomy system in the treatment of symptomatic CVT.[80] An AngioJet catheter (Possis Medical, Minneapolis, MN) was directed over the micro–guide wire to the thrombus. The AngioJet catheter was activated, and partial sinus thrombolysis was achieved using the hydrodynamic thrombolytic action of the catheter as it was slowly withdrawn to the jugular bulb. Concomitant infusion of urokinase was performed as well, and the patient had only minimal neurological deficit at 6 months' follow-up.

Local infusion of thrombolytics can be achieved by transfemoral venous catheterization and cannulation of the cerebral venous system. This is usually done after the diagnostic cerebral arterial angiogram demonstrating venous thrombosis. A small catheter is navigated to the venous channel where the clot resides, and a thrombolytic agent is infused at a predetermined rate (Fig. 104–7). An exact regimen for local thrombolytic treatment has not been definitively determined. Current trends at major centers with neurointerventional capability advocate the administration of urokinase initially by bolus (100,000 IU or less if the patient has a hemorrhagic infarct present on CT), followed by a constant infusion of 40,000 to 80,000 IU/hour for up to 72 hours.[62] Response to thrombolytic therapy is assessed by means of serial venograms obtained approximately every 6 hours and ultimately by means of arteriography when therapy is stopped. Although three groin hematomas and one retroperitoneal hematoma were reported by Horowitz and coauthors in their series of 12 patients,[75] no intracranial hemorrhage as a direct result of endovascular urokinase treatment has been reported in the previously cited series.

Although there are no conclusive data regarding the efficacy of local thrombolytic agents in the treatment of CVT, it appears that endovascular local thrombolysis is generally safe and effective in opening venous occlusions and that patients treated successfully have a better clinical outcome than can be achieved with the use

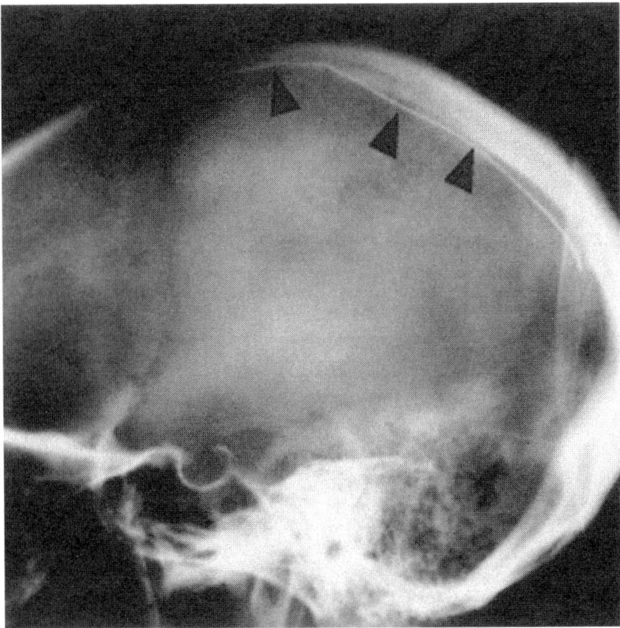

FIGURE 104–7. Lateral skull radiograph showing an endovascular catheter located in the superior sagittal sinus *(arrowheads)*.

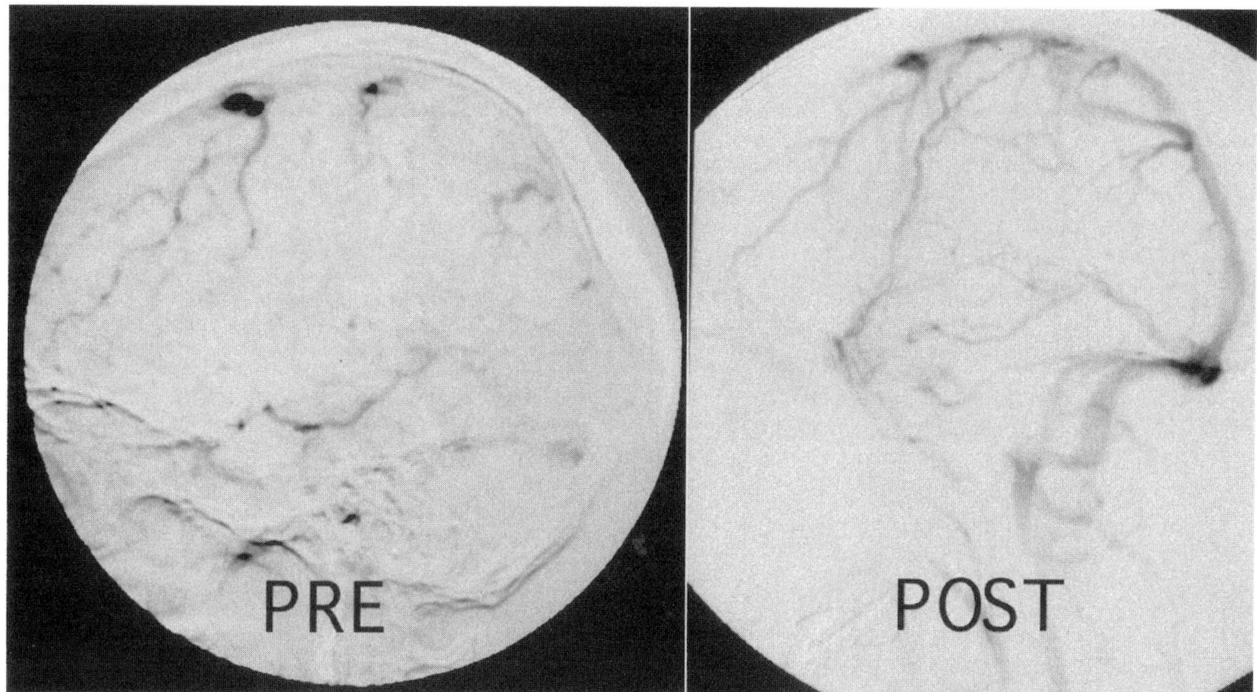

FIGURE 104–8. Lateral view of the venous phase of a cerebral arteriogram demonstrating thrombosis of the superior sagittal sinus *(left)* and a patent superior sagittal sinus after local thrombolytics *(right)*.

of other available agents (Fig. 104–8). Currently, only recombinant tissue plasminogen activator is available in the United States; urokinase has been withdrawn from the market. There are no defined guidelines for the use of this drug in the treatment of CVT.

Surgery

Surgical treatment may be indicated in CVT complicated by malignant intracranial hypertension, acute visual loss, or intracranial hemorrhage. Ventriculostomy can serve as a method for cerebrospinal fluid diversion and intracranial pressure monitoring. Direct thrombectomy can be done through a craniotomy, opening of the dural sinus, and embolectomy, although the results have not been particularly promising.[29, 81]

OUTCOME

Like its clinical presentation, the outcome of patients with CVT is highly variable. Earlier series reported mortality rates ranging from 30% to 80%.[47] More recent series have reported mortality rates of less than 20%.[14] Extreme cases exist in which patients either die acutely or recover rapidly. However, the mortality of CVT (an entity that was once thought to be almost invariably lethal) has been drastically decreased by thrombolytic therapy and antithrombotic treatment. Factors that suggest a bad prognosis are the presence of coma, extremes of age (high mortality in infants and in the elderly),[50] site of thrombosis in the deep venous system or cerebellar system,[82] severely increased intracranial pressure, and underlying sepsis or malignancy.[14]

Preter and colleagues conducted a retrospective follow-up of 77 patients with CVT evaluated from 1975 through 1990.[83] The age of the patients ranged from 18 to 77 years (mean, 38.5 years). Sixty-six patients (87%) had no neurological sequelae during follow-up. Eleven patients (14.3%) remained neurologically impaired. Two who initially presented with isolated intracranial hypertension had blindness due to optic atrophy. The other nine had focal signs at the time of CVT and were left with various cognitive or focal deficits. Four of 28 patients (14.3%) who had seizures during the acute stage had recurrent seizures. One of the 51 patients with lateral sinus thrombosis developed a dural arteriovenous fistula. Nine of the 77 patients (11.7%) suffered a second CVT, all but one in the first year. Noncerebral thrombotic events occurred in 11 patients (14.3%). No recurrence of CVT occurred during later pregnancies, but one patient had a postpartum deep vein thrombosis. The authors concluded that CVT has an essentially good long-term prognosis. The frequency of long-standing epilepsy was low, suggesting that long-term anticonvulsant treatment is not necessary in most cases. A second CVT or another thrombotic episode occurred in 20% of patients, stressing the need in a minority of cases for long-term anticoagulation.

Long-term changes in venous hemodynamics may lead to the development of collateral venous outflow channels. Extension of these channels to the external jugular venous system can lead to the development of dural arteriovenous fistula.

The functional prognosis is much better in CVT than in arterial thrombosis. About two thirds of patients recover rapidly without sequelae, particularly when the initial presentation is that of isolated intracranial hypertension. Optic atrophy and blindness have been reported in a few cases. Focal or cognitive deficits occur as sequelae of CVT that initially presented with focal signs or with a diffuse encephalopathy. Recurrent seizures occur in less than 10% of cases, and only in patients who suffered seizures during the acute stage. The recurrence rate of CVT is 10% to 15%; recurrence is especially prevalent when the patient has an underlying prothrombotic condition, but it occasionally occurs in the absence of a known cause.

CONCLUSION

CVT is a relatively rare entity. Its clinical presentation and outcome have a wide spectrum. A high level of suspicion is necessary for clinicians to make an accurate diagnosis. Recent advances in diagnostic and therapeutic modalities have changed the detection and prognosis of this entity. MRI and MRV have been used as standards in diagnostic modalities.

Although the results are nonconclusive, antithrombotic agents have been used with success to treat this condition. More recently, interventional neuroradiologic techniques have been used to locally deliver thrombolytic agents, with initial success.

Endovascular techniques offer local delivery of thrombolytic agents; thus, superior clot lysis is achieved selectively in the venous sinuses, and systemic morbidity from hemorrhagic complications is minimized. These techniques will undoubtedly be used with increasing frequency in the future for the treatment of CVT.

REFERENCES

1. Ribes MF: Des rescherches faites sur la phlébite. Revue Médicale Française et Etrangère et Journal de Clinique de l'Hôtel-Dieu et de la Charité de Paris 3:5, 1825.
2. Sanders MD, Hoyt WF: Hypoxic ocular sequelae of carotid-cavernous fistulae: Study of the causes of visual failure before and after neurosurgical treatment in a series of 25 cases. Br J Ophthalmol 53:82, 1969.
3. Kuether TA, O'Neill O, Nesbit GM, Barnwell SL: Endovascular treatment of traumatic dural sinus thrombosis: Case report. Neurosurgery 42:1163–1167, 1998.
4. Seegers WH, Marlar RA, Walz DA: Anticoagulant effects of autoprothrombin II-A and prothrombin fragment 1. Thromb Res 13: 233, 1978.
5. Dusser A, Boyer-Neumann C, Wolf M: Temporary protein C deficiency associated with cerebral arterial thrombosis in childhood. J Pediatr 113:849, 1988.
6. Pugliese D, Nicoletti G, Andreula C, et al: Combined protein C deficiency and protein C activated resistance as a cause of caval, peripheral, and cerebral venous thrombosis—a case report. Angiology 49:399–401, 1998.
7. Dulli DA, Luzzio CC, Williams EC, Schutta HS: Cerebral venous thrombosis and activated protein C resistance. Stroke 27:1731–1733, 1996; see comments.
8. Martinelli I, Landi G, Merati G, et al: Factor V gene mutation is a risk factor for cerebral venous thrombosis. Thromb Haemost 75:393–394, 1996; see comments.
9. Vuillier F, Moulin T, Tatu L, et al: Isolated cortical vein thrombosis and activated protein C resistance [letter]. Stroke 27:1440–1441, 1996.
10. Deschiens MA, Conard J, Horellou MH, et al: Coagulation studies, factor V Leiden, and anticardiolipin antibodies in 40 cases of cerebral venous thrombosis. Stroke 27:1724–1730, 1996; see comments.
11. Biousse V, Conard J, Brouzes C, et al: Frequency of the 20210 G→A mutation in the 3′-untranslated region of the prothrombin gene in 35 cases of cerebral venous thrombosis. Stroke 29:1398–1400, 1998.
12. Levine SR, Kieran S, Puzio K, et al: Cerebral venous thrombosis with lupus anticoagulants: Report of two cases. Stroke 18:801–804, 1987.
13. Carhuapoma JR, Mitsias P, Levine SR: Cerebral venous thrombosis and anticardiolipin antibodies. Stroke 28:2363–2369, 1997.
14. Bousser MG, Chiras J, Sauron B: Cerebral venous thrombosis: A review of 38 cases. Stroke 16:199–213, 1985.
15. Karabudak R, Caner H, Oztekin N: Thrombosis of intracranial venous sinuses: Aetiology, clinical findings and prognosis of 56 patients. J Neurosurg Sci 34:117, 1990.
16. Wechsler B, Vidailhet M, Piette JC: Cerebral venous thrombosis in Behçet's disease: Clinical study and long-term follow-up of 25 cases. Neurology 42:614, 1992.
17. Bridger S, Evans N, Parker A, Cairns SR: Multiple cerebral venous thromboses in a child with inflammatory bowel disease. J Pediatr Gastroenterol Nutr 25:533–536, 1997.
18. Derdeyn CP, Powers WJ: Isolated cortical venous thrombosis and ulcerative colitis. AJNR Am J Neuroradiol 19:488–490, 1998.
19. Johns DR: Cerebrovascular complications of inflammatory bowel disease. Am J Gastroenterol 86:367, 1991.
20. Hammans SR, Ginsberg L: Superior sagittal sinus thrombosis in Wegener's granulomatosis. J Neurol Neurosurg Psychiatry 52: 287, 1989.
21. Gilbert WS, Talbot FJ: Cogan's syndrome: Signs of periarteritis nodosa and cerebral venous sinus thrombosis. Arch Ophthalmol 82:633, 1969.
22. Ameri A, Bousser M-G: Cerebral venous thrombosis. Neurol Clin 10:87–111, 1992.
23. Dinubile MJ: Septic thrombosis of the cavernous sinuses: Neurological review. Arch Neurol 45:567–574, 1988.
24. Sekhar LN, Dujovny M, Rao GR: Carotid cavernous sinus thrombosis caused by *Aspergillus fumugatus*. J Neurosurg 52:120–125, 1980.
25. Bousser MG: Cerebral Venous Thrombosis. New York, Academic Press, 1997, pp 385–389.
26. Wakhloo A, Johnson B, Kraus G, Spetzler R: Cerebral sinus and venous thrombosis. In Carter P, Spetzler R, Hamilton M (eds): Neurovascular Surgery. New York, McGraw-Hill, 1995, pp 1337–1363.
27. Toms SA, Chyatte D: Cerebral Venous Thrombosis: Primer on Cerebrovascular Diseases. New York, Academic Press, 1997, pp 528–532.
28. Fisher W III: Intracranial venous occlusive diseases. In Tindall G, Cooper P, Barrow D (eds): The Practice of Neurosurgery. Baltimore, Williams & Wilkins, 1996, pp 1907–1919.
29. Estanol B, Rodriguez A, Conte G: Intracranial venous thrombosis in young women. Stroke 10:680–684, 1979.
30. Hommet CD, Toffol BD, Cottier JP, et al: Cerebral venous thrombosis and estrogen-progesterone therapy. Eur Neurol 39:245–247, 1998.
31. Chiras J, Bousser MG, Meder JF: CT in cerebral thrombophlebitis. Neuroradiology 27:145, 1985.
32. Diaz JM, Schiffman JS, Urban ES, Maccario M: Superior sagittal sinus thrombosis and pulmonary embolism: A syndrome rediscovered. Acta Neurol Scand 86:390–396, 1992.
33. Ehler H, Courville CB: Thrombosis of internal cerebral veins in infancy and childhood: Review of literature and report of five cases. J Pediatr 8:600, 1936.
34. Barnett HJM, Hyland HH: Non-infective intracranial venous thrombosis. Brain 76:36, 1953.
35. Erez N, Babuna C, Uner A: Low incidence of thromboembolic disease: An evaluation of obstetric and gynecologic patients in Istanbul. Obstet Gynecol 27:833, 1966.
36. Towbin A: The syndrome of latent cerebral venous thrombosis. Stroke 4:419, 1973.
37. Scotti LN, Goldman RL, Hardman DR, Heinz ER: Venous thrombosis in infants and children. Radiology 112:393, 1974.
38. Cantú C, Barinagarrementeria F: Cerebral venous thrombosis associated with pregnancy and puerperium: Review of 67 cases. Stroke 24:1880–1884, 1993.

39. Buchanan DS, Brazinsky JH: Dural sinus and cerebral venous thrombosis: Incidence in young women receiving oral contraceptives. Arch Neurol 22:440–444, 1970.
40. Crawford SC, Digre KB, Palmer CA, et al: Thrombosis of the deep venous drainage of the brain in adults. Arch Neurol 52: 1101–1108, 1995.
41. Daif A, Awada A, Al-Rajeh S, et al: Cerebral venous thrombosis in adults: A study of 40 cases from Saudi Arabia. Stroke 26: 1193–1195, 1995.
42. Perkin GD: Cerebral venous thrombosis: Developments in imaging and treatment. Neurol Neurosurg Psychiatry 59:1–3, 1995.
43. Krayenbühl H: Cerebral venous and sinus thrombosis. Clin Neurosurg 14:1, 1967.
44. Jacobs K, Moulin T, Bogousslavsky J, et al: The stroke syndrome of cortical vein thrombosis. Neurology 47:376–382, 1996.
45. Ford K, Sarwar M: Computed tomography of dural sinus thrombosis. AJNR Am J Neuroradiol 2:539–543, 1981.
46. Rao KCVG, Knipp HC, Wagner EJ: CT findings in cerebral sinus and venous thrombosis. Radiology 140:391–398, 1981.
47. Buonanno FS, Moody DM, Ball RM: CT scan finding in cerebral sinovenous occlusion. Neurology 12:288–292, 1982.
48. Buonnano FS, Moody DM, Ball MR: Computed cranial tomographic findings in cerebral sinovenous occlusion. J Comput Assist Tomogr 2:281, 1979.
49. Shinohara Y, Yosmitoshi M, Yoshii F: Appearance and disappearance of empty delta sign in superior sagittal sinus thrombosis. Stroke 17:1282–1284, 1986.
50. Virapongse C, Cazenave C, Quisling R: The empty delta sign: Frequency and significance in 76 cases of dural sinus thrombosis. Radiology 162:779, 1987.
51. Padayachee TS, Bingham JB, Graves MJ, et al: Dural sinus thrombosis: Diagnosis and follow-up by magnetic angiography and imaging. Neuroradiology 33:165–167, 1991.
52. Rippe DJ, Boyko OB, Spritzer CE, et al: Demonstration of dural sinus occlusion by the use of MR angiography. AJNR Am J Neuroradiol 11:199–201, 1990.
53. Tsai FY, Wang A-M, Matovich VB, et al: MR staging of acute dural sinus thrombosis: Correlation with venous pressure measurements and implications for treatment and prognosis. AJNR Am J Neuroradiol 16:1021–1029, 1995.
54. Tsuruda JS, Shimakawa A, Pelc NJ, Saloner D: Dural sinus occlusion: Evaluation with phase-sensitive gradient-echo MR imaging. AJNR Am J Neuroradiol 12:481–488, 1991.
55. Yuh WTC, Simonson TM, Wang A-M, et al: Venous sinus occlusive disease: MR findings. AJNR Am J Neuroradiol 15:309–316, 1994.
56. Halbach VV, Higashida RT, Hieshima GB, et al: Venography and venous pressure monitoring in dural sinus meningiomas. AJNR Am J Neuroradiol 10:1209–1213, 1989.
57. Canhão P, Batista P, Ferro JM: Venous transcranial Doppler in acute dural sinus thrombosis. J Neurol 245:276–279, 1998.
58. Hanley DF, Feldman E, Borel CO, et al: Treatment of sagittal sinus thrombosis associated with cerebral hemorrhage and intracranial hypertension. Stroke 19:903–909, 1988.
59. Stansfield FR: Puerperal cerebral thrombophlebitis treated by heparin. BMJ 4:436, 1942.
60. Dorndorf D, Wessel K, Kessler C, Kömpf D: Thrombosis of the right vein of Labbé: Radiological and clinical findings. Neuroradiology 35:202, 1993.
61. Einhäupl KM, Villringer A, Meister W, et al: Heparin treatment in sinus venous thrombosis. Lancet 338:597–600, 1991.
62. Barnwell SL, Nesbit GM, Clark WM: Local thrombolytic therapy for cerebrovascular disease: Current Oregon Health Sciences University experience (July 1991 through April 1995). J Vasc Intervent Radiol 6:78S–82S, 1995.
63. Levine SR, Twyman RE, Gilman S: The role of anticoagulation in cavernous sinus thrombosis. Neurology 38:517–522, 1988.
64. Alexander LF, Yamamoto Y, Ayoubi S: Efficacy of tissue plasminogen activator in the lysis of thrombosis of the cerebral venous sinus. Neurosurgery 26:559–564, 1990.
65. Castaigne P, Laplace D, Bousser MG: Superior sagittal sinus thrombosis [letter]. Arch Neurol 34:788, 1977.
66. Di Rocco C, Iannelli A, Leone G: Heparin-urokinase treatment in aseptic dural sinus thrombosis. Arch Neurol 38:431, 1981.
67. Fletcher AP, Alkjaersig N, Lewis M: A pilot study of urokinase therapy in cerebral infarction. Stroke 7:135, 1976.
68. Meyer JS, Gilory J, Barnhart MI, Johnson JF: Therapeutic thrombolysis in cerebral thromboembolism: Double-blind evaluation of intravenous plasmin therapy in carotid and middle cerebral artery occlusion. Neurology 13:927, 1963.
69. Vines FS, Davis DO: Clinical-radiological correlation in cerebral venous occlusive disease. Radiology 98:9, 1971.
70. Scott JA, Pascuzzi RM, Hall PV, Becker GJ: Treatment of dural sinus thrombosis with local urokinase infusion. J Neurosurg 68: 284–287, 1988.
71. Higashida RT, Helmer E, Halbach VV, Hieshema GB: Direct thrombolytic therapy for superior sagittal sinus thrombosis. AJNR Am J Neuroradiol 10:S4–S6, 1989.
72. Barnwell SL, Higashida RT, Halbach VV: Direct endovascular thrombolytic therapy for dural sinus thrombosis. Neurosurgery 28:135–142, 1991.
73. Tsai FY, Higashida RT, Matovich V, Alferi K: Acute thrombosis of the intracranial dural sinus: Direct thrombolytic therapy. AJNR Am J Neuroradiol 13:1137–1141, 1992.
74. Smith TP, Higashida RT, Barnwell SL: Treatment of dural sinus thrombosis by urokinase infusion. AJNR Am J Neuroradiol 15: 801–807, 1994.
75. Horowitz M, Purdy P, Unwin H, et al: Treatment of dural sinus thrombosis using selective catheterization and urokinase. Ann Neurol 38:58–67, 1995.
76. Spearman MP, Jungreis CA, Wehner JJ, et al: Endovascular thrombolysis in deep cerebral venous thrombosis. AJNR Am J Neuroradiol 18:502–506, 1997.
77. Holder CA, Bell DA, Lundell AL, et al: Isolated straight sinus and deep cerebral venous thrombosis: Successful treatment with local infusion of urokinase. J Neurosurg 86:704–707, 1997.
78. Rael JR, Orrison WW Jr, Baldwin N, Sell J: Direct thrombolysis of superior sagittal sinus thrombosis with coexisting intracranial hemorrhage. AJNR Am J Neuroradiol 18:1238–1242, 1997.
79. Smith AG, Cornblath WT, Deveikis JP: Local thrombolytic therapy in deep cerebral venous thrombosis. Neurology 48:1613–1619, 1997.
80. Dowd CF, Malek AM, Phatouros CC, Hemphill JC III: Application of a rheolytic thromboectomy device in the treatment of dural sinus thrombosis: A new technique. AJNR Am J Neuroradiol 20:568–570, 1999.
81. Ray BS, Dunbar HS: Thrombosis of the dural venous sinuses as a cause of "pseudotumor cerebri." Ann Surg 134:376, 1951.
82. Eick JJ, Miller KD, Bell KA: Computed tomography of deep cerebral venous thrombosis in children. Radiology 140:399, 1981.
83. Preter M, Tzourio C, Ameri A, Bousser M-G: Long-term prognosis in cerebral venous thrombosis: Follow-up of 77 patients. Stroke 27:243–246, 1995.
84. Gerszten PC, Welch WC, Spearman MP, et al: Isolated deep cerebral venous thrombosis treated by direct endovascular thrombolysis. Surg Neurol 48:261–266, 1997.

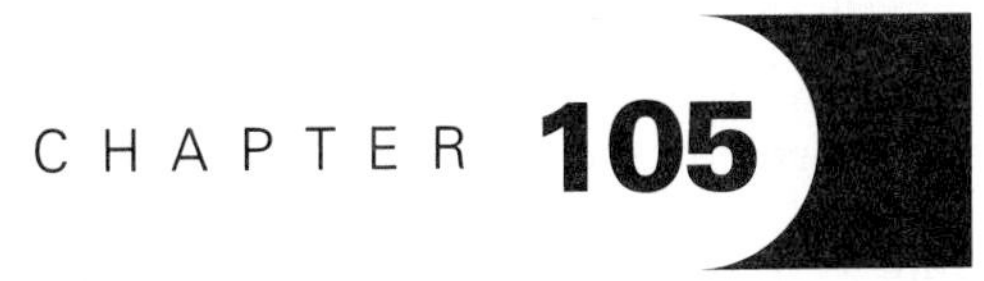

Spontaneous Intracerebral Hemorrhage: Non–Arteriovenous Malformation, Nonaneurysm

RAN VIJAI P. SINGH ■ CHAD J. PRUSMACK ■ JACQUES J. MORCOS

The management of spontaneous intracerebral hemorrhage (ICH) has aroused much controversy over the years. The relative merits of medical and surgical treatments and their relationship to outcome have been debated since McKissock and coworkers[1] published the results of a clinical trial in 1961. Based on the few clinical trials published since then, it has been difficult to draw definitive conclusions about the best mode of treatment. Numerous contributing variables such as age, sex, and premorbid neurological status; location, size, and cause of the resulting hematoma; and method, timing, and extent of evacuation have led to this difficulty.

Spontaneous ICH, defined as hemorrhage in brain parenchyma in the absence of immediate trauma, can be divided into primary and secondary types. Primary ICH occurs in the absence of a structural disease process; secondary ICH is associated with a congenital or acquired lesion. This chapter reviews the biologic, pathologic, and clinical characteristics of ICH and critically evaluates current methods of management. Hemorrhages from aneurysms and arteriovenous malformations (AVMs) are not discussed here.

HISTORICAL REVIEW

Magladery[2] states that the first recorded evidence of ICH and subarachnoid hemorrhage dates to Hippocrates (400 BC), who alluded to "sanguineous apoplexy." According to Walton,[3] Avicenna (AD 980–1037) described apoplexy due to "sanguineous humour effused suddenly about the ventricle" in the book *Al Quanoun Fi'l Tibb* (The Canon of Medicine).

As discussed by Donley,[4] John James Wepfer in 1658 first described the relationship between circulating blood and cerebral function and the consequences of effusion of blood in the head in *De Apoplexia*. In their historical reviews, Clarke[5] and Fazio[6] note that Hoffman (1660–1742) first introduced the concept of ICH. They also indicate that Morgagni (1682–1771) described the difference between apoplexy associated with hemorrhage into the cerebral parenchyma and into the ventricular system in *De Sedibus*.

In 1888, Macewen[7] described the first successful operation for spontaneous ICH. In 1903, Cushing[8] reported the first surgical evacuation of a cerebral hematoma and attributed increased intracranial pressure (ICP) to the mass effect caused by the hematoma. During the next 3 decades, the surgical treatment of ICH was occasionally reported.

Bagley[9] first described surgical indications based on the location of the hematoma. He suggested that surgical treatment was ineffective for hemorrhages in the basal ganglia and was best reserved for subcortical hematomas associated with increased ICP. He also hypothesized that a ruptured aneurysm or rupture of an atherosclerotic or congenitally weak blood vessel wall without an aneurysm often caused spontaneous ICH. In 1932, Robinson[10] suggested the possibility of spontaneous recovery in patients with small hemorrhages.

In a review of nine cases, Craig and Adson[11] suggested the possibility of ICH caused by Charcot-Bouchard aneurysms. Penfield[12] suggested that ICH should be evacuated via a craniotomy and cortical incision rather than aspirated through a bur hole.

The advent of cerebral angiography in 1929 provided an impetus for the surgical treatment of hematomas and resulted in multiple publications in the French literature in the 1940s and 1950s.[13, 14] In 1959, Lazorthes[13] reported the results of his 52 cases, sparking a resurgence of interest in the surgical management of ICH.

In 1961, McKissock and colleagues[1] reported no difference in outcome after either surgical or medical management and cast serious doubt on the benefit of surgical treatment. The advent of computed tomography (CT) in 1973 and magnetic resonance imaging (MRI) in 1982 has allowed a much better recognition and understanding of the occurrence, evolution, and precise localization of ICH.

EPIDEMIOLOGY

Although the relative frequency of ICH varies with race and geography, it has been reported to account for 10% to 13% of all strokes.[15, 16] It is associated with a disproportionately high mortality rate, which ranges from 20% to 70%.[17–20] The advent of CT permitted the early recognition of less severe cases, leading to improved prognosis.[21–25] Thus, the 30-day survival rate has increased from 8% to 44%.[26] Further, the more aggressive management of hypertension has lessened the incidence of ICH.

The overall incidence of ICH in North America is approximately 10 to 15 per 100,000 population per year, which is about twice the incidence of subarachnoid hemorrhage.[16] A higher incidence is reported among Japanese,[27] Chinese,[28] and African Americans.[29] In Japan, approximately 90,000 persons die each year from hypertensive hemorrhage.[30] The influence of gender is unclear, with various investigators reporting a higher incidence in women[31–33] or in men.[20, 27, 29]

ICH is rare before age 45 years and becomes increasingly more frequent with advancing age. Among those 80 years and older, ICH affects 350 per 100,000 population per year—about 25 times the occurrence within the total population.[34] The primary causes of spontaneous parenchymal bleeding in the young are vascular malformations, aneurysms, and drug abuse (cocaine, amphetamines, alcohol). Among the elderly, hypertension, tumors (primary and metastatic), vasculopathy, and coagulopathy (warfarin, heparin, aspirin, fibrinolytic agents) are the major contributing factors. In children, leukemia is a significant factor.

TABLE 105–1 ■ **Causes of Spontaneous Intracerebral Hemorrhage**

Trauma
Environmental
Postoperative, iatrogenic

Hypertension
Chronic
Acute
  Cold related
  Trigeminal nerve stimulation
  Posterior fossa surgery
  Cardiac surgery
  Scorpion bite
  Electroconvulsive therapy
  After carotid endarterectomy
  After migraine attack

Coagulopathy
Anticoagulants
Antiplatelet agents
Fibrinolytics
Blood dyscrasias

Structural Vascular Lesions
Aneurysms (infectious and noninfectious)
Arteriovenous malformations
Cavernous angiomas
Vasculopathy
  Chronic amyloid angiopathy
  Moyamoya syndrome
Collagen vascular disease
  Polyarteritis nodosa
Vasculitis

Drug Related
Sympathomimetics
Substance abuse
  Alcohol
  Tobacco
  Cocaine

Tumors
Primary
Metastatic

Postoperative Cerebrovascular Accident
Arterial
  Atherosclerotic
  Embolic
  Arterial dissection
Venous
  Cerebral venous thrombosis

Miscellaneous
Neonatal
Secondary brainstem
Cerebral endometriosis

CAUSES

Overall, trauma is the most common cause of ICH. In the nontraumatic group, chronic arterial hypertension is the most common cause, accounting for about 50% of cases (Table 105–1).

Anticoagulant Therapy

ICH is one of the most devastating complications of anticoagulant therapy and is associated with a high mortality rate.[35] In the first 6 months of anticoagulation therapy, 61% of intracerebral hemorrhages would have occurred.[36] Long-term anticoagulation therapy increases the risk of ICH 8- to 11-fold.[37] The incidence of ICH in patients taking warfarin after myocardial infarction is 1% per year.[35]

A number of factors contribute to the increased risk of ICH in this group of patients, including advanced age, prior cerebrovascular disease, hypertension, and concomitant use of aspirin.[35, 38] In the Reversible Ischemia Trial, which evaluated stroke prevention, patients were randomized to a warfarin or an aspirin group. The study was terminated early because the warfarin group, which had an international normalized ratio between 3 and 4.5, sustained 24 ICHs, compared with none in the aspirin group.[39] Some studies have suggested a higher frequency of cerebellar and lobar hemorrhage in patients on anticoagulation therapy.[36, 40]

Although the evolution of hematomas in patients on anticoagulation therapy is protracted, their hematomas are about twice the size of those in patients not on anticoagulation therapy, and their mortality rate increases to 60% to 65%.[35] The pathophysiology of ICH in patients on anticoagulation therapy is not well known, but various factors have been hypothesized: enlargement of small, spontaneous hemorrhages that would be of no consequence in normal individuals; local vascular disease processes, such as lipohyalinosis or fibrinoid necrosis; and inhibition of normal vascular repair.

ICH during treatment with heparin is rare and occurs mostly in patients being treated for acute embolic cerebral infarction and uncontrolled hypertension. In most patients, the activated partial thromboplastin time is prolonged excessively.[41, 42]

ICH during treatment with aspirin and other antiplatelet agents is less common. In a review of eight placebo-controlled clinical trials for the prevention of stroke, Mayo and colleagues[43] found that the risk of hemorrhagic stroke was 0.7% among 2981 patients on anticoagulation therapy, compared with 0.37% among 2187 patients receiving a placebo.

The efficacy of fibrinolytic agents in the treatment of myocardial infarction is well known. ICH has been reported in 0.4% to 1.3% of patients with acute myocardial infarction treated with the single-chain tissue plasminogen activator (t-PA) alteplase.[44] In an initial pilot study on the management of acute ischemic stroke, intra-arterial use of urokinase and t-PA resulted in a 55% rate of reperfusion, at the cost of an 11% rate of ICH and neurological deterioration.[45] Intravenous t-PA was used in two studies, the European Cooperative Acute Stroke Study[46] and the National Institutes of Neurological Disorders and Stroke rt-PA Stroke Study,[47] with a therapeutic window of 6 and 3 hours, respectively. The rate of symptomatic ICH was 6.3%, compared with 0.6% in the placebo group; however, the functional outcome at 3 months was better in the t-PA–treated group.

Drug Use

ICH has been associated with the use of multiple sympathomimetic drugs: amphetamines, pseudoephedrine, phenylpropanolamine, cocaine, heroin, phencyclidine, and chymopapain.[48–51] Typically, these hemorrhages are lobar and are attributed to either a transient elevation of blood pressure or arteritis-like vascular changes caused by the drug that unmask an underlying lesion, such as an aneurysm, AVM, or brain tumor.[48] The arteritis-like changes in the vessel wall are thought to be the effects of either direct drug toxicity or hypersensitivity.

In the younger age group, cocaine is increasingly reported as a cause of subarachnoid hemorrhage and ICH. ICH usually occurs within hours of use and can be lobar or deep ganglionic. The use of cocaine is related to a higher incidence of aneurysmal and AVM rupture compared with other sympathomimetics.[49]

Cerebral Amyloid Angiopathy

Cerebral amyloid angiopathy is associated with the deposition of amyloid in the media and adventitia of medium-sized and small cortical and leptomeningeal arteries.[52] Although it occurs only sporadically, familial forms have been found in Iceland and Holland. The incidence of this disease rises steeply after age 70 years; it reportedly ranges from 23% to 48.8% in the 8th decade, from 37% to 46.4% in the 9th decade, and from 57% to 58% in the 10th decade.[52, 53]

Cerebral amyloid angiography is associated with dementia and features of Alzheimer's disease (neuritic plaques and neurofibrillary tangles) in more than 30% of cases.[54] Hypertension is present in only a small percentage of cases. Histologically, deposits are found in the media and adventitia of small and medium-sized cortical and leptomeningeal arteries and show characteristic Congo red birefringence in polarized light.[54] The histologic features most consistently associated with ICH seem to be a severe degree of amyloid deposition in vessel walls and the coexistence of fibrinoid necrosis, with or without microaneurysm formation.[55]

The hematoma is usually subcortical or lobar and is predominantly in the occipital and parietal lobes.[54, 55] Another characteristic is multiplicity over time and location (Fig. 105–1).

Intracranial Tumors

Intracranial tumors are an uncommon but well-recognized cause of ICH. The primary brain tumors associated with ICH are pituitary adenoma, glioblastoma multiforme, meningioma, oligodendroglioma, and ependymoma.[56, 57] The most common metastatic tumors presenting with ICH are melanoma, choriocarcinoma, renal cell carcinoma, bronchogenic carcinoma, and germ cell tumors. The bleeding tendency of tumors is related to their vascularity, but metastatic choriocarcinomas tend to invade the blood vessel wall. ICH may be the first manifestation of a brain tumor.

Patients with multiple metastases and one hemorrhage are easily diagnosed by CT, but the diagnosis of patients with a single metastasis may be more difficult. Helpful diagnostic features are the presence of perilesional edema, contrast enhancement, unusual location (such as in the corpus callosum), clinical findings of papilledema, and an antecedent history of cognitive decline, seizures, and progressive focal deficits. MRI and angiography may further assist in identifying a tumor. If the results are still inconclusive, a biopsy of the hematoma cavity at the time of evacuation should always be obtained in an attempt to establish the diagnosis.

PATHOLOGY AND PATHOGENESIS

Spontaneous ICH occurs predominantly in deep locations in the brain. The most common location is the

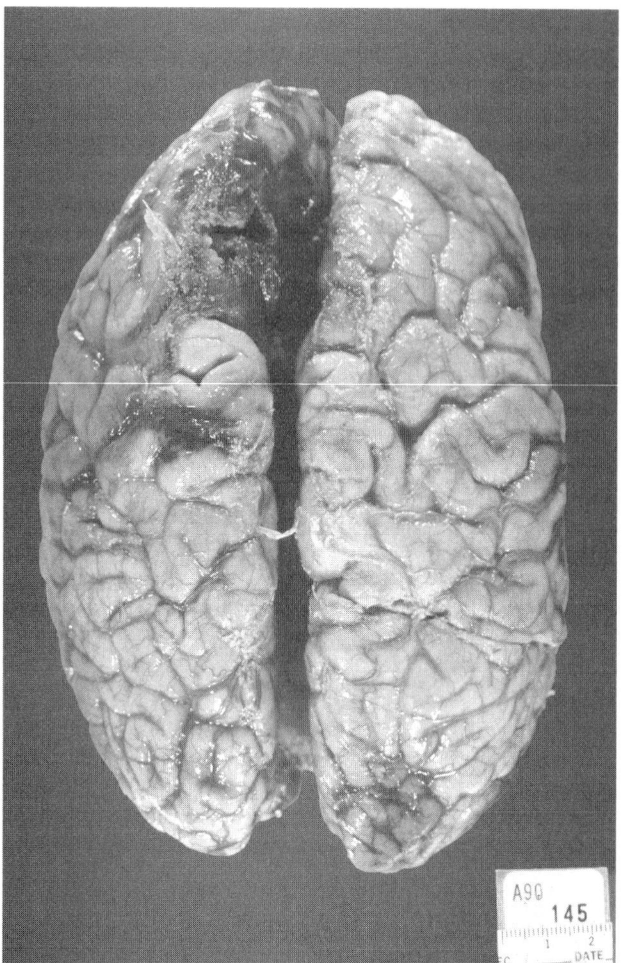

FIGURE 105–1. Autopsy examination of a patient with recent frontal intracerebral hematoma and older hemorrhages in the posterior frontal and occipital lobes is typical of senile amyloid angiopathy.

putamen, followed by the subcortical white matter, cerebellum, and thalamus. In 100 unselected cases, Kase and associates[38] found putaminal hemorrhage in 34, lobar hemorrhage in 24, thalamic hemorrhage in 20, cerebellar hemorrhage in 7, and pontine hemorrhage in 6 cases.

Hemorrhages in the caudate nucleus, putamen, thalamus, brainstem, and cerebellum occur in the distribution of small perforating arteries with a diameter of 50 to 200 μm. Various causative mechanisms have been proposed. Because chronic arterial hypertension is the most common cause of ICH, various pathologic changes in the vessel wall have been implicated. Charcot and Bouchard[58] described miliary aneurysms in the brain specimens of patients with ICH. Ellis[59] then showed that these lesions were not true aneurysmal dilatations and attributed ICH to dissection of the vessel wall. Ross-Russell[60] found miliary aneurysms in 15 of 16 brains of hypertensive patients in an autopsy study involving angiography and histology. These findings were substantiated by Cole and Yates,[61, 62] who described miliary aneurysms in 85% of cases of massive hypertensive ICH. However, a direct relationship between the miliary aneurysms and bleeding sites was not established.

CLINICAL AND DIAGNOSTIC EVALUATION

ICH can manifest with a wide spectrum of symptoms and signs, depending on the location and size of the hematoma. Most ICHs occur during activity and manifest with the sudden onset of a neurological deficit, followed by a gradual progression. One third of the cases in the Harvard Cooperative Stroke Registry had maximal deficits from the onset of symptoms.[63]

The evaluation of a patient suspected of having an ICH should start with a thorough history and physical examination. Additional information from witnesses to the ictus can be helpful. Patients may present with the sudden onset of headache, with or without vomiting. In a series reported by Mohr and coworkers,[63] only 36% of the 54 awake patients presented with headache, and 44% presented with vomiting, stressing that the absence of these symptoms does not rule out ICH. Seizures at the onset of ICH are rare. The history of chronic arterial hypertension should alert physicians to the possibility of hypertensive ICH, which must be differentiated from the acute hypertension present in patients with elevated ICP. A history of previous stroke, seizures, liver disease, coagulopathy, primary or metastatic brain tumor, or valvular heart disease may suggest an underlying cause for the ICH.

The most relevant neurological sign is the degree of impairment of consciousness, subject to the location, size, and extension of the hematoma (deep structures and ventricles). Some degree of altered consciousness was present in 60% of the cases reported by Mohr and coworkers.[63] Patients with peripherally located hematomas are more alert and have appropriate focal deficits. Patients with hematomas in deep locations present with a significant decrease in the level of consciousness and dense, lateralized neurological deficits. The hallmark of brainstem involvement is a mixture of coma, long tract signs, and cranial nerve deficits. The presentation of cerebellar hemorrhage is unique, and the classic symptoms and signs are well summarized by Heros[64] (Table 105–2).

Baseline laboratory studies should include a complete blood count, prothrombin time, partial thromboplastin time, liver and renal function tests, serum glucose, electrocardiography, and chest radiography.

The initial radiologic study should be a plain computed tomographic scan of the brain. This demonstrates the location and size of the hematoma and the presence or absence of mass effect, perilesional edema, and ventricular extension. Contrast enhancement offers the possibility of diagnosing associated abnormalities such as AVMs, aneurysms, and tumors. CT within 4 hours shows a hyperdense lesion. In severely anemic patients, the lesion may appear iso- or hypodense to the brain. After about 7 to 10 days, the high attenuation values of the hematoma start decreasing peripherally. Depending on its size, the whole hematoma may become isodense

TABLE 105–2 ■ **Clinical Features of Cerebellar Hemorrhage**

SYMPTOMS	SIGNS
Early	
Headache Nausea Dizziness Lack of balance Vomiting	Truncal or appendicular ataxia Dysarthria Nystagmus Stiff neck
Intermediate	
Confusion Somnolence, stupor	Abducens palsy Gaze paresis Peripheral facial palsy Depressed corneal reflex Horner's syndrome Babinski's sign Mild hemiparesis
Late	
Stupor Coma	Pinpoint pupils Ataxic respirations Decerebrate posture

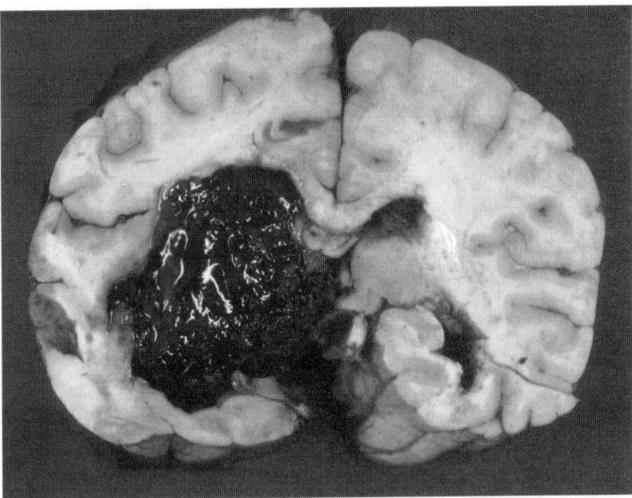

FIGURE 105–2. Extension of a primarily putaminal hemorrhage into the rest of the basal ganglia, internal capsule, thalamus, and ventricle was evident at autopsy.

in 2 to 3 weeks and resolve completely to an area of decreased density within 2 months. Occasionally, a resolving hematoma may give the appearance of ring enhancement, due to either increased vascularity at the periphery or disruption of the blood-brain barrier.

Although it offers superior resolution, MRI is rarely instrumental in the acute evaluation of patients with ICH. The presence of blood and its confusing signal characteristics can mask an underlying structural lesion. MRI, however, often reveals associated multiple lesions that may not be detected by CT. Thus, MRI in the acute setting should be reserved for highly atypical cases in which the clinical presentation, a conflicting CT study, or both are unusual.

HEMATOMA LOCATION AND CLINICAL PROFILE

Putaminal Hemorrhage

Putaminal hemorrhage is the most common form of ICH and can manifest in different ways, depending on the size and extent of the hematoma. The typical presentation is the abrupt onset of headache, with or without vomiting, followed by the gradual progression of focal neurological signs and worsening level of consciousness. A dense deficit from the beginning is unusual. Common neurological signs are hemiparesis, hemisensory syndrome, homonymous hemianopsia, horizontal gaze palsy, aphasia (in the dominant hemisphere), and hemineglect (in the nondominant hemisphere).[65, 66] Dense neurological deficits associated with coma usually suggest large hematomas and are associated with a poor prognosis. Intraventricular extension also implies extensive parenchymal dissection or destruction (Fig. 105–2).[67, 68] Patients who present with partial motor deficits, an alert neurological status, normal extraocular movements, full visual fields, and no lateral or upward extension of the hematoma have a better prognosis on the basis of reversible compression of capsular fibers.[68]

Caudate Hemorrhage

Caudate hematomas represent approximately 5% to 7% of cases of ICH.[67] The bleeding vessels are perforating branches of the anterior and middle cerebral arteries. The presentation is that of abrupt headache and vomiting, followed by decreased level of consciousness. Patients are usually disoriented, with evidence of neck stiffness.[67] Occasional patients have seizures and horizontal gaze paresis.

On CT, ventricular extension of the hematoma into the frontal horn is common, with secondary hydrocephalus. Occasionally, the hemorrhage extends into the anterior portion of the thalamus. Such patients present with transient but significant short-term memory deficits.[68] Most patients recover fully, with no significant neurological deficits.[67]

Thalamic Hemorrhage

Thalamic hemorrhages account for 10% to 15% of all ICHs (Fig. 105–3).[66, 69] The clinical presentation depends on the size and pattern of extension of the hematoma. Bleeding occurs in an area supplied by thalamic perforators arising from the posterior cerebral arteries and may extend laterally into the internal capsule, medially into the ventricles, superiorly into the corona radiata, and inferiorly into subthalamus and midbrain.[70]

Thalamic hemorrhage typically manifests with the acute onset of a usually dense sensorimotor deficit, vomiting with or without headache, and occasionally coma.[69, 71, 72] The characteristic ocular findings include upward gaze palsy; convergence; miotic, unreactive pupils due to compression of the midbrain tectum;

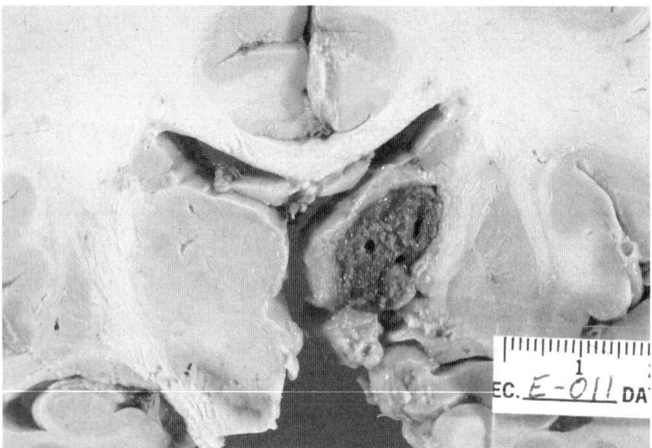

FIGURE 105–3. This medium-sized hypertensive thalamic hemorrhage, which spared the capsular fibers laterally, is well confined.

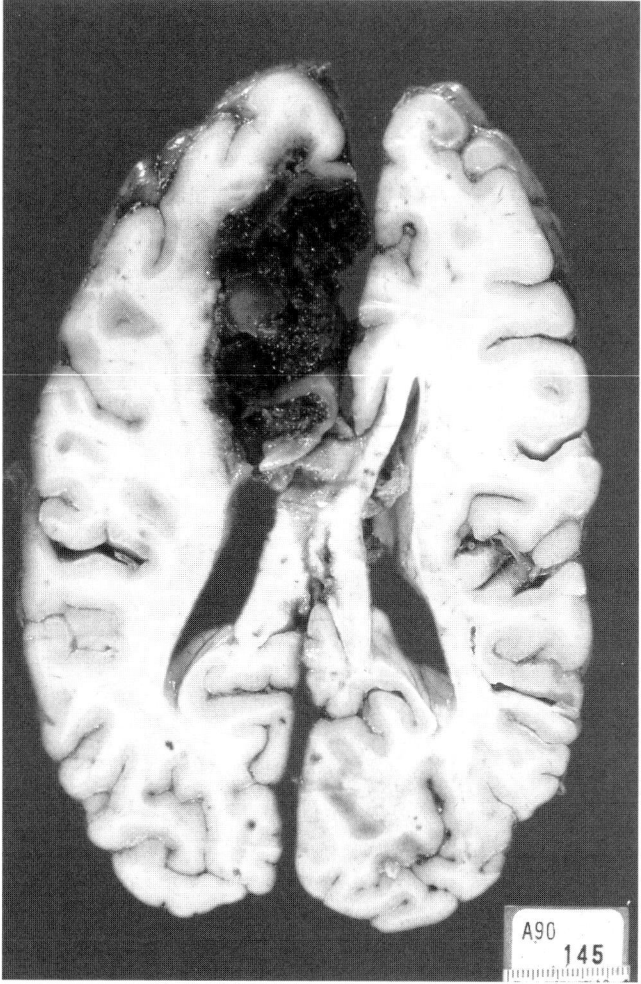

FIGURE 105–4. An extensive medial frontal intracerebral hematoma due to amyloid angiopathy caused this patient's death.

and, less commonly, retraction nystagmus on upward gaze and skew deviation.[66, 69, 71, 72]

Lobar Hemorrhage

Lobar hemorrhages (Fig. 105–4) usually occur in the subcortical white matter and have a predilection for the parietal, temporal, and occipital lobes.[73, 74] The frequent occurrence of lobar hemorrhages in the parieto-occipital lobes has been attributed to the higher concentration of intracerebral microaneurysms reported in anatomic studies.[61]

Hypertension as a cause of lobar hemorrhage is unusual.[73–75] Only 31% of the patients reported by Ropper and Davis[74] had chronic hypertension. Kase and associates[73] reported elevated blood pressure in only 50% of their patients on admission. In a series reported by Broderick and colleagues,[16] hypertension contributed almost equally to lobar and deep hemispheric, cerebellar, and pontine hemorrhages. Other causes of lobar hemorrhages are AVMs, tumors, anticoagulation therapy, blood dyscrasias, and amyloid angiopathy.[54, 76, 77] In a significant number of cases, no definite cause can be found.[73] Cerebral amyloid angiopathy is probably the most common cause in nonhypertensive patients 70 years and older.

The clinical manifestations of lobar ICH depend on the location and size of the hematoma.[74] Compared with other forms of ICH, the frequency of associated hypertension and coma on admission is lower. The low incidence of coma is probably related to the peripheral location of the hematoma.[74] Most patients complain of headache and vomiting. Seizures are also frequent.[15, 73, 78] Hemiparesis is seldom pronounced.

The prognosis of lobar ICH is relatively better than that of other forms of ICH. Mortality rates range from 11% to 29%.[73, 74, 79] The functional outcome for survivors also tends to be better.[79] In their series of 22 patients, Kase and associates[73] reported good outcomes in those with hematoma volumes less than 20 cm^3. Seventy percent survived after the surgical removal of hematomas that were 20 to 60 cm^3. No patient with a hematoma volume greater than 60 cm^3 survived.

Cerebellar Hemorrhage

The frequency of cerebellar hemorrhage ranges between 5% and 10%.[41, 66, 80, 81] Unlike with hemorrhages at other locations, coma does not imply irreversible deterioration, as long as the diagnosis is made early and surgical intervention is prompt.[64, 82–84] The dentate nuclei are the most common substrate. The hematoma extends into the hemispheric white matter and often into the fourth ventricle, causing either brainstem compression or direct invasion (Fig. 105–5). Rarely, cerebellar hemorrhage involves only the vermis. Hypertension and anticoagulation are the two most important causative factors in cerebellar hemorrhage.[83, 84]

Patients usually present with headache and an inability to walk or stand. Vomiting is common and may or may not be associated with headache.[83, 84] Other symptoms are dizziness, neck stiffness, dysarthria, tinnitus, and hiccups. Loss of consciousness at the onset is rare. On admission to the hospital, about one third of patients are obtunded.[84]

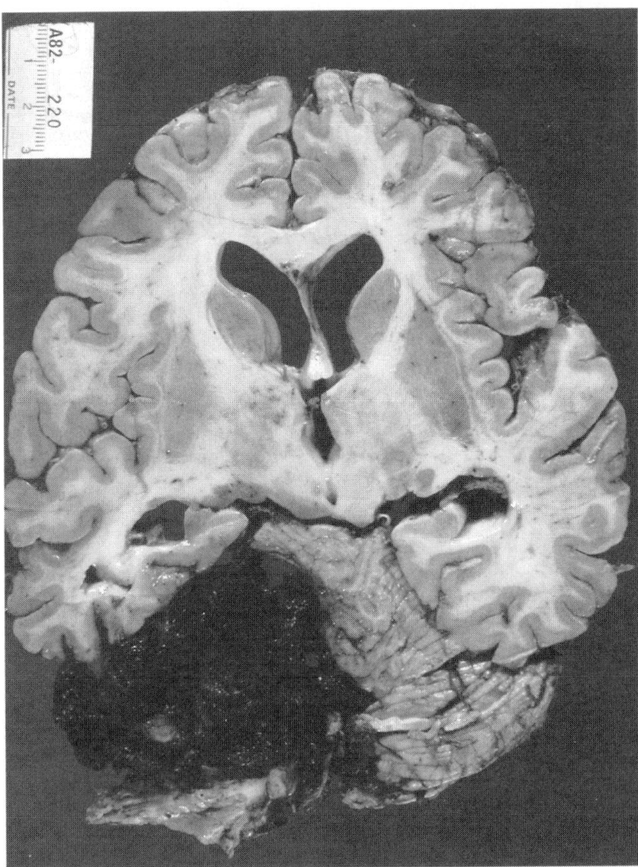

FIGURE 105–5. This extensive hypertensive cerebellar hemisphere hematoma started in the deep nuclei and extended, causing brainstem compression, hydrocephalus, and death.

The early physical signs are appendicular or truncal ataxia, dysarthria, ipsilateral horizontal gaze palsy, peripheral facial palsy, nystagmus, and sixth nerve palsy. At least two of the three characteristic clinical signs—appendicular ataxia, ipsilateral gaze palsy, and peripheral facial palsy—were present in 73% of the cases reported by Ott and coworkers.[84]

The clinical course of cerebellar hemorrhage is unpredictable. These patients, whether alert or lethargic on admission, can deteriorate quickly to coma and die with no warning.[84, 85] Although prognosis and final outcome are largely related to the patient's initial preoperative condition, even comatose patients can make a good recovery.[86]

Little and colleagues[87] reported two groups of patients with cerebellar hemorrhage. The first group presented with an abrupt onset, progressive course, and low level of consciousness. CT in this group of patients, who required surgery, showed cerebellar hematomas 3 cm or greater in diameter, obstructive hydrocephalus, and extension of hemorrhage into the fourth ventricle.[88, 89] The second group of patients was awake and stable and had hematomas smaller than 3 cm in diameter. They were treated medically, with good outcomes.[87]

Brainstem Hemorrhage

The pons is the most common location for nonvascular causes of ICH in the brainstem. Spontaneous nontraumatic midbrain and medullary hematomas are rare. On the basis of an autopsy study of 77 subjects with pontine hemorrhages, Attwater[90] was able to differentiate primary and secondary brainstem hemorrhages in 1911. He attributed some pontine hemorrhages to elevated ICP. Several years later in a monograph, Duret[91] also described this phenomenon.

The location of pontine hematomas depends on the location of perforating arteries (direct from the basilar or short or long circumferential arteries). Thus, these hematomas can be dividied into paramedian, basal pontine, and lateral tegmental hemorrhages.

In an autopsy review of 30 cases of pontine hemorrhages among 511 cases of ICH at Boston City Hospital, two thirds of the patients were comatose on presentation and had massive hemorrhages that extended into the midbrain or fourth ventricle. Within 48 hours, 78% of the patients died. Fisher[85] suggested that primary hemorrhage, by virtue of a pressure effect, caused the surrounding vessels to rupture, initiating a cascade of gradual enlargement of the hematoma. The bleeding in hypertensive patients was attributed to leakage from tiny penetrating vessels damaged by lipohyalinosis and containing small microaneurysms.[41, 61, 62, 85]

The rupture of the paramedian perforating branches of the basilar artery is thought to be the cause of massive pontine hematomas (Fig. 105–6). The lesion usually begins in the midpons at the junction of the tegmentum and basis pontis and extends along the longitudinal axis of the brainstem into the midbrain, middle cerebellar peduncle, or fourth ventricle.[80]

The clinical presentation of a hypertensive patient is typically one of rapid onset of coma. Awake patients may become symptomatic with headache, vomiting, and focal pontine signs such as facial or limb numbness, deafness, diplopia, quadriparesis, paraparesis, or hemiparesis. Occasionally, seizure (which can be a true convulsive episode), spasmodic decerebrate posturing, or violent shivering associated with autonomic dysfunction and rapidly developing hypothermia is de-

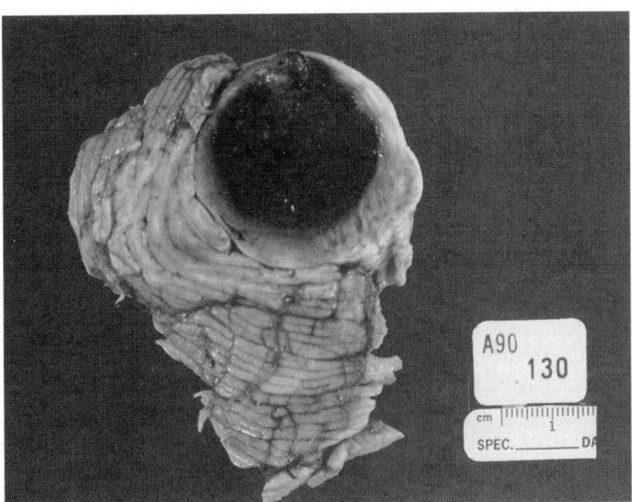

FIGURE 105–6. Large hypertensive pontine hematoma expanding and distorting the pons.

scribed. On examination, patients have an abnormal breathing pattern, apnea, cranial nerve and long tract deficits, occasional decerebrate posturing, and multiple oculomotor findings.[80, 92, 93] Weakness of the pontine and bulbar musculature is invariably associated with large median pontine hemorrhages, but it is seldom appreciated, owing to the depressed level of consciousness. The various ophthalmic findings are reactive, miotic, pinpoint pupils; absent horizontal gaze movement (with bilateral damage of the parapontine reticular formation); one-and-a-half syndrome (with unilateral pontine involvement); and ocular bobbing.

Massive pontine hemorrhages are always fatal, but death may not be instantaneous.[93] Some patients with medium-sized hematomas and most patients with small basal or lateral tegmental hematomas survive, with various degrees of residual neurological deficits.

MEDICAL MANAGEMENT

The natural history of ICH after medical management can be dismal. Mortality rates range from 27% to 77%.[79, 94–96] However, optimizing medical care with regard to managing blood pressure, controlling ICP, and stabilizing the cardiorespiratory system can have important effects on outcome and help prevent deterioration.

The single most important factor in determining rapid expansion of an ICH is blood pressure. In studies of patients with hypertensive ICH, persistently elevated blood pressure increased the risk of hematoma progression.[97–99] In a retrospective review of 320 patients with hypertensive ICH, 10 patients showed rapid expansion of the hematoma on serial CT.[97] The consecutive scans were obtained an average of 1.7 and 48.9 hours after hemorrhage. Of the 10 patients with radiographic evidence of expansion, all had persistent hypertension, and half deteriorated neurologically. The average blood pressure of this group on admission was 179/110 mm Hg, and the average blood pressure recorded before deterioration was 190/121 mm Hg. The first 24 hours seem to be particularly critical.

The degree to which blood pressure should be controlled is controversial. Patients with a history of chronic hypertension have impaired autoregulation, and overzealous lowering of blood pressure can lower cerebral perfusion pressure, producing secondary ischemic damage. This is especially true of patients with a decreased level of consciousness who may have elevated ICP. Some authors recommend lowering systolic blood pressure to less than 160 mm Hg[100]; others recommend lowering it to normotensive levels but not below.[101] In a prospective, randomized trial of putaminal ICH that compared craniotomy with medical therapy, patients were initially treated with sodium nitroprusside (Nipride) to decrease systolic blood pressure 25% during the first 24 hours. During the next 48 to 72 hours, blood pressure decreased to normotensive levels.[94] In this study, mean admission systolic blood pressure was 234 mm Hg. Despite the tight control of blood pressure, the 6-month mortality rate was 77%. Because this study did not report the cause of death or the time of deterioration, it is difficult to determine whether the degree of blood pressure control was adequate.

Experimental rat studies suggest that although transient alterations in blood flow occur within minutes of hemorrhage, the severe alterations of perihematoma microcirculation that cause ischemia are not maximal until 4 hours thereafter.[102, 103] In addition, the formation of edema is not maximal for 6 to 8 hours.[104] However, the period associated with the maximal risk of hemorrhage progression in the presence of persistent hypertension is 3 to 6 hours.[34, 97, 105, 106] Therefore, an argument can be made to reduce blood pressure dramatically during the first 4 hours after hemorrhage to reduce the risk of rehemorrhage and then to raise the blood pressure slowly to perfuse ischemic areas.

The use of steroids in patients with ICH is controversial. Batjer and associates[94] used steroids (4 mg dexamethasone intravenously every 6 hours) in their protocol. The rationale of using steroids in the treatment of ICH is that they might lessen the damaging effects of cerebral edema, increased ICP, a disrupted blood-brain barrier, and stress. The first randomized study followed 40 patients with ICH but showed no statistical difference in outcome associated with the use of steroids.[107] This study, however, lacked case uniformity and appropriate, relevant stratification. Therefore, a well-designed, randomized, placebo-controlled study of 93 patients receiving dexamethasone (10 mg intravenously and then 5 mg every 6 hours) was performed in 1987.[108] The study was terminated early because the steroid group showed no benefit, and their rate of complications (hyperglycemia, septicemia, gastrointestinal bleeding) was 11 times higher than that of the control group. This study suggests that steroids have no role in the treatment of ICH, at least not in comatose or stuporous patients.

Elevated ICP should be treated vigorously with diuretics.[109] Mannitol effectively and safely decreases ICP and can be used alone or with urea to potentiate its effect. In a study following ICP-monitored patients, aggressive medical treatment with urea, mannitol, or both adequately controlled ICP and was associated with better outcomes and lower mortality rates.[110] A double-blind, randomized, placebo-controlled study of 216 patients examined the use of glycerol for the treatment of ICH.[111] In experimental animals, glycerol reduces cerebral edema without a rebound effect and increases cerebral perfusion. In this study, however, glycerol had no effect on outcome and caused subclinical hemolysis in some patients.

Hemodilution has also been studied in patients with ICH, because it increases cerebral blood flow (CBF) and decreases blood viscosity in experimental animals. One study showed no differences in outcome when hematocrit level was decreased an average of 13% with dextran and venesection.[112]

There has been some interest in the use of neuroprotective agents. Because ICH causes focal cerebral ischemia,[103, 113, 114] neuroprotectants could interrupt the excitotoxic cascade and prevent neuronal death. In an experimental rat model of ICH, muscimol (GABA antagonist) and MK 801 (NMDA antagonist) increased the rats' tolerance to larger hematomas. The area of white matter around the basal ganglia was also better preserved. In another study,[103] pretreatment with nimodipine (Ca^{2+} channel blocker) and D-CPP-ene (NMDA-receptor blocker) significantly reduced the ischemic volume and brain edema, respectively, at 24 hours, compared with no treatment.

General measures to control blood pressure, reduce ICP, prevent seizures, and maintain systemic health are important in preventing the progression of hemorrhage, edema, and brain ischemia. Despite disappointing results thus far, these parameters should be controlled aggressively. The optimal reduction of blood pressure needed to perfuse the brain adequately yet prevent rebleeding or progression is controversial. However, the patient's state of consciousness is the best guide to prognosis[1, 115, 116] and may help determine the degree of blood pressure and ICP control that should be instituted. If neurological deterioration occurs or ICP cannot be controlled, surgical evacuation should be considered.

SURGICAL MANAGEMENT

Experimental Rationale

The physiologic effect of ICH on the brain is multifactorial. In clinical practice, patients are particularly susceptible to neurological deterioration within the first 24 hours after hemorrhage,[34, 117] particularly the first 4 to 6 hours.[34, 105, 106] However, neurological status is often affected disproportionately to the anatomic extent of the lesion. Further, studies have failed to correlate elevated ICP with clinical condition.[118] Animal models suggest that the hematoma's effect on local rather than global CBF is responsible for progressive ischemia.[102, 103, 113, 119, 120] Interest in the progressive effect of this local "intracerebral squeeze" focuses on its potential reversibility and the possible efficacy of early evacuation in clinical practice.

Nath and coworkers[113] studied the effect of various volumes of blood injected into the caudate nucleus of rats. Larger volumes produced larger areas of ischemia at 1 minute, and CBF decreased significantly in areas near the hematoma and ipsilateral frontal lobe. Cerebral perfusion pressure, however, remained unchanged, implying the presence of a local squeezing effect on the microcirculation rather than a generalized alteration in perfusion pressure.

Nehls and colleagues[102] studied the amount of ipsilateral caudate blood flow that was below ischemic levels. At 5 minutes, 11.5% of caudate volume was associated with blood flow of less than 25 mL/kg per minute. The ischemic area increased to a maximum of 38.9% at 4 hours. This time course suggested that interventions that reduce hematoma size might decrease ischemia. Therefore, in a subsequent study, the caudate balloon was deflated after 10 minutes in group 1 and after 24 hours in group 2. Group 1 had a higher mean CBF in the caudate nucleus and cortex and smaller areas of ischemia than did group 2. Group 1 also had a better neurological outcome. In further studies, this potential for limiting local ischemia was found to be less if the balloon was deflated after 2.5 hours.[103] A pig model using a clot rather than a balloon showed that removal of the clot at 3 hours markedly reduced perihematoma edema and mass effect at 24 hours.[104] Eliminating the hematoma prevented its serum proteins from diffusing into the adjacent white matter, thereby preventing subsequent edema. These experiments imply that early evacuation of ICH may decrease the ischemia caused by the hematoma by improving local blood flow, preventing the formation of edema, and preventing local mass effect.

Ropper and Zervas[119] compared lesions made from whole blood, centrifuged blood, and inert plastic in the caudate nucleus. In all animals, regional CBF about the hematoma decreased. Relative hyperperfusion was associated with one or both cortices on the second and third days with whole blood, immediately with centrifuged blood, and never with inert plastic. These findings imply that sheer destruction of the caudate nucleus is not entirely responsible for changes in blood flow, whereas certain elements within blood may be.

Jenkins and associates[120] compared equal volumetric caudate injections of blood, oil (equal to blood's viscosity), and cerebrospinal fluid. They evaluated CBF and ischemic cell damage by light microscopy. CBF was immediately reduced adjacent to the lesion in all groups. With blood, however, CBF was reduced over a greater radius and throughout the ipsilateral cortex. In addition, at 4 hours, ischemic damage was present with both blood and oil but not with cerebrospinal fluid. This finding implies that both tissue pressure and vasoactive substances are components in decreased regional CBF and that both play a role in ischemia at 4 hours.

In rats whose hematomas were "contained" within the caudate nucleus, global cerebral perfusion pressure was unaffected, whereas "unconfined" extension into the ventricles or subarachnoid space reduced cerebral perfusion pressure globally. This finding may explain the poorer outcome in this subgroup and may indicate a need to monitor ICP.[103]

In summary, ICH causes alterations in CBF. Larger hematomas produce a stronger, immediate effect. The effect of both vasoactive substances and local tissue pressure increases during the first 4 hours, and the effect persists for 24 hours. This change in regional CBF produces histologic ischemia and poorer neurological outcome, which is reversible to some extent. Animal studies suggest that early surgery may help limit secondary ischemia and improve outcome.

Effect of Age

Age has a predictive role in the outcome and mortality rate of patients with ICH.[106, 121–124] In a prospective outcome study of conservatively treated patients, old age was the most important predictor of a poor outcome.[123] In a prospective, randomized trial that compared surgical and conservative treatment, surgically treated patients younger than 60 years had a significantly lower mortality rate than those older than 60 years (25% versus 65%).[124] In surgically treated patients older than 60 years, 67% had poor outcomes (activities of daily living [ADL] score >3), compared with 50% of patients younger than 60 years old.[122] The relationship between age and outcome is even more pronounced with thalamic hemorrhages. Among patients who were younger than 59, 60 to 69, and older than 70 years, 59%, 33%, and 17%, respectively, had good or excellent outcomes. In a retrospective study of patients identified as having a "rapidly progressive" hematoma by serial CT, age older than 65 years was associated with 100% mortality in patients whose deterioration prompted surgery. Age is thus an important element in any treatment decision, and age older than 60 years implies a poor prognosis, regardless of treatment.

Effect of Hematoma Volume

In the era before CT, the volume of ICH could only be inferred from the angiographic distortion of vessels, yielding imprecise estimates of the size and quality of the hematoma. CT made it possible to quantify the volume of hematomas and to elucidate their characteristics, helping to delineate their natural history and clinical outcome. In experimental animal models of ICH, larger volumes were associated with larger areas of ischemia and poorer outcomes.[113] In many retrospective[27, 34, 68, 69, 71, 105, 117, 121, 122, 125–129] and prospective studies,[124] the volume of hematomas based on CT measurements is a strong predictor of functional outcome and death in humans. The progression of hematomas has been examined by serial computed tomographic imaging, which helps predict further growth and potential clinical deterioration.[34, 117]

Hematomas can be measured by direct computer imaging or estimated using simple calculations. The volume can be calculated by recording the largest diameter seen on CT, the diameter orthogonal to it, and the number of 1-cm slices on which the hemorrhage can be seen. The total volume can be estimated by using the formula for an ellipsoid, $V = 4 \div 3 \times \pi \times ABC \div 8$, where A, B, and C represent the respective diameters of the three dimensions.[105] Simplified, this equation yields an approximation of $ABC/2$, which has proved to be quite accurate.[127]

SUPRATENTORIAL HEMATOMAS

In 1977, Hier and colleagues[68] reviewed 5000 computed tomographic scans to correlate the volume of putaminal hematomas with presentation and prognosis. The authors defined three groups. Patients with small hematomas (<35 cm^3) showed mild to moderate hemiparesis or hemisensory loss, preservation of higher cortical function, and a good prognosis, regardless of treatment. Patients with moderate hematomas (mean, 120 cm^3) had classic flaccid hemiplegia, hemisensory defect, lateral gaze preference, homonymous hemianopsia, and either aphasia or apractagnosia. Massive hemorrhages (>200 cm^3) produced coma, fixed and dilated pupils, papilledema, absent eye movements, bilateral fixed plantar response, and rapid death. These correlations suggested that patients with moderate hematomas might be candidates for a controlled clinical comparison of surgical and conservative treatments.

In a retrospective review of 188 cases of supratentorial ICH, Broderick and coworkers[105] showed that hematoma volume was the strongest predictor of the 30-day mortality rate and functional outcome for all locations (putaminal, thalamic, and subcortical). The 30-day mortality rates for deep hemorrhages less than 30 cm^3, between 30 and 60 cm^3, and greater than 60 cm^3 were 23%, 64%, and 93%, respectively. Mortality rates for lobar hemorrhages at these volumes were 7%, 60%, and 71%, respectively. Half the patients who died did so within the first 2 days. Of 71 patients surviving with hematoma volumes larger than 30 cm^3, only 1 (1.4%) was independent at 30 days. In contrast, of the 91 patients who survived with hematoma volumes less than 30 cm^3, 16 (18%) were independent. Combining hematoma volumes with admission Glasgow Coma Scale (GCS) scores proved to be a 97% sensitive and 97% specific test for 30-day mortality. For patients with GCS scores less than 8 and hematoma volumes greater than 60 cm^3, the probability of death at 30 days was 91%, whereas it was 19% for those with GCS scores higher than 9 and hematoma volumes less than 30 cm^3 (Fig. 105–7). Although this study did not aim to evaluate the effectiveness of treatment, operative removal was associated with a decreased 30-day mortality rate, although overall surgical morbidity and mortality rates were not significantly different from those associated with conservative treatment.

Volpin and associates[128] retrospectively reviewed the outcome of medical treatment and craniotomy in 132 supratentorial ICHs with respect to hematoma volume, regardless of location. Compared with conservative treatment, surgery decreased the mortality rate of comatose patients with hematoma volumes between 26 and 85 cm^3, but the probability of discharge with a severe deficit was high. All patients with hematoma volumes greater than 85 cm^3 died, irrespective of treatment, and all patients with hematoma volumes less than 26 cm^3 survived without surgery.

In contrast, a retrospective comparison of surgery and conservative therapy in 182 patients with putaminal hemorrhage showed that the size of the hematoma on CT was a statistically significant predictor of outcome, despite treatment modality.[27] Localized hematomas or those extending into either limb of the internal capsule (groups I–III) were compared with those that extended into both limbs of the internal capsule, the thalamus, or both (groups IV and V). The 30-day mortality rate was significantly lower in groups I–III than in groups IV and V (12% versus 57%).

A randomized, prospective study comparing endoscopic removal of supratentorial ICH with medical management found surgery to be beneficial for hematomas of all volumes, especially subcortical hematomas.[124] Interestingly, patients with hematoma volumes less than 50 cm^3 had better outcomes after surgery than after conservative treatment (25% versus 0% ADL score

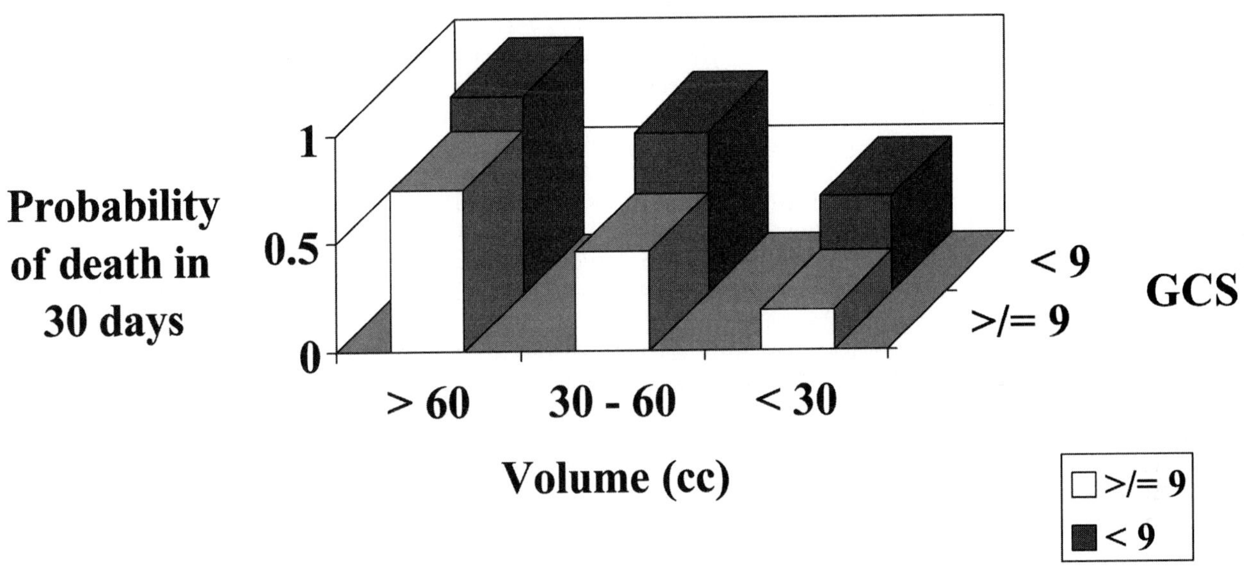

FIGURE 105–7. Graphic representation of outcome data from Broderick and colleagues[105] showing how admission Glasgow Coma Scale score and intracerebral hematoma volume combine independently to influence the 30-day mortality rate.

of 1), although the mortality rate was the same. For large hematomas (>50 cm^3), there was no difference in functional outcome between the two groups, but the mortality rate was lower in the surgical group than in the conservative group (48% versus 90%). This study suggests that surgical evacuation may play a life-saving role in patients with large hematomas by sparing viable local brain function by decreasing mass effect, progressive edema, or impaired cerebral perfusion. The overall lower surgical mortality rate (30%) in this study compared with others may reflect surgical technique and is discussed later in this chapter.

Large-volume thalamic hematomas are more devastating than similarly sized subcortical or putaminal hematomas. Of 29 patients with thalamic hemorrhages, those with volumes greater than 10 cm^3 or with a maximal diameter greater than 3 cm had ADL scores of 4 or 5.[127] Thalamic hematomas with a long axis greater than 3 cm are associated with poor outcomes.[69, 71, 129] In a comparison of 75 patients with thalamic hemorrhages who underwent either stereotactic aspiration or conservative treatment, 31 of 40 (78%) surgical patients with hematoma diameters larger than 3.3 cm returned to useful activity in 6 months.[121] This finding suggests that the less invasive nature of stereotactic aspiration may improve therapeutic outcomes, despite the size and location of the hematoma.

Hematoma volume also seems to be related to the risk of deterioration. In a retrospective study of 182 African Americans, the presence of an ICH greater than 30 cm^3 increased the risk of deterioration and death in the first 24 hours by 6.78 and 6.66 times, respectively.[117] Of 46 noncomatose patients, 15 deteriorated during the initial 24 hours. In this study, hematoma volume was a better early predictor of poor outcome than was admission GCS score.

INFRATENTORIAL HEMATOMAS

With cerebellar hemorrhages, identifying the appropriate clinical progression is paramount to guiding surgical evacuation. When hematomas are near the brainstem, however, irreversible deterioration can occur without warning. Most studies recommend surgery for all hematomas greater than 3 cm in diameter.[84, 130, 131] Smaller lesions have a more benign course. However, the patient's clinical profile must still be followed carefully, because spatial accommodation is, by necessity, more limited here than supratentorially.

Progression

SUPRATENTORIAL HEMATOMAS

Understanding the natural time course of an acute ICH and its effect on clinical deterioration is critical to therapeutic decision making. Before CT was available, the period of active bleeding was thought to be brief.[132]

The radiographic progression of a hematoma and its correlation with clinical course have been well studied. Rehemorrhage typically occurs within the first 6 hours of the primary ictus.[105, 106] Most of the extravasation of contrast in the angiograms of patients with ICH is seen within 3 to 6 hours of onset.[133, 134] If deterioration occurs later than 6 hours after hemorrhage, other factors—edema, hydrocephalus, a new intraventricular hemorrhage, or a metabolic abnormality—must be contributing.

One retrospective study of putaminal ICH on serial computed tomographic studies obtained over a precise time line in 180 patients revealed that most hemorrhages were completed within 6 hours.[106] Secondary thalamic hemorrhage or ventricular rupture caused deterioration between 6 and 12 hours after the original ICH. Finally, clinical severity at 6 hours most accurately represented the severity of the ictus. Patients who were comatose or obtunded with herniation signs were classified as "fulminant." Their outcomes were poor, despite treatment. Patients who were obtunded or stuporous without herniation signs were classified as "rapidly progressive." Their outcomes improved if the hematoma was evacuated before irreversible damage occurred. One third of the conservatively treated group in this class deteriorated by day 3. Patients lethargic at 6 hours were classified as "slowly progressive," and they showed no significant difference in outcome based on treatment. A small group of these patients, however, deteriorated with conservative therapy; thus, surgery may need to be limited to this undefined subgroup. Considering the rapidity as well as the extent of deterioration at 6 hours after ictus may help in planning surgery for individual patients.

In a study of 419 patients, Fujii and coworkers[135] obtained the first computed tomographic scan within 24 hours of onset and a follow-up scan 24 hours after admission. They found that hematomas had enlarged in 14.3% of patients. In another study, Kazui and colleagues[136] obtained sequential computed tomographic scans from 204 patients with acute ICH. Hematomas enlarged 40% in 20% of the patients. This was seen when the scans were obtained early; none of the patients showed an increase in hematoma size after 24 hours.

To define the progression over time more closely, Brott and associates[34] prospectively studied 103 patients with ICH at all locations who underwent CT within 3 hours of onset. The patients were rescanned 1 and 20 hours after the first scan. On the 1-hour follow-up scan, 26% of patients exhibited hematoma growth (>33% enlargement). An additional 12% showed growth between 1 and 20 hours. Therefore, 38% of patients exhibited hematoma progression within 24 hours of hemorrhage. Of these patients, 33% deteriorated within the first hour, and an additional 25% deteriorated within the next 20 hours. Therefore, the clinical condition of more than 50% of all patients showing progression on serial CT deteriorated. This finding implies that early hematoma evacuation may not only reduce perihematoma ischemia[103, 113, 114] and the toxic effect of blood products[103, 119, 120] but also contain potential hemorrhagic progression.

Bae and colleagues[97] reported similar results from their retrospective study of 320 patients who underwent serial CT for ICH. Three percent of patients showed rapid hematoma progression. The mean follow-up scan was obtained at 48.9 hours (range, 10.5 to 149 hours), and 50% of the patients showing progression deteriorated before 24 hours had elapsed. In this study, the most important risk factor for progression was persistent hypertension.

Qureshi and coworkers[117] retrospectively reviewed 182 African American patients to identify independent predictors of early deterioration and death. Of the patients with GCS scores higher than 12, 23% showed early deterioration (mean, 7.9 hours). An ICH volume greater than 30 cm^3 and ventricular extension were independent predictors of early deterioration (odds ratios of 6.78 and 4.67, respectively) and death (odds ratios of 6.66 and 4.23, respectively). These findings suggest that a prospective, randomized trial of early surgery (within 6 hours) is needed to support this evidence-based hypothesis that early surgery may prevent secondary deterioration.

INFRATENTORIAL HEMATOMAS

Cerebellar hemorrhage tends to progress rapidly and to cause death because of its proximity to the brainstem. It has been recommended that patients with GCS scores of 13 or less or hemorrhages of 4 cm or greater should undergo surgical evacuation.[137] Other authors, however, contend that rapid progression of particular cerebellar and cranial nerve syndromes (see earlier) represents a surgical emergency, despite these criteria.[64, 138]

The review by Ott and associates[84] of 56 cases of cerebellar hemorrhage showed that 9 of 28 patients treated conservatively died precipitously from misdiagnosis and rapid progression. Additionally, 50% of awake or drowsy patients deteriorated within 2 days of onset, and an additional 25% deteriorated within 7 days.

Death ususally occurs within the first 2 days, but it can occur later. Progressive hematomas produce consistent clinical findings that must be recognized promptly. With the first sign of deterioration, patients must undergo immediate surgical evacuation.

Timing of Surgery

Credible experimental evidence indicates that early evacuation of hematomas improves CBF,[102, 103, 114, 119, 120] histologic changes,[139] brain edema,[104] ischemia,[103] and outcome.[114] The natural history of ICH reveals that 50% of related deaths occur within 48 hours of hemorrhage,[105] and radiographic expansion or rebleeding occurs maximally within 3 to 4 hours but for as long as 24 hours thereafter.[34] Therefore, early surgery may improve the outcome for many reasons.

Extensive clinical evidence also supports early surgery.[140–142] A single lenticulostriate branch rupture that bleeds for a brief time creates a significant hypertensive hematoma.[143] Consequently, direct early vessel coagulation seems to be advantageous. Exacerbation occurs suddenly and most often within 4 to 6 hours of bleeding[34]; thus, early surgery may prevent clinical progression. Because secondary changes such as edema occur 7 to 8 hours after a hemorrhage, evacuation before that time may prevent these changes.

In an important retrospective study of ultra-early surgery, Kaneko and colleagues[140] reviewed 100 putaminal hemorrhages, all of which were operated on within 7 hours. All patients were hemiplegic, with GCS scores between 6 and 12 and hematoma volumes greater than 20 to 30 cm^3. The mortality rate was 7%, and the 6-month rate of "useful recovery" was 83%. Two patients died of rapid exacerbation before surgery, and two died from reaccumulation of hematoma. These results are favorable when compared with the series of Yukawa and Kanaya,[144] which did not emphasize early surgery (28.6% mortality rate and 62.8% rate of useful recovery). The patients of Kaneko and colleagues[140] had better immediate preoperative neurological grades, implying that earlier surgery limited the time available for further deterioration. Their study, however, did not address patients with GCS scores of 13 and hematoma volumes between 20 and 30 cm^3.

These results are supported by a retrospective analysis that showed that a subgroup of patients with moderate-sized putaminal hematomas had better outcomes when operated on within 6 hours of hemorrhage.[141] In a prospective study by Juvela and associates,[145] 52 patients with GCS scores between 7 and 10 did not benefit from surgery performed after 24 hours, but mortality rates improved when surgery occurred within 13 hours.

A recent randomized, controlled, prospective trial evaluated the feasibility of early surgery.[146] The median onset from time of hemorrhage to hospitalization was 3.3 hours, and time to surgery was 8.5 hours (beyond the range of <6 hours). There was no difference in outcome between surgery and medical treatment, but there was a trend toward a lower 3-month morbidity rate with surgery. This study suggests that there are logistical barriers to ultra-early surgery, and this is where the bulk of the "brain attack" effort is directed (i.e., educating primary physicians, paramedics, and the public).

With cerebellar hemorrhage, ultra-early surgery is vital in patients with signs of brainstem compression. At the earliest sign of clinical change, immediate evacuation without CT can be life saving. Without brainstem signs, however, the timing of surgery is controversial. Ott and associates[84] studied the natural history of cerebellar hemorrhage and found that 9 of 28 patients died precipitously up to 2 weeks after hemorrhage. Fifty percent deteriorated within 2 days, and an additional 25% deteriorated within 1 week. Only after 8 days did awake or drowsy patients treated conservatively have a lower mortality rate than those undergoing surgery. Therefore, patients presenting in the first week of hemorrhage may still benefit from surgery.

A well-designed, randomized, controlled study is needed to fully reveal the benefits (if any) of early surgery. Until then, we continue to favor ultra-early surgical treatment for moderate-sized putaminal hematomas causing obtundation, stupor, or significant motor deficits.

Surgical Techniques

In 1903, Cushing[8] first removed an intracerebral hematoma by craniotomy. In 1932, Bagley[9] first described indications for removal based on location. In 1950, Fazio,[147] a neurologist, suggested surgical removal based on pathologic studies.

In 1961, McKissock and coworkers[1] published the first pessimistic view of surgical treatment for ICH. They reported a 51% mortality rate in 244 operated cases and a 100% mortality rate for comatose patients. Since then, outcome studies have yielded controversial results. Operative mortality can range from 20% to 90% in comatose patients with deep ganglionic or thalamic bleeds.[1, 94, 148, 149] Most studies, however, have either failed or lacked the power to stratify patients appropriately or to identify the optimal timing of surgery in a well-designed, randomized, prospective manner. Because of this controversy, various less invasive methods of removal are practiced around the world: simple aspiration, stereotactic aspiration, fibrinolytic treatment, mechanically assisted aspiration, and endoscopy.[150] In particular circumstances, some of these techniques may be more efficacious for deep putaminal or thalamic hemorrhages. Others are beneficial for subcortical hematomas. These techniques and the use of standard craniotomy for ICH are detailed in this section.

CRANIOTOMY

Several technical points must be considered when planning a craniotomy for ICH. In the preoperative period, an arterial line, intravenous fluids, and correction of electrolytes are crucial. During intubation, hypertension must be avoided, and medical therapy must be maximized based on the patient's neurological condition.

For putaminal hematomas, three general approaches have been used: transtemporal, transfrontal, and transsylvian.[151] We treat a surgical putaminal hemorrhage as a microsurgical lesion requiring meticulous technique to avoid adding insult to injury. We favor a transcisternal-transsylvian-transinsular approach. The hematoma often extends to within millimeters of the insular cortex, and a small 2-cm insular corticotomy is often all that is needed to evacuate the largest hematoma. The operating microscope is used routinely, and the improved illumination and magnification make the identification and bipolar coagulation of cavity wall bleeders straightforward. We rely on a malleable graduated sucker to suction and handle tissue alternately.

For several reasons, we rarely use self-retaining retractors. First, steady retraction is deleterious to brain parenchyma. Second, the "static" retraction provided is nonergonomic and ignores the fact that the evacuation process relies on constant change of angle, depth, and orientation. The center of the hematoma is removed first. The remaining marginal clot then collapses and can likewise be evacuated, with particular attention to bleeding points and possible subtle pathologic findings such as small tumors, cryptic AVMs, and cavernous angiomas. All tissue is sent for histologic analysis.

Extreme caution is used to avoid traumatic manipulation of the capsular fibers at the depth of the surgical cavity. Hemostasis is ensured by elevating systolic pressure temporarily to identify potential rebleeding sites.[151] Otherwise, blood pressure is maintained postoperatively in the normal range for the *specific* patient. If the hematoma extends significantly into the temporal lobe, the transtemporal approach can be used. The transfrontal approach is rarely used and is almost obsolete because the surgical tract is, by necessity, deep. Suzuki and Sato[152] reported that the functional prognosis was better when the transsylvian rather than the transcortical approach was used. Kanaya and Kuroda[153] advocate transcortical approaches for large hematomas. The general surgical principles for evacuating hematomas at other locations also follow commonsense strategies: corticotomies are placed near the epicenter of the ICH, their length is minimized, and, above all, eloquent tissue is avoided.

For infratentorial hematomas, a suboccipital craniotomy with the patient in the prone or lateral position is standard. Most commonly (i.e., for unilateral deep cerebellar nuclei hemorrhage), a paramedian straight incision is used. We strongly advocate a bone flap craniotomy rather than a craniectomy; the latter is slower, produces less cosmetic results, and may cause craniectomy headaches. A ventriculostomy is often necessary to relieve hydrocephalus.[154]

■ CASE HISTORY 1

A 60-year-old hypertensive man had an acute headache for a few hours and left hemiparesis (1/5) on admission. He was somnolent, and his blood pressure was 220/95. A putaminal hemorrhage mildly encroached on the internal capsule (Fig. 105–8*A*). He underwent an emergent standard transsylvian-transinsular approach for microsurgical evacuation. On postoperative day 1, CT showed a good evacuation, with decreased capsular mass effect (see Fig. 105–8*B*). He improved to grade 3/5 within 4 weeks.

■ CASE HISTORY 2

A 54-year-old hypertensive patient arrived at the hospital 2.5 hours after the onset of a grade 1/5 hemiparesis with mild confusion. His condition improved dramatically to antigravity strength 3/5 within 4 hours of surgical evacuation performed 4.5 hours after the ictus (Fig. 105–9). He subsequently achieved grade 4+/5 strength 6 weeks after surgery.

■ CASE HISTORY 3

A 71-year-old man on warfarin (Coumadin) suffered a coagulopathy-related ICH, best described as putaminal, with extension into the globus pallidus and claustrum, sparing the internal capsule (Fig. 105–10). On arrival, he was lethargic, and his strength was grade 0/5. During the ensuing 5 hours, his coagulopathy was reversed with fresh frozen plasma. Surgical evacuation followed. By postoperative day 8, he was grade 2/5, with a satisfactory computed tomographic scan. At 6 months, he had improved to 4/5.

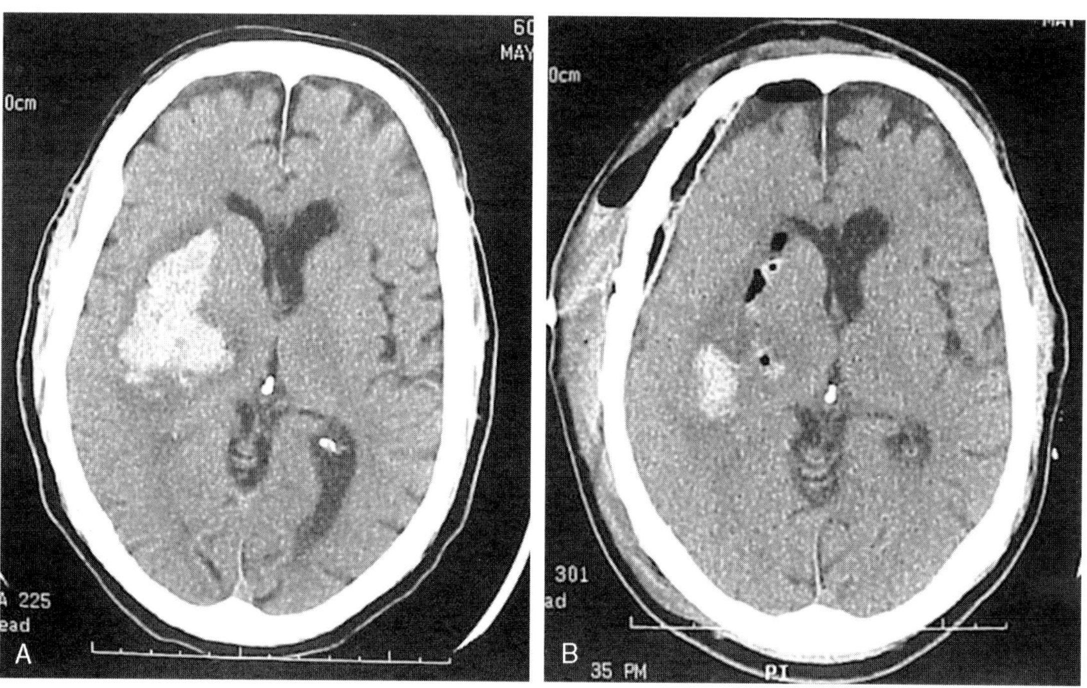

FIGURE 105–8. *A*, Admission computed tomographic scan of a somnolent patient with an acute hypertensive putaminal hemorrhage and grade 1/5 hemiparesis. *B*, Computed tomographic scan of the same patient on postoperative day 1.

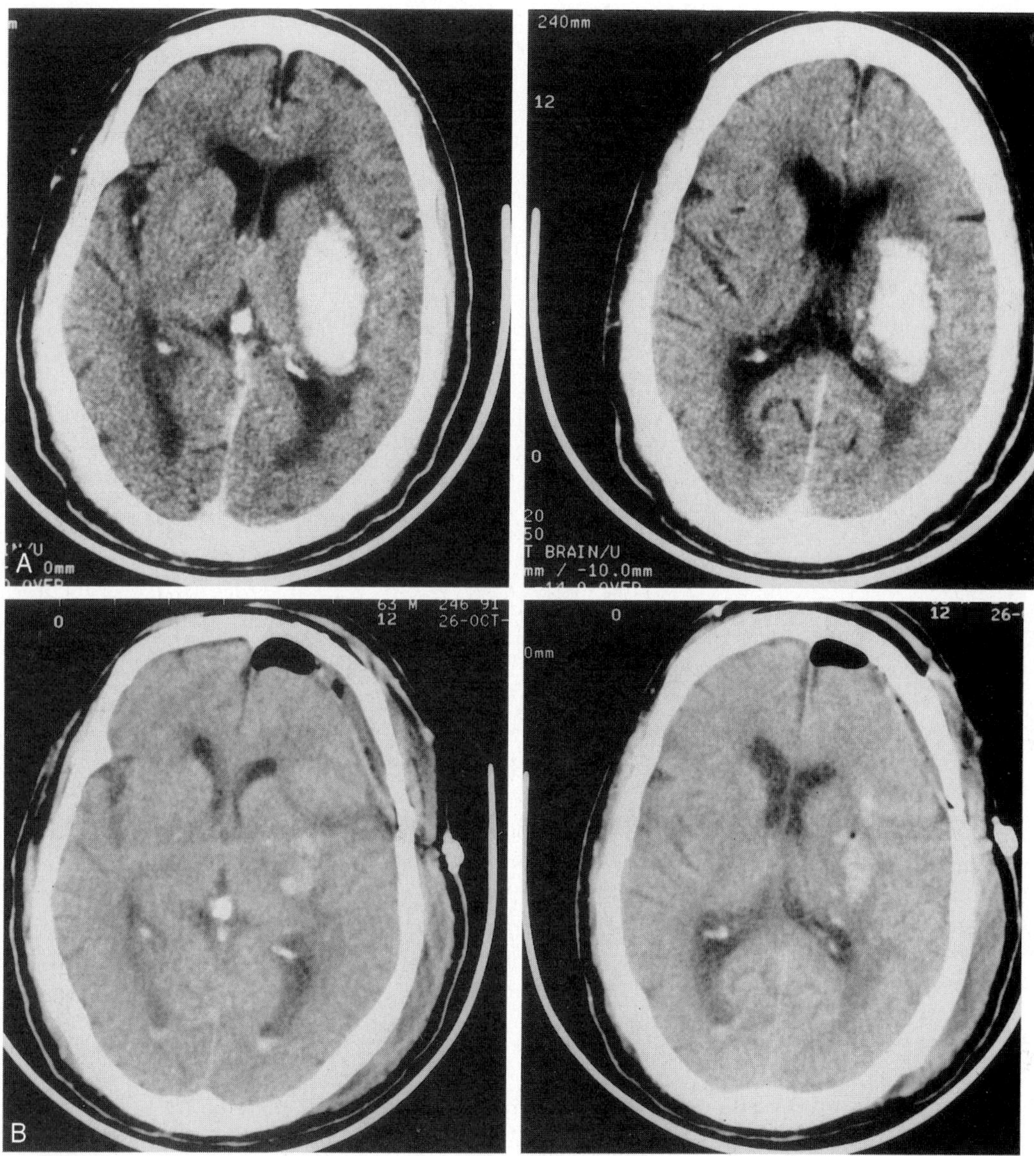

FIGURE 105–9. *A*, Admission computed tomographic scans of a 54-year-old patient with an acute hypertensive putaminal hemorrhage, grade 1/5 hemiparesis, and mild confusion. *B*, Computed tomographic scans of the same patient on postoperative day 1.

■ CASE HISTORY 4

In contrast, a 73-year-old woman on warfarin experienced an extensive striatocapsular intraventricular hemorrhage (Fig. 105–11*A* and *B*). She herniated clinically and failed to recover from coma after emergency evacuation. Despite an adequate evacuation (see Fig. 105–11*C* and *D*), she died of sepsis within 8 days.

Typically, lobar hemorrhages are the most rewarding to treat surgically, particularly when addressed early. This is only a generalization, however. Age, medical history, and neurological grade at admission are among the most powerful prognosticators, as discussed earlier.

■ CASE HISTORY 5

A 78-year-old homeless hypertensive man arrived almost stuporous with a grade 1/5 hemiparesis. A large, deep, left temporal lobe hematoma encroached on the striatum (Fig. 105–12). After an emergency transinsular microsurgical evacuation, he improved to opening his eyes spontaneously, with global aphasia on postoperative day 1. Within 1 week, he developed pulmonary sepsis, bilateral occipital infarcts, and a bleeding gastric ulcer (not on steroids). After 2 months of hospitalization, he could open his eyes to voice, remained 1/5 hemiparetic, and was transferred to a nursing home.

■ CASE HISTORY 6

A 62-year-old man had chronic renal failure requiring hemodialysis. On admission, he was obtunded and coagulopathic hours after dialysis but could move all limbs symmetrically (Fig. 105–13*A* to *C*). The possibility of a ruptured anterior communicating artery aneurysm was ruled out by emergency magnetic resonance angiography,

Text continued on page 1753

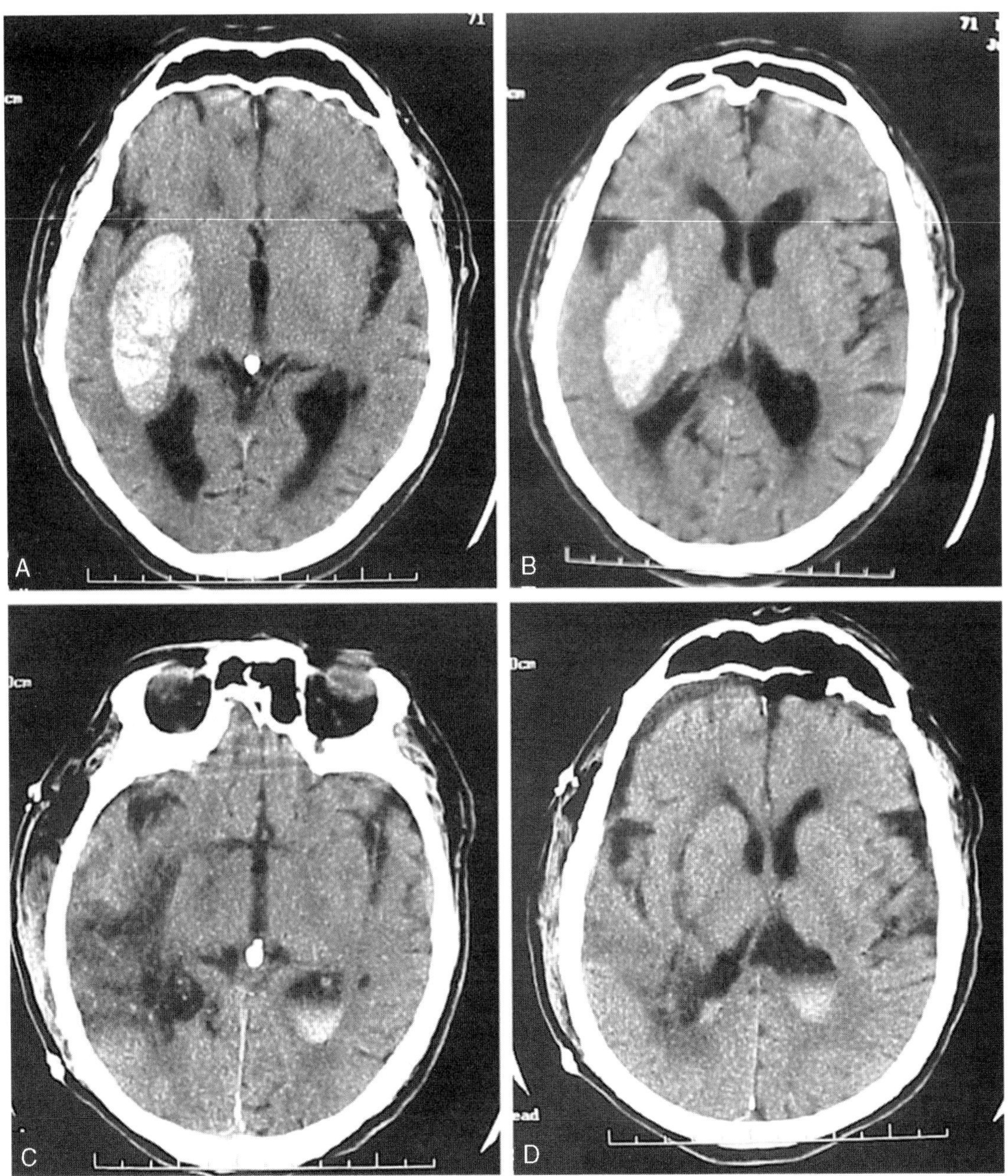

FIGURE 105–10. *A* and *B*, Admission computed tomographic scans of a 71-year-old patient with warfarin-induced hemorrhage into the putamen, globus pallidus, and claustrum. He was completely hemiplegic and lethargic. *C* and *D*, Computed tomographic scans of the same patient 8 days after surgery.

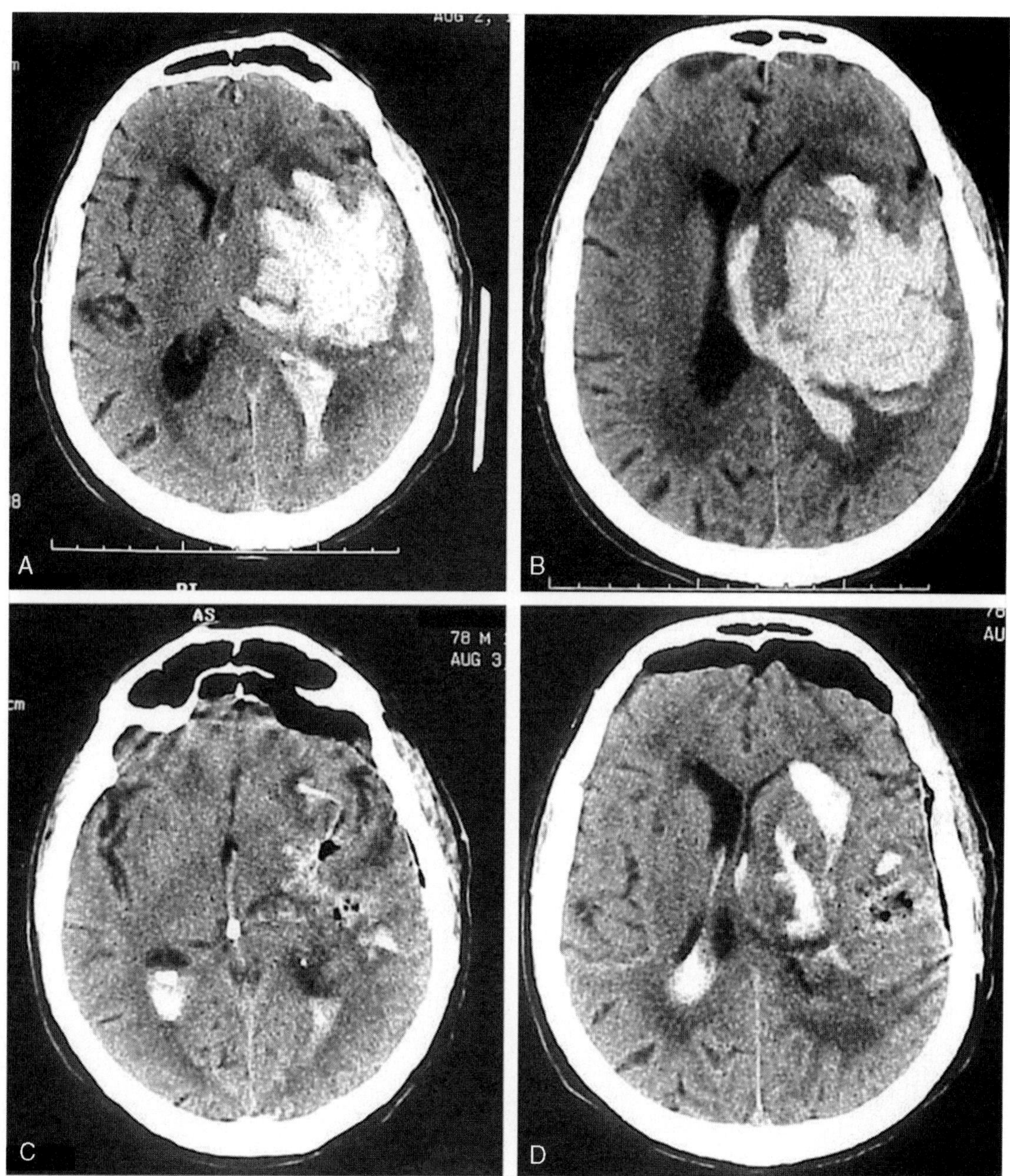

FIGURE 105–11. *A* and *B*, Admission computed tomographic scans of a 73-year-old woman who suffered a warfarin-induced striatocapsular hemorrhage with clinical herniation. *C* and *D*, Computed tomographic scans of the same patient on postoperative day 1 showing good evacuation, but she died of sepsis 8 days later.

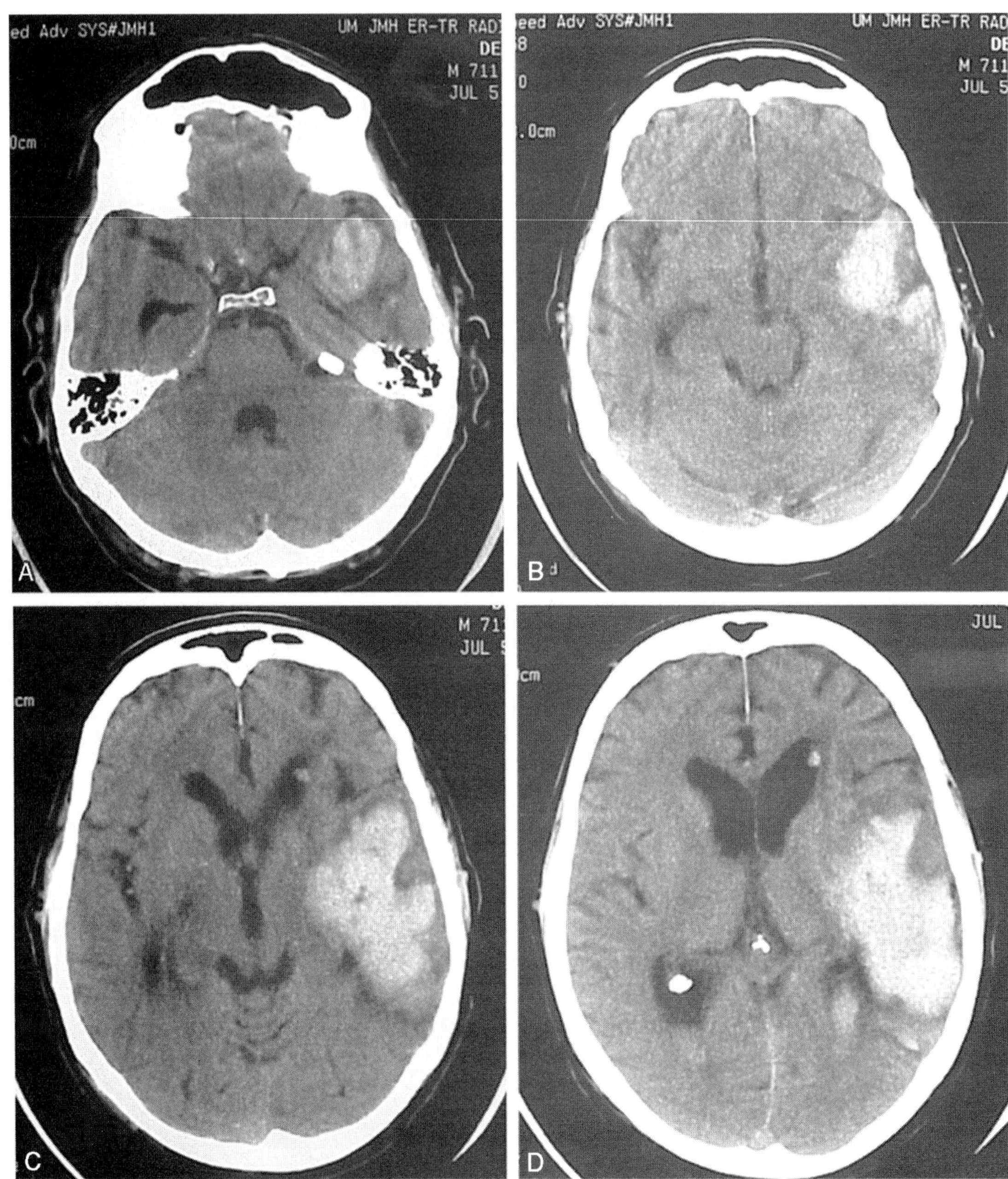

FIGURE 105–12. *A–D*, Admission computed tomographic scans of a 78-year-old hypertensive man with an intracerebral hematoma in the temporal lobe, grade 1/5 hemiparesis, and stupor.

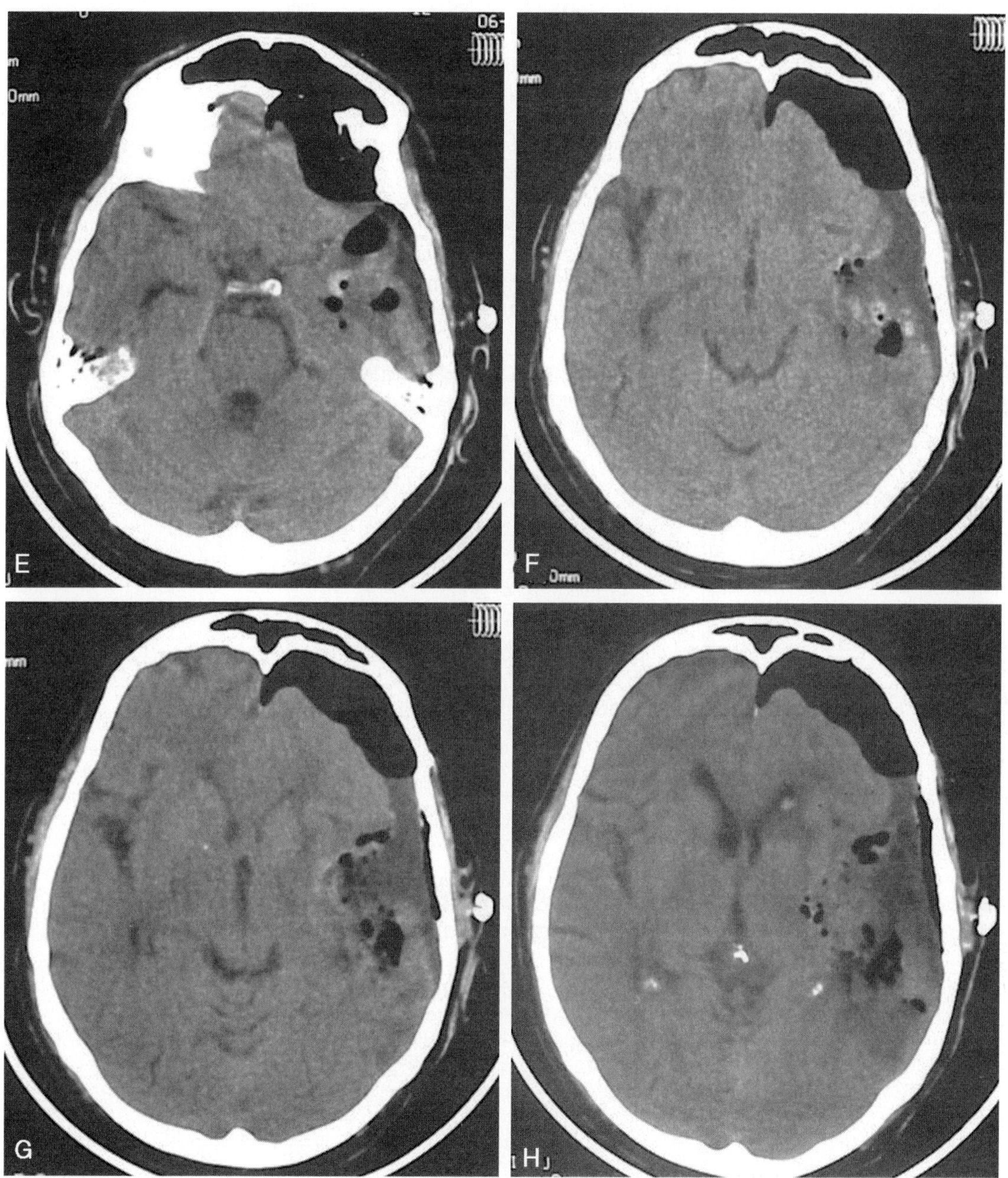

FIGURE 105–12 *Continued. E–H,* Computed tomographic scans of the same patient on postoperative day 1.

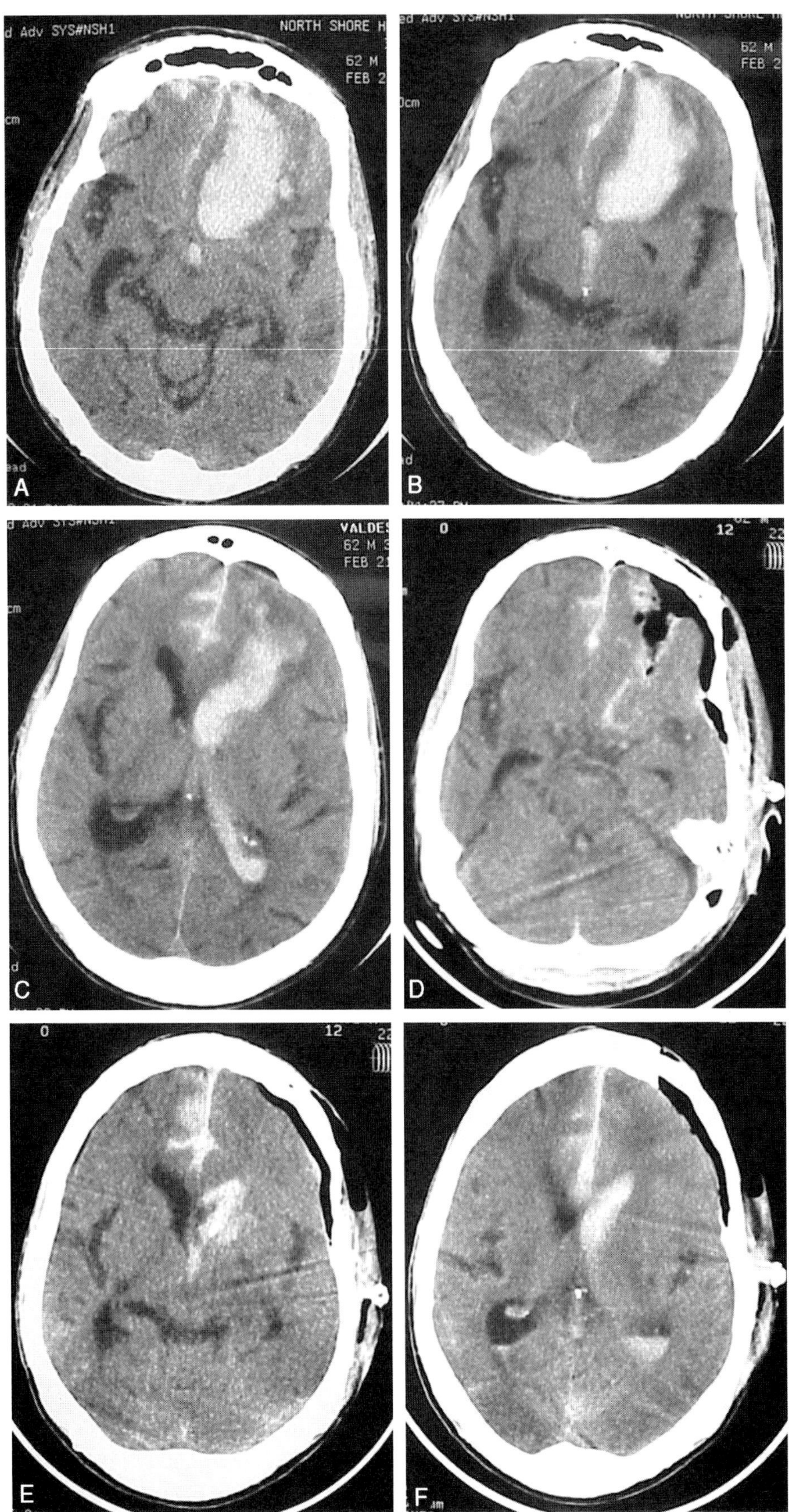

FIGURE 105–13. *A–C,* Admission computed tomographic scans of a 62-year-old coagulopathic man who developed renal failure on dialysis and was found obtunded. The scans show intraventricular and subarachnoid hemorrhage, in addition to the frontal intracerebral hematoma. Angiography failed to reveal an aneurysm. *D–F,* Computed tomographic scans of the same patient on postoperative day 1.

while his coagulation profile was normalized. After 4 hours, and as his level of consciousness declined, a left frontal craniotomy for evacuation was performed. His postoperative computed tomographic scans were satisfying (see Fig. 105–13*D* to *F*). Clinically, however, he developed multisystem organ failure, a "do not resuscitate" order was given, and he died on day 4.

BUR HOLE ASPIRATION

Theoretically, if evacuation is adequate, an expedient and simple procedure such as bur hole aspiration would be the optimal treatment approach. However, the unpredictable consistency of hematomas makes aspiration difficult. There is also a propensity to rebleed, which makes the lack of visualization riskier. Experimentally, within only hours of clot genesis, 80% of the clot becomes dense fibrous tissue.[126] In 175 patients treated with stereotactic aspiration, 134 (75%) had more than 50% of the clot removed, and 13 (7.4%) had postoperative rebleeding.[155] These stereotactic results show the major limitations of simple aspiration: low effectiveness and high rates of recurrence.

STEREOTACTIC ASPIRATION

Benes and coworkers[156] first reported the use of stereotactic techniques in 1965, obtaining limited success in nontraumatic hematomas. In 1978, Backlund and von Holst[157] performed the first successful stereotactic aspiration of an acute hemorrhage. As interest in this technique increased, it was realized that certain shapes, consistencies, and locations made hematoma evacuation difficult. Therefore, adding fibrinolytics and mechanically assisted devices to simple aspiration under CT and MRI guidance improved the evacuation of hematomas and patient outcomes. Although no randomized, prospective, controlled studies have compared stereotactic aspiration with craniotomy and conservative therapy, studies show favorable outcomes, especially with deep-seated lesions. Honda and associates[158] retrospectively compared stereotactic aspiration and medical therapy for thalamic hemorrhages. Patients with hematomas smaller than 2.5 cm in diameter had significantly higher ADL scores with aspiration. In addition, patients whose lesions were CT grade IIB or better had better outcomes with aspiration. Despite these favorable results, the lack of direct visualization and the risk of rebleeding may limit this technique's utility, especially during the hyperacute phase of hemorrhage.

FIBRINOLYTIC THERAPY

Fibrinolysis is used to facilitate clot dissolution by activating plasminogen, which dissolves fibrin. In experimental animal models, adding fibrinolysis to stereotactic removal significantly improved CBF at 24 hours compared with placebo.[159, 160] In this method, the hematoma is first evacuated with simple needle aspiration using CT guidance through a bur hole. The localization procedure using CT can be done with a stereotactic device or by projecting the hematoma onto the scalp itself with a radiopaque marker derived from the images. Direct-image projection can be done on any CT scanner, and no special apparatus is needed. The disadvantage of the projection method is an approximately 5-mm error compared with stereotaxy.[161]

After localization, a bur hole is made with the patient under local anesthesia, and a 3- to 4-mm silicone tube is passed into the clot. The hematoma is aspirated with a syringe repeatedly until no more clot is removed. Then, a Dandy ventricular catheter is placed into the hematoma bed, and urokinase (6000 U in 3 mL) is infused.[162] Most studies use 6000 U of urokinase two to four times a day for 1 to 6 days until CT documents clot dissolution. In a canine model of intraventricular hemorrhage, urokinase caused clot lysis within 3 to 6 days, whereas in control groups, lysis took more than 7 days.[163–165]

Both urokinase and t-PA have been studied, but urokinase is used much more often. Urokinase is less expensive than t-PA and has a longer half-life, and it has both fibrinolytic and fibrinogenolytic activity. Therefore, urokinase not only dissolves existing clot but also inhibits the formation of new clot.[150] However, in an experimental animal study, the rate of hematoma dissolution after 6 hours of either t-PA or urokinase was 89% for the former and 16.4% for the latter, suggesting that t-PA is more effective.[134] Whether t-PA is more beneficial clinically has yet to be studied in a controlled setting.

An additional risk of fibrinolysis is rebleeding. Fibrinolytics cannot distinguish between hematoma and protective fibrin clot. Therefore, in most studies, stereotactic aspiration is performed no earlier than 6 hours after hemorrhage. A study of serial computed tomographic scans suggested that primary hemorrhage is completed within 6 hours,[106] implying that hemostasis can be achieved by 6 hours and that the likelihood of inducing rebleeding can be reduced.

In Japan, interest in the stereotactic evacuation of hematomas is high because its clinical incidence is so high in that country. Niizuma and coworkers published three consecutive retrospective reports on the effectiveness and potential pitfalls of stereotaxy and fibrinolysis.[121, 155, 166] In 1985, 97 patients with ICH at all locations (cortex, thalamus, basal ganglia, cerebellum) and of all neurological grades were retrospectively reviewed within 24 hours of presentation.[166] Only 58% of patients had 50% or more of the hematoma volume evacuated by initial aspiration before urokinase was administered. After urokinase infusion, the hematomas were 80% resolved in more than 70% of patients. The rebleeding rate was 7% (4% major, 3% minor), and the mortality rate was 3%.

In 1989, the same authors reported on 241 consecutive putaminal hematomas, 175 of which were evacuated stereotactically.[155] Results showed that 77% of patients had 50% of the hematoma volume evacuated during initial aspiration, and 82% of patients had 80% or better resolution after treatment with urokinase. Notably, 52 patients did not require fibrinolysis because their initial evacuation volumes were greater than 80%.

The rebleeding rate of 7.4% (4% major, 3.4% minor) most likely underestimates the true rebleeding rate after fibrinolysis, because 30% of the patients did not require infusion. This improvement on initial aspiration of the hematoma may reflect improved technique and the particularity of the putaminal location.

In 1989, Niizuma and coworkers[155] published a refined variation of stereotactic removal called "double track aspiration." This technique enabled the evacuation of a larger proportion of the hematoma. The authors suggested that a hematoma is somewhat harder at its center, which is therefore more difficult to aspirate than its periphery. Therefore, the authors made two passes, aspirating anteriorly and then posteriorly. During the initial aspiration, a mean of 77% of hematoma volume was evacuated, and 44% of patients did not require treatment with urokinase. There were only nine patients in the study, but no one rebled.

The same authors also retrospectively compared stereotactic aspiration with craniotomy and conservative therapy in 241 cases of putaminal hematomas.[155] Patients who were more than 6 hours beyond ictus with more than an 8-cm^3 hemorrhage and who lacked antigravity strength in the contralateral limb underwent stereotactic aspiration. Patients with stupor or semicoma, a hematoma larger than 40 cm^3, and clinical progression or those who presented within 6 hours underwent a craniotomy. The remainder received medical therapy. With stereotactic aspiration, more than 50% of the hematoma volume was aspirated in 77% of the patients. The rebleeding rate was 7.4% (3.4% major, 4% minor); 26% had bleeding diathesis. There was no overall difference in outcome at 6 months between stereotaxis and craniotomy, and 80% of all stereotactic patients returned to useful lives. These findings suggest that stereotactic aspiration is an effective treatment for deep-seated lesions, but it should probably be avoided in coagulopathic patients.

The outcome of patients undergoing stereotactic aspiration with fibrinolysis is comparable to that of patients undergoing craniotomy and medical therapy. Without randomized, prospective, controlled studies, however, controversy persists. Because outcome strongly depends on neurological grade and the location and volume of hematoma, it is difficult to compare retrospective studies, given the inconsistencies in patient stratification and operator bias.

Nonetheless, deep-seated lesions in the thalamus may respond to stereotactic aspiration better than to medical or surgical therapy. A review of 75 patients with thalamic hemorrhages treated with stereotactic evacuation showed that 44% were living independently at 6 months, and 32% needed assistance.[121] The mortality rate of 13% compared favorably with the 38% to 50% mortality rate associated with conservative treatment.[69, 71, 167] This finding is consistent with a previous review of 99 cases of stereotactically aspirated thalamic hemorrhages, which were associated with a mortality rate of 23%.[158] The study of Niizuma and coworkers,[166] which included all locations, showed that 70% of patients lived independently at 6 months. The mortality rate was 3%.

In the study of 175 putaminal hematomas by Niizuma and coworkers,[155] 52% of the stereotactically aspirated group achieved independent outcomes (excellent or good grades) at 6 months, whereas only 7% of the craniotomy group achieved similar recoveries. The mortality rate was 6% and 7% in the stereotactic and craniotomy groups, respectively. Notably, patients undergoing immediate craniotomies had larger hematomas and worse neurological grades. All cases of stereotactic aspiration performed between 1980 and 1982 were compared retrospectively with surgically treated historical controls.[161] Among 51 patients, 34 had putaminal hematomas; 41% were living independently (excellent or good grade) at 6 months, and the mortality rate from neurological causes was 11%. The authors compared craniotomy with stereotactic aspiration and evaluated outcome stratified by preoperative neurological grade. There were no significant differences in mortality, but prognosis at 6 months for poor-grade groups was better with craniotomy than with aspiration. This difference probably reflects early hematoma evacuation in the craniotomy cases.

Fibrinolytic stereotactic evacuation may be associated with outcomes that are comparable to those achieved with other methods of treatment, and it is particularly advantageous for deep-seated lesions. No clear advantage, however, can be delineated until a prospective study compares stereotactic, surgical, and medical treatments and patients are stratified according to their neurological grades and hematoma locations.

MECHANICALLY ASSISTED ASPIRATION

Devices that can physically fragment a hematoma are used to facilitate aspiration. In 1978, Backlund and von Holst[157] first described aspiration of an acute hemorrhage using a "screw and suction" technique. This concept is based on the Archimedes water screw principle. It involves inserting a long twist drill through a cannula where suction is applied. The rotating helical mandrel cuts portions of the clot, which are sucked into the cannula. This maneuver facilitates suctioning of hard clot. In 1982, Broseta and colleagues[168] applied the technique to ICH in 16 patients and obtained a 13% rebleeding rate and a postoperative mortality rate of 81%. Using a thinner screw and a walled cannula and adding a motor, Kandel and Peresedov[169] treated 32 patients in "grave condition." Clot was removed completely in 88% of the patients, but the rebleeding rate was 16% and the mortality rate was 22%. These results suggest that mechanical removal of hematomas is associated with relatively high rates of rebleeding and excessive fibrinolysis and is notably time-consuming, while the degree of clot removal is variable and unpredictable.

One study of 28 putaminal and 18 thalamic hematomas evacuated by the Archimedes screw yielded good results.[170] The average initial hematoma volume was 23 cm^3 (range, 6 to 37 cm^3), with an average aspiration volume of 81% (range, 54% to 100%). Only one patient hemorrhaged immediately after surgery. In general, the motor function of patients with thalamic hematomas improved, regardless of their preoperative functional condition or extension of blood into the internal capsule. Among the patients with putaminal hematomas, two thirds of those with severe preoperative motor weakness remained hemiplegic. This study contradicted previous data and suggested that use of the Archimedes screw is associated with low rates of rebleeding and good motor recoveries, especially with thalamic hemorrhages. This difference may reflect relatively smaller hematoma volumes and better preoperative neurological function.

Other less widely accepted devices include water-irrigation systems, ultrasonic aspirators, and oscillating cutters. The stereotactic "aquastream" and aspirator is an automatic irrigator that effectively aspirates clot in vitro.[171] In 1987, Matsumoto and associates[172] used an ultrasonic aspiration device similar to the Cavitron on 375 patients and reported better outcomes compared with either medical management or conventional craniotomy. Oscillating cutters contain a guillotine blade oriented parallel to the surface of the hematoma and encased in a suctioning, irrigating cannula. The tip is closed, with an open side port for aspiration of clot, which is amputated and removed with saline through a reservoir. The irrigation rate, vacuum pressure, and cutting speed are adjustable.[150] An in vitro clot model with a vacuum pressure of 150 mm Hg dissolved 75% of a 4-hour-old clot in 15 minutes.[150] However, the device was cumbersome and the procedure was time-consuming, and the U.S. trial was terminated.

NEUROENDOSCOPIC TECHNIQUES

Endoscopy has not been used extensively to treat ICH. One randomized, prospective study compared endoscopy and best medical treatment. The 6-mm-diameter neuroendoscope (manufactured by Storz, Tuttliger, West Germany) was placed through a bur hole and guided by intraoperative ultrasonography. Once the cavity was reached, it was rinsed intermittently with artificial cerebrospinal fluid at body temperature at 10 to 15 mm Hg through one channel whie interval suctioning was performed through another. Hemostasis was achieved using a neodymium:yttrium-aluminum-garnet laser. An external drain was placed and left for days.

The procedure was associated with good outcomes. Evacuation volume exceeded 50% in all patients and exceeded 70% in 45% of patients. There were no early deaths from the primary procedure and only a 4% rate of rebleeding. Forty percent of endoscopically treated patients with subcortical hematomas had good 6-month outcomes, compared with 25% treated medically. There were no differences in outcome for putaminal or thalamic hemorrhages. Certain subgroups particularly benefited from endoscopy. Patients with subcortical hemorrhages larger than 50 cm^3 had a significantly lower mortality rate but no difference in functional outcome, whereas patients with hemorrhages less than 50 cm^3 had better outcomes. There was, however, no significant difference in mortality rate. These findings imply that in patients with severe hemorrhage, endoscopy is merely a life-saving procedure, but it could improve function in patients with moderate hematomas.

INTRACRANIAL PRESSURE MONITORING

Patients with ICH have a propensity to deteriorate rapidly from hemorrhage progression, edema formation, intraventricular hemorrhage, and alterations in regional CBF. Overall, treating patients conservatively, especially those with poor neurological grades, has produced poor outcomes. The role of ICP monitoring in predicting this progression and in guiding medical therapy has been studied, but the results are mixed.

Papo and coworkers[118] retrospectively reviewed a mixture of 66 conservatively and surgically treated patients who underwent either intermittent or continuous ICP monitoring. In all patients with a normal level of consciousness, ICP was less than 20 mm Hg; all comatose patients had very high ICP. In patients with intermediate levels of consciousness, however, there was no correlation between ICP and clinical course. Surgical treatment had mixed effects on ICP. If surgery was performed early, ICP decreased but did not return to preoperative levels. If surgery was performed late, either there was no change in ICP or it dropped initially and later returned to preoperative levels. These findings imply that ICP correlates poorly with outcome and that the secondary destruction of brain tissue by the hematoma may be reversible if it is addressed early enough.

To further investigate the destructive effect of the hematoma and the optimal timing of its evacuation, Nakayama and colleagues[173] studied ICP in surgically treated patients with putaminal ICHs who presented with severe neurological deficits (semicomatose). Patients with smaller hematomas evacuated before 8 hours had lower ICP than those with larger hematomas evacuated after 8 hours (Fig. 105–14). In this setting, high ICP correlated with death and poor outcome. In this group, elevated ICP may reflect the secondary effects of the hematoma-induced alterations in microcirculation, because experimentally, these effects are more pronounced when larger hematomas are evacuated late.[102, 103, 113, 114] ICP monitoring may help define a subgroup of comatose patients with elevated ICP who will benefit from early evacuation. Ropper and King[174] also studied ICP in 10 comatose patients; none of the three patients with ICP less than 20 mm Hg died. Despite best medical treatment, there were four brain deaths among the seven patients whose ICP was greater than 20 mm Hg. All conservatively treated patients died, whereas three patients with refractory ICP who underwent surgery survived. Therefore, ICP monitoring may guide therapy in deeply comatose patients whose ICP is elevated, and thereby help prevent death.

In terms of response to medical treatment in a similar subgroup, Duff and associates[110] showed that ICP monitoring resulted in improved outcome when treat-

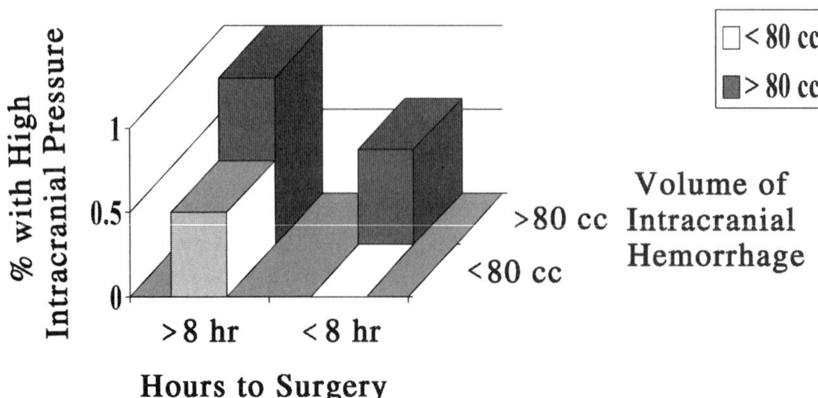

FIGURE 105–14. Graph illustrating the dependence of postevacuation intracranial pressure on the volume of an intracerebral hematoma and the time to evacuation. (Adapted from Nakayama K, Miyasaka Y, Sato K, et al: Postoperative intracranial pressure in severe cases with hypertensive intracerebral hematoma. No To Shinkei 41:1149–1154, 1989.)

ment was guided by elevated pressures. Elevated ICP readings in patients with ICH also correlate with CT findings of lateral ventricular compression, intraventricular hemorrhage, and compression of the basal cisterns.[175]

It seems that ICP monitoring is useless in intermediate-grade patients but may have a role in guiding therapy for comatose patients. It may help maximize medical management to control elevated ICP optimally, and it may be a guide for deciding on early surgery.

OUTCOME OF MANAGEMENT: META-ANALYSIS OF THE LITERATURE

Retrospective Studies

An exhaustive search of the literature addressing the outcome of ICH reveals a huge variability among individual management methodologies, study populations, and other more specific relevant factors. Not surprisingly, discrepant conclusions have been reached. Table 105–3 lists retrospective studies performed since 1957. It would be impossible to critique each study individually, but notwithstanding the usual limitations of retrospective analysis—not the least of which is selection bias in both treatment arms—certain trends can be observed. Overall, mortality rates range from 7% to 58%. Admission neurological grade heavily influences final outcome. Surgery tends to lower the mortality rate in severe cases but does not improve outcome in mild cases. The Japanese Cooperative Study published in 1990 found that outcome, regardless of medical or surgical treatment, is heavily dependent on admission grade (Fig. 105–15).[176] The collective outcomes of the studies listed in Table 105–3, based on admission ADL score, mirror this finding (Fig. 105–16). Table 105–4 addresses retrospective studies related to the stereotactic evacuation of hematomas. Mortality rates range from 0% to 27%—undoubtedly a reflection of the preselection of milder cases. This group cannot be compared with medical management unless historical controls are considered.

Prospective Studies

In an effort to overcome the biases and confounding variables of retrospective methodology, several prospective trials have attempted to define the optimal therapy for ICH. To date, six randomized, prospective trials have compared surgical and medical management of ICH.[1, 94, 124, 145, 146, 177] This section compares and contrasts those study designs and results in an effort to determine guidelines for planning more conclusive studies.

In the first prospective study of ICH, McKissock and coworkers[1] stratified 180 of a series of 303 patients, aged 32 to 76 years, presenting to two hospitals between 1959 and 1960. Angiography diagnosed 60% of the cases, and ventriculography the remainder. All locations of ICH except the posterior fossa were included. Eighty-two patients were excluded because they died; recovered rapidly; or had a hemorrhage referable to a tumor, AVM, or aneurysm. The end point was death or level of independence among survivors at 6 months. Independence was defined as the ability to resume a prior occupation. The overall mortality rate was 51%, with an insignificant difference between surgical and conservative management groups (75% and 62%, respectively, at 6 months). Surgical treatment, however, was associated with increased odds of being dead or dependent at 6 months (odds ratio [OR] 2.04; 95% confidence interval [CI] 1.04 to 3.98).[178] This study, however, had several potential biases. The overall accuracy of the angiographic or ventriculographic diagnosis was a concern. Was the randomization concealed, and was the evaluator blinded? Further, the relatively high mortality rate may reflect the selection of severe cases unlikely to benefit from intervention.

In the study of Juvela and colleagues,[145] 52 patients

TABLE 105–3 ■ Summary of Retrospective Trials: Surgery versus Medical Therapy for Intracerebral Hemorrhage

AUTHORS	YEAR	TOTAL CASES		PREOPERATIVE NEUROLOGICAL GRADE		GOOD OUTCOME (ADL 1, 2) (%)		FAIR OUTCOME (ADL 3) (%)		POOR OUTCOME (ADL 4, 5) (%)		GROUP STRATIFIED MORTALITY (%)		OUTCOME	OVERALL MORTALITY (%)
		Surgical	Medical	Surgical	Medical	Surgical	Medical	Surgical	Medical	Surgical	Medical	Surgical	Medical		
Guillaume et al	1957	128	—	N/A		N/A		N/A		N/A		N/A			41 (32)
McKissock et al	1961	89	91	N/A		10 (11)	12 (13)	8 (9)	21 (23)	13 (15)	15 (17)	58 (65)	46 (51)		89 (58)
Cuatico et al	1965	99	—	2.6	—	35 (35)		23 (23)		33 (33)					8 (8)
Mitsuno et al	1966	43	—	N/A		N/A		N/A		N/A		N/A			19 (43)
Luessenhop et al	1967	37	27	N/A		N/A		N/A		N/A		12 (32)	12 (44)		24 (38)
Scott & Werthan	1970	17	25	3.2	2.8	3 (18)	4 (16)	3 (18)	2 (8)	0 (0)	3 (12)	11 (65)	15 (60)		23 (55)
Mitsuno et al	1971	514	436	N/A		N/A		N/A		N/A		N/A			180 (35)
Mizukami et al	1972	72	—	N/A		N/A		N/A		N/A		N/A			19 (26)
Paillas & Alliez	1973	137	—	N/A		N/A		N/A		N/A		N/A			64 (47)
Kanaya & Handa	1974	1558	—	N/A		N/A		N/A		N/A		N/A			476 (31)
Tedeschi et al	1975	57	14	N/A		8 (14)	0 (0)	13 (23)	2 (14)	14 (25)	6 (43)	22 (39)	6 (43)		28 (39)
Kanaya et al	1976	174	—	N/A		N/A		N/A		N/A		N/A			59 (33.9)
Kanaya et al	1978	410	204	1		(89)	(89)	N/A		N/A		(2.7)	(2.0)	At 6 mo	(25.9)
				2		(59)	(59)					(9.3)	(9.3)		
				3		(33)	(5)					(17.8)	(52.7)		
				4A		(47)	(8)					(28.2)	(58.2)		
				4B		(0)	(0)					(57.1)	(100.0)		
				5		(0)	(0)					(87.5)	(100.0)		
Matsumoto et al	1980	94	—	1		(92)	—	(0)	—	(0)	—	(8)	—		(13)
				2		(50)	—	(50)	—	(0)	—	(0)	—		
				3		(58)	—	(38)	—	(0)	—	(4)	—		
				4A		(0)	—	(25)	—	(50)	—	(25)	—		
				4B		(0)	—	(0)	—	(50)	—	(50)	—		
				5		(0)	—	(0)	—	(0)	—	(0)	—		
Kanaya et al	1981	3216	—	1		(61.6)	—	(34.7)	—	(3.7)	—	(5.3)	—	At 6 mo	(20.7)
				2		(55.9)	—	(37.2)	—	(6.9)	—	(9.4)	—		
				3		(38.7)	—	(45.4)	—	(15.9)	—	(16.8)	—		
				4A		(27.2)	—	(44.0)	—	(28.8)	—	(29.3)	—		
				4B		(16.2)	—	(47.6)	—	(36.2)	—	(57.8)	—		
				5		(0)	—	(15.4)	—	(84.6)	—	(75.9)	—		
Kaneko et al*	1983	100	87	1		(0)	(81)	(0)	(19)	(0)	(0)	(0)	(0)	Overall:	(22)
				2		(70)	(47)	(20)	(33)	(0)	(13)	(10)	(7)	Total surgical:	(7)
				3		(53)	(8)	(37)	(39)	(6)	(31)	(4)	(23)	Total medical:	(39)
				4A		(39)	(0)	(28)	(0)	(33)	(50)	(0)	(50)		
				4B		(0)	(0)	(25)	(0)	(0)	(0)	(75)	(100)		
				5		(0)	(0)	(0)	(0)	(0)	(4)	(0)	(96)		
Zuccarello et al	1983	167	139	N/A		N/A		N/A		N/A		(52.1)	(21.5)		
Bolander et al[†]	1983	39	35	N/A		(16)	(16)	(19)	(28)	(38)	(25)	(27)	(29)	At 3 mo	
Brambilla et al	1983	37	49	N/A		N/A		N/A		N/A		(52)	(43)	At 30 days	
Volpin et al	1984	32	34	1		(100)	(67)	(0)	(33)	(0)	(0)	(0)	(0)		(16) (32)
				2		(100)	(71)	(0)	(21)	(0)	(0)	(0)	(7)		
				3		(20)	(16.7)	(60)	(33)	(0)	(0)	(0)	(50)		
				4A, 4B, 5		(18)	(0)	(50)	(0)	(9)	(0)	(23)	(100)		
Kanno et al*	1984	154	305	Mild		(84.4)	(83)	(7.4)	(7.5)	(7.4)	(9.4)				
				Moderate		(36.6)	(30)	(30.0)	(5.0)						
				Severe		(41.0)	(45)	(33.0)	(54.0)						
				Fulminant		N/A		N/A							
				Very severe		(0)	(0)	(0)	(0)						
Coraddu et al[‡]	1990	31	28	N/A		N/A		N/A		N/A		(17)	(0)	At 30 days	

* Putamen.
[†] All locations.
[‡] Supra- and infratentorial.
ADL, activities of daily living; N/A, data not available.
Neurological grades: 1, alert or confused; 2, somnolent; 3, stuporous; 4A, semicomatose without herniation signs; 4B, semicomatose with herniation signs; 5, deep coma.

Japanese Cooperative Study - Retrospective

Surgical Treatment

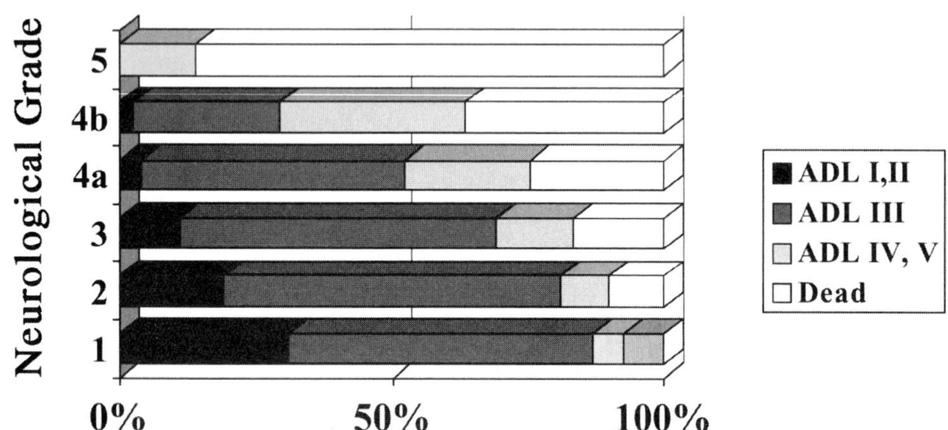

Medical Treatment

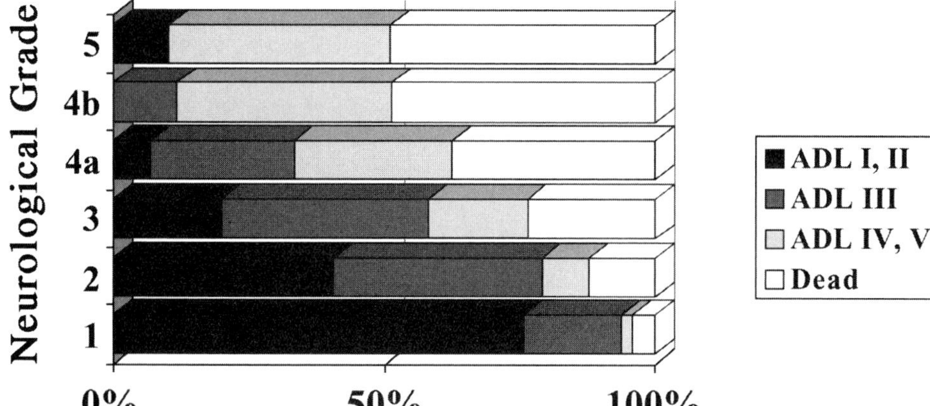

FIGURE 105–15. Outcome data calculated from the retrospective Japanese Cooperative Study[176] indicate that outcome after medical or surgical treatment is heavily dependent on admission grade. Survival is improved in the surgical group.

aged 15 to 65 years, admitted to one hospital between 1982 and 1985, were randomized for surgery or conservative therapy. CT established the diagnosis in all cases. Patients were included if they presented within 24 hours of the onset of symptoms. Patients were not stratified by hematoma location, but cerebellar hemorrhages were excluded. Patients were included if they were unconscious but reacting to pain or if they had severe hemiparesis or dysphasia. Patients were excluded if they were improving rapidly or not responding to pain and if they had a poor medical prognosis or a tumor, AVM, or aneurysm. Patients were "randomly allocated" (method of randomization not described) to surgery ($n = 26$) within 48 hours or to medical therapy ($n = 26$). Medical therapy was not described, except that corticosteroids were not given. An investigator who did not perform the surgery assessed outcomes. The end points were level of dependence at 1, 6, and 12 months using the Glasgow Outcome Scale. The results suggested a trend toward a higher level of dependence with surgical treatment (OR 5.95; 95%).[178] Subgroup analysis, however, showed that patients with admission GCS scores between 7 and 10 who underwent surgery had a significantly lower mortality rate than those treated conservatively (0% versus 80%). Groups were not well balanced. The surgical group had significantly lower preoperative GCS scores and a higher number of patients with intraven-

Retrospective Series - Metanalysis

Surgical Treatment

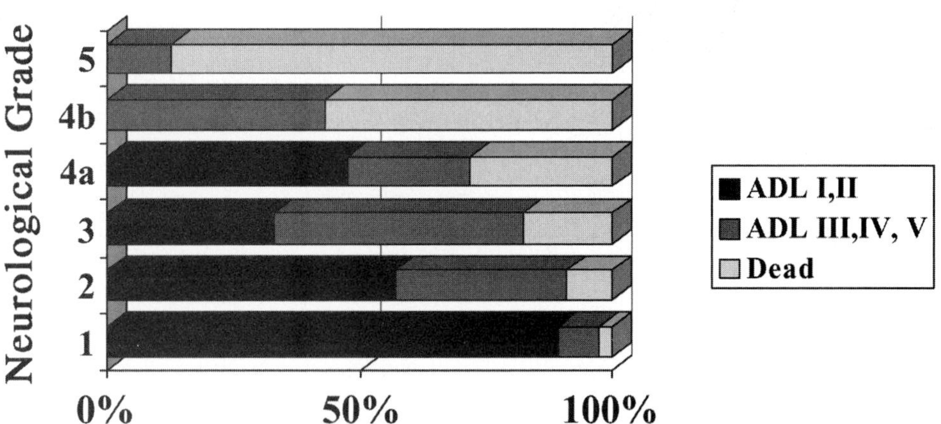

Medical Treatment

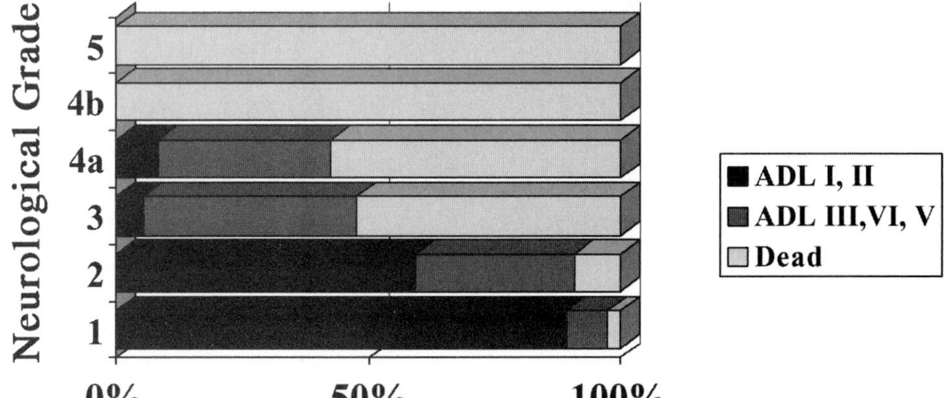

FIGURE 105–16. Outcome data calculated from a meta-analysis of published retrospective trials echo the Japanese experience illustrated in Figure 105–15.

TABLE 105–4 ■ **Summary of Retrospective Stereotactic Evacuation Studies**

AUTHOR	YEAR	TOTAL CASES	AVERAGE VOLUME EVACUATED	MEAN PREOPERATIVE CT GRADE	MEAN TIME OF ONSET TO ASPIRATION (hr)	MEAN PREOPERATIVE NEUROLOGICAL STATUS	ADL (1,2,3) INDEPENDENT AT 6 MO (%)	ADL (4,5) DEPENDENT AT 6 MO (%)	DEAD AT 6 MO (%)	REBLEED (%)
All locations										
Niizuma	1985	97	>50% in 56 30%–49% in 29 <29% in 12	N/A	N/A	1.7	41 (71)	17 (26)	3 (3)	(7)
Kanaya	1990	569	N/A	N/A	N/A	2.0	447 (79)	57 (10)	65 (11)	(11)
Putamen										
Matsumoto	1984	34	33.9%	IIIa	64.6 (4–672)	2.7	24 (71)	4 (11)	6 (18)	(5.9)
Tanikawa	1985	28	N/A	II	N/A	1.5	26 (93)	2 (7.2)	0 (0)	(3.6)
Niizuma	1988	9	>80%	IIIb	14.6	2.2	9 (100)	0 (0)	0 (0)	(0)
Niizuma	1989	175	>80% in 75 (43) 50%–79% in 59 (34) 30%–49% in 30 (17)	III	6–24 hr in 87 24–48 hr in 42 48–72 hr in 21 96–168 hr in 15 >168 hr in 10	1.6	151 (86)	12 (6.9)	10 (5.7)	(7.4)
Hondo	1990	258	N/A	N/A	N/A	N/A	N/A	N/A	69 (27)	N/A
Thalamus										
Matsumoto	1984	3	29.1%	IIIa	18.7	3.3	2 (66)	1 (33)	0 (0)	(0)
Hondo	1990	99	N/A	N/A	N/A	N/A	N/A	N/A	23 (23)	N/A
Niizuma	1990	75	>80% in 30 50%–70% in 36 <40% in 9 61 of 77 IVH	N/A	N/A	1.8	60 (80)	10 (13)	5 (7)	(3)

ADL, activities of daily living; CT, computed tomography; IVH, intraventricular hemorrhage; N/A, data not available.

tricular hemorrhages. Further, increased ICP was reported as the cause of death in 68% of the patients,[179] raising several questions: Was ICP monitored continuously? What was ICP before randomization? How was elevated ICP treated?

Batjer and coworkers[94] prospectively randomized 21 patients with putaminal ICH, aged 30 to 75 years, to receive medical therapy, medical therapy and ICP monitoring, or surgery. Patients were admitted to one hospital between 1983 and 1989. Patients were included if they had a CT diagnosis of putaminal hemorrhage at least 3 cm in diameter; a history of hypertension; and were alert with hemiparesis (≤2/5), lethargic with hemiparesis (≤2/5), or obtunded or stuporous but with purposeful movement on the unaffected side. Patients were excluded if they had end-stage systemic disease, coagulopathy, positive angiography (aneurysm, AVM, tumor), or unassociated neurological disease. Outcomes were assessed by one of the investigators (unknown whether the assessor was blind to treatment modality). The end points were levels of independence at 3 and 6 months. The study was stopped prematurely because of "miserable" functional outcomes. No patients were able to return to their prestroke activities. There were no significant differences among treatment outcomes. Only 22% and 28% in the medically and surgically treated groups, respectively, had "favorable" outcomes. There was a trend toward a lower rate of death or dependence with surgery (OR 0.86; CI 0.09 to 8.1).[178]

Auer and associates[124] randomized 100 patients with supratentorial ICH (subcortical, thalamic, or putaminal), aged 30 to 80 years, to receive either medical therapy or endoscopic evacuation of the hematoma. Patients were admitted to one hospital between 1983 and 1986. Inclusion criteria were as follows: hematoma less than 10 cm^3, neurological deficit or impaired consciousness, less than 48 hours elapsed from onset of symptoms, medical clearance, and negative unilateral angiography. The outcome event was death or level of dependence at 6 months. Results of this study are summarized in Table 105–5.

Based on a meta-analysis of four prospective randomized trials, Hankey and Hon[178] suggested that endoscopic evaluation is associated with less chance of death or dependence at 6 months. The results also suggest that surgery in patients with *subcortical* hematomas yields significantly lower mortality rates and more favorable outcomes than medical treatment does (40% versus 70% and 40% versus 25%, respectively, at 6 months). Subgroup analysis suggests that surgery affects outcome differently with respect to hematoma volume. Patients with subcortical hematomas larger than 50 cm^3 who underwent surgery had a lower mortality rate than their medically treated counterparts but showed no difference in terms of functional outcome. In contrast, patients with subcortical hematomas less than 50 cm^3 who underwent surgery had better functional outcomes, but there was no difference in mortality rate. In addition, patients who were younger than 60 years had a higher incidence of good outcome and a lower mortality rate. No differences with regard to mortality or independence were cited for treatment modalities for thalamic or putaminal hemorrhages. Hankey and Hon concluded that "patients with subcortical hematomas <50 cm^3, >60 years old who were alert or somnolent significantly benefited from surgery."[178]

A critical analysis of Hankey and Hon's study, however, labeled their results a statistical "misinterpretation." Prasad and colleagues[179] noted that using multiple significance tests on multiple outcome categories unavoidably results in inappropriate subgroup analysis. In their reanalysis using the single outcome of "independence at 6 months," surgery was found to reduce the proportion of dead or dependent patients by 18%. Their stratified analysis using the Brelow-Day technique showed that functional outcome in patients with hematomas larger than 50 cm^3 (*not* <50 cm^3, as suggested by the original authors) was strongly affected by surgery. The role of surgery is therefore inconclusive.

Zucarrello and coworkers[146] prospectively randomized 20 patients to either medical therapy or craniotomy or stereotactic evacuation to evaluate the feasibility of early surgery. The patients included in the study were diagnosed by CT; had ICHs greater than 10 cm^3, a focal neurological deficit, and a GCS score less than 4; and were treated within 24 hours. The median time from onset of symptoms to surgery was 8.5 hours. There was no significant difference in mortality rates between the surgical and medical treatment groups (22% versus 27%). At 3 months, however, there was a significant trend toward decreased morbidity in patients undergoing surgery compared with those receiving conservative treatment (National Institutes of Health Stroke Survey score of 14 versus 4; $P = 0.04$). Despite evidence that early surgery (within 6 hours) may prevent progression of hemorrhage or secondary insults, the results of this study suggest that there may be limitations. Conclusions are also biased by the use of stereotactic evacuation based on location (deep versus superficial).

Morgenstern and colleagues[177] prospectively randomized 34 patients within 12 hours of symptom onset. Patients were diagnosed by CT and had ICHs less than 9 cm^3, lobar or putaminal hematomas without thalamic extension, GCS scores between 5 and 15, and Rankin scores greater than 2 (before hemorrhage). Patients with hematomas between 10 and 19 cm^3 with GCS scores of 15 and antigravity strength on the affected side were excluded. At 6 months, the mortality rates associated with surgical or medical treatment were not significantly different (17% versus 24%). There was a slight increase in the length of survival of surgically treated patients with hematoma volumes between 26 and 85 cm^3. The study, however, had a small sample and was conducted at a single site. The study population was biased, with more cases of lobar ICHs and patients with poor neurological grades in the surgical group.

Table 105–5 summarizes the salient features of the studies discussed earlier. Based on available data, we calculated the individual OR that medical therapy is

TABLE 105-5 ■ **Summary of Prospective Randomized Controlled Trials: Surgery versus Medical Therapy in Intracerebral Hemorrhage**

AUTHOR	YEAR	LOCATION	INCLUSION CRITERIA	TOTAL CASES	MEAN HEMATOMA SIZE	PREOPERATIVE NEUROLOGICAL STATUS	INDEPENDENT AT 6 MO (%)	DEPENDENT AT 6 MO	DEAD AT 6 MO (%)	TIME (hr) FROM ONSET TO SURGERY (MEAN)	ODDS RATIO (95% CI)	COMMENTS
Open Craniotomy												
McKissock	1961	All	Not clear	S 89 M 91	N/A	Equal groups	S 18 (20) M 31 (34)	S 13 (15) M 14 (15)	S 58 (65) M 46 (51)	72	2.04 (1.04–3.98)	Method of randomization not described Pre-CT era
Juvela	1989	All	"Unconscious and/or severe hemiparesis or dysphasia" Excluded patients "not responding to pain"	S 26 M 26	S 56.2 cc M 66.7 cc	S 9 M 12 (mean GCS)	S 1 (4) M 5 (19)	S 13 (50) M 11 (42)	S 12 (46) M 10 (39)	48 (14.5)	5.95	Surgical group with overall lower pretreatment GCS and increased incidence of IVH ($P < 0.05$) 4 patients in ICP and medically managed group
Batjer	1990	Putamen	>3 cm diameter ICH, alert & ≤2/5, lethargic & ≤2/5, obtunded, or stuporous but purposeful with hemiplegia	S 8 M 9	> 3 cm	S 2 M 2 (# of patients in grade 3)	S 2 (25) M 2 (22)	S 2 (25) M 0 (0)	S 4 (50) M 7 (78)	24	0.86 (0.09–8.09)	Not clear if assessor blinded Exact time to surgery not mentioned

Morgenstern	1998	Lobe Putamen	GCS 5–15 ICH > 9 cc Exclude: Large IVH, GCS 15 & 10–20 cc & antigravity strength	S 17 M 17	S 49.0 cc M 43.8 cc	S 10 M 11 (mean GCS)	S 6 (35) M 7 (41)	S 8 (47) M 6 (35)	S 3 (18) M 4 (24)	12 (8.3)	1.28	Single site Small sample size Surgical group mostly lobar ICH Surgical group worse pretreatment neurological grade
Zucarrello	1999	All	Age > 18 yr ICH > 10 cc & focal neurological deficit GCS > 4 <24 hr from onset	S 9 M 11	S 35.0 cc M 30.0 cc (median)	S 12.2 M 10.2 (mean GCS)	S 5 (56) M 4 (36)	S 2 (22) M 4 (36)	S 2 (22) M 3 (18)	24 (8.5)	0.45	4/9 cases done stereotactically
Subtotal				S 149 M 154			S 32 (22) M 49 (32)	S 38 (26) M 35 (23)	S 79 (53) M 71 (46)		*1.71*	
Endoscopic												
Auer	1989	All	>10 cc ICH <48 hr from onset Age 30–80 yr "With neurological deficit and/or disturbance of consciousness"	S 50 M 50	S 44% M 48% (>50 cc)		S 22 (44) M 13 (26)	S 7 (14) M 2 (4)	S 21 (42) M 35 (70)	48	0.45 (0.19–1.98)	Did not use valid statistical subgroup analysis No statistical adjustments made for multiple testing of multiple outcome categories
Total				S 199 M 204			S 54 (27) M 62 (44)	S 45 (23) M 37 (18)	S 100 (50) M 106 (62)		1.21	

CI, confidence interval; CT, computed tomography; GCS, Glasgow Coma Scale; ICH, intracerebral hematoma; IVH, intraventricular hemorrhage; M, medical group; S, surgical group.

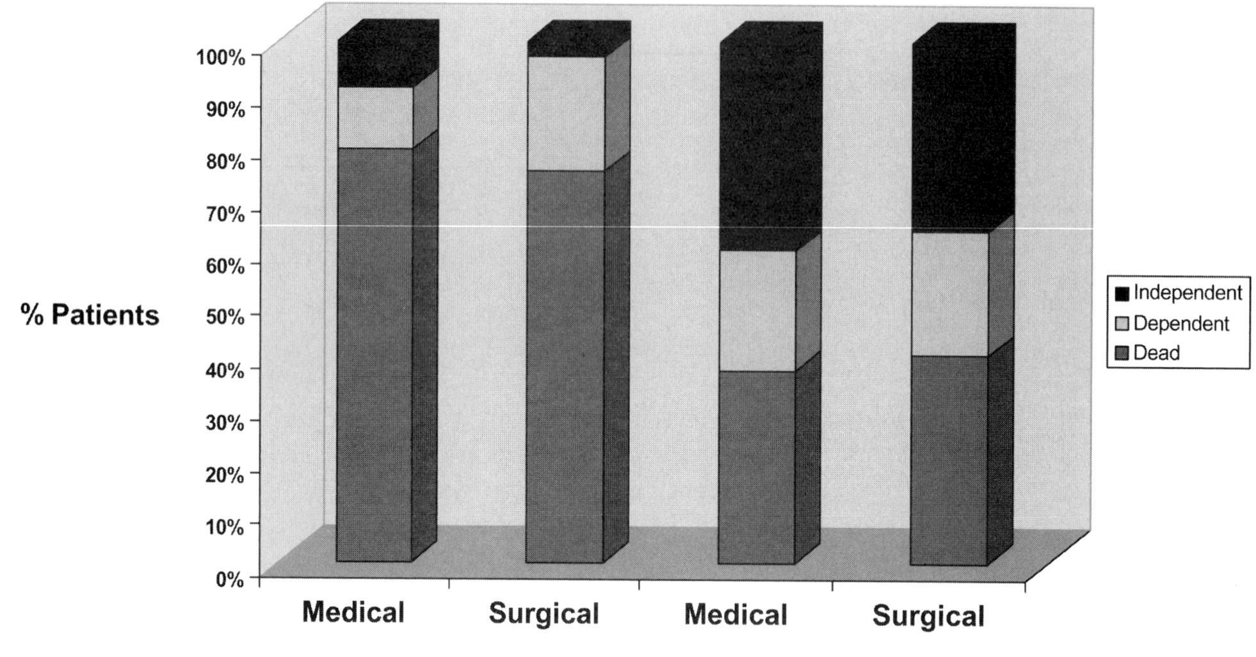

FIGURE 105–17. Outcome data pooled from prospective published reports. At best, there is a weak trend in favor of surgical evacuation in patients with Glasgow Coma Scale scores less than 11, and no advantage for better-grade patients. Very few patients, however, underwent "hyperacute" evacuation.

superior to surgery and included our comments. Figure 105–17 illustrates the collective outcome from these studies for both treatment groups based on admission GCS scores (<11 or >11).

CONCLUSION

Spontaneous ICH not related to an AVM or aneurysm (i.e., predominantly hypertensive) remains a perplexing clinical problem. The avenues already explored regarding best management have yielded controversial results. It may hold true that *immediate* and *aggressive* medical care in an intensive care unit setting, emphasizing the control of blood pressure, offers the best chance of recovery for mildly disabled patients at ictus. It may also hold true that emergency surgical evacuation of a large hematoma offers devastated patients the best chance of survival, but without much recovery of function over and above what medical management might have achieved. The fate of "middle-grade" patients, however, remains unclear. One of the most pressing questions that must be answered in a rigorous prospective fashion is whether hyperacute surgical intervention benefits any or all patients. Without such a trial, we have chosen to rely on level 2 evidence and continue to assume and to advocate that a hypertensive putaminal, lobar, or subcortical ICH large enough to cause moderate deficits is an acute "brain attack" that needs to be evacuated emergently by standard open microsurgical techniques.

REFERENCES

1. McKissock W, Richardson A, Taylor J: Primary intracerebral hemorrhage: A controlled trial of surgical and conservative treatment in 180 unselected cases. Lancet 2:221–226, 1961.
2. Magladery JW: The natural course of cerebrovascular hemorrhage. Clin Neurosurg 9:106–113, 1963.
3. Walton J: Subarachnoid Hemorrhage. Baltimore, Williams & Wilkins, 1956.
4. Donley J: John James Wepfer: A renaissance student of apoplexy. Bull Johns Hopkins Hosp 20:1–2, 1909.
5. Clarke E: Cerebrovascular system—historical aspects. In Newton T, Potts D (eds): Radiology of the Skull and Brain, vol 2, book 1. Great Neck, NY, Mosby, 1974, pp 875–889.
6. Fazio C: Clinical pathology of hypertensive intracerebral hemorrhage: Historical aspects. In Mizukami M, Kogure K, Kanaya H, Yamori Y (eds): Hypertensive Intracerebral Hemorrhage. New York, Raven Press, 1983, pp 105–113.
7. MacEwen W: An address on the surgery of the brain and spinal cord. BMJ 2:302–309, 1888.
8. Cushing H: The blood-pressure reaction of acute cerebral compression, illustrated by cases of intracranial hemorrhage. Am J Med Sci 125:1017–1044, 1903.
9. Bagley CJ: Spontaneous cerebral hemorrhage: Discussion of four

types, with surgical considerations. Arch Neurol Psychiatry 27: 1133–1174, 1932.

10. Robinson G: Encapsulated brain hemorrhages: A study of their frequency and pathology. Arch Neurol Psychiatry 27:1441–1444, 1932.
11. Craig W, Adson A: Spontaneous intracerebral hemorrhage: Etiology and surgical treatment with a report of nine cases. Arch Neurol Psychiatry 35:701–714, 1936.
12. Penfield W: The operative treatment of spontaneous intracerebral hemorrhage. Can Med Assoc J 28:369–379, 1933.
13. Lazorthes G: Surgery of cerebral hemorrhage: Report on the results of 52 surgically treated cases. J Neurosurg 16:355–364, 1959.
14. Guillaume J, Roger R, Maxars G, et al: Indications chirurgicales dans les hemorragies cerebrales. Presse Med 63:827–829, 1957.
15. Massaro AR, Sacco RL, Mohr JP, et al: Clinical discriminators of lobar and deep hemorrhages: The Stroke Data Bank. Neurology 41:1881–1885, 1991.
16. Broderick JP, Brott T, Tomsick T, et al: Intracerebral hemorrhage more than twice as common as subarachnoid hemorrhage. J Neurosurg 78:188–191, 1993.
17. Bogousslavsky J, Van Melle G, Regli F: The Lausanne Stroke Registry: Analysis of 1000 consecutive patients with first stroke. Stroke 19:1083–1092, 1988.
18. Bozzola F, Gorelick P, Jensen J: Epidemiology of intracranial hemorrhage. Neuroimaging Clin N Am 2:1–14, 1992.
19. Portenoy RK, Lipton RB, Berger AR: Intracerebral haemorrhage: A model for the prediction of outcome. J Neurol Neurosurg Psychiatry 50:976–979, 1987.
20. Sacco RL, Wolf PA, Bharucha NE: Subarachnoid and intracerebral hemorrhage: Natural history, prognosis, and precursive factors in the Framingham study. Neurology 34:847–854, 1984.
21. Drury I, Whisnant JP, Garraway WM: Primary intracerebral hemorrhage: Impact of CT on incidence. Neurology 34:653–657, 1984.
22. Fieschi C, Carolei A, Fiorelli M: Changing prognosis of primary intracerebral hemorrhage: Results of a clinical and computed tomographic follow up study of 104 patients. Stroke 19:192–195, 1988.
23. Garraway WM, Whisnant JP, Furlan AJ: The declining incidence of stroke. N Engl J Med 300:449–452, 1979.
24. Schutz H, Bodeker RH, Damian M, et al: Age-related spontaneous intracerebral hematoma in a German community. Stroke 21: 1412–1418, 1990.
25. Whisnant JP, Cartlidge NE, Elveback LR: Carotid and vertebral-basilar transient ischemic attacks: Effect of anticoagulants, hypertension and cardiac disorders on survival and stroke occurrence—a population study. Ann Neurol 3:107–115, 1978.
26. Weiner M, Piepgras D: Surgical management of primary intracerebral hemorrhage. In Schmidek HH, Sweet WH (eds): Operative Neurosurgical Techniques: Indications, Methods and Results, 3rd ed. Philadelphia, WB Saunders, 1995, pp 929–936.
27. Waga S, Miyazaki M, Okada M, et al: Hypertensive putaminal hemorrhage: Analysis of 182 patients. Surg Neurol 26:159–166, 1986.
28. Shi FL, Hart RG, Sherman DG, et al: Stroke in the People's Republic of China. Stroke 20:1581–1585, 1989.
29. Kunitz SC, Gross CR, Heyman A, et al: The Pilot Stroke Data Bank: Definition, design, and data. Stroke 15:740–746, 1984.
30. Mizukami M, Nishijima M, Kin H: Computed tomographic findings of good prognosis for hemiplegia in hypertensive putaminal hemorrhage. Stroke 12:648–652, 1981.
31. Matsumoto N, Whisnant JP, Kurland L, et al: Natural history of stroke in Rochester, Minnesota, 1955 through 1969: An extension of a previous study, 1945 through 1954. Stroke 4:20–29, 1973.
32. Abu-Zied HA, Choi NW, Maini KK: Relative role of factors associated with cerebral infarction and cerebral hemorrhage: A matched pair case-control study. Stroke 8:106–112, 1977.
33. Robins M, Baum HM: The National Survey of Stroke: Incidence. Stroke 12(Pt 2, Suppl 1):I45–I57, 1981.
34. Brott T, Broderick J, Kothari R, et al: Early hemorrhage growth in patients with intracerebral hemorrhage. Stroke 28:1–5, 1997.
35. Hart RG, Boop BS, Anderson DC: Oral anticoagulants and intracranial hemorrhage: Facts and hypotheses. Stroke 26:1471–1477, 1995.
36. Kase CS, Robinson RK, Stein RW, et al: Anticoagulant-related intracerebral hemorrhage. Neurology 35:943–948, 1985.
37. Franke CL, de Jonge J, van Swieten JC, et al: Intracerebral hematomas during anticoagulant treatment. Stroke 21:726–730, 1990.
38. Kase C, Mohr J, Caplan L: Intracerebral hemorrhage. In Barnett HH (ed): Stroke: Pathophysiology, Diagnosis and Management. New York, Churchill Livingstone, 1999, pp 649–700.
39. Algra A: Bleeding complications in patients after cerebral ischemia treated with anticoagulant drugs [abstract]. Stroke 28:231–235, 1997.
40. Radberg JA, Olsson JE, Radberg CT: Prognostic parameters in spontaneous intracerebral hematomas with special reference to anticoagulant treatment. Stroke 22:571–576, 1991.
41. Caplan L: Intracerebral hemorrhage. In Tyler H, Dawson D (eds): Current Neurology, vol 2. Boston, Houghton Mifflin, 1979, pp 185–205.
42. Charmorro A, Vila N, Saiz A, et al: Early anticoagulation after large cerebral embolic infarction: A safety study. Neurology 45: 861–865, 1995.
43. Mayo NE, Levy AR, Goldberg MS: Aspirin and hemorrhagic stroke. Stroke 22:1213–1214, 1991.
44. Camerlingo M, Casto L, Censori B, et al: Immediate anticoagulation with heparin for first-ever ischemic stroke in the carotid artery territories observed within 5 hours of onset. Arch Neurol 51:462–467, 1994.
45. Pessin MS, Del Zoppo GJ, Estol CJ: Thrombolytic agents in the treatment of stroke. Clin Neuropharmacol 13:271–289, 1990.
46. Hacke W, Kaste M, Fieschi C, et al: Intravenous thrombolysis with recombinant tissue plasminogen activator for acute hemispheric stroke: The European Cooperative Acute Stroke Study. JAMA 274:1017–1025, 1995.
47. National Institutes of Neurological Disorders and Stroke rt-PA Stroke Study Group: Tissue plasminogen activator for acute ischemic stroke. N Engl J Med 333:1581–1587, 1995.
48. Norrving B: Cerebral hemorrhage. In Ginsberg M, Bogousslavsky J (eds): Cerebrovascular Disease: Pathophysiology, Diagnosis and Management. Cambridge, Mass, Blackwell Science, 1999, pp 1447–1473.
49. Levine SR, Brust JC, Futrell N, et al: Cerebrovascular complications of the use of the "crack" form of alkaloidal cocaine. N Engl J Med 323:699–704, 1990.
50. Kase CS, Foster TE, Reed JE, et al: Intracerebral hemorrhage and phenylpropanolamine use. Neurology 37:399–404, 1987.
51. Delaney P, Estes M: Intracranial hemorrhage with amphetamine abuse. Neurology 30:1125–1128, 1980.
52. Gilbert JJ, Vinters HV: Cerebral amyloid angiopathy: Incidence and complications in the aging brain. I. Cerebral hemorrhage. Stroke 14:915–923, 1983.
53. Vinters HV: Cerebral amyloid angiopathy: A critical review. Stroke 18:311–324, 1987.
54. Gilles C, Brucher JM, Khoubesserian P, et al: Cerebral amyloid angiopathy as a cause of multiple intracerebral hemorrhages. Neurology 34:730–735, 1984.
55. Vonsattel JP, Myers RH, Hedley-Whyte ET, et al: Cerebral amyloid angiopathy without and with cerebral hemorrhages: A comparative histological study. Ann Neurol 30:637–649, 1991.
56. Little JR, Dial B, Bellanger G, et al: Brain hemorrhage from intracranial tumor. Stroke 10:283–288, 1979.
57. Wakai S, Yamakawa K, Manaka S, et al: Spontaneous intracranial hemorrhage caused by brain tumors: Its incidence and clinical significance. Neurosurgery 10:437–444, 1982.
58. Charcot J, Bouchard C: Nouvelles recherches sur la pathogenie de l'hemorragie cerebrale. Arch Physiol Norm Pathol 1:110–127, 643–665, 725–734, 1868.
59. Ellis A: The pathogenesis of spontaneous cerebral hemorrhage. Proc Pathol Soc 12:197–235, 1909.
60. Ross-Russell RW: Observations on intracerebral aneurysms. Brain 86:425–442, 1963.
61. Cole FM, Yates P: Intracerebral microaneurysms and small cerebrovascular lesions. Brain 90:759–768, 1967.
62. Cole FM, Yates PO: The occurrence and significance of intracerebral microaneurysms. J Pathol Bacteriol 93:393–411, 1967.
63. Mohr JP, Caplan LR, Melski JW, et al: The Harvard Cooperative Stroke Registry: A prospective registry. Neurology 28:754–762, 1978.

64. Heros R: Cerebellar hemorrhage and infarction. Stroke 13:106–109, 1982.
65. Ojemann RG, Heros RC: Spontaneous brain hemorrhage. Stroke 14:468–475, 1976.
66. Fisher C: Clinical syndromes in cerebral hemorrhage. In Fields W (ed): Pathogenesis and Treatment of Cerebrovascular Disease. Springfield, Ill, Charles C Thomas, 1961, p 318.
67. Stein RW, Kase CS, Hier DB, et al: Caudate hemorrhage. Neurology 34:1549–1554, 1984.
68. Hier DB, Davis KR, Richardson EP Jr, et al: Hypertensive putaminal hemorrhage. Ann Neurol 1:152–159, 1977.
69. Walshe TM, Davis KR, Fisher CM: Thalamic hemorrhage: A computed tomographic–clinical correlation. Neurology 27:217–222, 1977.
70. Ojemann RG, Mohr JP: Hypertensive brain hemorrhage. Clin Neurosurg 23:220–244, 1976.
71. Barraquer-Bordas L, Illa I, Escartin A, et al: Thalamic hemorrhage: A study of 23 patients with diagnosis by computed tomography. Stroke 12:524–527, 1981.
72. Fazio C, Sacco G, Bugiani O: The thalamic hemorrhage: An anatomo-clinical study. Eur Neurol 9:30–43, 1973.
73. Kase CS, Williams JP, Wyatt DA, et al: Lobar intracerebral hematomas: Clinical and CT analysis of 22 cases. Neurology 32: 1146–1150, 1982.
74. Ropper AH, Davis KR: Lobar cerebral hemorrhages: Acute clinical syndromes in 26 cases. Ann Neurol 8:141–147, 1980.
75. McCormick WF, Rosenfield DB: Massive brain hemorrhage: A review of 144 cases and an examination of their causes. Stroke 4:946–954, 1973.
76. Tyler KL, Poletti CE, Heros RC: Cerebral amyloid angiopathy. J Neurosurg 57:286–289, 1982.
77. Finelli PF, Kessimian N, Bernstein PW: Cerebral amyloid angiopathy manifesting as recurrent intracerebral hemorrhage. Arch Neurol 41:330–333, 1984.
78. Weisberg LA: Subcortical lobar intracerebral haemorrhage: Clinical–computed tomographic correlations. J Neurol Neurosurg Psychiatry 48:1078–1084, 1985.
79. Helweg-Larsen S, Sommer W, Strange P, et al: Prognosis for patients treated conservatively for spontaneous intracerebral hematomas. Stroke 15:1045–1048, 1984.
80. Dinsdale HB: Spontaneous hemorrhage in the posterior fossa: A study of primary cerebellar and pontine hemorrhages with observations on their pathogenesis. Arch Neurol 10:200–217, 1964.
81. Freeman RE, Onofrio BM, Okazaki H, et al: Spontaneous intracerebellar hemorrhage: Diagnosis and surgical treatment. Neurology 23:84–90, 1973.
82. Brennan RW, Bergland RM: Acute cerebellar hemorrhage: Analysis of clinical findings and outcome in 12 cases. Neurology 27: 527–532, 1977.
83. Fisher CM, Picard EH, Polak A, et al: Acute hypertensive cerebellar hemorrhage: Diagnosis and surgical treatment. J Nerv Ment Dis 140:38–57, 1965.
84. Ott KH, Kase CS, Ojemann RG, et al: Cerebellar hemorrhage: Diagnosis and treatment. A review of 56 cases. Arch Neurol 31: 160–167, 1974.
85. Fisher CM: Pathological observations in hypertensive cerebral hemorrhage. J Neuropathol Exp Neurol 30:536–550, 1971.
86. Yoshida S, Sasaki M, Oka H, et al: Acute hypertensive cerebellar hemorrhage with signs of lower brainstem compression. Surg Neurol 10:79–83, 1978.
87. Little JR, Tubman DE, Ethier R: Cerebellar hemorrhage in adults: Diagnosis by computerized tomography. J Neurosurg 48:575–579, 1978.
88. Elkind MS, Mohr JP: Cerebellar hemorrhage. New Horiz 5: 352–358, 1997.
89. Pollack L, Rebey JM, Gur R, et al: Indications to surgical management of cerebellar hemorrhage. Clin Neurol Neurosurg 100: 99–103, 1998.
90. Attwater H: Pontine hemorrhage. Guys Hosp Rep 65:339–389, 1911.
91. Duret H: Traumatismes Cranio-Cerebraux. Paris, Librairie Felix Alcan, 1919.
92. Silverstein A: Primary pontile hemorrhage: A review of 50 cases. Confin Neurol 29:33–46, 1967.
93. Steegmann A: Primary pontile hemorrhage. J Nerv Ment Dis 114:35–65, 1951.
94. Batjer HH, Reisch JS, Allen BC, et al: Failure of surgery to improve outcome in hypertensive putaminal hemorrhage: A prospective randomized trial. Arch Neurol 47:1103–1106, 1990.
95. Kutsuzawa T, Ito K, Kawakami H: [Conservative treatment of hypertensive cerebral hemorrhage: Results of 104 patients in the acute stage.] Neurol Med Chir (Tokyo) 16(Pt 2):29–36, 1976.
96. Scott M, Werthan M: The fate of hypertensive patients with clinically proven spontaneous intracerebral hematomas treated without intracranial surgery. Stroke 1:286–300, 1970.
97. Bae HG, Lee KS, Yun IG, et al: Rapid expansion of hypertensive intracerebral hemorrhage. Neurosurgery 31:35–41, 1992.
98. Kase C: Pathophysiology, diagnosis and management. In Kase C (ed): Stroke, vol 1. New York, Churchill Livingstone, 1986, pp 497–523.
99. Kelley RE, Berger JR, Scheinberg P, et al: Active bleeding in hypertensive intracerebral hemorrhage: Computed tomography. Neurology 32:852–856, 1982.
100. Zabramski JM, Hamilton MG: Intracerebral hematomas. In Spetzler RF, Carter LP, Hamilton MG (eds): Neurovascular Surgery. New York, McGraw-Hill, 1995, pp 477–496.
101. Crowell RM, Ojemann RG, Ogilvy CS: Brain hemorrhage. In Bucheit WA, Truex RCJ (eds): Surgery of the Posterior Fossa. New York, Raven Press, 1979, pp 562–576.
102. Nehls DG, Mendelow AD, Graham DI, et al: Experimental intracerebral hemorrhage: Progression of hemodynamic changes after production of a spontaneous mass lesion. Neurosurgery 23:439–444, 1988.
103. Mendelow AD: Mechanisms of ischemic brain damage with intracerebral hemorrhage. Stroke 24(Suppl):I115–I119, 1993.
104. Wagner KR, Xi G, Hua Y, et al: Lobar intracerebral hemorrhage model in pigs: Rapid edema development in perihematomal white matter. Stroke 27:490–497, 1996.
105. Broderick JP, Brott TG, Duldner JE, et al: Volume of intracerebral hemorrhage: A powerful and easy-to-use predictor of 30-day mortality. Stroke 24:987–993, 1993.
106. Fujitsu K, Muramoto M, Ikeda Y, et al: Indications for surgical treatment of putaminal hemorrhage: Comparative study based on serial CT and time-course analysis. J Neurosurg 73:518–525, 1990.
107. Tellez H, Bauer RB: Dexamethasone as treatment in cerebrovascular disease. 1. A controlled study in intracerebral hemorrhage. Stroke 4:541–546, 1973.
108. Poungvarin N, Bhoopat W, Viriyavejakul A: Effects of dexamethasone in primary supratentorial intracerebral hemorrhage. N Engl J Med 316:1229–1233, 1987.
109. Janny P, Papo I, Chazal J, et al: Intracranial hypertension and prognosis of spontaneous intracerebral haematomas: A correlative study of 60 patients. Acta Neurochir (Wien) 61:181–186, 1982.
110. Duff TA, Ayeni S, Levin AB, et al: Nonsurgical management of spontaneous intracerebral hematoma. Neurosurgery 9:387–393, 1981.
111. Yu YL, Kumana CR, Lauder IJ, et al: Treatment of acute cerebral hemorrhage with intravenous glycerol: A double-blind, placebo-controlled, randomized trial. Stroke 23:967–971, 1992.
112. Italian Acute Stroke Study Group: Haemodilution in acute stroke: Results of the Italian haemodilution trial. Lancet 1:318–321, 1988.
113. Nath FP, Jenkins A, Mendelow AD, et al: Early hemodynamic changes in experimental intracerebral hemorrhage. J Neurosurg 65:697–703, 1986.
114. Nehls DG, Mendelow DA, Graham DI, et al: Experimental intracerebral hemorrhage: Early removal of a spontaneous mass lesion improves late outcome. Neurosurgery 27:674–682, 1990.
115. Pia H: Spontaneous Intracerebral Hematomas. New York, Springer-Verlag, 1980.
116. Benes V, Koukolik F, Obrovska D: Two types of spontaneous intracerebral hemorrhage due to hypertension. J Neurosurg 37: 509–513, 1972.
117. Qureshi AI, Safdar K, Weil J, et al: Predictors of early deterioration and mortality in black Americans with spontaneous intracerebral hemorrhage. Stroke 26:1764–1767, 1995.
118. Papo I, Janny P, Caruselli G, et al: Intracranial pressure time

course in primary intracerebral hemorrhage. Neurosurgery 4: 504–511, 1979.
119. Ropper AH, Zervas NT: Cerebral blood flow after experimental basal ganglia hemorrhage. Ann Neurol 11:266–271, 1982.
120. Jenkins A, Mendelow AD, Graham DI, et al: Experimental intracerebral haematoma: The role of blood constituents in early ischaemia. Br J Neurosurg 4:45–51, 1990.
121. Niizuma H, Yonemitsu T, Jokura H, et al: Stereotactic aspiration of thalamic hematoma: Overall results of 75 aspirated and 70 nonaspirated cases. Stereotact Funct Neurosurg 55:438–444, 1990.
122. Hosaka Y, Kaneko M, Muraki M, et al: [Re-evaluation of the effect of the operation in the per-acute stage: Review of 166 cases of hypertensive intracerebral hemorrhage (the lateral type).] Neurol Med Chir (Tokyo) 20:907–913, 1980.
123. Daverat P, Castel JP, Dartigues JF, et al: Death and functional outcome after spontaneous intracerebral hemorrhage: A prospective study of 166 cases using multivariate analysis. Stroke 22:1–6, 1991.
124. Auer LM, Deinsberger W, Niederkorn K, et al: Endoscopic surgery versus medical treatment for spontaneous intracerebral hematoma: A randomized study. J Neurosurg 70:530–535, 1989.
125. Durward QJ, Barnett HJ, Barr HW: Presentation and management of mesencephalic hematoma: Report of two cases. J Neurosurg 56:123–127, 1982.
126. Kaufman HH, Schochet S: Pathology, pathophysiology, and modeling. In Kaufman HH (ed): Intracerebral Hematomas. New York, Raven Press, 1992, p 240.
127. Kwak R, Kadoya S, Suzuki T: Factors affecting the prognosis in thalamic hemorrhage. Stroke 14:493–500, 1983.
128. Volpin L, Cervellini P, Colombo F, et al: Spontaneous intracerebral hematomas: A new proposal about the usefulness and limits of surgical treatment. Neurosurgery 15:663–666, 1984.
129. Weisberg LA: Caudate hemorrhage. Arch Neurol 41:971–974, 1984.
130. Ojemann RG, Heros RC: Spontaneous brain hemorrhage. Stroke 14:468–475, 1983.
131. Almaani WS, Awidi AS: Spontaneous intracranial bleeding in hemorrhagic diathesis. Surg Neurol 17:137–140, 1982.
132. Herbstein DJ, Schaumberg HH: Hypertensive intracerebral hematoma: An investigation of the initial hemorrhage and rebleeding using chromium Cr 51–labeled erythrocytes. Arch Neurol 30:412–414, 1974.
133. Takada I: [On the phenomenon of extravasation of contrast media during cerebral angiogram for hypertensive intracerebral hematoma: Clinical significance and analysis of 14 cases.] No Shinkei Geka 4:471–478, 1976.
134. Ebina K, Okabe S, Manabe H, et al: [Experimental study of the liquefaction of intracranial hematoma: Usefulness of tissue plasminogen activator (t-PA), a hematolytic agent, and their combination.] No Shinkei Geka 18:927–934, 1990.
135. Fujii Y, Tanaka R, Takeuchi S, et al: Hematoma enlargement in spontaneous intracerebral hemorrhage. J Neurosurg 80:51–57, 1994.
136. Kazui S, Naritomi H, Yamamoto H, et al: Enlargement of spontaneous intracerebral hemorrhage: Incidence and time course. Stroke 27:1783–1787, 1996.
137. Kobayashi S, Sato A, Kageyama Y, et al: Treatment of hypertensive cerebellar hemorrhage: Surgical or conservative management? Neurosurgery 34:246–251, 1994.
138. Heros RC: Surgical treatment of cerebellar infarction. Stroke 23: 937–938, 1992.
139. Takasugi S, Ueda S, Matsumoto K: Chronological changes in spontaneous intracerebral hematoma—an experimental and clinical study. Stroke 16:651–658, 1985.
140. Kaneko M, Tanaka K, Shimada T, et al: Long-term evaluation of ultra-early operation for hypertensive intracerebral hemorrhage in 100 cases. J Neurosurg 58:838–842, 1983.
141. Kanno T, Sano H, Shinomiya Y, et al: Role of surgery in hypertensive intracerebral hematoma: A comparative study of 305 nonsurgical and 154 surgical cases. J Neurosurg 61:1091–1099, 1984.
142. Mizukami M, Araki G, Mihara H, et al: Surgical treatment of hypertensive cerebral hemorrhage. 4. The prognosis based on cerebral angiography. No To Shinkei 24:579–583, 1972.
143. Takebayashi S, Kaneko M: Electron microscopic studies of ruptured arteries in hypertensive intracerebral hemorrhage. Stroke 14:28–36, 1983.
144. Yukawa H, Kanaya H: Indication for surgery in hypertensive intracerebral hemorrhage—a statistical study. Neurol Med Chir (Tokyo) 18:361–365, 1978.
145. Juvela S, Heiskanen O, Poranen A, et al: The treatment of spontaneous intracerebral hemorrhage: A prospective randomized trial of surgical and conservative treatment. J Neurosurg 70:755–758, 1989.
146. Zuccarello M, Brott T, Derex L, et al: Early surgical treatment for supratentorial intracerebral hemorrhage: A randomized feasibility study. Stroke 30:1833–1839, 1999.
147. Fazio C: A neurologist's study of problems concerning surgical treatment of spontaneous cerebral hemorrhage. Sc Med Ital 1: 101–110, 1950.
148. Luessenhop AJ, Kachmann R: Surgical treatment of surgical primary spontaneous intracerebral hemorrhage. Georgetown Univ Med Cent Bull 18:117–119, 1964.
149. Paillas JE, Alliez B: Surgical treatment of spontaneous intracerebral hemorrhage: Immediate and long-term results in 250 cases. J Neurosurg 39:145–151, 1973.
150. Kopitnik TJ: Spontaneous cerebral hemorrhage: Innovative new techniques for decompression. In Batjer H (ed): Cerebrovascular Disease. Philadelphia, Lippincott-Raven, 1997, pp 641–647.
151. Mizukami M: Hypertensive Intracerebral Hemorrhage. New York, Raven Press, 1983.
152. Suzuki J, Sato S: The new transinsular approach to the hypertensive intracerebral hematoma. Jpn J Surg 2:47–52, 1972.
153. Kanaya H, Kuroda K: Development in neurosurgical approaches to hypertensive intracerebral hemorrhage in Japan. In Kaufman H (ed): Intracerebral Hematomas. New York, Raven Press, 1992, pp 197–209.
154. Crowell RM, Ojemann RG: Cerebellar hemorrhage. In Bucheit WA, Truex RCJ (eds): Surgery of the Posterior Fossa. New York, Raven Press, 1979, pp 135–142.
155. Niizuma H, Shimizu Y, Yonemitsu T, et al: Results of stereotactic aspiration in 175 cases of putaminal hemorrhage. Neurosurgery 24:814–819, 1989.
156. Benes V, Vladyka V, Zverina E: Stereotaxic evacuation of typical brain haemorrhage. Acta Neurochir (Wien) 13:419–426, 1965.
157. Backlund EO, von Holst H: Controlled subtotal evacuation of intracerebral haematomas by stereotactic technique. Surg Neurol 9:99–101, 1978.
158. Honda E, Hayashi T, Shimamoto H, et al: A comparison between stereotaxic operation and conservative therapy for thalamic hemorrhage. No Shinkei Geka 16(Suppl):665–670, 1988.
159. Deinsberger W, Vogel J, Fuchs C, et al: Fibrinolysis and aspiration of experimental intracerebral hematoma reduces the volume of ischemic brain in rats. Neurol Res 21:517–523, 1999.
160. Deinsberger W, Hartmann M, Vogel J, et al: Local fibrinolysis and aspiration of intracerebral hematomas in rats: An experimental study using MR monitoring. Neurol Res 20:349–352, 1998.
161. Matsumoto K, Hondo H: CT-guided stereotaxic evacuation of hypertensive intracerebral hematomas. J Neurosurg 61:440–448, 1984.
162. Doi E, Moriwaki H, Komai N, et al: Stereotactic evacuation of intracerebral hematomas. Neurol Med Chir (Tokyo) 22:461–467, 1982.
163. Pang D, Sclabassi RJ, Horton JA: Lysis of intraventricular blood clot with urokinase in a canine model. Part 3. Effects of intraventricular urokinase on clot lysis and posthemorrhagic hydrocephalus. Neurosurgery 19:553–572, 1986.
164. Pang D, Sclabassi RJ, Horton JA: Lysis of intraventricular blood clot with urokinase in a canine model. Part 2. In vivo safety study of intraventricular urokinase. Neurosurgery 19:547–552, 1986.
165. Pang D, Sclabassi RJ, Horton JA: Lysis of intraventricular blood clot with urokinase in a canine model. Part 1. Canine intraventricular blood cast model. Neurosurgery 19:540–546, 1986.
166. Niizuma H, Otsuki T, Johkura H, et al: CT-guided stereotactic aspiration of intracerebral hematoma—result of a hematomalysis method using urokinase. Appl Neurophysiol 48:427–430, 1985.

167. Weisberg LA: Thalamic hemorrhage: Clinical-CT correlations. Neurology 36:1382–1386, 1986.
168. Broseta J, Gonzalez-Darder J, Barcia-Salorio JL: Stereotactic evacuation of intracerebral hematomas. Appl Neurophysiol 45: 443–448, 1982.
169. Kandel EI, Peresedov VV: Stereotaxic evacuation of spontaneous intracerebral hematomas. J Neurosurg 62:206–213, 1985.
170. Tanikawa T, Amano K, Kawamura H, et al: CT-guided stereotactic surgery for evacuation of hypertensive intracerebral hematoma. Appl Neurophysiol 48:431–439, 1985.
171. Ito H, Mukai H, Higashi S, et al: [Removal of hypertensive intracerebral hematoma with stereotactic aqua-stream and aspirator.] No Shinkei Geka 17:939–943, 1989.
172. Matsumoto K, Hondo H, Tomida K: Aspiration surgery for hypertensive brain hemorrhage in the acute stage. In Suzuki J (ed): Advances in Surgery for Cerebral Stroke: Proceedings of the International Symposium on Surgery for Cerebral Stroke. Tokyo, Springer-Verlag, 1987.
173. Nakayama K, Miyasaka Y, Sato K, et al: Postoperative intracranial pressure in severe cases with hypertensive intracerebral hematoma. No To Shinkei 41:1149–1154, 1989.
174. Ropper AH, King RB: Intracranial pressure monitoring in comatose patients with cerebral hemorrhage. Arch Neurol 41:725–728, 1984.
175. Hara M, Kadowaki C, Shiogai T, et al: Correlation between intracranial pressure (ICP) and changes in CT images of cerebral hemorrhage. Neurol Res 20:225–230, 1998.
176. Kanaya H: Results of conservative and surgical treatment in hypertensive intracerebral hemorrhage: Cooperative study in Japan. Jpn J Stroke 12:509–524, 1990.
177. Morgenstern LB, Frankowski RF, Shedden P, et al: Surgical treatment for intracerebral hemorrhage (STICH): A single-center, randomized clinical trial. Neurology 51:1359–1363, 1998.
178. Hankey GJ, Hon C: Surgery for primary intracerebral hemorrhage: Is it safe and effective? A systematic review of case series and randomized trials. Stroke 28:2126–2132, 1997.
179. Prasad K, Browman G, Srivastava A, et al: Surgery in primary supratentorial intracerebral hematoma: A meta-analysis of randomized trials. Acta Neurol Scand 95:103–110, 1997.

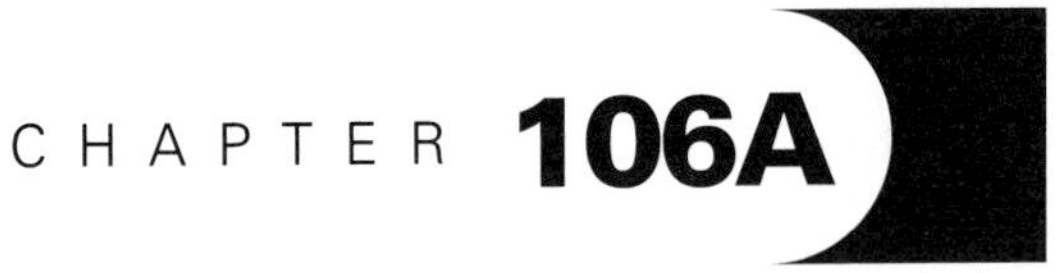

Genetics of Intracranial Aneurysms

WOUTER I. SCHIEVINK

The exact etiology and pathogenesis of intracranial aneurysms remain unclear. Several lines of evidence implicate acquired risk factors such as smoking or hypertension,[1] whereas others support the role of genetic factors.[2] The two main lines of evidence supporting the role of genetic factors are the association of intracranial aneurysms with heritable connective tissue disorders and the familial occurrence of intracranial aneurysms.

HERITABLE CONNECTIVE TISSUE DISORDERS

Numerous heritable connective tissue disorders have been associated with intracranial aneurysms, including polycystic kidney disease, Ehlers-Danlos syndrome type IV, Marfan's syndrome, neurofibromatosis type 1, pseudoxanthoma elasticum, and α_1-antitrypsin deficiency (Table 106A–1).[2, 3] To what extent these specific heritable disorders contribute to the entire population of patients with intracranial aneurysms is unknown. In one series of 100 consecutive hospitalized patients with intracranial aneurysms, 5 had an identifiable heritable connective tissue disorder.[4] The true frequency of heritable connective tissue disorders in patients with aneurysms is probably higher because these disorders often remain undiagnosed, reflecting the substantial variability in their phenotypic expression. Family history also may be negative because the disease can be caused by a new mutation. Nevertheless, identifiable heritable connective tissue disorders contribute to a relatively small percentage of intracranial aneurysms.

Autosomal Dominant Polycystic Kidney Disease

Autosomal dominant polycystic kidney disease (ADPKD) affects about 1 in 400 to 1000 persons and is the most common monogenetic disease in humans.[5] It is inherited as an autosomal dominant trait with almost complete penetrance but with variable expression. Family history is negative in about 20% of patients, suggesting a fairly high spontaneous mutation rate.

ADPKD is a systemic disease, and cysts are present in the kidneys, liver, pancreas, spleen, ovaries, and seminal vesicles.[5] Moreover, ADPKD should be included among the heritable connective tissue disorders.[3] A wide variety of connective tissues may be involved,[5] including the heart valves (mitral valve prolapse), vasculature (aneurysms and dissections), and meninges (arachnoid cysts). Patients with ADPKD are at increased risk for the development of gastrointestinal diverticula and inguinal hernias.[5]

Neurosurgical disorders that have been associated with ADPKD include intracranial aneurysms, cervicocephalic arterial dissections, intracranial dolichoectasia, intracranial arachnoid cysts, spinal meningeal diverticula, and chronic subdural hemorrhages.[5–10] Intracranial aneurysms have long been known to be associated with ADPKD. Until the underlying connective tissue defect of the disease became well known, however, aneurysms frequently were attributed to the arterial hypertension that usually accompanies ADPKD. Intracranial aneurysms are detected in approximately one fourth of patients with ADPKD at autopsy; in most of these patients, aneurysmal rupture was the cause of death.[8] Conversely, ADPKD accounts for 2% to 7% of all patients with intracranial aneurysms.[8, 11] Using magnetic resonance angiography or, less commonly, catheter angiography in patients with good renal function, several groups have screened adult ADPKD patients for asymptomatic intracranial aneurysms. The detection rate has ranged between 5% and 10%.[12–17] Familial clustering of intracranial aneurysms occurs in ADPKD; the yield of screening increases to 10% to 25% in such families.[13, 14, 16, 17] The presence of polycystic

TABLE 106A–1 ■ **Heritable Disorders That Have Been Associated with Intracranial Aneurysms**

DISORDER	MIM NO.*	INHERITANCE PATTERN	LOCUS	GENE	GENE PRODUCT
Achondroplasia	100800	AD	4p16.3	*FGFR3*	Fibroblast growth Factor receptor 3
Alagille syndrome	118450	AD	20p12	*JAG1*	?
Alkaptonuria	203500	AR	3q2	*AKU*	?
Autosomal dominant polycystic kidney disease	173900 173910	AD	16p13.3 4q21	*PKD1* *PKD2*	Polycystin-1 Polycystin-2
Autosomal dominant polycystic liver disease	174050	AD	?	?	?
Cohen's syndrome	216550	AR	8q22	*CHS1*	?
Ehlers-Danlos syndrome type I	130000	AD	9q34.2	*COL5A1*	Collagen type V†
Ehlers-Danlos syndrome type IV	130050	AD	2q31	*COL3A1*	Collagen type III†
Fabry's disease	301500	XL-R	Xq22.1	*GLA*	α-Galactosidase A
Kahn's syndrome‡	210050	AR	?	?	?
Marfan's syndrome	154700	AD	15q21.1	*FBN1*	Fibrillin-1
Neurofibromatosis type 1	162200	AD	17q11.2	*NF1*	Neurofibromin
Noonan's syndrome	163950	AD	12q22	*NS1*	?
Osler-Rendu-Weber disease	187300	AD	9q34.1 12q	*HHT1* *HHT2*	Endoglin ?
Osteogenesis imperfecta type 1	166200	AD	17q22.1 7q22.1	*COL1A1* *COL1A2*	Collagen type 1† Collagen type I§
Pompe's disease	232300	AR	17q23	*GAA*	α-Glucosidase
Pseudoxanthoma elasticum	177850 264800	AD and AR	16p13.1	?	?
Rambaud's syndrome‡	277175	AR	?	?	?
Seckel's syndrome	210600	AR	?	?	?
Tuberous sclerosis	191100 191092	AD	9q34 16p13.3	*TSC1* *TSC2*	? Tuberin
Wermer's syndrome	131100	AD	11q13	*MEN1*	?
3M syndrome	273750	AR	?	?	?
α_1-Antitrypsin deficiency	107400	ACoD	14q32.1	*PI*	α_1-Antitrypsin

*McKusick VA: Mendelian Inheritance in Man: Catalogs of Human Genes and Genetic Disorders. Baltimore, Johns Hopkins University Press, 1994, ed 11. Online Mendelian Inheritance in Man. Center for Medical Genetics, Johns Hopkins University (Baltimore, MD), and National Center for Biotechnology Information, National Library of Medicine (Bethesda, MD). World Wide Web: http://www.ncbi.nlm.nih.gov/omim/.
†α_1-Polypeptide.
‡Syndromes associated with idiopathic nonarteriosclerotic cerebral calcifications.
§α_2-Polypeptide.
AD, autosomal dominant; AR, autosomal recessive; XL-R, X-linked recessive; ACoD, autosomal codominant.

liver disease in ADPKD patients may also increase the development of intracranial aneurysms.[13]

Screening patients with ADPKD for asymptomatic aneurysms remains controversial but should certainly be considered for those with a family history of intracranial aneurysms. Most asymptomatic intracranial aneurysms detected with screening are less than 6 mm in diameter. In one study, none of these small aneurysms ruptured during 500 months of cumulative follow-up.[14] It has been suggested that ADPKD patients are at an increased risk of developing *de novo* aneurysms some time after their first intracranial aneurysm is discovered, but the exact significance of this risk remains to be determined.[14, 18] Compared with the general population, aneurysmal subarachnoid hemorrhage in patients with ADPKD occurs at an earlier age but the mortality rate is similar.[8]

ADPKD is a genetically heterogeneous disease. Several loci are involved, and mutations, which are responsible for at least 85% of cases, have been identified on a gene on chromosome 16 *(PKD1)* as well as on a gene on chromosome 4 *(PDK2)*.[19–21] In general, patients with mutations in the *PKD1* gene are more severely affected than those with mutations in the *PKD2* gene, but intracranial aneurysms are a manifestation of both types of ADPKD.[20–22] Polycystin-1 and polycystin-2 are the proteins encoded by the *PKD1* and *PKD2* genes, respectively.[19] Both proteins are integral membrane proteins with large extracellular domains, which probably play a role in maintaining the structural integrity of the connective tissue extracellular matrix.[19]

Autosomal dominant polycystic liver disease (ADPLD) is a familial form of isolated polycystic liver disease that is distinct from ADPKD.[23] Patients with ADPLD also may be at high risk for the development of intracranial aneurysms.[23]

Ehlers-Danlos Syndrome Type IV

Ehlers-Danlos syndrome type IV is potentially one of the most deadly heritable connective tissue disorders that neurosurgeons may encounter. It is uncommon, with a prevalence of approximately 1 in 50,000 to 500,000 persons.[24] It is inherited in an autosomal dominant fashion, but family history frequently is noncontributory because of the high spontaneous mutation rate (approximately 50%).

Ehlers-Danlos syndrome type IV can be life threatening because spontaneous rupture, dissection, or aneurysmal formation on large and medium-sized arteries occurs in all areas of the body.[3, 24–26] These arterial complications cause death in most patients. Other well-described life-threatening complications of Ehlers-Danlos syndrome type IV are spontaneous rupture of the bowel or gravid uterus and spontaneous pneumothorax.[24, 26]

An intracranial aneurysm may be the initial manifestation of Ehlers-Danlos syndrome type IV. Consequently, neurosurgeons may be the first physicians involved in these patients' medical care. The syndrome often is difficult to recognize because external features can be subtle.[3, 24–26] The more salient features of Ehlers-Danlos syndrome type IV are summarized in Table 106A–2. The characteristic facial appearance was first described by Graf, a neurosurgeon[27]; many striking examples have since been published.[25, 26] The facial features consist of (1) large expressive eyes with the sclera clearly visible around the iris, (2) a thin nose, (3) thin lips, and (4) lobeless ears. Many patients with Ehlers-Danlos syndrome type IV, however, do not exhibit this facial appearance. The characteristic cutaneous features include thin and fragile skin that is almost transparent, allowing the subcutaneous veins to be clearly visible. Patients bruise easily, and multiple ecchymoses are common. Scars are often papyraceous and wide, or they may be complicated by keloid formation. The skin of some patients with Ehlers-Danlos syndrome type IV, however, appears normal. The joint hypermobility is often mild and limited to the fingers and toes. Identifying Ehlers-Danlos syndrome type IV in any patient with an intracranial aneurysm is important because vascular fragility can make any invasive procedure a hazardous undertaking.

Intracranial aneurysms and spontaneous carotid-cavernous fistulas are well-described vascular complications of Ehlers-Danlos syndrome type IV.[3, 25–27] In some patients the carotid-cavernous fistula is due to the rupture of a cavernous-carotid aneurysm, although the fistula may be caused by a simple tear in the artery in other patients. The importance of intracranial aneurysmal disease in this group of patients is well described. For example, in a cohort of 202 patients with Ehlers-Danlos syndrome type IV, 4 had ruptured intracranial aneurysms, 4 suffered an intracranial hemorrhage of undetermined cause, and 6 had carotid-cavernous fistulas.[28] The exact incidence of intracranial aneurysms in Ehlers-Danlos syndrome type IV is unknown because screening for asymptomatic intracranial aneurysms is limited and systematic autopsy studies are unavailable. Screening for asymptomatic intracranial aneurysms in these patients is not recommended because safe treatment options are limited; arteriography, endovascular intervention, and surgical treatment are all associated with high complication rates.

TABLE 106A–2 ■ Characteristic Features of Ehlers-Danlos Syndrome Type IV

HISTORY	EXAMINATION
Easy bruisability	Face
Vascular rupture, dissection, or aneurysm	Expressive eyes
	Thin nose
	Thin lips
Gastrointestinal perforation	Lobeless ears
	Skin
Uterine rupture	Thin and fragile
Pneumothorax	Ecchymoses
	Abnormal scarring
	Subcutaneous veins easily visible
	Joints
	Hypermobility (often just of fingers)

Mutations in the gene encoding the pro-α_1-(III) chain of collagen type III *(COL3A1)* on chromosome 2 are the cause of Ehlers-Danlos syndrome type IV.[24–26, 29] This type of collagen is the major structural component of distensible tissues, including arteries, veins, hollow viscera, and the uterus. In addition, collagen type III may play an important role in the fibrillogenesis of collagen type I.[30] Several studies have reported evidence of abnormal collagen type III metabolism in up to 50% of patients with intracranial aneurysms who do not have Ehlers-Danlos syndrome type IV.[31–37] Mutations in the *COL3A1* gene, however, are rare. For example, in a study of 40 patients with intracranial aneurysms, *COL3A1* mutations were found in only two patients, and the functional consequences of these mutations were considered insignificant.[38] The reasons for these conflicting data are unclear.

α_1-Antitrypsin Deficiency

The structural integrity of the arterial wall depends on a wide variety of interrelated extracellular matrix proteins such as collagen and elastin. The degradation of these proteins by proteolytic enzymes (proteases) is regulated by protease inhibitors (antiproteases). Recently, several studies have focused on an imbalance between proteases and antiproteases as a possible risk factor for the development of intracranial aneurysms.[4, 39–42] α_1-Antitrypsin, a powerful and abundant circulating antiprotease, is a small glycoprotein that is synthesized in the liver.[43] The primary target of an α_1-antitrypsin is not trypsin but neutrophil elastase. Consequently, α_1-antitrypsin deficiency (a codominantly inherited disorder) is characterized by damage of elastic tissues such as the lungs, resulting in emphysema.[43] α_1-Antitrypsin deficiency may also cause a breakdown of subcutaneous septa, resulting in cutis laxa.[44] Several vascular disorders have been associated with α_1-antitrypsin deficiency, including arterial aneurysms, spontaneous arterial dissections, and arterial fibromuscular dysplasia.[4, 42, 45–50] Patients with α_1-antitrypsin deficiency are at increased risk for the development of intracranial aneurysms, but it remains to be determined how clinically significant this risk is. Among 362 consecutive patients with α_1-antitrypsin deficiency, 3 had suffered an aneurysmal subarachnoid hemorrhage (SAH), a considerably higher number than would be expected by chance.[42] Some studies have shown that α_1-antitrypsin deficiency is more common in patients with intracranial aneurysms than in the general population.[4, 50] By contrast, other studies have not found a statistically significant excess of α_1-antitrypsin deficiency in patients with intracranial aneurysms.[50, 51] These conflicting data may be explained by differences in the genetic background of the patient populations. For example, the common α_1-antitrypsin deficiency alleles *PiZ* and *PiS* are typically (North)-Western European marker genes.[52] Screening for asymptomatic intracranial aneurysms in patients with α_1-antitrypsin deficiency generally is not advocated.

The α_1-antitrypsin gene is located on chromosome 14.[43] It is a highly polymorphic gene, and more than 75 allelic variants have been identified. The locus has been designated "*Pi*" for protease inhibitor. The most common allele is *PiM*, and more than 95% of the white population carry the homozygous PiMM phenotype. Patients who are homozygous for the deficient PiZ phenotype have low serum levels of α_1-antitrypsin (approximately 15% of normal), whereas only moderately reduced levels of α_1-antitrypsin are found in individuals with the heterozygous PiMZ phenotype (approximately 65%) or PiMS phenotype (approximately 80%). Patients who are homozygous for PiZ usually develop pulmonary emphysema; in our experience, this occurs before they present with an intracranial aneurysm. Heterozygous patients tend to remain asymptomatic if they refrain from smoking cigarettes. Although the Pi phenotype is the major contributor to α_1-antitrypsin levels, α_1-antitrypsin is also an acute phase protein and its levels increase after injury (e.g., SAH and craniotomy) or infection. Thus, quantification of the serum α_1-antitrypsin level in isolation may give a false-negative result. Cigarette smoking has been observed to lower the inhibitory capacity of α_1-antitrypsin, but it does not affect α_1-antitrypsin levels.

Marfan's Syndrome

Marfan's syndrome affects approximately 1 in 10,000 to 20,000 people and is characterized by abnormalities of the skeleton, cardiovascular system, eye, and spinal meninges.[53, 54] Aortic and mitral valve insufficiency are the most frequent causes of death in children with Marfan's syndrome, and spontaneous aortic rupture and dissection are the most frequent causes of death in adults with the syndrome.[53, 54] Dissections of medium-sized arteries, however, are much less common.[55] Although Marfan's syndrome is easily recognized in patients who display the main features of the syndrome (particularly the skeletal manifestations of tall stature, dolichostenomelia, arachnodactyly, and anterior chest deformity), the variability of phenotypic expression is great and the diagnosis is seldom straightforward.[53, 54] For example, if the parents of a patient with Marfan's syndrome are short, the affected person's habitus may be comparatively normal.[53] Ectopia lentis, the classic ocular manifestation of Marfan's syndrome, is observed in only about half the cases.[53] Dural ectasia, another major diagnostic criterion of the syndrome, is usually asymptomatic and requires computed tomography or magnetic resonance imaging for diagnosis.[56, 57] Other manifestations of Marfan's syndrome include spontaneous pneumothorax, striae distensae, and retinal detachment.[53, 54]

Intracranial aneurysms in patients with Marfan's syndrome may be saccular or fusiform, and intracranial dissecting aneurysms have also been described.[3, 58–60] Similar to Ehlers-Danlos syndrome type IV, there is a propensity for proximal intracranial carotid artery involvement although carotid-cavernous fistulas seem to be rare.[3] Connective tissue fragility is seldom a major problem in the neurosurgical treatment of patients with Marfan's syndrome. The frequently observed ectasia and tortuosity of the extracranial carotid and vertebral arteries, however, may render endovascular treatment of intracranial aneurysms impossible. The association of Marfan's syndrome and intracranial aneurysms has not been firmly established. In an autopsy series of 7 patients with Marfan's syndrome collected during a 25-year period at the Mayo Clinic, intracranial aneurysms, one ruptured and one unruptured aneurysm, were observed in 2 patients.[59] Combining this autopsy study with one performed at Johns Hopkins University,[61] but excluding the one ruptured aneurysm, incidental aneurysms were found in 2 (6.5%) of 31 patients.[62] This frequency is higher than would be expected in the general population, particularly considering the young age of the patients.[62] Results of screening for asymptomatic intracranial aneurysms in patients with Marfan's syndrome have not been reported.

Mutations in the gene encoding fibrillin-1 *(FBN-1)* cause Marfan's syndrome.[63] Fibrillin-1 is a recently diagnosed glycoprotein that is one of the major components of microfibrils.[63, 64] These microfibrils are important constituents of the extracellular matrix and are distributed throughout the body in elastic tissues (e.g., skin, aorta) and nonelastic tissues (e.g., the ciliary zonules of the ocular lens). In elastic arteries, such as the aorta, fibrillin-1 is found in all three layers of the arterial wall. It is thought that fibrillin-1 plays an important role in maintaining the structural integrity of connective tissues, in part by providing a scaffolding for elastic fibers. Mutations in the *FBN1* gene or abnormal fibrillin metabolism ("fibrillinopathy") have also been detected in patients with isolated features of Marfan's syndrome but without the classic syndrome.[65–68]

Neurofibromatosis Type 1

Neurofibromatosis type 1 is a progressive systemic disease affecting approximately 1 in 3000 to 5000 persons.[69] The principal clinical features of neurofibromatosis type 1 are café-au-lait spots, neurofibromas, and Lisch nodules (hamartomas) of the iris.[69] Although these features each occur in more than 90% of adults with neurofibromatosis type 1, the number of lesions is variable. Patients with neurofibromatosis type 1 are also at increased risk of developing optic glioma, pheochromocytoma, dural ectasia, and skeletal abnormalities such as scoliosis and sphenoid wing dysplasia.[69] Vascular complications of neurofibromatosis type I have been recognized since 1945 and are characterized by stenosis, rupture, and aneurysm or fistula formation of large- and medium-sized arteries.[69–72]

Intracranial aneurysms in patients with neurofibromatosis type 1 may be saccular or fusiform, and some have the appearance of dissecting aneurysms.[73–78] Surgical repair of these aneurysms may be complicated by excessive vascular fragility or distortion of anatomic landmarks caused by sphenoid wing dysplasia.[77] The intracranial aneurysms associated with neurofibromatosis type 1 often coexist with intracranial arterial occlusive disease,[79] increasing the risks of their surgical and particularly endovascular treatment. An increased probability of developing intracranial aneurysms has not been clearly established for patients with neurofibromatosis type 1, but the number of reported cases continues to increase and some have advocated screening patients with neurofibromatosis for asymptomatic intracranial aneurysms.[74] Among a group of 100 consecutive patients with intracranial aneurysms, one patient was revealed to have neurofibromatosis type 1.[4]

Neurofibromatosis type 1 is caused by mutations in the gene *(NF1)* encoding neurofibromin, a protein with a centrally located domain homologous to guanosine triphosphatase–activating protein (GAP) that is similar to other tumor suppressor gene products.[80, 81] The GAP domain of neurofibromin colocalizes with cytoplasmatic microtubules, and it has been postulated that neurofibromin may have a regulatory role in the development of various connective tissues, including vascular connective tissue, through an effect on microtubular function. In a mouse model of mutations in *GAP* and *NF1* genes, Henkemeyer and associates[82] demonstrated thinning and rupture of large and medium-sized arteries during embryonic development. The GAP domain of neurofibromin, however, encompasses only about 10% of the protein, and neurofibromin may have a variety of undiscovered functions.

Pseudoxanthoma Elasticum

Pseudoxanthoma elasticum (PXE) is a disorder affecting elastic fibers in the skin, ocular system, and cardiovascular system.[83, 84] The characteristic skin lesions consist of round, oval, or linear yellow-orange papules, resembling xanthomas. The skin lesions are often associated with laxity and thickening of the skin and preferentially involve flexoral areas, such as the neck, axilla, groin, and antecubital and popliteal spaces.[83, 84] Angioid streaks are the characteristic ocular findings and occur in about 85% of affected patients.[85, 86] Angioid streaks are caused by breaks in the thickened and calcified membrane of Bruch.[83, 84] The number and prominence of angioid streaks increase with age. Retinal hemorrhage occurs in about one third of patients. The cardiovascular changes associated with PXE are those of stenotic, occlusive, or (less frequently) aneurysmal disease primarily affecting medium-sized peripheral arteries.[83, 84, 87–91] The aorta is usually spared. Intermittent claudication of the lower extremities, hypertension, and abdominal angina are the most frequent sequelae of the vascular involvement. The arteries in the extremities may become palpably hard, and plain radiographs often reveal arterial calcification. Gastrointestinal hemorrhage may be a presenting symptom of PXE and is believed to be the result of visceral arterial degeneration or general fragility of the submucosal arteries.[83, 84] Myocardial infarction is not particularly common, although it has been described as early as adolescence in patients with PXE and occasionally requires coronary artery bypass procedures. Mitral valve prolapse is the most common cardiac valvular abnormality of PXE.[92]

The prevalence of PXE has been estimated to be about 1 in 100,000 population. PXE is genetically heterogeneous; two autosomal recessive and two autosomal dominant types have been described.[93, 94] One of the autosomal dominant forms appears to be associated with the most significant vascular changes.[94] There is no generally accepted classification of these types of PXE, and one cannot determine the type in an individual case because of clinical variability even within families.

Cerebral infarction caused by (presumed) premature stenotic and occlusive disease of the carotid and vertebral arteries is the most frequently reported neurovascular manifestation of PXE.[95–98] Both the intracranial and extracranial vessels may be involved, and the cerebral infarctions are often multiple. Cerebral ischemic symptoms may occur as early as the third decade of life but usually are not noted until the fifth or sixth decade. Many of these older patients also have hypertension or other risk factors for cardiovascular disease. Cervical spinal cord ischemia can also be associated with PXE.[99]

Josien[100] reported a 17-year-old boy with PXE who suffered a spontaneous dissection of the cervical vertebral artery. Mokri and colleagues[101] mentioned a 40-year-old man with a spontaneous extracranial internal carotid artery dissection who was found to have at least one angioid streak but no cutaneous abnormalities. Their patient may have had a mild form of PXE, although angioid streaks are also associated with Ehlers-Danlos syndrome and Marfan's syndrome. Tortuosity and ectasia of the cervical arteries with or without distinct aneurysm formation have been described in some patients with PXE.[102]

Several cases of intracranial aneurysm associated with PXE have been reported since its first description in 1951.[87, 103–106] In 100 patients with PXE attending a dermatologic clinic, the only neurovascular complication was aneurysmal SAH.[105] SAH, however, may not be the most common presenting symptom of intracranial aneurysms associated with PXE because the aneurysms are often located within the cavernous sinus, causing ocular motor nerve palsies. Kito and coworkers[107] reported the unique case of a 37-year-old woman with PXE who suffered an SAH caused by the rupture of an anterior spinal artery aneurysm. No symptomatic aneurysms have been observed in some groups of patients with PXE[98]; however, such studies have had relatively small numbers of patients with a mean age in the fourth decade of life.

The pathogenesis of PXE appears to involve abnormalities of elastic fibers, but the basic molecular defect of PXE is unknown. Both the autosomal recessive and dominant variants of PXE have been mapped to chromosome 16p13.1.[108]

FAMILIAL INTRACRANIAL ANEURYSMS

With the exception of ADPKD and, rarely, Ehlers-Danlos syndrome type IV, Pompe's disease, or syndromes associated with idiopathic nonarteriosclerotic cerebral calcifications, familial intracranial aneurysms have not been associated with any of the known heritable connective tissue disorders. The familial aggregation of intracranial aneurysms was first described in 1954 by Chambers and colleagues.[109] Since then, hundreds of families have been reported. During the past decade, interest in familial intracranial aneurysms has been renewed. Several studies have been focused on their epidemiologic features, clinical characteristics, and presymptomatic detection with noninvasive screening methods.

TABLE 106A–4 ■ **Risk of Subarachnoid Hemorrhage in First-Degree Relatives of Patients with Subarachnoid Hemorrhage**

STUDY	LOCATION	RISK RATIO*
Wang et al, 1995†	King County, Washington	1.8 (0.9–3.7)
Bromberg et al, 1995†	The Netherlands	2.7 (1.4–5.5) 6.6 (2.0–21)
Schievink et al, 1995‡	Rochester, Minnesota	4.1 (2.1–7.4)
de Braekeleer et al, 1996‡	Quebec, Canada	4.7 (3.1–7.5)
Gaist et al, 2000‡	Denmark	2.9 (1.9–4.6) 4.5 (2.7–7.3)

*Confidence interval, 95%.
†Includes aneurysmal and nonaneurysmal subarachnoid hemorrhage.
‡Includes aneurysmal subarachnoid hemorrhage only.

Epidemiology

Familial intracranial aneurysms are much more common than has generally been appreciated. Four epidemiologic studies have examined the frequency of familial intracranial aneurysms and revealed that 7% to 20% of patients with aneurysmal SAH had first- or second-degree relatives with intracranial aneurysms (Table 106A–3).[110–113] However, this familial aggregation could have been fortuitous because at least 1% of adults harbor intracranial aneurysms and most of the reported families have included only two affected members. Whether relatives of patients with intracranial aneurysms have an increased risk of developing SAH was therefore unknown.

To address these issues, five independently conducted studies examined the risk of SAH in relatives of patients with SAH and have reported comparable results despite widely differing analytical methods and patient populations (Table 106A–4).[110, 113–116] Among the population of King County, Washington, Wang and associates[114] compared the frequency of familial SAH in patients with SAH to that of a control population.

TABLE 106A–3 ■ **Frequency of Familial Intracranial Aneurysms among Patients with Aneurysmal Subarachnoid Hemorrhage**

STUDY	LOCATION	FREQUENCY OF FAMILIAL DISEASE % (RANGE)*
Norrgård et al, 1987†	Sweden	6.6 (4.6–9.2)
Ronkainen et al, 1993†	East Finland	9.8 (8.2–11.7)
Schievink et al, 1995‡	Rochester, Minnesota	20.0 (11.5–30.5)
de Braekeleer et al, 1996†	Quebec, Canada	17.4 (14.2–20.6)

*Confidence interval, 95%.
†Includes one or more probands per family.
‡Includes one proband per family only.

Patients with SAH were almost twice as likely to have an affected first-degree relative. However, this difference did not reach statistical significance and a family history of SAH was never verified. Bromberg and coworkers[115] compared the frequency of SAH in first-degree relatives to that of second-degree relatives of patients with SAH who were admitted to several hospitals in the Netherlands. Depending on how well certain diagnostic criteria for SAH were met, they observed a threefold to sevenfold increased risk. Among a group of patients with aneurysmal SAH from Rochester, Minnesota, Schievink and colleagues[113] compared the observed and expected number of first-degree relatives with aneurysmal SAH using the well-established incidence rates of SAH in this community and observed about a fourfold increased risk. Despite this significantly increased risk, the overall absolute risk of first-degree relatives for developing aneurysmal SAH did not reach 2% until the age of 70 years. Among the inhabitants of the Saguenay Lac/Saint-Jean region of Quebec, Canada, de Braekeleer and associates[110] compared the frequency of familial intracranial aneurysms in patients with ruptured and unruptured intracranial aneurysms with that of a control population and observed an approximately fivefold increased risk for first-degree relatives. Using data from two Danish national registries, Gaist and coworkers compared the incidence of SAH in first-degree relatives of patients with an SAH to the incidence in the general population and found a threefold to fivefold increased risk.[116]

Pattern of Inheritance

The inheritance pattern of familial intracranial aneurysms is unknown. The main difficulty in establishing the mode of transmission is that intracranial aneurysms are acquired lesions and often remain asymptomatic. At visual inspection, some pedigrees support autosomal dominant inheritance and others support autosomal recessive or multifactorial transmission; in most, however, the inheritance pattern is unclear.[111–113, 116–122] In a segregation analysis of published pedigrees, no single mendelian model was the overall best fitting.

However, several possible patterns of inheritance were identified and autosomal transmission was the most likely.[117] This finding suggests that genetic heterogeneity is important in the genetics of intracranial aneurysms.[117] Genetic heterogeneity had been suspected on the basis of the large number of heritable disorders that have been associated with intracranial aneurysms (see Table 106A–1).

Although the Saguenay Lac/Saint-Jean region is well known for its large number of consanguineous marriages, de Braekeleer and associates[110] observed that the coefficient of inbreeding was no higher in patients with intracranial aneurysms than in a control population. They also noted a decrease in the frequency of intracranial aneurysms among first-, second-, and third-degree relatives of affected patients. These observations suggest the presence of dominant instead of recessive genes in their reported kinships.

Among families with two affected generations, children suffer SAH at a significantly younger age than the parents.[118, 119] Although this age difference could be explained by ascertainment bias, disease onset at earlier ages in later generations (genetic anticipation) is increasingly recognized as an expression of unstable deoxyribonucleic acid trinucleotide repeats expanding in subsequent generations. This genetic mechanism has been demonstrated in several dominantly inherited neurodegenerative diseases and may also underlie the inheritance of intracranial aneurysms in some families.

Are Familial Aneurysms Different?

Numerous studies have compared the characteristics of familial intracranial aneurysms with those of nonfamilial (sporadic) aneurysms. These studies have consistently shown that familial aneurysms rupture, on average, about 5 years earlier than sporadic aneurysms.[111, 113, 118–120, 122] In several populations of siblings, aneurysms more commonly rupture within the same decade of life.[121, 122] Aneurysms of the anterior communicating artery complex are underrepresented in patients with familial aneurysms.[111, 113, 118–120] Although prospective studies are unavailable, two studies suggest that familial aneurysms rupture at a smaller size than sporadic aneurysms.[121, 122] The observed differences are small (1 to 2 mm) but may be important, particularly for the treatment of small asymptomatic aneurysms. Patients with familial aneurysms also may develop *de novo* aneurysms more often than patients with sporadic aneurysms, although the number of observed cases is small.[117, 123, 124] An increased proportion of multiple aneurysms is also found in patients with familial aneurysms.[111, 113, 118–120, 122] One hospital-based study suggests that the case-fatality rate of SAH is worse in patients with familial aneurysms[125]; however, other studies do not support this observation.[126, 127] At autopsy, patients with familial intracranial aneurysms have had changes in the media of the intracranial and extracranial artery that were not present in patients with sporadic aneurysms.[128] Together, these clinical and pathologic data suggest that familial intracranial aneurysms are different from nonfamilial intracranial aneurysms.

Screening

The benefits of screening for asymptomatic intracranial aneurysms have never been quantified. Several groups, however, have extensive experience with screening for familial intracranial aneurysms using MR angiography (Table 106A–5). In the absence of any clinical feature or biologic marker that can identify individuals who are most likely to develop intracranial aneurysms, screening for asymptomatic familial intracranial aneurysms may be recommended for first-degree relatives in families with two or more affected members.[17, 117, 129–131] With this screening strategy, approximately 10% of individuals are found to have an intracranial aneurysm.[17, 129–131] In approximately a third of these patients, the aneurysms are larger than 5 mm in diameter.[17] Some investigators have recommended screening individuals with only a single family member with an intracranial aneurysm.[115, 118] The absolute lifetime risk for first-degree relatives to suffer an aneurysmal SAH when there is only a single family member with an aneurysm is modest,[113] however. Furthermore, the yield of such a screening strategy is fairly low (2% to 4%).[132–135] Therefore, screening is seldom recommended for those patients.[77, 117, 130]

There are no guidelines for determining when aneurysm screening should be performed. Several investigators have used sophisticated decision-making analytic models using similar data to determine the optimum age for screening. Widely differing age ranges have been suggested (e.g., Obuchowski and associates, <30 years[135]; Leblanc and colleagues, 20–50 years[136]; ter Berg and coworkers, 35–65 years[137]). Ronkainen and colleagues[138] limit their screening to individuals older than 30 years of age. To detect *de novo* aneurysms, repeat screening has been suggested at 6-month to 5-year intervals after the initial study.[139]

Evaluation of Patients With a Familial Aneurysm

Patients with an intracranial aneurysm and a family history of intracranial aneurysm or SAH warrant fur-

TABLE 106A–5 ■ **Yield of Screening for Asymptomatic Intracranial Aneurysms**

POPULATION	RANGE OF YIELD (%)
General population	0.5–2.0
First-degree relatives in families with one affected member	2–4
First-degree relatives in families with two or more affected members	10
Polycystic kidney disease	5–10
Polycystic kidney disease and family history of intracranial aneurysm	10–25

TABLE 106A–6 ■ Evaluation of Patients with Familial Intracranial Aneurysms

Medical history
Family history
Physical examination
Review of medical/autopsy records
Medical genetics consultation
Renal ultrasonography
Collagen analysis
Screening of first-degree relatives

ther evaluation (Table 106A–6). This evaluation primarily consists of obtaining a detailed medical and family history supplemented by a review of the available medical or autopsy records. A review of these records is important because a self-reported family history alone may not prove or refute a diagnosis of intracranial aneurysm or SAH. Consultation by a medical geneticist is often valuable in constructing a pedigree, obtaining records, and evaluating the patient for the presence of heritable disorders that have been associated with intracranial aneurysms. Apart from ADPKD[8, 13, 17] and, occasionally, Ehlers-Danlos syndrome type IV,[25, 140] however, the heritable connective tissue disorders are rarely identified in families with intracranial aneurysms. Familial intracranial aneurysms may be the first manifestation of ADPKD.[141] Renal ultrasonography is a noninvasive and reliable technique and should therefore be considered to rule out ADPKD. At least one study has reported a low yield of screening for ADPKD in patients with familial intracranial aneurysms.[17] When Ehlers-Danlos syndrome type IV is suspected, collagen type III analyses should be performed on cultured skin fibroblasts to confirm this diagnosis. Finally, adult first-degree relatives should be contacted and advised about the possibilities and uncertainties of invasive and noninvasive screening for asymptomatic intracranial aneurysms.

Gene-Environment Interactions

The etiology and pathogenesis of intracranial aneurysms are clearly multifactorial, and acquired (environmental) factors play a major role. Cigarette smoking is the most important modifiable environmental risk factor.[1] Smokers are at a 3- to 10-fold increased risk of aneurysmal SAH.[1] Those who continue to smoke may be at a particularly high risk for developing *de novo* aneurysms.[1] Other risk factors include hypertension and excessive alcohol use. The gene–environment interactions underlying the development of intracranial aneurysms are complex and poorly understood, but genetic components may predominate in younger patients and environmental components may predominate in the older population. It is possible, at least partially, that the familial aggregation of intracranial aneurysms can be explained by certain environmental factors that are shared by affected family members, such as cigarette smoking. For example, a Dutch study suggested that hypertension is a familial factor contributing to the increased risk of aneurysmal SAH in first-degree relatives but it could not explain the entire excess risk.[142]

Intracranial Aneurysm Gene?

Before the burgeoning capabilities of molecular genetic linkage, several allelic association studies were conducted in patients with intracranial aneurysms using classic markers such as human lymphocyte antigens, red blood cell types, and serum group systems. These studies failed to show any convincing associations.[77]

Recent advances in molecular genetics have made linkage studies possible to map the chromosomal locus of a putative intracranial aneurysm gene mutation. One approach is to screen the human genome for intracranial aneurysm genes by testing linkage of a large number of distinct highly polymorphic genetic markers. Such linkage analysis is classically performed in large families with multiple affected members. However, this method (as applied to intracranial aneurysms) is hampered by the genetic heterogeneity, the paucity of well-documented multiple case families, and the uncertainties in designating family members as unaffected if screening does not show an aneurysm.

Another method for studying linkage is to analyze variations in the sharing of marker alleles among affected sibling pairs only. Although this method requires no knowledge of the mode of transmission and only affected family members are studied, very large sample sizes are often required. An alternative approach to locate intracranial aneurysm genes is candidate gene sequence analysis. This analysis involves evaluating the sequence of a gene for a protein plausibly involved in intracranial aneurysm development (e.g., *PKD1* or *COL3A1;* see Table 106A–2) and determining whether a mutant sequence variation occurs more frequently among affected patients than is predicted by chance. Several laboratories are currently directing their efforts at locating intracranial aneurysm genes using one or more of these approaches.

Polymorphisms of several genes have now been investigated in patients with intracranial aneurysms.[143–145] Certain polymorphisms of the angiotensin I–converting enzyme[144] and endoglin[144] genes may be associated with an increased risk for aneurysm development, but these findings need to be confirmed in other groups of patients with aneurysms.

Olson and colleagues[146] performed a sibling-pair linkage analysis in Finnish patients with intracranial aneurysms and identified a susceptibility locus at 19q13.1–13.3. One of the candidate genes in this region is *uPAR* (urokinase-type plasminogen activator receptor) at 19q13.2.

REFERENCES

1. Schievink WI: Intracranial aneurysms. N Engl J Med 336:28–40, 1997.
2. Schievink WI: Genetics and aneurysm formation. Neurosurg Clin N Am 9:485–495, 1998.
3. Schievink WI, Michels VV, Piepgras DG: Neurovascular mani-

festations of heritable connective tissue disorders: A review. Stroke 25:889–903, 1994.

4. Schievink WI, Katzmann JA, Piepgras DG, et al: Alpha-1-antitrypsin phenotypes among patients with intracranial aneurysms. J Neurosurg 84:781–784, 1996.
5. Fick GM, Gabow PA: Natural history of autosomal dominant polycystic kidney disease. Annu Rev Med 45:23–29, 1994.
6. Schievink WI, Huston J III, Torres VE, et al: Intracranial cysts in autosomal dominant polycystic kidney disease. J Neurosurg 83:1004–1007, 1995.
7. Schievink WI, Torres VE: Spinal meningeal diverticula in autosomal dominant polycystic kidney disease. Lancet 349:1223–1224, 1997.
8. Schievink WI, Torres VE, Piepgras DG, et al: Saccular intracranial aneurysms in autosomal dominant polycystic kidney disease. J Am Soc Nephrol 3:88–95, 1992.
9. Schievink WI, Torres VE, Wiebers DO, et al: Intracranial arterial dolichoectasia in autosomal dominant polycystic kidney disease. J Am Soc Nephrol 8:1298–1303, 1997.
10. Wijdicks EFM, Torres VE, Schievink WI: Chronic subdural hematoma in autosomal dominant polycystic kidney disease. Am J Kidney Dis 35:40–43, 2000.
11. Suter W: Das kongenitale Aneurysma der basalen Hirnarterien und Cystennieren. Schweiz Med Wochenschr 79:471–476, 1949.
12. Chapman AB, Rubinstein D, Hughes R, et al: Intracranial aneurysms in autosomal dominant polycystic kidney disease. N Engl J Med 327:916–920, 1992.
13. Huston J III, Torres VE, Sulivan PP, et al: Value of magnetic resonance angiography for the detection of intracranial aneurysms in autosomal dominant polycystic kidney disease. J Am Soc Nephrol 3:1871–1877, 1993.
14. Huston J III, Torres VE, Wiebers DO, et al: Follow-up of intracranial aneurysms in autosomal dominant polycystic kidney disease by magnetic resonance angiography. J Am Soc Nephrol 7:2135–2141, 1996.
15. Iida H, Naito T, Hondo H, et al: Intracranial aneurysms in autosomal dominant polycystic kidney disease detected by MR angiography: Screening and treatment. Nippon Jinzo Gakkai Shi 40:42–47, 1998.
16. Ruggieri PM, Poulos N, Masaryk TJ, et al: Occult intracranial aneurysms in polycystic kidney disease: Screening with MR angiography. Radiology 191:33–39, 1994.
17. Ronkainen A, Hernesniemi J, Puranen M, et al: Familial intracranial aneurysms. Lancet 349:380–384, 1997.
18. Hughes R, Chapman A, Rubinstein D, et al: Recurrent intracranial aneurysms (ICA) in autosomal dominant polycystic kidney disease (ADPKD). Stroke 27:178, 1996.
19. Harris PC: Autosomal dominant polycystic kidney disease: Clues to pathogenesis. Hum Mol Genet 8:1861–1866, 1999.
20. Kimberling WJ, Fain PR, Kenyon JB, et al: Linkage heterogeneity of autosomal dominant polycystic kidney disease. N Engl J Med 319:913–918, 1988.
21. Ong AC, Harris PC: Molecular basis of renal cyst formation—one hit or two? Lancet 349:1039–1040, 1997.
22. van Dijk MA, Chang PC, Peters DJM, et al: Intracranial aneurysms in polycystic kidney disease linked to chromosome 4. J Am Soc Nephrol 6:1670–1673, 1995.
23. Schievink WI, Spetzler RF: Screening for intracranial aneurysms in patients with isolated polycystic liver disease. J Neurosurg 89:719–721, 1998.
24. Byers PH: Ehlers-Danlos syndrome type IV: A genetic disorder in many guises. J Invest Dermatol 105:311–313, 1995.
25. Pope FM, Kendall BE, Slapak GI, et al: Type III collagen mutations cause fragile cerebral arteries. Br J Neurosurg 5:551–574, 1991.
26. Pope FM, Narcisi P, Nicholls AC, et al: COL3A1 mutations cause variable clinical phenotypes including acrogeria and vascular rupture. Br J Dermatol 135:163–181, 1996.
27. Graf CJ: Spontaneous carotid-cavernous fistula: Ehlers-Danlos syndrome and related conditions. Arch Neurol 13:662–672, 1965.
28. North KN, Whiteman DA, Pepin MG, et al: Cerebrovascular complications of Ehlers-Danlos syndrome type IV. Ann Neurol 38:960–964, 1995.
29. Pope FM, Martin GR, Lichtenstein JR, et al: Patients with Ehlers-Danlos syndrome type IV lack type III collagen. Proc Natl Acad Sci U S A 72:1314–1316, 1975.
30. Liu X, Wu H, Byrne M, et al: Type III collagen is crucial for collagen I fibrillogenesis and for normal cardiovascular development. Proc Natl Acad Sci U S A 94:1852–1856, 1997.
31. Brega KE, Seltzer WK, Munro LG, et al: Genotypic variations of type III collagen in patients with cerebral aneurysms. Surg Neurol 46:253–257, 1996.
32. Majamaa K, Savolainen E-R, Myllalä VV: Synthesis of structurally unstable type III procollagen in patients with cerebral artery aneurysm. Biochim Biophys Acta 138:191–196, 1992.
33. Neil-Dwyer G, Bartlett JR, Nicholls AC, et al: Collagen deficiency and ruptured cerebral aneurysms: A clinical and biochemical study. J Neurosurg 59:16–20, 1983.
34. Østergaard JR, Oxlund H: Collagen type III deficiency in patients with rupture of intracranial saccular aneurysms. J Neurosurg 67:690–696, 1987.
35. Pope FM, Limburg M, Schievink WI: Familial cerebral aneurysms and type III collagen deficiency. J Neurosurg 72:156–158, 1990.
36. Pope FM, Nicholls AC, Narcisi P, et al: Some patients with cerebral aneurysms are deficient in type III collagen. Lancet 1: 973–975, 1981.
37. van den Berg JS, Pals G, Arwert F, et al: Type III collagen deficiency in saccular intracranial aneurysms. Defect in gene regulation? Stroke 30:1628–1631, 1999.
38. Kuivaniemi H, Prockop DJ, Wu Y, et al: Exclusion of mutations in the gene for type III collagen (COL3A1) as a common cause of intracranial aneurysms or cervical artery dissections: Results from sequence analysis of the coding sequences of type III collagen from 55 unrelated patients. Neurology 43:2652–2658, 1993.
39. Baker CJ, Fiore A, Connolly ES Jr, et al: Serum elastase and alpha-1-antitrypsin levels in patients with ruptured and unruptured cerebral aneurysms. Neurosurgery 37:56–62, 1995.
40. Chyatte D, Bruno G, Desai S, et al: Inflammation and intracranial aneurysms. Neurosurgery 45:1137–1147, 1999.
41. Connolly ES Jr, Fiore AJ, Winfree CJ, et al: Elastin degradation in the superficial temporal arteries of patients with intracranial aneurysms reflects changes in plasma elastase. Neurosurgery 40:903–909, 1997.
42. Schievink WI, Prakash UBS, Piepgras DG, et al: α_1-Antitrypsin deficiency in intracranial aneurysms and cervical artery dissection. Lancet 343:452–453, 1994.
43. Cox DW: α_1-Antitrypsin deficiency. In Scriver CR, Beaudet AL, Sly WS, et al (eds): The Metabolic and Molecular Bases of Inherited Disease, vol 3, 7th ed. New York, McGraw-Hill, 1995, pp 4125–4158.
44. Corbett E, Glaisyer H, Chan C, et al: Congenital cutis laxa with a dominant inheritance and early onset emphysema. Thorax 49: 836–837, 1994.
45. Cohen JR, Sarfati I, Ratner L, et al: α_1-Antitrypsin phenotypes in patients with abdominal aortic aneurysms. J Surg Res 49: 319–321, 1990.
46. Cox DW: α_1-Antitrypsin: A guardian of vascular tissue. Mayo Clin Proc 69:1123–1124, 1994.
47. Mitchell MB, McAnena OJ, Rutherford RB: Ruptured mesenteric artery aneurysm in a patient with alpha$_1$-antitrypsin deficiency: Etiologic implications. J Vasc Surg 17:420–424, 1993.
48. Schievink WI, Björnsson J, Parisi JE, et al: Arterial fibromuscular dysplasia associated with severe α_1-antitrypsin deficiency. Mayo Clin Proc 69:1040–1043, 1994.
49. Schievink WI, Katzmann JA, Piepgras DG: Alpha-1-antitrypsin deficiency in spontaneous intracranial arterial dissections. Cerebrovasc Dis 8:42–44, 1998.
50. St. Jean P, Hart B, Webster M, et al: α_1-Antitrypsin deficiency in aneurysmal disease. Hum Hered 46:92–97, 1996.
51. Broderick J, Sauerbeck L, Khoury J, et al: S and Z mutations in the alpha-1-antitrypsin gene are not associated with an increased risk of ruptured intracranial aneurysm. Stroke 31:285, 2000.
52. Beckman L, Sikstrom C, Mikelsaar A, et al: Alpha1-antitrypsin (PI) alleles as markers of West European influence in the Baltic Sea region. Hum Hered 49:52–55, 1999.
53. Godfrey M: The Marfan syndrome. In Beighton P (ed): McKusick's Heritable Disorders of Connective Tissue, 5th ed. St. Louis, CV Mosby, 1993, pp 51–135.

54. Pyeritz RE: The Marfan syndrome. In Royce PM, Steinmann B (eds): Connective Tissue and Its Heritable Disorders: Molecular, Genetic, and Medical Aspects. New York, Wiley-Liss, 1993, pp 437–468.
55. Schievink WI, Björnsson J, Piepgras DG: Coexistence of fibromuscular dysplasia and cystic medial necrosis in a patient with Marfan's syndrome and bilateral carotid artery dissections. Stroke 25:2492–2496, 1994.
56. Pyeritz RE, Fishman EK, Bernhardt BA, et al: Dural ectasia is a common feature of the Marfan syndrome. Am J Hum Genet 43: 726–732, 1988.
57. Fattori R, Nienaber CA, Descovich B, et al: Importance of dural ectasia in phenotypic assessment of Marfan's syndrome. Lancet 354:910–913, 1999.
58. Rose BS, Pretorius DL: Dissecting basilar artery aneurysm in Marfan syndrome: Case report. AJNR Am J Neuroradiol 12: 503–504, 1991.
59. Schievink WI, Parisi JE, Piepgras DG, et al: Intracranial aneurysms in Marfan's syndrome: An autopsy study. Neurosurgery 41:866–871, 1997.
60. Sekhar LN, Bucur SD, Bank WO, et al: Venous and arterial bypass grafts for difficult tumors, aneurysms, and occlusive vascular lesions: Evolution of surgical treatment and improved graft results. Neurosurgery 44:1207–1224, 1999.
61. Conway JE, Hutchins GM, Tamargo RJ: Marfan syndrome is not associated with intracranial aneurysms. Stroke 30:1632–1636, 1999.
62. Schievink WI: Intracranial aneurysms and Marfan syndrome. Stroke 30:2767–2768, 1999.
63. Ramirez F, Gayraud B, Pereira L: Marfan syndrome: New clues to genotype-phenotype correlations. Ann Med 31:202–207, 1999.
64. Sakai LY, Keene DR, Engvall E: Fibrillin, a new 350-kD glycoprotein, is a component of extracellular microfibrils. J Cell Biol 103: 2499–2509, 1986.
65. Aoyama T, Francke U, Gasner C, et al: Fibrillin abnormalities and prognosis in Marfan syndrome and related disorders. Am J Med Genet 58:169–176, 1995.
66. Francke U, Berg MA, Tynan K, et al: A Gly1127Ser mutation in an EGF-like domain of the fibrillin-1 gene is a risk factor for ascending aortic aneurysm and dissection. Am J Hum Genet 56:1287–1296, 1995.
67. Milewicz DM, Grossfield J, Cao S-N, et al: A mutation in *FBN1* disrupts profibrillin processing and results in isolated skeletal features of the Marfan syndrome. J Clin Invest 95:2373–2378, 1995.
68. Schievink WI, Meyer FB, Schrijver I, et al: A syndrome of spontaneous spinal cerebrospinal fluid leaks and skeletal features of Marfan syndrome. Ann Neurol 44:458, 1998.
69. Riccardi VM: Neurofibromatosis: Phenotype, Natural History and Pathogenesis, 2nd ed. Baltimore, Johns Hopkins University, 1992.
70. Greene JF Jr, Fitzwater JE, Burgess J: Arterial lesions associated with neurofibromatosis. Am J Clin Pathol 62:481–487, 1974.
71. Reubi F: Neurofibromatosis et lésions vasculaires. Schweiz Med Wochenschr 75:463–465, 1945.
72. Schievink WI, Piepgras DG: Cervical vertebral artery aneurysms and arteriovenous fistulae in neurofibromatosis type 1: Case reports. Neurosurgery 29:760–765, 1991.
73. Benatar MG: Intracranial fusiform aneurysms in von Recklinghausen's disease: Case report and literature review. J Neurol Neurosurg Psychiatry 57:1279–1280, 1994.
74. Poli P, Peillon C, Lahda E, et al: Anéurysmes intracraniens multiples en rapport avec une maladie de Recklinghausen: A propos d'un cas. J Mal Vasc 19:253–255, 1994.
75. Sasaki J, Miura S, Ohishi H, et al: Neurofibromatosis associated with multiple intracranial vascular lesions: Stenosis of the internal carotid artery and peripheral aneurysm of the Huebner's artery; report of a case [Japanese]. No Shinkei Geka 23:813–817, 1995.
76. Urashini R, Ochiai C, Okuno S, et al: Cerebral aneurysms associated with von Recklinghausen neurofibromatosis: Report of two cases [Japanese]. No Shinkei Geka 23:237–242, 1995.
77. Schievink WI: Genetics of intracranial aneurysms. Neurosurgery 40:651–663, 1997.
78. Zhao JZ, Han XD: Cerebral aneurysm associated with von Recklinghausen's neurofibromatosis: A case report. Surg Neurol 50:592–596, 1998.
79. Sobata E, Ohkuma H, Suzuki S: Cerebrovascular disorders associated with von Recklinghausen's neurofibromatosis: A case report. Neurosurgery 22:544–549, 1988.
80. Gutmann DH, Collins FS: The neurofibromatosis type 1 gene and its protein product, neurofibromin. Neuron 10:335–343, 1993.
81. Shen MH, Harper PS, Upadhyaya M: Molecular genetics of neurofibromatosis type 1 (NF1). J Med Genet 33:2–17, 1996.
82. Henkemeyer M, Rossi DJ, Holmyard DP, et al: Vascular system defects and neuronal apoptosis in mice lacking *ras* GTPase-activating protein. Nature 377:695–701, 1995.
83. Viljoen D. Pseudoxanthoma elasticum. In Beighton P (ed): McKusick's Heritable Disorders of Connective Tissue, 5th ed. St. Louis, CV Mosby, 1993, pp 335–365.
84. Neldner KH: Pseudoxanthoma elasticum. In Royce PM, Steinmann B (eds): Connective Tissue and Its Heritable Disorders: Molecular, Genetic, and Medical Aspects. New York, Wiley-Liss, 1993, pp 425–436.
85. Connor PJ, Juergens JL, Perry HO, et al: Pseudoxanthoma elasticum and angioid streaks: A review of 106 cases. Am J Med 30:537–543, 1961.
86. Carlborg U: Studies of circulatory disturbances, pulse wave velocity and pressure pulses in larger arteries in cases of pseudoxanthoma elasticum and angioid streaks. Acta Med Scand 151 Suppl):1–209, 1944.
87. Scheie HG, Hogan TF: Angioid streaks and generalized arterial disease. Arch Ophthalmol 57:855–868, 1957.
88. Di Matteo J, Heulin A, Jaubert F, et al: Les manifestation cardiovasculaires de l'élastorrhexie systématisée (syndrome Grønblad-Strandberg-Touraine). Ann Med Interne (Paris) 134:470–474, 1983.
89. Lebwohl M, Halperin J, Phelps RG: Brief report: Occult pseudoxanthoma elasticum in patients with premature cardiovascular disease. N Engl J Med 329:1237–1239, 1993.
90. Heno P, Fourcade L, Duc HN, et al: [Aorto-coronary dysplasia and pseudoxanthoma elastica]. Arch Mal Coeur Vaiss 91:415–418, 1998.
91. Bete JM, Banas JS Jr, Moran J, et al: Coronary artery disease in an 18-year-old girl with pseudoxanthoma elasticum: Successful surgical therapy. Am J Cardiol 36:515–520, 1975.
92. Lebwohl MG, Distefano D, Prioleau PG, et al: Pseudoxanthoma elasticum and mitral-valve prolapse. N Engl J Med 307:228–231, 1982.
93. Pope FM: Autosomal dominant pseudoxanthoma elasticum. J Med Genet 11:152–157, 1974.
94. Pope FM: Historical evidence for the genetic heterogeneity of pseudoxanthoma elasticum. Br J Dermatol 92:493–509, 1975.
95. Iqbal A, Alter M, Lee SH: Pseudoxanthoma elasticum: A review of neurological complications. Ann Neurol 4:18–20, 1978.
96. Fasshauer K, Reimers CD, Gnau H-J, et al: Neurological complications of Grønblad-Strandberg syndrome. J Neurol 231:250–252, 1984.
97. Bennis A, Mehadji BA, Soulami S, et al: Les manifestations cardio-vasculaires des dyplasies héréditaires du tissu conjonctif. Ann Cardiol Angeiol (Paris) 42:173–181, 1993.
98. van den Berg JSP: Prevalence of symptomatic intracranial aneurysms and ischaemic strokes in pseudoxanthoma elasticum. In Intracranial Aneurysms and Connective Tissue Disorders [thesis]. University of Amsterdam, Benda, Nijmegen, 1999, pp 33–41.
99. Beurey J, Weber M, Picard L, et al: Myélopathie cervicale ischémique au cours d'une élastorrhexie systématisée. Bull Soc Fr Dermatol Syphiligr 78:509–511, 1971.
100. Josien E: Extracranial vertebral artery dissection: Nine cases. J Neurol 239:327–330, 1992.
101. Mokri B, Sundt TM Jr, Houser OW: Spontaneous internal carotid dissection, hemicrania, and Horner's syndrome. Arch Neurol 36:677–680, 1979.
102. Mikol F, Mikol J, Leclere J: Dilatations anéurysmales des carotides internes et calcinose cutanée au cours d'une élastorhexie systématisée: Essai de traitement par la calcitonine. Ann Med Interne (Paris) 125:225–238, 1974.
103. Dixon JM: Angioid streaks and pseudoxanthoma elasticum:

With aneurysm of the internal carotid artery. Am J Ophthalmol 34:1322–1323, 1951.
104. Munyer TP, Margulis AR: Pseudoxanthoma elasticum with internal carotid artery aneurysm. AJR Am J Roentgenol 136:1023–1024, 1981.
105. Neldner KH: Pseudoxanthoma elasticum. Clin Dermatol 6:1–159, 1988.
106. Miller NR. Walsh and Hoyt's Clinical Neuro-Ophthalmology, 4th ed. Baltimore, Williams & Wilkins, 1991.
107. Kito K, Kobayashi N, Mori N, et al: Ruptured aneurysm of the anterior spinal artery associated with pseudoxanthoma elasticum: Case report. J Neurosurg 58:126–128, 1983.
108. Struk B, Neldner KH, Rao VS, et al: Mapping of both autosomal recessive and dominant variants of pseudoxanthoma elasticum to chromosome 16p13.1. Hum Mol Genet 6:1823–1828, 1997.
109. Chambers WR, Harper BF Jr, Simpson JR: Familial incidence of congenital aneurysms of cerebral arteries. JAMA 155:358–359, 1954.
110. De Braekeleer M, Pérusse L, Cantin L, et al: A study of inbreeding and kinship in intracranial aneurysms in the Saguenay Lac-Saint-Jean region (Quebec, Canada). Ann Hum Genet 60: 99–104, 1996.
111. Norrgård Ö, Ångquist K-A, Fodstad H, et al: Intracranial aneurysms and heredity. Neurosurgery 20:236–239, 1987.
112. Ronkainen A, Hernesniemi J, Ryynänen M: Familial subarachnoid hemorrhage in east Finland, 1977–1990. Neurosurgery 33: 787–797, 1993.
113. Schievink WI, Schaid DJ, Michels VV, et al: Familial aneurysmal subarachnoid hemorrhage: A community-based study. J Neurosurg 83:426–429, 1995.
114. Wang PS, Longstreth WT Jr, Koepsell TD: Subarachnoid hemorrhage and family history. A population-based case-control study. Arch Neurol 52:202–204, 1995.
115. Bromberg JEC, Rinkel GJE, Algra A, et al: Subarachnoid haemorrhage in first and second degree relatives of patients with subarachnoid haemorrhage. BMJ 311:288–289, 1995.
116. Gaist D, Vaeth M, Tsiropoulos I, et al: Risk of subarachnoid haemorrhage in first-degree relatives of patients with subarachnoid haemorrhage: Follow up study based on national registries in Denmark. BMJ 320:141–145, 2000.
117. Schievink WI, Schaid DJ, Rogers HM, et al: On the inheritance of intracranial aneurysms. Stroke 25:2028–2037, 1994.
118. Bromberg JEC, Rinkel GJE, Algra A, et al: Familial subarachnoid hemorrhage: Distinctive features and patterns of inheritance. Ann Neurol 38:929–934, 1995.
119. Bailey JC: Familial subarachnoid haemorrhage: Ulster Med J 62: 119–126, 1993.
120. Leblanc R, Melanson D, Tampieri D, et al: Familial cerebral aneurysms: A study of 13 families. Neurosurgery 37:633–639, 1995.
121. Lozano AM, Leblanc R: Familial intracranial aneurysms. J Neurosurg 66:522–528, 1987.
122. Ronkainen R, Hernesniemi J, Tromp G: Special features of familial intracranial aneurysms: Report of 215 familial aneurysms. Neurosurgery 37:43–47, 1995.
123. Motuo Fotso MJ, Brunon J, Outhel R, et al: Anéurysmes familiaux, anéurysmes multiples et anéurysmes "de novo": A propos de deux observations. Neurochirurgie 39:225–230, 1993.
124. Leblanc R: De novo formation of familial cerebral aneurysms: Case report. Neurosurgery 44:871–877, 1999.
125. Bromberg JE, Rinkel GJ, Algra A, et al: Outcome in familial subarachnoid hemorrhage. Stroke 26:961–963, 1995.
126. Schievink WI, Schaid DJ: The prognosis of familial versus nonfamilial aneurysmal subarachnoid hemorrhage. Stroke 27:340–341, 1996.
127. Ronkainen A, Niskanen M, Piironen R, et al: Familial subarachnoid hemorrhage: Outcome study. Stroke 30:1099–1102, 1999.
128. Schievink WI, Parisi JE, Piepgras DG: Familial intracranial aneurysms: An autopsy study. Neurosurgery 41:1247–1252, 1997.
129. Brown BM, Soldevilla F: MR angiography and surgery for unruptured familial intracranial aneurysms in persons with a family history of cerebral aneurysms. AJR Am J Roentgenol 173: 133–138, 1999.
130. Ronkainen A, Puranen MI, Hernesniemi JA, et al: Intracranial aneurysms: MR angiographic screening in 400 asymptomatic individuals with increased familial risk. Radiology 195:35–40, 1995.
131. Raaymakers TW, Rinkel GJ, Ramos LM: Initial and follow-up screening for aneurysms in families with familial subarachnoid hemorrhage. Neurology 51:1125–1130, 1998.
132. Ronkainen A, Miettinen H, Karkola K, et al: Risk of harboring an unruptured intracranial aneurysm. Stroke 29:359–362, 1998.
133. Raaymakers TW: Aneurysms in relatives of patients with subarachnoid hemorrhage: Frequency and risk factors. MARS Study Group. Magnetic resonance angiography in relatives of patients with subarachnoid hemorrhage. Neurology 53:982–988, 1999.
134. The Magnetic Resonance Angiography in Relatives of Patients with Subarachnoid Hemorrhage Study Group: Risks and benefits of screening for intracranial aneurysms in first-degree relatives of patients with sporadic subarachnoid hemorrhage. N Engl J Med 341:1344–1350, 1999.
135. Obuchowski NA, Modic MT, Magdinec M: Current implications for the efficacy of noninvasive screening for occult intracranial aneurysms in patients with a family history of aneurysms. J Neurosurg 83:42–49, 1995.
136. Leblanc R, Worsley KJ, Melanson D, et al: Angiographic screening and elective surgery of familial cerebral aneurysms: A decision analysis. Neurosurgery 35:9–19, 1994.
137. ter Berg HW, Dippel DW, Limburg M, et al: Familial intracranial aneurysms: A review. Stroke 23:1024–1030, 1992.
138. Ronkainen A, Hernesniemi J, Kuivaniemi H, et al: Current implications for the efficacy of noninvasive screening for occult intracranial aneurysms in patients with a family history of aneurysms. J Neurosurg 84:534–536, 1996.
139. Schievink WI, Limburg M, Dreissen JJR, et al: Screening for unruptured familial intracranial aneurysms: Subarachnoid hemorrhage 2 years after angiography negative for aneurysms. Neurosurgery 29:434–438, 1991.
140. Pollack JS, Custer PL, Hart WM, et al: Ocular complications in Ehlers-Danlos syndrome type IV. Arch Ophthalmol 115:416–419, 1997.
141. McConnell RS, Hughes AE, Rubinsztein DEC, et al: Gene-environment interactions in familial clustering of cerebral aneurysm formation. J Neurol Neurosurg Psychiatry 63:128, 1997.
142. Bromberg JEC, Rinkel GJE, Algra A, et al: Hypertension, stroke, and coronary heart disease in relatives of patients with subarachnoid hemorrhage. Stroke 27:7–9, 1996.
143. Takenaka K, Sakai H, Yamakawa H, et al: Polymorphism of the endoglin gene in patients with intracranial saccular aneurysms. J Neurosurg 90:935–938, 1999.
144. Takenaka K, Yamakawa H, Sakai N, et al: Angiotensin I-converting enzyme gene polymorphism in intracranial saccular aneurysm individuals. Neurol Res 20:607–611, 1998.
145. Yoon S, Tromp G, Vongpunsawad S, et al: Genetic analysis of MMP3, MMP9, and PAI-1 in Finnish patients with abdominal aortic or intracranial aneurysms. Biochem Biophys Res Commun 265:563–568, 1999.
146. Olson J, Vongpunsawad S, Kuivaniemi H, et al: Genome scan for intracranial aneurysm susceptibility loci using Finnish families. Am J Hum Genet 63:A17, 1998.

CHAPTER **106B**

The Natural History of Unruptured Saccular Cerebral Aneurysms

GAVIN W. BRITZ ■ H. RICHARD WINN

The natural history of any disease is defined as the outcome of the disease in the absence of any intervention. With the knowledge of the natural history of a disease, the physician and surgeon can assess the effectiveness of treatment options. When evaluating the natural history of cerebral aneurysms, intact and ruptured aneurysms should be considered separately, because results obtained from epidemiologic studies have determined that the natural history of unruptured and ruptured cerebral aneurysms are different.

Unruptured intracranial aneurysms (UIAs) are aneurysms with no recent or remote history of subarachnoid hemorrhage (SAH) or symptoms that may be related to a previous hemorrhage. An increasing number of unruptured and often incidental intracranial aneurysms are being diagnosed because of the increasing age of the population and the improvement in imaging techniques. The management of these patients is controversial and is one of the most important issues confronting neurosurgeons today.[1] The risk of a UIA is related to hemorrhage, which is a potentially devastating disease; 45% to 80% of patients die of SAH.[2–10]

Prevention of this rupture with surgical or endovascular treatment is believed to be the most effective strategy for lowering these mortality rates. However, all current treatments carry some risks, and in formulating recommendations for treatment of the patient, the natural history of UIAs must be considered carefully with the patient's life expectancy. Assessing the patient's life expectancy includes consideration of the patient's age, medical condition, and family history. This allows the neurosurgeon to make a calculated judgment about the lifetime risk of a UIA compared with the risk of treatment. For example, a relatively benign natural history makes observation a reasonable or even preferred choice, particularly in the older population, whereas a more malignant natural history in the younger patient makes treatment more urgent. Life expectancy tables can provide an estimate of the patient's life expectancy. Table 106B–1 provides the average number of years of life remaining for different age groups. At the age of 50 years, patients have, on average, 29 years of life remaining for both sexes, whereas patients who are 85 years of age have only an estimated 6 years of life remaining.[11] This complex assessment is further complicated by having two modes of therapy: surgical and endovascular. Each mode of therapy has its own advantages, disadvantages, and complications.

Before addressing the data on the natural history of UIAs, we discuss the prevalence of UIA and the incidence of SAH.

PREVALENCE OF ANEURYSMS

Prevalence is defined as the number of affected persons present in the population at a specific time divided by the number of persons in the population at that time. Prevalence is a sample of the population at a point in time and indicates the frequency of the disease process in the population. In respect to unruptured cerebral aneurysms, prevalence is the number of people with unruptured aneurysms at a specific time. These individuals define the population at risk for a hemorrhage. The prevalence of UIA has largely been determined in autopsy and radiologic studies.

In a review by Fox and colleagues[12] of 20 autopsy series published between 1926 and 1973, each of which covered more than 5000 cases, there was a total of 164,764 autopsies during which 1289 aneurysms were found, yielding a prevalence rate of 0.8%.[12] In nine studies published between 1918 and 1973, each of which covered between 2 and 5000 cases, there were 30,150 autopsies during which 603 aneurysms were found, for a rate of aneurysm occurrence of 2%.[12] In Stehbens' series[13] of 1364 autopsies conducted at a large hospital in Australia between 1952 and 1954, at least one cerebral aneurysm was found in 5.6% of cadavers. Stehbens[14] also reviewed the literature of autopsy studies (14 studies published between 1890 and 1966) and found a prevalence of 2.4% (range, 0.2% to 9%). In the autopsy series conducted by McCormick and Nofzinger,[15] 153 patients were identified as harboring saccular intracranial aneurysms among 7650 patients, giving a prevalence of 2%.

TABLE 106B-1 ■ **Modified U.S. Life Table, 1995**

AGE INTERVAL	NUMBER LIVING PER 100,000 BORN ALIVE	NUMBER DYING DURING AGE INTERVAL PER 100,000	AVERAGE REMAINING LIFETIME AT BEGINNING OF AGE INTERVAL
0–1	100,000	757	75.8
1–5	99,243	159	75.4
5–10	99,084	98	71.5
10–15	98,986	125	66.6
15–20	98,861	410	61.6
20–25	98,451	527	56.9
25–30	97,924	583	52.2
30–35	97,341	779	47.5
35–40	96,562	1,013	42.8
40–45	95,549	1,315	38.3
45–50	94,234	1,755	33.8
50–55	92,479	2,586	29.3
55–60	89,893	3,844	25.1
60–65	86,049	5,770	21.1
65–70	80,279	7,888	17.4
70–75	72,391	10,573	14.1
75–80	61,818	13,140	11
80–85	48,678	15,520	8.3
85+	33,158	33,158	6

From Mon Vital Stat Rep 45:18, 1997.

Rosenorn and colleagues[16] estimated a prevalence of unruptured aneurysms of 0.6% (range, 0.1% to 2.9%) based on data from autopsy studies and a prevalence of 0.4% (range, 0.18% to 6.01%) based on data from radiologic studies. Rinkel and colleagues[17] performed a systematic review of retrospective and prospective autopsy and radiologic data. In the retrospective study of 43,676 autopsies, 191 aneurysms were found (prevalence of 0.4%; 95% CI, 0.4% to 0.5%). In the prospective study of 5493 autopsies, the prevalence was 3.6% (95% CI, 3% to 4.4%). In a retrospective study of 2934 angiographic examinations, the prevalence was 3.7% (95% CI, 3% to 4.4%). The highest rate of prevalence was 6% (95% CI, 5.3% to 6.8%) for 3751 patients studied prospectively by angiography. In angiographic studies, the prevalence per 100 male patients was 3.5 (95% CI, 2.7 to 4.5), and for female patients, it was 4.6 (95% CI, 3.5 to 5.9).[17]

Ujie and associates [18] studied 1612 Japanese patients undergoing four-vessel angiography for suspected nonaneurysmal diseases, and the prevalence of aneurysms was 2.7%; among 463 patients with ischemic stroke, it was 2.8%; and among 127 cases of intracerebral hematomas, it was 7.8%. Yoshimoto and coworkers[19] studied a total of 375 presumably healthy people in Japan undergoing routine magnetic resonance angiography (MRA), and there were 10 cases, giving a prevalence of 2.7% in which an unruptured aneurysm was present. A report by Winn and colleagues[20] of 4568 arteriograms described 24 cases of asymptomatic aneurysms, yielding a prevalence rate of 0.65%.

Based on autopsy and radiologic data, the prevalence of intracranial aneurysms ranges from 0.2% to 9%, and the frequently quoted prevalence rate of 5% reported by Sekhar and Heros[21] on the basis of a literature review must be interpreted with caution and may be an overestimation of the true prevalence of UIA. This wide prevalence range for UIAs may be related to several factors, such as the inherent biases and inherent errors in the collection of the data. For example, the presence of a neurosurgical unit and expert neuropathologists with an interest in aneurysms may lead to higher rates of lesions discovered at autopsy. In the radiologic data, patients' disease may cause selection bias. The sensitivity and specificity of aneurysm detection by radiologic techniques is less than 100%. The definition of what constitutes an aneurysm in autopsy series may differ from that used in radiologic studies. In autopsy reports, the age range of the patient may be greater than in radiographic series and the normal population.

INCIDENCE OF SUBARACHNOID HEMORRHAGE

The incidence of a disease is defined as the number of new cases of a disease that occur during a specified period in a population at risk for developing the disease. This is usually expressed as an incidence per x number of persons. The incidence of SAH is often expressed as the number of aneurysm ruptures per 100,000 persons per year. The reported incidence of SAH depends on the following factors: the nature of the population (i.e., Finnish and Japanese persons may be particularly prone to develop aneurysms)[8–10]; the quality of diagnostic techniques (i.e., industrialized countries record higher rates of unruptured aneurysms than developing ones); the size of the population (i.e., a small town with high autopsy rates have a higher incidence than the larger, less populated region in which the small town is located); the diagnostic criteria (i.e., blood in the cerebrospinal fluid or evidence based on computed tomography [CT] scans, magnetic resonance imaging [MRI], digital substraction angiography, or clinical impressions); the age distribution of the population (i.e., a younger population has a lower incidence); the sophistication of data collection and analysis (i.e., ability to differentiate spontaneous from aneurysmal intracerebral hematomas and the ability to capture these distinctions among hospital deaths); and factors that may increase the likelihood of occurrence of the disease (i.e., cigarette addiction and hypertension).[22]

The available data on the incidence of SAH suggests a range that depends on geography. For example, in the United States, two large studies have been performed. The first was reported from Framingham, Massachusetts, and yielded a rate of 28 cases per 100,000 adults (30 to 88 years old) per year.[23] The second study was from Rochester, Minnesota, which gave a rate of 10.8 cases per 100,000 persons per year between 1945 and 1974 for all ages.[24] In patients in Greenland, Denmark, the incidence of SAH was 9.3 per 100,000 for all ages.[25] In the city of Izumo in Japan, the incidence was 18.3 per 100,000 for the general population, but for men in the eighth decade, it is 92.3 per 100,000 persons per year.[26] In Shimane Prefecture, it was 11 per 100,000 persons.[26] The incidence of SAH in New Zealand was 14.6 per 100,000 persons from 1981 to 1983 and was lower from 1991 to 1993 (11.3 per 100,000 persons).[27]

The Finnish population appears to have a high incidence of SAH. An early study by Pakarinen demonstrated an annual incidence of SAH of 16.8 per 100,000 in the population of Helsinki during the years between 1954 and 1961.[28] In a later Finnish study, the age-standardized annual incidence of SAH was 33 per 100,000 Finnish men and 25 per 100,000 Finnish women.[29] SAH was responsible for 11% of all strokes reported between 1983 and 1985.[29] These rates were higher than those previously reported in Finland and were thought to be an example of changes in diagnostic classification and improvements in detection, rather than a real increase in the incidence of SAH. The studies reviewed were prospective and population based. CT was considered to be the definitive diagnostic method for SAH because lumbar puncture can be traumatic or provide false-positive results in the presence of nonaneurysmal lesions such as intracerebral hematomas. Reliance on angiographic series can lead to underestimates of the incidence of aneurysmal SAH because angiography is not performed in patients who die outside of institutions or who are very old or moribund.[30] The more frequently CT was used, the lower the incidence of aneurysmal SAH.

In conclusion, most studies suggest the incidence of aneurysmal SAH is 10 to 11 cases per 100,000 persons per year. However, in the Finnish and Japanese population, the incidence may be higher.

NATURAL HISTORY OF UNRUPTURED INTRACRANIAL ANEURYSMS

Although understanding the natural history of UIA is critical, it is not perfectly defined (Table 106B–2). In a 1966 report, Locksley[31] followed 34 patients with 34 UIAs for 47 months. During this time, nine cases of SAH were documented, giving a rupture rate of 7% per year.

Zacks and colleagues[32] reported data from 10 patients with 12 incidental aneurysms. Five of these lesions were smaller than 3 mm, three were 3 to 6 mm, and one was 10 mm in diameter. One of the patients died of a pulmonary embolus 2 months after treatment. Three of the nine survivors underwent follow-up angiography 12 to 16 months later, and no change in the appearance of the aneurysm was observed. The nine patients were observed for a mean of 37 months (maximum, 90 months) during which no SAH occurred.[32]

Heiskanen and associates[33] presented a follow-up review of 61 patients with 129 unruptured aneurysms who had undergone previous treatment for ruptured aneurysms and who were followed for 10 years. Dur-

TABLE 106B–2 ■ **Natural History Studies of Unruptured Intracronial Aneurysms**

STUDY	CASE NO.	UIA NO.	NO. OF SAH	MEAN FOLLOW-UP	RISK PER YEAR (%)	RISK PER YEAR (%) <10 mm	RISK PER YEAR (%) >10 mm	PRIOR SAH (%)	RISK PER YEAR (%) MA
Locksley, 1966	34	34	9	47	7			100	
Heiskanen, 1981	61	129	7	120	~1.1			100	~1.1
Wiebers, 1981	65	81	8	98.5		0	~1.7	0	Increased
Wiebers, 1987	130	161	15	99.6		0	~2	0	
Juvela, 1993	142	181	27	166.8	1.4	≅	≅	92	1.3
Asari, 1993	54	72	11	43.7	1.9				
Taylor, 1995 (1, 2)	7113, 11066	7113, 11066	119, 98	2.5	(2, 1.3)				
Yasui, 97	234	303	34	75.1	2.3				Increased
ISUIA, 1998 (NH, PH)	727, 722	977, 960	12, 20	99.6		0.05	0.5, 1.9 (>20 mm)		
Juvela, 2000	142	181	33	236.4	~1.3	≅		92	
Tsutsumi, 2000	62	62	7	52.6		1.3	2.1		

MA, multiple aneurysms; NH, no prior history of SAH; PH, prior history of SAH; SAH, subarachnoid hemorrhage; UIA, unruptured intracranial aneurysm.

ing this period, seven patients bled from a previously unruptured aneurysm, yielding a rupture risk of approximately 1.1% per year. Wiebers and coworkers[34] reported a selected group of 65 patients with 81 unruptured intracranial saccular aneurysms who did not undergo surgery. Eight of the 65 patients subsequently had SAH due to aneurysmal rupture over a mean follow-up interval of slightly more than 8 years, yielding an approximate risk of rupture of 1%. This study was particularly important in that is was first to stratify the lesions by size and to assess the value of aneurysm size in the risk of rupture. Weibers and colleagues[34] reported a zero risk of rupture for aneurysms less than 10 mm in diameter and an approximate risk for aneurysms larger than 10 mm of 1.7% per year. Their data also suggested that patients with multiple aneurysms had an increased risk for rupture.

In 1983, Winn and colleagues[35] reported the long-term (10-year) outcomes of patients with multiple aneurysms. All patients had a history of SAH with surgical treatment of the ruptured aneurysm. The investigators evaluated the fate of the intact aneurysms and found an approximately 1% per year risk of hemorrhage.

In 1987, Weibers and associates[36] further reported their results of a long-term follow-up study of 130 patients with 161 unruptured intracranial saccular aneurysms. This study also included follow-up data on the patients from the prior study. The findings suggest that unruptured saccular aneurysms less than 10 mm in diameter have a very low probability of subsequent rupture; no patients who had aneurysms less than 10 mm in diameter rebled. However, 15 of the 59 aneurysms larger than 10 mm ruptured, producing a rupture rate of approximately 2% per year for that group.

Easton and coworkers[37] speculated on the natural history by assuming a frequency of 5% (based on autopsy rates) and a population-based incidence of aneurysmal SAH of 10 per 100,000 persons per year. These investigators concluded that most aneurysms never rupture. Moreover, Easton and colleagues[37] concluded that most aneurysms tend to rupture shortly after formation. They also suggested that patients with unruptured aneurysms who have not undergone treatment could reasonably be studied at yearly intervals for 3 years, particularly those harboring lesions between 6 and 9 mm in diameter. The investigators also speculated that, even if aneurysm enlargement occurred and no symptoms developed after 3 years, it might be adequate to rely on follow-up examinations performed at 5-year intervals. They also postulated that a history of SAH from a different source increases the likelihood that a patient with an unruptured aneurysm will experience a later SAH from the untreated lesion.[37]

In 1993, Juvela and colleagues[8] reported 181 aneurysms in 142 patients with a mean follow-up 166.8 months. They stated that the overall risk of rupture for an unruptured aneurysm was 1.4% annually, a value based on the 27 first aneurysm ruptures during the follow-up period. If considering aneurysms rather than cases, the annual risk was 1.1% (27 events during 2434 aneurysm-years). This population was somewhat different from that of Wiebers in that 92% of the patients had had a previous SAH from another aneurysm but was similar to the population studied by Winn and colleagues.[35]

Another study in 1993 by Asari and Ohmoto[38] followed 54 patients with 72 unruptured cerebral aneurysms. Twenty-two patients died during the observation period, which averaged 43.7 months. The 5-year survival rate was 56%. Aneurysms ruptured in 11 patients (20.4%), 10 of whom died without undergoing surgery. The annual bleeding rate was 1.92%, and the average size of the 11 ruptured aneurysms was 13.1 mm. In four patients, however, bleeding occurred in unruptured cerebral aneurysms of 4 to 5 mm.[38]

Taylor and coworkers[39] reported a large study involving 20,767 Medicare patients who were admitted to a hospital and were diagnosed with unruptured cerebral aneurysms. The average age of these patients was 73.8 years, and 70% were women. In that cohort, 2648 patients were excluded from the follow-up study because of a concurrent diagnosis of SAH or in-hospital death, and therefore 18,119 patients were identified with the diagnosis of unruptured cerebral aneurysms. These patients were divided into two populations. Group 1 consisted of patients with UIA as a primary diagnosis; group 2 consisted of patients with UIA as a secondary diagnosis. The first group consisted of 7113 patients, and the second group consisted 11,066 patients. Follow-up treatment (surgical or endovascular) occurred for 13.5% of women and 10.5% of men and for 27.2% of group 1 and 3.1% of group 2. After 2.5 years of follow-up, the risk of hemorrhage was 2% per year for the first group and 1.3% for the second group.[39]

In 1997, Yasui and colleagues[40] reported results of a follow-up study of 303 unruptured aneurysms in 234 patients. Single aneurysms were present in 171 patients and multiple aneurysms in 63. The mean follow-up period was 75 months (range, 3 to 270 months). Of the 234 patients, 132 (56.4%) survived, 59 (25.2%) died of other diseases, 9 (3.8%) underwent surgery, and 34 (14.5%) had bleeding from unruptured aneurysms, which was fatal for 18 of the patients. The annual rupture rate was 2.3%.[40] There were no significant differences among the patients according to underlying disease or aneurysm site. The cumulative rate of bleeding for all patients was 20% at 10 years after diagnosis and 35% at 15 years. The cumulative probability of rupture was significantly higher for the multiple aneurysms than the single aneurysms.

In their review of the literature, Rinkel and associates[17] evaluated 356 patients with UIAs. Ninety-three percent of these patients harbored lesions that were 10 mm in diameter or smaller. The investigators assumed that, in a cohort of 100,000 persons, only the 75,000 persons older than 20 years would be at risk for aneurysm rupture. Most patients did not have a family history of aneurysm, adult polycystic kidney disease, or other risk factors. Rinkel and colleagues[17] found a prevalence rate of approximately 2.3% for 1725 patients harboring aneurysms. Of these, based on their original data, 93% would harbor lesions smaller than 10 mm in diameter. Of the total population with UIAs (1725 patients), 1605 patients would harbor small aneurysms (<10 mm), and 120 patients would harbor aneurysms larger than 10 mm in diameter. The annual risk of rupture was assumed to be 0.7% in the cohort with small aneurysms and 4% in the group with larger ones.

This continued debate was significantly highlighted by the landmark report from the International Study of Unruptured Intracranial Aneurysms (ISUIA), which suggested a yearly rate of hemorrhage of 0.05% per year for aneurysms less than 10 mm in diameter.[3] The ISUIA is the first and largest systematic study on the natural history of UIAs. The ISUIA had two objectives. The first was to evaluate the natural history of UIA, and the second was to establish the risk of treatment. To achieve these objectives, the study consisted of retrospective and prospective components; 2621 patients were enrolled in 53 participating centers worldwide. In the retrospective component, the natural history of UIAs was evaluated, and in the prospective component, the morbidity and mortality related to treatment were evaluated. The data for the retrospective component were obtained from the medial records of patients who were diagnosed with intracranial aneurysms between 1970 and 1991 and for whom hard copy angiograms and medical records were available in 53 centers. This cohort included patients with symptomatic and asymptomatic aneurysms and those with a history of SAH from another aneurysm. Mycotic, fusiform, and traumatic aneurysms and aneurysms smaller than 2 mm in diameter were excluded. The aneurysms were assessed in regard to the size and the location of the aneurysm to the parent artery.

A total of 1449 patients with 1937 UIAs were included in the retrospective cohort. They were divided into two groups: the 727 patients of group 1 who had no prior history of SAH from another aneurysm and the 722 patients of group 2 who had a history of SAH. Follow-up information was obtained from an annual standard questionnaire and medical records. The mean duration of follow-up was 8.3 years, with a total of 12,023 patient-years follow-up.

Of the 1449 patients, 32 had documented aneurysmal ruptures. In group 1, the cumulative rate of rupture was 0.05% per year for aneurysms less than 10 mm and about 1% in those over 10 mm in diameter. Aneurysms larger than 25 mm had a 6% rupture rate in the first year. In group 2, the cumulative rate of rupture was about 0.5% per year for lesions smaller than 10 mm and about 1% for those larger than 10 mm in diameter. In group 1, in addition to size, location was related to hemorrhage risk, with basilar tip, vertebrobasilar, posterior cerebral, and posterior communicating artery aneurysms having a higher risk of rupture. In group 2, only location (i.e., basilar tip) and increasing age predicted an increased risk of hemorrhage.

The ISUIA is an ongoing study and has influenced contemporary thinking on the natural history of UIA. The strengths of the ISUIA include its multicenter design, which minimizes referral and treatment bias, and its size, which provides robust statistical power to formulate conclusions. The study, however, has been challenged on a number of points that are largely related to selection bias, the retrospective nature of the study, and the inclusion of patients with cavernous aneurysms in the study population.

The most significant criticism of the study is related to the possibility of selection bias: Does the population studied truly represent a population of patients with UIA, or has some selection bias created a population that has inherent less risk of rupture? This concern is particularly significant because selection bias cannot be corrected with any statistical methods. In regard to selection bias, all patients were selected for observation or surgery after consultation with a neurosurgeon.[41–43] If it is assumed that most experienced neurosurgeons have an intuitive concept of what constitutes a aneurysm at high risk for rupture (e.g., size, configuration, family history), it is reasonable to presume that high-risk patients were treated and removed from the study pool. Removal of these high-risk patients skewed downward the risk of rupture.

The possibility of selection bias is supported by the fact that the patients in the retrospective component were significantly older than in the prospective component. Some studies suggest a higher rate of aneurysm rupture in the elderly.[26]

The retrospective nature of the study might have introduced unrecognized bias because, as in all retrospective studies, patients might have been excluded from follow-up by death, relocation, patient noncompliance, and subsequent surgical treatment.[42]

Another concern about the ISUIA study is the inclusion of intracavernous sinus aneurysms in the study population. These aneurysms are located outside the subarachnoid space. Intracavernous aneurysms may not manifest with SAH during rupture and thereby skew downward the rate of rupture. However, the investigators,[44] after excluding intracavernous aneurysms, concluded that the risk of hemorrhage was only slightly increased from 0.05% to 0.066% per year for small aneurysms and from 0.95% to 1.38% in patients with large aneurysms.[44]

However, as outlined by Winn and associates,[1] the ISUIA rupture rate of 0.05% to 0.066% per year is in conflict with the prevalence rate of UIA and the incidence of aneurysmal SAH (30,000 SAH in North America per year). The investigators reasoned that 30,000 people in North America suffer from aneurysmal SAH each year. Based on ISUIA data, which revealed that 49% of group 1 (i.e., no history of SAH) and 73% of group 2 (i.e., history of SAH from a different aneurysm) harbored aneurysms less than 1 cm in diameter, approximately one half of the 30,000 SAHs, or 15,000 SAHs per year, were from aneurysms smaller than 1 cm (bearing in mind that the critical size for rupture of an aneurysm remains in dispute).[45, 46] Using the ISUIA yearly rupture rate of 0.05% (0.0005), the prevalence of UIA can be calculated by solving the equation $15{,}000/x = 0.0005$. Such a calculation yields 30 million persons per year in North America who harbor unruptured aneurysms that are smaller than 1 cm, or approximately 10% of the population of all ages. However, it would be appropriate to exclude that portion of the population for which there is a very low likelihood of aneurysm occurrence— those younger than 30 years of age, or 42% of the population according to the United States 2000 census. These 30 million people harboring unruptured aneurysms would be concentrated within approximately 180 million individuals in North America older than 30 years, which yields a one in six chance (30,000/180,000, or 16.6%) that a person older than 30 years of age would harbor an intact aneurysm smaller than 1 cm.[1] A similar number of individuals should have UIAs larger than 1 cm in diameter.

Such a high prevalence is not supported by clinical experience or the rate of discovery of aneurysms on routine MRI or MRA. Five millimeters is the critical size for prospective detection of an aneurysm by using MRA, with which 87% of aneurysms are detected.[47] In the ISUIA, 67% of aneurysms smaller than 1 cm were larger than 5 mm. MRA would detect 60% (0.067 × 87%) of unruptured aneurysms smaller than 1 cm. Following this formula, 10% (0.6 × 16.6%) of the population of North America should harbor aneurysms with diameters less than 1 cm but that are detectable using MRA. At a busy imaging center, 100 MRI or MRA examinations of the brain may be performed within a week. The discovery of unruptured aneurysms of any size is much less frequent than 10 patients in a single week, even in the busiest centers. Using angiography, the gold standard, the detection rate for aneurysms is better than that provided using MRI or MRA.[47] In the setting of angiography performed for nonaneurysmal indications, approximately 16.6% of patients older than 30 years of age could be expected to harbor unruptured aneurysms smaller than 1 cm if the ISUIA rate (0.05%) is correct. As with MRA series, angiography performed for non-SAH patients revealed a 0.65% rate of discovery of UIA, significantly below 16.6%.[1]

Natural history studies by Juvela and colleagues[9] and Tsutsumi and associates[10] differed in their conclusions from the ISUIA. Juvela and coworkers[9] studied 142 Finnish patients, 131 (92%) of whom had suffered a prior SAH by the time of diagnosis of their unruptured aneurysms and whose mean duration of follow-up in the study was 19.7 years (range, 0.8 to 38.9 years). The investigators found a risk of hemorrhage of 10.5% at 10 years, 23% at 20 years, and 30.3% at 30 years, resulting in an annual incidence of about 1.3% (95% CI, 0.9% to 1.7%). Seventy percent of the aneurysms that ruptured were also smaller than 6 mm, and the aneurysm rupture rate was found to increase linearly with lesion size. Advancing age and cigarette smoking also increased the risk for rupture, as did female gender. Female gender and smoking also increased the risk of new aneurysm formation.

The study by Juvela and colleagues[9] is unique in that there was no bias introduced by surgery; before 1979, patients with unruptured aneurysms were not treated surgically in Finland. Until the late 1960s, Helsinki was the only neurosurgical center in Finland. In the time between 1970 and 1975, this center was responsible for the neurosurgical services of 88% of the Finnish people and for 60% between 1975 and 1978. This study has the further advantage that it does not represent the typical single-referral neurosurgical tertiary center with a highly selected patient population.[42] The confined catchments area and stable Finnish population made possible a long and maximally complete follow-up.

As with other studies, the study by Juvela and colleagues[9] has inherent flaws, and the results must be interpreted with caution. First, it has a relatively small sample size. Second, although the study generally lacked selection bias, as pointed out by ISUIA investigators, the detection of aneurysms before the advent of CT and MRI 30 to 50 years ago in Finland may represent a different group of patients than seen today.[48] Third, the data were derived from a single center with the inherent single-center bias.[49] Fourth, a potential does exists for genetic bias because the Finnish population is known to have a different aneurysm distribution, with a higher percentage of middle cerebral artery aneurysms than other populations.[43, 50] Finland has a higher incidence of SAH (13 to 16/100,000 persons per year)[29, 51] compared with other western countries(10/100,000 persons per year).[24] Most importantly, in regard to the validity of the natural history of UIA, the study had insufficient numbers of truly incidental asymptomatic aneurysms; only 5 (4%) of the 142 patients had no history of prior SAH.[9] The patients in the study by Juvela and colleagues[9] were similar to the patients in group 2 in the ISUIA study, and it is therefore not surprising that the rupture rates approximate that of the group 2 patients from the ISUIA.

In a second natural history study, Tsutsumi and colleagues[10] reported 62 patients treated conservatively for more than 6 months for saccular, nonthrombotic, noncalcified, unruptured aneurysms at locations not related to the cavernous sinus. These aneurysms were detected by cerebral angiographic studies performed for causes other than SAH. Clinical follow-up data for the 62 patients were reviewed to identify the risk of SAH. All patients were followed for a period ranging from 6 months to 17 years (mean, 4.3 years). Seven patients (11.3%) developed SAH confirmed by CT at a mean interval of 4.8 years; six died, and one recovered with a major deficit. One patient died of the mass effect of the aneurysm, and another died after sudden onset of headache and vomiting. The 5- and 10-year cumulative risks of CT-confirmed SAH calculated by the Kaplan-Meier method were 7.5% and 22.1%, respectively, for total cases; 33.5% and 55.9%, respectively, for large (>10 mm) aneurysms; and 4.5% and 13.9%, respectively, for small (<10 mm) aneurysms.[10]

The study by Tsutsumi and colleagues[10] must be interpreted with caution because the sample population was small and the power of the statistical analysis is therefore in question. Moreover, the follow-up period is relatively short, and the data were derived from a single center, with the associated single-center bias. Most importantly, a potential existed for selection bias because the investigators excluded low-risk cases such as thrombosed or calcified aneurysms, which would increase the calculated rate of rupture of unruptured aneurysms. The patients were obtained from a population of patients undergoing cerebral angiography that were older (mean age, 70.8 years) and had a high concomitant rate of ischemic and hemorrhagic events.

In summary, we conclude that the natural history on UIA has yet to be clearly defined.

CONFOUNDING FACTORS

The rate of rupture of UIA may be affected by other factors, such as aneurysm size, aneurysm location, multiplicity of aneurysms, aneurysmal growth, symptomatic aneurysms, and patient factors such as age, gender, and history of hypertension or smoking.

Aneurysm Size

Aneurysm size has long been considered to be an important independent variable in the risk of rupture. This was first clearly demonstrated in the study by Weibers and coworkers[34] in 1981, when they reported a zero risk of rupture for aneurysms less than 10 mm in diameter compared with an approximate risk for aneurysms larger than 10 mm of 1.7% per year. These findings were supported in their later study reported in 1987.[36] Further studies have also supported this finding. Winn and associates[35] observed that aneurysms larger than 10 cm had a higher risk of hemorrhage in a long-term follow-up of 127 multiple aneurysm patients whose ruptured aneurysm was surgically treated. In 1995, Mizoi and coworkers[52] reported results of a retrospective review of 139 consecutively managed, incidental unruptured aneurysms. Conservative management was chosen for 49 patients (35%). During the follow-up period (mean, 4.3 years), 16% of these patients experienced aneurysm rupture, and 88% of the patients died of hemorrhage. The mean size of aneurysms with late hemorrhage was significantly larger than that of lesions without subsequent rupture. The mean diameter of aneurysms that subsequently ruptured was 18 mm, compared with a mean diameter of 7 mm for lesions that remained clinically asymptomatic. None of 26 tiny aneurysms (4 mm) bled, but one of the 5-mm aneurysms bled.[52]

In a literature review, Rinkel and colleagues[17] assessed 27 ruptures in 3742 patients with aneurysms 10 mm in diameter or smaller and 27 ruptures in 675 patients with larger aneurysms. The relative risk of rupture for larger aneurysms was 5.5% (95% CI, 3.3 to 9.5), with an incidence of 4% (95% CI, 2.7% to 5.8%), compared with 0.7% (95% CI, 0.5% to 1%) for the smaller aneurysms.[17] The ISUIA data demonstrated that, in group 1, the cumulative rate of rupture was 0.05% per year for aneurysms less than 10 mm and about 1% for those larger than 10 mm in diameter. Aneurysms larger than 25 mm had a 6% rupture rate in the first year. In group 2, the cumulative rate of rupture was about 0.5% per year for those smaller than 10 mm and about 1% for those larger than 10 mm in diameter. Patients with giant aneurysms, (>25 mm) have a particularly grave prognosis, with a rupture rate of 6% in the first year and 45% within 7.5 years.[3]

Juvela and coworkers[9] found that the aneurysm rupture rate increased linearly with lesion size. The relative risk for rupture per millimeter of aneurysm diameter was 1.11 (95% CI, 1 to 1.23; $P = .05$). Seventy percent of the aneurysms that ruptured were smaller than 6 mm. Aneurysm size remained a significant independent predictor for subsequent rupture after adjustment for the sex, hypertension, and aneurysm group of the patient. The estimated relative risk of aneurysm rupture for lesions measuring 7 mm or larger was 2.19 compared with smaller lesions. The average annual risk of aneurysm rupture for lesions 7 mm or larger was 2.5% (i.e., 9 first ruptures during 364 patient-years) and 1.1% (i.e., 18 ruptures during 1580 patient-years) for aneurysms smaller than 7 mm in diameter.[9]

Tsutsumi and associates[10] reported the 5- and 10-year cumulative risks of CT-confirmed SAH. They were calculated by the Kaplan-Meier method as 7.5% and 22.1%, respectively, for total cases; 33.5% and 55.9%, respectively, for large (>10 mm) aneurysms; and 4.5% and 13.9%, respectively, for small (<10 mm) aneurysms. In summary, size (i.e., largest diameter) is a determinant in the rupture rate, but whether a threshold or critical size for rupture exists is not clearly defined.

Aneurysm Location

Data suggest that aneurysm location is an independent variable in the risk of rupture, with higher risks for posterior circulation aneurysms, posterior communicator aneurysms, and anterior communicator aneurysms.[3] In the study by Wiebers and colleagues,[34] 42% of the basilar artery aneurysms ultimately ruptured, whereas the rates for inferior cerebellar artery (ICA), anterior communicating artery (ACoA), and anterior cerebral artery (ACA) aneurysms were all less than 7%. Location was also found to be important in the 1992 report by Inagawa and colleagues[53] on their series of 769 aneurysms; 67% were ruptured, and 33% were unruptured. Eighty-nine percent of ACoA aneurysms were ruptured, compared with 62% of middle cerebral artery (MCA), 58% of ICA, and 53% of vertebrobasilar aneurysms. Of the lesions 9 mm in diameter or smaller, ACoA aneurysms were more than twice as likely to be ruptured as MCA aneurysms and more than 1.5 times as likely as ICA aneurysms. Aneurysms located at the vertebrobasilar junction were slightly less likely to be ruptured than ICA lesions and slightly more likely to be ruptured than MCA aneurysms.[53] The same investigator evaluated 22 patients with 24 unruptured petrous and cavernous ICA aneurysms, in contrast to aneurysms lying in the subarachnoid space. The male-to-female ratio was 1:4.5, and the mean age was 63 years. Fifty-five percent of the patients harbored multiple, unruptured aneurysms. Sixteen unruptured lesions with a mean diameter of 5 mm (range, 2 to 17 mm) were followed for 11 months to 10.5 years (mean, 4.7 years). None of these 16 aneurysms ruptured, and 94% remained asymptomatic.[51]

The well-designed ISUIA trial showed location to be important, with posterior circulation lesions, particularly basilar tip, vertebrobasilar, posterior cerebral, and posterior communicating artery aneurysms, having a higher risk of rupture.[3] In their review of the literature, Rinkel and associates[17] demonstrated that the relative risk of aneurysm rupture was higher for aneurysms located in the posterior circulation, with a relative risk of 4.1.

In summary, UIAs located at the basilar bifurcation, in anterior and posterior communicating artery locations, appear to have a higher risk of rupture compared with other sites. In contrast, aneurysms within the cavernous sinus appear to have a lower likelihood of bleeding.

Multiple Aneurysms

Multiple aneurysms are present in approximately 15% to 20% of all aneurysm patients. The literature suggests that patients with UIAs are at increased risk for hemorrhage. In 1974, Mount and colleagues[55] reviewed 158 cases of unruptured, multiple aneurysms that were followed for less than 11 years and found a bleeding rate of at least 10%. In 1981 and 1987, Wiebers and associates[36] also found that unruptured lesions that are part of multiple aneurysm constellations might have a greater propensity for rupture than solitary aneurysms. This was consistent with the data by Winn and colleagues,[35] who reported that the minimum risk of rupture for this group of intact aneurysms was 1% per year.

The Finnish data support the concept that patients with multiple aneurysms have a higher likelihood of UIA rupture. Heiskanen and coworkers[56] described 84 patients with multiple aneurysms in whom the ruptured lesion was definitely identified and treated surgically. Of the 84 patients, 8 had a recurrent hemorrhage from the unruptured aneurysm during follow-up periods ranging from 4 months to 11 years, with a rupture rate of more than 1% per year. The same investigators reported a 10-year follow-up study of 61 patients with UIAs who had surgery for prior ruptured aneurysms,[33] and a rupture rate of more than 1% per year was demonstrated. In a study conducted in Helsinki by Juvela and colleagues[8] with 14 years of follow-up, the percentage of UIAs that ruptured was as follows: 20% (five cases) with incidental unruptured aneurysms, 33% (six cases) with symptomatic unruptured lesions, but only 18% (131 cases) with multiple, intact aneurysms.[8] In these investigators' latest report,[9] published in 2000, the percentage of patients without SAH was 65% to 80% at 20 of years of follow-up, and the percentages did not seem to differ significantly when multiple, symptomatic, and incidental aneurysms were compared.

The Japanese data also support an increased risk of hemorrhage in patients with multiple aneuryms. A study conducted by Yasui and associates[40] demonstrated an annual rupture rate of 6.8% for multiple aneurysms and 1.9% for single lesions.

A meta-analysis by Rinkel and associates[17] found the risk of rupture was higher for patients with multiple aneurysms, with a relative risk of rupture of a multiple lesion compared with an asymptomatic lesion of 1.7.

In summary, most studies support the concept that multiple UIAs have a higher risk of hemorrhage than solitary aneurysms.

Aneurysm Growth

Aneurysm growth is defined as an increase in size of the aneurysm as determined on repeat studies. In 1962, Björkesten and colleagues[57] described changes in the size of intracranial aneurysms. The report was based on 19 patients with aneurysms who underwent repeated angiography sessions performed at intervals of 2 weeks to 10 years without intervening surgical procedures. All patients had initially experienced aneurysmal SAH, and the mean age was 40 years. Among 10 patients in whom aneurysm growth was definitely established at intervals between 2 weeks and 10 years, 6 patients suffered recurrent SAH. In eight patients in whom the size of the aneurysm was unchanged at intervals between 4 and 88 months after the first angiogram, none experienced a second SAH.

The report by Juvela and colleagues[8] in 1993 is consistent with the observations of Björkesten.[57] In their large series of UIA with a median follow-up period of 14 years, the initial mean diameter of aneurysms that ruptured or remained intact during the follow-up period was 4 mm. The aneurysms that subsequently ruptured (17 patients) displayed a significant increase in size. Among the 14 patients for whom angiographic follow-up was available and in whom there was no sign of rupture, there was no significant increase in aneurysm size.

A contrary conclusion was reported by Sampei and associates[58] in 1991. These investigators described the growth of aneurysms between successive angiographic examinations in 25 patients.[58] In 11 patients, the interval was less than 1 month, and in 14, it was longer, ranging up to 15 years or longer. For patients who underwent short-term follow-up, all initial angiograms were obtained because a rupture had occurred. Four of the 11 patients had experienced repeated hemorrhages, and in all of them, aneurysm enlargement or development of an aneurysmal loculus was demonstrated on angiograms. Rebleeding did not appear to be affected by the growth rate or by the initial size of the aneurysm.[58]

In summary, there exist insufficient data in the literature to conclusively document a relationship between aneurysm growth and risk of rupture.

Symptomatic Aneurysms

Symptomatic aneurysms are aneurysms that manifest with signs and symptoms related to the lesion, excluding clinical features related to a hemorrhage. These aneurysms, in common with incidental aneurysms, are unruptured but come to medical attention because of symptoms directly related to the aneurysm. Symptoms may be mild, such as headaches, or manifestation may be more severe, such as cranial nerve palsies and brainstem signs. In a relatively small clinical series, 20% of the unruptured aneurysms were symptomatic, 32% were asymptomatic and components of multiple aneurysm constellations, and 48% were true incidental lesions.[59] Symptomatic aneurysms may be at increased risk for hemorrhage, but not all the data are congruent.

In the 1969 Cooperative Aneurysm Study, there were 165 patients with symptomatic, unruptured aneurysms who were at risk for SAH. Seventy-nine percent of these unruptured aneurysms were treated surgically, and 34 cases were left untreated and the natural course of the disease was studied. Thirty-five percent of untreated, unruptured aneurysms were followed for 20 months to 12 years, during which time 26% of the patients harboring these lesions died of SAH.[60] This rate was significantly higher than the rupture rate for incidental aneurysms (0.8%/year), but selection bias and variation in follow-up might have skewed the results.

Stronger evidence for a higher rupture rate for symptomatic lesions was provided by Rinkel and coworkers,[17] who found that the relative risk of rupture of a symptomatic aneurysm was 8.2 times that of an asymptomatic lesion.

However, in a multivariate analysis by Wiebers and associates,[34] no correlation could be found between risk of hemorrhage and symptoms. This was also the case for Juvela and coworkers,[9] who found that the percentage of patients without SAH was between 65% and 80% at 20 years of follow-up, which did not differ significantly when multiple, symptomatic, and incidental aneurysms were compared.

Many of the symptomatic aneurysms arise from the posterior communicating artery. This location has been found to have a higher rate of rupture of UIAs. This location may be the explanation for the perception that symptomatic aneurysms have a higher rate of rupture.

Age

Increasing age has been considered to increase the risk of hemorrhage. However, a protective effect of age was suggested by the earlier autopsy data by McCormick,[61] in which the rate of rupture was 81% for aneurysms in patients 30 and 39 years old, 60% for those 40 to 49 years old, 42% for those 50 to 59 years old, 25% in those 60 to 69 years old, and 21% in those 70 to 79 years old.[61] Of the 15 aneurysms in patients older than 79 years, none was proved to have ruptured. In a study by Taylor and colleagues,[39] advanced age produced a small but statistically significant protective effect against subsequent hemorrhage.

Wier,[62] in a comprehensive review of the literature, stated that the rate of aneurysm rupture progressively increased with age and that the protective effect was seen only in extreme old age.[62] Increasing age and an associated increased risk of hemorrhage was also demonstrated by Wiebers and coworkers.[36] These investigators found no significant correlation between patient age and aneurysm size. However, in patients older than 59 years, the rupture rate was 48% after diagnosis of an unruptured aneurysm, which was twice the rate (24%) found in younger patients.[36] These figures were, however, only applicable for patients harboring aneurysms 10 mm or larger.

In a series conducted in Finland, Juvela and associates[8] reported similar findings. In 142 patients with 181 unruptured aneurysms, the only variable that tended to predict rupture was the age of the patient, with increasing age correlating with a higher risk of hemorrhage.[8, 9] Another report by Yasui and colleagues[63] in 1998 followed 14 patients older than 70 years who harbored incidental unruptured aneurysms. Of the 10 patients who did not undergo surgery, 2 patients (20%) experienced aneurysm rupture during a follow-up period ranging from 3 months to 7 years. Age as a predictor of rupture was also demonstrated in the ISUIA in patients with a history of SAH (group 2).[3]

In summary, most of the literature supports the concept of increasing age being associated with an increased risk of rupture, except in the very elderly.

Hypertension

The role of systemic hypertension in aneurysm formation and rupture has been controversial. The concept of hypertension increasing the risk for hemorrhage is attractive, because it is known that intracranial hemorrhage is associated with hypertension. Stehbens,[13, 14] however, in a review of the pathology data, concluded that no association existed between hypertension and SAH, and other studies have had similar conclusions. Philips and coworkers[64] reviewed the medical records of residents of Rochester, Minnesota, over a 30-year period and found no correlation between hypertension and SAH. Wiebers and associates[34] followed 65 patients with 81 unruptured aneurysms. A multivariate analysis demonstrated no relationship between hypertension and the risk of rupture. A follow-up study with an additional 65 patients and 80 unruptured aneurysms did not change the result.[36] Juvela and colleagues[8] described 142 patients with 181 unruptured aneurysms who were followed for at least 10 years, and hypertension was not found to be a predictor of subsequent rupture.

However, other studies have found that hypertension increases the risk of SAH. For example, the study by Sacco and assocaites,[23] which considered the data on 5184 residents in Framingham, Massachusetts, demonstrated a significantly higher risk of SAH for patients with hypertension. Winn and colleagues[35] evaluated the long-term outcome (average follow-up period of 7.7 years) of 182 patients with multiple aneurysms who suffered SAH to document the incidence of late bleeding. Of the 182 patients, 132 were treated by bed rest and 50 by surgery (i.e., craniotomy) directed only at the ruptured aneurysm. Seventy of the patients on bed rest were alive after 6 months, and 21 (30%) of them suffered a late hemorrhage. Of the 50 craniotomy patients, 38 were alive after 6 months. Hypertension increased the risk of late hemorrhage in both groups of patients. Asari and coworkers[38] analyzed data from 54 patients with 72 unruptured aneurysms and found that hypertension was significant in predicting future rupture.

In 1995, Taylor and colleagues[39] described the demographics and prevalence of hypertension in 20,767 Medicare patients with unruptured aneurysms and compared these results to a random sample of the hospitalized Medicare population. The prevalence of hypertension in patients with unruptured aneurysms was 43.2%, compared with 34.4% in the random sample. Patients who survived their initial hospitalization were separated into two groups: those with an unruptured cerebral aneurysm as the primary diagnosis and those with an unruptured cerebral aneurysm as a secondary diagnosis. Follow-up data for 18,119 patients were examined. For patients with an unruptured cerebral aneurysm as the primary diagnosis, hypertension was found to be a significant risk factor for future SAH (risk ratio = 1.46; 95% CI, 1.01 to 2.11).

In summary, most data are unclear about whether hypertension increases the risk for subsequent SAH, but the large study by Taylor and colleagues[39] does suggest an association.

Cigarette Smoking

Cigarette smoking has been associated with aneurysmal SAH. In a multicenter study,[65] prospective data revealed that patients with SAH reported current smoking rates 2.5 times higher than expected based on U.S. and European national surveys ($P < .0001$). Cigarette smoking was also associated with younger age at onset of SAH (5 to 10 years, $P < .0001$).[65]

Matsumoto and colleagues[66] followed 182 patients with SAH and 123 patients with an unruptured cerebral aneurysm incidentally detected during investigation of other diseases. Sixty-nine patients with other diseases served as a control population, and they were shown to be free of cerebral aneurysms with MRA. Smoking significantly increased the risk of aneurysm formation and SAH. The odds ratio for SAH was 2.4, and the odds ratio for unruptured cerebral aneurysm was 1.7. Smoking especially increased the occurrence of SAH in women and in youngsters.[66]

In 2000, Juvela and associates[9] followed 87 patients with 111 unruptured aneurysms and 7 patients with de novo aneurysms for 18.9 years. In more than one third (36%) of patients with unruptured aneurysms, impressive lesion growth (≥3 mm) was observed.[66] Of several potential risk factors, only cigarette smoking (odds ratio = 3.48; 95% CI, 1.14 to 10.64; $P < .05$) was associated with this magnitude of growth.

In 2000, Qureshi and coworkers[67] analyzed prospectively collected data from the placebo-treated group in a multicenter clinical trial conducted at 54 neurosurgical centers in North America. Smoking at any time (odds ratio = 2.2; 95% CI, 1.1 to 4.5) was independently associated with large aneurysms. Intracranial aneurysm size is an important determinant of risk of rupture and outcome after treatment. Pobereskin and colleagues[68] found smoking to be positively associated with survival after aneurysmal SAH.

In summary, the preponderance of the literature reports a strong association between cigarette smoking and aneurysmal SAH.

Gender

Cerebral aneurysms have been observed more frequently in women than in men.[13, 15, 61] In respect to gender and rupture rate, several studies suggest that female gender increases the risk of rupture. For example, the meta-analysis by Rankle and colleagues[17] of nine studies found a higher rupture rate in women, with a relative risk of 2.1, and Juvela and coworkers[69] found that female gender was an independent risk factor. However, in the large analysis of hospital data, Taylor and associates[39] found that gender was not a predictor for risk of hemorrhage.

In summary, women may have an increased likelihood for UIA rupture, but the data are inconclusive.

CONCLUSIONS

The numbers of UIAs will continue to increase as the age of the population increases and as imaging techniques improve. In deciding on the management of patients with UIAs, the treating physician must understand the natural history to assess the effectiveness of treatment options. Although the natural history is not absolutely defined, the data suggest that the rupture rate is between 0.066% and 2% per year. Other factors influencing this risk include aneurysm size, location, multiplicity, growth rate, and symptoms and patient factors such as age, sex, history of hypertension, and smoking.

Until the natural history is clarified, patients should have a management plan that is individualized and considers the age of the patient, life expectancy, comorbidities, and characteristics of the aneurysm.

REFERENCES

1. Winn HR: Section overview: Unruptured aneurysms. J Neurosurg 96:1–2, 2002.
2. Bederson J, Awad IA, Wiebers DO, et al: Recommendations for the management of patients with unruptured intracranial aneurysms. Circulation 102:2300–2308, 2000.
3. International Study of Unruptured Intracranial Aneurysm Investigators: Unruptured intracranial aneurysms—risk of rupture and risks of surgical intervention. N Engl J Med 339:1725–1733, 1998.
4. Broderick JP, Thoma GB, Dudler JE, et al: Initial and recurrent bleeding are the major causes of death following subarachnoid hemorrhage. Stroke 25:1342–1347, 1994.
5. Kassell NF, Torner JC, Haley C, et al: The international cooperative study on the timing of aneurysm surgery. Part 1. Overall management results. J Neurosurg 73:18–36, 1990.
6. Kassell NF, Torner JC, Jane J, et al: The international cooperative study on the timing of aneurysm surgery. Part 2. Surgical results. J Neurosurg 73:37–47, 1990.
7. Ljunggren B, Saveland H, Brandt L, et al: Aneurysmal subarachnoid hemorrhage: Total annual outcome in a 1.46 million population. Surg Neurol 22:435–438, 1984.
8. Juvela S, Porras M, Heiskanen O: Natural history of unruptured intracranial aneurysms: A long-term follow-up study. J Neurosurg 79:174–182, 1993.
9. Juvela S, Porras M, Poussa K: Natural history of unruptured aneurysms: Probability of and risk factors for aneurysm rupture. J Neurosurg 93:379–387, 2000.
10. Tsutsumi K, Ueki K, Morita A: Risk of rupture from incidental cerebral aneurysms. J Neurosurg 93:550–553, 2000.
11. Mon Vital Stat Rep 45:18, 1997.
12. Fox JL (ed): Intracranial Aneurysms. New York, Springer-Verlag, 1983, pp 15–18.

13. Stehbens WE: Aneurysmal and anatomical variation of cerebral arteries. Arch Pathol 75:45–64, 1963.
14. Stehbens WE: Pathology of the Cerebral Blood Vessels. St. Louis, CV Mosby, 1972, pp 351–470.
15. McCormick WF, Nofzinger JD: Saccular intracranial aneurysms: An autopsy study. J Neurosurg 22:155–159, 1965.
16. Rosenorn J, Eskesen V, Schmidt K: Unruptured intracranial aneurysms: An assessment of the annual risk of rupture based on epidemiological and clinical data. Br J Neurosurg 2:369–377, 1988.
17. Rinkel GJ, Djibuti M, Algra A: Prevalence and risk of rupture of intracranial aneurysms: A systematic review. Stroke 29:251–256, 1998.
18. Ujiie H, Sato K, Onda H: Clinical analysis of incidentally discovered unruptured aneurysms. Stroke 24:1850–1856, 1993.
19. Yoshimoto T, Mizoi K: Importance of management of unruptured cerebral aneurysms. Surg Neurol 47:522–526, 1997.
20. Winn HR, Jane JA Sr, Taylor J, et al: Prevalence of asymptomatic incidental aneurysms: Review of 4568 arteriograms. J Neurosurg 96:43–49, 2002.
21. Sekhar LN, Heros RC: Origin, growth, and rupture of saccular aneurysms: A review. Neurosurgery 8:248–260, 1981.
22. Weir B: Unruptured aneurysms. J Neurosurg 97:1011–1012, 2002, discussion 1012–1013, 2002.
23. Sacco RL, Wolf PA, Bharucha NE: Subarachnoid and intracerebral hemorrhage: Natural history, prognosis, and precursive factors in the Framingham Study. Neurology 34:847–854, 1984.
24. Ingall TJ, Whisnat JP, Wiebers DO, et al: Has there been decline in subarachnoid hemorrhage mortality? Stroke 20:718–724, 1989.
25. Ostergaard Kristensen M: Increased incidence of bleeding intracranial aneurysms in Greenlandic Eskimos. Acta Neurochir 67: 37–43, 1983.
26. Inagawa T, Ishikawa S, Aoki H: Aneurysmal subarachnoid hemorrhage in Izumo City and Shimane Prefecture of Japan, Incidence. Stroke 19:170–175, 1988.
27. Truelsen T, Bonita R, Duncan J: Changes in subarachnoid hemorrhage mortality, incidence, and case fatality in New Zealand between 1981–1983 and 1991–1993. Stroke 29:2298–2303, 1998.
28. Pakarinen S: Incidence, etiology, and prognosis of primary subarachnoid hemorrhage: A study based on 589 cases diagnosed in a defined urban population in a defined period. Acta Neurol Scand 43(Suppl 29):1–28, 1967.
29. Sarti C, Tuomilehto J, Salomaa V: Epidemiology of subarachnoid hemorrhage in Finland from 1983 to 1985. Stroke 22:848–853, 1991.
30. Linn FHH, Rinkel GJ, Algra A: Incidence of subarachnoid hemorrhage: role of region, year, and rate of computed tomography: A meta-analysis. Stroke 27:625–629, 1996.
31. Locksley HB: Natural history of subarachnoid hemorrhage, intracranial aneurysms and arteriovenous malformations. J Neurosurg 25:321–368, 1966.
32. Zacks DJ, Russell DB, Miller JD: Fortuitously discovered intracranial aneurysms. Arch Neurol 37:39–41, 1980.
33. Heiskanen O: Risk of bleeding from unruptured aneurysm in cases with multiple intracranial aneurysms. J Neurosurg 55:524–526, 1981.
34. Wiebers DO, Whisnant JP, O'Fallon WM: The natural history of unruptured intracranial aneurysms. N Engl J Med 304:696–698, 1981.
35. Winn HR, Almaani WS, Berga SL: The long-term outcome in patients with multiple aneurysms: Incidence of late hemorrhage and implications for treatment of incidental aneurysms. J Neurosurg 59:642–651, 1983.
36. Wiebers DO, Whisnant JP, Sundt TM Jr, O'Fallon M: The significance of unruptured intracranial saccular aneurysms. J Neurosurg 66:23–29, 1987.
37. Easton JD, Castel JP, Wiebers DO: Management of unruptured aneurysms. Cerebrovasc Dis 3:60–64, 1993.
38. Asari S, Ohmoto T: Natural history and risk factors of unruptured cerebral aneurysms. Clin Neurol Neurosurg 95:205–214, 1993.
39. Taylor CL, Yuan Z, Selman WR: Cerebral arterial aneurysm formation and rupture in 20,767 elderly patients: Hypertension and other risk factors. J Neurosurg 83:812–819, 1995.
40. Yasui N, Suzuki A, Nishimura H: Long-term follow-up of unruptured intracranial aneurysms. Neurosurgery 40:1155–1160, 1997.
41. Piepgras DG: Unruptured aneurysms [editorial]. J Neurosurg 96: 63, 2002.
42. Juvela S: Unruptured aneurysms [editorial]. J Neurosurg 96:58–60, 2002.
43. Dumont AS, Lanzino G, Kassell KF: Unruptured aneurysms [editorial]. J Neurosurg 96:52–56, 2002.
44. Piepgras DG, Kassell NF, Torner J: A response from the ISUIA. Surg Neurol 52:428–429, 1999.
45. Kassell NF, Torner JC: Aneurysmal rebleeding: A preliminary report from the cooperative aneurysm study. Neurosurgery 13: 479–481, 1983.
46. Rosenorn J, Eskesen V: Does a safe size-limit exist for unruptured intracranial aneurysms? Acta Neurochir 121:113–118, 1993.
47. Huston J III, Nichols DA, Luetmer PH: Blinded prospective evaluation of sensitivity of MR angiography to known intracranial aneurysms: Importance of aneurysms size. AJNR Am J Neuroradiol 15:1607–1614, 1994.
48. Wiebers DO, Piepgras DG, Brown RD, et al: Unruptured aneurysms [editorial]. J Neurosurg 96:50–51, 2002.
49. Riina HA, Spetzler RF: Editorial: Unruptured aneurysms. J Neurosurg 96:61–62, 2002.
50. Rinne J, Hernesniemi J, Niskanen M: Analysis of 561 patients with 690 middle cerebral artery aneurysms: Anatomical and clinical features as correlated to management outcome. Neurosurgery 38:2–11, 1996.
51. Fogelholm R, Hernesniemi J, Vapalahti M: Impact of early surgery outcome after aneurysmal subarachnoid hemorrhage: A population-based study. Stroke 24:1649–1654, 1993.
52. Mizoi K, Yoshimoto T, Nagamine Y: How to treat incidental cerebral aneurysms: A review of 139 consecutive cases. Surg Neurol 44:114–121, 1995.
53. Inagawa T, Hada H, Katoh Y: Unruptured intracranial aneurysms in elderly patients. Surg Neurol 38:364–370, 1992.
54. Inagawa T: Surgical treatment of multiple intracranial aneurysms. Acta Neurochir 108:22–29, 1991.
55. Mount LA, Brisman R: Treatment of multiple aneurysms—symptomatic and asymptomatic. Clin Neurosurg 21:166–170, 1974.
56. Heiskanen O, Marttila I: Risk of rupture of a second aneurysm in patients with multiple aneurysms. J Neurosurg 32:295–299, 1970.
57. Björkesten G, Troupp H: Changes in the size of intracranial arterial aneurysms. J Neurosurg 19:583–588, 1962.
58. Sampei T, Mizuno M, Nakajima S: Clinical study of growing up aneurysms: Report of 25 cases [in Japanese]. No Shinkei Geka 19:825–830, 1991.
59. Dix GA, Gordon W, Kaufmann AM: Ruptured and unruptured intracranial aneurysms—surgical outcome. Can J Neurol Sci 22: 187–191, 1995.
60. Graf CJ: Prognosis for patients with nonsurgically treated aneurysms. Analysis of the Cooperative Study of Intracranial Aneurysms and Subarachnoid Hemorrhage. J Neurosurg 35:438–443, 1971.
61. McCormick WF: The natural history of intracranial saccular aneurysms: An autopsy study. Neurol Neurosurg 1:1–8, 1978.
62. Weir B: Aneurysms Affecting the Nervous System. Baltimore, Williams & Wilkins, 1987, pp 19–53.
63. Yasui T, Sakamoto H, Kishi H, et al: Management of elderly patients with incidentally discovered unruptured aneurysms. No Shinkei Geka 26:679–684, 1998.
64. Philips LH, Whisnant JP, O'Fallon WM, et al: The unchanging pattern of subarachnoid hemorrhage in a community: Influence of arterial hypertension and gender. Neurology 30:1034–1040, 1980.
65. Weir BK, Kongable GL, Kassell NF, et al: Cigarette smoking as a cause of aneurysmal subarachnoid hemorrhage and risk for vasospasm: A report of the Cooperative Aneurysm Study. J Neurosurg 89:405–411, 1998.
66. Matsumoto K, Akagi K, Abekura M, et al: Cigarette smoking increases the risk of developing a cerebral aneurysm and of subarachnoid hemorrhage. No Shinkei Geka 27:831–835, 1999.
67. Qureshi AI, Sung GY, Suri MF, et al: Factors associated with aneurysm size in patients with subarachnoid hemorrhage: Effect of smoking and aneurysm location. Neurosurgery 46:44–50, 2000.
68. Pobereksin LH: Incidence and outcome of subarachnoid hemorrhage: A retrospective population based study. J Neurol Neurosurg Psychiatry 70:340–343, 2001.
69. Juvela S: Natural history of unruptured intracranial aneurysms: Risks for aneurysm formation, growth, and rupture. Acta Neurochir Suppl 82:27–30, 2002.

CHAPTER **107**

Surgical Decision Making for the Treatment of Cerebral Aneurysms

PETER D. LE ROUX ■ H. RICHARD WINN

The primary goal of intracranial aneurysm treatment is complete, permanent, and safe aneurysm occlusion. Aneurysms can be occluded by surgical or endovascular means or by a combination of both techniques. Some aneurysms, however, may not be amenable to direct occlusion and may be better treated by parent vessel sacrifice or vascular reconstruction. Choosing the treatment modality that is safest and most efficient for each patient is an important therapeutic decision. A variety of factors, such as aneurysm size and location, the patient's age and medical condition, and associated factors such as intracerebral hemorrhage (ICH), intraventricular hemorrhage (IVH), and clinical grade after aneurysm rupture, can all influence the outcome of attempted aneurysm occlusion. It is important to consider these factors before treating each patient.

This chapter reviews surgical decision making in the treatment of cerebral aneurysms and highlights the natural history and treatment risk of unruptured aneurysms; treatment of the ruptured aneurysm, including timing of surgery and management of the poor-grade patient or those who present with ICH, IVH, or hydrocephalus; and special circumstances, including pregnancy, aneurysms in children or the elderly, aneurysms associated with infection, trauma, arteriovenous malformations, carotid artery disease, microaneurysms, and fusiform, giant, or residual aneurysms. We discuss the appropriate use of endovascular or surgical techniques to occlude the aneurysm and consider surgical strategies that require special preoperative planning, such as intraoperative angiography, parent vessel occlusion, revascularization, or hypothermic circulatory arrest.

THE UNRUPTURED ANEURYSM

Natural History

Several long-term follow-up studies demonstrate that the overall risk of subarachnoid hemorrhage (SAH) from an unruptured aneurysm is between 1% and 2% each year; between 50% and 60% of these ruptures are fatal.[1–5] The annual risk of rupture, however, may vary from 0.05% to 6% each year, depending on factors such as aneurysm size or location and whether the individual has suffered an SAH from another aneurysm.[2, 4] The median time between discovery of an unruptured aneurysm and SAH is estimated to be 9.6 years.[3]

Factors Associated with Rupture of Unruptured Aneurysms

The risk of SAH from an unruptured aneurysm depends largely on aneurysm characteristics rather than the patient (Table 107–1). Several factors, including increased aneurysm size, posterior circulation aneurysm, symptomatic aneurysms, aneurysms associated with arteriovenous malformations, unruptured aneurysms that increase in size on follow-up imaging, and previous SAH from another aneurysm, are thought to be associated with an increased risk of rupture.[1–4, 6] Population-based studies after SAH suggest that factors such as cigarette smoking, hypertension, and binge alcohol drinking are associated with aneurysm rupture.[7–10] Whether these factors influence the natural history of unruptured aneurysms is unclear.

Increased aneurysm size appears to be an important factor associated with rupture of unruptured aneurysms. In the International Study of Unruptured Intracranial Aneurysms (ISUIA),[2] a retrospective, multicenter study of 1449 patients, the annual risk of hemorrhage among patients who had previously not had SAH was 0.05% if the lesion was less than 10 mm in diameter. Among the same group of patients, the annual risk of rupture was increased 11-fold when the lesion was larger than 10 mm in diameter. Small aneurysms (5 to 6 mm in diameter), however, can rupture.[3, 11, 12] For example, Yasui and colleagues[12] retrospectively identified 25 patients with unruptured aneurysms who, on average, suffered SAHs 5 years later. Sixteen of the aneurysms were less than 5 mm in diameter when first diagnosed. Similarly, Juvela and coworkers[13] followed 142 patients with 181 aneurysms for a median follow-up of 13.9 years; 27 patients (19%)

TABLE 107–1 ■ **Natural History and Risk of Rupture from Unruptured Aneurysms**

FACTORS ASSOCIATED WITH UNRUPTURED ANEURYSM RUPTURE	RELATIVE RISK (95% CI)*
Female	2.1 (1.1–3.9)
Symptomatic	8.2 (3.9–17)
>10 mm	5.5 (3.3–9.5)
Posterior circulation	4.1 (1.5–11)
60–79 years	1.7 (0.7–4.0)
Overall risk	1.9%/yr (1.5–2.4%)

Data are from nine studies, including 3907 patients years, that followed patients between 1955 and 1996.

Adapted from Rinkel GJE, Djibuti M, Algra A, van Gijn J: Prevalence and risk of rupture of intracranial aneurysms: A systematic review. Stroke 29:251–256, 1998.

subsequently suffered aneurysm rupture. The median aneurysm size at initial diagnosis was 4 mm in diameter; 63% of the aneurysms that ruptured increased in size during follow-up. These findings are consistent with retrospective analysis of ruptured aneurysms that demonstrate that more than one half of the lesions are less than 10 mm in diameter.[13, 14]

Efficacy of Aneurysm Surgery

Aneurysm surgery is effective; overall, more than 90% of aneurysms undergoing surgical clip occlusion are completely obliterated at surgery.[15–20] However, very few studies report the routine use of postoperative angiography, suggesting that many patients may not undergo postoperative evaluation. This may be important because several clinical series suggest that, even when a surgeon believes the operative result is satisfactory, vessel occlusion or aneurysm remnants may be found on 5% of postoperative angiograms.[19, 21–23]

What factors are associated with failure to occlude the aneurysm? Aneurysmal remnants and vessel occlusion are more likely when a large aneurysm or cerebrovascular atherosclerosis is identified or when multiple attempts to place aneurysm clips are made.[19] For example, Solomon and associates,[24] describing the surgical treatment of 202 unruptured aneurysms, observed that increased aneurysm size is associated with poor technical results. Among giant aneurysms, only 60% underwent clip occlusion at surgery. In contrast, clip occlusion was achieved in 85% of lesions larger than 10 mm in diameter and 93% of lesions less than 10 mm in diameter. Postoperative angiographs were obtained in two thirds of the patients; complete aneurysm occlusion was observed in more than 90% of the small aneurysms but in only 54% of the giant aneurysms. During surgery, inadequate brain relaxation is associated with poor technical results. For example, Giannotta and Litofsky[25] retrospectively reviewed 524 patients, including 20 who required reoperation for inadequately treated aneurysms. Fourteen of the reoperations were attributed to failure to obtain a slack brain or inadequate bone exposure at the initial surgery.

Surgical Risk

Surgical outcome after repair of unruptured aneurysms has been described in several case series dealing with unruptured aneurysms. Most case series[24, 26–30] demonstrate that the morbidity and mortality associated with surgical treatment of unruptured aneurysms are very low; about 5% of patients die or are disabled. In contrast, findings from the ISUIA, a prospective study including 1172 patients, 85% of whom underwent surgery, suggested that overall surgical risk was much higher; the combined morbidity and mortality rate approached 15% at 1 year.[2] The surgical risk was greater than the risk of hemorrhage among patients with incidental aneurysms less than 10 mm in diameter. Several investigators have performed meta-analysis of surgical series to clarify surgical risk (Table 107–2); most suggest that the combined morbidity and mortality rate is between 3% and 7%. For example, King and colleagues[31] performed meta-analysis of 28 clinical series containing 733 patients; overall, 4.1% of patients were disabled, and 1% died. Raaymakers and coworkers[32] performed a meta-analysis from a MEDLINE search between 1966 and 1996 and identified 61 studies involving 2460 patients. The surgical morbidity rate was 10.9%, and the mortality rate was 2.6%; the risk of a poor outcome decreased in later years. It is difficult, however, to derive meaningful conclusions by combing the various surgical series for several reasons. Most are reported by surgeons with an inherent bias. Unruptured aneurysms of various sizes and location are included in each series, and the technique of aneurysm occlusion such as wrapping or clip is not always de-

TABLE 107–2 ■ **Summary of Published Reviews or Meta-analysis Describing Surgical Risk for Unruptured Aneurysms**

STUDY	NUMBER OF PATIENTS/STUDIES	MORTALITY (95% CI)	MORBIDITY (95% CI)
G. Wirth et al, 1983[30]	260/7	0 (0–1)	6.5 (3.9–10.3)
Rosenorn et al, 1988[215]	354/10	0 (0–4)	4 (0–12)
Piepgras, 1989[216]	234/5	0 (0–1.3)	7.3 (4.3–11.4)
Pertuiset et al, 1991[217]	293/10	1 (0.2–3)	2 (0.8–4.4)
King et al, 1994[31]	733/28	1 (0.4–20)	4.1 (2.8–5.8)
Raaymakers et al, 1998[32]	2460/61	2.6 (2–3.3)	10.9 (9.6–12.2)

scribed. The effectiveness of surgery is rarely described because postoperative angiography is rarely performed. The description of outcome measures is lacking, as are neuropsychological and quality of life assessments.

Factors Associated with Surgical Outcome

Increased aneurysm size is the most important factor associated with surgical complications and poor outcome[24, 30, 32, 33] (Fig. 107– 1). Overall, aneurysms larger than 25 mm in diameter have a fourfold increased risk compared with 5-mm aneurysms.[34] Wirth and associates[30] demonstrated that significant operative morbidity complicated surgery for 2% of unruptured aneurysms smaller than 5 mm, 7% of aneurysms between 6 and 15 mm, and 14% of aneurysms larger than 16 mm in diameter. Similarly, Solomon and colleagues[24] observed a favorable outcome for 83% of patients who underwent surgical repair of giant, unruptured aneurysms. In contrast, 99% of patients who had aneurysms less than 10 mm in diameter experienced good outcomes. The association between increased aneurysm size and poor outcome may be explained in part by the aneurysm's intimate association with small perforators, the broad aneurysm neck, intraluminal thrombosis, or atherosclerosis in the aneurysm neck or dome.

Repair of unruptured posterior circulation aneurysms, particularly giant basilar bifurcation aneurysms, is associated with increased surgical risk[32, 34] (see Fig. 107–1). Solomon and coworkers[24] observed that giant, unruptured basilar aneurysms were associated with a 50% surgical morbidity and mortality rate. In contrast, the combined morbidity and mortality rate for giant, unruptured aneurysms with anterior circulation was 13%. Reasonable surgical results can be expected with nongiant, unruptured posterior circulation aneurysms.[29] However, when compared with similar-sized lesions in the anterior circulation, there is a nearly 10-fold increase in risk.[34, 35] In the anterior circulation, anterior communicating artery and internal carotid artery (ICA) bifurcation lesions appear to have the greatest risk.[30]

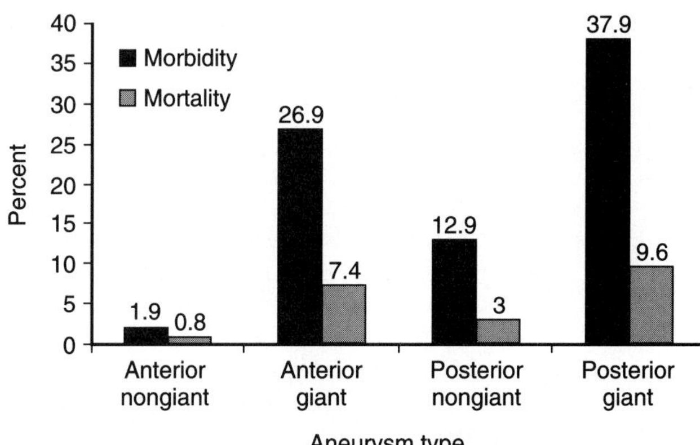

FIGURE 107–1. Surgical risk for unruptured intracranial aneurysms. (Data from 61 studies, including 2460 patients treated between 1966 and 1996, from Raaymakers TW, Rinkel G, Limburg M, Algra A: Mortality and morbidity of surgery for unruptured intracranial aneurysms: A meta-analysis. Stroke 29:1531–1538, 1998.)

Several other aneurysm features identified on angiograms, such as aneurysm orientation, a wide aneurysm neck, atherosclerosis, and calcification in the aneurysm neck, are associated with increased risk. For example, we have observed a significant increase in surgical complications among posteriorly oriented basilar bifurcation aneurysms.[36] Similarly, there is an increased risk among posterosuperiorly oriented anterior communicating artery aneurysms. Calcification in the aneurysm neck often is associated with poor outcome, in part because many of these lesions are large or giant aneurysms. Multiple clips frequently are necessary to occlude the aneurysm, increasing the incidence of cerebral embolism. Calcification may be removed by endarterectomy, but surgical results remain poor because the remaining wall for clip placement is often very friable and thin. Preoperative computed tomography (CT) can help identify neck calcification. Hypothermic circulatory arrest should be considered in the reconstruction of some heavily calcified aneurysms.

Patient-related factors include advanced age, ischemic cerebrovascular disease, and medical conditions such as diabetes mellitus, which increase the risk of unruptured aneurysm surgery.[24, 30, 33, 34] For some patients, such as those with severe cardiac or pulmonary disease, anesthesia may carry a great immediate risk, whereas for others, such as patients with advanced malignancy, any potential benefit is negated by a reduced life expectancy.

Who Should Be Treated?

In 1994, the American Heart Association published guidelines for the treatment of cerebral aneurysms. Although there was no level I or level II evidence, they recommended clipping unruptured aneurysms larger than 5 to 7 mm in diameter in patients with acceptable surgical risk.[37] Since then, several studies have improved our understanding of the natural history and surgical risk, and alternate treatments for unruptured aneurysms have evolved. Intradural, unruptured, saccular aneurysms should be referred to an experienced cerebrovascular surgeon for evaluation. Complex lesions such as large basilar bifurcation aneurysms or giant aneurysms should be referred to cerebrovascular centers with the ability to perform hypothermic circulatory arrest if necessary. Management should be tailored to the individual based on the patient's risk and the physician's experience. Khana and associates[34] have attempted to do this by creating a grading scale for unruptured aneurysms (Table 107–3 and Fig. 107–2). This scale was derived from a retrospective analysis of 172 patients who underwent treatment of unruptured aneurysms and then validated prospectively in 50 patients. The incidence of poor outcome progressively increased from 0% for grade 0 to 66% in grade IV patients. Based on the available literature, we believe

TABLE 107-3 ■ **Point Values for Grading Surgical Risk for Unruptured Aneurysms**

RISK FACTOR	POINT VALUE
Patient age (yr)	
<40	0
40–60	1
>60	2
Aneurysm size (mm)	
≤10 mm	0
11–25 mm	1
>25 mm	2
Aneurysm location	
Simple anterior	0
Complex anterior	1
Simple posterior	1
Complex posterior	2

Adapted from Khanna RK, Malik GM, Qureshi N: Predicting outcome following surgical treatment of unruptured intracranial aneurysms: A proposed grading system. J Neurosurg 84:49–54, 1996.

that patients with unruptured aneurysms and with the following characteristics should be treated: SAH from another aneurysm, symptomatic aneurysm, aneurysm larger than 10 mm in diameter, and aneurysms between 6 and 9 mm in diameter if the patient is young or middle-aged. Patient with aneurysms less than 6 mm in diameter should undergo a follow-up angiogram within 2 years and be treated if the lesion enlarges. The decision to use surgical or endovascular occlusion should be based on aneurysm morphology and on the patient's age and medical condition. Because of the unknown risk of recanalization with current interventional techniques, surgical occlusion is preferred if the patient is in reasonable medical condition.

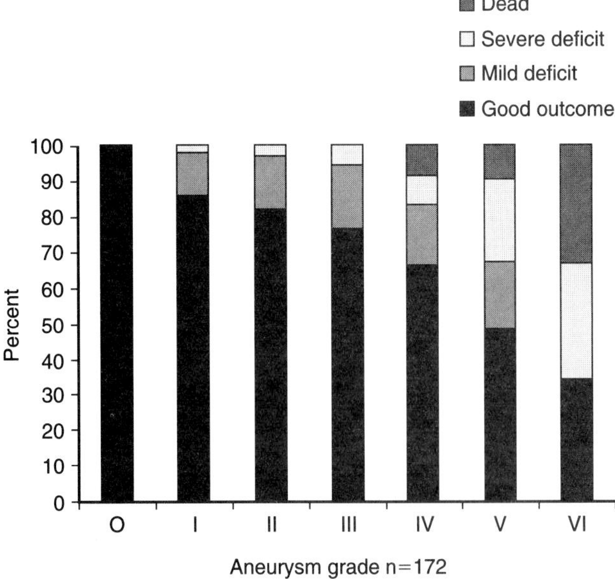

FIGURE 107-2. Histogram illustrating that aneurysm grade (see Table 107-3), which is determined by adding the point value for each factor, is strongly associated with surgical outcome of unruptured aneurysms. (Adapted with permission from Khanna RK, Malik GM, Qureshi N: Predicting outcome following surgical treatment of unruptured intracranial aneurysms: A proposed grading system. J Neurosurg 84:49–54, 1996.)

THE RUPTURED ANEURYSM

Each year, approximately 30,000 Americans suffer intracranial aneurysm rupture. Epidemiologic studies demonstrate that 60% of these patients die or are severely disabled.[38–41] Among the remaining patients, one half have significant neuropsychological and cognitive deficits and are unable to return to work. The primary causes of death or disability are the effect of the initial hemorrhage, subsequent rebleeding, and vasospasm.[38, 39, 42, 43] Aneurysm obliteration to prevent rebleeding is therefore central to successful management of SAH. Important surgical decisions include the timing of surgery to prevent rebleeding, appropriate use of endovascular or surgical aneurysm occlusion, and management of factors such as poor clinical grade, ICH, IVH, or vasospasm, which can all adversely affect outcome.

Aneurysm Rebleeding

After SAH, 20% to 30% of ruptured aneurysms rebleed within 30 days and then at a rate of approximately 3% per year.[44, 45] Rebleeding is most likely on day 1 (4%) and occurs at a constant rate of 1% to 2% per day during the next 4 weeks.[46, 47] Poor clinical grade, posterior circulation aneurysms, excess ventricular drainage, and abnormal hemostatic parameters appear to be associated with an increased risk of rebleeding.[48–50] More than 70% of patients who rebleed die. Aneurysm rebleeding can be prevented only by occluding the aneurysm by direct surgery or endovascular techniques. There are two important questions to consider. When should surgery be performed? Which patients should undergo surgical or endovascular aneurysm occlusion?

Timing of Aneurysm Obliteration

Early surgery eradicates the risk of rebleeding and appears to be associated with improved outcome. For example, among the 722 patients treated at 27 North American centers in the International Cooperative Study on the Timing of Aneurysm Surgery, a prospective, epidemiologic, nonrandomized study found that early surgery significantly improved outcome.[51] Adjusted overall outcome demonstrated that 70.9% of patients undergoing surgery between 0 and 3 days after aneurysm rupture experienced good recovery, whereas 62.9% of patients enjoyed a similar outcome if surgery was performed after 14 days.

For each patient with a ruptured aneurysm, aneurysm-related, hemorrhage-related, and patient-related factors influence whether to operate immediately or to delay surgery. Among patient-related factors, neurological grade and age are the most important. Poor-grade patients are at greater risk for rebleeding and vasospasm.[49, 52] Early aneurysm occlusion should therefore be achieved. Although cerebral swelling is more common in this group, early surgery in poor-grade patients is not associated with a greater risk of surgical complications than in good-grade patients.[18] Alternatively, patients who demonstrate significant swelling on admission CT may be excellent candidates for endovascular occlusion. Advanced age is associated with poor outcome, but it should not exclude the patient from early surgery, in part because elderly patients are more likely to have intracerebral hematomas and a decreased cerebrovascular reserve that increases their risk for delayed ischemia.[53] Similarly, these patients may be excellent candidates for endovascular aneurysm occlusion. Early surgery may be useful in patients at high risk for vasospasm, such as those with thick SAH on CT, in part because hypervolemic therapy and angioplasty may be most beneficial when the aneurysm is secured. Delayed surgery may be preferable for complex lesions such as giant aneurysms or those in which prolonged periods of temporary occlusion are expected to achieve occlusion.

Several lines of evidence demonstrate that surgery within 3 days of SAH is associated with improved outcome among patients with ruptured, anterior circulation aneurysms. A single randomized study addressed surgical timing in good clinical grade (Hunt and Hess I through III) patients after anterior circulation aneurysm rupture.[54] At 3 months, independent outcomes were observed in 91.5% of patients undergoing surgery within 3 days, 78.6% between 4 and 7 days, and 80% undergoing surgery more than 8 days after SAH. Nonrandomized studies, describing concurrent cohorts or historical controls, and large clinical series[40, 51, 55–60] have observed a tendency for patients undergoing early surgery to experience better outcomes.

The timing of aneurysm obliteration for posterior circulation aneurysms is less well defined. Much early information favoring delayed surgery came from referral centers. This may bias results, because epidemiologic studies demonstrate that patients with posterior circulation aneurysms are three times more likely to die before reaching the hospital or within the first 48 hours of SAH than patients with anterior circulation lesions.[61, 62] Several studies suggest that early surgery may reduce morbidity and mortality.[63–65] Hillman and colleagues[64] prospectively reviewed 59 cases of ruptured posterior fossa aneurysms treated during 1 year. Fifty percent of 26 patients scheduled for late surgery made a good recovery, whereas 72% of the 23 patients scheduled for early surgery made a good recovery. Intraoperative complications were equally common in the early- or delayed-surgery groups. We recommend early surgery for ruptured posterior circulation aneurysms except for lesions that may present technical difficulties, such as large posteriorly oriented basilar bifurcation aneurysms.

Poor-Grade Patients

Between 20% and 40% of patients admitted to hospital after aneurysm rupture are in poor clinical condition (Hunt and Hess grades IV and V). The association between poor outcome and poor clinical grade after SAH has been well described. However, the published data suggest that an aggressive policy may provide these patients their best chance of recovery (Fig. 107–3). Treatment includes rapid resuscitation and transport to hospital, intracranial pressure (ICP) control, early aneurysm occlusion, and prophylaxis against delayed cerebral ischemia. The use of noninvasive physiologic assessment such as transcranial Doppler, single photon emission computed tomography (SPECT), and invasive monitoring of ICP and cardiac hemodynamics are necessary to guide therapy. Epidemiologic studies show that up to 15% of the patients die before reaching hospital and that 30% die within the first 48 hours of aneurysm rupture.[38, 43, 61, 62] To be successful, an aggressive approach requires organized, multidisciplinary, proactive critical care that starts with resuscitation in the field and immediate ICP control. Alternate, but less successful, strategies include treatment of selected patients or delayed treatment when clinical improvement is observed.[49, 66, 67]

Aggressive management requires a large commitment of resources. Should all poor-grade patients be treated? For the individual poor-grade patient, clinical and radiographic findings on admission are often insufficient to accurately predict outcome.[49, 66–70] For example, predicting outcome based only on admission findings may result in withholding treatment from 30% of the grades IV and V patients who subsequently experience favorable outcomes.[68] Consequently, we believe that management should be initiated for most patients. Continued observation, including ICP monitoring and follow-up CT, help define outcome. Most poor-grade patients who do well are able to follow commands within 5 days of an aneurysm rupture, whereas those who die generally do so within the same time frame.[66, 67, 70] Patients who do poorly frequently develop intractable intracranial hypertension and progressive low-density changes on follow-up CT.[49, 67] Our management algorithm for poor-grade patients is illustrated in Figure 107–4.

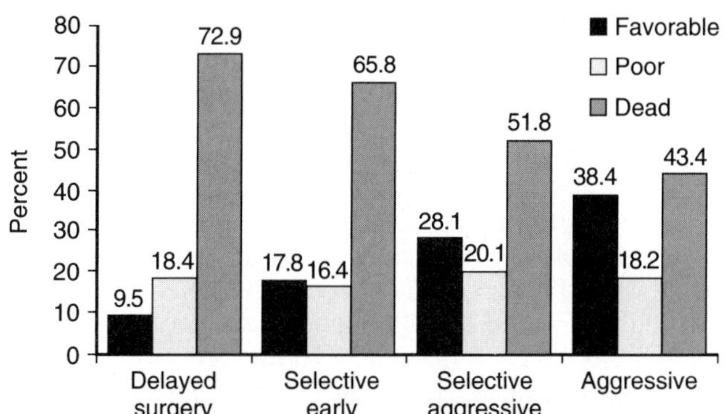

FIGURE 107–3. Overall management outcome for Hunt and Hess grade IV or V patients. (Modified with permission from Le Roux P, Elliott JP, Newell DW, et al: Predicting outcome in poor grade subarachnoid hemorrhage: A retrospective review of 159 aggressively managed patients. J Neurosurg 85:39–49, 1996.)

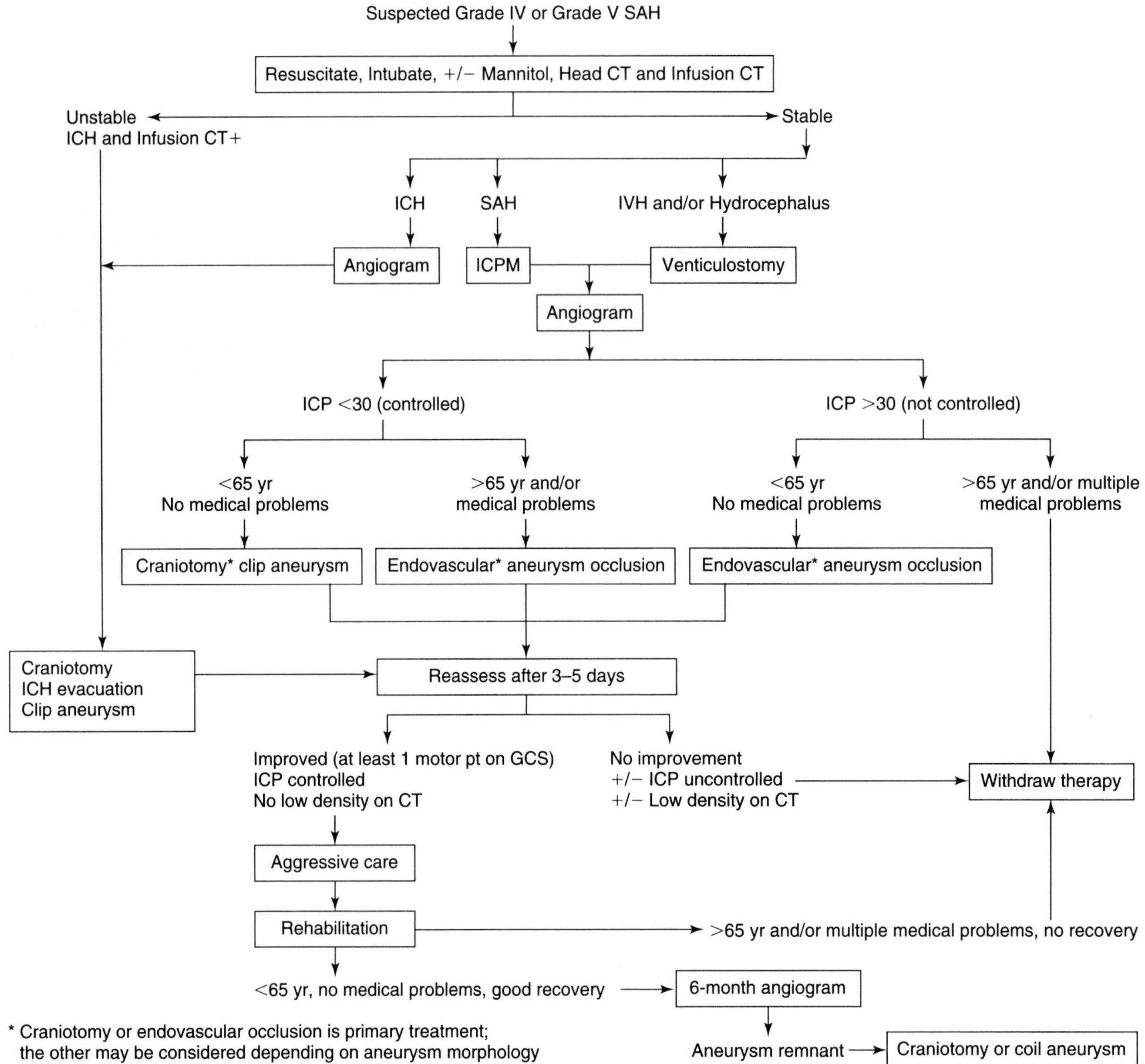

FIGURE 107–4. Algorithm for the management of poor-grade aneurysm patients. CT, computed tomography; ICH, intracerebral hemorrhage; ICP, intracranial pressure; ICPM, intracranial pressure monitor; IVH, intraventricular hemorrhage; SAH, subarachnoid hemorrhage. (From Le Roux P, Winn HR: The poor grade aneurysm patient. Acta Neurochir Suppl (Wien) 72:7–26, 1999.)

Intracerebral Hemorrhage

ICH increases the likelihood of mortality after SAH.[71, 72] A single randomized study[74] and several clinical series[68, 74, 75] found a tendency for improved patient outcome when emergency ICH evacuation was performed, particularly when simultaneous aneurysm obliteration was achieved. Factors such as young age, better clinical grade, and small ICH volume (<25 mL) are associated with better outcomes. However, many comatose patients, including those with brainstem compression and large ICH, can have favorable outcomes if rapidly resuscitated and operated on within a few hours of aneurysm rupture.[68] We perform angiography on patients with suspected aneurysmal ICH if they are neurologically stable. In the unstable patient, even single-vessel angiography may cause a life-threatening delay. Infusion CT or CT angiography[76–79] done immediately after the computed tomographic head scan is useful in these patients; both techniques are rapid and can detect more than 90% of aneurysms larger than 3 to 5 mm in diameter. For the neurologically unstable patient, we then proceed to craniotomy, ICH evacuation, and aneurysm obliteration based on the computed tomographic infusion study or CT-angiography (CTA) alone (see Fig. 107–4). Using this strategy, we have found that 30% of moribund patients with clinical and computed tomographic evidence of brainstem compression after aneurysmal ICH are independent and living at home with only mild disability 6 months later.[68]

During surgery for aneurysmal ICH, large bone flaps are preferable to prevent brain herniation and strangulation, and they provide easy access to the hemorrhage. Brain relaxation using mannitol is important. Similarly, the sphenoid wing and orbital roof should be drilled down to reduce brain retraction. In some patients, this may not be possible. Instead, the ICH distant from the aneurysm can be partially removed before proceeding with vascular dissection. The aneurysm should be occluded using standard microvascular techniques and magnification before complete ICH evacuation. During closure, lobectomy, ventriculostomy, or dural augmentation without bone replacement may be necessary if cerebral swelling persists.

Acute Intraventricular Hemorrhage and Hydrocephalus

Acute hydrocephalus and IVH are often observed after aneurysm rupture, particularly in poor-grade patients and those with thick subarachnoid blood on CT.[80–85] External ventricular drainage (EVD) is recommended, particularly when the patient has depressed consciousness. Several clinical series describe good results using EVD for hydrocephalus or IVH after aneurysm rupture, provided early aneurysm occlusion is achieved.[81, 84] Attempts to remove casted intraventricular blood through a craniotomy or the infusion of urokinase do not appear to improve outcome.[85, 86] Clinical improvement within 24 hours of starting EVD suggests a favorable outcome, but clinical improvement after ventricular drainage is not always associated with a favorable outcome.[69, 70, 82, 83] Many patients who do not improve can undergo surgery with satisfactory results. Several surgeons have observed that EVD increases the risk of aneurysm rebleeding[50, 80, 84, 87] or impairs natural mechanisms that arrest aneurysm rupture.[88] Ventricular drainage should therefore be performed carefully to avoid altering aneurysm transmural pressure that may precipitate rebleeding. Acute hydrocephalus is often associated with vasospasm[89]; ventricular drainage should therefore be accompanied by early aneurysm occlusion to allow effective use of hyperdynamic therapy and angioplasty.

Chronic hydrocephalus is observed in 20% of patients after SAH.[90] One half of patients with acute clinical hydrocephalus eventually require a ventriculoperitoneal shunt. Factors associated with hydrocephalus include increased ventricular size and IVH at admission, poor clinical grade, preexisting hypertension, alcoholism, female sex, increased aneurysm size, pneumonia, and meningitis.[90] The need for a permanent shunt can be reduced by EVD, including long, tunneled catheters; serial lumbar punctures; and perhaps by lamina terminalis fenestration at craniotomy.[80, 91] Whether an aneurysm is occluded using surgery or endovascular techniques does not influence the subsequent risk for hydrocephalus.[92]

Ruptured Aneurysms and Early Vasospasm

Vasospasm is associated with poor outcome, and 10% to 15% of patients present with angiographic evidence of vasospasm within 48 hours of aneurysm rupture.[93] What management is appropriate for these patients? Experimental and clinical observations suggest that surgical manipulation of blood vessels does not exacerbate the arterial narrowing seen after SAH.[94–97] For example, in patients undergoing preoperative and postoperative angiography, surgical timing does not alter the incidence of angiographic vasospasm[95] or correlate with infarction, provided prophylactic hypervolemia is instituted early.[97] Quershi and coworkers,[93] in an analysis of 296 patients in the placebo arm of a multicenter trial, found that early vasospasm was associated with subsequent poor outcome and an increased risk of symptomatic vasospasm. However, early surgery reduced the risk of poor outcome in these patients. We found that prompt aneurysm obliteration, followed by immediate angioplasty for patients presenting with symptomatic vasospasm and an unsecured aneurysm, was feasible and offered a reasonable chance of neurological recovery to these patients who might otherwise progress to cerebral infarction.[98] The outcome of angioplasty depends less on angiographic success than on early intervention.[99, 100] In poor-grade patients who cannot be reliably evaluated clinically, prophylactic angioplasty may be feasible in selected patients with severe vasospasm.[101] These patients may be selected for treatment based on cerebral blood flow studies or microdialysate analysis of extracellular metabolites for delayed ischemia.[102]

Surgical Complications after Subarachnoid Hemorrhage

Surgical complications, such as intraoperative aneurysm rupture, major vessel occlusions, cerebral contusion, or ICH are associated with about 10% of the morbidity and mortality after SAH.[18, 23, 40, 103–109] Factors such as inexperience or poor surgical technique may play a role.[104, 108] However, several series suggest that surgical complications after SAH are primarily associated with aneurysm location, size, and morphology.[19, 22, 105–107, 109, 110] Large or giant aneurysms, aneurysms with atherosclerotic necks, or aneurysms located at the basilar bifurcation or anterior communicating artery are more frequently associated with surgical complications. The International Cooperative Study on the Timing of Aneurysm Surgery and several studies comparing patient cohorts with historical controls suggest that, although brain swelling is more common during early surgery, surgical timing is not associated with surgical complications.[55, 56, 58, 106] Similarly, we found that the incidence of surgical complications is not influenced by clinical grade.[18] However, it is not clear whether the impact of a surgical complication in a poor-grade patient has greater adverse effect than the same complication in a good-grade patient. Similarly, whether retraction of the swollen brain results in neuropsychological or cognitive deficits that may not occur in delayed surgery when the brain is less swollen is not defined. However, data using neuropsychological testing demonstrate no association between timing of surgery and neuropsychological outcome.[111]

SPECIAL CIRCUMSTANCES

The approach to management of patients harboring cerebral aneurysms may be altered by a variety of special circumstances, including pregnancy; extremes of age (i.e., children or the elderly); associated infection, trauma, arteriovenous malformations, or carotid artery disease; and certain types of lesions, such as microaneurysms or fusiform, giant, and residual aneurysms. Some of these circumstances are the subject of separate chapters (see Chapter 121, Giant Aneurysms, Chapter 122, Infectious Intracranial Aneurysms, Chapters 219 and 220 on pediatric Vascular Issues, and Chapter 143, Pregnancy and Treatment of Vascular Disease).

Advanced Age and Cerebral Aneurysms

Many studies suggest advanced age is associated with a poor outcome after SAH. However, other studies demonstrate that young and old people in the same clinical condition experience similar outcomes.[40, 42, 57, 112–117] There are several important caveats when examining the association between age and outcome. Older patients are frequently excluded from active treatment, which influences outcome; older patients are more often in a poor clinical grade category, which has a greater impact on outcome than age[115, 118, 119]; and other variables such as hypertension or atherosclerosis are common in elderly patients. These factors may have independent adverse effects on outcome or replace the effect of age in multivariate analyses.[40, 67, 114, 120] Although no randomized trial has specifically addressed the role of active treatment in elderly patients, several lines of evidence suggest that surgically treated patients do better than conservatively treated patients after aneurysm rupture.[116, 121] Consequently, we believe that withholding treatment on the grounds of advanced age may not always be justified. Instead, the decision to treat an elderly patient after SAH should be considered in light of the natural history of the disease and the patient's overall physiologic condition and associated risk factors. Atherosclerosis in the aneurysm and associated vessels frequently increases the technical risk of aneurysm occlusion in the elderly, and these patients may be best treated at specialized centers.[122]

Although good results among patients older than 60 years of age undergoing surgical repair of unruptured aneurysms are reported, advanced age is a risk factor.[2, 24, 26, 34] This increased risk in part results from more medical complications among older patients. Older patients are more likely to have atherosclerotic or calcified aneurysms or adjacent vessels, both of which increase surgical risk.[18] Very old patients may not benefit from unruptured aneurysm treatment. Decision-analysis studies suggest that surgical treatment of unruptured aneurysms is beneficial if the patient's life expectancy is longer than 13 years.[123, 124] Quality-of-life studies suggest that quality life is lengthened by 4 years in 40-year-old patients, 2.4 years in 50-year-old patients, 1.3 years in 60-year-old patients, and 0.6 years in 70-year-old patients.[125] These various studies make certain assumptions about surgical risk and risk of aneurysm rupture but suggest overall that surgery may be appropriate in a 64-year-old man or a 68-year-old woman.[124] Patients older than 70 years, particularly those with small, asymptomatic aneurysms or giant, posterior circulation aneurysms associated with few symptoms, should probably be followed with serial magnetic resonance imaging (MRI), magnetic resonance angiography (MRA), and CTA. For these patients, treatment probably offers little over the natural history of these lesions and should be considered only if symptoms progress or aneurysm growth is documented.

Pregnancy

The management of intracranial aneurysms during pregnancy is complicated by the physiologic changes that accompany pregnancy and by potential risks to the fetus when investigating and treating the mother. Intracranial aneurysms are not commonly discovered during pregnancy, in part because the risk of hemorrhage is greatest during the late third trimester and delivery.[126] Investigation of the pregnant woman with an aneurysm is similar to that for a nonpregnant woman. However, the abdomen should be shielded with lead to reduce the risk of ionizing radiation to the fetus. In general, pregnant patients with ruptured aneurysms are treated the same as nonpregnant women, with certain caveats. For example, during surgery, temporary clips rather than hypotension are preferred to reduce the risk of fetal hypoperfusion. Care should be taken when mannitol is administered because its use can lead to maternal hypoperfusion and subsequent uterine hypoperfusion or fetal hyperosmolality. Hyperventilation can cause acid-base shifts and decreased oxygen delivery to the fetus. After the aneurysm is occluded, pregnancy is allowed to proceed to term. If the patient is in good neurological condition, the baby should be delivered vaginally. When labor begins or is expected to begin immediately after aneurysm occlusion, cesarean section is preferred. If aneurysm rupture occurs during labor, simultaneous craniotomy and cesarean section may be necessary; the cesarean section should be performed first so that the fetus is not exposed to prolonged anesthesia.[127] Surgery should be deferred until the second trimester, when an unruptured aneurysm is discovered during the first trimester to reduce potential drug teratogenic effects during treatment. Other medications such as anticonvulsants or calcium channel blockers should be avoided or used cautiously. A cesarean section may be preferable when an unruptured aneurysm is discovered late in pregnancy, particularly if the aneurysm becomes symptomatic or has enlarged. A vaginal delivery, using epidural anesthesia to shorten the second stage of labor, is acceptable for an asymptomatic patient with an unruptured aneurysm.

Pediatric Aneurysms

Aneurysms in children are rare. In contrast to adults, posterior circulation, giant, infectious, or traumatic aneurysms are more common.[128, 129] For small children, the operating room should be warmed and care taken to avoid intraoperative rupture, because the total blood volume is relatively small.

Infective Aneurysms

Mycotic or infective aneurysms account for 2% to 6% of intracranial aneurysms in adults. These lesions often are associated with infective endocarditis or immunologic compromise.[130] Fungal infections, particularly aspergillosis and candidal disease, may be associated with proximal aneurysms. Aneurysms associated with bacterial infections, most commonly streptococci and *Staphylococcus aureus*, usually are located on distal middle cerebral artery (MCA) branches. All infective aneurysms require 4 to 6 weeks of culture-directed antimicrobial therapy, whether the aneurysm is occluded or not. Antimicrobial therapy alone may be used to treat some infective aneurysms, and 30% to 50% resolve or decrease in size. The lesions require close follow-up with serial angiography and blood cultures. When aneurysm surgery is required, any hemodynamically significant cardiac lesion should be corrected before aneurysm obliteration. However, when the aneurysm is associated with an abscess or a hematoma, aneurysm surgery may be necessary first. During surgery, the surgeon must be prepared for aneurysm excision and parent vessel anastomosis, bypass, or a ligation procedure. A short course of preoperative antibiotics may make the aneurysm and parent vessels less friable. The role of endovascular techniques to occlude infective aneurysms is not defined, in part because of concerns about placing a foreign body in an infected, friable sac.

Traumatic Aneurysms

Less than 1% of all intracranial aneurysms are traumatic. Traumatic aneurysms usually are associated with penetrating head injury or contiguous skull fracture and are most common in the MCA region after low-velocity shrapnel injuries or stab wounds. However, basal skull fractures may be associated with basal traumatic aneurysms.[131, 132] Most traumatic aneurysms manifest within 2 to 3 weeks of the original injury and are false aneurysms.[130] A definable neck is rare, and the lesions are prone to intraoperative rupture. Consequently, the surgeon should be prepared to trap or excise the lesion. Encircling clips may also be useful. The surgical approach must provide proximal and distal control and access to the superficial temporal artery or saphenous vein for a bypass, if required.

Aneurysms and Arteriovenous Malformations

Between 3% and 14% of arteriovenous malformations (AVMs) are associated with an aneurysm. In some instances, the aneurysms may arise because of hemodynamic stress. Several types of aneurysms are associated with AVMs. Type I dysplastic or remote aneurysms are located at some distance from the AVM and appear structurally unrelated to major inflow vessels. Type II proximal aneurysms arise from the circle of Willis or proximal portion of a major feeding vessel. Type III pedicular aneurysms are located on the middle portion of a major feeding pedicle, whereas type IV intranidal lesions are found within the AVM. The natural history of these various aneurysms may be different, and they may therefore require different treatment strategies.[133] A management protocol for AVMs and associated aneurysms manifesting with hemorrhage is provided in Figure 107–5. In general, when the lesions come to attention in the absence of hemorrhage, the aneurysm should be treated first because of the higher morbidity associated with aneurysm rupture.

Coexistent Carotid Artery Disease

Most physicians recommend treatment of the symptomatic lesion first when a patient presents with carotid artery disease and an intracranial aneurysm.[122] When both lesions are asymptomatic, treatment should be directed at the lesion with a worse natural history.[134] An association between carotid endarterectomy and an increased risk of aneurysm rupture has not been clearly demonstrated.

Fusiform Aneurysms

Fusiform intracranial aneurysms occur most frequently at the skull base, particularly in the vertebrobasilar system. These aneurysms are characterized by circumferential dilatation and by elongation and tortuosity of cerebral arteries. They are associated with atherosclerosis and dolichoectasia. The vessel dilatation can cause turbulence, damage branching vessels, and precipitate thrombus formation. Most patients with fusiform aneurysms present with ischemic symptoms. Provided there is no SAH, anticoagulation may improve the outcome of these patients. Some fusiform aneurysms, however, require surgery, which can usually be accomplished by circumferential wrapping techniques.[135, 136] Aneurysm wrapping should be followed by anticoagulation. Fusiform aneurysms of the vertebral artery may be best treated with endovascular hunterian ligation under full heparinization or by surgical hunterian ligation when precise ligation is necessary to avoid inclusion of vital perforators.

Microaneurysms

Microaneurysms are smaller than 3 mm in diameter. They are often broad based relative to their height and so do not lend themselves to clipping or to the use of

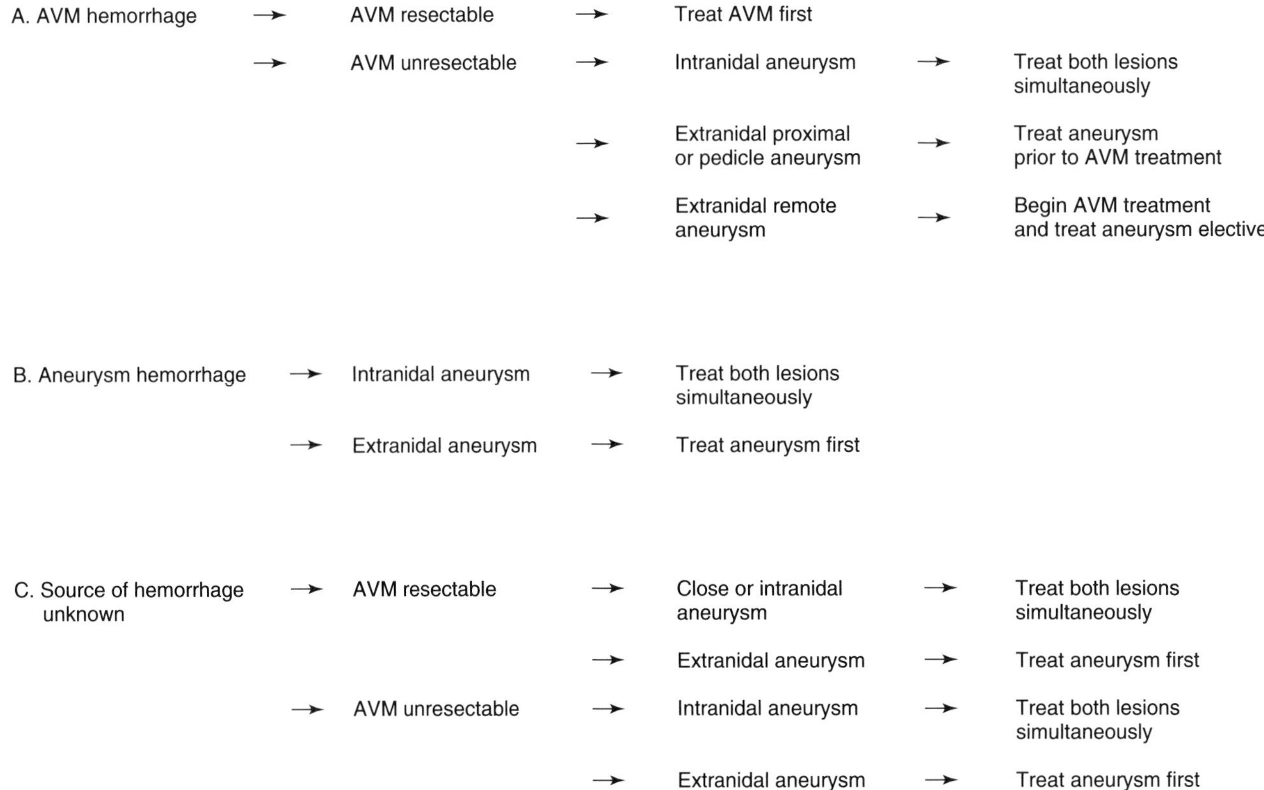

FIGURE 107–5. Suggested treatment algorithm for patients with intracranial hemorrhage, arteriovenous malformation, and aneurysm. (Adapted from Cockroft K, Thompson RC, Steinberg GK: Aneurysms and arteriovenous malformations. Neurosurg Clin North Am 9:565–576, 1998.)

Guglielmi detachable coils (GDCs). Unruptured microaneurysms, particularly if asymptomatic, require close follow-up. Treatment of ruptured microaneurysms is uncertain. Short-term angiographic follow-up suggests that bipolar electrocoagulation and reinforcement with muslin gauze may be a reasonable treatment.[137]

Giant Aneurysms

Giant aneurysms represent approximately 4% of intracranial aneurysms. Untreated, the 2-year mortality rate for persons with giant aneurysms is between 60% and 100%. This poor prognosis warrants aggressive management, preferably in tertiary referral centers. There are two treatment goals: preventing aneurysm rupture and relief of mass effect. Direct clipping is the preferred treatment method; however, surgical results by direct clipping for giant aneurysms are worse than for small aneurysms, even when using sophisticated techniques such as bypass or cardiac standstill.[40, 138–142] Overall, surgery on giant aneurysms is associated with a procedure-related mortality rate of 5% to 15%, whereas 70% to 86% of patients have favorable outcomes.[138–140, 143–145] The best surgical option for many giant aneurysms, particularly serpentine lesions or those with wide necks, may be aneurysm trapping, aneurysmorrhaphy, or parent vessel occlusion and bypass, if needed.[140, 144] In some instances, the mass effect can be alleviated by parent vessel occlusion. Surgery should be delayed after aneurysm rupture to evaluate the cerebral circulation and hemodynamic reserve and to allow disturbed autoregulation to recover.[144]

There are three important technical considerations during surgery for giant aneurysms: wide exposure, proximal and distal control, and clip reconstruction. Wide exposure can be obtained using skull base techniques. For giant, anterior circulation aneurysms, an orbitozygomatic approach may be preferable to the pterional approach. The orbitozygomatic approach can be useful for lesions such as proximal, giant ICA (e.g., ophthalmic, superior hypophyseal, paraclinoid) aneurysms that may require anterior clinoidectomy, for cavernous lesions, or when an upward viewing angle is required for lesions such as giant, anterior communicating or ICA bifurcation aneurysms that tend to project upward. Deep bypass procedures also are facilitated by the orbitozygomatic approach. For posterior circulation aneurysms, exposures such as the orbitozygomatic, various transpetrosal approaches (i.e., retrolabyrinthine, presigmoid, translabyrinthine, or transcochlear), the far lateral or extreme lateral approach, or a combination of approaches, depending on aneurysm location, may be needed.[138] Dividing the basilar artery into fifths helps determine which approach is suitable. An orbitozygomatic approach is reasonable for lesions involving the upper two fifths of the basilar artery. For lesions involving the middle fifth, transpetrosal approaches are preferable, whereas far or extreme lateral approaches are suitable for aneurysms of the lower two fifths of the basilar artery and the intradural vertebral artery. When the lesion straddles these zones, a combination of approaches is recommended.

Proximal and distal vascular control is important during repair of giant aneurysms; it permits reduction of aneurysm size and improves visualization of the surrounding anatomy. Similarly, an aneurysm with intraluminal thrombosis can be opened and the clot removed. Cerebral protection, as with the use of barbiturates, is necessary. Skull base techniques facilitate vascular control. For some giant, proximal ICA aneurysms, exposure of the cervical or petrous carotid artery may be helpful, whereas endovascular techniques or hypothermic circulatory arrest may be useful for giant, posterior circulation aneurysms. Surgical aneurysm clipping requires a favorable neck; many giant aneurysms have wide necks, whereas fusiform aneurysms have no intervening neck.[146] Clip reconstruction to recreate the normal anatomy, rather than clip occlusion, often is required to occlude giant aneurysms. Single clips may be inadequate; instead, several shorter clips or fenestrated clips placed serially along the aneurysm neck may be a better choice.

Residual Aneurysm

What should be done with a residual aneurysm found on postoperative angiogram? Although some residual aneurysms may thrombose, even small residual aneurysms may regrow and bleed. Overall, the incidence of rebleeding from residual, ruptured aneurysms is estimated to be less than 0.5% per year.[16, 17, 22, 147, 148] However, aneurysms with broad-based residua frequently enlarge and appear to have a nearly fourfold greater risk of subsequent hemorrhage.[16] These lesions should therefore be repaired when identified on postoperative angiograms. Small, residual dog-ear remnants may be observed, but careful, long-term follow-up is important. For example, Giannotta and Litofsky[25] reported an average interval of 10.5 years between the original surgery and subsequent rebleeding among inadequately treated ruptured aneurysms. How small, residual, unruptured aneurysms should be managed is less certain. The lesions may be followed using angiography or spiral CTA; aneurysm obliteration is necessary when aneurysm growth is observed.[3] Risk factors for aneurysm growth or rupture, such as hypertension or cigarette smoking, should be treated.[149]

ENDOVASCULAR TECHNIQUES FOR ANEURYSM OCCLUSION

Surgical clip ligation remains the preferred therapy for many aneurysms. In the past, endovascular techniques were used to occlude aneurysms because of "anticipated surgical difficulty," "medical contraindications," or "failed surgery." Today, endovascular techniques, particularly GDCs, should be considered as a complement to surgical techniques and, in some instances, the primary treatment for selected aneurysms. The appropriate selection of surgical or endovascular aneurysm occlusion requires a collaborative approach between neurosurgeons and interventional radiologists and an understanding of the anatomic, physical, and physiologic characteristics of both techniques. The selection of one treatment over the other requires careful consideration of patient- and aneurysm-specific factors. Anecdotal reports suggest that collaboration between neurosurgeons and interventional radiologists increases the number of patients who can safely be treated de novo or after one technique fails.[150–152] In the following sections, we review factors that influence selection of endovascular techniques for aneurysm occlusion. Detailed information concerning endovascular aneurysm treatment is provided in Chapter 120.

Safety and Results of Endovascular Aneurysm Occlusion

Several clinical series have established that endovascular aneurysm occlusion is feasible and safe.[153–159] In expert hands, complete aneurysm occlusion or more than 90% occlusion is observed in approximately 50% or 90% of aneurysms, respectively, using endovascular techniques.[150, 154, 159–161] In contrast, more than 90% of aneurysms are completely occluded using surgical techniques.[16, 19, 20] Technical complications, including aneurysm perforation, distal embolization, parent vessel occlusion, or coil migration, may be observed in 9% to 30% of patients. Overall, permanent complications of embolization occur in 4% to 7% of patients.[153, 155, 156, 158–160, 162–166]

Long-Term Stability and the Implications of Residual Aneurysms

The clinical relevance of partial aneurysm occlusion by coils is not clear because few patients have undergone long-term follow-up. Limited short-term studies (6 to 24 months) suggest that aneurysm remnants lead to recurrence and that there are an increasing number of suboptimal results with time.[153, 154, 158, 163, 167] Malisch and associates[164] published the longest follow-up, averaging 3.5 years for 100 patients, including 53 who had SAH and who underwent coil occlusion of their aneurysm. Seventeen patients required subsequent surgery, and three needed repeat embolizations. Recurrences may also be seen in patients with completely occluded aneurysms, but this appears to be rare.[154, 168]

Aneurysm occlusion using endovascular techniques or surgery is very different, and this difference may have significant implications for residual aneurysms. In the clipped aneurysm, the walls are closely apposed, and the remaining aneurysm is completely excluded from the circulation. In contrast, using endovascular techniques, the coils keep the remnant's walls apart. Although experimental models of coiled aneurysms demonstrate that the aneurysm neck becomes entirely occluded by organized thrombus and that the free luminal surface is covered by endothelium,[169, 170] endothelialization is not observed in coiled aneurysms inspected at autopsy or surgery.[171, 172] These various factors mean that any intra-aneurysmal thrombus or coil is exposed to circulating blood, which may allow compaction of the coils or flow around the coil's periphery into the aneurysm sac.

Patients with incompletely occluded coiled aneurysms consequently require repeat angiography, coil embolization, or surgery. Is this safe or cost effective? Angiography is relatively safe in patients harboring cerebral aneurysms; less than 1% suffer a stroke.[19] However, in the presence of atherosclerotic disease, the stroke risk is increased fourfold. Spiral CTA may prove useful for following aneurysm remnants.[174] There is limited experience with surgical treatment of coiled aneurysms. Small clinical series suggest that a coiled aneurysm is not a simple surgical lesion.[172, 174, 175] Aneurysm obliteration may be easily obtained if the aneurysm is partially packed with coils, but it is difficult with more complete packing, in part because there is insufficient space between the coils and the parent vessel for clip placement.[150, 174]

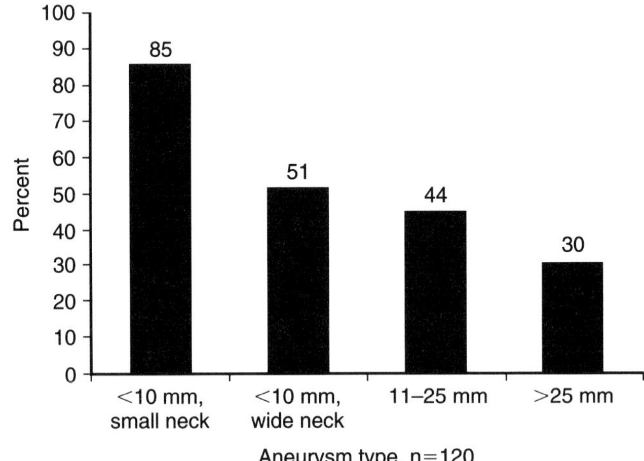

FIGURE 107–6. Complete occlusion of incidental unruptured aneurysms using Guglielmi detachable coils (n = 120). (Adapted from Murayama Y, Vinuela F, Duckwiler G, et al: Embolization of incidental cerebral aneurysms by using the Guglielmi detachable coil system. J Neurosurg 90:207–214, 1999.)

Which Aneurysms Can Be Successfully Occluded?

In general, when using endovascular techniques, morphologic results are good in small aneurysms with small necks and those at a right angle to blood flow (Table 107–4 and Fig. 107–6). Endovascular procedures appear less effective in large or wide-necked aneurysms.[150, 158–160, 163, 164, 168, 176, 177] Zubillga and colleagues[177] treated 79 aneurysms with GDCs; complete occlusion was observed in 85% of small-necked aneurysms but in only 15% of large-necked aneurysms. An aneurysm neck less than 4 mm in diameter appears to be the desired size for endovascular occlusion. Wide aneurysm necks generally play a less significant role in surgery, because the parent vessel can be reconstructed using fenestrated and angled clips. Newer techniques such as balloon remodeling appear to improve the results of endovascular occlusion of wide-necked aneurysms; initial case series suggest that more than 80% of wide-necked aneurysms can be occluded using this technique.[178, 179]

Aneurysm location may also influence the success of the procedure. For example, superior hypophyseal aneurysms are more amenable to coils than carotid-ophthalmic aneurysms because the catheter tends to follow the curve of the siphon into the aneurysm because of its location within the concavity of the carotid artery.[180] MCA aneurysms may also be difficult to treat because of inability to separate out the aneurysm neck and surrounding vessels.[181, 182]

TABLE 107–4 ■ **Factors That Limit Successful Endovascular Aneurysm Occlusion**

Dome-to-neck ratio < 2
Neck width > 4 mm
Inadequate endovascular access
Unstable intraluminal thrombus
Arterial branch incorporated in neck
Middle ± cerebral artery aneurysms

Endovascular Techniques after Subarachnoid Hemorrhage

Observational studies suggest that GDC occlusion of ruptured aneurysms is comparable to that of conventional microsurgery in the short term and can prevent early rebleeding.[53, 155, 156, 159, 163, 183] These studies suggest that endovascular techniques provide protection against rebleeding in the first few months, when rebleeding occurs most frequently.[153, 159, 183] Vinuela and coworkers[159] described short-term follow-up after coil occlusion of 401 ruptured aneurysms. One half of the aneurysms were incompletely occluded; overall, 4.5% of patients rebled within 6 months. Although these results are worse than surgery, they may represent an improvement on the natural history, because 75% of the aneurysms were treated within 7 days of SAH. Clinical data suggest a procedure-related permanent morbidity rate between 3% and 9% and mortality rate between 0% and 8%.[153, 155, 156, 158–160, 163, 166, 183, 184] Angiographic data demonstrate that 50% of ruptured aneurysms can be completely occluded using endovascular techniques. Large aneurysms or aneurysms with wide necks, however, are difficult to occlude.[153, 159, 177] The use of endovascular techniques does not appear to alter the risk of vasospasm.[185]

What are the long-term results of using GDCs for ruptured aneurysms? Overall, recurrent filling is seen in 15% of aneurysms on angiograms obtained 6 months after treatment.[153] Aneurysm recurrence is generally observed in wide-necked aneurysms and is related to coil compaction. Greater packing at the initial procedure may improve long-term results but at the potential risk of increased complications, such as vessel occlusion or thromboembolism, during the procedure. Patients undergoing endovascular procedures require heparin. The impact of heparin in patients shortly after SAH has not been studied, but the use of long-term anticoagulation doubles the risk of a poor outcome after aneurysm rupture.[186] It is uncertain, however, whether these findings apply to short-term heparinization. The incidence of aneurysm rebleeding after coil occlusion is between 1% and 3% per year.[153, 155, 156, 158–160, 163, 165] Aneurysm size significantly influences rebleeding, ranging from 0% for small and 4% for large to 33% for giant aneurysms.[163] Rebleeding is usual from recurrent aneurysms but rare from completely occluded or stable aneurysms. Byrne and associates[153] treated 317 patients within 30 days of SAH; the median follow-up was 22.3 months. Thirty-eight aneurysm recurrences were observed; 3 (8%) rebled. In contrast, 1 (0.4%) of 221 aneurysms that appeared angiographically stable after at least 11 months rebled. These findings suggest that complete occlusion is protective and that regrowth and rebleeding are inevitable consequences of incomplete aneurysm occlusion.

Endovascular occlusion of the acutely ruptured aneurysm may be an attractive alternative to surgery for some poor-grade patients, but the role of endovascular therapy in these patients has only been described in limited clinical series. Malisch and colleagues[163] treated nine poor-grade patients using coils; all nine patients died or had a poor outcome. In contrast, Kinugasa and coworkers[187] used cellulose acetate polymer and cisternal tissue plasminogen activator (t-PA) in 12 patients with grades III through V lesions. Eight patients experienced favorable outcomes, but seven had partially thrombosed aneurysms that required subsequent surgery. Kremer and associates[184] described 40 poor-grade patients whose aneurysms were occluded using GDCs. Sixteen (40%) patients had good outcomes; there was a tendency for better outcomes among those with posterior circulation aneurysms. The potential advantage of endovascular therapy is that it is physiologically less stressful, because brain retraction and vessel dissection are not required. Consequently, endovascular therapy may be the preferable treatment of some poor-grade patients when extensive cerebral swelling is seen on CT or when ICP is not controlled. Endovascular therapy may be useful in elderly patients, for whom long-term coil stability may be less relevant (see Fig. 107–4). Surgery should be the primary treatment in young patients when the ruptured aneurysm is associated with ICH, the aneurysm is associated with mass effect, or the aneurysm, such as a wide-necked lesion, is not suitable for coil occlusion.

Endovascular Techniques for Incidental Unruptured Aneurysms

The existing literature suggests that endovascular aneurysm occlusion may play a limited role in the treatment of unruptured aneurysms, particularly in younger patients, in large part because complete aneurysm occlusion is achieved in only one half of the aneurysms, and aneurysm recurrence rates are high.[155, 159, 160, 168] Murayama and colleagues[168] treated 115 patients with 120 incidentally found aneurysms using GDCs. Complete aneurysm occlusion was achieved in 63% of the lesions, but 5% could not be treated (see Fig. 107–6). Five patients developed a permanent neurological deficit from a periprocedural complication. Follow-up angiograms were obtained for 77 patients; one third of the aneurysms that were incompletely occluded had recanalized at median follow-up of 16.3 months.

Endovascular Techniques for Giant Aneurysms

The various clinical series describing endovascular treatment of giant aneurysms suggest that most lesions require multiple procedures and that the immediate neurological results are similar to those of surgery.[159, 161, 162, 188] Gruber and coworkers[188] treated 31 giant or large aneurysms in 30 patients; mortality and morbidity rates for the procedure were 6.7% and 13.3%, respectively. There are several disadvantages to using endovascular techniques for giant aneurysms. First, morphologic results are poor because very few giant aneurysms can be completely occluded,[162, 163, 177, 188] in large part because many have wide necks. Second, symptoms from the aneurysm are improved in only one half of the patients, and the mass effect can be aggravated in some.[161, 163, 175, 188] Third, more than one half of the giant aneurysms occluded using endovascular techniques recur during follow-up and require recoiling.[163, 188] Rebleeding complicates one third of giant aneurysms that have been coiled.[163] These observations suggest that surgery remains the first-line treatment for giant aneurysms. Alternatively, endovascular techniques may be used for parent vessel occlusion with or without bypass.

In the future, intravascular stents may improve endovascular treatment of giant aneurysms. Stents may uncouple the aneurysm from the circulation, leading to thrombosis, or may aid in packing coils in wide-necked aneurysms by providing a scaffold to prevent coil herniation.[189]

Collaboration and Comparison

Few studies have directly compared surgical and endovascular aneurysm occlusion. Results of a single, small, retrospective comparative study suggest that, in selected patients, basilar bifurcation aneurysms may be best treated using endovascular techniques rather than surgery.[190] However, larger case series of patients undergoing coil occlusion of basilar bifurcation aneurysms demonstrate that one half of the patients may suffer a periprocedural adverse event, that nearly one third require a second procedure to occlude the aneurysm, and that permanent deficits due to stroke complicate up to 10% of GDC procedures.[155, 191] Only one half of the basilar bifurcation aneurysms can be completely occluded using coils, whereas more than 90% can be occluded with surgery.[29, 65, 155, 158, 165, 190–193] A single, randomized study of 109 patients compared GDC with surgical aneurysm occlusion within 72 hours of SAH; there was no difference in the 3-month outcome when the analysis was controlled for grade.[166] Better angiographic results were observed for anterior circulation aneurysms with surgery, whereas posterior circulation lesions demonstrated better angiographic results with GDCs. In a prospective series of 103 patients, coil embolization was considered the first treatment option, provided aneurysm morphology was favorable.[181] Sixty-four aneurysms underwent coil occlusion, 63 aneurysms were treated surgically, and 12 coiled aneurysms required subsequent surgery. Residual aneurysms were identified in 31% of coiled aneurysms, 1.6% of surgically treated lesions, and none of the lesions that underwent coil occlusion and then surgery. Poor outcomes were experienced by 13% of the patients treated using coils, 6% who underwent surgery, and 8% who underwent both procedures.

Taken together, these study results suggest that neurovascular surgeons and interventionists must cooperate to determine which procedure or combination of procedures is most likely to succeed for each patient. Aneurysm morphology appears to be closely associated with the success and risk of endovascular and surgical techniques. Careful collaborative study of imaging studies is essential to determine aneurysm size and configuration, presence of intra-aneurysmal thrombosis, relationship between the aneurysm and surrounding structures, aneurysm wall thickness, and neck morphology.[194] This information is provided by conventional, two-dimensional angiography, but additional information can be obtained from computer-assisted delineation of the geometric design of aneurysms and surrounding structures from conventional angiography,[196] MRA, three-dimensional CT, spiral CTA,[173, 195] and computer-assisted "virtual reality" reconstruction of vascular anatomy.[195]

TECHNICAL CONSIDERATIONS

Intraoperative Angiography and Endoscopy

Several investigators advocate the use of intraoperative angiography to prevent incomplete aneurysm occlusion or inadvertent vessel occlusion. When used, intraoperative angiography can lead to clip readjustment in 10% to 30% of patients because of incomplete aneurysm occlusion or parent vessel occlusion.[197–199] Most clip readjustments occur for giant, basilar apex, or superior hypophyseal aneurysms.[198, 199] We have studied 637 aneurysms with routine postoperative angiograms; aneurysmal remnants and vessel occlusion are more likely when a large aneurysm or cerebrovascular atherosclerosis is identified or when multiple attempts are made to place aneurysm clips.[19] Although useful in selected patients, intraoperative angiography may not be cost effective in routine use.[197, 200–202] Instead, intraoperative angiography should be considered for patients undergoing repair of giant aneurysms or those with cerebrovascular atherosclerosis. A radiolucent operating table and head holder and sterile groin access should be planned for preoperatively. For some patients with complex lesions, an endoscope may be used to help confirm regional anatomy before and after clip application.[203, 204] In the future, by providing an endoluminal view of the aneurysm, angioscopy-assisted aneurysm surgery may reduce the need for intraoperative angiography for complex cases.[205]

Alternate Techniques of Surgical Aneurysm Occlusion

The goals of intracranial aneurysm treatment are isolation of the lesion from the circulation and parent vessel preservation. These goals can usually be accomplished using clip ligation or endovascular coils. However, in some lesions that have unique anatomic features, aneurysm occlusion using either technique is dangerous or impossible. These factors include large or giant aneurysm size, particularly when the aneurysm has a wide neck and incorporates the parent vessels or perforating arteries; calcification at the aneurysm base; and fusiform or dissecting aneurysms. Treatment of these complex aneurysms may be accomplished using parent vessel occlusion, aneurysm trapping, aneurysm excision and arterial reconstruction, or revascularization using interposition or extracranial-to-intracranial bypass grafting. Parent vessel occlusion reduces blood flow to the aneurysm, which may lead to aneurysm thrombosis. Similarly, revascularization procedures divert blood flow to the circulation distal to the aneurysm, which leads to aneurysm thrombosis in some instances.

Parent vessel occlusion or hunterian ligation is an excellent treatment option for some symptomatic cavernous sinus aneurysms, giant proximal ICA aneurysms, serpentine MCA aneurysms, wide-necked basilar aneurysms that incorporate the P1 origins, selected vertebral artery lesions, and dissecting aneurysms. When parent vessel occlusion is considered, patients must be carefully evaluated by endovascular surgeons and neurosurgeons. To determine whether revascularization or a bypass procedure is necessary, the adequacy of the collateral circulation and the patient's ability to tolerate parent vessel sacrifice must be examined. If the collateral circulation is adequate, endovascular parent artery occlusion is preferable. This technique requires heparinization to prevent thromboembolism or progressive local thrombosis that may occlude perforators. Heparinization may influence the timing of aneurysm occlusion if other procedures, such as ventricular drainage or hematoma evacuation, are required after SAH. Surgical occlusion is indicated if the occlusion point must be precise to spare perforators. For example, surgical occlusion is preferred to ligate the basilar artery between the posterior cerebral and superior cerebellar arteries. Vascular augmentation and bypass are necessary before parent vessel occlusion in patients who have inadequate collateral circulation.

Aneurysm trapping completely eliminates an aneurysm from the circulation. This technique is reserved for lesions that have a good collateral supply or that can be revascularized. The clips are placed as close to the aneurysm as possible to reduce the size of the vessel segment that is sacrificed. When important branch vessels are located along the trapped segment, it is better to perform only proximal occlusion. Aneurysm excision and aneurysmorrhaphy are alternatives for lesions that cannot be clip occluded. This technique is especially useful for MCA aneurysms because the sylvian fissure provides adequate room to perform vessel suturing and because there usually is enough redundant artery for the proximal and distal stumps to be mobilized and approximated without excess tension on the anastomosis.

Patient Selection for Bypass Procedures

When it is probable or certain that the parent artery will be sacrificed or severely compromised by proximal ligation or aneurysm trapping, revascularization procedures may be necessary. These techniques are described in Chapter 116. In this section, we review patient selection for these bypass procedures. There are three approaches: sacrifice the parent vessel without bypass and rely on the collateral circulation, perform routine bypass to provide collateral blood flow before or at the time of parent vessel occlusion or trapping, and select patients for bypass based on the results of preoperative testing.

Careful evaluation of the angiogram may predict whether a bypass is necessary. For example, the presence of an adequately sized contralateral vertebral artery or posterior communicating arteries suggests that occlusion of a single vertebral artery will be tolerated. In other patients, preoperative endovascular balloon occlusion tests may identify vessels that cannot be sacrificed. Temporary occlusion tests are often used with some measure of cerebral perfusion such as xenon-enhanced cerebral blood flow, SPECT, or transcranial Doppler measurements and can be augmented by temporarily reducing blood pressure during balloon occlusion.[206–209] When patients develop a neurological deficit during balloon occlusion, parent artery sacrifice should be augmented with a bypass graft or a vessel replacement graft. A bypass is usually not needed in patients who maintain cerebral perfusion (>30 mL/100 g per minute) and are neurologically intact during balloon occlusion. In patients who remain neurologically intact but have reduced cerebral perfusion (<30 mL/100 g per minute), a bypass should be considered to augment blood flow and prevent ischemia. The value of bypass procedures in patients who remain neurologically intact but develop reduced cerebral perfusion is not clearly defined,[207] in part because some postocclusion ischemic deficits may be embolic rather than hemodynamic in nature.

Complete Circulatory Arrest and Deep Hypothermia

Hypothermic circulatory arrest can completely devascularize an aneurysm and is particularly useful for complex, giant aneurysms.[141, 210] Chapter 90 provides a detailed discussion of this topic. Careful planning is required when using this technique, because it is a major undertaking that requires a dedicated multidisciplinary team and poses additional risks to the patient that can be justified only in selected cases.[141, 211–213] Before selecting appropriate cases for circulatory arrest, aneurysm-specific, parent artery–related, and patient-related factors must be considered. Surgical occlusion of giant basilar aneurysms or aneurysms larger than 3 cm in diameter in other locations is usually enhanced with hypothermic circulatory arrest. These patients are identified from preoperative neuroradiologic studies, including CT, CTA, MRI, MRA, and conventional angiography, or at surgery, when an aneurysm that is too difficult to occlude using standard techniques is found. Surgery can then be stopped and the patient returned within 1 week for a circulatory arrest procedure. Patient-related factors such as age, clinical grade, and time after aneurysm rupture do not contraindicate using circulatory arrest.[143] However, preexisting disease, particularly cardiopulmonary disease, may contraindicate circulatory arrest surgery, and a thorough preoperative medical evaluation is therefore necessary.

REFERENCES

1. Asari S, Ohmoto T: Natural history and risk factors of unruptured cerebral aneurysms. Clin Neurol Neurosurg 95:205–214, 1993.
2. International Study of Unruptured Intracranial Aneurysms Investigators: Unruptured intracranial aneurysms—risk of rupture and risks of surgical intervention. N Engl J Med 339; 1725–1733, 1998.
3. Juvela S, Porras M, Heiskanen O: Natural history of unruptured intracranial aneurysms: A long-term follow-up study. J Neurosurg 79:174–182, 1993.
4. Rinkel GJE, Djibuti M, Algra A, van Gijn J: Prevalence and risk of rupture of intracranial aneurysms: A systematic review. Stroke 29:251–256, 1998.
5. Wiebers DO, Whisnant JP, Sundt TM Jr, O'Fallon M: The significance of unruptured intracranial saccular aneurysms. J Neurosurg 66:23–29, 1987.
6. Brown RD, Wiebers DO, Forbes GS: Unruptured intracranial aneurysms and arteriovenous malformations: Frequency of intracranial hemorrhage and relationship of lesions. J Neurosurg 73:859–863, 1990.
7. Bonita R: Cigarette smoking, hypertension and the risk of subarachnoid hemorrhage: A population-based case-control study. Stroke 17:831–835, 1986.
8. Juvela S, Hillbom M, Numminen H, Koskinen P: Cigarette smoking and alcohol consumption as risk factors for aneurysmal subarachnoid hemorrhage. Stroke 24:639–646, 1993.
9. Longstreth WT Jr, Nelson LM, Koepsell TD, van Belle G: Cigarette smoking, alcohol use, and subarachnoid hemorrhage. Stroke 23:1242–1249, 1992.
10. Teunissen LL, Rinkel GJE, Algra A, van Gijn J: Risk factors for subarachnoid hemorrhage—a systematic review. Stroke 27: 544–549, 1996.
11. Schievink W, Piepgras DG, Wirth FP: Rupture of previously documented small asymptomatic saccular intracranial aneurysms: Report of three cases. J Neurosurg 76:1019–1024, 1992.
12. Yasui N, Magarisawa S, Suzuki A, et al: Subarachnoid hemorrhage caused by previously diagnosed, previously unruptured intracranial aneurysms: A retrospective analysis of 25 cases. Neurosurgery 39:1096–1101, 1996.
13. Kassell NF, Torner JC: Size of intracranial aneurysms. Neurosurgery 12:291–297, 1983.
14. Rosenørn J, Eskesen V: Does a safe size-limit exist for unruptured intracranial aneurysms? Acta Neurochir (Wien) 121:113–118, 1993.
15. Acevedo JC, Turjman F, Sindou M: Postoperative angiography in surgery for intracranial aneurysm: Prospective study in consecutive series of 267 operated cases. Neurochirurgie 43:275–284, 1997.

16. David CA, Vishteh G, Spetzler RF, et al: Late angiographic follow-up of surgically treated aneurysms. J Neurosurg 91:396–401, 1999.
17. Feuerberg I, Lindquist C, Lindqvist M: Natural history of postoperative aneurysm rests. J Neurosurg 66:30–34, 1987.
18. Le Roux P, Elliott JP, Winn HR: The incidence of surgical complications is similar in good and poor grade patients undergoing repair of ruptured anterior circulation aneurysms: A retrospective review of 355 patients. Neurosurgery 38:887–895, 1996.
19. Le Roux P, Elliott JP, Eskridge JM, et al: Risks and benefits of diagnostic angiography following aneurysm surgery: A retrospective analysis of 597 studies. Neurosurgery 42:1248–1255, 1998.
20. Rauzzino MJ, Quinn CM, Fischer W: Angiography after aneurysm surgery: Indications for selective angiography. Surg Neurol 49:32–41, 1998.
21. Drake CG, Allcock JM: Postoperative angiography and the slipped clip. J Neurosurg 39:683–689, 1973.
22. Drake CG, Friedman AH, Peerless SJ: Failed aneurysm surgery: Reoperation in 115 cases. J Neurosurg 61:848–856, 1984.
23. MacDonald RL, Wallace C, Kestle JRW: Role of angiography following aneurysm surgery. J Neurosurg 79:826–832, 1993.
24. Solomon RA, Fink ME, Pile-Spellman J: Surgical management of unruptured intracranial aneurysms. J Neurosurg 80:440–446, 1994.
25. Giannotta SL, Litofsky NS: Reoperative management of intracranial aneurysms. J Neurosurg 83:387–393, 1995.
26. Deruty R, Gelissou-Guyotat I, Mottolese C, et al: Surgical management of unruptured intracranial aneurysms: Personal experience with 37 cases and discussion of the indications. Acta Neurochir (Wien) 119:35–41, 1992.
27. Eskesen V, Rosenørn J, Schmidt K, et al: Clinical features and outcome in 48 patients with unruptured intracranial saccular aneurysms: A prospective consecutive study. Br J Neurosurg 1: 47–52, 1987.
28. Heiskanen O: Risks of surgery for unruptured intracranial aneurysms. J Neurosurg 65:451–453, 1986.
29. Rice BJ, Peerless SJ, Drake, CG: Surgical treatment of unruptured aneurysms of the posterior circulation. J Neurosurg 73: 165–173, 1990.
30. Wirth FP, Laws ER Jr, Piepgras D, Scott RM: Surgical treatment of intracranial aneurysms. Neurosurgery 12:507–511, 1983.
31. King JT, Berlin JA, Flamm ES: Morbidity and mortality from elective surgery for asymptomatic, unruptured, intracranial aneurysms: A meta-analysis. J Neurosurg 81:837–842, 1994.
32. Raaymakers TW, Rinkel G, Limburg M, Algra A: Mortality and morbidity of surgery for unruptured intracranial aneurysms: A meta-analysis. Stroke 29:1531–1538, 1998.
33. Connolly ES, Solomon RA: Management of symptomatic and asymptomatic unruptured aneurysms. Neurosurg Clin North Am 9:509–524, 1998.
34. Khanna RK, Malik GM, Qureshi N: Predicting outcome following surgical treatment of unruptured intracranial aneurysms: A proposed grading system. J Neurosurg 84:49–54, 1996.
35. Drake CG: Management of cerebral aneurysm Stroke 12:273–283, 1981.
36. Le Roux P, Sethi R, Grant G, et al: Factors associated with surgical complications for basilar bifurcation aneurysms: An analysis of 101 patients [abstract]. J Neurosurg 88:391A, 1998.
37. Mayberg MR, Batjer HH, Dacey R, et al: Guidelines for the management of aneurysmal subarachnoid hemorrhage. Stroke 25:2315–2338, 1994.
38. Broderick JP, Thoma GB, Dudler JE, et al: Initial and recurrent bleeding are the major causes of death following subarachnoid hemorrhage. Stroke 25:1342–1347, 1994.
39. Fogelholm R, Hernesniemi J, Vapalahti M: Impact of early surgery on outcome after aneurysmal subarachnoid hemorrhage: A population-based study. Stroke 24:1649–1654, 1993.
40. Kassell NF, Torner JC, Haley C, et al: The international cooperative study on the timing of aneurysm surgery. Part 1. Overall management results. J Neurosurg 73:18–36, 1990.
41. Ljunggren B, Saveland H, Brandt L, et al: Aneurysmal subarachnoid hemorrhage: Total annual outcome in a 1.46 million population. Surg Neurol 22:435–438, 1984.
42. Longsteth WT Jr, Nelson LM, Koepsell TD, van Belle G: Clinical course of spontaneous subarachnoid hemorrhage: A population based study in King County, Washington. Neurology 43:712–718, 1993.
43. Pakarinen S: Incidence, etiology and prognosis of primary subarachnoid hemorrhage: A study based on 589 cases diagnosed in a defined population during a defined period. Acta Neurol Scand 43(Suppl 29):1–128, 1967.
44. Alvord EC, Loeser JD, Bailey WL, Copass MK: Subarachnoid hemorrhage due to ruptured aneurysms: A simple method of estimating prognosis. Acta Neurol 27:273–284, 1972.
45. Winn HR, Richardson AE, Jane JA: The long-term prognosis in untreated cerebral aneurysms. I. The incidence of late hemorrhage in cerebral aneurysm: A 10-year evaluation of 364 patients. Ann Neurol 1:358–370, 1977.
46. Kassell NF, Torner JC: Aneurysmal rebleeding: A preliminary report from the cooperative aneurysm study. Neurosurgery 13: 479–481, 1983.
47. Rosenørn J, Eskesen V, Schmidt K, et al: The risk of rebleeding from ruptured intracranial aneurysms. J Neurosurg 67: 329–332, 1987.
48. Fujii Y, Takeuchi S, Sasaki O, et al: Ultra-early rebleeding in spontaneous subarachnoid hemorrhage. J Neurosurg 84:35–42, 1996.
49. Le Roux P, Winn HR: The poor grade aneurysm patient. Acta Neurochir Suppl 72:7–26, 1999.
50. Paré L, Delfino R, Leblanc R: The relationship of ventricular drainage to aneurysmal rebleeding. J Neurosurg 76:422–427, 1992.
51. Haley EC Jr, Kassell NF, Torner JC: The International Cooperative Study on the timing of aneurysm surgery: The North American experience. Stroke 23:205–214, 1992.
52. Richardson AE, Jane JA, Yashon D: Prognostic factors in the untreated course of posterior communicating aneurysms. Arch Neurol 14:172–176, 1966.
53. Lanzino G, Kassell N, Germanson T: Age and outcome after aneurysmal subarachnoid hemorrhage: Why do elderly patients fare worse? J Neurosurg 85:410–418, 1996.
54. Öhman J, Heiskanen O: Timing of operation for ruptured supratentorial aneurysms: A prospective randomized study. J Neurosurg 70:55–60, 1989.
55. Chyatte D, Forde N, Sundt T: Early versus late intracranial aneurysm surgery in subarachnoid hemorrhage. J Neurosurg 69:326–331, 1988.
56. Disney L, Weir B, Petruk K: Effect on management mortality of a deliberate policy of early operation on supratentorial aneurysms. Neurosurgery 20:695–701, 1987.
57. Hernesniemi J, Vapalahti M, Niskanen M, et al: One-year outcome in early aneurysm surgery: A 14-year experience. Acta Neurochir (Wien) 122:1–10, 1993.
58. Milhorat TH, Krautheim M: Results of early and delayed operations for ruptured intracranial aneurysms in two series of 100 consecutive patients. Surg Neurol 26:123–128, 1986.
59. Miyaoka M, Sato K, Ishii S: A clinical study of the relationship of timing to outcome of surgery for ruptured cerebral aneurysms: A retrospective analysis of 1622 cases. J Neurosurg 79: 373–378, 1993.
60. Rosenørn J, Eskesen V, Schmidt K, et al: Clinical features and outcome in 1076 patients with ruptured intracranial saccular aneurysms: A prospective consecutive study. Br J Neurosurg 1: 33–46, 1987.
61. Schievink WI, Wijdick EFM, Piepgras DG, et al: The poor prognosis of ruptured intracranial aneurysms of the posterior circulation. J Neurosurg 82:791–795, 1995.
62. Schievink WI, Wijdicks EFM, Parisi JE, et al: Sudden death from aneurysmal subarachnoid hemorrhage. Neurology 45:871–874, 1995.
63. Hernesniemi J, Vapalahti M, Niskanen M, Kari A: Management outcome for vertebrobasilar artery aneurysms by early surgery. Neurosurgery 31:857–862, 1992.
64. Hillman J, Saveland H, Jakobsson K-E, et al: Overall management outcome of ruptured posterior fossa aneurysms. J Neurosurg 85:33–38, 1996.
65. Peerless SJ, Hernesniemi JA, Gutman FB, Drake CG: Early surgery for ruptured vertebrobasilar aneurysms. J Neurosurg 80: 643–649, 1994.

66. Bailes JE, Spetzler RF, Hadley MN, Baldwin ME: Management morbidity and mortality of poor grade aneurysm patients. J Neurosurg 72:559–566, 1990.
67. Le Roux P, Elliott JP, Newell DW, et al: Predicting outcome in poor grade subarachnoid hemorrhage: A retrospective review of 159 aggressively managed patients. J Neurosurg 85:39–49, 1996.
68. Le Roux P, Dailey AT, Newell DW, et al: Emergent aneurysm clipping without angiography in the moribund patient with intracerebral hemorrhage: The use of infusion computed tomography scans. Neurosurgery 33:189–197, 1993.
69. Nowak G, Schwachenwald R, Arnold H: Early management in poor grade aneurysm patients. Acta Neurochir (Wien) 126: 33–37, 1994.
70. Steudel WI, Reif J, Voges M: Modulated surgery in the management of ruptured intracranial aneurysm in poor grade patients. Neurol Res 16:49–53, 1994.
71. Hauerberg J, Eskesen V, Rosenorn J: The prognostic significance of intracerebral hematoma as shown on CT scanning after aneurysmal subarachnoid hemorrhage. Br J Neurosurg 8:333–339, 1994.
72. O'Sullivan MG, Sellar R, Statham PF, Whittle IR: Management of poor grade patients after subarachnoid haemorrhage: The importance of neuroradiological findings on clinical outcome. Br J Neurosurgery 10:445–452, 1996.
73. Heiskanen O, Poranen A, Kuurne T, et al: Acute surgery for intracerebral hematomas caused by rupture of an intracranial arterial aneurysm: A prospective randomized study. Acta Neurochir (Wien) 90:81–83, 1988.
74. Pasqualin A, Bazzan A, Cavazzani P, et al: Intracranial hematomas following aneurysmal rupture: Experience with 309 cases. Surg Neurol 25:6–17, 1986.
75. Wheelock B, Weir B, Watts R, et al: Timing of surgery for intracerebral hematomas due to aneurysm rupture. J Neurosurg 58:476–481, 1983.
76. Anderson G, Steinke D, Petruk K, et al: Computed tomographic angiography versus digital subtraction angiography for the diagnosis and early treatment of ruptured intracranial aneurysms. Neurosurgery 45:1315–1322, 1999.
77. Hsiang JNK, Liang EY, Lam JMK, et al: The role of computed tomographic angiography in the diagnosis of intracranial aneurysms and emergent aneurysm clipping. Neurosurgery 38:481–487, 1996.
78. Murai Y, Takagi R, Ikeda Y, et al: Three-dimensional computerized tomography angiography in patients with hyperacute intracerebral hemorrhage. J Neurosurg 91:424–431, 1999.
79. Newell DW, Le Roux PD, Dacey RG, et al: CT infusion scanning for the detection of cerebral aneurysms. J Neurosurg 71:175–179, 1989.
80. Hasan D, Vermeulen M, Wijdicks EFM, et al: Management problems in acute hydrocephalus after subarachnoid hemorrhage. Stroke 20:747–753, 1989.
81. Milhorat TH: Acute hydrocephalus after aneurysmal subarachnoid hemorrhage. Neurosurgery 20:15–20, 1987.
82. Mohr G, Ferguson G, Khan M, et al: Intraventricular hemorrhage from ruptured aneurysm: Retrospective analysis of 91 cases. J Neurosurg 58:482–487, 1983.
83. Rajshekhar V, Harbaugh RE: Results of routine ventriculostomy with external ventricular drainage for acute hydrocephalus following subarachnoid haemorrhage. Acta Neurochir (Wien) 115: 8–14, 1992.
84. Raimondi AJ, Torres H: Acute hydrocephalus as a complication of subarachnoid hemorrhage. Surg Neurol 1:23–26, 1973.
85. Shimoda M, Oda S, Shibata M, et al: Results of early surgical evacuation of packed intraventricular hemorrhage from aneurysm rupture in patients with poor grade subarachnoid hemorrhage. J Neurosurg 91:408–414, 1999.
86. Todo T, Usui M, Takakura K: Treatment of severe intraventricular hemorrhage by intraventricular infusion of urokinase. J Neurosurg 74:81–86, 1991.
87. Van Gijn J, Hijdra A, Wijdicks E, et al: Acute hydrocephalus after aneurysmal subarachnoid hemorrhage. J Neurosurg 63: 355–362, 1985.
88. Voldby B, Enevoldsen E: Intracranial pressure changes during aneurysm rupture: Recurrent hemorrhages. J Neurosurg 56:784–789, 1982.
89. Black P: Hydrocephalus and vasospasm after subarachnoid hemorrhage from ruptured intracranial aneurysms. Neurosurgery 18:12–16, 1986.
90. Sheehan JP, Polin RS, Sheehan JM, et al: Factors associated with hydrocephalus after aneurysmal subarachnoid hemorrhage. Neurosurgery 45:1120–1128, 1999.
91. Tomasello F, d'Avella D, de Divitiis O: Does lamina terminalis fenestration reduce the incidence of chronic hydrocephalus after subarachnoid hemorrhage? Neurosurgery 45:827–832, 1999.
92. Gruber A, Reinprecht A, Bavinski G, et al: Chronic shunt dependent hydrocephalus after early surgery and early endovascular treatment of ruptured intracranial aneurysms. Neurosurgery 44: 503–512, 1999.
93. Qureshi A, Sung G, Suri MA, et al: Prognostic value and determinants of ultra-early vasospasm after aneurysmal subarachnoid hemorrhage. Neurosurgery 44:967–974, 1999.
94. Findlay JM, MacDonald RL, Weir BKA, Grace MGA: Surgical manipulation of primate cerebral arteries in established vasospasm. J Neurosurg 75:425–532, 1991.
95. MacDonald RL, Wallace MC, Coyne TJ: The effect of surgery on the severity of vasospasm. J Neurosurg 80:433–439, 1994.
96. Origitano TC, Wascher TM, Reichman OH, Anderson DE: Sustained increased cerebral blood flow with prophylactic hypertensive hypervolemic hemodilution (triple-H therapy) after subarachnoid hemorrhage. Neurosurgery 27:729–740, 1990.
97. Solomon RA, Onesti ST, Klebanoff L: Relationship between the timing of aneurysm surgery and the development of delayed cerebral ischemia. J Neurosurg 75:56–61, 1991.
98. Le Roux P, Newell DW, Eskridge J, et al: Severe symptomatic vasospasm: The role of immediate postoperative angioplasty. J Neurosurg 80: 224–229, 1994.
99. Eskridge J, McAuliffe W, Song JK, et al: Balloon angioplasty for the treatment of vasospasm: Results of the first 50 cases. Neurosurgery 42:510–517, 1998.
100. Rossenwasser R, Armonda R, Thomas J, et al: Therapeutic modalities for the management of cerebral vasospasm: Timing of endovascular options. Neurosurgery 44:975–980, 1999.
101. Muizelaar JP, Zwienenberg M, Rudisill N, Hecht S: The prophylactic use of transluminal balloon angioplasty in patients with Fischer grade 3 subarachnoid hemorrhage: A pilot study. J Neurosurg 91:51–58, 1999.
102. Nilsson O, Brandt L, Ungerstedt U, Saveland H: Bedside detection of brain ischemia using intracerebral microdialysis: Subarachnoid hemorrhage and delayed ischemic deterioration. Neurosurgery 45:1176–1185, 1999.
103. Allcock JM, Drake CG: Postoperative angiography in cases of ruptured intracranial aneurysm. J Neurosurg 20:752–759, 1963.
104. Batjer H, Samson D: Intraoperative aneurysmal rupture: Incidence, outcome, and suggestions for surgical management. Neurosurgery 18:701–707, 1986.
105. Giannotta SL, Oppenheimer JH, Levy ML, Zelman V: Management of intraoperative rupture of aneurysm without hypotension. Neurosurgery 28:531–536, 1991.
106. Kassell NF, Torner JC, Jane J, et al: The international cooperative study on the timing of aneurysm surgery. Part 2. Surgical results. J Neurosurg 73:37–47, 1990.
107. Ljunggren B, Saveland H, Brandt L: Causes of unfavorable outcome after early aneurysm operation. Neurosurgery 13:629–633, 1983.
108. Maurice-Williams R, Kitchen ND: Ruptured intracranial aneurysms—learning from experience. Br J Neurosurg 8:519–527, 1994.
109. Schramm J, Cedzich C: Outcome and management of intraoperative aneurysm rupture. Surg Neurol 40:26–30, 1993.
110. Sundt TM, Whisnant JP: Subarachnoid hemorrhage from intracranial aneurysms: Surgical management and natural history of disease. N Engl J Med 299:116–122, 1978.
111. Mavaddat N, Sahakian B, Hutchinson PJ, Kirkpatrick PJ: Cognition following subarachnoid hemorrhage from anterior communicating artery aneurysm: Relation to timing of surgery. J Neurosurg 91:402–407, 1999.
112. Brouwers PJAM, Dippel DWJ, Vermeulen M, et al: Amount of blood on computed tomography as an independent predictor after aneurysm rupture. Stroke 24:809–814, 1993.
113. Hugosson R: Intracranial arterial aneurysms: Consideration on

the upper age limit for surgical treatment. Acta Neurochir (Wien) 28:157–164, 1973.
114. Niskanen MM, Hernesniemi JA, Vapalahti MP, Kari A: One-year outcome in early aneurysm surgery: Prediction of outcome. Acta Neurochir 123:25–32, 1993.
115. O'Sullivan MG, Dorwartod N, Whittle IR, et al: Management and long-term outcome following subarachnoid haemorrhage and intracranial aneurysm surgery in elderly patients: An audit of 199 consecutive cases. Br J Neurosurg 8:23–30, 1994.
116. Rosenorn J, Eskesen V, Schmidt K: Age as a prognostic factor after intracranial aneurysm rupture. Br J Neurosurg 1:335–341, 1987.
117. Taylor B, Harries P, Bullock R: Factors affecting outcome after surgery for intracranial aneurysm in Glasgow. Br J Neurosurg 5:591–600, 1991.
118. Gerber CJ, Lang DA, Neil-Dwyer G, et al: A simple scoring system for accurate prediction of outcome within four days of a subarachnoid hemorrhage. Acta Neurochir (Wien) 122: 11–22, 1993.
119. Inagawa T: Management outcome in the elderly patient following subarachnoid hemorrhage. J Neurosurg 78:554–561, 1993.
120. Le Roux P, Elliott JP, Downey L, et al: Improved outcome following rupture of anterior circulation aneurysms: A retrospective 10-year review of 224 good grade patients. J Neurosurg 83:394–402, 1995.
121. Fridikson SM, Hillman J, Saveland H, et al: Intracranial aneurysm surgery in the 8th and 9th decades of life: Impact on population-based management outcome. Neurosurgery 37:627–632, 1995.
122. Elliott JP, Le Roux P: Cerebral aneurysms in the elderly. Neurosurg Clin North Am 9:587–594, 1998.
123. King JT, Glick HA, Mason TJ, Flamm ES: Elective surgery for asymptomatic, unruptured, intracranial aneurysms: A cost-effectiveness analysis. J Neurosurg 83:403–412, 1995.
124. Leblanc R, Worsley KJ: Surgery for unruptured asymptomatic aneurysms: A decision analysis. Can J Neurol Sci 22:30–35, 1995.
125. Chang HS, Kirino T: Quantification of operative benefit for unruptured aneurysms: A theoretical approach. J Neurosurg 83: 413–420, 1995.
126. Stoodley M, MacDonald RL, Weir BKA: Pregnancy and intracranial aneurysms. Neurosurg Clin North Am 9:549–556, 1998.
127. Kriplani A, Relan S, Misra NK: Ruptured intracranial aneurysm complicating pregnancy. Int J Gynaecol Obstet 48:201–206, 1995.
128. Meyer F, Sundt T, Fode N: Cerebral aneurysms in childhood and adolescence. J Neurosurg 70:420–425, 1989.
129. Norris JS, Wallace MC: Pediatric intracranial aneurysms. Neurosurg Clin North Am 9:557–563, 1998.
130. Kumar M, Kitchen ND: Infective and traumatic aneurysms. Neurosurg Clin North Am 9:577–586, 1998.
131. Haddad FS, Haddad GF, Taha J: Traumatic intracranial aneurysms caused by missiles: Their presentation and management. Neurosurgery 28:1–7, 1991.
132. Kieck CF, de Villiers JC: Vascular lesions due to transcranial stab wounds. J Neurosurg 60:42–46, 1984.
133. Perata HJ, Tomsick TA, Tew JM: Feeding artery pedicle aneurysms: Association with parenchymal hemorrhage and arteriovenous malformations. J Neurosurg 8:631–634, 1994.
134. Mackey WC, O'Donnell TF, Callow AD: Carotid endarterectomy in patients with intracranial vascular disease: Short-term risk and long-term outcome. J Vasc Surg 10:432–438, 1989.
135. Bederson J, Zambramski J, Spetzler RF: Treatment of fusiform intracranial aneurysms by circumferential wrapping with clip reinforcement: Technical note. J Neurosurg 77:478–480, 1992.
136. Sugita K, Kobayashi S, Inoue T: New angled fenestrated clips for fusiform vertebral artery aneurysms. J Neurosurg 54:346–350, 1981.
137. Nussbaum ES, Erickson DL: The fate of intracranial microaneurysms treated with bipolar electrocoagulation and parent vessel reinforcement. Neurosurgery 45:1172–1175, 1999.
138. Lawton MT, Daspit CP, Spetzler RF: Technical aspects and recent trends in the management of large and giant midbasilar artery aneurysms. Neurosurgery 41:513–520, 1997.
139. Lawton MT, Spetzler R: Surgical strategies for giant intracranial aneurysms. Neurosurg Clin North Am 9:725–742, 1998.
140. Solomon RA, Baker CJ: Direct surgical approaches to giant intracranial aneurysms. Neurosurg Q 2:1–27, 1992.
141. Spetzler RF, Hadley MN, Rigamonti D, et al: Aneurysms of the basilar artery treated with circulatory arrest, hypothermia, and barbiturate cerebral protection. J Neurosurg 68:868–879, 1988.
142. Symon L, Vajda J: Surgical experience with giant intracranial aneurysms. J Neurosurg 61:1009–1028, 1984.
143. Drake CG: Giant intracranial aneurysms: Experience with surgical treatment in 174 patients. Clin Neurosurg 26:12–96, 1979.
144. Piepgras DG, Khurana VG, Whisnant J: Ruptured giant intracranial aneurysms: A retrospective analysis of timing and outcome of surgical treatment. J Neurosurg 88:430–435, 1998.
145. Sundt T, Piepgras D, Fode N, Meyer F: Giant intracranial aneurysms. Clin Neurosurg 37:116–154, 1991.
146. Anson J, Lawton M, Spetzler R: Characteristics and surgical treatment of dolichoectatic and fusiform aneurysms J Neurosurg 84:185–193, 1996.
147. Drake CG, Vanderlinden RG: The late consequences of incomplete surgical treatment of cerebral aneurysms. J Neurosurg 27: 226–238, 1967.
148. Lin T, Fox AT, Drake CG: Regrowth of aneurysm sacs from residual neck following aneurysm clipping. J Neurosurgery 70: 556–560, 1989.
149. Le Roux P, Winn HR: Management of cerebral aneurysms: How can current management be improved? Neurosurg Clin North Am 9:421–433, 1998.
150. Gurian JH, Martin NA, King WA, et al: Neurosurgical management of cerebral aneurysms following unsuccessful or incomplete endovascular embolization. J Neurosurg 83:843–853, 1995.
151. Khayata MH, Spetzler RF, Moov JJA, et al: Combined surgical and endovascular treatment of a giant vertebral artery aneurysm in a child. J Neurosurg 81:304–307, 1994.
152. Thielen KR, Nichols DA, Fulcham JR, Piepgras DG: Endovascular treatment of cerebral aneurysms following incomplete clipping. J Neurosurg 87:184–189, 1997.
153. Byrne JV, Sohn MJ, Molyneux AJ: Five-year experience in using coil embolization for ruptured intracranial aneurysms: Outcomes and incidence of late rebleeding. J Neurosurg 90:656–663, 1999.
154. Casasco AE, Aymard A, Gobin P, et al: Selective endovascular treatment of 71 intracranial aneurysms with platinum coils. J Neurosurg 79:3–10, 1993.
155. Eskridge J, Song J: Endovascular embolization of 150 basilar tip aneurysms with Guglielmi detachable coils: Results of the Food and Drug Administration multicenter clinical trial. J Neurosurg 89:81–86, 1998.
156. Graves, VB, Strother CM, Duff TA, Perl J II: Early treatment of ruptured aneurysms with Guglielmi detachable coils: Effect on subsequent bleeding. Neurosurgery 37:640–648, 1995.
157. Guglielmi G, Viñuela F, Dion J, Duckwiler G: Electrothrombosis of saccular aneurysms via endovascular approach. Part 2. Preliminary clinical experience. J Neurosurg 75:8–14, 1991.
158. Raymond J, Roy D, Boianowski M, et al: Endovascular treatment of acutely ruptured and unruptured aneurysms of the basilar bifurcation. J Neurosurg 86:211–219, 1997.
159. Vinuela F, Duckwiler G, Mawad M: Guglielmi detachable coil embolization of acute intracranial aneurysm: Perioperative anatomical and clinical outcome in 403 patients. J Neurosurg 86: 475–482, 1997.
160. Brilstra E, Rinkel G, van der Graaf Y, et al: Treatment of intracranial aneurysms by embolization with coils: A systematic review. Stroke 30:470–476, 1999.
161. Halbach VV, Higashida RT, Down CF, et al: The efficacy of endosaccular aneurysm occlusion in alleviating neurological deficits produced by mass effect. J Neurosurg 80:659–666, 1994.
162. Bryne J, Adams CBT, Kerr R, Molyneux A: Endosaccular treatment of inoperable intracranial aneurysms with platinum coils. Br J Neurosurg 9:585–592, 1995.
163. Malisch T, Guglielmi G, Vinuela F, et al: Intracranial aneurysms treated with Guglielmi detachable coil: Midterm clinical results in a consecutive series of 100 patients. J Neurosurg 87:176–183, 1997.
164. Nelson PK. Neurointerventional management of intracranial aneurysms. Neurosurg Clin North Am 9:879–875, 1998.
165. Pierot L, Boulin A, Castainhs L, et al: Selective occlusion of basilar artery aneurysms using controlled detachable coils: Report of 35 cases. Neurosurgery 38:948–954, 1996.

166. Vanninen R, Kovisto T, Saari T, et al: Ruptured intracranial aneurysms: Acute endovascular treatment with electrolytically detachable coils—a prospective randomized study. Radiology 211:325–336, 1999.
167. McDougall C, Halbac VV, Dowd CF, et al: Endovascular treatment of basilar tip aneurysms using electrolytically detachable coils. J Neurosurg 84:393–399, 1996.
168. Murayama Y, Vinuela F, Duckwiler G, et al: Embolization of incidental cerebral aneurysms by using the Guglielmi detachable coil system. J Neurosurg 90:207–214, 1999.
169. Dawson RC, Krisht AF, Barrow DL, et al: Treatment of experimental aneurysms using collagen-coated microcoils. Neurosurgery 36:133–140, 1995.
170. Guglielmi G, Viñuela F, Sepetka I, Macellari V: Electrothrombosis of saccular aneurysms via endovascular approach. Part 1. Electrochemical basis, technique, and experimental results. J Neurosurg 75:1–7, 1991.
171. Kwan ESK, Heilman CB, Shucart WA: Enlargement of basilar artery aneurysms following balloon occlusion: "Water-hammer effect"—report of two cases. J Neurosurg 75;963–968, 1991.
172. Mizoi K, Yoshimoto T, Takahashi A, Nagamine Y: A pitfall in the surgery of a recurrent aneurysm after coil embolization and its histological observation: Technical case report. Neurosurgery 39:165–169, 1996.
173. Dorsch NWC, Young N, Kingston RJ, Compton JS: Early experience with spiral CT in the diagnosis of intracranial aneurysms. Neurosurgery 36:230–238, 1995.
174. Civit T, Auque J, Marchal JC, et al: Aneurysm clipping after endovascular treatment with coils: A report of eight patients. Neurosurgery 38:955–961, 1996.
175. Litofsky NS, Vinuela F, Giannotta SL: Progressive visual loss after electrothrombosis treatment of a giant intracranial aneurysm: Case report. Neurosurgery 34:548–551, 1994.
176. Rufenacht D, Mandai S, Levrier O: Endovascular treatment of intracranial aneurysms. AJNR Am J Neuroradiol 17:1658–1660, 1996.
177. Zubillaga AF, Guglielmi G, Vinuela F, Duckwiler GR: Endovascular occlusion of intracranial aneurysms with electrically detachable coils: Correlation of aneurysm neck size and treatment results. AJNR Am J Neuroradiol 15:815–820, 1994.
178. Lefkowitz M, Gobin P, Akiba Y, et al: Balloon-assisted Guglielmi detachable coiling of wide-necked aneurysms. Part II. Clinical results. Neurosurgery 45:531–538, 1999.
179. Moret J, Cognard C, Weill A: La technique de reconstruction dans la traitment des anevrismes intracranies a collet large. Resultats angiographiques et cliniques a long terms: A propose de 56 cas. J Neuroradiol 24:30–44, 1997.
180. Gurian JH, Vinuela F, Guglielmi G, et al: Endovascular embolization of superior hypophyseal artery aneurysms. Neurosurgery 39:1150–1156, 1996.
181. Raftopoulos C, Mathurin P, Boscherini D, et al: Prospective analysis of aneurysm treatment in a series of 103 consecutive patients when endovascular embolization is considered the first option. J Neurosurgery 93:175–182, 2000.
182. Regli L, Uske A, De Tribolet N: Endovascular coil placement compared with surgical clipping for the treatment of unruptured middle cerebral artery aneurysms: A consecutive series. J Neurosurg 90:1025–1030, 1999.
183. Byrne JV, Molyneaux AJ, Brennan RP, Renowden SA: Embolization of recently ruptured intracranial aneurysms. J Neurol Neurosurg Psychiatry 59:616–620, 1995.
184. Kremer C, Groden C, Hansen HC, et al: Outcome after endovascular treatment of Hunt and Hess grade IV or V aneurysms: Comparison of anterior versus posterior circulation. Stroke 30: 2617–2622, 1999.
185. Murayama Y, Malisch T, Guglielmi G, et al: Incidence of cerebral vasospasm after endovascular treatment of acutely ruptured aneurysms: Report of 69 cases. J Neurosurg 87:830–835, 1997.
186. Rinkel GJE, Prins NEM, Algra A: Outcome of aneurysmal subarachnoid hemorrhage in patients on anticoagulant treatment. Stroke 28:6–9, 1997.
187. Kinugasa K, Kamata I, Hirotsune N, et al: Early treatment of subarachnoid hemorrhage after preventing rerupture of an aneurysm. J Neurosurg 83:34–41, 1995.
188. Gruber A, Killer M, Bavinzski G, Richling BL: Clinical and angiographic results of endosaccular coiling treatment of giant and very large intracranial aneurysms: A 7-year single-center experience. Neurosurgery 45:793–804, 1999.
189. Lanzino G, Wakhloo A, Fessler R, et al: Efficacy and current limitations of intravascular stents for intracranial internal carotid, vertebral and basilar artery aneurysms. J Neurosurg 91: 538–546, 1999.
190. Gruber DP, Zimmerman G, Tomsick TA, et al: A comparison between endovascular and surgical management of basilar apex aneurysms. J Neurosurg 90:868–874, 1999.
191. Bavinski G, Killer M, Gruber A, et al: Treatment of basilar artery bifurcation aneurysms by using Guglielmi detachable coils: A 6-year experience. J Neurosurg 90:843–852, 1999.
192. Redekop GJ, Durity FA, Woodhurst WB: Management related morbidity in unselected aneurysms of the upper basilar artery. J Neurosurg 87:836–842, 1997.
193. Samson D, Batjer H, Kopitnik T: Current results of the surgical management of aneurysms of the basilar apex. Neurosurgery 44:697–704, 1999.
194. Melgar MA, Zamorano L, Jiang Z, et al: Three-dimensional magnetic resonance angiography in the planning of aneurysm surgery. Comput Aided Surg 2:11–24, 1997.
195. Koyama T, Okudera H, Gibo H, Kobayashi S: Computer generated microsurgical anatomy of the basilar artery bifurcation. J Neurosurg 91:145–152, 1999.
196. Harbaugh RE, Schlusselberg DS, Jeffery R, et al: Three-dimensional computed tomographic angiography in the preoperative evaluation of cerebrovascular lesions. Neurosurgery 36:320–327, 1995.
197. Alexander TD, MacDonald RL, Weir B, Kowalczuk A: Intraoperative angiography in cerebral aneurysm surgery: A prospective study of 100 craniotomies. Neurosurgery 39:10–18, 1996.
198. Origitano TC, Schwartz K, Anderson D, et al: Optimal clip application and intraoperative angiography for intracranial aneurysms. Surg Neurol 51:117–128, 1999.
199. Payner T, Horner T, Leipzig TJ, et al: Role of intraoperative angiography in the surgical treatment of cerebral aneurysms. J Neurosurg 88:441–448, 1998.
200. Barrow DL, Boyer KL, Joseph GJ: Intraoperative angiography in the management of neurovascular disorders. Neurosurgery 30:153–159, 1992.
201. Derdeyn CP, Moran CJ, Cross DT, et al: Intraoperative digital subtraction angiography: A review of 112 consecutive examinations. Am J Neuroradiol 16:307–318, 1995.
202. Martin NA, Bentson J, Viñuela F, et al: Intraoperative digital subtraction angiography and the surgical treatment of intracranial aneurysms and vascular malformations. J Neurosurg 73: 526–533, 1990.
203. Menovsky T, Grotenhuis A, de Vries J, Bartels R: Endoscope assisted supraorbital craniotomy for lesions of the interpeduncular fossa. Neurosurgery 44:106–112, 1999.
204. Taniguchi M, Takmoto H, Yoshimine T, et al: Application of rigid endoscope to the microsurgical management of 54 cerebral aneurysms: Results in 48 patients. J Neurosurg 91:231–237, 1999.
205. Lanzino G, Miskolci L, Guterman L, Hopkins LN: Angioscopy assisted aneurysm clipping. Neurosurgery 45:609–613, 1999.
206. Giller CA, Mathews D, Walker B, et al: Prediction of tolerance to carotid artery occlusion using transcranial Doppler ultrasound. J Neurosurg 81:15–19, 1994.
207. Linskey ME, Jungreis CA, Yonas H, et al: Stroke risk after abrupt internal carotid artery sacrifice: Accuracy of preoperative assessment with balloon test occlusion and stable xenon-enhanced CT. Am J Neuroradiol 15:829–843, 1994.
208. Segal DH, Sen C, Bederson J, et al: Predictive value of balloon test occlusion of the internal carotid artery. Skull Base Surg 5: 97–107, 1995.
209. Standard SC, Ahuja A, Guterman LR, et al: Balloon test occlusion of the internal carotid artery with hypotensive challenge. AJNR Am J Neuroradiol 16:1453–1458, 1995.
210. Solomon RA, Smith CR, Raps EC, et al: Deep hypothermic circulatory arrest for the management of complex anterior and posterior circulation aneurysms. Neurosurgery 29:732–77; 1991.
211. Gonski A, Acedillo AT, Stacey RB: Profound hypothermia in the treatment of intracranial aneurysms. Aust N Z J Surg 56: 639–643, 1986.

212. Richards PG, Marath A, Edwards JM, et al: Management of difficult intracranial aneurysms by deep hypothermia and elective cardiac arrest using cardiopulmonary bypass. Br J Neurosurg 1:261–269, 1987.
213. Silverberg GD: Giant aneurysms: Surgical treatment. Neurol Res 6:57–63, 1984.
214. Cockroft K, Thompson RC, Steinberg GK: Aneurysms and arteriovenous malformations. Neurosurg Clin North Am 9:565–576, 1998.
215. Rosenorn J, Eskesen V, Schmidt K: Unruptured intracranial aneurysms: An assessment of the annual risk of rupture based on epidemiological and clinical data. Br J Neurosurg 2:369–377, 1988.
216. Piepgras DG: Management of incidental intracranial aneurysms. Clin Neurosurg 35:511–518, 1989.
217. Pertuiset B, Mahdy M, Sichez J, et al: Unruptured intracranial saccular aneurysms less than 20 mm in diameter in adults: Surgery in 89 cases. Rev Neurol (Paris) 147:111–120, 1991.

CHAPTER **108**

Perioperative Management of Subarachnoid Hemorrhage

R. LOCH MACDONALD ■ BRYCE WEIR

There has been no change in the incidence of aneurysmal subarachnoid hemorrhage (SAH) over the past 40 years.[1] It remains at about 11 cases per 100,000 population per year and accounts for 6% to 8% of all strokes. Despite a constant incidence, there has been a decline in the mortality. In Rochester, Minnesota, mortality fell from 6.8 per 100,000 for patients managed between 1955 and 1964 to 4.3 per 100,000 for patients managed between 1975 and 1984.[1] This was thought to be due to decreased case-fatality rate. Although many aspects of medical care have changed over this time, prominent changes were the decrease in average time from SAH to surgery from 12 to 2 days and the institution of more aggressive medical management over these same years. Medical aspects that are believed to be important are reviewed in this chapter.

SAH is the pathologic condition that exists when there is blood in the subarachnoid space. The most common cause overall is head injury. The incidence of SAH in head-injured patients increases with increasing severity of injury and with penetrating injuries. Thirty-nine percent of 753 patients with severe head injury (Glasgow Coma Scale score of 8 or less) had SAH on admission computed tomography (CT); and in another study, about a third of patients with a head injury and a Glasgow Coma Scale score less than 14 had SAH.[2, 3] The presence of SAH doubled the mortality. The most common cause of spontaneous SAH is aneurysm rupture (Table 108–1). Not all SAH is due to aneurysm rupture, and not all aneurysm ruptures are primarily into the subarachnoid space. In autopsy series of patients with ruptured aneurysms, the location of hemorrhage may be biased because the sample population is composed of fatalities and there often is a short duration of survival, but in general SAH is almost universal. Intracerebral and intraventricular hemorrhages are common and subdural hemorrhage is uncommon.

PATHOPHYSIOLOGY

Intracranial Pressure Response

The volume of blood escaping during aneurysm rupture varies from a negligible amount that constitutes a "warning leak" to massive amounts that are associated with immediate death. A massive SAH is probably more than 150 mL. The pathophysiologic consequences will depend on the volume and location of the bleeding as well as on the preexisting size of the cerebrospinal fluid (CSF) space into which the aneurysm ruptures and the patient's age and premorbid condition. A general correlation can be expected between the volume of SAH and the clinical grade, risk of vasospasm, risk of other complications (e.g., increased intracranial pressure [ICP], seizures, and hydrocephalus), and the magnitude of physiologic changes (e.g., reduced cerebral blood flow [CBF] and metabolism), systemic alterations (e.g., hyponatremia, hypovolemia, and hypermetabolism), catabolic state, cardiac arrhythmia, and cardiac wall motion abnormalities.

The ICP response to aneurysm rebleeding is known in the subset of patients with SAH who have ICP monitors in place during their rebleed. These changes may not be representative of those occurring with the first hemorrhage. During rebleeding, ICP rises to diastolic blood pressure and CBF occurs only during systole.[4, 5] The temporary circulatory arrest may help stop the aneurysm bleeding. It also is associated with transient global ischemia that would cause loss of consciousness. Because many patients do not lose consciousness, however, normal clotting probably also contributes to hemorrhage arrest in many cases. In addition, animal experiments show that the flow rate of blood into the subarachnoid space determines the volume of SAH.[6] High flow rates, which would theoretically occur with large aneurysm tears, produced a large-volume SAH in a short time, whereas low flow rates that might result from a small hole in the aneurysm produce slow accumulation of a small volume of SAH. ICP increases did not stop the bleeding.

Results of ICP monitoring for a mean of 8 days after SAH in 52 patients showed that mean ICP rose as clinical grade worsened.[7] Mean ICP was 10 mm Hg in patients in clinical grade 1 and 2, 18 mm Hg in patients in clinical grade 2 and 3, and 29 mm Hg in patients in clinical grade 3 to 5. Vasospasm, which was more common in patients with a poor clinical grade with larger

TABLE 108–1 ■ **Causes of Subarachnoid Hemorrhage (SAH)**

CATEGORY	CAUSES
Idiopathic	Benign perimesencephalic SAH
Infections	Bacterial, tuberculous, and fungal meningitis; syphilis; herpes simplex or other viral encephalitis; leptospirosis; listeriosis; brucellosis; yellow fever; typhoid fever; dengue; malaria; anthrax
Trauma	Closed head injury, electrical injury, gunshot wounds and other penetrating cranial trauma, heat injury, strangulation, high altitude, caisson disease, radiation, germinal matrix hemorrhage in neonates
Toxins	Amphetamines, cocaine, monoamine oxidase inhibitors, epinephrine, alcohol, ether, carbon monoxide, morphine, nicotine, lead, quinine, phosphorus, pentylenetetrazol, hydrocyanic acid, insulin, snake venom
Vascular	Atherosclerosis, rupture of hypertensive, amyloid or other type of intracerebral hemorrhage into the cerebrospinal fluid, hemorrhagic transformation of ischemic infarction, ruptured arteriovenous or other vascular malformation, vasculitis from systemic lupus erythematosus, polyarteritis nodosa, eclampsia, intracranial venous thrombosis secondary to pregnancy, oral contraceptives, volume depletion, hypercoagulable states, trauma or infection
Blood diseases	Leukemia, hemophilia, sickle cell anemia, pernicious anemia, aplastic anemia, agranulocytosis, thrombocytopenic purpura, polycythemia vera, Waldenström's macroglobulinemia, lymphoma, myeloma, hereditary spherocytosis, afibrinogenemia, liver diseases associated with coagulopathy, disseminated intravascular coagulation, acquired coagulopathies due to anticoagulant drugs
Neoplasms	Glioma, meningioma, hemangioblastoma, choroid plexus papilloma, chordoma, hemangioma, pituitary adenoma, sarcoma, osteochondroma, ependymoma, neurofibroma, bronchogenic carcinoma, choriocarcinoma, melanoma

(Modified from Weir B: Aneurysms Affecting the Nervous System. Baltimore, Williams & Wilkins, 1987.)

SAH, was associated with a significant rise in ICP from a mean of 16 mm Hg in patients without vasospasm to 29 mm Hg in patients with vasospasm. This fact should be considered carefully in patients experiencing deterioration from vasospasm days after SAH. Substantial improvement in cerebral perfusion pressure can be achieved by ventricular drainage. Cerebral perfusion pressure is equal to mean arterial blood pressure minus ICP. There are no specific data regarding optimal cerebral perfusion pressures for patients with aneurysmal SAH, but the guidelines for head injuries suggest that it be maintained above 70 mm Hg. ICP is related to outcome; patients with pressures below 15 mm Hg do well in over 80% of cases, as opposed to good outcome in only 15% of patients whose ICPs exceed this.[8]

Cerebral Blood Flow, Volume, and Metabolism

Numerous studies of CBF, blood volume, and metabolism have been conducted in patients with ruptured aneurysms. Almost all studies agree that CBF is globally decreased after SAH.[8] For example, among 30 patients with SAH, mean regional CBF decreased from a mean of 54 mL/100 g/min in normal individuals to 42 mL/100 g/min in patients with grade 1 to 2 without vasospasm, 35 mL/100 g/min in patients with grade 3 to 4 without vasospasm, 36 mL/100 g/min in patients with grade 1 to 2 with vasospasm, and 33 mL/100 g/min in patients with grade 3 to 4 with vasospasm.[9] Cerebral metabolic rate for oxygen ($CMRO_2$) showed a similar pattern with progressive reductions associated with deteriorating clinical grade and worsening vasospasm. Cerebral blood volume was markedly increased in patients with severe neurologic deficits associated with severe vasospasm. It was concluded that vasospasm produced narrowing of the large, angiographically visible arteries at the base of the brain and that this was accompanied by a compensatory dilation of distal, intracerebral arterioles. Few of the early studies examined the time course of blood flow and metabolism changes after SAH, but once the importance of time from SAH was identified, it could be demonstrated that mean CBF decreased with time, reaching a nadir 10 to 14 days after SAH, after which CBF slowly increased toward normal.[8, 10] There is relative hyperemia in relation to the reduced $CMRO_2$ immediately after SAH.[11, 12] In patients with poor grade disease, CBF and metabolism may remain depressed for weeks. In addition to global reductions in CBF and $CMRO_2$, regional perfusion defects can develop after SAH and can be correlated with areas of angiographically demonstrated severe vasospasm and ventricular dilation. Areas of low CBF around intracerebral hematomas are also present, although their size and importance may be overestimated.[13] Regions of brain irrigated by vasospastic arteries have elevated oxygen extraction fractions. Positron emission tomography shows that, as long as the area is ischemic and infarction has not developed, $CMRO_2$ remains normal, although flow is reduced. Development of infarction is heralded by a fall in $CMRO_2$ with relatively increased CBF (relative hyperemia[11]). The degree to which reduced blood flow after SAH has been due to hypovolemia and hypotension is unclear, but there is some evidence that the alterations in flow can be prevented by maintenance of normovolemia or hypervolemia with or without induced hypertension.[14, 15]

There is little information on the pathogenesis of CBF and metabolism changes after SAH. In patients without vasospasm, intracerebral clots, or hydrocephalus studied in the first 4 days after SAH, $CMRO_2$ is decreased without accompanying changes in oxygen extraction fraction, suggesting that the primary alteration is a reduction in $CMRO_2$ and that CBF falls due to decreased demand.[11] This is usually attributed to a toxic effect of the subarachnoid blood, but a neural mechanism or an effect of global ischemia may be important. There is usually a relative hyperemia, which is postulated to be due to intracranial circulatory arrest, transient global cerebral ischemia, and lactic acidosis occurring at the time of rupture. Mitochondrial respiration, sodium-potassium adenosine triphosphatase activity, extracellular potassium, and calcium are altered in brain tissue of experimental animals exposed to subarachnoid blood, although the relationship of these changes to CBF and $CMRO_2$ is not fully clarified.[16–18]

The relationship of CBF to blood pressure and $Paco_2$ is also altered after SAH. The response of CBF to changes in blood pressure at different times after SAH was studied in 38 patients.[19] Autoregulation was intact in good-grade patients but became progressively impaired in poor-grade patients and with development of vasospasm. Autoregulation is not lost in an all-or-none fashion. The degree of impairment tends to be worse as consciousness is more impaired, as vasospasm becomes more severe, and as the patient enters the 5- to 10-day post-SAH interval. Loss of CBF response to changes in $Paco_2$ occurs with more severe brain damage than is required to disturb autoregulation, and the combined loss of autoregulation and variation of CBF with changes in $Paco_2$ is termed *vasomotor paralysis*. After SAH, this is relatively uncommon but may be observed in patients with clinical grade 4 and 5 disease, usually with severe vasospasm. Measurements of CBF with intra-arterial xenon-133 in 38 cases of aneurysmal SAH found responses to alteration in $Paco_2$ were generally preserved, although they were reduced.[19] Impaired CO_2 reactivity was associated with increased ICP and high lactate levels in CSF. Poor clinical grade and vasospasm were associated with impaired CO_2 responsiveness. Transcranial Doppler studies have demonstrated impairment of CO_2 reactivity even in patients with good clinical grade after SAH.[20] This tends to appear during vasospasm and then subsequently resolve. Hyperventilation should be used with caution in patients with SAH. It may be useful for reducing increased ICP and increasing $CMRO_2$ but also may increase the risk of ischemia by causing vasoconstriction.[21]

PATIENT EVALUATION

Symptoms and Signs of Subarachnoid Hemorrhage

Among 1752 patients with aneurysm rupture from three series, 340 (20%, range: 15% to 37%) had a history of sudden, severe headache before the event leading to admission.[22–24] Such premonitory symptoms (warning leaks or sentinel hemorrhages), typically an unusually severe headache of sudden onset, sometimes associated with nausea, vomiting, and dizziness, are usually attributed to small hemorrhages from the aneurysm. Other possible mechanisms include hemorrhage into the aneurysm wall, acute expansion of the aneurysm sac, or ischemia. The importance of recognition of warning leaks has been repeatedly emphasized, because diagnosis may be delayed until catastrophic SAH occurs. Hauerberg and associates studied 99 patients who presented with major SAH but who had warning leaks that were misdiagnosed.[23] Outcome in these patients probably would have been significantly better had they been diagnosed at their initial presentation.

All patients with headaches that are unusually severe or sudden in onset should be investigated for SAH. Other ominous features include vomiting, onset with exertion, alteration in level of consciousness, meningism, or focal neurologic deficit. The absence of these clinical features, however, does not rule out SAH. Numerous unusual presentations are reported; a classic one is acute chest pain.[25] Sudden severe headaches are relatively uncommon in the general population, although they are not uncommon in patients attending the emergency department. Abbott and van Hille studied 49 patients presenting to the emergency department with sudden severe headache and found 35 had SAH (71%).[26] In another study, 15% of 27 patients with sudden severe headache were found to have SAH on CT. An additional 19% had SAH detectable only by lumbar puncture.[27]

A variety of other symptoms and signs can develop before aneurysm rupture. They depend on the site and size of the aneurysm and include hemiparesis, dysphasia, extraocular muscle impairment, visual loss, visual field defect, and localized headache.[8]

The hallmark of SAH is sudden, usually severe headache, although at most about 80% of patients who can give a history will recount such a story.[8] There is brief loss of consciousness in about 45%. Fontanarosa retrospectively studied 109 patients with proven SAH and found headache in 74%, nausea or vomiting in 77%, loss of consciousness in 53%, and nuchal rigidity in 35%.[28] Aneurysm rupture results in sudden death in 12% to 15% of patients.[29, 30] In the most recent cooperative study on the timing of surgery, 41% of patients admitted within 3 days of SAH were alert, 67% had normal speech, 52% were oriented, 69% had normal motor responses, 66% had headache, 74% had a stiff neck, 9% had a third nerve palsy, and 4% had another cranial nerve deficit.[31, 32] The type of headache from SAH is sufficiently variable, however, as to render misdiagnosis common. The most common incorrect diagnoses are, in order of decreasing frequency, systemic infection or viral illness, migraine, hypertensive crisis, cervical spine disorders such as arthritis or herniated disk, brain tumor, aseptic meningitis, sinusitis, and alcohol intoxication.[33]

Ruptured aneurysms at specific sites may produce distinct clinical features. Transient bilateral lower extremity weakness may be due to anterior cerebral artery aneurysm rupture. SAH from a middle cerebral artery aneurysm is more likely to produce hemiparesis, paresthesia, hemianopsia, and dysphasia. Sarner and Rose found no particular aneurysm site had a higher propensity to produce coma.[34] Seizures occur more commonly with anterior circulation aneurysms and probably with middle cerebral artery lesions. Third nerve palsy or unilateral retro-orbital pain suggests an aneurysm arising at the internal carotid/posterior communicating artery junction. Third nerve lesions also occur with aneurysms at the origin of the superior cerebellar artery. Carotid-ophthalmic artery aneurysms may produce unilateral visual loss or visual field defect. Focal neurologic deficit after SAH may be due to mass effect from the aneurysm, vasospasm, seizures, or hematomas in the brain or subdural spaces.

Terson reported vitreous hemorrhages and hemiparesis in association with SAH.[8] Vitreous hemorrhage may be seen on ophthalmoscopic examination in up to 25% of patients either immediately after SAH or days later. Opinions differ about the prognosis for visual recovery. Vitrectomy is sometimes performed after an observation period of several months.

Numerous exertional activities have been reported to be temporally associated with aneurysm rupture. In the first cooperative study, roughly a third of 2288 aneurysm ruptures occurred during sleep, a third during unspecified circumstances, and a third during various exertional activities, including lifting, emotional strain, defecation, coitus, coughing, and parturition.[35] Schievink and associates found SAH occurred during stressful events in 43% of cases, nonstressful events in 34%, rest or sleep in 12%, and uncertain circumstances in 11%.[36] If one takes into account that exertional activities probably occupy a small percentage of one's lifetime, then it seems likely that blood pressure fluctuations, changes in venous and CSF pressure, and possibly movement of brain structures in relation to one another that may occur with these activities increase the risk of aneurysm rupture.

Diagnosis

COMPUTED TOMOGRAPHY

Nonenhanced cranial CT is the first step in investigation of patients with suspected SAH. The probability of detecting the hemorrhage is proportional to the clinical grade, the time after the hemorrhage, and the quality of the scan (Fig. 108–1). Three percent of 1553 patients had normal scans within 24 hours of confirmed SAH.[31] CT on the day of the ictus showed SAH in 92%, intraventricular hemorrhage in 20%, intracerebral hemorrhage in 19%, subdural hemorrhage in 2%, hypodense areas in 1%, mass effect in 8%, hydrocephalus in 16%, and an aneurysm in 5%. With time, the incidence of normal CT and hypodense areas increased, whereas hydrocephalus and hemorrhage decreased. By 5 days after SAH, 27% of scans were normal and 58% showed hemorrhage. Intracerebral hemorrhages took longer to resolve than SAH. Alert patients were significantly more likely than drowsy patients to have a normal scan or a thin, local collection of blood, and all other abnormalities evident on CT were more common in patients with a poor clinical grade. We have not routinely infused scans acutely after SAH, although some neurosurgeons are using helical CT angiography and not catheter-based angiography. The patient is taken to surgery if the CT angiogram shows an aneurysm in a location that is compatible with the SAH on CT and any clinical findings are also consistent.[37] This may be useful to detect an aneurysm when emergency craniotomy is required in patients with intracerebral hemorrhage.[38]

Enlargement of the temporal horns may occur after SAH in the absence of increases in other parts of the ventricular system.[39] This change is quite sensitive to small amounts of SAH; if the temporal horns are visible on CT in a patient with a history compatible with SAH, then lumbar puncture or angiography or both may be indicated.

The volume and location of subarachnoid blood on CT gives important prognostic information about vasospasm and outcome after SAH. A widely used system of grading SAH on CT was proposed by Fisher and coworkers (Fig. 108–2).[40,41] In a prospective study, these authors reported a good correlation between the location and volume of the blood and the subsequent development of vasospasm. The degree of SAH on CT

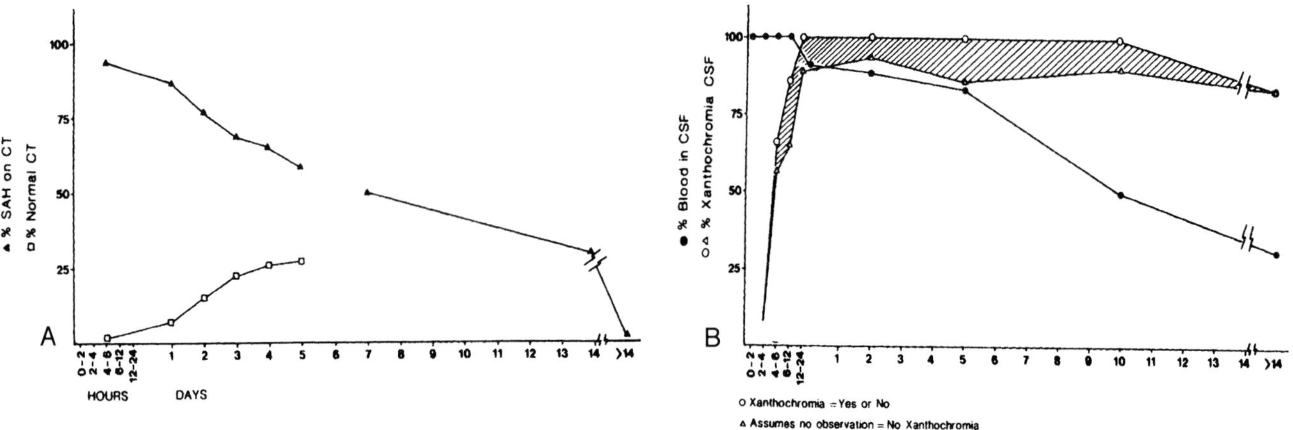

FIGURE 108–1. *A*, Changes on computed tomography (CT) in patients with aneurysm rupture in relation to time after subarachnoid hemorrhage. The incidence of CT abnormalities is highest initially and decreases thereafter so that at 5 days about 27% of patients have normal findings. *B*, Changes in the cerebrospinal fluid in patients with aneurysm rupture in relation to time after subarachnoid hemorrhage. Xanthochromia appears within hours and is found almost universally after 12 hours. (From Weir B: Headaches from aneurysms. Cephalalgia 14:79–87, 1994.)

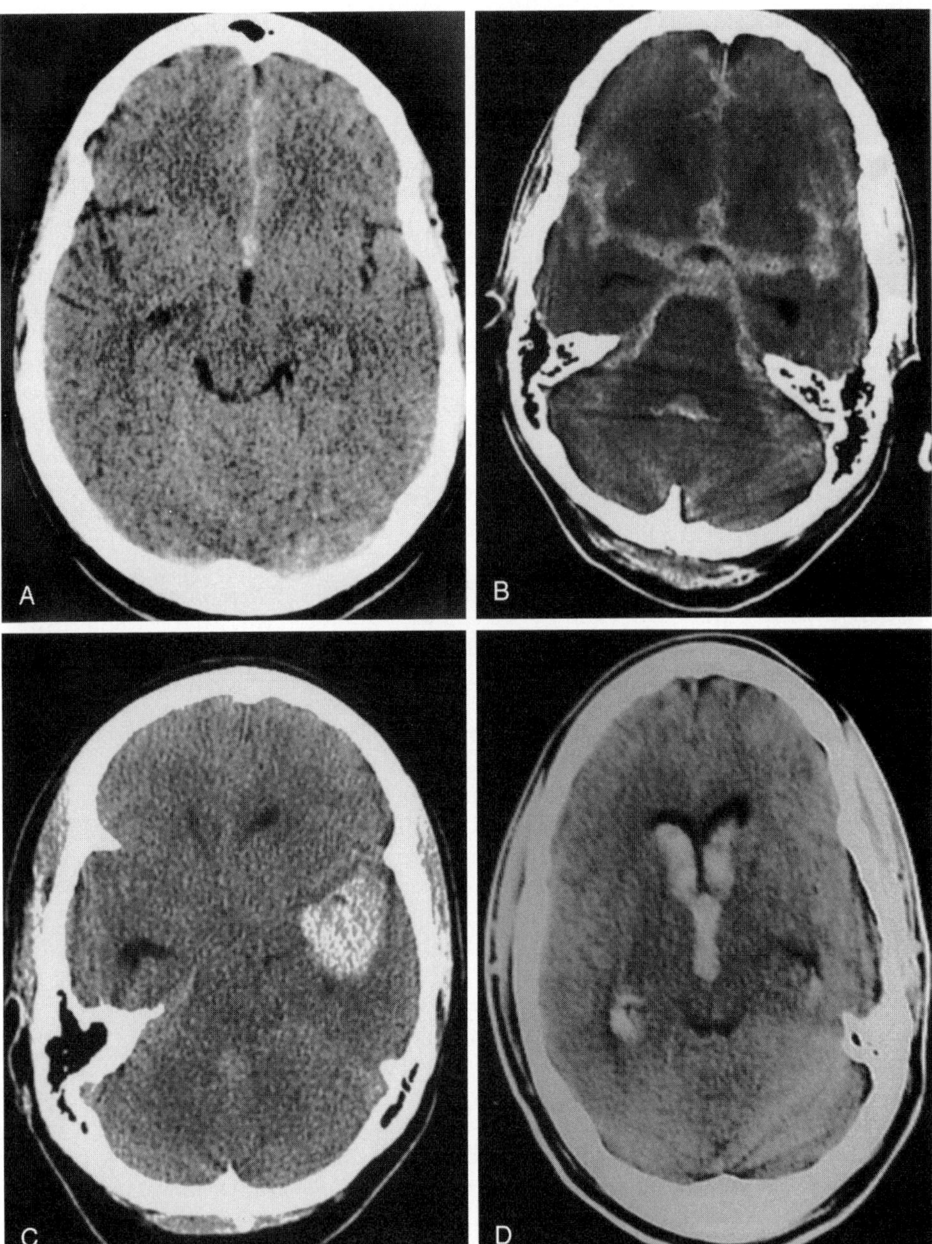

FIGURE 108–2. Computed tomography shows different grades of subarachnoid hemorrhage according to the scale of Fisher and colleagues.[40] Grade 1 is a scan with no subarachnoid hemorrhage. *A,* Grade 2 is a scan showing a thin layer of subarachnoid blood less than 1 mm thick. *B,* Grade 3 is a scan showing focal or diffuse thick subarachnoid blood more than 3 mm thick. Grade 4 is a scan showing intracerebral *(C)* or intraventricular *(D)* blood with or without subarachnoid blood.

was an independent risk factor for death and disability in the cooperative timing of surgery study.[31] CT also is invaluable for detecting complications of SAH and surgery, including intracranial clots, low-density areas, infarcts, and hydrocephalus.

LUMBAR PUNCTURE

Lumbar puncture is indicated to diagnose SAH when CT is normal. The scan may be normal because only a very small SAH occurred or because an inordinate amount of time has elapsed between the SAH and the first scan. Contraindications to lumbar puncture include abnormal blood clotting, increased ICP due to a space-occupying lesion, suspected spinal arteriovenous malformation, and infection at the puncture site. The risks include neurologic deterioration from aneurysm rebleeding or from cerebral herniation. Data from two studies reported that 17 (10%) of 165 patients with SAH who underwent lumbar puncture experienced deterioration within 24 hours.[42, 43] Duffy recommended that CT always be performed before lumbar puncture in the setting of suspected SAH.[43] Limited accessibility to a CT scanner and a high level of suspicion for infectious meningitis may make lumbar puncture the initial diagnostic test in patients who do not have focal neurologic deficits or a depressed level of consciousness. A review of literature on lumbar puncture and meningitis concluded that there was no evidence to recommend CT before lumbar puncture in suspected acute meningitis unless the patient had atypical features or focal neurologic findings.[44]

Theoretically, any erythrocytes in the CSF represent hemorrhage. It is possible that a small hemorrhage from an aneurysm could occur directly into the brain parenchyma or into a loculated CSF space and that erythrocytes would not be detected in the lumbar CSF, although this must be very rare. During CSF access, however, erythrocytes may be introduced artifactually into the CSF sample (traumatic tap). There are many criteria for differentiating a traumatic tap from SAH (Table 108–2). None are without exception. The observation of a declining erythrocyte count in subsequent tubes is an unreliable indicator of traumatic tap.[45] Xanthochromia is yellow discoloration of a centrifuged CSF sample due to hemoglobin and its breakdown products released by hemolysis of erythrocytes. It is a very reliable sign of SAH in CSF obtained more than 12 hours after SAH. The most sensitive test for its detection is spectrophotometry. Most laboratories, however, only visually inspect the CSF. If the CSF is not centrifuged, it may be discolored by erythrocytes that are present either as a result of SAH or a traumatic tap. Furthermore, when erythrocytes are introduced into the CSF sample during a traumatic tap, they will eventually lyse and produce xanthochromia. Therefore, CSF samples should be kept at 4°C, centrifuged immediately, and examined for xanthochromia in a timely fashion. The time taken for xanthochromia to appear after SAH is variable, but it persists for longer than intact erythrocytes do (see Fig. 108–1). If spectrophotometry for hemoglobin and bilirubin is negative on CSF obtained more than a few hours after the onset of symptoms, then angiography probably is not necessary except under unusual circumstances. If CT is normal with erythrocytes but no xanthochromia and 12 or more hours have elapsed from the ictus, we generally perform at least magnetic resonance angiography (MRA) and occasionally catheter angiography. About 70% of patients presenting 3 or more weeks after a suspected SAH have xanthochromia. CT will usually be normal, and if the CSF is clear at this time then magnetic resonance or catheter-based angiography should be obtained.

MAGNETIC RESONANCE IMAGING

The signal characteristics of acute blood on magnetic resonance imaging (MRI) studies make it difficult to detect with conventional image acquisition sequences. Other disadvantages of MRI are difficulties scanning critically ill patients, sensitivity to motion artifact, greater cost, and longer time required. Benefits are that more information may be obtained about the brain and MRA may be used to image the aneurysm without having to administer any contrast medium. In general, we obtain MRI and MRA in patients with SAH who have negative angiography and in those with normal results of CT and equivocal CSF analysis when the suspicion of ruptured aneurysm is low. MRA has not replaced catheter-based angiography as the initial test because of inadequate sensitivity and difficulty scanning critically ill patients. Technical advances will undoubtedly require revision of these practices.

There is concern about obtaining postoperative MRI in patients with aneurysm clips. Fatalities have been reported.[46] Rebleeding may occur even after reportedly successful aneurysm surgery, so a complete evaluation of such cases requires evaluation of postclipping angiography and probably a detailed autopsy. Modern aneurysm clips are made of alloys of cobalt, nickel, molybdenum, and chromium with or without small amounts of iron.[47] They are not ferromagnetic and therefore should not move in an MR magnet. Titanium clips are either pure titanium or alloys of titanium, vanadium, and aluminum and are not ferromagnetic. Some institutions test the clips by seeing if they move in the magnet before they are implanted. Stainless steel clips should not be used.

CATHETER-BASED ANGIOGRAPHY

Catheter-based cerebral angiography remains the diagnostic test of choice for patients with spontaneous SAH and should be performed in patients who are candidates for further treatment. The incidence of multiple aneurysms, as well as of coincident arteriovenous malformations, suggests that four-vessel angiography

TABLE 108–2 ■ **Characteristics of Cerebrospinal Fluid after Subarachnoid Hemorrhage and Traumatic Lumbar Puncture***

FEATURE	TRAUMATIC TAP	SAH
Erythrocyte count	Decreasing with sequential tubes	Constant count between tubes, usually thousands per cubic millimeter but may be as few as 350 cells/mm^3
Clotting	Clots	Does not clot
Xanthochromia	None	Xanthochromia on spectrophotometry of centifuged sample
Erythrocyte to leukocyte ratio	Normal	May be decreased
Protein	Normal or increased in direct relation to number of erythrocytes	May be increased
Hemosiderin-laden macrophages	Absent	Present within days of SAH
Cerebrospinal fluid pressure	Normal	Elevated
Repeat tap at another level	Normal	Consistent with SAH

*The presence of any erythrocytes or xanthochromia should lead to the tentative diagnosis of ruptured aneurysm.

should generally be performed in all cases. A rapidly deteriorating neurologic condition may preclude this, and even angiography at all, in patients with large intracerebral hematomas or acute ventricular dilation. Magnification, subtraction, and stereoscopic techniques will delineate the cause of bleeding in most cases. When no lesion is immediately apparent, selective injection of the external carotid arteries may reveal a dural arteriovenous fistula. Views of the anterior communicating artery complex with cross-compression and injections of the vertebral artery with carotid compression may show aneurysms at the anterior or posterior communicating arteries, respectively.[48] If neck or back pain or lower extremity neurologic deficit is prominent, then search for a spinal arteriovenous malformation, aneurysm, or neoplasm with spine MRI or angiography or both may be indicated. If the initial angiogram is negative and the clinical and CT pattern is not consistent with benign perimesencephalic hemorrhage, then we usually obtain another angiogram about 7 days later. Angiogram-negative benign perimesencephalic hemorrhage typically presents as a noninstantaneous onset of severe headache, and blood on CT is symmetric about the midline and localized primarily to the prepontine, interpeduncular, crural, and ambient cisterns.

The risks of angiography were documented in a prospective study of 1002 consecutive cerebral angiograms performed in 1983 and 1984.[49] Ischemic events occurred in 1.3% (0.1% permanent) in the first 24 hours after angiography. There was a statistically insignificant increase in these events to 2.5% in patients investigated for cerebrovascular disease. Neurologic deterioration occurred between 24 and 72 hours after angiography in 1.8% (0.3% permanent). Complications were related to increased volumes of contrast medium, increased serum creatinine levels, when transient ischemic attacks or strokes were the indication for angiography, increased numbers of catheters used, longer duration of the procedure, and increased patient age. Allergic reactions to contrast medium occur in less than 1 in 50,000 studies, and death from such a reaction happens in about 1 in 1 million patients.

Rupture of an aneurysm during angiography is uncommon. In the first Cooperative Study, in which there were 5484 cases studied by angiography, 7 patients (0.13%) rebled during angiography and 12 (0.22%) rebled 10 minutes to 24 hours later.[35] In two other studies, about 3% of patients showed dye extravasation when angiography was being performed for investigation of SAH.[50] At least 216 cases have been reported.[50–57] The average age was 50, and 66% of patients were female. Angiography was performed within 24 hours of SAH in 78% and within 1 week in 91%. The aneurysms were located on the anterior communicating artery (24%), middle cerebral artery (33%), and internal carotid artery (34%) and on the posterior circulation (6%). Less than 1% of patients were in clinical grade 1; 9% were grade 2, 23% were grade 3, 32% were grade 4, and 35% were grade 5. If dye extravasation was observed on an angiogram, then the patient died in 70% of cases. Overall, therefore, there is probably an increased risk in poor-grade patients with internal carotid artery aneurysms undergoing angiography within 6 hours of SAH. Some of these circumstances, however, are associated with an increased risk of rebleeding, and it cannot be determined whether the rate of rebleeding during angiography differs substantially from that of the natural history of aneurysmal SAH. It has been suggested that this complication can be avoided by delaying angiography for more than 6 hours after the SAH.[58, 59] Many cases were attributed to pressure changes with angiography performed by direct carotid puncture, but the incidence does not seem to have decreased substantially with the widespread use of transfemoral angiography.

Twenty to 30 percent of patients have multiple aneurysms.[8, 30] A combination of clinical and radiologic features can identify the ruptured aneurysm in 90% to 95% of cases.[60–64] A review of 69 patients with multiple aneurysms generated the following algorithm to predict which aneurysm bled: (1) exclude extradural aneurysms, (2) study CT for presence of focal SAH, (3) look for focal spasm or mass effect on angiogram, (4) pick the larger or more irregularly shaped aneurysm, (5) examine the patient for focal neurologic signs, (6) consider repeating the angiogram at a later date to look for change in aneurysm size or for focal angiographic signs, and (7) choose the aneurysm that has the highest chance of rupture (anterior communicating artery aneurysm).[62] Overall, the most proximal and largest aneurysm usually ruptures. If there are two aneurysms on the same artery, then usually it is the proximal one that is ruptured. In some cases, MRI has provided additional evidence of localizing value. In about two thirds of patients with multiple aneurysms, all lesions will be clippable through a single craniotomy, and it may be advisable to do this depending on the age and condition of the patient and the location of the aneurysms. Under exceptional circumstances and despite the best diagnostic aids, it may not be possible to determine preoperatively which aneurysm bled. The literature contains cases in which recurrent SAH occurred in patients with multiple aneurysms after the wrong one was clipped.

No cause will be found for SAH in 9% to 30% of patients undergoing angiography for SAH. There are numerous other causes for SAH (see Table 108–1). We obtain cranial MRI and MRA in such patients, but the yield is low. Among 15 series published between 1978 and 1988, 253 of 1218 patients underwent repeat angiography after an initially negative study and an aneurysm was found in 11%.[65] The aneurysm may be missed initially if it thromboses totally after bleeding. Review of the initial studies by another neuroradiologist may be helpful. The anterior communicating artery complex probably harbors the most missed aneurysms. Studies have shown that there is a subgroup of patients with angiogram-negative SAH in whom blood is located predominately in the prepontine and perimesencephalic cisterns. Repeat angiography is probably unnecessary in this situation if a good quality initial angiogram does not show a posterior circulation aneurysm.[66]

Should intraoperative or postoperative angiography be performed? Residual aneurysm was detected on 8% of postoperative angiograms obtained on 2416 patients reported in nine series.[67] Residual portions of aneurysms hemorrhage at about 0.5% per year.[68] Rarely, second undetected aneurysms may be seen on such studies. The advantage of knowing about an unexpected residual portion of aneurysm intraoperatively is that an attempt can be made to obliterate it at the time. This must be weighed against the risk of further clip manipulations and of angiography itself. The incidence of unexpected major arterial occlusion is about 6% among the series just reviewed.[67] These are best detected by intraoperative angiography before permanent ischemia develops. Several series have identified characteristics that increase the yield of intraoperative angiography, such as giant aneurysms and those arising at the ophthalmic, anterior communicating, middle cerebral artery, or basilar bifurcation.[67, 69] We use intraoperative angiography routinely in most of these cases.

Clinical Grading

It is important to assign a neurologic grade to the patient on admission and to repeatedly document this over time.[70] This is useful for estimation of prognosis and standardization of patient condition to facilitate communication between neurosurgeons and so that multicenter studies can be conducted. Finally, repeated standardized assessments using some type of semiquantitative neurologic scale are essential to detect deterioration in the patient's condition. The neurologic grade is best determined after the patient is resuscitated and undergone ventricular drainage if necessary. Clinical grade is an independent predictor of outcome after aneurysmal SAH.[31] Numerous grading scales have been developed, the most popular include the Botterell, Hunt and Hess, and World Federation of Neurological Surgeons' scales (Table 108–3). It is a prerequisite for any grading scale that it have minimal interobserver variability. Lindsay and coworkers noted that the Botterell and Hunt and Hess scales displayed considerable interobserver variability, although there was agreement above that which would be expected on the basis of chance alone.[71] Assessment of level of consciousness using the Glasgow Coma Scale, which is used in the World Federation scale,[72] showed less interobserver variability.[73] The World Federation scale was based on the observation that, in a large clinical trial, the clinical features that best predicted outcome were level of consciousness and focal neurologic deficit. Unqualified application of the Glasgow Coma Scale may be as useful or more so than the classic aneurysm scales.

GENERAL MANAGEMENT

General Care

A complete history and physical and neurologic examination should be obtained at some point. The initial emergency care may include assessment of adequacy of the airway, breathing, and circulatory function. A brief neurologic assessment of level of consciousness, the cranial nerves, and motor function will determine if emergent surgical interventions (placement of an external ventricular drain and evacuation of an intracerebral hematoma) are required emergently. Other than lifesaving procedures such as these to reduce severely increased ICP, treatment of the aneurysm has the main goal of reducing the risk of rebleeding. Secondary purposes are to facilitate use of other treatments that might increase the risk of rebleeding unless the aneurysm is secured, such as intrathecal tissue plasminogen activator or induced hypertension for vasospasm. The decision to treat is based on multiple factors, including neurologic grade, age, location and size of the aneu-

TABLE 108–3 ■ **Clinical Grading Scales for Aneurysmal Subarachnoid Hemorrhage**

GRADE	BOTTERELL ET AL[197]	HUNT AND HESS[198]	WORLD FEDERATION OF NEUROLOGICAL SURGEONS[70]
1	Conscious with or without signs of blood in the subarachnoid space	Asymptomatic or minimal headache and slight nuchal rigidity	Glasgow Coma Scale score 15, no motor deficit
2	Drowsy without significant neurological deficit	Moderate to severe headache, nuchal rigidity, no neurological deficit other than cranial nerve palsy	Glasgow Coma Scale score 13 to 14, no motor deficit
3	Drowsy with neurological deficit and probably intracerebral clot	Drowsy, confusion or mild focal deficit	Glasgow Coma Scale score 13 to 14 with motor deficit
4	Major neurological deficit, deteriorating because of large intracerebral clots or older patients with less severe neurological deficit but preexisting cerebrovascular disease	Stupor, moderate to severe hemiparesis, possibly early decerebrate rigidity and vegetative disturbances	Glasgow Coma Scale score 7 to 12, with or without motor deficit
5	Moribund or near moribund with failing vital centers and extensor rigidity	Deep coma, decerebrate rigidity, moribund appearance	Glasgow Coma Scale score 3 to 6, with or without motor deficit

rysm, and the medical condition of the patient. The family history should be documented. Screening of other family members may be indicated if there are first-degree relatives with aneurysms. Diseases associated with aneurysms (see Chapter 106), such as coarctation of the aorta, polycystic kidney disease, fibromuscular dysplasia, and sickle cell disease, cocaine use, and smoking should be searched for.

Typical admitting orders are shown in Table 108–4. Most patients are admitted to an intensive care unit. Good-grade patients can be cared for in less vigilant settings. Bed rest, a dark room, limited visitors, and minimal stimulation are recommended. We remove these restrictions and allow patients up as long as they tolerate it once the aneurysm is obliterated. Mobilizing the patient early may decrease complications of bed rest.[74] Adequate analgesia should be administered and excessive painful stimuli avoided because this can increase cerebral oxygen use by up to 30%.[25] Intermittent pneumatic compression devices are used routinely as well as low-dose subcutaneous heparin starting after the aneurysm is obliterated.

Monitoring includes hourly vital signs and neurologic assessment. The flow velocities in the intracranial arteries, the rate of change over 24 hours, and the ratio of intracranial to extracranial velocities are monitored by transcranial Doppler ultrasound obtained every or every other day. It is an imperfect surrogate for angiographically demonstrated vasospasm and by itself changes in velocities should not be the basis for therapeutic decisions. Some centers monitor CBF as well. A central venous catheter may be useful for monitoring volume status and administering medications, fluids, and blood products. A Swan-Ganz catheter may be inserted immediately in those with severe cardiac or pulmonary disease or advanced age. We usually do not insert one immediately unless absolutely necessary. We wait until the patient is several days out from the SAH and is being treated with hemodynamic therapy and requires one for more invasive monitoring. An indwelling urinary catheter is often needed and is preferable to intermittent catheterizations before the aneurysm is obliterated.

Patients who are obtunded may require intubation and ventilation. Unplanned self-extubation increases the risk of pneumonia and neurologic complications

TABLE 108–4 ■ Admitting Orders for Patients with Aneurysmal Subarachnoid Hemorrhage

Investigations

Computed tomography; chest radiography; complete catheter-based cerebral angiogram, repeated as necessary; magnetic resonance imaging and angiography for giant aneurysms, associated vascular abnormalities, and negative initial angiogram

Complete blood cell count including platelet count, prothrombin time, partial thromboplastin time, and bleeding time if history of recent aspirin ingestion

Electrolytes; blood urea nitrogen; creatinine

Urinalysis; urine toxicology screen particularly for cocaine

Daily cerebrospinal fluid cell count; glucose and protein; culture and sensitivity when ventricular drain in place

Monitoring

Vital signs; neurological assessment (brainstem reflexes, Glasgow Coma Scale score as indicated); fluid intake and output every hour

Maintain body temperature and avoid fever

Daily body weight

Arterial catheter (for blood pressure measurement generally only for poor grade patients preoperatively) inserted after adequate sedation and anesthesia in all patients for surgery and left in place postoperatively

Central venous line for fluid management when required

Nursing Care

Bed rest until the aneurysm is obliterated or until several days from the hemorrhage

Elevate head of bed 30 degrees especially in patients with marginal airway and intubated, ventilated patients

Restricted visitors; avoidance of unnecessary stimulation

Graduated compression stockings or intermittent pneumatic compression devices on lower extremities

Foley catheter for poor-grade patients or those unable to void

Nasogastric tube for intubated patients; replace with nasoduodenal tube for nutritional support if unable to eat

Medications

Stool softeners

- Dioctyl sodium sulfosuccinate, 50–400 mg/day orally in one to four divided doses

Medications *(Continued)*

Laxatives

- Bisacodyl, 5 mg/day orally, 5–10 mg/day rectally
- Extract of senna concentration, 1–4 tablets orally one to four times a day

Analgesics such as acetaminophen or morphine

Intravenous fluids, at least 3 L per day

Antiemetics

Sucralfate or omeprazole to reduce risk of gastrointestinal bleeding

Sedatives such as lorazepam 1–2 mg every 8 hours for agitation

Anticonvulsants such as phenytoin (Dilantin), 15–19 mg/kg intravenous loading dose at not greater than 50 mg/min followed by 100 mg intravenous or orally every 8 hours, or phenobarbital

Antihypertensives to reduce blood pressure predominantly within the first 4 days after subarachnoid hemorrhage when the aneurysm is not obliterated: nifedipine, 10–20 mg orally, may repeat after 30 minutes (use with caution in aortic stenosis); captopril, 25 mg orally, repeat as required (use with caution in renal artery stenosis); labetalol, 200–400 mg orally, repeat every 2 to 3 hours (may cause bronchoconstriction or heart block), or intravenous 20- to 80-mg boluses every 10 minutes to a maximum of 300 mg until desired blood pressure reached, then infusion of 2 mg/min (contraindicated in heart failure, bronchospastic disease); nicardipine, 5 to 15 mg/hr intravenously until desired blood pressure reached, then reduced to 3 mg/hr, or nitroprusside, 0.25 to 10 μg/kg/min intravenously, maximal dose for 10 minutes only and titrate to desired blood pressure

Other Medical Care

Ventricular drain for patients with neurologic compromise from ventricular dilation or for postoperative monitoring, drain for pressure $>$ 20 mm Hg until aneurysm obliterated and then for pressure $>$ 5–10 mm Hg

Culture and sensitivity of respiratory secretions, urine, blood, cerebrospinal fluid, or other sources if fever or signs of infection and should be avoided by pharmacologic and/or mechanical restraint. Ventriculomegaly associated with depressed or deteriorating level of consciousness should be treated with ventriculostomy. The only other common indication for emergency surgery is the patient with a large intracerebral hematoma.

Daily fluid intake should be at least 3 L. Fluid intake of less than 2 L/day combined with the use of antihypertensive drugs increases the risk of cerebral ischemia in patients with SAH compared with patients not treated with antihypertensive drugs who receive more than 3 L of fluid per day.[75] A discussion of hemodynamic manipulations of blood volume, blood pressure, and hematocrit is contained in Chapter 109. The optimal hematocrit for CBF in humans after SAH is not known.[76, 77] We generally transfuse patients to maintain a hematocrit over 30% to maintain oxygen-carrying capacity. The average aneurysm case treated by surgery has a fall in hematocrit of around 10% during hospitalization. Trials of hemodilution for ischemic stroke have not shown benefit over untreated controls even when hemodilution was instituted within 6 hours of symptom onset.[77] The other important principles in the management of patients with vasospasm are the administration of nimodipine and the avoidance of hyperthermia, hypotension, hypovolemia, increased ICP, and hyponatremia. Nimodipine usually is administered enterally (60 mg every 4 hours) to all patients with SAH, although it is approved for use in patients in grades 1 to 3 in North America. The recommended duration of treatment is 21 days, although delayed cerebral ischemia is rare more than 14 days after SAH. Side effects include headache, hypotension, and intestinal pseudo-obstruction. Hypotension can be avoided by giving 30 mg every 2 hours or by reducing the dose. Patients with liver failure also may require a lower dose.

The use of corticosteroids is controversial.[78] They have not been shown to improve outcome after aneurysmal SAH, and even a short course is associated with hyperglycemia and an increased risk of infection.[79] Morbid long-term complications such as avascular necrosis of the femur are reported even after short-term use.[80]

Management of Blood Pressure

The optimal blood pressure depends on many factors that include the time after SAH, whether or not the aneurysm has been clipped or coiled, the ICP, and the patient's premorbid blood pressure. It is theoretically that which optimizes perfusion to the brain while minimizing the transmural pressure gradient across the aneurysm. Clearly, these goals run counter to one another, and the information necessary to determine an optimal blood pressure may not be available clinically. Unless a ventricular catheter is in place, the ICP may not be known exactly. Optimal perfusion pressure also depends on the premorbid blood pressure. If the patient had uncontrolled hypertension before the hemorrhage, reducing the blood pressure below "normal" levels may compromise cerebral perfusion. Treating elevated blood pressure after SAH has been shown to increase the risk of cerebral ischemia and to have no effect on outcome.[81] Specific numbers cannot be given. Rapid variations in blood pressure may be more important than the overall level of blood pressure.[82] In general, blood pressure should be reduced to decrease the risk of rebleeding in patients who are within 3 or 4 days of SAH and who have yet not had their aneurysms obliterated. Analgesia with drugs such as morphine and sedation with drugs such as midazolam are often adequate to achieve this. Propofol may be used in intubated patients. Antihypertensive medications such as sodium nitroprusside, esmolol, nicardipine, and labetalol may be useful. Hypertension should be avoided particularly in the early hours after SAH during transport and angiography. Once the aneurysm is obliterated, elevated blood pressure is not treated except at extreme elevations or when infarction has already occurred because CBF may be pressure dependent because of loss of autoregulation. It should be kept in mind that at any time after SAH the blood pressure may be elevated as a homeostatic response to increased ICP or vasospasm. In patients with unsecured aneurysms who are in the time during which vasospasm develops from 4 to 14 days after SAH, a much more conservative approach to blood pressure reduction can be taken because the risk of rebleeding is lower and reduction in blood pressure may precipitate ischemia and infarction from vasospasm.

COMPLICATIONS SPECIFIC TO SUBARACHNOID HEMORRHAGE

Rebleeding

The risk of rebleeding can be definitively reduced by surgical clipping of the aneurysm. Alternatively, endovascular treatment with Guglielmi detachable coils may also reduce rebleeding, but this has not been proven in a randomized trial. Medical means such as antifibrinolytic drugs and reduction of blood pressure are less reliable methods. In our opinion, timing of surgery is seldom an issue and ruptured aneurysms should be obliterated by clipping or coiling as soon as feasible. Early surgery reduces the risk of rebleeding and facilitates the treatment of vasospasm by increasing the safety of hemodynamic manipulations. Theoretical advantages are that the subarachnoid blood may be drained away surgically or removed by intrathecal fibrinolytics, reducing the risk of delayed cerebral vasospasm; the patient can be mobilized quickly, avoiding the complications of bed rest; acute subarachnoid clots are easier to dissect than firm clots that are days old; and the hospital stay may be shortened.[83] The risks of early surgery include increased risk of retraction injury, intraoperative aneurysm rupture, and possibly an increased risk of brain ischemia. The benefits of early endovascular treatment are the reduction in rebleeding risk without the risks of surgery. The disadvantage of coiling is the lower likelihood of achieving complete aneurysm obliteration, the higher risk of early rebleeding from the aneurysm, and the lack of long-term data on the risk of aneurysm re-formation and bleeding. Both treatments carry similar risks of stroke, vasospasm, and other morbidity related to the aneurysm rupture itself.[32, 84]

Antifibrinolytic drugs (tranexamic acid) reduce the risk of rebleeding but increase the risk of cerebral infarction and as a result have no overall effect on outcome.[85, 86] Among 479 patients with SAH randomly allocated to tranexamic acid or to placebo, there was no difference in outcome at 3 months. Rebleeding was reduced from 24% in the control group to 9% in the treated group at the expense of an increase in ischemic complications from 15% in the control group to 24% in the treated group. Combining antifibrinolytics with more effective antivasospasm treatments[87] or using a shorter course of treatment[88, 89] has been studied to try to overcome the increased risk of ischemia but have not been subjected to randomized clinical trials. Antifibrinolytic drugs increase the risk of chronic hydrocephalus and venous thromboembolic complications.[90] They may be indicated in selected cases where the risk of vasospasm is low and the aneurysm cannot be obliterated early. If no loading dose is given, then adequate CSF levels are not reached for 36 hours. If a loading dose is given (5 g of ϵ-aminocaproic acid followed by 1 to 1.5 g/hr), then a therapeutic effect is reached rapidly. There is evidence, however, that antifibrinolytics increase mortality even in good-grade patients with small-volume SAH[91] and that they are harmful even when given for as little as 4 days.[88]

In a cooperative study on the timing of aneurysm surgery, the peak risk of rebleeding was within the first 24 hours of the first SAH.[92] Four percent of patients rebled within 24 hours of SAH. The rate declined thereafter to 1.5% per day, with a cumulative risk of 19% in the first 2 weeks. Prior studies suggested that the risk of rebleeding was maximal about 7 days after SAH,[93] but it is probably highest within the first hours after SAH. In another series, 17% of patients rebled in the first 24 hours after the initial SAH despite maintenance of systolic blood pressure under 150 mm Hg.[94] The risk of rebleeding was maximal immediately after the SAH, with 39% of patients who rebled within 24 hours rebleeding within 2 hours. The risk of rebleeding may be increased in patients with poor clinical grade, high blood pressure,[94, 95] short interval from SAH to admission, large aneurysm size, advanced age, and female sex.[25] Rebleeding is an unmitigated disaster that was associated with a mortality in excess of 75% in several series.[25] Accordingly, it would seem worthwhile to reduce blood pressure in the acute setting after SAH when ischemia from vasospasm is not a risk (see earlier), although the efficacy of this maneuver has not been scientifically documented.[96] Performance of angiography within 6 hours of SAH was associated with rebleeding in one series, leading to the suggestion that diagnostic angiography be delayed until after this.[94] It should be recognized that patients who have a poor clinical grade tend to be admitted earlier, increasing the chances that early rebleeding would be identified.

The risk of rebleeding after coil embolization was 3% among 509 patients.[97] Three hundred eighty-nine (80%) were Hunt and Hess grade 1 to 3 before embolization, 36% were treated within 3 days of SAH, and 97% were treated within 2 weeks. This included patients bleeding within 36 months of treatment. The risk of rebleeding after surgical clipping appears to be less and varies from 0.14% of 715 patients followed for an average of 8 years[68] to about 1% in Yasargil's series of over 1350 aneurysms.[98]

Hydrocephalus

The frequency of acute ventricular dilation after SAH is 20%.[31, 99] Ventricular drainage may be required emergently as a lifesaving measure to relieve acute hydrocephalus in patients with depressed level of consciousness or increased ICP or both with or without signs of herniation. Clinically significant hydrocephalus within the first days after SAH is more likely to occur with increasing age, preexisting or postoperative hypertension, intraventricular hemorrhage, diffuse SAH, focal thick SAH, posterior circulation aneurysms, use of antifibrinolytic drugs, hyponatremia, and depressed level of consciousness (equivalent to worsening clinical grade).[100] Another series showed the most important predictors of acute hydrocephalus were intraventricular hemorrhage and larger volumes of subarachnoid clot.[101] The pathogenesis of ventricular dilation probably is multifactorial and related to blockade of CSF circulation either within the ventricular system (aqueduct of Sylvius, outlets of the fourth ventricle) or in the subarachnoid space (tentorial incisura or basal cisterns) or to increased resistance to CSF outflow at the arachnoid granulations. Acutely, these blockages must be due to blood clots; this gives way to proliferation of macrophages, arachnoid cells, and fibroblasts after several weeks.

It is worthwhile quantifying the degree of hydrocephalus by measuring the ventriculocranial ratio and determining whether the ventricles are larger than the 95th percentile for age (Fig. 108–3 and Table 108–5). Insertion of a ventricular drain is usually indicated in patients with a ventriculocranial ratio 20% to 25% greater than the 95th percentile for age who have depressed level of consciousness. This applies to most grade 4 and 5 patients.[102] Decisions must be individualized depending on the clinical situation. Risks of ven-

TABLE 108–5 ■ **Upper 95% Confidence Value for Ventriculocranial Ratio, by Age**

AGE (yr)	UPPER 95% CONFIDENCE VALUE
<30	0.16
<50	0.18
<60	0.19
<80	0.21
<100	0.25

Data from van Gijn J, Hijdra A, Wijdicks EFM, et al: Acute hydrocephalus after aneurysmal subarachnoid hemorrhage. J Neurosurg 63:355–362, 1985.

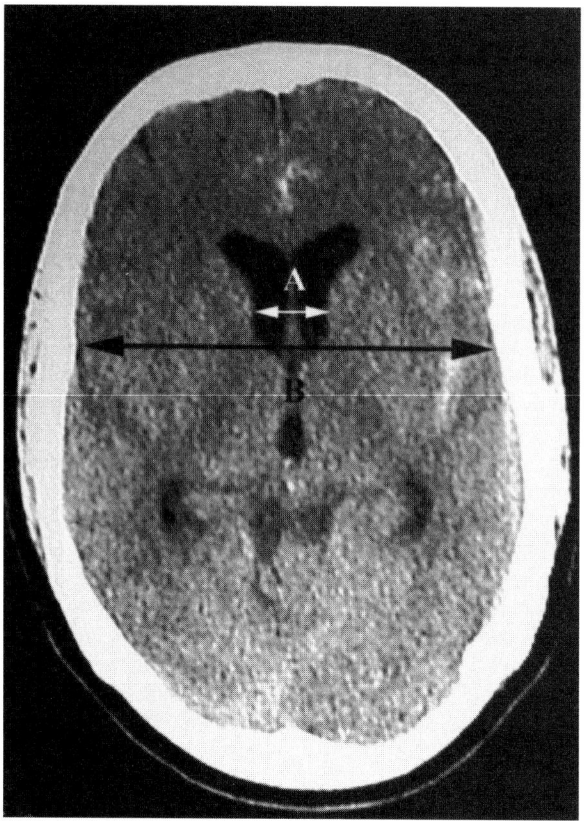

FIGURE 108–3. Computed tomography showing ventriculomegaly. The ventriculocranial ratio (A/B) is calculated by taking the ratio of the width of the ventricles over the width of the inner diameter of the skull at the level of the foramen of Monro at a point behind the head of the caudate nuclei where the lateral walls of the ventricles are roughly parallel.[196]

tricular drainage include rebleeding, infection, and intracerebral hematoma along the catheter tract. The risk of rebleeding with ventricular drainage may be higher in poor-grade patients and those with larger aneurysms.[103] If a drain is not in place preoperatively, we usually insert one at the time of surgery to achieve optimal brain relaxation.[104] The catheter is left in place postoperatively to monitor ICP, drain CSF as necessary, and administer fibrinolytic agents if indicated. We generally change the catheter or convert it to a permanent shunt if it cannot be removed within 5 to 7 days unless there is substantial intraventricular blood.

Chronic hydrocephalus develops in 10% to 20% of patients surviving aneurysmal SAH.[105] Patients should have CT 1 month after SAH to rule this out as a cause of persistent or progressive neurologic deficit. Multivariate analysis shows that the need for a shunt is increased with worsening neurologic grade and when intraventricular hemorrhage is present.[105] Prolonged cisternal or ventricular drainage may increase the chances that chronic hydrocephalus will develop.[106, 107] Permanent diversion of CSF with a ventriculoperitoneal shunt is usually performed, although the indications remain subjective and include lack of improvement from a neurologic plateau or deterioration in the presence of ventricular dilation, often with periventricular lucencies, rounding of the frontal horns, and obliteration of the cortical sulci. The ICP may be normal or elevated.

Intraventricular Hemorrhage

A major intraventricular hemorrhage complicates aneurysm rupture in 13% to 28% of clinical series and 37% to 54% of autopsy series.[31, 102] Small amounts of intraventricular blood, for example, blood layered in the occipital horns, are seen even more commonly. In 91 cases of intraventricular hemorrhage, the aneurysm was located on the anterior cerebral artery in 40%, the internal carotid artery in 25%, and the middle cerebral artery in 21%.[102] Anterior communicating and basilar termination aneurysms are the most common to cause large, primarily intraventricular hemorrhages. Intraventricular hemorrhage was an independent risk factor for disability but not death[31] and for development of acute and chronic hydrocephalus after SAH.[100, 101] Vasospasm is less common when blood is primarily intraventricular, as opposed to when it fills the basal cisterns.

Over 50% of patients with large intraventricular hemorrhage are admitted in poor grades, and the mortality in such cases exceeds 64%.[102] Ventricular size predicts survival, in addition to known prognostic factors such as age, clinical grade, and hypertension. A fourth ventricle that is dilated and packed with clot is a particularly ominous sign.[108]

Intraventricular administration of tissue plasminogen activator (t-PA) has been reported for treatment of intraventricular hemorrhage.[109, 110] Twenty-two patients were given from to 2 to 31 mg of t-PA in single or divided doses through intraventricular catheters. The ruptured aneurysm should be clipped before giving t-PA; otherwise there would be potential for lysis of the clot in the ruptured aneurysm with catastrophic rebleeding. Only one patient died, and the outcome seemed better than what would be expected for patients with severe intraventricular hemorrhage. Although further study is required to determine whether this therapy is efficacious, we use intraventricular t-PA after the aneurysm is obliterated in patients with marked intraventricular hemorrhage who have increased ICP and in whom there is difficulty keeping the ventricular drain patent.

Increased Intracranial Pressure

Some patients with acute hydrocephalus have markedly increased ICP and require ventricular drainage as a lifesaving measure.[99, 111] Increased ICP may occur in the absence of ventricular dilation.[112] Advantages of placing a ventricular drain include the ability to measure ICP and thus optimize cerebral perfusion pressure. Risks include infection, hematoma, and precipitating aneurysm rebleeding.[99, 103, 107] Paré and colleagues reported that ventricular drainage increased the risk of rebleeding only in patients with hydrocephalus after SAH. Although they did not find that the level of the ICP was predictive, others have suggested that the risk of rebleeding was not increased as long as drainage was only for pressures over 25 mm Hg.[113] Ventricular drainage may increase the risk of rebleeding by increasing the transmural pressure gradient across the aneurysm wall or because patients who need ventricular drainage are predisposed as part of their natural history to have had larger tears in their aneurysms that produced more SAH and more hydrocephalus and that are more prone to rebleed.[103]

The etiology of increased ICP acutely after SAH includes acute hydrocephalus, intraventricular or intracerebral hemorrhage, brain swelling, ischemic brain edema, and increased resistance to CSF outflow probably due to blockade of the arachnoid villi by blood.[114] There is some evidence that the blood-brain barrier is disrupted after SAH, although some studies have not found this. Blood-brain barrier leakiness may produce vasogenic edema; in the absence of this most brain edema after SAH probably is due to ischemia.[25]

Treatment of increased ICP after SAH includes removal of sizable intracranial hematomas, ventricular drainage, assisted ventilation, sedation, pharmacologic paralysis, maintenance of normal body temperature and sodium, prevention of seizures, intravenous mannitol boluses with or without concomitant furosemide, and short periods of hyperventilation to overcome acute pressure elevations. Increased ICP associated with endotracheal suctioning can be avoided by pretreatment with 100% oxygen and intravenous lidocaine, 1 to 1.5 mg/kg.

Intracerebral Hemorrhage

Aneurysms arising from the distal anterior cerebral arteries are the most likely to produce intracerebral hematomas. Owing to the relative rarity of these aneurysms, however, intracerebral hematomas are more commonly seen with aneurysms of the middle and anterior communicating arteries, which are associated with clots in autopsy series in about 67% and 62% of cases, respectively. These percentages are lower in patients surviving their aneurysm ruptures. Intracerebral hematomas complicated 34% of aneurysm cases reported by Pasqualin and associates.[115] The sites of hemorrhage vary depending on the location of the aneurysm and the direction of rupture of the aneurysm into the brain parenchyma. The pattern is usually distinctive but does not always differ sufficiently from that of hypertensive intracerebral hemorrhage to allow an accurate diagnosis based on CT or MRI. Indications for angiography must be based on clinical suspicion.

A retrospective review of patients from 11 medical centers identified 132 patients with intracerebral hematoma due to ruptured aneurysm.[116] Discriminant function analysis showed that, in order of importance, size and location of hematoma, aneurysm location, and size of midline shift were factors contributing to prediction of survival. Hematoma size was also a strong predictor of clinical grade. About 40% of clots were frontal and 40% were temporal. Patients with temporal lobe clots have the greatest capacity for clinical recovery.

Craniotomy for hematoma evacuation is generally indicated in patients with depressed or deteriorating level of consciousness, with or without signs of herniation. The aneurysm should be obliterated at the time of clot removal.

Seizures

Seizures occur at or around the time of SAH in about 20% of patients.[117] These are not usually witnessed by medical personnel, so it is difficult to differentiate these episodes from posturing or movements precipitated by acutely increased ICP. Similar events, however, occurred with the same frequency at the time of aneurysm rebleeding and were often witnessed and still classified as seizures. They usually followed the rebleed, leading to the generally accepted conclusion that seizures are the result but not the cause of aneurysm rupture in most cases. Patients who have seizures should be investigated to rule out an underlying new event, such as new bleeding into the subarachnoid, subdural, intracerebral, or intraventricular spaces, cerebral ischemia, or metabolic disturbances such as hyponatremia. Risk factors for seizures at the time of SAH have not been identified. Common neurosurgical practice in North America is to administer anticonvulsants to patients with SAH for at least a week after SAH or until the ruptured aneurysm is obliterated.[118] There is no compelling scientific evidence that this is efficacious. The brain swells due to increased cerebral blood volume during a seizure. This may be tolerated under normal circumstances, but in the setting of SAH when intracranial compliance may be low, severe increases in ICP may result in transient cerebral ischemia, permanent infarction, and death. Seizures increase cerebral oxygen consumption and may cause hypoxemia, hypercarbia, acidosis, aspiration, and pneumonia. Despite evidence to suggest that seizures follow rather than precipitate aneurysm rupture, the increase in blood pressure that may accompany a seizure may increase the risk of bleeding. In addition, early prevention of seizures might reduce the risk of late epilepsy by preventing kindling, although this has generally not been demonstrable clinically after SAH[119, 120] or head injury.[121] Early seizures within a week of SAH are not a risk factor for late epilepsy.[119, 122]

The incidence of epilepsy, defined as two or more seizures at least 1 week after SAH, in patients who survived after surgery for ruptured aneurysms was 10% to 27% in series reported up to 1973.[120] More recent series report an incidence of 3% to 10%.[119, 123–125] In one large series, 72% of seizures began within 1 year and 94% within 2 years.[122] Risk factors for development of late epilepsy have been determined in several series and commonly include younger age, middle cerebral artery aneurysms, intracerebral hematoma, poor initial grade, postoperative focal neurologic deficit due to cortical infarction, medial temporal lobe retraction, history of seizures, and shunt-dependent hydrocephalus.[119, 122, 125, 126] Independent risk factors in multivariate analysis produced conflicting results (Table 108–6).[125, 127] Treatment with anticonvulsants is recommended for most SAH patients in the first days until the aneurysm

TABLE 108–6 ■ **Results of Multivariate Analysis of Factors Associated with Epilepsy after Aneurysmal Subarachnoid Hemorrhage (SAH)**

FEATURE	OHMAN, 1990[125]	HASAN ET AL, 1993[127]
Patient population	307 patients with aneurysmal SAH; mean follow-up 1.4 years; surgery a mean of 6 days after SAH; no antifibrinolytics	381 patients with SAH, most due to aneurysms; operations planned for day 12 post SAH; some received antifibrinolytics
Incidence of epilepsy	9%	9%
Risk factors	History of hypertension; presence of infarction on late computed tomographic scan; duration of coma after SAH	High cisternal blood score; rebleeding

is obliterated and increased ICP is not present.[96] We discontinue anticonvulsants after this except in patients at high risk for epilepsy, such as those with prior epilepsy, intraparenchymal hematoma, cortical infarcts, and concomitant arteriovenous malformation.[120]

MEDICAL COMPLICATIONS

The only common premorbid medical illness in patients with aneurysmal SAH is hypertension, which is present in 20% to 40% of patients.[31, 118, 128] Medical complications, however, are very frequent complications of the disease and contribute substantially to morbidity and mortality. Among 457 patients in the placebo group of a clinical trial, almost every patient had at least one, 40% had at least one life-threatening complication, and one fourth of the deaths were due to medical complications (Table 108–7).[118] The most common medical complications are anemia, hypertension, cardiac arrhythmias, fever, electrolyte disturbances, elevated liver enzymes, pulmonary edema, pneumonia, and atelectasis. Medical complications are significantly more common in poor-grade patients and in those with diffuse, thick SAH.[118] Death due to medical complications equals that due to neurologic complications, with about a fifth of patients dying of vasospasm, rebleeding, direct effects of the SAH, and medical complications (see Tables 108–7 and 108–8).

Respiratory Complications

Respiratory complications are more common with advancing age and poor clinical grade. They cause almost 50% of deaths from medical causes.[118] The most common respiratory complications are pulmonary edema, pneumonia, atelectasis, aspiration, pneumothorax, asthma, and pulmonary emboli.

The indications for intubation and controlled respiration in patients with aneurysmal SAH include gross abnormalities of respiratory rate, decreased tidal volume, decreased inspiratory force, hypoxia, and hypercapnia. Depressed level of consciousness is an indication because of inability to protect the airway and clear secretions, inability to breathe deeply or sigh to prevent atelectasis, and loss of protective pharyngeal reflexes that normally prevent atelectasis. Most grade 4 and all grade 5 patients require intubation and ventilation. An obvious trend in patient condition may warrant prophylactic intubation. For example, in patients who deteriorate during vasospasm and become obtunded with rising ICP, early institution of ventilatory and respiratory support may lessen or even reverse deterioration and promote more rapid recovery.

A small number of patients with SAH suffer immediate respiratory arrest or life-threatening arrhythmias from which they die unless emergency life support is instituted. In a series of 245 SAH patients, 15% required emergency intubation and ventilation. Aggressive measures are indicated early on because the outlook is reasonable; about half eventually recovered, occasionally completely.[129]

Pulmonary edema may complicate the course of aneurysmal SAH patients at any time and may be cardiogenic (increased pulmonary venous pressure secondary to left-sided heart failure) or noncardiogenic (neurogenic or secondary to pulmonary insults such as aspiration and shock). Delayed cases are usually cardiogenic and secondary to fluid overload during hemodynamic therapy for vasospasm.[130] Among patients dying of SAH, pulmonary edema is more common and was diagnosed clinically in 34% and at autopsy in 71%.[131] The mean age of patients with aneurysmal SAH who develop acute pulmonary edema is 48, which is about a decade younger than the average age for aneurysm rupture and the severity of the SAH is worse, with two thirds of patients being grade 4 or 5.[132, 133] Survival can be achieved in about 50% of cases. A sudden increase in ICP is probably a prerequisite in all cases. SAH may be associated with marked sympathetic hyperactivity that causes systemic hypertension and pulmonary vasoconstriction. If the constriction extends to the pulmonary veins, then there will be increased pressure in the pulmonary capillaries that will, by a hydrostatic mechanism, cause transudation of low-protein fluid into the lungs.[131, 134] A second theory is that there is a primary increase in lung capillary permeability that allows protein-rich plasma to leak into the lungs. The cause of increased capillary permeability may involve neural pathways from the central nervous system or pressure changes in the lung, thus creating some overlap with the hydrostatic theory. In any case, neurogenic pulmonary edema is characterized by rapid onset, association with severe neurologic injury often involving the hypothalamus, suppression by adrenergic blockers, high protein content in the edema fluid, and resemblance to epinephrine-induced pulmonary edema. The treatment includes immediate

TABLE 108–7 ■ **Frequency of Causes of Morbidity and Mortality in Patients with Aneurysmal Subarachnoid Hemorrhage (SAH)***

	PATIENT POPULATION		
COMPLICATION	**Weir[199]**	**Kassell et al[31]**	**Solenski et al[118]**
	100 ruptured aneurysms, treated before 1979	3521 patients admitted within 3 days of aneurysmal SAH, 1980–1983	457 patients admitted within 7 days of aneurysmal SAH, 1987–1989
Respiratory	54		
Pneumonia	17	7.0	22
Pulmonary edema	11	1.7	23
Hypoventilation	9		
Respiratory arrest	3		
Pulmonary embolus	1	0.8	<1
Pneumothorax	1		3
Atelectasis		2.3	16
Adult respiratory distress syndrome		2.0	4
Cardiovascular	23		
Arrhythmia	14	3.6	35
Hypotension	3	3.0	18
Thrombophlebitis	3	1.4	2
Myocardial infarction	3	0.7	1
Hypertension		18.3	36
Cardiac failure		2.0	4
Peripheral edema			20
Genitourinary	26		
Cystitis	16		16
Renal failure	1	1.4	7
Vaginitis	9		
Gastrointestinal	3		
Hemorrhage	3	3.7	2
Miscellaneous	3		
Other infections	3		14
Hepatic failure/hepatitis		3.0	24
Bleeding disorder		1.0	4
Hematologic			
Anemia		4.9	37
Fluid and electrolytes			28
Hyponatremia		3.6	9
Diabetes insipidus			7
Hyperglycemia			21

*Values are percent of patients in the series.

TABLE 108–8 ■ **Neurologic Complications in a Series of Patients with Aneurysmal SAH***

	RESULT	
COMPLICATION	**Death**	**Disability**
Rebleeding	6.7	0.8
Vasospasm	7.2	6.3
Hydrocephalus	0.3	1.4
Direct effect of SAH	7.0	3.6
Intracerebral hemorrhage	1.0	1.0
Complications of intracranial surgery	1.7	2.3
Other	2.0	1.2

*Patient population: 3521 patients with aneurysmal SAH, admitted within 3 days.
Data from Kassell NF, Torner JC, Haley ECJ, et al: The international cooperative study on the timing of aneurysm surgery: I. Overall management results. J Neurosurg 73:18–36, 1990.

intubation and ventilation, adequate oxygenation, positive end-expiratory pressure, furosemide, and measures to reduce increased ICP.

Most pneumonia occurs in intubated patients. Prevention of pneumonia in these cases should include removal of nasogastric and endotracheal tubes as soon as indicated, avoidance of unanticipated extubation and gastric overdistention, strict hand washing procedures, semirecumbent positioning of the patient, maintenance of adequate nutrition, oral intubation and proper ventilator care.[135] Gastrointestinal stress ulcer prophylaxis with sucralfate does not remove the protective antibacterial effect of acidic gastric acid secretions. This may decrease gastric bacterial growth and reduce the risk of pneumonia. Exposure to antibiotics is a risk factor for ventilator-associated pneumonia because it results in colonization of the patient with antibiotic-resistant bacteria. The use of antibiotics for inappropriate or unproven indications or for prophylactic purposes should be considered carefully.

In patients with head injury, tracheostomy and percutaneous feeding gastrostomy shorten the duration of mechanical ventilation.[136] We generally perform a tracheostomy when the patient has been intubated for 10 to 14 days and extubation is not imminent.

Venous Thromboembolism

About 2% of patients with SAH develop symptomatic deep vein thrombosis. Up to 50% of these develop pulmonary embolism, which is fatal in half. Asymptomatic deep vein thrombosis occurs in 19% to 50% of patients undergoing neurosurgical procedures. Risk factors for venous thromboembolism include increased age, heart failure, previous venous thromboembolism, direct trauma to the lower limb, varicose veins, use of oral contraceptives, pregnancy and the puerperium, obesity, malignancy, infection, duration of surgery over 4 hours, and limb weakness or paralysis.[137, 138] Patients with deficiencies of antithrombin III, protein C, or protein S and with various genetic clotting factor abnormalities, such as factor 5 Leiden, are also at risk for venous thromboembolism.[138] Graduated compression stockings and pneumatic compression devices decrease the incidence of deep vein thrombosis in neurosurgical patients, as detected by the radiolabeled fibrinogen technique and are recommended for all patients.[139, 140] They work by intermittently squeezing the lower limbs, compressing the veins, and preventing thrombosis from venous stasis. There is evidence that they induce a systemic fibrinolytic state. Other proven methods of prophylaxis include low-dose subcutaneous heparin, adjusted-dose subcutaneous heparin, low-molecular-weight heparins, and oral anticoagulants. It is reasonable to assume that these drugs have a low therapeutic index in patients undergoing craniotomy. As the dose is increased, the risk of venous thromboembolism will decrease but the risk of catastrophic intracranial bleeding will increase. We routinely place patients on heparin, 5000 U subcutaneously every 12 hours, starting after aneurysm obliteration, although this practice is subject to continuing study.[141] Platelet counts should be monitored at least once every 2 days.

If deep vein thrombosis or pulmonary embolism develops, options include anticoagulation or placement of an inferior vena cava filter. It is usually considered to be safe to anticoagulate patients when a week or more has passed since craniotomy, although this is based on a very limited number of patients described in the medical literature.[142] A filter may still be a better temporizing measure if the need for other invasive procedures, such as further angiography or shunting, has not been determined. Filters reduce the risk of pulmonary embolism, although whether they reduce mortality is less certain.[143]

Cardiovascular Complications

Almost all patients with SAH develop some type of cardiovascular abnormality. The most common are electrocardiographic (ECG) changes, cardiac rhythm disturbances, and alterations in blood pressure. SAH was suggested to be associated with sympathetic hyperactivity that may predispose to or cause arrhythmias, ECG changes, and reversible subendocardial heart damage.[144]

ECG abnormalities occurred in 98% of SAH patients in one series. Changes included peaked P waves; pathologic Q waves; increased QRS voltages; ST segment depression or elevation; peaked, flattened, diphasic or inverted T waves; sinus bradycardia or tachycardia; prolonged QTc interval; and large U waves.[145, 146] If only one ECG is examined, the chances of finding abnormalities will be lower—it increases if daily electrocardiography is done. The ECG changes themselves are serious in less than 4% of cases.[118, 147] They may, however, be associated with underlying cardiac damage manifest as contraction band necrosis and elevated cardiac enzymes. Contraction band necrosis is a reversible cardiac pathology often found in patients who die after SAH and that is characteristic of heart muscle exposed to excessive catecholamines and intracellular calcium, leading to a hypercontracted state. Echocardiography showed left ventricular wall motion abnormalities with moderately to severely reduced ejection fractions in 8% of 57 patients studied within 6 days of SAH,[145] an incidence consistent with other studies.[148, 149] These patients usually were poor grade, had episodes of pulmonary edema and hypotension requiring intravenous pressors, and had elevated cardiac enzymes.[145, 148, 149] Symmetric T-wave inversion and severe QT prolongation may be specifically associated with the subpopulation of SAH patients with ventricular dysfunction.[145, 148] It was postulated that sympathetic hyperactivity after SAH leads to a hyperdynamic cardiovascular state with increased left ventricular performance and that elevations in cardiac enzymes indicated inability of the left ventricle to respond to the sympathetic stress. Wall motion abnormalities are rare in the absence of marked ECG changes or elevated cardiac enzymes or both, and it would be unusual for a patient with a normal ECG to have an abnormal echocardiogram.[149] Echocardiography is recommended for SAH patients with hypotension, pulmonary edema, acute ECG changes (Q waves, ST segment elevation, or other changes of acute ischemia), or symmetric T-wave inversions or severe QT prolongations.[145] It is important to maintain normokalemia and to be aware of the possibility of left ventricular function when instituting hemodynamic measures for vasospasm. Hypokalemia and preexisting cardiac disease may aggravate ECG abnormalities and cardiac dysfunction after SAH.[147] Impaired left ventricular function may increase the likelihood of asymptomatic vasospasm becoming symptomatic.[146]

Almost any cardiac arrhythmia can occur after SAH.[118] Vidal and associates prospectively monitored 100 patients with SAH and found that every patient developed an arrhythmia at some time, usually in the absence of preexisting heart disease, hypoxemia, or electrolyte abnormalities.[150] In another series of 52 patients with SAH who had continuous cardiac monitoring for a mean of 5 days, 98% developed arrhythmias at some time, most commonly on the first day after SAH or 7 to 8 days later.[151] The most common arrhythmias were sinus tachycardia (85%), multifocal ventricular extrasystoles (54%), couplets (40%), supraventricular extrasystoles (33%), nonsustained ventricular tachycardia (29%), sinus bradycardia (23%), asystole (27%), and sinus arrhythmia (25%). Other series reported arrhythmias in about a third of SAH patients, which probably reflects less diligent monitoring. Factors predicting which patients would develop arrhythmias could not be identified in one study,[118] although another study showed that they were more common in patients with preexisting heart disease.[151]

Patients with SAH should have continuous monitoring of cardiac rhythm, as well as baseline and follow-up ECGs and frequent monitoring of electrolytes, particularly potassium. Hypokalemia should be avoided because it may aggravate arrhythmias and has been associated with prolonged QT interval, ventricular fibrillation, and torsades de pointes.[150, 152] A double-blind, randomized, placebo-controlled trial of patients with SAH showed that patients treated with the adrenergic blocker propranolol with or without phentolamine were less likely to die and had a better outcome than those receiving placebo.[153] The patients were operated on late after SAH and blood pressures were not reported, but this treatment has not seen widespread use, probably because it is at variance with other reports showing that antihypertensive treatments worsen outcome after SAH.[75]

Fluid and Electrolyte Disturbances

The most common electrolyte disturbances after aneurysmal SAH are hyponatremia, hypernatremia, and hypokalemia.[154] Hypokalemia should be corrected by potassium administration because it may predispose to cardiac arrhythmias. Ruptured anterior communicating artery aneurysms are the most likely aneurysms to be associated with electrolyte abnormalities.[154] The mortality in cases with hypernatremia was 42%, compared with 15% with hyponatremia, 25% with diabetes insipidus, and 6% for all patients.

Most patients with SAH seem to become hypovolemic even if maintenance fluid requirements are met. Maroon and Nelson measured red blood cell mass and total blood volume in 15 patients with SAH and found that both parameters decreased significantly when measured on average 10 days after SAH.[155] Causes were postulated to include bed rest, supine diuresis, pooling in peripheral vascular beds, negative nitrogen balance, inadequate erythropoiesis, and iatrogenic blood loss. Wijdicks and coworkers found that plasma volume also decreased in about 50% of patients with SAH when maintenance fluids (about 1.5 L/day) were administered.[156] Plasma volume probably decreases earlier after SAH and is followed by a reduction in red cell and blood volume.[157] The incidence of volume depletion increases with decreasing Glasgow Coma Scale score.[158] About half of patients developed hyponatremia, but this was not related to changes in plasma volume. SAH was associated with an acute increase in plasma antidiuretic hormone (ADH), but this decreased within 3 days whereas hyponatremia developed on average 7 days after SAH.[159] Decreased plasma volume was usually associated with negative sodium balance, decreased body weight, and increased blood urea nitrogen. These findings suggested that SAH was associated with natriuresis. It had been assumed that hyponatremia in SAH patients was due to the syndrome of inappropriate secretion of ADH (SIADH) because this condition had been reported in association with other neurologic illnesses and the hormone responsible for it had been identified. In SIADH, however, there are high levels of plasma ADH with normal or increased total body water. Hyponatremia is dilutional. There is reduced renin and aldosterone and increased atrial natriuretic peptide secretion, which maintains urinary sodium excretion.[158] Urinary sodium is high, probably because the sodium intake must be excreted in a lower volume of urine. Normally, ADH is secreted in response to increased plasma osmolarity, decreased plasma volume, stress, severe pain, increased ICP, and hypotension and suppressed by decreased plasma osmolarity and increased plasma volume. In SIADH, there is inappropriate ADH secretion when the decreased plasma osmolarity (and sodium) should completely suppress it. The acute ADH increase after SAH is probably a response to stress. That patients with SAH were volume depleted was more consistent with cerebral salt wasting, a condition described before SIADH but ignored perhaps because the natriuretic substances responsible for it were not identified. In salt wasting, there is natriuresis with volume depletion and sodium deficiency. Serum sodium is often low, but it varies depending on the composition of fluid intake. The natriuresis is therefore inappropriate, leading some authors to call it the syndrome of inappropriate secretion of atrial natriuretic peptide.[159]

Natriuretic hormones (peptides, factors) were eventually discovered, and measurements in plasma and CSF after SAH showed that they were indeed elevated after SAH.[158, 160–162] They may be increased within hours of SAH but then decrease and rise again on day 3 and remain elevated for a week or more. Most studies have not found a correlation between elevated atrial natriuretic factor and hyponatremia,[159, 163, 164] probably because serum sodium can be maintained by sodium replacement independent of overall volume status. Atrial natriuretic factor is synthesized in and released from the heart in response to atrial stretch and increased blood volume, factors that did not seem to be present after SAH, suggesting the increase was due to neural mechanisms.[159, 161–163] In support of this, elevations in atrial natriuretic factor correlated with the presence of suprasellar or intraventricular blood that was postulated to disturb the function of the hypothalamus, a structure that is known to be important in regulation of sodium and water balance.[163] Serial measurements of serum atrial natriuretic factor, antidiuretic hormone, sodium, and overall sodium balance confirmed these observations and showed that SAH tended to be associated with an acute increase in atrial natriuretic factor and ADH.[164] The concomitant increase in ADH tended to prevent early volume loss and hyponatremia. Days later, however, transient marked increases in atrial natriuretic factor occurred without a concomitant increase in ADH, leading to natriuresis and water loss. This often precipitated neurologic deterioration. In some cases, ADH also is elevated; so in addition to inappropriate natriuresis there is SIADH.[158]

Other natriuretic peptides are brain and C-type natriuretic peptides. Brain natriuretic peptide is derived principally from the cardiac ventricles and also was elevated after SAH in a manner that seemed independent of atrial natriuretic factor.[165] This may contribute to natriuresis and fluid loss in aneurysmal SAH patients.[166]

Hyponatremia develops in about one third of patients with aneurysmal SAH on average about a week after the ictus.[158, 167, 168] Hyponatremia was associated with enlargement of the third ventricle but not with the amount of intraventricular or subarachnoid blood.[169] The cause should be accurately diagnosed. Symptoms and signs include deterioration in level of consciousness, onset of or exacerbation of focal neurologic deficits, seizures, and asterixis. Possible causes include SIADH, inhibition of the sodium-potassium adenosine triphosphatase by endogenous digoxin-like substances causing decreased extracellular sodium and increased extracellular potassium, and cerebral salt wasting. Most will be due to salt wasting, and fluid restriction may be harmful, increasing the risk of cerebral ischemia and fatal infarction.[167] Even if fluid restriction was not applied, more patients with hyponatremia after SAH developed cerebral ischemia compared with patients who were not hyponatremic.[168] These investigators did not assess volume status, and they postulated that most of the hyponatremic patients were hypovolemic as a result of natriuresis. Preventing volume depletion may decrease the risk of ischemia[75]; it is unclear as to whether hyponatremia per se is harmful or whether it is due to the associated hypovolemia. It also is not clear whether restoring normovolemia is as effective as induced hypervolemia at preventing ischemia. Most studies of induced hypervolemia have reported ventricular filling pressures as measures of hypervolemia, although these are notoriously unreliable.[76] Hypervolemia can be associated with morbid complications such as pulmonary and cerebral edema.[170] Furthermore, SIADH should be reversed slowly because rapid salt and water replacement may lead to fatal osmotic demyelination.[166] Inhibition of the sodium-potassium adenosine triphosphatase is probably not common after SAH; this should be associated with hyperkalemia and digoxin-like immunoreactivity in the serum, both of which are uncommon.[166]

The first principle of fluid and sodium management is to make an accurate diagnosis (Table 108–9). The key differentiating feature between SIADH and salt wasting is volume status. Acute change in body weight is a good measure of volume status. There are numerous others, including changes in hematocrit, blood urea nitrogen to creatinine ratio, and cardiac filling pressures.[171] The primary treatment for salt wasting is adequate water and sodium replacement to maintain at least normovolemia and normal serum sodium. Natriuresis can be prevented by administering mineralocorticoids such as fludrocortisone acetate but a randomized, controlled trial showed that this had no effect on the risk of cerebral ischemia or on outcome, probably because administering large quantities of sodium and water are equally effective.[158, 172] Volume replacement should be guided by measures of total body water such as weight. Ventricular filling pressures are less reliable. In cases of SIADH, fluid restriction may be appropriate.

Diabetes insipidus complicates about 0.04% of aneurysmal SAH cases.[154] Most cases are associated with ruptured anterior communicating artery aneurysms. The treatment is replacement of fluid losses with hypotonic solutions such as 5% dextrose in water or 0.45% sodium chloride. In the chronic phase, exogenous ADH replacement may be administered as desmopressin (1-deamine-8-D-arginine vasopressin), which is a synthetic analogue of ADH that can be given intravenously, subcutaneously, or intranasally starting as 1- or 2-μg boluses.

TABLE 108–9 ■ **Features of SIADH, Cerebral Salt Wasting, and Diabetes Insipidus**

FEATURE	SIADH	CEREBRAL SALT WASTING	DIABETES INSIPIDUS
Serum sodium	<135 mEq/L	<135 mEq/L	Variable, may be elevated
Plasma osmolarity	<280 mOsmol/L	<280 mOsmol/L	Variable, may be elevated
Urine sodium	>20 mEq/L	>20 mEq/L	Variable
Urine osmolarity	>Plasma osmolarity	>Plasma osmolarity	50–150 mOsmol/L
Serum potassium	Decreased or normal	Increased or normal	Normal
Blood volume	Increased	Decreased	Normal or decreased
Sodium balance	Variable	Negative	
Body weight	Increased	Decreased	Normal or decreased
Cardiac filling pressures	Increased or normal	Decreased	Normal or decreased
Hematocrit	Decreased	Increased	Normal or decreased
Blood urea nitrogen/creatine	Decreased or normal	Increased	Normal or decreased
Blood pressure	Normal	Postural hypotension	Normal or decreased
Heart rate	Normal	Tachycardia	Normal or tachycardia
Other criteria	Normal thyroid, adrenal and renal function, no peripheral edema, no dehydration	Signs and symptoms of volume depletion	Urine volume >3 L/day

SIADH, syndrome of inappropriate diuretic hormone.

Gastrointestinal Complications

There is a marked increase in urinary catecholamine excretion within the first 3 days after SAH that is probably due to sympathetic hyperactivity. These two features as well as increased cortisol, glucagon, and cytokine release probably contribute to the increased oxygen consumption, carbon dioxide production, and metabolic expenditure noted in SAH patients.[173] In addition to a hypermetabolic state, patients with SAH have a catabolic response marked by negative nitrogen balance and impaired ability to use exogenous nitrogen. It is difficult to normalize nitrogen balance even by administration of exogenous nitrogen.[174] These changes are similar to those found in patients with other acute, severe neurologic illnesses such as head injury.[175] This response causes weight loss and may increase the risk of infection and impair wound healing.[176] The primary therapy to counteract it is early nutritional support. There are few studies investigating patients with SAH, but after stroke there is evidence that early institution of nutritional support improves survival.[177] In patients who cannot swallow because of impaired consciousness or focal neurologic deficits, this is best achieved by gastrostomy or jejunostomy tubes rather than by nasogastric tubes.[177] It is probably preferable to feed enterally rather than parenterally because parenteral nutrition may be associated with loss of the intestinal mucosal bacterial barrier and an increased risk of sepsis. Enteral feeding avoids the risk of sepsis from central venous catheters, reduces the incidence of hyperglycemia, and is less expensive. Hyperglycemia aggravates neurologic injury at least in experimental models.[178] Parenteral nutrition is indicated for the occasional patient who cannot meet nutritional needs with enteral feeding and in whom this situation is likely to persist for at least 5 days.

Mucosal ulceration (stress ulceration) in the stomach and upper gastrointestinal tract may occur after SAH and can cause serious and sometimes fatal bleeding. Studies specific to patients with SAH are limited but suggest that such lesions occur after SAH just as they do after other serious neurologic injuries. Accepted treatments included neutralization of gastric acid secretion with antacids or drugs that block acid production such as histamine receptor antagonists (cimetidine, ranitidine). The use of drugs to prevent gastrointestinal bleeding remains controversial and some studies have failed to show that they are efficacious.[179] Furthermore, loss of gastric acidity may be associated with an increased risk of pneumonia. Sucralfate is an attractive drug for stress ulcer prophylaxis because it does not reduce gastric acidity and appears to be effective.[180]

Stool softeners are administered routinely to prevent straining and to prevent impaction and abdominal pain. Nimodipine may be associated with gastrointestinal pseudo-obstruction and ileus.[181] This usually resolves with conservative measures but may progress to perforation requiring surgery.

Up to 24% of patients with SAH develop increased hepatic enzymes and 4% develop severe liver dysfunction.[118] The etiology is unclear but may relate to passive liver congestion, systemic inflammation, or exogenous drugs.

Miscellaneous Complications

Subarachnoid hemorrhage causes an inflammatory process in the subarachnoid space that may be accompanied by fever and leukocytosis. An initial elevation of both on admission to hospital tends to be associated with an increased risk of mortality and of vasospasm, as is an increase during the subsequent hospital course.[182, 183]

POSTOPERATIVE DETERIORATION

Peerless listed 39 causes for deterioration in patients after SAH (Table 108–10).[184] Multiple causes were often found for each episode of worsening. Although he found vasospasm to account for 30% of cases of deterioration, systemic abnormalities and neurologic complications must be detected before neurologic decline can be attributed to vasospasm. Any factor that disrupts perfusion of brain tissue with well-oxygenated, glucose-rich blood can cause patients with aneurysmal SAH to worsen. Particularly important systemic factors were hyponatremia, hypoxemia, hypercarbia, hypotension, and cardiac arrhythmias.

TABLE 108–10 ■ **Causes of Neurological Deterioration After Subarachnoid Hemorrhage**

NEUROLOGICAL	SYSTEMIC
Related to SAH or aneurysm	Systemic infection
Vasospasm	Hepatic, renal failure
Hydrocephalus	Drug related
Rebleeding	Corticosteroid psychosis
Intracerebral hematoma	Sedative overdose
Subdural hematoma	Alcohol withdrawal
Cerebral edema	Other drug reactions
Enlargement of aneurysm	Metabolic
Arterial thromboembolism	Hyponatremia, SIADH, or cerebral salt wasting
Seizures	Hypernatremia, diabetes insipidus
Postoperative complications	Metabolic alkalosis
Major arterial occlusion	Metabolic acidosis
Venous occlusion	Hypocalcemia
Perforator injury	Hypomagnesemia
Intracranial hematoma	Pulmonary
Cerebral edema	Hypoxemia
Retraction injury	Respiratory alkalosis
Hypotensive, hypoxic brain damage	Respiratory acidosis
Aseptic meningitis	Pulmonary embolism
Bacterial meningitis	Cardiovascular
Aneurysm thrombosis	Hypotension
Seizures	Hypertension
Complications of angiography	Arrhythmias

SIADH, syndrome of inappropriate diuretic hormone.
Data from Peerless SJ: Pre- and postoperative management of cerebral aneurysms. Clin Neurosurg 26:209–231, 1979.

SPECIAL CONSIDERATIONS

The urine should be checked for cocaine metabolites, which remain detectable for up to 72 hours after use depending on the frequency and doses used. Cocaine use is associated with aneurysm rupture, although about half of cases of intracranial hemorrhages in cocaine-positive patients have no underlying vascular anomalies and 15% of SAHs show no aneurysm. There are at least 32 cases reported.[185–187] The mean age is 32 years, which is much younger than the SAH population as a whole, although the distribution of aneurysms is the same. The pathophysiology is believed to involve hypertension induced by sympathetic hyperactivity secondary to blockade of norepinephrine reuptake into neurons. The outcome tends to be worse than in patients who have not used cocaine.[187] Cocaine use is associated with myocardial ischemia and arrhythmias; the clinician should be even more vigilant for these.

Sickle cell anemia may be associated with aneurysmal SAH, although it is a less common neurologic complication of sickle cell anemia than cerebral infarction or intracerebral hemorrhage.[188–191] There are about 46 reported cases. Most patients have sickle cell disease, although aneurysmal SAH may occur in the setting of sickle cell trait. Most patients present in the third and fourth decades of life. The pathogenesis of aneurysm formation may involve repeated sickle cell–induced endothelial injury with eventual damage to and destruction of the internal elastic lamina, degeneration of the tunica media, and aneurysm formation. Aneurysms are more likely to be multiple (up to 40% to 60% of reported cases) and tend to be small. Numerous stimuli can induce sickling and should be avoided including hypoxia, acidosis, infection, volume depletion, hypothermia, and contrast media. Recommended management is to perform exchange transfusion until the level of hemoglobin S is below 30% to 40% and the hematocrit is over 30% before angiography and then throughout the hospital stay. Supplemental oxygen should be used liberally. Preanesthetic sedation carries the risk of causing respiratory acidosis and hypoxemia and should be avoided. Mannitol and furosemide increase the risk and must therefore be used cautiously and only when brain relaxation cannot be achieved by other measures such as ventricular drainage. Mild hyperventilation is acceptable but carries a risk of excess vasoconstriction that may precipitate sickling. The patient should not be allowed to become hypothermic. Dehydration and hemoconcentration are to be avoided. Temporary clipping for aneurysm dissection and hemorrhage control may be preferable to induced hypotension, although both carry increased risks. During anesthesia, adequate oxygenation, prevention of respiratory acidosis (hypercarbia), maintenance of adequate circulating blood volume, and prevention of hypothermia and of venous stasis must be ensured. When adhering to such measures, good outcomes may be achieved.

Aneurysmal SAH is progressively less common with decreasing age. The clinical presentation in older children is no different from adults, although neonates and infants may present with irritability or other vague symptoms that suggest a diagnosis of meningitis.[25] Children with aneurysms may be more likely to be associated with an underlying disorder predisposing to or causing the aneurysm,[192] although, in most series, no cause for the aneurysm was found in the majority of patients. There are few studies specifically addressing the treatment of children with aneurysmal SAH; and, at this time, the management of pediatric patients with SAH should follow the same general guidelines as for adults.

ESTIMATION OF OUTCOME

About 12% of patients die of aneurysmal SAH before coming to medical attention.[30] In surgical series, about 25% of those who reach the hospital alive die and 60% recover.[31] Epidemiologic studies estimate that about 40% of those reaching hospital die.[30] Many studies have assessed outcome using the Glasgow Outcome Scale score.[193] This scale was developed for measuring outcome from head injury and has limitations in patients with SAH.[96] Patients with SAH often have no gross neurologic deficits but are disabled because of disordered higher cortical function.

Factors that affect outcome after SAH include characteristics of the patient, the pathology, and the treatments that are rendered. Results of several multivariate analyses are provided in Table 108–11. The most consistently identified prognostic factors are age, neurologic grade, amount of SAH on CT, preoperative hypertension, vasospasm, presence of intracerebral or intraventricular hemorrhage or both, and the location and size of the aneurysm. The timing of admission to hospital after SAH is important and must be considered when comparing outcomes between different published series.[59] The earlier the patient is admitted after SAH, the higher the risk of rebleeding and that an unsalvageable patient has been admitted and, therefore, the higher the risk of poor outcome.

When is the outcome of a patient with SAH hopeless? In one study, the oldest patient to achieve a good outcome after Hunt and Hess grade 3 SAH was 77 and after grade 4 SAH the oldest patient was 66.[194] No grade 5 patient achieved good outcome. It is important to assess the clinical grade after resuscitation.

CONCLUSION

The nonoperative management of patients with aneurysmal SAH has been outlined, excluding measures pertaining to cerebral vasospasm that are discussed in a separate chapter. Surgery to obliterate the aneurysm effectively prevents rebleeding, but the neurosurgical team must continue to monitor the patient closely. The majority of patients will develop at least one neurologic or medical complication, and the optimization of outcome requires ongoing vigilance to facilitate early detection and institution of appropriate treatment of complications. It is hoped that optimal neurological and medical care and attendant advances in these areas will

TABLE 108–11 ■ **Results of Multivariate Analyses of Factors Affecting Outcome after Aneurysmal Subarachnoid Hemorrhage***

FACTOR ANALYZED	WEIR ET AL[200]	TORNER ET AL[95]	ARTIOLA I FORTUNY AND PRIETO-VALIENTE[201]	DISNEY ET AL[194]	KASSELL ET AL[31]
No. of patients	135 surgically treated	1117 admitted within 7 days of SAH, treated with delayed surgery, antifibrinolytics	265 good-grade aneurysmal SAH, including 3% unruptured aneurysms	184 poor-grade aneurysmal SAH patients admitted within 96 hours	3521 admitted within 3 days
Years of study	1968–1973	1970–1977	1972–1977	1984–1986	1980–1983
Outcome measure	Mortality at 2 months	Mortality at 14 days	Mortality at 5 years	Glasgow Outcome Scale score at 3 months	Mortality, Glasgow Outcome Scale score at 6 months
Factors (numbers refer to rank order of importance within series)					
Age	4	No	4	Yes	Yes
Clinical grade	1	1	2	Yes	Yes
Grade at surgery	7	No	Not assessed	Not assessed	Not assessed
Vasospasm	2	4	1	No	Yes
Mass lesion	5	No	Not assessed	No	Yes
Hypertension	3	2	3	Yes	Yes
Short interval from SAH to surgery	6	3	4	No	No
Medical illnesses	Not assessed	5	Not assessed	Not assessed	Yes
Aneurysm side	Not assessed	Not assessed	5	Not assessed	No
Aneurysm size	Not assessed	No	Not assessed	Yes	No
Aneurysm location	Not assessed	No	Not assessed	No	Yes
Other	Variables assessed accounted for only 25% of the variance in outcome		Hydrocephalus was an adverse factor, males had better outcome than females, aneurysm clipping was better than wrapping	Aneurysm treated surgically was a significant favorable prognostic factor	Amount of SAH on computed tomography also important

*Not assessed: factor was not entered into multivariate analysis; no: factor was entered into analysis but was not of prognostic importance; yes: factor was important determinant of outcome in analysis. Numbers refer to rank order of prognostic importance within series. For example, 1 means this was the most important factor predicting outcome in the multivariate analysis in that series.

improve the outcome of patients with aneurysmal SAH.

REFERENCES

1. Ingall TJ, Whisnant JP, Wiebers DO, et al: Has there been a decline in subarachnoid hemorrhage mortality? Stroke 20:718–724, 1989.
2. Eisenberg HM, Gary HE Jr, Aldrich EF, et al: Initial CT findings in 753 patients with severe head injury: A report from the NIH Traumatic Coma Data Bank. J Neurosurg 73:688–698, 1990.
3. European Study Group on Nimodipine in Severe Head Injury: A multicenter trial of the efficacy of nimodipine on outcome after severe head injury. J Neurosurg 80:797–804, 1994.
4. Hassler W, Steinmetz H, Pirschel J: Transcranial Doppler study of intracranial circulatory arrest. J Neurosurg 71:195–201, 1989.
5. Nornes H: The role of intracranial pressure in the arrest of hemorrhage in patients with ruptured intracranial aneurysm. J Neurosurg 39:226–234, 1973.
6. McCormick PW, McCormick J, Zabramski JM, et al: Hemodynamics of subarachnoid hemorrhage arrest. J Neurosurg 80: 710–715, 1994.
7. Kaye AH, Brownbill D: Postoperative intracranial pressure in patients operated on for cerebral aneurysms following subarachnoid hemorrhage. J Neurosurg 54:726–732, 1981.
8. Weir B: Aneurysms Affecting the Nervous System. Baltimore, Williams & Wilkins, 1987, pp 1–671.
9. Grubb RLJ, Raichle ME, Eichling JO, et al: Effects of subarachnoid hemorrhage on cerebral blood volume, blood flow, and oxygen utilization in humans. J Neurosurg 46:446–453, 1977.
10. Meyer CHA, Lowe D, Meyer M: Progressive change in cerebral blood flow during the first three weeks after subarachnoid hemorrhage. Neurosurgery 12:58–76, 1983.
11. Carpenter DA, Grubb RLJ, Tempel LW, et al: Cerebral oxygen metabolism after aneurysmal subarachnoid hemorrhage. J Cereb Blood Flow Metab 11:837–844, 1991.
12. Voldby B, Enevoldsen EM, Jensen FT: Regional CBF, intraventricular pressure, and cerebral metabolism in patients with ruptured intracranial aneurysms. J Neurosurg 62:48–58, 1985.
13. Videen TO, Dunford-Shore JE, Diringer MN, et al: Correction for partial volume effects in regional blood flow measurements adjacent to hematomas in humans with intracerebral hemorrhage: Implementation and validation. J Comput Assist Tomogr 23:248–256, 1999.
14. Origitano TC, Wascher TM, Reichman OH: Sustained increased cerebral blood flow with prophylactic hypertensive hypervolemic hemodilution ("Triple-H" therapy) after subarachnoid hemorrhage. Neurosurgery 27:729–740, 1990.
15. Rosenstein J, Suzuki M, Symon L, et al: Clinical use of a portable bedside cerebral blood flow machine in the management of aneurysmal subarachnoid hemorrhage. Neurosurgery 15:519–525, 1984.
16. Fein JM: Brain energetics and circulatory control after subarachnoid hemorrhage. J Neurosurg 45:498–507, 1976.
17. Hubschmann OR, Nathanson DC: The role of calcium and cellular membrane dysfunction in experimental trauma and subarachnoid hemorrhage. J Neurosurg 62:698–703, 1985.
18. Marzatico F, Gaetani P, Rodriguez y Baena R: Experimental subarachnoid hemorrhage: Lipid peroxidation and Na^+,K^+-ATPase in different rat brain areas. Mol Chem Neuropathol 11: 99–107, 1989.
19. Voldby B, Enevoldsen EM, Jensen FT: Cerebrovascular reactivity in patients with ruptured intracranial aneurysms. J Neurosurg 62:59–67, 1985.
20. Dernback PD, Little JR, Jones SC: Altered cerebral autoregulation and CO_2 reactivity after aneurysmal subarachnoid hemorrhage. Neurosurgery 22:822–826, 1988.
21. Voldby B, Enevoldsen EM: Intracranial pressure changes following aneurysm rupture: I. Clinical and angiographic correlations. J Neurosurg 56:186–196, 1982.
22. Bassi P, Bandera R, Loiero M: Warning signs in subarachnoid hemorrhage: A cooperative study. Acta Neurol Scand 84:277–281, 1991.
23. Hauerberg J, Andersen BB, Eskesen V: Importance of recognition of a warning leak as a sign of a ruptured intracranial aneurysm. Acta Neurol Scand 83:61–64, 1991.
24. Juvela S: Minor leak before rupture of an intracranial aneurysm and subarachnoid hemorrhage of unknown etiology. Neurosurgery 30:7–11, 1992.
25. Weir B: Subarachnoid Hemorrhage: Causes and Cures. New York, Oxford, 1998, pp 1–301.
26. Abbott RJ, van Hille P: Thunderclap headache and unruptured cerebral aneurysm. Lancet 2:1459, 1986.
27. Lledo A, Calandre L, Martinez-Menendez B, et al: Acute headache of recent onset and subarachnoid hemorrhage: A prospective study. Headache 34:172–174, 1994.
28. Fontanarosa PB: Recognition of subarachnoid hemorrhage. Ann Emerg Med 18:1199–1205, 1989.
29. Pakarinen S: Incidence, aetiology, and prognosis of primary subarachnoid hemorrhage. Acta Neurol Scand 43(Suppl 29): 1–151, 1967.
30. Schievink WI: Intracranial aneurysms. N Engl J Med 336:28–40, 1997.
31. Kassell NF, Torner JC, Haley ECJ, et al: The international cooperative study on the timing of aneurysm surgery: I. overall management results. J Neurosurg 73:18–36, 1990.
32. Kassell NF, Torner JC, Jane JA, et al: The international cooperative study on the timing of aneurysm surgery: II. Surgical results. J Neurosurg 73:37–47, 1990.
33. Adams HP Jr, Jergenson DD, Kassell NF, et al: Pitfalls in the recognition of subarachnoid hemorrhage. JAMA 244:794–796, 1980.
34. Sarner M, Rose FC: Clinical presentation of ruptured intracranial aneurysm. J Neurol Neurosurg Psychiatr 30:67–70, 1967.
35. Locksley HB: Natural history of subarachnoid hemorrhage, intracranial aneurysms, and arteriovenous malformations: Based on 6368 cases in the cooperative study: I. In Sahs AL, Perret GE, Locksley HB (eds): Intracranial Aneurysms and Subarachnoid Hemorrhage. Philadelphia, JB Lippincott, 1969, pp 37–57.
36. Schievink WI, Karemaker JM, Hageman LM: Circumstances surrounding aneurysmal subarachnoid hemorrhage. Surg Neurol 32:266–272, 1989.
37. Velthuis BK, van Leeuwen MS, Witkamp TD, et al: Computerized tomography angiography in patients with subarachnoid hemorrhage: From aneurysm detection to treatment without conventional angiography. J Neurosurg 91:761–767, 1999.
38. Le Roux PD, Dailey AT, Newell DW, et al: Emergent aneurysm clipping without angiography in the moribund patient with intracerebral hemorrhage: The use of infusion computed tomography scans. Neurosurgery 33:189–197, 1993.
39. Johansson I, Bolander HG, Kourtopoulos H: CT showing early ventricular dilatation after subarachnoidal hemorrhage. Acta Radiol 33:333–337, 1992.
40. Fisher CM, Kistler JP, Davis JM: Relation of cerebral vasospasm to subarachnoid hemorrhage visualized by computerized tomographic scanning. Neurosurgery 6:1–9, 1980.
41. Kistler JP, Crowell RM, Davis KR, et al: The relation of cerebral vasospasm to the extent and location of subarachnoid blood visualized by CT scan: A prospective study. Neurology 33: 424–436, 1983.
42. Patel MK, Clarke MA: Lumbar puncture and subarachnoid hemorrhage. Postgrad Med J 62:1021–1024, 1986.
43. Duffy GP: Lumbar puncture in spontaneous subarachnoid haemorrhage. BMJ 285:1163–1164, 1982.
44. Archer BD: Computed tomography before lumbar puncture in acute meningitis: A review of the risks and benefits. Can Med Assoc J 148:961–965, 1993.
45. Vermeulen M, van Gijn J: The diagnosis of subarachnoid haemorrhage. J Neurol Neurosurg Psychiatry 53:365–372, 1990.
46. Klucznik RP, Carrier DA, Pyka R, et al: Placement of a ferromagnetic intracerebral aneurysm clip in a magnetic field with a fatal outcome. Radiology 187:855–856, 1993.
47. Payner TD, Tew JM Jr, Steiger HJ: Aneurysm clips. In Wilkins RH, Rengachary SS (eds): Neurosurgery, 2nd ed, vol 2. New York, McGraw-Hill, 1996, pp 2271–2276.
48. Chui M, Muller P, Tucker W: Angiographic diagnosis of small aneurysms of the posterior communicating artery. Am J Neuroradiol 11:1165, 1990.
49. Dion JE, Gates PC, Fox AJ, et al: Clinical events following

neuroangiography: A prospective study. Stroke 18:997–1004, 1987.
50. Sampei T, Yasui N, Mizuno M, et al: Contrast medium extravasation during cerebral angiography for ruptured intracranial aneurysm—clinical analysis of 26 cases. Neurol Med Chir 30: 1011–1015, 1990.
51. Aoyagi N, Hayakawa I: Rerupture of intracranial aneurysms during angiography. Acta Neurochir 98:141–147, 1989.
52. Behr R, Agnoli AL, Zierski J: Rupture of giant cerebral aneurysms during angiography: Case report and review of literature. J Neurosurg Sci 32:195–202, 1988.
53. Gelmers HJ, Simons AJ, Loew F: Rupture of intracranial aneurysms and ventricular opacification during carotid angiography. Acta Neurochir 70:43–51, 1984.
54. Henry MMP, Guerin J, Vallat JM, et al: Extravasation per angiographique du produit de contraste au cours des ruptures d'aneurysmes (à propos de 2 cas). Neurochirurgia 14:121–126, 1971.
55. Noda S, Tamaki N, Yamaguchi M, et al: Giant suprasellar aneurysm with extravasation of contrast medium into the ventricular system. Surg Neurol 13:208–210, 1980.
56. Palmieri A, Liguori R, De Rosa R: A propos d'un cas de rupture d'anéurysme artériel sacculaire intracranien au cours d'une artériographie. Ann Radiol 14:943–947, 1971.
57. Komiyama M, Tamura K, Nagata Y, et al: Aneurysmal rupture during angiography. Neurosurgery 33:798–803, 1993.
58. Inagawa T: Effect of ultra-early referral on management outcome in subarachnoid haemorrhage. Acta Neurochir 136:51–61, 1995.
59. Inagawa T: Timing of admission and management outcome in patients with subarachnoid hemorrhage. Surg Neurol 41: 268–276, 1994.
60. Almaani WS, Richardson AE: Multiple intracranial aneurysms: Identifying the ruptured lesion. Surg Neurol 9:303–305, 1978.
61. Marttila I, Heiskanen O: Value of neurological and angiographic signs as indicators of the ruptured aneurysm in patients with multiple intracranial aneurysms. Acta Neurochir 23:95–102, 1970.
62. Nehls DG, Flom RA, Carter LP, et al: Multiple intracranial aneurysms: Determining the site of rupture. J Neurosurg 63: 342–348, 1985.
63. Sakamoto T, Kwad R, Mizoi K, et al: Angiographical study of ruptured aneurysm in the multiple aneurysm patients. No Shinkei Geka 6:549–553, 1978.
64. Wood EH: Angiographic identification of the ruptured lesion in patients with multiple cerebral aneurysms. J Neurosurg 21: 182–198, 1964.
65. Friedman AH: Subarachnoid hemorrhage of unknown etiology. In Wilkins RH, Rengachary SS (eds): Neurosurgery Update II. New York: McGraw-Hill, 1991, pp 73–77.
66. Rinkel GJE, Wijdicks EFM, Vermeulen M, et al: Nonaneurysmal perimesencephalic subarachnoid hemorrhage: CT and MR patterns that differ from aneurysmal rupture. Am J Neuroradiol 157:829–834, 1991.
67. Alexander TD, Macdonald RL, Weir B, et al: Intraoperative angiography in cerebral aneurysm surgery: A prospective study of 100 craniotomies. Neurosurgery 39:10–17, 1996.
68. Feuerberg I, Lindquist C, Lindqvist M, et al: Natural history of postoperative aneurysm rests. J Neurosurg 66:30–34, 1987.
69. Origitano TC, Schwartz K, Anderson D, et al: Optimal clip application and intraoperative angiography for intracranial aneurysms. Surg Neurol 51:117–124, 1999.
70. Drake CG, Hunt WE, Sano K, et al: Report of World Federation of Neurological Surgeons Committee on a Universal Subarachnoid Hemorrhage Grading Scale. J Neurosurg 68:985–986, 1988.
71. Lindsay KW, Teasdale G, Knill-Jones RP, et al: Observer variability in grading patients with subarachnoid hemorrhage. J Neurosurg 56:628–633, 1982.
72. Teasdale G, Jennett B: Assessment of impaired consciousness and coma: A practical scale. Lancet 2:81–84, 1974.
73. Lindsay KW, Teasdale GM, Knill-Jones RP: Observer variability in assessing the clinical features of subarachnoid hemorrhage. J Neurosurg 58:57–62, 1983.
74. Vroomen PCAJ, De Krom MCTFM, Wilmink JT, et al: Lack of effectiveness of bed rest for sciatica. N Engl J Med 340: 418–423, 1999.
75. Hasan D, Vermeulen M, Wijdicks EFM, et al: Effect of fluid intake and antihypertensive treatment on cerebral ischemia after subarachnoid hemorrhage. Stroke 20:1511–1515, 1989.
76. Oropello JM, Benjamin E: Critical care of patients with subarachnoid hemorrhage. In Bederson JB (ed): Subarachnoid hemorrhage: Pathophysiology and management. Park Ridge, IL, American Association of Neurosurgery, 1997, pp 173–188.
77. Asplund K, Israelsson K, Schampi I: Haemodilution for acute ischaemic stroke (Cochrane review). Cochrane Library 2, 1–22. Oxford, Update Software, 1999.
78. Lee SH, Heros RC: Principles of management of subarachnoid hemorrhage: Steroids. In Ratcheson RA, Wirth FP (eds): Ruptured Cerebral Aneurysms: Perioperative Management, vol 6. Baltimore: Williams & Wilkins, 1994, pp 77–85.
79. DeMaria EJ, Reichman W, Kenney PR, et al: Septic complications of corticosteroid administration after central nervous system trauma. Ann Surg 202:248–252, 1985.
80. Pfeiffer M, Griss P: Craniocerebral trauma and aseptic osteonecrosis: Steroid-induced sequelae after therapy of brain edema. Unfallchirurg 95:284–287, 1992.
81. Wijdicks EF, Vermeulen M, Murray GD, et al: The effects of treating hypertension following aneurysmal subarachnoid hemorrhage. Clin Neurol Neurosurg 92:111–117, 1990.
82. Stornelli SA, French JD: Subarachnoid hemorrhage factors in prognosis and management. J Neurosurg 21:769–781, 1964.
83. Friedman AH: Timing of aneurysm surgery. In Wilkins RH, Rengachary SS (eds): Neurosurgery, 2nd ed. New York, McGraw-Hill, 1996, pp 2255–2260.
84. Vinuela F, Duckwiler G, Mawad M: Guglielmi detachable coil embolization of acute intracranial aneurysm: Perioperative anatomical and clinical outcome in 403 patients. J Neurosurg 86: 475–482, 1997.
85. Vermeulen M, Lindsay KW, Murray GD, et al: Antifibrinolytic treatment in subarachnoid hemorrhage. N Engl J Med 31:432–437, 1984.
86. Tsementzis SA, Hitchcock ER, Meyer CH: Benefits and risks of antifibrinolytic therapy in the management of ruptured intracranial aneurysms: A double-blind placebo-controlled study. Acta Neurochir 102:1–10, 1990.
87. Beck DW, Adams HP, Flamm ES, et al: Combination of aminocaproic acid and nicardipine in treatment of aneurysmal subarachnoid hemorrhage. Stroke 19:63–67, 1988.
88. Wijdicks EF, Hasan D, Lindsay KW, et al: Short-term tranexamic acid treatment in aneurysmal subarachnoid hemorrhage. Stroke 20:1674–1679, 1989.
89. Leipzig TJ, Redelman K, Horner TG: Reducing the risk of rebleeding before early aneurysm surgery: A possible role for antifibrinolytic therapy. J Neurosurg 86:220–225, 1997.
90. Kassell NF, Torner JC, Adams HPJ: Antifibrinolytic therapy in the acute period following aneurysmal subarachnoid hemorrhage: Preliminary observations from the Cooperative Aneurysm Study. J Neurosurg 61:225–230, 1984.
91. Beguelin C, Seiler R: Subarachnoid hemorrhage with normal cerebral panangiography. Neurosurgery 13:409–411, 1983.
92. Kassell NF, Torner JC: Aneurysm rebleeding: A preliminary report from the cooperative aneurysm study. Neurosurgery 13: 479–481, 1983.
93. Locksley HB: Report of the cooperative study of intracranial aneurysms and subarachnoid hemorrhage: Section V, Part II. Natural history of subarachnoid hemorrhage, intracranial aneurysms, and arteriovenous malformation. Based on 6368 cases in the cooperative study. J Neurosurg 25:321–368, 1966.
94. Fujii Y, Takeuchi S, Sasaki O, et al: Ultra-early rebleeding in spontaneous subarachnoid hemorrhage. J Neurosurg 84:35–42, 1996.
95. Torner JC, Kassell NF, Wallace RB, et al: Preoperative prognostic factors for rebleeding and survival in aneurysm patients receiving antifibrinolytic therapy: Report of the cooperative aneurysm study. Neurosurgery 9:506–513, 1981.
96. Mayberg MR, Batjer HH, Dacey R, et al: Guidelines for the management of aneurysmal subarachnoid hemorrhage: A statement for health care professionals from a special writing group of the Stroke Council, American Heart Association. Stroke 25: 2315–2328, 1994.
97. Brilstra EH, Rinkel GJ, van der Graaf Y, et al: Treatment of

intracranial aneurysms by embolization with coils: A systematic review. Stroke 30:470–476, 1999.
98. Yasargil MG, Smith RD, Young PH, et al: Microneurosurgery: II. Clinical considerations, surgery of the intracranial aneurysms and results. Stuttgart, Thieme, 1984, pp 1–386.
99. Hasan D, Vermeulen M, Wijdicks EF, et al: Management problems in acute hydrocephalus after subarachnoid hemorrhage. Stroke 20:747–753, 1989.
100. Graff-Radford NF, Torner J, Adams HP Jr, et al: Factors associated with hydrocephalus after subarachnoid hemorrhage: A report of the cooperative aneurysm study. Arch Neurol 46: 744–752, 1989.
101. Hasan D, Tanghe HL: Distribution of cisternal blood in patients with acute hydrocephalus after subarachnoid hemorrhage. Ann Neurol 31:374–378, 1992.
102. Mohr G, Ferguson G, Khan M, et al: Intraventricular hemorrhage from ruptured aneurysm: Retrospective analysis of 91 cases. J Neurosurg 58:482–487, 1983.
103. Paré L, Delfino R, Leblanc R: The relationship of ventricular drainage to aneurysmal rebleeding. J Neurosurg 76:422–427, 1992.
104. Paine JT, Batjer HH, Samson D: Intraoperative ventricular puncture. Neurosurgery 22:1107–1109, 1988.
105. Vale FL, Bradley EL, Fisher WS: The relationship of subarachnoid hemorrhage and the need for postoperative shunting. J Neurosurg 86:462–466, 1997.
106. Ogura K, Hara M, Tosaki F, et al: Effect of cisternal drainage after early operation for ruptured intracranial aneurysms. Surg Neurol 30:441–444, 1988.
107. Kasuya H, Shimizu T, Kagawa M: The effect of continuous drainage of cerebrospinal fluid in patients with subarachnoid hemorrhage: A retrospective analysis of 108 patients. Neurosurgery 28:56–59, 1991.
108. Shapiro SA, Campbell RL, Scully T: Hemorrhagic dilation of the fourth ventricle: An ominous predictor. J Neurosurg 80: 805–809, 1994.
109. Findlay JM, Grace MG, Weir BK: Treatment of intraventricular hemorrhage with tissue plasminogen activator. Neurosurgery 32:941–947, 1993.
110. Mayfrank L, Lippitz B, Groth M, et al: Effect of recombinant tissue plasminogen activator on clot lysis and ventricular dilatation in the treatment of severe intraventricular hemorrhage. Acta Neurochir 122:32–38, 1993.
111. Suzuki J, Yoshimoto T, Hori S: Continuous ventricular drainage to lessen surgical risk in ruptured intracranial aneurysm. Surg Neurol 2:87–90, 1974.
112. Bailes JE, Spetzler RF, Hadley MN, et al: Management morbidity and mortality in poor-grade aneurysm patients. J Neurosurg 72: 559–566, 1990.
113. Voldby B, Enevoldsen EM: Intracranial pressure changes following aneurysm rupture: III. Recurrent hemorrhage. J Neurosurg 56:784–789, 1982.
114. Gjerris F, Borgesen SE, Sorensen PS, et al: Resistance to cerebrospinal fluid outflow and intracranial pressure in patients with hydrocephalus after subarachnoid hemorrhage. Acta Neurochir 88:79–86, 1987.
115. Pasqualin A, Bazzan A, Cavanazzi P, et al: Intracranial hematomas following aneurysmal rupture: Experience with 309 cases. Surg Neurol 25:6–17, 1986.
116. Benoit RG, Cochrane DD, Durity F, et al: Clinical-radiological correlates in intracerebral hematomas due to aneurysmal rupture. Can J Neurol Sci 9:409–414, 1982.
117. Hart RG, Byer JA, Slaughter JR, et al: Occurrence and implications of seizures in subarachnoid hemorrhage due to ruptured intracranial aneurysms. Neurosurgery 8:417–421, 1981.
118. Solenski NJ, Haley ECJ, Kassell NF, et al: Medical complications of aneurysmal subarachnoid hemorrhage: A report of the multicenter, cooperative aneurysm study. Participants of the Multicenter Cooperative Aneurysm Study. Crit Care Med 23: 1007–1017, 1995.
119. Sbeih I, Tamas LB, O'Laoire SA: Epilepsy after operation for aneurysms. Neurosurgery 19:784–788, 1986.
120. Baker CJ, Prestigiacomo CJ, Solomon RA: Short-term perioperative anticonvulsant prophylaxis for the surgical treatment of low-risk patients with intracranial aneurysms. Neurosurgery 37: 863–870, 1995.
121. Temkin NR, Dikmen SS, Wilensky AJ, et al: A randomized, double-blind study of phenytoin for the prevention of post-traumatic seizures. N Engl J Med 323:497–502, 1990.
122. Rose FC, Sarner M: Epilepsy after ruptured intracranial aneurysm. BMJ 1:18–21, 1965.
123. Fabinyi GCA, Artiola-Fortuny L: Epilepsy after craniotomy for intracranial aneurysm. Lancet 1:1299–1300, 1980.
124. Notani M, Kawamura H, Amano K, et al: The incidence of postoperative epilepsy and prophylactic anticonvulsants in patients with intracranial aneurysm. No Shinkei Geka 12:269–274, 1984.
125. Ohman J: Hypertension as a risk factor for epilepsy after aneurysmal subarachnoid hemorrhage and surgery. Neurosurgery 27:578–581, 1990.
126. Keränen T, Tapaninaho A, Hernesniemi J, et al: Late epilepsy after aneurysm operations. Neurosurgery 17:897–900, 1985.
127. Hasan D, Schonck RS, Avezaat CJ, et al: Epileptic seizures after subarachnoid hemorrhage. Ann Neurol 33:286–291, 1993.
128. Toftdahl DB, Torp-Pedersen C, Engel UH, et al: Hypertension and left ventricular hypertrophy in patients with spontaneous subarachnoid hemorrhage. Neurosurgery 37:235–239, 1995.
129. Hijdra A, Vermeulen M, van Gijn J, et al: Respiratory arrest in subarachnoid hemorrhage. Neurology 34:1501–1503, 1984.
130. Medlock MD, Dulebohn SC, Elwood PW: Prophylactic hypervolemia without calcium channel blockers in early aneurysm surgery. Neurosurgery 30:12–16, 1992.
131. Weir BK: Pulmonary edema following fatal aneurysm rupture. J Neurosurg 49:502–507, 1978.
132. Kondoh T, Kuwamura K, Miyata M, et al: Early surgery for ruptured intracranial aneurysms associated with neurogenic pulmonary edema: Report of 2 cases. Neurol Med Chir 28: 1107–1112, 1988.
133. Niikawa S, Nokura H, Uno T, et al: Neurogenic pulmonary edema following aneurysmal subarachnoid hemorrhage: Report of 9 cases. Neurol Med Chir 28:157–163, 1988.
134. Smith WS, Matthay MA: Evidence for a hydrostatic mechanism in human neurogenic pulmonary edema. Chest 111:1326–1333, 1997.
135. Kollef MH: The prevention of ventilator-associated pneumonia. N Engl J Med 340:627–634, 1999.
136. D'Amelio LF, Hammond JS, Spain DA, et al: Tracheostomy and percutaneous endoscopic gastrostomy in the management of the head-injured trauma patient. Am Surg 60:180–185, 1994.
137. Collins R, Scrimgeour A, Yusuf S, et al: Reduction in fatal pulmonary embolism and venous thrombosis by perioperative administration of subcutaneous heparin: Overview of results of randomized clinical trials in general, orthopedic, and urologic surgery. N Engl J Med 318:1162–1173, 1988.
138. Hirsh J, Hoak J: Management of deep vein thrombosis and pulmonary embolism: A statement for healthcare professionals—Council on Thrombosis (in consultation with the Council on Cardiovascular Radiology). Circulation 93:2212–2245, 1996.
139. Bucci MN, Papadopoulos SM, Chen JC, et al: Mechanical prophylaxis of venous thrombosis in patients undergoing craniotomy: A randomized trial. Surg Neurol 32:285–288, 1989.
140. Turpie AGG, Hirsh J, Gent M, et al: Prevention of deep vein thrombosis in potential neurosurgical patients: A randomized trial comparing graduated compression stockings alone or graduated compression stockings plus intermittent pneumatic compression with control. Arch Intern Med 149:679–681, 1989.
141. Macdonald RL, Amidei C, Lin G, et al: Safety of perioperative subcutaneous heparin for prophylaxis of venous thromboembolism in patients undergoing craniotomy. Neurosurgery 45:245–252, 1999.
142. Lazio BE, Simard JM: Anticoagulation in neurosurgical patients. Neurosurgery 45:838–848, 1999.
143. Decousus H, Leizorovicz A, Parent F, et al: A clinical trial of vena caval filters in the prevention of pulmonary embolism in patients with proximal deep-vein thrombosis. N Engl J Med 338:409–415, 1998.
144. Marion DW, Segal R, Thompson ME: Subarachnoid hemorrhage and the heart. Neurosurgery 18:101–106, 1986.

145. Mayer SA, LiMandri G, Sherman D, et al: Electrocardiographic markers of abnormal left ventricular wall motion in acute subarachnoid hemorrhage. J Neurosurg 83:889–896, 1995.
146. Mayer SA, Lin J, Homma S, et al: Myocardial injury and left ventricular performance after subarachnoid hemorrhage. Stroke 30:780–786, 1999.
147. Andreoli A, Di Pasquale G, Pinelli G, et al: Subarachnoid hemorrhage: Frequency and severity of cardiac arrhythmias: A survey of 70 cases studied in the acute phase. Stroke 18:558–564, 1987.
148. Pollick C, Cujec B, Parker S, et al: Left ventricular wall motion abnormalities in subarachnoid hemorrhage: An echocardiographic study. J Am Coll Cardiol 12:600–605, 1988.
149. Davies KR, Gelb AW, Manninen PH, et al: Cardiac function in aneurysmal subarachnoid haemorrhage: A study of electrocardiographic and echocardiographic abnormalities. Br J Anaesth 67:58–63, 1991.
150. Vidal BE, Dergal EB, Cesarman E, et al: Cardiac arrhythmias associated with subarachnoid hemorrhage: Prospective study. Neurosurgery 5:675–680, 1979.
151. Stober T, Anstätt T, Sen S, et al: Cardiac arrhythmias in subarachnoid hemorrhage. Acta Neurochir 93:37–44, 1988.
152. Brouwers PJAM, Wijdicks EFM, Hasan D, et al: Serial electrocardiographic recording in aneurysmal subarachnoid hemorrhage. Stroke 20:1162–1167, 1989.
153. Walter P, Neil-Dwyer G, Cruickshank JM: Beneficial effects of adrenergic blockade in patients with subarachnoid haemorrhage. BMJ 284:1661–1664, 1982.
154. Takaku A, Shindo K, Tanaka S, et al: Fluid and electrolyte disturbances in patients with intracranial aneurysms. Surg Neurol 11:349–356, 1979.
155. Maroon JC, Nelson PB: Hypovolemia in patients with subarachnoid hemorrhage: Therapeutic implications. Neurosurgery 4: 223–226, 1979.
156. Wijdicks EFM, Vermeulen M, ten Haaf JA, et al: Volume depletion and natriuresis in patients with a ruptured intracranial aneurysm. Ann Neurol 18:211–216, 1985.
157. Nelson RJ: Blood volume measurement following subarachnoid haemorrhage. Acta Neurochir Suppl 47:114–121, 1990.
158. Diringer MN, Wu KC, Verbalis JG, et al: Hypervolemic therapy prevents volume contraction but not hyponatremia following subarachnoid hemorrhage. Ann Neurol 31:543–550, 1992.
159. Shimoda M, Yamada S, Yamamoto I, et al: Atrial natriuretic polypeptide in patients with subarachnoid haemorrhage due to aneurysmal rupture: Correlation to hyponatremia. Acta Neurochir 97:53–61, 1989.
160. Dóczi T, Joó F, Vecsernyés M, et al: Increased concentration of atrial natriuretic factor in the cerebrospinal fluid of patients with aneurysmal subarachnoid hemorrhage and raised intracranial pressure. Neurosurgery 23:16–19, 1988.
161. Diringer M, Ladenson P, Stern BJ, et al: Plasma atrial natriuretic factor and subarachnoid hemorrhage. Stroke 19:1119–1124, 1988.
162. Rosenfeld JV, Barnett GH, Sila CA, et al: The effect of subarachnoid hemorrhage on blood and CSF atrial natriuretic factor. J Neurosurg 71:32–37, 1989.
163. Diringer M, Lim JS, Kirsch JR, et al: Suprasellar and intraventricular blood predict elevated plasma atrial natriuretic factor in subarachnoid hemorrhage. Stroke 22:577–581, 1991.
164. Wijdicks EFM, Pooer AH, Hunnicutt EJ, et al: Atrial natriuretic factor and salt wasting after aneurysmal subarachnoid hemorrhage. Stroke 22:1519–1524, 1991.
165. Wijdicks EF, Schievink WI, Burnett JC Jr: Natriuretic peptide system and endothelin in aneurysmal subarachnoid hemorrhage. J Neurosurg 87:275–280, 1997.
166. Berendes E, Walter M, Cullen P, et al: Secretion of brain natriuretic peptide in patients with aneurysmal subarachnoid haemorrhage. Lancet 349:245–249, 1997.
167. Wijdicks EFM, Vermeulen M, Hijdra A, et al: Hyponatremia and cerebral infarction in patients with ruptured intracranial aneurysms: Is fluid restriction harmful? Ann Neurol 17:137–140, 1985.
168. Hasan D, Wijdicks EFM, Vermeulen M: Hyponatremia is associated with cerebral ischemia in patients with aneurysmal subarachnoid hemorrhage. Ann Neurol 27:106–108, 1990.
169. Wijdicks EFM, van Dongen KJ, van Gijn J, et al: Enlargement of the third ventricle and hyponatremia in aneurysmal subarachnoid hemorrhage. J Neurol Neurosurg Psychiatr 51:516–520, 1988.
170. Shimoda M, Oda S, Tsugane R, et al: Intracranial complications of hypervolemic therapy in patients with a delayed ischemic deficit attributed to vasospasm. J Neurosurg 78:423–429, 1993.
171. Harrigan MR: Cerebral salt wasting syndrome: A review. Neurosurgery 38:152–160, 1996.
172. Hasan D, Lindsay KW, Wijdicks EFM, et al: Effect of fludrocortisone acetate in patients with subarachnoid hemorrhage. Stroke 20:1156–1161, 1989.
173. Toho H, Sawada T, Karasawa J, et al: Metabolic response to hypertensive intracerebral hemorrhage and ruptured intracranial aneurysm. Neurol Med Chir 26:683–688, 1986.
174. Hersio K, Vapalahti M, Kari A, et al: Impaired utilization of exogenous amino acids after surgery for subarachnoid haemorrhage. Acta Neurochir 106:13–17, 1990.
175. Gadisseux P, Ward JD, Young HF, et al: Nutrition and the neurosurgical patient. J Neurosurg 60:219–232, 1984.
176. Touho H, Karasawa J, Shishido H, et al: Hypermetabolism in the acute stage of hemorrhagic cerebrovascular disease. J Neurosurg 72:710–714, 1990.
177. Norton B, Homer-Ward M, Donnelly MT, et al: A randomised prospective comparison of percutaneous endoscopic gastrostomy and nasogastric tube feeding after acute dysphagic stroke. BMJ 312:13–21, 1996.
178. Voll CL, Auer RN: The effect of postischemic blood glucose levels on ischemic brain damage in the rat. Ann Neurol 24: 638–646, 1988.
179. Irwin LR: Can we really prevent gastrointestinal bleeding after head injury? Results of a recent audit. J R Coll Surg Edinburgh 39:292–294, 1994.
180. Yu WY, Rhoney DH, Boling WB, et al: A review of stress ulcer prophylaxis in the neurosurgical intensive care unit. Neurosurgery 41:416–426, 1997.
181. Wadworth AN, McTavish D: Nimodipine: A review of its pharmacological properties and therapeutic efficacy in cerebral disorders. Drugs Aging 2:262–286, 1992.
182. Weir B, Disney L, Grace M, et al: Daily trends in white blood cell count and temperature after subarachnoid hemorrhage from aneurysm. Neurosurgery 25:161–165, 1989.
183. Spallone A, Acqui M, Pastore FS, et al: Relationship between leukocytosis and ischemic complications following aneurysmal subarachnoid hemorrhage. Surg Neurol 27:253–258, 1987.
184. Peerless SJ: Pre- and postoperative management of cerebral aneurysms. Clin Neurosurg 26:209–231, 1979.
185. Wojak JC, Flamm ES: Intracranial hemorrhage and cocaine use. Stroke 18:712–715, 1987.
186. Simpson RK Jr, Fischer DK, Narayan RK, et al: Intravenous cocaine abuse and subarachnoid hemorrhage: Effect on outcome. Br J Neurosurg 4:27–30, 1990.
187. Oyesiku NM, Colohan ART, Barrow DL, et al: Cocaine-induced aneurysmal rupture: An emergent negative factor in the natural history of intracranial aneuryms? Neurosurgery 32:518–526, 1993.
188. Portnoy BA, Herion JC: Neurological manifestations in sickle-cell disease: With a review of the literature and emphasis on the prevalence of hemiplegia. Ann Intern Med 76:643–652, 1972.
189. Oyesiku NM, Barrow DL, Eckman JR, et al: Intracranial aneurysms in sickle-cell anemia: Clinical features and pathogenesis. J Neurosurg 75:356–363, 1991.
190. Anson JA, Koshy M, Ferguson L, et al: Subarachnoid hemorrhage in sickle-cell disease. J Neurosurg 75:552–558, 1991.
191. Batjer HH, Adamson T, Bowman GW: Sickle cell disease and aneurysmal subarachnoid hemorrhage. Surg Neurol 36:145–149, 1991.
192. Meyer FB, Sundt TM Jr, Fode NC, et al: Cerebral aneurysms in childhood and adolescence. J Neurosurg 70:420–425, 1989.
193. Jennett B, Bond M: Assessment of outcome after severe brain damage: A practical scale. Lancet 1:480–484, 1975.
194. Disney L, Weir B, Grace M: Factors influencing the outcome of aneurysm rupture in poor grade patients: A prospective series. Neurosurgery 23:1–9, 1988.

195. Weir B: Headaches from aneurysms. Cephalalgia 14:79–87, 1994.
196. van Gijn J, Hijdra A, Wijdicks EFM, et al: Acute hydrocephalus after aneurysmal subarachnoid hemorrhage. J Neurosurg 63: 355–362, 1985.
197. Botterell EH, Lougheed WM, Scott JW, et al: Hypothermia and interruption of carotid, or carotid and vertebral, circulation in the surgical management of intracranial aneurysms. J Neurosurg 13:1–42, 1956.
198. Hunt WE, Hess RM: Surgical risk as related to time of intervention in the repair of intracranial aneurysms. J Neurosurg 28: 14–20, 1968.
199. Weir B: Medical aspects of the preoperative management of aneurysms: A review. Can J Neurol Sci 6:441–450, 1979.
200. Weir B, Rothberg C, Grace M, et al: Relative prognostic significance of vasospasm following subarachnoid hemorrhage. Can J Neurol Sci 2:109–114, 1975.
201. Artiola I, Fortuny L, Prieto-Valiente L: Long-term prognosis in surgically treated intracranial aneurysms: I. Mortality. J Neurosurg 54:26–34, 1981.

CHAPTER **109**

Cerebral Vasospasm

J. MAX FINDLAY

Although cerebral arteries can transiently constrict in response to a number of physiologic, pharmacologic, and mechanical stimuli, *cerebral vasospasm* has become a clinical term referring to a different and specific type of cerebral arterial vasoconstriction. Cerebral vasospasm is a prolonged, sometimes severe, but ultimately reversible cerebral arterial narrowing that occurs days after bleeding into the subarachnoid space. Other terms have appeared in the literature referring to the same condition, including *post–subarachnoid hemorrhage (SAH) vasculopathy* and *constrictive angiopathy of subarachnoid hemorrhage.* SAH significant enough to cause vasospasm is usually due to the rupture of a saccular cerebral aneurysm, but vasospasm can complicate traumatic SAH and the rare occasion when vascular malformations or tumors bleed massively into the subarachnoid space.

Angiographic vasospasm is arterial narrowing demonstrated on arteriography after SAH, which is common (Fig. 109–1), whereas *clinical* or *symptomatic vasospasm* is narrowing that has resulted in cerebral ischemia with corresponding symptoms and signs, sometimes referred to as *delayed ischemic neurological deficits*, which is less common. The progression to symptomatic cerebral ischemia is dependent on a number of factors, including the patient's circulating blood volume and arterial blood pressure, but the most important factor is the degree of arterial narrowing. Vasospasm can be focal or diffuse in distribution and mild, moderate, or severe in severity. Vasospasm affects only intradural cerebral arteries and primarily those larger vessels at the base of the brain. The distribution and severity of vasospasm parallels the location and thickness of subarachnoid hematoma, which underlies the pathogenesis of vasospasm through a number of interrelated and complex extracellular and intracellular mechanisms affecting the entire cerebral artery wall and which are still being defined.

The delayed onset and the relative predictability of vasospasm provide a unique therapeutic window of opportunity lacking in other types of ischemic stroke. Over the past 2 decades, improvements in our understanding and ability to manage vasospasm, and SAH in general, have resulted in an important decline in patient morbidity and mortality due to vasospasm. Minimizing the harm caused by vasospasm through judicious management of blood volume and pressure, timely intervention with endovascular treatment such as balloon angioplasty, and reducing the risk of ischemic injury with cerebroprotectants such as nimodipine remains one of the most important goals of SAH management. Trying to determine the precise pathogenesis of vasospasm in the hope this will provide a simple and complete pharmacologic preventative strategy continues to be an elusive goal in neurosurgical research.

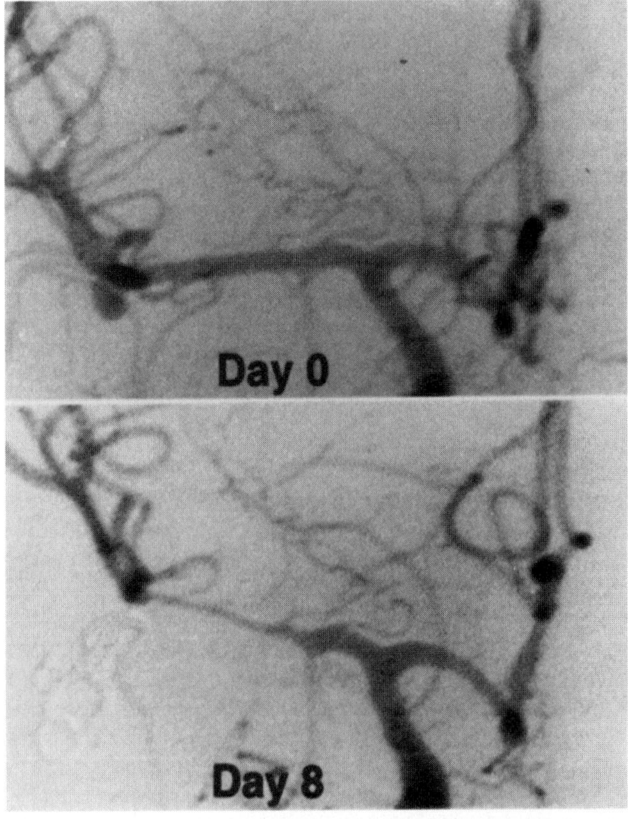

FIGURE 109–1. Severe angiographic vasospasm of the main trunk of the right middle cerebral artery 8 days after the rupture and repair of a small middle cerebral artery bifurcation aneurysm.

VASOSPASM: HISTORICAL HIGHLIGHTS

Angiographic vasospasm was first described by a neurosurgeon, Ecker, along with a radiologist, Riemenschneider, in Syracuse, New York, in 1951.[1] From their analysis these authors accurately concluded that vasospasm, when it occurs, is only seen within several weeks of hemorrhage, is maximal near the aneurysm but extends along adjacent intracranial arteries in lesser degree, and plays an important role in determining outcome after aneurysm rupture. Acceptance of this concept was slow, however. Although the clinical picture of progressive hemiparesis days after hemorrhage without clear evidence of aneurysm rebleeding (i.e., fresh blood in cerebrospinal fluid [CSF]) was recognized as a common occurrence, repeat cerebral angiography was seldom performed in the early years of aneurysm surgery. As well, many argued that cerebral arteries lacked a sufficient muscle layer in their coats to cause a prolonged and deleterious spasm (PA Riemenschneider, personal communication, 1999). It was approximately 10 years after Ecker's report that sufficient evidence was provided by authors such as Pool,[2, 3] Maspes and Marini,[4] Du Boulay,[5] Allcock and Drake,[6] and Wilkins and associates[7] to convince the neurosurgical community that vasospasm was a true entity and was a main cause of morbidity and mortality in patients with ruptured intracranial aneurysms.

Beginning in the 1960s, neurosurgical research laboratories became busy creating animal models of SAH to determine the cause of vasospasm (i.e., the underlying "spasmogen") and to test a wide variety of invariably ineffective drugs for the prevention and reversal of vasospasm.[8] On the clinical side, the usefulness of induced hypertension to treat ischemic neurological deficits associated with vasospasm was first reported by Kosnik and Hunt in 1976[9] and by Giannotta and colleagues the following year,[10] although the benefit of deliberate hypertension in cerebral ischemia due to other causes was first proposed by Farhat and Schneider 10 years earlier.[11] The effectiveness of a standard protocol of intravascular volume expansion and induced hypertension in a series of patients with delayed vasospastic ischemia was convincingly demonstrated by Kassell and coworkers in 1982.[12] Supported by a growing understanding of ischemic thresholds and acceptance of Astrup and Symon's theory of ischemic "penumbral" brain, which could potentially be saved if blood flow into the region could be augmented,[13, 14] hypervolemic, hypertensive therapy became a standard treatment for patients with symptomatic vasospasm (and surgically secured aneurysms) by the late 1980s.

In 1980, C. Miller Fisher and colleagues clearly described the relationship between subarachnoid clots seen on computed tomography (CT) soon after SAH and the relative risk for vasospasm[15] and provided a useful predictive grading scale based on the location and thickness of clot. Aaslid and associates introduced transcranial Doppler ultrasound testing in 1984,[16] which subsequently became adopted by many neurosurgical units around the world as a practical, noninvasive method of monitoring the cerebral circulation for developing vasospasm.

In 1983, Allen and coworkers published the first controlled trial of the calcium antagonist nimodipine after SAH, which showed that in patients in good neurological condition after aneurysm rupture nimodipine significantly reduced the occurrence of severe neurological deficits.[17] This somewhat controversial result (the clinical effect not readily perceived by clinicians hoping for a pharmacologic "silver bullet" for vasospasm) was subsequently supported by a number of other larger trials.[18] Although the beneficial effect of nimodipine is probably unrelated to arterial narrowing as originally intended, and instead more likely due to neuronal protection, nimodipine has won an established role in SAH management.

Zubkov and colleagues were the first to use transluminal balloon angioplasty to dilate vasospastic cerebral arteries; and although it sounded to most of the world as almost an impossibly difficult and dangerous treatment when first described in 1984,[19] it is now a relatively safe, effective, and even standard part of vasospasm treatment in a growing number of neurosurgical centers around the world.

Contributors to the clinical and basic science of cerebral vasospasm are far too numerous to list, but some of the important figures over the past several decades have included Wilkins in Durham, North Carolina; White and Robertson in Memphis, Tennessee; Zervas and Peterson in Boston, Massachusetts; Rosemary and John Bevan in Burlington, Vermont; Smith in Jackson, Mississippi; Cook in Edmonton, Alberta; Sano and Sasaki in Tokyo and Asano in Saitama, Japan; Pickard in Southampton, England; Seifert and Stolke in Hannover, Germany; and Dorsch in Sydney, Australia. Bryce Weir in Edmonton (and later Chicago) and Neal Kassell in Charlottesville, Virginia, have made especially important and frequent laboratory and clinical investigations in cerebral vasospasm over several decades.

VASOSPASM IN CONDITIONS OTHER THAN ANEURYSM RUPTURE

Post-traumatic Vasospasm

A number of studies have indicated that vasospasm can sometimes complicate traumatic brain injury. Although several of these have been transcranial Doppler studies in which post-traumatic vasoparalysis and hyperemia may have been difficult to distinguish from vasospasm,[20, 21] others have included angiography or cerebral blood flow (CBF) measurements, or both, that confirmed either vasospasm or cerebral hypoperfusion in a number of patients.[22–25] Delayed-onset post-traumatic vasospasm appears to correlate with the presence of thick traumatic subarachnoid blood clots in the basal subarachnoid cisterns and has a time course similar to aneurysmal vasospasm. Because the aneurysmal pattern of thick SAH in cisterns surrounding the circle of Willis is both uncommon after closed-head injury (seen in less than 10% of patients with severe head injury)[26] and correlates strongly with poor neurological condition on presentation,[27] clinically significant post-traumatic vasospasm appears to be relatively rare and difficult to recognize when it does occur. The value of monitoring head-injured patients for vasospasm (i.e., with transcranial ultrasound or CBF studies) may exist but has not been demonstrated. Several studies have indicated that the L-type calcium channel blocker nimodipine started within 12 hours of traumatic brain injury with CT-identifiable SAH has a modest but significantly beneficial effect on patient outcome.[28, 29]

Vasospasm and Arteriovenous Malformations, Brain Tumors, and Unruptured Intracranial Aneurysms

Vasospasm rarely complicates arteriovenous malformation (AVM) rupture, probably because the common locations of these lesions do not allow for the deposition of a large volume of blood clot into the basal subarachnoid cisterns.[30, 31] There have been several reports of severe vasospasm in the setting of intraventricular hemorrhage from AVMs[32, 33] and from an intraventricular hemorrhage of undetermined etiology,[34] which appear to be exceptional because the cause of vasospasm is difficult to explain in this situation.

There have been a number of reports of vasospasm complicating brain tumor surgery,[35–37] although in most cases recognized or unrecognized bleeding into the subarachnoid space can be implicated as the cause.

There have also been scattered reports of vasospasm complicating surgery for unruptured intracranial aneurysms,[38, 39] although again it is difficult to completely exclude the possibility of surgical bleeding into the subarachnoid space or vessel injury as the cause of these rare instances of vasospasm and/or cerebral ischemia.

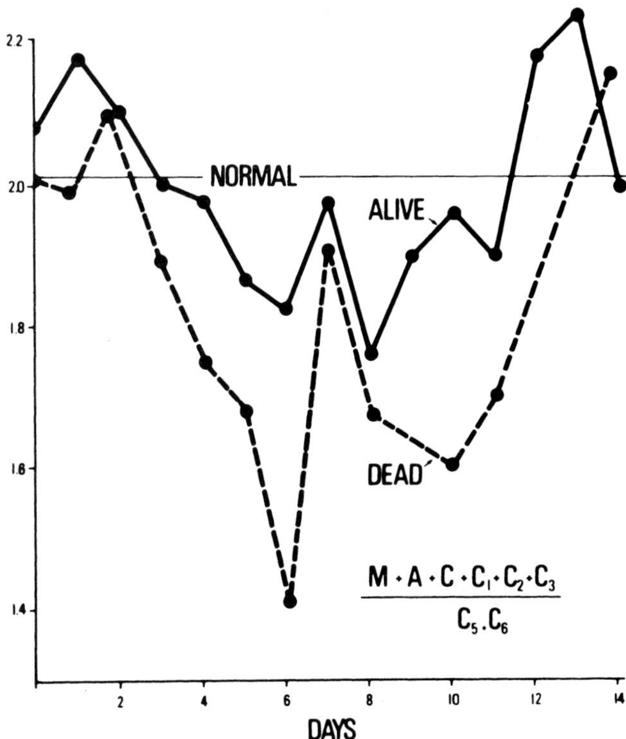

FIGURE 109–2. Curve for reduction in ratio of the caliber of vessels within the subarachnoid space to those without versus time, based on data from 429 angiograms done post SAH and preoperatively. There is more constriction in the angiograms in the 120 patients who died *(broken line)* than in the 309 who survived *(solid line)*. (From Weir B, Grace M, Hansen J, Rothberg C: Time course of vasospasm in man. J Neurosurg 48:173–178, 1979.)

THE EPIDEMIOLOGY OF VASOSPASM

Incidence and Time Course of Vasospasm after Subarachnoid Hemorrhage

A review of the literature found that the overall incidence of angiographic vasospasm after SAH was roughly 50%, although the estimates ranged from 20% to nearly 100%.[40] The variation appeared due to inconsistencies in the timing of cerebral angiography and definitions of vasospasm used. It is probable that if all degrees of narrowing were considered, and angiograms performed daily, the majority of SAH patients with blood visible on initial CT would at some point have evidence of angiographic vasospasm. Vasospasm begins during the first week after initial hemorrhage, peaks in severity during the second week, and generally lasts until the third or fourth week (Fig. 109–2).[40, 41] The presence of angiographic vasospasm within 48 hours of aneurysm rupture (i.e., at admission and detected on diagnostic angiography), although difficult to establish with certainty without a baseline study, has been correlated with a higher risk for later symptomatic vasospasm and poor outcome.[42]

Risk Factors for Vasospasm

A number of studies have found a relationship between the amount and location of subarachnoid blood seen on admission CT and the risk and distribution of angiographic vasospasm.[15, 43–49] Fisher's grading system, or modifications of it, have been widely adopted.[15] This system classifies SAH on CT into four groups: group 1, no blood detected (very low risk for vasospasm); group 2, thin layers of clot, less than 1 mm thick (low risk); group 3, thick clots greater than 1 mm (moderate to high risk); and group 4, intracerebral or intraventricular clots with no or little subarachnoid blood (low risk). The important group to note in terms of vasospasm risk are those with localized or diffuse thick clots. In a recent study that carefully assessed the amount of subarachnoid clot on the admission CT scan, almost 60% of patients with thick clots developed moderate to severe angiographic vasospasm in at least one major cerebral artery.[50] Related to this subject is the demonstration that reducing the subarachnoid clot burden at the time of early surgery (within 48 hours of rupture) reduces the risk of severe angiographic vasospasm.[50]

TABLE 109–1 ■ **Risk Factors for Symptomatic Vasospasm**

Thick subarachnoid clots on computed tomography
Poor neurological condition on admission
Cigarette smoking
Age younger than 35 and older than 65
Preexisting hypertension
Incomplete circle of Willis

Risk factors have also been identified for symptomatic vasospasm. Poor clinical grade (related to more severe hemorrhage), age younger than 35, and cigarette smoking have been shown to be independent risk factors for clinical vasospasm (Table 109–1).[51–53] There is some evidence that the elderly have a lower incidence of angiographic vasospasm, perhaps due to impaired reactivity to spasmogens,[54] but that they have a higher incidence of symptomatic vasospasm and infarcts due to vasospasm, perhaps due to decreased cerebrovascular reserve.[55] Other, less robust risk factors for clinical vasospasm include preexisting hypertension and an incomplete circle of Willis.

Nonaneurysmal Perimesencephalic Subarachnoid Hemorrhage and Vasospasm

Roughly 15% of patients presenting with SAH will have no demonstrable source of the bleeding identified on initial cerebral angiography, and the majority of this group will have a distinctive pattern of bleeding into the perimesencephalic and prepontine cisterns. These patients have a typical SAH clinical presentation of sudden severe headache, although they usually remain conscious and alert. Cerebral angiography is normal, and the cause of the usually small to moderate volume clot around the upper brainstem near the tentorial hiatus is unknown. These patients have a low incidence of complications, including clinical vasospasm. One study found angiographic vasospasm in 5 of 12 patients with this type of hemorrhage, although in 4 the narrowing was localized, and it was not mentioned if it was severe or if any of the patients became symptomatic.[56] In a larger series of 65 patients, none suffered symptomatic vasospasm[57]; and in a review of the literature on perimesencephalic SAH, only 3 patients were identified who possibly experienced deterioration from vasospasm.[58] It would appear that spontaneous perimesencephalic SAH has a quite benign natural history, including a low risk for vasospasm. Thick, diffuse, and nonperimesencephalic types of SAHs with negative angiography need to be followed closely for both the appearance of an aneurysm on follow-up angiography and the development of clinical vasospasm.

Effect of Aneurysm Treatment on Vasospasm

It had been suspected for some time that surgery for aneurysm clipping during the interval of peak vasospasm was more hazardous,[59–61] and this was verified in two separate studies on the timing of aneurysm surgery in which patients who underwent surgery toward the end of the first week from the initial hemorrhage had significantly poorer outcomes than earlier or later surgery groups.[62, 63] Although a prevalent theory is that surgical manipulation of vasospastic arteries exacerbates the arterial narrowing, this was not found in a primate experiment in which manipulation of vasospastic monkey cerebral arteries did not increase vasospasm 24 hours later.[64] A multivariate analysis of the factors predisposing to vasospasm found that the time of surgery did not affect the development of vasospasm.[65] The possibility remains that the increased risk of surgery-related ischemia during the peak vasospasm period may be due to other mechanisms, including increased susceptibility to intraoperative or postoperative hypotension or brain retraction and manipulation during surgery. Surgery in the face of established vasospasm must be undertaken with due caution.

It remains uncertain as to whether endovascular treatment of aneurysms is associated with a different vasospasm risk than microsurgical clipping.[66] Early aneurysm clipping does afford the surgeon the opportunity to reduce the subarachnoid clot burden both mechanically and with thrombolysis, which may be useful in reducing the vasospasm risk in patients with large-volume SAHs.

Vasospasm as a Cause of Morbidity and Mortality after Aneurysmal Subarachnoid Hemorrhage

Whereas it was formerly estimated that roughly one half of patients with SAH developed angiographic vasospasm, one half of this group would become symptomatic, and one half of these symptomatic patients would die of cerebral infarction,[67] modern perioperative care of SAH has clearly improved this situation. Understanding the need to avoid hypovolemia, hypotension, and antifibrinolytic agents, use of the calcium antagonist nimodipine, and deliberate hypervolemia with induced hypertension to treat symptomatic vasospasm have reduced the combined risk of all morbidity and mortality due to vasospasm to between 10% and 15% in more recent SAH patient series.[68–74] That having been said, vasospasm remains an important clinical problem, a leading cause of preventable death and disability after SAH, and one of the most important independent predictors of poor outcome when it occurs.

EXPERIMENTAL VASOSPASM MODELS

Studies of the pathology, pathogenesis, and treatment of vasospasm often involve animal models, so it is useful to consider the differences, strengths, and weaknesses of these models when evaluating the vasospasm literature (Table 109–2).

In vitro studies of vasospasm require removal of cerebral arteries for testing immediately after an animal

TABLE 109–2 ■ **Animal Models of Vasospasm: Summary of Features, Comparisons to Human Vasospasm, and Suggested Best Uses**

MODEL	COST (U.S. DOLLARS)	DIAMETER OF ARTERY (OF HUMAN)	TIME COURSE (OF HUMAN)		ANGIOGRAPHIC VASOCONSTRICTION	MORPHOLOGIC VASOCONSTRICTION	ASSOCIATED CEREBRAL ISCHEMIA	PATHOLOGY	OVERALL CORRELATION WITH HUMAN VASOSPASM	BEST USE: PATHOGENESIS	BEST USE: TREATMENT
			Onset	Resolution							
Rat, intracranial	2–20	Much smaller	Sooner (minutes)	Sooner (5 days)	Yes	Yes	No	Good	Fair	Fair	Screening for pharmacologic prevention and reversal
Rabbit intracranial	20–80	Much smaller	Similar (~3 days)	Similar (~14 days)	Yes	Yes	No	Good	Good	Good	Screening for pharmacologic prevention and reversal
Cat, intracranial	100–500	Much smaller	Sooner (hours)	Sooner (7 days)	Yes	Yes	No	Good	Fair	Fair	Screening for pharmacologic prevention and reversal
Pig, intracranial	50–500	Similar	Similar (2–10 days)	Not determined	Yes	Yes	No	Good	Good	Good	Screening for pharmacologic/angioplasty prevention and reversal
Dog, intracranial	150–1000	Smaller	Similar (2–7 days)	Similar (14 days)	Yes	Yes	No	Very good	Very good	Very good	Screening and preclinical trials for pharmacologic angioplasty prevention and reversal
Primate, intracranial	500–several thousand	Smaller	Similar (4–7 days)	Similar (14 days)	Yes	Yes	Yes, but low incidence	Excellent	Excellent	Excellent	Preclinical trials for pharmacologic angioplasty prevention and reversal
Rat, femoral	2–20	Much smaller	Similar (2 days)	Similar (20 days)	Yes	Yes	Not applicable	Good	Good	Good	Screening for pharmacologic prevention and reversal
Rabbit, extracranial carotid	20–80	Smaller	Sooner (1 day)	Sooner (6 days)	Yes	Yes	No	Good	Fair	Fair	Screening for pharmacologic/angioplasty prevention and reversal
Dog, extracranial carotid	150–1000	Similar	Similar (7 days)	Similar (14–21 days)	Yes	Yes	No	Good	Good	Good	Screening for pharmacologic/angioplasty prevention and reversal

is killed and suspending segments or strips of those arteries in organ baths held by fixation devices so they can be exposed to test substances. Normal arteries or arteries rendered vasospastic in vivo with induced SAH can be used. Arterial specimens can be observed to determine if contraction or relaxation occurs; and then various physiologic, pharmacologic, and morphologic properties can be studied, depending on the focus of the experiment. Using in vitro techniques, researchers have studied putative spasmogens, as well as potential vasospasm therapies (for examples of this methodology, see references 75–77).

In vivo models of SAH and vasospasm require induction or placement of a blood clot around a vessel in a living animal, which then results in a consistent narrowing that is angiographically and/or morphologically detectable and measurable and lasts a period of days before resolution. It is desirable that the time course of the vasospasm be similar to that observed in humans, but it is acknowledged that animals very rarely develop vasospasm-related ischemic neurological deficits, probably because of ample collateral CBF in animals. Because most vasospasm experiments study vessel constriction, with their end points either its prevention or reversal, the absence of clinically identifiable cerebral ischemia in animal models of vasospasm is probably of little significance. However, the optimal animal model of vasospasm would include a measurable reduction in CBF associated with severe vasospasm.

In vivo models of SAH and vasospasm have been developed using intracranial arteries whereby autologous blood is introduced into cisternal spaces to surround the basal cerebral arteries. Models of this type have been developed in the rat,[78, 79] rabbit,[80] cat,[81, 82] pig,[83, 84] dog,[85, 86] and primate.[87–89] Most models of intracranial vasospasm use a technique in which autologous blood is injected or placed around blood vessels to induce vasospasm, rather than puncturing or tearing the artery with a needle or ligature to induce a higher pressure SAH. Whereas the latter method has been thought to induce more severe vasospasm,[89, 90] no doubt related to the more severe SAH that ensues, it is a more difficult technical procedure and is associated with a significantly higher animal mortality rate.

Because primates are phylogenetically closest to humans, these models have provided results that have been most applicable to vasospasm in humans. However, the cost and ethical issues surrounding primate experimentation have become considerable. Rat and rabbit models are relatively inexpensive, and SAH is technically easy to induce in these animals, but angiography in small animals is difficult. In these models greater reliance is placed on morphologic evidence of vasospasm. The applicability of results from rabbits, where vasospasm is relatively easy to both induce and prevent, is less certain. The most widely used experimental model of vasospasm is the double-hemorrhage canine model, which involves two injections of autologous blood in the dog's cisterna magna over 2 days and the measurement of angiographic and morphologic vasospasm on the seventh day.[86] This model produces moderate to severe vasospasm in the basilar artery in over 90% of animals and is associated with little animal morbidity and mortality, and angiography in the dog is relatively easy to perform and the basilar artery readily visualized. At least for basic pathogenetic and drug screening experiments, the dog model is believed to be satisfactory and may be especially useful before advancing to primate experiments.

A number of in vivo animal models of vasospasm that use extracranial arteries have also been developed. The advantages of these models include the easy application and maintenance of blood clot around peripheral arteries (usually within silicone tubes or Silastic cuffs), the simplicity of animal handling and negligible animal morbidity, the accessibility of the arteries for in vivo manipulations (i.e., transluminal angioplasty), and the relatively low cost of the experiments. However, the disadvantage is that the arteries under study are noncerebral, with important structural and physiologic differences.[91–95] The extracranial carotid arteries of rabbits,[96, 97] femoral arteries of rats,[98] and extracranial carotid arteries of dogs[76, 77] have been used. Bearing in mind the just-mentioned limitations, these models would appear to have a role in specific areas of vasospasm research.

PATHOLOGY: ARTERIAL WALL CHANGES IN VASOSPASM

There have been a number of published studies on the pathologic arterial wall changes after experimental SAH in animals and after aneurysmal hemorrhage in humans who demonstrated angiographic vasospasm before death or biopsy. Animal studies have included both light and electron microscopic findings after perfusion fixation, whereas human studies have been histologic after immersion fixation. A review of these studies determined that electron microscopy frequently reveals early degenerative changes in the endothelial cell layer, including vacuolization, disruption of interendothelial tight junctions, and occasionally endothelial desquamation and luminal microthrombosis.[99] The tunica intima, like the underlying internal elastic lamina, is convoluted due to contraction of the media. Seventeen of the 27 studies reviewed reported some degree of intimal thickening variously ascribed to edema, polymorph infiltration, granulation tissue, migration (presumably from the media) and proliferation of smooth muscle cells, or fibroplasia and collagenization. Intimal thickening significant enough to be appreciated histologically is usually not seen in the first week after hemorrhage and when it occurs is usually most noticeable after several weeks. One human study found that in those patients surviving 17 days or fewer from aneurysm rupture the tunica intima was only slightly swollen, whereas in those surviving longer the intima became the most abnormal component of the arterial wall.[100] In another autopsy study where no specific arterial changes other than arterial contraction were found, and the intima was considered normal, all patients had died within 16 days of rupture.[101] It would appear, therefore, that ultrastructural changes in the endothelium demonstrated in animal models and mentioned earlier precede any significant hyperplastic intimal changes evident on light microscopy. Pathologic changes in the endothelium, perhaps surprising given that it is the cell layer farthest from the subarachnoid clot, are especially relevant given the role the endothelium has in the pathogenesis of vasospasm, to be discussed in the next section.

Characteristic of both experimental and human vasospastic vessels is a markedly thickened media, a change that was speculated by some to be due to an inflammatory or hypertrophic reaction in the vessel wall after SAH. However, whereas wall thickness in severe experimental vasospasm increases up to fivefold, it is accompanied by only a small increase in cross-sectional area of the vessel wall in monkeys[99, 102] dogs,[103] and pigs[84]; and this is similar to what is observed when normal cerebral arteries are pharmacologically vasoconstricted in vitro.[99, 102] Vessel wall thickening is therefore primarily related to vascular contraction, and the increase in the wall area that has been noted is secondary to inflammatory infiltration of the blood-coated adventitia (Fig. 109–3). Vasospasm is accompanied by a variable amount of patchy myonecrosis in the tunica media[99] (Fig. 109–4) and at least in some animal models an increase in extracellular matrix, presumably elaborated by myointimal cells in the same arterial wall layer.[84, 104]

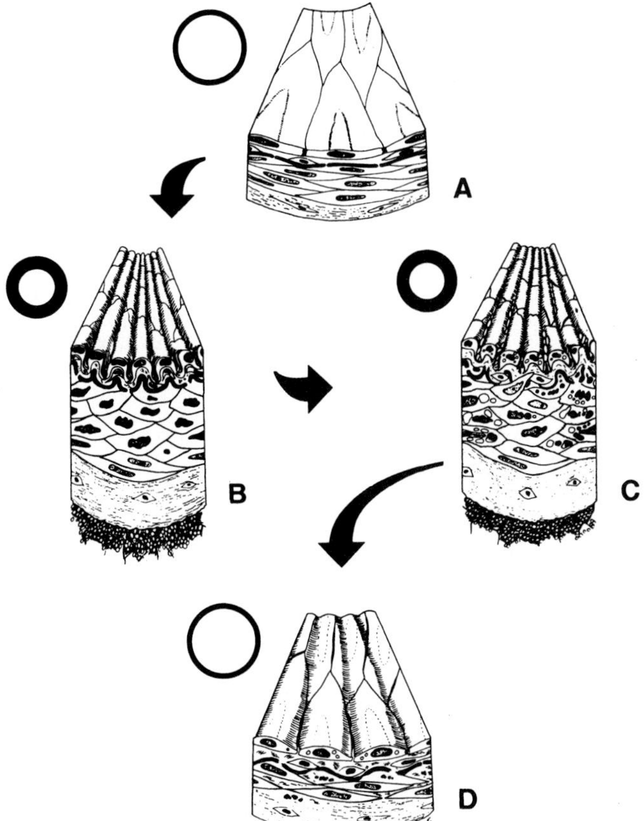

FIGURE 109–3. Cerebral arterial wall changes in cerebral vasospasm. Normal cerebral artery wall *(A)*. After subarachnoid hemorrhage (SAH) the artery is coated in blood clot, which over several days induces vasoconstriction associated with medial thickening and corrugation of the internal elastic lamina and intima *(B)*. Sustained constriction leads to functional impairment of the arterial wall associated with ultrastructural damage: endothelial vacuolization, loss of tight junctions, breakage of the internal elastic lamina, and medial myonecrosis *(C)*. Within several weeks most vessels resume normal luminal caliber, although ultrastructural morphologic abnormalities persist for a longer period of time *(D)*. (Modified from Findlay JM, Weir BKA, Kanamaru K, Espinosa F: Arterial wall changes in cerebral vasospasm. Neurosurgery 25:736–746, 1989.)

Cerebral arteries do not have an external elastic lamina, but the adventitia after SAH is generally thickened by granulation tissue admixed with adherent fibrin and erythrocytes.

In a study of the long-term effects of experimental canine vasospasm it was found that carotid arteries returned to their normal morphologic appearance and pharmacologic responsiveness by 21 to 28 days after clot placement.[77] Additionally, in a series of patients examined many years after suffering SAH and proven vasospasm, blood flow velocities in the circle of Willis and cerebrovascular reserve capacities tested with acetazolamide challenge were found to be normal.[105] Vasospasm therefore appears to have no long-term effects on the cerebral vasculature.

Vasospasm has, from its first recognition, been appreciated as primarily affecting the larger muscular arteries within the subarachnoid space and exposed to the greatest concentration of subarachnoid blood clot. Depending on the extent of SAH, it can also reach to the more distal arteries.[106] Involvement of penetrating intraparenchymal arterioles not easily appreciated on angiography is debated, with conflicting experimental evidence.[107, 108] The intraparenchymal course of these arteries protects them from thick coats of blood clot, and isolated lenticulostriate or thalamoperforating infarcts complicating human vasospasm are rare. If these vessels do become involved in vasospasm, it is probably not common.

ETIOLOGY AND PATHOGENESIS OF VASOSPASM

Etiology of Vasospasm: Blood Clots in the Subarachnoid Space

Over the past several decades a large number of molecules and chemicals released or potentially released from subarachnoid clots were considered as possible "spasmogens," but a series of studies in the late 1980s and 1990s seemed to establish that red blood cells,[109, 110] the hemoglobin released as the red blood cells hemolyze,[111] and specifically oxyhemoglobin were primarily responsible for vasospasm, including experimental primate vasospasm.[112–114] The more recent demonstration that more highly purified hemoglobin may be less vasospastic than previous experiments suggested has reopened the question of whether several products of clots and hemolysis must be present and act in concert to cause more severe vasospasm with myonecrosis.[115, 116] The possible mechanisms through which blood clots induce vasospasm are discussed next.

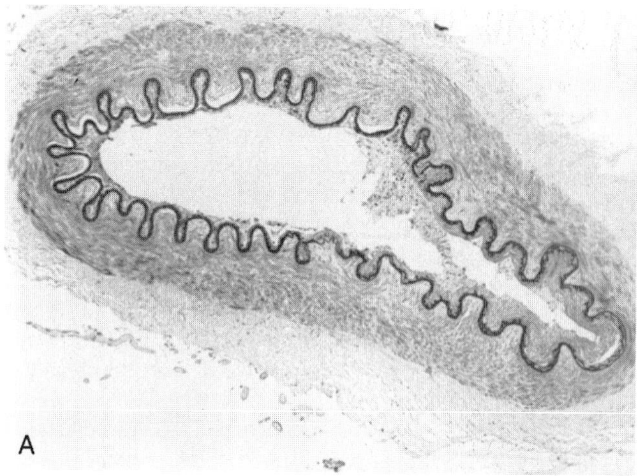

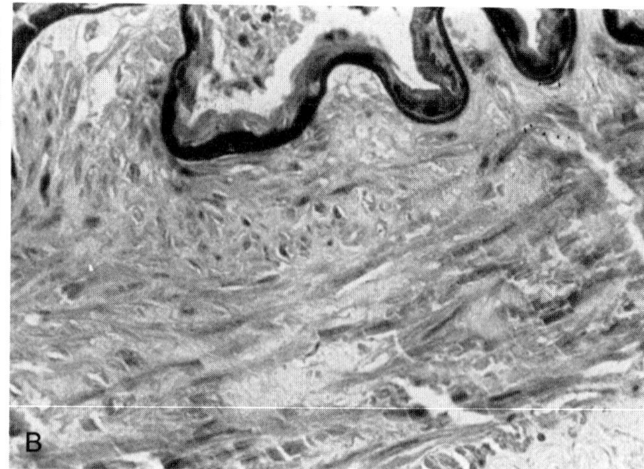

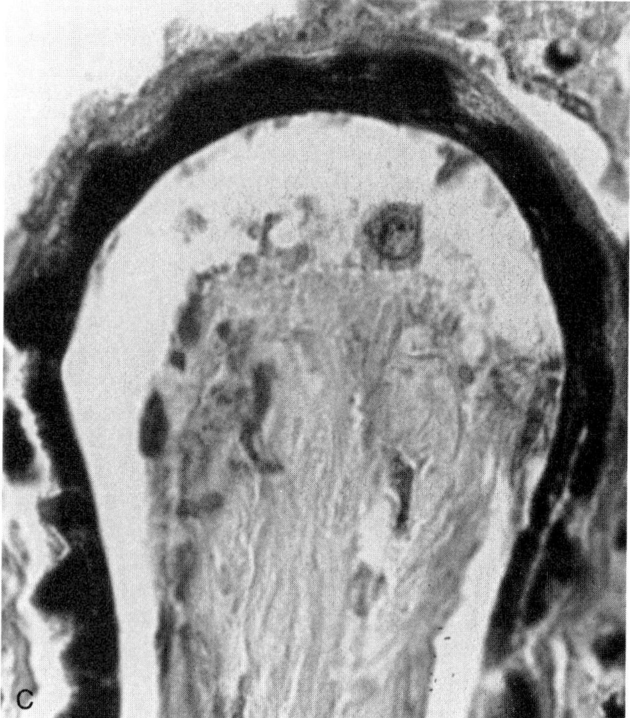

FIGURE 109–4. A 46-year-old woman died 10 days after the rupture of a right internal carotid artery aneurysm, due to severe symptomatic vasospasm, and autopsy and cerebral artery examination was performed within hours of death. *A,* A transverse section of the right middle cerebral artery shows luminal narrowing and an irregular tunica elastica (H&E, ×25). Details from the same section shows that the tunica intima is swollen and the tunica media is disorganized with smooth muscle cell necrosis (H&E, ×100). *C,* Higher magnification shows the tunica media beneath the tunica elastica is edematous and contains a prominent "plump" cell, probably a phagocyte (H&E, ×150). Note the absence of cellular invasion or proliferation at this stage. (Photomicrographs courtesy of Dr. Charlie Hao, University of Alberta.)

Pathogenesis of Vasospasm

A number of theories of the pathogenesis of vasospasm have been explored over the years, many finding some measure of support in animal experiments (Table 109–3). That, along with the apparent complexity of the vasospastic process that has been so difficult to entirely prevent and/or reverse across species, continues to support the notion that vasospasm has a multifactorial and complex pathogenesis involving each of the artery wall layers and cell types. With that in mind, the theories discussed here should not be considered as competitive but instead potentially additive or even synergistic (Fig. 109–5).

Experimental evidence exploring particular theories has been of several different types. Evidence has been obtained by probing some aspect of the vasospastic process in animals or in man, such as for example measuring the vessel wall, subarachnoid blood clot, or

TABLE 109–3 ■ **Theories of the Pathogenesis of Cerebral Vasospasm**

Structural (Non–Smooth Muscle Cell) Theories
Proliferative vasculopathy
Immune vasculopathy
Vessel wall inflammation
Extracellular lattice contraction
Vasoconstriction Theories
Free radical lipid peroxidation
Derangement in eicosanoid production
Nitric oxide deficit
Endothelin excess
Neurogenic factors

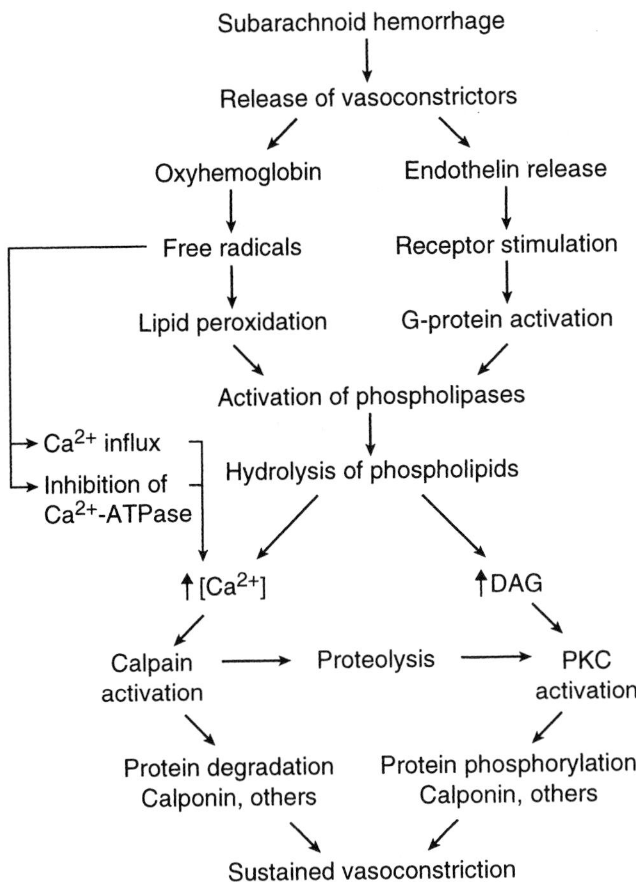

FIGURE 109–5. Processes likely to be involved in the production of cerebrovascular spasm after subarachnoid hemorrhage. The figure shows possible mechanisms by which cerebral vasospasm might arise. Oxyhemoglobin-induced generation of free radicals results in lipid peroxidation and activation of phospholipases C, D, and A_2. Endothelin activates phospholipases and subsequent lipid hydrolysis by acting on ET_A and ET_B receptors present in vascular tissue. The phospholipases hydrolyze phospholipids, phosphatidylinositol 4,5-biphosphate, and phosphatidylcholine to give inositol triphosphate, diacylglycerol (DAG), and arachidonic acid. Inositol triphosphate stimulates release of intracellular calcium from the sarcoplasmic reticulum. This is followed by an influx of calcium from the extracellular space through channels that seem to be different from dihydropyridine-sensitive, voltage-dependent calcium channels. Free radicals can also cause plasma membrane perturbation, which can result in the inhibition of calcium extrusion from the cell by the calcium pump. Resulting high levels of intracellular calcium activate calpains, which are responsible for proteolytic cleavage of cytoskeletal proteins, thin filament proteins (calponin and caldesmon), and protein kinases (PKC, Ca^{2+}-CaM kinase II, MLCK). Transient formation of diacylglycerol from inositol phospholipids is followed by a sustained generation of this lipid from phosphatidylcholine in a process catalyzed by phospholipase D. Sustained activation of PKC and phosphorylation of calponin removes an inhibitory effect of this protein on actomyosin ATPase and contributes to vasoconstriction. The key process involves a prolonged elevation of intracellular calcium, which ultimately becomes a self-perpetuating process resulting in prolonged clinical vasospasm. See text for details. (From Cook DA, Vollrath B: Free radicals and intracellular events associated with cerebrovascular spasm. Cardiovasc Res 30:493–500, 1995.)

CSF for a putative mediator of vasospasm. Proposed spasmogens have been administered to animals in vivo or to arterial strips in vitro and the results compared with what is known about blood-induced vasospasm. And finally the inhibitory effect of agents has been used to support a pathogenetic process in which that agent is thought to interfere (these experiments also therefore suggesting possible treatments), although this evidence alone is circumstantial and best includes some measure that the agent under investigation is having the biochemical effect intended.

Structural Theories: Proliferative, Immune, and Inflammatory Mechanisms and Vasospasm

The observation that vasospastic arterial walls are thick compared with normal arteries led to the suggestion that vasospasm might represent inflammatory cell infiltration into the vessel wall and/or migration and proliferation of cells native to the wall (i.e., a "response to injury" reaction) somehow related to the effect of SAH.[117–119] Subsequent studies have demonstrated, however, that vasoconstriction alone results in marked arterial wall thickening with a much smaller change in overall vessel wall area,[84, 99, 102, 104] and a labeling study in primates showed relatively little cell division after SAH and through the vasospastic interval.[120] Intimal thickening, due partly to cell proliferation in this layer, appears to occur late in vasospasm and does not contribute significantly to luminal narrowing.[121]

Related to this, immune mechanisms have been implicated in vasospasm, including the complement cascade,[121–124] humoral immunity,[125] and cellular immunity.[126, 127] A number of immunosuppressants and modulators have been tested in experimental and human vasospasm.[128–137] Although effective in animals, cyclosporin A did not prevent vasospasm in a small pilot study in humans at high risk,[137] whereas the nonspecific protease inhibitor FUT-175, also effective in animals, did appear to have a preventative effect in an uncontrolled clinical trial.[132]

Nonimmune inflammatory processes have been considered in vasospasm. Periarterial inflammation,[138–140] cytokines,[141, 142] and intercellular adhesion molecules[142–144] have been examined. Monoclonal antibodies directed against several adhesion molecules responsible for the attachment of leukocytes to endothelial cells were effective in reducing experimental vasospasm in rats (anti–intercellular adhesion molecule [CAM] 1)[145] and rabbits (anti-ICAM-1 and anti-CD18).[146]

Structural Theories, Extracellular Lattice Contraction, and Vasospasm

It has been suggested that the stiffness and pharmacologic unresponsiveness of established vasospasm[147, 148] is due to arterial wall fibrosis and that myofibroblast cells in the tunica media rearrange and contract the collagen extracellular matrix of the arterial wall, locking the artery into prolonged, chronic vasospasm.[149–153] A study in primates, however, did not find evidence of gross collagenization of vasospastic vessels.[154] Even if this mechanism does not increase the extracellular protein content of the arterial wall significantly but rather just remodels it, it remains unclear how an arterial reaction of this sort could be activated by SAH and how it could be transient, as vasospasm is known to be. Interest in this proposed mechanism continues, however, and its participation in the established and most resistant phase of vasospasm remains possible.

Vasoconstriction and Vasospasm

The majority of vasospasm research has explored smooth muscle contractile mechanisms and, related to this, interactions between the endothelium and vascular smooth muscle.

Physiologic smooth muscle contraction begins with cell membrane depolarization and an increase in intracellular calcium.[155] Vascular smooth muscle depends more on extracellular than intracellular calcium stores, which enter through voltage-gated and receptor-operated calcium channels. Intracellular calcium binds the protein calmodulin that then activates myosin light chain kinase (MLCK), and this enzyme phosphorylates and activates the myosin light chain, allowing actin and myosin cross-linkage and mechanical shortening. This process of contraction requires adenosine triphosphate (ATP) in addition to calcium. Phosphorylation of MLCK, triggered through the adenylate and guanylate second messenger systems that elevate intracellular cyclic nucleotides adenosine monophosphate (AMP) and guanosine monophosphate (GMP) levels, results in a decreased affinity for the calcium-calmodulin complex, dephosphorylation of myosin light chain, and smooth muscle cell relaxation.

Although vasospasm after SAH may commence through the receptor-mediated (i.e., "spasmogen"-triggered) calcium-calmodulin pathway and myofilament activation summarized earlier, tonic contraction (chronic vasospasm) may not depend on it. Both animal[156–158] and human[159] cerebral arteries exposed to subarachnoid blood show progressively diminished reactivity to vasoactive agents over time, and this may be despite intact second messenger systems and the capacity to generate cyclic nucleotides.[160] CSF from SAH patients induces induction of cytosolic free calcium in vascular smooth muscle cells,[161] but there is conflicting evidence regarding intracellular calcium homeostasis in chronic vasospasm, with some work suggesting that intracellular calcium levels decline.[162–169] In addition, a progressive decrease in intracellular high-energy phosphates has been noted in chronic vasospasm in the dog model, indicating metabolic failure in close association with the development of fixed arterial narrowing.[170, 171] It has also been shown that hemoglobin and its metabolites lead to a significant decline in energy metabolism of cultured smooth muscle cells.[172] Perhaps related to this, myosin light-chain phosphorylation declines markedly in rat femoral artery vasospasm[173] and does not occur in response to vasoconstrictors in spastic canine basilar artery.[174] Myosin light-chain phosphorylation remained elevated, however, in another dog experiment.[167]

Although not all experiments agree, the foregoing indicates that chronic, more irreversible vasospasm is the result of a less energy-requiring and more tonic contraction, perhaps also independent of elevated intracellular calcium concentrations. Activation of the protein kinase C (PKC) system through accumulations of intracellular diacylglycerol (DAG) has been a suggested mechanism in a number of studies[166, 175–178] but not all.[179] A high-force, low-phosphorylation, and low–energy consumption state named "latch," about which not a great deal is known, has also been discussed.[174] Reduced expression or degradation of actinomysin regulatory proteins (inhibitors of actinomysin interaction) such as calponin and caldesmon has been another proposal.[174, 180–182] A protein tyrosine kinase–based mechanism has also been described as yet another possible cause of chronic vasospasm.[183]

Free Radicals, Lipid Peroxidation, and Vasospasm

From the foregoing, it is apparent that the intracellular contractile processes in vasospasm may change as the condition progresses and have not yet been fully clarified. Unfortunately, the extracellular events in the pathogenesis of vasospasm are also not yet fully known and they, too, are almost certainly complex.

The auto-oxidation of oxyhemoglobin, producing methemoglobin and superoxide anion radical, occurs in the subarachnoid space and leads to lipid peroxidation.[184, 185] Both hydroxyl radicals and lipid peroxides permeate the vessel wall layers and are both directly vasoactive[186, 187] and harmful, injuring endothelial and smooth muscle cells.[188, 189] Because iron released from hemoglobin catalyzes lipid peroxidation, a number of animal and tissue-culture studies have examined the preventative effect of iron-chelation with deferoxamine,[190–194] deferiprone,[195] and 2,2′-dipyridyl[196]; and these agents ameliorated vasospasm in a variety of animal models, including primates.[196] Free radical scavenger superoxide dismutase prevented vasospasm in one experiment in rabbits[197] but not in another using primates.[198]

The nonglucocorticoid 21-aminosteroid lipid peroxidation inhibitor U74006F (one of the "lazaroids" and later known as tirilazad mesylate) was applied in vasospasm models first in the late 1980s, with overall beneficial effects.[199–205] This agent has come to clinical trials, which are discussed later. Other 21-aminosteroids have been tested in animal models, once again with some success, although their advantage over tirilazad mesylate, if any, is not clear.[206–208]

Eicosanoids and Vasospasm

Eicosanoids are compounds derived from 20-carbon unsaturated fatty acid precursors, usually membrane phospholipids. Certain stimuli, including SAH, trigger the metabolism of phospholipids into either prostaglandins (via the cyclooxygenase pathway) or leukotrienes (via the lipoxygenase pathway), which are the two main classes of eicosanoids. Because some of the prostaglandins possess vasoactive properties, it was postulated that vasospasm is the result of vessels synthesizing less vasodilating prostaglandins, such as prostaglandin I_2, and more vasoconstricting prostaglandins and/or leukotrienes, such as prostaglandin E_2, 15-hydroperoxyeicosatetraenoic acid, and thromboxane A_2.[209–211] Again, these are effects on the endothelial cell layer in particular. Inhibitors of prostaglandin and thromboxane synthesis have had only modest success in experimental and clinical vasospasm prevention,[212–215] and experimental[216] and clinical[217] studies found no clear SAH-induced CSF prostaglandin profile that correlated with angiographic vasospasm or delayed cerebral ischemia, respectively.

Related to this discussion is the known role of thromboxane A_2 as a promotor of platelet aggregation and the possibility that SAH, through increases in thromboxane A_2 synthesis as well as reduced endothelial antiplatelet activity, leads to thrombosis as part of the vasospastic process.[218–220]

Nitric Oxide and Vasospasm

Experimental SAH causes a loss of what was formerly called "endothelium-derived relaxation factor" (EDRF)[221–225] and what is now known to be the simple molecule nitric oxide (NO).[226] NO is made from the amino acid arginine by various forms of the enzyme NO synthase in a number of different central nervous system locations, including endothelial cells, vascular smooth muscle cells, adventitial perivascular nerves, neurons, glia, and macrophages. NO appears to play a role in modulating cerebrovascular tone and blood flow,[227, 228] and it vasodilates via the vascular smooth muscle cyclic GMP second messenger system.[229] Loss of NO synthase immunoreactivity has been noted in the adventitia of vasospastic primate arteries,[230] and intracarotid NO and NO donors were found to reverse and prevent primate vasospasm.[231, 232] Finally, NO synthase gene transfer has been effected ex vivo into vasospastic canine basilar arteries using an adenovirus vector, resulting in partial restoration of NO-mediated vascular relaxations.[233]

Endothelin and Vasospasm

Vascular endothelium expresses endothelin-1 (ET-1), which acts primarily as an autocoid, binding to ET receptors of adjacent vascular smooth muscle cells of the vessel wall and causing a powerful sustained contraction. First discovered in 1988, it was soon after suspected a possible participant in the pathogenesis of vasospasm.[234, 235] Several lines of evidence support a role of ET-1 in vasospasm, although not all experiments have demonstrated a clear connection. Thrombin and hemoglobin stimulate ET production in vitro,[236–239] and ET-1 causes a dose-dependent and long-lasting vasoconstriction when applied to arterial strips in vitro and, when administered into the CSF of animals in vivo,[240–244] a contraction that resembles the nature of vasospasm in humans. ET-1 may induce contraction via the PKC pathway mentioned previously.

In animal models, SAH causes increased arterial wall levels of ET-1. Several conflicting reports may have resulted from different experimental designs, types of measurements, and the timing of the various ET-1 assays.[245–247] Similarly, not all clinical reports have shown increased ET-1 levels in the CSF of patients who develop vasospasm,[248–251] but intra-arterial levels may not be accurately reflected in the CSF. Indirect evidence for a causative role for ET in vasospasm comes from animal trials that have shown that some ET antagonists or inhibitors prevent or reverse vasospasm.[245, 252–262] Finally, unique and compelling evidence for the role of the ET-1 in the pathogenesis of vasospasm has come from genetic interventions in rats[263] and dogs,[264] where blocking the expression of the ET-1 gene using antisense techniques significantly reduced vasospasm.

Neurogenic Factors and Vasospasm

Cerebral arteries are innervated by adrenergic, cholinergic, and peptidergic nerves.[265] Periadventitial adrenergic nerve endings in cerebral arteries degenerate after experimental SAH, and this finding, in conjunction with data suggesting noradrenaline levels increase after SAH, led to suggestions that denervation hypersensitivity might contribute to vasospasm.[266] However, and as discussed previously, pharmacologic studies have shown that vasospastic arteries usually have impaired rather than heightened responses to catecholamines or other vasoconstrictors. Despite ongoing interest and research,[267] at present there is limited evidence supporting a prominent neurogenic or neuropeptidergic role in vasospasm pathogenesis.[268]

CLINICAL FEATURES AND DIAGNOSIS OF VASOSPASM

Symptoms, Signs, and Differential Diagnosis

Delayed neurological deterioration after aneurysmal SAH can have a number of causes (Table 109–4), and

TABLE 109–4 ■ Causes of Delayed-Onset Neurological Worsening after Aneurysmal Subarachnoid Hemorrhage

Symptomatic vasospasm
Hydrocephalus
Increased cerebral edema or swelling around an intracerebral clot, contusion, or infarct
Aneurysm or aneurysm remnant rebleeding
Seizure(s)
Hyponatremia from elevated arterial natriuretic factor or less commonly the syndrome of inappropriate secretion of antidiuretic hormone
Hypoxia or hypotension from cardiopulmonary complications
Systemic sepsis
Bacterial meningitis or ventriculitis

all other causes of worsening should be ruled out before making a diagnosis of symptomatic vasospasm. Clinical vasospasm does not occur in the first few days after SAH, and if truly present this early suggests that the patient experienced an unrecognized SAH before the presenting rupture. The development of cerebral ischemia is dependent on a number of factors, including the patient's intravascular volume, blood pressure, the presence of anatomical collaterals in the cerebrovasculature (i.e., a patent circle of Willis), and the presence of brain injury resulting from the SAH itself. The most important factor, however, is the severity and distribution of arterial narrowing.

Symptomatic vasospasm usually has a gradual onset, sometimes heralded by increased headache and decreased alertness, and then a progressive course if untreated. A smaller group of patients will have a more precipitous deterioration.[269] Patients who do not present with SAH itself (i.e., classic sudden severe headache) can present primarily with cerebral ischemia due to vasospasm, emphasizing the need for a careful history and correct diagnosis in ischemic stroke before undertaking thrombolytic or anticoagulant therapy.[270]

Signs of symptomatic vasospasm are referable to the territory that has become ischemic and are most easily distinguished when they lateralize to a middle cerebral artery (MCA) territory with monoparesis or hemiparesis and, when the dominant hemisphere is affected, with dysphasia. Anterior cerebral artery vasospasm can be marked by leg weakness, but because it is often bilateral in distribution it is usually more noticeably associated with confusion, drowsiness, poverty of speech, and, eventually, abulia. Vertebrobasilar vasospasm can also cause a more generalized deterioration, with a reduced level of consciousness being an early sign.

Vasospastic ischemia can be difficult to detect in patients who remain in poor neurological condition after SAH. Head-injured patients with traumatic SAH are another group of patients in whom the clinical signs of ischemia may be obscured by the effects of the primary cerebral injury. The only clues of ischemia in these patients may be the failure to improve when expected or the appearance of a new cortical infarction on CT. Monitoring of patients with a significantly decreased level of consciousness with ancillary techniques may be particularly important.

Diagnosis

The diagnosis of symptomatic vasospasm requires that the other causes of delayed worsening mentioned earlier be ruled out with CT and appropriate clinical and laboratory examinations, that the neurological deficit be appropriate to the artery(ies) affected, and that the deficit onset is delayed. If vasospasm remains the probable cause of deterioration and appropriate treatment, such as induced hypertension, promptly reverses the deficit, then the diagnosis can be safely assumed without further testing. Failure to respond, however, or contemplation of invasive vasospasm reversal treatments usually requires corroboration of the clinical diagnosis with additional testing.

Transcranial Doppler

Introduced by Aaslid and colleagues in the 1980s, transcranial Doppler (TCD) works on the principle that as an artery narrows, blood flow velocity within it increases.[16] Because the examinations are noninvasive and at the bedside, and can be performed on a daily basis, TCD is frequently used to monitor post-SAH patients for increases in intracranial blood flow velocities suggestive of developing vasospasm.[271–279] The literature supports a good general correlation between TCD velocities and vasospasm,[280] with velocities in the MCA greater than 120 cm/s indicative of some degree of vasospasm and those greater than 200 cm/s consistent with severe vasospasm. Because other factors can influence velocities, including blood pressure and overall CBF, distinguishing vasospastic from hyperemic increases in MCA blood velocities has been reported to be facilitated by measuring the cervical internal carotid artery (ICA) velocities in addition to the intracranial blood velocities.[272] A "Lindegaard ratio" of Vmca/Vica greater than 3 is consistent with vasospasm (hyperemia is associated with increased velocities in both the MCA and ICA, so the ratio remains the same).

Despite the good overall correlation, a recent study that carefully correlated TCD velocities with not just the presence or absence of angiographic vasospasm but also its degree found that the clinical dependability of TCD (using predictive values and likelihood ratios) was limited.[280] The positive predictive value of velocities of more than 200 cm/s for clinically significant moderate to severe angiographic vasospasm was 87%, but that of lower velocities was only approximately 50%. The negative predictive value of velocities less than 120 cm/s was 94%, but that of higher velocities was approximately 75%. Only the likelihood ratios for velocities of less than 120 cm/s or greater than 200 cm/s were clinically useful in individual patients, and, overall, 57% of patients exhibited maximum velocities in the indeterminate range between 120 and 199 cm/s. Lindegaard ratios and daily trends did not improve the predictive value of TCD in that study. Transcranial color-coded ultrasonography, which allows visualization of the arteries and permits registration of angle-corrected flow velocities, may be more accurate than conventional TCD,[281] but calculation of predictive values for clinically significant vasospasm using this technique is needed for verification.

TCD is attractive because it is simple, noninvasive, and relatively inexpensive. It has a good overall correlation with the presence or absence of all degrees of vasospasm, but it is relatively inaccurate in the intermediate range into which at least one half SAH patients fall. Invasive treatment decisions should probably not be based on TCD measurements alone. It has not been shown that routine TCD monitoring significantly improves patient outcome, but it may be especially useful in the group of patients developing severe vasospasm in whom clinical testing is difficult, such as those who are being treated with pharmacologic muscle paralysis and patients in poor clinical neurological condition.

Cerebral Blood Flow Measurements, Magnetic Resonance Imaging, and Angiography

Both single photon emission computed tomography (SPECT)[282–284] and quantitative stable xenon-enhanced computed tomography (XeCT)[285, 286] have been used to detect cerebral ischemia due to vasospasm and guide SAH management. XeCT requires a motionless patient during the scan, during which they inhale gaseous 27% to 33% xenon in oxygen, which can result in agitation in some patients. Quantitative CBF information is displayed tomographically in conjunction with CT anatomy. A strong argument can be made for its use in certain confusing clinical situations, for example, the comatose patient with high TCD velocities in whom invasive anti-vasospasm treatment is being considered.

Diffusion- and perfusion-weighted magnetic resonance imaging is sensitive in detecting early ischemia (and certainly more sensitive than plain CT),[287] and magnetic resonance angiography[288] as well as CT angiography[289] can detect vasospasm (Fig. 109–6).

The most practical method of imaging cerebral vessels at this time remains cerebral angiography. Cerebral angiography is occasionally required to clarify the cause of neurological deterioration and will establish the diagnosis with certainty in those patients being considered for endovascular treatment of vasospasm. Vasospasm appears as a concentric narrowing that can be focal, segmental, or diffuse. It is commonly graded

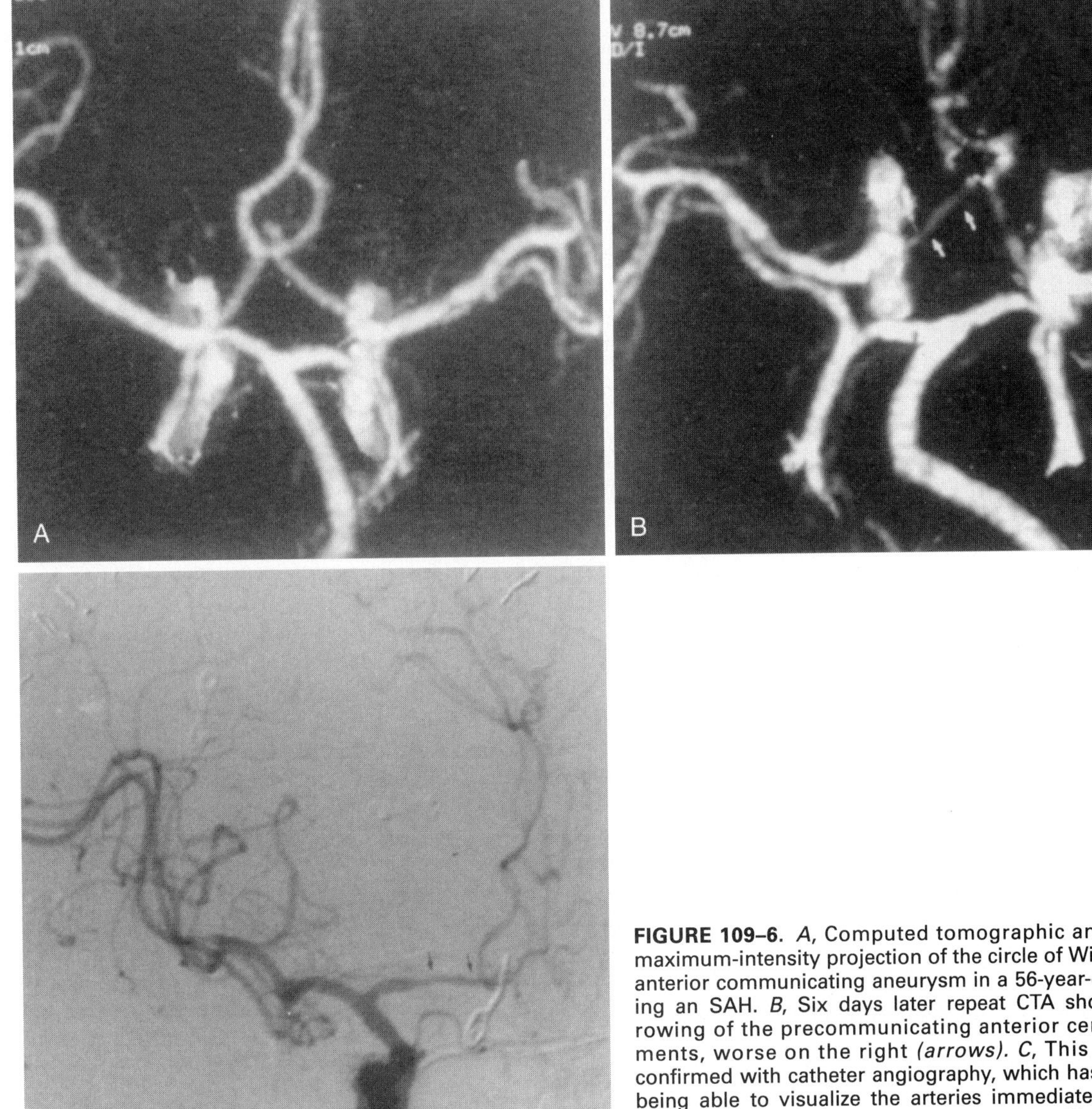

FIGURE 109–6. *A*, Computed tomographic angiography (CTA), maximum-intensity projection of the circle of Willis, shows a small anterior communicating aneurysm in a 56-year-old woman suffering an SAH. *B*, Six days later repeat CTA shows localized narrowing of the precommunicating anterior cerebral artery segments, worse on the right *(arrows)*. *C*, This observation was confirmed with catheter angiography, which has the advantage of being able to visualize the arteries immediately adjacent to the aneurysm clip. (Radiographs courtesy of Dr. Glenn Anderson, University of Alberta.)

as mild (<25%), moderate (25% to 50%), or severe (>50%).

VASOSPASM PREVENTION AND CEREBRAL PROTECTION

Fluid Management

The most important measure in preventing vasospastic ischemia is preventing post-SAH hypovolemia and anemia with adequate hydration and red blood cells and avoiding antihypertensive and antifibrinolytic drugs, because they, too, can aggravate ischemia.[290–292] Patients should receive at least 3 L of isotonic fluids daily because there is a tendency toward volume contraction after SAH, and the systemic blood pressure should be maintained in the high normotensive to slightly hypertensive range (120 to 160 mm Hg), providing the aneurysm has been repaired. Cerebral perfusion pressure (CPP) is a more important parameter to follow and maintain greater than 70 mm Hg in poor-grade patients with elevated intracranial pressure (ICP) that must be treated usually in part with ventricular drainage.[293] Deliberate, prophylactic hypervolemia has not been proven to reduce symptomatic ischemia and can precipitate cardiopulmonary decompensation in older patients and those with fragile cardiopulmonary systems. A reasonable approach to fluid management is to aim toward slight hypervolemia in postoperative patients in the prevasospastic interval (i.e., the first 4 days) and increase fluid administration as well as commence colloidal infusions in those patients who have an increase of TCD blood velocities (if this test is being performed) into the pathologic range greater than 200 cm/s. In such patients, a central venous line is advantageous.

Subarachnoid Blood Clot Removal and Lysis

Clinical,[294, 295] followed by experimental,[296, 297] evidence suggested that surgical removal of subarachnoid clot within several days of hemorrhage reduces vasospasm. Although this result was intuitive and appealing, the difficulty in accomplishing this at the time of aneurysm clipping led to the testing of fibrinolytic agents injected into the subarachnoid space to clear clot from around the arteries and prevent vasospasm.[298–300] The success of recombinant tissue-type plasminogen activator (rt-PA) in the primate model[301] led to a number of phase 1 clinical studies, which again suggested that subarachnoid clot thrombolysis reduced vasospasm.[302–306]

The only randomized controlled trial of cisternal fibrinolysis (using 10 mg rt-PA administered intraoperatively and intracisternally immediately after aneurysm clipping) showed that angiographic vasospasm (the primary end point of the trial) prevention was significant only in patients with thick, Fisher group 3 SAHs on CT (which was the target population).[50] This did not translate into a statistically significant improvement in clinical outcome in this relatively small study of 100 patients. Cisternal fibrinolysis, whether given intraoperatively or postoperatively via cisternal or ventricular catheters, appears to be effective in clearing the central basal cisterns and reducing proximal vasospasm particularly. Some use rt-PA in the situation of large volume SAHs, but only when it can be established with certainty that the aneurysm has been fully repaired (Fig. 109–7).

Calcium Channel Blockers

Nimodipine prevents intracellular calcium increases by blocking dihydropyridine-sensitive (L-type) calcium channels and in a series of randomized controlled trials has had a modest but statistically significant beneficial impact on clinical outcome after aneurysmal SAH.[17, 307–311] The largest and most compelling study was the British Aneurysm Nimodipine Trial (BRANT),[310] which recruited 554 patients of all grades to begin treatment within 96 hours of hemorrhage, consisting of either placebo or nimodipine 60 mg every 4 hours for 21 days. Cerebral infarction occurred in 22% of nimodipine-treated patients versus 33% of those who received placebo, and poor outcomes (death, vegetative state, and severe disability) were also significantly reduced in the nimodipine group: 20% versus 33% for placebo. A number of meta-analyses of the published data[312–315] have also concluded that nimodipine is efficacious (Fig. 109–8). The precise mechanism of nimodipine's effect is unknown, because it does not reduce angiographic vasospasm.[310] Other suggestions include neuronal protection, arteriolar vasodilation, and increased blood flow in the brain "microcirculation" and reduced platelet aggregation.[316]

The dosage of nimodipine is 60 mg every 4 hours by mouth or through a nasogastric tube (in North America the intravenous formulation is not available). Nimodipine can cause temporary depression of blood pressure, which can be problematic during hypertensive therapy for symptomatic vasospasm, and it must be given cautiously to patients with either congestive heart failure or hepatic insufficiency. It should be continued until either the time of discharge from the hospital in good condition or for 21 days, whichever comes first. The possible efficacy of nimodipine after traumatic SAH has already been mentioned.[28, 29]

Nicardipine is another dihydropyridine calcium antagonist, with virtually equivalent pharmacologic activity to nimodipine, but with the advantage of being available for study in an intravenous preparation, which can be more easily titrated in response to hypotension. Nicardipine was compared with placebo in a multicenter randomized trial of 906 patients and was associated with a decreased incidence of both clinical and moderate or severe angiographic vasospasm, each occurring in about one third of the nicardipine-treated patients and about one half of the placebo-treated patients.[317–318] Despite this, overall outcome did not differ between the two groups, and it was postulated that increased use of hypertensive/hypervolemic therapy in the placebo group prevented vasospasm from progressing to infarction, thus compensating for what was

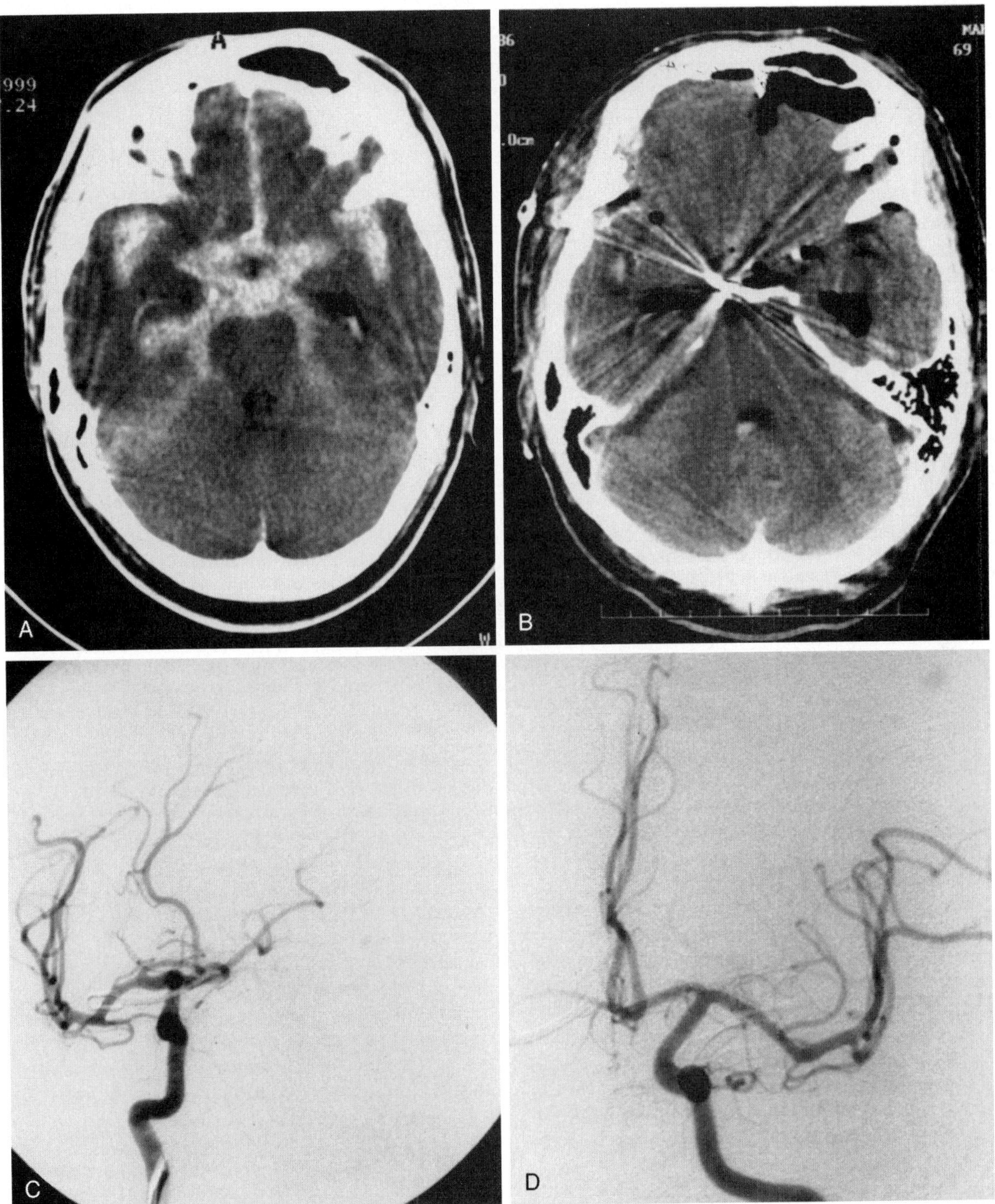

FIGURE 109–7. *A*, A 69-year-old man presented in poor neurological condition (grade IV) after a severe right posterior communicating artery aneurysm rupture and thick, diffuse SAH. *B*, At the time of aneurysm clipping 10 mg of rt-PA solution was injected into the basal cisterns, resulting in computed tomographic evidence of good subarachnoid clot clearance roughly 24 hours later (note air in subarachnoid space and ventricles). *C* and *D*, The patient's condition improved slowly over several weeks, and angiography 9 days from rupture showed little to no angiographic vasospasm (*C*, right internal carotid artery injection; *D*, left internal carotid artery injection).

not prevented by nicardipine in this patient group. Nicardipine has not subsequently been made available for clinical use.

Tirilazad Mesylate

The rationale and mechanism of action of the 21-aminosteroid tirilazad mesylate has been discussed previously in this chapter. Generally effective in animal studies,[199–205] this agent has been tested by its manufacturer in a series of multicenter randomized, controlled trials.[319–323] Tirilazad is already in use in a number of foreign countries, and it may become available in North America. Like nimodipine, tirilazad was developed to prevent cerebral vasospasm but may have

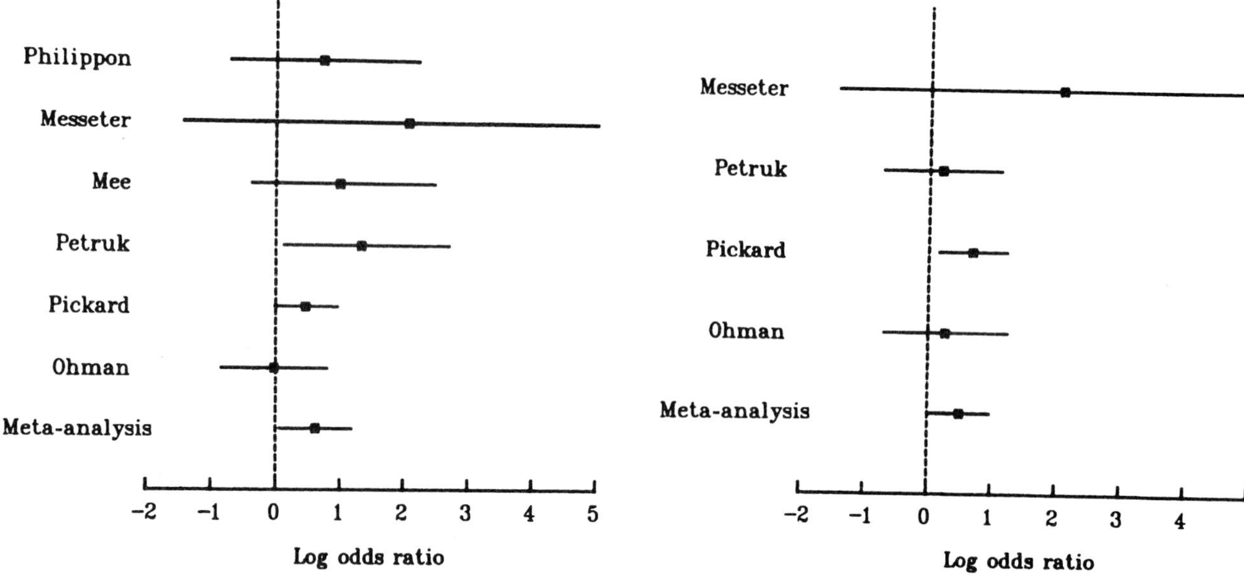

FIGURE 109–8. Charts displaying comparisons of results of trials testing the effects of prophylactic nimodipine. Horizontal lines depict results of analyses of raw data from individual studies. The central black square indicates the estimated treatment effect of nimodipine for each study, with 99% confidence intervals (CIs) shown by the extent of the horizontal lines. Where the line does not overlap the dotted vertical line at the origin, the study has shown a significant difference between nimodipine and placebo at the $P < .01$ level. *Left*, Chart showing the principal meta-analysis results (good versus all other outcomes). An advantage of nimodipine over placebo is indicated by a positive treatment effect (greater odds of good outcome in the treated group). The last line shows the treatment effect (odds ratio 1.86%) and 99% CI (1.07–3.25) for the meta-analysis. Nimodipine is favored over placebo ($P = .004$). *Right*, Chart showing the results of the meta-analysis of good plus fair versus all other outcomes. A positive treatment effect denotes greater chance of good or fair outcome with nimodipine treatment. The last line shows the treatment effect (odds ratio 1.67) and 99% CI (1.13–2.46) for the meta-analysis. Nimodipine is favored over placebo ($P = .0007$). (From Barker FG II, Ogilvy CS: Efficacy of prophylactic nimodipine for delayed ischemic deficit after subarachnoid hemorrhage: A meta-analysis. J Neurosurg 84:405–414, 1996.)

several sites of action in the central nervous system and appears to have no clearly significant effect on large artery vasospasm. Its clinical efficacy has not been entirely consistent and appears modest and only significant in poorer grade patients (Hunt and Hess grades 4 and 5). Higher dosages may be necessary in women, who appear to benefit less than men. The drug is given intravenously every 6 hours for 10 days after SAH, can be given safely with nimodipine, and appears to have very few side effects.

Other Preventative Treatments

Other drugs have been tested for vasospasm prevention include nizofenone, a possible neuroprotectant (effective in a controlled clinical trial[324]), high-dose methylprednisolone (effective in a cohort clinical trial[325]), vasodilator calcitonin gene-related peptide (CGRP) slow-release tablets given intrathecally (effective in a primate model[326]), the hydroxyl radical scavenger nicaraven (effective in a controlled clinical trial[327]), the combination inotrope and vasodilator drug milrinone (effective in a controlled dog study[328]), vasodilator papaverine slow-release pellets (effective intrathecally in a dog model[329]), the neuroprotectant ebselen (effective in a controlled clinical trial[330]), a variety of ET-1 inhibitors and antagonists (effective in the majority of animal models[245, 252-264]), and "prophylactic" balloon angioplasty (effective in a case series[331]). This is a far from comprehensive list, but it still emphasizes the breadth of ongoing research seeking a better way to prevent either vasospastic arterial narrowing or the ischemic damage it can cause (Table 109–5). The foregoing suggests a publication bias toward successful treatments, so the true measure of efficacy is often best determined

TABLE 109–5 ■ Strategies for Vasospasm or Cerebral Ischemia Prevention after Aneurysmal Subarachnoid Hemorrhage

Avoidance of hypovolemia, hypotension, antihypertensive and antifibrinolytic drugs, and raised intracranial pressure (prevents ischemia)
Subarachnoid clot removal or lysis with fibrinolytic agents (prevents vasospasm)
Calcium channel blockers and other potential calcium-based neuroprotectants (probably prevents ischemic damage)
21-Aminosteroids and other antioxidants, lipid peroxidation inhibitors, and free radical scavengers (probably prevents ischemic damage)
Intrathecally administered slow-release vasodilators (prevents vasospasm—experimental treatment)
Endothelin inhibitors and antagonists (prevents vasospasm—experimental treatment)

from the willingness to investigate a study drug more rigorously after a successful preliminary result.

VASOSPASM REVERSAL OR "RESCUE" TREATMENTS

Augmentation of CBF through and around vasospastic vessels by elevating systemic blood volume and pressure can reverse cerebral ischemia, and either pharmacologic or balloon dilatation of narrowed arteries can reverse vasospasm itself (Table 109–6). When and how these two "reversal" or "rescue" treatments should be implemented and combined is the subject of a great deal of variation and discussion and is an unsettled matter in the literature.

Induced Hypervolemia and Hypertension, "Hyperdynamic" or "Triple-H" Therapy

This refers to some combination of hypervolemia, hemodilution, and induced hypertension that is intended to improve cardiac output, optimize hemorheology for oxygen transport, and increase CPP, respectively. There is considerable variation on how to achieve and monitor these hemodynamic goals.[12, 332–336] A degree of hemodilution accompanies any deliberate intravascular volume expansion, and reduced viscosity may in fact contribute to an improvement in oxygen delivery providing the hematocrit (i.e., the oxygen-carrying capacity) does not fall below 30 to 35 and the hemoglobin concentration is kept over 10 g/dL.[336, 337]

Although now widely accepted as being important, if not essential, treatment for symptomatic vasospasm, the use of "triple-H" therapy has never been confirmed in a randomized or even nonrandomized trial. Given its apparent efficacy, however, it is unlikely that this treatment will ever be withheld in a randomized study.

A common way of commencing hyperdynamic therapy is to quickly treat newly recognized symptomatic vasospasm with additional volume expansion with an isotonic crystalloid infusion supplemented with a colloid. The colloid chosen is usually albumin because there is both experimental and clinical evidence that this is beneficial under these circumstances.[338, 339] A replete intravascular volume, beyond which additional expansion is probably of no further benefit, is central venous pressure between 8 and 10 mm Hg or pulmonary capillary wedge pressure in the range of 14 to 16 mm Hg.

Providing the ruptured aneurysm has been repaired, symptomatic vasospasm should also be treated with induced hypertension. This is often sought first with administration of either dobutamine or dopamine, which at low-to-moderate doses have mainly beta-agonist, inotropic effects. Blood pressure rises with elevations in cardiac output, which increases the CPP. If inotrope fails to reverse symptoms within 1 to 2 hours, and especially if the blood pressure has failed to respond (i.e., to dopamine at 10–15 μg/kg/min), more purely alpha-agonist vasopressor, such as either phenylephrine (titrated to maximal dose of 180 μg/min) or norepinephrine (titrated to maximal dose of 20 μg/min) or their combination, should be added. A systolic blood pressure of 200 to 220 mm Hg is sometimes required to reverse ischemic symptoms and is generally safe, providing the ruptured aneurysm is repaired and the patient does not have underlying heart disease.

The significant risks of hypervolemic, hypertensive therapy are cardiac failure and infarction, pulmonary edema, the complications of central vein or pulmonary artery catheter placement, and possibly cerebral edema and a type of hypertensive encephalopathy.[340–342] Cardiopulmonary risks of hypervolemia and hypertension are considerable in the elderly and in those patients with either congestive heart failure or chronic lung disease.

TABLE 109–6 ■ Strategies for Vasospasm and/or Cerebral Ischemia Reversal after Aneurysmal Subarachnoid Hemorrhage

Hypervolemia, hemodilution, and hypertension (reverses ischemia)
Intra-arterial papaverine administration (reverses vasospasm)
Percutaneous transluminal balloon angioplasty (reverses vasospasm)
Intraventricular nitroprusside (reverses vasospasm—experimental)

Intra-aortic Balloon Counterpulsation

There have been several reports on the use of intra-aortic balloon counterpulsation treatment for patients with symptomatic vasospasm and concomitant heart failure refractory to hypervolemic, hypertensive therapy,[343, 344] which was based on some previous experimental work in dogs.[345] In the patients described, both cardiac and cerebral function were improved and this treatment is an option for the rare critically ill patient with this combination of problems. However, in such patients endovascular treatment of vasospasm (discussion to follow) would have to be considered as well.

Endovascular Reversal of Vasospasm

If hemodynamic goals of hypervolemic, hypertensive therapy are not easily met in a patient with persistent symptoms of cerebral ischemia, or if symptoms do not reverse within several hours of induced hypertension into the desired range, or if the patient has a fragile cardiopulmonary status, it is now a widespread practice to proceed directly to endovascular treatment of vasospasm, providing it is available at the treating institution. Endovascular therapy might also be preferred over extreme hypertensive treatment in any patient possessing additional unruptured and unrepaired aneurysms. An important caveat is that prior to endovascular therapy the presence of a large cerebral infarct should be ruled out with CT, since dilation therapy would be both unsuccessful and dangerous if it augmented perfusion into newly infarcted brain. CBF studies might be particularly helpful in this circumstance.

Intra-arterial Papaverine for Vasospasm

There has been experimental interest in intrathecally administered papaverine to reverse vasospasm for some time (the drug administered to the abluminal surface of the vessel),[329, 346–348] but it was first reported to be effective in reversing angiographic vasospasm in humans when administered intra-arterially in 1992.[349, 350] Superselective intra-arterial papaverine infusions (200 to 400 mg over 30 minutes) are relatively easy to administer, but "chemical" or pharmacologic reversibility of chronic vasospasm is variable; and when it does occur, it is usually partial.[351, 352] In addition, the vasorelaxation is relatively short lived, with vasospasm usually recurring within 24 hours[353, 354] (Fig. 109–9). Although it can clearly dilate some vasospastic vessels and at least transiently improve CBF to the distal parenchyma, its efficacy in improving patient outcome has not been established.[355–357] Notably, intra-arterial papaverine can cause transient ipsilateral pupillary dilatation (as it can when given intracisternally[358]), transient elevations in ICP,[359] and severe but reversible thrombocytopenia.[360] The greatest drawback for this treatment is that the effect, when it occurs, is transient (which is what one would expect), whereas vasospasm lasts days and sometimes weeks.

Percutaneous Transluminal Balloon Angioplasty for Vasospasm

First used in Russia in the 1980s,[19] this technique has now gained widespread acceptance around the world.[361–368] Specially trained interventional radiologists are able to dilate all of the proximal major cerebral arteries, and the angiographic response is immediate and appears to be durable. Owing to the sharp angle of the anterior cerebral artery origin from the internal carotid artery, this vessel is difficult to catheterize and dilate, although an "over-the-wire" navigation system has been developed to overcome this problem.[369] Second- and third-order branches are not generally dilatable owing to their smaller size, although dilatation of proximal arteries is sometimes sufficient to improve flow into these vessels, especially with continued hypertensive treatment.

Like hypervolemic, hypertensive treatment, balloon angioplasty has not been proven to result in better outcomes when vasospasm complicates SAH, but the evidence suggests that it can help individual patients, even dramatically, on occasion. Published series from experienced neurovascular teams suggest that an angiographic result is uniform: providing the balloon can reach the affected artery, early symptomatic improvement is seen in one half to two thirds of patients selected for treatment (failure to improve presumably due to established infarction at the time of the procedure), and complications such as vessel rupture and

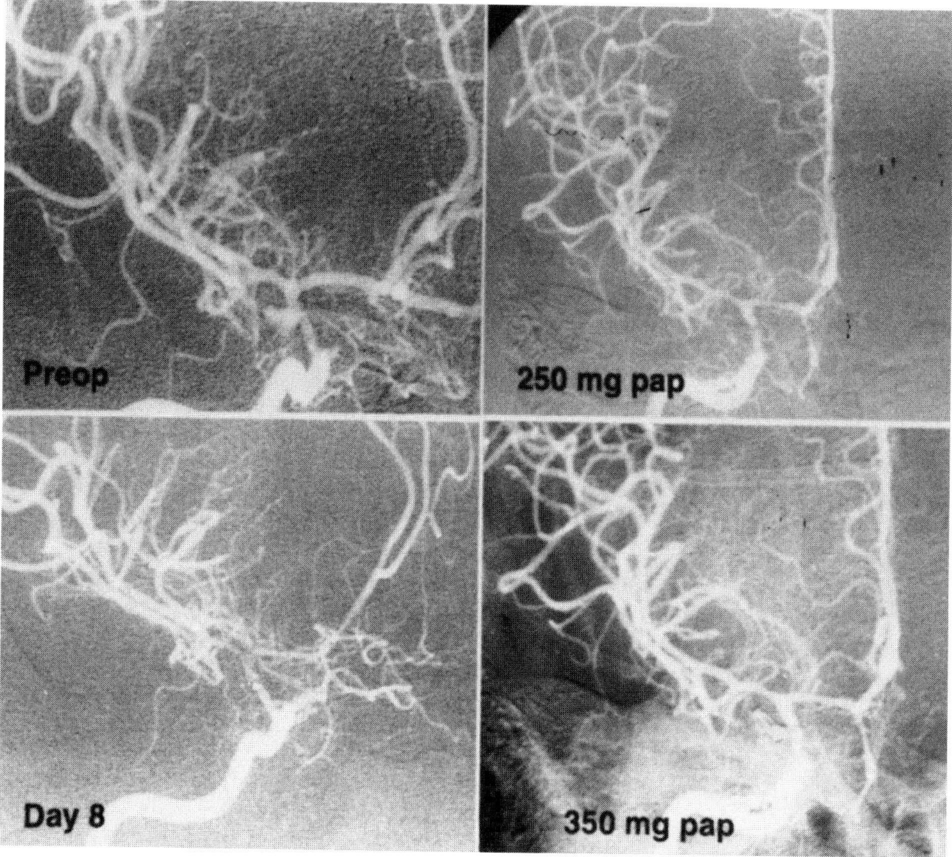

FIGURE 109–9. Eight days after rupture of a right posterior communicating artery aneurysm *(upper left)* severe angiographic vasospasm *(lower left)* responded partially to 250 mg of intra-arterially administered papaverine solution *(upper right)*, and more fully to 350 mg *(lower right)*. The following day the patient's condition was unimproved, and repeat angiography showed recurrent, severe vasospasm (not shown).

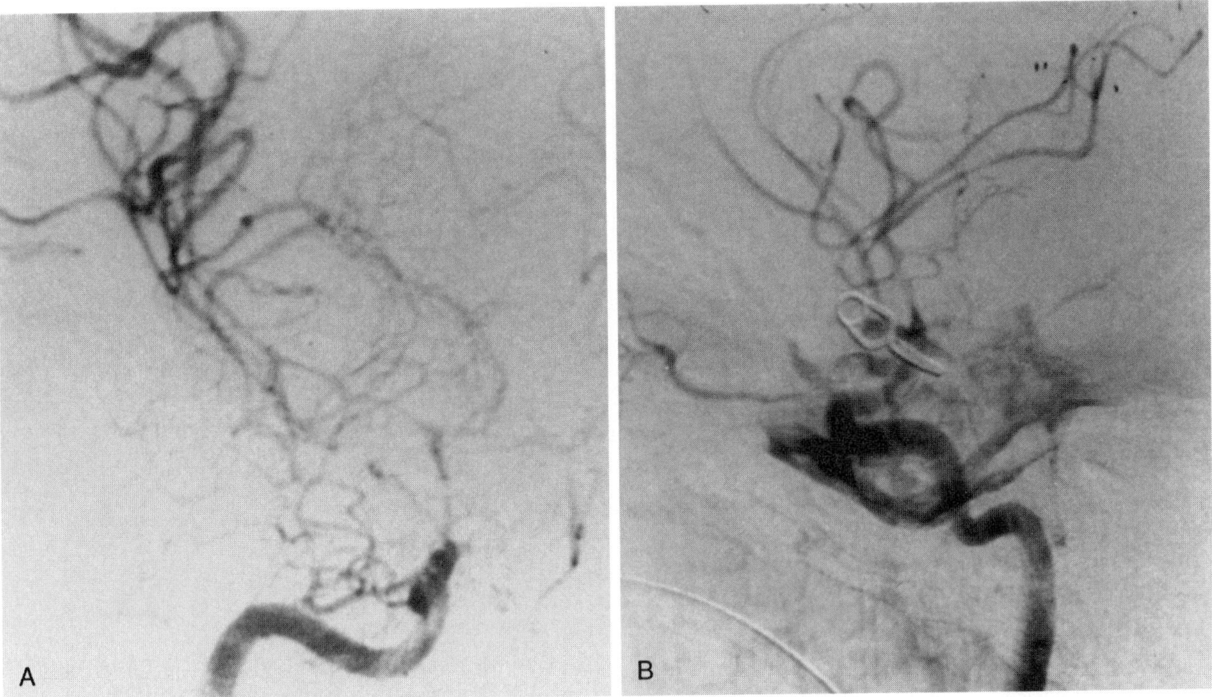

FIGURE 109–10. Early in my experience with transluminal balloon angioplasty, overdilatation of severe, symptomatic right internal carotid artery vasospasm *(A)* resulted in vessel rupture *(B)* and the patient's death.

occlusion are rare, in the order of several percent[361–368] (Fig. 109–10). The results of balloon angioplasty are best when it is performed within several hours of deficit onset[368] and earlier in the course of angiographic vasospasm when the vessels are less stiff.[366] Dilatation proximal to an infarcted territory should be avoided, as should angioplasty proximal to an unrepaired ruptured aneurysm unless it is going to be treated immediately with surgery or coiling.[366]

In vitro and in vivo experiments in dogs suggest that angioplasty results in arterial stretching with an immediate and profound functional impairment in vascular smooth muscle,[75, 76] and a time-course study demonstrated that this impairment lasted 2 to 3 weeks after angioplasty of vasospastic vessels, with morphologic alterations that had mostly resolved over the same time.[77] In normal vessels, angioplasty causes functional impairment and morphologic alterations that are not as severe or as long lasting as those seen in vasospastic arteries.

As experience with balloon angioplasty increases, there has become an increased tendency in many units to perform angioplasty earlier in the course of vasospasm, before extreme or exhaustive hypertensive therapy when infarction is imminent and the procedure more hazardous. Many also recommend dilatation of accessible but asymptomatic vasospastic vessels after dilatation of the symptomatic arteries (Fig. 109–11).

Other Reversal Therapies for Vasospasm

Once again the list of agents tested for the reversal of established vasospasm is too great for a comprehensive review, but intravenous CGRP was unsuccessful in a small clinical trial,[370] whereas intraventricular sodium nitroprusside has been reported effective in a growing series of patients from one center.[371, 372] In an interesting series of experiments, pulse-dye laser, delivered via an endovascular catheter, was shown to reverse vasospasm.[373–375] Intracisternally administered papaverine will likely receive greater attention in the future, although it has not, in my small and unpublished experience, had any angiographic effect on severe vasospasm.

Approach to the Prevention and Treatment of Cerebral Vasospasm

Whenever possible, I prefer early surgery or endovascular occlusion of ruptured aneurysms; and for patients with thick, diffuse subarachnoid clots (usually patients in poorer neurological condition) at high risk for severe angiographic vasospasm, my first choice is surgical clipping with intraoperative administration of 5 to 10 mg of rt-PA for subarachnoid clot lysis. Intraoperative inspection or angiography must first make completely certain that the aneurysm is completely repaired before intracisternal fibrinolysis. If good overnight clot lysis is obtained, the patient is at low risk for significant, proximal (circle of Willis) vasospasm.

Patients are kept well hydrated with isotonic crystalloid and intermittent albumin infusions (at least 3 L/day altogether), ICPs are kept normal, often facilitated by ventricular drainage (which I am liberal with), and CPPs are optimized for approximately 14 days (Fig. 109–12). I monitor daily with transcranial Doppler, but only velocities over 200 cm/s are considered

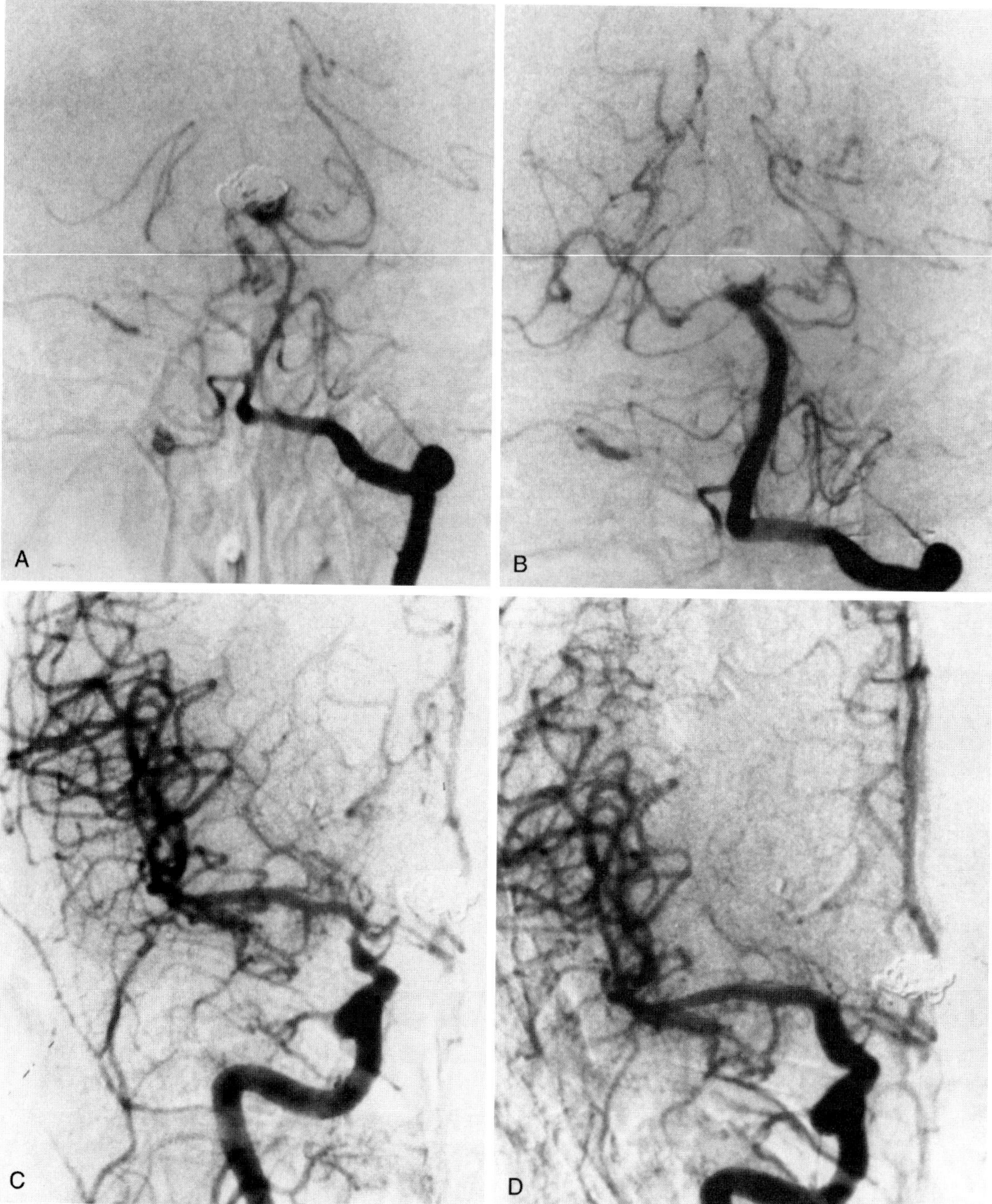

FIGURE 109–11. *A*, Severe basilar artery vasospasm resulted in a marked deterioration in consciousness in a 36-year-old woman with a ruptured and partially coiled, basilar tip aneurysm. *B*, Transluminal balloon angioplasty resulted in marked angiographic and clinical responses. As well, more moderate and localized vasospasm of the right internal carotid artery, believed to be asymptomatic at the time *(C)*, was treated successfully *(D)* during the same session. The patient went on to make a full clinical recovery, has undergone further aneurysm coiling, and is being followed for a small aneurysm remnant. There has been no subsequent evidence of arterial renarrowing over time. (Angiograms courtesy of Dr. David Pelz, Department of Radiology, University of Western Ontario.)

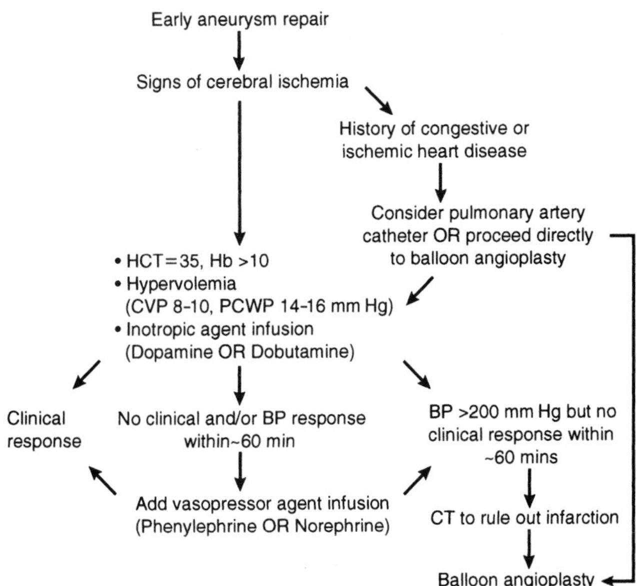

FIGURE 109–12. Algorithm for the management of symptomatic cerebral vasospasm. HCT, hematocrit; Hb, hemoglobin; CVP, central venous pressure; BP, blood pressure, CT, computed tomography.

likely indicative of significant vasospasm: values between 120 and 200 cm/s are not helpful. Clinical observation is most important. All patients with aneurysmal SAH receive nimodipine.

Symptomatic vasospasm is managed with extra volume administration and inotrope, followed by vasopressor infusion; but if the patient does not respond quickly and completely to these measures with reversal of neurological deficits or an increase in blood pressure into the target range, or if the patient has a fragile cardiopulmonary status, I will move quickly to endovascular treatment with balloon angioplasty. Intra-arterial papaverine is occasionally administered for distal vasospasm, unreachable with standard balloon catheters, although its effect, when seen, is recognized to be transient. In general, I prefer not to wait until "medical" treatment of symptomatic vasospasm has utterly failed over many hours before opting for endovascular treatment, because under those circumstances balloon angioplasty is more often inconvenient, dangerous, and unsuccessful.

If the health regulatory agency approves the use of tirilazad mesylate in this country I will prescribe it for those poor-grade (IV) patients selected for active treatment.

In the future it is anticipated that better vasospasm prevention will be possible, likely through combined treatments because of the complexity of the vasospastic process. Unless a safer and more complete means of subarachnoid clot removal can be discovered, methods of neutralizing clot effects will be pursued. Because rescue treatment with hypervolemia, hypertension, and angioplasty is effective in reversing ischemia and preventing vasospasm-related morbidity and mortality, it is difficult to establish outcome efficacy with new preventative strategies. As in animal studies, arterial narrowing is a simpler and more practical end point for prevention trials in humans.

ACKNOWLEDGMENT

The author would like to thank Ms. Laurie Arneson for expert assistance in the preparation of this chapter.

REFERENCES

1. Ecker A, Riemenschneider PA: Arteriographic demonstration of spasm of the intracranial arteries: With special reference to saccular arterial aneurysm. J Neurosurg 8:660–667, 1951.
2. Pool JL: Cerebral vasospasm. N Engl J Med 259:1259–1264, 1958.
3. Fletcher TM, Taveras JM, Pool JL: Cerebral vasospasm in angiography for intracranial aneurysm: Incidence and significance in one hundred consecutive angiograms. Arch Neurol 1:38–47, 1959.
4. Maspes PE, Marini G: Intracranial arterial spasm related to supraclinoid ruptured aneurysms. Acta Neurochir 10:630–638, 1962.
5. Du Boulay G: Distribution of spasm in the intracranial arteries after subarachnoid haemorrhage. Acta Radiol Diagn 1:257–266, 1963.
6. Allcock JM, Drake CG: Ruptured intracranial aneurysm—the role of arterial spasm. J Neurosurg 22:21–29, 1965.
7. Wilkins RH, Alexander JA, Odom GL: Intracranial arterial spasm: A clinical analysis. J Neurosurg 29:121–134, 1968.
8. Wilkins RH: Attempts at treatment of intracranial arterial spasm in animals and human beings. Surg Neurol 1:148–159, 1973.
9. Kosnik EJ, Hunt WE: Postoperative hypertension in the management of patients with intracranial arterial aneurysms. J Neurosurg 45:148–154, 1976.
10. Giannotta SL, McGillicuddy JE, Kindt GW: Diagnosis and treatment of postoperative cerebral vasospasm. Surg Neurol 8:286–290, 1977.
11. Farhat SM, Schneider RC: Observations on the effect of systemic blood pressure on intracranial circulation in patients with cerebrovascular insufficiency. J Neurosurg 27:441–445, 1967.
12. Kassell NF, Peerless SJ, Durward QJ, et al: Treatment of ischemic deficits from vasospasm with intravascular volume expansion and induced arterial hypertension. Neurosurgery 11:337–343, 1982.
13. Astrup J, Symon L, Branston NM, Lassen NA: Cortical evoked potential and extracellular K^+ and H^+ at critical levels of brain ischemia. Stroke 8:51–57, 1977.
14. Astrup J: Thresholds in cerebral ischemia—the ischemic penumbra. Stroke 12:723, 1981.
15. Fisher CM, Kistler JP, Davis JM: Relation of cerebral vasospasm to subarachnoid hemorrhage visualized by computerized tomographic scanning. Neurosurgery 6:1–9, 1980.
16. Aaslid R, Huber P. Nornes H: Evaluation of cerebrovascular spasm with transcranial Doppler ultrasound. J Neurosurg 60: 37–41, 1984.
17. Allen GS, Ahn HS, Preziosi TJ, et al: Cerebral arterial spasm—a controlled trial of nimodipine in patients with subarachnoid hemorrhage. N Engl J Med 308:619–624, 1983.
18. Robinson MJ, Teasdale GM: Calcium antagonists in the management of subarachnoid haemorrhage. Cerebrovasc Brain Metab Rev 2:205–226, 1990.
19. Zubkov YN, Nikiforov BM, Shustin VA: Balloon catheter technique for dilatation of constricted cerebral arteries after aneurysmal SAH. Acta Neurochir (Wien) 70:65–79, 1984.
20. Weber M, Grolimund P, Seiler RW: Evaluation of posttraumatic cerebral blood flow velocities by transcranial Doppler ultrasonography. Neurosurgery 27:106–112, 1990.
21. Gomez CR, Backer RJ, Bucholz RD: Transcranial Doppler ultrasound following closed head injury: Vasospasm or vasoparalysis? Surg Neurol 35:30–35, 1991.
22. Martin NA, Doberstein C, Zane C, et al: Posttraumatic cerebral arterial spasm: Transcranial Doppler ultrasound, cerebral blood flow, and angiographic findings. J Neurosurg 77:575–583, 1992.
23. Taneda M, Kataoka K, Akai F, et al: Traumatic subarachnoid

hemorrhage as a predictable indicator of delayed ischemic symptoms. J Neurosurg 84:762–768, 1996.

24. Martin NA, Patwardhan RV, Alexander MJ, et al: Characterization of cerebral hemodynamic phases following severe head trauma: Hypoperfusion, hyperemia, and vasospasm. J Neurosurg 87:9–19, 1997.
25. Lee JH, Martin NA, Alsina G, et al: Hemodynamically significant cerebral vasospasm and outcome after head injury: A prospective study. J Neurosurg 87:221–233, 1997.
26. Fukuda T, Hasue M, Ito H: Does traumatic subarachnoid hemorrhage caused by diffuse brain injury cause delayed ischemic brain damage? Comparison with subarachnoid hemorrhage caused by ruptured intracranial aneurysms. Neurosurgery 43: 1040–1049, 1998.
27. Greene KA, Marciano FF, Johnson BA, et al: Impact of traumatic subarachnoid hemorrhage on outcome in nonpenetrating head injury: I. A proposed computerized tomography grading scale. J Neurosurg 83:445–452, 1995.
28. The European Study Group on Nimodipine in Severe Head Injury, Department of Neurosurgery, University Hospital Dijkzigt, Erasmus University Rotterdam, Rotterdam, The Netherlands; and Central Data Office, Biometric Department, Bayer Pharamceutical Research Centre, Wuppertal, Germany: A multicenter trial of the efficacy of nimodipine on outcome after severe head injury. J Neurosurg 80:797–804, 1994.
29. Harders A, Kakarieka A, Braakman R, and the German tSAH Study Group: Traumatic subarachnoid hemorrhage and its treatment with nimodipine. J Neurosurg 85:82–89, 1996.
30. Nishimura K, Hawkins TD: Cerebral vasospasm with subarachnoid haemorrahge from arteriovenous malformations of the brain. Neuroradiology 8:201–207, 1975.
31. Sasaki T, Mayanagi Y, Yano K: Cerebral vasospasm with subarachnoid hemorrhage from cerebral arteriovenous malformations. Surg Neurol 16:183–187, 1981.
32. Yanaka K, Hyodo A, Tsuchida Y, et al: Symptomatic cerebral vasospasm after intraventricular hemorrhage from ruptured arteriovenous malformation. Surg Neurol 38:63–67, 1992.
33. Maeda K, Kurita H, Nakamura T, et al: Occurrence of severe vasospasm following intraventricular hemorrhage from an arteriovenous malformation. J Neurosurg 87:436–439, 1997.
34. Grady MS, Cooper GW, Kassell NF, Login IS: Profound cerebral vasospasm without radiological evidence of subarachnoid hemorrhage: Case report. Neurosurgery 18:653–659, 1986.
35. Mawk JR, Ausman JI, Erickson DL, Maxwell RE: Vasospasm following transcranial removal of large pituitary adenomas: Report of three cases. J Neurosurg 50:229–232, 1979.
36. Machado de Almeida G, Bianco E, Souza AS: Vasospasm after acoustic neuroma removal. Surg Neurol 23:38–40, 1985.
37. LeRoux PD, Haglund MM, Mayberg MR, Winn HR: Symptomatic cerebral vasospasm following tumor resection: Report of two cases. Surg Neurol 36:25–31, 1991.
38. Raynor RB, Messer HD: Severe vasospasm with an unruptured aneurysm: Case report. Neurosurgery 6:92–95, 1980.
39. Bloomfield SM, Sonntag VKH: Delayed cerebral vasospasm after uncomplicated operation on an unruptured aneurysm: Case report. Neurosurgery 17:792–796, 1985.
40. Dorsch NWC, King MT: A review of cerebral vasospasm in aneurysmal subarachnoid haemorrhage: I. Incidence and effects. J Clin Neuroscience 1:19–26, 1994.
41. Weir B, Grace M, Hansen J, Rothberg C: Time course of vasospasm in man. J Neurosurg 48:173–178, 1978.
42. Qureshi AI, Sung GY, Suri MAK, et al: Prognostic value and determinants of ultra-early angiographic vasospasm after aneurysmal subarachnoid hemorrhage. Neurosurgery 44:967–974, 1999.
43. Bell BA, Kendall BE, Symon L: Computed tomography in aneurysmal subarachnoid haemorrhage. J Neurol Neurosurg Psychiatry 43:522–524, 1980.
44. Davis JM, Davis KR, Crowell RM: Subarachnoid hemorrhage secondary to ruptured intracranial aneurysm: Prognostic significance of cranial CT. AJNR Am J Neuroradiol 1:17–21, 1980.
45. Mizukami M, Takemae T, Tazawa T, et al: Value of computed tomography in the prediction of cerebral vasospasm after aneurysm rupture. Neurosurgery 7:583–586, 1980.
46. Suzuki J, Komatsu S, Sato T, Sakurai Y: Correlation between CT findings and subsequent development of cerebral infarction due to vasospasm in subarachnoid haemorrhage. Acta Neurochir (Wien) 55:63–70, 1980.
47. Sano H, Kanno T, Shinomiya Y, et al: Prospection of chronic vasospasm by CT findings. Acta Neurochir (Wien) 63:23–30, 1982.
48. Pasqualin A, Da Pian R: An analysis of vasospasm following early surgery for intracranial aneurysms. Acta Neurochir (Wien) 63:153–159, 1982.
49. Kistler JP, Crowell RM, Davis KR, et al: The relation of cerebral vasospasm to the extent and location of subarachnoid blood visualized by CT scan: A prospective study. Neurology (NY) 33:424–436, 1983.
50. Findlay JM, Kassell NF, Weir BKA, et al: A randomized trial of intraoperative, intracisternal tissue plasminogen activator for the prevention of vasospasm. Neurosurgery 37:168–178, 1995.
51. Rabb CH, Tang G, Chin LS, Giannotta SL: A statistical analysis of factors related to symptomatic cerebral vasospasm. Acta Neurochir (Wien) 127:27–31, 1994.
52. Lasner TM, Weil RJ, Riina HA, et al: Cigarette smoking–induced increase in the risk of symptomatic vasospasm after aneurysmal subarachnoid hemorrhage. J Neurosurg 87:381–384, 1997.
53. Weir BKA, Kongable GL, Kassell NF, et al: Cigarette smoking as a cause of aneurysmal subarachnoid hemorrhage and risk for vasospasm: A report of the Cooperative Aneurysm Study. J Neurosurg 89:405–411, 1998.
54. Inagawa T: Cerebral vasospasm in elderly patients with ruptured intracranial aneurysms. Surg Neurol 36:91–98, 1991.
55. Lanzino G, Kassell NF, Germanson TP, et al: Age and outcome after aneurysmal subarachnoid hemorrhage: Why do older patients fare worse? J Neurosurg 85:410–418, 1996.
56. Tatter SB, Crowell RM, Ogilvy CS: Aneurysmal and microaneurysmal "angiogram-negative" subarachnoid hemorrhage. Neurosurgery 37:48–55, 1995.
57. Rinkel GJE, Wijdicks EFM, Vermeulen M, et al: The clinical course of perimesencephalic non-aneurysmal subarachnoid hemorrhage. Ann Neurol 29:463–468, 1991.
58. Schwartz TH, Solomon RA: Perimesencephalic nonaneurysmal subarachnoid hemorrhage: Review of the literature. Neurosurgery 39:433–440, 1996.
59. Lougheed WM: Selection, timing and technique of aneurysm surgery of the anterior circle of Willis. Clin Neurosurg 16: 95–113, 1968.
60. Sundt TM Jr: Cerebral vasospasm following aneurysmal subarachnoid hemorrhage: Evolution, management, and relationship to timing of surgery. Clin Neurosurg 24:228–239, 1977.
61. Drake CG: On the surgical treatment of intracranial aneurysms. Ann R Coll Phys Sur Can 11:185–195, 1978.
62. Öhman J, Heiskanen O: Timing of operation for ruptured supratentorial aneurysms: A prospective randomized study. J Neurosurg 70:55–60, 1989.
63. Kassell NF, Torner JC, Jane JA, et al: The International Cooperative Study on the timing of aneurysm surgery: II. Surgical results. J Neurosurg 73:37–47, 1990.
64. Findlay JM, Macdonald RL, Weir BKA, Grace MGA: Surgical manipulation of primate cerebral arteries in established vasospasm. J Neurosurg 75:425–432, 1991.
65. Macdonald RL, Wallace MC, Coyne TJ: The effect of surgery on the severity of vasospasm. J Neurosurg 80:433–439, 1994.
66. Gruber A, Ungersböck K, Reinprecht A, et al: Evaluation of cerebral vasospasm after early surgical and endovascular treatment of ruptured intracranial aneurysms. Neurosurgery 42:258–268, 1998.
67. Heros RC, Zervas NT, Varsos V: Cerebral vasospasm after subarachnoid hemorrhage: An update. Ann Neurol 14:599–608, 1983.
68. Hijdra A, Braakman R, van Gijn J, et al: Aneurysmal subarachnoid hemorrhage: Complications and outcome in a hospital population. Stroke 18:1061–1067, 1987.
69. Kassell NF, Torner JC, Haley EC Jr, et al: The international cooperative study on the timing of aneurysm surgery: I. Overall management results. J Neurosurg 73:18–36, 1990.
70. Säveland H, Hillman J, Brandt L, et al: Overall outcome in aneurysmal subarachnoid hemorrhage. J Neurosurg 76:729–734, 1992.

71. Haley EC Jr, Kassell NF, Torner JC, and Participants: The International Cooperative Study on the timing of aneurysm surgery: The North American experience. Stroke 23:205–214, 1992.
72. Broderick JP, Brott TG, Duldner JE, et al: Initial and recurrent bleeding are the major causes of death following subarachnoid hemorrhage. Stroke 25:1342–1347, 1994.
73. Proust F, Hannequin D, Langlois O, et al: Causes of morbidity and mortality after ruptured aneurysm surgery in a series of 230 patients: The importance of control angiography. Stroke 26: 1553–1557, 1995.
74. Findlay JM, Deagle GM: Causes of morbidity and mortality following intracranial aneurysm rupture. Can J Neurol Sci 25: 209–215, 1998.
75. Chan PDS, Findlay JM, Vollrath B, et al: Pharmacological and morphological effects of in vitro transluminal balloon angioplasty on normal and vasospastic canine basilar arteries. J Neurosurg 83:522–530, 1995.
76. Megyesi JF, Findlay JM, Vollrath B, et al: In vivo angioplasty prevents the development of vasospasm in canine carotid arteries: Pharmacological and morphological analyses. Stroke 28: 1216–1224, 1997.
77. Megyesi JF, Vollrath B, Cook DA, et al: Long-term effects of in vivo angioplasty in normal and vasospastic canine carotid arteries: Pharmacological and morphological analyses. J Neurosurg 91:100–108, 1999.
78. Delgado TJ, Brismar J, Svendgaard NA: Subarachnoid haemorrhage in the rat: Angiography and fluorescence microscopy of the major cerebral arteries. Stroke 16:595–602, 1985.
79. Solomon RA, Antunes JL, Chen RYZ, et al: Decrease in cerebral blood flow in rats after experimental subarachnoid hemorrhage: A new animal model. Stroke 16:58–64, 1985.
80. Takahashi S, Kassell NF, Toshima M, et al: Effect of U88999E on experimental cerebral vasospasm in rabbits. Neurosurgery 32: 281–288, 1993.
81. Mahaley MS, Kapp J: The effect of Isordil and Cyclospasmol on vascular spasm induced in the basilar artery of the cat. Stroke 1:325–329, 1970.
82. Duff TA, Louie J, Feilbach JA, Scott G: Erythrocytes are essential for development of cerebral vasculopathy resulting from subarachnoid hemorrhage in cats. Stroke 19:68–72, 1988.
83. Takemae T, Branson J, Alksne JF: Intimal proliferation of cerebral arteries after subarachnoid blood injection in pigs. J Neurosurg 61:494–500, 1984.
84. Mayberg MR, Okada T, Bark DH: The significance of morphological changes in cerebral arteries after subarachnoid hemorrhage. J Neurosurg 72:626–633, 1990.
85. Kuwayama A, Zervas NT, Belson R, et al: A model of experimental cerebral arterial spasm. Stroke 3:49–56, 1972.
86. Varsos VG, Liszczak TM, Han DH, et al: Delayed cerebral vasospasm is not reversible by aminophylline, nifedipine, or papaverine in a "two-hemorrhage" canine model. J Neurosurg 58:11–17, 1983.
87. Frazee JG: A primate model of chronic cerebral vasospasm. Stroke 13:612–614, 1982.
88. Espinosa F, Weir B, Overton T, et al: A randomized placebo-controlled double-blind trial of nimodipine after SAH in monkeys: I. Clinical and radiologic findings. J Neurosurg 60:1167–1175, 1984.
89. Clower BR, Smith RR, Haining JL, Lockard J: Constrictive endarteropathy following experimental subarachnoid hemorrhage. Stroke 12:501–508, 1981.
90. Simeone FA, Trepper PJ, Brown DJ: Cerebral blood flow evaluation of prolonged experimental vasospasm. J Neurosurg 37: 302–311, 1972.
91. Boullin DJ, Hunt TM, Rogers AT: Models for investigating the aetiology of cerebral arterial spasm: Comparative responses of the human basilar artery with rat colon, anococcygeus, stomach fundus, and aorta and guinea-pig ileum and colon. Br J Pharmacol 63:251–257, 1978.
92. Dahl E: Microscopic observations on cerebral arteries. In Cervos-Navarro J (ed): The Cerebral Wall. New York, Raven Press, 1976, pp 15–21.
93. Edvinsson L: The blood vessel wall: Endothelial and smooth muscle cells. In Edvinsson L (ed): Cerebral Blood Flow and Metabolism. New York, Raven Press, 1993, pp 40–56.
94. Rhodin JAG: Architecture of the vessel wall. In Bohr DF, Somlyo AP, Sparks HV (eds): Handbook of Physiology, section 2, vol 2. Philadelphia, WB Saunders, 1980, pp 1–31.
95. Vanhoutte PM, Katuši ZS, Shepherd JT: Vasopressin induces endothelium-dependent relaxations of cerebral and coronary, but not of systemic arteries. J Hypertens 2(Suppl 3):421–422, 1984.
96. Pickard JD, Walker V, Perry S, et al: Arterial eicosanoid production following chronic exposure to a periarterial haematoma. J Neurol Neurosurg Psychiatry 47:661–667, 1984.
97. Macdonald RL, Wallace MC, Montanera WJ, Glen JA: Pathological effects of angioplasty on vasospastic carotid arteries in a rabbit model. J Neurosurg 83:111–117, 1995.
98. Okada T, Harada T, Bark DH, Mayberg MR: A rat femoral artery model for vasospasm. Neurosurgery 27:349–356, 1990.
99. Findlay JM, Weir BKA, Kanamaru K, Espinosa F: Arterial wall changes in cerebral vasospasm. Neurosurgery 25:736–746, 1989.
100. Hughes JT, Schianchi PM: Cerebral artery spasm: A histological study of necropsy of the blood vessels in cases of subarachnoid hemorrhage. J Neurosurg 48:515–525, 1978.
101. Eldevik OP, Kristiansen K, Torvik A: Subarachnoid hemorrhage and cerebrovascular spasm: Morphological study of intracranial arteries based on animal experiments and human autopsies. J Neurosurg 55:869–876, 1981.
102. Macdonald RL, Weir BKA, Grace MGA, et al: Morphometric analysis of monkey cerebral arteries exposed in vivo to whole blood, oxyhemoglobin, methemoglobin, and bilirubin. Blood Vessels 28:498–510, 1991.
103. Seifert V, Stolke D, Reale E: Ultrastructural changes of the basilar artery following experimental subarachnoid haemorrhage. Acta Neurochir (Wien) 100:164–171, 1989.
104. Macdonald RL, Weir BKA, Grace MGA, et al: Mechanism of cerebral vasospasm following subarachnoid hemorrhage in monkeys. Can J Neurol Sci 19:419–427, 1992.
105. Szabo S, Sheth RN, Novak L, et al: Cerebrovascular reserve capacity many years after vasospasm due to aneurysmal subarachnoid hemorrhage: A transcranial Doppler study with acetazolamide test. Stroke 28:2479–2482, 1997.
106. Newell DW, Grady MS, Eskridge JM, Winn HR: Distribution of angiographic vasospasm after subarachnoid hemorrhage: Implications for diagnosis by transcranial Doppler ultrasonography. Neurosurgery 27:574–575, 1990.
107. Nihei H, Kassell NF, Dougherty DA, Sasaki T: Does vasospasm occur in small pial arteries and arterioles of rabbits? Stroke 22: 1419–1425, 1991.
108. Ohkuma H, Itoh K, Shibata S, Suzuki S: Morphological changes of intraparenchymal arterioles after experimental subarachnoid hemorrhage in dogs. Neurosurgery 41:230–236, 1997.
109. Duff TA, Louie J, Feilbach JA, Scott G: Erythrocytes are essential for development of cerebral vasculopathy resulting from subarachnoid hemorrhage in cats. Stroke 19:68–72, 1988.
110. Harada T, Suzuki Y, Satoh S, et al: Blood component induction of cerebral vasospasm. Neurosurgery 27:252–256, 1990.
111. Mayberg M, Okada T, Bark DH: The role of hemoglobin in arterial narrowing after subarachnoid hemorrhage. J Neurosurg 72:634–640, 1990.
112. Macdonald RL, Weir BKA, Runzer TD, et al: Etiology of cerebral vasospasm in primates. J Neurosurg 75:415–424, 1991.
113. Macdonald RL, Weir BKA: A review of hemoglobin and the pathogenesis of cerebral vasospasm. Stroke 22:971–982, 1991.
114. Pluta RM, Afshar JKB, Boock RJ, Oldfield EH: Temporal changes in perivascular concentrations of oxyhemoglobin, deoxyhemoglobin, and methemoglobin after subarachnoid hemorrhage. J Neurosurg 88:557–561, 1998.
115. Macdonald RL, Zhang J, Weir B, et al: Adenosine triphosphate causes vasospasm of the rat femoral artery. Neurosurgery 42: 825–833, 1998.
116. Macdonald RL, Weir B, Zhang J, et al: Adenosine triphosphate and hemoglobin in vasospastic monkeys. Neurosurg Focus 3: Article 3 1997.
117. Alksne JF, Branson PJ: A comparison of intimal proliferation in experimental subarachnoid hemorrhage and atherosclerosis. Angiology 27:712:720, 1976.
118. Peerless SJ, Kassell NF, Komatsu K, Hunter JG: Cerebral vasospasm: Acute proliferative vasculopathy? II. Morphology. In

Wilkins RH (ed): Cerebral Arterial Spasm. Baltimore, Williams & Wilkins, 1980, pp 88–96.
119. Smith RR, Clower BR, Peeler DR Jr, Yoshioka J: The angiography of subarachnoid hemorrhage: Angiographic and morphologic correlates. Stroke 14:240–245, 1983.
120. Pluta RM, Zauner A, Morgan JK, et al: Is vasospasm related to proliferative arteriopathy? J Neurosurg 77:740–748, 1992.
121. Kasuya H, Weir BKA, Shen Y, et al: Insulin-like growth factor-1 in the arterial wall after exposure to periarterial blood. Neurosurgery 35:99–105, 1994.
122. Kasuya H, Shimizu T: Activated complement components C3a and C4a in cerebrospinal fluid and plasma following subarachnoid hemorrhage. J Neurosurg 71:741–746, 1989.
123. German JW, Gross CE, Giclas P, et al: Systemic complement depletion inhibits experimental cerebral vasospasm. Neurosurgery 39:141–146, 1996.
124. Park CC, Shin ML, Simard JM: The complement membrane attack complex and the bystander effect in cerebral vasospasm. J Neurosurg 87:294–300, 1997.
125. Handa Y, Kabuto M, Kobayashi H, et al: The correlation between immunological reaction in the arterial wall and the time course of the development of cerebral vasospasm in a primate model. Neurosurgery 28:542–549, 1991.
126. Mathiesen T, Fuchs D, Wachter H, von Holst H: Increased CSF neopterin levels in subarachnoid hemorrhage. J Neurosurg 73: 69–71, 1990.
127. Kubota T, Handa Y, Tsuchida A, et al: The kinetics of lymphocyte subsets and macrophages in subarachnoid space after subarachnoid hemorrhage in rats. Stroke 24:1993–2001, 1993.
128. Peterson JW, Nishizawa S, Hackett JD, et al: Cyclosporine A reduces cerebral vasospasm after subarachnoid hemorrhage in dogs. Stroke 21:133–137, 1990.
129. Ryba M, Iwanska K, Walski M, Pastuszko M: Immunomodulators interfere with angiopathy but not vasospasm after subarachnoid haemorrhage in rabbits. Acta Neurochir (Wien) 108: 81–84, 1991.
130. Handa Y, Hayashi M, Takeuchi H, et al: Effect of cyclosporine on the development of cerebral vasospasm in a primate model. Neurosurgery 28:380–386, 1991.
131. Yanamoto H, Kikuchi H, Okamoto S, Nozaki K: Preventive effect of synthetic serine protease inhibitor, FUT-175, on cerebral vasospasm in rabbits. Neurosurgery 30:351–357, 1992.
132. Yanamoto H, Kikuchi H, Sato M, et al: Therapeutic trial of cerebral vasospasm in the serine protease inhibitor, FUT-175, administered in the acute stage after subarachnoid hemorrhage. Neurosurgery 30:358–363, 1992.
133. Nagata K, Sasaki T, Iwama J, et al: Failure of FK-506, a new immunosuppressant, to prevent cerebral vasospasm in a canine two-hemorrhage model. J Neurosurg 79:710–715, 1993.
134. Ryba M, Grieb P, Pastuszko M, et al: Successful prevention of neurological deficit in SAH patients with 2-chlorodeoxyadenosine. Acta Neurochir 124:61–65, 1993.
135. Yanamoto H, Kikuchi H, Okamoto S, Nozaki K: Cerebral vasospasm caused by cisternal injection of polystyrene latex beads in rabbits is inhibited by a serine protease inhibitor. Surg Neurol 42:374–381, 1994.
136. Yanamoto H, Kikuchi H, Okamoto S: Effects of protease inhibitor and immunosuppressant on cerebral vasospasm after subarachnoid hemorrhage in rabbits. Surg Neurol 42:382–387, 1994.
137. Manno EM, Gress DR, Ogilvy CS, et al: The safety and efficacy of cyclosporine A in the prevention of vasospasm in patients with Fisher Grade 3 subarachnoid hemorrhages: A pilot study. Neurosurgery 40:289–293, 1997.
138. Peterson JW, Kwun B, Hackett JD, Zervas NT: The role of inflammation in experimental cerebral vasospasm. J Neurosurg 72:767–774, 1990.
139. Hirashima Y, Endo S, Ohmori T, et al: Platelet-activating factor (PAF) concentration and PAF acetylhydrolase activity in cerebrospinal fluid of patients with subarachnoid hemorrhage. J Neurosurg 80:31–36, 1994.
140. Hirashima Y, Endo S, Kato R, Takaku A: Prevention of cerebrovasospasm following subarachnoid hemorrhage in rabbits by the platelet-activating factor antagonist, E5880. J Neurosurg 84: 826–830, 1996.
141. Mathiesen T, Andersson B, Loftenius A, von Holst H: Increased interleukin-6 levels in cerebrospinal fluid following subarachnoid hemorrhage. J Neurosurg 78:562–567, 1993.
142. Mathiesen T, Edner G, Ulfarsson E, Andersson B: Cerebrospinal fluid interleukin-1-receptor antagonist and tumor necrosis factor-alpha following subarachnoid hemorrhage. J Neurosurg 87: 215–220, 1997.
143. Sills AK Jr, Clatterbuck RE, Thompson RC, et al: Endothelial cell expression of intercellular adhesion molecule 1 in experimental posthemorrhagic vasospasm. Neurosurgery 41:453–361, 1997.
144. Polin RS, Bavbek M, Shaffrey ME, et al: Detection of soluble E-selectin, ICAM-1, VCAM-1, and L-selectin in the cerebrospinal fluid of patients after subarachnoid hemorrhage. J Neurosurg 89:559–567, 1998.
145. Oshiro EM, Hoffman PA, Dietsch GN, et al: Inhibition of experimental vasospasm with anti-intercellular adhesion molecule-1 monoclonal antibody in rats. Stroke 28:2031–2038, 1997.
146. Bavbek M, Polin R, Kwan A, et al: Monoclonal antibodies against ICAM-1 and CD18 attenuate cerebral vasospasm after experimental subarachnoid hemorrhage in rabbits. Stroke 29: 1930–1936, 1998.
147. Kim P, Sundt TM Jr, Vanhoutte PM: Alterations of mechanical properties in canine basilar arteries after subarachnoid hemorrhage. J Neurosurg 71:430–436, 1989.
148. Vorkapic P, Bevan RD, Bevan JA: Pharmacologic irreversible narrowing in chronic cerebrovasospasm in rabbits is associated with functional damage. Stroke 21:1478–1484, 1990.
149. Yamamoto Y, Bernanke DH, Smith RR: Accelerated non-muscle contraction after subarachnoid hemorrhage: Cerebrospinal fluid testing in a culture model. Neurosurgery 27:921–928, 1990.
150. Yamamoto Y, Smith RR, Bernanke DH: Accelerated nonmuscle contraction after subarachnoid hemorrhage: Culture and characterization of myofibroblasts from human cerebral arteries in vasospasm. Neurosurgery 30:337–345, 1992.
151. Iwasa K, Bernanke DH, Smith RR, Yamamoto Y: Nonmuscle arterial constriction after subarachnoid hemorrhage: Role of growth factors derived from platelets. Neurosurgery 32:619–624, 1993.
152. Shiota T, Bernanke DH, Parent AD, Hasui K: Protein kinase C has two different major roles in lattice compaction enhanced by cerebrospinal fluid from patients with subarachnoid hemorrhage. Stroke 27:1889–1895, 1996.
153. Kasuya H, Weir B, Shen Y, et al: Procollagen types I and III and transforming growth factor-beta gene expression in the arterial wall after exposure to periarterial blood. Neurosurgery 33:716–722, 1993.
154. Macdonald RL, Weir BKA, Young JD, Grace MGA: Cytoskeletal and extracellular matrix proteins in cerebral arteries following subarachnoid hemorrhage in monkeys. J Neurosurg 76:81–90, 1992.
155. Rembold CM: Regulation of contraction and relaxation in arterial smooth muscle. Hypertension 20:129–137, 1992.
156. Krueger C, Weir B, Nosko M, et al: Nimodipine and chronic vasospasm in monkeys: II. Pharmacological studies of vessel in spasm. Neurosurgery 16:137–140, 1985.
157. Bevan JA, Bevan RD, Frazee JG: Functional arterial changes in chronic cerebrovasospasm in monkeys: An in vitro assessment of the contribution to arterial narrowing. Stroke 18:472–481, 1987.
158. Saito A, Handa J, Toda N: Reactivity to vasoactive agents of canine basilar arteries exposed to experimental subarachnoid hemorrhage. Surg Neurol 35:461–467, 1991.
159. Onoue H, Kaito Nobuyoshi K, Akiyama M, et al: Altered reactivity of human cerebral arteries after subarachnoid hemorrhage. J Neurosurg 83:510–515, 1995.
160. Sutter B, Suzuki S, Arthur AS, et al: Effects of subarachnoid hemorrhage on vascular responses to calcitonin gene-related peptide and its related second messengers. J Neurosurg 83: 516–521, 1995.
161. Takenaka K, Yamada H, Sakai N, et al: Induction of cytosolic free calcium elevation in rat vascular smooth-muscle cells by cerebrospinal fluid from patients after subarachnoid hemorrhage. J Neurosurg 75:452–457, 1991.
162. Sakaki S, Ohue S, Kohno K, Takeda S: Impairment of vascular reactivity of changes in intracellular calcium and calmodulin levels of smooth muscle cells in canine basilar arteries after subarachnoid hemorrhage. Neurosurgery 25:753–761, 1989.

163. Takanashi Y, Weir BKA, Vollrath B, et al: Time course of changes in concentration of intracellular free calcium in cultured cerebrovascular smooth muscle cells exposed to oxyhemoglobin. Neurosurgery 30:346–350, 1992.
164. Yamada T, Tanaka Y, Fujimoto K, et al: Relationship between cystosolic Ca^{2+} level and contractile tension in canine basilar artery of chronic vasospasm. Neurosurgery 34:496–504, 1994.
165. Wang J, Ohta S, Sakaki S, et al: Changes in Ca^{++}-ATPase activity in smooth-muscle cell membranes of the canine basilar artery with experimental subarachnoid hemorrhage. J Neurosurg 80: 269–275, 1994.
166. Matsui T, Kaizu H, Itoh S, Asano T: The role of active smooth-muscle contraction in the occurrence of chronic vasospasm in the canine two-hemorrhage model. J Neurosurg 80:276–282, 1994.
167. Butler WE, Peterson JW, Zervas NT, Morgan KG: Intracellular calcium, myosin light chain phosphorylation, and contractile force in experimental cerebral vasospasm. Neurosurgery 38: 781–788, 1996.
168. Zuccarello M, Boccaletti R, Tosun M, Rapoport RM: Role of extracellular Ca^{2+} in subarachnoid hemorrhage-induced spasm of the rabbit basilar artery. Stroke 27:1896–1902, 1996.
169. Iwabuchi S, Marton LS, Zhang JH: Role of protein tyrosine phosphorylation in erythrocyte lysate-induced intracellular free calcium concentration elevation in cerebral smooth-muscle cells. J Neurosurg 90:743–751, 1999.
170. Kim P, Jones JD, Sundt TM Jr: High-energy phosphate levels in the cerebral artery during chronic vasospasm after subarachnoid hemorrhage. J Neurosurg 76:991–996, 1992.
171. Yoshimoto Y, Kim P, Sasaki T, Takakura K: Temporal profile and significance of metabolic failure and trophic changes in the canine cerebral arteries during chronic vasospasm after subarachnoid hemorrhage. J Neurosurg 78:807–812, 1993.
172. Nagatani K, Masciopinto JE, Letarte PB, et al: The effect of hemoglobin and its metabolites on energy metabolism in cultured cerebrovascular smooth-muscle cells. J Neurosurg 82:244–249, 1995.
173. Harada T, Seto M, Sasaki Y, et al: The time course of myosin light-chain phosphorylation in blood-induced vasospasm. Neurosurgery 36:1178–1183, 1995.
174. Sun H, Kanamaru K, Ito M, et al: Myosin light chain phosphorylation and contractile proteins in a canine two-hemorrhage model of subarachnoid hemorrhage. Stroke 29:2149–2154, 1998.
175. Suzuki Y, Shibuya M, Takayasu M, et al: Protein kinase activity in canine basilar arteries after subarachnoid hemorrhage. Neurosurgery 22:1028–1031, 1988.
176. Matsui T, Sugawa M, Johshita H, et al: Activation of the protein kinase C–mediated contractile system in canine basilar artery undergoing chronic vasospasm. Stroke 22:1183–1187, 1991.
177. Nishizawa S, Nezu N, Uemura K: Direct evidence for a key role of protein kinase C in the development of vasospasm after subarachnoid hemorrhage. J Neurosurg 76:635–639, 1992.
178. Nishizawa S, Peterson JW, Shimoyama I, Uemura K: Relation between protein kinase C and calmodulin systems in cerebrovascular contraction: Investigation of the pathogenesis of vasospasm after subarachnoid hemorrhage. Neurosurgery 31:711–716, 1992.
179. Yokota M, Peterson JW, Kaoutzanis MC, et al: Protein kinase C and diacylglycerol content in basilar arteries during experimental cerebral vasospasm in the dog. J Neurosurg 82:834–840, 1995.
180. Doi M, Kasuya H, Weir B, et al: Reduced expression of calponin in canine basilar artery after subarachnoid haemorrhage. Acta Neurochir 139:77–81, 1997.
181. Lee KS, Foley PL, Vanderklish P, et al: The role of calcium-activated proteolysis in vasospasm after subarachnoid hemorrhage. In Findlay JM (ed): Cerebral Vasospasm. Amsterdam, Elsevier Science, 1993, pp 85–88.
182. Yamaura I, Tani E, Maeda Y, et al: Calpain-calpastatin system of canine basilar artery in vasospasm. In Findlay JM (ed): Cerebral Vasospasm. Amsterdam, Elsevier Science, 1993, pp 137–140.
183. Vollrath B, Cook D, Megyesi J, et al: Novel mechanism by which hemoglobin induces constriction of cerebral arteries. Eur J Pharmacol 361:311–319, 1998.
184. Sasaki T, Wakai S, Asano T, et al: The effect of a lipid hydroperoxide of arachidonic acid on the canine basilar artery: An experimental study on cerebral vasospasm. J Neurosurg 54:357–365, 1981.
185. Macdonald RL, Weir BKA, Runzer TD, Grace MGA: Malondialdehyde, glutathione peroxidase, and superoxide dismutase in cerebrospinal fluid during cerebral vasospasm in monkeys. Can J Neurol Sci 19:326–332, 1992.
186. Steele JA, Stockbridge N, Maljkovic G, Weir B: Free radicals mediate actions of oxyhemoglobin on cerebrovascular smooth muscle cells. Circ Res 68:416–423, 1991.
187. Cook DA, Vollrath B: Free radicals and intracellular events associated with cerebrovascular spasm. Cardiovasc Res 30:493–500, 1995.
188. Ohta T, Satoh G, Kuroiwa T: The permeability change of major cerebral arteries in experimental vasospasm. Neurosurgery 30: 331–336, 1992.
189. Foley PL, Takenaka K, Kassell NF, Lee KS: Cytotoxic effects of bloody cerebrospinal fluid on cerebral endothelial cells in culture. J Neurosurg 81:87–92, 1994.
190. Vollmer DG, Hongo K, Ogawa H, et al: A study of the effectiveness of the iron-chelating agent deferoxamine as vasospasm prophylaxis in a rabbit model of subarachnoid hemorrhage. Neurosurgery 28:27–32, 1991.
191. Harada T, Mayberg MR: Inhibition of delayed arterial narrowing by the iron-chelating agent deferoxamine. J Neurosurg 77:763–767, 1992.
192. Comair YG, Schipper HM, Brem S: The prevention of oxyhemoglobin-induced endothelial and smooth muscle cytoskeletal injury by deferoxamine. Neurosurgery 32:58–65, 1993.
193. Luo Z, Harada T, London S, et al: Antioxidant and iron-chelating agents in cerebral vasospasm. Neurosurgery 37:1154–1159, 1995.
194. Vollrath B, Chan P, Findlay JM, Cook D: Lazaroids and deferoxamine attenuate the intracellular effects of oxyhaemoglobin in vascular smooth muscle. Cardiovasc Res 30:619–626, 1995.
195. Arthur AS, Fergus AH, Lanzino G, et al: Systemic administration of the iron chelator deferiprone attenuates subarachnoid hemorrhage–induced cerebral vasospasm in the rabbit. Neurosurgery 41:1385–1392, 1997.
196. Horky LL, Pluta RM, Boock RJ, Oldfield EH: Role of ferrous iron chelator 2,2′-dipyridyl in preventing delayed vasospasm in a primate model of subarachnoid hemorrhage. J Neurosurg 88: 298–303, 1998.
197. Shishido T, Suzuki R, Qian L, Hirakawa K: The role of superoxide anions in the pathogenesis of cerebral vasospasm. Stroke 25:864–868, 1994.
198. Macdonald RL, Weir BKA, Runzer TD, et al: Effect of intrathecal superoxide dismutase and catalase on oxyhemoglobin-induced vasospasm in monkeys. Neurosurgery 30:529–539, 1992.
199. Steinke DE, Weir BKA, Findlay JM, et al: A trial of the 21-aminosteroid U74006F in a primate model of chronic cerebral vasospasm. Neurosurgery 24:179–186, 1989.
200. Vollmer DG, Kassell NF, Hongo K, et al: Effect of the nonglucocorticoid 21-aminosteroid U74006F on experimental cerebral vasospasm. Surg Neurol 31:190–194, 1989.
201. Zuccarello M, Anderson DK: Protective effect of a 21-aminosteroid on the blood-brain barrier following subarachnoid hemorrhage in rats. Stroke 20:367–371, 1989.
202. Zuccarello M, Marsch JT, Schmitt G, et al: Effect of the 21-aminosteroid U-74006F on cerebral vasospasm following subarachnoid hemorrhage. J Neurosurg 71:98–104, 1989.
203. Kanamaru K, Weir BKA, Findlay JM, et al: A dosage study of the effect of the 21-aminosteroid U74006F on chronic cerebral vasospasm in a primate model. Neurosurgery 27:29–38, 1990.
204. Kanamaru K, Weir BKA, Simpson I, et al: Effect of 21-aminosteroid U-74006F on lipid peroxidation in subarachnoid clot. J Neurosurg 74:454–459, 1991.
205. Matsui T, Asano T: Effects of new 21-aminosteroid tirilazad mesylate (U74006F) on chronic cerebral vasospasm in a "two-hemorrhage" model of beagle dogs. Neurosurgery 34:1035–1039, 1994.
206. Takahashi S, Kassell NF, Toshima M, et al: Effect of U88999E on experimental cerebral vasospasm in rabbits. Neurosurgery 32: 281–288, 1993.
207. Smith SL, Scherch HM, Hall ED: Protective effects of tirilazad mesylate and metabolite U-89678 against blood-brain barrier

damage after subarachnoid hemorrhage and lipid peroxidative neuronal injury. J Neurosurg 84:229–233, 1996.

208. Macdonald RL, Bassiouny M, Johns L, et al: U74389G prevents vasospasm after subarachnoid hemorrhage in dogs. Neurosurgery 42:1339–1346, 1998.
209. Maeda Y, Tani E, Miyamoto T: Prostaglandin metabolism in experimental cerebral vasospasm. J Neurosurg 55:779–785, 1981.
210. Nosko M, Schulz R, Weir B, et al: Effects of vasospasm on levels of prostacyclin and thromboxane A_2 in cerebral arteries of the monkey. Neurosurgery 22:45–50, 1988.
211. Sasaki T, Murota S, Wakai S, et al: Evaluation of prostaglandin biosynthetic activity in canine basilar artery following subarachnoid injection of blood. J Neurosurg 55:771–778, 1981.
212. White RP, Robertson JT: Comparison of piroxicam, meclofenamate, ibuprofen, aspirin, and prostacyclin efficacy in a chronic model of cerebral vasospasm. Neurosurgery 12:40–46, 1983.
213. Tokiyoshi K, Ohnishi T, Nii Y: Efficacy and toxicity of thromboxane synthetase inhibitor for cerebral vasospasm after subarachnoid hemorrhage. Surg Neurol 36:112–118, 1991.
214. Yokota M, Tani E, Fukumori T, et al: Effects of subarachnoid hemorrhage and a thromboxane A_2 synthetase inhibitor on intracranial prostaglandins. Surg Neurol 35:345–349, 1991.
215. Kobayashi H, Ide H, Handa Y, et al: Effect of leukotriene antagonist on experimental delayed cerebral vasospasm. Neurosurgery 31:550–556, 1992.
216. Seifert V, Stolke D, Kunz U, Resch K: Influence of blood volume on cerebrospinal fluid levels of arachidonic acid metabolites after subarachnoid hemorrhage: Experimental study on the pathogenesis of cerebral vasospasm. Neurosurgery 23:313–321, 1988.
217. O'Neill P, Walton S, Foy PM, Shaw MDM: Role of prostaglandins in delayed cerebral ischemia after subarachnoid hemorrhage. Neurosurgery 30:17–22, 1992.
218. Juvela S, Öhman J, Servo A, et al: Angiographic vasospasm and release of platelet thromboxane after subarachnoid hemorrhage. Stroke 22:451–455, 1991.
219. Ohkuma H, Suzuki S, Kimura M, Sobata E: Role of platelet function in symptomatic cerebral vasospasm following aneurysmal subarachnoid hemorrhage. Stroke 22:854–859, 1991.
220. Ohkuma H, Ogane K, Fujita S, et al: Impairment of anti–platelet-aggregating activity of endothelial cells after experimental subarachnoid hemorrhage. Stroke 24:1541–1546, 1993.
221. Kim P, Sundt TM Jr, Vanhoutte PM: Alterations in endothelium-dependent responsiveness of the canine basilar artery after subarachnoid hemorrhage. J Neurosurg 69:239–246, 1988.
222. Hongo K, Kassell NF, Nakagomi T, et al: Subarachnoid hemorrhage inhibition of endothelium-derived relaxing factor in rabbit basilar artery. J Neurosurg 69:247–253, 1988.
223. Kim P, Lorenz RR, Sundt TM Jr, Vanhoutte PM: Release of endothelium-derived relaxing factor after subarachnoid hemorrhage. J Neurosurg 70:108–114, 1989.
224. Kanamaru K, Weir BKA, Findlay JM, et al: Pharmacological studies on relaxation of spastic primate cerebral arteries in subarachnoid hemorrhage. J Neurosurg 71:909–915, 1989.
225. Hatake K, Wakabayashi I, Kakishita E, Hishida S: Impairment of endothelium-dependent relaxation in human basilar artery after subarachnoid hemorrhage. Stroke 23:111–1117, 1992.
226. Palmer RMJ, Ferrige AG, Moncada S: Nitric oxide release accounts for the biological activity of endothelium-derived relaxing factor. Nature 327:524–526, 1987.
227. Faraci FM, Brian JE Jr: Nitric oxide and the cerebral circulation. Stroke 25:692–703, 1994.
228. Miranda FJ, Alabadí JA, Torregrosa G, et al: Modulatory role of endothelial and nonendothelial nitric oxide in 5-hydroxytryptamine-induced contraction in cerebral arteries after subarachnoid hemorrhage. Neurosurgery 39:998–1004, 1996.
229. Kasuya H, Weir BKA, Nakane M, et al: Nitric oxide synthase and guanylate cyclase levels in canine basilar artery after subarachnoid hemorrhage. J Neurosurg 82:250–255, 1995.
230. Pluta RM, Thompson BG, Dawson TM, et al: Loss of nitric oxide synthase immunoreactivity in cerebral vasospasm. J Neurosurg 84:648–654, 1996.
231. Afshar JKB, Pluta RM, Boock RJ, et al: Effect of intracarotid nitric oxide on primate cerebral vasospasm after subarachnoid hemorrhage. J Neurosurg 83:118–122, 1995.
232. Pluta RM, Oldfield EH, Boock RJ: Reversal and prevention of cerebral vasospasm by intracarotid infusions of nitric oxide donors in a primate model of subarachnoid hemorrhage. J Neurosurg 87:746–751, 1997.
233. Onoue H, Tsutsui M, Smith S, et al: Expression and function of recombinant endothelial nitric oxide synthase gene in canine basilar artery after experimental subarachnoid hemorrhage. Stroke 29:1959–1966, 1998.
234. Shigeno T, Mima T: A new vasoconstrictor peptide, endothelin: Profiles as vasoconstrictor and neuropeptide. Cerebrovasc Brain Metab Rev 2:227–239, 1990.
235. Zimmerman M, Seifert V: Endothelin and subarachnoid hemorrhage: An overview. Neurosurgery 43:863–876, 1998.
236. Cocks TM, Malta E, King SJ, et al: Oxyhaemoglobin increases the production of endothelin-1 by endothelial cells in culture. Eur J Pharmacol 196:177–182, 1991.
237. Kasuya H, Weir BKA, White DM, Stefansson K: Mechanism of oxyhemoglobin-induced release of endothelin-1 from cultured vascular endothelial cells and smooth-muscle cells. J Neurosurg 79:892–898, 1993.
238. Ohlstein EH, Storer BL: Oxyhemoglobin stimulation of endothelin production in cultured endothelial cells. J Neurosurg 77: 274–278, 1992.
239. Schini VB, Hendrickson H, Heublein DM: Thrombin enhances the release of endothelin from porcine aortic endothelial cells. Eur J Pharmacol 165:333–334, 1989.
240. Cosentino F, Katuši ZS: Does endothelin-1 play a role in the pathogenesis of cerebral vasospasm? Stroke 25:904–908, 1994.
241. Kobayashi H, Hayashi M, Kobayashi S, et al: Cerebral vasospasm and vasoconstriction caused by endothelin. Neurosurgery 28:673–679, 1991.
242. Mima T, Yanagisawa M, Shigeno T, et al: Endothelin acts in feline and canine cerebral arteries from the adventitial side. Stroke 20:1553–1556, 1989.
243. Papadopoulos SM, Gilbert LL, Webb RC, D'Amato CJ: Characterization of contractile responses to endothelin in human cerebral arteries: Implications for cerebral vasospasm. Neurosurgery 26:810–815, 1990.
244. Pluta RM, Boock RJ, Afshar JK, et al: Source and cause of endothelin-1 release into cerebrospinal fluid after subarachnoid hemorrhage. J Neurosurg 87:287–293, 1997.
245. Hino A, Weir BKA, Macdonald RL, et al: Prospective, randomized, double-blind trial of BQ-123 and bosentan for prevention of vasospasm following subarachnoid hemorrhage in monkeys. J Neurosurg 83:503–509, 1995.
246. Kobayashi M, Nishikibe M, Maruyama H, et al: Localization and alteration of immunoreactive endothelin-1 in canine basilar arteries following aneurysmal subarachnoid hemorrhage. Acta Histochem Cytochem 28:129–136, 1995.
247. Yamaura I, Tani E, Maeda Y, et al: Endothelin-1 of canine basilar artery in vasospasm. J Neurosurg 76:99–105, 1992.
248. Gaetani P, Rodriguez Y, Baena R, et al: Endothelin and aneurysmal subarachnoid haemorrhage: A study of subarachnoid cisternal cerebrospinal fluid. J Neurol Neurosurg Psychiatry 57:66–72, 1994.
249. Hamann G, Isenberg E, Strittmatter M, Schimrigk K: Absence of elevation of big endothelin subarachnoid hemorrhage. Stroke 24:383–386, 1993.
250. Seifert V, Löffler BM, Zimmermann M, et al: Endothelin concentrations in patients with aneurysmal subarachnoid hemorrhage: Correlation with cerebral vasospasm, delayed ischemic neurological deficits, and volume of hematoma. J Neurosurg 82:55–62, 1995.
251. Suzuki H, Sato S, Suzuki Y, et al: Increased endothelin concentration in CSF from patients with subarachnoid hemorrhage. Acta Neurol Scand 81:554–554, 1990.
252. Cosentino F, McMahon EG, Carter JS, Katušic ZS: Effect of endothelinA-receptor antagonist BQ-123 and phosphoramidon on cerebral vasospasm. J Cardiovasc Pharmacol 22:S332–335, 1993.
253. Clozel M, Watanabe H: BQ-123, a peptidic endothelin ETA receptor antagonist, prevents the early cerebral vasospasm following subarachnoid hemorrhage after intracisternal but not intravenous injection. Life Sci 52:825–834, 1993.
254. Foley PL, Caner HH, Kassell NF, Lee KS: Reversal of subarach-

noid hemorrhage–induced vasoconstriction with an endothelin receptor antagonist. Neurosurgery 34:108–112, 1994.
255. Itoh S, Sasaki T, Ide K, et al: A novel endothelin ET_A receptor antagonist, BQ-485, and its preventative effect on experimental cerebral vasospasm in dogs. Biochem Biophys Res Commun 195:969–975, 1993.
256. Matsumura Y, Ikegawa R, Suzuki Y, et al: Phosphoramidon prevents cerebral vasospasm following subarachnoid hemorrhage in dogs: The relationship to endothelin-1 levels in the cerebrospinal fluid. Life Sci 49:841–848, 1991.
257. Nirei H, Hamanda K, Shoubo M, et al: An endothelin ETA receptor antagonist, FR139317, ameliorates cerebral vasospasm in dogs. Life Sci 52:1869–1874, 1993.
258. Shigeno T, Clozel M, Sakai S, et al: The effect of bosentan, a new potent endothelin receptor antagonist, on the pathogenesis of cerebral vasospasm. Neurosurgery 37:87–90, 1995.
259. Shigeno T, Mima T, Yanagisawa M, et al: Prevention of cerebral vasospasm by actinomycin D. J Neurosurg 74:940–943, 1991.
260. Zimmermann M, Seifert V, Löffler BM, et al: Prevention of cerebral vasospasm after experimental subarachnoid hemorrhage by RO 47-0203, a newly developed orally active endothelin receptor antagonist. Neurosurgery 38:115–120, 1996.
261. Kwan A, Bavbek M, Jeng AY, et al: Prevention and reversal of cerebral vasospasm by an endothelin-converting enzyme inhibitor, CGS 26303, in an experimental model of subarachnoid hemorrhage. J Neurosurg 87:281–286, 1997.
262. Zuccarello M, Boccaletti R, Romano A, Rapoport RM: Endothelin B receptor antagonists attenuate subarachnoid hemorrhage–induced cerebral vasospasm. Stroke 29:1924–1929, 1998.
263. Onoda K, Ono S, Ogihara K, et al: Inhibition of vascular contraction by intracisternal administration of preproendothelin-1 mRNA antisense oligoDNA in a rat experimental vasospasm model. J Neurosurg 85:846–852, 1996.
264. Ohkuma H, Parney I, Megyesi J, et al: Antisense preproendothelin-oligoDNA therapy for vasospasm in a canine model of subarachnoid hemorrhage. J Neurosurg 90:1105–1114, 1999.
265. Edvinsson L: Innervation of cerebral circulation. Ann N Y Acad Sci 519:334–348, 1987.
266. Duff TA, Feilbach JA, Scott G: Does cerebral vasospasm result from denervation supersensitivity? Stroke 18:85–91, 1987.
267. Juul R, Hara H, Gisvold SE, et al: Alterations in perivascular dilatory neuropeptides (CGRP, SP, VIP) in the external jugular vein and in the cerebrospinal fluid following subarachnoid haemorrrhage in man. Acta Neurochir 132:32–41, 1995.
268. Pluta RM, Deka-Starosta A, Zauner A, et al: Neuropeptide Y in the primate model of subarachnoid hemorrhage. J Neurosurg 77:417–432, 1992.
269. Fisher CM, Roberson GH, Ojemann RG: Cerebral vasospasm with ruptured saccular aneurysm—the clinical manifestations. Neurosurgery 1:245–258, 1977.
270. Nussbaum ES, Sebring LA, Wen DYK: Intracranial aneurysm rupture presenting as delayed stroke secondary to cerebral vasospasm. Stroke 28:2078–2080, 1997.
271. Seiler RW, Grolimund P, Aaslid R, et al: Cerebral vasospasm evaluated by transcranial ultrasound correlated with clinical grade and CT-visualized subarachnoid hemorrhage. J Neurosurg 64:594–600, 1986.
272. Lindegaard KF, Bakke SJ, Sorteberg W, et al: A non-invasive Doppler ultrasound method for the evaluation of patients with subarachnoid hemorrhage. Acta Radiol 369:96–98, 1986.
273. DeWitt LD, Weschler LR: Transcranial Doppler. Stroke 19:915–921, 1988.
274. Hutchison K, Weir B: Transcranial Doppler studies in aneurysm patients. Can J Neurol Sci 16:411–416, 1989.
275. Ekelund A, Saveland H, Romner B, Brandt L: Is transcranial Doppler sonography useful in detecting late cerebral ischaemia after aneurysmal subarachnoid hemorrhage? Br J Neurosurg 10: 19–25, 1996.
276. Grosset DG, Straiton J, McDonald I, et al: Use of transcranial Doppler sonography to predict development of a delayed ischemic deficit after subarachnoid hemorrhage. J Neurosurg 78: 183–187, 1993.
277. Burch CM, Wozniak MA, Sloan MA, et al: Detection of intracranial internal carotid artery and middle cerebral artery vasospasm following subarachnoid hemorrhage. J Neuroimag 6: 8–15, 1996.
278. Eskridge JM, Song JK: A practical approach to the treatment of vasospasm. AJNR Am J Neuroradiol 18:1653–1660, 1997.
279. Wardlaw JM, Offin R, Teasdale GM, Teasdale EM: Is routine transcranial Doppler ultrasound monitoring useful in the management of subarachnoid hemorrhage? J Neurosurg 88:272–276, 1998.
280. Vora YY, Suarez-Almazor M, Steinke DE, et al: Role of transcranial Doppler monitoring in the diagnosis of cerebral vasospasm after subarachnoid hemorrhage. Neurosurgery 44:1237–1248, 1999.
281. Proust F, Callonec F, Clavier E, et al: Usefulness of transcranial color-coded sonography in the diagnosis of cerebral vasospasm. Stroke 30:1091–1098, 1999.
282. Shinoda J, Kimura T, Funakoshi T, et al: Acetazolamide reactivity on cerebral blood flow in patients with subarachnoid hemorrhage. Acta Neurochir 109:102–108, 1991.
283. Lewis DH, Loyd D, Grothaus-King A, et al: Brain SPECT and the effect of cerebral angioplasty in delayed ischemia due to vasospasm. J Nucl Med 33:1789–1796, 1992.
284. Kimura T, Shinoda J, Funakoshi T: Prediction of cerebral infarction due to vasospasm following aneurysmal subarachnoid haemorrhage using acetazolamide-activated ^{123}I-IMP SPECT. Acta Neurochir 123:125–128, 1993.
285. Yonas H, Sekhar L, Johnson DW, Gur D: Determination of irreversible ischemia by xenon-enhanced computed tomographic monitoring of cerebral blood flow in patients with symptomatic vasospasm. Neurosurgery 24:368–372, 1989.
286. Clyde BL, Resnick DK, Yonas H, et al: The relationship of blood velocity as measured by transcranial Doppler ultrasonography to cerebral blood flow as determined by stable xenon computed tomographic studies after aneurysmal subarachnoid hemorrhage. Neurosurgery 38:896–905, 1996.
287. Rordorf G, Koroshetz WJ, Copen WA, et al: Diffusion- and perfusion-weighted imaging in vasospasm after subarachnoid hemorrhage. Stroke 30:599–605, 1999.
288. Tamatani S, Sasaki O, Takeuchi S, et al: Detection of delayed cerebral vasospasm, after rupture of intracranial aneurysms, by magnetic resonance angiography. Neurosurgery 40:748–754, 1997.
289. Ochi RP, Vikeco PT, Gross CE: CT angiography of cerebral vasospasm with conventional angiographic comparison. AJNR Am J Neuroradiol 18:265–269, 1997.
290. Hasan D, Vermeulen M, Wijdicks EFM, et al: Effect of fluid intake and antihypertensive treatment on cerebral ischemia after subarachnoid hemorrhage. Stroke 20:1511–1515, 1989.
291. Vermeulen M, Lindsay KW, Murray GD, et al: Antifibrinolytic treatment of subarachnoid hemorrhage. N Engl J Med 311: 432–437, 1984.
292. Kassell NF, Torner JC, Adams HP Jr: Antifibrinolytic therapy in the acute period following aneurysmal subarachnoid hemorrhage. J Neurosurg 61:225–230, 1984.
293. Bailes JE, Spetzler RF, Hadley MN, Baldwin HZ: Management and morbidity of poor-grade aneurysm patients. J Neurosurg 72:559–566, 1990.
294. Mizukami M, Kawase T, Usami T, Tazawa T: Prevention of vasospasm by early operation with removal of subarachnoid blood. Neurosurgery 10:301–307, 1982.
295. Taneda M: Effect of early operation for ruptured aneurysms on prevention of delayed ischemic symptoms. J Neurosurg 57: 622–628, 1982.
296. Nosko M, Weir BKA, Lunt A, et al: Effect of clot removal at 24 hours on chronic vasospasm after SAH in the primate model. J Neurosurg 66:416–422, 1987.
297. Handa Y, Weir BKA, Nosko M, et al: The effect of timing of clot removal on chronic vasospasm in a primate model. J Neurosurg 67:558–564, 1987.
298. Alksne JF, Branson PJ, Bailey M: Modification of experimental post-subarachnoid hemorrhage vasculopathy with intracisternal plasmin. Neurosurgery 19:20–25, 1986.
299. Findlay JM, Weir BKA, Steinke D, et al: Effect of intrathecal thrombolytic therapy on subarachnoid clot and chronic vasospasm in a primate model of SAH. J Neurosurg 69:723–735, 1988.
300. Seifert V, Eisert WG, Stolke D, Goetz C: Efficacy of single intracisternal bolus injection of recombinant tissue plasminogen

activator to prevent delayed cerebral vasospasm after experimental subarachnoid hemorrhage. Neurosurgery 25:590–598, 1989.

301. Findlay JM, Weir BKA, Kanamaru K, et al: Intrathecal fibrinolytic therapy after subarachnoid hemorrhage: Dosage study in a primate model and review of the literature. Can J Neurol Sci 16:28–40, 1989.
302. Findlay JM, Weir BKA, Kassell NF, et al: Intracisternal recombinant tissue plasminogen activator after aneurysmal subarachnoid hemorrhage. J Neurosurg 75:181–188, 1991.
303. Mizoi K, Yoshimoto T, Fujiwara S, et al: Prevention of vasospasm by clot removal and intrathecal bolus injection of tissue-type plasminogen activator: Preliminary report. Neurosurgery 28:807–813, 1991.
304. Öhman J, Servo A, Heiskanen O: Effect of intrathecal fibrinolytic therapy on clot lysis and vasospasm in patients with aneurysmal subarachnoid hemorrhage. J Neurosurg 75:197–201, 1991.
305. Zabramski JM, Spetzler RF, Lee KS, et al: Phase I trial of tissue plasminogen activator for the prevention of vasospasm in patients with aneurysmal subarachnoid hemorrhage. J Neurosurg 75:189–196, 1991.
306. Stolke D, Seifert V: Single intracisternal bolus of recombinant tissue plasminogen activator in patients with aneurysmal subarachnoid hemorrhage: Preliminary assessment of efficacy and safety in open clinical study. Neurosurgery 30:877–881, 1992.
307. Philippon J, Grob R, Dagreou F, et al: Prevention of vasospasm in subarachnoid hemorrhage: A controlled study with nimodipine. Acta Neurochir 82:110–114, 1986.
308. Mee E, Dorrance D, Lowe D, Neil-Dwyer G: Controlled study of nimodipine in aneurysm patients treated early after subarachnoid hemorrhage. Neurosurgery 22:484–491, 1988.
309. Petruk KC, West M, Mohr G, et al: Nimodipine treatment in poor-grade aneurysm patients. J Neurosurg 68:505–517, 1988.
310. Pickard JD, Murray GD, Illingworth R, et al: Effect of oral nimodipine on cerebral infarction and outcome after subarachnoid haemorrhage: British aneurysm nimodipine trial. BMJ 298: 636–642, 1989.
311. Ohman J, Servo A, Heiskanen O: Long-term effects of nimodipine on cerebral infarcts and outcome after aneurysmal subarachnoid hemorrhage and surgery. J Neurosurg 74:8–13, 1991.
312. Robinson MJ, Teasdale GM: Calcium antagonist in management of subarachnoid hemorrhage. Cerebrovasc Brain Metab Rev 2: 205–226, 1990.
313. Di Mascio R, Marchioli R, Tognoni G: From pharmacological promises to controlled clinical trials to meta-analysis and back: The case of nimodipine in cerebrovascular disorders. Clin Trials Meta-Analysis 29:57–79, 1994.
314. Dorsch NWC: A review of cerebral vasospasm in aneurysmal subarachnoid haemorrhage. J Clin Neurosci 1:78–92, 1994.
315. Barker FG, Ogilvy CS: Efficacy of prophylactic nimodipine for delayed ischemic deficit after subarachnoid hemorrhage: A meta-analysis. J Neurosurg 84:405–414, 1996.
316. Wong MCW, Haley EC Jr: Calcium antagonist: Stroke therapy coming of age. Stroke 24:31–36, 1989.
317. Haley EC Jr, Kassell NF, Torner JC: A randomized controlled trial of high-dose intravenous nicardipine in aneurysmal subarachnoid hemorrhage. A report of the Cooperative Aneurysm Study. J Neurosurg 78:537–547, 1993.
318. Haley EC Jr, Kassell NF, Torner JC: A randomized trial of nicardipine in subarachnoid hemorrhage: Angiographic and transcranial Doppler ultrasound results. A report of the Cooperative Aneurysm Study. J Neurosurg 78:548–553, 1993.
319. Haley EC Jr, Kassell NF, Alves WM, et al: Phase II trial of tirilazad in aneurysmal subarachnoid hemorrhage. J Neurosurg 82:786–790, 1995.
320. Kassell NF, Haley EC Jr, Apperson-Hansen C, et al: Randomized, double-blind, vehicle-controlled trial of tirilazad mesylate in patients with aneurysmal subarachnoid hemorrhage: A cooperative study in Europe, Australia, and New Zealand. J Neurosurg 84:221–228, 1996.
321. Haley EC Jr, Kassell NF, Apperson-Hansen C, et al: A randomized, double-blind, vehicle-controlled trial of tirilazad mesylate in patients with aneurysmal subarachnoid hemorrhage: A cooperative study in North America. J Neurosurg 86:467–474, 1997.
322. Lanzino G, Kassell NF, Dorsch NWC, et al: Double-blind, randomized, vehicle-controlled study of high-dose tirilazad mesylate in women with aneurysmal subarachnoid hemorrhage: I. A cooperative study in Europe, Australia, New Zealand, and South Africa. J Neurosurg 90:1011–1017, 1999.
323. Lanzino G, Kassell NF, and the Participants: Double-blind, randomized, vehicle-controlled study of high-dose tirilazad mesylate in women with aneurysmal subarachnoid hemorrhage: II. A cooperative study in North America. J Neurosurg 90:1018–1024, 1999.
324. Ohta T, Kikuchi H, Hashi K, Kudo Y: Nizofenone administration in the acute stage following subarachnoid hemorrhage. J Neurosurg 64:420–426, 1986.
325. Chyatte D, Fode NC, Nichols DA, Sundt TM Jr: Preliminary report: Effects of high dose methylprednisolone on delayed cerebral ischemia in patients at high risk for vasospasm after aneurysmal subarachnoid hemorrhage. Neurosurgery 21:157–160, 1987.
326. Inoue T, Shimizu H, Kaminuma T, et al: Prevention of cerebral vasospasm by calcitonin gene-related peptide slow-release tablet after subarachnoid hemorrhage in monkeys. Neurosurgery 39:984–990, 1996.
327. Asano T, Takakura K, Sano K, et al: Effects of hydroxyl radical scavenger on delayed ischemic neurological deficits following aneurysmal subarachnoid hemorrhage: Results of a multicenter, placebo-controlled double-blind trial. J Neurosurg 84:792–803, 1996.
328. Khajavi K, Ayzman I, Shearer D, et al: Prevention of cerebral vasospasm in dogs with milrinone. Neurosurgery 40:354–363, 1997.
329. Shiokawa K, Kasuya H, Miyajima M, et al: Prophylactic effect of papaverine prolonged-release pellets on cerebral vasospasm in dogs. Neurosurgery 42:109–116, 1998.
330. Saito I, Asano T, Sano K, et al: Neuroprotective effect of an antioxidant, ebselen, in patients with delayed neurological deficits after aneurysmal subarachnoid hemorrhage. Neurosurgery 42:269–278, 1998.
331. Muizelaar JP, Zwienenberg M, Rudisill NA, Hecht ST: The prophylactic use of transluminal balloon angioplasty in patients with Fisher grade 3 subarachnoid hemorrhage: A pilot study. J Neurosurg 91:51–58, 1999.
332. Awad IA, Carter P, Spetzler RF, et al: Clinical vasospasm after subarachnoid hemorrhage: Response to hypervolemic hemodilution and arterial hypertension. Stroke 18:365–372, 1987.
333. Solomon RA, Fink ME, Lennihan L: Early aneurysm surgery and prophylactic hypervolemic hypertensive therapy for treatment of aneurysmal subarachnoid hemorrhage. Neurosurgery 23:699–704, 1988.
334. Origitano TC, Wascher TM, Reichman OH, Anderson DE: Sustained increased cerebral blood flow with prophylactic hypertensive hypervolemic hemodilution ("Triple-H" therapy) after subarachnoid hemorrhage. Neurosurgery 27:729–740, 1990.
335. Levy ML, Giannotta SL: Cardiac performance indices during hypervolemic therapy for cerebral vasospasm. J Neurosurg 75: 27–31, 1991.
336. Pritz MB: Treatment of cerebral vasospasm due to aneurysmal subarachnoid hemorrhage: Past, present, and future of hyperdynamic therapy. Neurosurg Q 7:273–285, 1997.
337. Wood JH, Snyder LL, Simeone FA: Failure of intravascular volume expansion without hemodilution to elevate cortical blood flow in region of experimental focal ischemia. J Neurosurg 56:80–91, 1982.
338. Matsui T, Asano T: The hemodynamic effects of prolonged albumin administration in beagle dogs exposed to experimental subarachnoid hemorrhage. Neurosurgery 32:79–84, 1993.
339. Mayer SA, Solomon RA, Fink ME, et al: Effect of 5% albumin solution on sodium balance and blood volume after subarachnoid hemorrhage. Neurosurgery 42:759–768, 1998.
340. Rosenwasser RH, Jallo JI, Getch CC, Liebman KE: Complications of Swan-Ganz catheterization for hemodynamic monitoring in patients with subarachnoid hemorrhage. Neurosurgery 37:872–876, 1995.
341. Miller JA, Dacey RG Jr, Diringer MN: Safety of hypertensive hypervolemic therapy with phenylephrine in the treatment of delayed ischemic deficits after subarachnoid hemorrhage. Stroke 26:2260–2266, 1995.

342. Amin-Hanjani S, Schwartz RB, Sathi S, Stieg PE: Hypertensive encephalopathy as a complication of hyperdynamic therapy for vasospasm: Report of two cases. Neurosurgery 44:1113–1116, 1999.
343. Apostolides PJ, Greene KA, Zambramski JM, et al: Intra-aortic balloon pump counterpulsation in the management of concomitant cerebral vasospasm and cardiac failure after subarachnoid hemorrhage: Technical case report. Neurosurgery 38:1056–1060, 1996.
344. Nussbaum ES, Sebring LA, Ganz WF, Madison MT: Intra-aortic balloon counterpulsation augments cerebral blood flow in the patient with cerebral vasospasm: A xenon-enhanced computed tomography study. Neurosurgery 42:206–214, 1998.
345. Nussbaum ES, Heros RC, Solien EE, et al: Intra-aortic balloon counterpulsation augments cerebral blood flow in a canine model of subarachnoid hemorrhage-induced cerebral vasospasm. Neurosurgery 36:879–886, 1995.
346. Kuwayama A, Zervas NT, Shintani A, Pickren KS: Papaverine hydrochloride and experimental cerebral arterial spasm. Stroke 3:27–33, 1972.
347. Ogata M, Marshall BM, Lougheed WM: Observations on the effects of intrathecal papaverine in experimental vasospasm. J Neurosurg 38:20–25, 1973.
348. Heffez DS, Leong KW: Sustained release of papaverine for the treatment of cerebral vasospasm: In vitro evaluation of release kinetics and biological activity. J Neurosurg 77:783–787, 1992.
349. Kaku Y, Yonekawa Y, Tsukahara T, Kazekawa K: Superselective intra-arterial infusion of papaverine for the treatment of cerebral vasospasm after subarachnoid hemorrhage. J Neurosurg 77: 842–847, 1992.
350. Kassell NF, Helm G, Simmons N, et al: Treatment of cerebral vasospasm with intra-arterial papaverine. J Neurosurg 77:848–852, 1992.
351. Nakagomi T, Kassell NF, Hongo K, Sasaki T: Pharmacological reversibility of experimental cerebral vasospasm. Neurosurgery 27:582–586, 1990.
352. Macdonald RL, Zhang J, Sima B, Johns L: Papaverine-sensitive vasospasm and arterial contractility and compliance after subarachnoid hemorrhage in dogs. Neurosurgery 37:962–968, 1995.
353. Milburn JM, Moran CJ, Cross DT III, et al: Increase in diameter of vasospastic intracranial arteries by intraarterial papaverine administration. J Neurosurg 88:38–42, 1998.
354. Elliott JP, Newell DW, Lam DJ, et al: Comparison of balloon angioplasty and papaverine infusion for the treatment of vasospasm following aneurysmal subarachnoid hemorrhage. J Neurosurg 88:277–284, 1998.
355. Polin RS, Apperson-Hansen C, Stat M, et al: Intra-arterially administered papaverine for the treatment of symptomatic cerebral vasospasm. Neurosurgery 42:1256–1267, 1998.
356. Fandino J, Kaku Y, Schuknecht B, et al: Improvement of cerebral oxygenation patterns and metabolic validation of super-selective intra-arterial infusion of papaverine for the treatment of cerebral vasospasm. J Neurosurg 89:93–100, 1998.
357. Firlik KS, Kaufmann AM, Firlik AD, et al: Intra-arterial papaverine for the treatment of cerebral vasospasm following aneurysmal subarachnoid hemorrhage. Surg Neurol 51:66–74, 1999.
358. Pritz MB: Pupillary changes after intracisternal injection of papaverine. Surg Neurol 41:281–283, 1994.
359. McAuliffe W, Townsend M, Eskridge JM, et al: Intracranial pressure changes induced during papaverine infusion for treatment of vasospasm. J Neurosurg 83:430–434, 1995.
360. Miller JA, DeWitte TC, Moran CJ, et al: Severe thrombocytopenia following intra-arterial papaverine administration for treatment of vasospasm. J Neurosurg 83:435–437, 1995.
361. Barnwell SL, Higashida RT, Halbach VV, et al: Transluminal angioplasty of intracerebral vessels for cerebral arterial spasm: Reversal of neurological deficits after delayed treatment. Neurosurgery 25:424–429, 1989.
362. Coyne TJ, Montanera WJ, Macdonald RL, Wallace MC: Percutaneous transluminal angioplasty for cerebral vasospasm after subarachnoid hemorrhage. Can J Surg 37:391–396, 1994.
363. Zubkov YN: Treatment of patients with intracranial arterial aneurysms in the haemorrhagic period. Neurol Res 16:6–8, 1994.
364. Livingstone K, Guterman LR, Hopkins LN: Intraarterial papaverine as an adjunct to transluminal angioplasty for vasospasm induced by subarachnoid hemorrhage [published erratum appears in AJNR Am J Neuroradiol 1993;14:1025]. AJNR Am J Neuroradiol 14:346–347, 1993.
365. Firlik AD, Kaufmann AM, Jungreis CA, Yonas H: Effect of transluminal angioplasty on cerebral blood flow in the management of symptomatic vasospasm following aneurysmal subarachnoid hemorrhage. J Neurosurg 86:830–839, 1997.
366. Eskridge JM, McAuliffe W, Song JK, et al: Balloon angioplasty for the treatment of vasospasm: Results of first 50 cases. Neurosurgery 42:510–517, 1998.
367. Bejjani GK, Bank WO, Olan WJ, Sekhar LN: The efficacy and safety of angioplasty for cerebral vasospasm after subarachnoid hemorrhage. Neurosurgery 42:979–987, 1998.
368. Rosenwasser RH, Armonda RA, Thomas JE, et al: Therapeutic modalities for the management of cerebral vasospasm: Timing of endovascular options. Neurosurgery 44:975–980, 1999.
369. Eskridge JM, Song JK, Elliott JP, et al: Balloon angioplasty of the A_1 segment of the anterior cerebral artery narrowed by vasospasm. J Neurosurg 91:153–156, 1999.
370. European CGRP in Subarachnoid Haemorrhage Study Group: Effect of calcitonin gene–related peptide in patients with delayed postoperative cerebral ischaemia after aneurysmal subarachnoid haemorrhage. Lancet 339:831–834, 1992.
371. Thomas JE, Rosenwasser RH: Reversal of severe cerebral vasospasm in three patients after aneurysmal subarachnoid hemorrhage: Initial observations regarding the use of intraventricular sodium nitroprusside in humans. Neurosurgery 44:48–58, 1999.
372. Thomas JE, Rosenwasser RH, Armonda RA, et al: Safety of intrathecal sodium nitroprusside for the treatment and prevention of refractory cerebral vasospasm and ischemia in humans. Stroke 30:1409–1416, 1999.
373. Teramura A, MacFarlane R, Owen CJ, et al: Application of the 1-μsec pulsed-dye laser to the treatment of experimental cerebral vasospasm. J Neurosurg 75:271–276, 1991.
374. Macfarlane R, Teramura A, Owen CJ, et al: Treatment of vasospasm with a 480-nm pulsed-dye laser. J Neurosurg 75:613–622, 1991.
375. Kaoutzanis MC, Peterson JW, Anderson RR, et al: Basic mechanism of in vitro pulsed-dye laser-induced vasodilation. J Neurosurg 82:256–261, 1995.

CHAPTER 110

Surgical Approaches for Anterior Circulation Aneurysms

KOJI IIHARA ■ GOPAL CHOPRA ■ MICHAEL TYMIANSKI

Aneurysms of the anterior circulation represent more than 85% of all intracranial aneurysms and arise from the internal carotid artery (ICA) or its two terminal branches, the anterior cerebral artery and middle cerebral artery (MCA). Major advances in microneurosurgical techniques and neuroanesthesiology have increased the safety and feasibility of surgery for many anterior circulation aneurysms. Their management continues to be challenging, however, especially given that the population is aging and an increasing number of patients present with intracranial pathology aggravated by systemic comorbidities. Other significant changes that affect the contemporary treatment of aneurysms include progress in awareness of the natural history of ruptured and unruptured aneurysms, an increasingly well-informed patient population, and improving endovascular approaches.

These developments have increased the capacity of neurosurgeons to select appropriate patients for surgical treatment and to provide an overall management strategy that results in the safest, most effective long-term solution for the patient's illness. This solution should be the goal of the surgical management of anterior circulation aneurysms. It is achieved by following two key principles: (1) a strategic approach to management optimized by advanced knowledge and understanding of the disease and (2) a technical component focused on the optimal use of microsurgical operative technique and ancillary technology. At present, surgical treatment, which is the focus of this chapter, is the most widely applied method for securing an aneurysm. In many centers, however, increasing experience with endovascular therapies for ruptured and unruptured aneurysms could alter the choice of primary treatment modality. A collaborative relationship between neurosurgeons and colleagues who are expert in neurointerventional techniques is necessary to maximize the chances of patients making a good recovery after subarachnoid hemorrhage (SAH).

The surgical approach for specific aneurysms is detailed in other chapters; this chapter provides the rationale for using specific surgical approaches to various aneurysms. The surgical options available to approaching aneurysms of the anterior circulation have been affected by advances in microsurgical techniques, a better understanding of microsurgical anatomy, and skull base approaches that minimize brain retraction with concomitant increase in surgical exposure. These all have led to an overall decline in rates of morbidity and mortality. It is impossible to weigh the risks and benefits of surgical treatment without knowledge of the risks associated with the disease, however.

STRATEGIC PRINCIPLES: PREPARATION FOR SURGERY

The most important aspect of the development of competency in vascular neurosurgery is appropriate training and mentorship. The purpose of such training is to endow trainees with the three elements essential to providing SAH patients with the best possible clinical outcomes: (1) a strategic approach to the overall management of aneurysmal SAH based on an understanding of the natural history of the disease, (2) experience in selecting the appropriate surgical approach for individual aneurysms, and (3) technical competency in microsurgical operative technique. The last two elements follow patient selection and are the topics of this chapter.

Medical Considerations

Many patients who suffer an SAH experience systemic and central nervous system complications that affect their outcome. Among the most common acute medical problems related to SAH are cardiac and pulmonary complications. Approximately 20% to 25% of patients with SAH have electrocardiographic (ECG) or cardiac enzyme abnormalities consistent with myocardial ischemia or myocardial infarction.[1–3] The pathophysiology of these abnormalities involves an imbalance in autonomic cardiovascular control and an increase in circulating and local myocardial tissue catecholamines. Only a small fraction of patients have clinically abnormal cardiac function, however, as shown by the presence of congestive heart failure or ECG abnormalities. In a large study of patients with SAH and ECG readings consistent with ischemia or myocardial infarction, the risk of death from cardiac causes was found to be low, with or without aneurysm surgery. ECG abnormalities were associated with more severe neurological injury but were not independently predictive of death or poor clinical outcomes. The advent of improved biochemical markers of myocardial ischemia[4] may be identifying an increasing fraction of SAH patients who exhibit abnormalities but whose significance in this patient population is uncertain. Such a trend could lead to unnecessary delays in the surgical treatment of aneurysms and could reduce the use of aggressive hypertensive-hemodynamic hemodilutional support after surgery. It is relatively uncommon to lose patients because of cardiac compromise and more common to lose patients because of vasospasm and other central nervous system complications.

Neurogenic pulmonary edema complicates the management of a large proportion of poor-grade SAH patients. The underlying pathophysiology consists of an increase in the permeability of pulmonary capillaries or a hydrostatic mechanism related to pulmonary venoconstriction or transient elevation in left-sided cardiovascular pressures after a catecholamine surge.[5] When severe, this complication can delay definitive surgical treatment of an aneurysm and in our experience has delayed surgery more frequently than cardiac compromise.

Operative Positioning

Almost all aneurysms of the anterior circulation can be approached with the patient in the supine position. Appropriate care is taken to pad all pressure points, with particular attention to elbows (ulnar nerves), knees (common peroneal nerves), and heels. Some surgeons advocate positioning the head with the neck flexed forward so that the cranial cavity is above the level of the heart (to facilitate venous return). We prefer to leave the head in a neutral position along the axis of the body so that the surgeon or anesthesiologist can rotate the bed along its long axis to alter the operative angle, while minimizing the lateral excursion of the intracranial contents.

The degree of lateral rotation of the head varies according to the aneurysm and the approach selected. It ranges from 0 degrees for pericallosal lesions to about 45 degrees for lesions of the MCA. Other authors have stressed the importance of positioning the head at specific, exact angles for surgery directed at specific anterior circulation aneurysms. We have found that the precise angle of the head has become less crucial since the advent of contemporary neurosurgical operating room beds. It is relatively easy to make small to moderate adjustments of the operative angle by tilting the bed along its long axis. Such adjustments obviate the surgeon's need to maintain his or her head in uncomfortable positions at any point during the operation.

Operating Microscope

The microscope is the most essential tool in aneurysm surgery and should provide no more hindrance to the progress of a procedure than wearing a pair of glasses. By providing magnification and illumination, this instrument allows microsurgeons to function at a level of technical proficiency that once was impossible. Microsurgeons must be aware of all of the capabilities of their particular microscope and be able to adjust and modify the instrument throughout the procedure.

Before each aneurysm surgery, the microscope must be balanced on its stand. Nothing is more frustrating when an aneurysm ruptures intraoperatively than an out-of-balance microscope. It is an equally good habit to learn to control the zoom and focus with a foot pedal rather than with hand-held controls to obviate the need to remove the hands from the operative site. Many microsurgeons prefer a microscope mouth switch, which permits precise orthogonal adjustments in the position of the microscope. The combination of foot controls for zoom and focus, bed controls for tilting the head angle, and mouth switch permits total control over the operating field and facilitates the surgery.

Intraoperative Angiography

Adjuncts for evaluating the patency of vessels when an aneurysm has been clipped are useful. Patency can be evaluated by visual inspection or by intraoperative Doppler ultrasonography.[6] Intraoperative angiography offers the most effective early evaluation of the surgical result, although its use in the treatment of aneurysms is controversial. It is used routinely in some centers and rarely in others. Large case series indicate that findings from intraoperative angiograms prompt a change in intraoperative strategy, such as clip repositioning, in about 15% of patients.[7] In one study,[8] unexpected angiographic findings necessitated at least one clip adjustment in 11% of cases. Clip readjustments restored blood flow through 6 major arterial occlusions (6%) and completely obliterated 10 persistently filling aneurysms (10%). Factors predicting unexpected arterial occlusion were the presence of a giant aneurysm and location at the basilar apex. Unexpected residual aneurysm was predicted by the presence of a giant aneurysm and a location on the posterior communicating artery (PCoA).

Such data confirm that intraoperative angiography detects unexpected arterial occlusions and residual aneurysms. It is unclear, however, whether this information decreases complications and improves clinical outcomes or whether the anticipation of immediate angiographic evaluation affects the surgeon's intraoperative strategy. Postoperative angiographic evaluation of 107 consecutive anterior circulation aneurysms operated at our institution by the senior author (M.T.) revealed only one clinically silent unexpected arterial occlusion, no residual aneurysms, and no findings that prompted reoperation. The yield from routine intraoperative angiography in unselected patients must be low, although it may be advantageous in selected cases

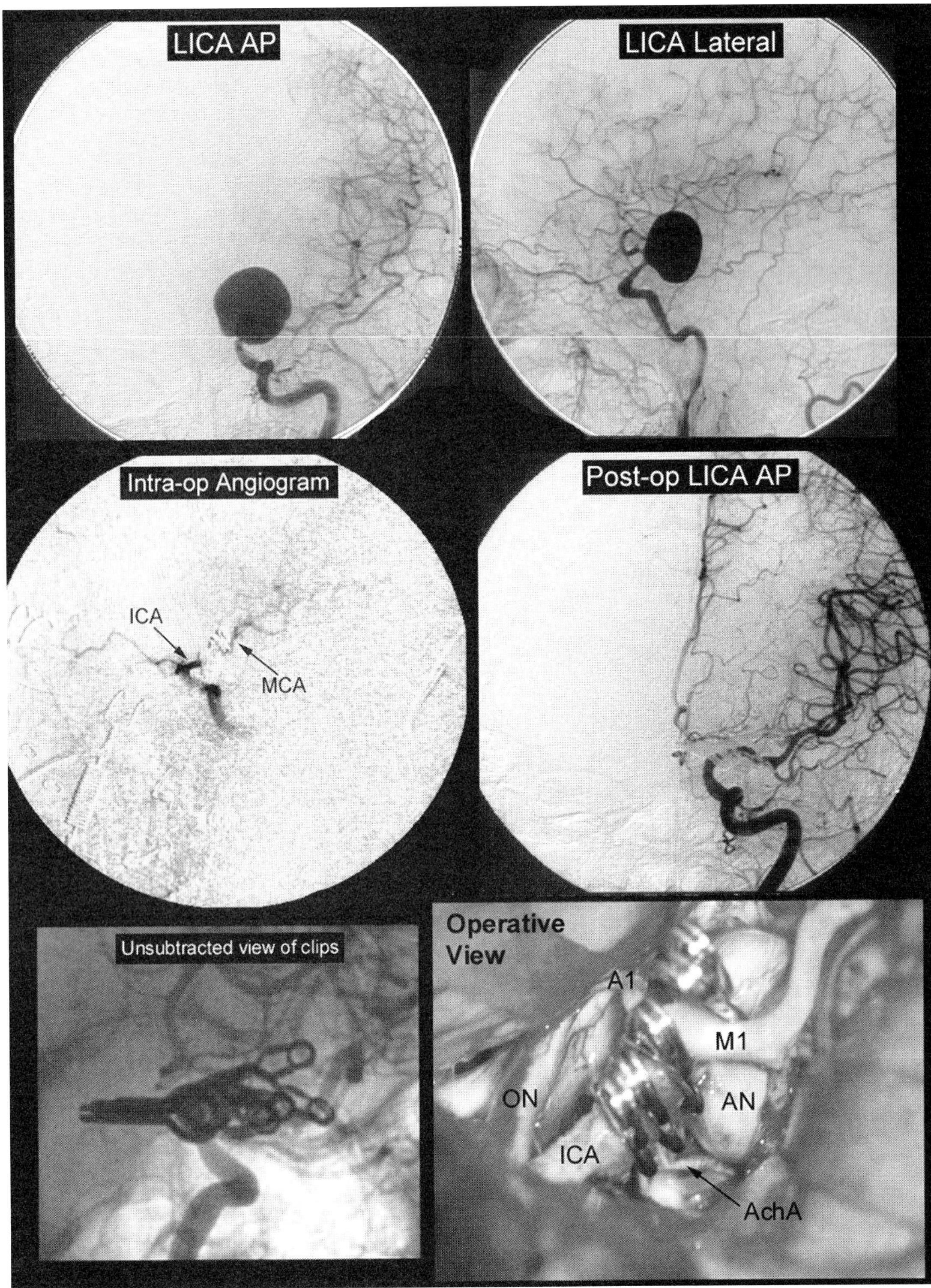

FIGURE 110–1. A 52-year-old man presented with headaches. Angiography revealed a giant carotid aneurysm. Initially the lesion was explored at another institution and found to be difficult to treat. The patient was transferred to our institution for further care. The lesion was exposed through a pterional approach with an orbitozygomatic extension and deflated using hypothermic circulatory arrest. Careful dissection revealed that it was an aneurysm of the anterior choroidal artery. Reconstruction of the internal carotid artery (ICA) required five aneurysm clips. Intraoperative angiography performed to evaluate the ICA after initial clipping revealed poor blood flow distal to the fifth clip. The clip was repositioned and the patient's angiographic and clinical outcomes were excellent. ON, optic nerve; AN, aneurysm.

(Fig. 110–1).[7, 8] An analysis of cost-effectiveness supports the use of intraoperative angiography, especially in selected patients harboring complex aneurysms.[9]

Stereotaxy

Standard stereotaxy and the increasingly popular technology of intraoperative frameless stereotaxy seldom are required for surgery of anterior circulation aneurysms.[10] Most lesions are located easily intraoperatively using standard anatomic landmarks. We have found stereotaxy to be useful in planning approaches to aneurysms of the pericallosal artery, however, because the location of such lesions can vary along the longitudinal course of the artery. In these instances, stereotaxy can minimize the size of the craniotomy flap, while optimizing the surgical approach (Fig. 110–2).

Neuroanesthesia, Monitoring, and Brain Relaxation

Advances in neuroanesthetic techniques have been important developments in aneurysm surgery. Discussion

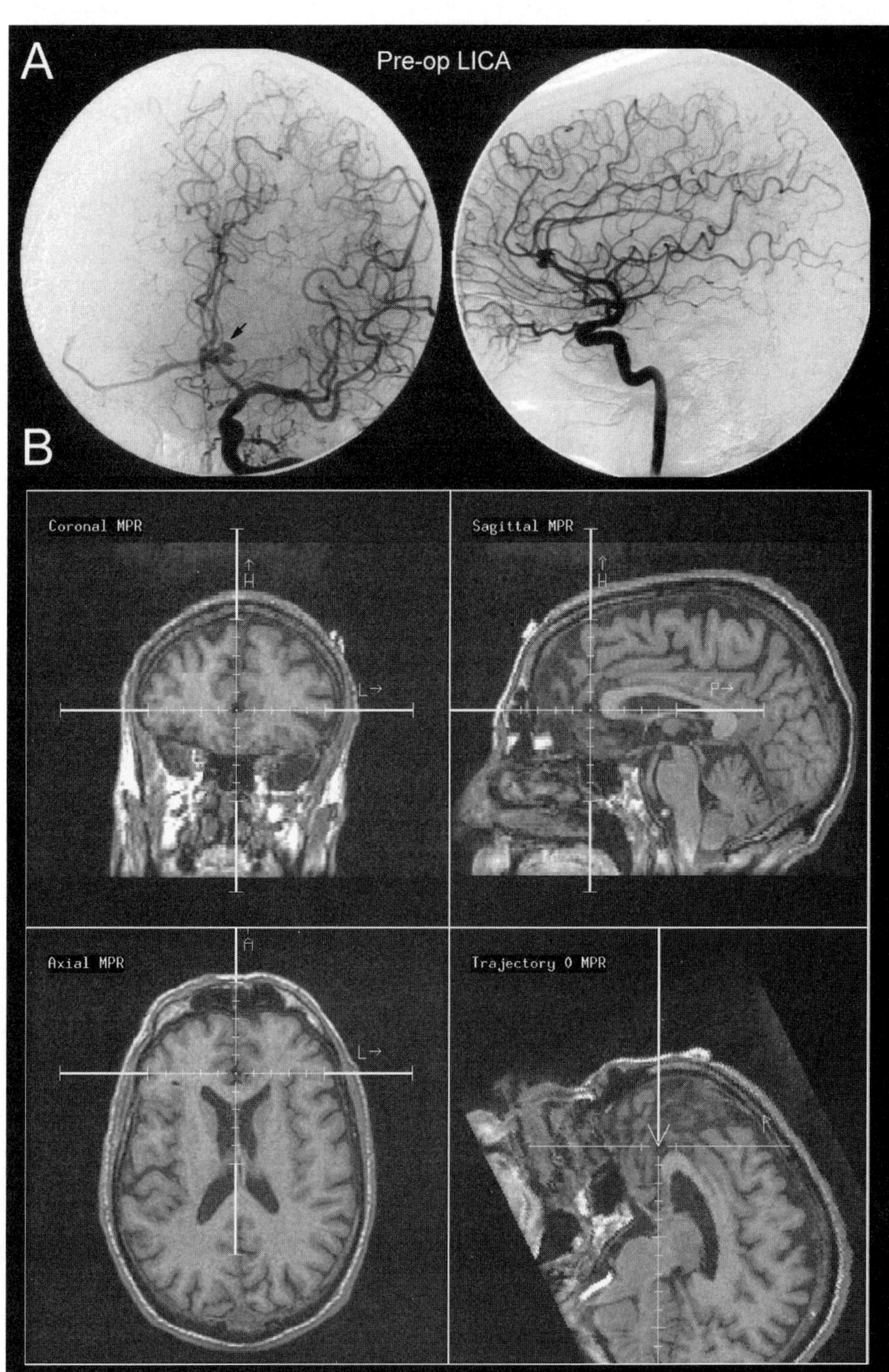

FIGURE 110–2. A 64-year-old man presented with a minor stroke resulting from distal emboli from a partially thrombosed aneurysm of the distal anterior cerebral (pericallosal) artery. The aneurysm was approached through a 2.5-cm craniotomy using intraoperative frameless stereotaxy to plan the craniotomy and trajectory.

of the range of inhalational and intravenous agents available is beyond the scope of this chapter. Appropriate agents must be chosen to maintain anesthesia, while appropriately controlling intracranial pressure, cerebral blood flow, and metabolism. The surgeon and the neuroanesthesiologist must participate in minimizing the likelihood of aneurysmal rupture during induction and in maximizing brain relaxation to enhance exposure during surgery.

Attention should be given to the patient's blood pressure during positioning in the surgical head frame. Pin sites should be infiltrated with local anesthetic, and the anesthesiologist should be aware when pins are tightened so that additional intravenous agents can be used to prevent hypertension. Osmotic agents, such as mannitol, should be given early so that brain relaxation is optimal near the end of the craniotomy and for the duration of the intracranial procedure.

A ventriculostomy is useful to achieve brain relaxation. This procedure often is performed before the patient arrives in the operating room for definitive surgery. If not, ventriculostomy should be kept in mind as an option whenever brain swelling might compromise the surgical exposure. Although the risk of causing an aneurysm to rupture when a ventriculostomy is inserted exists, the amount of damage that can be caused by operating on a swollen brain without proper diversion of the cerebrospinal fluid often outweighs this concern.

Intraoperative monitoring of brain function and specific protocols vary greatly among institutions. Widely available modalities include intraoperative electroencephalography, somatosensory and motor evoked potentials, brain oxygen saturation and pH probes, and temperature monitors. Discussion of the utility of these adjuncts to outcomes and their cost-effectiveness is beyond the scope of this chapter. Electroencephalography and somatosensory and motor evoked potentials monitoring often are used to gauge the depth of anesthesia, especially when neuroprotective agents (e.g., barbiturates) are used. Monitors also are used to gauge brain function during surgery that might compromise the blood supply.

Strategic Considerations of Computed Tomography and Angiography

Surgeons likely have reviewed a patient's computed tomography (CT) and angiography studies on several occasions while deciding whether to operate on a patient's aneurysm. When the decision has been made, however, some issues that relate specifically to operative strategy remain. All but the most distal aneurysms of the anterior circulation can be reached through either a transsylvian or interhemispheric approach. The choice depends on the site and size of the lesion and is covered in the discussion of specific aneurysms subsequently. Some general principles apply. From CT and angiography studies, most experienced aneurysm surgeons can predict with relative accuracy what they will find at surgery using a given surgical approach, how to deal with it, and how to avoid complications. It is a useful exercise to attempt to predict the intraoperative appearance of an aneurysm and the surrounding structures and what type of clipping strategy would be appropriate. Forethought assists in planning a clipping strategy, in the preparation and availability of specialty clips, and in anticipating a need for temporary clipping or an extracranial-intracranial (EC-IC) bypass (Figs. 110–3 and 110–4). The details of a surgical approach might be modified based on the presence of an intracerebral hematoma, the suspicion of thrombus within the aneurysm, or a suspected site of rupture as shown on CT and angiography. If case clipping an aneurysm is not as straightforward as anticipated or desired, a backup plan must be devised beforehand.

CRANIOTOMY

Many neurosurgeons have the technical skill to clip an aneurysm without damaging the brain or surrounding arterial or venous structures perceptibly and to attain excellent neurological outcomes. In such cases, many problems perceived by patients relate to their craniotomy site, including the appearance of the hair and underlying scar, pulling sensations at the incision site, wasting of the ipsilateral temporalis muscle, and defects or bumps at the craniotomy edge. Such matters may seem trivial to neurosurgeons who have cared for their patient through grave illness, but these issues are increasingly relevant now that treatment outcomes are evaluated based on patients' perceptions of quality of life. These issues also have gained importance now that advanced imaging increasingly detects asymptomatic aneurysms whose natural history is uncertain and endovascular treatment alternatives exist. Patients often may choose a treatment based on their perception of morbidity or inconvenience rather than on sound scientific judgment. Attention to surgical technique during opening and closing of a craniotomy must be meticulous to achieve the most satisfactory results, and the technical issues of maximizing hair preservation and minimizing blood loss and craniotomy defects should be considered carefully.

Hair preservation is a surprisingly rare practice, given the paucity of scientific data supporting the need to shave the scalp. Patients highly desire retaining their hair, and the adverse psychologic consequences of a shaved scalp coupled with a neurological illness are self-evident. Several large patient series indicate that it is safe to preserve the hair rather than to shave it off. Several studies suggest that infection rates are higher with shaving.[11–13] In contrast to surgery for malignant brain tumors, in which hair loss often follows adjuvant radiotherapy and chemotherapy, the sole threat to the external appearance of aneurysm patients is the surgeon. Given the previous arguments, all neurosurgeons should consider preserving the hair of patients undergoing aneurysm surgery.

Aneurysm surgery should cause little or no blood loss. In most cases, blood is lost when the scalp is incised. Consequently, blood loss can be minimized by infiltrating the scalp beforehand with a vasopressor,

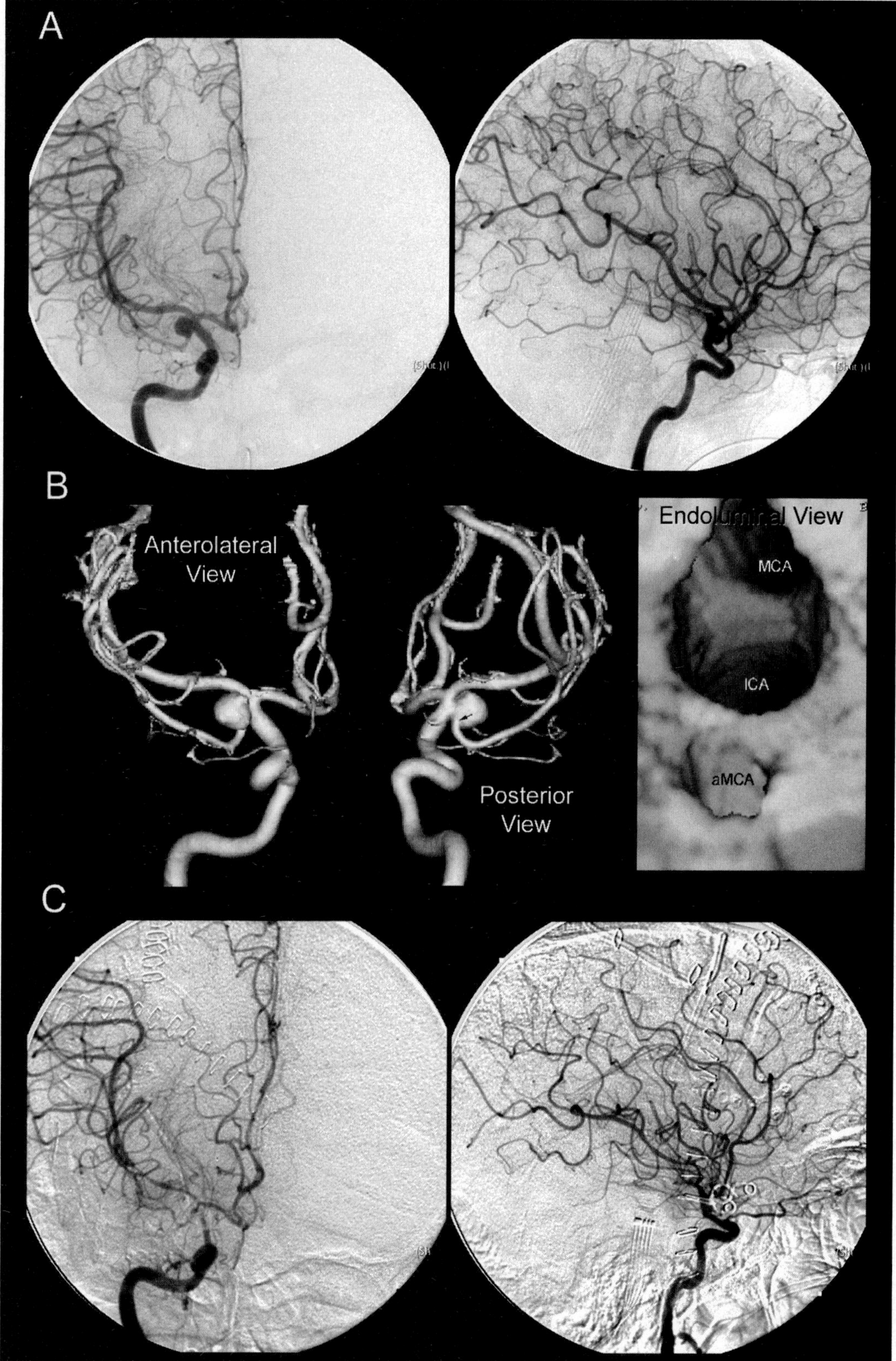

FIGURE 110–3. A 64-year-old woman presented with a grade IV subarachnoid hemorrhage from a carotid aneurysm. Deemed to be a poor surgical candidate at another institution, she was transferred to ours for endovascular therapy. *A,* Angiography revealed her lesion to be an aneurysm of an accessory middle cerebral artery (aMCA), however. *B,* Three-dimensional angiography with endoluminal views of the neck showed that the aMCA originated from the proximal aspect of the dome *(arrow)*. Endovascular treatment was abandoned because of concerns about losing the aMCA. *C,* The patient was treated surgically through a pterional craniotomy with reconstruction of the aneurysm using fenestrated clips.

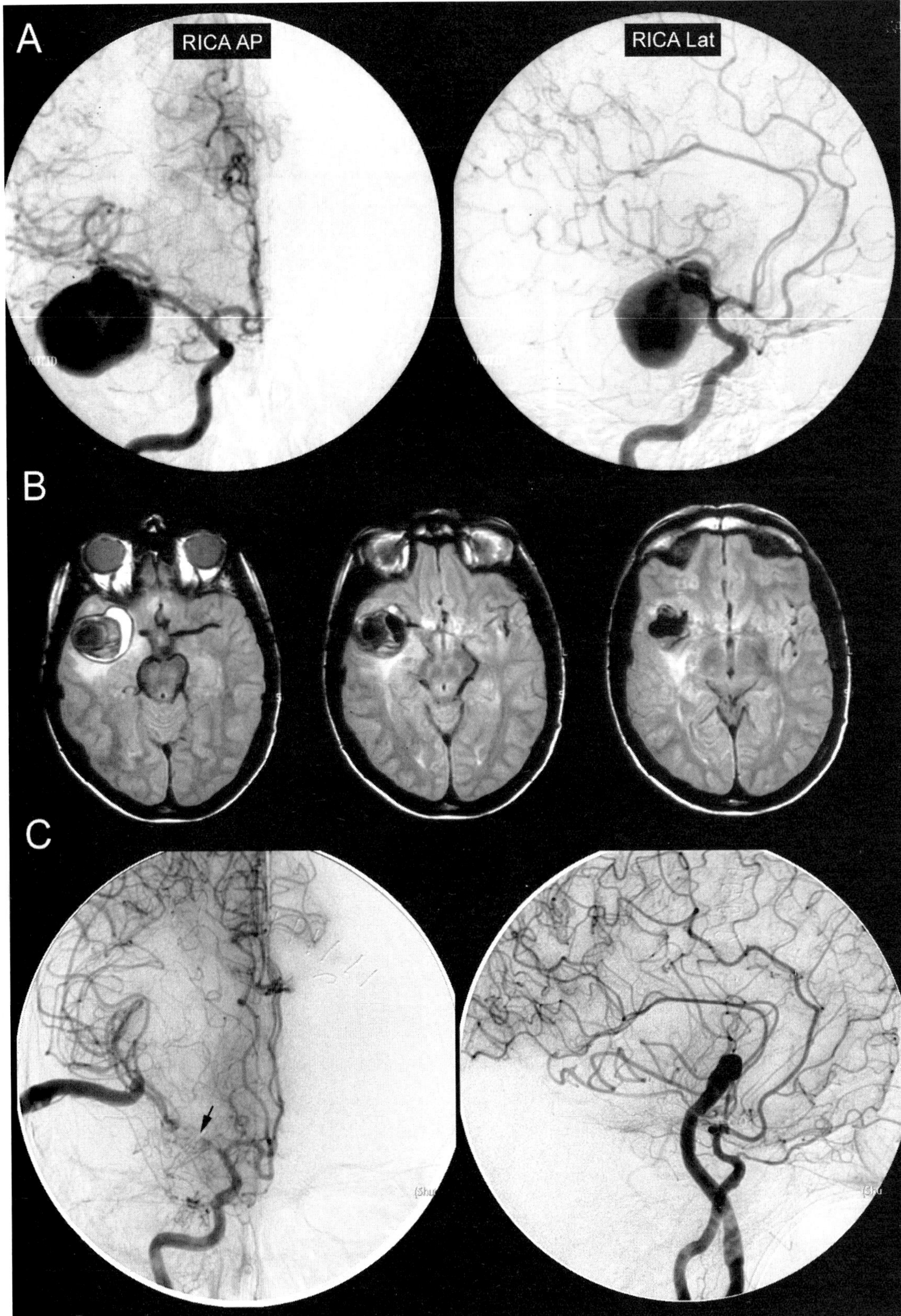

FIGURE 110–4. A 50-year-old woman presented with headaches. *A,* Investigations revealed a giant, partially thrombosed middle cerebral artery (MCA) aneurysm. *B,* Surgical exploration revealed that the aneurysm's neck could not be clipped safely. *C,* The lesion was treated with proximal occlusion using a clip on M1 *(arrow)* and an extracranial-intracranial bypass to maintain the MCA circulation.

such as epinephrine, or with saline alone to cause a tamponade effect at the surgical site. Meticulous attention to hemostasis throughout the procedure is essential to avoid a transfusion (which should be rare in aneurysm surgery) and opacification of the surgical field with blood, which reduces visibility and increases the risk of neurological injury.

The use of high-speed drills has made the opening of a bony craniotomy a simple matter. The apparent ease of using a drill can lead the uninitiated to create a larger than necessary bone flap, however, or, more frequently, a flap lacking beveled edges that fail to overlap with surrounding bone. The motion of the repaired flap may be increased, causing the flap to *sink*. The latter complication most often is avoided by rigidly fixating the craniotomy with one of the diverse craniofacial plating systems, but it still occurs when simple sutures are used to replace the craniotomy flap. Defects in the craniotomy bone, such as those resulting from drilling the sphenoid wing of the temporal bone, can be filled with cranioplasty material. This practice is not essential but prevents the sunken appearance at the pterion caused by a combination of bone defect and atrophy of the temporalis muscle.

Pterional Craniotomy

The pterional transsylvian approach, popularized by Yasargil and colleagues,[15–17] provides excellent exposure of the anterior circulation as well as the upper basilar artery and its bifurcations. This approach, a standard for many neurosurgeons dealing with aneurysms of the anterior circulation, is described briefly.

In Yasargil's description, the patient's head is rotated about 30 degrees to the opposite side, and the vertex is directed 10 degrees down. The neck is extended slightly so that the zygoma is positioned as the highest point in the field. These guidelines have become less crucial with the advent of modern neurosurgical beds that allow the head to be turned along its long axis, as long as the head remains at least in a neutral degree of flexion as discussed earlier. A curvilinear incision is extended from the temporal process of the zygoma, about 1 cm anterior to the tragus of the ear, to the midforehead hairline. If a patient has a receding hairline, a better cosmetic result is achieved by extending the incision posteriorly and beyond the midline to avoid producing a visible scar.

The skin flap is reflected anteriorly, along with the underlying temporalis muscle. A variation on this theme is the interfascial temporalis flap, popularized by Yasargil and colleagues[18] and intended to preserve the frontalis branch of the facial nerve, while maximizing exposure. The scalp, including the galea, is reflected downward by opening the plane between the pericranium and the galea. The temporal fascia is incised just above the fat pad containing the branches of the facial nerve to the forehead so that the fat pad and facial branches can be reflected downward with the scalp flap. The possibility of damaging these branches of the facial nerve is reduced. A cuff of pericranium and temporalis fascia is preserved along the anterior part of the temporal line to facilitate closure of the temporalis muscle and fascia. The temporalis muscle and its fascia are reflected into the posteroinferior margin of the exposure.

Next, a free frontotemporal bone flap with the center of its base at the pterion is elevated and removed. This maneuver usually can be achieved with a single drill or bur hole that permits the craniotome footplate to be introduced into the correct plane. Making several bur holes in a craniotomy is preferable to tearing the dura, however. The anteromedial extent of the flap depends on the aneurysm, ranging from 1 cm anterior to the pterion for aneurysms of the MCA to almost to the midline for aneurysms of the anterior communicating complex. The surgeon must individualize the size of the flap, being aware of variations in the degree of pneumatization of the frontal sinus among individual patients. If the frontal sinus is breached, it should be exenterated and sealed with a pericranial flap before definitive closure. The remainder of the lateral wall of the sphenoid wing is removed. This maneuver is achieved most elegantly with a high-speed drill but often is performed in a piecemeal fashion with a rongeur until the bone is flush with the floor of the anterior cranial fossa. The sphenoid wing can be drilled to varying extents, even beyond the superior orbital fissure and, when necessary, to the anterior clinoid process.

The dura is tacked up, opened in a curvilinear fashion based on the pterion, and retracted. Although the precise technique of opening the dura is unimportant, the intent should be to create flaps that serve as gutters, draining any extradural bleeding from the operative site. Meticulous attention to hemostasis during the opening phase of the operation greatly facilitates the intradural portion of the operation by preventing the surgical field from becoming obscured by blood.

Pterional-Orbitozygomatic Craniotomy

The pterional-orbitozygomatic approach illustrates the philosophy of applying skull base techniques to enhance a surgical exposure, while minimizing brain retraction.[19, 20] Variations on the orbitozygomatic osteotomy most often have been used to expose lesions such as meningiomas and fibrous dysplasia of the sphenoid ridge. This approach has been applied to widen the exposure angle of aneurysms of the anterior and posterior circulation.[21, 22]

Patient positioning is similar to that used for the pterional approach. The curvilinear skin incision is similar but continues about 1 cm inferior to the zygomatic arch. As the skin flap is reflected, the superior orbital foramen is opened with a bone chisel, and the supraorbital nerve is turned over with the scalp for protection. The temporalis muscle is reflected inferiorly along with the pericranium to expose the temporal fossa. Use of the interfascial temporalis flap described earlier helps the surgeon to remain in the subperiosteal plane while exposing the zygoma. The periosteum is elevated over the entire extent of the zygomatic arch, the superolateral orbital rim, and the upper lateral

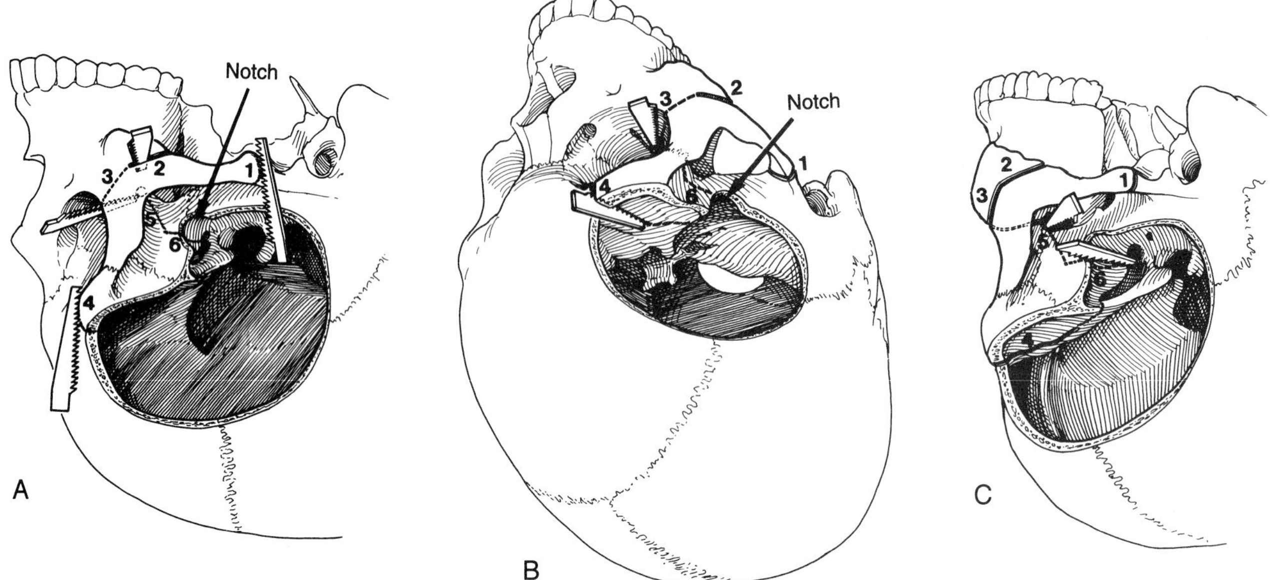

FIGURE 110–5. The orbitozygomatic extension. Osteotomies are performed as described in the text, initially along the root and maxillary buttress of the zygoma *(A)*, followed by the orbital osteotomies *(B)*, and ending by connecting the superior and inferior orbital fissures *(C)*. (From Zabramski JM, Kiris T, Sankhla SK, et al: Orbitozygomatic craniotomy: Technical note. J Neurosurg 89:336–341, 1998. With permission from Journal of Neurosurgery.)

surface of the maxilla. The periorbita is dissected free superiorly and laterally. A standard pterional bone flap is elevated, and then the frontal lobe is elevated along with the overlying dura to expose the orbital roof.

The osteotomy cuts (Fig. 110–5) begin with the base of the zygomatic process of the temporal bone. An angled cut through the maxillary process of the zygoma extending medially through the lateral orbital wall to the inferior orbital fissure follows. Next, the supraorbital rim is cut, as is the orbital roof with the periorbita protected, back toward the sphenoid ridge, and then laterally. This last cut is joined to the osteotomy in the lateral orbital wall at the inferior orbital fissure. The bone segment is mobilized and removed. The anterior clinoid process and the lateral wall and roof of the orbit can be resected if additional exposure is needed. The dura is opened using a wide curvilinear incision based on the pterion and reflected inferiorly along with the globe. When combined with resection of the orbital rim, as described earlier, this is a key maneuver that increases the exposure by depressing the globe and widening the angle of approach to the basal frontal lobe and the interhemispheric fissure. Improved exposure of lesions that traditionally were exposed through the pterional route can be obtained (Fig. 110–6). The operating microscope is brought into the field, and microdissection of appropriate structures is performed according to the principles outlined earlier for the pterional approach.

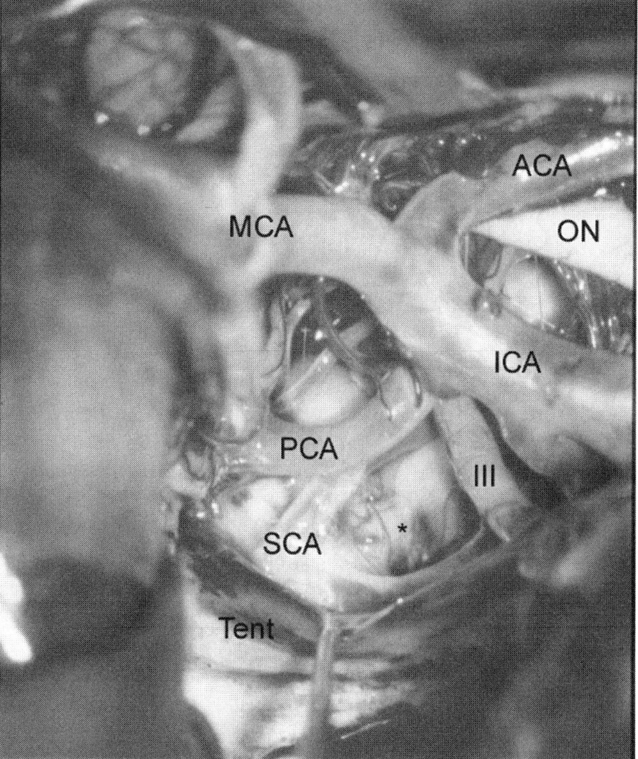

FIGURE 110–6. Intraoperative view of anterior circulation vessels through the orbitozygomatic approach. ICA, internal carotid artery; ACA, anterior cerebral artery; MCA, middle cerebral artery; PCA, posterior cerebral artery; SCA, superior cerebellar artery; Tent, medial edge of tentorium cerebelli; III, third cranial nerve; ON, optic nerve. Asterisk indicates cerebral peduncle.

A modification of the orbitozygomatic approach that achieves a similar degree of anterior exposure is the orbital osteotomy, in which the rim of the orbit and the superior and lateral orbital walls are removed. The anterior osteotomy cuts are identical to those described earlier. The osteotomy line typically performed along the maxillary process of the zygoma is replaced, however, by one that extends from the intraorbital inferior orbital fissure, along the base of the lateral orbital rim. The osteotomy at the base of the zygomatic process is omitted. This modification produces a free bone fragment that encompasses the orbital rims and walls but leaves the zygomatic arch in place. This approach requires less subperiosteal dissection along the zygoma, causing less trauma to the temporalis muscle. Potentially, however, it permits less access to basal structures and the middle fossa floor because the zygomatic arch limits the capacity to reflect the temporalis muscle inferiorly. This disadvantage is rarely a concern with anterior circulation aneurysms.

Compared with the pterional approach, the orbitozygomatic osteotomy and its variations add considerably wider access to relevant structures and reduce the depth of the exposure. The enhanced angle of approach obtainable by removing the orbital roof and depressing the globe increases the superior limits of the angle of exposure, easing access to aneurysms of the anterior communicating complex with minimal brain retraction.[21] Reducing the need for brain retraction shortens the intracranial portion of the operation. For aneurysms of the anterior communicating complex, we have found it unnecessary to resect the gyrus rectus in most cases, a maneuver sometimes necessary to reach the aneurysm through the pterional craniotomy. Although the more extensive craniotomy has the potential to increase morbidity in a case, the orbitozygomatic osteotomy is tolerated extremely well, and no untoward morbidity is attributable to it in trained hands.

Frontal Craniotomy

Aneurysms arising in the midline, particularly those of the distal anterior cerebral artery, can be reached through an anterior interhemispheric approach. More proximal lesions at the anterior communicating complex and carotid ophthalmic aneurysms also were approached in this manner before the pterional approach became popular. Large surgical series have shown the feasibility and efficacy of obliterating aneurysms of the anterior communicating artery (ACoA) using the anterior interhemispheric route, with excellent results.[23–25] This approach has been associated with a higher frequency of venous injury, neuropsychological sequelae, and anosmia, however.[26, 27] For proximal anterior circulation aneurysms, frontal craniotomy largely has been supplanted by the pterional variations.

Originally, ACoA aneurysms were approached through a trephine craniotomy made through a limited transverse incision performed in a forehead crease as described by Lougheed[28] and modified by others.[29] Salient features of the operative technique include a low anterior frontal midline trephine (about 4 cm), a unilateral dural opening (2.5 cm), opening of the anterior interhemispheric fissure, and exposure of the aneurysm and anterior cerebral vessels through a phased dissection. Anatomic orientation is retained because the entire procedure was performed in the midline (interhemispheric fissure) along rigid structures, such as the superior sagittal sinus and falx cerebri.[30]

Proponents of the anterior interhemispheric approach suggest that it has the following benefits: The retraction pressure on the brain is thought to be less than that of the standard pterional route; various types of aneurysms, especially those located high and in a posterior direction, can be clipped; and clots can be removed adequately from the interhemispheric fissure, the chiasmatic and prepontine cisterns, and the frontal lobe. Interarterial anastomosis between both anterior cerebral arteries can be applied if necessary to ease the clipping of unusual aneurysms. Finally, temporary occlusion of the A1 and A2 branches and external decompression can be achieved easily. Most of these benefits apply equally well to the pterional route, however, especially with the orbitozygomatic variation. The anterior interhemispheric approach to anterior communicating aneurysms should be used only by experienced hands and in selected patients.

The patient is placed in a supine position with the head immobilized and facing forward. The jaw protrudes slightly to facilitate an approach to the frontal lobes. A bicoronal skin incision is made behind the hairline, and a bur hole is drilled. A bifrontal craniotomy is performed with its inferior extent as close to the upper ridge of the orbita as possible. In most cases, the frontal sinus is opened, requiring that it be exenterated, packed, and covered with a pericranial flap at closure. The ostium communicating with the nasal passage is closed with bone chips produced during the craniotomy, and a small amount of bone is smeared firmly over the chips to block all communication with the nasal passage. The dura is opened bilaterally along the anterior bone edge as far forward as possible to minimize damage to the bridging veins. Through this dural opening, the falx cerebri is cut as far forward as possible. Bleeding from the severed end of the superior sagittal sinus is stopped by ligation, electrocoagulation, or both. Alternatively the dura can be cut unilaterally, sparing the superior sagittal sinus and protecting the contralateral olfactory tract and bulb. A variation on the bone approach consists of a more basal interhemispheric exposure that removes additional bone, extending down to the nasion to reduce further the extent of frontal lobe retraction.[26] The operating microscope then is brought into the field for the remainder of the intracranial procedure.

In the case of aneurysms of the distal ACoA, the anteroposterior location of the craniotomy is determined according to the site of the aneurysm. Intraoperative stereotaxy (conventional or frameless; see Fig. 110–2) can be used to optimize the location of the opening and to minimize its size. Most distal aneurysms operated on through this route can be clipped successfully with a well-placed flap that is 3 to 4 cm at its greatest diameter. In this approach, the dura is opened in a U-shaped fashion on one side of the superior sagittal sinus and reflected medially with the sinus itself. An operating microscope is used for the remaining portion of the approach, and care should be taken to avoid surface bridging veins.

INTRADURAL OPERATION

When the craniotomy is completed and the dura is opened, the operating microscope is brought into the field. Many general surgical principles apply, regardless of the aneurysm and the chosen approach.

Strategic Principles

Hemostasis of the extradural portion of the operation should be meticulous. Self-retaining retractors, instrument holders, hand rests, and other items that need to be attached in the vicinity of the head should be tested and in place before the operating microscope is brought into the surgical field. The operating microscope should be balanced, draped, and positioned so that it is easy to use. A microscope draped too tightly can be thrown out of balance. The surgeon should be comfortable and have access to all appropriate controls (usually for the microscope and bipolar cauterization). The aneurysm clip applier should be tested. Based on the angiographic appearance of the aneurysm, a permanent aneurysm clip should be chosen early. Temporary clips should be available before the aneurysm is reached.

Anatomic Principles of Surgery

BRAIN RETRACTION

Each operation should use the least amount of brain retraction as possible. A good principle to begin with is the assumption that all aneurysms, including those of poor-grade patients with swollen brains, can be approached with little retraction. If significant retraction is being applied, the operative strategy should be reconsidered. Frequently a modification of the approach, the extent of exposure, cerobrospinal fluid drainage, and patience permit the amount of retraction to be reduced.

With an appropriate strategy, most anterior circulation aneurysms can be clipped using a single brain retractor. It is not the number of retractors, but their position on the brain and the pressure they apply that count. The face of a brain spatula should be parallel to the surface of the brain to avoid injuries from the edges of a retractor. At the beginning of the operation and as the arachnoid dissection proceeds, the retractor should be adjusted frequently to permit relevant structures to be separated from adhesions.

ARACHNOID DISSECTION

Arachnoid dissection is the key to a successful aneurysm operation. To some degree, the direction and sequence of cisternal openings depend on the location of the lesion. The neurosurgeon must be familiar with the anatomy of the subarachnoid cisterns, however. The arachnoid membrane should be dissected extensively and completely. This translucent membrane is surprisingly strong and often limits the mobility of any brain structure to which it is attached, be it the frontal lobe, an artery, or a cranial nerve. Opening the arachnoid cisterns permits cerebrospinal fluid to escape, a subarachnoid hematoma to be drained, and the brain to be retracted evenly to maximize exposure. Ignoring this principle uniformly leads to increased injury of the brain and vascular structures.

Navigation through the subarachnoid space requires few microsurgical instruments. Almost every aneurysm can be exposed using suction, bipolar cauterization, microscissors, and a single microdissector. Sharp dissection takes more practice than blunt dissection but places less stress on arachnoid-bound structures. Straight instruments are preferable to sharply curved ones (such as hooks), whose tips are easier to lose sight of in tight spots. Rather than reaching for a hook, it might be more prudent to open the overlying arachnoid more widely under direct vision.

ANEURYSM DISSECTION

Proximal and distal control should be obtained. The parent artery should be exposed proximal to the aneurysm to permit the application of a temporary clip. The distal artery must be exposed to permit visualization of the distal aneurysm neck. If possible, the side of the parent vessel opposite the side on which the aneurysm arises should be exposed before the neck of the aneurysm is dissected, and the aneurysm neck should be dissected before the fundus. All perforating arterial branches should be separated from the aneurysm neck before the clip is passed around the aneurysm.

Dissection should not be impeded by a fear of intraoperative rupture. Typically, morbidity caused by a suboptimal exposure and insufficient microdissection outweigh morbidity caused by a rupture. When appropriate preoperative and operative strategies are applied, all intraoperative ruptures can be controlled. Small hemorrhages caused by pinhole ruptures should be controlled by applying a small cotton pledget to the bleeding point, by concomitantly reducing mean arterial pressure, and by patience. If the hemorrhage does not stop, a temporary clip can be applied to the proximal and distal blood supply as needed. Definitive clipping of the aneurysm can proceed at the usual pace.

ANEURYSM CLIPPING

The surgeon must be familiar with the available varieties of clips. Clipping strategies that result in the blind application of one or both clip blades should be avoided. In most cases, both clip blades can be visualized by extending the dissection to expose the neck and fundus, by selecting a different clipping strategy using an angled or fenestrated clip, or by using multiple clips. Clips can be removed and reapplied as many times as necessary to obliterate the aneurysm optimally, while preserving the parent vessels. After the aneurysm is secured, the entire length of the clip should be inspected to ensure that only the aneurysm neck, not adjacent structures, is obliterated. The area should be inspected to make certain that the clip does not kink or obstruct a major vessel and that no perforating branches are included in it. Some aneurysms cannot be clipped in a straightforward manner. The surgeon must be able to recognize these situations and to consider alternative strategies, such as wrapping,[31] trapping, and proximal occlusion. One of the most difficult and personal decisions for a surgeon is when to stop and back out.

Transsylvian Exposure of Aneurysms of the Carotid and Middle Cerebral Arteries

For most lesions approached through a pterional craniotomy, the sylvian cistern between the basal frontal and temporal lobes and the whole lamina terminalis cistern adhering the frontal lobes to the optic nerves and chiasms are opened. The landmarks for identifying the optic nerve are at the intersection of the olfactory tract and the sphenoid wing. A wide opening permits cerebrospinal fluid to be removed and slackens the brain. Using sharp dissection with a blade or arachnoid knife, the surgeon enters the sylvian cistern at the level of the opercular frontal gyrus.

The arachnoid of the sylvian cistern may be thin and transparent, allowing good visualization of structures within the cistern. Often, however, it is mildly yellow or completely opaque after an SAH. In the latter case, gentle suction and irrigation can remove hematoma. All that is needed is a 1- to 2-mm space on the surface between the frontal and temporal lobes to allow easy entry into the cistern and rapid identification of the major vessels. Often the arachnoid and pia of the frontal and temporal lobes are only superficially adherent. After the cistern has been entered a few millimeters, separation becomes easy. In some cases, the direction of the cistern is obscured from the surface. The orientation of the cistern can be discovered by following a superficial artery into the fissure toward the main trunk of the MCA.

Meticulous dissection that avoids any injury to the MCA candelabra and the superficial middle cerebral venous system is essential. The superficial middle cerebral veins are one or more large venous channels that course on the temporal side of the sylvian fissure. Typically, they empty into the sphenoparietal or cavernous sinuses but occasionally continue around the temporal pole to the superior petrosal sinus. The arachnoid of the sylvian cistern should be opened on the frontal side of these veins so that they do not cross the sylvian fissure when the frontal lobe is retracted. Occasionally two or three fronto-orbital venous tributaries that cross the sylvian fissure to enter the middle cerebral vein must be sacrificed to complete the dissection. With experience, however, it is possible to split the entire sylvian fissure without sacrificing veins.

After an SAH, arachnoidal and pial attachments may be apparent within the sylvian fissure. The frontal and temporal lobes are seldom so tightly adherent to the MCA, however, that the fissure cannot be opened without incurring damage to the frontal or temporal surfaces.

Because the most anteromesial portion of the temporal lobe adheres tightly to the frontal lobe, the final stages of this dissection often are the most tenuous. The orbitofrontal gyrus sharply indents the corresponding temporal lobe, distorting this portion of the sylvian cistern. To avoid damaging the gyrus, the cistern must be followed laterally around it. The frontal lobe can be retracted away from the M1 segment of the MCA with relative ease because M1 never supplies branches to it.

When dissection of this division of the sylvian cistern is completed, the frontal and temporal lobes fall apart away from the sphenoid ridge and orbital roof, enlarging the overall angle of the exposure. When the carotid and lamina terminalis cisterns are opened bilaterally, a large empty pyramidal space is created. Its base is bordered by the flattened sphenoid ridge and orbital roof and its upper and lower margins by the separated frontal and temporal operculi (with its apex directed into the limen insulae). An orbitozygomatic extension with depression of the eyeball enhances the angle of this pyramid further while reducing its depth. Extensive visualization of the relevant structures is achieved with less brain retraction.

Interhemispheric Exposure

ANEURYSMS OF THE ANTERIOR COMMUNICATING COMPLEX

The olfactory tract is dissected from the orbital surface of the frontal lobes bilaterally as far as the olfactory trigone. With this method, the olfactory tract, and olfactory function are preserved because traction is not applied to the olfactory tract, even if the frontal lobe is elevated during surgery. Unilateral variations aimed at preserving the contralateral olfactory nerve also have been described.[24, 26] After ICA has been exposed, the arachnoid membrane is opened over the base of the sylvian fissure, starting proximally. Although subarachnoid blood clots are being removed, dissection proceeds in a distal direction. Removal of clots reduces brain volume, facilitating elevation of the frontal lobes and exposure of both A1 segments to obtain proximal control.

Next, dissection proceeds to the interhemispheric fissure. At this stage, the aneurysm is not approached directly. Instead the distal A2 segments beneath the genu of the corpus callosum are approached and exposed. From that point, blunt dissection is used to proceed toward the ACoA complex. Damage to the medial surface of the cerebral hemispheres is minimized, the entire length of the A2 segment is exposed, and subsequent management of the aneurysm becomes easy.

As the aneurysm is approached, a temporary clip should be available for the surgeon to place on the dominant A1 segment. In the event of aneurysm rupture during dissection, temporary clips applied to the subdominant A1 and both A2 segments allow treatment of the aneurysm in a bloodless field.

The direction that an aneurysm projects should be considered, and an aneurysm never should be dissected from its dome. Particularly in the case of a superiorly projecting aneurysm, dissection starting from the A2 segments initially leads to the aneurysm's dome, with a higher risk of rupture. In such a case, dissection of the proximal A2 segments should be halted. After temporary clipping of the dominant A1 segment, both frontal lobes should be dissected from the optic nerves, proceeding medially until the terminal portions of both A1 segments are identified. In this manner, the ACoA complex can be visualized without brain resection. Laterally projecting aneurysms should be dissected toward the ACoA complex along the lateral wall of the A2 segments in a direction opposite that to which the aneurysm points.

The aneurysm is freed from the surrounding vessels, brain tissue, dura mater, and optic chiasm, and the neck is exposed. Sometimes the presence of either small arteries (such as the hypothalamic perforating vessels) behind the neck or a fibrous adhesion makes it possible to kink a feeding or draining vessel inadvertently or to overlook the presence of a small aneurysm behind the larger one. Consequently, it is best to dissect the aneurysm completely from all surrounding structures until it *hangs loose,* allowing a direct view of the neck of the aneurysm during clipping. Then a clip is placed on the neck.

The ACoA complex is the site of frequent anatomic variations. Larger variations (such as an azygos anterior cerebral artery)[32] may be detected on preoperative angiography, but smaller variations may be detected only by direct inspection during surgery. Consequently the arteries leading to and leaving the aneurysm must be dissected completely. Fenestrations[33] or a small aneurysm located behind a large one is common in this region.

ANEURYSMS OF THE DISTAL ANTERIOR CEREBRAL ARTERY

After the bone flap is elevated, the dura is opened as a U-shaped or triangular flap based on the superior sagittal sinus. The topography of the draining veins in this region is variable, but only a 2- to 3-cm gap between two veins is necessary, and one can be developed with careful microdissection. The medial surface of the frontal lobe is retracted away from the falx, and a small tunnel is established. Frontal branches of the pericallosal artery are followed toward the corpus callosum. A false impression of having reached the corpus callosum may be gained as the falx ends and adherent cingulate gyri are encountered. Gentle separation of the cingulate gyri reveals the white corpus callosum hidden beneath, however. The pericallosal arteries are seen on top of the corpus callosum. Most proximal pericallosal aneurysms are located proximal to the section of artery first encountered. The artery is followed anteriorly 1 to 2 cm to reach the aneurysm. The aneurysm is dissected and clipped according to the principles outlined previously.

SPECIFIC ANEURYSMS

As discussed earlier, the principles of meticulous opening, adequate surgical exposure, opening of the arachnoid cisterns and sylvian fissure, and optimal brain relaxation apply to all intracranial operations. The following discussion highlights strategic and technical matters related to specific aneurysms.

Aneurysms of the Cervical and Intrapetrous Carotid Artery

PRESENTATION AND DECISION MAKING

Basal ICA aneurysms can arise at any level from the carotid bifurcation in the neck to the dural ring where the ICA enters the subarachnoid space. During evaluation, these aneurysms should be categorized as symptomatic or incidental, and the type of risk that they pose to the patient (discussed further subsequently) should be considered. It is useful to classify the aneurysms according to cause; straightforward saccular aneurysms are rare below the level of the cavernous sinus. The most common aneurysmal lesions of the intrapetrous ICA are pseudoaneurysms caused by spontaneous or traumatic carotid dissections or those caused by iatrogenic vessel injury.

Dissecting aneurysms rarely rupture, and acute symptoms are produced by reduced blood flow or distal emboli. When patients present with an established, stable neurological deficit, initial treatment typically is conservative because about 70% of dissecting ICA aneurysms recanalize spontaneously.[34] Symptomatic lesions may require more urgent surgical treatment, which should be individualized (Figs. 110–7 and 110–8). As discussed earlier, decision making is more difficult with completely asymptomatic lesions.

Iatrogenic aneurysms likely require treatment or close observation because their risk of rupturing is higher than dissecting aneurysms.[35, 36] Dissecting pseudoaneurysms most frequently are observed in patients with collagen-vascular disorders or fibromuscular dysplasia. Although they rarely resolve spontaneously (see Figs. 110–7 and 110–8), symptoms should be stable.[37] Whether asymptomatic dissections of the cervical carotid artery require prophylactic surgical correction has not been established.

Aneurysms arising from the petrous carotid artery are extremely rare. They almost always are pseudoaneurysms associated with an erosive process of the skull base, such as a tumor, or they are iatrogenic.[36, 38] It is difficult to comment about their natural history because they are so rare. Pseudoaneurysms caused by an erosive process often progress, resulting in parent vessel rapture or occlusion. Enthusiasm for managing lesions conservatively is low. Most require close observation and treatment, even when they are asymptomatic (Fig. 110–9).

TREATMENT

Primary reconstruction of cervical ICA pseudoaneurysms is difficult because the vessel giving rise to the lesion often is abnormal. Surgical options include aneurysm excision with reanastomosis of the ICA, reimplantation of the ICA onto the external carotid artery, and

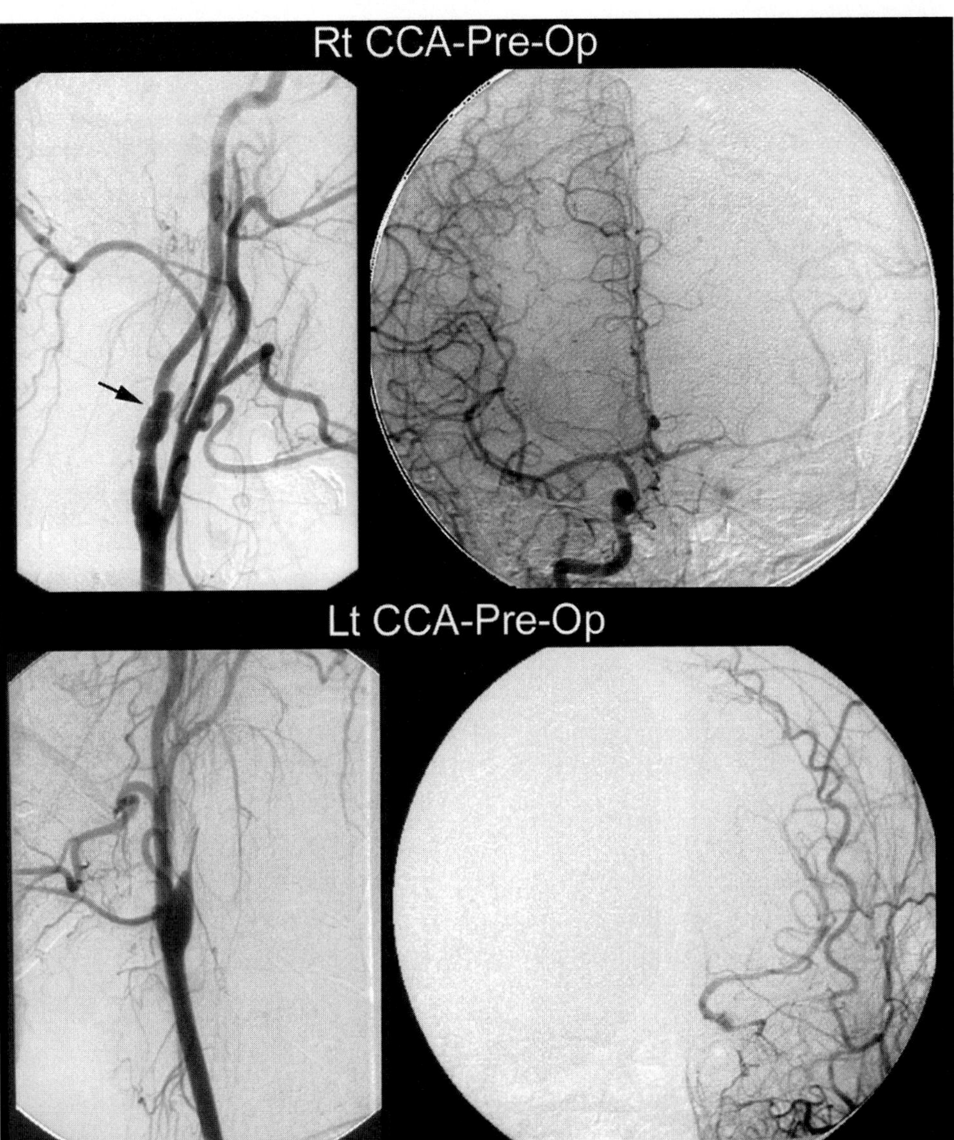

FIGURE 110–7. Angiograms of a 30-year-old woman who suffered bilateral spontaneous carotid dissections with right internal carotid artery (ICA) pseudoaneurysm formation *(arrow)*, and complete left ICA occlusion. Cross-flow from the right to the left was poor. The patient presented with rapidly progressive right hemiplegia and aphasia. A decision was made to revascularize the left hemisphere emergently with an extracranial-intracranial bypass using a saphenous vein graft.

placement of an interposition graft. Simple aneurysmectomy and closure of the wall defect with or without a patch are options in only about 20% of cases.[35] Reconstruction of pseudoaneurysms of the intrapetrous ICA is rarely possible. Operative management most often consists of trapping the diseased segment with or without reconstruction or a bypass procedure (see Fig. 110–9). Indications for different bypass procedures vary with diverse aneurysms and are discussed in the following sections.

Intracavernous Aneurysms

PRESENTATION AND DECISION MAKING

About 20% of intracavernous ICA aneurysms are large (>1 cm), and about 20% are giant (>2.5 cm). With modern imaging, an increasing proportion of saccular aneurysms is being discovered incidentally or concomitantly with other intracranial aneurysms. Although infectious or traumatic aneurysms often require treatment, the natural course of many intracavernous saccular lesions is benign.[39] Neurosurgeons must be familiar with how these aneurysms present, the risks they can pose, and their indications for treatment.

Asymptomatic cavernous aneurysms have an uncertain but likely small risk of becoming symptomatic. The most important issue is to determine whether the patient is at risk for a subarachnoid rupture. In select cases, extension beyond the dural ring can be determined by diagnostic imaging. Many cases require surgical exploration to ascertain this detail, however. In the event of rupture, aneurysms confined to the cavernous sinus pose little danger because they do not cause SAH. Treatment can be deferred until they become symptomatic.

Compression most often is caused by large or giant aneurysms. The aneurysms often are partially thrombosed, causing a cavernous sinus syndrome. Patients may experience any combination of symptoms involving cranial nerves III, IV, and VI and less often facial

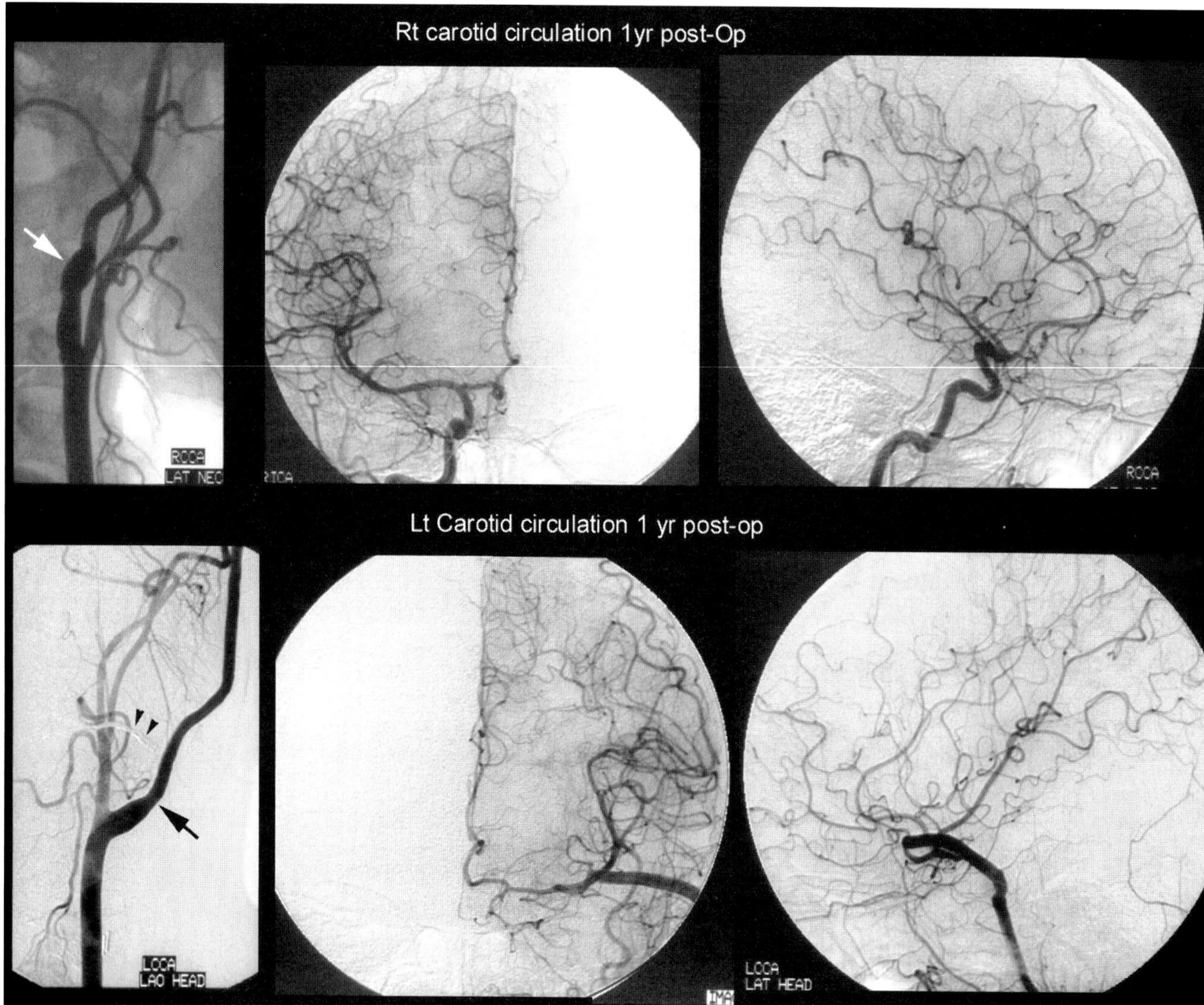

FIGURE 110–8. Angiograms from the same patient as shown in Figure 110–7, 1 year later. The patient made an excellent clinical recovery. She had no motor deficits and a mild expressive dysphasia. The configuration of the right pseudoaneurysm did not change, exemplifying stability of these lesions over time *(white arrow)*. The saphenous vein graft from the cervical internal carotid artery (ICA) proximal to the dissection *(black arrow)* fills the entire middle cerebral artery territory on the left. A clip is visible *(arrowheads)* on the ICA stump distal to the proximal anastomosis site.

sensory symptoms in the V_2 distribution. Sizable aneurysms enlarge the cavernous sinus and can impinge on the optic apparatus to cause visual symptoms.[40] Acute enlargement or thrombosis can cause painful ophthalmoplegia, prompting a more urgent need for treatment. Indications should be individualized, however. Expectant therapy of a painless cavernous sinus syndrome in elderly patients who might not tolerate aggressive treatment often is associated with partial or complete resolution of symptoms within several weeks to months. We reserve treatment for young individuals with progressive symptoms, visual symptoms, or pain.

The rupture of an aneurysm restricted to the cavernous sinus produces a carotid-cavernous fistula. Almost uniformly, the fistulas are high flow and unlikely to regress spontaneously. Patients always present with a dramatic pulsatile exophthalmos and conjunctival injection associated with a rise in intraocular pressures that can damage vision. The increased venous pressure can cause reflux into cortical veins through the sphenoparietal sinus anteriorly and the superior or inferior petrosal sinuses posteriorly. Such patients are at high risk for an intracranial hemorrhage.[80] Consequently, all high-flow carotid-cavernous fistulas require treatment.

Larger intracavernous aneurysms and aneurysms located near the dural ring can erode through the dura and manifest with an SAH (Fig. 110–10). Indications for treatment are similar to those associated with other aneurysms within the subarachnoid space.

TREATMENT

Intracavernous ICA aneurysms can be treated by direct clipping, trapping, proximal ICA occlusion, or bypass.

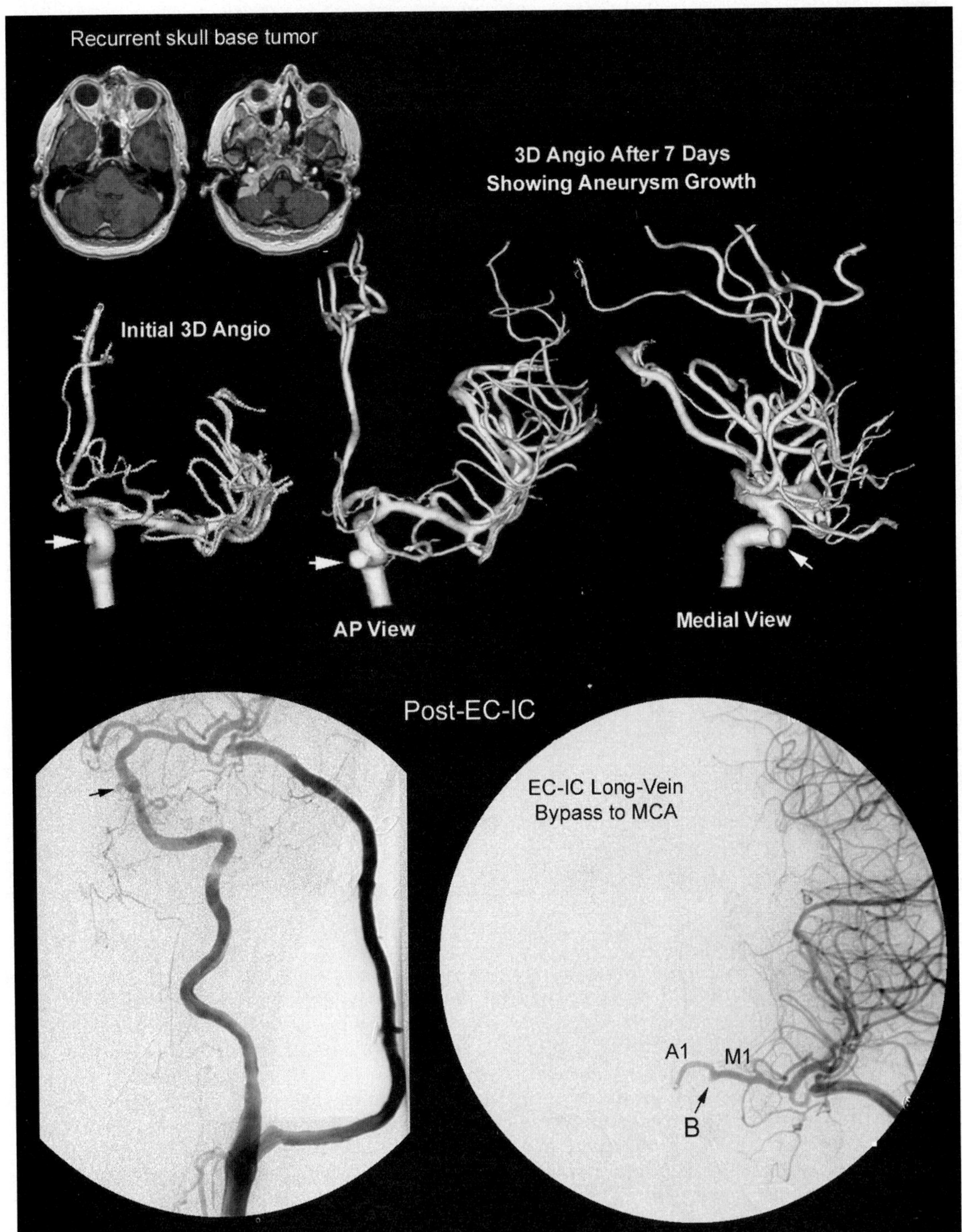

FIGURE 110–9. A 49-year-old woman with a recurrent skull base tumor (esthesioneuroblastoma) initially underwent surgery at another institution and was reoperated at our own. The operating surgeon reported brisk bleeding that prompted the initial three-dimensional angiogram, which revealed a small pseudoaneurysm at the C2 portion of the internal carotid artery (ICA, *white arrow*). Seven days later, another three-dimensional angiogram revealed aneurysmal growth *(white arrow)*. Concern that the aneurysm would rupture prompted a test balloon occlusion of the left ICA, which the patient failed clinically. The aneurysm was treated by performing a long cervical external carotid artery–to–M2 long saphenous vein bypass. A postoperative angiogram obtained immediately revealed patency of the bypass and the aneurysm *(black arrow)*. The ICA above and below the aneurysm was trapped with balloons, leaving the middle cerebral artery to fill via the bypass. B, Site of distal ICA balloon occlusion.

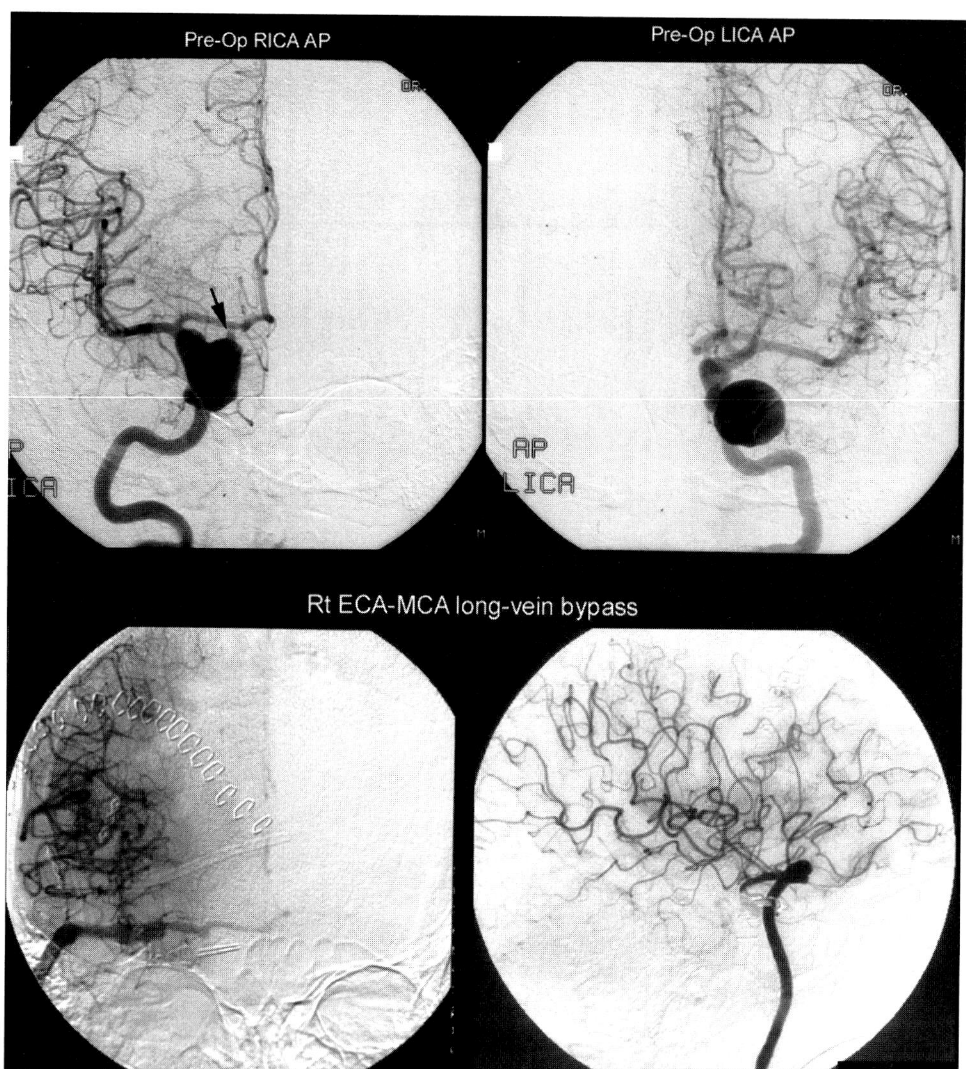

FIGURE 110–10. A 50-year-old woman presented with a grade III subarachnoid hemorrhage. Angiography revealed bilateral giant cavernous carotid aneurysms. The right aneurysm had eroded the roof of the cavernous sinus and ruptured into the subarachnoid space *(arrow)*. The aneurysm was treated by trapping with clips placed proximally on the internal carotid artery and distally below the posterior communicating artery. Concern that the patient might suffer vasospasm and concern about the contralateral aneurysm prompted the addition of a long vein bypass.

The specific treatment should be tailored to the patient, the symptoms, and the aneurysm. Surgical therapy for these lesions is more difficult than for other aneurysms of the anterior circulation. Although direct clipping remains the best philosophical approach to treatment, it can be achieved safely only by the most experienced surgeon.[42] Even then, morbidity to cranial nerves should be expected. Consequently, endovascular techniques offer significant advantages for some patients. The large caliber of the intracavernous ICA allows endovascular access with coils and balloons. In the future, stenting devices will enable endoluminal reconstitution of the parent vessel. Treatment decisions should be made in a multidisciplinary fashion when endovascular and surgical treatments are available.

Depending on the severity and progression of symptoms and the patient's condition, treatment options for aneurysms presenting with compression include proximal occlusion or trapping with or without a bypass. Aneurysms treated in this fashion almost uniformly thrombose, which reduces their size and pulsatility. A small reduction in volume often suffices to reverse cranial nerve abnormalities in ensuing months. When these lesions are trapped surgically, the intracranial ICA is exposed and clipped below the level of the PCoA, which always should be preserved. Proximal trapping is achieved most easily by ligating the ICA in the neck. It also is possible to ligate the ICA proximal to the aneurysm in the petrous bone, but this strategy is used rarely unless combined with a petrous carotid–to–intradural carotid saphenous vein graft.[43]

In most centers, the surgical treatment of high-flow carotid-cavernous fistulas has been relegated to a second-line strategy. The original method of direct surgical attack, pioneered by Parkinson,[44–46] required direct opening of the cavernous sinus under cardiopulmonary bypass, visualization of the fistula site, and direct repair. This approach has been supplanted by endovascular treatment using combined transarterial and transvenous approaches with coils and detachable balloons, which cures most cases. An endovascular cure is not feasible without carotid sacrifice in patients who fail a test occlusion or patients who harbor complex lesions. A surgical approach to trapping the aneurysm is required with or without an EC-IC bypass.

When a high-flow carotid-cavernous fistula is approached directly, the patient's head is fixed in a radiolucent head rest, and the fistula site is identified by intraoperative angiography. The dura of the cavernous sinus is exposed through a pterional approach, and the sinus is filled with thrombogenic material through multiple small punctures under direct visualization. The most effective material is cotton shaped into small pledgets that can be introduced through direct punctures with a microinstrument. The site of rupture along the course of the ICA must be identified on preoperative angiography. The cotton pledgets can be directed preferentially toward this site during the procedure. Progress in obliterating the fistula is gauged intermittently by intraoperative angiography. The procedure continues until the fistula is obliterated. A high rate of carotid preservation can be obtained. The procedure is associated, however, with a high probability of producing third nerve palsy, most cases of which resolve within several weeks.

Cavernous aneurysms that manifest with SAH pose a special treatment problem because most are giant lesions that erode the dura of the cavernous sinus to reach the subarachnoid space (see Fig. 110–10). Treatments involving carotid sacrifice alone (proximal occlusion or trapping) should be avoided if possible. Even if carotid occlusion is tolerated at presentation, these patients are at risk of delayed ischemic sequelae caused by vasospasm. During vasospasm, patients treated with carotid occlusion have a high risk of cerebral infarction because the cerebral circulation already is compromised. Trapping cavernous ICA aneurysms in SAH patients should be combined with a vascular bypass procedure.

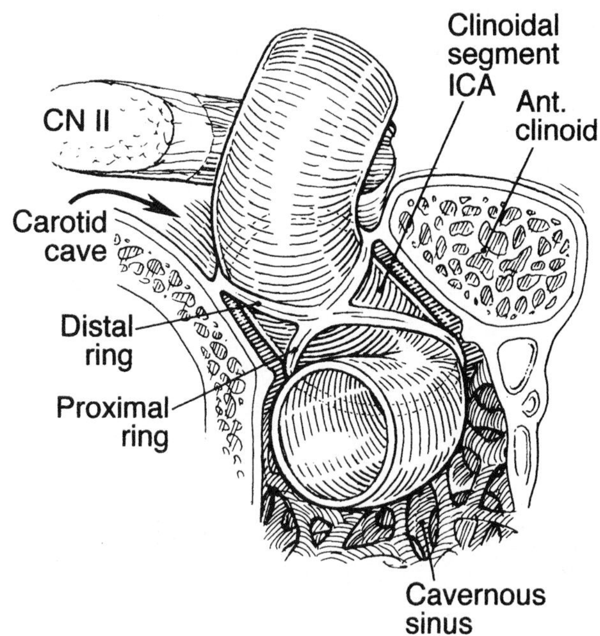

FIGURE 110–11. Schematic representation of cross-sectional view of anterior cavernous sinus, with posteroanterior view of paraclinoid portion of the internal carotid artery (ICA). Note the carotid cave, a potential dural space on the ventromedial side of the carotid artery. Note also the distal and proximal rings and their point of fusion on the posterior aspect of the ICA at its outlet from the cavernous sinus roof; the rings are defined better along the lateral and anterior margins of the ICA and less so medially. The clinoidal segment of ICA is within a collar surrounded by the rings of dura and the dura lining the anterior clinoid process. (Courtesy of Barrow Neurological Institute, Phoenix, Arizona.)

Carotid Cave Aneurysms

ANATOMY

Aneurysms of the carotid cave arise from the medial side of the juxtadural ring. The carotid cave is present in approximately 70% of anatomic specimens.[47, 48] It usually is located in the posteromedial aspect of the carotid dural ring and was originally described as lying in the 1 to 6 o'clock position in a recess bounded by the sphenoid bone (carotid sulcus) medially and ICA laterally (Fig. 110–11).[49] It has been classified into three types according to the topographic microanatomy: (1) the slit type, which shows a small, thin recess of the dura mater with fine connective tissue loosely adhered to the carotid wall; (2) the pocket type, which has a definite dural pouch with the apex attached to the vessel wall; and (3) the mesh type, which forms a slit-type or pocket-type dural cave covered with a meshlike dural roof. In about 30% of the cases, there is a tight dural attachment without any caval structure around the dural ring. The posteromedial portion of the carotid dural ring has no contact with any bone structure, and this feature appears to facilitate the formation of the carotid cave and extension of the aneurysm into the cavernous sinus space. The carotid cave contains or abuts the subarachnoid space in 80% of the cases,[47] resulting in its presentation with SAH. Its availability and the closely situated origin of the superior hypophyseal artery may allow for aneurysms to develop. The clinoidal segment on the medial aspect of the anterior clinoid segment is quite distinct from the carotid cave.

PRESENTATION AND DECISION MAKING

On diagnostic imaging, aneurysms arising in the carotid cave are difficult to differentiate from aneurysms arising from the distal ICA entirely within the cavernous sinus. Their access to the subarachnoid space poses a risk of SAH, however. Similar to distal or giant cavernous sinus aneurysms, surgical exploration of asymptomatic lesions is necessary to determine their exact location in relation to the subarachnoid space. Treatment decisions for cave aneurysms associated with SAH or mass effect are made similarly to those for other paraclinoid aneurysms.

TREATMENT

These aneurysms usually are small and project medially on an anteroposterior angiographic view. At surgery, they are located intradurally, where the ICA penetrates the dura on the ventromedial side. The aneurysms appear to be buried in the dural pouch (carotid cave; see Fig. 110–11) and often are difficult to find, dissect, and clip. The aneurysm extends into the cavernous sinus space, and the parent ICA penetrates the dural ring obliquely. An ipsilateral pterional approach can be used, and fenestrated clips are needed because of their ventromedial location. Several technical steps are required to obliterate these aneurysms successfully. First, the cervical ICA must be exposed for proximal control. Second, the optic canal must be unroofed and the anterior clinoid process removed to permit lateral retraction of the optic nerve and ICA. Third, the ICA should be explored around the dural ring and opening of the cavernous sinus to identify the proximal neck. Finally, ring clips that conform to the natural curvature of the carotid artery should be applied.[49]

The ipsilateral approach is associated with a significant risk to the optic nerve because the nerve and artery must be retracted laterally. An alternative strategy is to approach these aneurysms from the contralateral side. When approached through a contralateral pterional craniotomy, these aneurysms can be visualized directly without undue retraction of the optic nerve. They often can be clipped with a straight aneurysm clip via the prechiasmatic root.[50–52]

Carotid-Ophthalmic Aneurysms

ANATOMY

Comprising approximately 10% of intracranial aneurysms,[53] aneurysms of the ophthalmic artery arise from the ICA just distal to the ophthalmic artery and point superiorly or superomedially. When they are large, they deflect the carotid artery posteriorly and inferiorly, closing the siphon. Abnormalities related to vision seldom are identified until the aneurysm reaches giant proportions. The optic nerve typically is displaced superomedially, restricting contralateral extension until late in the clinical course and causing unilateral nasal field loss. About 10% of patients have bilateral ophthalmic artery aneurysms. Aneurysms of the superior hypophyseal artery arise just above the dural ring from the medial bend of the ICA, at the origin of the perforator on the superior aspect of the hypophysis. They have no direct association with the ophthalmic artery. The carotid artery usually is located lateral or superolateral relative to the aneurysm. These lesions can extend medially beneath the chiasm (suprasellar variant), producing a clinical and CT picture similar to a pituitary adenoma. They also can extend ventrally, burrowing beneath the anterior clinoid process (paraclinoid variant). Preoperative categorization of these lesions according to their likely branch of origin provides excellent correlation with visual deficits and operative findings.[54]

PRESENTATION AND DECISION MAKING

In several series, 25% to 50% of carotid ophthalmic aneurysms are large or giant, and 50% manifest without SAH with minimal or no symptoms. Usually, female predominance is marked, and the incidence of multiple aneurysms is high (20% to 45%).[55–58] Consequently, this area must be scrutinized on preoperative angiography, and additional oblique views should be obtained. The presence and size of the superficial temporal artery should be noted in case revascularization is needed. The topography of the aneurysm and projection of the dome must be examined carefully. Dorsally projecting aneurysms can be embedded in the inferior aspect of the frontal lobe, leading to early operative rupture when the frontal lobe is retracted. Large paraclinoid aneurysms may be partially thrombosed and have thick walls. CT scans should be scrutinized for calcium in the aneurysm wall and laminated clots within the dome. Attention should be given to pneumatization of the anterior clinoid process, which, if ignored, can lead to postoperative cerebrospinal fluid rhinorrhea.

TREATMENT

The craniotomy and initial exposure require little modification of the principles outlined previously. Small aneurysms are approached through a pterional craniotomy, whereas larger lesions may be better approached with an orbitozygomatic extension.[59] The carotid should be exposed in the neck for proximal control. The sylvian fissure is opened to minimize brain retraction. Careful attention must be given to dorsally placed aneurysms that may be vulnerable to disruption by the deep placement of retractors or retraction of the frontal lobe.

The anterior clinoid process must be removed to obtain proximal control intracranially and to reach the proximal neck of the aneurysm. A high-speed drill is used. It should be held comfortably in one hand, have excellent balance, and be unencumbered by a heavy hose. Drilling the clinoid is preceded by opening the dura that is reflected over the proximal carotid artery. Experienced surgeons can use a 2-mm steel cutting bur to begin the removal of large clinoid processes. As the aneurysm, dura, or optic nerve is approached, a diamond-tipped drill should be used. The entire clinoid process should be removed to expose the proximal cavernous sinus and the most distal carotid ring. The optic nerve should be unroofed completely, especially the bone on the medial border, so that the optic nerve can be deflected medially. Pneumatized clinoids must be packed with bone wax to avoid cerebrospinal fluid rhinorrhea.

During dissection of the aneurysm, suction tips that have been used to remove the clinoid should be exchanged for tips that have not been damaged inadvertently by touching the drill tip. The inner layer of the dura (dura propria) is opened along the lateral aspect of the optic nerve. If the neck of the aneurysm is more proximal, the carotid ring is opened with dissection of the superiormost aspect of the cavernous sinus. The ophthalmic artery, superior hypophyseal perforators, and perforators to the optic chiasm should be dissected free from the neck of the aneurysm. The optic nerve should be retracted only as much as necessary and intermittently. Before the clip is applied, an instrument should be passed completely behind the neck of the aneurysm to ensure an unobstructed passage for both clip blades. A faulty or aborted attempt to place aneurysm clips before the aneurysm has been dissected completely is a common cause of intraoperative rupture. Distally the most appropriate place for temporary occlusion is between the aneurysm and the PCoA. Proximally, there are three potential sites for temporary clip occlusion: (1) the ICA in the neck, (2) extradural exposure of the petrous ICA, and (3) the short distance on the carotid between the two dural rings.

Several issues need to be considered in terms of clip application. Aneurysms with narrow necks can be clipped directly with a straight clip. Otherwise the clip should be placed parallel with the long axis of the parent vessel. Perforators should be preserved and the orientation of the overlying optic nerve considered carefully. It often is necessary to use one or more angled fenestrated clips that encircle the parent ICA (Fig 110–12).[60] Clips should not be placed too close to the base of the aneurysm to avoid compromising the parent vessel. For globular and large aneurysms, temporary occlusion with deflation of the aneurysm may be needed before the clip can be placed.[61–63] Large aneurysms with an intraluminal clot require gaining complete control of the carotid so that the sac can be opened, the thrombus removed, and the vessel reconstructed. Contralateral clip application should be considered for smaller aneurysms that project medially or dorsally from the ICA.[50, 51]

Suction decompression[62] can help deflate large aneurysms without exposing the proximal ICA intracranially. After the aneurysm has been trapped temporarily distally and proximally in the neck, a No. 18 angiocatheter is inserted into the cervical ICA. The catheter is connected to a wall suction point, allowing rapid aneurysm deflation. Final dissection and clipping then are performed. Occasionally a clip slightly deflects the optic nerve from its normal course. If so, the position of the clip needs to be altered only if the nerve is unduly angulated.

Paraophthalmic aneurysms may be treated by trapping or proximal occlusion with or without an EC-IC bypass. This treatment should never be the first choice, however, and each aneurysm should be explored to determine whether it can be clipped.

Midcarotid Artery (Posterior Communicating Artery) Aneurysms

ANATOMY

Aneurysms of the PCoA and anterior choroidal artery (AchA) constitute approximately 25% and 5% of intracranial aneurysms, respectively.[53] PCoA aneurysms arise distal to the artery in 85% to 90% of cases. Of these, 10% to 15% are associated with a fetal posterior cerebral artery. In 10% to 15% of cases, the PCoA is visualized on the distal side of the aneurysm neck, suggesting that the aneurysm actually arises from a more proximal, unnamed perforating branch of the ICA that was not appreciated on preoperative angiography. Rarely, aneurysms arise from the PCoA directly from branches that supply the optic chiasm and tract, pituitary stalk, and hypothalamus.[16, 64]

AchA aneurysms arise distal to their named parent vessel. Duplications and early branchings of the AchA are common and give rise to aneurysms associated with choroidal branches proximal and distal to the neck of the lesion.

PRESENTATION AND DECISION MAKING

SAH is the most common mode of presentation. The close association of the PCoA and the third cranial nerve also can cause partial or complete third nerve palsy, which sometimes is painful because of pressure on adjacent dura. This palsy almost always involves the pupil, although a few instances of pupillary sparing have been reported.[65–67] Because of their close association with the dura, PCoA aneurysms can rupture through the arachnoid to produce a subdural hematoma.

Patients with large PCoA or AchA aneurysms can present with headaches, signs and symptoms of cranial nerve dysfunction, and pituitary dysfunction. Less commonly, these lesions are associated with temporal lobe epilepsy. Similar to all large aneurysms, these lesions can present with embolic events related to stasis of the blood in the aneurysmal sac and partial thrombosis. Treatment decisions for asymptomatic lesions and for lesions presenting with SAH follow the general principles outlined previously. A new onset of third nerve palsy usually indicates that the aneurysm has grown and is an indication for expedient therapy.

TREATMENT

Typically, aneurysms are treated through a pterional craniotomy. For PCoA aneurysms, it is important to extend the medial bone opening to allow the medial side of the ICA to be visualized. Then the PCoA artery distal to the aneurysm's neck, the medial aspect of the aneurysmal dome, and the PCoA perforators can be seen. Only giant aneurysms require an orbitozygomatic craniotomy. For PCoA and AchA aneurysms, both arteries must be identified. These lesions are discussed together.

Several key steps are involved in securing these aneurysms. We believe that the sylvian fissure should be split appropriately to reveal the medial border of the temporal lobe and to appreciate the PCoA artery and the course and number of AchA vessels. We recognize, however, that many surgeons do not split the fissure for access to the PcoA artery and gain exposure through careful temporal and frontal retraction. The surgeon should create a mental picture of the aneurysm's neck during an early stage of the operation. Microsurgical dissection follows the principles of the transsylvian exposure described in the previous sections. It is essential to avoid the temptation to open the arachnoid cisterns inadequately when the aneurysm becomes visible early in the exposure. The relationship

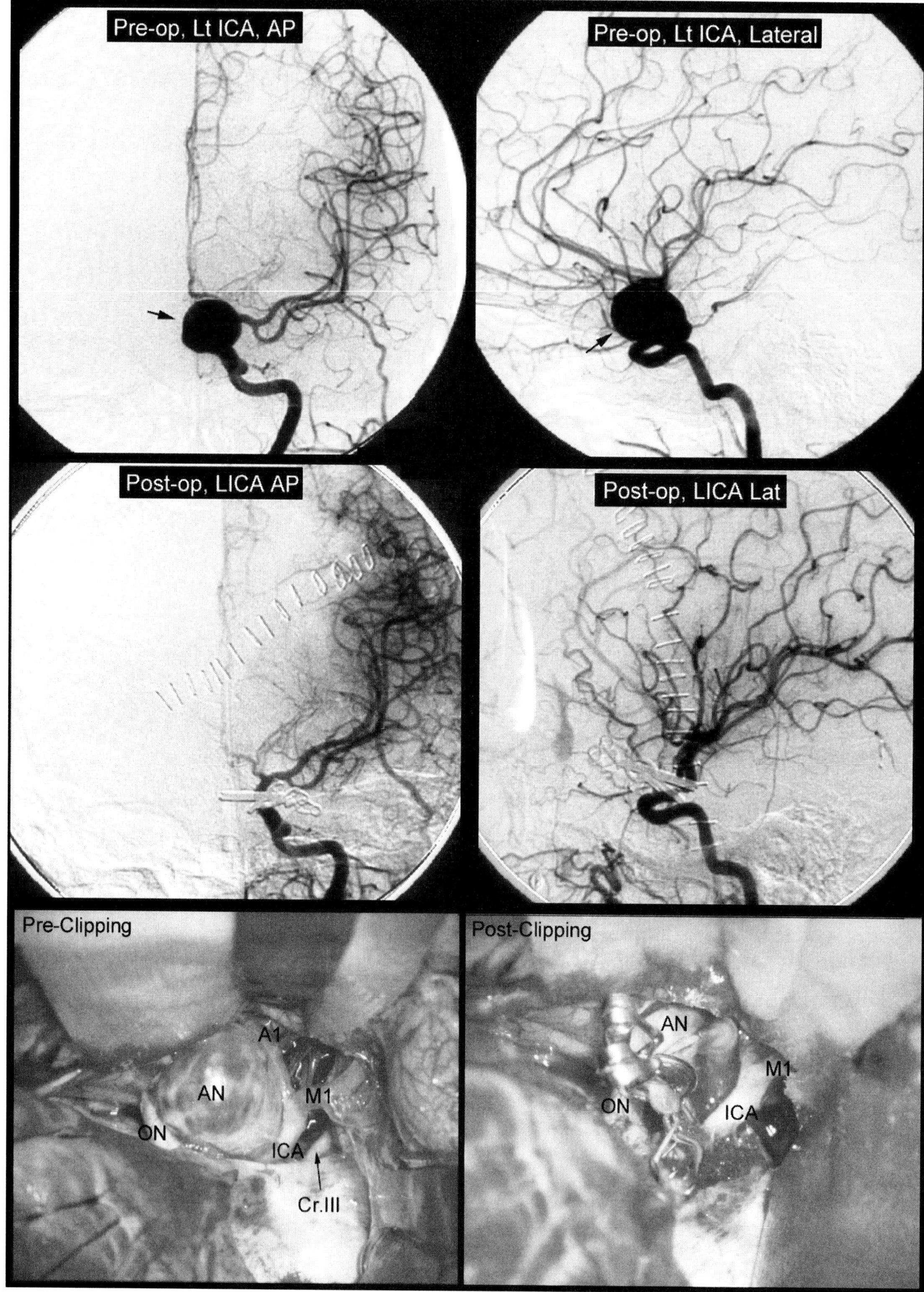

FIGURE 110–12. A 59-year-old woman presented with visual difficulties and pituitary dysfunction from a large paraophthalmic aneurysm *(arrows)*. The lesion was treated by deflating the aneurysm using the suction decompression technique and by reconstructing the internal carotid artery with three aneurysm clips. The intraoperative picture shows the view afforded through an orbitozygomatic transsylvian approach. AN, aneurysm; ON, optic nerve; ICA, internal carotid artery; and Cr. III, third cranial nerve.

between the dome of aneurysm and the medial temporal lobe should not be disturbed before the arachnoid has been dissected adequately and proximal control has been obtained. The two most common causes of intraoperative rupture are medial retraction of the carotid artery and lateral retraction of the temporal lobe while the aneurysm dome is still adherent to the temporal lobe.

Sometimes a PCoA aneurysm may be quite proximal or partially covered by the anterior clinoid process. This situation may necessitate removing the clinoid or exposing the carotid artery in the neck. The AchA should be visualized and preserved in all instances. Adequate opening of the sylvian fissure facilitates this task by revealing the course of the AchA. The artery may travel medial to the aneurysm, making it necessary to separate the vessel from the aneurysm's neck before clipping. Every effort should be made to identify the origin of the artery itself.[64] It should be possible to clip a PCoA aneurysm without clipping the artery itself. This strategy is essential when the aneurysm arises from a fetal posterior cerebral artery. Preservation of the parent vessel is more crucial in the case of an AchA aneurysm. Of giant aneurysms, 14% arise in the vicinity of the PCoA or AchA.[53] Proximal and distal control of these aneurysms must be obtained, and the dome must be deflated to permit meticulous visualization of medial perforators and the AchA (see Fig. 110–1).

Rarely, giant aneurysms of the midcarotid artery may contain organized thrombus and calcified plaque along the neck where the clip is to be applied. The aneurysm must be trapped, the dome opened, and the clot removed. Often the body of the aneurysm shares the wall of the ICA and the neck is wide. Closing the aneurysm requires reconstructing the carotid artery itself, either with multiple fenestrated clips (see Fig. 110–1) or, rarely, with interrupted stitches. Trapping or hunterian ligation may be an option for low-lying or difficult-to-clip PCoA aneurysms if the PCoA is small. This never should be considered as a first option, however. All of these aneurysms should be explored surgically to determine whether clipping the neck is feasible.

Carotid Bifurcation Aneurysms

ANATOMY

Composing 4% to 15% of aneurysms in most large series,[53, 68] lesions of the carotid bifurcation typically point in one of three directions. Most commonly, they point superiorly (medially), impinging on the orbitofrontal gyrus or olfactory tract. The dome projects along the A1 vessel. Others point posteriorly, occupying the sylvian cistern and accompanying the MCA. Least commonly, the lesions point inferiorly, and the dome drapes over the posteromesial aspect of the ICA and may enter the interpeduncular cistern. The most crucial anatomy around the aneurysm's neck is related to medial lenticulostriate perforators arising from the ICA bifurcation, deep branches from the PCoA and AchA, and the recurrent artery of Heubner from the anterior cerebral artery complex. On exposing the carotid bifurcation, the surgeon encounters the medial sylvian veins, which should be preserved. Deep to the aneurysm lies the basal vein of Rosenthal and its tributaries.

PRESENTATION AND DECISION MAKING

The most common presentation is SAH. Isolated cranial nerve abnormalities are rare, but symptoms related to mass effect, distal emboli, and ischemia can arise with giant lesions. The treatment morbidity of carotid bifurcation aneurysms is higher than that of PCoA or MCA aneurysms because the former are associated with crucial perforating vessels.

TREATMENT

The craniotomy and initial exposure follow the principles outlined earlier. How the dissection of the arachnoid begins depends on the projection of the aneurysm. For example, the initial approach in anteriorly projecting lesions might be through the sylvian fissure instead of following the ICA to avoid the dome, which often adheres to the ICA. Posteriorly projecting aneurysms can be approached through the ICA route but still necessitate a wide sylvian exposure of parent and perforator vessels near the aneurysm.

The strategy for retraction, similar to the arachnoid dissection, depends on the direction of the aneurysm's dome. If it points along the anterior cerebral artery (superiorly), only temporal retraction is used until the lesion is in view. If it points along the MCA (posteriorly), frontal retraction alone is used to start. If it points back down to the mesial ICA, frontal and temporal retraction may be used from the start.

The aneurysm's neck must be prepared by separating it from the surrounding perforating vessels. This dissection can be difficult when the neck is expanded because perforators can be incorporated into the neck. Temporary clipping with attention to clearing the AchA is helpful in the final portion of the dissection. Collapsing the aneurysm may require a clip on the A1 and M1 vessels as well. For clipping the neck, an excessively long clip should be avoided, and its tips should be visualized at all times. Occasionally the neck is broad, and application of a straight clip can crimp the parent vessels, incompletely clip the aneurysm, or both. To avoid these problems, a fenestrated clip can be placed in the axis of the A1 and M1 vessels, with the fenestration placed around the MCA or ICA.

Hunterian ligation is not a viable option for these aneurysms even if the patient appears to tolerate sacrifice of the ICA. The lesion continues to fill with blood at high pressure because blood must cross from the contralateral hemisphere to supply the ipsilateral brain. Aneurysms that are deemed unclippable can be treated with a combination of ipsilateral carotid sacrifice, a clip on A1 distal to the medial aneurysm neck, and a bypass procedure to revascularize the MCA territory. Then the aneurysm becomes a terminal sac fed by the bypass and thromboses.

Middle Cerebral Artery Aneurysms

ANATOMY

Surgery for MCA aneurysms requires a thorough understanding of the anatomy of the sylvian fissure. The most common reason that the fissure is opened inadequately is a lack of understanding of the topology of the brain and associated veins. In the medial extent of the fissure, the proximal part of the fronto-orbital gyrus and the superior temporal gyrus often indent each other and interlock inside the fissure, causing confusion in novice hands. Adding further difficulty are the surface veins that appear to adhere tightly to each other and not to follow a predetermined course. This is not the case, however. The superficial sylvian veins empty into the sphenoparietal sinus and cavernous sinus and often anastomose with the transverse sinus via the vein of Labbé. The deeper vein receives lenticulostriate venous branches and courses medially to join the basal vein of Rosenthal. Great care must be taken to preserve the large venous trunks to avoid venous infarcts. The surface veins always can be separated from each other to allow access to the fissure, even when it is filled with subarachnoid blood.

The sylvian fissure hosts the course of the MCA. The M1 segment averages 15 mm in length and gives rise to 5 to 30 lateral lenticulostriate perforators that arise almost exclusively from its superior and posterior surfaces. It is safest to dissect the M1 segment from the inferior (temporal) side. M1 ends in a bifurcation in 70% to 80% of the cases, a trifurcation in 20%, and a quadrifurcation in 1%. In a bifurcated M1, the M2 branches exhibit equal dominance in 25%, inferior trunk dominance in 35%, and superior trunk dominance in 40% of cases. The M2 vessels average 11 mm in length and may give rise to a few lenticulostriate perforators. They terminate in the M3 segments that course over the frontoparietal and temporal opercula. M4 branches spread out over the cortical surface. Named branches of the M1 segment include early cortical branches that originate from the temporal (lateral or anterior) surface, the uncal artery, the polar and anterior temporal arteries, and, occasionally, an orbitofrontal artery. Unusual variations of the MCA include a fenestration or complete duplication of M1 beginning at or near the terminal ICA or an *accessory MCA* (i.e., a vessel originating from the anterior cerebral artery that follows a recurrent path to reach the sylvian cistern; see Fig. 110–3). Although a detailed description of the MCA anatomy is beyond the scope of this chapter, its course and branchings are described to provide the appreciation that aneurysms can arise at any branch point. Branches of M1 host up to 85% of MCA aneurysms.

PRESENTATION AND DECISION MAKING

Unless they are giant, MCA aneurysms rarely are symptomatic until they bleed. Because of their location, the incidence of intracerebral hematoma is as high as 50%. Giant lesions may present with mass effect, distal emboli, or seizures. The principles and timing of surgery are as described previously.

TREATMENT

MCA aneurysms are treated through a pterional craniotomy. The posterior aspect of the bone opening may be extended to allow easier access to large lesions or to aneurysms in the distal sylvian fissure. A skull base variation rarely is necessary. Before surgery, the surgeon should note the length of the M1, which can indicate whether the aneurysm should be approached through the proximal or distal fissure. The location of the aneurysm in relation to branch points and dominance of the branches should be appreciated. The lobularity of the lesion should be determined, and the neurosurgeon should create a mental picture of the neck. Up to 50% of lesions are bilobular or multilobular. Even small MCA aneurysms may require reconstruction with multiple clips. The presence of a collateral circulation from the anterior cerebral territory is important in the event that temporary clipping becomes necessary.

The initial approach to the aneurysms follows the principles of a transsylvian dissection, beginning with opening the optic and carotid cisterns to release cerebrospinal fluid. The sylvian fissure then is opened. In one strategy, M1 dissection begins at the ICA bifurcation to provide proximal control. The difficulty of the surgical dissection correlates with the width, length, and depth of the sylvian cistern. Alternatively, except in the case of an unusually short M1 segment, MCA aneurysms can be approached through a purely sylvian exposure that begins laterally and proceeds in a proximal direction.

When a cortical artery has been identified within the fissure, it can be followed down to the MCA, which often is tucked into the medial aspect of the sylvian cistern as one descends through the fissure. M1 is followed distally on its superior and lateral surface to stay clear of lenticulostriate vessels arising on the opposite side of the artery. In patients with a temporal lobe hematoma, patients with considerable brain swelling, and patients with large aneurysms that project laterally, anteriorly, or inferiorly, the aneurysm can be approached via the superior or middle temporal gyrus (or both).

As MCA aneurysms grow, they become structurally complex and tend to carry the origins of cortical and lenticulostriate branches up onto their walls. An aneurysm's neck almost always can be found with smaller lesions if arachnoid dissection is meticulous. The need to dissect the neck fully from all sides cannot be overemphasized. Temporary clipping of the M1 often helps to soften the dome and facilitates the final steps of dissection.

With large or giant lesions, a clot partially filling the aneurysm and atheroma within its wall can interfere with clip application. In such cases, several treatment options exist. The aneurysmal sac can be wrapped with gauze in the hope of strengthening its wall. The proximal vessel can be occluded with a distal bypass to promote thrombosis of the aneurysm without distal infarction (see Fig. 110–4). Finally, the aneurysm can be excised and an end-to-end reanastomosis of the parent vessels performed.

Anterior Communicating Artery Aneurysms

ANATOMY

The microsurgical anatomy and variations associated with the ACoA complex[64, 69, 70] make this a challenging area for microneurosurgeons. The ACoA complex is the last to be tackled solo by microsurgical trainees. Apart from the arterial variations, it is essential to become familiar with the anatomy of the interhemispheric fissure that hosts the ACoA complex. This fissure is least well appreciated during microsurgical dissection of a swollen brain but must be entered to reach the aneurysm.

Typically the anterior cerebral artery is the smaller of the two arteries leaving the ICA bifurcation, although it may be equal to or larger than the MCA when the contralateral A1 is hypoplastic. Several small perforators arise along the inferoposterior aspect of the proximal A1 segment, supplying the septum pellucidum, the medial portion of the anterior commissure, the pillars of the fornix, the optic chiasm, the paraolfactory area, the anterior limb of the internal capsule, the anteroinferior part of the striatum, and the anterior hypothalamus. Hypothalamic branches exhibit numerous variations. In 65% of cases, they originate from the ACoA even if it is quite small because a single-stem vessel divides into many fine branches after 2 to 5 mm. In other instances, hypothalamic branches may arise from the proximal A2 branches.

The diameter of the recurrent artery of Heubner varies from 0.2 to 3 mm. It usually runs anterior to the A1 segment (60%) but also frequently courses posterosuperior to it (40%). The artery supplies the anterior third of the putamen, a small portion of the outer segment of the globus pallidus, and the anterior limb of the internal capsule. Occlusion of this vessel can result in a clinical syndrome of aphasia (dominant), hemiparesis, and paralysis of the face and tongue. In most cases, this artery originates at or distal to the ACoA.

In 90% of cases, the distal anterior cerebral arteries (A2) are equal in size, and each vessel supplies only the ipsilateral hemisphere. There also are many variations, such as unpaired A2 (0.5%) and a median callosal artery. Aneurysms in this location are rare.

ACoA aneurysms are associated with a dominant A1 in about 70% to 85% of cases, confirming the role of hemodynamic stress in their development. On anteroposterior projections, the dome points in the direction of blood flow along the A1. From a strategic perspective, ACoA aneurysms can be classified as pointing anteriorly, superiorly, or posteriorly. This feature dictates presentation, surgical approach, and potential morbidity associated with SAH and treatment (discussed further subsequently).

PRESENTATION AND DECISION MAKING

SAH is the most common presentation except in large or thrombosed aneurysms that can produce mass effect. Ruptures from superiorly and posteriorly pointing lesions frequently are associated with intracerebral and intraventricular hemorrhage, causing the patient to become acutely ill from mass effect and hydrocephalus. For this reason, poor-grade patients must be resuscitated aggressively and provided with a ventriculostomy. Many patients improve given the opportunity. The presence of an interhemispheric hematoma can obscure the aneurysm on early cerebral angiography. In the presence of a negative angiogram, an appropriate history and CT confirmation of an interhemispheric clot suffice to support the decision to explore the ACoA complex, which almost invariably reveals an aneurysm.[71] The surgical approach should be chosen on the basis of the side of the clot and the dominance and direction of the A1 vessel that is most likely to give rise to the lesion.

TREATMENT

The choice of surgical approach depends on the surgeon's preference and the aneurysm's configuration. Many lesions can be approached through an interhemispheric approach, as discussed earlier. Most surgeons use the pterional exposure, however. The need for an orbitozygomatic extension is not absolute, although it undeniably affords increased basal exposure with less brain retraction (see earlier). At our institution, the orbitozygomatic transsylvian approach has become increasingly popular for treating most ruptured ACoA aneurysms and unruptured superiorly and posteriorly pointing lesions (Fig. 110–13). Anteriorly pointing aneurysms can be treated with minimal brain retraction without the orbitozygomatic extension. The side of the pterional craniotomy is usually on the right to avoid retraction of the dominant hemisphere. Exceptions are cases in which the dome of the aneurysm projects directly to the right, when the left frontal lobe already is damaged by hematoma or infarction, or another aneurysm is located on the left carotid circulation. The side of dominance of the A1 segment does not determine the side of the craniotomy because both A1 vessels can be identified and secured early in the dissection.

The ACoA complex can be approached by following the ICA distally to its bifurcation, and then along the A1 vessel. Alternatively, both A1 branches can be identified directly by following the course of the optic nerves to the chiasm, without dissecting out the ICA. The latter strategy, however, does not preclude the need for a wide arachnoid dissection and appropriate splitting of the sylvian fissure to minimize brain retraction.

The sequence of arachnoid opening depends on the aneurysm's configuration. Anteriorly pointing lesions may adhere to the chiasmatic cisterns and optic nerve. Arachnoid dissection should begin laterally. Superiorly and posteriorly pointing lesions are separated from the

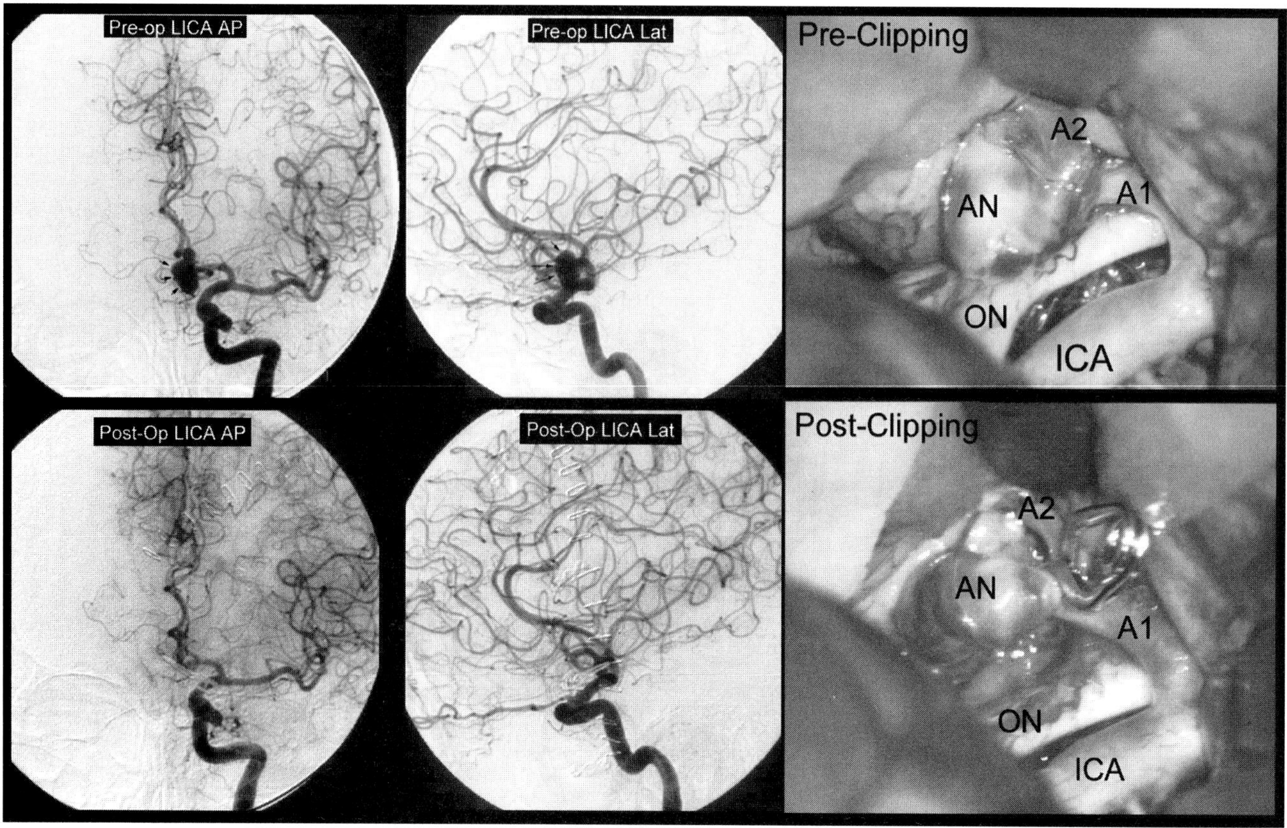

FIGURE 110–13. A 61-year-old man presented with an incidental, 1.2-cm aneurysm of the anterior communicating artery *(arrows)*. It was exposed and clipped through an orbitozygomatic pterional approach. Note the basal exposure and minimal retraction needed to show the anatomy. AN, aneurysm; ON, optic nerve; ICA, internal carotid artery.

ICA and chiasmatic cisterns. These lesions should be opened widely early in the operation to reveal both A1 vessels and to obtain proximal control.

Meticulous attention should be given to preserving perforating vessels that arise from the Al and A2 segments, especially the recurrent artery of Heubner. In this region, blind application of a clip is associated with enormous morbidity. Clipping the aneurysm should not be attempted until the entire H complex is dissected and the anatomy is understood. The most frequent difficulties arise in identifying the contralateral A2 segment and the posterior extent of the aneurysm neck. The ACoA gives rise to multiple perforators to the lamina terminalis and hypothalamus. Clip placement with inadequate dissection places the A2, contralateral Heubner, and perforators at risk. The clipping strategy always should be designed to preserve the ACoA. This point is critical when both A2 branches are supplied by a dominant A1. Despite the apparent complexity of the ACoA complex, ACoA aneurysms can be clipped with a single straight clip if the aneurysm's neck has been dissected adequately.

Aneurysms of the Distal Anterior Cerebral Artery

Aneurysms of the distal anterior cerebral artery arise at anterior cerebral artery branches distal to the ACoA complex. Presentation and decision making follow the basic principles outlined previously. The surgical approach is through an interhemispheric exposure, as already described (see Fig. 110–2). Reported series suggest that these lesions have a higher rate of intraoperative rupture than other aneurysms.[72–74]

Carotid Sacrifice Versus Extracranial-Intracranial Bypass

An EC-IC bypass is required if a patient cannot tolerate sacrifice of the carotid artery. The definition of tolerance is controversial, however. Surgeons debate whether sacrificing a carotid artery at any time constitutes optimal treatment. Whether any preoperative test can reliably predict a patient's long-term ability to tolerate ICA sacrifice also is controversial. When carotid sacrifice is initially well tolerated, it is associated with several potential disadvantages: an early risk of stump emboli, a risk of delayed stroke because of hemodynamic factors, and the theoretical risk of a "loss of reserve" if the remaining ICA were compromised in the future. Hemodynamic stresses related to ICA sacrifice have been associated with the development of de novo aneurysms and with the growth and rupture of aneurysms from increased blood flow through the remaining collateral segments.[75] A scholarly discussion of the controversies surrounding patient selection for carotid sacrifice versus EC-IC bypass is beyond the scope of this chapter. Opinions about selection criteria range from a need for EC-IC bypass in every case of carotid sacrifice to selection based on multimodality testing, including one or more of the following: cerebral angiography, test balloon occlusions, ultrasonography, magnetic resonance imaging, single photon emission or positron emission tomography scanning, and other methodologies for assessing cerebral blood flow and oxygen extraction.[76–82]

Our protocol begins with a cerebral angiogram obtained under local anesthesia and test occlusion of the ICA with an inflatable balloon. The patient is examined clinically with the ICA occluded, under normotensive conditions and during a 15-minute hypotensive challenge. Angiographic injections through the contralateral common carotid artery and then through the ICA show arterial and venous phases. These studies are examined for cross-flow to the ipsilateral (test) hemisphere, for collateral flow via the ophthalmic artery and anterior cerebral arteries, and for symmetry of venous filling. A vertebral angiogram is obtained to determine the extent of collateral blood flow through the PCoA. In most cases, failure to tolerate the test balloon occlusion clinically or angiographic demonstration of poor arterial or venous filling is the chief criterion for considering EC-IC bypass. We are reluctant to sacrifice an ICA in young patients because the natural history of this approach is uncertain.

CONCLUSIONS

Advances in understanding the natural history of ruptured and unruptured aneurysms and a critical evaluation of the role of operative intervention have improved the treatment of anterior circulation aneurysms. Surgery for these lesions is a technically demanding task. The key to success in treating these aneurysm patients is strategic decision making to select patients who would benefit from surgical treatment and to select the surgical strategy that would yield the best clinical outcomes with the lowest rates of morbidity.

REFERENCES

1. Horowitz MB, Willet D, Keffer J: The use of cardiac troponin-I (cTnI) to determine the incidence of myocardial ischemia and injury in patients with aneurysmal and presumed aneurysmal subarachnoid hemorrhage. Acta Neurochir (Wien) 140:87–93, 1998.
2. Marion DW, Segal R, Thompson ME: Subarachnoid hemorrhage and the heart. Neurosurgery 18:101–106, 1986.
3. Zaroff JG, Rordorf GA, Newell JB, et al: Cardiac outcome in patients with subarachnoid hemorrhage and electrocardiographic abnormalities. Neurosurgery 44:34–40, 1999.
4. Adams J III: Impact of troponins on the evaluation and treatment of patients with acute coronary syndromes. Curr Opin Cardiol 14:310–313, 1999.
5. Smith WS, Matthay MA: Evidence for a hydrostatic mechanism in human neurogenic pulmonary edema. Chest 111:1326–1333, 1997.
6. Bailes JE, Tantuwaya LS, Fukushima T, et al: Intraoperative microvascular Doppler sonography in aneurysm surgery. Neurosurgery 40:965–972, 1997.
7. Derdeyn CP, Moran CJ, Cross DT III, et al: Intracranial aneurysm: Anatomic factors that predict the usefulness of intraoperative angiography. Radiology 205:335–339, 1997.
8. Alexander TD, Macdonald RL, Weir B, et al: Intraoperative angiography in cerebral aneurysm surgery: A prospective study of 100 craniotomies. Neurosurgery 39:10–18, 1996.
9. Kallmes DF, Kallmes MH: Cost-effectiveness of angiography performed during surgery for ruptured intracranial aneurysms. AJNR Am J Neuroradiol 18:1453–1462, 1997.
10. Frazee JG, King WA: Endoscopy and stereotaxy for aneurysms. Neurosurg Clin N Am 9:869, 1998.
11. Sheinberg MA, Ross DA: Cranial procedures without hair removal. Neurosurgery 44:1263–1265, 1999.
12. Ratanalert S, Saehaeng S, Sripairojkul B, et al: Nonshaved cranial neurosurgery. Surg Neurol 51:458–463, 1999.
13. Horgan MA, Piatt JH Jr: Shaving of the scalp may increase the rate of infection in CSF shunt surgery. Pediatr Neurosurg 26: 180–184, 1997.
14. Braun V, Richter HP: Shaving the hair—is it always necessary for cranial neurosurgical procedures? Acta Neurochir (Wien) 135: 84–86, 1995.
15. Yasargil MG, Gasser JC, Hodosh RM, et al: Carotid-ophthalmic aneurysms: Direct microsurgical approach. Surg Neurol 8:155–165, 1977.
16. Krayenbuhl HA, Yasargil MG, Flamm ES, et al: Microsurgical treatment of intracranial saccular aneurysms. J Neurosurg 37: 678–686, 1972.
17. Yasargil MG, Antic J, Laciga R, et al: Microsurgical pterional approach to aneurysms of the basilar bifurcation. Surg Neurol 6: 83–91, 1976.
18. Yasargil MG, Reichman MV, Kubik S: Preservation of the frontotemporal branch of the facial nerve using the interfascial temporalis flap for pterional craniotomy: Technical article. J Neurosurg 67:463–466, 1987.
19. Fujitsu K, Kuwabara T: Zygomatic approach for lesions in the interpeduncular cistern. J Neurosurg 62:340–343, 1985.
20. Zabramski JM, Kiris T, Sankhla SK, et al: Orbitozygomatic craniotomy: Technical note. J Neurosurg 89:336–341, 1998.
21. Fujitsu K, Kuwabara T: Orbitocraniobasal approach for anterior communicating artery aneurysms. Neurosurgery 18:367–369, 1986.
22. Sekhar LN, Kalia KK, Yonas H, et al: Cranial base approaches to intracranial aneurysms in the subarachnoid space. Neurosurgery 35:472–483, 1994.
23. Diraz A, Kobayashi S, Toriyama T, et al: Surgical approaches to the anterior communicating artery aneurysm and their results. Neurol Res 15:273–280, 1993.
24. Fukushima T, Miyazaki S, Takusagawa Y, et al: Unilateral interhemispheric keyhole approach for anterior cerebral artery aneurysms. Acta Neurochir (Wien) 53 (suppl):42–47, 1991.
25. Suzuki J, Mizoi K, Yoshimoto T: Bifrontal interhemispheric approach to aneurysms of the anterior communicating artery. J Neurosurg 64:183–190, 1986.
26. Fujiwara H, Yasui N, Nathal-Vera E, et al: Anosmia after anterior communicating artery aneurysm surgery: Comparison between the anterior interhemispheric and basal interhemispheric approaches. Neurosurgery 38:325–328, 1996.
27. Tsutsumi K, Shiokawa Y, Sakai T, et al: Venous infarction following the interhemispheric approach in patients with acute subarachnoid hemorrhage. J Neurosurg 74:715–719, 1991.
28. Lougheed WM: Selection, timing, and technique of aneurysm surgery of the anterior circle of Willis. Clin Neurosurg 16:95–113, 1969.
29. Ito Z: The microsurgical anterior interhemispheric approach suitably applied to ruptured aneurysms of the anterior communicating artery in the acute stage. Acta Neurochir (Wien) 63:85–99, 1982.
30. Keogh AJ, Sharma RR, Vanner GK: The anterior interhemispheric trephine approach to anterior midline aneurysms: Results of treatment in 72 consecutive patients. Br J Neurosurg 7:5–12, 1993.
31. Cudlip SA, Kitchen ND, McKhahn GM, et al: Wrapping of solitary ruptured intracranial aneurysms, outcome at five years. Acta Neurochir (Wien) 140:1167–1170, 1998.
32. Nardi PV, Esposito S, Greco R, et al: Aneurysms of azygous anterior cerebral artery: Report of two cases treated by surgery. J Neurosurg Sci 34:17–20, 1990.

33. Sanders WP, Sorek PA, Mehta BA: Fenestration of intracranial arteries with special attention to associated aneurysms and other anomalies. AJNR Am J Neuroradiol 14:675–680, 1993.
34. Steinke W, Rautenberg W, Schwartz A, et al: Noninvasive monitoring of internal carotid artery dissection. Stroke 25:998–1005, 1994.
35. Faggioli GL, Freyrie A, Stella A, et al: Extracranial internal carotid artery aneurysms: Results of a surgical series with long-term follow-up. J Vasc Surg 23:587–595, 1996.
36. Kinugasa K, Yamada T, Ohmoto T, et al: Iatrogenic dissecting aneurysm of the internal carotid artery. Acta Neurochir (Wien) 137:226–231, 1995.
37. Friedman WA, Day AL, Quisling RG, et al: Cervical carotid dissecting aneurysms. Neurosurgery 7:207–214, 1980.
38. Bavinzski G, Killer M, Knosp E, et al: False aneurysms of the intracavernous carotid artery—report of 7 cases. Acta Neurochir (Wien) 139:37–43, 1997.
39. Jafar JJ, Huang PP: Surgical treatment of carotid cavernous aneurysms. Neurosurg Clin N Am 9:755–763, 1998.
40. Date I, Ohmoto T: Long-term outcome of surgical treatment of intracavernous giant aneurysms. Neurol Med Chir (Tokyo) 38: 62–69, 1998.
41. Davies MA, TerBrugge K, Willinsky R, et al: The validity of classification for the clinical presentation of intracranial dural arteriovenous fistulas. J Neurosurg 85:830–837, 1996.
42. Dolenc VV: Extradural approach to intracavernous ICA aneurysms. Acta Neurochir (Wien) 72:99–106, 1999.
43. Spetzler RF, Fukushima T, Martin N, et al: Petrous carotid-to-intradural carotid saphenous vein graft for intracavernous giant aneurysm, tumor, and occlusive cerebrovascular disease. J Neurosurg 73:496–501, 1990.
44. Parkinson D, Downs AR, Whytehead LL, et al: Carotid cavernous fistula: Direct repair with preservation of carotid. Surgery 76: 882–889, 1974.
45. Parkinson D: Carotid cavernous fistula: Direct repair with preservation of the carotid artery: Technical note. J Neurosurg 38: 99–106, 1973.
46. Parkinson D: Transcavernous repair of carotid cavernous fistula: Case report. J Neurosurg 26:420–424, 1967.
47. Oikawa S, Kyoshima K, Kobayashi S: Surgical anatomy of the juxta-dural ring area. J Neurosurg 89:250–254, 1998.
48. Hitotsumatsu T, Natori Y, Matsushima T, et al: Micro-anatomical study of the carotid cave [published erratum appears in Acta Neurochir (Wien) 1998;140(1):106]. Acta Neurochir (Wien) 139: 869–874, 1997.
49. Kobayashi S, Kyoshima K, Gibo H, et al: Carotid cave aneurysms of the internal carotid artery. J Neurosurg 70:216–221, 1989.
50. Nakao S, Kikuchi H, Takahashi N: Successful clipping of carotid-ophthalmic aneurysms through a contralateral pterional approach: Report of two cases. J Neurosurg 54:532–536, 1981.
51. Milenkovic Z, Gopic H, Antovic P, et al: Contralateral pterional approach to a carotid-ophthalmic aneurysm ruptured at surgery: Case report. J Neurosurg 57:823–825, 1982.
52. Kato Y, Sano H, Hayakawa M, et al: Surgical treatment of internal carotid siphon aneurysms. Neurol Res 18:409–415, 1996.
53. Flamm ES: Midcarotid (posterior communicating and anterior choroidal artery) aneurysms. In Apuzzo MLJ (ed): Brain Surgery. New York, Churchill Livingstone, 1993, pp 958–970.
54. Day AL: Aneurysms of the ophthalmic segment: A clinical and anatomical analysis. J Neurosurg 72:677–691, 1990.
55. Drake CG, Vanderlinden RG, Amacher AL: Carotid-ophthalmic aneurysms. J Neurosurg 29:24–31, 1968.
56. Guidetti B, La Torre E: Management of carotid-ophthalmic aneurysms. J Neurosurg 42:438–442, 1975.
57. Ferguson GG, Drake CG: Carotid-ophthalmic aneurysms: Visual abnormalities in 32 patients and the results of treatment. Surg Neurol 16:1–8, 1981.
58. Nutik SL: Ventral paraclinoid carotid aneurysms. J Neurosurg 69:340–344, 1988.
59. Origitano TC, Anderson DE, Tarassoli Y, et al: Skull base approaches to complex cerebral aneurysms. Surg Neurol 40:339–346, 1993.
60. Sugita K, Kobayashi S, Kyoshima K, et al: Fenestrated clips for unusual aneurysms of the carotid artery. J Neurosurg 57: 240–246, 1982.
61. Flamm ES: Suction decompression of aneurysms: Technical note. J Neurosurg 54:275–276, 1981.
62. Batjer HH, Samson DS: Retrograde suction decompression of giant paraclinoidal aneurysms: Technical note. J Neurosurg 73: 305–306, 1990.
63. Scott JA, Horner TG, Leipzig TJ: Retrograde suction decompression of an ophthalmic artery aneurysm using balloon occlusion: Technical note. J Neurosurg 75:146–147, 1991.
64. Rhoton AL Jr, Saeki N, Perlmutter D, et al: Microsurgical anatomy of common aneurysm sites. Clin Neurosurg 26:248–306, 1979.
65. Good EF: Ptosis as the sole manifestation of compression of the oculomotor nerve by an aneurysm of the posterior communicating artery. J Clin Neuroophthalmol 10:59–61, 1990.
66. Kissel JT, Burde RM, Klingele TG, et al: Pupil-sparing oculomotor palsies with internal carotid-posterior communicating artery aneurysms. Ann Neurol 13:149–154, 1983.
67. Kwan ES, Laucella M, Hedges TR 3d, et al: A cliniconeuroradiologic approach to third cranial nerve palsies. AJNR Am J Neuroradiol 8:459–468, 1987.
68. Ogilvy CS, Crowell RM: Carotid bifurcation aneurysms. In Apuzzo MLJ (ed): Brain Surgery. New York, Churchill Livingstone, 1993, pp 970–983.
69. Rhoton AL Jr: Microsurgical anatomy of saccular aneurysms. In Wilkins RH, Rengachary SS (eds): Neurosurgery, vol II. New York, McGraw-Hill, 1996, pp 2215–2228.
70. Rhoton AL Jr, Perlmutter D: Microsurgical anatomy of anterior communicating artery aneurysms. Neurol Res 2:217–251, 1980.
71. Jafar JJ, Weiner HL: Surgery for angiographically occult cerebral aneurysms. J Neurosurg 79:674–679, 1993.
72. de Sousa AA, Dantas FL, de Cardoso GT, et al: Distal anterior cerebral artery aneurysms. Surg Neurol 52:128–135, 1999.
73. Inci S, Erbengi A, Özgen T: Aneurysms of the distal anterior cerebral artery: Report of 14 cases and a review of the literature. Surg Neurol 50:130–139, 1998.
74. Proust F, Toussaint P, Hannequin D, et al: Outcome in 43 patients with distal anterior cerebral artery aneurysms. Stroke 28:2405–2409, 1997.
75. Fujiwara S, Fujii K, Fukui M: De novo aneurysm formation and aneurysm growth following therapeutic carotid occlusion for intracranial internal carotid artery (ICA) aneurysms. Acta Neurochir (Wien) 120:20–25, 1993.
76. Linskey ME, Jungreis CA, Yonas H, et al: Stroke risk after abrupt internal carotid artery sacrifice: Accuracy of preoperative assessment with balloon test occlusion and stable xenon-enhanced CT. AJNR Am J Neuroradiol 15:829–843, 1994.
77. Giller CA, Mathews D, Walker B, et al: Prediction of tolerance to carotid artery occlusion using transcranial Doppler ultrasound. J Neurosurg 81:15–19, 1994.
78. Sen C, Segal D: Is carotid artery reconstruction mandatory? Clin Neurosurg 42:135–153, 1995.
79. Mathis JM, Barr JD, Jungreis CA, et al: Temporary balloon test occlusion of the internal carotid artery: Experience in 500 cases. AJNR Am J Neuroradiol 16:749–754, 1995.
80. McIvor NP, Willinsky RA, TerBrugge KG, et al: Validity of test occlusion studies prior to internal carotid artery sacrifice. Head Neck 16:11–16, 1994.
81. Mathews D, Walker BS, Purdy PD, et al: Brain blood flow SPECT in temporary balloon occlusion of carotid and intracerebral arteries. J Nucl Med 34:1239–1243, 1993.
82. Schomer DF, Marks MP, Steinberg GK, et al: The anatomy of the posterior communicating artery as a risk factor for ischemic cerebral infarction. N Engl J Med 330:1565–1570, 1994.

CHAPTER 111

Surgical Treatment of Intracavernous and Paraclinoid Internal Carotid Artery Aneurysms

GREGORY J. ZIPFEL ■ ARTHUR L. DAY

Proximal internal carotid artery (ICA) aneurysms encompass a heterogeneous group of vascular lesions in proximity to the skull base and anterior clinoid process (ACP). Using the broadest definition, such aneurysms include those arising from the intracavernous, clinoidal, ophthalmic, and posterior communicating segments of the ICA. This chapter addresses only the lesions arising proximal to the origin of the posterior communicating artery, and the more distal aneurysm variants are discussed in later chapters.

Proximal carotid aneurysms have been variously classified over the years, but advances in microsurgical anatomy have permitted a more specific categorization scheme based on traditional aneurysm nomenclature.[1–3] These distinct aneurysm subtypes have unique anatomic relationships, clinical features, and risks of intracranial hemorrhage, largely related to their site of origin, direction of projection, and association with a particular arterial branch. Appropriate indications for intervention, treatment options, and detailed descriptions and illustrations of applicable surgical technique are provided in this chapter.

ANATOMY AND TERMINOLOGY

Osseous Relationships

The ACP, formed by the medial extension of the lesser wing of the sphenoid bone, provides a bony roof to the superior orbital fissure (SOF) and the anterior cavernous sinus (Fig. 111–1). The optic strut extends from the inferomedial surface of the ACP to the body of the sphenoid bone, separating the optic canal and its contents from the SOF. The ACP and optic strut define and obstruct access to the anterior and lateral borders of the ascending ICA as it exits the cavernous sinus, an anatomic arrangement often obligating ACP removal for exposure of proximal ICA lesions.

Dural Relationships

Various dural folds converge at or near each ACP, forming the paired cavernous sinuses that extend alongside the sella turcica and body of the sphenoid bone from the SOF anteriorly to the apex of the petrous bone posteriorly (Fig. 111–2).[4] Two dural sheaths are particularly important to proximal carotid artery aneurysm terminology: the dural ring and the carotid-oculomotor membrane. The *dural ring* is a circular aperture that marks the point of ICA penetration through the medial continuation of the dural layer off the superior ACP surface that merges with the dura of the diaphragma sella and optic canal floor.[5–9] The dural ring marks the exact point where the ascending ICA enters into the subarachnoid space. The oblique anterior-to-posterior and lateral-to-medial, downward-sloping orientation of the dural ring produces a small subarachnoid pocket medial to the ICA called the *carotid cave*.[6, 7, 10] The *carotid-oculomotor membrane* (COM) is formed by a merging of the dura off the inferior surface of the ACP with the venous lining of the cavernous sinus.[4] This membrane extends laterally from the point where the clinoid abuts the ICA inferiorly to the oculomotor nerve. This thin, dural-venous membrane marks the true exit of the ascending ICA from the major cavernous sinus venous lumen.

Vascular Relationships

ARTERIAL SEGMENTS

The ICA is traditionally divided into four segments: cervical, petrous, cavernous, and supraclinoid (see Fig. 111–2).[11] The cavernous segment begins as the ICA ascends from the carotid canal of the petrous bone at the foramen lacerum. The vessel briefly continues upward toward the posterior clinoid process and then turns forward to travel horizontally alongside the sphenoid bone. After traveling a distance of approximately 2 cm, the artery bends superiorly and ascends just medial to the ACP to enter the subarachnoid space.

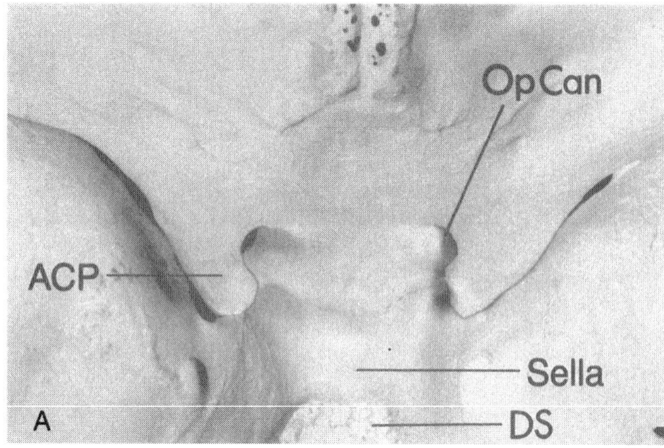

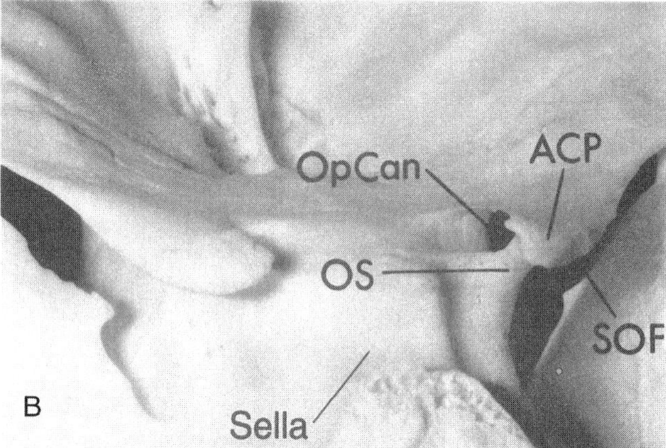

FIGURE 111–1. Paraclinoid osseous anatomy. *A*, Dorsal view. *B*, Posterior oblique view. The anterior clinoid process (ACP) is the most medial extension of the lesser wing of the sphenoid bone. Notice the relationship of the ACP to the superior orbital fissure (SOF), the ascending internal carotid artery, the anterior cavernous sinus, and the optic strut (OS). DS, dorsum sella; OpCan, optic canal.

The cavernous segment includes the portion of the ICA associated with the cavernous venous compartment and has been typically apportioned into five divisions: posterior vertical segment, posterior genu, horizontal segment, anterior genu, and anterior vertical segment.[12] The first four divisions lie completely within the venous plexus of the cavernous sinus (Fig. 111–3) and are collectively referred to as the *true cavernous segment* (CavSeg).[4, 8, 9]

The distal portion of the fifth division (i.e., anterior vertical segment) is located above the major venous lumen of the cavernous sinus, just beyond the COM. Corresponding to the distal anterior vertical segment, this region of the ICA, called the *clinoidal segment* (ClinSeg), is a transitional ICA division found medial to the ACP between the COM and the dural ring.[4, 8, 9] The ClinSeg is located neither within the venous channels of the cavernous sinus nor within the subarachnoid space and is essentially interdural.[4, 8, 9]

The remaining distal portion of the ICA (i.e., supraclinoid segment) lies entirely within the subarachnoid space, beginning at the dural ring and extending to the vessel's terminal bifurcation. Three subdivisions of the supraclinoid carotid have been delineated,[11] but only the first, the *ophthalmic segment* (OphSeg), is considered here. This segment extends from the dural ring to the origin of the posterior communicating artery and represents the longest subarachnoid segment of the ICA.[11]

ARTERIAL BENDS AND BRANCHES

Saccular aneurysms typically form at points of hemodynamic stress where a bend in the vessel and a branch site coincide.[13] Three major bends in the proximal ICA predispose this region to aneurysm formation. The first bend, seen best on lateral angiogram, is the prominent forward turn of the posterior genu of the cavernous ICA. This arterial turn primarily places a superior hemodynamic force on the CavSeg wall at the proximal end of the horizontal portion. The second bend, also seen best on a lateral angiogram, is the posteriorly projecting turn that begins at the anterior genu of the CavSeg and continues as the vessel ascends through the dural ring. This bend creates a strong superior vector on the anterior and dorsal wall of the clinoidal and ophthalmic ICA segments. A less conspicuous third bend, seen best from an anteroposterior or dorsal view, is the gentle lateral-to-medial-to-lateral curve beginning at the anterior genu of the CavSeg and continuing as the ICA travels toward its terminal bifurcation. This medially projecting hemodynamic vector places significant stress on the medial aspect of the clinoidal and ophthalmic ICA segments.

Two branches consistently arise from the CavSeg. The first, called the *meningohypophyseal trunk,* projects posteriorly from the posterior genu of the CavSeg and ramifies into three endarteries: the tentorial artery (or artery of Bernasconi-Cassinari), which supplies the tentorium; the inferior hypophyseal artery, which supplies the inferior pituitary gland; and the dorsal meningeal artery, which supplies the dura of the upper clivus.[4, 12] The second branch, called the *inferolateral trunk* or *artery of the inferior cavernous sinus,* projects laterally from the horizontal portion of the CavSeg above the abducens nerve to supply the nearby cranial nerves and dura of the inferior cavernous sinus and middle fossa floor.[4, 12] McConnell's capsular artery is an inconstant branch (found in about 8% of cadaveric specimens) of the CavSeg, and it projects medially from the anterior genu or distal horizontal segment to supply the capsule of the pituitary gland.[4]

The OphSeg harbors several prominent arterial branches that predispose this region to aneurysm formation. The *ophthalmic artery* (OphArt) is the most prominent and clinically significant branch from this region, and it typically arises from the dorsomedial carotid surface just above the dural ring and below the inferolateral portion of the optic nerve.[14, 15] This branch projects anterolaterally to accompany the optic nerve through the optic canal, supplying the retina and orbit. The *superior hypophyseal artery* (SupHypArt) is the second major branch (or series of branches), usually arising from the medial or inferomedial ICA surface just distal to the takeoff of the OphArt along the medial-to-lateral ICA bend within the OphSeg.[16, 17] This artery

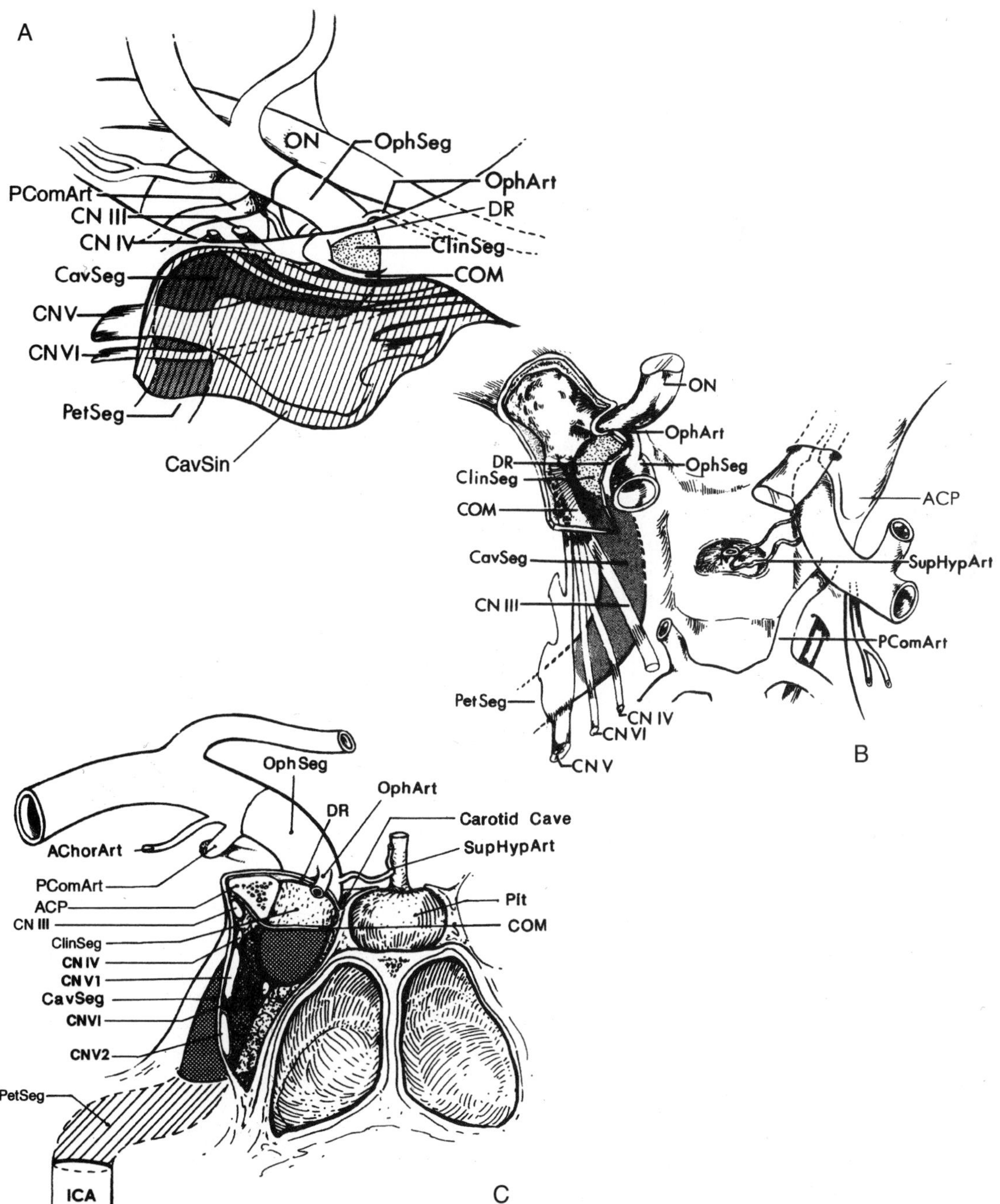

FIGURE 111–2. Paraclinoid osseous, dural, vascular, and neural anatomy (schematic). *A,* Lateral view. *B,* Dorsal view. *C,* Anteroposterior view. The cavernous (CavSeg), clinoidal (ClinSeg), and ophthalmic (OphSeg) segments of the internal carotid artery (ICA) are close to the anterior clinoid process (ACP). The true CavSeg lies within the venous channels of the cavernous sinus (CavSin), the ClinSeg has an interdural location between the dural ring (DR) and the carotid-oculomotor membrane (COM), and the OphSeg is entirely subarachnoid. Notice the location of the oculomotor (CN III), trochlear (CN IV), and first division of the trigeminal (CN V_1) cranial nerves within the lateral sinus wall and the abducens nerve (CN VI) within the venous channels between the CavSeg and CN V_1. Care during ACP removal is critical to avoid injury to the nearby oculomotor and trochlear nerves, which exit the cavernous sinus immediately below the ACP. AChorArt, anterior choroidal artery; ON, optic nerve; OphArt, ophthalmic artery; PComArt, posterior communicating artery; PetSeg, petrous segment; Pit, pituitary gland; SupHypArt, superior hypophyseal artery.

(or arteries) projects medially to supply the superior aspect of the pituitary stalk and gland, a portion of the cavernous sinus dura, and the posterior optic nerve and chiasm.

The ClinSeg is usually devoid of arterial perforators. Occasionally, the ophthalmic and superior hypophyseal arteries originate from this segment, typically reaching their end-organs through alternate anatomic pathways. The OphArt, for example, can originate from the distal CavSeg or ClinSeg in up to 10% of cadaveric specimens, usually entering the orbit through the SOF or an orifice within the optic strut.[4, 12, 18]

Neural Relationships

The *oculomotor nerve* is located within the superior lateral cavernous sinus wall and courses anteriorly just beneath the ACP to enter the orbit through the

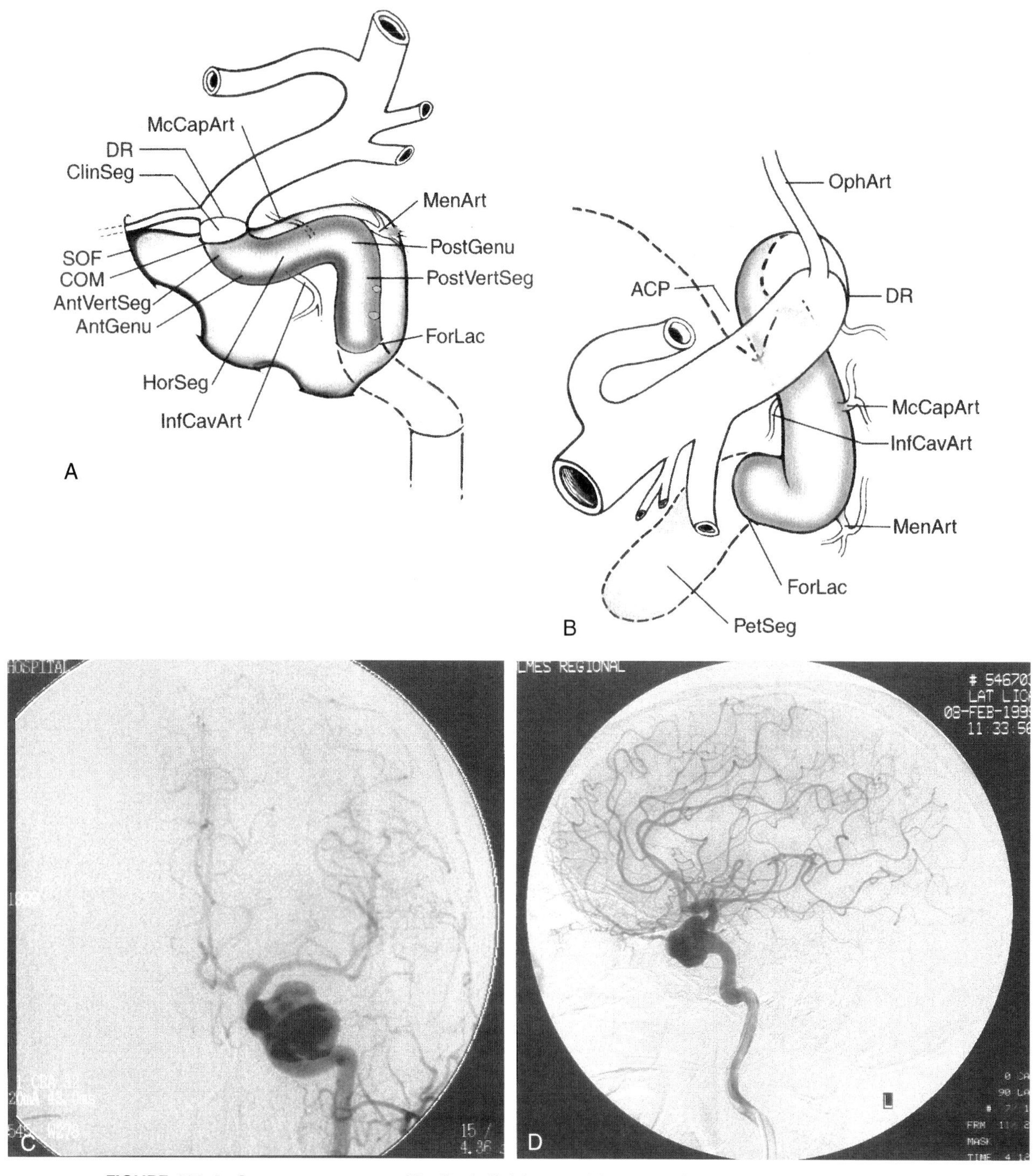

FIGURE 111–3. Cavernous segment (CavSeg) divisions and branches (schematic). *A,* Lateral view. *B,* Dorsal view. *C,* Arteriogram, anteroposterior view. *D,* Arteriogram, lateral view.

Illustration continued on following page

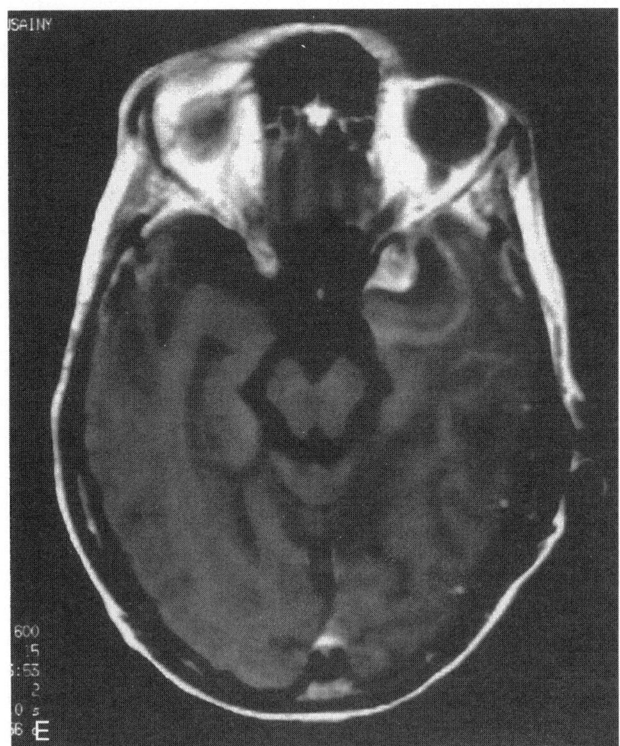

FIGURE 111–3. *Continued. E,* Magnetic resonance imaging. The CavSeg of the internal carotid artery begins at the foramen lacerum (ForLac) and ends as the vessel ascends near the anterior clinoid process (ACP). The CavSeg is traditionally divided into five portions: posterior vertical segment (PostVertSeg), posterior genu (PostGenu), horizontal segment (HorSeg), anterior genu (AntGenu), and anterior vertical segment (AntVertSeg). The distal portion of the AntVertSeg has been separately called the *clinoidal segment* (ClinSeg), because it represents a unique "interdural" internal carotid artery (ICA) segment that resides between the carotid-oculomotor membrane (COM) and dural ring (DR). The three prominent CavSeg branches include the meningohypophyseal trunk (MenArt), the artery of the inferior cavernous sinus (InfCavArt), and McConnell's capsular artery (McCapArt). Aneurysms originating from the true CavSeg (i.e., portion of the ICA residing entirely within the venous confines of the cavernous sinus) are usually located along the HorSeg or AntGenu and typically project beneath the ACP toward the superior orbital fissure (SOF). With enlargement, CavSeg aneurysms project anterolaterally beneath the lesser wing of the sphenoid bone. *C* to *E,* Notice the aneurysm origin from the anterior portion of the horizontal segment, and its expansion below the sphenoid ridge toward the SOF.

SOF (see Fig. 111–2). The *trochlear nerve* is also located within the lateral cavernous sinus wall, traveling just beneath and parallel to the oculomotor nerve. The *first division of the trigeminal nerve* (V_1) courses several millimeters below the oculomotor and trochlear nerves within the lateral sinus wall, and the *abducens nerve* courses within the cavernous venous compartment itself between the CavSeg and V_1. The *sympathetic fiber bundles* course as a plexus along the cavernous and clinoidal ICA, eventually departing the carotid proximal to the dural ring to project into the orbit.

ANEURYSM TYPES

Three distinct aneurysm locations are discussed in this chapter: CavSeg, ClinSeg, and OphSeg, all of which share several common features. Aneurysms from each of these carotid segments are much more common in women, with a female-to-male predominance as high as 9:1.[2, 19, 20] Most manifest during the fifth and sixth decades of life, usually discovered as incidental lesions or because of a mass effect.[2, 19, 21] Approximately two thirds of CavSeg and three fourths of OphSeg lesions are 1 cm or larger in diameter at time of initial diagnosis.[2, 21] These segments have a striking propensity for aneurysm multiplicity; approximately one third of CavSeg aneurysm patients and nearly one half of OphSeg aneurysm patients harbor at least one additional intracranial aneurysm.[2, 22, 23] Despite these similarities, each segment also has its own peculiarities relative to external shape and factors contributing to their cause (i.e., saccular and fusiform varieties), clinical features at time of presentation, radiographic features, and indications and type of treatment.

Computed tomography (CT) is the best imaging modality for diagnosing subarachnoid hemorrhage, and it may also diagnose the aneurysm, especially if the lesion is large or giant. Bony details delineated by CT, such as focal erosion of the ACP or sella, can help differentiate particular proximal aneurysm subtypes. CT may also reveal aneurysm features that potentially increase treatment complexity (i.e., intraluminal thrombus and aneurysm wall calcification) and factors that may prompt further studies such as awake trial balloon occlusion testing before intervention. CT–angiography is becoming increasingly useful in the evaluation of intracranial aneurysms, including those emanating from the carotid siphon.[24, 25]

Magnetic resonance imaging (MRI) often provides adjunctive anatomic detail that can help determine the relationship between the aneurysm and the soft tissue structures such as the optic apparatus and pituitary gland or whether a portion of a CavSeg or ClinSeg lesion enters the subarachnoid space. Magnetic resonance angiography (MRA) is capable of delineating the topographic anatomy of paraclinoid aneurysms[26] and may be useful (as may CT–angiography) for noninvasively screening high-risk patient populations such as those with Ehlers-Danlos syndrome, Marfan's disease, or polycystic kidney disease and those with a strong family history of aneurysms.

Four-vessel transfemoral cerebral angiography remains the gold standard for aneurysm diagnosis and is generally recommended for all patients harboring proximal carotid artery aneurysms if intervention is being considered. The cervical carotid artery should be carefully inspected for atherosclerotic plaque that may make proximal temporary clamping hazardous, and the superficial temporary artery should be evaluated for its applicability as a bypass conduit. An awake trial balloon occlusion test with induced hypotension or cerebral blood flow studies (i.e., single photon emission CT or xenon–CT) should be considered for complex lesions that may require long temporary or permanent ICA occlusion during aneurysm obliteration.

Intracavernous Segment Aneurysms

CLINICAL AND RADIOGRAPHIC FEATURES

Cavernous sinus region aneurysms account for approximately 3% to 5% of all angiographically identified intracranial aneurysms, and up to 15% of all aneurysms originating from the ICA.[27, 28] CavSeg aneurysms may originate anywhere along the cavernous carotid artery, but most clinically significant lesions arise from the horizontal segment and project forward and laterally toward the SOF below the ACP (see Fig. 111–3).[21–23] Other less common locations include the anterior and posterior genu, both of which may project superiorly and erode the dural roof of the cavernous sinus to enter the subarachnoid space. These aneurysm locations correspond well to the three most common CavSeg arterial branches—McConnell's capsular artery, the inferolateral trunk, and the meningohypophyseal trunk—suggesting that hemodynamic stress at arterial branch sites may contribute to the formation of some CavSeg aneurysms.[4, 29] Most CavSeg aneurysms, however, originate apart from branch sites and arterial bends, prompting considerations of alternate pathogenetic mechanisms such as arteriosclerosis and spontaneous or traumatic dissection.[21]

Traumatic dissections frequently affect the infraclinoid ICA, particularly at the anterior genu, and usually manifest in boys and young men after a head injury with the triad of anterior skull base fracture, unilateral visual loss, and epistaxis, or the typical signs of a carotid-cavernous fistula.[30, 31] Most intracavernous aneurysms, however, have no clear association with trauma during their formation or clinical evolution.

Most spontaneous (nontraumatic) CavSeg aneurysms remain asymptomatic until reaching giant proportions (approximately 2.5 cm), at which point symptoms are caused by a local mass effect against adjacent structures. Symptom onset may be insidious or explosive and may include isolated or combined deficits of the oculomotor, trochlear, abducens, trigeminal, and sympathetic nerves. Most symptomatic patients exhibit a combination of ophthalmoplegia and facial pain or numbness, constituting a cavernous sinus syndrome.[19, 21, 22] Other presentations include retro-orbital pain (usually in a V_1 distribution), nonspecific headaches, or incidental discoveries during workup for other lesions or symptoms. Even less common presentations include thrombotic or embolic phenomenon, hypopituitarism, visual loss, or rupture into the cavernous sinus producing signs and symptoms of a spontaneous carotid-cavernous fistula.

Any life-threatening risks attributed to true spontaneous CavSeg aneurysms are rare, because these lesions, in addition to their own arterial wall, are covered by the venous structures within the sinus and by the overlying dura and surrounding bony structures. Epistaxis or secondary extension into the subarachnoid space can occur, but it is becoming increasingly uncommon with the application of modern diagnostic studies.[32–35] Although some reports indicate a subarachnoid hemorrhage risk as high as 7% to 40%, these studies are confounded by the inclusion of aneurysms that originated within (OphSeg) or extended into (ClinSeg) the subarachnoid compartment.[21, 29, 36] When including only the aneurysms whose necks originated within the cavernous sinus (as described earlier), the risk of subarachnoid hemorrhage is found to be extremely low.[19, 23, 29]

In the symptomatic patient, CT or MRI invariably demonstrates a round or oblong, extradural, parasellar mass expanding anteriorly toward the SOF and laterally into the middle cranial fossa beneath the sphenoid ridge and ACP.[21–23] The bone of the adjacent skull base inhibits identification of small lesions with CT, but MRI and MRA can usually demonstrate the aneurysm. The definitive diagnosis is established by arteriography, and when performed, it should include a lateral view of the ipsilateral external carotid artery for potential donor vessels in the event that carotid ligation and extracranial-intracranial bypass is considered. Mural thrombosis often occurs in large lesions, causing the aneurysm lumen to appear smaller on angiogram than its actual size. Most true CavSeg aneurysms arise along the horizontal segment unassociated with an obvious arterial branch. Many appear fusiform, a shape that makes clip or coil obliteration with sparing of the parent vessel quite difficult. Lesions arising at or just beyond the anterior genu can be difficult to discern radiographically from ClinSeg lesions.

INDICATIONS AND METHODS OF TREATMENT

Asymptomatic CavSeg aneurysms without radiographic extension into the subarachnoid space are treated conservatively regardless of aneurysm size, because these lesions have such a low risk for life-threatening problems. When symptoms are mild and confined to oculomotor or painless trigeminal dysfunction in the typical 65-year-old woman, operative intervention is often not advised, because many patients have a benign clinical course.[19] Visual loss (rare with this lesion type), severe intractable facial pain, and radiographic evidence of subarachnoid extension (e.g., dural "waisting" on arteriography[37]) are stronger indications for operative intervention. Subarachnoid hemorrhage and epistaxis should obviously be treated aggressively.

With intractable or progressive symptoms, treatment through surgical or endovascular means is recommended based on aneurysm characteristics and location. CavSeg lesions originating along the anterior genu can be treated with direct surgical obliteration using the techniques described for ClinSeg and OphSeg lesions. More proximal lesions are usually best treated with platinum coils (especially if the aneurysm has a clearly defined neck) or with surgical or endovascular ICA occlusion (with an arterial bypass as needed).[22, 38–43] Figure 111–4 outlines the treatment algorithm for these lesions.

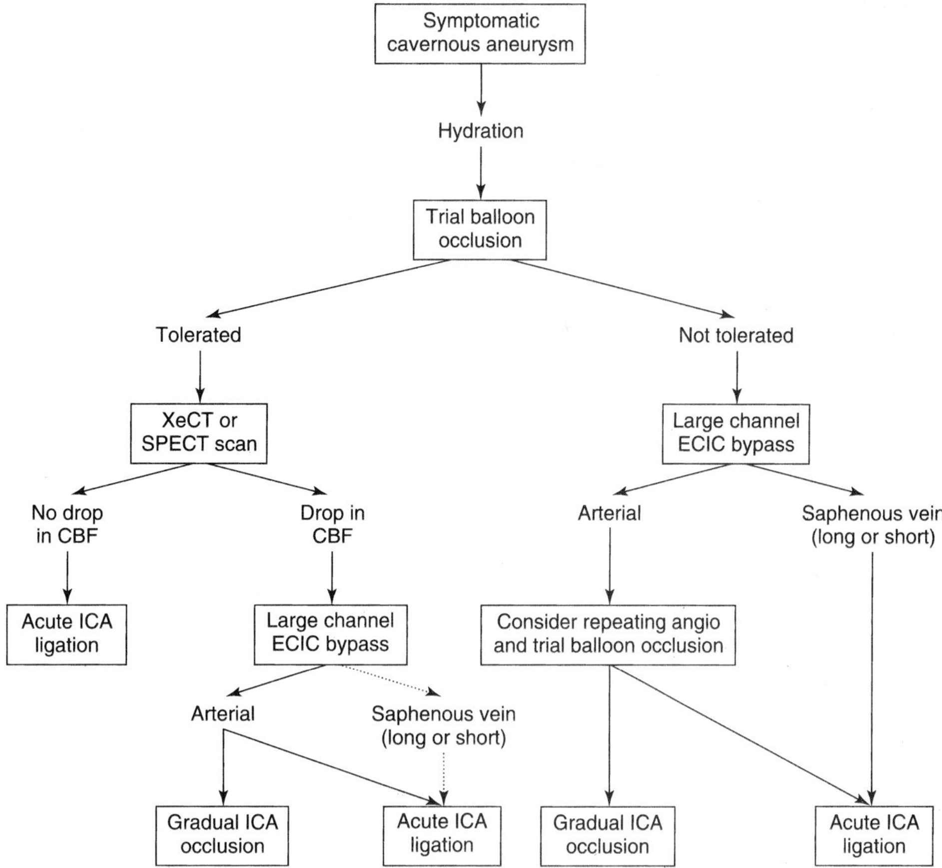

FIGURE 111–4. Treatment algorithm for internal carotid artery ICA) ligation. angio, angiography; CBF, cerebral blood flow; ECIC, extracranial-intracranial; SPECT, single photon emission computed tomography; XeCT, xenon–computed tomography.

Clinoidal Segment Aneurysms

CLINICAL AND RADIOGRAPHIC FEATURES

Two ClinSeg aneurysm variants can be differentiated according to their site of origin and direction of projection (Fig. 111–5). Each variant is influenced by the arterial bends and branches within the segment and the adjacent dural and osseous structures. The *anterolateral variant* arises from the anterolateral surface of the ClinSeg as it obliquely ascends toward the dural ring underneath the ACP.[1] The superiorly and slightly medially directed hemodynamic vector and the occasional presence of a proximal ophthalmic artery origin promote a superiorly projecting aneurysm that expands lateral and anterior to the ascending ICA. When small, the anterolateral variant may erode the optic strut and undersurface of the ACP to cause monocular visual loss from ipsilateral optic nerve compression within the optic canal. Larger lesions may secondarily compress the visual system (nerve or chiasm) within the subarachnoid space after extension through the dura adjacent to the dural ring.

The *medial variant* extends from the medial surface of the ClinSeg, and enlarges toward the sphenoid sinus and sella.[1] The projection of these lesions arises from the more subtle medially directed hemodynamic vector created as the ICA turns from lateral to medial to lateral during its ascent toward and through the dural ring. Initially, this aneurysm type expands beneath the diaphragma sella into the pituitary fossa, and gradual enlargement may cause hypopituitarism. Rarely, aneurysm rupture into the pituitary gland itself may simulate pituitary apoplexy, or extension and rupture into the sphenoid sinus may cause life-threatening epistaxis. Large or giant lesions may extend through the diaphragma sella to enter the subarachnoid space. Visual loss from this aneurysm type does not occur with small lesions, but field cuts resembling those of pituitary tumors may occur with large or giant lesions.

Because both ClinSeg variants are located interdurally below the dural ring and subarachnoid space, the risk of hemorrhage associated with small lesions (<1 cm) is extremely low. After this size is exceeded, however, these lesions may erode through the dura adjacent to the dural ring and extend into the subarachnoid space, where they assume the same or greater hemorrhage risk as those of the OphSeg. In addition to subarachnoid hemorrhage, ClinSeg aneurysms also manifest with visual disturbance or headaches and as incidentally discovered lesions. Headaches from ClinSeg aneurysms are generally limited to the ipsilateral V_1 and retro-orbital regions and are presumably caused by pulsatile distortion of the dura overlying this segment. Much less commonly, ClinSeg lesions may produce facial numbness or diplopia from compression against the lateral cavernous sinus wall, but a full-blown cavernous sinus syndrome is rare from these lesions.

The anterolateral variant lesion can often closely

resemble an OphArt aneurysm, and differentiation between these two lesions can sometimes be challenging. Dorsal expansion of the anterolateral ClinSeg aneurysm variant beneath the ACP and optic strut often produces focal bony erosion evident on CT or MRI scanning. Several angiographic features also help with appropriate classification:

- Origination proximal to the typical takeoff of the OphArt
- A subtle "double density" along the anterolateral ICA wall dictates this lesion's proximal nature
- Aneurysm projection dorsal and lateral to the ICA (in contrast to the dorsal or dorsomedial projection of an OphArt aneurysm)
- An angiographic "waist" marking the penetration of the lesion through the overlying dural coverings into the subarachnoid space

Differentiating a medial variant ClinSeg from a SupHypArt aneurysm can also be difficult. MRI can often define the intimate association of the medial variant with the pituitary gland. Neither produces significant bony erosion seen on CT. Both lesions project medially: the ClinSeg subtype beneath the diaphragma sella and SupHypArt type above the diaphragma sella into the parasellar or suprasellar space. This origin beneath the diaphragma sella often displaces the medial variant downward and flattens its superior margin. Medial variant ClinSeg lesions typically have a narrow neck, because of the origin between the COM and the dural ring, whereas SupHypArt aneurysms, free of such dural restraints, usually have a wide neck. On a lateral view, the ClinSeg medial variant lesion originates proximal to the OphArt and creates a subtle double density along the anterior genu below the plane of the ACP, indicating the lesion's proximal origin. SupHypArt le-

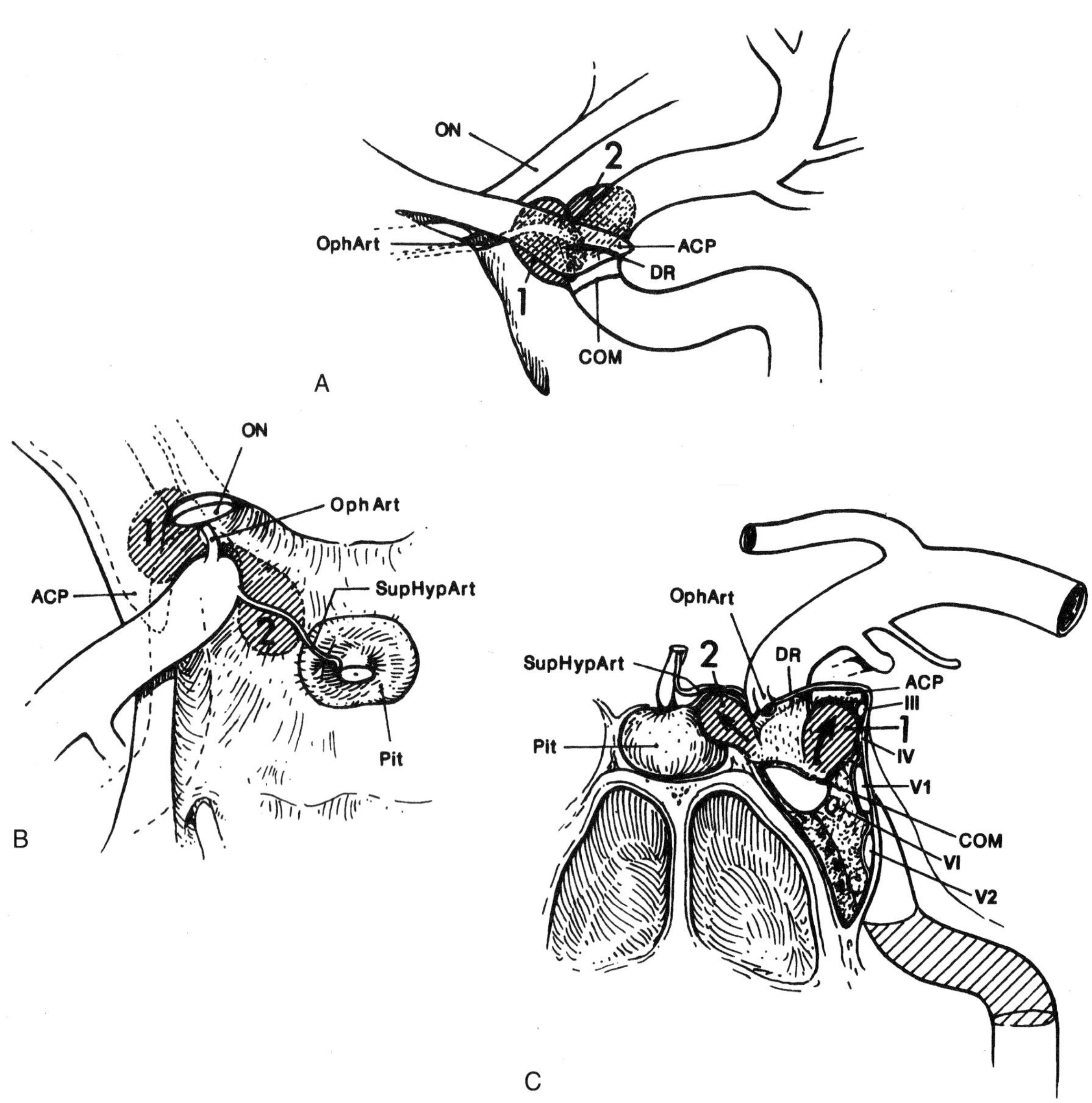

FIGURE 111–5. Clinoidal segment (ClinSeg) aneurysm types. *A,* Lateral view (schematic). *B,* Dorsal view (schematic). *C,* Anteroposterior (AP) view (schematic).

Illustration continued on following page

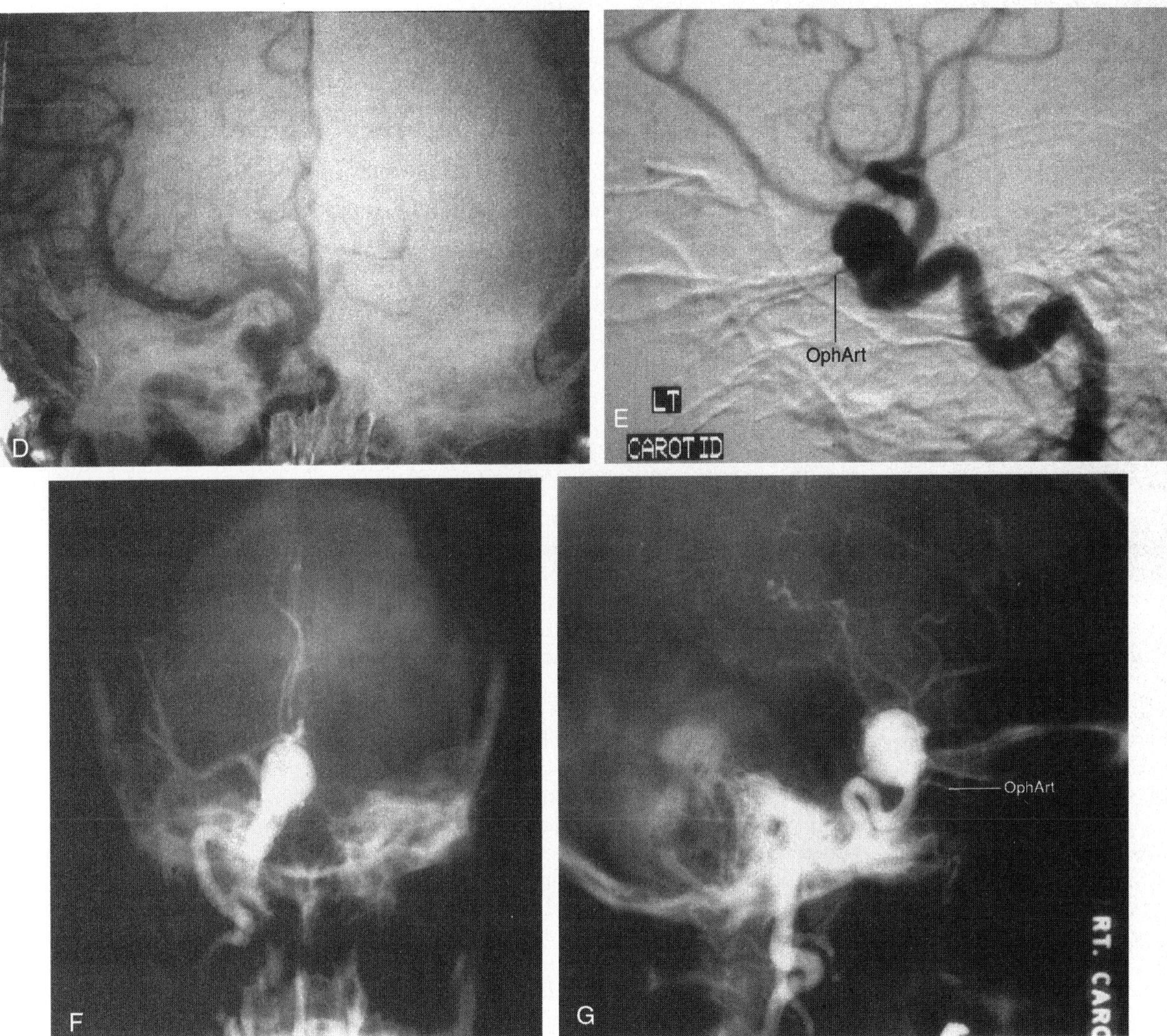

FIGURE 111–5. *Continued. D,* Anterolateral variant: arteriogram, AP view. *E,* Anterolateral variant: arteriogram, lateral view. *F,* Medial variant: arteriogram, AP view. *G,* Medial variant: arteriogram, lateral view. Anterolateral variant ClinSeg aneurysms *(hatched area 1, A* to *C)* originate from the dorsolateral aspect of the ClinSeg and project upward and laterally toward the anterior clinoid process (ACP). Medial variant ClinSeg aneurysms *(hatched area 2, A* to *C)* originate from the medial aspect of the ClinSeg and project upward and medially toward the sella beneath the diaphragma sella. *D* and *E,* Notice the double density of the aneurysm origin from the clinoidal segment below the plane of the ophthalmic artery and the superolateral projection toward and through the anterior clinoid process. *F* and *G,* Notice the similar double density of aneurysm origin below the ophthalmic artery but with its projection medial to the internal carotid artery (ICA) into the sella. COM, carotid-oculomotor membrane; DR, dural ring; ON, optic nerve; OphArt, ophthalmic artery; Pit, pituitary gland; SupHypArt, superior hypophyseal artery.

sions appear to arise on the posterior or posteromedial ICA wall opposite the OphArt origin.

INDICATIONS AND METHODS OF TREATMENT

Indications for treatment of ClinSeg aneurysm are largely dictated by the size of the offending lesion and its associated symptoms. Small, asymptomatic aneurysms (<1 cm) are interdural below the subarachnoid space and are therefore generally treated conservatively with periodic clinical and radiographic follow-up. Small symptomatic lesions (e.g., visual deficits or focal, unrelenting headaches) or those whose protective ACP roof has been removed for treatment of another aneurysm in the region should be treated. Most large (≥1 cm) ClinSeg aneurysms have extended through the overlying dural coverings into the subarachnoid space and carry a significant risk for intracranial hemorrhage. Strong consideration for intervention is given to such lesions, even if they are asymptomatic. Small ClinSeg aneurysms may be the most ideal lesion to treat with endovascular therapy, because most have a narrow neck-to-fundus ratio. We generally treat large ClinSeg lesions with direct surgical obliteration although endovascular therapy can be considered, particularly if the aneurysm characteristics are favorable. Lesions presenting with subarachnoid hemorrhage or epistaxis should be obliterated urgently.

Ophthalmic Segment Aneurysms

CLINICAL AND RADIOGRAPHIC FEATURES

About one half of patients harboring OphSeg aneurysms present with visual symptoms or subarachnoid hemorrhage, and the remaining patients have incidentally discovered lesions (Fig. 111–6).[2, 3] Ruptured or incidental lesions coincide with aneurysms of various sizes, whereas lesions producing visual symptoms are almost always giant (≥2.5 cm), suggesting that considerable mass effect must take place before visual defects occur and are noticed by the patient.[2, 3]

Three aneurysm subtypes arise from the OphSeg: OphArt, SupHypArt, and dorsal carotid wall lesions. Aneurysms with a clear association with the OphArt are called *OphArt aneurysms*.[1–3, 20, 44, 45] These lesions typically arise along the posterior bend of the ICA just distal to the OphArt and dural ring. OphArt aneurysms project dorsally or dorsomedially toward the latter half of the optic nerve. OphArt aneurysms cause visual field deficits by elevating the ipsilateral optic nerve superiorly and medially into the sharp edge of the falciform ligament, preferentially damaging the superolateral portion of the nerve. A monocular inferior nasal field defect is initially produced but may go unnoticed by the patient. As the lesion enlarges, however, the entire nasal field can become affected, followed by a superior temporal field loss in the contralateral eye. If the clinical course is protracted, ipsilateral blindness with marked contralateral deficits can occur.

SupHypArt aneurysms arise from the inferior or inferomedial surface of the ICA along the gentle lateral-to-medial-to-lateral ICA bend in close association with the takeoff of the SupHypArt and separate from the OphArt origin.[1–3] Most arise just above the dural ring, but some may arise more distally along the OphSeg. Many small lesions burrow inferiorly and medially toward and below the diaphragma sella, expanding the carotid cave. These lesions, called *parasellar variant SupHypArt aneurysms*, have also been called *carotid cave aneurysms*.[1–3, 7, 46] When small, the fundus of this variant is invested by adjacent lateral parasellar dura, and the risk of subarachnoid hemorrhage is quite low. With growth, however, these lesions expand superomedially above the diaphragma sella into the suprasellar space, where the hemorrhage risk becomes greater.

Another variety of SupHypArt aneurysm projects medially above a shallow carotid cave, encountering little resistance from the lateral sellar wall and expanding into the medial suprasellar space above the diaphragm without investment by the parasellar dura. These lesions with primary suprasellar projection or the enlarged parasellar variants with secondary suprasellar extension are called *suprasellar variant SupHypArt aneurysms*. In contrast to OphArt aneurysms, SupHypArt lesions cause their visual compression by expansion into the suprasellar space and elevation of the optic chiasm, producing superior bitemporal or other patterns of visual loss more suggestive of pituitary tumors.

Some OphSeg aneurysms arise along the dorsal surface of the ICA distinctly distal to the OphArt origin.[1–3, 44] Many of these lesions, called *dorsal variant OphSeg aneurysms*, appear to be pure hemodynamically induced saccular lesions unassociated with a branch point that arise from an accentuated bend in the ICA as the vessel approaches the posterior communicating artery. Others appear more like blisters and probably represent dissections.[47] The thickened or arteriosclerotic anterior walls characteristic of large or giant OphArt aneurysms may create a gap between the aneurysm origin and the OphArt takeoff on the lateral arteriogram, mimicking a true dorsal variant lesion. Because dorsal variant lesions arise more distally along the ICA, they often are situated lateral to the visual system and uncommonly manifest with visual apparatus.[12, 15]

A ruptured OphSeg (or ClinSeg) aneurysm typically produces hemorrhage within the chiasmatic and parasellar cisterns, occasionally producing an additional focal clot within the orbitofrontal gyri. Because OphSeg lesions arise distal to the dural ring, bony erosion is not seen on imaging studies, in contrast to the image seen with the more proximal anterolateral ClinSeg variant. MRI is often useful in defining the relationship between the aneurysm and the visual system.

On arteriography, OphArt aneurysms arise from the dorsal ICA surface just distal to the OphArt takeoff. The ipsilateral optic nerve stretched by the dorsal expansion of the aneurysm often flattens the superomedial aneurysm surface and inhibits aneurysm growth across the midline. This optic nerve tethering also produces inferior deflection of the OphSeg and "closing" of the carotid siphon.

The inferior slant of the dural ring from anterior to posterior often places the origin of SupHypArt aneurysms, as seen on a lateral view, below the plane of the ACP. As the lesion expands and fills the parasellar space or carotid cave (usually about 1 cm), it begins to enlarge into the suprasellar space, and often ventures across midline unimpeded by the visual system. The ICA is often deflected laterally and superiorly, leading to an "opening" of the carotid siphon.

Dorsal variant OphSeg aneurysms project superiorly similar to OphArt aneurysms, but the aneurysm origin is clearly separate (usually by 2 to 4 mm) from the OphArt takeoff.

INDICATIONS AND METHODS OF TREATMENT

All OphSeg aneurysms are located within the subarachnoid space and have at least some risk for rupture and intracranial hemorrhage. Those presenting with subarachnoid hemorrhage or visual loss should be treated urgently, either by surgical or endovascular

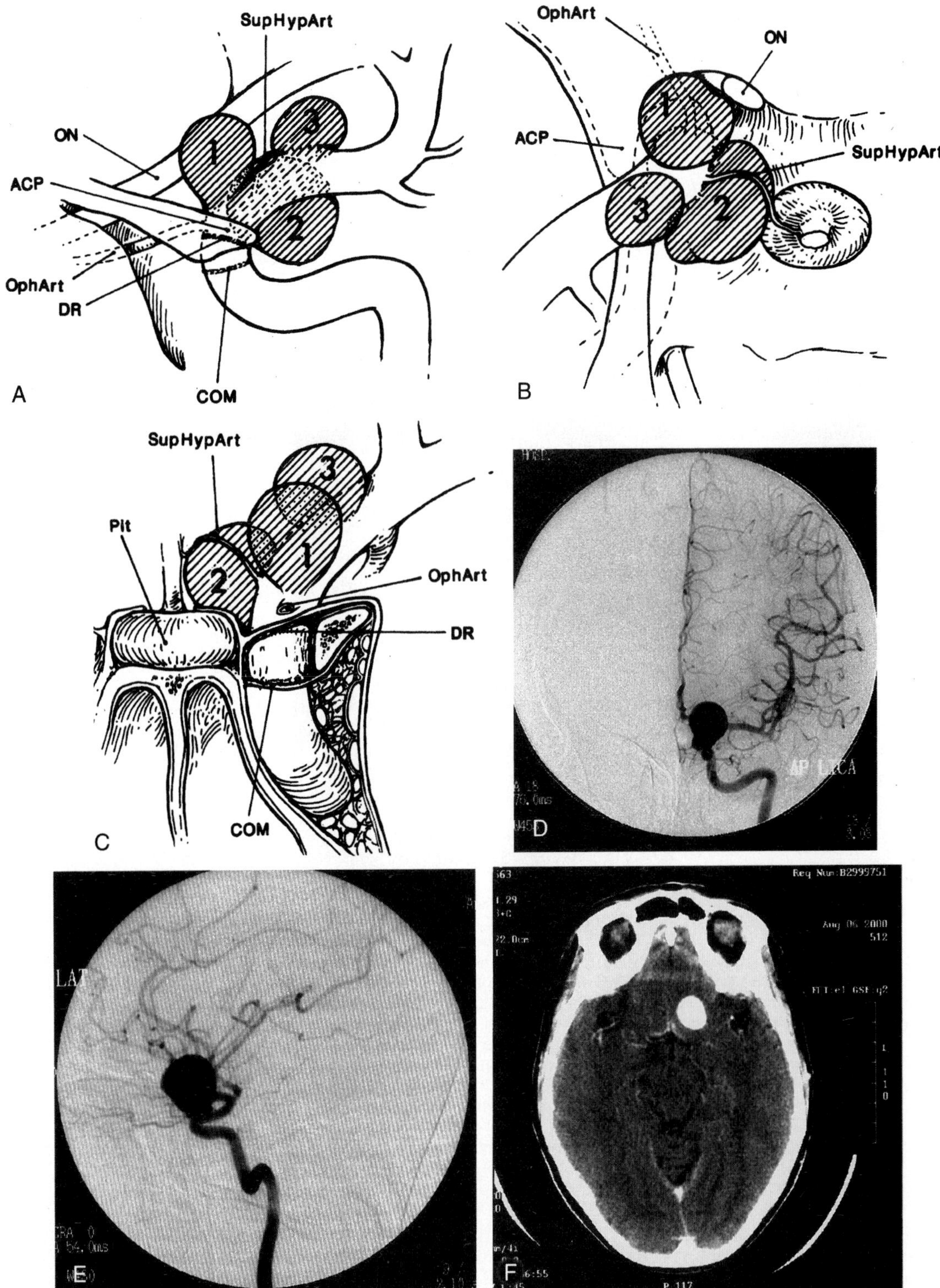

FIGURE 111–6. Ophthalmic segment (OphSeg) aneurysm types. *A,* Lateral view (schematic). *B,* Dorsal view (schematic). *C,* Anteroposterior (AP) view (schematic). *D,* Ophthalmic artery (OphArt) aneurysm: arteriogram, AP view. *E,* Ophthalmic artery (OphArt) aneurysm: arteriogram, lateral view. *F,* Magnetic resonance imaging (MRI).

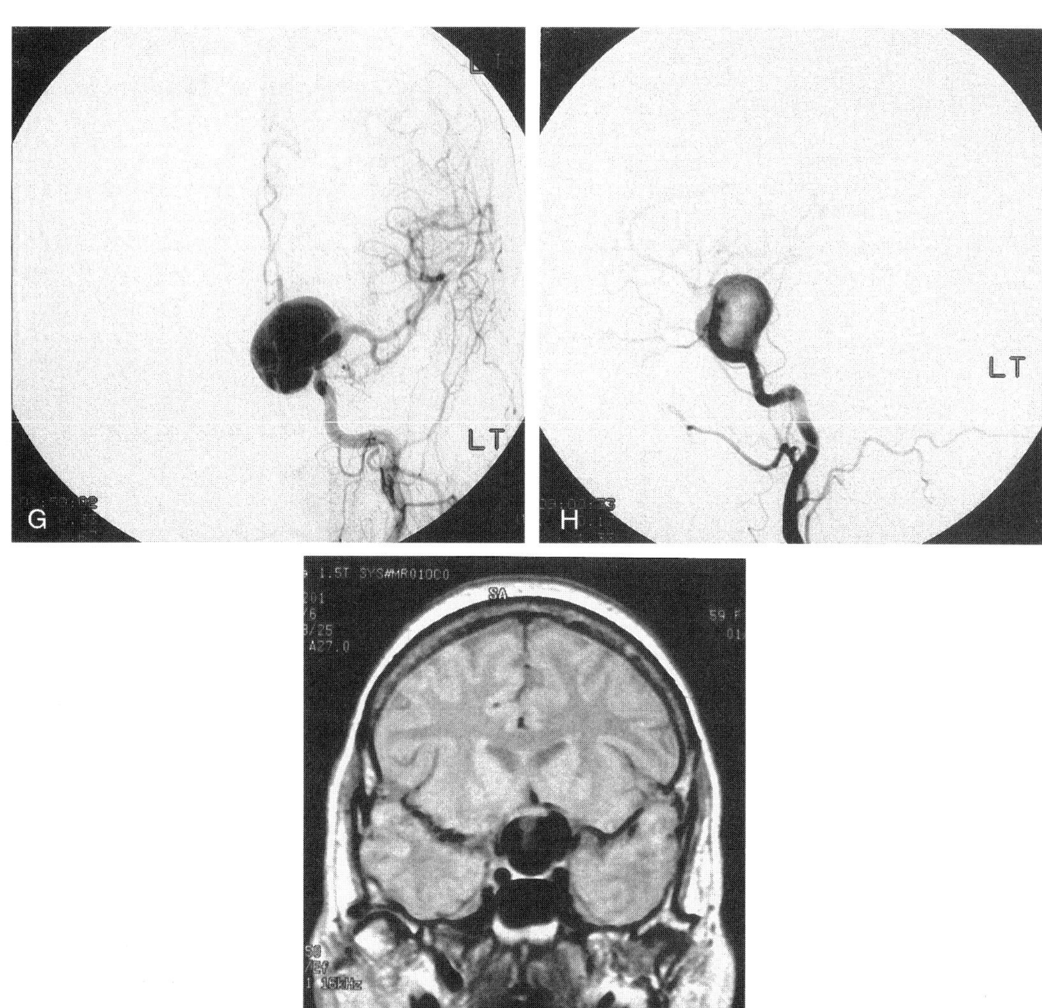

FIGURE 111–6. *Continued. G,* Superior hypophyseal artery (SupHypArt) aneurysm: arteriogram, AP view. *H,* Superior hypophyseal artery (SupHypArt) aneurysm: arteriogram, lateral view. I, MRI. OphArt aneurysms *(hatched area 1, A* to *C)* arise from the dorsomedial internal carotid artery (ICA) surface just distal to the OphArt origin. SupHypArt aneurysms *(hatched area 2, A* to *C)* arise from the inferomedial ICA surface independent of the OphArt origin, in close association with the arterial perforators that supply the optic chiasm and parasellar dura. SupHypArt aneurysms project medially, burrowing within the carotid cave above the dural ring (DR) alongside the lateral sellar dura (parasellar variant) or expanding beyond the carotid cave into the suprasellar space below the optic chiasm (suprasellar variant). Dorsal OphSeg aneurysms *(hatched area 3, A* to *C)* are rare, often pure hemodynamic lesions, which arise from the dorsal ICA surface well distal to the OphArt origin and overlying ON. *D* to *F,* Notice the aneurysm origin just distal to OphArt origin, closing carotid siphon, and remaining ipsilateral, tethered from further medial growth by the superomedially optic nerve displacement. *G* to *I,* Notice the giant aneurysm projecting medially into suprasellar space with chiasm distortion. ACP, anterior clinoid process; AN, aneurysm; COM, carotid-oculomotor membrane; ON, optic nerve; Pit, pituitary gland.

means depending on the patient's risk factors and the experience of the treatment team. With a firm understanding of paraclinoid anatomy, proper skull base exposure, and strict adherence to general aneurysm surgical principles, direct operative obliteration of nearly all OphSeg and ClinSeg aneurysms can be accomplished with low rates of cranial nerve and brain morbidity.

Some small, unruptured lesions (e.g., parasellar SupHypArt aneurysms) appear to have a very low risk of rupture and are often treated conservatively, particularly in older patients with higher surgical risks. Alternative therapeutic modalities include indirect surgical treatment and endovascular techniques. Indirect surgery seeks to proximally ligate or trap the aneurysm with or without a superficial temporal artery–middle cerebral artery anastomosis or interposition saphenous vein graft,[31] whereas endovascular methods use detachable balloons or coils to selectively obliterate the aneurysm or proximally occlude the ICA (sometimes in conjunction with a blood flow augmentation procedure).[30, 48]

DIRECT OPERATIVE TECHNIQUES

Preoperative Preparation

Preoperative management of patients harboring paraclinoid aneurysms is similar to that for patients with aneurysms at other sites. Patients presenting with epistaxis or subarachnoid hemorrhage are admitted to the intensive care unit and treated on an urgent basis. Patients with unruptured aneurysms are evaluated and treated electively unless there is a rapid progression of compressive symptoms. The preoperative neurologic assessment should place special emphasis on the extraocular movements, facial sensation, visual field and visual acuity, and endocrine status. The most appropriate method of treatment is selected after the patient is stabilized and the radiographic workup is complete, which may include a preoperative trial balloon occlusion test.

Anesthesia And Neurophysiologic Monitoring

Prophylactic antibiotics, intravenous steroids, mild hypothermia, an indwelling radial arterial line for blood pressure monitoring, and continuous evoked potential and electroencephalographic (EEG) monitoring are routinely used during surgery for these types of aneurysms. Brain relaxation is achieved by modest $PaCO_2$ reduction, wide sylvian fissure splitting, and in cases of ruptured aneurysms, intravenous mannitol administered 20 minutes before dural opening. When temporary regional circulatory arrest is employed, mild hypertension is induced and intravenous barbiturates are titrated to EEG burst suppression.

Patient Positioning

The patient is placed on the operating table in the supine position with a shoulder roll underneath the ipsilateral shoulder. The head is fixed in a radiolucent rigid fixation system (allowing for intraoperative angiography if needed), turned 45 degrees toward the contralateral side, and elevated above the heart (promoting venous drainage). The vertex is lowered so that the maxilla is the highest bony landmark, allowing gravity to gently retract the frontal and temporal lobes.

Initial Exposure

CERVICAL INTERNAL CAROTID ARTERY EXPOSURE

The ipsilateral neck is prepared and draped into the sterile field, allowing access to the carotid bifurcation for proximal ICA control, retrograde suction decompression, or saphenous vein bypass grafting as needed. Proximal control is obtained at the cervical ICA before craniotomy for all giant or complicated aneurysms and for ruptured ClinSeg lesions.

SCALP FLAP AND CRANIOTOMY

The scalp incision extends behind the hairline from midline to zygoma, carefully sparing the superficial temporal artery that may later be needed as a bypass conduit (Fig. 111–7). A Yasargil-type interfascial temporalis dissection is performed, allowing low basal frontal exposure, and a frontotemporal bone flap is constructed with at least 2 cm of frontal fossa floor exposed.[20] The lesser wing of the sphenoid bone is then extensively removed extradurally, allowing excellent exposure and removal of the posterior orbital roof, orbital lateral wall, and greater wing of the sphenoid bone to further decompress the SOF.

ANTERIOR CLINOID PROCESS REMOVAL

Removal of the ACP and optic strut is essential for safe surgical obliteration of CavSeg, ClinSeg, and most OphSeg aneurysms. Anterolateral variant ClinSeg aneurysms have an intimate association with the ACP and are often adherent to or erode through this bony landmark, a relationship that makes extradural removal of the ACP hazardous. OphSeg aneurysms can usually be safely exposed through an extradural anterior clinoid removal, particularly when unruptured. We generally advocate an intradural clinoid removal for all ClinSeg lesions and for OphSeg lesions that are large, complex, or ruptured.

When the ACP is to be removed extradurally, the posterior half of the roof and lateral wall of the orbit and the sphenoid ridge covering the SOF are resected until the orbital portion of the optic nerve is clearly identified. The ACP is then internally hollowed out with a high-speed diamond drill, and the remaining thin remnants are carefully removed with small rongeurs. Bleeding is easily controlled with bone wax and Gelfoam (Pharmacia & Upjohn, Peapack, NJ).

When the ACP is removed intradurally, the orbital roof and ridge are similarly resected extradurally, but the ACP is left in place. After the dural is opened, the sylvian fissure is split widely from lateral to medial aspects, gaining exposure to the middle cerebral and internal carotid arteries down to the ACP. A 3- to 4-cm-long dural incision is made from the ACP tip to well beyond the resected edge of the medial sphenoid ridge. An additional relaxing incision is made through the falciform ligament to decompress the optic nerve. The ACP and optic canal roof and lateral wall are thinned with a high-speed diamond drill, and the remaining bony shell is carefully removed with small rongeurs. The optic strut is drilled down to expose the anterior border of the ClinSeg. Dorsal wall carotid aneurysms usually do not require ACP removal for effective clipping.

Temporary Circulatory Arrest

Complex or giant paraclinoid aneurysms often require methods designed to decompress the internal aneurysm pressure, enabling the surgeon to clearly identify all aspects of the aneurysm neck and nearby perforators for safe and accurate clip application. A clamp is placed across the cervical ICA to relax the aneurysm enough to allow clipping without trapping in many cases. For OphSeg aneurysms, a proximal temporary

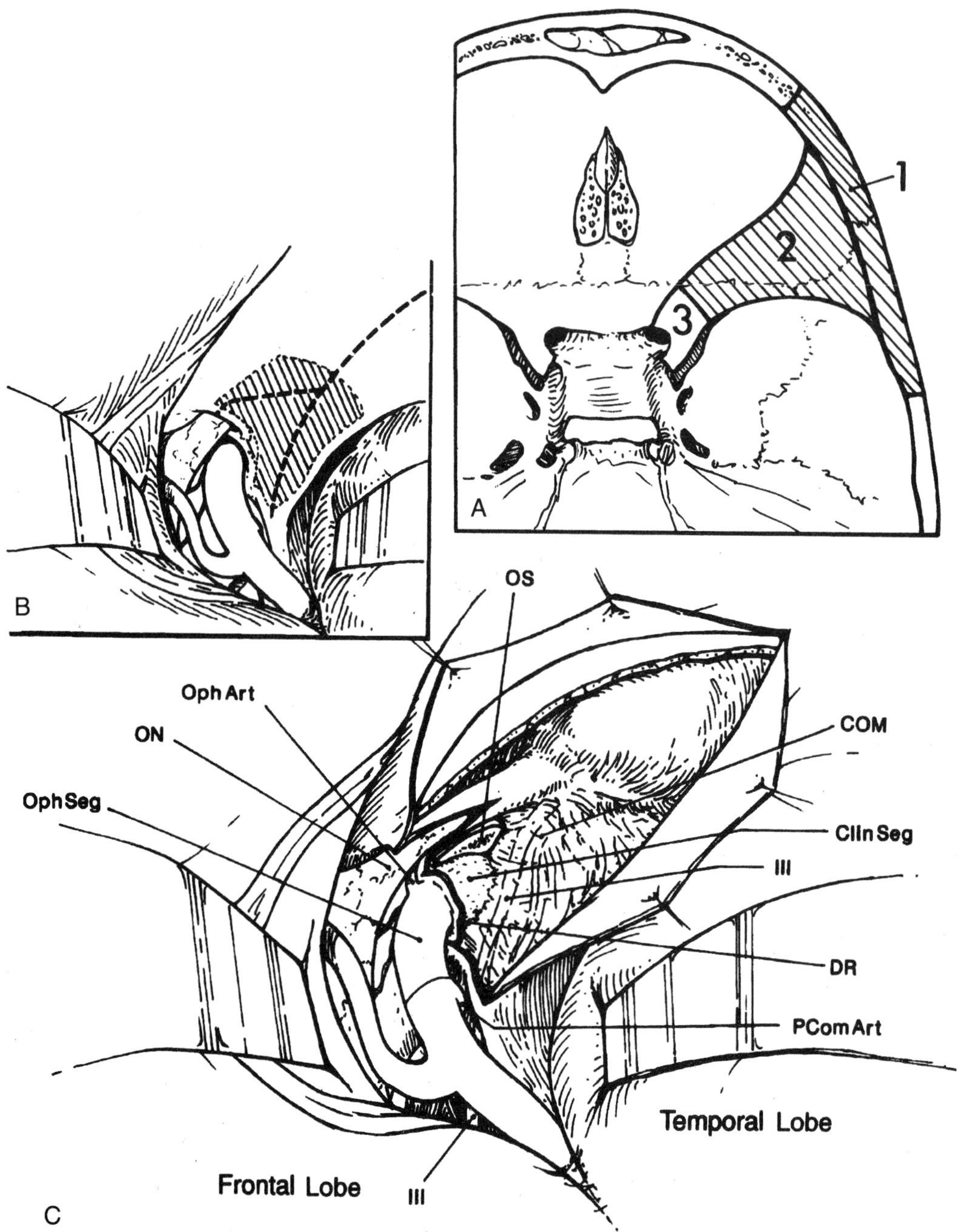

FIGURE 111–7. Bony resection for paraclinoid aneurysm surgery (schematic). *A,* Extradural bone removal includes a frontotemporal craniotomy *(hatched area 1)* and resection of the sphenoid ridge, posterior orbital roof, and medial floor of the superior orbital fissure *(hatched area 2).* Intradural bone removal includes resection of the remaining medial sphenoid wing and the anterior clinoid process (ACP) and optic strut (OS) *(area 3). B,* The *dashed lines* represent the dural incisions used during intradural anterior clinoidectomy. The *hatched area* represents the residual ACP prior to dural incision. The incision is extended to include the falciform ligament; the optic nerve (ON) sheath can be opened laterally as needed to decompress and mobilize the ON. *C,* Final exposure after intradural ACP removal and drilling of the OS. Aneurysms arising from the clinoidal segment (ClinSeg) and ophthalmic segment (OphSeg) of the internal carotid artery (ICA) are easily accessed through this approach. Opening through the carotid-oculomotor membrane (COM) allows superior entry into the cavernous sinus and access to the anterior genu and horizontal segment of the cavernous ICA. DR, dural ring; OphArt, ophthalmic artery; PComArt, posterior communicating artery.

clip can be alternatively placed on the exposed ClinSeg, obviating the need for cervical exposure.

When trapping is required, temporary clips may also be placed across the ICA just proximal to the posterior communicating artery and on the ophthalmic artery. To promote further aneurysm collapse, retrograde suction decompression techniques[49–53] or direct aneurysm puncture can be added. All temporary clipping or trapping procedures, whether surgical or endovascular, are performed under barbiturate-induced EEG suppression and mild hypertension. Cardiac standstill and global circulatory arrest techniques are rarely required for lesions in this location.

Aneurysm Dissection and Clipping

INTRACAVERNOUS SEGMENT ANEURYSMS

Although lateral entry into the cavernous sinus through Parkinson's triangle allows the widest access to the CavSeg, we favor superior entry into the sinus through the anteromedial triangle. This approach allows excellent access to aneurysms arising from the anterior genu, which are generally the best intracavernous lesions for direct surgery. In contrast, we generally favor endovascular or indirect surgical treatment for more proximal CavSeg lesions, because cranial nerve morbidity after direct obliteration is often unacceptably high.

To access the CavSeg through the anteromedial triangle, the ACP is removed, and the dural ring is circumferentially sectioned. An incision through the COM between the ClinSeg and the oculomotor nerve is extended posterolaterally along the medial aspect of the third nerve in the direction of the posterior clinoid. Lateral retraction of the lateral sinus wall provides excellent exposure to the anterior and lateral surfaces of the anterior genu and the superior and lateral surface of the horizontal segment. With posterolateral retraction of the ICA, the medial surface of the anterior bend is also well visualized. Gentle packing with Gelfoam and Surgicel (Johnson & Johnson, Arlington, TX) easily controls venous bleeding. After hemostasis and adequate exposure are obtained, appropriate aneurysm clip application ensues.

CLINOIDAL SEGMENT ANEURYSMS

Because these aneurysms can burrow into the ACP and adhere to the adjacent dura and cavernous sinus, the decision about whether to gain proximal control in the cervical region is made early in the dissection. Great care is taken to extensively remove the ACP and optic strut, followed by circumferential sectioning of the dural ring to allow complete mobilization of the ICA and viewing of the entire ClinSeg (Fig. 111–8). Sectioning the ring also allows unimpeded clip blade passage from the OphSeg to the COM, thereby spanning the entire ClinSeg. Using these preparations, most premature aneurysm ruptures can be avoided. The anterolateral variant lies on the anterolateral surface of the ClinSeg. To eliminate the proximal neck, the clip blades must be passed proximal to the COM, most frequently using a gently curved or side-angled clip that runs parallel to the ICA. Opening the COM and gentle packing of the cavernous sinus lumen with Gelfoam or Surgicel achieve the desired meticulous hemostasis and gently displace the cranial nerves away from the plane of the advancing clip blade. The medial variant projects beneath the diaphragma sella into the pituitary fossa. Circumferential section of the dural ring allows placement of a fenestrated clip whose blades run parallel to the curvature of the ClinSeg medial wall. Care must be taken to spare the ophthalmic and any superior hypophyseal or other perforating vessels that arise from the ClinSeg or OphSeg.

OPHTHALMIC SEGMENT ANEURYSMS

For OphArt aneurysms, the falciform ligament is sectioned and the cut extended along the lateral aspect of the optic nerve to allow exposure to the junction of the proximal neck and OphArt (Fig. 111–9). The distal neck is usually easily identified and is typically free of perforators. A gently curved or side-angled clip directed parallel to the plane of the ICA, sparing the OphArt, obliterates most lesions. Dorsal carotid wall aneurysms are clipped in a similar fashion, with easier identification of the proximal neck.

For SupHypArt aneurysms, the most difficult part of the dissection is inferior and medial, where the burrowing nature of the aneurysm has adhered the aneurysm wall to the parasellar dura. ICA mobilization through circumferential sectioning of the dural ring typically allows separation of the two structures and identification of the perforators supplying the optic apparatus and hypophysis. One or more right-angled and fenestrated clips with blades parallel to and encircling the ICA can then reconstruct the ICA lumen, sparing the SupHypArt perforators. The posterior communicating artery and other ICA perforator vessels must also be identified and preserved.

GIANT AND COMPLEX ANEURYSMS

Paraclinoid aneurysms are frequently giant, and specific techniques must often be used to ensure safe and complete surgical obliteration. Proximal ligation or trapping of the arterial segment harboring the giant lesion is accomplished under barbiturate-induced EEG burst suppression and mild hypertension. Further aneurysm collapse may be achieved through retrograde suction decompression as needed. The lesion is then opened, allowing removal of intraluminal thrombus and partial resection of the often-calcified aneurysm wall. The ICA lumen is then reconstructed using one or more clips appropriate to the type of paraclinoid lesion being addressed, being sure to eliminate all debris and air from the parent vessel before flow restoration.

Many large or giant paraclinoid aneurysms are complicated by significant atherosclerotic plaque within the aneurysm wall or neck that can cause an initial aneurysm clip to migrate downward and partially occlude the vessel lumen or prevent complete occlusion of the

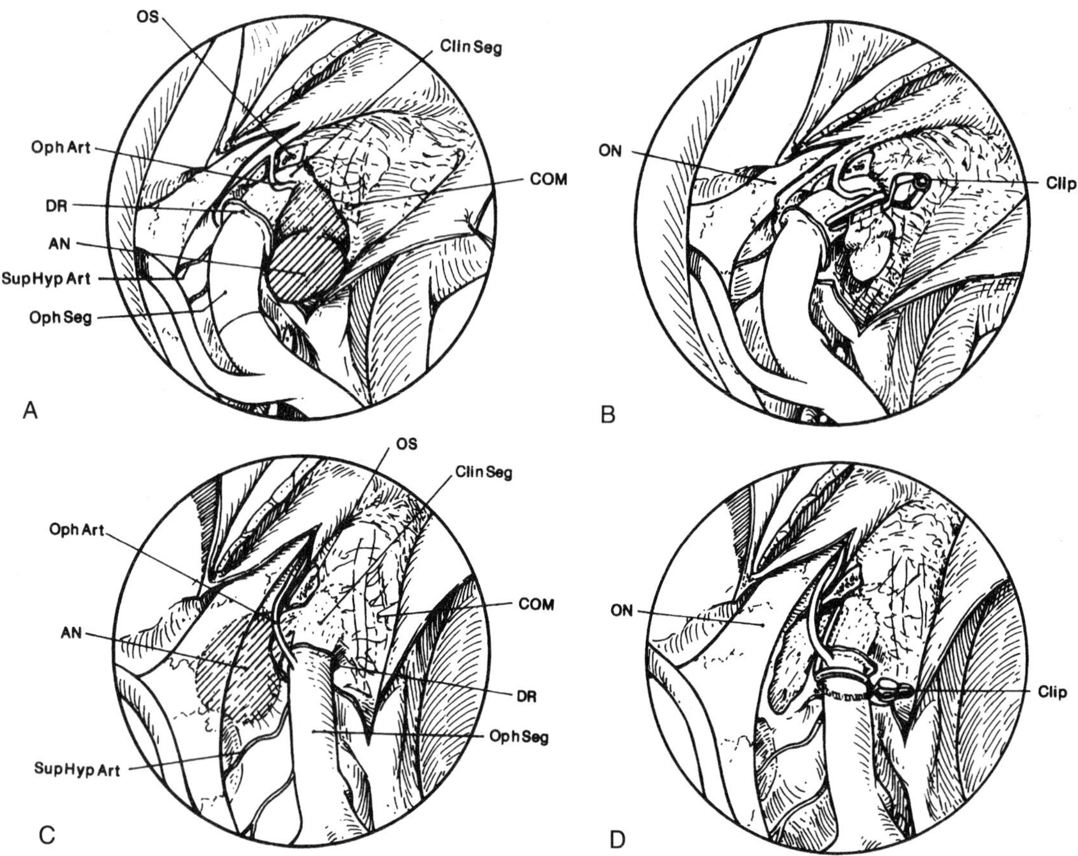

FIGURE 111–8. Operative view of clinoidal segment (ClinSeg) aneurysms: anterolateral and medial variants (schematic). The ipsilateral neck is prepared and draped into the sterile field in all cases. Proximal control at the cervical internal carotid artery (ICA) is obtained before craniotomy for all giant, complicated, or ruptured ClinSeg aneurysms. *A* and *B*, Exposure and clipping of anterolateral variant aneurysm. After frontotemporal craniotomy and extradural removal of the sphenoid ridge, the anterior clinoid process (ACP) and optic strut (OS) are extensively removed intradurally to expose the ClinSeg. Notice the constriction of the aneurysm, where it has eroded through the dura and entered the subarachnoid space. The anterolateral variant is generally best obliterated using a gently curved clip placed along the long axis of the ICA, paralleling the curve of the clinoidal ICA. *C* and *D*, Exposure and clipping of a medial variant aneurysm. Notice that the medial variant projects beneath the diaphragma sella into the pituitary fossa. Medial variant aneurysms usually require a fenestrated clip placed parallel to the ICA with the tips abutting or extending past the carotid-oculomotor membrane (COM). In each case, the ophthalmic and superior hypophyseal arteries must be carefully spared. AN, aneurysm; DR, dural ring; OphArt, ophthalmic artery; OphSeg, ophthalmic segment; SupHypArt, superior hypophyseal artery.

aneurysm neck altogether. Sequential application and fastidious readjustment of aneurysm clips can often remedy both scenarios. If the ICA lumen is compromised, two additional clips are placed distal to the original clip, which then allows removal of the original proximal clip and restores parent artery patency. If atherosclerotic plaque prevents complete aneurysm neck obliteration, a booster clip can promote aneurysm neck occlusion through affixing additive closing pressure. A fenestrated clip can also facilitate aneurysm neck collapse by encircling the atheroma.

Closure

After apparently successful aneurysm clipping, it may be difficult to determine ICA patency with certainty through direct inspection alone. An intraoperative angiogram through direct common carotid artery puncture (if the cervical carotid is already exposed) or through a preoperatively placed transfemoral catheter is invaluable in these circumstances. After ICA patency is ensured, dural closure begins. First, any communication between the optic strut and the sphenoid sinus is identified and sealed with muscle, Gelfoam, and methylmethacrylate. The dural leaves covering the medial sphenoid wing are then closed primarily, followed by a watertight closure of the more superficial dural opening. The bone flap is returned and secured, the temporalis muscle reapproximated, a subgaleal drain placed, and the skin closed.

Postoperative Care

The postoperative care for patients with paraclinoid aneurysms is similar to that provided to patients with aneurysms in general. If the aneurysm was unrup-

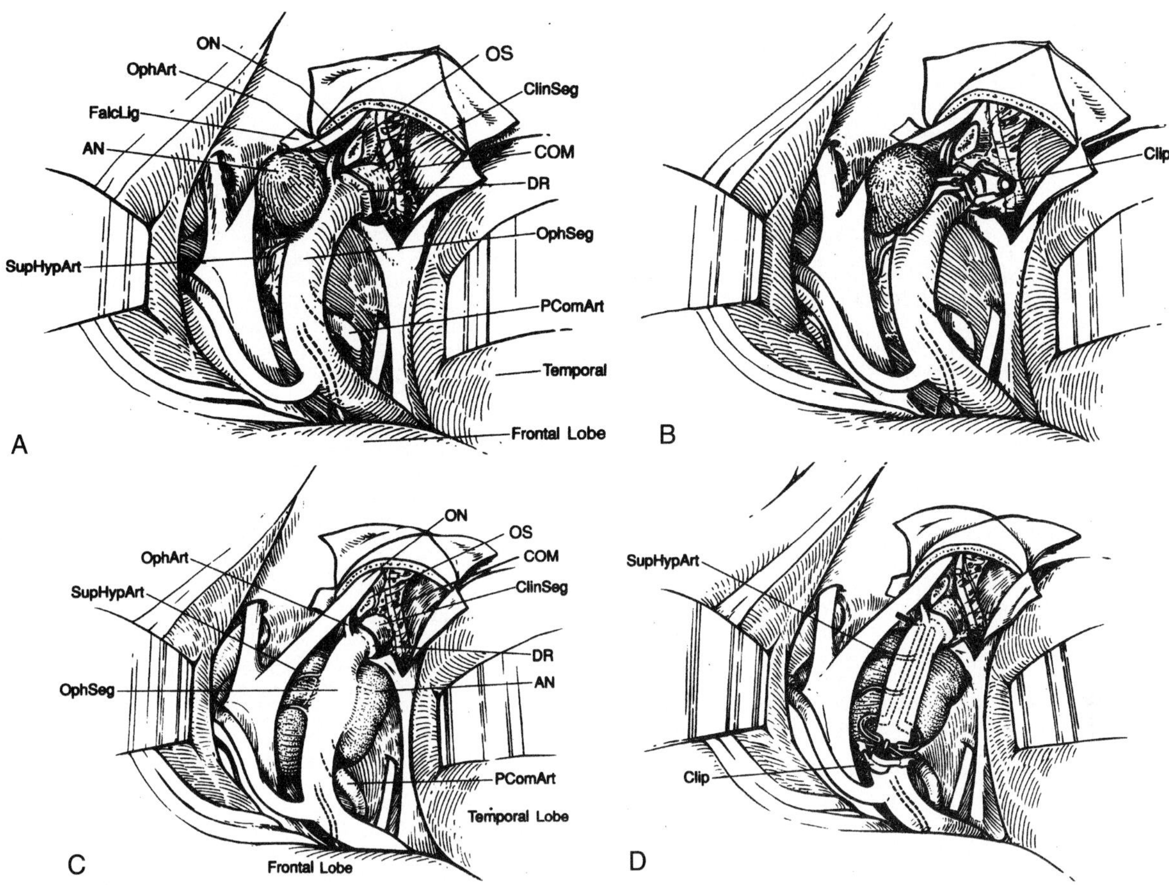

FIGURE 111–9. Operative view of ophthalmic segment (OphSeg) aneurysms (schematic). The ipsilateral neck is prepared and draped into the sterile field in all cases, and proximal control at the cervical internal carotid artery (ICA) is obtained before craniotomy for giant or complicated ophthalmic artery (OphArt) and superior hypophyseal artery (SupHypArt) aneurysms. Proximal control for the more distally located dorsal variant OphSeg aneurysms (not pictured) is typically accomplished intracranially. *A* and *B,* Exposure and clipping of an OphArt aneurysm. After frontotemporal craniotomy and extradural sphenoid ridge removal, the anterior clinoid process (ACP) is extensively removed, providing excellent visualization of the clinoidal segment (ClinSeg) and proximal OphSeg. The deep blade of a side-angled or curved clip is placed into the interval between the OphArt and the aneurysm and is then rotated medial to the aneurysm, ending in a plane closely parallel to the long axis of the ICA. *C* and *D,* Exposure and clipping of a SupHypArt aneurysm. The skull base is exposed, similar to that obtained for the OphArt aneurysm. For SupHypArt aneurysm clipping, a fenestrated clip is placed parallel to the ICA to reconstruct the carotid lumen. The SupHypArt must be visualized and spared. Notice that the dural ring (DR) has been circumferentially sectioned, allowing access of the clip blades to the ClinSeg. The butt of the clip must spare the posterior communicating artery (PComArt). AN, aneurysm; COM, carotid-oculomotor membrane; FalcLig, falciform ligament; ON, optic nerve; OS, optic strut; III, oculomotor nerve.

tured, the patient generally has a 1-day intensive care unit stay, followed by early mobilization and normalization of diet and medications. If the aneurysm was ruptured, standard protocols for management of subarachnoid hemorrhage include aggressive hydration and monitoring for vasospasm during the window of risk.

Potential Operative Complications and Their Management

The complications specific to paraclinoid aneurysm surgery generally revolve around the anatomic structures present within the region: the ICA, arterial perforators, and neighboring cranial nerves. Even though intraoperative angiography may demonstrate initial ICA patency, delayed stenosis or thrombosis can still occur. Any evidence of hemibody neurologic deficits should be emergently addressed with CT and angiography, with a return trip to the operating room for emergent re-exploration and clip adjustment strongly considered.

Visual deterioration after paraclinoid aneurysm surgery is usually attributable to excessive optic nerve manipulation or arterial perforator compromise during aneurysm exposure. Re-exploration and clip adjustment should be entertained if intraoperative events do not adequately explain any postoperative visual deficit. Oculomotor, trochlear, and abducens palsies, as well as ptosis and miosis resulting from sympathetic fiber disruption, are generally the result of surgical trauma during anterior clinoidectomy, clip blade advancement, cranial nerve manipulation, or cavernous sinus packing. These deficits are usually partial and transient in nature, and they are best avoided through careful dissection and retraction of these nerves.

REFERENCES

1. Cawley CM, Zipfel GJ, Day AL: Surgical treatment of paraclinoid and ophthalmic aneurysms. Neurosurg Clin N Am 9:765–783, 1998.
2. Day AL: Aneurysms of the ophthalmic segment. A clinical and anatomical analysis. J Neurosurg 72:677–691, 1990.
3. Day AL: Clinicoanatomic features of supraclinoid aneurysms. Clin Neurosurg 36:256–274, 1990.
4. Inoue T, Rhoton AL Jr, Theele D, et al: Surgical approaches to the cavernous sinus: A microsurgical study. Neurosurgery 26: 903–932, 1990.
5. Dolenc VV: A combined epi- and subdural direct approach to carotid-ophthalmic artery aneurysms. J Neurosurg 62:667–672, 1985.
6. Knosp E, Muller G, Perneczky A: The paraclinoid carotid artery: Anatomical aspects of a microneurosurgical approach. Neurosurgery 22:896–901, 1988.
7. Kobayashi S, Kyoshima K, Gibo H, et al: Carotid cave aneurysms of the internal carotid artery. J Neurosurg 70:216–221, 1989.
8. Nutik SL: Removal of the anterior clinoid process for exposure of the proximal intracranial carotid artery. J Neurosurg 69:529–534, 1988.
9. Perneczky A, Knosp E, Vorkapic P, et al: Direct surgical approach to infraclinoidal aneurysms. Acta Neurochir (Wien) 76:36–44, 1985.
10. Nutik SL: Ventral paraclinoid carotid aneurysms. J Neurosurg 69:340–344, 1988.
11. Gibo H, Lenkey C, Rhoton AL Jr: Microsurgical anatomy of the supraclinoid portion of the internal carotid artery. J Neurosurg 55:560–574, 1981.
12. Harris FS, Rhoton AL Jr: Anatomy of the cavernous sinus. A microsurgical study. J Neurosurg 45:169–180, 1976.
13. Rhoton AL Jr: Anatomy of saccular aneurysms. Surg Neurol 14: 59–66, 1980.
14. Hayreh S: The ophthalmic artery. In Newton TH, Potts DG, (eds): Radiology of the Skull and Brain. St. Louis, CV Mosby, 1974, pp 1333–50.
15. Nishio S, Matsushima T, Fukui M, et al: Microsurgical anatomy around the origin of the ophthalmic artery with reference to contralateral pterional surgical approach to the carotid-ophthalmic aneurysm. Acta Neurochir (Wien) 76:82–89, 1985.
16. Dawson BH: The blood vessels of the human optic chiasma and their relation to those of hypophysis and hypothalamus. Brain 81:207–217, 1958.
17. Gibo H, Kobayashi S, Kyoshima K, et al: Microsurgical anatomy of the arteries of the pituitary stalk and gland as viewed from above. Acta Neurochir (Wien) 90:60–66, 1988.
18. Kyoshima K, Oikawa S, Kobayashi S: Interdural origin of the ophthalmic artery at the dural ring of the internal carotid artery. Report of two cases. J Neurosurg 92:488–489, 2000.
19. Kupersmith MJ, Hurst R, Berenstein A, et al: The benign course of cavernous carotid artery aneurysms. J Neurosurg 77:690–693, 1992.
20. Yasargil MG, Gasser JC, Hodosh RM, et al: Carotid-ophthalmic aneurysms: Direct microsurgical approach. Surg Neurol 8:155–165, 1977.
21. Linskey ME, Sekhar LN, Hirsch WL Jr, et al: Aneurysms of the intracavernous carotid artery: Natural history and indications for treatment. Neurosurgery 26:933–937, discussion 937–938, 1990.
22. Al-Rhodan N, Piepgras DG: Aneurysms within the Cavernous Sinus and Transitional Cavernous Aneurysms. In Wilkins RH, Rengachary SS (eds): Neurosurgery, 2nd ed. New York, McGraw-Hill, 1996, pp 2283–2289.
23. Al-Rodhan NR, Piepgras DG, Sundt TM Jr: Transitional cavernous aneurysms of the internal carotid artery. Neurosurgery 33: 993–996, 1993.
24. Ochi T, Shimizu K, Yasuhara Y, et al: Curved planar reformatted CT angiography: Usefulness for the evaluation of aneurysms at the carotid siphon. AJNR Am J Neuroradiol 20:1025–1030, 1999; see comments.
25. Teasdale E: Curved planar reformatted CT angiography: Utility for the evaluation of aneurysms at the carotid siphon. AJNR Am J Neuroradiol 21:985, 2000.
26. Nagasawa S, Deguchi J, Arai M, et al: Topographic anatomy of paraclinoid carotid artery aneurysms: Usefulness of MR angiographic source images. Neuroradiology 39:341–343, 1997.
27. Inagawa T: Follow-up study of unruptured aneurysms arising from the C3 and C4 segments of the internal carotid artery. Surg Neurol 36:99–105, 1991.
28. Locksley HB: Natural history of subarachnoid hemorrhage, intracranial aneurysms and arteriovenous malformations. J Neurosurg 25:321–368, 1966.
29. Barr HW, Blackwood W, Meadows SP: Intracavernous carotid aneurysms. A clinical-pathological report. Brain 94:607–622, 1971.
30. Masana Y, Taneda M: Direct approach to a traumatic giant internal carotid artery aneurysm associated with a carotid-cavernous fistula: Case report. J Neurosurg 76:524–527, 1992.
31. Reddy SV, Sundt TM Jr: Giant traumatic false aneurysm of the internal carotid artery associated with a carotid-cavernous fistula: Case report. J Neurosurg 55:813–818, 1981.
32. Ding MX: Traumatic aneurysm of the intracavernous part of the internal carotid artery presenting with epistaxis: Case report. Surg Neurol 30:65–67, 1988.
33. Sudhoff H, Stark T, Knorz S, et al: Massive epistaxis after rupture of intracavernous carotid artery aneurysm: Case report. Ann Otol Rhinol Laryngol 109:776–778, 2000.
34. Teitelbaum GP, Halbach VV, Larsen DW, et al: Treatment of massive posterior epistaxis by detachable coil embolization of a cavernous internal carotid artery aneurysm. Neuroradiology 37: 334–336, 1995.
35. Yang X, Saari T, Kansanen M, et al: Epistaxis from nontraumatic intracavernous carotid aneurysm: Endovascular treatment with detachable coils and electrothrombosis. Am J Otolaryngol 16: 255–259, 1995.
36. Diaz FG, Ohaegbulam S, Dujovny M, et al: Surgical alternatives in the treatment of cavernous sinus aneurysms. J Neurosurg 71: 846–853, 1989.
37. White JA, Horowitz MB, Samson D: Dural waisting as a sign of subarachnoid extension of cavernous carotid aneurysms: A follow-up case report. Surg Neurol 52:607–609, discussion 609–610, 1999.
38. Arnautovic KI, Al-Mefty O, Angtuaco E: A combined microsurgical skull-base and endovascular approach to giant and large paraclinoid aneurysms. Surg Neurol 50:504–518, discussion 518–520, 1998.
39. Bavinzski G, Killer M, Ferraz-Leite H, et al: Endovascular therapy of idiopathic cavernous aneurysms over 11 years. AJNR Am J Neuroradiol 19:559–565, 1998.
40. Halbach VV, Higashida RT, Dowd CF, et al: Cavernous internal carotid artery aneurysms treated with electrolytically detachable coils. J Neuroophthalmol 17:231–239, 1997.
41. Higashida RT, Halbach VV, Dowd C, et al: Endovascular detachable balloon embolization therapy of cavernous carotid artery aneurysms: Results in 87 cases. J Neurosurg 72:857–863, 1990.
42. Larson JJ, Tew JM Jr, Tomsick TA, et al: Treatment of aneurysms of the internal carotid artery by intravascular balloon occlusion: Long-term follow-up of 58 patients. Neurosurgery 36:26–30, discussion, 30, 1995.
43. Roy D, Raymond J, Bouthillier A, et al: Endovascular treatment of ophthalmic segment aneurysms with Guglielmi detachable coils. AJNR Am J Neuroradiol 18:1207–1215, 1997.
44. Batjer HH, Kopitnik TA, Giller CA, et al: Surgery for paraclinoidal carotid artery aneurysms. J Neurosurg 80:650–658, 1994.
45. Drake CG, Vanderlinden RG, Amacher AL: Carotid-ophthalmic aneurysms. J Neurosurg 29:24–31, 1968.
46. Nutik SL: Carotid cave aneurysms. J Neurosurg 71:302–303, 1989.
47. Miyazawa N, Nukui H, Mitsuka S, et al: Treatment of intradural paraclinoidal aneurysms. Neurol Med Chir (Tokyo) 39:727–732, discussion 732–724, 1999.
48. Liu MY, Shih CJ, Wang YC, et al: Traumatic intracavernous carotid aneurysm with massive epistaxis. Neurosurgery 17:569–573, 1985.

49. Batjer HH, Samson DS: Retrograde suction decompression of giant paraclinoidal aneurysms: Technical note. J Neurosurg 73: 305–306, 1990.
50. Fahlbusch R, Nimsky C, Huk W: Open surgery of giant paraclinoid aneurysms improved by intraoperative angiography and endovascular retrograde suction decompression. Acta Neurochir 139:1026–1032, 1997.
51. Fan YW, Chan KH, Lui WM, et al: Retrograde suction decompression of paraclinoid aneurysm—a revised technique. Surg Neurol 51:129–131, 1999.
52. Mizoi K, Yoshimoto T, Takahashi A: Direct clipping of paraclinoid large aneurysms using retrograde balloon suction decompression. No Shinkei Geka 21:981–989, 1993.
53. Scott JA, Horner TG, Leipzig TJ: Retrograde suction decompression of an ophthalmic artery aneurysm using balloon occlusion: Technical note. J Neurosurg 75:146–147, 1991.

CHAPTER 112

Intracranial Internal Carotid Artery Aneurysms

MAHMOUD AL-YAMANY ■ M. CHRISTOPHER WALLACE

Saccular aneurysms of the internal carotid artery (ICA) trunk represent approximately 30% to 50% of all intracranial aneurysms.[1-4] Although these aneurysms are usually considered easier to approach surgically than posterior circulation lesions, they may have a complex anatomy and relationship to surrounding neurovascular structures in the subarachnoid space. Therefore, an intimate understanding of the aneurysm's relationship to these structures is necessary and can be achieved by careful assessment with preoperative diagnostic imaging. In this chapter we discuss aneurysms arising from the ICA trunk, posterior communicating artery, anterior choroidal artery, and carotid artery bifurcation. Their specific anatomic characteristics, current diagnostic evaluation methods, general management, and surgical techniques, including complications and outcome, are reviewed.

DIAGNOSTIC EVALUATION

Computed tomography (CT) of the brain following subarachnoid hemorrhage (SAH) is the investigation of choice to detect blood in the subarachnoid space. It is capable of detecting subarachnoid blood in up to 92% of cases.[1] It also provides clues about the possible location of the aneurysm, which may be helpful in determining which aneurysm has ruptured in a patient with multiple intracranial aneurysms. It may also aid in recognizing nonaneurysmal SAH. Magnetic resonance angiography and CT–angiography have proved to be reliable in detecting small aneurysms less than 5 mm.[5, 6]

Conventional transfemoral cerebral angiography remains the standard in planning the management of these aneurysms. It is superior to any other diagnostic modality in determining certain characteristics of the aneurysm, such as its neck width and size, and in detecting intra-aneurysmal calcification and atherosclerotic changes in the parent vessel. It helps assess the possibility of sacrificing the posterior communicating artery during clipping of the aneurysm, which is extremely dangerous in patients with a fetal origin of the artery. It demonstrates some of the perforating arteries in and around the aneurysm and the parent vessel. It also accurately determines the aneurysm's relation to the bony structures intracranially. The surgeon's confidence in the diagnosis and orientation of the projection of the angiographic pictures is extremely important in deciding how to position the patient on the operating table and in determining the need for additional bone removal. We recommend performing four-vessel cerebral angiography before deciding on treatment. We do not rely on magnetic resonance angiography or CT–angiography for operative planning or management strategies for aneurysms greater than 4 mm in diameter. However, at many institutions, CT–angiography is used to accurately delineate aneurysm geometry and anatomy.

PREOPERATIVE MANAGEMENT

Based on the presentation of the patient, preoperative preparations vary. In patients with SAH, after ensuring adequate breathing, the patient is assessed neurologically to determine the SAH clinical grade using either the Hunt and Hess or the World Federation of Neurological Surgeons grading system (Table 112–1). The four major issues to be addressed before planning a strategy to obliterate the aneurysm are rebleeding, vasospasm, hydrocephalus, and electrolyte abnormalities.

The rebleeding rate can be as high as 6% in the first 48 hours and may be associated with devastating results. Vasospasm peaks at days 3 through 14 and kills or severely disables about 14% of patients.[1] Hydrocephalus may occur as early as a few hours after the hemorrhage. In a patient with a poor-grade SAH or one who has deteriorated, an external ventricular drain may improve the clinical status. Therefore, it is important to closely observe these patients in the intensive care unit and, if necessary, perform serial computed tomographic scans.

Serum electrolyte disturbances are also seen following SAH and must be corrected before any management plans are made. It has been our practice to oper-

TABLE 112–1 ■ **Clinical Grading Systems for Patients with Subarachnoid Hemorrhage**

GRADE	HUNT AND HESS	WORLD FEDERATION OF NEUROLOGICAL SURGEONS	
		Glasgow Coma Score	Motor Deficit
1	No symptoms or minimal headache and slight nuchal rigidity	15	No
2	Moderate to severe headache, no neurological deficit other than cranial nerve palsy	13–14	No
3	Drowsiness, confusion, or mild focal deficit	13–14	Yes
4	Stupor, moderate to severe hemiparesis, possible early decerebrate rigidity and vegetative disturbances	7–12	Yes or no
5	Deep coma, decerebrate rigidity, moribund	3–6	Yes or no

ate on favorable-grade aneurysms within the first 24 to 48 hours after the SAH. Poor-grade patients are allowed to recover in the intensive care unit with optimization of their electrolytes and volume status. If they demonstrate an improvement in clinical grade, surgery is considered. Calcium channel blockers, specifically, nimodipine administered orally in a dose of 60 mg every 4 hours, are used, and patients are kept euvolemic to slightly hypervolemic if their cardiac status permits. This approach allows us to treat patients with hypervolemia both preoperatively and postoperatively without increasing the risk of rehemorrhage. It also allows us to use balloon angioplasty and institute hypertensive and hemodilution therapy in patients who show clinical signs of cerebral vasospasm. Hypertension is controlled with the use of beta-blockers or calcium channel blockers, especially preoperatively, and blood pressure is allowed to rise slightly postoperatively. We do not use steroids in the perioperative management of patients with SAH unless they were taking these drugs for other reasons, in which case we replace them with a stress dose of hydrocortisone 100 mg twice daily. Anticonvulsants are used in patients who develop seizures following SAH and in high-grade patients who have normal serum electrolytes and no evidence of hydrocephalus on CT. Broad-spectrum antibiotics are given 1 hour before the operation to reduce the risk of wound infection.

Patients with unruptured aneurysms are admitted on the same day of surgery after a preoperative assessment by the neurosurgeon and the neuroanesthesiologist. Patients are discharged from the hospital within 3 to 4 days after a postoperative angiogram if there are no complications.

INTRAOPERATIVE AIDS

To maximize exposure of subarachnoid vessels with limited brain retraction, we use 20% mannitol 0.5 g/kg body weight, infused shortly before the skin incision. The partial pressure of carbon dioxide ($Paco_2$) is allowed to drift down to approximately 30 mm Hg. Lumbar cerebrospinal fluid (CSF) drains are rarely used. A microscope should be used in every case. Intraoperative somatosensory evoked potentials or electroencephalograms can be useful adjuncts if the surgeon decides to clip the aneurysm under local flow arrest. Dexamethasone is used preoperatively by some neurosurgeons, although we have not found it beneficial in relaxing or protecting the brain during surgery.

POSTOPERATIVE CARE

The major postoperative concerns in patients with SAH from ruptured aneurysms are vasospasm, hydrocephalus, electrolyte imbalance, seizures, brain swelling, and rebleeding from a residual portion of the aneurysm. The patient is kept in the intensive care unit in a hypervolemic state, with central venous pressure kept at 7 to 10 mm H_2O. The blood pressure is allowed to rise to the patient's high normal pressure without the use of ionotropes or vasopressors unless the patient shows clinical evidence of vasospasm. Serum sodium is kept at 135 to 148, and broad-spectrum antibiotics are continued for 2 postoperative days or as long as the patient has an external ventricular drain. Patients with SAH-induced seizures are maintained on phenytoin (Dilantin) postoperatively for 6 months to 1 year. CT of the head is done routinely on the second postoperative day unless the patient deteriorates before that. If symptomatic hydrocephalus is documented, a ventriculoperitoneal shunt is inserted to divert the CSF. Routine cerebral angiography is done on postoperative day 7 to ensure complete obliteration of the aneurysm unless the patient shows clinical evidence of vasospasm, in which case an angiogram is done and balloon angioplasty or intra-arterial papaverine infusion is considered. If clipping is incomplete, surgical as well as endovascular options are discussed to obliterate the aneurysm remnant.

SPECIFIC ANEURYSM SITES

Posterior Communicating Artery

ANATOMY

The communicating segment of the ICA (C7 segment) begins just below the posterior communicating artery and ends at the bifurcation. Two major arterial branches, the posterior communicating artery and the anterior choroidal artery, arise from this segment.[7] In the old classification system, the posterior communicating segment ends at the origin of the anterior choroidal artery. This is a short segment that has two bends. The first is an upward curve above the ophthalmic artery, and the second bend is a continuum of the medial to lateral curve that begins in the clinoidal segment and ends at the bifurcation. The posterior communicating artery arises from the posteromedial surface of the ICA and courses medially and inferiorly, through the membrane of Liliquest above and medial to the oculomotor nerve, to join the posterior cerebral artery at the junction of the P1 and P2 segments. Multiple perforators arising from the posterior communicating artery, the anterior thalamic perforators, are at risk of injury during aneurysm dissection and clipping. In 15% to 22% of people, the P1 segment of the posterior cerebral artery is hypoplastic, and the posterior cerebral artery arises directly from the posterior communicating artery. This is termed a fetal origin of the posterior cerebral artery,[8] and when it is present, the posterior communicating artery cannot be clipped with the aneurysm, and the aneurysm has to be repaired in a way that guarantees the patency of the parent vessel. The typical posterior communicating aneurysm arises just distal to the origin of the artery off the wall of the ICA. It projects posteriorly, laterally, and slightly inferiorly and may pinch the oculomotor nerve as it enters the dural fold of the cavernous sinus. An acute third nerve palsy can occur with an acutely expanding posterior communicating artery aneurysm. It usually does not point medially and thus does not bleed into the sella, because it is pushed out by the curve of the ICA laterally.

PRESENTATION

Aneurysms of this segment of the ICA constitute about 50% of ICA aneurysms[9, 10] and are more common in females. They usually become symptomatic at a size smaller than 10 mm by SAH with a lateral suprasellar and ambient cistern pattern. Intraparenchymal hemorrhage into the uncus of the temporal lobe, intraventricular hemorrhage into the temporal horn, or hemorrhage into the subdural space can also occur. As noted earlier, these aneurysms can expand and compress the third cranial nerve, causing a painful, non–pupil-sparing oculomotor nerve palsy. SAH can also irritate the dura and cause retro-orbital pain (Table 112–2).[10–13]

OPERATIVE TECHNIQUE

Under general anesthesia and endotracheal intubation, the patient is placed in the supine position with the head secured in three- or four-point fixation. The ipsilateral shoulder is raised using a gel roll, and the patient is strapped to the table to allow intraoperative rotation of the operating table. The head is then slightly extended and tilted to the opposite side. The neck is slightly flexed to allow proper venous drainage. This head position allows the brain to fall away from the base of the skull, minimizing brain retraction. A 'C'-shaped, 1 inch–wide line is shaved, and the skin is prepped and draped along that line. The skin incision is made starting at the ipsilateral zygoma and curving forward and medially to the forehead at the midline. The skin flap is reflected forward, leaving the pericranium on the bone. The pericranium is then reflected as a vascularized flap based frontally, and the temporalis fascia is opened with scissors, leaving a cuff of fascia to suture at closure. The muscle is cut using monopolar cautery, and the myocutaneous flap is reflected together to prevent injury to the frontalis branch of the facial nerve and to maintain blood supply to the muscle. The flap is retracted using fishhooks, and the "keyhole" region behind the frontozygomatic junction is exposed.

The large bur of the drill is used to make a bur hole in the keyhole region, and the dura is stripped away from the bone to allow placement of the footplate epidurally. The drill is used to cut the craniotomy. The bone may need to be carefully cracked at the sphenoid ridge, protecting the underlying brain. The dura is then separated from the sphenoid wing medially, and the wing is either drilled or rongeured, keeping in mind that the limiting factor to inferior exposure is the bulk of the temporalis muscle. The frontal inner table is beveled with the drill. If the frontal air sinus is opened, it is exonerated, packed with Gelfoam, and covered with the vascularized pericranial flap and fibrin adhesive at the end of the procedure. The dura at the edge of the craniotomy is then tacked up to the bone through tangential holes. A curvilinear incision is made

TABLE 112–2 ■ **Presentation Patterns of Supraclinoid Internal Carotid Artery Aneurysms**

SITE	SAH	ICH	IVH	SDH	SPECIAL FEATURES
Posterior communicating artery	Lateral suprasellar, ambient cistern	Medial temporal (uncal)	Temporal horn	Inferior lateral convexity	Painful pupil involving oculomotor palsy, retro-orbital pain
Anterior choroidal artery	Lateral suprasellar, ambient cistern	Rare	Temporal horn	Rare	None; may be similar to above
Internal carotid bifurcation	Lateral suprasellar, proximal sylvian fissure	Basal ganglia	Lateral ventricle	Rare	Optic tract signs, contralateral deficit, aphasia

ICH, intracerebral hemorrhage; IVH, intraventricular hemorrhage; SAH, subarachnoid hemorrhage; SDH, subdural hematoma.

in the dura, and the dural flap is reflected inferiorly over the muscle to further aid hemostasis.

If the brain is still full despite mannitol and hyperventilation to a Pa_{CO_2} of 25 to 30, and especially if the patient has hydrocephalus, a catheter is passed into the frontal horn of the lateral ventricle 1 inch above the base of the frontal lobe and 1 inch anterior to the sylvian fissure.[14] Some surgeons prefer to use frontal lobe retraction and drainage of CSF from the optic and carotid cisterns and then proceed with splitting the fissure from medial to lateral, which requires some temporal lobe retraction. We recommend splitting the fissure properly for any giant or complex aneurysm in the anterior circulation.

Under the microscope, the sylvian fissure is divided from lateral to medial. Splitting the sylvian fissure is possible and advantageous for any anterior circulation aneurysm. During splitting of the fissure, gentle frontal lobe retraction allows proper visualization of the proximal end of the fissure, the optic nerve, and the proximal ICA. The optic and carotid cisterns are then opened. The optic nerve is separated from the undersurface of the frontal lobe using sharp dissection to allow the frontal lobe to fall away with minimal retraction.

Dissection of the ICA should be done on the anterosuperior surface until proximal and distal controls are achieved. The opticocarotid triangle is opened, and dissection is continued on the medial aspect of the ICA unless the aneurysm is pointing medially on the preoperative angiogram. The clot on the base of the aneurysm is swiped away from the neck to visualize it better. The posterior communicating artery, its anterior thalamic perforators, and the anterior choroidal artery are identified. Anteromedial retraction on the ICA is dangerous, because it may pull on the dome of the aneurysm and tear it. Occasionally, the dome may be stuck to the third nerve, and traction may cause permanent damage to this nerve. After identifying the proximal and distal ends of the neck, a straight clip can usually be used to occlude the neck completely. Occasionally, a right-angle fenestrated clip, keeping the ICA in the fenestration and the blades parallel to it, may be necessary. After applying the clip, the tips must be inspected to ensure complete closure around the aneurysm and patency of the posterior communicating artery, thalamoperforators, and, most importantly, anterior choroidal artery. A small residual neck can be left to maintain the caliber of the parent vessel (ICA). Sometimes the proximal posterior communicating artery is blown into the aneurysm. In this case, if the preoperative angiogram ensures the absence of an ipsilateral fetal origin of the posterior cerebral artery and confirms filling of the artery from the posterior circulation, the artery can be included in the clip, followed by a second clip applied between the aneurysm and the first thalamoperforator. Temporary clipping of the parent artery may be used in large aneurysms to reduce the flow to reconstruct the parent vessel. When used, temporary clipping is done for no longer than 3 minutes at a time, allowing 10 minutes between the application of temporary clips.

After clipping of the aneurysm, the dome may be pulled and punctured with a 25-gauge needle to ensure obliteration. Blood clots are then thoroughly washed out. In patients with large clots and no clotting disorder, recombinant tissue plasminogen activator in the dose of 10 mL of 1 mg/mL can be injected in the basal cisterns after obliteration of the aneurysm. This may have some effect in resolving the subarachnoid blood clot and hence prevent the occurrence of severe vasospasm postoperatively.[15]

Anterior Choroidal Artery

ANATOMY

According to the new classification of the carotid artery segments, the anterior choroidal artery arises from the C7 segment, which is also called the posterior communicating segment.[7] In the older classification, it arises from the choroidal segment, which begins at the takeoff of the anterior choroidal artery and ends at the carotid bifurcation.[16] This artery is the only named branch that arises from this segment. It arises distal and lateral to the posterior communicating artery and has a characteristic course, swinging initially laterally and then posteriorly, following the optic tract, and supplying a branch to the mesial temporal structures.[17] The main trunk then continues posteriorly, inferior to the optic tract, to enter the choroid fissure. The size of this artery is quite variable, and duplication occurs in as many as 30% of normal autopsy specimens.[13]

PRESENTATION

Aneurysms of this segment may be difficult to differentiate radiographically from those arising from the posterior communicating segment. On CT, the SAH is in the lateral suprasellar region and ambient cisterns, rarely causing intraparenchymal or subdural hematomas. When present, intraventricular hematomas usually involve the temporal horn (see Table 112–2). Because of the high location of the aneurysm above the tentorium, cranial nerve deficits are uncommon. The aneurysm may be buried within the uncus of the temporal lobe.[11]

OPERATIVE TECHNIQUE

Following standard positioning and a pterional craniotomy, as described previously, the sylvian fissure is split under the microscope using a single frontal lobe retractor. Excessive temporal lobe retraction must be avoided because of the potential of ripping the dome of the aneurysm, which is frequently adherent to the mesial temporal lobe. In 70% of cases, the anterior choroidal artery arises as a single trunk from the inferior aspect of the neck of the aneurysm.[18] It runs in a lateral course, making it visible from a temporal line of sight. It can be duplicated or, rarely, triplicated. When there is more than one artery, the aneurysm arises in relation to the largest branch. The key to this operation is preserving the anterior choroidal artery, because its occlusion may lead to contralateral hemiparesis, hemianopia, and hemisensory deficit. Dissection on the carotid artery is done on the lateral aspect, moving toward the proximal aspect of the neck of the aneurysm. It is usually easier to start the dissection on the proximal aspect of the neck to define the anterior choroidal artery and the plane between it and the aneurysm. The carotid artery is dissected free from the arachnoid early to obtain proximal control. Medial carotid artery retraction should be avoided to prevent tearing of the aneurysm.

After defining the proximal aneurysm neck, the surgeon moves distally, along the underside of the ICA bifurcation. Not infrequently, a bit of the medial aspect of the temporal lobe may be resected, leaving some brain on the aneurysm to allow retraction of the temporal lobe in order to visualize the top part of the aneurysm neck, the distal ICA, and its bifurcation. If present, the second anterior choroidal artery should also be preserved. With a large, superiorly projecting aneurysm, the recurrent artery of Heubner may be on the medial aspect of the aneurysm and must be preserved. Once the two aspects of the aneurysm are defined, a proper length clip—usually a straight one—is slowly applied with the lower blade above the anterior choroidal artery and the upper blade against the superior aspect of the neck of the aneurysm. Unnecessarily long clips should be avoided to prevent clipping perforators arising from the ICA, posterior communicating artery, or recurrent artery of Heubner. After securing the aneurysm, the surgeon must check to ensure the patency of the anterior choroidal artery and the absence of perforators between the blades of the clip. Finally, the aneurysm is punctured with a 25-gauge needle to ensure its obliteration, and closure is done following meticulous hemostasis.

Internal Carotid Artery Bifurcation

ANATOMY

The bifurcation of the ICA into the anterior and middle cerebral arteries takes place underneath the basal forebrain. The anterior cerebral artery passes forward and medially over the optic nerve to meet its counterpart in the midline through the anterior communicating artery. It sends perforating branches to the basal forebrain and gives rise to the recurrent artery of Heubner, which passes medial to the carotid bifurcation and its lenticulostriate perforators. The middle cerebral artery passes laterally and then posteriorly, dividing under cover of the frontal and parietal opercula. Aneurysms of the ICA bifurcation therefore tend to point up in the direction of the jet of blood inside the vessel, toward the anterior perforated substance.[16, 19] The aneurysm usually points anterosuperiorly, straight superiorly, or posterosuperiorly. In most cases, the lenticulostriate perforators off the ICA are displaced posteriorly and may be adherent to the aneurysm. These perforators usually supply the basal ganglia but may also supply the optic apparatus, hypothalamus, and mesial temporal lobe.

PRESENTATION

ICA bifurcation aneurysms account for approximately 5% to 15% of all intracranial aneurysms.[20, 21] They most commonly present with SAH but may present with intraparenchymal hemorrhage into the basal ganglia, simulating hypertensive hemorrhage (see Table 112–2). They may enlarge to a giant size and compress the optic apparatus.

OPERATIVE TECHNIQUE

Patient positioning and the standard pterional craniotomy are performed as described for posterior communicating artery aneurysms. With the aid of the microscope, the sylvian fissure is widely divided. Before approaching the aneurysm, proximal control must be obtained. Following that, the inferior aspects of both the anterior and the middle cerebral arteries are exposed; only then can the arachnoid membrane around the bifurcation be rolled up to expose the neck of the aneurysm and the perforating vessels. The dome of the aneurysm, which is usually buried in the substance of the basal forebrain, should not be disturbed. A small frontal corticotomy may be performed to facilitate visualization of the lenticulostriates and the recurrent artery of Heubner. Some surgeons open the lamina terminalis for CSF drainage and better visualization of the anterior communicating complex and its perforators, but we do not think this is necessary. The aneurysm neck is then dissected from the superior aspect of the anterior cerebral artery anteriorly and from the middle cerebral artery posteriorly. The recurrent artery of Heubner is then identified running medial to and behind the bifurcation. The type and direction of the clip to be used are dictated by the configuration of the aneurysm. Usually a straight clip is applied perpendicular to the direction of the anterior and middle cerebral arteries. The clip should not exceed the size of the aneurysm, to avoid clipping the lenticulostriate perforators, recurrent artery of Heubner, basal vein of Rosenthal, or deep sylvian vein. After clip placement, the vessels are inspected, and the aneurysm is punctured with a 25-gauge needle to ensure obliteration. Meticulous hemostasis is secured, followed by dural closure and closure of the craniotomy and the soft tissues.

Ventral Internal Carotid Artery Trunk

Aneurysms off the ventral wall of the supraclinoid ICA are not common, but they pose special problems, including the fact that the ICA stands between the surgeon and the neck of the aneurysm. They are usually seen in the setting of atherosclerotic changes in the wall of the carotid artery, which may not allow proper placement of the clip. The dome may project anteromedially, displacing the anterior perforators or the pituitary stalk in a medial direction.[10] Clipping of these aneurysms should be done very carefully after tailoring the positioning and the approach to each individual case based on the angiographic features. Proximal control remains the key issue in preventing intraoperative disasters, and proper visualization of medial structures is vital.

Paraclinoid aneurysms of the ICA and giant intracranial aneurysms are discussed in Chapters 111 and 121, respectively.

Infundibulum

Dilatation of the takeoff of a branch of the ICA (usually the posterior communicating artery) of 3 mm or less is termed an *infundibulum.* Radiographic and autopsy series suggest an incidence of 6% to 16%, increasing with older age.[10, 22, 23] The argument about whether this is a preaneurysmal phenomenon continues,[10] but it is generally accepted that, by itself, an infundibulum does not need to be treated.

INTRAOPERATIVE ANEURYSM RUPTURE

Intraoperative aneurysm rupture is a dreadful complication that every neurosurgeon should anticipate and be prepared to deal with before bringing the patient to the operating room. The appropriate reaction to intraoperative rupture is determined by when it happens. Proximal control is crucial, and the ability to apply a temporary clip on the parent vessel must be ensured before dealing with the aneurysm.

If the rupture occurs before exposing the aneurysm, two large-bore suctions should be placed in the wound immediately. One of them should be placed on the hole of the aneurysm to help visualize the proximal vessel, which is temporarily clipped. Following that, another temporary clip can be applied to the distal vessel. The dissection is then done in the setting of high blood pressure and barbiturate administration to reduce the ischemic insult. If the rupture occurs after completing the dissection of the aneurysm neck, with proper suctioning, the clip can be applied safely across the neck of the aneurysm. If the rupture takes place before completing the dissection, there is no point in trying to clip the aneurysm. Temporary clips must be applied to the parent vessel proximally and distally, and the aneurysm is repaired under local flow arrest. Hemorrhage that occurs while inspecting the vessels after applying the clip means that the aneurysm has not been completely obliterated. In this case, opening and blindly advancing the clip may tear the aneurysm or artery, further compromising repair. Again, temporary clips are probably the best option. Having a strategy for dealing with an intraoperative rupture is the only way to ensure a nonpanicked, stepwise approach to handling this complication.

CLOSURE

Following obliteration of the aneurysm, the operative field is thoroughly irrigated to wash out any residual blood clots. The microscope is used to inspect the surgical field to secure hemostasis. Surgicel is applied over any violated pial surface. The surgeon should avoid leaving Gelfoam in the basal cisterns, because it allows blood products to remain around basal vessels, which may aggravate vasospasm. The dural opening is then closed using interrupted 4–0 sutures, and the center of the dura is tacked up to holes in the bone flap. The flap is then fixed back in place using miniplates and screws. The bone may be slightly grooved to settle the plate for a better cosmetic result. Because the temporalis muscle usually atrophies following this approach, the surgeon may use a small amount of acrylic cement under the temporalis muscle in the pterion; this may lead to early swelling and bulging of the surgical side for 1 to 2 weeks, but the long-term results are satisfactory. Some acrylic may also be used to cover the miniplates. Screws should not be placed in the frontal sinus unless cranialized. If an opening into the frontal air sinus is made, it is exonerated, packed with Gelfoam, covered with a vascularized pericranial flap extradurally, and sealed with fibrin adhesive before putting the bone flap back. The temporalis muscle is reapproximated, and the fascia is closed using interrupted 3–0 Vicryl sutures, especially over the keyhole region. The galea is then closed with 3–0 Vicryl sutures, and the skin is closed with staples or nonabsorbable monofilament sutures.

TABLE 112–3 ■ **Surgical Results of Ruptured Internal Carotid Artery Aneurysms**

AUTHOR	FAVORABLE (%)	MORBIDITY (%)	MORTALITY (%)
Flamm	86.7	7.9	5.4
Ogilvy	94	2	4
Heros	95	4.2	0.8

OUTCOME

The surgical outcome for ICA aneurysms is generally very good (Table 112–3). Poor results are usually related to poor preoperative patient grade and severe, persistent vasospasm. Third nerve palsy following SAH or rapid expansion of a posterior communicating artery aneurysm usually resolves completely over a 3-month period in up to 90% of patients, and it resolves partially in the remaining 10%.[3]

CONCLUSION

Surgical clipping of aneurysms of the supraclinoid ICA is relatively less complex than that of other aneurysms. However, unless the neurosurgeon has a good understanding of the angiographic anatomy of the aneurysm, the parent vessel, and associated perforators, clipping of these aneurysms can be extremely difficult, and the results may not be ideal. Underestimation of the angiographic features of associated conditions such as severe atherosclerosis may create difficulties during temporary clipping. It is crucial to avoid aggressive manipulation of the ICA to reduce the chance of intraoperative rupture and postoperative vasospasm. Finally, no matter how successful the surgical procedure is, it has to be complemented by vigilant perioperative care of these critically ill patients to ensure good results.

REFERENCES

1. Kassell NF, Torner JC, Haley EC, et al: The international cooperative study on the timing of aneurysm surgery. Part I. Overall management results. J Neurosurg 73:18–36, 1990.
2. Kassell NF, Torner JC, Jane JA, et al: The international cooperative study on the timing of aneurysm surgery. Part II. Surgical results. J Neurosurg 73:37–47, 1990.
3. Pikus HJ, Heros RC: Surgical treatment of internal carotid and posterior communicating artery aneurysms. Neurosurg Clin N Am 9:785–795, 1998.
4. The International Study of Unruptured Intracranial Aneurysms investigators: Unruptured intracranial aneurysms—risk of rupture and risk of surgical intervention. N Engl J Med 339:1725–1733, 1998.
5. Korogi Y, Takahashi M, Mabuchi N, et al: Intracranial aneurysms: Diagnostic accuracy of MR angiography with evaluation of maximum intensity projection and source images. Radiology 199: 199–207, 1996.
6. Hope JKA, Wilson JL, Thomson FJ: Three dimensional CT angiography in the detection and characterization of berry aneurysms. AJNR Am J Neuroradiol 17:439–445, 1996.
7. Bouthillier A, Van Loveren HR, Keller JT: Segments of the internal carotid artery: A new classification. Neurosurgery 38:425–433, 1996.
8. Saeki N, Rhoton AL Jr: Microsurgical anatomy of the upper basilar artery and the posterior circle of Willis. J Neurosurg 46: 563–578, 1977.
9. Sundt TMJ, Wisnant JP: Subarachnoid hemorrhage from intracranial aneurysms: Surgical management and natural history of disease. N Engl J Med 229:116–122, 1978.
10. Fox JL: Techniques of aneurysm surgery: Internal carotid artery aneurysms. In Intracranial Aneurysms, vol 1. New York, Springer-Verlag, 1983, pp 949–1011.
11. Day AL, Morcos JJ, Revilla F: Management of aneurysms of the anterior circulation. In Youmans JR (ed): Neurological Surgery, 4th ed. Philadelphia, WB Saunders, 1996, pp 1272–1309.
12. Lanzino G, Andreoli A, Tognetti F, et al: Orbital pain and unruptured carotid–posterior communicating artery aneurysms: The role of sensory fibers of the third cranial nerve. Acta Neurochir (Wien) 120:7–11, 1993.
13. Yasargil MG: Microneurosurgery, vols 1, 2. New York, Thieme-Stratton, 1987.
14. Paine JT, Batjer HH, Samson D: Intraoperative ventricular puncture. Neurosurgery 22:1107–1109, 1988.
15. Findlay JM, Kassell NF, Weir BKA, et al: A randomized trial of intraoperative intracisternal tissue plasminogen activator for the prevention of vasospasm. Neurosurgery 37:168–176, 1995.
16. Gibo H, Lenkey C, Rhoton AL Jr: Microsurgical anatomy of the supraclinoid portion of the internal carotid artery. J Neurosurg 55:560–574, 1981.
17. Rosner SS, Rhoton AL Jr, Ono M, et al: Microsurgical anatomy of the anterior perforating arteries. J Neurosurg 61:468–485, 1984.
18. Ogilvy CS: Internal carotid artery aneurysms associated with the posterior communicating and anterior choroidal arteries. In Ojeman RG, Ogilvy CS, Crowell RN, Heros RC (eds): Surgical Management of Neurovascular Disease. Philadelphia, Williams & Wilkins, 1995, pp 214–226.
19. Grand W: Microsurgical anatomy of the proximal middle cerebral artery and the internal carotid artery bifurcation. Neurosurgery 7:215–218, 1980.
20. Sahs AL, Perret GE, Locksley HB, et al: Intracranial Aneurysms and Subarachnoid Hemorrhage: A Cooperative Study. Philadelphia, JB Lippincott, 1969.
21. Weir B: Surgery: Specific sites and results of series. In Aneurysms Affecting the Nervous System. Baltimore, Williams & Wilkins, 1987, pp 438–504.
22. Watanabe M, In S, Kuramoto S: Junctional dilation of the posterior communicating artery. Neurol Surg (Tokyo) 3:917–924, 1975.
23. Wollschlaeger G, Wollschlaeger PB, Lucas FV, et al: Experience and results with postmortem cerebral angiography performed as routine procedure of the autopsy. AJR Am J Roentgenol 101: 68–87, 1967.

CHAPTER **113**

Anterior Communicating Artery and Anterior Cerebral Artery Aneurysms

RAFAEL J. TAMARGO ■ RAYMOND I. HAROUN ■ DANIELE RIGAMONTI

SURGICAL MANAGEMENT OF ANTERIOR COMMUNICATING ARTERY AND PROXIMAL ANTERIOR CEREBRAL ARTERY ANEURYSMS

Based on clinical studies, the anterior communicating artery (ACoA) region is the most common site for intracranial aneurysms. In the original Cooperative Study of Intracranial Aneurysms and Subarachnoid Hemorrhage (1958–1965), 30.3% of 2349 aneurysms were located in the ACoA region.[1] Also in this study, the incidence of anterior cerebral artery (ACA) aneurysms proximal to the ACoA junction (on the A1 segment) was 1.5%, and the incidence of aneurysms distal to the ACoA junction was 2.8%. The total incidence of A1–ACoA–distal ACA aneurysms in the original Cooperative Study was 34.6%. This incidence has remained fairly constant over the years. In the more recent International Cooperative Study on the Timing of Aneurysm Surgery (1980–1983), the incidence of ACoA-ACA aneurysms was 39.0%.[2] In this chapter, we discuss the microsurgical treatment of ACoA aneurysms and distal ACA aneurysms.

Embryology of the Anterior Communicating Artery Region

A basic understanding of the embryologic development of the ACoA region allows us to anticipate its most common congenital anomalies. Current understanding of the developmental anatomy of the intracranial arteries is based on Hager Padget's 1948 article on this subject.[3] At 35 days (12- to 14-mm stage), the primitive anterior division of the internal carotid artery (ICA) develops a distinct distal branch that is the stem of the ACA. By 40 days (16- to 18-mm stage), the stem of the ACA elongates medially toward its counterpart. At this stage, a midline cluster of plexiform anastomoses begins to form between the adjacent and elongating ACAs. At 44 days (20- to 24-mm stage), the channels of the midline cluster of plexiform anastomoses coalesce and form one or more ACoAs. The coalescing channels of the midline cluster of plexiform anastomoses give rise to a median ACA that originates from the ACoA.

In humans, the median ACA, also known as the *median artery of the corpus callosum,* subsequently regresses and disappears, but it persists in other vertebrates. The development of this artery may result in regression and dissolution of the paired ACAs. With the formation of the ACoA at 44 days (20- to 24-mm stage), the adult configuration of the intracranial arteries is established, and the circle of Willis is complete.

Given this description, the most common congenital anomalies of this region can be predicted: (1) multiple or fenestrated ACoAs, (2) triplicate A2 segments, and (3) the azygous A2 segment. Perlmutter and Rhoton[4] found two or three ACoAs in 30% and 10% of 50 cadaver brain dissections. They confirmed that absence of the ACoA is exceedingly rare.[4] Hager Padget[5] calculated that the ACoA is absent in only 0.2% of cases (3 of 1803). Persistence of the median artery of the corpus callosum creates three A2s. Baptista[6] identified triplicate ACAs in 13.1% of his specimens (50 of 381), but Perlmutter and Rhoton[4] found triplicate ACAs in only 2% of their specimens (1 of 50). An azygous or solitary A2 segment arises when the paired ACAs regress after formation and enlargement of the median artery of the corpus callosum.[3] An azygous A2 has been identified in only 0.26% of general autopsies[6] and in only 0.22% of unselected angiograms.[7] The higher incidence of azygous A2 segments in aneurysm series results from the fact that 41.1% of azygous A2 segments have a terminal aneurysm.[7]

Microsurgical Anatomy of the A1–Anterior Communicating Artery–A2 Region

The anatomy of this region is reviewed in detail elsewhere in this book. Here we discuss only a few definitions and anatomic details that serve as a background for the subsequent surgical discussion. The ACA is divided into five anatomic segments, A1 through A5.[8]

The A1 segment starts at the ICA termination and ends at the ACoA junction. The A2 segment starts at the ACoA junction, follows the course of the rostrum of the corpus callosum, and terminates at the junction of the rostrum and genu of the corpus callosum. It commonly is referred to as the *pericallosal artery.* The A3 segment follows the curve of the genu of the corpus callosum and terminates where the ACA turns posteriorly above the genu. The A4 and A5 segments run over the body of the corpus callosum; the transition from A4 to A5 is set arbitrarily at the level of the plane defined by the coronal suture.[8]

A1 SEGMENT

The average diameter of the A1 segment is 2.6 mm (range 0.9 to 4.0 mm),[4] about two thirds that of the middle cerebral artery at the ICA bifurcation and about half that of the supraclinoid ICA at its origin (Fig. 113–1). Although absence of the A1 segment is extremely rare, hypoplasia of the A1 segment is recognized in about 10% of cases.[4] Perlmutter and Rhoton[4] chose a diameter of 1.5 mm as the threshold for labeling the A1 segment as hypoplastic, but there is no agreed-on threshold below which an artery is labeled *hypoplastic.* They found 10% of their specimens had A1 segments that were 1.5 mm or less in diameter, and 2% had A1 segments 1 mm or less in diameter.[4] Another rare but surgically important anatomic variant is the duplication of the A1 segment (2%), which when present occurs only unilaterally.[4]

The paired A1 segments are of equal diameter in only half of cases. In 50% of cases, there is a difference of 0.5 mm or more between the diameters of the A1 segments. In 12% of cases, the difference is 1 mm or more.[4] This discrepancy in diameter between the paired A1 segments is even more prevalent when one considers cases with an ACoA aneurysm. In the presence of an ACoA aneurysm, the paired A1 segments are of unequal diameter in 85% of cases.[9] Typically the base of the aneurysm arises on the side of the larger A1, and the dome points toward the side of the hypoplastic A1.

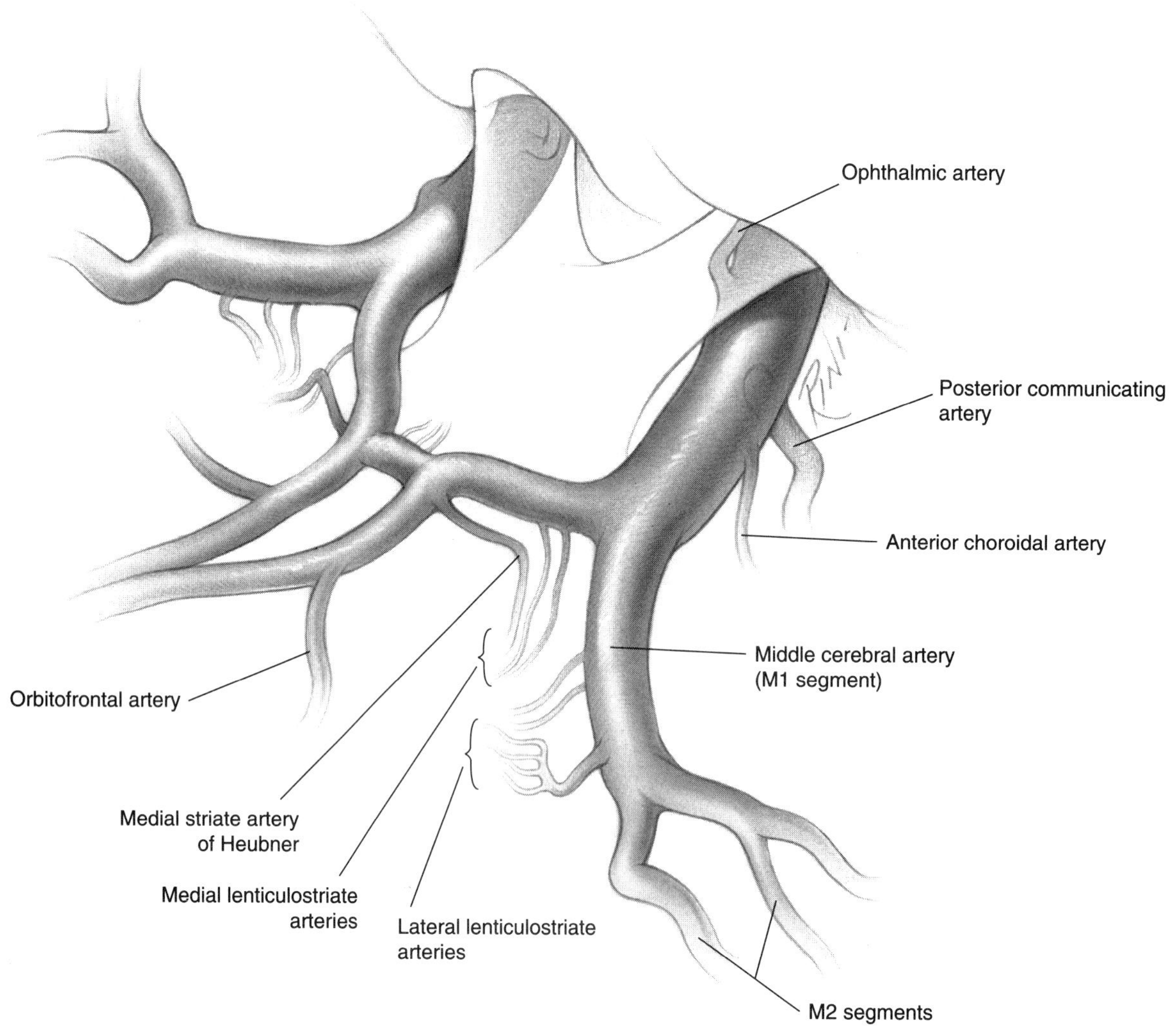

FIGURE 113–1. Anatomy of the anterior circulation with the major branches and perforators of the internal carotid artery (ICA), of the M1 segment of the middle cerebral artery (MCA), of the A1 and A2 segments of the anterior cerebral artery (ACA), and of the anterior communicating artery (ACoA).

ANTERIOR COMMUNICATING ARTERY

The diameter of the ACoA is on average about half that of the A1 segment (see Fig. 113–1). Although the average diameter of the A1 segment is 2.6 mm, that of the ACoA is 1.5 mm (range 0.2 to 3.4 mm).[4] There is a constant relationship between the diameter of the ACoA and the difference in the diameters of the A1 segments: The larger the difference between the A1 segments, the larger the ACoA.[4] Because unequal A1 segments typically are found in the presence of an aneurysm and because unequal A1 segments typically are associated with a larger ACoA, one can expect essentially always to find a patent ACoA when exploring an aneurysm in this region, even when it is not shown angiographically.

The ACoA rarely is oriented in a strictly transverse plane, as depicted in most non-neurosurgical textbooks. At the level of the ACoA junction, the left ACA courses anterior to the right in 48% of cases, and the right ACA courses anterior to the left in 34% of cases; only in 18% of cases do they enter the interhemispheric fissure side by side.[4] Because of the course of the ACAs, the ACoA usually is oriented in an oblique or sagittal plane. As described earlier, two ACoAs are present in 30% of cases and three ACoAs are present in 10% of cases.[4] Absence of the ACoA is exceedingly rare (only 0.2% of cases).[5]

A2 SEGMENT

Although most neurosurgeons refer to the A2 segment as the *pericallosal artery* and consider the callosomarginal artery a branch of the pericallosal artery, some use the term *pericallosal artery* to define one of the two branches at the bifurcation of the distal A2 segment, the other branch being the callosomarginal artery. The main problem with this alternative nomenclature is that because the callosomarginal artery is absent in 18% of cases, it makes it difficult to define where the pericallosal artery starts.[8] The callosomarginal artery originates most frequently (60% of cases) from the A3 segment, an average of 43 mm (range 12 to 47 mm) from the ACoA junction, which places it beyond the junction of the rostrum and genu of the corpus callosum. It originates more proximally (from the A2 segment) in 10% of cases and more distally (from the A4 segment) in 12% of cases.[8]

PERFORATORS OF THE A1, ANTERIOR COMMUNICATING ARTERY, AND A2 SEGMENTS

The A1 segment gives rise to an average of 8 perforators (range 2 to 15), 41% of which terminate in the anterior perforated substance.[4] These perforators sometimes are identified as the medial lenticulostriate arteries to distinguish them from the lateral lenticulostriate arteries, which originate from the M1 segment and terminate in the anterior perforated substance.[10, 11] Typically the proximal half of A1 gives rise to twice as many perforators as the distal half. Another way of stating this is that of all the perforators of the A1 segment, two thirds arise from the proximal half, and one third arise from the distal half. Although the proximal half gives rise to an average of 5.3 perforators (range 1 to 11), the distal half gives rise to an average of 2.5 perforators (range 0 to 6).[4] Most (86%) of the A1 perforators arise from the superior (54%) and posterior (32%) surfaces of this segment. Only rarely (14%) do they arise from the inferior (9%) and anterior (5%) surfaces of A1.[4] Of all the A1 perforators, 41% terminate in the anterior perforated substance. These perforators branch into as many as 49 vessels as they reach the anterior perforated substance.[12] Most enter the medial portion of the anterior perforated substance and typically course posterior to the branches of the medial striate artery of Heubner.[12] The remaining A1 perforators terminate in the dorsal optic chiasm or suprachiasmatic hypothalamus (29%), the inferior frontal lobe (10%), the optic tract (11%), the sylvian fissure (5%), the dorsal optic nerve (2%), or the interhemispheric fissure (2%).[4]

There have been conflicting anatomic reports concerning the number of ACoA perforators. Perlmutter and Rhoton[4] in their study of 50 brains found that the ACoA may have no perforators or four.[4] By contrast, Dunker and Harris[13] and Crowell and Morawetz[14] examined 20 and 10 brains, and both concluded that the ACoA always has at least 3 perforators.

In a pattern similar to that seen on the A1 segment, most (90%) of the ACoA perforators arise from its superior (54%) and posterior (36%) surfaces and only rarely (10%) from its anterior (7%) and inferior (3%) surfaces.[4] Most ACoA perforators are hidden from the surgeon's view. Of all the ACoA perforators, 51% terminate in the suprachiasmatic region, 21% terminate on the dorsal optic chiasm, and 15% reach the anterior perforated substance.[4]

MEDIAL STRIATE ARTERY (RECURRENT ARTERY OF HEUBNER)

The most important perforator from the proximal A2 segment is the medial striate artery, better known as the *recurrent artery of Heubner* (see Fig. 113–1). We have reviewed elsewhere the anatomy of this vessel and the life and accomplishments of its discoverer, Heubner (1843–1926), a German pediatrician who described it in an article published in 1872.[15] The medial striate artery of Heubner arises from the A2 segment in 78% of cases, from the A1 segment in 14% of cases, and at the level of the ACoA in 8% of cases.[4] Perlmutter and Rhoton[4] found that it originates within 4 mm of the ACoA junction (either proximal or distal to it) in 95% of cases.[4] They also found this artery to be absent (only on one side) in 2% of cases and duplicated (also only on one side) in 2% of cases.[4] Gomes and colleagues[16] found this artery to be absent in 3% of cases but duplicated in 12% of cases.

The medial striate artery of Heubner courses anterior to the A1 segment in 60% of cases and superior to the A1 segment in 40% of cases.[4] This artery is encountered before the A1 segment on initial retraction of the frontal lobe during surgery in most (60%) cases. The length of the medial striate artery of Heubner is on average twice that of the A1 segment. Although the average length of the A1 segment is 12.7 mm,[4] that of the medial striate artery is 23.4 mm (range 12 to 38 mm).[16] Its length increases its exposure to injury during surgery.

The medial striate artery of Heubner should not be confused during surgery with the orbitofrontal artery, which is typically the second major branch of the A2 segment (see Fig. 113–1). The medial striate artery of Heubner is usually the first branch of the A2 segment immediately after the ACoA junction. It also is typically the largest vessel arising from the A2 segment. The orbitofrontal artery originates on average 5 mm (range 0 to 15 mm) from the ACoA junction and has an average diameter of 0.9 mm (range 0.4 to 2.0 mm).[8] Based on diameter alone, the orbitofrontal artery can be mistaken for the medial striate artery of Heubner, which has an average diameter of 1 mm (range 0.2 to 2.9 mm).[4] Their courses are different, however. Although the medial striate artery of Heubner follows the course of the A1 segment, the orbitofrontal artery courses perpendicularly over the gyrus rectus and across the olfactory tract.[11] (The subfrontal gyral and sulcal anatomy is depicted in Fig. 113–2.) Another important anatomic distinction of the orbitofrontal artery is that it typically demarcates the boundary of the lamina terminalis cistern (where it originates) and the beginning of the callosal cistern.[11]

After the orbitofrontal artery, the third major branch of the A2 segment is the frontopolar artery. The frontopolar artery is a cortical branch that originates on average 14 mm (range 2 to 30 mm) from the ACoA junction and has an average diameter of 1.3 mm (range 0.6 to 1.8 mm).[8] It courses anteriorly along the medial surface of the frontal lobe and crosses the subfrontal sulcus (see Fig. 113–2).[8]

The medial striate artery of Heubner supplies the anterior striatum (caudate nucleus and putamen), a portion of the outer segment of the globus pallidus, and the anterior limb of the internal capsule.[4] Injury to this vessel typically results in a moderate paresis of the contralateral upper extremity and mild paresis of the contralateral face. It also causes dysfunction of the tongue and palate, which can be documented only during a careful swallowing evaluation. If the dominant hemisphere is involved, an expressive aphasia may be evident. In most patients, these deficits tend to resolve completely in a matter of months.

In addition to the medial striate artery of Heubner, the orbitofrontal artery, and the frontopolar artery, the proximal A2 segment gives rise to an average of 4.8 (range 0 to 10) basal perforating branches. These branches supply the optic chiasm, anterior hypothalamus, medial portion of the anterior commissure, pillars of the fornix, and anterior-inferior portion of the striatum (caudate nucleus and putamen).[8]

ARACHNOID CISTERNS OF THE A1–ANTERIOR COMMUNICATING ARTERY–A2 REGION

The sequential recognition and opening of three arachnoid cisterns (carotid, chiasmatic, and lamina terminalis) leads to the ACoA junction (Fig. 113–3). The A1 segment originates within the confines of the carotid cistern. It courses within the lamina terminalis cistern over the optic chiasm (70% of the time) or, less fre-

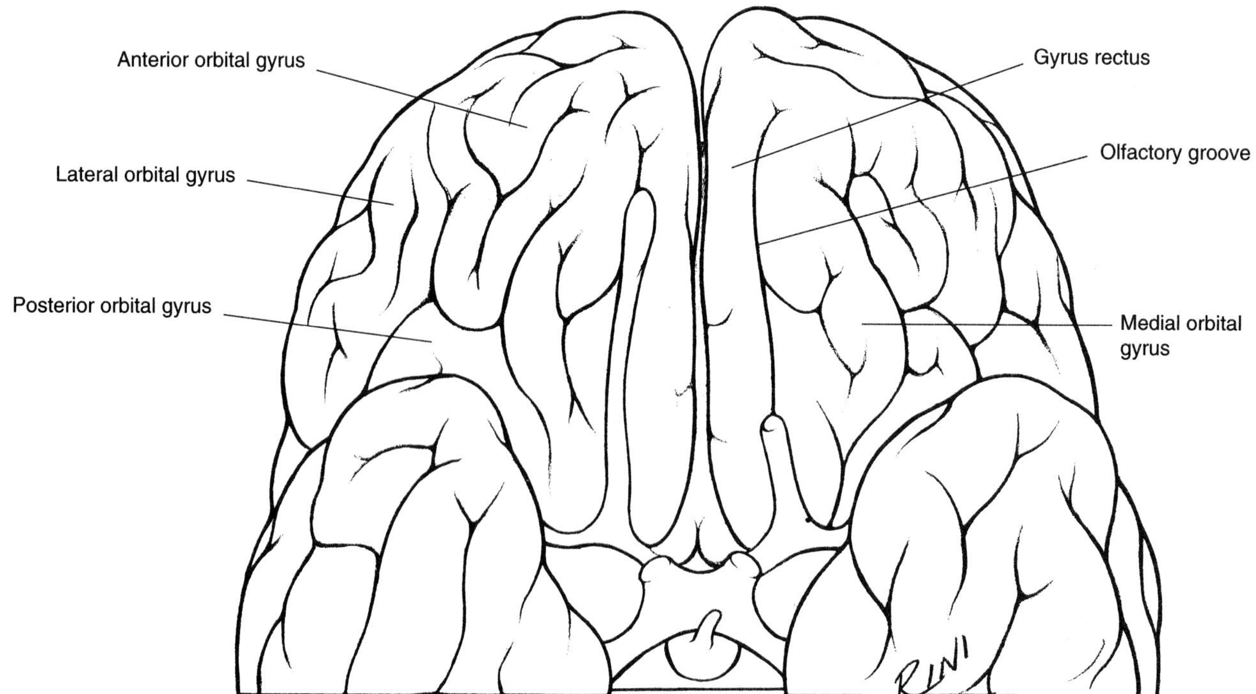

FIGURE 113–2. Anatomy of the subfrontal gyri and sulci in relation to the course of the olfactory nerve.

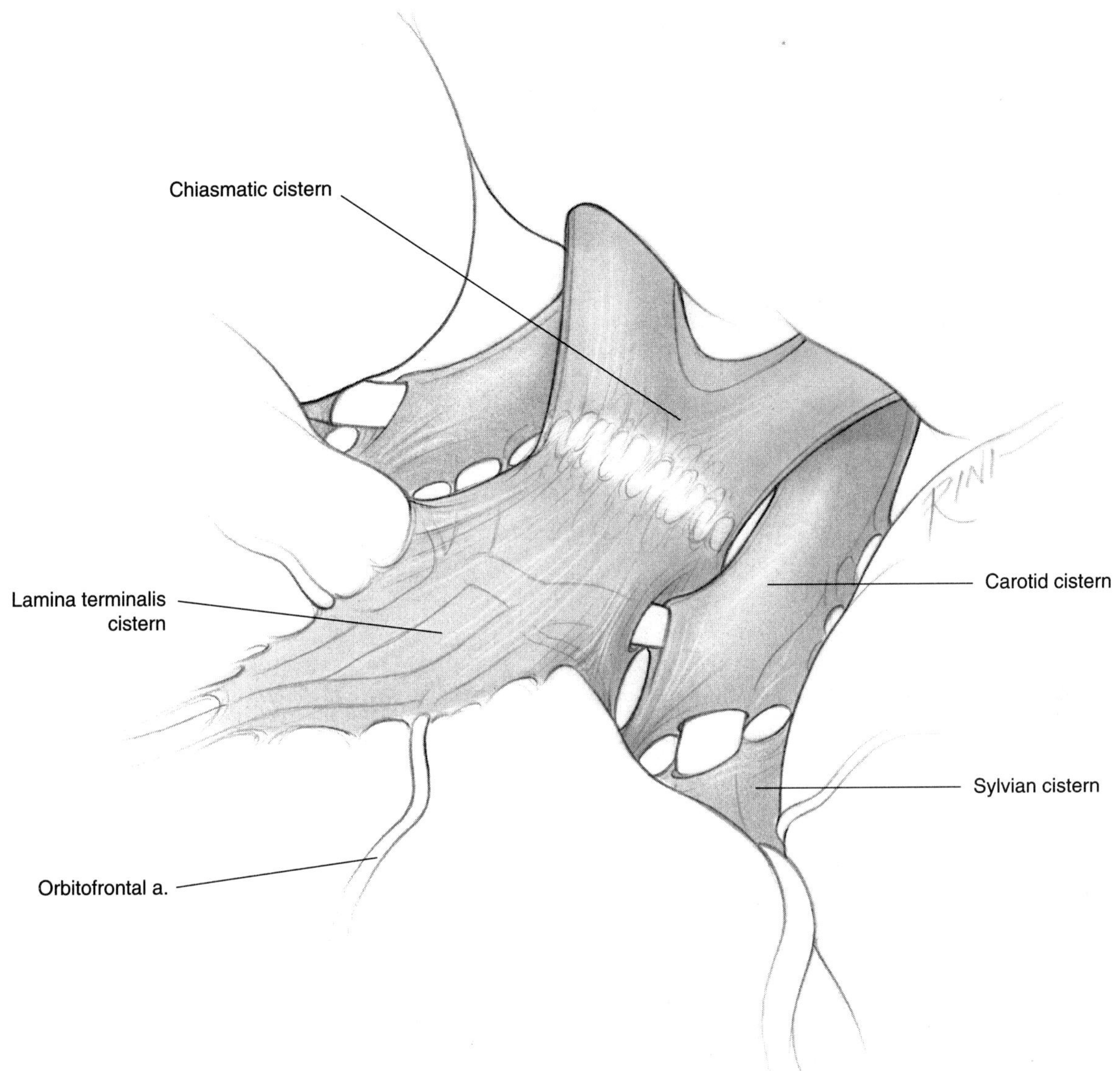

FIGURE 113–3. The arachnoid cisterns of the anterior circulation. Anterior communicating artery aneurysms originate within the lamina terminalis cistern.

quently, over the optic nerve (30% of the time).[4] It enters into the interhemispheric fissure still within the confines of the lamina terminalis cistern.[11] In addition to the origin of the A1 segment, the carotid cistern contains the supraclinoid ICA and the origins of its branches. The carotid cistern shares its medial wall with the chiasmatic cistern, which contains the optic nerves, optic chiasm, and infundibulum, but does not contain any major arteries. The lamina terminalis cistern is a midline structure that contains the paired A1 and proximal A2 segments, the ACoA, and the medial striate arteries of Heubner.[11]

Because the lamina terminalis cistern contains the A1-ACoA-A2 complex, ACoA aneurysms by definition arise within the confines of this cistern (see Fig. 113–3). A clear understanding of the boundaries of this cistern is important microsurgically. Inferiorly the lamina terminalis cistern stretches over the surface of the optic chiasm, where it apposes the chiasmatic cistern. Posteriorly, it is bounded by the lamina terminalis. Superiorly, it stretches into the interhemispheric fissure, where it is bounded by the rostrum of the corpus callosum. Its anterior surface stretches free over the A1-ACoA-A2 complex. Laterally the lamina terminalis cistern surrounds the entire A1 segment after it emerges from the carotid cistern. Yasargil[11] pointed out that the lateral boundary of the lamina terminalis cistern is a thickened band of arachnoid fibers that stretch between the area immediately medial to the olfactory nerve and the optic nerve. The A1 segment enters the lamina terminalis cistern below this thickened band of arachnoid fibers. The medial striate artery of Heubner and the orbitofrontal artery originate within the confines of the lamina terminalis cistern.

For the purpose of the arachnoid dissection during the approach to an ACoA aneurysm, it is important to

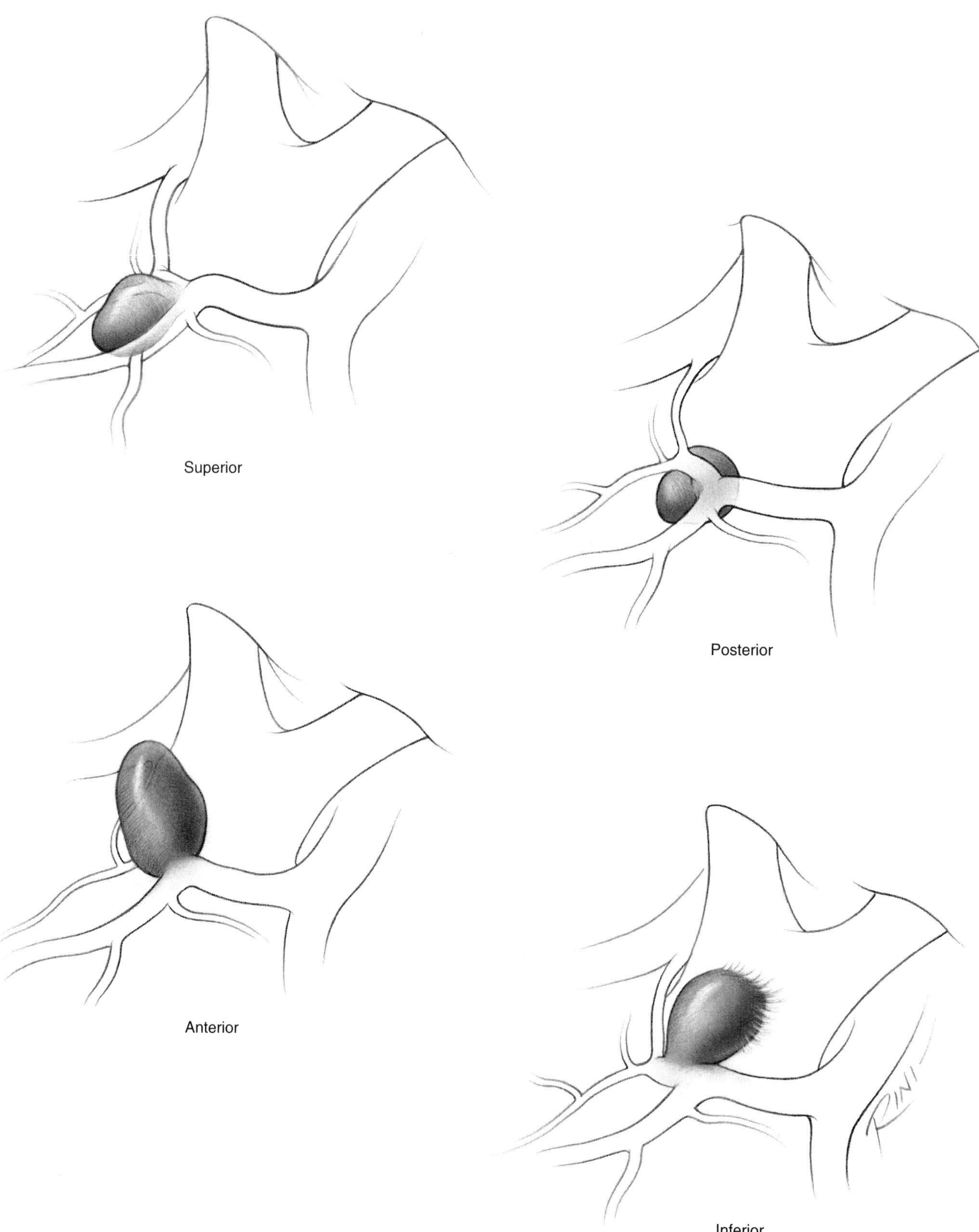
Superior
Posterior
Anterior
Inferior
RINI

TABLE 113–1 ■ Chronology of Landmark Surgical Contributions Pertinent to Microsurgery of Anterior Communicating Artery Aneurysms

DATE	SURGEONS	CONTRIBUTION
1918	Heuer Dandy	First description of frontotemporal craniotomy for lateral subfrontal approach to the circle of Willis[22]
1931	Dott	First direct surgical attack of an aneurysm (ICA bifurcation)[73]
1935	Tonnis	Anterior interhemispheric approach first used for ACoA aneurysms[26]
1937	Dandy	First clipping of an aneurysm (PCoA)[19]
1941	Dandy	Frontotemporal approach first used for ACoA aneurysms[20,21]
1953	Norlen Barnum	Transfrontal approach (partial frontal lobectomy) first used for ACoA aneurysms[24]
1956	Logue	Proximal ligation of AI[74]
1961	Pool	Bilateral anterior subfrontal/interhemispheric approach for large series of ACoA aneurysms[27,28]
1962	French	Transfrontal approach (partial frontal lobectomy) for large series of ACoA aneurysms[50]
1968	Kempe	Sphenoid extension of frontotemporal craniotomy and gyrus rectus resection[23]
1971	Kempe VanderArk	Gyrus rectus approach first used for ACoA aneurysms[25]
1975	Yasargil Fox	Frontolateral, spheno-orbital or pterional craniotomy for aneurysms[17,18]

ACoA, anterior communicating artery; ICA, internal carotid artery; PCoA, posterior communicating artery.

remember that the optic nerves and chiasm are found in a separate cistern, the chiasmatic cistern. This means that if the aneurysm dome is oriented superiorly or posteriorly (Fig. 113–4), one can dissect along the anterior edge of the optic chiasm and the optic nerves without entering the lamina terminalis cistern and potentially disturbing the aneurysm.

History of Surgical Approaches for Anterior Communicating Artery Aneurysms

The history of surgical treatment of aneurysms is reviewed in detail elsewhere in this book. Table 113–1 provides a chronology of the landmark surgical contributions pertinent to microsurgery of ACoA aneurysms. The modern frontosphenotemporal or *pterional* craniotomy as described by Yasargil and Fox[17, 18] is the culmination of a 40-year neurosurgical refinement of a safe and efficient craniotomy to approach ACoA aneurysms. It is based on Dandy's lateral subfrontal approach through a frontotemporal craniotomy,[19–22] it incorporates elements of Kempe's sphenoid wing removal,[23] and it acknowledges the need to resect a portion of the frontal lobe as advocated by Norlen and Barnum[24] but only in a limited fashion (gyrus rectus resection) as advocated by Kempe and VanderArk.[23, 25] The pterional craniotomy currently is favored by most

FIGURE 113–4. Aneurysms of the anterior communicating artery (ACoA) region have a predictable orientation in the coronal and sagittal planes. As described in the text, in the presence of an ACoA aneurysm, there is usually a marked discrepancy between the diameter of the A1 segments. In the coronal plane, ACoA aneurysms typically arise from the side of the larger A1 segment, and their domes project toward the side of the smaller A1 segment. This is probably because the higher hydrodynamic pressures generated by the dominant A1 segment drive the growth of the aneurysm.

In the sagittal plane, ACoA aneurysms may project superiorly, anteriorly, inferiorly, or posteriorly. Although most ACoA aneurysms do not fall neatly into one of these four categories, the recognition of the predominant sagittal projection of these aneurysms is useful in anticipating the complications associated with each projection. This helpful classification scheme for ACoA aneurysms was formulated by Yasargil.[40] Our anterior/posterior and superior/inferior nomenclature refers to the standard anatomic orientation, not the surgical orientation of the lesion, as originally described by Yasargil.

Most ACoA aneurysms (71.2%) project into the interhemispheric fissure, and only a few (12.8%) project inferiorly into the chiasmatic cistern (16% of all ACoA aneurysms have complex, multilobulated projections).[40] Although superior-pointing and posterior-pointing aneurysms are found entirely within the interhemispheric fissure, anterior-pointing aneurysms typically are found only partially inside the interhemispheric fissure. Inferior-pointing aneurysms—the most treacherous of ACoA aneurysms—are almost entirely outside the interhemispheric fissure and are typically adherent to the optic chiasm, the optic nerves, or the dura of the interoptic space. In terms of the initial subfrontal exposure of ACoA aneurysms, superior-pointing and posterior-pointing aneurysms are the most favorable because they rarely rupture at this stage. By contrast, inferior-pointing aneurysms are the worst in this respect because elevation of the frontal lobes may avulse the dome from the optic chiasm, optic nerves, or the dura of the interoptic space early in the subarachnoid dissection.

Anterior-pointing aneurysms have the most favorable orientation in relation to the hypothalamic and infundibular perforators, and posterior-pointing aneurysms have the worst orientation in this respect. For this reason, anterior-pointing aneurysms are usually easier to clip, and posterior-pointing aneurysms are usually the most difficult.

The specific anatomic relationships of the four types of ACoA aneurysms to the arteries of the ACoA region are discussed in the text in the surgical dissection section.

neurosurgeons around the world. A few neurosurgeons still advocate a frontal interhemispheric approach (as originally advocated by Tonnis[26] and Pool[27, 28]), however, through a frontal parasagittal craniotomy for some ACoA aneurysms.[29–31]

Clinical and Radiographic Presentation of Anterior Communicating Artery Aneurysms

The clinical presentation of aneurysmal subarachnoid hemorrhage (SAH) is reviewed in another chapter and elsewhere.[32] Because the clinical presentation of ruptured ACoA aneurysms is in general not different from that of aneurysms in other locations, we do not discuss this issue in this chapter.

The radiographic evaluation of ACoA aneurysms warrants further discussion because there are two radiographic issues that are unique to ACoA aneurysms. The first is that frequently the diagnosis of an ACoA aneurysm can be made on the basis of the computed tomographic (CT) scan alone because the CT scan may reveal either subarachnoid blood only in the interhemispheric fissure or a thicker clot in the interhemispheric fissure (Fig. 113–5*A*). Similarly an intraparenchymal hemorrhage in the region of the gyrus rectus indicates an ACoA aneurysm (Fig. 113–6*A*).

The second radiographic issue is that angiography of ACoA aneurysms has the highest false-negative rate of any intracranial aneurysm. Iwanaga and colleagues[33] performed repeat angiograms in 38 of 469 patients with SAH whose initial angiograms did not show an aneurysm. Of the 38 studies, 8 (21%) revealed an aneurysm, and of the 8 positive repeat studies, 7 were ACoA aneurysms. The reason for the higher false-negative rate in angiography of ACoA aneurysms is probably the balanced flow into the ACoA from the paired A1 segments, which may prevent filling of the aneurysm by the dye. It is crucial that a cross compression study be carried out routinely during angiography for SAH to visualize the ACoA region completely.

Operative Technique for Anterior Communicating Artery and Proximal Anterior Cerebral Artery Aneurysms

ACoA aneurysms remain surgically challenging lesions mainly because of three anatomic features: (1) their bilateral anterograde arterial supply; (2) their deep, midline location; and (3) their intimate relationship to 11 crucial arteries. In contrast to most other intracranial aneurysms, which typically have only one parent artery, ACoA aneurysms are supplied anterogradely by two arteries, the paired A1 segments. During surgery for ACoA aneurysms, both A1 segments have to be exposed early in the dissection to obtain proximal control. Although ACoA aneurysms are midline structures, they nevertheless are approached best through a lateral craniotomy. Although the lateral subfrontal approach is the shortest route to the ACoA region, it

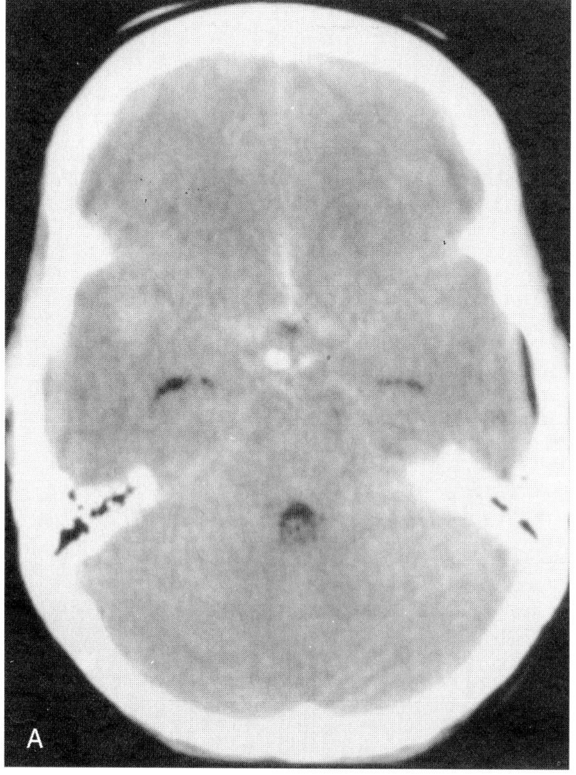

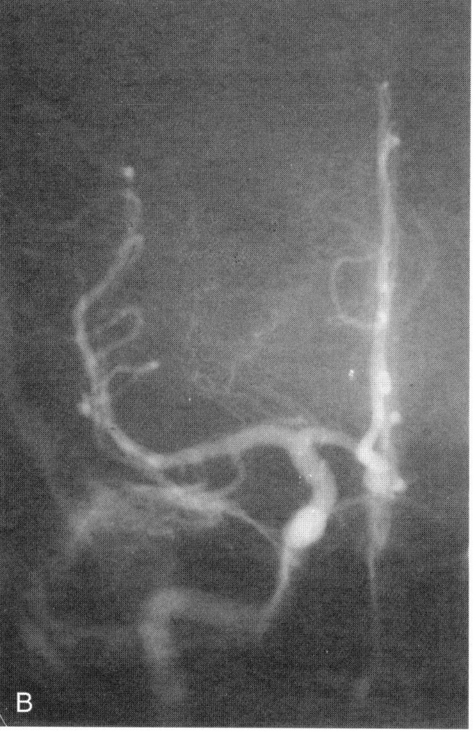

FIGURE 113–5. *A,* Subarachnoid hemorrhage with a slightly thicker clot in the interhemispheric fissure, which is characteristic of an anterior communicating artery (ACoA) aneurysm. *B,* Inferior/anterior-pointing ACoA aneurysm responsible for the hemorrhage.

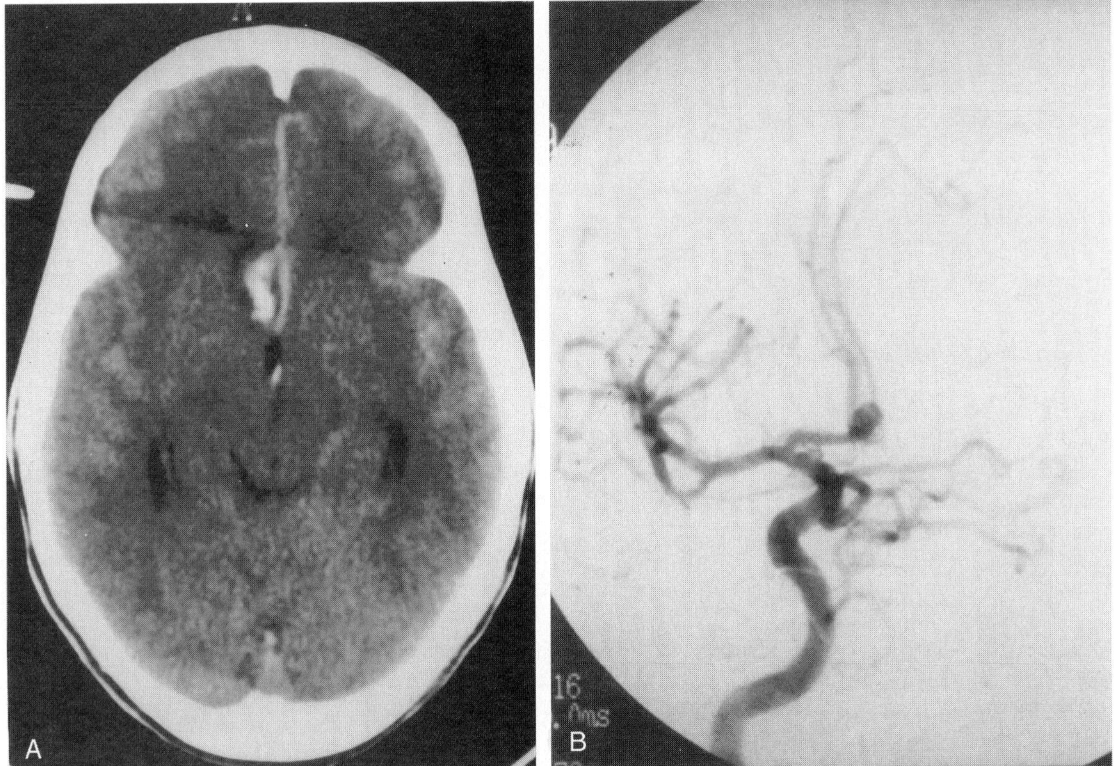

FIGURE 113–6. *A,* Subarachnoid hemorrhage accompanied by an intraparenchymal hemorrhage in the gyrus rectus, which is characteristic of an anterior communicating artery (ACoA) aneurysm. *B,* Superior-pointing ACoA aneurysm responsible for the hemorrhage.

has the disadvantage of requiring early retraction of the ipsilateral frontal lobe, which may decompress the aneurysm dome before identification of the paired A1 segments. Finally, there is an increased risk of ischemic injury during surgery of ACoA aneurysms because these lesions are associated intimately with 11 vessels and their perforators: the paired A1 segments, the paired A2 segments, the 2 medial striate arteries of Heubner, the 2 orbitofrontal arteries, the 2 frontopolar arteries, and the ACoA. There is no other aneurysm intimately associated with as many vessels. In this section, we expand the previous description of our microsurgical approach to midline and contralateral aneurysms,[34] which is ideal for ACoA aneurysms.

SURGICAL ADJUNCTS

Currently at our institution, we routinely use (1) mild hypothermia, (2) intraoperative electroencephalography and somatosensory evoked potential monitoring, (3) temporary clipping, (4) mild hypertension, (5) electroencephalographic burst suppression, and (6) intraoperative angiography during surgery of most aneurysms. Brain relaxation is obtained with a mannitol infusion, mild hyperventilation, drainage of the arachnoid cisterns, and fenestration of the lamina terminalis. In the case of some ACoA aneurysms, opening of the lamina terminalis may have to be delayed after the aneurysm is clipped because an inferior-pointing aneurysm may obstruct access to the lamina terminalis, or the dome of a posterior-pointing aneurysm may be prematurely decompressed with this maneuver. Opening the lamina terminalis may have the additional benefit of reducing the incidence of post-SAH chronic hydrocephalus.[35] Cerebrospinal fluid (CSF) drainage with an intraoperative intraventricular catheter (IVC) sometimes is necessary. The best insertion point for an intraoperative IVC is the one described by Paine and colleagues[36]: the apex of an isosceles right-angle triangle with a 3.54-cm base that starts at the sphenoid ridge and overlies the sylvian fissure and with 2.5-cm sides. A perpendicular pass of the IVC through this point enters the frontal horn just anterior to the foramen of Monro.

The approach described subsequently for ACoA aneurysms is also the best approach for A1 segment aneurysms and for A2 segment aneurysms that arise at the level of the orbitofrontal artery or 10 mm from the ACoA junction. Aneurysms that arise immediately inferior, anterior, or superior to the genu of the corpus callosum are approached best interhemispherically through a right anterior, frontal parasagittal craniotomy and are discussed later. These aneurysms typically are associated with either the frontopolar or callosomarginal arteries, which originate on average 14 mm and 43 mm from the ACoA junction.[8]

CHOICE OF THE SIDE OF THE CRANIOTOMY

We approach the aneurysm from the side of the dominant A1 segment. The paired A1 segments are of un-

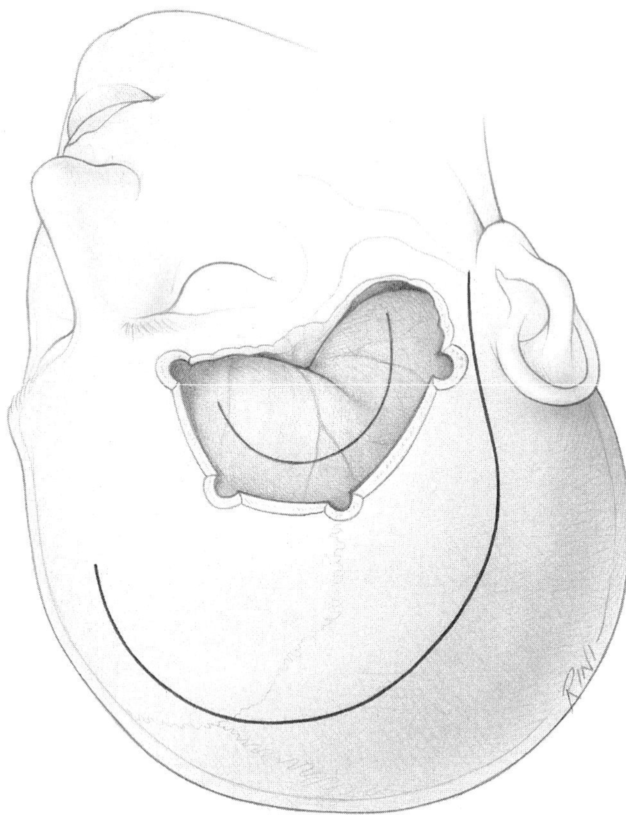

FIGURE 113–7. The frontosphenotemporal craniotomy. The incision is started a few millimeters anterior to the tragus at the upper border of the root of the zygoma and extended superiorly to the linea temporalis. At the linea temporalis, it is curved anteriorly to the midline, ending at the edge of the hairline.

Five bur holes are made. The anterior frontal bur hole should be about 2 cm off the midline in the midpupillary line and as low on the forehead as the skin flap allows. The keyhole bur hole should be positioned inferior to the linea temporalis and posterior to the frontozygomatic process to preserve the aesthetically important contours of these prominences. The temporal bur hole is made above the root of the zygoma. The stretch between the keyhole and the temporal bur hole is drilled. This stretch crosses the frontosphenoidal and the temporosphenoidal sutures and encompasses the lateral aspect of the greater wing of the sphenoid bone and the anterior inferior portion of the squamous portion of the temporal bone, just superior to the root of the zygoma. The fourth bur hole is made below the linea temporalis slightly on the coronal plane of the temporal bur hole. The fifth posterior frontal temporal hole is placed equidistant from the two adjacent bur holes.

After the bone flap is removed, the edge of the remaining temporal squamosal bone is removed with a Leksell rongeur starting above the root of the zygoma and proceeding anteriorly until the greater wing of the sphenoid is encountered. The frontal and temporal dura is peeled off the surface of the sphenoid wing. The greater wing of the sphenoid is drilled medially. This bulky, pyramidal structure gradually leads to a more slender structure, which is the lesser wing of the sphenoid. This is drilled until the dural sleeve of the orbitomeningeal artery is reached. Removal of these bony structures allows for a tangential approach to the circle of Willis along the posterior curve of the lesser wing of the sphenoid. The orbital roof and inner table of the frontal bone also are drilled at this stage. The roof of the orbit has several ridges that should be smoothed with the drill. It is important not to drill through the orbital roof into the periorbita because this technical error invariably results in a swollen, ecchymotic eye. The inner table of the frontal ledge should be drilled extensively. If the frontal sinus is entered, it should be exenterated, packed with muscle, and sealed with fibrin glue. Before replacing the

bone flap toward the end of the procedure, a pedicled galeal graft is reflected over the opening into the sinus, sutured to the dura, and pinched in place between the edges of the bone flap and frontal ledge.

The dura is opened in a curvilinear fashion from the medial edge of the craniotomy in the frontal region to the lateral edge of the craniotomy in the temporal region and reflected anteriorly. Three sutures are placed over the region of the sphenoid wing, the anterior fossa ledge, and the middle fossa ledge to retract the base of the dural flap, which otherwise may obstruct the view along the skull base.

equal diameter in 85% of cases of ACoA aneurysms.[9] The neck of the aneurysm typically originates on the side of the larger A1, and the dome is associated more closely with the side of the smaller A1. Approaching the aneurysm from the side of the dominant A1 has no significant benefit in terms of proximal control, but it is advantageous in the sense that the aneurysm neck is exposed before its dome. If the A1 segments are of equal diameter or the aneurysm dome is truly midline, we prefer a right (nondominant) craniotomy. Some surgeons advocate approaching all ACoA aneurysms from the nondominant side.

HEAD POSITION

The head is rotated 30 to 45 degrees away from the operative site. This maneuver, if done correctly, should render the malar or zygomatic eminence the highest point on the head as seen from the side. This head position allows the frontal lobe to fall away from the orbital roof and facilitates the microsurgical exposure.

INCISION

The incision is shown in Figure 113–7 and described in the legend. This incision is more aesthetic than one placed anteriorly along the edge of the hairline.

DISSECTION OF THE TEMPORALIS MUSCLE

The superficial fascia of the temporalis muscle is incised vertically about 1 cm anterior to the ascending limb of the skin incision and horizontally about 1 cm inferior to the linea temporalis and separated from the underlying temporalis fibers as described by Yasargil.[37] This protects the frontal branch of the facial nerve, which runs along the surface of this superficial temporalis fascia.[38] To reflect the temporalis muscle, it is divided superiorly with a monopolar cautery, leaving a 1.5-cm cuff attached to the skull.[39]

FRONTOSPHENOTEMPORAL (PTERIONAL) CRANIOTOMY

Five bur holes are made as shown in Figure 113–7 and described in the legend.

DRILLING THE GREATER AND LESSER SPHENOID WINGS

Drilling the lateral aspects of the greater and lesser wings of the sphenoid bone is one of the key features and crucial technical steps of this craniotomy, as shown in Figure 113–7 and described in the legend.

DURAL OPENING

The dura is opened as shown in Figure 113–7 and described in the legend. Sutures are placed over the region of the sphenoid wing, the anterior fossa ledge, and the middle fossa ledge to retract the base of the dural flap, which otherwise may obstruct the view along the skull base.

SYLVIAN FISSURE DISSECTION

Opening the sylvian fissure is an important maneuver even for midline aneurysms. Freeing the anterior frontal lobe from the burden of the temporal lobe allows for easier retraction of the frontal lobe. The sylvian fissure is on average 6 cm long and can be divided into three 2-cm portions or thirds. It is best to enter the fissure in its middle third (i.e., 2 to 4 cm measured from the curve of the lesser sphenoid wing). After opening the fissure in its middle third for a stretch of about 5 mm, the tip of a microirrigator is inserted into this opening, and the cistern is insufflated with several cycles of irrigation. This maneuver partially clears the hemorrhage and expands the subarachnoid space. Through the same 5-mm opening, the surgeon identifies an artery emerging from the fissure and follows it down, dissecting around it into the depth of the fissure.

The sylvian cistern consists of a shallow superficial space and a more capacious deep space. These two chambers are separated by approximation of the pia-arachnoid of the frontal and temporal opercula. When the deep sylvian cistern is opened, the larger M2 branches of the middle cerebral artery are seen coursing along the axis of the fissure. The most difficult portion of the fissure to open is the horizontal portion in its anterior third in front of the limen of insula. When the sylvian fissure is opened wide, the optic nerve and ICA can be reached with only minimal retraction of the frontal lobe.

This initial approach entirely through the sylvian fissure is particularly important in the case of an inferior-pointing ACoA aneurysm, which may have its dome attached to the optic chiasm, optic nerve, or dura of the interoptic space (see Fig. 113–4). With this type of ACoA aneurysm, the standard initial maneuver of retracting the frontal lobe until the olfactory nerve is seen may result in avulsion of the dome and a catastrophic hemorrhage too early in the exposure.

EXPOSURE OF THE OPTIC NERVE AND INTERNAL CAROTID ARTERY

The chiasmatic cistern envelops the optic nerve and is opened along the junction between the optic nerve and the frontal lobe. The carotid cistern envelops the ICA and is opened along the axis of the ICA. The ICA is followed distally to its bifurcation to expose the origin of the A1 segment. In addition to opening the chiasmatic and carotid cisterns, the interpeduncular cistern should be opened at this stage through either the optico-carotid triangle or the carotico-oculomotor triangle by incising Liliequist's membrane.

EXPOSURE OF THE IPSILATERAL AND CONTRALATERAL A1 SEGMENTS

Reaching the ipsilateral A1 segment is the first step in accomplishing proximal control of the aneurysm (Fig. 113–8). Only when both A1 segments are exposed can proximal control be accomplished, however, because the ACoA is almost always present (99.8% of cases[5]), and the aneurysm can be filled by either A1 segment. There is usually retrograde flow through the A2 segments when the A1 segments are occluded.

After the origin of the ipsilateral A1 segment is reached, it is dissected distally off the inferior surface of the frontal lobe. The medial striate artery of Heubner is identified either anterior or superior to the A1 segment.

The dissection of the A1 segment is continued distally beyond where most of the medial lenticulostriate perforators arise (see Fig. 113–8). The midpoint of the A1 segment is a good position to place a temporary clip because placement of a temporary clip on the A1 segment too close to the ACoA region may compromise placement of the permanent clip. Particular care

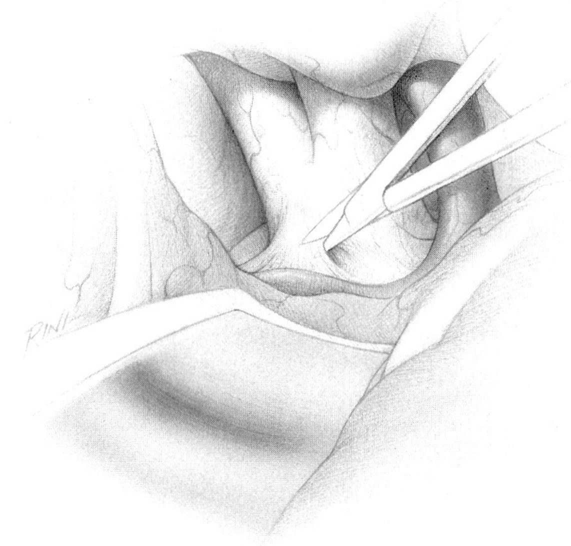

FIGURE 113–8. Initial microsurgical approach to the anterior communicating artery (ACoA) region. After dissecting the ipsilateral A1 segment and preparing its midportion for temporary clipping, the contralateral A1 segment is exposed. The ipsilateral opening of the chiasmatic cistern is extended over the anterior edge of the optic chiasm and over the distal contralateral optic nerve by following the anterior curve of the optic chiasm. This maneuver usually does not disturb most ACoA aneurysms, most of which (71.2%) project superiorly, anteriorly, or posteriorly into the interhemispheric fissure.[40] The contralateral optic nerve is dissected posteriorly until the A1 segment is seen draping over it. The contralateral A1 segment is dissected distally toward the interhemispheric fissure.

must be taken to avoid pinching the medial striate artery of Heubner with the temporary clip.

After dissecting the ipsilateral A1 segment and preparing its midportion for temporary clipping, the contralateral A1 segment is exposed as follows. The ipsilateral opening of the chiasmatic cistern is extended over the anterior edge of the optic chiasm and over the distal contralateral optic nerve (see Fig. 113–8). This is done by following the anterior curve of the optic chiasm. This maneuver usually does not disturb most ACoA aneurysms, most of which (71.2%) project superiorly, anteriorly, or posteriorly into the interhemispheric fissure.[40] Most ACoA aneurysms are found within the confines of the lamina terminalis cistern, which is separate from the chiasmatic cistern. At this point, if the aneurysm orientation permits it, it is usually helpful to fenestrate the lamina terminalis, which makes the remainder of the contralateral dissection easier. Fenestration of the lamina terminalis at this stage is not possible with an inferior-pointing aneurysm and may be risky with a posterior-pointing aneurysm.

The contralateral optic nerve is dissected posteriorly until the A1 segment is seen draped over it (see Fig. 113–8). The contralateral A1 segment is dissected distally toward the interhemispheric fissure. The midportion of the A1 segment is cleared, and a temporary clip is applied. This temporary clip application eliminates temporarily the second ACoA aneurysm feeder and leaves the ipsilateral A1 segment as the only feeder of the aneurysm. Because the ipsilateral A1 segment is usually dominant and because the ACoA is almost always present, temporary clipping of the contralateral A1 segment rarely results in significant somatosensory evoked potential changes.

In the case of an inferior-pointing or anterior-pointing aneurysm, it may be prudent to place a temporary clip on the ipsilateral A1 segment before initiating the contralateral dissection in search of the opposite A1 segment. These aneurysms have a propensity to rupture with slight retraction. When the contralateral A1 segment is identified and its temporary clip is applied, the temporary clip on the ipsilateral A1 segment is removed. The A1 segments are followed into the interhemispheric fissure to determine the location of the ACoA and the aneurysm.

GYRUS RECTUS RESECTION

Resection of the gyrus rectus is essential for adequate exposure of most ACoA aneurysms (Fig. 113–9). To resect the gyrus rectus, the retractor is repositioned over the medial orbital gyrus just lateral to the olfactory nerve aiming toward the estimated level of the ACoA junction in the interhemispheric fissure. The pia is cauterized with the bipolar forceps. At this point, the mean arterial pressure is raised about 10% above baseline, burst suppression is initiated, and if appropriate, a temporary clip is applied to the ipsilateral A1 segment. An incision is made longitudinally along the lateral aspect of the gyrus rectus. Using the suction and the bipolar cautery simultaneously, the gyrus rectus resection is accomplished rapidly until the medial pia-arachnoid of the gyrus rectus is recognized draped over the aneurysm and the ipsilateral A1 and A2 segments (see Fig. 113–9). This pial-arachnoidal remnant is resected, entering into the interhemispheric fissure and fully exposing the A1-ACoA-A2 complex.

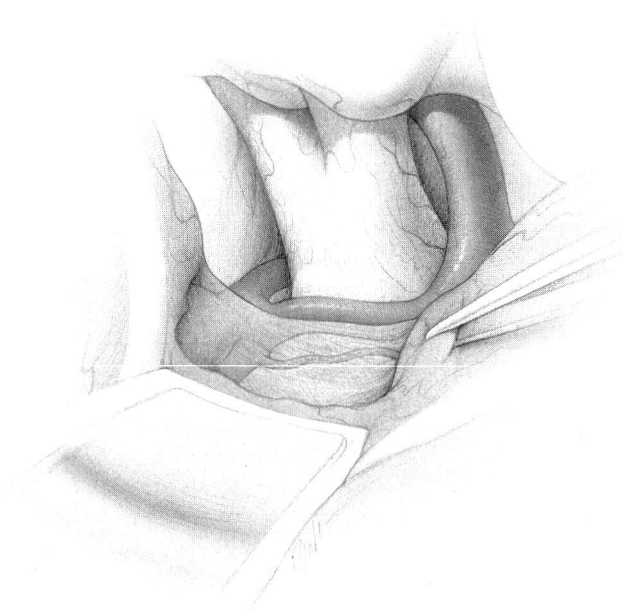

FIGURE 113–9. Resection of the gyrus rectus is essential for adequate exposure of most anterior communicating artery (ACoA) aneurysms. To resect the gyrus rectus, the retractor is repositioned over the medial orbital gyrus just lateral to the olfactory nerve aiming toward the estimated level of the ACoA junction in the interhemispheric fissure. The pia of the gyrus rectus segment to be resected is cauterized with the bipolar forceps. At this point, burst suppression is initiated, and if appropriate, a temporary clip is applied to the ipsilateral A1 segment. An incision is made longitudinally along the lateral aspect of the gyrus rectus. Using the suction and the bipolar cautery simultaneously, the gyrus rectus resection is accomplished rapidly until the medial pia-arachnoid of the gyrus rectus is recognized draped over the aneurysm and the ipsilateral A1 and A2 segments. This pial-arachnoidal remnant is resected, entering into the interhemispheric fissure and fully exposing the A1-ACoA-A2 complex.

IDENTIFICATION OF THE A1–ANTERIOR COMMUNICATING ARTERY–A2 COMPLEX VESSELS

The dissection is continued along the lateral aspect of the ipsilateral A1 segment to identify the ipsilateral A2 segment (Fig. 113–10). The ipsilateral medial striate artery of Heubner and the orbitofrontal artery are identified. From this point on, the dissection varies depending on the orientation of the aneurysm (see Fig. 113–4). In the case of superior-pointing aneurysms, the contralateral A1 segment can be exposed, and the distal course of the contralateral medial striate artery of Heubner can be identified, but the contralateral A2 segment is usually hidden. In the case of inferior-pointing aneurysms, the contralateral A2 segment and origin of the contralateral medial striate artery of Heubner can be exposed, but the contralateral A1 segment usually is hidden and may have to be traced backward following the course of the A2 segment from distal to proximal. Posterior-pointing aneurysms may or may not obstruct the view of the contralateral A2 segment, depending on the course of this vessel and the size of the aneurysm. Anterior-pointing aneurysms may obstruct partially the view of the contralateral A2 segment or the contralateral A1 segment. In any case, further sharp dissection of the neck and either displacement or mobilization of the aneurysm body usually are required to visualize the vessels initially hidden from view. Frequently the clip has to be applied without complete visualization of the hidden vessel and repositioned after decompression of the sac and further dissection.

Because the A2 segments enter the interhemispheric fissure one anterior to the other, the ACoA usually is oriented in an oblique or sagittal plane. It is crucial to keep this fact in mind when one is attempting to reconstruct mentally the anatomy of the complex during dissection and clipping.

After identifying the entering A1 segments, the exiting A2 segments, the ACoA, the medial striate arteries of Heubner, the orbitofrontal arteries, and the frontopolar arteries, the crucial perforators of the ACoA and A2 segments must be identified and cleared out of the path of the clip blades (see Fig. 113–10). Inadvertent occlusion or injury to these perforators can result in dramatic neurological, endocrine, or cognitive deficits. Meticulous preservation of all these vessels is the supreme challenge of clipping ACoA aneurysms.

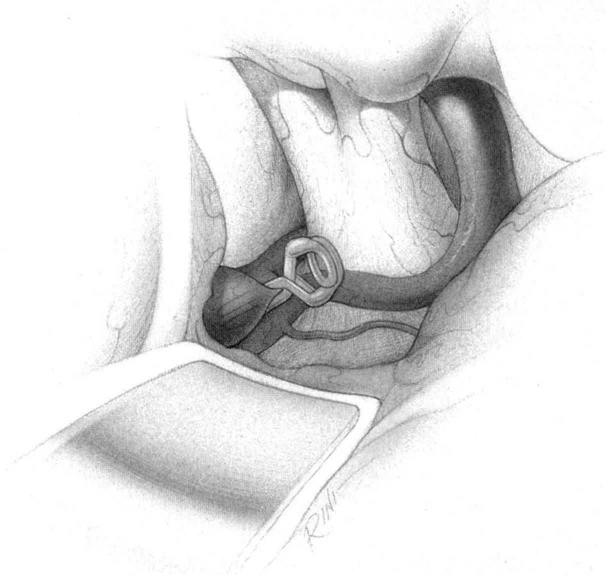

FIGURE 113–10. Clipping of a superior-pointing anterior communicating artery (ACoA) aneurysm. After identifying the entering A1 segments, the exiting A2 segments, the ACoA, the medial striate arteries of Heubner, the orbitofrontal arteries, and the frontopolar arteries, the critical perforators of the ACoA and A2 segments must be identified and cleared out of the path of the clip blades. Most ACoA aneurysms project superiorly (34.4% in Yasargil's series of 375 ACoA aneurysms[40]). Few ACoA aneurysms have necks that are ready to be clipped on initial exposure. With ACoA aneurysms, it is usually the case that an extended analysis of the neck, the lobes of the aneurysm, and their relationship to the critical vessels is necessary to figure out a safe clipping strategy. It is also not unusual that after application of the initial clip, the body and fundus of the aneurysm have to be reshaped with the bipolar forceps (aneurysmoplasty), and even part of the dome has to be resected to inspect the complex fully. This inspection often reveals the need either to reposition the clip or to apply a second or third clip. Superior-pointing aneurysms grow between the A2 segments. The posterior wall of their neck usually is associated intimately with the infundibular and hypothalamic perforators, which must be cleared and displaced below the path of the clip blade. Frequently, superior-pointing aneurysms have an additional complicating feature, which is that either one or both A2 segments may be densely adherent to the body of the aneurysm. When the ipsilateral A2 segment is not separated easily from the aneurysm neck, it is prudent to use a fenestrated clip around the ipsilateral A2 origin. Otherwise, if the neck can be separated from the adjacent A2 segments, a straight clip almost perpendicular to the ACoA may be adequate, as shown.

DISSECTION OF THE ANEURYSM NECK

The early dissection of superior-pointing and posterior-pointing aneurysms differs from that of the inferior-pointing and anterior-pointing aneurysms (see Fig. 113–4). Most ACoA aneurysms project superiorly, anteriorly, or posteriorly into the interhemispheric fissure, and a few project inferiorly out of the interhemispheric fissure and into the chiasmatic cistern.[18] In Yasargil's series of 375 ACoA aneurysms,[40] 34.4% projected superiorly, 22.7% projected anteriorly, 14.1% projected posteriorly, 12.8% projected inferiorly, and 16% had complex, multilobulated projections.

Superior-pointing and posterior-pointing aneurysms have the advantage of being buried in the interhemispheric fissure but have the disadvantage of being more intimately associated with the hypothalamic and infundibular perforators (see Fig. 113–4). Because they are contained within the interhemispheric fissure, they usually do not rupture when the retractor is placed across the interhemispheric fissure during the exposure of the contralateral A1 segment. By contrast, inferior-pointing aneurysms have the disadvantage of being usually adherent to the optic chiasm, optic nerves, or the interoptic space but the advantage of a more favorable relation to the hypothalamic and infundibular perforators. Similarly the dome of anterior-pointing aneurysms may be adherent to the gyrus rectus and may rupture during early subfrontal retraction.

Few ACoA aneurysms have necks that are ready to be clipped on initial exposure. With ACoA aneurysms more so than with other aneurysms, it is usually the case that an extended analysis of the neck, the lobes of the aneurysm, and their relationship to the crucial vessels is necessary to figure out a safe clipping strategy. It also is not unusual that either before or after application of the initial clip, the body and fundus of the aneurysm have to be reshaped with the bipolar forceps (aneurysmoplasty) and even part of the dome resected (after clip application) to inspect the complex fully.

This inspection often reveals the need to reposition the clip or to apply a second or third clip. If an aneurysmoplasty with the bipolar cautery is attempted, the surgeon must (1) rehydrate the sac with plenty of irrigation, (2) wax the tips of the bipolar forceps to prevent sticking, and (3) reduce the bipolar current to as low as possible and increase it as necessary until it starts to shrink the wall.

When exposed, anterior-pointing and inferior-pointing aneurysms are easier to clip than superior-pointing and posterior-pointing aneurysms because of their more favorable relationship to the infundibular and hypothalamic perforators (see Fig. 113–4). Anterior-pointing aneurysms have the most favorable anatomy in this respect because the crucial infundibular and hypothalamic perforators course in a direction opposite the aneurysm. A straight clip placed parallel to the ACoA typically spares these perforators. A complicating feature of interior-pointing aneurysms is, however, that the orbitofrontal or a proximal frontopolar artery is often adherent to the wall of the aneurysm and may have to be sacrificed during the clipping. A complicating feature of inferior-pointing aneurysms is that they often have infundibular and hypothalamic perforators adherent to the posterior aneurysmal wall. In the case of inferior-pointing aneurysms, the posterior wall always should be displaced anteriorly to visualize and separate the perforators before application of a straight clip. The orientation of the ACoA can be helpful with inferior-pointing and posterior-pointing aneurysms because a straight clip oriented exactly parallel to the course of the ACoA is usually ideal for these two types of aneurysms.

Superior-pointing aneurysms—the most common type of ACoA aneurysm—grow between the A2 segments. The posterior wall of their neck usually is associated intimately with the infundibular and hypothalamic perforators, which must be cleared and displaced below the path of the clip blade. Frequently, superior-pointing aneurysms have an additional complicating feature that either one or both A2 segments may be densely adherent to the body of the aneurysm. When the ipsilateral A2 segment is not separated easily from the aneurysm neck, it is prudent to use a fenestrated clip encircling the ipsilateral A2. Otherwise, if the neck can be separated from the adjacent A2 segments, a straight clip almost perpendicular to the ACoA may be adequate (see Fig. 113–10).

Posterior-pointing aneurysms are the most difficult and treacherous to clip because the crucial infundibular and hypothalamic perforators characteristically surround the neck of this aneurysm (see Fig. 113–4). The perforators may be found over the inferior wall or less commonly the superior wall of posterior-pointing aneurysms. An extended dissection of the perforators and more creative clip configurations usually are required for posterior-pointing aneurysms.

When the neck has been cleared completely of all perforators, a No. 7 microdissector is passed gently into the spaces where the clip blades will be inserted. It is important to ensure that the entire neck is cleared and that there is not a secondary lobe of the aneurysm that could be punctured with the clip blade. When dissecting right on the aneurysm, sharp dissection with either an arachnoid knife or microscissors is better than blunt dissection. Blunt dissection of the aneurysm neck can result in wide tears that are difficult to seal.

Although most aneurysm necks can be dissected and cleared with only one temporary clip on the dominant A1 segment, difficult aneurysms may require temporary clips on both A1 segments. There is usually adequate retrograde flow through the A2 segments. On rare occasions, the ACoA complex has to be isolated completely with temporary clips on the A1 and A2 segments for extensive dissection in preparation for clipping.

CLIP SELECTION AND APPLICATION

In selecting a clip, it is important to anticipate the final dimensions of the clipped aneurysm neck. The length of the selected clip should be *at least* 1.5 times the diameter of the aneurysm neck. This rule is derived from the fact that the circumference of the neck is its diameter multiplied by π or 3.1416 (circumference of a circle $= 2\pi r = \pi d$, where r = radius and d = diameter). As the neck is flattened by the clip blades, the length of the closed neck will be half that of its circumference, expressed as $1/2\pi d = 1.5d$ (because $\pi \simeq 3$ and $3 \div 2 = 1.5$). A 10-mm neck requires at least a 15-mm clip. In the case of a particularly broad neck, which often is encountered in ACoA aneurysms, the clip should be applied well above the origin of the aneurysm so that the tension on closure does not tear the origin of the aneurysm.

ASPIRATION OF THE DOME

After final clip placement, the dome is punctured and aspirated with a 25-gauge spinal needle attached to a short segment of intravenous tubing and a 5-mL syringe filled with saline. The intraoperative angiogram is not a substitute for a thorough microsurgical inspection of the aneurysm neck and the surrounding vessels. Refilling of the aneurysm, the telltale sign of partial clipping, often may be slow and subtle. It is evaluated best with puncture and aspiration of the aneurysm followed by an extended period of direct observation of the sac.

PAPAVERINE APPLICATION

At the end of the microsurgical portion of the procedure, papaverine is applied to all the exposed and manipulated arteries.

Complications of Anterior Communicating Artery Aneurysms

The general postoperative complications of aneurysm patients are reviewed in another chapter and elsewhere[32] and are not discussed here in detail. There are, however, two complications that are more common in patients with ACoA aneurysms that warrant further discussion: electrolyte abnormalities and cognitive dysfunction.

Patients with ruptured ACoA aneurysms have a high incidence of electrolyte abnormalities. The most common electrolyte abnormality in these patients is hyponatremia. In Yasargil's series of 371 ruptured ACoA aneurysms,[40] hyponatremia was present in 18.1% of patients preoperatively and in 40.5% postoperatively. It lasted 1 to 5 days in most patients (about 84%) and was more common in the higher grade patients. By contrast, hypernatremia was present in this series in only 1.6% of patients preoperatively and in 6.7% postoperatively. Although originally thought to be uniformly a manifestation of the syndrome of inappropriate antidiuretic hormone secretion,[41] post-SAH hyponatremia more commonly may be due to cerebral salt wasting.[42] Cerebral salt wasting first was described in 1950[43] and consists of the inability of the kidneys to retain sodium in the presence of central nervous system pathology, which results in hyponatremia and obligatory water loss during natriuresis.

Another common complication of patients with ruptured ACoA aneurysms is cognitive dysfunction. Logue and colleagues[44] were the first to document in a large series (79 patients) the cognitive and emotional sequelae associated specifically with ruptured ACoA aneurysms. In a later study of cognitive impairment in aneurysmal SAH patients without neurological deficits, Ljunggren and colleagues[45] also documented an association between ACoA aneurysms and marked cognitive dysfunction. Although only 14% of patients with no or mild cognitive dysfunction had ACoA aneurysms, 43% of patients with marked cognitive dysfunction had aneurysms in this location. A similar study by Bornstein and colleagues[46] reached the same conclusion. In this study, 28% of patients in the good cognitive outcome group had ACoA aneurysms, and 57% of patients in the poor outcome group had aneurysms in this location. Numerous studies have confirmed the association of ACoA aneurysm rupture or repair with cognitive dysfunction. This association occasionally has been referred to as the *ACoA syndrome*.[47] The characteristic deficits of this syndrome are impaired memory, personality changes, and confabulation. It generally is assumed that these deficits are the result of a "focal lesion" in the basal forebrain.[47]

OUTCOMES OF ANTERIOR COMMUNICATING ARTERY ANEURYSMS

This section reviews the improving outcomes of ACoA aneurysm patients over the past 5 decades by comparing surgical and overall mortality figures as reported in the literature. To assess the outcomes of aneurysm patients after treatment, we currently take into account not only mortality and neurological morbidity, but also the cognitive and emotional sequelae of the treatment. Earlier studies of aneurysm patients emphasized mortality figures, however, as the major, and sometimes the only, outcome measure. Even among modern studies, direct comparisons of outcomes are difficult because different groups use diverse neurocognitive outcome measures. We discuss in this section surgical and overall mortality figures but recognize the need to incorporate detailed neurocognitive outcome measures in all current studies.

Before the 1970s, the outcome of patients with ruptured ACoA aneurysms was dismal. Between 1958 and 1963, McKissock and colleagues[48] conducted a prospective randomized trial of 300 patients with ruptured ACoA aneurysms assigned to either medical (153 patients) or surgical (147 patients) treatment. The overall mortality for this group of patients was even higher than that documented for either treatment group because the exclusion criteria for the trial included, among others, irreversible neurological damage, coma, inoperable lesion, death before angiography, and obligatory surgery for a life-threatening hematoma. Outcomes were assessed 6 months after admission. Surgical treatment consisted of common carotid artery ligation in 21% of cases, ACA ligation in 40%, wrapping of the aneurysm in 25%, and clipping of the aneurysmal neck in only 14% of cases. Medical treatment was associated with a 40% mortality, and surgical treatment was associated with a 44% mortality. The mortality of the patients who underwent clipping of the aneurysmal neck was 37%. The proportion of patients who returned to full work was 41% in the medical group and 37% in the surgical group. These results reported by McKissock and colleagues[48] were typical for the period, as evidenced by the fact that similar operative mortality figures for the same period were reported in the original Cooperative Study of Intracranial Aneurysms and Subarachnoid Hemorrhage (1958–1965), in which the mortality associated with surgery for ACoA aneurysms was 36%.[49]

A few early neurosurgeons reported excellent surgical results in small series of selected patients with ruptured ACoA aneurysms. French and colleagues[50] reported a series of 25 patients with a 4% mortality, Hook and Norlen[51] reported 67 patients with a 7% mortality, and Pool[52] reported 56 patients with a 7% mortality. These encouraging results indicated that maybe better surgical techniques could produce better outcomes.

The surgical series of ACoA aneurysms reported by Yasargil and colleagues[18] in 1975 is arguably the first modern series for the treatment of these lesions. They reported 203 cases of ruptured ACoA aneurysms (grades I through IV) operated on by Yasargil between 1967 and 1974. All patients were operated on using Yasargil's microsurgical pterional approach. In 1984, Yasargil[40] published a detailed analysis of this extended ruptured ACoA aneurysm series, which at that point consisted of 371 cases with a total surgical mortality of 5.9%. Although these outstanding results established the standard against which surgical outcomes since have been measured, this series included only patients selected for surgery and does not provide an overall management mortality for each grade. This selection bias, which is described by the authors, is apparent in the relatively high proportion of good grade patients in this series (grades I and II = 298 of 374 [80%]) compared with that reported in the International Cooperative Study on the Timing of Aneurysm Surgery (1980–1983), which is the largest, most recent hospital-based series (fully alert = 1723 of 3521 [48.9%]).[2] A review of our own published series of ruptured aneurysms and that of other centers showed that 49.5% to 59.3% (average 54.4%) of patients were either grade I or II (Hunt and Hess scale) on admission.[53]

The most representative current figures on the specific surgical outcome and the overall management outcome of patients with ruptured ACoA aneurysms are found in the International Cooperative Study on the Timing of Aneurysm Surgery (1980–1983).[2, 54] In the Cooperative Study, ACoA and ACA aneurysms were reported together, and specific outcome figures for ACoA aneurysms were not provided. It is reasonable to assume, however, that most of these aneurysms (>95%[1]) were ACoA lesions and that the specific mortality statistics for ACoA aneurysms might be only slightly worse than those for the ACoA-ACA group as a whole. In the Cooperative Study, the surgical mortality for ACoA-ACA aneurysms was 16.8%, and the overall management mortality was 30.1%.[2] These mortality figures for ACoA aneurysms were slightly higher than the mortality figures for all aneurysms in this study, which had a 14.3% surgical mortality and a 26% overall management mortality.[2, 54]

In the 1990s, these outcome figures improved further in neurosurgical centers with dedicated cerebrovascular programs. Although there are currently few large published series of exclusively ACoA aneurysms treated in the 1990s,[55] it is reasonable to consider that the trend in outcomes of ACoA aneurysms has been similar to the trend in outcomes documented for all aneurysms. It is apparent that the aneurysm treatment outcomes in the 1990s are better than those reported in the International Cooperative Study on the Timing of Aneurysm Surgery (1980–1983).[2, 54] The Johns Hopkins Hospital rate of 17.8% overall management mortality of ruptured aneurysms treated between 1992 and 1996[53] represents an improvement over the 26% overall management mortality of the International Cooperative Study.[2] These improved statistics are typical for most major centers with dedicated cerebrovascular programs.

SURGICAL MANAGEMENT OF DISTAL ANTERIOR CEREBRAL ARTERY ANEURYSMS

Aneurysms that arise beyond the ACoA junction are referred to as *distal ACA aneurysms.* In the original Cooperative Study of Intracranial Aneurysms and Subarachnoid Hemorrhage (1958–1965), the incidence of distal ACA aneurysms was 2.8% of a total 2349 aneurysms.[1] A review of 17 large series of distal ACA aneurysms (each with ≥10 patients) reported in the literature between 1960 and 1990 provided a slightly higher average incidence of 4.8% (range 2% to 9.2%).[56] Distal ACA aneurysms are considered separately in this section because they have several unique features. Most importantly, they are the only aneurysms that routinely are approached interhemispherically.

Most distal ACA aneurysms are found in association with the major branches of the distal ACA—the orbitofrontal, frontopolar, and callosomarginal arteries. The anatomy of these arteries was discussed earlier. In relation to the corpus callosum, the orbitofrontal artery typically is found anterior to the rostrum of the corpus callosum, the frontopolar artery is found inferior to the genu, and the callosomarginal artery is found superior to the genu. Aneurysms associated with the frontopolar or callosomarginal arteries (14 to 43 mm from the ACoA junction) are approached best interhemispherically through a right frontal parasagittal craniotomy. By contrast, aneurysms associated with the orbitofrontal artery (5 mm from the ACoA junction) are approached best through a frontosphenotemporal craniotomy with a generous gyrus rectus resection, as described in the previous section for ACoA aneurysms. In this section, we discuss the microsurgical treatment of distal ACA aneurysms.

Clinical Series of Distal Anterior Cerebral Artery Aneurysms

The first report of a direct surgical treatment of a distal ACA aneurysm is probably that of Whalley from Newcastle-upon-Tyne, who performed the operation on June 5, 1947.[57] He carried out a right frontal craniotomy and a partial frontal lobectomy and trapped the aneurysm by applying two silver clips to the right ACA. He then excised the 2.4-cm lesion.[57]

Since the 1960s, several series of distal ACA aneurysms have been published. The largest series is that of Ohno and colleagues[56] from Tokyo, Japan (42 patients). They included in their report a comprehensive review of the literature.[56] Several characteristic features of distal ACA aneurysms are documented in their series and in most other representative series. Most patients (71%) presented with ruptured aneurysms. Most of the ruptured aneurysms were small; in 67% of cases, the aneurysms were less than 5 mm in diameter, and in only 10% of cases were they larger than 10 mm. A high proportion of patients (42.9%) had more than one aneurysm. Their review of the literature shows that on average 37.5% of distal ACA aneurysms present with other aneurysms. Most distal ACA aneurysms (81%) were located in the region of the genu of the corpus callosum, near the frontopolar or the callosomarginal arteries. They approached all lesions interhemispherically. Since the report of Ohno and colleagues,[56] only one other large series of distal ACA aneurysms (11 patients) has been published[58] with conclusions similar to those described earlier.

Clinical and Radiographic Presentations of Distal Anterior Cerebral Artery Aneurysms

The clinical presentation of distal ACA aneurysms includes two important scenarios that warrant discussion here. In a few cases, distal ACA aneurysms have either an infectious or a traumatic cause. It is important to recognize these two scenarios because they require different treatments.

The distal ACA is a common site for infectious aneurysms. Weir's review[59] of two large series revealed that the most common site for infectious aneurysms is the middle cerebral artery (39%) and that the ACA is a distant second (5%). Most of these lesions occur in patients with either acute or subacute bacterial endocarditis.[60] In 49.3% of cases, infectious aneurysms are found distal to the first bifurcation of a major cerebral artery. In the case of the distal ACA, this point is beyond the takeoff of the callosomarginal artery. It is important to recognize infectious aneurysms as such because they are treated best with an extended course of intravenous antibiotics and not with surgery. These lesions typically are fusiform, inflammatory dilatations of the vessel wall that do not tolerate clipping well and, if surgery is attempted, often end up requiring excision.

Traumatic aneurysms also are found often on the distal ACA. Of all traumatic aneurysms, 36.7% are found on the distal ACA and its branches.[61] The most common location of this type of aneurysm is, however, the middle cerebral artery (58% of cases).[61] It has been postulated that some distal ACA aneurysms arise from indirect trauma to the vessel wall from the free edge of the falx.[62, 63] Traumatic distal ACA aneurysms typically are found on the peripheral segments of the distal ACA branches, along the free edge of the falx. They most often are irregular and lack a neck. Contrary to infectious aneurysms, which are treated best medically with antibiotics, traumatic aneurysms have to be treated urgently with surgery, even if they have not ruptured. If left untreated, the natural history of these lesions is invariably one of growth and rupture.[64] In their review of the literature of 41 cases of traumatic aneurysms, Fleischer and colleagues[64] documented a 41% mortality for patients treated expectantly but an 18% mortality for those treated surgically.

Two features of the radiographic presentation of distal ACA aneurysms warrant special mention. First, these lesions may present on CT scan with either a contained SAH or a hematoma entirely within the interhemispheric fissure (Fig. 113–11*A*).[55, 56] There may be little or no SAH in the basal cisterns. This may happen because often the interhemispheric fissure is sealed by tight adhesions between the frontal lobes, particularly if the inferior edge of the falx is incompetent. Second, rarely ruptured distal ACA aneurysms may present with a convexity subdural hematoma, usually in association with an interhemispheric hematoma. We found eight such cases reported in Japanese abstracts.[66–69]

Operative Technique for Distal Anterior Cerebral Artery Aneurysms

The microsurgical approach to distal ACA aneurysms is the most interesting aspect of these lesions because they are the only aneurysms routinely approached interhemispherically (Fig. 113–12). These aneurysms present with aneurysms in other locations in 37.5% of cases.[56] Under these circumstances, the parasagittal craniotomy flap may be fashioned as an extension of a frontosphenotemporal flap. In this section, we describe the right anterior (precoronal) frontal parasagittal cra-

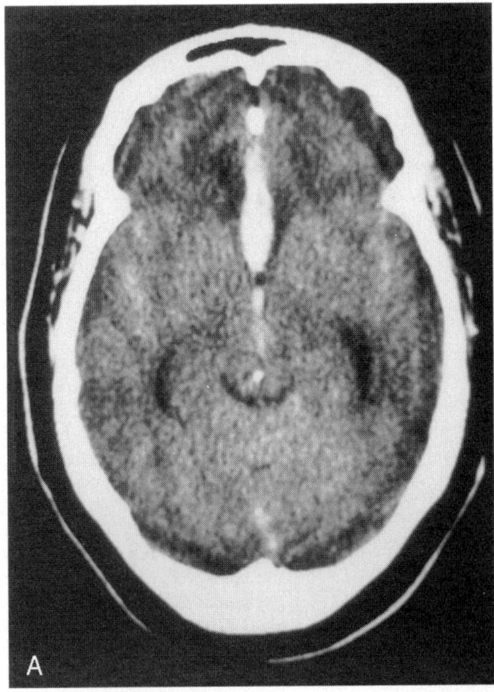

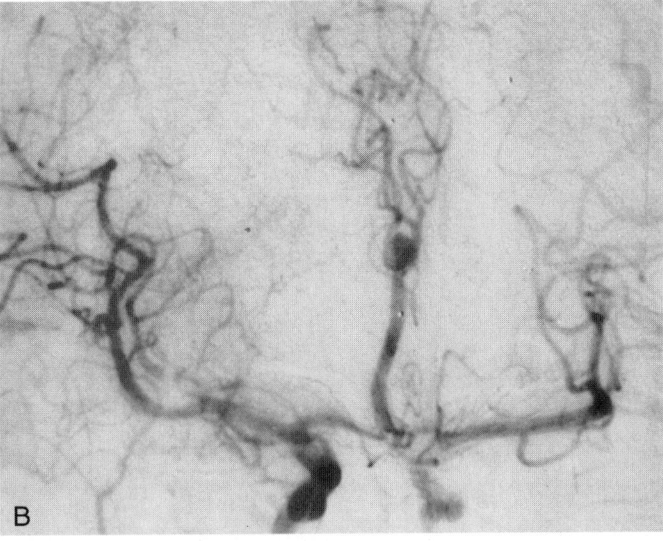

FIGURE 113–11. *A*, Contained interhemispheric fissure subarachnoid hematoma is common with distal anterior cerebral artery (ACA) aneurysms. *B*, Distal ACA aneurysm arising from an azygous A2 segment and responsible for the contained interhemispheric fissure subarachnoid hematoma.

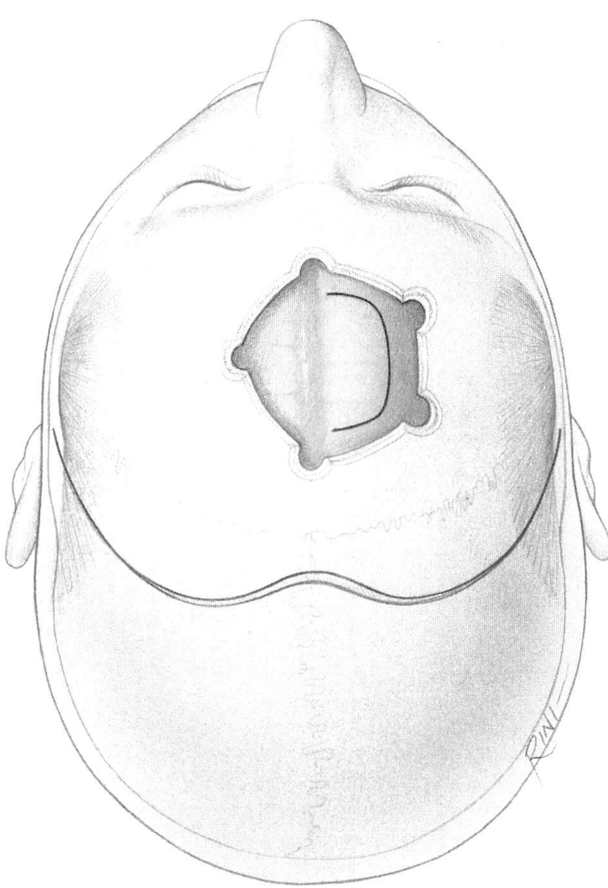

FIGURE 113–12. The anterior (precoronal) frontal parasagittal craniotomy for the interhemispheric approach to distal anterior cerebral artery (ACA) aneurysms is a pentagonal craniotomy with five bur holes. A bicoronal incision is made well beyond the horizon of the head (about 2 cm posterior to the coronal suture) from the root of the zygoma on the right to the same point on the left. The scalp is reflected anteriorly by carrying out a subfascial dissection of the temporalis musculature bilaterally to avoid injury to the frontal branch of the facial nerve. For most aneurysms of the distal ACA at the level of the callosomarginal artery origin, the following craniotomy is carried out. This craniotomy can be shifted slightly anteriorly for aneurysms at the level of the frontopolar artery or posteriorly for A4 or A5 segment aneurysms.

The right anterior (precoronal) frontal parasagittal craniotomy is a pentagonal craniotomy with five bur holes. Two lateral bur holes are placed 4 cm to the right of the midline (on the midpupillary line) and 2 and 6 cm anterior to the coronal suture. The posterior lateral bur hole (Kocher's point) can be used for placement of an intraventricular catheter. Two midline bur holes are placed over the superior sagittal sinus 2 and 7 cm anterior to the coronal suture. A single bur hole is placed 1.5 cm to the left of the midline and 4.5 cm anterior to the coronal suture, halfway between the midline bur holes. The bur holes are connected with the Gigli saw, creating a pentagonal flap 6 cm at its widest point along the midline. The dura is opened medially in a horseshoe pattern based on the sinus. There may be draining veins attached to the dural flap or bridging the interhemispheric cleft. These may need to be sacrificed for the approach, but in general it is best to preserve them.

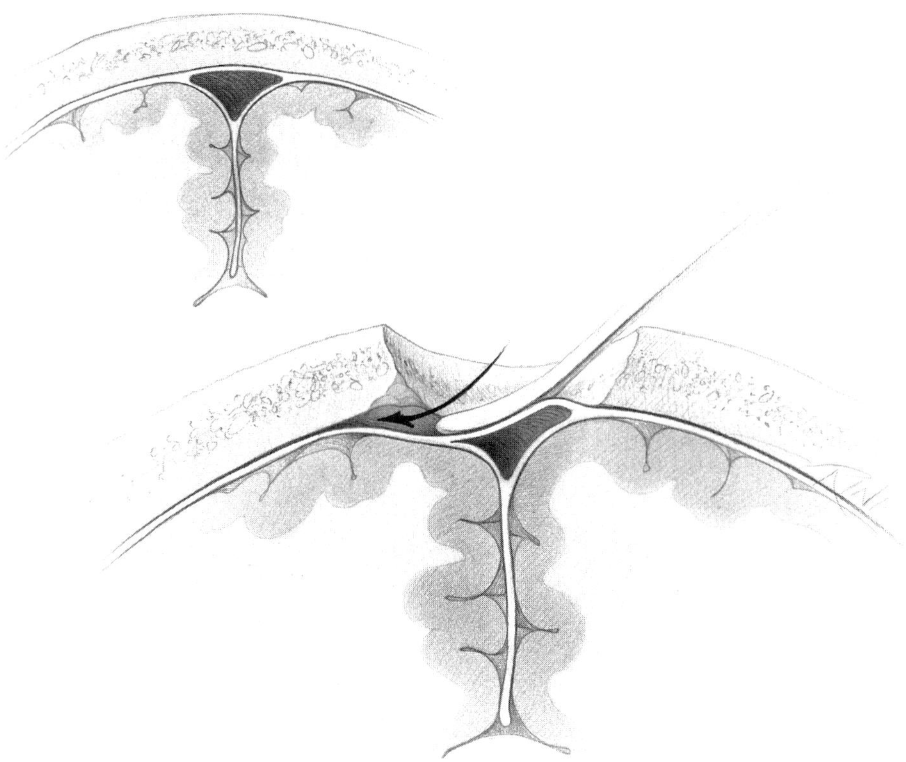

FIGURE 113–13. It is safer to place a midline bur hole directly over the sagittal sinus than to place paired bur holes astride the sinus, then connect them across the midline over the sinus. The midline bur hole should be made with a 5- or 6-mm cutting drill bit and not with the perforator, which has a higher probability of lacerating the sinus. Because the roof of the superior sagittal sinus often bows slightly into the inner table, working *toward* the midline from the paired parasagittal bur holes has a higher probability of tearing the sinus wall than working out laterally *from* the midline bur holes, as shown. The inner table of the midline bur hole is undermined laterally from the midline with 2- or 3-mm Kerrison punches.

niotomy for an aneurysm of the A2-A3 segments. If the aneurysm is found on the A4 or A5 segments, the same type of craniotomy is made further posteriorly.

SURGICAL ADJUNCTS

The same adjuncts described for ACoA aneurysms are used for distal ACA aneurysms with the following exception. Lumbar CSF drainage is important in distal ACA aneurysms because the interhemispheric approach provides access to at the most two arachnoid cisterns, the callosal cistern and rarely the lamina terminalis cistern. The callosal cistern is entered late in the interhemispheric approach, after most of the dissection has been completed, and has only a small amount of CSF. An alternative to a lumbar drain is passing an IVC. The IVC should be inserted through the right lateral posterior bur hole of the frontal parasagittal craniotomy (Fig. 113–12), which is placed at Kocher's point (4 cm from the midline on the midpupillary line and 1 to 2 cm anterior to the coronal suture) (Fig. 113–13).

HEAD POSITION

The head is secured in the Mayfield skull clamp with the single pin on the midline 1 to 2 cm superior to the glabella and the paired pins on the occipital region equidistant from the midline. The arm of the Mayfield skull clamp is swung toward the patient's left shoulder below the level of the external acoustic meatus. The head is positioned in the midline and extended about 15 degrees below the horizontal. The head can be tilted slightly to the right to allow the dependent frontal lobe to be retracted by gravity. It is important to raise the back of the table about 15 degrees to place the head above the level of the heart to promote venous drainage.

INCISION

A bicoronal incision is illustrated in Figure 113–12 and described in the legend.

CRANIOTOMY AND DURAL OPENING

The craniotomy and dural opening are illustrated in Figure 113–12 and described in the legend.

INTERHEMISPHERIC DISSECTION

The interhemispheric dissection can be difficult and tedious, particularly after SAH. Where the falx is incompetent, the medial surfaces of the frontal lobes often are fused. We favor starting the interhemispheric dissection as anteriorly as possible, where the frontal lobes are clearly apart. When the interhemispheric fissure is identified clearly, the dissection can be carried posteriorly and inferiorly aiming toward the most anterior point of the genu of the corpus callosum. At this location, the paired ACAs can be identified as they emerge from the infracallosal region and proximal control can be established. The ACAs then can be traced posteriorly to the region of the aneurysm. It is not unusual that a subpial dissection has to be pursued and that the aneurysm is "sculpted" out of the medial frontal parenchyma where it is often embedded.

In the case of distal ACA aneurysms at the level of the prefrontal artery and below the genu of the corpus callosum, it may be advantageous to split and resect the genu. This maneuver is associated rarely with cognitive morbidity.[70, 71]

ANEURYSM DISSECTION AND CLIPPING

Distal ACA aneurysms often incorporate the origin of their branch of origin (Fig. 113–14). Sharp dissection of the neck and temporary clipping with deflation of the aneurysm may be necessary to clear the neck for clip-

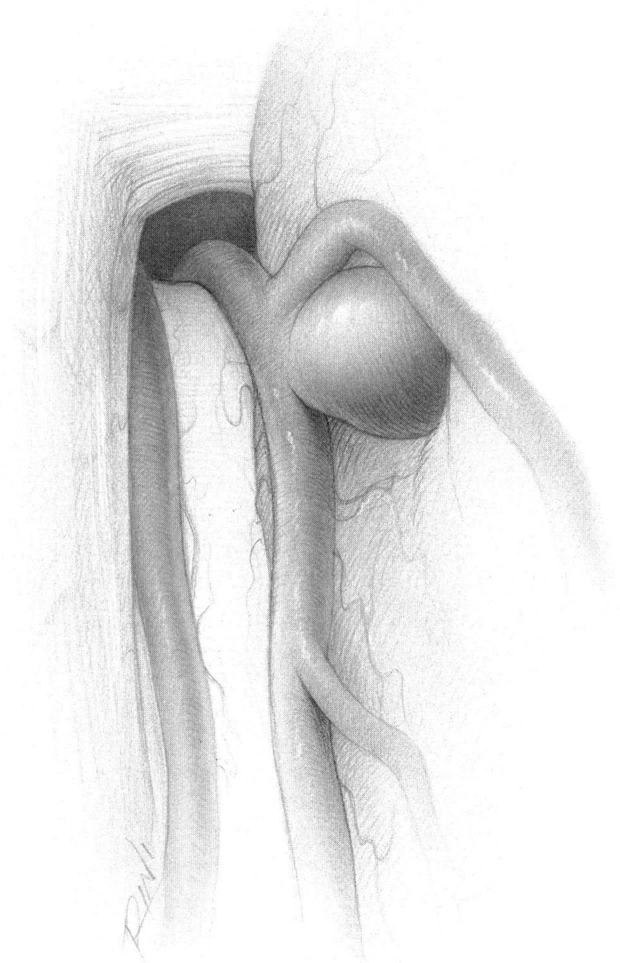

FIGURE 113–14. Distal anterior cerebral artery (ACA) aneurysm associated with the right callosomarginal artery. Distal ACA aneurysms often incorporate the origin of their branch of origin. Sharp dissection of the neck and temporary clipping with deflation of the aneurysm may be necessary to clear the neck for clipping, which often requires reconstruction of the main vessel and the involved branch with the clip. It is important to apply papaverine to these delicate vessels.

ping, which often requires reconstruction of the main vessel and the involved branch with the clip. It is important to apply papaverine to these delicate vessels. Traumatic and infectious distal ACA aneurysms are particularly difficult to clip because they are often fusiform dilatations of the vessel wall and may require either resection or reconstruction of the segment of origin.

Outcomes of Distal Anterior Cerebral Artery Aneurysms

The outcomes of distal ACA aneurysms have improved dramatically. Currently the outcomes of distal ACA aneurysms are better than for most other aneurysms. Hamilton and Falconer[72] reported the first series of distal ACA aneurysms in 1959. Of their six patients, two died (33%), three remained disabled (50%), and only one had a good result (17%). Ohno and colleagues[56] reported in 1990 good outcomes in most of their patients. Of their 42 patients, 4 died (9.5%), 2 had a poor outcome (4.8%), but 36 had a good outcome (85.7%), which represents a reversal of Hamilton and Falconer's figures.

REFERENCES

1. Locksley HB: Report on the Cooperative Study of Intracranial Aneurysms and Subarachnoid Hemorrhage. Section V, Part I: Natural history of subarachnoid hemorrhage, intracranial aneurysms and arteriovenous malformations: Based on 6368 cases in the Cooperative Study. J Neurosurg 25:219–249, 1966.
2. Kassell NF, Torner JC, Clark Haley J, et al, and participants: The International Cooperative Study on the Timing of Aneurysm Surgery. Part I: Overall management results. J Neurosurg 73: 18–36, 1990.
3. Hager Padget D: The development of the cranial arteries in the human embryo. Contrib Embryol 32:205–261, 1948.
4. Perlmutter D, Rhoton AL: Microsurgical anatomy of the anterior cerebral-anterior communicating-recurrent artery complex. J Neurosurg 45:259–272, 1976.
5. Hager Padget D: The circle of Willis: Its embryology and anatomy. In Dandy WE (ed): Intracranial Arterial Aneurysms. Ithaca, NY, Comstock Publishing Company, 1944, pp 67–90.
6. Baptista AG: Studies of the arteries of the brain: II. The anterior cerebral artery: Some anatomic features and their clinical implications. Neurology 13:825–835, 1963.
7. Huber P, Braun J, Hirschmann D, Agyeman JF: Incidence of berry aneurysms of the unpaired pericallosal artery: Angiographic study. Neuroradiology 19:143–147, 1980.
8. Perlmutter D, Rhoton AL: Microsurgical anatomy of the distal anterior cerebral artery. J Neurosurg 49:204–228, 1978.
9. Wilson G, Riggs HE, Rupp C: The pathologic anatomy of ruptured cerebral aneurysms. J Neurosurg 11:128–134, 1954.
10. Truex R, Carpenter M: Human Neuroanatomy. Baltimore, Williams & Wilkins, 1969.
11. Yasargil MG: Microneurosurgery: I. Microsurgical Anatomy of the Basal Cisterns and Vessels of the Brain, Diagnostic Studies, General Operative Techniques and Pathological Considerations of the Intracranial Aneurysms. New York, Georg Thieme Verlag/Thieme Stratton, 1984.
12. Rosner SS, Rhoton AL, Ono M, Barry M: Microsurgical anatomy of the anterior perforating arteries. J Neurosurg 61:468–485, 1984.
13. Dunker RO, Harris AB: Surgical anatomy of the proximal anterior cerebral artery. J Neurosurg 44:359–367, 1976.
14. Crowell RM, Morawetz RB: The anterior communicating artery has significant branches. Stroke 8:272–273, 1977.
15. Haroun RI, Rigamonti D, Tamargo RJ: Recurrent artery of Heubner: Otto Heubner's description of the artery and his influence on pediatrics in Germany. J Neurosurg 93:1084–1088, 2000.
16. Gomes F, Dujovny M, Umansky F, et al. Microsurgical anatomy of the recurrent artery of Heubner. J Neurosurg 60:130–139, 1984.
17. Yasargil MG, Fox JL: The microsurgical approach to intracranial aneurysms. Surg Neurol 3:7–14, 1975.
18. Yasargil MG, Fox JL, Ray MW: The operative approach to aneurysms of the anterior communicating artery. In Krayenbuhl HA (ed): Advances and Technical Standards in Neurosurgery. New York, Springer-Verlag, 1975, pp 113–170.
19. Dandy WE: Intracranial aneurysm of the carotid artery cured by operation. Ann Surg 107:654–659, 1938.
20. Dandy WE: Aneurysm of the anterior cerebral artery. JAMA 119: 1253–1254, 1942.
21. Dandy WE: Intracranial Arterial Aneurysms. Ithaca, NY, Comstock Publishing Company, 1944.
22. Heuer GJ, Dandy WE: A new hypophysis operation. Johns Hopkins Hosp Bull 29:154–155, 1918.
23. Kempe LG: Operative Neurosurgery. New York, Springer-Verlag, 1968.
24. Norlen G, Barnum AS: Surgical treatment of aneurysms of the anterior communicating artery. J Neurosurg 10:634–650, 1953.
25. Kempe LG, VanderArk GD: Anterior communicating artery aneurysms: Gyrus rectus approach. Neurochirurgia (Stuttg) 14:63–70, 1971.
26. Tonnis W: Erfolgreiche Behandlung eines Aneurysma der Art. commun. ant. cerebri. Zentralblatt fur Neurochirurgie 1:39–42, 1936.
27. Pool JL: Early treatment of ruptured intracranial aneurysms of the circle of Willis with special clip technique. Bull N Y Acad Med 35:357–369, 1959.
28. Pool JL: Aneurysms of the anterior communicating artery: Bifrontal craniotomy and routine use of temporary clips. J Neurosurg 18:98–112, 1961.
29. Fukushima T, Miyazaki S, Takusagawa Y, Reichman M: Unilateral interhemispheric keyhole approach for anterior cerebral artery aneurysms. Acta Neurochir Suppl 53:42–47, 1991.
30. Suzuki J, Mizoi K, Yoshimoto T: Bifrontal interhemispheric approach to aneurysms of the anterior communicating artery. J Neurosurg 64:183–190, 1986.
31. Yeh H-S, Tew JT: Anterior interhemispheric approach to aneurysms of the anterior communicating artery. Surg Neurol 23: 98–100, 1985.
32. Tamargo RJ, Walter KA, Oshiro EM: Aneurysmal subarachnoid hemorrhage: Prognostic features and outcomes. New Horiz 5: 364–375, 1997.
33. Iwanaga H, Wakai S, Ochiai C, et al. Ruptured cerebral aneurysms missed by initial angiographic study. Neurosurgery 27: 45–51, 1990.
34. Oshiro EM, Rini DA, Tamargo RJ: Contralateral approaches to bilateral cerebral aneurysms: A microsurgical anatomical study. J Neurosurg 87:163–169, 1997.
35. Tomasello F, d'Avella D, deDivitis O: Does lamina terminalis fenestration reduce the incidence of chronic hydrocephalus after subarachnoid hemorrhage? Neurosurgery 45:827–832, 1999.
36. Paine JT, Batjer HH, Ray MW: Intraoperative ventricular puncture: Technical note. Neurosurgery 22:1107–1109, 1988.
37. Yasargil MG, Reichman MD, Kubik S: Preservation of the frontotemporal branch of the facial nerve using the interfascial temporalis flap for pterional craniotomy. J Neurosurg 67:463–466, 1987.
38. Ammirati M, Spallone A, Ma J, et al: An anatomicosurgical study of the temporal branch of the facial nerve. Neurosurgery 33: 1038–1044, 1993.
39. Spetzler RF, Lee KS: Reconstruction of the temporalis muscle for the pterional craniotomy: Technical note. J Neurosurg 73: 636–637, 1990.
40. Yasargil MG: Microneurosurgery: II. Clinical Considerations, Surgery of the Intracranial Aneurysms and Results. New York, Georg Thieme Verlag/Thieme Stratton, 1984.
41. Doczi T, Bende J, Huszka E, Kiss J: Syndrome of inappropriate secretion of antidiuretic hormone after subarachnoid hemorrhage. Neurosurgery 9:394–397, 1981.
42. Harrigan MR: Cerebral salt wasting: A review. Neurosurgery 38: 152–160, 1996.
43. Peters JP, Welt LG, Sims EAH, et al: A salt wasting syndrome associated with cerebral disease. Trans Assoc Am Physicians 63: 57–64, 1950.

44. Logue V, Durward M, Pratt RTC, et al: The quality of survival after rupture of an anterior cerebral aneurysm. Br J Psychiatry 114:137–160, 1968.
45. Ljunggren B, Sonesson B, Saveland H, Brandt L: Cognitive impairment and adjustment in patients without neurological deficits after aneurysmal SAH and early operation. J Neurosurg 62: 673–679, 1985.
46. Bornstein RA, Weir BKA, Petruk KC, Disney LB: Neuropsychological function in patients after Subarachnoid hemorrhage. Neurosurgery 21:651–654, 1987.
47. DeLuca J: Cognitive dysfunction after aneurysm of the anterior communicating artery. J Clin Exp Neuropsychol 14:924–934, 1992.
48. McKissock W, Richardson A, Walsh L: Anterior communicating aneurysms: A trial of conservative and surgical treatment. Lancet 1:873–876, 1965.
49. Skultety FM, Nishioka H: Report on the Cooperative Study of Intracranial Aneurysms and Subarachnoid Hemorrhage. Section VIII, Part 2: The results of intracranial surgery in the treatment of aneurysms. J Neurosurg 25:683–704, 1966.
50. French LA, Zarling ME, Schultz EA: Management of aneurysms of the anterior communicating artery. J Neurosurg 19:870–876, 1962.
51. Hook O, Norlen G: Aneurysms of the anterior communicating artery. Acta Neurol Scand 40:219–240, 1964.
52. Pool JL: Bifrontal craniotomy for anterior communicating artery aneurysms. J Neurosurg 36:212–220, 1972.
53. Oshiro EM, Walter KA, Piantadosi S, et al: A new subarachnoid hemorrhage grading system based on the Glasgow Coma Scale: A comparison with the Hunt and Hess and World Federation of Neurological Surgeons Scales in a clinical series. Neurosurgery 41:140–148, 1997.
54. Kassell NF, Torner JC, Jane JA, et al, and participants: The International Cooperative Study on the Timing of Aneurysm Surgery. Part 2: Surgical results. J Neurosurg 73:37–47, 1990.
55. Lin CL, Kwan AL, Howng SL: Surgical outcome of anterior communicating artery aneurysms. Kaohsiung J Med Sci 14:561–568, 1998.
56. Ohno K, Monma S, Suzuki R, et al: Saccular aneurysms of the distal anterior cerebral artery. Neurosurgery 27:907–913, 1990.
57. Whalley N: Ruptured congenital aneurysm of anterior cerebral artery: Report of a case with successful surgical removal. J Neurol Neurosurg Psychiatry 12:322–324, 1949.
58. Martines F, Blundo C, Chiappetta F: Surgical treatment of the distal anterior cerebral artery aneurysms. J Neurosurg Sci 40: 189–194, 1996.
59. Weir B: Special aneurysms (nonsaccular and saccular): Part I. Nonsaccular. Infective. Bacterial. In Aneurysms Affecting the Nervous System. Baltimore, Williams & Wilkins, 1987, pp. 159–168.
60. Bohmfalk GL, Story JL, Wissinger JP, Brown WE: Bacterial intracranial aneurysm. J Neurosurg 48:369–382, 1978.
61. Asari S, Nakamura S, Yamada O, et al: Traumatic aneurysm of peripheral cerebral arteries: Report of two cases. J Neurosurg 46: 795–803, 1977.
62. Benoit BG, Wortzman G: Traumatic cerebral aneurysms: Clinical features and natural history. J Neurol Neurosurg Psychiatry 36: 127–138, 1973.
63. Smith KR, Bardenheier JA: Aneurysm of the pericallosal artery caused by closed cranial trauma. J Neurosurg 29:551–554, 1968.
64. Fleischer AS, Patton JM, Tindall GT: Cerebral aneurysms of traumatic origin. Surg Neurol 4:223–239, 1975.
65. Fein J, Rovit R: Interhemsipheric subdural hematoma secondary to hemorrhage from a calloso-marginal artery aneurysm. Neuroradiology 1:183–186, 1970.
66. Ban S, Sato S, Yamamoto T, Ogata M: Distal anterior cerebral artery aneurysm causing acute subdural hematoma. No Shinkei Geka 13:911–916, 1985.
67. Hashizume K, Nukui H, Horikoshi T, et al: Giant aneurysm of the azygos anterior cerebral artery associated with acute subdural hematoma—case report. Neurol Med Chir (Tokyo) 32:693–697, 1992.
68. Kamiya K, Inagawa T, Yamamoto M, Monden S: Subdural hematoma due to ruptured intracranial aneurysm. Neurol Med Chir (Tokyo) 31:82–86, 1991.
69. Watanabe K, Wakai S, Okuhata S, Nagai M: Ruptured distal anterior cerebral artery aneurysms presenting as acute subdural hematoma—report of three cases. Neurol Med Chir (Tokyo) 31: 514–517, 1991.
70. Dickey PS, Bloomgarden GM, Arkins TJ, Spencer DD: Partial callosal resection for pericallosal aneurysms. Neurosurgery 30: 136–137, 1992.
71. Traynelis VC, Dunker RO: Interhemispheric approach with callosal resection for distal anterior cerebral artery aneurysms. J Neurosurg 77:481–483, 1992.
72. Hamilton JG, Falconer MA: Immediate and late results of surgery in cases of saccular intracranial aneurysms. J Neurosurg 16: 514–541, 1959.
73. Dott NM: Intracranial aneurysms: Cerebral arterio-radiography: Surgical treatment. Edinburgh Med J 40:219–234, 1933.
74. Logue V: Surgery in spontaneous subarachnoid hemorrhage. 1:473–479, 1956.

CHAPTER **114**

Distal Anterior Cerebral Artery Aneurysms

DAVID A. STEVEN ■ GARY G. FERGUSON

Aneurysms of the distal anterior cerebral artery (ACA) arise on the ACA or its branches distal to the anterior communicating artery (ACoA). Aneurysms in this location are relatively uncommon, representing approximately 5% of all intracranial aneurysms.[1–7] Distal ACA aneurysms most commonly occur at the bifurcation of the callosomarginal artery and the main trunk of the distal ACA and are frequently associated with other intracranial aneurysms. Their location in the interhemispheric fissure and frequent association with intraparenchymal hemorrhage present the neurosurgeon with a considerable technical challenge.

HISTORICAL BACKGROUND

In 1948, Sugar and Tinsley[8] reported the first attempt to treat a distal ACA aneurysm surgically. Their patient, a 19-year-old woman, presented with subarachnoid hemorrhage (SAH). The aneurysm was approached using an interhemispheric route. Although they were able to identify the dorsal surface of the corpus callosum, they were unable to locate the aneurysm and therefore clipped the feeding ACA. The patient survived with a left-sided hemiparesis. This case illustrates the difficulties faced by neurosurgeons managing these aneurysms before the development of microsurgical techniques for aneurysm surgery.

In the premicrosurgical era, intracranial surgery for distal ACA aneurysms was associated with a high perioperative mortality, comparable to that for aneurysms at other sites. In one cooperative study,[9] ruptured aneurysms in this location carried a perioperative mortality of 32%, compared with an overall mortality rate of 31% for all patients in the study subjected to an intracranial procedure. In 1973, Snyckers and Drake[10] reported a series of 20 operative cases with a perioperative mortality of 10% and major perioperative morbidity of 15%. The only series in the premicrosurgical era with a low perioperative mortality was that of Yoshimoto and colleagues,[11] who reported a rate of 2.9% in a series of 34 cases. However, this series differed from the other early reports in that 79% of the patients had a favorable preoperative clinical grade.

Since the advent of the microsurgical era,[12] the reported perioperative mortality rate for distal ACA aneurysms has declined significantly, in keeping with the rates for aneurysms at most other sites. In eight reports since 1984,[2–7, 13, 14] the average perioperative mortality rate was 7.1% (0% to 14%). The major perioperative morbidity rate in these eight reports remained relatively high, averaging 9.7% (0% to 17.9%). It is evident that these aneurysms represent a continuing challenge.

ANATOMY

The complex anatomy of the distal ACA is presented in Figure 114–1. The ACA distal to the ACoA passes anterior to the lamina terminalis to enter the longitudinal (interhemispheric) fissure. The vessel then courses tightly around the corpus callosum in the pericallosal cistern, giving rise to a number of central and cortical branches. It continues as a fine branch behind the splenium of the corpus callosum, terminating in the choroid plexus of the third ventricle. The distal ACA receives collateral flow from cortical branches of the middle cerebral artery and the posterior pericallosal branch of the posterior cerebral artery.

There have been a number of proposals to describe the anatomy of the distal ACA; most accepted is that of Perlmutter and Rhoton.[15] They divided the ACA into five segments (A1 to A5). A1 is the segment proximal to the ACoA. The remaining segments (A2 to A5) constitute the distal ACA. A2 extends from the ACoA to the junction of the rostrum and the genu of the corpus callosum. A3 ascends superiorly around the genu, ending where the vessel takes a sharp turn posteriorly. The A4 and A5 segments are located above the corpus callosum, the point of division occurring just posterior to the line of the coronal suture.

The branches of the distal ACA are either central or cortical. The central (basal perforating) branches terminate in the suprachiasmatic area, anterior diencephalon, septum pellucidum, and corpus callosum. In the anatomic study of Perlmutter and Rhoton,[15] there was great variability in the number of central branches

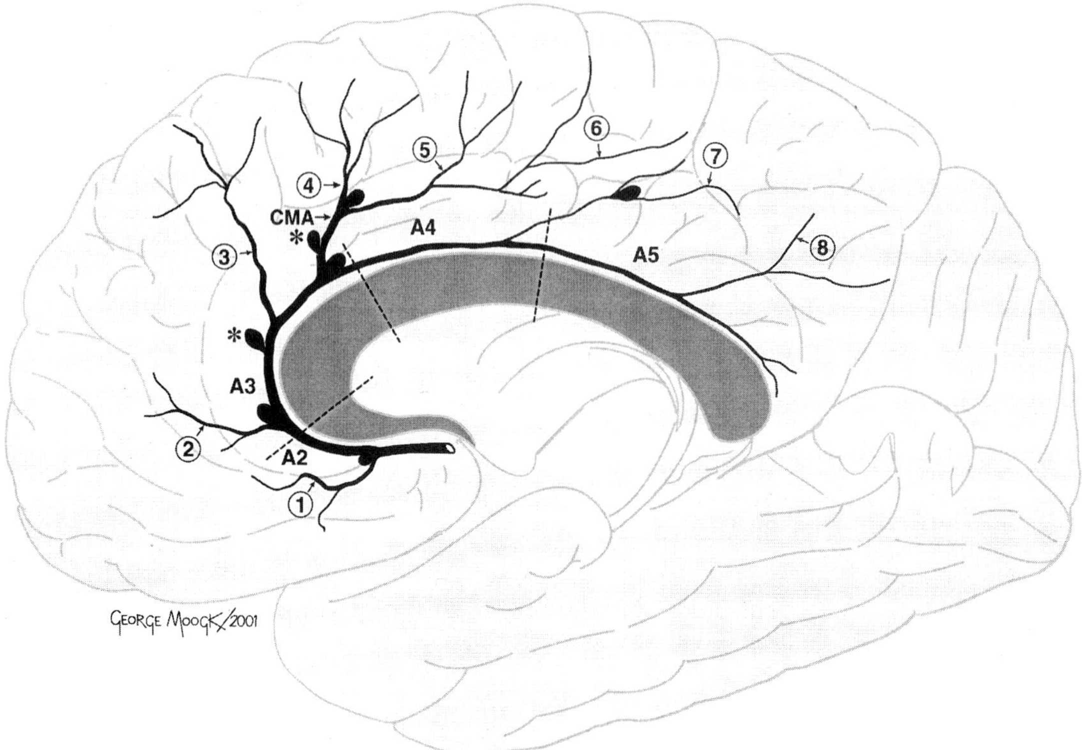

FIGURE 114–1. Schematic representation of the anatomy of the distal anterior cerebral artery (ACA) and possible sites for aneurysms. 1, orbitofrontal artery; 2, frontopolar artery; 3, anterior internal frontal artery; 4, middle internal frontal artery and callosomarginal artery (CMA); 5, posterior internal frontal artery; 6, paracentral artery; 7, superior parietal artery; 8, inferior parietal artery. The most common sites for distal ACA aneurysms are at the origins of the CMA and frontopolar artery. (* denotes typical sites for traumatic aneurysms of the distal ACA.)

(an average of five arose from the A2 segment, and approximately three arose from each of the A3, A4, and A5 segments).

The eight cortical branches of the distal ACA are the orbitofrontal, frontopolar, anterior internal frontal, middle internal frontal, posterior internal frontal, paracentral, and superior and inferior parietal arteries. The largest branch of the distal ACA, the callosomarginal artery (CMA), usually arises from the A3 segment, at an average distance of 43 mm from the ACoA.[15] The CMA is the most common site for distal ACA aneurysms. The CMA gives rise to a variable number of cortical branches—most commonly, the middle internal frontal artery, followed by posterior and anterior internal frontal arteries and the paracentral artery, and less commonly the superior parietal artery. The frontopolar artery usually arises from the A2 segment and is the second most common site of distal ACA aneurysms.

The term *pericallosal artery* has been used variably in the literature. Some authors define the pericallosal artery as that segment of the distal ACA continuing beyond the origin of the CMA, and others use the term to describe the ACA distal to the ACoA. Because the CMA is not always present, to avoid confusion, Perlmutter and Rhoton recommended that the term *pericallosal artery* refer to the ACA beginning at the ACoA, in which case, it is synonymous with the term *distal ACA.*

Anomalies of the distal ACA are common (Fig. 114–2). Baptista,[16] in a detailed anatomic study of 381 specimens, recognized three common variations in addition to the usual pattern of the distal ACA. In the usual pattern, both A2 segments arise from the ipsilateral A1 segment to supply the ipsilateral hemisphere. Baptista found this pattern in 75% of his specimens. In the type I (unpaired, or azygous) variation, a single A2 segment arises from the junction of both A1 segments, which subsequently divides to supply both hemispheres. Baptista found this variation in only one of his specimens. In the type II (bihemispheric) variation, one A2 segment supplies a significant portion of the contralateral hemisphere; the other A2 segment is hypoplastic, giving rise to the most proximal cortical branches only. In the type III (accessory) variation, there is a triplication of the A2 vessels, with a smaller median artery supplying a portion of either or both hemispheres. Although type I variations are rare, they are relatively commonly associated with distal ACA aneurysms, with a reported incidence of 7% to 10% (Fig. 114–3).[3, 6, 13]

Although aneurysms may arise at any bifurcation formed by the distal ACA and its branches (see Fig. 114–1), the origin of the CMA is the most common site, representing 50% to 60% of all cases.[17] The second most common site is at the origin of the frontopolar artery, accounting for 10% to 20% of cases. Aneurysms that

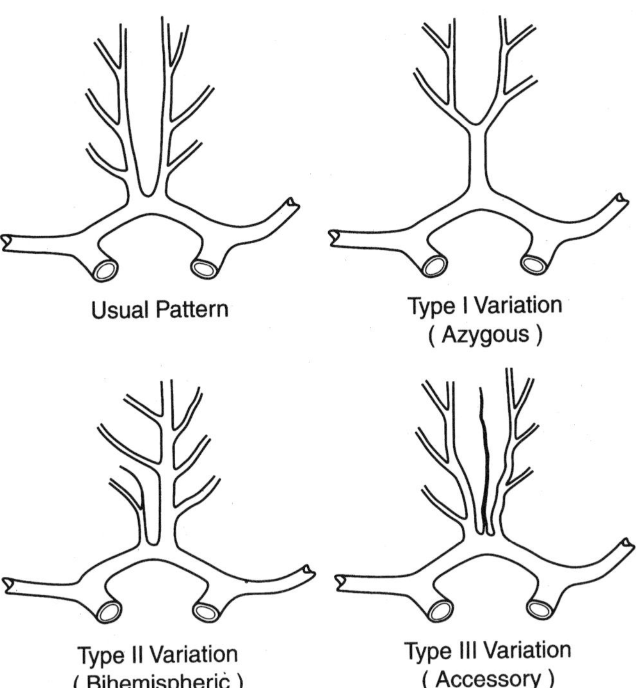

FIGURE 114–2. The usual pattern and common variations of the anatomy of the distal anterior cerebral artery based on the anatomic studies of Baptista[16] and adapted from Royand and colleagues.[17]

develop in association with an azygous A2 segment form at the bifurcation of that vessel into bilateral A3 segments.

In general, ruptured aneurysms of the distal ACA are smaller than ruptured intracranial aneurysms at other sites. Ohno and coworkers[6] found that in 67% of their cases, the ruptured aneurysm was less than 5 mm in diameter. The mean size of distal ACA aneurysms in the series of Hernesniemi and associates[5] was 8.1 mm, whereas that of 1002 aneurysms in other locations was 11.3 mm.

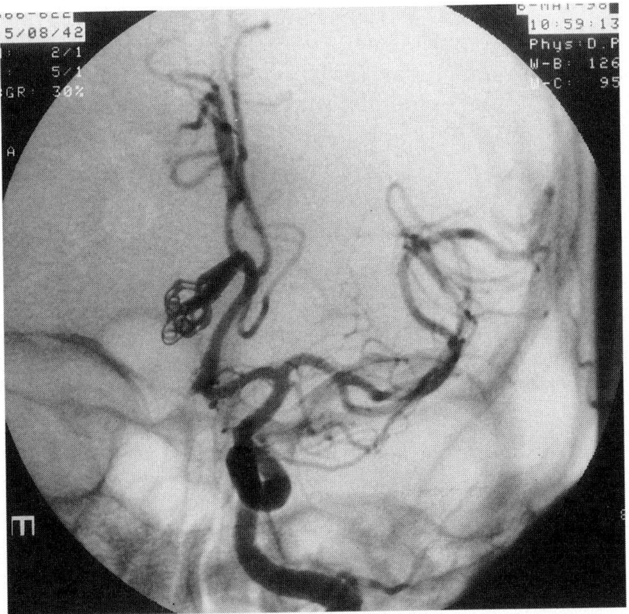

FIGURE 114–3. Postoperative angiogram of a successfully clipped distal anterior cerebral artery aneurysm that arose at the bifurcation of an azygous A2 segment.

CLINICAL CHARACTERISTICS

A detailed analysis of the incidence of aneurysms by site, based on a database of 5808 intracranial aneurysms derived from the world literature to 1978, demonstrated an incidence of 4.8%.[1] The average incidence derived from more recent major reports of distal ACA aneurysms is 5.4% (Table 114–1). In an unpublished review of 1109 cases of anterior circulation aneurysms managed at our institution since 1973, 59 patients (5.3%) with distal ACA aneurysms were identified. It therefore seems reasonable to conclude that distal ACA aneurysms represent approximately 5% of all intracranial aneurysms. The average age at presentation is approximately 50 years, and there appears to be a slight female preponderance (see Table 114–1), findings that are not significantly different from those for intracranial aneurysms at other sites.[1]

Patients with ruptured distal ACA aneurysms present with symptoms and signs typical of SAH. Some patients demonstrate monoparesis of a lower extremity, paraparesis, or hemiparesis in association with an intraparenchymal hemorrhage. A hemispheric disconnection syndrome may occur if there has been a significant intracallosal hemorrhage.[18] Some authors have reported an unusually high incidence of poor clinical grades in patients presenting with ruptured distal ACA aneurysms in comparison to those with aneurysmal ruptures at other sites. Hernesniemi and associates[5] noted that 60% of their patients presenting with SAH had a Hunt and Hess[19] clinical grade of 3 or higher. Snyckers and Drake[10] reported that 63% of their patients presented with an unfavorable clinical grade. Intracerebral hemorrhage is a common complication of ruptured distal ACA aneurysms and may be seen in as many as 50% of cases.[3, 10] The small size of the pericallosal cistern and the close approximation of the corpus callosum and frontal lobe to these aneurysms have been proposed as explanations for this phenomenon.[10, 13] The majority of patients presenting with poor clinical grades (Hunt and Hess grade 4 or 5) are harboring significant intracerebral hematomas.[10, 13]

Although the majority of patients with distal ACA aneurysms present with SAH, in 20% of 317 patients described in eight major reports from the microsurgical era, the findings were incidental.[2–7, 13, 14] Distal ACA aneurysms are commonly associated with other intracranial aneurysms and may be identified in patients investigated for SAH from aneurysms at other sites. In 269 patients with distal ACA aneurysms published in eight major reports, 41% had one or more additional intracranial aneurysm (Table 114–2). The most frequent site was the middle cerebral artery (43%). Another distal ACA aneurysm was present in 22% of cases.

The distal ACA is a common site for traumatic intra-

TABLE 114–1 ■ **Clinical Characteristics of Patients with Distal Anterior Cerebral Artery Aneurysms**

AUTHOR	YEAR	NUMBER OF PATIENTS	PERCENTAGE OF ALL CASES	PERCENTAGE RUPTURED	FEMALE	MALE	MEAN AGE/ RANGE (YR)
de Sousa et al[2]	1999	72	5.3	90	51	21	44 (26–69)
Inci et al[3]	1998	14	2.8	86	8	6	44 (7–63)
Proust et al[4]	1997	43	5.7	81	27	16	49 (17–77)
Hernesniemi et al[5]	1992	84	7.3	77	41	43	49 (22–72)
Ohno et al[6]	1990	42	9.2	71	24	18	54 (29–71)
Sindou et al[14]	1988	19	N/A	95	12	7	49 (29–65)
Wisoff & Flamm[13]	1987	20	N/A	60	13	7	51 (36–66)
Yasargil[7]	1984	23	2.3	100*	15	8	42 (24–60)
		317	5.4	83	184(58%)	133(42%)	48 (7–77)

*This report excluded seven incidental distal anterior cerebral artery aneurysms from analysis.
N/A, data not available.

cranial aneurysms. Asari and colleagues[20] reviewed 60 such cases, 30% of which occurred on the distal ACA. Fleischer and coworkers[21] reviewed 41 cases of traumatic intracranial aneurysms, 25% of which were on the distal ACA. These aneurysms are particularly common in the pediatric age group and, in their report, four of nine pediatric patients had traumatic aneurysms of the distal ACA. Nakstad and colleagues[22] identified three traumatic distal ACA aneurysms, all occurring in children. Most of these aneurysms arise along the anterior border of the genu of the corpus callosum, either from the main trunk of the distal ACA, and not in relationship to a bifurcation, or from the CMA (see Fig. 114–1). These vessels are in close apposition to the free edge of the falx cerebri at this point and are presumably injured by that structure as a result of sudden brain shift at the moment of impact during head injury. Patients typically present with SAH days to weeks following the head injury. The inciting head injury is usually significant, most commonly the result of a motor vehicle accident or a fall, but a case resulting from a seemingly minor head injury has been reported.[23] The shaken baby syndrome has been identified as a possible cause of traumatic distal ACA aneurysm in infants.[24]

INVESTIGATIONS

Preoperative computed tomographic findings are similar to those seen with ACoA aneurysms. However, high-density areas are more frequently seen in the interhemispheric fissure, cingulate sulcus, pericallosal cistern, and cistern of the lamina terminalis in ruptured distal ACA aneurysms (Fig. 114–4).[6, 25] Intraparenchymal frontal hematomas are common and are usually ipsilateral to the ruptured aneurysm. Hemorrhage into the corpus callosum may occur with both ACoA and distal ACA aneurysms. Jackson and coworkers[25] reviewed the pattern of hemorrhage as seen on computed tomographic scans in 17 patients with callosal hematomas caused by these two types of aneurysms. In the 12 callosal hematomas caused by distal ACA aneurysms, the hemorrhage originated in the pericallosal cistern and passed posteriorly into the genu of the corpus callosum. Within the corpus callosum, the hematoma extended posteriorly along its dorsal aspect, displacing it and the ventricles inferiorly. In contrast, callosal hematomas arising from ACoA aneurysms arose from the passage of blood up through the cistern of the lamina terminalis into the septum pellucidum and then into the ventral aspect of the anterior corpus

TABLE 114–2 ■ **Incidence of Multiple Aneurysms in Patients with Distal Anterior Cerebral Artery Aneurysms**

AUTHOR	YEAR	NUMBER OF PATIENTS	NUMBER OF PATIENTS WITH MULTIPLE ANEURYSMS (%)	NUMBER OF ADDITIONAL ANEURYSMS	MCA	DISTAL ACA	OTHER ICA	ACOA	POSTERIOR CIRCULATION
Inci et al[3]	1998	14	5 (36)	7	3	1	—	2	1
Proust et al[4]	1997	43	12 (28)	12	3	7	2	—	—
Hernesniemi et al[5]	1992	84	39 (46)	78	37	8	20	9	4
Ohno et al[6]	1990	42	18 (43)	23	12	7	4	—	—
Sindou et al[14]	1988	19	7 (37)	8	4	2	2	—	—
Wisoff & Flamm[13]	1987	20	11 (55)	17	8	2	5	1	1
Yasargil[7]	1984	23	11 (48)	12	1	9	—	1	1
Snyckers & Drake[10]	1973	24	6 (25)	9	3	1	2	3	—
		269	109 (41)	166	71 (43%)	37 (22%)	35 (21%)	16 (10%)	7 (4%)

ACA, anterior cerebral artery; ACoA, anterior communicating artery; ICA, internal carotid artery; MCA, middle cerebral artery.

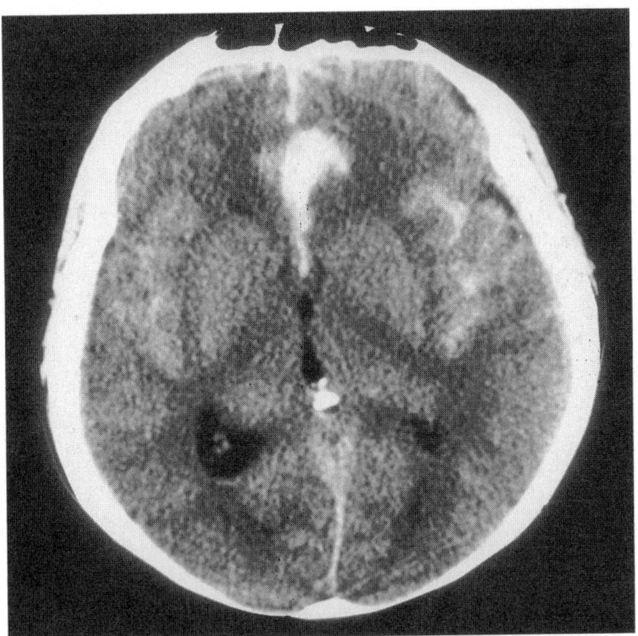

FIGURE 114–4. Axial computed tomographic scan in a 50-year-old woman presenting with a ruptured distal anterior cerebral artery aneurysm arising at the origin of the right callosomarginal artery. As well as a diffuse subarachnoid hemorrhage, there is a thick clot in the interhemispheric fissure that has extended into the left mesial frontal lobe.

callosum. Lau and colleagues[26] noted that callosal hemorrhages may masquerade as enhancing callosal gliomas if imaging has been delayed for more than 1 week. Calcified, incidental, supracallosal distal ACA aneurysms may be confused with midline supracallosal meningiomas. Wisoff and Flamm[13] remarked that three of six incidental aneurysms in their series had an initial radiologic diagnosis of meningioma. They cautioned that distal ACA aneurysms must be part of the differential diagnosis of any calcified midline supracallosal lesion.

Intraventricular hemorrhage is a less common manifestation of a ruptured distal ACA aneurysm. When present, it generally results from extension of a frontal lobe hematoma into the ipsilateral frontal horn, rather than downward extension into the third ventricle. If intraventricular hemorrhage is seen in association with a callosal hematoma or hemorrhage into the septum pellucidum, a ruptured ACoA aneurysm is more likely.

Retrospectively, magnetic resonance angiography may demonstrate cerebral aneurysms with a diameter of 3 mm or greater, but prospectively, 5 mm is the critical size for detection.[27] Although magnetic resonance angiography has successfully detected a distal ACA aneurysm prospectively,[28] there is a significant risk that these aneurysms will not be seen by this technique because they are often less than 5 mm in diameter at the time of rupture.

Four-vessel digital subtraction angiography remains the investigation of choice for the evaluation of SAH from distal ACA aneurysms. In most cases, the aneurysm is readily demonstrated on standard anteroposterior and lateral projections (Fig. 114–5). Confusion may arise in determining the laterality of the aneurysm. This is particularly true if a unilateral injection opacifies both A2 segments through a dominant A1 segment. Even with multiple projections, occasionally it is impossible to determine the site of origin of the aneurysm with certainty. Given the high incidence of multiple aneurysms in these patients, a meticulous angiographic examination is mandatory to identify additional aneurysms if a distal ACA aneurysm is identified.

SURGICAL CONSIDERATIONS

Patient Selection

In patients with ruptured distal ACA aneurysms, decisions regarding the timing of surgery are based primarily on the clinical grade of the patient on admission.[19] Patients with favorable clinical grades (Hunt and Hess grades 1 and 2) are candidates for early surgical intervention. When the admission grade is poor, the timing of surgical intervention is more problematic, and most would advise delaying surgery until the patient's clinical status improves. An important exception is a patient with a poor clinical grade and a large parenchymal hemorrhage, a situation not uncommon in patients with ruptured distal ACA aneurysms. If a large hematoma is present and the patient's condition is judged to be deteriorating because of it, urgent craniotomy, evacuation of the clot, and clipping of the aneurysm are indicated. It should be recognized, however, that the operating conditions in such a situation may be very difficult. An alternative strategy to be considered to prevent recurrent hemorrhage in poor-grade cases is early endovascular treatment of the ruptured aneurysm using detachable platinum coils.[29]

The decision to treat an unruptured, incidentally discovered distal ACA aneurysm is not straightforward. The report of the initial results of the International Study of Unruptured Intracranial Aneurysms[30] demonstrated that incidental intracranial aneurysms less than 10 mm in diameter have a remarkably benign natural history. However, this finding may not be true in the case of distal ACA aneurysms, which appear to rupture on average at a smaller size than do aneurysms at most other sites.[3, 6, 7, 17] Accordingly, conservative management of incidental aneurysms at this site may not be appropriate.

Surgical Techniques

Distal ACA aneurysms present special difficulties for the surgeon, which have been summarized by Yasargil.[7] The interhemispheric fissure and the callosal cistern are narrow, and exposure is difficult unless the brain is adequately relaxed. The cingulate gyri may be densely adherent, making exposure of the pericallosal arteries and corpus callosum awkward. Thick clot in the interhemispheric fissure obscures the normal vascular anatomy, which may disorient the surgeon and make the dissection slow and tedious. There may be

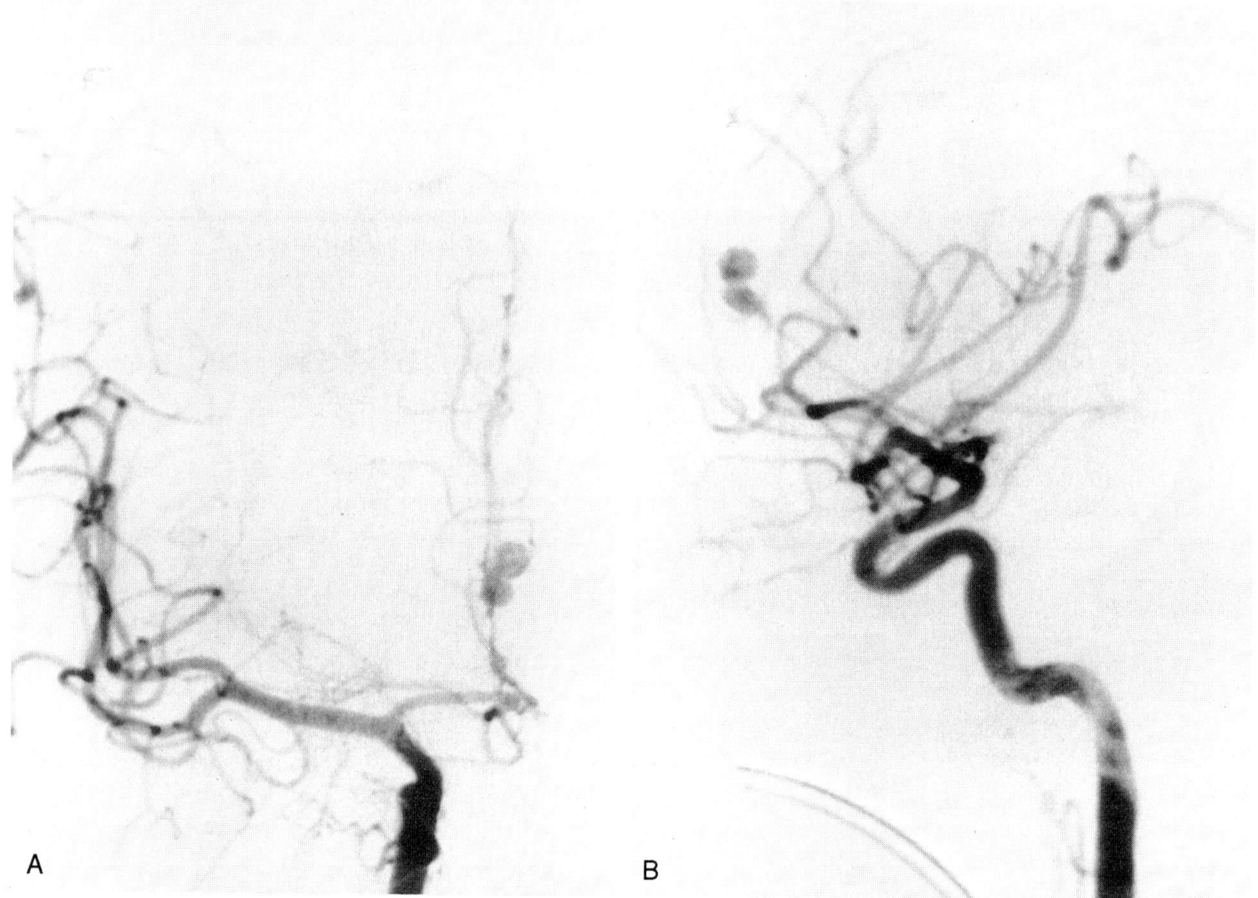

FIGURE 114–5. Standard anteroposterior *(A)* and lateral *(B)* right carotid angiogram revealing a bilobed distal anterior cerebral artery aneurysm arising at the origin of the right callosomarginal artery. This 55-year-old woman had suffered an initial hemorrhage 10 days earlier from a second coma-producing hemorrhage. Note the severe vasospasm of the A2 segment, reflecting the earlier unrecognized hemorrhage.

uncertainty about whether one is proximal or distal to the aneurysm once the pericallosal arteries have been identified. Most commonly, one is distal to the aneurysm, and by necessity, the fundus of the aneurysm will be exposed, at least in part, before the proximal artery can be seen, increasing the risk of premature rupture of the aneurysm during the dissection. At times, it is difficult to ascertain from the preoperative angiogram which distal ACA the aneurysm arises from. The dome of the aneurysm may be densely adherent to the pia of the cingulate gyrus, risking premature rupture with anything but the most gentle retraction of the frontal lobe. The neck of the aneurysm may be broad based and sclerotic, and the fundus may be densely adherent to branches of the opposite pericallosal artery, increasing the difficulty of the final dissection of the neck of the aneurysm.

We routinely use prophylactic intravenous antibiotics in patients undergoing craniotomy (cefazolin, 1 g on call to the operating room, followed by 1 g every 8 hours for three doses postoperatively; vancomycin is the alternative for patients with a penicillin allergy). To achieve adequate brain relaxation, mannitol (0.5 to 1 g/kg) is routinely infused during the opening; intravenous furosemide (20 to 40 mg) may be required as well. Moderate hyperventilation to achieve a $Pa{CO_2}$ of 30 to 35 is routine. Some surgeons recommend the use of lumbar spinal drainage,[7, 13] but others find it unnecessary.[5, 17] As a rule, we have a lumbar spinal drain positioned, to be used if necessary. Although we no longer routinely use profound systemic hypotension in aneurysm surgery, some degree of systemic hypotension is an important consideration, as it may lessen the risk of premature rupture if dissection of the aneurysm itself must be undertaken before there is adequate exposure of the parent artery.

The majority of distal ACA aneurysms arise either at the level of the genu of the corpus callosum or more distally in a supracallosal location.[6] Such aneurysms are best approached through the interhemispheric fissure using a right frontal parasagittal craniotomy sited anterior to the coronal suture.[2, 3, 5–7, 10, 13–15, 17] The patient is positioned supine with the head secured by three-point skeletal fixation in a neutral position, with slight hyperextension of the neck. The exact siting of the craniotomy is dictated by the location of the aneurysm (Fig. 114–6). If the aneurysm is relatively proximal, in front of the genu, a low frontal parasagittal craniotomy

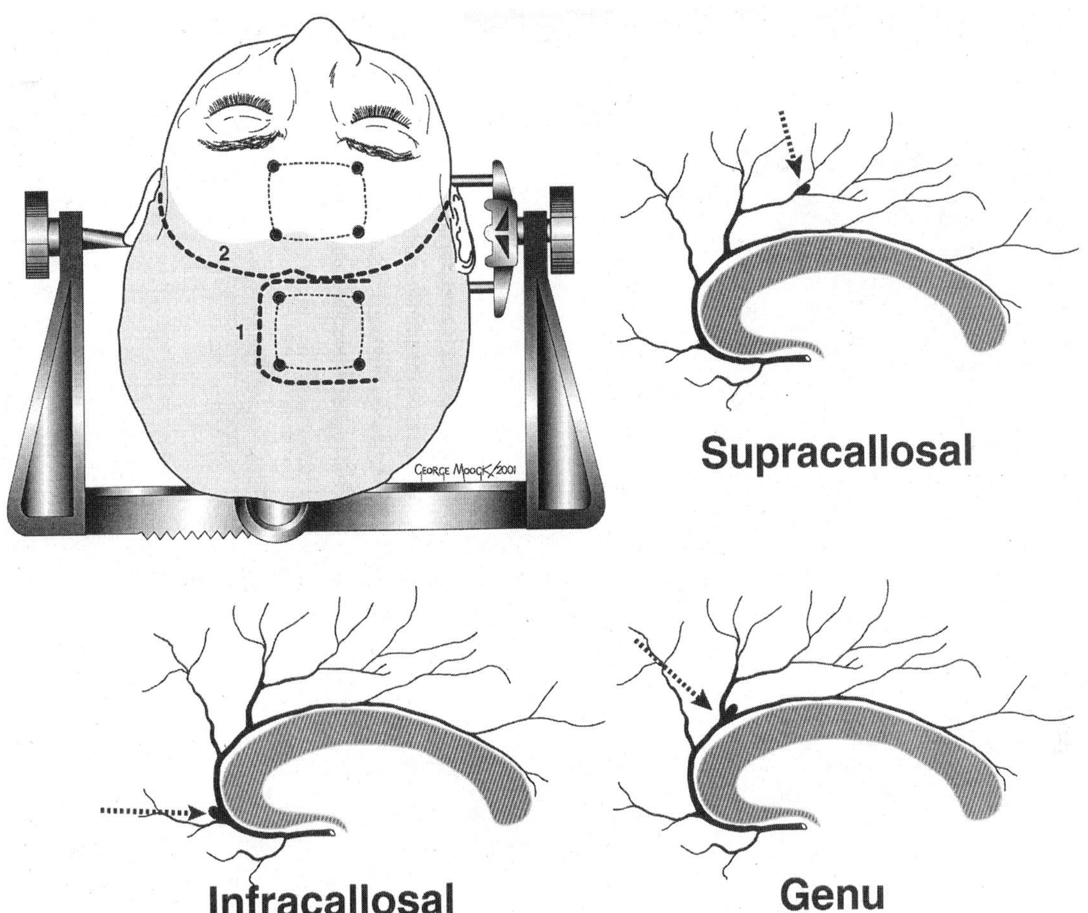

FIGURE 114–6. Surgical approaches to distal anterior cerebral artery aneurysms. 1, Approach for supracallosal aneurysms; 2, approach for proximal aneurysms.

is required, and a bicoronal scalp flap behind the hairline is used. If the aneurysm is supracallosal, the craniotomy is more posteriorly positioned, and a small horseshoe- or L-shaped scalp flap can be used. We usually raise a rectangular craniotomy flap, although some surgeons prefer a triangular flap.[17] Most surgeons prefer the craniotomy exposure to extend across the midline to fully expose the sagittal sinus. This allows efficient control of any hemorrhage from the sinus and guarantees adequate midline exposure and ease of retraction of the falx.

The dura is opened in a curvilinear or horseshoe fashion and retracted medially, with the opening taken as close to the sinus as possible, which minimizes the need for retraction of the frontal lobe. Bridging cortical veins to the sinus may make exposure of the interhemispheric fissure awkward. Large veins should be preserved. One or two small bridging veins may be divided without risk.[7, 10] The length of the interhemispheric exposure needs to be at least 2 cm.

Dissection of the interhemispheric fissure and the approach to the distal ACA aneurysm are undertaken using the operating microscope. Self-retaining retractors allow gentle retraction of the mesial aspect of the frontal lobe and of the falx. Gentle retraction minimizes the risk of inadvertent tearing of stretched bridging veins. Retraction must be especially gentle in the region of the cingulate gyri, as the fundus of the aneurysm is often embedded in one or the other, making premature rupture of the aneurysm a significant risk if retraction is excessive. Premature aneurysmal rupture was common in the premicrosurgical era[10] but is less common today.[5] Premature rupture of these aneurysms is particularly vexing, as exposure of the proximal feeding artery may be difficult or impossible to achieve in the face of active bleeding. If a large frontal intracerebral hematoma is present, its partial evacuation should be undertaken early in the dissection to allow adequate exposure of the interhemispheric fissure. Hematoma in the region of the fundus should be left undisturbed. Clot in the interhemispheric fissure obscures the normal anatomy, making the dissection slow and tedious. The longitudinal exposure of the interhemispheric fissure should be as extensive as possible, with particular attention to proximal exposure in the hope of obtaining control of the proximal vessels before exposure of the aneurysm. This is often not possible, however, and one must approach the aneurysm from a distal orientation. The aim is to identify the pericallosal arteries that lie directly on the corpus callosum, which is recognized by its transversely running, parallel white fibers. The corpus callosum is usually a centimeter or more deep to the free edge of the falx. The anatomy can be confusing even to the most experienced surgeon. The cingulate gyri may be densely adherent and mistaken for the corpus callosum initially. If exposure of the pericallosal arteries proves difficult, dissection of the CMA or other medial frontal artery, proximally, will ultimately lead to the pericallosal arteries.

On identification of the pericallosal arteries, dissection continues in the cistern of the corpus callosum until the site of the aneurysm is identified. If one is distal to the aneurysm, as is usually the case, attention is directed toward exposure of the proximal pericallosal arteries. Because the fundus of the aneurysm is often directed laterally, the proximal arteries are best exposed by dissecting along the contralateral cingulate gyrus. Alternatively, but with greater risk of premature rupture, the proximal arteries may be exposed by subpial dissection around the fundus of the aneurysm within the ipsilateral cingulate gyrus. Once adequate exposure of both the right and left pericallosal arteries proximal and distal to the aneurysm has been achieved, final dissection of the neck of the aneurysm is undertaken using fine, blunt microdissectors. Further confusion can arise at this stage if the preliminary dissection of the pericallosal arteries was not thorough. The arteries may be overlapping and crossed, and the wrong artery may be chosen in search of the neck of the aneurysm. Based on the preoperative angiogram, there may be uncertainty as to which of the pericallosal arteries gives rise to the aneurysm. Occasionally, small bilateral aneurysms are mistaken for a single aneurysm on the preoperative angiogram. This may be identified intraoperatively, or it may be missed and recognized only on the postoperative angiogram (Fig. 114–7).

The aneurysm is prepared for clipping by thoroughly clearing arachnoid and hematoma from both sides of the neck. Use of a temporary proximal clip during final dissection of the neck and clipping of the aneurysm may be considered, but the narrow confines of the interhemispheric fissure may make the use of a temporary clip awkward, if not impossible. Successful clip placement may be hampered by the small size of the aneurysm, a relatively broad neck,[5] and atheroma within the aneurysm.[7] Occasionally, an aneurysm is so small that it cannot safely accept even the smallest clip. Chopped muslin gauze can be used to wrap the fundus and neck of such aneurysms. Once the aneurysm has been clipped, the branches and parent artery are carefully inspected to ensure their patency. The fundus may be aspirated and collapsed. Unless an aneurysm has been collapsed, we routinely perform postoperative angiography to confirm that the aneurysm has been adequately treated.

Chritchley[31] described the syndrome of infarction of the distal ACA with preservation of the recurrent artery of Heubner. Such infarction may result in contralateral monoparesis of the leg, hemiparesis, contralateral sensory loss, psychomotor phenomena, impaired memory, incontinence, and visual agnosia and apraxia. A transient aphasia may occur if the dominant supplementary motor area is involved.[15] Bilateral deficits are possible if a bihemispheric branch is occluded. Occlusion of the distal ACA or a major branch does not invariably lead to neurological deficit, as this vessel territory has rich collateral potential from both the middle cerebral artery and the posterior cerebral artery.[5, 10]

A variety of approaches have been described for those aneurysms arising proximal to the genu of the corpus callosum (infracallosal aneurysms). If the aneurysm is very proximal (e.g., at the orbitofrontal artery origin), a standard pterional approach with adequate resection of the gyrus rectus and dissection of the proximal interhemispheric fissure allows proximal control of the A2 segments and good exposure of the aneurysm.[5, 7, 13] This approach is particularly useful if there are multiple ipsilateral aneurysms that can be clipped through the same craniotomy. Yoshimoto and coworkers[11] described a proximal interhemispheric approach through a very low bifrontal craniotomy. They recommend initial exposure of both A1 segments. The proximal superior sagittal sinus and falx can be divided if necessary, and the interhemispheric fissure is entered as far inferiorly and anteriorly as possible. Others[32, 33] described the use of a small anterior corpus callosotomy through a standard interhemispheric approach as a means of securing exposure of the A2 segments proximal to infracallosal aneurysms and those arising anterior to the genu.

We have had some experience with endovascular therapy to treat distal ACA aneurysms using detachable platinum coils (Fig. 114–8). Although it can be difficult to access all distal aneurysms using the endovascular techniques presently available, experience and success with such techniques are certain to increase in the future.

RESULTS

Table 114–3 summarizes the surgical results in patients with distal ACA aneurysms from eight major reports in the microsurgical era. Results of series from the premicrosurgical era are of historical interest but are not relevant to the current practice standards for these aneurysms. The reported surgical results and overall management results are quite variable, reflecting the particular case mix of each series in relationship to the percentage of ruptured versus unruptured aneurysms, the clinical grades of the patients at the time of surgery, and the timing of surgery. None of the reports has a large number of patients, and most represent an evolving experience gathered over many years by surgeons with a particular interest in aneurysm surgery. Most neurosurgeons have relatively little experience with these aneurysms and would probably be unable to duplicate the results reflected in Table 114–3. In 289 operative cases, the reported perioperative mortality was 7.1% (0% to 14%), and the major perioperative morbidity was 9.7% (0% to 17.9%), with an overall satisfactory operative outcome of 83% (70% to 94%). Many of these reports include a significant number of patients with unruptured aneurysms, which improves and distorts the apparent surgical results as they relate

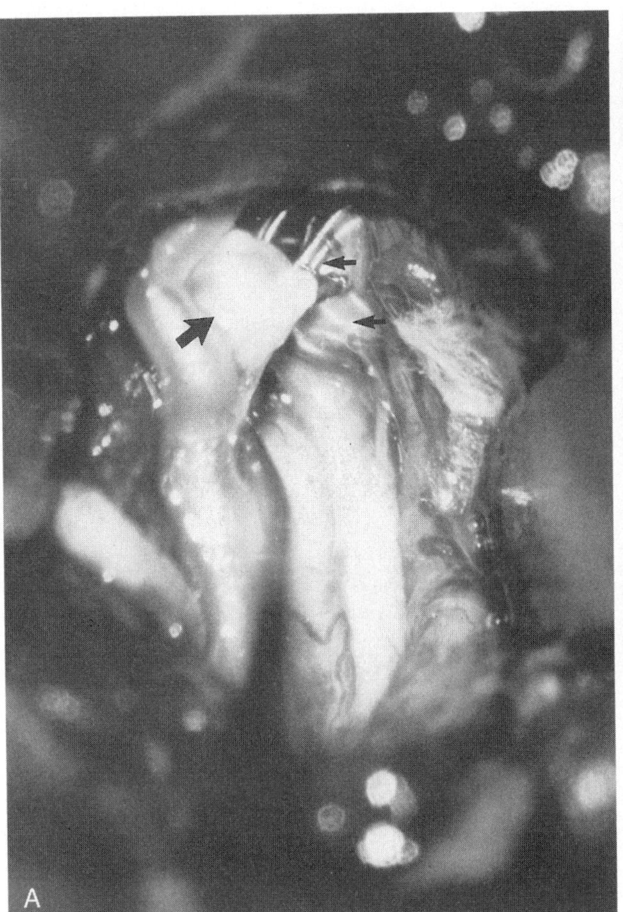

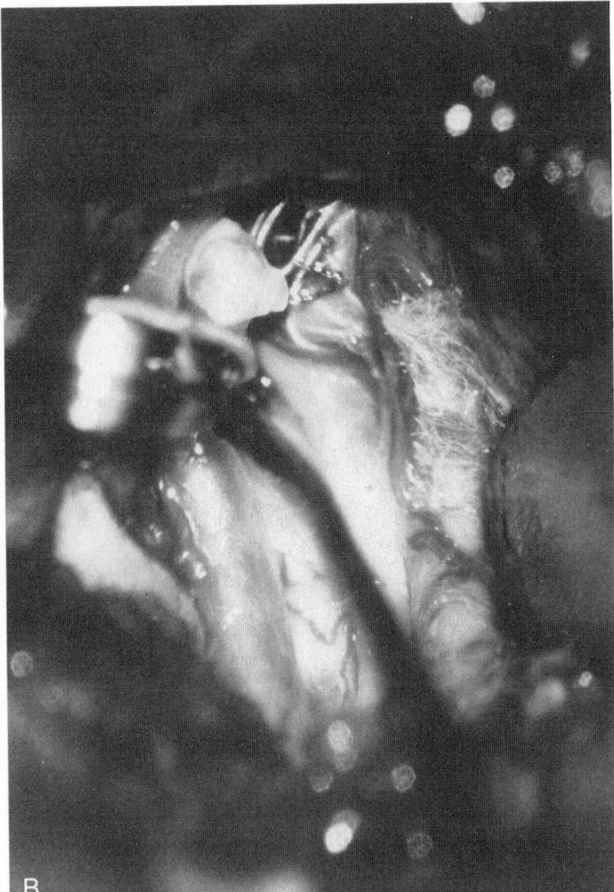

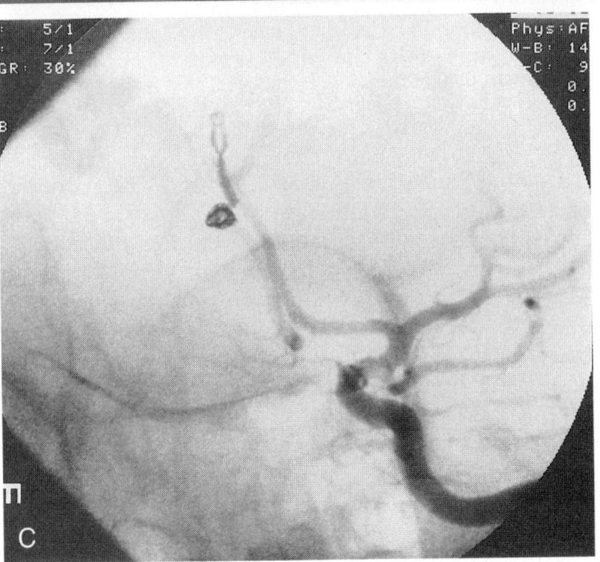

FIGURE 114–7. *A*, Intraoperative photograph of an unruptured distal anterior cerebral artery (ACA) aneurysm arising at the origin of the left callosomarginal artery (CMA) *(large arrow)*. This patient had previously been treated for a ruptured distal ACA aneurysm arising at the origin of the right CMA using detachable platinum coils. The coils can be seen through the thin wall of that aneurysm *(small arrows)*. *B*, A curved Sugita clip has been placed across the neck of the left-sided aneurysm. *C*, Postoperative left carotid angiogram showing successful obliteration of the left-sided aneurysm and the platinum coil mass in the right-sided aneurysm. (*A* and *B*, Courtesy of Dr. S. P. Lownie.)

to ruptured distal ACA aneurysms. Until the 1990s, relatively few patients were operated on soon after hemorrhage. Some of these series have had a disproportionate number of patients with poor clinical grade and, as a result, poorer surgical outcomes.

In 1984, Yasargil published his experience with 23 patients with ruptured aneurysms at this site.[7] In 16 cases, the aneurysm arose at the CMA, and in 6, it arose at the origin of the frontopolar artery. Intracerebral hematomas were present in 14 patients (60.9%), half of which were large frontal or callosal hemorrhages. Thirteen patients (57%) had a good preoperative clinical grade, and 10 had a poor grade. The timing of surgery varied from 3 days to 9 months, with an average delay of 3 weeks from the time of the most recent hemorrhage. In 19 cases, the aneurysm was approached by the interhemispheric route. Pterional craniotomies were used in four cases—once for an aneu-

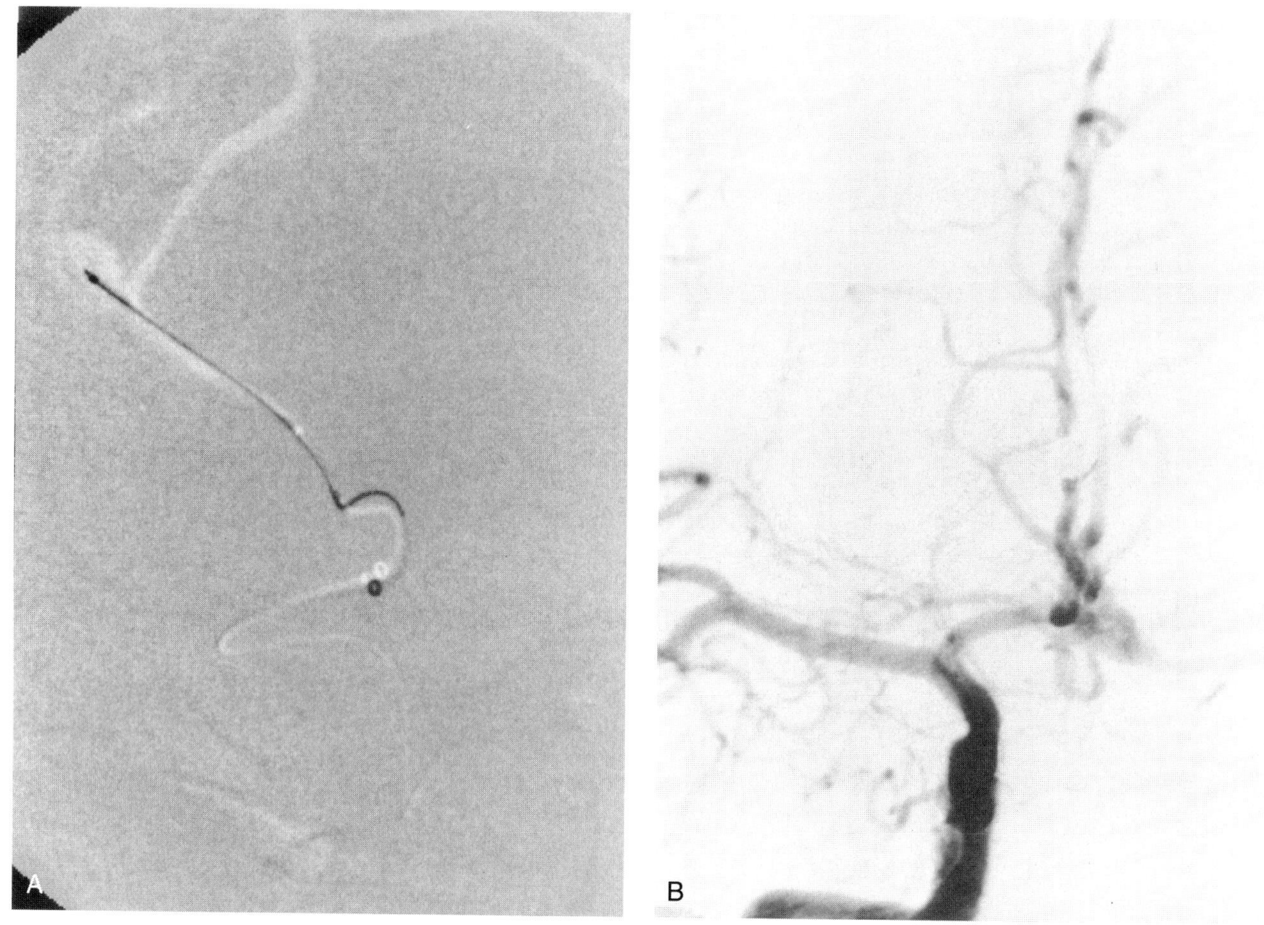

FIGURE 114–8. Embolization of the right distal anterior cerebral artery aneurysm illustrated in Figure 114–5. *A*, Microcatheter positioned in the sac of the aneurysm through the left A2 segment. *B*, Successful obliteration of the aneurysm by detachable platinum coils.

rysm arising very proximally at the orbitofrontal artery, and in the other cases to deal with additional aneurysms. The results in this series were remarkable. Despite 43% of the patients having a poor clinical grade, there were no deaths. A satisfactory operative outcome was achieved in 87% of the patients. The three unsatisfactory outcomes occurred in patients with poor clinical grade disease. Although this was a relatively small series, these outstanding results established the standard for the microsurgical era.

Wisoff and Flamm[13] reported a series of 20 patients with 24 distal ACA aneurysms in 1987. Fourteen of these patients had ruptured aneurysms—12 from a distal ACA aneurysm, and 2 from another aneurysm. Seven of the 12 patients (58%) with ruptured distal ACA aneurysms had a Hunt and Hess clinical grade

TABLE 114–3 ■ **Surgical Results in Patients with Distal Anterior Cerebral Artery Aneurysms**

AUTHOR	YEAR	NUMBER OF OPERATIVE CASES	NUMBER RUPTURED (%)	POSTOPERATIVE MORTALITY (%)	MAJOR POSTOPERATIVE MORBIDITY (%)	SATISFACTORY OPERATIVE OUTCOME (%)
de Sousa et al[2]	1999	72	65 (90)	6.9	8.3	85
Inci et al[3]	1998	14	12 (86)	7.1	0	93
Proust et al[4]	1997	43	35 (81)	14	16.3	70
Hernesniemi et al[5]	1992	67	54 (81)	7.5	17.9	75
Ohno et al[6]	1990	34	25 (74)	5.9	5.9	88
Sindou et al[14]	1988	16	16 (100)	0	6.3	94
Wisoff & Flamm[13]	1987	20	12 (60)	15	10	75
Yasargil[7]	1984	23	23 (100)	0	13	87
		289	242 (84)	7.1 (0–14)	9.7 (0–17.9)	83 (70–94)

of 3 or 4, which in each case was associated with an intracerebral or intraventricular hematoma and the subsequent development of vasospasm. All 20 patients were operated on using an interhemispheric approach. There was no instance of intraoperative aneurysmal rupture. There were three perioperative deaths (15%), all in patients with grade 4 disease. Two patients with poor preoperative grades suffered major, persisting disability. The outcome was favorable in 15 of 20 (75%) of the patients overall, but in only 9 of the 14 patients (64%) with ruptured aneurysms.

In 1988, Sindou and associates[14] reported a series of 19 patients with distal ACA aneurysms, 18 of whom had ruptured aneurysms. Two patients died of recurrent hemorrhage before surgery, and the patient with an incidental aneurysm refused surgery. In the 16 operated cases, there were no deaths. The overall management mortality was 10.5%. Major postoperative morbidity occurred in one patient with a good clinical grade (6.3%), and some degree of postoperative morbidity occurred in four others. Overall, a satisfactory operative outcome occurred in 94% of their patients, with a satisfactory management outcome in 16 of 19 (84%).

Ohno and colleagues[6] reported their experience with 42 patients with distal ACA aneurysms in 1990. Thirty patients presented with ruptured aneurysms, 83% with a clinical grade of 1 or 2. Nine patients had unruptured distal ACA aneurysms. Only 13 patients were operated on within 48 hours of bleeding; the remainder had delayed surgery. An interhemispheric approach was used in every case, with the parasagittal craniotomy site based on whether the aneurysm was infracallosal, anterior to the genu, or supracallosal in location. There were two deaths (5.9%) and two poor outcomes (5.9%) in the surgical patients, with an overall satisfactory outcome in 30 of 34 patients (88%). There were two preoperative deaths, resulting in an overall satisfactory management outcome in 36 of 42 (85.7%). These impressive results probably reflect the unusually high percentage of patients presenting with a good clinical grade in this series. Of the 25 patients with grade 1 and grade 2 disease who had ruptured distal ACA aneurysms operated on, there was one death and one poor outcome, resulting in a satisfactory outcome in 92%. The authors concluded that excellent results were possible with early surgery in patients who presented with a favorable clinical grade.

In 1992, Hernesniemi and coworkers[5] published the largest series of patients with distal ACA aneurysms to date, consisting of 84 patients with 92 distal ACA aneurysms. A distal ACA aneurysm had ruptured in 65 patients and was incidental in 19. Surgery was undertaken for 54 of the 65 ruptured aneurysms. The aneurysms were approached by an interhemispheric route, except for the most proximal aneurysms, which were approached by an extended pterional route. The majority of the patients were operated on within 3 days of hemorrhage (31 of 54, or 57%). Premature intraoperative rupture occurred in 10 of 54 cases (18.5%). Twenty-four patients (44%) were Hunt and Hess grades 1 and 2 preoperatively, in whom there were three poor outcomes (12.5%). Thirty patients (56%) were grade 3 or worse (grade 3, 28 patients; grade 4, 2 patients), in whom there were five postoperative deaths and nine poor outcomes. In these 54 patients, the overall postoperative mortality was 5 of 54 (9.3%), and the major postoperative morbidity was 12 of 54 (22%), with a satisfactory outcome in 37 of 54 (68.5%). Thirteen of the 19 incidental aneurysms were operated on without incident. The overall postoperative mortality in this series was 5 of 67 (7.5%), and the major postoperative morbidity was 12 of 67 (17.9%), with a satisfactory outcome in 75% of the patients. The overall management results in the 65 patients with ruptured aneurysms were as follows: death, 12 of 65 (18.5%); poor results, 15 of 65 (23%); satisfactory results, 38 of 65 (58.5%). Mortality and poor outcomes correlated with poor clinical grade related to the severity of the initial hemorrhage and the presence of intracerebral hematomas. The results reported in this large series are likely representative of the results that can be achieved presently when a significant percentage of patients present with a poor clinical grade. The authors concluded that satisfactory results can be achieved with early surgery in patients with favorable clinical grades.

Proust and associates[4] published a retrospective analysis of 43 patients with 50 distal ACA aneurysms. A distal ACA aneurysm had ruptured in 35 patients and was incidental in 8. The purpose of the study was to determine the incidence and cause of unfavorable outcomes. An interhemispheric approach was used in the majority of these cases (83%). Surgery was undertaken within 2 days of admission to the neurosurgical unit but, on average, occurred 8 days from the day of bleeding. Postoperative angiography was undertaken in all cases. Outcome at 6 to 12 months was scored according to the Glasgow Outcome Scale (GOS).[34] Of the 35 ruptured aneurysms, 26 were regarded as good grade (Hunt and Hess grades 1, 2, and 3), and 9 were regarded as poor grade (Hunt and Hess grades 4 and 5). Among the 26 good-grade cases, the results were as follows: GOS 1 (good recovery), 18 (69.2%); GOS 2 (moderate disability but independent), 2 (7.7%); GOS 3 (severe disability), 2 (7.7%); GOS 5 (death), 4 (15.4%). Among the nine poor-grade cases, the results were as follows: GOS 1, 11.1%; GOS 2, 22.2%; GOS 3, 55.6%; GOS 5, 11.1%. The overall surgical results in the 35 patients with ruptured distal ACA aneurysms were as follows: GOS 1, 54.3%; GOS 2, 11.4%; GOS 3, 11.4%; GOS 5, 22.9%, for an overall satisfactory outcome of 65.7%. Unsatisfactory outcomes were attributed to the initial hemorrhage in 4 of 35 (11.4%), unanticipated occlusion of a parent or major branch artery in 4 of 35 (11.4%), prolonged temporary proximal artery occlusion in 3 of 35 (8.7%), and rebleeding because of incomplete clipping in 1 of 35 (2.8%). There was a very high rate of premature, intraoperative aneurysmal rupture in this series (40%), which was thought to be the direct cause of the poor outcomes in all cases except for those in which the poor outcome was attributed to the effects of the initial hemorrhage. Eight patients with incidental distal ACA aneurysms were also treated surgically (six of whom had a hemorrhage from another aneurysm).

Including the results among those patients, the overall postoperative mortality in the 43 patients was 14%, and the major postoperative morbidity was 16.3%, with an overall satisfactory surgical outcome in 70%.

Inci and coworkers[3] reported a series of 14 patients in 1998. All the aneurysms were at the genu of the corpus callosum and were approached by an interhemispheric route. In two patients, the aneurysm was unruptured. Early surgery was considered in patients with Hunt and Hess grades 1 and 2, of whom there were nine. Thirteen of the 14 aneurysms were successfully clipped. The patient whose incidental aneurysm could not be clipped died as a result of right frontal hemorrhagic infarction attributed to excessive retraction and disruption of bridging veins. There was no major postoperative morbidity, and a satisfactory outcome was achieved in 93% of the cases.

The largest surgical report to date is that of de Sousa and colleagues[2] published in 1999. This series included 72 patients with distal ACA aneurysms (65 ruptured, 7 unruptured). Forty patients had a single distal ACA aneurysm; 32 had multiple aneurysms at various sites. Only three patients were operated on early; the others were treated at least 10 days after hemorrhage. The majority of patients (69%) with ruptured aneurysms were well at the time of surgery (Hunt and Hess grades 1 and 2). All the aneurysms were approached by an interhemispheric route. There was no instance of premature rupture of a distal ACA aneurysm. The perioperative mortality was 6.9%. All the deaths occurred in patients with multiple aneurysms. One death resulted from the intraoperative rupture of another aneurysm, one from an anesthetic complication, one from a postoperative hematoma, and two from severe postoperative swelling. The rate of major postoperative morbidity was 8.3%. A satisfactory outcome was noted in 85% of the patients. Most of the poor results occurred in patients with a poor clinical grade at the time of surgery.

SUMMARY

It appears that satisfactory surgical results can be achieved in patients with ruptured distal ACA aneurysms who have a good clinical grade at the time of surgery (Hunt and Hess grades 1 and 2). There is a strong trend to operate on such patients early. Premature intraoperative rupture of these aneurysms is a distinct risk and is associated with worse outcomes, but this risk can be minimized with meticulous microsurgical technique. The management of patients with a poor clinical grade remains a significant challenge and is associated with a high rate of permanent disability and death. Delayed surgery has been the rule in such cases, unless there is a life-threatening hematoma requiring evacuation. It is likely that endovascular treatment will play an increasingly important role in the management of these aneurysms, especially in patients with poor clinical grades who do not harbor life-threatening clots.

REFERENCES

1. Ferguson G: Intracranial arterial aneurysms—a surgical perspective. In Vinken P, Bruyn G, Klawans H (eds): Handbook of Clinical Neurology, vol 11. New York, Elsevier Science, 1989, pp 41–87.
2. de Sousa A, Dantas F, de Cardosa G, et al: Distal anterior cerebral artery aneurysms. Surg Neurol 52:128–136, 1999.
3. Inci S, Erbengi A, Özgen T: Aneurysms of the distal anterior cerebral artery: A report of 14 cases and a review of the literature. Surg Neurol 50:130–140, 1998.
4. Proust F, Toussaint P, Hannequin D, et al: Outcome in 43 patients with distal anterior cerebral artery aneurysms. Stroke 28:2405–2409, 1997.
5. Hernesniemi J, Tapaninaho A, Vapalahti M, et al: Saccular aneurysms of the distal anterior cerebral artery and its branches. Neurosurgery 31:994–999, 1992.
6. Ohno K, Monma S, Suzuki R, et al: Saccular aneurysms of the distal anterior cerebral artery. Neurosurgery 27:907–913, 1990.
7. Yasargil G: Distal anterior cerebral artery aneurysms. In Yasargil G: Microneurosurgery, vol 2. Stuttgart, Georg Thieme Verlag, 1984, pp 224–231.
8. Sugar O, Tinsley M: Aneurysm of the terminal portion of anterior cerebral artery. Arch Neurol Psychiatry 60:81–85, 1948.
9. Skultety F, Nishioka H: Report on the cooperative study of intracranial aneurysms and subarachnoid hemorrhage. Section VIII, part 2. The results of intracranial aneurysm surgery in the treatment of aneurysms. J Neurosurg 25:683–704, 1966.
10. Snyckers F, Drake C: Aneurysms of the distal anterior cerebral artery: A report on 24 verified cases. S Afr Med J 47:1787–1791, 1973.
11. Yoshimoto T, Uchida K, Suzuki J: Surgical treatment of distal anterior cerebral artery aneurysms. J Neurosurg 50:40–44, 1979.
12. Yasargil G, Carter P: Saccular aneurysms of the distal anterior cerebral artery. J Neurosurg 39:218–223, 1974.
13. Wisoff J, Flamm E: Aneurysms of the distal anterior cerebral artery and associated vascular anomalies. Neurosurgery 20:735–741, 1987.
14. Sindou M, Pelissou-Guyotat I, Mertens P, et al: Pericallosal aneurysms. Surg Neurol 30:434–440, 1988.
15. Perlmutter D, Rhoton A: Microsurgical anatomy of the distal anterior cerebral artery. J Neurosurg 49:204–228, 1978.
16. Baptista A: Studies on the arteries of the brain. II. The anterior cerebral artery: Some anatomic features and their clinical implications. Neurology (Minneap) 13:825–835, 1963.
17. Royand F, Carter P. Guthkelch N: Distal anterior cerebral artery aneurysms. In Carter P, Spetzler R, Hamilton M (eds): Neurovascular Surgery. New York, McGraw-Hill, 1995, pp 717–728.
18. Levine H, Goldstein F, Ghostine S, et al: Hemispheric disconnection syndrome persisting after anterior cerebral artery aneurysm rupture. Neurosurgery 21:831–838, 1987.
19. Hunt W, Hess R: Surgical risk as related to time of intervention in the repair of intracranial aneurysms. J Neurosurg 28:14–20, 1968.
20. Asari S, Nakamura S, Yamada O, et al: Traumatic aneurysm of peripheral cerebral arteries: Report of two cases. J Neurosurg 46: 795–803, 1977.
21. Fleischer A, Patton J, Tindall G: Cerebral aneurysms of traumatic origin. Surg Neurol 4:233–239, 1975.
22. Nakstad P, Nornes H, Hauge H: Traumatic aneurysms of the pericallosal arteries. Neuroradiology 28:335–338, 1986.
23. Senegor M: Traumatic pericallosal aneurysm in a patient with no major trauma. J Neurosurg 75:475–477, 1991.
24. Lam C, Montes J, Farmer J-P, et al: Traumatic aneurysm from shaken baby syndrome: Case report. Neurosurgery 39:1252–1255, 1996.
25. Jackson A, Fitzgerald J, Hartley R, et al: CT appearances of hematomas in the corpus callosum in patients with subarachnoid hemorrhage. Neuroradiology 35:420–423, 1993.
26. Lau L, Bannan E, Tress B: Pseudotumor of the corpus callosum due to subarachnoid hemorrhage from pericallosal aneurysm. Neuroradiology 26:67–69, 1984.
27. Houston J, Nichols D, Luetmer P, et al: Blinded prospective evaluation of sensitivity of MR angiography to known intracranial aneurysms: Importance of aneurysm size. AJNR Am J Neuroradiol 15:1607–1614, 1994.
28. Cinnamon J, Zito J, Chalif D, et al: Aneurysm of the azygos

pericallosal artery: Diagnosis by MR imaging and MR angiography. AJNR Am J Neuroradiol 13:280–282, 1992.
29. Viñuela F, Duckwiller G, Mawad N: Guglielmi detachable coil embolization of acute intracranial aneurysms: Perioperative, anatomical and clinical outcome in 403 patients. J Neurosurg 86: 475–482, 1997.
30. The International Study of Unruptured Intracranial Aneurysm Investigators: Unruptured intracranial aneurysms—risk of rupture and risks of surgical intervention. N Engl J Med 339:1725–1733, 1998.
31. Chritchley M: The anterior cerebral artery, and its syndrome. Brain 53:120–165, 1930.
32. Traynelis V, Dunker R: Interhemispheric approach with callosal resection for distal anterior cerebral artery aneurysms. J Neurosurg 77:481–483, 1992.
33. Dickey P, Bloomgarden G, Arkins T, et al: Partial callosal resection for pericallosal aneurysms. Neurosurgery 30:136–137, 1992.
34. Jennett B, Bond M: Assessment of outcome after severe brain damage: A practical scale. Lancet 1:480–484, 1975.

CHAPTER **115**

Middle Cerebral Artery Aneurysms

JONATHAN A. FRIEDMAN ■ DAVID G. PIEPGRAS

Aneurysms of the middle cerebral artery (MCA) are common, constituting 20% of all intracranial aneurysms.[1,2] Damage to frontal and temporal parenchyma from the initial hemorrhage is common; this accounts for the worse clinical grade at presentation in patients with MCA aneurysms compared with patients with ruptured supratentorial aneurysms at other sites.[3,4] In part because of the patients' worse clinical condition on admission, MCA aneurysms were associated with worse management outcomes than other anterior circulation aneurysms in some series.[4] Additionally, outcomes for these aneurysms are adversely affected by the large volume of eloquent cortex supplied exclusively by the MCA, the limited collateral arterial supply to this territory, and the intimate relationships of conducting and perforating endarteries to the aneurysm. Indeed, Dandy once considered these aneurysms inoperable.[5] In spite of these challenges, modern microneurosurgical management has proved to be a reasonably low risk and highly effective treatment for MCA aneurysms. MCA aneurysms in general have proved to be difficult to access and treat effectively with endovascular techniques; craniotomy with direct aneurysm repair thus remains the primary therapy for these difficult lesions.[6]

EPIDEMIOLOGY

In the largest operative series of MCA aneurysms—561 patients reported by Rinne and colleagues[4]—the familial occurrence of intracranial aneurysms among patients with a single MCA aneurysm was 11%. MCA aneurysms were associated with a 39% incidence of additional intracranial aneurysms, a 20% incidence of additional MCA aneurysms, and an 11% incidence of mirror aneurysms of the contralateral MCA. Similarly, Yasargil's series of 184 patients with MCA aneurysms demonstrated a 32% incidence of multiple intracranial aneurysms.[7] However, only 4% of patients in Yasargil's series had mirror aneurysms. Because the frequency of MCA aneurysms, the male predominance, and the number of patients with multiple intracranial aneurysms differed substantially in the Finnish study compared with findings reported in other series, it is likely that the epidemiology varies somewhat among genetically distinct populations.

ANATOMY AND DISTRIBUTION

A brief review of MCA anatomy is appropriate for an understanding of MCA aneurysm location and the fundamentals of operative management. The MCA trunk, designated the M1 segment, arises at the carotid bifurcation and follows a horizontal course from its origin at the most medial aspect of the sylvian fissure laterally to its bifurcation near the limen insulae. Along this course, the M1 segment travels below the anterior perforated substance and gives rise to a variable number of lenticulostriate branches, which can be conveniently grouped into medial, intermediate, and lateral branches. Additionally, the M1 segment may give off cortical branches, particularly to the anterior temporal and operculofrontal regions, which follow laterally into the insular compartment of the sylvian fissure. At times, these branches, particularly the temporopolar and anterior temporal branches arising from the inferior aspect of the M1 segment, may be quite large and on angiography give the false impression of a proximal MCA bifurcation.

The postbifurcation branches of the MCA arise in the lateral aspect of the sylvian fissure and, by convention, have been designated M2 branches. In nearly 80% of cases, the MCA trunk forms a true bifurcation, giving rise to two M2 branches; in approximately 12% of cases, there is a trifurcation; and in the remainder, there are multiple branches. Lateral lenticulostriate branches commonly arise in close proximity to the MCA bifurcation, from either M1 or M2 segments, and proceed into the lateral anterior perforated substance to nourish an extensive area of the deep structures of the cerebral hemisphere, including the corpus striatum, external and internal capsule, thalamus, and portions of the corona radiata. In the usual bifurcation anatomy, the M2 branches are best characterized as superior and inferior trunks that variably tend to be distributed to the orbitofrontal, precentral frontal and temporal, and temporal occipital areas. The angular branches of the MCA may arise from either the superior or the inferior division, varying with the dominance of the division. For a detailed description of the surgical anatomy, readers are referred to Yasargil.[8] Further studies have been carried out by Gibo and colleagues[9] that emphasize the highly variable patterns of the MCA. Additionally, these authors have cited a variation in the designation of the MCA segments, with M2 segments being characterized as insular segments, M3 as opercular, and M4 as cortical branches beginning at the sylvian fissure surface.

Approximately 10% to 15% of MCA aneurysms arise from the M1 segment.[4, 10] Hosoda and colleagues reviewed their series of 21 M1 aneurysms, dividing them into superior and inferior wall types.[10] Superior wall aneurysms arise off the dorsal or frontal lobe surface of the M1 segment in association with lenticulostriate or fronto-orbital arterial origins. These aneurysms typically project posterosuperiorly, and with rupture, they are more likely to be associated with frontal hematomas. Inferior wall types arise in conjunction with the early temporal branch arterial origins and project anteroinferiorly. With subarachnoid hemorrhage, aneurysms in these locations are more likely to cause anterior temporal hematomas. Noteworthy in Hosoda and colleagues' report, as in most other series, is a gender predilection for MCA aneurysms in women. The incidence of multiple intracranial aneurysms is higher in patients with M1 segment aneurysms.[4, 10]

The vast majority of MCA aneurysms are located at the division of the main (M1) trunk, accounting for 80% to 85% of cases.[1, 7, 11] These aneurysms tend to project laterally and inferiorly, although any projection is possible. Giant MCA aneurysms are more common than giant aneurysms at other sites and may grow large before becoming symptomatic through brain compression. Nevertheless, giant MCA aneurysms are relatively rare—constituting 15 of 174 giant aneurysms in Drake's series[12] and 12 of 80 giant aneurysms in the series of Sundt and Piepgras[13]; giant aneurysyms constituted 12% of the MCA aneurysms in the latter series. In Yasargil's series, only 3 of 184 MCA aneurysms were giant.[7] Aneurysms of the M2, M3, and M4 segments are uncommon, accounting for only 5% of MCA aneurysms. These have a higher likelihood of being mycotic or inflammatory and are not included in this discussion.[14]

CLINICAL PRESENTATION AND IMAGING

More than 90% of MCA aneurysms present with rupture.[4, 7] The presentation is typical of subarachnoid hemorrhage, but patients with ruptured MCA aneurysms frequently lose consciousness at the time of rupture.[15] In addition, MCA aneurysms have a propensity to present with intracerebral hematomas and, consequently, with focal neurological deficits (Figs. 115–1 and 115–2).[3, 15–17] The frequency of intracerebral hematomas in ruptured MCA aneurysms is near 40%.[3, 4] Up to 80% of patients with ruptured MCA aneurysms have focal neurological findings, compared with only 30% of patients with aneurysms at other sites.[15] One third of patients with ruptured MCA aneurysms report headache that localizes to the side of the aneurysm.[15] Intraventricular hemorrhage and hydrocephalus are less common in ruptured MCA aneurysms than in other aneurysms, probably because of MCA aneurysms' greater distance from the ventricular system.[18, 19]

Unruptured MCA aneurysms may present with symptoms of mass effect on the frontal and temporal lobes, including hemiparesis and aphasia.[7, 15] Seizures secondary to unruptured MCA aneurysms have also been described.[11, 20] Cortical stroke from aneurysmal thrombus formation and distal embolization is rare, but it occurs more commonly with MCA aneurysms than with aneurysms at other locations.[11, 14] Giant aneurysms are more likely to present with distal embolization or seizures than are smaller aneurysms.

Adequate demonstration of aneurysm anatomy is essential before proceeding with elective repair. In almost all cases, this should include at least a computed tomographic scan and routine cerebral angiography. In some circumstances, computed tomography–angiography with three-dimensional reconstruction may be helpful, and for unruptured giant or partially thrombosed MCA aneurysms, magnetic resonance imaging and magnetic resonance angiography may be helpful in demonstrating the local and pathologic anatomy.

SURGICAL TREATMENT

Timing of Operation and Preoperative Planning

As for other aneurysms, the timing of the operation in patients with aneurysmal subarachnoid hemorrhage due to MCA aneurysms is dependent on the condition of the patient, the presence of hematoma with major mass effect, and the complexity of the aneurysm. In good-grade patients with uncomplicated MCA aneurysms, aneurysm repair should be carried out as soon as possible by a skilled surgical team.

Peculiar to MCA aneurysms is their more frequent presentation with subarachnoid hemorrhage and associated major intracerebral hemorrhage, often in the temporal lobe. This occurs in 5% to 40% of patients, half of whom show symptoms and signs of mass effect.[4] Patients who present with severe or progressive depressed level of consciousness due to hematoma mass effect may require emergency operation for hematoma evacuation and relief of increased intracranial pressure, at which time definitive treatment of the aneurysm should also be carried out. In most cases, computed tomography and cerebral angiography are accomplished before operation to allow optimal surgical planning. Rarely, however, if a patient presents in the emergency room with acute obtundation or progressive deterioration due to temporal hematoma, emergent intervention is required before angiography can be car-

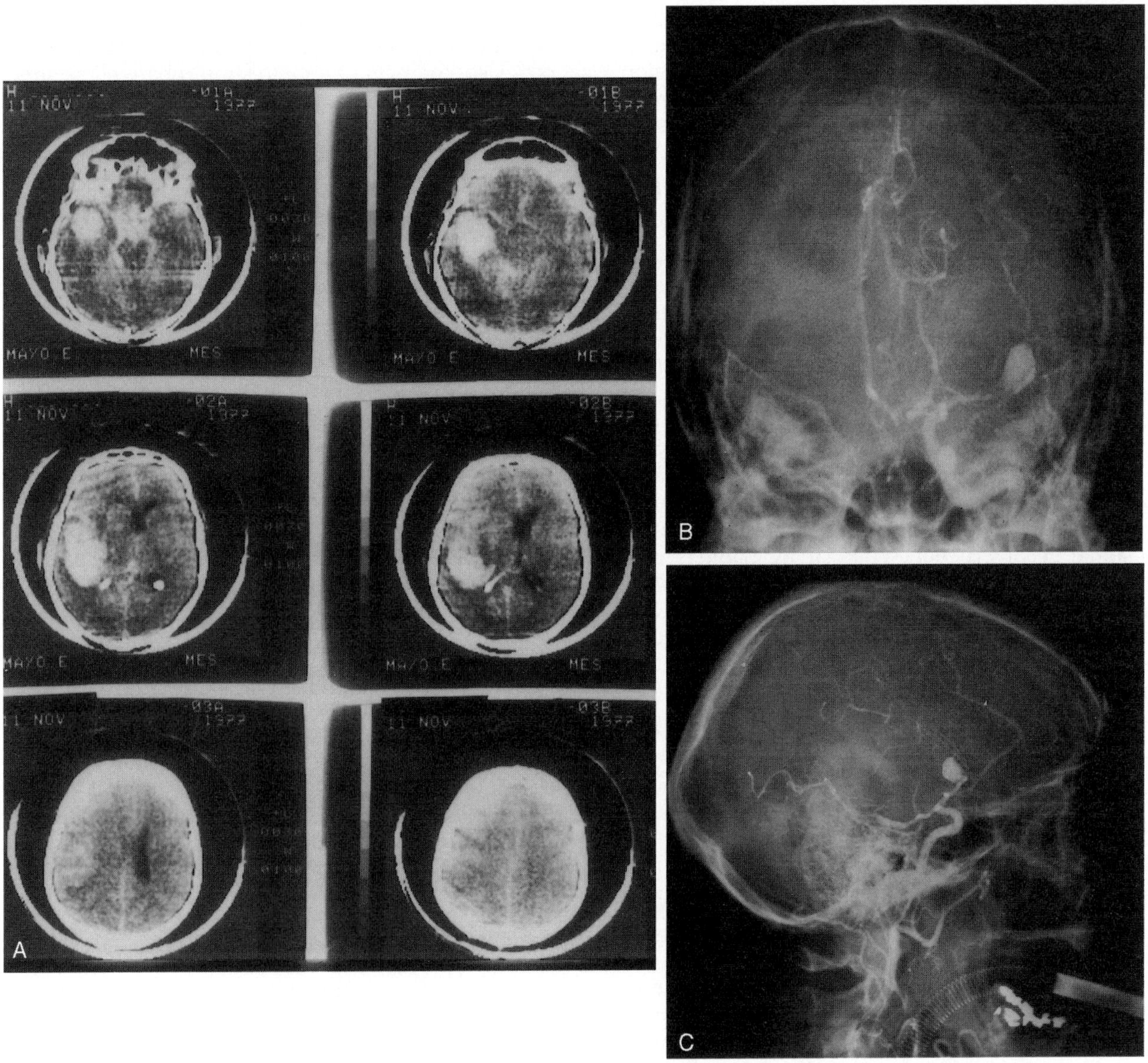

FIGURE 115–1. *A*, Noncontrast computed tomographic scan of a patient with a ruptured middle cerebral artery (MCA) aneurysm shows the classic appearance of left temporal hematoma (sides reversed on older scanners) and diffuse subarachnoid hemorrhage. *B* and *C*, Anteroposterior and lateral views of left internal carotid angiogram demonstrate the 1.5-cm MCA bifurcation aneurysm.

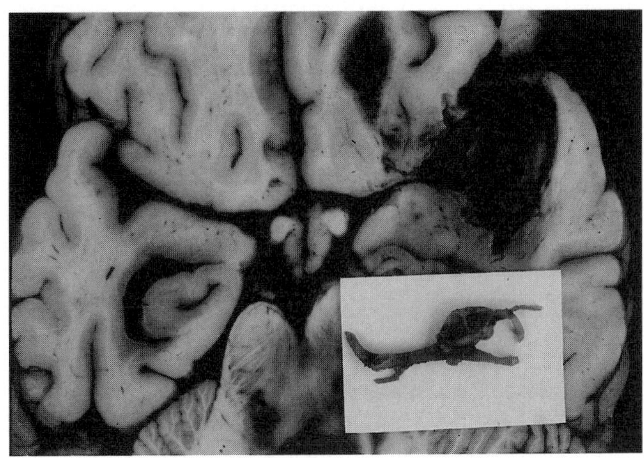

FIGURE 115–2. Gross pathologic specimen from a patient with left temporal and frontal hematoma from a ruptured middle cerebral artery bifurcation aneurysm (*inset*).

ried out. In these cases, computed tomographic definition of a parasylvian hematoma should raise suspicion of an underlying MCA aneurysm, and rapid-infusion contrasted computed tomography (if possible) may demonstrate the aneurysm within the hemorrhage. Although morbidity and mortality are high in these cases, emergency surgery for removal of the clot and repair of the aneurysm can be lifesaving and is sometimes rewarded by satisfactory outcome.[21]

Occasionally, among stable and good-grade patients with subarachnoid hemorrhage or those presenting with unruptured intracranial aneurysms, studies demonstrate a complex or giant aneurysm arising from the MCA. Often, these aneurysms arise at the MCA bifurcation and have broad necks that encompass the origins of the major MCA divisions; this makes the prospect of definitive clipping uncertain and risky. In these cases, operative intervention may best be delayed to allow thorough evaluation of the aneurysm anatomy with computed tomography–angiography and three-dimensional reconstruction. Also, if available, three-dimensional angiography may be helpful in evaluating aneurysm anatomy. Such detailed definition of the aneurysm facilitates surgical planning and optimizes outcome in these difficult cases,[22] which may include microsurgical reconstruction of the aneurysm base or revascularization of jeopardized branches with superficial temporal artery (STA)–MCA anastomosis.[23]

Operative Technique

Most MCA aneurysms, whether proximal on the M1 trunk or at the MCA bifurcation in the lateral sylvian fissure, are best approached through a standard frontotemporal (pterional) craniotomy as espoused by Yasargil.[7, 24] For patients with associated intracerebral hemorrhage (and, in the opinion of some surgeons, for all cases of aneurysm clipping), preoperative loading with anticonvulsant medication is advisable.[25] For patients with recent subarachnoid hemorrhage and in whom a ventricular catheter has not been established, placement of a lumbar drain for intraoperative cerebrospinal fluid (CSF) removal to facilitate cerebral relaxation during dural opening seems advantageous. For patients with major intracerebral hemorrhage, CSF drainage is unnecessary because clot evacuation usually provides adequate relaxation for exposure, and lumbar puncture may be contraindicated owing to the increased risk of herniation secondary to hematoma mass effect. For most cases of unruptured MCA aneurysms, we consider lumbar drainage unnecessary and possibly disadvantageous, because a full cisternal volume facilitates dissection down the sylvian fissure.

Patient positioning for craniotomy and clipping of the MCA aneurysm is also as classically described by Yasargil,[7, 24] with the head turned to the opposite side approximately 30 degrees and slightly extended to position the malar eminence at the highest point. Securing the head in a pinion head holder is considered mandatory. Care should be taken to ensure that the pinion sites are infiltrated with local anesthetic before their application to minimize reflex hypertension and the risk of induced aneurysm rupture during clamp application. Also, the patient's torso should be well secured on the operating table with straps and padding to allow side-to-side rotation of the table to optimize intraoperative visualization down the sylvian fissure while minimizing cerebral retraction.

The standard pterional craniotomy is carried out. The craniotomy must extend at least 2 cm into the supraorbital area to provide adequate exposure of the proximal sylvian fissure and room for placement of a frontal self-retaining retractor, which is often necessary to expose either the aneurysm or the proximal middle cerebral trunk. The pterion and lateral sphenoid wing are fully drilled away with a diamond or semisharp bit down to the superior orbital fissure, which also facilitates the view down the sylvian fissure and minimizes cerebral retraction.

Approaches to Middle Cerebral Artery Aneurysms

Although there are three basic approaches to MCA aneurysms, the fundamental concepts of providing proximal control and adequate exposure while protecting critical structures remain inviolate. Particular aspects of each case dictate which approach is most appropriate. The reader is referred to the authoritative prescriptions of Yasargil[7] and the more recent contribution of Chyatte and Porterfield,[26] the latter of which provides a web-based video for further elaboration of these techniques.

LATERAL TRANS-SYLVIAN APPROACH

The lateral trans-sylvian approach is preferred by many neurosurgeons for unruptured or uncomplicated MCA aneurysms located at the MCA bifurcation, particularly when the MCA stem (M1 segment) has the usual configuration, which places the aneurysm very near the surface in the anterior third of the sylvian fissure. The lateral trans-sylvian approach is less desirable for large or complicated MCA aneurysms, particularly after subarachnoid hemorrhage, and in the hands of less experienced surgeons, because this approach brings the surgeon to the aneurysm dome before exposure of the M1 segment.

The sylvian fissure is opened, beginning in its anterior third, using microsurgical technique. Care should be taken to keep the dissection within the sylvian fissure and avoid straying into a subpial plane. In cases of subarachnoid hemorrhage with clot in the fissure, meticulous removal of the clot with suction and irrigation can facilitate the approach to the aneurysm. Sacrifice of one or more sylvian veins is often necessary and can usually be done without consequence. Nevertheless, attempts should be made to preserve those veins that lie lateral or medial to the dissection. Early identification of M3 branches within the fissure provides reference for further proximal dissection to M2 divisions and the aneurysm dome. At this juncture, with the patient often under mild induced hypotension, a self-retaining retractor is placed on the frontal sylvian surface; gentle retraction and opening of the fissure proximal to the aneurysm permit exposure of the M1 trunk, which is prepared for temporary clipping should that become necessary. Only after proximal control is assured should the dissection return to the aneurysm for identification of every branch in the aneurysm field, including the critical lenticulostriate branches, which may be closely approximated to the aneurysm neck or dome, even when arising at the typical MCA bifurcation region.

Clipping of MCA aneurysms requires careful dissection of branches away from the aneurysm neck and dome to avoid their compromise during clip application. Not infrequently, in cases of ruptured and occasionally unruptured aneurysms, this dissection is most safely accomplished under periods of temporary M1 occlusion, which we limit to less than 10 minutes, followed by equal or greater periods of reperfusion should repetition be necessary. Once the branches are freed, we have found that shrinking of the aneurysm dome with bipolar cautery (after the technique of Yasargil) is helpful in reducing the irregular or bulbous aneurysm sac to a more easily clipped configuration. The initial coagulation may also be best accomplished with temporary proximal occlusion or under relative hypotension. The operative approach and techniques for clipping are presented in Figures 115–3 to 115–6. Once clipping has been achieved, confirmation of flow in each adjacent branch or MCA division can be confirmed with the micro-Doppler probe. Topical application of dilute papaverine solution to the MCA branches is often desirable to reverse mechanically induced or aggravated spasm.

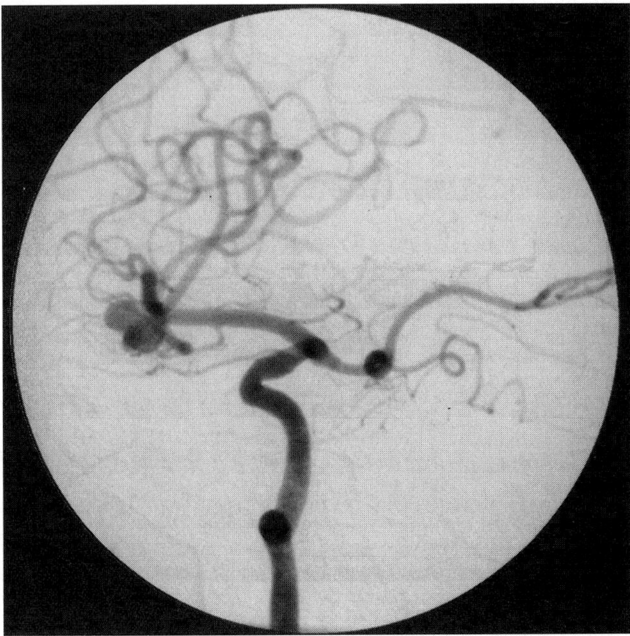

FIGURE 115–3. Oblique view of a right internal carotid angiogram demonstrates a bilobed middle cerebral artery bifurcation aneurysm.

MEDIAL TRANS-SYLVIAN APPROACH

The medial trans-sylvian approach may be the approach of choice for aneurysms that arise along the proximal M1 trunk, in those patients with very short M1 segments, or for aneurysms that have ruptured and have a complicated configuration based on either size or suspected fragility of the sac. Such aneurysms may carry an increased risk of rerupture at the time of exposure, or they may hinder identification of the M1 trunk, making proximal control more difficult to achieve. In these cases, it may be especially helpful to provide intraoperative CSF drainage and adequate low frontal extension of the pterional craniotomy to allow a subfrontal exposure to the carotid cistern and most proximal sylvian fissure. Alternatively, the initial dissection may be carried through the thick arachnoidal bands between the anterior temporal and frontal lobes down to the anterior sylvian base, where the arachnoid is opened to allow exposure of, in turn, the optic nerve, internal carotid artery, internal carotid artery bifurcation, and M1 trunk. In either case, the sylvian fissure is opened medially to laterally by sharply dissecting the arachnoid bands between the mesial anterior temporal and frontal lobes, to allow gentle frontal lobe retraction. Brain relaxation may be facilitated by CSF drainage from a lumbar catheter, from the carotid and basal cisterns, or, if necessary, through opening of the lamina terminalis. Dissection is carried laterally along the anterior and inferior surface of the M1 trunk so as to avoid injury to the lenticulostriate and recurrent perforating branches. This dissection proceeds until the aneurysm and adjacent branches are adequately exposed for thorough visualization of the pathologic anatomy and aneurysm clipping.

SUPERIOR TEMPORAL GYRUS APPROACH

The transcortical approach through the superior temporal gyrus has been advocated by Heros and colleagues[27] as the preferred approach to MCA bifurcation aneurysms whether associated with intracerebral hemorrhage or not. In this technique, the anterior aspect of the superior temporal gyrus is opened parallel to the sylvian fissure for 2 to 3 cm, and brain resection is carried down to the vertical segment of the fissure over the insula. The middle cerebral branches, bifurcation, and aneurysm are then identified through a transpial extension into the sylvian fissure. Although good results may be achieved with this variation, it has little advantage over the lateral trans-sylvian approach in our minds. One notable exception in which the superior temporal gyrus approach is clearly advantageous is the case of associated intracerebral hemorrhage, where opening of the superior temporal gyrus provides access for evacuation of the clot, cerebral relaxation, and then access to the MCA and the aneurysm, as illustrated in Figure 115–7. In keeping with basic principles, after partial evacuation of the hematoma, exposure should be directed to the MCA trunk proximal to the aneurysm before removing the clot overlying the site of aneurysm rupture. The second situation in

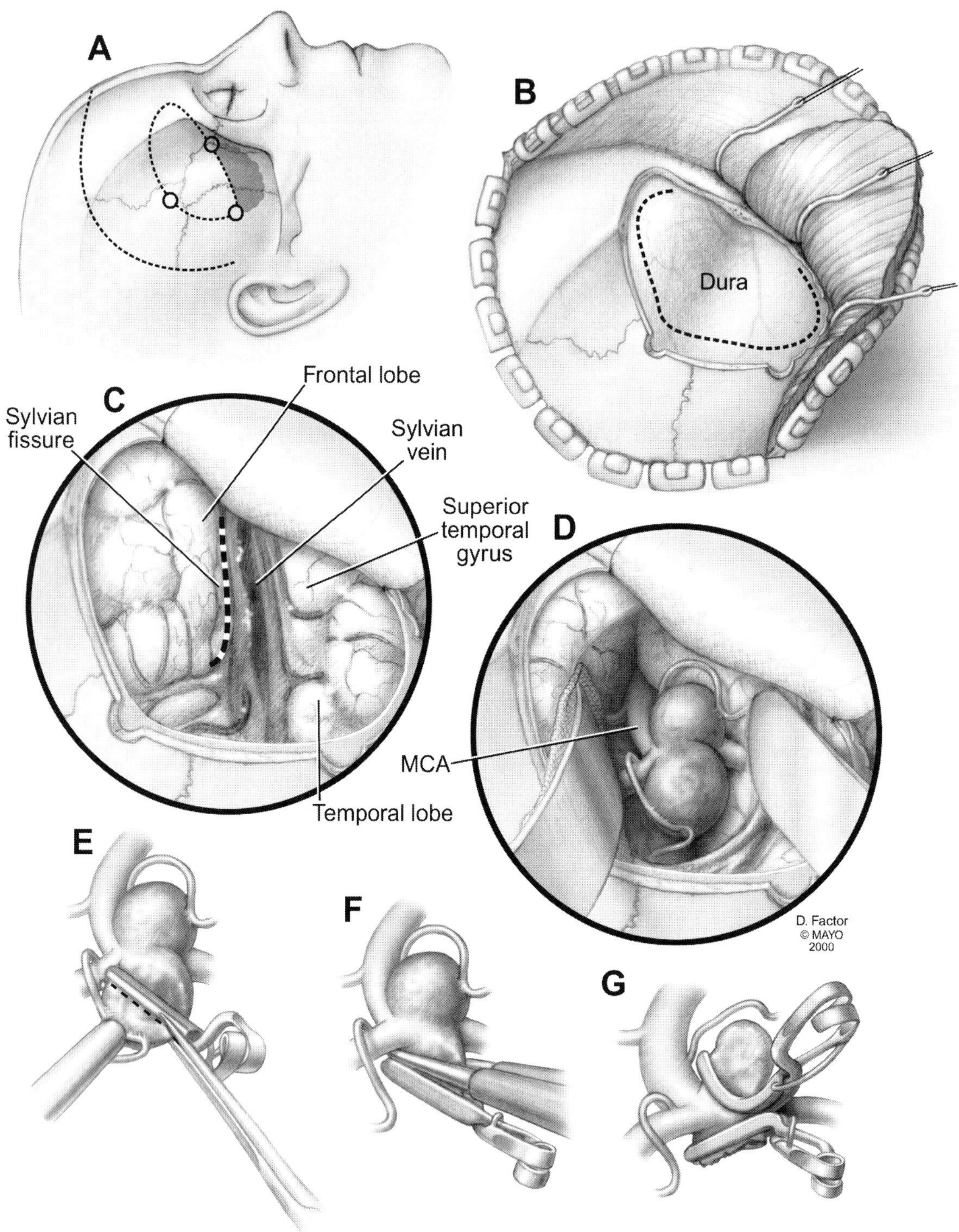

FIGURE 115–4. Operative approach to the aneurysm shown in Figure 115–3. *A* and *B*, Standard frontotemporal incision and craniotomy. *C* and *D*, Dura is opened and reflected anteriorly, exposing the sylvian fissure. The sylvian fissure is dissected and retracted, exposing the proximal M1 segment, the middle cerebral artery (MCA) bifurcation, and the lobes of the aneurysm. *E*, One lobe of the aneurysm is partially clipped to allow transection of a segment of the aneurysm dome, which is adherent to a perforating artery. *F* and *G*, Bipolar cautery is used to shrink the aneurysm. Both lobes of the aneurysm are clipped at their respective bases, preserving both M2 branches.

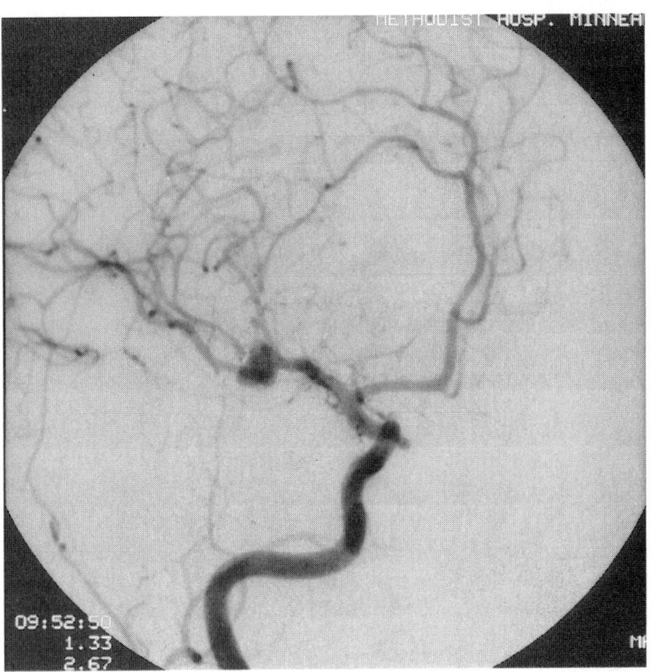

FIGURE 115–5. Oblique view of a right internal carotid angiogram demonstrates a middle cerebral artery bifurcation aneurysm with a different morphology than the one depicted in Figure 115–3.

which the superior temporal gyrus approach may be the best alternative is when the brain is full and CSF drainage has not been provided for or cannot be achieved by ventricular puncture. In this case, superior temporal gyrus dissection may provide the best access to an MCA aneurysm or the basal cisterns by extending

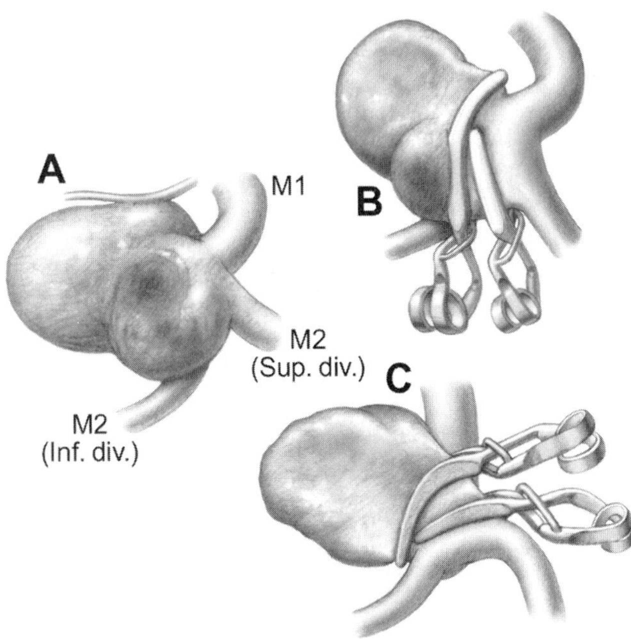

FIGURE 115–6. Two clips are stacked to completely occlude the aneurysm neck while preserving both M2 branches.

the dissection through the temporal polar and uncal gyri.

Complex Aneurysms and Alternatives to Clipping

Perhaps more than at any other site, aneurysms arising along the MCA, and particularly at the MCA bifurcation, may have complicated anatomy that precludes straightforward clipping or may jeopardize the patency of one of the major MCA branches. Such situations can be anticipated in cases of large aneurysms (>15 mm) or those with a poorly defined base or neck on angiography (Fig. 115–8). Additionally, special considerations may be necessary when computed tomographic scanning indicates the presence of heavy calcification at the aneurysm base. In these situations, it is advisable to obtain the necessary preoperative studies and surgical expertise to plan for operative alternatives, such as microvascular reconstruction of the aneurysm base or reconstitution of flow to a compromised division by STA or, rarely, interposition venous bypass.[23, 28, 29] When the feasibility of aneurysm clipping is in question, the scalp incision should be constructed to preserve the STA (Fig. 115–9). The aneurysm should be thoroughly dissected, and repair options considered. If it appears that the aneurysm base cannot be clipped with preservation of flow in each of the major branches, STA-MCA anastomosis can be carried out into one or even two branches before trapping the aneurysm for evacuation and clipping (Fig. 115–10). Such management minimizes the risk of intraoperative or postoperative ischemia but requires preoperative planning and confidence in one's microsurgical skills.

We firmly believe such an approach is preferable to the "fallback," nondefinitive treatment options such as aneurysm wrapping or coating, which were employed by previous generations of neurosurgeons who lacked the ability to perform microsurgical reconstructions.

Postoperative Care

Postoperative care of patients with MCA aneurysms is similar to that for other aneurysm patients. In those who have suffered a major intracerebral hemorrhage, long-term anticonvulsant therapy has been recommended, but its use is at the discretion of the surgeon.[25] For complicated aneurysms, such as large or giant aneurysms, or when clip obliteration appears suboptimal, a postoperative angiogram is advised. Also, if the patient wakes from surgery with new, unexplained neurological deficits, an immediate angiogram is advised to facilitate management decisions.

Outcomes

In spite of the poor results in early surgical series,[15] reports since the mid-1980s suggest that MCA aneurysms can be treated by craniotomy and clipping with good outcomes. In Yasargil's series of 184 patients, 84% returned to their former activities with no deficits, including 4 of 9 Hunt-Hess grade IV patients.[7] Among

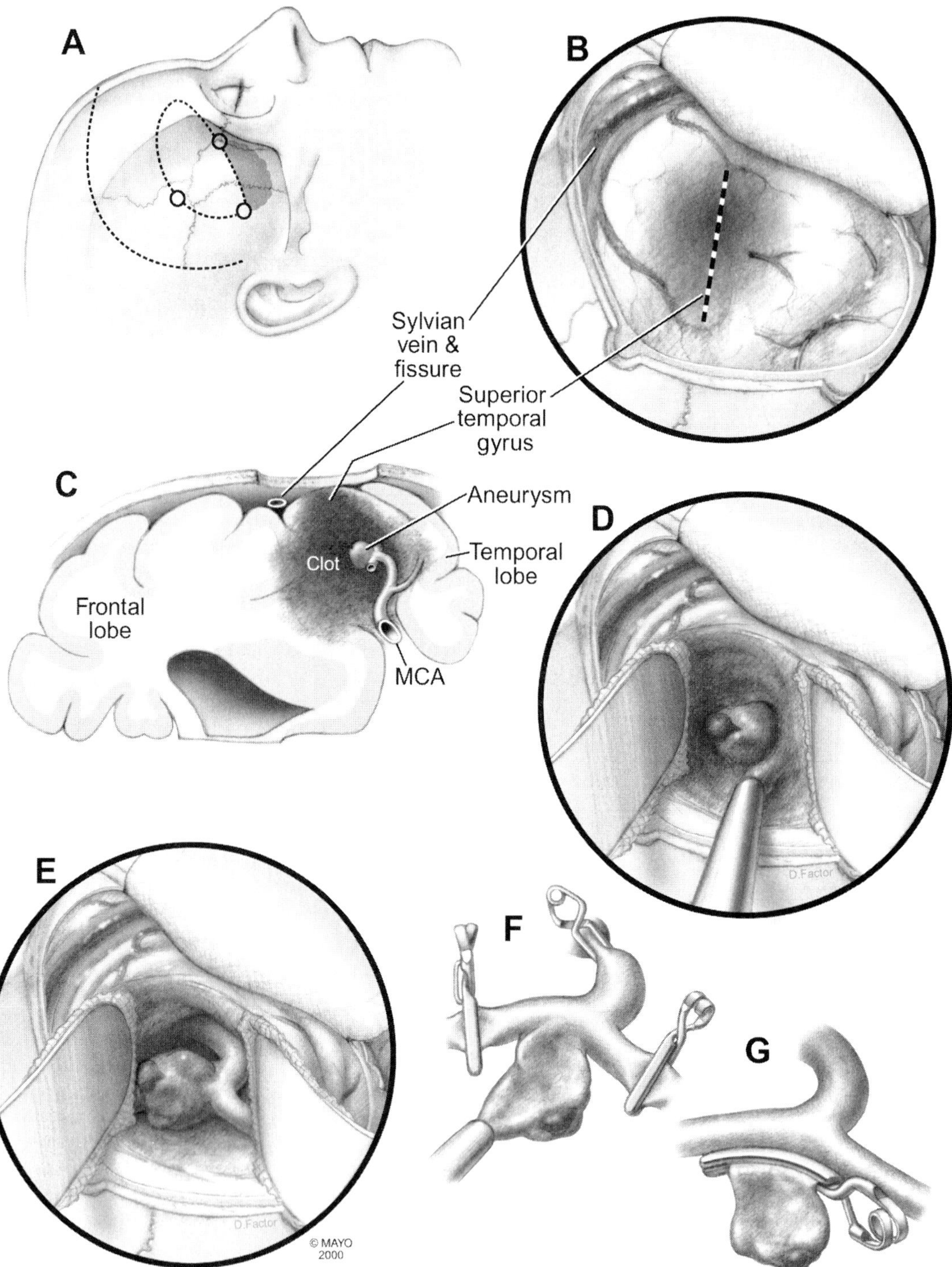

FIGURE 115–7. Operative approach to a middle cerebral artery bifurcation aneurysm in a patient with a large hematoma in the temporal lobe. *A–C*, Standard frontotemporal incision and craniotomy. The sylvian fissure is displaced superiorly by the temporal hematoma. *D* and *E*, The aneurysm is approached and exposed through the hematoma cavity in the superior temporal gyrus. *F*, Temporary clips are applied to M1 and both M2 branches. *G*, The aneurysm is clipped at its base.

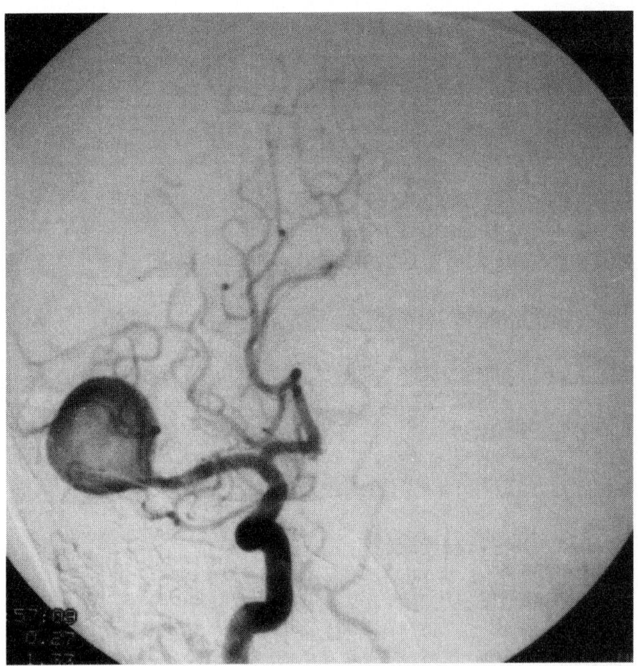

FIGURE 115–8. Anteroposterior angiographic view of a large right middle cerebral artery bifurcation aneurysm with M2 branches draped over the aneurysm dome. The origins of these branches in relationship to the aneurysm neck cannot be well defined.

the patients in this series, 8% were left in poor condition or died. Hunt-Hess grade was a strong predictor of poor outcome and death in operated patients. Suzuki and colleagues reported an excellent or good outcome in 82% of their 265 patients with single MCA aneurysms at an average follow-up of 3 years[30]; 4% of patients were independent but could not return to work, and 13% had poor outcomes or died. A subgroup of 91 patients treated at the end of the series, when the surgical approach and technique had been refined, had significantly better outcomes—92% of patients were in good or excellent condition postoperatively.

Pasztor and colleagues reported a favorable outcome in 82% and a poor outcome in 18% of 265 patients treated surgically for ruptured MCA aneurysms at the National Institute of Neurosurgery in Budapest.[31] Glasgow Coma Scale score and Hunt-Hess grade were the most important preoperative predictors of outcome. Although patients treated within 48 hours did significantly better overall, most patients were treated more than a week after hemorrhage, and preoperative vasospasm was a significant predictor of outcome. Interestingly, aneurysm size did not play a significant role in outcome in this study; nor did age for patients with low clinical grades. Among 113 patients operated on for MCA aneurysms reported by Sundt and colleagues,[1] 14% had a poor outcome, which is consistent with the results of other series.

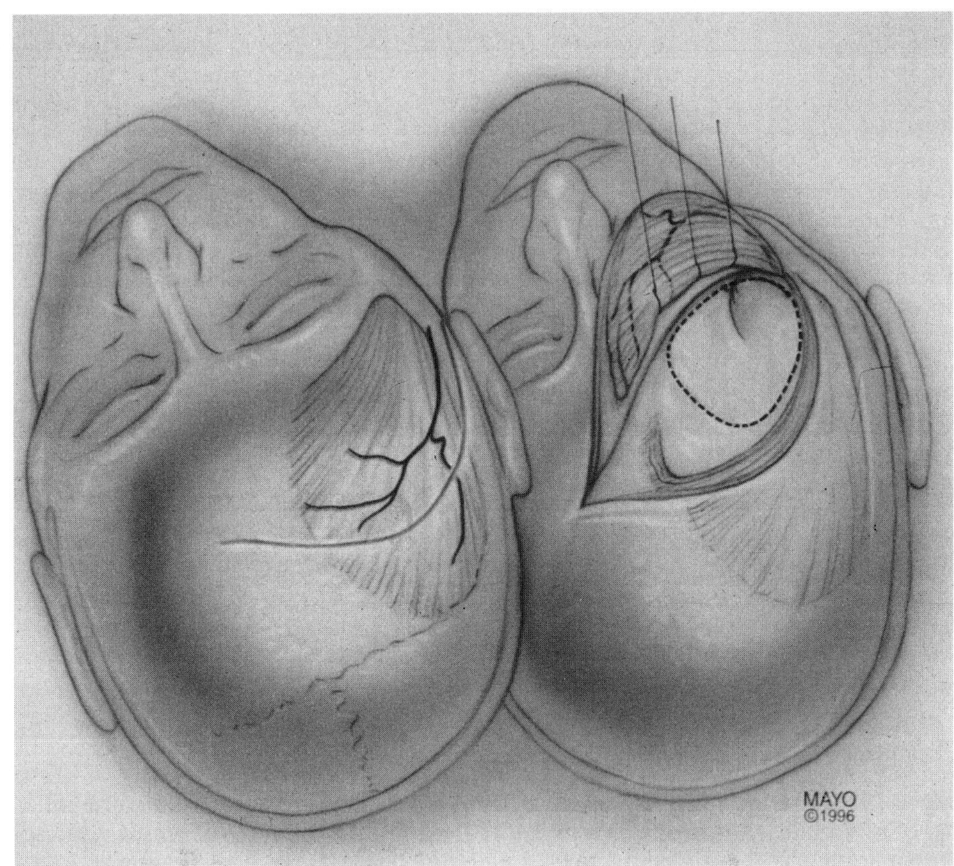

FIGURE 115–9. Illustration of the scalp incision that preserves the anterior branch of the superficial temporal artery (STA) for pterional craniotomy. A more posterior incision can be made, if necessary, to preserve the posterior STA branch as well.

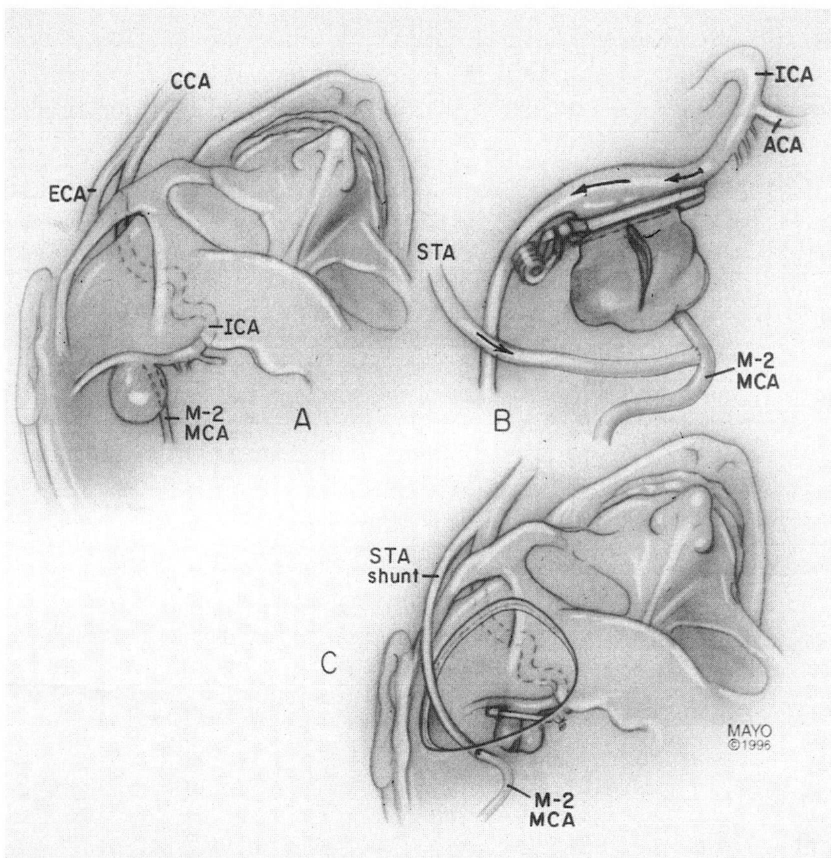

FIGURE 115–10. *A*, Schematic diagram of a large, broad-based, middle cerebral artery (MCA) bifurcation aneurysm in which the M2 divisions are incorporated in the aneurysm dome and base. Clipping is accomplished after reconstruction of a superior temporal artery (STA) anastomosis to the superior M2 division. *B*, The end-to-side technique is preferred. *C*, Alternative end-to-end anastomosis technique. ACA, anterior cerebral artery; CCA, common carotid artery; ECA, external carotid artery; ICA, internal carotid artery.

More recently, Heros reported a good outcome in 69% of his 108 patients treated for MCA aneurysms.[11] In this series, more patients had poor clinical grades than in earlier series; only 1 of 11 patients with preoperative clinical grades of IV or V achieved a good outcome. Diaz and colleagues described their experience with 48 MCA aneurysms larger than 20 mm or of complex configuration.[32] Of these aneurysms, 29 were directly clipped, 5 were trapped, 5 were trapped and underwent extracranial-intracranial vascular bypass, 5 were resected with primary anastomosis of the MCA, and 1 was wrapped with muslin. In this high-risk subgroup of patients, 35% had significant new neurological deficits postoperatively, yet 81% of the total operated group had full functional recovery at long-term follow-up (minimum 1 year).

In the largest published series of surgically treated MCA aneurysms, Rinne and coworkers cataloged their outcomes in 561 patients with 690 lesions.[4] Despite low surgical morbidity and mortality, 30% of patients had poor outcome scores at 1 year, defined as a Glasgow Outcome Scale score of 3 or less. The same surgeons reported a 23% rate of poor outcome in patients operated on for other anterior circulation aneurysms. The frequency of poor outcome was higher when multiple aneurysms were present, with larger MCA aneurysms, and with irregularly shaped MCA aneurysms. There was no significant difference in overall management outcome for MCA aneurysms at proximal, bifurcation, and distal sites. However, among patients with a good clinical grade, those with ruptured proximal MCA aneurysms had a higher likelihood of poor outcome than did similar-grade patients with aneurysms at the MCA bifurcation or distally. Multivariate analysis of these results indicated that the most important predictors of outcome were admission clinical grade, postoperative vasospasm, postoperative hematoma, and age.

In summary, the published experience of the surgical treatment of ruptured MCA aneurysms suggests that the overall management outcome is largely determined by the clinical grade of subarachnoid hemorrhage on admission. Because of the frequency of intracerebral hemorrhage, there is a high incidence of persistent neurological deficits and seizure disorders. Although the largest series suggests a worse overall management outcome for MCA aneurysms than for other anterior circulation aneurysms, this unquestionably pertains to the consequences of hemorrhage in these patients.

Concerning the outcome of treatment for unruptured MCA aneurysms, few studies report the treatment risks of unruptured aneurysms by aneurysm location. Wirth and colleagues found that the treatment risk associated with incidental MCA aneurysms was approximately half that of aneurysms at anterior communicating and carotid bifurcation sites, but twice that of internal carotid artery and posterior communicating artery aneurysms.[33] The International Study of Unruptured Intracranial Aneurysms (ISUIA) provided unique data on the risks of treating unruptured intracranial aneurysms. In the preliminary (phase I) analysis, overall treatment mortality and major morbidity (including dementia) for aneurysms of all sizes and at all locations was approximately 15%. Outcome was strongly related to patient age.[34] More robust data on the entire ISUIA series, including phase I and phase II patients, permitted an analysis of outcome and the risks of repair by aneurysm site and size. These results, soon to be published, show a clear relationship between outcome and aneurysm size, with increased risks related to the clipping of large and giant aneurysms at all locations. Important to this discussion is the finding that the outcome of clipping MCA aneurysms was comparable to that of clipping internal carotid–posterior communicating artery aneurysms, and the MCA was among the lowest risk sites for repair.[35]

ENDOVASCULAR TREATMENT

Although the long-term efficacy of Guglielmi detachable coil (GDC) embolization of cerebral aneurysms is uncertain, the technique has gained acceptance as an alternative to surgery in certain cases.[36, 37] However, the angioanatomy of MCA aneurysms is less conducive to treatment with GDC embolization than is that of aneurysms at other sites. In 34 consecutive unruptured MCA aneurysms reviewed by Regli and colleagues,[6] all were initially considered for endovascular treatment by the interventional neuroradiologist. In 21 patients, the angiographic configuration of the aneurysms was thought to be unfavorable for GDC embolization. In the remaining 13 patients, GDC embolization was attempted but was successful in only 2 patients. The reasons for embolization failure were wide aneurysm neck or an arterial branch originating from the base of the aneurysm. Until new endovascular technologies are introduced, surgical clipping will likely remain the standard treatment modality for most MCA aneurysms.

ACKNOWLEDGMENTS

The authors are indebted to David Factor for his excellent medical illustrations and to Mary Soper for secretarial assistance.

REFERENCES

1. Sundt T, Kobayashi S, Fode NC, et al: Results and complications of surgical management of 809 intracranial aneurysms in 722 cases: Related and unrelated to grade of patient, type of aneurysm, and timing of surgery. J Neurosurg 56:753–765, 1982.
2. Kassell N, Torner JC, Haley EC, et al: The International Cooperative Study on the Timing of Aneurysm Surgery. Part I. Overall management results. J Neurosurg 73:18–36, 1990.
3. Tokuda Y, Inagawa T, Katoh Y, et al: Intracerebral hematoma in patients with ruptured cerebral aneurysms. Surg Neurol 43: 272–277, 1995.
4. Rinne J, Hernesniemi J, Niskanen M, et al: Analysis of 561 patients with 690 middle cerebral artery aneurysms: Anatomical and clinical features as correlated to management outcome. Neurosurgery 38:2–11, 1996.
5. Dandy W: Surgical treatment of aneurysms of the middle cerebral artery. In Intracranial Arterial Aneurysms. Ithaca, NY, Comstock, 1945, pp 129–132.
6. Regli L, Uske A, deTribolet N: Endovascular coil placement compared with surgical clipping for the treatment of unruptured middle cerebral artery aneurysms: A consecutive series. J Neurosurg 90:1025–1030, 1999.
7. Yasargil M: Middle cerebral artery aneurysms. In Yasargil M (ed): Microneurosurgery II: Clinical Considerations, Surgery of the Intracranial Aneurysms and Results. Stuttgart, Georg Thieme Verlag, 1984, pp 124–164.
8. Yasargil MG: Operative anatomy. In Microneurosurgery: Microsurgical Anatomy of the Basal Cisterns and Vessels of the Brain, Diagnostic Studies, General Operative Techniques and Pathological Considerations of Intracranial Aneurysms, vol 1. Stuttgart, Georg Thieme Verlag, 1984, pp 72–91.
9. Gibo H, Carver C, Rhoton A, et al: Microsurgical anatomy of the middle cerebral artery. J Neurosurg 54:151–169, 1981.
10. Hosoda K, Fujita S, Kawaguchi T, et al: Saccular aneurysms of the proximal (M1) segment of the middle cerebral artery. Neurosurgery 36:441–446, 1995.
11. Heros R: Middle cerebral artery aneurysms. In Wilkins R, Rengachary SS (eds): Neurosurgery. New York, McGraw-Hill, 1996, pp 2311–2316.
12. Drake CG: Giant intracranial aneurysms: Experience with surgical treatment in 174 patients. Clin Neurosurg 26:12–95, 1979.
13. Sundt TM Jr, Piepgras D: Surgical approach to giant intracranial aneurysms. J Neurosurg 51:731–742, 1979.
14. Stoodley M, Macdonald RL, Weir BK: Surgical treatment of middle cerebral artery aneurysms. Neurosurg Clin N Am 9:823–834, 1998.
15. Hook O, Norlen G: Aneurysms of the middle cerebral artery. Acta Chir Scand Suppl 235:1–39, 1958.
16. Graf C, Nibbelink DW: Cooperative Study of Intracranial Aneurysms and Subarachnoid Hemorrhage: Report on a randomized treatment study. III. Intracranial surgery. Stroke 5:559–601, 1974.
17. Lougheed W, Marshall BM: Management of aneurysms of the anterior circulation by intracranial procedures. In Youmans JR (ed): Neurological Surgery. Philadelphia, WB Saunders, 1973, pp 731–767.
18. Pietila T, Heimberger KC, Palleske H, et al: Influence of aneurysm location on the development of chronic hydrocephalus following SAH. Acta Neurochir (Wien) 137:70–73, 1995.
19. Vale F, Bradley EL, Fisher WS: The relationship of subarachnoid hemorrhage and the need for postoperative shunting. J Neurosurg 86:462–466, 1997.
20. Tanaka K, Hriayama K, Hattori H, et al: A case of cerebral aneurysm associated with complex partial seizures. Brain Dev 16:233–237, 1994.
21. LeRoux PD, Daily AT, Newell DW, et al: Emergent aneurysm clipping without angiography in the moribund patient with intracerebral hemorrhage: The use of infusion computed tomography scans. Neurosurgery 79:826–832, 1993.
22. Piepgras D, Khurana GV, Whisnant J: Ruptured giant intracranial aneurysms. Part II. A retrospective analysis of timing and outcome of surgical treatment. J Neurosurg 88:430–435, 1998.
23. Lawton MT, Hamilton MG, Marcos JJ, et al: Revascularization and aneurysm surgery: Current techniques, indications, and outcome. Neurosurgery 38:83–94, 1996.
24. Yasargil MG: Operative anatomy. In Microneurosurgery: Microsurgical Anatomy of the Basal Cisterns and Vessels of the Brain, Diagnostic Studies, General Operative Techniques and Pathological Considerations of Intracranial Aneurysms, vol 1. Stuttgart, Georg Thieme Verlag, 1984, pp 208–271.
25. Mayberg MR, Batjer H, Dacey R, et al: Guidelines for the management of aneurysmal subarachnoid hemorrhage. Stroke 25: 2315–2328, 1994.
26. Chyatte D, Porterfield R: Nuances of middle cerebral artery aneurysm microsurgery. Neurosurgery 48:339–346, 2001.
27. Heros RC, Ojemann RG, Crowell RM: Superior temporal gyrus approach to middle cerebral artery aneurysms: Technique and results. Neurosurgery 10:308–313, 1982.
28. Drake C, Peerless SJ, Ferguson CG: Hunterian proximal arterial occlusion for giant aneurysms of the carotid circulation. J Neurosurg 81:656–665, 1994.
29. Sundt TM Jr: Surgical Techniques for Saccular and Giant Intracranial Aneurysms. Baltimore, Williams & Wilkins, 1990, pp 179–210.

30. Suzuki J, Yoshimoto T, Kayama T: Surgical treatment of middle cerebral artery aneurysms. J Neurosurg 61:17–23, 1984.
31. Pasztor E, Vajda J, Johasz J, et al: The surgery of middle cerebral artery aneurysms. Acta Neurochir (Wien) 82:92–101, 1986.
32. Diaz F, Guthikonda M, Guyot L, et al: Surgical management of complex middle cerebral artery aneurysms. Neurol Med Chir (Tokyo) 38(Suppl):50–57, 1998.
33. Wirth FP, Laws ER, Piepgras D, et al: Surgical treatment of incidental intracranial aneurysms. Neurosurgery 12:507–511, 1983.
34. International Study of Unruptured Intracranial Aneurysms investigators: Unruptured intracranial aneurysms—risk of rupture and risks of surgical intervention. N Engl J Med 339:1725–1733, 1998.
35. International Study of Unruptured Intracranial Aneurysms investigators: Personal communication.
36. Malisch T, Guglielmi G, Vinuela F, et al: Intracranial aneurysms treated with Guglielmi detachable coil: Midterm clinical results in a consecutive series of 100 patients. J Neurosurg 87:176–183, 1997.
37. Vinuela F, Duckwiler G, Mawad M, et al: Guglielmi detachable coil embolization of acute intracranial aneurysms: Perioperative anatomical and clinical outcome in 403 patients. J Neurosurg 86: 475–482, 1997.

CHAPTER **116**

Surgical Approaches for Posterior Circulation Aneurysms

MICHAEL T. LAWTON ■ G. EDWARD VATES ■ ROBERT F. SPETZLER

Exposure is everything. This statement captures the essence of successful aneurysm surgery. Only with adequate exposure can neurosurgeons directly visualize vascular anatomy, obtain proximal and distal control of afferent and efferent arteries, apply meticulous microsurgical technique, and maneuver a clip to occlude an aneurysm successfully with a good outcome. In the posterior circulation, exposure is elusive. The deep midline location of vertebrobasilar aneurysms, the bony enclosure of the clivus and petrous pyramids, and the complex intertwining of neural and arterial structures in the posterior fossa all conspire to make posterior circulation aneurysms more difficult to access and thus more difficult to treat compared with their anterior circulation counterparts.

Neurosurgeons have fought to overcome these disadvantages in the posterior fossa. Rather than defy the inherent anatomic constraints, early efforts sought alternatives to direct clipping, and proximal or hunterian ligation of the basilar artery became an acceptable treatment for some basilar tip aneurysms.[1, 2] The introduction of the operating microscope, combined with a more thorough understanding of skull base anatomy, led to the development of techniques for removing the bony impediments of the skull base and increasing operative exposure. This resulted in more direct approaches and improved outcomes.[3] Hypothermic circulatory arrest allowed complete vascular control of complex aneurysms where limited exposure otherwise would have precluded temporary proximal and distal clipping of parent arteries.[4]

These surgical advances have rendered posterior circulation aneurysms treatable, but at a price. With these techniques, surgical complications are unavoidable and sometimes even planned. The ability to tackle these formidable aneurysms must be weighed against the operative risks and the risks of less invasive therapies such as endovascular coiling, making the treatment of posterior circulation aneurysms both intellectually and technically challenging. It has been suggested that surgery for posterior circulation aneurysms will become obsolete as endovascular technologies evolve, making this chapter a historical piece. If current practices at multidisciplinary cerebrovascular centers provide a glimpse of the future, then endovascular techniques will become established in the treatment armamentarium of posterior circulation aneurysms. However, they too will be associated with their own insurmountable limitations. Thus, the surgical techniques described in this chapter will be essential for managing a subset of patients with complex aneurysms that cannot be treated by endovascular obliteration or that recur after coiling. This challenging subset will increase the technical demands on vascular neurosurgeons.

The list of surgical approaches to posterior circulation aneurysms is long (Table 116–1), technical differences are often subtle, and the nomenclature can be confusing. Nonetheless, approaches fall into three categories defined by the exposed vascular territory and surgical trajectory (Fig. 116–1).[5] The three vascular territories are the basilar apex, basilar trunk, and vertebral trunk. The surgical trajectories to these territories are anterosuperior, lateral, and posteroinferior, respectively. Within each category, technical differences can be reduced to variations in the "outer" cranial exposure (Table 116–2) and the "inner" skull base exposure

TABLE 116–1 ■ **Surgical Approaches to Posterior Circulation aneurysms**

Subtemporal approach
Pterional-transsylvian approach
Orbitozygomatic-pterional approach
Extended orbitozygomatic approach
Retrosigmoid approach
Transpetrosal approaches
Retrolabyrinthine
Translabyrinthine
Transcochlear
Combined supra- and infratentorial approach
Extended middle fossa approach
Transoral approach
Midline suboccipital approach
Far-lateral approach
Extended far-lateral approach
Combined-combined approach (far-lateral combined supra- and infratentorial approach)

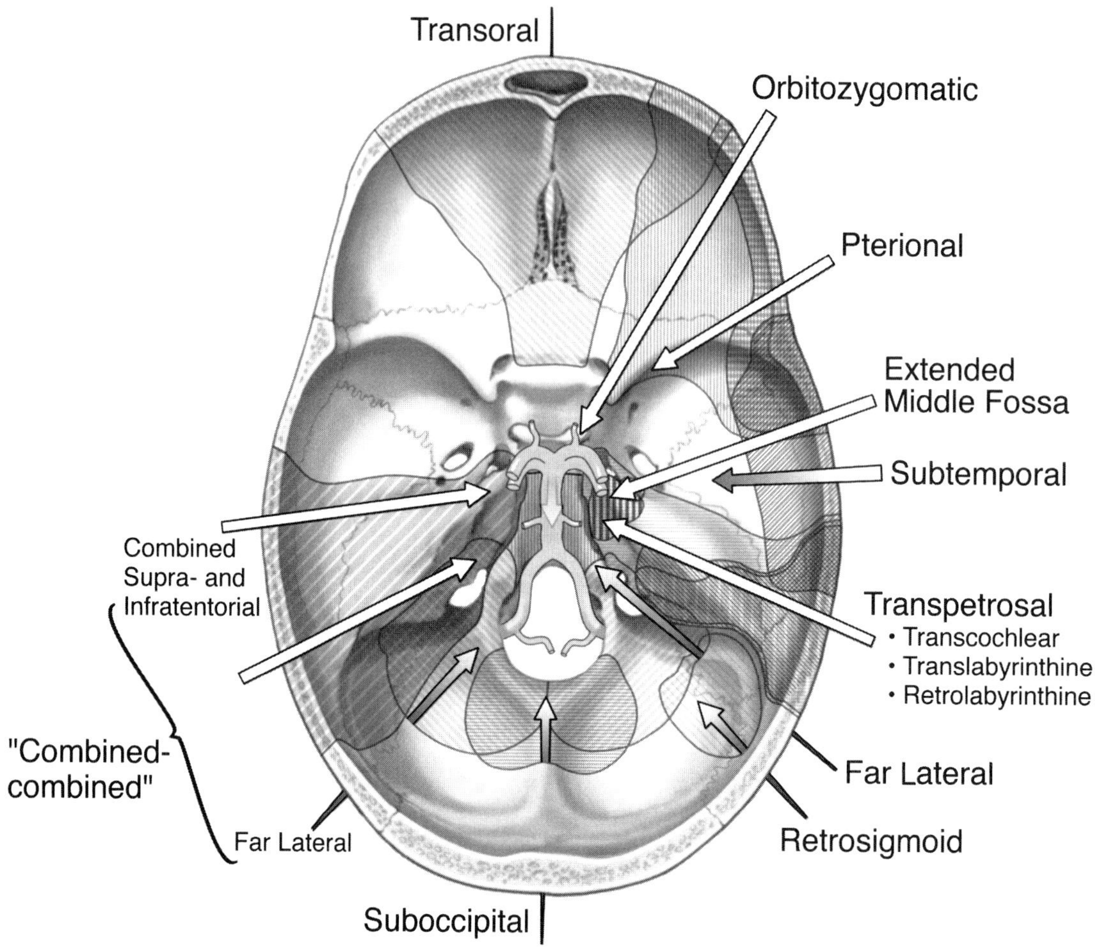

FIGURE 116–1. Illustration of the skull base showing surgical approaches to posterior circulation aneurysms and their associated trajectories. (Courtesy of Barrow Neurological Institute, Phoenix, Arizona.)

TABLE 116–2 ■ **"Outer" Cranial Approaches for Posterior Circulation Aneurysms**

VASCULAR TERRITORY	TRAJECTORY	ANEURYSMS	OUTER CRANIAL EXPOSURE
Basilar apex	Anterosuperior	Basilar tip Posterior cerebral artery Superior cerebellar artery Upper basilar artery	Subtemporal approach Pterional approach Orbitozygomatic approach Extended orbitozygomatic approach*
Basilar trunk	Lateral	Anterior inferior cerebellar artery Midbasilar artery	Transpetrosal approach* Combined supra- and infratentorial approach* Extended middle fossa approach Transoral approach
Vertebral trunk	Posteroinferior	Vertebral artery Posterior inferior cerebellar artery Vertebrobasilar junction	Midline suboccipital approach Far-lateral approach* Extended far-lateral approach Combined-combined approach

* Preferred approach.

TABLE 116–3 ■ "Inner" Skull Base Exposures for Posterior Circulation Aneurysms

VASCULAR TERRITORY	SKULL BASE RESECTION	TRANSCRANIAL ROUTE
Basilar apex	Posterior clinoid process Anterior clinoid process Dorsum sellae Clivus Medial petrous apex	Transsylvian Transclinoidal-extracavernous Transclinoidal-transcavernous Transtentorial
Basilar trunk	Posterior petrous bone Semicircular canals Cochlea Medial petrous apex	Retrolabyrinthine Translabyrinthine Transcochlear Medial transpetrous Transsigmoid
Vertebral trunk	Occipital condyle Jugular tubercle Transverse foramen of C1 Mastoid bone	Transcondylar Transcondylar-retrosigmoid

(Table 116–3). The result is slightly different transcranial routes to aneurysms. This chapter reviews the relevant posterior fossa anatomy, the clinical presentation of posterior circulation aneurysms, and the diagnostic studies needed to plan an attack on these aneurysms. The available approaches are catalogued, and our preferences are discussed.

SURGICAL ANATOMY

The anatomy of the posterior circulation and its relationship to adjacent neural structures are best thought of as three neurovascular complexes in the posterior fossa: the basilar apex, the basilar trunk, and the vertebral trunk.[6] As noted, surgical approaches to posterior circulation aneurysms are also best categorized within this thematic trinity.

Anatomy of the Vertebral Trunk

After their exit from the subclavian arteries, the vertebral arteries ascend through the transverse processes of the upper six cervical vertebrae, swing posterior to the lateral masses of the atlas, pass anterior to the lateral border of the atlanto-occipital membrane, and pierce the dura behind the occipital condyles.[7, 8] Just before passing through the dura, each vertebral artery gives off a posterior meningeal artery that supplies the dura of the occipital surface of the posterior fossa. The initial intradural segment of each vertebral artery passes over the dorsal and ventral roots of the first cervical nerve and then crosses anterior to the dentate ligament and spinal portion of the accessory nerve. Each vertebral artery courses from the lower lateral to upper anterior surface of the medulla and gives rise to numerous perforating arteries that supply the medulla. In the process, each vertebral artery passes across the pyramid to join with its contralateral mate at or near the pontomedullary sulcus to form the vertebrobasilar junction and basilar artery. The vertebral trunk is the intradural portion of the artery from its dural ring to the vertebrobasilar junction.

Intracranially, the first branch to exit from each vertebral artery is the posterior spinal artery.[7, 8] Sometimes this artery arises from the extradural portion of the vertebral artery and travels with it through its dural sheath into the subarachnoid space. Here, the posterior spinal artery courses medially behind the dentate ligament and divides into ascending and descending branches to supply the dorsal columns and the superficial portion of the dorsal half of the cervical spinal cord.

The next branch, the posterior inferior cerebellar artery (PICA), is the largest and most clinically significant branch of the vertebral artery. The PICA can be considered as having four segments as it winds around the medulla to reach the posterior surface of the cerebellar hemispheres[9]: the anterior medullary, lateral medullary, tonsillomedullary, and telovelotonsillary segments. These segments are defined by their relationship to adjacent cranial nerves (CNs), as described later.

The last branch to exit from the vertebral artery just proximal to the vertebrobasilar junction is the anterior spinal artery, which joins its contralateral mate to form a single midline anterior spinal artery.[7] This artery descends in the midline through the foramen magnum on the ventral surface of the medulla and spinal cord in or near the anterior median fissure. It supplies the pyramids and their decussation, the medial lemniscus, and the hypoglossal nuclei and nerves.

The key anatomic landmarks in the inferior neurovascular complex are the rootlets of the glossopharyngeal (CN IX), vagus (CN X), and accessory (CN XI) nerves.[6, 7, 10] The most recognizable member of this trio is CN XI, whose spinal rootlets ascend through the foramen magnum and drape across the intracranial portion of the vertebral artery as they course anterolaterally toward the jugular foramen. CN XI can be followed rostrally to identify its partners in the jugular foramen, CNs IX and X. The rootlets of CNs IX, X, and

XI originate in the groove between the lateral surface of the olive and the posterolateral medulla. In contrast, the rootlets of the hypoglossal nerve (CN XII) originate more anteromedially in the groove between the medial edge of the olive and the medullary pyramids. The rootlets of CN XII course laterally to the hypoglossal canal, which runs above the anterior third of the occipital condyle. The vertebral arteries always pass anterior to the rootlets of CNs IX, X, XI, and XII.

The four segments of the PICA are defined by the artery's relationship to the lower cranial nerves.[9] The anterior medullary segment begins at the origin of the PICA, lies anterior to the medulla, and extends posteriorly past the hypoglossal rootlets at the medial edge of the inferior olive. The second lateral medullary segment extends from the olive along the lateral surface of the medulla to the rootlets of CNs IX, X, and XI at the lateral edge of the olive. The third tonsillomedullary segment passes under or between the rootlets of the CN IX, X, XI triad and around the cerebellar tonsil; it then makes an inferomedial turn, called the caudal or infratonsillar loop. The fourth segment of the PICA, the telovelotonsillar segment, passes along the medial surface of the tonsil, ascends toward the roof of the fourth ventricle, and curves downward again, forming a cranial or supratonsillar loop. The telovelotonsillar segment ends as it branches into numerous cortical vessels that exit the fissures between the vermis, tonsil, and hemisphere of the cerebellum to reach the suboccipital surface of the cerebellum.

Anatomy of the Basilar Trunk

The basilar artery originates at the junction of the vertebral arteries at the level of the pontomedullary sulcus[8] and ascends anterior to the pons toward its apex in the interpeduncular fossa. Along its course, numerous branches of various sizes exit. The largest is the anterior inferior cerebellar artery (AICA), which originates from the basilar artery near the pontomedullary sulcus and courses around the pons toward the cerebellopontine angle (CPA).[8, 11] It can arise as a single or duplicate vessel and occasionally arises from the PICA below to create an AICA-PICA complex. Along its course, the AICA sends branches to the upper anterolateral medulla, the facial (CN VII) and vestibulocochlear (CN VIII) nerves as they enter the internal auditory canal, the middle cerebellar peduncle, and the petrous surface of the cerebellum, the terminal target of the AICA.

Intermediate branches exit the basilar artery throughout its course from the vertebrobasilar junction to the apex. The most proximal branch is the pontomedullary artery, which arises between the vertebrobasilar junction and the origin of the AICA. The pontomedullary artery courses laterally in the pontomedullary sulcus and supplies the olivary complex.[11] Two long lateral pontine arteries exit the basilar artery and course laterally to supply the paramedian and lateral pons.[12] Finally, the posterolateral artery arises from the basilar artery just inferior to the superior cerebellar artery and supplies the superolateral pons.

The most delicate and arguably the most vital branches of the basilar trunk are its numerous small perforators. These end arteries, which supply cranial nerve nuclei, input and output pathways to the cerebrum and cerebellum, and the reticular centers for arousal, have been divided into three groups: caudal, middle, and rostral perforators.[13] Their diameters range from 100 to 500 μm. They occur along the entire course of the basilar artery and arise from its posterior and lateral surfaces, not from its anterior surface. Occasionally, some perforators arise from the larger branches of the basilar artery such as the AICA.

This middle complex has its own trio of related cranial nerves: the abducent nerve (CN VI), CN VII, and CN VIII.[6] CN VI serves as a landmark for the AICA.[11] The AICA begins at the basilar artery in the pontomedullary sulcus and almost always courses below or between the abducent fascicles in the pontomedullary sulcus until it reaches the region of the acoustic meatus. Then the AICA passes between or around CNs VII and VIII as these nerves head toward the acoustic meatus. The AICA sends branches to these nerves and also supplies the choroid plexus, where it protrudes laterally from the foramen of Luschka. From here, the AICA courses posterolaterally to supply the petrous surface of the cerebellum.

Anatomy of the Basilar Apex

The basilar artery terminates at its apex, giving rise to the posterior cerebral arteries (PCAs) and superior cerebellar arteries in the anterior incisural space between the posterior perforated substance and the clivus.[8] The apex of the basilar artery is located within 1 cm of the dorsum sellae in almost 90% of patients,[14, 15] but this configuration means that the basilar artery can bifurcate as far caudally as 10 mm below the pontomesencephalic junction or as far rostrally as the mamillary bodies. The location of the basilar apex in relation to the dorsum sellae and posterior clinoid processes can dramatically affect the visibility of the basilar apex and related aneurysms from a chosen approach.

The basilar apex and its bifurcation into the left and right PCAs constitute the posterior portions of the circle of Willis.[12, 14] The PCAs can be subdivided into a series of segments. The P1 segment extends from the basilar bifurcation to the posterior communicating artery (PCoA). The P2 segment starts at the PCA-PCoA junction and extends to the posterior aspect of the midbrain. Subsequently, the P3 branch climbs over the free edge of the tentorium and continues posteriorly above the tentorium to supply the occipital and posterior temporal lobes.

The basilar apex and PCAs give rise to a large number of essential perforating arteries (Fig. 116–2) with variable branching patterns that have been described in detail.[12, 14, 16–18] These perforators can be divided into three categories. The first group of perforators originates from the apex of the basilar artery itself, typically arising from the last 2 to 3 mm of the artery. These branches supply the posterior perforated substance, cerebral peduncles, and lateral pons. Perforators in the second group are less numerous and arise from the superior and posterior aspects of the P1 segments of the PCA, along with the long and short circumflex

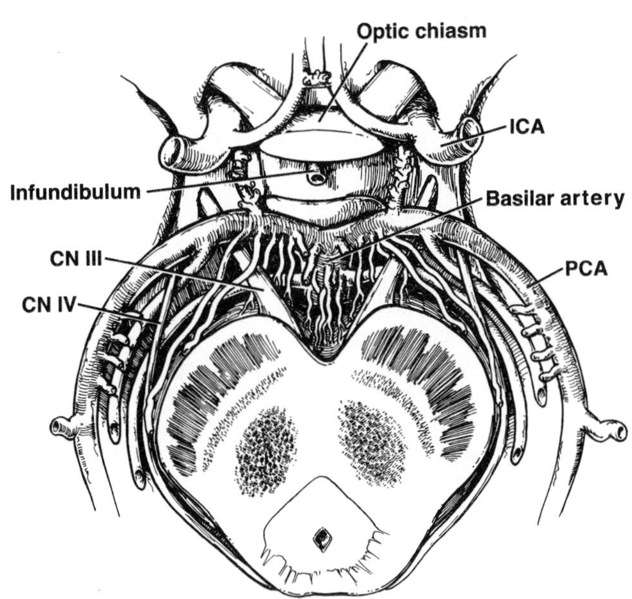

FIGURE 116-2. Preservation of perforating arteries originating from the basilar apex is critical to safe surgical clipping. CN III, oculomotor nerve; CN IV, trochlear nerve; ICA, internal carotid artery; PCA, posterior cerebral artery. (From Wascher TM, Spetzler RF: Saccular aneurysms of the basilar bifurcation. In Carter LP, Spetzler RF, Hamilton MG [eds]: Neurovascular Surgery. New York, McGraw-Hill, 1995, pp 729–752.)

arteries. Together, these vessels supply the medial and lateral geniculate nuclei (posterior thalamoperforating arteries), interpeduncular fossa, mamillary bodies, cerebral peduncles, and posterior mesencephalon. The third group of perforators originates from the PCoA, typically from the superior and lateral surfaces of the artery, and courses either anteriorly to perfuse the hypothalamus and posterior optic chiasm or posteriorly to perfuse the posterior perforated substance and thalamus (anterior thalamoperforating arteries).

The superior cerebellar artery originates just below the PCA[19] and encircles the midbrain in the pontomesencephalic sulcus. It supplies the cerebral peduncles and brainstem through multiple perforating branches. The superior cerebellar artery then curves medially and superiorly to supply the tentorial surface of the cerebellum.

The basilar apex is located in the interpeduncular cistern. This cistern is located within the posterior portion of the anterior incisural space and communicates anteriorly with the chiasmatic cistern located below the optic chiasm.[20] The interpeduncular and chiasmatic cisterns are separated by Liliequist's membrane,[21] a dense arachnoid sheet that extends between the dorsum sellae and the anterior border of the mamillary bodies, around the infundibulum and the pituitary stalk. The free edge of the tentorium is attached anteriorly to the medial petrous apices and to the anterior and posterior clinoid processes.

The oculomotor (CN III), trochlear (CN IV), and trigeminal (CN V) nerves constitute the cranial nerve triad that serves as a guidepost in this region.[6] CN III emerges from the brainstem between the cerebral peduncles and courses anterolaterally in the anterior incisural space toward the free edge of the tentorium. CN III invariably passes through the crux made by the ipsilateral PCA and superior cerebellar arteries. Therefore, CN III can be followed from the free edge of the tentorium back through the interpeduncular cistern to identify the PCA and superior cerebellar arteries when the basilar apex is being approached.[8, 22] As the PCAs sweep around the cerebral peduncles and midbrain, they pass above the oculomotor nerves medially and the trochlear nerves laterally. The PCAs then exit the anterior incisural space and enter the midline incisural space by coursing between the uncus and the cerebral peduncle.[14] After passing under CN III, the superior cerebellar artery passes medially to the free edge of the tentorium and inferiorly to CN IV, which runs from the lateral edge of the brainstem toward its dural sheath in the tentorium.[19] Finally, the superior cerebellar artery winds around the brainstem, passes over CN V, and courses in the cerebellomesencephalic fissure to supply the tentorial surface of the cerebellum.

ANATOMIC DISTRIBUTION OF POSTERIOR CIRCULATION ANEURYSMS

Like anterior circulation aneurysms, posterior circulation aneurysms follow three basic anatomic principles[23]: (1) they arise from branch sites on the parent artery, (2) they arise at turns or curves in the artery, and (3) they point in the direction that blood would flow if the curve at the aneurysm site was not present (i.e., in the direction of maximal hemodynamic thrust). Aneurysms of the posterior circulation account for as many as 15% of all intracranial aneurysms.[22, 24–26] They most often occur at the basilar apex, followed by the origins of the superior cerebellar artery and PICA. Saccular aneurysms of the PCA and AICA are the least common. The epidemiology of saccular aneurysms in the posterior circulation is similar to that in the anterior circulation: they manifest in the fifth and sixth decades of life, most often in females.

Giant aneurysms (>25 mm in diameter)[26, 27] occur in the posterior circulation as frequently as in the anterior circulation, and their anatomic distribution is similar to that of smaller aneurysms. Dissections and fusiform aneurysms are more common in the posterior circulation than in the anterior circulation.[28–32] Vertebral artery dissections account for 31% of all vertebral artery lesions. These lesions, once thought to be due almost exclusively to trauma, are being discovered with increasing frequency in the absence of trauma as modern imaging techniques evolve. Fusiform aneurysms constitute 9% of all posterior circulation aneurysms. Peerless and Drake[26] postulated that large, fusiform, S-shaped aneurysms of the vertebrobasilar system arise in the setting of intracranial atherosclerosis and that large bulbous and giant globular aneurysms result from enlargement of small saccular aneurysms originating from small or intermediate perforating branches. Dolichoectatic aneurysms of the vertebral and basilar arteries may result from dissections that produce fusiform degeneration of the artery, progressive enlargement, and luminal thrombosis.[33, 34] In contrast to saccular aneurysms, fusiform aneurysms involving the basilar artery tend to occur in younger males.[28, 32, 35, 36]

Aneurysms in the posterior circulation are associated with anatomic variations and vascular abnormalities. Arteriovenous malformations in the occipital lobes or the cerebellum have been observed with aneurysms at the basilar apex.[22, 26] Hypoplastic or fetal PCAs are often associated with aneurysms.[2, 15, 37] Fenestration of the vertebrobasilar junction is also associated with an increased incidence of aneurysms there.[38–40] Persistent carotid-to-basilar anastomoses are associated with aneurysms in the posterior circulation, in part because these anastomoses can overtake the vertebral arteries to become the primary vascular supply of the posterior fossa. The result is aberrant blood-flow dynamics within the vertebrobasilar system.[41–45] Likewise, vertebrobasilar aneurysms are often associated with Moyamoya syndrome because these vessels become the primary inflow track for cerebral blood flow as the internal carotid arteries (ICAs) become progressively narrowed.[46, 47] Connective tissue disorders (e.g., polycystic kidney disease, Marfan's syndrome, Ehlers-Danlos syndrome) can increase the likelihood of aneurysms in the posterior circulation, as they do in the anterior circulation.[17, 37]

CLINICAL PRESENTATION

The clinical presentation of posterior circulation aneurysms depends on whether the aneurysm has ruptured. Almost 80% of posterior fossa aneurysms manifest with the signs and symptoms of acute subarachnoid hemorrhage, and these symptoms do not differ significantly from those of aneurysmal rupture in the anterior circulation.[22, 26, 48] In fact, in one third of patients with ruptured posterior circulation aneurysms, the signs and symptoms are too nonspecific to suggest the site of the lesion. Headache, nuchal pain and rigidity, nausea, vomiting, and altered mental status are the most common manifestations of rupture. Intraparenchymal bleeding is often associated with aneurysms of the anterior circulation but rarely occurs with posterior circulation aneurysms,[22, 26, 27] perhaps because of the tough pial envelope of the brainstem. Upward-pointing basilar tip aneurysms, however, often rupture through the floor of the third ventricle, causing intraventricular hemorrhage and obstructive hydrocephalus.

Cranial nerve deficits are seldom associated with the rupture of posterior circulation aneurysms, despite the tight quarters that these aneurysms share with the brainstem.[22, 26] Occasionally, however, a cranial nerve deficit points to the origin of a particular aneurysm. Aneurysms of the basilar apex, superior cerebellar artery, and upper basilar artery can be associated with CN III dysfunction. The rupture of an AICA aneurysm can cause hearing loss or CN VII palsy. Aneurysms of the vertebrobasilar junction or lower basilar trunk can cause CN VI dysfunction.

Unruptured posterior circulation aneurysms announce themselves through mass effect on the adjacent cranial nerves and brainstem.[22, 26, 48] These signs can range from isolated cranial neuropathies to brainstem compression syndromes that mimic posterior fossa tumors. Hydrocephalus results when an aneurysm is large enough to obstruct the flow of cerebrospinal fluid (CSF) through the cerebral aqueduct or fourth ventricle. The spectrum of findings associated with a particular aneurysm is dictated by its location. Basilar tip, PCA, and superior cerebellar artery aneurysms can be associated with CN III palsy and contralateral hemiparesis due to compression of the cerebral peduncle. Forward-pointing basilar tip aneurysms can mimic pituitary tumors with compression of the optic chiasm. AICA aneurysms can cause CN VI palsy or, if very large, pontine compression. PICA aneurysms can cause palsies of CNs IX through XII. In addition, unruptured fusiform or dolichoectatic aneurysms can manifest with transient or permanent ischemic symptoms due to showering of emboli from within the sac of the aneurysm or intraluminal thrombosis that leads to the occlusion of small perforators emanating from the aneurysm wall.

DIAGNOSTIC STUDIES

The initial evaluation of a patient with suspected subarachnoid hemorrhage invariably includes computed tomography, which cinches the diagnosis. The distribution of blood occasionally gives clues to the location of the aneurysm. Basilar tip aneurysms can cause a large amount of clot in the interpeduncular cistern. If the jet of rupture is directed through the floor of the third ventricle, intraventricular hemorrhage results.[22] When PICA aneurysms rupture, the resultant subarachnoid blood may be limited to the lower regions of the posterior fossa.[48] More often than not, however, the distribution of blood seen on computed tomographic scans is not a reliable indicator of an aneurysm's location; it simply confirms that subarachnoid hemorrhage has occurred. If the patient's history strongly suggests subarachnoid hemorrhage and the computed tomographic scan is negative, a lumbar puncture may be indicated.

High-quality four-vessel angiography in multiple projections remains the gold standard for diagnosis and surgical planning. Preoperative angiographic studies determine five key features: (1) the aneurysm's vessel of origin; (2) the aneurysm's size, shape, and relationship to parent and adjacent arteries; (3) the presence and location of vasospasm; (4) the displacement of adjacent vessels, suggesting mass effect from hematoma or partial thrombosis of an aneurysmal sac whose dimensions are much larger than that seen on angiography; and (5) the presence of other aneurysms or vascular abnormalities.

Four-vessel angiography also delineates features of the underlying circulatory supply to the posterior fossa that may affect surgical strategy. The presence and size of the PCoAs or the presence of a fetal PCA must be understood before approaching basilar tip aneurysms. The presence of persistent carotid-basilar anastomoses must be identified preoperatively. The origin of the AICAs and PICAs must be visualized bilaterally, because one side may be dominant, or the AICA and PICA on one or both sides may be fused into an AICA-

PICA complex.[9, 11, 37] Likewise, the origin of both vertebral arteries must be assessed, because one vertebral artery is often dominant and the other small or nonexistent.[49] The nondominant vertebral artery often terminates in the ipsilateral PICA.

Magnetic resonance imaging can be a helpful adjunct in the evaluation of giant aneurysms of the posterior circulation.[22, 48] Many of these aneurysms are partially thrombosed, and the internal dimensions of the lumen appreciated on angiography do not accurately reflect the true size of the aneurysm. Magnetic resonance imaging also allows exquisite identification of the mass as it relates to the brainstem and cranial nerves. It helps delineate the extent of preoperative brain injury due to intraparenchymal hematoma or ischemia related to early vasospasm. Computed tomography and computed tomography–angiography may better define an aneurysm's relationship to the bony anatomy of the skull base.

SURGICAL APPROACHES TO THE BASILAR APEX

The first category of surgical approaches targets aneurysms of the basilar apex from an anterosuperior trajectory. The craniotomy-transcranial route can be subtemporal, pterional-transsylvian, or orbitozygomatic-pterional, a sequence that reflects both the genealogy of surgical approaches and an increasingly anterior trajectory. Combining these cranial exposures provides the flexibility to vary the trajectory as needed. Removing adjacent bony obstructions (e.g., anterior and posterior clinoid processes, dorsum sellae and upper clivus, medial petrous apex) or working through the cavernous sinus or tentorium increases inner exposure.

Subtemporal Approach

Peerless and Drake developed the subtemporal approach and, in the process, established basilar tip aneurysms as surgically treatable lesions.[26, 27, 47, 50–54] This approach proceeds from a lateral trajectory that elevates the temporal lobe. Dissection is directed between the medial temporal lobe and the tentorial edge. In many cases, the subtemporal trajectory parallels the long axis of the aneurysm's neck, which is the optimal direction for placing a clip on these aneurysms. The posterior perforating arteries, whose preservation is perhaps the most crucial aspect of the procedure, can be visualized best from this vantage point. However, this approach provides poor visualization of the contralateral anatomy (PCA, superior cerebellar artery, perforating arteries, and CN III), puts the ipsilateral CN III in the center of the operative field, and demands potentially dangerous retraction of the temporal lobe.

In most cases, a right-sided approach is used unless mitigating factors are present, such as aneurysmal anatomy that favors a left-sided approach, a preexisting left CN III palsy, right hemiparesis, or known right hemispheric dominance. Patients are placed in either the lateral decubitus or the supine position with a shoulder roll. The head is rotated until the midline plane parallels the floor, and the head is angled 15 degrees downward to achieve a line of sight parallel to the floor of the middle fossa (Fig. 116–3*A*). A lumbar

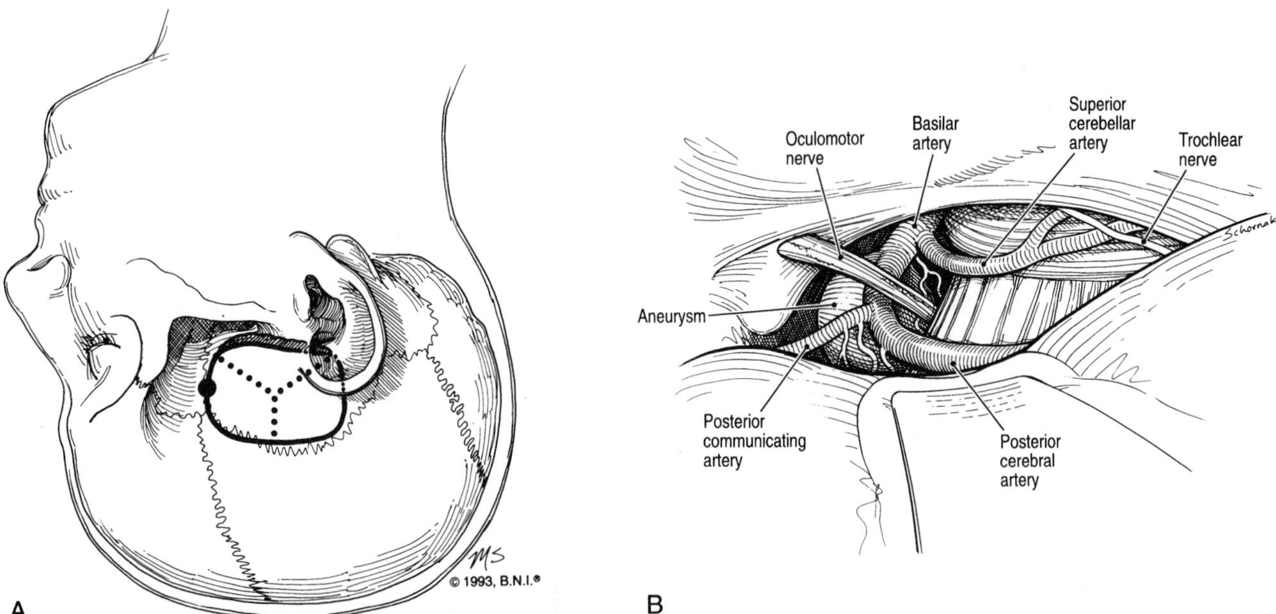

FIGURE 116–3. Subtemporal approach. *A*, Lateral head position and craniotomy for the subtemporal approach. Additional temporal bone is drilled inferiorly to make the cranial exposure flush with the middle fossa floor *(cross-hatching)*. *B*, Microsurgical anatomy of the tentorial incisura. From this trajectory, the posterior perforating arteries and the back of the aneurysm's neck are well visualized. (Courtesy of Barrow Neurological Institute, Phoenix, Arizona.)

subarachnoid drain permits CSF drainage and brain relaxation, which facilitate temporal lobe retraction during the approach to the tentorial incisura. Afterward, CSF can be removed directly from opened cisterns.

A linear incision that extends 7 cm up from the zygomatic arch and 1 cm anterior to the tragus, or a horseshoe-shaped flap based over the ear, is used. Depending on the skin incision, the temporalis muscle is either divided and held apart or flapped inferiorly. A 4 cm × 4 cm craniotomy is made in the temporal bone. Additional temporal squamosal bone is drilled inferiorly until the cranial exposure is flush with the floor of the middle fossa. The dura is opened by a Y-shaped incision with an inferiorly based flap.

Under the operating microscope, a self-retaining retractor is positioned to elevate the temporal lobe and expose the tentorial incisura (see Fig. 116–3*B*). The arachnoid is opened to enter the interpeduncular and ambient cisterns, and CN III is identified. The opening into the interpeduncular cistern can be enlarged by pulling the edge of the tentorium laterally with a tacking suture placed between CNs III and IV. Additional inferior exposure in the posterior fossa can be gained by dividing the tentorium behind the entry of CN IV. Manipulation of CN III is minimized, and superior retraction of the nerve is often afforded by its adhesions to the medial temporal lobe. The superior cerebellar arteries and PCA are then followed medially to the basilar apex, and the aneurysm is dissected and clipped.

Pterional-Transsylvian Approach

The pterional craniotomy, popularized by Yasargil and colleagues, is an excellent approach to basilar apex aneurysms.[26, 37, 54–56] It is familiar to most neurosurgeons because it is the standard approach for most anterior circulation aneurysms. Compared with the subtemporal trajectory, the pterional trajectory is more anterolateral, which provides a better overall survey of the anatomy. The contralateral anatomy is well visualized, but the posterior perforating arteries are not; this disadvantage necessitates increased manipulation of the aneurysm. The more anterior approach also places the ICA in the center of the operative field, making it an obstacle between the surgeon and the basilar apex.

The patient is positioned supine, with the head rotated approximately 30 degrees to the opposite side and extended approximately 20 degrees to make the maxillary bone the highest point in the field. Lumbar subarachnoid drainage is not used, because CSF in the basal cisterns can be readily accessed before brain retraction is needed. A curvilinear skin incision is made, beginning at the zygomatic arch 1 cm anterior to the tragus and arcing to the midline just behind the hairline (Fig. 116–4*A*). The bone flap need not extend to the midline, but the skin incision is extended so that the scalp flap can be retracted enough inferiorly to drill the pterion thoroughly. The scalp and temporalis muscle are flapped anteriorly, leaving a cuff of muscle along the superior temporal line for reapproximation during closure. Retraction of these soft tissue flaps with fishhooks on rubber bands pulls them out of the way of the pterional opening.

A frontotemporal craniotomy (see Fig. 116–4*B*) is made through a single temporal bur hole, with the frontal cut extending medially to the foramen of the supraorbital nerve and inferiorly to the floor of the anterior cranial fossa. By centering the craniotomy on the pterion, this approach facilitates further resection of the pterion, exposes the sylvian fissure, and creates a corridor down to the ICA. The pterion is drilled extensively (see Fig. 116–4*C* to *E*) to remove the lesser wing of the sphenoid bone, the base of the anterior clinoid process, the bony ridges of the orbital roof, the inner table of the inferior frontal bone over the superior orbital rim, and the squamosal portion of the temporal bone inferiorly to the middle fossa floor. After the drilling is complete, the dural fold of the superior orbital fissure is skeletonized. The removal of bone around the pterion creates a flat corridor with ample space under the frontal and temporal lobes in the sylvian fissure. The dura is then incised to create a curvilinear flap based over the orbit (see Fig. 116–4*F* and *G*). If the deep drilling is adequate, the bony prominence at the base of the anterior clinoid process that typically blocks the optic nerve (CN II) and carotid artery is eliminated, and these structures can be seen with minimal brain retraction.

Exposure of the basilar apex through this approach requires splitting the sylvian fissure, widely opening the cisterns around CN II and the carotid artery, and gently retracting the frontal and temporal lobes (see Fig. 116–4*H*). Division of some temporal bridging veins is often necessary to mobilize the temporal pole, and this is well tolerated. The PCoA is followed back through Liliequist's membrane to the PCA, which is then followed medially to the basilar apex (see Fig. 116–4*I*). Following the anterior choroidal artery posteriorly as it courses along the optic tract to the choroidal fissure enables deeper separation of the frontal and temporal lobes and better visualization of high-lying aneurysms. The anterior temporal artery sometimes

FIGURE 116–4. Pterional approach. *A*, Head position, scalp flap, and temporalis muscle flap for the pterional approach. Anterior retraction on the scalp and temporalis muscle exposes the pterion without having to divide the muscle. A muscle cuff is created to reattach the muscle at closure. *B*, The craniotomy is made with a single bur hole (1), two craniotomy cuts that end at the pterion (2 and 3), and drilling of the pterion (4 and 5). *C*, Surgical view showing the bone flap removed and drilling of the sphenoid wing. Axial *(D)* and coronal *(E)* views showing the bone to be removed (1). The pterion and medial sphenoid wing are drilled extensively until the superior orbital fissure and its contents are reached (2). The inferior temporal bone is also drilled to the floor of the middle fossa (3). (*figure continues*)

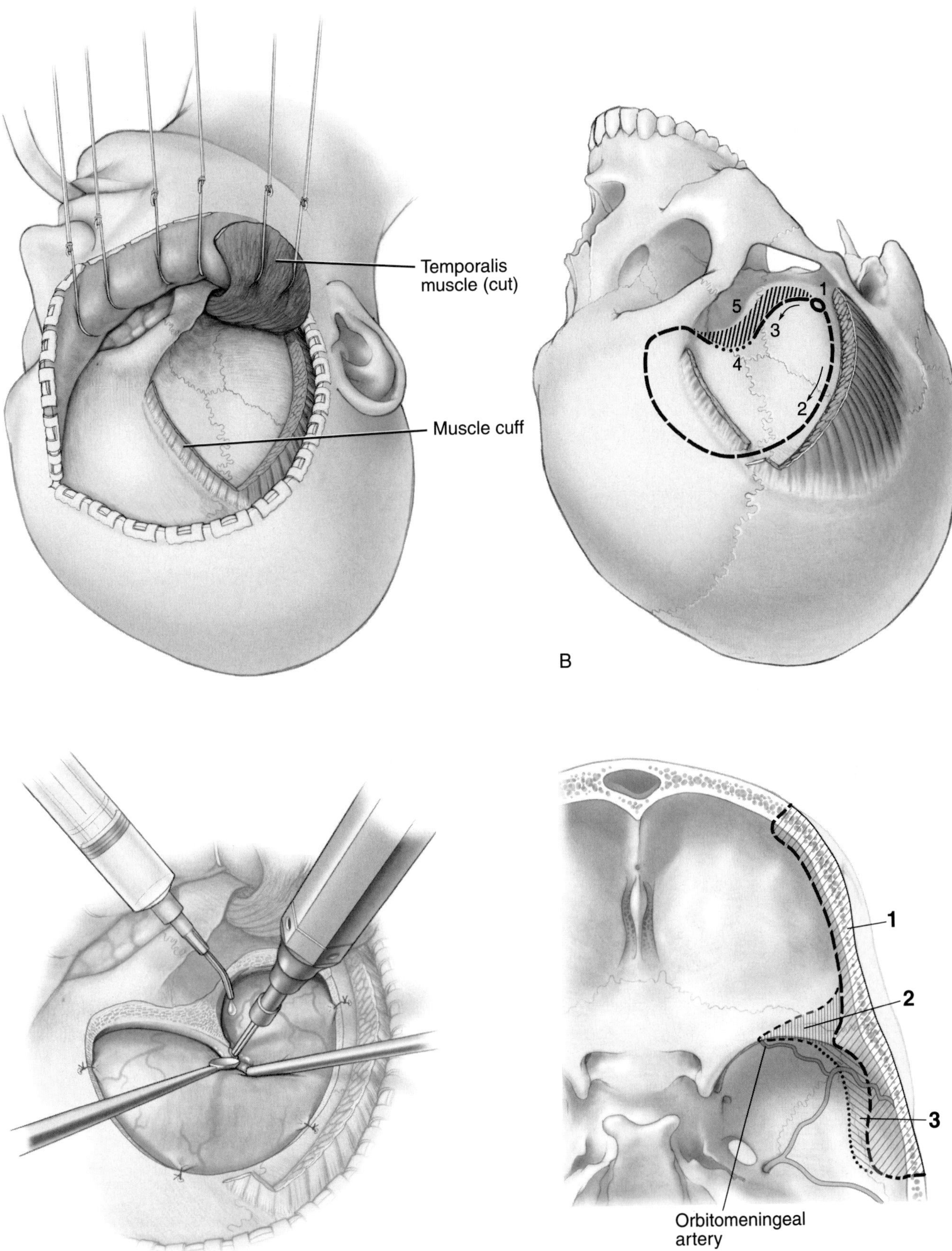
Temporalis
muscle (cut)
Muscle cuff
1
5
3
4
2
B
1
2
3
Orbitomeningeal
artery
C
D

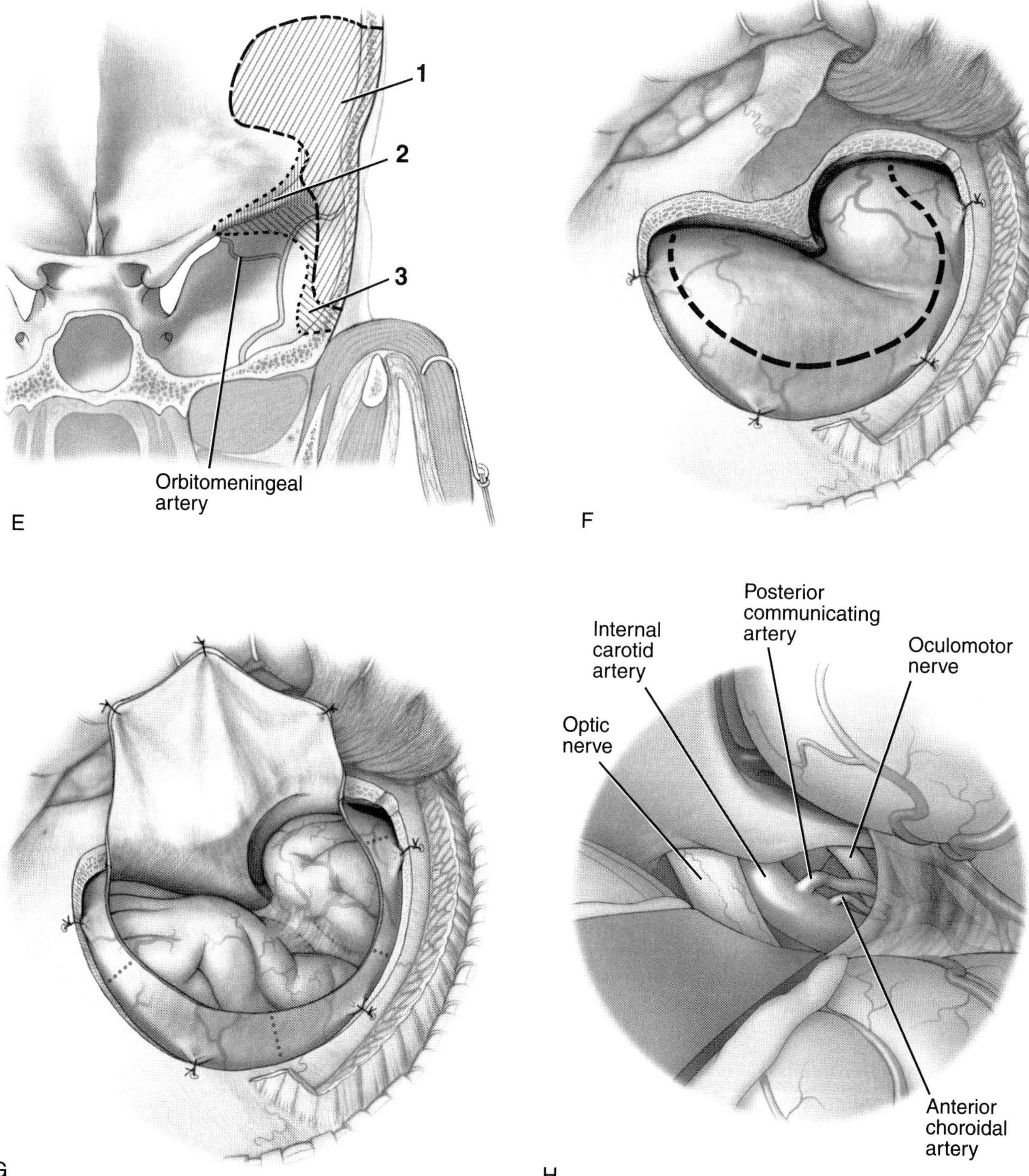

FIGURE 116–4. *Continued. F,* The dural flap is based on the pterion. *G,* The dural flap is pulled flat against the bone with tacking sutures. *H,* Intraoperative view showing the microsurgical anatomy of the pterional approach. (*figure continues*)

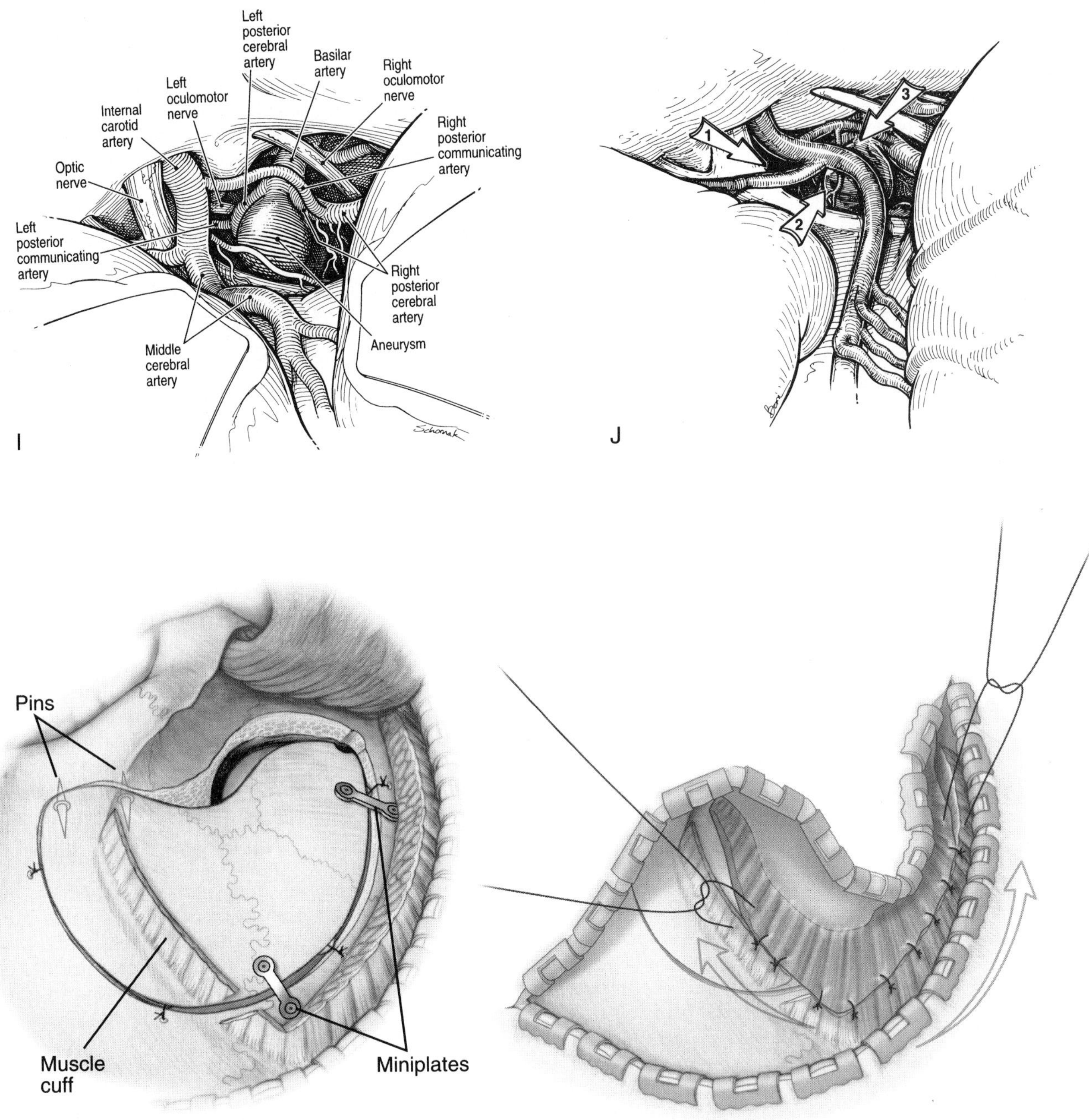

FIGURE 116–4. *Continued. I,* Splitting the sylvian fissure allows the frontal and temporal lobes to be mobilized and the deep anatomy around the basilar apex to be visualized. *J,* The basilar apex can be approached through routes medial to the carotid artery (1), superior to the carotid bifurcation (2), or lateral to the carotid artery, centered on the third cranial nerve (3). *K,* For optimal cosmetic results, the bone flap is positioned anteriorly to smoothly recontour the lateral forehead. *L,* The temporalis muscle is pulled forward to fill the keyhole. (*A–I, K,* and *L,* Courtesy of Barrow Neurological Institute, Phoenix, Arizona; *J,* From Wascher TM, Spetzler RF: Saccular aneurysms of the basilar bifurcation. In Carter LP, Spetzler RF, Hamilton MG [eds]: Neurovascular Surgery. New York, McGraw-Hill, 1995, pp 729–752.)

limits temporal lobe retraction posteriorly, especially when the artery arises proximally on the middle cerebral artery. Its division can dramatically enhance exposure.

With the pterional approach, the ICA becomes an obstacle in the operative field and can obscure access to the basilar apex. Three routes around the ICA are available (see Fig. 116–4*J*). A medial route runs through the triangle formed by the lateral edge of CN II, the medial ICA, and the A1 segment of the anterior cerebral artery (optic-carotid triangle). A superior route runs through the triangle formed by A1, M1, and the optic tract. A lateral route runs through the interval between the lateral ICA and CN III. The lateral route is preferred, because the optic-carotid triangle is typically narrow, and the superior triangle is obscured by small but crucial perforating arteries from the ICA. The lateral route usually provides ample access and can be expanded by mobilizing the ICA further medially if necessary. Sometimes, multiple routes of exposure are needed to dissect different parts of the aneurysm, or separate triangles are needed to pass the instrument in one hand and the suction in the other hand.

Orbitozygomatic-Pterional Approach

This approach expands on the pterional approach by removing the superior and lateral portions of the orbit (Fig. 116–5*A*), thereby creating more space in the operative corridor and providing a more anterior trajectory than the standard pterional approach. This modification allows an extended upward view of the basilar apex (see Fig. 116–5*B*).[3, 57–69] Consequently, it has become our preferred approach for basilar apex aneurysms. The approach requires additional work to remove the orbitozygomatic unit and poses additional risks, including frontalis nerve injury; pulsatile enophthalmos; orbital entrapment; diplopia from extraocular muscle or nerve injury; blindness; communication with the frontal sinus, with potential routes of infection or CSF leakage; and increased periorbital bruising postoperatively. The incidence of these complications, however, is low, and the advantages gained by the increased exposure far outweigh the disadvantages.

The orbitozygomatic approach adds two steps to the pterional approach: soft tissue dissection to expose the orbitozygomatic unit, and osteotomies to free it. The zygoma and orbital rim are ensheathed in two layers of the temporalis fascia, which are elevated to expose the bone (see Fig. 116–5*C* and *D*). Exposure can be accomplished either by an interfascial dissection that peels apart the layers or by a subfascial dissection that cuts the inner layer as it passes under the zygoma, thereby releasing the fascia. The subfascial dissection is simple, fast, and preferred; it leaves the frontalis branch of CN VII, which runs superficial to the outer fascial layer, undisturbed. The periorbita, which is continuous with the outer layer of temporal fascia, is carefully stripped from the orbit because its integrity helps contain the periorbital fat and facilitates the orbital osteotomies. Once the orbitozygomatic unit is exposed, the temporalis muscle is mobilized inferiorly, a frontotemporal craniotomy is made, and the dura of the frontal lobe is elevated. Removing the orbit obviates the need for drilling the pterion.

The orbitozygomatic unit consists of the orbital rim, orbital roof, lateral orbital wall, and zygomatic arch. It is released by a series of six osteotomies (see Fig. 116–5*E*) made with a reciprocating saw (to minimize bone loss from the cuts). The first cut is made across the zygomatic root, with care taken to avoid the temporomandibular joint. A fixation plate is placed in the zygoma and registered to improve the cosmesis of the repair (see Fig. 116–5*H*). The second and third cuts are made across the zygomatic bone—first from the inferolateral margin of the zygomatic bone halfway across to the lateral orbital rim, and then from the inferior orbital fissure to the same end point. With these two cuts, the resulting V in the zygomatic bone allows the fragment to be secured into position when replaced. The fourth cut is along the medial orbital roof, just lateral to the supraorbital notch. Care is taken to protect the frontal dura during these cuts (see Fig. 116–5*F*). The fifth cut crosses the posterior orbital roof, approximately 2.5 cm posterior to the inner table of frontal bone (to preserve the orbital roof), and finishes laterally in the thick bone of the sphenoid ridge and pterion. The sixth cut crosses the lateral orbital wall, connecting the previous cut with the inferior orbital fissure. The orbitozygomatic unit can then be removed as a single piece, and additional bone is removed over the orbital apex around the superior orbital fissure. A dural flap based over the orbit is tented forward with tacking sutures to depress the globe gently and thereby gain a wide exposure of the sylvian region (see Fig. 116–5*G*).

The intradural exposure of the orbitozygomatic approach is the same as that of the pterional approach. The difference is the amount of space created and the ability to view the basilar region more freely, particularly in an upward direction. The fulcrum of the trajectory drops lower across the orbit, resulting in a higher view above the posterior clinoid process. Opening the choroidal fissure and mobilizing the temporal pole laterally are important maneuvers that widen this view. Occasionally, an anterior temporal artery that originates proximally on the M1 may tether the temporal lobe and need to be divided to mobilize the temporal lobe.

Extended Orbitozygomatic Approach

The different cranial exposures achieved by the subtemporal, pterional, and orbitozygomatic approaches create dramatically different trajectories to the basilar apex. Often, the optimal angle for dissecting the aneurysm cannot be predicted from the preoperative studies. Other factors, such as the course of the ICA, the axis of the aneurysm's neck, and the aneurysm's relationship to the posterior clinoid processes, influence the optimal surgical trajectory and are best appreciated intraoperatively. Consequently, an approach that provides a full range of trajectories (Fig. 116–6) gives the surgeon the flexibility to shift trajectories during the

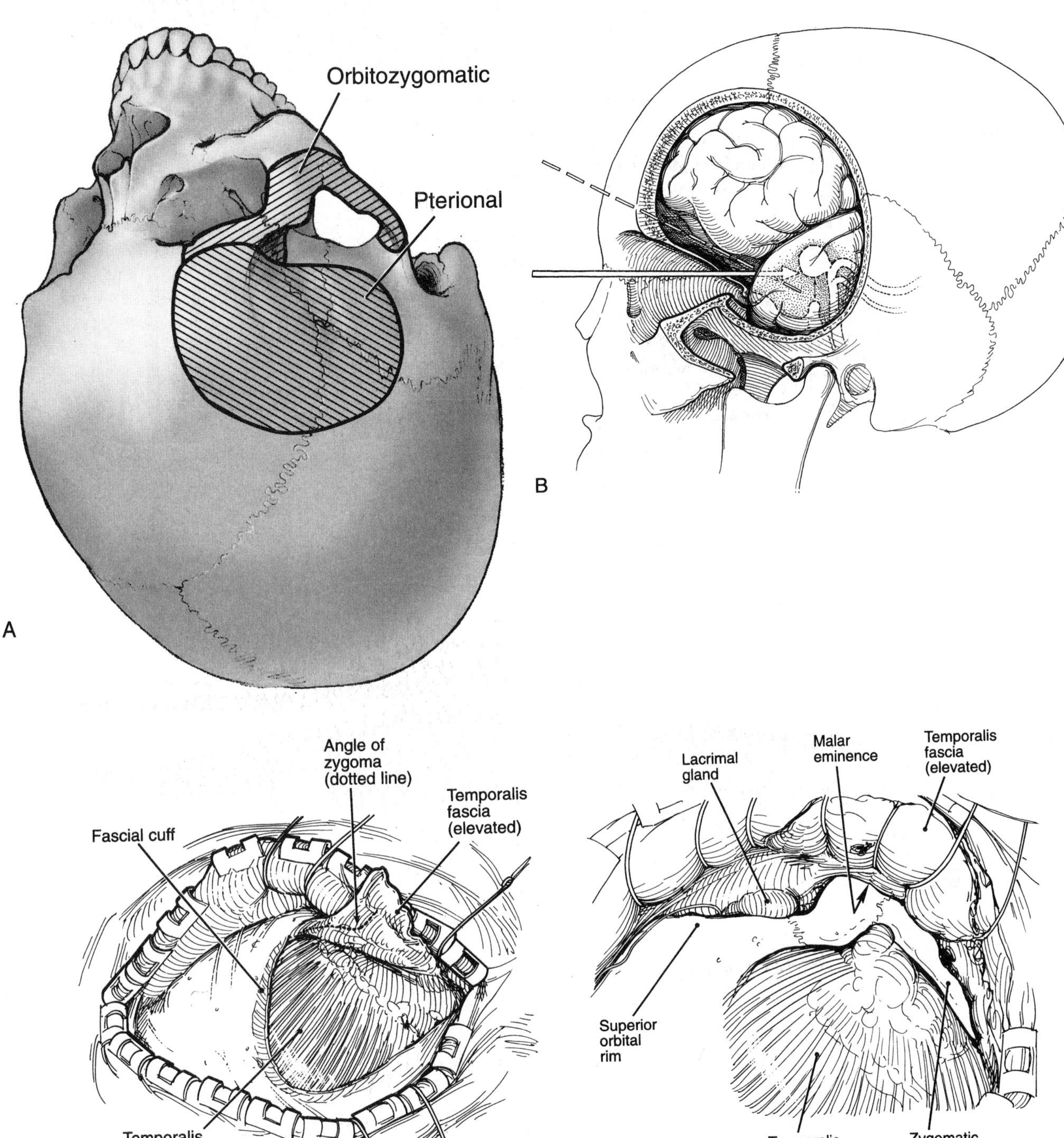

FIGURE 116–5. Orbitozygomatic approach. *A*, The orbitozygomatic approach increases the exposure associated with the pterional approach by removing the superolateral orbit and the zygomatic arch as a unit, separate from the bone flap. *B*, This additional maneuver changes the trajectory of the approach to allow better visualization of high-lying basilar apex aneurysms *(arrow)* than would be possible with a pterional approach *(dashed line)*. *C*, Temporalis fascia is elevated away from the muscle. *D*, The inner fascial layer that runs under the zygomatic arch is cut to mobilize the fascia over the malar eminence. (*figure continues*)

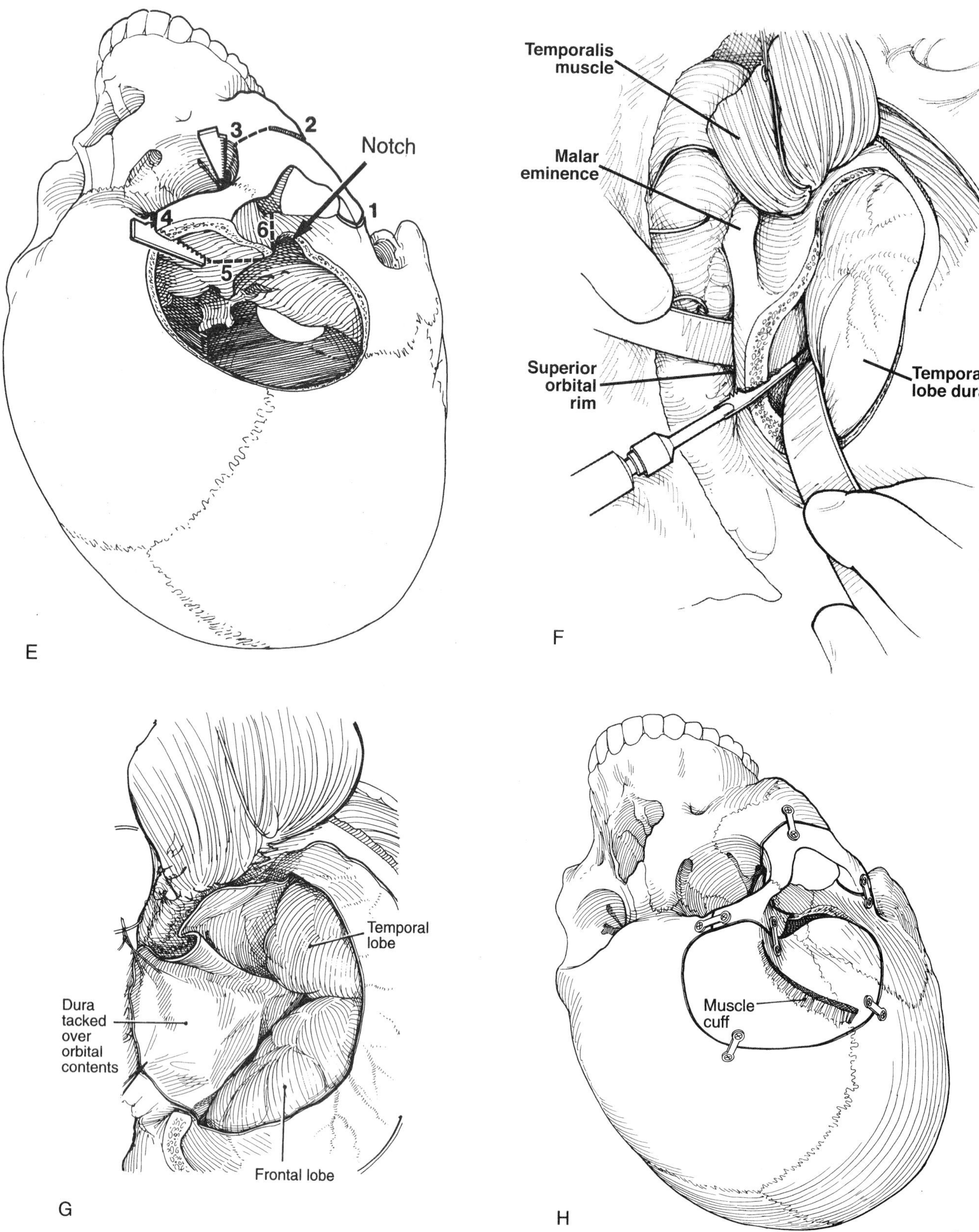

FIGURE 116–5. *Continued. E,* Six osteotomies are made across the zygomatic root (1), malar eminence (2), inferolateral orbit (3), medial orbital roof (4), posterior orbital roof (5), and lateral orbit (6). *F,* The frontal lobe and orbital contents are protected during these osteotomy cuts with malleable retractors. *G,* After the orbitozygomatic unit is removed, the dural flap retracts the orbit inferiorly. *H,* Registering the reconstruction plates before making the osteotomies helps restore the skull anatomy. (*A–G,* Courtesy of Barrow Neurological Institute, Phoenix, Ariz.; *H,* From Zabramski JM, Kiris T, Sankhla SK, et al: Orbitozygomatic craniotomy: Technical note. J Neurosurg 89:336–341, 1998.)

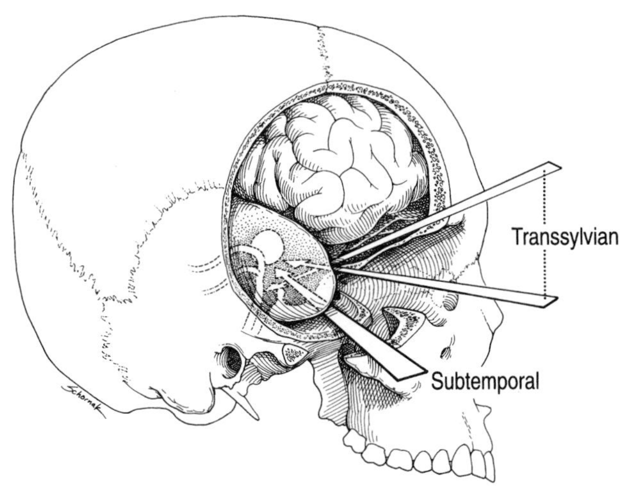

FIGURE 116–6. The extended orbitozygomatic approach provides the surgeon the full range of trajectories to the basilar apex. (Courtesy of Barrow Neurological Institute, Phoenix, Arizona.)

dissection, without interrupting the microsurgery for additional extradural work. A combination of the subtemporal, pterional, and orbitozygomatic approaches can be accomplished by simply extending the posteroinferior cranial exposure of the orbitozygomatic approach.[3]

The extended orbitozygomatic approach is analogous to the combined subtemporal and pterion approach that has been called the "half-and-half" or "one-and-a-half" approach. All that is required is a slightly larger craniotomy that extends more posteriorly. Then, the inferior margin of this craniotomy is drilled flush with the middle fossa floor. During the microdissection of a large aneurysm, the anatomy of the basilar apex and dissection of the contralateral arteries and nerves can be surveyed from an orbitozygomatic angle. Perforators can be separated from the back of the aneurysm, and the clip can be applied from a subtemporal angle. Taking advantage of multiple views within this 90-degree window of exposure can significantly improve the definition of anatomy, making the clipping easier and safer.

Skull Base Exposures

The outer cranial exposure brings the aneurysm within reach, but variations in basilar artery anatomy often draw parts of the skull base (e.g., posterior clinoid process, dorsum sellae, clivus) into the surgeon's view. Neurovascular structures such as the ICA, CN II, and CN III can block access to the neck of a basilar aneurysm if the artery lies too high. Dural structures such as the tentorium and cavernous sinus can block access to the neck of a basilar aneurysm if the artery lies too low. Ultimately, the success or failure of an operation can be determined by the manner in which these small inner obstacles are conquered.

Access to the basilar artery inferior to the superior cerebellar artery is crucial to gain proximal control of an apical aneurysm. In most cases, this access is available without additional maneuvers. For low-lying aneurysms, however, the posterior clinoid process may be in the way. Drilling the posterior clinoid process is sometimes all that is needed to expose the artery and gain proximal control.[70–72] The posterior clinoid process is bordered laterally by CN III and the cavernous sinus and medially by the sella, dorsum, and clivus. When the posterior clinoid process is large or only minimal additional exposure is needed, the bone can be resected without encroaching on the cavernous sinus and clival venous plexus.

An alternative route to the proximal basilar artery is laterally through the tentorium. A pretemporal or subtemporal trajectory under CN III sometimes offers the exposure needed for proximal control without cutting the tentorium at all. A tacking suture in the tentorium can pull it inferolaterally and enlarge this window. When these maneuvers are inadequate, the tentorium can be incised, providing a wider corridor into the posterior fossa. An incision in the tentorium that begins medially behind the dural sleeve of CN IV protects this nerve and avoids the cavernous sinus (transtentorial-retrocavernous) but may be far enough posterior that it can only be reached subtemporally.[73] An incision in the tentorium that begins medially between CNs III and IV can be reached from a pretemporal trajectory, but it risks transecting CN IV and violating the cavernous sinus (transtentorial-transcavernous). Most patients tolerate sacrifice of CN IV, and cavernous sinus bleeding can be controlled easily with packing. Although neither transtentorial approach provides an optimal solution, either can be used to gain the exposure needed to obtain control of the proximal basilar artery.

For basilar tip aneurysms that lie even lower in the posterior fossa, a more extensive transclinoidal approach is needed. Two transclinoidal approaches exist: inferolaterally through the cavernous sinus (transclinoidal-transcavernous),[70, 74, 75] or inferomedially through the dorsum and upper clivus outside the cavernous sinus (transclinoidal-extracavernous).[3]

The transclinoidal-transcavernous approach includes anterior clinoidectomy, posterior clinoidectomy, and entrance into the cavernous sinus. Anterior clinoidectomy only marginally increases exposure of the basilar artery, but it enables the distal dural ring around the ICA to be dissected and the ICA to be mobilized medially. This maneuver increases the opening into and through the cavernous sinus. An incision is made in the roof of the cavernous sinus, or carotid-oculomotor membrane, medial to CN III, and venous bleeding is controlled by packing the cavernous sinus. Working in the bend of the anterior loop of the ICA, the surgeon can resect the posterior clinoid and lateral clivus. An incision in the clival dura then exposes the basilar trunk inferior to the superior cerebellar arteries. This approach creates a deep corridor into the posterior fossa through the cavernous sinus and rostral clivus.

The transclinoidal-extracavernous approach aims medially to the medial wall of the cavernous sinus. The posterior clinoid process, dorsum, and upper clivus are drilled away (Fig. 116–7), and the clival venous plexus is cauterized or tamponaded. This approach avoids entry into the cavernous sinus. In addition, resection of the anterior clinoid process and dissection of the carotid dural rings are not always required. The disadvantage of this approach is that the course of the basilar artery intersects the cavernous sinus, and a transclinoidal-extracavernous approach may open a medial corridor of exposure that does not parallel the course of the basilar artery. Still, it is an easy method of gaining exposure and can be attempted before committing to the bloodier transcavernous route.

Medial petrosectomy is another skull base addition that can augment the standard subtemporal approach. In the next section, the details of the technique are discussed as it applies to the extended middle fossa approach. Extradural removal of petrous bone in Kawase's triangle allows the trigeminal ganglion to sag inferiorly and the medial tentorium to be incised,

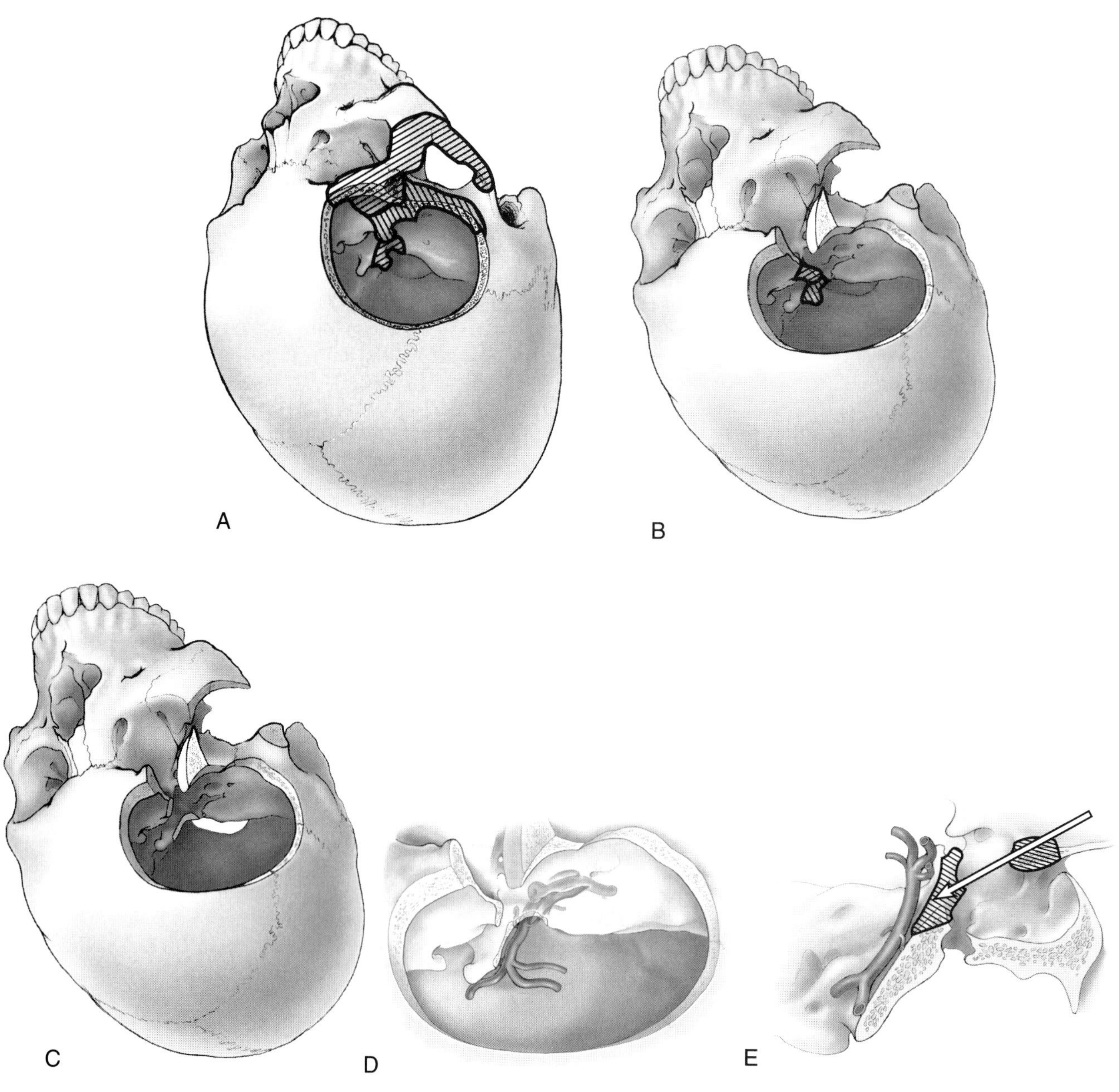

FIGURE 116–7. Transclinoidal-extracavernous approach. *A*, The bone flap has been removed. Removing the superolateral orbit and zygomatic arch *(cross-hatching)* creates the orbitozygomatic exposure. *B*, The anterior and posterior clinoid processes, dorsum sellae, and upper clivus *(cross-hatching)* are then removed *(C)*. *D*, Drilling away these bony obstacles creates a window in the upper clivus through which the upper basilar artery can be accessed. *E*, The trajectory of this approach is aligned with the axis of the basilar artery. (Courtesy of Barrow Neurological Institute.)

thereby creating an opening into the posterior fossa. These additional maneuvers can be used for low-lying basilar apex aneurysms that are approached from the subtemporal trajectory.

SURGICAL APPROACHES TO THE BASILAR TRUNK

The second category of surgical approaches targets aneurysms of the basilar trunk from a lateral trajectory, and the principal obstacle to the aneurysm is the petrous bone. Lateral approaches to the basilar trunk require a presigmoid corridor made by drilling through the temporal bone. The extent of bone removal varies from a retrolabyrinthine resection to a radical transcochlear petrosectomy. Transpetrous routes in front of the labyrinth (extended middle fossa approach through Kawase's triangle) involve removing the medial petrous apex to arrive at the lower basilar trunk through a narrow window; the approach is suited only for small vertebrobasilar aneurysms. More extensive approaches combine transpetrous and subtemporal exposures, dividing the intervening tentorium to widen the CPA significantly. Transoral approaches, which access the midbasilar artery, are mentioned for completeness; however, these approaches have been replaced because they are associated with high rates of CSF leakage, meningitis, and other complications.

Transpetrosal Approaches

Transpetrosal approaches expose the basilar trunk from a lateral trajectory through presigmoid surgical corridors excavated in the petrous bone. These lateral approaches provide good vascular control (proximal and distal) of the basilar artery but often place the aneurysm's dome between the surgeon and the neck of the aneurysm, where the clip is applied. Although this relationship can be disadvantageous, the approach typically is from the same side as the aneurysm. Approaches on the side away from the dome typically require more complicated clipping techniques, such as with fenestrated clips. Lateral approaches also interpose the cranial nerves in the foreground of the operative field, which places them at risk for injury and limits operative maneuverability.

The petrous drilling required for these approaches is usually outside the neurosurgeon's expertise and therefore necessitates a skull base team with readily available neuro-otologists.

Temporal bone dissection is categorized into three variations, based on the increasing extent of resected bone: retrolabyrinthine, translabyrinthine, and transcochlear (Fig. 116–8*A*). The retrolabyrinthine approach removes temporal bone between the semicircular canals anteriorly and the posterior fossa dura on the posterior aspect of the temporal bone.[67, 76–78] The semicircular canals are skeletonized, but not violated, to increase the working space. The translabyrinthine approach removes more bone than the retrolabyrinthine approach. In the process, the semicircular canals are removed, and hearing is sacrificed.[67, 78–81] Exposure increases anteriorly to the internal auditory canal. CN VII is left in its bony sheath, thereby protecting the function of the nerve. The transcochlear approach opens the canal of the facial nerve, transposes the nerve posteriorly, and thereby provides access to the cochlea, which is then removed.[67, 78, 82, 83] This approach almost completely removes the petrous bone, maximizing exposure of the brainstem, clivus, and basilar trunk.

The three types of temporal bone dissections repre-

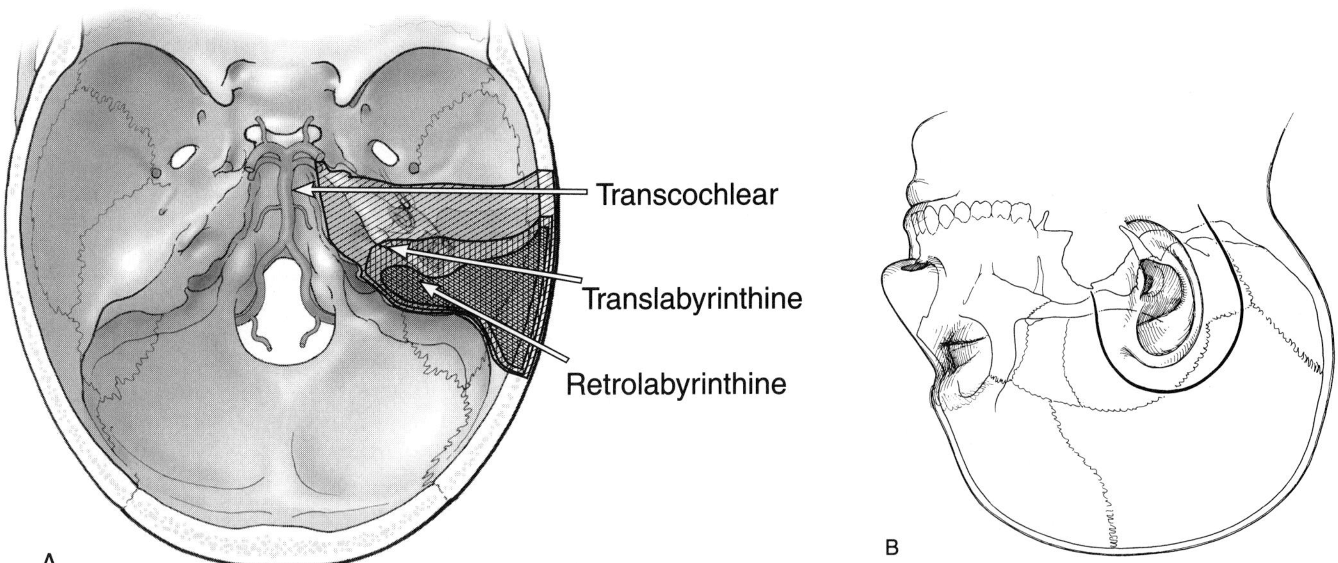

FIGURE 116–8. Transpetrosal approaches. *A*, The three types of presigmoid transpetrosal approaches. *B*, The head is positioned laterally, and the C-shaped skin incision is the same for all three approaches. (*figure continues*)

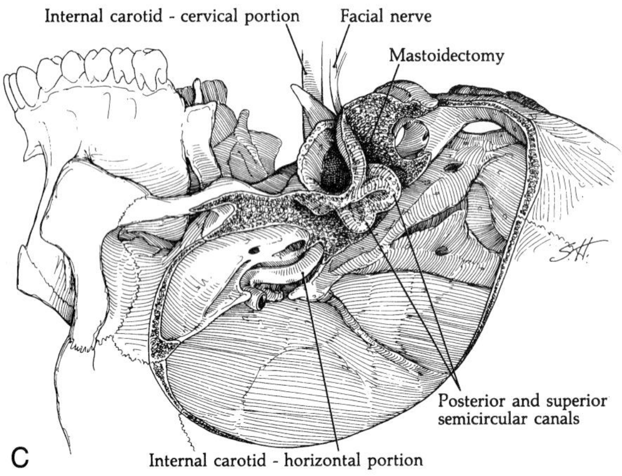

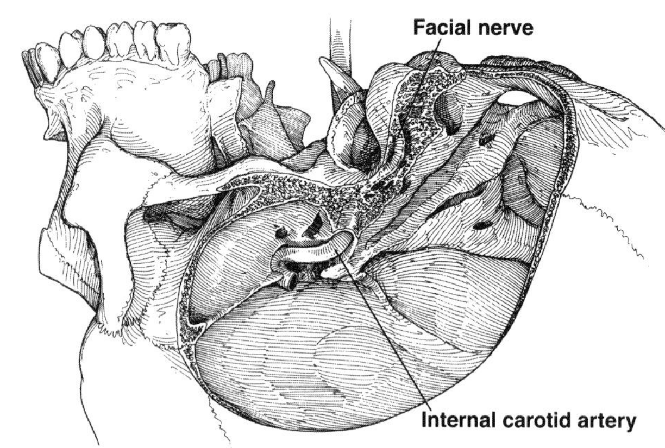

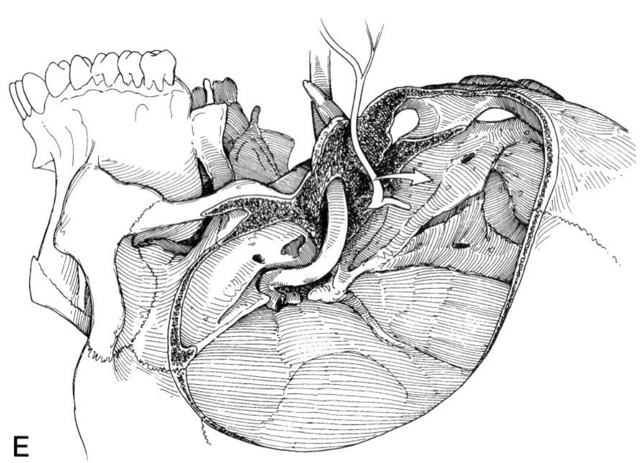

FIGURE 116–8. *Continued. C,* The retrolabyrinthine approach consists of a mastoidectomy and removal of the temporal bone anteriorly to the posterior semicircular canal. *D,* The translabyrinthine approach removes the semicircular canals and skeletonizes the internal auditory canal and the descending segment of the facial nerve. *E,* The transcochlear approach transposes the facial nerve posteriorly to allow complete removal of temporal bone anteriorly to the petrous internal carotid artery. (Courtesy of Barrow Neurological Institute, Phoenix, Arizona.)

sent a graduated increase in the amount of petrous bone that is resected, with a corresponding increase in anterior exposure. The price of this increased exposure is progressively greater sacrifice of CN VII and CN VIII function (Table 116–4). Preservation of the inner ear with the retrolabyrinthine approach leaves these nerves intact. Violation of the inner ear with the translabyrinthine and transcochlear approaches sacrifices hearing. The function of CN VII is protected if the nerve remains in its bony canal (translabyrinthine approach) but is at risk if the nerve is transposed from its canal (transcochlear approach).

EXTENDED RETROLABYRINTHINE APPROACH

The patient is positioned supine with a shoulder roll to minimize neck rotation, and the head is positioned in a Mayfield head holder with the midline parallel to the floor and inclined slightly downward. Because the surgeon works from the tight quarters of the patient's side, the head should be flexed slightly and the shoulder taped caudally to provide additional room. The mastoid bone becomes the highest point in the operative field. The skin is incised 1 cm anterior to the tragus and 2 cm above the zygoma, curving gently around the ear to the mastoid tip (see Fig. 116–8*B*), and the scalp flap is retracted anteriorly.

The drilling begins with an initial cut along the temporal line, the bony ridge that continues from the superior border of the zygomatic arch posteriorly to the mastoid cortex. The temporal line marks both the inferior limit of temporalis muscle insertion and the floor of the middle fossa. A second cut is made perpendicularly, running inferiorly to the mastoid tip. A large cutting bur is used to perform a rapid, simple mastoidectomy. Bone in the sinodural angle and covering the sigmoid sinus is removed completely to allow identification of the sigmoid sinus, which is the critical anatomic landmark. Posterior retraction of the sinus and presigmoid dura exposes the middle fossa dura and sinodural angle between them. The superior petrosal sinus lies deep to the sinodural angle and represents the posterior-superior margin of the petrous bone. Dissection into the mastoid antrum reveals the horizontal

TABLE 116–4 ■ **Preservation of Cranial Nerve Function Associated with Transpetrosal Approaches**

APPROACH	HEARING	FACIAL NERVE
Retrolabyrinthine	Preserved	Preserved
Translabyrinthine	Sacrificed	Preserved
Transcochlear	Sacrificed	Transient paralysis or paresis

semicircular canal, which leads to other anatomic guideposts, including the external genu of CN VII medially and inferiorly, the posterior semicircular canal posteriorly, and the epitympanum and superior semicircular canal anteriorly. The posterior and superior semicircular canals are skeletonized, and drilling continues as far anteriorly as possible (see Fig. 116–8*C*). Resection of the temporal bone above and below the otic capsule exposes the medial dura of the middle fossa floor, the superior petrosal sinus, and the jugular bulb. A large dural surface is thereby exposed that, when opened, allows access to the CPA.

The retrolabyrinthine approach provides excellent exposure of the CPA but rarely provides enough exposure to access aneurysms on the basilar trunk. Other maneuvers are needed if the petrosectomy is limited to a retrolabyrinthine approach. One such maneuver involves ligation and division of the sigmoid sinus.[84] A transsigmoid dural opening eliminates the restraint of the sigmoid sinus and allows the cerebellum to be retracted more posteriorly than is possible with an intact sigmoid sinus. Nonetheless, this retrolabyrinthine-transsigmoid approach should be used only with smaller aneurysms of the basilar trunk. Another useful modification of the retrolabyrinthine approach is tentoriotomy in conjunction with a subtemporal exposure. This modification constitutes the "combined" approach, which is discussed later.

TRANSLABYRINTHINE APPROACH

The translabyrinthine approach is used when more exposure is needed than a simple retrosigmoid approach can provide. The initial part of this approach is the same as the retrolabyrinthine approach, but then all three semicircular canals are drilled away, thereby exposing the posterior half to two thirds of the internal auditory canal (see Fig. 116–8*D*). The medial walls of the vestibule and the superior semicircular canal ampulla represent the lateral wall of the fundus of the internal auditory canal, and minimal bone removal at this location exposes the internal auditory canal. The dura lining the internal auditory canal is not opened when this approach is used for aneurysm surgery, but the location of CN VII is kept in mind to protect it during the approach. CN VII lies anterosuperiorly in the internal auditory canal and is separated from the superior vestibular nerve posterosuperiorly by a shelf of bone (Bill's bar). Monitoring CN VII helps protect the nerve throughout the drilling.

The distal segment of CN VII is skeletonized with a diamond bit along its horizontal (tympanic) segment, external or second genu, and descending (mastoid) segment. The nerve is left in its thinned bony canal to minimize the risk of injury to it. Additional exposure is gained by removing petrous bone anteriorly and medially above the internal auditory canal in Kawase's quadrangle. Inferiorly, the sigmoid sinus is unroofed to the jugular bulb to maximize inferior exposure beneath the internal auditory canal.

The translabyrinthine exposure extends farther anterior than the retrolabyrinthine approach does. The CPA, anterolateral brainstem, and inferior clivus are better visualized, but the surgical corridor is still narrow and suitable only for small aneurysms of the basilar trunk unless maneuvers such as division of the sigmoid sinus or tentorium are added.

TRANSCOCHLEAR APPROACH

The transcochlear approach is a forward extension of the translabyrinthine approach that unsheathes and mobilizes CN VII, removes the cochlea, and opens the CPA to expose the anterolateral brainstem, clivus, and basilar trunk. This approach provides the maximal exposure that can be achieved from a transpetrosal approach by resection of essentially the entire petrous bone.

The initial procedure is the same as for the translabyrinthine approach, except that the external auditory canal is transected and oversewn in two layers. CN VII is skeletonized along its course from its entrance into the internal auditory canal to its exit from the stylomastoid foramen. The facial recess is a tract of air cells bounded medially by the descending segment of CN VII, laterally by the chorda tympani, and superiorly by the fossa incudis. Opening the facial recess exposes the middle ear space, the stapes and incus, the promontory of the cochlea, Jacobson's nerve, and the horizontal segment of CN VII. Through this opening into the epitympanum, the ossicles are removed. The chorda tympani is sectioned inferiorly at its origin from the descending portion of CN VII to allow the facial recess to be extended inferiorly to the hypotympanum and retrofacial area. The greater superficial petrosal nerve is sectioned anteriorly at its origin from the geniculate ganglion. These maneuvers free CN VII, which is transposed posteriorly after it is dissected from its bony canal.

The cochlea is then drilled out completely, beginning with the promontory that houses the basal turn of the cochlea. Bone is removed forward to the septum between the basal turn and the petrous ICA. The ICA and internal jugular vein leave the carotid sheath and enter the skull base near each other. The jugulocarotid septum—a ridge of bone that separates the carotid artery as it turns anteriorly from the jugular vein, which turns posteriorly—is removed to expose the jugular bulb completely. The close relationship among CNs IX, X, and XI within the jugular foramen must be remembered to avoid injuring them. During the extensive drilling of the temporal bone, the dura of the internal auditory canal is kept intact to protect this part of CN VII.

When the drilling is completed, the entire temporal bone is gone (see Fig. 116–8*E*). The superior petrosal sinus, stretching from the sinodural angle laterally to Meckel's cave medially, forms the superior boundary of this exposure. The inferior petrosal sinus and jugular bulb are the inferior border. Bone removal extends medially to the clivus and anteriorly to the ICA and periosteum of the temporomandibular joint. The bone surrounding the ICA can be removed superiorly to the middle fossa floor. Of the transpetrosal approaches, the transcochlear approach provides the greatest exposure. A wide triangular corridor is opened and leads directly to the basilar trunk, through which even large aneurysms can be exposed adequately for dissection, proximal and distal control, and clipping. The maneuvers added to the retrolabyrinthine and translabyrinthine approaches (i.e., division of the sigmoid sinus or tentorium) are seldom necessary to make the transcochlear approach suitable for basilar trunk aneurysms.

Combined Supra- and Infratentorial Approach

The transpetrosal approaches described previously are sometimes inadequate to expose the basilar trunk fully for successful clipping of large or giant aneurysms. When petrous-sparing approaches such as the retrolabyrinthine and even the translabyrinthine approaches are used to preserve hearing or CN VII function, the surgical corridor is squeezed by residual petrous bone anteriorly, the tentorium superiorly, and the sigmoid sinus posteriorly to the extent that aneurysm dissection and clipping may still be unsafe. Two maneuvers dramatically enhance exposure after petrosectomy: division of the tentorium, and posterior mobilization of the sigmoid sinus.[67, 78, 83, 85, 86] The petrosectomy then becomes the cornerstone of a combination approach that relaxes these confining superior and posterior barriers. The two critical additions to the transpetrosal approaches are, first, a supra- and infratentorial craniotomy that crosses the transverse sinus, and second, a tentoriotomy that permits free communication between the supra- and infratentorial compartments. Extensive exposure of the medial petrous and clival regions and associated neurovascular structures is obtained with minimal brain retraction.

When the temporal bone drilling is completed, an edge of middle fossa dura is exposed above the petrosectomy defect, and an edge of posterior fossa dura is exposed behind the sigmoid sinus. These epidural locations serve as bur holes for a subtemporal-suboccipital craniotomy that crosses the transverse sinus. After the bone flap has been removed, a large dural surface is exposed, and the transverse, sigmoid, and superior petrosal sinuses are visible (Fig. 116–9*A*). Before the dura is opened, the brain is relaxed with hyperventilation, mannitol, and removal of CSF through a lumbar drain. The dura is incised anteriorly over the temporal lobe and curves posteriorly and inferiorly to the superior petrosal sinus below, where it enters the sigmoid sinus. A second dural incision is made inferiorly in front of the sigmoid sinus, curving up to the superior petrosal sinus. The superior petrosal sinus is cauterized or clipped and divided. The surgeon should beware of low-lying veins of Labbé, which need to be preserved when the dura is opened.

The sigmoid sinus can be sacrificed if the contralateral transverse and sigmoid sinuses are patent and communicate with the ipsilateral transverse and sagittal sinuses through a patent torcular Herophili. As an added assurance, sigmoid sinus pressure can be measured before and after test occlusion of the sigmoid sinus to document that pressure does not increase more than 10 mm Hg. These measurements are made after the superior petrosal sinus has been divided. When these angiographic and hemodynamic criteria are met, the sigmoid sinus can be sacrificed safely. It is divided below its confluence with the superior petrosal sinus. The vein of Labbé consistently and reliably enters the transverse sinus above this junction and therefore drains contralaterally. Notwithstanding these safety concerns, division of the sigmoid sinus is rarely necessary, because a presigmoid dural opening is usually adequate to expose the tentorium and mobilize the sigmoid sinus.

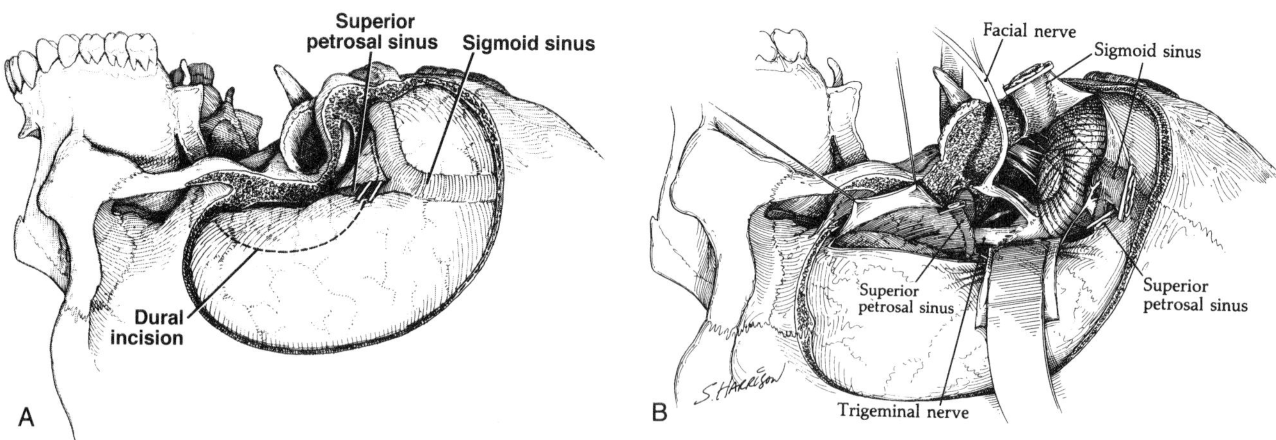

FIGURE 116–9. The combined supra- and infratentorial approach is a combination of the subtemporal and transpetrosal approaches. *A*, The approach begins with temporal bone resection, which then serves as a bur hole for a craniotomy that crosses the transverse sinus and exposes the dura of the temporal lobe and cerebellum. A dural incision can then be made across the superior petrosal sinus. *B*, Division of the tentorium from the transverse-sigmoid junction to the incisura exposes the cranial nerves, brainstem, clivus, and basilar artery. (Courtesy of Barrow Neurological Institute, Phoenix, Arizona.)

When the dural incisions are completed and the superior petrosal sinus has been divided, the tentorium is incised medially to the tentorial hiatus, posterior to CN IV (see Fig. 116–9*B*). This crucial maneuver connects the supra- and infratentorial compartments and relaxes neural structures. The posterior temporal lobe is elevated with care to avoid traction on the vein of Labbé, which is tethered to the transverse sinus. The petrous region, clivus, brainstem, cranial nerves, and vessels of the posterior circulation are now easily visualized, and the aneurysm can be accessed by working between cranial nerve bundles.

This approach provides wide exposure along the skull base from the foramen magnum to the dorsum sellae with minimal brain retraction. The combined approach works with any of the three variations of petrosectomy. Typically, it is used with a retrolabyrinthine approach instead of a more radical transcochlear approach when a decision has been made to conserve petrous bone and to preserve the function of CNs VII and VIII. The added maneuvers of the combined approach are designed to compensate for less presigmoid exposure.

Extended Middle Fossa Approach

The middle fossa approach was developed to remove small, intracanalicular acoustic neuromas that extend less than 5 mm into the CPA. This approach provides a direct route to the internal auditory canal, keeps the hearing apparatus intact, and offers patients with useful preoperative hearing a good chance at preserving their hearing.[87–89] The approach has been adapted for use with basilar aneurysms not only by skeletonizing the internal auditory canal but also by resecting the medial petrous apex. This approach has several names, including the extended middle fossa approach, Kawase's approach, and rhomboid approach.[71, 90, 91] The anterior subtemporal–medial transpetrosal approach is similar, but the surgeon works intradurally in the middle fossa instead of extradurally.[92] The extended middle fossa approach differs from the other lateral transpetrosal approaches by reaching the basilar artery from a more anterolateral and superior trajectory in front of the otic capsule and by leaving the posterolateral temporal bone intact.

Kawase described the extended middle fossa approach to basilar aneurysms, which requires resection of bone in the triangle that bears his name (Fig. 116–10*A* and *B*). Kawase's triangle is really a quadrangle formed by the internal auditory canal posteriorly, the greater superficial petrosal nerve laterally, the lateral margin of the trigeminal nerve and ganglion anteriorly, and the medial edge of the petrous bone medially.[90] The quadrangle extends inferiorly to the inferior petrosal sinus. Between these neurovascular boundaries are temporal bone and air cells. Resection of Kawase's quadrangle opens a corridor through which the basilar artery can be reached (see Fig. 116–10*C*). The trajectory of this narrow bony corridor and the orientation of the nerve bundles of CNs V, VII, and VIII limit the view of the vertebrobasilar junction and provide minimal working space, thereby making the approach impractical for most basilar trunk aneurysms. The approach is described because it can be used for selected small aneurysms and because the relevant anatomy is important.

The patient is positioned supine, with the head fixated as for a subtemporal approach. A question mark or horseshoe-shaped incision is used, and the skin and temporalis muscle flaps are reflected anteriorly. A 5- by 5-cm craniotomy is made in the squamosal portion of the temporal bone, two thirds anterior and one third posterior to the external auditory canal. The edge of the inferior bone is drilled inferiorly to the middle fossa floor. The dura is elevated from the middle fossa floor medially to the petrous ridge, where a self-retaining retractor is placed with its tip over the lip of the ridge. The middle meningeal artery is followed along the dura to the foramen spinosum, where it is coagulated and divided. The greater superficial petrosal nerve is identified approximately 1 cm medially. The greater superficial petrosal nerve originates from the geniculate ganglion of CN VII and runs superficially along the middle fossa floor in an anteromedial direction. The greater superficial petrosal nerve and geniculate ganglion are often dehiscent and vulnerable to injury during dissection. Lateral to the greater superficial petrosal nerve is Glasscock's triangle, through which the petrous ICA can be exposed as it runs horizontally toward the cavernous sinus.

The arcuate eminence, a bony prominence along the middle fossa floor that is almost perpendicular to the petrous ridge and that marks the underlying superior semicircular canal, is identified next. The greater superficial petrosal nerve and arcuate eminence form a 120-degree angle that is bisected by a line that parallels the internal auditory canal. The internal auditory canal can be exposed by drilling along this line medially where there are no adjacent neurovascular structures. Bone is removed around the porus acusticus and internal auditory canal, working medially to laterally. The lateral internal auditory canal (fundus) is surrounded by important anatomy. The cochlea is immediately anterior. Its basal turn is particularly vulnerable to violation when drilling in the angle between the greater superficial petrosal nerve and the internal auditory canal. Perforation of the cochlea causes complete hearing loss. The vestibule and ampulla of the superior semicircular canal are immediately posterior to the fundus. As drilling proceeds laterally, the exposure is narrowed to avoid the cochlea and superior semicircular canal. The dura of the internal auditory canal is exposed laterally to Bill's bar.

The medial petrous apex is removed, drilling between the borders of Kawase's quadrangle. The horizontal segment of the petrous ICA is identified laterally in Glasscock's triangle and skeletonized to increase the exposure anteriorly and inferiorly. After drilling is completed, the petrous dural exposure extends from the superior petrosal sinus to the inferior petrosal sinus. The superior petrosal sinus is coagulated and divided just lateral to the trigeminal ganglion. The posterior dura is opened to enter the posterior fossa.

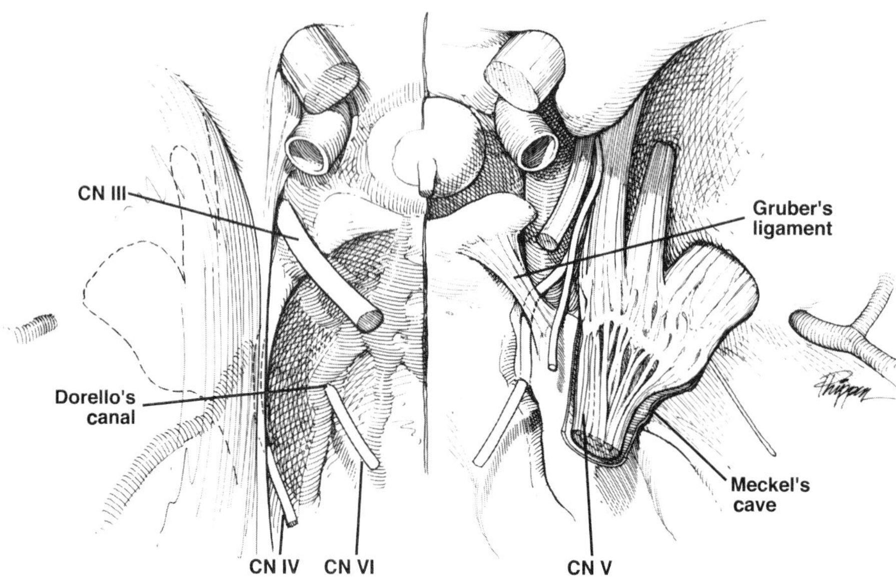

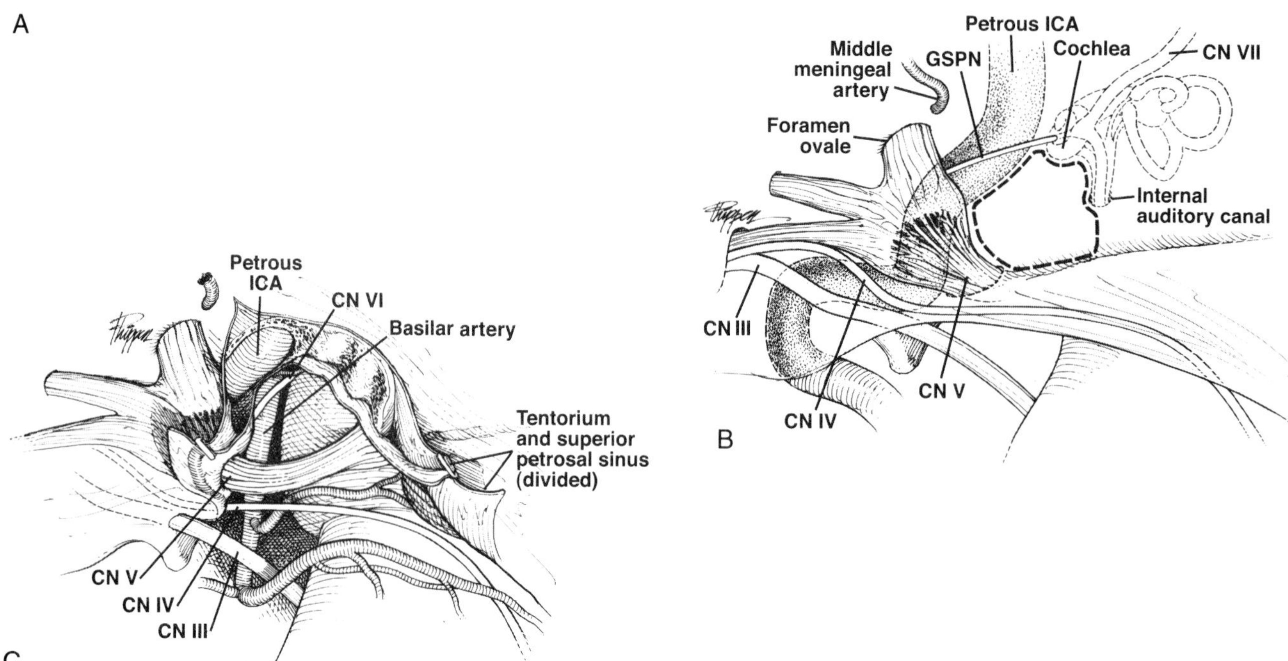

FIGURE 116–10. Extended middle fossa approach. *A*, Overview from above of the middle fossa anatomy, with *(left)* and without *(right)* overlying middle fossa and tentorial dura. *B*, Bone removal within Kawase's quadrangle *(dashed line)* opens the corridor to the basilar artery (right-sided approach, surgeon's view). *C*, The dura is opened with a lateral incision in the middle fossa dura, a medial incision in the tentorium, and an inferior incision in the posterior fossa dura. Note that the superior petrosal sinus is divided, and the petrous carotid artery forms the anterior border of the exposure. The trajectory leads to the vertebrobasilar junction. CN III, oculomotor nerve; CN IV, trochlear nerve; CN V, trigeminal nerve; CN VI, abducent nerve; CN VII, facial nerve; GSPN, greater superficial petrosal nerve; ICA, internal carotid artery. (Courtesy of Barrow Neurological Institute, Phoenix, Arizona.)

The middle fossa dura is incised laterally, and the tentorium is incised medially to the incisura, just behind the entrance of CN IV in its dural canal. The lower basilar artery is then dissected through this opening. The dissection proceeds between CNs V and VII.

Transoral Approaches

The transoral approach (Fig. 116–11*A*) to basilar trunk aneurysms is used with great reluctance and is mentioned only for completeness.[93–96] This approach is associated with a high incidence of postoperative CSF leakage and meningitis, and the surgical corridor is long and limiting. For these reasons, it is not recommended.

The patient is positioned supine. Unless the oral retraction system (see Fig. 116–11*B*) adequately depresses the tongue and endotracheal tube out of the surgical field, a tracheostomy and gastrostomy are performed. A lumbar subarachnoid drain is also inserted. The pharyngeal cavity is prepared with povidone-iodine (Betadine), and a midline incision is made in the pharyngeal mucosa. After the soft tissues have been elevated and the proper trajectory has been confirmed fluoroscopically, the clivus is drilled to create a rectangular opening in the midline. The clival dura is opened in the midline, and the basilar trunk is exposed. Closure requires packing the clival defect with abdominal fat and closing the pharyngeal mucosa in layers. CSF drainage and prophylactic antibiotics are used postoperatively.

SURGICAL APPROACHES TO THE VERTEBRAL TRUNK

The third category of surgical approaches targets aneurysms of the intradural vertebral artery. These approaches provide posteroinferior trajectories along the axis of the vertebral trunk and include the midline suboccipital approach, the far-lateral approach, and the extended far-lateral approach. The inner exposure of a lateral suboccipital approach is increased by resection of the occipital condyle and jugular tubercle and, occasionally, by mobilization of the extradural vertebral artery—all skull base techniques that are the hallmarks of the far-lateral approach. This approach can be combined with a transpetrous approach in the "combined-combined" approach to gain even greater exposure of the vertebral and basilar arteries.

Midline Suboccipital Approach

The suboccipital approach, a standard approach to cerebellar lesions and the fourth ventricle, is sometimes used to deal with posterior circulation aneurysms, notably those that arise from the distal PICA after it courses around the anterior and lateral medulla.[7, 47, 73] Bilateral proximal vertebral artery lesions are sometimes best accessed through a midline approach that permits equal access to both sides. Bypass procedures involving the distal PICA are also performed through a midline suboccipital approach. The midline approach does not provide good exposure of aneurysms located

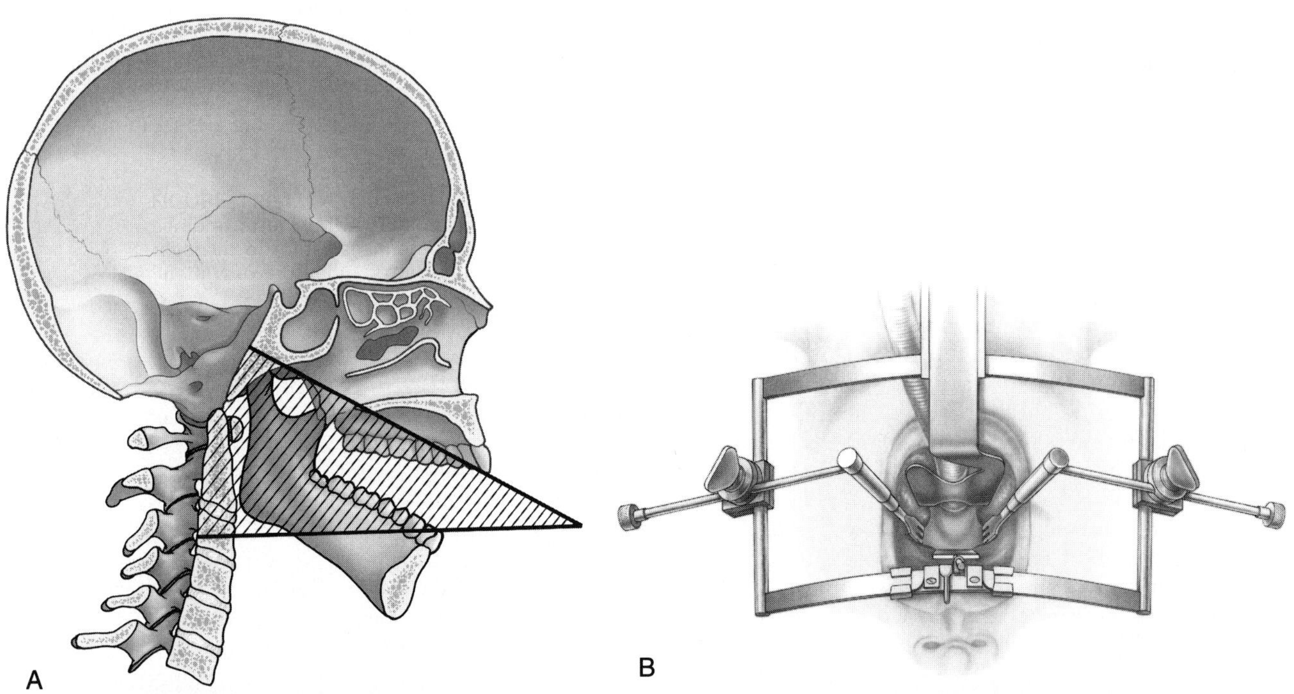

FIGURE 116–11. Transoral approach. *A*, This approach to the basilar artery is deep and long, and the nasopharyngeal and subarachnoid compartments are in communication. *B*, A retraction system that depresses the tongue and endotracheal tube spares the patient a tracheostomy. For aneurysm surgery, the transoral approach is avoided. (Courtesy of Barrow Neurological Institute, Phoenix, Arizona.)

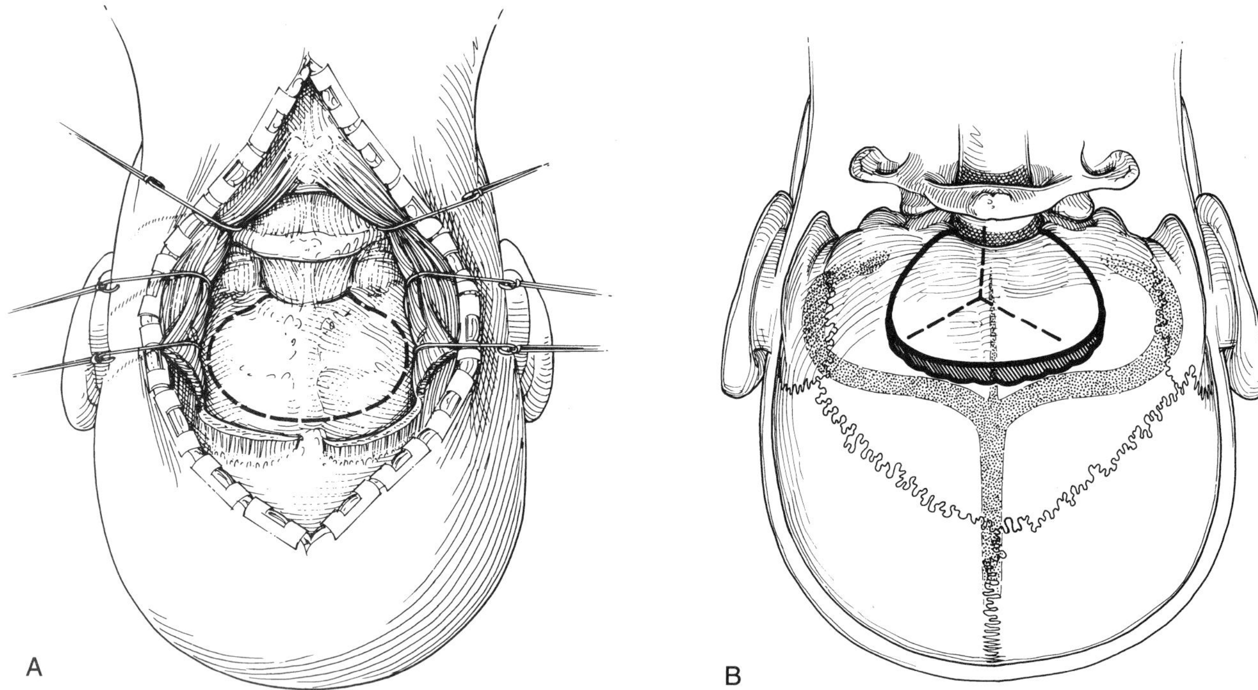

FIGURE 116–12. Midline suboccipital approach. *A*, The patient is positioned prone, with the head flexed to open the suboccipital-cervical angle. A midline linear skin incision is used, and the superior nuchal ligament is left as a cuff to reattach the muscles at closure. *B*, The craniotomy extends from the foramen magnum to the torcula and as far laterally as a linear midline incision allows. The Y-shaped dural incision (inverted on figure) is shown *(dashed line)*. (Courtesy of Barrow Neurological Institute, Phoenix, Arizona.)

distally on the vertebral artery near the typical origin of PICA.

The patient is positioned prone with the chin tucked, to open the interval between the foramen magnum and the posterior arch of C1 (Fig. 116–12*A*). In this position, the surgeon can operate while seated over the patient's head. A midline skin incision is made from the vertex to the spinous process of C4. The superior nuchal line and posterior cervical fascia are exposed approximately 3 cm to each side of the midline to enable a Y-cut in the fascia. Incising the fascia in this manner readily exposes the midline nuchal ligament, enables the posterior cervical musculature to be separated in an avascular plane, and creates fascial flaps that can be reapproximated during closure to prevent CSF leakage. The paraspinous muscles are mobilized laterally to expose the occiput, foramen magnum, C1, and C2. Complete exposure of the C2 spinous process facilitates soft tissue retraction. The dural adhesions around the foramen magnum are stripped with an angled curet, and a craniotomy can be performed using the lip of the foramen magnum as the epidural access for the drill (see Fig. 116–12*B*). In elderly patients with adherent dura, a suboccipital bur hole with subsequent cuts down to the foramen magnum may help preserve the dura. Additional lateral bone around the foramen magnum is rongeured off to widen the exposure.

The dura is opened in a Y-shaped fashion, with care taken to control bleeding from the circular sinus. The arachnoid of the cisterna magna is opened, and the cervicomedullary junction is exposed. The vertebral arteries can be identified anterior to the dentate ligaments coursing anteromedially. Dissection in the tonsillomedullary fissure exposes the PICA distally along its course. To gain more distal exposure, the interhemispheric fissure can be split between the tonsils, and its course through the cranial loop can be followed.

Far-Lateral Approach

The far-lateral approach is the most common approach to aneurysms of the vertebral trunk.[67, 97–101] Most such aneurysms are unilateral and extend beyond the region that can be accessed through a midline suboccipital exposure. Therefore, the craniotomy can be limited to one side, and the patient's position can be changed from prone to three-quarters prone. These modifications substantially improve exposure of the vertebral artery by shifting the corridor of exposure laterally. The outer cranial exposure is enhanced by resection of the posterior arch of the first cervical vertebra and the posteroinferior skull base (including the posterolateral foramen magnum, posterior half of the occipital condyle, and jugular tubercle). Together, these maneuvers constitute the far-lateral approach. Synonyms for the far-lateral approach include the lateral suboccipital approach, extreme lateral approach, and extreme lateral inferior transcondylar exposure (ELITE).[71] Resection of bone in the angle between the lower medulla and cerebellum creates a surgical corridor along the axis of the vertebral artery through which aneurysms can be exposed with minimal cerebellar retraction.

An important element of the far-lateral approach is the patient's position (Fig. 116–13*A* and *B*). A modified park-bench or three-quarters prone position is used, with the side of the patient's lesion placed upward. The operating table is extended by placing a 3/4-inch-thick plastic board under the mattress and pulling both the mattress and the board 6 inches beyond the edge of the table. This extender creates a gap between the Mayfield head holder and its attachment to the table, allowing the dependent arm, cradled in a padded sling, to hang comfortably over the extended end of the table. When the arm and shoulder are dropped downward, the head can be rotated effectively into position. This position minimizes brachial plexus compression and allows better venous return compared with the full prone position.

Three maneuvers are essential to position the head optimally: (1) *flexion* in the anteroposterior plane until the chin is one fingerbreadth from the sternum, (2) *rotation* 45 degrees away from the side of the lesion, and (3) lateral flexion 30 degrees *down* toward the floor. These maneuvers place the clivus perpendicular to the floor, allowing the surgeon to look down the axis of the vertebral and basilar arteries and to work between the horizontally arrayed cranial nerves. The ipsilateral mastoid process becomes the highest point in the operative field, and the posterior cervical-suboccipital angle is opened maximally to increase the surgeon's operating space. The patient's superior shoulder may need to be taped to keep the cervical-suboccipital angle open.

A hockey-stick incision is made (see Fig. 116–13C) beginning in the cervical midline over the C5 spinous process. It extends cephalad to the inion, courses laterally along the superior nuchal line to the mastoid bone, and finishes inferiorly at the mastoid tip. The midline nuchal ligament is identified to split the paraspinous musculature in this avascular plane. A cut just below the superior nuchal line detaches the paraspinous muscles, which are then mobilized inferolaterally to expose the occipital bone and foramen magnum while also creating a cuff for reattaching the muscle during closure. Mobilization of the paraspinous musculature in this manner provides adequate exposure of the lateral foramen magnum and eliminates the need to dissect or transect these muscles, thereby eliminating a significant source of postoperative pain. Retraction of soft tissue is facilitated by exposure down to and around the C2 spinous process. Care must be taken to identify and protect the vertebral artery as it courses from the transverse foramen of the lateral mass of C1, through the sulcus arteriosus of the C1 vertebral arch, to its dural entry point. The lateral epidural venous plexus can cause troublesome bleeding; it is best preserved by blunt dissection.

Bone removal consists of three parts: a C1 laminotomy, a lateral occipital craniotomy, and a condylectomy. The arch of C1 is removed with the drill; a cut is made just lateral to the sulcus arteriosus, and another is made across the contralateral arch. Additional atlantal bone can be removed under the vertebral artery lateral to the transverse foramen. The foramen can be opened dorsally and the artery mobilized, but this maneuver is rarely needed for intradural aneurysms. A suboccipital craniotomy (see Fig. 116–13*D*) is extended unilaterally from the foramen magnum in the midline to as far laterally as possible and then back around to the foramen magnum. The rim of the foramen magnum is rongeured to extend the opening across the midline and laterally toward the condyle.

Finally, the lateral aspect of the foramen magnum, the posteromedial two thirds of the occipital condyle, and the jugular tubercle are removed with a drill, using a diamond bit to minimize injury to adjacent emissary veins. The anterior extent of condylar resection is defined by the hypoglossal canal, the condylar emissary vein, or bone removal that exposes dura as it begins to curve anteromedially. Condylar resection to this extent enables the dural flap that is centered on the condyle to be completely flat. The dural incision (see Fig. 116–13*E*) curves from the cervical midline, across the circular sinus, and laterally to the edge of the craniotomy. An inferior cut laterally under C1 mobilizes the flap farther laterally against the margin of the craniotomy. The cisterna magna is opened under the microscope, and the arachnoid layers are reflected.

Just beyond its point of dural penetration, the proximal vertebral artery is prepared for proximal control of the aneurysm. Exposure here keeps temporary clips out of the deep corridor and typically requires division of the dentate ligament. The corridor along the vertebral artery is exposed by dissecting the tonsillomedullary fissure and mobilizing the ipsilateral cerebellar tonsil away from the medulla. The vertebral artery is dissected proximally to distally, and the PICA is dissected distally to proximally. These converging lines lead to the origin of the PICA, where most of the aneurysms treated with this approach are located. The vertebral artery can be followed distally to the vertebrobasilar junction. The approach requires operating around and through the lower cranial nerves.

The far-lateral approach provides wide exposure of the vertebral trunk and anterolateral brainstem, with minimal retraction on the cerebellum. It is the preferred approach to this region and is suitable for most aneurysms located there.

Extended Far-Lateral Approach

The exposure of the far-lateral approach can be extended superiorly by removing occipital bone to the junction of the transverse and sigmoid sinuses.[102] This retrosigmoid addition enables the CPA to be entered, and large vertebral artery aneurysms and their efferent arteries can be accessed. The trajectories from the far-lateral and retrosigmoid approaches are almost perpendicular; consequently, the retrosigmoid extension does not improve the exposure of the far-lateral approach. It does, however, provide an additional vantage of anatomy, which can help clarify the anatomy and operative strategy.

The approach is identical to the far-lateral technique,

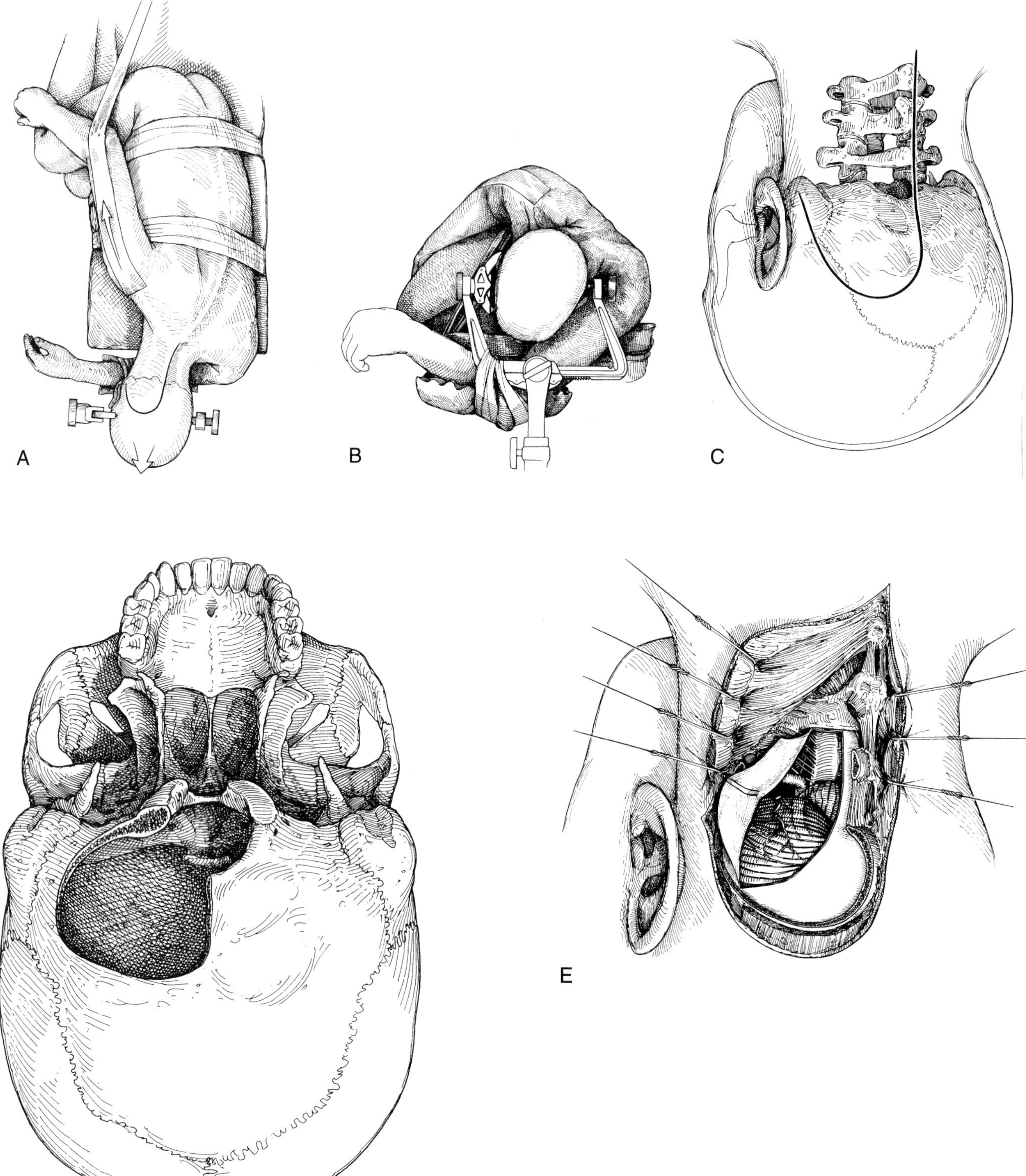

FIGURE 116–13. Far-lateral approach. *A*, The park-bench or three-quarters prone position is shown from above, with the shoulder pulled down to create space for the microscope. *B*, The arm is cradled in a sling between the edge of the bed and the Mayfield head holder. *C*, A hockey-stick skin incision extends from the mastoid tip, along the superior nuchal line to the inion, and down to the spinous process of C5. *D*, The extent of bone resection from the skull base. *E*, The dural incision. (Courtesy of Barrow Neurological Institute, Phoenix, Arizona.)

but the superolateral edge of the craniotomy is defined by drilling through the mastoid bone to define the transverse-sigmoid junction. The sigmoid sinus is skeletonized down to the jugular bulb. The subsequent far-lateral craniotomy then connects to this exposed dura, and the craniotomy flap is enlarged. The dura is opened with a flap based along the sigmoid sinus. When tacked anteriorly, the flap pulls the sinus forward to open the route into the CPA. The standard far-lateral dural flap then connects with this flap.

Far-Lateral Combined Supra- and Infratentorial (Combined-Combined) Approach

Occasionally, giant aneurysms involving the vertebrobasilar junction or lower basilar trunk require an exposure that spans the entire length of the posterior fossa from the petrous apex to the foramen magnum. The far-lateral approach, when used with the combined supra- and infratentorial approach, exposes the entire petroclival region.[83, 103, 104] Such an approach joins the transpetrosal, subtemporal, and far-lateral approaches, overcoming the limitations of a transpetrosal approach or an extended far-lateral approach alone. This approach is the most extensive of the combination approaches and is referred to as the "combined-combined" approach.

The patient is placed in the park-bench position (Fig. 116–14*A*), with the head fixated as it would be for the far-lateral approach. The hockey-stick incision is enlarged, beginning anteriorly at the zygoma, coursing superiorly around the ear toward the inion, and ending inferiorly in the midline at C5 (see Fig. 116–14*B*). A myocutaneous flap is elevated to expose the lateral temporal bone, mastoid, posterior cranium, and laminae of C1 and C2. A cuff of nuchal fascia is left to reattach the cervical muscles at the end of the procedure.

Bone removal consists of four parts: a petrosectomy, a C1 laminotomy, a craniotomy, and a condylectomy. The neuro-otologist first drills the temporal bone. Rotation of the patient's head can be adjusted during the petrosectomy to bring the head parallel to the floor to facilitate drilling. The arch of C1 is exposed, the vertebral artery is identified, and a C1 laminotomy is performed. The craniotomy cut then connects the midline foramen magnum with the anterior margin of the petrosectomy overlying the inferior temporal lobe, crossing the transverse sinus just lateral to the torculum. A second cut connects the lateral foramen magnum with the posteroinferior margin of the petrosectomy, immediately behind the sigmoid sinus. The underlying dural sinuses are dissected carefully from the bone flap, which is then removed. A large dural surface is exposed (see Fig. 116–14C), with the transverse and sigmoid sinuses in the middle. Finally, the lateral aspect of the foramen magnum, posteromedial two thirds of the occipital condyle, and jugular tubercle are removed.

The dura can be opened either in two flaps in front of and behind the sigmoid sinus to preserve it or in a single flap that sacrifices the sigmoid sinus. The two dural flaps are simply the standard openings for the combined approach plus the standard opening for the far-lateral approach. The flaps create two windows of exposure on either side of the preserved sigmoid sinus. In contrast, sacrificing the sigmoid sinus and crossing it below the sinodural angle joins these two incisions to create a single flap extending from the anterior margin of the craniotomy over the temporal lobe, across the sigmoid sinus, and down to C1 (see Fig. 116–14*D*). When the tentorium is incised to the hiatus, a large unobstructed opening is created that exposes the anterolateral brainstem from the midbrain to the upper cervical spinal cord (see Fig. 116–14*E*). Arachnoid dissection reveals CNs II through XII, both vertebral arteries, the PICA, the anterior spinal artery, the vertebrobasilar junction, the basilar artery, and the entire length of the clivus. The exposure of this approach is unsurpassed, but it is needed only rarely for unusual giant aneurysms.

SELECTION OF SURGICAL APPROACH

As this review of surgical approaches demonstrates, the choices can be overwhelming. In the authors' practices, however, several approaches stand out as clear favorites.[3] For aneurysms at the basilar apex, the approach that provides the greatest exposure and flexibility of trajectories is the extended orbitozygomatic approach. This cranial exposure eliminates the need to decide among a pterional, subtemporal, or orbitozygomatic approach by combining them. Removal of the orbitozygomatic piece enhances the pterional approach by creating room and upward viewing angles to high-lying aneurysms. The extended orbitozygomatic approach also enhances the subtemporal approach by removing the zygomatic arch and mobilizing the temporalis muscle more inferiorly.

For aneurysms of the midbasilar trunk, the choice is between a radical transpetrous approach (e.g., the transcochlear approach) and a petrous-sparing combined approach. The radical transpetrous approach provides the most direct corridor to the aneurysm, with the cone of exposure focused at the aneurysm. However, the labyrinthectomy and transposition of CN VII sacrifice hearing and cause at least transient facial paresis. In patients with preexisting complications from hemorrhage or brainstem compression, such sacrifices may be acceptable, and the decision to resect the petrous bone radically may be simplified. In minimally symptomatic patients with unruptured aneurysms, however, a petrous-sparing approach may be more appropriate. The approach is less direct and requires an additional subtemporal craniotomy, tentoriotomy, and retraction of the cerebellum to compensate for the more posterior trajectory. The surgeon must decide whether the exposure associated with an inferior approach is enough to even make it an option. Other approaches to the midbasilar territory (extended middle fossa approach, retrolabyrinthine-transsigmoid approach, and transoral approach) are not recommended

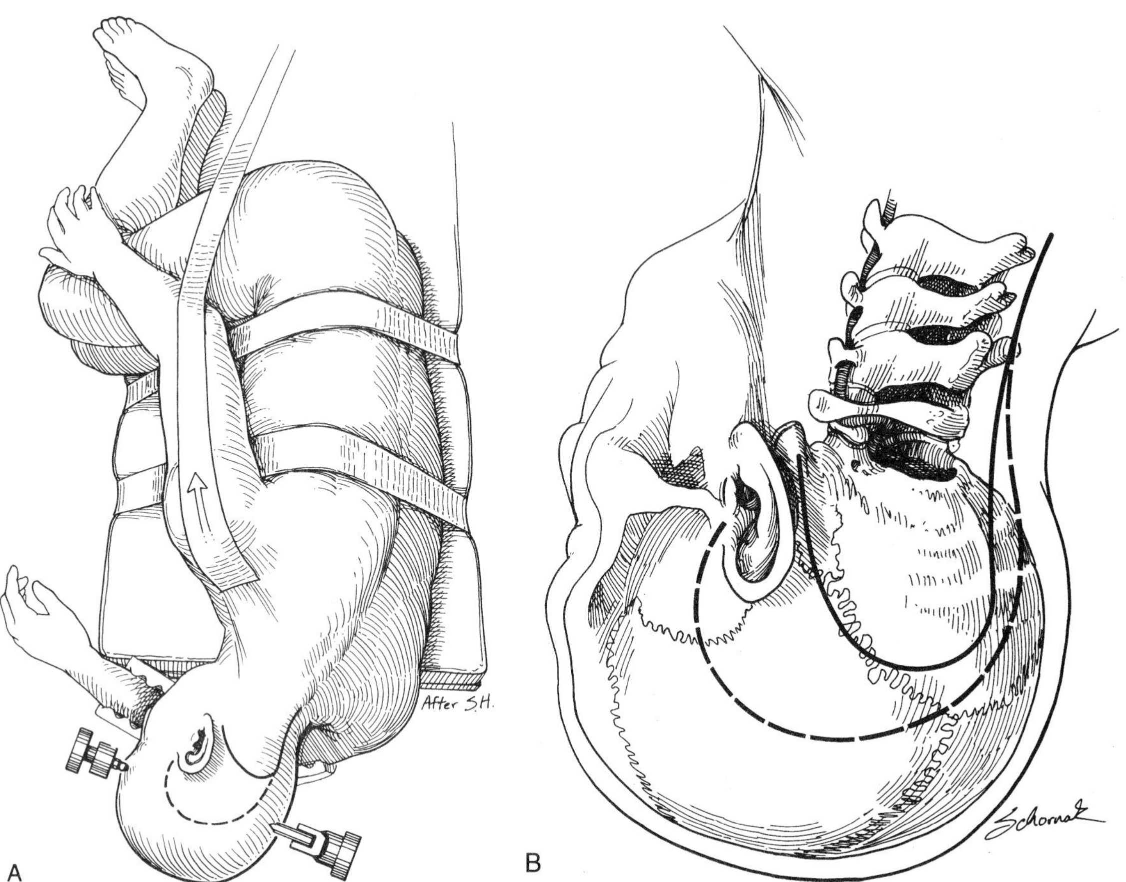

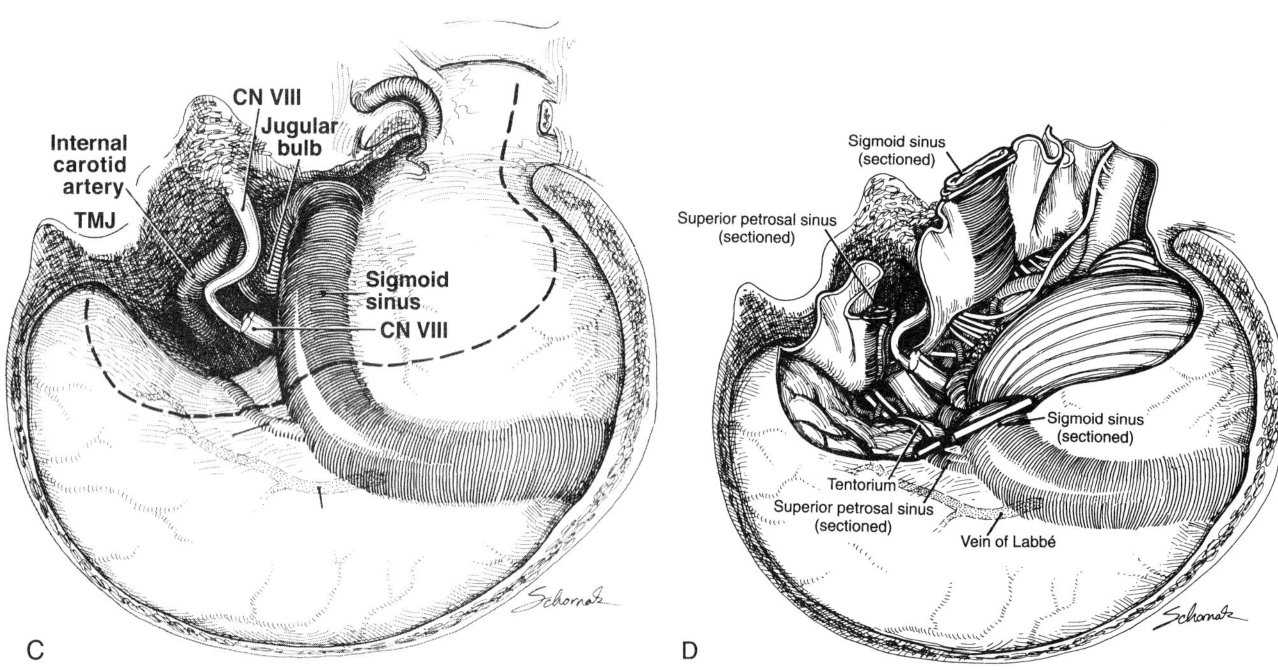

FIGURE 116–14. Far-lateral combined supra- and infratentorial ("combined-combined") approach. *A*, The park-bench position used for the far-lateral approach is also used for this approach. *B*, Instead of the hockey-stick incision used with the far-lateral approach *(solid line)*, the incision is extended anteriorly and superiorly to the zygoma *(dashed line)*. Bone resection includes a petrosectomy, condylectomy, C1 laminectomy, and large suboccipital-temporal craniotomy. *C*, When this bone exposure is completed, a transsigmoid dural incision is made. *D*, With the dura opened, the vertebrobasilar system is accessible by working in between cranial nerve bundles. *(Figure continues)*

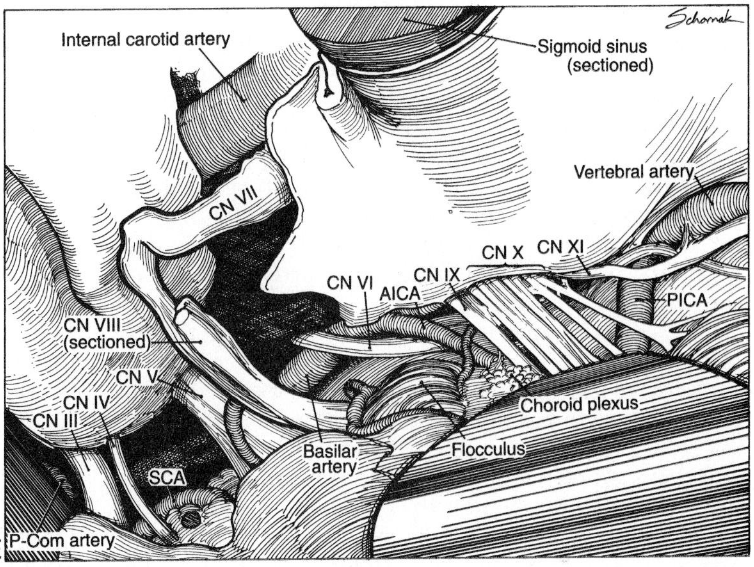

FIGURE 116–14. *Continued. E,* The microsurgical anatomy of the basilar artery, its branches, and the cranial nerves. AICA, anterior inferior cerebellar artery; CN III, oculomotor nerve; CN IV, trochlear nerve; CN V, trigeminal nerve; CN VI, abducent nerve; CNVII, facial nerve; CN VIII, vestibulocochlear nerve; CN IX, glossopharyngeal nerve; CN X, vagus nerve; CN XI, spinal accessory nerve; P-Com, posterior communicating artery; PICA, posterior inferior cerebellar artery; SCA, superior cerebellar artery; TMJ, temporomandibular joint. (From Baldwin HZ, Miller CG, Van Loveren HR, et al: The far lateral/combined supra- and infratentorial approach: A human cadaveric prosection model for routes of access to the petroclival region and ventral brain stem. J Neurosurg 81:60–68, 1994.)

unless warranted by specific features of a particular aneurysm.

The selection of an approach to vertebral trunk aneurysms is straightforward: the far-lateral approach. The approach provides excellent access to the region and an ideal trajectory through which to work. The overlying cranial nerves make it challenging at times, but no approach overcomes this obstacle. The midline suboccipital approach is only rarely applicable to select distal PICA aneurysms. The retrosigmoid extension is easily performed. It is valuable in selected large and giant aneurysms but is used only occasionally. The combined-combined approach is spectacular, offering almost complete exposure of the posterior skull base. However, it is more applicable for petroclival tumors than for aneurysms and is only rarely used to access vascular lesions.

Therefore, most posterior circulation aneurysms can be approached through one of four routes: an extended orbitozygomatic approach, the transcochlear approach, the combined supra- and infratentorial approach, or the far-lateral approach. The other approaches offer subtle differences in exposure and trajectory that seldom apply. The surgeon must be comfortable with the gamut of "inner" skull base maneuvers that provide that extra millimeter or two of exposure immediately adjacent to an aneurysm and make the difference in surgical outcomes. These skull base techniques vary from case to case, and their use cannot be predicted from preoperative diagnostic studies. The surgeon must select among these techniques carefully.

OTHER TECHNIQUES FOR TREATING UNUSUAL POSTERIOR CIRCULATION ANEURYSMS

The surgical approaches described earlier are selected with the goal of clipping an aneurysm directly. Direct clipping remains the optimal surgical technique for treating aneurysms. It closes the aneurysm's orifice, approximates the normal arterial walls to promote endothelialization that seals the orifice, and preserves blood flow in parent and branch arteries around the base of the aneurysm. Giant saccular aneurysms and complex fusiform or dolichoectatic aneurysms that lack a clippable neck require alternative techniques that can alter the selection of surgical approach. In the posterior circulation, these alternative techniques include proximal occlusion of the parent artery (hunterian ligation), aneurysmal trapping, revascularization procedures, aneurysmal excision with reanastomosis, use of hypothermic circulatory arrest, and endovascular techniques.

Revascularization

Proximal artery occlusion can be considered when blood flow in the collateral arteries is adequate. For example, distal occlusion of the basilar artery is one way to treat a complex basilar tip aneurysm and is tolerated by patients with large PCoAs. Similarly, an aneurysm of the midbasilar trunk can be occluded either proximally or distally if the PCoAs are large. At best, the size of the PCoAs on angiography is a crude predictor of a patient's tolerance of basilar artery occlusion. One technique for assessing the safety of such a maneuver is the basilar tourniquet used by Steinberg and colleagues.[105] Postoperatively, the tourniquet is gradually tightened while the patient is observed carefully. Balloon test occlusions also have been used to assess clinical tolerance. Other arteries, such as a vertebral artery, can be sacrificed proximally with little concern about tolerance, except when the contralateral anatomy is aberrant (e.g., a vertebral artery that terminates at the PICA or is hypoplastic distally).

Patients often do not tolerate surgical or endovascular arterial occlusion, or their tolerance cannot be determined reliably. In such cases, a bypass procedure is needed. Revascularization procedures are designed to reconstitute blood flow in a major artery before or immediately after surgical occlusion to minimize the risk of ischemic damage.[106–113] Therefore, the surgical approach to a giant or complex posterior circulation aneurysm may be determined not by the exposure needed to dissect the aneurysm but by the exposure needed to perform the bypass and arterial occlusion. In many cases, the exposure needed to accomplish these objectives is significantly less than that needed for direct clipping, making the overall surgery less traumatic for patients. Furthermore, arterial occlusion can often be accomplished endovascularly, reducing the exposure required to only that needed for the bypass.

The surgical approaches required to perform these technically demanding revascularizations are no different from the ones discussed already. The surgical strategy depends on what part of the posterior circulation requires revascularization (basilar apex, basilar trunk, or vertebral trunk) and how much blood flow is required. The list of possible posterior circulation bypasses is short (Table 116–5) compared with anterior circulation bypasses, partially because the tight confines of the posterior fossa limit the options.

The extended orbitozygomatic approach is used to revascularize the upper basilar artery because it provides highly valued extra room. The trajectory to the recipient artery (PCA and superior cerebellar artery) is subtemporal (Fig. 116–15*A* and *B*); the orbit is removed for the sole purpose of increasing maneuverability in a narrow surgical corridor that is approximately 8 cm deep. The PCA is accessible at the tentorial incisura. The superior cerebellar artery is accessible more distally in the ambient cistern at the lateral midbrain. Typically, the tentorium is incised behind the dural sheath of CN IV to increase the exposure in this tight corner.

Bypass procedures to the basilar trunk are performed much less frequently. In such cases, the AICA is the recipient artery in the CPA, just lateral to CN VIII. Typically, only a standard retrosigmoid approach is required. Removal of petrous bone anteriorly (i.e., a retrolabyrinthine approach) provides more room or accommodates a swollen cerebellum. The skin incision and patient position for these approaches favor the use of the occipital artery, but the superficial temporal artery can be used.

Several good options exist for revascularization of the vertebral trunk or PICA (see Fig. 116–15*C* to *E*). The PICAs converge in the posterior midline; therefore, the contralateral PICA can serve as a donor artery in a side-to-side anastomosis. The vertebral artery is widely accessible for high-flow saphenous vein grafts and offers excellent protection from ischemia during temporary occlusion of the contralateral vertebral artery. Again, the occipital artery is easily mobilized into the surgical field as a donor artery. The midline suboccipital approach is adequate for PICA-PICA bypasses when lateral exposure of the aneurysm is not needed. For all other bypasses, extra room and more favorable views of the vertebral artery are provided by the far-lateral approach.

Some of the most challenging posterior circulation aneurysms are dolichoectatic aneurysms that involve a significant portion of the basilar artery and often its entire length.[33, 34] These aneurysms have no necks or separate inflow and outflow zones. Major arteries and perforators arise from them, and they have calcified and atherosclerotic walls and thrombus within the lumen. Furthermore, patients typically have compelling histories of progressive neurological deterioration from ischemic events or brainstem compression. Bypass techniques can play a role in the management of these challenging patients. Strategies are designed to change the blood flow within an aneurysm to remove degenerative hemodynamic stresses, such as creating retrograde perfusion of the basilar artery after proximal occlusion. Revascularization of the upper basilar artery is often required as an initial step in the treatment plan. These interventions are difficult and risky, but the associated surgical approaches are the same as discussed earlier.

Hypothermic Circulatory Arrest

Hypothermic circulatory arrest is a useful technique for giant and complex posterior circulation aneurysms that cannot be treated by conventional surgical or endovascular approaches.[4, 114–117] Circulatory arrest converts a large, hard aneurysm into a collapsed, soft sac that is easily manipulated. Consequently, the critical anatomy of the aneurysm's neck can be visualized, the perforators can be dissected off the aneurysm, and a

TABLE 116–5 ■ **Surgical Bypasses for Posterior Circulation Aneurysms**

VASCULAR TERRITORY	EC-IC, LOW FLOW	EC-IC, HIGH-FLOW	IC-IC, LOW-FLOW	APPROACH
Basilar apex	STA-SCA STA-PCA	ECA-SCA ECA-PCA	PCA-SCA	Extended orbitozygomatic
Basilar trunk	OA-AICA	ECA-AICA	AICA-PICA	Retrosigmoid Retrolabyrinthine
Vertebral trunk	OA-PICA	VA-VA VA-PICA	PICA-PICA	Far-lateral Midline suboccipital

Where ECA is indicated, the external carotid artery can be substituted for the proximal anastomosis.
AICA, anterior inferior cerebellar artery; EC, extracranial; IC, intracranial; ECA, external carotid artery; OA, occipital artery; PCA, posterior cerebral artery; PICA, posterior inferior cerebellar artery; STA, superior cerebellar artery; STA, superficial temporal artery; VA, vertebral artery.

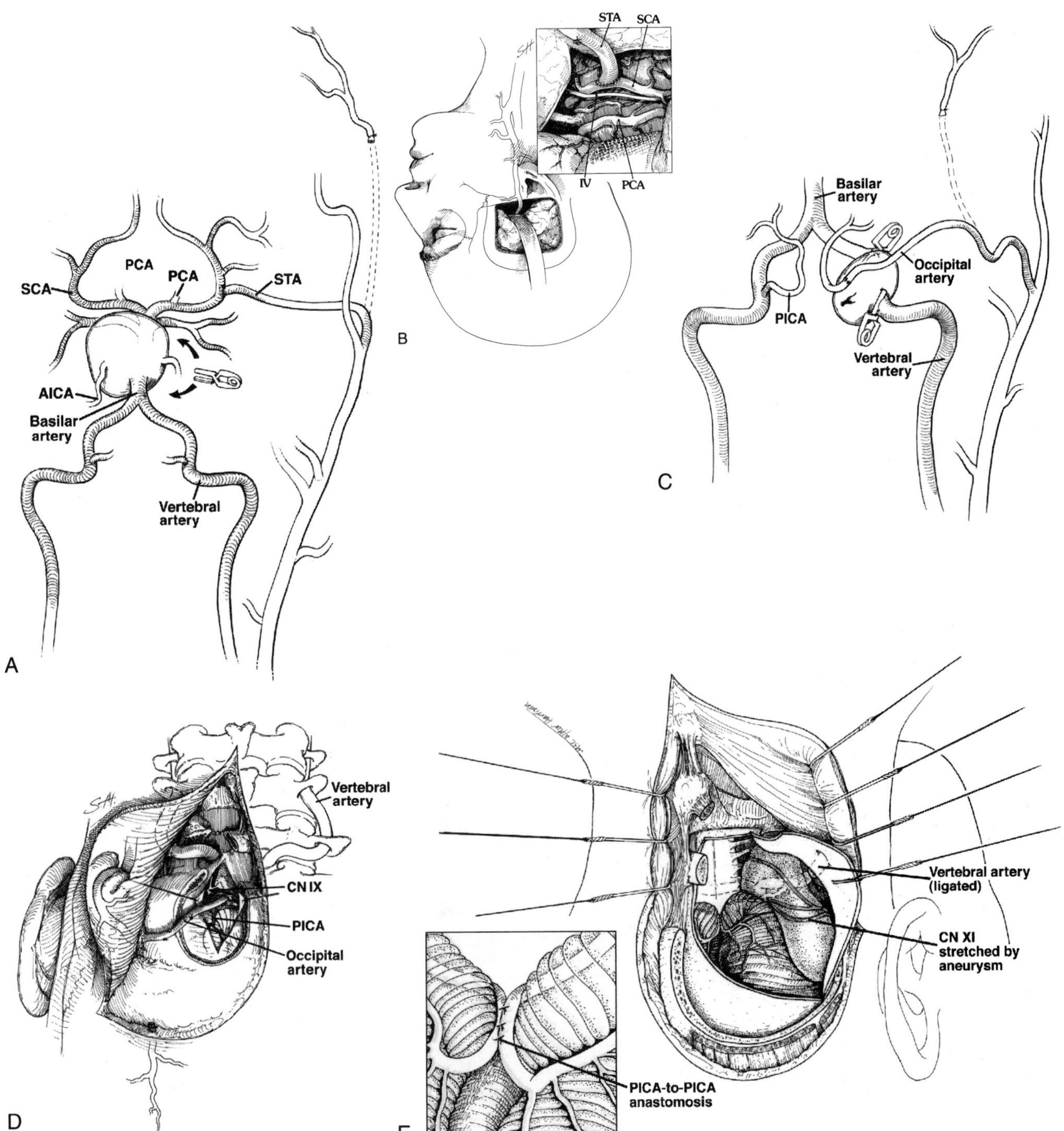

FIGURE 116–15. Revascularization of the posterior circulation. *A*, The upper brainstem can be revascularized with a superficial temporal artery–to–posterior cerebral artery (or superior cerebellar artery) bypass when the posterior communicating arteries do not provide adequate collateral blood flow for proximal occlusion of the aneurysm. *B*, The craniotomy and microsurgical anatomy *(inset)* of these bypasses. *C* and *D*, Schematic and surgical views showing revascularization of the posterior inferior cerebellar artery (PICA) with an occipital artery–to–PICA bypass. *E*, A PICA-to-PICA bypass, typically performed with a far-lateral approach, can also be used. AICA, anterior inferior cerebellar artery; CN IV, trochlear nerve; CN IX, glossopharyngeal nerve; CN XI, spinal accessory nerve; PCA, posterior cerebral artery; SCA, superior cerebellar artery; STA, superficial temporal artery. (*A–D*, Courtesy of Barrow Neurological Institute, Phoenix, Ariz.; *E*, From Khayata MH, Spetzler RF, Mooy JJA, et al: Combined surgical and endovascular treatment of giant vertebral artery aneurysm in a child: Case report. J Neurosurg 81:304–307, 1994.)

clip can be maneuvered across the neck. The risk of operative rupture is eliminated, as is the need for proximal control or bulky temporary clips in an already limited surgical field. Thrombus-filled aneurysms can be opened to remove thrombus and create a collapsible neck. For these reasons, it is possible to clip many aneurysms directly through a particular surgical approach accompanied by hypothermic circulatory arrest that could not be clipped through the same surgical approach without it. Therefore, hypothermic circulatory arrest improves a particular approach by enabling the surgeon to use the space once occupied by the inflated aneurysm. Central exposure is increased, and the peripheral exposure does not have to be broadened to gain vascular control. Consequently, hypothermic circulatory arrest has allowed some aneurysms of the upper and lower basilar artery to be clipped through extended orbitozygomatic and far-lateral approaches, respectively, that otherwise would have required more extensive transpetrosal approaches. Both approaches provide the surgeon with a direct view along the barrel of the basilar artery and the aneurysm's neck, thereby enabling a straight clip to be applied along this line of sight, parallel to the parent artery. This view contrasts with that provided by lateral transpetrous approaches, where the surgeon must look around the dome of the aneurysm to visualize its neck and must shift the aneurysm during clip application to see both sides of the neck and both blades sliding onto it.

Hypothermic circulatory arrest, however, is a technique that should be used with extreme caution. It is associated with significant morbidity and mortality rates related to systemic heparinization, cardiopulmonary bypass, cardiac arrest, and prolonged ischemia. It was once considered a therapy of last resort, to be used when surgical and endovascular options were exhausted. As the use of endovascular treatment for posterior circulation aneurysms increases, however, the number of patients requiring further surgical therapy to treat recurrent aneurysms already packed with coils may also increase. Typically, these aneurysms must be opened to clear the neck of coils and to prepare it to accept a clip. The advantage of circulatory arrest—namely, the aneurysm's collapse—is lost after coiling, but the complete vascular control and cerebral protection afforded by profound hypothermia are critical for these difficult and sometimes lengthy repairs.

Endovascular Options

As students of neurosurgery, we dedicate years to learning the approaches described in this chapter. As practitioners of neurosurgery, we often try hard to avoid using them. For some posterior circulation aneurysms, surgical techniques cannot compete with newer endovascular technologies in terms of procedural morbidity and mortality rates, associated costs, and appeal to patients. For some posterior circulation aneurysms, endovascular techniques may be the better option, and they belong in the new neurosurgical armamentarium.

Determining the best treatment strategy for posterior circulation aneurysms is a challenge best handled by a team of neurovascular and endovascular surgeons. The risks and efficacies of the different techniques can be compared, and the advantages and disadvantages of various treatment options can be discussed with patients and their families. Endovascular options in the posterior circulation include luminal obliteration with Guglielmi detachable coils and coils with three-dimensional shapes.[118–120] Stents can be used to cover the orifice of an aneurysm and to serve as a buttress to keep coils within the aneurysm from herniating into the lumen of the parent artery.[121] Stents can be used to channel blood flow through giant and dolichoectatic aneurysms, with the surrounding aneurysm obliterated by coils.[121] Multimodality strategies, such as a surgical bypass with subsequent endovascular occlusion of the aneurysm, can also be designed. A poor-grade patient can be treated by partially coiling the aneurysm, obliterating its dome to protect against rehemorrhage, and leaving the neck for definitive clipping later. Alternatively, broad-necked aneurysms that cannot be clipped completely might be clipped partially to create a narrower neck that would be more amenable to coiling. The promise of endovascular technology is enormous, and the management of patients with posterior circulation aneurysms will be improved by strategies that combine surgical and endovascular techniques.

CONCLUSIONS

Like Sirens that lure mariners at sea, posterior circulation aneurysms have engaged neurosurgery's technical innovators in a treacherous seduction. These lesions have spawned the development of skull base techniques that require surgeons to operate in deep holes, navigate complex neural and vascular anatomy, and accomplish delicate maneuvers in tight quarters. The territory is unforgiving, and technical errors can have devastating consequences. In the pursuit of better techniques, the skull has been disassembled and reassembled in every conceivable way; at this point, there is little room for surgical innovation. Future improvements in the treatment of posterior circulation aneurysms will likely come from the endovascular arena—a technology that is in its infancy and has enormous potential. The challenge for vascular neurosurgeons is to embrace and integrate endovascular techniques into the management of posterior circulation aneurysms while still maintaining technical proficiency in all the skull base approaches. Endovascular therapy will someday encounter its outer limits, and it will not replace open surgical clipping of aneurysms. Instead, surgeons will have to contend with giant aneurysms, fusiform aneurysms, broad-necked aneurysms, or recurrent aneurysms already packed with coils. Therefore, the future challenge for neurosurgeons is not to develop new surgical techniques but to maintain the technical mastery needed to keep pace with increasingly challenging aneurysms.

REFERENCES

1. Dandy WE: Intracranial Arterial Aneurysms. Ithaca, NY, Comstock, 1944.

2. Schwartz HG: Arterial aneurysm of the posterior fossa. J Neurosurg 5:312–316, 1948.
3. Lawton MT, Daspit CP, Spetzler RF: Technical aspects and recent trends in the management of large and giant midbasilar artery aneurysms. Neurosurgery 41:513–521, 1997.
4. Lawton MT, Raudzens PA, Zabramski JM, et al: Hypothermic circulatory arrest in neurovascular surgery: Evolving indications and predictors of patient outcome. Neurosurgery 43:10–21, 1998.
5. Lawton MT, Spetzler RF: Surgical strategies for giant intracranial aneurysms. Neurosurg Clin N Am 9:725–742, 1998.
6. Rhoton AL Jr: The three neurovascular complexes in the posterior fossa and vascular compression syndromes [honored guest lecture]. Clin Neurosurg 41:112–149, 1994.
7. de Oliveira E, Rhoton AL Jr, Peace D: Microsurgical anatomy of the region of the foramen magnum. Surg Neurol 24:293–352, 1985.
8. de Oliveira E, Tedeschi H, Rhoton AL Jr, et al: Microsurgical anatomy of the posterior circulation: Vertebral and basilar arteries. In Carter LP, Spetzler RF (eds): Neurovascular Surgery. New York, McGraw-Hill, 1995, pp 25–34.
9. Lister JR, Rhoton AL Jr, Matsushima T, et al: Microsurgical anatomy of the posterior inferior cerebellar artery. Neurosurgery 10:170–199, 1982.
10. Rhoton AL Jr, Buza R: Microsurgical anatomy of the jugular foramen. J Neurosurg 42:541–550, 1975.
11. Martin RG, Grant JL, Peace D, et al: Microsurgical relationships of the anterior inferior cerebellar artery and the facial-vestibulocochlear nerve complex. Neurosurgery 6:483–507, 1980.
12. Saeki N, Rhoton AL, Jr.: Microsurgical anatomy of the upper basilar artery and the posterior circle of Willis. J Neurosurg 46: 563–578, 1977.
13. Marinkovic SV, Gibo H: The surgical anatomy of the perforating branches of the basilar artery. Neurosurgery 33:80–87, 1993.
14. Zeal AA, Rhoton AL Jr: Microsurgical anatomy of the posterior cerebral artery. J Neurosurg 48:534–559, 1978.
15. Krayenbuhl HA, Yasargil MG: Cerebral Angiography, 2nd ed. London, Butterworths, 1968.
16. Milisavljevic MM, Marinkovic SV, Gibo H, et al: The thalamogeniculate perforators of the posterior cerebral artery: The microsurgical anatomy. Neurosurgery 28:523–530, 1991.
17. Yasargil MG: Microsurgical Anatomy of the Basal Cisterns and Vessels of the Brain, vol 1. In Yasargil MG (ed): Microneurosurgery. Stuttgart, Germany, Georg Thieme Verlag Stuttgart, 1984.
18. Ono M, Ono M, Rhoton AL Jr, et al: Microsurgical anatomy of the region of the tentorial incisura. J Neurosurg 60:365–399, 1984.
19. Hardy DG, Peace DA, Rhoton AL Jr: Microsurgical anatomy of the superior cerebellar artery. Neurosurgery 6:10–28, 1980.
20. Yasargil MG, Kasdaglis K, Jain KK, et al: Anatomical observations of the subarachnoid cisterns of the brain during surgery. J Neurosurg 44:298–302, 1976.
21. Liliequist B: The subarachnoid cisterns: An anatomic and roentgenologic study. Acta Radiol Suppl 185:1–24, 1959.
22. Wascher TM, Spetzler RF: Saccular aneurysms of the basilar bifurcation. In Carter LP, Spetzler RF (eds): Neurovascular Surgery. New York, McGraw-Hill, 1995, pp 729–752.
23. Rhoton AL Jr, Saeki N, Perlmutter D, et al: Microsurgical anatomy of common aneurysm sites. Clin Neurosurg 26:248–306, 1979.
24. Duvoisin RC, Yahr MD: Posterior fossa aneurysms. Neurology 15:231–241, 1965.
25. McCormick WF, Nofzinger JD: Saccular intracranial aneurysms: An autopsy study. J Neurosurg 22:155–159, 1965.
26. Peerless SJ, Drake CG: Management of aneurysms of the posterior circulation. In Youmans JR (ed): Neurological Surgery: A Comprehensive Guide to the Diagnosis and Management of Neurosurgical Problems. Philadelphia, WB Saunders, 1990, pp 1764–1806.
27. Drake CG: The treatment of aneurysms of the posterior circulation. Clin Neurosurg 26:96–144, 1979.
28. Andoh T, Shirakami S, Nakahhima T, et al: Clinical analysis of a series of vertebral aneurysm cases. Neurosurgery 31:987–993, 1992.
29. Friedman AH, Drake CG: Subarachnoid hemorrhage from intracranial dissecting aneurysm. J Neurosurg 60:325–334, 1984.
30. Tiyaworabun S, Wanis A, Schirmer M, et al: Aneurysms of the vertebro-basilar system: Clinical analysis and follow-up results. Acta Neurochir (Wien) 63:221–229, 1982.
31. Yamaura A: Diagnosis and treatment of vertebral aneurysms. J Neurosurg 69:345–349, 1988.
32. Yamaura A, Watanabe Y, Saeki N: Dissecting aneurysms of the intracranial vertebral artery. J Neurosurg 72:183–188, 1990.
33. Mizutani T, Aruga T: "Dolichoectatic" intracranial vertebrobasilar dissecting aneurysm. Neurosurgery 31:765–773, 1992.
34. Anson JA, Lawton MT, Spetzler RF: Characteristics and surgical treatment of dolichoectatic and fusiform aneurysms. J Neurosurg 84:185–193, 1996.
35. Berger MS, Wilson CB: Intracranial dissecting aneurysms of the posterior circulation: Report of six cases and review of the literature. J Neurosurg 61:882–894, 1984.
36. Tanaka K, Waga S, Kojima T, et al: Non-traumatic dissecting aneurysms of the intracranial vertebral artery: Report of six cases. Acta Neurochir (Wien) 100:62–66, 1989.
37. Yasargil MG: Clinical Considerations, Surgery of Intracranial Aneurysms, and Results, vol 2. In Yasargil MG (ed): Microneurosurgery. New York, Georg Thieme Verlag, Stuttgart, 1984.
38. Andrews BT, Brant-Zawadzki M, Wilson CB: Variant aneurysms of the fenestrated basilar artery. Neurosurgery 18:204–207, 1986.
39. Campos J, Fox AJ, Viñuela F, et al: Saccular aneurysms in basilar artery fenestration. AJNR Am J Neuroradiol 8:233–236, 1987.
40. Lupret V, Vidovic D, Negovetic L, et al: Surgical approach to a large basilar artery bifurcation and upper basilar trunk aneurysm: Case report. Surg Neurol 33:404–406, 1990.
41. Anderson M: Persistent primitive hypoglossal artery with basilar aneurysm. J Neurol 213:377–381, 1976.
42. Wolpert SM: The trigeminal artery and associated aneurysms. Neurology 16:610–614, 1966.
43. Yeh H, Heiss JD, Tew JM Jr: Persistent hypoglossal artery associated with basilar artery aneurysm. Neurochirurgia (Stuttg) 30: 158–159, 1987.
44. Naruse S, Odake G: Primitive trigeminal artery associated with an ipsilateral intracavernous giant aneurysm—a case report. Neuroradiology 17:259–264, 1979.
45. Agnoli AL: Vascular anomalies and subarachnoid haemorrhage associated with persisting embryonic vessels. Acta Neurochir (Wien) 60:183–199, 1982.
46. Weir B: Aneurysms Affecting the Nervous System. Baltimore, Williams & Wilkins, 1987.
47. Wright DC, Wilson CB: Surgical treatment of basilar aneurysms. Neurosurgery 5:325–333, 1979.
48. Batjer HH, Kopitnik TA, Purdy PD, et al: Vertebral and PICA aneurysms. In Carter LP, Spetzler RF (eds): Neurovascular Surgery. New York, McGraw-Hill, 1995, pp 763–776.
49. Osborn AG: Diagnostic Cerebral Angiography, 2nd ed. Philadelphia, Lippincott-Raven, 1999.
50. Drake CG: Bleeding aneurysms of the basilar artery: Direct surgical management in four cases. J Neurosurg 18:230–238, 1961.
51. Drake CG: Surgical treatment of ruptured aneurysms of the basilar artery. J Neurosurg 23:457–473, 1965.
52. Drake CG: Further experience with surgical treatment of aneurysm of the basilar artery. J Neurosurg 29:372–392, 1968.
53. Drake CG: The surgical treatment of aneurysms of the basilar artery. J Neurosurg 29:436–446, 1968.
54. Peerless SJ, Drake CG: Posterior circulation aneurysms. In Wilkins RH, Rengachary SS (eds): Neuurosurgery. New York, McGraw-Hill, 1985, pp 1422–1436.
55. Yasargil MG, Fox JL: The microsurgical approach to intracranial aneurysms. Surg Neurol 3:7–14, 1975.
56. Yasargil MG, Antic J, Laciga R, et al: Microsurgical pterional approach to aneurysms of the basilar bifurcation. Surg Neurol 6:83–91, 1976.
57. Al-Mefty O: Supraorbital-pterional approach to skull base lesions. Neurosurgery 21:474–477, 1987.
58. Al-Mefty O, Anand VK: Zygomatic approach to skull-base lesions. J Neurosurg 73:668–673, 1990.
59. Fujitsu K, Kuwabara T: Zygomatic approach for lesions in the interpeduncular cistern. J Neurosurg 62:340–343, 1985.
60. Hakuba A, Liu S, Nishimura S: The orbitozygomatic infratemporal approach: A new surgical technique. Surg Neurol 26: 271–276, 1986.

61. Hakuba A, Tanaka K, Suzuki T, et al: A combined orbitozygomatic infratemporal epidural and subdural approach for lesions involving the entire cavernous sinus. J Neurosurg 71:699–704, 1989.
62. Ikeda K, Yamashita J, Hashimoto M, et al: Orbitozygomatic temporopolar approach for a high basilar tip aneurysm associated with a short intracranial internal carotid artery: A new surgical approach. Neurosurgery 28:105–110, 1991.
63. Jane JA, Park TS, Pobereskin LH, et al: The supraorbital approach: Technical note. Neurosurgery 11:537–542, 1982.
64. Lee JP, Tsai MS, Chen YR: Orbitozygomatic infratemporal approach to lateral skull base tumors. Acta Neurol Scand 87: 403–409, 1993.
65. McDermott MW, Durity FA, Rootman J, et al: Combined frontotemporal-orbitozygomatic approach for tumors of the sphenoid wing and orbit. Neurosurgery 26:107–116, 1990.
66. Sano K: Temporo-polar approach to aneurysms of the basilar artery at and around the distal bifurcation: Technical note. Neurol Res 2:361–367, 1980.
67. Sekhar LH, Kalia KK, Yonas H, et al: Cranial base approaches to intracranial aneurysms in the subarachnoid space. Neurosurgery 35:472–483, 1994.
68. Uttley D, Archer DJ, Marsh HT, et al: Improved access to lesions of the central skull base by mobilization of the zygoma: Experience with 54 cases. Neurosurgery 28:99–104, 1991.
69. Zabramski JM, Kiris T, Sankhla SK, et al: Orbitozygomatic craniotomy: Technical note. J Neurosurg 89:336–341, 1998.
70. Dolenc VV: Anatomy and Surgery of the Cavernous Sinus. New York, Springer-Verlag, 1989.
71. Day JD, Fukushima T, Giannotta SL: Cranial base approaches to posterior circulation aneurysms. J Neurosurg 87:544–554, 1997.
72. Day JD, Giannotta SL, Fukushima T: Extradural temporopolar approach to lesions of the upper basilar artery and intrachiasmatic region. J Neurosurg 81:230–235, 1994.
73. Kopitnik TA: Temporary arterial occlusion for giant intracranial aneurysms: Indications and limitations. Tech Neurosurg 4:99–108, 1998.
74. Dolenc VV, Skrap M, Sustersic J, et al: A transcavernous-transsellar approach to the basilar tip aneurysms. Br J Neurosurg 1:251–259, 1987.
75. Nutik SL: Pterional craniotomy via a transcavernous approach for the treatment of low-lying distal basilar artery aneurysms. J Neurosurg 89:921–926, 1998.
76. Spetzler RF, Hamilton MG, Daspit CP: Petroclival lesions. Clin Neurosurg 41:62–82, 1994.
77. Brackmann DE, Hitselberger WE: Retrolabyrinthine approach: Technique and newer indications. Laryngoscope 88:286–297, 1978.
78. Sekhar LN, Bucur SD: Cranial base approaches to large and giant aneurysms. Tech Neurosurg 4:133–152, 1998.
79. Brackmann DE, Green JD: Translabyrinthine approach for acoustic tumor removal. Otolaryngol Clin North Am 25:311–329, 1992.
80. House WF: Translabyrinthine approach. In House WF, Luetje CM (eds): Acoustic Tumors. Baltimore, University Park Press, 1979, pp 43–87.
81. Morrison AW, King TT: Experiences with a translabyrinthine-transtentorial approach to the cerebellopontine angle: Technical note. J Neurosurg 38:382–390, 1973.
82. House WF, Hitselberger WE: The transcochlear approach to the skull base. Arch Otolaryngol 102:334–342, 1976.
83. Lawton MT, Daspit CP, Spetzler RF: Transpetrosal and combination approaches to skull base lesions. Clin Neurosurg 43:91–112, 1996.
84. Giannotta SL, Maceri R: Retrolabyrinthine transsigmoid approach to basilar trunk and vertebrobasilar artery junction aneurysms: Technical note. J Neurosurg 69:461–466, 1988.
85. Spetzler RF, Daspit CP, Pappas CTE: The combined supra- and infratentorial approach for lesions of the petrous and clival regions: Experience with 46 cases. J Neurosurg 76:588–599, 1992.
86. Hitselberger WE, House WF: A combined approach to the cerebellopontine angle: A suboccipital-petrosal approach. Arch Otolaryngol 84:267–285, 1966.
87. House W: Surgical exposure of the internal auditory canal and its contents through the middle cranial fossa. Laryngoscope 71: 1363–1385, 1961.
88. Brackmann DE, House JR III, Hitselberger WE: Technical modifications to the middle fossa craniotomy approach in removal of acoustic neuromas. Am J Otol 15:614–619, 1994.
89. House WF, Shelton C: Middle fossa approach for acoustic tumor removal. Otolaryngol Clin North Am 25:347–359, 1992.
90. Kawase T, Toya S, Shiobara R, et al: Transpetrosal approach for aneurysms of the lower basilar artery. J Neurosurg 63:857–861, 1985.
91. Day JD, Fukushima T, Giannotta SL: Microanatomical study of the extradural middle fossa approach to the petroclival and posterior cavernous sinus region: Description of the rhomboid construct. Neurosurgery 34:1009–1016, 1994.
92. MacDonald JD, Antonelli P, Day AL: The anterior subtemporal, medial transpetrosal approach to the upper basilar artery and ponto-mesencephalic junction. Neurosurgery 43:84–89, 1998.
93. Crockard HA: The transoral approach to the base of the brain and upper cervical cord. Ann R Coll Surg Engl 67:321–325, 1985.
94. Hadley MN, Spetzler RF, Sonntag VKH: The transoral approach to the superior cervical spine: A review of 53 cases of extradural cervicomedullary compression. J Neurosurg 71:16–23, 1989.
95. Menezes AH, VanGilder JC: Transoral-transpharyngeal approach to the anterior craniocervical junction: Ten-year experience with 72 patients. J Neurosurg 69:895–903, 1988.
96. Ogilvy CS, Barker FG 2nd, Joseph MP, et al: Transfacial transclival approach for midline posterior circulation aneurysms. Neurosurgery 39:736–742, 1996.
97. Heros RC: Lateral suboccipital approach for vertebral and vertebrobasilar artery lesions. J Neurosurg 64:559–562, 1986.
98. Spetzler RF, Grahm TW: The far-lateral approach to the inferior clivus and the upper cervical region: Technical note. BNI Q 6: 35–38, 1990.
99. Sen CN, Sekhar LN: An extreme lateral approach to the intradural lesions of the cervical spine and foramen magnum. Neurosurgery 27:197–204, 1990.
100. Wen HT, Rhoton AL Jr, Katsuta T, et al: Microsurgical anatomy of the transcondylar, supracondylar, and paracondylar extensions of the far-lateral approach. J Neurosurg 87:555–585, 1997.
101. George B, Dematons C, Cophignon J: Lateral approach to the anterior portion of the foramen magnum. Application to surgical removal of 14 benign tumors: Technical note. Surg Neurol 29:484–490, 1988.
102. Tedeschi H, Rhoton AL Jr: Lateral approaches to the petroclival region. Surg Neurol 41:180–216, 1994.
103. Baldwin HZ, Miller CG, van Loveren HR, et al: The far lateral/combined supra- and infratentorial approach: A human cadaveric prosection model for routes of access to the petroclival region and ventral brain stem. J Neurosurg 81:60–68, 1994.
104. Baldwin HZ, Spetzler RF, Wascher TM, et al: The far-lateral combined supra- and infratentorial approach: Clinical experience. Acta Neurochir (Wien) 134:155–158, 1995.
105. Steinberg GK, Drake CG, Peerless SJ: Deliberate basilar or vertebral artery occlusion in the treatment of intracranial aneurysms: Immediate results and long-term outcome in 201 patients. J Neurosurg 79:161–173, 1993.
106. Lawton MT, Spetzler RF: Surgical management of giant intracranial aneurysms: Experience with 171 patients [honored guest lecture]. Clin Neurosurg 42:245–266, 1995.
107. Lawton MT, Hamilton MG, Morcos JJ, et al: Revascularization and aneurysm surgery: Current techniques, indications, and outcome. Neurosurgery 38:83–94, 1996.
108. Martin NA: Arterial bypass for the treatment of giant and fusiform intracranial aneurysms. Tech Neurosurg 4:153–178, 1998.
109. Hopkins LN, Grand W: Extracranial-intracranial arterial bypass in the treatment of aneurysms of the carotid and middle cerebral arteries. Neurosurgery 5:21–31, 1979.
110. Peerless SJ, Hampf CR: Extracranial to intracranial bypass in the treatment of aneurysms. Clin Neurosurg 32:114–154, 1985.
111. Sundt TM Jr, Piepgras DG, Marsh WR, et al: Saphenous vein bypass grafts for giant aneurysms and intracranial occlusive disease. J Neurosurg 65:439–450, 1986.
112. Spetzler RF, Carter LP: Revascularization and aneurysm surgery: Current status. Neurosurgery 16:111–116, 1985.
113. Onesti ST, Solomon RA, Quest DO: Cerebral revascularization: A review. Neurosurgery 25:618–629, 1989.

114. Baumgartner WA, Silverberg GD, Ream AK, et al: Reappraisal of cardiopulmonary bypass with deep hypothermia and circulatory arrest for complex neurosurgical operations. Surgery 94: 242–249, 1983.
115. Solomon RA, Smith CR, Raps EC, et al: Deep hypothermic circulatory arrest for the management of complex anterior and posterior circulation aneurysms. Neurosurgery 29:732–738, 1991.
116. Ausman JI, Malik GM, Tomecek FJ, et al: Hypothermic circulatory arrest and the management of giant and large cerebral aneurysms. Surg Neurol 40:289–298, 1993.
117. Spetzler RF, Hadley MN, Rigamonti D, et al: Aneurysms of the basilar artery treated with circulatory arrest, hypothermia, and barbiturate cerebral protection. J Neurosurg 68:868–879, 1988.
118. Lempert TE, Malek AM, Halbach VV, et al: Endovascular treatment of ruptured posterior circulation cerebral aneurysms: Clinical and angiographic outcomes. Stroke 31:100–110, 2000.
119. Vinuela F, Duckwiler G, Mawad M: Guglielmi detachable coil embolization of acute intracranial aneurysm: Perioperative, anatomical and clinical outcome in 403 patients. J Neurosurg 86: 475–482, 1997.
120. McDougall CG, Halbach VV, Dowd CF, et al: Endovascular treatment of basilar tip aneurysms using electrolytically detachable coils. J Neurosurg 84:393–399, 1996.
121. Phatouros CC, Sasaki TYJ, Higashida RT, et al: Stent-supported coil embolization: The treatment of fusiform and wide-neck aneurysms and pseudoaneurysms. Neurosurgery 47:107–115, 2000.

CHAPTER **117**

Vertebral Artery, Posterior Inferior Cerebellar Artery, and Vertebrobasilar Junction Aneurysms

BRIAN L. HOH ■ CHRISTOPHER S. OGILVY

CLINICAL SIGNIFICANCE

Vertebral artery, posterior inferior cerebellar artery (PICA), and vertebrobasilar junction aneurysms can pose significant challenges to the neurovascular surgeon. They arise at a region of the skull base that can be difficult to access surgically. Avoiding injury to the brainstem and the lower cranial nerves, which are in direct close proximity, can prove to be technically challenging. Additionally the anatomy of the vertebral artery and PICA can be variable, adding further complexity to their surgical management. Surgical series for vertebral and vertebrobasilar aneurysms carry a much higher morbidity and mortality than for anterior circulation aneurysms. These lesions cannot be left untreated, however, because they are known to bear a high risk of rehemorrhage—in one series, vertebrobasilar aneurysms had a fatal rebleeding rate three times that of anterior circulation aneurysms.[1] For this reason, neurosurgeons have worked since the 1980s to improve surgical management of aneurysms of this location with the development of advanced skull base approaches, pharmacologic brain protection, and new microsurgical techniques. The advent of endovascular treatment of aneurysms has added another treatment strategy to the armamentarium of the neurovascular surgeon to treat patients with aneurysms in this difficult anatomic location.

Cruveilhier[2] in 1829 was the first to report a vertebral aneurysm when he described a spherical aneurysm arising from the vertebral artery–PICA junction. Krayenbuhl[3] was the first to show a vertebrobasilar aneurysm by positive contrast angiography in 1941. Dandy[4] in 1944 described his surgical experience with treating three vertebrobasilar aneurysms. In 1947, Rizzoli and Hayes[5] performed trapping of a vertebral aneurysm between two silver clips (reported in 1953), and in 1948, Schwartz[6] described a suboccipital approach for direct surgical treatment of a posterior fossa aneurysm. Early surgical experience with aneurysms of the vertebrobasilar system met with varied success, however. High morbidity and mortality and complications plagued early neurovascular surgeons. These surgeons were reluctant to treat aggressively vertebral and vertebrobasilar aneurysms surgically.

The introduction of the microscope to neurosurgical operations ushered in a new era of microneurosurgery, and after this, direct approaches to posterior circulation aneurysms became more frequent.[7] Drake[8] was the first to report a successful large series of surgically treated vertebral and vertebrobasilar aneurysms. Advances in skull base approaches to this region of the posterior circulation as well as improvements in microneurosurgical technique and pharmocologic brain protection have contributed to better outcomes in more recent reported surgical series. A variety of approaches have been developed to attack lesions at the different locations in the vertebrobasilar system.[9–12]

Vertebral, PICA, and vertebrobasilar junction aneurysms are relatively uncommon lesions. Pia[13] classified these aneurysms and found that posterior circulation aneurysms account for approximately 8% to 9% of all intracranial aneurysms. Of these, 25% originate from the proximal vertebral artery, the vertebral artery–PICA junction, the distal PICA, or the distal vertebral artery. These aneurysms of the vertebral artery or PICA account for only 2% of all intracranial aneurysms.[13, 14] The Cooperative Study of Intracranial Aneurysms and Subarachnoid Hemorrhage[15] found 21 (0.8%) vertebral artery aneurysms, 4 (0.1%) vertebrobasilar junction aneurysms, and 13 (0.5%) PICA aneurysms from a total of 2672 single-site aneurysms; thus, vertebral artery, PICA, and vertebrobasilar junction aneurysms accounted for 1.4% of all intracranial aneurysms. In a Japanese 30-year autopsy study[16] of 1230 consecutive cases, 73 intracranial aneurysms were found in 57 cases (4.6%). Seven of the aneurysms were located at the vertebral artery or PICA locations, accounting for 9.6% of all intracranial aneurysms.

There is a high incidence of fusiform nonsaccular aneurysms at the vertebrobasilar locations, much more frequent than in the anterior circulation. Many of the fusiform aneurysms that occur at the vertebral artery are due to dissections and carry with them a high risk of bleeding. Yamaura and colleagues[17] found vertebral dissections to account for 28% of posterior circulation aneurysms in their series. The rebleeding rate from ruptured vertebral dissecting aneurysms has been reported to be 21% to 71%,[17–20] with the highest risk in the acute stage after initial bleeding. Many neurovascular surgeons believe that they cannot be left untreated. Because of their morphology, however, fusiform aneurysms, dissecting or nondissecting, often are unamenable to standard aneurysm clipping techniques. Neurovascular surgeons have been forced to devise alternative treatment strategies for these lesions. One surgical strategy has been deliberate therapeutic occlusion of the parent vertebral or basilar artery, otherwise known as proximal *hunterian* ligation.[21–23] Occlusion of the vertebral artery has been performed endovascularly with balloons or coils.[24–26]

INDICATIONS

Although vertebral artery and vertebrobasilar aneurysms are rare relative to intracranial aneurysms found at other locations, ruptured vertebral artery and vertebrobasilar aneurysms carry a high risk of rebleeding and a high morbidity and mortality. Hernesniemi and colleagues[1] reported fatal rebleeding in 10% of vertebrobasilar aneurysms, three times the number (3.4%) in their anterior circulation aneurysm group. Two-month mortality for untreated ruptured vertebrobasilar aneurysms in their series was 63% compared with 8% to 11% for the surgically treated group. At 1 year, mortality for untreated ruptured vertebrobasilar aneurysms was 83.3%. Schievink and associates[27] reported their series of 136 aneurysmal subarachnoid hemorrhage (SAH) patients and found that mortality within the first 48 hours was 80% in patients with ruptured vertebral artery aneurysms compared with 23% in patients with anterior circulation aneurysms. For these reasons, it is generally believed that ruptured vertebral artery and vertebrobasilar aneurysms cannot be left untreated (Fig. 117–1).

Ruptured vertebral dissecting aneurysms carry a worse prognosis than saccular aneurysms of the same location. Kawaguchi and associates[18] reported in their series of vertebral dissecting aneurysms a 21% rebleeding rate in the first 72 hours with 100% mortality. Yamaura and coworkers[17] reported a 24% rebleeding rate within 17 days of the initial bleed with 80% mortality. Aoki and Sakai[19] reported 30% rebleeding with 80% mortality occurring in the first few hours. Mizutani and colleagues[20] reported 71% rebleeding, with the mortality of the rebleeding group being 46.7% and the mortality of the nonrebleeding group being 8.3%. Some authors have advocated a conservative approach of anticoagulation and serial angiography in managing vertebral dissections. Kitanaka and associates[28] managed six patients with unruptured vertebral dissections conservatively and followed them with serial angiography. There was no episode of SAH, and there was *angiographic cure* in four of the patients. All the patients had unruptured vertebral dissections, however, with no cases of ruptured vertebral dissections.

Because there is such a high morbidity and mortality in the acute period after the rupture of a vertebral artery and vertebrobasilar aneurysm, one might expect that neurovascular surgeons would treat these lesions aggressively with early surgery. The timing of surgery for ruptured vertebral artery and vertebrobasilar aneurysms is still debated, however. The International Cooperative Study on the Timing of Aneurysm Surgery[29, 30] did not include enough vertebrobasilar aneurysms to make any significant conclusions about the timing of surgery for aneurysms at this location. Posterior circulation aneurysms differ from anterior circulation aneurysms in that rarely are emergent lifesaving operations for hematoma evacuation necessary, whereas they more commonly are necessary with rupture of aneurysms in the anterior circulation. Ventricular drainage can be a necessary emergent procedure, however, because many patients with rupture of vertebral artery or verebrobasilar aneurysms have SAH complicated by hydrocephalus. The high management morbidity and mortality associated with surgical treatment of aneurysms in this location have made neurovascular surgeons reluctant to treat these lesions aggressively in the acute setting. Early surgery often is confounded by a brain that is frequently more swollen and with a confining exposure. The delicate vascular anatomy of perforating branches can be difficult to visualize. It is also thought that in the acute period, the aneurysm dome may be more friable and at greater risk for intraoperative rupture with manipulation. Although the general trend in the 1990s for anterior circulation aneurysms was early surgery, for posterior circulation aneurysms, most centers have adopted a protocol of delayed surgery. A few authors have advocated early surgery, however.[1, 31, 32] Early aneurysm clipping facilitates more aggressive vasospasm management and reduces the risk of early rebleeding in the acute period, which carries with it high morbidity and mortality. Hernesniemi and colleagues[1] reported 63 patients operated on for ruptured vertebrobasilar aneurysms—36 patients in the first 6 days after SAH and 27 patients in 7 or more days after SAH. Outcome at 1 year in the early surgery group was 55.6% good recovery, 16.7% moderate disability, 19.4% severe disability, and 8.3% dead. Outcome at 1 year in the late surgery group was 59.3% good recovery, 11.1% moderate disability, 7.4% severe disability, and 22.2% dead. In an untreated group of 30 patients, 1-year outcome was 6.7% good recovery, 6.7% moderate disability, 3.3% severe disability, and 83.3% dead. Lanzino and associates[33] reported their results with a protocol for delayed surgery for vertebrobasilar aneurysms and concluded that early surgery would be preferable. Although they achieved 87% excellent/good surgical outcome and 8% surgical mortality, an additional 41% died under the delayed treatment protocol before reaching surgery. Peerless and Hernesniemi[31] reported an extensive series from 1959 to 1992 of 1767 patients with vertebrobasilar aneurysms. Because of their referral pattern,

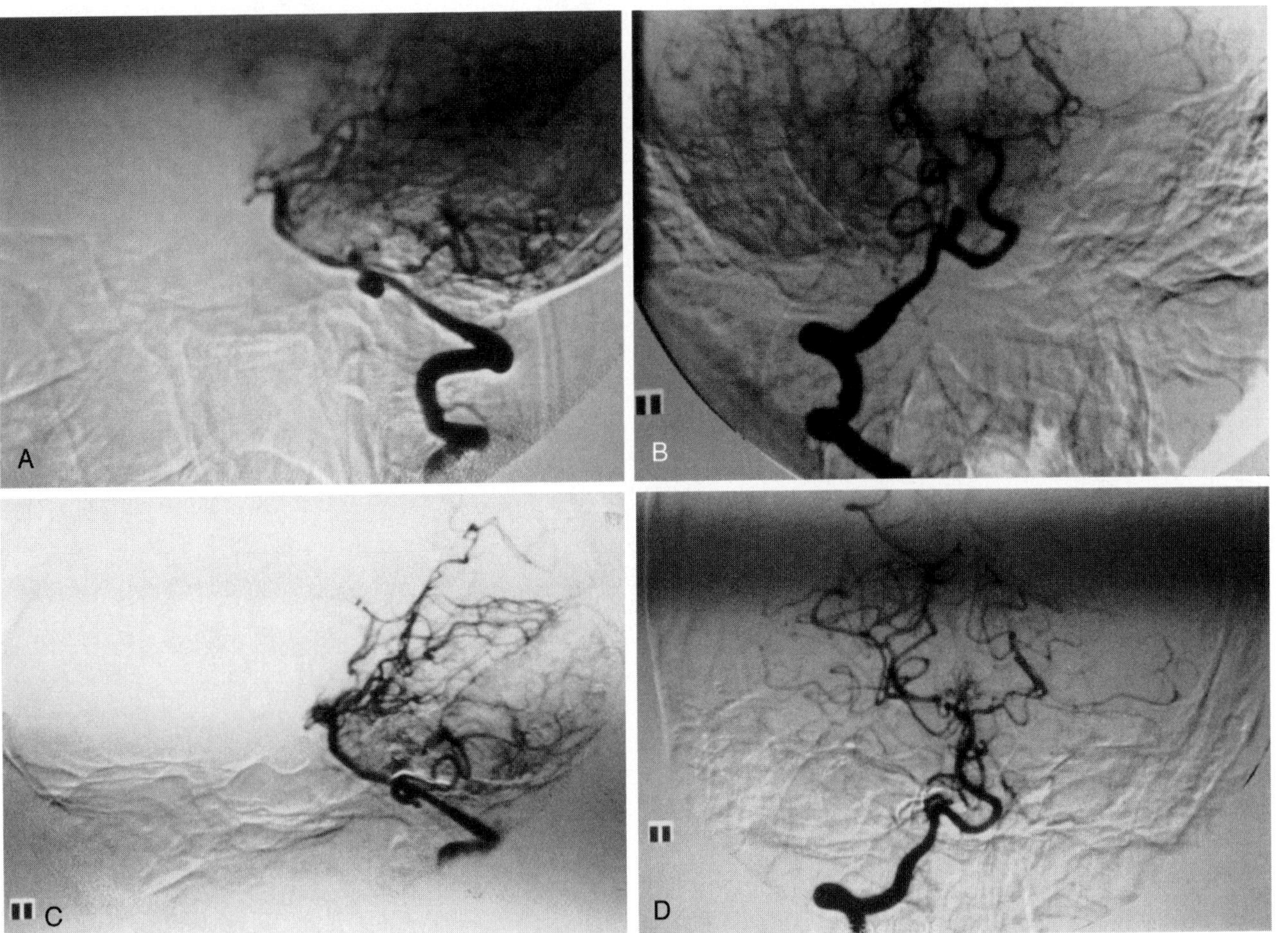

FIGURE 117–1. A 50-year-old woman suffered a Hunt and Hess grade I subarachnoid hemorrhage. Lateral *(A)* and oblique *(B)* right vertebral artery injection angiograms show a right vertebral–posterior inferior cerebellar artery (PICA) aneurysm. A far lateral suboccipital craniectomy was performed, and the aneurysm was surgically clipped with no complication. Postoperative lateral *(C)* and oblique *(D)* right vertebral artery injection angiograms show satisfactory clip occlusion of the aneurysm with preservation of the PICA.

most of these aneurysms were operated on in 14 or more days after SAH. Since 1970, these investigators operated on 206 ruptured vertebrobasilar aneurysms in 7 days or less after SAH. In the 206 early operated patients, outcome was 62.6% excellent, 18.9% good, 8.7% poor, and 9.7% dead. Bertalanffy and coworkers[32] reported that their group operated on ruptured vertebrobasilar aneurysms in the *acute stage.* Of 17 vertebrobasilar aneurysms, they reported a 94% good result and 5.9% mortality.

Whether early or late, for the reasons outlined previously, there is not much question that ruptured vertebral artery, PICA, and vertebrobasilar junction aneurysms should not be left untreated except in the extenuating circumstances of a medically unstable patient or in the case of an unacceptably high treatment risk. The natural history for unruptured vertebral artery, PICA, or vertebrobasilar junction aneurysms without treatment is less clear, however. Nevertheless, an international cooperative study[34] of 1937 unruptured intracranial aneurysms found a 13.6 relative risk of rupture in the group of patients with vertebrobasilar artery and posterior cerebral artery aneurysms that had never had a history of SAH compared with patients with intracranial aneurysms of other locations ($P = .007$). It is our conviction that unruptured aneurysms as well as ruptured aneurysms of this location must be treated.

PRESENTATION

The most frequent clinical presentation of vertebral artery, PICA, or vertebrobasilar junction aneurysms is SAH. SAH was the primary presentation for all or most aneurysms at these locations in the published series in Table 117–1. The clinical condition of patients with SAH from ruptured vertebral artery, PICA, or vertebrobasilar aneurysms can range from relatively good condition (Hunt and Hess[35] grade 1 or 2) to poor or comatose (Hunt and Hess grade 4 or 5). In the report by Peerless and Hernesniemi[31] of 206 ruptured vertebrobasilar aneurysms (this included basilar bifurcation, basilar trunk, and posterior cerebral artery an-

TABLE 117–1 ■ **Some Previously Reported Series of Vertebral, Posterior Inferior Cerebellar Artery, and Vertebrobasilar Aneurysms**

AUTHORS	CENTER	SAH (%)	ANEURYSM LOCATION	APPROACH	EXCELLENT/ GOOD	FAIR/POOR	DEAD	COMMENTS
Drake, 1969[8]	London, Canada	100	VA-PICA, 3	SO	3 (75%)	0	1 (25%)	
			VBJ, 1	TO-TC				
Hammon and Kempe, 1972[91]	Washington, DC	100	VA, 5	SO	1 (20%)	4 (80%)	0	
			VA-PICA, 7[1]	SO	5 (71.4%)	1 (14.3%)	0	
			PICA, 9	SO	7 (77.8%)	1 (11.1%)	1 (11.1%)	Outcome in one patient unreported
			VBJ, 3	SO	0	3 (100%)	0	
Sharr, 1973[92]	Southampton, UK	100	VA and BR, 7	Operated, 4[2]	3 alive (75%)	0	1 (25%)	Approach unreported
				Unoperated, 3	3 alive (100%)	0	0	
Chou and Ortiz-Suarez, 1974[59]	Minneapolis, MN	100	VA-PICA, 5	SO, 4	3 (60%)	0	2 (40%)	
				RM, 1				
Sano, 1979[93]	Tokyo, Japan	100	VA, 1	TO-TP	2 (100%)	0	0	
			VBJ, 2	TO-TP	0	0	1 (100%)	
Saito et al, 1980[94]	Tokyo, Japan	100	VA, 1	TO-TP	1 (100%)	0	0	
			VBJ, 1	TO-TP	0	0	1 (100%)	
Tiyaworabun et al, 1982[95]	Dusseldorf, Germany	100	PICA, 4	MSO, PSO	84.6%[3]	0	15.4%	Reported on all posterior circulation aneurysms as a group (n = 13 treated)
			VBJ, 3	MSO, PSO				
Gacs et al, 1983[96]	London, Canada	100	PICA, 8	Unreported	7 (87.5%)	0	1 (12.5%)	
Hudgins et al, 1983[57]	Gainesville, FL	100	VA-PICA, 17	SO, 20	14 (66.7%)	5 (23.8%)	2 (9.5%)	
			PICA, 4	ST, 1				
Yamamoto et al, 1984[97]	Ischara and Ichinomiya, Japan	83.3	PICA, 6	SO	5 (83.3%)	0	1 (16.7%)	
Yamada et al, 1984[23]	Osaka and Kobe, Japan	50	VA, 6[4]	SO	3 (50%)	1 (16.7%)	2 (33.3%)	All were unclippable aneurysms treated with parent VA clip occlusion
Yasargil, 1984[39]	Zurich, Switzerland	83.3	VA, 13	PSO	11 (84.6%)	1 (7.7%)	1 (7.7%)	
			PICA, 5	MSO	4 (80%)	1 (20%)	0	
			VBJ, 2	TO-TP	0	0	2 (100%)	
Archer et al, 1987[77]	London, UK	100	VA, 1	TM-TC	1 (100%)	0	0	
			PICA, 2	TM-TC	2 (100%)	0	0	
Gianotta and Maceri, 1988[62]	Los Angeles, CA	100	VBJ, 1	RL-TS	1 (100%)	0	0	
Solomon and Stein, 1988[98]	New York City, NY	77.3	VA, 5	SO	84.1%[5]	13.6%	2.3%	Reported on all posterior circulation aneurysms as a group (n = 44)
			PBA/VBJ, 9	SO				
Sugita et al, 1988[38]	Matsumoto, Japan	40	VA, 5[6]	LSO	5 (100%)	0	0	All were giant vertebral aneurysms
Yamaura, 1988[37]	Chiba, Japan	67	VA-PICA, 77	LSO	Operated: 64 (94.1%)	4 (5.9%)	0	
			PICA, 13	LSO				
			VBJ, 4	LSO	Unoperated: 13 (50%)	0	13 (50%)	
Lee et al, 1989[99]	Winston-Salem, NC	100	VA-PICA, 10	LSO	11 (78.6%)	1 (7.1%)	2 (14.3)	
			PICA, 4	MSO				
Salcman et al, 1990[55]	Baltimore, MD	100	VA-PICA, 10	LSO	11 (64.7%)[7]	2 (11.8%)	4 (23.5%)	Operative (n = 14), nonoperative (n = 3)
			PICA, 3	MSO				
			VBJ, 4	LSO				

Roux, 1990[14]	Montreal, Canada	100	VA, 3	MSO	7 (87.5%)	0	1 (12.5%)	
			VA-PICA, 3	MSO				
			PICA, 2	MSO				
Yamaura et al, 1990[17]	Chiba, Japan	87.5	VA, 17[8]	Unreported	13 (76.5%)	4 (23.5%)	0	All were dissecting aneurysms
			PICA, 2	Unreported	2 (100%)	0	0	
Aymard et al, 1991[24]	Paris, France	71.4	VA, 3	BO-VA	3 (100%)	0	0	
			PICA, 1	BO-VA	1 (100%)	0	0	
			VBJ, 3	BO-VA	3 (100%)	0	0	
Pritz, 1991[100]	Orange, CA	80	VA, 2	LSO 4	4 (80%)	1 (20%)	0	
			VA-PICA, 2	BO-VA, 1				
			VBJ, 1					
Hernesniemi et al, 1992[1]	Kuopio, Finland	100	VA and BR, 27	LSO, MSO	52.7%[9]	10.8%	36.6%	Reported on all posterior circulation aneurysms as a group (n = 93)
Andoh et al, 1992[40]	Gifu, Japan	86.8	VA, 10	LSO	26 (68.4%)	2 (5.3%)	10 (26.3%)	
			VA-PICA, 26	LSO				
			VBJ, 2					
Guglielmi et al, 1992[88]	Multicenter trial	50	PICA, 3	GDC	3 (100%)	0	0	One patient had two VBJ aneurysms treated
			VBJ, 5	GDC	4 (100%)[10]	0	0	
Steinberg et al, 1993[21]	Stanford, CA; London, Canada; Miami, FL	43.8	VA, 37	Unreported[11]	86.5%	5.5%	8%	All aneurysms were treated with parent VA occlusion (surgically or endovascularly)
			VBJ, 35		74%	3%	23%	
Lanzino et al, 1993[33]	Bologna, Italy	100	VA and BR, 16	VA: LSO	87%[12]	0	8%	Reported on all posterior circulation aneurysms as a group (n = 24 operated, n = 22 unoperated)
			VBJ, 2	PICA: MSO				
				VBJ: ST				
Lang and Gailbraith, 1993[58]	Glasgow, Scotland	80.2	VA, 5	ST, PT[13]	58%[14]	13%	29%[15]	Used ST early in series, later PT
			PICA, 27	SO				Reported on all posterior circulation aneurysms as a group (n = 121)
			VBJ, 4	ST, PT				Reported vegetative and dead together
Peerless and Hernesniemi, 1994[31]	Miami, FL; Kuopio, Finland; London, Canada	100	VA, 31	Unreported	26 (83.9%)	3 (9.7%)	2 (6.5%)	
			VBJ, 14	Unreported	12 (85.7%)	1 (7.1%)	1 (7.1%)	
Sekhar et al, 1994[9]	Washington, DC; Pittsburgh, PA	Unreported	VA, 5	EL-TC-TJ	5 (83.3%)	0	1 (16.7%)	
			VBJ, 1	ST-IT				
Bertalanffy et al, 1995[32]	Aachen, Germany; Tokyo, Japan	Unreported	VA, 6	TC	5 (83.3%)	0	1 (16.7%)	
			VA-PICA, 9	TC	9 (100%)	0	0	
			VBJ, 2	TC	2 (100%)	0	0	
Heros, 1995[60]	Miami, FL	Unreported	VA, 6	FLSO	33 (84.6%)	3 (7.7%)	3 (7.7%)	
			VA-PICA, 17	FLSO				
			PICA, 5	CLMSO				
			VBJ, 11	FLSO				
Seifert and Stolke, 1996[61]	Essen, Germany	55.6	VA, 2	SIT-PT	7 (77.8%)	1 (11.1%)	1 (11.1%)	
			VBJ, 3	SIT-PT				
			Lower BA, 4	SIT-PT				
Kawase et al, 1996[11]	Tokyo, Japan	80	VA, 2	SO-TC, PS-TP	2 (100%)	0	0	
			VA-PICA, 5	SO-TC, LSO	5 (100%)	0	0	
			VBJ, 3	ATP, SO-TC	3 (100%)	0	0	

Table continued on following page

TABLE 117–1 ■ **Some Previously Reported Series of Vertebral, Posterior Inferior Cerebellar Artery, and Vertebrobasilar Aneurysms** ***Continued***

AUTHORS	CENTER	SAH (%)	ANEURYSM LOCATION	APPROACH	EXCELLENT/ GOOD	FAIR/POOR	DEAD	COMMENTS
Day et al, 1997[12]	Los Angeles, CA	92.9	VA, 8	ELITE	8 (100%)	0	0	
			VBJ, 6	RLTS	5 (83.3%)	0	1 (16.7%)	
Nichols et al, 1997[89]	Rochester, MN	100	VA-PICA, 1	GDC	80.8%[16]	3.8%	15.4%	Reported on all posterior circulation aneurysms as a group (n = 26)
			VBJ, 3	GDC				
Bertalanffy et al, 1998[36]	Marburg, Germany	81.5	VA, 9	TC, LSO[17]	23 (85%)	2 (7.5%)	2 (7.5%)	Surgery (n = 21), endovascular occlusion of parent VA (n = 2), no treatment (n = 4)
			VA-PICA, 7	TC, LSO				
			PICA, 11	PSO				
Fukasawa et al, 1998[22]	Kofu, Japan; Yamanashi, Japan	100	VA, 20[18]	LSO	18 (90%)	1 (5%)	1 (5%)	All were ruptured dissecting VA aneurysms
Han et al, 1998[46]	Seoul, Korea	53.3	VA, 15[19]	Operative or coil, 7	6 (85.7%)	0	1 (14.3%)	All were dissecting VA aneurysms
				Nonoperative, 8	5 (62.5%)	1 (12.5%)	2 (25%)	
Seifert, 1998[63]	Leipzig, Germany	63.6	VA, 2	CTP	7 (63.6%)	3 (27.2%)	1 (9%)	
			VBJ, 3	CTP				
			Lower BA, 6	CTP				
Collice et al, 1998[64]	Milan, Italy	83.3	VBJ, 6	TM-TL-LSO, 1	5 (83.3%)	0	1 (16.7%)	
				TM-RL-LSO, 5				
Yonekawa et al, 1999[65]	Zurich, Switzerland	100	VA-PICA, 17	LSO-PC	15 (88.2%)	1 (5.9%)	1 (5.9%)	
			VBJ, 3	LSO-PC	2 (66.7%)	1 (33.3%)	0	
Ogilvy, 1999*	Boston, MA	76.6	PICA, 29	FLSO, TF-TC, BO-VA, GDC	27 (93.1%)	2 (6.9%)	0	
			VBJ, 17	CLMSO, TF-TC, BO-VA, GDC	12 (70.6%)	1 (5.9%)	4 (23.5%)	
			VA dissection, 18	BO-VA, GDC	14 (77.8%)	1 (5.6%)	3 (16.7%)	

*Personal communication.

ATP, anterior transpetrosal; BO-VA, balloon occlusion (endovascular) of vertebral artery; CLMSO, combined lateral and medial suboccipital; CTP, combined transpetrosal; ELITE, extreme-lateral inferior transtubercular exposure: EL-TC-TJ, extreme lateral, transcondylar, transjugular; FLSO, far lateral suboccipital; GDC, Guglielmi detachable coil embolization; LSO, lateral suboccipital; LSO-PC, lateral suboccipital and partial condylectomy without laminectomy; MSO, midline suboccipital; PBA, proximal basilar artery; PICA, distal posterior inferior cerebellar artery; PSO, paramedian suboccipital; PS-TP, presigmoid transpetrosal; PT, pterional; RLTS, retrolabyrinthine transsigmoid; RM, retromastoid; SAH, subarachnoid hemorrhage; SIT-PT, supra/infratentorial-posterior transpetrosal; SO, suboccipital; SO-TC, suboccipital transcondylar; ST, subtemporal; ST-IT, subtemporal-infratemporal; TC, transcondylar; TF-TC, transfacial transclival; TM-RL-LSO, transmastoid-retrolabyrinthine (retrosigmoid) plus lateral suboccipital; TM-TC, transmandibular transclival; TM-TL-LSO, transmastoid-translabyrinthine (transsigmoid) plus lateral suboccipital; TO-TC, transoral transclival; TO-TP, transoral transpalatal; VA, vertebral artery; VA and BR, vertebral artery and branches; VA-PICA, vertebral artery–posterior inferior cerebellar artery junction; VBJ, vertebrobasilar junction.

eurysms), 51.9% presented in Hunt and Hess grade 1, 30.1% presented in Hunt and Hess grade 2, 10.7% presented in Hunt and Hess grade 3, 4.9% presented in Hunt and Hess grade 4, and 2.4% presented in Hunt and Hess grade 5. In the series by Bertalanffy and coworkers of 27 patients with vertebral artery–PICA complex aneurysms, 22 (81.5%) presented with SAH. Of these patients, 2 presented in Hunt and Hess grade 1 (9.1%), 2 presented in Hunt and Hess grade 2 (9.1%), 11 presented in Hunt and Hess grade 3 (50%), 4 presented in Hunt and Hess grade 4 (18.1%), and 3 presented in Hunt and Hess grade 5 (13.6%). A patient with a ruptured vertebral artery, PICA, or vertebrobasilar aneurysm requires urgent management because of the high incidence of rebleeding and accompanying high mortality in the acute period after initial bleeding (Fig. 117–2).

Unruptured vertebral artery, PICA, or vertebrobasilar aneurysms can present with signs and symptoms of mass effect, most notably lower cranial nerve deficits, brainstem compression, or posterior fossa symptoms. In Yamaura's[37] series of 94 vertebral artery aneurysms, 63 (67%) presented with SAH, 16 presented among multiple aneurysms (17%), 6 (6%) presented as mass lesions, 3 (3%) presented with ischemic symptoms, and 6 (6%) presented incidentally during the evaluation of unrelated disease. In Yamaura and coworkers'[17] separate series of 24 vertebral dissections, 87.5% presented with SAH, and 12.5% presented with ischemic symptoms. In the series by Sugita and associates[38] of giant vertebral artery aneurysms, the patients that did not present with SAH presented with lower cranial nerve deficits (dysarthria, dysphagia), cerebellar symptoms (ataxia), hemiparesis, or a combination of these. In Yasargil's[39] series, the patients with unruptured vertebral artery aneurysms presented with lower cranial nerve deficits (V through XII), hemiparesis, and bulbar deficits.

DIAGNOSTIC EVALUATION

SAH in these patients is diagnosed first clinically, by history and examination, followed by confirmation with computed tomography (CT). As with the diagnostic evaluation for other forms of SAH, a CT scan that does not reveal hemorrhage must be followed by a lumbar puncture (except when contraindicated) with analysis of cerebrospinal fluid for the presence of blood. Andoh and colleagues[40] performed CT in 38 patients with vertebral artery aneurysms. They found intraventricular hemorrhage (IVH) in addition to diffuse SAH in the basal cisterns in 14 (78%) of the 18 patients with ruptured saccular vertebral artery aneurysms. Hydrocephalus was found in 8 of these 18 patients (44%). These investigators found IVH in addition to diffuse SAH in 9 (90%) of the 10 patients with ruptured fusiform vertebral artery aneurysms. Hydrocephalus was seen in 3 of these 10 patients (30%). All five patients with ruptured dissecting aneurysms had IVH with SAH. In the three patients who had unruptured dissecting aneurysms, pontine infarction was seen in two and lacunar infarction of the occipital lobe in the other. A neuroradiologic review of CT scans[41] of

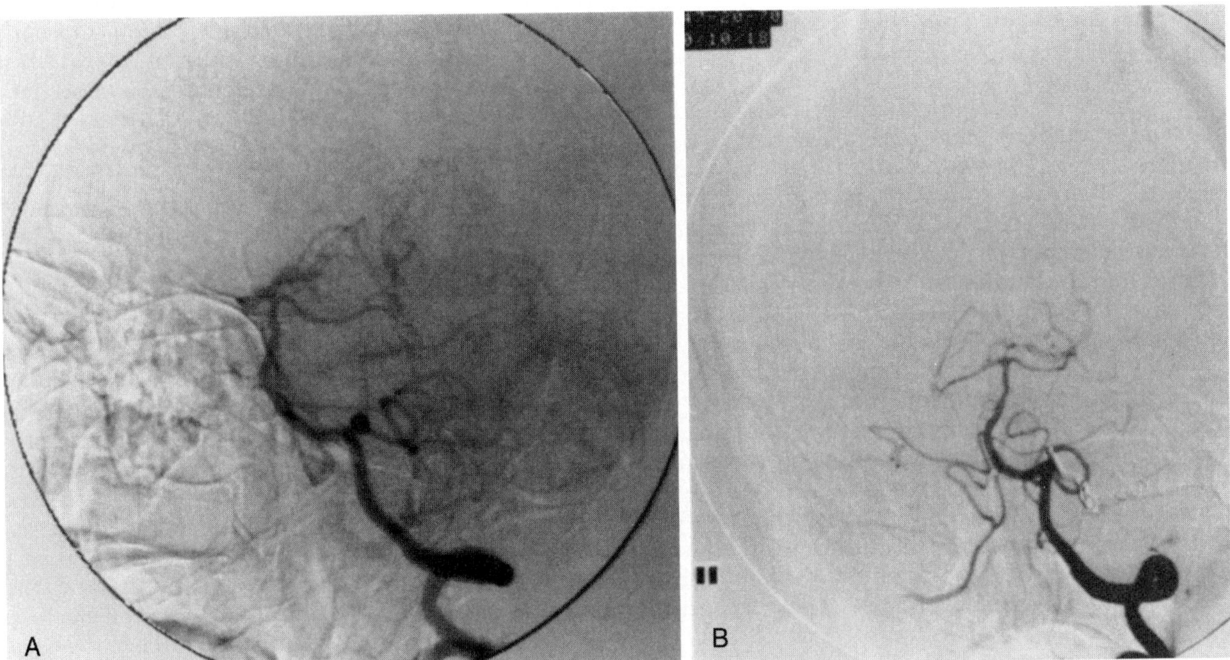

FIGURE 117–2. A 77-year-old woman suffered a Hunt and Hess grade I subarachnoid hemorrhage. *A*, Oblique left vertebral artery injection angiogram shows a left vertebral–posterior inferior cerebellar artery aneurysm. A far lateral suboccipital craniectomy was performed, and the aneurysm was surgically clipped. *B*, Postoperative left verterbal artery injection angiogram shows satisfactory clip occlusion of the aneurysm with preservation of the posterior inferior cerebellar artery. Postoperatively the patient suffered a left sixth cranial nerve palsy and swallowing difficulty that improved over time.

44 ruptured PICA aneurysms showed that 95% were associated with radiologic hydrocephalus, and 95% were associated with IVH. Supratentorial SAH was present in 70% of patients (isolated posterior fossa SAH occurred in only 30% of patients). An essential part of the diagnostic and pretreatment evaluation is conventional four-vessel cerebral angiography. Angiography is necessary to show details about the precise site, shape, and size of the aneurysm as well as nearby perforators. Although CT-angiography is being used increasingly in the preoperative planning for aneurysm surgery, its sensitivity for detecting intracranial aneurysms is best for aneurysms larger than 3 mm[42–45]; in almost all cases, conventional angiography still is essential in the diagnostic evaluation to eliminate the possibility of small (<3 mm) aneurysms. The diagnosis of vertebral dissection relies on the angiographic findings of a *string sign, rosette sign, pearl and string sign*, tapered narrowing, occlusion, double lumen, or pseudoaneurysm.[46] With increased experience, magnetic resonance (MR) angiography and CT-angiography are becoming increasingly useful in this diagnosis.

PREOPERATIVE EVALUATION

Current surgical management for vertebral artery and vertebrobasilar aneurysms involves considerable preoperative assessment and planning. Careful patient selection is crucial and depends on consideration of all factors, such as aneurysm morphology, surgical anatomy, and medical stability of the patient. The importance of endovascular treatments demands an interdisciplinary team approach between neurosurgeons and endovascular interventionalists in the clinical decision-making process to devise management strategies for these patients.

Careful attention to angiographic detail should be given to the orientation and projection of the neck and dome. The surgical approach to the aneurysm should be planned such that the dome is not encountered first with the neck obscured behind it. The size of a vertebrobasilar aneurysm is particularly important to assess not only because it affects natural history, but also because it can influence treatment strategy. Giant vertebrobasilar aneurysms can be difficult to treat, with many of them unamenable to standard surgical clipping. Drake and others[21, 47, 48] reported that clipping was impossible in 66% of their 354 giant vertebrobasilar aneurysms. Additionally, giant aneurysms of the posterior circulation have been associated with significantly worse outcomes.[47, 49, 50] The finding of a giant aneurysm on angiography may necessitate further evaluation by CT-angiography or MR angiography. In greater than 50% of cases of giant vertebral artery aneurysms, there are varying degrees of intraluminal thrombosis, and the angiographic opacity may not show the actual full size of the aneurysm appreciated on CT scan.[47, 51–54]

Preoperative planning should include careful attention to angiographic details, such as whether the PICA is reduplicated; whether the contralateral artery is present; whether the PICA territory is supplied by an alternative vessel (such as the anterior inferior cerebellar artery); and whether the posterior communicating arteries are filling and, if they are, whether they are fetal in nature and their size.[55] The angiographic size of the posterior communicating artery has been found to be associated significantly with outcome in patients who have unclippable vertebrobasilar artery aneurysms treated by vertebral artery or basilar occlusion. The presence of a small posterior communicating artery was associated with worse outcome in these cases; the presence of two small posterior communicating arteries was associated with an even worse outcome.[21, 56]

We have been using three-dimensional reconstructed CT-angiographic images increasingly in our preoperative planning. The three-dimensional anatomy of the aneurysm is elucidated nicely, particularly in the projections on the computer workstation monitor, and have been helpful in planning the surgical strategy. Thin-slice CT images of the bone structures are particularly important in planning skull base approaches. The shape of the clivus and posterior fossa can be assessed accurately preoperatively in the planning of surgery.

TECHNIQUE

For vertebral artery, PICA, and vertebrobasilar aneurysms, various surgical approaches have been described. Most authors have used the lateral suboccipital or the far lateral suboccipital approaches for vertebral artery, vertebral artery–PICA, and vertebrobasilar junction aneurysms and have used midline suboccipital or paramedian suboccipital approaches for peripheral PICA aneurysms (see Table 117–1). Subtemporal,[33, 57, 58] retromastoid,[59] pterional,[58] extreme lateral-transcondylar-transjugular,[9] subtemporal-infratemporal,[9] transcondylar,[32, 36] combined lateral medial suboccipital,[60] supra/infratentorial-posterior transpetrosal,[61] suboccipital transcondylar,[11] presigmoid transpetrosal,[11] anterior transpetrosal,[11] extreme-lateral inferior transtubercular exposure,[12] retrolabyrinthine transsigmoid,[12, 62] combined transpetrosal,[63] transmastoid-translabyrinthine (trans-sigmoid) and lateral suboccipital,[64] transmastoid-retrolabyrinthine (retrosigmoid) and lateral suboccipital,[64] and lateral subocciptal and partial condylectomy without laminectomy[65] also have been used.

Each approach has advantages and disadvantages. Some standard surgical approaches are hampered by a long working distance and having to work around the brainstem and through the lower cranial nerve rootlets. Considerable medullary retraction often is required with the risk of stretching of the lower cranial nerves. These approaches at times can be hazardous in instances in which the surgeon comes upon the dome of the aneurysm in the approach with the neck directly behind it. The anterior midline approaches (transfacial or transoral transclival) are hampered by high rates of complications, particularly cerebrospinal fluid leak and meningitis. A review of the literature[66] found a 50% incidence of cerebrospinal fluid leak, meningitis, or both in all published series using transclival approaches for aneurysms.

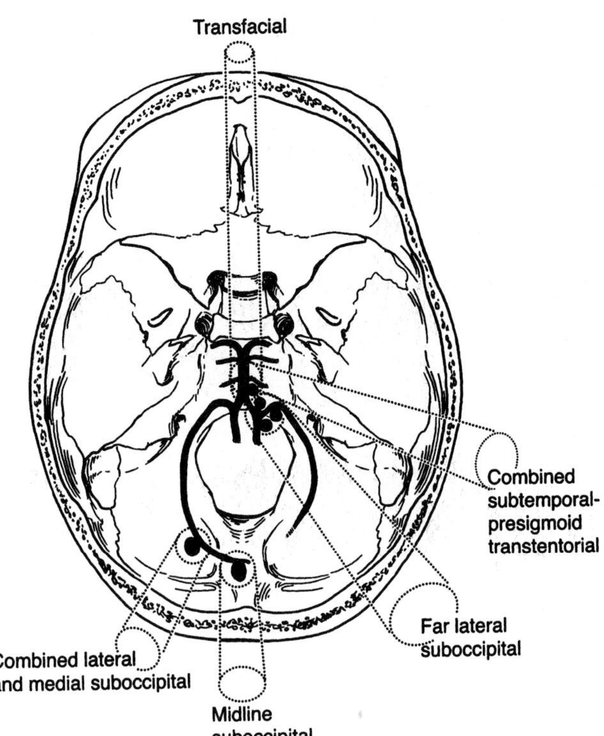

FIGURE 117–3. Surgical approaches to aneurysms of the vertebral artery, posterior inferior cerebellar artery (PICA), and vertebrobasilar junction. The far lateral suboccipital approach gains access to most vertebral artery, proximal PICA, and vertebrobasilar junction aneurysms. For midline lesions, a transfacial transclival approach can be used. Vertebrobasilar junction aneurysms that are unusually high can be accessed by a combined subtemporal-presigmoid transtentorial approach. For distal peripheral PICA aneurysms in the tonsillomedullary segment, a combined lateral and medial suboccipital approach is used, and for PICA aneurysms more distal, a standard midline suboccipital approach is used.

Based on the clinical experience at our institution, we use a handful of surgical approaches to gain access to various lesions of the vertebral artery, PICA, and vertebrobasilar junction. Figure 117–3 depicts the approaches we use. We have used the far lateral suboccipital approach described by Heros[60, 67] for most vertebral artery, proximal segment PICA, and vertebrobasilar junction aneurysms.[68] In certain circumstances with midline vertebrobasilar junction aneurysms, we have used the transfacial transclival approach (Fig. 117–4).[69] In unusually high vertebrobasilar junction aneurysms, we have used the combined subtemporal-presigmoid transtentorial approach.[70] For distal peripheral PICA aneurysms located in the tonsillomedullary segment, we have used the combined lateral and medial suboccipital approach.[60, 68] For PICA aneurysms in the segments distal to this in the cerebellotonsillar and cortical segments, we have used a standard midline suboccipital craniectomy extending through the foramen magnum.[60]

Far Lateral Suboccipital Approach

For most vertebral, vertebral artery–PICA, and vertebrobasilar junction aneurysms, we use a modification of the far lateral suboccipital approach described previously in detail by Heros[60, 67] (Fig. 117–5). Briefly, the patient is placed in the straight lateral position with the operative side upward and the head higher than the heart and slightly angled toward the ipsilateral shoulder. An S-shaped skin incision is made from the level of the superior aspect of the pinna, medial to the mastoid, down to the C2 spinous process. The muscular attachments and soft tissues are dissected using standard electrocautery technique, and the subperiosteum is exposed with sharp dissection with careful attention so as not to injure the vertebral artery. A teardrop craniectomy is fashioned from the transverse–sigmoid sinus junction to beyond the midline and through the foramen magnum, followed by a C1 laminectomy. Generous bone removal from the foramen magnum is crucial and should extend from the occipital condyle laterally to the entry of the vertebral artery into the dura superiorly. The dural exposure should follow a gentle curve after which point the microscope is brought into the field, bringing the vertebral artery immediately into view. The cerebellar tonsil and the caudal hemisphere are retracted gently superiorly and medially, revealing the origin of the PICA. The vertebrobasilar junction can be reached by following the vertebral artery rostrally through a window formed by the ninth and tenth cranial nerves superiorly, the eleventh nerve inferiorly, and the medulla medially. An alternative window above it is formed by the seventh and eighth cranial nerves superiorly, the ninth and tenth cranial nerves inferiorly, and the medulla medially. This window is smaller, but it may be necessary in cases of a high vertebrobasilar junction. Heros also suggests that in certain instances it may be necessary to direct the line of vision through the upper window while working through the wider space provided by the lower window.[60, 67]

Transfacial Transclival Approach

For rare vertebral artery or vertebrobasilar aneurysms with midline locations, we have used a modification of transfacial approach by deFries and colleagues[71] and have described it in detail previously (Fig. 117–6).[69] Briefly, a lumbar drain should be placed if ventriculostomy is not already present. The patient should be placed in a supine position. Doppler probe should be used at the beginning and throughout the procedure to locate and preserve the left facial artery. A skin incision is made from the glabella around the right lateral alar margin into the piriform aperture. Osteotomy of the nasal bones and disarticulation of the septal cartilage from the ethmoid allow for reflection of the nose laterally. The medial wall of one or both maxillary sinuses, the bony septum, the turbinates, the ethmoid air cells, and the floor the sphenoid sinuses should be removed. A large triangular exposure of the clivus is revealed by a midline incision in the retropharyngeal mucosa. A rectangular window of approximately 2 cm superior-inferior × 1.2 to 2.5 cm left-right is drilled in the anterior clivus with lateral margins determined superiorly by preoperative MR imaging assessment of

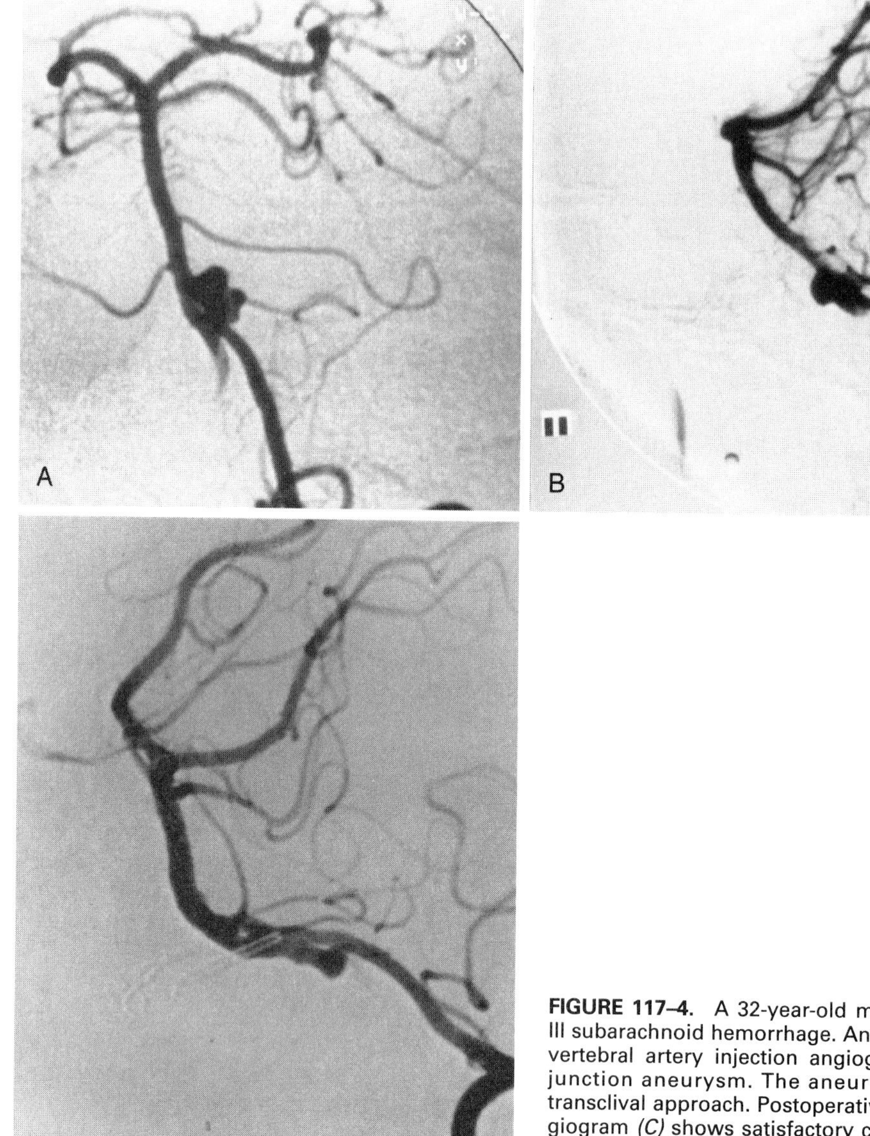

FIGURE 117–4. A 32-year-old man suffered a Hunt and Hess grade III subarachnoid hemorrhage. Anteroposterior *(A)* and lateral right *(B)* vertebral artery injection angiograms show a right vertebrobasilar junction aneurysm. The aneurysm was clipped via a transfacial transclival approach. Postoperative right vertebral artery injection angiogram *(C)* shows satisfactory clip occlusion of the aneurysm. Postoperatively the patient developed a cerebrospinal fluid leak and meningitis requiring a surgical procedure for repair but suffered no permanent neurologic morbidity from it.

the carotid arteries and inferiorly by the hypoglossal canals. A curet may be useful after drilling to finish bone removal. Opening of the dura should reveal the basilar and vertebral arteries. The dural exposure should be generous to allow for proximal and distal control of the vessels as needed. A variety of clip appliers have been developed with a long shank and angulation to reach the clivus by this route.[72, 73]

Closure of the clival trough should consist of fascia lata and a free fat graft (we usually take these from the thigh), which are held in place with fibrin glue. A plate of bone or cartilage from the nasal septum kept from the opening is glued in place. Finally a split-thickness skin graft (also from the thigh) is placed over the entire area from the roof of the ethmoid and sphenoid sinuses down to the posterior oropharyngeal wall below the palate and laterally to the lateral walls of the sphenoid sinus and nasopharynx. The inferior edge is sutured to the posterior pharyngeal wall through the mouth. The nasal complex is closed, and a nasal splint is applied. Cerebrospinal fluid diversion by lumbar drain or ventriculostomy and prophylactic antibiotics should be maintained (we continue these for 2 weeks postoperatively) to prevent cerebrospinal fluid leak or meningitis.

Combined Subtemporal-Presigmoid Transtentorial Approach

Rarely, for vertebrobasilar junction aneurysms that are relatively high in location, we use a combined subtemporal-presigmoid transtentorial approach, which we have described previously (Fig. 117–7).[70] The patient should be placed in a supine position with the head rotated in the straight lateral position, elevated, and tilted slightly backward. When this is not possible from

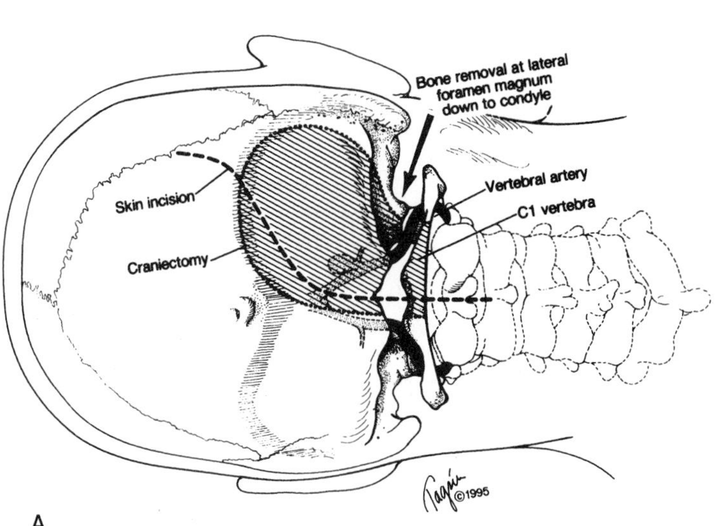

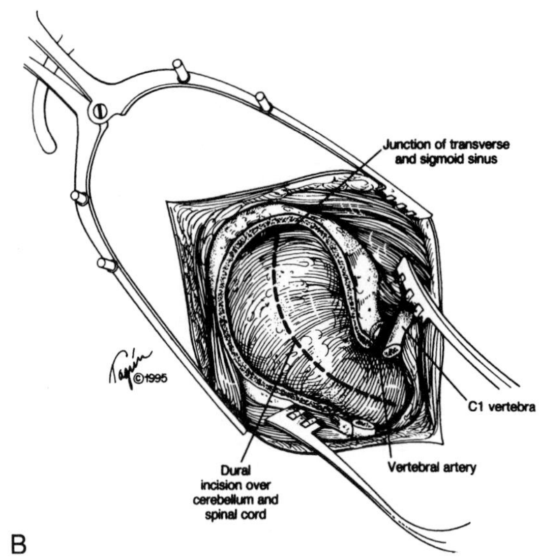

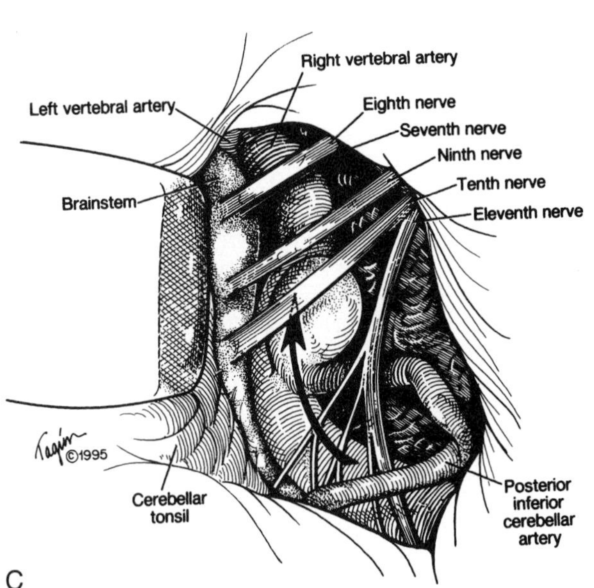

FIGURE 117–5. Far lateral suboccipital approach. *A,* Skin incision *(dashed line)* and craniectomy *(dotted line).* Once the extracranial vertebral artery has been exposed, the rim of the foramen magnum is removed laterally to the occipital condyle *(arrow).* The posterior arch of C1 is removed between the arterial sulcus of the vertebral artery laterally to just beyond the midline *(hatched area). B,* The dura is opened in a gentle curve from the junction of the sigmoid and transverse sinuses superiorly to the midline just below C1. *C,* After the dura and the arachnoid are opened, the preferred direction of approach is in the space between the eleventh cranial nerve inferiorly and the ninth and tenth cranial nerves superiorly *(arrow).* (*A–C* from Heros RC: Lateral suboccipital approach for vertebral and vertebrobasilar artery lesions. J Neurosurg 64:555–562, 1986.)

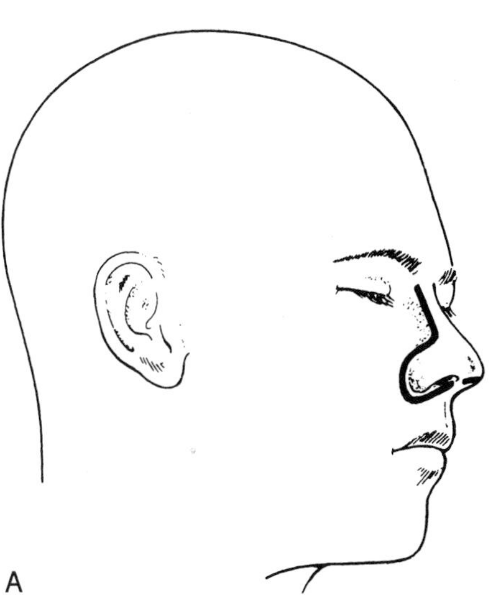

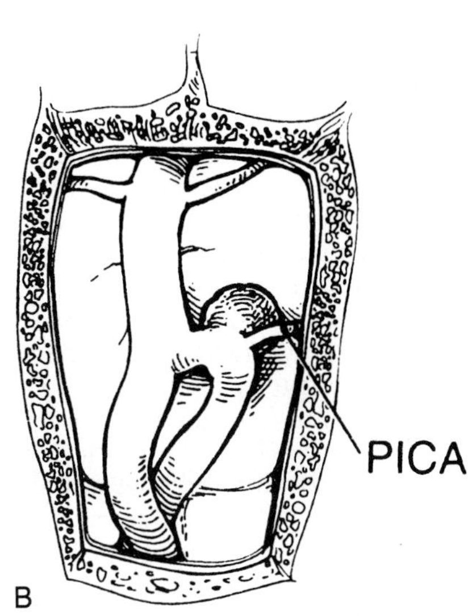

FIGURE 117–6. Transfacial transclival approach. *A,* Skin incision. *B,* Intraoperative exposure of vertebrobasilar region providing direct access to a proximal posterior inferior cerebellar artery (PICA) aneurysm. (*A* from Ogilvy CS, Crowell RM, Heros RC: Basilar and posterior cerebral artery aneurysms. In Ojemann RG, Ogilvy CS, Crowell RM, et al [eds]: Surgical Management of Neurovascular Disease, Baltimore, Williams & Wilkins, 1995, pp 269–290. *B* from Ogilvy CS, Barker FG II, Joseph MP, et al: Transfacial transclival approach for midline posterior circulation aneurysms. Neurosurgery 39:736–741, 1996.)

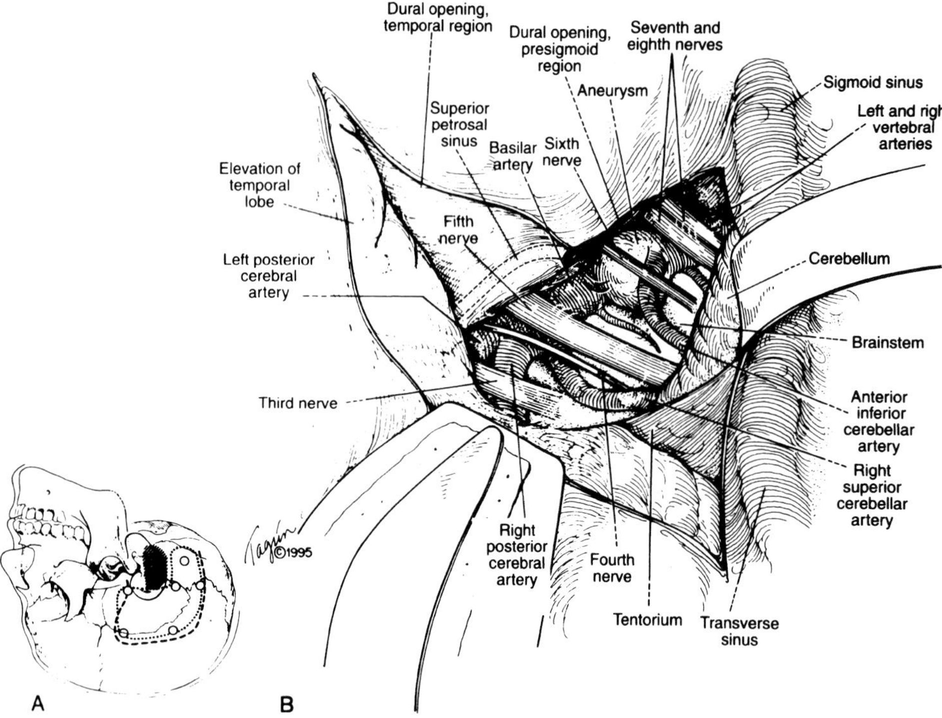

FIGURE 117–7. Combined subtemporal-presigmoid transtentorial approach. *A*, Skin incision *(dashed line)* and craniectomy *(dotted line)*. A complete mastoidectomy is drilled along with extensive removal of the posterior superior petrous pyramid anteriorly to but not exposing the facial canal and the lateral and posterior semicircular canals *(hatched area)*. *B*, The dura is opened linearly in the low subtemporal region and vertically anterior to the sigmoid sinus. The superior petrosal sinus is divided, and the tentorium is opened from lateral to medial, carefully preserving the trochlear nerve. (*A* and *B* from Ogilvy CS, Crowell RM, Heros RC: Basilar and posterior cerebral artery aneurysms. In Ojemann RG, Ogilvy CS, Crowell RM, et al [eds]: Surgical Management of Neurovascular Disease, Baltimore, Williams & Wilkins, 1995, pp 269–290.)

the supine position, the patient alternatively can be placed in the lateral position with the ipsilateral shoulder retracted. A U-shaped skin incision is made just anterior to the tragus at the level of the zygoma, circling above the pinna and descending behind the pinna to a point approximately 1.5 to 2 cm behind (medial) to the mastoid. The temporal muscle and the insertion of the sternocleidomastoid muscle are reflected to reveal the mastoid. Bur holes are placed such that the dura over the transverse sinus and the sigmoid-transverse junction can be evaluated. If the dura can be separated easily, a small combined temporal/suboccipital (retrosigmoid) craniotomy is fashioned. If the dura does not separate easily, it is safer to fashion a small subtemporal craniotomy initially, separate the transverse and upper portions of the sigmoid sinuses carefully under direct vision, then proceed with the suboccipital craniotomy as a separate bone flap. A complete mastoidectomy is drilled along with extensive removal of the posterior superior petrous pyramid anteriorly to but not exposing the facial canal and the lateral and posterior semicircular canals. The sigmoid sinus should be skeletonized down to the beginning of the jugular bulb. A linear dural incision is made parallel to the floor of the middle fossa anteriorly and to the transverse sinus posteriorly. A vertical dural incision is made in the presigmoid region continuing up toward the tentorium. The temporal lobe is elevated gently, and under direct vision of the tentorium from above and below, the superior petrosal sinus is divided. The tentorium is divided in a direction parallel to the posterior aspect of the petrous pyramid, toward the incisura. As the incisura is approached, careful attention should be directed so as not to injure the fourth cranial nerve.

Working from posteriorly, attention is turned toward the front of the superior aspect of the cerebellum where the arachnoid is opened. The cerebellum is allowed to fall naturally backward by lysis of adhesions holding the cerebellum anteriorly, coagulation and division of the superior petrosal vein, and dissection of the arachnoid investing the fifth cranial nerve. An excellent exposure of the basilar trunk and the vertebrobasilar junction is obtained. The vertebrobasilar junction can be accessed by a window formed between the seventh and eighth nerves superiorly and the lower cranial nerves inferiorly.

Combined Lateral and Medial Suboccipital Approach

For distal peripheral PICA aneurysms located in the tonsillomedullary segment, we have used the combined lateral and medial suboccipital approach.[60, 68] The patient position, skin incision, and craniectomy are as described for the far lateral suboccipital approach with bone removal extending well past the midline in the inferior aspect of the occipital bone and the foramen magnum as well as the arch of C1. Proximal control of the PICA with temporary clips is gained from a lateral approach. Then in most instances, we prefer to resect the tonsil but can, depending on the aneurysm location, retract the tonsil upward, medially, or laterally. After temporary clipping of the PICA distal to its medullary branches, the aneurysm is approached by subpial dissection.

Midline Suboccipital Approach

For PICA aneurysms in the segments distal to the tonsillomedullary segment (the cerebellotonsillar and cortical segments), we have used a standard midline suboccipital craniectomy extending through the foramen magnum.[60] The cerebellar tonsil can be resected with subpial dissection to the aneurysm, or both tonsils can be retracted gently laterally to approach the aneurysm between them.

Endovascular Embolization

The advent of endovascular techniques, particularly detachable coil embolization of aneurysms, has added a new treatment strategy to the armamentarium of the neurovascular surgeon in the management of intracranial aneurysms. Endovascular treatment strategies appear to be useful in circumstances in which surgical risk is unacceptably high or in a medically unstable patient. In the short-term, endovascular coil embolization may secure a ruptured vertebrobasilar aneurysm during the acute period in which the risk of rebleeding is the highest. Much remains to be elucidated, however, about the efficacy and the long-term clinical and radiographic outcome with these technologies.

Treatment for Vertebral Dissecting and Fusiform Aneurysms

Vertebral artery dissecting aneurysms, particularly ruptured ones, carry a high risk of rebleeding in the acute period after initial bleed and require early management. If their shape and morphology are such that direct surgical clipping is possible, we have used the far lateral suboccipital approach. These aneurysms often can take on a fusiform morphology, however, and pose the same treatment dilemmas as that of fusiform vertebral artery aneurysms. Because of their shape and morphology, fusiform vertebral artery aneurysms and vertebral artery dissecting aneurysms with a fusiform appearance often are unamenable to standard surgical clipping techniques, and neurovascular surgeons have been forced to devise alternative treatment strategies. One such strategy has been proximal *hunterian* ligation, occlusion of the ipsilateral vertebral artery proximal to the aneurysm.[21–23] This occlusion can be accomplished by a direct surgical approach by clipping of the vertebral artery, or endovascular occlusions have been performed with balloons or coils (Fig. 117–8).[24–26] Detailed temporary occlusion testing should be performed before permanent occlusion to ensure that adequate retrograde or collateral flow would supply the cerebellar territories if flow to the ipsilateral PICA is compromised. With balloon or coil proximal occlusion, we typically have used heparin to minimize thromboembolic complications.

COMPLICATIONS

A major cause of morbidity in the surgical treatment of vertebral artery, PICA, and vertebrobasilar junction aneurysms is inadvertent injury to the lower cranial nerves (ninth through twelfth). Some of the standard approaches to these locations require working through the lower cranial nerve rootlets, which are at particular risk of injury. At times, considerable retraction is necessary, causing injury secondary to stretching of the nerve rootlets. Additionally the PICA is variable in its course through the lower cranial nerves and often can be quite tortuous.[13, 57, 74, 75] Injury to the lower cranial nerves can result in dysphagia, dysarthria, dysphonia, and inadequate airway protection. Occasionally the sixth cranial nerve is located close to a high vertebrobasilar junction and can be subject to injury. Gentle

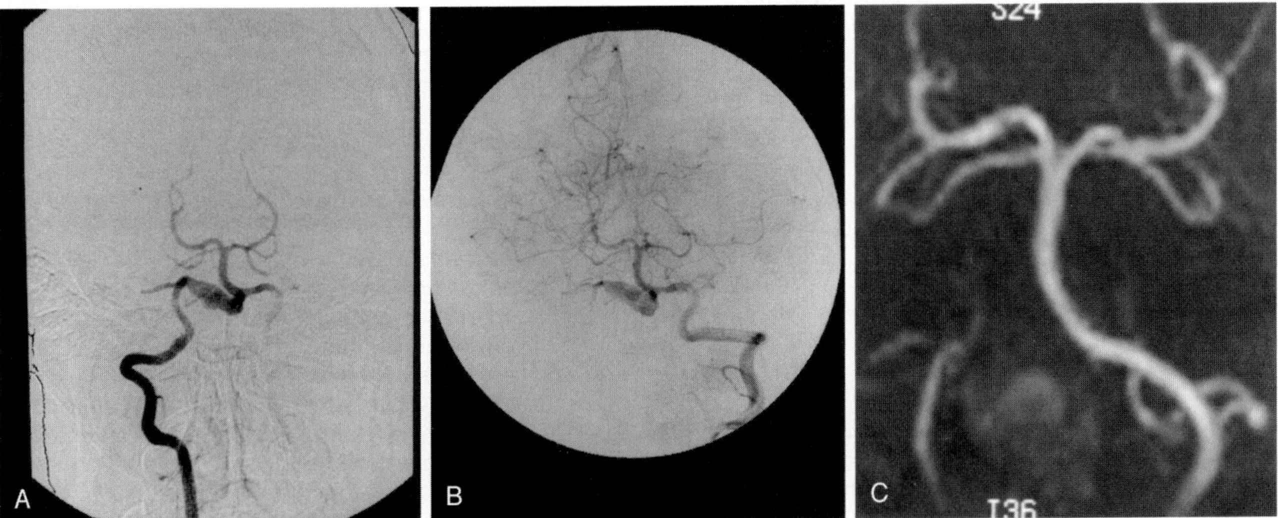

FIGURE 117–8. A 14-year-old boy who presented with left hemiplegia, left facial weakness, and dysarthria. *A*, Right vertebral artery injection angiogram shows a fusiform dissecting aneurysm of the right vertebral artery. Endovascular balloon occlusion of the right vertebral artery was performed proximal to the aneurysm. *B*, Left vertebral artery injection angiogram shows sluggish retrograde flow to the right vertebral artery aneurysm. *C*, Magnetic resonance angiogram 1 month later shows thrombosis of the fusiform dissecting aneurysms. The patient made an excellent recovery.

retraction and sharp dissection are essential in preventing cranial nerve complications.

There is the risk of postoperative lateral medullary (Wallenberg) syndrome if the PICA is occluded inadvertently or with cases of deliberate occlusion of the vertebral artery for fusiform or dissecting vertebral artery aneurysms. The variable and tortuous anatomy of the PICA can make it susceptible to injury.[13, 57, 74, 75] Careful preoperative planning and meticulous attention to the complex vascular anatomy are crucial. In the case of deliberate therapeutic vertebral occlusion for fusiform or dissecting vertebral aneurysms, detailed temporary occlusion testing beforehand is essential.

Transclival approaches have been plagued by particularly high rates of complications, especially cerebrospinal fluid leak and meningitis. A review of all the published reports in the literature[66] using transclival approaches for aneurysms revealed a 50% rate of cerebrospinal fluid leak, meningitis, or both. These rates remained high despite the efforts of various groups to devise techniques to prevent cerebrospinal fluid leak and meningitis, including permanent lumboperitoneal shunt,[72, 76] fibrin glue,[72, 77, 78] a bone baffle,[79] various oropharyngeal flaps,[80–82] and various techniques for watertight dural closure.[83]

In Yamaura's[37] series of 94 vertebral artery, vertebral artery–PICA, PICA, and vertebrobasilar junction aneurysms, surgical complications included sixth cranial nerve palsy (three patients [4.4% of 68 operated cases]) and ninth or tenth cranial nerve paresis (eight patients [11.8%]; all improved except for one patient who had a persistent hoarse voice [1.5%]). Lateral medullary syndrome developed in 3 of the 12 patients (25%) treated with proximal vertebral occlusion for vertebral dissection. In the series by Peerless and Hernesniemi[31] of 45 patients with vertebral artery, vertebral artery–PICA, and vertebrobasilar junction aneurysms, lower cranial nerve deficits occurred in 14 patients (31%); in 6 patients, these were persistent (13.3%). In the series by Salcman and colleagues[55] of 14 patients with vertebral artery–PICA, PICA, and vertebrobasilar junction aneurysms, complications were sixth nerve palsy (4 patients [29%]), seventh nerve palsy (3 patients [21%]), ninth and tenth nerve palsy requiring tracheostomy (4 patients [29%]), hemiparesis (2 patients [14%]), ataxia (1 patient [7%]), and meningitis (1 patient [7%]).

OUTCOMES

Surgical Outcome

Direct surgical treatment for vertebral artery, PICA, and vertebrobasilar junction aneurysms has improved since the 1980s as a result of several advances in operative microneurosurgery. Early neurovascular surgeons met with varied success and high rates of morbidity and mortality. Drake[8] was the first to report a large series of vertebral artery, PICA, and vertebrobasilar aneurysms with good results. Since then, many authors have reported their surgical experiences with these difficult lesions as well as a variety of different surgical approaches. Table 117–1 provides the surgical approaches and clinical outcomes reported from a number of authors with experience treating vertebral artery, PICA, and vertebrobasilar junction aneurysms. Although outcomes have improved as surgical treatment for these lesions has become more sophisticated, they still have not equaled that produced by surgical treatment for anterior circulation aneurysms.

Endovascular Outcome

Endovascular detachable coil embolization was designed to secure ruptured aneurysms in the acute period in which they are at highest risk for rebleeding. Good clinical outcomes in the short-term appear to be possible with endovascular treatment of intracranial aneurysms; however, the long-term clinical and radiographic outcome from these technologies remains to be elucidated. The angiographic rate of complete aneurysm occlusion fails to meet the results produced with surgical clipping. In an eight-center prospective trial[84] with 403 patients treated with endovascular detachable coil embolization for ruptured intracranial aneurysms of all locations, complete occlusion was seen in only 192 patients (47.6%). The rate of occlusion appears to be related to the size of the aneurysm and the aneurysm neck. Complete occlusion in the eight-center trial was seen in 70.8% of small aneurysms with a small neck (aneurysm, ≤10 mm; neck, ≤4 mm), 31.2% of small aneurysms with a wide neck, 35% of large aneurysms (11 to 25 mm), and 50% of giant aneurysms (>25 mm). In another study[85] in which the aneurysm necks were measured and analyzed for radiographic outcome in 79 aneurysms treated with detachable coil embolization, complete aneurysm occlusion was seen in 85% of small-neck aneurysms (≤4 mm) and 15% of wide-neck aneurysms. The long-term angiographic outcome can be altered by the effects of coil compaction over time resulting in incomplete aneurysm occlusion. In a study of 63 aneurysms in 58 patients treated with coil embolization,[86] follow-up angiograms showed coil compaction in 28%, and there was aneurysm growth in 11%. In a study of 45 basilar bifurcation aneurysms treated by coil embolization,[87] there was coil compaction seen in 38.7% and a 57% recanalization rate in large aneurysms.

Several authors reported their results using endovascular embolization to treat vertebral artery, PICA, and vertebrobasilar junction aneurysms. Guglielmi et al[88] reported a multicenter series of posterior circulation aneurysms treated with coil embolization. Of 43 posterior circulation aneurysms, there were 5 vertebrobasilar junction aneurysms and 3 PICA aneurysms (one patient had 2 vertebrobasilar junction aneurysms). Complete occlusion of the aneurysm was seen in two (40%) of the five vertebrobasilar junction aneurysms and two (66.7%) of the three PICA aneurysms. Clinical outcome was good in all seven patients. In the eight-center prospective trial[84] of 403 ruptured aneurysms treated with detachable coil embolization, 21 (5.2%) were vertebral artery aneurysms, and 15 (3.7%) were vertebrobasilar junction aneurysms. The clinical outcome for the 230 (57%) posterior circulation aneurysms (outcome was not reported by further specified anatomic site) was 84.3% unchanged, 9.6% deterioration, and 6.1% death. Radiographic outcome was not analyzed according to aneurysm site. Nichols et al[89] reported their series of 26 posterior circulation aneurysms treated by coil embolization, 3 of which were at the vertebrobasilar junction and 1 at the origin of PICA. These authors did not report clinical outcome by anatomic site of the aneurysm, but overall outcome for the group of posterior circulation aneurysms was 80.8% excellent or good, 3.8% poor, and 15.4% dead. Six-month follow-up angiography was performed in 19 of the 26 patients (73.1%), in which there was complete occlusion in 12 of 20 aneurysms (60%). New endovascular techniques, such as balloon remodeling, have led to advances in the field.[90]

Outcome After Deliberate Vertebral Artery Occlusion

Vertebral dissections and fusiform vertebral aneurysms often are unamenable to standard clipping techniques because of their shape and morphology. One strategy to treat these lesions has been proximal hunterian ligation, deliberate therapeutic occlusion of the parent vertebral artery. This strategy has been fraught with complications, however, such as thromboembolic ischemia, inadvertent occlusion of PICA with resulting lateral medullary syndrome, and failure of intra-aneurysm thrombosis. Steinberg and colleagues[21] reported their experience with 201 such hunterian ligations in the treatment of unclippable vertebrobasilar aneurysms. Their overall outcome was 73% successful, 3% poor, and 24% dead. Yamada and associates[23] elucidated the various complications associated with this treatment strategy, among which were failure of intra-aneurysm thrombosis and thromboembolic ischemia. Deliberate occlusion of the vertebral or basilar arteries for the treatment of unclippable aneurysms has been performed endovascularly. Aymard and coworkers[24] reported their series of 21 patients with posterior circulation aneurysms treated by endovascular occlusion of either unilateral or bilateral vertebral arteries. Of the 21 posterior circulation aneurysms, 3 were vertebral artery aneurysms, 1 was a PICA aneurysm, and 3 were vertebrobasilar aneurysms. All seven had normal outcomes with radiographic cure of their aneurysms, with one patient suffering transient ischemia as a complication. Of the overall group of 21 posterior circulation aneurysms, 13 patients had good outcomes with radiographic cure of their aneurysms (61.9%), 2 patients died (9.5%), and 1 patient suffered a transient stroke (4.8%). The remaining patients had partial thrombosis of their aneurysms. Although endovascular occlusion of the parent vertebral artery may be the best possible option in certain cases of fusiform vertebral aneurysms, it can be accompanied by a significant rate of complications, such as rehemorrhage, balloon migration, recanalization, thromboembolic ishemia, or aneurysm enlargement.[24, 25]

CONCLUSIONS

Treatment for vertebral artery, PICA, and vertebrobasilar junction aneurysms continues to advance with improvements in microsurgical technique, innovative skull base approaches, preoperative imaging and planning, and advances in endovascular treatment. Treatment of these difficult lesions still is associated with high management morbidity and mortality, however, relative to anterior circulation aneurysms. Aneurysms at these locations cannot be left untreated because they have an ominous natural history, and ruptured aneurysms at these locations have a particularly high incidence of fatal rebleeding in the acute period after initial bleed.

REFERENCES

1. Hernesniemi J, Vapalahti M, Niskanen M, et al: Management outcome for vertebrobasilar artery aneurysms by early surgery. Neurosurgery 31:857–861, 1992.
2. Cruveilhier J: Anatomie Pathologique de Corps Humain. Vol 2. Paris, JB Bailliere, 1829. Cited in Schwartz HG: Arterial aneurysms of the posterior fossa. J Neurosurg 5:312–316, 1948.
3. Krayenbuhl H: Das Hirnaneurysma. Schweiz Arch Neurol Psychiatry 47:155–236, 1941.
4. Dandy WE: Intracranial Arterial Aneurysms. Ithaca, NY, Comstock, 1944.
5. Rizzoli HV, Hayes GJ: Congenital berry aneurysm of the posterior fossa: Case report with successful operative excision. J Neurosurg 10:550–551, 1953.
6. Schwartz HG: Arterial aneurysms of the posterior fossa. J Neurosurg 5:312–316, 1948.
7. Rand RW, Janetta PJ: Micro-neurosurgery for aneurysms of the vertebral-basilar artery system. J Neurosurg 27:330–335, 1967.
8. Drake CG: The surgical treatment of vertebral-basilar aneurysms. Clin Neurosurg 16:114–169, 1969.
9. Sekhar LN, Kalia KK, Yonas H, et al: Cranial base approaches to intracranial aneurysms in the subarachnoid space. Neurosurgery 35:472–481, 1994.
10. Sekhar LN, Estonillo R: Transtemporal approach to the skull base: An anatomical study. Neurosurgery 19:799–808, 1986.
11. Kawase T, Bertalanffy H, Shiobara R: Surgical approaches for vertebro-basilar trunk aneurysms located in the midline. Acta Neurochir (Wien) 138:402–410, 1996.
12. Day JD, Fukushima T, Gianotta SL: Cranial base approaches to posterior circulation aneurysms. J Neurosurg 87:544–554, 1997.
13. Pia HW: Classification of vertebro-basilar aneurysms. Acta Neurochir (Wien) 47:3–30, 1979.
14. Roux A: Vertebro-PICA aneurysms: Midline suboccipital approach and laminectomy of the atlas. Br J Neurosurg 4:113–121, 1990.
15. Locksley HB: Report on the Cooperative Study of Intracranial Aneurysms and Subarachnoid Hemorrhage: Section V, part I. Natural history of subarachnoid hemorrhage, intracranial aneurysms, and arteriovenous malformations: Based on 6368 cases in the cooperative study. J Neurosurg 25:219–239, 1966.
16. Iwamoto H, Kiyohara Y, Fujishima M, et al: Prevalence of intracranial saccular aneurysms in a Japanese community based on a consecutive autopsy series during a 30-year observation period: The Hisayama study. Stroke 30:1390–1395, 1999.
17. Yamaura A, Watanabe Y, Saeki N: Dissecting aneurysms of the intracranial vertebral artery. J Neurosurg 72:183–188, 1990.
18. Kawaguchi S, Sasaki T, Tsunoda S, et al: Management of dissecting aneurysms of the posterior circulation. Acta Neurochir (Wien) 131:26–31, 1994.
19. Aoki N, Sakai T: Rebleeding from intracranial dissecting aneurysm in the vertebral artery. Stroke 21:1623–1631, 1990.
20. Mizutani T, Aruga T, Kirino T: Recurrent subarachnoid hemorrhage from untreated ruptured vertebrobasilar dissecting aneurysms. Neurosurgery 36:905–911, 1995.

21. Steinberg GK, Drake CG, Peerless SJ: Deliberate basilar or vertebral artery occlusion in the treatment of intracranial aneurysms: Immediate results and long-term outcome in 201 patients. J Neurosurg 79:161–173, 1993.
22. Fukasawa I, Sasaki H, Nukui H: Surgical treatment for ruptured vertebral artery dissecting aneurysms. Neurol Med Chir Suppl (Tokyo) 38:104–106, 1998.
23. Yamada K, Hayakawa T, Ushio Y: Therapeutic occlusion of the vertebral artery for unclippable vertebral aneurysm: Relationship between site of occlusion and clinical outcome. Neurosurgery 15:834–888, 1984.
24. Aymard A, Gobin P, Hodes JE: Endovascular occlusion of vertebral arteries in the treatment of unclippable vertebrobasilar aneurysms. J Neurosurg 74:393–398, 1991.
25. Hodes JE, Aymard A, Gobin P: Endovascular occlusion of intracranial vessels for curative treatment of unclippable aneurysms: Report of 16 cases. J Neurosurg 75:694–701, 1991.
26. Halbach VV, Higashida RT, Dowd CF: Endovascular treatment of vertebral artery dissections and pseudoaneurysms. J Neurosurg 79:183–191, 1993.
27. Schievink WI, Wijdicks EFM, Peipgrass DG, et al: The poor prognosis of ruptured intracranial aneurysms of the posterior circulation. J Neurosurg 82:791–795, 1995.
28. Kitanaka C, Tanaki JI, Kuwahara M: Nonsurgical treatment of unruptured intracranial vertebral artery dissection with serial follow-up angiography. J Neurosurg 80:667–674, 1994.
29. Kassell NF, Torner JC, Haley EC Jr, et al: The International Cooperative Study of the Timing of Aneurysm Surgery: Part 2. Surgical results. J Neurosurg 73:37–47, 1990.
30. Kassell NF, Torner JC, Haley EC Jr, et al: The International Cooperative Study on the Timing of Aneurysm Surgery: Part 1. Overall management results. J Neurosurg 73:18–36, 1990.
31. Peerless SJ, Hernesniemi J: Early surgery for ruptured vertebrobasilar aneurysms. J Neurosurg 80:643–649, 1994.
32. Bertalanffy H, Gilsbach JM, Mayfrank L, et al: Planning and surgical strategies for early management of vertebral artery and vertebrobasilar junction aneurysms. Acta Neurochir (Wien) 134: 60–65, 1995.
33. Lanzino G, Andreoli A, Limoni P, et al: Vertebro-basilar aneurysms: Does delayed surgery represent the best surgical strategy? Acta Neurochir (Wien) 125:5–8, 1993.
34. International Study of Unruptured Intracranial Aneurysms Investigators: Unruptured intracranial aneurysms—risk of rupture and risks of surgical intervention. N Engl J Med 339: 1725–1733, 1998.
35. Hunt WE, Hess RM: Surgical risks as related to time of intervention in the repair of intracranial aneurysms. J Neurosurg 28: 14–20, 1968.
36. Bertalanffy H, Sure U, Petermeyer M, et al: Management of aneurysms of the vertebral artery–posterior inferior cerebellar artery complex. Neurol Med Chir (Tokyo) 38(suppl):93–103, 1998.
37. Yamaura A: Diagnosis and treatment of vertebral aneurysms. J Neurosurg 69:345–349, 1988.
38. Sugita K, Kobayashi S, Takemae T, et al: Giant aneurysms of the vertebral artery: Report of five cases. J Neurosurg 68:960–966, 1988.
39. Yasargil MG: Microneurosurgery: II. Clinical Considerations, Surgery of the Intracranial Aneurysms and Results. New York, Georg Thieme Verlag, 1984.
40. Andoh T, Shirakami S, Nakashima T, et al: Clinical analysis of a series of vertebral aneurysm cases. Neurosurgery 31:987–993, 1992.
41. Kallmes DF, Lanzino G, Dix JE, et al: Patterns of hemorrhage with ruptured posterior inferior cerebellar artery aneurysms: CT findings in 44 cases. AJR Am J Roentgenol 169:1169–1171, 1997.
42. Harbaugh RE, Schlusselberg DS, Jeffery R, et al: Three-dimensional computerized tomography angiography in the diagnosis of cerebrovascular disease. J Neurosurg 76:408–414, 1992.
43. Katz DA, Marks MP, Napel SA, et al: Circle of Willis: Evaluation with spiral CT angiography, MR angiography, and conventional angiography. Radiology 195:445–449, 1995.
44. Nakajima Y, Yoshimine T, Yoshida H, et al: Computerized tomography angiography of ruptured cerebral aneurysms: Factors affecting time to maximum contrast concentration. J Neurosurg 88:663–669, 1998.
45. Tampieri D, Leblanc R, Oleszek J, et al: Three-dimensional computed tomographic angiography of cerebral aneurysms. Neurosurgery 36:749–755, 1995.
46. Han DH, Kwon OK, Oh CW: Clinical characteristics of vertebrobasilar artery dissection. Neurol Med Chir Suppl (Tokyo) 38: 107–113, 1998.
47. Drake CG: Giant intracranial aneurysms: Experience with surgical treatment in 176 patients. Clin Neurosurg 26:12–95, 1979.
48. Peerless SJ, Wallace MC, Drake CG: Giant intracranial aneurysms. In Youmans JR (ed): Neurological Surgery, Vol 3, Philadelphia, WB Saunders, 1990, pp 1764–1806.
49. Ogilvy CS, Carter BS: A proposed comprehensive grading system to predict outcome for surgical management of intracranial aneurysms. Neurosurgery 42:959–970, 1998.
50. Kempe LG: Aneurysms of the vertebral artery. In Pia HW, Langmaid C, Zierski J (eds): Cerebral Aneurysms: Advances in Diagnosis and Therapy. Berlin, Springer-Verlag, 1979, pp 119–120.
51. Beck DW, Boarini DJ, Kassell NF: Surgical treatment of giant aneurysm of vertebral-basilar junction. Surg Neurol 12:283–285, 1979.
52. Ganti SR, Steinberger A, McMurtry JG 3rd, et al: Computed tomographic demonstration of giant aneurysms of the vertebrobasilar system: Report of eight cases. Neurosurgery 9:261–267, 1981.
53. Ishii R, Tanaka R, Koike T, et al: Computed tomographic demonstration of the effect of proximal parent artery ligation for giant intracranial aneurysms. Surg Neurol 19:532–540, 1983.
54. Schubiger O, Valavanis A, Hayek J: Computed tomography in cerebral aneurysms with special emphasis on giant intracranial aneurysms. J Comput Assist Tomogr 4:24–32, 1980.
55. Salcman M, Rigatoni D, Numaguchi Y, et al: Aneurysms of the posterior inferior cerebellar artery–vertebral artery complex: Variations on a theme. Neurosurgery 27:12–20, 1990.
56. Pelz DM, Vinuela F, Fox AJ, et al: Vertebrobasilar occlusion therapy of giant aneurysms: Significance of angiographic morphology of the posterior communicating arteries. J Neurosurg 60:560–565, 1984.
57. Hudgins RJ, Day AL, Quisling RG, et al: Aneurysms of the posterior inferior cerebellar artery: A clinical and anatomical analysis. J Neurosurg 58:381–387, 1983.
58. Lang DA, Gailbraith SL: The management outcome of patients with a ruptured posterior circulation aneurysm. Acta Neurochir (Wien) 125:9–14, 1993.
59. Chou SN, Ortiz-Suarez HJ: Surgical treatment of arterial aneurysms of the vertebrobasilar circulation. J Neurosurg 41:671–680, 1974.
60. Heros RC: Aneurysms of the vertebral artery and its branches. In Ojemann RG, Ogilvy CS, Crowell RM, et al (eds): Surgical Management of Neurovascular Disease. Baltimore, Williams & Wilkins, 1995, pp 291–304.
61. Seifert V, Stolke D: Posterior transpetrosal approach to aneurysms of the basilar trunk and vertebrobasilar junction. J Neurosurg 85:373–379, 1996.
62. Giannotta SL, Maceri DR: Retrolabyrinthine transsigmoid approach to basilar trunk and vertebrobasilar artery junction aneurysms: Technical note. J Neurosurg 69:461–466, 1988.
63. Seifert V: Direct surgery of basilar trunk and vertebrobasilar junction aneurysms via the combined transpetrosal approach. Neurol Med Chir (Tokyo) 38(suppl):86–92, 1998.
64. Collice M, Arena O, D'Aliberti G, et al: Transbasal approaches to aneurysms of the vertebro-basilar junction. J Neurosurg Sci 42:81–86, 1998.
65. Yonekawa Y, Kaku Y, Imhof HG, et al: Posterior circulation aneurysms: Technical strategies based on angiographic anatomical findings and the results of 60 recent consecutive cases. Acta Neurochir Suppl (Wien) 72:123–140, 1999.
66. Hoh BL, Ogilvy CS: Midline approaches to cerebrovascular lesions. Operat Techn Neurosurg 3:44–52, 2000.
67. Heros RC: Lateral suboccipital approach for vertebral and vertebrobasilar artery lesions. J Neurosurg 64:559–562, 1986.
68. Ogilvy CS, Quinones-Hinjosa A: Surgical treatment of vertebral and posterior inferior cerebellar artery aneurysms. Neurosurg Clin N Am 9:851–860, 1998.
69. Ogilvy CS, Barker FG II, Joseph MP, et al: Transfacial transclival

approach for midline posterior circulation aneurysms. Neurosurgery 39:736–741, 1996.
70. Ogilvy CS, Crowell RM, Heros RC: Basilar and posterior cerebral artery aneurysms. In Ojemann RG, Ogilvy CS, Crowell RM, et al (eds): Surgical Management of Neurovascular Disease. Baltimore, Williams & Wilkins, 1995, pp 269–290.
71. deFries HO, Deeb ZE, Hudkins CP: A transfacial approach to the nasal-paranasal cavities and anterior skull base. Arch Otolaryngol Head Neck Surg 114:766–769, 1988.
72. Crockard HA, Koksel T, Watkin N: Transoral transclival clipping of anterior inferior cerebellar artery aneurysm using new rotating applier: Technical note. J Neurosurg 75:483–485, 1991.
73. Sano K: A multipurpose all-angle clip applier for aneurysm surgery: Technical note. J Neurosurg 53:260–261, 1980.
74. Lister JR, Rhoton AL Jr, Matsushima T, et al: Microsurgical anatomy of the posterior inferior cerebellar artery. Neurosurgery 10:170–199, 1982.
75. Shrontz C, Dujovny M, Ausman JI, et al: Surgical anatomy of the arteries of the posterior fossa. J Neurosurg 65:540–544, 1986.
76. Crockard HA, Bradford R: Transoral transclival removal of a schwannoma anterior to the craniocervical junction: Case report. J Neurosurg 62:293–295, 1985.
77. Archer DJ, Young S, Uttley D: Basilar aneurysms: A new transclival approach via maxillotomy. J Neurosurg 67:54–58, 1987.
78. Hadley MN, Martin NA, Spetzler RF, et al: Comparative transoral dural closure techniques: A canine model. Neurosurgery 22:392–397, 1988.
79. Bonkowski JA, Gibson RD, Snape L: Foramen magnum meningioma: Transoral resection with a bone baffle to prevent CSF leakage: Case report. J Neurosurg 72:493–496, 1990.
80. Hayakawa T, Kamikawa K, Ohnishi T, et al: Prevention of postoperative complications after a transoral transclival approach to basilar aneurysms: Technical note. J Neurosurg 54: 699–703, 1981.
81. Litvak J, Summers TC, Barron JL, et al: A successful approach to vertebrobasilaraneurysms: Technical note. J Neurosurg 55: 491–494, 1981.
82. Hayakawa T, Yamada K, Yoshimine T: Transoral transclival approach: Anatomical and technical notes. No Shinkei Geka 17: 609–614, 1989.
83. Guity A, Young PH: A new technique for closure of the dura following transsphenoidal and transclival operations: Technical note. J Neurosurg 72:824–828, 1990.
84. Vinuela F, Duckwiler G, Mawad M: Guglielmi detachable coil embolization of acute intracranial aneurysm: Perioperative anatomical and clinical outcome in 403 patients. J Neurosurg 86: 475–482, 1997.
85. Zubillaga AF, Guglielmi G, Vinuela F, et al: Endovascular occlusion of intracranial aneurysms with electrically detachable coils: Correlation of aneurysm neck size and treatment results. AJNR Am J Neuroradiol 15:815–820, 1994.
86. Hope JK, Byrne JV, Molyneux AJ: Factors influencing successful angiographic occlusion of aneurysms treated by coil embolization. AJNR Am J Neuroradiol 20:391–399, 1999.
87. Bavinzski G, Killer M, Gruber A, et al: Treatment of basilar bifurcation aneurysms by using Guglielmi detachable coils: A 6-year experience. J Neurosurg 90:843–852, 1999.
88. Guglielmi G, Vineula F, Duckwiler G, et al: Endovascular treatment of posterior circulation aneurysms by electrothrombosis using electrically detachable coils. J Neurosurg 77:515–524, 1992.
89. Nichols DA, Brown RD Jr, Thielen KR, et al: Endovascular treatment of ruptured posterior circulation aneurysms using electrolytically detachable coils. J Neurosurg 87:374–380, 1997.
90. Lefkowitz MA, Gobin YP, Akiba Y, et al: Balloon-assisted Guglielmi detachable coiling of wide-necked aneurysms: Part II. Clinical results. Neurosurgery 45:531–537, 1999.
91. Hammon WM, Kempe LG: The posterior fossa approach to aneurysms of the vertebral and basilar arteries. J Neurosurg 37: 339–347, 1972.
92. Sharr MM: Vertebrobasilar aneurysms: Experience with 27 cases. Eur Neurol 10:129–143, 1973.
93. Sano K: Basilar artery aneurysms: Transoral-transclival approach. In Pia HW, Langmaid C, Zierski J (eds): Cerebral Aneurysms: Advances in Diagnosis and Therapy. New York, Springer-Verlag, 1979, pp 326–328.
94. Saito I, Takahashi H, Joshita H, et al: Clipping of vertebrobasilar aneurysms by the transoral transclival approach. Neurol Med Chir (Tokyo) 20:753–758, 1980.
95. Tiyaworabun S, Takahashi H, Joshita H, et al: Aneurysms of the vertebro-basilar system: Clinical analysis and follow-up results. Acta Neurochir (Wien) 63:221–229, 1982.
96. Gacs G, Vinuela F, Fox AJ, et al: Peripheral aneurysms of the cerebellar arteries: Review of 16 cases. J Neurosurg 58:63–68, 1983.
97. Yamamoto I, Tsugane R, Ohya M, et al: Peripheral aneurysms of the posterior inferior cerebellar artery. Neurosurgery 15:839–845, 1984.
98. Solomon RA, Stein BM: Surgical approaches to aneurysms of the vertebral and basilar arteries. Neurosurgery 23:203–208, 1988.
99. Lee KS, Gower DJ, Branch CL Jr, et al: Surgical repair of aneurysms of the posterior inferior cerebellar artery—a clinical series. Surg Neurol 31:85–91, 1989.
100. Pritz MB: Evaluation and treatment of aneurysms of the vertebral artery: Different strategies for different lesions. Neurosurgery 29:247–256, 1991.

CHAPTER **118**

Basilar Trunk Aneurysms

SEAN D. LAVINE ■ J. DIAZ DAY ■ FELIPE C. ALBUQUERQUE ■ STEVEN L. GIANNOTTA

Posterior circulation aneurysms represent approximately 15% of all intracranial aneurysms. The most common of these are the basilar apex aneurysms, followed by those of the basilar–superior cerebellar artery (SCA) and vertebral–posterior inferior cerebellar artery (PICA) regions. In their series of nearly 1200 posterior circulation aneurysms, Peerless and Drake reported that 16% were located in the upper basilar trunk, 8% in the lower basilar trunk, and 7% at the vertebrobasilar junction.[1] Aneurysms of the basilar trunk present some of the most difficult challenges in neurovascular surgery. Surgical access, perforator anatomy, the specter of daunting complications, and the use of endovascular techniques underscore the need for studied decision making. The relative paucity of basilar aneurysms below the apex makes for a steep learning curve.

Aneurysms of the basilar trunk are those arising between the vertebrobasilar junction and the SCA. The majority of these rare lesions are located at the origin of the anterior inferior cerebellar artery (AICA) along the lower and middle thirds of the clivus.[2] These aneurysms usually project laterally in association with the AICA. True trunk aneurysms arising at the origin of one of the long lateral pontine arteries or other perforating branches may project posteriorly, into the pons, or anteriorly, pressing against the clivus. They tend to have a close relationship to the sixth cranial nerve. Upper trunk lesions originate between the AICA and the SCA and may have a variable relationship to the clivus, depending on their size. Larger lesions may project superiorly above the clivus, making them amenable to approaches from an anterolateral trajectory.

The transsylvian (pterional) and subtemporal approaches have been used with great success for those lesions near the basilar apex.[3–5] For more caudally situated lesions, including those near the origin of the PICA, the retrosigmoid craniectomy is a common and effective strategy. For lesions of the basilar trunk and AICA, however, a combined supra- and infratentorial approach, as originally proposed by Drake, provides an innovative strategy and has served as a foundation for several technical advances.[3] The evolving field of cranial base surgery has provided additional operative strategies for the management of aneurysms in this region.

The principles underlying cranial base surgical techniques include the following: (1) obtaining the shortest trajectory to the lesion, (2) bone removal in lieu of brain retraction, (3) maximization of extradural exposure, (4) skeletonization and decompression of cranial nerves and vascular structures, and (5) reconstitution of all dural openings. Using these principles, we have expanded on existing strategies and, in certain circumstances, developed alternative approaches to large and complex aneurysms of the basilar trunk.[6–8]

CLINICAL PRESENTATION

The majority of aneurysms of the posterior circulation, including those of the basilar trunk, manifest through symptoms and signs of subarachnoid hemorrhage.[2] Rarely can the clinical picture be differentiated from that associated with rupture of an anterior circulation aneurysm. Headache, nuchal pain and rigidity, nausea, and vomiting are frequent presenting complaints. Intraparenchymal hemorrhage and lower cranial neuropathies are not common presenting problems. Rupture of a basilar trunk aneurysm may be suggested by abrupt loss of consciousness, coma, middle and lower cranial neuropathies, crossed hemiparesis, pulmonary edema, and cardiac arrest. Less than a third of patients, however, present with this constellation of symptoms.[1, 9]

Occasionally, a cranial nerve deficit elucidates a specific posterior circulation lesion. Oculomotor dysfunction may be associated with rupture of lesions affecting the basilar apex, SCA, and upper basilar trunk. Ruptured peripheral aneurysms of the AICA may present with acute hearing loss or facial paresis, and lesions of the lower trunk frequently present with abducens palsy. With giant aneurysms affecting the basilar trunk, subarachnoid hemorrhage less often dominates the clinical picture compared with similar lesions affecting the anterior circulation.[3] Because of their close association with the brainstem, however, these larger lesions more often present with signs and symptoms of mass effect. Obstructive hydrocephalus is another presenting feature in this scenario. Large or giant dolichoectasias of the basilar artery typically present with symptoms referable to brainstem or cranial nerve compression. Ischemic syndromes may also occur because of intermittent but progressive compression of perforating arteries to the brainstem.[1, 10] Trigeminal neuralgia and hemifacial spasm are also frequently seen in patients with dolichoectasias.

Direct surgical approaches to basilar trunk aneurysms are best performed in cases of saccular aneurysms presenting with subarachnoid hemorrhage, mass effect, or embolic complications. In such cases, however, the timing of surgical intervention may be problematic. Although we prefer to address these lesions early in their posthemorrhagic course, optimal results are obtained when the patient's neurological status and systemic health have been stabilized. Large or giant aneurysms are best approached only by surgeons who are completely familiar with the various approaches, and only when anesthetic and other support teams, including endovascular and cardiac bypass services, are available.

ANATOMY OF THE BASILAR TRUNK

The basilar artery begins at the vertebrobasilar junction and courses superiorly in the basilar sulcus of the pons toward the interpeduncular fossa.[2] The artery has several major and intermediate branches, all of which provide a point of origin for an aneurysm. The first major branch of the basilar artery is the AICA, which arises several millimeters distal to the vertebrobasilar junction and courses laterally and posteriorly to supply the inferior surface of the cerebellum. The SCA originates just proximal to the bifurcation and courses laterally in the pontomesencephalic sulcus to supply the superior cerebellar hemisphere. The basilar artery terminates in the region of the interpeduncular fossa as it bifurcates to form the posterior cerebral arteries.

In addition to these major arterial branches, the basilar artery gives rise to several intermediate-sized vessels.[11] The most proximal is the pontomedullary artery, which originates between the vertebrobasilar junction and the takeoff of the AICA. This vessel travels laterally in the pontomedullary sulcus and terminates in the retro-olivary fossa. The long lateral pontine arteries are the next major branches. Usually consisting of a superolateral and an inferolateral artery, these vessels arise at about the level of the trigeminal nerve and course laterally to supply the paramedian and lateral pontine surface. The posterolateral artery is the most distal intermediate branch, arising just proximal to the takeoff of the SCA. This vessel is responsible for supplying the superolateral pontine surface.

Critical to reducing surgical morbidity is the preservation of the perforating branches of the basilar artery. Perforators can arise either directly from the basilar artery or from its branches. These vessels may be divided into three groups: caudal, middle, and rostral.[11] The caudal group originates from the dorsal surface of the initial segment of the basilar artery, between the vertebrobasilar junction and the takeoff of the AICA. This group, comprising from one to four vessels, descends along the basilar sulcus and enters the foramen caecum medullae oblongatae. Occasionally, one or more of these vessels arise from the pontomedullary artery or the AICA. The middle group of perforators arises from the segment of the basilar artery between the origins of the AICA and the posterolateral artery. They also arise from the dorsal surface and course rostrally or caudally for a short distance before penetrating the pons in the basilar sulcus. Some of these vessels may also originate from the AICA, long lateral, posterolateral, and pontomedullary arteries. The rostral perforator group usually numbers from one to five vessels and originates from the dorsal surface of the terminal basilar artery. These vessels course rostrally to enter the caudal posterior perforated substance. In a small percentage of patients, these perforators may arise from the SCA or the posterolateral artery.[11]

SURGICAL APPROACHES

Subtemporal Transtentorial Approach

The subtemporal transtentorial approach is a modification of the standard subtemporal approach popularized by Drake for exposure of basilar apex aneurysms.[3, 12] The addition of tentorial sectioning and ligation of

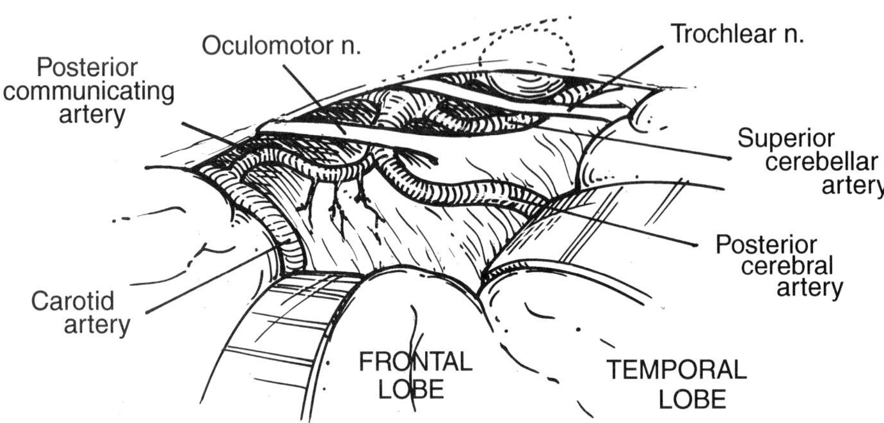

FIGURE 118–1. With the frontal and temporal lobes retracted, the tentorial edge, upper basilar complex, and oculomotor nerve are exposed.

the superior petrosal sinus provides exposure of the upper basilar trunk. This technique provides a rather limited view of the middle and lower portions of the trunk, however. It also requires excessive manipulation of the cranial nerves and retraction of the brainstem and cerebellum when addressing these more caudally situated lesions. Nonetheless, this approach can be combined with petrous resection to provide better access to the middle and lower basilar trunk, as described in a subsequent section.

The patient is placed in a lateral decubitus position with the head positioned parallel to the floor. A lumbar drain is inserted to provide maximal brain relaxation during temporal lobe retraction. A question mark–shaped incision, beginning just below the zygomatic arch and not more than a centimeter anterior to the tragus of the ear, is made. The incision is extended about 2 to 3 cm posterior to the external auditory canal, reaching approximately 3 cm above the pinna and ending inside the hairline. A scalp flap is then elevated, exposing the origin of the zygomatic arch. The temporalis muscle is reflected inferiorly with the scalp flap. A temporal craniotomy is then performed, exposing the dura to a point approximately 2 to 3 cm posterior to the external auditory canal. The temporal squama is drilled flush with the floor of the middle cranial fossa to reduce the amount of temporal lobe retraction.

The dura is opened along the inferior surface of the temporal lobe, while draining cerebrospinal fluid from the lumbar catheter. Mannitol and furosemide (Lasix) are routinely used for relaxation in all aneurysm surgery, but when the temporal lobe will be retracted intradurally, lumbar catheter or ventriculostomy drainage is added. The temporal lobe is gently elevated to expose the tentorium. Retraction of the tentorial edge exposes the trochlear nerve (Fig. 118–1). The superior petrosal sinus is coagulated and then divided. The dural incision is extended over the area of Meckel's cave, allowing anterior retraction of the tentorium. The tentorial flap may be retracted anterolaterally to expose the ventrolateral pons, trigeminal root entry zone, and upper basilar trunk up to 2 cm below the origin of the SCA (Fig. 118–2). In general, clip application is performed between the seventh-eighth nerve complex laterally and the fifth nerve medially. This space can be quite narrow. Standard clip appliers may be too wide to maneuver in this space, necessitating the use of narrow-profile, extended-length appliers. Alternatively, longer clips may be used in such a fashion that only the blades of the clip are placed between the cranial nerves during application.

It is unlikely that the origin of the AICA will be seen without excessive retraction of the fifth nerve, seventh-eighth nerve complex, and brainstem. For access below the upper basilar trunk, the approaches described later are preferable. The major benefit of the subtemporal transtentorial route is the avoidance of injury to the lower cranial nerves. This route is shorter for upper basilar trunk and high AICA–basilar junction aneurysms than traditional posterior fossa approaches are. Peerless and Drake emphasize the difficulty of deep dissection in a narrow corridor. Nonetheless, they

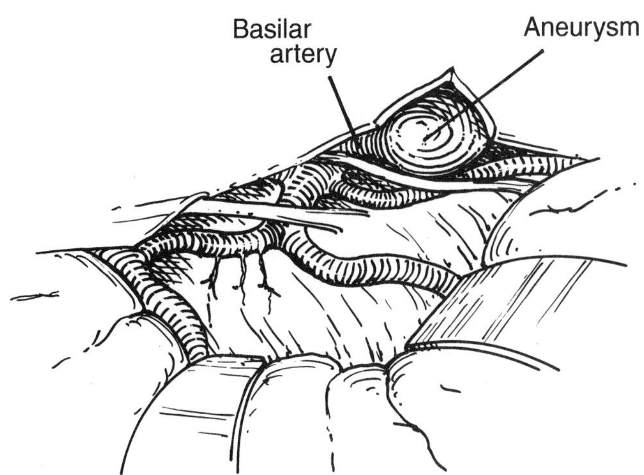

FIGURE 118–2. To access the upper basilar trunk, the tentorium is incised toward Meckel's cave.

prefer the subtemporal approach for most aneurysms of the upper basilar region and reported a success rate of 82% in their series of more than 1000 vertebrobasilar aneurysms.[1] The need for temporal lobe retraction and concomitant injury to vital venous structures is another risk one must consider when undertaking this approach. Given the limited exposure of the mid to lower basilar trunk from this approach, we use it only to address small aneurysms of the superior trunk and SCA. Occasionally, high-lying AICA region aneurysms may be amenable to clipping via this approach as well.

Transsylvian Approaches, Including Zygomatic and Temporopolar Modifications

The traditional transsylvian approach to posterior circulation aneurysms, popularized by Yasargil, is of limited use for aneurysms of the basilar trunk. Only lesions near the basilar apex or in the region of the SCA are amenable to treatment by this approach. The original technique is not described here, as it was addressed in previous chapters.

The transsylvian strategy can be conceptualized as an inverted cone. The base of the cone is represented by the cranial flap and sphenoid wing removal. The apex is the aperture bordered by the carotid artery from the clinoid to the bifurcation and by the edge of the tentorium and oculomotor nerve. For the transsylvian approach to be successful as a cranial base strategy, either the base or the apex of the cone, or both, must be expanded (Figs. 118–3 and 118–4).

In an effort to expand the base of the cone, Fujitsu and Kuwabara recognized the theoretical advantages of removing the zygoma to increase access to the central cranial base.[13] Chief among these advantages was redirection of the bulky temporalis muscle. Additionally, the interpeduncular fossa, containing the upper third of the basilar artery, is better visualized along a trajectory that closely parallels the clivus. The orbitozygomatic approaches and their variations are now used

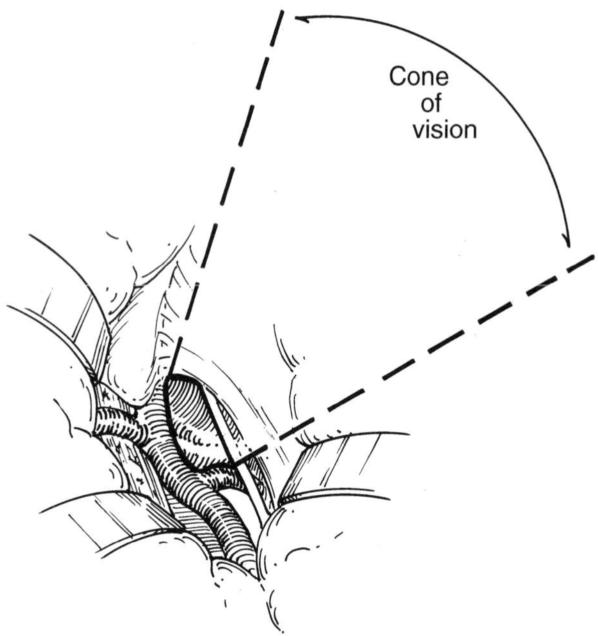

FIGURE 118–3. Despite a luxurious exposure afforded by the various cranial base approaches, access to the basilar trunk is severely limited.

for upper trunk aneurysms. The greatest advantage of this trajectory is that it parallels the path of the basilar artery. From this trajectory, clip application is facilitated in select cases, and the incidence of parent artery narrowing is reduced.

Various names have been used to describe these zygomatic modifications, including orbitozygomatic infratemporal, supraorbital, orbitocranial, modified supraorbital, and extended orbitozygomatic.[13–18]

This orbitozygomatic modification allows a more lateromedial, rostrocaudal trajectory when compared with traditional pterional techniques. It is limited by the need to work through the sylvian fissure. Once again, a lumbar catheter is placed to facilitate retraction. The patient is placed supine on the operating table with the head turned 45 degrees away from the side of incision. The vertex is oriented in a downward trajectory about 15 to 20 degrees. This places the malar eminence as the highest point in the field.

An incision is made beginning 0.5 cm anterior to the tragus and approximately 1 cm below the posterior zygomatic root. The incision is curved gently behind the hairline, ending at the midline. The scalp is opened in two layers to preserve the frontalis branch of the facial nerve. The lateral orbital rim and the entire length of the zygomatic arch are exposed in a subperiosteal fashion. The scalp is then reflected anteriorly and inferiorly over the zygoma and malar eminence via fishhooks attached to a Leyla bar. The temporalis muscle is incised posteriorly to the periosteum and forward 3 to 4 mm below the superior temporal line, leaving a cuff of muscle and fascia for later reattachment. A final incision is made in the temporal fascia and muscle along the supraorbital rim to the frontozygomatic junction, leaving an attachment to the coronoid process of the mandible. This exposes the frontozygomatic recess and the temporal squama (Fig. 118–5).

Titanium microplates are placed across the root of the zygoma, the junction of the zygoma and the frontal bone, and the malar eminence as templates for proper

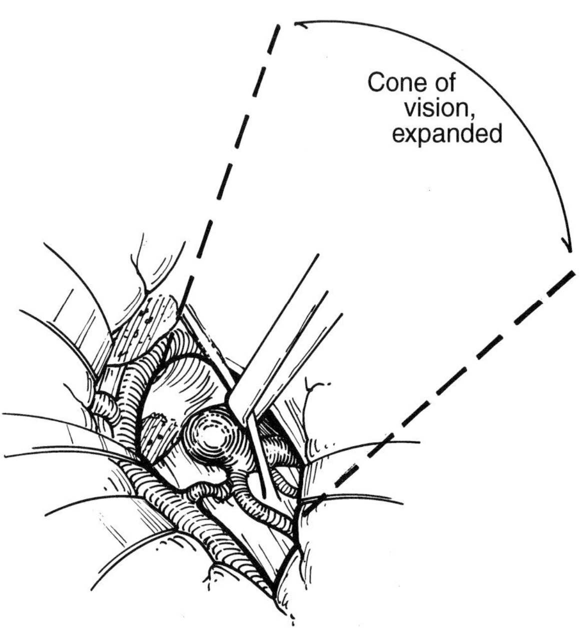

FIGURE 118–4. The apex of the cone can be dramatically expanded by removing both clinoids, retracting the carotid artery, opening the porous oculomotorius, and retracting the third nerve.

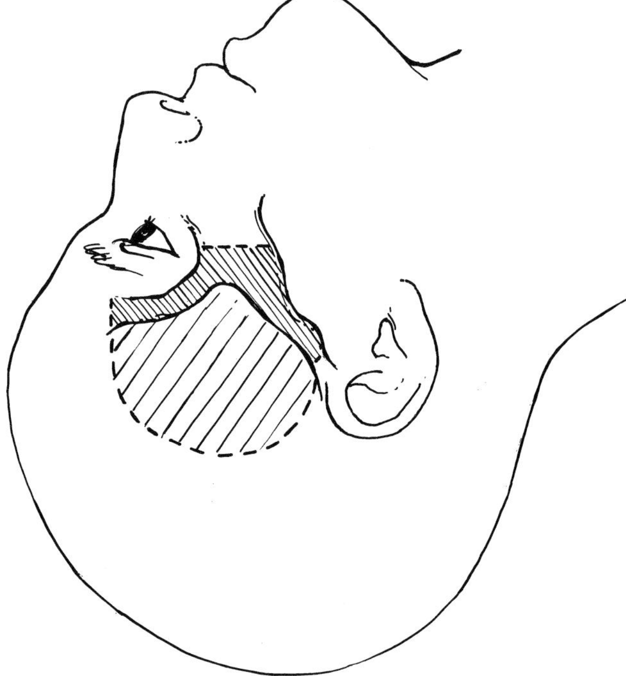

FIGURE 118–5. The orbitozygomatic construct can be removed in continuity with the craniotomy flap or as a separate piece.

screw position for eventual reattachment. After drilling these holes, the plates are removed and stored for future use. Three osteotomies are then performed, with either a sagittal oscillating saw or an osteotome. The first incorporates the posterior portion of the lateral rim of the orbit, including the bone overhanging the frontozygomatic recess. The second is parallel to the temporal squama at the root of the zygoma. The third splits the malar eminence in half. The oscillating saw is used to undercut the entire construct. The orbitozygomatic piece is removed for future replacement. The temporalis muscle and fascia posterior and inferior can then be reflected with additional fishhooks (Fig. 118–6).

A frontotemporal craniotomy, with the inferior cuts as close as possible to the frontal and temporal floors, is performed. The sphenoid wing is flattened, as in a standard pterional craniotomy, with removal of any bony excrescences of the middle and frontal floors with rongeurs and a high-speed drill. Next, the dura is opened in a semilunar flap based anteriorly. A "T" cut is made in this flap down to the region of the optic nerve to provide additional intradural exposure. The sylvian fissure is opened widely under the microscope before opening the lumbar drain. Removal of the anterior and posterior clinoid processes expands exposure of the basilar cistern. The temporal lobe is retracted laterally so that the oculomotor nerve is in the center of the exposure. Expansion of the midportion of the cone is accomplished by coagulating the temporal tip veins and retracting the temporal tip.

Orbital roof removal in conjunction with zygoma resection, the standard orbitozygomatic craniotomy, provides additional exposure of this region, allowing

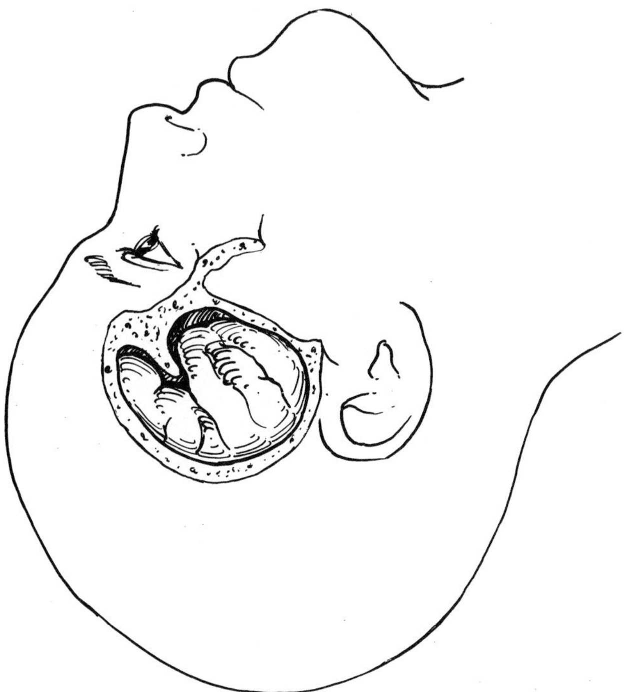

FIGURE 118–6. The bony removal, in conjunction with deflection of the temporalis muscle inferiorly, provides a widened arc of visual access.

multidirectional viewing of the upper basilar trunk and surrounding structures. Lawton and colleagues proposed the extended orbitozygomatic craniotomy as the preferred approach to lesions of the upper two fifths of the basilar artery.[17]

Extradural Temporopolar Approach

To further expand both the base and the apex of the cone represented by the transsylvian trajectory, we use a modified version of the temporopolar strategy.[6,7] This approach involves extensive bone removal and extradural dissection to minimize retraction injury to the frontal and temporal lobes. The essential components of the temporopolar exposure are (1) extradural drilling of the sphenoid wing and exposure of the superior orbital fissure (SOF) and foramen rotundum, (2) removal of the anterior clinoid process via the anterolateral route, (3) decompression of the optic canal, (4) extradural retraction of the temporal tip, (5) transcavernous mobilization of the carotid artery and third cranial nerve, and (6) removal of the posterior clinoid process. This approach may be combined with removal of the zygoma alone or both the zygoma and the orbital rim. The main advantage of this approach is the widened visual arc afforded by the temporal tip retraction. This maneuver exaggerates the basal trajectory afforded by the orbitozygomatic approach.

The patient is placed in the supine position with the head rotated 45 degrees. The neck is moderately extended to orient the vertex slightly downward. The standard skin incision used for a pterional approach is made, with the inferior aspect extending over the root of the zygoma. The scalp is elevated in two layers, preserving a frontal, vascularized pericranial flap for use in the dural closure. The temporalis muscle is reflected posteroinferiorly to accomplish maximal exposure of the anterior temporal base. A frontotemporal craniotomy is performed, with removal of the temporal squama inferiorly, to allow a flat viewing angle along the floor of the middle fossa. When anterior orbital retraction is desired to enhance the inferosuperior viewing angle from a more frontal direction, the orbital rim may be removed with the bone flap as a single unit, as described previously.

The dura is elevated from the anterolateral middle fossa to expose the foramen rotundum and SOF, and it is opened medially to expose the floor of the anterior cranial fossa. The limits of dural elevation are the foramen ovale laterally and the anterior superior ethmoidal artery medially. A high-speed drill with cutting and diamond burs is used to flatten the sphenoid ridge along with all the irregularities of the orbital roof and anterior middle cranial fossa floor. To provide some mobility of the SOF contents, the lateral dural wall of the SOF is skeletonized with meticulous drilling. The foramen rotundum is unroofed to expose the second trigeminal branch and the optic canal, thereby achieving modest mobility of the optic nerve. The anterior clinoid process is resected by drilling the center of the process and removing the thin shell of bone with microrongeurs. Constant cooling irrigation minimizes thermal damage to surrounding structures during drilling.

After the extradural bone is removed, the dura propria of the temporal tip is elevated from the inner cavernous membrane. The meningo-orbital vessels are divided, beginning at the apex of the SOF. A cleavage plane is developed from the junction of the temporal dura and the periorbital fascia, elevating the dura from the true cavernous membrane. This plane is elaborated from the SOF along the second trigeminal branch, continuing posteriorly to the foramen ovale. The true (or "inner") cavernous membrane is composed of the thin connective tissue and sheaths of the third, fourth, and fifth cranial nerves and surrounds the venous plexus of the cavernous sinus. Judicious packing of Surgicel in this region may be required to effect hemostasis. The limits of the dural reflection are the third trigeminal branch posteriorly and the tentorial edge medially. It is necessary to incise the medial tentorial incisura by opening the porous oculomotorius all the way to the SOF, separating it from the inner cavernous membrane near the third cranial nerve. Retraction of the temporal lobe is accomplished by intermittently positioning a self-retaining retractor blade over the temporal fossa dura during exposure of the cavernous sinus membrane.

The dura is incised over the sylvian fissure until reaching the optic nerve sheath. An L-shaped incision is completed by extending along the frontal base for 2 to 3 cm. Perneczky's fibrous ring is then opened laterally to free the carotid artery of its dural attachment. The temporal lobe is retracted posterolaterally with dural protection, and the frontal lobe is retracted posteromedially in a similar fashion. In this manner, the temporal tip veins are preserved with the anterior temporal dura (Fig. 118–7).

The anterior 2 cm of the sylvian fissure is opened to widen the exposure of the superior clival area; the internal carotid artery and the proximal A1 and M1 segments are well exposed at this point. The superior triangle of the cavernous sinus (between the oculomotor and trochlear nerves) and the porous oculomotorius are opened to mobilize the oculomotor and trochlear nerves. Thus, the oculomotor nerve is exposed from its origin at the midbrain to its dural entrance into the SOF. The third cranial nerve may be covered with a soft cottonoid and gently retracted laterally. The internal carotid artery may be mobilized medially or laterally, because it has been freed from its anterior dural attachment. This gentle retraction widens the aperture to the sella, posterior clinoid, and membrane of Liliequist (Fig. 118–8). The arachnoid membrane lateral to the internal carotid artery is incised, exposing the basilar artery. Removal of the posterior clinoid process with a high-speed drill may be completed to expose the basilar artery below the sella. The combination of medial carotid retraction, lateral tentorial and oculomotor retraction, and posterior clinoid removal enlarges the apex of the exposure, allowing a sight line parallel to the trunk of the basilar artery.

At the conclusion of the procedure, the dura is closed in a watertight fashion, using a dural patch graft or the previously harvested section of pericranium. Titanium microplates are used to secure the zygoma and cranial bone flap for maximal cosmesis.

Similar to the subtemporal transtentorial approaches, the transsylvian approach and its zygomatic variations are best suited to treat aneurysms of the basilar apex and upper basilar trunk in proximity to the SCA. Occasionally, high-lying AICA region or mid-trunk aneurysms can be treated with these approaches as well.

Combined Petrosal Approach

For large lesions of the mid or upper basilar trunk when a transverse trajectory is desired for simultaneous proximal and distal control, the transpetrosal ap-

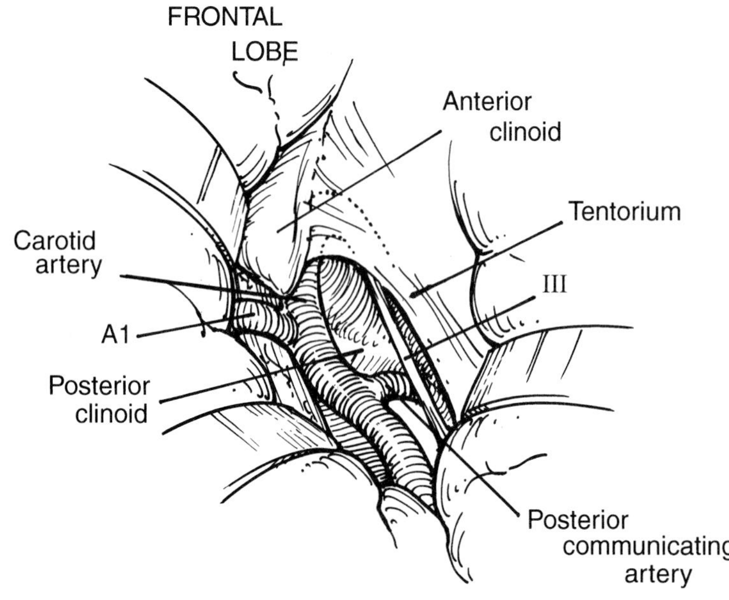

FIGURE 118–7. Retraction of the temporal lobe expands the cone of vision to the level of the tentorial incisura.

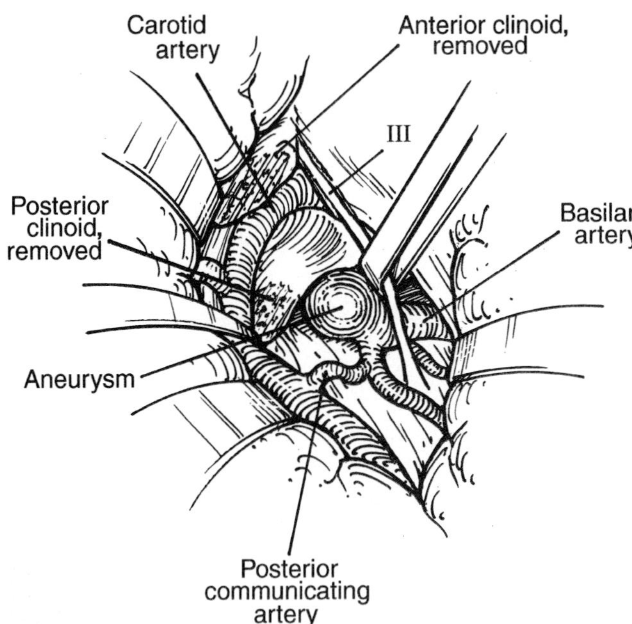

FIGURE 118–8. Mobilizing the carotid and third nerve deepens the exposure and provides access to the basilar trunk with a trajectory parallel to the parent vessel.

proach is ideal. The combined petrosal strategy is actually an infratentorial-supratentorial trajectory that modifies the original subtemporal transtentorial approach described by Drake and Peerless. Variations of this approach have been described previously, especially for use in cranial base neoplasms.[19–27] Accessible structures include the basilar complex, SCA, AICA, and, in many circumstances, vertebrobasilar junction. Essential features for appropriate exposure of pathology in this region include the following: (1) retrolabyrinthine presigmoid mastoid removal; (2) modest temporal craniotomy, with gentle superior retraction of the midportion of the temporal lobe; (3) ligation of the superior petrosal sinus, with division of the tentorium to the tentorial hiatus; and (4) posterior retraction of the sigmoid sinus. Thus, this approach is best termed a subtemporal craniotomy with posterior petrosectomy.[25] A number of authors have contributed to the development of this approach. Both Drake and Malis identified and promulgated the reasons for a combined supratentorial-infratentorial approach to aneurysms in this region.[3, 24, 28] Hashi and colleagues eloquently detailed the nuances of this approach.[21] Samii and colleagues further refined the technique for use in managing petroclival tumors.[26] The benefit of such an approach is limitation of brain retraction due to a more lateral-to-medial and superior-to-inferior trajectory. Further, the sigmoid sinus is not sacrificed. By using a retrolabyrinthine technique, hearing may also be preserved. Radical removal of the petrous apex is usually not necessary for treatment of vascular lesions, making the approach not only relatively quick to accomplish but also easy to learn.

The patient is placed on the operating table in the lateral decubitus position. A small question mark–shaped skin incision is made starting at the root of the zygoma just anterior to the tragus. This incision is extended around the ear, approximately 5 cm above the external auditory meatus and curving gently posteriorly to below the retromastoid region. The incision is extended about 1 cm behind the body of the mastoid and 1 cm below the tip. The galeal-cutaneous flap is elevated and reflected inferiorly. The pericranium and temporalis muscle are elevated in a single layer, fashioning a superior and inferior flap. The superior flap is composed of the temporalis muscle and fascia. The inferior flap of muscle and fascia may be retracted anteriorly.

A partial mastoidectomy is performed by skeletonizing the bony labyrinth, posterior fossa and middle fossa dura, sigmoid sinus, sinodural angle, and superior petrosal sinus. It is not necessary to skeletonize the fallopian canal when using this approach for the treatment of aneurysms. An L-shaped craniotomy is raised around the ear, exposing the temporal and posterior fossa dura. The temporal portion of the craniotomy should lie flush with the floor of the middle fossa (Fig. 118–9). The dura is then opened beginning over the inferior temporal lobe and continuing to the transverse-sigmoid junction. The superior petrosal sinus is ligated as it enters the transverse-sigmoid junction, and the dural opening is continued inferiorly in front of the sigmoid sinus toward the jugular bulb. The key maneuver involves opening the presigmoid posterior fossa dura in conjunction with ligation of the superior petrosal sinus and incising the tentorium to the tentorial incisura parallel to the petrous ridge. This allows for simultaneous gentle retraction of the sigmoid sinus and cerebellum posteriorly and the temporal lobe superiorly. The arachnoid may then be opened, exposing cranial nerves V through X. This results in a panoramic view of the mid to upper basilar trunk and its ipsilateral branches (Fig. 118–10). For improved lateral exposure, an incision in the retrosigmoid dura can be made, thereby effectively skeletonizing the sigmoid sinus. This allows for reflection of the sigmoid sinus in both

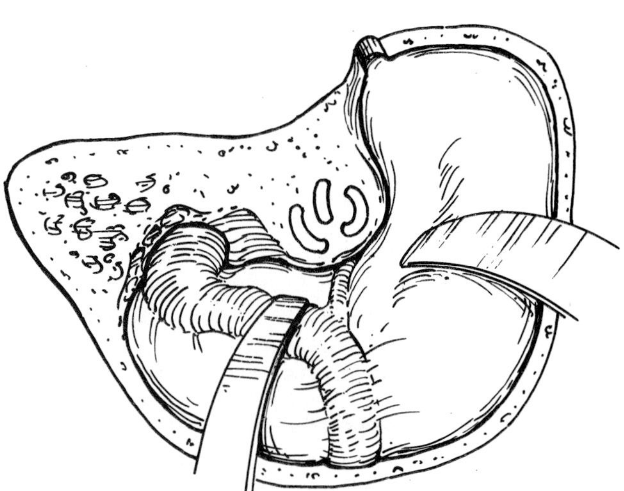

FIGURE 118–9. Extent of exposure completed before dural opening and ligation of the superior petrosal sinus.

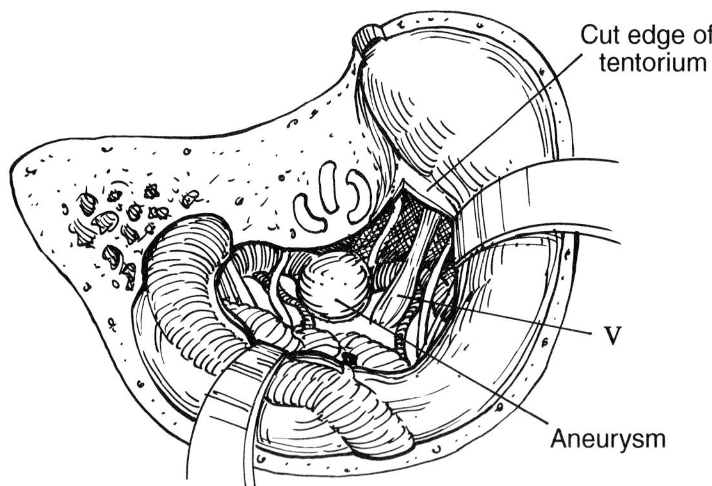

FIGURE 118–10. The tentorium is divided to the incisura, exposing the entire length of the trigeminal nerve and distal portion of the basilar trunk.

the anterior and posterior directions and provides access to the lower cranial nerve structures and upper vertebral artery. In addition, exposure can be enhanced by removal of the bony labyrinth. This affords a more laterally situated basal trajectory that further eliminates the need for brainstem retraction. Unfortunately, this maneuver sacrifices hearing and the ipsilateral balance apparatus. Because watertight dural repair is difficult, an autologous adipose graft harvested from either the lateral thigh or abdomen is placed in the mastoid defect. The bone flap is then secured, and the scalp is closed in a multilayer fashion.

The benefits of the approach include the opportunity to control the basilar artery both proximally and distally. The exposure is quite luxurious and allows for both a wide lateral trajectory and a wide cephalocaudad approach (Figs. 118–11 and 118–12). Further, the sigmoid sinus can be preserved, which may be mandatory when there is a dominant ipsilateral sigmoid sinus or incomplete communication of the transverse sinuses with the torcular. Aneurysms best treated by this approach include those of the basilar trunk originating near the takeoff of the AICA up to and including the origin of the SCA. The approach is particularly useful for large or giant lesions.

Retrolabyrinthine Transsigmoid Approach

The vertebrobasilar junction is typically located near the midline of the clivus, at the level of the pontomedullary junction. A routine lateral suboccipital approach may not adequately expose the lower basilar trunk without an unacceptable amount of cerebellar or brainstem retraction. In addition, a tortuous vertebral artery may place the lesion at a relatively long distance from the surgeon when using a suboccipital or transcondylar approach. Therefore, for trunk lesions above the vertebral bifurcation, the retrolabyrinthine transsigmoid approach provides increased rostral exposure and decreased operative distance to the pathology. This approach was originally described in 1990 as a method to open a lateral corridor to the lower basilar trunk, vertebrobasilar junction, and distal portion of the vertebral artery.[8] It is based on the traditional retrolabyrinthine transmastoid strategy used by otologists to gain limited access to the cochlear and vestibular nerves in the cerebellopontine angle.[29, 30] Although the retrolabyrinthine technique affords a basolateral trajectory to the vertebrobasilar junction, the exposure needs to be expanded to deal with larger pathologies such as aneu-

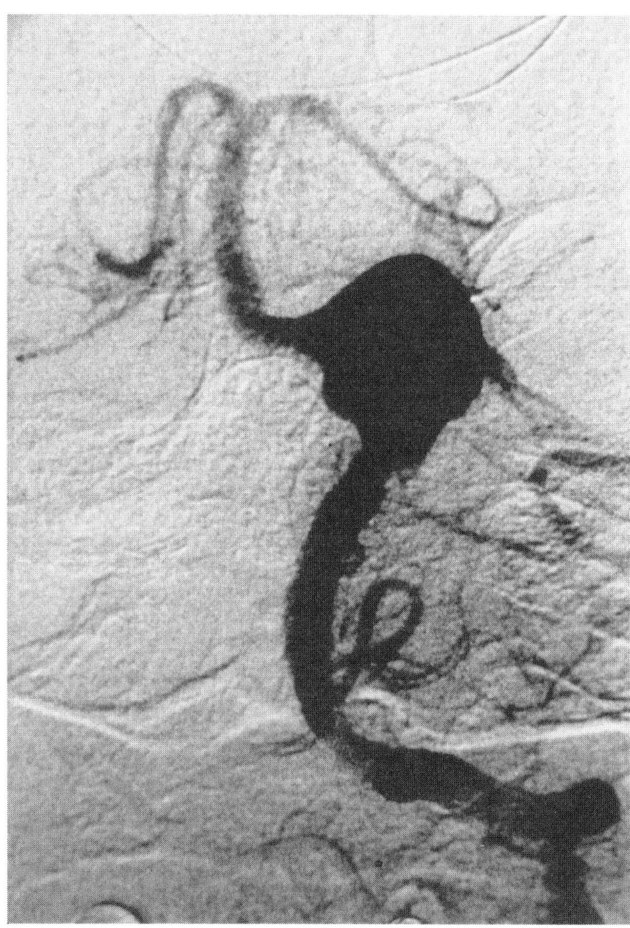

FIGURE 118–11. Large fusiform aneurysm of the vertebrobasilar junction causing subarachnoid hemorrhage in a 70-year-old man.

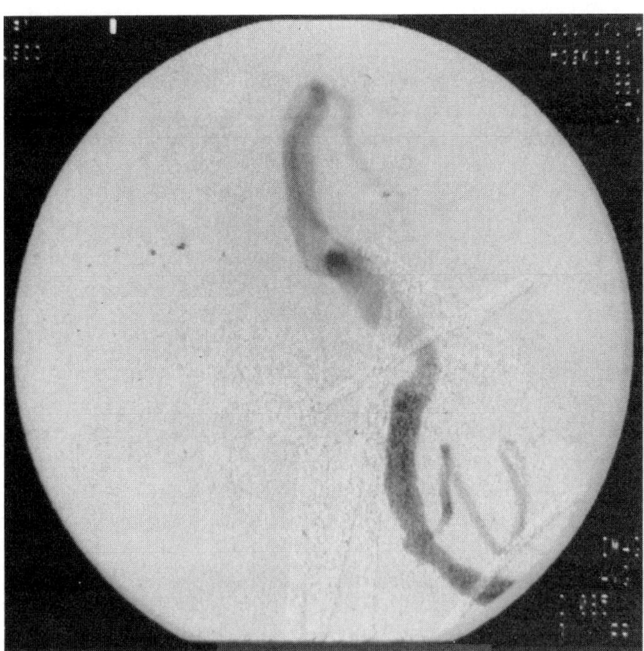

FIGURE 118–12. Intraoperative angiogram showing the majority of the sac obliterated by stacking multiple clips through the transpetrosal approach.

rysms of the lower trunk. Hence, in selected individuals, ligation of the sigmoid sinus is added.

To determine the preferred side of the approach, preoperative venous-phase angiography must be scrutinized to evaluate collateral venous outflow and the side of the dominant sigmoid sinus and to confirm the presence of an internal jugular vein on the ipsilateral side. In midline lesions, those that project either dorsally or ventrally, the approach is carried out on the side of the smallest sigmoid sinus. In lateralized lesions, those that point to the right or left, the aneurysm is approached on the side of the aneurysm neck. This allows the most versatility in terms of clip placement, as well as avoidance of injury to surrounding perforating vessels.

An approach on the side of dominant venous drainage often necessitates preservation of the sinus. In these cases, temporary occlusion of the sinus with measurement of the venous sinus pressure by direct puncture manometry has been used to predict tolerance. A rise in sinus pressure of less than 5 mm Hg likely conveys a reasonable margin of safety for sinus ligature. When temporary occlusion of the sinus produces a rise of more than 5 mm Hg in venous pressure, we resort to a variation of the extreme lateral transcondylar or transpetrosal approach to preserve the sigmoid sinus.

The patient is placed either supine with the head in a lateral position away from the side of approach or in the lateral position. These positions enlist the aid of gravity as the cerebellum falls away from the petrous bone and clivus, thereby reducing the need for retraction. Facial nerve electromyography and brainstem auditory evoked response leads should be placed before sterile prepping and draping. A curvilinear retroauricular incision is made from just above the nuchal line to the level of C1. The skin and subcutaneous tissue are taken down in separate layers from the muscle and fascia and reflected laterally with fishhooks. Next, a mastoidectomy with retrolabyrinthine exposure is performed, skeletonizing the sigmoid sinus from its junction with the superior petrosal sinus down to the jugular bulb. The limits of the mastoidectomy include the middle fossa dura (superior), jugular bulb (inferior), posterior semicircular canal (anterior), and 2 cm of retrosigmoid dura (posterior) (Fig. 118–13). This exposure allows ligation of the sigmoid sinus at the sigmoid-jugular and sigmoid-petrosal junctures and facilitates reflection of the dural flap over the intact labyrinth. The center of the operative field should include the seventh-eighth cranial nerve complex and the flocculus of the cerebellum. The superior portion of the field includes the fifth cranial nerve, spanning the subarachnoid space until its entrance into Meckel's cave. Inferiorly, cranial nerves IX, X, and XI are in view as they enter the pars nervosa of the jugular foramen (Fig. 118–14). Fully skeletonizing the posterior semicircular canal widens the exposure. Accessible structures include the upper vertebral artery, vertebrobasilar junction, and lower basilar trunk, up to and including the origin of the AICA.

The arachnoid of the cerebellopontine angle is then opened to clearly expose the vertebral artery as it meets its contralateral counterpart. Dissection of the arachnoid membrane enclosing the relevant cranial nerves is completed with microinstruments. The space between the nerves may be very tight, and delicate, sharp dissection is mandatory. The retrolabyrinthine transsigmoid approach affords the surgeon a line of sight parallel to the course of cranial nerves V through X. Once the arachnoid has been dissected, proximal and distal exposure of the vertebral and basilar vessels is now available, facilitating control of these arteries in preparation for clip ligation of the aneurysm. Because of the narrow corridor between the cranial nerves, low-profile clip appliers are necessary. In their absence, the use of elongated clips may obviate the need to force a large

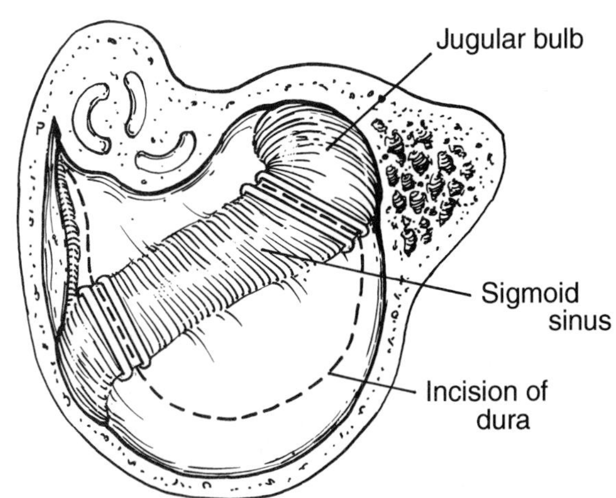

FIGURE 118–13. Retrolabyrinthine exposure of the entire sigmoid sinus allows clipping and division at the jugular bulb and junction of the superior petrosal sinus.

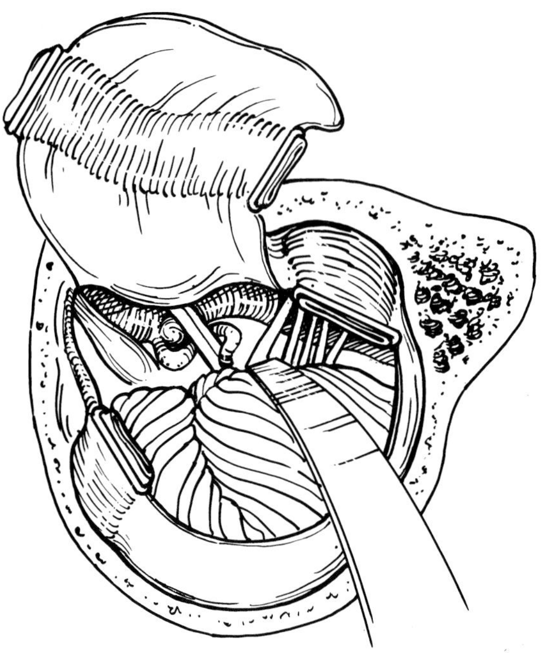

FIGURE 118–14. Exposure is centered on the seventh-eighth nerve complex with access to the lower basilar trunk and vertebrobasilar junction.

clip applier between two delicate cranial nerves. After clip ligation of the aneurysm, the dura is closed tightly, with interposition of an abdominal or lateral thigh fat graft if necessary. The muscle and fascia layer are closed separately from the skin.

Since developing this approach in 1990, we have continued to validate its simplicity and its efficacy in obtaining a virtually straight lateral-to-medial trajectory to the vertebrobasilar junction and lower basilar trunk.[8] As with any approach to this region, morbidity relates not only to brain retraction but also to injury to the lower cranial nerves. Aneurysms of the AICA origin, lower basilar trunk, and vertebrobasilar junction can be approached via this trajectory. However, this approach should be limited to lesions less than 2 cm in diameter so that proximal and distal control can be more easily effected (Figs. 118–15 and 118–16).

Extreme Lateral Inferior Transtubercular Exposure

For giant aneurysms in the region of the distal vertebral artery and lower basilar trunk, a more expanded corridor is necessary. The extreme lateral inferior transtubercular exposure (ELITE) approach is an expansion of the far-lateral approach described by Heros.[31] The trajectory is anterolateral to the medulla and upper cervical spinal cord, sacrificing bone of the mastoid and rim of the foramen magnum in lieu of lower brainstem and upper cervical spinal cord retraction. This exposure is facilitated by resection of the jugular tubercle as the defining maneuver to effect exposure anterior to the brainstem.[32–34] A far-lateral suboccipital craniotomy coupled with extradural removal of the jugular tubercle allows a dural incision parallel to the inferior sigmoid sinus. Resultant dural reflection and sigmoid sinus retraction allow visualization along a sight line parallel to the course of the intracranial vertebral artery.

Such an expanded approach allows one to view superior to the vertebrobasilar junction and lower basilar trunk. Further, the extradural exposure of the vertebral artery above the C1 posterior arch allows proximal vascular control. One unavoidable drawback is the necessity of working through the network of lower cranial nerves. The major morbidity associated with this approach involves vocal cord paralysis and the possibility of aspiration pneumonia.

The key features of the approach include a lateral suboccipital craniectomy in conjunction with a limited mastoidectomy, exposing the inferior sigmoid sinus and jugular bulb. The patient is positioned in a three-quarter lateral decubitus position with the vertex oriented slightly downward. The shoulder is moved out of the way by pulling it caudally, rotating it anteriorly, and fixing it with adhesive tape. Care is taken not to pull excessively on the joint and risk injuring the brachial plexus. A lateral retromastoid incision beginning 2 to 3 cm behind the ear at the level of the external auditory meatus is carried inferiorly along the poste-

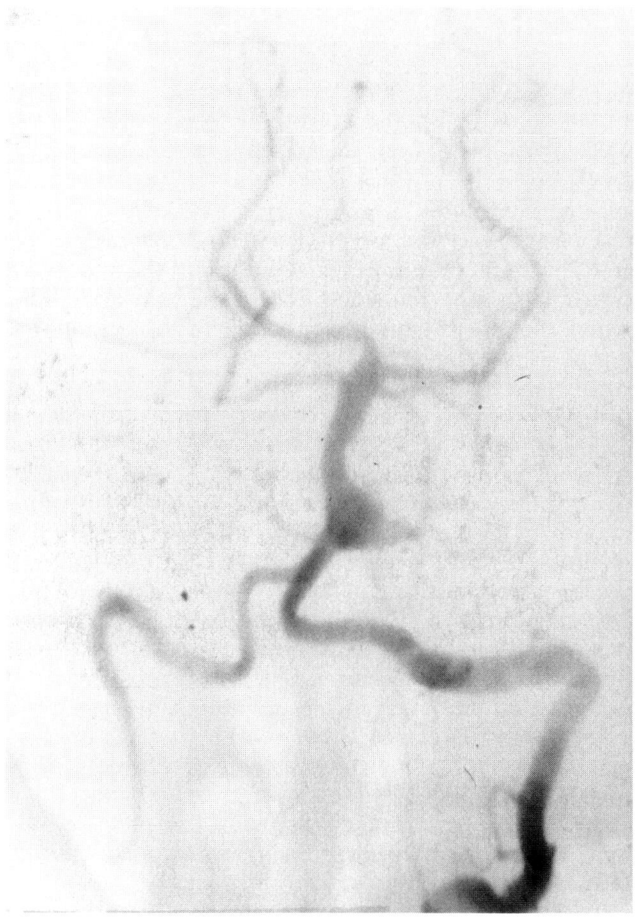

FIGURE 118–15. Wide-based aneurysm of the basilar trunk near the takeoff of the anterior inferior cerebellar artery.

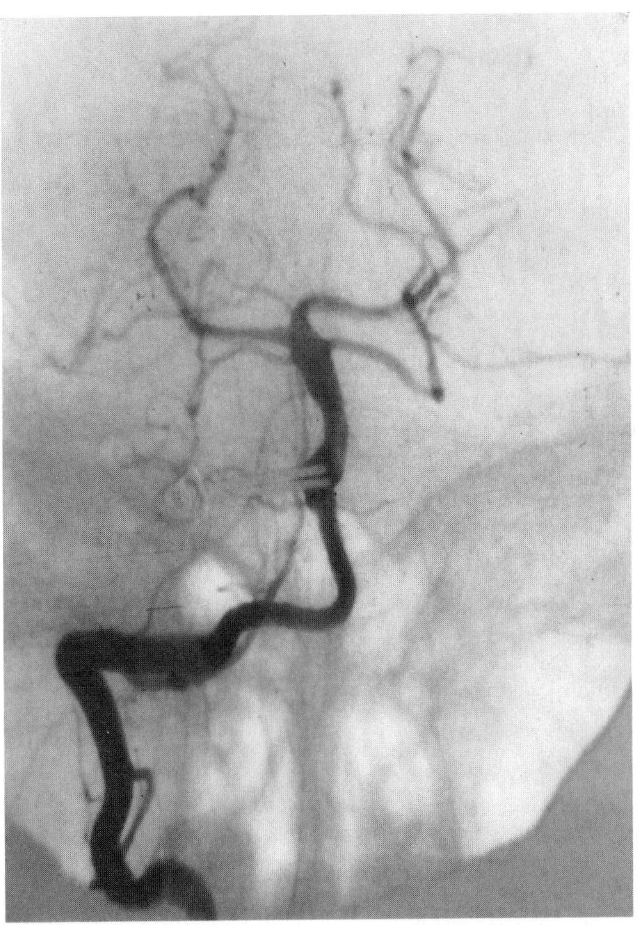

FIGURE 118–16. Postoperative angiogram demonstrating obliteration of the sac with preservation of the anterior inferior cerebellar artery using the retrolabyrinthine transsigmoid exposure.

rior body of the mastoid and the posterior aspect of the sternocleidomastoid to approximately the level of the C4 transverse process. The incision should take the shape of a lazy S. The superficial and intermediate muscle layers of the lateral neck are reflected with monopolar cautery and retracted laterally with fishhooks. The superficial layer is composed of the trapezius and sternocleidomastoid muscles. The intermediate layer includes the splenius capitis, longissimus capitis, and semispinalis capitis muscles. The deep layer of muscles includes the superior and inferior obliques and the rectus capitis major and minor.

Precise localization of the vertebral artery as it arches over C1 to pierce the atlanto-occipital membrane is essential. The vertebral artery is found in the suboccipital triangle, defined by the superior and inferior obliques and the rectus capitis major muscles. This artery's course may be quite variable, and it may have significant extension lateral to the arch of C1, where it is vulnerable to injury with this approach. Once the surrounding venous plexus is encountered, it is coagulated with bipolar cautery, and the connective tissue is removed. The posterior meningeal artery originates just proximal to the dural entrance of the vertebral artery and can be divided if necessary. One must recall that the posterior spinal artery typically arises just distal to the dural entrance of the artery within the subarachnoid space. The oblique muscles are then detached and reflected from the transverse process of C1.

A retromastoid craniectomy down through the foramen magnum is performed. The anterolateral margin of the craniectomy is the sigmoid sinus. Using a high-speed drill, one can skeletonize the sigmoid sinus and undersurface of the jugular bulb. Removal of the rim of the foramen magnum, including the posterior one third of the occipital condyle, is also necessary. By drilling anteriorly, one is able to expose the hypoglossal canal. The jugular tubercle is then reduced by removing bone between and medial to the hypoglossal canal and the jugular bulb. This allows exposure of the lower brainstem (Fig. 118–17).

The dura is then opened starting at the transverse–sigmoid sinus junction, paralleling the entire length of the exposed sigmoid sinus, inferior to the level of C2 and posterior to the vertebral artery's dural entrance. A second, short incision superior to the vertebral artery's dural entrance is then made. Preservation of a dural margin around the vertebral artery facilitates a tight closure. The dura is reflected anterolaterally, carrying with it the inferior portion of the sigmoid sinus. The line of sight is parallel to the intracranial course of the vertebral artery and anterior surface of the medulla, obviating the need for brainstem retraction. The hypoglossal nerve is seen crossing over the vertebral artery within the subarachnoid space. The spinal portion of cranial nerve XI should be clearly seen as it travels rostrally toward the vagus and glossopharyngeal nerves. Here, it is joined by its cranial portion. The nerve roots exit the jugular foramen along with the

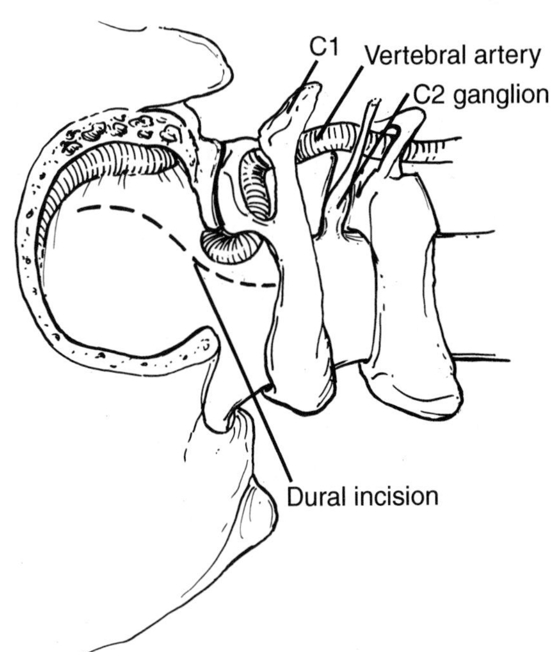

FIGURE 118–17. The vertebral artery is exposed extradurally, and the lower sigmoid is skeletonized down to the undersurface of the jugular bulb.

vagus nerve. The line of sight can be adjusted to visualize the vertebrobasilar junction and lower basilar trunk (Fig. 118–18). Proximal and distal control of the vertebral artery is feasible through this trajectory. At the completion of the intradural portion of the procedure, the dura is closed in a watertight fashion. The muscular layers of the neck are reapproximated, and the fascia and skin are closed in separate layers.

The transcondylar approaches can be expanded in a number of ways to attack large or complex lesions. Removal of up to half the condyle and all of the jugular tubercle further enhances visualization anterior to the brainstem. In selected cases, hemilaminectomy of the lateral portion of the C1 or C2 posterior arch provides a more caudal-to-rostral trajectory and, if necessary, the vertebral artery can be transposed from the C1 or C2 transverse foramina. The extended ELITE adds the mastoidectomy described in the previous retrolabryrinthine transsigmoid section to provide further rostral exposure, such as that needed for midbasilar aneurysms. The rostrocaudal limits of this exposure are from the point at which the trigeminal nerve enters Meckel's cave superiorly to the vertebral artery's dural entrance inferiorly.

The ELITE approach is best suited for giant vertebral, giant PICA, distal vertebral, giant vertebrobasilar junction, and giant lower basilar trunk lesions. This strategy is also a useful alternative to the retrolabyrinthine transsigmoid approach when aneurysms are giant or are strongly lateralized to the side of a dramatically dominant sigmoid sinus (Figs. 118–19 and 118–20).

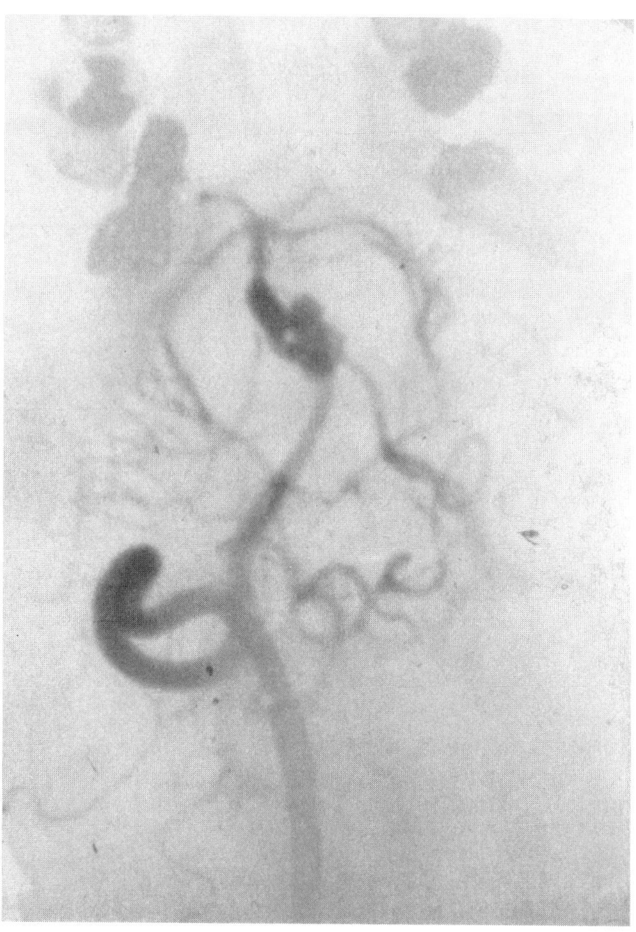

FIGURE 118–19. Multilobulated aneurysm of the lower basilar trunk associated with basilar fenestration.

COMPLICATIONS AND RESULTS

Ischemia remains the major source of complications in the surgical treatment of aneurysms of the basilar trunk.[2] Because of the critical nature of the neural structures supplied by the perforating branches of the basilar artery, perforator occlusion is often dramatically symptomatic. For this reason, the anatomy of these vessels and the techniques necessary for their meticulous preservation must be mastered. Maneuvers that ensure the identification and liberation of all perforating branches from the aneurysm sac before clip placement are of paramount importance. Inspection after clip positioning is also crucial to ensure that any proximal vessels continue to fill. Major arterial branch occlusions, although much less common, have staggering consequences as well. These problems are most often secondary to poor clip placement. The selective use of intraoperative angiography can significantly reduce the incidence of this complication. In the case of large or giant lesions or when temporary occlusion is likely, a femoral artery sheath is positioned as part of the anesthetic induction and positioning. The normal Mayfield headrest is used but is positioned such that reasonably unobstructed lateral and oblique views can be obtained. The process is facilitated by the fact that all aneurysm surgery is done on radiographically transparent tables and that the interventional neuroradiologic team can obtain images within minutes of entering the suite.

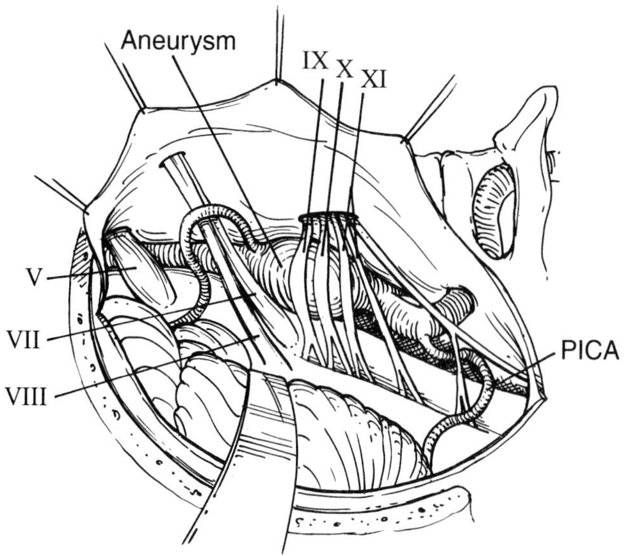

FIGURE 118–18. Removal of the foramen magnum ring and the jugular tubercle, if necessary, provides adequate exposure of the proximal vertebral artery and vertebrobasilar junction behind the lower cranial nerves.

Ischemic complications from intraoperative events may be ameliorated in part by the use of pharmacologic brain protection, the maintenance of euvolemia and normal blood pressure, and the use of technical strategies to decrease retractor pressure.[2] Electroencephalograms and somatosensory evoked potentials are routinely monitored in all aneurysm cases in the event temporary occlusion may be necessary. Brainstem auditory evoked potentials are added in the case of trunk aneurysms. Before planned temporary parent vessel occlusion, propofol is infused in doses sufficient to induce a 10-second-interval burst-suppression pattern on the electroencephalogram. The infusion is continued until well after flow has been restored. In many cases, temporary occlusion of vessels is not required, although ischemia is better tolerated if the protective agent is infused before it is needed. Propofol has the added benefit of rapid emergence from the anesthetic, allowing appropriate evaluation.

The use of hypothermic circulatory arrest is a valuable adjunct to the treatment of large and giant basilar trunk aneurysms, particularly when petrous-sparing approaches are chosen.[17] The ability to collapse aneurysms creates additional room for both dissection and clip application. It should be emphasized that the surgical and anesthetic teams must be experienced and comfortable with hypothermic circulatory arrest to reduce the morbidity directly related to this technique, such as brainstem ischemia, cranial nerve injuries, and intracranial hematomas. Case selection for hypothermic circulatory arrest is a matter of individual judgment. For aneurysms at the basilar apex, those 2 cm or larger are typical candidates. Because of the restricted working room surrounding basilar trunk lesions, even lesions approaching 1.5 cm may be appropriate for this technique.

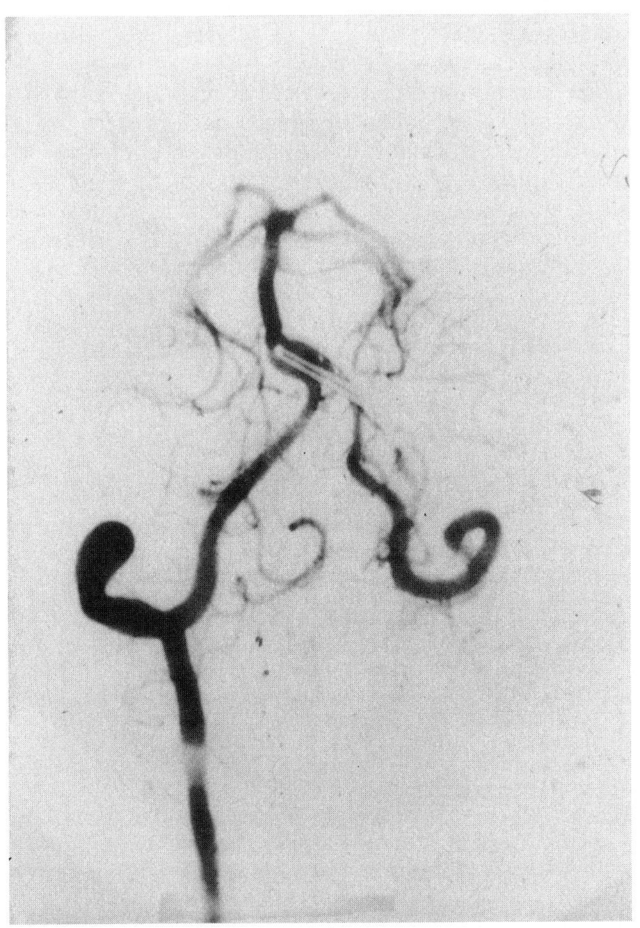

FIGURE 118–20. Successful clip ligation performed through the extreme lateral inferior transtubercular exposure (ELITE). The sigmoid sinus was dominant on the planned side of exposure.

Perhaps the most devastating complication is intraoperative rupture.[2] The morbidity and mortality rates of such events are exceedingly high. It is critical for the operator to adopt a practiced set of steps, not only to avoid this complication but also to treat it as quickly and efficiently as possible. Complete dissection of the lesion before attempting clip ligation reduces the incidence of premature rupture. Should intraoperative rupture occur, tamponade is usually the quickest and most effective method for initial management. Should this technique fail, temporary arterial occlusion should be considered. Only in the most dire circumstances should hypotension be induced, and typically only for the brief period required to gain control of the hemorrhage.

Cranial nerve deficits are a well-recognized sequela of surgery in this region.[2] Operative manipulation, poor clip placement, and occlusion of perforating arteries are all causes of these neuropathies. The third cranial nerve is vulnerable in cases involving the basilar apex, and the fourth nerve is at particular risk during use of the subtemporal approach. Sixth nerve injury is most often produced following surgery in the region of the midbasilar trunk, whereas compromise of function of the seventh and eighth cranial nerves is usually related to approaches for vertebrobasilar junction, AICA, and upper trunk lesions. The most common cause of hearing loss is retraction injury to the cochlear nerve, although it can also occur from injury to the labyrinth or cochlea during the bony exposure. Peculiar to the middle fossa approaches is the occurrence of postoperative trigeminal distribution dysesthetic pain. This symptom is typically self-limited and is undoubtedly secondary to extradural trigeminal manipulation.

Ischemic and hemorrhagic complications are reduced by employing strategies that reduce the need for excessive or prolonged retraction of nervous tissue.[2] The obstruction of venous drainage is another consequence of excessive retraction or the use of methods that interrupt major venous drainage outlets. Procedures that use retraction on the inferior temporal lobe place the temporal basal veins—most importantly, the vein of Labbé—at risk. Using strategies of extradural bone removal, such as making the subtemporal craniotomy flush with the middle fossa floor or using a posterior transpetrosal approach, reduces the stress placed on this critical venous structure. Careful assessment of preoperative angiographic studies may also inform the surgeon of anatomic anomalies in venous drainage. For example, approaching a lesion contralateral to the side of a dominant sigmoid sinus may spare the patient the risk of severely impaired venous drainage by either inadvertent injury or intentional sacrifice of the sinus.

Drake and Peerless reported the largest series of posterior circulation aneurysms, including basilar trunk lesions, treated primarily through the subtemporal transtentorial route or petrosal approaches.[1, 3] Overall, of 1767 patients with vertebrobasilar aneurysms of all sizes and grades treated surgically, 84% had either excellent or good outcomes; the remaining 16% either died or did poorly. Further, of 295 patients with aneurysms involving the basilar trunk, 88.5% had either excellent or good outcomes. The authors argue that better results are seen with lesions involving the trunk, despite the somewhat more challenging operative approaches, because of the potential for injury to the P1 perforating branches frequently encountered during surgery for basilar apex aneurysms.

These results are supported by the work of Sugita and colleagues, who reported satisfactory outcomes in 70% of patients with basilar trunk aneurysms treated through a subtemporal approach.[35] Seifert and Stolke reported a morbidity rate of 30%—specifically, the accentuation of cranial neuropathies—using the combined petrosal approach for the treatment of lesions involving the basilar trunk and vertebrobasilar junction.[36] In Solomon and Stein's series of 44 patients with vertebrobasilar aneurysms (15 located along the basilar trunk), 32 patients were able to return to their previous occupations, 11 had neurological deterioration, and 1 died.[37] The lesions, which included aneurysms involving the basilar trunk and superior cerebellar artery, were treated through either a subtemporal or a combined petrosal approach. Day and coworkers, detailing a series of 30 patients with posterior circulation aneurysms, reported the results of several different approaches, including the extradural temporopolar, combined petrosal, retrolabyrinthine transsigmoid, and ELITE trajectories.[7] The authors offered a treatment paradigm that included the subtemporal approach for lesions of the upper trunk, the retrolabyrinthine transsigmoid or combined petrosal route for midtrunk lesions, and the ELITE exposure for aneurysms involving the lower basilar artery. Overall, 2 patients in this series died, 5 were left with moderate deficits, 1 had a severe deficit, and 22 were normal following treatment.

In a comprehensive review of morbidity from basilar aneurysm surgery, Batjer and Samson divided the causes of poor outcomes into seven different groups that included such factors as the initial effects of hemorrhage, timing of surgery, technical errors, and effects of delayed cerebral ischemia.[38] Specific technical errors adversely affecting the results of surgery included perforator artery injury, inadequate clip ligation, and inappropriate approach (e.g., selection of the transsylvian exposure in cases involving the midtrunk that would be more adequately attacked through a combined petrosal or retrolabyrinthine transsigmoid approach). Intraoperative rupture and venous injuries, particularly to the vein of Labbé during the subtemporal approach, were other technical difficulties that complicated surgical outcomes.[38] Hernesniemi and colleagues echoed the difficulties associated with treating this patient population, reporting a daunting 37% rate of management mortality in a series of 93 patients with vertebrobasilar aneurysms.[39] As one would suspect, complications were significantly less frequent among patients with good clinical grade.

The results of the foregoing series confirm the practical assessment that surgery in this region is complicated by a number of factors, including patient condition, selection of the appropriate operative approach, and posthemorrhagic sequelae such as vasospasm. Because selection and performance of the operative approach are within the control of the surgeon, facility with these factors is of paramount importance in achieving the goal of improved patient outcome.

CONCLUSION

The approaches described in this chapter provide alternative strategies for the treatment of complex aneurysms of the basilar trunk. They allow the surgeon to take advantage of the tenets underlying contemporary cranial base surgery to protect cranial nerve function and reduce brainstem retraction. For the most part, these exposures are relatively luxurious, allowing satisfactory exposure of large and giant aneurysms. From the standpoint of both trajectory and breadth of exposure, they complement and expand on the three traditional approaches, namely, the transsylvian, subtemporal, and lateral suboccipital.

The success of direct surgical approaches to basilar trunk aneurysms relies on several factors. The use of skull base approaches, the appropriate choice of approach based on the location and size of the lesion, and the experience and training of the surgical and anesthetic teams are essential components for achieving therapeutic goals.

REFERENCES

1. Peerless SJ, Drake CG: Posterior circulation aneurysms. In Wilkins RH, Rengachary SS (eds): Neurosurgery, vol 2. New York, McGraw-Hill, 1996, pp 2341–2356.
2. Day JD, Giannotta SL: Posterior circulation aneurysms. In Youmans JR (ed): Neurological Surgery, 4th ed. Philadelphia, WB Saunders, 1996, pp 1335–1353.
3. Drake CG: The treatment of aneurysms of the posterior circulation. Clin Neurosurg 26:96–144, 1979.
4. Yasargil G, Antic J, Laciga R, et al: Microsurgical pterional approach to aneurysms of the basilar bifurcation. Surg Neurol 6: 83–91, 1976.
5. Yasargil MG, Fox JL: The microsurgical approach to intracranial aneurysms. Surg Neurol 3:7–14, 1975.
6. Day JD, Giannotta SL, Fukushima T: Extradural temporopolar approach to lesions of the upper basilar artery and infrachiasmatic region. J Neurosurg 81:230-250, 1994.
7. Day JD, Fukushima T, Giannotta, SL: Cranial base approaches to posterior circulation aneurysms. J Neurosurg 87:544–554, 1997.
8. Giannotta SL, Maceri DR: Retrolabyrinthine transsigmoid approach to basilar trunk and vertebrobasilar artery junction aneurysms. J Neurosurg 69:461–466, 1988.
9. Duvoisin RC, Yahr MD: Posterior fossa aneurysms. Neurology 15:231–241, 1965.
10. Mizutani T, Aruga T: "Dolichoectatic" intracranial vertebrobasilar dissecting aneurysms. Neurosurgery 31:765–773, 1992.
11. Marinkovic S, Gibo H: The surgical anatomy of the perforating branches of the basilar artery. Neurosurgery 33:80–87, 1993.

12. Schneider JH, Giannotta SL: Basilar trunk and vertebrobasilar junction aneurysms. In Carter LP, Spetzler RF (eds): Neurovascular Surgery. New York, McGraw-Hill, 1995, pp 753–762.
13. Fujitsu K, Kuwabara T: Zygomatic approach for lesions in the interpeduncular cistern. J Neurosurg 62:340–343, 1985.
14. Delashaw JB, Tedeschi H, Rhoton AL: Modified supraorbital craniotomy: Technical note. Neurosurgery 30:954–956, 1992.
15. Hakuba A, Liu SS, Nishimura S: The orbitozygomatic infratemporal approach: A new surgical technique. Surg Neurol 26:271–276, 1986.
16. Jane JA, Park TS, Pobereskin LH, et al: The supraorbital approach: Technical note. J Neurosurg 11:537–542, 1982.
17. Lawton MT, Daspit CP, Spetzler RF: Technical aspects and recent trends in the management of large and giant midbasilar artery aneurysms. Neurosurgery 41:513–521, 1997.
18. Smith RR, Al-Mefty O, Middleton TH: An orbitocranial approach to complex aneurysms of the anterior circulation. Neurosurgery 24:385–391, 1989.
19. Al-Mefty O, Fox J, Smith R: Petrosal approach for petroclival meningiomas. Neurosurgery 22:510–516, 1988.
20. Hakuba A, Nishimura S, Inove Y: Transpetrosal-transtentorial approach and its application in the therapy of retrochiasmatic craniopharyngiomas. Surg Neurol 24:405–415, 1985.
21. Hashi K, Nin K, Shimotake K: Transpetrosal combined supratentorial and infratentorial approach for midline vertebro-basilar aneurysms. In Brock M (ed): Modern Neurosurgery I. Berlin, Springer-Verlag, 1982, pp 442–448.
22. Kadson DL, Stein BM: Combined supratentorial and infratentorial exposure for low-lying basilar aneurysms. Neurosurgery 4: 422–426, 1979.
23. Kawase T, Shiobara R, Toaya S: Anterior transpetrosal-transtentorial approach for sphenopetroclival meningiomas: Surgical method and results in 10 patients. Neurosurgery 28:869–876, 1991.
24. Malis LI: Surgical resection of tumors of the skull base. In Wilkins RH, Rengachary SS (eds): Neurosurgery, vol 1. New York, McGraw-Hill, 1985, pp 1011–1021.
25. Miller CG, van Loveren HR, Keller JT, et al: Transpetrosal approach: Surgical anatomy and technique. Neurosurgery 33:461–469, 1993.
26. Samii M, Ammirati M, Mahran A, et al: Surgery of petroclival meningiomas: Report of 24 cases. Neurosurgery 24:358–365, 1988.
27. Spetzler RF, Daspit CP, Pappas CTE: The combined supra- and infratentorial approach for lesions of the petrous and clival regions: Experience with 46 cases. J Neurosurg 76:588–599, 1992.
28. Decker RE, Malis LI: Surgical approaches to midline lesions at the base of the skull: A review. Mt Sinai J Med 37:84–102, 1970.
29. Brackmann DE, Hitselberger WE: Retrolabyrinthine approach: Technique and newer indications. Laryngoscope 88:286–297, 1978.
30. Silverstein H, Norrell H: Retrolabyrinthine surgery: A direct approach to the cerebellopontine angle. Otolaryngol Head Neck Surg 88:462, 1980.
31. Heros RC: Lateral suboccipital approach for vertebral and vertebrobasilar artery lesions. J Neurosurg 64:559–562, 1986.
32. Bertalanffy H, Seeger W: The dorsolateral, suboccipital, transcondylar approach to the lower clivus and anterior portion of the craniocervical junction. Neurosurgery 29:816–821, 1991.
33. George B, Dematons C, Cophigon J: Lateral approach to the anterior portion of the foramen magnum. Surg Neurol 29:484–490, 1988.
34. Sen CN, Sekhar LN: An extreme lateral approach to intradural lesions of the cervical spine and foramen magnum. Neurosurgery 27:197–204, 1990.
35. Sugita K, Kobayashi S, Takemae T, et al: Aneurysms of the basilar artery trunk. J Neurosurg 66:500–505, 1987.
36. Seifert V, Stolke D: Posterior transpetrosal approach to aneurysms of the basilar trunk and vertebrobasilar junction. J Neurosurg 85:373–379, 1996.
37. Solomon RA, Stein BM: Surgical approaches to aneurysms of the vertebral and basilar arteries. Neurosurgery 23:203–208, 1988.
38. Batjer HH, Samson DS: Causes of morbidity and mortality from surgery of aneurysms of the distal basilar artery. Neurosurgery 25:904–916, 1989.
39. Hernesniemi J, Vapalahti M, Niskanen M, Kari A: Management outcome for vertebrobasilar artery aneurysms by early surgery. Neurosurgery 31:857–861, 1992.

CHAPTER **119**

Basilar Apex and Posterior Cerebral Artery Aneurysms

BERNARD R. BENDOK ■ MIR JAFER ALI ■ CHRISTOPHER C. GETCH
H. HUNT BATJER

There has been a trend in recent years to lump all posterior circulation aneurysms into one category when analyzing outcomes and comparing treatment methodologies. This approach conceals the unique features, management strategies, and outcomes that distinguish the various types of posterior circulation aneurysms. In this chapter, we summarize the body of knowledge and our perspectives on basilar apex and posterior cerebral artery (PCA) aneurysms.

The management of basilar apex aneurysms remains one of the most challenging areas of neurosurgery. The technical challenge involved with clipping these aneurysms has inspired several generations of surgeons to push the limits of technical achievements. Advances in neuroanesthesia, cerebral protection paradigms, and critical care management have enhanced the care and probably the outcome for the patient harboring a basilar apex aneurysm. Endovascular techniques have improved to the point of offering an alternative to open surgery for some aneurysms in this location.

Patients with PCA aneurysms have benefited from similar advances. PCA aneurysms require a special understanding of their unique anatomy and pathophysiology. Their management and outcome differ from those for other aneurysms in the posterior circulation.

BASILAR APEX ANEURYSM SURGERY: CLINICAL EXPERIENCE

Dr. Charles Drake generously shared his insight into basilar apex aneurysm surgery throughout his career in multiple publications and lectures.[1–8] In an update on his experience in 1990, he described 545 patients who had been treated, with good outcomes achieved in 475 patients (87%).[9] During the past 40 years, other experienced surgeons have courageously tackled basilar apex aneurysms and contributed to our knowledge regarding this challenging area of neurosurgery.[1, 9–19] One report suggests that well-trained young individuals with intense dedication to neurovascular surgery and sufficient experience can also achieve successful results when treating basilar apex aneurysms.[20]

In a review of their experience with 303 basilar apex aneurysms, Samson and colleagues[21] demonstrated a statistical correlation between poor outcome and various factors: poor admission grade (Hunt and Hess grades IV and V), patient age older than 65 years, computed tomographic demonstration of thick basal cistern clot, aneurysm diameter larger than 20 mm, and symptoms attributable to brainstem compression. In a review of all series published between 1980 and 1989, Wascher and Spetzler[22] found that, for a total of 957 patients, the rate of good outcomes was 82.4% and that the mortality rate was 5.1%. These series include results for a heterogeneous group of aneurysm sizes, patient ages, and clinical presentations. In a report focusing on the management outcomes of 179 unruptured posterior circulation aneurysms, of which 99 were bifurcation aneurysms, Rice and colleagues[1] found a 4.2% combined morbidity and mortality rate. This variability in morbidity and mortality based on clinical factors and aneurysmal morphology must be considered when comparing clip ligation with endovascular options and when counseling specific patients. An important issue to consider when assessing the efficacy of a treatment modality for aneurysms is the rate of complete aneurysm occlusion that can be achieved. In the series reported by Samson and colleagues,[21] postoperative angiography was performed in 246 patients. Residual aneurysm was identified in 6% (i.e., complete aneurysm occlusion in 94%). This rate of complete aneurysm occlusion is superior to the current results achieved with endovascular treatment.[23–27]

MICROSURGICAL ANATOMY OF THE INTERPEDUNCULAR CISTERN

The technical challenges of clipping basilar apex aneurysms are related to the complex anatomy in and around the interpeduncular cistern and the depth of dissection through narrow corridors that is required to safely secure aneurysms in this location. The subarachnoid space within the interpeduncular cistern is enclosed by the clivus and posterior clinoid process anteriorly, the mesial aspects of the temporal lobes and tentorial edges laterally, the cerebral peduncles posteriorly, and the mamillary bodies and posterior perforated substance superiorly. The terminal basilar artery has a normal diameter of 2.7 to 4.3 mm and lies 15 to 17 mm posterior to the posterior aspect of the internal carotid arteries.[19, 28, 29] This proximity to the internal carotid artery provided a basis for seeking a trans-sylvian approach to basilar apex aneurysms. A point proximal to the bifurcation of the basilar artery gives rise to bilateral superior cerebellar arteries (SCAs), which may be duplicated. Blood flow through the SCAs is approximately 50 mL per minute. The dentate nuclei are irrigated by these vessels.[30]

The PCAs originate at the basilar bifurcation. They are usually 2 to 3 mm in diameter. The size of the segment of the PCA from the basilar bifurcation to the junction with the posterior communicating artery (i.e., P1 segment) depends on the extent to which the posterior communicating artery contributes to blood flow in the distal PCA. A fetal PCA implies that the P1 is a vestigial band, with all PCA blood flow originating in the posterior communicating artery.

Respect for the thalamoperforating arteries is an essential technical nuance of basilar apex aneurysm surgery. These critical perforators arise from the posterior aspect of the basilar trunk, the proximal P1 segments, and the posterior communicating arteries. The cranial nerve most intimately associated with this region is the oculomotor nerve that traverses the space between the PCA and the SCA within the interpeduncular cistern. The membrane of Liliequist forms an anterior "curtain" for the interpeduncular cistern. This membrane is a thick layer of arachnoid that anchors from the mamillary bodies superiorly and extends anteriorly and inferiorly before folding posteriorly to form the roof of the prepontine cistern. The basilar apex can be located above, below, or at the level of the dorsum sellae.

SURGICAL STRATEGIES

Basilar apex aneurysms account for approximately one half of posterior circulation aneurysms. The anatomic complexity of the interpeduncular cistern makes basilar apex aneurysm surgery one of the most technically challenging operations in our specialty. Posteriorly located perforators must be protected, or disabling neurological deficits will result. Optimal surgical results and outcomes require excellent technical skill, superb knowledge of operative anatomy, and familiarity with operative nuances accumulated by Dr. Drake, Dr. Yasargil, and a generation of surgeons they trained.

The two pure approaches for basilar apex aneurysms are the subtemporal approach and the trans-sylvian approach. In our practice, we employ both approaches but are increasingly relying on a new modification or hybrid approach. We emphasize the importance of tailoring the operation to the patient's particular anatomy. Considering the key assets and liabilities of each approach allows a more rational design of operative strategies for each patient. The pure trans-sylvian approach has several assets:

1. Neurosurgeons are familiar with this approach because it is used for more common aneurysms and tumors.
2. Proximal control is straightforward.
3. Exposure of both P1 segments for temporary trapping is uncomplicated.
4. Wide exposure is possible.

The trans-sylvian exposure also has liabilities:

1. Exposure of posteriorly located perforators is difficult.
2. Inspection of distal aspect of clip blade is difficult.
3. Technical features make treatment of directly anteriorly or directly posteriorly projecting aneurysms very difficult.

The subtemporal approach offers the surgeon many assets:

1. Proximal control is easy.
2. The lateral view facilitates dissection of the perforators.
3. Tentorial division allows exposure of the upper one third of the clivus for low-lying bifurcations.
4. Fenestrated clips can be placed with excellent visualization of the thalamoperforators.
5. Exposure and clipping of anteriorly or posteriorly directed aneurysms are uncomplicated.

The subtemporal exposure also has liabilities:

1. The field is narrow.
2. Access to the contralateral P1 for temporary trapping is poor.
3. The temporal lobe often is damaged in fresh subarachnoid hemorrhage in poor-grade or obese patients.
4. Cranial nerve III palsy often occurs postoperatively.
5. Intraoperative bleeding is difficult to control.

Pure Trans-sylvian Approach

The trans-sylvian exposure provides excellent visualization for aneurysms with necks at the level between the middle depth of the sella turcica and a line 1 cm superior to the posterior clinoid process (Fig. 119–1). Aneurysms with necks lying inferior to the midsellar level are better approached through the subtemporal corridor or a "half-and-half" conversion with tentorial division. Extremely high aneurysms are difficult to approach but are probably best tackled through a trans-sylvian approach above the carotid bifurcation. The orbitozygomatic osteotomy is very helpful when tackling high aneurysms because the surgeon's line of sight passes from the globe and angles superiorly. Several maneuvers, including drilling the posterior clinoid for

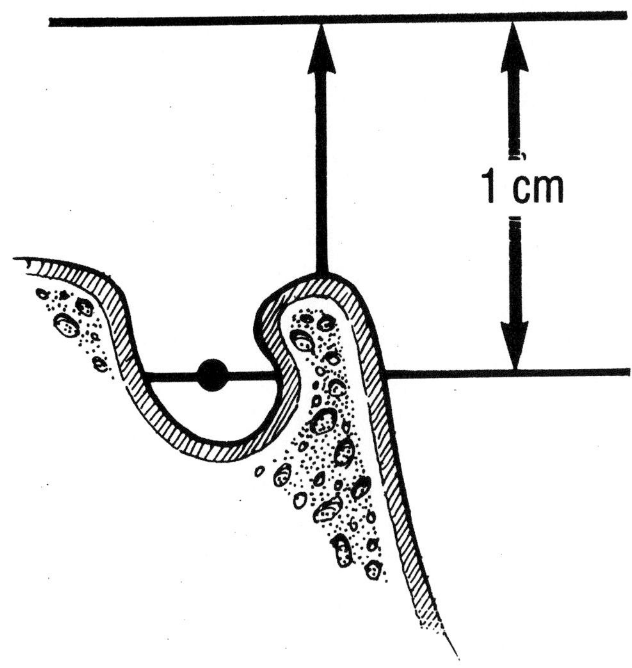

FIGURE 119–1. The pterional exposure provides excellent visualization of the neck of basilar bifurcation aneurysms that originate between the midsellar depth and a line 1 cm superior to the posterior clinoid process. (From Apuzzo MLJ [ed]: Brain Surgery: Complications, Avoidance and Management. New York, Churchill Livingstone, 1993.)

low-lying lesions, have been described to tackle anatomic problems encountered during trans-sylvian exposure.[5, 6]

OPERATIVE TECHNIQUE

Dr. Yasargil[30] pioneered the trans-sylvian approach for basilar apex aneurysms. The advantages of this approach include its familiarity to neurosurgeons, the proximity of the basilar artery to the carotid artery, and the wide exposure of the interpeduncular cistern that can be achieved by opening the membrane of Liliequist. We typically approach midline basilar apex aneurysms from the right side. A left-sided approach is valid when the patient has a right hemiparesis or left third nerve palsy. Some anatomic variants also warrant a left-sided approach. For example, an aneurysm that tilts to the left side makes it difficult to dissect the left PCA off the aneurysm from the right. Occasionally, the entire basilar artery is displaced to the left, which would make a right-sided trans-sylvian approach difficult.

Positioning

Precise positioning is critical to optimize exposure of the basilar apex. Excellent positioning can be achieved with four steps after the Mayfield-Kees skull fixation device is placed with two pins on the contralateral side of the frontal bone and the single pin placed superior to the mastoid process (Fig. 119–2). First, the head is elevated above the long access of the body to maximize venous drainage. Second, the head is rotated away from the operative side by 20 degrees. Third, flexion of the neck brings the chin toward the contralateral shoulder and ensures the plane of the floor of the anterior cranial fossa is perpendicular to the long axis of the body. Fourth, the head is extended until the maxillary eminence is well above the orbital rim.

Scalp Incision

The incision is begun at the zygoma and carried superiorly in a straight line for about 10 cm above the superior temporal line and then curved gently forward toward the midline (Fig. 119–3). Care is taken to ensure that the incision is within 1 cm of the tragus to avoid damage to the frontalis branch of the facial nerve. We preserve at least one branch of the superficial temporal artery. In addition to maximizing scalp healing potential, preservation of this vessel may prove useful if a revascularization procedure is needed. We retract the scalp flap with fishhooks and perform an interfascial dissection of the temporalis muscle. Using a knife, we incise the temporalis fascia from the area of the zygoma to just 1 cm below the muscle attachment to the temporal bone and then to the area of the keyhole. We use cautery to cut the muscle through the opening made with the knife and then peel the muscle off the temporal squama and retract it over the scalp flap with fishhooks (Fig. 119–4).

Craniotomy

We perform a three- or four-hole craniotomy (Fig. 119–5). The fourth hole is reserved for older patients with presumed adherent dura. The first bur hole is placed just above the zygomatic arch. The second bur hole is superior to the first bur hole and just inferior to the superior temporal line. The third bur hole is placed at the anatomic key. The optional fourth bur hole is placed medial and anterior to the second bur hole. A power-driven craniotome is used to incise the bone. After elevating the bone flap, we perform a generous temporal craniectomy, exposing the middle fossa from the temporal tip to the zygomatic root. This degree of temporal exposure can be critical if conversion to a half-and-half or subtemporal approach is needed. We then perform an aggressive resection of the sphenoid ridge with rongeurs and a cutting bur on an air-driven drill (Fig. 119–6). Preferably, the bony exposure is carried to the lateral aspect of the superior orbital fissure. We remove the inner table of the frontal bone for a distance of 2 cm from the bur hole at the anatomic key. After adequate bony exposure, we find it to be very rewarding to spend extra time obtaining excellent hemostasis with bone wax, oxidized cellulose, and tack-up sutures. This approach avoids the dangerous obstruction of the view from run-down later in the case.

We then incise the dura in a semilunar fashion, with the medial limb extending to the frontal bone 1 cm below the medial edge of the craniotomy. The lateral limb crosses the sylvian fissure and extends anteriorly to a point 1 cm below the sylvian fissure at the edge

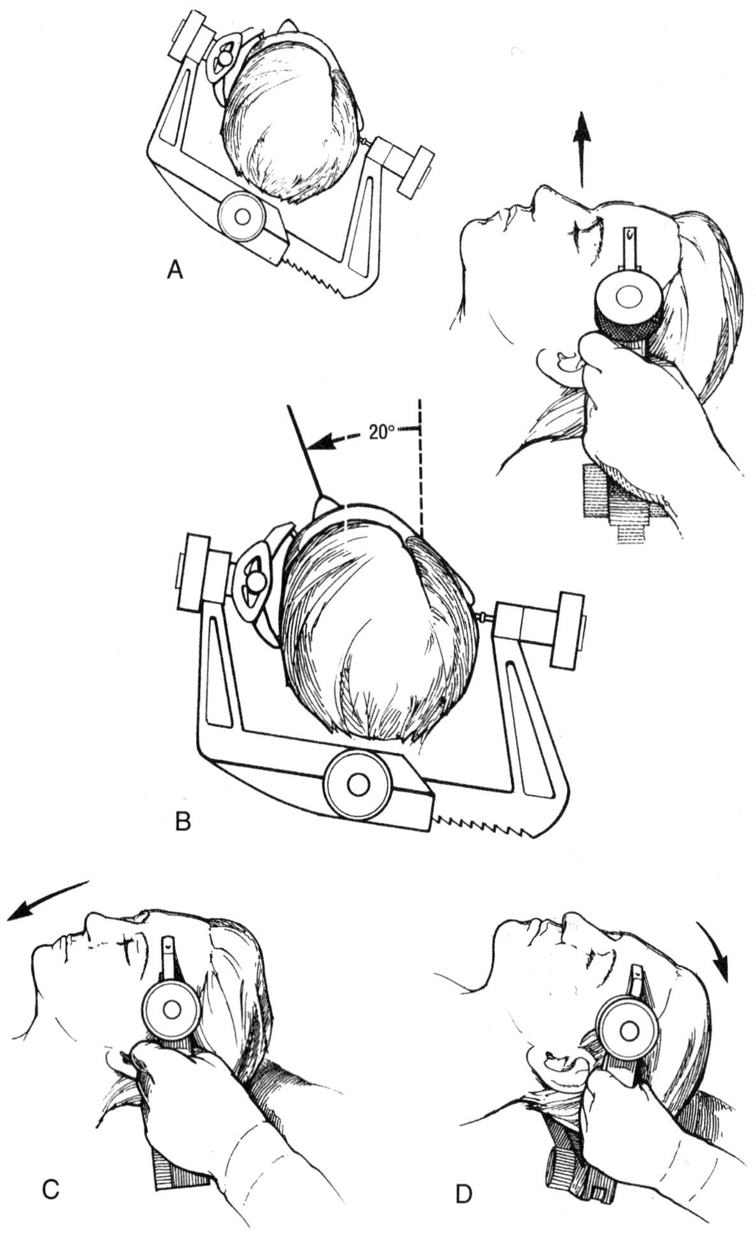

FIGURE 119–2. Positioning for a pterional approach. *A,* The Mayfield-Kees skull fixation device is placed with two pins anteriorly across the midline and the single pin posteriorly to facilitate a flat, unobtrusive surgical field. The head is elevated slightly from the long axis of the body. *B,* Rotation of the head to the contralateral side by 20 degrees minimizes subsequent temporal lobe encroachment on the operative field. *C,* Flexion of the neck brings the chin toward the contralateral shoulder and ensures that the plane of the floor of the anterior cranial fossa is perpendicular to the long axis of the body. This maneuver allows maximal surgical comfort and flexibility and prevents encroachment of the surgeon's arms and microscope onto the ipsilateral shoulder. *D,* Extension of the head is then achieved in a somewhat exaggerated degree compared with anterior circulation surgery to minimize subsequent diencephalic retraction. The maxillary eminence is elevated well above the superior orbital ridge. (From Apuzzo MLJ [ed]: Brain Surgery: Complications, Avoidance and Management. New York, Churchill Livingstone, 1993.)

of the craniectomy. At this point, for ruptured aneurysms, we place a ventriculostomy catheter using anatomic points defined by Dr. Paine[34] if the brain appears to be tight. The point of entry is the vertex of an isosceles right triangle whose hypotenuse overlies the sylvian fissure and whose sides are 2.5 cm long (Fig. 119–7). A ventricular catheter is used to puncture the frontal lobe at this point. We have reliably tapped the frontal horn using this technique. We suture the catheter posterior to the dura, and we let it drain continuously until aneurysm clipping is completed. We then bring in the operative microscope.

Subarachnoid Exposure

During the initial subarachnoid dissection, two goals were kept in mind: maximizing brain relaxation by generous arachnoidal opening, allowing for egress of cerebrospinal fluid (CSF), and extensive dissection of the sphenoidal portion of the sylvian fissure. CSF released from the subarachnoid space results in further brain relaxation, even after spinal or ventricular drainage and particularly when subarachnoid hemorrhage has produced loculated pockets of CSF. Because of the significant amount of traction that may be needed on the frontal and temporal lobes, the middle cerebral artery may kink near its origin because of the dense arachnoid adhesions in this area. For this reason, we begin the sylvian dissection laterally after placing a retractor at the posterior inferior surface of the frontal lobe just anterior to the sylvian vein for a distance of 3 cm along the sphenoid ridge. Placing retraction on the orbital surface of the frontal lobe creates gentle traction on the superficial sylvian fissure, which we incise with an arachnoid knife.

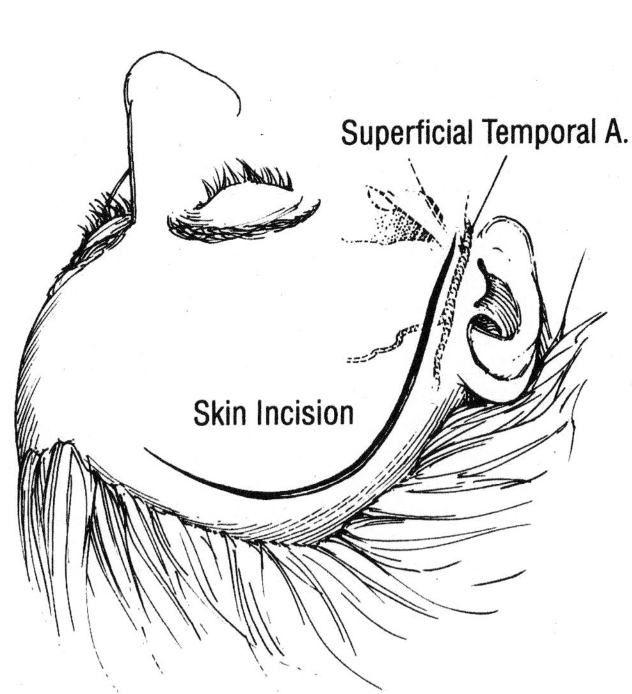

FIGURE 119–3. Scalp incision for a pterional approach. (From Apuzzo MLJ [ed]: Brain Surgery: Complications, Avoidance and Management. New York, Churchill Livingstone, 1993.)

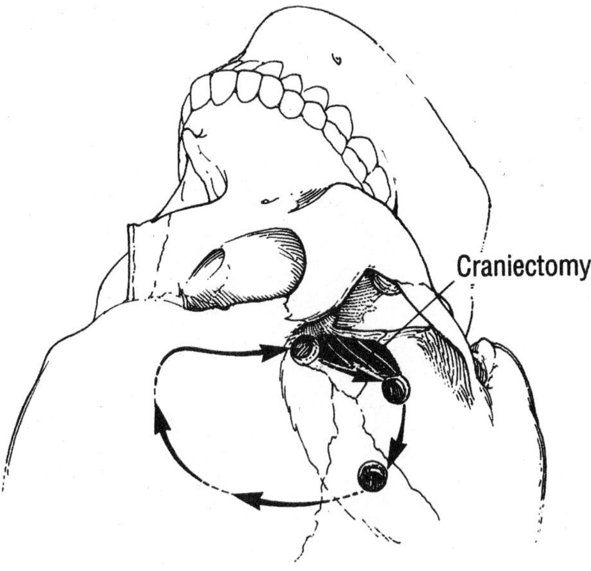

FIGURE 119–5. Pterional craniotomy. A critical aspect of the craniotomy is a generous anterior temporal craniectomy. (From Apuzzo MLJ [ed]: Brain Surgery: Complications, Avoidance and Management. New York, Churchill Livingstone, 1993.)

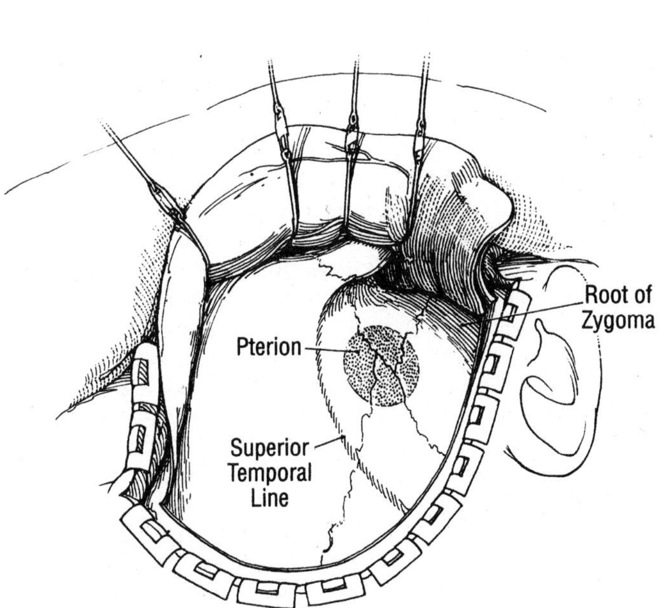

FIGURE 119–4. The temporalis fascia and muscle are incised with the cutting cautery with care to avoid injury to the deep neurovascular bundle in the muscle. The resultant single-layer flap is dissected from the underlying bone and retained with fishhook retractors. (From Apuzzo MLJ [ed]: Brain Surgery: Complications, Avoidance and Management. New York, Churchill Livingstone, 1993.)

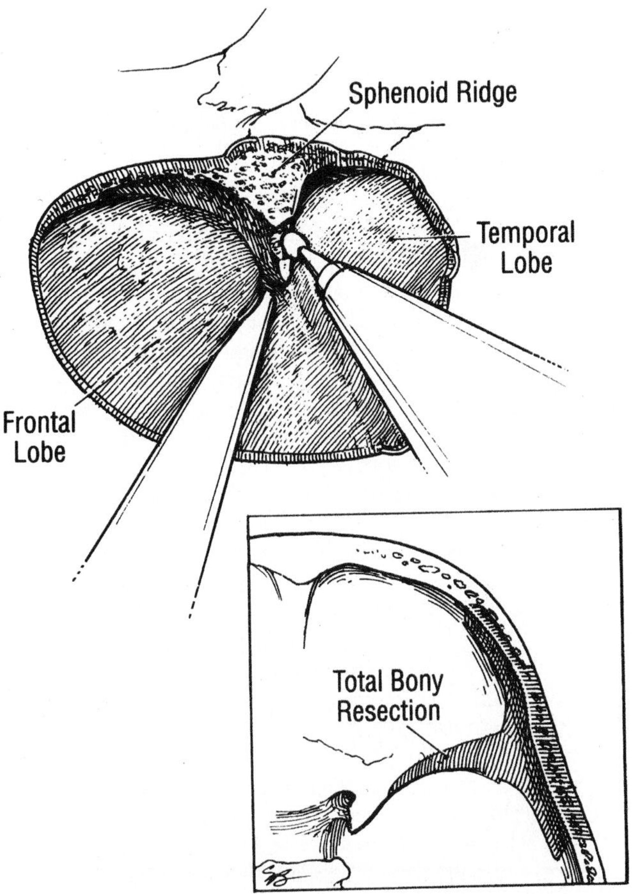

FIGURE 119–6. Aggressive resection of the sphenoid ridge. (From Apuzzo MLJ [ed]: Brain Surgery: Complications, Avoidance and Management. New York, Churchill Livingstone, 1993.)

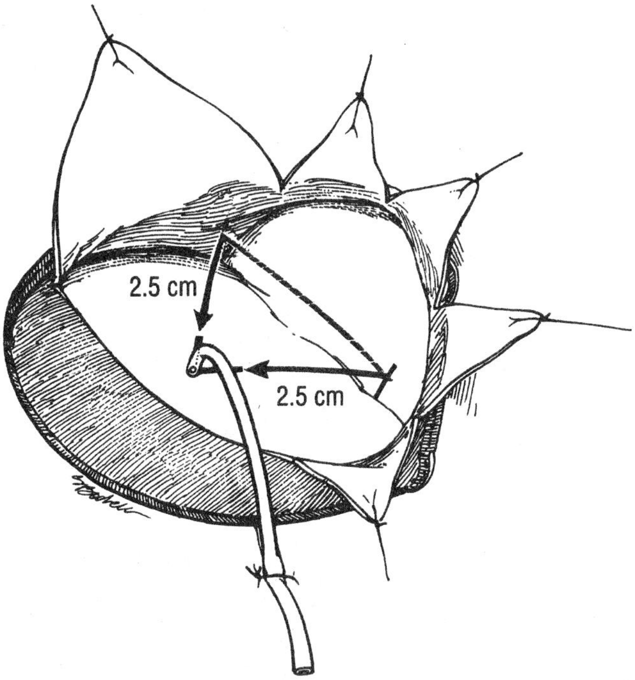

FIGURE 119–7. Reliable access to the frontal horn of the lateral ventricle may be obtained during a pterional craniotomy employing Paine's point. The landmarks for this point involve the creation of a 2.5-cm isosceles right triangle whose anterior limb abuts on the dura overlying the sphenoid ridge and whose posterior limb touches the sylvian fissure. The hypotenuse overlies the sylvian fissure. A Silastic brain catheter is used to enter the frontal cortex perpendicularly at the vertex of the triangle. (From Apuzzo MLJ [ed]: Brain Surgery: Complications, Avoidance and Management. New York, Churchill Livingstone, 1993.)

The dissection is begun into the opercular insular fissure about 2 cm posterior to the sphenoid ridge. We carry this dissection medially to incorporate the carotid cistern. A T-shaped incision is made in a posterolateral direction toward the insertion of cranial nerve III into the cavernous sinus. We then return to the lateral sylvian fissure and dissect the arachnoid down to the carotid bifurcation, effectively liberating the entire segment of the middle cerebral artery (i.e., MI segment). When necessary, bridging veins are coagulated and cut to facilitate the separation of the frontal and temporal lobes. In effect, this exposure allows for generous retraction on the frontal lobes without placing undue traction on the carotid segment of the anterior cerebral artery (i.e., A1), or M1.

We then turn our attention to the arachnoid, which tethers the gyrus rectus with the optic nerve. Dissecting the arachnoid further frees the frontal lobe and opens the prechiasmatic cistern. At this point, the temporal lobe is usually found to be displaced posteriorly, which can result in uncal tissue spreading medially and obstructing the view of the interpeduncular cistern. Although retraction of this tissue is an option, we have occasionally performed a subpial uncal resection with good results. For this approach, we routinely use frontal and temporal lobe retractors. When a significant amount of posterior temporal lobe retraction is needed, with or without conversion to a half-and-half or extended lateral approach, it is wise to coagulate and cut the veins that drain the temporal lobe into the sphenoparietal sinus. Rupture of one of these veins later could obstruct the view during a critical part of the procedure.

After temporal and frontal lobe retraction is optimal, we turn our attention to the three corridors that allow access to the interpeduncular cistern from this vantage point: the space between the carotid and the optic nerve, the retrocarotid space, and the area superior to the carotid bifurcation. Ideally, we dissect through each of these corridors to maximize the routes of access to the interpeduncular cistern. Individual anatomic variations may make one of these spaces more or less accessible. A medially displaced carotid, for example, makes the retrocarotid space more relevant for access. With these three windows in mind, we then identify the posterior communicating artery and dissect along its inferior surface toward its junction with the PCA. This is the safest approach to the basilar apex, because it avoids injury to the anterior thalamoperforating vessels and ensures that the dissection can lead to the inferior aspect of the P1-P2 junction (the P2 segment represents the PCA from the junction with the posterior communicating artery to where the artery passes the posterior midbrain). This prevents dissection superior to the P1 segment, which could result in perforator injury and an inadvertent and premature encounter with the aneurysm. After the P1-P2 junction is defined, we turn our attention to sharply opening the membrane of Liliequist inferiorly and medially. We then go back to the internal carotid artery and follow the posterior communicating artery posteriorly, further dissecting the membrane of Liliequist open. The described maneuvers widely expose the P1-P2 junction.

Our dissection then turns medially along the inferior edge of P1, across the front of the basilar apex toward the contralateral SCA and the inferior aspect of the contralateral P1. The inferior aspect is favored because perforators are spared and inadvertent aneurysmal rupture is avoided. At this point, we define an area on the basilar artery that can safely and comfortably accommodate a temporary clip. Occasionally, this area is below the SCA if the space between the PCAs and the SCAs is too narrow for a clip. After this is done, attention is turned to the superior aspect of the contralateral P1, where we dissect arachnoid adhesions and free perforators that may be adherent to the neck or dome. We then do the same for the ipsilateral P1.

After both P1s have been adequately dissected, we address the critical perforators that stream up the posterior aspect of the basilar artery and frequently adhere to the back wall of the aneurysm. Safe clipping should not be attempted until all these perforators are seen and freed. Using the suction tip, the aneurysmal dome can be gently moved forward to create a plane for the clip blade behind the basilar artery. This maneuver can be done more easily for most aneurysms if a temporary clip is on the basilar artery. We typically employ 10 to 15 minutes of temporary occlusion with the patient in burst suppression and mild hypothermia. When there is a need to access the aneurysm from above the carotid bifurcation, a space can be created by dissecting through the arachnoid that adheres to the perforators emanating from the M1 and A1 segments and gently elevating the optic tract.

Clip Application

The narrow confines of the interpeduncular cistern make adequate visualization during clip placement challenging. The clip applier can easily obstruct visualization. During clip application, it is useful to insert the ipsilateral blade gently along the neck while leaving the contralateral blade wide open. After the ipsilateral blade is in position, the mouthpiece can be used to shift the scope to see the contralateral neck. We have found several maneuvers to be extremely helpful in maximizing visualization during clipping. The first maneuver takes advantage of the wide dissection medial and lateral to the carotid, which was described earlier. A right-handed surgeon operating from the right-hand side can insert the clip and clip applier lateral to the carotid and insert the suction medial to the carotid. This prevents the loss of vision, which can be caused by the clip applier. A left-handed surgeon can similarly insert the clip applier and clip medial to the carotid while inserting the suction tip lateral to the carotid. Another maneuver involves using an inverted bayoneted clip to avoid visual obstruction. Great care must be exercised to avoid using a clip that is too long, because this risks perforator and brainstem injury. After the clip is applied, vigilant inspection of the clip blades must be performed to ensure complete neck clipping and to make sure that no perforators were enclosed in the clips.

The pterional view can be enhanced by the orbitozygomatic approach.[31] We have found that this approach works for extremely high aneurysms, but for most other basilar apex aneurysms, this approach does not contribute significantly.

Subtemporal Approach

Most basilar apex aneurysms that were treated in London, Ontario, by Dr. Drake were treated with a subtemporal approach.[8] Several situations make this approach preferable to the trans-sylvian route. Aneurysms arising below the middle depth of the sella turcica are not easily clippable from a trans-sylvian view. Aneurysms with a posterior projection pose special risks, because it is extremely difficult to see the perforators when approaching these aneurysms from the trans-sylvian corridor. The subtemporal approach allows the surgeon to dissect the perforators off the posterior wall of the aneurysm and visualize the clip placement across the neck. Large aneurysms that project anteriorly may be difficult to clip from a trans-sylvian route because of the limited working space and restricted visualization imposed by the aneurysm. These situations are managed well from a subtemporal approach. For this reason, detailed familiarity with this approach is important for the basilar apex aneurysm surgeon.

A right-sided approach usually is preferable to prevent damaging the dominant temporal lobe. Several circumstances make a left-sided approach more reasonable. A left cranial nerve III palsy or right hemiparesis mandates a left-sided approach to avoid injury to the right cranial nerve III and cerebral peduncle. Occasionally, a tilt of the basilar apex can elevate one P1 significantly above the other. If the left PCA is significantly higher than the right PCA, a right-sided approach could risk trapping the left PCA in the clip blades.

CSF drainage is paramount to the success of this approach. When the subtemporal approach is used, we place lumbar drains routinely in the operating room before positioning the patient. CSF drainage is particularly important after subarachnoid hemorrhage. When positioning the Mayfield fixation device, the surgeon should always consider the possibility of needing to convert to a trans-sylvian approach; the ability to do this without redraping is obviously advantageous. After the Mayfield head frame has been positioned with one pin over the forehead and two pins over the occiput, we place the patient on her or his side and allow the dependent arm to rest in a sling. We use gel pads to protect the axilla. The chest area, hips, and legs are appropriately padded and taped to the operating table (Fig. 119–8). After the body is well positioned, we elevate the head slightly and then tilt the vertex 10 to 20 degrees below horizontal to allow the temporal lobe to fall away from the middle fossa floor, minimizing retraction and maximizing the working space.

For unruptured aneurysms, we use a straight incision, which extends 10 cm up from a point 1 cm anterior to the tragus (Fig. 119–9). The craniotomy is then based over the zygomatic root and has a diameter of approximately 3.5 cm. For patients with recent subarachnoid hemorrhage, we favor a larger craniotomy.

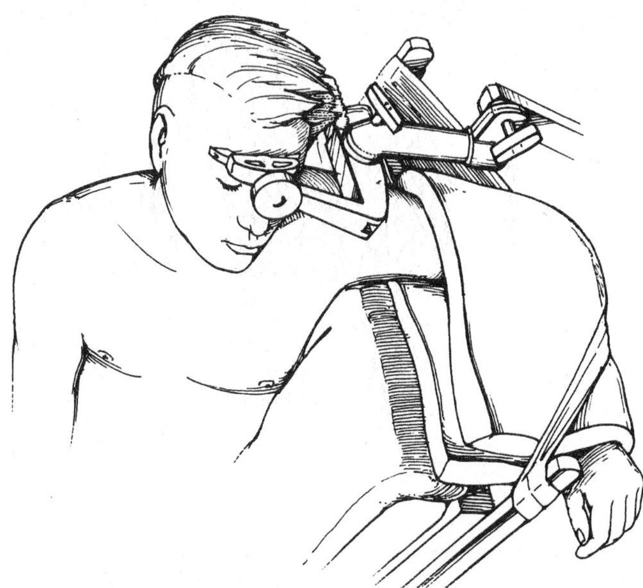

FIGURE 119–8. Positioning for a subtemporal approach. (From Apuzzo MLJ [ed]: Brain Surgery: Complications, Avoidance and Management. New York, Churchill Livingstone, 1993.)

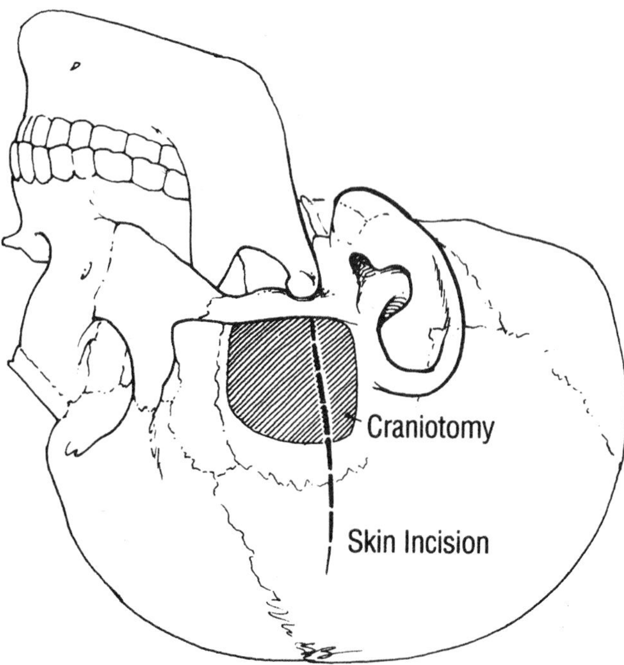

FIGURE 119–9. Skin incision and craniotomy for a subtemporal approach for an unruptured aneurysm. (From Apuzzo MLJ [ed]: Brain Surgery: Complications, Avoidance and Management. New York, Churchill Livingstone, 1993.)

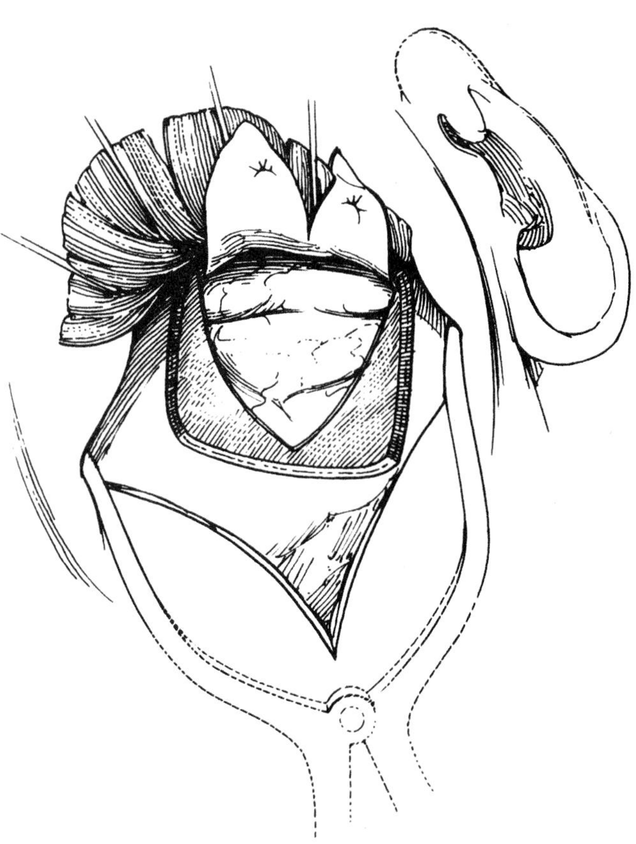

FIGURE 119–11. Dura tacked up for a subtemporal exposure. (From Apuzzo MLJ [ed]: Brain Surgery: Complications, Avoidance and Management. New York, Churchill Livingstone, 1993.)

We use an upside-down horseshoe incision and then perform a craniotomy in addition to an anterior craniectomy (Fig. 119–10). The wider exposure allows temporal lobe resection if it is needed for further exposure. Resection of bone down to the floor of the middle fossa minimizes the need for brain retraction. After the craniotomy, the dura is opened in a cruciate fashion such that the inferior limb can be secured inferiorly to minimize extradural bleeding and maximize exposure (Fig. 119–11). Hyperventilation, diuresis, and lumbar drainage often result in sufficient brain relaxation to maneuver subtemporally. In patients with a recent hemorrhage, these maneuvers may not be sufficient. In this situation, we have frequently resected the inferior temporal gyrus with the fusiform and parahippocampal gyri. We have not noticed any increased morbidity associated with this method, and the resulting exposure is usually excellent. When resorting to this resection, we have found it helpful to leave the medial pia-arachnoid tissue to serve as an anchor for the retractor. When the uncus is elevated, cranial nerve III elevates with the uncus. To further enhance exposure, we place a tentorial stitch as advocated by Drake.[8] This stitch is placed posterior to the dural insertion of cranial nerve IV. For extremely low-lying aneurysms, splitting the tentorium may be necessary. Bleeding can be minimized by aggressively coagulating the tentorium over the incision site and by placing small pieces of cotton in the leaflets of the dura with a nerve hook.

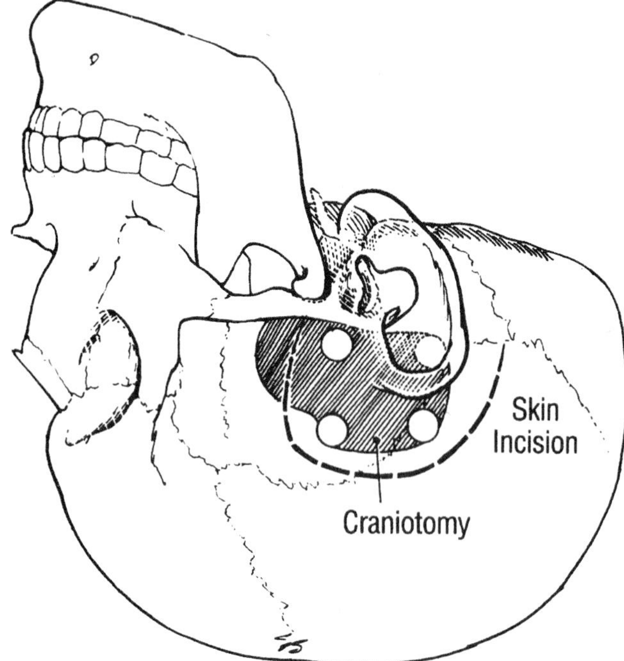

FIGURE 119–10. Skin incision and craniotomy for a subtemporal approach for a ruptured aneurysm. (From Apuzzo MLJ [ed]: Brain Surgery: Complications, Avoidance and Management. New York, Churchill Livingstone, 1993.)

After adequate exposure is achieved, the arachnoid between cranial nerve III and the uncus should be excised. The next structure to be identified is the SCA as it curves back around the cerebral peduncle into the ambient cistern. The surgeon then follows the SCA medially toward the basilar artery. The basilar artery can be cleared anteriorly and posteriorly for a temporary clip. The inferior margin of the ipsilateral P1 is then identified, and dissection is carried across the anterior aspect of the basilar artery to the contralateral P1. Mistaking the contralateral SCA for the P1 can lead to occlusion of the contralateral P1 and its perforators with a clip. The SCA is differentiated from the PCA by remembering that the PCA is usually larger and invested with thicker tissue, whereas the SCA is usually red. The surgeon can be definitive about this decision by continuing the dissection across to the P1-P2 junction and identifying the posterior communicating artery and cranial nerve III passing between the SCA and the P1.

After the anterior aspect of the basilar artery and both P1 origins have been identified and dissected of arachnoid adhesions and blood, attention is turned to the posterior aspect of the aneurysm complex. Perforators emanating from the posterior wall of the basilar artery are often adherent to the neck and must be dissected free. This dissection is best started at the ipsilateral P1 and carried to the contralateral P1. The goal of this dissection is to create room for safe application of an aneurysm clip. Clip length should match the neck length as closely as possible because excessively long clips risk occluding medial perforators emanating from the contralateral P1. Although anteriorly projecting aneurysms may obscure the contralateral P1, the contralateral P1 occasionally can be visualized during the final phases of clip closure. Control of the microscope with the mouthpiece allows subtle maneuvering that can enhance visualization on both sides of the aneurysm during clip closure.

The subtemporal approach provides excellent simultaneous access of posterior carotid wall aneurysms. After a basilar apex aneurysm has been addressed, the microscope can be redirected anteriorly to address other carotid artery aneurysms.

Pterional Approach Through the Extended Lateral Corridor

The main limitation of the subtemporal approach is the limited ability to see the contralateral P1 and its medial perforators. In contrast, the trans-sylvian approach is limited by poor visualization of the posterior perforators of the basilar artery. In an effort to combine the advantages of the subtemporal and trans-sylvian approaches while minimizing the limitations of each we have developed a modified approach, the pterional approach via the extended lateral corridor (PAVEL).[32] This extended lateral exposure has eliminated most of the risks and liabilities of the pure trans-sylvian and the subtemporal approaches, and we employ it for the treatment of most patients with upper basilar aneurysms. The essential elements of PAVEL include the following:

1. It is performed from the surgeon's dominant side, which facilitates a due lateral dissection plane and clipping.
2. Thorough dissection of the sylvian fissure is possible.
3. The surgical field is centered on cranial nerve III.
4. Mesial temporal lobe structures are elevated out of the incisura to the level of the cerebral peduncle.
5. Posterior dissection is performed behind and below ipsilateral P1, not through the neck.
6. The initial clip is fenestrated with a very small blade to close the contralateral neck.
7. The final clip is a short, conventional clip to eliminate residual neck filling through fenestration.

The patient is positioned as for a pterional craniotomy. The head is rotated no more than 30 degrees away from the operative side to minimize the temporal lobe falling into the surgical field. A frontotemporal scalp incision is extended down to the zygoma. The scalp is incised to the subgaleal plane but not through the temporalis fascia. As the scalp is reflected anteriorly in the subgaleal plane, we use an interfascial technique to identify the fat pad containing the frontalis branch of the fascial nerve. This tissue is dissected away from the temporalis fascia to minimize retraction on the nerve. The temporalis muscle is divided along the zygoma, the anterior temporal squama, and the superior temporal line and reflected posteriorly, as described by Heros.[33] These maneuvers minimize obstruction of the view along the skull base and usually obviate the need for a skull base approach such as the orbitozygomatic approach.

The craniotomy is performed with bur holes in the keyhole, at the posterior exposure of the superior temporal line, and at the root of the zygoma. A power craniotome is used to connect the bur holes and to extend the flap anteriorly to the mid-supraorbital ridge, yielding a rectangular free bone flap. An extensive subtemporal craniectomy is then performed to provide generous exposure of the anterior temporal tip. Gentle elevation of the temporal lobe opens a lateral view of the interpeduncular cistern. A Micro-Aire drill and rongeurs are used to remove the inner table and thin the diploë of the frontal bone from the sphenoid ridge to the anterior extent of the flap. This provides additional exposure along the skull base and limits frontal lobe retraction. The sphenoid ridge is then drilled down to a degree that creates a continuous, unobstructed view along the skull base from the middle fossa floor to the floor of the frontal fossa. This extensive bony resection is essential to providing an unobstructed view of the basal cisterns while minimizing the need for brain retraction.

DURAL OPENING

After the bony resection is complete, the dura is opened with a semilunar incision extending from the anterior extent of the exposed frontal floor superiorly across the sylvian fissure to the posteroinferior extent of the exposed middle fossa floor. The dural flap can then be reflected anteroinferiorly with its base flush against the skull base.

CEREBROSPINAL FLUID DRAINAGE, HYPERVENTILATION, AND DIURESIS

As with the traditional approaches, CSF drainage, hyperventilation, and diuresis are critical for maximizing the view of the basilar apex without excessive brain retraction. CSF drainage can be accomplished by lumbar drainage or intraoperative ventricular puncture. We use the previously described Paine's point to accurately tap the ventricle.[34]

MICRODISSECTION

Initial attention is given to the opercular-insular segment and then to the sphenoidal segment of the sylvian fissure. A brain microretractor is used to elevate the frontal lobe and stretch the arachnoid of the sylvian fissure. Completely dissecting M1 free after widely opening the fissure prevents kinking of M1 or its branches during subsequent frontal and temporal lobe retraction. The dissection is carried medially with the goal of opening the optic carotid and prechiasmatic cisterns and further freeing the frontal lobe.

Attention is then focused on elevating the temporal lobe out of the middle fossa. The bridging veins connecting the temporal lobe and the floor of the middle fossa are cauterized and cut. The arachnoid connecting cranial nerve III and the uncus is divided. These maneuvers facilitate mobilizing the uncus out of the tentorial incisura. The dissection is continued posteriorly until the P2 segment of the PCA is seen passing superior to cranial nerve III. During dissection, the microsurgical field is centered on cranial nerve III, and the anterior choroidal artery is followed to the choroidal fissure. A microretractor is then brought in at a 90-degree angle to retract the uncus laterally. In this way, the tentorial incisura is cleared of any obstruction as far posteriorly as the cerebral peduncle.

Arachnoidal microdissection is completed in the optic carotid triangle, the retrocarotid space along the posterior communicating artery, and the supracarotid space above the bifurcation. At this stage, the membrane of Liliequist comes into view and is opened to reveal the contents of the interpeduncular cistern. The SCA is then identified below cranial nerve III. Dissection is carried medially to the basilar trunk, where a temporary clip site is identified. Cranial nerve III is used to identify the P1-P2 junction, and the P1 segment is followed medially to the basilar apex. The arachnoid anterior to the apex is dissected until the contralateral P1 segment is identified.

The safest and most effective way to clear the posteriorly located perforators is to begin the dissection proximal to the ipsilateral P1, not through the original neck of the aneurysm. As all aneurysm surgeons know, there is always some expansion of the basilar artery inferior to the P1 as a transition into the neck. The anteroposterior Towne's view is misleading in this regard, and this posterior tissue is a common site of residual aneurysm, which may regrow over the years. As the P1 is mobilized anteriorly with suction, the surgeon's dominant hand can enter from a due lateral trajectory to sharply dissect the ipsilateral and then contralateral thalamoperforators from posterior to the complex. This dissection occurs exactly as it would during a subtemporal approach. With experience, it is possible to recognize the difference in course between the ipsilateral and contralateral perforators. This is critical because the contralateral P1 is rarely seen from behind the complex. The initial course of each P1 almost always runs anteriorly. Clearing of the contralateral perforators marks the definitive posterior neck and dissection.

Clipping is performed to maximally use the advantages of the exposure. We typically perform clipping in two stages. The first stage has the goal of closing the contralateral neck and gathering the broad neck. This can be done using a fenestrated clip with a very short blade and keeping the ipsilateral P1 and part of the ipsilateral neck in the fenestration. If performed from the surgeon's dominant side, the clip applier can be brought in from a true lateral trajectory. The posterior blade is passed first, and exposure is maintained with the suction tube. After the posterior blade is in position, the mouthpiece is used to shift the scope anteriorly to benefit from the anterior trans-sylvian portion of the exposure. The contralateral P1 is seen, and the anterior blade is closed to perfectly seal the contralateral neck. At this point, residual filling often can be seen through the fenestration. This residual aneurysm neck is clipped superior to the P1 with a short, conventional blade that kisses the end of the fenestration of the primary clip.

Timing of Treatment

The peak incidence of repeat hemorrhage after subarachnoid hemorrhage occurs in the first 48 hours.[35] The peak incidence of vasospasm occurs 7 to 10 days after subarachnoid hemorrhage.[36] Early surgery after subarachnoid hemorrhage avoids the morbidity and mortality associated with repeat hemorrhage and allows aggressive medical management of vasospasm.[37] However, certain patients with basilar apex aneurysms may be harmed by early surgery. It has been our practice to delay surgery in the high-grade patient (i.e., Hunt and Hess grades 4 and 5) for a few days. We have frequently considered partial or complete endovascular treatment for patients with high clinical grades. Of the various approaches, we have found that the subtemporal approach is particularly not well tolerated soon after hemorrhage in the high-grade patient. We have occasionally used aminocaproic acid for patients for whom we delay surgery, particularly if the subarachnoid portion of the bleeding is modest.

Temporary Occlusion

Proximal occlusion and trapping have important roles in basilar apex aneurysm surgery. The application of cerebral protectants such as etomidate or propofol to achieve burst suppression coupled with mild hypothermia (32°C to 34°C) has increased the safety of temporary occlusion.[38, 39] Temporary occlusion allows the surgeon to soften the sac sufficiently to visualize the posterior perforators and safely place a clip and to mobilize the sac out of the interpeduncular cistern for posteriorly projecting aneurysms. Proximal occlusion often is insufficient, and complete trapping is needed, as in the case of thrombotic giants. In this situation, an anterior approach is advantageous because the contralateral P1 can be well visualized. The amount of time available for temporary occlusion is not entirely clear and may vary and depend on complex parameters, which are not yet easily decipherable. In a study considering 121 patients, patient age older than 61 years and poor neurological grade (i.e., Hunt and Hess grades 3 to 4) were associated with decreased tolerance for temporary occlusion compared with younger and better grade patients.[39] In this study, patients occluded for less than 14 minutes did not develop infarcts, whereas those occluded for greater than 31 minutes routinely developed an infarct. Although not statistically significant, there was a trend toward more infarction for occlusions proximal to perforator segments of the M1 and basilar artery and for increasing episodes of temporary occlusion.

Complication Avoidance

As for any other surgery, approaching the operation with a clear understanding of all complications and strategies for avoidance is paramount to achieving good results. However, with surgery in this area, even technical perfection can result in complications. One of the earliest technical challenges of surgery in the interpeduncular cistern was described by Drake: preservation of the perforators. Even transient occlusion of a perforator with a temporary clip can injure the vessel permanently. Temporary occlusion should be used when it can result in better visualization of the posterior perforators. This is particularly true of large aneurysms. Sharp dissection, maximal illumination, and the microscope mouthpiece are essential to safe and effective perforator visualization and dissection.

Leaving neck remnants can result in delayed aneurysm growth and hemorrhage.[40–43] Whenever feasible, a second, small "baby clip" should be used to occlude neck remnants or "dog ears." When these remnants cannot be tackled safely, the patient should be followed with serial angiography. The follow-up interval has not been determined. Computed tomography–angiography may serve this purpose well. Clear distinction should be made between neck remnants and residual aneurysm fundus. The latter represents a much more dangerous and unstable situation. Such situations should be managed promptly with reoperation[42, 44, 45] if deemed feasible or with endovascular coiling.[46–49]

Intraoperative rupture is perhaps the most notorious intraoperative complication in aneurysm surgery.[50] This complication is particularly dangerous for basilar apex aneurysms. When rupture does occur, the patient should be placed in burst suppression if this has not already been done. Gentle tamponade with a small piece of cotton is often effective. If tamponade fails within 5 minutes, temporary occlusion should be seriously considered. Prophylactic temporary occlusion in our opinion also reduces the incidence of intraoperative rupture.[39]

The different approaches have their own complications. The subtemporal approach can be associated with temporal lobe swelling and herniation postoperatively. Serious consideration should be given to partial or complete anterior temporal lobectomy when the temporal lobe appears "boggy." We think the subtemporal approach should be avoided in the acute setting in the high-grade patient. The vein of Labbé should be respected with this approach. We have found that placing moist Gelfoam and cottonoids on the vein and its connection with the transverse or sigmoid sinus before retraction helps avoid injury. The trans-sylvian approach can be associated with kinking of the M1 and its branches, with resulting postoperative infarction.[51] In treating giant aneurysms, we avoid overly aggressive evacuation of the sac because collapse of the large sac may injure perforators due to an "accordion" phenomenon.

ENDOVASCULAR MANAGEMENT OF BASILAR APEX ANEURYSMS

Since 1990, aneurysm coiling for some aneurysms has improved the natural history of subarachnoid hemorrhage during short-term follow-up.[27, 52] The effect on long-term hemorrhage rates of ruptured and unruptured aneurysms remains to be determined. During the same period, experience has accumulated regarding the use of Guglielmi detachable coils (GDCs) in the management of basilar apex aneurysms. Lessons have been learned regarding the safety, efficacy, limitations, and durability of coiling in this area. In a multicenter study of coiling for basilar apex aneurysms,[53] the periprocedural mortality rate was 2.7%. During follow-up, mortality rates of 23% for ruptured aneurysms and 12% for unruptured aneurysms were seen. Rebleeding occurred for 3.3% of ruptured aneurysms and 4.1% of unruptured aneurysms. These statistics imply that, although procedural morbidity and mortality may be competitive with surgery, the durability and efficacy of this approach are still in question. Although multiple other studies have demonstrated short-term safety and efficacy, long-term data continue to be lacking in the literature.[23, 24, 54] In the following sections, we consider three strategies: coiling as a curative modality, coiling as a temporizing measure, and coiling as an adjunct to surgery.

Coiling As a Curative Strategy

The word *cure* should be used with caution when addressing coil embolization of cerebral aneurysms because long-term results have not been determined. Experience with aneurysms at the basilar apex and elsewhere has demonstrated that the efficacy, safety, and durability of endovascular treatment are mainly a function of the morphology of the aneurysm. The three most important factors are aneurysm neck size, aneurysm size, and the relationship of the PCAs to the aneurysm.[26, 54–56] Recurrence and suboptimal treatment have been demonstrated in large, giant, and wide-necked aneurysms.[25, 57] In a study by Raymond and colleagues of 31 patients treated with GDCs for basilar apex aneurysms, 29% of wide-necked aneurysms had a significant rate of recurrence.[57] For patients with aneurysm necks less than 4 mm, 77% had complete aneurysm occlusion.[57] The relationship of the posterior communicating arteries to the aneurysm is a significant determinant of whether complete aneurysm occlusion can be achieved. In a nonselected study population with basilar apex aneurysms, Klein and colleagues[23] produced PCA occlusion in 5 patients (24%). This study highlights the fact that PCA anatomy can prevent complete aneurysm occlusion in a significant number of aneurysms. To achieve complete aneurysm occlusion safely in a high percentage of patients, GDC coiling should be limited to small aneurysms with neck sizes less than 4 mm and PCAs that do not originate from the dome.

Guglielmi Detachable Coils As a Temporizing Measure

When an aneurysm is not suitable for complete endovascular cure by the previously mentioned criteria or surgery is not safe in an acute situation (e.g., high-grade patient), partial treatment can be performed to reduce the risk of repeat hemorrhage. It is important when using this strategy to balance the protective effect with the need to clip the aneurysm in the future. Overpacking the dome may make surgery more difficult,[54] but underpacking may not be protective. Although our center and others have used this strategy, sufficient data are lacking to validate this approach.

Coiling As an Adjunct to Surgery

Coiling can be used to treat aneurysm remnants or recurrences. Remnants are usually the result of anatomic limitations in experienced hands. If the remnant is larger than 2 mm and is at least as deep as it is wide, coiling may be feasible.[47–49, 58–60] Although reoperation is an option for some recurrences, scarring can be a prohibitive factor.[45]

POSTERIOR CEREBRAL ARTERY ANATOMY

The PCA supplies portions of the temporal, parietal, and occipital lobes; the thalamus midbrain; and other deep structures, such as the choroid plexus of the third and lateral ventricles. The PCA irrigates several centers that play integral roles in vision. Although various classifications have been used to describe the PCA, the one used and popularized by Rhoton's laboratory is the most widely used.[61] In this classification, the PCA is divided into P1, P2A, P2B, and P3 segments. The P1 segment extends from the PCA origin to the posterior communicating artery. The P2 segment, which represents the PCA to the area where it passes the posterior midbrain, is bisected equally into the P2A and P2B segments. The P3 segment extends posteriorly from the pulvinar into the lateral aspect of the quadrigeminal cistern and ends at the anterior limit of the calcarine fissure. The point where the PCAs from each side are nearest is referred to as the collicular or quadrigeminal point.

The main branches of the P1 segment are the anatomically variable and highly critical posterior thalamoperforators (the anterior thalamoperforators originate on the posterior communicating artery). The thalamoperforators almost invariably arise from the posterior and superior surface of the P1s.[62] It is for this reason that dissection of the P1 during basilar apex surgery should commence on the inferior surface of P1, as was often advocated by Drake.[6, 8, 63] The P2 segment, also called the *ambient segment,* sweeps around the cerebral peduncle above the level of the tentorium. The P2 segment has brainstem branches, ventricular branches, and cortical branches. The brainstem branches consist of one to seven thalamogeniculate arteries, which supply the thalamus, posterior limb of the internal capsule, geniculate bodies, and optic tract. Peduncular perforating branches also arise from P2. The medial and lateral posterior choroidal branches emanate from P2. The inferior temporal group of arteries is one of four PCA cortical branches, and they arise from the P2, whereas other cortical branches originate more distally. The cortical branches consist of the parieto-occipital artery, the calcarine artery, and the splenial arteries. Greater anatomic detail on the PCA if offered in the classic manuscript by Zeal and Rhoton.[61]

ANEURYSMS OF THE POSTERIOR CEREBRAL ARTERY

PCA aneurysms are rare lesions comprising 0.7% to 2.2% of published series.[64–75] Most older published series probably underestimated the incidence of PCA aneurysms because posterior circulation angiography was not performed routinely for aneurysm workups in earlier series. Of 118 PCA aneurysms identified in the literature by Zeal and Rhoton,[61] 55 could be localized to a specific PCA segment. Fifteen percent arose on the P1 segment, 16% at the P1-P2 junction, 20% on the proximal P2A, 36% on the distal P2A and P2B, and 13% further distally. Compared with other types of aneurysms, a larger proportion of PCA aneurysms tend to be giant. Of 14 PCA aneurysms reported by Yasargil, 7 (50%) were giant.[65] In Drake's report on his experience with PCA aneurysms, 13 (42%) of 31 aneurysms were giant.[72] We have found that PCA aneurysms that appear to be irregular may be dissecting aneurysms. In a 20-year experience at the Mayo Clinic, which was reviewed by Meyer and coworkers,[76] 24 of 1387 aneurysms were in patients younger than 18 years of age.

Of these 24 aneurysms, 4 were in the PCA and all 4 were giant aneurysms.[76] Fusiform and serpentine aneurysms are also seen in the PCA distribution.[74] These may result from atherosclerosis or "healing" dissections.

Surgical Approaches

The various approaches discussed earlier for basilar apex aneurysms can be used to approach aneurysms of the P1 segment. Aneurysms of the P2 can be approached subtemporally. P2 aneurysms that are high in relation to the tentorium can be accessed by opening the occipitotemporal sulcus, entering the temporal horn of the lateral ventricle, and reaching the ambient cistern through the choroidal fissure.[77] P3 aneurysms usually require an occipital interhemispheric approach. The tentorium may need to be cut to better visualize P3 aneurysms. Computed tomography–angiography combined with three-dimensional angiography can be extremely helpful in mapping a comfortable route of access to these aneurysms.

Because a large proportion of PCA aneurysms are giant or fusiform, clipping is often not an option. Controversy exists regarding the need for revascularization when hunterian ligation or trapping is performed for PCA aneurysms. Early in the history of treating PCA aneurysms, it was noticed that excellent collateral circulation often protects the PCA distribution from infarction. In nine cases that required P1 or P2 occlusion without revascularization, only one in Drake's series of PCA aneurysms suffered ischemic complications.[72] PCA revascularization, although possible, is technically challenging and carries definite risks. We have used trial balloon occlusion as a way to determine tolerance to proximal PCA occlusion, and although we are encouraged by the result of this technique, the sensitivity and specificity of this test have not been determined. Most PCA aneurysm trapping or proximal ligations reported in the literature have been treated without revascularization.[74] When trapping these lesions, clear visualization of adjacent perforators is critical during clip placement. Although not foolproof, a patent posterior communicating artery usually implies tolerance to P1 occlusion. The overall outcome of patients with PCA aneurysms is significantly better than for others with aneurysms in the posterior circulation.[67, 72]

Endovascular Management of Posterior Cerebral Artery Aneurysms

Three main factors make surgery a superior option for most PCA aneurysms. First, the surgery has a proven efficacy and relatively low morbidity in treating these aneurysms. Second, the morphology of these aneurysms is often not amenable to coiling; a large proportion of these aneurysms are giant or fusiform. Third, the plethora of critical perforators on the PCA makes precise occlusion mandatory. Clipping continues to be more precise in this regard. However, there are several scenarios in which coiling may be on par or better suited for the patient:

1. Patients who cannot tolerate surgery because of medical conditions
2. Poor-grade patients, although the risks of repeat hemorrhage must be weighed against the perceived efficacy and safety of the endovascular option
3. Small saccular aneurysms with narrow necks (i.e., dome-to-neck ratio greater than or equal to 2 or neck size smaller than 5 mm)
4. Patients who have arteriovenous malformations and diminished flow-related PCA aneurysms

Endovascular options such as surgery depend on the morphology of the aneurysm. Small aneurysms with suitable necks can be coiled. Occlusion of the parent vessel can be achieved by coiling the aneurysm and the parent vessel at the level of the neck. Encouraging results using these strategies have been reported.[78] In our opinion, trial balloon occlusion of the PCA should be studied further as a helpful tool in determining treatment options and need for revascularization.

CONCLUSIONS

Successful management of PCA and basilar apex aneurysms can be achieved with a clear understanding of the anatomy of the respective vessels and the areas surrounding the aneurysm. These aneurysms require well-designed strategies and carefully executed plans. A clear understanding of the advantages and disadvantages of surgical and endovascular options should lead to better clinical decision making. Although the rhetoric has focused on determining the superiority of one technique over another, the future will likely reveal that both methodologies will find wide applications that will be determined on a case-by-case basis.

Patients with these conditions are optimally managed by a cerebrovascular team with substantial experience. Over time, most teams will be serving tertiary or quaternary referral centers. Necessary components of such teams include cerebrovascular neurosurgeons, diagnostic neuroradiologists, endovascular surgeons, critical care physicians, internists, and highly experienced neuroanesthesiologists.

REFERENCES

1. Rice B, Peerless S, Drake C: Surgical treatment of unruptured aneurysms of the posterior circulation. J Neurosurg 73:165–173, 1990.
2. Peerless S, Hernesniemi J, Gutman C, Drake C: Early surgery for ruptured posterior circulation aneurysms. J Neurosurg 80: 643–649, 1994.
3. Drake C: Bleeding aneurysms of the basilar artery: Direct surgical management in four cases. J Neurosurg 18:230, 1961.
4. Drake C: Surgical treatment of ruptured aneurysms of the basilar artery: Experience with 14 cases. J Neurosurg 23:457, 1965.
5. Drake CG: Further experience with surgical treatment of aneurysm of the basilar artery. J Neurosurg 29:372–392, 1968.
6. Drake C: The surgical treatment of aneurysms of the basilar artery. J Neurosurg 29:436–446, 1968.
7. Drake C: The surgical treatment of the vertebral-basilar aneurysms. Clin Neurosurg 16:114–169, 1969.
8. Drake CG: The treatment of aneurysms of the posterior circulation. Clin Neurosurg 26:96–144, 1979.
9. Peerless S, Drake C: Management of aneurysms of the posterior

circulation. In Youmans J (ed): Neurological Surgery. A Comprehensive Reference Guide to the Diagnosis and Management of Neurosurgical Problems, 3rd ed. Philadelphia, WB Saunders, 1990, pp 1764–1806.
10. Batjer HH, Samson DS: Causes of morbidity and mortality from surgery of aneurysms of the distal basilar artery. Neurosurgery 25:904–915, discussion 915–916, 1989.
11. Chou SN, Ortiz-Suarez HJ: Surgical treatment of arterial aneurysms of the vertebrobasilar circulation. J Neurosurg 41:671–680, 1974.
12. Dolenc V: A transcavernous-transsellar approach to the basilar tip aneurysms. Br J Neurosurg 1:251, 1987.
13. Hakuba A, Liu S, Nishimura S: The orbitozygomatic infratemporal approach: A new surgical technique. Surg Neurol 26:271, 1986.
14. Jamieson K: Aneurysms of the vertebrobasilar system: surgical intervention in 19 cases. J Neurosurg 21:781, 1968.
15. Kodama N, Kamiyama K, Mineura K, et al: [Surgical treatment of vertebrobasilar aneurysms (author's translation)]. No Shinkei Geka 7:321–329, 1979.
16. MacFarlane M, McAllister V, Whitby D, Sengupta R: Posterior circulation aneurysms: Results of direct operations. Surg Neurol 20:399, 1983.
17. McMurtry JG, Housepian EM, Bowman FO Jr, Matteo RS: Surgical treatment of basilar artery aneurysms. Elective circulatory arrest with thoracotomy in 12 cases. J Neurosurg 40:486–494, 1974.
18. Ojemann R, Crowell R: Surgical Management of Cerebrovascular Disease. Baltimore, Williams & Wilkins, 1988.
19. Samson DS, Hodosh RM, Clark WK: Microsurgical evaluation of the pterional approach to aneurysms of the distal basilar circulation. Neurosurgery 3:135–141, 1978.
20. Lawton MT: Basilar apex aneurysms: Surgical results and perspectives from an initial experience. Neurosurgery 50:1–10, 2002.
21. Samson D, Batjer HH, Kopitnik TA Jr: Current results of the surgical management of aneurysms of the basilar apex. Neurosurgery 44:697–702, discussion 702–704, 1999.
22. Wascher T, Spetzler R: Saccular aneurysms of the basilar bifurcation. In Carter LP, Spetzler RF, Hamilton MG (eds): Neurovascular Surgery. New York, McGraw-Hill, 1995, pp 729–752.
23. Klein GE, Szolar DH, Leber KA, et al: Basilar tip aneurysm: Endovascular treatment with Guglielmi detachable coils—midterm results. Radiology 205:191–196, 1997.
24. Tateshima S, Murayama Y, Gobin YP, et al: Endovascular treatment of basilar tip aneurysms using Guglielmi detachable coils: Anatomic and clinical outcomes in 73 patients from a single institution. Neurosurgery 47:1332–1339, discussion 1339–1342, 2000.
25. Malisch TW, Guglielmi G, Vinuela F, et al: Intracranial aneurysms treated with the Guglielmi detachable coil: Midterm clinical results in a consecutive series of 100 patients. J Neurosurg 87: 176–183, 1997.
26. Turjman F, Massoud TF, Sayre J, Vinuela F: Predictors of aneurysmal occlusion in the period immediately after endovascular treatment with detachable coils: A multivariate analysis. AJNR Am J Neuroradiol 19:1645–1651, 1998.
27. Vinuela F, Duckwiler G, Mawad M: Guglielmi detachable coil embolization of acute intracranial aneurysm: Perioperative anatomical and clinical outcome in 403 patients. J Neurosurg 86: 475–482, 1997.
28. Wollschlaeger G, Wollschlaeger PB, Lucas FV, Lopez VF: Experience and result with postmortem cerebral angiography performed as routine procedure of the autopsy. Am J Roentgenol Radium Ther Nucl Med 101:68–87, 1967.
29. Krayenbuhl H, Yasargil M: Cerebral Angiography. Philadelphia, JB Lippincott, 1968.
30. Yasargil M: Operative anatomy. In Yasargil M (ed): Microneurosurgery. Stuttgart, George Thieme Verlag, 1984, p 5.
31. Zabramski JM, Kiris T, Sankhla SK, et al: Orbitozygomatic craniotomy: Technical note. J Neurosurg 89:336–341, 1998.
32. Ciacci J, Bendok B, Getch C, Batjer H: Pterional approach to distal basilar aneurysms via the extended lateral corridor: PAVEL. Tech Neurosurg 6:221–227, 2000.
33. Heros RC, Lee SH: The combined pterional/anterior temporal approach for aneurysms of the upper basilar complex: Technical report. Neurosurgery 33:244–250, discussion 250–251, 1993.
34. Paine JT, Batjer HH, Samson D: Intraoperative ventricular puncture. Neurosurgery 22:1107–1109, 1988.
35. Kassell NF, Torner JC: Aneurysmal rebleeding: A preliminary report from the Cooperative Aneurysm Study. Neurosurgery 13: 479–481, 1983.
36. Kwak R, Niizuma H, Ohi T, Suzuki J: Angiographic study of cerebral vasospasm following rupture of intracranial aneurysms. Part I. Time of the appearance. Surg Neurol 11:257–262, 1979.
37. Bendok BR, Getch CC, Malisch TW, Batjer HH: Treatment of aneurysmal subarachnoid hemorrhage. Semin Neurol 18:521–531, 1998.
38. Batjer HH, Frankfurt AI, Purdy PD, et al: Use of etomidate, temporary arterial occlusion, and intraoperative angiography in surgical treatment of large and giant cerebral aneurysms. J Neurosurg 68:234–240, 1988.
39. Samson D, Batjer HH, Bowman G, et al: A clinical study of the parameters and effects of temporary arterial occlusion in the management of intracranial aneurysms. Neurosurgery 34:22–28, discussion 28–29, 1994.
40. Lin T, Fox AJ, Drake CG: Regrowth of aneurysm sacs from residual neck following aneurysm clipping. J Neurosurg 70:556–560, 1989.
41. Ebina K, Suzuki M, Andoh A, et al: Recurrence of cerebral aneurysm after initial neck clipping. Neurosurgery 11:764–768, 1982.
42. Drake CG, Friedman AH, Peerless SJ: Failed aneurysm surgery. Reoperation in 115 cases. J Neurosurg 61:848–856, 1984.
43. Feuerberg I, Lindquist C, Lindqvist M, Steiner L: Natural history of postoperative aneurysm rests. J Neurosurg 66:30–34, 1987.
44. Batjer HH, Samson DS: Reoperation for aneurysms and vascular malformations. Clin Neurosurg 39:140–171, 1992.
45. Giannotta SL, Litofsky NS: Reoperative management of intracranial aneurysms. J Neurosurg 83:387–393, 1995.
46. Bendok BR, Ali M, Malisch T, et al: Coiling of cerebral aneurysm remnants after clipping. Neurosurgery 51:693–697, discussion 697–698, 2002.
47. Cekirge HS, Islak C, Firat MM, et al: Endovascular coil embolization of residual or recurrent aneurysms after surgical clipping. Acta Radiol 41:111–115, 2000.
48. Cockroft KM, Marks MP, Steinberg GK: Planned direct dual-modality treatment of complex broad-necked intracranial aneurysms: four technical case reports. Neurosurgery 46:226–230, discussion 230–231, 2000.
49. Forsting M, Albert FK, Jansen O, et al: Coil placement after clipping: Endovascular treatment of incompletely clipped cerebral aneurysms. Report of two cases. J Neurosurg 85:966–969, 1996.
50. Batjer H, Samson D: Intraoperative aneurysmal rupture: Incidence, outcome, and suggestions for surgical management. Neurosurgery 18:701–707, 1986.
51. Hua SE, Gluckman TJ, Batjer HH: Middle cerebral artery occlusion after pterional approach to basilar bifurcation aneurysm: Technical case report. Neurosurgery 39:1050–1053, discussion 1053–1054, 1996.
52. Graves VB, Strother CM, Duff TA, Perl J 2nd: Early treatment of ruptured aneurysms with Guglielmi detachable coils: Effect on subsequent bleeding. Neurosurgery 37:640–647, discussion 647–648, 1995.
53. Eskridge JM, Song JK: Endovascular embolization of 150 basilar tip aneurysms with Guglielmi detachable coils: Results of the Food and Drug Administration multicenter clinical trial. J Neurosurg 89:81–86, 1998.
54. Gruber DP, Zimmerman GA, Tomsick TA, et al: A comparison between endovascular and surgical management of basilar artery apex aneurysms. J Neurosurg 90:868–874, 1999.
55. Debrun GM, Aletich VA, Kehrli P, et al: Selection of cerebral aneurysms for treatment using Guglielmi detachable coils: the preliminary University of Illinois at Chicago experience. Neurosurgery 43:1281–1295, discussion 1296–1297, 1998.
56. Hayakawa M, Murayama Y, Duckwiler GR, et al: Natural history of the neck remnant of a cerebral aneurysm treated with the Guglielmi detachable coil system. J Neurosurg 93:561–568, 2000.
57. Raymond J, Roy D, Bojanowski M, et al: Endovascular treatment of acutely ruptured and unruptured aneurysms of the basilar bifurcation. J Neurosurg 86:211–219, 1997.

58. Bavinzski G, Talazoglu V, Killer M, et al: Coiling of recurrent and residual cerebral aneurysms after unsuccessful clipping. Minim Invasive Neurosurg 42:22–26, 1999.
59. Fraser KW, Halbach VV, Teitelbaum GP, et al: Endovascular platinum coil embolization of incompletely surgically clipped cerebral aneurysms. Surg Neurol 41:4–8, 1994.
60. Thielen KR, Nichols DA, Fulgham JR, Piepgras DG: Endovascular treatment of cerebral aneurysms following incomplete clipping. J Neurosurg 87:184–189, 1997.
61. Zeal A, Rhoton A: Microsurgical anatomy of the posterior cerebral artery. J Neurosurg 48:534–559, 1978.
62. Pedroza A, Dujovny M, Ausman JI, et al: Microvascular anatomy of the interpeduncular fossa. J Neurosurg 64:484–493, 1986.
63. Drake CG: Giant intracranial aneurysms: experience with surgical treatment in 174 patients. Clin Neurosurg 26:12–95, 1979.
64. Spetzler R, Carter L: Neurovascular Surgery. New York, McGraw-Hill, 1995.
65. Yasargil MG: Microneurosurgery. Stuttgart, Thieme, 1984.
66. Simpson RK Jr, Parker WD: Distal posterior cerebral artery aneurysm. Case report. J Neurosurg 64:669–672, 1986.
67. Sakata S, Fujii K, Matsushima T, et al: Aneurysm of the posterior cerebral artery: Report of eleven cases—surgical approaches and procedures. Neurosurgery 32:163–167, discussion 167–168, 1993.
68. Pia HW, Fontana H: Aneurysms of the posterior cerebral artery: Locations and clinical pictures. Acta Neurochir (Wien) 38:13–35, 1977.
69. Gerber CJ, Neil-Dwyer G, Evans BT: An alternative surgical approach to aneurysms of the posterior cerebral artery. Neurosurgery 32:928–931, discussion 931, 1993.
70. Gerber CJ, Neil-Dwyer G: A review of the management of 15 cases of aneurysms of the posterior cerebral artery. Br J Neurosurg 6:521–527, 1992.
71. Fukamachi A, Hirato M, Wakao T, Kawafuchi J: Giant serpentine aneurysm of the posterior cerebral artery. Neurosurgery 11:271–276, 1982.
72. Drake CG, Amacher AL: Aneurysms of the posterior cerebral artery. J Neurosurg 30:468–474, 1969.
73. Chang HS, Fukushima T, Miyazaki S, Tamagawa T: Fusiform posterior cerebral artery aneurysm treated with excision and end-to-end anastomosis: Case report. J Neurosurg 64:501–504, 1986.
74. Chang HS, Fukushima T, Takakura K, Shimizu T: Aneurysms of the posterior cerebral artery: Report of ten cases. Neurosurgery 19:1006–1011, 1986.
75. Awasthi D, Leclerq T: Distal posterior cerebral aneurysms: Anatomical and surgical considerations. Contemp Neurosci 16:1–6, 1994.
76. Meyer FB, Sundt TM Jr, Fode NC, et al: Cerebral aneurysms in childhood and adolescence. J Neurosurg 70:420–425, 1989.
77. Seoane ER, Tedeschi H, de Oliveira E, et al: Management strategies for posterior cerebral artery aneurysms: A proposed new surgical classification. Acta Neurochir (Wien) 139:325–331, 1997.
78. Ciceri EF, Klucznik RP, Grossman RG, et al: Aneurysms of the posterior cerebral artery: Classification and endovascular treatment. AJNR Am J Neuroradiol 22:27–34, 2001.

CHAPTER **120**

Endovascular Treatment of Aneurysms

GIUSEPPE LANZINO ■ LEE R. GUTERMAN ■ L. NELSON HOPKINS

Interest in endovascular techniques for the treatment of intracranial aneurysms has exploded in the past decade. Not too long ago, endovascular aneurysm occlusion was considered a second-line treatment, but it has rapidly become the primary therapeutic option at some centers.[1, 2]

Additional impetus for the application of endovascular techniques arises from its popularity among patients. The "minimally invasive" nature of this microcatheter-based approach allows the treatment of an intracranial aneurysm through a small groin incision. This approach is understandably more appealing to patients than open surgery involving craniotomy, brain retraction, and dissection. Other factors favoring the rapid spread of this technology include the ease of endovascular access to surgically difficult and demanding areas, such as the basilar trunk or bifurcation, and the ability to visualize angiographically the patency of adjacent vessels during the procedure.

ENDOVASCULAR ANEURYSM OBLITERATION: DECONSTRUCTIVE VERSUS RECONSTRUCTIVE APPROACH

Endovascular therapy of intracranial aneurysms is generally aimed toward occlusion or thrombosis of the aneurysm sac. The approaches can be classified into two broad categories. Deconstructive approaches involve occlusion of the parent vessel, with the aim of thrombosing both the parent vessel and its aneurysm, or occlusion of one or two major afferent vessels by diminishing and changing the direction of flow in the parent vessel, with resultant stasis of blood inside the aneurysm. Reconstructive approaches involve selective occlusion of the aneurysm lumen, with sparing of the parent artery.[3–5] The method of aneurysm obliteration depends primarily on the site, size, and morphologic features of the aneurysm.

Deconstructive Approach

BALLOON OCCLUSION OF THE PARENT VESSEL

As Home[6] recounts, in 1784 Hunter first occluded the parent artery proximal to an aneurysm to treat a popliteal aneurysm; thus, this type of therapy is often referred to as hunterian ligation. According to Nishioka,[7] it was applied to intracranial aneurysms by Horsley, who reportedly ligated the carotid artery to treat an intracranial aneurysm in 1885. With advances in endovascular techniques, surgical ligation of the parent vessel has been replaced by endovascular balloon occlusion.[8]

Currently, parent artery occlusion is considered for the treatment of large, giant (Fig. 120–1), and fusiform aneurysms; for select aneurysms distal to the circle of Willis; and for some post-traumatic pseudoaneurysms and infectious aneurysms that have fragile walls and are subject to perforation during endovascular packing.[5, 9] Parent artery occlusion should be avoided in the acute period after aneurysmal subarachnoid hemorrhage (SAH), because the development of vasospasm may result in ischemic deficits in the presence of marginal flow secondary to vessel occlusion. In such cases, parent artery occlusion can be performed in a delayed fashion after recovery from SAH.

BALLOON TEST OCCLUSION

Occluding the parent artery of an intracranial aneurysm causes cessation of blood flow, leading to thrombosis of the aneurysm–parent vessel complex. In aneurysms involving the basilar trunk, occlusion of one or both vertebral arteries produces the same result. Infarction in the vascular territory of the sacrificed vessel does not occur if collateral circulation is adequate. Thus, there is a need to test the adequacy of the collateral blood supply from the cerebral vasculature, as originally recognized by Matas and Allen in 1911.[10] Before the parent artery (either the cervical carotid or vertebral artery) harboring an aneurysm is occluded permanently, it is temporarily occluded with a balloon to test the patient's tolerance of occlusion.

Protocols for testing tolerance before permanent occlusion of the internal carotid artery (ICA) vary greatly from institution to institution.[11] Our protocol consists of 20 minutes of occlusion under normotension with repeated neurological assessment.[12] If the patient remains without neurological deficit, the mean arterial pressure is reduced to two thirds of the resting value

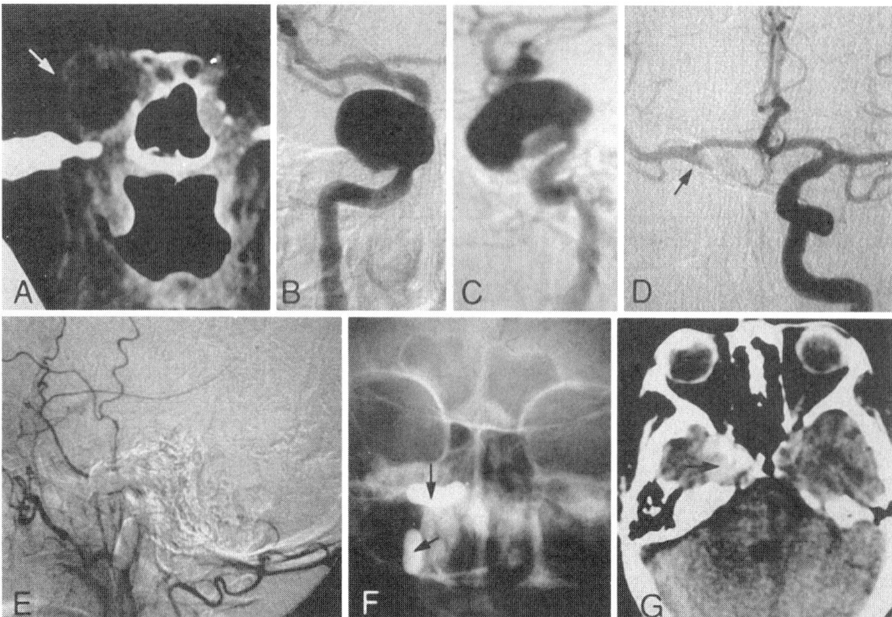

FIGURE 120–1. A 68-year-old woman suffered the sudden onset of severe headache and complete ophthalmoplegia. *A*, Cranial computed tomographic scan shows a parasellar mass consistent with a giant, calcified, partially thrombosed aneurysm *(arrow)* of the intracavernous portion of the internal carotid artery (ICA). *B* and *C*, Cerebral angiography—anteroposterior (AP) *(B)* and lateral *(C)* views—confirms these findings. Balloon test occlusion of the right ICA was performed. Because of the extreme proximal tortuosity of the great vessels, a transfemoral approach was unsuccessful; direct puncture of the common carotid artery (CCA) was performed after surgical exposure of the vessel with the patient under local anesthesia. *D*, Selective left ICA injection, AP view, performed during temporary balloon test occlusion of the right ICA. There is excellent collateralization through the anterior communicating artery, with good filling of the contralateral middle cerebral artery (MCA) territory, partial reconstitution of the supraclinoid right ICA *(arrow)*, but no angiographic evidence of aneurysm filling. Because the patient tolerated temporary occlusion with hypotensive challenge, the right ICA was occluded permanently by delivering two detachable balloons in tandem, proximal to the aneurysm. *E*, Right CCA injection, lateral view, after balloon detachment. The external carotid artery branches fill, but not the aneurysm. Two balloons are in place within the right ICA. The patient tolerated permanent occlusion with no new neurological deficits. *F*, The next day, a plain skull radiograph (AP view) confirmed that the position of the balloons was stable *(arrows)*. *G*, Noncontrast axial computed tomographic scan obtained 48 hours after permanent balloon occlusion and 24 hours after discontinuation of intravenous heparin administration shows evidence of aneurysm thrombosis *(arrow)*. Six months after the procedure, the patient is maintained on antiplatelet drugs, and her headaches are much improved. She has regained 90% of her sixth cranial nerve function, and the ptosis has resolved. She continues to have diplopia as a result of incomplete recovery of third cranial nerve function.

using intravenous vasodilators, beta-blockers, or both. Repeated neurological evaluation continues for another 20 minutes. If the patient tolerates balloon occlusion under this hypotensive challenge, arterial sacrifice can proceed with a low risk of stroke.[12–14] If the patient's neurological status changes, the balloon is immediately deflated, and the procedure is terminated.

In our experience, neurological changes from baseline are usually observed immediately after inflation of the balloon or a few minutes thereafter in patients who fail test occlusion. During balloon occlusion, we evaluate the collateral circulation by catheterizing the contralateral carotid artery and vertebral arteries with a diagnostic catheter placed through the contralateral femoral artery. Potential sites of collateral circulation are injected with contrast while the main artery feeding the aneurysm is occluded (see Fig. 120–1*D*). These injections are also helpful in assessing potential collateral pathways leading to persistent filling of the aneurysm. In patients who fail the balloon occlusion test, a surgical bypass is performed before proceeding with endovascular occlusion. The balloon test occlusion provides vital information, and if it is performed correctly and cautiously, the complication rate is quite low.[15, 16]

During test occlusion, periodic contrast-saline injections are performed to confirm continued occlusion of the vessel. At the conclusion of the test, the balloon is deflated, and repeat angiography is performed. Particular attention is paid to the distal distribution of the occluded vessel to rule out any evidence of thromboemboli. After the balloon catheter is withdrawn more proximally, another angiogram is obtained, with particular attention paid to the condition of the tested vessel at the point of balloon occlusion.

PERMANENT BALLOON OCCLUSION

Permanent occlusion of the target vessel can be performed immediately after the test occlusion if the criteria for tolerance have been satisfied. The balloon is prepared and advanced through a guide catheter to the appropriate location. The placement site of a balloon or balloons for permanent occlusion depends on the aneurysm's location and test occlusion findings relative to the presence or absence of aneurysm reperfusion from collateral flow. Ideally, the aneurysm sac should be trapped (with a first balloon placed distal to the aneurysm neck and a second balloon placed proximal to it). Possibly, the aneurysm neck should be covered by the balloon that is placed to occlude the parent vessel. In practice, however, this maneuver is very difficult to achieve because of the balloon's propensity to follow blood flow into large and giant aneurysms. At times, a combination of balloons and coils can be used for this purpose. In most cases, however, the proximal parent artery is occluded. In an aneurysm below the origin of the ophthalmic artery, there is little possibility of reperfusion, and the balloon is positioned just proximal to the aneurysm neck. In a carotid-ophthalmic aneurysm, the potential exists for reperfusion of the aneurysm by the ophthalmic artery. In this situation, the balloon is positioned (1) over the aneurysm neck, between the aneurysm and the ophthalmic artery, if there is more than a 5-mm segment in which to deposit the balloon; (2) in front of the orifice of the ophthalmic artery if there is a functional anastomosis with the external carotid artery; or (3) below the ophthalmic artery if there is no reperfusion of the aneurysm by collateral circulation.[17] For distal supraophthalmic aneurysms, occlusion is preferably performed at the level of the aneurysm, taking care to preserve the posterior communicating artery. If this approach is not possible, occlusion can be performed proximal to the posterior communicating artery (to reduce blood flow in the aneurysm) in conjunction with partial embolization with detachable coils (to induce further thrombosis).

The criteria for balloon placement in the vertebrobasilar system are also based on the dual goals of inducing thrombosis of the aneurysm lumen and maintaining collateral blood flow. These goals are somewhat contradictory, because thrombosis is best achieved by placing the occluding balloon as close as possible to the aneurysm, whereas preservation of adequate collateral flow may demand maintenance of blood flow through or past the aneurysm orifice. In most cases, unilateral occlusion of the dominant vertebral artery is sufficient to induce thrombosis in the aneurysm. If not, occlusion of the contralateral vertebral artery can be performed 3 or 4 weeks later, following a new test occlusion of this artery to verify adequate retrograde flow from the posterior communicating artery.[17] Preferably, the level of the occlusion is distal to the origin of the posterior inferior cerebellar artery (PICA) if a 5-mm or greater arterial segment is available between the PICA origin and the aneurysm for placement of either coils or a balloon while preserving the PICA. In such a case, only one balloon is detached distal to the PICA. This method allows flow reduction as well as parent artery occlusion in aneurysms of the intracranial vertebral artery or at the vertebrobasilar junction. Alternatively, the vertebral artery can be occluded more proximally, although this method permits potential anterograde flow from muscular collateral branches of the external carotid artery.[18] If clinically tolerated, the proximal basilar artery can be occluded to treat basilar trunk aneurysms.[19]

After optimal balloon size and position have been determined, detachment should proceed with a short, rapid pull on the microcatheter. A single balloon may not provide enough resistance to axial forces produced by arterial pressure to prevent the balloon from migrating. Even an inflated balloon can migrate. To prevent distal balloon migration, a "safety" balloon is detached proximally to the distal one (see Fig. 120–1*E* and *F*). Two detachable balloons are delivered through a single guide catheter. After the distal balloon has been positioned and inflated, the proximal balloon is partially inflated, producing proximal flow arrest. The distal balloon is detached, and then the proximal balloon is fully inflated and detached as well.

RESULTS AND COMPLICATIONS OF PERMANENT BALLOON OCCLUSION

The goal of endovascular treatment by parent artery occlusion is to induce intra-aneurysmal thrombosis and subsequent permanent involution of the aneurysm. Clot organization and fibrosis, as well as elimination of local hemodynamic factors responsible for aneurysm growth, then cause the sac to shrink, relieving symptoms due to neural compression while preventing rupture and further aneurysm growth. Involution of large or giant aneurysms may take months or years, particularly if the walls are very thick and calcified.[16] However, pressure symptoms and signs are usually alleviated soon after either parent artery occlusion or flow reversal within the parent artery, because pulsation of the sac is immediately reduced, and small reductions in the size of the aneurysm may be sufficient to relieve pressure on adjacent neural structures. However, transient swelling can occur acutely after thrombosis of the sac and exacerbate symptoms such as cranial nerve palsies[20] or hydrocephalus.

The ability of proximal endovascular parent artery occlusion to induce complete thrombosis of large and giant aneurysms is related to the likelihood of persistent reperfusion from collateral flow, as mentioned. In the anterior circulation, carotid artery occlusion below the origin of the ophthalmic artery is usually effective.[16, 20–22] Higashida and coworkers[21] reported stable, complete thrombosis in 100% of 68 cavernous aneurysms after endovascular parent artery occlusion. Symptoms of local compression caused by giant aneurysms improved, despite no evidence of shrinkage on follow-up scans. Efficacy of the procedure decreases in the anterior circulation when it is performed for aneurysms located distal to the ophthalmic artery. In their series, Fox and colleagues[20] observed that although all aneurysms of the cavernous-carotid region were completely thrombosed after proximal parent artery occlusion, only 47% of 21 aneurysms located above the ophthalmic artery origin became thrombosed without an additional trapping procedure. Similarly, vertebral artery occlusion is very effective for aneurysms of the intracranial vertebral artery, vertebrobasilar junction, and midbasilar artery; it is less effective for aneurysms of the basilar bifurcation, superior cerebellar artery, and other more distal sites.[18]

After parent carotid artery occlusion for cavernous sinus aneurysms, headaches and cranial neuropathies involving cranial nerves II, IV, V, and VI improve in most patients.[23] Normal function of the oculomotor nerve is less likely to be regained.[23] As mentioned, cranial nerve palsies can worsen transiently after successful aneurysm thrombosis.[20] In posterior circulation aneurysms, symptoms related to mass effect can improve dramatically after parent artery sacrifice, even in patients with severe preoperative neurological compromise.[19]

Despite a negative preoperative test occlusion, neurological deficits can occur after parent artery sacrifice. After endovascular sacrifice of the ICA, the rate of permanent postprocedural deficits varies from 0% to 10%.[20, 21, 23–25] In a series of 21 patients with giant and fusiform aneurysms of the vertebrobasilar system, no permanent deficits resulted; however, one patient (4%) had a fatal stroke.[18] When neurological worsening is related to hemodynamic factors, deficits can resolve after the initiation of aggressive hyperdynamic therapy.[23]

Several concerns exist regarding the possible long-term sequelae of elective parent artery sacrifice. This method may cause ischemic symptoms in a delayed fashion by reducing cerebrovascular reserve. Roski and associates[26] reported a 16.6% occurrence of ischemic neurological deficits in 39 patients 1 to 19.5 years after sacrifice of the carotid artery. By increasing blood flow in neighboring arteries providing collateral flow, parent artery sacrifice may cause de novo aneurysms to form.[27] Whether these de novo aneurysms are due to the same pathologic process (e.g., atherosclerosis) that caused the original aneurysm or are related to increased blood flow in the intact carotid artery remains speculative.

Although it is an established treatment, endovascular parent artery sacrifice cannot be considered a definitive treatment for large, giant, or fusiform aneurysms. Aneurysms can recanalize, regrow, or rupture if the potential for revascularization from a collateral source exists.[18, 28, 29] Diligent follow-up with axial imaging studies is therefore recommended. Given all these limitations and the ongoing refinements in endovascular techniques, parent artery sacrifice will likely be used less often in the future for the treatment of these challenging aneurysms.

Reconstructive Approach

The next major step in the endovascular treatment of aneurysms came with the introduction of endovascular coils. Coils had been available for endovascular embolization for some time,[30] but not until the 1980s did Hilal and Solomon[31] extend their use to the treatment of intracranial aneurysms. Several other authors subsequently reported occlusion of intracranial aneurysms with "pushable" platinum coils.[32, 33] The major disadvantage of these systems, however, was that an advanced coil could not be retrieved.

The persistence and ingenuity of Guglielmi, an Italian neurosurgeon, led to the major advancement represented by detachable coils, thus beginning a new era in the endovascular treatment of aneurysms. In the early 1980s, while applying current to a stainless steel electrode introduced into an experimental aneurysm to promote electrothrombosis, Guglielmi observed accidental electrolytic detachment of the electrode tip. Several years later, in conjunction with Sepetka and others, Guglielmi worked to combine the two processes of endovascular electrolysis and electrothrombosis, an undertaking that eventually led to the development of the Guglielmi detachable coil (GDC) as we know it today.[34, 35]

With the GDC system, an aneurysm can be excluded from the intracranial circulation while preserving the patency of the parent vessel, thus giving a more physiologic result than parent artery sacrifice. Different types of coils have been used successfully for endovascular occlusion of intracranial aneurysms.[36–39] This chapter focuses on the use of the GDC system, because these coils are used almost universally. The availability of detachable coils has revolutionized the endovascular approach to intracranial aneurysms.

Previous occlusive agents such as pushable coils and endosaccular balloons were associated with two major shortcomings: lack of control over delivery, and lack of compliance between the agent and the aneurysm. The GDC design combines the advantages of very soft, compliant platinum and retrievability, resulting in markedly improved safety and efficacy. An improperly fitting coil can be withdrawn, repositioned, or replaced with a coil of another size before detachment. Controlled delivery is the primary advantage of the GDC; the coil is detached only when the correct position is demonstrated by angiography. A further advantage is the flexibility and softness of the coils; this enables the filling of an aneurysmal outpouching to minimize the risk of rupture and allows them to absorb the systolic pulse pressure.

GUGLIELMI DETACHABLE COIL SYSTEM

GDCs are platinum spiral coils with a circular memory, soldered to a stainless steel delivery wire (Fig. 120–2). The coil consists of a thin, spiral-woven platinum wire formed in the shape of a helix. Coil softness refers to the ease with which a GDC can compress and expand and is influenced primarily by the wire diameter. Soft GDCs are made of a thinner platinum wire than are standard GDCs. Soft and standard coils are available in a range of sizes and lengths so that aneurysms can be packed piecemeal with appropriately sized coils. When positioned within a microcatheter, the coil assumes a straight shape and can easily be advanced into the aneurysm.

More elaborate designs have become available, including the two-diameter GDC, in which the helix of

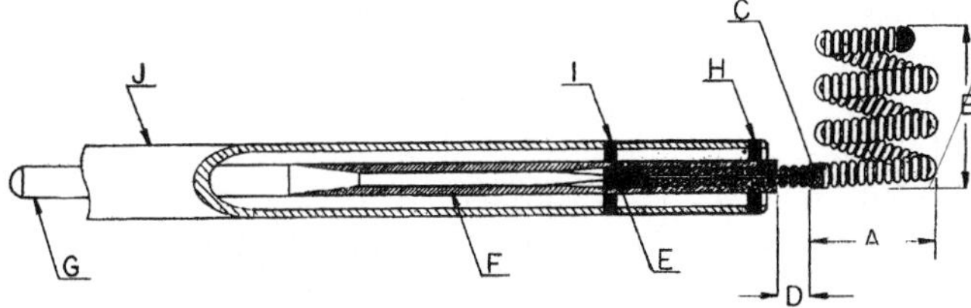

FIGURE 120–2. Schematic drawing of the Guglielmi detachable coil (GDC). *A*, Diameter of the circular memory. *B*, Platinum component of the GDC. *C*, Junction between platinum and stainless steel. *D*, Uninsulated portion of the delivery wire (this is the portion that undergoes electrolysis, detaching the coil in the aneurysm). *E*, Proximal platinum marker on the delivery wire. *F*, Insulated delivery wire. *G*, Proximal, uninsulated end of the delivery wire. *H*, Distal radiopaque marker microcatheter on the double-marker microcatheter. *I*, Proximal radiopaque marker on the double-marker microcatheter. *J*, Microcatheter. (From Byrne JV, Guglielmi G: Endovascular Treatment of Intracranial Aneurysms. New York, Springer-Verlag, 1998, p 137.)

the initial coil segment defines a smaller diameter than the remaining helices. With two-diameter coils, the first, or leading, coil loop tends to remain inside the aneurysm sac while avoiding contact between the advancing coil tip and the aneurysm wall, because of the smaller loop diameter. This design also reduces the predisposition of the first coil to herniate from the aneurysm during deployment. In an attempt to decrease the incidence and degree of coil compaction,[40] another novel GDC configuration has been developed in which the secondary coil structure consists of a series of omega-like loops. This three-dimensional GDC spontaneously forms a complex three-dimensional configuration during delivery and has been used successfully to occlude aneurysms with an unfavorable geometry for conventional GDC embolization.[41] Thrombogenic coils are designed either to be simply pushed out of the microcatheter tip with a delivery wire or to be detachable, with the capability of retrieving and repositioning the coil. In fibered coils, the thrombogenicity of the platinum coil is enhanced by attached Dacron fibers.

The coil delivery wire is insulated except for the most distal part, the detachment zone (see Fig. 120–2*D*). Three centimeters proximal to the detachment zone, a radiopaque marker is incorporated in the delivery wire. During detachment, this marker aligns with the proximal marker on the microcatheter. By checking the position of the proximal markers, the operator can ensure that the coil has advanced outside the microcatheter tip, even though the distal marker on the catheter tip may be obscured by overlying, previously placed coils, and avoid advancing the stiff delivery wire into the lumen of the aneurysm. When the coil has been placed in a satisfactory position, a positive, low-voltage, direct current is applied to the delivery wire. The current induces electrolysis at the solder junction between the coil and the delivery wire, and the coil is gradually detached. This technique allows delivery of the coil without displacement from its location.

TECHNIQUE OF ANEURYSM EMBOLIZATION WITH THE GUGLIELMI DETACHABLE COIL SYSTEM

Although cooperative patients can tolerate embolization of an aneurysm under conscious sedation, we prefer to administer general endotracheal anesthesia to minimize problems related to patient movement. The quality of roadmapping is thereby improved, and possible intraprocedural hemorrhagic or ischemic complications can be controlled and managed better.[42, 43] After a femoral sheath has been placed in the right groin, a diagnostic angiogram is obtained. Appreciation of the aneurysm neck and its relationship to adjacent perforating and major arteries is a prerequisite to the embolization procedure. It is particularly important to isolate the aneurysm neck from the parent vessel angiographically, so that any coil prolapse into the parent vessel can easily be detected. This often requires the acquisition of multiple oblique views. Once a "working projection" is identified, it is recorded for use during the embolization procedure. In some cases, the complex three-dimensional geometry of the aneurysm and surrounding vessels or the overlapping of different structures prevents the acquisition of an adequate view for safe embolization of the aneurysm. The future use of three-dimensional magnetic resonance imaging and rotational angiography will improve the visualization of local anatomy and be a great aid.

A coaxial system consisting of a guide catheter and delivery microcatheter is used to catheterize the aneurysm selectively. Once the selected microcatheter has been prepared, it is navigated through the guide catheter over a steerable micro–guide wire. The entire procedure is performed under full heparinization, and the coaxial system is flushed continuously with a solution of saline and heparin (1000 IU of heparin per 1000 mL of saline) to prevent thrombus formation caused by friction between the two catheters or while the coils are being advanced through the microcatheter.

The aneurysm is negotiated with the micro–guide wire. Roadmapping is helpful during this part of the procedure. Care is taken to avoid touching the aneurysm wall with the tip of the wire or microcatheter. An appropriately sized GDC is chosen by matching the helix radius of the coil to the estimated diameter of the aneurysm. The best choice for the first coil is one that bridges the aneurysm neck and allows dense, homogeneous packing of the aneurysm. In principle, the longest coil available to fill as much of the aneurysm sac as possible should be used.[42] The first and second coils are critical for achieving complete occlusion. The first coil must be placed in a basket-like configuration within the aneurysm. The occlusion is stable when the first coil covers the neck of the aneurysm. If possible, the first coil should be delivered away from angiographically identifiable bleeding sites.[43]

After placement and before electrolytic detachment of each GDC, a control angiogram is obtained with manual injection through the guide catheter to confirm proper placement of the coil, as well as to demonstrate patency of the adjacent arteries. After the first coil is detached, the remaining cavity is filled with smaller diameter coils, which are placed within the loops of the first coil to prevent bulging into the parent artery. The procedure is terminated when dense packing is achieved or when the aneurysm accepts no more coils. Although some authors suggest packing the aneurysm as much as possible and stopping the procedure only when the last coil cannot be introduced inside the sac (thus, the last coil is always wasted),[44] we prefer to individualize the degree of packing to an aneurysm's morphology and the procedural goals.

BALLOON-REMODELING TECHNIQUE

To overcome the problem presented by wide-necked aneurysms, a balloon can be inflated across the neck of an aneurysm and inflated during coil delivery through a microcatheter positioned within the aneurysm sac (Fig. 120–3).[45–50] The balloon functions as an external (to the aneurysm) mechanical barrier that allows tighter packing of the aneurysm while preventing coil herniation into the parent artery during coil delivery. In addition, as stressed by Lefkowitz and coworkers,[45] the balloon stabilizes the microcatheter during coil delivery and forces the coils to conform to the three-dimensional shape of the aneurysm. This technique, originally pioneered and popularized by Moret and colleagues,[49] is often referred to as the balloon-remodeling technique because it enables temporary remodeling of the aneurysm's neck during GDC deposition. This technique is most suitable and less technically challenging for proximal aneurysms of the ICA or the vertebrobasilar tree. However, it has also been used successfully to treat aneurysms originating from smaller vessels, such as the posterior cerebral artery,[48, 49] anterior communicating artery,[46, 49] and middle cerebral artery (MCA),[49] owing to the availability of balloon microcatheters that can be used with a micro–guide wire.

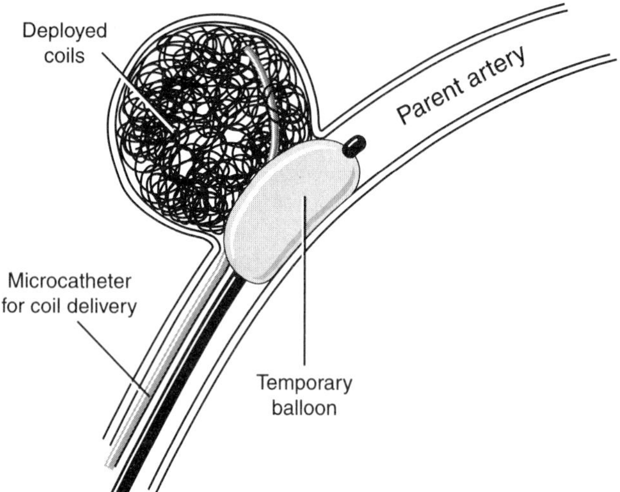

FIGURE 120–3. Schematic drawing of the balloon-remodeling technique. With the balloon inflated, Guglielmi detachable coils (GDCs) are delivered through the microcatheter placed within the aneurysm. This technique allows for tighter coil packing, even in wide-necked aneurysms with unfavorable geometry for GDC embolization alone. (From Mericle RA, Wakhloo AK, Rodriguez R, et al: Temporary balloon protection as an adjunct to endosaccular coiling of wide-necked cerebral aneurysms: Technical note. Neurosurgery 41:975–978, 1997.)

To avoid undesired movements of the microcatheter within the aneurysm when the remodeling technique is used, the nondetachable balloon must be placed first in the parent vessel, in front of the aneurysm neck.[45, 49] Superselective microcatheterization of the aneurysm is then performed. Inflation of the nondetachable balloon in front of the aneurysm neck temporarily occludes both the neck and the parent vessel. Under the protection of the balloon, microcoils are then deposited into the aneurysm sac. After each coil is positioned but before detachment, the balloon is deflated to test the stability of the coil. If no displacement of the coil is observed, the coil is detached. If movement of the coil is detected after balloon deflation, the coil is not well anchored within the sac, and the coil is never detached.

In experienced hands, application of the remodeling technique has been associated with complete angiographic obliteration in 77% to 83% of the aneurysms treated.[45, 49] However, the technique has several drawbacks. Technical demands on the operator are increased by the need to use two microcatheters simultaneously. The dangers of local thrombus formation and distal embolization are increased by temporary interruption of blood flow in the parent vessel, and thromboembolic complications have been observed in 5% to 8% of treated patients.[45, 49] The need to inflate and deflate the balloon repeatedly risks intimal damage. Finally, a broader mass of coil is exposed to the bloodstream after successful obliteration of wide-necked aneurysms.[45]

There is also concern that an increase in intra-aneurysmal pressure during balloon inflation across the aneurysm neck,[51] coupled with forceful placement of coils in a closed space,[49] may increase the risk of bleeding, especially during treatment of acutely ruptured aneurysms. The incidence of intraprocedural rupture with the remodeling technique can be as high as 5%, double that encountered with simple GDC embolization.[49] In the event of rupture, however, the balloon can be inflated immediately to stop the hemorrhage and allow placement of another coil to occlude the breach. In this way, bleeding is rapidly managed, and clinical consequences are minimized.[49]

Despite these limitations, this technique is a valid part of the armamentarium of endovascular surgeons and has been used by experienced teams to treat between 17% and 20% of the total number of GDC-embolized aneurysms.[45, 49] Although the long-term effectiveness of this technique in promoting stable occlusion of wide-necked aneurysms is unknown, short-term outcomes are promising. In their series of 56 patients, Moret and coworkers[49] reported that 20 of 21 totally occluded aneurysms remained totally occluded at follow-up angiography 3 to 6 months later. In another series of 23 aneurysms treated with the balloon-remodeling technique, no aneurysm required further treatment after a mean follow-up of 10 months.[45]

STENT-COIL TECHNIQUE

Owing to the recent availability of flexible intravascular stents, a new therapeutic approach to complex wide-necked aneurysms originating from the ICA and vertebrobasilar complex is possible (Fig. 120–4).[52–56] Experimentally, a stent has been deployed across an aneurysm neck, in conjunction with GDC embolization, to improve the density of coil packing.[57–62] In this situation, the stent acts as an endoluminal scaffold to prevent coil herniation. After the stent has been placed, the aneurysm sac can be filled with coils by introducing a microcatheter through the stent mesh. Placement of an endovascular stent within the parent artery across the aneurysm neck may also divert blood from the aneurysm inflow tract and promote intra-aneurysmal stasis and thrombosis.[61–65] Further, at least in an experimental setting, stents appear to provide a luminal matrix for endothelial growth[60–62] and also may prevent coil compaction by changing intra-aneurysmal flow dynamics.[65] Thus, the combination stent-coil technique permits the dense packing of even complex, large, wide-necked, fusiform aneurysms that are notoriously difficult to approach surgically.[57, 60–62] Reports of a few clinical cases involving the ICA[54, 66] or the vertebrobasilar system[52–56] that have been successfully treated with the stent-coil technique suggest that this approach is a feasible and safe alternative to the surgical exclusion of these challenging lesions.

In a clinical setting, placement of an intravascular stent across an aneurysm neck seems to have a limited ability to induce stasis and thrombosis, for a variety of reasons. The need for systemic anticoagulation to lessen the risk of thromboembolic complications during endovascular procedures, as well as the need to reduce the risk of subacute stent thrombosis caused by prolonged postprocedural antiplatelet therapy, may interfere with and delay aneurysm thrombosis in clinical practice, despite the hemodynamic changes observed after stent placement in experimental aneurysms. The high porosity of the intravascular stents currently used is another factor limiting aneurysm thrombosis after primary stent placement.

Although there are several theoretical concerns about the use of intracranial stents,[65] preliminary clinical experience suggests that some of these concerns are unjustified. For example, stents are known to induce intimal hyperplasia,[67] and it has been argued that excessive neointimal proliferation after stent placement can result in hemodynamically significant stenosis, especially of the smaller intracranial branches.[65] The occurrence of neointimal hyperplasia is usually evident in the first few months after treatment as a consequence of the vessel reacting to the presence of a foreign body. However, in a series of six patients undergoing follow-up angiograms after stent placement for the treatment of intracranial aneurysms, we observed evidence of intimal hyperplasia in only one patient.[54] In this patient, despite the presence of in-stent stenosis on follow-up angiography at 5 months, the 10-month study

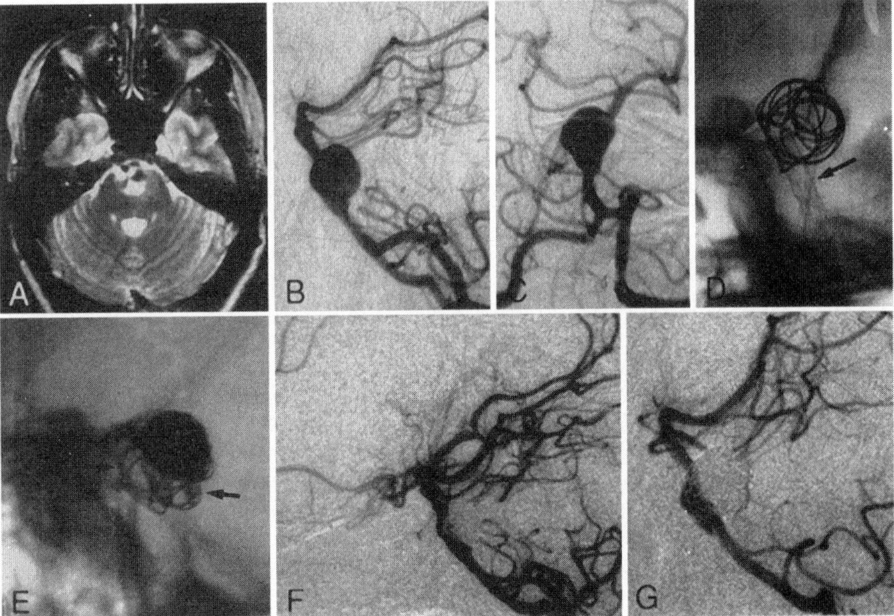

FIGURE 120–4. *A,* Magnetic resonance T2-weighted image demonstrates a mass in the ventral pons, with intraluminal flow voids consistent with an aneurysm. *B* and *C,* Digital subtraction angiograms—lateral *(B)* and anteroposterior *(C)* projections—demonstrate a giant aneurysm arising from the basilar trunk. *D,* Plain skull radiography, lateral view. An intravascular stent is in place *(arrow).* The stent allows tight packing of this giant, irregularly shaped aneurysm. *E,* Radiograph shows coils filling the aneurysm on each side of the stent *(arrows). F,* Digital subtraction angiogram, right vertebral artery injection, lateral view. Final result after stent placement and deployment of 22 Guglielmi detachable coils, showing satisfactory aneurysm obliteration and excellent distal flow, with even filling of the anterior circulation. *G,* Five-month follow-up digital subtraction angiogram, lateral projection, demonstrating mild aneurysm recanalization, with no evidence of aneurysm growth.

revealed remodeling of the stented segment, with resolution of the stenosis and improvement of flow (Hopkins, unpublished data, 1999).

Concerns also exist that occlusion of the ostia of small side branches and perforating arteries by stent placement may result in ischemia or infarction in the territory of these vessels. However, experimental evidence in dogs suggests that small lateral carotid branches, which approximate intracranial perforating vessels relative to their diameter and angle of origin, tend to stay patent if less than 50% of the ostial diameter is covered by the stent struts.[62] These canine study results were mirrored by our observations and those of other authors that no difficulties involving perforating branch occlusion were encountered after treatment of basilar trunk aneurysms.[53, 54] It is also possible that in patients with fusiform aneurysms of critical segments, such as the basilar trunk, the involved perforating vessels have become "nonfunctional," thus explaining the absence of permanent neurological sequelae following stent placement with or without secondary coil placement. Because of the high porosity of the stents used, lateral branches such as the ophthalmic artery and the anterior inferior cerebellar artery remain patent after a stent is placed across their origins.

Current imaging techniques limit complete coil packing of some irregularly shaped fusiform aneurysms. In such cases, after the first few coils are placed, it becomes very difficult (and sometimes impossible) to determine whether any coil loop has herniated into the parent vessel because the coil-packed aneurysm is superimposed over the parent artery in all angiographic projections. This situation can prevent further tight packing. Advances in novel imaging techniques such as intravascular ultrasonography and endovascular angioscopy may afford a solution. Additionally, the use of less porous stents in the future may facilitate tighter coil packing. Given these limitations, long-term follow-up of these patients is of utmost importance.

OUTCOMES OF GUGLIELMI DETACHABLE COIL EMBOLIZATION

At this stage of the technology, the results obtained with GDC aneurysm embolization are still being assessed. Reported series are often difficult to compare because of different selection criteria for treatment, inclusion of ruptured as well as unruptured aneurysms, and different definitions used to assess the degree of angiographic occlusion. In particular, it is difficult to assess the aneurysm occlusion rate after endovascular embolization. Such evaluation is subjective, and it is impossible to compare what authors define as complete or successful occlusion among series.

The immediate clinical and angiographic results after GDC embolization of ruptured intracranial aneurysms were assessed by Vinuela and coworkers.[68] They reported 403 patients treated at eight U.S. institutions participating in the Food and Drug Administration study that eventually led to approval of the device in 1995. All aneurysms were treated within 15 days of rupture. The most common reasons for selecting endovascular treatment in this series included high surgical risk because of aneurysm size and location (69%), failed surgical exploration (12.7%), and poor neurological (12.2%) or medical (4.7%) status. Because of this preselection, the majority of the aneurysms (57%) were in the posterior circulation. Immediate angiographic results varied, primarily according to the size of the aneurysm neck and sac. Complete aneurysm occlusion at the end of the embolization procedure was observed in 70.8% of the small aneurysms (4 to 10 mm at largest diameter) with small necks (<4 mm). In this subgroup, technical failures (inability to place coils because of technical difficulties such as vessel tortuosity or wide neck) were uncommon (3.6% of cases). In contrast, complete occlusion was achieved in only 31% of the small aneurysms with wide necks, and technical failure occurred in 16.9%. Despite the high-risk preselected population, overall rates of morbidity (8.9%) and mortality (6.2%) were low and were not significantly influenced by aneurysm location when anterior and posterior circulation aneurysms were compared (morbidity, 8.1% versus 9.6%; mortality, 6.4% versus 6.1%, respectively). In critically assessing these results, it must be recalled that the aneurysms treated represent the early experience of the participating centers. Current success rates can be expected to be higher because of improved selection criteria and treatment strategies, along with the availability of a greater range of coil sizes and types.

As more experience has been accumulated, several centers have reported their results after GDC embolization of intracranial aneurysms.[5, 34, 69–75] These series have confirmed the overall safety of this technique; however, in the absence of long-term follow-up data, concern exists that GDC embolization permits complete angiographic obliteration of only a fraction of treated aneurysms. In addition, the stability of the consequent occlusion is unknown, as some aneurysms recanalize[76] (Fig. 120–5) and even rupture,[77, 78] despite initial satisfactory packing. Further, the current GDC technology has several limitations in the treatment of a significant number of aneurysms encountered in clinical practice. Raftopoulos and coworkers[79] analyzed a prospective series of 103 patients harboring 132 aneurysms treated with a therapeutic paradigm in which endovascular embolization was considered the first option. In this study, surgical clipping was performed only when endovascular embolization was deemed unlikely based on the aneurysm's characteristics or when embolization failed. Three groups were defined: group A consisted of aneurysms (N = 64) that were treated by endovascular embolization (these aneurysms had a neck-to-sac ratio of 1:3); group B included those aneurysms (N = 63) that were not considered suitable for endovascular treatment and were surgically clipped; group C encompassed those aneurysms that failed to be satisfactorily embolized (>95%) and were successively clipped. The incidence of residual aneurysm was 31.2% in group A, 1.6% in group B, and 0% in group C. Poor outcomes (Glasgow Outcome Scale score 1 to 3) in patients with good clinical status before treatment

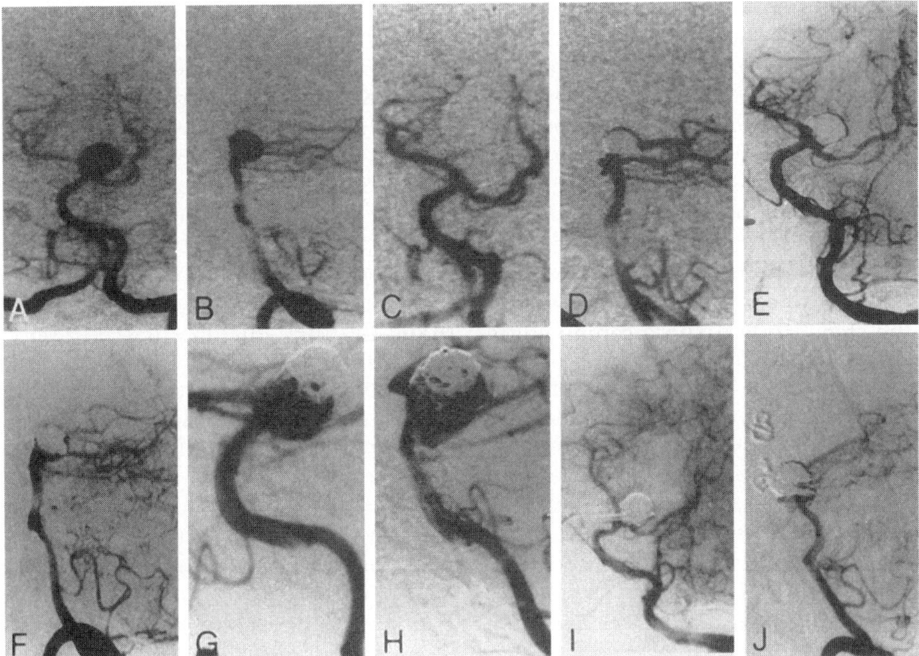

FIGURE 120–5. Digital subtraction angiogram of a basilar apex aneurysm. Towne's *(A)* and lateral *(B)* views demonstrate the wide neck and anatomy of the lesion. Digital subtraction angiograms (*C, D*) after Guglielmi detachable coil (GDC) treatment in two similar projections. The aneurysm is at least 95% occluded. Follow-up angiogram 1 year after GDC treatment in Towne's *(E)* and lateral *(F)* projections, suggesting possible minimal loosening of the coil loops in the proximal portion of the coil mass. Repeat angiogram 2 years after treatment in Towne's *(G)* and lateral *(H)* views. At the base of the mass, coils have loosened and unraveled, and aneurysm regrowth is evident. Postoperative angiograms *(I, J)* after surgical clipping. The aneurysm is completely obliterated by the combination of aneurysm clip and coils. (From Mericle RA, Wakhloo AK, Lopes DK, et al: Delayed aneurysm regrowth and recanalization after Guglielmi detachable coil treatment. J Neurosurg 89:142–145, 1998.)

occurred in 10.7% of patients in group A, 0% in group B, and 8.3% in group C.

Recent reports have concentrated on follow-up angiographic results.[44, 80] Cognard and associates[44] reported their observations in 169 aneurysms (ruptured and unruptured) in which at least one follow-up angiogram was obtained a minimum of 3 months after treatment. At the end of the initial procedure, occlusion was judged to be total in 95 cases (56%), subtotal in 66 (39%), and incomplete in 8 (5%). Because of initial subtotal or incomplete occlusion, a second procedure was performed in 18 patients, with subsequent total occlusion achieved in 14. The first follow-up angiogram confirmed total occlusion in an additional 39 aneurysms that initially had been considered subtotally occluded. Overall, total occlusion was obtained in 148 aneurysms (88%). This study underscores the importance of long-term follow-up studies. Recurrence was observed in 5% of totally occluded aneurysms after 3 months and in 9% of 99 aneurysms that were totally occluded on the first follow-up angiogram and underwent a second follow-up study a mean of 18 months later. Of 39 aneurysms totally occluded on the second follow-up angiogram, 3 (8%) had recurred when a third angiogram was obtained an average of 38 months later. Recurrence was more frequent in ruptured than in unruptured aneurysms (17% versus 7%) and in large than in small aneurysms, but there was no difference in the frequency of recurrence relative to aneurysm location.

The importance of angiographic follow-up was also underscored by Byrne and colleagues,[80] who reviewed their 5-year experience at Oxford (United Kingdom) with GDC treatment of ruptured intracranial aneurysms. Surviving patients were followed for a median of 22 months. Angiographic occlusion was assessed in 259 aneurysms in 250 patients. After treatment, 64% of the aneurysms were completely occluded. At angiographic follow-up, usually obtained between 6 and 12 months later, the degree of occlusion observed at the end of the embolization procedure remained stable in 86.4% of small aneurysms and in 85.2% of large aneurysms. In 38 aneurysms (14.7%), a remnant had enlarged to some degree. In 8.5% of cases, improvement of occlusion was observed at follow-up angiography due to thrombosis subsequent to the completion of packing.

There is no agreement about the timing and duration of angiographic follow-up. In general, we obtain a first follow-up angiogram at 6 months in patients with totally occluded aneurysms or with minimal rests. In patients with residual sacs, an earlier study (usually at 3 months) is indicated to assess the stability and size of the remnant and the possible need for additional treatment. The necessity and timing of additional follow-up are determined on an individual basis; however, all patients, even those with a stable occlusion on the first follow-up angiogram, should undergo a 1-year follow-up study. The need for repeated angiographic follow-up, which exposes patients to the low but definite risk of an invasive procedure, is one of the current limits of GDC embolization of intracranial aneurysms. Encouraging experience with magnetic resonance angiography shows that this imaging technology has the potential to replace angiographic follow-up.[81–83] The coils create a very low level of magnetic resonance artifact and no ferromagnetism.[84] Thus, they are compatible with magnetic resonance angiography in terms of both safety and image quality.[81]

Several factors affect the degree and stability of angiographic occlusion. The importance of aneurysm geometry has been demonstrated by Fernandez Zubillaga and coworkers,[85] who observed complete aneurysm occlusion in 85% of small-necked (≦4 mm) aneurysms and in only 15% of aneurysms with necks measuring greater than 4 mm. This observation has been confirmed by other authors.[9, 68] The importance of the ratio between maximal sac diameter and neck diameter (dome-to-neck ratio) has been debated.[44, 49, 86] It has been suggested that when this ratio is less than 2, the aneurysm has a so-called wide neck,[73] and that optimal results are obtained when this ratio is at least 2.[86] When aneurysms are selected for endovascular treatment on the basis of this favorable anatomic-geometric consideration, complete angiographic occlusion can be achieved in 72% of acutely ruptured aneurysms and in 80% of unruptured ones.[86] Small-sized aneurysms with wide necks present the greatest technical challenge.[68]

Randomized Trials of Embolization versus Surgery

So far, only one randomized trial has assessed the role and efficacy of GDC embolization compared to surgical clipping. Vanninen and coworkers[87] in 1999 reported the results of a single-center, prospective, randomized study of GDC embolization versus surgery for the treatment of recently (<72 hours) ruptured intracranial aneurysms. The study was conducted in Finland between February 1995 and August 1997. Fifty-two patients were assigned to the endovascular treatment group and 57 to the surgical treatment group. The two groups were well matched for age, sex, Hunt-Hess grade,[88] Fisher grade,[89] and site or size of the ruptured aneurysm. Interestingly, despite relatively broad inclusion criteria, 70 patients treated in the same period were not randomized for the following reasons: endovascular treatment was deemed anatomically infeasible (33 patients), surgical evacuation of a large hematoma was required (35 patients), or cranial nerve compression was present (2 patients). There were no differences in 3-month clinical outcomes, as determined by the Glasgow Outcome Scale,[90] between the two treatment groups: 81% of the patients initially assigned to endovascular treatment and 79% of the patients assigned to surgery showed a good or moderate recovery.

Because there is no need for brain retraction and dissection, endovascular treatment may be associated with a lower incidence of neuropsychological sequelae than is observed after surgical clipping. In the aforementioned Finnish trial, however, no differences were observed between the two groups when neuropsychological outcome was assessed at 12 months, and the scores were significantly improved in both groups 3 to 12 months after treatment (Koivisto and coworkers, unpublished data). In the same study, magnetic resonance imaging of the brain was performed according to protocol at 12 months. Patients in the surgical group had more ischemic lesions in the parent artery territory of the ruptured aneurysm, in addition to signs of brain retraction injury. Although this trial showed equivalent outcomes with current endovascular embolization techniques and with surgery, it did not answer questions about long-term durability of the treatment.

A large multicenter, prospective, randomized, controlled clinical trial, the International Subarachnoid Aneurysm Trial, is comparing surgical clipping with endovascular coiling of ruptured intracranial aneurysms.[91, 92] The primary objective of the trial is to determine whether endovascular or surgical treatment reduces by 25% the proportion of patients in an eligible population with moderate or poor outcomes at 1 year. The secondary objectives are to determine the following for endovascular therapy: whether it is as effective as surgery in preventing rebleeding, whether it results in a better quality of life than surgery at 1 year, whether it is more cost effective than surgery, and whether it improves neuropsychological outcomes at 1 year. The tertiary objectives are to determine the long-term outcomes of both treatments and to determine the significance of angiographic results. To achieve statistical significance, about 2500 patients must be enrolled.

By January 1998, almost 800 patients had been randomized at the 20 participating centers. Among this population, 88% were of good grade after SAH, and almost all had anterior circulation aneurysms. The blinded outcome data show that about 25% of patients had a poor outcome at both 2 months and 1 year. The study is in progress, and a report should be available in the near future. The hope is that it will answer many of the outstanding questions about the management of SAH.[91] The trial began as a pilot study in 1994 and became a full study in January 1997. Preliminary data from the participating centers also indicate a trend to treat patients with posterior circulation aneurysms of poor grade endovascularly rather than enter them in the trial. Patients with anterior circulation aneurysms of good grade tend to be either managed surgically or enrolled in the trial.

Large and Giant Aneurysms

Aneurysm size is another limiting factor of GDC technology. If the results of GDC embolization are deemed satisfactory for small aneurysms with small necks, the same is not true for large and giant aneurysms. In a review of the University of Vienna experience, Gruber and associates[93] reported complete occlusion of 68% of large and giant aneurysms achieved immediately after the first session of GDC embolization. However, recanalization was observed on the first follow-up angiogram in most of these cases, and additional treatment by repeat embolization, parent artery occlusion, or surgery was required. A single embolization session resulted in definitive occlusion in only 12.5% of the giant and 31% of the large aneurysms. The procedure-related morbidity and mortality rates were not negligible (13.3% and 6.7%, respectively).

Giant aneurysms have a high recurrence rate not only because of their relatively large necks but also because their sacs are frequently lined with soft thrombus in which the coil may eventually become embedded.[94] At this time, indications for the use of GDC in large and giant aneurysms are for palliation or as a complementary therapy in more complicated lesions.[95, 96] With new coil shapes (three-dimensional) and theballoon-remodeling technique, better results may beobtained, but significant limitations remain. When feasible, the combination of stenting and coiling is a valid alternative for these challenging cases.

Unruptured Incidental Aneurysms and Unruptured Aneurysms Presenting with Mass Effect

GDCs have been used to embolize aneurysms in patients who presented with symptoms of mass effect,[5, 93, 97, 98] even though thrombus formation after embolization and the volume of the coil mass may exacerbate symptoms.[99] After coil embolization, symptoms of mass effect can improve in as many as 66% of patients.[5] In a series of 31 patients with large and giant aneurysms treated by GDC embolization, Gruber and associates[93] reported improvement in 45% of cases, whereas symptoms remained unchanged in 27% and worsened in another 27%. In an assessment of longer-term results following GDC embolization in 19 patients who presented with cranial nerve deficits caused by aneurysm compression, symptoms completely resolved in 32%, improved in 42%, remained the same in 21%, and worsened in 5%, despite worsening of symptoms immediately after GDC packing in 22% of cases.[97] Worsening of symptoms at follow-up is usually related to aneurysm regrowth.[93] Immediately or soon after embolization, such deterioration can be related to excessive intravascular thrombosis or mechanical neural compression by the coils. Surgical decompression may be required to relieve symptoms.[99] In successful cases, shrinkage of aneurysm size or resolution of perianeurysmal edema can be documented on follow-up magnetic resonance imaging.[5]

The results of GDC embolization for incidentally discovered, unruptured aneurysms were assessed in a series of 120 patients treated at UCLA by Murayama and colleagues.[100] Thirty-nine percent of the aneurysms were ophthalmic segment aneurysms, and 18% were located at the basilar bifurcation. Complete GDC occlusion could be achieved in only 63% of cases (76 aneurysms), and procedure-related morbidity was 5.2%. Follow-up angiograms were available in only 77 patients (79 aneurysms) of the original 120-patient cohort. After the original embolization, complete occlusion was observed in 52 aneurysms, and a small neck remnant was visualized in 22 aneurysms. At follow-up angiography, none of the 52 completely occluded aneurysms had recanalized. In the 22 aneurysms with small neck remnants, 8 (36%) showed aneurysmal recanalization due to coil compaction. Among these recanalized aneurysms, additional embolization completely occluded the aneurysms in three patients. One patient underwent successful surgical clipping, and three patients were treated conservatively. The degree of occlusion failed to improve in the five incompletely treated aneurysms. In one of these patients, a partially embolized large posterior communicating artery aneurysm ruptured 3 years later, causing a debilitating, permanent neurological deficit.

The outcomes of GDC embolization and surgery for both symptomatic and incidental unruptured aneurysms were compared by Johnston and coworkers[101] in a cohort of patients treated at 60 university hospitals from January 1994 through June 1997 using the University Health System Consortium database. In this study, adverse outcomes were defined as in-hospital deaths and discharges to nursing homes or rehabilitation hospitals. Adverse outcomes were significantly more common in surgical cases (18.5%) than in endovascular cases (10.6%), and this difference remained after adjusting for age, sex, race, transfer admissions, emergency room admissions, and year of treatment. The in-hospital mortality rate was also higher for surgical cases (2.3% versus 0.4%). Length of stay and hospital charges were significantly greater for surgical cases.

The cost-effectiveness of endovascular obliteration of unruptured aneurysms in nonsurgical candidates was also assessed by Kallmes and colleagues,[102] who concluded that in such cases, cost-effectiveness is markedly affected by the natural course of unruptured, untreated aneurysms. Rates of spontaneous rupture higher than 2% per year resulted in favorable cost-utility ratios that were relatively unaffected by variations in GDC efficacy. In contrast, rates of rupture less than 1% per year resulted in unfavorable ratios that were highly dependent on GDC efficacy. Given the low incidence of rupture in unruptured aneurysms[103] and the lack of long-term data on the efficacy of GDC embolization for unruptured aneurysms, this novel therapy should be recommended with caution in patients with unruptured aneurysms, despite the encouraging results reported.

Aneurysms at Specific Sites

The morbidity associated with endovascular treatment is less dependent on aneurysm site than is that observed with conventional neurosurgery techniques. For this reason, much attention has been focused on the endovascular treatment of aneurysms in locations that notoriously represent surgical challenges, such as the basilar artery[104–113] and the ophthalmic segment of the ICA.[114, 115]

Eskridge and Song[106] summarized the results of the 159-patient subgroup with basilar bifurcation aneurysms enrolled in the Food and Drug Administration multicenter trial. There were nine technical failures, leaving 150 patients who underwent GDC embolization. All patients were referred for endovascular treatment because they were considered high-risk surgical candidates or because they had already failed surgical treatment. Eighty-three patients presented with aneurysmal SAH, and 67 had unruptured aneurysms. Of the patients with ruptured aneurysms, 46% were Hunt-Hess grade III, IV, or V. There were four periprocedural deaths (2.7%), and the overall mortality rate was 23% in the ruptured group and 12% in the unruptured group. Although embolic events were noted in 23% of all cases, only 5% of the patients with ruptured aneurysms and 9% of the patients with unruptured aneurysms had permanent deficits due to stroke. Importantly, two patients with ruptured aneurysms and two others with unruptured aneurysms developed episodes of rebleeding within the first year of treatment. These results represent the initial experience of a large pool of interventionists at the beginning of their learning curve. As expected, more recent single-center series have reported improved results with GDC treatment of basilar artery aneurysms.[104, 105, 107–113]

At the University of Vienna, Bavinzski and coworkers[105] reported the largest single-center experience with GDC treatment of basilar bifurcation aneurysms: 45 patients. Initially, these authors used GDC embolization only in patients with basilar aneurysms who were considered high surgical risks.[116] However, after observing good outcomes in their first 13 patients treated, they broadened their indications to include all patients with basilar aneurysms considered suitable for coiling, regardless of clinical status. In this series, the mortality and permanent morbidity rates directly related to intervention were 2.2% and 4.4%, respectively.[105] Angiographic occlusion rates, both immediately and at follow-up, were much better in small-necked aneurysms. One patient suffered a rebleed on the second day after treatment.

Similar results were reported by Klein and coworkers[108] in a series of 21 patients with ruptured (16 patients) and unruptured (5 patients) basilar bifurcation aneurysms that were considered solely for GDC embolization. Initially, 100% occlusion of the aneurysm was achieved in 14 patients (67%). In the remaining seven patients (33%), all with wide-necked aneurysms, 90% occlusion was achieved. In three of these patients, angiographic follow-up at 6 months revealed evidence of intra-aneurysmal coil compaction and recanalization requiring retreatment. In each of the remaining four patients who underwent partial treatment, the residual aneurysm was stable at follow-up and was considered too small for repeat embolization. No change in the rate of occlusion was noted 6 months after the initial treatment in any of the 12 patients with completely occluded aneurysms who were available for angiographic follow-up. In the three patients who required retreatment, occlusion of the aneurysm remained stable after a mean angiographic follow-up of 30 months. No rebleeding occurred after a mean follow-up of more than 2 years in the 16 patients who were treated after acute SAH. The overall permanent morbidity rate in this series was 5% (one patient with a permanent neurological deficit secondary to posterior communicating artery occlusion), and no procedure-related deaths occurred. An excellent or good outcome was observed in 15 of the 16 patients treated acutely after SAH, even though 9 patients were classified as Hunt-Hess grade III, IV, or V at presentation. Analysis of angiographic follow-up data also suggests that basilar bifurcation aneurysms tend to maintain a more stable angiographic appearance compared with aneurysms in other locations.[117, 118]

Given the low mortality and permanent morbidity rates observed after GDC embolization of posterior circulation aneurysms, some authors have compared the results of endovascular embolization with those obtained at surgery.[104, 119] Gruber and colleagues[104] compared the outcome of 41 patients with basilar bifurcation aneurysms; 20 underwent surgery, and 21 underwent GDC embolization. Patients in the two groups had aneurysms with comparable dimensions and configurations. Overall, 75% of the surgical patients and 95% of the embolized patients had a good outcome. Among patients treated in the acute phase after SAH, 73% of the surgical group and 91% of the endovascular group had a good outcome. There were two deaths in the surgical group and none in the endovascular group. Patients treated surgically were hospitalized twice as long as those who underwent endovascular treatment and incurred twice the expense. These results suggest that endovascular treatment of basilar bifurcation aneurysms is competitive with surgical treatment and could be the preferred mode of treatment if long-term follow-up shows protracted protection. At several institutions, GDC embolization is already considered the first therapeutic choice for patients with basilar artery aneurysms. Because patients harboring these aneurysms are considered primarily for endovascular treatment, only a few patients with basilar aneurysms have been enrolled in the ongoing International Subarachnoid Aneurysm Trial.

Because of the proximity of the optic nerve, the difficulty in obtaining proximal control, and the often partial intracavernous extension that results in a high frequency of failed or incomplete clipping, aneurysms of the ophthalmic segment represent one of the most common lesions treated by endovascular technique in several series.[115] Location of the aneurysm proximally in the circle of Willis is advantageous for catheterization, and the presence of a large parent vessel carries less risk of major vessel occlusion.[114]

Roy and coworkers[115] reported 28 consecutive GDC embolizations for ophthalmic segment aneurysms, of which 14 were ophthalmic and 14 were superior hypophyseal. Complete occlusion was achieved in 11 superior hypophyseal aneurysms (79%) but in only 3 ophthalmic aneurysms (21%); the superior hypophyseal aneurysms more frequently had small necks. All complete occlusions persisted at a mean angiographic follow-up of 14 months. No hemorrhagic episodes occurred at follow-up. In two patients, an MCA embolus occurred during treatment; both patients were treated with urokinase and recovered completely, with no detectable deficits. Another patient suffered a permanent neurological deficit that resulted from a loop of coil herniating into the ICA lumen and causing distal occlusion. These outcomes were echoed by Gurian and coworkers,[114] who reported successful embolization of 22 patients with superior hypophyseal aneurysms. On the basis of these series, it seems reasonable to consider GDC embolization for the treatment of small-necked aneurysms of the ICA ophthalmic segment. In large-necked aneurysms, the results with GDC alone are less optimal, with a significant rate of incomplete angiographic occlusion. Such cases may be better treated with the balloon-remodeling or combination stent-GDC technique.

Aneurysms arising at the bifurcation or trifurcation of the MCA are the least amenable to coil embolization because of an unfavorable neck-dome ratio, a relatively wide neck, and the possibility that one of the branches might be incorporated in the aneurysm's neck.[120] In a study of 30 consecutive patients harboring 34 unruptured aneurysms of the MCA in which coil embolization was considered the first option, only 2 aneurysms (6%) were successfully embolized, and 32 (94%) were clipped.[120] Although in this study 13 aneurysms were initially considered suitable for endovascular treatment, this treatment failed in 11 (85%).[120] The authors concluded that for unruptured MCA aneurysms, surgical clipping appears to be the most efficient treatment option.[120]

Rebleeding

The mechanisms of protection from aneurysm rupture after GDC embolization are largely unknown. Unlike surgical clipping, which permits immediate exclusion of the aneurysm sac from the parent artery (when successful), partial filling of the aneurysm may persist after GDC embolization despite complete angiographic obliteration.[121–123] True anatomic exclusion of the aneurysm from the circulation secondary to the formation of an endothelialized membrane across the aneurysm neck occurs in few patients. Further, when the endothelialization process occurs, it takes time for the membrane to become complete.[121] Despite these limitations, satisfactory (though not absolute) protection from further rebleeding occurs after GDC embolization of acutely ruptured intracranial aneurysms. Several series of patients treated in the acute phase after aneurysm rupture with GDC embolization have confirmed that the rate of rebleeding is lower than that indicated by the natural history of untreated ruptured aneurysms.[1, 44, 68, 71, 74, 80, 87, 124]

It is also obvious that even incomplete coiling offers protection during the acute or subacute phase after SAH. This protection has been related to the observation that clot organization and subsequent fibrosis are present in autopsy specimens, even in incompletely obliterated aneurysms, primarily at the periphery of the aneurysm wall (sac) ("endosaccular wrapping"; Richling, unpublished data). As mentioned, however, protection from further bleeding is not absolute, especially in incompletely coiled aneurysms.[80, 93, 124] In 317 patients treated by coil embolization soon after SAH and followed clinically for a median period of 22.3 months, Byrne and coworkers[80] reported annual rebleeding rates of 0.8% in the first year, 0.6% in the second year, and 2.4% in the third year. No further episodes of bleeding occurred in the 67 patients who were observed beyond 3 years. In this same series, rebleeding occurred in 3 of 38 recurrent aneurysms (7%) and in 1 of 221 aneurysms (0.4%) that appeared stable on angiography. In a series of 75 patients with acutely ruptured aneurysms treated with GDCs, Raymond and Roy[74] observed early subsequent bleeding in 3 aneurysms in 12 patients (25%) when the immediate angiographic results indicated residual aneurysm, compared with a 1.7% occurrence when there was no opacification of the aneurysm sac.

In assessing the midterm (>2 years) clinical follow-up of 61 patients who underwent GDC embolization as definitive aneurysm treatment, Malisch and colleagues[124] reported four deaths in patients with previously unruptured, partially thrombosed giant aneurysms that bled 12 to 20 months after incomplete GDC treatment. In addition, two nonfatal bleeding episodes were associated with one giant and one large aneurysm 33 and 30 months, respectively, after incomplete GDC treatment. Thus, the hemorrhage rate was 0% in small aneurysms, 4% in large aneurysms, and 33% in giant aneurysms. Rebleeding has also been observed after incomplete GDC embolization[100] and after complete endovascular occlusion[77] of a previously unruptured aneurysm. Again, these reports stress the importance of close long-term clinical and angiographic follow-up. The long-term clinical outcome of endovascular treatment remains to be validated.[125]

Vasospasm and Shunt-Dependent Hydrocephalus

One potential limitation of the endovascular approach in patients treated acutely after aneurysm rupture is the inability to remove cisternal clot, with a theoretical risk of increasing the likelihood of vasospasm. Early series, however, suggested that the risk of delayed cerebral ischemia after endovascular treatment of acutely ruptured intracranial aneurysms is no higher than that encountered after surgical clipping.[87, 126] It may even be lower, because mechanical injury is decreased by endovascular treatment.[127, 128]

In 69 patients classified as Hunt-Hess grades I, II, or III who underwent GDC occlusion of intracranial aneurysms within 72 hours of rupture, symptomatic vasospasm occurred in 23% of patients, resulting in an overall combined morbidity and mortality rate of 5.6% at 6 months.[126] In a comparison of surgical and endovascular treatment relative to the development of vasospasm and delayed cerebral ischemia, Gruber and associates[129] observed that when hemorrhage was confined to the subarachnoid space (Fisher computed tomographic grades I to III), the incidence of infarction was similar for both treatment groups. In the presence of intracerebral clot (Fisher grade IV), however, patients receiving endovascular treatment sustained a significantly higher rate of ischemic infarction than did their surgical counterparts.[129] A negligible difference in the occurrence rate of clinically symptomatic vasospasm was observed in the Finnish randomized trial that compared surgery with GDC embolization for the treatment of acutely ruptured intracranial aneurysms.[87]

Preliminary clinical evidence seems to suggest that shunt-dependent hydrocephalus might occur less frequently in patients undergoing GDC embolization than in patients treated with surgical clipping. In the Finnish randomized trial, shunt insertion was required significantly more often in the surgical group.[87] Similarly, in a retrospective series, Gruber and coworkers[130] observed that shunt-dependent hydrocephalus developed in 23.2% of patients undergoing surgery and in 17.7% of those undergoing early endovascular treatment. The reasons for these differences are unknown.

Aneurysms in Particular Situations

The successful use of detachable coils has been reported in a variety of unusual situations, such as in vertebrobasilar junction aneurysms associated with fenestration,[131] intracranial serpentine aneurysms,[132, 133] pseudoaneurysms,[134] aneurysms in patients with Moyamoya disease,[135] and multiple intracranial aneurysms.[136–138] GDCs have also been used to achieve parent vessel occlusion of dissecting aneurysms,[139, 140] giant and fusiform aneurysms,[141] and aneurysms involving distal branches.[142, 143]

Aneurysm Histopathology

Experimental studies,[35, 94, 122, 123, 144–147] autopsies,[121, 148–155] and pathology reports[156] have attempted to characterize the sequential histopathologic changes observed in intracranial aneurysms after GDC treatment. Dense packing with coils alters the local flow dynamics and favors intra-aneurysmal thrombus formation. The role of electrothrombosis in the formation of intra-aneurysmal clot is subject to debate.

The principle of electrothrombosis is based on the rationale that thrombus formation results from the attraction between negatively charged blood elements (such as red blood cells, white blood cells, platelets, and fibrinogen) and positively charged electrodes or metal wires. However, experimental and clinical evidence has questioned the role and importance of electrothrombosis in the mechanism of action of the GDC system. The small electrical current (1 mA) applied for coil detachment causes minimal electrothrombosis in vivo, especially if heparin is given.[35, 94] Experimental studies following Guglielmi's initial report demonstrated that the electricity used to detach the coils appears to have little effect on thrombus formation.[151] Further, the rate of occlusion is similar with mechanically detachable coils in which no electrothrombosis occurs.[157]

Horowitz and colleagues[158] reported a patient who underwent GDC treatment of a ruptured pericallosal aneurysm with no residual angiographic filling. No heparin was administered perioperatively. Two hours later, the aneurysm was explored surgically, and swirling blood was seen in the sac around the coils. After the aneurysm was opened, no thrombus was seen. These findings suggest that electrothrombosis has limited, if any, importance in the process of aneurysm thrombosis, and the GDCs' mechanism of action consists primarily of filling the space within the aneurysm, altering the local hemodynamics, and eventually promoting thrombosis.

After GDC delivery and thrombus formation, the thrombus undergoes a variable degree of organization. Thrombus organization involves invasion of the clot by thin-walled capillaries[122] arising from the aneurysm neck,[148] the aneurysm wall,[151] or both. Histologically, as soon as 16 hours after embolization, the coils within the aneurysm cavity are coated with fibrin,[152] which contains enmeshed red blood cells.[121] The process of thrombus organization proceeds centripetally, and a denser infiltration of the fibrin layer by polymorphonuclear neutrophilic leukocytes is present near the periphery of the dome along the aneurysm wall.[121, 151, 153] The presence of relatively dense scar formation at the aneurysm dome soon after coiling may explain the protective effect of incomplete coil packing and the consequent reduced rebleeding rate in patients treated acutely after SAH.

After GDC treatment, a thin fibrin membrane contiguous with the parent vessel occasionally covers the coils completely at the level of the aneurysm neck. This membrane has been reported to be complete in human specimens obtained as soon as 36 hours after GDC treatment,[154] as well as at different time intervals.[121, 148, 150, 155] Histologically, this membrane is composed primarily of fibrin, with thicker fibrils in the proximity of the neck.[121, 154] Such a thin membrane at the aneurysm entrance is most often observed 9 to 14 days after embolization. At this stage, the fibrin mesh that coated the coil fragments appears to be infiltrated by a large number of leukocytes and, to a lesser extent, by macrophages. Some centripetally invading fibroblasts are seen in the fibrin mesh at sites where the coils appose the aneurysm wall. Long-term autopsic observations have shown the presence of endothelial cells covering this fibrin membrane on the side of the parent vessel.[155]

Experimental and clinical studies have clearly shown that angiography is of little value in estimating the degree of aneurysm occlusion observed on pathologic examination[121–123] and actually overestimates the degree of occlusion. In a clinicopathologic study,[121] only five of seven small aneurysms that had been considered 100% occluded on angiography were completely covered by a membrane and therefore anatomically excluded from the parent vessel.

Given the variability in the degree of occlusion observed in animal studies (whether a side-wall or bifurcation aneurysm model was used), as well as the variability in human autopsy cases, it can be speculated that different factors, including local flow dynamics, density of coil packing, and size of the aneurysm and neck, all play an important role in determining the final degree of aneurysm occlusion after GDC embolization. More work is needed to characterize the factors that lead to the formation of such a complete membrane with consequent endothelialization. When a large sample of treated aneurysms is analyzed pathologically, this membrane seems to be the exception rather than the rule.[121]

COMPLICATIONS: AVOIDANCE AND MANAGEMENT

Ischemic Complications

Thromboembolic complications have been observed in as many as 24% of patients during GDC embolization.[108] Different stages of the procedure can trigger thrombus formation with or without consequent distal embolization. Meticulous attention to detail and extreme caution are recommended when trying to position the guide catheter in a stable position (see the section on GDC technique). This portion of the procedure can be the most challenging and time-consuming, especially in elderly patients with tortuous, atherosclerotic proximal vessels. During coil placement, thromboembolic complications can be a consequence of either thrombus dislodged from within the aneurysm (more likely while trying to embolize a partially thrombosed aneurysm) or thrombus formation around the coil mass during or even after the embolization procedure. This risk is especially high in the case of coils herniating through the neck into the parent vessel or, even worse, into distal branches arising near the aneurysm neck, as is often the case with aneurysms of the MCA or basilar bifurcation.

When coils herniate, several options are available, depending on the specific situation. The herniation of one or even several coils into the parent vessel is not necessarily associated with thromboembolic complications. As long as the herniation is well tolerated clinically, observation alone is a valid option. In such cases, we prefer to maintain the patient on full anticoagulation for 24 to 48 hours and then on antiplatelet therapy for 6 to 8 weeks. If the coil is floating within the parent artery and is considered a potential cause of secondary thromboembolism, a stent can be deployed to force the herniated coil against the parent vessel wall,[159] which may promote secondary endothelialization. If necessary, as in the case of secondary ischemia directly related to the occluding effects of the migrated coil or coils, an emergency craniotomy with coil and thrombus extraction can restore vessel patency and reverse the ongoing ischemia.[160]

When distal embolism is suspected or documented, superselective thrombolytic therapy can reestablish patency and reverse otherwise disabling neurological deficits.[161] Cronqvist and coworkers[161] reported 19 patients with intracranial aneurysms who suffered thromboembolic events during either catheterization or insertion of embolic material (both GDC and detachable spirals) or within the first few hours of intervention. All patients were fully heparinized during the procedure. The clot was distributed in the MCA territory in 14 cases, the anterior communicating artery in 3, and the basilar trunk in 2. A continuous intra-arterial injection of urokinase was immediately administered superselectively distal to the thrombus, within the thrombus, or closely proximal to it. In nine cases, pharmacologic lysis was combined with mechanical clot fragmentation by using the micro–guide wire. The occluded vessel segment recanalized completely in 10 patients and partially in 9 others. Fourteen patients experienced a good clinical recovery, one patient was moderately disabled, and two were severely disabled. Two of these patients died—one as a result of the original SAH, and the other when a hematoma developed after thrombolysis. In two additional patients, the aneurysm ruptured during fibrinolytic therapy, causing severe disability in one of them.

To prevent or minimize the risk of aneurysm rerupture and catastrophic consequences, these authors suggest that fibrinolysis be considered only if the aneurysm has been sufficiently embolized. As evidenced by this series, prompt fibrinolysis is not always successful, and its success depends on clot composition. An embolus consisting of fresh thrombus that develops during the procedure is much more likely to be dissolved by thrombolysis than is an embolus consisting of an atherosclerotic plaque fragment dislodged during catheterization of the proximal vessels.

Ischemic complications occur predominantly in patients undergoing treatment of aneurysms of the MCA or anterior communicating artery.[161, 162] This tendency is most likely related to the complex branching pattern of the vessels adjacent to the aneurysm neck. Additionally, the relationships between an aneurysm of the MCA or anterior communicating artery and the parent artery and its branches are often poorly defined on angiography, especially in the final stages of GDC embolization of these aneurysms. Parent artery compromise and clot formation can then occur. Before an aneurysm is catheterized or a coil is placed within an aneurysm, great effort should be devoted to obtaining an angiographic projection that delineates these relationships at all stages of the procedure.[162]

Intraprocedural Rupture

Intraprocedural aneurysm rupture is reported to occur in 2% to 8% of patients treated by GDC embolization.[43, 68, 74, 80, 163, 164] Rupture seems to be more common in the treatment of small aneurysms,[68, 74, 164] especially in the acute phase immediately following SAH.[43] Operator experience is also an important factor, with intraprocedural aneurysm rupture being most common in the early phase of the learning curve. In 75 patients treated during the acute phase after SAH, Raymond and Roy[74] experienced five ruptures in the first 25 patients, one in the next 25, and none in the last 25 patients treated.

Intraprocedural rupture can occur during several phases of the embolization procedure. Microcatheter-related ruptures occur while trying to catheterize the aneurysm and obtain stable and optimal placement of the microcatheter within the aneurysm. During this maneuver, it is important to avoid excessive slack in the microcatheter, which can cause it to move forward suddenly and perforate the aneurysm.[42, 43, 163] When catheterizing the aneurysm sac, the guide wire precedes the catheter's entry into the aneurysm. Using roadmapping techniques, the microcatheter is slowly advanced and placed at the center of the aneurysm sac. Distal placement of the microcatheter against the aneurysm wall can be associated with aneurysm perforation.[42] Undesirable forward movements are avoided when positioning the microcatheter by relieving any forward tension that might remain within the microcatheter–guide wire system before withdrawing the guide wire. Slack from the microcatheter is removed by making several passes with the guide wire.[43] After ensuring that no residual forward tension is present, the guide wire is slowly withdrawn under direct fluoroscopic control.[163]

While the first coil is delivered, excessive stress against the aneurysm wall is avoided. This maneuver is greatly enhanced by the availability of two-diameter coils and soft coils of different sizes. In acute aneurysms, the hemorrhage site can usually be identified as a small bleb on the aneurysm fundus. When possible, the first coil should be delivered away from these sites.[43] Rupture occurs less often during delivery or after detachment of subsequent coils.[164] A disturbing but often asymptomatic occurrence is the penetration of coil loops through the aneurysm sac, as observed during surgical exploration of previously embolized aneurysms.[165]

The clinical manifestations of intraprocedural rupture are variable. Although in some cases minimal extravasation of blood may not produce symptoms, awake patients tend to have headaches of varying severity. Neurological focal deficits and impairment of the level of consciousness may follow, depending on the severity of the hemorrhage. When an intraprocedural rupture occurs in anesthetized patients, hemodynamic monitoring reveals an otherwise unexplained increase in systemic blood pressure and heart rate.[43, 164] Prompt management of the rupture is of utmost importance to minimize its consequences. Intraprocedural heparinization is promptly reversed by the administration of intravenous protamine.

It is critical to avoid withdrawing the device responsible for the rupture (micro–guide wire, microcatheter, or coil). In such a situation, the offending device plugs the ruptured site, limiting the amount of extravasated blood. When the microcatheter is responsible for the rupture, a coil can be delivered within the subarachnoid space as the microcatheter is slowly removed in an attempt to seal the leak. Similarly, if a rupture occurs with a coil, it is important to continue to deliver the coil. In general, once a rupture has occurred, the remaining aneurysm sac is packed as quickly as possible. In refractory situations, temporary or permanent balloon occlusion of the parent artery can be performed.[166] The outcome of an intraprocedural rupture can be variable and is related primarily to the severity of the bleed. Prompt control of increased intracranial pressure by immediate placement of an external ventricular drain in the angiography suite can be a life-saving maneuver in severe ruptures.[164]

Infection

Although infection is a concern after the placement of any endovascular implant, it is extremely uncommon after GDC embolization of intracranial aneurysms. However, this possibility should be considered when coils are placed in an aneurysm extending into or adjacent to a potentially contaminated space, such as the sphenoid sinus, or when they are used in the treatment of mycotic aneurysms. In such cases, prophylactic antibiotic coverage has been suggested before and after coil placement.[167] Some authors recommend that all patients with endovascular implants receive appropriate prophylactic coverage during any invasive procedure in case of bacteremia, but no consensus exists regarding this practice.[167]

Unraveling or Fracture

Coils can unravel or fracture if there is friction between the coil and the delivery catheter or when there is significant resistance to placement of a coil within the aneurysm sac. In such cases, several techniques have been described for removal of the responsible coil.[168, 169] This complication should not be encountered if a "stretch-resistant" coil design is used.

COMBINED APPROACHES

In selected cases, endovascular aneurysm embolization and surgery can be used as complementary therapeutic modalities. For example, in poor-grade patients, GDC embolization can be attempted even when the geometry of the aneurysm is not ideal for coiling. Vasospasm can be treated aggressively. If the patient recovers, the aneurysm can be treated definitively by surgery, thereby allowing the surgeon to operate on a more relaxed brain (Fig. 120–6).[95, 160, 170] Alternatively, in a wide-necked aneurysm, if neither primary coiling nor complete surgical clipping of the neck can be accomplished, partial clipping can be pursued to transform the aneurysm into one with a smaller neck that is more amenable to coil packing (Fig. 120–7). Experience has shown that the clinical application of these approaches is quite limited, despite their appeal. Nevertheless, embolization after incomplete surgical clipping or, conversely, surgery after incomplete embolization of intracranial aneurysms provides definitive treatment in a large percentage of complicated cases.[95, 96, 160, 165, 170–174]

As the number of aneurysms treated with GDC embolization grows, neurosurgeons will increasingly confront the challenge represented by residual or recurring aneurysms. Several reports have addressed this issue and described the associated difficulties.[76, 156, 160, 165, 170] There is consensus that additional coiling should be considered when feasible.[165] In cases that are not amenable to further GDC embolization, the major considerations when attempting surgery are the degree of oc-

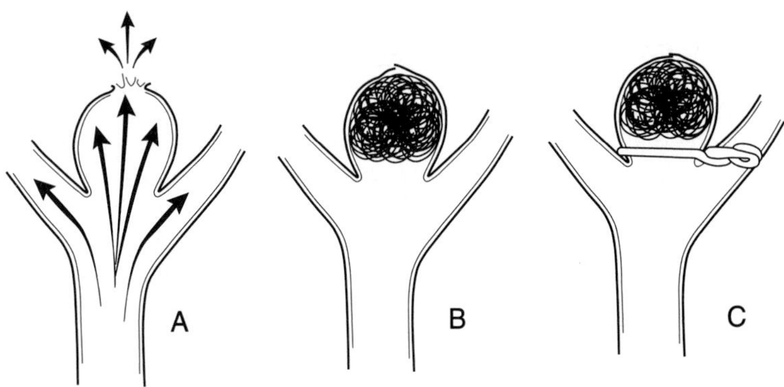

FIGURE 120–6. *A*, Schematic drawing of a ruptured aneurysm whose geometry is not ideal for endovascular treatment. *B*, At least temporarily, the aneurysm can be partially coiled if the patient is in poor neurological condition. This option allows aggressive management of vasospasm with an acceptably low risk of rerupture. *C*, After the patient improves neurologically, definitive surgical clipping can be performed, thus allowing the surgeon to operate on a more relaxed brain. (From Borchers DJ, Mericle RA, Wakhloo AK, et al: Endovascular management of intracranial aneurysms. Neurosurg Q 8:1–15, 1998.)

clusion of the aneurysm neck and the time elapsed since the last embolization.[160]

Aneurysms without coils at the base are easier to treat with primary clipping; those with coils massed in the neck are difficult to clip without removing the coils from the sac.[160, 165, 170] Clipping large, partially coiled aneurysms can pose additional difficulties because the coiled, relatively immobile mass makes visualization around the lesion difficult.[76, 160] In such cases, intraprocedural angiography permits viewing of the clip's position and assessment of parent vessel patency. If a coil loop is found at surgery to herniate into the parent vessel, the coils should not be extracted, because the loop might be incorporated within the parent vessel wall.[160] One or two loops of coil in a parent vessel may be harmless in terms of generating thrombus or embolus, whereas attempts at coil extraction might tear the vessel if the coil is incorporated in the vessel wall or the aneurysm fundus or neck. Coil incorporation may be seen as early as 2 weeks after embolization.[160] If a partially coiled aneurysm or recurrent lesion is to be treated surgically, obtaining proximal and distal control of the parent artery is of utmost importance, especially if coil extraction is required to obliterate the lesion. If the aneurysm neck can be clipped without compromising the parent vessel, clip application without coil removal should be attempted.[165]

Problems can also be encountered while attempting endovascular embolization after incomplete surgery.[171–174] Thielen and colleagues[171] detailed the endovascular treatment of eight patients with residual aneurysms treated at different intervals after surgical clipping. There were no deaths or permanent complications. Four patients, however, experienced transient neurological deficits that resolved without sequelae. Complete angiographic aneurysm occlusion was observed on the last control angiogram in six patients, and there was near occlusion in the remaining two patients. No clinical episodes of rebleeding were encountered in this small group of patients after a mean follow-up of 28 months.

Technical challenges encountered during endovascular treatment of previously clipped cerebral aneurysms (but not observed with previously untreated aneurysms) include the following: (1) The configuration of the aneurysm remnant is seldom saccular. It is more likely to have a straight or truncated side because of the previously placed clip, thereby making coil selection difficult at times. (2) Surgical clips can make angiographic delineation of the aneurysm neck more prob-

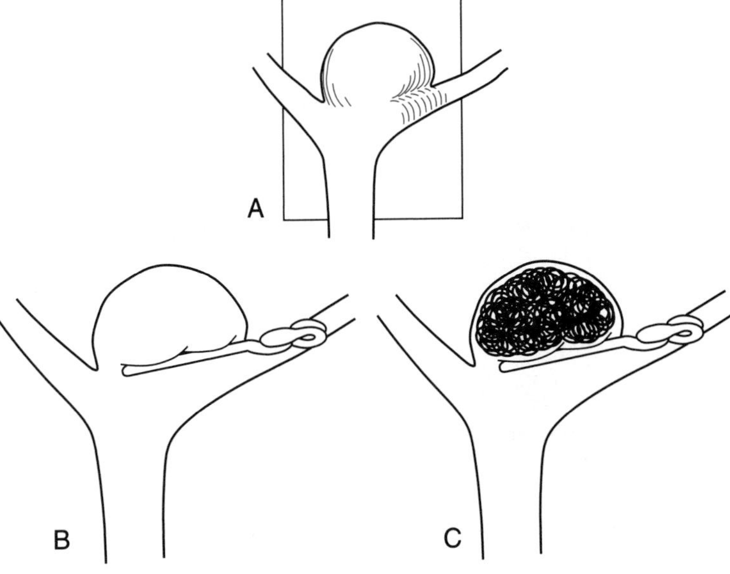

FIGURE 120–7. *A*, Schematic drawing of a combined surgical-endovascular approach that takes advantage of both techniques. *B*, In the case of a wide-necked aneurysm that is difficult to cure with either approach alone, the lesion can be initially approached surgically, and the neck partially clipped. *C*, This strategy transforms a wide-necked aneurysm into an aneurysm with favorable geometry for definitive coiling. (From Borchers DJ, Mericle RA, Wakhloo AK, et al: Endovascular management of intracranial aneurysms. Neurosurg Q 8:1–15, 1998.)

lematic.[171, 174] Consequently, positioning the microcatheter and coils under fluoroscopic control is more difficult. (3) If the clip extends across the neck and along the rigid wall of the aneurysm, delivering the coils can be problematic. The wall pushes the coils back, resisting stabilization within the sac.[174] Despite these limitations, as shown by the experience of Thielen and colleagues[171] and other authors,[174] embolization can be performed safely in most incompletely clipped aneurysms, with good immediate and follow-up angiographic results.

In our personal experience, surgical approaches to cervical carotid or vertebral arteries for endovascular access to otherwise unreachable aneurysms (because of proximal arterial disease or tortuosity) are another example of the effective combination of surgical and endovascular techniques.

FUTURE DIRECTIONS

During the past decade, tremendous advances have occurred in the endovascular treatment of cerebrovascular disorders and of intracranial aneurysms in particular, and it is likely that other innovations will occur in the next few years. Compared with current surgical techniques for the treatment of intracranial aneurysms, one of the major advantages of the endovascular approach is the great potential for improvements in the technologies and devices used. Several attempts have been made and are in progress to improve the thrombogenicity of GDCs.[175–183] Further developments in novel materials such as liquid embolic agents may dramatically change the endovascular approach to intracranial aneurysms by permitting the aneurysm sac to be filled with such agents.[184–186] It may also be possible to deploy a covered stent across a wide-necked aneurysm,[187–190] thus immediately excluding the aneurysm from the parent vessel flow. Alternatively, with improved knowledge of the molecular basis of aneurysm thrombosis following endovascular embolization,[191, 192] coils can be used to deliver biologic factors locally and in a controlled fashion to facilitate such a process.[177, 178]

REFERENCES

1. Cognard C, Weill A, Castaings L, et al: Intracranial berry aneurysms: Angiographic and clinical results after endovascular treatment. Radiology 206:499–510, 1998.
2. Lot G, Houdart E, Cophignon J, et al: Combined management of intracranial aneurysms by surgical and endovascular treatment: Modalities and results from a series of 395 cases. Acta Neurochir (Wien) 141:557–562, 1999.
3. Nelson PK: Neurointerventional management of intracranial aneurysms. Neurosurg Clin N Am 9:879–895, 1998.
4. Nichols DA, Meyer FB, Piepgras DG, et al: Endovascular treatment of intracranial aneurysms. Mayo Clin Proc 69:272–285, 1994.
5. van Rooij WJJ: Endovascular treatment of cerebral aneurysms [thesis]. Utrecht, The Netherlands, 1998.
6. Home E: An account of Mr. Hunter's method for performing the operation for the popliteal aneurysms. London Med J 7: 391–406, 1786.
7. Nishioka H: Results of treatment of intracranial aneurysms by occlusion of the carotid artery in the neck. J Neurosurg 25: 660–704, 1966.
8. Drake CG, Peerless SJ, Ferguson GG: Hunterian proximal arterial occlusion for giant aneurysms of the carotid circulation. J Neurosurg 81:656–665, 1994.
9. Byrne JV, Guglielmi G: Endovascular Treatment of Intracranial Aneurysms. New York, Springer-Verlag, 1998.
10. Matas R, Allen CW: Occlusion of large surgical arteries with removable metallic bands to test the efficiency of the collateral circulation: Experimental and clinical observations. JAMA 56: 233–237, 1911.
11. Connors JJ: Temporary test occlusion of the internal carotid artery. In Connors JJ, Wojak JC (eds): Interventional Neuroradiology, Strategies and Practical Techniques. Philadelphia, WB Saunders, 1999, pp 377–390.
12. Standard SC, Ahuja A, Guterman LR, et al: Balloon test occlusion of the internal carotid artery with hypotensive challenge. AJNR Am J Neuroradiol 16:1453–1458, 1995.
13. Standard SC, Guterman LR, Chavis TD, et al: Endovascular management of giant intracranial aneurysms. Clin Neurosurg 42:267–293, 1995.
14. Guterman LR, Hopkins LN: Endovascular treatment of giant intracranial aneurysms. Tech Neurosurg 4:179–184, 1998.
15. Mathis JM, Barr JD, Jungreis CA, et al: Temporary balloon test occlusion of the internal carotid artery: Experience with 500 cases. AJNR Am J Neuroradiol 16:749–754, 1995.
16. Vasquez Anon V, Aymard A, Gobin YP, et al: Balloon occlusion of the internal carotid artery in 40 cases of giant intracavernous aneurysm: Technical aspects, cerebral monitoring, and results. Neuroradiology 34:245–251, 1992.
17. Valee JN, Aymard A, Casasco AE, et al: Endovascular test and permanent occlusion of extracranial and intracranial cerebral vessels: Indications, techniques, and management. In Connors JJ, Wojak JC (eds): Interventional Neuroradiology, Strategies and Practical Techniques. Philadelphia, WB Saunders, 1999, pp 394–408.
18. Aymard A, Gobin YP, Hodes JE, et al: Endovascular occlusion of vertebral arteries in the treatment of unclippable vertebrobasilar aneurysms. J Neurosurg 74:393–398, 1991.
19. Aymard A, Hodes JE, Rufenacht, et al: Endovascular treatment of a giant fusiform aneurysm of the entire basilar artery. AJNR Am J Neuroradiol 13:1143–1146, 1992.
20. Fox AJ, Vinuela F, Pelz DM, et al: Use of detachable balloons for proximal artery occlusion in the treatment of unclippable cerebral aneurysms. J Neurosurg 66:40–46, 1987.
21. Higashida RT, Halbach VV, Dowd C, et al: Endovascular detachable balloon embolization therapy of cavernous carotid artery aneurysms: Results in 87 cases. J Neurosurg 72:857–863, 1990.
22. Bavinzski G, Killer M, Ferraz-Leite H, et al: Endovascular therapy of idiopathic cavernous aneurysms over 11 years. AJNR Am J Neuroradiol 19:559–565, 1998.
23. Polin RS, Shaffrey ME, Jensen ME, et al: Medical management in the endovascular treatment of carotid-cavernous aneurysms. J Neurosurg 84:755–761, 1996.
24. Larson JJ, Tew JM Jr, Tomsick TA, et al: Treatment of aneurysms of the internal carotid artery by intravascular balloon occlusion: Long-term follow-up of 58 patients. Neurosurgery 36:26–30, 1995.
25. Linskey ME, Sekhar LN, Horton JA, et al: Aneurysms of the intracavernous carotid artery: A multidisciplinary approach to treatment. J Neurosurg 75:525–534, 1991.
26. Roski RA, Spetzler RF, Nulsen FE: Late complications of carotid ligation in the treatment of intracranial aneurysms. J Neurosurg 54:583–587, 1981.
27. Hodes JE, Fox AJ, Pelz DM, et al: Rupture of aneurysms following balloon embolization. J Neurosurg 72:567–571, 1990.
28. Chang SD, Marks MP, Steinberg GK: Recanalization and rupture of a giant vertebral artery aneurysm after hunterian ligation: Case report. Neurosurgery 44:1117–1121, 1999.
29. Gurian JH, Vinuela F, Gobin YP, et al: Aneurysm rupture after parent vessel sacrifice: Treatment with Guglielmi detachable coil embolization via retrograde catheterization: Case report. Neurosurgery 37:1216–1221, 1995.
30. Gianturco C, Anderson JH, Wallace S: Mechanical devices for arterial occlusion. AJR Am J Roentgenol 124:428–435, 1975.
31. Hilal SK, Solomon RA: Endovascular treatment of aneurysms with coils. J Neurosurg 76:337–339, 1992.

32. Dowd CF, Halbach VV, Higashida RT, et al: Endovascular coil embolization of unusual posterior inferior cerebellar artery aneurysms. Neurosurgery 27:954–961, 1990.
33. Higashida RT, Halbach VV, Dowd CF, et al: Interventional neurovascular treatment of a giant intracranial aneurysm using platinum microcoils. Surg Neurol 35:64–68, 1991.
34. Guglielmi G, Vinuela F, Dion J, et al: Electrothrombosis of saccular aneurysms via endovascular approach. Part 2. Preliminary clinical experience. J Neurosurg 75:8–14, 1991.
35. Guglielmi G, Vinuela F, Sepetka I, et al: Electrothrombosis of saccular aneurysms via endovascular approach. Part 1. Electrochemical basis, technique, and experimental results. J Neurosurg 75:1–7, 1991.
36. Casasco AE, Aymard A, Gobin YP, et al: Selective endovascular treatment of 71 intracranial aneurysms with platinum coils. J Neurosurg 79:3–10, 1993.
37. Cekirge HS, Saatci I, Firat MM, et al: Interlocking detachable coil occlusion in the endovascular treatment of intracranial aneurysms. AJNR Am J Neuroradiol 17:1651–1657, 1996.
38. Cognard C, Pierot L, Boulin A, et al: Intracranial aneurysms: Endovascular treatment with mechanical detachable spirals in 60 aneurysms. Radiology 202:783–792, 1997.
39. Tournade A, Courtheoux P, Sengel C, et al: Saccular intracranial aneurysms: Endovascular treatment with mechanical detachable spiral coils. Radiology 202:481–486, 1997.
40. Guglielmi G: Treatment of an intracranial aneurysm using a new three-dimensional-shape Guglielmi detachable coil: Technical case report [letter]. Neurosurgery 45:959–961, 1999.
41. Malek AM, Higashida RT, Phatouros CC, et al: Treatment of an intracranial aneurysm using a new three-dimensional-shape Guglielmi detachable coil: Technical case report. Neurosurgery 44:1142–1145, 1999.
42. Mena F, Vinuela F, Duckwiler G, et al: Pitfalls of GDC embolization of intracranial aneurysms. Intervent Neuroradiol 4:231–240, 1998.
43. Watson V, Coumans JV, McGrail K, et al: Rupture of cerebral aneurysms during endovascular treatment with electrolytically detachable coils: Incidence, management, and outcome. J Neurovasc Dis 3:269–275, 1998.
44. Cognard C, Weill A, Spelle L, et al: Long-term angiographic follow-up of 169 intracranial berry aneurysms occluded with detachable coils. Radiology 212:348–356, 1999.
45. Lefkowitz MA, Gobin YP, Akiba Y, et al: Balloon-assisted Guglielmi detachable coiling of wide-necked aneurysms. Part II. Clinical results. Neurosurgery 45:531–538, 1999.
46. Levy DI: Embolization of wide-necked anterior communicating artery aneurysm: Technical note. Neurosurgery 41:979–982, 1997.
47. Levy DI, Ku A: Balloon-assisted coil placement in wide-necked aneurysms: Technical note. J Neurosurg 86:724–727, 1997.
48. Mericle RA, Wakhloo AK, Rodriguez R, et al: Temporary balloon protection as an adjunct to endosaccular coiling of wide-necked cerebral aneurysms: Technical note. Neurosurgery 41: 975–978, 1997.
49. Moret J, Cognard C, Weill A, et al: The "remodeling technique" in the treatment of wide neck intracranial aneurysms: Angiographic results and clinical follow-up in 56 cases. Intervent Neuroradiol 3:21–35, 1997.
50. Takahashi A, Ezura M, Yoshimoto T: Broad neck basilar tip aneurysm treated by neck plastic intra-aneurysmal GDC embolization with protective balloon. Intervent Neuroradiol 3:167–170, 1997.
51. Akiba Y, Murayama Y, Vinuela F, et al: Balloon-assisted Guglielmi detachable coiling of wide-necked aneurysms. Part I. Experimental evaluation. Neurosurgery 45:519–530, 1999.
52. Bracard S, Anxionnat R, Da Costa E, et al: Combined endovascular stenting and endovascular coiling for the treatment of a wide-necked intracranial vertebral aneurysm: Technical case report. Intervent Neuroradiol 5:245–249, 1999.
53. Higashida RT, Smith W, Gress D, et al: Intravascular stent and endovascular coil placement for a ruptured fusiform aneurysm of the basilar artery: Case report and review of the literature. J Neurosurg 87:944–949, 1997.
54. Lanzino G, Wakhloo AK, Fessler RD, et al: Efficacy and current limitations of intravascular stents for intracranial internal carotid, vertebral, and basilar artery aneurysms. J Neurosurg 91: 538–546, 1999.
55. Lylyk P, Ceratto R, Hurvitz D, et al: Treatment of a vertebral dissecting aneurysm with stents and coils: Technical case report. Neurosurgery 43:385–388, 1998.
56. Sekhon LHS, Morgan MK, Sorby W, et al: Combined endovascular stent implantation and endosaccular coil placement for the treatment of a wide-necked vertebral artery aneurysm: Technical case report. Neurosurgery 43:380–384, 1998.
57. Massoud TF, Turjman F, Ji C, et al: Endovascular treatment of fusiform aneurysms with stents and coils: Technical feasibility in a swine model. AJNR Am J Neuroradiol 16:1953–1963, 1995.
58. Szikora I, Guterman LR, Wells KM, et al: Combined use of stents and coils to treat experimental wide-necked carotid aneurysms: Preliminary results. AJNR Am J Neuroradiol 15:1091–1102, 1994.
59. Turjman F, Massoud TF, Ji C, et al: Combined stent implantation and endosaccular coil placement for treatment of experimental wide-necked aneurysms: A feasibility study in swine. AJNR Am J Neuroradiol 15:1087–1090, 1994.
60. Wakhloo AK, Lieber BB, Divani AA, et al: Parent vessel remodeling after stenting of broad-based canine carotid artery aneurysms. Intervent Neuroradiol 3(Suppl 1):81, 1997.
61. Wakhloo AK, Schellhammer F, de Vries J, et al: Self-expanding and balloon-expandable stents in the treatment of carotid aneurysms: An experimental study in a canine model. AJNR Am J Neuroradiol 15:493–502, 1994.
62. Wakhloo AK, Tio FO, Lieber BB, et al: Self-expanding nitinol stents in canine vertebral arteries: Hemodynamics and tissue response. AJNR Am J Neuroradiol 16:1043–1051, 1995.
63. Geremia G, Haklin M, Brennecke L: Embolization of experimentally created aneurysms with intravascular stent devices. AJNR Am J Neuroradiol 15:1223–1231, 1994.
64. Lieber BB, Stancampiano AP, Wakhloo AK: Alteration of hemodynamics in aneurysm models by stenting: Influence of stent porosity. Ann Biomed Eng 25:460–469, 1997.
65. Wakhloo AK, Lanzino G, Lieber BB, et al: Stents for intracranial aneurysms: The beginning of a new endovascular era? Neurosurgery 43:377–379, 1998.
66. Mericle RA, Lanzino G, Wakhloo AK, et al: Stenting and secondary coiling of intracranial internal carotid artery aneurysm: Technical case report. Neurosurgery 43:1229–1234, 1998.
67. Bai H, Masuda J, Sawa Y, et al: Neointima formation after vascular stent implantation: Spatial and chronological distribution of smooth muscle cell proliferation and phenotypic modulation. Arterioscler Thromb 14:1846–1853, 1994.
68. Vinuela F, Duckwiler G, Mawad M: Guglielmi detachable coil embolization of acute intracranial aneurysm: Perioperative anatomical and clinical outcome in 403 patients. J Neurosurg 86: 475–482, 1997.
69. Byrne JV, Adams CB, Kerr RS, et al: Endovascular treatment of inoperable intracranial aneurysms with platinum coils. Br J Neurosurg 9:585–592, 1995.
70. Byrne JV, Molyneux AJ, Brennan RP, et al: Embolisation of recently ruptured intracranial aneurysms. J Neurol Neurosurg Psychiatry 59:616–620, 1995.
71. Graves VB, Strother CM, Duff TA, et al: Early treatment of ruptured aneurysms with Guglielmi detachable coils: Effects on subsequent bleeding. Neurosurgery 37:640–647, 1995.
72. Kuether TA, Nesbit GM, Barnwell SL: Clinical and angiographic outcomes, with treatment data, for patients with cerebral aneurysms treated with Guglielmi detachable coils: A single-center experience. Neurosurgery 43:1016–1025, 1998.
73. Martin D, Rodesch G, Alvarez H, et al: Preliminary results of embolisation of nonsurgical intracranial aneurysms with GD coils: The 1st year of their use. Neuroradiology 38 (Suppl 1): S142–S150, 1996.
74. Raymond J, Roy D: Safety and efficacy of endovascular treatment of acutely ruptured aneurysms. Neurosurgery 41:1235–1246, 1997.
75. Scotti G, Righi C, Simionato F, et al: Endovascular therapy of intracranial aneurysms with Guglielmi detachable coils (GDC). Riv Neuroradiol 7:723–733, 1994.
76. Mericle RA, Wakhloo AK, Lopes DK, et al: Delayed aneurysm regrowth and recanalization after Guglielmi detachable coil treatment. J Neurosurg 89:142–145, 1998.

77. Hodgson TJ, Carroll T, Jellinek DA: Subarachnoid hemorrhage due to late recurrence of a previously unruptured aneurysm after complete endovascular occlusion. AJNR Am J Neuroradiol 19:1939–1941, 1998.
78. Manabe H, Fujita S, Hatayama T, et al: Rerupture of coil-embolized aneurysm during long-term observation: Case report. J Neurosurg 88:1096–1098, 1998.
79. Raftopoulos C, Mathurin P, Boscherini D, et al: Prospective analysis of aneurysm treatment in a series of 103 consecutive patients when endovascular embolization is considered the first option. J Neurosurg 93:175–182, 2000.
80. Byrne JV, Sohn MJ, Molyneux AJ: Five-year experience in using coil embolization for ruptured intracranial aneurysms: Outcomes and incidence of late rebleeding. J Neurosurg 90:656–663, 1999.
81. Adams WM, Laitt RD, Jackson A: Time of flight 3D magnetic resonance angiography in the follow-up of coiled cerebral aneurysms. Intervent Neuroradiol 5:127–137, 1999.
82. Derdeyn CP, Graves VB, Turski PA, et al: MR angiography of saccular aneurysms after treatment with Guglielmi detachable coils: Preliminary experience. AJNR Am J Neuroradiol 18:279–286, 1997.
83. Kahara VJ, Seppanen SK, Ryymin PS, et al: MR angiography with three-dimensional time-of-flight and targeted maximum-intensity-projection reconstructions in the follow-up of intracranial aneurysms embolized with Guglielmi detachable coils. AJNR Am J Neuroradiol 20:1470–1475, 1999.
84. Hartman J, Nguyen T, Larsen D, et al: MR artifacts, heat production, and ferromagnetism of Guglielmi detachable coils. AJNR Am J Neuroradiol 18:497–501, 1997.
85. Fernandez Zubillaga A, Guglielmi G, Vinuela F, et al: Endovascular occlusion of intracranial aneurysms with electrically detachable coils: Correlation of aneurysm neck size and treatment results. AJNR Am J Neuroradiol 15:815–820, 1994.
86. Debrun GM, Aletich VA, Kehrli P, et al: Selection of cerebral aneurysms for treatment using Guglielmi detachable coils: The preliminary University of Illinois at Chicago experience. Neurosurgery 43:1281–1297, 1998.
87. Vanninen R, Koivisto T, Saari T, et al: Ruptured intracranial aneurysms: Acute endovascular treatment with electrolytically detachable coils—a prospective randomized study. Radiology 211:325–336, 1999.
88. Hunt WE, Hess RM: Surgical risk as related to time of intervention in the repair of intracranial aneurysms. J Neurosurg 28: 14–20, 1968.
89. Fisher CM, Kistler JP, Davis JM: Relation of cerebral vasospasm to subarachnoid hemorrhage visualized by computerized tomographic scanning. Neurosurgery 6:1–9, 1980.
90. Jennett B, Bond M: Assessment of outcome after severe brain damage. Lancet 1:480–484, 1975.
91. Molyneux AJ: Surgery or coiling for intracranial aneurysms: The current position and future prospects. Neurointerventionist 1:12–15, 1999.
92. Molyneux A, Kerr R: International Subarachnoid Aneurysm Trial. J Neurosurg 91:352–353, 1999.
93. Gruber A, Killer M, Bavinzski G, et al: Clinical and angiographic results of endosaccular coil treatment of giant and very large intracranial aneurysms: A 7-year, single-center experience. Neurosurgery 45:793–804, 1999.
94. Byrne JV, Hope JK, Hubbard N, et al: The nature of thrombosis induced by platinum and tungsten coils in saccular aneurysms. AJNR Am J Neuroradiol 18:29–33, 1997.
95. Cockroft KM, Marks MP, Steinberg GK: Planned direct dual-modality treatment of complex broad-necked intracranial aneurysms: Four technical case reports. Neurosurgery 46:226–231, 2000.
96. Hacein-Bey L, Connolly ES Jr, Mayer SA, et al: Complex intracranial aneurysms: Combined operative and endovascular approaches. Neurosurgery 43:1304–1313, 1998.
97. Malisch TW, Guglielmi G, Vinuela F, et al: Unruptured aneurysms presenting with mass effect symptoms: Response to endosaccular treatment with Guglielmi detachable coils. Part I. Symptoms of cranial nerve dysfunction. J Neurosurg 89:956–961, 1998.
98. Vargas ME, Kupersmith MJ, Setton A, et al: Endovascular treatment of giant aneurysms which cause visual loss. Ophthalmology 101:1091–1098, 1994.
99. Litofsky NS, Vinuela F, Giannotta SL: Progressive visual loss after electrothrombosis treatment of a giant intracranial aneurysm: Case report. Neurosurgery 34:548–551, 1994.
100. Murayama Y, Vinuela F, Duckwiler GR, et al: Embolization of incidental cerebral aneurysms by using the Guglielmi detachable coil system. J Neurosurg 90:207–214, 1999.
101. Johnston SC, Dudley RA, Gress DR, et al: Surgical and endovascular treatment of unruptured cerebral aneurysms at university hospitals. Neurology 52:1799–1805, 1999.
102. Kallmes DF, Kallmes MH, Cloft HJ, et al: Guglielmi detachable coil embolization for unruptured aneurysms in nonsurgical candidates: A cost-effectiveness exploration. AJNR Am J Neuroradiol 19:167–176, 1998.
103. International Study of Unruptured Aneurysms Investigators: Unruptured intracranial aneurysms—risk of rupture and risks of surgical intervention. N Engl J Med 339:1725–1733, 1998.
104. Gruber DP, Zimmerman GA, Tomsick TA, et al: A comparison between endovascular and surgical management of basilar artery apex aneurysms. J Neurosurg 90:868–874, 1999.
105. Bavinzski G, Killer M, Gruber A, et al: Treatment of basilar artery bifurcation aneurysms by using Guglielmi detachable coils: A 6-year experience. J Neurosurg 90:843–852, 1999.
106. Eskridge JM, Song JK: Endovascular embolization of 150 basilar tip aneurysms with Guglielmi detachable coils: Results of the Food and Drug Administration multicenter clinical trial. J Neurosurg 89:81–86, 1998.
107. Guglielmi G, Vinuela F, Duckwiler G, et al: Endovascular treatment of posterior circulation aneurysms by electrothrombosis using electrically detachable coils. J Neurosurg 77:515–524, 1992.
108. Klein GE, Szolar DH, Leber KA, et al: Basilar tip aneurysm: Endovascular treatment with Guglielmi detachable coils—midterm results. Radiology 205:191–196, 1997.
109. Lempert TE, Malek AM, Halbach VV, et al: Endovascular treatment of ruptured posterior circulation cerebral aneurysms: Clinical and angiographic outcomes. Stroke 31:100–110, 2000.
110. McDougall CG, Halbach VV, Dowd CF, et al: Endovascular treatment of basilar tip aneurysms using electrolytically detachable coils. J Neurosurg 84:393–399, 1996.
111. Nichols DA, Brown RD Jr, Thielen KR, et al: Endovascular treatment of ruptured posterior circulation aneurysms using electrolytically detachable coils. J Neurosurg 87:374–380, 1997.
112. Pierot L, Boulin A, Castaings L, et al: Selective occlusion of basilar artery aneurysms using controlled detachable coils: Report of 35 cases. Neurosurgery 38:948–954, 1996.
113. Raymond J, Roy D, Bojanowski M, et al: Endovascular treatment of acutely ruptured and unruptured aneurysms of the basilar bifurcation. J Neurosurg 86:211–219, 1997.
114. Gurian JH, Vinuela F, Guglielmi G, et al: Endovascular embolization of superior hypophyseal artery aneurysms. Neurosurgery 39:1150–1156, 1996.
115. Roy D, Raymond J, Bouthillier A, et al: Endovascular treatment of ophthalmic segment aneurysms with Guglielmi detachable coils. AJNR Am J Neuroradiol 18:1207–1215, 1997.
116. Bavinzski G, Richling B, Gruber A, et al: Endosaccular occlusion of basilar artery bifurcation aneurysms using electrically detachable coils. Acta Neurochir (Wien) 134:184–189, 1995.
117. Hope JKA, Byrne JV, Molyneux AJ: Factors influencing successful angiographic occlusion of aneurysms treated by coil embolization. AJNR Am J Neuroradiol 20:391–399, 1999.
118. Richling B, Gruber A, Bavinzski G, et al: GDC-system embolization for brain aneurysms: Location and follow-up. Acta Neurochir (Wien) 134:177–183, 1995.
119. Nakabayashi K, Negoro M, Itou Y, et al: Endovascular approach vs microsurgical approach for posterior circulation aneurysms. Intervent Neuroradiol 3(Suppl 2):171–176, 1997.
120. Regli L, Uske A, de Tribolet N: Endovascular coil placement compared with surgical clipping for the treatment of unruptured middle cerebral artery aneurysms: A consecutive series. J Neurosurg 90:1025–1030, 1999.
121. Bavinzski G, Talazoglu V, Killer M, et al: Gross and microscopic histopathological findings in aneurysms of the human brain treated with Guglielmi detachable coils. J Neurosurg 91:284–293, 1999.

122. MacDonald RL, Mojtahedi C, Johns L, et al: Randomized comparison of Guglielmi detachable coils and cellulose acetate polymer for treatment of aneurysms in dogs. Stroke 29:478–486, 1998.
123. Reul J, Weis J, Spetzger U, et al: Long-term angiographic and histopathologic findings in experimental aneurysms of the carotid bifurcation embolized with platinum and tungsten coils. AJNR Am J Neuroradiol 18:35–42, 1997.
124. Malisch TW, Guglielmi G, Vinuela F, et al: Intracranial aneurysms treated with the Guglielmi detachable coil: Midterm clinical results in a consecutive series of 100 patients. J Neurosurg 87:176–183, 1997.
125. Mawad M: Subarachnoid hemorrhage due to late recurrence of a previously unruptured aneurysm after complete endovascular occlusion. AJNR Am J Neuroradiol 19:1810–1811, 1998.
126. Murayama Y, Malisch T, Guglielmi G, et al: Incidence of cerebral vasospasm after endovascular treatment of acutely ruptured aneurysms: Report on 69 cases. J Neurosurg 87:830–835, 1997.
127. Strother CM: Does reduction in vascular trauma during treatment of acutely ruptured saccular aneurysms reduce the incidence of vasospasm? [editorial]. AJNR Am J Neuroradiol 19: 592, 1998.
128. Yalamanchili K, Rosenwasser RH, Thomas JE, et al: Frequency of cerebral vasospasm in patients treated with endovascular occlusion of intracranial aneurysms. AJNR Am J Neuroradiol 19:553–558, 1998.
129. Gruber A, Ungersbock K, Reinprecht A, et al: Evaluation of cerebral vasospasm after early surgical and endovascular treatment of ruptured intracranial aneurysms. Neurosurgery 42:258–268, 1998.
130. Gruber A, Reinprecht A, Bavinzski G, et al: Chronic shunt-dependent hydrocephalus after early surgery and early endovascular treatment of ruptured intracranial aneurysms. Neurosurgery 44:503–512, 1999.
131. Graves VB, Strother CM, Weir B, Duff TA: Vertebrobasilar junction aneurysms associated with fenestration: Treatment with Guglielmi detachable coils. AJNR Am J Neuroradiol 17:35–40, 1996.
132. Duong H, Lycette C, Pile-Spellman J, et al: Guglielmi detachable coil treatment of a serpentine middle cerebral artery aneurysm. J Neurovasc Dis 1:33–38, 1996.
133. Mawad ME, Klucznik RP: Giant serpentine aneurysms: Radiographic features and endovascular treatment. AJNR Am J Neuroradiol 16:1053–1060, 1995.
134. Lempert TE, Halbach VV, Higashida RT, et al: Endovascular treatment of pseudoaneurysms with electrolytically detachable coils. AJNR Am J Neuroradiol 19:907–911, 1998.
135. Massoud TF, Guglielmi G, Vinuela F, et al: Saccular aneurysms in Moyamoya disease: Endovascular treatment using electrically detachable coils. Surg Neurol 41:462–467, 1994.
136. Massoud TF, Guglielmi G, Vinuela F, et al: Endovascular treatment of multiple aneurysms involving the posterior intracranial circulation. AJNR Am J Neuroradiol 17:549–554, 1996.
137. Pierot L, Boulin A, Castaings L, et al: The endovascular approach in the management of patients with multiple intracranial aneurysms. Neuroradiology 39:361–366, 1997.
138. Solander S, Ulhoa A, Vinuela F, et al: Endovascular treatment of multiple intracranial aneurysms treated by using Guglielmi detachable coils. J Neurosurg 90:857–864, 1999.
139. Tikkakoski T, Leinonen S, Siniluoto T, et al: Isolated dissecting aneurysm of the left posterior inferior cerebellar artery: Endovascular treatment with a Guglielmi detachable coil. AJNR Am J Neuroradiol 18:936–938, 1997.
140. Yamaura I, Tani E, Yokota M, et al: Endovascular treatment of ruptured dissecting aneurysms aimed at occlusion of the dissected site by using Guglielmi detachable coils. J Neurosurg 90: 853–856, 1999.
141. Gobin YP, Vinuela F, Gurian JH, et al: Treatment of large and giant fusiform intracranial aneurysms with Guglielmi detachable coils. J Neurosurg 84:55–62, 1996.
142. Cloft HJ, Kallmes DF, Jensen ME, et al: Endovascular treatment of ruptured, peripheral cerebral aneurysms: Parent artery occlusion with short Guglielmi detachable coils. AJNR Am J Neuroradiol 20:308–310, 1999.
143. Suzuki K, Meguro K, Wada M, et al: Embolization of a ruptured aneurysm of the distal anterior inferior cerebellar artery: Case report and review of the literature. Surg Neurol 51:509–512, 1999.
144. Graves VB, Strother CM, Rappe AH: Treatment of experimental canine carotid aneurysms with platinum coils. AJNR Am J Neuroradiol 14:787–793, 1993.
145. Mawad ME, Mawad JK, Cartwright J Jr, et al: Long-term histopathologic changes in canine aneurysms embolized with Guglielmi detachable coils. AJNR Am J Neuroradiol 16:7–13, 1995.
146. Spetzger U, Reul J, Weis J, et al: Microsurgically produced bifurcation aneurysms in a rabbit model for endovascular coil embolization. J Neurosurg 85:488–495, 1996.
147. Tenjin H, Fushiki S, Nakahara Y, et al: Effect of Guglielmi detachable coils on experimental carotid artery aneurysms in primates. Stroke 26:2075–2080, 1995.
148. Castro E, Fortea F, Villoria F, et al: Long-term histopathologic findings in two cerebral aneurysms embolized with Guglielmi detachable coils. AJNR Am J Neuroradiol 20:549–552, 1999.
149. Gewirtz RJ, Geissler RH: Post mortem ultrastructural analysis of a small aneurysm treated with Guglielmi detachable coils and clipped secondarily: A case report. J Neurovasc Dis 3: 31–35, 1998.
150. Horowitz MB, Purdy PD, Burns D, et al: Scanning electron microscopic findings in a basilar tip aneurysm embolized with Guglielmi detachable coils. AJNR Am J Neuroradiol 18:688–690, 1997.
151. Molyneux AJ, Ellison DW, Morris J, et al: Histological findings in giant aneurysms treated with Guglielmi detachable coils: Report of two cases with autopsy correlation. J Neurosurg 83: 129–132, 1995.
152. Padolecchia R, Puglioli M, Collavoli PL, et al: Acute histopathologic and ultrastructural study in one case of human basilar tip aneurysm embolised with Guglielmi detachable coils. Intervent Neuroradiol 5:257–260, 1999.
153. Shimizu S, Kurata A, Takano M, et al: Tissue response of a small saccular aneurysm after incomplete occlusion with a Guglielmi detachable coil. AJNR Am J Neuroradiol 20:546–548, 1999.
154. Stiver SI, Porter PJ, Willinsky RA, et al: Acute human histopathology of an intracranial aneurysm treated using Guglielmi detachable coils: Case report and review of the literature. Neurosurgery 43:1203–1208, 1998.
155. Suda Y, Kikuchi K, Shioya H, et al: Long-term histopathology of intracranial aneurysms after endovascular treatment with coils: Report of two cases with ultrastructural evaluations by scanning electron microscopy. Intervent Neuroradiol 5(Suppl 1): 225–231, 1999.
156. Mizoi K, Yoshimoto T, Takahashi A, et al: A pitfall in the surgery of recurrent aneurysm after coil embolization and its histological observation: Technical case report. Neurosurgery 39:165–169, 1996.
157. Sadato A, Taki W, Ikada Y, et al: Effect of electrical thrombosis on coil embolization of experimental aneurysms. J Neurovasc Dis 2:235–245, 1997.
158. Horowitz M, Samson D, Purdy P: Does electrothrombosis occur immediately after embolization of an aneurysm with Guglielmi detachable coils? AJNR Am J Neuroradiol 18:510–513, 1997.
159. Fessler RD, Ringer AJ, Qureshi AI, et al: Intracranial stent placement to trap an extruded coil during endovascular aneurysm treatment: Technical note. Neurosurgery 46:248–253, 2000.
160. Gurian JH, Martin NA, King WA, et al: Neurosurgical management of cerebral aneurysms following unsuccessful or incomplete endovascular embolization. J Neurosurg 83:843–853, 1995.
161. Cronqvist M, Pierot L, Boulin A, et al: Local intraarterial fibrinolysis of thromboemboli occurring during endovascular treatment of intracerebral aneurysms: A comparison of anatomic results and clinical outcome. AJNR Am J Neuroradiol 19:157–165, 1998.
162. Strother CM: Continued progress in the evolution of endovascular therapy [editorial]. AJNR Am J Neuroradiol 19:190, 1998.
163. McDougall CG, Halbach VV, Dowd CF, et al: Causes and management of aneurysmal hemorrhage occurring during embolization with Guglielmi detachable coils. J Neurosurg 89:87–92, 1998.
164. Ricolfi F, Le Guerinel C, Blustajn J, et al: Rupture during treatment of recently ruptured aneurysms with Guglielmi electrodetachable coils. AJNR Am J Neuroradiol 19:1653–1658, 1998.

165. Horowitz M, Purdy P, Kopitnik T, et al: Aneurysm retreatment after Guglielmi detachable coil and nondetachable coil embolization: Report of nine cases and review of the literature. Neurosurgery 44:712–720, 1999.
166. Aymard A, Gobin YP, Casasco A, et al: Multiple intracranial aneurysms: Endovascular treatment by coils [French]. Neurochirurgie 38:353–357, 1992.
167. Teitelbaum GP, Halbach VV, Larsen DW, et al: Treatment of massive posterior epistaxis by detachable coil embolization of a cavernous internal carotid artery aneurysm. Neuroradiology 37: 334–336, 1995.
168. Prestigiacomo CJ, Fidlow K, Pile-Spellman J: Retrieval of a fractured Guglielmi detachable coil with use of the goose neck snare "twist" technique. J Vasc Interv Radiol 10:1243–1247, 1999.
169. Standard SC, Chavis TD, Wakhloo AK, et al: Retrieval of a Guglielmi detachable coil after unraveling and fracture: Case report and experimental results. Neurosurgery 35:994–999, 1994.
170. Civit T, Auque J, Marchal C, et al: Aneurysm clipping after endovascular treatment with coils: A report of eight patients. Neurosurgery 38:955–961, 1996.
171. Thielen KR, Nichols DA, Fulgham JR, et al: Endovascular treatment of cerebral aneurysms following incomplete clipping. J Neurosurg 87:184–189, 1997.
172. Forsting M, Albert FK, Jansen O, et al: Coil placement after clipping: Endovascular treatment of incompletely clipped cerebral aneurysms: Report of two cases. J Neurosurg 85:966–969, 1996.
173. Fraser KW, Halbach VV, Teitelbaum GP, et al: Endovascular platinum coil embolization of incompletely surgically clipped cerebral aneurysms. Surg Neurol 41:4–8, 1994.
174. Pierot L, Boulin A, Visot A, et al: Postoperative aneurysm remnants: Endovascular treatment as an alternative to further surgery. Neuroradiology 41:315–319, 1999.
175. Abrahams JM, Diamond SL, Hurst RW, et al: Topic review: Surface modifications enhancing biological activity of Guglielmi detachable coils in treating intracranial aneurysms. Surg Neurol 5:34–41, 2000.
176. Ahuja AA, Hergenrother RW, Strother CM, et al: Platinum coil coatings to increase thrombogenicity: A preliminary study in rabbits. AJNR Am J Neuroradiol 14:794–798, 1993.
177. Kallmes DF, Borland MK, Cloft HJ, et al: In vitro proliferation and adhesion of basic fibroblastic growth factor–producing fibroblasts on platinum coils. Radiology 206:237–243, 1998.
178. Kallmes DF, Williams AD, Cloft HJ, et al: Platinum coil–mediated implantation of growth factor–secreting endovascular tissue grafts: An in vivo study. Radiology 207:519–523, 1998.
179. Murayama Y, Suzuki Y, Vinuela F, et al: Development of a biologically active Guglielmi detachable coil for the treatment of cerebral aneurysms. Part 1. In vitro study. AJNR Am J Neuroradiol 20:1986–1991, 1999.
180. Murayama Y, Vinuela F, Suzuki Y, et al: Development of the biologically active Guglielmi detachable coil for the treatment of cerebral aneurysms. Part II. An experimental study in a swine aneurysm model. AJNR Am J Neuroradiol 20:1992–1999, 1999.
181. Murayama Y, Vinuela F, Suzuki Y, et al: Ion implantation and protein coating of detachable coils for endovascular treatment of cerebral aneurysms: Concepts and preliminary results in swine models. Neurosurgery 40:1233–1244, 1997.
182. Szikora I, Wakhloo AK, Guterman LR, et al: Initial experience with collagen-filled Guglielmi detachable coils for endovascular treatment of experimental aneurysms. AJNR Am J Neuroradiol 18:667–672, 1997.
183. Tamatani S, Ozawa T, Minakawa T, et al: Radiologic and histopathologic evaluation of canine artery occlusion after collagen-coated platinum microcoil delivery. AJNR Am J Neuroradiol 20: 541–545, 1999.
184. Cognard C, Weill A, Tovi M, et al: Treatment of distal aneurysms of the cerebellar arteries by intraaneurysmal injection of glue. AJNR Am J Neuroradiol 20:780–784, 1999.
185. Nishi S, Taki W, Nakahara I, et al: Embolization of cerebral aneurysms with a liquid embolus, EVAL mixture: Report of three cases. Acta Neurochir (Wien) 138:294–300, 1996.
186. Murayama Y, Vinuela F, Tateshima S, et al: Endovascular treatment of experimental aneurysms by use of a combination of liquid embolic agents and protective devices. Am J Neuroradiol 21:1726–1735, 2000.
187. Iwakoshi T, Negoro M, Okamoto T, et al: Intra-arterial vein bypass using a vein-loaded stent system to occlude wide-necked aneurysms: An experimental study in dogs. Neuroradiology 41:214–220, 1999.
188. Link J, Feyerabend B, Grabener M, et al: Dacron-covered stent-grafts for the percutaneous treatment of carotid aneurysms: Effectiveness and biocompatibility—experimental study in swine. Radiology 200:397–401, 1996.
189. Schellhammer F, Walter M, Berlis A, et al: Polyethylene terephthalate and polyurethane coatings for endovascular stents: Preliminary results in canine experimental arteriovenous fistulas. Radiology 211:169–175, 1999.
190. Singer RJ, Dake MD, Norbash A, et al: Covered stent placement for neurovascular disease. AJNR Am J Neuroradiol 18:507–509, 1997.
191. Berenstein A: Tissue response to Guglielmi detachable coils: Present implications and future developments. AJNR Am J Neuroradiol 20:533–534, 1999.
192. Raymond J, Desfaits AC, Roy D: Fibrinogen and vascular smooth muscle cell grafts promote healing of experimental aneurysms treated by embolization. Stroke 30:1657–1664, 1999.

Giant Aneurysms

G. MICHAEL LEMOLE, JR. ■ JEFFREY S. HENN ■ ROBERT F. SPETZLER ■
HOWARD A. RIINA

By definition, cerebral aneurysms are classified as giant when they attain a dimension of 25 mm or more. The very nature and the associated anatomic complexity of these aneurysms make them among the most challenging lesions a neurosurgeon can address, and their poor natural history necessitates treatment. Like other cerebral aneurysms, giant aneurysms can become symptomatic with subarachnoid hemorrhage (SAH); however, they are more likely to do so with signs and symptoms of mass effect on surrounding neural structures. Although cerebral angiography remains the gold standard for the diagnosis of all cerebral aneurysms, modalities such as magnetic resonance imaging (MRI) and computed tomography (CT)–angiography are important in the assessment of giant intracranial lesions to determine their true size and relationship to surrounding neural and skull base structures. Effective treatment of these lesions requires a multimodality approach involving neurosurgical, neuroendovascular, neuroradiologic, and neuroanesthesia subspecialties. Since the 1970s, the advent of skull base approaches and endovascular techniques has greatly improved treatment. It is hoped that this trend will continue, minimizing the risks associated with the management of giant intracranial aneurysms.

HISTORICAL CONSIDERATIONS

Cerebral aneurysms were not recognized as a pathologic entity until the mid-18th century, when Biumi of Milan identified a ruptured aneurysm during an autopsy in 1765. Throughout the 19th century, several investigators described the appearance of aneurysms along the vascular tree. Some even suggested a connection between sudden apoplexy in young persons and aneurysmal rupture.[1] In 1875, Hutchinson[2] described the first giant intracranial aneurysm, which was diagnosed by an audible bruit. Although Hutchinson recommended hunterian ligation of the carotid artery, the patient refused. His diagnosis was confirmed 11 years later when the patient died of an aortic aneurysm. At autopsy, he found a partially calcified aneurysm the size of a bantam hen's egg in the middle fossa.

In the next century, as Standard and colleagues[3] have noted, the diagnosis of cerebral aneurysms improved significantly when Moniz developed cerebral angiography. Nonetheless, these lesions were still sometimes mistaken for brain tumors. In the early part of the 20th century, treatment included hunterian ligation of the internal carotid artery (ICA).[4] According to Laws and Udvarhelyi,[1] Dandy was the first to actually expose a cerebral aneurysm and ligate its neck by clipping.

Based on 6368 cases in a cooperative study, Locksley[5] classified aneurysms that were 25 mm or greater as giant. The study noted that a high rate of morbidity and mortality was associated with these lesions. The first two significant studies of giant aneurysms were reported by Morley and Barr[6] and Bull.[7] The size of the aneurysms in these series may well have been underestimated, because diagnosis was based solely on plain radiography and angiography. At that time, the natural history of these lesions was beginning to be understood, and surgical treatment was fraught with hazards. Morley and Barr[6] concluded that "direct surgical attack on extracavernous giant aneurysms is seldom possible or successful except in the case of middle cerebral artery aneurysms."

During the next several decades, several large series confirmed that significant morbidity and mortality rates were associated with these lesions. Peerless and associates[8] reported mortality rates of 68% and 85% at 2 and 5 years, respectively, for untreated giant aneurysms. In that series, even the survivors suffered marked neurological dysfunction. Michel[9] noted a 100% mortality rate at 2 years in this patient population, and Kodama and Suzuki[10] reported that 75% of their untreated hospitalized patients died of SAH. In contrast to this dismal natural history, several large surgical series demonstrated excellent to good outcomes in 61% to 87% of all patients treated surgically; the rate of surgical mortality ranged from 5% to 22% (Table 121–1).

The improved outcomes associated with surgical intervention resulted from a variety of factors, including the development of microneurosurgery and skull base approaches. Alternatives to direct surgical attack, such

TABLE 121–1 ■ **Comparison of Outcomes in Surgical Series of Giant Intracranial Aneurysms**

AUTHOR	NO. OF PATIENTS	OUTCOME: Excellent/ Good (%)	Fair/ Poor (%)	Dead (%)
Sundt[18]	315	80	6	15
Peerless et al[8]	305	67	22	11
Lawton & Spetzler[21]	171	87	8	5
Hosobuchi[19]	82	84	9	7
Ausman et al[15]	62	84	11	5
Kodama & Suzuki[10]	49	61	16	22
Symon & Vajda[20]	36	86	6	8
Yasargil[17]	30	67	23	10
Heros[118]	28	82	7	5

Adapted from Lawton MT, Spetzler RF: Surgical management of giant intracranial aneurysms: Experience with 171 patients. Clin Neurosurg 42:245–266, 1995.

as parent vessel ligation, aneurysm trapping, aneurysmorrhaphy and aneurysmectomy, and extracranial-to-intracranial bypass procedures, have also increased the surgical options for the treatment of these challenging lesions. Since the 1990s, endovascular techniques have proved to be valuable surgical adjuncts. Given the improvement in surgical outcomes and the otherwise dismal natural history of giant aneurysms, their aggressive surgical treatment is warranted.

EPIDEMIOLOGY AND INCIDENCE

Giant aneurysms represent 2% to 5% of all intracranial aneurysms.[6, 11–14] As with small aneurysms, most series show a female prevalence, although Kodama and Suzuki[10] found an equal sex distribution. Most patients become symptomatic in the fourth through sixth decades of life.[4, 13, 15, 16]

Giant aneurysms are found in all locations throughout the intracranial vascular tree; however, their distribution is somewhat different from that of smaller aneurysms (Table 121–2). In general, 34% to 67% of giant intracranial aneurysms are associated with the ICA, 11% to 40% with the anterior cerebral artery and middle cerebral artery (MCA), and 13% to 56% with the vertebral and basilar arteries.[4, 8, 13, 14, 17–22] In the senior author's (RFS) experience, most aneurysms of the posterior circulation (70%) are located on the basilar tip, the P1 segment of the posterior cerebral artery, or the superior cerebellar artery.[23] In contrast to the percentage of giant aneurysms associated with the posterior circulation, small aneurysms of the posterior circulation constitute 10% to 20% of all aneurysms.[4] Peerless and colleagues[8] reported that 56% of their surgical series consisted of giant aneurysms of the vertebrobasilar system, most likely reflecting a referral bias to their institution.[13]

PATHOPHYSIOLOGY

The purported mechanisms underlying the formation of giant aneurysms are similar to those of their smaller counterparts. As early as 1930, Forbus[24] proposed that aneurysms developed from defects in the medial layers of the vessel. Pathologic evaluation of giant aneurysms often demonstrates a lack of a muscular layer and degeneration of the elastic laminar layers.[25] Because most aneurysms are saccular and occur at arterial bifurcations, it is believed that hemodynamic factors must be involved in the formation of cerebral aneurysms. Stehbens[26] was a proponent of acquired defects rather than congenital vessel defects contributing to the formation of cerebral aneurysms. Vessel weaknesses could be accelerated by flow-related phenomena or degenerative disease such as atherosclerosis. Some authors have postulated that giant aneurysms grow from repeated intramural hemorrhage of the aneurysm wall,[11, 13, 27] followed by thrombus formation and neovascularization.[28, 29] Giant aneurysms developing de novo or from smaller aneurysms have been described.[13, 25, 30, 31] They have also been associated with underlying systemic arteriopathies.[11, 32] Giant aneurysms can result directly from trauma.[33] More than one aneurysm may be present in 10% to 36% of cases.[17, 22, 34]

Giant aneurysms can be either fusiform or saccular. Given the complexity of these lesions and their involvement with multiple vessels, it is not always possible to differentiate these two morphologic conditions. Saccular lesions most often occur at arterial bifurcations, likely the result of continuous hemodynamic

TABLE 121–2 ■ **Distribution of Giant Aneurysms in the Cerebral Circulation**

AUTHOR	NO. OF ANEURYSMS	ICA (%)	MCA (%)	ACA (%)	VERTEBROBASILAR (%)
Lawton & Spetzler[21]	171	94 (55)	27 (16)	13 (8)	39 (23)
Sundt[18]	323*	182 (56)	58 (18)	16 (5)	49 (15)
Peerless et al[8]	635	213 (34)	49 (8)	9 (3)	354 (56)
Hosobuchi[19]	84	56 (67)	4 (5)	9 (11)	15 (18)
Symon & Vajda[20]	55	26 (47)	10 (18)	7 (13)	12 (22)
Yasargil[17]	31	14 (45)	4 (13)	1 (3)	12 (39)
Onuma & Suzuki[14]	32	15 (47)	3 (9)	10 (31)	4 (13)

*Some patients with multiple giant aneurysms.
ACA, anterior cerebral artery; ICA, internal carotid artery; MCA, middle cerebral artery.

stresses. Fusiform or dolichoectatic lesions may result from atherosclerosis, congenital arteriopathies, or traumatic dissections.[11, 16, 35, 36] Numerous factors have been linked to the formation and rupture of aneurysms, including female sex, age, hypertension, connective tissue disease, and tobacco use.[26, 37, 38]

As aneurysms grow, wall tension must increase to maintain vessel integrity, as can be calculated from Laplace's law. This equation relates the stresses over the aneurysmal wall to the radius of the lesion.[4] The same hemodynamic forces that prompt an aneurysm to grow may be responsible for its ultimate rupture.

A significant portion of giant aneurysms have associated intraluminal thromboses—as many as 60% in some series.[4, 11, 13] Intra-aneurysmal thromboses may develop in areas where blood outside the turbulent flow stream stagnates, thereby promoting thrombosis. The presence of a partially thrombosed aneurysm does not appear to lower the risk of aneurysmal rupture.[28, 39]

CLINICAL PRESENTATION

Although patients with giant intracranial aneurysms may become symptomatic with SAH, most develop signs and symptoms related to aneurysmal mass effect. Only about a third of patients present with SAH,[15, 23] although Onuma and Suzuki[14] reported that 80% of the patients in their series presented with SAH. One third to two thirds manifest with signs and symptoms of neural compression related to aneurysmal mass.[23, 34] As many as 50% of patients with giant fusiform aneurysms present with signs of mass effect, compared with 20% who present with SAH.[36]

The symptoms related to aneurysmal mass effect depend on the aneurysm's location. In the anterior circulation, mass effect can manifest as pain, visual field and acuity defects, and extraocular dysfunction. Dementia and mental disturbances, as well as hemiparesis and epilepsy, have also been described.[11] Lownie and coworkers[40] reported that an aneurysm had to be 3.5 cm to produce dementia, whereas those between 2.7 and 3.2 cm compressed the optic apparatus. In the posterior circulation, cranial nerve dysfunctions may be present. If brainstem compression is significant, bulbar palsies and hemiparesis also can occur.[11] The remainder of patients may present with headache, syncope, sinusitis, epistaxis, confusion, or cerebrovascular accidents or after head trauma.[11, 23]

The risk of thromboembolism to distal vascular territories from a partially thrombosed giant aneurysm must be emphasized. Lawton and Spetzler[21] reported that 8% of patients with giant aneurysms presented with symptoms of distal thromboembolism, including transient ischemic attack and stroke. Sano and colleagues[41] noted that five conservatively treated patients all died of infarction. Naturally, only complete isolation of an aneurysm from the cerebral circulation eliminates the risk of rupture, continued enlargement, and thromboembolic phenomena.

Even though SAH is less commonly associated with giant intracranial aneurysms than with small ones, it can have a devastating effect. In fact, the annual rate of hemorrhage for giant intracranial aneurysms appears to be higher than that of smaller aneurysms. In several studies,[42–44] the annual risk rate of aneurysmal rupture appeared to correlate with increasing size of the aneurysm. This finding was confirmed by a recent analysis of aneurysm natural history,[45] in which the annual rupture rate for giant intracranial aneurysms was higher than the 1% to 3% quoted for smaller aneurysms.[21] In fact, in a multicenter study,[46] the annual risk of rupture of giant intracranial aneurysms was 6%.

SAH from giant aneurysms may be associated with more severe neurological deficits. According to Laplace's law, the higher stress over the giant aneurysmal wall could result in a greater amount of SAH during rupture.[3, 13] As with smaller intracranial aneurysms, once a SAH has occurred, more than 50% of patients die or experience significant complications.[22, 47] The goal is to diagnose aneurysms before they rupture or become irreversibly symptomatic.

DIAGNOSIS

High-quality four-vessel cerebral angiography has long been considered the gold standard for the diagnosis of cerebral aneurysms (Fig. 121–1). This modality provides information about an aneurysm's location, anatomy, adjacent branch vessels, collateral circulation, and distal cerebral perfusion.[23] It can also reveal multiple intracranial aneurysms. Anteroposterior, lateral, and oblique views can help define the exact relationship of inflow and outflow vessels to the aneurysm. Superselective injections and manual compression techniques may provide information about the vessels involved and collateral blood flow patterns. The disadvantage is that traditional angiography shows only luminal filling. Consequently, it may fail to reveal the aneurysm's true size if part of the lumen is occupied by laminated thrombus. Other portions of a giant aneurysm may not be visualized properly if areas of stagnant blood flow preclude the even distribution of contrast medium.

CT can define the dimensions of an aneurysm. Often a lesion demonstrates a calcified eggshell border.[11] When contrast is administered, this border may appear as a "target sign," with contrast filling the center while the calcified rim appears hyperdense.[4] CT is the diagnostic modality of choice for SAH because it best visualizes acute blood. CT also helps define the precise relationship between the aneurysm and the skull base. Calcification of the wall of the aneurysm, which can influence surgical technique, can also be demonstrated. Advances in high-speed scanners permitted the development of CT-angiography (Fig. 121–2), which avoids some of the risks of stroke associated with cannulation of the head and neck vessels during traditional angiography. Three-dimensional reconstruction techniques often exquisitely demonstrate an aneurysm, as well as all the associated inflow and outflow vessels.[48] This modality is capable of improved anatomic and hemo-

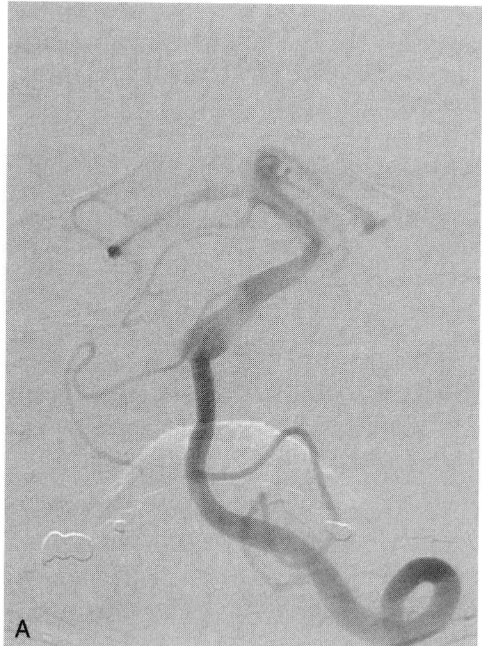

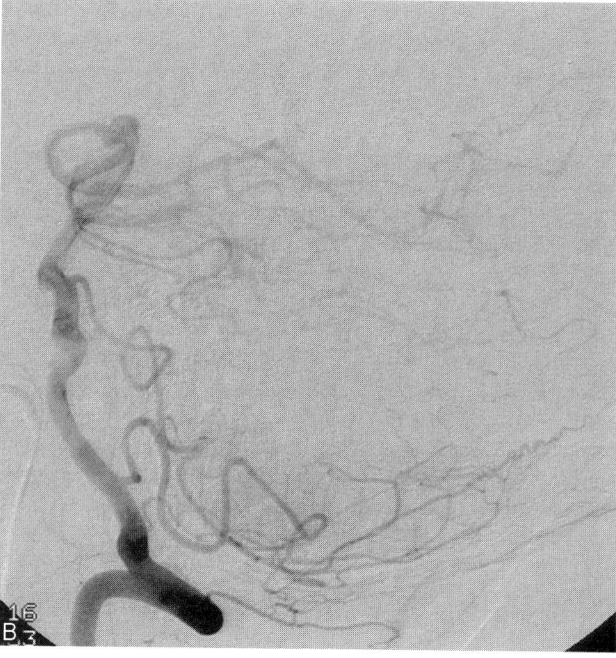

FIGURE 121–1. Anteroposterior *(A)* and lateral *(B)* angiographic views of a left vertebral artery injection show aneurysmal pathology at the basilar apex, along with a dolichoectatic basilar artery. (Courtesy of Barrow Neurological Institute, Phoenix, AZ.)

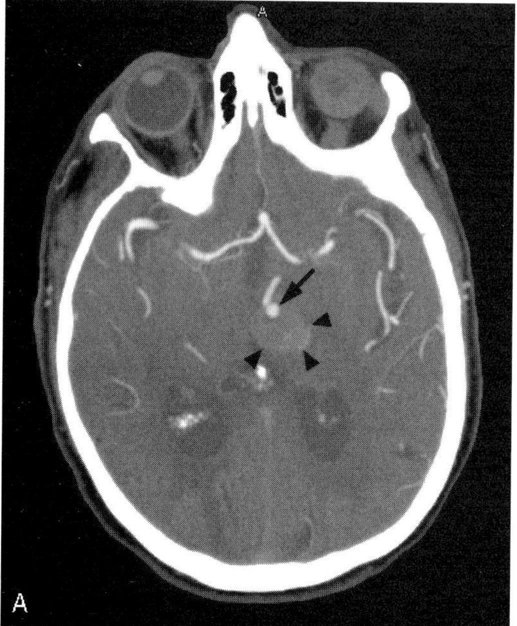

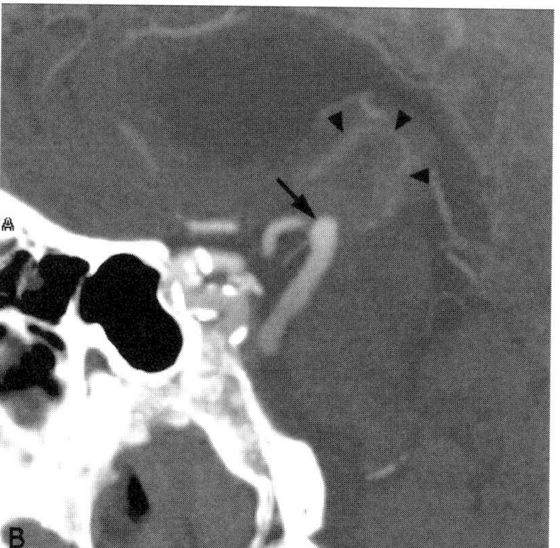

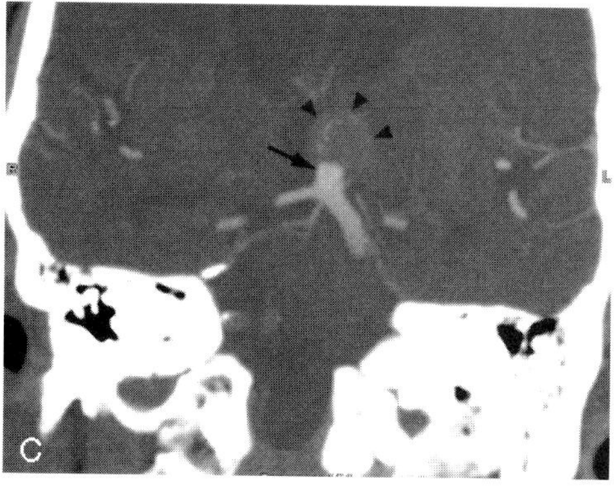

FIGURE 121–2. Axial *(A)*, sagittal *(B)*, and coronal *(C)* reconstructed computed tomography–angiography images show the aneurysm in Figure 121–1. Note the true dimensions of the aneurysm *(arrowheads)*, even though only a small portion of the aneurysm fills with contrast *(arrows)*. (Courtesy of Barrow Neurological Institute, Phoenix, AZ.)

dynamic resolution, but its exact role in the evaluation of giant aneurysms has yet to be defined.

MRI offers a noninvasive technique for identifying and defining giant cerebral aneurysms. The breakdown products of blood, including deoxyhemoglobin, methemoglobin, and hemosiderin, are associated with distinct signal characteristics on both T1- and T2-weighted imaging. Consequently, intraluminal clots can be visualized, and their ages estimated. Signal flow voids, which indicate active blood flow within aneurysms, help define the filling component of an aneurysm. As a result, MRI provides excellent information about actual and luminal anatomy.[49] Magnetic resonance angiography can take advantage of the flow-void phenomenon to reconstruct excellent anatomic models of the vascular tree.[50] Postoperative follow-up may be difficult with magnetic resonance angiography, however, owing to clip or coil metal artifact.[51] As with other newer imaging techniques, however, the precise role of MRI and magnetic resonance angiography in the diagnosis of giant cerebral aneurysms has yet to be determined.

MANAGEMENT

Given the dismal natural history of giant cerebral aneurysms, a conservative or expectant approach should be considered only if there are mitigating factors (e.g., poor medical grade, patient's refusal of intervention). Once the decision for intervention has been made, several treatment options are available in the neurosurgeon's arsenal, including both direct and indirect surgical attacks, as well as endovascular procedures. Once a giant aneurysm has been diagnosed, several perioperative issues must be addressed. If the patient presented with SAH, the complications of aneurysmal rupture should be managed according to accepted principles and protocols. In particular, we recommend aggressive control of hypertension, prompt institution of calcium channel blockers (e.g., nimodipine), and ventriculostomy, if indicated.[23] It is preferable that all patients undergo definitive treatment for ruptured aneurysms within 48 hours.[52]

Other considerations include the use of intraoperative electrophysiologic monitoring, intraoperative angiography, and specialized anesthesia techniques. Because of the potential for massive blood loss, all patients must be typed and crossmatched, and central venous access should be available. If hypothermic circulatory arrest is considered, a Swan-Ganz catheter should be placed for cardiac monitoring. Cerebral protective anesthetics such as isoflurane should be employed. Cerebral protective agents such as barbiturates or propofol can be used during temporary vessel occlusion, and their efficacy can be monitored using electroencephalographic techniques.[53, 54] Intraoperative angiography may help determine whether residual luminal filling is present after the aneurysm is clipped and can be useful to assess the patency of bypass procedures. Further, any stenosis or kinking associated with a clipped vessel or reconstructed vessel can be confirmed immediately. Microvascular Doppler ultrasonography

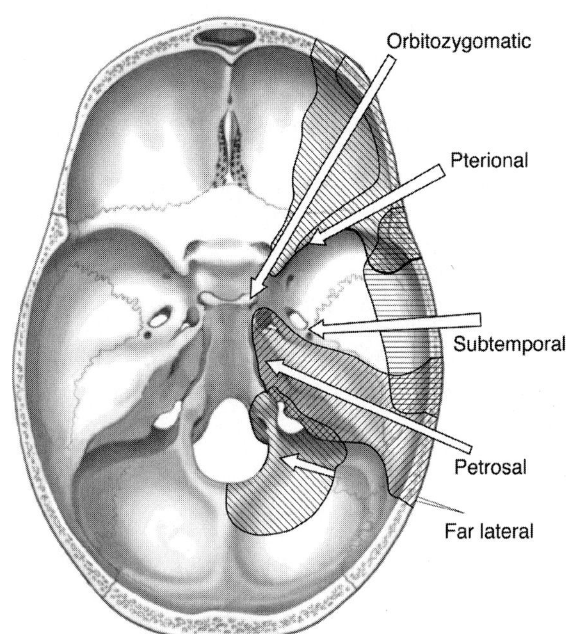

FIGURE 121–3. Specific skull base approaches to aneurysms are shown by shaded areas. Selection of the proper approach can provide access to almost any skull base lesion. (Courtesy of Barrow Neurological Institute, Phoenix, AZ.)

may be used to determine hemodynamically significant vessel stenosis.

The optimal skull base approach to a giant aneurysm offers a wide degree of exposure with full visualization of the aneurysm's origin, outflow, associated perforators, adjacent vessels, and nearby neural structures (Fig. 121–3). The location of the aneurysm dictates the most appropriate skull base approach (Table 121–3). The basic principles of minimal brain retraction with maximal bone exposure apply. Increasingly, endovas-

TABLE 121–3 ■ **Selection of Surgical Approach Based on Location of Giant Aneurysm**

SITE OF ANEURYSM	SKULL BASE APPROACH
Proximal internal carotid artery	Pterional, orbitozygomatic
Bifurcation of internal carotid artery	Pterional, orbitozygomatic
Proximal anterior cerebral artery	Pterional, orbitozygomatic
Distal anterior cerebral artery	Pterional, orbitozygomatic, interhemispheric
Middle cerebral artery	Pterional, orbitozygomatic
Vertebral artery	Far-lateral
Vertebrobasilar junction	Far-lateral
Midbasilar artery	Petrosal, far-lateral, orbitozygomatic
High basilar artery	Orbitozygomatic
Posterior inferior cerebellar artery	Far-lateral, suboccipital
Anterior inferior cerebellar artery	Petrosal, far-lateral, orbitozygomatic
Superior cerebellar artery	Orbitozygomatic

From Lemole GM Jr, Henn J, Spetzler RF, Riina HA: Surgical management of giant aneurysms. Operative Techn Neurosurg 3:239–254, 2000.

cular techniques are being combined with operative techniques to achieve impressive outcomes.[55–60]

Anterior Circulation Approaches

Orbitozygomatic Pterional Approach. The pterional transsylvian approach is one of the most commonly used approaches to aneurysms of the anterior circulation. It provides access to the entire circle of Willis and its constituent branches. Exposure can be further enhanced by drilling the pterion and the bony ridges over the floor of the frontal fossa.[23] When combined with a transsylvian pterional approach, the orbitozygomatic osteotomy can greatly increase the amount of exposure.[61–64] Removal of the orbital rim, orbital roof, lateral wall, and zygomatic arch significantly enhances access to anterior skull base and upper clival lesions. Removing the orbitozygomatic bar provides the surgeon's hands a wider corridor of access to the lesion and a shallower depth of field. Deep bypass procedures at the skull base are often technically difficult, and the added exposure can be essential for vessel suturing. This is particularly true for giant MCA aneurysms that must be excised with parent vessel reanastomosis. In addition, the orbitozygomatic approach provides a lower trajectory along the skull base, reducing the need for cerebral retraction (Fig. 121–4).

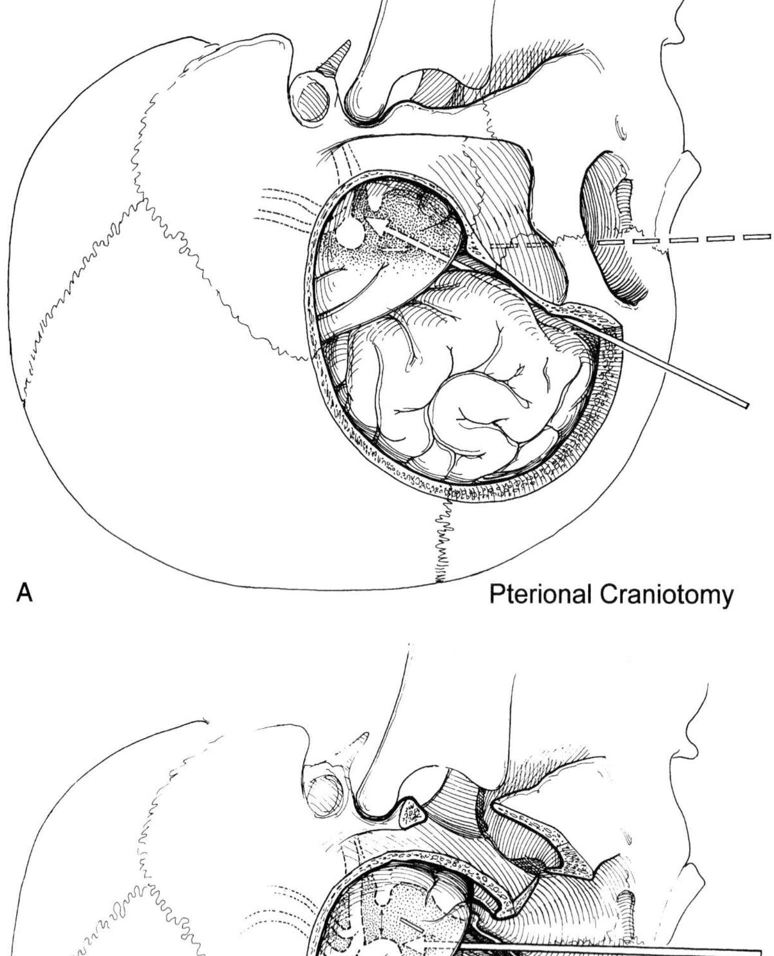

FIGURE 121–4. Orbitozygomatic approach. *A*, Standard pterional craniotomy. *B*, Removing the orbitozygomatic bar provides a wider degree of access and a more shallow surgical field. Further, less cerebral retraction is required to reach deep brain structures. (Courtesy of Barrow Neurological Institute, Phoenix, AZ.)

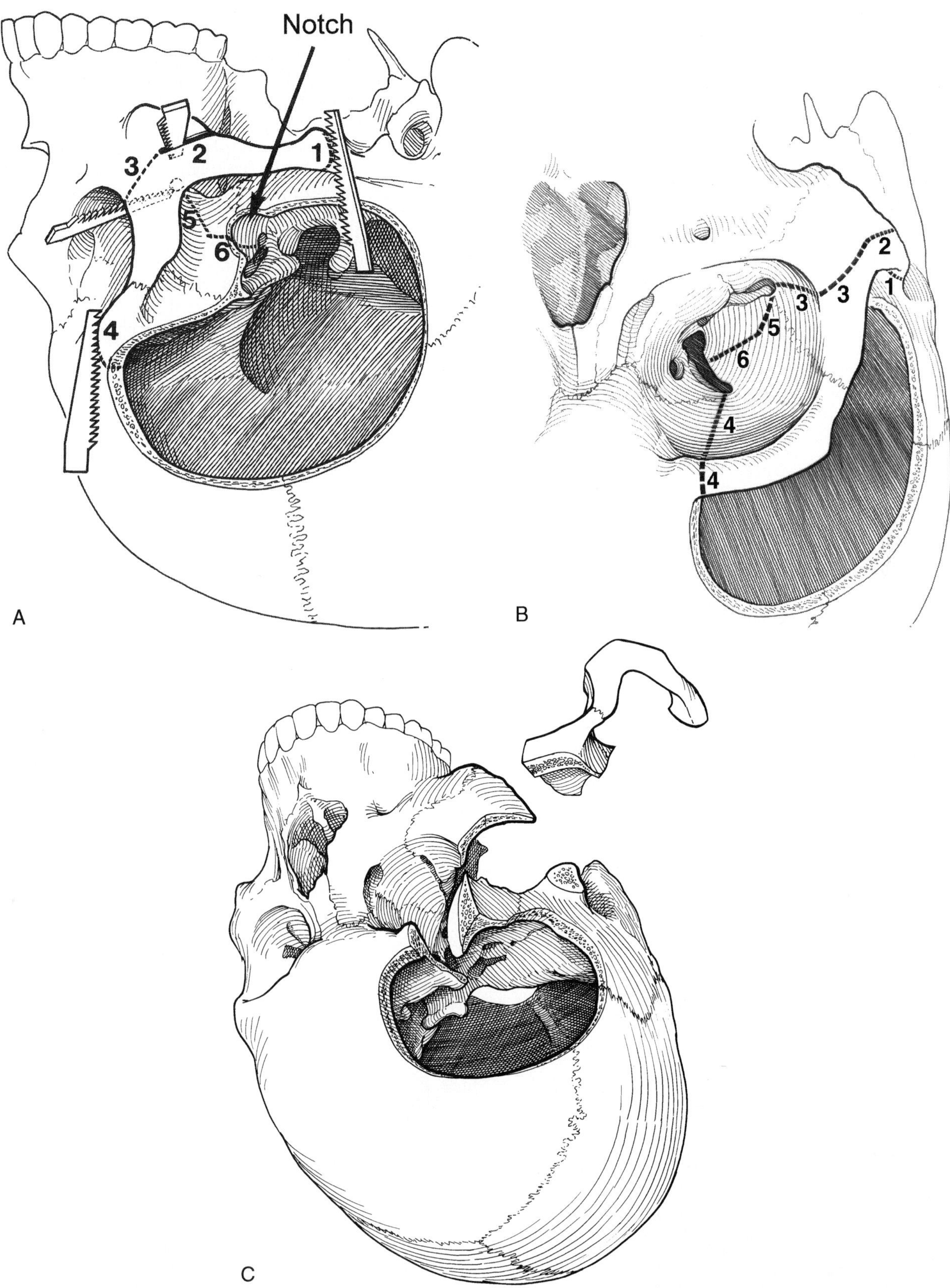

FIGURE 121–5. Orbitozygomatic osteotomy. *A* and *B*, The orbitozygomatic bar is freed from the skull base with a series of cuts, including those through the zygomatic root (1), the malar eminence (2 and 3), and the orbital roof just lateral to the supraorbital notch, extending back to the superior orbital fissure (4), and finally connecting the superior and inferior orbital fissures (5 and 6). *C*, The resulting orbitozygomatic bar can then be freed as one piece. (Courtesy of Barrow Neurological Institute, Phoenix, AZ.)

The orbitozygomatic osteotomy is usually performed after a traditional pterional craniotomy is completed.[65] A series of cuts through the lateral orbit, orbital roof, and maxillary and zygomatic roots frees the orbital bar from the adjacent skull base (Fig. 121–5). This piece of bone is preserved for later reinsertion. In addition, bone surrounding the superior orbital fissure can be removed with a high-speed drill or microrongeurs. Opening the dura with its flap based inferiorly allows the dural flap to gently depress the globe inferiorly and laterally, again enhancing exposure.[23] In preparation for the orbitozygomatic osteotomy, we also recommend a subfascial or interfascial dissection of the temporalis fascia to protect the frontalis branch of the facial nerve.[65, 66]

The risks associated with the orbitozygomatic osteotomy include periorbital bruising and swelling, pulsatile enophthalmos, frontalis nerve injury, orbital entrapment, diplopia from an extraocular muscle or nerve injury, and blindness. However, the overall incidence of these complications is low. Typically, the advantages provided by the orbitozygomatic approach more than offset its theoretical risks.[65, 67]

The orbitozygomatic osteotomy may be ideal for almost all giant and complex aneurysms originating from the circle of Willis, including ophthalmic, paraclinoid, superior hypophysial, posterior communicating, anterior choroidal, and ICA bifurcation aneurysms. Sometimes, additional exposure by drilling the anterior clinoid process and exposing the carotid artery in Glasscock's triangle further enhances the exposure of certain lesions. At our institution, we also use the orbitozygomatic osteotomy to approach giant and complex lesions of the MCA, because the approach trajectory to the proximal M1 segment and the aneurysm neck is optimized (Fig. 121–6).

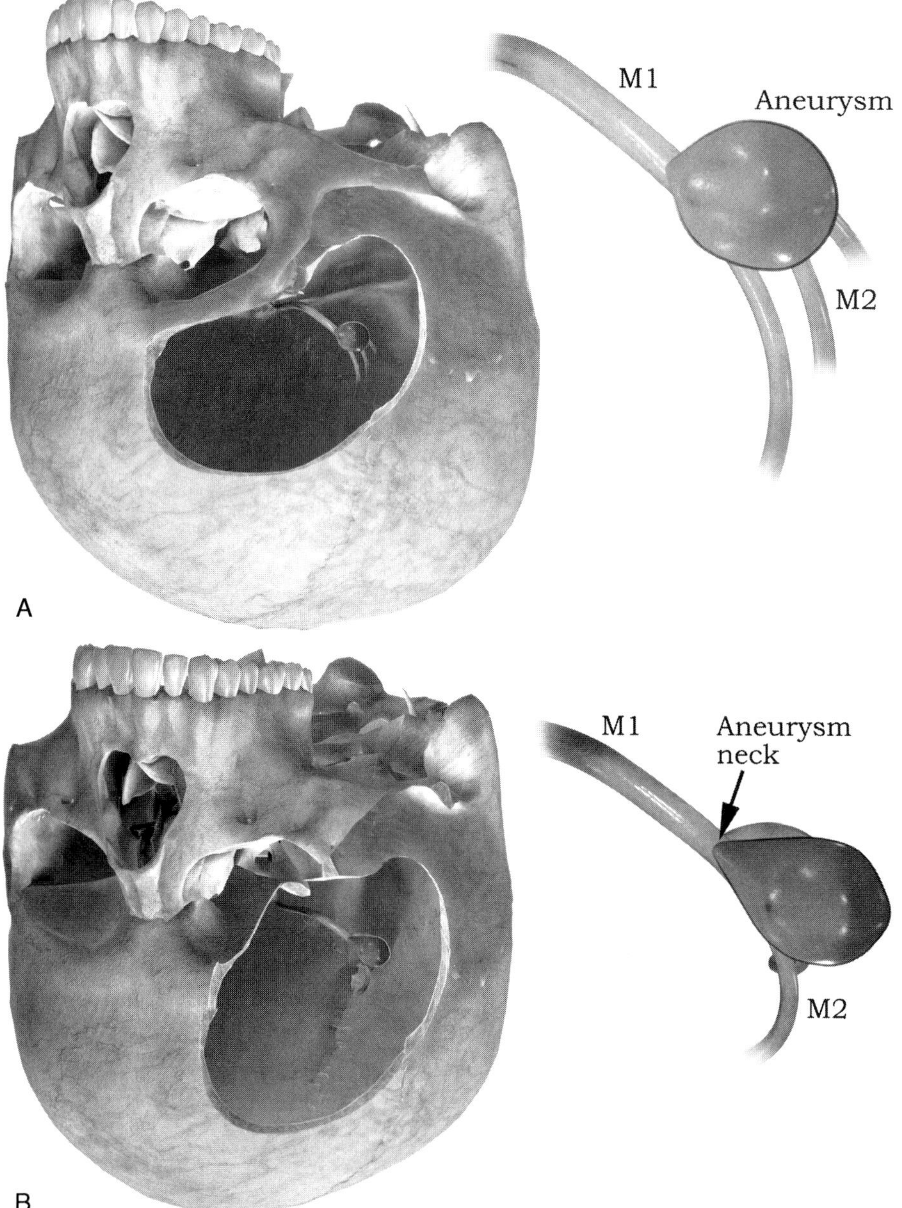

FIGURE 121–6. Computer reconstruction of pterional *(A)* and orbitozygomatic *(B)* approaches for middle cerebral artery (MCA) aneurysms. Compared with the pterional approach, the orbitozygomatic approach provides a lower trajectory along the skull base floor, and the supraorbital trajectory facilitates proximal control of giant and complex MCA aneurysms. The approach provides a perpendicular trajectory to the M1 segment and aneurysmal neck (compare insets).

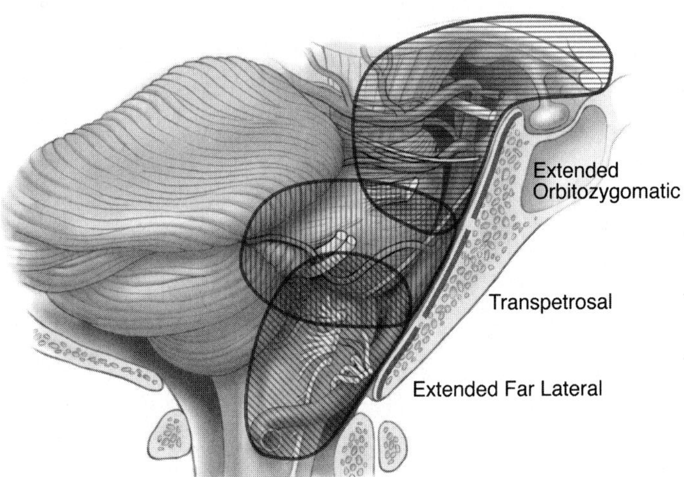

FIGURE 121–7. Skull base approaches to posterior circulation aneurysms. Access to the basilar artery zones and brainstem is provided by the skull base approaches shown here. The shaded areas demonstrate the degree of exposure provided by each approach. (Courtesy of Barrow Neurological Institute, Phoenix, AZ.)

Interhemispheric Approach. To access lesions involving the distal anterior cerebral arteries, a bifrontal interhemispheric approach may be necessary. This approach can be combined with pterional and orbitozygomatic osteotomies to widen the degree of proximal control, as well as to secure distal control.

Posterior Circulation Approaches

The skull base approaches used for giant aneurysms of the posterior fossa include the orbitozygomatic approach, the transpetrosal approach, and the far-lateral approach. Combinations of these approaches can be used for more extensive lesions. Selection of the appropriate skull base approach depends on the location of the giant aneurysm (Fig. 121–7). Conceptually, the basilar artery can be divided into fifths.[70] The upper two fifths define the upper basilar zone, the middle fifth defines the midbasilar zone, and the lower two fifths define the vertebrobasilar zone. The orbitozygomatic approach is optimal for lesions of the upper basilar zone, and the vertebrobasilar area is best accessed with the far-lateral approach. Lesions involving only the midbasilar zone may require transpetrosal approaches.

Orbitozygomatic Approach. The particulars of the orbitozygomatic osteotomy were described previously, but modifications can improve access to the upper basilar artery. Drilling the anterior and posterior clinoid processes and the clivus itself[68] allows visualization down toward the midbasilar zone (Fig. 121–8). The orbitozygomatic approach is also useful with high-riding giant aneurysms of the basilar artery because it provides exposure into the upper interpeduncular space without requiring excessive frontal lobe traction. Important with any approach to aneurysms in this area is adequate visualization of all inflow and outflow vessels, including the bilateral posterior cerebral arteries and superior cerebellar arteries, as well as the proximal basilar artery.

Transpetrosal Approaches. The anterior clivus and brainstem can be accessed by progressive removal of the petrous ridge. Depending on the degree of removal, the approaches can be defined as retrolabyrinthine, translabyrinthine, and transcochlear (Fig. 121–9).[69–74] The amount of petrosal drilling dictates the degree of exposure of the anterior brainstem and clivus. Drilling the semicircular canals sacrifices hearing, whereas drilling the facial canal and transposition of the facial nerve may produce temporary facial nerve palsy. With the more aggressive petrosal approaches, their expected morbidities involving cranial nerves VII and VIII must be weighed against the advantages of increasing exposure in the posterior fossa. At our institution, transpetrosal approaches are reserved for complex lesions of the midbasilar zone. If possible, we prefer to use the orbitozygomatic or far-lateral approach or a combination to access lesions that extend into the midbasilar zone.

Far-Lateral Approach. The far-lateral approach provides excellent exposure from the midbasilar zone down to the intradural vertebral artery.[53, 77–79] A lateral suboccipital craniotomy is modified in three ways to create the far-lateral approach: (1) the arch of C1 is

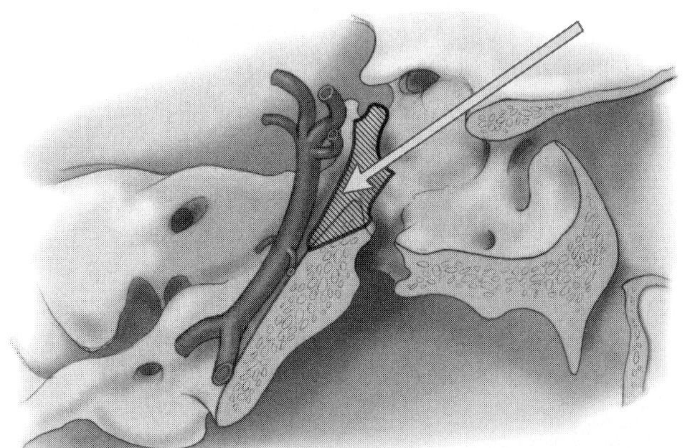

FIGURE 121–8. Modified orbitozygomatic approach to the upper basilar region. The orbitozygomatic approach can be modified to improve access to the upper basilar area. These modifications consist of removing the posterior clinoid processes and upper clivus with a high-speed drill *(cross-hatch)*. (Courtesy of Barrow Neurological Institute, Phoenix, AZ.)

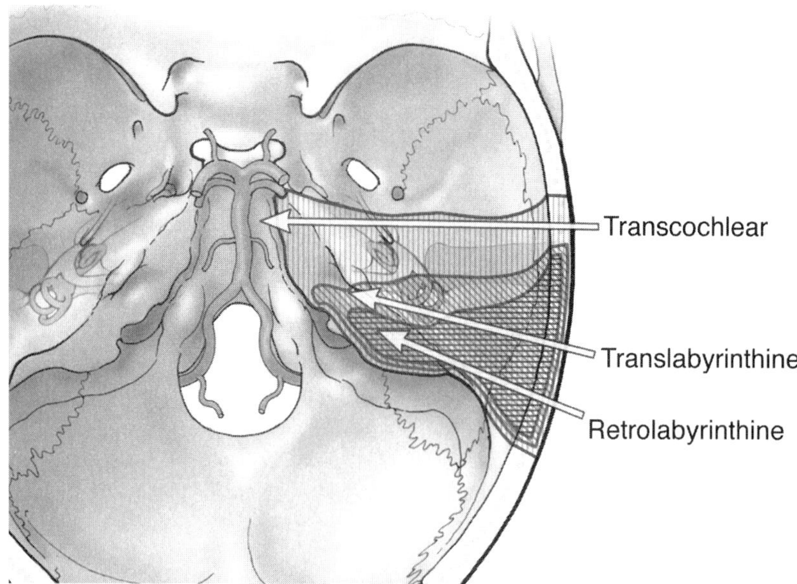

FIGURE 121–9. Transpetrosal skull base approaches. The degree of bony removal defines the transpetrosal approach. The retrolabyrinthine approach preserves middle ear structures. The translabyrinthine approach removes the semicircular canals, thereby sacrificing hearing. The transcochlear approach offers the greatest exposure to the anterior brainstem by removing the cochlea and transposing the facial nerve. (Courtesy of Barrow Neurological Institute, Phoenix, AZ.)

removed to the sulcus arteriosus, (2) the bony rim of the foramen magnum is resected to the occipital condyle, and (3) the posterior third of the occipital condyle is removed (Fig. 121–10). Removing less than half of the occipital condyle should not affect spinal stability,[80] nor should it pose a risk to cranial nerve XII as it courses through the hypoglossal canal. The extracranial vertebral artery may be freed from its course in the sulcus arteriosus and transverse foramen and transposed laterally to improve operative exposure. The far-lateral approach is best used to access lesions of the vertebrobasilar junction, including giant aneurysms of the vertebrobasilar, vertebral, and proximal posterior inferior cerebellar arteries.

Combined Approaches. Several approaches can be combined to treat complex lesions involving multiple basilar zones or when anatomic complexity necessitates wider access and control (Fig. 121–11).[70] A combined supra- and infratentorial approach merges a subtemporal craniotomy with a transpetrosal approach. It can be extended farther inferiorly if a far-lateral approach is added to it.[81] Sometimes, the tentorium and lateral sinus can be transected to facilitate exposure.[82] As al-

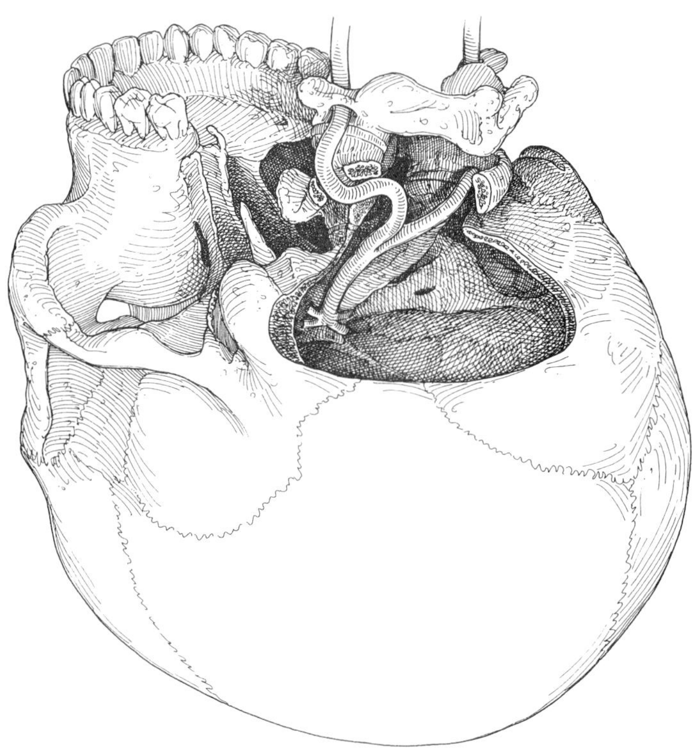

FIGURE 121–10. A far-lateral suboccipital craniotomy is combined with a C1 hemilaminectomy and posterior condylectomy. This exposure provides excellent access to the vertebrobasilar junction as far rostrally as the mid-basilar zone. (Courtesy of Barrow Neurological Institute, Phoenix, AZ.)

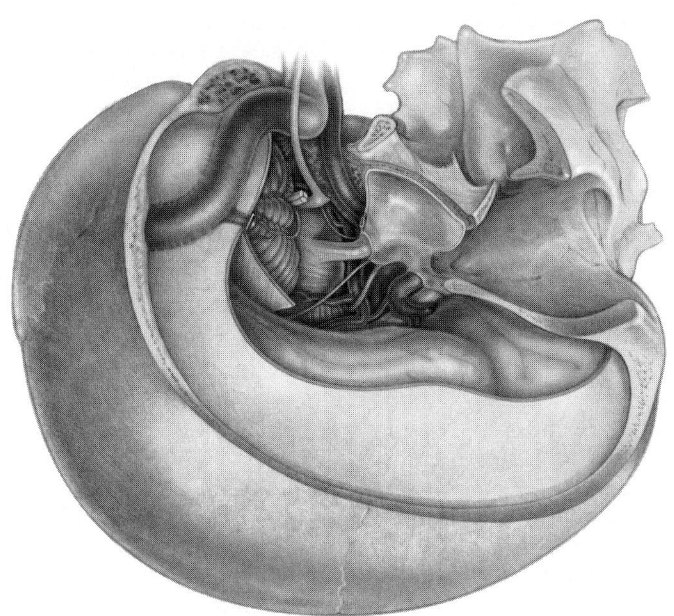

FIGURE 121–11. Combined approaches. In this example, the combined-combined approach is shown, with the orbitozygomatic craniotomy coupled with transpetrosal drilling and a far-lateral exposure. The entire brainstem is exposed from the foramen magnum to the circle of Willis. (Courtesy of Barrow Neurological Institute, Phoenix, AZ.)

ways with skull base approaches, the risks of extensive bony drilling are offset by minimized brain retraction.

Subtemporal Approach. Historically, the subtemporal approach was routinely used for aneurysms involving the upper basilar artery.[62–64, 68, 69] The transsylvian pterional approach has now supplanted it to a large degree. The subtemporal approach can still be useful with posteriorly projecting upper basilar aneurysms[21] and those located around the lateral edge of the tentorium.

Operative Techniques

The basic tenets of aneurysm surgery apply to giant intracranial aneurysms. These include adequate vascular control, aneurysm exposure, clip application, and use of adjuvant techniques. If an aneurysm cannot be directly attacked surgically and clipped, parent vessel occlusion, aneurysmorrhaphy and aneurysmectomy, and trapping and bypass procedures must be considered.

Vascular Control. Adequate vascular control is imperative for the surgical treatment of giant cerebral aneurysms. Vascular control helps the neurosurgeon maintain hemostasis, should the aneurysm rupture intraoperatively. Gaining vascular control may be particularly important if the aneurysm must be dissected free from surrounding neural structures and the dome manipulated or if aggressive clip reconstruction is warranted. For aneurysmorrhaphy and aneurysmectomy, vascular control is essential. Further, vascular control may facilitate visualization of the feeding, draining, and perforating vessels by allowing more aggressive repositioning of the aneurysm dome.

In the anterior circulation, obtaining vascular control may be routine. However, when aneurysms are located at the skull base, particularly where the carotid artery exits the cavernous sinus, proximal control may be more difficult to achieve. In these instances, the aneurysm itself may obstruct the view of a proximal vessel. Alternative techniques of proximal control may be essential for giant paraclinoid, ophthalmic, and superior hypophysial artery aneurysms. In these cases, several options exist.[23] The artery can be controlled in the neck through a surgical incision or along its petrous course by drilling Glasscock's triangle. Intracranial exposure can be facilitated by drilling the anterior clinoid and possibly by bisecting the distal dural ring. Recently, endovascular balloon techniques have been used to gain proximal control of the ICA.[60]

Proximity to the skull base and complex vascular anatomy make control of the posterior circulation crucial and difficult to achieve. Skull base approaches can provide excellent access to these areas, but several issues predominate. Extreme caution must be exercised when placing temporary clips along the middle portion of the basilar artery, because the brainstem perforating vessels there are susceptible to injury. With adequate exposure, proximal control along the lower basilar and vertebral arteries can be achieved. Gaining control more distally along the basilar artery can be problematic. Bilateral control of the superior cerebellar arteries and posterior cerebral arteries must be secured. If these vessels are incorporated within the dome of the aneurysm, it may be impossible to achieve complete distal control.

Endovascular temporary balloon occlusion techniques can also be useful in the posterior circulation, particularly in the proximal basilar and vertebral artery regions.[56] Distal balloon occlusion of the middle basilar artery may obstruct brainstem perforator vessels, with devastating consequences. Retrograde placement of a temporary occlusion balloon into the upper basilar artery from the anterior circulation is usually difficult.[23] As with all temporary occlusion techniques, the risk of cerebral ischemia can be lessened by using cerebral protective agents, minimizing clip occlusion time, and providing alternative sources of circulation through appropriate bypass procedures, if necessary. Mild hypertension can also be induced to maximize circulation through collateral pathways.

When all other forms of vascular control prove insufficient, hypothermic circulatory arrest can be considered. Circulatory arrest permits complete vascular control, and the risk of intraoperative aneurysmal rupture is eliminated. Hypothermic circulatory arrest can facilitate surgical technique by allowing more aggressive manipulation of the aneurysm dome without fear of rupture. Systemic vascular control greatly facilitates aneurysmal debulking and clip reconstruction. During circulatory arrest, adequate cerebral protection is imperative and may take the form of cerebral anesthetics as well as cerebral protective agents such as barbiturates. The use of systemic hypothermia also reduces the brain's metabolic requirements for oxygen.[54] The risks associated with hypothermic circulatory arrest are well described and include coagulopathies associated with hypothermia[83] and those associated with hemodilution after blood products and intravenous fluids are replaced.[84] Systemic heparinization is needed to place the percutaneous bypass catheter required for bypass procedures, but this can subject patients to hemorrhagic complications.[85] Finally, even when cerebral protective agents and hypothermia are used, the total length of circulatory arrest must be minimized to avoid ischemic complications. In our surgical series, hypothermic circulatory arrest was associated with a morbidity rate of 13% and a mortality rate of 8%.[86] These numbers, in part, reflect the complexity of aneurysms that require hypothermic circulatory arrest for adequate vascular control.

Surgical Techniques for Clipping. Successful clipping of a giant aneurysm depends on the anatomic complexity and morphologic features of the lesion. Successful clipping of saccular aneurysms typically requires a favorable and well-defined aneurysm neck. The clip is positioned to bring the vessel walls together at the neck of the aneurysm while the patency of the parent vessel is preserved. Fusiform or dolichoectatic giant aneurysms have no definable neck, and efferent vessels may arise at various points along the aneurysm.[35] Simple clipping of these lesions is often impossible, and clip reconstruction techniques are often necessary to exclude these aneurysms from the circulation. In these instances, clips must be used to reconstruct vessel lumina to connect all inflow and outflow vessels. These techniques require an exquisite comprehension of vascular anatomy and spatial creativity.

The technical aspects of direct clipping of giant aneurysms must not be overlooked. Aneurysm clips have mechanical limitations. Notably, the lowest closing force along the clip is located at its tip.[4] Consequently, several smaller clips placed in tandem may be a better solution than placing one long clip (Fig. 121–12). Clips also may be stacked on top of one other to guard against clip migration or slippage.[68, 69] Aneurysms with atherosclerotic changes within their walls may prevent clips from closing completely. The surgeon must then be careful not to loosen plaque into the parent vessel, where it can embolize to distal vascular territories.[20] In these cases, some authors use crushing instruments to make aneurysm necks more malleable.[87]

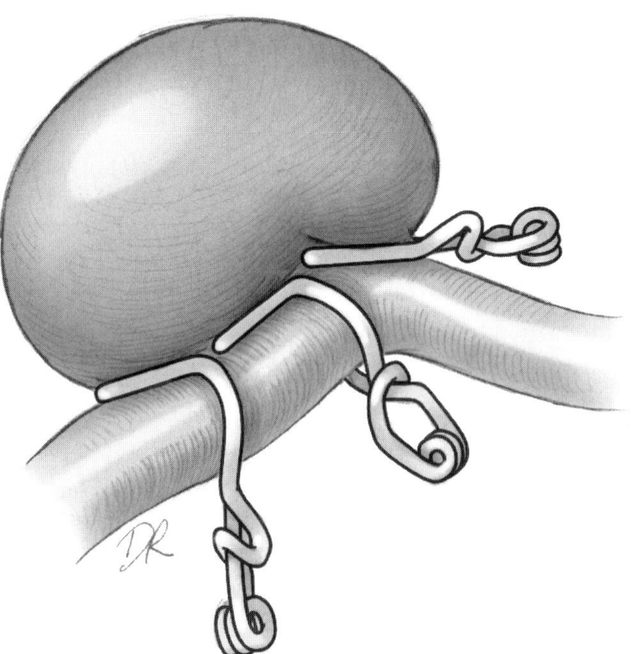

FIGURE 121–12. Tandem clip placement. Tandem clips can be used to reinforce one another to cover a wide aneurysm neck. This construct takes advantage of the fact that the clips' greatest closing force is along the more proximal portion of their tines. (From Lemole GM Jr, Henn J, Spetzler RF, Riina HA: Surgical management of giant aneurysms. Operative Techn Neurosurg 3: 239–254, 2000.)

Once a clip has been placed, the neurosurgeon should inspect the parent vessel and any associated neural and vascular structures. Hemodynamically significant stenoses may result if vessels kink after clips are placed.[13] The neurosurgeon must also ascertain that no small perforating vessels are caught within the clip blades, particularly brainstem and thalamic perforators associated with basilar tip aneurysms or lenticulostriate perforators associated with ICA bifurcation and proximal MCA aneurysms. Vessel patency and blood flow can be assessed intraoperatively with micro-Doppler probes or intraoperative angiography.

Alternative Occlusion Techniques. Because of their size, location, or morphologic features, certain giant aneurysms cannot be clipped directly. The neurosurgeon must then consider other options, which include parent vessel occlusion, trapping with or without bypass, aneurysmorrhaphy, and aneurysmectomy.[23, 88] Aneurysm trapping and aneurysmectomy can exclude the lesion from the cerebral circulation. The goal of parent vessel occlusion or aneurysmorrhaphy may be to divert and redirect blood flow from the aneurysm to minimize its risk of rupture. These latter techniques are inferior to direct clipping and are usually considered only for aneurysms that are likely to fail direct clipping but that need to be treated, given their poor natural history.

Parent vessel occlusion can involve sacrifice of the giant aneurysm's parent artery, either proximal or distal to the lesion. Hunterian ligation of parent vessels harboring giant aneurysms is a viable surgical alternative.[89] These techniques are particularly useful for aneurysms with no definable necks, such as fusiform or dolichoectatic aneurysms. Surgical or spontaneous alteration of the blood flow dynamics through these lesions may result in thrombosis and resolution,[90–92] but spontaneous revascularization of a previously thrombosed aneurysm is possible.[93–95] Collateral blood flow upstream of the parent vessel occlusion must be available through either naturally occurring sources or surgical augmentation. In the latter case, several appropriate bypass procedures may be able to provide blood flow to the distal circulation (Fig. 121–13). Preoperatively, collateral circulation can be assessed by cerebral angiography and temporary balloon occlusion tests that measure neurological status and cerebral blood flow. None of these studies, however, are completely reliable in determining which patients will tolerate permanent vessel occlusion without a bypass.[22, 87, 89, 96]

Trapping an aneurysm removes it from the cerebral circulation and, by definition, involves occlusion of the parent vessel proximal and distal to the giant aneurysm. Again, collateral circulation distal to the trapped aneurysm must be guaranteed. Further, trapping may be impossible if important vascular territories are fed by branches incorporated in the giant aneurysm itself. For example, brainstem perforators intrinsically involved in a giant fusiform midbasilar artery aneurysm will have no blood supply if that lesion is trapped, and brainstem infarction will ensue. In such cases, proximal or distal parent vessel occlusion may be considered.

Revascularization procedures and bypass techniques must be used when naturally occurring collateral circulation is insufficient to support upstream blood flow after permanent vessel occlusion.[19, 97, 98] Various bypass techniques have been described for both the anterior and posterior circulations. Sometimes, altering hemodynamics with a bypass alone may result in aneurysm thrombosis and resolution.[91, 92] In many cases, bypass procedures involve supplying the intracranial circulation through a mobilized pedicle of the external carotid circulation. The superficial temporal arteries and occipital arteries have been used this way to supply blood to branches of the MCA, posterior cerebral artery, and superior cerebellar artery (Fig. 121–14).[15, 99] With these techniques, the neurosurgeon must be cognizant of the potential for mismatches in blood flow, because some bypass techniques are limited by the absolute amount of blood available through small-caliber vessels. For example, if the ICA is to be sacrificed, superficial temporal artery–to–MCA bypass may provide inadequate blood flow to compensate for the input lost from the sacrificed vessel. Blood flow through a bypass can be augmented through the use of interposition saphenous vein grafts[91, 100] or "double-barrel" bypasses that connect several branches of the feeding vessel to the recipient vessels.[23] Likewise, interposition vein grafts can be used to bypass diseased segments of large-caliber vessels (Fig. 121–15), such as petrous-to-supraclinoid bypass procedures of the ICA. The radial artery has also been used for this purpose.[101] Finally, certain vascular

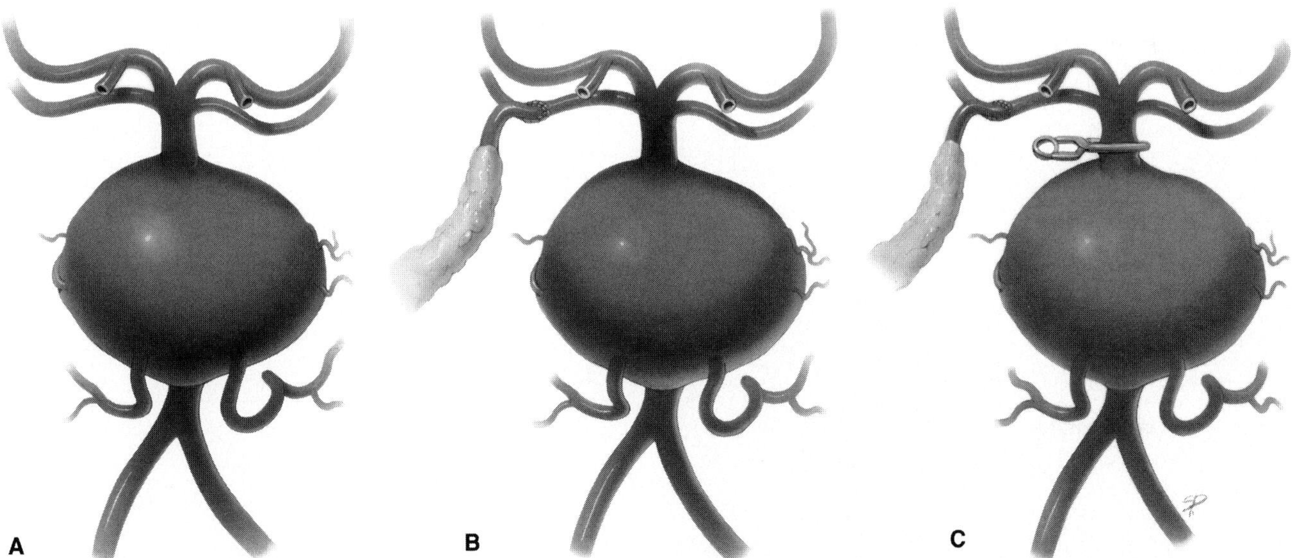

FIGURE 121–13. Parent vessel occlusion with bypass. *A*, A giant fusiform aneurysm in the midbasilar region is seldom amenable to direct surgical clipping or trapping. Blood flow must be directed away from the aneurysm while blood flow to the midbrain stem perforators and distal vasculature is preserved. *B*, Distal blood supply is augmented surgically by performing a superficial temporal artery–to–superior cerebellar artery bypass. Blood flow through the posterior communicating arteries from the anterior circulation represents the naturally occurring collateral source. *C*, Distal occlusion of the basilar artery directs blood flow from the aneurysm while still supplying the brainstem perforators involved within the aneurysm itself. (Courtesy of Barrow Neurological Institute, Phoenix, AZ.)

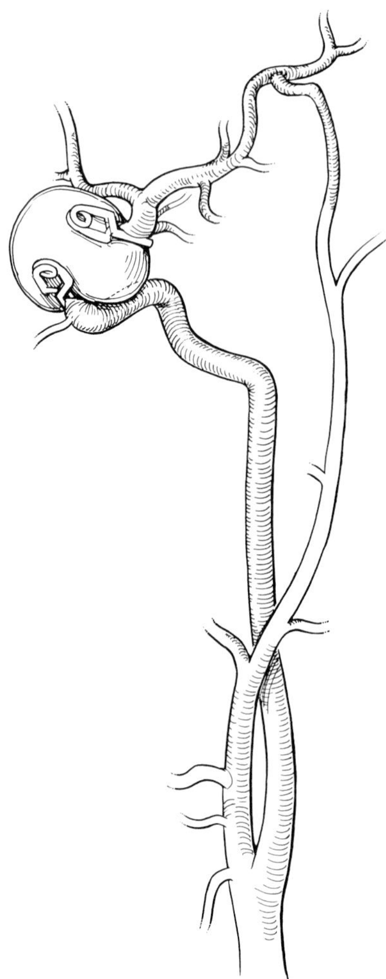

FIGURE 121–14. Extracranial-to-intracranial bypass. The mobilized pedicle of one superficial temporal artery is anastomosed with a distal branch of the middle cerebral artery (MCA) distribution. In this manner, blood flow to the ipsilateral MCA distribution and ipsilateral hemisphere is augmented. (Courtesy of Barrow Neurological Institute, Phoenix, AZ.)

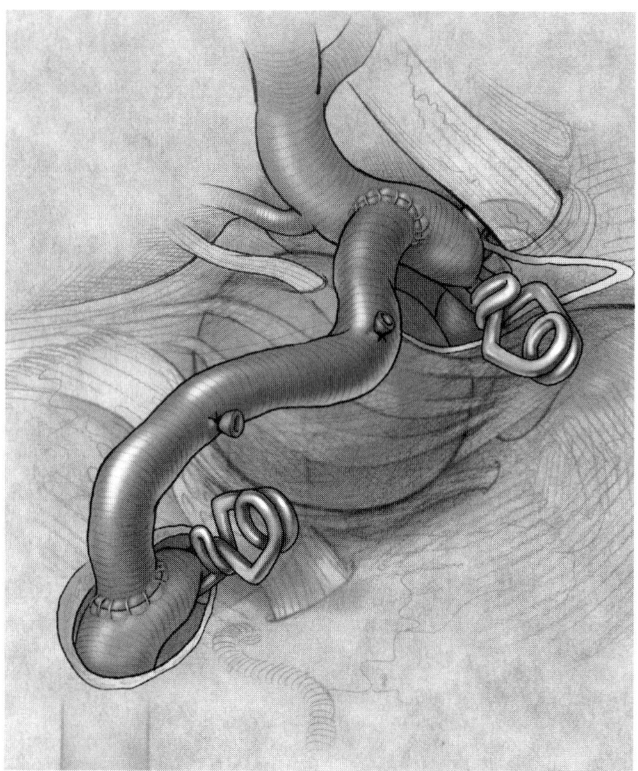

FIGURE 121–15. Vein bypass. When large intracranial vessels such as the internal carotid artery must be sacrificed, the caliber of the bypassing vessel must approximate the caliber of the original artery to avoid ischemia from a perfusion mismatch. The saphenous vein is readily harvested and anastomosed proximal and distal to the diseased artery segment. (Courtesy of Barrow Neurological Institute, Phoenix, AZ.)

territories within the brain are amenable to revascularization using in situ anastomoses, particularly the paired anterior cerebral and posterior inferior cerebellar arteries (Fig. 121–16). In this situation, blood flow distal to the trapped aneurysm can be augmented with a side-to-side anastomosis from the contralateral circulation. The anterior temporal branch of the MCA can sometimes be mobilized to bypass diseased segments just distal to it.

Aneurysmectomy may be considered for giant intracranial aneurysms that involve vessels that can be mobilized and reanastomosed after aneurysm excision (Fig. 121–17), such as giant aneurysms involving the MCA bifurcation.[102, 103] Excision is precluded if the aneurysm directly involves significant perforators or outflow vessels.

When an aneurysm cannot be clipped directly or the parent vessel cannot be reconstructed, it may be possible to reduce the mass effect of the aneurysm by needle aspiration[13] or by directly incising the lesion and reducing its associated thrombus. The vessel can then be sutured or clip-reconstructed to minimize the resulting mass effect and achieve a more physiologically appropriate morphology (Fig. 121–18).[40, 104]

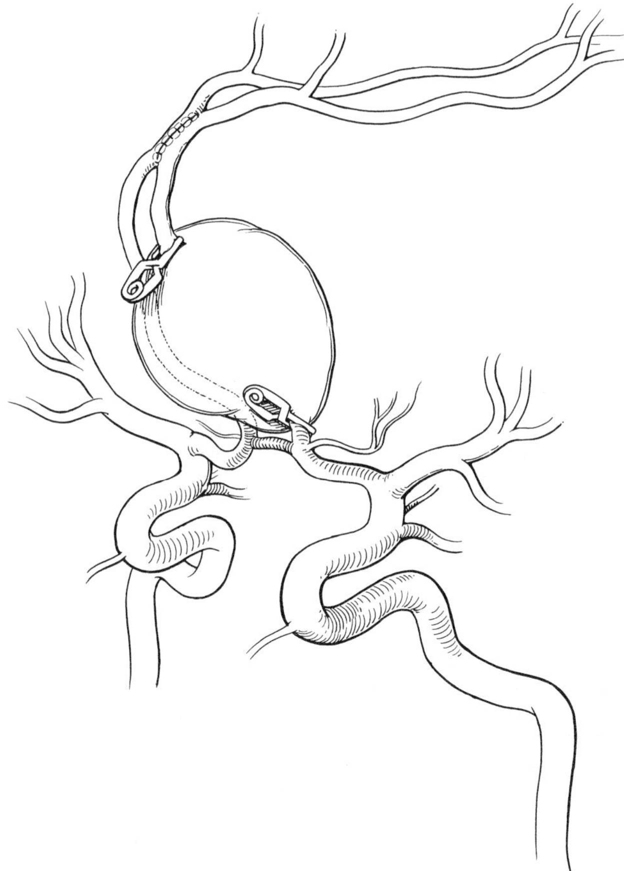

FIGURE 121–16. In situ bypass. At certain intracranial locations, paired arterial branches coexist that are amenable to side-to-side bypass techniques. Here, the A2 segment of the anterior cerebral artery is anastomosed to the contralateral vessel to provide distal flow once the parent vessel and the associated giant aneurysm are sacrificed. (Courtesy of Barrow Neurological Institute, Phoenix, AZ.)

Endovascular Treatment

Endovascular techniques, which include the use of detachable balloons, embolic polymers, and detachable thrombogenic coils,[3, 105–107] have been used to occlude giant intracranial aneurysms directly and to exclude them from the cerebral circulation. Two studies have used stents along with detachable coils to isolate and control aneurysmal thrombosis.[3, 108] Significant improvements have made it possible to exclude some aneurysms completely from the cerebral circulation using endovascular techniques alone. Often, the lesions most amenable to endovascular treatment are also those that are best treated by surgical techniques, namely, those with well-defined, small, narrow necks.[3, 109]

Unfortunately, occlusion is incomplete in a considerable percentage of endovascular treatments.[3, 109, 110] Even if a significant portion of an aneurysm's lumen is embolized or thrombosed, the patient is still subject to the risk of SAH from that lesion.[3, 105] In fact, endothelialization of the aneurysm orifice does not always follow coil occlusion.[111] Further, follow-up studies have demonstrated refilling and recurrence of aneurysms thought to have been completely occluded.[3]

There are a number of hypotheses about how the lumen of an aneurysm is recanalized (Fig. 121–19). The water-hammer effect proposes that the pulsatile hemodynamic blood flow compacts the thrombus and coil mass within the lumen, impacting them up toward the dome and allowing filling around the neck. Other mechanisms might include recanalization of a blood flow channel around the outer surface of the coil and thrombus mass next to the aneurysmal wall.[3] In contrast, the recurrence rates associated with large surgical series are low.[112] Endovascular techniques must be measured against this standard when their overall efficacy is assessed. The morbidity and mortality rates associated with either surgical or endovascular procedures must include the risks of the procedure itself weighed against the risks of the natural history of partially treated or recurrent aneurysms.

Endovascular techniques are associated with their own complications. Embolization and infarction from cerebral catheterization are risks.[58, 60] Coil migration into a parent vessel lumen with subsequent thrombosis or embolization is a rare but real risk.[3] Further, a partially treated, coiled aneurysm poses a greater surgical challenge to the neurosurgeon than if no endovascular intervention had been undertaken.

Endovascular techniques are often inadequate to address the mass effect of a giant aneurysm, the likely manifestation in most patients. Parent vessel sacrifice using detachable endovascular balloons can promote thrombosis and resolution of the aneurysm. Endovascular studies have demonstrated resolution of mass effect symptoms with aneurysmal coiling. Coil occlusion of the aneurysm may reduce the hemodynamic pulsations of the aneurysm on surrounding neural structures.[105, 107, 113] Nonetheless, deterioration after coiling procedures and signs of worsening mass effect have been described.[113, 114]

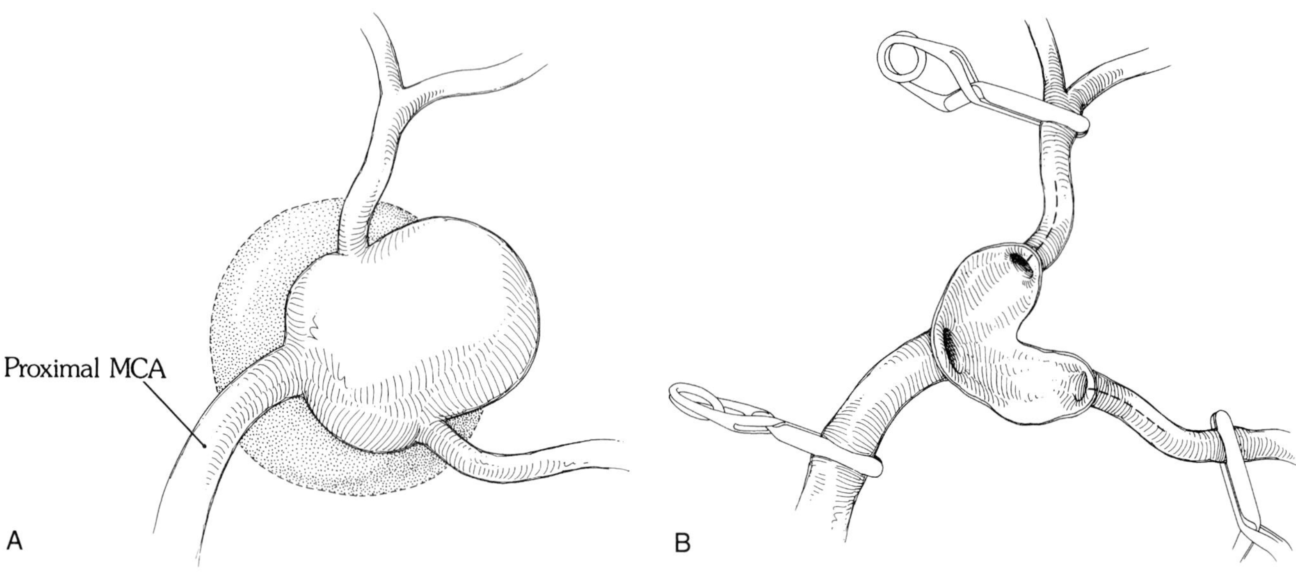

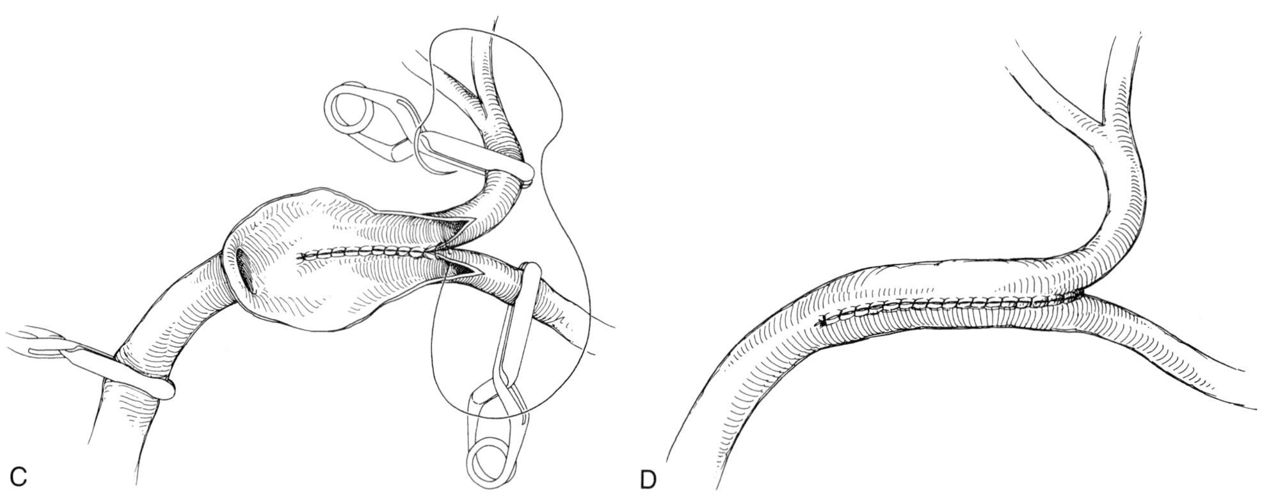

FIGURE 121–17. Aneurysmectomy. *A,* Giant aneurysms of the middle cerebral artery (MCA) can sometimes be excised directly with vessel reanastomosis. *B,* Complete vascular control of all outflow and tributary vessels must be obtained. *C,* After the aneurysm dome is excised, enough tissue must be preserved to perform a suture vessel or clip vessel reconstruction. *D,* The resulting anastomosis preserves the blood supply to all the original territory subserved by the aneurysm. (From Bojanowski WM, Spetzler RF, Carter LP: Reconstruction of the MCA bifurcation after excision of a giant aneurysm. J Neurosurg 68:974–977, 1988.)

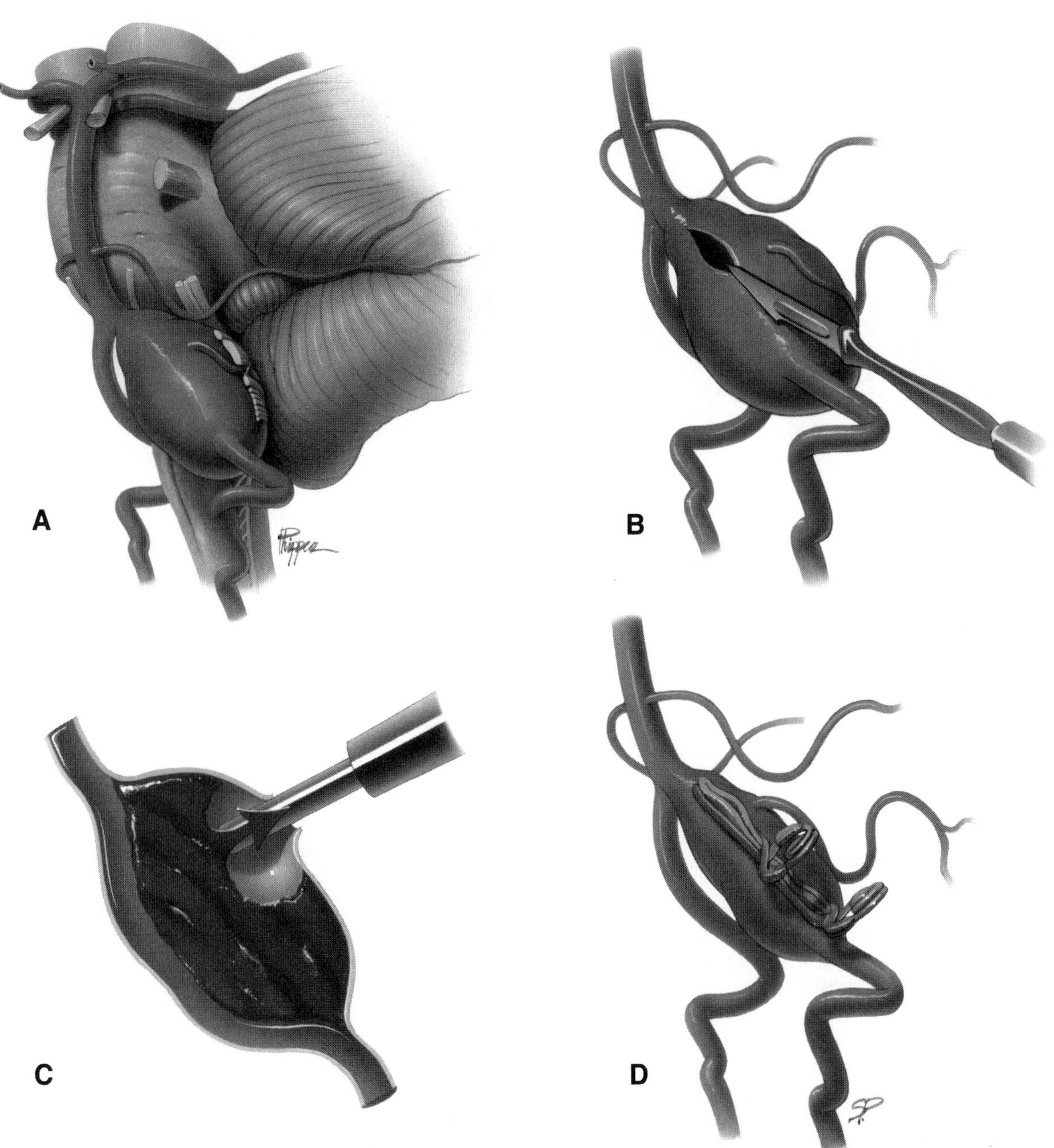

FIGURE 121–18. Aneurysmorrhaphy. *A,* A giant fusiform aneurysm of the vertebral artery exerts mass effect and must be decompressed. *B,* The lesion is incised directly to remove thrombus. *C,* The thrombus in the aneurysm is removed with an ultrasonic aspirator. *D,* The aneurysmorrhaphy site is clip-reconstructed, thereby lessening the local mass effect of the aneurysm. (Courtesy of Barrow Neurological Institute, Phoenix, AZ.)

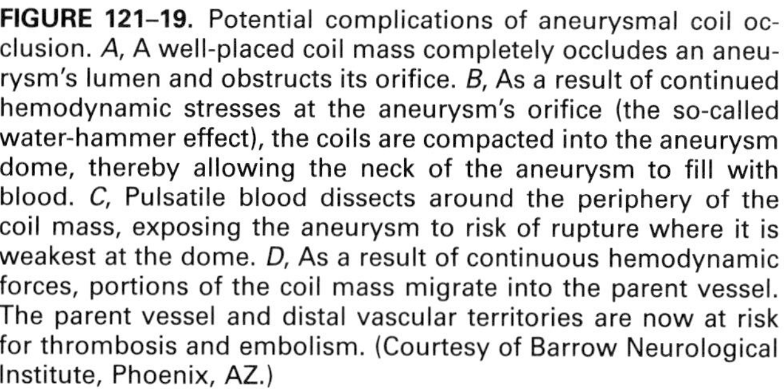

FIGURE 121–19. Potential complications of aneurysmal coil occlusion. *A*, A well-placed coil mass completely occludes an aneurysm's lumen and obstructs its orifice. *B*, As a result of continued hemodynamic stresses at the aneurysm's orifice (the so-called water-hammer effect), the coils are compacted into the aneurysm dome, thereby allowing the neck of the aneurysm to fill with blood. *C*, Pulsatile blood dissects around the periphery of the coil mass, exposing the aneurysm to risk of rupture where it is weakest at the dome. *D*, As a result of continuous hemodynamic forces, portions of the coil mass migrate into the parent vessel. The parent vessel and distal vascular territories are now at risk for thrombosis and embolism. (Courtesy of Barrow Neurological Institute, Phoenix, AZ.)

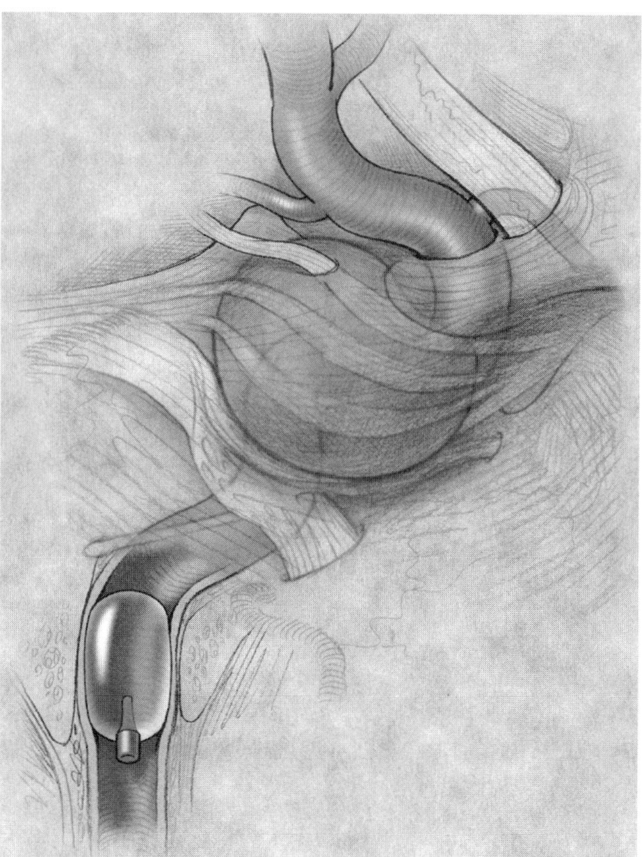

FIGURE 121–20. Parent vessel sacrifice with detachable balloon occlusion techniques. If parent vessel occlusion techniques are considered for complex giant aneurysms, one alternative is to perform this procedure endovascularly with detachable balloons or coil occlusion of the parent vessel. Distal vascular territories must be supplied through naturally occurring collaterals or surgical augmentation. (Courtesy of Barrow Neurological Institute, Phoenix, AZ.)

Endovascular techniques have revolutionized the treatment of giant aneurysms of the cavernous sinus. Direct surgical approaches through the cavernous sinus can be associated with significant morbidity,[87] and endovascular coiling of the lesion or sacrifice of the parent vessel by balloon occlusion, if tolerated, has reduced the need for such aggressive surgeries.[115, 116] Further, the need to completely occlude aneurysms outside the subarachnoid space is less pronounced, because the morbidity and mortality rates associated with their rupture are much lower.

Endovascular techniques are rapidly becoming an indispensable adjunct to microsurgical attacks on giant cerebral aneurysms. Proximal or distal parent vessel occlusion can be performed with detachable endovascular balloons if an amenable vascular territory is involved (Fig. 121–20).[3, 59, 106] Likewise, proximal vascular control is sometimes readily achieved with endovascular balloon occlusion techniques.[57, 58, 60] Results are impressive when endovascular techniques are combined with direct surgical attack of giant cerebral aneurysms.[55, 56, 117] For example, endovascular balloon occlusion has been combined with aneurysmal suction decompression to facilitate surgical manipulation and clipping of paraclinoid aneurysms.[57, 58, 60] No doubt as endovascular technology advances, less invasive surgical and endovascular options will be applied to the treatment of these problematic lesions.

SUMMARY

Giant intracranial aneurysms have a poor natural history that demands intervention. These lesions can present anywhere along the cerebral vascular tree and may manifest with SAH. As aneurysms reach giant proportions, they also manifest with signs and symptoms of neurological compromise related to mass effect. The most efficacious form of treatment involves the complete elimination of these lesions from the cerebral circulation, thereby eliminating their risk of rupture and continued enlargement. Lesions that are symptomatic with aneurysmal mass effect may need to be debulked. Surgical techniques require selection of the appropriate skull base approach to minimize brain retraction while maximizing surgical exposure. The basic tenets of aneurysm surgery, including vascular control and surgical clipping, as well as adjuncts such as parent vessel occlusion, trapping and bypass procedures, aneurysmectomy, and aneurysmorrhaphy, are applicable to the treatment of giant intracranial lesions. Endovascular procedures must also be considered, both as adjuncts to traditional surgical techniques and, in certain situations, as stand-alone procedures. Whatever intervention is undertaken, the neurosurgeon must compare the risks of the invasive procedure with its efficacy over the patient's remaining functional lifetime.

REFERENCES

1. Laws ER Jr, Udvarhelyi GB: The Genesis of Neuroscience by A. Earl Walker, MD. Park Ridge, Ill, American Association of Neurological Surgeons, 1998.
2. Hutchinson J: Aneurysms of the internal carotid within the skull diagnosed 11 years before patient's death: Spontaneous cure. Trans Clin Soc (Lond) 8:127, 1875.
3. Standard SC, Guterman LR, Chavis TD, et al: Endovascular management of giant intracranial aneurysms. Clin Neurosurg 42:267–293, 1995.
4. Atkinson JLD, Piepgras DG: Giant aneurysms: Supratentorial. In Carter LP, Spetzler RF (eds): Neurovascular Surgery. New York, McGraw-Hill, 1995, pp 815–828.
5. Locksley HB: Natural history of subarachnoid hemorrhage, intracranial aneurysms and arteriovenous malformations: Based on 6368 cases in the cooperative study. J Neurosurg 25:219–239, 1966.
6. Morley TP, Barr HW: Giant intracranial aneurysms: Diagnosis, course, and management. Clin Neurosurg 16:73–94, 1969.
7. Bull J: Massive aneurysms at the base of the brain. Brain 92: 535–570, 1969.
8. Peerless SJ, Wallace MC, Drake CG: Giant intracranial aneurysms. In Youmans JR (ed): Neurological Surgery: A Comprehensive Reference Guide to the Diagnosis and Management of Neurological Problems. Philadelphia, WB Saunders, 1990, pp 1742–1763.
9. Michel WF: Posterior fossa aneurysms simulating tumours. J Neurol Neurosurg Psychiatry 37:218–223, 1974.
10. Kodama N, Suzuki J: Surgical treatment of giant aneurysms. Neurosurg Rev 5:155–160, 1982.
11. Pia HW, Zierski J: Giant cerebral aneurysms: A review of clinical picture, diagnosis, and management with illustrative cases. Neurosurg Rev 5:117–148, 1982.
12. Weir B: Special aneurysms: Saccular. In Weir B (ed): Aneurysms Affecting the Nervous System. Baltimore, Williams & Wilkins, 1987, pp 185–208.
13. Shibuya M, Sugita K: Intracranial giant aneurysms. In Youmans JR (ed): Neurological Surgery: A Comprehensive Reference Guide to the Diagnosis and Management of Neurological Problems. Philadelphia, WB Saunders, 1996, pp 1310–1319.
14. Onuma T, Suzuki J: Surgical treatment of giant intracranial aneurysms. J Neurosurg 51:33–36, 1979.
15. Ausman JI, Diaz F, Sadasivan B, et al: Giant intracranial aneurysm surgery: The role of microvascular reconstruction. Surg Neurol 34:8–15, 1990.
16. Nakayama Y, Tanaka A, Kumate S, et al: Giant fusiform aneurysm of the basilar artery: Consideration of its pathogenesis. Surg Neurol 51:140–145, 1999.
17. Yasargil MG: Giant intracranial aneurysms. In Yasargil MG (ed): Microneurosurgery II: Clinical Considerations, Surgery of the Intracranial Aneurysms and Results. New York, Thieme-Stratton, 1984, pp 296–304.
18. Sundt TM Jr: Results of surgical management. In Sundt TM Jr (ed): Surgical Techniques for Saccular and Giant Intracranial Aneurysms. Baltimore, Williams & Wilkins, 1990, pp 19–23.
19. Hosobuchi Y: Giant intracranial aneurysms. In Wilkins RH, Rengachary SS (eds): Neurosurgery. New York, McGraw-Hill, 1985, pp 1404–1414.
20. Symon L, Vajda J: Surgical experiences with giant intracranial aneurysms. J Neurosurg 61:1009–1028, 1984.
21. Lawton MT, Spetzler RF: Surgical management of giant intracranial aneurysms: Experience with 171 patients. Clin Neurosurg 42:245–266, 1995.
22. Barrow DL, Alleyne C: Natural history of giant intracranial aneurysms and indications for intervention. Clin Neurosurg 42: 214–244, 1995.
23. Lawton MT, Spetzler RF: Surgical strategies for giant intracranial aneurysms. Neurosurg Clin N Am 9:725–742, 1998.
24. Forbus WD: On the origin of miliary aneurysms of the superficial cerebral arteries. Bull Johns Hopkins Hosp 47:239–284, 1930.
25. Sekhar LN, Heros RC: Origin, growth, and rupture of saccular aneurysms: A review. Neurosurgery 8:248–260, 1981.
26. Stehbens WE: Etiology of intracranial berry aneurysms. J Neurosurg 70:823–831, 1989.
27. Koyama S, Kotani A, Sasaki J: Giant basilar artery aneurysm with intramural hemorrhage and then disastrous hemorrhage: Case report. Neurosurgery 39:174–178, 1996.
28. Khurana VG, Wijdicks EFM, Parisi JE, et al: Acute deterioration from thrombosis and rerupture of a giant intracranial aneurysm. Neurology 52:1697–1699, 1999.
29. Maruishi M, Shima K, Chigasaki H, et al: Giant intracranial aneurysm with rapid thrombus formation and intramural hemorrhage—case report. Neurol Med Chir (Tokyo) 34:829–831, 1994.
30. Barth A, de Tribolet N: Growth of small saccular aneurysms to giant aneurysms: Presentation of three cases. Surg Neurol 41: 277–280, 1994.
31. Johnston SC, Halbach VV, Smith WS, et al: Rapid development of giant fusiform cerebral aneurysms in angiographically normal vessels. Neurology 50:1163–1166, 1998.
32. Schievink WI, Puumala MR, Meyer FB, et al: Giant intracranial aneurysm and fibromuscular dysplasia in an adolescent with alpha 1-antitrypsin deficiency. J Neurosurg 85:503–506, 1996.
33. Casey AT, Moore AJ: A traumatic giant posterior cerebral artery aneurysm mimicking a tentorial edge meningioma. Br J Neurosurg 8:97–99, 1994.
34. Whittle IR, Dorsch NW, Besser M: Giant intracranial aneurysms: Diagnosis, management, and outcome. Surg Neurol 21:218–230, 1984.
35. Anson JA, Lawton MT, Spetzler RF: Characteristics and surgical treatment of dolichoectatic and fusiform aneurysms. J Neurosurg 84:185–193, 1996.
36. Drake CG, Peerless SJ: Giant fusiform intracranial aneurysms: Review of 120 patients treated surgically from 1965 to 1992. J Neurosurg 87:141–162, 1997.
37. Baker CJ, Fiore A, Connolly ES Jr, et al: Serum elastase and alpha-1-antitrypsin levels in patients with ruptured and unruptured cerebral aneurysms: Clinical study. Neurosurgery 37:56–62, 1995.
38. Connolly ES Jr, Choudhri TF, Mack WJ, et al: Influence of smoking, hypertension, and sex on the phenotypic expression of familial intracranial aneurysms in siblings. Neurosurgery 48: 65–69, 2001.
39. Khurana VG, Piepgras DG, Whisnant JP: Ruptured giant intracranial aneurysms. Part I. A study of rebleeding. J Neurosurg 88:425–429, 1998.
40. Lownie SP, Drake CG, Peerless SJ, et al: Clinical presentation and management of giant anterior communicating artery region aneurysms. J Neurosurg 92:267–277, 2000.
41. Sano H, Kato Y, Shankar K, et al: Treatment and results of partially thrombosed giant aneurysms. Neurol Med Chir Suppl (Tokyo) 38:58–61, 1998.
42. McCormick WF, Acosta-Rua GJ: The size of intracranial saccular aneurysms: An autopsy study. J Neurosurg 33:422–427, 1970.
43. Wiebers DO, Whisnant JP, Sundt TM Jr, et al: The significance of unruptured intracranial saccular aneurysms. J Neurosurg 66: 23–29, 1987.
44. Orz Y, Kobayashi S, Osawa M, et al: Aneurysm size: A prognostic factor for rupture. Br J Neurosurg 11:144–149, 1997.
45. Juvela S, Porras M, Poussa K: Natural history of unruptured intracranial aneurysms: Probability of and risk factors for aneurysm rupture. J Neurosurg 93:379–387, 2000.

46. The International Study of Unruptured Intracranial Aneurysms Investigators: Unruptured intracranial aneurysms—risk of rupture and risks of surgical intervention. N Engl J Med 339: 1725–1733, 1998.
47. Pakarinen S: Incidence, aetiology, and prognosis of primary subarachnoid haemorrhage: A study based on 589 cases diagnosed in a defined urban population during a defined period. Acta Neurol Scand 43:1–28, 1967.
48. Tanabe S, Ohtaki M, Uede T, et al: Diagnosis of ruptured and unruptured cerebral aneurysms with three-dimensional CT angiography (3D-CTA). No Shinkei Geka 23:787–795, 1995.
49. Lang EW, Steffens JC, Link J, et al: The utility of contrast-enhanced MR-angiography for posterior fossa giant cerebral aneurysm management. Neurol Res 20:705–708, 1998.
50. Brugieres P, Blustajn J, Le Guerinel C, et al: Magnetic resonance angiography of giant intracranial aneurysms. Neuroradiology 40:96–102, 1998.
51. Anzalone N, Righi C, Simionato F, et al: Three-dimensional time-of-flight MR angiography in the evaluation of intracranial aneurysms treated with Guglielmi detachable coils. AJNR Am J Neuroradiol 21:746–752, 2000.
52. Symon L: Management of giant intracranial aneurysms. Clin Neurosurg 36:21–47, 1990.
53. Spetzler RF, Hadley MN: Protection against cerebral ischemia: The role of barbiturates. Cerebrovasc Brain Metab Rev 1:212–229, 1989.
54. Connolly ES Jr, Solomon RA: Hypothermic cardiac standstill for cerebral aneurysm surgery. Neurosurg Clin N Am 9:681–695, 1998.
55. Ewald C, Kühne D, Hassler W: Giant basilar artery aneurysms incorporating the posterior cerebral artery: Bypass surgery and coil occlusion. Two case reports. Neurol Med Chir Suppl (Tokyo) 38:83–85, 1998.
56. Hacein-Bey L, Connolly ES Jr, Mayer SA, et al: Complex intracranial aneurysms: Combined operative and endovascular approaches. Neurosurgery 43:1304–1313, 1998.
57. Arnautovic KI, Al-Mefty O, Anguaco E: A combined microsurgical skull-base and endovascular approach to giant and large paraclinoid aneurysms. Surg Neurol 50:504–520, 1998.
58. Fahlbusch R, Nimsky C, Huk W: Open surgery of giant paraclinoid aneurysms improved by intraoperative angiography and endovascular retrograde suction decompression. Acta Neurochir (Wien) 139:1026–1032, 1997.
59. Taki W, Nakahara I, Sakai N, et al: Large and giant middle to lower basilar trunk aneurysms treated by surgical and interventional neuroradiological methods. Neurol Med Chir (Tokyo) 38: 826–834, 1998.
60. Ng P-Y, Huddle D, Gunel M, et al: Intraoperative endovascular treatment as an adjunct to microsurgical clipping of paraclinoid aneurysms. J Neurosurg 93:554–560, 2000.
61. Al-Mefty O: The cranio-orbital zygomatic approach for intracranial lesions. Contemp Neurosurg 14:1–6, 1992.
62. Sano K: Temporo-polar approach to aneurysms of the basilar artery at and around the distal bifurcation: Technical note. Neurol Res 2:361–367, 1980.
63. Sano K, Asano T, Tamura A: Surgical technique. In Sano K, Tamura A (eds): Acute Aneurysm Surgery: Pathophysiology and Management. New York, Springer-Verlag, 1987, pp 194–246.
64. Diaz FG: Vertebrobasilar aneurysms: Surgical management. Crit Rev Neurosurg 2:146–158, 1992.
65. Zabramski JM, Kiris T, Sankhla SK, et al: Orbitozygomatic craniotomy: Technical note. J Neurosurg 89:336–341, 1998.
66. Salas E, Ziyal IM, Bejjani GK, et al: Anatomy of the frontotemporal branch of the facial nerve and indications for interfascial dissection: Anatomical report. Neurosurgery 43:563–569, 1998.
67. Lawton MT, Spetzler RF: Surgical strategies for giant intracranial aneurysms. Acta Neurochir (Wien) 72:141–156, 1999.
68. Drake CG: Giant intracranial aneurysms: Experience with surgical treatment in 174 patients. Clin Neurosurg 26:12–96, 1979.
69. Drake CG: The treatment of aneurysms of the posterior circulation. Clin Neurosurg 26:96–144, 1979.
70. Lawton MT, Daspit CP, Spetzler RF: Technical aspects and recent trends in the management of large and giant midbasilar artery aneurysms. Neurosurgery 41:513–521, 1997.
71. Hitselberger WE, House WF: A combined approach to the cerebellopontine angle: A suboccipital-petrosal approach. Arch Otolaryngol 84:49–67, 1966.
72. House WF: Translabyrinthine approach. In House WF, Luetje CM (eds): Acoustic Tumors. Baltimore, University Park, 1979, pp 43–87.
73. House WF, Hitselberger WE: The transcochlear approach to the skull base. Arch Otolaryngol 102:334–342, 1976.
74. Malis LI: Surgical resection of tumors of the skull base. In Wilkins RH, Rengachary SS (eds): Neurosurgery. New York, McGraw-Hill, 1985, pp 1011–1021.
75. Spetzler RF, Grahm TW: The far-lateral approach to the inferior clivus and upper cervical region: Technical note. BNI Q 6: 35–38, 1990.
76. Lawton MT, Daspit CP, Spetzler RF: Transpetrosal and combination approaches to skull base lesions. Clin Neurosurg 43:91–112, 1996.
77. Heros RC: Lateral suboccipital approach for vertebral and vertebrobasilar artery lesions. J Neurosurg 64:559–562, 1986.
78. Sen CN, Sekhar LN: An extreme lateral approach to intradural lesions of the cervical spine and foramen magnum. Neurosurgery 27:197–204, 1990.
79. Hammon WM, Kempe LG: The posterior fossa approach to aneurysms of the vertebral and basilar arteries. J Neurosurg 37: 339–347, 1972.
80. Vishteh AG, Crawford NR, Melton MS, et al: Stability of the craniovertebral junction after unilateral occipital condyle resection: A biomechanical study. J Neurosurg 90:91–98, 1999.
81. Baldwin HZ, Miller CG, van Loveren HR, et al: The far lateral/combined supra- and infratentorial approach: A human cadaveric prosection model for routes of access to the petroclival region and ventral brain stem. J Neurosurg 81:60–68, 1994.
82. Hamilton MG, Kraus GE, Daspit CP, et al: Giant aneurysms: Infratentorial. In Carter LP, Spetzler RF (eds): Neurovascular Surgery. New York, McGraw-Hill, 1995, pp 829–850.
83. Baumgartner WA, Silverberg GD, Ream AK, et al: Reappraisal of cardiopulmonary bypass with deep hypothermia and circulatory arrest for complex neurosurgical operations. Surgery 94: 242–249, 1983.
84. Morgan H, Nofzinger JD, Robertson JT, et al: Hemorrhagic studies with severe hemodilution in profound hypothermia and cardiac arrest. J Surg Res 14:459–464, 1973.
85. Doutremepuich C: Haemostasis defects following cardio-pulmonary by-pass based on a study of 1350 patients. Thromb Haemost 39:539–541, 1978.
86. Lawton MT, Raudzens PA, Jacobowitz R, et al: Hypothermia-induced circulatory arrest in neurovascular surgery: Evolving indications and predictors of patient outcome. J Neurosurg 86: 401A, 1997.
87. Batjer HH, Kopitnik TA Jr, Purdy PD, et al: Giant intracranial aneurysms. In Wilkins RH, Rengachary SS (eds): Neurosurgery. New York, McGraw-Hill, 1996, pp 2361–2376.
88. Cantore GP, Santoro A: Treatment of aneurysms unsuitable for clipping or endovascular therapy. J Neurosurg Sci 42:71–75, 1998.
89. Drake CG, Peerless SJ, Ferguson GG: Hunterian proximal arterial occlusion for giant aneurysms of the carotid circulation. J Neurosurg 81:656–665, 1994.
90. Gerber S, Dormont D, Sahel M, et al: Complete spontaneous thrombosis of a giant intracranial aneurysm. Neuroradiology 36:316–317, 1994.
91. Cantore G, Santoro A, Da Pian R: Spontaneous occlusion of supraclinoid aneurysms after the creation of extra-intracranial bypasses using long grafts: Report of two cases. Neurosurgery 44:216–220, 1999.
92. Yeh H, Tomsick TA: Obliteration of a giant carotid aneurysm after extracranial-to-intracranial bypass surgery: Case report. Surg Neurol 48:473–476, 1997.
93. Lee KC, Joo JY, Lee KS, et al: Recanalization of completely thrombosed giant aneurysm: Case report. Surg Neurol 51:94–98, 1999.
94. Numagami Y, Ezura M, Takahashi A, et al: Antegrade recanalization of completely embolized internal carotid artery after treatment of a giant intracavernous aneurysm: A case report. Surg Neurol 52:611–616, 1999.
95. Chang SD, Marks MP, Steinberg GK: Recanalization and rupture

of a giant vertebral artery aneurysm after hunterian ligation: Case report. Neurosurgery 44:1117–1121, 1999.
96. Standard SC, Ahuja A, Guterman LR, et al: Balloon test occlusion of the internal carotid artery with hypotensive challenge. AJNR Am J Neuroradiol 16:1453–1458, 1995.
97. Spetzler RF, Selman W, Carter LP: Elective EC-IC bypass for unclippable intracranial aneurysms. Neurol Res 6:64–68, 1984.
98. Peerless SJ, Ferguson GG, Drake CG: Extracranial-intracranial (EC/IC) bypass in the treatment of giant intracranial aneurysms. Neurosurg Rev 5:77–81, 1982.
99. Ausman JI, Diaz FG, Vacca DF, et al: Superficial temporal and occipital artery bypass pedicles to superior, anterior inferior, and posterior inferior cerebellar arteries for vertebrobasilar insufficiency. J Neurosurg 72:554–558, 1990.
100. Ramina R, Meneses MS, Pedrozo AA, et al: Saphenous vein graft bypass in the treatment of giant cavernous sinus aneurysms: Report of two cases. Arq Neuropsiquiatr 58:162–168, 2000.
101. Sekhar LN, Bucur SD, Bank WO, et al: Venous and arterial bypass grafts for difficult tumors, aneurysms, and occlusive vascular lesions: Evolution of surgical treatment and improved graft results. Neurosurgery 44:1207–1224, 1999.
102. Hadley MN, Spetzler RF, Martin NA, et al: Middle cerebral artery aneurysm due to *Nocardia asteroides:* Case report of aneurysm excision and extracranial-intracranial bypass. Neurosurgery 22:923–928, 1988.
103. Ceylan S, Karakus A, Duru S, et al: Reconstruction of the middle cerebral artery after excision of a giant fusiform aneurysm. Neurosurg Rev 21:189–193, 1998.
104. Bojanowski WM, Spetzler RF, Carter LP: Reconstruction of the MCA bifurcation after excision of a giant aneurysm: Technical note. J Neurosurg 68:974–977, 1988.
105. Gruber A, Killer M, Bavinzski G, et al: Clinical and angiographic results of endosaccular coiling treatment of giant and very large intracranial aneurysms: A 7-year, single-center experience. Neurosurgery 45:793–804, 1999.
106. Ross IB, Weill A, Piotin M, et al: Endovascular treatment of distally located giant aneurysms. Neurosurgery 47:1147–1153, 2000.
107. Gobin YP, Vinuela F, Gurian JH, et al: Treatment of large and giant fusiform intracranial aneurysms with Guglielmi detachable coils. J Neurosurg 84:55–62, 1996.
108. Lanzino G, Wakhloo AK, Fessler RD, et al: Efficacy and current limitations of intravascular stents for intracranial internal carotid, vertebral, and basilar artery aneurysms. J Neurosurg 91: 538–546, 1999.
109. Zubillaga AF, Guglielmi G, Vinuela F, et al: Endovascular occlusion of intracranial aneurysms with electrically detachable coils: Correlation of aneurysm neck size and treatment results. AJNR Am J Neuroradiol 15:815–820, 1994.
110. Klein GE, Szolar DH, Leber KA, et al: Basilar tip aneurysm: Endovascular treatment with Guglielmi detachable coils—midterm results. Radiology 205:191–196, 1997.
111. Bavinzski G, Talazoglu V, Killer M, et al: Gross and microscopic histopathological findings in aneurysms of the human brain treated with Guglielmi detachable coils. J Neurosurg 91:284–293, 1999.
112. David CA, Vishteh AG, Spetzler RF, et al: Late angiographic follow-up review of surgically treated aneurysms. J Neurosurg 91:396–401, 1999.
113. Vargus ME, Kupersmith MJ, Setton A, et al: Endovascular treatment of giant aneurysms which cause visual loss. Ophthalmology 101:1091–1098, 1994.
114. Ushikoshi S, Kikuchi Y, Houkin K, et al: Aggravation of brainstem symptoms caused by a large superior cerebellar artery aneurysm after embolization by Guglielmi detachable coils. Neurol Med Chir (Tokyo) 39:524–529, 1999.
115. Higashida RT, Halbach VV, Dowd C, et al: Endovascular detachable balloon embolization therapy of cavernous carotid artery aneursyms: Results in 87 cases. J Neurosurg 72:857–863, 1990.
116. Bavinzski G, Ferraz-Leite H, Gruber A, et al: Endovascular therapy of idiopathic cavernous aneurysms over 11 years. AJNR Am J Neuroradiol 19:559–565, 1998.
117. Pluchino F, Giombini S, Broggi G, et al: Surgical management of giant anterior aneurysms. J Neurosurg 42:65–69, 1998.
118. Heros RC: Management of giant paraclinoid aneurysms. In Kikuchi H, Fukushima T, Watanabe K (eds): Intracranial Aneurysms. Niigata, Japan, Nishimura, 1986, pp 273–282.

CHAPTER **122**

Infectious Intracranial Aneurysms

KEVIN C. YAO ■ JOSHUA B. BEDERSON

In 1869 Church[1] described the first intracranial aneurysm of infectious origin. In 1885 Osler[2] coined the term *mycotic aneurysm* in his description of an aortic aneurysm that arose in the setting of bacterial endocarditis. This term has since been applied to all aneurysms of infectious origin, including those found in the intracranial circulation. Eppinger[3] acknowledged the significance of infected emboli in the development of these lesions by calling them mycotic-embolic aneurysms. In 1923 Stengel and Wolforth[4] published the first review of intracranial bacterial aneurysms, which included 34 cases. Ojemann and coworkers[5] then reviewed 81 cases of infectious intracranial aneurysms associated with bacterial endocarditis reported between 1959 and 1980. Subsequent reviews and case reports have brought the total number of reported cases to more than 200.[6, 7]

The term *mycotic* has been used inaccurately to label all intracranial aneurysms of infectious origin. Mycotic is synonymous with fungal, incorrectly discounting bacteria as a common cause of these aneurysms. Several alternative terms have been proposed, including *infected, infectious, infective,* and *inflammatory.* This chapter uses the terms *aneurysms of infectious origin, bacterial aneurysms, fungal aneurysms,* and *infectious aneurysms* and reviews the underlying pathophysiology, natural history, diagnosis, treatment, and outcomes of these lesions.

EPIDEMIOLOGY

Intracranial aneurysms of infectious origin are rare, constituting approximately 2% to 6% of all intracranial aneurysms.[8–10] Their incidence is higher in children, where they represent 10% of all intracranial aneurysms.[11] In fact, the true incidence of these lesions is unknown. Their propensity to grow or regress rapidly and asymptomatically suggests that they are often undetected and that reported rates underestimate their true incidence. In 1916 Fearnsides's autopsy review reported that 30% of all intracranial aneurysms were infectious.[12] Based on autopsies, McDonald and Korb[10] reported an incidence of 6.2%, which has been upheld by more recent reports.[8, 9] This relative decline in the incidence of infectious aneurysms over time has been attributed to the introduction of antibiotic therapy. However, the emergence of more virulent organisms and increasing rates of immunosuppression have also created the potential for a resurgence of these lesions in certain populations.

Endocarditis predisposes patients, especially those with left-sided cardiac valve disease, to infectious aneurysms and neurological complications. More than 80% of patients with intracranial infectious aneurysms carry an underlying diagnosis of endocarditis.[13] Twenty percent to 40% of patients with endocarditis suffer neurological sequelae. Cerebral infarction is most common, afflicting as many as 31%.[14] Intracranial hemorrhage occurs in 5%.[15] Overall, 2% of patients with endocarditis are clinically diagnosed with an infectious intracranial aneurysm.[16] In autopsy series, the incidence is higher (5% to 10%),[14] suggesting that many of these aneurysms are clinically silent.

Intracranial infectious aneurysms can also develop in the absence of endocarditis or intravascular infection. Extravascular infections such as meningitis, cavernous sinus thrombophlebitis, osteomyelitis of the skull, and sinus infections can extend into the arterial wall, inducing arteritis and the formation of an aneurysm.[13, 17–23] The infectious process is usually focused at the base of the brain and may be bacterial or fungal. The relative number of bacterial intracranial aneurysms attributable to extravascular infection is small; about 40 cases have been reported.[5, 24]

Fungal or "true" mycotic aneurysms are rare. Approximately 40 well-documented cases have been reported.[6, 25, 26] However, the incidence of these lesions has increased.[7] Unlike their bacterial counterparts, fungal intracranial aneurysms arise almost exclusively in the setting of an extravascular infection in an immunocompromised host. Prolonged use of steroids, immunosuppressive therapy, and exposure to broad-spectrum antibiotics have been implicated in their development.[27, 28] More prevalent application of these therapies combined with an increasing population of patients with immunocompromising diseases may explain the resurgence of fungal intracranial aneurysms.[7]

PATHOPHYSIOLOGY

As mentioned, infectious intracranial aneurysms can be divided into those derived from an intravascular infection and those with an infectious origin in the extravascular space. Intravascularly derived infectious aneurysms are usually bacterial; rarely, they may be fungal.[28] Because of their embolic cause, intravascularly derived infectious aneurysms tend to form in locations where blood flow is maximal and vascular anatomy favors the lodging of embolic particles, such as vessel branch points in the distal vasculature. The most common location is the distal middle cerebral artery, where more than 60% of emboli lodge.[29] Showers of emboli may give rise to the formation of multiple lesions, which are found in as many as 20% of patients.[30] In contrast, saccular aneurysms tend to form as solitary lesions on large basal vessels.

Unlike infectious aneurysms derived from an intravascular source, those arising from an extravascular source tend to form proximally, owing to the predilection for infection at the base of the brain. Usual locations include the intracavernous internal carotid artery, the midbasilar artery, and the vertebral artery. Whereas most bacterial aneurysms arise from intravascular infections, almost all fungal aneurysms originate in the extravascular space. These true mycotic aneurysms tend to be solitary, larger, and more saccular or fusiform than their bacterial counterparts.[28]

The precise mechanism of aneurysm formation in the setting of infection has not been elucidated completely. Several animal models have provided clues to key pathogenetic events. Nakata and coworkers[31] induced aneurysms to form in canine aortas by infusing bacteria directly into aortic segments. The rate at which infectious aneurysms formed was higher when peripheral branches were occluded. This finding implicated stasis and septic involvement of nutrient vasa vasorum as the predisposing events leading to vessel wall destruction. The relative paucity of vasa vasorum in the cerebral vasculature, however, casts doubt on this theory.

Molinari and colleagues[32] provided a more realistic model by injecting bacteria-coated catheters directly into canine carotid arteries. Confirming the results of others, they observed the spread of infection from the adventitia inward. The muscular intimal layer and inner elastic membrane were affected last. This pattern of infectious dissemination is counterintuitive in the setting of intravascular infection, where septic emboli are delivered to the intimal surface. The authors postulated that infectious dissemination from the intravascular space directly into the Virchow-Robin spaces of small penetrating vessels leads to this apparently paradoxical pattern.

The pathologic changes produced by either septic embolization or the contiguous spread of infection are similar. Infiltration of the adventitia and media by polymorphonuclear leukocytes is accompanied by marked intimal proliferation. Thrombosis of the involved vessel may occur but is unnecessary for an aneurysm to form. Focal arteritis gives rise to a severely weakened and necrotic vessel wall. Aneurysmal dilatation or frank disintegration and perforation of the vessel wall are the result. Consequently, intracranial infectious aneurysms are typically friable and seldom separable from the surrounding parenchyma. Antibiotic treatment may reverse this damage by inducing reparative fibrosis of the aneurysmal wall and parent artery,[9, 32] but it does not necessarily preclude aneurysmal rupture.

Intracranial aneurysms of infectious origin demonstrate dynamic cycles of formation, enlargement, regression, and resolution. In their canine model, Molinari and coworkers demonstrated the rapidity with which an infected embolus can cause an aneurysm to form.[32] On average, aneurysms formed and ruptured within 3 days of inoculation. Pathologic aneurysmal dilatation was detectable as early as 24 hours after embolization. Antibiotic therapy slowed the rate at which aneurysms formed (7 days) and also made the aneurysms tough, fibrotic, and less likely to rupture. Clinical studies have further underscored the dynamic manner in which infectious aneurysms develop and resolve.[33, 34] The behavior of an individual lesion can range from abrupt rupture, despite organism-directed antibiotic treatment, to spontaneous resolution within weeks to years.

MICROBIOLOGY

The most common organism cultured from aneurysms attributable to bacterial endocarditis is *Streptococcus*, which is documented in 25% to 44% of cases.[6, 30] The second most common organism, *Staphylococcus aureus*, is found in 14% to 18% of cases.[6, 30] Other bacterial organisms that have been cultured include enterococci, *Pseudomonas*, and corynebacteria. Multiple organisms are found in less than 5% of patients.[30] An organism fails to grow despite multiple blood or cerebrospinal fluid cultures in at least 12% to 19% of patients.[6, 30]

Extravascular infections that predispose to intracranial aneurysms include meningitis, cavernous sinus thrombophlebitis, osteomyelitis, tonsillitis, pharyngitis, sinusitis, and wound infections; drug abuse is also implicated. Bacterial organisms cultured from these infections include *S. aureus*, *Mycobacterium tuberculosis*, pneumococcus, *Pseudomonas*, brucella, *Neisseria*, and other species that inhabit potential portals to the intracranial space.

As mentioned, aneurysms of fungal origin usually develop in immunocompromised hosts. *Aspergillus* is the most common fungus cultured, followed by Phycomycetes and *Candida albicans*. Intracranial fungal aneurysms due to cryptococcus, coccidioidomycosis, *Petriellidium boydii*, *Pseudallescheria boydii*, *Nocardia asteroides*, and chromoblastomycosis have also been reported.[25, 26, 35, 36] Aspergillosis of the central nervous system usually occurs from direct infection via the paranasal sinus or indirectly by hematogenous infectious spread, most commonly from the lung.[37] Other reported routes of fungal infection include previous neurosurgical, gynecologic, or dental procedures.

CLINICAL MANIFESTATIONS

The initial encounter with a patient harboring an intracranial infectious aneurysm cannot be stereotyped. Patients may exhibit clinical manifestations referable to numerous underlying disease processes. Diagnosis is therefore often challenging.

Most patients with infectious intracranial aneurysms also have subacute bacterial endocarditis. They are typically septic with fever, weight loss, and generalized malaise. About 40% of patients ultimately diagnosed with an intracranial infectious aneurysm and endocarditis report a history of congenital or rheumatic heart disease.[38] Forty percent also describe a neurological prodrome.[38] The most common complaint is a focal neurological deficit occurring 2 days to 18 months before presentation. Not all neurological complaints signify the presence of an aneurysm. Although neurological manifestations are common in endocarditis, only a minority are ultimately referable to an infectious aneurysm.[14] Manifestations of subarachnoid or intracranial hemorrhage associated with endocarditis should raise strong suspicion of an infectious aneurysm. Signs and symptoms of hemorrhage are present in 57% of patients with an infectious aneurysm and are otherwise uncommon in patients with endocarditis.[38] Symptoms may include focal neurological deficits, headaches, meningismus, seizures, or a change in mental status.

Patients with intracranial aneurysms caused by extravascular infection exhibit a wide array of symptoms and signs referable to the site of infection. Patients are usually immunocompromised. Underlying disease processes include systemic lupus erythematosus, near drowning, Burkitt's lymphoma, meningitis, sinusitis, tonsillitis, pharyngitis, osteomyelitis, and infection from prior intracranial surgery. Intracavernous internal carotid aneurysms associated with cavernous sinus thrombophlebitis cause stereotypical exophthalmos, ophthalmoplegia, and ocular pain.

NATURAL HISTORY

Little information exists regarding the true incidence of infectious aneurysms, and their natural history is uncertain as well. The discrepancy in reported incidence rates between autopsy and clinical series indicates that many infectious aneurysms remain clinically dormant and undiscovered. Dynamic cycles of growth and regression hinder efforts to obtain reliable incidence rates and limit the reliability of clinical prediction. Clinical series confirm these findings. Serial angiographic imaging of infectious aneurysms reveals unpredictable cycles of growth and regression. Ojemann retrospectively reviewed 27 patients who underwent follow-up angiography while being treated medically: 30% of the aneurysms resolved, 19% decreased in size, 15% did not change, and 22% enlarged; 15% of patients demonstrated a new aneurysm.[30] Bohmfalk and coworkers[13] reported similar figures in their review of 25 patients who were treated conservatively and underwent repeat angiography.

Previous reports of infectious intracranial aneurysms indicate that their prognosis is poor. In one study the mortality rate for all bacterial intracranial aneurysms was 32%.[6] Multiple aneurysms do not portend a worse prognosis.[30] The most important prognostic factor for outcome is the presence of hemorrhage. Based on a review by Bohmfalk and colleagues,[13] the mortality rate after rupture of a bacterial intracranial aneurysm is 80%, compared with a mortality rate of 30% without rupture. Many patients who suffer hemorrhage die before reaching the hospital. Of patients presenting to the hospital with evidence of subarachnoid hemorrhage due to an intracranial bacterial aneurysm, 42% die.[13] Intracranial fungal aneurysms have an even worse prognosis, with a mortality rate greater than 90% despite medical or surgical therapy.[6]

DIAGNOSTIC EVALUATION

The diagnosis of an intracranial aneurysm of infectious origin requires a high index of clinical suspicion accompanied by thorough clinical, laboratory, and radiographic examinations. Prompt diagnosis is crucial to the timely institution of appropriate medical and surgical therapy. A thorough history documents cardiac disease and preexisting conditions that predispose to intracranial infection. As in patients with aneurysms of a noninfectious cause, the neurological examination centers on the presence of focal and generalized neurological deficits.

The diagnosis of endocarditis is often suggested by the patient's physical examination. Fever, heart murmur, Roth's spots, and subungual petechiae are all suggestive. Fever associated with a neurological deficit also suggests endocarditis and mandates an evaluation for infection. Blood cultures are crucial because they may confirm the presence of bacteremia or fungemia and identify the pathogen. Normocytic normochromic anemia, microhematuria, and positive serology for rheumatoid factor also corroborate the diagnosis of endocarditis. Echocardiography and transesophageal Doppler ultrasonography confirm the presence of cardiac vegetations in as many as 90% of patients with endocarditis.

Computed tomography (CT) is the most useful initial diagnostic tool for evaluating a patient suspected of harboring an intracranial aneurysm of infectious origin. Rupture of an intracranial infectious aneurysm often causes subarachnoid or intraparenchymal hemorrhage demonstrable on CT. Other findings readily identified by noncontrast CT are infarction, edema, and hydrocephalus. Contrast infusion extends the utility of CT by accentuating the cerebral vasculature and infectious processes, such as abscess. Almost 50% of endocarditis patients with a neurological deficit demonstrate abnormalities on CT. Infarction due to septic embolization is the most common finding.[14] Intracranial hemorrhage in the setting of endocarditis is a strong indication for cerebral angiography. Some authors advocate using cerebral infarction as an indication for angiography because of its association with subsequent aneurysm formation. A normal computed tomographic scan does not preclude the presence of an intracranial aneurysm of infectious origin. When performed on the day of aneurysm rupture, CT identifies 95% of subarachnoid hemorrhages,[39] but if imaging is delayed or the hemorrhage is mild, CT may be normal.

CT–angiography is a relatively new technique that permits imaging of the intracranial vasculature by rapid-sequence CT after a patient is administered a bolus of intravenous contrast medium. CT–angiography is less invasive, quicker, and more cost-efficient than conventional digital subtraction angiography. Furthermore, studies have demonstrated its emerging efficacy in detecting intracranial aneurysms. However, the ability of CT–angiography to identify small or distal intracranial infectious aneurysms is limited. Undoubtedly, further refinement of CT–angiography will increase its utility and efficacy in the diagnosis of intracranial infectious aneurysms.

Magnetic resonance imaging (MRI) and magnetic resonance angiography (MRA) are evolving techniques that have become increasingly useful in the diagnosis of aneurysms. MRI can demonstrate intracranial hemorrhage, edema, and infection. MRA is a blood flow–dependent technique that can illustrate vascular anatomy and identify intracranial aneurysms. Current limitations include the relative insensitivity of MRI to acute intracranial hemorrhage compared with CT, as well as the inability of MRA to identify small, peripherally located aneurysms.[40]

Lumbar puncture is performed to rule out the presence of subarachnoid hemorrhage in patients with normal CT or MRI studies. Cerebrospinal fluid sampling also permits cell count, Gram stain, and culture analysis for possible infection. Cerebrospinal fluid cultures from a large percentage of patients with intracranial aneurysms of infectious origin fail to grow the offending organism.

Digital subtraction angiography is the gold standard for the diagnosis of intracranial aneurysms. Cerebral angiography is warranted in patients with intracranial hemorrhage, infarction, or focal neurological deficit in the setting of endocarditis or suspected intracranial infection. Complete four-vessel angiography must be performed, because the likelihood of multiple aneurysms is high. Attention to distal and proximal cerebral vessels is indicated. Intracranial infectious aneurysms display unpredictable cycles of growth and regression despite appropriate medical therapy. Consequently, serial follow-up angiography is indicated. The inherent risk of angiography has prompted debate about the appropriate timing and duration of follow-up angiography. Frazee and coworkers[41] recommend serial angiography every 7 to 10 days during antibiotic therapy. Alternatively, Morawetz and Karp[34] recommend serial angiography at 6 weeks, 3 months, 6 months, and 1 year after the onset of symptoms. Digital subtraction angiography can be correlated with a less invasive study such as CT–angiography performed contemporaneously. Once correlation has been confirmed, CT–angiography can be performed serially to follow treatment, allowing less frequent follow-up with digital subtraction angiography.

TREATMENT

The prompt initiation of medical and surgical therapy is paramount to avoid the potentially devastating consequences of aneurysmal rupture. Nevertheless, the optimal treatment modality and the timing of surgical intervention are controversial issues.

Cardiac Considerations

Patients with intracranial aneurysms of infectious origin often have compromised cardiac function. The goals of endocarditis therapy are to eradicate microorganisms from cardiac vegetations and to stabilize the patient's hemodynamic status. Occasionally, a patient's cardiac status is so compromised that surgical intervention is warranted. Indications for cardiac surgery in endocarditis are as follows: acute heart failure due to severe valvular regurgitation, bacteremia refractory to appropriate antibiotic therapy, and recurrent septic embolization despite adequate antibiotic therapy. In these situations, cardiac surgery is often performed before the aneurysm is obliterated. The principal neurological concerns during cardiac surgery are perioperative stroke and hemorrhage. In some instances, an intracranial hematoma or abscess mandates emergent evacuation despite severe cardiac dysfunction. In such cases, simultaneous intracranial and cardiac surgery can be considered. However, neurosurgical decompression and aneurysm obliteration are complicated by the heparinization required during cardiac valve replacement. In the absence of acute intracranial hemorrhage or stroke, cardiac valves can be replaced before surgical or medical treatment of an infectious intracranial aneurysm. Intraoperative heparinization during cardiac surgery does not appear to increase the risk of perioperative hemorrhage from an unruptured infectious aneurysm. However, a bioprosthetic rather than synthetic cardiac replacement valve should be used to obviate the need for long-term postoperative anticoagulation.[34]

Medical Therapy

The objectives in treating an intracranial infectious aneurysm are obliteration of the aneurysm and eradication of microorganisms from both the aneurysm and the underlying infectious process. Several authors have demonstrated the efficacy of antimicrobial therapy without surgery, especially in cases of unruptured aneurysms.[5, 17] All patients suspected of harboring an intracranial aneurysm should be promptly started on antibiotic therapy. Antibiotics should be targeted toward the most common infectious organisms—staphylococcal and streptococcal species—until a specific organism is identified by culture. Antibiotic dosages must be adequate to penetrate the blood-brain barrier and should be continued for a minimum of 4 to 6 weeks or until cultures are consistently sterile.

Initially, unruptured aneurysms should be treated conservatively without surgery unless the lesion enlarges during antibiotic therapy or fails to regress after a full course of antibiotics.[7, 26, 30] Additional relative indications for continued conservative, nonsurgical management of ruptured or unruptured intracranial infectious aneurysms include the following: (1) aneurysms arising from the proximal cerebral vessels, (2) aneurysms whose surgical obliteration would result in a serious neurological deficit, (3) aneurysms that regress during antibiotic therapy, and (4) fungal aneurysms.[30] Despite adequate antibiotic therapy, aneurysms of infectious origin may remain the same size, enlarge, or even rupture. Consequently, follow-up angiography is important to monitor intracranial infectious aneurysms during antibiotic treatment.

Surgical and Endovascular Treatment

Indications for surgical intervention include (1) the presence of a significant symptomatic mass such as a hematoma or abscess, (2) a ruptured aneurysm located distally, (3) enlargement of an aneurysm during appropriate antibiotic treatment, (4) failure of an aneurysm to resolve despite a full course of appropriate antibiotic therapy, and (5) neurological deterioration during antibiotic therapy. Surgical manipulation of recently ruptured or newly developed intracranial bacterial or fungal aneurysms is often difficult because both the lesion and the parent vessel are friable and necrotic. Clinical and experimental studies have shown that antimicrobial therapy can induce reparative fibrosis in the walls of aneurysms.[9, 26] Therefore, a short course of antibiotics should be instituted before surgery whenever possible.

When planning surgical repair of an intracranial infectious aneurysm, the surgeon must be prepared to use a variety of techniques and alternative tactics if the planned surgical strategy is unsuccessful. Clipping is not always possible because of the aneurysm's friable nature and adherence to surrounding parenchyma. An alternative technique that is particularly useful for distally located lesions is surgical excision of the aneurysm along with a short segment of the parent vessel. For peripheral aneurysms, the morbidity rate associated with this procedure is usually low. Excision has been combined successfully with revascularization techniques to treat proximal aneurysms.[42] Examples include excision of a proximal middle cerebral artery aneurysm with primary anastomosis of the parent vessel, and excision of a proximal middle cerebral artery aneurysm with a concomitant superficial temporal artery–middle cerebral artery bypass.[35] Similarly, carotid ligation with or without distal revascularization has been successful in the treatment of intracavernous infectious aneurysms.[43]

Multiple intracranial infectious aneurysms are often encountered and can create a surgical dilemma. Some authors recommend an aggressive approach to multiple aneurysms, including elective surgical obliteration of all unilateral aneurysms during one operation when possible or, in the case of bilateral aneurysms, elective obliteration of the largest aneurysm or the one most likely to have bled.[41] Given the equivalent prognosis and hemorrhage rate of patients with multiple and single aneurysms, we recommend identical treatment programs and surgical guidelines for each individual aneurysm. When surgery is indicated for a patient with multiple aneurysms, an attempt should be made to obliterate the lesion most likely to have bled, as well as any easily accessible aneurysms whose obliteration will not unnecessarily increase the risk of surgical complications. Remaining aneurysms should be treated individually based on radiographic and clinical follow-up.

Infectious intracranial aneurysms are often difficult to locate surgically because of their preference for the peripheral vasculature. Stereotaxy may be useful in the intraoperative localization of these lesions. CT and angiographic-guided stereotactic techniques have been used to minimize cortical disruption and vessel dissection during surgical obliteration.[44, 45] Frameless MRI or MRA stereotaxy may likewise prove useful in the management of these lesions.

Endovascular obliteration is a recently developed treatment for infectious intracranial aneurysms.[46, 47] Intravascular embolization may be suitable for lesions that require treatment but pose an unacceptable surgical risk. Reports have demonstrated the safety and efficacy of these methods in the treatment of intracranial infectious aneurysms.[46, 47] The same authors, however, note that the fragile nature of these aneurysms and the surrounding vasculature may increase the risk associated with endovascular procedures.[47]

OUTCOME AFTER TREATMENT

The paucity of large series of intracranial infectious aneurysms has led to a retrospective meta-analysis of smaller series to assess outcomes. In Ojemann's analysis of cases reported through 1980, a 42% mortality rate was associated with antibiotic treatment alone, whereas the mortality rate associated with antibiotics and surgery was 19%.[30] A patient selection bias influences these rates, in that the most critically ill patients are often deemed unfit for surgery. Outcomes after surgery are significantly better when the operation is performed electively (5% mortality rate) rather than emergently (52% mortality rate).

Fungal aneurysms bear a poorer prognosis, with a mortality rate of 90% despite medical or surgical therapy.[6] Conversely, infectious aneurysms of the intracavernous carotid artery respond well to conservative or surgical treatment. Only one death and one poor outcome were reported in a retrospective review of 18 patients.[43]

CONCLUSION

Intracranial infectious aneurysms are rare lesions that usually develop in the setting of endocarditis. Their natural history is unpredictable. An aggressive approach consisting of organism-directed antibiotic therapy, serial angiographic monitoring, and, when these fail, surgical intervention is indicated.

REFERENCES

1. Church WS: Aneurysm of the right cerebral artery in a boy of thirteen. Trans Pathol Soc Lond 20:109–110, 1869.
2. Osler W: Gulstonian lectures on malignant endocarditis. Lancet 1:415–418, 459–464, 505–508, 1885.
3. Eppinger H: Pathogenesis (Histogenesis und Aetiologie) der Aneurysmen einschliesslich des Aneurysma equi verminosum. Arch Klin Chir 35:1–553, 1887.
4. Stengel A, Wolforth CC: Mycotic (bacterial) aneurysms of intravascular origin. Arch Intern Med 31:527–554, 1923.
5. Ojemann RG: Infectious intracranial aneurysms. In Ojemann RG, Ogilvy CS, Crowell RM, Heros RC (eds): Surgical Management of Neurovascular Disease. Baltimore, Williams & Wilkins, 1995, pp 369–376.
6. Kojima Y, Saito A, Kim I: The role of serial angiography in the management of bacterial and fungal intracranial aneurysms —report of two cases and review of the literature. Neurol Med Chir (Tokyo) 29:202–216, 1989.
7. Baldwin HZ, Zabramski JM, Spetzler RF: Infectious intracranial aneurysms. In Carter LP, Spetzler RF, Hamilton MG (eds): Neurovascular Surgery. New York, McGraw-Hill, 1995, pp 777–788.
8. Roach MR, Drake CG: Ruptured cerebral aneurysms caused by micro-organisms. N Engl J Med 273:240–244, 1965.
9. Cantu RC, LeMay M, Wilkinson HA: The importance of repeated angiography in the treatment of mycotic-embolic intracranial aneurysms. J Neurosurg 25:189–193, 1966.
10. McDonald CA, Korb M: Intracranial aneurysms. Arch Neurol Psychiatry 42:298–328, 1939.
11. Lee KS, Liu SS, Spetzler RF, et al: Intracranial mycotic aneurysm in an infant: Report of a case. Neurosurgery 26:129–133, 1990.
12. Fearnsides EG: Intracranial aneurysms. Brain 39:224, 1916.
13. Bohmfalk GL, Story JL, Wissinger JP, et al: Bacterial intracranial aneurysm. J Neurosurg 48:369–382, 1978.
14. Tunkel AR, Kaye D: Neurological complications of infective endocarditis. Neurol Clin 11:419–440, 1993.
15. Hart RG, Kagan-Hallet K, Joerns SE: Mechanisms of intracranial hemorrhage in infective endocarditis. Stroke 18:1048–1056, 1987.
16. Lerner PI: Neurological complications of infective endocarditis. Med Clin North Am 69:385–398, 1985.
17. Bingham WF: Treatment of mycotic intracranial aneurysms. J Neurosurg 46:428–437, 1977.
18. Morriss FH Jr, Spock A: Intracranial aneurysm secondary to mycotic orbital and sinus infection: Report of a case implicating *Penicillium* as an opportunistic fungus. Am J Dis Child 119: 357–362, 1970.
19. Ojemann RG, New PF, Fleming TC: Intracranial aneurysms associated with bacterial meningitis. Neurology 16:1222–1226, 1966.
20. Shibuya S, Igarashi S, Amo T, et al: Mycotic aneurysms of the internal carotid artery: Case report. J Neurosurg 44:105–108, 1976.
21. Suwanwela C, Suwanwela N, Charuchinda S, et al: Intracranial mycotic aneurysms of extravascular origin. J Neurosurg 36:552–559, 1972.
22. Tomita T, McLone DG, Naidich TP: Mycotic aneurysm of the intracavernous portion of the carotid artery in childhood: Case report. J Neurosurg 54:681–684, 1981.
23. Weisman AD: Cavernous-sinus thrombophlebitis: Report of a case with multiple cerebral infarcts and necrosis of the pituitary body. N Engl J Med 231:118–122, 1944.
24. Clare CE, Barrow DL: Infectious intracranial aneurysms. Neurosurg Clin N Am 3:551–566, 1992.
25. Mielke B, Weir B, Oldring D, et al: Fungal aneurysm: Case report and review of the literature. Neurosurgery 9:578–582, 1981.
26. Barrow DL, Prats AR: Infectious intracranial aneurysms: Comparison of groups with and without endocarditis. Neurosurgery 27:562–573, 1990.
27. Kikuchi K, Watanabe K, Sugawara A, et al: Multiple fungal aneurysms: Report of a rare case implicating steroid as predisposing factor. Surg Neurol 24:253–259, 1985.
28. Takeda S, Wakabayashi K, Yamazaki K, et al: Intracranial fungal aneurysm caused by *Candida* endocarditis. Clin Neuropathol 17: 199–203, 1998.
29. Gacs G, Merei FT, Bodosi M: Balloon catheter as a model of cerebral emboli in humans. Stroke 13:39–42, 1982.
30. Ojemann RG: Surgical management of bacterial intracranial aneurysms. In Schmidek HH, Sweet WH (eds): Operative Neurosurgical Techniques. New York, Grune & Stratton, 1988, pp 997–1001.
31. Nakata Y, Shionoya S, Kamiya K: Pathogenesis of mycotic aneurysm. Angiology 19:593–601, 1968.
32. Molinari GF, Smith L, Goldstein MN, et al: Pathogenesis of cerebral mycotic aneurysms. Neurology 23:325–332, 1973.
33. Pootrakul A, Carter LP: Bacterial intracranial aneurysm: Importance of sequential angiography. Surg Neurol 17:429–431, 1982.
34. Morawetz RB, Karp RB: Evolution and resolution of intracranial bacterial (mycotic) aneurysms. Neurosurgery 15:43–49, 1984.
35. Hadley MN, Spetzler RF, Martin NA, et al: Middle cerebral artery aneurysm due to *Nocardia asteroides*: Case report of aneurysm excision and extracranial-intracranial bypass. Neurosurgery 22: 923–928, 1988.
36. Hadley MN, Martin NA, Spetzler RF, et al: Multiple intracranial aneurysms due to *Coccidioides immitis* infection: Case report. J Neurosurg 66:453–456, 1987.
37. Kurino M, Kuratsu J, Yamaguchi T, et al: Mycotic aneurysm accompanied by aspergillotic granuloma: A case report. Surg Neurol 42:160–164, 1994.
38. Salgado AV, Furlan AJ, Keys TF: Mycotic aneurysm, subarachnoid hemorrhage, and indications for cerebral angiography in infective endocarditis. Stroke 18:1057–1060, 1987.
39. Adams HP Jr, Kassell NF, Torner JC, et al: Predicting cerebral ischemia after aneurysmal subarachnoid hemorrhage: Influences of clinical condition, CT results, and antifibrinolytic therapy. A report of the Cooperative Aneurysm Study. Neurology 37: 1586–1591, 1987.
40. Ahmadi J, Tung H, Giannotta SL, et al: Monitoring of infectious intracranial aneurysms by sequential computed tomographic/magnetic resonance imaging studies. Neurosurgery 32:45–50, 1993.
41. Frazee JG, Cahan LD, Winter J: Bacterial intracranial aneurysms. J Neurosurg 53:633–641, 1980.
42. Day AL: Extracranial-intracranial bypass grafting in the surgical treatment of bacterial aneurysms: Report of two cases. Neurosurgery 9:583–588, 1981.
43. Rout D, Sharma A, Mohan PK, et al: Bacterial aneurysms of the intracavernous carotid artery. J Neurosurg 60:1236–1242, 1984.
44. Elowiz EH, Johnson WD, Milhorat TH: Computerized tomography (CT) localized stereotactic craniotomy for excision of a bacterial intracranial aneurysm. Surg Neurol 44:265–269, 1995.
45. Steinberg GK, Guppy KH, Adler JR, et al: Stereotactic, angiography-guided clipping of a distal, mycotic intracranial aneurysm using the Cosman-Roberts-Wells system: Technical note. Neurosurgery 30:408–411, 1992.
46. Khayata MH, Aymard A, Casasco A, et al: Selective endovascular techniques in the treatment of cerebral mycotic aneurysms: Report of three cases. J Neurosurg 78:661–665, 1993.
47. Frizzell RT, Vitek JJ, Hill DL, et al: Treatment of a bacterial (mycotic) intracranial aneurysm using an endovascular approach. Neurosurgery 32:852–854, 1993.

CHAPTER **123**

Revascularization Techniques for Complex Aneurysms and Skull Base Tumors

NEIL A. MARTIN ■ INAM KURESHI ■ DOMINGOS COITEIRO

In 1967, Donaghy and Yasargil[1] introduced the technique of intracranial arterial bypass after extensive experimental work. Initially, extracranial-intracranial (EC-IC) bypass was envisioned as a surgical strategy for preventing stroke in patients with carotid and intracranial arterial occlusion, but the results of the EC-IC Bypass Study Group[2] failed to establish that the procedure reduced the risk of stroke. Nevertheless, when combined with parent artery occlusion, this procedure plays a key role in the management of unclippable complex aneurysms and cranial base tumors involving the major cerebral arteries. Sundt and colleagues,[3] Ausman and coworkers,[4] Ito,[5] Peerless and Hampf,[6] Lawton and colleagues,[7] Sen and Sekhar,[8] and others pioneered and refined surgical revascularization techniques for the treatment of aneurysms and tumors.

WHEN IS A BYPASS NECESSARY WITH PARENT ARTERY OCCLUSION?

In which patients does the cerebral collateral circulation permit occlusion of major intracranial arteries without causing cerebral ischemia? This question most often arises when occlusion of the internal carotid artery (ICA) is planned as a component of surgical treatment for intracavernous aneurysms or for head and neck or skull base tumors that involve this artery. Elective occlusion or resection of the ICA has been associated with complications in 30% to 45% of cases, but experience with carotid test occlusion suggests that 80% to 90% of patients tolerate ICA occlusion (at least acutely).[9, 10] Many clinicians advocate a *selective approach* to surgical revascularization when therapeutic ICA occlusion is planned.[11] This approach involves angiographic evaluation of the competence of the circle of Willis and balloon test occlusion coupled with measurement of cerebral blood flow or a hypotensive challenge to identify patients with inadequate or marginal collateral circulation who require bypass in conjunction with parent artery occlusion. Others argue for a *universal approach*, calling for a bypass in all patients who undergo ICA occlusion.[7] This strategy is intended to avoid the risk of the balloon test occlusion itself, to minimize the risk of delayed or chronic cerebral ischemia, and to avoid inducing new aneurysms on collateral vessels. Given the safety of balloon test occlusion using contemporary endovascular technique, however, most centers reserve the use of bypass for patients with demonstrably insufficient or marginal collateral circulation in the ICA territory.[10, 12, 13]

Vertebral artery occlusion may be required to treat unclippable posterior circulation aneurysms. Typically, unilateral vertebral artery occlusion is well tolerated when the contralateral vertebral artery is not hypoplastic and does not terminate in the posterior inferior cerebellar artery (PICA). Bilateral vertebral artery or basilar artery occlusion is associated with a much higher risk of ischemia and should be considered only if blood flow through both posterior communicating arteries is sufficient (>1 mm).[14]

Occlusion of proximal major arterial branches, such as the middle cerebral artery (MCA), PICA, or anterior inferior cerebellar artery (AICA), is associated with a substantial risk of ischemia. Branch artery revascularization should be considered when these vessels must be occluded. The posterior cerebral artery appears to have relatively good collateral potential, however, from leptomeningeal interconnections with the distal temporal and occipital MCA branches. Proximal occlusion of this artery for giant or fusiform aneurysms usually is well tolerated; only a few cases develop an ischemic deficit (hemianopsia).[15]

Revascularization for the Treatment of Aneurysms

Intracranial aneurysms optimally are treated by surgical clipping. Clipping giant or fusiform aneurysms, which may incorporate the parent artery or adjacent arterial branches into the aneurysm base, may be impossible, however.[3, 4, 6, 7, 14–19] Calcification or atherosclerotic thickening can make clipping hazardous or impossible. Aneurysms that have recurred after coil embolization may be unclippable because of the stenting effect of coils near the aneurysm base.[20] Such aneurysms can be treated by proximal arterial (hunterian) ligation to induce aneurysmal thrombosis or by trapping (proximal and distal occlusion) to isolate the aneurysm completely. Both techniques interrupt the normal pattern of the cerebral circulation and carry the risk of cerebral hypoperfusion. If collateral circulation is inadequate, arterial bypass is required to avoid cerebral ischemia from proximal occlusion or trapping.

Hypothermic circulatory arrest first was used as a surgical adjunct for difficult giant intracranial aneurysms in the 1960s and was refined dramatically in the 1980s.[21–24] Hypothermic circulatory arrest has been a particularly useful strategy for managing giant posterior circulation aneurysms by allowing the aneurysm to collapse, then reconstructing the neck with clips. Hypothermic circulatory arrest is a complex procedure, however, with its own risks.[22, 23] Even with profound hypothermia, it may be impossible to reconstruct the aneurysm satisfactorily and to preserve the parent artery. Parent artery occlusion and distal bypass often may be a superior alternative.

Revascularization for the Treatment of Skull Base Tumors

The petrous and cavernous portions of the ICA can be involved with anterior skull base or lateral skull base tumors. Because most anterior skull base tumors, such as meningiomas, schwannomas, pituitary adenomas, angiofibromas, or chordomas, are benign, the carotid artery is more likely to be encased than frankly invaded.[25] Meningiomas, particularly recurrent meningiomas, can be so densely adherent to the carotid artery, however, that total resection is impossible unless the involved carotid artery is resected along with the neoplasm. Malignant skull base tumors are substantially more likely to invade the carotid artery wall than benign tumors. In such cases, carotid artery occlusion and resection, with or without revascularization, may be required for radical oncologic surgical resection.[26]

The issue whether to occlude and resect the carotid artery to maximize tumor removal for benign and malignant tumors is controversial. In the case of skull base or cavernous sinus meningiomas, some surgeons argue for aggressive tumor resection with preservation of the carotid artery. Others advocate resection of the ICA when the tumor is densely adherent. Representative contemporary surgical series with and without carotid preservation show only small differences, however, in the rates of gross total resection or recurrence.[8, 27]

The availability of stereotactic radiosurgery to control residual tumor further argues against sacrificing the carotid artery during the treatment of benign lesions. There is a developing consensus that the carotid artery should not be resected in most nonmalignant tumors.[25, 27] In a review of ICA sacrifice for the resection of skull base tumors, Lawton and Spetzler[25] indicated that they sacrificed the ICA and performed revascularization in only 10 of more than 300 anterior skull base tumors.

The poor prognosis of most head and neck cancers that involve the anterior skull base and carotid artery has prompted some surgeons to consider radical tumor resection with removal of the involved segment of the carotid artery.[8, 26] Angiographic evaluation and balloon test occlusion (with or without provocative testing or cerebral blood flow measurements) may identify patients who can tolerate carotid artery sacrifice. The rate of morbidity related to carotid artery sacrifice during skull base tumor surgery (and the modest but significant rate of morbidity associated with balloon test occlusion alone) suggests, however, that carotid revascularization should be considered when resection of the carotid artery is essential to achieve an oncologically meaningful resection.[26]

A revascularization procedure may be performed as a preliminary, separate surgical stage before tumor and carotid artery resection or as one step in a single definitive operation. The type of revascularization may involve replacing the carotid artery with an interposition saphenous vein graft (type I), with a saphenous vein graft between the extracranial carotid artery and MCA (type II), or with a superficial temporal artery (STA)–to–MCA anastomosis (type III) (Fig. 123–1).

All series of cerebral revascularization associated with carotid artery sacrifice for the treatment of skull base tumors have reported complications associated with the bypass procedures,[7, 8] particularly procedures that involve a saphenous vein graft. The rate of ischemic complications and graft occlusion typically exceeds 10% in these cases. It is unclear whether aggressive carotid artery resection results in a meaningful improvement in the control of malignant tumors. In some cases, however, it may be reasonable to consider carotid artery resection and revascularization when the carotid artery is the only structure that stands in the way of a potentially curative tumor resection. Carotid occlusion and bypass would be indicated most strongly in patients whose carotid artery has ruptured (or appears impending) secondary to tumor invasion, radionecrosis, or surgical arterial injury.

SURGICAL TECHNIQUE

Preoperative Planning and Preparation for Bypass Procedures

Preoperative imaging studies must be planned to define thoroughly the optimal site of arterial occlusion, the collateral circulation, and the size and location of the intended bypass recipient and donor vessels. Carotid artery compression during the angiographic study optimally shows the integrity of the circle of Willis.[14, 17]

Typically, patients are given standard perioperative steroids and anticonvulsants when a cerebral hemisphere is to be exposed or retracted. Preoperatively, all patients are given aspirin (325 mg daily) to minimize the risk of postoperative thrombosis and occlusion at the anastomotic site.

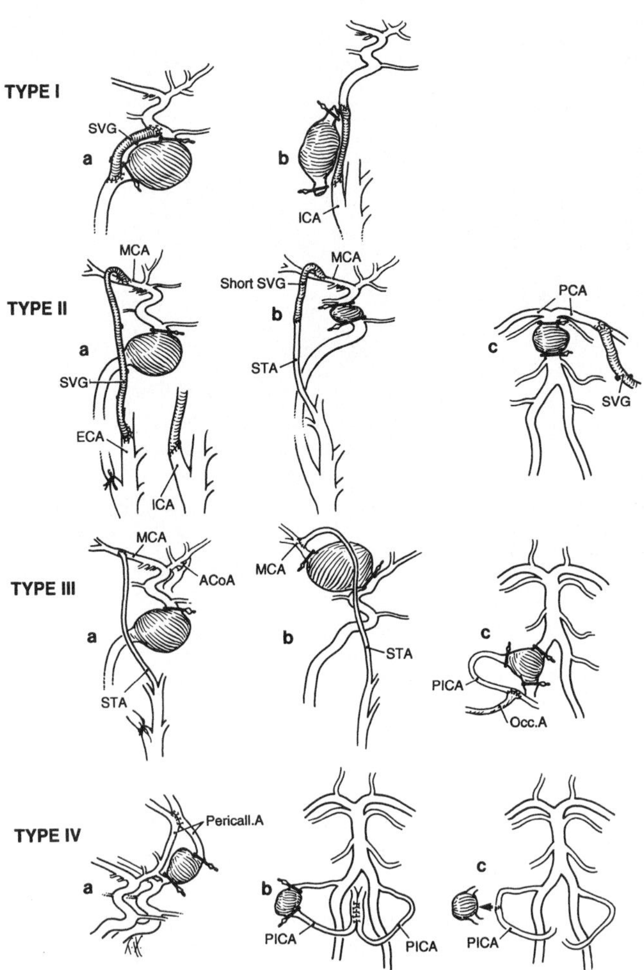

FIGURE 123–1. Types of arterial bypasses. *Type I:* Saphenous vein interposition graft for carotid artery replacement. *Type II:* Saphenous vein bypass graft from the extracranial carotid artery to the middle (*a* and *b*) or posterior (*c*) cerebral artery. *Type III:* Superficial temporal (*a* or *b*) or occipital (*c*) artery bypass to intracranial arterial branch. *Type IV:* Anastomosis of one intracranial artery to an adjacent intracranial artery (*a* and *b*) or primary reanastomosis (*c*) after aneurysm excision. (From Martin NA: Arterial bypass for the treatment of giant and fusiform intracranial aneurysms. Tech Neurosurg 4:153–178, 1998.)

Intraoperative Monitoring and Management

Electroencephalographic activity and evoked potentials are monitored in every case. The electroencephalogram is used to monitor burst suppression during the infusion of metabolic suppressive agents (e.g., barbiturates, etomidate, or propofol). Evoked potential monitoring reflects the activity of the sensory cortex and subcortical and brainstem pathways during bypass procedures.

The patient is allowed to become mildly hypothermic (32°C to 34°C).[28] Metabolic suppressive therapy provides cerebral protection during the period of cerebral artery occlusion during the bypass anastomosis.[28] We typically use thiopental rather than propofol or etomidate. The efficacy of barbiturates for cerebral protection during transient focal ischemia is supported strongly by laboratory and clinical evidence.[7, 28, 29] The barbiturates are administered until the anastomosis is complete, and the recipient vessels are deoccluded.

We do not use systemic heparinization during bypass procedures. The combination of preoperative aspirin, mild hypothermia, and systemic heparin administration causes a problematic degree of intraoperative and postoperative coagulopathy. The bypass vessel simply is flushed with heparinized saline.

Types of Revascularization Procedures

Strategies for cerebral revascularization after parent artery occlusion (see Fig. 123–1) include the use of various vessels as the bypass conduit (e.g., STA, occipital artery, or long or short saphenous vein) and the selection of various arterial sites for the distal anastomosis. These variations can be classified into four types of bypass.[30] A type I bypass involves an interposition graft from the parent artery proximal to the site of occlusion immediately distal to the parent artery (Figs. 123–2 and 123–3). The primary example of this type of revascularization is the purely intracranial petrous carotid–to–supraclinoid carotid saphenous vein interposition graft. It is used primarily to reconstruct the carotid artery when it must be resected to remove skull base tumors and to treat giant intracavernous carotid aneurysms.[8, 31–33] This graft has the disadvantages of

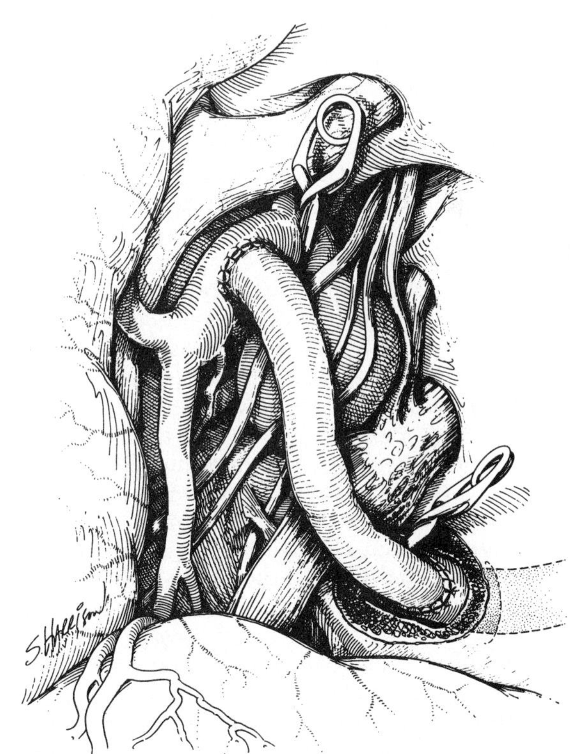

FIGURE 123–2. A petrous-to-supraclinoid carotid skull base bypass showing a saphenous interposition graft from the petrous segment of the carotid artery (exposed by drilling the middle cranial fossa floor) to the supraclinoid carotid artery (in this case for treatment of an intracavernous aneurysm). (From Spetzler RF, Fukushima T, Martin NA, et al: Petrous carotid-to-intradural carotid saphenous vein graft for intracavernous giant aneurysm, tumor, and occlusive disease. J Neurosurg 73:496–501, 1990.)

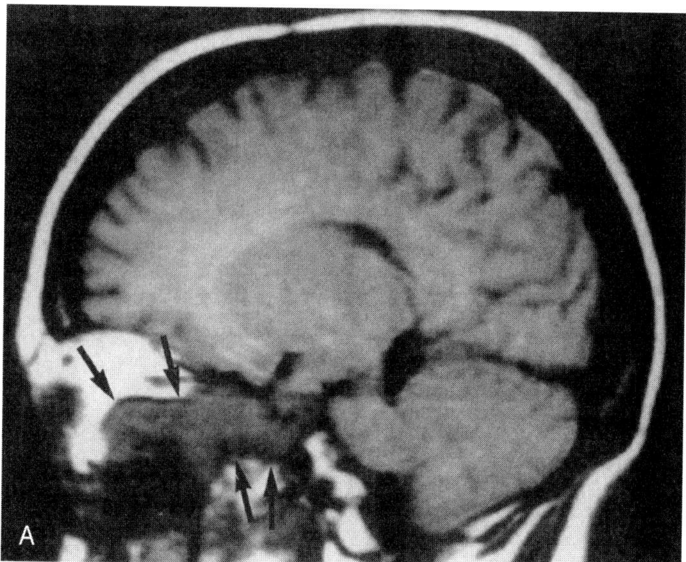

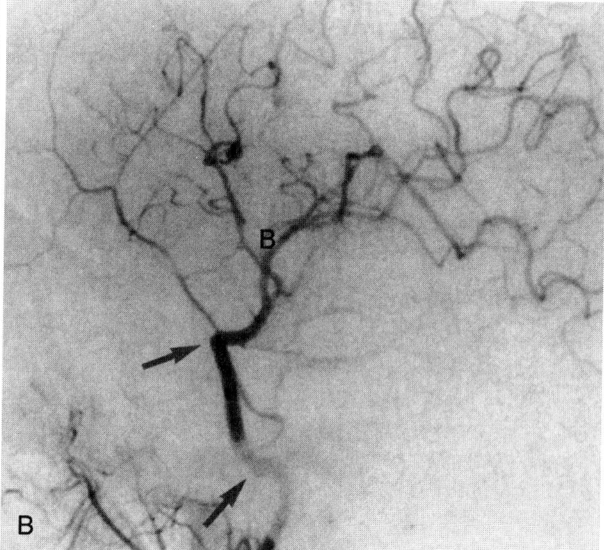

FIGURE 123–3. Type I bypass for intracavernous tumor. *A*, Preoperative magnetic resonance image shows squamous cell carcinoma involving the orbit and cavernous sinus *(arrows)*. *B*, Carotid angiogram after resection of the orbital and cavernous sinus contents (including the involved carotid artery) shows a type I saphenous vein graft *(between arrows)* from the petrous to the supraclinoid carotid artery. (From Spetzler RF, Fukushima T, Martin NA, et al: Petrous carotid-to-intradural carotid saphenous vein graft for intracavernous giant aneurysm, tumor, and occlusive disease. J Neurosurg 73:496–501, 1990.)

being technically complex and, most important, requires a prolonged period of ICA occlusion. It is associated with a significant complication rate related to graft occlusion and perioperative ischemic brain damage.[7, 8] The procedure is difficult and lengthy, and occlusion of the carotid artery is prolonged. A comprehensive description of this procedure is not included because we prefer to use a type II procedure for this operation. Readers are referred to technical descriptions elsewhere.[32, 33]

A type II bypass consists of a saphenous vein interposition graft between the extracranial carotid artery and a major intracranial branch vessel (Figs. 123–4 and 123–5).[34] This procedure is employed when a major arterial trunk must be occluded to treat a tumor or giant aneurysm, and the distal-collateral circulation is grossly inadequate (evidenced by the absence of communicating arteries seen angiographically or by the rapid onset of a deficit during balloon test occlusion).[3, 7] In such cases, the bypass must replace all of the circulation to a major arterial territory. A large conduit is needed. The normal blood flow of the MCA is about 250 mL/minute to the cerebral hemisphere; the blood flow of the posterior cerebral artery is only moderately less. Although the average STA graft provides blood flow of only 10 to 70 mL/minute, blood flow through a saphenous vein graft typically ranges from 50 to 150 mL/minute. The blood flow through the saphenous vein graft is high enough to support the circulation in an entire major arterial territory at a level well above the ischemic threshold (particularly when added to the variable contribution through leptomeningeal collateral vessels). A type II bypass can be a substitute for an STA-MCA bypass when the scalp artery is hypoplastic, diseased, or occluded.

EXTRACRANIAL CAROTID ARTERY–TO–MIDDLE CEREBRAL ARTERY SAPHENOUS VEIN INTERPOSITION GRAFT

The saphenous vein graft typically is connected end-to-end to the proximal stump of the ICA or end-to-side to the external carotid artery (ECA) (Figs. 123–4 and 123–5). For the distal anastomosis, we prefer a larger, more proximal MCA branch (M2 or M3 segment) in the sylvian fissure. These vessels better match the size of the saphenous vein and provide a more direct conduit to the entire MCA territory.

After the carotid bifurcation is exposed and a pterional craniotomy opened, the sylvian fissure is opened widely. The ideal M2 or M3 arterial recipient site, free of perforating vessels, is exposed. Next, the saphenous vein is exposed and isolated but left in situ in continuity until just before it is used for the bypass. Meticulous care is exerted while exposing the vein to avoid trauma that might cause the bypass to thrombose.[35–37] Before excision, the alignment of the vein should be marked with a 6–0 Prolene suture (Ethicon, Johnson & Johnson Professionals, Inc, Somerville, NJ) through the adventitia to define the proper orientation of the vein. This maneuver avoids twisting the vein as it is positioned for the bypass. The vein is ligated proximally and distally, excised, and flushed without overdistention with cool, heparinized saline.

The vein graft then is passed from the cervical incision to the cranial incision through a large chest tube. The orientation of the vein is observed carefully to keep it from twisting as it is passed through the chest tube. The tube is pulled from the subcutaneous tunnel, leaving the vein in place. The graft is filled with cool, heparinized saline and occluded proximally and distally with temporary clips.

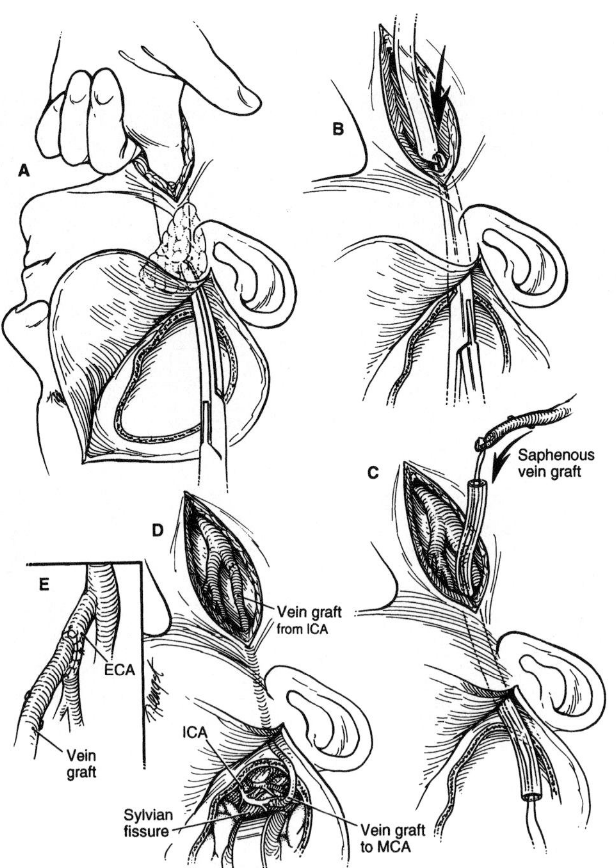

FIGURE 123–4. Extracranial carotid artery–to–middle cerebral artery (MCA) saphenous vein bypass graft. *A*, A clamp is passed from the cranial incision behind the root of the zygomatic arch to the cervical incision. *B*, A chest tube is pulled from the cervical incision to the cranial incision. *C*, The harvested saphenous vein graft is passed through the chest tube, which is removed leaving the graft in its subcutaneous tunnel. *D*, The completed bypass after end-to-end anastomosis to the internal carotid artery and end-to-side anastomosis to the MCA. *E*, Alternative technique showing end-to-side anastomosis to the external carotid artery. (From Martin NA: Arterial bypass for the treatment of giant and fusiform intracranial aneurysms. Tech Neurosurg 4:153–178, 1998.)

As suggested by Sundt and associates,[3] the intracranial anastomosis is performed first. This sequence allows the surgeon to take advantage of slack in the graft, which can be manipulated freely while the back and front walls of the anastomosis are sutured. The terminal 7- to 8-mm portion of the vein graft is trimmed of loose adventitia, and the end is beveled to create an orifice 5 to 6 mm in diameter. After barbiturates are administered and blood pressure is stabilized, a 10- to 15-mm length of MCA is occluded between temporary clips. A linear arteriotomy is matched to the diameter of the vein graft orifice. The vein graft is fixed to the MCA branch using 8–0 monofilament nylon sutures, which are used to complete a running closure. After the anastomosis is completed, blood flow is restored, and the barbiturates can be stopped.

The vein graft is pulled gently into the cervical incision to remove slack and redundancy. The proximal anastomosis can be constructed end-to-end to the ICA or end-to-side to the ECA. The vein-carotid anastomosis is completed with 6–0 Prolene sutures. If the proximal and distal anastomoses are widely patent, a bounding pulse should be visible and palpable in the vein graft. If there is any doubt about the integrity of the graft, intraoperative angiography should be considered.

The craniotomy is closed with care to avoid compromising the vein graft with dura or temporalis muscle. A notch for the graft is cut in the bone flap. The cervical incision is closed in routine fashion. A short vein graft can be placed between the STA trunk (exposed at the zygomatic arch) and a proximal M2 or M3 branch of the MCA.[38] This procedure is useful when only a short segment of saphenous vein is available or when the cervical carotid artery cannot be used as the site of the proximal anastomosis.

EXTERNAL CAROTID ARTERY–TO–POSTERIOR CEREBRAL ARTERY SAPHENOUS VEIN INTERPOSITION GRAFT

The ECA–to–posterior cerebral artery saphenous vein interposition graft is used when the basilar artery or bilateral vertebral arteries are occluded to treat an unclippable basilar artery aneurysm.[3, 19] Bypass is necessary when collateral circulation through the posterior communicating arteries is inadequate.[14] Because of its difficulty and the substantial associated risks, this procedure is considered only for unclippable basilar aneurysms associated with subarachnoid hemorrhage or intractable progressive symptoms related to mass effect.

The subtemporal approach is used to expose the posterior cerebral artery. Cerebrospinal fluid is drained through a lumbar subarachnoid catheter to relax the brain enough to evaluate the temporal lobe safely. The posterior cerebral artery is dissected from the arachnoid as it passes around the lateral surface of the cerebral peduncle. The proximal 20 to 25 mm of the P2 segment are isolated, and a segment free of brainstem-perforating vessels is chosen for the anastomosis.

The cervical carotid artery is exposed, and the vein graft is tunneled just as the grafts are for the carotid-to-MCA procedure. After barbiturates are administered, the posterior cerebral artery is occluded proximally and distally with temporary aneurysm clips. After the posterior cerebral artery is arteriotomized, the tip and base of the beveled orifice of the saphenous vein are fixed to the posterior cerebral artery using 8–0 monofilament nylon sutures. The front and back wall closures usually are completed with a running suture. Closure of the lateral or front wall of the anastomosis is facilitated by bringing the vein under the blade of the self-retaining retractor on the temporal lobe.

After the intracranial anastomosis is completed, an end-to-side anastomosis is fashioned to the ECA. Sundt and coworkers[3] observed that a large percentage of patients develop subdural hygromas after this procedure. Sundt and coworkers[3] suggested routinely placing a subtemporal subdural-peritoneal (or atrial) shunt to avoid this complication.

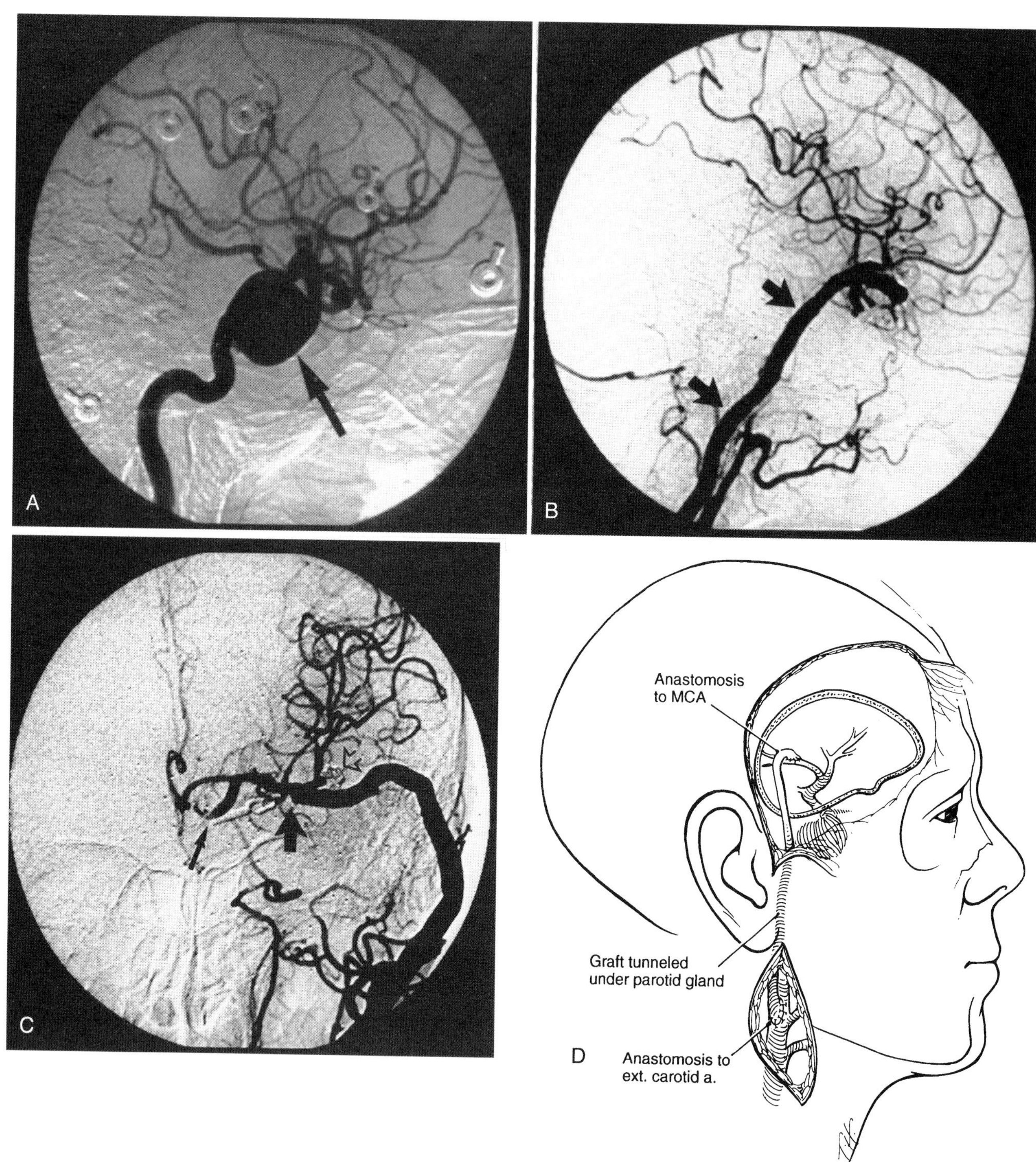

FIGURE 123–5. Giant intracavernous carotid aneurysm. *A*, Lateral carotid angiogram shows intracavernous aneurysm *(arrow)*. *B*, After the surgical procedure, the lateral carotid angiogram shows occlusion of the internal carotid artery (ICA) and filling of the intracranial circulation to the external carotid–to–middle cerebral artery (MCA) saphenous vein graft *(arrows)*. *C*, Anteroposterior postoperative arteriogram shows end-to-side anastomosis between the vein graft and the proximal MCA *(large black arrow)*, the site of intracranial occlusion of the ICA *(small arrow)*, and clip on second small MCA aneurysm *(open arrow)*. *D*, Illustration of completed bypass. (From Martin NA: Arterial bypass for the treatment of giant and fusiform intracranial aneurysms. Tech Neurosurg 4:153–178, 1998.)

A type III bypass uses a scalp artery as the donor vessel.[4, 6, 39, 40] This procedure is used when a giant aneurysm requires occlusion of a single, crucial arterial branch or when carotid occlusion is required (for an aneurysm or tumor) and the circle of Willis is only marginally inadequate.[41–43] Because the arterial territory at risk is smaller, a lower flow bypass is required than in the case of the type II procedure. The STA or occipital artery can be used for the bypass.

SUPERFICIAL TEMPORAL ARTERY–TO–MIDDLE CEREBRAL ARTERY BYPASS

The STA branches are identified with a Doppler probe and marked on the scalp (Figs. 123–6 and 123–7). The largest temporal artery branch, as identified on the preoperative angiogram, is selected as the donor vessel. After a linear incision is made over the artery distally, spreading with a small curved hemostat permits the STA, which is located just superficial to the galea, to be identified. The artery is exposed to the zygomatic arch, separated from the adjacent subcutaneous tissue with an adventitial cuff, and left in continuity until detached for the anastomosis.

If the parietal branch of the STA is used, the cutdown incision over this vessel can be used for the craniotomy. The craniotomy is centered 6 cm above the external auditory meatus (Chater's point), where several large MCA branches emerge from the distal sylvian fissure. If the frontal branch of the STA is selected, a second, vertically oriented incision above the ear is required over Chater's point. The two incisions are unconnected, but the frontal branch of the STA can be tunneled from one to the other in the subgaleal plane.

Anterior and posterior temporal muscle flaps are developed, and a small oval craniotomy flap is made. A larger (e.g., pterional) craniotomy may be used to expose the aneurysm. After the dura is opened, and an appropriate recipient artery ($\geq$1.0 mm in diameter) is selected, the arachnoid over this vessel is opened, and a 10-mm length of the vessel is prepared. The anesthesiologist administers barbiturates, while the distal end of the STA is prepared for the bypass. The STA is occluded. The vessel is divided distally and flushed with heparinized saline. The orifice of the STA is beveled to fit a 3- to 4-mm arteriotomy.

The MCA branch is occluded proximally and distally with small, low-pressure clips, and a 3- to 4-mm linear arteriotomy is made. The proximal and distal ends of the STA orifice are fixed in place with 9–0 or 10–0 monofilament nylon sutures, and the anastomosis is completed with about six 10–0 sutures on the front and back walls. The dura is reapproximated loosely, the bone flap is trimmed to leave an opening for the bypass vessel, and the temporalis muscle is closed loosely. The scalp is closed carefully to insure a watertight closure.

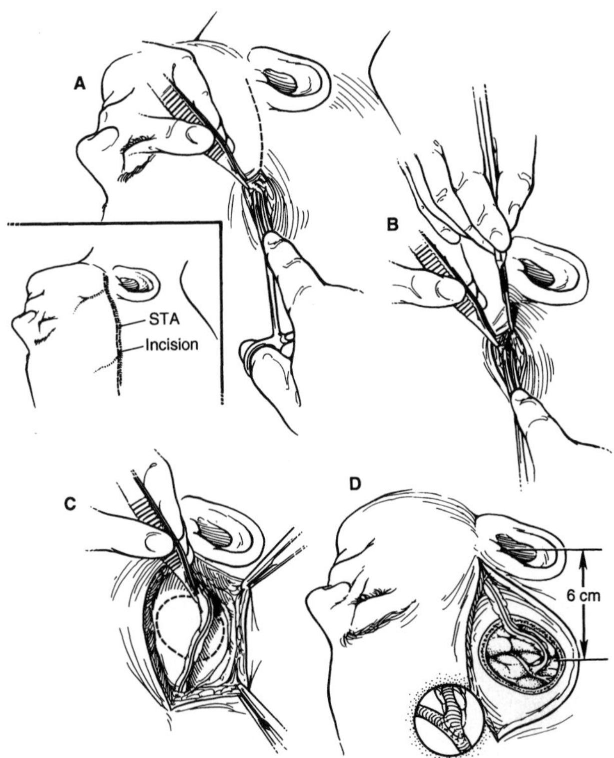

FIGURE 123–6. Superficial temporal artery (STA)–to–middle cerebral artery (MCA) bypass. *A*, After Doppler identification of the STA, a linear incision is made over its distal aspect. *B*, The STA is exposed by cutdown technique. *C*, After the temporalis muscle is incised, an oval or circular craniotomy is made over the posterior aspect of the sylvian fissure. *D*, The completed anastomosis is shown. (From Martin NA: Arterial bypass for the treatment of giant and fusiform intracranial aneurysms. Tech Neurosurg 4: 153–178, 1998.)

OCCIPITAL ARTERY–TO–POSTERIOR INFERIOR CEREBELLAR ARTERY BYPASS

The patient is placed in the lateral position with the operative side up (Figs. 123–8 and 123–9). The head is fixed in moderate flexion. The course of the occipital artery is identified with the Doppler probe. A hockey-stick incision, with the transverse limb located 2 cm above the superior nuchal line, is made. The occipital artery is dissected from the subcutaneous tissue and suboccipital musculature. The vessel is left in continuity until just before it is required for the anastomosis. The occiput, the arch of C1, and the laminae of C2 are exposed. To provide access to the caudal loop of the PICA, the craniotomy is extended from just beyond the midline almost to the region of the occipital condyle. If the vertebral artery is to be exposed intradurally, for instance, for trapping a fusiform aneurysm of the vertebral artery, the craniotomy is extended into a far-lateral transcondylar exposure. It often is helpful to remove the posterior arch of C1 unilaterally. After the dura is opened, PICA ordinarily can be mobilized by carefully dividing numerous small arachnoid fibers that fix it to the dorsal surface of the medulla. After the PICA loop is exposed and the distal end of the occipital artery is prepared, the patient is given barbiturates. The PICA is occluded, and the anastomosis is completed in a fashion similar to that for the

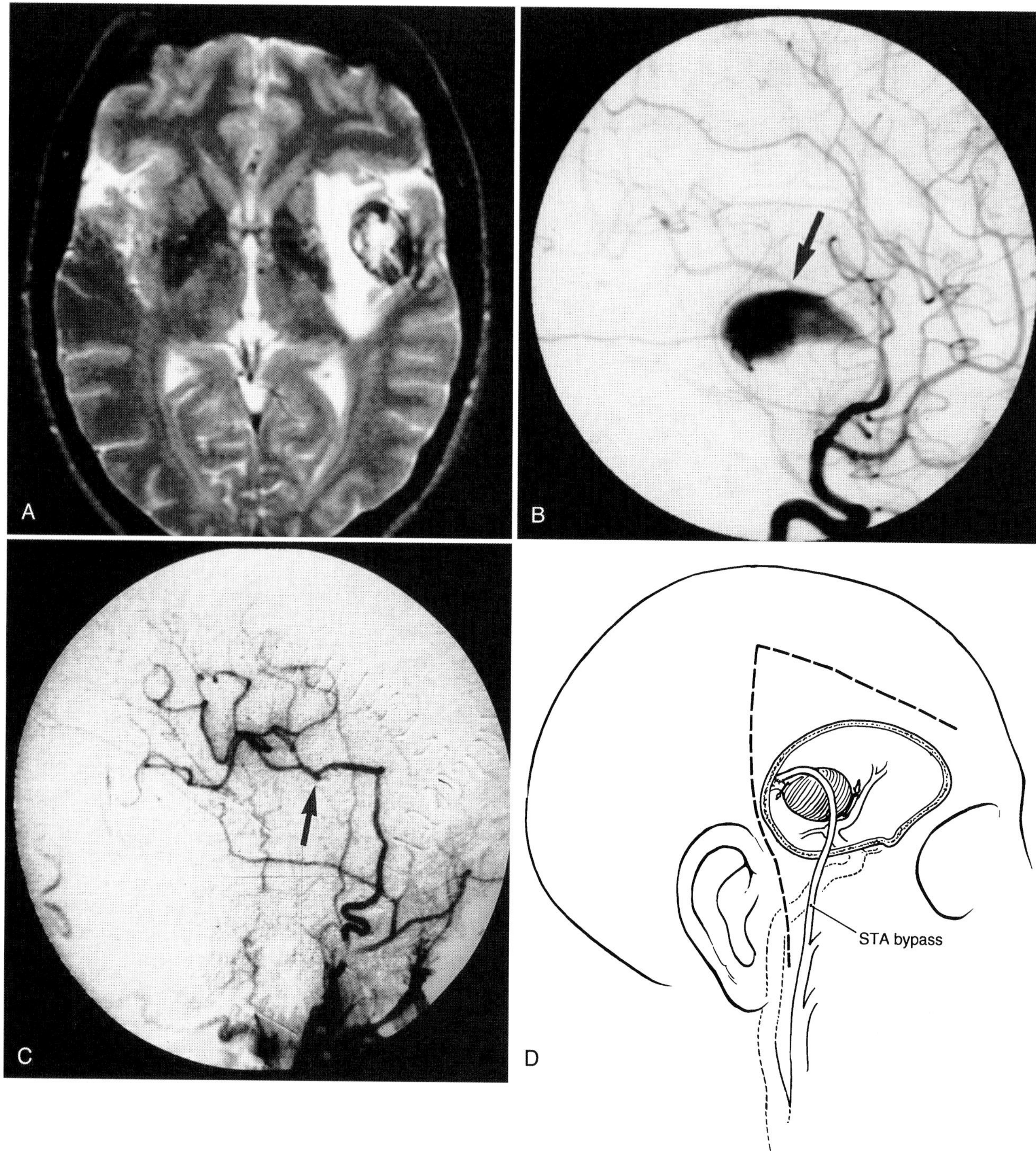

FIGURE 123–7. Giant fusiform middle cerebral artery (MCA) aneurysm. *A*, Magnetic resonance image shows a large aneurysm within the left sylvian fissure. *B*, Lateral carotid angiogram shows the fusiform, partially thrombosed aneurysm. The *arrow* indicates the exit of the distal aspect of the angular branch of the MCA from the aneurysm. *C*, The aneurysm was trapped, and the angular branch was occluded as it exited the aneurysm. Selective injection of the external carotid artery shows the superficial temporal artery (STA) graft that fills the distal trunk of the angular artery *(anastomosis at the arrow)*. *D*, Aneurysm trapping and STA bypass. (From Martin NA: Arterial bypass for the treatment of giant and fusiform intracranial aneurysms. Tech Neurosurg 4:153–178, 1998.)

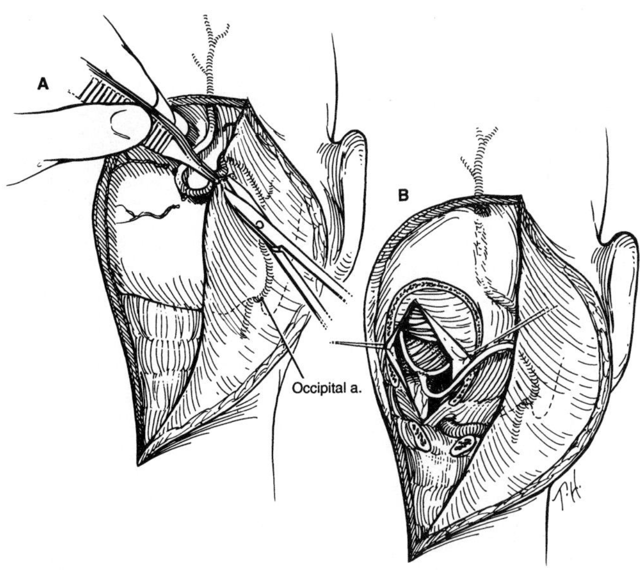

FIGURE 123–8. Technique for occipital–to–posterior inferior cerebellar artery (PICA) bypass. *A*, The scalp flap and isolation of the occipital artery. *B*, The suboccipital craniotomy and completed occipital-to-PICA bypass is apparent. (From Martin NA: Arterial bypass for the treatment of giant and fusiform intracranial aneurysms. Tech Neurosurg 4:153–178, 1998.)

STA-MCA bypass. A multilayer meticulous muscle closure is essential because a watertight dural closure cannot be achieved. During the muscle closure, the occipital artery must not become kinked or severely compressed.

SUPERFICIAL TEMPORAL ARTERY–TO–SUPERIOR CEREBELLAR ARTERY BYPASS

An STA-to-superior cerebellar artery bypass may be substituted for the saphenous vein graft–to–posterior cerebral artery when some collateral blood flow is available through small posterior communicating arteries.[44] After the STA is isolated, the incision is extended posteriorly above and behind the ear for the temporal craniotomy. After the temporal lobe is elevated, the superior cerebellar artery is exposed lateral to the brainstem. An unbranched length of this vessel is isolated and occluded after barbiturates are administered, and a 3- to 4-mm arteriotomy is made along its lateral surface. A sufficiently long length of the STA is isolated and brought down to the superior cerebellar artery. The anastomosis is completed in the same fashion as the STA-MCA anastomosis.

A type IV bypass involves an anastomosis between two adjacent cerebral arteries. This type of procedure can involve end-to-end primary reanastomosis after excision of an aneurysm, side-to-side anastomosis of two adjacent intracranial arteries, or an end-to-side anastomosis between two cerebral arteries.[4, 5, 7, 45–49]

PRIMARY REANASTOMOSIS

The simplest form of intracranial arterial reconstruction involves aneurysm excision with primary reconstruction of the parent artery. This procedure is possible only when the excised segment of the parent artery is short, and the remaining proximal and distal segments of the vessel are redundant enough to allow primary reanastomosis.

PERICALLOSAL-TO-PERICALLOSAL BYPASS

Pericallosal-to-pericallosal bypass can be used to treat fusiform aneurysms of the proximal pericallosal artery or for giant anterior communicating artery aneurysms that require trapping.[5] Interhemispheric exposure of the pericallosal arteries on the dorsal surface of the corpus callosum requires medial expansion of the pterional craniotomy or a separate parasagittal approach. After barbiturates are administered, temporary clips are placed on each pericallosal artery just beyond the genu of the corpus callosum. A 5-mm linear arteriotomy is made along the medial surface of each pericallosal artery. The back walls of the two pericallosal arteries are joined first with running 10–0 nylon suture, followed by closure of the front wall with a second suture. This side-to-side anastomosis serves as a communicating artery.

POSTERIOR INFERIOR CEREBELLAR ARTERY–TO–POSTERIOR INFERIOR CEREBELLAR ARTERY ANASTOMOSIS

The PICA-to-PICA anastomosis can be used when the occipital artery is small or has been damaged during a prior surgical procedure. This type of anastomosis requires a wider craniotomy than the occipital-to-PICA procedure. After the dura is opened and the cerebellar tonsil elevated, both caudal loops of the PICAs are freed of arachnoidal adhesions. The two distal vertical midline segments are approximated and occluded proximally and distally after burst suppression has been achieved. The side-to-side anastomosis is performed as described for the pericallosal-to-pericallosal anastomosis.

OTHER VARIATIONS OF INTRACRANIAL ARTERIAL RECONSTRUCTION

Sundt and Piepgras,[18] Ausman and colleagues,[4] Bederson and Spetzler,[45] and others[46, 48] have described variations of intracranial arterial reconstruction or transposition for the treatment of giant aneurysms. Most such cases have involved large MCA aneurysms, which tend to incorporate distal branches into the base of the aneurysm.

Techniques for Occluding or Trapping an Aneurysm after Bypass

It is often possible to occlude an aneurysm surgically by trapping it (combined proximal and distal parent artery occlusion) immediately after the bypass procedure is completed. Trapping is preferable because it isolates the aneurysm from the circulation, avoids the risk of rupture from retrograde filling (reported in rare

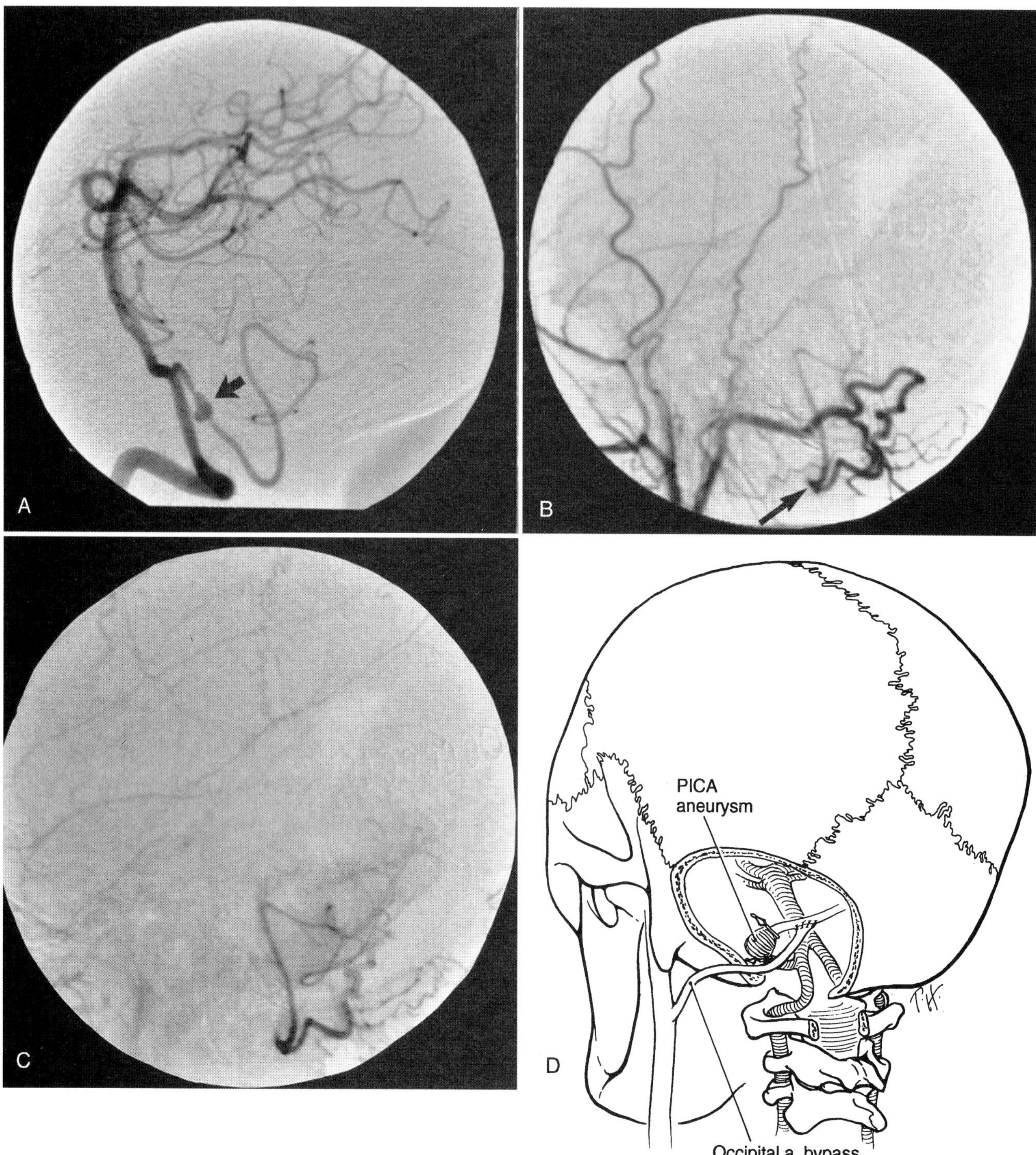

FIGURE 123–9. Distal fusiform posterior inferior cerebellar artery (PICA) aneurysm. *A,* Lateral vertebral angiogram shows a small fusiform aneurysm on the PICA (arrow) that had ruptured. *B,* The early phase of the external carotid injection shows the anastomosis *(large arrow)* between the occipital artery and proximal PICA. *C,* A later angiographic phase shows filling of distal branches of the PICA. *D,* Trapping of the PICA aneurysm and the occipital-PICA bypass. (From Martin NA: Arterial bypass for the treatment of giant and fusiform intracranial aneurysms. Tech Neurosurg 4: 153–178, 1998.)

cases), and allows immediate decompression of the aneurysm to relieve mass effect.

Proximal parent artery occlusion alone tends to be adequate to induce aneurysmal thrombosis. Proximal ICA occlusion often is used to treat giant intracavernous aneurysms. Direct surgical occlusion of the proximal ICA in the neck typically is performed immediately after construction of the bypass. This maneuver should be done in the operating room if patency of the bypass is certain and with electroencephalography or evoked potential monitoring to verify that bypass flow is adequate to prevent ischemia. In some cases, the parent artery proximal to a giant aneurysm cannot be exposed easily during the same procedure used for the bypass. In such cases, balloon or coil occlusion of the parent artery can be used.

Postoperative Management

Postoperatively, aspirin is continued without interruption. Careful maintenance of euvolemia and normal systolic blood pressure are key components of postoperative care. A new focal neurological deficit or a delay in postoperative reawakening (even in patients who have received substantial doses of barbiturates) should be evaluated by computed tomography scan to rule out the presence of a subdural or epidural hematoma.

Postoperative patency often can be confirmed by palpating the bypass pulse or by using a Doppler probe. Given the safety of modern contrast angiography, it is reasonable to use this test after surgery to evaluate graft patency, to rule out anastomotic stenoses, and to confirm aneurysm thrombosis.

OUTCOMES

Complications

The most serious acute complication is that of early graft occlusion. In almost all cases, patency of arterial and venous grafts can be ensured by gentle and meticulous surgical technique; careful avoidance of twisting, kinking, or stretching of the graft; avoidance of graft spasm by adventitial papaverine irrigation; and administration of perioperative antiplatelet therapy. In our experience with 58 bypass procedures for intracranial aneurysms, three grafts became occluded acutely. Two scalp artery bypass occlusions were related to acute angulation and kinking of the graft; the other was an idiopathic vein graft occlusion. If there is any question intraoperatively about the patency of the bypass, angiography should be performed. If the graft is found to be severely stenotic or occluded, the bypass vessel or anastomosis should be revised. Sometimes simply repositioning the bypass vessel is adequate. Other cases require undoing at least one of the anastomoses, removing thrombus, then resuturing.

Another devastating postoperative complication is that of aneurysmal rupture associated with the hemodynamic changes that accompany arterial reconstruction with a bypass. In our experience, two patients with a giant fusiform basilar trunk aneurysm died from aneurysmal rupture after vein grafts to the posterior cerebral artery were placed.[30] In both cases, hemodynamic stress associated with the presence of the distal high-flow bypass apparently caused the aneurysm to rupture. Other surgeons have reported ruptured giant intracranial aneurysms after distal bypass procedures.[50] This complication emphasizes the need to isolate the aneurysm completely from the circulation by trapping whenever possible.

Ischemic neurological deficits may be evident postoperatively. In some cases, their presence reflects the prolonged period of temporary arterial occlusion while the bypass anastomosis was constructed. Cerebral protection with moderate hypothermia, induced arterial hypertension, and barbiturate administration ordinarily minimizes this risk, however. One of our patients who developed an occlusion of the STA bypass sustained an ischemic deficit that caused mild dysphasia, and one patient died from a massive stroke caused by early occlusion of the vein graft.

A few of our patients developed subdural and epidural hematomas postoperatively. Both patients who developed postoperative subdural hematomas had been given heparin in addition to aspirin when the carotid-to-MCA bypass procedure was performed with a long saphenous vein graft. We no longer use systemic heparinization for saphenous vein bypass procedures. Instead, we use local anticoagulation by filling the saphenous vein with heparinized saline.

Long-Term Graft Patency

The International Cooperative EC-IC Bypass Study of 1985 found that the postoperative patency rate of 663 STA-MCA bypasses was 96%.[2, 51] Schick and associates[51] reported a 91% patency rate with a mean follow-up of 2.8 years. Clinical and experimental data from the cardiac and vascular literature indicate that occlusion of vein grafts increases over time. Ten years after surgery, thrombosis occurs in about 40% of aortocoronary grafts and in more than 50% of femoropopliteal bypasses. When Regli and coworkers[35] used long saphenous vein grafts for cerebral revascularization, they found that the early patency rate (0 to 30 days from surgery) was 88% and that the 1-year cumulative patency rate was 86%. At 5 years, the patency rate was 82%; at 13 years, it was 73%. These rates correspond to a mean annual graft failure rate of 1% to 1.5%.

Results of Extracranial-to-Intracranial Bypass for Giant and Fusiform Aneurysms

In our series, 21 of 22 saphenous vein bypass grafts were patent, and 31 of 33 STA or occipital grafts were patent. All five type IV bypasses were patent. Altogether, 54 patients (some with more than one bypass) underwent a combination of arterial bypass and parent artery occlusion (36 in the anterior circulation, 18 in the posterior circulation). Forty-three patients (80%) had excellent or good outcomes. Eight patients died from perioperative complications (two of whom were Hunt/Hess grade V preoperatively).[30,*]

Using saphenous vein graft bypasses for giant aneurysms, Sundt and coworkers[3] reported an acute graft patency rate of 94% in their more recent experience. Excellent or good outcomes were achieved in 80% of anterior circulation aneurysms and in 44% of posterior circulation aneurysms. Lawton and colleagues[7] reported that 93% of 61 patients had good outcomes after revascularization for intracranial aneurysms. Sen and Sekhar[8] reported results in 30 patients who underwent vein grafting with carotid occlusion or resection (primarily for tumors). Their rate of graft patency was 86% at 18 months; four patients sustained ischemic injury related to the bypass procedure.

SUMMARY

Several types of EC-IC bypass procedures are available for the treatment of unclippable aneurysms or skull base tumors that have invaded the carotid artery. The selection of the type of revascularization procedure depends on the demand for blood flow through the bypass and the anatomy of the vessels associated with the lesion. Parent artery occlusion (or preferably trapping) combined with EC-IC bypass is an effective strategy for treating aneurysms that are difficult or impossible to clip and still allows the parent artery to be preserved. Careful attention to technique yields a high rate of bypass patency and good clinical outcomes in most patients.

REFERENCES

1. Donaghy R, Yasargil MG: Microvascular Surgery. St. Louis, CV Mosby, 1967.
2. EC/IC Bypass Study Group: Failure of extracranial-intracranial arterial bypass to reduce the risk of ischemic stroke: Results of an international randomized trial. N Engl J Med 313:1191–1200, 1985.
3. Sundt TM Jr, Piepgras D, Marsh WR, et al: Saphenous vein bypass grafts for giant aneurysms and intracranial occlusive disease. J Neurosurg 65:439–450, 1986.
4. Ausman JI, Diaz FG, Sadasivan B, et al: Giant intracranial aneurysm surgery: The role of microvascular reconstruction. Surg Neurol 34:8–15, 1990.
5. Ito Z: A new technique of intracranial interarterial anastomosis between distal anterior cerebral arteries (ACA) for ACA occlusion and its indications [Japanese]. Neurol Med Chir (Tokyo) 21: 931–939, 1981.
6. Peerless SJ, Hampf CR: Extracranial to intracranial bypass in the treatment of aneurysms. Clin Neurosurg 32:114–154, 1985.
7. Lawton MT, Hamilton MG, Morcos JJ, et al: Revascularization and aneurysm surgery: Current techniques, indications, and outcome. Neurosurgery 38:83–94, 1996.
8. Sen C, Sekhar LN: Direct vein graft reconstruction of the cavernous, petrous, and upper cervical internal carotid artery: Lessons learned from 30 cases. Neurosurgery 30:732–743, 1992.
9. Brennan JA, Jafek BW: Elective carotid artery resection for advanced squamous cell carcinoma of the neck. Laryngoscope 104: 259–263, 1994.
10. Higashida RT, Halbach VV, Dowd C, et al: Endovascular detachable balloon embolization therapy of cavernous carotid artery aneurysms: Results in 87 cases. J Neurosurg 72:857–863, 1990.

*Updated from Martin.[30]

11. Hacein-Bey L, Connolly ES Jr, Duong H, et al: Treatment of inoperable carotid aneurysms with endovascular carotid occlusion after extracranial-intracranial bypass surgery. Neurosurgery 41:1225–1234, 1997.
12. Heros RC (Comment to: Lawton MT, Hamilton MV, Morcos JJ, et al): Revascularization and aneurysm surgery: Current techniques, indications, and outcome. Neurosurgery 38:83–94, 1996.
13. Piepgras D (Comment to Lawton MT, Hamilton MV, Morcos JJ, et al): Revascularization and aneurysm surgery: Current techniques, indications, and outcome. Neurosurgery 38:83–94, 1996.
14. Steinberg GK, Drake CG, Peerless SJ: Deliberate basilar or vertebral artery occlusion in the treatment of intracranial aneurysms: Immediate results and long-term outcome in 201 patients. J Neurosurg 79:161–173, 1993.
15. Drake CG, Peerless SJ: Giant fusiform intracranial aneurysms: Review of 120 patients treated surgically from 1965 to 1992. J Neurosurg 87:141–162, 1997.
16. Anson JA, Lawton MT, Spetzler RF: Characteristics and surgical treatment of dolichoectatic and fusiform aneurysms. J Neurosurg 84:185–193, 1996.
17. Drake CG, Peerless SJ, Ferguson CG: Hunterian proximal arterial occlusion for giant aneurysms of the carotid circulation. J Neurosurg 81:656–665, 1994.
18. Sundt TM Jr, Piepgras DG: Surgical approach to giant intracranial aneurysms: Operative experience with 80 cases. J Neurosurg 51: 731–742, 1979.
19. Sundt TM Jr, Piepgras D, Houser OW, et al: Interposition saphenous vein grafts for advanced occlusive disease and large aneurysms in the posterior circulation. J Neurosurg 56:205–215, 1982.
20. Gurian JH, Martin NA, King WA, et al: Neurosurgical management of cerebral aneurysms following unsuccessful or incomplete endovascular embolization. J Neurosurg 83:843–853, 1995.
21. Drake CG, Barr HW, Coles JC, et al: The use of extracorporeal circulation and profound hypothermia in the treatment of ruptured intracranial aneurysms. J Neurosurg 21:575–581, 1964.
22. Silverberg GD, Reitz BA, Ream AK: Hypothermia and cardiac arrest in the treatment of giant aneurysms of the cerebral circulation and hemangioblastoma of the medulla. J Neurosurg 55: 337–346, 1981.
23. Solomon RA, Smith CR, Raps EC, et al: Deep hypothermic circulatory arrest for the management of complex anterior and posterior circulation aneurysms. Neurosurgery 29:732–737, 1991.
24. Spetzler RF, Hadley MN, Rigamonti D, et al: Aneurysms of the basilar artery treated with circulatory arrest, hypothermia, and barbiturate cerebral protection. J Neurosurg 68:868–879, 1988.
25. Lawton MT, Spetzler RF: Internal carotid artery sacrifice for radical resection of skull base tumors. Skull Base Surg 6:119–123, 1996.
26. Brisman MH, Sen C, Catalano P: Results of surgery for head and neck tumors that involve the carotid artery at the skull base. J Neurosurg 86:787–792, 1997.
27. DeMonte F, Smith HK, Al-Mefty O: Outcome of aggressive removal of cavernous sinus meningiomas. J Neurosurg 81:245–251, 1994.
28. Solomon RA: Principles of aneurysm surgery: Cerebral ischemic protection, hypothermia, and circulatory arrest. Clin Neurosurg 41:351–363, 1994.
29. Batjer HH: Cerebral protective effects of etomidate: Experimental and clinical aspects. Cerebrovasc Brain Metab Rev 5:17–32, 1993.
30. Martin NA: Arterial bypass for the treatment of giant and fusiform intracranial aneurysms. Tech Neurosurgery 4:153–178, 1998.
31. Linskey ME, Sekhar LN, Sen C: Cerebral revascularization in cranial base surgery. In Sekhar LN, Janeck IP (eds): Surgery of Cranial Base Tumors. New York, Raven, 1993, pp 45–68.
32. Sekhar LN, Sen CN, Jho HD: Saphenous vein graft bypass of the cavernous internal carotid artery. J Neurosurg 72:35–41, 1990.
33. Spetzler RF, Fukushima T, Martin NA, et al: Petrous carotid-to-intradural carotid saphenous vein graft for intracavernous giant aneurysm, tumor, and occlusive cerebrovascular disease. J Neurosurg 73:496–501, 1990.
34. Lougheed WM, Marshall BM, Hunter M, et al: Common carotid to intracranial internal carotid bypass venous graft: Technical note. J Neurosurg 34:114–118, 1971.
35. Regli L, Piepgras D, Hansen KK: Late patency of long saphenous vein bypass grafts to the anterior and posterior cerebral circulation. J Neurosurg 83:806–811, 1995.

36. Sundt TM 3rd, Sundt TM Jr: Maximizing patency and saphenous vein bypass grafts: Principles of preparation learned from coronary and peripheral vascular surgery. In Meyer FB (eds): Sundt's Occlusive Cerebrovascular Disease. Philadelphia, WB Saunders, 1994, pp 479–488.
37. Sundt TM 3rd, Sundt TM Jr: Principles of preparation of vein bypass grafts to maximize patency. J Neurosurg 66:172–180, 1987.
38. Little JR, Furlan AJ, Bryerton B: Short vein grafts for cerebral revascularization. J Neurosurg 59:384–388, 1983.
39. Yasargil MG, Krayenbuhl HA, Jacobson JH 2nd: Microneurosurgical arterial reconstruction. Surgery 67:221–233, 1970.
40. Yasargil MG, Yonekawa Y: Results of microsurgical extra-intracranial arterial bypass in the treatment of cerebral ischemia. Neurosurgery 1:22–24, 1977.
41. Khodadad G, Singh RS, Olinger CP: Possible prevention of brain stem stroke by microvascular anastomosis in the vertebrobasilar system. Stroke 8:316–321, 1977.
42. Roski RA, Spetzler RF, Hopkins LN: Occipital artery to posterior inferior cerebellar artery bypass for vertebrobasilar ischemia. Neurosurgery 10:44–49, 1982.
43. Sundt TM Jr, Piepgras DG: Occipital to posterior inferior cerebellar artery bypass surgery. J Neurosurg 48:916–928, 1978
44. Ausman JI, Diaz FG, de los Reyes RA, et al: Posterior circulation revascularization: Superficial temporal artery to superior cerebellar artery anastomosis. J Neurosurg 56:766–776, 1982.
45. Bederson JB, Spetzler RF: Anastomosis of the anterior temporal artery to a secondary trunk of the middle cerebral artery for treatment of a giant M1 segment aneurysm: Case report. J Neurosurg 76:863–866, 1992.
46. Dolenc V: End-to-end suture of the posterior inferior cerebellar artery after the excision of a large aneurysm: Case report. Neurosurgery 11:690–693, 1982.
47. Ito Z: The microsurgical anterior interhemispheric approach suitably applied to ruptured aneurysms of the anterior communicating artery in the acute stage. Acta Neurochir (Wien) 63:85–99, 1982.
48. Madsen JR, Heros RC: Giant peripheral aneurysm of the posterior inferior cerebellar artery treated with excision and end-to-end anastomosis. Surg Neurol 30:140–143, 1988.
49. Smith RR, Parent AD: End-to-end anastomosis of the anterior cerebral artery after excision of a giant aneurysm: Case report. J Neurosurg 56:577–580, 1982.
50. Heros RC, Ameri AM: Rupture of a giant basilar aneurysm after saphenous vein interposition graft to the posterior cerebral artery: Case report. J Neurosurg 61:387–390, 1984.
51. Schick U, Zimmermann M, Stolke D: Long-term evaluation of EC-IC bypass patency. Acta Neurochir (Wien) 138:938–943, 1996.

CHAPTER **124**

Multimodality Management of Complex Cerebrovascular Lesions

BRUCE E. POLLOCK ■ JAY J. SCHINDLER ■
DOUGLAS A. NICHOLS ■ FREDRIC B. MEYER

The treatment of patients with complex vascular disorders is among the most challenging for neurologists, neurosurgeons, and interventional neuroradiologists. Proper clinical management must balance the risk of conservative therapy against the potential morbidity and mortality of any proposed intervention. Natural history studies emphasize the high lifetime risk associated with intracranial vascular lesions.[1–7] A 40-year-old patient with an arteriovenous malformation (AVM) has a 50% to 70% chance of sustaining an intracranial hemorrhage.[8] The morbidity and mortality associated with bleeding ranges from approximately 50% for AVMs[3–5] to greater than 70% for aneurysms[1, 2] depending on anatomic factors, such as size and configuration. Advances in microsurgery, endovascular embolization techniques, and radiosurgery now enable physicians to treat most patients with intracranial vascular disease safely, decreasing future risk of intracranial hemorrhage. Nonetheless, some patients have either complex or multiple vascular lesions that cannot be managed effectively with any single therapeutic intervention. Referral to regional centers of excellence equipped with experienced personnel and state-of-the-art equipment can maximize patient outcomes for this difficult subgroup of vascular patients. This chapter outlines several multimodality management approaches for patients with complex cerebrovascular lesions.

PATIENTS WITH CEREBRAL ANEURYSMS

Surgical repair has been the standard of care for treatment of patients with intracranial aneurysms.[2] Detachable microcoils have been used increasingly for the management of ruptured and unruptured aneurysms[9] and now may be preferred over surgical clipping for select patients. If a patient's medical or neurologic condition is unfavorable for general anesthesia, a direct surgical approach may be judged high risk, and coil embolization may be preferred. Endovascular therapy may be used initially to allow adequate time for the patient's medical or neurologic condition to improve sufficiently to allow for surgical treatment if coiling does not achieve full thrombosis and occlusion.[10, 11] In this setting, endovascular treatment may decrease the risk of rebleeding after acute subarachnoid hemorrhage (SAH), facilitating volume expansion and hypertensive therapy to reduce the incidence of symptomatic vasospasm. Aneurysm location is an important factor when determining whether endovascular intervention is appropriate. In a nonrandomized comparison, Gruber and associates[12] found that patients with basilar caput aneurysms with a definable neck and not involving the P-1 segments appeared to have less morbidity after endovascular treatment compared with surgical repair. Whether such an observation is true would depend on the results of a randomized trial and long-term follow-up.

There are restrictions to the endovascular treatment of aneurysms. A narrow neck is optimal—the ratio of aneurysm neck to aneurysm diameter must be adequate to allow safe placement of coils.[10, 13] Complete aneurysm occlusion can be accomplished in 85% of aneurysms with a small neck, whereas only 15% of large-necked aneurysms can be eliminated. If the aneurysm cannot be removed completely from the circulation, concern remains for continued risk of bleeding. Because endovascular aneurysm treatment is relatively new, follow-up data of treated patients are limited. Indications for combined surgical and endovascular therapy include early coil embolization of high-risk SAH patients to protect from rebleeding before definitive management, multiple aneurysms, and temporary balloon occlusion of proximal vessels intraoperatively to facilitate repair.[14]

Multiple Aneurysms

Intracranial aneurysms are multiple in approximately 15% to 20% of all cases of SAH.[15] Multiple aneurysms occur more frequently in women, and bilaterally symmetrical aneurysms (mirror aneurysms) are common. For patients with SAH, it is crucial to determine which aneurysm ruptured. The location of the SAH or intracerebral hemorrhage, aneurysm size, and aneurysm morphology all are important factors in deciding which aneurysm must be treated. Numerous management options exist for patients with multiple aneurysms. One option is to repair surgically or treat endovascularly the ruptured or symptomatic lesion and manage conservatively the remaining lesions. This approach may be appropriate for elderly patients or for patients with more than three small aneurysms. A second option is to repair surgically all aneurysms. This option is reasonable if the aneurysms can be approached safely through a single craniotomy or if it is unclear which aneurysm has ruptured and exploration is necessary. A third option is to combine surgical repair of the symptomatic aneurysm with endovascular treatment of the remaining lesions. A fourth option is to treat endovascularly the ruptured or symptomatic aneurysm followed by elective surgical repair of the remaining aneurysms. Finally, endovascular treatment of all aneurysms can be considered.

Treating multiple aneurysms solely by endovascular means may be an appropriate method of approaching this problem, especially if the aneurysm shapes and sizes are conducive to achieving total aneurysm occlusion. Coiling can be accomplished safely in the acute phase of SAH. Treating multiple aneurysms in a single session eliminates the risk of mistaking the wrong aneurysm as the site of rupture. It also reduces the risk of rupture from other incidental aneurysms, which would remain vulnerable to rupture during the treatment of vasospasm. A report reviewed 38 consecutive patients with a total of 101 aneurysms.[16] Of these patients, 25 (66%) received embolization of more than one aneurysm in a single session. Fifteen of 21 patients who presented with SAH underwent treatment of all aneurysms in a single session. Three additional patients (18 of 21 [86%]) underwent coiling of all aneurysms within 3 days of admission. Excellent or good outcomes were achieved in 35 of 38 patients (92%), 1 patient had a fair outcome, and 2 patients died.

Surgery after Failed Aneurysm Embolization

Surgery often is required if attempts at coil embolization have failed to eliminate the aneurysm completely (Fig. 124–1). Because greater than 80% of aneurysms rupture at the dome, however, partial aneurysm embolization and thrombosis of the dome may decrease the rupture rate until definitive treatment can be undertaken. Subtotal aneurysm embolization is common. Of 126 patients managed initially by coil embolization at Texas Southwestern Medical Center, 11 (9%) had to be retreated: 6 by direct surgery and 5 with repeat embolization.[11] Another report of aneurysm patients embolized with coils through 1995 found that 9% required later surgical clipping of aneurysm remnants.[17] All 11 patients had good to excellent outcomes.

Many factors have been reported to be important regarding surgery after incomplete aneurysm coiling. First, repeat embolization should be considered before surgical management. In many cases, coil impaction facilitates additional coil placement, and complete aneurysm obliteration may be feasible. Second, the amount of time between the embolization and the surgical procedure must be considered. After 2 or more weeks, coils often become embedded within the wall of the aneurysm, making coil removal difficult at surgery. This situation increases the risk of tearing the aneurysm or parent vessel, and surgical clipping may become technically impossible. To minimize complica-

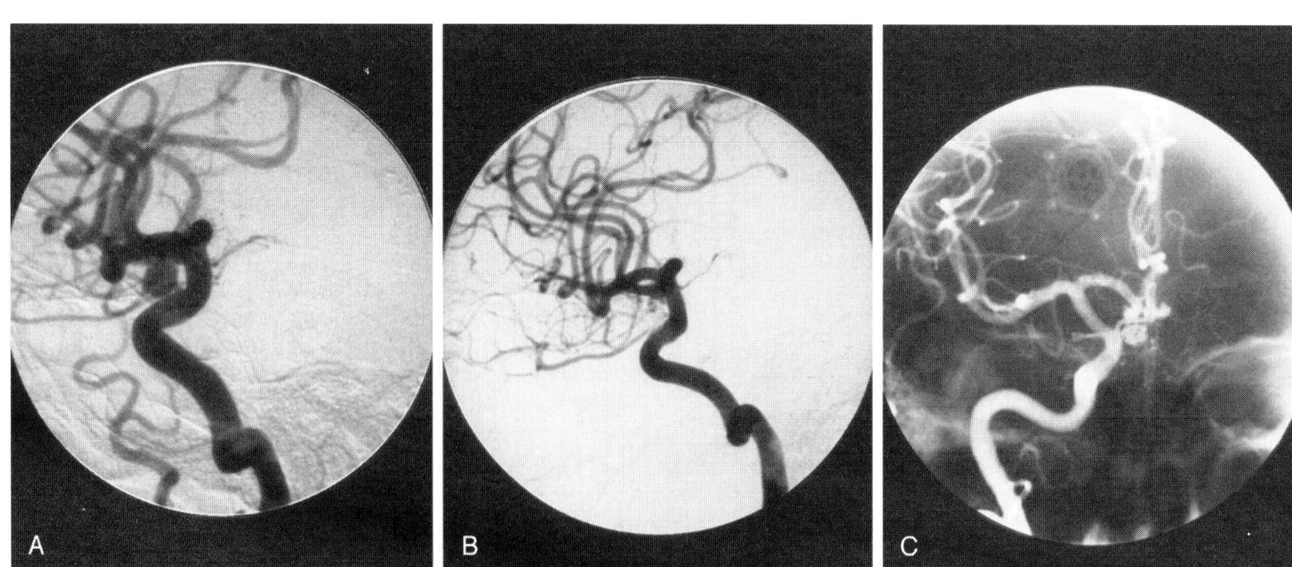

FIGURE 124–1. A 41-year-old man who sustained a subarachnoid hemorrhage and underwent primary coil embolization of an anterior communicating artery aneurysm. *A*, Lateral right internal carotid artery injection showing aneurysm. *B*, Lateral right internal carotid artery injection showing residual aneurysm neck measuring 1.5 mm × 3.0 mm. *C*, Anteroposterior right internal carotid artery injection after patient underwent craniotomy and clip ligation of aneurysm neck.

tions in this setting, some surgeons recommend that coils never should be extracted but that the goal of surgery should be simply to occlude any remaining aneurysm neck rest.[18] It is important to recognize that partially coiled aneurysms frequently are less mobile, making three-dimensional visualization more difficult at surgery.

Embolization after Failed Aneurysm Surgery

If satisfactory clip ligation of an aneurysm is not technically feasible at surgery, coil embolization can be a useful adjunct to promote progressive aneurysm thrombosis (Fig. 124–2). In addition to difficulties encountered at initial clip placement, aneurysm regrowth after incomplete clipping and clip slippage can occur, and the patient remains at risk for future hemorrhage. This regrowth occurs in approximately 4% of patients undergoing aneurysm surgery.[19] In such circumstances, partial clipping of the aneurysm may result in a smaller neck, improving the likelihood of complete occlusion after coil embolization.

Thielen and colleagues[19] treated eight patients with incompletely clipped necks and aneurysm rests measuring 5 to 14 mm with detachable platinum microcoils. No permanent treatment-related neurologic or medical morbidity occurred. Six of the eight aneurysms were obliterated completely on follow-up angiography. The two other patients had small remaining remnants. In both of these cases, the aneurysm had a wide neck, making complete coil occlusion technically unfeasible. The combined surgical morbidity and mortality has been reported to be higher for repeat surgery after initial unsuccessful aneurysm surgery.[20] Embolization may be safer than repeat surgery for patients with incompletely clipped aneurysms.

PATIENTS WITH ANEURYSMS AND ARTERIOVENOUS MALFORMATIONS

The coexistence of cerebral aneurysms and AVMs has been well described.[21–25] The cause of these aneurysms most likely is related to abnormal hemodynamic stresses secondary to the increased blood flow of the AVM. Flow-related aneurysms can occur proximal on the circle of Willis or more distal on the feeding vessels. Intranidal aneurysms have been reported in 58% of patients examined with superselective angiography[26] and are discovered in many patients who present with an AVM hemorrhage.[27] Management of a patient presenting with an AVM and an associated aneurysm or multiple aneurysms is complicated by the fact that each entity has a different natural history. Treatment initially should be directed toward the symptomatic lesion. As a general rule, SAH generally arises from the aneurysm, and intraparenchymal blood generally arises from the AVM. Determining the site of hemorrhage can be difficult, however, in many cases because of close proximity of the lesions. Both lesions should be treated simultaneously whenever possible. Simultaneous treatment often is not feasible, and a decision regarding which lesion to treat first is necessary. Aneurysm disappearance and enlargement have been reported in cases in which the AVM was managed initially.[23, 28] This unpredictable behavior of associated

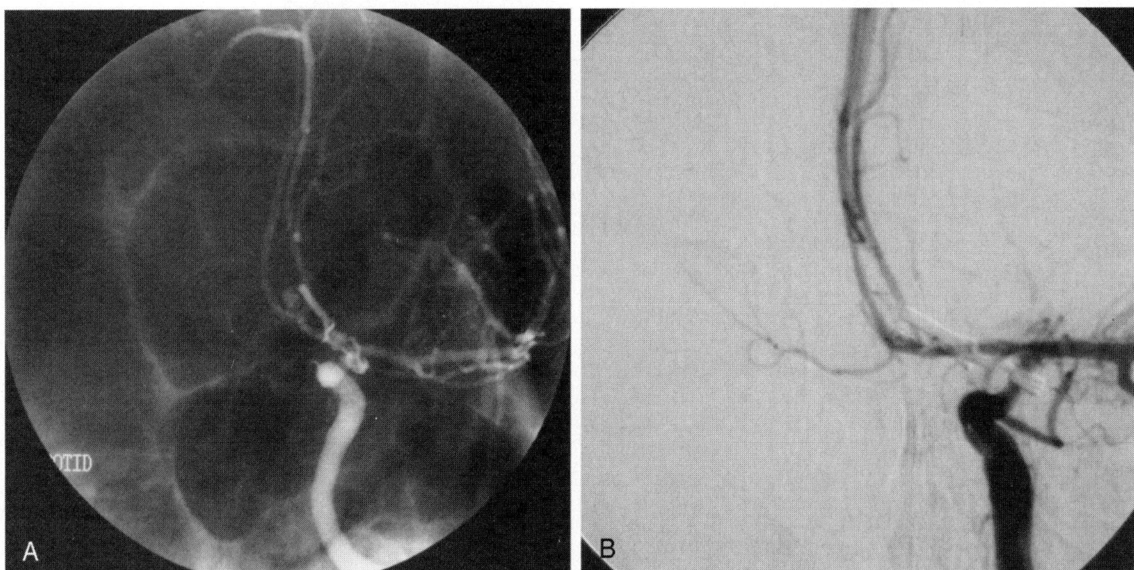

FIGURE 124–2. Anteroposterior left internal carotid artery angiograms of a 42-year-old woman who sustained a subarachnoid hemorrhage and was discovered to have an aneurysm involving the anterior communicating artery. The patient underwent craniotomy and clip ligation of the aneurysm. No postoperative angiogram was performed. One month later, the patient had a repeat subarachnoid hemorrhage. *A*, Angiogram at the time of rebleeding shows persistent aneurysm. Note clip placement on dome of aneurysm. *B*, Angiogram after endovascular coil embolization of aneurysm remnant shows complete aneurysm obliteration.

aneurysms reflects complex AVM-aneurysm blood flow relationships.

Microsurgery

Patients with AVMs and aneurysms can be treated with microsurgery alone. When surgery is performed, it should be approached with the attitude of treating both lesions definitively. This treatment is possible in select cases in which the AVM and aneurysm are on the same side and can be reached through a single craniotomy. For patients who present with aneurysm SAH, it may be prudent to repair the aneurysm initially followed by AVM treatment in a delayed fashion after the patient has recovered. If the site of hemorrhage is from the AVM and the patient does not require urgent clot evacuation, it is reasonable to delay surgical resection of the AVM 4 to 6 weeks permitting the adjacent edema to subside. During this period, the risk of repeat hemorrhage is considered low. In such cases, consideration should be given to securing the aneurysm before excising the AVM. A sudden increase in arterial resistance can occur after AVM resection, leading to aneurysm enlargement and rupture.[22, 24] This concern should be greatest for patients with aneurysms on feeding pedicles to the AVM and less for patients with more proximal aneurysms.

Microsurgery and Embolization

When aneurysms associated with AVMs are distant, staged multimodality therapy is reasonable to consider. This is especially true for patients harboring multiple aneurysms not within surgical proximity of the AVM (Fig. 124–3). The primary decision is to treat the symptomatic lesion initially and manage the remaining vascular lesions in a delayed manner. The risk of procedural morbidity and mortality may be lower with endovascular treatment for such patients. In this manner, a patient would have to undergo only a single craniotomy to reduce the future risk of hemorrhage.

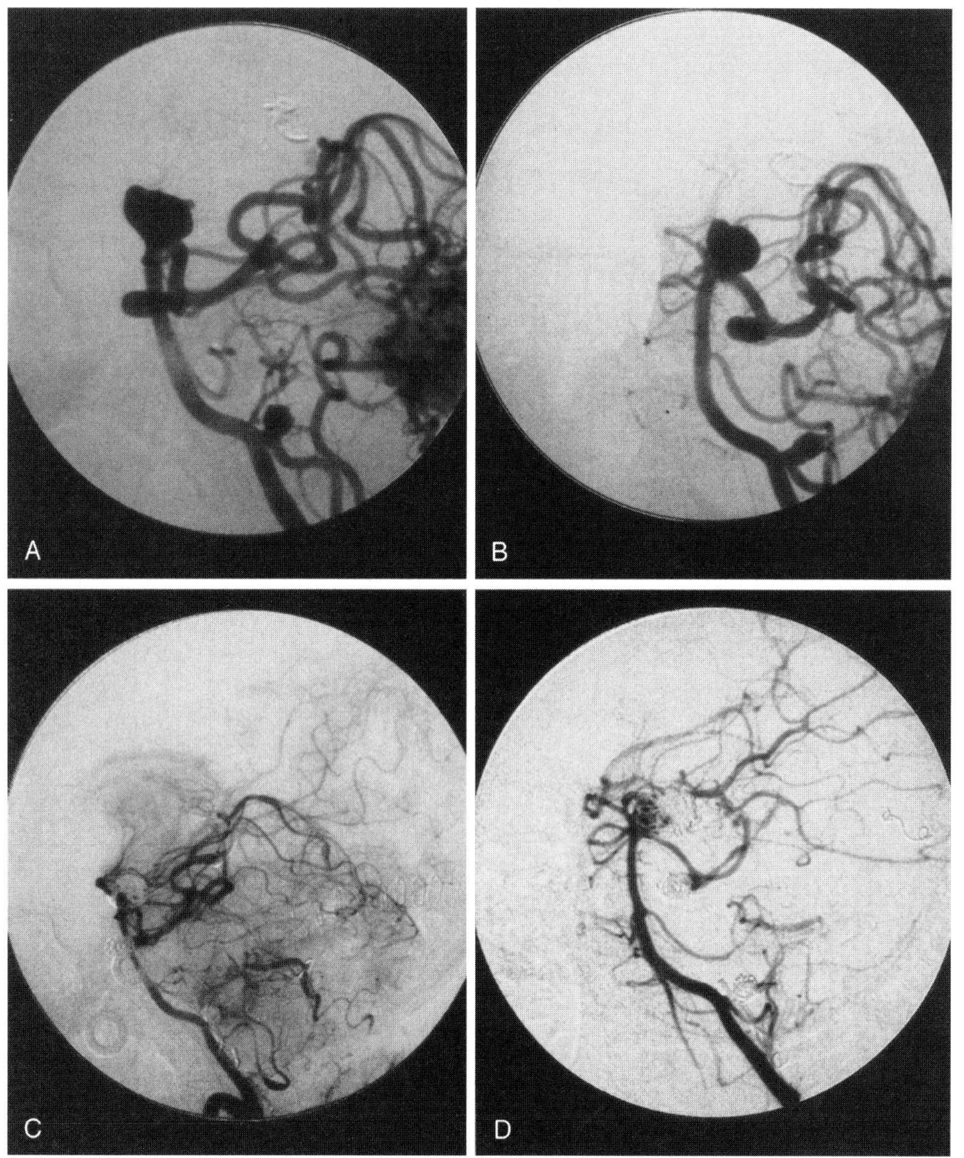

FIGURE 124–3. Lateral and anteroposterior vertebral artery angiograms of a 42-year-old woman who sustained a subarachnoid hemorrhage and was discovered to have multiple aneurysms and a left cerebellar arteriovenous malformation. *A* and *B*, Angiogram at the time of the patient's initial evaluation. The patient also had a right intracavernous artery aneurysm. *C* and *D*, Angiogram after the patient underwent staged coil embolization of multiple aneurysms (basilar artery, left superior cerebellar artery, left posterior inferior cerebellar artery), followed by embolization and resection of the arteriovenous malformation.

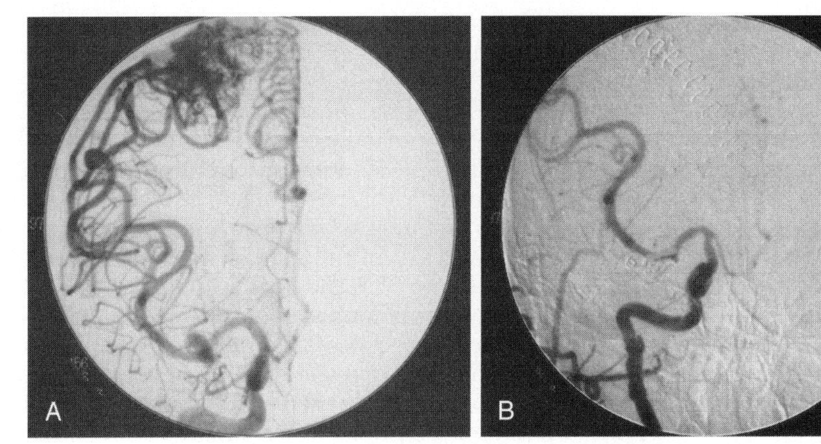
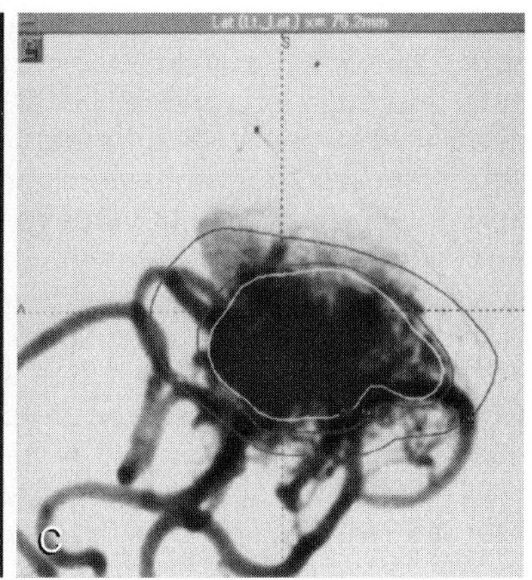

FIGURE 124–4. A 52-year-old man who sustained a right frontal, subarachnoid, and intraventricular hemorrhage. *A*, Anteroposterior right internal carotid artery injection revealed a bilobed middle cerebral artery aneurysm. Note the incidental right parietal arteriovenous malformation. *B*, Anteroposterior right internal carotid artery injection after clip ligation of the aneurysm. *C*, Lateral right internal carotid artery injection at the time of radiosurgery for the arteriovenous malformation. The volume of the arteriovenous malformation was 6 cm^3 and was covered with a margin radiation dose of 16 Gy.

Microsurgery or Embolization and Radiosurgery

Stereotactic radiosurgery is effective and safe for properly selected AVM patients.[29–33] Radiosurgery causes injury to the vessel walls, resulting in progressive closure of the lumens and obliteration of the malformation.[34] For patients with deep AVMs (basal ganglia, thalamus, brainstem), radiosurgery is preferred over surgical resection to minimize neurologic injury.[35–37] Consequently, for most patients that present with a symptomatic aneurysm and are found to have an incidental AVM, it is reasonable to manage the aneurysm with surgery (Fig. 124–4) or endovascular therapy (Fig. 124–5) initially and perform radiosurgery of the AVM in a delayed manner. The timing and order of management of patients having an intracerebral hemorrhage from an AVM in a location associated with high morbidity for removal and a related aneurysm should consider the morphology and relationship of the aneurysm to the AVM. If the aneurysm is directly proximal, is large, or contains any daughter sacs, strong consideration is given to early treatment of the aneurysm before AVM radiosurgery.

PATIENTS WITH LARGE ARTERIOVENOUS MALFORMATIONS

The morbidity associated with any treatment of large AVMs is high. For patients with AVMs greater than 3 cm, the reported significant morbidity in the early postoperative period ranges from 40% to 75%, with

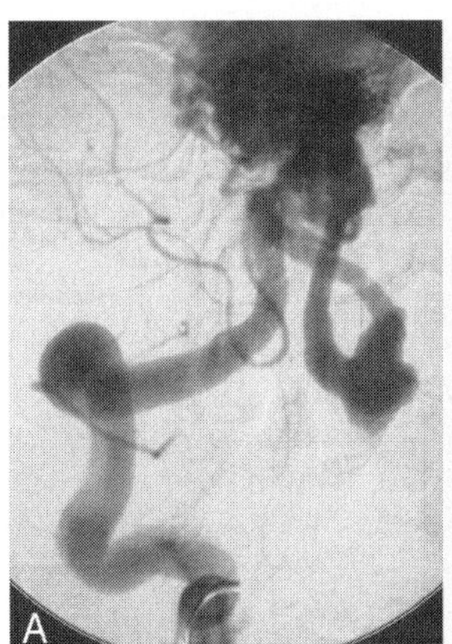
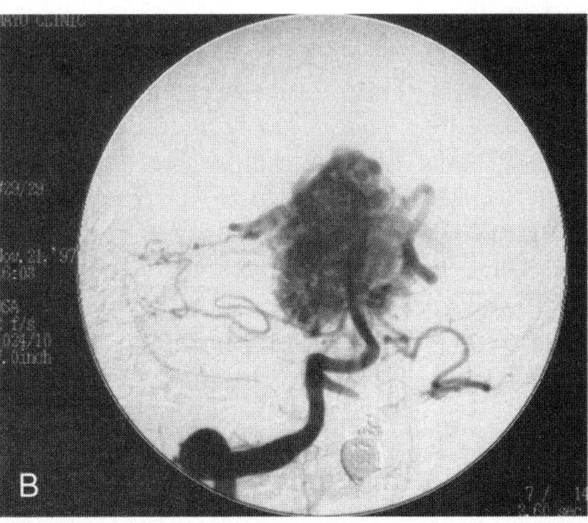
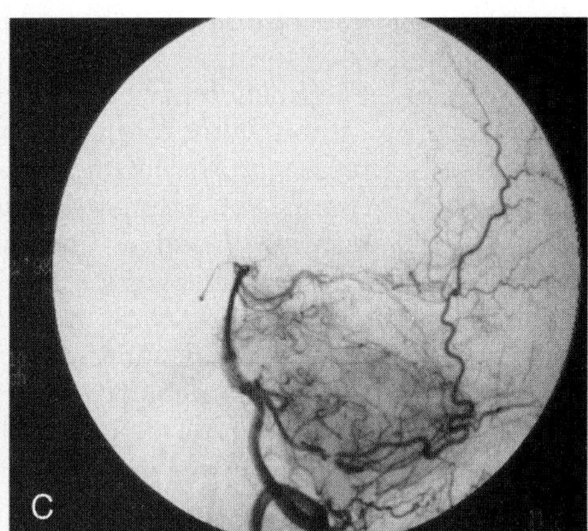

FIGURE 124–5. A 50-year-old man with a history of subarachnoid hemorrhage. Cerebral angiography revealed a right posterior inferior cerebellar artery aneurysm and a 5.5-cm arteriovenous malformation. *A*, Anteroposterior right vertebral artery injection showing fusiform aneurysm and the arteriovenous malformation. *B*, Anteroposterior right vertebral angiogram after occlusion of the artery with microcoils. *C*, Lateral left vertebral angiogram 1 year after staged-volume radiosurgery shows complete obliteration of the cerebellar arteriovenous malformation.

approximately 30% of patients having a moderate-to-severe disability at late follow-up.[38–40] It is believed that hyperemia occurs in the adjacent brain after the removal of large AVMs secondary to cerebral dysautoregulation, resulting in hemorrhage and neurologic injury.[41, 42] An alternative hypothesis is that venous occlusion, not cerebral dysautoregulation, is the cause of local hyperemia.[43] Because of the high risk of neurologic injury in treating large AVMs, Hamilton and Spetzler[38] concluded that only when a patient has a prior hemorrhage or progressive neurologic disability should intervention be considered. The natural history of such AVMs is probably less dangerous than attempts at resection, embolization, or radiosurgery.

Embolization and Microsurgery

Embolization can be used before removal of large AVMs to reduce postoperative neurologic deficits.[44–49] Preferably, embolization is performed preoperatively, but it can be done intraoperatively, with the goal being flow reduction and elimination of deep or inaccessible feeding vessels. Preoperative embolization results in reduced operating time and less blood loss and often allows clear delineation of the AVM margins. The postoperative complication rates are reported to be lower because of a reduction in the amount of perilesional hyperemia. Cost analyses found preoperative embolization to be cost-effective in the treatment of patients with large AVMs when compared with surgery alone.[50]

Vinuela and coworkers[49] reported on 101 patients managed with embolization and surgical resection. Of patients, 60 (59%) had Spetzler-Martin grade IV or V AVMs. Preoperative embolization achieved 50% to 75% size reduction in 50 cases and 75% to 90% size reduction in 31 cases. Complete AVM removal was accomplished in 97 of 101 patients. Spetzler and colleagues[45] presented the results of 20 patients with giant (>6 cm) grade V (eloquent brain and deep venous drainage) AVMs who underwent staged embolization followed by surgical resection. Complete excision was possible in 18 of the 20 patients after embolization. Although AVMs meeting these criteria were associated with a 50% combined major morbidity and mortality without embolization as an adjunct, there was no mortality and only one case of disabling morbidity associated with the 20 patients presented. DeMeritt and colleagues[48] reported on 71 patients and compared the results of patients treated with preoperative embolization followed by surgery with surgery alone. At last follow-up, 86% of patients undergoing combined embolization and surgery were independent without significant disability compared with 66% of patients managed with surgery alone.

Embolization and Radiosurgery

The goal of AVM radiosurgery is complete AVM obliteration with minimal morbidity. Obliteration rates of greater than 70% have been documented when the radiation dose to the AVM margin is at least 16 Gy.[51] Although higher radiation doses appear to correlate directly with AVM obliteration, dose prescription must take into account the likelihood of radiation-related complications.[52, 53] As a result of the dose-volume relationship for AVM postradiosurgical radiation-related complications,[30, 54] radiosurgery generally is recommended only for AVMs with an average maximum diameter of 3 cm or less (approximately 15 cm^3).

Embolization frequently has been used in conjunction with radiosurgery in the management of patients with larger AVMs.[36, 37, 55–58] The goal of preradiosurgical embolization is permanent volume reduction of the nidus. Gobin and associates[55] reported on 96 patients undergoing acrylate embolization followed by radiosurgery. Of 90 evaluable patients, 53 (59%) had total AVM obliteration. Preradiosurgical embolization is not without risk. New neurologic deficits occurred in 4% to 40% of reported AVM patients undergoing embolization before radiosurgery.[35, 56–58] The high rate of morbidity is at least partially due to the critical location of most AVMs undergoing radiosurgery. Recanalization has been reported in approximately 15% of patients after particle and glue embolization procedures.[55, 59] Embolization may make radiosurgery more difficult if the resultant shape of the AVM is irregular or if it has been divided into multiple compartments.

Staged-Volume Radiosurgery

Recognition of the limitations of embolization as an adjunct to radiosurgery has led some radiosurgical centers to manage patients with large AVMs with staged-volume radiosurgery.[60] Staged-volume radiosurgery consists of dividing an AVM into separate components and covering each region during multiple radiosurgical procedures. This technique allows a higher radiation dose to be delivered to the entire AVM volume (increasing the likelihood of AVM obliteration), while respecting the dose-volume relationships that predict radiation-induced complications after AVM radiosurgery. The goal of staged-volume radiosurgery is no different than other management strategies for intracranial AVMs: elimination of the patient's future risk of bleeding at an acceptable risk of morbidity and mortality. Because the procedure itself may span 12 to 24 months, and the patient remains at risk for bleeding during the latency interval after radiosurgery, any benefit is likely to be conferred only on patients with extended life expectancies. The primary drawback of this technique is the same as single-stage AVM radiosurgery: The patients remain at risk for bleeding until the malformation obliterates. Publications have shown that the annual risk of AVM bleeding after radiosurgery is either unchanged[28, 61] or reduced, however, compared with the natural history of untreated AVMs.[62] Follow-up is needed to determine whether this technique is able to obliterate large AVMs at an acceptable rate of radiation-related complications.

PATIENTS WITH DURAL ARTERIOVENOUS FISTULAS

Dural arteriovenous fistulas (DAVFs) are thought to be acquired lesions and comprise approximately 10% to

15% of intracranial vascular malformations. The cause of DAVFs is thought to be secondary to thrombosis or stenosis of a venous sinus with subsequent recruitment of shunting dural arteries.[63] Patients with DAVFs often complain of pulsatile tinnitus, headaches, seizures, or ocular symptoms. Intracranial hemorrhage is less common as the presenting symptom for patients with DAVFs compared with patients with pial AVMs. The most frequent sites of involvement are the transverse and sigmoid sinuses, but DAVFs may occur at the cavernous sinus, anterior cranial base, and tentorium. Untreated DAVFs have an annual hemorrhage rate of 1.6%.[7] A meta-analysis of the published literature on DAVFs found cortical venous drainage, venous dilations, and galenic drainage as predisposing factors for hemorrhage.[6] Several classifications exist to predict the clinical behavior of DAVFs based on the direction and type of venous drainage.[64–66] Treatment typically is reserved for patients with cortical venous drainage or persistent severe symptoms regardless of the nature of the venous outflow from the fistula.

Embolization

DAVFs may be treated primarily with embolization alone.[67] The treatment protocol depends on location of the lesion, the complexity of the associated vascular channels, the clinical presentation, and the associated risk of treatment. Because many DAVFs have a relatively benign natural history, the treatment options must be tailored to have acceptably low risks. Although surgical approaches have been used to resect the involved sinus and adjacent dura to devascularize the lesion, most patients today can be managed without the need for surgery. Transarterial embolization is effective at decreasing the blood flow of DAVFs and relieving symptoms in a rapid, safe fashion.[68, 69] Recanalization occurs frequently, however, and DAVFs typically recruit new collateral arterial supply to maintain fistula patency. Most arterial approaches result in subtotal fistula obliteration. In these cases as well as cases in which the feeding arteries have been altered with previous treatment, transvenous embolization may prove a safer option.[70–75] Transvenous embolization results in a higher cure rate and lower rate of recurrence than transarterial embolization.[71]

Embolization and Surgical Resection

Surgical resection of DAVFs typically is reserved for patients who have failed prior attempts at endovascular therapy or who are symptomatic but have poor venous access to the lesion. Goto and associates[76] used three angiographic categories to determine appropriate treatment for high-risk DAVFs of the transverse sinus. Category one was defined as having extremely high flow with no associated sinus occlusion or leptomeningeal retrograde venous drainage. These investigators reported that these are treated best by combined transarterial and transvenous embolization. Surgical resection of the involved sinus could be performed as needed. Category two consisted of localized DAVFs not involving a sinus and direct cortical venous drainage. These investigators recommended transarterial embolization followed by surgically disconnecting the leptomeningeal veins. The third category consisted of DAVFs with occlusion of some component of the venous sinus but with retrograde leptomeningeal venous drainage as well. For these patients, transarterial embolization together with sinus packing and surgical resection was recommended.

Another situation in which preoperative embolization followed by surgery may be beneficial is in the management of DAVFs involving the deep cerebral venous system. DAVFs of the tentorium traditionally are difficult to obliterate with endovascular techniques

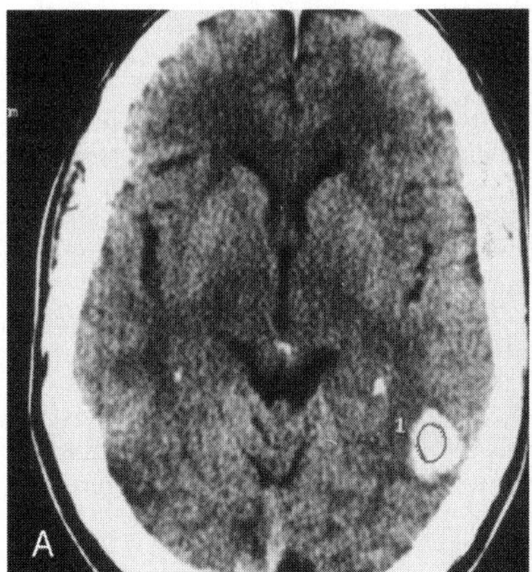

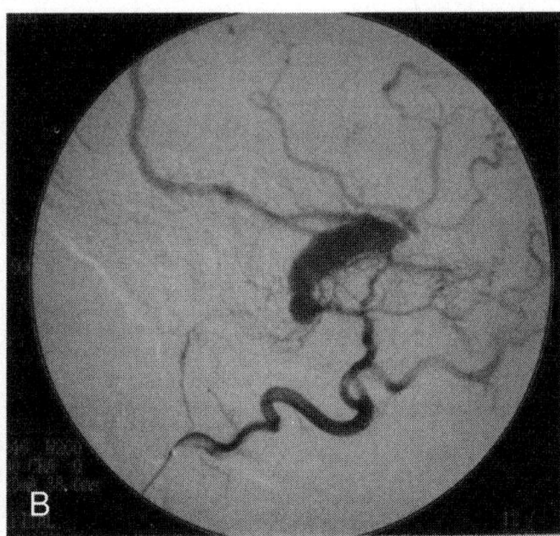

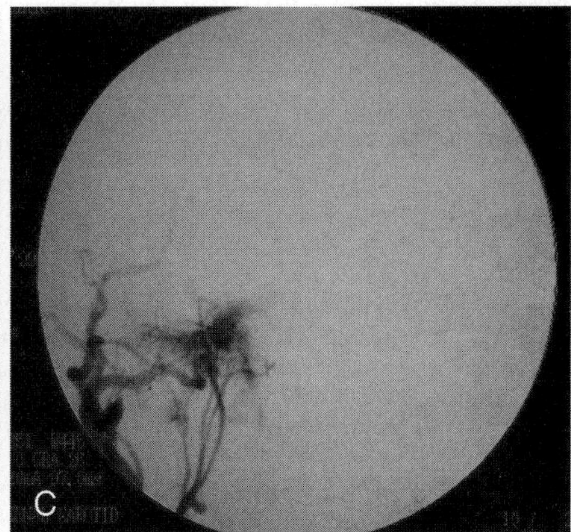

FIGURE 124–6. A 53-year-old man with sudden onset of expressive aphasia. *A*, CT scan shows a left posterior temporal intracranial hemorrhage. *B*, Lateral left occipital artery angiogram shows a dural arteriovenous fistula involving the transverse/sigmoid sinuses. Note the distal occlusion of the jugular sinus and the extensive cortical venous drainage. *C*, Anteroposterior right external carotid angiogram reveals a second dural arteriovenous fistula involving the jugular bulb. Venous drainage was anterograde through a patent jugular vein. The patient underwent transarterial embolization followed by excision of the left transverse sinus. Later, the patient had radiosurgery and transarterial embolization to the right jugular bulb fistula.

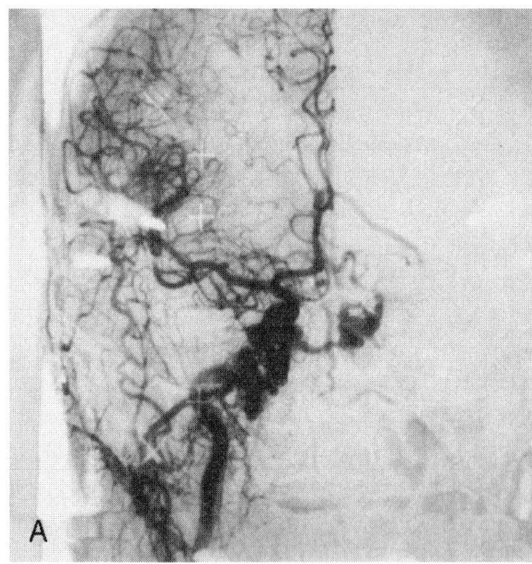

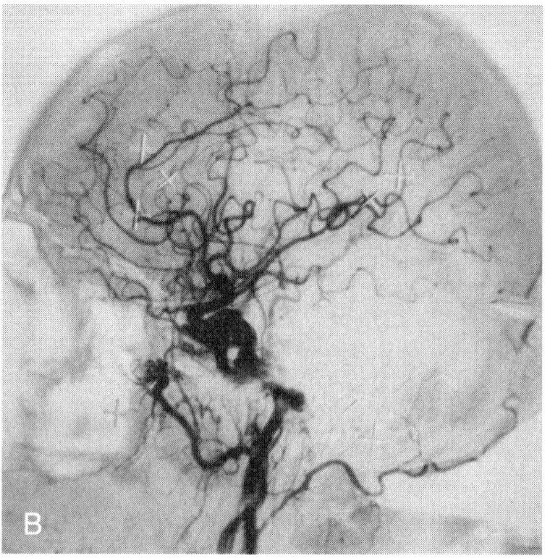

FIGURE 124–7. A 60-year-old woman with chemosis, headache, and diplopia. Workup revealed a dural arteriovenous fistula involving the left cavernous sinus. Prior attempts at transvenous embolization by inferior petrosal sinus and ophthalmic vein approaches were unsuccessful. The patient was managed with staged radiosurgery and transarterial embolization. Anteroposterior *(A)* and lateral *(B)* left common carotid angiograms at the time of radiosurgery. The fistula has arterial supply from the internal and external carotid arteries. Venous drainage is primarily retrograde through the deep venous system via the basal vein of Rosenthal.

because of the multiple small feeding arteries, which are difficult to visualize and often originate off the internal carotid arteries. Transarterial embolization of feeding arteries from the external carotid artery whenever possible followed by surgical resection has been reported (Fig. 124–6).[77]

Although rare, pediatric DAVFs present another clinical situation when combination therapy may be beneficial. Infants and small children have little vascular reserve so that preoperative embolization can be beneficial to reduce blood flow and intraoperative blood loss during surgical resection. An example is a 6-month-old boy who underwent 14 transarterial and transvenous embolizations before undergoing successful surgical resection of a large DAVF that involved the torcula, sagittal sinus, and right transverse sinus.[78]

Radiosurgery and Embolization

Radiosurgery has been used in the treatment of patients with DAVFs.[77, 79–84] A staged approach to intracranial DAVFs involving radiosurgery followed by planned transarterial embolization of 29 patients has been reported.[83] Staging in this manner allows complete radiosurgical coverage of the entire involved dural sinus for progressive long-term obliteration of any abnormal fistulous connections. Subsequent embolization provides rapid symptom relief or elimination of cortical venous drainage (or both). In our experience, greater than 90% of patients have a rapid improvement in symptoms after the embolization. Follow-up angiography has confirmed complete obliteration of the DAVFs in approximately 80% of patients. This staged approach has been especially effective for patients with DAVFs of the cavernous sinus (Fig. 124–7).[84] Although this subgroup of patients can present with significant visual symptoms requiring urgent intervention to reduce intraocular pressures, the hemorrhage risk for these patients is low. Improvement of symptoms occurs in greater than 95% of patients, and all 16 patients having follow-up angiography to date have achieved either total (n = 15) or near-total (n = 1) obliteration of the fistula. Accordingly, combined radiosurgery and embolization provides a minimally invasive alternative to microsurgery[85–87] and may be the treatment of choice for cavernous sinus DAVFs.

REFERENCES

1. Jane JA, Kassell NF, Torner JC, Winn HR: The natural history of aneurysms and arteriovenous malformations. J Neurosurg 62: 321–323, 1985.
2. Kassell NF, Torner JC, Jane JA, et al: The international cooperative study on the timing of aneurysm surgery: Part 1. Overall management results. J Neurosurg 73:18–36, 1990.
3. Brown RD, Wiebers DO, Forbes G, et al: The natural history of unruptured intracranial arteriovenous malformations. J Neurosurg 68:352–357, 1988.
4. Ondra SL, Troupp H, George ED, Schwab K: The natural history of symptomatic arteriovenous malformations of the brain: A 24-year follow-up assessment. J Neurosurg 73:387–391, 1990.
5. Pollock BE, Flickinger JC, Lunsford LD, et al: Factors that predict the bleeding risk of cerebral arteriovenous malformations. Stroke 27:1–6, 1996.
6. Awad IA, Little JR, Akrawi WP, Ahl J: Intracranial dural arteriovenous malformations: Factors predisposing to an aggressive neurological course. J Neurosurg 72:839–850, 1990.
7. Brown RD, Wiebers DO, Nichols DA: Intracranial dural arteriovenous fistulae: Angiographic predictors of intracranial hemorrhage and clinical outcome in nonsurgical patients. J Neurosurg 81:531–538, 1994.
8. Kondziolka D, McLaughlin MR, Kestle JRW: Simple risk predictions for arteriovenous malformation hemorrhage. Neurosurgery 37:851–855, 1995.
9. Guglielmi G, Vinuela F, Dion J, et al: Electrothrombosis of saccular aneurysms via endovascular approach: Part II. Preliminary clinical experience. J Neurosurg 75:8–14, 1991.
10. Marks MP, Steinberg GK, Lane B: Combined use of endovascular coils and surgical clipping for intracranial aneurysms. AJNR Am J Neuroradiol 16:15–18, 1995.
11. Horowitz M, Purdy P, Kopitnik T, et al: Aneurysm retreatment after Guglielmi detachable coil and nondetachable coil embolization: Report of nine cases and review of the literature. Neurosurgery 44:712–720, 1999.
12. Gruber DP, Zimmerman GA, Tomsick TA, et al: A comparison between endovascular and surgical management of basilar artery apex aneurysms. J Neurosurg 90:868–874, 1999.
13. Zubillaga AF, Guglielmi G, Vinuela F, Duckwiler GR: Endovascular occlusion of intracranial aneurysms with electrically detachable coils: Correlation of aneurysm neck size and treatment results. AJNR Am J Neuroradiol 15:821–827, 1994.
14. Hacein-Bey L, Connolly ES, Mayer SA, et al: Complex intracranial aneurysms: Combined operative and endovascular approaches. Neurosurgery 43:1304–1313, 1998.

15. Ostergaard JR, Hog E: Incidence of multiple intracranial aneurysms: Influence of arterial hypertension and gender. J Neurosurg 63:49–55, 1985.
16. Solander S, Ulhoa A, Vinuela F, et al: Endovascular treatment of multiple intracranial aneurysms by using Guglielmi detachable coils. J Neurosurg 90:857–864, 1999.
17. Gurian JH, Maratin NA, King WA, et al: Neurosurgical management of cerebral aneurysms following unsuccessful or incomplete endovascular embolization. J Neurosurg 83:843–853, 1995.
18. Civit T, Auque J, Marchal JC, et al: Aneurysm clipping after endovascular treatment with coils: A report of eight patients. Neurosurgery 38:955–961, 1996.
19. Thielen KR, Nichols DA, Fulgham JR, Piepgras DG: Endovascular treatment of cerebral aneurysms following incomplete clipping. J Neurosurg 87:184–189, 1997.
20. Drake CG, Friedman AH, Peerless SJ: Failed aneurysm surgery: Reoperation in 115 cases. J Neurosurg 61:848–856, 1984.
21. Miyasaka K, Wolpert SM, Prager RJ: The association of cerebral aneurysms, infundibula, and intracranial arteriovenous malformations. Stroke 13:196–203, 1982.
22. Cunha e Sa MJ, Stein BM, Soloman RA, McCormick PC: The treatment of associated intracranial aneurysms and arteriovenous malformations. J Neurosurg 77:853–859, 1992.
23. Kondziolka D, Nixon BJ, Lasjaunias P, et al: Cerebral arteriovenous malformations with associated arterial aneurysms: Hemodynamic and therapeutic considerations. Can J Neurol Sci 15: 130–134, 1988.
24. Batjer H, Suss R, Samson D: Intracranial arteriovenous malformations associated with aneurysms. Neurosurgery 18:29–35, 1986.
25. Brown RD, Wiebers DO, Forbes GS: Unruptured intracranial aneurysms and arteriovenous malformations: Frequency of intracranial hemorrhage and relationship of lesions. J Neurosurg 73: 859–863, 1990.
26. Turjman F, Massoud TF, Vinuela F, et al: Aneurysms related to cerebral arteriovenous malformations: Superselective angiographic assessment in 58 patients. AJNR Am J Neuroradiol 15: 1601–1605, 1994.
27. Marks MP, Lane B, Steinberg GK, Snipes GJ: Intranidal aneurysms in cerebral arteriovenous malformations: Evaluation and endovascular treatment. Radiology 183:355–360, 1992.
28. Pollock BE, Flickinger JC, Lunsford LD, et al: Hemorrhage risk after stereotactic radiosurgery of cerebral arteriovenous malformations. Neurosurgery 38:652–661, 1996.
29. Friedman WA, Bova FJ, Mendenhall WM: Linear accelerator radiosurgery for arteriovenous malformations: The relationship of size to outcome. J Neurosurg 82:180–189, 1995.
30. Kjellberg RN, Hanamura T, Davis KR, et al: Bragg-peak protonbeam therapy for arteriovenous malformations. N Engl J Med 309:269–274, 1983.
31. Pollock BE, Flickinger JC, Lunsford LD, et al: Factors associated with successful arteriovenous malformation radiosurgery. Neurosurgery 42:1239–1247, 1998.
32. Steiner L, Lindquist C, Adler JR, et al: Clinical outcome of radiosurgery for cerebral arteriovenous malformations. J Neurosurg 77:1–8, 1992.
33. Yamamoto Y, Coffey RJ, Nichols DA, Shaw EG: Interim report on the radiosurgical treatment of cerebral arteriovenous malformations: The influence of size, dose, time, and technical factors on obliteration rate. J Neurosurg 83:832–837, 1995.
34. Schneider BF, Eberhard DA, Steiner LE: Histopathology of arteriovenous malformations after gamma knife radiosurgery. J Neurosurg 87:352–357, 1997.
35. Hurst RW, Berenstein A, Kupersmith MJ, et al: Deep central arteriovenous malformations of the brain: The role of endovascular treatment. J Neurosurg 82:190–195, 1995.
36. Lawton MT, Hamilton MG, Spetzler RF: Multimodality treatment of deep arteriovenous malformations: Thalamus, basal ganglia, and brain stem. Neurosurgery 37:29–36, 1995.
37. Paulsen RD, Steinberg GK, Norbash AM, et al: Embolization of basal ganglia and thalamic arteriovenous malformations. Neurosurgery 44:991–997, 1999.
38. Hamilton MG, Spetzler RF: The prospective application of a grading system for arteriovenous malformations. Neurosurgery 34:2–7, 1994.
39. Heros RC, Korosue K, Diebold PM: Surgical excision cerebral arteriovenous malformations: Late results. Neurosurgery 26:570–578, 1990.
40. Spetzler RF, Martin NA: A proposed grading system for arteriovenous malformations. J Neurosurg 65:476–483, 1986.
41. Batjer HH, Devous MD, Seibert B, et al: Intracranial arteriovenous malformation: Relationship between clinical factors and surgical complications. Neurosurgery 24:75–79, 1989.
42. Spetzler RF, Wilson CB, Weinstein P, et al: Normal perfusion pressure theory. Clin Neurosurg 25:651–672, 1978.
43. Al-Rodhan NRF, Sundt TM, Piepgras DG, et al: Occlusive hyperemia: A theory for the hemodynamic complications following resection of intracerebral arteriovenous malformations. J Neurosurg 78:167–175, 1993.
44. Deruty R, Pelissou-Guyotat I, Amat D, et al: Multidisciplinary treatment of cerebral arteriovenous malformations. Neurol Res 17:169–177, 1995.
45. Spetzler RF, Martin NA, Carter LP, et al: Surgical management of large AVM's by staged embolization and operative excision. J Neurosurg 67:17–28, 1987.
46. Andrews BT, Wilson CB: Staged treatment of arteriovenous malformations. Neurosurgery 21:314–323, 1987.
47. Purdy PD, Batjer JJ, Risser RC, Samson D: Arteriovenous malformations of the brain: Choosing embolic materials to enhance safety and ease of excision. J Neurosurg 77:217–222, 1992.
48. DeMeritt JS, Pile-Spellman J, Mast H, et al: Outcome analysis of preoperative embolization with N-butyl cyanoacrylate in cerebral arteriovenous malformations. AJNR Am J Neuroradiol 16:1801–1807, 1995.
49. Vinuela F, Dion JE, Duckwiler G, et al: Combined endovascular embolization and surgery in the management of cerebral arteriovenous malformations: Experience with 101 cases. J Neurosurg 75:856–864, 1991.
50. Jordan JE, Marks MP, Lane B, Steinberg GK: Cost-effectiveness of endovascular therapy in the surgical management of cerebral arteriovenous malformations. AJNR Am J Neuroradiol 17:247–254, 1996.
51. Flickinger JC, Pollock BE, Kondziolka D, Lunsford LD: A dose-response analysis of arteriovenous malformation obliteration by radiosurgery. Int J Radiat Oncol Biol Phys 36:873–879, 1996.
52. Flickinger JC, Kondziolka D, Lunsford LD, et al: Development of a model to predict permanent symptomatic post-radiosurgery injury for arteriovenous malformation patients. Int J Radiat Oncol Biol Phys 46:1143–1148, 2000.
53. Lax I, Karlsson B: Prediction of complications in gamma knife radiosurgery of arteriovenous malformations. Acta Oncol 35: 49–56, 1996.
54. Flickinger JC: An integrated logistic formula and prediction of complications from radiosurgery. Int J Radiat Oncol Biol Phys 17:879–885, 1989.
55. Gobin YP, Laurent A, Merienne L, et al: Treatment of brain arteriovenous malformations by embolization and radiosurgery. J Neurosurg 85:19–28, 1996.
56. Mathis JA, Barr JD, Horton JA, et al: The efficacy of particulate embolization combined with stereotactic radiosurgery for treatment of large arteriovenous malformations of the brain. AJNR Am J Neuroradiol 16:299–306, 1995.
57. Wikholm G, Lundqvist C, Svendsen P: Embolization of cerebral arteriovenous malformations: Part I. Technique, morphology, and complications. Neurosurgery 39:448–459, 1996.
58. Wikholm G, Lundqvist C, Svendsen P: Embolization of cerebral arteriovenous malformations: Part II. Aspects of complications and late outcome. Neurosurgery 39:460–469, 1996.
59. Pollock BE, Kondziolka D, Lunsford LD, et al: Repeat stereotactic radiosurgery of arteriovenous malformations: Factors associated with incomplete obliteration. Neurosurgery 38:318–324, 1996.
60. Pollock BE, Kline RW, Stafford SL, et al: The rationale and technique of staged-volume arteriovenous malformation radiosurgery. Int J Radiat Oncol Biol Phys 48:817–824, 2000.
61. Friedman WA, Blatt DL, Bova FJ, et al: The risk of hemorrhage after radiosurgery for arteriovenous malformations. J Neurosurg 84:912–919, 1996.
62. Karlsson B, Lindquist C, Steiner L: The effect of gamma knife surgery on the risk of rupture prior to AVM obliteration. Minim Invasive Neurosurg 39:21–27, 1996.
63. Mullan S: Reflections upon the nature and management of intra-

cranial and intraspinal vascular malformations and fistulae. J Neurosurg 80:606–616, 1994.
64. Borden JA, Wu JK, Shucart WA: A proposed classification for spinal and cranial dural arteriovenous fistulous malformations and implications for treatment. J Neurosurg 82:166–179, 1995.
65. Cognard C, Gobin YP, Pierot L, et al: Cerebral dural arteriovenous fistulas: Clinical and angiographic correlation with a revised classification of venous drainage. Neuroradiology 194:671–680, 1995.
66. Davies MA, TerBrugge K, Willinsky R, et al: The validity of classification for the clinical presentation of intracranial dural arteriovenous fistulas. J Neurosurg 85:830–837, 1996.
67. Lucas CP, Zabramski JM, Spetzler RF, Jacobowitz R: Treatment for intracranial dural arteriovenous malformations: A meta-analysis from the English language literature. Neurosurgery 40:1119–1132, 1997.
68. Grossman RI, Sergott RC, Goldberg HI, et al: Dural malformations with ophthalmic manifestations: Results of particulate embolization in seven patients. AJNR Am J Neuroradiol 6:809–813, 1985.
69. Kupersmith MJ, Berenstein A, Choi IS, et al: Management of nontraumatic vascular shunts involving the cavernous sinus. Ophthalmology 95:121–130, 1988.
70. Halvach VV, Higashida RT, Hieshima GB, et al: Transvenous embolization of dural fistulas involving the cavernous sinus. AJNR Am J Neuroradiol 10:377–383, 1989.
71. Halvach VV, Higashida RT, Hieshima GB, et al: Transvenous embolization of dural fistulas involving the transverse and sigmoid sinuses. AJNR Am J Neuroradiol 10:385–392, 1989.
72. Halbach VV, Higashida RT, Hieshima GB, et al: Treatment of dural fistulas involving the deep cerebral venous system. AJNR Am J Neuroradiol 10:393–399, 1989.
73. Dawson RC, Joseph GJ, Owens DS, Barrow DL: Transvenous embolization as the primary therapy for arteriovenous fistulas of the lateral and sigmoid sinuses. AJNR Am J Neuroradiol 19: 571–576, 1998.
74. McDougall CG, Halbach VV, Dowd CF, et al: Dural arteriovenous fistulas of the marginal sinus. AJNR Am J Neuroradiol 18:1865–1872, 1997.
75. Roy D, Raymond J: The role of transvenous embolization in the treatment of intracranial dural arteriovenous fistulas. Neurosurgery 40:1133–1144, 1997.
76. Goto, K, Sidipratomo P, Ogato N, et al: Combining endovascular and neurosurgical treatments of high-risk dural arteriovenous fistulas in the lateral sinus and the confluence of the sinuses. J Neurosurg 90:289–299, 1999.
77. Lewis AI, Tomsick TA, Tew JM Jr: Management of tentorial arteriovenous malformations: Transarterial embolization combined with stereotactic radiation or surgery. J Neurosurg 81: 851–859, 1994.
78. Morita A, Meyer FB, Nichols DA, Patterson MC: Childhood dural arteriovenous fistulae of the posterior dural sinuses: Three case reports and literature review. Neurosurgery 37:1193–1200, 1995.
79. Barcia-Salorio JL, Soler F, Hernandez G, Barcia JA: Radiosurgical treatment of low flow carotid-cavernous fistulae. Acta Neurochir 52:93–95, 1991.
80. Chandler HC Jr, Friedman WA: Successful radiosurgical treatment of a dural arteriovenous malformation: Case report. Neurosurgery 33:139–142, 1993.
81. Coffey RJ, Link MJ, Nichols DA, et al: Gamma knife radiosurgery and particulate embolization of dural arteriovenous fistulas, with a special emphasis on the cavernous sinus. In Lunsford LD, Kondziolka D, Flickinger JC (eds): Gamma Knife Brain Surgery. Basel, Karger, 1998, pp 60–77.
82. Guo W, Pan DHC, Wu H, et al: Radiosurgery as a treatment alternative for dural arteriovenous fistulas of the cavernous sinus. AJNR Am J Neuroradiol 19:1081–1087, 1998.
83. Link MJ, Coffey RJ, Nichols DA, Gorman DA: The role of radiosurgery and particulate embolization in the treatment of dural arteriovenous fistulas. J Neurosurg 84:804–809, 1996.
84. Pollock BE, Nichols DA, Garrity JA, et al: Stereotactic radiosurgery and particulate embolization of cavernous sinus dural arteriovenous fistulae. Neurosurgery 45:459–467, 1999.
85. Day JD, Fukushima T: Direct microsurgery of dural arteriovenous malformations type carotid-cavernous sinus fistulas: Indications, technique, and results. Neurosurgery 41:1119–1126, 1997.
86. Tu YK, Liu HM, Hu SC: Direct surgery of carotid cavernous fistulae and dural arteriovenous malformations of the cavernous sinus. Neurosurgery 41:798–806, 1997.
87. Miller NR, Monsein LH, Debrun GM, et al: Treatment of carotid-cavernous sinus fistulas using a superior ophthalmic vein approach. J Neurosurg 83:838–842, 1998.

Traumatic Cerebral Aneurysms Secondary to Penetrating Intracranial Injuries

GAVIN W. BRITZ ■ DAVID W. NEWELL ■ G. ALEXANDER WEST ■ H. RICHARD WINN

Traumatic intracranial aneurysms may be the result of either penetrating or nonpenetrating trauma.[1–3] Traumatic aneurysms were first described in 1895 by Guibert,[4] and despite the common occurrence of head trauma, they are rare entities, representing less than 1% of all intracranial aneurysms.[5–13] The risk of developing a traumatic intracranial aneurysm depends on the mechanism of injury, with aneurysm formation being much less likely following closed head injury than penetrating trauma. In addition to their occurrence after traditional trauma, traumatic aneurysms have been reported to occur iatrogenically, such as after transsphenoidal surgery,[14–18] sinus surgery,[17, 19] ventricular taps,[20, 21] stereotactic brain biopsy,[22] and endoscopic third ventriculostomy.[23]

Penetrating trauma can be divided into low-velocity injuries, such as those created by knives, screwdrivers, and shotgun pellets,[24] or high-velocity injuries caused by missiles such as bullets and shrapnel. South Africa has provided much of the literature with respect to low-velocity injuries, which are prevalent in this region, with stab wounds to the brain accounting for up to 6% of all trauma admissions.[7, 25] The incidence of aneurysm formation following this type of injury may be as high as 10% to 12%.[7, 25, 26]

With respect to missile injuries, conflicts in Lebanon, Iraq, and Iran have demonstrated aneurysm formation in 0.1% to 8% of patients sustaining this type of injury. The incidence is related to velocity, with lower-velocity shrapnel injuries having a higher incidence of aneurysm formation than higher-velocity bullet injuries.[1, 3, 5, 27] The American experience was obtained during the Vietnam War and reported by Ferry and Kempe, who demonstrated only 2 traumatic aneurysms in 2187 patients with penetrating head trauma, primarily gunshot wounds.[27]

Despite the rarity of traumatic intracranial aneurysms, they have a mortality rate of 30%.[5] This outcome is related more to the primary injury than to the aneurysm itself.[3] However, it is important to make the diagnosis and offer surgical treatment, because secondary insults affect the neurological outcome of patients.

PATHOLOGY

In penetrating trauma, the traumatic event disrupts the elements of the vessel wall, which may involve varying amounts of intima, media, and adventitia.[28] Depending on the degree of involvement of the different internal structures, a false aneurysm, true aneurysm, dissection, or fistula may occur.

Aneurysms are defined as true or false based on histologic findings. True aneurysms demonstrate outpouching of the intima through the media, with fragmentation of the internal elastic membrane, resulting in an aneurysm wall consisting of intima separated from the adventitia by fibrous tissue. True aneurysms account for the majority of saccular aneurysms associated with aneurysmal subarachnoid hemorrhage, but they are much less common after trauma. In contrast, false aneurysms, which form the majority of traumatic intracranial aneurysms, are essentially contained hematomas, with disruption of all three layers of the vessel wall. The distinction between a true aneurysm and a false one requires histologic analysis, so it is not always possible to distinguish them on angiography. The more inclusive term *pseudoaneurysm* is often used to describe aneurysms related to trauma.

Traumatic aneurysms occur distally in the vascular tree, in contrast to the proximal bifurcation site of saccular aneurysms. This peripheral location reflects the underlying mechanism of injury. The anterior circulation is most often affected, with the peripheral branches of the middle cerebral artery the most frequent site, followed by branches of the pericallosal vessels.[3]

In penetrating injuries, the velocity of the projectile correlates inversely with aneurysm formation; that is, the lower the velocity, the more likely aneurysm formation is. For example, traumatic aneurysms are 14 times more likely in shrapnel injuries than in bullet injuries, which are of a higher velocity.[3] Shotgun[29, 30] and low-caliber wounds[29, 31, 32] also have a higher incidence of traumatic aneurysm formation than do injuries caused by high-velocity missiles. Bullets having a higher velocity and thus greater kinetic injury are more likely to rupture a vessel rather than merely damage the wall.[3] Further support for this theory is the very high incidence of traumatic aneurysm after stab wounds to the brain in the South African experience.[7, 25, 26] Traumatic aneurysms have also been described in skull fractures, and in this type of penetrating trauma, it has been postulated that momentary herniation of the cerebral cortex and vessel through the fracture results in aneurysm formation.[33]

Traumatic fistulas are abnormal connections between the intracranial arterial and venous circulation that can occur after severe or even relatively minor nonpenetrating trauma. Occasionally they result from penetrating trauma, with the most common location being the cavernous sinus and the formation of a carotid cavernous fistula—an acquired communication 136between the intracranial carotid artery and the cavernous sinus.[34] This communication may occur at the time of trauma or in a delayed fashion if a false aneurysm is created that ruptures later. Dural fistulas may also occur after penetrating trauma; in this type of fistula, the abnormal communication between the intracranial arterial and venous circulation lies within the dura.[35] These dural fistulas may occur in relation to the cavernous sinus and other venous sinuses, including the transverse and sigmoid sinuses.[36–39]

Much less common is the formation of dissecting aneurysms following penetrating trauma. These may occur at the skull base and involve the internal carotid artery and vertebrobasilar system. Dissecting aneurysms occur when injury to one or more of the arterial layers allows blood to force its way between the vessel layers along a dissection plane,[9] creating an intimal flap.[40] This intimal flap may act as a nidus for embolic material or may occlude the arterial lumen. Occasionally, dissections originate within the media or adventitia, and in this situation, rupture may occur through the adventitia, with resultant subarachnoid hemorrhage or pseudoaneurysm formation.[41] Dissections are more common after nonpenetrating trauma[42–44] and may occur spontaneously.[45, 46]

CLINICAL PRESENTATION

The initial clinical presentation of patients with head injuries, regardless of whether they have traumatic intracranial aneurysms, is largely related to the primary brain injury, with the initial Glasgow Coma Scale score being a good predictor of outcome.[3, 47] Secondary presentations are related to the location and type of the vascular injury. In aneurysms involving the peripheral vascular tree, there is delayed neurological deterioration, usually within 3 weeks of injury.[7] Because most traumatic aneurysms are false aneurysms, intracranial hemorrhage is often the reason for this deterioration, but cerebral edema from the initial coexisting hemorrhage or stroke may be responsible. Patients with multiple episodes of hemorrhage tend to do poorly,[48] so it is best to have a high index of suspicion for traumatic aneurysm and make the diagnosis before its overt clinical presentation.

In patients with aneurysms involving the infraclinoid internal carotid artery, severe and life-threatening epistaxis can be the presenting event if the arterial injury communicates with a sphenoidal sinus fracture.[31, 49–53] Aneurysms in this location may also present with a bruit, chemosis, exophthalmos, visual loss, and cranial neuropathies referable to the cavernous sinus and formation of a carotid cavernous fistula.[15, 49, 50] The extent of these symptoms largely depends on the size of arterial injury and the adequacy of venous drainage.[35]

Dural fistulas often present in a delayed fashion, with pulsatile tinnitus or headaches as the only features. A less common presentation is neurological deterioration secondary to an embolic stroke, which occurs with dissecting aneurysms involving the intracranial vessels, or mass effect secondary to an enlarging unruptured pseudoaneurysm, particularly in children.[54]

DIAGNOSIS

The most common cause of subarachnoid hemorrhage is trauma, so the diagnosis of traumatic intracranial aneurysm requires a high index of suspicion. This diagnosis is important, because patients with multiple episodes of hemorrhage or neurological insults do poorly.[48] Computed tomography is usually the first investigation, and this may demonstrate nonspecific hemorrhages, infarctions, and skull base fractures. Penetrating trauma often has associated intracranial hemorrhage, and with missile injuries, concomitant intracerebral hemorrhage is found in 39% to 80% of cases,[3, 5] with 26% of patients having subdural hemorrhages.[3] In low-velocity penetrating injuries, de Trevou and van Dellen demonstrated that 50% of patients had evidence of an intracerebral hemorrhage.[26]

Cerebral angiography is the gold standard and should be obtained in the setting of all penetrating trauma.[7, 55, 56] This is particularly important in patients with orbitopterional injuries; penetrating fragments; and subarachnoid, intracerebral, or subdural hemorrhage.[3, 5, 26, 57] In penetrating trauma, traumatic aneurysms may be visualized on angiography as early as 2 hours after the injury, but the majority of aneurysms manifest angiographically in 2 to 3 weeks, with a mean of 20 days (median, 13 days).[5] Therefore, it has been suggested that the first angiogram should be obtained at the beginning of the second week after injury.[7] In patients with a higher probability of having or developing a traumatic aneurysm (e.g., those with stab wounds), angiography shortly after admission should be considered. Computed tomography–angiography can also be performed as a screening study and may reveal an unsuspected aneurysm. The timing of the angiogram is important, and it is not unusual for the first angiogram to be negative in those with penetrating trauma.[1, 31, 58] Twenty percent of traumatic aneurysms are multiple, and each individual aneurysm may regress, enlarge, or form in a delayed fashion.[3, 6] Therefore, most authors agree that a follow-up angiogram should be obtained even if the initial one was negative. The second angiogram should be performed at least 3 weeks after injury, and it could be argued that a third angiogram should be performed 6 weeks after injury.

TREATMENT

The treatment of a traumatic aneurysm depends on the location, type of vascular injury, and mode of presentation. In a patient with a large, life-threatening intracerebral hemorrhage, rapid removal of the hematoma is required, and the vascular injury needs to be dealt with. The outcome is generally worse following secondary brain insults, so it is important to diagnose a traumatic aneurysm early; treatment of these aneurysms may be complicated.

Surgery has been the traditional method of therapy, with ligation of the carotid artery in the neck historically used for traumatic aneurysms involving the intracranial internal carotid artery.[59] Traumatic intracranial aneurysms have been documented to disappear on repeat angiograms,[1, 3, 6] with Amirjamshidi and coworkers reporting that 19.4% of the aneurysms in their patients disappeared.[60] This finding has not been supported by all authors, and most recommend that once a traumatic aneurysm has been diagnosed, therapy should be instituted. The principle of managing a saccular aneurysm is to exclude the aneurysmal bulge from the circulation by clipping or coiling, with preservation of the parent vessel and its branches. Traumatic aneurysms, however, are mostly false aneurysms, so this approach is often not possible; successful clipping has been reported, but it is unusual.[23, 61, 62] Therefore, in traumatic aneurysms, the preoperative planning must include the possibility of excising the involved vessel, as well as the high probability of having an intraoperative rupture.

In very distal vessels, the likelihood of an ischemic event following resection of the aneurysm is small, and these aneurysms are often excised with no complications.[3, 5, 63] In more proximal vessels, preparation for a vascular bypass should be considered, with the surgical approach allowing for access to the superficial temporal artery, the saphenous vein, or both. In addition to a vascular bypass, an interposition graft using the superficial temporal artery can be placed.[64] Some aneurysms may not be amenable to either resection or bypass; in those cases, wrapping with Dacron mesh or muslin may be performed.

Over the last 3 decades, endovascular techniques have advanced, and intravascular embolization and occlusion now play a larger role in the management of intracranial traumatic arterial injuries.[65–67] Endovascular therapy has not been a mainstay of treatment for traumatic aneurysms in the peripheral vascular tree owing to the high incidence of false aneurysms and the risk of rupture. Recently, however, coils have successfully been placed in traumatic aneurysms.[68]

Endovascular therapy has become more important in vascular injuries involving the skull base.[69] Traumatic aneurysms involving the skull base are difficult to access and control surgically. In carotid injuries, the options include the endovascular occlusion of the carotid artery at the skull base, a bypass graft, or, rarely, direct repair of the vessel. Stenting may play an important role in the future. Before carotid occlusion, collateral circulation needs to be evaluated using balloon test occlusion. Adequate collateral circulation is defined as symmetrical angiographic filling of both hemispheres. Awake patients are also examined continuously for neurological deficits. In patients with evidence of adequate cross-flow and collateral flow based on transcranial Doppler studies, angiography, and balloon test occlusion, simple endovascular occlusion can be performed.[53, 70] Patients who deteriorate clinically or whose middle cerebral artery transcranial Doppler velocities decrease by 60% have inadequate collateral flow.[71] In these patients, alternative therapies have to be considered. These include a direct attack on the carotid artery in the skull base, including the cavernous sinus, which has had variable success.[72–74] Most authors would advocate an extracranial-to-intracranial bypass.[53] Saphenous vein bypass graft can be used, with sacrifice of the internal carotid artery surgically.[64] In some patients, both endovascular and surgical techniques can be used simultaneously to achieve optimal results.[64]

Intracranial dissections pose the risk of both hemorrhage and stroke. To prevent these complications, medical, surgical, and endovascular methods have been described. Medical therapy consists of anticoagulation with either antiplatelet therapy or warfarin (Coumadin) to prevent thrombotic and embolic complications, but it carries the risk of intracranial hemorrhage. Endovascular therapy now offers the alternatives of angioplasty and stent deployment to restore vessel patency. This method is based on using a balloon to dilate the restriction and then stenting back the intimal flap.

CONCLUSION

Traumatic intracranial aneurysms are a rare but important surgical problem in patients with penetrating intracranial trauma. Secondary neurological insults can impair recovery, so traumatic vascular injuries should be considered in all cases of penetrating injury. Angiography is required to make the diagnosis, and the test should be repeated even if the fist angiogram is negative, because traumatic vascular injuries can develop in a delayed fashion. Surgery is still the mainstay of treatment, but endovascular therapy is becoming an important aspect of care in patients with traumatic vascular injuries, particularly those involving the skull base.

REFERENCES

1. Aarabi B: Traumatic aneurysm of brain due to high velocity missile head wounds. Neurosurgery 22:1056, 1988.
2. Bostrom K, Helander CG, Lindgren SO: Blunt basilar head trauma: Rupture of posterior inferior cerebellar artery. Forensic Sci Int 53:61–68, 1992.
3. Han MH, Sung MW, Chang KH, et al: Traumatic pseudoaneurysm of the intracavernous ICA presenting with massive epistaxis: Imaging diagnosis and endovascular treatment. Laryngoscope 104:370, 1994.
4. Guibert J: Anevrisme arteriel de la carotide interne au niveau du sinus caverneux, communication avec le sinus sphenoidal droit, hemorrhagies nasales, mort, autopsie. Ann Oculist 113:314–318, 1895.
5. Aarabi B: Management of traumatic aneurysms caused by high-velocity missile head wounds. Neurosurg Clin N Am 6:775–796, 1995.
6. Fleisher AS, Patton JM, Tindall GT: Cerebral aneurysms of traumatic origin. Surg Neurol 4:233–239, 1975.
7. Kiek CF, de Villiers JC: Vascular lesions due to transcranial stab wounds. J Neurosurg 60:42–46, 1984.
8. McLaughlin MR, Wahlig JB, Kaufman AM, Albright AL: Traumatic basilar aneurysm after endoscopic third ventriculostomy: Case report. Neurosurgery 41:1400–1403, 1997.
9. Melvill RL, de Villiers JC: Peripheral cerebral arterial aneurysms caused by stabbing. S Afr Med J 51:471–473, 1977.
10. Mendel R, Carter L: Intracranial arterial injury. In Carter L, Spetzler R, Hamilton M (eds): Neurovascular Surgery. New York, McGraw-Hill, 1995, p 1301.
11. Shinoda S, Murata H, Waga S, Koijima T: Bilateral spontaneous dissection of the posteroinferior cerebellar arteries: Case report. Neurosurgery 43:357–359, 1998.
12. van Dellen JR: Intracavernous traumatic aneurysms. Surg Neurol 13:203–207, 1980.
13. Wortzman D, Tucker WS, Gershater R: Traumatic aneurysm in the posterior fossa. Surg Neurol 13:329–331, 1980.
14. Ali S, Bihari J: Intracranial traumatic aneurysm following hypophysectomy. J Laryngol Otol 95:749–755, 1981.
15. Awad I, Sawhny B, Little JR: Traumatic postsurgical aneurysm of the intracavernous carotid artery: A delayed presentation. Surg Neurol 18:54–57, 1982.
16. Dolenc VV, Lipovsek M, Slokan S: Traumatic aneurysm and carotid-cavernous fistula following transsphenoidal approach to pituitary adenoma: Treatment by transcranial operation. Br J Neurosurg 13:185–188, 1999.
17. Levy ML, Litofsky SN, Rezai A, et al: The significance of subarachnoid hemorrhage following penetrating craniocerebral injury: Correlation with angiography and outcome in a civilian population. Neurosurgery 32:532–540, 1993.
18. Morard M, de Tribolet N: Traumatic aneurysm of the posterior inferior cerebellar artery: Case report. Neurosurgery 29:438–441, 1991.
19. Barret JH, Lawrence VL: Aneurysm of the internal carotid artery as a complication of mastoidectomy. Arch Otolaryngol 72:366–368, 1960.
20. Lam CH, Montes J, Farmer JP, et al: Traumatic aneurysm from shaken baby syndrome: Case report. Neurosurgery 39:1252–1255, 1996.
21. Sahrakar K, Boggan JE, Salamat MS: Traumatic aneurysm: A complication of stereotactic brain biopsy: Case report. Neurosurgery 36:842–846, 1995.
22. Salar G, Mingrino S: Traumatic intracranial internal carotid aneurysms due to gunshot wounds: Case report. J Neurosurg 49: 100–102, 1978.
23. Lylyk P, Vianuela F, Campos J, et al: Diagnosis and endovascular therapy of vascular lesions in the cavernous sinus. Acta Radiol Suppl 369:584, 1986.
24. Courville CB: Traumatic aneurysm of an intracranial artery: Description of a lesion incident to a shotgun wound of the skull and brain. Bull LA Neurol Soc 25:48–54, 1960.
25. Meguro K, Rowed DW: Traumatic aneurysms of the posterior inferior cerebellar artery caused by fracture of the clivus. Neurosurgery 16:666–668, 1985.
26. de Trevou MD, van Dellen JR: Penetrating stab wounds to the brain: The timing of angiography in patients with weapon already removed. Neurosurgery 31:905, 1992.
27. Ferry DJ, Kempe LG: False aneurysm secondary to penetration of the brain through orbitofacial wounds. J Neurosurg 36:503, 1972.
28. Britz GW, Mayberg MR: Pathology of cerebral aneurysms and subarachnoid hemorrhage. In Welch KMA, Caplan LR, Reis DJ, et al (eds): Primer on Cerebrovascular Diseases. New York, Academic Press, 1997, pp 498–502.
29. Acosta C, Williams PE, Clark K: Traumatic aneurysms of the cerebral vessels. J Neurosurg 36:531–536, 1972.
30. Asari S, Nakamura S, Yamada O, et al: Traumatic aneurysm of peripheral cerebral arteries: Report of two cases. J Neurosurg 46: 795–803, 1977.
31. Rumbaugh CL, Bergerson RT, Talalla A, et al: Traumatic aneurysms of the cortical cerebral arteries. Radiology 96:49, 1970.
32. Sadar ES, Jane JA, Lewis LW, et al: Traumatic aneurysms of the intracranial circulation. Surg Gynecol Obstet 137:59–67, 1973.
33. Rahimizadeh A, Abtahi H, Daylami MS, et al: Traumatic cerebral aneurysms caused by shell fragments: Report of four cases and review of the literature. Acta Neurochir (Wien) 84:93–98, 1987.
34. Greatz KW, Imhof HG, Valavanis A: Traumatic carotid cavernous sinus fistula due to a gun shot injury. Int J Oral Maxillofac Surg 20:280, 1991.
35. Hemphill JC, Gress DR, Halbach VV: Endovascular therapy of traumatic injuries of the intracranial cerebral arteries. Crit Care Clin 15:811–829, 1999.
36. Halbach VV, Higashida RT, Hieshmima GB, et al: Dural fistulas involving the transverse and sigmoid sinuses: Results of treatment in 28 patients. Radiology 163:443, 1987.
37. Halbach VV, Hieshmima GB, Higashida RT, et al: Carotid cavernous fistulae: Indications for urgent treatment. AJR Am J Roentgenol 149:587, 1987.
38. Halbach VV, Higashida RT, Hieshmima GB, et al: Transvenous embolization of dural fistulas involving the cavernous sinus. AJNR Am J Neuroradiol 10:377, 1989.
39. Halbach VV, Higashida RT, Barnwell SL, et al: Transarterial platinum coil embolization of carotid-cavernous fistulas. AJR Am J Roentgenol 12:429, 1991.
40. Yokota H, Tazaki H, Murayama K, et al: Traumatic cerebral aneurysm: 94 cases from the literature and 5 cases observed by the authors. No Shinkei Geka 11:521–528, 1983.
41. Yonas H, Agamanolis D, Takaoka Y, et al: Dissecting intracranial aneurysms. Surg Neurol 8:407, 1977.
42. Auer RN, Kreck J, Butt JC: Delayed symptoms and death after minor head injury with occult vertebral injury. J Neurol Neurosurg Psychiatry 57:500–502, 1994.
43. Jafar JJ, Kamiryo T, Chiles BW, Nelson PK: A dissecting aneurysm of the posterior inferior cerebellar artery: Case report. Neurosurgery 43:353–356, 1998.
44. Kumar M, Kitchen ND: Infective and traumatic aneurysms. Neurosurg Clin N Am 9:577–586, 1998.
45. Paullus WS Jr, Norwood CW, Morgan HW: False aneurysm of the cavernous carotid artery and progressive external ophthalmoplegia after transsphenoidal hypophysectomy: Case report. J Neurosurg 51:707–709, 1979.
46. Schuster JM, Santiago P, Elliot JP, et al: Acute traumatic posteroinferior cerebellar artery aneurysms: Report of three cases. Neurosurgery 45:1465–1468, 1999.
47. Aarabi B, Koleini MK: Traumatic aneurysms due to missile head wounds: Report of twenty cases. Iran J Med Sci 14:26–32, 1989.
48. Buckingham MJ, Crone CR, Ball WS, et al: Traumatic intracranial aneurysms in childhood. Neurosurgery 22:398, 1988.
49. Bavinzski G, Killer M, Knosp E, et al: False aneurysms of the intracavernous carotid artery—report of 7 cases. Acta Neurochir (Wien) 139:37–43, 1997.
50. Bavinzski G, Killer M, Gruber A, et al: Treatment of post-traumatic carotico-cavernous fistula using electrolytically detachable coils: Technical aspects and preliminary experience. Neuroradiology 39:81, 1997.
51. Dial DL, Maurer GB: Intracranial aneurysms: Report of 13 cases. Am J Surg 35:2–21, 1937.
52. Jackson FE, Augusta FA, Sazima HJ, et al: Head injury and delayed epistaxis: Report of case of rupture of traumatic aneurysms of internal carotid artery due to grenade fragment wound received in Vietnam conflict. J Trauma 10:1158–1167, 1970.

53. Teitelbaum GP, Bernstein K, Choi S, et al: Endovascular coil occlusion of a traumatic basilar-cavernous fistula: Technical report. Neurosurgery 42:1394, 1998.
54. Endo S, Takaku A, Aihara H, et al: Traumatic cerebral aneurysm associated with widening skull fracture. Childs Brain 6:131, 1980.
55. Achram M, Rizk G, Haddad FS: Angiographic aspects of traumatic intracranial aneurysms following war injuries. Br J Radiol 53:1144–1149, 1980.
56. Haddad FS: Nature and management of penetrating head injuries during the civil war in Lebanon. Can J Surg 21:233–240, 1978.
57. Lempert TE, Halbach VV, Higashida RT, et al: Endovascular treatment of pseudoaneurysms with electrolytically detachable coils. AJNR Am J Neuroradiol 19:907, 1998.
58. Capanna AH: Traumatic intracranial aneurysms and Gradenigo's syndrome secondary to gunshot wound. Surg Neurol 22:263–266, 1984.
59. Cooper A: Account of the first successful operation performed on the common carotid artery for aneurysm in the year 1808: With the post-mortem examination, 1821. Guys Hosp Rep (Lond) 1:53, 1836.
60. Amirjamshidi A, Rahmat H, Abbassioun K: Traumatic aneurysms and arteriovenous fistulas of intracranial vessels associated with penetrating head injuries occurring during war: Principles and pitfalls in diagnosis and management. A survey of 31 cases and review of the literature. J Neurosurg 84:769–780, 1996.
61. Ding MX: Traumatic aneurysm of the intracavernous part of the internal carotid artery presenting with epistaxis: Case report. Surg Neurol 30:65–67, 1988.
62. Serbinenko FA, Lazarev VA: Use of balloon catheter in cases of traumatic pseudoaneurysm of the carotid artery complicated by profuse nosebleed. Zh Vopr Neirokhir 6:9–16, 1981.
63. Pozzati E, Gaist G, Poppi M: Resolution of occlusion in spontaneously dissected carotid arteries. J Neurosurg 56:857, 1982.
64. Horowitz MB, Kopitnik TA, Landreneau F, et al: Multidisciplinary approach to traumatic intracranial aneurysms secondary to shotgun and handgun wounds. Surg Neurol 51:31–42, 1999.
65. Chen D, Concus AP, Halbach VV, et al: Epistaxis originating from traumatic pseudoaneurysm of the internal carotid artery: Diagnosis and endovascular therapy. Laryngoscope 108:326, 1998.
66. Higashida RT, Halbach VV, Dowd C, et al: Interventional neurovascular treatment of traumatic carotid and vertebral artery lesions: Results in 234 cases. AJR Am J Roentgenol 153:577, 1989.
67. Sure U, Becker R, Petermeyer M, Bertalanffy H: Aneurysm of the posterior inferior cerebellar artery caused by a traumatic perforating artery tear-out mechanism in a child. Childs Nerv Syst 15:354–356, 1999.
68. Lassman LP, Ramani PS, Sengupta RP: Aneurysms of peripheral cerebral arteries due to surgical trauma. Vasc Surg 8:1–5, 1974.
69. Lister JR, Sypert GW: Traumatic false aneurysm and carotid-cavernous fistula: A complication of sphenoidotomy. Neurosurgery 5:473–475, 1979.
70. Scharfetter F, Fodisch HJ, Menardi G, et al: Falsches Aneurysma der Arteria gyri angularis durch Gefassverletzung bei einer Ventrikpunktion. Acta Neurochir (Wien) 33:123–132, 1976.
71. Hetzel A, von Reutern G, Wernz MG, et al: The carotid compression test for therapeutic occlusion of the internal carotid artery: Comparison of angiography with transcranial Doppler sonography. Cerebrovasc Dis 10:194–199, 2000.
72. Dolenc V: Direct microsurgical repair of intracavernous vascular lesions. J Neurosurg 58:824–831, 1983.
73. Fabian G: Traumatisches Aneurysma der Carotis interna in der Keilbeinhole. Hals-Nasen-Ohrenbeilk 3:346–349, 1952.
74. Uzan M, Cantasdemir M, Seckin MS, et al: Traumatic intracranial carotid tree aneurysms. Neurosurgery 43:1314–1320, 1998.

PART IX TRUE ARTERIOVENOUS MALFORMATIONS

CHAPTER 126

Hemorrhagic Disease: Arteriovascular Malformations

IAN G. FLEETWOOD ■ MARK G. HAMILTON

This chapter provides an overview of the various intracranial vascular malformations. Traditionally, these lesions are classified based on histopathologic features as (1) capillary telangiectasias, (2) developmental venous anomalies, (3) cavernous malformations, and (4) true arteriovenous malformations (AVMs).[1–3] The epidemiology, pathophysiology, clinical presentation, natural history, imaging studies, and treatment of each of these entities are reviewed (Table 126–1). Current controversies regarding the pathogenesis of these lesions and the so-called mixed malformations are discussed, followed by a brief review of syndromic vascular malformations, including those associated with Rendu-Osler-Weber syndrome (hereditary hemorrhagic telangiectasia) and Wyburn-Mason syndrome. Dural arteriovenous fistulas are not discussed in this chapter because they are considered acquired lesions; the arteriovascular malformations reviewed here are congenital.[1–3] Later chapters provide a more in-depth analysis of the surgical principles and techniques related to the more clinically significant arteriovascular malformations.

CAPILLARY TELANGIECTASIAS

Epidemiology

Capillary telangiectasias represent the second most common vascular malformations affecting the brain. They also have been referred to as *capillary malformations*. Based on large autopsy series, their estimated prevalence is 0.3%,[4] whereas that of all arteriovascular malformations is 0.1% to 4.0%.[5] Other general autopsy series quote a lower prevalence of 0.04% to 0.1%.[6] Capillary telangiectasias compose 12.4% of angiographically occult vascular malformations,[7] and no current evidence supports the presence of an underlying genetic abnormality that predisposes these lesions to form. Remote case reports of familial occurrence exist[8, 9]; however, whether these reports represented capillary telangiectasias or cavernous malformations is unclear.

Pathology and Pathophysiology

With the exception of their dilated nature, vessels in capillary telangiectasias are otherwise similar to normal cerebral capillaries. Their enlargement sets them apart pathologically. The number of capillaries does not increase.[10] These malformations are usually small (<2.0 cm in diameter)[11]; however, a case report described a capillary telangiectasia with a diameter of 5 cm.[12]

Capillary telangiectasias tend to be solitary (78%) and can affect any area of the brain. An analysis of autopsy data suggested that most capillary telangiectasias (71%) are located in the pons.[13] An older large autopsy series identified an equal distribution of these lesions within the supratentorial and infratentorial compartments, however.[2] The pons is probably the most common location. Other common locations include the middle cerebellar peduncle[3] and dentate nucleus of the cerebellum.[5]

Grossly the cut surface of the brain has small areas that resemble pink or brownish petechial hemorrhages. In 1941, Blackwood[10] provided the first classic histologic descriptions. Microscopically, there are small tufts of capillaries, which are not structurally different from normal capillaries. There is no smooth muscle and a noted absence of elastic fibers.[1, 3, 10] There are no feeding or draining vessels.[14] Normal parenchyma is present

TABLE 126–1 ■ **Review of Clinically Relevant Features of Arteriovascular Malformations**

MALFORMATION	PREVALENCE (%)	PATHOLOGY	COMMON SYMPTOMS	NATURAL HISTORY	ANGIOGRAPHY	MRI APPEARANCE	TREATMENT OPTIONS
Capillary telangiectasia	0.3	Dilated capillaries surrounded by normal parenchyma. No smooth muscle or elastic fibers. No evidence of hemorrage	Generally asymptomatic (often discovered incidentally on MR imaging or at autopsy)	Benign	Occult	Signal loss on GRE sequences	No treatment necessary unless patient experiences a rare hemorrhage, which may require surgery
DVA	0.5–0.7	Collateral venous channels coalesce to form physiologically normal venous outflow tract. Veins can be thickened or hyalinized. Surrounding parenchyma is normal	Generally asymptomatic. Nonspecific headaches in 67%. Seizures (but generally not attributable to DVA)	Benign. Annual hemorrhage risk of 0.22–0.68%	Classic appearance is caput medusae as medullary veins converge centrally	Linear or curvilinear hypointensity on T1- and T2-weighted images that enhances with gadolinium. Hyperintensity seen on T2-weighted images may correlate with region of venous hypertension	Treatment not recommended; in event of hemorrhage, clot should be evacuated but DVA left intact to avoid catastrophic venous infarction. Radiosurgery not recommended; does not obliterate and causes complications
Cavernous malformation	0.5	Mulberry appearance. Sinusoidal thin-walled vascular channels lined by single-cell endothelial layer. Vessel walls lack structural elements. Absence of parenchyma within lesion. Surrounding brain gliotic and hemosiderin stained	Most common presentation is seizures (80%). Subclinical hemorrhage seen in almost all patients. Clinical hemorrhage in 12.2%	Tend to grow through clinical and subclinical hemorrhage. Annual risks of developing seizures, 1.5%, and clinically significant hemorrhage, 0.3–0.7%	Occult	Central reticulated honeycomb pattern of T2-weighted MR images with surrounding hypointensity. GRE imaging more sensitive for small lesions	Asymptomatic lesions generally do not require treatment. Surgery undertaken for seizures in patients with EEG focus with good results. Surgery considered for hemorrhagic lesions. Stereotactic radiosurgery ineffective
AVM	0.1	Feeding arteries, nidus, and draining veins are major components. Secondary arterial dilation of muscular elastic walls and thin collagenous venous walls. Brain within AVM is gliotic and hemosiderin stained	Seizures are the initial symptom in 27–38%; 70% experience a seizure. Most common cause of nontraumatic intracranial hemorrhage in young people (<35 years old). Headache and neurologic deficits	Annual hemorrhage rate of 2–4%. AVM regresses spontaneously in small but undefined subgroup of patients	Definition of arterial supply, nidus, and venous drainage pattern. Identification of associated aneurysms, venous varices, and vasculopathic stenoses	Delineates relationships between AVM and brain anatomy	Surgery provides the best option for cure and prevention of hemorrhage. Low surgical risk in grade I–II patients. Seizures can be controlled medically, and surgery has better results than endovascular techniques for refractory epilepsy. Stereotactic radiosurgery obliterates approximately 80% of appropriately selected lesions; however, the risk of hemorrhage persists 2–3 years

AVM, arteriovenous malformation; DVA, developmental venous anomalies; EEG, electroencephalogram; GRE, gradient-echo.

between the dilated capillaries, and mild gliosis can surround the parenchyma. Hemosiderin and other evidence of prior hemorrhage are unusual. The rare case is calcified and referred to as *hemangioma calcificans*.[15] The pathogenesis of these lesions is unknown.

Clinical Presentation and Natural History

When vascular malformations are discussed in general, a distinction is made between symptomatic and asymptomatic lesions and between angiographically detectable and angiographically occult lesions. Capillary telangiectasias usually are asymptomatic and angiographically occult. They are found most commonly in adults in their 30s to 70s, although they can occur in infancy and at 5 months of gestational age.[13, 16] Capillary telangiectasias are thought to be clinically silent with a benign natural history and most often are identified incidentally at autopsy or with magnetic resonance imaging (MRI).[17–19] Based on a literature review, Rigamonti and coworkers[7] concluded that 2.6% of the symptomatic angiographically occult vascular malformations of the brain were capillary telangiectasias. Given that capillary telangiectasias compose more than one tenth (12.4%) of angiographically occult vascular malformations, they are associated with a disproportionately small incidence of symptoms. Not all lesions are completely silent, however.[7, 20] Various reports have indicated the presence of symptoms, including headache, seizures, hemorrhage, and progressive neurologic deficit.[7] In contrast, an earlier report suggested that these lesions do not produce epilepsy.[2] Only extremely rarely are these lesions associated with hemorrhage. Other causes for intracerebral hemorrhage must be sought before capillary telangiectasia is implicated.

If a hemorrhage does occur, its effects reflect the location of the capillary telangiectasia. Because the pons and middle cerebellar peduncle are common sites for capillary telangiectasias, the potential for devastation when they bleed is significant. Hemorrhage is so rare, however, that it is impossible to derive rates of risk from the available literature. Symptoms may manifest in the absence of hemorrhage or mass effect—possibly secondary to lesional growth or altered metabolism in the region of the telangiectasia.[20, 21]

Imaging

Capillary telangiectasias are not detectable on conventional cerebral angiography[11] or contrast-enhanced computed tomography (CT) studies. An article has characterized the MRI appearance of histopathologically unproven lesions thought to be capillary telangiectasia on clinical grounds.[11] Lee and associates[11] reported that these lesions tend to be small, homogeneously enhancing, hypointense to isointense on T1-weighted imaging, and isointense to hyperintense on T2-weighted and proton density–weighted imaging. They can be difficult to appreciate on these sequences and, when seen, can be mistaken for active demyelination, subacute infarction, or lymphoma. The most important finding was marked signal loss on susceptibility-sensitive gradient-echo (GRE) sequences. Lee and associates[11] concluded that the increased susceptibility on the GRE sequence is essential in diagnosing these lesions because this feature distinguishes them from other lesions that appear similar on conventional MRI sequences.

Treatment

Asymptomatic lesions are identified rarely, and when they are, surgery is not recommended. Several case reports have implicated hemorrhage from capillary telangiectasias. Only in a few cases has the cause of a hemorrhage been proved histopathologically to be from a capillary telangiectasia.[13, 16] When hemorrhage has occurred and the suspected cause is a capillary telangiectasia, the clinical decision-making process regarding surgical management is similar to that of any other intracerebral hemorrhage. If possible, a biopsy specimen of the wall of the clot cavity should be obtained to prove the etiologic diagnosis.

DEVELOPMENTAL VENOUS ANOMALIES

Epidemiology

Developmental venous anomalies (also called *venous angiomas* or *venous malformations*) are the most common intracranial vascular malformation. In some series, they represent the most common intracranial vascular abnormality of any kind. The evolution of the nomenclature of these lesions reflects an improved understanding of their pathophysiology. In an early series,[34] developmental venous anomalies composed 15% of vascular malformations; more recently, they have been said to compose 63%.[4] Their prevalence varies among studies but typically ranges from 0.5% to 0.7% in retrospective imaging studies[22] and is about 2.6% in autopsy studies.[4] They are congenital anomalies of the brain that occur equally in males and females. No evidence suggests that developmental venous anomalies are familial.[23]

Pathology and Pathophysiology

The cause of developmental venous anomalies is incompletely understood, but it has been proposed that they form in the late stages of fetal maturation. Saito and Kobayashi[24] and Toro and colleagues[25] implicated an intrauterine *accident* with resultant ischemia during the formation of perimedullary veins as leading to the development of collateral venous channels. Mullan and coworkers[26, 27] proposed a similar model. In both paradigms, the resulting venous anomaly represents the anatomically abnormal but physiologically normal venous outflow pathway for the involved portion of the brain.

In 1887, Pfannenstiel[28] published pathologic descriptions of developmental venous anomalies, but McCormick[1] presented the classic description in 1966. On gross examination, one finds a radially arranged pattern of medullary veins converging centrally on a single draining vein, which in turn drains either superficially or deeply. This configuration has been described as a *star cluster*.[26, 27] Microscopically the veins are thickened and hyalinized. There is minimal smooth muscle or elastic tissue, and the anomaly is found predictably within normal parenchyma.[1, 3, 29, 30] The number or size of the surrounding arteries does not increase.[25] Hemodynamically, these venous anomalies are low flow and low resistance and present only a small likelihood of hemorrhage.[31] They most often are unilateral and tend to occur in the frontal lobes and posterior fossa.[32]

Clinical Presentation and Natural History

Whether these anomalies produce symptoms has been debated. The clinician should investigate other causes of potential symptoms before implicating a developmental venous anomaly as the cause. Association is different from causality. Patients have presented with nonspecific symptoms, such as headache, nausea, and vomiting, as well as with seizures, progressive neurological deficit, and hemorrhage. Although most identified patients (67%) present with headache,[23] the headaches seldom are attributed to the developmental venous anomaly.[22] Likewise, with seizures, only a few patients have epileptiform activity in the region of the developmental venous anomaly.[33] In most patients, there is no correlation between the developmental venous anomaly and seizures.[22, 24] Patients with posterior fossa lesions have presented with ataxia, dizziness, and lower cranial nerve dysfunction but usually without direct cause attributed to the developmental venous anomaly.

The crucial issue in the presentation of these patients is the risk of hemorrhage, which once was thought to range from 8% to 43%.[34, 35] The increased utility of MRI and the discovery of large numbers of asymptomatic patients have modified these statistics, however. In a retrospective study, Garner and associates[33] calculated the risk of hemorrhage to be 0.22% per year. McLaughlin and coworkers[31] found the risk to be 0.61% per year in the retrospective component of their study, whereas their prospective data estimated the risk of a hemorrhage to be 0.68% per year and the risk of a symptomatic hemorrhage to be 0.34% per year. No patient in either series died, suffered significant morbidity, or required an operation directed toward the developmental venous anomaly. The risk of hemorrhage was no greater in the posterior fossa, in contrast to previous suggestions that lesions in this location bleed more often.[18] These data emphasize that if a patient with a developmental venous anomaly presents with hemorrhage, a second lesion must be sought.

Imaging

Imaging of developmental venous anomalies is well described in the literature. The first angiographic description of these lesions was by Wolf and colleagues,[36] and the gold standard for diagnosing developmental venous anomalies is conventional cerebral angiography. Findings classically include normal circulation time and normal arterial and capillary phases of the study, with the venous anomaly visualized entirely during the late venous phase (Fig. 126–1). There is no early filling of a draining vein as with AVMs. The classic angiographic picture is described as a *caput medusae* lesion because of the lesion's resemblance to the snakes on the head of the mythical character. The images also have been likened to spiders, a hydra, spoked wheels, umbrellas, and a sunburst[14] and are referred to by Mullan and colleagues[26, 27] as *star clusters*.

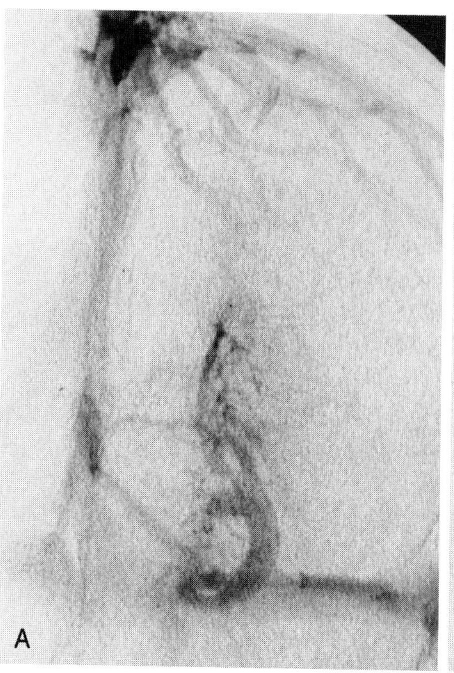

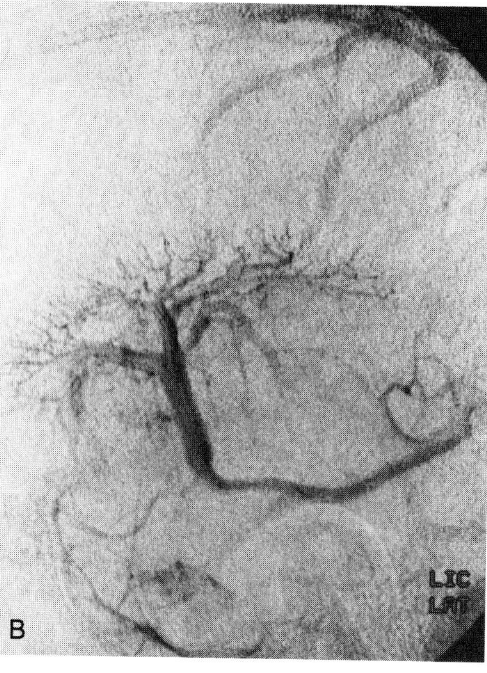

FIGURE 126–1. Conventional *(A)* anteroposterior and *(B)* lateral angiographic views show the classic appearance of a developmental venous anomaly in the frontal lobe. The perimedullary veins are described as a *star cluster* or *caput medusae* (see text). (Courtesy of Dr. W. Hu, Foothills Medical Centre, Calgary.)

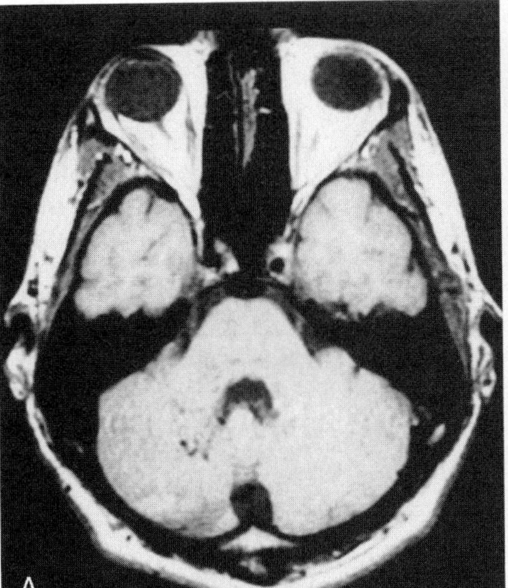

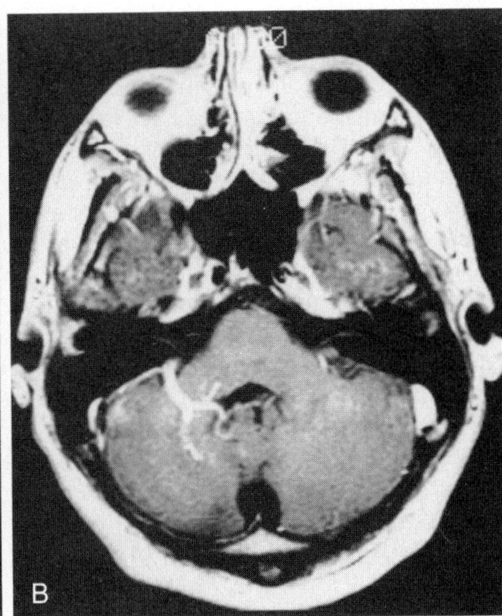

FIGURE 126–2. T1-weighted *(A)* and gadolinium-enhanced T1-weighted *(B)* magnetic resonance images of a developmental venous anomaly show hypointensity on the nonenhanced sequences. With administration of gadolinium, there is bright enhancement.

These findings are pathognomonic for a developmental venous anomaly.

Contemporary investigations do not always include conventional angiography. More commonly, patients undergo contrast-enhanced CT or MRI. On an infused CT scan, the most common finding is linear or curvilinear enhancement after contrast administration. Delineation of the medullary veins sometimes can be seen on these imaging studies. MRI is as sensitive and more specific than CT, with the important finding being a linear or curvilinear hypointensity on T1-weighted and T2-weighted images.[32, 37] The developmental venous anomaly enhances brightly with contrast administration (Fig. 126–2). The draining vein is seen better on T2-weighted sequences.[38, 39] Because of the slow flow, there is good definition of the draining vein and the perimedullary caput medusae veins. Although no specific literature reports the diagnostic accuracy of magnetic resonance angiography, these studies also identify developmental venous anomalies.[32]

Early reports suggested that the area of developmental venous anomaly was often hyperintense on T2-weighted images.[38] The hyperintensity subsequently was determined to be artifactual, however.[32] More recent reports have noted a hyperintensity surrounding a developmental venous anomaly in 50% of cases. This finding may have implications for the pathogenesis of mixed malformations (see later). It is possible that these areas represent regions of venous hypertension or ischemia. Not all studies report this hyperintensity, however.[25] Additionally, one report has documented a region of hyperintensity on MRI that was proved pathologically to be an area of acute demyelination surrounding a developmental venous anomaly.[40]

Treatment

Most patients with a developmental venous anomaly are asymptomatic. The anomaly is a functional and physiologic venous channel. Another source of symptoms should be sought in symptomatic patients. Specifically, high-field MRI has been advocated to rule out the possibility of an associated cavernous malformation.[23] Another angiographically occult arteriovascular malformation (cavernous malformation) typically causes the symptoms in such patients. In most patients with epilepsy and a developmental venous anomaly, the seizures can be well controlled with anticonvulsant medication alone. There are no cases reported more recently in which refractory epilepsy has been described as an indication for surgery. A few patients with developmental venous anomalies present with hemorrhage in the region of the vein. In these situations, it is tempting to attribute a hemorrhage to the developmental venous anomaly. The hemorrhage is most likely from a second lesion, however.

Many authors have described surgery to treat these hemorrhages. Although patients may do well after surgery, the potential for catastrophic complications or death exists if the normal venous drainage is interfered with.[29, 41–45] Some patients have been no worse after surgery despite the sacrifice of this normal-variant vessel.[35] Most surgeons would recommend a conservative approach, however.[7, 33, 41, 46–50] Experience has shown that the most prudent course of action for patients with symptomatic hemorrhages that require surgery is to evacuate the hematoma and to make every effort to preserve the developmental venous anomaly. Increased morbidity from cerebral edema, infarction, and hemorrhage has followed obliteration of these anomalies, much as one would expect based on reports of complications after spontaneous thrombosis of these lesions.[51, 52]

The presumed pathophysiology of neurological deterioration in patients who suffer morbidity from these operations is the sudden occlusion of the venous channel that drains normal brain. This occlusion leads to venous hypertension and eventually to venous infarction. Lindquist and colleagues[53] hypothesized that gradual occlusion of these channels through the use of radiosurgery would allow the slow recruitment of other venous channels and prevent this complication. In their study of 13 patients, however, most developmental venous anomalies were obliterated incompletely, and the incidence of neurological morbidity was high. Based on this study and its subsequent criticism,[46, 49, 50] stereotactic radiosurgery is not recommended for developmental venous anomalies.

Most authors now recommend that no intervention be directed at developmental venous anomalies. If hemorrhage has occurred, other causes for it must be sought. The clinical decision-making process regarding surgical management is similar to that associated with any other intracerebral hemorrhage, but the developmental venous anomaly must be preserved.

CAVERNOUS MALFORMATIONS

Epidemiology

Cavernous malformations compose a large proportion of what has been described as angiographically occult vascular malformations. Other terms used to describe these lesions include *cavernous angiomas, cavernomas,* and *cavernous hemangiomas.* Based on clinical series, the prevalence of cavernous malformations is estimated at 0.5%.[54] Similarly, it is 0.4% to 0.5% in large autopsy series.[4, 55] In autopsy series, cavernous malformations compose 16% of intracranial vascular malformations.[34] In contrast to developmental venous anomalies, which are the most common arteriovascular lesions and cause few symptoms, cavernous malformations are less common vascular malformations and can be symptomatic. They occur throughout life but are diagnosed more often in adults. Most lesions become symptomatic in adults in their 20s and 30s.[54, 56] The lesions tend to occur equally in men and women.[54, 56]

There are two subgroups of cavernous malformations. The first group includes patients with nonhereditary (sporadic) lesions, whereas the second group includes patients with familial lesions.[57] More than half of patients with cavernous malformations (54%) have the familial variant,[58] which occurs primarily in people of Hispanic descent, but also in Icelandic and French kindreds.[59–61] Zabramski and colleagues[57] showed that patients with the familial form of the disease are likely to have multiple lesions (84% versus 15% in sporadic disease) and that cavernous malformations in this group tend to be dynamic, as witnessed by an increased rate of growth and an increased number of de novo lesions. These lesions are more likely to become symptomatic if their appearance on MRI is hyperintense.

The genetic causes of familial cavernous malformation are being elucidated. These lesions are inherited in an autosomal dominant fashion with incomplete clinical penetrance. In Hispanic kindreds of Mexican descent, a mutation in the long arm of chromosome 7 (*CCM1*) has been identified.[62] Subsequently, it was shown that this mutation shows a founder effect accounting for almost all familial and many sporadic cases of familial cavernous malformation.[63] The inference is that the inherited mutation was likely from a common ancestor in a recent generation. Since this discovery, it has been shown that non-Hispanic kindreds with familial cavernous malformations do not harbor the mutation on 7q. They do share additional loci, however, for a mutation on the short arm of chromosome 7 (*CCM2*) and the long arm of chromosome 3 (*CCM3*).[64, 65]

At present, at least 109 families are known to harbor cavernous malformations,[66] and their presenting symptoms were similar to those previously described: seizures (43%), hemorrhage (28%), headache (23%), and focal neurological deficit (50%). In this population, 24% were asymptomatic. *Anticipation* is the term used to describe the earlier onset of an inherited disease in one generation when compared with the previous generation. A report has documented anticipation in familial cavernous malformation.[66] It was found that the onset of symptoms occurred at a mean age of 31.6 years in one generation, 17.8 years in the next, and 6.3 years in the youngest. In certain diseases, such as spinal cerebellar ataxia, myotonic dystrophy, and Huntington's disease, the biologic basis of anticipation is the occurrence of specific unstable trinucleotide repeats. Based on the statistically significant occurrence of anticipation in familial cavernous malformation, trinucleotide repeats may be identified as the underlying anomaly in the hereditary form of this disease.[67] These findings confirm the heterogeneity of these lesions but do not explain definitively their pathogenesis. The gene products and their function are unknown.

Pathology and Pathophysiology

The cause of cavernous malformations is uncertain. Some theories have implicated cavernous malformations as being derived from the same pathogenetic process as capillary telangiectasias or developmental venous anomalies. In contrast to these other malformations, cavernous malformations have a distinct tendency toward growth and repetitive occult hemorrhage. In contrast to capillary telangiectasia and developmental venous anomalies, cavernous malformations predominantly are located supratentorially. Series have reported these lesions above the tentorium cerebelli in 74% to 90% of patients.[34, 54, 56, 68–70] The distribution is probably equal throughout the central nervous system (proportional to central nervous system mass).

From a gross pathologic perspective, cavernous malformations have a mulberry appearance, and their size varies. Lesions measuring 8 cm have been reported,[71] but the average size tends to be 1 to 2 cm.[54] The vessels that comprise the lesion are sinusoidal, thin-walled, and dilated and have a single-cell endothelial layer (Fig. 126–3). The vessel walls lack structural elements, such as elastin or smooth muscle.[5, 72] The distinguishing feature of cavernous malformations is the absence of any parenchyma within the lesion (see Fig. 126–3) as opposed to the presence of normal tissue within capillary telangiectasias. Thrombus may be present within

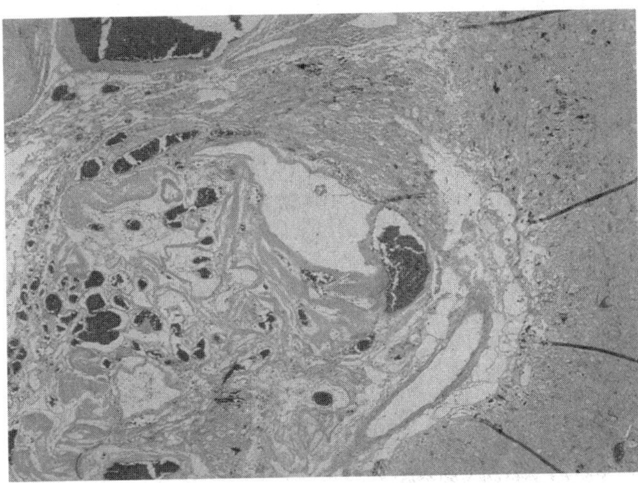

FIGURE 126–3. Histopathologic appearance of a cavernous malformation shows the dilated sinusoidal channels and single-cell endothelial layer. Areas of thrombosis can be seen. Intervening parenchyma within the lesion is absent. (Hematoxylin and eosin.)

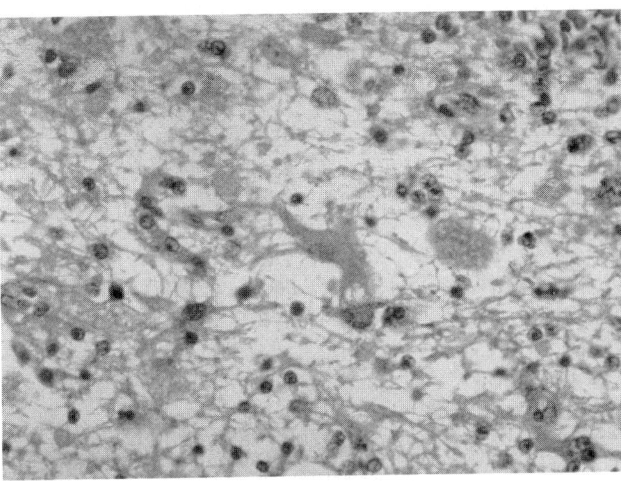

FIGURE 126–5. Representative area of gliosis from the parenchyma adjacent to a cavernous malformation. (Hematoxylin and eosin.)

the venous channels of a cavernous malformation, and the surrounding parenchyma can be iron-rich as a result of hemorrhage from it (Fig. 126–4). Typically a region of gliosis surrounds the cavernous malformation (Fig. 126–5). Blood pressure within cavernous malformations is low when measured intraoperatively.[73] It is greater than central venous pressure but less than mean arterial pressure. The pressure changes when the patient moves, suggesting that the lesion communicates directly with the venous system. Accordingly, there is no significant change in cortical blood flow in the surrounding brain.[73]

Cavernous malformations grow over time and can develop de novo after a previously normal MRI study. There are several theories regarding their mechanism of growth. Generally accepted factors include the processes of bleeding and thrombosis within the lesion. One theory is based on the routine evidence of previous hemorrhage around these lesions on imaging studies. Presumably the hemorrhage is a slow, low-pressure seepage of blood from the lesion (so-called erythrocyte diapedesis), possibly associated with transient rises in venous pressure.[73] If pressure is low, any bleeding from these lesions would be expected to be self-limited.[73]

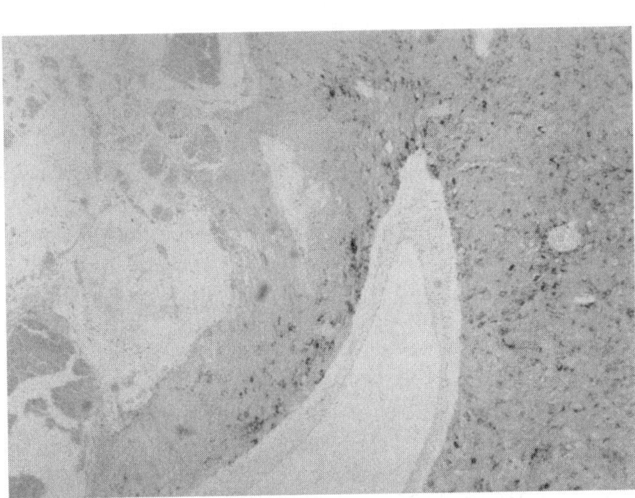

FIGURE 126–4. Prussian blue staining shows iron deposition in the region surrounding a cavernous malformation.

A second theory proposes that cavernous malformations expand by the same mechanism as chronic subdural hematomas. There is evidence that cavernous malformations endothelialize the small hematomas that they create.[74, 75] Noting similarities between membranes surrounding a chronic subdural hematoma and the organizing clot at the site of hemorrhage from a cavernous malformation, Frim and associates[76] studied the vascular endothelium of resected cavernous malformations. They found that immunohistochemical staining was positive for tissue plasminogen activator, which may contribute to the potential for hemorrhage.

A third theory, strongly supported by evidence, suggests that these lesions are dynamic by nature of the endothelial cells themselves. Pozzati and colleagues[77] suggest that the lesions are either induced to produce or spontaneously produce angiogenic factors that allow gradual propagation of vessels. This theory describes a proliferative vasculopathy, or what Awad and coworkers[46, 78] have referred to as *hemorrhagic dysangiogenesis* or *hemorrhagic angiogenic proliferation.*

Another hypothesis implicates hormonal influences on platelet-mediated thrombosis and is consistent with the tendency for disease to progress in women and during pregnancy.[79] The size of cavernous malformations is known to increase during pregnancy and to decrease after delivery.[80] Finally, some authors have noted the de novo formation of cavernous malformations after therapeutic radiation for various indications.[77, 81] The exact incidence after radiation exposure has not been determined, however.[81]

Many researchers argue that cavernous malformations represent one manifestation along a wide spectrum of disease, with capillary telangiectasias representing another variant and developmental venous anomalies being associated (see later). Most likely, the answer lies somewhere between these theories. To speculate conservatively, it is likely that once formed, the endothelium in these lesions responds to an external stimulus, possibly hormonal, resulting in self-limited microhemorrhages that induce angiogenic factors and endothelialization of the clot. As a result, the lesion grows and eventually recanalizes thrombosed areas. The opportunity to elucidate the pathogenesis of these lesions may follow the successful isolation and growth of endothelial cell cultures from cavernous malformations.[82]

Clinical Presentation and Natural History

In accordance with the presentation of patients with other vascular malformations, patients with cavernous malformations tend to be asymptomatic or to present with headaches, seizures, focal neurological deficits, or hemorrhage. In contrast to the other arteriovascular malformations, the most common clinical symptom is seizures, most of which arise from supratentorial lesions.[54, 56] Older patients tend to present with focal deficits, whereas younger patients are 5.6 times more likely to suffer from seizures.[71] The incidence of seizures in these patients ranges from 39% to 79%.[56, 57, 70] The average annual risk of developing seizures for patients with sporadic cavernous malformations is 1.5%. Patients with a single lesion have a lower risk of epilepsy (1.3%) and develop their seizures at a later age.[56] This risk is higher (2.5%) for patients known to harbor multiple lesions, and these patients tend to develop seizures at a younger age. Seizures are presumably the result of the gliosis that follows the deposition of ferric iron-containing hemosiderin in the parenchyma surrounding the lesion,[54, 74, 83, 84] but this proposal has been debated. Seizure types include complex partial (37%), simple partial (21%), and secondarily generalized seizures (43%). Generalized seizures are significantly more common with frontal lesions. Temporal and frontal lobe lesions tend to underlie intractable epilepsy.[70] Chronic intractable epilepsy can be present in almost half (44.7%) of the patients with a supratentorial cavernous malformation.[85]

MRI of almost all cavernous malformations shows evidence of prior hemorrhage. In a retrospective analysis of the natural history of cavernous malformations, Del Curling and coworkers[56] found that only 9% of patients in their series suffered from a clinically significant hemorrhage attributable to the cavernous malformation, whereas a further 19% had asymptomatic bleeds. In a similar analysis by Robinson and colleagues,[54] 12.2% of patients presented with hemorrhage. For patients with sporadic cavernous malformations, they calculated the annual risk of clinically significant hemorrhage to be 0.3% to 0.7%.[54, 56, 70] Kondziolka and associates[86] found this rate to be 0.6%, but the rate was 4.5% per year in patients who had suffered previous hemorrhage. The incidence of symptomatic hemorrhage for patients with familial disease, in contrast to the sporadic type, is 1.1% per year. Although Porter and colleagues[86a] found the overall annual event rate attributable to cavernous malformations to be 4.2%, the event rate from deep cavernous malformations was almost 11% per year.

In investigating the factors leading to *malignant* behavior, defined as lesion growth, recurrent overt bleeding, or de novo appearance, Pozzati and associates[77] found that pregnancy; familial disease; previous therapeutic radiation; incomplete resection; an associated venous malformation; and a location in the third ventricle, basal ganglia, or brainstem predicted aggressive tendencies. The association of certain locations of cavernous malformations with aggressive behavior probably represents their effect on *density of function* within these areas (similar to the motor or speech areas) rather than to a particular feature of the lesions. Patients with posterior fossa lesions are 6.8 times more likely to become symptomatic with focal neurological deficits.[71]

Neurologic disability has been associated significantly with previous hemorrhage.[71] Patients who suffer hemorrhage from a cavernous malformation that arises after therapeutic radiation are at a much higher risk of rehemorrhage.[77, 81] This rate might be 6.7% per year after radiation if the lesion is entirely radiation-induced.[81, 87] Women are known to be at higher risk for symptomatic hemorrhage,[54, 71] even though the incidence is not selective for either sex,[56] and men typically are diagnosed at a younger age.[88] After one hemorrhage, the interval to a second hemorrhage is briefer: 30.7% of patients suffer a repeat hemorrhage within 48 months.[65] Hemorrhages in these patients are seldom catastrophic or cause death. Although approximately 22% of patients present with focal deficits, many of the deficits resolve over time with no specific intervention.[56] Robinson and coworkers[54] found that gross hemorrhage had no significant effect on outcome.

Imaging

The imaging characteristics of cavernous malformations, which are known to be angiographically occult,[88] are well described. CT imaging often fails to delineate these lesions reliably.[88] When cavernous malformations do appear on CT, they most often appear as hyperdense or heterogeneous lesions that may enhance partially with contrast administration (Fig. 126–6*A* and *B*). MRI currently is the most sensitive and most specific method for imaging cavernous malformations.[73] Characteristic findings on MRI include a variable hyperintense signal centrally with a *reticulated* pattern on T2-weighted images representing degrading hemorrhage of various ages. A surrounding hypointense ring corresponds to the hemosiderin-containing region around the cavernous malformation (Fig. 126–6*C* and *D*). The central portion is said to have a *popcorn* or *honeycomb* appearance and should enhance with the administration of contrast medium.[88, 89] On T1-weighted MRIs, the region of low-intensity signal also is seen, along with a heterogeneous signal centrally. The absence of feeding and draining vessels on MRI allows cavernous malformations to be distinguished from true AVMs.[56] Gradient-echo (GRE) images are much more sensitive

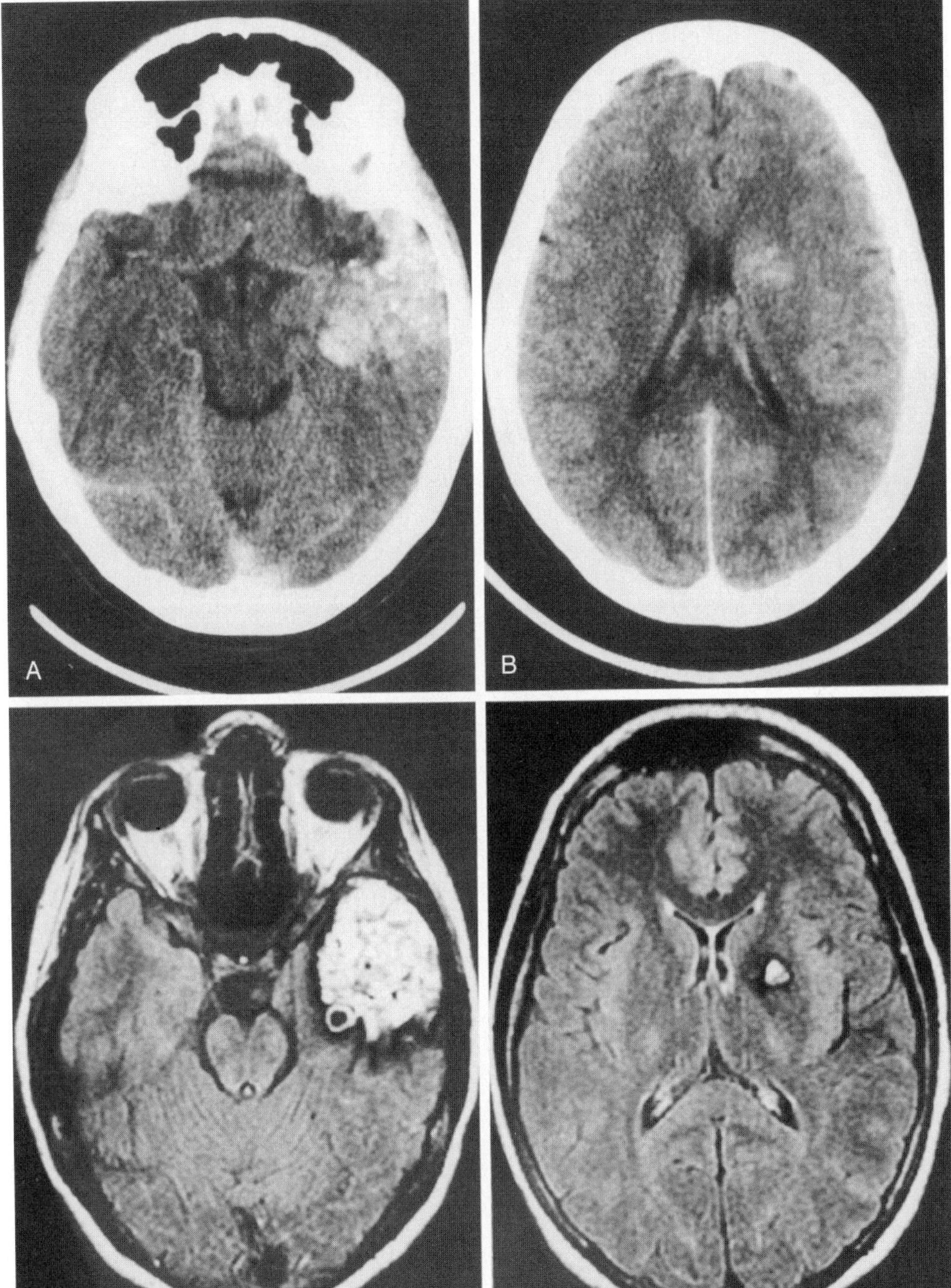

FIGURE 126–6. Comparison of typical findings of cavernous malformations on CT and MRI. A large left temporal lobe cavernous malformation is seen on a contrast-enhanced CT scan as a hyperdense area *(A)*, whereas a less notable abnormality is seen on a higher cut from the same study *(B)*. The corresponding fluid-attenuated inversion recovery images show the large cavernous malformation at the left temporal pole surrounded by a hypointense ring *(C)*. The second lesion, shown vaguely on the CT scan, is seen easily on the MR images with a characteristic reticulated central core surrounded by a ring of hypodensity representing the hemosiderin-stained parenchyma *(D)*.

than conventional sequences for detecting small cavernous malformations (Fig. 126–7).[65]

Based on the MRI appearance of cavernous malformations, Zabramski and coworkers[57] classified lesions into four types reflecting their dynamic nature. Type I lesions are associated with subacute hemorrhage and have a hyperintense central region on T1-weighted imaging. Initially, T2-weighted images also are hyperintense. Images become hypointense peripherally to centrally, however, as products of the hemorrhage degrade. Type II lesions contain loculated areas of thrombosis and hemorrhage of variable age. Hemosiderin stains the surrounding brain, which has become gliotic. These lesions show the typical reticulated pattern of mixed signal intensity in their core surrounded by a rim of hypointensity. Type III lesions show the imaging correlate of chronic hemorrhage. A profound hypointense signal occurs on T2-weighted and GRE images, whereas on T1-weighted images the lesion is isointense or hypointense. Finally, type IV lesions are difficult to detect on conventional imaging studies. When detected, their imaging characteristics are similar to those of capillary telangiectasias. Typically, lesions are small and hypointense on GRE sequences.

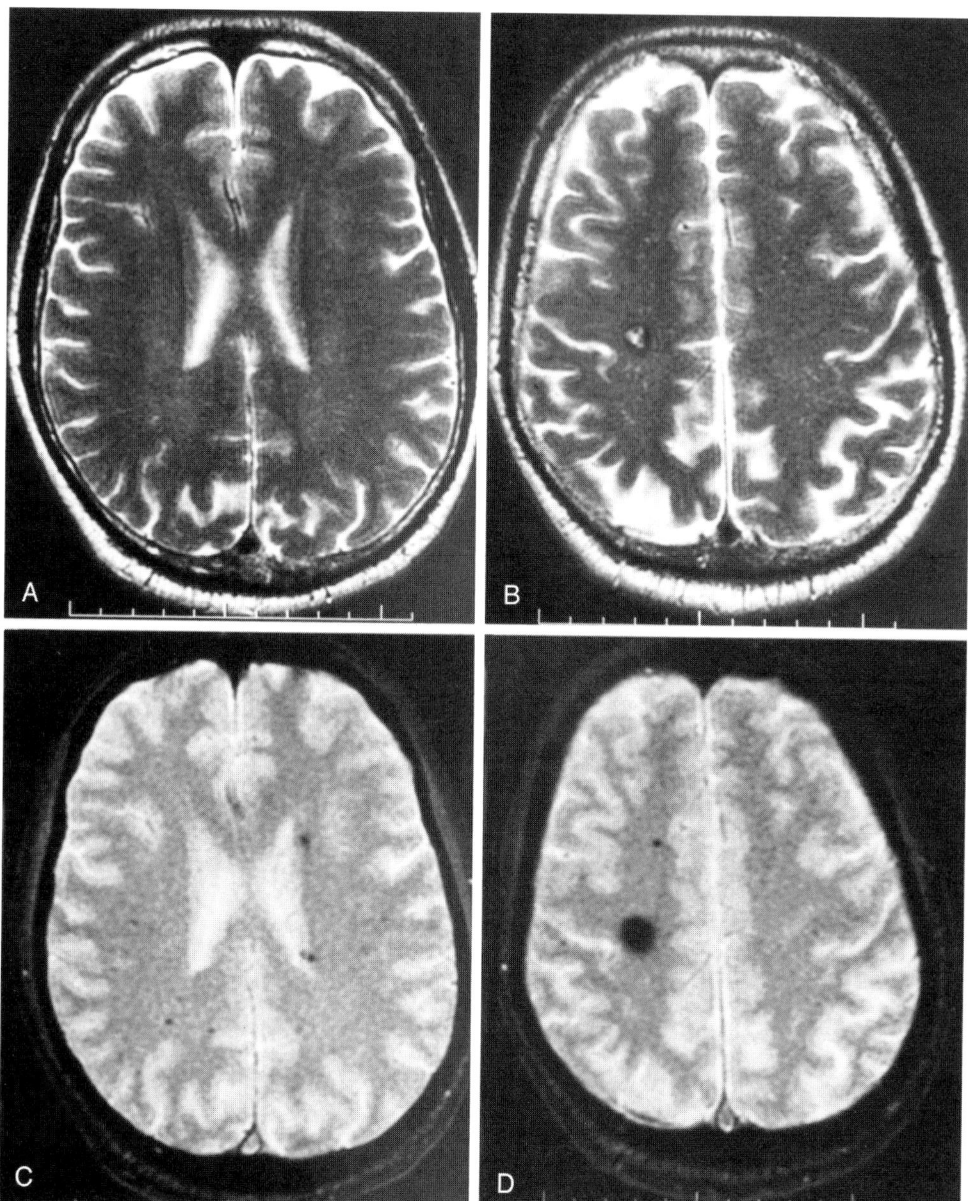

FIGURE 126–7. Comparison of T2-weighted and gradient-echo (GRE) images of cavernous malformations. *A*, On T2-weighted imaging, the left periventricular region appears normal. *B*, A typical type II cavernous malformation is seen in another area of the same study. Comparable images from the GRE sequence show multiple periventricular lesions *(C)* and identify the lesion previously seen in the right hemisphere *(D)*.

Treatment

With better clinical and imaging follow-up of patients with cavernous malformations, the decisions regarding treatment indications and treatment methods are under evaluation. Symptomatic lesions are less controversial and are discussed later. Asymptomatic lesions require further evaluation. The rate of fatal hemorrhage is low.[90] The threat of hemorrhage alone typically is not considered a surgical indication.[56] Some reports still recommend surgical management of accessible asymptomatic cavernous malformations in women contemplating pregnancy.[54] The gold standard of treatment, when initiated, is considered complete surgical excision of the cavernous malformation. The indications for surgical treatment can be classified according to the presenting symptoms: seizures, hemorrhage, or focal neurologic deficit.

In patients who are symptomatic with epilepsy, the primary question is whether the seizures are refractory to medical treatment. Although prospective trials of medical and surgical treatment are lacking, intractable epilepsy with concordant neuroimaging and electroencephalography is accepted widely as an indication for surgery.[54, 56, 70, 85] Giulioni and associates[91] recognized intractable seizures as a treatment indication but also advocated surgery for nonrefractory patients, citing the known tendency for these lesions to grow and possibly to enlarge the epileptogenic region.

One of the basic assumptions of seizure surgery for cavernous malformations is that the area of hemosiderin staining and gliosis around the lesion is the epileptogenic focus and must be resected.[84] Casazza and coworkers[85] found, however, that leaving the hemosiderin-containing ring behind (as evidenced by its persistence on postoperative MRI) did not worsen outcomes. Conversely, removing the hemosiderin ring did not improve outcomes. In terms of postoperative seizure cessation, another group found no advantage associated with removing glial scar tissue.[92] Although not all patients are completely seizure-free after surgery, seizure control is improved significantly in a good proportion by the continued use of anticonvulsant medication.[85] Risk factors for seizure relapse or worsening include the presence of multiple lesions and subtotal resection of the cavernous malformation.[85]

The information guiding a surgical treatment decision for a patient with medically controlled epilepsy is less dogmatic. Because most seizure disorders can be controlled medically,[56] the decision to proceed with surgery is multifactorial. Disability from seizures, tolerance of anticonvulsants, fitness for operation, accessibility of the lesion, and surgical risks all must be considered. Robinson and colleagues[54] noted that 50% of their patients were seizure-free after surgery. Zevgaridis and associates[92] reported a positive effect of surgery (seizure-free or reduction in frequency) in 94.8% of their patients with a superficial cavernous malformation. In one study, several different surgical management strategies were evaluated in all patients with epilepsy secondary to a cavernous malformation. At a minimum 1-year follow-up,[70] 84% were seizure-free, and a further 14% improved or were unchanged. The risks of this type of surgery typically are low, although patients with a cavernous malformation have died after epilepsy surgery.[93] For patients lacking a clear concordance between the lesion site and electroencephalography, preoperative ictal scalp recordings may improve outcomes.[92]

The indications for surgical treatment after hemorrhage are open to interpretation. These lesions are prone to repeated subclinical microhemorrhage as illustrated by the increasing hypointense ring around cavernous malformations shown on MRI.[56] This characteristic alone is not an indication for surgery. No good clinical evidence has documented the benefit of surgery as prophylaxis against hemorrhage in asymptomatic patients compared with the natural history of these lesions. When cavernous malformations become hyperintense on MRI, it suggests subacute bleeding.[57] The decision-making process then becomes similar to that for the treatment of an intracranial hemorrhage of any origin. If the patient is symptomatic and has proven hemorrhage on MRI, surgery should be considered. If the surgical option is explored, one must be vigilant concerning the possibility of an associated developmental venous anomaly because its occlusion or partial occlusion can be catastrophic. A large symptomatic hemorrhage is a strong indication for surgical treatment.[54, 71] A final note is made regarding pregnancy: Based on hemorrhage in two patients in the first trimester of pregnancy, Robinson and coworkers[54] recommended prophylactic surgery for asymptomatic women contemplating pregnancy as long as their lesion is accessible. This recommendation is controversial, however.

When patients with a focal neurological deficit related to a cavernous malformation without gross hemorrhage are evaluated, surgeons should remember that many of these patients recover to some degree over time. If the deficit is progressive, however, surgery is indicated.[71] For a patient with a static neurological deficit, considerations include the surgical accessibility of the lesion and the risks of surgery.[56] The surgical planning, approaches, and specific technical issues related to operations for cavernous malformations above and below the tentorium are the subjects of later chapters and are not discussed here.

Stereotactic radiosurgery has been used in the treatment of cavernous malformation for a variety of indications. The early results were not promising,[94] and additional experience has proved disappointing. Kondziolka and colleagues[95] reported their experience with hemorrhagic cavernous malformations in surgically inaccessible locations. They noted the difficulty associated with follow-up imaging and elected to use clinical outcomes and, specifically, hemorrhage rates as their measure of outcome. They found a significant reduction in the hemorrhage rate, but it was offset by a significant rate of treatment complications.

In a similar study, Karlsson and coworkers[96] confirmed the relative lack of a protective effect associated with radiosurgery and a high rate of post-treatment hemorrhage. Simultaneously, they documented neurologic deterioration related to treatment in 41% of the patients studied. They stated that microsurgery remains the standard of treatment for cavernous malformation until a prospective randomized clinical trial proves otherwise. Gewirtz and associates[97] found little in the way of pathologic change in their series of cavernous malformations excised after radiosurgical treatment had failed. The lesions had patent vascular channels 10 years after radiation treatment (mean interval, 3.5 years). In a smaller series, Seo and colleagues[98] reported similar findings and reached similar conclusions. In contrast, Kida and associates[99] reported a decrease in lesion size, reduction in hemorrhage rate, and minimal morbidity in their patients with angiographically occult vascular malformations that were treated with radiosurgery. They studied fewer patients than the previous authors, however.

ARTERIOVENOUS MALFORMATIONS

Epidemiology

True AVMs are abnormalities of the intracranial vessels that constitute a connection between the arterial and venous systems and that lack an intervening capillary bed. Approximately 2% of these lesions are multiple, and the remainder are solitary.[100] Both sexes are affected equally. It is estimated that 0.1% of the population harbors an AVM.[101, 102] According to autopsy studies, only 12% of these lesions become symptomatic during life.[103] Arteriovenous malformations are the leading cause of nontraumatic intracerebral hemorrhage in young people (<35 years old), and AVMs are the most common cause of neurological impairment or death in patients younger than 20 years old.[104] Most lesions reach attention in patients in their 40s, and 75% of the hemorrhagic presentations occur before the age of 50 years.[101]

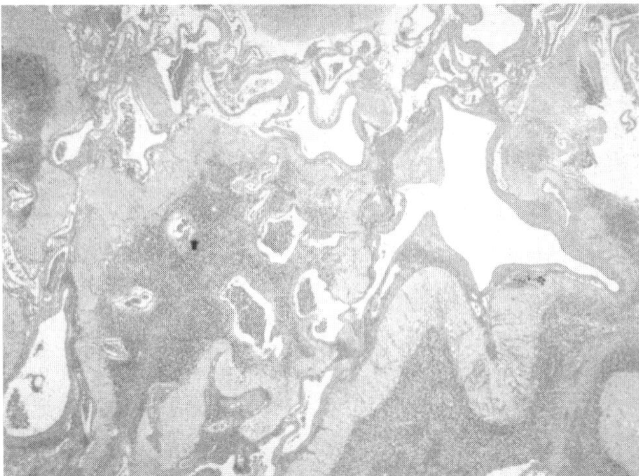

FIGURE 126–8. Histologic appearance of a resected arteriovenous malformation shows the relationship between the preserved cerebellar parenchyma and the abnormal vessels. (Courtesy of Dr. R. Auer, University of Calgary.)

Pathology and Pathophysiology

AVMs have three primary components: feeding arteries, nidus, and draining veins.[105] Gross features of an AVM include the absence of a capillary bed and single or multiple direct arteriovenous connections that permit high-flow arteriovenous shunting through small feeding arteries that lack a muscularis layer. Over time, this high-flow shunt produces secondary changes in the structure of the feeding and draining vessels—dilation of the feeding arteries and dilation and thickening of the draining veins.[105] The arteries develop smooth muscle hyperplasia associated with fibroblasts and connective tissue elements, known as *fibromuscular cushions*. Cushing and Bailey[21] described the nidus as a *snarl* based on its gross appearance. Microscopic features are variable and depend on which portion of the lesion is sampled. Venous elements have thin collagenous walls, whereas arterial feeders have muscular elastic walls (Fig. 126–8). There are parenchymal elements within the AVM, but they tend to be gliotic, hemosiderin stained, and nonfunctional (Fig. 126–9). Some lesions may exhibit vascular or interstitial calcification.[106]

Clinical Presentation and Natural History

Similar to the previously discussed arteriovascular malformations, AVMs tend to manifest with seizures, headache, focal neurological deficits, or hemorrhage. Learning disorders have been associated with AVMs.[102]

In a review of multiple patient series comprising 5191 patients managed conservatively by excision or multimodal treatment, Weinand[107] found that seizures were the initial symptom in 27% to 38% of the patients. Nonhemorrhagic seizures occur in 16% to 53% of patients.[108] Although seizures may be of any type, partial and partial complex are the most frequent types. Of patients with AVMs, 70% might be expected to develop seizures, and seizures are more common with superficial lesions involving the cortex or mesial temporal structures.[105, 109, 110]

Other presenting features include headache and focal neurological deficits. Headaches, the presenting feature in 7% to 48% of patients, typically lack pathognomonic features.[102, 108] An association has been drawn, however, between headache and AVMs that derive their blood supply from meningeal vessels or the posterior cerebral artery.[105]

Focal deficits occur in these patients, affecting 1% to 40%.[102] Only 4% to 8% manifest progressive deficits unrelated to hemorrhage.[105, 108] The pathogenesis of these deficits is likely multifactorial and variably includes a vascular steal phenomenon, venous hypertension, or both.[102] Response to treatment depends on the exact cause of the focal deficit and its chronicity.

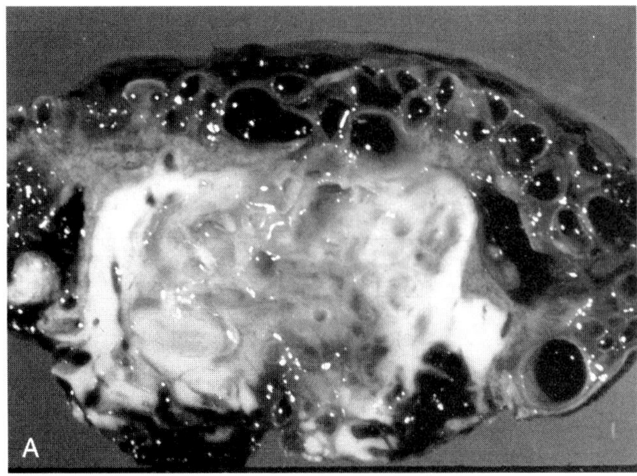

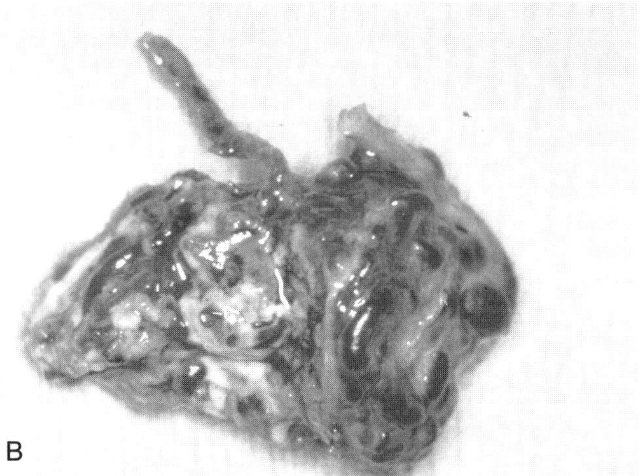

FIGURE 126–9. *A*, Gross pathologic appearance of a resected arteriovenous malformation shows tortuous dilated vessels around the periphery of the lesion and gliotic-appearing parenchyma within the lesion. *B*, A second specimen shows a 2.5-cm completely resected arteriovenous malformation with the same gross features as previously described. (*A* courtesy of Dr. Roland Auer, University of Calgary.)

Of the numerous clinical presentations that patients with AVMs can have, intracranial hemorrhage is the most catastrophic and feared. An AVM can hemorrhage into any compartment of the brain. A prospective review of patients suffering intracranial hemorrhage from AVMs found subarachnoid hemorrhage in 30% (Fig. 126–10), parenchymal hemorrhage in 23%, intraventricular hemorrhage in 16%, and combinations of the aforementioned in 31%.[111] Hartmann and colleagues[111] described the morbidity associated with these hemorrhages to be less than previously thought: 84% of patients suffered no deficit or a nondisabling deficit that allowed independent function. Despite this report, numerous previous accounts estimate the short-term mortality rate associated with AVM hemorrhage to be 10% to 29%.[101, 112–115]

The annual rate of hemorrhage from AVMs has been fairly well established by several authors and is thought to be 2% to 4% per year.[113, 114, 116, 117] Only about half of all patients who harbor an AVM present with a hemorrhage during their lifetime.[101, 105, 117] The factors that predispose a patient with an AVM to intracranial hemorrhage are not known definitively. Reasonable evidence supports a list of variables as possible risk factors for hemorrhage, however. The two most frequently reported risk factors are a history of a prior hemorrhage and deep venous drainage of the AVM. Mast and coworkers[118] found that after a hemorrhagic presentation, patients with AVMs had a 17.8% annual risk of hemorrhage, whereas patients presenting without hemorrhage had only a 2.2% annual risk. Pollock and associates[119] found prior hemorrhage to be an independent risk factor in a multivariate analysis and calculated the risk of recurrent hemorrhage to be 7.5% per year. Other authors have documented an increased risk of hemorrhage after a hemorrhagic presentation.[113, 114, 117, 120, 121]

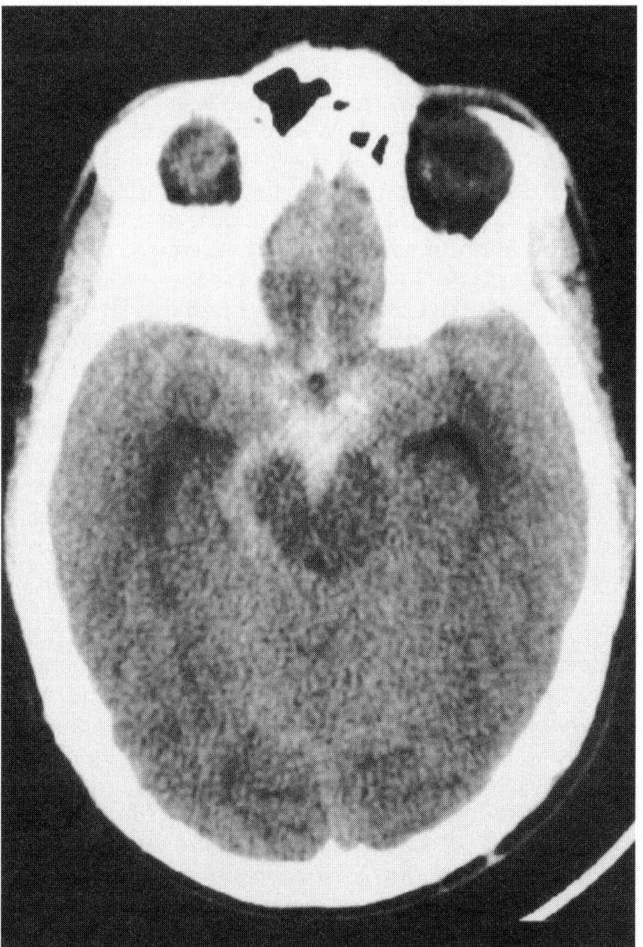

FIGURE 126–10. Non–contrast-enhanced CT scan of a healthy 26-year-old man who presented with a clinical history of headache shows subarachnoid hemorrhage in the interpeduncular and ambient cisterns.

Deep venous drainage of an AVM often is associated with hemorrhage and was found to be a significant independent risk factor by Mast,[118] Kader,[122] and Turjman[123] and their colleagues. High feeding artery pressures are thought to be predictive of risk and severity of hemorrhage and are thought to be associated inversely with the size of the AVM nidus.[122, 124] Other factors reported to lead to hemorrhage include male sex,[118] venous aneurysm or outflow compromise,[125] intranidal aneurysms or multiple aneurysms,[123] and feeding from perforating vessels.[123] A small AVM nidus has long been thought to represent an independent risk factor for intracranial hemorrhage.[117, 124, 126–128] Pollock and associates[119] studied the risk of AVM rehemorrhage, however, and found that a small AVM was not a predictor of increased risk of hemorrhage. This finding has been echoed in two other reports. The observation that small AVMs tend to present with hemorrhage may be a bias created by the fact that larger lesions tend to present with seizures.[129, 130]

Although most AVMs eventually are treated, a small, undefined population of patients experiences spontaneous resolution of their AVM. Abdulrauf and coworkers[131] reported 6 cases and identified another 24 cases in the literature. They could not identify definitively the factors leading to lesion regression, but histologic studies of their most recent specimen showed patent vascular channels and expression of antigens specific for endothelium and angiogenesis factor. They suggested that features predisposing patients to spontaneous AVM resolution might include a single draining vein, thrombosis secondary to mass effect of a clot, arteriosclerosis in AVM vessels, and kinking of vessels secondary to hemorrhage and gliosis.

Imaging

The imaging of intracranial AVMs is well documented and summarized by Osborn.[100] The salient imaging features basically relate to definition of the angioarchitecture. Conventional cerebral angiography shows three essential features: the feeding arteries, nidus, and draining veins. One of the important but not pathognomonic angiographic features is visualization of the AVM during the arterial phase of an early draining vein. This feature confirms the presence of an arteriovenous shunt. When the nidus is opacified completely, it is typically a wedge-shaped arrangement of tangled vessels with the base located superficially and the apex

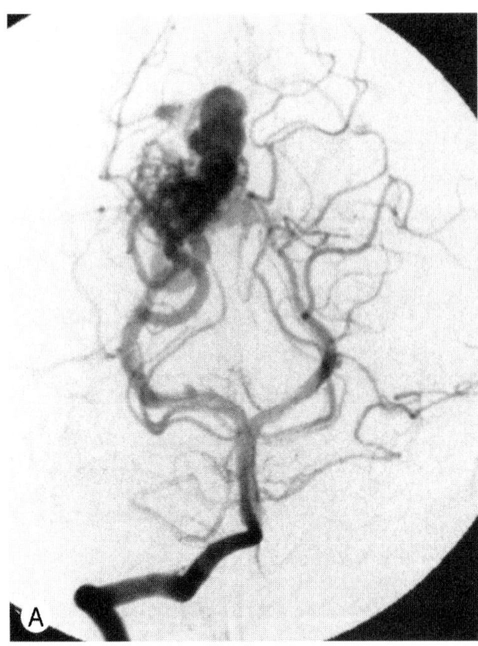

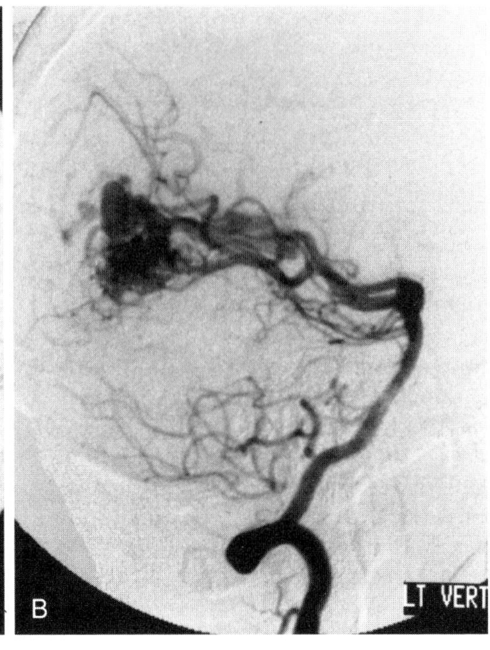

FIGURE 126–11. Conventional cerebral angiogram of the neurologically intact patient seen in Figure 126–10 shows an arteriovenous malformation (AVM). *A*, Anteroposterior view shows an AVM nidus filling from the posterior cerebral artery. A small distal flow-related aneurysm appears to arise just beyond the primary bifurcation of the posterior cerebral artery. A venous varix courses superomedially from the region of the nidus as well. *B*, Lateral projection also shows the nidus and the venous varix but not the aneurysm.

projecting toward the ventricular surface (accounting for the previously mentioned intraventricular hemorrhage). The angioarchitecture of the feeding and draining vessels is defined best using superselective injections of contrast material. Angiography is mandatory for the documentation of associated aneurysms (see later), venous varices, and vasculopathic stenotic segments on arteries and veins (Fig. 126–11). In the presence of a hemorrhage, mass effect also can be appreciated on angiography. In contemporary series, however, mass effect usually is documented first on CT or MRI. Although cavernous malformations comprise most angiographically occult vascular malformations, a thrombosed AVM can escape angiographic detection. The value of CT for the diagnosis and investigation of AVMs is limited. Hemorrhages of any type usually are identified on CT, however, and with contrast enhancement the images provide limited definition of the anatomy of the vascular malformation.

On MRI, hypointense signals, representing the tortuous feeding arteries, nidus, and draining veins, are seen in the region of the malformation. Hyperintense signals can represent thrombosed vessels. MRI also shows any associated hemorrhage at various stages of evolution. Similar to cavernous malformations, T2-weighted and GRE sequences are the most sensitive to breakdown products. Although magnetic resonance angiography can be performed and allows diagnosis of an AVM, its usefulness in surgical planning is limited. Conventional angiography is essential. MRI can be essential for preoperative planning in that it engenders an appreciation for the relationships between the lesion and important parenchymal and cortical areas and allows an appropriate surgical approach to be planned (Fig. 126–12).

Treatment

In approaching the treatment of AVMs, similar to any other disease, one must attempt to stratify the risks of treatment to compare the potential morbidity of a given treatment with the natural history of the disease. In 1986, Spetzler and Martin[132] introduced a grading scale for AVMs based on nidus size, location in relation to eloquent cortex, and venous drainage pattern (Table 126–2). Subsequently, this scale has been applied prospectively to a series of AVM patients and validated. Importantly, the use of all three variables in determining the patient's grade was the most accurate and statistically significant predictor of outcome.[133] The routine application of such a grading scheme is essential, especially given the results of Hartmann and colleagues[111] that suggest the initial morbidity associated with intracerebral hemorrhage is less than previously thought. Hartmann and colleagues[111] encourage a reevaluation of invasive treatments of patients with AVMs. All treatment modalities have risks that must be weighed carefully against the natural history risks during the treatment decision-making process.

The indications for surgical treatment can be classified according to the presenting symptoms: seizures, headache, focal neurological deficit, or hemorrhage. Anticonvulsant medications typically control seizures adequately,[134] and it is unusual for patients with AVMs to develop epilepsy refractory to medical treatment.[105] Of 118 patients who presented with seizures and who underwent excision of the AVM alone (without cortical resection), 56% were cured by surgery. The remainder had persistent seizures.[107] In contrast, 75% of patients were seizure-free after resection of the AVM plus cortical excision.[107] Results of both of these surgical techniques were superior to the results of embolization and ligation treatment strategies. If there is a strong suspicion that an AVM contributes to a patient's headache, the clinical response to AVM treatment may be good. In many patients, however, there is no causal association between the AVM and the headache.

Complete microsurgical resection of an AVM with

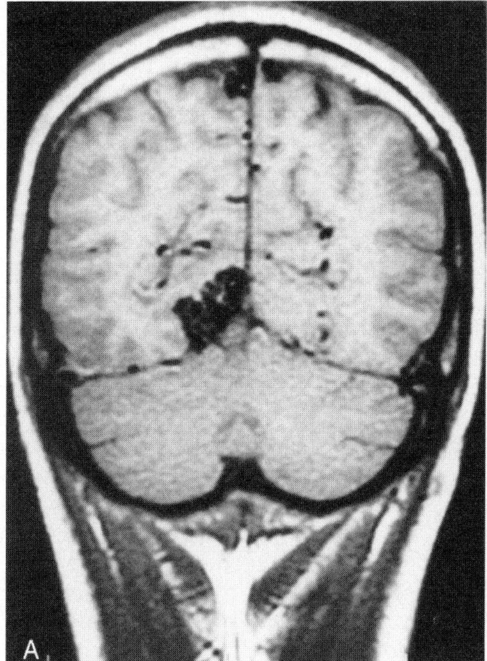

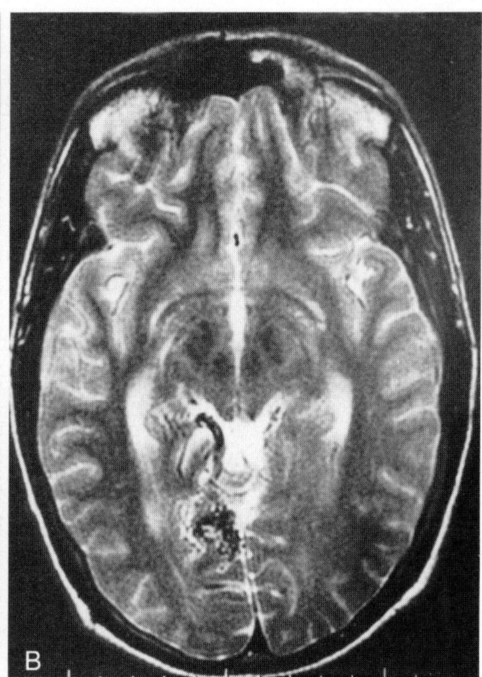

FIGURE 126–12. MRI scans of same patient shown in Figures 126–10 and 126–11 show the anatomic relationships of the AVM. *A*, Coronal T1-weighted image shows the arteriovenous malformation to be located entirely within the right occipital lobe. *B*, Axial T2-weighted image defines the relationship between the AVM and surrounding brain and shows the feeding artery as it courses through the ambient cistern.

angiographic confirmation of obliteration provides a cure with protection from hemorrhage in adult patients. The cure in children is less definitive. A growing body of literature suggests that AVMs are more dynamic in children and may have the ability to regenerate after negative angiography studies.[135, 136] In a review of surgical results, it was determined that the surgical risk of permanent neurological morbidity and mortality for grade 1 to grade 3 patients was low (0%). In higher grade patients, the risks were considerably higher: Grade 4 patients incurred a 21.9% risk, and grade V patients incurred a 16.7% risk.[133] Microsurgical adjuncts to help facilitate a better surgical outcome include the use of stimulation, mapping, corticography, and functional MRI.[137, 138] Microsurgery is the gold standard for the definitive treatment of AVMs. The risks of surgery and techniques of AVM resection are discussed in later chapters.

TABLE 126–2 ■ **Spetzler-Martin Scale of Evaluating the Risk of Surgery in Patients with Arteriovenous Malformation**

CHARACTERISTIC	POINTS
Lesion size	
Small (<3 cm)	1
Medium (3–6 cm)	2
Large (>6 cm)	3
Location	
Noneloquent site	0
Eloquent site	1
Venous drainage pattern	
Superficial only	0
Any deep drainage	1

From Spetzler RF, Martin NA: A proposed grading system for arteriovenous malformations. J Neurosurg 65:476–483, 1986; with permission from the *Journal of Neurosurgery.*

The use of stereotactic radiosurgery to treat these lesions has become fairly well established. Approximately 80% of the lesions less than 3 cm in diameter can be obliterated.[128, 139, 140] The time from treatment to obliteration ranges from 2 to 3 years. During that interval, the patient has no protection from hemorrhage because of the delay involved in achieving changes after radiation. Pollock and colleagues[129] reported that during the initial 2 years after radiosurgery the risk of hemorrhage was 4.8% per year. This finding compares favorably with the natural history but is less favorable than microsurgical removal, had it been possible. The risk of hemorrhage is slightly higher (5.0% per year) but not remarkably different from that of the natural history 2 to 5 years after radiosurgery. Friedman and associates[141] found no difference between the hemorrhage rate after radiosurgery and the natural history of the disease. Although these results compare favorably with the natural history of the disease, Pikus and coworkers[142] compared the results of grade I to III AVMs treated microsurgically with stereotactic radiosurgery. With microsurgical treatment, there were statistically significantly fewer postoperative hemorrhages, deaths, and neurological deficits and a higher incidence of obliteration. Additionally, these investigators reported a significant difference between the two groups in hemorrhage-free survival. Gallina and associates[143] identified several reasons for the failure of radiosurgical treatment. Primarily the failures reflected technical errors, including errors in evaluating the target's shape and size and missing the target. In several cases, the lesion intentionally was treated nonaggressively as a strategic choice (i.e., high perceived risk of complications). In one case, the AVM was reperfused by a previously embolized portion of the lesion.

Treatment of AVMs with embolization techniques is associated with a low rate of complete obliteration.

These strategies are used primarily as adjunctive treatment to reduce the size of the lesion before microsurgical or radiosurgical treatment. Gobin and coworkers[144] described the successful angiographic obliteration by embolization alone in only slightly more than 10% of the AVMs. They stated that there was almost no chance of completely occluding an AVM with more than three feeding arteries using endovascular therapy alone. Potential causes of complications in these procedures included occlusion of normal arteries by thrombi, technical difficulties with catheters and glue polymerization times, and occlusion of the draining vein while the nidus was being actively fed. As with radiosurgical treatment, the hemorrhage rate after embolization resulting in residual nidus mirrored the natural history of the disease.

Arteriovenous Malformation–Associated Aneurysms

As mentioned, a distinct group of AVM patients presents with an associated intracranial aneurysm. The pathophysiology of these lesions is not known definitively, but the predominant theory relates their development to a high-flow vasculopathy.[122, 145, 146] Aneurysms are associated with 2.3% to 16.7% of AVMs.[147, 148] With superselective angiography, however, Turjman and associates[149] found aneurysms in 58% of patients. Although their incidence may not be defined clearly, aneurysms are associated more frequently with AVMs than they are in the general population.

AVM-associated aneurysms are classified by location, which appears to be correlated with clinical behavior before and after treatment. AVM-associated aneurysms are categorized as being either flow-related or unrelated. The latter are located on remote vessels that bear no relation to the blood supply of the AVM.[130, 150] Flow-related aneurysms occur along vessels that supply the AVM and are classified as either proximal (from vessels on the circle of Willis or the proximal feeding vessels up to a primary bifurcation) or distal (from the feeding vessel distal to its origin from the parent artery at its primary bifurcation).[130, 150] Intranidal aneurysms occur within the nidus of the AVM and show filling early during angiography.[130] The incidence of aneurysms at each of these locations and which ones are most likely to be associated with an increased risk of hemorrhage are controversial issues. Flow-related aneurysms account for 85% of the aneurysms, whereas 15% are remote. Redekop and coworkers[130] found that 5.5% of flow-related aneurysms were intranidal.

Patients with an AVM and an aneurysm have a higher risk (7% per year) of intracranial hemorrhage than patients with AVMs alone.[115] Most eventually present after a hemorrhage that more often than not involves the aneurysm.[150] Redekop and coworkers[130] found that intranidal aneurysms posed a particularly high threat of rupture and calculated the risk at 9.8% per year. These authors found that distal flow-related aneurysms regressed 80% of the time with complete AVM obliteration. In contrast, proximal aneurysms rarely regressed completely (4%), and the size of only 17% more decreased. Pollock and coworkers[129] noted a statistically significant hemorrhage rate from flow-related aneurysms after radiosurgery for AVMs (proximal or distal location was not specified). No hemorrhages came from intranidal lesions. Thompson and colleagues[150] reported several deaths caused by aneurysm hemorrhage related to treatment of the AVM. Based on their experience, they recommend endovascular or microsurgical treatment of the aneurysm before treating the AVM.

The approaches to the management of AVM-associated aneurysms can be summarized as follows: First, symptomatic (ruptured) aneurysms should be treated according to standard management protocols for ruptured aneurysms. Two schools of thought exist concerning the management of unruptured AVM-associated aneurysms. One school suggests that AVM treatment constitutes a reasonably effective passive treatment for the aneurysm; the other suggests that a small but definable risk of aneurysm rupture after AVM treatment warrants primary treatment of the aneurysm.

MIXED ARTERIOVASCULAR MALFORMATIONS

With the increasingly sensitive and specific diagnostic yield of MRI and growing clinical experience with previously angiographically occult arteriovascular malformations, the number of patients reported to harbor multiple malformations is increasing.[11, 33, 91, 151–155] Concomitantly the body of literature dealing specifically with *mixed malformations* or *transitional forms* is enlarging.[12, 27, 43, 78, 152, 156, 157] It is becoming difficult to find a current sizable series of patients with arteriovascular malformations that lacks patients with mixed malformations. The natural history of these lesions is unknown because they have been described relatively recently and have not been studied in a longitudinal fashion. Little is known about their prevalence, their natural history, or, more importantly, their pathogenesis. Numerous interesting questions have been raised, however, about their pathogenesis based on the rare occurrence of mixed malformations in the same patient.

Capillary Telangiectasias and Developmental Venous Anomalies

Wolf and Brock[30] first observed the definite presence of a vein within a capillary telangiectasia, suggesting that developmental venous anomalies might have developed from the capillary telangiectasia. Blackwood[10] made an early observation regarding the similarity between capillary telangiectasias and developmental venous anomalies. Challa and associates[158] stated that the two cannot be distinguished unless a draining vein is seen. In a case report of a hemorrhage from a capillary telangiectasia associated with a developmental venous anomaly, McCormick and colleagues[159] suggested that the capillary telangiectasia may develop as a result of venous hypertension within the developmental venous anomaly and may be a transitional early form of cavernous malformation. Van Roost and coworkers[154] reported a patient with a coexisting developmental venous anomaly and capillary telangiectasia and discussed their findings in the context of mixed arteriovascular malformations. This association is speculative, and these pathophysiologic mechanisms are elaborated on further (see later).

Capillary Telangiectasias and Cavernous Malformations

Russell[160] first hypothesized that cavernous malformations may be derived from capillary telangiectasias. This theory was largely rejected until more recent reports provided substantiating evidence. Rigamonti and coworkers[157] studied the radiographic and histopathologic characteristics of these lesions and found that normal parenchyma exists between the dilated vascular channels within 35% of cavernous malformations, a feature traditionally assigned to capillary telangiectasia. These workers suggested that these two lesions be combined under the category *cerebral capillary malformations*. This categorization has not yet gained widespread acceptance, however.

Awad and colleagues[78] reported two such cases. In their patients, capillary telangiectasias were located in a zone of parenchyma surrounding the cavernous malformations. They suggested that these lesions may be two manifestations of the same disease process and that cavernous malformations may arise from capillary telangiectasias through the same processes that are proposed to cause cavernous malformations to grow. This pathogenetic concept first was elaborated when Rigamonti and associates[157] reported that 42% of the studied cavernous malformations had either a distinct capillary telangiectasia or a transitional form. In support of this theory, another group from the same institution later included capillary telangiectasia–like malformations as type IV lesions in their MRI classification of cavernous malformations.[57]

Theoretically, factors underlying the growth or de novo formation of cavernous malformations would be involved in the transformation of a capillary telangiectasia to a cavernous malformation. Various angiogenic factors, including basic fibroblast growth factor and platelet-derived growth factor, may be influential in the initiation and propagation of this change.[161, 162]

Cavernous Malformations and Developmental Venous Anomalies

Numerous authors have described this particular combination of vascular malformations.[151] Awad and colleagues[78] found that almost half of their mixed malformations were of this type. This particular combination of vascular malformations is likely the most common form of mixed malformation. Considering that developmental venous anomalies are the most common arteriovascular malformation and that 8% of these lesions have an associated cavernous malformation, it is intuitive that they should occur frequently.[163] Most importantly, a clinical presentation in any of these patients is related to the cavernous malformation. This particular combination of malformations is diagnosed easily with MRI, currently the diagnostic modality of choice for both lesions. An associated pathogenesis for cavernous malformations and developmental venous anomalies is speculative. Sasaki and coworkers[151] showed a direct connection between a developmental venous anomaly and cavernous malformation in their patient.

The most enticing theory predicts that brief episodes of mild venous hypertension at the site of a developmental venous anomaly cause microhemorrhages or obstruct venous outflow. These microhemorrhages may precipitate the development of a cavernous malformation through the release of angiogenic factors. If this were truly the case, however, one might expect to see cavernous malformations associated with more than the observed 8% of developmental venous anomalies.[163]

True Arteriovenous Malformations and Other Vascular Malformations

Mixed lesions that include a component of true AVM are relatively uncommon. It is unusual to encounter a mixed lesion that has a true arterial component, especially when the current theories regarding the pathogenesis of these other transitional lesions are considered.

ARTERIOVENOUS MALFORMATIONS AND CAPILLARY TELANGIECTASIAS

A case was reported in which a capillary telangiectasia grew and became symptomatic approximately 1 month after the resection of an adjacent AVM.[12] The authors postulated that the growth of the capillary telangiectasia may have been caused by the decompressive effect or changes in hemodynamics associated with the AVM resection or by the release of angiogenic factors after surgery. This is the only report of such an association. It is difficult to explain the coexistence of these two lesions from the perspective of a unified pathogenesis. The association may represent random chance.

ARTERIOVENOUS MALFORMATIONS AND DEVELOPMENTAL VENOUS ANOMALIES

The coexistence of developmental venous anomalies and AVMs is described better, despite being one of the rarer combinations. The earliest description may have been that of Hirata and colleagues.[164] This case did not show an AVM nidus, however, and may have represented an arteriovenous fistula. In the series by Awad and coworkers,[78] three lesions clearly had components of AVMs and developmental venous anomalies. The clinical presentation of these three patients was considered secondary to the AVM, not to the developmental venous anomaly.

These combined lesions preserve the appearance of the developmental venous anomaly on angiography with the exception of arteriovenous shunting during the arterial phase of the injection. Consequently the venous lesion is identified earlier. In contrast to some of the other vascular malformation combinations, it is difficult to appreciate the developmental venous anomaly separate from the AVM on MRI. Conventional cerebral angiography is more sensitive. Meyer and associates[43] emphasized the pitfall of obliterating the developmental venous anomaly when approaching the AVM component when a hemorrhage is symptomatic.[43]

This combination is probably the simplest of all of the mixed malformations to explain from a pathophysiologic perspective. Mullan and colleagues[27] reviewed four such patients and discussed the pathophysiology in context of embryologic development of the cerebral venous system. They suggested that in these situations, the AVM might form in a fashion similar to a dural arteriovenous fistula: Thrombosis of the star cluster would allow the developmental venous anomaly to become arterialized, forming the basis of an AVM. In reviewing their patient with a combined AVM and developmental venous anomaly, Nussbaum and associates[156] acknowledged that venous hypertension may increase directly (through erythrocyte diapedesis) or indirectly (through tissue ischemia) the levels of angiogenic factors as previously suggested by Wilson.[165] This venous hypertension may be chronic at the site of drainage of the developmental venous anomaly, with an acute increase reflecting an increase in intracranial venous pressure or as a result of acute thrombosis.[165] Comey and associates[152] mentioned an unpublished series of patients who showed so-called collector vein stenosis, which would serve to create venous hypertension and strengthen this hypothesis further. Wilson[165] speculated that venous hypertension may force open previously diminutive arteriovenous shunts, which then could enlarge over time. In support of these theories, the literature has described areas of hyperintensity surrounding some developmental venous anomalies associated with cavernous malformations. The finding may indicate that in some patients there is legitimate hypertension and disruption of the blood-brain barrier.[152] This concept is supported by a case reported by Ciricillo and coworkers.[166] An angiographically occult AVM in association with a developmental venous anomaly was resected from a child who later developed new angiographically occult lesions, presumably cavernous malformations.

ARTERIOVENOUS MALFORMATIONS AND CAVERNOUS MALFORMATIONS

AVMs have been described in association with cavernous malformations. Garner and coworkers[33] reported one such patient, and Awad and coworkers[78] reported three. The latter group suggested that the AVM portion of the lesion tends to be angiographically and radiographically occult, making preoperative diagnosis extremely difficult. With respect to pathogenesis, smooth muscle may develop in the wall of the cavernous malformation as a reaction to angiogenic factors. An alternative theory suggests that microhemorrhage from an occult AVM precipitates development of the cavernous malformation.

SYNDROMIC VASCULAR MALFORMATIONS

Although rare, there is a genetic predisposition for certain arteriovascular malformations to develop in association with two syndromes.[100] Multiple AVMs occur in Rendu-Osler-Weber syndrome (hereditary hemorrhagic telangiectasia) and Wyburn-Mason syndrome, which are described briefly here.

Rendu-Osler-Weber Syndrome

Rendu-Osler-Weber syndrome first was described about 100 years ago and is the most common form of familial AVMs. It has been determined that Rendu-Osler-Weber syndrome represents a collection of autosomal dominant disorders. Its prevalence ranges geographically from 1 in 2351 to 1 in 39,216.[167] The disorder has been linked to areas on chromosomes 9q and 12q.[168–170] The mutation is presumed to affect a membrane glycoprotein that binds transforming growth factor-β with resultant abnormalities of endothelial cell adhesion, proliferation, and migration.[167] Structurally the vessels are abnormal with dilation of venules into telangiectasias and loss of elastic fibers. True AVMs also occur, although they are rare.

Non-neurological manifestations include epistaxis from telangiectasias of the nasal mucosa; skin lesions that represent cutaneous telangiectasia; pulmonary arteriovenous fistulas, which can lead to brain abscess or stroke; and recurrent upper and lower gastrointestinal hemorrhage from telangiectasias, AVMs, or angiodysplasias.[167] Cerebral manifestations predominantly reflect ischemia or infection.

AVMs occur in about 5% of patients with Rendu-Osler-Weber syndrome, and about a third of patients become symptomatic with hemorrhage or seizure secondary to an intracranial AVM.[171–174] In a review of patients with multiple AVMs, five of the seven patients with a family history of vascular disease had Rendu-Osler-Weber syndrome.[173] The management of these lesions should consider all the principles of vascular malformation management outlined in this and other chapters. Unaffected family members of patients with Rendu-Osler-Weber syndrome have an increased risk of having a cerebral AVM, suggesting a potential role for screening with MRI.[167]

Wyburn-Mason Syndrome

Encephaloretinofacial angiomatosis, or Wyburn-Mason syndrome, is a rare condition involving unilateral vascular malformations of the diencephalon or mesencephalon, ipsilateral retina, and face.[105, 175] Mental changes also have been noted.[175] The underlying genetic defect is unknown.[176] The clinical presentation varies depending on the site of the AVM and can include hemiparesis, cognitive changes, seizures, cerebellar dysfunction, or Parinaud's syndrome.[177] Subarachnoid or intracerebral hemorrhages can occur. These vascular malformations tend to follow the optic tracts and radiations.[173] Because of the deep-seated nature of these AVMs, treatment is complicated and frequently multimodal.

CONCLUSION

Although clinicians are gaining a better understanding of how arteriovascular malformations look and, to a certain extent, behave, we are only beginning to understand their pathogenesis and pathophysiology. Advances in imaging technology now allow clinicians to follow these lesions in a prospective and analytic fashion. As we acquire a greater understanding of their natural history, treatment issues become defined more clearly. Only recently have clinicians begun to understand their genetic basis.

Theories that attempt to unify the cause of arteriovascular malformations raise as many questions as they answer. If cavernous malformations are truly manifestations of the same pathophysiologic process as capillary telangiectasias, why has the familial occurrence of the latter not been documented? If developmental venous anomalies and AVMs represent the same spectrum of disease, what is the inciting factor that triggers differentiation into an AVM? If the theories of mixed malformations are correct and cavernous malformations, developmental venous anomalies, and capillary telangiectasias are truly manifestations of a single pathophysiologic process, what determines when these lesions stop differentiating? Alternatively, these theories suggest that cavernous malformations and AVMs can arise from developmental venous anomalies, but what determines the path that will be followed? Much remains to be learned of the pathogenetic mechanisms underlying the formation of arteriovascular malformations.

REFERENCES

1. McCormick WF: The pathology of vascular ("arteriovenous") malformations. J Neurosurg 24:807–816, 1966.
2. McCormick WF, Nofzinger JD: "Cryptic" vascular malformations of the central nervous system. J Neurosurg 24:865–875, 1966.
3. Russell DS, Rubenstein LJ: Pathology of Tumours of the Nervous System, 3rd ed. Baltimore, Williams & Wilkins, 1971.
4. Sarwar M, McCormick WF: Intracerebral venous angioma: Case report and review. Arch Neurol 35:323–325, 1978.
5. Russell DS, Rubenstein LJ: Pathology of Tumours of the Nervous System, 5th ed. Baltimore, Williams & Wilkins, 1989.
6. White RJ, Kernohan JW, Wood MW: A study of fifty intracranial vascular tumours found incidentally at autopsy. J Neuropathol Exp Neurol 17:392–398, 1958.
7. Rigamonti D, Hsu FPK, Huhn S: Angiographically occult vascular malformations. In Carter LP, Spetzler RF, Hamilton MG (eds): Neurovascular Surgery. New York, McGraw-Hill, 1995, pp 521–540.
8. Michael JC, Levin PM: Multiple telangiectasias of the brain: A discussion of hereditary factors in their development. Arch Neurol Psychiatry 36:514, 1936.
9. Kufs H: Über heredofamiliare angiomatose des Gehirns und der Retina, ihre Bexiehungen Zueinander und ur angiomatose der haut. Z Neurol Psychiatr 113:651, 1928.
10. Blackwood W: Two cases of benign cerebral telangiectasis. J Pathol Bacteriol 52:209, 1941.
11. Lee RR, Becher MW, Benson ML, et al: Brain capillary telangiectasia: MR imaging appearance and clinicohistopathologic findings. Radiology 205:797–805, 1997.
12. Chang SD, Steinberg GK, Rosario M, et al: Mixed arteriovenous malformation and capillary telangiectasia: A rare subset of mixed vascular malformations: Case report. J Neurosurg 86: 699–703, 1997.
13. Bland LI, Lapham LW, Ketonen L, et al: Acute cerebellar hemorrhage secondary to capillary telangiectasia in an infant: A case report. Arch Neurol 51:1151–1154, 1994.
14. Rengachary SS, Kalyan-Raman UP: Telangiectasias and venous angiomas. In Wilkins RH, Rengachary SS (eds): Neurosurgery. New York, McGraw-Hill, 1996, pp 2509–2514.
15. Vaquero J, Manrique M, Oya S, et al: Calcified telangiectatic hamartomas of the brain. Surg Neurol 13:453–457, 1980.
16. Thrash AM: Vascular malformations of the cerebellum. Arch Pathol 75:65–69, 1963.
17. Sahs A: Intracranial Aneurysm and Subarachnoid Hemorrhage: A Cooperative Study. Philadelphia, JB Lippincott, 1969.
18. Moritake K, Handa H, Mori K, et al: Venous angiomas of the brain. Surg Neurol 14:95–105, 1980.
19. Handa H: Venous angiomas of the brain. In Fein JM (ed): Cerebrovascular Surgery. New York, Springer Verlag, 1985, pp 1139–1149.
20. Farrell DF, Forno LS: Symptomatic capillary telangiectasis of the brainstem without hemorrhage: Report of an unusual case. Neurology 20:341–346, 1970.
21. Cushing H, Bailey P: Tumours Arising from the Blood Vessels of the Brain. Springfield, IL, Charles C Thomas, 1928, pp 9–102.
22. Töpper R, Jürgens E, Reul J, et al: Clinical significance of intracranial developmental venous anomalies. J Neurol Neurosurg Psychiatry 67:234–238, 1999.
23. Rigamonti D, Spetzler RF, Medina M, et al: Cerebral venous malformations. J Neurosurg 73:560–564, 1990.
24. Saito Y, Kobayashi N: Cerebral venous angiomas: Clinical evaluation and possible etiology. Radiology 139:87–94, 1981.
25. Toro VE, Geyer CA, Sherman JL, et al: Cerebral venous angiomas: MR findings. J Comput Assist Tomogr 12:935–940, 1988.
26. Mullan S, Mojtahedi S, Johnson DL, et al: Embryological basis of some aspects of cerebral vascular fistulas and malformations. J Neurosurg 85:1–8, 1996.
27. Mullan S, Mojtahedi S, Johnson DL, et al: Cerebral venous malformation-arteriovenous malformation transition forms. J Neurosurg 85:9–13, 1996.
28. Pfannenstiel J: Apoplexie als todlicher Ausgang von Eklampsie. Zentrabl Gynakol 11:601–606, 1887.
29. Pak H, Patel SC, Malik GM, et al: Successful evacuation of a pontine hematoma secondary to rupture of a venous angioma. Surg Neurol 15:164–167, 1981.
30. Wolf A, Brock S: The pathology of cerebral angiomas. Bull Neurol Inst New York 4:144, 1935–1936.
31. McLaughlin MR, Kondziolka D, Flickinger JC, et al: The prospective natural history of cerebral venous malformations. Neurosurgery 43:195–201, 1998.
32. Truwit CL: Venous angioma of the brain: history, significance, and imaging findings. AJR Am J Roentgenol 159:1299–1307, 1992.
33. Garner TB, Del Curling O Jr, Kelly DL Jr, et al: The natural history of intracranial venous angiomas. J Neurosurg 75:715–722, 1991.
34. McCormick WF, Hardman JM, Boulter TR: Vascular malformations ("angiomas") of the brain, with special reference to those occurring in the posterior fossa. J Neurosurg 28:241–251, 1968.
35. Malik GM, Morgan JK, Boulos RS, et al: Venous angiomas: An underestimated cause of intracranial hemorrhage. Surg Neurol 30:350–358, 1988.
36. Wolf PA, Rosman NP, New PF: Multiple small cryptic venous angiomas of the brain mimicking cerebral metastases: A clinical, pathological, and angiographic study. Neurology 17:491–501, 1967.
37. Rigamonti D, Spetzler RF, Drayer BP, et al: Appearance of

venous malformations on magnetic resonance imaging. J Neurosurg 69:535–539, 1988.
38. Augustyn GT, Scott JA, Olson E, et al: Cerebral venous angiomas: MR imaging. Radiology 156:391–395, 1985.
39. Cammarata C, Han JS, Haaga JR, et al: Cerebral venous angiomas imaged by MR. Radiology 155:639–643, 1985.
40. Jung G, Schröder R, Lanfermann H, et al: Evidence of acute demyelination around a developmental venous anomaly: Magnetic resonance imaging findings. Invest Radiol 32:575–577, 1997.
41. Biller J, Toffol GJ, Shea JF, et al: Cerebellar venous angiomas: A continuing controversy. Arch Neurol 42:367–370, 1985.
42. Lobato RD, Perez C, Rivas JJ, et al: Clinical, radiological, and pathological spectrum of angiographically occult intracranial vascular malformations: Analysis of 21 cases and review of the literature. J Neurosurg 68:518–531, 1988.
43. Meyer B, Stangl AP, Schramm J: Association of venous and true arteriovenous malformation: A rare entity among mixed vascular malformations of the brain: Case report. J Neurosurg 83:141–144, 1995.
44. Sadeh M, Shacked I, Rappaport ZH, et al: Surgical extirpation of a venous angioma of the medulla oblongata simulating multiple sclerosis. Surg Neurol 17:334–337, 1982.
45. Senegor M, Dohrmann GJ, Wollmann RL: Venous angiomas of the posterior fossa should be considered as anomalous venous drainage. Surg Neurol 19:26–32, 1983.
46. Awad IA: Radiosurgery and venous malformations [letter]. J Neurosurg 80:171–175, 1994.
47. Goulao A, Alvarez H, Garcia Monaco R, et al: Venous anomalies and abnormalities of the posterior fossa. Neuroradiology 31: 476–482, 1990.
48. Lasjaunias P, Burrows P, Planet C: Developmental venous anomalies (DVA): The so-called venous angioma. Neurosurg Rev 9:233–242, 1986.
49. Spetzler RF, Hamilton MG: Radiosurgery and venous malformations [letter] J Neurosurg 80:173–175, 1994.
50. Stein BM, Sisti MB, Mohr JP, et al: Radiosurgery and venous malformations [letter] J Neurosurg 80:175–177, 1994.
51. Yamamoto M, Inagawa T, Kamiya K, et al: Intracerebral hemorrhage due to venous thrombosis in venous angioma—case report. Neurol Med Chir (Tokyo) 29:1044–1046, 1989.
52. Kim P, Castellani R, Tresser N: Cerebral venous malformation complicated by spontaneous thrombosis. Childs Nerv Syst 12: 172–175, 1996.
53. Lindquist C, Guo WY, Karlsson B, et al: Radiosurgery for venous angiomas. J Neurosurg 78:531–536, 1993.
54. Robinson JR, Awad IA, Little JR: Natural history of the cavernous angioma. J Neurosurg 75:709–714, 1991.
55. Otten P, Pizzolato GP, Rilliet B, et al: 131 cases of cavernous angioma (cavernomas) of the CNS, discovered by retrospective analysis of 24,535 autopsies [Fr]. Neurochirurgie 35:82–83, 1989.
56. Del Curling O Jr, Kelly DL Jr, Elster AD, et al: An analysis of the natural history of cavernous angiomas. J Neurosurg 75: 702–708, 1991.
57. Zabramski JM, Wascher TM, Spetzler RF, et al: The natural history of familial cavernous malformations: Results of an ongoing study. J Neurosurg 80:422–432, 1994.
58. Rigamonti D, Hadley MN, Drayer BP, et al: Cerebral cavernous malformations: Incidence and familial occurrence. N Engl J Med 319:343–347, 1988.
59. Hayman LA, Evans RA, Ferrell RE, et al: Familial cavernous angiomas: Natural history and genetic study over a 5-year period. Am J Med Genet 11:147–160, 1982.
60. Kidd HA, Cumings JN: Cerebral angiomata in an Icelandic family. Lancet 1:747–748, 1947.
61. Labauge P, Laberge S, Brunereau L, et al: Hereditary cerebral cavernous angiomas: Clinical and genetic features in 57 French families. Société Française de Neurochirurgie. Lancet 352:1892–1897, 1998.
62. Dubovsky J, Zabramski JM, Kurth J, et al: A gene responsible for cavernous malformations of the brain maps to chromosome 7q. Hum Mol Genet 4:453–458, 1995.
63. Gunel M, Awad IA, Finberg K, et al: A founder mutation as a cause of cerebral cavernous malformation in Hispanic Americans. N Engl J Med 334:946–951, 1996.
64. Gunel M, Awad IA, Finberg K, et al: Genetic heterogeneity of inherited cerebral cavernous malformation. Neurosurgery 38: 1265–1271, 1996.
65. Craig HD, Günel M, Cepeda O, et al: Multilocus linkage identifies two new loci for a Mendelian form of stroke, cerebral cavernous malformation, at 7p15-13 and 3q25.2-27. Hum Mol Genet 7:1851–1858, 1998.
66. Siegel AM: Familial cavernous angioma: An unknown, known disease. Acta Neurol Scand 98:369–371, 1998.
67. Siegel AM, Andermann F, Badhwar A, et al: Anticipation in familial cavernous angioma: Ascertainment bias or genetic cause. Acta Neurol Scand 98:372–376, 1998.
68. Voigt K, Yasargil MG: Cerebral cavernous haemangiomas or cavernomas: Incidence, pathology, localization, diagnosis, clinical features and treatment: Review of the literature and report of an unusual case. Neurochirurgia (Stuttg) 19:59–68, 1976.
69. Giombini S, Morello G: Cavernous angiomas of the brain: Account of fourteen personal cases and review of the literature. Acta Neurochir (Wien) 40:61–82, 1978.
70. Moran NF, Fish DR, Kitchen N, et al: Supratentorial cavernous haemangiomas and epilepsy: A review of the literature and case series. J Neurol Neurosurg Psychiatry 66:561–568, 1999.
71. Robinson JR Jr, Awad IA, Magdinec M, et al: Factors predisposing to clinical disability in patients with cavernous malformations of the brain. Neurosurgery 32:730–736, 1993.
72. Jellinger K: Vascular malformations of the central nervous system: A morphological overview. Neurosurg Rev 9:177–216, 1986.
73. Little JR, Awad IA, Jones SC, et al: Vascular pressures and cortical blood flow in cavernous angioma of the brain. J Neurosurg 73:555–559, 1990.
74. Steiger HJ, Markwalder TM, Reulen HJ: Clinicopathological relations of cerebral cavernous angiomas: Observations in eleven cases. Neurosurgery 21:879–884, 1987.
75. Scott RM, Barnes P, Kupsky W, et al: Cavernous angiomas of the central nervous system in children. J Neurosurg 76: 38–46, 1992.
76. Frim DM, Zec N, Golden J, et al: Immunohistochemically identifiable tissue plasminogen activator in cavernous angioma: Mechanism for re-hemorrhage and lesion growth. Pediatr Neurosurg 25:137–142, 1996.
77. Pozzati E, Acciarri N, Tognetti F, et al: Growth, subsequent bleeding, and de novo appearance of cerebral cavernous angiomas. Neurosurgery 38:662–670, 1996.
78. Awad IA, Robinson JR Jr, Mohanty S, et al: Mixed vascular malformations of the brain: Clinical and pathogenetic considerations. Neurosurgery 33:179–188, 1993.
79. Comair Y, LeBlanc R, Robitaille Y: Effects of estrogen on cerebral arteriovenous malformations in vitro: Towards a new paradigm [abstract]. J Neurosurg 72:337A, 1990.
80. Katayama Y, Tsubokawa T, Maeda T, et al: Surgical management of cavernous malformations of the third ventricle. J Neurosurg 80:64–72, 1994.
81. Larson JJ, Ball WS, Bove KE, et al: Formation of intracerebral cavernous malformations after radiation treatment for central nervous system neoplasia in children. J Neurosurg 88:51–56, 1998.
82. Baev NI, Awad IA: Endothelial cell culture from human cerebral cavernous malformations. Stroke 29:2426–2434, 1998.
83. Kraemer DL, Awad IA: Vascular malformations and epilepsy: Clinical considerations and basic mechanisms. Epilepsia 35(Suppl 6):S30–43, 1994.
84. Rigamonti D, Hsu FPK, Monstein LH: Cavernous malformations and related lesions. In Wilkins RH, Rengachary SS (eds): Neurosurgery. New York, McGraw-Hill, 1996, pp 2503–2508.
85. Casazza M, Broggi G, Franzini A, et al: Supratentorial cavernous angiomas and epileptic seizures: Preoperative course and postoperative outcome. Neurosurgery 39:26–34, 1996.
86. Kondziolka D, Lunsford LD, Kestle JR: The natural history of cerebral cavernous malformations. J Neurosurg 83:820–824, 1995.
86a. Porter PJ, Willinsky RA, Harper W, Wallace MC: Cerebral cavernous malformations: Natural history and prognosis after clinical deterioration with or without hemorrhage. J Neurosurg 87:190–197, 1997.

87. Detwiler PW, Porter RW, Zabramski JM, et al: Radiation-induced cavernous malformation [letter]. J Neurosurg 89:167–169, 1998.
88. Requena I, Arias M, López-Ibor L, et al: Cavernomas of the central nervous system: Clinical and neuroimaging manifestations in 47 patients. J Neurol Neurosurg Psychiatry 54:590–594, 1991.
89. Rigamonti D, Drayer BP, Johnson PC, et al: The MRI appearance of cavernous malformations (angiomas). J Neurosurg 67:518–524, 1987.
90. Margolis G, Odom GL, Woodhall B: Further experiences with small vascular malformations as a cause of massive intracerebral bleeding. J Neuropathol Exp Neurol 20:161–167, 1961.
91. Giulioni M, Acciarri N, Padovani R, et al: Results of surgery in children with cerebral cavernous angiomas causing epilepsy. Br J Neurosurg 9:135–141, 1995.
92. Zevgaridis D, van Velthoven V, Ebeling U, et al: Seizure control following surgery in supratentorial cavernous malformations: A retrospective study in 77 patients. Acta Neurochir (Wien) 138: 672–677, 1996.
93. Cohen DS, Zubay GP, Goodman RR: Seizure outcome after lesionectomy for cavernous malformations. J Neurosurg 83:237–242, 1995.
94. Well S, Tew JM, Steiner L: Comparison of radiosurgery and microsurgery for treatment of cavernous malformations of the brainstem [abstract]. J Neurosurg 72:336A, 1990.
95. Kondziolka D, Lunsford LD, Flickinger JC, et al: Reduction of hemorrhage risk after stereotactic radiosurgery for cavernous malformations. J Neurosurg 83:825–831, 1995.
96. Karlsson B, Kihlström L, Lindquist C, et al: Radiosurgery for cavernous malformations. J Neurosurg 88:293–297, 1998.
97. Gewirtz RJ, Steinberg GK, Crowley R, et al: Pathological changes in surgically resected angiographically occult vascular malformations after radiation. Neurosurgery 42:738–743, 1998.
98. Seo Y, Fukuoka S, Takanashi M, et al: Gamma Knife surgery for angiographically occult vascular malformations. Stereotact Funct Neurosurg 64(Suppl 1):98–109, 1995.
99. Kida Y, Kobayashi T, Tanaka T: Treatment of symptomatic AOVMs with radiosurgery. Acta Neurochir Suppl (Wien) 63: 68–72, 1995.
100. Osborn AG: Intracranial vascular malformations. In Osborn AG (ed): Diagnostic Neuroradiology. St Louis, Mosby-Year Book, 1994, pp 284–301.
101. Brown RD Jr, Wiebers DO, Torner JC, et al: Frequency of intracranial hemorrhage as a presenting symptom and subtype analysis: A population-based study of intracranial vascular malformations in Olmsted Country, Minnesota. J Neurosurg 85:29–32, 1996.
102. Arteriovenous Malformation Study Group: Arteriovenous malformations of the brain in adults. N Engl J Med 340:1812–1818, 1999.
103. McCormick WE: Classification, pathology and natural history of angiomas of the central nervous system. Wkly Update Neurol Neurosurg 14:2–7, 1978.
104. Ruiz-Sandoval JL, Cantu C, Barinagarrementeria F: Intracerebral hemorrhage in young people: Analysis of risk factors, location, causes, and prognosis. Stroke 30:537–541, 1999.
105. Martin NA, Vinters HV: Arteriovenous malformations. In Carter LP, Spetzler RF, Hamilton MG (eds): Neurovascular Surgery. New York, McGraw-Hill, 1995, pp 875–903.
106. Burger PC, Sheithauer BW, Vogel FS: Cerebrovascular disease. In Burger PC, Sheithauer BW, Vogel FS (eds): Surgical Pathology of the Nervous System and its Coverings. New York, Churchill Livingstone, 1991, pp 439–467.
107. Weinand ME: Arteriovenous malformations and epilepsy. In Carter LP, Spetzler RF, Hamilton MG (eds): Neurovascular Surgery. New York, McGraw-Hill, 1995, pp 933–956.
108. Mast H, Mohr JP, Osipov A, et al: "Steal" is an unestablished mechanism for the clinical presentation of cerebral arteriovenous malformations. Stroke 26:1215–1220, 1995.
109. Heros RC: Arteriovenous malformations of the medial temporal lobe: Surgical approach and neuroradiological characterization. J Neurosurg 56:44–52, 1982.
110. Heros RC, Korosue K, Diebold PM: Surgical excision of cerebral arteriovenous malformations: Late results. Neurosurgery 26: 570–578, 1990.
111. Hartmann A, Mast H, Mohr JP, et al: Morbidity of intracranial hemorrhage in patients with cerebral arteriovenous malformation. Stroke 29:931–934, 1998.
112. Brown RD Jr, Wiebers DO, Forbes G, et al: The natural history of unruptured intracranial arteriovenous malformations. J Neurosurg 68:352–357, 1988.
113. Crawford PM, West CR, Chadwick DW, et al: Arteriovenous malformations of the brain: Natural history in unoperated patients. J Neurol Neurosurg Psychiatry 49:1–10, 1986.
114. Graf CJ, Perret GE, Torner JC: Bleeding from cerebral arteriovenous malformations as part of their natural history. J Neurosurg 58:331–337, 1983.
115. Wilkins RH: Natural history of intracranial vascular malformations: A review. Neurosurgery 16:421–430, 1985.
116. Ondra SL, Troupp H, George ED, et al: The natural history of symptomatic arteriovenous malformations of the brain: A 24-year follow-up assessment. J Neurosurg 73:387–391, 1990.
117. Fults D, Kelly DL Jr: Natural history of arteriovenous malformations of the brain: A clinical study. Neurosurgery 15:658–662, 1984.
118. Mast H, Young WL, Koennecke HC, et al: Risk of spontaneous haemorrhage after diagnosis of cerebral arteriovenous malformation. Lancet 350:1065–1068, 1997.
119. Pollock BE, Flickinger JC, Lunsford LD, et al: Factors that predict the bleeding risk of cerebral arteriovenous malformations. Stroke 27:1–6, 1996.
120. Forster DM, Steiner L, Håkanson S: Arteriovenous malformations of the brain: A long-term clinical study. J Neurosurg 37: 562–570, 1972.
121. Itoyama Y, Uemura S, Ushio Y, et al: Natural course of unoperated intracranial arteriovenous malformations: Study of 50 cases. J Neurosurg 71:805–809, 1989.
122. Kader A, Young WL, Pile-Spellman J, et al: The influence of hemodynamic and anatomic factors on hemorrhage from cerebral arteriovenous malformations. Neurosurgery 34:801–808, 1994.
123. Turjman F, Massoud TF, Viñuela F, et al: Correlation of the angioarchitectural features of cerebral arteriovenous malformations with clinical presentation of hemorrhage. Neurosurgery 37:856–862, 1995.
124. Spetzler RF, Hargraves RW, McCormick PW, et al: Relationship of perfusion pressure and size to risk of hemorrhage from arteriovenous malformations. J Neurosurg 76:918–923, 1992.
125. Vinuela F, Dion JE, Duckwiler G, et al: Combined endovascular embolization and surgery in the management of cerebral arteriovenous malformations: Experience with 101 cases. J Neurosurg 75:856–864, 1991.
126. Parkinson D, Bachers G: Arteriovenous malformations: Summary of 100 consecutive supratentorial cases. J Neurosurg 53: 285–299, 1980.
127. Waltimo O: The relationship of size, density and localization of intracranial arteriovenous malformations to the type of initial symptom. J Neurol Sci 19:13–19, 1973.
128. Colombo F, Pozza F, Chierego G, et al: Linear accelerator radiosurgery of cerebral arteriovenous malformations: An update. Neurosurgery 34:14–21, 1994.
129. Pollock BE, Flickinger JC, Lunsford LD, et al: Hemorrhage risk after stereotactic radiosurgery of cerebral arteriovenous malformations. Neurosurgery 38:652–661, 1996.
130. Redekop G, TerBrugge K, Montanera W, et al: Arterial aneurysms associated with cerebral arteriovenous malformations: Classification, incidence, and risk of hemorrhage. J Neurosurg 89:539–546, 1998.
131. Abdulrauf SI, Malik GM, Awad IA: Spontaneous angiographic obliteration of cerebral arteriovenous malformations. Neurosurgery 44:280–288, 1999.
132. Spetzler RF, Martin NA: A proposed grading system for arteriovenous malformations. J Neurosurg 65:476–483, 1986.
133. Hamilton MG, Spetzler RF: The prospective application of a grading system for arteriovenous malformations. Neurosurgery 34:2–7, 1994.
134. Osipov A, Koennecke HC, Hartmann A, et al: Seizures in cerebral arteriovenous malformations: Type, clinical course and medical management. Intervent Neuroradiol 3:37–41, 1997.
135. Kader A, Goodrich JT, Sonstein WJ, et al: Recurrent cerebral

arteriovenous malformations after negative postoperative angiograms. J Neurosurg 85:14–18, 1996.
136. Gabriel EM, Sampson JH, Wilkins RH: Recurrence of a cerebral arteriovenous malformation after surgical excision: Case report. J Neurosurg 84:879–882, 1996.
137. Burchiel KJ, Clarke H, Ojemann GA, et al: Use of stimulation mapping and corticography in the excision of arteriovenous malformations in sensorimotor and language-related neocortex. Neurosurgery 24:322–327, 1989.
138. Latchaw RE, Hu X, Ugurbil K, et al: Functional magnetic resonance imaging as a management tool for cerebral arteriovenous malformations. Neurosurgery 37:619–626, 1995.
139. Friedman WA, Bova FJ, Mendenhall WM: Linear accelerator radiosurgery for arteriovenous malformations: The relationship of size to outcome J Neurosurg 82:180–189, 1995.
140. Lunsford LD, Kondziolka D, Flickinger JC, et al: Stereotactic radiosurgery for arteriovenous malformations of the brain. J Neurosurg 75:512–524, 1991.
141. Friedman WA, Blatt DL, Bova FJ, et al: The risk of hemorrhage after radiosurgery for arteriovenous malformations. J Neurosurg 84:912–919, 1996.
142. Pikus HJ, Beach ML, Harbaugh RE: Microsurgical treatment of arteriovenous malformations: Analysis and comparison with stereotactic radiosurgery. J Neurosurg 88:641–646, 1998.
143. Gallina P, Merienne L, Meder JF, et al: Failure in radiosurgery treatment of cerebral arteriovenous malformations. Neurosurgery 42:996–1004, 1998.
144. Gobin YP, Laurent A, Merienne L, et al: Treatment of brain arteriovenous malformations by embolization and radiosurgery. J Neurosurg 85:19–28, 1996.
145. Gao E, Young WL, Pile-Spellman J, et al: Cerebral arteriovenous malformation feeding artery aneurysms: A theoretical model of intravascular pressure changes after treatment. Neurosurgery 41:1345–1358, 1997.
146. Kondziolka D, Nixon BJ, Lasjaunias P, et al: Cerebral arteriovenous malformations with associated arterial aneurysms: Hemodynamic and therapeutic considerations. Can J Neurol Sci 15: 130–134, 1988.
147. Patterson JH, McKissock WA: A clinical survey of intracranial angiomas with special reference to their mode of progression and surgical treatment: A report of 110 cases. Brain 79:233–266, 1956.
148. Miyasaka K, Wolpert SM, Prager RJ: The association of cerebral aneurysms, infundibula and intracranial arteriovenous malformations. Stroke 13:196–203, 1982.
149. Turjman F, Massoud TF, Viñuela F, et al: Aneurysms related to cerebral arteriovenous malformations: Superselective angiographic assessment in 58 patients. AJNR Am J Neuroradiol 15: 1601–1605, 1994.
150. Thompson RC, Steinberg GK, Levy RP, et al: The management of patients with arteriovenous malformations and associated intracranial aneurysms. Neurosurgery 43:202–212, 1998.
151. Sasaki O, Tanaka R, Koike T, et al: Excision of cavernous angioma with preservation of coexisting venous angioma: Case report. J Neurosurg 75:461–464, 1991.
152. Comey CH, Kondziolka D, Yonas H: Regional parenchymal enhancement with mixed cavernous/venous malformations of the brain: Case report. J Neurosurg 86:155–158, 1997.
153. Scamoni C, Dario A, Basile L: The association of cavernous and venous angioma: Case report and review of the literature. Br J Neurosurg 11:346–349, 1997.
154. Van Roost D, Kristof R, Wolf HK, et al: Intracerebral capillary telangiectasia and venous malformation: A rare association. Surg Neurol 48:175–183, 1997.
155. Kuroiwa T, Ohta T: Cavernous angioma associated with venous angioma—two case reports. Neurol Med Chir (Tokyo) 38:648–653, 1998.
156. Nussbaum ES, Heros RC, Madison MT, et al: The pathogenesis of arteriovenous malformations: Insights provided by a case of multiple arteriovenous malformations developing in relation to a developmental venous anomaly. Neurosurgery 43:347–352, 1998.
157. Rigamonti D, Johnson PC, Spetzler RF, et al: Cavernous malformations and capillary telangiectasia: A spectrum within a single pathological entity. Neurosurgery 28:60–64, 1991.
158. Challa VR, Moody DM, Brown WR: Vascular malformations of the central nervous system. J Neuropathol Exp Neurol 54: 609–621, 1995.
159. McCormick PW, Spetzler RF, Johnson PC, et al: Cerebellar hemorrhage associated with capillary telangiectasia and venous angioma: A case report. Surg Neurol 39:451–457, 1993.
160. Russell D: Discussions on vascular tumours of the brain and spinal cord. Proc Roy Soc Med 24:383, 1930–1931.
161. Rutka JT, Brant-Zawadzki M, Wilson CB, et al: Familial cavernous malformations: Diagnostic potential of magnetic resonance imaging. Surg Neurol 29:467–474, 1988.
162. Maraire JN, Awad IA: Intracranial cavernous malformations: Lesion behavior and management strategies. Neurosurgery 37: 591–605, 1995.
163. Rigamonti D, Spetzler RF: The association of venous and cavernous malformations: Report of four cases and discussion of the pathophysiological, diagnostic, and therapeutic implications. Acta Neurochir (Wien) 92:100–105, 1988.
164. Hirata Y, Matsukado Y, Nagahiro S, et al: Intracerebral venous angioma with arterial blood supply: A mixed angioma. Surg Neurol 25:227–232, 1986.
165. Wilson CB: Cryptic vascular malformations. Clin Neurosurg 38: 49–84, 1992.
166. Ciricillo SF, Dillon WP, Fink ME, et al: Progression of multiple cryptic vascular malformations associated with anomalous venous drainage: Case report. J Neurosurg 81:477–481, 1994.
167. Guttmacher AE, Marchuk DA, White RI Jr: Hereditary hemorrhagic telangiectasia. N Engl J Med 333:918–924, 1995.
168. Shovlin CL, Hughes JM, Tuddenham EG, et al: A gene for hereditary haemorrhagic telangiectasia maps to chromosome 9q3. Nat Genet 6:205–209, 1994.
169. McDonald MT, Papenberg KA, Ghosh S, et al: A disease locus for hereditary haemorrhagic telangiectasia maps to chromosome 9q33-34. Nat Genet 6:197–204, 1994.
170. Johnson DW, Berg JN, Gallione CJ, et al: A second locus for hereditary hemorrhagic telangiectasia maps to chromosome 12. Genome Res 5:21–28, 1995.
171. Jessurun GA, Kamphuis DJ, van der Zande FH, et al: Cerebral arteriovenous malformations in The Netherlands Antilles: High prevalence of hereditary hemorrhagic telangiectasia-related single and multiple cerebral arteriovenous malformations. Clin Neurol Neurosurg 95:193–198, 1993.
172. Román G, Fisher M, Perl DP, et al: Neurological manifestations of hereditary hemorrhagic telangiectasia (Rendu-Osler-Weber disease): Report of 2 cases and review of the literature. Ann Neurol 4:130–144, 1978.
173. Willinsky RA, Lasjaunias P, Terbrugge K, et al: Multiple cerebral arteriovenous malformations (AVMs): Review of our experience from 203 patients with cerebral vascular lesions. Neuroradiology 32:207–210, 1990.
174. White RI Jr, Lynch-Nyhan A, Terry P, et al: Pulmonary arteriovenous malformations: Techniques and long-term outcome of embolotherapy. Radiology 169:663–669, 1988.
175. Kikuchi K, Kowada M, Sakamoto T, et al: Wyburn-Mason syndrome: Report of a rare case with computed tomography and angiographic evaluations. J Comput Assist Tomogr 12:111–115, 1988.
176. Golfinos J, Zabramski JM: The genetics of intracranial vascular malformations. In Raffel C, Harsh GR (eds): The Molecular Basis of Neurosurgical Disease. Baltimore, Williams & Wilkins, 1996, pp 270–277.
177. Théron J, Newton TH, Hoyt WF: Unilateral retinocephalic vascular malformations. Neuroradiology 7:185–196, 1974.

CHAPTER 127

Natural History of Intracranial Vascular Malformations

KELLY D. FLEMMING ■ ROBERT D. BROWN, JR

Treatment options for intracranial vascular malformations continue to change as microsurgical, radiosurgical, and endovascular procedures evolve. However, before one can define the best management, the natural history of each malformation must be known. Natural history data allow proper counseling of patients on long-term outcome, complication anticipation, and management decision making.

The natural history of vascular malformations is complicated by a number of factors. First, there are many subtypes of vascular malformations, each with unique characteristics; however, the distinction among subtypes is not always clear, owing to transitional or mixed types of malformations. Second, because of the high frequency of asymptomatic lesions, the study population may not be representative of the general population. Third, patients found to have vascular malformations are often treated; therefore, selection bias is inherent in these studies. Finally, the length of follow-up is often inconsistent and thus not always representative of the general population.

Despite these limitations, epidemiologic studies have clarified the frequency of detection, clinical presentation, hemorrhagic risk, and prognosis of these vascular malformations. These features are often dependent on the type of malformation and its size, location, and angioarchitectural characteristics.

Classic pathoanatomic schemes divide vascular malformations into four categories: arteriovenous malformations, venous malformations, cavernous malformations, and capillary malformations. Although this classification scheme is widely used, it may be outdated by new information on the pathogenesis and evolution of these lesions. Reports of de novo lesions and of the evolution of lesions have challenged the conventional concept of congenital, static malformations. Also, mixed vascular malformations have been poorly reconciled with this conventional scheme. Finally, there are several important arteriovenous shunting malformations (dural arteriovenous fistula, carotid-cavernous fistula, galenic malformation) that clearly have distinctive pathoanatomic, radiologic, and natural history characteristics. An integrated classification scheme has been proposed to address the inadequacies of conventional pathoanatomic classifications (Table 127–1).[1]

This chapter addresses the natural history of several vascular malformation subtypes.

ARTERIOVENOUS MALFORMATION

Synonyms. Arteriovenous fistulous malformation, pial arteriovenous malformation, parenchymal arteriovenous malformation, arteriovenous anomaly, cryptic arteriovenous malformation, angiographically occult vascular malformation.*

Definition and Pathogenesis

Arteriovenous malformations (AVMs) are vascular abnormalities consisting of fistulous connections of arteries and veins without normal intervening capillary beds. Typically, they are triangular, with the base toward the meninges and the apex toward the ventricular system.[2] There is an abrupt transition between the arteries, which contain variable amounts of smooth muscle and elastic laminae, and the dilated veins. The veins have thickened walls that appear arterialized owing to the proliferation of fibroblasts. Within the arteries and veins, evidence of prior thrombosis and recanalization may be evident. Residua of prior hemorrhages such as dystrophic calcification and blood breakdown products may surround the AVM, with histologic evidence of hemosiderin-laden macrophages.[2] Marked surrounding gliosis due to the high-flow, low-resistance AVM shunt "stealing" blood away from surrounding tissue may also be present.[2, 3]

AVMs appear as serpiginous isointense or slightly hyperintense vessels that strongly enhance following contrast administration on computed tomographic scanning.[4–6] Calcification is identified in 25% to 30% of

*Although the majority of angiographically occult and cryptic vascular malformations are cavernous malformations, thrombosed arteriovenous malformations may look similar on imaging studies.

TABLE 127–1 ■ Classification Scheme for Central Nervous System Vascular Anomalies

Proliferating Vascular Tumor
Hemangioma
Nonproliferating Vascular Malformations (or Anomalies)
Capillary malformation (telangiectasia)
Venous malformation
Cavernous malformation
Arterial malformations (no arteriovenous shunting)
Congenital angiodysplasia
Intracranial aneurysm
Arteriovenous shunting malformations
Classic cerebral AVM
Pial AVF
Carotid-cavernous fistula
Dural AVF
Galenic AVM
Mixed malformations
Venous-cavernous
AVM-venous
Cavernous-AVM
Syndromic central nervous system malformations

AVF, arteriovenous fistula; AVM, arteriovenous malformation.

cases.[6, 7] In addition to identifying the AVM, computed tomographic scans are useful for demonstrating acute hemorrhage and may show mass effect or displacement of normal anatomic structures. Magnetic resonance imaging (MRI), however, is superior in sensitivity and specificity. MRI is useful for determining size, location, and evidence of prior symptomatic or subclinical hemorrhage, as well as secondary changes such as mass effect, edema, and ischemic changes in the adjacent brain.[8] The typical AVM appears as a tightly packed "honeycomb" of flow voids on T1- and T2-weighted images, caused by high flow velocity signal loss. Increased signal may be seen in thrombosed or low-flow vessels.[6] Phase-contrast magnetic resonance angiography can be useful in the depiction of flow, but complete definition of complex lesions and their internal angioarchitecture requires a cerebral angiogram.[9, 10]

On cerebral angiography, parenchymal AVMs appear as tightly packed masses of enlarged feeding arteries and dilated, tortuous veins with little or no intervening parenchyma within the nidus. There is little or no mass effect unless an associated hemorrhage or venous varix is present. Arteriovenous shunting with abnormal early filling of veins that drain the lesion is characteristic of AVM.[6] Angiography allows the identification of feeding and draining vessels, as well as associated vascular abnormalities such as aneurysms. Superselective angiography is preferred to delineate the internal angioarchitecture in detail.[11] Although angiography is highly sensitive, it may be negative after acute hemorrhage[12–14] or after spontaneous AVM thrombosis.[15]

AVMs are thought to be congenital in origin, owing to the lack of development of intervening capillary beds.[16–18] Although this may be part of the story, other influences may predispose to the development of AVMs. Recurrent AVMs have been documented after negative angiography, particularly in young adults.[19] In addition, AVMs may be associated with other vascular malformations.[20] These examples raise questions whether abnormalities of venous outflow,[21–24] angiogenic humoral factors, and hormonal influences play a role in pathogenesis.[19]

AVMs may also have a genetic basis in some populations. In addition to the association with hereditary hemorrhagic telangiectasia (Osler-Weber-Rendu disease), a few rare pedigrees of familial AVMs have been described, predominantly in the Asian population.[25] Some have shown an autosomal-dominant pattern of inheritance, although this is variable and no gene has yet been identified. No clinically distinguishing features have been found between familial and congenital AVMs, although the familial type may present at an earlier age.[25–29]

Epidemiology

The exact incidence of AVMs in unknown. Large autopsy series estimate the frequency of AVM detection to be 1.4% to 4.3%.[30] In the only population-based study, the sex- and age-adjusted incidence rate was 1.11 per 100,000 persons.[31] AVMs are the most frequently detected symptomatic vascular formation,[32] accounting for 2% of all strokes[33, 34] and 38% of all intracerebral hemorrhages in patients between 15 and 45 years.[35] AVMs are one seventh as common as aneurysms, and the prevalence has been estimated at 0.2% to 0.8% of the general population.[1, 31, 36, 37] The prevalence may be slightly higher in the Asian population.[38]

Patients typically present between 20 and 40 years of age.[39–58] Most studies report an equal gender predilection[34, 46] or a slight male predominance among patients presenting with AVMs.[39–42, 49, 50]

The majority of AVMs are located supratentorially.[34, 42, 45, 51, 52] Less common sites include the cerebellum, the brainstem, and within the ventricle. In the posterior fossa, the cerebellum is the most common site.[53] Extracranially, AVMs may be present in the spinal cord as well as in various organs and soft tissues.

Although AVMs are typically solitary, multiple AVMs have rarely been described.[54, 55] A cooperative study of intracranial aneurysms and subarachnoid hemorrhage reported a less than 1% incidence of multiple AVMs.[34] Willinsky and coworkers,[55] however, reported an incidence of 9% in 203 consecutive patients. Occasionally, embolization or definitive treatment of a larger, dominant AVM unmasks others as a result of changes in hemodynamics.[55] Multiple AVMs may be present without apparent cause or in association with hereditary hemorrhagic telangiectasia,[34, 54–57] Wyburn-Mason syndrome,[58] or soft tissue vascular malformations.[59] Cases of AVMs in the brain as well as the spinal cord have also been described.[46, 60]

AVMs may be associated with other vascular malformations.[20] Mixed vascular malformations are those that contain angiographic or imaging characteristics of more than one type of vascular malformation. Of 280 consecutive cases of vascular malformations, 14 were mixed lesions.[20] Although rare, their presence may generate hypotheses regarding a common pathogenesis or causation evolution among different types of lesions. AVMs have been reported in association with cavernous malformations,[20] venous angiomas,[20, 24, 34] and aneurysms.[43, 61–71] Nussbaum and colleagues reported a case of a patient with an AVM that drained into a developmental venous anomaly.[24] After regression of the initial AVM, new malformations that drained into the same venous anomaly appeared, suggesting the possible importance of venous outflow in the pathogenesis of AVMs. The association with arterial aneurysms is discussed later.

Clinical Presentation

Asymptomatic. In one large autopsy series, only 12% of patients harboring an AVM had symptoms related to it.[30] Although the exact number of asymptomatic patients is unknown, clinical studies report that 2% to 4% of detected AVMs are incidental findings.[44, 72] In a population-based study of patients with intracranial vascular malformations, 40% were asymptomatic.[31]

Hemorrhage. AVMs most commonly present with hemorrhage. In a population-based study, 65% of patients with AVMs presented with hemorrhage, with a peak occurrence in the fifth decade.[31] In the cooperative study, 72% of patients with hemorrhage presented before the age of 40.[34] Before the availability of computed tomography (CT), most studies reported a high incidence of subarachnoid hemorrhage.[34, 46, 49] Since the advent of CT, the distinction among hemorrhage types has become easier. Intraparenchymal hemorrhage is most common, followed by intraventricular hemorrhage and subarachnoid hemorrhage.[4, 73, 74] Of 50 consecutive cerebral angiograms in patients with AVMs and hemorrhage, 60% had intracerebral hemorrhage, 26% had intracerebral hemorrhage with intraventricular extension, 8% had intraventricular hemorrhage, 4% had subarachnoid hemorrhage, and 2% had evidence of subdural hemorrhage on presentation.[74] Subarachnoid hemorrhage is more common when the AVM is located cortically and is rarely associated with vasospasm, depending on the location and thickness of the blood.[46, 75, 76] Among patients presenting with primary subarachnoid hemorrhage, in 0.6% the hemorrhage was attributable to an AVM.[61]

Risk of Hemorrhage. The risk of bleeding from an AVM has been calculated in several studies. Retrospective risk is calculated by dividing the person-years of exposure from birth to hemorrhage or intervention by the number of patients with hemorrhage. The retrospective risk is based on the assumption that the lesion is congenital and has a constant risk over time, which may not be accurate. Prospective risk assessment is more useful, but surgical selection and referral bias are common. In addition, follow-up is often inconsistent. For instance, some studies do not require follow-up imaging to confirm a bleeding episode. Furthermore, the length of follow-up is highly variable.

The risk of hemorrhage has been estimated at 2% to 4% per year.[39, 42, 43, 50, 52, 77] Brown and associates studied 168 patients without a prior history of hemorrhage over 8.2 years.[52] Eighteen percent of the patients experienced a symptomatic hemorrhage during the follow-up period, yielding a crude risk of 2.2% per year. Using life-table analysis, the risk was 1.3% at 1 year, 1.7% at 5 years, 1.5% at 10 years, and 2.2% at 15 years. Graf and coworkers also evaluated the prospective rate of hemorrhage.[43] The risk of first hemorrhage in those patients presenting with seizures was 2% at 1 year, 13% at 5 years, and 30% at 10 years, for an overall rate of 2% to 3% per year. Similarly, other studies reported prospective hemorrhage risks of 1% to 3% per year.[41, 42, 78]

Ondra and colleagues studied 160 patients with AVMs, representing 90% of such lesions in Finland.[50] Patients presented with hemorrhage, seizure, or other symptoms and were followed over a 24-year period. This study found 147 new hemorrhage events in 64 patients during the follow-up period, for an overall hemorrhage risk of 4% per year that was constant over time. The mean interval between diagnosis and hemorrhage was 7.7 years. This study started during the pre-CT era, and some patients had multiple hemorrhages. It is important to note that if one considers the risk for only the first hemorrhage, the hemorrhagic risk is 1.7% per year, similar to the findings in other studies. Graf and Pollock found the initial hemorrhage risk to be approximately 2% per year.[43, 77] Pollock and colleagues studied predominantly small AVMs (<3 cm).[77] Of 315 patients, 196 presented with hemorrhage, yielding a retrospective risk of 1.89% per year. A crude overall rate of 2.4% per year was determined when multiple hemorrhages were included.

Using the multiplicative law of probability, the lifetime risk of AVM rupture can be assessed using the formula [1 − (risk of no hemorrhage)^n], where n is the number of expected years of life remaining obtained from life tables.[79] This formula assumes that the lesion is congenital and that the risk is constant over time. Assuming that the risk of hemorrhage is 3% per year, the formula becomes $(1 - 0.97)^n$. For example, a 35-year-old patient with 43 years of remaining life yields $(1 - 0.97)^{43} = 73\%$. The hemorrhage risk figures obtained with this formula are useful in clinical practice for counseling patients and their families regarding the lifetime risk of AVM hemorrhage. However, there is a simpler way of approximating this lifetime risk of hemorrhage for persons with intracranial AVMs. The following formula, based on a 3% annual risk of hemorrhage, closely approximates the multiplicative formula: 105 − patient's age in years = lifetime risk of hemorrhage.[80] For example, for a 35-year-old patient presenting with an AVM, the risk of hemorrhage is 105 − 35 = 70% (versus 73% using the complicated multiplicative formula).

Risk Factors for Hemorrhagic Presentation. Many studies have attempted to elucidate clinical and angiographic predictors for presentation with AVM hemorrhage to delineate which patients may be at higher risk. Some clinical risk factors for presentation with hemorrhage may include age,[34] sex,[78] pregnancy,[81] and hypertension.[82] Patients are most likely to present with hemorrhage before the age of 40. Hemorrhage in infants and children is distinctly uncommon, and before the age of 2 years, patients with AVMs typically present with congestive heart failure, hydrocephalus, or seizures.[34] In a multivariate analysis, Mast and associates reported that male sex is a risk factor for hemorrhagic presentation.[78] Conversely, another study showed a slight predominance of females presenting with hemorrhage (62 males; 72 females),[43] but this was not statistically significant, and others failed to confirm sex as a risk factor for hemorrhagic presentation. Pregnancy may increase the likelihood for rupture, but this concept is controversial and is discussed in more detail later. One study found a history of hypertension to be independently associated with a hemorrhagic presentation of AVM.[82] The association with recurrent hemorrhages, however, was unclear, and no other studies have confirmed this observation.

Angiographic risk factors for AVMs presenting with hemorrhage have also been studied, but there are certain biases. Angiography performed after acute hemorrhage must be interpreted carefully, because the hemorrhage may have changed the AVM's size and morphologic features.[13] Furthermore, patients undergoing angiography after hemorrhage have survived to that point, which means that patients who died were excluded from the population studied. Early mortality may also be excluded in some studies because the patients represent a selected subgroup referred to centers with angiography capabilities.

One large study of 168 patients with AVMs detected before rupture evaluated angiographic characteristics predictive of future rupture. Despite meticulous analysis of AVM size, site, and flow characteristics, no angioarchitectural features were found to be predictive of rupture in this multivariate analysis.[52]

Several studies indicate that location influences hemorrhagic risk. The presence of an AVM in a deep location,[47, 63] such as the basal ganglia,[11, 44] posterior fossa,[44] or intraventricular and periventricular areas,[83, 84] may predispose to hemorrhagic presentation. Some studies also report an increased risk of hemorrhage in cerebellar lesions.[70, 83–86] The higher risk in one study was attributed to the relatively high incidence of associated aneurysms.[85] In contrast to these studies, others found location to be inconsequential in predicting hemorrhagic risk.[48, 50, 52] Some hypothesize that deeply located AVMs may simply not cause symptoms other than hemorrhage until they reach a size at which cortical irritation is possible.

Size is a controversial factor. Several large studies, including one of unruptured AVMs at the start of follow-up,[52] found no difference in hemorrhage risk based on the size of the AVM.[11, 41, 48, 50, 52, 83] Others found that small AVMs (<3 cm) pose a higher risk of hemorrhagic presentation.[43–46, 49, 51, 82, 87–89] One study found that 90% of patients with small AVMs presented with hemorrhage.[44] Hemodynamic assessment of small AVMs revealed distinct differences in flow pattern and pressure. Spetzler and coworkers found higher intra-arterial pressures in smaller AVMs, suggesting a potential role in hemorrhage.[87] In addition, the transnidal pressure gradient is higher in smaller AVMs.[90] Others question whether such AVMs have simply not grown large enough to cause other symptoms, leading to a higher proportion presenting with hemorrhage. In contrast to these studies, however, Sadasivan and Hwang found that 12 of 27 patients with large (>5 cm) AVMs presented with rupture, and an additional 4 patients initially presenting with seizures went on to AVM rupture.[91] Furthermore, a study of predominantly small AVMs found a hemorrhage risk rate similar to that in other studies, suggesting that size may not make a difference.[77]

Feeding arteries and venous drainage have also been assessed. Norris and colleagues evaluated a number of angiographic features in 31 patients, including size and several arterial and venous parameters.[92] The studies were performed several months after hemorrhage to minimize changes due to acute hemorrhage. The only difference in those presenting with hemorrhage was slower arterial filling with contrast, suggesting high feeding arterial pressure. Mean feeding arterial pressure was confirmed to be an important factor in the pathophysiology of AVM hemorrhage by the Columbia AVM study group,[44] independent of size and location; however, mean arterial pressures were not assessed in patients with small AVMs. Patients may also be predisposed to hemorrhagic presentation depending on which artery feeds the nidus. Various arteries have been implicated, including perforating arteries[11, 44, 63] and the vertebrobasilar trunk.[11]

Many AVMs that rupture do so from the venous drainage system. Recent studies have focused on the venous drainage pattern of AVMs and its importance in the pathophysiology of hemorrhage. Contributing features include deep venous drainage, often with accompanying stenosis and occlusion; the number of draining veins; and turbulent venous flow, perhaps leading to enhanced platelet aggregation and thrombosis.[44]

Impaired venous drainage may lead to a higher risk of hemorrhage due to increased pressure transmitted through the shunt. This was mathematically evaluated[93] and clinically suggested by several studies.[46, 63, 94, 95] Vinuela and associates found that 21 of 41 patients presenting with intracranial hemorrhage due to deep AVMs had vessel wall irregularity, stenosis, or occlusion in the deep venous system.[95]

Deep venous drainage has frequently been shown to increase the risk of hemorrhagic presentation.[11, 44, 63, 78, 82, 83, 94] Because many lesions with deep venous drainage are noncortical and unlikely to cause seizures, some believe that hemorrhage is the only presentation possible. The Columbia AVM study group examined a large number of physiologic indices in 449 patients to determine the relationship of AVM hemorrhage and venous drainage, as well as other parameters.[96] A multivariate analysis revealed that size and deep venous drainage were *independent* risk factors for bleeding, arguing against the belief that deep venous drainage increases the risk due to deep location or size. In fact, even large cortical AVMs with deep venous drainage were more likely to hemorrhage. Further, equal draining pressures were found in both deep and superficial AVMs that bled. From this study, four groups of patients emerged, based on the model's prediction of probability of intracerebral hemorrhage using size and venous drainage: (1) small AVM size and the presence of deep venous drainage only, probability = 96%; (2) medium or large AVM and deep venous drainage only, probability = 80%; (3) small AVM and superficial venous drainage, probability = 69%; (4) medium or large AVM with superficial venous drainage, probability = 29%.

A single draining vein was predictive of hemorrhagic risk in some studies[86, 94] but was not confirmed by others.[11, 52, 77] This may reflect that smaller AVMs are more likely to have single draining veins.[44] The presence, but not the size, of fragile venous aneurysms was significantly associated with risk of hemorrhage in two studies,[63, 97] although this, too, is controversial.[11, 52, 94]

Seizure. Approximately 15% to 35% of patients with AVMs present with seizure.[34, 36, 37, 42, 43, 45, 52] Seizures may be the result of mass effect with cortical irritation; flow characteristics leading to steal, ischemia, and neuronal damage; or hemorrhage and gliosis.[37, 98] In a series by Morello and Borghi, 35% of patients presented with seizure.[45] Of these, 57% presented with seizures alone, and 43% presented with seizures associated with hemorrhage. The majority of these patients had fewer than six seizures per year. Seizures are most commonly focal (simple or partial complex) but may also be generalized.

Some risk factors have been delineated for predicting seizure presentation in patients with AVMs. Ninety percent of patients presenting with seizures had supratentorial AVMs. Superficial, large (>6 cm) AVMs[45, 72] and those in the frontal or temporal location[34, 45] are more likely to present with seizures. Turjman and coworkers identified six angioarchitectural features predictive of seizure presentation in a multivariate analysis of 100 patients with AVMs.[98] The predictive features were cortical location, feeding by the middle cerebral artery, a cortical feeding artery, absence of aneurysms, presence of varices in venous drainage, and the association of a varix in the absence of an intranidal aneurysm. Interestingly, AVM size and high-flow shunting failed to reach statistical significance and were not predictive.

Headache. Headaches are a common complaint in patients with AVMs, even in the absence of hemorrhage. Approximately 15% of unruptured AVMs present with headache.[52] The headache is typically located hemicranially (ipsilateral or contralateral to the lesion) or in the occipital region, and the quality is similar to migraine. The incidence of migraine headache in patients with AVMs does not exceed that in the general population,[99] making it difficult to know which headaches are related to the AVM unless treatment is performed. In fact, successful embolization of an AVM in patients presenting with headache has been reported. The pathologic cause of the headache is hypothesized to relate to long-standing meningeal artery involvement and recruitment of blood supply by the AVM. Occipital AVM location may be a risk factor for headache.[37]

Neurological Deficit. Less than 10% of patients present with transient, permanent, or progressive focal neurological deficits not ascribed to hemorrhage or seizure.[39, 42, 52, 100] Progression of neurological dysfunction may be the result of the long-term effects of recurrent small hemorrhages, mass effect of the AVM, hydrocephalus, or ischemic complications and steal. *Steal* is the term used to describe blood flow away from a region of the brain in order to flow toward the AVM shunt. This flow may cause hypoperfusion, ischemia, and symptoms in the region where the blood was "stolen." Consequently, this may lead to focal or more global neurological deficits. Learning disorders have been documented in 66% of adults with AVMs, suggesting that functional brain deficits may be present before other clinical signs appear.[37, 101]

Risk factors for progressive neurological deficits include size[87] and shunt characteristics.[102] Large AVMs are more likely to result in neurological symptoms attributed to steal. Spetzler and colleagues hypothesized that the low feeding artery pressure associated with large AVMs provides a low perfusion pressure to the surrounding cortex, thereby producing a relative ischemia.[87] Patients with progressive deficits are also more likely to have extremely fast shunts with higher flow volumes as evidenced by transcranial Doppler ultrasonography.[102] In contrast to these studies, Mast and colleagues believe that steal is a rare phenomenon.[100] They found no relationship between size or flow velocities and focal deficits. Furthermore, although positron emission tomographic studies have shown reduced cerebral blood flow around AVMs, oxygen extraction fractions remain normal, suggesting that the surrounding parenchyma compensates for reduced flow.[103]

Outcome

Morbidity and Mortality. The mortality associated with the initial symptomatic hemorrhage is approximately 6% to 29%.[31, 36, 43, 48, 50, 52, 104–106] Brown and coworkers reported a 29% 30-day mortality with initial hemorrhage and a long-term disability of 23%.[52] The annual risk of major morbidity or death was calculated at 2.7% per year.[50] Many studies report complete recovery or mild disability in more than 50% of patients after an initial hemorrhage.[43, 104, 105, 107] Outcome is dependent on the location and type of hemorrhage, but not on the size of the AVM.[42, 43] Patients were more likely to have neurological deficits if the hemorrhage was parenchymal rather than subarachnoid or intraventricular.[43, 105, 107] In addition, hemorrhages in the posterior fossa were associated with a higher mortality rate. The mortality was as high as 66.7% in patients with posterior fossa hemorrhage in one study.[42]

Recurrent Hemorrhage. Recurrent hemorrhage occurs in 23% to 44% of patients, and the risk may be higher in the first year after the initial hemorrhage.[42, 43, 78, 108] Because the average time from initial presentation to hemorrhage is 7 to 12 years,[43, 50, 52] few studies have assessed the risk of recurrent hemorrhage. Graf and associates followed 134 patients presenting with ruptured AVMs for a median of 2 years.[43] Twenty-four percent of patients had recurrent hemorrhage during the follow-up period, for an annual rebleed risk of 6% at 1 year and 2% thereafter. Although this study found size to be predictive of initial hemorrhage, size was not a predictor of subsequent hemorrhage.

Of 315 patients in one study, 196 presented with an initial hemorrhage.[77] Recurrent hemorrhage was found in 44% patients with 591 patient-years of follow-up, for an annual risk of recurrence of 7.45% per year. Four AVM groups were constructed to predict hemorrhage risk on the basis of three significant variables of the multivariate analysis. The low-risk group had no prior history of hemorrhage, more than one draining vein, and a compact nidus. The intermediate low-risk group had no prior history of hemorrhage, one draining vein, and a diffuse nidus. The intermediate high-risk group had a history of prior hemorrhage, more than one draining vein, and a compact nidus. The high-risk AVM group had a history of prior hemorrhage, one draining vein, and a diffuse nidus. The annual rates of hemorrhage were 1.31% for the low-risk group, 2.4% for both intermediate groups, and 8.99% for the high-risk group.

Other studies confirm that prior hemorrhage is a risk factor for subsequent hemorrhage.[34, 39, 42, 43, 78, 83, 104, 108, 109] The Columbia AVM study group found an 18% per year risk of hemorrhage in patients with prior hemorrhage, compared with 2% per year for all others.[96]

Mortality did not necessarily increase with subsequent hemorrhagic episodes.[42] The mortality associated with recurrent hemorrhage has been estimated at 12% to 15%.[34, 39, 48, 104] In a small population-based study, 4 of 17 patients had recurrent hemorrhage, with a mortality reaching 50%.[31]

Seizure. Information on the risk of de novo seizure development over time and the outcome of patients with epilepsy treated conservatively is scant. Crawford and associates followed 245 patients presenting with symptoms other than seizures for a median of 7 years.[72] Ninety-six patients were treated surgically, and they had a higher risk of developing epilepsy. The 20-year risk was 57% in the surgical group and 19% (<1% per year) in the conservatively treated group. Three fourths of the patients who developed seizures did so within 2 years of treatment. Members of the surgically treated group were more likely to develop seizures if they were younger at diagnosis and if the AVM was in the frontal or parietal lobe. Among the conservatively treated group, those presenting with hemorrhage at a younger age and those with temporally located AVMs were most likely to develop seizures. The size of the AVM did not play a significant role. None of the patients with nonhemorrhagic focal neurological deficits or who were initially asymptomatic developed seizures. The reason why the surgically treated patients had a higher risk of epilepsy is unclear. It may be the result of selection bias, as most patients who were selected for surgery had hemorrhage on presentation and their lesions were located superficially.

Piepgras and colleagues studied 280 patients over 7.5 years.[89] Fifty-six percent (156) patients presented with hemorrhage, 25% (70) presented with seizures, and 19% (54) presented with other symptoms. Sixty-nine patients (25%) presented with both seizures and hemorrhage. Patients were treated surgically mainly to reduce the risk of bleeding, not specifically because of seizures. Of the surviving 136 patients who had no history of preoperative seizures, 94% were seizure free, and only 6% developed new seizures after surgery. Of patients with preoperative seizures, 83% were seizure free after surgery (50% on antiepileptic medications), and 17% had intermittent seizures, although the majority had some improvement. The difference between this and older studies likely relates to improved diagnostic and surgical techniques.

In conservatively treated patients, the majority are well controlled on antiepileptic medication.[34, 110] Murphy found that only 16% of conservatively treated patients were incapacitated by seizures.[110] Similarly, Perret and Nishioka found that only 4 of 39 patients treated with medications alone were unable to work.[34]

Radiographic Features and Lesion Behavior. AVMs may increase in size, remain stable, decrease in size, or completely regress or thrombose over time.[14, 46, 48, 88, 111–116] Minikawa and coworkers found that patients with enlarging AVMs had their first angiograms at a young age (0 to 11 years).[112] Subsequently, three of the four patients in that study rebled. Those AVMs that regressed were relatively small and fed by few feeding arteries.

Spontaneous regression can be acute or gradual and occurs in approximately 2% to 3% of patients with AVMs.[15] Causes include low flow; occlusion of feeding vessels by atherosclerosis, emboli, or dissection; or hemorrhage due to mass effect or vasospasm.[14, 111, 113, 117] Thrombosis is thought to be protective. Thrombosed AVMs rarely cause hemorrhage, although the risk of seizures remains.[36, 115] Caution is suggested in concluding that an AVM is thrombosed after hemorrhage with negative angiography. Transient regression after acute hemorrhage may be secondary to vasospasm and not thrombosis.[13] Others have reported recanalization after thrombosis.[118]

Arteriovenous Malformation and Aneurysm

The relationship between AVMs and aneurysms has been established,[34, 43, 61–69, 71, 119–121] and numerous studies have attempted to classify the types of aneurysms associated with AVMs. In general, each classification system takes into account the distance and flow relationship to the AVM. Aneurysms may be flow related, intranidal, or unrelated.[63] Flow-related aneurysms are saccular aneurysms arising along the course of arteries that eventually supply the AVM. A proximal flow-related aneurysm is one located on the supraclinoid internal carotid artery, the circle of Willis, the middle cerebral artery up to the bifurcation, the anterior cerebral artery up to the anterior communicating artery, or the vertebrobasilar trunk. All flow-related aneurysms beyond these locations are distal flow-related aneurysms.[63] These distal aneurysms are generally on the main feeding artery of the AVM and are also known as pedicle artery aneurysms.[62] Some authors break down the classification to denote whether the feeding artery is deep or superficial.[68] Intranidal aneurysms lie within the AVM nidus. Unrelated or dysplastic aneurysms are remote to the AVM.

The pathogenesis of aneurysms associated with AVMs is unknown. Three theories have evolved. The first proposes that the association between aneurysms and AVMs is coincidental, without a causal relationship. This is probably not the case, as the prevalence of aneurysms in patients with AVMs exceeds that in the general population.[69, 71] The second theory hypothesizes that both AVMs and aneurysms are congenital vascular abnormalities. The third and more favored theory is that aneurysms result from hemodynamic factors as a result of the increased flow through the AVM.[67] Supporting this hypothesis are the increased occurrence of aneurysms on the feeding arteries,[71] evidence of endothelial changes and internal elastic lamina rupture proximal to the AVM shunt, and the observation that distal flow-related aneurysms often regress with definitive treatment of the AVM. Brown and colleagues, however, found that even patients with low-shunt AVMs harbored pedicle aneurysms.[71] They further hypothesized that the pathogenesis of aneurysms may be related to the size of the AVM, because all aneurysms associated with small AVM were noted at atypical locations. Thus the pathogenesis may relate to a combination of factors—an underlying vascular defect, hemodynamic stimuli, vasoactive substances, and locally generated growth factors.

Depending on the series, aneurysms are present in 2.7% to 23% of patients with AVMs.[34, 43, 61, 62, 64–71, 121] The average 8% to 10% exceeds the 0.5% to 2% prevalence of aneurysms in the general population.[69] The mean age at presentation may be slightly later than that of the general AVM population. Miyasaka and coworkers found that the mean age of presentation was 41 years in those with aneurysms, versus 31 in those without.[65] The male-to-female ratio is similar to that of the entire AVM population.[66] Males may be more likely to harbor flow-related and intranidal aneurysms, whereas females may be more likely to have associated dysplastic or remote aneurysms.[66]

As with AVMs in isolation, AVMs with associated aneurysms typically present with hemorrhage.[68, 70] Among 39 patients with 64 aneurysms, Cunha and colleagues found that intracerebral hemorrhage was the presentation in 63%.[68] Forty-six percent of these bleeds were secondary to the aneurysm, 33% were related to the AVM, and in 21% the site of hemorrhage was unclear. Redekop and colleagues reported that 36% of 632 patients with AVMs presented with hemorrhage.[63] Among those with intranidal aneurysms, 72% presented with hemorrhage. Similar to the overall group, 40% of patients with flow-related aneurysms presented with hemorrhage. Of the 29 patients with AVMs and flow-related aneurysms, 12 (41.4%) bled from the aneurysm (5 distal; 7 proximal), 15 (51.7%) bled from the AVM, and in 2 the origin was undetermined.

Aneurysms may be multiple in 30% to 50% of patients with AVMs and aneurysms.[65, 68, 70] The majority of studies reveal no difference in the size of the AVM and the type, number, and size of the associated aneurysm.[63, 68, 71] Only one study found that larger AVMs were more likely to be associated with aneurysms.[65] The size of the associated aneurysm ranges from 3 mm to 2.5 cm and averages approximately 7.2 to 8 mm.[63, 71] The frequency of aneurysm type varies according to the study. The majority are flow related.[34, 61, 63, 65, 66, 68] The frequency of distal, feeding artery aneurysms ranges from 37% to 69%.[34, 61, 63, 65, 120] Remote aneurysms are less common, found in 1.6% to 43%.[34, 63, 65, 66, 68] Intranidal aneurysms represent approximately 20% of aneurysms,[63] but this is variable, based on the type of study performed. Superselective angiography is more likely to detect intranidal aneurysms and was not uniformly used in these studies. Typical locations (artery bifurcations) were found in association with high-shunt malformations.[71] Atypical locations were noted in association with high- or low-flow and high- or low-shunt AVMs.

Several studies reported an increased risk of hemorrhage when an AVM is associated with an aneurysm.[63, 71, 119] Brown and coworkers studied 16 patients with 26 aneurysms associated with unruptured AVMs.[71] The risk of hemorrhage in a patient with a coexisting aneurysm was 7% per year at 5 years. In those without a coexisting aneurysm, the rate was 3% per year at 1 year and declined to 1.7% per year at 5 years.

Risk factors for hemorrhage in patients harboring both lesions have been evaluated. Neither the size of the AVM nor that of the aneurysm was important, although the series were small. Two studies reported an increased risk of presentation with hemorrhage and subsequent rebleed in patients with associated intranidal aneurysms.[63, 119] In another study, all patients with intranidal aneurysms presented with hemorrhage, versus 58% of those without.[119] As previously mentioned, 72% of those with intranidal aneurysms in the study by Redekop and associates presented with hemorrhage.[63] Thirteen of the patients with intranidal aneurysms in that study could not be treated with surgery. Fourteen subsequently hemorrhaged over 143 patient-years, for an annual rate of hemorrhage of 9.8%. This was compared with a risk of 5.3% per year for four flow-related aneurysms that could not be treated with surgery. The authors concluded that patients with intranidal aneurysms had a high risk of rupture and presentation with hemorrhage, as well as a high risk of rebleeding. In addition, for flow-related aneurysms, patients had an equal chance of bleeding from the aneurysm as from the AVM.

Pedicle artery aneurysms were also considered a

risk factor for hemorrhage in two other studies.[62, 70] Perata and coworkers demonstrated the significance of pedicle artery aneurysms in four cases.[62] They hypothesized that short perforators (thalamoperforate or lenticulostriate) are exposed to higher pressures and flow rates and are more likely to undergo aneurysm formation and rupture during the development of an aneurysm. Batjer and colleagues confirmed the danger of pedicle or feeding artery aneurysms.[70] Of nine patients presenting with intracranial hemorrhage, seven bled from the aneurysm. All seven aneurysms were atypical aneurysms located on the major feeding vessel.

Aneurysms may increase in size, remain the same, or regress over time. With definitive AVM treatment, distal flow-related aneurysms are the most likely to regress.[63] Proximal aneurysms on the circle of Willis or remote aneurysms are unlikely to change.[67, 69] Furthermore, in untreated patients with AVMs, new aneurysms may arise over time.

Arteriovenous Malformation in Pregnancy

Cerebral hemorrhage during pregnancy is the third leading cause of maternal death from nonobstetric causes. Maternal mortality with intracranial hemorrhage has been reported to be as high as 40% to 50%.[122] Intracerebral hemorrhage is most commonly caused by eclampsia but may also be due to AVM or aneurysm rupture, venous thrombosis, hypertension, or choriocarcinoma.[123] Although referral sources may bias the frequency, estimates of cerebral hemorrhage due to AVM or aneurysm during pregnancy range from 0.01% to 0.05%.[124]

Controversy exists whether pregnancy increases the risk of bleeding from an AVM.[41, 81, 122–127] Robinson and associates reported a 10% risk of subarachnoid hemorrhage from AVM in nonpregnant women of childbearing age and an 87% risk in association with pregnancy.[81] Hemorrhage "associated with pregnancy" was defined as hemorrhage during pregnancy or delivery or less than 2 years after pregnancy. While Robinson noted that there was an 87% risk of hemorrhage during pregnancy, the data actually indicate that among AVMs that presented during pregnancy, 87% will hemorrhage. With conservative treatment, the fetal death rate was 26%, and 29% of mothers were dead or disabled.

In contrast to this, Horton and colleagues studied 451 women (540 pregnancies) with AVMs.[125] In this study, 17 patients with AVMs had pregnancies complicated by hemorrhage. There was no difference in hemorrhage rate between the months of pregnancy and all other months of the women's lives. However, the pregnancy term used was somewhat arbitrary, and a definition of pregnancy that covered a slightly shorter period would have led to a statistically significant hemorrhage difference. Patients with no prior history of hemorrhage had a 3.5% risk of bleeding during pregnancy, which is similar to the risk of bleeding during the nongravid months in the same patients with unruptured AVMs. The risk increased to 5.8% in those patients with a prior history of hemorrhage. Of 17 pregnancies complicated by hemorrhage, 4 resulted in maternal disability, and there were 3 fetal deaths. This study selected patients chosen for proton beam therapy, thereby potentially eliminating early deaths, severely disabled women, or vascular malformations that would not have been proton beam candidates.

Several studies evaluated risk factors for hemorrhage from AVM during pregnancy. Compared with patients who hemorrhaged from aneurysms, patients with AVMs were more likely to be younger,[122, 123, 128] to have had fewer children,[128] and to present between 15 and 20 weeks.[128] Dias and Sekhar reviewed 154 cases of hemorrhage during pregnancy due to AVM or aneurysm.[122] They found that 77% of hemorrhages were due to aneurysmal rupture and 23% were due to AVMs. Patients with AVM rupture were more likely to be younger than those with aneurysms, but in this study, no difference in parity or gestational age was found. It was also noted in this and other studies[128] that there is an increasing frequency of hemorrhage with advancing gestational age, possibly due to a combination of hemodynamic, coagulation, and hormonal factors.

Recurrent hemorrhage is not uncommon and increases the rate of mortality.[124] Few patients suffer initial AVM rupture during labor and delivery.[41, 124] However, rebleeding may commonly occur during this time.[128] Subsequent pregnancies also carry an increased risk of rebleeding.[81, 123]

Arteriovenous Malformation in Children

In large clinical series, children (younger than 20 years) accounted for 15% to 33% of all patients presenting with AVM.[34, 43, 104] Symptomatic AVM hemorrhage during childhood is rare, although the most common cause of intracerebral hemorrhage in children is AVM.[29, 129] In the only population-based study, 3 of 20 patients presenting with hemorrhage due to a vascular malformation were younger than 20 years old.[31]

Hemorrhage is by far the most common initial manifestation of the lesion (50% to 79%),[130–135] followed by seizures (8% to 25%)[130, 132–134] and congestive heart failure (18%).[131, 136, 137] Symptoms of congestive heart failure due to high left-to-right shunting through the AVM and hydrocephalus predominate in newborns.[138] Hemorrhage and seizures occur more often in children older than 2 years.[34, 133, 134] In addition to these symptoms, patients may rarely present with mental deterioration or progressive neurological symptoms secondary to steal phenomena.[139]

D'Aliberti and colleagues compared the clinical and angiographic features of 19 children (mean age, 11 years) and 120 adults with AVM.[140] The main differences between the two groups were sex distribution and the size, depth, location, and complexity of the AVM. AVMs were more common in male pediatric patients, and AVMs in pediatric patients tended to be smaller and located superficially. Although 68% of pediatric patients presented with hemorrhage, only 6% had deep venous drainage.

AVMs can grow in size, and this is usually most prominent in the pediatric age group. In addition, AVM recurrence after resection and negative postoperative angiograms has been described.[130, 134, 141] Hldaky and coworkers hypothesized that persistent microshunts not evident on early postoperative angiograms may increase over time, predisposing the patient to recurrent hemorrhage.[130]

Morbidity and Mortality. Despite new diagnostic techniques and therapeutic interventions, the mortality associated with AVM hemorrhage in children remains high. Clinical studies of pediatric patients presenting with hemorrhage report a 6.5% to 35% mortality rate.[131, 133, 134, 142–144] Hemorrhage location and volume predict mortality.[134, 143] The mortality associated with posterior fossa hemorrhage was far greater than that associated with supratentorial lesions. In one study of cerebellar AVMs in children, 6 of 17 patients (35%) died.[143] In another series, the mortality was 67% in nine patients with brainstem AVMs.[141] The higher mortality in pediatric series may relate to the distribution of posterior fossa AVMs in some studies. In addition, the cumulative morbidity and mortality caused by AVMs in children are high owing to the prolonged risk period of potential hemorrhage. The risk of rebleeding has been reported to be between 22% and 29%[134, 144] and can increase mortality.[144]

Despite high mortality rates, children are more likely than adults to improve after intracerebral hemorrhage due to AVM.[140] D'Aliberti and colleagues found that 89% of children versus 79% of adults had good recovery based on the Glasgow Outcome Score.[140] Similarly, another study found satisfactory outcomes in 81% of children presenting with AVM hemorrhage followed over a mean period of 8.5 years.[130] In this study, 72% of patients presenting with hemiparesis recovered fully or were left with only mild residual effects. Neonates presenting with congestive heart failure, however, have a very poor prognosis. In the series of seven neonates described by Melville and associates, six died in the first 17 days or at the time of intervention.[138] Although some deaths were due to neurosurgical complications, poor prognosis may also relate to residual shunting following treatment.

CAVERNOUS MALFORMATION

Synonyms. Cavernous angioma, cavernous hemangioma, cryptic vascular formation,* occult vascular formation,* angiographically occult vascular malformation.*

Definition and Pathogenesis

Cavernous malformations (CMs) are well-circumscribed, multilobulated, angiographically occult vascular malformations. Pathologically, they are composed of sinusoidal vascular channels (caverns) lined by a single layer of endothelium. The caverns are separated by collagenous stroma devoid of elastin, smooth muscle, or other mature vascular wall elements. The lack of intervening brain parenchyma is a characteristic pathologic marker. Within the lesion, hyalinization, thrombosis with varying degrees of organization, calcification, cysts, and cholesterol crystals are common, leading CMs to be likened to mulberries. Surrounding parenchyma consistently exhibits evidence of prior microhemorrhage, hemosiderin discoloration, and hemosiderin-filled macrophages. A gliomatous reaction of surrounding parenchyma is characteristic and may form a capsule around the lesion.[2, 3, 15, 145–149]

CT is 70% to 100% sensitive but less than 50% specific in detecting CMs.[147, 150–152] The typical appearance is a well-circumscribed nodular lesion with calcification. Hemorrhage and cystic components may also be present, and faint enhancement may be seen with contrasted imaging. MRI is most sensitive in detecting CMs,[153] which appear as well-defined, lobulated lesions with a central core of mixed signal intensities surrounded by a rim of signal hypointensity.[147, 154–160] The mixed signal reflects the lesion behavior. The decreased rim of T2 intensity is related to repeated subclinical intralesional and perilesional hemorrhages. Low T2 signal within the lesion reflects intralesional calcification. The hyperintensity reflects acute and subacute hemorrhage in different stages. Residua of previously expanded cisterns that have involuted with thrombus organization and resolution are reflected by the presence of cysts. Some studies have further characterized the MRI appearance of CMs for clinical study (Table 127–2).[161, 162]

Although MRI is more specific than CT, the MRI appearance is not pathognomonic. The differential diagnosis should include thrombosed AVM, calcified tumor (e.g., oligodendroglioma), granuloma, and infectious and inflammatory nodules.[147, 151, 155, 157, 159, 163–165] The absence of systemic neoplasm and surrounding edema and the presence of multiple lesions, calcification, and ossification offer clues for distinguishing neoplasm from CM. A typical MRI appearance, family history, and multiple lesions may favor a diagnosis of CM.

Distinguishing CMs from other cryptic vascular malformations on imaging and even pathology studies may be more difficult. The term *cryptic* or *occult* refers

TABLE 127–2 ■ **Categories of Cavernous Malformation Based on Magnetic Resonance Imaging Characteristics**

TYPE	T1-WEIGHTED	T2-WEIGHTED	MARGIN
I	Hyperintense	Hyperintense	Hyper- or hypointense
II	Mixed	Reticulated	Hypointense rim
III-A	Hypointense with hyperintense core		Hypointense
III-B	Hypointense without hyperintense core		Hypointense
IV	Hyperintense beyond hypointense rim		Hypointense rim

*These terms encompass cavernous malformations as well as thrombosed AVMs and sometimes venous angiomas.

to vascular malformations that are angiographically occult. They include CMs but may also include thrombosed AVMs, mixed lesions, or rarely venous angiomas. The majority of cryptic malformations are CMs.[166, 167] In a study of 34 consecutive angiographically occult malformations undergoing surgical excision and pathology, there were 21 CMs, 3 AVMs, 3 venous malformations, 2 capillary telangectasias, and 5 mixed lesions.[15] One study attempted to find radiographic features distinguishing angiographically occult malformations. Vanefsky and colleagues found that cryptic malformations due to CM were more likely to have hemosiderin rings and absence of edema.[168] A compulsive subdivision of such malformations may be unnecessary, however, because angiographically occult vascular malformations of any type may not have a distinctive natural history.[15, 116, 163, 169]

Angiography is almost always negative.[148–150, 153, 158, 167, 170] Occasional abnormalities seen in association with CMs include avascular mass, capillary blush, and evidence of neovascularity.[149, 151, 153, 158, 159, 170–175] In addition, CMs are occasionally associated with other vascular malformations, such as AVMs or venous malformations, that can be detected by angiography.

The pathogenesis of CMs is unclear. Although CMs are thought to be congenital, cases of de novo formation have been documented[162, 176–179] in association with radiation therapy,[176, 177, 180, 181] along the path of stereotactic biopsy,[182] and in association with venous angiomas.[183] One hypothesis is that venous hypertension associated with venous angioma may lead to red cell diapedesis and angiogenic growth factor release, leading to the formation of a CM.[183, 184] Others are investigating the role of cytomegalovirus infection in patients with de novo CM formation after irradiation.[185]

There is also a genetic predisposition in some patients, particularly Hispanic individuals. An autosomal-dominant pattern of inheritance has been seen in some families. A gene (*CCM1*) responsible for familial CM has been mapped to chromosome 7q11.2-q21.[186, 187] The protein product of this gene has not yet been characterized. In addition, Gunel and colleagues studied both sporadic and familial CM in Hispanic Americans. They found that both sporadic and familial CMs share the same alleles, suggesting a founder mutation—inheritance of the same mutation from a common ancestor.[188] A separate CM gene (*CCM2*) has also been recognized, reflecting genetic heterogeneity.[189, 190] Craig and colleagues studied 20 non-Hispanic, white kindreds with familial CMs.[189] Linkage analysis demonstrated two new loci: *CCM2* at 7p13-15, and *CCM3* at 3q25.2-27. Recently, four families with CMs inherited in an autosomal-dominant fashion were noted to have associated hyperkeratotic cutaneous vascular malformations.[191]

Epidemiology

The exact incidence and prevalence of CMs are unknown, as many are asymptomatic. In a population-based study, the age- and gender-adjusted incidence was 0.15 per 100,000 persons.[31] Prior estimates of prevalence are available primarily through autopsy and MRI series. Berry and associates retrospectively found that in 6686 consecutive autopsies, 0.2% had CMs, but they were not specifically looking for vascular malformations and may have underestimated the prevalence.[192] Subsequent prospective autopsy series by McCormick[3] and by Otten and coworkers[193] revealed a prevalence of 0.4% (16 of 4069 autopsies) and 0.53% (131 of 24,535 autopsies), respectively. MRI series report similar prevalences, ranging from 0.39% to 0.9%.[161, 194–196] CMs account for approximately 5% to 10% of all vascular malformations[53, 150, 153, 197] and are the second most frequent intracranial vascular malformation responsible for hemorrhage in surgical series.[198]

Patients with CMs typically present between the second and fourth decades.[148, 149, 152, 161, 194, 196, 199–202] Among the pediatric age group there is a bimodal distribution, with typical presentations near the ages of 3 and 11 years.[200] The pediatric age group has a higher propensity for overt hemorrhage.[148, 171, 203–205] In contrast, CMs are rarely symptomatic in the elderly.

The overall prevalence among males and females is equal.[172, 194–197, 206] Differences arise when patients are stratified by age and the time of clinical presentation. Males typically present with symptoms before age 30 years, whereas females typically present between 30 and 60 years of age.[195] Above the age of 60, there appears to be an equal prevalence of male and female patients presenting with CMs. Females are more likely than males to have CMs in the middle fossa, to have mixed malformations, and to present with hemorrhage.[171, 195] Males, however, are more likely to present with seizures.

In one series, familial CMs accounted for 30% to 50% of patients presenting with CMs[153]; in other series, the figure is slightly lower owing to selection bias and aggressiveness in seeking relatives.[202] Most epidemiologic data are similar to those for sporadic cases of CMs.[162, 207] One difference is the tendency for multiple lesions—up to 84% in one series.[162] There is an increased prevalence among Hispanic populations, and some studies suggest that successive generations may manifest at earlier ages.

The majority of CMs are supratentorial[162, 194, 195, 202] and range in size from 0.1 to 9 cm, with a mean of 1.4 to 1.7 cm.[148–151, 161, 194, 195, 197] In the posterior fossa, the pons and cerebellum are the most common sites of involvement. Less common sites include the pineal gland, cerebellopontine angle, middle cerebral fossa, cavernous sinus, optic nerve or chiasm, and dura. CMs may also appear extracranially in the orbit or intraspinally. Most CMs are solitary. Multiple CMs may occur in 10% to 30% of sporadic cases and in up to 84% of familial cases.[162, 208] Symptoms, however, are usually due to a single dominant lesion.

CMs may be associated with other vascular malformations and central nervous system pathology such as central nervous system tumors, extracerebral soft tissue tumors, and visceral hamartoma.[156, 172, 201, 209] Association with venous malformations, capillary telangiectasias, and AVMs has also been described.[15, 20, 36, 151, 158, 195, 210–214]

Mixed vascular malformations are thought to be

uncommon but may be underrecognized. The co-occurrence of cavernous malformations and venous malformations has been reported most commonly, although the exact prevalence is not known. Clinical studies estimate that 2.1% to 36% of patients with CMs have associated venous angiomas.[20, 214–217] Occasionally the association is not discovered until the patient undergoes surgery.[214]

Abdulrauf and colleagues studied 55 patients with CMs over a 4-year period.[217] Forty-two patients (76%) had CMs alone, and 13 (24%) had CMs in association with venous malformations. The clinical profiles of those with and without associated venous malformations were compared. Patients with associated venous malformations were more likely to be female, have overt hemorrhage, and suffer repeated hemorrhages. These features were trends but did not reach statistical significance. A clinically significant finding was that mixed lesions were more common in the posterior fossa. Interestingly, those patients with mixed lesions were less likely to have familial histories. This may suggest different pathogenetic models for those with and without associated venous angiomas.

Clinical Presentation

Asymptomatic. There is a high incidence of asymptomatic lesions, up to 95% in autopsy series.[218, 219] In MRI series, 11% to 44% of patients referred for unrelated symptoms were found to have CMs.[153, 195, 196, 209] In familial patients with multiple CMs, few lesions are symptomatic. More males than females present with incidental lesions,[199] and all sizes and locations can be clinically silent. Small punctate lesions, designated type III by Kim and colleagues (see Table 127–2), were rarely symptomatic and were often found in familial cases.[161]

Seizure. Because most CMs are supratentorial, it is not surprising that seizures are the most common presenting symptom.[148, 149, 152, 153, 161, 162, 173, 194, 195, 206] CMs are more likely than AVMs and venous malformations to present with seizures secondary to recurrent microhemorrhages and local gliomatous reaction.[147, 153, 220, 221] Calcification, thick gliomatous capsule, temporal location, and extensive hemosiderin deposition are frequently associated with the clinical presentation of epilepsy.[149, 152, 172, 173, 222] Males more commonly present with seizures than do females.[195] All types of seizures have been described in association with CMs—simple partial, complex partial, and generalized tonic-clonic seizures.[149, 172, 197] Among 49 patients (30 male, 19 female) presenting with seizures, 20 had focal motor or complex partial, 15 had generalized, and 10 had both focal and generalized seizures.[149]

Hemorrhage. Evidence of previous hemorrhage is present in every lesion, regardless of clinical history. CMs have persistent intralesional microhemorrhages that occur over time.[150, 152, 153, 169, 171, 195, 197, 210, 223, 224] Hemorrhage within the area of the hemosiderin ring is rarely associated with symptoms. Overt hemorrhage is less common but more clinically significant. Overt hemorrhage has been defined as (1) MRI signal of acute or subacute blood outside the hemosiderin ring, (2) evidence of prior hemorrhage on lumbar puncture, and (3) fresh clot outside the confines of the lesion at surgery.[161, 195] Clinical series report that 8% to 37% of patients present with hemorrhage.[176] Although patients with CMs most commonly present with intraparenchymal hemorrhage, subarachnoid and intraventricular hemorrhages have also been described.[171, 210, 225, 226] Several clinical series reported a higher propensity for overt hemorrhages in women and children.[195, 205, 227, 228]

Risk of Hemorrhage. The natural history of CMs has been reported in numerous series, but they are difficult to compare because of methodologic differences. The definition of hemorrhage differs among studies. Some use overt, extra-lesional hemorrhage, whereas others include intralesional or perilesional hemorrhage. In addition, some retrospective studies may not require radiologically verified hemorrhage. Studies also differ in the method of measuring hemorrhagic rate, with some using person-years and others using lesion-years. Prospective hemorrhage rates are clearly superior to retrospective rates, as the latter assume that the lesion is congenital and the risk remains the same throughout life.

The annual prospective hemorrhage risk in patients with CMs has been estimated at between 0.7% and 4.2% per patient-year (Table 127–3). Suggested risk factors for hemorrhage include prior symptomatic bleed,[149–152, 160, 162, 169, 173, 195, 209, 210] female sex,[195, 202] and pregnancy.[195, 196, 223, 224] One study also found deep location to be a risk factor,[216] but other studies did not confirm this.[162, 195, 199, 202, 206] The size of the CM and multiple lesions were not found to be risk factors for subsequent hemorrhage.

Kondziolka and colleagues studied 122 patients over a mean of 34 months.[206] The retrospective hemorrhage risk was 1.3% per patient-year. Nine patients had hemorrhages during the prospective follow-up period. Patients with prior hemorrhage had a greater annual hemorrhage risk (4.5% per year) than did those without prior hemorrhage (0.6% per year). No difference was found with regard to location, sex, or presentation.

Aiba and coworkers also found prior hemorrhage to be a risk factor for recurrent bleeds.[199] This was especially true in younger females. In a retrospective study, 62 of 110 patients with intracranial CMs initially presented with hemorrhage. The hemorrhage risk in patients with prior hemorrhage was 22.9% per year per lesion over a 3.1-year follow-up. Recurrent hemorrhage due to the initial lesion was found in 23 patients, and 4 patients had recurrent hemorrhage involving another lesion or both the initial lesion and another lesion. In contrast, the hemorrhage rate in those patients initially presenting with seizures or other symptoms was only 0.39% per year per patient. The rate of recurrent hemorrhage may be higher in this study than in others because the definition of intracerebral hemorrhage included those with intralesional or perilesional hemorrhage.

Deep location was found to be a risk factor in only one study. Porter and colleagues studied 110 patients

TABLE 127–3 ■ **Prospective Hemorrhage Risk in Patients with Cavernous Malformations**

STUDY	NO. OF PATIENTS (NO. OF LESIONS)	MEAN FOLLOW-UP PERIOD	HEMORRHAGES	PROSPECTIVE INITIAL HEMORRHAGE RATE
Moriarity[202]	68 (228)	5.2 yr	11	3.1% per person-year
Kim[161]	62 (108)	22.4 mo	2 of 28 conservatively treated patients	3.8% per person-year
Porter[216]	173	46 mo	7	4.2% per person-year
Kondziolka[206]	122	34 mo	9	2.6% per person-year
No prior bleed	61		1	0.6% per person-year
Prior bleed	61		8	4.5% per person-year
Robinson[195]	66 (76)	26 mo	1	0.7% per year per lesion
Zabramski[162]	31 (128)	2.2 yr		1.1% per lesion per year 6.5% per person-year
Aiba[199]	110		28	
No prior bleed	25	4.17 yr	1	0.39% per patient-year
Prior bleed	62	3.12 yr	27	22.9% per year per lesion

over a mean of 46 months.[229] The overall reported risk of hemorrhage was 4.2% per patient-year (18 events in 427 patient-years of follow-up). Patients with deep CMs (basal ganglia, thalamus, cerebellar nuclei, brainstem) had a significantly higher rate of hemorrhage (10.6% per patient-year) than did those with superficially located lesions (0%).

Female sex was a risk factor for hemorrhage in two prospective studies. Moriarity and associates prospectively studied 68 patients with 228 lesions over a 5.2-year period.[202] The overall prospective risk of hemorrhage was 3.1% per patient-year. Female patients had a significantly higher risk (4.2% versus 0.9% per patient-year), even though a similar number of male and female patients initially presented with hemorrhage. This study did not find initial presentation, size, or location to be a risk factor. Robinson and colleagues also found a significant difference in the rate of hemorrhage between male and female patients.[195] Females made up 86% of the hemorrhage group, two members of which were in their first trimester of pregnancy.

Case reports suggest an aggressive clinical course during pregnancy.[169, 171, 195, 196, 230] In one series of patients presenting with hemorrhage, one third of women were in their first trimester of pregnancy. Sage and coworkers also reported a significant number of pregnant women presenting with acute onset of neurological deficits.[196] Other series did not find an increased risk in women, although the number of pregnancies was not always clear.[206] The specific risk factors for an aggressive course and recurrence during future pregnancies have not been assessed.

Zabramski and colleagues reported the natural history of CMs in familial cases.[162] Fifty-nine members of six families were prospectively followed at 6- to 12-month intervals. Thirty-one patients (53%) had CMs, 19 of which were symptomatic. The patients were followed over a mean of 2.2 years. The incidence of symptomatic hemorrhage during follow-up was 1.1% per lesion per year. Patients with prior hemorrhage were more likely to experience rebleeding.

Focal Deficit. Patients may present with acute or subacute focal deficits, usually due to an intralesional or perilesional hemorrhage. The frequency in clinical series is 15.4% to 46.6%.[149–153, 160, 162, 171, 173, 194, 195, 197, 209, 223] The deficit may be transient, progressive, recurrent, or fixed, depending on the location and size of the lesion. Recurrent symptoms may mimic the course of demyelinating disease and were often mistaken for multiple sclerosis before the advent of MRI. Rarely, patients present with cranial neuropathies (trigeminal neuralgia), hypothalamic symptoms, or hydrocephalus.[118, 148, 150, 153]

Outcome

Hemorrhage Morbidity and Mortality. Initial hemorrhages are rarely associated with deterioration or death.[195, 210] Patients generally achieve fair or good recovery after an initial bleed.[195, 210, 229] In one study, the mortality rate was 5.3%, and no deaths were due to the CM.[195] All conservatively treated patients had good or fair outcomes, including two with overt hemorrhage. Aiba and colleagues similarly reported good or excellent recovery in patients with hemorrhage treated surgically or conservatively.[199] The only death was due to repeated brainstem hemorrhages. Moderate or severe disability was noted in 10 of the 62 patients—6 with recurrent hemorrhage, 2 with initial hemorrhage, and 2 with operative complications. All lesions were in eloquent areas of the brain. All patients in the nonhemorrhagic group had good outcomes.

Infratentorial location, but not CM size or multiplicity, increases the risk of neurological disability from hemorrhage. Patients with infratentorial hemorrhage are 6.75 times more likely to be neurologically disabled than are those with supratentorial hemorrhage.[223] Thirty conservatively treated patients with brainstem CMs were followed over a mean of 35.7 months.[231] The mortality in this group was 20%. It is notable, however, that of the survivors, 66.6% had mild or no deficits.

Recurrent overt hemorrhage may occur days to years after an initial bleed and is associated with increased morbidity and cumulative disability.[150, 151, 153, 194–196, 210, 223, 232] In the series by Tung and coworkers, there was a correlation among the number of recurrent hemorrhages, the location of recurrent hemorrhages, and the occurrence of persistent neurological deficits.[226] In most cases (80%), the initial hemorrhage caused only a transient deficit; however, with each successive recurrent bleed, the likelihood of persistent deficit increased.[226]

Seizure Risk. Few studies have evaluated the prospective risk of seizures. Moriarity and associates reported an overall risk of 4.8% per patient-year over a 5.2-year mean follow-up period.[202] In the subgroup of patients without prior seizures, the risk was 2.4% per patient-year. Similarly, Kondziolka and colleagues reported a 4.3% risk of new seizure over a 34-month period.[206] The only risk factors determined for seizure occurrence are multiple CMs and supratentorial location. DelCurling and coworkers calculated the retrospective risk of developing seizures as 1.51% per person-year of exposure overall.[194] The rate was 1.34% per person-year for those with single lesions and 2.48% per person-year for those with multiple lesions. Neither size nor specific lobar location (frontal, parietal, temporal, occipital) has been shown to be a risk factor.

Data suggest that the majority of patients with seizures related to CMs are well controlled with medication.[172, 221] Some suggest that CMs in a temporal location may be more refractory to medication and cause greater disability in younger patients.[223] Patients younger than 40 years of age were 5.6 times more likely to have disability from seizures than were those presenting after the age of 40. Although multiplicity may be a risk factor for seizure, it was not found to be a risk factor for disability from seizure.[223]

Lesion Behavior. Progressive or new focal deficits may arise due to lesion growth, de novo CM formation, or hemorrhage. CMs are dynamic entities. Robinson and colleagues reported that 40% of initially silent lesions became symptomatic within 6 months to 2 years.[195] The risk factors for symptomatic transformation are not known, but changes are thought to be due to intralesional hemorrhage, thrombosis, organization, calcification, and involution of caverns.[151, 162, 210, 233] Neuroimaging has shown changes in lesion size and characteristics over time.[36, 149, 155, 162, 196, 210, 228, 233] In one study, up to 38% of patients had evidence of lesion growth.[160, 162, 195] Robinson and colleagues documented 3 cases of enlargement of CMs, and 31 of 35 had widening rings of hemosiderin.[195] Zabramski and associates documented 4 cases of increased growth, 1 case of regression, and 17 de novo lesions (0.4 lesion per patient-year).[162] Kim and coworkers found that some type II lesions changed to type IV, and vice versa.[161]

DURAL ARTERIOVENOUS FISTULA

Synonyms. Dural arteriovenous malformation,* dural arteriovenous fistulous malformation.

*Not a preferred term, because it implies that these lesions are congenital when the majority are actually idiopathic or acquired.

Definition and Pathogenesis

Dural arteriovenous fistulas (DAVFs) are arteriovenous shunts from a dural arterial supply to a dural venous drainage channel. Any dural vessel is a potential supply source, although most commonly the occipital and meningeal arteries are involved.[6] Venous drainage is through the dural sinus or other dural and leptomeningeal venous channels. DAVFs are often described according to the venous sinus they are related to or the anatomic location of the fistula. On gross pathologic examination, the dural arteries are thickened and the veins are dilated in an abnormal vascular network within the wall of a venous sinus.[234] Numerous microfistulas are seen on histologic examination. Fistulas may have high or low flow and unilateral or bilateral supply. Demyelination may be seen around leptomeningeal veins due to venous hypertension.[2]

Angiography is the gold standard of diagnosis. Injection must include the vertebral and internal and external carotid arteries, as DAVFs may be overlooked with conventional studies alone. The premature appearance during the early arterial phase of a venous structure within or adjacent to the dura mater is characteristic. Visualization of dilated pachymeningeal arteries lends supporting evidence.[235] CT is often normal, although it is most sensitive in evaluating acute subarachnoid, subdural, or intraparenchymal blood. If fistulas drain to cortical veins, contrasted CT may demonstrate serpiginous enhancement. MRI is able to characterize anatomy as well as areas of ischemia and chronic hemorrhage. In addition, evidence of dilated cortical veins may suggest a DAVF with venous hypertension. New magnetic resonance angiography and venography techniques may indicate the location and extent of the fistula but may have insufficient resolution to fully characterize the lesion. Both MRI and CT can miss DAVFs, especially if they are small or if they drain into the ipsilateral venous sinus.[236–238]

The vast majority of DAVFs are acquired, idiopathic lesions.[235, 238–243] In a minority of cases, a possible cause is found, and the site and characteristics of the fistula may provide clues. Possible causes include trauma,[244–246] cranial surgery,[245, 246] sinus infection,[243] and association with meningiomas.[247–249] Syndromes associated with vascular fragility such as Ehlers-Danlos, fibromuscular dysplasia, and neurofibromatosis type 1 may also be associated with DAVFs. In addition, many studies have shown an association with venous sinus thrombosis.[241, 242, 247–250] In some cases, the thrombosis precedes the formation of the DAVF. It is proposed that thrombosis enlarges the normally present microscopic arteriovenous shunts in the walls of the sinus or stimulates their development.[238, 251] In other cases, sinus thrombosis follows the formation of a DAVF.[252, 253] Here, it is believed that turbulence and epithelial damage predispose to clot. Chaloupka believes that various initiating events lead to a common path of angiogenesis within the dura, and the resulting budding and proliferation of microarterial or capillary vessels within the dura create numerous microvascular arteriovenous fistulas.[252, 253] In support of this theory are pathologic specimens of DAVFs that contain angiogenic growth factor and basic fibroblast growth factor. It is not clear whether this is the cause or the effect of DAVF formation.[254, 255] Whatever the inciting event, the final common path that evolves was described by Awad and colleagues.[251] The arteriovenous shunting vessels result in recruitment of arterial feeding vessels (sump effect), with secondary venous hypertension. Venous hypertension can lead to leptomeningeal retrograde drainage and predispose those channels to become varicose and potentially rupture.

Epidemiology

The prevalence of DAVF is unknown, as some remain asymptomatic for years. The estimated age- and sex-adjusted incidence from a population-based study is 0.17 per 100,000 persons, but this is likely an underestimate due to the number of asymptomatic, unreported lesions.[31] Based on imaging studies, DAVFs are found in 1.1% of consecutive angiograms and are one fifth as common as AVMs.[251] They represent approximately 10% to 15% of all intracranial vascular malformations,[106, 239, 240, 251, 256, 257] and patients typically present between the ages of 40 and 60 years. Carotid cavernous and transverse sigmoid DAVFs are more common in women,[258] whereas anterior fossa and tentorial DAVFs are more common in men.[258]

The transverse sigmoid location is the most common, representing more than 50% of DAVFs.[235] The majority are idiopathic, but they may occur with a linear fracture across the transverse venous sinus. Approximately 10% to 15% are located in the cavernous sinus. Women may be affected during pregnancy or after menopause, suggesting a possible hormonal relationship. In addition, prior history of sinusitis has been described in patients with carotid cavernous fistulas. The anterior fossa, tentorial incisura, sylvian or middle fossa, and sagittal sinus are less common locations.[235] DAVFs are usually solitary; multiplicity has been reported in less than 7% of cases.[259–261] The risk for multiplicity is not known, although some hypothesize that in the presence of a hypercoagulable state, venous thrombosis may lead to fistulization.

Clinical Presentation

The natural history of DAVFs is highly variable. Some patients have no symptoms or benign symptoms for many years, and the DAVF is an incidental finding on angiography performed for other reasons.[240, 241, 262–264] These are generally small or located near the occiput.[238] Others exhibit aggressive and catastrophic behaviors. Clinical behavior—including initial presentation, eventual behavior, and prognosis—is a complex function of multiple factors such as location, mode of venous drainage, and magnitude of flow, as well as host angiologic and hormonal factors.

Reversal of flow and venous hypertension in the leptomeningeal draining veins account for the majority of neurological manifestations.[265] Nonhemorrhagic symptoms most commonly include pulsatile tinnitus and headache. Other manifestations include global or focal neurological deficit that may be transient or progressive, seizure, and pseudotumor (papilledema with normal MRI). Rarely, patients present with hydrocephalus, dementia,[266, 267] cranial nerve palsies,[268] and cervical myelopathy.[269, 270] Cervical myelopathy may occur due to venous hypertension affecting the spinal cord through medullary veins distant from the cranial DAVF.

Pulsatile Tinnitus. Pulsatile tinnitus is the most common presenting symptom and is often associated with high-flow fistulas in the transverse sinus or sigmoid location.[235, 238, 243] This occurs because of the recruitment of arterial feeders and the close proximity to the middle ear.[251] A bruit can often be auscultated over the cranium. Compression of the carotid artery and jugular vein or occipital artery may result in reduction of bruit intensity, providing a clue to the diagnosis.

Headache. Headache is also a common presenting symptom. The headache may be unilateral on the side of the DAVF or generalized. It is frequently exacerbated by physical activity or position changes. Engorgement of innervated venous collaterals and dural sinus distention are thought to be the pathophysiologic mechanisms for head pain associated with DAVF. Other mechanisms include brain edema secondary to venous hypertension, compression of the trigeminal nerve, and inflammation due to venous thrombosis. More worrisome causes of headache include associated hemorrhage, hydrocephalus, or pseudotumor as a result of generalized venous hypertension.

Hemorrhage. Intraparenchymal hemorrhage, subarachnoid hemorrhage, and subdural hemorrhage may occur but are distinctly uncommon presentations of DAVF. The annual risk of hemorrhage from an unruptured DAVF was found to be 1.8% in a group of 54 patients followed over a mean of 6.6 years.[256] In this study, lesions of the petrosal or straight sinus had a higher incidence of hemorrhage, as did those with a venous varix. Sixty percent of DAVFs draining into a venous varix and none without this characteristic experienced DAVF-associated hemorrhage. The presence of leptomeningeal venous drainage showed a trend toward increased risk of hemorrhage, but this was not found to be significant.

Other studies assessed risk factors for the prediction of aggressive DAVFs—that is, those with hemorrhagic presentation or progressive neurological deficit. Most concluded that the risk of hemorrhagic presentation is directly related to the impedance of outflow. Lesions with anterograde flow through larger sinuses have a lower risk than those with restricted or retrograde flow into sinuses and cortical veins.[238, 257, 262, 271] Awad and colleagues found that leptomeningeal venous drainage, variceal or aneurysmal venous structure, and galenic venous drainage predicted an aggressive course.[251] In this meta-analysis of 17 personal patients and 360 cases from the literature, DAVFs associated with the tentorial incisura were more often associated with an aggressive course, but no location was immune.

TABLE 127–4 ■ **Classification and Grading of Dural Arteriovenous Fistulas**

GRADE	DESCRIPTION	NUMBER	HEMORRHAGE
Cognard[258]			
1	Dural venous sinus and meningeal vein outflow, anterograde	84	1 (1.2%)*
2a	Dural venous sinus and meningeal vein outflow, retrograde	27	10 (37%)*
2b	Dural venous sinus and meningeal vein outflow (anterograde) and retrograde leptomeningeal venous drainage	10	3 (30%)*
2a + b	Dural venous sinus and meningeal vein outflow (retrograde) and retrograde leptomeningeal venous drainage	18	12 (67%)*
3	Retrograde leptomeningeal venous drainage only (no ectasia)	25	19 (76%)*
4	Retrograde leptomeningeal venous drainage only (ectasia)	29	28 (97%)*
5	Retrograde leptomeningeal venous drainage only (spinal)	12	12 (100%)*
Border[273]			
1	Dural venous sinus and meningeal vein outflow	55	0 (0%)
2	Dural venous sinus and meningeal vein outflow and retrograde leptomeningeal venous drainage	18	2 (11%)
3	Retrograde leptomeningeal venous drainage	29	14 (48%)
Lalwani[271]			
1	Anterograde sinus drainage; no venous restrictive disease; no retrograde or cortical drainage	—	0
2	Anterograde and retrograde venous sinus drainage with or without cortical drainage	—	0
3	Retrograde and cortical drainage without anterograde sinus drainage	—	31%
4	Cortical venous drainage only	—	100%

*Classified as aggressive, denoting hemorrhage or focal deficit, excluding ophthalmoplegia.

Numerous classification systems have been proposed and are useful in determining which DAVF will have an aggressive course.[258, 272–274] Most classification and grading systems take into account the following: presence of venous stenosis or occlusion, direction of flow, presence of leptomeningeal venous drainage, aneurysm, and single or multiple fistulas. Table 127–4 demonstrates several classification systems and the associated risk of hemorrhage.

Little information is available on the risk of recurrent hemorrhage. Only case reports were available until recently.[251, 275] In one report,[276] 20 patients with DAVF-related hemorrhage were followed over a median of 10 months. Seven patients (35%) rebled within 2 weeks after the first hemorrhage. Three patients died, and one worsened after the recurrent hemorrhage.

Specific Symptoms and Location. Carotid cavernous fistulas may present with proptosis, chemosis, retro-orbital pain, and ophthalmoplegia. These symptoms are related to venous hypertension and reduced venous drainage from the orbits. Over time, this can result in choroid and retinal detachment, central retinal venous thrombosis, and reduction in visual acuity. Treatment is usually necessary. If the patient's sight has already been reduced to light perception only, the prognosis for return of vision is poor.[277]

Prognosis

In the study by Brown and colleagues,[256] 52 patients were available for follow-up. Pulsatile tinnitus improved or resolved in 50% of patients. Of 10 patients with headache, 5 worsened, 2 were unchanged, and 3 improved. Three patients (6%) had debilitating symptoms affecting their activities of daily living. Patients without associated sinus occlusion were more likely to improve or remain stable. Mortality associated with initial hemorrhage due to DAVF ranged from 20% to 30%.[251, 256]

DAVFs may change over time. A significant number of benign DAVFs spontaneously thrombose, occasionally after angiography or compression.[278–280] In addition, acute or gradual progression from one grade to the next has been documented. Patients may experience a new neurological deficit or a change in the nature of their symptoms. A sustained change in the character or intensity of the bruit may herald a change in the nature of the fistula. A change or reduction in the bruit does not necessarily mean obliteration of the fistula; in some cases, it may signal development of alternative paths, such as a leptomeningeal vein. Therefore, any change in the bruit or symptoms of a benign DAVF warrants re-evaluation of the lesion.

VENOUS MALFORMATION

Synonyms. Developmental venous anomaly, venous angioma.

Definition and Pathogenesis

Venous malformations (VMs) are congenital venous anomalies.[281–285] Saito and Kobayashi hypothesized that an intrauterine ischemic event occurs during the formation of medullary veins, resulting in collateral venous drainage.[281] Pathologically, these malformations are characterized by anomalous veins separated by normal brain tissue. On histologic section, the walls of the veins are thickened and hyalinized and usually lack elastic tissue and smooth muscle.[2, 286] Despite histologic abnormalities, venous angiomas drain normal cerebral tissue. Contrasted imaging studies reveal a stellate mass or linear enhancement of a transcerebral vein without parenchymal abnormalities.[287] Angiography is typically normal during the arterial and capillary phases. During the venous phase, however, arcades of veins or caput medusae are visualized converging into a large venous channel.[288, 289]

Epidemiology

The exact prevalence of VMs is unknown. In one autopsy series of 4069 consecutive patients, 105 patients (2.6%) were found to have venous angiomas.[53] Autopsy studies also reveal that VMs are the most common type of vascular malformation, accounting for up to 65% of cases.[30] Similarly, radiographic series show that VMs are common among vascular malformations. One series found that 50% of patients with vascular malformations diagnosed by MRI had venous angiomas.[290] In a population-based study,[31] the incidence of VMs was second only to that of AVMs, with an age- and sex-adjusted detection incidence rate of 0.41 per 100,000 person-years. The initial diagnosis is typically made in the third decade,[290–292] but VMs have been reported in children as well as in adults in the eighth decade. There is an equal prevalence in men and women.[290, 291]

VMs are typically located at the junction of superficial and deep venous systems. They may occur anywhere in the central nervous system but are most common within the cerebrum and cerebellum, typically adjacent to a cortical surface or near the ependymal surface of the ventricles. The converging veins of infratentorial VMs are deeply located near or in the choroid plexus and dentate nucleus in the inferior half of the cerebellum. Therefore, infratentorial VMs are virtually always in the cerebellum. Although some report a predominance of intracranial VMs in the posterior fossa,[257, 283, 292–295] other series dispute this.[287, 290, 291] In one large study,[290] the distribution of VMs was as follows: frontal (42%), parietal (24%), occipital (4%), temporal (2%), basal-ventricular (11%), cerebellum (14%), and brainstem (3%). They are most commonly solitary, but several cases of multiple VMs have been reported.[294]

The association of VM with other vascular malformations has been established.[183, 214, 288, 296–301] Association has been noted with AVMs[288, 298, 302, 303] as well as with CMs.[20, 151, 158, 195, 210, 211, 213, 214] Mullan and coworkers hypothesized that the association of VMs and AVMs may be related to failure of the development of the cortical venous mantle.[303] Komiyama and associates reviewed 31 patients with AVMs and VMs and found no difference in the prognosis of those with and without associated AVMs.[302] The association of VMs with CMs and occult vascular malformations is also well documented.[183, 214, 215, 294, 296, 300, 304, 305] Abe and colleagues found that 23% of patients with occult vascular malformations also had VMs.[301] Although some may represent a coexistent congenital abnormality, there may be a subgroup of CMs that arise de novo in the vicinity of a VM.[183, 296, 306] It is hypothesized that regional venous hypertension may facilitate CM formation by red cell diapedesis and angiogenic growth factor release.[183, 296, 306]

Other pathology, including infarct and tumor, is found in 10% to 20% of patients with VMs.[290, 292, 307] It is unclear whether the two are related or whether the selection of patients for scanning leads to this observation. In addition, a case report of venous anomaly associated with facial hemangiomas has been described.[308]

Clinical Presentation

The clinical relevance of VMs has been brought into question.[283, 287, 308] VMs rarely cause symptoms and are often incidental findings. They may be considered symptomatic if the location is consistent with signs and symptoms of the presenting illness or if hemorrhage occurs within the VM. Neurological symptoms leading to imaging studies that identified venous angiomas include headache, seizure, focal deficit, and intracerebral or subarachnoid hemorrhage. Rarely, trigeminal neuralgia and hydrocephalus have been described as presenting symptoms.[283, 306, 309] In large clinical series, less than 25% of symptoms are attributable to the venous angioma (Table 127–5), so other pathology should be sought.[287]

Hemorrhage. Before improved neurodiagnostic techniques, VMs were recognized only after catastrophic events, leading to the belief that complications related to VMs were frequent.[257, 283, 286, 288, 293, 297, 305, 310] Hemorrhage due to venous angiomas was reported in 8% to 43% of older clinical series. Prior studies also showed an increased risk of hemorrhage in posterior fossa lesions[36, 257, 283, 286, 295, 310–312] and in association with pregnancy.[257] Subsequently, several large studies evaluated the hemorrhagic risk and prognosis of these vascular malformations.

Garner and coworkers retrospectively reviewed 100 patients with radiographically diagnosed VMs.[290] Less than 20% were considered to be symptomatic. Six patients presented with hemorrhage, and in only one case was this attributed to the venous angioma. The hemorrhagic risk was calculated to be 0.22% per year

TABLE 127–5 ■ **Presenting Features Leading to Diagnosis of Venous Angioma**

SYMPTOM	GARNER[290] (N = 100)	MCLAUGHLIN[292] (N = 80)	KONDZIOLKA[291] (N = 27)
Headache	36 (4)	(9)	8
Seizure	23 (5)	(4)	(2)
Focal deficit	41 (8)	(6)	6 (1)
Hemorrhage	6 (1)	(1)	(10)
Other	15		(1)

Numbers in parentheses represent the number of cases thought to be related to the venous malformation.

(1 hemorrhage in 4498 person-years). The lower risk found in this study compared with older studies relates to the increased recognition of incidental venous angiomas on MRI. In addition, the authors believe that this estimate of risk is high, due to the nature of tertiary care referrals.

McLaughlin and associates retrospectively reviewed the charts of 80 patients with VMs and prospectively followed them over a mean of 3.6 years.[292] There were 16 hemorrhages at the time of initial registration and 2 additional hemorrhages in subsequent follow-up. They calculated a retrospective hemorrhage rate of 0.61% per year (18 bleeds in 2949 patient-years). In the prospective group, the annual rate was 0.34% (2 bleeds in 298 patient-years). Sex, location, and size did not influence the risk. The authors concluded that the rate of hemorrhage was similar to that of CMs, and perhaps unidentified CMs associated with the venous angiomas caused the hemorrhages.

Others agree that caution is advisable when attributing hemorrhage to VMs and that other pathologies should be searched for.[287, 295, 313] In one study, two patients sustained hemorrhages attributed initially to VMs. The presence of a CM was suggested on MRI in one case, but not clearly. Both patients underwent surgery for the hemorrhage and were found to have pathologically confirmed CMs associated with VMs.[214]

The risk of recurrent bleeding from venous angiomas has not been well defined. A review of 27 cases from the literature revealed that 5 cases (18.5%) had documented recurrence.[293, 295] No risk factors for recurrence were identified due to the small numbers. These cases were also reported before 1985, so other pathology may have been missed owing to the limitations of imaging at that time.

Seizure. The association of venous angiomas and seizures is controversial. In one study, 11 patients with VMs and no other lesions presented with seizures. Electroencephalographic localization was inconsistent in 8 of the 11 cases.[281] In a more recent study by Garner and coworkers, 5 of 23 patients presenting with seizures had electroencephalographic localization consistent with the VM.[290] All these patients were successfully treated with medication alone.

Focal Deficit. Rarely, venous anomalies thrombose, resulting in infarction.[314, 315] This may be the predisposing event before hemorrhage.[316]

It is difficult to ascertain the relationship of the venous angioma to a neurological deficit in the absence of hemorrhage or thrombosis. No pathologic evidence of ischemic changes or microhemorrhages has been demonstrated. In addition, MRI findings rarely show mass effect unless there is associated bleeding. Despite this, focal deficits are occasionally attributed to VMs. Eight patients in one series were found to have VMs potentially causing focal deficits in the absence of hemorrhage,[290] none of which was disabling. Kondziolka and colleagues found two patients with focal deficits potentially related to VMs.[291] One had hemiparesis and a venous angioma in the contralateral posterior internal capsule. The other presented with a movement disorder and had an associated contralateral caudate nucleus VM. Cerebellar lesions may be more likely to cause focal deficits. In one study, 10 of 12 patients with cerebellar VMs had signs or symptoms attributable to the lesion, such as ataxia, diplopia, or dizziness.[287]

Headache. Headache is a common symptom in patients undergoing imaging studies. The causal relationship of VMs is difficult to assess, as definitive proof would require treatment.

Morbidity and Mortality

VMs rarely lead to significant morbidity or mortality. In 14 patients with symptomatic VMs followed over a mean of 3.7 years, there was no death or significant morbidity attributed to the VMs.[291] Garner and coworkers followed 100 patients over a mean of 2.46 years.[290] Eleven patients died and six were disabled, but in no case was this related to the VM. In another series, only 4 of 30 patients had persistent symptoms (2 with seizure, 1 with ataxia, and 1 with headache). No new hemorrhage or focal deficit developed in the 45-month follow-up.[287]

Because VMs drain normal brain parenchyma, treatment may result in devastating venous infarcts.[282, 293] Therefore, surgery is not indicated for these benign lesions. It is not clear whether a subset exists that may require more aggressive treatment.

CAPILLARY TELANGIECTASIA

Synonym. Capillary malformation.

Definition and Pathogenesis

Capillary telangiectasias are vascular malformations composed of dilated capillaries with normal intervening neural tissue. Microscopically, they consist of ectatic individual vessels with thin capillary walls that course among normal architectural elements without adjacent gliosis or hemosiderin deposition.[2]

Imaging studies often miss capillary telangiectasias due to their size and the absence of hemorrhage. These lesions are nearly always angiographically occult.[6] CT is often normal[317] but may display variable enhancement without mass effect.[6] MRI may reveal small enhancing lesions with a brushlike pattern, particularly in the pons, but they are often undetectable on standard T1- and T2-weighted images.[318, 319] The differential diagnosis of an enhancing pontine lesion includes capillary telangiectasia, neoplasm, subacute infarction, and demyelinating or inflammatory disease. The lack of mass effect or increased T2 signal argues against other pathology. In addition, capillary telangiectasia is the only entity in this group of pathologies that is composed of sacs of stagnant blood with deoxyhemoglobin and therefore exhibits susceptibility dephasing, which is evident only on gradient echo images.[318]

Controversy exists regarding the pathogenesis of capillary telangiectasias.[213, 319, 320] Some believe that these lesions are congenital; others believe that their association with other vascular malformations and the age at presentation suggest an acquired lesion. Rigamonti and colleagues hypothesized that CMs and capillary telangiectasias have similar origins but are at opposite ends of a spectrum.[213] The only feature that distinguishes capillary telangiectasia from CM is the presence or absence of brain parenchyma between the vascular channels. Satellite telangiectasias have been found near CMs, and transitional vascular malformations have been described. Therefore, Rigamonti and colleagues suggested a single category of vascular malformation based on pathogenesis. The clear difference in the natural history of these two entities, however, argues against combining CMs and capillary telangiectasias.

Epidemiology

Little information exists on the incidence and prevalence of capillary telangiectasias. Autopsy studies reveal a prevalence of 0.06% to 0.4%.[30, 321] McCormick and colleagues found 60 capillary telangiectasias; 38 were in the posterior fossa, and 22 were supratentorial.[53] They were the second most commonly detected vascular malformation in that autopsy series.

Capillary telangiectasias are most commonly located in the pons[2, 3, 219] but may occur elsewhere in the central nervous system, as well as in other organs. Intracranially, they are most often solitary, but multiple lesions have been described.[322]

Coexistence of capillary telangiectasias and other vascular malformations has been described.[20, 213, 318] Telangiectasias may coexist with sporadic or syndromic central nervous system vascular malformations such as Osler-Weber-Rendu disease, ataxia-telangiectasia, or Wyburn-Mason syndrome. They have been described in association with all types of vascular malformations, but the association with CMs is of particular interest because of the potential common pathogenesis.[213]

Osler-Weber-Rendu disease (hereditary hemorrhagic telangiectasia) is a familial neurocutaneous syndrome with multisystem vascular malformations. Despite its name, malformations in the lung, liver, and mucocutaneous areas are often true AVMs. Between 5% and 11% of patients have associated central nervous system vascular malformations. Although AVM is the most frequent central nervous system accompaniment, DAVF, telangiectasia, CM, VM, and aneurysm have also been described.

Clinical Presentation

Capillary telangiectasias are common incidental findings at autopsy and are rarely symptomatic. In the series by Sarwar and McCormick, only 2 of 60 patients had symptoms related to capillary telangiectasia.[30] Vague, nonspecific neurological symptoms often lead to the incidental discovery of capillary telangiectasia.

Case reports of all types of neurological symptoms, including hemorrhage, seizure, cranial nerve palsy, extrapyramidal disorders, and focal hemispheric syndromes, have been described. Focal symptoms are thought to be secondary to hemorrhage, ischemic necrosis, or progression of the lesion.[219]

Hemorrhage. Patients with capillary telangiectasias may present with intraparenchymal or subarachnoid hemorrhage, although this is quite rare.[219, 322–325] In a population-based study of hemorrhage due to vascular malformations, no hemorrhage caused by capillary telangiectasia was found in a 27-year period.[31] Of the 60 patients described by Sarwar and McCormick, only 2 suffered hemorrhage (1 in the cerebellum, 1 in the diencephalon).[30] Wijdicks and Schievink reported a case of a perimesencephalic subarachnoid hemorrhage likely due to capillary telangiectasia, although this could not be proved.[325] Subsequent MRI follow-up in 20 patients with perimesencephalic hemorrhage failed to demonstrate further telangiectasias.[326] Caution should be used in attributing hemorrhage to capillary telangiectasia, and other pathology should be sought.[327]

The risk of hemorrhage is assumed to be low, but there are no large case series with extensive follow-up. In the study by Lee and coworkers, 18 patients were followed for a mean of 23 months, with no reported bleeds or neurological deficits.[318] Similarly, in another study of 12 patients, no initial symptoms were thought to be definitively related to capillary telangiectasias, and no new symptoms developed in a 3-week to 4-month follow-up.[319]

Focal Deficit. Several cases of focal neurological deficits in the absence of hemorrhage have been reported.[328, 329] Farrell and Forno described a 68-year-old patient presenting with progressive gait ataxia and bulbar dysfunction due to a large pontine capillary telangiectasia.[328] They proposed that the deficit was due to local oxygen deficiency caused by the abnormal blood vessels.

REFERENCES

1. Chaloupka J, Huddle D: Classification of vascular malformations of the central nervous system. Neuroimaging Clin N Am 8:295–321, 1998.
2. Kalimo H, Kase M, Haltia M: Vascular diseases. In Graham D, Lantos P (eds): Greenfield's Neuropathology, 6th ed. New York, Oxford University Press, 1997, pp 345–347.
3. McCormick W: The pathology of vascular malformations. J Neurosurg 24:807–816, 1966.
4. LeBlanc R, Ethier R, Little J: Computerized tomography findings in arteriovenous malformations of the brain. J Neurosurg 51:765–772, 1979.
5. Kumar A, Fox M, Vinuela F, Rosenbaum A: Revisited old and new findings in unruptured larger arteriovenous malformations of the brain. J Comput Assist Tomogr 8:648–655, 1984.
6. Osborn A: Diagnostic Radiology. Chicago, Mosby, 1994.
7. Rumbaugh C, Potts D: Skull changes associated with intracranial arteriovenous malformations. AJR Am J Roentgenol Radium Ther Nucl Med 98:525–534, 1966.
8. Prayer L, Wimberger D, Stigbauer R, et al: Haemorrhage in intracerebral arteriovenous malformations: Detection with MRI and comparison with clinical history. Neuroradiology 35:424–427, 1993.
9. Kesava P, Turski P: MR angiography of vascular malformations. Neuroimaging Clin N Am 8:349–370, 1998.
10. Huston J, Rufenacht D, Ehman R, Wiebers D: Intracranial aneurysms and vascular malformations: Comparison of time of flight

and phase contrast MR angiography. Radiology 181:721–730, 1991.

11. Turjman F, Massoud T, Vinuela F, et al: Correlation of the angioarchitectural features of cerebral arteriovenous malformations with clinical presentation of hemorrhage. Neurosurgery 37:856–862, 1995.
12. Wakai S, Kumakura N, Nagai M: Lobar intracerebral hemorrhage: A clinical, radiographic, and pathological study of 29 consecutive operated cases with negative angiography. J Neurosurg 76:231–238, 1992.
13. London D, Enzmann D: The changing angiographic appearance of an arteriovenous malformation after subarachnoid hemorrhage. Neuroradiology 21:281–284, 1981.
14. Wharen RJ, Scheithauer B, Laws EJ: Thrombosed arteriovenous malformations of the brain. J Neurosurg 57:520–526, 1982.
15. Robinson JJ, Awad I, Masaryk T, Estes M: Pathological heterogeneity of angiographically occult vascular malformations of the brain. Neurosurgery 33:547–555, 1993.
16. Dandy W: Venous abnormalities and angiomas of the brain. Arch Surg 17:715–793, 1928.
17. Padget D: The cranial venous system in man in reference to development, adult configuration and relation to arteries. Am J Anat 98:307–355, 1956.
18. Stein B, Wolpert S: Arteriovenous malformations of the brain. I. Current concepts and treatment. Arch Neurol 37:1–5, 1980.
19. Kader A, Goodrich J, Sonstein W, et al: Recurrent cerebral arteriovenous malformations after negative postoperative angiograms. J Neurosurg 85:14–18, 1996.
20. Awad I, Robinson JJ, Mohanty S, Estes M: Mixed vascular malformations of the brain: Clinical and pathogenetic considerations. Neurosurgery 33:179–188, 1993.
21. Deshpande D, Vidyasagar C: Histology of the persistent embryonic veins in arteriovenous malformations of brain. Acta Neurochir (Wien) 53:227–236, 1980.
22. Mullan S, Mojtahedi S, Johnson DL, Macdonald R: Embryological basis of some aspects of cerebral vascular fistulas and malformations. J Neurosurg 85:1–8, 1996.
23. Mullan S: Reflections upon the nature and management of intracranial and intraspinal vascular malformations and fistulae. J Neurosurg 80:606–616, 1994.
24. Nussbaum E, Heros R, Madison M, et al: The pathogenesis of arteriovenous malformations: Insights provided by a case of multiple arteriovenous malformations developing in relation to a developmental venous anomaly. Neurosurgery 43:347–352, 1998.
25. Yokoyama K, Asano Y, Murakawa T, et al: Familial occurrence of arteriovenous malformation of the brain. J Neurosurg 74: 585–589, 1991.
26. Snead O, Acker J, Morawetz R: Familial arteriovenous malformation. Ann Neurol 5:585–587, 1979.
27. Goto S, Abe M, Tsuji T, Tabuchi K: Familial arteriovenous malformations of the brain: Two case reports. Neurol Med Chir (Tokyo) 34:221–224, 1994.
28. Boyd M, Steinbok P, Paty D: Familial arteriovenous malformations: Report of four cases in one family. Neurosurgery 62: 597–599, 1985.
29. Brilli R, Sacchetti A, Neff S: Familial arteriovenous malformation in children. Pediatr Emerg Care 11:376–378, 1995.
30. Sarwar M, McCormick W: Intracerebral venous angioma: Case report and review. Arch Neurol 35:323–325, 1978.
31. Brown RJ, Do DW, Torner J, O'Fallon W: Frequency of intracranial hemorrhage as a presenting symptom and subtype analysis: A population based study of intracranial vascular malformation in Olmsted County, Minnesota. J Neurosurg 85:29–32, 1996.
32. Furlan A, Whisnant J, Elveback L: The decreasing incidence of primary intracerebral hemorrhage: A population study. Ann Neurol 5:367–373, 1979.
33. Gross C, Kase C, Mohr J, et al: Stroke in south Alabama: Incidence and diagnostic features—a population based study. Stroke 15:249–255, 1984.
34. Perret G, Nishioka H: Report on the cooperative study of intracranial aneurysms and subarachnoid hemorrhage. Section VI. Arteriovenous malformations. J Neurosurg 25:467–490, 1966.
35. Toffol G, Biller J, Adams HJ: Nontraumatic intracerebral hemorrhage in young adults. Arch Neurol 44:483–485, 1987.
36. Wilkins R: The natural history of intracranial vascular malformations: A review. Neurosurgery 16:421–430, 1985.
37. Michelson W: Natural history and pathophysiology of arteriovenous malformations. Clin Neurosurg 26:307–313, 1978.
38. Tay C, Oon C, Lai C, et al: Intracranial arteriovenous malformations in Asians. Brain 94:61–68, 1971.
39. Crawford P, West C, Chadwick D, Shaw M: Arteriovenous malformations of the brain: Natural history in unoperated patients. J Neurol Neurosurg Psychiatry 49:1–10, 1986.
40. Albert P: Personal experience in the treatment of 178 cases of arteriovenous malformations of the brain. Acta Neurochir (Wien) 61:207–226, 1982.
41. Forster D, Steiner L, Hakanson S: Arteriovenous malformations of the brain: A long-term clinical study. J Neurosurg 37:562–570, 1972.
42. Fults D, Kelly DJ: Natural history of arteriovenous malformations of the brain: A clinical study. Neurosurgery 15:658–662, 1984.
43. Graf C, Perret G, Torner J: Bleeding from cerebral arteriovenous malformations as part of their natural history. J Neurosurg 58: 331–337, 1983.
44. Kader A, Young W, Pile-Spellman J, et al: The influence of hemodynamic and anatomic features on hemorrhage from cerebral arteriovenous malformations. Neurosurgery 34:801–808, 1994.
45. Morello G, Borghi G: Cerebral angiomas: A report of 154 personal cases and a comparison between the results of surgical excision and conservative management. Acta Neurochir (Wien) 28:135–155, 1973.
46. Parkinson D, Bachers G: Arteriovenous malformations: Summary of 100 consecutive supratentorial cases. J Neurosurg 53: 285–299, 1980.
47. Troupp H, Marttila I, Halonen V: Arteriovenous malformations of the brain: Prognosis without operation. Acta Neurochir (Wien) 22:125–128, 1970.
48. Trumpy J, Eldevik P: Intracranial arteriovenous malformations: Conservative or surgical treatment? Surg Neurol 8:171–175, 1977.
49. Guidetti B, Delitala A: Intracranial arteriovenous malformations: Conservative and surgical treatment. J Neurosurg 53: 149–152, 1980.
50. Ondra S, Troupp H, George E, Schwab K: The natural history of symptomatic arteriovenous malformations of the brain: A 24-year follow-up assessment. J Neurosurg 73:387–391, 1990.
51. Houser O, Baker H, Svien H, Okazaki H: Arteriovenous malformations of the parenchyma of the brain: Angiographic aspects. Radiology 109:83–90, 1973.
52. Brown RJ, Wiebers D, Forbes G, et al: The natural history of unruptured intracraniaal arteriovenous malformations. J Neurosurg 68:352–357, 1988.
53. McCormick W, Hardman J, Boulter T: Vascular malformations (angiomas) of the brain with special reference to those occurring in the posterior fossa. J Neurosurg 28:241–251, 1968.
54. Reddy K, West M, McClarty B: Multiple intracerebral arteriovenous malformations: A case report and literature review. Surg Neurol 27:495–499, 1987.
55. Willinsky R, Lasjaunias P, Burrows P: Multiple cerebral arteriovenous malformations (AVMs): Review of our experience from 203 patients with cerebral vascular lesions. Neuroradiology 32: 207–210, 1990.
56. Yamashita K, Suzuki Y, Yshizumi J, et al: Multiple cerebral arteriovenous malformations. Neurol Med Chir (Tokyo) 33:24–27, 1993.
57. Putman C, Chaloupka J, Fulbright R, et al: Exceptional multiplicity of cerebral arteriovenous malformations associated with hereditary hemorrhagic telangiectasia (Osler Weber Rendu). AJNR Am J Neuroradiol 17:1733–1742, 1996.
58. Wyburn-Mason R: Arteriovenous aneurysm of mid-brain and retina, facial nevi, and mental changes. Brain 66:163–203, 1943.
59. Hanieh A, Blumbers P, Carney P: Multiple cerebral arteriovenous malformations associated with soft tissue vascular malformations: Case report. J Neurosurg 54:670–672, 1981.
60. Hasegawa S, Hamada J, Morioka M, et al: Multiple cerebral arteriovenous malformations (AVMs) associated with spinal AVM. Acta Neurochir (Wien) 141:315–319, 1999.

61. Suzuki J, Onuma T: Intracranial aneurysms associated with arteriovenous malformations. J Neurosurg 50:742–746, 1979.
62. Perata H, Tomsick T, Tew J Jr: Feeding artery pedicle aneurysms: Association with parenchymal hemorrhage and arteriovenous malformation in the brain. J Neurosurg 80:631–634, 1994.
63. Redekop G, TerBrugge K, Montanera W, Willinsky R: Arterial aneurysms associated with cerebral arteriovenous malformations: Classification, incidence, and risk of hemorrhage. J Neurosurg 89:539–546, 1998.
64. Paterson J, McKissock W: A clinical survey of intracranial angiomas with special reference to their mode of progression and surgical treatment: A report of 110 cases. Brain 79:233–266, 1956.
65. Miyasaka K, Wolpert S, Prager R: The association of cerebral aneurysms, infundibula, and intracranial arteriovenous malformations. Stroke 13:196–203, 1982.
66. Lasjaunias P, Piske R, TerBrugge K, Willinsky R: Cerebral arteriovenous malformations and associated arterial aneurysms. Acta Neurochir (Wien) 91:29–36, 1988.
67. Kondziolka D, Nixon B, Lasjaunias P, et al: Cerebral arteriovenous malformations and associated arterial aneurysms: Hemodynamic and therapeutic considerations. Can J Neurol Sci 15: 130–134, 1988.
68. Cunha E, Sa M, Stein B, et al: The treatment of associated intracranial aneurysms and arteriovenous malformations. J Neurosurg 77:853–859, 1992.
69. Hodgson T, Zaman S, Cooper J, Forster D: Proximal aneurysms in association with arteriovenous malformations: Do they resolve following obliteration of the malformation with stereotactic radiosurgery? Br J Neurosurg 12:434–437, 1998.
70. Batjer H, Suss R, Sampson D: Intracranial arteriovenous malformations associated with aneurysms. Neurosurgery 18:29–35, 1986.
71. Brown RJ, Wiebers D, Forbes G: Unruptured intracranial aneurysms and vascular malformations: Frequency of intracranial hemorrhage and relationship of lesions. J Neurosurg 73:859–863, 1990.
72. Crawford P, West C, Shaw M, Chadwick D: Cerebral arteriovenous malformations and epilepsy: Factors in the development of epilepsy. Epilepsia 27:270–275, 1986.
73. Jomin M, Lesoin F, Lozes G: Prognosis for arteriovenous malformations of the brain in adults based on 150 cases. Surg Neurol 23:362–366, 1985.
74. Aoki N: Do intracranial arteriovenous malformations cause subarachnoid haemorrhage? Review of computed tomography features of ruptured arteriovenous malformations in the acute stage. Acta Neurochir (Wien) 112:92–95, 1991.
75. Sasaki T: Cerebral vasospasm with subarachnoid hemorrhage from cerebral arteriovenous malformations. Surg Neurol 16: 183–187, 1981.
76. Nishimura K: Cerebral vasospasm with subarachnoid hemorrhage from arteriovenous malformations of the brain. Neuroradiology 8:201–207, 1975.
77. Pollock B, Flickinger J, Lunsford L, et al: Factors that predict the bleeding risk of cerebral arteriovenous malformations. Stroke 27:1–6, 1996.
78. Mast H, Young W, Koennecke H, et al: Risk of spontaneous haemorrhage after diagnosis of cerebral arteriovenous malformation. Lancet 350:1065–1068, 1997.
79. Kondziolka D, McLaughlin M, Kestle J: Simple risk predictions for arteriovenous malformation hemorrhage. Neurosurgery 37: 851–855, 1995.
80. Brown RD Jr: Personal communication, 1999.
81. Robinson J, Hall C, Sedzimir C: Arteriovenous malformations, aneurysms, and pregnancy. J Neurosurg 41:63–70, 1974.
82. Langer D, Lasner T, Hurst R, et al: Hypertension, small size, and deep venous drainage are associated with risk of hemorrhagic presentation of cerebral arteriovenous malformations. Neurosurgery 42:481–489, 1998.
83. Marks M, Lane B, Steinberg G, Chang P: Hemorrhage in intracerebral arteriovenous malformations: Angiographic determinants. Radiology 176:807–813, 1990.
84. Nagata S, Matsushima T, Fujii K, et al: Lateral ventricular arteriovenous malformations: Natural history and surgical indications. Acta Neurochir (Wien) 112:37–46, 1991.
85. Drake C, Friedman A, Peerless S: Posterior fossa arteriovenous malformations. J Neurosurg 64:1–10, 1986.
86. Albert P, Salgado H, Polaina M, et al: A study on the venous drainage of 150 cerebral arteriovenous malformations as related to haemorrhagic risks and size of the lesion. Acta Neurochir (Wien) 103:30–34, 1990.
87. Spetzler R, Hargraves R, McCormick P, et al: Relationship of perfusion pressure and size to risk of hemorrhage from arteriovenous malformations. J Neurosurg 76:918–923, 1992.
88. Waltimo O: The change in size of intracranial arteriovenous malformations. J Neurol Sci 19:21–27, 1973.
89. Piepgras D, Sundt TJ, Ragoowansi A, Stevens L: Seizure outcome in patients with surgically treated cerebral arteriovenous malformations. J Neurosurg 78:5–11, 1993.
90. Young W, Kader A, Pile-Spellman J, et al: Arteriovenous malformation draining vein physiology and determinants of transnidal pressure gradients. Neurosurgery 35:389–396, 1994.
91. Sadasivan B, Hwang P: Large cerebral arteriovenous malformations: Experience with 27 cases. Surg Neurol 45:245–249, 1996.
92. Norris J, Valiante T, Wallace M, et al: A simple relationship between radiological arteriovenous malformation hemodynamics and clinical presentation: A prospective, blinded analysis of 31 cases. J Neurosurg 90:673–679, 1999.
93. Hademenos G, Massoud T: Risk of intracranial arteriovenous malformation rupture due to venous drainage impairment: A theoretical analysis. Stroke 1996:1072–1083, 1996.
94. Miyasaka Y, Yada K, Ohwada T, et al: An analysis of the venous drainage system as a factor in hemorrhage from arteriovenous malformations. J Neurosurg 76:239–243, 1992.
95. Vinuela F, Nombela L, Roach M, et al: Stenotic and occlusive disease of the venous drainage system of deep brain AVMs. J Neurosurg 63:180–184, 1985.
96. Columbia AVM Study Group: Arteriovenous malformations of the brain in adults. N Engl J Med 340:1812–1818, 1999.
97. Pritz M: Ruptured supratentorial arteriovenous malformations associated with venous aneurysms. Acta Neurochir (Wien) 128: 150–162, 1994.
98. Turjman F, Massoud T, Sayre J, et al: Epilepsy associated with cerebral arteriovenous malformations: A multivariate analysis of angioarchitectural characteristics. AJNR Am J Neuroradiol 16:345–350, 1995.
99. Troost B, Newton T: Occipital lobe arteriovenous malformations: Clinical and radiologic features in 26 cases with comments on differentiation from migraine. Arch Ophthalmol 93:250–256, 1975.
100. Mast H, Mohr J, Osipov A, et al: "Steal" is an unestablished mechanism for the clinical presentation of cerebral arteriovenous malformations. Stroke 26:1215–1220, 1995.
101. Lazar R, Connaire K, Marshall R, et al: Developmental deficits in adult patients with arteriovenous malformations. Arch Neurol 56:103–106, 1999.
102. Manchola I, Salles AD, Foo T, et al: Arteriovenous malformation hemodynamics: A transcranial Doppler study. Neurosurgery 33: 556–562, 1993.
103. Fink G: Effects of cerebral angiomas on perifocal and remote tissue: A multivariate positron emission tomography study. Stroke 23:1099–1105, 1992.
104. Svien H, McRae J: Arteriovenous anomalies of the brain: Fate of patients not having definitive surgery. J Neurosurg 23:23–28, 1965.
105. Porter P, TerBrugge K, Montanera W, et al: Outcome following hemorrhage from brain arteriovenous malformations at presentation and during follow up: Is it worse than we think? J Neurosurg 88:184A, 1998.
106. Luessenhop A: Dural arteriovenous malformations. In Wilkins R, Rengachary S (eds): Neurosurgery. New York, McGraw-Hill, 1986, pp 1473–1477.
107. Hartmann A, Mast H, Mohr J, et al: Morbidity of intracranial hemorrhage in patients with cerebral arteriovenous malformation. Stroke 29:931–934, 1998.
108. Itoyama Y, Uemura S, Ushio Y, et al: Natural course of unoperated intracranial arteriovenous malformations: Study of 50 cases. J Neurosurg 71:805–809, 1989.
109. Aminoff M: Treatment of unruptured cerebral arteriovenous malformations. Neurology 37:815–819, 1987.
110. Murphy M: Long-term follow-up of seizures associated with cerebral arteriovenous malformations: Results of therapy. Arch Neurol 42:477–479, 1985.

111. Pasqualin A, Vivenza C, Rosta L, et al: Spontaneous regression of intracranial arteriovenous malformation. Surg Neurol 39:385–391, 1993.
112. Minikawa T, Tanaka R, Koike T: Angiographic follow-up study of cerebral arteriovenous malformation with reference to their enlargement and progression. Neurosurgery 24:68–74, 1989.
113. Marconi F, Parenti G, Puglioli M: Spontaneous regression of intracranial arteriovenous malformation. Surg Neurol 39:385–391, 1993.
114. Hook O, Johanson C: Intracranial arteriovenous malformations: A follow-up study with particular attention to their growth. Arch Neurol Psychiatry 80:39–54, 1958.
115. Guazzo E, Zuered J: Spontaneous thrombosis of an arteriovenous malformation. J Neurol Neurosurg Psychiatry 57:1410–1412, 1994.
116. Ebeling J, Tranmer B, Davis K: Thrombosed arteriovenous malformations: A type of occult vascular malformation. Magnetic resonance imaging and histopathological considerations. Neurosurgery 23:605–609, 1988.
117. Abdulrauf S, Malik G, Awad I: Spontaneous angiographic obliteration of cerebral arteriovenous malformations. Neurosurgery 44:280–287; discussion 287–288, 1999.
118. Mizutani T, Tanaka H, Aruga T: Total recanalization of a spontaneously thrombosed arteriovenous malformation: Case report. J Neurosurg 82:506–508, 1995.
119. Marks M, Lane B, Steinberg G, Snipes G: Intranidal aneurysms in cerebral arteriovenous malformations: Evacuation and endovascular treatment. Radiology 183:335–360, 1992.
120. Cronqvist S, Troupp H: The intracranial arteriovenous malformation and arterial aneurysm in the same patient. Acta Neurol Scand 42:307–316, 1966.
121. Thompson R, Steinberg G, Levy R, Marks M: The management of patients with arteriovenous malformations and associated intracranial aneurysms. Neurosurgery 43:202–212, 1998.
122. Dias M, Sekhar L: Intracranial hemorrhage from aneurysms and arteriovenous malformations during pregnancy and the puerperium. Neurosurgery 27:855–866, 1990.
123. Wiebers D: Subarachnoid hemorrhage in pregnancy. Semin Neurol 8:226–229, 1988.
124. Dias M: Neurovascular emergencies in pregnancy. Clin Obstet Gynecol 37:337–354, 1994.
125. Horton J, Chambers W, Lyons S, et al: Pregnancy and the risk of hemorrhage from cerebral arteriovenous malformations. Neurosurgery 27:867–872, 1990.
126. Sadasivan B, Malik G, Lee C, Ausman J: Vascular malformations and pregnancy. Surg Neurol 33:305–313, 1990.
127. Lanzino G, Jensen M, Cappelletto B, Kassell N: Arteriovenous malformations that rupture during pregnancy: A management dilemma. Acta Neurochir (Wien) 126:102–106, 1994.
128. Robinson J, Chir B, Hall C, Sedzimir C: Subarachnoid hemorrhage in pregnancy. J Neurosurg 36:27–33, 1972.
129. Sano K, Ueda Y, Saito I: Subarachnoid hemorrhage in children. Childs Brain 4:38–46, 1978.
130. Hldaky J, Lejeune J, Blond S, et al: Cerebral arteriovenous malformations in children: Report on 62 cases. Childs Nerv Syst 10:328–333, 1994.
131. Mori K, Murata T, Hashimoto N, Handa H: Clinical analysis of arteriovenous malformations in children: Clinical features and outcome of treatment in children and adults. Clin Neurol 22: 43–49, 1984.
132. Kelly JJ, Mellinger J, Sundt TJ: Intracranial arteriovenous malformations in childhood. Ann Neurol 3:338–343, 1978.
133. Suarez J, Viano J: Intracranial arteriovenous malformations in infancy and adolescence. Childs Nerv Syst 5:15–18, 1989.
134. Kondziolka D, Humphreys R, Hoffman J, et al: Arteriovenous malformations of the brain in children: A forty-year experience. Can J Neurol Sci 19:40–45, 1992.
135. Lasjaunias P, Hui F, Zerah M: Cerebral arteriovenous malformations in children: Management of 179 consecutive cases and review of the literature. Childs Nerv Syst 5:15–18, 1989.
136. Miller C, Bissonnette B, Humphreys R: Cerebral arteriovenous malformations in children. Childs Nerv Syst 7:43–47, 1991.
137. Hara H, Burrows P, Flodmark O, et al: Neonatal superficial cerebral arteriovenous malformations. Pediatr Neurosurg 20: 126–136, 1994.
138. Melville C, Walsh K, Sreeram N: Cerebral arteriovenous malformations in the neonate: Clinical presentation, diagnosis and outcome. Int J Cardiol 31:175–180, 1991.
139. Kurokawa T, Matsuzaki A, Hasuo K, et al: Cerebral arteriovenous malformations in children. Brain Dev 7:408–413, 1985.
140. D'Aliberti G, Talamonti G, Versari P, et al: Comparison of pediatric and adult cerebral arteriovenous malformations. J Neurosurg Sci 41:331–336, 1997.
141. Humphreys R, Hendrick E, Hoffman H: Arteriovenous malformations of the brainstem in childhood. Childs Brain 11:1–11, 1984.
142. Menovsky T, vanOverbeeke J: Cerebral arteriovenous malformations in childhood: State of the art with special reference to treatment. Eur J Pediatr 156:741–746, 1997.
143. Griffiths P, Blaser S, Armstrong D, et al: Cerebellar arteriovenous malformations in children. Neuroradiology 40:324–331, 1998.
144. Gerosa M, Cappellotto P, Licata C, et al: Cerebral arteriovenous malformations in children (56 cases). Childs Brain 8:356–371, 1981.
145. Johnson P, Wascher T, Golfinos J, Spetzler R: Definition and pathological features. In Awad I, Barrow D (eds): Cavernous Malformations. Park Ridge, Ill, AANS, 1993, pp 1–11.
146. Ramina R, Ingunza W, Vonofakos D: Cystic cerebral cavernous angioma with dense calcification: Case report. J Neurosurg 52: 259–262, 1980.
147. Rigamonti D, Drayer B, Johnson P, et al: The MRI appearance of cavernous malformations (angiomas). J Neurosurg 67:518–524, 1987.
148. Voigt K, Yasargil M: Cerebral cavernous haemangiomas or cavernomas: Incidence, pathology, localization, diagnosis, clinical features and treatment. Review of the literature and report of an unusual case. Neurochirurgia (Stuttg) 19:59–68, 1976.
149. Simard J, Garcia-Bengochea F, Ballinger WJ, et al: Cavernous angioma: A review of 126 collected and 12 new clinical cases. Neurosurgery 18:162–172, 1986.
150. Giombini S, Morello G: Cavernous angiomas of the brain: Account of fourteen personal cases and review of the literature. Acta Neurochir (Wien) 40:61–82, 1978.
151. Lobato R, Perez C, Rivas J, Cordobes F: Clinical, radiological, and pathological spectrum of angiographically occult intracranial vascular malformations: Analysis of 21 cases and review of the literature. J Neurosurg 68:518–531, 1988.
152. Vaquero J, Leunda G, Martinez R, Bravo G: Cavernomas of the brain. Neurosurgery 12:208–210, 1983.
153. Rigamonti D, Hadley M, Drayer B, et al: Cerebral cavernous malformations: Incidence and familial occurrence. N Engl J Med 319:343–347, 1988.
154. Bien S, Friedburg H, Harders A, Schumacher M: Intracerebral cavernous angiomas in magnetic resonance imaging. Acta Radiol Suppl (Stockh) 369:79–81, 1986.
155. Biondi A, Scotti G, Scialfa G, Landoni L: Magnetic resonance imaging of cerebral cavernous angiomas. Acta Radiol Suppl (Stockh) 369:82–85, 1986.
156. Bourgouin P, Tampieri D, Johnston W, et al: Multiple occult vascular malformations of the brain and spinal cord: MRI diagnosis. Neuroradiology 34:110–111, 1992.
157. Duong H, Carpio-O'Donovan RD, Pike B, Ethier R: Multiple intracerebral cavernous angiomas. Can Assoc Radiol J 42:329–334, 1991.
158. Rapacki T, Brantley M, Furlow TJ, et al: Heterogeneity of cerebral cavernous hemangiomas diagnosed by MR imaging. J Comput Assist Tomogr 14:18–25, 1990.
159. Perl J, Ross J: Diagnostic imaging of cavernous malformations. In Awad I, Barrow D (eds): Cavernous Malformations. Park Ridge, Ill, AANS, 1993, pp 37–48.
160. Sigal R, Krief O, Houtteville J, et al: Occult cerebrovascular malformations: Follow-up with MR imaging. Radiology 176: 815–819, 1990.
161. Kim D, Park Y, Choi J, et al: An analysis of the natural history of cavernous malformations. Surg Neurol 48:9–18, 1997.
162. Zabramski J, Wascher T, Spetzler R, et al: The natural history of familial cavernous malformations: Results of an ongoing study. J Neurosurg 80:422–432, 1994.
163. Ogilvy C, Heros R, Ojemann R, New P: Angiographically occult arteriovenous malformations. J Neurosurg 70:293, 1989.

164. Sze G, Krol G, Olsen W, et al: Hemorrhagic neoplasms: MR mimics of occult vascular malformations. AJR Am J Roentgenol 149:1223–1230, 1987.
165. Steinberg G, Marks M: Lesions mimicking cavernous malformations. In Awad I, Barrow D (eds): Cavernous Malformations. Park Ridge, Ill, AANS, 1993, pp 151–162.
166. Dillon W: Cryptic vascular malformations: Controversies in terminology, diagnosis, pathophysiology, and treatment. AJNR Am J Neuroradiol 18:1839–1846, 1997.
167. Tomlinson F, Houser O, Scheithauer B, et al: Angiographically occult vascular malformations: A correlative study of features on magnetic resonance imaging and histological examination. Neurosurgery 34:792–800, 1994.
168. Vanefsky M, Cheng M, Chang S, et al: Correlation of magnetic resonance characteristics and histopathological type of angiographically occult vascular malformations. Neurosurgery 44: 1174–1181, 1999.
169. Abe M, Kjellberg R, Adams R: Clinical presentations of vascular malformations of the brain stem: Comparison of angiographically positive and negative types. J Neurol Neurosurg Psychiatry 52:167–175, 1989.
170. Servo A, Porras M, Raininko R: Diagnosis of cavernous haemangiomas by computed tomography and angiography. Acta Neurochir (Wien) 71:273–282, 1984.
171. Yamasaki T, Handa H, Yamashita J, et al: Intracranial and orbital cavernous angiomas: A review of 30 cases. J Neurosurg 64: 197–208, 1986.
172. Weber M, Vespignani H, Bracard S, et al: Intracerebral cavernous angioma. Rev Neurol (Paris) 145:429–436, 1989.
173. Tagle P, Huete I, Mendez J, Villar SD: Intracranial cavernous angioma: Presentation and management. J Neurosurg 64:720–723, 1986.
174. Numaguchi Y, Kishikawa T, Fukui M, et al: Prolonged injection angiography for diagnosing intracranial cavernous hemangiomas. Radiology 131:137–138, 1979.
175. Numaguchi Y, Fukui M, Miyake E, et al: Angiographic manifestations of intracerebral cavernous hemangioma. Neuroradiology 14:113–116, 1977.
176. Maraire J, Awad I: Intracranial cavernous malformations: Lesion behavior and management strategies. Neurosurgery 37:591–605, 1995.
177. Wilson C: Cryptic vascular malformations. Clin Neurosurg 38: 49–84, 1992.
178. Tekkok I, Ventureyra E: De novo familial cavernous malformation presenting with hemorrhage 12.5 years after the initial hemorrhagic ictus: Natural history of an infantile form. Pediatr Neurosurg 25:151–155, 1996.
179. Detwiler P, Porter R, Zabramski J, Spetzler R: De novo formation of a central nervous system cavernous malformation: Implications for predicting risk of hemorrhage. Case report and review of the literature. J Neurosurg 87:629–632, 1997.
180. Larson J, Ball W, Bove K, et al: Formation of intracerebral cavernous malformations after radiation treatment for central nervous system neoplasia in children. J Neurosurg 88:51–56, 1998.
181. Chang S, Vanefsky M, Havton L, Silverberg G: Bilateral cavernous malformations resulting from cranial irradiation of a choroid plexus papilloma. Neurol Res 20:529–532, 1998.
182. Ogilvy C, Moayeri N, Golden J: Appearance of a cavernous hemangioma in the cerebral cortex after a biopsy of a deeper lesion. Neurosurgery 33:307–309, 1993.
183. Ciricillo S, Dillon W, Fink M, Edwards M: Progression of multiple cryptic vascular malformations associated with anomalous venous drainage: Case report. J Neurosurg 81:477–481, 1994.
184. Maeder P, Gudinchet F, Meuli R, Tribolet ND: Development of a cavernous malformation of the brain. AJNR Am J Neuroradiol 19:1141–1143, 1998.
185. Pozzati E, Musiani M: Cavernous hemangioma. J Neurosurg 89: 498, 1998.
186. Gunel M, Awad I, Anson J, Lifton R: Mapping a gene causing cerebral cavernous malformation to 7q11.2–q21. Proc Natl Acad Sci U S A 92:6620–6624, 1995.
187. Dubovsky J, Zabramski J, Kurth J, et al: A gene responsible for cavernous malformations of the brain maps to chromosome 7q. Hum Mol Genet 4:453–458, 1995.
188. Gunel M, Awad I, Finberg K, et al: A founder mutation as a cause of cerebral cavernous malformation in Hispanic Americans. N Engl J Med 334:946–951, 1996.
189. Craig H, Gunel M, Cepeda O, et al: Multilocus linkage identifies two new loci for a mendelian form of stroke, cerebral cavernous malformation, at 7p15–13 and 3q25.2–27. Hum Mol Genet 7: 1851–1858, 1998.
190. Gunel M, Awad I, Finberg K, et al: Genetic heterogeneity of inherited cerebral cavernous malformation. Neurosurgery 38: 1265–1271, 1996.
191. Labauge P, Enjolras O, Bonerandi J, et al: An association between autosomal dominant cerebral cavernomas and a distinctive hyperkeratotic cutaneous vascular malformation in 4 families. Ann Neurol 45:250–254, 1999.
192. Berry R, Alpers B, White J: The site, structure and frequency of intracranial aneurysms, angiomas and arteriovenous abnormalities. In Millikan C (ed): Research Publications: Association for Research in Nervous and Mental Disease. Baltimore, Williams & Wilkins, 1966, pp 4–72.
193. Otten P, Pizzolato G, Rilliet B, Berney J: 131 Cases of cavernous angioma (cavernomas) of the CNS, discovered by retrospective analysis of 24,535 autopsies. Neurochirurgie 35:128–131, 1989.
194. Del Curling O Jr, Kelly DL Jr, Elster A, Craven T: An analysis of the natural history of cavernous angiomas. J Neurosurg 75: 702–708, 1991.
195. Robinson J, Awad I, Little J: Natural history of the cavernous angioma. J Neurosurg 75:709–714, 1991.
196. Sage M, Brophy B, Sweeney C, et al: Cavernous haemangiomas (angiomas) of the brain: Clinically significant lesions. Australas Radiol 37:147–155, 1993.
197. Lonjon M, Roche J, George B, et al: Intracranial cavernoma: 30 cases. Presse Med 22:990–994, 1993.
198. Martin N, Vinters H: Pathology and grading of intracranial vascular malformations. In Awad I, Barrow D (eds): Intracranial Vascular Malformations. Park Ridge, Ill, AANS, 1990, pp 1–30.
199. Aiba T, Tanaka R, Koike T, et al: Natural history of intracranial cavernous malformations. J Neurosurg 83:56–59, 1995.
200. Edwards M, Baumgartner J, Wilson C: Cavernous and other cryptic vascular malformations in the pediatric age group. In Awad I, Barrow D (eds): Cavernous Malformations. Park Ridge, Ill, AANS, 1993, pp 163–183.
201. Hsu F, Rigamonti D, Huhn S: Epidemiology of cavernous malformations. In Awad I, Barrow D (eds): Cavernous Malformations. Park Ridge, Ill, AANS, 1993, pp 13–23.
202. Moriarity J, Clatterbuck R, Rigamonti D: The natural history of cavernous malformations. Neurosurg Clin N Am 10:411–417, 1999.
203. Bergeson P, Rekate H, Tack E: Cerebral cavernous angiomas in the newborn. Clin Pediatr 31:435–437, 1992.
204. Dobyns W, Michels W, Groover R, et al: Familial cavernous malformations of the central nervous system and retina. Ann Neurol 21:578–583, 1987.
205. Mazza C, Scienza R, Bernardin BD, et al: Cerebral cavernous malformations (cavernomas) in children. Neurochirurgie 35: 106–108, 1989.
206. Kondziolka D, Lunsford L, Kestle J: The natural history of cerebral cavernous malformations. J Neurosurg 83:820–824, 1995.
207. Hayman L, Evans R, Ferrell R, et al: Familial cavernous angiomas: Natural history and genetic study over a 5-year period. Am J Med Genet 11:147–160, 1982.
208. Gangemi M, Maiuri F, Donati P, et al: Familial cerebral cavernous angiomas. Neurol Res 12:131–136, 1990.
209. Requena I, Arias M, Lopez-Ibor L, et al: Cavernomas of the central nervous system: Clinical and neuroimaging manifestations in 47 patients. J Neurol Neurosurg Psychiatry 54:590–594, 1991.
210. Barrow D, Krisht A: Cavernous malformations and hemorrhage. In Awad I, Barrow D (eds): Cavernous Malformations. Park Ridge, Ill, AANS, 1993, pp 65–80.
211. Diamond C, Torvik A, Amundsen P: Angiographic diagnosis of telangiectasias with cavernous angioma of the posterior fossa: Report of two cases. Acta Radiol 17:281–288, 1976.
212. Hirsh L: Combined cavernous-arteriovenous malformation. Surg Neurol 16:135–139, 1981.

213. Rigamonti D, Johnson P, Spetzler R, et al: Cavernous malformations and capillary telangiectasia: A spectrum within a single pathological entity. Neurosurgery 28:60–64, 1991.
214. Rigamonti D, Spetzler R: The association of venous and cavernous malformations: Report of four cases and discussion of the pathophysiological, diagnostic, and therapeutic implications. Acta Neurochir (Wien) 92:100–105, 1988.
215. Wilms G, Bleus E, Demaerel P, et al: Simultaneous occurrence of developmental venous anomalies and cavernous angiomas. AJNR Am J Neuroradiol 15:1247–1254, 1994.
216. Porter R, Detwiler P, Spetzler R, et al: Cavernous malformations of the brainstem: Experience with 100 patients. J Neurosurg 90: 50–58, 1999.
217. Abdulrauf S, Kaynar M, Awad I: A comparison of the clinical profile of cavernous malformations with and without associated venous malformations. Neurosurgery 44:41–47, 1999.
218. McCormick W: Pathology of vascular malformations of the brain. In Wilson C, Stein B (eds): Intracranial Arteriovenous Malformations. Baltimore, Williams & Wilkins, 1984, pp 44–63.
219. Jellinger K: Vascular malformations of the central nervous system: A morphological overview. Neurosurg Rev 9:177–216, 1986.
220. Kraemer D, Awad I: Vascular malformations and epilepsy: Clinical considerations and basic mechanisms. Epilepsia 35(Suppl 6):S30–S43, 1994.
221. Awad I, Robinson J: Cavernous malformation and epilepsy. In Awad I, Barrow D (eds): Cavernous Malformations. Park Ridge, Ill, AANS, 1993, pp 49–63.
222. Fargueta J, Iranzo R, Garcia M, Jorda M: Hemangioma calcifications: A benign epileptogenic lesion. Surg Neurol 15:66–70, 1981.
223. Robinson JJ, Awad I, Magdinec M, Paranandi L: Factors predisposing to clinical disability in patients with cavernous malformations of the brain. Neurosurgery 32:730–736, 1993.
224. Robinson J: Clinical spectrum and natural course. In Awad I, Barrow D (eds): Cavernous Malformations. Park Ridge, Ill, AANS, 1993, pp 25–36.
225. Ueda S, Saito A, Inomori S, Kim I: Cavernous angioma of the cauda equina producing subarachnoid hemorrhage: Case report. J Neurosurg 66:134–136, 1987.
226. Tung H, Giannotta S, Chandrasoma P, Zee C: Recurrent intraparenchymal hemorrhages from angiographically occult vascular malformations. J Neurosurg 73:174–180, 1990.
227. Hubert P, Choux M, Houtteville J: Cerebral cavernomas in infants and children. Neurochirurgie 35:104–105, 1989.
228. Scott R, Barnes P, Kupsky W, Adelman L: Cavernous angiomas of the central nervous system in children. J Neurosurg 76: 38–46, 1992.
229. Porter P, Willinsky R, Harper W, Wallace M: Cerebral cavernous malformations: Natural history and prognosis after clinical deterioration with or without hemorrhage. J Neurosurg 87:190–197, 1997.
230. Zauberman H, Feinsod M: Orbital hemangioma growth during pregnancy. Acta Ophthalmol (Copenh) 48:929–933, 1970.
231. Fritschi J, Reulen H, Spetzler R, Zabramski J: Cavernous malformations of the brain stem: A review of 139 cases. Acta Neurochir (Wien) 130:35–46, 1994.
232. Duffau H, Capelle L, Sichez J, et al: Early radiologically proven rebleeding from intracranial cavernous angiomas: Report of 6 cases and review of the literature. Acta Neurochir (Wien) 139: 914–922, 1997.
233. Pozzati E, Giuliani G, Nuzzo G, Poppi M: The growth of cerebral cavernous angiomas. Neurosurgery 25:92–97, 1989.
234. Nishijima M, Takaku A, Endo S, et al: Etiological evaluation of dural arteriovenous malformations of the lateral and sigmoid sinuses based on histopathological examinations. J Neurosurg 76:600–606, 1992.
235. Awad I, Little J: Dural arteriovenous malformation. In Barrow D (ed): Intracranial Vascular Malformation. Park Ridge, Ill, AANS, 1990, pp 219–226.
236. Chen J, Tsurdua J, Halbach V: Suspected dural arteriovenous fistula: Results with screening MR angiography in seven patients. Radiology 183:265–271, 1992.
237. DeMarco J, Dillon W, Halbach V, Tsuruda J: Dural arteriovenous fistulas: Evaulation with MR imaging. Radiology 175:193–199, 1990.
238. Malek A, Halbach V, Dowd C, Higashida R: Diagnosis and treatment of dural arteriovenous fistulas. Neuroimaging Clin N Am 8:445–468, 1998.
239. Grady M, Pobereskin L: Arteriovenous malformations of the dura mater. Surg Neurol 28:135–140, 1987.
240. Aminoff M: Vascular anomalies in the intracranial dura mater. Brain 96:601–612, 1973.
241. Chaudhary M, Sachdev V, Cho S, et al: Dural arteriovenous malformation of the major venous sinuses: An acquired lesion. AJNR Am J Neuroradiol 3:13–19, 1982.
242. Houser O, Campbell J, Campbell R, Sundt TJ: Arteriovenous malformation affecting the transverse dural venous sinus: An acquired lesion. Mayo Clin Proc 54:651–661, 1979.
243. Little N, Piepgras D: Intracranial dural arteriovenous fistula. In Batjer H (ed): Cerebrovascular Disease. Philadelphia, Lippincott-Raven, 1997, pp 799–809.
244. Dennery J, Ignacio B: Post-traumatic arteriovenous fistula between the external carotid arteries and the superior longitudinal sinus: Report of a case. Can J Surg 10:333–336, 1967.
245. Nabors M, Azzam C, Albanna F, et al: Delayed postoperative dural arteriovenous malformations: Report of two cases. J Neurosurg 66:768–772, 1987.
246. Watanabe A, Takahara Y, Ibuchi Y, Mizukami K: Two cases of dural arteriovenous malformation occurring after intracranial surgery. Neuroradiology 26:375–380, 1984.
247. Davie J, Hodges F: Arteriovenous fistula after removal of meningioma: Case report. J Neurosurg 27:364–369, 1967.
248. Ugrinovski J, Vrcakovski M, Lozance K: Dural arteriovenous malformation secondary to meningioma removal. Br J Neurosurg 3:603–607, 1989.
249. Yokota M, Tani E, Maeda Y, Yamaura I: Meningioma in sigmoid sinus groove associated with dural arteriovenous malformation: Case report. Neurosurgery 33:316–319, 1993.
250. Picard L, Bracard S, Mallet J: Spontaneous arteriovenous fistulas. Semin Intervent Radiol 4:219–240, 1987.
251. Awad I, Little J, Akrawi W, Ahl J: Intracranial dural arteriovenous malformations: Factors predisposing to an aggressive neurological course. J Neurosurg 72:839–850, 1990.
252. Chaloupka J: Endovascular therapy of dural arteriovenous fistulae. Semin Intervent Radiol 11:1–13, 1994.
253. Chaloupka J, Putman C: Endovascular therapy for surgical diseases of the cranial base. Clin Plast Surg 22:417–450, 1995.
254. Lawton M, Jacobowitz R, Spetzler R: Redefined role of angiogenesis in the pathogenesis of dural arteriovenous malformations. J Neurosurg 87:267–274, 1997.
255. Terada T, Higashida R, Halbach V, et al: Development of acquired arteriovenous fistulas in rats due to venous hypertension. J Neurosurg 80:884–889, 1994.
256. Brown RJ, Wiebers D, Nichols D: Intracranial dural arteriovenous fistulae: Angiographic predictors of intracranial hemorrhage and clinical outcome in nonsurgical patients. J Neurosurg 81:531–538, 1994.
257. Malik G, Morgan J, Boulos R, Ausman J: Venous angiomas: An underestimated cause of intracranial hemorrhage. Surg Neurol 30:350–358, 1988.
258. Cognard C, Gobin Y, Peirot L, et al: Cerebral dural arteriovenous fistulas: Clinical and angiographic correlation with a revised classification of venous drainage. Radiology 194:671–680, 1995.
259. Nakamura M, Tamaki N, Hara Y, Nagashima T: Two unusual cases of multiple dural arteriovenous fistulas. Neurosurgery 41: 288–293, 1997.
260. Kuwayama N, Takaku A, Nishijima M, et al: Multiple dural arteriovenous malformations: Report of two cases. J Neurosurg 71:932–934, 1989.
261. Ushikoshi S, Kikuchi Y, Miyasaka K: Multiple dural arteriovenous shunts in a 5-year-old boy. AJNR Am J Neuroradiol 20: 728–730, 1999.
262. Fermand M, Reizine D, Melki J, et al: Long term follow-up of 43 pure dural arteriovenous fistulae (AVF) of the lateral sinus. Neuroradiology 29:348–353, 1987.
263. Obrador S, Gomez-Bueno J, Silvela J: Spontaneous carotid-cavernous fistula produced by ruptured aneurysm of the meningohypophyseal branch of the internal carotid artery: Case report. J Neurosurg 40:539–543, 1974.

264. Edwards M, Connolly E: Cavernous sinus syndrome produced by communication between the external carotid artery and cavernous sinus. J Neurosurg 46:92–96, 1977.
265. Lasjaunias P, Chiu M, Brugge KT, et al: Neurological manifestations of intracranial dural arteriovenous malformations. J Neurosurg 64:724–730, 1986.
266. Zeidman S, Monsein L, Arosarena O, et al: Reversibility of white matter changes and dementia after treatment of dural fistulas. AJNR Am J Neuroradiol 16:1080–1083, 1995.
267. Hurst R, Bagley L, Galetta S, et al: Dementia resulting from dural arteriovenous fistulas: The pathologic findings of venous hypertensive encephalopathy. AJNR Am J Neuroradiol 19:1267–1273, 1998.
268. Ito J, Imamura H, Kobayashi K, et al: Dural arteriovenous malformations of the base of the anterior cranial fossa. Neuroradiology 24:149–153, 1983.
269. Brunereau L, Gobin Y, Meder J, et al: Intracranial dural arteriovenous fistulas with spinal venous drainage: Relation between clinical presentation and angiographic findings. AJNR Am J Neuroradiol 17:1549–1554, 1996.
270. Wrobel C, Oldfield E, Chiro GD, et al: Myelopathy due to intracranial dural arteriovenous fistulas draining intrathecally into spinal medullary veins: Report of three cases. J Neurosurg 69:934–939, 1988.
271. Lalwani A, Dowd C, Halbach V: Grading venous restrictive disease in patients with dural arteriovenous fistulas of the transverse/sigmoid sinus. J Neurosurg 79:11–15, 1993.
272. Barrow D, Spector R, Braun I, et al: Classification and treatment of spontaneous carotid-cavernous sinus fistulas. J Neurosurg 62:248–256, 1985.
273. Borden J, Wu J, Shucart W: A proposed classification for spinal and cranial dural arteriovenous fistulous malformations and implications for treatment. J Neurosurg 82:166–179, 1995.
274. Djindjian R, Cophignon J, Theron JR, et al: Superselective arteriographic embolization by the femoral route in neuroradiology: Study of 50 cases. 3. Embolization in craniocerebral pathology. Neuroradiology 6:143–152, 1973.
275. Grisoli F, Vincentelli F, Fuchs S, et al: Surgical treatment of tentorial arteriovenous malformations draining into the subarachnoid space: Report of four cases. J Neurosurg 60:1059–1066, 1984.
276. Duffau H, Lopes M, Janosevic V, et al: Early rebleeding from intracranial dural arteriovenous fistulas: Report of 20 cases and review of the literature. J Neurosurg 90:78–84, 1999.
277. Halbach V, Hieshima G, Higashida R, Reicher M: Carotid cavernous fistulae: Indications for urgent treatment. AJR Am J Roentgenol 149:587–593, 1987.
278. Halbach V, Higashida R, Hieshima G, et al: Transvenous embolization of dural fistulas involving the cavernous sinus. AJNR Am J Neuroradiol 10:377–383, 1989.
279. Newton T, Cronqvist S: Involvement of dural arteries in intracranial arteriovenous malformations. Radiology 93:1071–1078, 1969.
280. Olutola P, Eliam M, Molot M, Talalla A: Spontaneous regression of a dural arteriovenous malformation. Neurosurgery 12:687–690, 1983.
281. Saito Y, Kobayashi N: Cerebral venous angiomas: Clinical evaluation and possible etiology. Radiology 139:87–94, 1981.
282. Senegor M, Dohrmann G, Wollmann R: Venous angiomas of the posterior fossa should be considered as anomalous venous drainage. Surg Neurol 19:26–32, 1983.
283. Numaguchi Y, Kitamura K, Fukui M, et al: Intracranial venous angiomas. Surg Neurol 18:193–202, 1982.
284. Lasjaunias P, Burrows P, Planet C: Developmental venous anomalies (DVA): The so-called venous angioma. Neurosurg Rev 9:232–242, 1994.
285. Huang Y, Robbins A, Patel S, Chaundhary M: Cerebral venous malformations and a new classification of cerebral vascular malformations. In Kapp J, Schmidek H (eds): The Cerebral Venous System and Its Disorders. New York, Grune & Stratton, 1984, pp 373–474.
286. Wolf A, Brock S: The pathology of cerebral angiomas: A study of nine cases. Bull Neurol Inst N Y 4:144–176, 1935.
287. Rigamonti D, Spetzler R, Medina M, et al: Cerebral venous malformations. J Neurosurg 73:560–564, 1990.
288. Valavanis A, Wellauer J, Yasargil M: The radiological diagnosis of cerebral venous angioma: Cerebral angiography and computed tomography. Neuroradiology 24:193–199, 1983.
289. Fierstien S, Pribram H, Hieshima G: Angiography and computed tomography in the evaluation of cerebral venous malformations. Neuroradiology 17:137–148, 1979.
290. Garner T, Del Curling O Jr, Kelly DL Jr, Laster DW: The natural history of intracranial venous angiomas. J Neurosurg 75:715–722, 1991.
291. Kondziolka D, Dempsey P, Lunsford L: The case for conservative management of venous angiomas. Can J Neurol Sci 18: 295–299, 1991.
292. McLaughlin M, Kondziolka D, Flickinger J, et al: The prospective natural history of cerebral venous malformations. Neurosurgery 43:195–201, 1998.
293. Biller J, Toffol G, Shea J, et al: Cerebellar venous angiomas. Arch Neurol 42:367–370, 1985.
294. Goulao A, Alvarez H, Monaco RG, et al: Venous anomalies and abnormalities of the posterior fossa. Neuroradiology 31: 476–482, 1990.
295. Rothfus W, Albright A, Casey K, et al: Cerebellar venous angioma: Benign entity? AJNR Am J Neuroradiol 5:61–66, 1984.
296. Comey C, Kondziolka D, Yonas H: Regional parenchymal enhancement with mixed cavernous/venous malformations of the brain: Case report. J Neurosurg 86:155–158, 1997.
297. Handa J, Suda K, Sato M: Cerebral venous angioma associated with varix. Surg Neurol 21:436–440, 1984.
298. Hirata Y, Matsukado Y, Nagahiro S, Kuratsu J: Intracerebral venous angioma with arterial blood supply: A mixed angioma. Surg Neurol 25:227–232, 1986.
299. Meyer B, Stangl A, Schramm J: Association of venous and true arteriovenous malformation: A rare entity among mixed vascular malformations of the brain. J Neurosurg 83:141–144, 1995.
300. Robinson JJ, Brown A, Spetzler R: Occult malformation with anomalous venous drainage. J Neurol 82:311–312, 1995.
301. Abe T, Singer R, Marks M, et al: Coexistence of occult vascular malformations and developmental venous anomalies in the central nervous system: MR evaluation. AJNR Am J Neuroradiol 19:51–57, 1998.
302. Komiyama M, Yamanaka K, Iwai Y, Yasui T: Venous angiomas with arteriovenous shunts: Report of three cases and review of the literature. Neurosurgery 44:1328–1335, 1999.
303. Mullan S, Oojtahedi S, Johnson D, Macdonald R: Cerebral venous malformation–arteriovenous malformation transition forms. J Neurosurg 85:9–13, 1996.
304. Scamoni C, Dario A, Basile L: The association of cavernous and venous angioma: Case report and review of the literature. Br J Neurosurg 11:346–349, 1997.
305. Abe M, Asfora W, DeSalles A, Kjellberg R: Cerebellar venous angioma associated with angiographically occult brain stem vascular malformation: Report of two cases. Surg Neurol 33: 400–403, 1990.
306. Avman N, Dincer C: Venous malformation of the aqueduct of Sylvius treated by interventriculostomy: 15 years follow-up. Acta Neurochir (Wien) 52:219–224, 1980.
307. Olson E, Gilmor R, Richmond B: Cerebral venous angiomas. Radiology 151:97–104, 1984.
308. Aagaard B, Song J, Eskridge J, Mayberg M: Complex right hemisphere developmental venous anomaly associated with multiple facial hemangiomas: Case report. J Neurosurg 90:766–769, 1999.
309. Oka K, Kumate S, Kibe M, et al: Aqueductal stenosis due to mesencephalic venous malformation: Case report. Surg Neurol 40:230–235, 1993.
310. Moritake K, Handa H, Mori K, et al: Venous angiomas of the brain. Surg Neurol 14:95–105, 1980.
311. Sadeh M, Shacked I, Rappaport Z, Tadmor R: Surgical extirpation of a venous angioma of the medulla oblongata simulating multiple sclerosis. Surg Neurol 17:334–337, 1982.
312. Wendling L, Moore JJ, Kieffer S, et al: Intracerebral venous angioma. Radiology 119:141–147, 1976.
313. Topper R, Jurgens E, Reul J, Thron A: Clinical significance of intracranial developmental venous anomalies. J Neurol Neurosurg Psychiatry 67:234–238, 1999.

314. Lai P, Chen P, Pan H, Yang C: Venous infarction from a venous angioma occurring after thrombosis of a drainage vein. AJR Am J Roentgenol 172:1698–1699, 1999.
315. Konan A, Raymond J, Bourgouin P, et al: Cerebellar infarct caused by spontaneous thrombosis of a developmental venous anomaly of the posterior fossa. AJNR Am J Neuroradiol 20: 256–258, 1999.
316. Merten C, Knitelius H, Hedde J, et al: Intracerebral haemorrhage from a venous angioma following thrombosis of a draining vein. Neuroradiology 40:15–18, 1998.
317. Gomori J, Grossman R, Goldberg H, et al: Occult cerebral vascular malformations: High-field MR imaging. Radiology 158:707–713, 1986.
318. Lee R, Becher M, Benson M, Rigamonti D: Brain capillary telangiectasia: MR imaging appearance and clinicohistopathologic findings. Radiology 205:797–805, 1997.
319. Barr R, Dillon W, Wilson C: Slow-flow vascular malformations of the pons: Capillary telangiectasias? AJNR Am J Neuroradiol 17:71–78, 1996.
320. Guibaud L, Pelizzari M, Guibal A, et al: Slow-flow vascular malformation of the pons: Congenital or acquired capillary telangiectasia. AJNR Am J Neuroradiol 17:1798–1800, 1996.
321. Courville C: Pathology of the Central Nervous System. Mountain View, CA, Pacific Press Publishing Association, 1950.
322. Milandre L, Pellissier J, Boudouresques G, et al: Non-hereditary multiple telangiectasias of the central nervous system: Report of two clinicopathological cases. J Neurol Sci 82:291–304, 1987.
323. McConnell T, Leonard J: Microangiomatous malformation with intraventricular hemorrhage. Neurology 17:618, 1967.
324. Teilman K: Hemangiomas of the pons. Arch Neurol Psychiatry 69:208, 1953.
325. Wijdicks E, Schievink W: Perimesencephalic nonaneurysmal subarachnoid hemorrhage: First hint of a cause? Neurology 49: 634–636, 1997.
326. Wijdicks E, Schievink W, Miller G: MR imaging in pretruncal nonaneurysmal subarachnoid hemorrhage: Is it worthwhile? Stroke 29:2514–2516, 1998.
327. VanRoost D, Kristof R, Wolf H, Keller E: Intracerebral capillary telangiectasia and venous malformation: A rare association. Surg Neurol 48:175–183, 1997.
328. Farrell D, Forno L: Symptomatic capillary telangiectasis of the brainstem without hemorrhage: Report of an unusual case. Neurology 20:341–346, 1970.
329. Cushing H, Bailey P: Tumors Arising from the Blood Vessels of the Brain. Springfield, Ill, Charles C Thomas, 1928.

CHAPTER **128**

Classification and Decision Making in Treatment and Perioperative Management, Including Surgical and Radiosurgical Decision Making

MICHAEL KERIN MORGAN

The outcome and management of arteriovenous malformations (AVMs) of the brain have changed dramatically since the reported surgical series by Cushing and Bailey[1] and Dandy[2] in 1928. Dandy[2] concluded from his experience that "the radical attempt at cure is attended by such supreme difficulties and is so exceedingly dangerous as to be contraindicated except in certain selected cases," and Cushing and Bailey[1] stated that to "extirpate one of these aneurysmal angiomas in its active state would be unthinkable." After the introduction of angiography, the preoperative identification and anatomic assessment of these lesions were easier. Surgical excision regained its ascendancy with the success reported by Olivecrona and Riives[3] and a follow-up report by Norlen[4] showing that in selected cases operative mortality and morbidity were considered acceptable given that the natural history was that "probably most, if not all, patients die of hemorrhage or are completely incapacitated." Olivecrona and Riives[3] further concluded that they "were unable to find any proof that Roentgen treatment . . . in any way alters the spontaneous course of the illness." Today, few adhere to the original statements of Cushing and Dandy on AVM treatment, and few adhere to the view of the natural history and the lack of the role of radiation therapy expressed by Olivecrona and Riives. Improvements in the surgical results, the expansion in treatment options, and a greater knowledge of the natural history have contributed to a more academic approach to managing AVM. The decision-making paradigms are much more complex, however, with the variations in the expected natural history and the risks of surgery, embolization, and focused irradiation having to be taken into account.

To make recommendations of best management for an individual patient harboring an AVM of the brain, a thorough knowledge of the risks of treatment and the tailored natural history of the pathology is needed. Factors cited as affecting the surgical risk for the development of complications with resection of AVMs include size, location in proximity to critical brain, deep venous drainage, angiographic evidence of steal, deep location, a less compact nidus, and feeding arteries from the deep perforating system.[5–18] Factors cited as a risk for the development of complications from focused irradiation include the dose-volume relationship, location of the target, target dose inhomogeneity, natural history of hemorrhage until ablation, and risks of repeat treatments if necessary.[19–29] The complexity of management paradigms is increasing because of the many treatment variables that need to be considered against the variables influencing the natural history. This chapter brings these variables together to develop a basis for individualizing management paradigms.

CLASSIFICATION SCHEMES

The first grading system of AVMs was introduced in 1977 by Luessenhop and Gennarelli.[30] Since then, many grading systems have been introduced.[13, 16, 31–33] However, the most widely used is the system proposed by Spetzler and Martin (Fig. 128–1).[33] They introduced a grading system by summing the points assigned to three variables—size, eloquence of adjacent brain, and presence of deep venous drainage (Table 128–1).

Eloquence was defined as the primary sensory, motor, language, and visual cortices; thalamus; hypothalamus; brainstem; and cerebellar peduncle. The graded features are easily understood and can be applied universally to all AVMs of the brain. The aim of this grading system was to determine operability. This system has gained wide favor and is the preferred classification system for most currently reported AVM series. When prospectively applied to patients undergoing surgery, there was no significant difference in the development

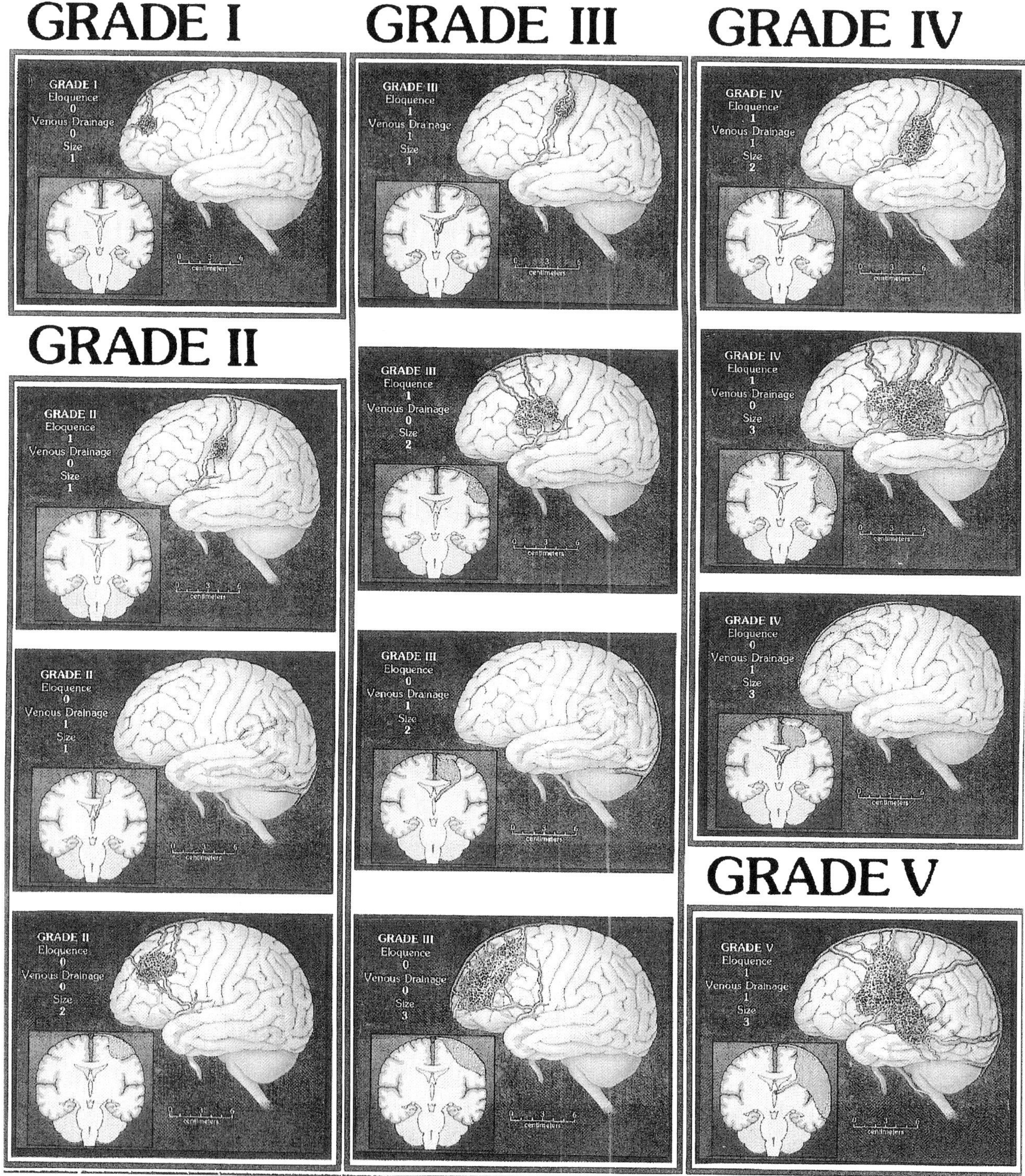

FIGURE 128–1. Spetzler-Martin grading system. These are the possible combinations of size, eloquent location, and deep venous drainage that determine classification between grades 1 and 5. (From Spetzler RF, Martin NA: A proposed grading system for arteriovenous malformations. J Neurosurg 65:476–483, 1986. With permission of the American Association of Neurological Surgeons.)

of new permanent deficits between grade 1 and 2 AVMs or between grade 4 and 5 AVMs.[6] The eloquence graded feature was a significant predictor of new transient neurological deficits but not of permanent deficits. This contrasts with the other two components of the grading system that significantly influence the development of permanent neurological deficits.

The Spetzler-Martin grading system has become adopted widely by surgical and focused irradiation series.[23, 27, 34–42] Criticisms of the Spetzler-Martin grading

TABLE 128–1 ■ **Spetzler and Martin Grading System**

GRADED FEATURE	CLASSIFICATION	POINTS ASSIGNED
Size	Small (<3 cm)	1
	Medium (3–6 cm)	2
	Large (>6 cm)	3
Eloquence of adjacent brain	Noneloquent	0
	Eloquent	1
Pattern of venous drainage	Superficial only	0
	Deep	1

From Spetzler RF, Martin NA: A proposed grading system for arteriovenous malformations. J Neurosurg 65:476–483, 1986. With permission of the American Association of Neurological Surgeons.

system have included the inclusion of deep venous drainage, the definition of eloquence, and the lack of consideration of nidus compactness.[9] Independent researchers established, however, that the Spetzler-Martin grading variables are significant in influencing surgical outcome.[14, 43] Of surprise was the lack of effect in long-term outcomes of eloquence.[6, 14, 43] This is counterintuitive, and it may be explained, first, by its importance in selecting patients for surgery, introducing a preoperative bias. Second, classifying eloquence also may be more prone to interobserver error. Third, the effects of preoperative deficits and developmental plasticity may diminish the importance of eloquence.[17]

The advantages of the Spetzler-Martin grading system are that it allows for interseries comparison; it defines a large group of patients that have a low risk of permanent deficits from surgery with little information; and it identifies a group of patients in which if treatment by surgery is to be considered, factors other than size, deep venous drainage, and eloquence need to be assessed.

FACTORS INFLUENCING THE PREDICTION OF COMPLICATIONS OF SURGERY

Complications leading to permanent or life-threatening disability can be attributed to embolization, intraoperative events (resection of functional brain, AVM rupture, aneurysm rupture, or myocardial infarction) or postoperative events (arterial-capillary-venous hypertensive syndrome or vasospasm), new seizure development, extracerebral hematomas, complications of blood product replacement, infections, and deep venous thrombosis.[11, 38] General complications (including serious infection and pulmonary embolism) may constitute 21% of all complications.[11] Their significance cannot be underemphasized because AVM surgery often takes longer, the large AVMs often require invasive monitoring after the surgery, blood products are often necessary, and prophylactic anticoagulants may be considered contraindicated in many patients. Of complications leading to permanent neurological deficits, 83% are present on emergence from anesthesia, and 17% develop later but within the first 9 days after surgery.[38]

Resection of Functional Brain and Intraoperative Arteriovenous Malformation Rupture

Resection of critical brain or damage caused by intraoperative hemorrhage (or its control) is easily understood as a cause for permanent neurological deficits. The size of the AVM, proximity to eloquent brain, and presence of a deep venous drainage each have been correlated with the development of new neurological deficits.[6, 14, 43] The effect of eloquence is less marked (as discussed earlier) but cannot be discounted because its effect may have been overcome by patient selection bias. Although it has been argued that the presence of deep venous drainage presents no great difficulty in and of itself,[9] its effect has been verified independently as important.[6, 14, 43] It is likely that deep venous drainage reflects the difficulty with the deep component of the nidus. Further evidence of this effect is found with the impact that deep perforating arteries have on the risk of surgical resection, particularly with the potential for hemorrhage.[10] This finding is important to Spetzler-Martin grades greater than 2.

Intraoperative Aneurysm Rupture

Hemodynamic stresses are likely to contribute to, or entirely explain, the 2.7% to 46.1%[44–53] incidence of aneurysms on the feeding artery of patients with AVMs. This compares with an incidence of 1% to 5% in the population screened without AVMs.[54] Some of the considerable variation may relate to the difficulties in identifying aneurysms angiographically on the distorted vasculature. Despite this variation in the reported incidence of aneurysms, there is a tendency for the higher incidence to be reported from more recent series and that the overall incidence of aneurysms is greater in the AVM population than in populations without. In AVM patients with aneurysms, the predilection for their occurrence on proximal or intranidal arteries is overwhelming. Angiographically and histologically, they are identical to other saccular aneurysms (the cause of which are thought to be based on hemodynamic stress).[55–57] The importance of this fact is the potential for aneurysm resolution with removal of the hemodynamic factors responsible for aneurysm genesis and resolution with AVM resection.[48, 51] Aneurysms may rupture on shunt ablation because of an increase in transmural pressure in the relevant feeding artery at this time.[45, 53, 58, 59] This situation has been reported to account for 7% of all complications leading to permanent deficits.[38]

For aneurysms on feeding arteries that cannot be exposed at the time of definitive AVM surgery, a separate procedure (either surgical or endovascular) preceding AVM ablation should be considered.[53, 58] This need is less pressing, however, in treatments by focused irradiation and is controversial for treatment by embolization.[48, 51]

Arterial-Capillary-Venous Hypertensive Syndromes

Clinical reports of hemorrhage or edema developing as a delayed neurological deficit (with the exception of reports of extracerebral hemorrhage and hemorrhage associated with anticoagulant therapy) have been ascribed to retained AVM rupture, rupture of the feeding arterial system, normal perfusion pressure breakthrough, or venous occlusive hyperemia.[10, 11, 15, 18, 38, 58, 60–64] Normal perfusion pressure breakthrough, first described by Spetzler and colleagues[63] in 1978 to account for some cases of hemorrhage and edema complicating AVM resection, has, as its central tenet, the loss of autoregulation with an inability for the capillary bed to be protected from a restoration of normal arterial pressure (from a previous low pressure) on arteriovenous shunt ablation.[65] This results in hyperemia.

Hyperemia associated with intracerebral hemorrhage is seen in other clinical states that produce a sudden reversal of noninfarctional cerebral hypoperfusion (after carotid endarterectomy and high-flow extracranial-intracranial bypass).[66–69] This mechanism is supported by experimental evidence by arteriovenous fistula ablation.[70–72] The mechanism for hyperemia after AVM has been ascribed variously to a loss of autoregulation,[63] a resetting of the upper limit of autoregulation downward,[73] and a neuropeptide-mediated disturbance.[74] The resetting of the upper limit of autoregulation to a lower blood pressure is an attractive hypothesis because of the evidence for this in other states with a chronic alteration in cerebral perfusion pressure.[75–77] In these conditions, vasodilatation of the larger caliber cerebral resistance vessels induces a shift of the upper and lower limit of autoregulation to the left.[78] Such chronic dilatation is also a feature of AVM feeding vessels.

Young and colleagues[79] performed intraoperative studies to assess pressure autoregulation after resection in AVM patients. Although blood flow remained unchanged despite an elevation in blood pressure, cerebral blood flow was measured more than 5 cm from the nidus, and the patients were hypocapnic, a condition known to cause a rise in the upper limit of autoregulation.[80] Autoregulation may not have been tested without knowledge of what the pressure difference between the pial arteries and pial veins was with respect to this change in blood pressure. Autoregulation cannot be assumed to have changed with the blood pressure in the presence of an AVM.

Despite the evidence for hyperemia to play a role in delayed hemorrhage or edema after AVM resection, many patients with hyperemia at the time of AVM excision do not develop edema or hemorrhage.[81–83] Hyperemia alone cannot account for the pathologic processes variously termed *normal perfusion pressure breakthrough*,[63] *congestive apoplexy*,[84] *overload*,[58] or *vasogenic turgescence of the brain*.[85] Higher cerebral blood flow values and more dramatic changes in cerebral blood flow have been found to occur during the study of seizures, a condition not characterized by brain swelling and hemorrhage.[86–88] Hyperemia may be an epiphenomenon of the malignant vascular process associated with the ability of the more proximal arterial system to withstand the rise in pressure or the redundant venous system thrombosing (occlusive hyperemia).[1]

Excision of an AVM removes the low-resistance circulation that exists in parallel with the normal circulation of the brain. The feeding artery pressure increases toward the systemic arterial pressure, and the pulsatility increases.[81, 89, 90] Because the radii of arteries feeding the AVM do not return immediately to normal after AVM ablation, the resistance to flow within these arteries is lower than normal (although their downstream resistance is higher) as predicted by the Poiseuille equation.[89] This results in the reduction in the degree of arterial pressure gradient normally occurring along the vessels before the arteriole. The pressure that occurs in these arteries, immediately after excision of the AVM, is greater than normal (Fig. 128–2). The larger than normal-diameter redundant feeding arterial system, with its normal downstream microcirculation, generates a larger reflected wave than a normal-diameter vessel, resulting in a greater than normal pulsatility and higher than normal peak pressures within the cardiac cycle.[91] The resulting increase in pressure and pulsatility after AVM excision may challenge the integrity of the arterial wall, particularly at sites of aneurysmal weakness or in vessels that are distal branches of the feeding artery that may have been extremely thin walled because of the chronic local hypotension.

The postsurgical state produces vascular redundancy (in terms of vessel diameters) that may have a propensity for stagnation and thrombosis.[92] This

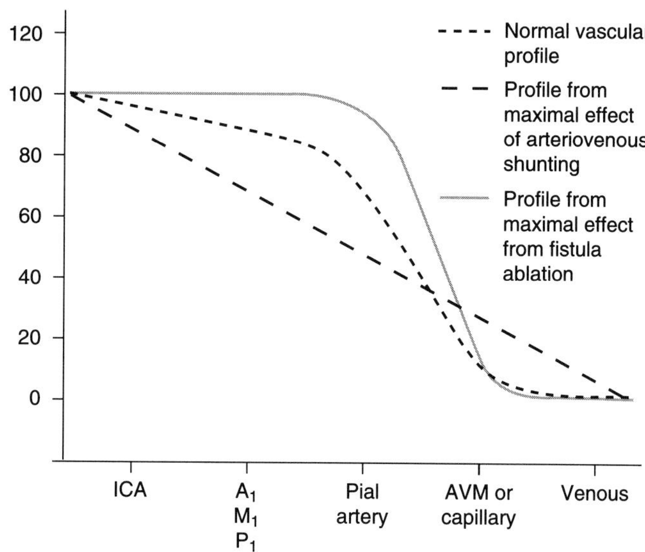

FIGURE 128–2. A schematic representation of the approximate relationships between pressure (as percentage of femoral artery pressure) and sites along the cerebrovascular profile. Three curves can be constructed reflecting the profile of the normal circulation, the theoretical pressure along a fistula, and the cerebral circulation after arteriovenous malformation resection.

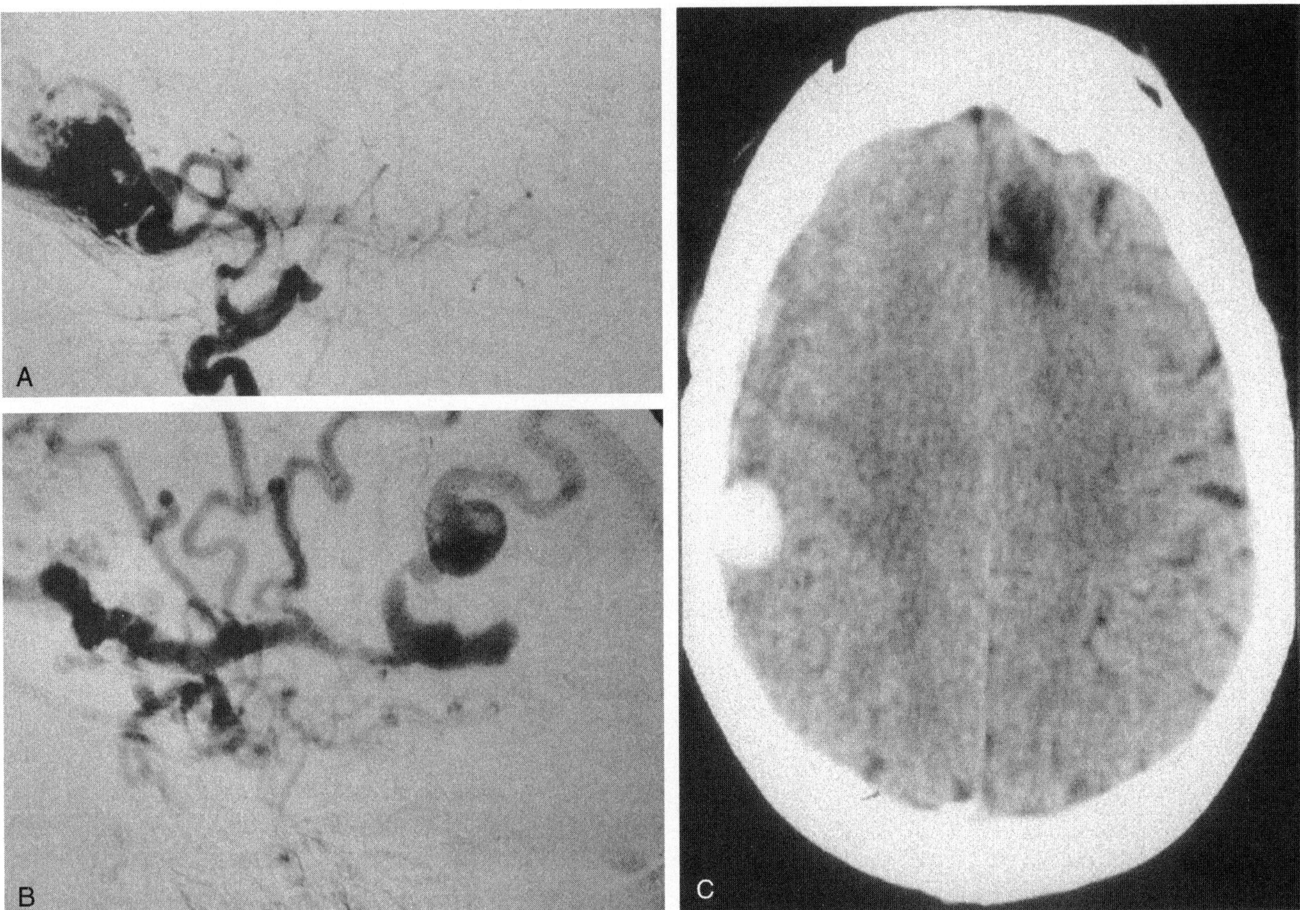

FIGURE 128–3. A 55-year-old woman presented with recurrent seizures and was found to have a small arteriovenous malformation in the left frontal lobe identified on this left lateral internal carotid angiogram *(A)* with extensive venous drainage over the left convexity surface *(B)*. Three days after surgery, she developed a hemiparesis and dysphasia that resolved over 2 weeks. The noncontrasted computed tomographic scan showed thrombosis of the venous drainage *(C)*.

thrombosis may develop in either arteries or veins. Propagated venous thrombosis of the major draining system is responsible for clinical deterioration in 1% to 3% of operated cases (Fig. 128–3).[1]

Differentiating the pathophysiologic mechanisms can be difficult, if not impossible, but they all have the common perturbation of local intravascular pressure rise to pathologic levels.[89] The term *arterial-capillary-venous hypertensive syndrome* (ACVH) is an appropriate classification to avoid considerable debate (Fig. 128–4).[89] The incidence of delayed ACVH has been reported to occur in 3% of operated cases.[38] This accounted for most of the delayed postoperative complications and is at greatest risk in AVM nidus size of at least 4 cm with postoperative hypertension or where markedly redundant draining veins are a feature of the AVM.[38, 60]

Vasospasm

Vasospasm occurs as a complication of AVM resection in only 2% of cases but is reported to occur in 27% of cases involving extensive dissection of the proximal middle and anterior cerebral arteries (Fig. 128–5).[38] The degree of vasospasm may not correlate with the degree of subarachnoid blood, and the mechanism for its development may be related to altered vasoreactivity of these vessels at this time. Management is confounded by the conflict with blood pressure control.[5, 38]

New Seizure Disorder

That new seizure disorder can follow supratentorial brain surgery is a known risk. Early authors reported an increase in seizure frequency after surgery for AVMs.[93–97] Patients with supratentorial AVMs present with a variable history of seizures (including none, single seizure, multiple seizures easily controlled by medications, and a major seizure disorder with poor medical control), hemorrhage (with its ability to predispose to epilepsy), or neither make analysis of reported series difficult to interpret, however. More recent large series have found an incidence of postoperative seizures of less than 40% in patients with a history of preoperative seizures and less than 10% in patients without such a history.[98–102]

Risk factors predicting the development of multiple postoperative seizures include multiple preoperative seizures, a neurological deficit at 12 months, presenta-

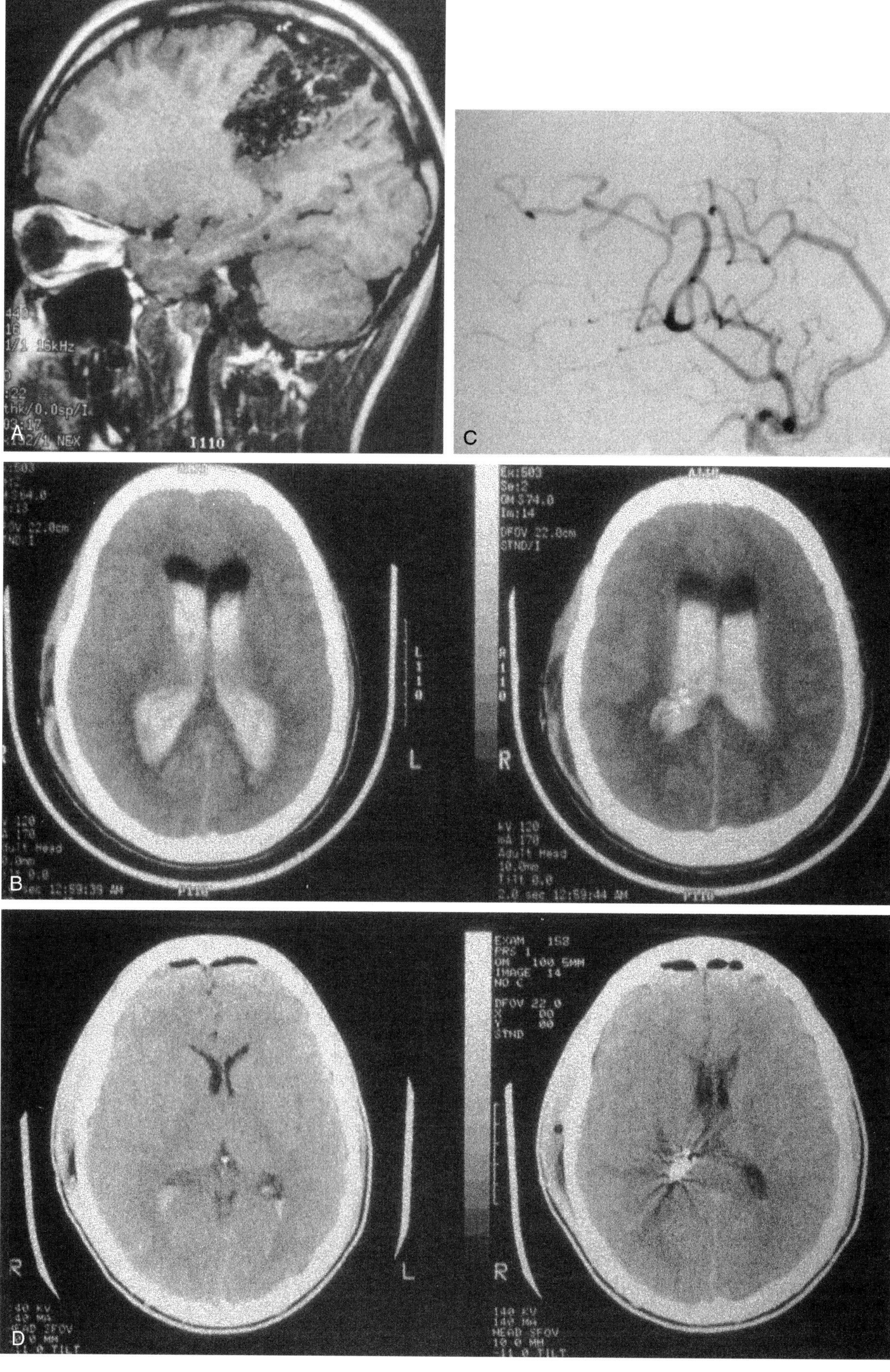
A
C
B
R
L
D
EXAM 153
140 KV
HEAD SFOV

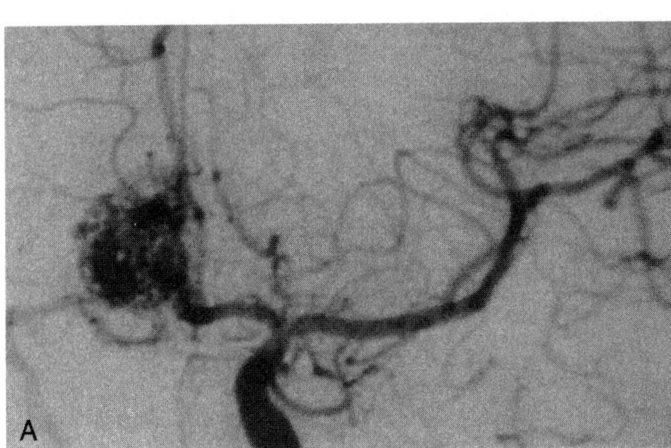

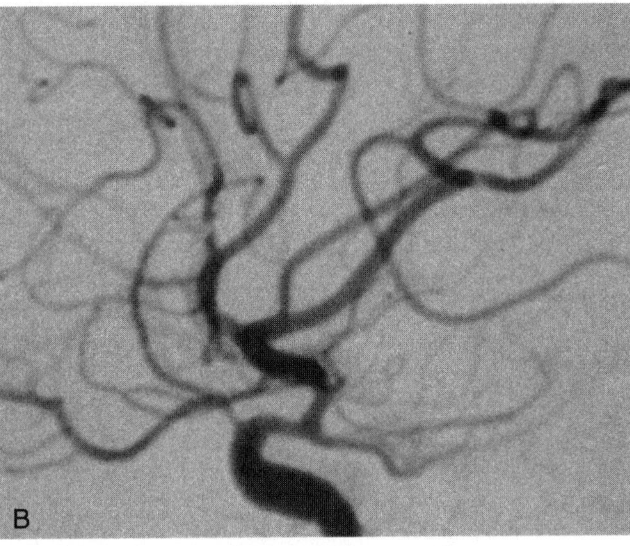

FIGURE 128–5. A 36-year-old patient presented with a seizure, and anteroposterior left internal carotid angiography showed a basal and medial frontal arteriovenous malformation *(A)*. Ten days after surgery, the patient became confused, and angiography at this time showed vasospasm *(B)*.

tion with hemorrhage, and size of nidus greater than 3 cm in a supratentorial location.[93, 100–103] Although location within some supratentorial sites (e.g., mesial temporal and rolandic) has been reported to be more epileptogenic, this has not been reported uniformly.[101]

RESULTS OF MANAGEMENT BY OBSERVATION ALONE

Annual Risk of Hemorrhage

The natural history of AVMs increasingly is understood despite being constrained by the difficulties expected of a disease presenting with an annual incidence of only 12 per 1 million population[104] and an annual incidence of hemorrhage of 8.2 per 1 million population per year.[105] Estimates of the annual risk for first hemorrhage is 2% to 4% and for recurrent hemorrhage is 6% to 18% in the initial year, declining to a prehemorrhage rate over 5 years.[106–110] A further discriminator of hemorrhage risk prediction is the presence of aneurysms.[46, 51] During the initial 5 years from diagnosis, the annual risk of hemorrhage in the presence of an aneurysm is 7% per year and in its absence is 1.7% per year.[46] If aneurysms are intranidal, the annual risk of hemorrhage is 9.8% per year.[51] Increasing age of patient may increase the risk of hemorrhage, with a risk of hemorrhage of 2% per year at 10 years of age, 4% at 20 years of age, 6% at 40 years of age, and 7% at 60 years of age reported.[111] Although this has not been uniformly supported,[106] it has been suggested independently as contributing to an increased likelihood of rebleeding.[108] An increased risk of bleeding has been suggested to occur with AVM outflow venous stenotic or occlusive pathology.[112, 113] Although factors may increase the risk of presentation with hemorrhage, they do not suggest an increase in the risk of hemorrhage (e.g., small deep AVMs are unlikely to present in any other way than hemorrhage, and AVMs in cortical border zone locations are more likely to present with neurological deficits). Site, size, presence of seizures, hypertension, and sex are unlikely to contribute to risk of hemorrhage.[106, 108]

The increased incidence of hemorrhage with aneurysms cannot be explained solely on the basis of a simple summation of the risk of hemorrhage from an AVM with the risk of hemorrhage from aneurysm. The origin of the hemorrhage is divided equally between the aneurysm and the AVM,[46, 47, 53, 108, 114] yet the risk of hemorrhage is approximately quadrupled when both lesions are present compared with when no aneurysm is present in association with an AVM.[46, 51] The presence of aneurysms may reflect a more advanced stage of vascular wear and tear from the shear stress of the high flow induced by the arteriovenous shunting and the more imminent threat of vascular integrity failure within the AVM nidus and at the site of aneurysm.

Consequences of Hemorrhage

The consequences of hemorrhage may lead to permanent neurological deficits or death in 50% of cases (death occurring in 30% of hemorrhagic epi-

FIGURE 128–4. A case illustration of complication by arterial-capillary-hypertensive syndrome after resection of a parietal arteriovenous malformation in a 21-year-old patient *(A)*. Hemorrhage occurred on day 6 *(B)* after an increase in blood pressure. Postoperative angiography before this event confirmed complete ablation of the arteriovenous malformation *(C)*, and computed tomographic scan was satisfactory *(D)*.

TABLE 128–2 ■ **Lifetime Risk for First Arteriovenous Malformation Hemorrhage When No Aneurysm Present (1.7% risk per year) and Aneurysm Present (7% risk per year)**

AGE AT INITIAL PRESENTATION, YR	ESTIMATED YEARS TO LIVE	RISK OF HEMORRHAGE AT 1.7% PER YEAR, %	RISK OF HEMORRHAGE AT 7% PER YEAR, %
0	76	73	99.6
15	62	65	99
25	52	59	98
35	43	52	96
45	34	44	92
55	25	35	84
65	18	27	73
75	11	17	55
85	6	10	35

sodes).[31, 106, 107] In a population-based study, AVMs with intracranial hemorrhage had an 18% mortality (with a 95% confidence interval of 3.8% to 43.4%).[105] Recurrent hemorrhage has been reported to have a higher mortality than initial hemorrhage, but this may reflect referral bias and sample size.[105, 107, 115] Because a patient with a recurrent hemorrhage is more likely to be under observation with a correct diagnosis of AVM, the higher mortality reports in comparison with initial hemorrhage may be more accurate. In support of this, Fults and Kelly[107] reported a 13.6% mortality for first hemorrhage and a 25% mortality for third or subsequent hemorrhage, a figure close to that of 29% reported by Brown and colleagues[105] after AVMs with a first hemorrhage.[107] There is some evidence that recurrent hemorrhage stereotypically may mimic the first hemorrhage, but this may be only in the short-term.[43, 116]

Nonhemorrhagic Causes for Decline in Function

In addition to hemorrhage, 1.5% of patients undergo a functional decline per year.[106] The basis for this decline is attributable to neurological deficits arising as a result of local microcirculation hypoperfusion (caused by the various combinations of local arterial hypotension and venous hypertension), often referred to by the term *steal*,[117] and seizures. AVMs most likely to have this course are large cortical lesions in border zone areas.[118, 119]

Influence of Age at Diagnosis on Long-Term Risk of Hemorrhage

Although the annual risk of hemorrhage seems to be increasingly understood, this needs to be placed into context for each individual patient. A major determinant of the likely chance for an event is age at initial diagnosis. Kondziolka and colleagues[120] approximated this by the equation:

$$\text{Risk of hemorrhage} = 1 - (\text{risk of no hemorrhage})^{\text{expected years of remaining life}}$$

A table can be constructed with the likelihood for lifelong first hemorrhage based on age at initial presentation and the estimated years to live (Table 128–2).[121]

RESULTS OF SURGICAL MANAGEMENT REGIMENS

Surgery may lead to new neurological deficits that are apparent and permanent on emergence from anesthesia, complications that can develop in the postoperative period, and the development of a seizure disorder. The significance and cause for each of these differs, and they are discussed separately.

New Neurological Deficits After Surgery

The results of surgery need to be considered from several viewpoints because AVMs can be classified into grades with defined surgical risks. Deep perforators enable Spetzler-Martin grade 3 lesions to be divided further; an AVM nidus less than 3 cm may be treated effectively by focused irradiation. Because there is no statistical difference between Spetzler-Martin grades 1 and 2 and between grades 4 and 5,[6, 14, 38] the Spetzler-Martin system can be simplified into three grades (1–2, 3, 4–5). The results of surgery are consistent in reported series using this classification, with grade 1–2 having a risk of new permanent disabling neurological deficits (a modified Rankin score of >2) in less than 1% of cases.[6, 37, 38, 122] No mortality is reported from these series. Reports with independent observation are rare, however. One study of 48 patients undergoing surgery with Spetzler-Martin grade 1–2 AVMs reported disabling persistent deficits in 6.25%.[43] Grade 3 AVMs also have been reported to have low complication rate.[6] It is possible, however, that case selection may contribute to this excellent result because it has been shown that grade 3 AVMs with deep perforating arteries have a similar complication rate to that of grade 4–5 AVMs, and in their absence the complication rate is similar to grade 1–2 (Fig. 128–6).[10] The rates of the new permanent neurological deficit leading to a downgrade in quality of life in grade 4–5 AVMs is 44% to 57%, and the rate of severe disability leading to loss of independence is 11% to 22%.[6, 37, 38] AVMs with nidus size less than 3 cm have a reported complication rate of new

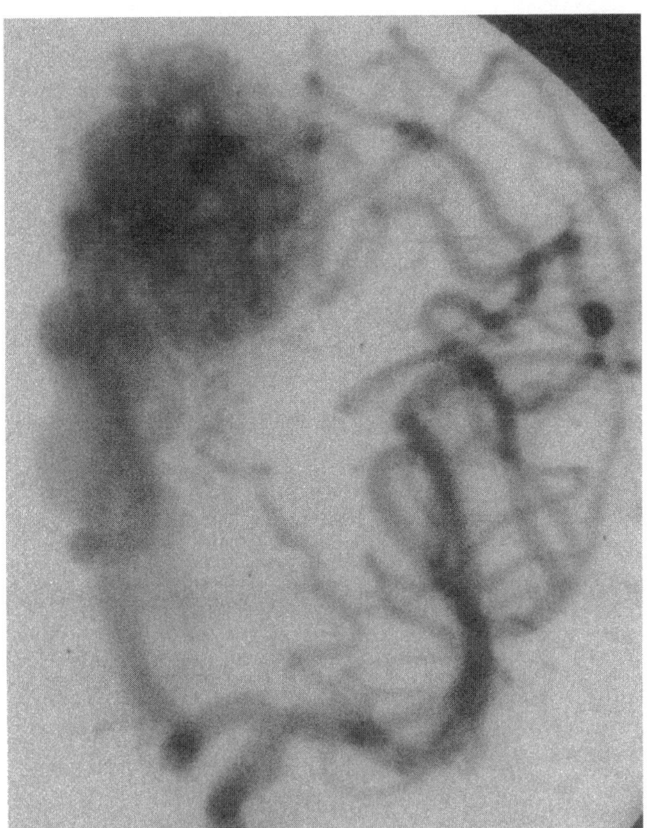

FIGURE 128–6. An example of an arteriovenous malformation that can be considered a grade 3–4 lesion by the presence of the lenticulostriate supply.

permanent neurological deficit of 1.5% to 2.7% with angiographically confirmed obliteration in 99% to 100%.[6, 42, 123, 124] Of these, 4.3% have worsening in eloquent brain and 1.6% in noneloquent brain.[123] Not all permanent neurological deficits are present on emergence from anesthesia. Although 83% of deficits occur during the surgery, 17% arise in a delayed fashion from the development of the ACVH within the first 8 days after surgery.[38] This condition has significant implications for postoperative management (see later).

Seizures After Surgery

In patients with no preoperative seizures and with a minimum follow-up of 2 years, 6% to 15% developed a new seizure disorder.[100, 101] When only multiple seizures are considered, this incidence is 5% to 6%.[100, 101] Overall, 68% of patients are without anticonvulsants.[100] In patients with preoperative seizures, 77% to 83% are seizure-free after surgery,[100, 101] and when multiple seizures have occurred preoperatively, this incidence is 70% to 76%.[100, 102] In patients with multiple seizures preoperatively, the incidence of being made worse is less than 2%.[100, 102] Timing of first seizure in the postoperative period was within the first 12 months in 75% of cases.[101] The expectations for seizure outcome are reported in Table 128–3.

RESULTS OF TREATMENT REGIMENS BY FOCUSED IRRADIATION

The role of radiotherapy in the management of AVMs has been under review for nearly as long as that of

TABLE 128–3 ■ **Postoperative Seizure Outcome**

POSTOPERATIVE MODIFIED ENGEL CLASSIFICATION	HISTORY OF MULTIPLE PREOPERATIVE SEIZURES,[102] %	HISTORY OF MULTIPLE PREOPERATIVE SEIZURES,[102] %	HISTORY OF PREOPERATIVE SEIZURES,[101] %	NO HISTORY OF PREOPERATIVE SEIZURES,[101] %	NO HISTORY OF PREOPERATIVE SEIZURES,[100] %
Class I Seizure-free, auras only or seizures only after withdrawal of antiepileptic drugs	70.4	76	77	87	94
Class II 90% reduction in seizure frequency or a single postoperative seizure	18.5		4	0	0
Class III No increase in seizure frequency but worse than class II	9.3		4	0	0
Class IV An increase in postoperative seizures	1.9	0	15	13 (5% multiple)	6

From Thorpe ML, Cordato DJ, Morgan MK, et al: Postoperative seizure outcome in a series of 114 patients with supratentorial arteriovenous malformations. J Clin Neurosci 7:107–111, 2000.

surgery.[4] Although the initial treatment by conventional fractionated radiotherapy was not promising, desperate attempts to offer some form of treatment in some cases continued its selective use and provided us with more recent data that reinforced the early opinion of its limited efficacy.[51, 125] With the introduction of focused irradiation, the role for radiation therapy became significant. This therapy results in damage to endothelial cells, followed by progressive thickening of the intimal layer caused by proliferation of smooth muscle cells that elaborate an extracellular matrix, leading to vessel occlusion.[126]

Ogilvy,[26] in a review of radiation therapy for AVMs in 1990, concluded, "there is convincing evidence that radiation therapy does have a role in obliterating carefully chosen inoperable lesions." That this conclusion should be presented by a cerebrovascular neurosurgeon after careful evaluation of the evidence is significant and has come to represent the common view with the exception that the word *inoperable* should be deleted and a risk-benefit evaluation should decide the appropriate mode of intervention. As with surgery, the concerns of treatment relate to the development of new problems and the additional risks associated with a delay to cure. As with surgery, the morbidity and mortality are likely to vary among treating centers, and, as with surgery, the literature reflects treatment in experienced hands, making it important to make decisions not only reflecting on these results, but also the results from individual treatment centers.

Failure to Cure by Focused Irradiation

Considerable variation exists in the potential for AVM cure by focused irradiation. The peripheral or marginal dose is the most significant factor determining obliteration rate, and the safe maximum marginal dose is related to the site and the 12-Gy volume irradiated.[127–131] At 10 Gy, Karlsson[111] reported a 43% chance of cure and at 22 Gy a 71% chance of cure from data collected from 1184 cases treated at Karolinska with 80% follow-up. These rates of cure seem to correlate well with reports from other treatment centers and from Linac centers. Concerns have been raised, however, that this cure rate is overestimated because of the nature of selective follow-up.[132] Heffez and colleagues,[132] comparing reporting techniques in the literature with data analysis by the Kaplan-Meier method, found the 2-, 3-, and 4-year obliteration rates were 37%, 73%, and 84% after a minimum 24-month follow-up when data analysis was limited to patients who had follow-up arteriography. Using Kaplan-Meier analysis, the 2-, 3-, and 4-year obliteration rates were 32%, 43%, and 55% (95% confidence interval = ±18%). The 2-year obliteration rate was 43% for AVMs less than 30 mm in diameter and 16% for AVMs greater than 30 mm in diameter. Despite this concern, the Karolinska data are from a large database with the likelihood of the 20% follow-up failure to be nonselective.

Karlsson and colleagues[128] examined the various predictive models for cure and found that applying four models to their own data of 1033 patients the prediction of cure was independent of volume and most closely related to the equation:

$$\text{Probability of obliteration} = 35.69 \times \ln(\text{marginal dose}) - 39.66$$

This represents an obliteration rate of 24% at a marginal dose of 6 Gy, 43% at 10 Gy, 55% at 14 Gy, 63% at 18 Gy, 71% at 22 Gy, and 77% at 28 Gy (Table 128–4).[128]

The probability of obliteration with a second treatment after a focused irradiation failure is no greater than that calculated for first treatment.[25, 133] The overall results for patients undergoing second treatments are a 60% to 70% complete obliteration rate at 2 years after repeat treatment with a 5% to 14% adverse radiation effect and 5% to 6% hemorrhage rate.[25, 133]

Delayed hemorrhage after angiographic cure has been reported. Most cases were children at the time of initial treatment, however, a finding that has been reported for microsurgical excision.[134] For patients younger than 18 years old undergoing focused irradiation, the late hemorrhage rate after angiographic obliteration is 3.4%,[134] a figure similar to the 3.5% reported after microsurgery.[135]

Delay in Cure

Crucial in the assessment of modality of treatment is the time taken from focused irradiation to AVM obliteration. At the time of Ogilvy's review,[26] data about the marginal dose necessary to produce obliteration and the safe dose to administer were lacking. The available reports suggested, however, the annual incidence of hemorrhage during the first 2 years after treatment with gamma knife, stereotactic linear accelerator, proton-beam therapy, and helium beam therapy is 2% to 2.6%, similar to the annual risk expected without treatment.[26] The time to cure was thought to average at least 2 years. Considerable knowledge has been gained from many large series using gamma knife and Linac therapies. The higher the marginal dose, the

TABLE 128–4 ■ **Marginal Dose and Probability of Cure**

MARGINAL DOSE, GY	PROBABILITY OF OBLITERATION, %
6	24
8	35
10	43
12	49
14	55
16	59
18	63
20	67
22	71
24	74
26	77
28	79

From Karlsson B, Lax I, Soderman M: Can the probability for obliteration after radiosurgery for arteriovenous malformations be accurately predicted Int J Radiat Oncol Biol Phys 43:313–319, 1999.

shorter the time to cure and the shorter the exposure of the natural history to hemorrhage. Although lower marginal doses may lead to late cures, these are unlikely after 4 years from treatment.[111]

Following patients with angiography has suggested that 44% of patients eventually obliterated have become so within 24 months and 87% by 36 months.[132] These data do not allow a calculation of when obliteration took place, however. The average AVM dose has been suggested to have a linear correlation with the time to cure, with an average AVM dose of 50 Gy taking 20 months to cure; 40 Gy, taking 22.5 months to cure; 30 Gy, taking 24 months to cure; and 20 Gy, taking 26.5 months to cure.[136] The range of average AVM dose in this study was 18 to 54 Gy. If cure occurred, the higher marginal dose used was likely to achieve this in 20 months and the lower marginal dose in a further 6.5 months. Yamamoto and colleagues[137] reported a similar pattern of time to cure, with AVMs no greater than 10 cm^3 having no cures in less than 6 months and 2-, 3-, and 4-year cure rates of 27%, 65%, and 82% compared with larger AVMs that had no cures before 18 months and 2- and 3-year cure rates of 13% and 71% by Kaplan-Meier plots. As expected, the smaller lesions received a higher marginal dose. In summary, on average the time to cure, if cure occurs, is 2 years from initial treatment.[134]

If AVMs remain unobliterated, regardless of time since treatment, the risk of bleeding does not deviate from the natural history of untreated AVMs.[28, 34, 138] This includes the increased risk associated with the presence of aneurysms.[138] Pollock and colleagues[39] calculated that the risk of hemorrhage is 4.8% per year (95% confidence interval = 2.4% to 7% per year) during the first 2 unobliterated years and 5% per year (95% confidence interval = 2.3% to 7.3% per year) for the third through the fifth unobliterated years. The relative risk associated with a proximal aneurysm was 4.56. The risk of death from hemorrhage in this study was 33%, similar to that of the natural history and similar to the mortality of bleeding reported by others.[39, 139] In patients receiving more than 25 Gy marginal dose not progressing to obliteration, there was no reduction in this risk of hemorrhage.[138]

It can be concluded that the natural history for the individual patient is unaltered until complete obliteration has occurred even after high marginal dose therapy (>25 Gy). As with the natural history, there is an increased risk associated with the presence of aneurysms. The outcome from hemorrhage occurring after focused irradiation is identical to the outcome from hemorrhage in the absence of treatment.

New Neurological Deficits After Focused Irradiation

Steiner and colleagues[140] reported that a risk of permanent radiation necrosis induced deficits after gamma knife treatment for AVMs of 3% (Fig. 127-7). A multicenter Arteriovenous Malformation Radiosurgery

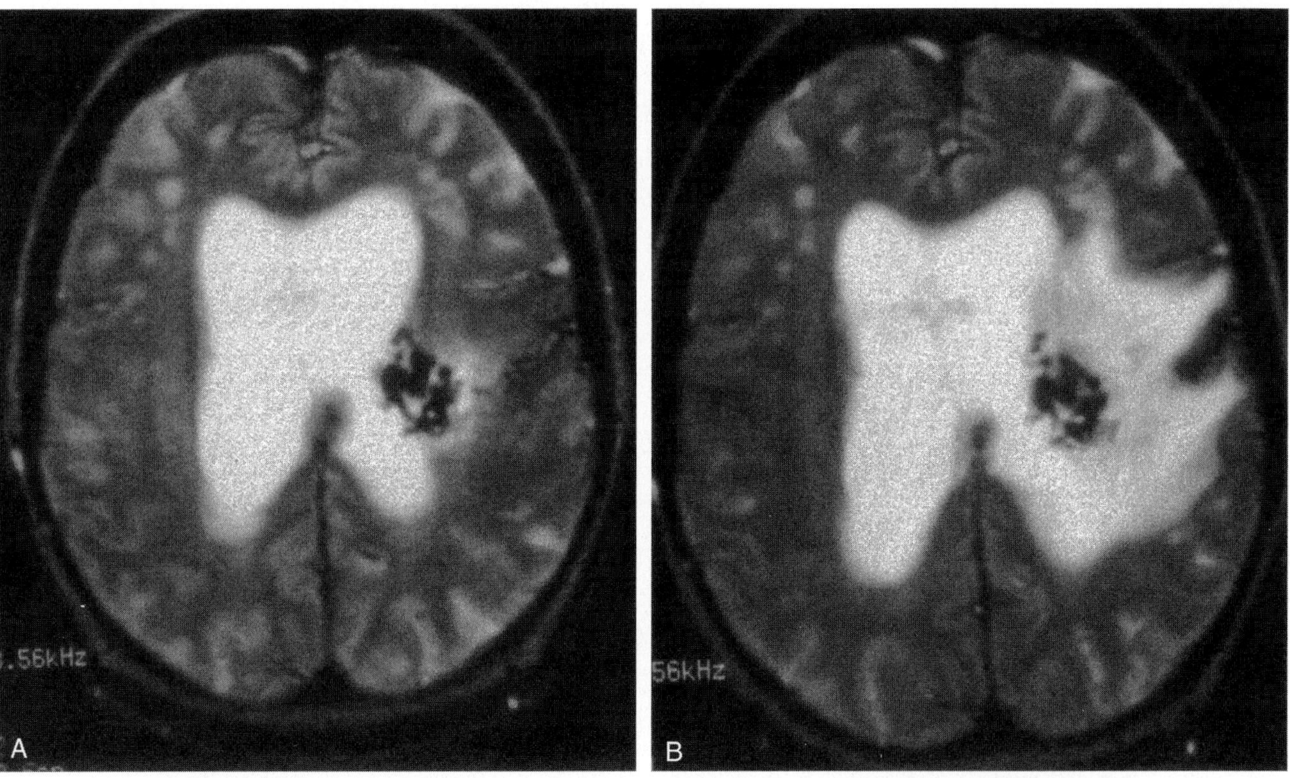

FIGURE 128–7. A 57-year-old patient presented having recurrent intraventricular hemorrhage and was treated with focused irradiation. Magnetic resonance imaging at the time of treatment *(A)* can be compared with imaging 2 years later *(B)* at the time the patient was dysphasic and hemiparetic.

Study Group carefully analyzed complications of gamma knife treatment.[141] At the University of Pittsburgh, the symptomatic radiosurgery complications occurred in 9%, but in total only 45% of these were permanent.[141] In the analysis of these patients with symptomatic radiation necrosis unresolved after 2 years of subsequent follow-up, a model was developed for the prediction of these complications. This two-step model involves first assigning a *significant postradiosurgery injury expression* score that depends on AVM location. Then each score has a unique plot on the graph: volume receiving no less than 12 Gy versus risk of symptomatic radiation necrosis. Because the 12-Gy volume cannot be calculated before completion of a radiosurgery treatment plan, it is useful to correlate what the likely volume receiving no less than 12 Gy is with the average AVM diameter.[141] A paradigm can be drawn predicting complications from AVM diameter location and size. An approximation of these risks is included in Table 128-5.

Complications have been reported to occur as a consequence of focused irradiation many years after the initial therapy.[29] Postmortem studies confirmed that intimal hypertrophy occurs in normal, AVM-unrelated, pial arteries as a result of irradiation of no less than 10 Gy, and the greater the dose the more extensive the damage. Complications reported at 2-year post-treatment may underestimate the final complication rate.

The development of further radiation-induced injury on repeat focused irradiation is greater than that of initial therapy and seems to be independent of the time elapsed between treatments.[25] This risk averages 12.5%.[25]

New Seizure Disorder

Of patients, 60% to 78% are seizure-free presenting with seizures before radiosurgery.[28, 98, 142, 143] Most report that this benefit seems to have a low or no risk for the development of new seizures.[28, 98, 143, 144] This is also the case in childhood treatments.[99] These results are similar to the seizure outcome after surgery.

TABLE 128–5 ■ **Approximation of Risks of Focused Irradiation–Induced Permanent Symptomatic Radiation Necrosis Developed from the Arteriovenous Malformation Radiosurgery Study Group**

DIAMETER (CM)	1.55	2.1	2.65	3.35	3.85	4.25
APPROXIMATE VOLUME (mL)	2	5	10	20	30	40
Frontal lobe, %	0	0	0	0	0	1
Temporal lobe, %	0	1	1	2	5	9
Intraventricular, %	1	2	2	5	9	19
Parietal lobe, %	1	2	3	7	12	21
Cerebellar, %	1	2	3	7	12	23
Corpus callosum or occipital, %	5	5	7	14	23	40
Medulla, %	8	9	13	23	38	56
Thalamus, %	12	14	20	35	53	69
Basal ganglia, %	15	18	24	41	58	74
Pons/midbrain, %	44	49	58	74	85	92

From Flickinger JC, Kondziolka D, Lunsford LD, et al: Development of a model to predict permanent symptomatic postradiosurgery injury for arteriovenous malformation patients. Int J Radiat Oncol Biol Phys 46:1143–1148, 2000.

RESULTS OF TREATMENT BY EMBOLIZATION

Embolization has proved a useful technique in the management of AVMs. This strategy has been used for 4 decades.[145] During this period, developments in catheters and embolic material have allowed application of embolization to palliation, cure, and reduction in intraoperative hemorrhage. With these advances, cure by embolization alone has been achieved in most patients with AVMs in some centers.[146] The most common application for embolization is preoperatively to attenuate intraoperative hemorrhage.[147, 148] Its application needs to be selective, however, because it is reported that 69% of patients embolized preoperatively achieved less than 75% obliteration, a level thought to be necessary to ameliorate operative bleeding.[148] Concern regarding the overall management risk reduction with preoperative embolization has been raised.[147, 149] AVMs treated in more recent times were cured in only 5% of cases (and these were mostly small AVMs), and 8% sustained permanent morbidity (including 1% mortality).[147] The most common causes for this morbidity with more recent technology were embolic infarction and hemorrhage (Fig. 128–8). The 4% morbidity from embolic infarction for embolization is likely to be the additional risk above that of surgery alone.[149]

Many factors need to be considered in conjunction with morbidity. In some cases, the morbidity might be regarded as "the price to pay" to avoid worse morbidity from the natural history or surgery alone. Included in this group of complications are quadrantanopic visual field deficits and other deficits that may not have a significant impact on quality of life for many individuals. The assessment of the options of management must take into account the patient's wishes regarding these anticipated deficits.

In addition to the risk of infarction from therapeutic embolization is the potential for structural changes and a compensatory increase in flow and diameter of unembolized feeding arteries. These arteries are the deep thin-walled perforators that increase surgical difficulties.[150] AVMs with a deep perforating contribution have been found to have a worse outcome with surgery as a result of hemorrhage.[10] Because of this, preoperative embolization might be hoped to improve outcome in larger AVMs with deep perforators. Complete ablation of the deep perforating system is difficult, however.[149] The lesions most suitable for preoperative embolization are large AVMs with feeding arteries arising from a deep perforating or meningeal supply or in large AVMs in which feeding arteries are not likely to be accessed easily early in the surgical procedure.

For appropriately selected cases, a benefit for embolization and surgery over surgery alone has been shown.[151, 152] Even when embolization is feasible, it has

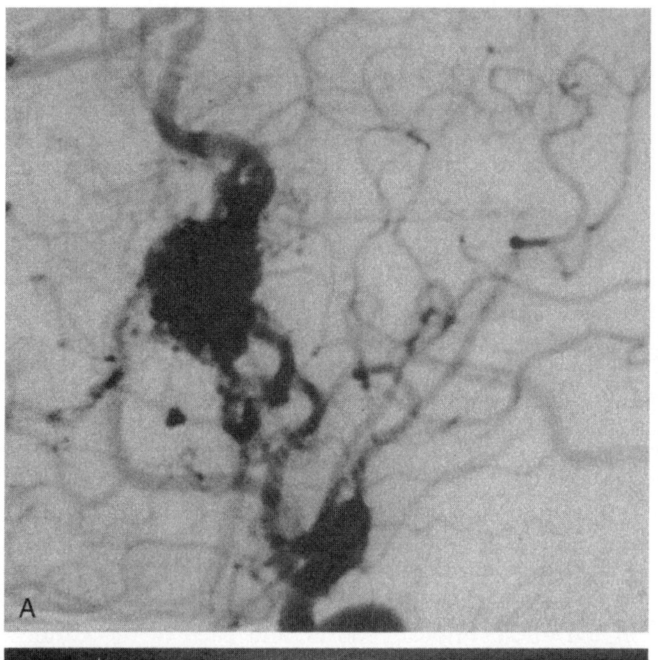

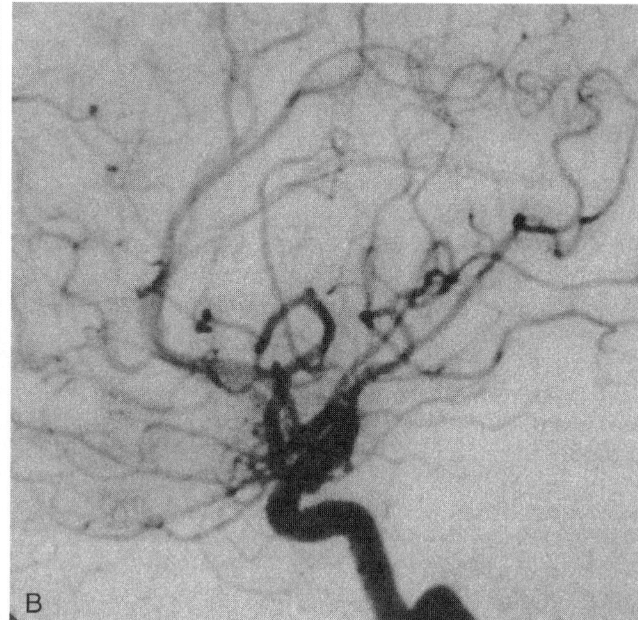

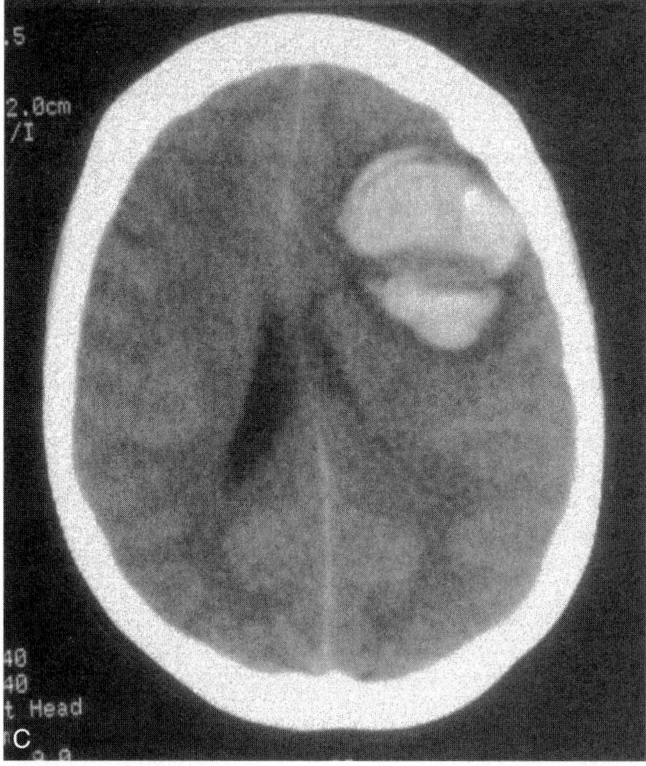

FIGURE 128–8. A 26-year-old patient presented with a seizure, and left lateral internal carotid artery angiography showed a frontal arteriovenous malformation *(A)* that was embolized with a good immediate postprocedure angiogram *(B)*. Eight hours after the procedure, while straining, the patient suddenly developed dysphasia and a hemiparesis. Computed tomographic scan showed intracerebral hemorrhage *(C)* that presumably reflects occlusion of the venous drainage with incomplete occlusion of the nidus.

been suggested that in low-grade AVMs surgery or focused irradiation be used alone rather than have the combined risks of multiple therapies.[153, 154] In addition to the therapeutic benefit, treatment with embolization and surgery in appropriately selected cases is likely to be cost-effective compared with surgery alone.[155]

Embolization as a prelude to focused irradiation also has been reported.[36] A cure rate of 73% has been reported in grades less than 4 and in 59% of grades greater than 3 with this combined therapy.[36] Overall the mortality was 1.6%, and the morbidity was 12.8%. It was thought that the reduction in AVM nidus size by the embolization increased the cure rate for these patients.

These results suggest that AVMs less than 3-cm maximum diameter rarely need preoperative embolization because of the lower morbidity from surgery alone compared with embolization followed by surgery in these lesions.[149] In larger AVMs, deep perforating arteries that cannot be embolized successfully possess a high risk of intraoperative or postoperative hemorrhage that is not likely to be ameliorated with embolization of other vessels.[149] If these deep perforating vessels can be embolized, there is likely to be a benefit from embolization. In large AVMs with feeding arteries arising from a deep meningeal supply, embolization of these vessels is likely to be of benefit, and when other feeding arteries are likely not to be accessed easily early in the surgical procedure, embolization may be of benefit. In the risk assessment of embolization, however, it must lower the morbidity of subsequent surgery by at least 5% to be justified based on the combined management morbidity. This is not likely for AVMs less than 3 cm in size, Spetzler-Martin grades 1 and 2 AVMs, or Spetzler-Martin grade 3 AVMs without deep perforating arteries. The role of embolization before focused irradiation is theoretically appealing, but embolization cannot be done without a significant morbidity and a potential for failure to cure in surgically more difficult cases.

COMBINATION TREATMENTS OF FOCUSED IRRADIATION AND MICROSURGERY

Experience in combining treatments to combat the difficult AVM is increasing with treatment failures in one therapy or the other. Steinberg and colleagues[156] reported that AVMs operated on 1 to 11 years after radiosurgical treatment are more easily resected. Of these 33 cases, 13 were grades less than 4, and a 10% mortality (from hemorrhage) occurred in grades greater than 3. These results show that combination therapy can work (in the same way that it has worked in the reverse order). The combined morbidity and mortality must be considered, however, in the overall risk assessment as has been discussed with the role of preoperative embolization.

INDIVIDUALIZING TREATMENT REGIMENS

Individualizing patient management is appropriate with the increasing knowledge of the variations in natural history that have been revealed (with an analysis of factors such as the presence of aneurysms and hemorrhagic presentation) along with the understanding of results expected from the range of treatment options available. It is readily apparent that the treatment options of microsurgery, focused irradiation, and embolization each can make significant contributions to the benefit of patients and that the task of the counseling medical practitioner is to plan a "best" patient management pathway. Because it is likely that there is a single best management pathway, it is important that this be presented to the patient and to make it clear that a naive consumer approach to this decision-making process can increase greatly the risks of management. Also important is the access to treatment centers with results that can be compared with reported series. As much, or more, variation exists among treating specialists of the same technique (i.e., microsurgeons, focused irradiation therapists, and interventional neuroradiologists) as between therapeutic techniques. The dramatic change in cases undergoing focused irradiation instead of microsurgery in one institution in Nagoya was attributed to the loss of one neurosurgeon.[157] The large case load treated at this institution went from almost totally surgical to almost totally therapy by focused irradiation in 1994 and was thought to relate more to a change in skill level than the relative merits of each form of treatment based on published series. The available skill level must influence the choice of management pathways. With this taken into account, the following discussion relates to published series and takes no account of individual therapists' abilities. Any recommended intervention must be weighed against the individualized risk of no treatment.

Several authors attempted to compare directly the patient suitable for either focused irradiation or microsurgery.[39, 42, 123, 124, 140, 158, 159] The outcome for patients chosen to undergo surgery for small lesions is excellent in the microsurgical reports, and each of the surgical studies reported no deaths and a maximum incidence of permanent morbidity of 0 to 2.7%. No study was randomized or large enough (with details of those not treated), however, to define unequivocally the best treatment option. In a report of AVMs less than 3 cm, 9% of cases did not undergo microsurgery, and in 2.5% of cases this was due to perceived operative difficulty. Referral bias before reaching centers reporting results of microsurgery prevents direct comparison between surgical and focused irradiation series.

Karlsson[111] reported that the combined risk of permanent neurological deficit and morbidity from recurrent hemorrhage was estimated to be 8% for marginal doses between 10 and 22 Gy. A greater contribution to this total comes from radiation necrosis at the higher marginal dose and a greater contribution by hemorrhage at the lower marginal dose. At 23 Gy, the risk was estimated to be 9%. This is an average and does not take into account variations in likelihood of hemorrhage with the presence of aneurysms or hemorrhagic presentation. Incorporating this study in forecasting schemes is useful, however, when preliminary decisions need to be made without the angioarchitectural or hemorrhagic history known (70% of 838 patients presenting with hemorrhage reported in 1999).[128]

Comparisons of focused irradiation with surgery have been reported using decision analysis modeling techniques.[158, 159] In a study from Toronto using probability estimates for surgery (95% cure, 5% neurological deficit, and 1% mortality) and focused irradiation (80% cure, 3% permanent neurological morbidity, 3% per year risk of hemorrhage for 2 years after treatment with a 15% mortality, and 30% permanent neurological morbidity from hemorrhage), it was found that for a 40-year-old with an AVM no greater than 3 cm surgery confers a large clinical benefit and had an excellent ratio of incremental cost per quality-adjusted life year gained.[159] Although this is a useful study for considering an "average lesion," the basis for probability estimates can be refined further (in light of current under-

TABLE 128–6 ■ **Assumptions on Which Decision-Making Strategies are Derived**

ITEM	DERIVED FIGURE USED
Risk of hemorrhage with aneurysm in unruptured AVM	7%/yr
Risk of hemorrhage without aneurysm in unruptured AVM	1.7%/yr
Risk of hemorrhage with hemorrhagic presentation	6–18% first year declining to unruptured rate over 5 yr
Death or permanent disability from rupture	50%
Death from rupture	25%
Time to cure if cure is to occur after focused irradiation	2 yr
Permanent symptomatic radiation damage	As per Table 128–5

AVM, arteriovenous malformation.

standing of AVM natural history and treatment risk factors). In a model using probability estimates for life expectancy, the natural history (unruptured AVM hemorrhage rate of 3% rising to 6% for 2 years after rupture with a 15% mortality and 40% disability arising from hemorrhage) and treatment with focused irradiation (0% mortality and 1% morbidity), a combined morbidity and mortality rate has been calculated for observation alone and focused irradiation.[158] For unruptured AVMs, the observed risk was 29% at 20 years of age, declining to 7% at 70 years of age, compared with focused irradiation at 7% for 20 years of age, declining to 3% at 70 years of age. For ruptured AVMs, the observed risk was 31% at 20 years of age, declining to 10% at 70 years of age, compared with focused irradiation at 8% for 20 years of age, declining to 5% at 70 years of age. Similar concerns exist with this study given the knowledge that angioarchitecture has a significant impact on the natural history. In addition, permanent radiation morbidity is underestimated in this study.

Management risks must take into account the variations in natural history, the site-specific and grading risks of treatment, and the risks of retreatment or multiple treatments. Although there is variation among studies, it is useful to have a figure that is likely best to reflect these results. To construct a decision-making regimen, the assumptions in Table 128–6 were used to calculate the risks of focused irradiation taking into account variations in the natural history and site and size of AVMs (Table 128-7).

Variations in the number of angiographic procedures for each treatment regimen do not appreciably affect the choice of treatment because when this is diagnostic and not interventional, the 0.07% risk is small compared with treatment risks[160] and does not significantly change the estimated morbidity and mortality.

Because of concerns regarding the disutility value of surgery, a definite advantage must be likely by surgery over focused irradiation for this to be the recommended therapeutic option. This advantage may be manifest in likelihood of cure or a lower disability rate. For certain lesions, it is difficult to be sure that the Spetzler-Martin classification accurately portrays the surgical risk because of limited surgical experience (e.g., thalamic and brainstem location). Ultimately, any forecasting scheme should be used as a guide rather than be followed blindly.

TABLE 128–7 ■ **Estimated Risks of Mortality and Permanent Morbidity from Treatment by Focused Irradiation***

LOCATION	SIZE, mL^3	ESTIMATED DIAMETER, CM	UNRUPTURED AND NO ANEURYSM, %	UNRUPTURED AND ANEURYSM, %	RUPTURED NO ANEURYSM, %	RUPTURED AND ANEURYSM, %
Frontal	<30	<3.85	2	7	11	12
Temporal	<10	<2.65	2	7	11	12
Temporal	10–20	2.65–3.35	4	9	13	14
Temporal	20–30	3.35–3.85	7	12	16	17
Intraventricular	<10	<2.65	3	8	12	13
Parietal or cerebellar	<10	<2.65	4	9	13	14
Parietal or cerebellar	10–20	2.65–3.35	9	14	18	19
Parietal or cerebellar	20–30	3.35–3.85	14	19	23	24
Corpus callosum or occipital	<10	<2.65	8	13	17	18
Corpus callosum or occipital	10–20	2.65–3.35	16	21	25	26
Corpus callosum or occipital	20–30	3.35–3.85	25	30	34	35
Medulla	<10	<2.65	12	17	21	22
Thalamus	<10	<2.65	17	22	26	27
Basal ganglia	<10	<2.65	21	26	30	31
Basal ganglia	10–20	2.65–3.35	43	48	52	53
Pons or midbrain	<10	<2.65	52	57	61	62

*Some lesion sizes have been excluded because of the unlikelihood of their eventuality, and the estimate for diameter is based on a spherical lesion.

PERIOPERATIVE MANAGEMENT DETERMINED BY INDIVIDUAL LESIONS AND ASSOCIATED FACTORS

Case selection with guidelines dictated by the aforementioned principles aims at minimizing the development of complications of treatment. Special consideration must be given, however, to perioperative management to avoid the development of delayed complications discussed earlier. These delayed complications include the development of the ACVH, vasospasm, and new seizure disorders. Of cases, 5% require postoperative intervention for the development of these delayed complications (excluding seizures).[38] Of complications of ACVH and vasospasm, 90% occur in Spetzler-Martin grade less than 4. A significant potential for morbidity and mortality can arise as a result of perioperative management in AVMs that are reported to have a low complication rate.

Each of these complications has identifiable risk factors that allow selective perioperative management tailored to the individual patient. In addition to the normal precautions needed for brain surgery (including dexamethasone and anticonvulsants when appropriate), lesions of size greater than 4 cm in diameter have an increased risk for the development of ACVH.[10, 38] Adjunctive therapeutic measures during surgery and in the early postoperative period for this group of patients include manipulation of the blood pressure (to, at least, avoid hypertension if not achieve hypotension), reducing the pulse pressure, and judicious use of antiplatelet and anticoagulant therapies. Controlling blood pressure includes the anticipation and prevention of sudden increases occurring because of pain or seizures. Because the risk period for ACVH is in the first 8 days after surgery,[38] consideration must be given to intensive monitoring during this time and aggressive blood pressure control when AVM nidus size is greater than 4 cm. Although anticonvulsants usually are indicated for AVM surgery, there is an acute need for seizure prevention in these larger lesions because of the potential for sudden blood pressure increases.

The use of anticoagulant or antiplatelet medications is controversial. In lesions thought to be especially prone to propagated venous thrombosis (e.g., an extensive redundant venous network on the convexity surface of the brain) that are less prone to hemorrhage (e.g., small and superficial), consideration should be given to the early introduction of these agents at a level that is appropriate for the surgery.[38] Vasospasm is an uncommon complication of AVM surgery, occurring in only 2% of all cases, but for patients undergoing extensive dissection of the proximal middle cerebral, internal carotid, or proximal anterior cerebral arteries, the incidence is 27%.[38] Given the restrictive control on blood pressure manipulation and angioplasty,[38, 161] it may well be that nimodipine is the treatment of choice.[38] This agent has the added benefit of lowering the blood pressure.

CONCLUSION

A summary of general treatment strategy recommendations is included in Table 128–8. As a general guide, surgery is recommended for Spetzler-Martin grade 1 and 2 AVMs. Many series report risks of permanent disability that are favorable in comparison with the aforementioned results for focused irradiation.[6, 37, 123] This is only for AVMs selected for surgery, however. An experienced cerebrovascular neurosurgeon should be included in the initial decision-making process for these AVMs.

Outcome for grade 3 AVMs may be influenced strongly by the presence of deep perforating arterial supply.[10] For AVMs without deep perforating supply, the outcome from surgery alone is similar to lower grade AVMs. When deep perforating supply is present, the grade 3 AVM has an outcome from surgery comparable to that of higher grade AVMs. From this finding, it can be concluded that grade 3 AVMs without deep perforating supply should do well with surgery alone and are not likely to benefit from combination therapy with embolization, and treatment by radiosurgery should be considered only when an experienced cerebrovascular neurosurgeon believes that the risks for the surgery would not be comparable to that of grade 1 and 2 AVMs. For grade 3 AVMs with deep perforating arteries that are less than 3 cm in diameter, consider-

TABLE 128–8 ■ **General Recommendations for Arteriovenous Malformation Treatment**

SPETZLER-MARTIN GRADE	DEEP PERFORATING ARTERIES	SIZE	FIRST CHOICE	SECOND CHOICE
1 and 2			Surgery	Focused irradiation
3	Absent		Surgery	Focused irradiation
3	Present	<3 cm	Focused irradiation	Palliation only
3	Present	>3 cm	Palliation only	Focused irradiation of deep perforators and delayed surgery ± embolization
4 and 5	Absent		Embolization and surgery	Palliation only
4 and 5	Present		Palliation only	Focused irradiation of deep perforators and delayed surgery ± embolization

ation must be given to radiosurgery as the first choice of treatment. Grade 3 AVMs larger than 3 cm and with deep perforating feeders should be considered as grade 4 and 5 AVMs.

In grade 4 and 5 AVMs undergoing surgery, many are treated with preoperative embolization. Also, an increasing number are being considered for multimodality therapy with surgery and focused irradiation. Firm recommendations regarding the best therapeutic options are limited by experience with these lesions.

Grades 4 and 5 AVMs present a difficult therapeutic challenge. These are, by definition, greater than 3 cm and likely to have a low cure rate by focused irradiation. The result of surgical resection is, on the whole, disappointing, however, with a range of permanent severe new deficits (modified Rankin score increase in follow-up of at least 2 points over preoperative score) or death in 9% to 44% in patients undergoing surgery.[6, 23, 37, 38, 43] The great variation in outcome may reflect surgical triaging. In reports in which the nonsurgical patients with grade 4 and 5 AVMs are included, many of these patients are counseled against treatment.[162] In one report in which 63% of referred patients underwent surgery, there was a significant bias against operating on patients with deep perforating arterial contribution.[163] Even with this bias, the major surgical morbidity was influenced significantly by the presence of deep perforating arteries. Of patients with grade 4 and 5 AVMs and no deep perforating contribution, 10% had significant permanent surgical morbidity compared with 44% when deep perforating supply was present. A group of approximately 22% of grade 4 and 5 AVMs are without deep perforating arterial supply and may be associated with a lower morbidity by surgery (or combined therapy) than conservative management (associated with a 27% decline in function over the average follow-up of 33 months).[163] In patients with deep perforating supply, it is theoretically appealing to treat the deep perforating component with focused irradiation and the remainder by surgery and embolization after a 2- to 3-year interval from focused irradiation. Whether or not this strategy is effective and beneficial is yet to be established.

REFERENCES

1. Cushing H, Bailey P: Tumours Arising from the Blood Vessels of the Brain: Angiomatous Malformations and Hemangioblastomas, vol III. Springfield, IL, Thomas, 1928.
2. Dandy WE: Arteriovenous aneurysm of the brain. Arch Surg 17:190–243, 1928.
3. Olivecrona H, Riives J: Arteriovenous aneurysms of the brain: Their diagnosis and treatment. Arch Neurol Psychiatry 59:567–602, 1948.
4. Norlen G: Arteriovenous aneurysms of the brain: Report of ten cases of total removal of the lesion. J Neurosurg 6:475–494, 1949.
5. Batjer HH, Devous MD Sr, Seibert GB, et al: Intracranial arteriovenous malformation: Relationships between clinical and radiographic factors and ipsilateral steal severity. Neurosurgery 23: 322–328, 1988.
6. Hamilton MG, Spetzler RF: The prospective application of a grading system for arteriovenous malformations. Neurosurgery 34:2–7, 1994.
7. Heros RC, Korosue K, Diebold PM: Surgical excision of cerebral arteriovenous malformations: Late results. Neurosurgery 26: 570–578, 1990.
8. Jomin M, Lesain F, Lozes G: Prognosis for arteriovenous malformations of the brain based on 150 cases. Surg Neurol 23:362–366, 1985.
9. Luessenhop AJ: AVM grading in assessing surgical risk. J Neurosurg 66:637, 1987.
10. Morgan MK, Drummond KJ, Sorby W, et al: Cerebral AVM surgery: Risks related to lenticulostriate arterial supply. J Neurosurg 86:801–805, 1997.
11. Morgan MK, Johnston IH, Hallinan JM, et al: Complications of surgery for arteriovenous malformations of the brain. J Neurosurg 78:176–182, 1993.
12. Pellettieri L, Carlsson C-A, Grevsten S, et al: Surgical versus conservative treatment of intracranial arteriovenous malformations. Acta Neurochir Suppl 29:1–85, 1980.
13. Shi YQ, Chen XC: A proposed scheme for grading intracranial arteriovenous malformations. J Neurosurg 65:484–489, 1986.
14. Steinmeier R, Schramm J, Müller H-G, et al: Evaluation of prognostic factors in cerebral arteriovenous malformations. Neurosurgery 24:193–200, 1989.
15. Sundt TM Jr, Piepgras DG, Stevens LN: Surgery for supratentorial arteriovenous malformations. Clin Neurosurg 37:49–115, 1990.
16. Tamaki N, Ehara K, Lim TK, et al: Cerebral arteriovenous malformations: Factors influencing the surgical difficulty and outcome. Neurosurgery 29:856–863, 1991.
17. Vkingstad EM, Cao Y, Thomas AJ, et al: Language hemispheric dominance in patients with congenital lesions of eloquent brain. Neurosurgery 47:562–570, 2000.
18. Yasargil MG, Curcic M, Kis M, et al: Microneurosurgery, vol IIIB. New York, Thieme Medical Publishers, 1988.
19. Coffey RJ, Nichols DA, Shaw EG: Stereotactic radiosurgical treatment of cerebral arteriovenous malformations. Mayo Clin Proc 70:214–222, 1995.
20. Colombo F, Pozza F, Chierego G, et al: Linear accelerator radiosurgery of cerebral arteriovenous malformations: An update. Neurosurgery 34:14–21, 1994.
21. Flickinger JC, Kondziolka D, Pollock BE, et al: Complications from arteriovenous malformation radiosurgery: Multivariate analysis and risk modeling. Int J Radiat Oncol Biol Phys 38: 485–490, 1997.
22. Flickinger JC, Kondziolka D, Lunsford LD: Radiobiology of vascular malformation radiosurgery. In Jafar JJ, Awad IA, Rosenwaser RH (eds): Vascular Malformations of the Central Nervous System. Philadelphia, Lippincott Williams & Wilkins, 1999, pp 455–462.
23. Friedman WA, Deshmukh V: Radiosurgery for arteriovenous malformations. In Jafar JJ, Awad IA, Rosenwaser RH (eds): Vascular Malformations of the Central Nervous System. Philadelphia, Lippincott Williams & Wilkins, 1999, pp 463–477.
24. Gallina P, Merienne L, Meder JF, et al: Failure in radiosurgery treatment of cerebral arteriovenous malformations. Neurosurgery 42:996–1004, 1998.
25. Karlsson B, Kihlström L, Lindquist C, et al: Gamma knife surgery for previously irradiated arteriovenous malformations. Neurosurgery 42:1–6, 1998.
26. Ogilvy CS: Radiation therapy for arteriovenous malformations: A review. Neurosurgery 26:725–735, 1990.
27. Seifert V, Stolke D, Mehdorn HM, et al: Clinical and radiological evaluation of long-term results of stereotactic proton beam radiosurgery in patients with cerebral arteriovenous malformations. J Neurosurg 81:683–689, 1994.
28. Steiner L, Lindquist C, Adler JR, et al: Clinical outcome of radiosurgery for cerebral arteriovenous malformations. J Neurosurg 77:1–8, 1992.
29. Yamamoto M, Jimbo M, Hara M, et al: Gamma knife radiosurgery for arteriovenous malformations: Long-term follow-up results focussing on complications occurring more than 5 years after irradiation. Neurosurgery 38:906–914, 1996.
30. Luessenhop AJ, Gennarelli TA: Anatomical grading of supratentorial arteriovenous malformations for determining operability. Neurosurgery 1:30–35, 1977.
31. Luessenhop AJ, Rosa L: Cerebral arteriovenous malformations: Indications for and results of surgery, and the role of intravascular techniques. J Neurosurg 60:14–22, 1984.
32. Pertuiset B, Ancri D, Kinuta Y, et al: Classification of supraten-

torial arteriovenous malformations: A score system for evaluation of operability and surgical strategy based on an analysis of 66 cases. Acta Neurochir 110:6–16, 1991.
33. Spetzler RF, Martin NA: A proposed grading system for arteriovenous malformations. J Neurosurg 65:476–483, 1986.
34. Friedman WA, Blatt DL, Bova FJ, et al: The risk of hemorrhage after radiosurgery for arteriovenous malformations. J Neurosurg 84:912–919, 1996.
35. Friedman WA, Bova FJ, Mendenhall WM: Linear accelerator radiosurgery for arteriovenous malformations: The relationship of size to outcome. J Neurosurg 82:180–189, 1995.
36. Gobin YP, Laurent A, Merienne L, et al: Treatment of brain arteriovenous malformations by embolization and radiosurgery. J Neurosurg 85:19–28, 1996.
37. Heros RC: Prevention and management of therapeutic complications. In Jafar JJ, Awad IA, Rosenwaser RH (eds): Vascular Malformations of the Central Nervous System. Philadelphia, Lippincott Williams & Wilkins, 1999, pp 363–373.
38. Morgan MK, Sekhon LHS, Finfer S, et al: Delayed neurological deterioration following resection of arteriovenous malformations of the brain. J Neurosurg 90:695–701, 1999.
39. Pollock BE, Lunsford LD, Kondziolka D, et al: Patient outcomes after stereotactic radiosurgery for "operable" arteriovenous malformations. Neurosurgery 35:1–8, 1994.
40. Pollock BE, Kondziolka D, Lunsford LD, et al: Repeat stereotactic radiosurgery of arteriovenous malformations: Factors associated with incomplete obliteration. Neurosurgery 38:318–324, 1996.
41. Pollock BE, Gorman DA, Schomberg PJ, et al: The Mayo Clinic gamma knife experience. Mayo Clin Proc 74:5–13, 1999.
42. Sisti MB, Kader A, Stein BM: Microsurgery for 67 intracranial arteriovenous malformations less than 3 cm in diameter. J Neurosurg 79:655–660, 1993.
43. Hartmann A, Stapf C, Hofmeister MS, et al: Determinants of neurological outcome after surgery for arteriovenous malformation. Stroke 31:2361–2364, 2000.
44. Anderson RMD, Blackwood W: The association of arteriovenous angioma and saccular aneurysm of the arteries of the brain. J Pathol Bacteriol 77:101–110, 1959.
45. Batjer H, Suss RA, Samson D: Intracranial arteriovenous malformations associated with aneurysms. Neurosurgery 18:29–35, 1986.
46. Brown RD, Wiebers DO, Forbes GS: Unruptured intracranial aneurysms and arteriovenous malformations: Frequency of intracranial hemorrhage and relationship of lesions. J Neurosurg 73:859–863, 1990.
47. Cunha e Sa MJ, Stein BM, Solomon RA, et al: The treatment of associated intracranial aneurysms and arteriovenous malformations. J Neurosurg 77:853–859, 1992.
48. Meisel HJ, Mansmann U, Alvarez H, et al: Cerebral arteriovenous malformations and associated aneurysms: Analysis of 305 cases from a series of 662 patients. Neurosurgery 46:793–802, 2000.
49. Okamoto S, Handa H, Hashimoto N: Location of intracranial aneurysms associated with cerebral AVM: Statistical analysis. Surg Neurol 22:335–340, 1984.
50. Perret G, Nishioka H: Arteriovenous malformations: An analysis of 545 cases of craniocerebral arteriovenous malformations and fistulae reported to the cooperative study. J Neurosurg 25: 467–490, 1966.
51. Redekop G, TerBrugge K, Montanera W, et al: Arterial aneurysms associated with cerebral arteriovenous malformations: Classification, incidence, and risk of hemorrhage. J Neurosurg 89:539–546, 1998.
52. Suzuki J, Onuma T: Intracranial aneurysms associated with arteriovenous malformations. J Neurosurg 50:742–746, 1979.
53. Thompson RC, Steinberg GK, Levy RP, et al: The management of patients with arteriovenous malformations and associated intracranial aneurysms. Neurosurgery 43:202–212, 1998.
54. Atkinson JLD, Sundt TM Jr, Houser OW, et al: Angiographic frequency of anterior circulation intracranial aneurysms. J Neurosurg 70:551–555, 1989.
55. Ferguson GG: Turbulence in human intracranial saccular aneurysms. J Neurosurg 33:485–497, 1970.
56. Ferguson GG: Physical factors in the initiation, growth and rupture of human intracranial saccular aneurysms. J Neurosurg 37:666–677, 1972.
57. Stehbens WE: Etiology of intracranial berry aneurysms. J Neurosurg 70:823–831, 1981.
58. Drake CG: Considerations for and experience with surgical treatment in 166 cases. Clin Neurosurg 26:145–206, 1979.
59. Fuwa I, Matsukado Y, Kaku M, et al: Enlargement of a cerebral aneurysm associated with ruptured arteriovenous malformation. Acta Neurochir 80:65–68, 1986.
60. Al-Rodhan NRF, Sundt TM Jr, Piepgras DG, et al: Occlusive hyperemia: A theory for the hemodynamic complications following resection of intracerebral arteriovenous malformations. J Neurosurg 78:167–175, 1993.
61. Batjer HH, Devous MD Sr, Meyer YJ, et al: Cerebrovascular hemodynamics in arteriovenous malformation complicated by normal perfusion pressure breakthrough. Neurosurgery 22:503–509, 1988.
62. Malis LI: Arteriovenous malformations of the brain. In Youmans JR (ed): Neurologic Surgery, vol 3. Philadelphia, WB Saunders, 1982, pp 1786–1806.
63. Spetzler RF, Wilson CB, Weinstein P, et al: Normal perfusion pressure breakthrough theory. Clin Neurosurg 25:651–672, 1978.
64. Young WL, Kader A, Ornstein E, et al: Cerebral hyperemia after arteriovenous malformation resection is related to "breakthrough" complications but not to feeding artery pressure. Neurosurgery 38:1085–1095, 1996.
65. Sekhon LHS, Morgan MK, Spence I, et al: Normal perfusion pressure breakthrough: The role of capillaries. J Neurosurg 86: 519–524, 1997.
66. Piepgras DG, Morgan MK, Sundt TM Jr, et al: Intracerebral hemorrhage after carotid endarterectomy. J Neurosurg 68:532–536, 1988.
67. Powers AD, Smith RR: Hyperperfusion syndrome after carotid endarterectomy: A transcranial Doppler evaluation. Neurosurgery 26:56–60, 1990.
68. Schroeder T, Sillesen H, Sorensen O, et al: Cerebral hyperperfusion following carotid endarterectomy. J Neurosurg 66:824–829, 1987.
69. Sundt TM Jr, Piepgras DG, Marsh WR, et al: Bypass vein grafts for giant aneurysms and severe intracranial occlusive disease in the anterior and posterior circulation. In Sundt TM Jr (ed): Occlusive Cerebrovascular Disease: Diagnosis and Surgical Management. Philadelphia, WB Saunders, 1987, pp 439–464.
70. Irikura K, Morii S, Miyasaka Y, et al: Impaired autoregulation in an experimental model of chronic cerebral hypoperfusion in rats. Stroke 27:1399–1404, 1996.
71. Morgan MK, Anderson RB, Sundt TM Jr: A model of the pathophysiology of cerebral arteriovenous malformations by a carotid-jugular fistula in the rat. Brain Res 496:241–250, 1989.
72. Morgan MK, Anderson RE, Sundt TM Jr: The effects of hyperventilation on cerebral blood flow in the rat with an open and closed carotid-jugular fistula. Neurosurgery 25:606–612, 1989.
73. Spetzler RF, Hamilton MG: Pressure autoregulation is intact after arteriovenous malformation resection. Neurosurgery 33: 772–773, 1993.
74. Macfarlane R, Moskowitz MA, Sakas DE, et al: The role of neuroeffector mechanisms in cerebral hyperperfusion syndromes. J Neurosurg 75:845–855, 1991.
75. Barry DI, Jarden JO, Paulson OB, et al: Cerebrovascular effects of converting enzyme inhibition: I. Effects of intravenous captopril in spontaneously hypertensive and normotensive rats. J Hypertens 2:589–597, 1984.
76. Bill A, Linder J: Sympathetic control of cerebral blood flow in acute arterial hypertension. Acta Physiol Scand 96:114–121, 1976.
77. Folkow B, Halbäck M, Lundgren Y, et al: Importance of adaptive changes in vascular design for establishment of primary hypertension, studied in man and in spontaneously hypertensive rats. Circ Res 32/33(Suppl 11):1-2–1-16, 1973.
78. Postiglione A, Bobkiewicz T, Vinholdt-Pedersen E, et al: Cerebrovascular effects of angiotensin converting enzyme inhibition involve large artery dilatation in rats. Stroke 22:1363–1368, 1991.
79. Young WL, Kader A, Prohovnik I, et al: Pressure autoregulation is intact after arteriovenous malformation resection. Neurosurgery 32:491–497, 1993.

80. Paulson OB, Strandgaard S, Edvinsson L: Cerebral autoregulation. Cerebrovasc Brain Metab Rev 2:161–192, 1990.
81. Barnett GH, Little JR, Ebrahim ZY, et al: Cerebral circulation during arteriovenous malformation operation. Neurosurgery 20: 836–842, 1987.
82. Rosenblum BR, Bonner RF, Oldfield EH: Intraoperative measurement of cortical blood flow adjacent to cerebral AVM using laser doppler velocimetry. J Neurosurg 66:396–399, 1987.
83. Young WL, Prohovnik I, Ornstein E, et al: Monitoring of intraoperative cerebral hemodynamics before and after arteriovenous malformation resection. Anesth Analg 67:1011–1014, 1988.
84. Gowers WR: A Manual of Disease of the Nervous System. Philadelphia, P Blakiston, 1888, pp 764–773.
85. Pertuiset B, Sichez JP, Philippon J, et al: Mortality and morbidity following the surgical excision of 162 intracranial arteriovenous malformations (1958–1978). Rev Neurol 135:319–327, 1979.
86. Nilsson B, Rehncrona S, Siesjö BK: Coupling of cerebral metabolism and blood flow in epileptic seizures, hypoxia and hypoglycaemia. Ciba Found Symp 56:199–218, 1978.
87. Nitsch C, Suzuki R, Fujiwara K, et al: Incongruence of regional cerebral blood flow increase and blood-brain barrier opening in rabbits at the onset of seizures induced by bicuculline, methoxypyridoxine, and kainic acid. J Neurol Sci 67:67–79, 1985.
88. Tenny RT, Sharbrough FW, Anderson RE, et al: Correlation of intracellular redox states and pH. Ann Neurol 8:564–573, 1980.
89. Morgan MK, Winder M: Haemodynamics of arteriovenous malformation of the brain and consequences of resection: A review. J Clin Neurosci 8:216–224, 2001.
90. Sorimachi T, Takeuchi S, Koike T, et al: Blood pressure monitoring in feeding arteries of cerebral arteriovenous malformations during embolization: A preventive role in hemodynamic complications. Neurosurgery 37:1041–1048, 1995.
91. Nichols WW, O'Rourke MF: McDonald's Blood Flow in Arteries: Theoretic, Experimental and Clinical Principles, 3rd ed. London, Edward Arnold, 1990.
92. Hassler W, Steinmetz H: Cerebral hemodynamics in angioma patients: An intraoperative study. J Neurosurg 67:822–831, 1987.
93. Crawford PM, West CR, Shaw MDM, et al: Cerebral arteriovenous malformations and epilepsy: Factors in the development of epilepsy. Epilepsia 27:270–275, 1986.
94. Forster DMC, Steiner L, Hakinson S: Arteriovenous malformations of the brain: A long-term clinical study. J Neurosurg 37: 562–570, 1972.
95. Foy PM, Copeland GP, Shaw MDM: The incidence of postoperative seizures. Acta Neurochir 55:253–264, 1981.
96. Murphy MJ: Long-term follow-up of seizures associated with cerebral arteriovenous malformations: Results of therapy. Arch Neurol 42:477–479, 1985.
97. Parkinson D, Bachers G: Arteriovenous malformations: Summary of 100 consecutive supratentorial cases. J Neurosurg 53: 285–299, 1980.
98. Falkson CB, Chakrabarti KB, Doughty D, et al: Stereotactic multiple arc radiotherapy: III-influence of treatment of arteriovenous malformations on associated epilepsy. Br J Neurosurg 11:12–15, 1997.
99. Gertzen PC, Adelson PD, Kondziolka D, et al: Seizure outcome in children treated for arteriovenous malformations using gamma knife radiosurgery. Pediatr Neurosurg 24:139–144, 1996.
100. Piepgras DG, Sundt TM Jr, Ragoowansi AT, et al: Seizure outcome in patients with surgically treated cerebral arteriovenous malformations. J Neurosurg 78:5–11, 1993.
101. Thorpe ML, Cordato DJ, Morgan MK, et al: Postoperative seizure outcome in a series of 114 patients with supratentorial arteriovenous malformations. J Clin Neurosci 7:107–111, 2000.
102. Yeh H, Tew JM, Gartner M: Seizure control after surgery on cerebral arteriovenous malformations. J Neurosurg 78:12–18, 1993.
103. Kraemer D, Awad IA: Vascular malformations and epilepsy: Clinical considerations and basic mechanisms. Epilepsia 35(Suppl 6):S30–S43, 1994.
104. Bagga RS: New York Islands arteriovenous malformation prospective study: Feasibility and initial results. The Fourth Annual Meeting of the AANS/CNS Section of Cerebrovascular Surgery and the American Society of Interventional and Therapeutic Neuroradiology. The Big Island Hawaii, Feb 9–12, 2001.
105. Brown RD Jr, Wiebers DO, Torner JC, et al: Frequency of intracranial hemorrhage as a presenting symptom and subtype analysis: A population-based study of intracranial vascular malformations in Olmsted County, Minnesota. J Neurosurg 85:29–32, 1996.
106. Brown RD, Wiebers DO, Forbes G, et al: The natural history of unruptured intracranial arteriovenous malformations. J Neurosurg 68:352–357, 1988.
107. Fults D, Kelly DL Jr: Natural history of arteriovenous malformations of the brain: A clinical study. Neurosurgery 15:658–662, 1984.
108. Graf CJ, Perrett GE, Torner JC: Bleeding from cerebral arteriovenous malformations as part of their natural history. J Neurosurg 58:331–337, 1983.
109. Itoyama Y, Uemura S, Ushio Y, et al: Natural course of unoperated intracranial arteriovenous malformations: Study of 50 cases. J Neurosurg 71:805–809, 1989.
110. Ondra SL, Troupp H, George ED, et al: The natural history of symptomatic arteriovenous malformations of the brain: A 24-year follow-up assessment. J Neurosurg 73:387–391, 1990.
111. Karlsson B: Angiography long term follow up data for arteriovenous malformations previously proven to be obliterated after gamma knife radiosurgery. The third ISAVM. Tokyo, April 23–24, 2000.
112. Dobbelaere P, Jomin M, Clarrisse J, et al: Interet pronostique de l'etude du drainage verneux de aneurysms arterio-veneux cerebraux. Neurochirurgie 25:178–184, 1979.
113. Vinuela F, Nombela L, Roach MR, et al: Stenotic and occlusive disease of the venous drainage system of deep brain AVM's. J Neurosurg 63:180–184, 1985.
114. Redekop GJ, Elisevich KV, Gaspar LE, et al: Conventional radiation therapy of intracranial arteriovenous malformations: Long-term results. J Neurosurg 78:413–422, 1993.
115. Luessenhop AJ: Natural history of cerebral arteriovenous malformations. In Wilson CB, Stein BM (eds): Intracranial Arteriovenous Malformations. Baltimore, Williams & Wilkins, 1984, pp 12–23.
116. Morgan MK, Sekhon L, Rahman Z, et al: Morbidity of intracranial hemorrhage in patients with cerebral arteriovenous malformation. Stroke 29:2001, 1998.
117. Murphy JP: Cerebrovascular Disease. Chicago, Year Book Medical Publishers, 1954, p 408.
118. Langer DJ, Lasner TM, Hurst RW, et al: Hypertension, small size, and deep venous drainage are associated with risk of hemorrhagic presentation of cerebral arteriovenous malformations. Neurosurgery 42:481–489, 1998.
119. Stapf C, Mohr JP, Sciacca RR, et al: Incident hemorrhage risk of brain arteriovenous malformations located in the arterial border zones. Stroke 31:2365–2368, 2000.
120. Kondziolka D, McLaughlin MR, Kestle JR: Simple risk predictions for arteriovenous malformation hemorrhage. Neurosurgery 37:851–855, 1995.
121. Arnold CD: Record high life expectancy. Stat Bull 74:28–35, 1993.
122. Jafar JJ, Huang PP: Surgical approaches: Convexity and sylvian lesions. In Jafar JJ, Awad IA, Rosenwaser RH (eds): Vascular Malformations of the Central Nervous System. Philadelphia, Lippincott Williams & Wilkins, 1999, pp 277–295.
123. Pik J, Morgan MK: Microsurgery for small arteriovenous malformations of the brain: Results of 110 consecutive cases. Neurosurgery 47:571–577, 2000.
124. Pikus HJ, Beach ML, Harbaugh RE: Microsurgical treatment of arteriovenous malformations: Analysis and comparison with stereotactic radiosurgery. J Neurosurg 88:641–646, 1998.
125. Laing RW, Childs J, Brada M: Failure of conventionally fractionated radiotherapy to decrease the risk of hemorrhage in inoperable arteriovenous malformations. Neurosurgery 30:872–875, 1992.
126. Schneider BF, Eberhard DA, Steiner LE: Histopathology of arteriovenous malformations after gamma knife radiosurgery. Neurosurg 87:352–357, 1997.
127. Flickinger JC, Pollock BE, Kondziolka D, et al: A dose-response analysis of arteriovenous malformation obliteration after radiosurgery. Int J Radiat Oncol Biol Phys 36:873–879, 1996.
128. Karlsson B, Lax I, Soderman M: Can the probability for obliteration after radiosurgery for arteriovenous malformations be ac-

curately predicted? Int J Radiat Oncol Biol Phys 43:313–319, 1999.
129. Miyawaki L, Dowd C, Wara W, et al: Five year results of LINAC radiosurgery for arteriovenous malformations: Outcome for large AVMs. Int J Radiat Oncol Biol Phys 44:1089–1106, 1999.
130. Schlienger M, Atlan D, Lefkopoulos D, et al: Linac radiosurgery for cerebral arteriovenous malformations: Results in 169 patients. Int J Radiat Oncol Biol Phys 46:1135–1142, 2000.
131. Touboul E, Al Halabi A, Buffat L, et al: Single-fraction stereotactic radiotherapy: A dose-response analysis of arteriovenous malformation obliteration. Int J Radiat Oncol Biol Phys 41: 855–861, 1998.
132. Heffez DS, Osterdock RJ, Alderete L, et al: The effect of incomplete patient follow-up on the reported results of AVM radiosurgery. Surg Neurol 49:373–381, 1998.
133. Maesawa S, Flickinger JC, Kondziolka D, et al: Repeated radiosurgery for incompletely obliterated arteriovenous malformations. J Neurosurg 92:961–970, 2000.
134. Lindqvist M, Karlsson B, Guo WY, et al: Angiographic long-term follow-up data for arteriovenous malformations previously proven to be obliterated after gamma knife radiosurgery. Neurosurgery 46:803–808, 2000.
135. Kader A, Goodrich JT, Sonstein WJ, et al: Recurrent cerebral arteriovenous malformations after negative postoperative angiograms. J Neurosurg 85:14–18, 1996.
136. Karlsson B, Lindquist C, Steiner L: Prediction of obliteration after gamma knife surgery for cerebral arteriovenous malformations. Neurosurgery 40:425–431, 1997.
137. Yamamoto Y, Coffey RJ, Nichols DA, et al: Interim report on the radiosurgical treatment of cerebral arteriovenous malformations: The influence of size, dose, time, and technical factors on obliteration rate. J Neurosurg 83:832–837, 1995.
138. Pollock BE, Flickinger JC, Lunsford LD, et al: Hemorrhage risk after stereotactic radiosurgery of cerebral arteriovenous malformations. Neurosurgery 38:652–659, 1996.
139. Betti OO, Munari C, Rosler R: Stereotactic radiosurgery with the linear accelerator: Treatment of arteriovenous malformations. Neurosurgery 24:311–321, 1989.
140. Steiner L, Lindquist C, Cail W, et al: Microsurgery and radiosurgery in brain arteriovenous malformations. J Neurosurg 79: 647–652, 1993.
141. Flickinger JC, Kondziolka D, Lunsford LD, et al: Development of a model to predict permanent symptomatic postradiosurgery injury for arteriovenous malformation patients. Int J Radiat Oncol Biol Phys 46:1143–1148, 2000.
142. Eisenschenk S, Gilmore RL, Friedman WA, et al: The effect of LINAC stereotactic radiosurgery on epilepsy associated with arteriovenous malformations. Stereotact Funct Neurosurg 71: 51–61, 1998.
143. Sutcliffe JC, Forster DM, Walton L, et al: Untoward clinical effects after stereotactic radiosurgery for intracranial arteriovenous malformations. Br J Neurosurg 6:177–185, 1992.
144. Kurita H, Kawamoto S, Suzuki I, et al: Control of epilepsy associated with cerebral arteriovenous malformations after radiosurgery. J Neurol Neurosurg Psychiatry 65:648–655, 1998.
145. Luessenhop AJ, Spence WT: Artificial embolization of cerebral arteries: Report of use in a case of arteriovenous malformation. JAMA 172:1153–1155, 1960.
146. Debrun GM, Aletich V, Ausman JI, et al: Embolization of the nidus of brain arteriovenous malformations with n-butyl cyanoacrylate. Neurosurgery 40:112–120, 1997.
147. Frizzel RT, Fisher WS III: Cure, morbidity, and mortality associated with embolization of brain arteriovenous malformations: A review of 1246 patients in 32 series over a 35-year period. Neurosurgery 37:1031–1040, 1995.
148. Vinuela F, Dion JE, Duckwiler G, et al: Combined endovascular embolization and surgery in the management of cerebral arteriovenous malformations: Experience with 101 cases. J Neurosurg 75:856–864, 1991.
149. Morgan MK, Zurin AAR, Harrington T, et al: Changing role for preoperative embolisation in the management of arteriovenous malformations of the brain. J Clin Neurosci 7:527–530, 2000.
150. Morgan MK, Sundt TM Jr: The case against staged operative resection of cerebral arteriovenous malformations. Neurosurgery 25:429–436, 1989.
151. DeMeritt JS, Pile-Spellman J, Mast H, et al: Outcome analysis of preoperative embolization with N-butyl cyanoacrylate in cerebral arteriovenous malformations. AJNR Am J Neuroradiol 16:1801–1807, 1995.
152. Westphal M, Cristante L, Grzyska U, et al: Treatment of cerebral arteriovenous malformations by neuroradiological intervention and surgical resection. Acta Neurochir 130:20–27, 1994.
153. Deruty R, Pelissou-Guyotat I, Amat D, et al: Complications after multidisciplinary treatment of cerebral arteriovenous malformations. Acta Neurochir 138:119–131, 1996.
154. Nussbaum ES, Heros RC, Camarata PJ: Surgical treatment of intracranial arteriovenous malformations with an analysis of cost-effectiveness. Clin Neurosurg 42:348–369, 1995.
155. Jordan JE, Marks MP, Lane B, et al: Cost-effectiveness of endovascular therapy in the surgical management of cerebral arteriovenous malformations. AJNR Am J Neuroradiol 17:247–254, 1996.
156. Steinberg GK, Chang SD, Levy RP, et al: Surgical resection of large incompletely treated intracranial arteriovenous malformations following stereotactic radiosurgery. J Neurosurg 84:920–928, 1996.
157. Negoro M: Management of cortical AVMs. The Fourth Annual Meeting of the AANS/CNS Section of Cerebrovascular Surgery and the American Society of Interventional and Therapeutic Neuroradiology. The Big Island Hawaii, Feb 9–12, 2001.
158. Chang HS, Nihei H: Theoretical comparison of surgery and radiosurgery in cerebral arteriovenous malformations. J Neurosurg 90:709–719, 1999.
159. Porter PJ, Shin AY, Detsky AS, et al: Surgery versus stereotactic radiosurgery for small, operable cerebral arteriovenous malformations: A clinical and cost comparison. Neurosurgery 41:757–766, 1997.
160. Cloft HJ, Joseph GJ, Dion JE: Risk of cerebral angiography in patients with subarachnoid hemorrhage, cerebral aneurysm, and arteriovenous malformation: A meta-analysis. Stroke 30: 317–320, 1999.
161. Morgan MK, Day MJ, Little N, et al: The use of intra-arterial papaverine in the management of vasospasm complicating the resection of arteriovenous malformations of the brain: A report of two cases. J Neurosurg 82:296–299, 1995.
162. de Oliveira E, Tedeschi H, Raso J: Comprehensive management of arteriovenous malformations. Neurol Res 20:673–683, 1998.
163. Ferch RD, Morgan MK: High grade arteriovenous malformations and their management. J Clin Neurosci 9:37–40, 2002.

CHAPTER **129**

Endovascular Management of Brain Arteriovenous Malformations

AVI SETTON ■ ALEJANDRO BERENSTEIN ■ ROBIN ALBERT

CLINICAL SIGNIFICANCE AND TREATMENT PLAN

The natural history and classification of brain arteriovenous malformations (BAVMs) are discussed elsewhere in this textbook, and other chapters address surgical and radiosurgical management. This chapter focuses on the endovascular management of BAVMs.

The three major treatment modalities for BAVMs are endovascular embolization, microsurgical resection, and stereotactic radiosurgery. Each method may be used as the sole treatment or may be used in combination with the other modalities. Endovascular embolization may be used as the sole mode of treatment if complete obliteration of the malformation is obtained with a permanent agent or, for incurable lesions, as a palliative treatment with targeted embolization. Embolization may be used as a preoperative adjunct, before microsurgical resection or radiosurgical treatment, as part of a combination therapy. Although combination therapy allows treatment of lesions previously considered untreatable, the patient is subject to the combined risk of each treatment. For each case, a unique treatment plan with specific goals and potential risks and benefits must be established and understood by the treating team of health professionals, the patient, and family.

To formulate the best plan of treatment for BAVMs, a complete clinicomorphologic analysis of each case is required. It includes knowledge about the clinical history and present clinical status, the cross-sectional imaging characteristics, and the angioarchitecture of the AVM and the normal brain circulation. The angioarchitecture of the AVM often determines the approach to the lesion and the probability of reaching the therapeutic goal. Only after this analysis is complete can a treatment plan be developed. Treatment of a particular patient with a BAVM should be considered if the therapy will result in an improved outcome compared with the expected natural history of the lesion considering the risk factors specific for that patient's condition. Under certain circumstances, a complete cure may not be possible or necessary.

Treatment of BAVMs often requires a multidisciplinary approach, with a team consisting of an interventional neuroradiologist, a vascular neurosurgeon, vascular neurologist, and a stereotactic radiosurgeon.[1, 2] Such a team offers the patient a balanced approach in the management of the AVM.

PATIENT SELECTION

The discovery of a BAVM in a patient does not represent an immediate indication for treatment. There is increasing evidence in the surgical and endovascular literature that all BAVMs do not behave the same and do not carry the same risk for future hemorrhage as aneurysms do.[3] An incidentally discovered cortical micro-BAVM in a young patient does not have the same prognosis and natural history as a large thalamic AVM in a young patient presenting with progressive neurological deficit. In 1986, Crawford[4] reported that none of the patients in his series with an incidentally discovered AVM bled during the 20-year follow-up period.

An important part of the management of incidentally discovered BAVMs is to educate the patient and provide information regarding the natural history and influencing factors that may apply to the specific situation, considering that the true natural history of asymptomatic BAVMs is not well defined. Treatment options and associated risks that exist within the treating team's experience must be explained. It is important to reassure the patient that he or she is expected to lead a normal, productive life with minimal restrictions.

A complete clinicomorphologic analysis of each case is required to determine if and when treatment is indicated and to determine which treatment modalities can best serve the patient with the lowest risk of morbidity.

CLINICOMORPHOLOGIC ANALYSIS

Clinical Factors

AGE

In general, the younger the patient is at the time of presentation, the more likely treatment should be considered. Presentation at a young age represents an early imbalance between the patient (i.e., host) and the BAVM. Patients older than 60 years of age are at a higher risk of bleeding[4] and have a greater risk of hemorrhage-associated morbidity and mortality than younger individuals. Treatment should be therefore considered in the elderly.

GENDER

The gender of the patient should not influence the decision to treat a BAVM. Although there has been some controversy about the increased risk of hemorrhage or other symptoms during pregnancy, this association has not been well established. Our observations concur with those of Yasargil[5] and Horton and colleagues[6] that pregnancy does not seem to increase the risk of hemorrhage or the risk of progression of neurological symptoms.

LIFESTYLE AND OCCUPATION

The decision to treat a patient with a BAVM should include an analysis of lifestyle and the impact of symptoms and potential complications of therapy in trying to achieve cure. Consideration of side dominance, stage of education, and occupation should have a role in therapeutic decisions.

PRESENTING SYMPTOMS

The initial presentation plays a significant role in the timing of treatment and choice of the treatment modality.

Hemorrhage

Most patients presenting with hemorrhage tolerate it well, and immediate therapy is usually unnecessary. Although some controversy exists regarding the rebleed rate during the first year after hemorrhage,[7, 8] it is generally believed to be similar or just slightly higher than the natural history risk of 3% to 4% per year. The study by Ondra and coworkers[7] analyzes the outcome of symptomatic AVMs. They reported a severe morbidity rate of 1.7%, annual mortality rate of 1%, and a mean rebleed interval of more than 6 years. There is seldom a need for urgent treatment after BAVM hemorrhage, and a treatment strategy can be planned accordingly. Conversely, in patents with recurrent hemorrhages, the likelihood of permanent neurological deficit and death increases with each hemorrhagic episode.[4, 9] In these individuals, the angioarchitecture of the AVM must be meticulously analyzed in search of areas of anatomic weakness. If such an abnormality is discovered, targeted embolization should be performed (Figs. 129–1 to 129–3).[3, 10] If embolization is technically impossible or unsuccessful, surgical resection should be considered. Although the type of treatment may vary among medical centers depending on local expertise, the universal goal should be to reduce or eliminate the risk of future hemorrhage in the patient with an acceptable treatment risk.

Seizures

Most patients presenting with a seizure disorder can be successfully treated with antiepileptic medications and rarely require immediate intervention. Patients who present with seizures carry the same future risk for hemorrhage as those with other symptomatic BAVMs.[7]

Headaches

Headache is a nonspecific symptom. Some patients with BAVMs with dural or posterior cerebral artery supply complain of headaches that resolve or improve after embolization.[3] Other patients with parietal lobe AVMs complain of worsening of headache after embolization of anterior and middle cerebral artery feeders if there is a compensatory increased supply through the posterior cerebral arteries. Although headaches by themselves do not represent an indication for treatment of patients with BAVMs, a role exists for partial targeted embolization if headaches are disabling and significant dural and posterior cerebral artery supplies are angiographically demonstrated. Certain characteristics of recurrent headaches represent a symptomatic lesion and share the same natural history as any other symptomatic AVM, indicating similar treatment strategies.

Neurological Deficit

Only 6% of patients with BAVMs present with nonhemorrhagic neurological deficit,[4] and in our experience and in the reports of others, progression of deficit occurs in less than one half.[8] Although arterial steal and mass effect have been implicated as possible causes,[11] we believe that venous congestion and ischemia are more probable mechanisms (Fig. 129–4).[3] Magnetic resonance imaging (MRI) has demonstrated changes in the venous drainage patterns of the adjacent brain with associated edema and partial thrombosis of draining veins of the AVM. If treated with partial embolization, these changes may be reversible in lobar AVMs manifesting with progressive neurological deficit. Partial embolization of deep thalamic and basal ganglia AVMs in patients presenting with progressive neurological deficits resulted in stabilization in 27% of cases and reversal of symptoms in 64% (see Fig. 129–3).[12]

Morphologic Factors: Cerebral Angiography

Careful analysis of the imaging studies and complete selective angiography is of great importance in making decisions about treatment. The angiogram must delineate the characteristics of the BAVM, including its arterial feeders, venous drainage, and its internal angioarchitecture and associated vascular lesions, and it must define the collateral circulation and venous drainage pathways of the normal brain. A decision to treat in part depends on the demonstration of area of weakness in the angioarchitecture indicating potential instability. If there is an associated arterial aneurysm on the feed-

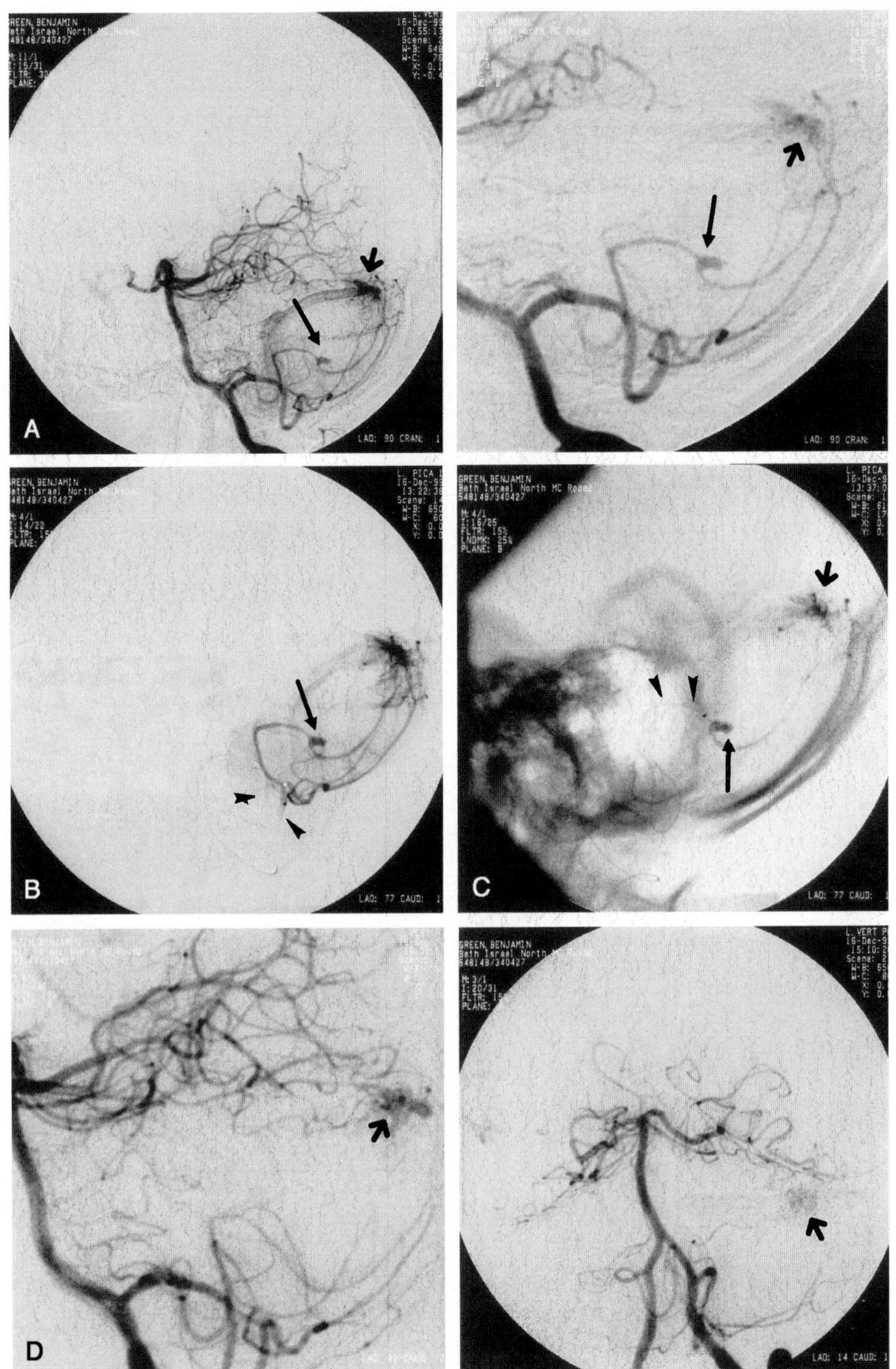

FIGURE 129–1. Targeted embolization. A patient with a left, high cerebellar micro–arteriovenous malformation presented with an off-midline, low cerebellar parenchymal hematoma. *A,* Lateral and magnified lateral views of a left vertebral angiogram demonstrate the malformation's small nidus *(small arrow)*, left posterior inferior cerebellar artery (PICA) pial supply with a proximal irregular aneurysm *(arrow)* anatomically correlated with the hematoma, and indirect left superior cerebellar pial supply. *B,* In the superselective angiographic study performed through a microcatheter *(arrowheads)* in the left PICA, notice the PICA branch with mild irregularity and the proximal aneurysm leading to the malformation *(arrow)*. Normal cortical branches are seen posteriorly. *C,* Angiographic superselective study before *n*-butyl-2-cyanoacrylate (NBCA) embolization. The microcatheter was navigated to the irregular aneurysm entrance. Embolization of the distal nidus *(small arrow)* with obliteration of the proximal aneurysm *(arrow)* is the goal to prevent an early repeat hemorrhage. *D,* Lateral and anteroposterior views during left vertebral angiography after embolization. Notice the obliteration of the PICA aneurysm and preservation of the normal cerebellar cortical branches and small residual nidus *(small arrow)* supplied by the left superior cerebellar distal branches. This residual malformation was resected surgically.

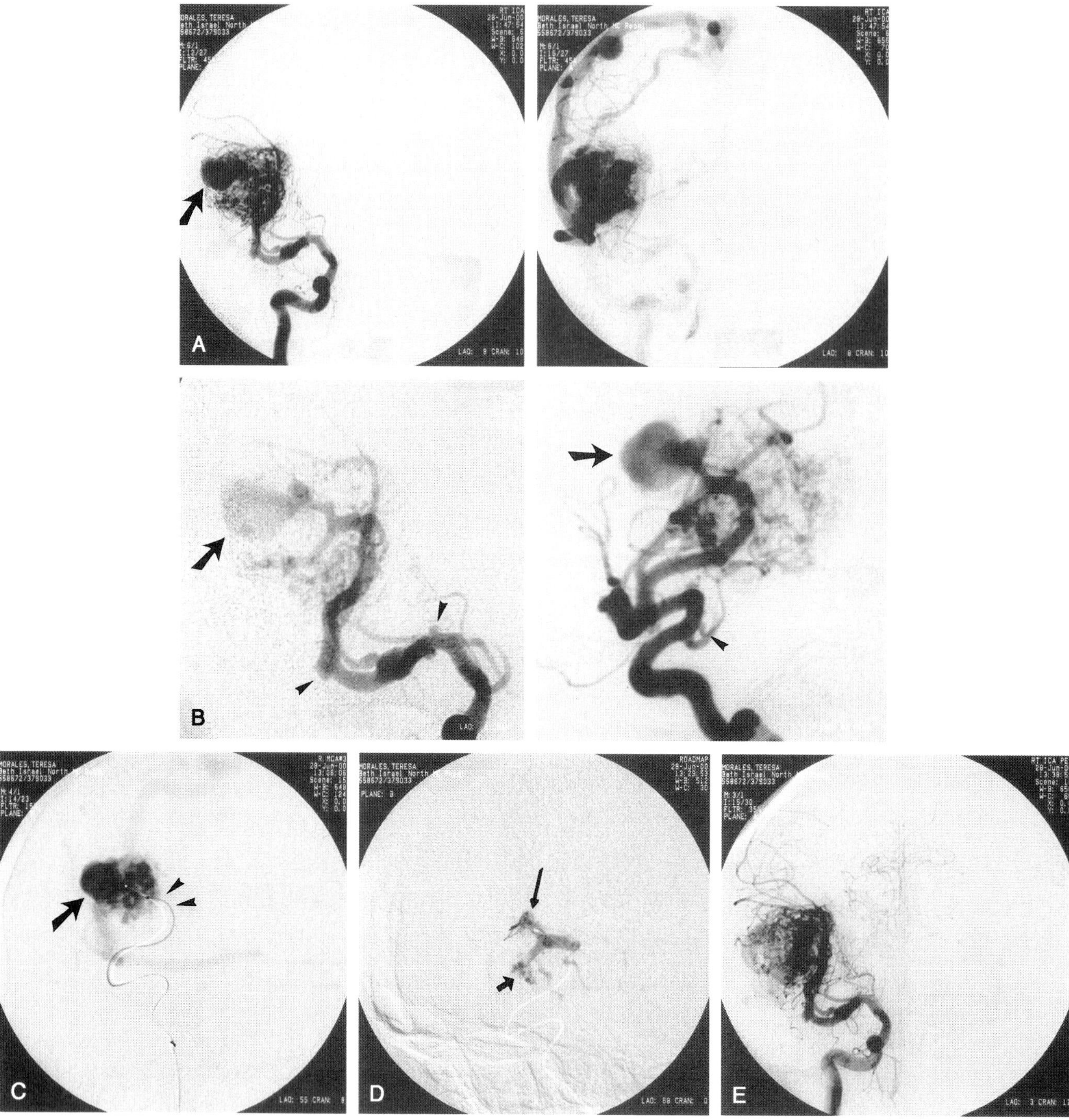

FIGURE 129–2. Targeted embolization of a symptomatic right insular arteriovenous malformation. *A,* Angiographic anteroposterior views of the right internal carotid artery (ICA) in arterial and venous phases show an insular malformation with predominantly cortical venous drainage. Notice the distal arterial aneurysm *(arrow). B,* In the magnified early arterial phases of the anteroposterior and lateral views of a global right ICA angiogram, notice the large, distal arterial aneurysm at the entrance to the nidus *(arrow)* and the proximal, small flow-related aneurysms *(arrowheads). C,* The lateral view of a superselective angiographic study performed through a microcatheter *(arrowheads)* positioned at the level of the aneurysm *(arrow)* shows high-flow fistulization distal to the aneurysm in combination with a proximal nidus. Occluding this area of angioarchitecture weakness was a high priority. *D,* A lateral subtracted fluoroscopic image shows a combination of microcoils and acrylic obliterating the base of the aneurysm and the leading pedicle *(arrow)* as well as a portion of the nidus *(small arrow). E,* In the anteroposterior view of a control angiographic study of the right ICA, notice the elimination of the large aneurysm and occlusion of the lateral portion of the nidus. The patient underwent second-stage embolization before radiosurgery.

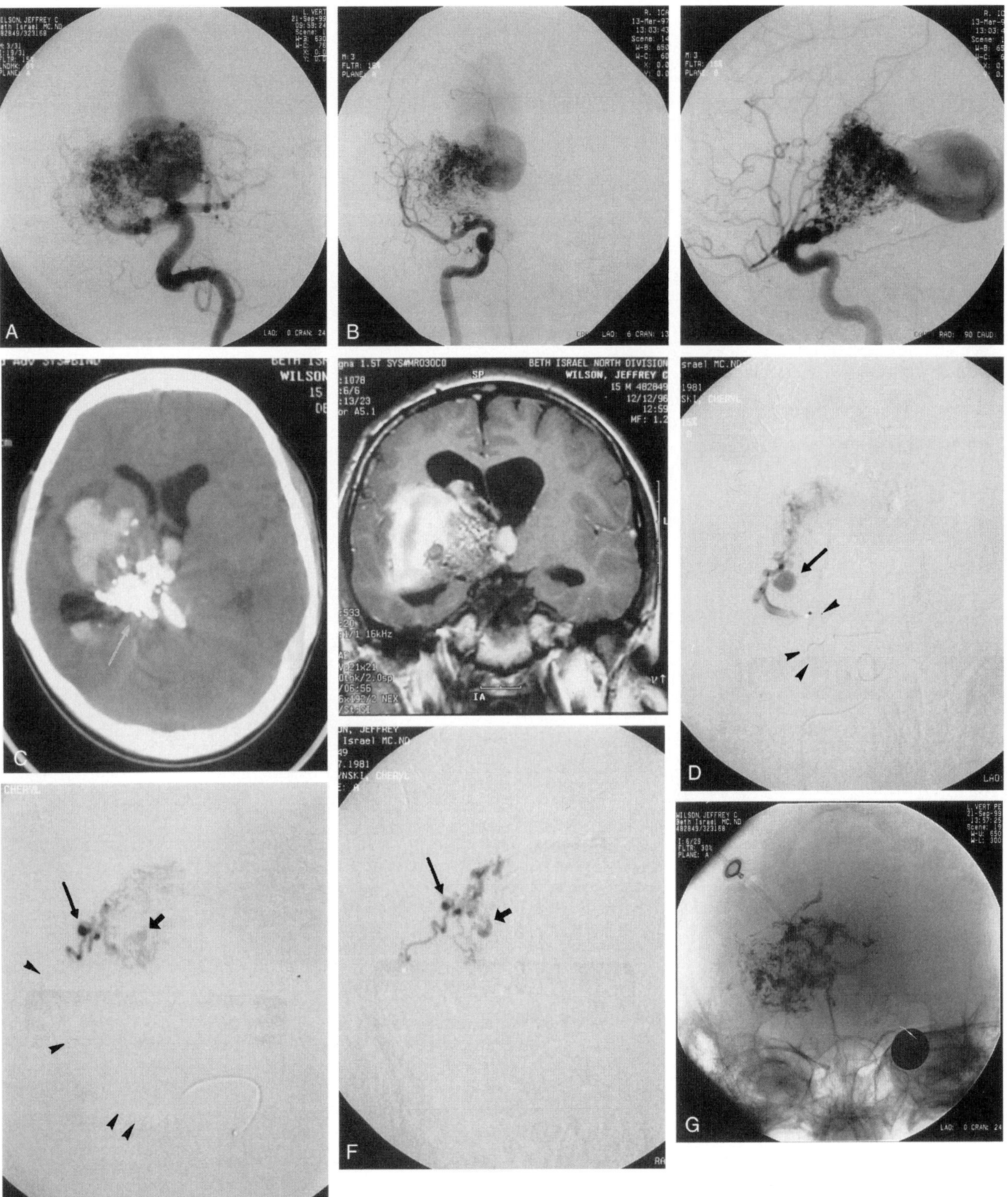

FIGURE 129–3. Palliative targeted embolization of a large basal ganglia and thalamic arteriovenous malformation (AVM) manifesting with recurrent hemorrhages and hemipareses. *A,* Anteroposterior view of a vertebral angiogram shows multiple, enlarged, right posterior thalamoperforators and posterior choroidal arteries supplying the malformation in the posterior thalamic region and draining to the aneurysmally dilated vein of Galen. *B,* The anteroposterior and lateral views of a right internal carotid artery angiogram show multiple, enlarged, medial and lateral lenticulostriate arteries that supply the widespread AVM in the basal ganglia and drain into the aneurysmally dilated vein of Galen and straight sinus. *C,* Axial computed tomography (CT) and coronal, T1-weighted magnetic resonance imaging (MRI) were completed a short period after the patient presented with combined parenchymal and intraventricular hemorrhage with neurological deterioration. Notice the acrylic cast *(arrow)* from previous embolization procedures. *D* and *E,* Anteroposterior views of the superselective

Legend continued on following page

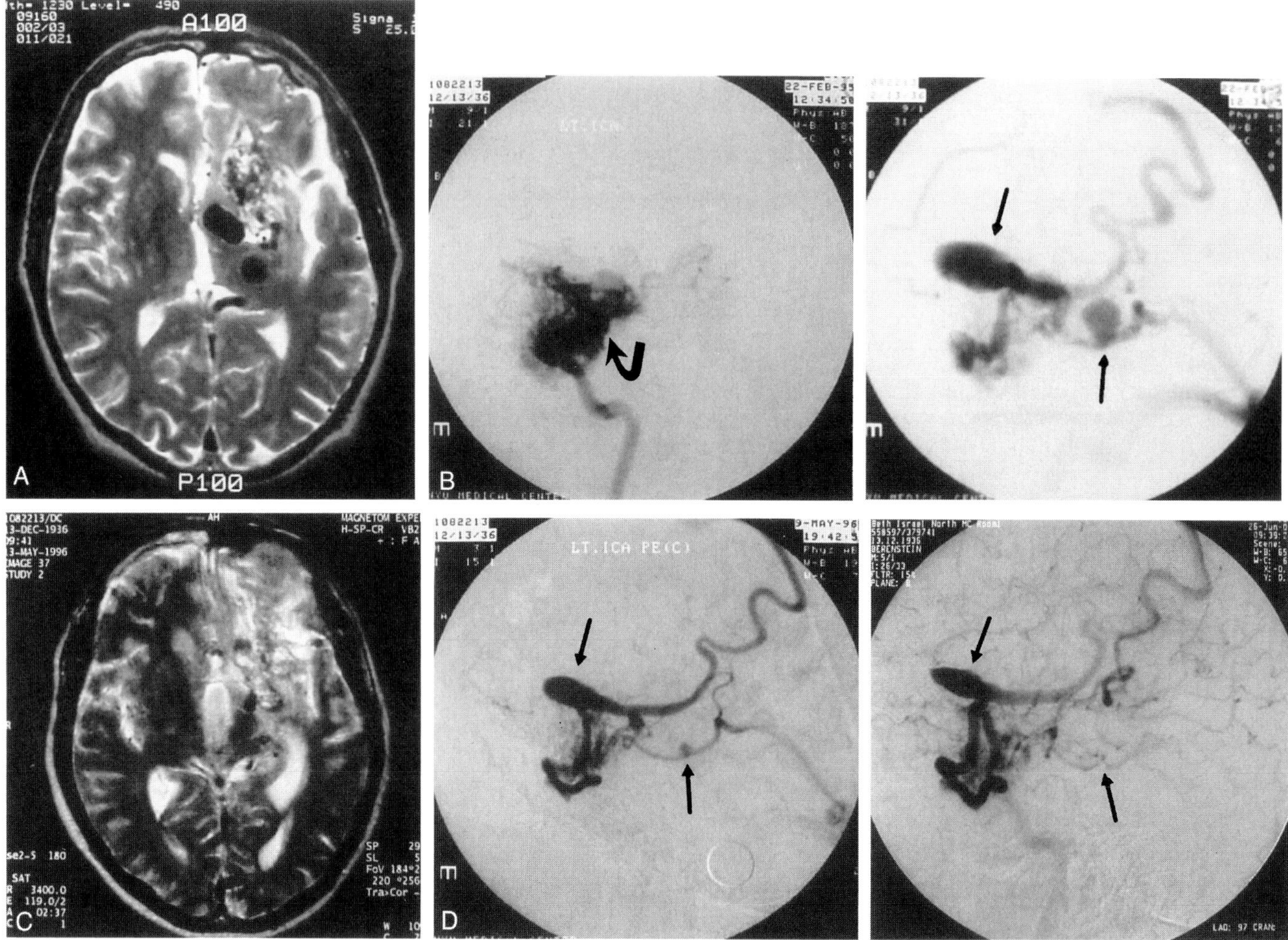

FIGURE 129–4. Palliative embolization of a left frontal and basal ganglia arteriovenous malformation in a patient with hemipareses and uncontrolled seizures. *A,* On axial, T2-weighted magnetic resonance imaging (MRI), notice the malformation and the large draining veins. *B,* In the early and late phases of the lateral view of the left internal carotid angiogram, notice the malformation nidus *(curved arrow)* and multiple venous aneurysms (*arrows,* correlated with the MRI scan) in the deep venous drainage into the basal vein of Rosenthal and in the superficial drainage pathway into the sylvian vein leading through the vein of Trolard to the superior sagittal sinus. *C,* Axial, T2-weighted MRI shows the area after multistage embolization. Notice the marked reduction of the nidus size and the venous outflow structures (compare with *A*). *D,* In the lateral views of the venous phases of repeated carotid angiograms, notice the progressive size reduction of the venous aneurysm in the basal vein of Rosenthal *(arrow)*, size reduction of the venous aneurysm close to the nidus *(arrow)*, and size reduction of the vein of Trolard. After palliative treatment, the patient had clinical improvement with medical control of his seizures.

FIGURE 129–3 *Continued.*
angiographic studies were obtained through a microcatheter *(arrowheads)* positioned distally in two separate lateral lenticulostriate arteries supplying a malformation in the basal ganglia in the territory of the hematoma seen on CT and MRI. Notice the arterial pseudoaneurysms *(long arrows)* and intranidal pseudoaneurysm *(short arrow)*, which could not be identified in the global angiographic studies. *F,* The anteroposterior view of a subtracted fluoroscopic study shows the acrylic cast deposited after the superselective study in *E.* Notice the obliteration with acrylic of the arterial *(long arrow)* and the intranidal *(short arrow)* pseudoaneurysm. *G,* An anteroposterior skull x-ray film demonstrates the radiopaque acrylic cast in the malformation after the last embolization stage. Multiple stages were performed as part of a prolonged palliative treatment targeting weaknesses in the angioarchitecture and reducing the malformation size and flow.

ing pedicle or in the nidus, evidence of venous thrombosis, outflow restriction, venous hypertension, venous pouches or dilatations, venous pseudoaneurysm, or venous outflow compromise, treatment is indicated and can achieve cure in certain circumstances or targeted treatment and partial cure in others (Fig. 129–5; see also Figs. 129–1 to 129–4).

The role of the newer imaging modalities, such as three-dimensional rotational angiography, may further advance our understanding of these complex lesions.

LOCATION, SIZE, AND DEEP VENOUS DRAINAGE

Although the location, size, and deep venous drainage of a malformation are important factors in determining the risks of surgical therapy,[13] these factors are a minor

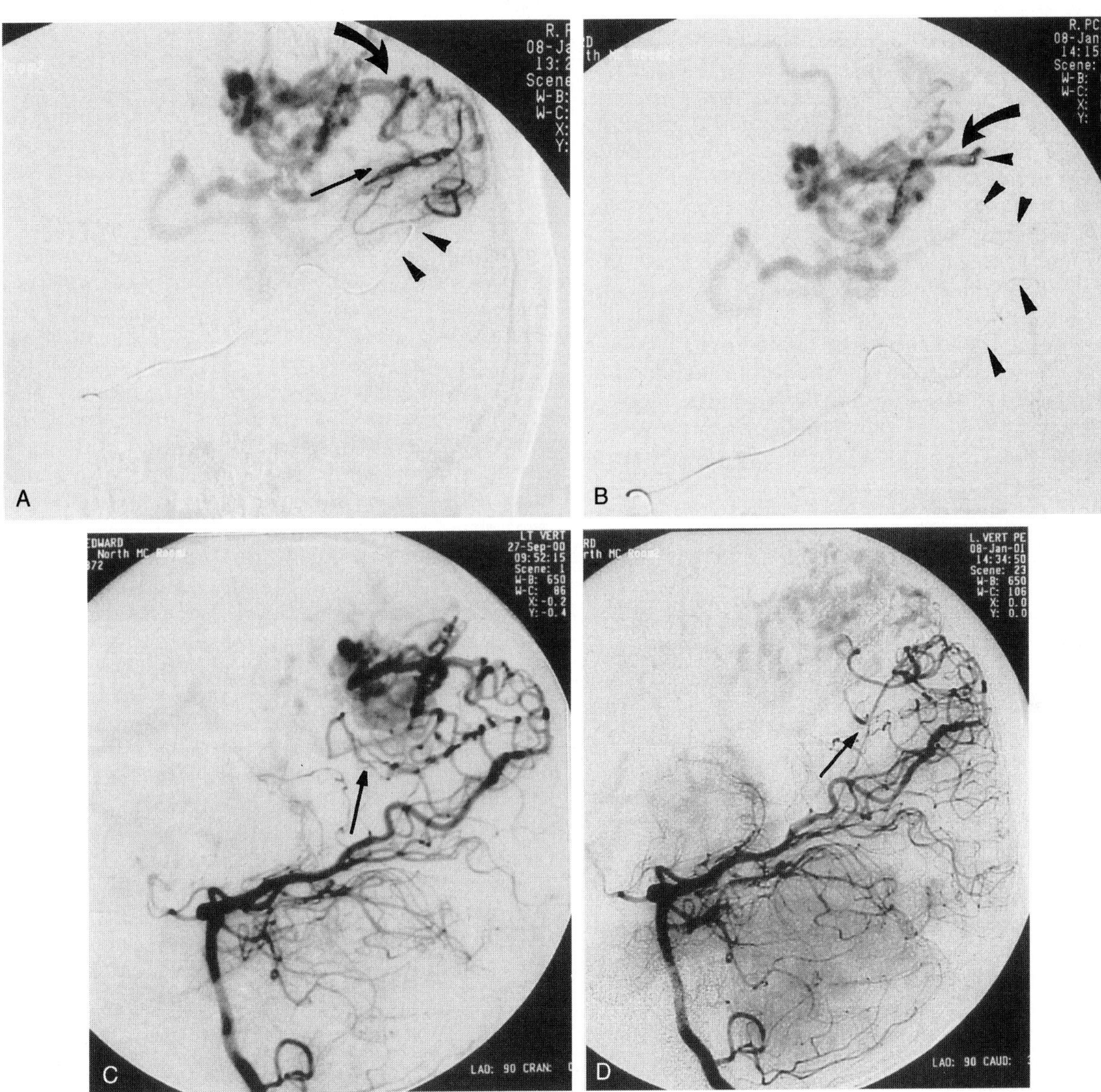

FIGURE 129–5. Angiographic studies were undertaken to define safe embolization in a right parietal arteriovenous malformation. *A,* The lateral view of a superselective angiogram was performed through a microcatheter *(arrowheads)* introduced through the left vertebral artery (VA) to the right posterior cerebral artery (PCA) and into a distal parietal occipital cortical branch. Normal branching arteries supply the cortex with a normal parenchymal blush *(arrow).* The angiogram shows the distal supply to the malformation *(curved arrow).* Acrylic embolization will induce ischemia in the surrounding normal cortex. *B,* The microcatheter was navigated distally, directly to the vessel leading to the malformation *(curved arrow)* beyond the normal cortex. There is no parenchymal blush. Embolization of the nidus was performed without neurological deficit or diffusion abnormality, as assessed by follow-up magnetic resonance imaging. Precise anatomic studies may eliminate the need for functional testing before acrylic deposition. *C,* On the lateral vertebral angiogram, before *(right)* and after *(left)* embolization, notice the obliteration of the whole posterior compartment of the malformation, preservation of normal cortical branches (as in *A*), and immediate regression of collateral circulation to the nidus *(arrow).*

concern for the endovascular treatment of BAVMs. In performing embolization of BAVMs, meticulous technique and sparing of all normal noncontributing arteries are essential, regardless of the location of the malformation (see Fig. 129–5).

ASSOCIATED LESIONS

Aneurysms associated with AVMs may be flow related (i.e., proximal or distal on a feeder vessel), intranidal, or remote and apparently unrelated (Figs. 129–6 and 129–7; see also Fig. 129–2). They represent the host's response to the AVM and a weakness in the vascular system. This weakness represents a marker for future hemorrhage and increases the hemorrhage risk from 3% to 7%.[14] In the presence of acute subarachnoid hemorrhage, the more likely source of the hemorrhage is an aneurysm. Patients presenting with subarachnoid hemorrhage or intracerebral hemorrhage, or both, and an angiographically demonstrated BAVM with an associated aneurysm should have therapy directed first toward the lesion that is suspected to be the source of hemorrhage. When only subarachnoid hemorrhage is present, the aneurysm should be treated first. When an intracerebral hematoma exists, the more likely source of hemorrhage is the AVM, and it should be targeted first (see Fig. 129–3). Enlarging pseudoaneurysms represent an unstable situation and deserve special attention to prevent early hemorrhage.

In our experience, proximal aneurysms are rarely responsible for hemorrhage in patients with BAVMs. Although remote, non–flow-related aneurysms may occur in patients with BAVMs, their presence may not alter the natural history. We have not experienced a rupture of a proximal flow-related aneurysm during or immediately after endovascular treatment of the AVM. Proximal flow-related aneurysm regression may occur after complete or partial obliteration of the AVM by endovascular embolization and is more likely to occur the closer the aneurysm is to the nidus of the AVM.[15] If the aneurysm is located close to the AVM, it should be obliterated at the time of embolization. If, on follow-up angiography 6 to 12 months after AVM embolization, there is no regression of the associated aneurysm, active treatment of the aneurysm should be considered. We recommend treating large, irregular, proximal aneurysms early as part of a global treatment plan (see Figs. 129–4 and 129–5). However, the treatment-associated morbidity must be low to justify the procedure in light of the unknown natural history of the aneurysm in the absence of the AVM.

TREATMENT GOALS

Endovascular embolization can be performed as the only treatment (curative or palliative), or it may be used in combination with surgery or stereotactic radiosurgery.

Curative Embolization

Curative embolization is a complete anatomic obliteration of the malformation by endovascular embolization, occluding the nidus and early venous shunting, and it therefore requires the use of a permanent, nonbiodegradable embolic agent to form a cast within the pathologic angioarchitecture (Fig. 129–8). In a direct pial arteriovenous fistula, detachable balloons, coils, or acrylic may accomplish a cure by obliterating the direct arteriovenous connection.[16–18] Particles or resorbable agents should not be used for curative embolization.

In addition to the immediate postembolization angiogram, 6-month and, preferably, 12- to 24-month postprocedural angiograms are needed to confirm the stability of the treatment. Long-term follow-up angiography is needed to detect small remnants that may not have been appreciated on the immediate postembolization angiogram and to exclude recanalization caused by the mixture of radiopaque embolic material with nonopaque autologous blood at the time of embolization.[19–21] Another important reason for obtaining long-term angiographic follow-up is to rule out the potential recruitment of arterial collaterals. These collaterals probably develop by a mechanism of nonsprouting angiogenesis because of insufficient embolic agent penetration and lack of obliteration of the nidal-venous junction, with occlusion of only the proximal feeding vessel. Although delayed thrombosis may occur, it must be confirmed on long-term angiographic follow-up.[19] After thrombosis of the venous outlets has occurred, no new veins can be recruited, and a cure has been achieved. In general, when long-term follow-up angiography demonstrates complete obliteration of the malformation without residual opacification of the lesion, no arteriovenous shunting, and no stasis in the nidus, future recanalization is not expected.

The complete cure rate for AVMs by embolization alone varies between 10% and 40%.[3, 20, 22, 23] Valavanis and Yasargil[23] noticed that, in addition to small size and limited number of arterial feeders, certain topographic locations (e.g., sulcal, deep extrinsic) favored complete obliteration with embolization alone. Total obliteration is related to the anatomic arrangement of the feeding vessels. Direct feeders ending in the AVM, feeders "en passage," or indirect leptomeningeal collaterals reconstituting the nidus influence our capability to reach the malformation and embolize safely. A high yield of total obliteration is expected in a single-pedicle, small lesion with a terminal feeder (see Fig. 129–8), but only partial palliative occlusion can be expected in holohemispheric AVMs.

Our experience is limited in total obliteration of small malformations. We emphasize the need for late angiographic follow-up to confirm the lack of residual small shunts. With the development of permanent embolic agents that are nonpolymerizing in nature, a higher cure rate may be achieved. Conversely, a high rate of complete obliteration is expected for surface pial fistulas or vein of Galen malformations (Fig. 129–9).

Palliative Targeted Embolization

To understand the rationale for partial embolization, the surgeon must accept the concept that the host will remain asymptomatic as long as equilibrium exists be-

Text continued on page 2217

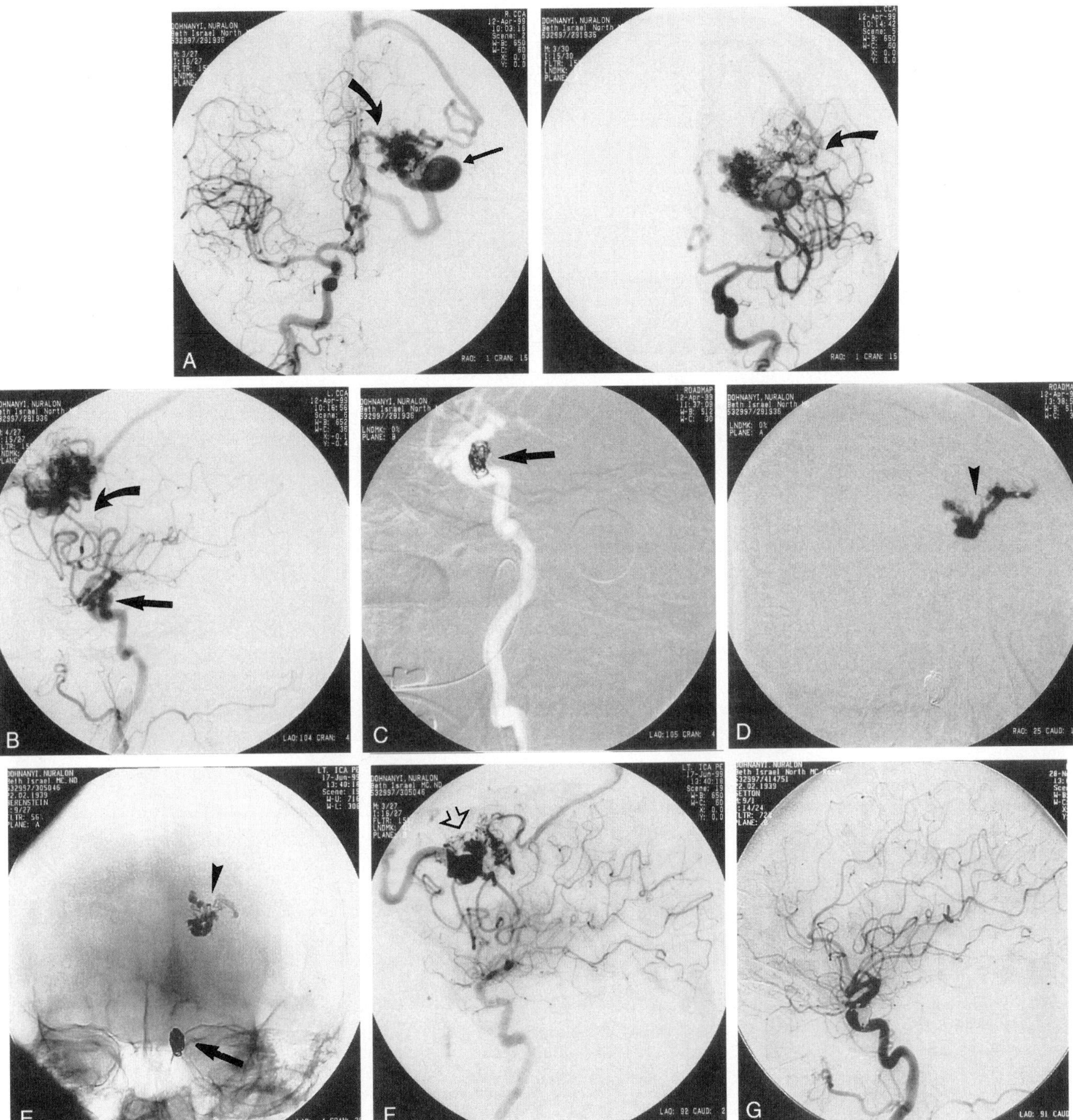

FIGURE 129–6. Preoperative embolization of a right frontal arteriovenous malformation (AVM) with a proximal left superior hypophyseal aneurysm. *A,* Anteroposterior angiographic views of the right and left internal carotid arteries (ICAs) demonstrate the malformation. A large, proximal venous aneurysm *(arrow)* and pial supply by the left anterior cerebral artery (ACA) and left middle cerebral artery (MCA) *(curved arrows)* cortical branches are seen. *B,* In the lateral angiographic view of the left common carotid, notice a left superior hypophyseal aneurysm *(arrow)* and the left MCA pial supply *(curved arrow). C,* A roadmap lateral view was obtained during endovascular occlusion of the aneurysm using Guglielmi detachable coils (GDCs) *(arrows). D,* A live fluoroscopic, subtracted anteroposterior oblique view demonstrates the acrylic cast *(arrowhead)* achieved by embolizing the malformation through a left ACA feeding cortical branch. *E,* The final radiopaque acrylic cast *(arrowhead)* is seen on an x-ray film of the skull. Notice the GDCs in the aneurysm *(arrow). F,* The lateral angiographic view of the left ICA after embolization but before surgery shows a small, residual malformation *(open arrow)* supplied by MCA frontal branches. The left hypophyseal aneurysm is completely obliterated by the coils. *G,* The patient underwent an uneventful microsurgical resection of the residual AVM. A follow-up lateral angiogram of the left ICA confirms complete removal and stable occlusion of the aneurysm.

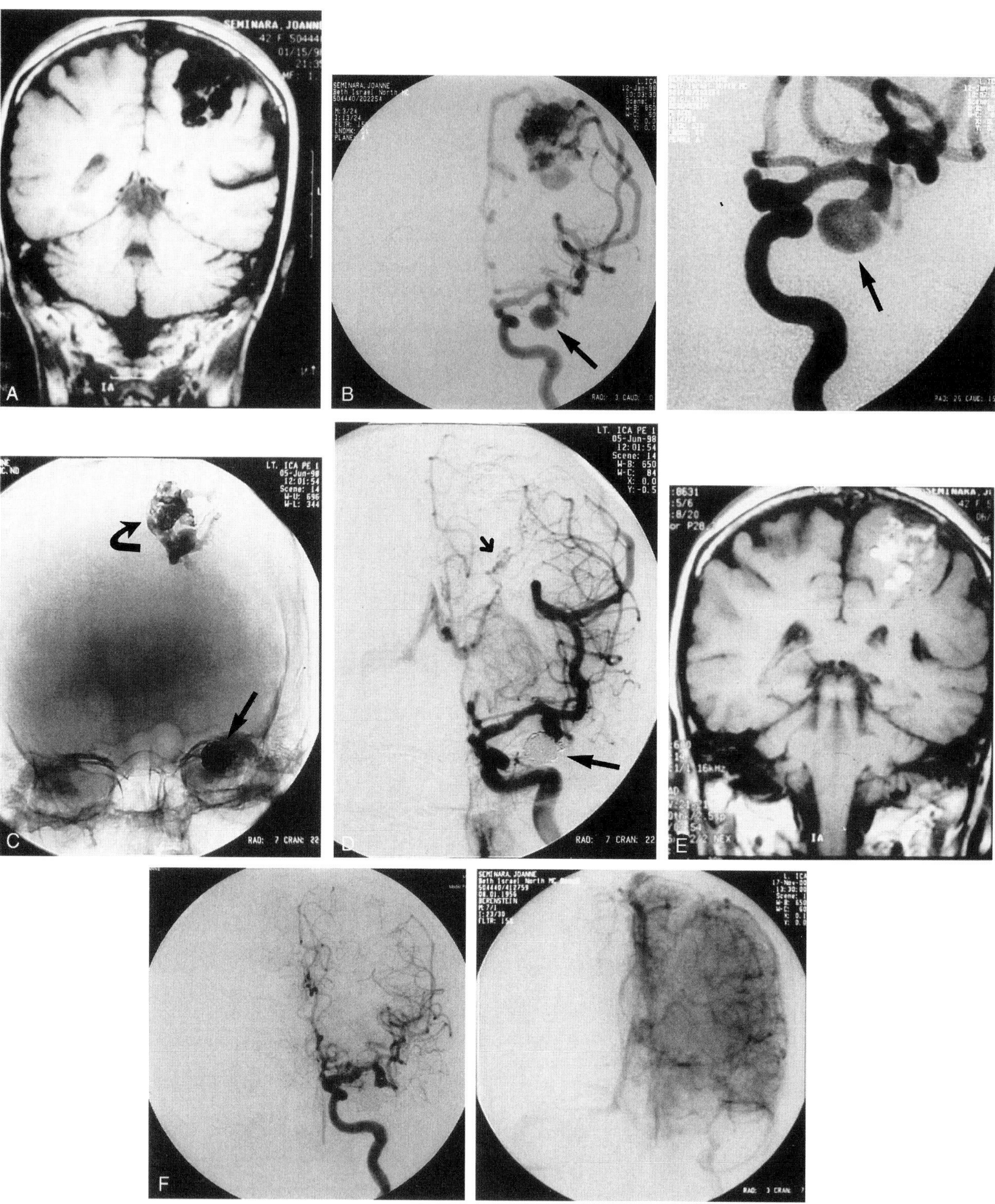

FIGURE 129–7. A left, posterior-frontal arteriovenous malformation (AVM) and a large, proximal aneurysm. Combined endovascular occlusion of the aneurysm and malformation nidus was achieved before radiosurgery. *A,* On coronal, T1-weighted magnetic resonance imaging (MRI), notice the high-flow cortical-gyral AVM. *B,* On global and magnified views of the anteroposterior angiogram of the left internal carotid artery (ICA), notice a proximal middle cerebral artery (MCA) aneurysm *(arrow)* and the cortical wedge shape of the malformation supplied by the left MCA and anterior cerebral artery distal branches. *C,* On the anteroposterior skull x-ray film obtained after the last endovascular procedure, notice the radiopaque acrylic cast in the nidus *(curved arrow)* and coils in the proximal aneurysm *(arrow)*. *D,* On the anteroposterior angiogram of the left ICA after the last endovascular procedure, notice the small, residual nidus deep within the white matter that drains to the deep venous system *(small arrow)*. Complete occlusion of the MCA aneurysm *(large arrow)* was achieved, and the patient was treated by radiosurgery for the residual malformation. *E,* Postembolization, T1-weighted, coronal MRI shows the acrylic casting of the nidus as a bright signal due to Lipiodol in the acrylic mixture. *F,* In the follow-up study after radiosurgery, the anteroposterior arterial and venous phases of a left ICA angiogram confirm complete obliteration.

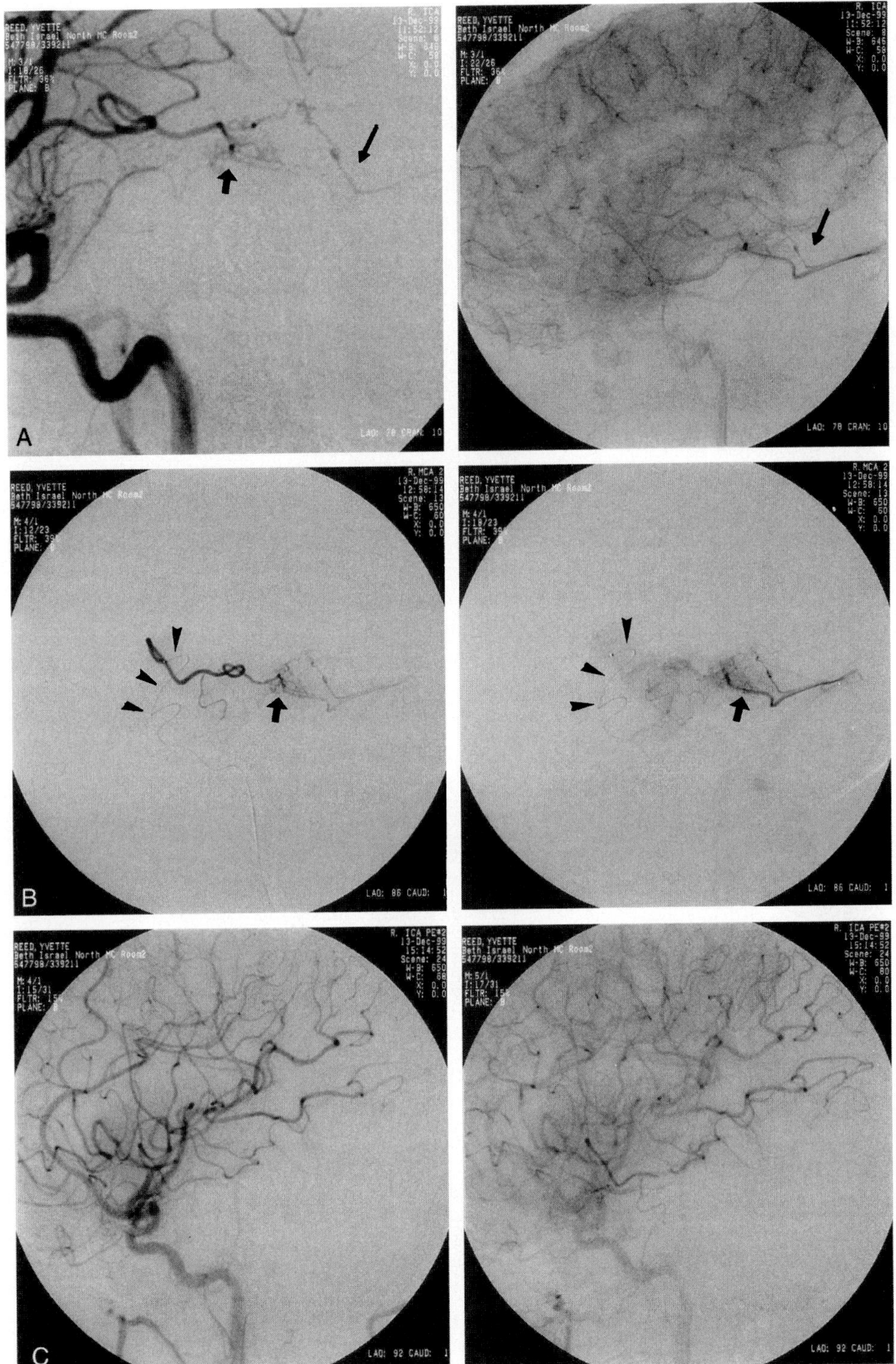

FIGURE 129–8. A right temporal micro–arteriovenous malformation (micro-AVM) in a patient presenting with a large parenchymal hematoma. *A,* On the early arterial and capillary phases of a lateral angiogram of the right internal carotid artery (ICA), notice the posterior temporal micro-AVM *(small arrow)* with early cortical venous drainage *(large arrow). B,* On the early and late phases of a lateral superselective angiogram performed through a microcatheter *(arrowheads)* in a minimally enlarged superior temporal branch, notice the normal proximal cortical branches with a parenchymal blush and distal cortical supply to the malformation *(arrow). C,* The early and late arterial phases of a lateral postembolization angiogram of the right ICA show that complete obliteration was achieved without residual nidus or early venous shunting.

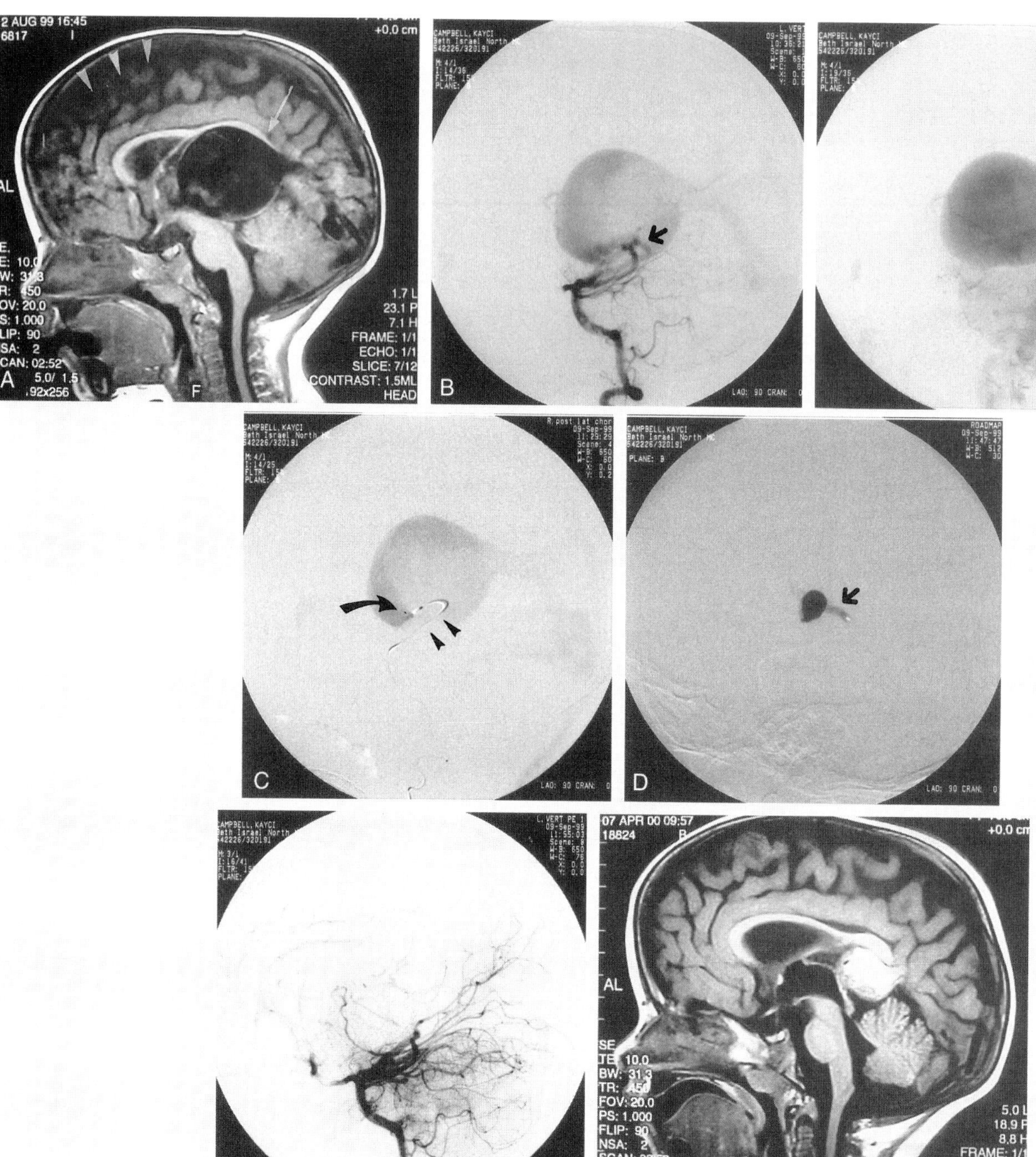

FIGURE 129–9. Vein of Galen malformation in a 1-year-old child presenting with macrocephaly. *A,* On sagittal, midline, T1-weighted magnetic resonance imaging (MRI), notice a very large, ballooned vein of Galen *(arrow)* and large cortical cerebrospinal fluid spaces *(arrowheads). B,* The arterial and late venous phases of the lateral angiographic views of the left vertebral artery show direct fistulization by a posterior choroidal branch *(arrow)* into the ballooned vein of Galen, draining to a straight and falcine sinuses. This is a characteristic mural-type malformation of the vein of Galen. *C,* On the lateral view of a superselective angiogram performed through a microcatheter *(arrowheads)* in the right posterior choroidal artery leading pedicle, notice the fistula site *(curved arrow)* in the wall of the ballooned vein. *D,* The fluoroscopic subtracted lateral view shows the acrylic cast occluding the leading pedicle and the fistula site *(arrow)* and protruding to the vein. *E,* After embolization, the lateral view of a left vertebral angiogram shows obliteration of the mural fistula, which achieved an anatomic cure without residual, early venous shunting and a normal arterial tree. *F,* Sagittal, midline, T1-weighted MRI (without contrast) was obtained 7 months after embolization. Notice the major size reduction of the ballooned vein. The high signal intensity in the venous lumen is compatible with residual thrombus. Further shrinkage is expected as the child develops normally.

tween the host and the BAVM. Only when the patient becomes symptomatic should treatment be considered to reestablish this equilibrium. Reestablishment of equilibrium may be attained without curative treatment because partial targeted embolization may be sufficient. Embolization should be used to occlude weakness in the angioarchitecture, mainly in cases of nidal pseudoaneurysms (see Fig. 129–3), distal arterial aneurysms, and venous aneurysms with decreased venous pressure and mostly in patients with outflow venous restriction and venous hypertension (see Fig. 129–4).

After partial embolization, clinical assessment and imaging follow-up are used to verify the results. If the intended goal of the embolization was obliteration of angioarchitectural weakness deemed responsible for a recent hemorrhage, follow-up angiography should be performed within days of the procedure to confirm that the therapeutic goal was achieved, thereby confirming the reduction of future hemorrhage risk.

If embolization was performed to reverse a progressive neurological deficit, clinical and MRI assessments in 3 to 6 months are recommended to determine whether the goal has been achieved and whether additional treatment stages are necessary (see Fig. 129–4). We believe that reduction of venous pressure and venous hypertension are the goals of this mode of treatment and can be documented by angiography and MRI. This management strategy should be discussed with the patient before treatment because it can facilitate patient compliance during the treatment and follow-up stages.

Combination Treatments

Anatomic cure can be accomplished by a combination of two or more modalities, one of which usually is endovascular embolization. A multimodality treatment plan can minimize risk and improve outcome.

PREOPERATIVE EMBOLIZATION

During the past 2 decades, the role of presurgical embolization of BAVMs has become well accepted and firmly established.[24–27] Facilitation of the surgical removal of the BAVM is the goal of preoperative embolization (see Fig. 129–6). To provide the best outcome with the lowest overall morbidity to the patient, communication between the neurointerventionalist and the vascular neurosurgeon regarding the specific goals of embolization is imperative.

The goals of preoperative BAVM embolization usually include one or more of the following: elimination of deep arterial feeders, occlusion of intranidal high-flow arteriovenous fistulas, overall size reduction, and obliteration and diminution of flow through the nidus. In recent years, obliteration of remote aneurysms and staged AVM occlusion, permitting gradual hemodynamic adaptation, have widened the use of staged presurgical procedures (see Fig. 129–6).

The choice of embolic agent used for preoperative BAVM embolization has varied over the past several decades. In the early 1960s, silicone spheres were used.[28–31, 32] Later, silk and polyethylene threads[33, 34] and polyvinyl alcohol (PVA) particles[35, 36] were used. Since the late 1970s and early 1980s, liquid adhesives—isobutyl-2-cyanoacrylate (IBCA) followed by *n*-butyl-2-cyanoacrylate (NBCA)—have been used as embolic agents.[37] PVA and NBCA have been the most widely used agents for presurgical embolization, and their safety and efficacy have been established.[25–27, 38–40] NBCA was shown to be superior to PVA for the purpose of presurgical embolization when outcome and combined endovascular and neurosurgical morbidity were considered.[27] A randomized study of presurgical embolization of BAVMs documented equivalence between NBCA and PVA microparticles. Primary and secondary efficacy endpoints and clinical safety endpoints were met and led to U.S. Food and Drug Administration approval of NBCA for presurgical use.[40]

We believe that, whenever possible, surgical resection, mostly in large lesions, should be delayed for 1 to 3 weeks after embolization to allow progressive thrombosis, which may occur after presurgical embolization, and stabilization of local and regional hemodynamic changes.

EMBOLIZATION AND RADIOSURGERY

The two major goals of embolization before stereotactic radiosurgery are overall size reduction and targeted embolization of specific angioarchitectural abnormalities (see Fig. 129–7). Preradiosurgical embolization of BAVM may be performed to decrease the size of the lesion to a volume suitable for radiosurgery. The volume of the AVM is one of the most important indicators predicting the success of stereotactic radiosurgery in achieving complete obliteration.[41–43] However, global size reduction by endovascular embolization of large-volume AVMs is not always possible. Volume diminution is most difficult to attain in lesions with feeders from multiple territories and in lesions located in areas with marked potential for collateral supply (i.e., occipital and temporal lobes). In such cases, to avoid the induction of collateral supply, intranidal deposition of embolic material is mandatory (see Fig. 129–7). Although limited data are available concerning the success rate of embolization for size reduction as the primary goal of treatment,[22] it remains the only method available to reduce BAVM size to within the range amenable by radiosurgery. At our institution, approximately 10% of patients undergoing planned preradiosurgical BAVM embolization required no further therapy because the embolization procedure achieved total obliteration.

Targeted preradiosurgical BAVM embolization may be performed in cases of angioarchitectural abnormalities believed to increase the risk of hemorrhage. Distal flow-related aneurysms, intranidal pseudoaneurysms, venous aneurysms, and venous outflow restriction should be targeted using a liquid adhesive. Large, irregular, multilobulated, proximal aneurysms should be occluded using Guglielmi detachable coils (GDCs) to eliminate the risk of future rupture and subarachnoid hemorrhage (see Figs. 129–6 and 129–7). We believe that a permanent embolic agent such as NBCA should be used for preradiosurgery embolization, regardless of the indication (i.e., size reduction or targeted embolization). There is no role for embolization with PVA or coils, because no permanent nidus obliteration can be achieved. Conversely, permanent occlusive agents such as NBCA should not be used for only proximal feeder occlusion, because it leads to induction of a collateral supply and destabilization of the lesion.[21, 44]

We advocate a waiting period between the embolization procedure and stereotactic radiosurgery. Repeat angiography may be performed before radiosurgery (within 2 to 3 months) to confirm the stability nidus occlusion and to delineate final size and volume.

TECHNIQUES OF EMBOLIZATION

Selective cerebral angiography that follows a protocol that includes bilateral carotid and vertebral angiography as well as mapping the pial and dural territories is mandatory for angioarchitecture evaluation. Correlation of the axial imaging (MRI) and angiographic studies is important in planning a global treatment, including endovascular goals and possible microsurgery or radiosurgery by a multidisciplinary group. The diagnostic angiographic studies are performed most commonly as elective outpatient studies or before the first therapeutic procedure. The use of small-caliber diagnostic catheters (4 or 5 Fr), roadmapping, and high-quality angiographic equipment (preferably biplane) helps to reduce risk and complications. The introduction of three-dimensional rotational angiography may further advance our appreciation of nidus architecture, flow dynamics, and compartmental structure.

For embolization procedures, we advocate general anesthesia, rarely with neurophysiologic monitoring for functional provocative testing. In our experience, high-quality angiography and knowledge of the functional vascular anatomy are the most important factors in differentiating normal from abnormal vasculature (see Fig. 129–5). Awake patients under local sedation and anesthesia stand-by with functional testing have been used by other groups with no clear advantages.

Superselective catheterization of the intracranial circulation is performed using microcatheters inserted coaxially through a guiding catheter in the parent vessel. Our group prefers flow-guided catheters, but over-the-guide wire microcatheters are used less often. We find the softer, flexible flow-guided catheters are advantageous in distal navigation along tortuous arterial loops. They have a reduced risk of vessel penetration, dissection, or spasm, and they are beneficial in entering the malformation nidus or leading pedicles to it. New hydrophilic micro–guide wires and microcatheters enhance the safety of distal navigation in cortical and deep penetrating branches.

With the goal of permanently occluding the malformation nidus and fistulization, not merely proximal pedicle occlusion, the use of liquid embolic material is mandatory to enable distal penetration. The use of microcoils is only supplementary to slow flow or to protect normal territory before acrylic deposition.

Achieving distal microcatheter position in the nidus or close to it offers the possibility of delivering embolic material under complete or partial flow control and the use of a lower concentration of acrylic. Prolongation of the injection period and improvement of permeation into the malformation nidus can be achieved without increasing the risk of gluing the microcatheter.

For fluoroscopic visualization, the acrylic (i.e., NBCA) is mixed with Lipiodol, an oily contrast material. The mixture is radiopaque, enabling accurate detection of acrylic deposition under live fluoroscopic monitoring and visualization on plain skull films (see Figs. 129–6 and 129–9). In addition to radiopacity, the Lipiodol retards the polymerization pace of acrylic. Changes in the mixture are adjusted according to flow conditions. In high-flow conditions, a high concentration of acrylic mixture can achieve early polymerization and occlusion. In flow-control situations, a low concentration of an acrylic-Lipiodol mixture can prolong the polymerization and may enable distal penetration into the malformation nidus. Tantalum powder is another agent used to opacify acrylic, mainly when pure acrylic is needed. In high-flow conditions, mainly with direct fistulization, induced systemic hypotension (by the anesthesiologist) for the acrylic injection period and the use of high acrylic concentrations are means to prevent untoward venous occlusion.

Our experience favors staging the malformation occlusion. The amount of fistulous and nidus occlusion, change in size and flow in venous drainage pathways, and malformation location (cortical versus deep AVM) are general considerations influencing our decision. Repeated interim angiographic studies help in assessing the procedure's progress and indicate staging.

Careful postoperative monitoring in the intensive care unit is a cornerstone in postoperative management. Monitoring vital signs and neurological status is essential in preventing and detecting hemodynamic or neurological changes. We advocate axial imaging, even without any detectable neurological deficit, to visualize the residual malformation and surrounding parenchymal signal change, to follow the venous drainage pathways, and to detect silent unexpected hemorrhage (see Figs. 129–4 and 129–7).

OUTCOMES AND COMPLICATIONS

Treatment of BAVM is a multidisciplinary team effort combining several stages and modalities. In accordance

TABLE 129–1 ■ **Morbidity and Mortality, January 1992 to December 1994, for 699 Patients (744 Procedures)**

	MORBIDITY		MORTALITY	
PROCEDURES	**%**	**No.**	**%**	**No.**
Total	2.1	16/744	0.53	4/744
Brain arteriovenous malformations	2	4/180	0.5	1/180
Aneurysms	9	9/98	1	1/98
Angiograms	0.16	2/1232	—	—

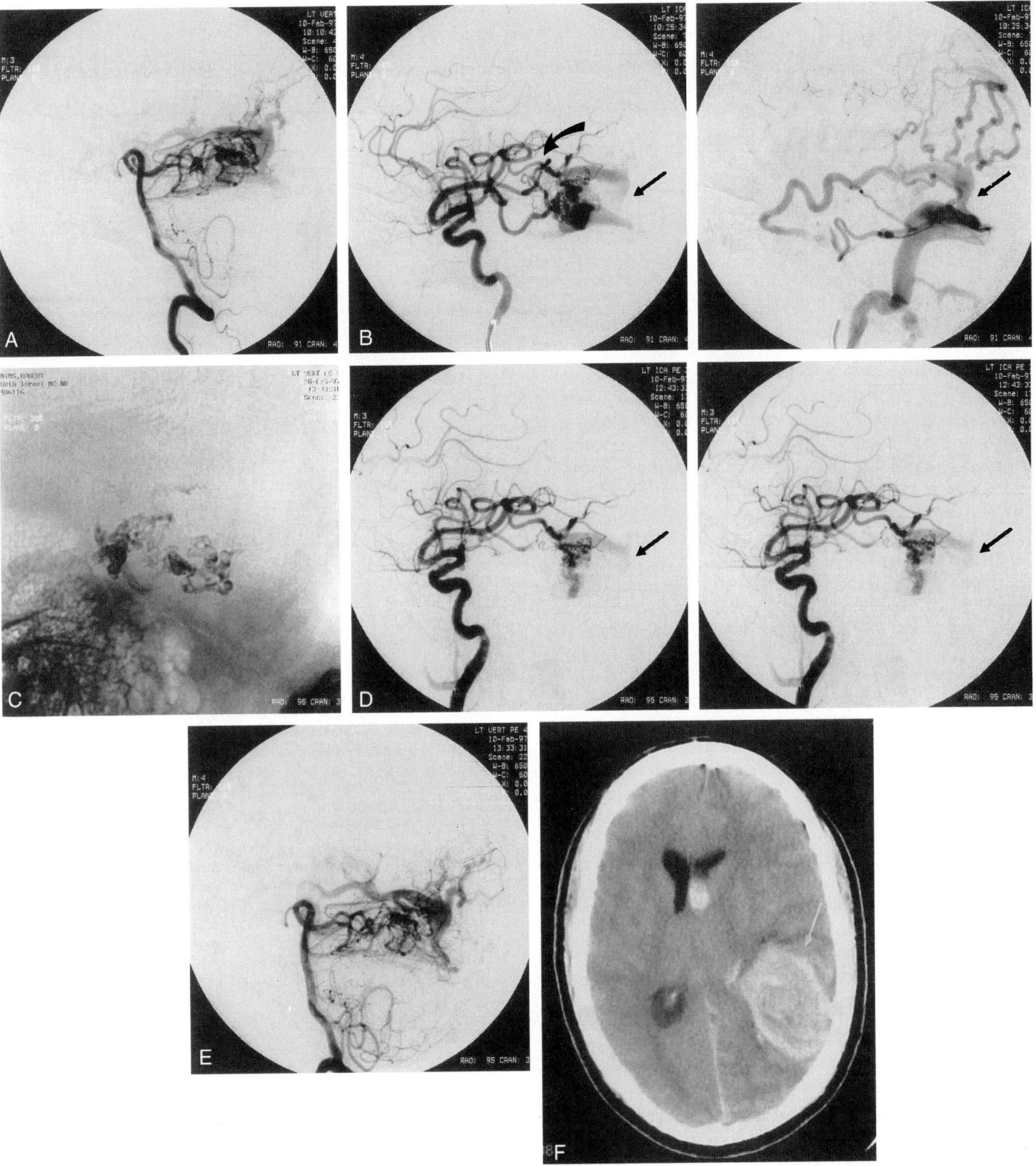

FIGURE 129–10. Late complications after endovascular embolization of a symptomatic left temporal arteriovenous malformation. *A,* The lateral view of the left vertebral angiogram demonstrates posterior temporal branches off the left posterior cerebral artery that supply the posterior compartment of the malformation with cortical venous drainage. *B,* The arterial and late venous phases of the lateral view of the left internal carotid artery (ICA) angiogram show that the left middle cerebral artery (MCA) temporal branches *(curved arrow)* supply the anterior compartment. Notice the multiple ectasias in the nidus, with cortical venous drainage by the vein of Labbé *(arrow)* and secondary venous reflux to the parietal and temporal cortical veins. *C,* As shown on a lateral view, a radiopaque acrylic cast was achieved by embolization through the temporal branches. *D,* The arterial and late venous phases of the lateral view of the left ICA angiogram show embolization of the anterior compartment. Reduction of the malformation size and shunting and maintaining a patent venous outflow *(arrow). E,* After embolization, the lateral angiographic view of the left vertebral artery demonstrates, as in the baseline study, the posterior compartment with patent venous outflow. *F,* A computed tomographic scan 8 hours after the procedure demonstrates an acute, large, left temporal hematoma *(arrow)*, intraventricular hemorrhage, a mass effect, and a midline shift. The patient who was neurologically intact immediately after embolization experienced delayed, acute deterioration. He was operated on emergently for clot evacuation and decompression.

TABLE 129–2 ■ **Brain Arteriovenous Malformations: Morbidity and Mortality, January 1998 to September 1999, for 90 Patients (144 Procedures)**

NEUROLOGIC DEFICIT					
Transient	**Permanent**	**DEATHS**	**SILENT/IMAGING**	**TECHNICAL**	**PUNCTURE SITE**
3	1 severe (late hemorrhage) 4 mild (2 late hemorrhages, 2 infarcts)	1	2 hemorrhages 11 infarcts	2	1
3.3%	5.5%	1.1%	14.4%	2.2%	1.1%

with the experience reported in the literature, only complete obliteration of a malformation can be considered a cure, abolishing future risk. Because the rate of total angiographic obliteration is still variable and relatively small, combined-therapy outcome reports are not readily available and difficult to compile.[45] Rates up to 16% were reported for combined-treatment–related complications among 1510 patients; 7% had permanent neurological deficits, and the mortality rate was 1%. Additional information regarding complementary treatment methods can be found in other chapters. We assessed our experience and complication rate for brain AVM treatment as part of a review of intracranial procedures. Two distinct periods were studied. During an early period, from 1992 to 1994 (Table 129–1), the permanent morbidity rate was 2%, and the mortality rate was 0.5% for 180 procedures. A periodic review from 1998 to 1999 (Table 129–2) revealed a permanent morbidity rate of 5.5% and a mortality rate of 1.1% for 144 procedures. In recent years, we regularly obtain early imaging, even without clinical deterioration or neurological changes. MRI can reveal signal changes around the malformation and adjacent parenchyma in 14.4%. In most cases, no clinical expression was found. Our accumulated experience in endovascular therapy highlights early neurological deficit and delayed postembolization hemorrhages (within 12 to 48 hours) as the main events influencing outcome after partial or complete embolization (Fig. 129–10).

Continuous technical developments and advancements in microcatheters and micro–guide wires with miniaturization, increased flexibility, and hydrophilic coating enhance the safety of endovascular approaches to malformations. Distal cortical and deep perforator territories are accessible while reducing the complications of vascular injury and retaining glued catheters.

We emphasize the use of permanent liquid embolic agent (i.e., acrylic) for obliteration of the malformation core and shunts within the nidus-venous junction. Future development of nonadhesive permanent agents may improve the success rate for total nidus obliteration, achieving angiographic anatomic cure. Permanent effective occlusion of the AVM nidus is instrumental in facilitating microsurgical resection or stereotactic radiosurgery, improving the success rate and reducing complications and procedural risks.

ACKNOWLEDGMENTS

We would like to give special thanks to Geum Joo Hwang, M.D., and Angel Arce for their contributions in the preparation of this manuscript and to Mary Madrid, R.N., Ph.D., for her contribution as Director of Patient Care.

REFERENCES

1. Gentili F, Schwartz M, TerBrugge K, Wallace M: A multidisciplinary approach to the treatment of brain vascular malformations. Adv Tech Stand Neurosurg 19:179–207, 1992.
2. Deruty R, Pelissou-Guyotat I, Morel C, et al: Reflections on the management of cerebral arteriovenous malformations. Surg Neurol 50:245–255, 1998.
3. Berenstein A, Lasjaunias P: Surgical Neuroangiography: Endovascular Treatment of Cerebral Lesions, vol 4. Berlin, Springer-Verlag, 1992, p 317.
4. Crawford P, West C, Chadwick DW, Shaw M: Arteriovenous malformations of the brain: Natural history in unoperated patients. J Neurol Neurosurg Psychiatry 49:1–10, 1986.
5. Yasargil M: Pathologic considerations. In Yasargil M (ed): Microneurosurgery, AVM of the Brain: History, Embryology, Pathologic Considerations, Hemodynamics, Diagnostic Studies, Microsurgical Anatomy, vol 3A. New York, Thieme, 1987, pp 49–211.
6. Horton J, Chambers W, Lyons S, et al: Pregnancy and the risk of hemorrhage from cerebral arteriovenous malformations. Neurosurgery 27:867–871, 1990.
7. Ondra S, Troupp H, George E, Schwab K: The natural history of symptomatic arteriovenous malformations of the brain: A 24-year follow-up assessment. J Neurosurg 73:387–391, 1990.
8. Mast H, Young W, Koennecke H, et al: Risk of spontaneous haemorrhage after diagnosis of cerebral arteriovenous malformation. Lancet 350:1065–1068, 1997.
9. Graf C, Perret G, Torner J: Bleeding from cerebral arteriovenous malformations as part of their natural history. J Neurosurg 58: 331–337, 1983.
10. Meisel H, Mansmann U, Alvarez H, et al: Cerebral arteriovenous malformations and associated aneurysms: Analysis of 305 cases from a series of 662 patients. Neurosurgery 46:793–800, 2000.
11. Carter L, Gumerlock M: Steal and cerebral arteriovenous malformations. Stroke 26:2371–2372, 1995.
12. Hurst R, Berenstein A, Kupersmith M, et al: Deep central arteriovenous malformations of the brain: The role of endovascular treatment. J Neurosurg 82:190–195, 1995.
13. Spetzler R, Martin N: A proposed grading system for arteriovenous malformations. J Neurosurg 65:476–483, 1986.
14. Brown R, Wiebers D, Forbes G, et al: The natural history of unruptured intracranial arteriovenous malformations. J Neurosurg 68:352–357, 1988.
15. Redekop G, TerBrugge K, Montanera W, Willinsky R: Arterial aneurysms associated with cerebral arteriovenous malformations: Classification, incidence, and risk of hemorrhage. J Neurosurg 1998; 89:539–546.
16. Vinuela F, Drake C, Fox A, et al: Giant intracranial varices secondary to high-flow arteriovenous fistulae. J Neurosurg 66:198–203, 1982.
17. Halbach V, Higashida R, Hieshima G, Hardin C: Transarterial occlusion of solitary intracerebral arteriovenous fistulas. AJNR Am J Neuroradiol 10:747–752, 1989.
18. Berenstein A, Choi I, Neophytides A, Benjamin V: Endovascular treatment of spinal cord arteriovenous malformations (SCAVMs). AJNR Am J Neuroradiol 10:898, 1990.

19. Lasjaunias P, Berenstein A: Surgical Neuroangiography: Endovascular Treatment of Craniofacial Lesions, vol 2. Berlin, Springer-Verlag, 1987, p 397.
20. Fournier D, Rodesch G, Terbrugge K, Flodmark R: Acquired mural (dural) arteriovenous shunts of the vein of Galen: Report of 4 cases. Neuroradiology 33:52–55, 1991.
21. Gruber A, Mazal P, Bavinzski G, Killer M: Repermeation of partially embolized cerebral arteriovenous malformations: A clinical, radiologic, and histologic study. AJNR Am J Neuroradiol 17:1323–1331, 1996.
22. Gobin Y, Laurent A, Merienne L, et al: Treatment of brain arteriovenous malformations by embolization and radiosurgery. J Neurosurg 85:19–28, 1996.
23. Valavanis A, Yasargil M: The endovascular treatment of brain arteriovenous malformations. Adv Tech Stand Neurosurg 24: 131–214, 1998.
24. Pelz D, Lownie S, Fox A: Thromboembolic events associated with the treatment of cerebral aneurysms with Guglielmi detachable coils. AJNR Am J Neuroradiol 19:1541–1547, 1998.
25. Vinuela F, Dion J, Duckwiler G, Martin N: Combined endovascular embolization and surgery in the management of cerebral arteriovenous malformations: experience with 101 cases. J Neurosurg 75:856–864, 1991.
26. Jafar J, Davis AJ, Berenstein A, et al: The effect of embolization with N-butyl cyanoacrylate before surgical resection of cerebral arteriovenous malformations. J Neurosurg 78:60–69, 1993.
27. Wallace R, Flom RA, Khayata M, et al: The safety and effectiveness of brain arteriovenous malformation embolization using acrylic and particles: The experience of a single institution. Neurosurgery 37:608–618, 1995.
28. Luessenhop A, Gibbs M, Velasquez A: Cerebrovascular response to emboli: Observations in patients with arteriovenous malformations. Arch Neurol 7:264–274, 1962.
29. Luessenhop A, Kachmann R, Shevlin W, et al: Clinical evaluation of artificial embolization in the management of large cerebral arteriovenous malformations. J Neurosurg 23:400–417, 1965.
30. Kricheff I, Madayag M, Braunstein P: Transfemoral catheter embolization of cerebral and posterior fossa arteriovenous malformations. Radiology 103:107–111, 1972.
31. Wolpert S, Stein B: Catheter embolization of intracranial arteriovenous malformations as an aid to surgical excision. Neuroradiology 10:73–85, 1975.
32. Hilal S, Michelson W: Therapeutic percutaneous embolization for extraaxial vascular lesions of head, neck and spine. J Neurosurg 43:275–287, 1975.
33. Benati A, Beltramello A, Maschio A, Perini S: Combined embolization of intracranial AVMs with multi-purpose mobile-wing microcatheter system; indications and results in 71 cases. AJNR Am J Neuroradiol 8, 1987.
34. Benati A, Beltramello A, Colombari R, et al: Preoperative embolization of arteriovenous malformations with polyethylene threads: Techniques with wing microcatheter and pathologic results. AJNR Am J Neuroradiol 10:579–586, 1989.
35. Latchaw R, Gold L: Polyvinyl foam embolization of vascular and neoplastic lesions of the head, neck and spine. Radiology 131: 669–679, 1979.
36. Scialfa G, Scotti G: Superselective injection of polyvinyl alcohol microemboli for the treatment of cerebral arteriovenous malformations. AJNR Am J Neuroradiol 6:957–960, 1985.
37. Cromwell D, Kerber C: Modification of cyanoacrylate for therapeutic embolization: Preliminary experience (a). AJNR Am J Neuroradiol 1:113, 1980.
38. DeMeritt J, Pile-Spellman J, Mast H, Moohan N: Outcome analysis of preoperative embolization with N-butyl cyanoacrylate in cerebral arteriovenous malformations. AJNR Am J Neuroradiol 16:1801–1807, 1995.
39. Jordan J, Marks M, Lane B, Steinberg G: Cost-effectiveness of endovascular therapy in the surgical management of cerebral arteriovenous malformations. AJNR Am J Neuroradiol 17:247–254, 1996.
40. U.S. Food and Drug Administration CfDaRH. PMA: P990040 TRUFILL® n-Butyl Cyanoacrylate (n-BCA) Liquid Embolic System. Washington, DC, U.S. Food and Drug Administration, 2001.
41. Steinberg G, Fabrikant J, Marks M, Levy R: Stereotactic heavy-charged-particle Bragg-peak radiation for intracranial arteriovenous malformations. N Engl J Med 323:96–101, 1990.
42. Lunsford L, Kondziolka D, Flickinger J, Bissonette D: Stereotactic radiosurgery for arteriovenous malformations of the brain. J Neurosurg 75:512–524, 1991.
43. Karlsson B, Lindquist C, Steiner L: Prediction of obliteration after gamma knife surgery for cerebral arteriovenous malformations. Neurosurgery 40:425–430, 1997.
44. Fournier D, Terbrugge K, Rodesch G, Lasjaunias P: Revascularization of brain arteriovenous malformations after embolization with bucrylate. Neuroradiology 32:497–501, 1990.
45. Group TAMS: Current Concepts: Arteriovenous Malformations of the Brain in Adults. N Engl J Med 340:1812–1818, 1999.

CHAPTER 130

Embolization of Arteriovenous Malformations as a Primary Treatment Modality

BERND RICHLING ■ MONIKA KILLER ■ ANDREAS GRUBER

Brain arteriovenous malformations (AVMs) are challenging cerebrovascular lesions. As Yasargil[1] reported, Dandy[2] stated that "the radical attempt at cure is attended by such supreme difficulties and is so exceedingly dangerous as to be contraindicated except in certain selected cases." Cushing and Bailey[3] found that "the surgical history of most of the reported cases shows not only the futility of an operative attack upon one of these angiomas, but the extreme risk of serious cortical damage which is entailed."

Because of these early surgical results, alternative treatment modalities were developed. Endovascular therapy was adopted as an adjunctive measure to overcome the obvious problems of open AVM surgery. Early results were disappointing. Medium and large AVMs could not be occluded totally and permanently, and the procedure-related complication rate was significant. Since then, increased understanding of AVM pathomorphology and significant refinements in endovascular technique have improved the risk-to-benefit ratio, and endovascular treatment has become a cornerstone in the therapeutic management of brain AVMs. Notwithstanding, total permanent occlusion (i.e., definitive cure of the brain AVM by endovascular embolization as the primary treatment modality) is achieved in only selected cases. The prerequisite to curing an AVM definitively with endovascular techniques alone is angioarchitecture that permits solid casting of the AVM nidus with a permanent embolizing material.

MORPHOLOGIC CRITERIA

Brain AVMs are cerebrovascular anomalies with a fistulous connection between feeding arteries and draining veins in the absence of a normal intervening capillary bed. Superselective microangiography discloses the angioarchitecture of the AVM (i.e., the morphology of the feeding arteries, the nidus, the draining veins, and the associated vascular anomalies). These parameters influence the outcome of endovascular therapy because they determine the accessibility of the lesion with microcatheter systems, the size of the AVM nidus, and its hemodynamic properties.

Accessibility

Accessibility of the nidus with the microcatheter is crucial. If an AVM feeder cannot be catheterized superselectively, embolization carries a high risk of inadvertently occluding physiologic arteries branching off the feeder between the microcatheter tip and the nidus. The resultant ischemia can damage physiologic brain parenchyma. If the subselective microcatheter position is not used, embolization remains incomplete.

The angioarchitectonic parameters that predict the accessibility of an AVM nidus with a microcatheter are the length, tortuosity, and diameter of the individual feeder. The arterial supply of brain AVMs can be derived from pial and dural arteries as well as from perforating and choroidal branches. Pial AVM feeders often are accessible with flow-directed and flow-independent microcatheter systems. In larger and longstanding lesions, arterial high-flow angiopathy can elongate significantly the tortuosity of the arterial AVM supply, which may be difficult to overcome with either microcatheter system. Only superselective microangiography can determine whether the feeders terminate in the AVM nidus (i.e., end-standing feeders) or continue distal to the AVM and supply normal brain parenchyma (i.e., feeders *en passage*). Although selective injection usually can be performed in the former, embolization endangers the distal normal brain parenchyma in the latter case.

Dural contributions are encountered in approximately 30% of brain AVMs.[4, 5] In most cases, these feeders require guidewire-supported microcatheter systems to permit selective approaches. AVMs with dural feeders particularly tend to recur either from recanalization of the branch that was cast initially or from dural collateralization. Perforating arteries and choroidal feeders can supply deep-seated brain AVMs and lesions in the vicinity of the ventricular system. In some cases, selective microcatheter approaches to perforating arteries are possible, but they carry a considerable risk of embolization-related permanent morbidity. The risk-to-benefit ratio of such injections must be scrutinized in light of the expected therapeutic benefits. In the spirit of combined management for brain AVMs, radiosurgery should be considered in most of these cases.

Size

In 1971, Doppman and coworkers[6] introduced the term *nidus*, which refers to the AVM segment where the arteriovenous shunt occurs (i.e., the area between the distal segment of the feeding arteries and the proximal segment of the draining veins). According to Yasargil's work,[1] the AVM nidus can be occult (not seen angiographically and not found at surgery), cryptic (invisible at angiography and surgery but recognized histologically), micro (just visible on angiography), small (1 to 2 cm), moderate (2 to 4 cm), large (4 to 6 cm), and giant (>6 cm).

The size of an AVM nidus apparently influences the difficulty of surgical resection and has been included in most surgical classifications of AVMs. Likewise, the size of an AVM is a crucial factor that determines whether the nidus can be obliterated totally and permanently by endovascular embolization.

Usually, only small brain AVMs with easily accessible feeders can be occluded totally and permanently without increasing the rate of procedure-related complications. The number of completely occluded brain AVMs is small in most reported endovascular series. In their series, Vinuela and colleagues[7] completely occluded 9.9% of small and medium-sized AVMs. Wikholm and associates[8] completely obliterated 71% of AVMs smaller than 4 mL but only 15% of AVMs whose volume ranged from 4 to 8 mL. In these two series, the overall rate of obliteration was 13.3%.[7, 8] In the 1996 series of Gobin and colleagues,[9] the overall rate of complete obliteration was 11.2%. In 1998, Valavanis and Yasargil[10] reported complete obliteration of 60% of sulcal AVMs but only 12.5% of gyral AVMs with endovascular therapy.

Large lesions tend to have additional dural and perforating arterial feeders. The therapeutic result of their embolization may be limited by the accessibility of the perforating arterial supply and the durability of the occlusion of the dural feeders. Larger AVMs may have many tortuous pial contributions, which may be difficult to approach even with current sophisticated microcatheter systems.

Hemodynamic Properties

In addition to the angioarchitectonic characteristics of the nidus and its feeders, the hemodynamic properties of an individual AVM nidus are crucial for successful endovascular embolization. The number and morphology of the arteriovenous shunts and the velocity of the arteriovenous shunting determine whether embolic material can be deposited selectively in the nidus.

The nidus of a brain AVM can be compact or diffuse, although the diffuse angiographic appearance of a perinidal hypervascularity often is related to high-flow arterial angiopathy rather than to diffuse segments of the AVM nidus. An AVM nidus can have one or more compartments, and it can be plexiform, fistulous, or mixed. In a plexiform nidus, selective angiography discloses a multitude of intranidal arteriovenous shunts. The diameter of the vessels is usually small, and the velocity of arteriovenous shunting is usually low. In contrast, fistulous lesions lack the plexiform area of the nidus but usually involve a single-hole, high-flow arteriovenous fistula. This pattern of arteriovenous shunting can be found in conjunction with a plexiform nidus in larger, so-called mixed lesions. The angioarchitecture of the AVM nidus and the velocity of arteriovenous shunting are crucial determinants of whether lesions can be embolized totally and permanently. Although particles and liquid embolic agents often can be deployed safely in low-flow plexiform lesions, fistulous-type lesions and high-velocity arteriovenous shunts are associated with the risk of losing embolic material on the venous side of the AVM.

TECHNICAL ASPECTS

As outlined, the endovascular accessibility of a brain AVM greatly reflects the angioarchitecture of its feeding arteries. Significant improvements in the field of microcatheter technology now permit the superselective catheterization of most pial AVM feeders.

Choice of Catheter

The first microcatheters that allowed a selective approach to AVM feeders were flow directed and occasionally mounted with *calibrated leak balloons* that controlled flow during injection.[11] The obvious advantage of flow control was outweighed, however, by the difficulty and sometimes unpredictability of handling the catheter. Later, a new generation of microcatheters with progressive softness was developed,[12–14] and these microcatheters combined the mechanical properties of different catheter designs in one tool. The proximal stiff, thick-walled catheter segment controls torque and transmits longitudinal movements without delay. The intermediate catheter segment is flexible but still transmits torque; the distal segment is soft and thin-walled. Depending on the type of catheter used, the distal section can be soft (i.e., flow-guided catheters [Magic, Balt, Paris]), or it can provide torque stability (i.e., flow-independent, microguidewire-supported systems [Tracker series, Boston Scientific/Target Therapeutics, Fremont, CA]).

Progressive catheter softness, guidewires suitable for cerebral vasculature (0.010 to 0.016), and hydrophilic microcatheter surface coatings (e.g., FasTRACKER series, Boston Scientific/Target Therapeutics, Fremont, CA) have improved significantly the performance of current microcatheter systems. Elongated and tortuous feeders can be approached and navigated with flow-dependent microcathers, and small arteries that branch at acute angles from large arterial stems can be approached with flow-independent, microguidewire-supported systems.

Flow Control

When a superselective microcatheter has been positioned in an AVM feeder, an individual compartment can be cast if flow can be controlled. Ideally, a solid column of embolic material is injected from a superselective microcatheter position in the AVM feeder.

As mentioned, high-velocity arteriovenous shunting, unsuitable nidal angiomorphology (i.e., fistulous single-hole compartments), or both can frustrate these attempts. This situation occurs if the angiogram shows *congestion* of the nidus (i.e., slow or stationary dye) during the endovascular procedure. Stenotic narrowing of draining veins is another risk factor because small amounts of glue passing through the shunt can occlude the stenotic portion of the draining vein. A special risk can arise with multicompartmental AVMs with multiple feeders and one draining vein. Under these circumstances, the casting of one compartment, including the venous outlet, can obstruct the draining system for the other compartments.

To overcome these difficulties, several techniques have been proposed. First, some microcatheter designs permit flow control in the feeder during embolization (calibrated leak balloon catheter). Second, soft platinum wires (available straight and coiled) can be injected through the microcatheter in high-flow fistulas before glue embolization.[15, 16] These *liquid coils* (Boston Scientific/Target Therapeutics, Fremont, CA) remain in the fistula site and prevent a large amount of glue from migrating through the fistula. Finally, embolization can be performed with the patient under induced systemic arterial hypotension or transient cardiac arrest.

Embolizing Material

After the description of free-flow embolization techniques using Silastic pellets[17]; blood clots[18]; and finely cut dura, Gelfoam, or polyvinyl-alcohol particles (Ivalon),[19] Zanetti and Sherman[20] introduced polymerizing cyanoacrylates as liquid embolic agents for endovascular embolization. Because of their low viscosity, cyanoacrylates can be injected through microcatheters, and their resistence to in vivo biodegradation is high.[21–23] The currently used Histoacryl-blue (*n*-butyl-2-cyanoacrylate [NBCA]) hardens immediately on contact with free hydrogen ions and is mixed with low-viscosity oily contrast media (e.g., Lipiodol ultrafluid) or tantalum powder for radiologic visualization. To prevent the Histoacryl-blue from hardening prematurely during injection, the catheter is rinsed with glucose (33%).

In general, solid casting of the entire nidus with cyanoacrylate can occlude totally and permanently an AVM in one of two ways. The embolic material can fill the nidus solidly, or it can block selectively the strategic sites of arteriovenous shunting inside the AVM nidus, which resembles the radiographic pattern of a *spotted distribution* of cast material inside the nidus.

Long-term follow-up studies support the notion that total solid casting of brain AVMs with cyanoacrylates is permanent; similar data are lacking for other embolic materials. Polyvinyl alcohol particles of defined sizes (150 to 500 μ) have been used for endovascular embolization of brain AVMs, but they provide only transient occlusion in the preoperative setting. This problem was overcome partially by the addition of 95% alcohol and collagen (Avitene). This so-called LA mixture permits a more stable occlusion than particles alone, presumably because of the marked inflammatory tissue reaction elicited by the alcohol added to the compound. Because balloons and microcoils usually occlude vessels proximally rather than distally, these tools are considered adjunctive measures only.

RISK ASSESSMENT

The first report addressing the risk associated with intra-arterial embolization was published by Wolpert and Stein,[24] who described neurological deficits from *aberrant emboli*. In 1981, Samson and colleagues[25] reported the intravascular use of isobutyl 2-cyanoacrylate and found no permanent treatment-related morbidity. Endovascular embolization of brain AVMs using cyanoacrylates has been associated consistently with an 8% to 22% rate of treatment-related morbidity and a 1.6% to 6.9% rate of treatment-related mortality.[8, 26–33]

Rates of treatment-related morbidity and mortality have not improved significantly in the past 15 years. Despite enormous improvements in the field of microcatheter technology and in x-ray equipment, the risk of suffering a technical complication during embolization has remained almost unchanged. In 1982, Debrun and coworkers[26] reported a 22% rate of morbidity and a 2.2% rate of mortality. In 1996, Gobin and associates[9] reported a 12.8% rate of morbidity and a 1.6% rate of mortality. In most cases, technical factors related to the procedure itself are assumed to underlie the complication rate. Most of these treatment-related technical complications resulted in intracerebral hemorrhages, ischemic strokes, or both; pulmonary embolism from dislodged embolic material or intranidal pyogenic infections are considered rare procedural complications.

Additionally a patient's age and general medical condition can alter the expected procedural risks. Atherosclerotic vessel wall disease increases the risk of embolic complications from dislodged atherosclerotic plaque, of incomplete embolization caused by atherosclerotic elongations of the AVM feeders that limit the endovascular accessibility of the nidus, and of thromboembolic complications from the manipulation of prolonged endovascular catheters. Additional risks from inappropriate endovascular technique and insufficient neurointerventional equipment are evident and not discussed.

Given the therapeutic options available for patients harboring a brain AVM (i.e., open surgery and radiosurgery), the potential procedure-related risks of embolization must be compared closely with the expected risk-to-benefit ratio. If total endovascular occlusion of the AVM can be attained only with a high risk of procedural complication, combined treatment strategies must be considered (i.e., embolization in conjunction with surgery or radiosurgery).

LONG-TERM ASPECTS

Histopathologic Findings

Endovascular embolization of brain AVMs leads to a definitive cure if the nidus is obliterated completely and patients remain stable at follow-up angiography. Repermeation of a previously embolized AVM represents a major threat to the quality of treatment. The results of embolization usually are estimated from postinterventional angiograms and long-term follow-up examinations.

Reliable angiographic follow-up studies showed stable total and solid casting of the AVM nidus in patients embolized with Histoacryl. Because AVMs totally embolized with Histoacryl-blue are considered cured, these lesions seldom are resected, and histopathologic data are sparse. We studied embolization-related lesions in tissue and the degree of intranidal cast repermeation in the surgical specimens of 26 AVM patients subtotally embolized with Histoacryl-blue who subsequently underwent open surgical resection.[34] The pattern and time course of embolization-related tissue lesions were typical. Structures did not repermeate during the first 3 months after embolization. In contrast, repermeation was shown in every case operated on later than 3 months after the first embolization (Fig. 130–1). Only the interval between the first embolization and surgery related to repermeation of the cast. Although the resistance to biodegradation may be altered by changing the Histoacryl-to-Lipiodol ratio of the compound, we found no evidence that either the Histoacryl-to-Lipiodol ratio or the addition of glacial acetic acid influenced the onset of repermeation. The location of the AVM, degree of preoperative nidus reduction, and Spetzler-Martin grade did not correlate with repermeation.

The tissue responses induced by the embolizing substance must be relatively mild because the cast is intended to remain in vivo for a lifetime. Heat production during the initial exothermic polymerization and the formaldehyde released during the breakdown process of cyanoacrylates have been proposed as causative factors underlying embolization-related tissue lesions. Some degree of mural inflammation seems to act synergistically, however, with the embolizing substance to occlude the nidus permanently by forming scars and fibrosis.

Among the embolization-related tissue lesions that we found, inflammation (Fig. 130–2) occurred in 25 cases (96%). Acute inflammation, comprising predominantly polymorphonuclear cells, occurred 24 hours after embolization. Chronic inflammation, marked by the appearance of transmural lymphocytic infiltration and foreign body giant cells within the cast areas, was detected in 23 cases (88.5%). Lymphocytic infiltration occurred 1 week after the intervention. Foreign body giant cells were not detected until 1 month after embolization but were detectable for 52 months thereafter. Mural angionecrosis (Fig. 130–3) began 2 days after embolization and reached a maximum after 1 week. Because of fibrosis of the vessel wall, angionecrosis was visible only 2 months after embolization. Intima loss, shrinking and calcification of the media, intramural hemorrhage, extravasation of the glue, and inflammation of neuronal tissue after embolization with cyanoacrylates other than Histoacryl-blue were not encountered in our series.

Altogether, our data indicate that the tissue re-

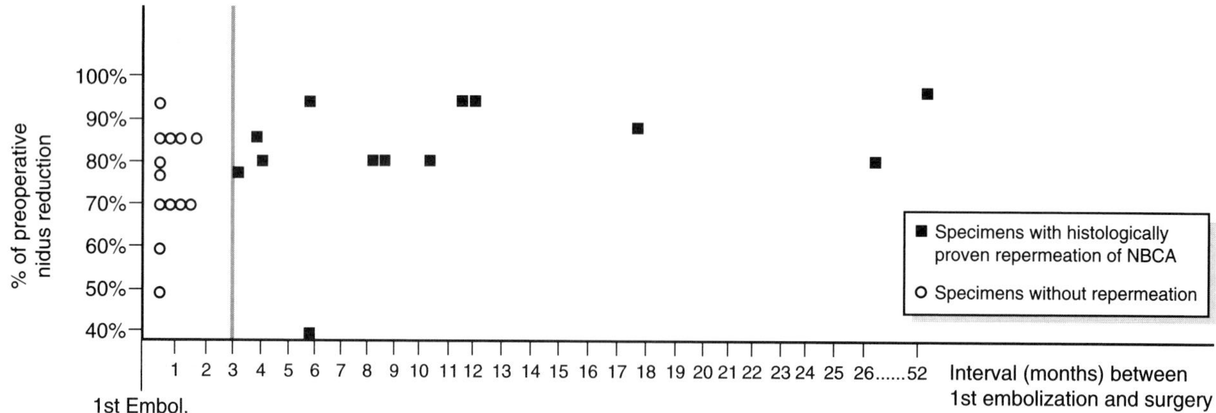

FIGURE 130–1. Repermeation of intranidal NBCA. Specimens are plotted according to their interval between first embolization and surgery (months) and according to the extent of preoperative endovascular nidus reduction (%). The graph shows the positive correlation between repermeation and the interval between the first embolization and surgery and the lack of correlation between repermeation and the extent of preoperative endovascular nidus reduction. Repermeation did not occur before 3 months after the first embolization. *Specimens with histologically proven repermeation of NBCA; °specimens without repermeation.

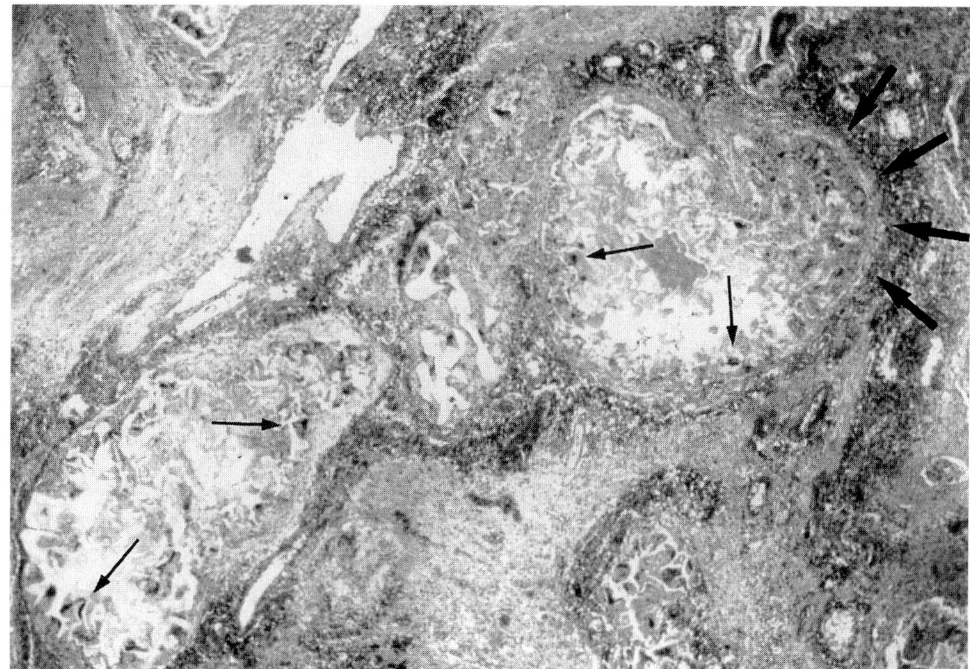

FIGURE 130–2. Photomicrograph of vascular channel containing embolic material. Intraluminal NBCA is surrounded by foreign body giant cells *(small arrows)* and a transmural inflammatory infiltration of the vessel wall *(large arrows)*. (Hematoxylin and eosin, ×40.)

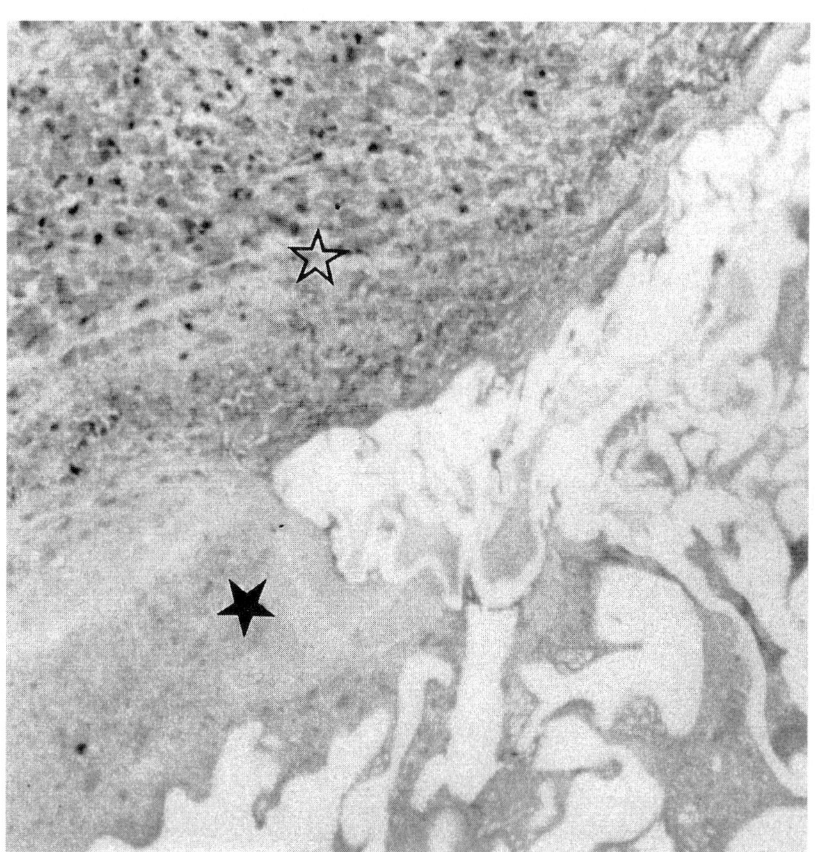

FIGURE 130–3. Photomicrograph shows an area of marked mural angionecrosis *(open star)* in proximity to the intraluminal cast *(black star)*. (Hematoxylin and eosin, ×20.)

sponses to Histoacryl-blue can be considered relatively benign. Angionecrosis is replaced by fibrosis of the vessel wall within 2 months, and acute inflammation develops into a chronic lesion within 1 month of embolization. Intranidal repermeation of the cast tends to occur longer than 3 months after embolization with Histoacryl-blue if the nidus is not obliterated completely.

OUTCOMES

In the Department of Neurosurgery at the University Hospital of Vienna, 34 AVMs were treated between 1985 and 1997 (unpublished data).[34, 35] Nineteen (55.9%) patients were male, and 15 (44.1%) were female. Their ages ranged from 1 to 69 years (mean age, 30.2 years). The presenting symptom was hemorrhage in 13 (38.2%) cases, seizures in 8 (23.5%) cases, and headache in 13 (38.2%) cases.

Nine (26.5%) AVMs were grade 1, 11 (32.4%) were grade 2, 10 (29.4%) were grade 3, and 4 (11.7%) were grade 4 according to the Spetzler-Martin classification.[36] In 26 cases (76.4%), the size of the AVM nidus was smaller than 3 cm, and in 8 (23.6%) AVMs, it was between 3 and 6 cm.

Fifteen (44.1%) AVMs were located on the right side, 12 (35.3%) were on the left, and 7 (20.6%) were in the midline. Five AVMs each were located in the frontal, temporal, and occipital lobes; central region; and basal ganglia. Three AVMs were in the posterior fossa. Five patients had a vein of Galen malformation.

Thirty-one (91.1%) AVMs had only one or two feeding arteries; the remaining 3 (8.9%) AVMs had more than two feeders. Thirty (88.2%) AVMs had pial feeders only; 2 (5.9%) AVMs had pial and perforating feeding arteries; and 2 (5.9%) AVMs had only perforating feeding arteries. In two patients (5.9%), an additional arterial aneurysm was found on the selective diagnostic angiogram (a flow-related aneurysm on the feeding artery and an intranidal aneurysm). Nine (26.5%) patients had venous ectasias.

Seventeen (50%) AVMs had a single superficial draining vein. Seven (20.6%) drained through a single deep vein. Six (17.6%) AVMs had multiple deep and superficial draining veins. Three (8.8%) AVMs had

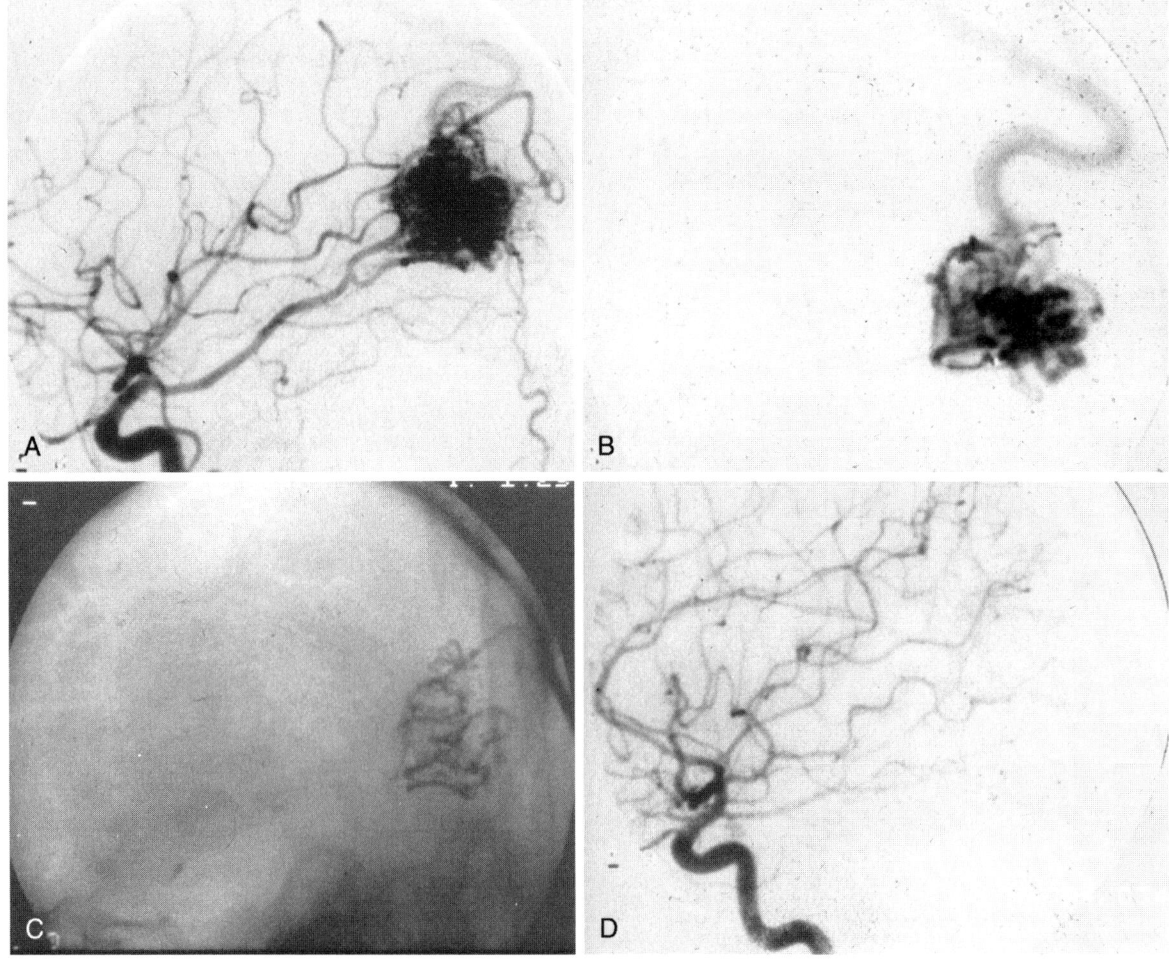

FIGURE 130–4. *A*, Left internal carotid artery angiogram in lateral view shows a parieto-occipital arteriovenous malformation (Spetzler-Martin grade 2). *B*, Superselective approach of one of the two compartments before embolization. *C*, Final cast in lateral view. *D*, Left internal carotid artery angiogram in lateral view after total embolization of the arteriovenous malformation.

multiple superficial draining veins, and one (3%) AVM had multiple deep draining veins.

In 34 patients, total AVM occlusion was achieved with embolization only (Fig. 130–4).[31–34] Only one embolization was necessary to occlude the AVM totally in 26 (76.4%) patients. Seven (20.6%) patients needed a second embolization to achieve total AVM occlusion, and one patient needed a third procedure.

Three patients underwent an additional operation. One patient underwent embolization 5 years after the initial operation because a follow-up angiogram showed revascularization of the AVM nidus. One patient underwent surgery the day after the endovascular procedure despite angiographic confirmation of total occlusion because only one feeder could be cast during the embolization. The third patient underwent surgery immediately after embolization because of hemorrhage during that procedure. This is the only patient in the series whose condition worsened after the endovascular procedure.

Three patients underwent radiosurgery as an additional treatment. One patient developed thrombosis in the remaining AVM after one of the two main feeders was embolized. Although angiography showed total occlusion of the AVM, radiosurgery was performed for security. One patient underwent radiosurgery twice as the primary treatment of AVM. On the 1-year follow-up angiogram after the second radiosurgical procedure, the patient's AVM was still perfused. A recurrent hemorrhage was the indication for endovascular treatment in this patient's case. The third patient underwent radiosurgery 3 months after embolization because the 3-month follow-up magnetic resonance imaging study and angiography showed that the AVM was reperfused.

Twenty-five (73.5%) patients had perfect clinical outcomes, and 8 (23.5%) had good clinical outcomes (i.e., their symptoms improved or their clinical course was stable). The one patient (3%) who worsened after embolization had a bad clinical outcome and died from pneumonia during rehabilitation.

CONCLUSION

To cure brain AVMs by endovascular embolization, the arteriovenous shunt must be occluded permanently. Typically, AVMs can be excluded from the brain vasculature by casting the AVM nidus with a rapidly polymerizing liquid. Partial casting of the AVM, especially if feeding arteries are occluded, may lead to the angiographic disappearance of the AVM. The angiogenetic capacity of the AVM reconstitutes perfusion to nonembolized arteriovenous shunts, however. The recurrent AVM is fed by multiple collaterals, making any further therapy more difficult.

Ideally, each endovascular approach through an AVM feeding artery to the nidus can lead to total casting of the vascular compartment involved. Factors such as the size of the nidus and vascular compartment, the angioarchitecture of the compartment, and the flow conditions and difficulties associated with positioning a catheter close to or inside the nidus hinder therapists from achieving a total cast. After medium or large AVMs are treated by a *feeder-by-feeder* approach, some components may be solidly cast, whereas others are partially cast. Postprocedural angiography may show remnants fed by branches too small or too tortuous to be used as an approach to the lesion.

In most published series, the number of totally and permanently embolized AVMs is small (unpublished data).[7, 9, 34] AVMs cured by endovascular therapy tend to be small with relatively simple architecture. There is no doubt that this kind of lesion can be cured by surgery or radiosurgery. For small, deep-seated AVMs with one or two feeding arteries, however, especially those in the basal ganglia, endovascular embolization offers an excellent treatment option with immediate protection from new or recurrent hemorrhage. For embolization of medium-sized and more complex AVMs, the strategic decision to consider is whether the target of total occlusion and endovascular cure is associated with a higher therapeutic risk than (eventually staged) preoperative embolization with subsequent surgery.

Endovascular therapy of brain AVMs can effect cures or help to effect cures. How aggressive endovascular therapy should be pursued must be decided by an endovascular therapist who can assess the individual risk factors of the endovascular treatment and the need for subsequent therapies.

REFERENCES

1. Yasargil MG: Microneurosurgery: Vol IIIA. AVM of the Brain. New York, Thieme Medical Publisher, 1987.
2. Dandy WE: Venous abnormalities and angiomas of the brain. Arch Surg (Chicago) 17:715–793, 1928.
3. Cushing HP, Bailey P: Tumours Arising from the Blood Vessels of the Brain: Vol III. Angiomatous Malformations and Hemangioblastomas. Springfield, IL, Charles C Thomas, 1928.
4. Newton TH, Cronqvist ST: Involvement of dural arteries in intracranial arteriovenous malformations. Radiology 93:1071–1078, 1969.
5. Willinsky RH, Lasjaunias P, TerBrugge K, et al: Brain arteriovenous malformations: Analysis of the angio-architecture in relationship to hemorrhage (based on 152 patients explored and/or treated at the hospital de Bicetre between 1981 and 1986). J Neuroradiol 15:225–237, 1988.
6. Doppman JL, Zapol W, Pierce J: Transcatheter embolization with silicone rubber preparation: Experimental observation. Invest Radiol 6:304–309, 1971.
7. Vinuela F, Duckwiler G, Gugliemi G, et al: Intravascular embolization of brain arteriovenous malformations. In Maciunas RJ (ed): Endovascular Neurological Intervention. American Association of Neurological Surgeons, Park Ridge, IL, 1995, pp 189–199.
8. Wikholm G, Lundqvist C, Svendsen P: Embolization of cerebral arteriovenous malformations: Part I. Technique, morphology, and complications. Neurosurgery 39:448–459, 1996.
9. Gobin YP, Laurent A, Merienne L, et al: Treatment of brain arteriovenous malformations by embolization and radiosurgery. J Neurosurg 85:19–28, 1996.
10. Valavanis A, Yasargil MG: The endovascular treatment of brain arteriovenous malformations. Adv Tech Stand Neurosurg 24: 131–214, 1998.
11. Kerber C: Balloon catheter with a calibrated leak: A new system for superselective angiography and occlusive catheter therapy. Radiology 120:547–550, 1976.
12. Berenstein A: Technique of catheterization and embolization of the lenticulostriate arteries. J Neurosurg 54:783–789, 1981.
13. Latchaw RE, Gold LHA: Polyvinyl foam embolization of vascular

and neoplastic lesions of the head, neck, and spine. Radiology 131:669–679, 1979.

14. Luessenhop AJ, Kachmann R, Shevlin W, Ferrero AA: Clinical evaluation of artificial embolization in the management of large cerebral arteriovenous malformations. J Neurosurg 23:400–417, 1965.
15. Berenstein A, Lasjaunias P: Surgical Neuroangiography, vol 4. New York, Springer, 1991, p 93.
16. Richling B, Knosp E: Ein führungsdrahtgesteuertes Kathetersystem zur Begehung und Embolisation intrazerebraler Arterien. In Schneider GH, Vogler E (eds): Digitale bildgebende Verfahren, Interventionelle Verfahren, Integrierte digitale Radiologie. Berlin, Springer, 1988, pp 348–351.
17. Luessenhop AJ, Rosa L: Cerebral arteriovenous malformations: Indications for and results of surgery, and the role of intravascular techniques. J Neurosurg 60:14–22, 1984.
18. Rösch J, Dotter CT, Brown MJ: Selective arterial embolization: A new method for control of acute gastrointestinal bleeding. Radiology 102:303–306, 1972.
19. Porstmann W, Wierny L, Warnke H, et al: Catheter closure of patent ductus arteriosus: 62 cases treated without thoracotomy. Radiol Clin North Am 9:203–218, 1971.
20. Zanetti PH, Sherman FE: Experimental evaluation of a tissue adhesive as an agent for the treatment of aneurysms and arteriovenous anomalies. J Neurosurg 36:72–79, 1972.
21. Richling B: Homologous controlled-viscosity fibrin for endovascular embolization: Part I. Experimental development of the medium. Acta Neurochir (Wien) 62:159–170, 1982.
22. Richling B: Homologous controlled-viscosity fibrin for endovascular embolization: Part II. Catheterization technique, animal experiments. Acta Neurochir (Wien) 64:109–124, 1982.
23. Richling B: The current state in endovascular treatment of cerebral arteriovenous malformations. In Aichinger F, Gerstenbrand F, Grcevic N (eds): Neuroimaging II. New York, Gustav Fischer, 1988, pp 309–315.
24. Wolpert SM, Stein BM: Catheter embolization of intracranial arteriovenous malformations as an aid to surgical excision. Neuroradiology 10:73–85, 1975.
25. Samson D, Ditmore QM, Beyer CW Jr: Intravascular use of isobutyl 2-cyanoacrylate: Part 1. Treatment of intracranial arteriovenous malformations. Neurosurgery 8:43–51, 1981.
26. Debrun G, Vinuela F, Fox A, Drake C: Embolization of cerebral arteriovenous malformations with bucrylate. J Neurosurg 56: 615–627, 1982.
27. Deruty R, Lapras C, Pierluca P, et al: Preoperative embolization of cerebral arteriovenous malformations with butylcyanoacrylate (18 cases) [French]. Neurochirurgie 31:21–29, 1985.
28. Lasjaunias P, Manelfe C, Terbrugge K, Lopez Ibor L: Endovascular treatment of cerebral arteriovenous malformations. Neurosurg Rev 9:265–275, 1986.
29. Merland JJ, Rufenacht D, Laurent A, Guimaraens L: Endovascular treatment with isobutyl cyano acrylate in patients with arteriovenous malformation of the brain: Indications, results and complications. Acta Radiol 369(suppl):621–622, 1986.
30. Berthelsen B, Lofgren J, Svendsen P: Embolization of cerebral arteriovenous malformations with bucrylate: Experience in a first series of 29 patients. Acta Radiol 31:13–21, 1990.
31. Schumacher M, Horton JA: Treatment of cerebral arteriovenous malformations with PVA: Results and analysis of complications. Neuroradiology 33:101–105, 1991.
32. Benati A: Interventional neuroradiology for the treatment of inaccessible arterio-venous malformations. Acta Neurochir (Wien) 118:76–79, 1992.
33. Bartholdy NJ, Haase J: Interventional neuroradiology: A presentation with preliminary results [Danish]. Ugeskr Laeger 156: 6541–6548, 1994.
34. Gruber A, Mazal PR, Bavinzski G, et al: Repermeation of partially embolized cerebral arteriovenous malformations: A clinical, radiologic, and histologic study. AJNR Am J Neuroradiol 17:1323–1331, 1996.
35. Richling B, Bavinzski G: Arterio-venous malformations of the basal ganglia: Surgical versus endovascular treatment. Acta Neurochir Suppl (Wien) 53:50–59, 1991.
36. Spetzler RF, Martin NA: A proposed grading system for arteriovenous malformations. J Neurosurg 65:476–483, 1986.

CHAPTER 131

Surgical Management of Supratentorial Arteriovenous Malformation

MICHAEL J. FRITSCH ■ ROBERTO C. HEROS

In few instances in neurosurgery are the management decisions as difficult as in the treatment of cerebral arteriovenous malformations (AVMs). This chapter reviews pathogenesis, diagnostic evaluation, treatment paradigms, and surgical approaches for supratentorial AVMs. The complications and outcome after surgical intervention are analyzed. Although a thorough understanding of the natural history of AVMs is essential for intelligent treatment decisions, this topic is discussed at length in another chapter.

PATHOGENESIS

AVMs are believed to be congenital, developmental malformations rather than angiomas or true vascular neoplasms. The structure of the lesions suggests an aberration in the development of the fetal circulation and persistence of primitive artery-to-vein shunts without intervening capillaries that normally occur during the early stages of central nervous system vascularization.[1] AVMs consist of a nidus, feeding arteries, and draining veins. The direct anastomosis of arteries and veins creates a high-flow, low-resistance shunt. The nidus is built by a complex of arteries, veins, and cavernous channels. Histologic studies have shown that there is mainly gliotic tissue within the malformation, with little or no normal neural tissue. The feeding arteries lack normal smooth musculature and elastica. Hyalinization and calcification of the vessels are common. The arteries do not exhibit normal patterns of autoregulation to changes in blood flow and pressure. Laboratory studies have revealed limited or no contraction of the proximal feeding arteries to agents that stimulate contraction of smooth muscle.[2]

Draining veins typically are dilated and thin walled secondary to the arterial pressure transmitted directly into the venous system. Segmental dilation and venous aneurysms commonly are found, and occasionally these venous *varices* are responsible for focal neurological deficits from direct neural compression or for hydrocephalus from compression and obstruction of cerebrospinal fluid pathways.

Because most AVMs do not become symptomatic until the patient is in his or her 20s, it is reasonable to assume some dynamic progression regarding size and hemodynamics of the lesion. Recurrence of an AVM after a negative postoperative angiogram has been reported in children.[3, 4] This finding might be secondary to the relatively immature cerebral vasculature and may involve active angiogenesis promoted by an unrecognized humoral factor. Another possible mechanism could be low resistance driven by the direction of blood flow from the surrounding tissue to the AVM, recruiting adjacent vessels that initially were not involved in the lesion. Spontaneous intermittent thrombosis within the AVM and development of collateral flow may be part of the angiographically demonstrable proven dynamic changes in morphology and hemodynamics of AVMs. It is clear that AVMs in infants and children tend to be *simpler* and frequently pure arteriovenous fistulas rather than the more complicated angioarchitecture found in the usual adult AVM. These findings speak against the assumption that AVMs are strictly congenital lesions.

Spontaneous obliteration of cerebral AVMs is rare; the incidence is estimated to be less than 1%.[15] It is proposed that the occlusion of a single draining vein may lead to total venous outflow obstruction and secondary lesion thrombosis. Immunohistochemical and histologic analysis of an angiographically completely thrombosed AVM revealed possible neovascularization and patent vessels within the AVM.[5] The clinical significance of these observations is unclear. Rarely, strokes develop from spontaneous thrombosis with retrograde occlusion of feeding arteries. More rarely, a moyamoya-like angiographic picture develops because of gradual spontaneous stenosis and eventual occlusion of large arteries and gradual revascularization with hypertrophied anastomotic vessels.

The importance of venous outflow changes in the pathogenesis of AVMs has received greater attention.[6] Some of the progressive symptoms that traditionally have been attributed to arterial *steal* may be due at least partially to venous hypertension because the venous outflow system of many AVMs also is responsible for venous drainage of healthy brain parenchyma. Dynamic changes such as stenosis and occlusion of major draining veins and sinuses may be responsible not only for hemorrhage and the development of venous varices, but also for venous hypertension, increased intracranial pressure, and progressive neural dysfunction.

DIAGNOSTIC EVALUATION

A computed tomography (CT) scan can identify most patients harboring an AVM. An unenhanced CT scan frequently shows irregular hyperdense areas with frequent calcification. With the addition of contrast material, the nidus and feeding vessels or dilated draining veins can be visualized. The study can determine the localization of the lesion and the presence of acute hemorrhage, hydrocephalus, and old areas of encephalomalacia.

Magnetic resonance imaging (MRI) is superior to CT in showing the exact anatomic relationships of the nidus, feeding arteries, and draining veins as well as in showing topographic relationships between AVM and adjacent brain.[7] MRI is sensitive in revealing subacute hemorrhage.[8] The lesion frequently appears as a spongelike structure with low signal intensity on T1-weighted sequence secondary to the flow with associated enlarged vessels, which could be feeding arteries or draining veins. MRI and angiography in combination provide complementary information that facilitates understanding the three-dimensional anatomy of the malformation, its feeding arteries, and the draining veins. Although magnetic resonance angiography is able to provide three-dimensional images, it currently cannot replace transfemoral cerebral angiography.

Functional MRI is a technique that uses the local increase of oxyhemoglobin concentration as a result of increase in blood flow and volume to identify and localize eloquent cortex in relation to an AVM.[9, 10] The information provided by functional MRI can be helpful in determining whether a specific malformation is operable or not (Fig. 131–1).

Complete transfemoral cerebral angiography with multiple projections is mandatory for preoperative determination of localization of the nidus and the feeding arteries and venous drainage pattern as well as for assessment of hemodynamics of the AVM. The search for associated aneurysms is part of the preoperative evaluation. External carotid injections to determine the presence of an external supply are necessary in cases of large-convexity AVMs. It is important that the angiogram is performed or repeated near the time of surgical excision because AVMs can change in size and configuration with time. Vessels that were not seen secondary to compression from a hemorrhage may appear on a follow-up arteriogram weeks later.

TREATMENT

Indication for Surgical Treatment

The decision-making process involved in recommending surgical treatment for a patient with an AVM must be supported by an understanding of the risks related to the natural history and the treatment of that particular AVM. Patient-related factors, lesion-related factors, and surgeon-related factors need to be considered in the process of risk evaluation.

PATIENT-RELATED FACTORS

The patient's age is one of the most crucial factors in decision making and determines the number of years at risk for hemorrhage if the lesion remains untreated. If surgery is successful in a young patient, a long disease-free survival is achieved. If significant disability results, however, it may be lifelong. A young patient tolerates better an extended surgical procedure and has a superior capacity for neurological recovery from deficits that may result from surgery. AVMs tend to enlarge over time, reach a stable size, and occasionally decrease in size after middle age. How this behavior relates to the risk of hemorrhage is unclear.

The general medical and neurological condition of the patient is important in the decision-making process. Patients with a possibly life-limiting medical condition have fewer years at risk than healthy individuals of the same age. The risk of prolonged general anesthesia has to be considered. The neurological condition of the patient is important because the patient and the physician determine the success of an operation based on the neurological status preoperatively and postoperatively.

Another important consideration is whether or not patients are symptomatic from their lesion. A patient with a progressive neurological deficit, with frequent seizures, or who has had repeated hemorrhages would accept the risk of morbidity from surgery better than patients who are asymptomatic. A potential important source of misjudgment in the preoperative evaluation is to underestimate the capacity for recovery after a recent hemorrhage from an AVM. A patient with a hemorrhage from a thalamic AVM may be hemiplegic initially, and the surgeon may be tempted to operate at that stage because the patient probably would not be worse after surgery. Significant spontaneous recovery after such hemorrhages can occur, however, and it may be advisable to delay surgery in these patients for several weeks to allow time to determine whether improvement would occur or not. After that time period, a more rational judgment can be made regarding the potential for additional damage by surgical excision.

The psychological impact must be considered; patients can be devastated psychologically by the knowledge that they have a potentially dangerous lesion that could bleed at any time. This problem frequently is brought about or exacerbated if physicians have used the terms *bomb in the head* or *cocked pistol* to refer to the AVM.

LESION-RELATED FACTORS

The most reliable grading scale cannot include all possible factors that influence surgical risk. Judgment of the surgical risk always is an individual and subjective matter. Nevertheless, grading scales are helpful to en-

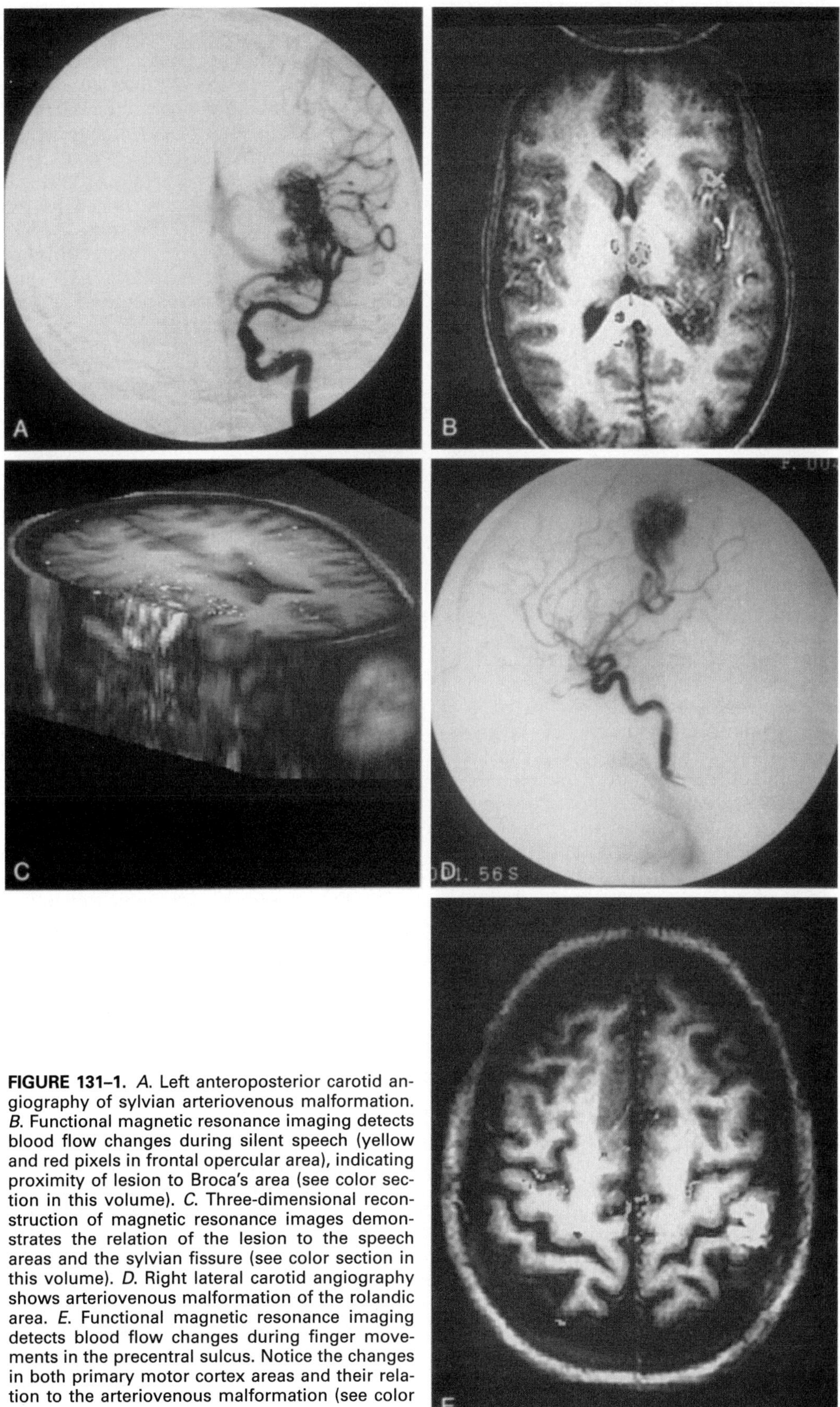

FIGURE 131–1. *A.* Left anteroposterior carotid angiography of sylvian arteriovenous malformation. *B.* Functional magnetic resonance imaging detects blood flow changes during silent speech (yellow and red pixels in frontal opercular area), indicating proximity of lesion to Broca's area (see color section in this volume). *C.* Three-dimensional reconstruction of magnetic resonance images demonstrates the relation of the lesion to the speech areas and the sylvian fissure (see color section in this volume). *D.* Right lateral carotid angiography shows arteriovenous malformation of the rolandic area. *E.* Functional magnetic resonance imaging detects blood flow changes during finger movements in the precentral sulcus. Notice the changes in both primary motor cortex areas and their relation to the arteriovenous malformation (see color section in this volume).

able a more precise evaluation of the risks of surgical treatment and to allow comparison of results. Several grading scales have been proposed by different authors to enable evaluation of lesion-related factors in AVM surgery. The predictive values of grading scales and of single clinical and radiographic factors were tested by Steinmeier and coworkers retrospectively.[11] The Spetzler-Martin grading system showed the best correlation for all tested outcome parameters and offered the best predictive value for operative difficulty and postoperative neurological condition.[12, 13] The system of Luessenhop and Rosa[14] was the best for predicting psychosocial outcome at 6 months after surgery. The most important single independent factor in predicting outcome at 6 months after surgery is the size of the AVM. Outcome correlates also with eloquence, deep venous drainage, number of feeding arteries, hemispheric dominance, and preoperative deficit.

The size of an AVM is responsible for much of the technical difficulty encountered in surgical resection. AVMs generally are considered to be small if they are less than 3 cm in diameter (1 point on the Spetzler-Martin grading scale); medium, if between 3 and 6 cm in diameter (2 points); and large, if more than 6 cm in diameter (3 points). The pattern of venous drainage is considered superficial if all draining veins are cortical (0 points). In contrast, the venous pattern is considered to be deep if all or part of the drainage is through the deep venous system (1 point). Following the classification proposed by Spetzler and Martin, lesions are considered eloquent (1 point) if they involve or are immediately adjacent to the sensorimotor, language, and visual cortex; the hypothalamus and thalamus, the internal capsule, the brainstem, the cerebellar peduncles, and the deep cerebellar nuclei. To assign a grade to an AVM, the size, the venous drainage, and the eloquence of the adjacent brain are determined on the basis of neuroradiologic studies, such as MRI and arteriography. Adding the points of each category derives the grade of the lesion.[13]

In terms of the relationship between size of the AVM and the tendency to bleed, almost every large series indicates that small AVMs present with hemorrhage significantly more often than large AVMs. Whether this finding indicates a higher propensity to bleed or a lesser likelihood to present with seizures, progressive neurological deficit, or headaches of small AVMs is not clear. In a study analyzing this issue, small AVMs were found to have a relatively higher feeding artery pressure, which was measured to be close to the mean arterial pressure of the patient during surgery. In patients with large AVMs, the feeding artery pressure was noted to be significantly lower than the mean arterial pressure. It was thought that this difference in arterial feeding pressure may be responsible for the greater size and severity of hemorrhage from small AVMs, as compared with larger lesions in this study.

It also was hypothesized that this difference could account for a presumed increase in tendency to hemorrhage in small AVMs.[15] Whether or not a patient has bled in the past should be only one and not the major factor influencing therapeutic considerations. Six months after hemorrhage, the risk of future hemorrhage is not different between patients who have bled and patients who have not.

One error in the preoperative assessment of an AVM is to misjudge the topographic relationships of the lesion, especially the deeper component of the lesion within projecting white matter tracts. If that happens and the AVM involves functioning cortical or subcortical areas, postoperative deficits generally result. Cortical mapping may be helpful during AVM surgery to determine the eloquence of a certain region, but it is unproven whether it facilitates AVM resection with decreased morbidity. Preoperative functional studies such as MRI also may be helpful.

SURGEON-RELATED FACTORS

It is the responsibility of the neurosurgeon who encounters a patient with a cerebral AVM to decide if he or she has enough experience with these lesions to evaluate the patient, to make appropriate recommendations, and to carry out the treatment if such is recommended. Surgical treatment of AVMs is rare enough that sufficient experience to deal with the more difficult lesions probably is gained only in referral centers that have particular expertise in the treatment of complex cerebrovascular lesions.

COST-EFFECTIVENESS

Surgical excision of AVMs smaller than 3 cm that are judged to be operable by an experienced cerebrovascular surgeon is highly efficacious in prolonging quality life expectancy when compared with radiosurgery or observation. Surgical excision of these AVMs with or without embolization is highly cost-effective compared with observation alone or radiosurgery when one considers the long-term costs, which include not only the actual immediate cost of treatment, but also the cost of caring for future hemorrhages and complications.[16]

Embolization

Selective preoperative embolization is an adjunct to surgical resection and may contribute positively to the outcome after AVM surgery.[6, 17–23] Endovascular embolization has the potential to reduce flow to the AVM and to obliterate deep vascular pedicles that are not accessible easily through the planned surgical approach. The reduction of flow allows the surgeon to stay closer to the margin of the AVM during surgical resection of the nidus. The preoperative embolization of feeders to which the surgeon could have access only by significant brain retraction can eliminate the need for such retraction and the risk of parenchymal damage or damage to draining veins as a result of retraction.[24] Repetitive staged embolization is a valuable strategy in the prevention of normal perfusion pressure breakthrough in large, high-flow lesions.[25]

Embolization, similar to any interventional procedure, is not without risk and has a certain morbidity and mortality on its own.[26, 27] In one study, the combined procedural rate of mortality and morbidity affecting lifestyle was 8%.[28] The presumed morbidity of embolization and surgical resection should be lower than the presumed morbidity of surgery alone if embolization is recommended as a surgical adjunct. Embolization should not be recommended solely to make the operation *easier* for the surgeon, to decrease operative time, or to reduce the possible need for blood transfusion, which is infrequent even in large nonembolized AVMs.

Radiosurgery

Radiosurgery is a valid alternative for the treatment of selected patients affected by cerebral AVMs. The idea of obtaining progressive obliteration of nidus vessels by highly focused radiation delivered with stereotactic guidance has proved to be effective, regardless of the device employed (i.e., Gamma knife, Cyclotron, or Linear Accelerator). Radiosurgery leads to complete angiographic obliteration in a high proportion of smaller lesions (<3 cm) at 2 years.[29–34] AVMs that had been shown histologically to be obliterated angiographically completely after radiosurgery still can show patent vascular channels, however.[35] The clinical significance of this is unclear. The patient treated by radiosurgery remains at risk for hemorrhage until the AVM is obliterated completely, and this risk appears to be the same as the risk of hemorrhage in untreated AVMs.[36] According to Kaplan-Meier life-table estimates, radiosurgery does not appear to confer any significant protection against bleeding or rebleeding in nonobliterated AVMs, at least during the first 5 years after treatment.[37]

Most, but not all, of the AVMs suitable for radiosurgical treatment are suitable for surgical resection. Microsurgery for small accessible AVMs seems to be superior to radiosurgery because of its proven high rate of efficacy and low rate of permanent morbidity.[16, 38] Immediate cure of the AVMs can be achieved in most of these patients, and they should not be offered radiosurgery as an equivalent alternative to neurosurgical excision. The ideal candidates for radiosurgery are patients whose AVM is less than 3 cm in diameter and is located in an area that is surgically inaccessible or only accessible with a high risk for a serious neurological deficit.

Partial obliteration of an AVM is considered to be a failure of radiosurgical therapy, independent of the percentage of obliterated volume.[39] Some results seem to indicate a bleeding rate in radiosurgery patients with only partially obliterated AVMs that is higher than in untreated patients.[29, 30, 33] One explanation is that radiosurgical treatment induces partial inhomogeneous obliteration of an AVM, leading to hemodynamic changes, such as disproportional occlusion of venous outflow in relation to arterial inflow, which could lead to hemorrhage.[40]

The latency period between irradiation and complete angiographic obliteration is the major shortcoming of radiosurgery in comparison with microsurgical resection. Embolization and radiotherapy should not be considered as a definitive therapy for AVMs unless the procedures have a high likelihood of resulting in complete obliteration of the lesion. Patients remain at risk for rebleeding as long as the malformation is still patent.

Coexisting Intracranial Aneurysm

It is estimated that about 7.5% of patients with AVMs have coexisting intracranial aneurysms.[41, 42] Typically, all of such patients have high-flow AVMs. Approximately 50% of the patients harbor multiple aneurysms. Most of these aneurysms (85%) are located either on a feeding vessel to the AVM or on a proximal major artery that participates in the arterial supply to the AVM.

The hypothetical explanation for the coexistence of AVMs and aneurysms is that hemodynamic stress in arteries feeding the AVM may lead to aneurysm formation. Support for this theory is provided by reports of aneurysms diminishing in size or disappearing after elimination of the shunt flow through the AVM.[43] The risk of intracranial hemorrhage in patients with AVMs and aneurysms is estimated to be around 7% per year,[44] which is higher than in patients without associated aneurysms. It was found that the risk of intracranial hemorrhage from either source—AVM or aneurysm—is higher in female patients.[42] The risk of rupture for aneurysms located on vessels remote from the AVM seems to be low.

When the pattern of the hemorrhage suggests that the aneurysm has bled, we recommend treatment of the aneurysm before treatment of the AVM. In cases in which the AVM has bled or in which it remains unclear which lesion has bled, some authors recommend aggressive treatment for the aneurysm before administering therapy for the AVM.[42, 45] Additionally, if embolization is to be considered in the treatment of the AVM, most endovascular surgeons fear passing the catheter through a feeding vessel bearing an aneurysm, and surgical or endovascular occlusion of the aneurysm or aneurysms is recommended before embolization. The treatment of patients with these complex vascular lesions needs to be individualized and predicated on a number of factors, such as the surgical accessibility of the aneurysm, the ease of resectability of the AVM, and the patient's age and general health.

Microsurgical Technique

TIMING

Surgery for cerebral AVMs generally should be elective. Occasionally, emergency surgery is required to remove a life-threatening hematoma. In these cases, a conservative evacuation of the clot without disturbing the AVM should be performed, unless the AVM is relatively small and simple and can be removed without significant morbidity.

Patients with hemorrhage resulting from an AVM tend to improve substantially, particularly young patients; as discussed earlier, it is improper to advise surgery of an AVM that normally would be predicted to lead to a major neurological deficit on the basis that the patient already has that kind of deficit. By waiting, a better sense can be gained of the degree of neurological recovery. The surgery should be planned and carried out in a way that most likely would not result in additional damage to the brain.

PREOPERATIVE MEASURES

A four-vessel angiogram is essential to evaluate the lesion and determine a surgical strategy. MRI is especially useful to determine the topography of the lesion and its relation to functioning regions of the brain. Depending on the localization of the AVM, neuro-ophthalmic evaluation, speech function evaluation, and neuropsychological testing might be indicated. The use of steroids, lumbar drainage, and mannitol is individualized depending on the specific lesion and the condition of the patient. Maintenance of normotension during surgery is recommended.

POSITIONING AND CRANIOTOMY

The patient is positioned depending on the location of the lesion. Generally, with convexity lesions, the surface of the lesion is placed parallel to the floor to allow a perpendicular approach with no brain retraction. With deep lesions, the positioning should be performed in a way that brain retraction during surgery is minimal and aided by gravity when possible. The cisterns and the subarachnoid space should be used for dissection. Specific approaches are discussed later in this chapter.

The head is fixed in a rigid device and, if intraoperative angiography is planned, in a radiolucent frame. When a certain degree of head flexion or rotation is required, sufficient jugular venous return has to be ensured. A well-placed, wide enough craniotomy contributes to minimize brain retraction. A large bone flap allows identification of surface veins and arterial feeders as they come along the convexity before they become hidden in a sulcus to approach the AVM. A wide craniotomy allows the surgeon to deal adequately with intraoperative parenchymal hemorrhage, which at times can extend well beyond the immediate operative field. After craniotomy, the dura is opened toward the adjacent major draining sinus, paying particular attention to the pattern of venous drainage to avoid premature damage to arterialized venous drainage.

General Principles of Microsurgical Dissection

The process of excision of the AVM after dural opening generally follows certain stages:

- Identification of the malformation
- Elimination of superficial feeding arteries
- Circumferential dissection of the nidus
- Dissection of the apex and control of the deep arterial pedicles
- Transection of the deep venous drainage and removal of the lesion
- Hemostasis

IDENTIFICATION OF THE MALFORMATION

After introduction of the microscope, the superficial venous and arterial anatomy is compared with the angiogram to identify the malformation. The visible arterial supply and the venous drainage pattern provide the most useful road map for defining the lesion. If the nidus does not reach the cortical surface, a red arterialized vein may be present and can be followed back to the AVM. MRI in combination with angiography sometimes is helpful in understanding the three-dimensional topography of the nidus, the feeding arteries, and the draining veins. Intraoperative ultrasound or frameless stereotactic guidance may be useful to identify the nidus in deep lesions.

ELIMINATION OF SUPERFICIAL FEEDING ARTERIES

Feeding arteries are identified over the cortex, then followed into a sulcus by carefully opening the arachnoid and spreading the adjacent gyri. If feeding arteries are not visible on the surface of the brain, but the arteriogram indicates that there are superficial feeders, the sulci around the AVM can be opened, and usually the feeders are identified deep in the sulci and can be followed to the nidus by progressive opening of the sulci.[46] Each single vessel should be inspected to see if it contributes to the perfusion of the normal surrounding brain. It is always desirable to take feeders only at the point where they enter the nidus.

Sometimes it is difficult to distinguish feeding arteries from arterialized draining veins. For differentiation, a temporary clip can be placed on the vessel. A vein often collapses distally to the nidus, and a feeding artery continues to pulsate.

Dealing with vessels of passage is a problem that is most significant with lesions of the sylvian fissure and the corpus callosum. Lesions of these two locations tend to be supplied by small branches of sylvian and pericallosal vessels, which pass adjacent to or through the AVM and go on to supply normal eloquent brain. These vessels must be skeletonized as they pass through the AVM, taking the small side branches supplying the nidus and preserving the main trunk. It might be helpful to use a proximal temporary clip on vessels on passage, then continue dissection through the AVM. When using a temporary clip, one must be extremely careful to ensure hemostasis for avoidance of bleeding when the clip is removed and normal perfusion pressure is restored.

CIRCUMFERENTIAL DISSECTION OF THE NIDUS

The plane of resection should be as close as possible to the AVM and should follow the nidus in a circumferential pattern.[47, 48] A gliotic plane may exist around AVMs that have bled previously, and some authors recommend dissection within this plane. In most unruptured AVMs, there is no such gliotic plane, and dissection should be performed staying as close as possible to the AVM. A too extensive margin of resection can lead to unnecessary parenchymal damage.

Vessels are coagulated with the bipolar cautery. A permanent hemoclip is applied before dividing any vessel larger than 1.5 mm in diameter. Large arteries sometimes do not shrink with bipolar coagulation. The use of a temporary aneurysm clip may aid in making the vessel amenable to coagulation. The aneurysm clip is removed after coagulation and replaced with a permanent hemoclip.

DISSECTION OF THE APEX AND THE DEEP ARTERIAL PEDICLES

Deep feeding vessels supplying the AVM are one of the major problems in AVM surgery. Small subependymal arteries often resist initial attempts to coagulate them. With persistence and patience and by taking one vessel at a time, dissection can be continued. It is important not to pack bleeding from these vessels because this simply allows the arteries to retract and to continue to bleed with consequent development of intraparenchymal or ventricular hematomas. We have found the small microclips designed by Sundt for this specific purpose useful for controlling these tiny vessels when everything else fails.

Substantial parenchymal damage can occur as deep perforators bleed and retract into the parenchyma. This is especially true when small perforating arteries that come through the substance of the basal ganglia, thalamus, or brainstem feed the AVM. Surgery on lesions that are substantially supplied by lenticulostriate and thalamoperforating vessels and by direct branches of the basilar artery to the brainstem carries a significant risk of serious morbidity. When these lesions are small enough, radiosurgery may be a preferable alternative.

TRANSECTION OF THE DEEP VENOUS DRAINAGE AND REMOVAL OF THE LESION

Venous drainage is sacrificed only as necessary, and the major draining veins are left as a pedicle. It sometimes is difficult to work around superficial veins, but those should be taken only if remaining sufficient deep venous outflow is present. If hemorrhage occurs from an important draining vein, it is preferable to stop the bleeding with a hemostatic agent and gentle pressure rather than to sacrifice the vein. One potential way of injuring important draining veins is by extensive retraction, especially in parasagittal lesions that drain to the superior sagittal sinus, in temporal and occipital lesions that drain to the transverse sinus, and in cerebellar lesions that drain superiorly into the tentorium.

After all arterial supply is controlled and the lesion is dissected circumferentially, frequently the remaining venous pedicle is still arterialized. This is secondary to small arterial feeders that lie directly underneath or adjacent to the major draining vein. Finally the venous drainage is occluded, and the nidus is removed.

HEMOSTASIS

Complete hemostasis at all times and after each single step of the dissection is absolutely necessary. After removal of the nidus, the cavity of resection is irrigated and inspected carefully. Systolic blood pressure is raised for about 10 to 15 minutes by 15 to 20 mm Hg above the normal mean pressure for the patient. The wall of the resection cavity is inspected under the microscope. Bleeding, spontaneous or induced by gently rubbing the wall of the resection cavity with a cottonoid, usually means residual malformation, which must be removed. After complete hemostasis, the bed of the AVM resection is lined with a single layer of absorbable knitted fabric (Surgicel). After this, the blood pressure is not allowed to rise above the normal mean pressure throughout the rest of the operation and the first 24 hours postoperatively.

Specific Surgical Management of Arteriovenous Malformations in Certain Locations

For convenience, the location of supratentorial AVMs is divided according to the schema shown in Figure 131–2.

CONVEXITY LESIONS

The positioning of the patient is dictated by the location of the lesion and its arterial supply. For small lesions, the general principles of microsurgical dissection apply. The head is elevated, and the plane of the lesion is kept parallel to the floor, to allow a perpendicular approach.

Large lesions usually are supplied by two or three major vascular pedicles and have superficial and deep venous drainage. Preoperative embolization can be helpful in decreasing the flow and reducing the risk of intraoperative or postoperative complications. In cases with external carotid supply, extreme caution must be used when turning the craniotomy. The use of multiple bur holes, careful stripping of the dura, and dural opening away from the surface presentation of the AVM are recommended to avoid bleeding from meningeal vascular pedicles.

SYLVIAN AND INSULAR LESIONS

Sylvian and insular lesions are located within the sylvian fissure or on the cortical surface of the insula and have their venous drainage into sylvian veins. The AVMs of this location are peculiar in that they tend to be supplied by *en passage* branches of the middle cerebral artery, which pass adjacent to or frequently right through the lesion, then go on to supply normal brain (Fig. 131–3).

For anterior sylvian malformations, a pterional or combined pterional and anterior temporal craniotomy is used to access the anterior sylvian fissure. The carotid artery is exposed and the median sylvian fissure is opened. Care is taken to preserve any arterialized

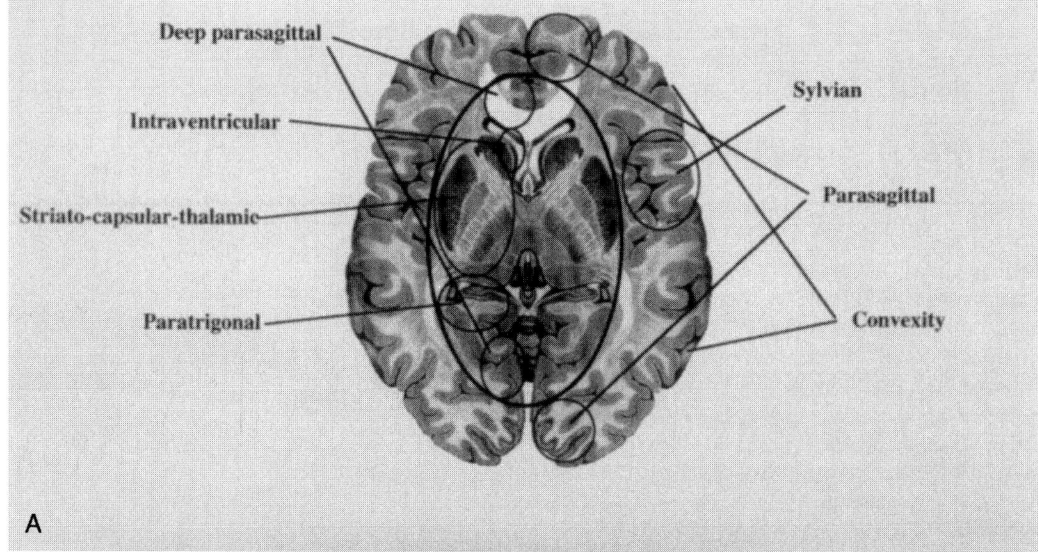

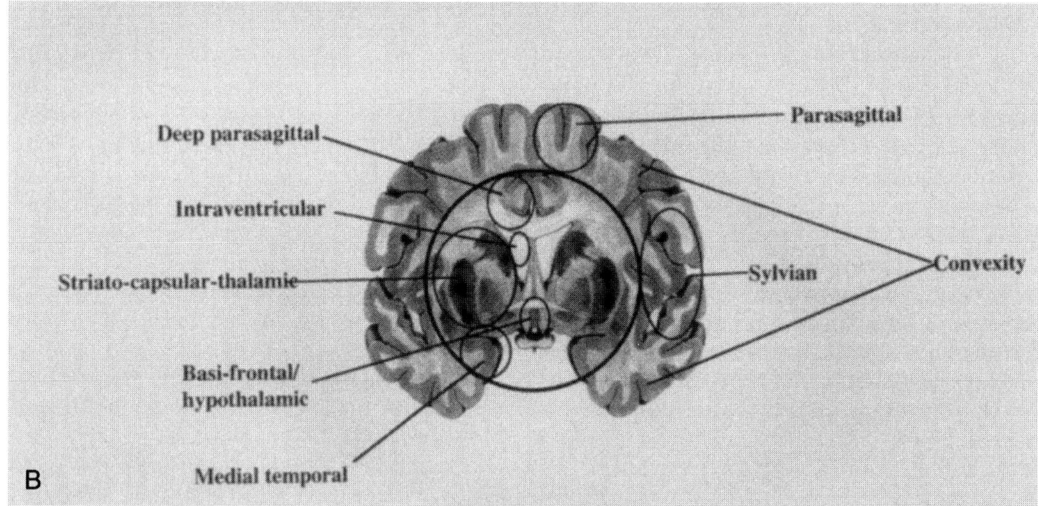

FIGURE 131–2. Anatomic classification of arteriovenous malformations: axial *(A)* and coronal *(B)*. (Adapted from Nieuwenhuys R, Voogd J, vanHuijzen C: The Human Central Nervous System: A Synopsis and Atlas, 3rd rev. ed. Berlin, Springer-Verlag, 1988, pp 70 and 91. Reprinted by permission.)

draining veins initially. Small veins draining across the fissure may be coagulated and divided. Dissection then proceeds along the M2 and M3 branches of the middle cerebral artery. Only vessels entering the malformation are divided. The senior author (R.C.H.) applies temporary clips to these vessels, while continuing distal dissection until it is assured that the vessel enters the malformation.

A specific problem with these lesions is bleeding from deep lenticulostriate feeders. These vessels are fragile and difficult to coagulate, and the temptation to pack them away must be resisted.

For more posterior malformations, a straight lateral position with a horseshoe-shaped incision over the ear is preferred. The sylvian fissure must be opened carefully, but in this location it may be difficult to identify the fissure. Sometimes it is helpful to trace arterialized veins in a retrograde fashion back to the malformation.

The vein of Labbé frequently can be used in correlation with the angiogram as a guide to the location of the AVM. Feeding arteries are skeletonized, taking only those branches that enter the lesion. The use of temporary clipping can be helpful in reducing turgency and bleeding from the malformation as the surgeon follows vessels en passage through the lesion, taking only the small branches that go exclusively to the AVM.

PARASAGITTAL LESIONS

Anterior frontal parasagittal lesions are approached best through a frontal craniotomy extending to the midline. If the lesion comes to the surface only on the medial aspect of the hemisphere, we prefer the lateral position with the ipsilateral side down to allow the brain to fall away from the falx by gravity. With larger lesions that come to the surface of the convexity, the supine position with the head looking straight ahead and flexed is preferred. This position allows control of both middle cerebral artery surface feeders and the deep anterior cerebral artery interhemispheric supply.

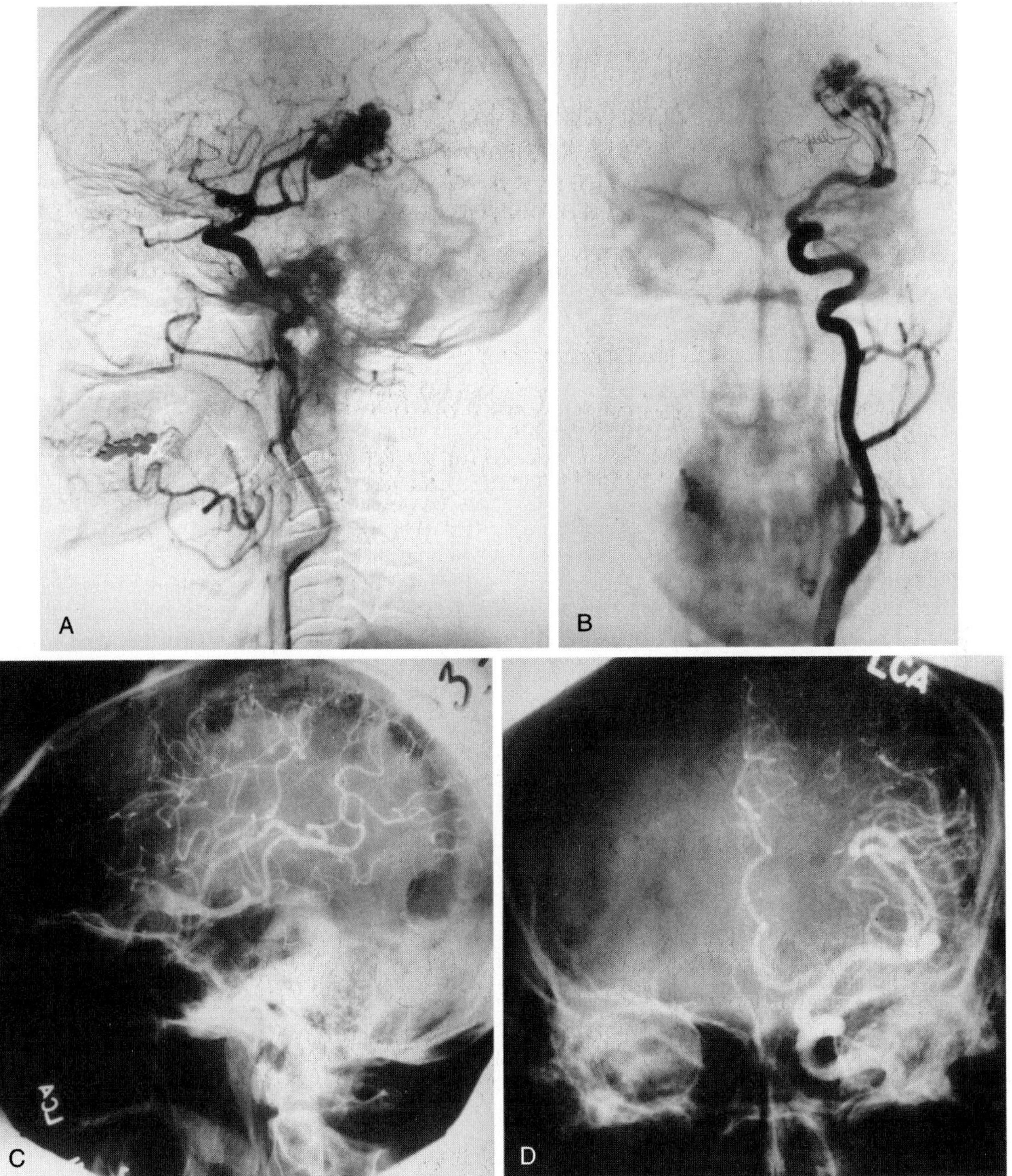

FIGURE 131–3. Left posterior sylvian anteriovenous malformations. *A* and *B*. Preoperative angiography. *C* and *D*. Postoperative angiography demonstrates no residual malformation.

Posterior frontal and parietal lesions often have blood supply from more than one major artery distribution and have large arterialized veins draining into the superior and inferior sagittal sinus limiting entry into the interhemispheric fissure. A broad-based bone flap is used to tailor the approach to the interhemispheric fissure between these veins. Preoperative embolization to control the anterior cerebral artery supply, when successful, can obviate the need for early parasagittal retraction.

Occipital parasagittal lesions are approached best through a craniotomy extending to the sagittal and transverse sinus with the patient either prone or in semisitting position. The lateral position with the ipsilateral side down, as described earlier, is preferred for small lesions that do not reach the convexity. Embolization can be helpful in eliminating medial feeders in the interhemispheric fissure from the anterior cerebral artery and the posterior cerebral artery systems.

MEDIAL TEMPORAL LESIONS

Medial temporal lesions can be subdivided conveniently into anterior, middle, and posterior medial temporal lesions. *Anterior medial temporal lesions* generally involve the uncus, amygdala, and anterior hippocam-

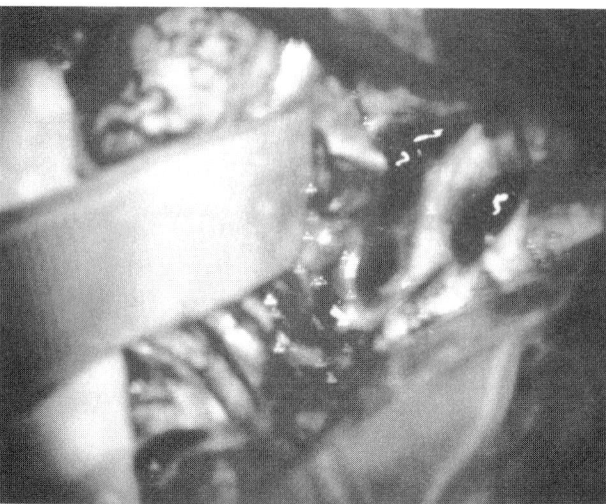

FIGURE 131–4. AVM of the left anterior temporal lobe. After a combined pterional (subfrontal) and anterior temporal craniotomy, the sylvian fissure has been opened. Feeders to the AVM come from the posterior communicating artery, the anterior choroidal artery and the middle cerebral artery.

pus and parahippocampus area. They are supplied primarily by anterior choroidal branches, anterior temporal branches of the middle cerebral artery, and branches of the posterior communicating and posterior cerebral arteries. Venous drainage is primarily into the basal vein, but also occasionally into the sphenoparietal sinus or sylvian veins. These lesions are approached best through a combined pterional (subfrontal) and anterior temporal craniotomy. The sylvian fissure is opened widely to control sequentially first the middle cerebral feeders, then the anterior choroidal feeders, and finally the feeders from the posterior communicating and posterior cerebral arteries (Fig. 131–4).

Deep midtemporal lesions involve the midhippocampus, the temporal horn with the choroid plexus, and the middle parahippocampal region. The head is positioned parallel to the floor with the vertex slightly down to allow the temporal lobe to fall away by gravity. A lumbar drain is helpful to this effect. A horseshoe-shaped incision extending over the ear with a low temporal craniotomy is used. Small lesions can be approached subtemporally to gain early control of the posterior cerebral feeders. Large lesions can be approached through the inferior temporal gyrus with a cortisectomy anterior or posterior to the vein of Labbé, sometimes in combination with a subtemporal approach. An approach through the superior or middle temporal gyrus seems to be more direct but carries the higher risk of leaving the patient with a visual field defect or dysphasia in the dominant temporal lobe. After the temporal horn has been entered, the anterior choroidal feeders are controlled through the choroidal fissure, and the lesion is removed gradually in an anterior-to-posterior fashion, until the draining venous pedicle at the basal vein is reached. With large lesions, the operation frequently results in quadrantanopsia owing to damage to the inferior optic radiation.[49]

Paratrigonal or deep posterior temporal lesions are lesions that involve the superior, medial, and inferior wall of the trigone and occasionally the pulvinar of the thalamus. The supply is from posterior cerebral and posterolateral choroidal artery branches. The venous drainage is into the basal vein of Rosenthal.

The surgical approach to these lesions depends on

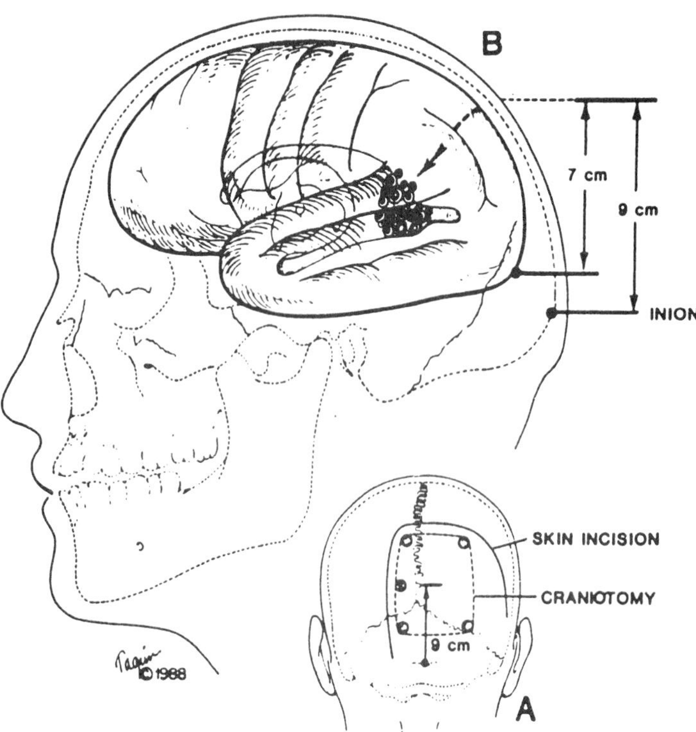

FIGURE 131–5. Diagram of approach to paratrigonal lesions that are primarily superior and medial to the trigone. The approach is through the posterior parietal lobule *(B)*. The craniotomy is centered at a point approximately 9 cm above the inion, and the point of cortical entry is located 7 cm above the occipital pole and about 3 cm off midline *(A)*. (From Heros RC: Brain resection for exposure of deep extracerebral and paraventricular lesions. Surg Neurol 34: 188–195, 1990. Copyright 1990 by Elsevier Science Inc. Reprinted by permission.)

where the lesion is located in reference to the trigone. In lesions superior and medial to the trigone, a transcortical approach through the posterior parietal area with the patient in a semisitting or prone position is preferred. The cortical incision is made at a point 2 cm lateral to the falx and 9 cm above the inion. The approach is directed from the cortical incision toward the ipsilateral pupil (Fig. 131–5).

Ultrasound or frameless stereotactic guidance to the trigone is helpful. If the bone flap is extended to the midline, the splenium can be visualized through the interhemispheric fissure and used as a guide to the location of the atrium, which is 3 cm lateral in the same axial plane. The feeding vessels come mainly from the anterior-inferior direction and can be interrupted by working in a plane anterior to the malformation (Fig. 131–6).

The senior author has found this approach preferable to the interhemispheric approach through the precuneus because there is essentially no retraction of the brain, and the approach is in a direct line rather than tangential as with the interhemispheric approach; with the latter, control of the laterally located feeders from the posterolateral choroidal arteries is difficult.[47]

For lesions located lateral and inferior to the trigone, a subtemporal-transtemporal approach is preferred. The patient is in the lateral position; the head is parallel to the floor with the vertex slightly tilted down. A temporal occipital craniotomy is performed. The initial approach is subtemporal to locate and divide the posterior cerebral feeders. The vein of Labbé is preserved by working anterior and posterior to it if necessary. Dissection through the inferior temporal gyrus is used to arrive at the nidus and is continued circumferentially. The difficulty with these lesions is the posterolateral choroidal artery feeding vessels, which are encountered late and deep in the dissection.

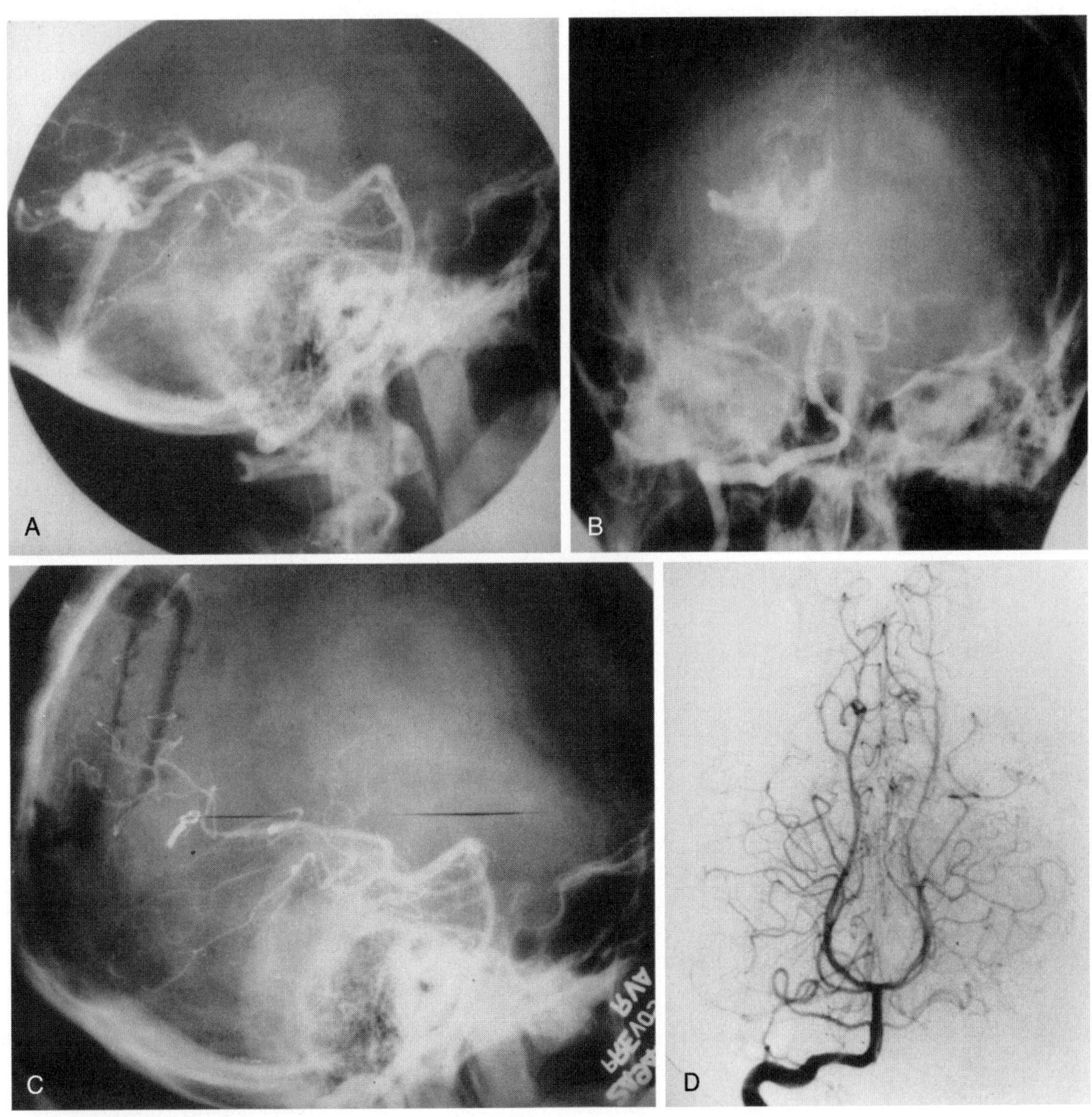

FIGURE 131–6. Paratrigonal arteriovenous malformation approached through the posterior parietal lobule. Preoperative *(A* and *B)* and postoperative *(C* and *D)* vertebral angiography.

ANTERIOR CORPUS CALLOSUM LESIONS

The smaller malformations involve only the corpus callosum, the cingulate gyrus, and the ventricular ependyma. The blood supply comes from the pericallosal and callosal marginal arteries. Venous drainage occurs superiorly into the sagittal sinus and intraventricularly into the septal, thalamostriate, and eventually internal cerebral veins. The approach uses a unilateral frontal craniotomy extending to the midline. These lesions can be resected by skeletonizing the pericallosal arteries as they pass through the lesion and taking only the side branches to the malformation. We prefer the lateral position with the ipsilateral side down for the interhemispheric approach to these AVMs. Larger lesions can involve the medial aspect of the striatum and anterior hypothalamus as well as the septal and preseptal regions. With lateral extension, these malformations recruit feeders from the recurrent artery of Heubner and from medial lenticulostriate arteries (Fig. 131–7). Blood supply also comes from perforators of the anterior cerebral artery and anterior communicating artery. With further lateral extension, the AVMs may obtain lateral lenticulostriate supply, which increases the surgical risk markedly because of the involvement of the internal capsule, making these larger lesions that extend laterally to the internal capsule inoperable in the senior author's opinion.

The approach to the larger lesions is through a large frontal craniotomy extending across the midline from the low frontal area to the coronal suture. The subfrontal approach allows identification and division of the feeding vessels from the anterior communicating complex and the anterior cerebral arteries. This can be followed by an anterior interhemispheric approach to follow the A2 vessels distally. The dissection of the medial and intraventricular planes of the lesion is completed using an approach through the corpus callosum.

POSTERIOR CORPUS CALLOSUM (SPLENIAL) AND POSTERIOR THIRD VENTRICLE LESIONS

AVMs of the splenium are supplied primarily by pericallosal branches of the posterior cerebral artery and distal pericallosal branches of the anterior cerebral artery as well as by medial and lateral choroidal branches of the posterior cerebral artery. Drainage is usually into the internal cerebral veins and the vein of Galen (Fig. 131–8).

The surgical approach is parasagittal interhemispheric on the side with the greater lateral extension of the lesion. Others prefer an approach from the opposite side with division of the falx to have a more direct, rather than tangential access to the lateral aspect of the lesion. The position is either semisitting with a generous parietal occipital craniotomy that crosses the midline or lateral with the head parallel to the floor and the ipsilateral side down to allow the occipital lobe to be retracted by gravity. Others have used the prone position preferentially.

The anterior pericallosal blood supply is approached along the posterior part of the corpus callosum. The posterior pericallosal and posteromedial choroidal supply is identified coming from the quadrigeminal cistern, below the lesion. The anterior and superior limits of the AVM are identified by an incision through the posterior cingulate gyrus. Delineation of the medial extent of the AVM is aided by dividing the falx.

The lateral extent of the lesion is defined by splitting the splenium in the direction of its fibers. With significant lateral extension of the lesion, there is important arterial supply from posterolateral choroidal feeders that come to the AVM with the choroidal plexus of the trigone of the ventricle. Control of these feeders may be difficult and may require considerable retraction. We prefer to access this lateral extent of the malformation through an incision in the precuneus, in front of the

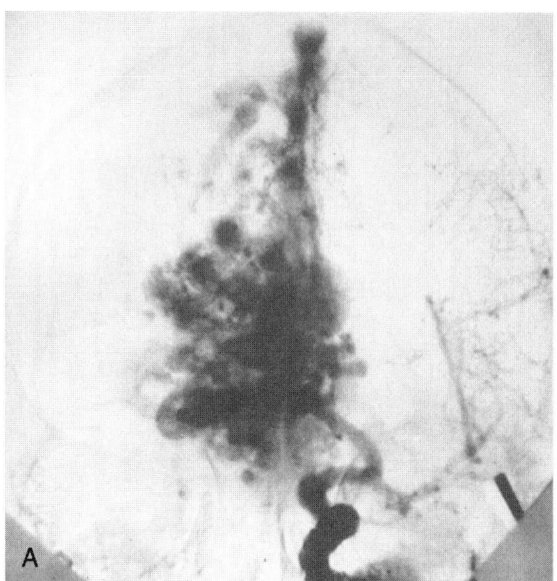

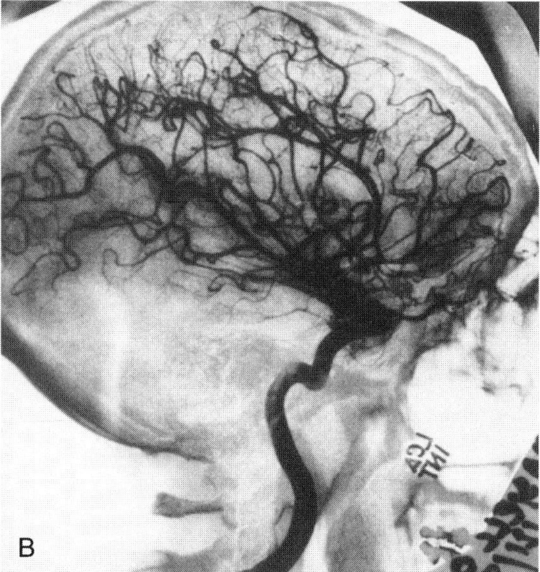

FIGURE 131–7. Large anterior callosal arteriovenous malformation extending into the basal ganglia. Preoperative *(A)* and postoperative *(B)* carotid angiography.

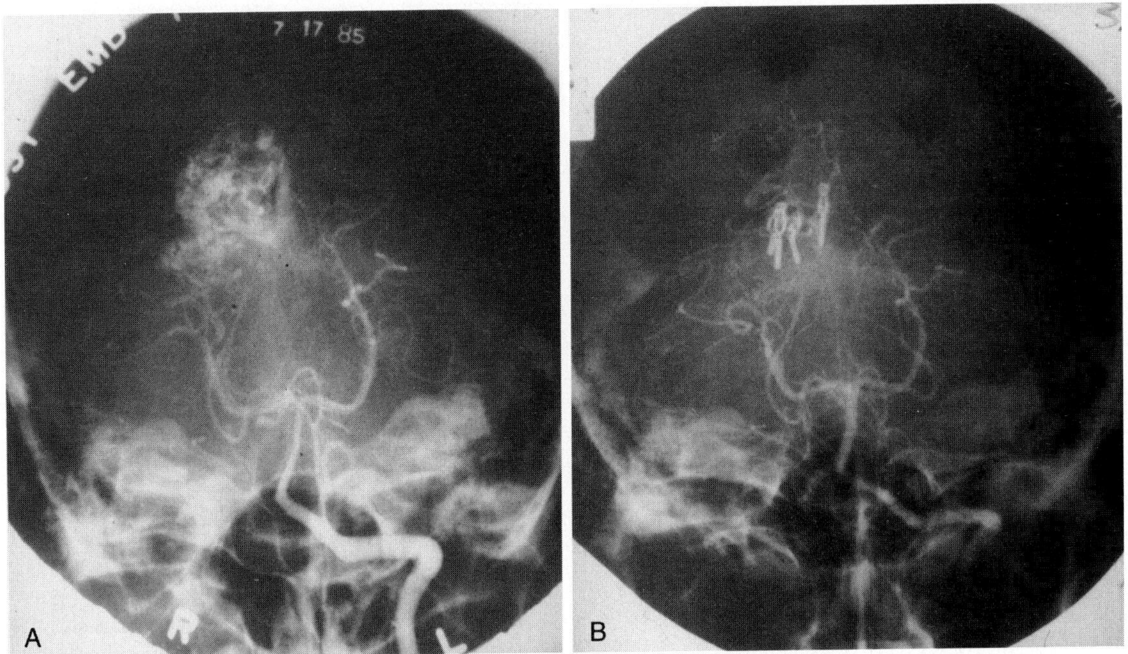

FIGURE 131–8. Preoperative *(A)* and postoperative *(B)* vertebral angiography of a right parasplenial arteriovenous malformation.

calcarine fissure. The venous drainage must be preserved until the end of the resection.

HYPOTHALAMIC AND INFERIOR FRONTAL LESIONS

Hypothalamic and inferior frontal lesions are usually small and involve the septal, anterior hypothalamic, and medial subfrontal regions with feeding vessels from the anterior communicating complex. They are operated using a pterional subfrontal approach, which provides direct access to the feeding vessels.

INTRAVENTRICULAR LESIONS

Although many AVMs have some ependymal representation, purely intraventricular lesions are rare. The operability of these lesions is determined by the relative contribution of feeding vessels from perforating as opposed to choroidal arteries. Lesions mostly fed by deep perforating vessels involve the deep substance of the basal ganglia and thalamus. During dissection of the deeper aspect of these lesions, perforators may retract into critical brain tissue, and deep hemorrhage or parenchymal damage in an attempt to control them can cause significant neurological deficit.

Conversely, choroidal supply can be controlled at the ependymal surfaces of the lesion. Although the lesions supplied mostly by choroidal vessels usually are selected for surgical excision, lesions in which the supply is predominantly by deep perforators generally should be considered for radiosurgery if small enough or for conservative therapy if too large for radiosurgery.

The intraventricular lesions, in part, have been discussed under other categories. AVMs of the head of the caudate are supplied by choroidal branches, Heubner's artery, and medial lenticulostriate vessels. They are approached through the anterior corpus callosum or, if there is significant hydrocephalus, through the lateral frontal horn. The anterior callosal approach can be used for small lesions of the anterior forniceal and septal region.

The approach to lesions of the dorsal thalamus depends on the primary arterial supply. AVMs of the dorsal thalamus medial to the fornix are supplied by medial posterior choroidal branches. An interhemispheric approach through a callosal incision just in front of the splenium is used in these lesions. Dorsal thalamic and pulvinar lesions that are lateral to the fornix are supplied by posterior lateral choroidal branches, and a transcortical posterior parietal approach to the atrium of the ventricle is preferred.

Purely intraventricular lesions are essentially AVMs of the choroid plexus (Fig. 131–9). These lesions are usually approached through the corpus callosum or transcortically through the middle frontal gyrus if there is significant hydrocephalus. If the lesion is located primarily in the anterior temporal horn, it is approached through the inferior temporal gyrus. If it is located in the atrium, a posterior parietal approach is used.

Large lesions of the medial temporal lobe can involve the entire distribution of the choroid plexus from the temporal tip to the trigone (Fig. 131–10). In these cases, a wide exposure is used to work through the sylvian fissure to control the middle cerebral artery branches. Dissection of these lesions is continued across the isthmus of the insula and into the ambient cistern, where posterior cerebral and choroidal branches can be controlled.

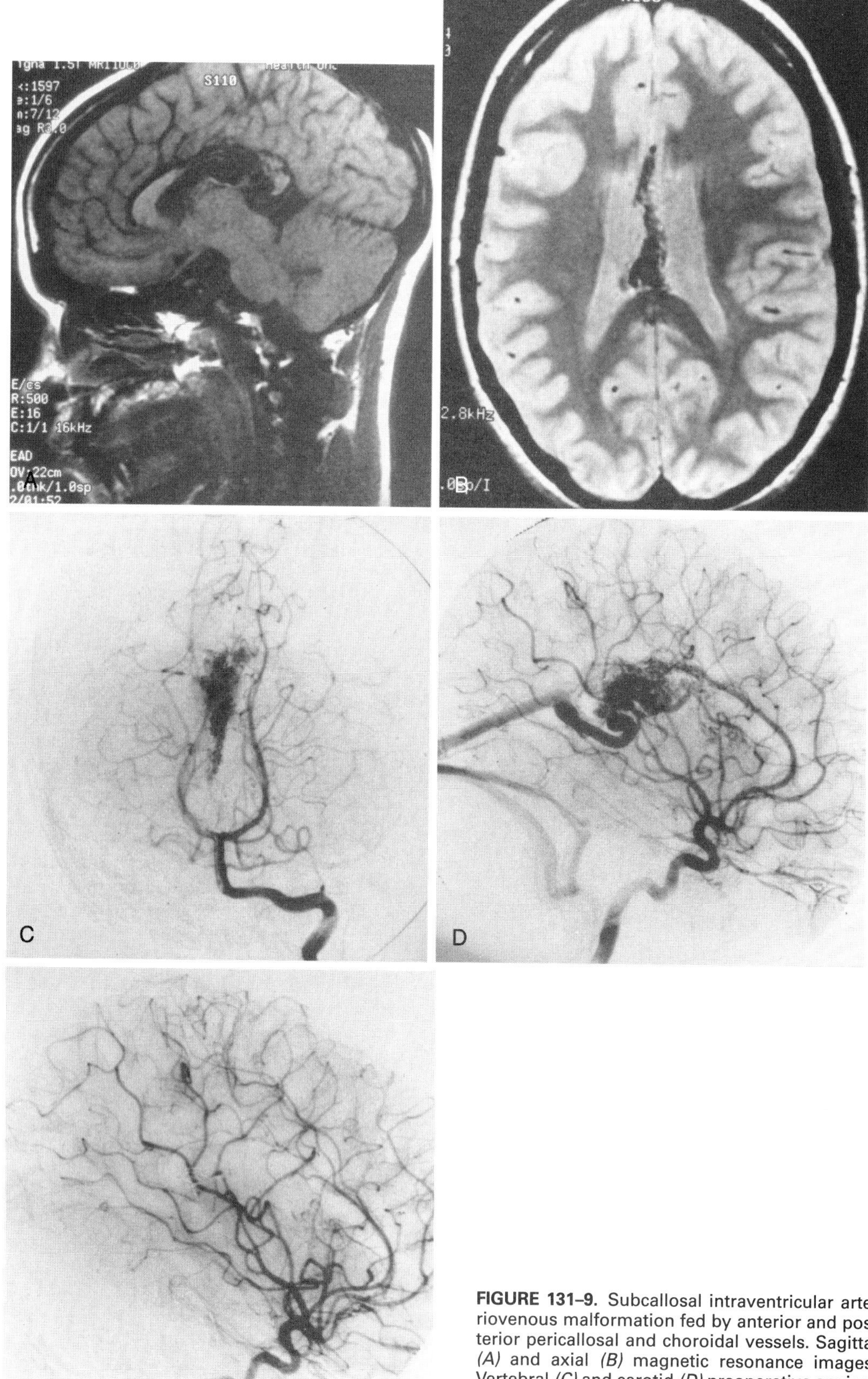

FIGURE 131–9. Subcallosal intraventricular arteriovenous malformation fed by anterior and posterior pericallosal and choroidal vessels. Sagittal *(A)* and axial *(B)* magnetic resonance images. Vertebral *(C)* and carotid *(D)* preoperative angiography. Postoperative angiography demonstrates complete excision *(E)*.

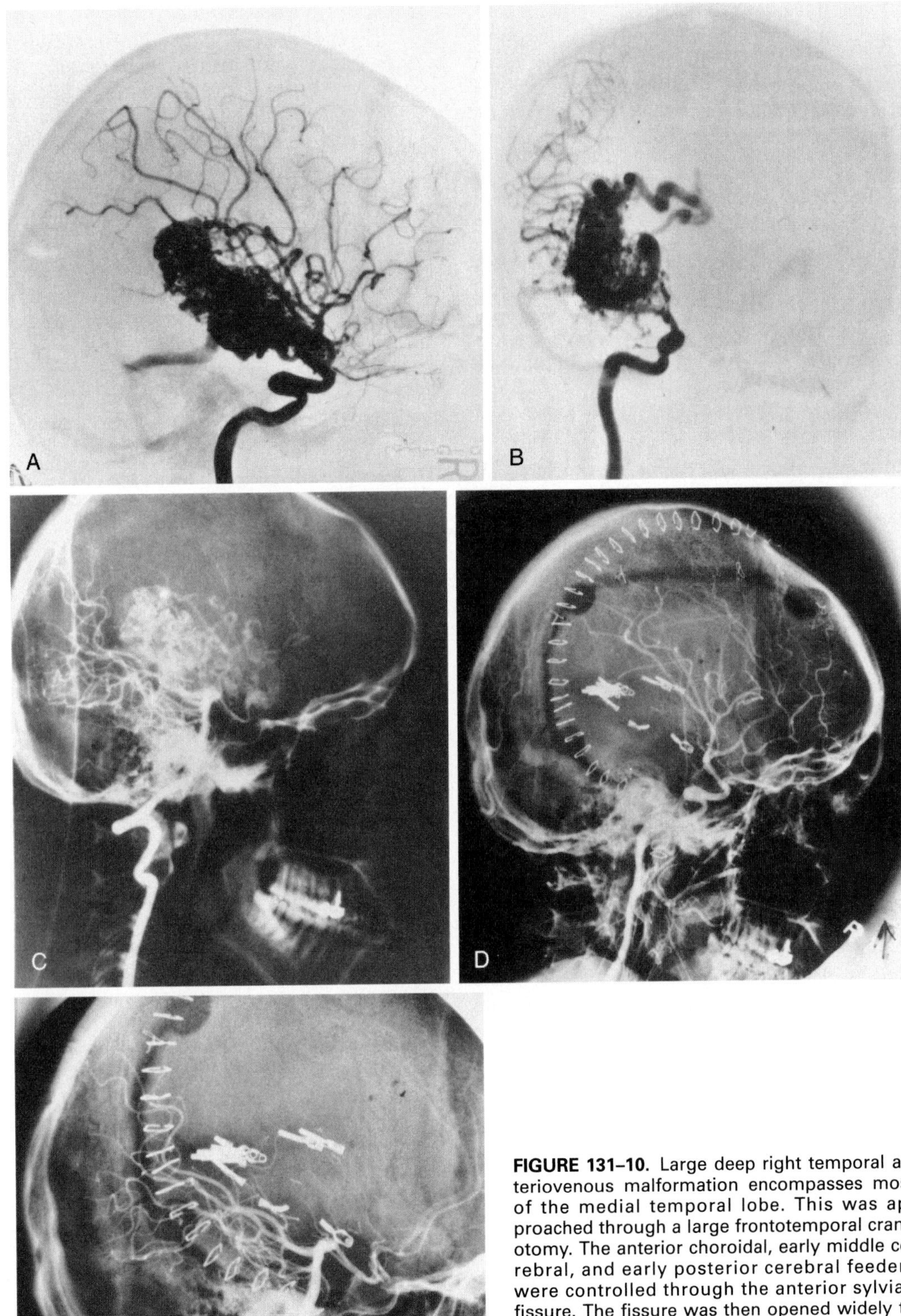

FIGURE 131–10. Large deep right temporal arteriovenous malformation encompasses most of the medial temporal lobe. This was approached through a large frontotemporal craniotomy. The anterior choroidal, early middle cerebral, and early posterior cerebral feeders were controlled through the anterior sylvian fissure. The fissure was then opened widely to control the more distal middle cerebral feeders, and an incision was made through the isthmus of the insula to gain access to the cisterna ambiens and the distal posterior cerebral and posterolateral choroidal feeders. Preoperative carotid *(A* and *B)* and vertebral *(C)* angiography. Postoperative carotid *(D)* and vertebral *(E)* angiography demonstrates complete resection.

Subcallosal lesions can be resected by an interhemispheric transcallosal approach. Lesions located primarily in the third ventricle can be resected through an anterior transcallosal approach with an interforniceal or subchoroidal extension, depending on the anatomy and, particularly, the venous drainage.

LESIONS OF THE CAUDATE, PUTAMEN, THALAMUS, AND INTERNAL CAPSULE

Lesions of the caudate, putamen, thalamus, and internal capsule are located lateral to the third ventricle and medial to the insula. If they are large and have supply primarily from deep perforators, they have a significant risk for surgical complications.[50] As stated previously, most of these lesions should not be resected and should be considered for radiosurgery if the size allows it.

Other lesions, such as small AVMs of the head of the caudate and the lateral aspect of the basal ganglia, can be removed with relatively low morbidity.[51] This removal is achievable if lenticulostriate vessels supply them, provided that these vessels do not come through the internal capsule. Lesions that can be resected with low morbidity fall into the following categories:

- Small lesions with primarily choroidal supply
- Small lesions of the head of the caudate nucleus
- Small lesions located lateral to the internal capsule (lateral basal ganglia)
- Small lesions of the dorsal aspect of the pulvinar
- Small lesions of the inferolateral thalamus supplied primarily by circumferential branches of the posterior cerebral artery and posterolateral choroidal vessels

Intraoperative Angiography

Intraoperative angiography is recommended in all but the most straightforward (small, superficial) AVMs.[52] Frequently an introducing catheter must be placed in the groin before craniotomy, especially when the patient is in any position other than supine. Before the routine use of intraoperative angiography, we experienced two major immediate postoperative hemorrhages that undoubtedly were due to residual AVM that most likely would have been detected by an intraoperative angiogram.

Postoperative Intensive Care

It is essential to keep the systolic blood pressure at normal or, preferably, slightly below normal level for the first 24 hours after surgery. Close neurological monitoring in an intensive care unit setting at least overnight is recommended.

Follow-Up

Postoperative angiographic confirmation of complete AVM resection is mandatory unless a good intraoperative angiogram has been obtained. The senior author is aware of cases in which the intraoperative angiogram was negative and a postoperative angiogram showed residual AVM; the conservative approach is always to perform postoperative angiography, regardless of the results of the intraoperative angiogram.

If there is a small residual AVM, it is preferable to go back and resect the lesion immediately. If the small residual is nonaccessible, radiosurgery or rarely observation may be recommended.

We have not recommended further angiographic follow-up when there has been complete obliteration shown by postoperative angiography. This recommendation still may be reasonable in adult patients. There have been several reports of children or young adolescents, however, who experienced recurrence of an AVM that had been shown by immediate postoperative angiography to be obliterated completely.[4] We now recommend at least one late angiogram, perhaps 3 to 5 years after excision, and MRI scans at more frequent intervals in children or young adolescents.

Complications

INTRAOPERATIVE COMPLICATIONS

Intraoperative hemorrhage results most frequently from bleeding from the AVM or from early occlusion of venous drainage. It is essential to preserve venous drainage to the AVM until the arterial supply to the lesion has been occluded completely.

Parenchymal damage can occur in a variety of ways. Injury occurs when the surgeon uses a too wide margin of resection around the AVM. A plane of resection millimeters away from the lesion reduces bleeding, but also damages surrounding eloquent brain. Another possible source of parenchymal damage is to take feeders too far away from the AVM. Feeders should be taken only at the point where they enter the nidus. This is important to prevent damage to arterial branches that contribute to the perfusion of the normal surrounding brain. Deep perforators are fragile vessels that are difficult to coagulate and that tend to retract into the white matter. Parenchymal damage can occur when they have to be followed into normal brain to stop bleeding. It is important not to pack this type of deep bleeding because packing can result in deep hemorrhage, which may not be recognized immediately and can result in significant damage. Retraction injury can be prevented with adequate positioning and a wide enough craniotomy, including a *skull base* approach to gain access to deeper lesions or to deep arterial supply with a minimum of brain retraction.

POSTOPERATIVE COMPLICATIONS

Hemorrhage

The most serious complication after AVM surgery is hemorrhage from residual fragments of an AVM or from insecure hemostasis. The former problem usually can be prevented by intraoperative angiography, as discussed previously. To avoid the second problem, we prefer to perform the entire operation under normotension. The use of hypotension possibly could reduce the amount of bleeding during surgical dissection but may increase the risk of postoperative hemorrhage from insecure hemostasis. After resection of the nidus, we routinely elevate the blood pressure by approximately 20 to 30 mm Hg over the pressure throughout the operation. With this maneuver, we have encountered spontaneous bleeding within a few minutes in several patients; most frequently the source of the bleeding has been an unrecognized small piece of residual AVM.

Seizures

We have encountered de novo postoperative seizures in about 15% of patients who had no seizures preoperatively. Among patients who had seizures preoperatively, seizure frequency improved in about 55%, remained unchanged in about 33%, and worsened in about 12%.[55] We recommend anticonvulsant prophylaxis for at least 6 months in all patients after surgical excision of a supratentorial parenchymal AVM.

Normal Perfusion Pressure Breakthrough

Reduction or elimination of blood flow through a high-flow AVM normalizes and redistributes blood flow to the adjacent normal brain tissue, which may have impaired autoregulation because of chronic relative ischemia. If the reestablishment of normal perfusion pressure exceeds the autoregulatory capacity of the surrounding brain, edema and hemorrhage may occur.[53] Although currently we do not observe this problem frequently because of the routine use of preoperative embolization in large, high-flow AVMs, we are convinced of the validity of this theory. Angiographic features that may be associated with normal perfusion pressure breakthrough are large-sized, high-flow, large-caliber long feeding arteries and diminished perfusion of adjacent brain (angiographic steal). Other features that would lead the surgeon to expect development of this problem are rapid early venous drainage and diffuse margins of the nidus. As insinuated previously, the problem usually can be avoided by a staged reduction in flow to the malformation, which currently is achieved by preoperative endovascular embolization.[54]

OUTCOME

The immediate postoperative (at the time of discharge from the hospital) results of a consecutive series of 441 patients who underwent surgical excision of a cerebral AVM by the senior author are shown in Table 131–1. Two obvious conclusions can be reached from a glance at this table. The first is that the morbidity and mortality are minimal for patients with Spetzler-Martin grades I and II AVMs and is acceptably low for patients with grade III AVMs. The second obvious conclusion is that the morbidity and mortality for patients with grade V AVMs are unacceptable. Given these results, we currently operate only rarely on patients with grade V AVMs who usually are progressively symptomatic or have had multiple hemorrhages; most of our patients in this group were operated during our earlier surgical experience. Careful judgment is required with grade IV AVMs because the morbidity of this group, although not nearly as high as with grade V AVMs, is still significant. Results similar to ours have been reported by other experienced cerebrovascular surgeons.[2, 11–13, 46]

Several authors documented that early postoperative deficits resulting from excision of a cerebral AVM tend to improve significantly within a 3- to 6-month period.[11, 55] In an early group of 153 patients included in Table 131–1, we obtained late follow-up at an average of 3 years after surgery. The late (in other words, permanent) major morbidity rate for patients with grades I, II, and III AVMs was 1.9% with an additional 1.9% mortality rate. Of patients with grade V AVMs, only 61% were in good condition at follow-up.[3] Overall morbidity of AVM surgery is similar in patients with ruptured or unruptured AVMs.[55]

CONCLUSION

The objective of AVM surgery is to eliminate the risk of hemorrhage and to stop seizures and neurological deterioration in a patient. Patients come to a physician for recommendations and advice. Nowadays patients are better informed and educated about specific diseases and the risks and benefits of each single treat-

TABLE 131–1 ■ **Early* Surgical Results**

GRADE S-M†	NO. PATIENTS	GOOD	FAIR	POOR	DEAD	MORBIDITY AND MORTALITY (%)
I	51	50	1	0	0	1.9
II	104	98	6	0	0	5.7
III	143	117	16	9	1‡	18.1
IV	98	70	18	9	1§	28.5
V	45	15	10	19	1	66.6
Total	441	350 (79.3%)	51 (11.5%)	37 (8.3%)	3 (0.7%)	20

*At the time of discharge from the hospital.
†Spetzler-Martin grading scale.
‡Died from massive infarction caused by carotid dissection from preoperative embolization.
§Died from pulmonary infarction caused by preoperative embolization.
Unpublished data from RC Heros, 1981–March 1999.

ment option. The decision of how to treat or not to treat an AVM is still influenced significantly by the way the neurosurgeon presents current data and his or her personal opinion to the patient. The neurosurgeon's decision to recommend surgical intervention should derive from a comparison of the long-term risks presented by an untreated AVM and the risk of invasive treatment, including embolization, radiosurgery, or microsurgical resection.

Surgical excision of AVMs classified as Spetzler-Martin grades I to III is generally advisable. Exceptions to that recommendation include patients with a limited life expectancy that are neurologically intact and have no seizure disorder. In patients who harbor grade IV lesions, the decision to operate or not is based on the individual circumstances. The patient's age and general medical condition as well as the clinical presentation influence the decision. Surgery can be recommended if the AVM is not located in an eloquent area or if the AVM is located in eloquent brain but the patient is suffering progressive neurological deterioration, has had recurrent hemorrhages, or already has a significant neurological deficit. Young patients deserve a more aggressive approach and generally make a good functional recovery from their predictable postoperative deficit.

As stated earlier, we believe that most AVMs classified as grade V should be treated conservatively. Surgery, usually preceded by endovascular embolization, can be considered in patients who have had multiple hemorrhages with a significant neurological deficit, patients with a progressive significant neurological deficit secondary to steal, and patients who have suffered a major hemorrhage that has left them already with the kind of major deficit that could be expected from excision of the AVM.

We are skeptical about the role of radiosurgery, preceded by embolization "to make the lesion smaller" in patients with large inoperable AVMs. Our impression is that currently there is no substantial data that indicate that this approach reduces the future incidence of hemorrhage when compared with the natural history of the disease. The significant risk of embolization in these patients that frequently undergo several sessions of embolization must be taken into account. We await further data before recommending this approach to our patients with large AVMs that we judge to be inoperable.

Radiosurgery alone or in combination with embolization seems to be indicated for the treatment of small AVMs that are located in deep eloquent areas of the brain where surgical resection likely would result in significant neurological deficit. The most important factor in minimizing morbidity is careful preoperative selection with avoidance of surgery in patients who are likely to experience serious morbidity from an operation. An understanding of the natural history of untreated lesions allows responsible selection of appropriate candidates for surgical treatment.

REFERENCES

1. Marin-Padilla M: Vascular malformation of the central nervous system: Embryological considerations. In Yasargil MG (ed): Microneurosurgery, vol III A. Thieme, Stuttgart, 1987, pp 23–47.
2. Stein BM, Solomon RA: Arteriovenous malformation of the brain. In Youmans JR (ed): Neurological Surgery. Philadelphia, WB Saunders, 1990, pp 1831–1863.
3. Heros RC: Prevention and management of therapeutic complications. In Jafar JJ, Awad IA, Rosenwasser RH (eds): Vascular Malformations of the Central Nervous System. Baltimore, Williams & Wilkins, 1999, pp 363–373.
4. Kader A, Goodrich JT, Sonstein WJ, et al: Recurrent cerebral arteriovenous malformations after negative postoperative angiograms. J Neurosurg 85:14–18, 1996.
5. Abdulrauf SI, Malik GM, Awad IA: Spontaneous angiographic obliteration of cerebral arteriovenous malformations. Neurosurgery 44:280–288, 1999.
6. Vinuela F, Dion JE, Duckwiler G, et al: Combined endovascular embolization and surgery in the management of cerebral arteriovenous malformations: Experience with 101 cases. J Neurosurg 75:856–864, 1991.
7. Leblanc R, Levesque M, Comair Y, Ethier R: Magnetic resonance imaging of cerebral arteriovenous malformations. Neurosurgery 21:15–20, 1987.
8. Smith HJ, Strother CM, Kikuchi Y, et al: MR imaging in the management of supratentorial intracranial AVMs. AJR Am J Roentgenol 150:1143–1153, 1988.
9. Latchaw RE, Hu X, Ugurbil K, et al: Functional magnetic resonance imaging as a management tool for cerebral arteriovenous malformations. Neurosurgery 37:619–625, 1995.
10. Maldjian J, Atlas SW, Howard RS, et al: Functional magnetic resonance imaging of regional brain activity in patients with intracerebral arteriovenous malformations before surgical or endovascular therapy. J Neurosurg 84:477–483, 1996.
11. Steinmeier R, Schramm J, Mueller HG, Fahlbusch R: Evaluation of prognostic factors in cerebral arteriovenous malformations. Neurosurgery 24:193–200, 1989.
12. Hamilton MG, Spetzler RF: The prospective application of a grading system for arteriovenous malformations. Neurosurgery 34:2–6, 1994.
13. Spetzler RF, Martin NA: A proposed grading system for arteriovenous malformations. J Neurosurg 65:476–483, 1986.
14. Luessenhop AJ, Rosa L: Cerebral arteriovenous malformations: Indications for and results of surgery, and the role of intravascular techniques. J Neurosurg 60:14–22, 1984.
15. Spetzler RF, Hargraves RW, McCormick PW, et al: Relationship of perfusion pressure and size to risk of hemorrhage from arteriovenous malformations. J Neurosurg 76:918–923, 1992.
16. Nussbaum ES, Heros RC, Camarata PJ: Surgical treatment of intracranial arteriovenous malformations with an analysis of cost-effectiveness. Clin Neurosurg 42:348–369, 1994.
17. DeMeritt JS, Pile-Spellman J, Mast H, et al: Outcome analysis of preoperative embolization with N-butyl cyanoacrylate in the treatment of cerebral arteriovenous malformations. AJNR Am J Neuroradiol 16:1801–1807, 1995.
18. Deruty R, Pelissou Guyotat I, Mottolese C, et al: The combined management of cerebral arteriovenous malformations: Experience with 100 cases and review of the literature. Acta Neurochir 123:101–112, 1993.
19. Frizzel RT, Fisher WS: Cure, morbidity and mortality associated with embolization of brain arteriovenous malformations: A review of 1246 patients in 32 series over a 35-year period. Neurosurgery 37:1031–1040, 1995.
20. Jafar JJ, Davis AJ, Berenstein A, et al: The effect of embolization with N-butyl cyanoacrylate before surgical resection of cerebral arteriovenous malformations. J Neurosurg 78:60–69, 1993.
21. Paulsen RD, Steinberg GK, Norbash AM, et al: Embolization of basal ganglia and thalamic arteriovenous malformations. Neurosurgery 44:991–997, 1999.
22. Tokunaga K, Kinugasa K, Kawada S, et al: Embolization of cerebral arteriovenous malformations with cellulose acetate polymer: A clinical, radiological, and histological study. Neurosurgery 44: 981–990, 1999.
23. Wallace RC, Flom RA, Khayata MH, et al: The safety and effectiveness of brain arteriovenous malformation embolization using acrylic and particles: The experience of a single institution. Neurosurgery 37:606–618, 1995.
24. Camarata PJ, Heros RC: Arteriovenous malformations of the brain. In Youmans JR (ed): Neurological Surgery. Philadelphia, WB Saunders, 1996, pp 1372–1404.

25. Spetzler RF, Martin NA, Carter LP, et al: Surgical management of large AVMs by staged embolization and operative excision. J Neurosurg 67:17–28, 1987.
26. Deruty R, Pelissou Guyotat I, et al: Reflections on the management of cerebral arteriovenous malformations. Surg Neurol 50: 255–256, 1998.
27. Gobin Y, Laurent A, Merienne L, et al: Treatment of brain arteriovenous malformation by embolization and radiosurgery. J Neurosurg 85:19–28, 1996.
28. Wikholm G, Lundkvist C, Svendsen P: Embolization of cerebral arteriovenous malformations: Part I. Technique, morphology, and complications. Neurosurgery 39:457–459, 1996.
29. Colombo F, Pozza E, Chierego G, et al: Linear accelerator radiosurgery of cerebral arteriovenous malformations: An update. Neurosurgery 34:14–21, 1994.
30. Colombo F, Pozza E, Chierego G, et al: Linear accelerator radiosurgery of cerebral arteriovenous malformations: Current status. Acta Neurochir 62(suppl):5–9, 1994.
31. Friedman WA, Bova FJ, Mendenhall WM: Linear accelerator radiosurgery for arteriovenous malformations: The relationship of size to outcome. J Neurosurg 82:180–189, 1995.
32. Lunsford LD, Kondziolka D, Flickinger JC, et al: Stereotactic radiosurgery for arteriovenous malformations of the brain. J Neurosurg 75:512–524, 1991.
33. Pollock BE, Lunsford LD, Kondziolka DK, et al: Stereotactic radiosurgery for postgeniculate visual pathway arteriovenous malformations. J Neurosurg 84:437–441, 1996.
34. Yamamoto Y, Coffey RJ, Nichols DA, Shaw EG: Interim report on the radiosurgical treatment of cerebral arteriovenous malformations. J Neurosurg 83:832–837, 1995.
35. Yamamoto M, Jimbo M, Kobayashi M: Long term results of radiosurgery for arteriovenous malformations: Neurodiagnostic imaging and histological studies of angiographically confirmed nidus obliteration. Surg Neurol 37:219–230, 1992.
36. Heros RC, Korosue K: Radiation treatment of cerebral arteriovenous malformation. N Engl J Med 323:127–129, 1990.
37. Steiner L, Lindquist CH, Adler JR, et al: Clinical outcome of radiosurgery for cerebral arteriovenous malformations. J Neurosurg 77:1–8, 1992.
38. Schaller C, Schramm J: Microsurgical results for small arteriovenous malformations accessible for radiosurgical or embolization treatment. Neurosurgery 40:644–672, 1997.
39. Gallina P, Merienne L, Meder JF, et al: Failure in radiosurgery treatment of cerebral arteriovenous malformations. Neurosurgery 42:996–1004, 1998.
40. Lo EH, Fabrikant JI, Levy RP, et al: An experimental compartmental flow model for assessing the hemodynamic response of intracranial arteriovenous malformations to stereotactic radiosurgery. Neurosurgery 28:251–259, 1991.
41. Deruty R, Mottolese C, Soustiel JF, Pelissou Guyotat I: Association of cerebral arteriovenous malformation and cerebral aneurysm: Diagnosis and management. Acta Neurochir 107:133–139, 1990.
42. Thompson RC, Steinberg GK, Levy RP, Marks MP: The management of patients with arteriovenous malformations and associated intracranial aneurysms. Neurosurgery 43:202–212, 1998.
43. Lasjaunias P, Piske R, Terbrugge K, Willinsky R: Cerebral arteriovenous malformations (C.AVM) and associated arterial aneurysms (AA): Analysis of 101 C.AVM cases, with 37 AA in 23 patients. Acta Neurochir 91:29–36, 1988.
44. Brown RD, Wiebers DO, Forbes GS: Unruptured intracranial aneurysms and arteriovenous malformations: Frequency of intracranial hemorrhage and relationship of lesions. J Neurosurg 73: 859–863, 1990.
45. Cunha e Sa MJ, Stein BM, Solomon RA, McCormick PC: The treatment of associated intracranial aneurysms and arteriovenous malformations. J Neurosurg 77:853–859, 1992.
46. Yasargil MG: Microneurosurgery, vol III B. Stuttgart, Thieme, 1988.
47. Heros RC, Korosue K: Parenchymal cerebral arteriovenous malformations. In Appuzzo MLJ (ed): Brain Surgery: Complication Avoidance and Management. New York, Churchill Livingstone, pp 1175–1192, 1993.
48. Morcos JJ, Heros RC: Supratentorial arteriovenous malformation. In Carter LP, Spetzler RF (eds): Neurovascular Surgery. New York, McGraw-Hill, 1995, pp 979–1004.
49. Bartolomei J, Wecht DA, Chaloupka J, et al: Occipital lobe vascular malformations: Prevalence of visual field deficits and prognosis after therapeutic intervention. Neurosurgery 43:415–423, 1998.
50. Morgan MK, Drummond KJ, Grinnell V, Sorby W: Surgery for cerebral arteriovenous malformations: Risk related to lenticulostriate arterial supply. J Neurosurg 86:801–805, 1997.
51. De Oliveira E, Tedischi H, Siqueira MG, et al: Arteriovenous malformations of the basal ganglia region: Rationale for surgical management. Acta Neurochir 139:487–506, 1997.
52. Anegawa S, Hayashi T, Torigoe R, et al: Intraoperative angiography in the resection of arteriovenous malformations. J Neurosurg 80:73–78, 1994.
53. Spetzler RF, Wilson CB, Weinstein PR: Normal perfusion pressure breakthrough theory. Clin Neurosurg 25:651–672, 1978.
54. Spetzler RF, Zabramski JM: Grading and staged resection of cerebral arteriovenous malformations. Clin Neurosurg 36:318–337, 1990.
55. Heros RC, Korosue K, Diebold PM: Surgical excision of cerebral arteriovenous malformations: Late results. Neurosurg 26:570–578, 1990.

CHAPTER **132**

Posterior Fossa Arteriovenous Malformations

THOMAS A. KOPITNIK ■ ZEENA DORAI ■ JONATHAN WHITE ■ DUKE SAMSON

Arteriovenous malformations (AVMs) of the central nervous system are uncommon lesions, with an estimated incidence of approximately 3 per 100,000 people in the general population.[1–5] The prevalence of these vascular lesions is difficult to estimate because many remain asymptomatic for long periods before becoming symptomatic. AVMs specifically confined to the posterior fossa are a unique subset of cerebral AVMs that are relatively uncommon compared with supratentorial lesions. Infratentorial AVMs were first reported as a clinical entity by Clingenstein[6] in 1908, although the first removal of a cerebellar AVM was not accomplished successfully until 1932 by Olivecrona.[7] Before the advent of computed tomography (CT), it was not uncommon to misdiagnose posterior fossa AVMs as tumors, frequently with disastrous results if surgical removal was attempted.[6]

Posterior fossa AVMs account for 10% to 20% of all intracranial intraparenchymal AVMs.[6–12] In the Cooperative Study of Intracranial Aneurysms and Subarachnoid Hemorrhage, 32 (7%) of 453 AVMs were located in the posterior fossa, and in Drake's series of 600 AVMs, 116 (20%) were located in the posterior fossa.[4, 11] It is probable that published clinical series before the widespread use of magnetic resonance imaging (MRI) significantly underestimated the prevalence of infratentorial AVMs. Based on pathologic studies, McCormick[13] classified cerebral vascular malformations into five groups: AVMs, capillary telangiectasias, cavernous malformations, venous angiomas, and cerebral varices. In his large autopsy series, McCormick found that approximately one half of all vascular malformations found within the cerebellum were AVMs.

AVMs of the cerebellum and brainstem were previously considered to be similar lesions because of their shared infratentorial location and common vascular supply patterns. Before the advent of MRI, it was difficult to clearly differentiate AVMs of the cerebellum from those that involved the brainstem based solely on angiography and CT. With the advent of high-resolution MRI and superselective digital subtraction angiography, cerebellar AVMs could be considered as separate and distinct entities from vascular lesions involving the brainstem. Cerebellar AVMs have a different natural history and clinical presentation compared with similarly sized AVMs involving the brainstem. AVMs involving only the cerebellum are relatively common compared with AVMs confined to the brainstem. For reasons probably related to embryologic vascular development, AVMs within the posterior fossa typically involve the cerebellum or the brainstem, but involvement of both is rare.[14] Large AVMs of the posterior fossa often compress but do not specifically involve the dorsal aspect of the brainstem (Fig. 132–1). For this reason, cerebellar and brainstem AVMs should be considered as separate pathologic, radiologic, and clinical entities.

CLINICAL PRESENTATION

AVMs of the posterior fossa usually manifest with hemorrhage or headache or are an incidental finding.

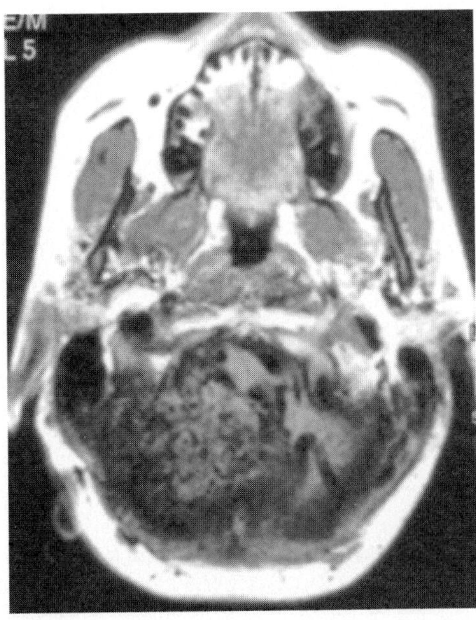

FIGURE 132–1. Magnetic resonance image of a large right cerebellar arteriovenous malformation compressing the dorsal and lateral aspects of the medulla.

Unlike supratentorial vascular lesions, seizure as the presenting symptom of a cerebellar AVM is rare and is usually related to global nervous system dysfunction from secondary effects of hemorrhage or cerebrospinal fluid (CSF) circulation abnormalities. A higher reported rate of hemorrhage in posterior fossa AVMs compared with supratentorial lesions is possibly explained by their small size relative to supratentorial AVMs and the propensity for smaller AVMs to hemorrhage.[4, 6, 10–12, 15–17] Guidetti and Delitala[18] reported that 89% of patients with small AVMs presented with symptoms related to hemorrhage, compared with 74% of patients with medium-sized AVMs and 58% of patients with large AVMs. In Drake's series[11] of 116 posterior fossa AVMs, only 13 (11%) were larger than 5 cm in diameter. In a series of 10 patients, Fults and Kelly[19] found that hemorrhage from posterior fossa AVMs is more frequent and more often fatal than hemorrhage from supratentorial AVMs. Batjer and Samson[10] reported that 11 of 23 patients who presented initially with hemorrhage from posterior fossa AVMs subsequently rebled. Although some contemporary reports suggest that posterior fossa AVMs have no higher hemorrhage rate than comparably sized supratentorial lesions,[6, 11, 20] the fact remains that, because of the paucity of other clinical symptoms at presentation, hemorrhage is the major presentation of most posterior fossa AVMs, with the rate of hemorrhage as the presenting event approaching 90%.[21–25]

We observed that posterior fossa AVMs were frequently associated with aneurysms on the feeding arterial pedicles to the nidus and were often the cause of hemorrhage[26] (Fig. 132–2). Between 5% and 8% of all intracranial AVMs are found to have coexisting aneurysms, whereas the incidence of aneurysms associated with infratentorial AVMs may be as high as 25%.[10, 26–34] In patients who have experienced a hemorrhage and harbor a posterior fossa AVM and an associated aneurysm, it is more likely in our experience that the aneurysm is the source of the hemorrhage. Arterial aneurysms associated with AVMs are usually flow related and occur on feeding vessels or are intranidal. In our experience, most accompanying aneurysms are flow related and tend to occur on AVM feeding vessels. We usually treat saccular aneurysms associated with posterior fossa AVMs before or during surgical resection of the AVM to ensure that increased pressure and decreased flow in the feeding artery during AVM resection does not rupture the aneurysm. In contradistinction to associated saccular aneurysms, preaneurysmal dilatations of the intracranial vertebral or basilar artery are frequently seen with moderate to large AVMs, especially at the origin of the posterior inferior cerebellar artery (PICA). If there is no saccular component to these aneurysms, we do not feel that treatment is necessary.

There is no convincing evidence that infratentorial AVMs cause seizures. Of 68 patients with posterior fossa AVMs, Yasargil[6] described 2 patients who presented with a history of seizures. Both patients also had evidence of massive hydrocephalus that he felt accounted for their epileptic symptoms (Yasargil, personal communication, 2001). Rarely, posterior fossa AVMs may present with progressive neurologic dysfunction or cranial neuropathies similar to that seen with a demyelinating process. Patients can present with deficits related to the cerebellum, brainstem, and cranial nerves, including symptoms of trigeminal neuralgia and hemifacial spasm. These deficits result from tortuous feeding arteries and draining veins exerting a

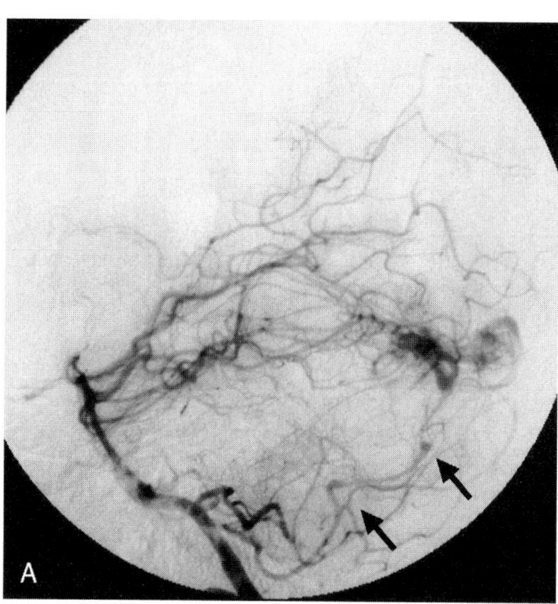

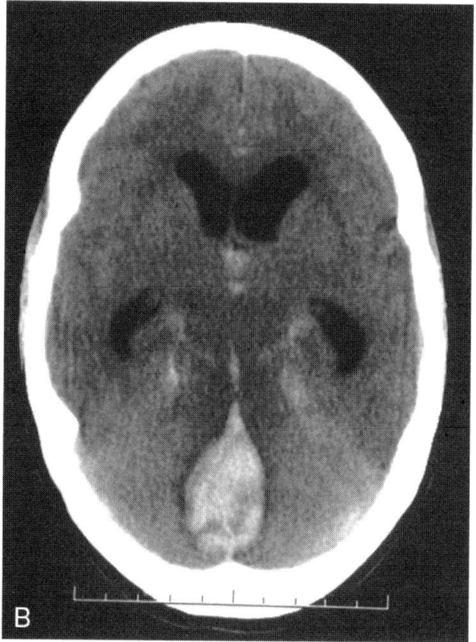

FIGURE 132–2. *A,* Lateral vertebral arteriogram demonstrating a small vermian arteriovenous malformation with flow-related aneurysms on distal feeding branches of the posterior inferior cerebellar artery *(arrows)*. *B,* Computed tomographic scan shows a large vermian hemorrhage.

mass effect on the cranial nerves or nerve root entry (exit) sites on the surface of the brainstem. It is possible but unlikely that cranial neuropathies may be produced from occult hemorrhage or from a vascular steal phenomenon. In our practice, we have frequently evaluated patients who were found to harbor posterior fossa AVMs on screening MRI scans performed for headache evaluation or for minimal neurologic symptoms. AVMs are frequently discovered as incidental findings without clear radiographic evidence of prior hemorrhage, giving credence to the assertion that the prevalence of such lesions was probably underrepresented in past studies because of the difficulty in confirming the diagnosis in the era before MRI.

PATIENT SELECTION AND TIMING OF INTERVENTION

Because of the high potential morbidity associated with hemorrhage in the posterior fossa, we recommend surgical treatment and resection of all AVMs in this region, with the exception of patients medically unable to withstand a surgical procedure or who are much older than 70 years. With contemporary advancements in the fields of microsurgical instrumentation, neuroanesthesia, interventional neuroradiology, and critical care management, AVMs located within the cerebellum can be successfully removed with excellent patient outcomes in most cases. AVMs involving the brainstem merit special discussion regarding the patients who are optimally suited for surgical treatment and those for whom surgical treatment should be avoided.

Because most patients with posterior fossa AVMs present with hemorrhage, initial patient management is directed at treatment of the mass effect, obstructive hydrocephalus, and any related aneurysms that may pose a risk of early rebleeding in the initial phases of management. The technical removal of a posterior fossa AVM is better executed by the surgeon and better tolerated by the patient if surgical resection is not performed immediately after presentation but rather deferred, if possible, for 4 to 6 weeks after the initial hemorrhage. Others and we believe that, for patients who present with or develop life-threatening posterior fossa hematoma associated with AVMs, optimal initial management is limited hematoma evacuation without AVM resection. Although this is our stated position, we often have found it necessary to remove the entire vascular malformation at the time of emergent clot evacuation, and the surgeon should be prepared for this contingency. Over a 12-year period, we have resected AVMs from 397 patients, and 53 of the AVMs were in the posterior fossa. We have emergently operated on 15 patients with posterior fossa AVMs because of life-threatening hematoma, and in every case, the malformation was removed at the time of the initial clot evacuation (Fig. 132–3). This experience emphasizes the fact that the initial radiologic evaluation should be as complete as possible and the surgeon should be prepared for AVM resection if necessary during emergent evacuation of hematoma in a patient harboring a posterior fossa AVM.

RADIOLOGIC EVALUATION

To formulate a cohesive and rational plan for treating any AVM, particularly an AVM of the posterior fossa, high-quality radiographic images much be obtained. CT is useful as a preliminary diagnostic tool for AVMs that have recently hemorrhaged (Fig. 132–4*A*). Mass effect from hematoma and early identification of hydrocephalus can determine whether external ventricular drainage or immediate surgical clot evacuation is required. When significant hemorrhage has occurred within the substance of the cerebellum, limited topographic information regarding the AVM can be ob-

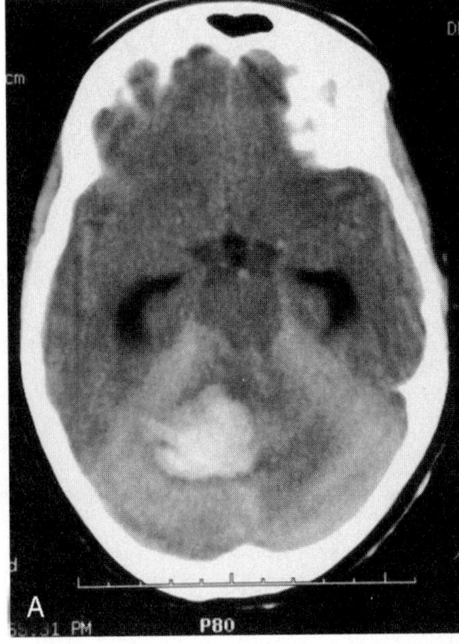

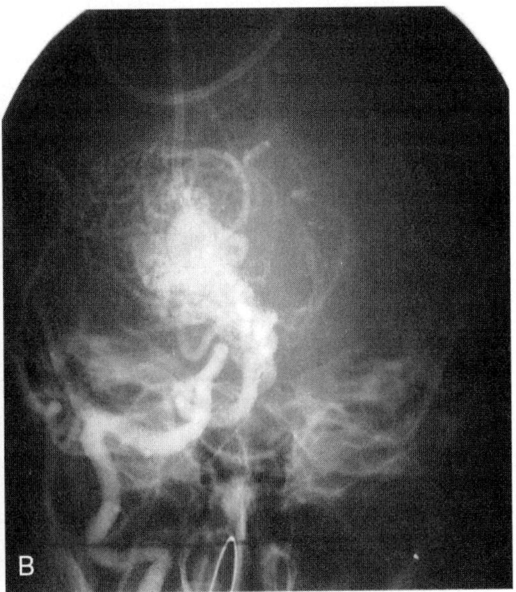

FIGURE 132–3. Computed tomographic scan *(A)* and anteroposterior, right arteriogram *(B)* of a patient with an acute posterior fossa hemorrhage from a hemispheric arteriovenous malformation. On the scan, notice the brainstem compression and acute obstructive hydrocephalus.

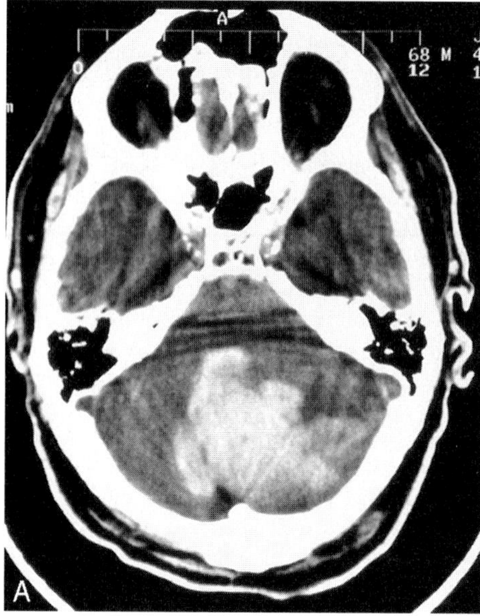

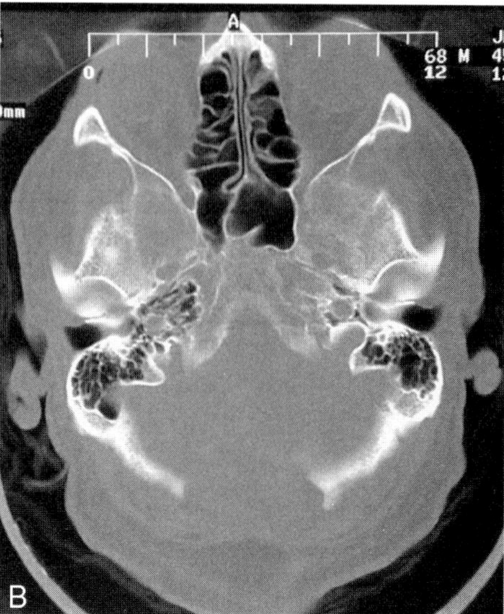

FIGURE 132–4. *A,* Computed tomographic scan of patient requiring acute clot evacuation because of a cerebellar hematoma from a small vermian arteriovenous malformation. *B,* The postoperative computed tomographic scan delineates the limits of the bony craniotomy.

tained from the preliminary computed tomographic scan because of distortion from the hematoma. The initial scan can allow the surgeon to form a general impression of the position of the nidus relative to the hematoma cavity after an acute hemorrhage. This information helps to determine the optimal corridor of approach and the size and position of the craniotomy if emergency hematoma evacuation is required (see Fig. 132–4*B*).

Complete cerebral angiography is required in the evaluation of AVMs and involves selective injection of the carotid and vertebral arteries. In evaluating the carotid circulation, injection of the common carotid arteries is usually sufficient, and we reserve selective injection of the external carotid arteries for when there is evidence of a dural component to the vascular malformation. Up to 10% of posterior fossa AVMs have significant dural feeding from the carotid circulation, which may be very amenable to preoperative embolization.[25, 26] With posterior fossa AVMs, it is essential to study each vertebral artery individually through a separate catheter injection.

Meticulous attention to the size and number of arterial feeders, venous drainage patterns, and associated aneurysms is of paramount importance for surgical planning and for determining the need and benefit of adjunctive preoperative embolization. Often, the complete picture regarding the feeding and drainage of a large cerebellar AVM is not clearly understood until the malformation has been partially embolized before

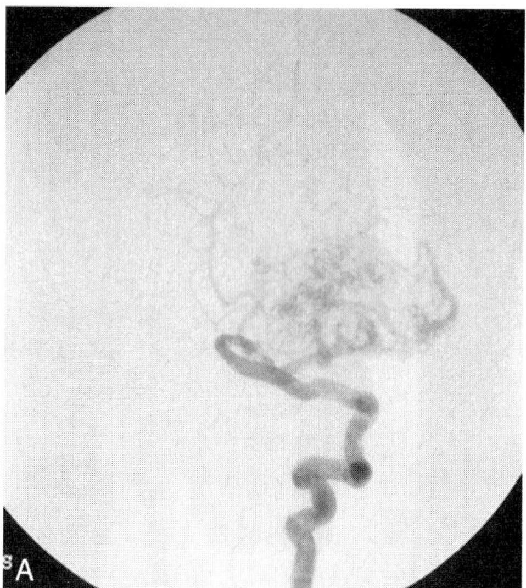

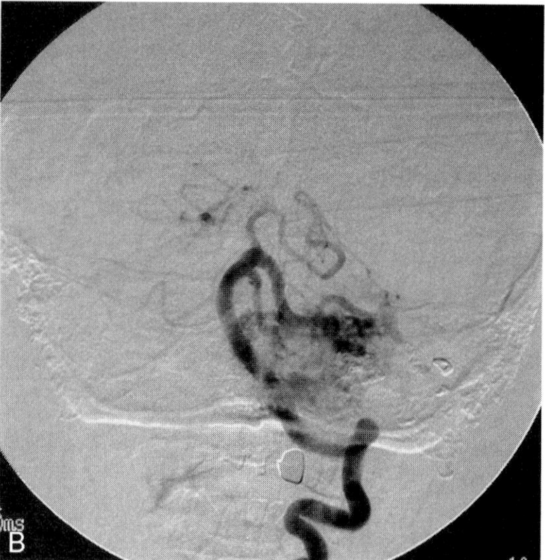

FIGURE 132–5. *A,* The anteroposterior left vertebral arteriogram demonstrates poor visualization of the anterior inferior cerebellar artery (AICA) feeding to a large cerebellar hemispheric arteriovenous malformation. *B,* After embolization of the posterior inferior cerebellar artery (PICA), the AICA feeding is clearly seen.

surgery because significant feeding from dilated proximal vessels may cause poor radiographic opacification of significant but more distally located feeders to the AVM. For example, the anterior inferior cerebellar artery (AICA) feeding to a large AVM of the cerebellar hemisphere may not significantly opacify during the initial diagnostic arteriogram (Fig. 132–5*A*). The contrast material preferentially flows into the PICA, which is typically the prominent feeder in most large AVMs involving the cerebellar hemisphere. After the PICA is embolized, previously underappreciated AICA feeding may become easier to visualize (see Fig. 132–5*B*). If PICA feeding to a cerebellar AVM originates proximal on the vertebral artery after it penetrates the dural ring adjacent to the occipital condyle, contrast injection of the contralateral vertebral artery may opacify and define AICA feeding without significant obscuration by or contrast runoff into the PICA ipsilateral to the malformation.

The presence of acute parenchymal hematomas can obscure or distort the angiographic appearance of an AVM nidus on the arterial and venous sides of the lesion due to mass effect. For this reason, if we have not removed a posterior fossa AVM immediately after a hemorrhage because of neurological deterioration, we repeat the angiographic studies after the hematoma has resolved over a period of 4 to 6 weeks and before any planned surgical intervention.

High-resolution MRI scans are obtained for all patients harboring AVMs shortly after presentation unless emergency hematoma evacuation is immediately required. Multiplanar MRI can provide valuable anatomic information regarding the AVM that influences the approach, intraoperative positioning, and craniotomy required to adequately expose and resect the lesion. MRI is useful to determine on which neural surface the malformation is most represented, the association and relationship of the malformation to the fourth ventricle, and the involvement or distortion of the brainstem surface (Fig. 132–6).

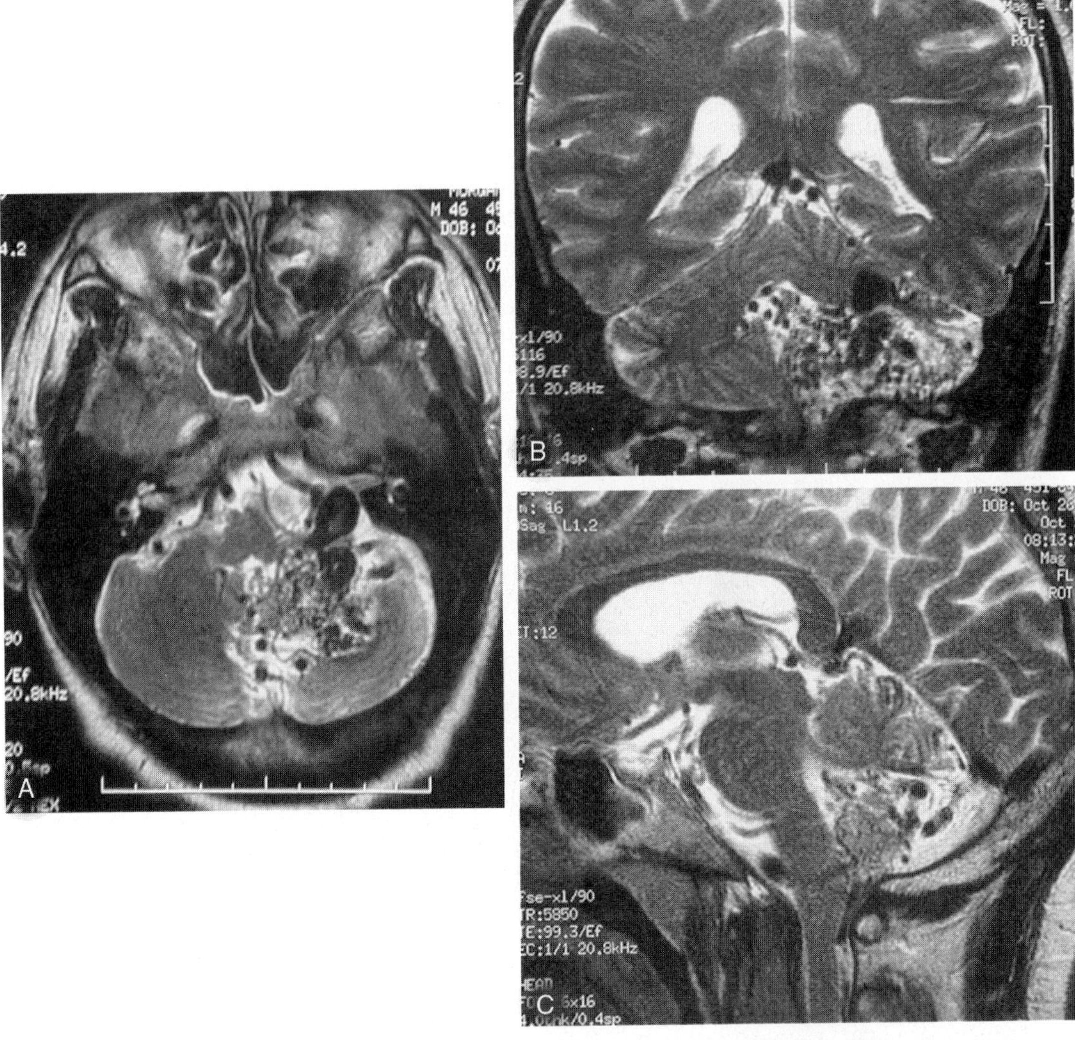

FIGURE 132–6. Axial *(A)*, coronal *(B)*, and sagittal *(C)* magnetic resonance imaging scans show a large tonsillohemispheric arteriovenous malformation extending into the fourth ventricle.

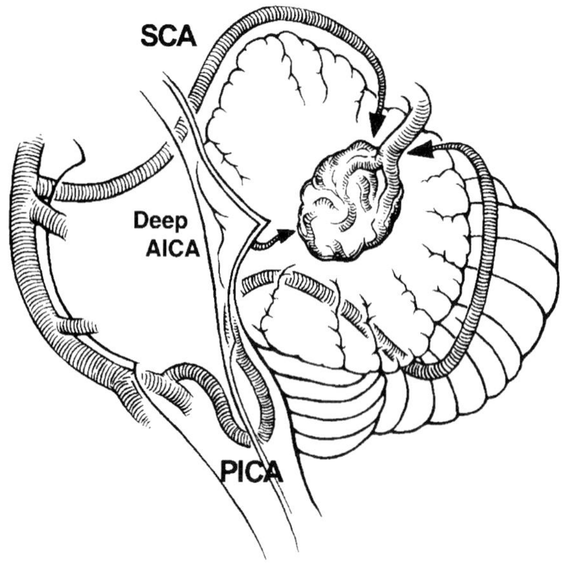

FIGURE 132–7. Schematic drawing of the arterial supply and venous outflow of a vermian arteriovenous malformation. Notice the deep anterior inferior cerebellar artery feeding through the ventricular roof. PICA, posterior inferior cerebellar artery; AICA, anterior inferior cerebellar artery; SCA, superior cerebellar artery.

CLASSIFICATION

A classification system for posterior fossa AVMs facilitates developing an operative approach, predicts blood supply to the AVM, and aids in determining the need for preoperative adjunctive embolization. We have categorized AVMs in the posterior fossa as located in the cerebellar vermis, cerebellar hemisphere, cerebellar tonsil, superficial pial brainstem, or deep parenchymal brainstem.[6, 11, 26] AVMs involving the cerebellar vermis and cerebellar hemispheres are the most commonly encountered AVMs within the posterior fossa because of the large geographic area represented by the cerebellar hemisphere and vermis compared with the size of the cerebellar tonsils and brainstem, which comprise only 5% of posterior fossa AVM locations.[6, 10, 11, 15, 26]

By classifying posterior fossa AVMs by specific locations, arterial supply and venous drainage can be reliably predicted before angiography. Vermian AVMs typically derive their arterial input primarily from distal branches of the superior cerebellar artery (SCA) and distal branches of the PICAs bilaterally (Fig. 132–7). If a vermian AVM is large or approaches the roof of the fourth ventricle, deep feeding from the AICA is typically seen. Deep AICA branches enter the foramen of Luschka, provide blood to the lateral roof of the fourth ventricle, and constitute the deep arterial irrigation to larger vermian AVMs. Vermian lesions located within the superior vermis involving the folium, declive, culmen, central lobule, and lingula derive arterial supply primarily from the SCA. When the lesion is located below the horizontal fissure and involves the tuber, pyramid, uvula, and nodulus, arterial input from the PICA usually predominates (Fig. 132–8*A*). The arterial input to vermian AVMs is bilaterally represented in most cases, and the venous drainage of vermian AVMs is usually directed superiorly into the galenic system by superior vermian veins bridging into the tentorium through the precentral cerebellar vein (see Fig. 132–8*B*).

The cerebellar hemisphere comparatively occupies a large region within the posterior fossa and is proportionately represented in the incidence of AVMs. Unlike vermian AVMs, hemispheric AVMs typically receive unilateral arterial supply from the SCA, AICA, and PICA (Fig. 132–9), unless the lesions are very large, in which case the PICA and, rarely, the SCA may be bilaterally represented. This principle can help distinguish vermian from hemispheric lesions when the malformation is medially located and abuts the cerebellar vermis. The dominant arterial supply is contingent on the specific location of the AVM within the cerebellar

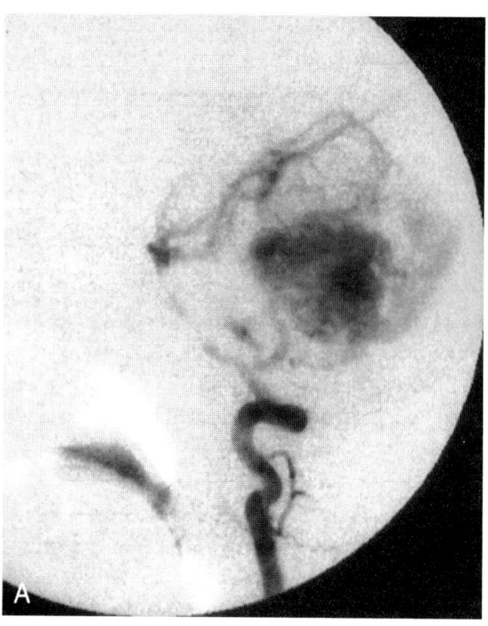

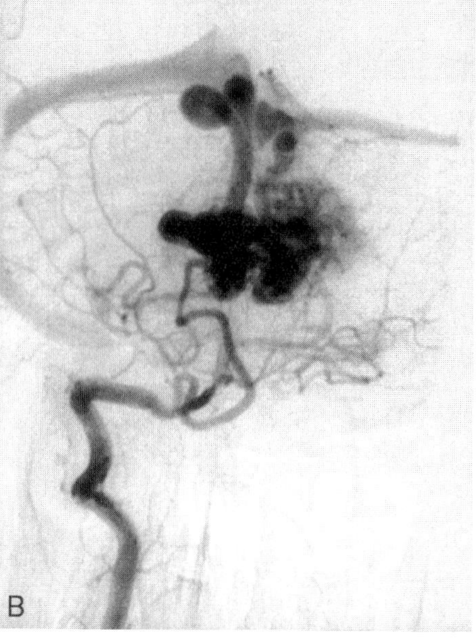

FIGURE 132–8. Lateral *(A)* and anteroposterior *(B)* vertebral arteriograms show a vermian arteriovenous malformation fed by branches of the superior cerebellar artery and posterior inferior cerebellar artery, with venous drainage superiorly into the galenic system.

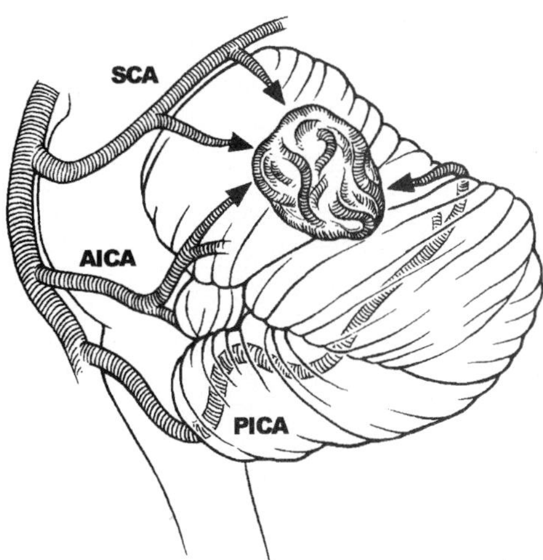

FIGURE 132–9. Schematic drawing of the typical arterial supply to arteriovenous malformations of the cerebellar hemisphere. AICA, anterior inferior cerebellar artery; PICA, posterior inferior cerebellar artery; SCA, superior cerebellar artery.

hemisphere. AVMs manifesting near the cerebellopontine angle (CPA) cistern or involving the lateral aspect of the ventricular wall and middle cerebellar peduncle typically receive significant feeding from AICA branches. With superiorly located hemispheric AVMs, the SCA is the dominant vascular supply (Fig. 132–10). AVMs situated superiorly within the cerebellar hemisphere typically drain into the petrosal vein laterally and into the galenic system superiorly.

Because of anatomic size constraints, AVMs involving or confined to the cerebellar tonsils are small and less frequently encountered lesions. AVMs strictly confined to the tonsil commonly receive unilateral PICA arterial feeding as the sole arterial input, although lesions that extend into the cerebellar hemisphere can have some blood supply from the AICA. Venous drainage of tonsillar AVMs is usually into the inferior vermian veins or lateral into the sigmoid sinus (Fig. 132–11).

Although large, cerebellar AVMs may encroach on structures of the brainstem, including the middle cerebellar peduncle, the lesions are usually distinctly marginated from the structures of the brainstem proper. We subgroup brainstem AVMs into two categories strictly related to pial or parenchymal involvement of the brainstem: superficial and deep lesions. This classification of brainstem AVMs has treatment implications, because superficial pial AVMs of the brainstem can be removed with reasonable safety, but deep parenchymal brainstem AVMs carry an extremely high risk with attempted microsurgical treatment. The arterial feeding of superficial brainstem AVMs is usually from SCA and AICA branches, and the venous drainage is invariably into the prepontine and petrosal venous system. Deep parenchymal brainstem AVMs typically receive arterial blood supply directly from vertebrobasilar perforators penetrating directly into the ventral portion of the brainstem. Venous drainage of deep parenchymal AVMs involving the brainstem is through periependymal venous channels into the galenic system.

TREATMENT

Preoperative Embolization

With the sole exception of very small AVMs, embolization is beneficial before surgical treatment of most AVMs in the posterior fossa. Technical advances in endovascular treatment techniques has increased the facility with which feeding pedicles leading to AVMs can be catheterized. Whether increasingly aggressive

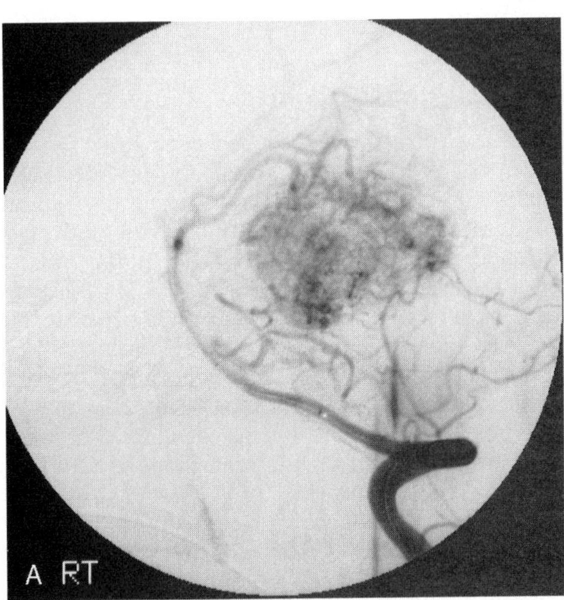

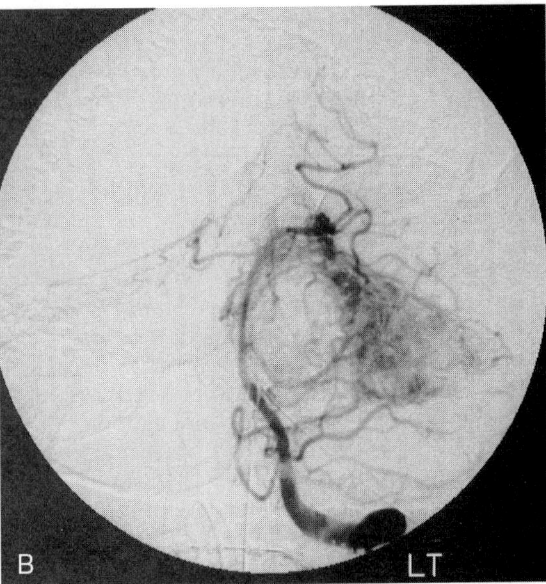

FIGURE 132–10. Lateral *(A)* and anteroposterior *(B)* vertebral arteriograms show a large arteriovenous malformation (AVM) involving the left cerebellar hemisphere. The AVM is supplied by branches of the superior cerebellar artery, anterior inferior cerebellar artery, and posterior inferior cerebellar artery.

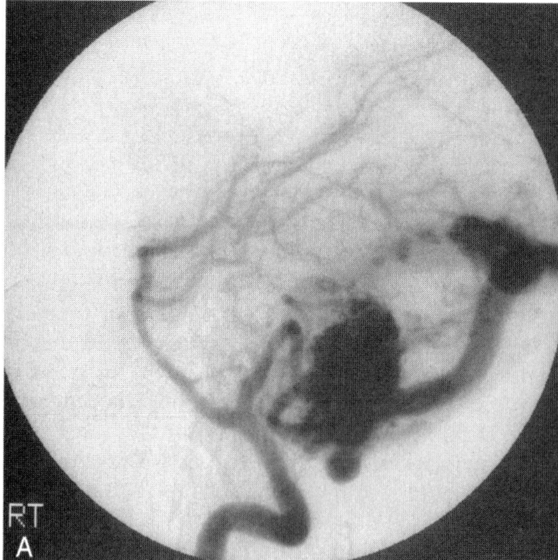

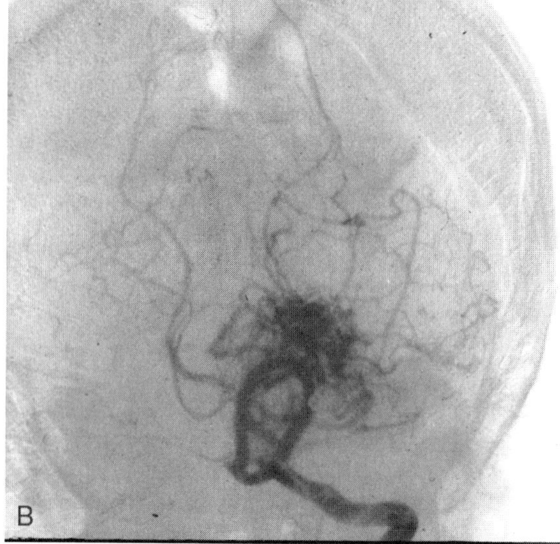

FIGURE 132–11. Lateral *(A)* and anteroposterior *(B)* vertebral arteriograms show a tonsillar arteriovenous malformation. The arterial supply is from the posterior inferior cerebellar artery, and the venous drainage is through the inferior vermian vein into the torcula.

embolization of vascular malformations significantly increases the overall management morbidity remains to be seen.[35–41] In a series of 150 patients who underwent embolization for treatment of intracranial AVMs, Wikhom and colleagues[42] reported a 1.3% mortality rate and severe and moderate complication rates of 6.7% and 15.3%, respectively. Because embolization is an adjunct to definitive surgical resection of the lesion, embolization should be primarily focused on feeding vessels that are very large or are difficult to expose early in the operative procedure. The preponderance of PICA feeding in most sizable AVMs of the cerebellum makes preoperative embolization of the PICA feeding helpful to decrease overall blood flow through the nidus. Because the PICA is easily exposed during the operative procedure, unnecessarily proximal embolization should be avoided because of the risk of brainstem or cerebellar infarction of uninvolved neural tissue.

Deep feeding from ventricular branches of the AICA is difficult to expose early in any posterior fossa operation, and embolization of these vessels are helpful. Embolization of feeding from SCA branches may be indicated if the SCA is dilated from increased blood flow and provides significant arterial supply to the lesion. If the feeding vessels to the malformation from the SCA are small, however, it may be difficult or impossible to selectively catheterize distal SCA feeding arteries. In this circumstance, proximal embolization of the SCA should be avoided, because unnecessary infarction of cerebellum not involved with the malformation will occur. The distal SCA feeders to the malformation can always be surgically accessed adjacent to the nidus during the operative resection of the AVM. The venous drainage of AVMs in this location is usually directed superiorly into the galenic system through the precentral cerebellar vein, and preoperative embolization of SCA branches to the malformation can help the surgical dissection on the tentorial surface of the cerebellum around the arterialized venous drainage.

Preoperative embolization has not been of significant utility in treating brainstem AVMs because of the high risk of brainstem infarction.[25, 26] We have surgically treated 25 patients with AVMs primarily confined to the brainstem. Of these, nine patients underwent attempted preoperative embolization, with minimal perceived benefit in seven and significant procedural morbidity in two patients. Because these patients were treated before the introduction of some of the newer liquid embolic agents, embolization of brainstem vascular malformations may have lower morbidity than these numbers reflect.

Radiosurgical Treatment

Stereotactic radiosurgery has been effective in a subgroup of patients with small AVMs. Successful treatment of AVMs by this modality requires that complete obliteration of the AVM be achieved with acceptable morbidity and mortality. Traditionally, radiosurgery was the treatment of choice for AVMs located in eloquent regions associated with high surgical morbidity such as the deep brain nuclei and brainstem. Obliteration rates of 64% to 81% over several months have been reported for AVMs measuring less than 3 cm in average diameter.[43] A strong correlation between AVM size and obliteration rate was demonstrated, showing a 100% obliteration rate for AVMs less than 1 cm^3 but only a 58% obliteration rate for AVMs between 4 and 10 cm^3.[44, 45] With cerebral AVMs treated exclusively by radiosurgery, complete obliteration rates for small, medium, and large AVMs were 92%, 80%, and 50%, respectively.[46–48] The obliteration rate for AVMs with volumes larger than 15 cm^3 increased to 58% when follow-up was extended to 50 months. Apart from small size, Pollock and coworkers[43, 46, 47] showed that other factors associated with successful radiosurgery included younger age, hemispheric AVM location, and fewer draining veins.

With radiosurgery, the latency interval until complete nidus obliteration may be 2 to 5 years, and during this time, no protective benefit is conferred.[49, 50] For patients with incomplete nidus obliteration, the reported hemorrhage rate until AVM obliteration is 4.8% during the first 2 years after radiosurgery and 5.0% per year during the third to fifth years after radiosurgery. In an analysis comparing microsurgical and stereotactic surgical treatment of AVMs, Pikus and colleagues[51] showed that, for AVMs with Spetzler-Martin grades of 1 to 3, patients treated with surgery had fewer postoperative hemorrhages, fewer deaths, fewer postoperative neurological deficits, and a higher incidence of obliteration.

Massager and associates[52] studied the results of 87 patients with brainstem AVMs treated with gamma knife radiosurgery and showed that 95% of the patients improved or remained neurologically stable, with an AVM obliteration rate of 63% at 2 years and 73% at 3 years. This result implies that, if the surgeon is experienced with AVM surgery, microsurgery is an excellent option for superficial pial AVMs of the brainstem, whereas radiosurgery is a better treatment for deep parenchymal vascular malformations within the brainstem.[26, 48]

Surgical Treatment

The basic tenets for surgical technique in posterior fossa AVM removal are similar to those for AVMs in other intracranial locations. The principles of optimal patient positioning, adequate bony exposure, extensive dural opening, meticulous attention to sharp microdissection, and compulsive hemostasis are critically important during surgical resection of posterior fossa AVMs.

POSITIONING

Special attention must be paid to the positioning of a patient for resection of a posterior fossa AVM. Because of the cramped confines of the posterior fossa, suboptimal positioning leads to poor exposure and surgeon fatigue and may compromise the entire procedure. The patient should be positioned in such a manner as to allow maximum brain relaxation with gravity and avoid mechanical retraction of the cerebellum. The selected patient position should be comfortable for the surgeon because the procedure may be of long duration. If the AVM presents to the CPA surface, a lateral position that allows optimal exposure of the CPA cistern and control of the feeding artery branches of the PICA and AICA is optimal. We use the body supine–head lateral position for AVMs involving the lateral aspect of the cerebellar hemisphere, the quadrangular lobule, the cerebellar tonsil, the flocculus, and the superficial aspect of the ventrolateral brainstem (Fig. 132–12). To resect AVMs involving the midline of the posterior fossa, such as vermian lesions or medial hemispheric lesions, we prefer the prone concord position (Fig. 132–13). With proper positioning, the cortical representation of the AVM should be readily accessible, the position should facilitate or minimize the degree of required brain retraction, provide the shortest corridor to the AVM, and be a comfortable position for the surgeon.[26]

1

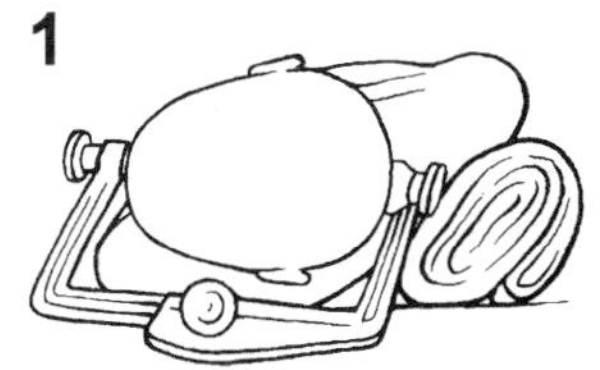

2

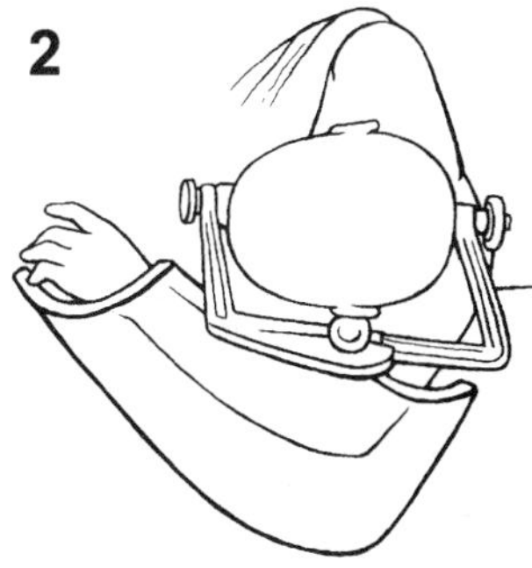

FIGURE 132–12. The supine head lateral position *(1)* and park-bench lateral position *(2)* are used for lateral posterior fossa exposures.

BONE REMOVAL AND CRANIOTOMY

For operative resection of a posterior fossa AVM, we create a generous bony opening that ensures adequate exposure of the entire AVM and helps identify feeding arteries and draining veins at some distance from the nidus. The opening should be large enough to allow room for AVM mobilization and address possible bleeding from several different corridors of approach. The dura must be adequately stripped before elevation of the bone flap because draining veins are often incor-

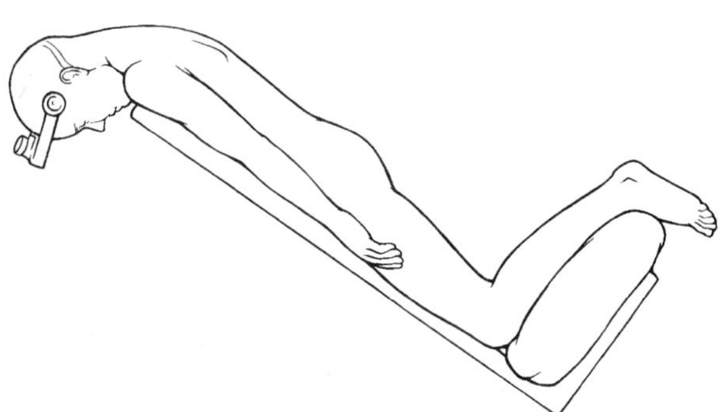

FIGURE 132–13. The prone concord position is used for midline posterior fossa exposures.

porated within the dura and can be injured during the opening of the craniotomy and produce torrential bleeding. When crossing an arterialized dural venous sinus with the bony craniotomy, the use of many perforator holes along with extensive dural stripping typically maximizes the safety of the opening and exposure of the lesion. The dura should be opened to the widest extent of the bony craniotomy to maximize AVM exposure.

DISSECTION TECHNIQUES

After opening the dura, the surface topography of the AVM is inspected and the approximate margins determined to be adequately within the bony opening. If the bone opening needs to be extended, it is better to perform the bone work at this stage of the operative procedure before any significant hemorrhaging from the AVM occurs. The AVM margin is then circumferentially demarcated by bipolar cautery, and any superficial arterial feeders to the AVM are transected at this time. The initial AVM dissection is focused on arterial supply that was not preoperatively embolized, and all venous drainage is carefully preserved. Early compromise of venous drainage leads to increased friability and swelling of the AVM and may result in AVM hemorrhage. It has been our experience that significant arterial feeding to supratentorial and infratentorial AVMs can be found hidden adjacent to significantly sized venous drainage. It is advantageous to dissect brain tissue completely away from the venous drainage to locate possible arterial feeding early in the operative procedure, taking care to avoid injuring the draining veins of the malformation. Before sacrificing any veins from the malformation, it is prudent to temporarily occlude them with bipolar forceps or temporary aneurysm clips and observe the AVM for swelling, increased turgor, or hemorrhage. Swelling of the malformation with temporary venous occlusion suggests that significant arterial supply to the AVM has not been completely eradicated.

As arterial feeding is eliminated to the AVM, we use a circumferential dissection technique beginning at the edge of the nidus and develop a dissection plane within a rim of gliotic tissue surrounding the nidus. Some vascular neurosurgeons have stated that infratentorial AVMs might have a much more indistinct margin compared with supratentorial AVMs or might be of racemose consistency. We and Yasargil[6] have not found any significant difference in the compactness of an AVM nidus within the posterior fossa compared with AVMs elsewhere in the brain, although this point merits mentioning for completeness (Yasargil, personal communication, 2001). It is important that the circumferential dissection of the nidus be performed evenly around the perimeter of the malformation. Symmetrical dissection of the AVM prevents inadvertent exposure of deep arterial feeding before adequate mobilization of the nidus. The deep feeding vessels to the malformation should not be dissected until the AVM nidus can be extensively mobilized and the deep, friable feeding arteries can be adequately exposed and controlled from several directions. This is best accomplished when the mass of the AVM has been well mobilized and is not significantly tethered in situ. As the AVM is mobilized, it is important not to undermine the AVM prematurely, especially when the malformation extends to the ventricle, because significant hemorrhaging typically results from periependymal feeders.

ANESTHETIC AND POSTOPERATIVE MANAGEMENT

We use a general anesthesia for surgical resection of all AVMs. After induction of anesthesia, central venous and arterial pressure monitoring lines are placed to provide close hemodynamic monitoring during the operative procedure and the postoperative period. During the operative procedure, the systemic blood pressure is kept at low normotensive levels, with systolic pressures typically between 100 and 120 mm Hg. Osmotic diuretics are administered on skin incision to facilitate brain retraction, and mild hyperventilation to P_{CO_2} levels of 30 mm Hg is used during the procedure. Perioperative medications include corticosteroids, antibiotics, and antihypertensive medications, if necessary. During the operative procedure and in the immediate postoperative period, invasive hemodynamic monitors, a Foley catheter, and lower extremity pneumatic compression devices are used.

The goal of surgery is complete removal of the malformation. Any residual AVM, regardless of size, carries a risk of hemorrhage. For this reason, we routinely perform immediate postoperative or intraoperative arteriograms on patients undergoing AVM resection before termination of the general anesthesia. If a residual AVM is visualized on the postoperative arteriogram, the patient is immediately returned to surgery for reopening of the craniotomy and total removal of the lesion.

SURGICAL RESECTION OF ARTERIOVENOUS MALFORMATIONS BY LOCATION

Arteriovenous Malformations of the Cerebellar Vermis

Lesions of the cerebellar vermis are best resected by a midline exposure using the prone concord position, regardless of the location of the AVM within the vermis. Chest rolls are employed, and the neck is flexed as much as tolerated. With the head in three-point fixation, the lower extremities are padded and flexed, and the operating table is angled into a reverse Trendelenburg position to bring the patient's nuchal region horizontal with the operating room floor (see Fig. 132–13). We employ a midline incision from above the inion to approximately the C3-4 spinous process. The craniotomy is fashioned for maximum exposure of the entire AVM, as previously described. For caudal lesions of the vermis, the bony opening is extended inferiorly to include opening of the foramen magnum. For AVMs involving the superior aspect of the vermis, we expose the transverse sinus and torcula to maximize superior exposure but typically do not resect and open the foramen magnum, except for extremely large malformations. For very caudally positioned AVMs, it may be necessary to remove the foramen magnum and the posterior arch of the first cervical vertebra to adequately expose the malformation. With the bone removed, a wide stellate durotomy further maximizes exposure.

Before beginning AVM dissection, we open the arachnoid overlying the cisterna magna and evacuate CSF from within the fourth ventricle to provide brain relaxation of the posterior fossa contents. During the initial microdissection, we locate both PICAs at the midline within the subarachnoid space. Dissection is performed distally along both PICAs until their entrance into the malformation can be visualized. The PICA feeding vessel is then ligated as close to the nidus as possible to prevent infarction of normal tissue (Fig. 132–14). After elimination of the main PICA feeding source is accomplished, we begin superficial circumferential dissection of the pial AVM margin from an inferior to superior direction. This usually eliminates the superficial AICA feeders that emanate from the CPA cistern and course over the hemispheric surface. Attention is turned to the SCA feeders that are exposed on the superior surface of the cerebellum and transected close to the AVM; they are often closely associated with superiorly directed venous drainage of the AVM. After dissection and transection of the PICA and SCA supply to vermian AVMs, a persistently turgid malformation is usually found among deep SCA or AICA feeders. When vermian AVMs approach the superior medullary velum or the lateral roof of the fourth ventricle, deep AICA branches are often involved and are clip ligated when the base of the malformation is dissected. It is often necessary to open the roof of the fourth ventricle because vermian AVMs commonly present to the fourth ventricular surface. After arterial supply has been completely eliminated, the draining veins are transected, and the nidus is delivered from the operative field.

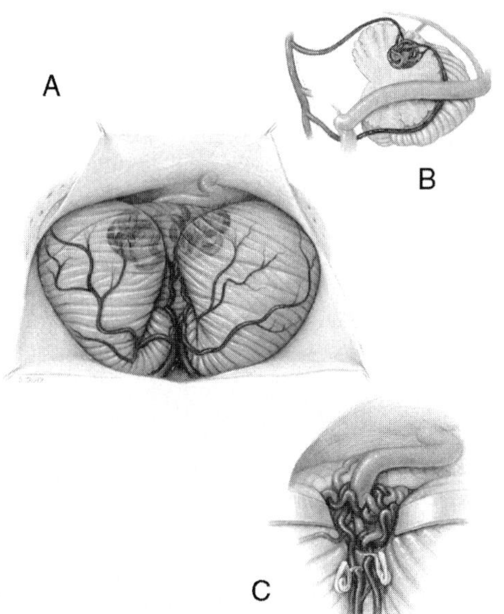

FIGURE 132–14. Artist's conception of the exposure *(A)*, blood supply *(B)*, and preliminary posterior inferior cerebellar artery dissection and ligation *(C)* for a vermian arteriovenous malformation.

Arteriovenous Malformations of the Cerebellar Hemisphere

The optimal approach for surgical resection of AVMs involving the cerebellar hemisphere depends on the size and location of the malformation, the need to expose the CPA cistern, and surgeon preference. When the patient is in the prone concord position, exposure and access to the CPA cistern are limited; we therefore place most patients in the supine or lateral position for resection of AVMs involving the lateral cerebellar hemisphere. With the patient in the supine position, a large roll is placed under the ipsilateral shoulder, and the head is rotated parallel to the floor of the operating room (see Fig. 132–12). Occasionally, patients are placed in the park-bench lateral position if they are large or have limited cervical spine mobility, although we try to avoid this position because the ipsilateral shoulder partially obstructs the working room for the surgeon. If a cerebellar hemispheric AVM is large or approaches the midline, we use the prone concord position.

For lateral exposures, a large, C-shaped incision centered over the mastoid area is used. After a subgaleal skin flap is elevated, the cervical muscles are detached from the occiput and reflected laterally and inferiorly. The bone is then removed as a craniectomy with the pneumatic drill to ensure adequate exposure of the malformation (Fig. 132–15). If access to the CPA cistern is needed to expose and control arterial supply to the malformation from the AICA, the bony craniectomy is performed to the margin of the transverse and sigmoid sinuses. As with vermian AVMs, after a cerebellar hemispheric AVM is exposed, the preliminary microsurgical dissection is focused on identification and division of the main arterial feeding vessels to the AVM. AVMs involving the cerebellar hemispheres can be fed by vessels of all three territories: SCA, AICA, and PICA (Fig. 132–16). PICA branches are identified adjacent to the cerebellar tonsils and are followed distally to their entry into the AVM. Similar to vermian lesions, dissection of the SCA branches can be difficult because they are often neighboring the engorged venous structures of the malformation and are usually encountered during dissection of the superior pial margin of the lesion. The blood supply from the AICA is identified in the CPA cistern as the branches course over the flocculus or enter the foramen of Luschka to supply the roof of the fourth ventricle. Unlike AVMs of the vermis, unless the hemispheric AVM is very large and without periependymal involvement of the AVM, it is usually not necessary to enter the fourth ventricle. Preoperative MRI demonstrates involvement of the roof of the fourth ventricle or middle cerebellar peduncle and helps to direct operative planning (Fig. 132–17). After the main arterial feeders are ligated adjacent to the

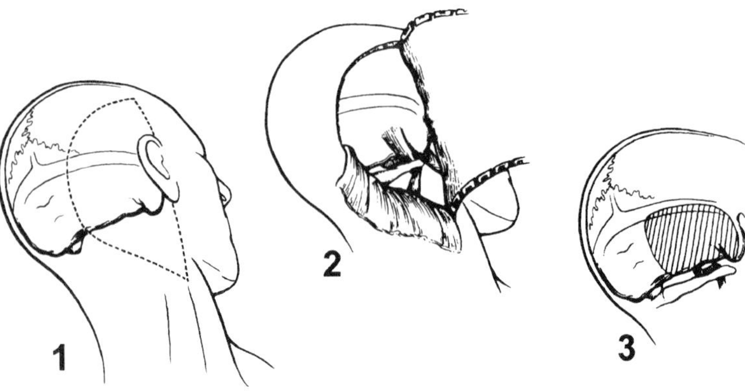

FIGURE 132–15. The C-shaped skin incision *(1)*, muscle reflection *(2)*, and bony craniotomy *(3)* are used to expose lateral posterior fossa vascular malformations.

nidus, the lesion is circumferentially dissected and elevated out of the uninvolved brain in the direction of the venous drainage, which is usually into the petrosal system or the galenic system, or both.

Arteriovenous Malformations of the Cerebellar Tonsils

The cerebellar tonsils occupy a relatively small geographic region within the posterior fossa. Consequently, AVMs confined to the cerebellar tonsil are not as frequently encountered as vermian or hemispheric malformations and are typically small lesions fed only by the ipsilateral PICA. Larger malformations involving the tonsil are described as tonsillohemispheric AVMs and typically glean their arterial blood supply from both PICAs and distal to the hemispheric branches of the AICA. Because of the small size and discrete arterial supply of AVMs confined to the cerebellar tonsil, surgical resection is relatively straightforward and uncomplicated.

For resection of tonsillar AVMs, patients are usually operated on in the supine position with a shoulder bolster under the ipsilateral shoulder and the head rotated laterally to obtain a true horizontal position. A curved, C-shaped skin incision is used, similar to that used for lateral hemispheric lesions, and the bony craniectomy is extended inferiorly to include the foramen magnum and laterally to the margin of the sigmoid sinus. It is occasionally necessary to remove the posterior arch of the first cervical vertebra to fully expose an AVM within a caudally located cerebellar tonsil. After the dura is opened and CSF is evacuated from the cisterna magna to facilitate relaxation of the cerebellar hemisphere, microsurgical dissection in the CPA cistern is performed to locate and control the PICA. The lateral or posterior medullary segment of this artery is dissected in the subarachnoid space and followed to the AVM. The PICA is then clip ligated and divided as it enters the nidus of the AVM (Fig. 132–18). Complete AVM removal can be expediently accomplished by simple resection or amputation of the involved cerebellar tonsil. Generally, venous drainage is routed into

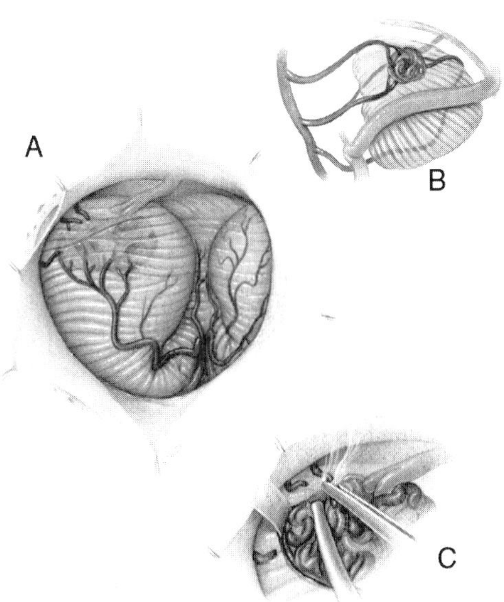

FIGURE 132–16. Artist's conception of the exposure *(A)*, blood supply *(B)*, and preliminary superior cerebellar artery dissection and ligation *(C)* for a hemispheric cerebellar arteriovenous malformation.

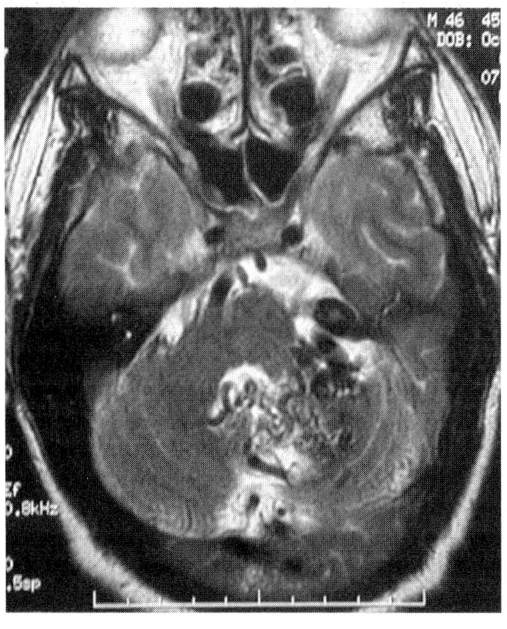

FIGURE 132–17. Axial magnetic resonance imaging shows a tonsillohemispheric arteriovenous malformation with involvement of the fourth ventricle and middle cerebellar peduncle.

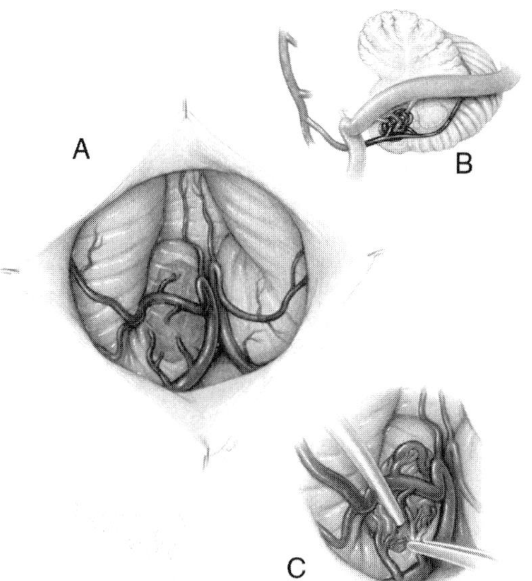

FIGURE 132–18. Artist's conception of exposure *(A)*, blood supply *(B)*, and preliminary posterior inferior cerebellar artery dissection and ligation *(C)* for an arteriovenous malformation involving the cerebellar tonsil.

the inferior vermian system but may also involve the sigmoid sinus laterally.

Arteriovenous Malformations of the Brainstem

AVMs of the brainstem are rare.[53, 54] In the cooperative study of subarachnoid hemorrhage, they represented 2% of all intracranial AVMs, and in Soloman and Stein's series[55] of 250 intracranial AVMs, only 12 (4.8%) involved the brainstem. These lesions may involve the mesencephalon, pons, medulla, tectal plate, floor of the fourth ventricle, or CPA cistern. Like most posterior fossa AVMS, brainstem malformations often manifest with hemorrhage as the initial symptom. Brainstem AVMs can cause subarachnoid or intraparenchymal hemorrhage and may be associated with venous or arterial aneurysms. Deep parenchymal AVMs of the brainstem are more likely to cause progressive neurological dysfunction that mimics a demyelinating process than superficial pial lesions. Superficial brainstem AVMs may manifest with hemorrhage but are also commonly associated with cranial neuropathies, typically involving the trigeminal, facial, or abducens nerves. The natural history of brainstem AVMs is ominous, with recurrent hemorrhages occurring in untreated lesions. We recommend surgical removal of all superficial brainstem AVMs in younger patients and removal of deep parenchymal malformations only in patients experiencing relentless neurological decline with conservative management.

The outcome of patients undergoing surgery for treatment of brainstem malformations largely depends on the location of the malformation and the skill and experience of the surgeon. We divide brainstem AVMs into those occurring in superficial and deep locations. Superficial brainstem AVMs are closely associated with the pia and are clearly represented within the subarachnoid space. They are most commonly situated in the anterolateral aspect of the brainstem surface, are associated with the CPA angle, and typically receive direct feeding from a dilated AICA or SCA branch (Fig. 132–19). These AVMs may involve surrounding parenchyma and sometimes extend into the adjacent foramen of Luschka. When located on the ventral surface of the brainstem, superficial pial AVMs can also be fed by deep, perforating arterial vessels from the basilar artery. Venous drainage typically occurs through the lateral pontine vein into the petrosal or galenic system.

AVMs associated with the CPA angle are approached laterally. Patients are placed in the supine or lateral position described previously for approaching lateral hemispheric AVMs of the cerebellum. An extensive bony craniotomy is performed from the transverse and sigmoid sinus above to the foramen magnum be-

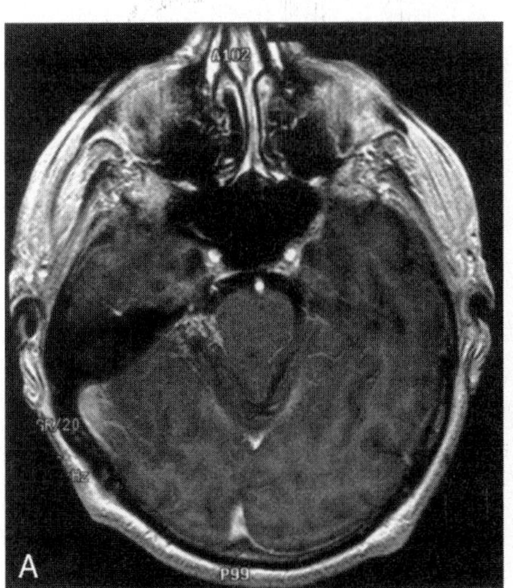

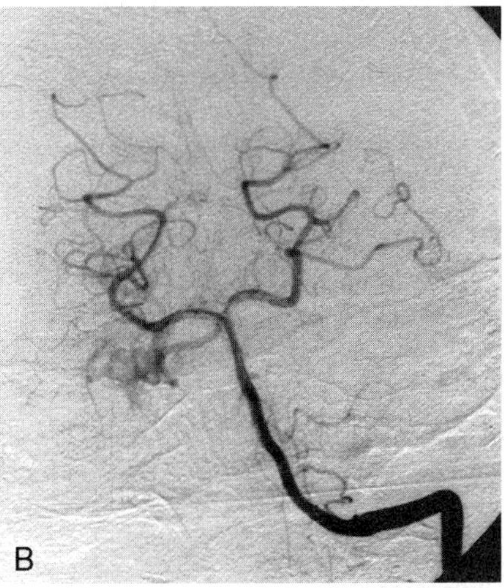

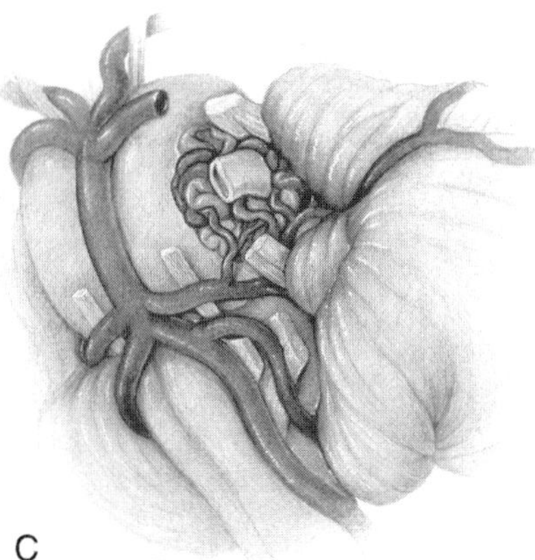

FIGURE 132–19. Magnetic resonance image *(A)*, anteroposterior vertebral arteriogram *(B)*, and artist's rendering *(C)* of the typical location and vascular supply of a ventral brainstem arteriovenous malformation involving the nerve root entry (exit) zones of cranial nerves V and VII.

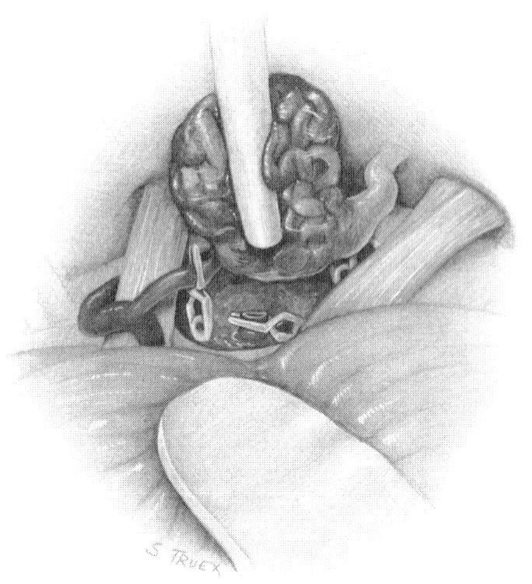

FIGURE 132–20. In the artist's depiction of a preliminary resection of a superficial pial brainstem arteriovenous malformation, notice that the malformation must be elevated away from the brainstem.

low. The lateral aspect of the sigmoid sinus is uncovered, allowing elevation of the posterior part of the sinus to optimize exposure of the CPA cistern. The cisterns are then opened widely from the vertebral artery to the petrosal vein, and CSF is evacuated to facilitate relaxation of the cerebellum. The typical circumferential dissection of the AVM nidus, although preferable, is limited because of the confines of working in the CPA cistern ventral to the cerebellum. The AVM must be elevated away from the pial surface and retracted laterally (Fig. 132–20). It can then be excised by performing a subpial dissection in a shallow plane from a posterolateral to anteromedial direction. By undercutting the malformation from the pial surface, arterial feeders are sequentially ligated.

A similar approach may be employed for superficial AVMs of the tectal plate, lateral medulla, and anterior and lateral cerebral peduncles. AVMs associated with the quadrigeminal plate and dorsal midbrain are operated on with patients positioned in a prone concord position and with an extensive suboccipital craniotomy extending from the transverse sinus to the foramen magnum. AVMs involving the fourth ventricle are best approached from the midline with patients in the prone

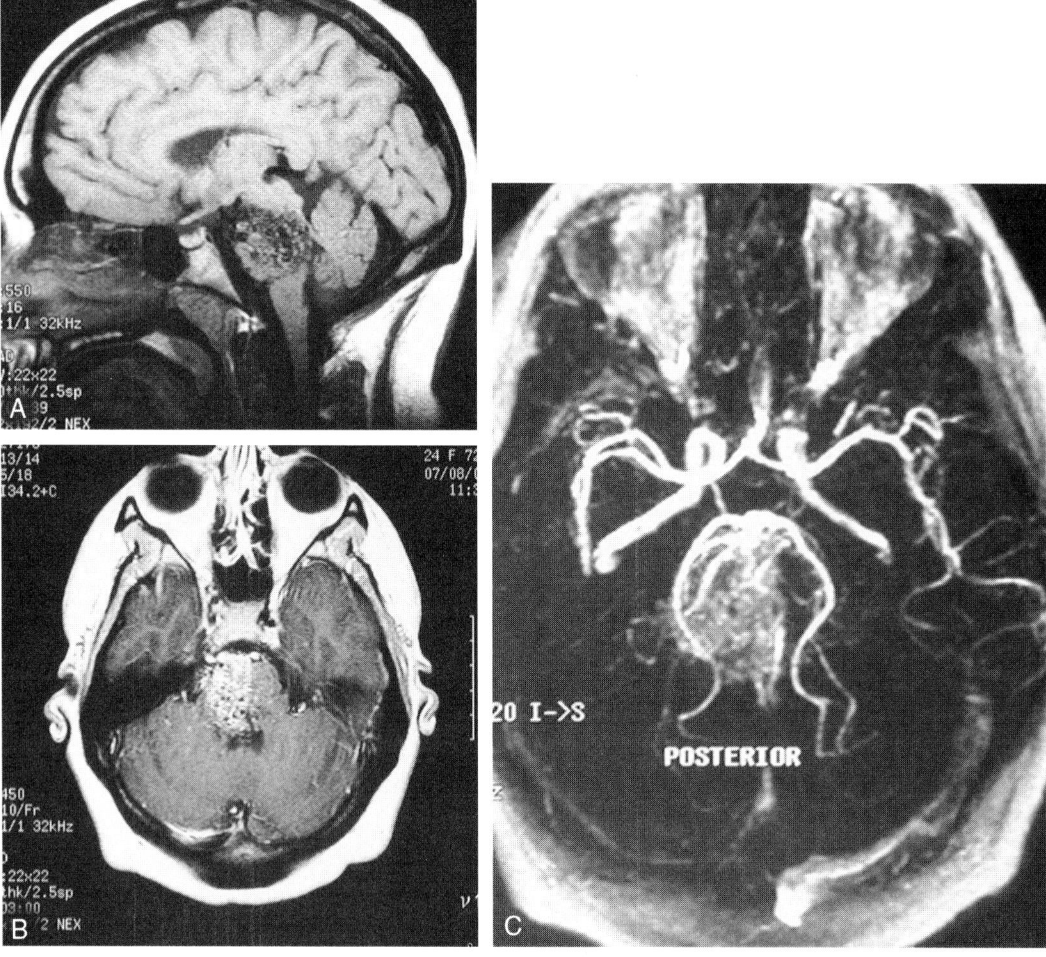

FIGURE 132–21. Sagittal magnetic resonance imaging (MRI) *(A)*, axial MRI *(B)*, and magnetic resonance angiography *(C)* show a deep parenchymal arteriovenous malformation of the brainstem.

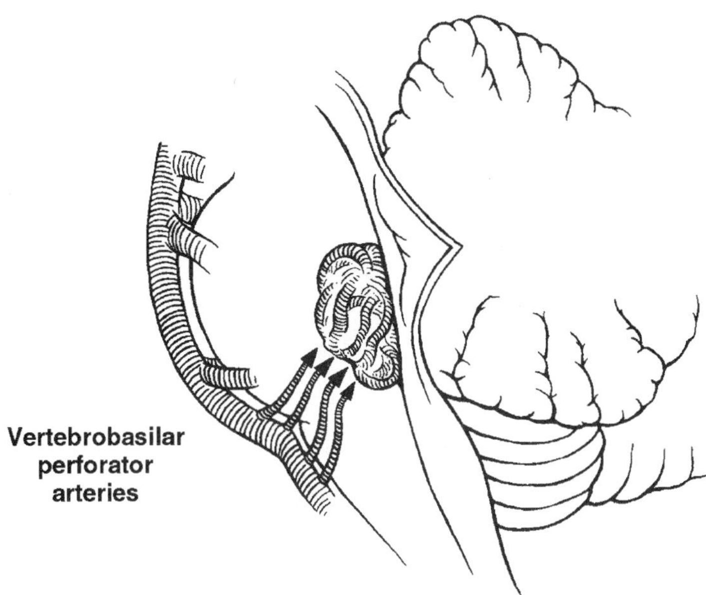

FIGURE 132–22. The schematic drawing shows the typical arterial supply to deep parenchymal arteriovenous malformations of brainstem.

concord position as well. Depending on the location of the AVM and the experience of the surgeon, even superficial pial AVMs of the brainstem should be considered as candidates for radiosurgical treatment if lower morbidity and durable treatment will result from nonmicrosurgical management.

Deep brainstem AVMs pose a greater risk of surgical morbidity and mortality because they are often intimately associated with surrounding midbrain, pontine, and medullary structures (Fig. 132–21). Arterial feeders are deep and usually arise from the vertebrobasilar system (Fig. 132–22). They enter from the ventral aspect of the lesion through normal brainstem tissue. Venous drainage is usually periependymal into the petrosal or galenic system. Embolization of these lesions is contraindicated because of the small size of the vessels that also supply normal brain.

For the most part, patients with deep brainstem AVMs are poor surgical candidates because of the high risk involved with operative excision of these lesions. However, if the lesion is small and surrounded by a resolving hematoma cavity, successful surgical resection is possible. The basic tenet of surgery in this area is to conserve the maximal amount of surrounding normal tissue by tolerating bleeding within the depths of the dissection cavity until bleeding can be controlled by precise bursts of bipolar cautery or application of very small AVM clips. Because patients with deep parenchymal AVMs of the brainstem are poor candidates for surgical resection, gamma irradiation of deep, small, and unruptured brainstem AVMs is generally advocated.

REFERENCES

1. Stein BM, Kadrer A: Intracranial arteriovenous malformations. Clin Neurosurg 39:76–113, 1992.
2. Wilkins RH: Natural history of intracranial vascular malformations: A review. Neurosurgery 16:421–430, 1985.
3. Berman MF, Sciacca RR, Spellman JP, et al: The epidemiology of brain arteriovenous malformations. Neurosurgery 47:389–397, 2000.
4. Perret G, Nishioka H: Arteriovenous malformations: An analysis of 545 cases of cranio-cerebral arteriovenous malformations and fistulae reported to the cooperative study. J Neurosurg 25:467–490, 1966.
5. Luessenhop AJ, Rosa L: Cerebral arteriovenous malformations. J Neurosurg 60:14–22, 1984.
6. Yasargil MG: Microsurgery, vol IIIB. New York, Thieme, 1998, pp 168–203, 358–366.
7. Olivecrona H, Rives J: Arteriovenous aneurysms of the brain: Their diagnosis and treatment. Arch Neurol Psychiatry (Chicago) 59:567, 1948.
8. Drake CG: Cerebral arteriovenous malformations: Considerations for and experience with surgical treatment in 166 cases. Clin Neurosurg 26:145–208, 1979.
9. Troupp H, Marttila I, Halonen V: Arteriovenous malformations of the brain. Prognosis without operation. Acta Neurochir (Wien) 22:125–128, 1970.
10. Batjer H, Samson D: Arteriovenous malformations of the posterior fossa. J Neurosurg 64:849–856, 1986.
11. Drake CG, Friedman AH, Peerless SJ: Posterior fossa arteriovenous malformations. J Neurosurg 64:1–10, 1986.
12. Garcia MR, Alvarez H, Eoulou A: Posterior fossa arteriovenous malformations: Angioarchitecture in relation to their hemorrhagic episodes. Neuroradiology 31:471–475, 1990.
13. McCormick WF: The pathology of vascular ("arteriovenous") malformations. J Neurosurg 24:807–816, 1966.
14. Nussbaum ES, Heros RC, Madison MT, et al: The pathogenesis of arteriovenous malformations: Insights provided by a case of multiple ateriovenous malformations developing in relation to a developmental venous anomaly. Neurosurgery 43:347–352, 1998.
15. Martin N, Stein B, Wilson C: Arteriovenous malformations of the posterior fossa. In Wilson C, Stein B (eds): Intracranial Arteriovenous Malformations. Baltimore, Williams & Wilkins, 1984, pp 209–221.
16. Matsumura H, Makita Y, Someda K, et al: Arteriovenous malformations in the posterior fossa. J Neurosurg 47:50–56, 1977.
17. McCormick W, Hardman J, Boutler T: Vascular malformations ("angiomas") of the brain, with special reference to those occurring in the posterior fossa. J Neurosurg 28:241–251, 1968.
18. Guidetti B, Delitala A: Intracranial arteriovenous malformations, conservative and surgical treatment. J Neurosurg 53:149–152, 1980.
19. Fults D, Kelly DL: Natural history of arteriovenous malformations of the brain: A clinical study. Neurosurgery 15:658–662, 1984.
20. Crawford P, West C, Chadwick D, Shaw M: Arteriovenous mal-

formations of the brain: Natural history in unoperated patients. J Neurol Neurosurg Psychiatry 49:1–10, 1986.
21. Brown RD, Weibers DO, Forbes G, et al: The natural history of unruptured intracranial arteriovenous malformations. J. Neurosurg 68:352–357, 1988.
22. Brown RD, Weibers DO, Forbes GS: Unruptured intracranial aneurysms and arteriovenous malformations: Frequency of intracranial hemorrhage and relationship of lesions. J Neurosurg 73: 859–863, 1990.
23. Itoyama Y, Uemura S, Ushio Y, et al: Natural course of unoperated intracranial arteriovenous malformations: Study of 50 cases. J Neurosurg 71:805–809, 1989.
24. Ondra SL, Troupp H, George ED: The natural history of symptomatic arteriovenous malformations of the brain: A 24-year follow-up assessment. J Neurosurg 73:387–391, 1990.
25. Samson D, Batjer H: Posterior fossa arteriovenous malformations. In Carter L, Spetzler R (eds): Neurovascular Surgery. New York, McGraw-Hill, 1995, pp 1005–1015.
26. Samson DS, Kopitnik TA, Batjer H, Purdy PD: Technical features of the management of arteriovenous malformations of the brainstem and cerebellum. In Batjer H, Caplan L, Friberg L, et al (eds): Cerebrovascular Disease. Philadelphia, Lippincott-Raven, 1997, pp 811–821.
27. Kaptain GJ, Lanzino G, Do HM, et al: Posterior inferior cerebellar artery aneurysms associated with posterior fossa arteriovenous malformation: Report of five cases and review of the literature Surg Neurol 51:146–152, 1999.
28. Mabuchi S, Kamiyama H, Abe H: Distal aneurysms of the superior cerebellar artery and posterior inferior cerebellar artery feeding an associated arteriovenous malformation: Case report. Neurosurgery 30:284–287, 1992.
29. Meisel HJ, Mansmann U, Alvarez H, et al: Cerebral arteriovenous malformations and associated aneurysms: Analysis of 305 cases from a series of 662 patients. Neurosurgery 46:793–802, 2000.
30. Noterman J, Georges, Brotchi J: Arteriovenous malformation associated with multiple aneurysms in the posterior fossa: A case report with review of the literature. Neurosurgery 21:387–391, 1987.
31. Cunha MJ, Stein BM, Solomon RA, et al: The treatment of associated intracranial aneurysms and arteriovenous malformations. J Neurosurg 77:853–859, 1992.
32. Redekop G, TerBrugge K, Montanera W, et al: Arterial aneurysms associated with cerebral arteriovenous malformations: Classification, incidence, and risk of hemorrhage. J Neurosurg 89:539–546, 1998.
33. Westphal M, Grzyska U: Clinical significance of pedicle aneurysms on feeding vessels, especially those located in infratentorial arteriovenous malformations. J Neurosurg 92:995–1001, 2000.
34. Thompson RC, Steinberg GK, Levy RP, et al: The management of patients with arteriovenous malformations and associated intracranial aneurysms. Neurosurgery 43:202–212, 1998.
35. Purdy PD, Batjer H, Samson D: Management of hemorrhagic complications from preoperative embolization of arteriovenous malformations. J Neurosurg 74:205–211, 1991.
36. Vinuela F, Dion JE, Duckwiler G, et al: Combined endovascular embolization and surgery in the management of cerebral arteriovenous malformation: Experience with 101 cases. J Neurosurg 75:856–864, 1991.
37. Latchaw RE, Harris RD, Chou SN, et al: Combined embolization and operation in the treatment of cervical arteriovenous malformations. Neurosurgery 6:131–137, 1980.
38. Luessenhop AJ, Presper JH: Surgical embolization of cerebral arteriovenous malformations through internal carotid and vertebral arteries. J Neurosurg 42:443–451, 1975.
39. Lundqvist C, Wikholm G, Svendsen P: Embolization of cerebral arteriovenous malformations: Part II—Aspects of complications and late outcomes. Neurosurgery 39:460–469, 1996.
40. Debrun GM, Aletich V, Ausman JI, et al: Embolization of the nidus of brain arteriovenous malformations with n-butyl cyanoacrylate. Neurosurgery 40:112–121, 1997.
41. Dion JE, Duckwiler GR, Lylyk P, et al: Progressive suppleness catheter: A new tool for superselective angiography and embolization. Neuroradiology 10:1068–1070, 1989.
42. Wikholm G, Lundqvist C, Svendsen P: Embolization of cerebral arteriovenous malformations. Part 1. Technique, morphology, and complications. Neurosurgery 39:448–459, 1996.
43. Pollock BE, Flickinger JC, Lundsford LD, et al: Factors associated with successful arteriovenous malformation radiosurgery. Neurosurgery 42:1239–1247, 1998.
44. Chang JH, Chang JW, Park YG, et al: Factors related to complete occlusion of arteriovenous malformations after gamma knife radiosurgery. J Neurosurg 93(Suppl 3):96–101, 2000.
45. Friedman WA, Bova FJ, Mendenhall WM: Linear accelerator radiosurgery for arteriovenous malformations: The relationship of size to outcome. J Neurosurg 82:180–189, 1995.
46. Pollock BE, Flickinger JC, Lunsford LD, et al: Hemorrhage risk after stereotactic radiosurgery of cerebral arteriovenous malformations. Neurosurgery 38:652–661, 1996.
47. Pollock BE, Lunsord LD, Kondziolka D, et al: Patient outcomes after stereotactic radiosurgery for "operable" arteriovenous malformations. Neurosurgery 35:1–8, 1994.
48. Schaller C, Schramm J: Microsurgical results for small arteriovenous malformations accessible for radiosurgical or embolization treatment. Neurosurgery 40:664–674, 1997.
49. Gobin PY, Laurent A, Merienne L, et al: Treatment of brain arteriovenous malformation by embolization and radiosurgery. J Neurosurg 85: 19–28, 1996.
50. Hung-chi Pan D, Guo W, Chung W, et al: Gamma knife radiosurgery as a single treatment modality for large cerebral arteriovenous malformations. J Neurosurg 93(Suppl 3):113–119, 2000.
51. Pikus HJ, Beach ML, Harbaugh RE: Microsurgical treatment of arteriovenous malformations: Analysis and comparison with stereotactic radiosurgery. J Neurosurg 88:641–646, 1998.
52. Massager N, Regis J, Kondziolka D, et al: Gamma knife radiosurgery for brainstem arteriovenous malformations: Preliminary results. J Neurosurg 93(Suppl 3):102–103, 2000.
53. Drake CG: Surgical removal of arteriovenous malformations from the brain stem and cerebellopontine angle. J Neurosurg 43: 661–670, 1975.
54. Chyatte D: Vascular malformations of the brain stem. J Neurosurg 70:847–852, 1989.
55. Solomon RA, Stein BM: Management of arteriovenous malformations of the brain stem. J Neurosurg 64:857–864, 1986.

CHAPTER 133

Surgical and Radiosurgical Management of Giant Arteriovenous Malformations

STEVEN D. CHANG ■ GARY K. STEINBERG

The successful treatment of arteriovenous malformations (AVMs) is a challenging problem faced by neurosurgeons. Giant AVMs represent a rare, but excessively difficult group of AVMs, which often carry a higher treatment morbidity and mortality than their smaller counterparts. Giant AVMs are high-flow, angiographically visible vascular malformations that are greater than 6 cm in maximal diameter. The size alone results in a Spetzler-Martin[1] grade of at least III, and most giant AVMs are classified as a Spetzler-Martin grade IV or V. The size of giant AVMs almost invariably results in at least a portion of the malformations being located within or immediately adjacent to eloquent regions of the brain, and these lesions often have deep and superficial venous drainage. These giant AVMs often have an arterial supply from multiple vascular distributions from the anterior as well as posterior circulation, and in many cases, the arterial supply is bilateral.

Many of these giant AVMs previously were considered untreatable by neurosurgeons based on their size. Since the 1980s, however, neurosurgeons have developed novel approaches that allow treatment of these lesions with an acceptable risk. The use of microinstrumentation and neurosurgical microscopes along with the aid of stereotaxis, electrophysiologic monitoring, and preoperative embolization has enabled neurosurgeons to resect some giant AVMs safely. Stereotactic radiosurgery has allowed treatment of many giant AVMs, either by decreasing the size of the nidus after radiosurgery and facilitating resection of a smaller AVM or by treating residual AVM after surgery, embolization, or both. The optimal management of these giant AVMs must include a detailed understanding of the hemodynamics and anatomy of each particular vascular malformation as well as familiarity with the various methods of AVM treatment.

PRESENTATION AND PREOPERATIVE EVALUATION

Presenting Symptoms

The size of giant AVMs and the large amount of arteriovenous shunting within these lesions often result in a symptom unique from smaller AVMs. Small vascular malformations typically present with headaches,[2, 3] seizures,[4–6] or hemorrhage.[4, 5, 7–9] Giant AVMs can manifest not only with any of the aforementioned symptoms, but also can cause transient and progressive neurological dysfunction through cerebrovascular *steal*. The large blood volume shunting through the malformations can cause a relative hypoperfusion in the surrounding neurological tissue resulting in ischemia.[10–13] This ischemia is due to lower blood pressure within the arterial feeders of the AVM than the surrounding brain, resulting in preferential shunting of blood to the AVM away from the normal brain.

AVMs have initial hemorrhage rates of 2% to 4% and annual rebleed rates of approximately 4% to 18%.[7, 14–17] Mortality from each hemorrhage approximates 10% to 15%,[4, 5, 7, 8] and 50% of patients suffer some form of neurological deficit as a result of AVM bleeding.[9] Some authors believe that larger AVMs have bleed rates slightly lower than their smaller counterparts.[7, 18, 19] Other studies have shown no consistent relationship between size and risk of hemorrhage,[15, 20] and feeding artery pressure (believed to be a factor in AVM hemorrhage risk) was not correlated with AVM size.[21] Giant AVMs with components in the basal ganglia, thalamus, and pineal region may be associated with increased morbidity if they bleed, however, with more than 60% of these patients suffering significant morbidity or death from hemorrhage.[22] Angiographic factors that have been shown to correlate with risk of AVM hemorrhage are central venous drainage, periventricular location, and intranidal aneurysms[23, 24] as well as a single draining vein[24] and stenotic venous drainage.[25] By their size alone, giant AVMs are more likely to have a component of central venous drainage and have a portion of the AVM adjacent to or within the ventricle.

Indications and Contraindications for Surgery

Indications for resection of giant AVMs must include the natural history of the AVM as well as the combined risks of multimodality treatment for a particular patient.[26, 27] Most angiographically documented giant AVMs are candidates for treatment, particularly if they have hemorrhaged or are causing significant progressive neurological deficits, disabling headaches, or medically intractable seizures. The risk of surgical resection generally is related to AVM size, location, and complexity of arterial feeders and venous drainage,[1] factors that make these giant AVMs a higher risk than smaller AVMs to treat with surgery alone. Larger lesions may require staged surgical resection or multimodality therapy combining microsurgery, embolization, and stereotactic radiosurgery.[27–29] Other factors affecting treatment risk include patient clinical condition and age and surgeon experience.

The location of the giant AVM under consideration significantly affects the risk of surgical resection.[26–28, 30–32] Because of their size, giant AVMs often involve eloquent cortex, significantly increasing risk on resection. Resection of giant cortical AVMs may cause motor or sensory deficits (frontal/parietal), visual field defects (occipital), or memory deficits and changes in cognition and personality (cingulate gyrus and corpus callosum). Treatment of deep portions of giant AVMs within the basal ganglia and thalamus can cause hemiplegia, sensory deficits, dysphasia, and cognitive and memory deficits.[22, 33, 34] The clinical condition of the patient has a bearing on surgical resection, with poor-grade patients usually experiencing poor outcome.[29] Younger patients have a better benefit-to-risk ratio for treatment of giant AVMs for two reasons. First, the brain of a young patient can tolerate better resection of the vascular malformation and has improved recovery after surgery.[35] Second, a young patient translates into longer AVM-free survival on completion of resection.[35] Likewise, patients with significant mass effect from a hemorrhagic clot resulting from AVM rupture should undergo emergent evacuation of the hemorrhage, with AVM resection reserved for a later date. The timing of resection of giant AVMs is similar to that of other AVMs in that resection should be planned under nonemergent conditions. Resection of the AVM 4 to 6 weeks after hemorrhage, when the blood is liquefied, may improve the ease of resection.[8, 22, 28, 36] In many cases, the hematoma cavity has performed a portion of the dissection around the nidus of the AVM. This short interval allows the patient to have stabilization or improvement in any neurological deficit.[37]

Failure of stereotactic radiosurgery and embolization are other indications for surgical resection,[26–29, 31, 32] although in the case of giant AVMs, these treatment modalities generally are used as adjuncts in reducing the AVM size before planned microsurgical resection. Partial obliteration after radiosurgery does not confer protection from AVM rehemorrhage,[22, 29, 33, 38, 39] and an alternative therapy should be sought for residual AVMs presenting more than 3 years after radiosurgical treatment. Embolization is a useful treatment for giant cortical AVMs,[40] but it is less useful in the treatment of deeper arterial feeders (thalamoperforating arteries, choroidal arteries, and lenticular striate arteries) within the basal ganglia and thalamus. These vessels primarily arise from parent vessels at right angles and have small lumens and are difficult to canulate.[22, 33, 34] Nonetheless, in selected cases, embolization has been extremely helpful in partially obliterating basal ganglia and thalamic arterial feeders.[28, 29, 41]

Contraindications to treatment of giant AVMs include poor clinical condition of the patient as a result of AVM hemorrhage, medical conditions precluding surgery, and very elderly AVM patients. Often, patients in poor neurological condition may improve over time or with minor procedural interventions, such as a ventriculostomy or ventriculoperitoneal shunt for hydrocephalus, and may become candidates for treatment. Other patients with significant neurological deficits as a result of hemorrhage can make dramatic improvements with time and would qualify for treatment. Patients having giant AVMs but with minimal symptoms sometimes are best followed clinically rather than treated.

GIANT ARTERIOVENOUS MALFORMATION HEMODYNAMICS

All AVMs serve as a shunt between arterial and venous systems. Pressure within the arterial feeders of AVMs has been shown to be lower than normal brain arteries, whereas pressure within the venous channels draining the AVM has been shown to be higher than normal venous pressure. As a result of this low pressure on the arterial side, blood that normally would supply the cortex adjacent to the AVM may flow preferentially to the AVM. This cerebrovascular steal, which may be more pronounced in giant AVMs, is hypothesized to cause ischemic symptoms within the cortex adjacent to the AVM. The arteries within the adjacent cortex respond to this steal phenomenon by dilating their lumen to maintain flow secondary to autoregulation. The extended interval in which these cortical arteries remain dilated results in the loss of their rapid ability to constrict should the blood pressure within these cortical arteries change. When these vessels are subjected to a higher pressure head, as when the low-resistance, high-flow giant AVM is removed, they may not have adequate autoregulatory compensation, resulting in surrounding brain edema and hemorrhage. Angiographic characteristics found to be correlated with cerebrovascular steal were angiomatous change, AVM size, and pattern of peripheral venous drainage.[42]

The process of impaired autoregulation and hemorrhage from cortical vessels adjacent to an AVM after AVM resection is called *normal perfusion pressure breakthrough*.[43] Although this phenomenon is rare, it is believed to occur more frequently in giant AVMs because these malformations shunt a higher volume of blood and create more vascular steal from the surrounding cortex. AVM features associated with increased likelihood of normal perfusion pressure breakthrough (other than AVM size) include dilated feeding arteries, poor filling of the surrounding cerebral vasculature on angiograms, clinical symptoms of ischemia from cerebrovascular steal, and physiologic evidence of impaired autoregulation in the brain.[30, 44] Normal perfusion pressure breakthrough bleeding can be limited through careful control of blood pressure in the immediate postoperative period, through staging of the giant AVM resection, and through the judicious use of presurgical embolization or radiosurgery (or both) in an attempt to reduce the size of the arteriovenous shunt.

EVALUATION

Angiography

Angiography is the gold standard for evaluating AVMs. Because of the multiplicity of arterial feeders to these giant AVMs, it is important that a four-vessel angiogram be performed to document all of the arterial supply. Giant AVMs may have a portion of their blood supply from extracranial sources, so both external carotid arteries should be evaluated.[45] As with smaller AVMs, multiple views should be obtained to ensure that the neurosurgeon has a complete understanding regarding the origin of all the arterial feeders, the size and configuration of the AVM, and the number and direction of veins draining the AVM. A complete initial angiogram allows for better comparison with subsequent angiograms obtained during and after treatment. Angiography potentially can document patients with a substantial amount of cerebrovascular steal as a result of the giant AVM. In these cases, normal cortical vessels may show limited flow compared with other vessels at a distance from the AVM.

Post-treatment angiograms should be performed to ensure complete obliteration of the AVM, either soon after microsurgical resection of the final portion of the giant AVM or within several years after stereotactic radiosurgery if this modality is used as the final treatment within the staged approach to a giant AVM. It is crucial to confirm complete treatment of an AVM, particularly giant AVMs, because reports suggest that partial treatment does not protect against future hemorrhage.[38, 39, 46–49]

Angiography plays an important role in the treatment of AVMs with stereotactic radiosurgery. Current radiosurgical systems rely on a fusion of angiography and magnetic resonance imaging (MRI) or computed tomography (CT) as a basis for treatment planning. In these cases, angiography is performed with a stereotactic base ring (or bite-block) attached to the patient's head with a fiducial cage mounted to the base ring. The fusion of angiography and MRI/CT imaging allows improved targeting of the nidus, while avoiding extraneous radiation dose to the draining veins or the surrounding cortical tissue.

Magnetic Resonance Imaging

Although angiography remains the primary radiologic modality to evaluate giant AVMs, pretreatment MRI provides additional information. MRI shows the relationship of the giant AVM with respect to other intracranial structures, affording the neurosurgeon a better understanding of the anatomy surrounding the AVM. The size and direction of large draining veins can be noted, as can radiographic evidence of prior hemorrhage. MRI is crucial during the planning of stereotactic radiosurgery in conjunction with cerebral angiography. In select cases of giant AVMs with irregular shapes or deep components, intraoperative stereotaxis using MRI-based image guidance can be extremely useful.

Xenon Computed Tomography

Xenon CT is used rarely in the evaluation of smaller AVMs, but for larger AVMs with significant surrounding cortical ischemia as a result of steal, this modality may be useful in identifying the degree and distribution of the hypoperfusion.[50] Impaired augmentation indicates failure of autoregulation and may indicate patients at high risk for normal perfusion pressure breakthrough bleeding.

TREATMENT

Because of the relative infrequency of giant AVMs (which are thought to comprise 10% of all AVMs)[15] and the complexity of arterial feeders and venous drainage, treatment is individualized for each patient. It is rare for giant AVMs to be treated successfully at a single sitting through one modality, and the best patient outcomes often involve staged treatment using two or more of the treatment modalities available.

Embolization

Because giant AVMs are difficult to treat with microsurgery alone and are too large to represent optimal targets for stereotactic radiosurgery, embolization is generally the first course of treatment. This process consists of using either small polyvinyl alcohol (PVA) particles[30] or cyanoacrylate glue[51–54] to attempt occlusion of feeding arteries. *N*-butyl-cyanoacrylate has emerged as the main embolic agent of choice because its soft nature after occluding portions of the nidus does not interfere with later surgical resection of the AVM.[54] The primary goal of embolization is to reduce the volume and flow in the AVM to facilitate safer, more effective subsequent treatment with microsurgery, radiosurgery, or both. Embolization of deep feeders to the AVM or deep AVM components may help with later surgical resection. Occasionally, embolization alone is used for palliation of symptoms in giant AVMs with no intent of obliterating the entire lesion. Embolization usually is performed in several stages (often three or more) for giant AVMs.[45] Staged embolization allows the AVMs to adjust to changes in flow hemodynamics after each embolic treatment; attempts to embolize large portions of a giant AVM in a single stage often are associated with increasing hemorrhage risk. Giant AVMs can have a significant external carotid component, and embolization of these vessels often makes the craniotomy opening easier for the surgeon as well as reducing blood supply to the AVM. Many giant AVMs have arterial supplies from the anterior and posterior circulation and often from both hemispheres so that multiple vessels need to be cannulated in attempts to achieve optimal embolization. Care must be taken to avoid passing embolic glue or particles into normal cortical vessels to avoid the development of infarcts.

During embolization, patients with giant AVMs are monitored with electrophysiologic potentials, which provides several benefits.[40, 41] First, such monitoring is particularly useful in identifying when normal cortical vessels are occluded inadvertently. Second, electrophysiologic monitoring during embolization can provide some insight to the neurosurgeon regarding whether or not the patient's brain tolerates periods of relative hypotension (which may be used during later surgery to reduce bleeding). This insight is particularly relevant when treating an AVM presenting with *steal* or ischemic symptoms. When a particular vessel is in question, amobarbital sodium (Amytal Sodium) can be injected into the vessel before embolization to determine whether the vessel supplies an area of eloquent cortex and would cause a neurological deficit if occluded.[55]

Some institutions use intraoperative embolization extensively in treating giant AVMs.[30] The advantages of this technique are that the risk of reflux into normal vessels is decreased and the surgeon has the opportunity to inject numerous distal vessels unattainable to the neurointerventionalist in the angiography suite. Intraoperative embolization proceeds when the surgeon has performed the craniotomy and exposed the AVM. Injection of the embolic agent should be performed as close to the AVM nidus as possible to minimize reflux into normal vessels. After temporary occlusion of the proximal portion of the vessel, 27-gauge needles can be introduced and several milliliters of *N*-butyl-cyanoacrylate can be injected. This process can be repeated for various feeding arteries, until the flow to the AVM is reduced significantly. After embolization, each feeding artery can be sacrificed with either a small clip or bipolar coagulation.

Stereotactic Radiosurgery

Stereotactic radiosurgery is a successful treatment for certain intracranial AVMs, particularly for small or moderate-sized AVMs located in critical brain regions. Many clinical series using either heavy charged particles (protons and helium ions) or photons (Gamma knife or LINAC) have shown that AVMs less than 3 cm in diameter treated with 20 to 25 GyE have a 3-year obliteration rate of 80% to 95% with a low complication rate (2.5% to 4.5% permanent neurological deficits, 2.5% to 4.5% transient deficits).[29, 38, 39, 56–64] Various limitations of stereotactic focused radiosurgery have become apparent, however, after analyzing the results in treating AVMs larger than 3 cm. These AVMs have a much lower obliteration rate, even after 3 years (33% to 58%), and a higher complication rate (20% to 30%) using treatment doses of 15 to 20 GyE.[29, 39, 56–60, 65, 66]

The primary mechanism of AVM obliteration after radiosurgery involves hyperplasia of the vascular intima,[67] with progressive narrowing and ultimately occlusion. Such obliteration typically takes place during 2 to 3 years. There are three considerations when weighing surgery versus radiosurgery for treatment of AVMs. First, AVMs greater than 4 cm diameter have only a 33% to 50% rate of obliteration at 3 years after radiosurgery but a 20% to 30% complication rate after treatment doses of 15 to 20 Gy.[39, 60] The rate of obliteration is increased for larger AVMs by using higher doses (25 to 45 Gy); however, the risk of radiation-induced complications increases significantly. Second, the risk of intracranial hemorrhage persists during the interval between treatment and complete obliteration.[39, 60, 62] Third, serial radiographic studies, including cerebral angiograms, are necessary to confirm complete obliteration.

Despite these limitations, radiosurgery may have less morbidity than surgical resection in patients with portions of giant AVMs in eloquent brain.[27, 28] Radiosurgery can be used as a preoperative adjunct to obliterate portions of giant AVMs, decreasing the remaining nidus in size for later surgical resection.[29] Some authors recommended staged stereotactic radiosurgery when treating giant AVMs.[68] In these cases, multiple radiosurgery treatments are delivered to different portions of the AVM at various time intervals to avoid delivering treatment to a single large target. This approach theoretically reduces the risk of radiation necrosis.

Some patients with giant AVMs require more than one course of stereotactic radiosurgery, and this option has been used in selected patients.[29, 69] The disadvantages of such an approach are the second latency period of 1 to 3 years before obliteration occurs; the possibility that a second radiosurgery treatment still may not obliterate the AVM; and the risk of radiation-induced injury, which may be higher with a second radiosurgery treatment.

Microsurgery

Generally, microsurgical resection of giant AVMs is planned after staged embolization or radiosurgery (or both) has reduced significantly the size of the AVM and the number of feeding arteries to the nidus. We routinely use corticosteroids and prophylactic antibiotics during resection of all AVMs, and patients are operated on under mild hypothermia (32°C to 33°C) for neuroprotection. Patients are placed on therapeutic levels of anticonvulsants, which are maintained at least during the acute postoperative period or longer if patients have seizures as part of their initial presentation. The use of lumbar drainage or mannitol to achieve brain relaxation is individualized, but usually employed.

Patients are positioned in a manner to allow optimal exposure to the AVM, while maintaining adequate jugular venous drainage. A supine position is preferred because this allows the optimal patient position for maintaining any femoral groin sheaths required for intraoperative angiography, which is difficult in the lateral position, and impossible in the prone position. The head is elevated 15 degrees above the heart to improve venous outflow and to reduce intraoperative bleeding. The head is placed in three-point head fixation for stabilization, using a radiolucent head frame if intraoperative angiography is planned.

The orientation of the incision in the scalp varies with the location and approach to each particular giant AVM, but should be situated directly over the AVM whenever possible. The bone flap should be created large enough to allow access to the entire AVM even if staged resection is planned because this would permit the optimal exposure should any unexpected intraoperative bleeding occur. Hemostasis is obtained, dural tack-up sutures are placed, and the dura is opened in a curvilinear fashion. Veins adherent to the dura can be taken down with bipolar coagulation and sharp dissection as long as they are not the primary draining veins. At this point, superficial giant AVMs usually are visualized on the cortical surface. For deeper AVMs, which do not present to the cortical surface, draining veins can be followed back to the malformation. Careful correlations between the pattern of vessels noted intraoperatively and the prior angiograms usually allow determination of the major feeding arteries and draining veins.

When identified, the AVM is resected in a systematic fashion using the microscope, with systemic mean blood pressure lowered to 65 to 70 mm Hg to minimize bleeding. Feeding arteries are located first, then individually coagulated and cut. The larger feeding vessels are clipped using Sundt micro AVM or mini aneurysm clips in addition to coagulation. It is important to proceed with treating one vessel at a time because hemorrhage from multiple sources can lead rapidly to significant bleeding and loss of control by the surgeon. Draining veins often are encountered before the feeding arteries are identified. It is imperative to preserve the venous drainage until all the arterial feeders are transected and the nidus is dissected out. Before transecting a vein, it is useful first to occlude it with a temporary aneurysm clip and observe the nidus. If the nidus begins to swell or bleed, the vein must be preserved until the final stages of resection. Intraoperative, quantitative, and directional ultrasound (Charbel Micro-flowprobe, Transonic Systems, Inc, Ithaca, NY) can be used to differentiate arterialized veins from feeding arteries.

Dissection begins on the superficial border of the malformation, and circumferential dissection of feeding arteries is performed around the AVM, with care taken to stay within the gliotic plane immediately outside the AVM when working in noneloquent cortex. Gentle traction on the nidus with a moist cottonoid allows visualization of these feeding arteries. When dissecting adjacent to critical brain parenchyma, it is safer to dissect close to the AVM, even encroaching on the nidus, instead of risking injury to the surrounding brain. When the superficial borders of the malformation are free, the AVM can be retracted gently so that deep perforating arteries can be coagulated. Retractors should be adjusted frequently to allow optimal exposure for each particular surgical view. Meticulous hemostasis must be maintained throughout the resection. A self-irrigating or nonstick bipolar coagulation unit is extremely useful during the dissection. Fragile arteries resistant to coagulation can be occluded with Sundt micro AVM clips. Judicious use of Surgicel (Johnson & Johnson, New Brunswick, NJ), Gelfoam (Pharmacia & Upjohn, Kalamazoo, MI), Avitene (Davol, Inc, Cranston, RI), and small pieces of bulk cotton can be quite helpful in treating general oozing. Larger feeding arteries can be occluded permanently with Sundt mini aneurysm clips (Codman & Shurtleff, Inc, Raynham, MA), but care must be taken to preserve the *en-passage* vessels. These vessels are often difficult to identify at first, and care should be taken to follow each of these vessels and to cauterize them only when the surgeon is sure that no normal cortex is supplied by the vessel in question.

Deep ependymal feeding arteries usually are the last, but often the most problematic feeders to deal with. These vessels tend to be fragile, tear easily, and often are difficult to control with bipolar coagulation. These vessels tend to retract into the surrounding brain tissue, often requiring the surgeon to dissect deeper than desirable to find the source of the hemorrhage. Patience on the part of the operating surgeon is required when occluding these vessels with bipolar coagulation or small Sundt micro clips to halt bleeding.

Venous drainage for giant AVMs is usually superficial and deep but usually toward the midline. During AVM dissection, superficial draining veins can be retracted gently to increase exposure. When possible, draining veins should be sacrificed last, immediately before removal of the nidus; smaller draining veins may have to be sacrificed during AVM resection to facilitate removal. When working within the ventricular system, the ventricles should be protected against the accumulation of blood using cotton patties or bulk cotton. This protection minimizes the likelihood of developing postoperative hydrocephalus. On completion of AVM resection, the microscope should be used to inspect the resection bed for any signs of residual AVM, which is more likely to occur in giant AVMs with irregular shapes than for smaller AVMs, and to achieve hemostasis. It is important to check for hemostasis at normotension or mild hypertension. An intraoperative angiogram can be performed to ensure complete resection of the nidus, but because of the lower quality of these intraoperative images, a conventional angiogram in the radiology suite also should be performed in the postoperative period.

If the surgical procedure is staged, owing to the size of the AVM, extent of surgical hemorrhage, or risk of normal perfusion pressure breakthrough bleeding, the neurosurgeon needs to determine the optimal point at which to complete the initial stage. Giant AVMs often have irregular shapes, and often resecting one or more lobes of these larger AVMs represents an ideal point to cease surgery. In other cases of AVMs extending down toward the basal ganglia and thalamus, resection of the superficial component of the AVM can be followed by a second stage involving resection of the deeper portion. In the event that the residual portion of the giant AVM after staged surgical resection would place the patient at significant neurological risk, this residual potentially could be treated with stereotactic radiosurgery. When staging surgical resection of AVMs, it is crucial that the portion of the AVM exposed but not resected be inspected carefully to ensure hemostasis. When postoperative bleeding is noted, it is generally from the residual AVM.

Because giant AVMs usually involve several different lobes, a compartmental approach to resection may be required even if the AVM nidus is to be resected in a single operation. A giant AVM within the frontal and temporal lobes may be resected by removing the malformation first from the temporal compartment and, when this is complete, subsequently removing the AVM from the frontal lobe. Major sulci or fissures can assist the surgeon by serving as natural planes of dissection. Compartmentalizing the AVM resection allows the surgeon to operate on several discrete lobes of the AVM rather than on one giant malformation. Often, if staged surgeries are planned, the surgical resection of one of the compartments or lobes of the AVM may represent an ideal stopping point.

Another indication for surgery in giant AVMs would involve resection of radiation necrosis. Radiation injury after stereotactic radiosurgery may result in significant mass effect and edema, requiring prolonged treatment with high doses of corticosteroids. We have observed several patients with steroid dependence as a result of radiation injury who have been tapered off corticosteroids successfully after resecting areas of necrosis and some patients who have shown substantial neurological improvement.

Before operative closure, meticulous hemostasis is obtained in the resection bed of the AVM, and a final inspection is performed to ensure that the entire malformation has been removed completely. Transient induced mild hypertension (90 to 100 mm Hg) is used to test hemostasis, then the resection bed is lined with Surgicel. Often a ventricular catheter is placed and connected to an external drainage bag if the AVM resection exposed the ventricle. The dura is closed in the standard fashion using 4–0 nylon suture, and the bone is replaced to complete the craniotomy. A subgaleal drain is attached to light suction for 12 to 24 hours. The scalp incision is closed in two layers, with approximation of the galeal layer using 3–0 Dexon sutures and skin with staples. Patient extubation should be performed in a smooth and deliberate fashion to avoid any elevations in intracranial pressure or venous pressure. During emergence from anesthesia, the systemic blood pressure must be monitored carefully to avoid any hypertensive episodes.

In the intensive care unit, hypotension should be maintained for 24 to 48 hours to prevent rebleeding. Although we previously used prophylactic barbiturates postoperatively after resecting large or giant AVMs, we now use this technique only if uncontrollable bleeding is encountered. Coagulation studies should be checked, and coagulation problems should be corrected. Any changes in neurological examination should be evaluated with emergent CT. A postoperative angiogram is obtained in the first week after surgery unless an intraoperative angiogram was performed with adequate angiographic resolution to confirm complete AVM resection.

Multimodality Treatment

The complexity of giant AVMs often requires combinations of embolization, stereotactic radiosurgery, and microsurgery to achieve a complete cure. Our experience with large and complex AVMs has shown that such multimodality therapy can reduce patient morbidity and mortality.[28, 29] Embolization reduces the nidus volume requiring resection, but stereotactic radiosurgery delivered several years before surgical resection also produces a benefit. In some patients, partial AVM thrombosis significantly reduced the volume of residual AVM that required surgical resection. More importantly, at surgery the radiated (but patent) AVMs were found to be much less vascular even in nonembolized areas compared with AVMs not radiated previously. Radiosurgically treated AVM vessels were easier to coagulate with a bipolar, facilitating quicker and safer resection with less blood loss.[29] Although preoperative angiograms often showed significant residual AVM after radiosurgery, the observations at surgery suggested that prior radiosurgery obliterated the small vessel component of the AVM not visible on the angiogram.[67] Our success in obliterating completely several previously radiated AVMs with embolization alone suggests that prior radiosurgery may thrombose a small vessel component, leaving larger arteriovenous fistulous portions of the AVM.[70, 71]

SPECIAL PERIOPERATIVE EQUIPMENT AND TECHNIQUES

Intraoperative Monitoring

Electrophysiologic monitoring is an extremely valuable aid during procedures for midline or deep AVM resection and improves clinical results.[31, 32, 72] Monitoring routinely consists of bilateral somatosensory evoked potentials. Continuous monitoring of the sensory pathways has allowed early detection of excessive retraction, manipulation of critical structures, excessive hypotension, or sacrifice of critical nonfeeding arteries, all of which are more likely to occur during resection of giant AVMs than smaller malformations. We have found brainstem auditory evoked potentials useful during the resection of posterior fossa AVMs.[72] Electrophysiologic monitoring has proved useful in assisting in the determination of extent of AVM resection when staged procedures are planned. Often, changes in electrophysiologic monitoring result in cessation of further AVM resection. When these changes are detected early and surgery is halted, potentials usually return to baseline, and patients generally do not develop clinical worsening. Because giant AVMs often are located adjacent to motor and sensory cortex, intraoperative mapping has proved useful in assessing resectability of these lesions. Burchiel and colleagues[73] used corticography and stimulation mapping to evaluate motor, sensory, and language cortex, with excellent results.

Frameless Image-Guided Stereotaxis

Intraoperative stereotaxis helps localize portions of the deep AVMs not presenting directly to the ventricular or pial surface. The Cosman-Roberts-Wells frame (Radionics, Inc, Burlington, MA) was used previously but was found to restrict exposure. Image-guided navigation, such as the Radionics Optical Tracking System (Radionics, Inc, Burlington, MA) or the Elekta Viewscope (Elekta, Inc, Atlanta, GA), obviates the need for any frame or articulating arm system and maintains a precision of a few millimeters. This stereotactic approach has allowed better planning for exposure of deeper AVMs and has helped confirm complete resection of all components of giant AVMs that may have irregular configurations.

Mild Hypothermia

Mild brain hypothermia can be used for cerebroprotection, dropping the core body and brain temperature to 32°C to 33°C by applying a cooling blanket. This degree of mild brain hypothermia has been shown to provide excellent protection against experimental ischemic and traumatic cerebral injury,[74] and we have used it at Stanford in more than 1100 intracranial cases with good results. Under operative conditions of AVM resection, this hypothermic technique is safe, feasible, and economical with good clinical outcomes overall.

Intraoperative Angiogram

Intraoperative angiograms have been possible with the advent of high-resolution portable angiography and allow the surgeon to determine the completeness of AVM resection.[75] If residual AVM is present, the surgeon has an opportunity to complete the resection before wound closure. At least two studies have shown that patients are not protected from partial resection of AVMs[6, 76] so that complete resection remains the goal for all AVMs. In two other studies, 10% to 18% of surgical procedures for resection of AVMs were altered by the results of intraoperative angiography.[77, 78] We routinely use intraoperative angiography for most giant AVM resections to document completeness of resection and sometimes to assess extent of residual AVM for deliberate staged surgery.

Intraoperative Doppler Blood Flow Measurements and Ultrasound

Intraoperative ultrasound for measuring blood flow can have several uses. First, ultrasound can determine whether flow through veins is arterialized. This determination allows the surgeon to establish whether the nidus still has a significant arterial source and whether the vein in question can be transected safely. Second, directional and quantitative ultrasound can help distinguish feeding arteries from arterialized draining veins as well as establish flow rates through individual feeding arteries. Nornes and Grip[11] estimated total AVM flow in 9 of 16 patients (range, 150 to >900 mL/min; average, 490 mL/min).[11] They also made pressure recordings from feeding arteries at their entrance to the AVM, showing that this pressure was well below the systemic arterial blood pressure in all cases (range, 40 to 77 mm Hg; average, 56 mm Hg). For deep AVMs, ultrasound can be used to locate the malformation, which can facilitate the planning of cortical incisions, identification of vessels involved, and the surgical approach.[79]

SURGICAL OUTCOME

There are few published series exclusively consisting of giant AVMs because most authors have included these vascular malformations in larger series of general vascular malformations. Anson and Spetzler[30] reported a series of 32 giant AVMs (all were Spetzler-Martin grade V lesions). After combined therapy, 15 patients were improved clinically, 7 were unchanged, and 10 had worsening deficits, although 8 of these 10 deficits were either transient or mild.[30] Seven patients required two surgical stages and four patients required three surgical stages to complete AVM resection. Three of the four patients undergoing three operations also required presurgical embolization (three courses each) to reduce AVM size.

Heros and coworkers[80] reported 21 patients with giant AVMs in a series of 153 AVM patients. Early good or excellent results were achieved in 61% of grade IV patients and 29% of grade V patients. Patients improved with longer follow-up, showing a 12% morbidity and mortality rate for grade IV giant AVMs and a 38% rate for grade V malformations.

Fifteen patients with AVMs greater than 5 cm were reported in a series of 90 AVM patients by Hernesniemi and Keranen.[81] Of 90 patients, 5 had excellent outcomes, 6 had moderate disabilities, 1 had a severe disability, 1 died, and 2 were lost to follow-up. These authors recommended staged resections and several days of induced systemic hypotension to prevent breakthrough bleeding.

We have treated 28 patients (12 men and 16 women) at Stanford with giant AVMs greater than 6 cm.[82] Of these patients, 13 (46%) presented with hemorrhage, 7 (25%) presented with headache, 5 (18%) presented with seizures, and 3 (11%) presented with progressive neurological deficits. Treatment included embolization in 26 patients, stereotactic radiosurgery in 25 patients, and one or more surgical resections in 16 patients (Figs. 133-1 through 133-4). Twenty patients (71%) were cured completely of the giant AVM. Eight patients (29%) had residual AVM seen on their last angiogram, but three of these eight patients were less than 3 years postradiosurgery. Long-term outcome was excellent in 21 patients (75%) and good in 5 patients (18%), with 2 patients dying during the follow-up period.

COMPLICATIONS

Hemorrhage

The most devastating complication is postoperative hemorrhage (Fig. 133-5), which is extremely rare. This

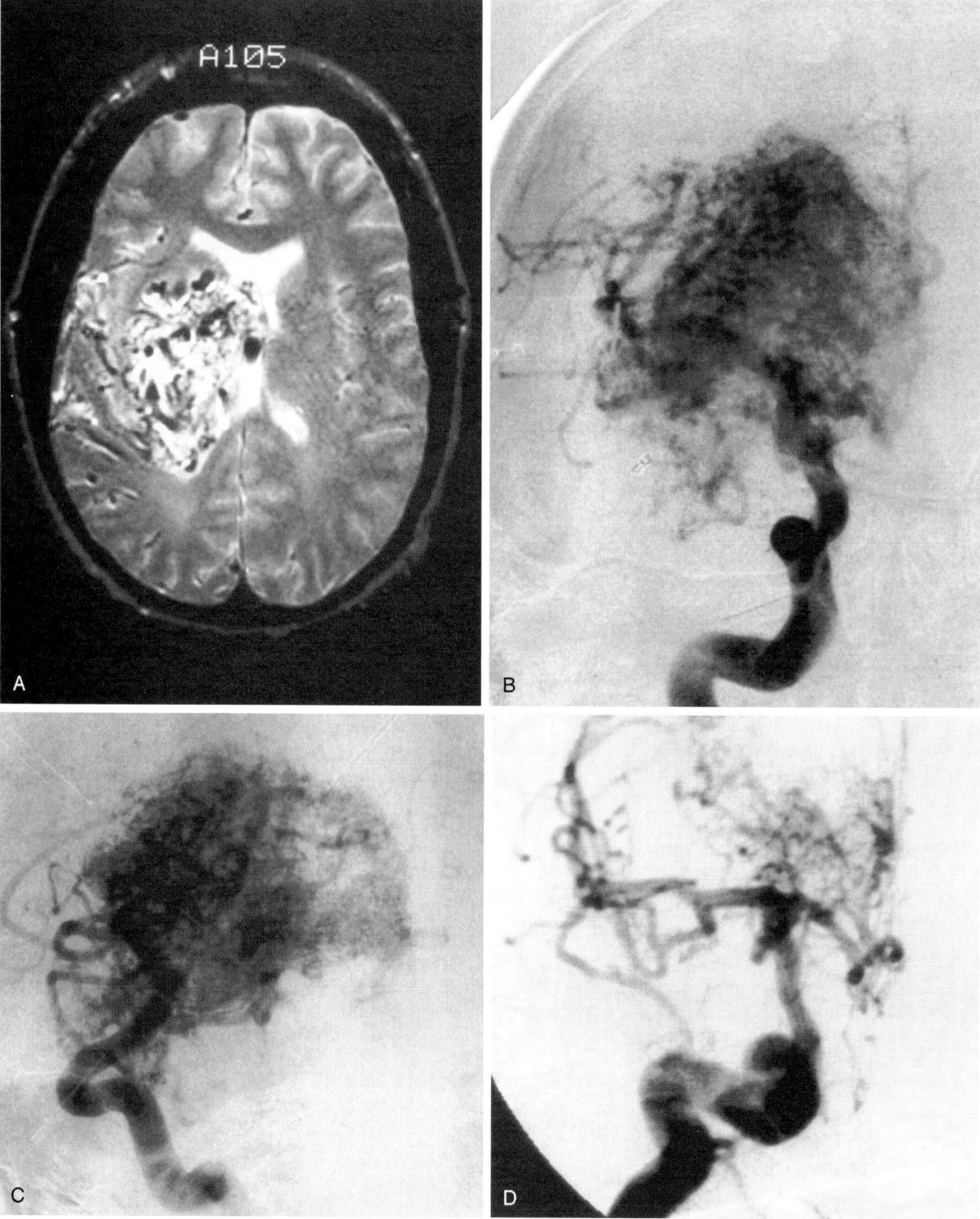

FIGURE 133–1. A 30-year-old man presented with headaches, intractable seizures, and a left hemiparesis as a result of a prior hemorrhage from a 7 × 4.5 × 4.5 cm right parietal arteriovenous malformation (AVM) extending into the basal ganglia and thalamus. Initial magnetic resonance imaging scan shows the AVM on an axial view (*A*). Initial angiography shows the AVM filling from the right internal carotid injection on anteroposterior (*B*) and lateral (*C*) views. The patient underwent heavy-particle radiosurgery with 17.5 GyE to a volume of 88,000 mm^3. Two years after radiosurgery, there was no change in the angiographic appearance of the AVM, so the patient underwent two courses of embolization, with postembolization right carotid angiography showing partial reduction in AVM volume, seen on anteroposterior (*D*) and lateral (*E*) views.

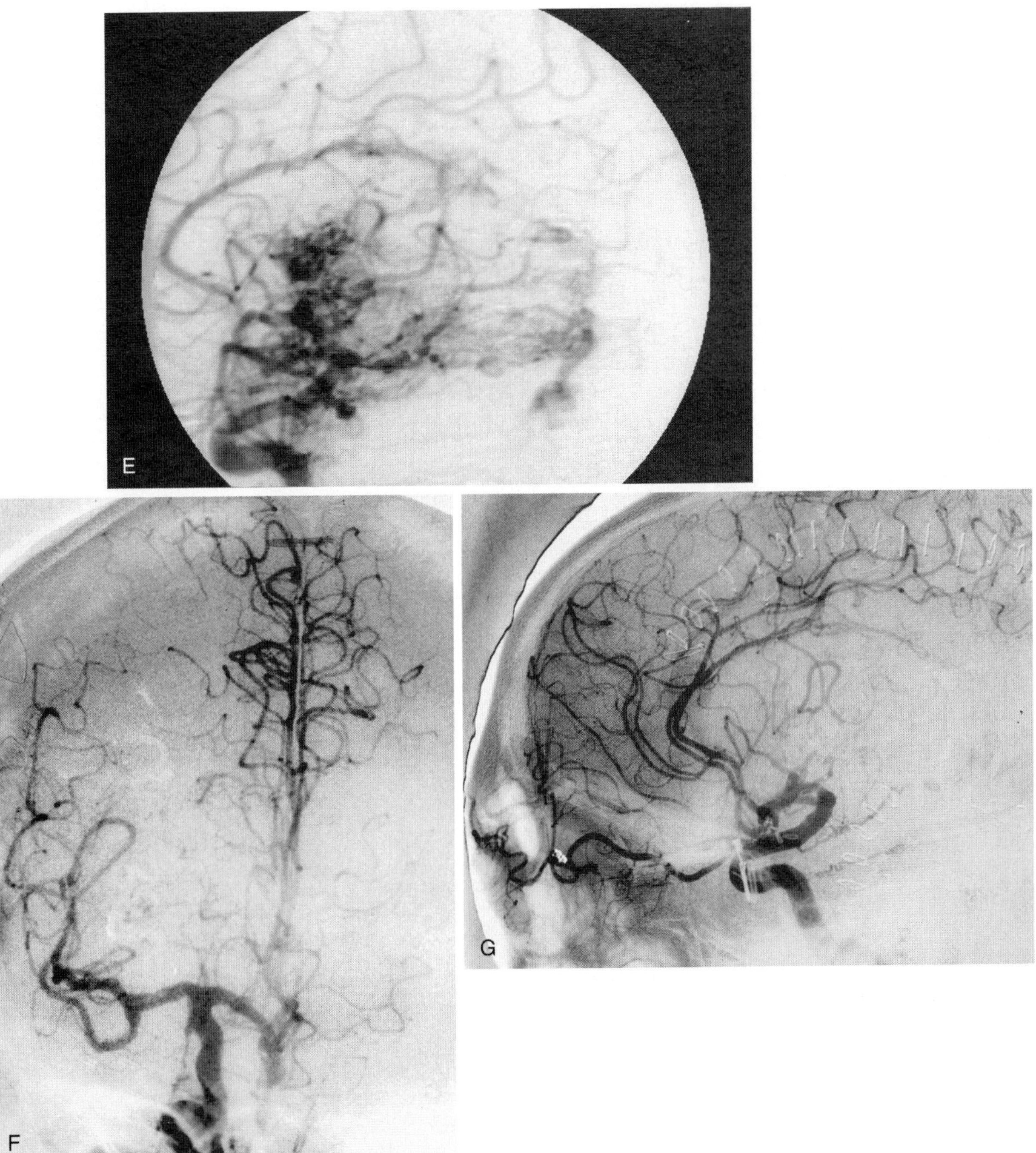

FIGURE 133–1. *Continued.* The patient underwent microsurgical resection of the residual AVM, with final right carotid angiography showing complete obliteration on anteroposterior (*F*) and lateral (*G*) views. The patient's headaches resolved, his seizures were improved significantly, and he had no new neurological deficits.

hemorrhage can be due to inadequate hemostasis, failure to resect the AVM completely, or normal perfusion pressure breakthrough. Postoperative hemorrhage can be minimized by careful inspection and hemostasis of the resection bed after AVM removal and by a short period of induced hypertension after resection but before closure to check for breakthrough bleeding. Intraoperative angiography and image-guided navigational systems can aid in confirming complete AVM resection. After surgery, hypotension is maintained in the intensive care unit for 1 to 2 days, to permit adjustment of the cerebral vasculature to the new hemodynamics. Normal perfusion pressure breakthrough bleeding can be minimized through staged surgical procedures, allowing for a gradual change in the cortical vasculature flow dynamics after each procedure, followed by

Text continued on page 2280

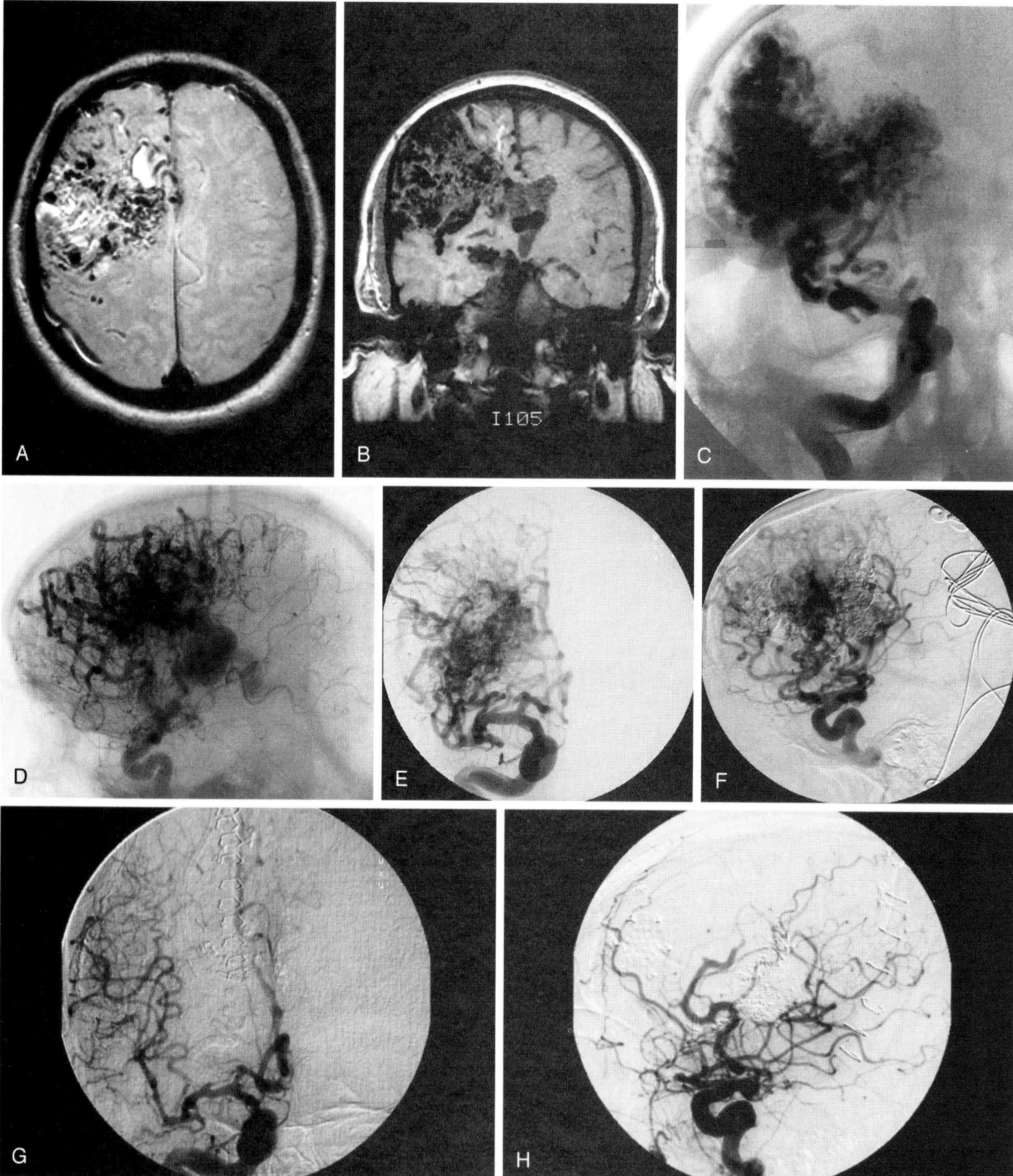

FIGURE 133–2. A 33-year-old man presented with three prior hemorrhages from a giant right fronto-temporal arteriovenous malformation (AVM), seen on pretreatment axial (*A*) and coronal (*B*) magnetic resonance images. Initial angiography shows the AVM filling from a right carotid injection, seen on anteroposterior (*C*) and lateral (*D*) views. The patient underwent two courses of embolization with a resultant 50% reduction in volume of the AVM. The patient was treated with heavy-particle stereotactic radiosurgery using a dose of 20 GyE to a volume of 72,000 mm^3. The patient underwent a third course of embolization, with further reduction in AVM volume, seen on anteroposterior (*E*) and lateral (*F*) right carotid views. The residual AVM was resected with microsurgery, with postoperative right carotid angiography showing complete obliteration of the AVM on anteroposterior (*G*) and lateral (H) views. The patient had some mild left-sided hemiparesis postoperatively, but this resolved completely during the next 6 months.

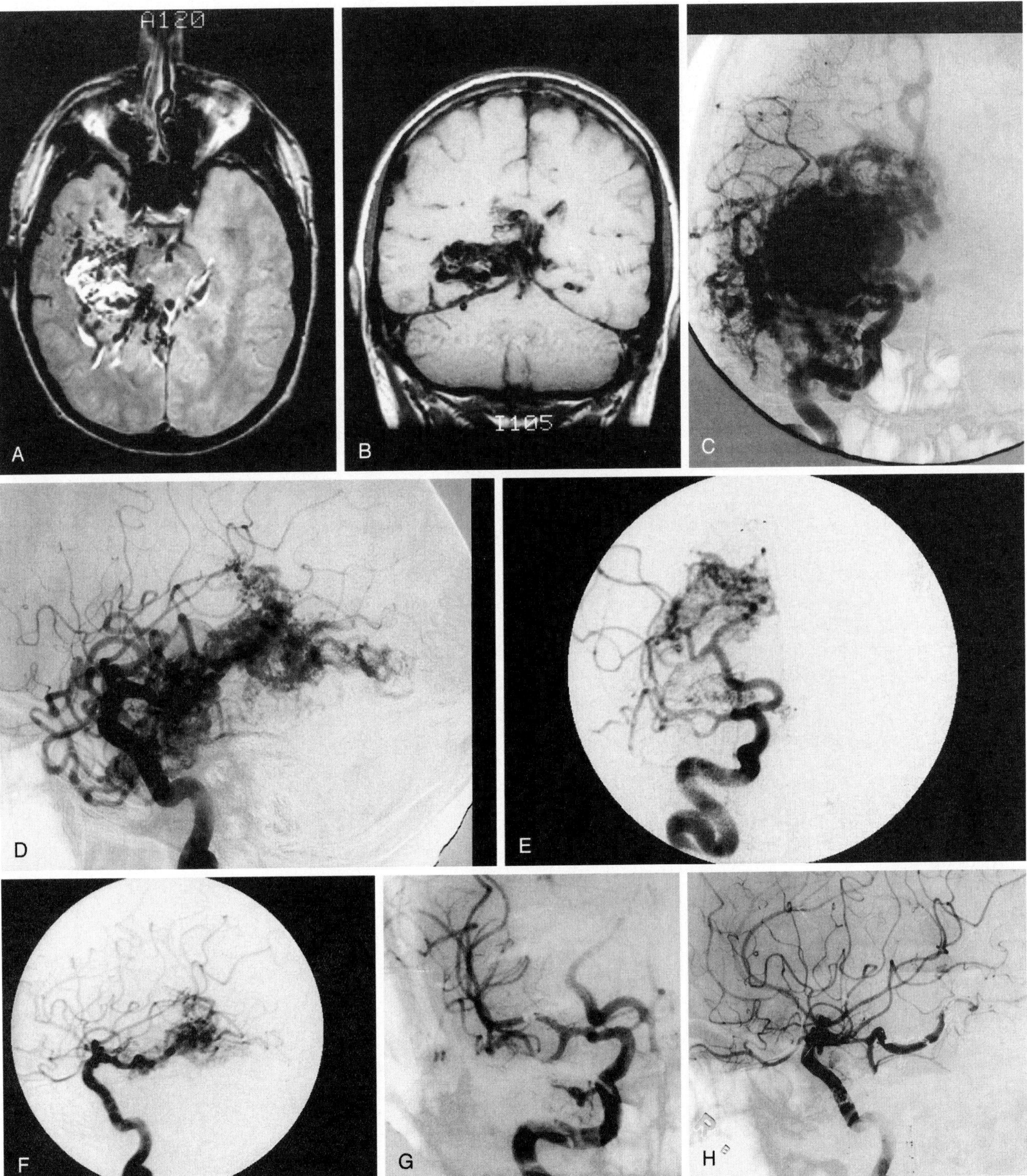

FIGURE 133–3. A 34-year-old man presented with a 2- to 3-year history of headaches that were precipitated with bending forward. Initial evaluation included a magnetic resonance imaging scan, which showed a giant arteriovenous malformation (AVM) in the right mesial temporal lobe on axial (*A*) and coronal (*B*) images. Initial angiography showed the AVM filling on anteroposterior (*C*) and lateral (*D*) carotid injections. The patient underwent three embolizations with a 40% reduction in AVM volume. This was followed by 15-GyE stereotactic radiosurgery to a volume of 47,500 mm^3. Three years after radiosurgery, there was still partial filling of the AVM, and a fourth course of embolization was performed, reducing the size of the AVM further, seen on anteroposterior (*E*) and lateral (*F*) carotid views. The residual AVM was resected with microsurgery, with postsurgical angiography confirming obliteration of the AVM, seen on anteroposterior (*G*) and lateral (*H*) carotid angiography. Clinically the patient remained neurologically intact with the exception of a new left upper quadrantanopsia.

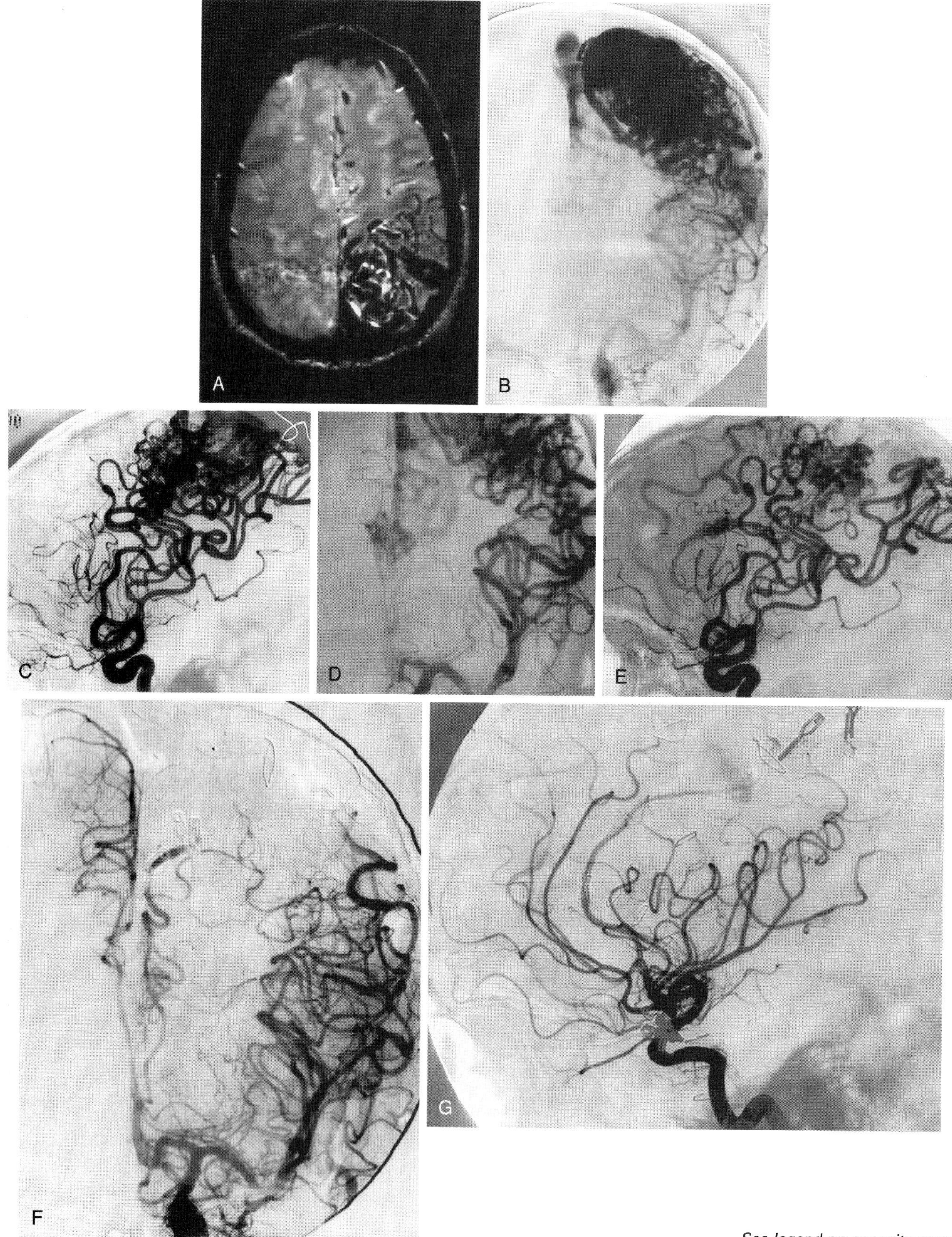

See legend on opposite page

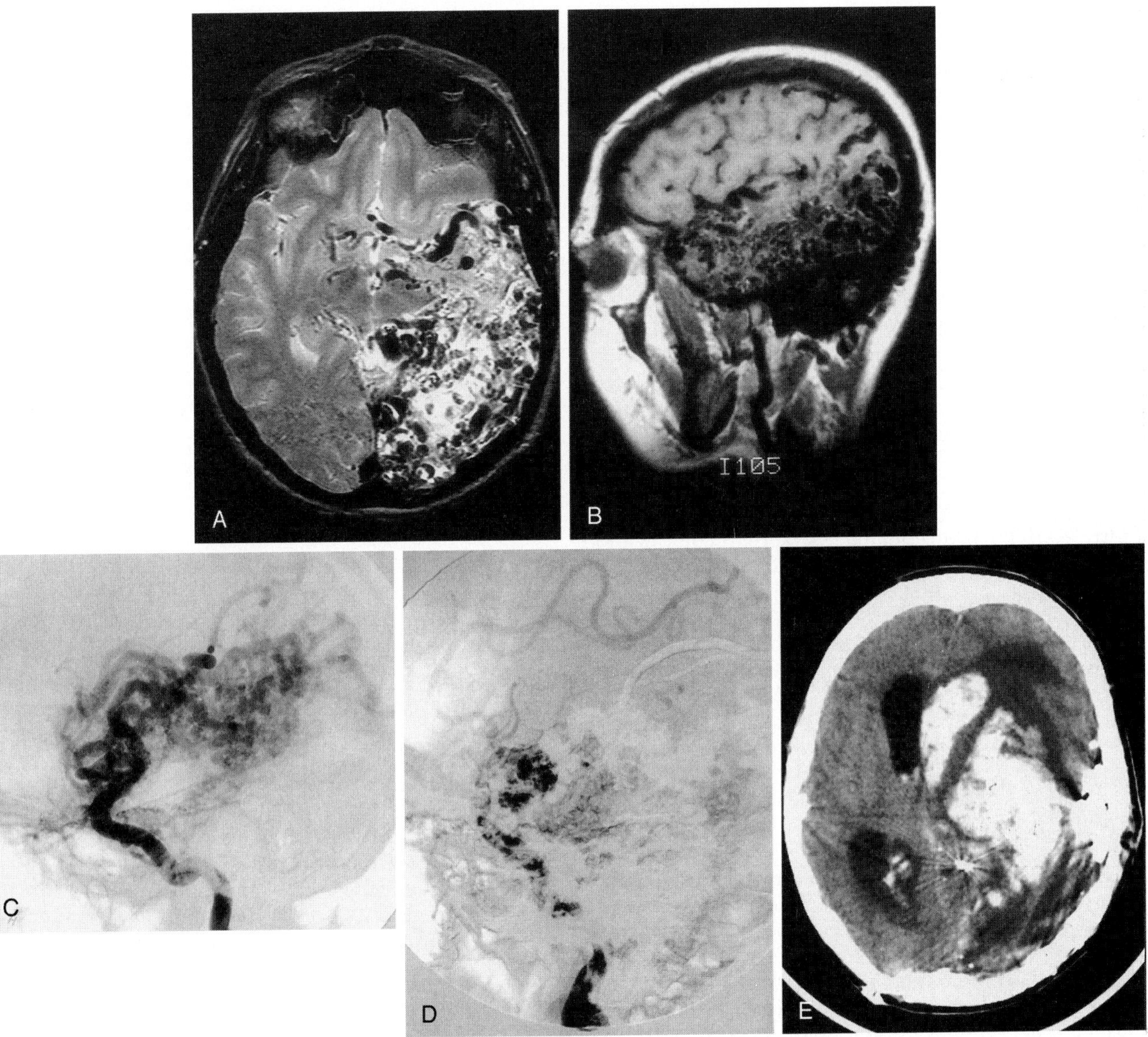

FIGURE 133–5. A 26-year-old woman with a giant left temporal-occipital arteriovenous malformation (AVM) underwent proton beam radiosurgery. She continued to deteriorate with medically intractable seizures, progressive memory impairment, and a right homonymous hemianopsia. Four years later, the AVM was unchanged angiographically from the preradiosurgery appearance, seen on axial (*A*) and sagittal (*B*) magnetic resonance imaging and on a lateral left internal carotid artery angiogram (*C*). The patient underwent four embolization procedures, with a postembolization lateral left carotid angiogram (*D*) showing significant reduction in AVM volume. The patient was then scheduled for repeat heavy-particle radiosurgery but suffered a fatal hemorrhage, shown on computed tomography (*E*), 1 week after her last embolization.

FIGURE 133–4. A 25-year-old man presented with headaches, a bruit, episodes of visual distortion, and memory difficulties. Evaluation revealed the presence of a giant left parietal arteriovenous malformation (AVM), seen on an axial magnetic resonance image (*A*). Initial left carotid angiography showed the AVM filling on anteroposterior (*B*) and lateral (*C*) views. The patient underwent stereotactic radiosurgery using 18 Gy as initial treatment. Three years after radiosurgery, there was no significant reduction in AVM volume, so two courses of embolization were administered with a 40% reduction in AVM volume, as seen on anteroposterior (*D*) and lateral (*E*) left carotid angiography. The patient was taken to the operating room, where intraoperative electrophysiologic mapping showed that the AVM was posterior to the somatosensory cortex. A total resection was achieved, as seen on anteroposterior (*F*) and lateral (*G*) left carotid angiography. The patient had an initial mild right hemiparesis and hemisensory deficit, which resolved completely during the next 6 months.

several days of deliberate hypotension after final resection of the AVM. Hemorrhage can occur after embolization of AVMs, occasionally resulting in the need for emergent craniotomy to remove blood clot.[83] This risk is reduced by staging embolization procedures and maintaining a 12-hour period of relative hypotension after the procedure.

Venous Thrombosis

Venous thrombosis may occur in the early postoperative period or occasionally after embolization. A sudden reduction of flow in the enlarged draining veins predisposes to this phenomenon, which may cause parenchymal swelling, hemorrhage, and severe neurological deficits. We avoid fluid restriction postoperatively in an attempt to minimize this problem.

Hydrocephalus

Postoperative hydrocephalus is a known complication in patients with significant intraventricular blood. Any intraventricular clot secondary to prior hemorrhage should be removed before AVM resection. Meticulous hemostasis should be maintained throughout the procedure to minimize any acute ventricular blood. If significant intraventricular blood is present, a ventriculostomy can be placed before closure. Long-term hydrocephalus is treated with a ventriculoperitoneal shunt.

Radiosurgical Complications

Adverse sequelae from radiation are classified broadly according to the time of appearance with respect to treatment.[84, 85] Complications from radiosurgery can be categorized similarly. Acute reactions are defined as occurring during, immediately after, or within the first several days of therapy and primarily consist of nausea and emesis. These symptoms occur in 10% to 16% of patients within 6 hours of treatment.[86] Preventive measures include pretreatment with antiemetics and steroids.[86] Late reactions occur more than 3 months after therapy and usually are associated with some degree of permanent neurological injury. Because of the large tissue volume of giant AVMs treated with stereotactic radiosurgery, the potential for adverse sequelae is greater than for smaller targets.

Although seizures can occur after stereotactic radiosurgery, they also are associated with the underlying pathology in many patients. Consequently, it is not always clear whether a seizure is related directly to treatment. Kjellberg and associates[87] reported a small increase in acute seizure risk in AVM patients treated with proton radiosurgery. Similarly, it has been our experience at Stanford that there is a slightly increased risk of seizures within the first 48 hours of radiosurgery, especially when treating large AVMs in eloquent cortex. Post-treatment seizures often correlate with subtherapeutic levels of anticonvulsants in patients who are receiving these agents. We regularly augment standard anticonvulsant doses on the day of radiosurgery to achieve a *high therapeutic* level in patients at risk for post-treatment seizures and have found that this minimized these adverse events during the immediate post-treatment period.

Symptomatic radiation necrosis and edema are the most debilitating of the late complications caused by stereotactic radiosurgery. Histologic changes in the affected brain consist of neuronal death, gliosis, and endothelial proliferation and hyalinization.[88] The reported incidence of radiation necrosis varies between 2.3% and 20%[39, 89–91] generally occurring 6 to 9 months after treatment, with larger AVM volumes likely to result in increased risk of injury. The current treatment for the edema that accompanies radiation necrosis is corticosteroids. The time course of symptoms and the need for steroids typically are quite protracted, lasting 1 year or longer before resolving. In severe cases of necrosis, surgical resection can ameliorate mass effect and improve clinical status significantly for some patients.

Ischemia

Embolization and microsurgical resection of AVMs can result in the inadvertent sacrifice of arteries that supply normal cortex. If these arteries are small, no obvious neurological deficit may occur. For larger vessel obliteration, however, patients may develop either transient or permanent neurological deficits as a result of ischemia. Series of patients undergoing embolizations have shown approximately 10% incidence of transient neurological events[40] and a 6% incidence of permanent neurological disorders.[41] In some instances, retrograde thrombosis of feeding arteries may be the cause of neurological deficits, with one report indicating that neurological deficits occurred in three of five patients in which retrograde thrombosis was noted on angiography.[92]

CONCLUSIONS

Many giant AVMs can be treated safely with current technology. With careful preoperative planning and embolization, stereotactic radiosurgery, advances in microsurgical technique, and compulsive perioperative management, excellent results overall can be obtained. The optimal management of patients with giant AVMs must include a detailed understanding of the hemodynamics and anatomy of each particular vascular malformation as well as familiarity with the various methods of AVM treatment. For many giant AVMs, multimodality treatment using embolization, stereotactic radiosurgery, and microsurgery may produce optimal results.

ACKNOWLEDGMENTS

We thank Beth Houle, for assistance with the figures. This chapter was supported in part by funding from Bernard and Ronnie Lacroute, the William Randolph Hearst Foundation, and John and Dodie Rosekrans.

REFERENCES

1. Spetzler RF, Martin NA: A proposed grading system for arteriovenous malformations. J Neurosurg 65:476–483, 1986.
2. Martin NA, Vinters HV: Arteriovenous malformations. In Carter LP, Spetzler RF, Hamilton MG (eds): Neurovascular Surgery. New York, McGraw-Hill, 1995, pp 875–903.
3. Troost BT, Newton TH: Occipital lobe arteriovenous malformations: Clinical and radiologic features in 26 cases with comment on differentiation and migraine. Arch Ophthalmol 93:250–254, 1956.
4. Mohr J: Neurological manifestations and factors related to therapeutic decisions. In Wilson CB, Stein BM (eds): Intracranial Arteriovenous Malformations. Baltimore, Williams & Wilkins, 1984, pp 32–41.
5. Luessenhop AJ: Natural history of cerebral arteriovenous malformations. In Wilson CB, Stein BM (eds): Intracranial Arteriovenous Malformations. Baltimore, Williams & Wilkins, 1984, pp 12–23.
6. Drake CG: Cerebral arteriovenous malformations: Considerations for and experience with surgical treatment in 166 cases. Clin Neurosurg 26:145–208, 1979.
7. Graf CJ, Perret GE, Torner JC: Bleeding from cerebral arteriovenous malformations as part of their natural history. J Neurosurg 58:331–337, 1983.
8. Perrit G, Nishioka H: Report on the cooperative study of intracranial aneurysms and subarachnoid hemorrhage: Section VI. Arteriovenous malformations: An analysis of 545 cases of craniocerebral arteriovenous malformations and fistulae reported to the cooperative study. J Neurosurg 25:467–490, 1966.
9. Wilkins RH: Natural history of intracranial vascular malformations: A review. Neurosurgery 16:421–430, 1985.
10. Spetzler RF, Selman WR: Pathophysiology of cerebral ischemia accompanying arteriovenous malformations. In Wilson CB, Stein BM (eds): Intracranial Arteriovenous Malformations. Baltimore, Williams & Wilkins, 1984, pp 24–31.
11. Nornes H, Grip A: Hemodynamic aspects of cerebral arteriovenous malformations. J Neurosurg 53:456–464, 1980.
12. Kusske JA, Kelly WA: Embolization and reduction of the "steal" syndrome in cerebral arteriovenous malformations. J Neurosurg 40:313–321, 1974.
13. Hachinski V, Norris JW, Cooper PW, et al: Symptomatic intracranial steal. Arch Neurol 34:149–153, 1977.
14. Hamilton MG, Spetzler RF: The prospective application of a grading system for arteriovenous malformations. Neurosurgery 34:2–7, 1994.
15. Brown RD Jr, Wiebers DO, Forbes G, et al: The natural history of unruptured intracranial arteriovenous malformations. J Neurosurg 68:352–357, 1988.
16. Ondra SL, Troupp H, George ED, et al: The natural history of symptomatic arteriovenous malformations of the brain: A 24-year follow-up assessment. J Neurosurg 73:387–391, 1990.
17. Group AMS: Arteriovenous malformations of the brain in adults. N Engl J Med 340:1812–1818, 1999.
18. Spetzler RF, Hargraves RW, McCormick PW, et al: Relationship of perfusion pressure and size to risk of hemorrhage from arteriovenous malformations. J Neurosurg 76:918–923, 1992.
19. Fults D, Kelly DL Jr: Natural history of arteriovenous malformations of the brain: A clinical study. Neurosurgery 15:658–662, 1984.
20. Crawford PM, West CR, Chadwick DW, et al: Arteriovenous malformations of the brain: Natural history in unoperated patients. J Neurol Neurosurg Psychiatry 49:1–10, 1986.
21. Hassler W, Steinmetz H: Cerebral hemodynamics in AVM patients: An intraoperative study. J Neurosurg 67:822–831, 1987.
22. Lewis AI, Tew JM Jr: Management of thalamic-basal ganglia and brain-stem vascular malformations. Clin Neurosurg 41:83–111, 1994.
23. Marks MP, Lane B, Steinberg GK, et al: Hemorrhage in intracerebral arteriovenous malformations: Angiographic determinants. Radiology 176:807–813, 1990.
24. Miyasaka Y, Yada K, Ohwada T, et al: An analysis of the venous drainage system as a factor of hemorrhage from arteriovenous malformations. J Neurosurg 76:239–243, 1992.
25. Miyasaka Y, Kurata A, Tokiwa K, et al: Draining vein pressure increases and hemorrhage in patients with arteriovenous malformation. Stroke 25:504–507, 1994.
26. Steinberg GK, Stoodley MA: Surgical management of arteriovenous malformations of the brain. In Schmidek HH (ed): Operative Neurosurgical Techniques. Philadelphia, WB Saunders, 2000, 1363–1379.
27. Steinberg GK, Marks MP, Levy RP, et al: Multimodality treatment of vascular malformations in functional brain areas using stereotactic radiosurgery, embolization and microsurgery. In Yamada S (ed): Arteriovenous Malformations in Functional Brain Areas. Mt Kisco, NY, Futura Publishing, 1999, pp 181–196.
28. Steinberg GK, Marks MP: Intracranial arteriovenous malformations: Therapeutic options. In Batjer HH (ed): Cerebrovascular Disease. New York, Lippincott-Raven Press, 1997, pp 727–742.
29. Steinberg GK, Chang SD, Levy RP, et al: Surgical resection of large incompletely treated intracranial arteriovenous malformations following stereotactic radiosurgery. J Neurosurg 84:920–928, 1996.
30. Anson JA, Spetzler RF: Giant arteriovenous malformations. In Carter LP, Spetzler RF, Hamilton MG (eds): Neurovascular Surgery. New York, McGraw-Hill, 1995, pp 1017–1028.
31. Chang SD, Steinberg GK: Surgical Approaches: Interhemispheric. In Awad IA, Jafar JJ, Rosenwasser RH (eds): Vascular Malformations of the Central Nervous System. New York, Lippincott-Raven, 1999, pp 297–308.
32. Chang SD, Steinberg GK: Infratentorial brainstem AVMs. In Steig PE, Batjer HH, Samson D (eds): Intracranial Arteriovenous Malformations. St Louis, Quality Medical Publishing, (in press).
33. Lee JP: Surgical treatment of thalamic arteriovenous malformations. Neurosurgery 32:498–503, 1993.
34. Solomon RA, Stein BM: Interhemispheric approach for the surgical removal of thalamocaudate arteriovenous malformations. J Neurosurg 66:345–351, 1987.
35. Heros RC, Tu Y-K: Unruptured arteriovenous malformations: A dilemma in surgical decision making. Clin Neurosurg 33:187–212, 1986.
36. Gewirtz RJ, Steinberg GK: AVMs of the posterior fossa: Evaluation and management. Contemp Neurosurg 18:1–6, 1996.
37. Martin NA, Wilson CB: Preoperative and post-operative care. In Wilson CB, Stein BM (eds): Intracranial Arteriovenous Malformations. Baltimore, Williams & Wilkins, 1984, pp 184–208.
38. Betti OO, Munari C, Rosler R: Stereotactic radiosurgery with the linear accelerator: Treatment of arteriovenous malformations. Neurosurgery 24:311–321, 1989.
39. Steinberg GK, Fabrikant JI, Marks MP, et al: Stereotactic heavy-charged-particle Bragg-peak radiation for intracranial arteriovenous malformations. N Engl J Med 323:96–101, 1990.
40. Paulson RD, Steinberg GK, Norbash AM, et al: Embolization of rolandic cortex arteriovenous malformations. Neurosurgery 44:479–484, 1999.
41. Paulson RD, Steinberg GK, Norbash AM, et al: Embolization of basal ganglia and thalamic arteriovenous malformations. Neurosurgery 44:996–997, 1999.
42. Marks MP, Lane B, Steinberg GK, et al: Vascular characteristics of intracerebral arteriovenous malformations in patients with clinical steal. AJNR Am J Neuroradiol 12:489–496, 1991.
43. Spetzler RF, Wilson CB, Weinstein P, et al: Normal perfusion pressure breakthrough theory. Clin Neurosurg 25:651–672, 1978.
44. Morcos JJ, Heros RC: Supratentorial arteriovenous malformations. In Carter LP, Spetzler RF, Hamilton MG (eds): Neurovascular Surgery. New York, McGraw-Hill, 1995, pp 979–1004.
45. Spetzler RF, Martin NA, Carter LP, et al: Surgical management of large AVMs by staged embolization and operative excision. J Neurosurg 67:17–28, 1987.
46. Steiner L: Radiosurgery in cerebral arteriovenous malformations. In Fein JM, Flamm ES (eds): Cerebrovascular Surgery, vol 4. New York, Springer-Verlag, 1985, pp 1161–1215.
47. Kjellberg RN, Hanamura T, Davis KR, et al: Bragg-peak proton-beam therapy for arteriovenous malformations of the brain. N Engl J Med 309:269–274, 1983.
48. Kjellberg RN, Candia GJ: Stereotactic proton beam therapy for cerebral AVMs. In Alexander E, Crowell RM, Loeffler J, Chapman P (eds): Harvard Radiology Update. Chestnut Hill, MA, Harvard Medical School, 1990, pp 1–3.
49. Kjellberg RN: Proton beam therapy for arteriovenous malforma-

tions of the brain. In Schmidek HH, Sweet WH (eds): Operative Neurosurgical Techniques: Indications, Methods, Results, vol 2, 2nd ed. Philadelphia, WB Saunders, 1988, pp 911–915.
50. Marks MP, O'Donahue J, Fabrikant JI, et al: Cerebral blood flow evaluation of arteriovenous malformations with stable xenon CT. AJNR Am J Neuroradiol 9:1169–1175, 1988.
51. Samson D, Ditmore QM, Beyer CW: Intravascular use of isobutyl 2-cyanoacrylate: Part I. Treatment of intracranial vascular malformations. Neurosurgery 8:43–51, 1981.
52. Cromwell LD, Harris AB: Treatment of cerebral arteriovenous malformations: A combined neurosurgical and neuroradiological approach. J Neurosurg 52:705–708, 1980.
53. Debrun G, Vinuela F, Fox A, et al: Embolization of cerebral arteriovenous malformations with bucrylate: Experience in 46 cases. J Neurosurg 56, 1982, pp 615–627.
54. Jafar JJ, Davis AJ, Berenstein A, et al: The effect of embolization with N-butyl cyanoacrylate prior to surgical resection of cerebral arteriovenous malformations. J Neurosurg 78:60–69, 1993.
55. Rauch RA, Vinuela F, Dion J, et al: Preembolization functional evaluation in brain arteriovenous malformations: The ability of superselective Amytal test to predict neurological dysfunction before embolization. AJNR Am J Neuroradiol 13:309–314, 1992.
56. Colombo F, Pozza F, Chierego G, et al: Linear accelerator radiosurgery of cerebral arteriovenous malformations: An update. Neurosurgery 34:14–20, 1994.
57. Fabrikant JI, Levy RP, Steinberg GK, et al: Charged-particle radiosurgery for intracranial vascular malformations. Neurosurg Clin N Am 3:99–139, 1992.
58. Friedman WA, Bova FJ: Linear accelerator radiosurgery for arteriovenous malformations. J Neurosurg 77:832–841, 1992.
59. Lunsford LD, Kondziolka D, Flickinger JC, et al: Stereotactic radiosurgery for arteriovenous malformations of the brain. J Neurosurg 75:512–524, 1991.
60. Steiner L, Lindquist C, Adler JR, et al: Clinical outcome of radiosurgery for cerebral arteriovenous malformations. J Neurosurg 77:1–8, 1992.
61. Leksell L: Stereotactic radiosurgery. J Neurol Neurosurg Psychiatry 46:797–803, 1983.
62. Lunsford LD, Kondziolka D, Bissonette DJ, et al: Stereotactic radiosurgery of brain vascular malformations. Neurosurg Clin N Am 3:79–98, 1992.
63. Alexander Ed, Loeffler JS: Radiosurgery using a modified linear accelerator. Neurosurg Clin N Am 3:167–190, 1992.
64. Colombo F, Benedetti A, Pozza F, et al: Linear accelerator radiosurgery of cerebral arteriovenous malformations. Neurosurgery 24:833–840, 1989.
65. Levy RP, Fabrikant JI, Frankel KA, et al: Charged-particle radiosurgery of the brain. Neurosurg Clin N Am 1:955–990, 1990.
66. Levy RP, Fabrikant JI, Frankel KA, et al: Stereotactic heavy-charged-particle Bragg peak radiosurgery for the treatment of intracranial arteriovenous malformations in childhood and adolescence. Neurosurgery 24:841–852, 1989.
67. Chang SD, Shuster DL, Steinberg GK, et al: Stereotactic radiosurgery of arteriovenous malformations: Pathologic changes in resected tissue. Clin Neuropathol 16:111–116, 1997.
68. Firlik AD, Levy EI, Kondziolka D, et al: Staged volume radiosurgery followed by microsurgical resection: A novel treatment for giant cerebral arteriovenous malformations: Technical case report. Neurosurgery 43:1223–1228, 1998.
69. Pollack BE, Kondziolka D, Lunsford LD, et al: Repeat stereotactic radiosurgery of arteriovenous malformations: Factors associated with incomplete obliteration. Neurosurgery 38:318–324, 1996.
70. Marks MP, Lane B, Steinberg GK, et al: Endovascular treatment of cerebral arteriovenous malformations following radiosurgery. AJNR Am J Neuroradiol 14:297–303, 1993.
71. Steinberg GK, Levy RP, Marks MP, et al: Vascular malformations: Charged-particle radiosurgery. In Alexander E, Loeffler JS, Lunsford L (eds): Stereotactic Radiosurgery. New York, McGraw-Hill, 1993, pp 122–135.
72. Chang SD, Lopez JR, Steinberg GK: The usefulness of electrophysiologic monitoring during resection of central nervous system vascular malformations. J Stroke Cerebrovasc Dis 8:412–422, 1999.
73. Burchiel KJ, Clarke H, Ojemann GA, et al: Use of stimulation mapping and corticography in the excision of arteriovenous malformations in sensorimotor and language related neocortex. Neurosurgery 24:322–327, 1989.
74. Steinberg GK, Grant G, Yoon EJ: Deliberate hypothermia. In Andrews RJ (ed): Intraoperative Neuroprotection. Baltimore, Williams & Wilkins, 1996, pp 65–84.
75. Anegawa S, Hayashi T, Torigoe R, et al: Intraoperative angiography in the resection of arteriovenous malformations. J Neurosurg 80:73–78, 1994.
76. Forster DMC, Steiner L, Hakanson S: Arteriovenous malformations of the brain: A long term clinical study. J Neurosurg 37: 562–570, 1972.
77. Barrow DL, Boyer KL, Joseph GJ: Intraoperative angiography in the management of neurovascular disorders. Neurosurgery 30: 153–159, 1992.
78. Martin N, Doberstein C, Benston J: Intraoperative angiography in cerebrovascular surgery. Clin Neurosurg 37:312–331, 1991.
79. Nornes H, Grip A, Wikeby P: Intraoperative evaluation of cerebral hemodynamics using directional Doppler techniques: Part I. Arteriovenous malformations. J Neurosurg 50:145–151, 1979.
80. Heros RC, Korosue K, Diebold PM: Surgical excision of cerebral arteriovenous malformations: Late results. Neurosurgery 26:570–577, 1990.
81. Hernesniemi J, Keranen T: Microsurgical treatment of arteriovenous malformations of the brain in a defined population. Surg Neurol 33:384–390, 1990.
82. Chang SD, Levy RP, Marks MP, et al: Multimodality treatment of giant intracranial arteriovenous malformations. J Neurosurg 92:554, 2000.
83. Purdy PD, Batjer HH, Samson D: Management of hemorrhage complications from preoperative embolization of arteriovenous malformations. J Neurosurg 74:205–211, 1991.
84. Sheline GE, Wara WM, Smith V: Therapeutic irradiation and brain injury. Int J Radiat Oncol Biol Phys 6:1215–1228, 1980.
85. Chang SD, Adler JR: Management of the radiosurgery patient: Causes and treatment of adverse sequalae. In Meyer J (ed): Radiation Injury: Advancements in Management and Prevention. New York, Karger Medical, 1999, pp 155–165.
86. Loeffler JS, Siddon RL, Wen PY, et al: Stereotactic radiosurgery of the brain using a standard linear accelerator: A study of early and late effects. Radiother Oncol 17:311–321, 1990.
87. Kjellberg RN, Davis KR, Lyons S, et al: Bragg peak proton beam therapy for arteriovenous malformation of the brain. Clin Neurosurg 31:248–290, 1983.
88. Adams JH, Graham DI: An Introduction to Neuropathology. London, Churchill Livingstone, 1988.
89. Sutcliffe JC, Forster DM, Walton L, et al: Untoward clinical effects after stereotactic radiosurgery for intracranial arteriovenous malformations. Br J Neurosurg 6:177–185, 1992.
90. Steiner L: Stereotactic radiosurgery with the Cobalt-60 gamma unit in the surgical treatment of intracranial tumors and arteriovenous malformations. In Schmidek HH, Sweet WH (eds): Operative Neurosurgical Techniques: Indications, Methods, and Results. Philadelphia, WB Saunders, 1988, pp 515–529.
91. McKenzie MR, Souhami L, Caron JL, et al: Early and late complications following dynamic stereotactic radiosurgery and fractionated stereotactic radiotherapy. Can J Neurol Sci 20:279–285, 1993.
92. Miyasaka Y, Yada K, Ohwada T, et al: Retrograde thrombosis of feeding arteries after removal of arteriovenous malformations. J Neurosurg 72:540–545, 1990.

CHAPTER 134

Treatment of Lateral-Sigmoid and Sagittal Sinus Dural Arteriovenous Malformations

C. MICHAEL CAWLEY ■ DANIEL L. BARROW ■ JACQUES E. DION

Dural arteriovenous malformations (DAVMs) are characterized by abnormal arteriovenous shunting confined to a region of pachymeninges. DAVMs manifest with a wide variety of clinical manifestations that relate to the location of the lesion and the pattern of venous drainage. DAVMs may be asymptomatic or associated with distressing subjective symptoms, overt neurological symptoms, or life-threatening hemorrhage. These clinical manifestations have been attributed to venous hypertension, local mass effect, cerebrovascular steal, and frank exsanguination. This chapter focuses on two specific locations for DAVMs: within the wall of the transverse-sigmoid sinus, the most common location of DAVMs (63%), and within the wall of the superior sagittal sinus, a relatively uncommon site for DAVMs (7%).[1, 2]

ETIOLOGY

Knowledge of the etiologic factors leading to the development of DAVMs is incomplete. Some fistulas within the dura are the result of trauma, and a few are clearly congenital. The precise cause of most DAVMs remains enigmatic, however. Host-related factors that are likely associated with the development of DAVMs include sinus thrombosis, infection, and vascular dysplasia. Primitive arteriovenous communications within the embryonic dura mater are known to involute as the dura matures and as dural venous channels develop. Microscopic remnants of these arteriovenous channels are found in the adult dura, particularly near major venous sinuses. It has been hypothesized that these channels may dilate in response to certain pathologic conditions and create a zone of regional dural arteriovenous shunting.[3] Numerous factors have been postulated to predispose individuals to this condition, including adjacent venous sinus thrombosis, infection, and trauma. Hormonal or hemostatic mechanisms may play a role.

When the fistula is formed, several unpredictable courses may ensue. The lesion may thrombose or regress spontaneously. Alternatively, it may acquire additional arterial sources that converge into the same region of involved dura. On the venous side of the lesion, transmission of arterial pressure may result in venous hypertension. In the presence of venous outflow obstruction, intracranial hypertension may result. Reversal of blood flow in leptomeningeal channels may produce venous dilation, varicosities, and venous aneurysms.

CLINICAL MANIFESTATIONS AND NATURAL HISTORY

The clinical course and natural history of DAVMs range from benign to aggressive and have been described most clearly by Davies and colleagues in Toronto.[4, 5] Some individual symptoms and signs, such as pain, cranial neuropathies, and pulsatile tinnitus, are related to lesion location. The pattern of venous drainage correlates well with the behavior of the lesion. DAVMs that drain into major dural venous sinuses are associated with a benign natural history. In contrast, DAVMs associated with leptomeningeal venous drainage or drainage into the galenic system have an aggressive course and a high likelihood of hemorrhage or progressive neurological deficit. These venous drainage patterns tend to be characteristic for DAVMs at particular locations. DAVMs at the tentorial incisura or the anterior cranial fossa are highly likely to be associated with leptomeningeal venous drainage and are predisposed to an aggressive natural history. DAVMs of the cavernous and lateral-sigmoid sinuses are unlikely to have leptomeningeal venous drainage, however, and usually are associated with a benign clinical course. Any DAVM may have leptomeningeal venous drainage, which, if present, portends an aggressive course, regardless of the location of the lesion.

Transverse-Sigmoid Dural Arteriovenous Malformations

The clinical course for most DAVMs of the lateral-sigmoid sinuses is benign. In the comprehensive analysis by Awad and coworkers[2] of 377 DAVMs reported in the literature, transverse-sigmoid lesions composed 62.6% of all DAVMs. Aggressive behavior was associated with only 1 DAVM for every 8.8 that were nonaggressive.[2, 6] Most manifest with pulsatile tinnitus; headache is the second most common presenting symptom. Patients usually describe the tinnitus as a *swishing* noise that coincides with the heartbeat; the tinnitus tends to become more prominent when patients go to bed in a quiet room. Patients frequently complain of discomfort in the retroauricular region and occasionally have some tenderness there. Most transverse-sigmoid DAVMs drain exclusively into the sinus and are not associated with leptomeningeal venous drainage. These DAVMs are unlikely to hemorrhage or to manifest with progressive neurological deficits. On occasion, DAVMs may produce venous hypertension and present with papilledema and visual obscurations. In the rare situation in which DAVMs of the lateral-sigmoid sinuses are associated with leptomeningeal venous drainage, progressive neurological deficits and frank hemorrhage are more likely occurrences.

Superior Sagittal Sinus Dural Arteriovenous Malformations

DAVMs involving the superior sagittal sinus are much less common than lateral-sigmoid sinus lesions. In the analysis of DAVMs by Awad and coworkers,[2] these lesions accounted for 7.4% of all DAVMs. Aggressive and nonaggressive behavior was exhibited equally among the reported lesions. The symptoms from these lesions, similar to other DAVMs, depend on the pattern of venous drainage. We have seen lesions in this area that were incidental findings in asymptomatic patients. If drainage is solely into the superior sagittal sinus, patients may present with headache, a bruit, or symptoms of venous hypertension. If the venous drainage is shared by cortical veins, there is a high incidence of hemorrhage or neurological deficits.

IMAGING

Although now rarely used in the diagnosis of DAVMs, plain skull radiographs may show increased vascular markings created by dilated draining veins or meningeal arterial feeders. In some long-standing cases, the thickness of the calvaria and bone sclerosis is increased.

Computed tomography (CT) rarely can show the fistulas themselves but more often reveals epiphenomena associated with the DAVM. Noncontrast-enhanced studies may show the bone thickening, sclerosis, and grooving mentioned earlier. Hemorrhage of various types, including intraparenchymal, subdural, and subarachnoid, may be visualized. When venous pressure is increased (either locally or globally), edema, hydrocephalus, or both may be apparent on CT. Contrast-enhanced studies allow dilated pial veins and varices to be visualized. A negative CT scan does not exclude the diagnosis of a DAVM in the proper clinical setting.

Magnetic resonance imaging (MRI) affords more sensitive visualization of the same epiphenomena seen on CT (Fig. 134–1). In addition, the ability of MRI sequences to visualize flow, or the lack thereof, allows thrombosed sinuses to be identified. In some cases, gadolinium-enhanced studies may have abnormal signal adjacent to a thrombosed sinus, the DAVM nidus, or both. The resolution and detail of MRI angiography have improved markedly. Such studies show thrombosed sinuses, sinus narrowing, and, in some cases, dilated cortical venous structures. A normal MRI examination cannot rule out a DAVM, however, so this modality should not be used as a screening tool.

When a DAVM is suspected on the basis of clinical characteristics and radiographic screening studies, high-resolution selective angiography, including studies of the external carotid arteries, must be performed to describe and classify a specific lesion (Fig. 134–2). Such description narrows the therapeutic choices to be offered the patient. Most centers now offer digital subtraction technology, which provides excellent resolution with less radiation than conventional cut films. If the latter are to be used, meticulous masking must enable clear subtraction of bone artifact because DAVMs often occur near areas of bony prominence.

We routinely use nonionic contrast material to minimize allergic reactions and the discomfort caused by large volumes of ionic contrast material injected into the external carotid artery system. Various dilutions of contrast material minimize the renal load and generate *two-dimensional* images with vessels of varying opacity. Fast sequencing (three or more images per second) is required to generate adequate anatomic detail, as are selective catheterizations aimed at defining the exact site of the fistula and patterns of venous drainage. In general, a comprehensive study should include selective injections of both external carotid arteries, both internal carotid arteries, and at least one vertebral artery. In many cases, studies of the subclavian branches, specifically the thyrocervical and costocervical trunks, must be included.

CLASSIFICATION

Perhaps paramount to the classification and ultimately to the treatment of DAVMs is the venous phase of a selective angiogram. The films must be obtained late in the venous phase, and meticulous attention must be directed at anatomic details, such as direction of venous flow, narrowing or obstruction of venous sinuses, presence of cortical venous drainage, and structural venous abnormalities. These variations have become the basis of most classification schemes relating the specific anatomic patterns seen on angiography with natural history. Initial classification schemes, such as that proposed by Aminoff,[7] separated lesions based on their topographic location. The schemes proposed by

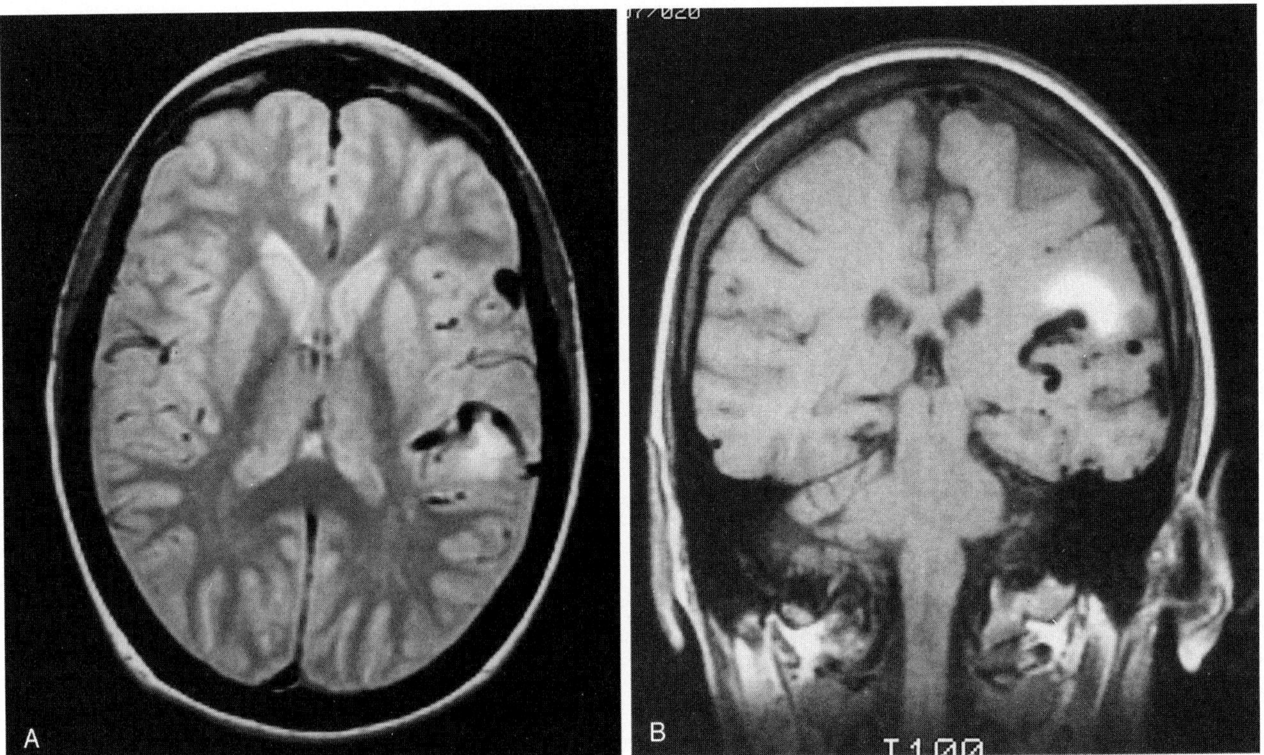

FIGURE 134–1. The typical appearance of a dural arteriovenous malformation on axial *(A)* and coronal *(B)* magnetic resonance images, in this case a superior sagittal sinus lesion with extensive cortical venous drainage. Intraparenchymal hemorrhage is evident.

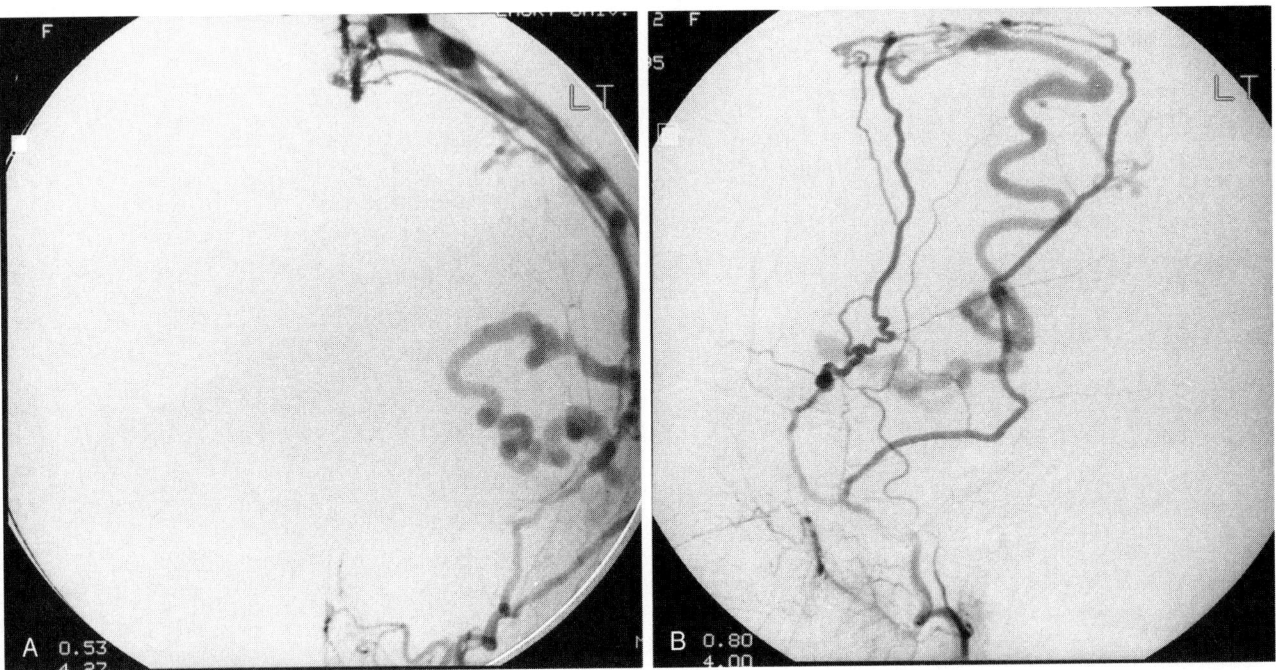

FIGURE 134–2. Anteroposterior *(A)* and lateral *(B)* angiograms of the same patient show meningeal arterial feeding vessels entering the wall of the superior sagittal sinus, then draining through dilated cortical veins.

Castaigne and associates,[8] Djindjian and coworkers,[9] Cognard and colleagues,[10] Lalwani and associates,[11] and Davies and coworkers[12] have clarified, however, that the pattern of venous drainage is the common factor that predicts the behavior of a DAVM in any location.

In our opinion, the system proposed by Borden and colleagues,[13] which focuses on venous drainage patterns, is the most elegant and streamlined classification to date. Borden type I DAVMs have no venous sinus outflow restrictions and drain only through sinuses in an anterograde fashion. Type II lesions have some degree of venous restriction that causes some anterograde or retrograde flow *and* subarachnoid venous drainage. Type III fistulas drain only through subarachnoid veins. In general, only Borden types II and III follow an aggressive course and are associated with a high rate of hemorrhage. It is apparent that some degree of obstruction to venous sinus outflow and subarachnoid venous drainage are the most ominous angiographic signs relative to the natural history of any DAVM. The variously aggressive nature of lesions stratified by location reflects each lesion's proclivity toward developing outflow obstruction and subarachnoid venous drainage. As mentioned, transverse-sigmoid sinus DAVMs seldom show such ominous features, whereas superior sagittal sinus fistulas are more likely to do so.

Transverse-Sigmoid Dural Arteriovenous Malformations

Transverse-sigmoid sinus DAVMs present aggressively in only 11% of cases. It is unusual that CT or MRI would show hemorrhage, hydrocephalus, or edema.[6] The utility of these studies is limited largely to the identification of large varices and abnormal flow-void patterns and to the elimination of neoplastic lesions from the differential diagnosis. Most often a bruit suggests the presence of some type of fistula and ultimately leads to cerebral angiography.

Selective angiography may reveal many potential feeders to DAVMs in this location (Fig. 134–3). Branches of the external carotid artery feeding a transverse-sigmoid DAVM often include transmastoid perforating vessels from the occipital, ascending pharyngeal, posterior auricular, middle meningeal, accessory meningeal, and superficial temporal arteries. Dural branches of the internal carotid artery, including the meningohypophyseal and inferolateral trunks, also frequently supply transverse-sigmoid sinus DAVMs. Less often, dural branches of the vertebral arteries (i.e., posterior meningeal, cerebellar falcine, muscular cervical anastomotic) and pial branches of the vertebrobasilar system (i.e., artery of Davidoff and Schecter, branches of the posterior cerebral arteries) are involved. When previous embolization or surgical obliteration has failed, the contralateral circulation must be investigated because branches from the external carotid artery and subclavian artery may cross over to feed recurrent or residual fistulas.

The veins associated with these specific fistulas may drain into a normal transverse or sigmoid sinus (or both) flowing in an anterograde fashion, into an obstructed sinus with anterograde or retrograde flow (with or without subarachnoid venous drainage), or purely into subarachnoid veins. Apart from the specific pattern of venous drainage (which helps determine *whether* any treatment is advocated), findings on the late venous phases of the angiogram are important in determining what *type* of treatment is advocated (Fig. 134–4). Attention to the late venous phase reveals the presence of normal venous structures (such as the vein

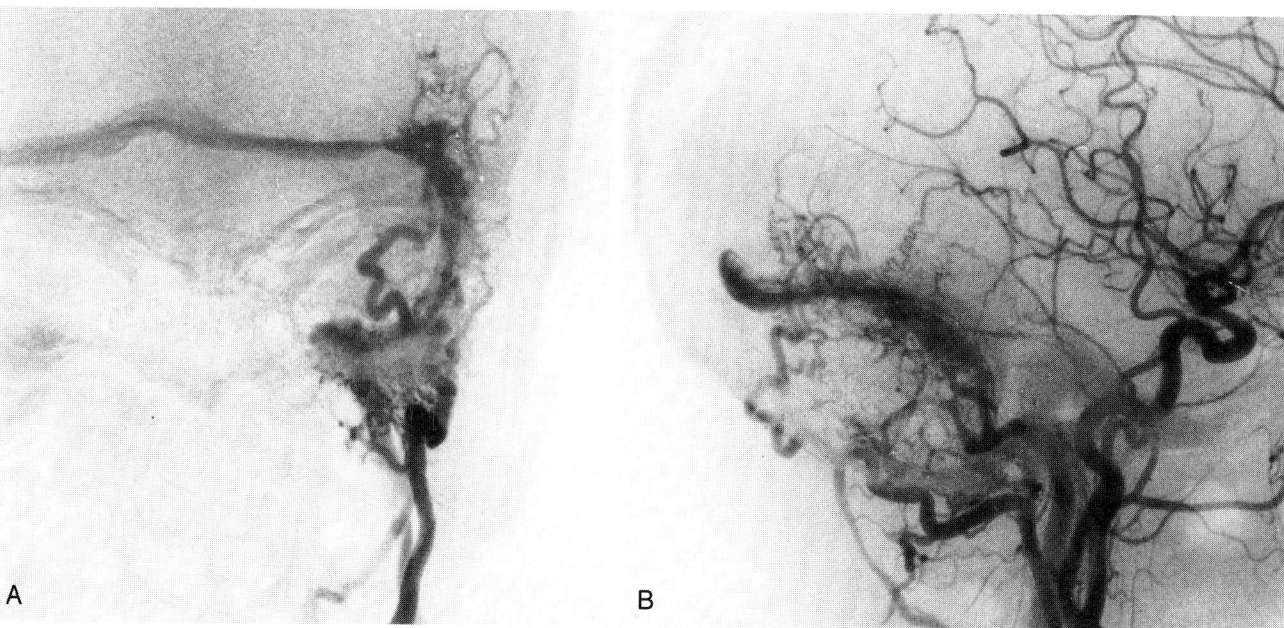

FIGURE 134–3. Anteroposterior *(A)* and lateral *(B)* angiograms of a typical lateral-sigmoid sinus dural arteriovenous malformation. Note the multiple feeding vessels from the occipital artery and other deep posterior cervical muscular branches.

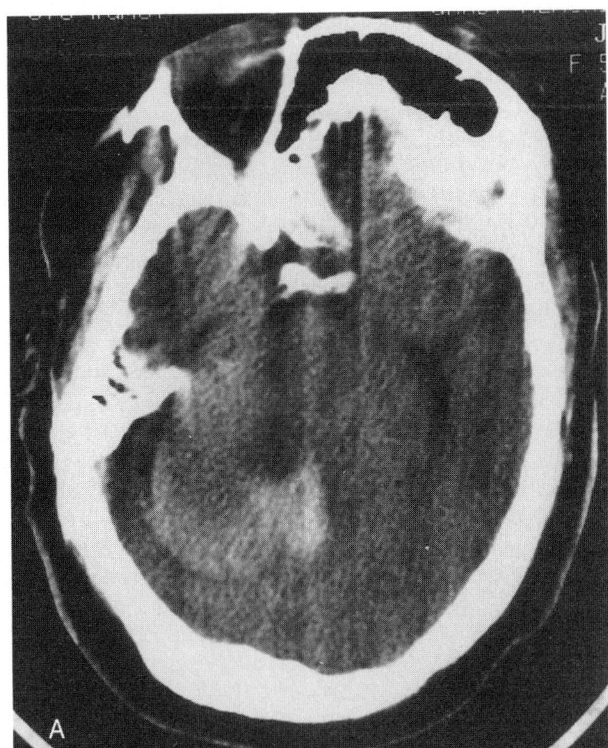

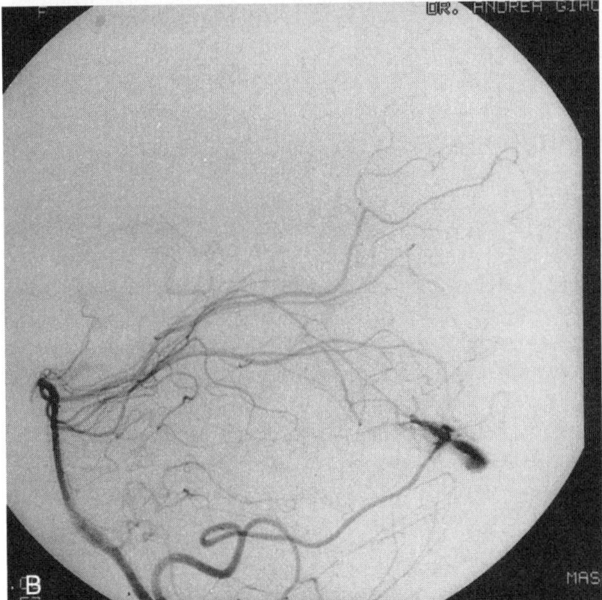

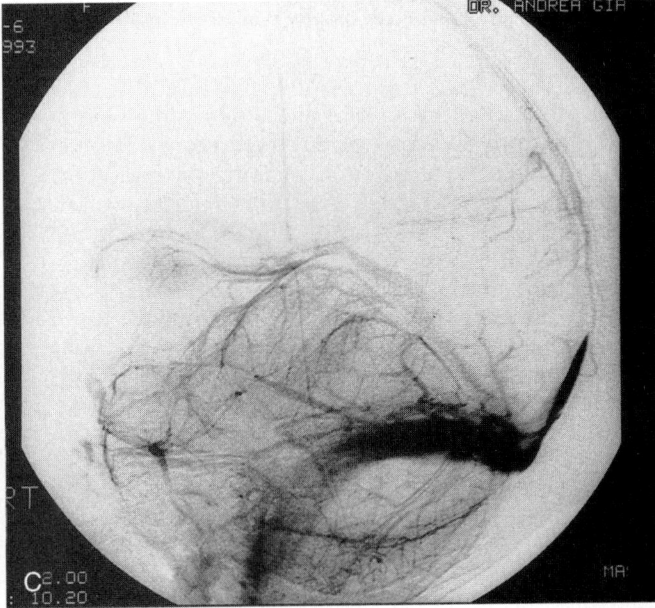

FIGURE 134–4. *A*, Axial computed tomography scan of a patient with a subdural hemorrhage along the tentorium. *B*, Early-phase angiogram reveals the fistula fed by the posterior meningeal artery. *C*, Late-phase study shows dural sinus stenosis at the transverse-sigmoid junction and, as a result, cortical venous drainage into the temporal and occipital lobes.

of Labbé) draining into the affected sinus. If the entire section of the transverse-sigmoid sinus is arterialized (as is usually the case), it may be sacrificed transvenously. If normal venous structures persist, a more focused (usually arterial) attack on the fistula must be planned.

Superior Sagittal Sinus Dural Arteriovenous Malformations

Plain radiographs may show prominent grooves secondary to enlarged branches of the middle meningeal artery. Long-standing hyperemia can cause sclerosis and thickening of overlying bone. CT scans show such abnormalities in addition to hydrocephalus and hemorrhage. In the special case of superior sagittal sinus DAVMs, CT with contrast enhancement often helps delineate patency of the sinus itself. The so-called empty delta sign is an indication that thrombus has occluded the sinus in the area through which the scan has imaged. MRI (especially MRI angiography) likewise shows hemorrhage, hydrocephalus, edema, and sinus thrombosis. Enlarged cortical veins also may be seen.

As described by Barnwell and colleagues,[14] there are two types of superior sagittal sinus DAVMs. In the

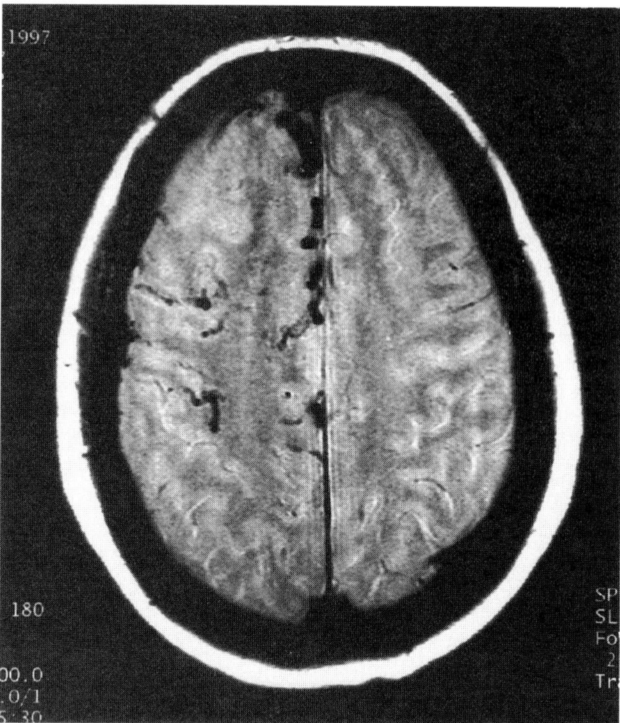

FIGURE 134–5. Superior sagittal sinus dural arteriovenous malformation with cortical venous drainage predominantly in the interhemispheric fissure.

first, vessels drain directly into the sagittal sinus; in the second, the sinus is disconnected, then reconnected via a cortical vein. The diagnostic imaging of choice for such complex lesions is high-resolution selective arteriography (Figs. 134–5 and 134–6). Such a study often reveals bilateral supply from the external carotid artery to the fistula through transosseous branches of the middle meningeal, superficial temporal, or occipital arteries. Lesser contributions may arise from the ophthalmic artery through the anterior falcine artery and from the vertebral artery through the posterior meningeal artery. In rarer cases, blood supply may arise from pial vessels of the anterior, middle, or posterior cerebral circulation or from the meningohypophyseal trunk through the artery of Bernasconi-Cassinari.

Similar to the evaluation of all DAVMs, rapid-sequence subtracted angiograms must be examined closely for the exact site of fistulization. The fistula itself may lie in the wall of the superior sagittal sinus, the falx, or an adjacent cortical vein. Fistulas that drain directly into the superior sagittal sinus rarely hemorrhage, although dementia has been reported as a result of chronically increased venous and intracranial pressure. Similar to dural arteriovenous fistulas in other locations, subarachnoid venous drainage is an ominous sign, especially when all anterograde drainage through the sinus has thrombosed, leaving only retrograde cortical venous routes.

TREATMENT

Therapies offered to patients harboring DAVMs must be tailored based on the location, vascular characteristics, and presentation of a particular lesion. In general, only fistulas deemed to be at high risk for severe neurological events as described previously or fistulas associated with intolerable, progressive symptoms should be considered for treatment. High-risk DAVMs often manifest with hemorrhage, venous infarcts, visual loss, or focal neurological deficits. Such lesions should be treated urgently and completely. As with aneurysms and arteriovenous malformations, partial treatment offers no protection from initial or recurrent hemorrhage. Any patient harboring a transverse-sigmoid or superior sagittal sinus DAVM with subarachnoid venous drainage should be considered for aggressive treatment, regardless of presentation.

Fistulas whose features are more consistent with a benign course, as outlined earlier, can be observed—if the patient is willing to live with the symptoms. In some cases, we have agreed to treat non–life-threatening lesions based on a patient's absolute intolerance of symptoms such as a constant bruit. When conservative therapy is chosen, the patient usually is advised to avoid medications that inhibit coagulation—although some physicians advocate aspirin therapy to limit further sinus thrombosis. Any change in symptoms, including abrupt disappearance, must be reported to the physician because such changes can herald a change in the venous drainage pattern (e.g., complete sinus thrombosis or shunting into subarachnoid veins).

Transverse-Sigmoid Dural Arteriovenous Malformations

COMPRESSION THERAPY

A significant percentage of DAVMs spontaneously thrombose without therapy. DAVMs that develop worrisome features can be treated in several ways. Rarely, transverse-sigmoid sinus DAVMs supplied only by the occipital artery can be treated effectively by manual self-compression. The patient is advised to compress the pulsatile occipital artery manually for 30 minutes, three times a day. In 25% of such simple fistulas, complete thrombosis may occur within several weeks.[15] If success is suspected clinically, an angiogram should be obtained to document the cure and to rule out any adverse change in venous drainage patterns.

TRANSARTERIAL THERAPY

Although embolization through the transarterial route formerly was the most common endovascular treatment of transverse-sigmoid sinus DAVMs, it now is reserved for selected cases in which venous access is unobtainable and as a preoperative adjunct. A historic disadvantage of attempting to obliterate a DAVM via a transarterial avenue includes a low rate of cure because of the myriad of feeders, some below the resolution of angiography, which often leads to the re-establishment of fistulous flow. In some such cases, symptoms such as bruit might resolve temporarily but often return remotely, accompanied by a more ominous angioarchitecture than before treatment. Arterial embolization can cause thrombosis of important venous ac-

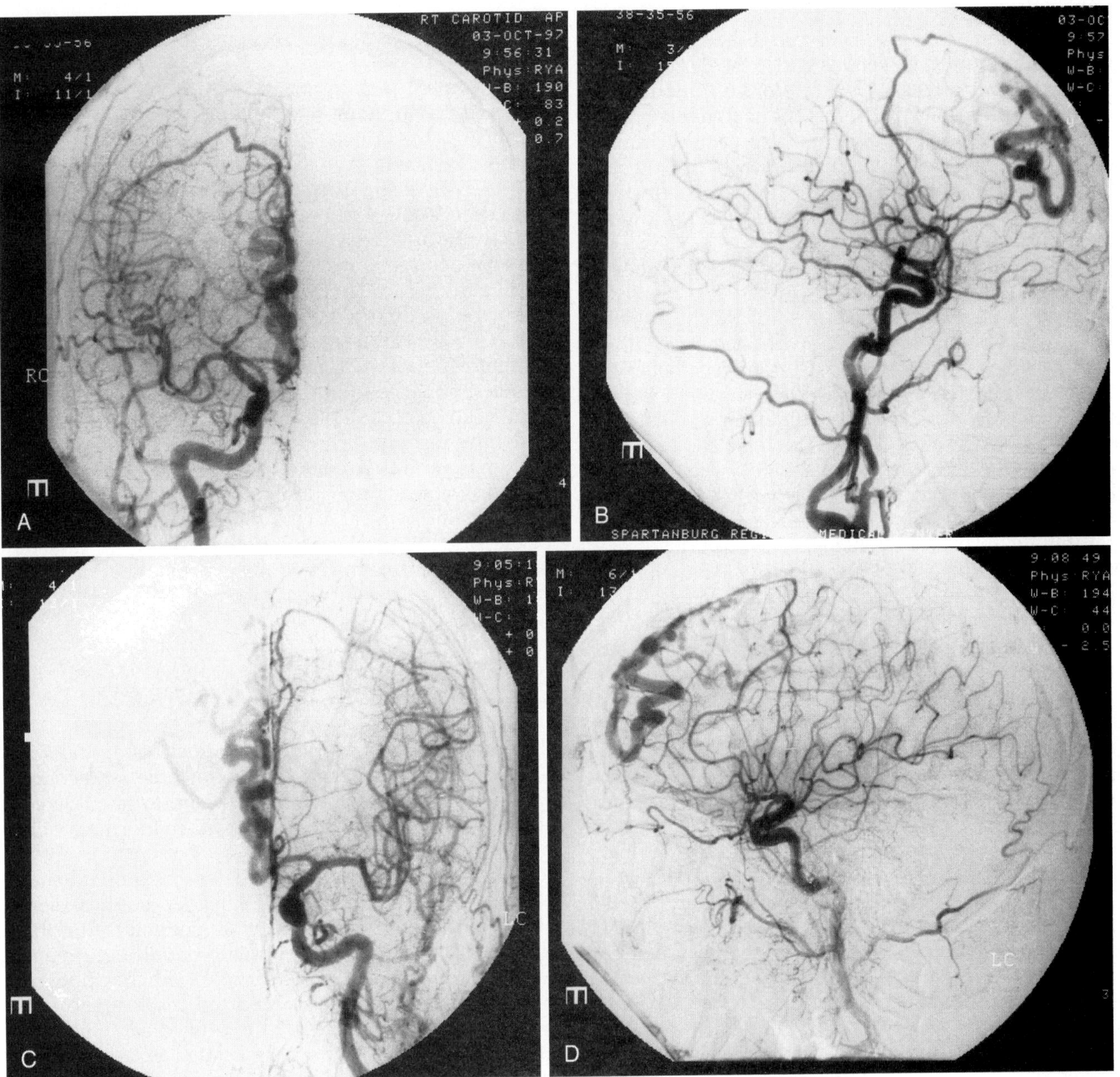

FIGURE 134–6. Anteroposterior *(A)* and lateral *(B)* angiograms of the patient in Figure 134–4 show two arterial feeders from the middle meningeal artery from both sides. Anteroposterior *(C)* and lateral *(D)* angiograms show that the cortical venous drainage is confined to the right side.

cess channels, while failing to cure the lesion. Such an occurrence occasionally precludes the possibility of definitive transvenous treatment and may lead to the recruitment of pial collaterals that make any subsequent therapy more complicated.

Transarterial embolization may be appropriate in selected cases. The agents most often used are polyvinyl alcohol (PVA) particulates and glues (such as *n*-butyl cyanoacrylate [NBCA]), although alcohol and silk strands also have been used. In general, we prefer PVA particles, which seem to be the safest embolization material. We deploy the particulates close to the site of the fistula because proximal occlusion universally leads to a recurrence. Occasionally, we test with lidocaine injections to ensure that the blood supply to the cranial nerves is not compromised. Glues usually are avoided because of the higher risk of downstream venous obstruction, which may result in an unfavorable change in the venous drainage pattern of a specific lesion. We most often use solely transarterial embolization to decrease flow through a particular DAVM to prepare for surgical excision or transvenous coil embolization or to reach the proximal venous outflow vessel to occlude it.

TRANSVENOUS THERAPY

Occlusion of the precise site of the fistula or of its immediate recipient vein is the only way to cure a transverse-sigmoid sinus or any other type of DAVM. In our opinion, occlusion is accomplished most efficaciously through a transvenous endovascular approach. Such treatment offers a high rate of cure, with a low risk of complications as long as the segment of vein or sinus to be occluded does not also serve as a drainage route for normal venous structures. Most of these sinuses are arterialized completely and are effectively nonfunctional; they may be sacrificed with a low risk of venous infarction.

Access most often is gained via the transfemoral approach. Occasionally, access to the transverse-sigmoid sinus may require a bur hole directly over the sinus, which then is entered with an angiocatheter through which embolic materials or microcatheters and guidewires may be advanced. When transfemoral percutaneous access is used, the guidewire and catheters are advanced through the inferior and superior vena cava, then through the internal jugular vein to enter the sigmoid sinus. If the sinus is occluded ipsilateral to the fistula, contralateral access across the torcular Herophili is relatively simple since the advent of modern high-performance, hydrophilic microcatheters and guidewires. When the segment of vein or sinus to be occluded is cannulated, we prefer a combination of the control of placement inherent in the Guglielmi detachable coil system and the thrombogenicity of Dacron-fibered platinum coils. With judicious use of each of these coils, thrombosis is usually immediate. When some filling through the coil pack is evident, thrombosis can be enhanced by a short course of ϵ-aminocaproic acid followed by angiography in 48 hours.

Transvenous embolization of DAVMs can be accomplished via a transarterial route. In such cases, a microcatheter is placed in the arterial side of the fistula. The embolization material, usually NBCA diluted with iodized oil (Lipiodol), is pushed into the fistula itself and the immediate recipient vein. In this way, a simple DAVM with few fistulous sites can be cured selectively, while the sinus itself is spared.

SURGICAL THERAPY

The first attempts to cure transverse-sigmoid sinus DAVMs employed surgical excision alone. These procedures were notoriously bloody ventures. Sundt and Piepgras[16] estimated that 300 mL of blood per minute could be lost until the resection was completed. These authors recommended prophylactic blood transfusions before turning the craniotomy.[16] Currently, surgery for such lesions usually is limited to gaining access to the sinuses to introduce the embolization material as described earlier. We continue to recommend surgical excision after arterial preoperative embolization, however, when occlusion of the fistula and immediate recipient vein is impossible by any other means. In the case of transverse-sigmoid DAVMs, such surgery requires a supratentorial and infratentorial exposure of the involved sinus segments and their complete isolation from the surrounding dura, which harbors real and potential feeders. This surgery is rendered much less bloody by preoperative embolization.

Superior Sagittal Sinus Dural Arteriovenous Malformations

The treatment paradigms and options offered to a patient with a superior sagittal sinus DAVM are almost identical to the options described earlier for transverse-sigmoid lesions. In the rare cases in which the fistula is fed solely by a superficial temporal artery, compression may be effective. More often, the feeding vessels are multiple and deep and require more invasive approaches. Surgery for these usually simple fistulas is an elegant, typically straightforward exercise in identifying and occluding the site of the fistula through some variation of an interhemispheric approach. Modern catheters permit a much less invasive endovascular option. Similar to transverse-sigmoid DAVMs, a simple fistula can be occluded by accessing the feeding arteries and injecting glue through the fistulous site into the proximal venous recipient vessel. As described earlier for transverse-sigmoid lesions, more complex DAVMs may require surgical access to an arterialized segment of the sinus for occlusion with coils. Surgical resection of such malformations requires skeletonization of the sinus and may benefit from preoperative arterial embolization.

OUTCOMES AND COMPLICATIONS

Because transverse-sigmoid and superior sagittal sinus DAVMs typically are benign, the outcomes and complications associated with any intervention must be considered carefully. When a specific malformation has ominous angioarchitectonic features or becomes symptomatic with hemorrhage, the risk of treatment usually is outweighed by its benefits. Older surgical series show that a high percentage of patients with these fistulas is cured with surgery (with or without preoperative embolization). In a series of 67 patients, however, Sundt and Piepgras[16] also reported a 7% rate of poor outcomes, including 3 patients who died. Frequently encountered complications associated with the operative treatment of these lesions include excessive blood loss, venous hypertension or infarction (or both), cerebral edema, and, rarely, hydrocephalus.

Series that have reported outcomes and complications after either transvenous or transarterial embolization are less extensive.[15, 17, 18] In general, long-term cure rates with arterial embolization alone are less than 50%. In contrast, our experience has indicated that few, if any, fistulas treated with venous-side occlusion recur. The incidence of serious complications in our cases is low but includes the small risk of vessel perforation causing a subarachnoid hemorrhage and redirection of arterialized blood into subarachnoid veins if thrombosis is only partial.

CONCLUSION

A better understanding of the natural history of DAVMs and advances in endovascular therapies have resulted in the rapid evolution of treatments for these lesions. Most DAVMs requiring therapeutic intervention are managed safely and effectively by endovascular techniques. Optimal management requires complete angiographic evaluation of the angioarchitecture, careful assessment of the risks related to the lesion's natural history and treatment, the selection of appropriate fistulas for treatment, and an experienced multidisciplinary team of neurovascular surgeons and endovascular therapists.

REFERENCES

1. Awad IA: The diagnosis and management of intracranial dural arteriovenous malformations. Contemp Neurosurg 13:1–6, 1991.
2. Awad IA, Little JR, Akarawi WP, et al: Intracranial dural arteriovenous malformations: Factors predisposing to an aggressive neurological course. J Neurosurg 72:839–850, 1990.
3. Bederson JB: Pathophysiology and animal models of dural arteriovenous malformations. In Awad IA, Barrow DL (eds): Dural Arteriovenous Malformations. Park Ridge, IL, American Association of Neurological Surgeons, 1993, pp 23–35.
4. Davies MA, Saleh J, Ter Brugge K, et al: The natural history and management of intracranial dural arteriovenous fistulae: Part I. Benign lesions. Interventional Neuroradiology 3:295–302, 1997.
5. Davies MA, Ter Brugge K, Willinsky R, et al: The natural history and management of intracranial dural arteriovenous fistulae: Part II. Aggressive lesions. Interventional Neuroradiology 3:303–311, 1997.
6. Awad IA: Dural arteriovenous malformations with aggressive clinical course. In Awad IA, Barrow DL (eds): Dural Arteriovenous Malformations. Park Ridge, IL, American Association of Neurological Surgeons, 1993, pp 93–105.
7. Aminoff MJ: Vascular anomalies in the intracranial dura mater. Brain 96:601–612, 1973.
8. Castaigne P, Bories J, Brunet P, et al: Meningeal arterio-venous fistulas with cortical venous drainage [French]. Rev Neurol (Paris) 132:169–181, 1976.
9. Djindjian R, Merland JJ, Theron J: Super-Selective Arteriography of the External Carotid Artery. New York, Springer-Verlag, 1977, pp 606–628.
10. Cognard C, Gobin YP, Pierot L, et al: Cerebral dural arteriovenous fistulas: Clinical and angiographic correlation with a revised classification of venous drainage. Radiology 194:671–680, 1995.
11. Lalwani AK, Dowd CF, Halbach VV: Grading venous restrictive disease in patients with dural arteriovenous fistulas of the transverse/sigmoid sinus. J Neurosurg 79:11–15, 1993.
12. Davies MA, TerBrugge K, Willinsky R, et al: The validity of classification for the clinical presentation of intracranial dural arteriovenous fistulas. J Neurosurg 85:830–837, 1996.
13. Borden JA, Wu JK, Shucart WA: A proposed classification for spinal and cranial dural arteriovenous fistulous malformations and implications for treatment. J Neurosurg 82:166–179, 1995.
14. Barnwell SL, Halbach VV, Dowd CF, et al: A variant of arteriovenous fistulas within the wall of dural sinuses: Results of combined surgical and endovascular therapy. J Neurosurg 74:199–204, 1991.
15. Halbach VV, Higashida RT, Hieshima GB, et al: Dural fistulas involving the transverse and sigmoid sinuses: Results of treatment in 28 patients. Radiology 163:443–447, 1987.
16. Sundt TM Jr, Piepgras DG: The surgical approach to arteriovenous malformations of the lateral and sigmoid dural sinuses. J Neurosurg 59:32–39, 1983.
17. Halbach VV, Higashida RT, Hieshima GB, et al: Treatment of dural arteriovenous malformations involving the superior sagittal sinus. AJNR Am J Neuroradiol 9:337–343, 1988.
18. Dawson RC 3rd, Joseph GJ, Owens DS, et al: Transvenous embolization as the primary therapy for arteriovenous fistulas of the lateral and sigmoid sinuses. AJNR Am J Neuroradiol 19:571–576, 1998.

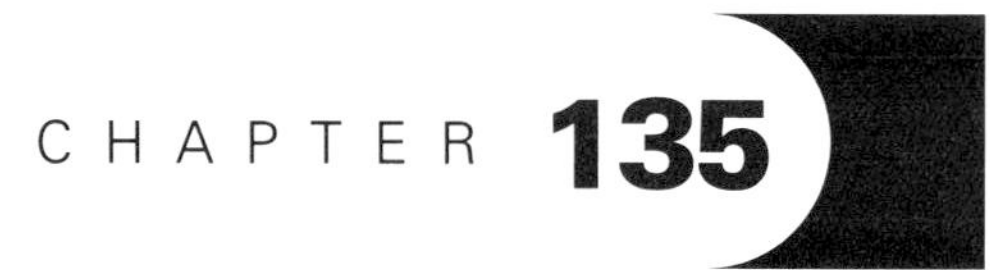

Epidemiology and Natural History of Cavernous Malformations

JOSEPH M. ZABRAMSKI ■ PATRICK P. HAN

Cerebrovascular malformations are developmental abnormalities that affect the blood vessels supplying the brain. Postmortem studies suggest that these cerebrovascular malformations affect approximately 4% of the population.[1–4] The most commonly used classification scheme divides these lesions into four categories: (1) venous malformations, (2) arteriovenous malformations, (3) cavernous malformations, and (4) telangiectases.[2, 5, 6] Although cavernous malformations constitute only 5% to 10% of cerebrovascular malformations, they are recognized increasingly as a cause of seizures and focal neurological deficits.[2–4, 7]

The introduction of magnetic resonance imaging (MRI) allowed cavernous malformations to be diagnosed without the need for pathologic confirmation, which, in turn, has enhanced greatly understanding of the natural history of these lesions. The growing availability of MRI has encouraged clinical interest in these lesions, and recognition that a large number of these cases had a familial component has stimulated research into the genetic basis of this disease. The gene responsible for the familial form of this disease recently was identified by two separate groups of investigators.[8, 9]

A logical approach to the management of these lesions requires that neurosurgeons understand the epidemiology and natural history of cavernous malformations. This chapter provides readers with an in-depth review of the available literature on these topics and examines the implications related to the treatment of these patients.

EPIDEMIOLOGY

Before the introduction of modern imaging technology, cavernous malformations were considered rare lesions. In 1976, Voigt and Yasargil[10] described their clinical experience with one case and thoroughly reviewed the world literature, finding only 126 reported cases. Soon after the publication of this article, computed tomography (CT) became widely available. Although CT was a significant step forward in neuroimaging, it lacked sensitivity and specificity for the diagnosis and imaging of cavernous malformations. Only partially calcified or recently hemorrhagic lesions could be visualized readily, and diagnosis required pathologic confirmation.

The introduction of MRI revolutionized understanding of these lesions and sparked interest in their management. The imaging characteristics of cavernous malformations are sufficiently unique to allow most of these lesions to be diagnosed on the basis of MRI findings alone (Fig. 135–1).[11–15] To obtain some idea of the impact that MRI has had on clinical interest in cerebral cavernous malformations, we reviewed the medical literature on this disease before and after the U.S. Food and Drug Administration approved MRI technology in 1986. We found 37 articles published on cerebral cavernous malformations during the 5-year period from 1981 to 1985 compared with 147 articles during the 5 years that followed (1987 to 1992). The number of publications has continued to increase; in 1999, more than 60 articles were published on this topic.

Cavernous malformations are more common than generally is suspected. Postmortem studies performed in the 1980s showed that cavernous malformations affect 0.37% to 0.5% of the population (Table 135–1).[1, 2] Remarkably similar results were reported by two groups reviewing more than 22,000 MRI examinations, with incidence rates of 0.4% to 0.5% (see Table 135–1).[16, 17] Based on these studies, it is estimated that 18 to 22 million people are affected by cavernous malformations worldwide.

Cavernous malformations occur in two forms: spon-

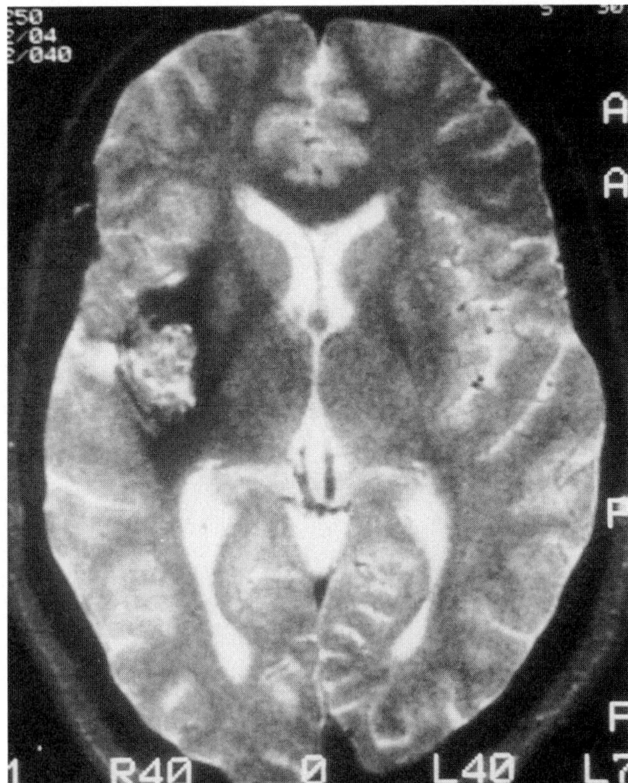

FIGURE 135–1. Axial T2-weighted magnetic resonance image shows the classic appearance of cavernous malformation: The core of the lesion has a reticulated *salt-and-pepper* pattern and is surrounded by a halo of low-intensity signal. Note the absences of mass effect and edema. This pattern is pathognomonic for cavernous malformation.

TABLE 135–1 ■ **Reported Incidence Rate of Cavernous Malformations**

AUTHOR, YEAR	NO. PATIENTS STUDIED	NO. LESIONS/ INCIDENCE RATE
McCormick,[2] 1984	5734	19/0.34%
Otten et al,[1] 1989	24,535	131/0.53%
Del Curling et al,[17] 1991	8131	32/0.39%
Robinson et al,[16] 1991	14,035	66/0.47%

taneous and familial. The spontaneous form occurs as an isolated case, most commonly with a single lesion. The familial form is characterized by multiple lesions (Fig. 135–2) and an autosomal dominant mode of inheritance.[18–21] Multiple lesions and a strong family history of seizures are pathognomonic for the familial form of cavernous malformations. With careful screening, more than 80% of patients with three or more lesions are found to have a history consistent with the familial form of this disease. Given the common occurrence of asymptomatic vascular lesions in patients affected with this disease, the masking of the autosomal dominant segregation pattern is a possibility, particularly in smaller families.

CLINICAL PRESENTATION

Cavernous malformations have been reported in infants and children, but most patients become symptomatic during the second to fifth decades of life.[16, 17, 20] Not all patients with cavernous malformations have clinical symptoms. Between 15% and 20% of lesions are discovered incidentally during an evaluation for headache or other unrelated neurological problem.[16, 17] In our experience, 40% of patients with the familial form of the disease remain asymptomatic despite the presence of multiple lesions.[20]

Evidence of prior hemorrhage is a constant feature of cavernous malformations whether or not lesions are symptomatic. Hemorrhage of varying ages, combined with the deposition of hemosiderin in the cerebral tissue surrounding the cavernous malformation, pro-

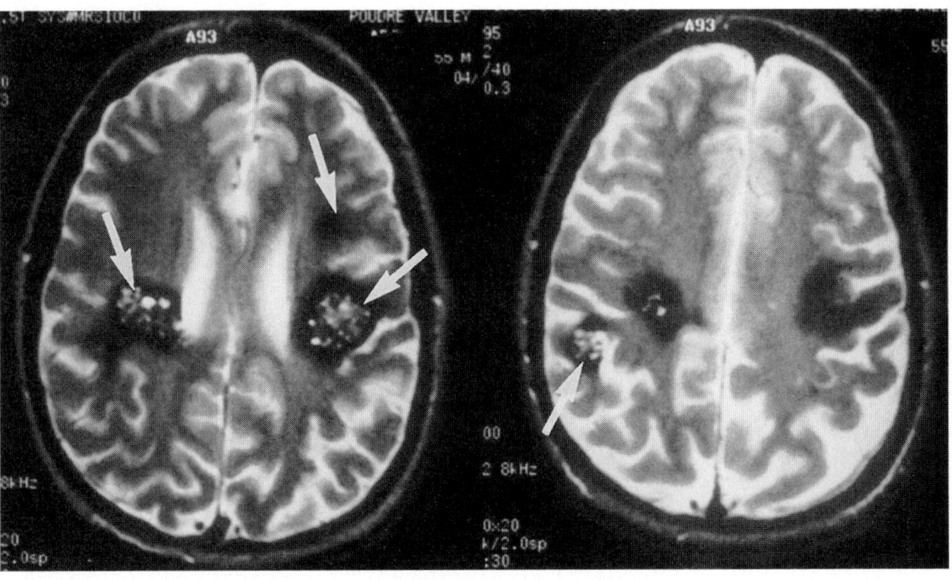

FIGURE 135–2. Axial T2-weighted magnetic resonance images in a patient with a strong familial history of seizures. Four distinct cavernous malformations are seen at these two levels *(arrows)*; a fifth cerebellar lesion also was identified. Multiple lesions and a family history of seizures are characteristic of the familial form of this disease.

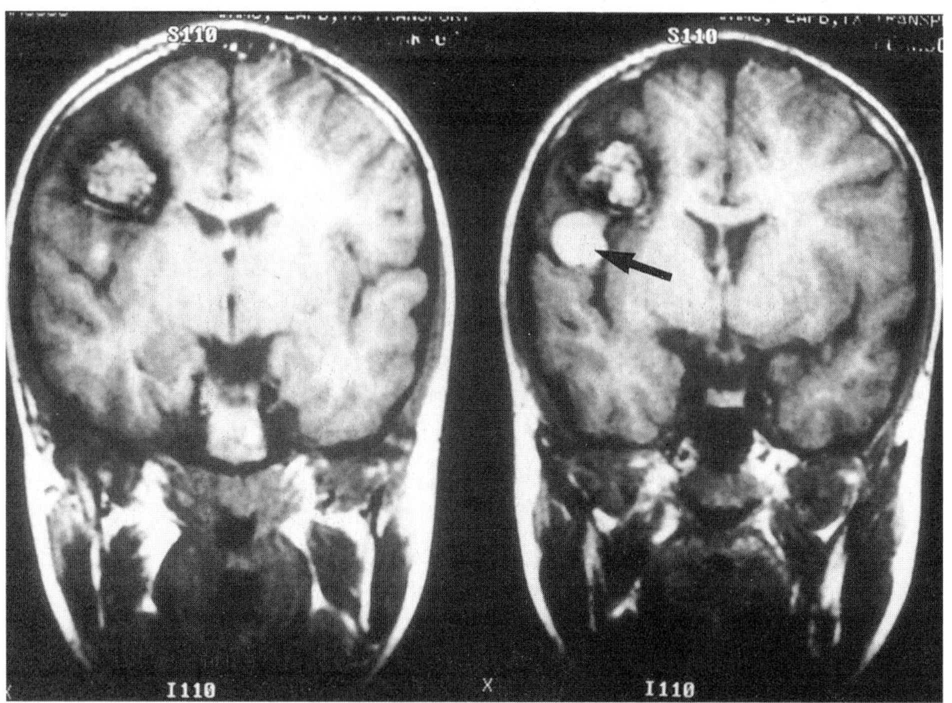

FIGURE 135–3. Coronal T1-weighted magnetic resonance images of a 10-year-old boy whose history was remarkable for an episode of seizure activity at 4 years of age with a negative computed tomography study. The patient presented with the sudden onset of mild weakness and decreased sensation in the left upper extremity. The focal area of subacute blood *(arrow)* extending outside the capsule of the lesion produces a so-called gross hemorrhage.

duces the unique MRI characteristics of these lesions (see Figs. 135–1 and 135–2). Increases in size appear to result from repeated small hemorrhages within the lesion, from spontaneous thrombosis of the blood-filled caverns, or both. Organization and endothelialization within these hemorrhagic and thrombotic cavities create the potential for further growth. Rarely, these lesions rupture outside their capsule, producing a *gross* hemorrhage into the surrounding brain (Fig. 135–3). Because cavernous malformations are low-flow, low-pressure lesions, hemorrhage (even gross hemorrhage outside the lesion) usually displaces and compresses adjacent neural tissue rather than destroying it.

Seizures are the most common manifestation of supratentorial cavernous malformations, accounting for 40% to 80% of the presenting symptoms.[7, 16, 17, 19, 20, 22] The onset or exacerbation of seizure activity in these patients often is associated with MRI evidence of acute or subacute hemorrhage (Fig. 135–4). Although the exact mechanism that leads to seizure activity in these lesions is unknown, it appears to be related to hemosiderin deposition. The iron present in hemosiderin is a well-known epileptogenic material used to induce seizures in laboratory models of epilepsy.[23, 24] Focal neurological deficits secondary to mass effect are associated rarely with supratentorial lesions, unless the lesion is located in the basal ganglia or thalamus.

In contrast, the sudden onset of focal neurological deficits is the most frequent presentation of patients with brainstem cavernous malformations (Fig. 135–5).[25–28] Porter and colleagues[28] reported 100 surgical cases of brainstem cavernous malformations. In their series, 97% of patients presented with focal neurological deficits from hemorrhage. In the brainstem where lesions may be adjacent to crucial tracts and nuclei, even small focal hemorrhages may be tolerated poorly.

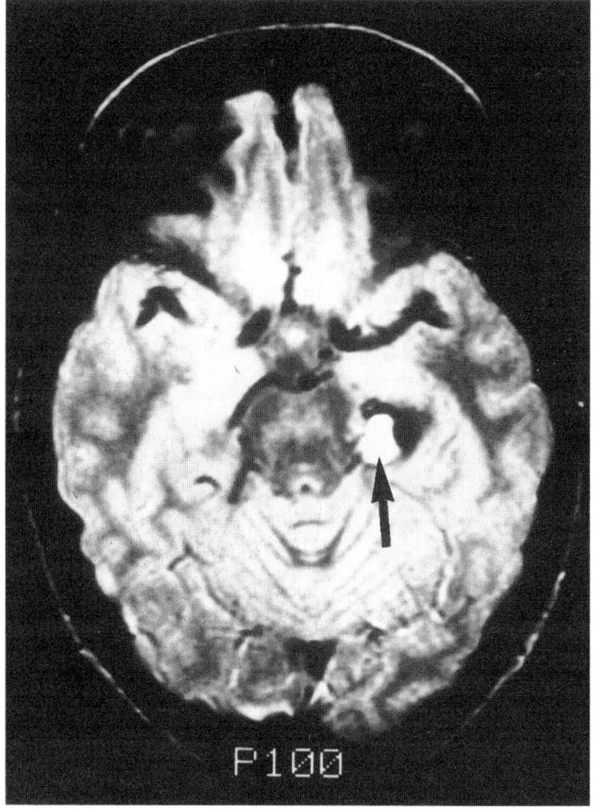

FIGURE 135–4. Intermediate-weighted, axial spin-echo magnetic resonance images of a 23-year-old man with an acute exacerbation of temporal lobe seizure activity. Note the focal area of high-intensity signal *(arrow)* compatible with subacute hemorrhage in the region of the left hippocampus. A ring of low-intensity signal surrounds this subacute collection of blood, consistent with hemosiderin deposition from previous remote episodes of hemorrhage. Surgical pathology confirmed the diagnosis of cavernous malformation.

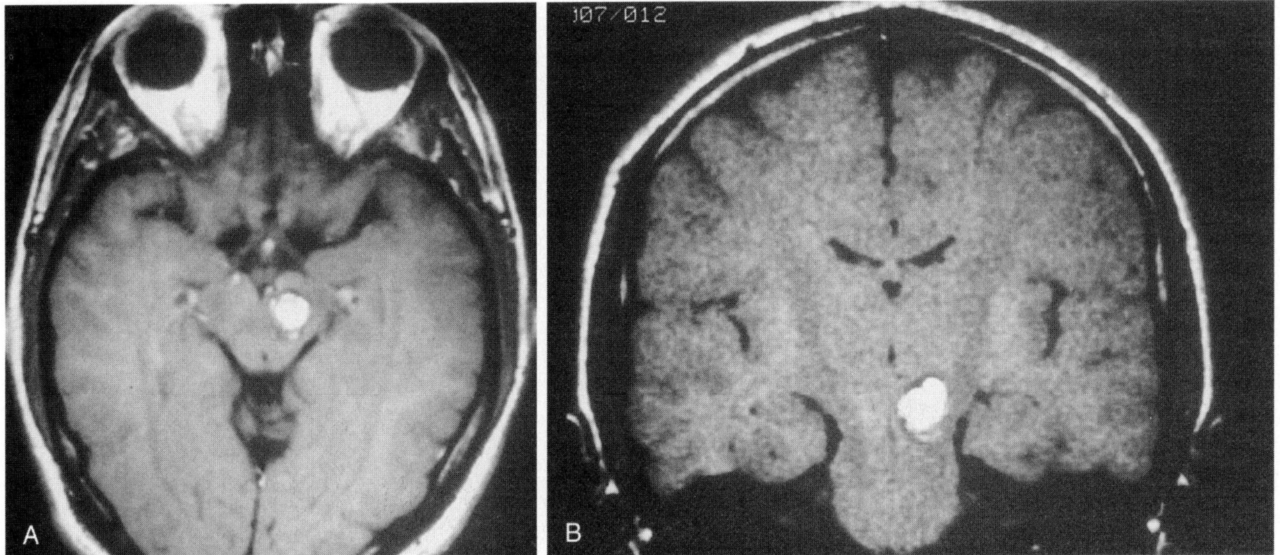

FIGURE 135–5. Axial *(A)* and coronal *(B)* T1-weighted magnetic resonance images of a 27-year-old woman who presented with a history of sudden onset of mild right-sided weakness and decreased coordination. The symptoms had resolved slowly during about 2 weeks. The patient was neurologically intact at the time of neurosurgical consultation. Resection of the lesion would require dissection through normal brainstem; nonoperative management was recommended.

The development of symptoms in patients with hemorrhage from brainstem cavernous malformations is characteristically acute and maximal at onset. Symptoms from the initial episode tend to resolve completely as the hemorrhage is organized and absorbed. Recurrent episodes of hemorrhage are associated with progressively more severe deficits and an increased risk of permanent neurological impairment (Figs. 135–5 and 135–6). Occasionally, large brainstem lesions develop associated with only minimal deficits, particularly in the pons, where the mass can displace gradually the densely packed ascending and descending fiber tracts (Fig. 135–7). Death is rare without multiple episodes of symptomatic hemorrhage.

NATURAL HISTORY

The management of cavernous malformations had been complicated by a lack of knowledge regarding their natural history. Although almost all cavernous malformations are associated with MRI or histologic evidence of hemorrhage, more recent studies suggest that the risk of clinically significant hemorrhage is low. Del Curling and coworkers[17] retrospectively reviewed the history of 32 patients with cavernous malformations documented by MRI. They estimated that the risk of symptomatic hemorrhage was 0.1% per lesion per year. This type of review, which depends on the patient's recall to define episodes of hemorrhage and assumes that all lesions are present from birth, is likely to underestimate the actual risk of significant bleeding. Growing evidence supports the idea that cavernous malformations are not necessarily congenital, but also may be acquired lesions. De novo lesions of familial and sporadic forms have been reported with increasing frequency in the literature.[5, 20, 21, 29–37] In prospective studies, the risk of symptomatic hemorrhage appears higher.

Robinson and colleagues[16] prospectively followed 57 patients for an average of 26 months and found a risk of symptomatic hemorrhage of 0.7% per lesion per year. This rate compares favorably with the risk of symptomatic hemorrhage reported by Zabramski and associates[20] in a group of patients with familial cavernous malformations: 21 patients with 128 MRI-documented cavernous malformations were followed for an average of 2.2 years (256 lesion-years of follow-up). Serial MRI studies and follow-up examinations at 6- to 12-month intervals documented hemorrhage in six lesions, for an overall rate of hemorrhage of 2.1% per lesion per year. Three of the six hemorrhages were clinically symptomatic, for a symptomatic hemorrhage rate of 1.2% per lesion per year.

Kondziolka and colleagues[38] reported a slightly higher hemorrhage rate of 2.6% per year but noted that the risk of hemorrhage was related strongly to clinical presentation. They followed 122 patients with cavernous malformations (mean, 34 months) and found that the hemorrhage rate was significantly lower in patients who presented with incidental lesions: 0.6% per year (n = 61) compared with 4.5% per year in patients with a history of previous symptomatic hemorrhage (n = 61). Aiba and associates[39] followed 110 patients with cavernous malformations for a mean of 4.5 years and reported a 0% hemorrhage rate for patients with incidental lesions versus 0.4% per year in patients who presented with seizures.

Porter and colleagues[28] reported an overall annual event rate of 4.2%. An *event* referred to neurological deterioration with or without radiologically proven hemorrhage. Location was the most important factor

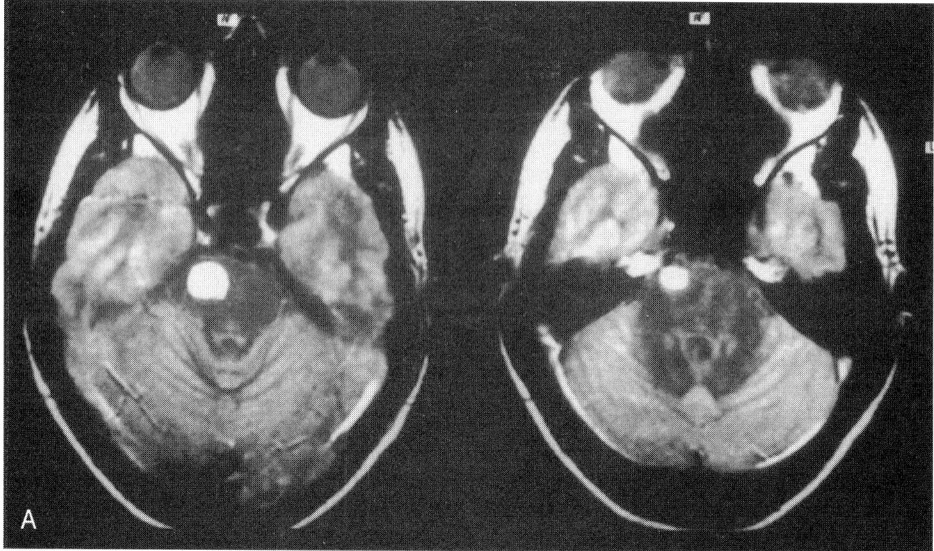

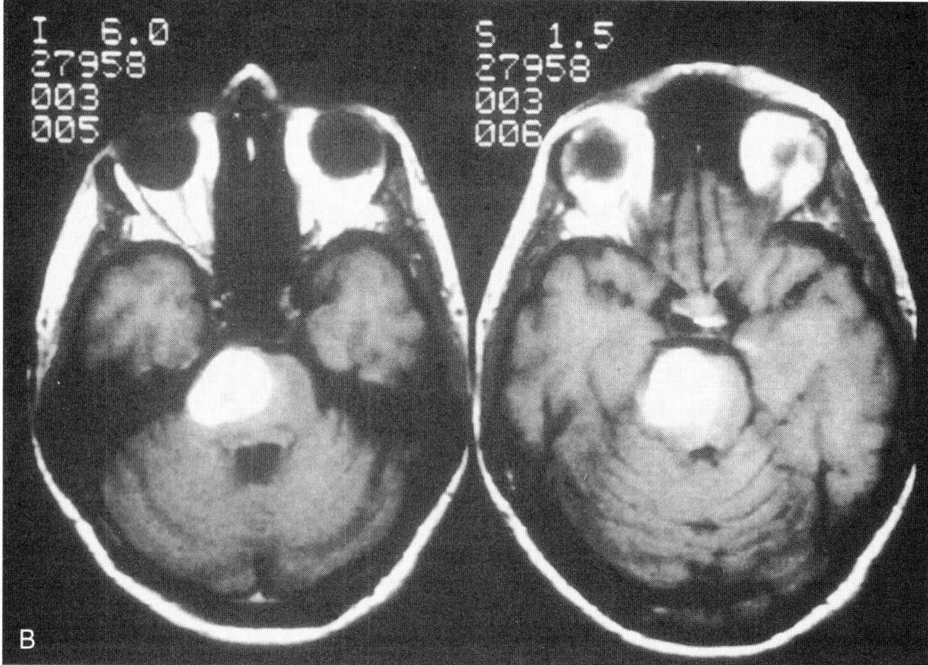

FIGURE 135–6. A 38-year-old woman was evaluated at an outside emergency department for complaints of severe headache and nausea. Basic head computed tomography revealed a questionable area of decreased density in the right pons. *A*, Follow-up axial T1-weighted magnetic resonance images revealed a 1.5-cm area of subacute blood consistent with recent hemorrhage from a cavernous malformation. The patient was seen for neurosurgical consultation about 1 month after this episode, when all symptoms had resolved. Conservative, nonoperative management was recommended. Two months after consultation, the patient presented with moderate left-sided weakness and hemisensory deficits. *B*, Repeat axial T1-weighted magnetic resonance images revealed a significant increase in the size of the lesion, which is composed almost entirely of acute and subacute blood. Surgical pathology confirmed the diagnosis of cavernous malformation.

for predicting future events, with significantly higher rates for deeply located lesions (10.6% per year) compared with superficially located lesions (0% per year).

Hemorrhage rates appear to be particularly high in patients who present after bleeding episodes that violate the lesion capsule, producing a gross extralesional hemorrhage into the surrounding brain (see Figs. 135–3 and 135–6). In this select group of patients, Aiba and associates[39] found a 22.3% per year rate of recurrent symptomatic hemorrhage. Similar rebleeding rates have been reported after incomplete resection of cavernous malformations.[26, 40, 41]

The risk of permanent neurological deficits caused by hemorrhage is related directly to the location of the lesion. Focal neurological deficits and death are associated almost exclusively with hemorrhage into lesions located in the brainstem or basal ganglia. Subcortical lesions rarely reach sufficient size to produce neurological deficits secondary to mass effect. Seizures are a significant cause of morbidity in patients with subcortical lesions, however.

CONCLUSIONS

Cavernous malformations of the central nervous system are relatively common lesions affecting 0.4% to 0.5% of the general population, or roughly 20 million people worldwide. They occur in two distinct forms: a sporadic form characterized by a single lesion and a familial form characterized by multiple lesions and an autosomal dominant mode of inheritance.

Symptoms result when a lesion grows from repeated episodes of hemorrhage and thrombosis. Seizures are

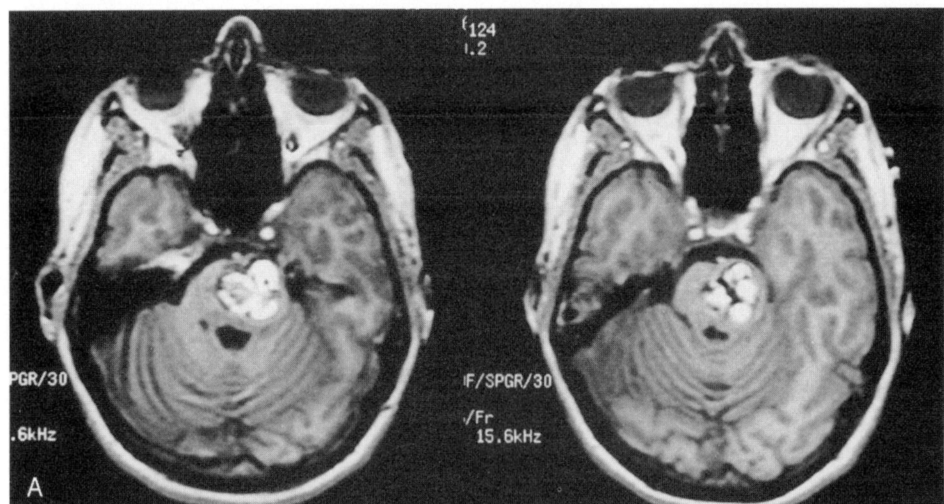

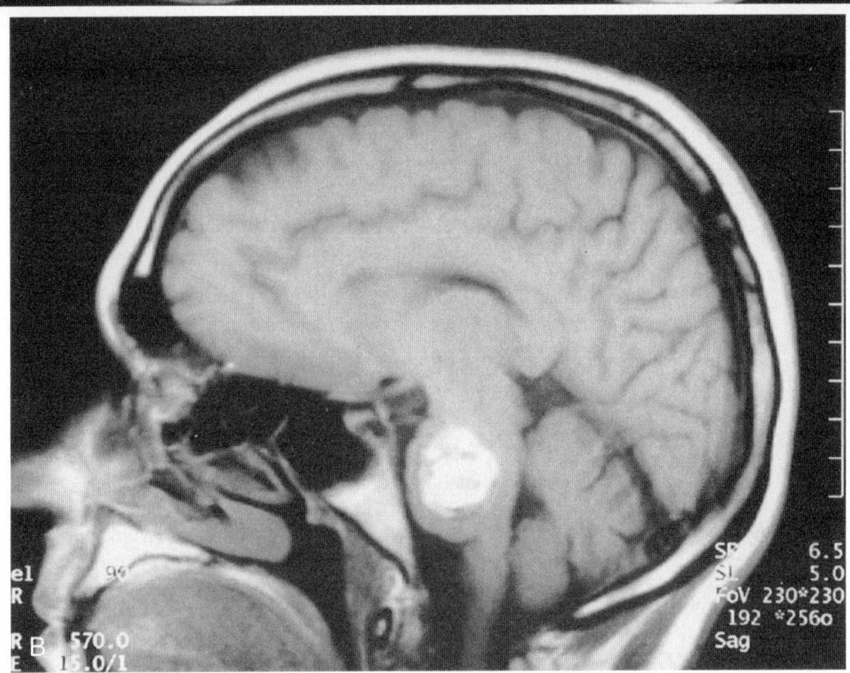

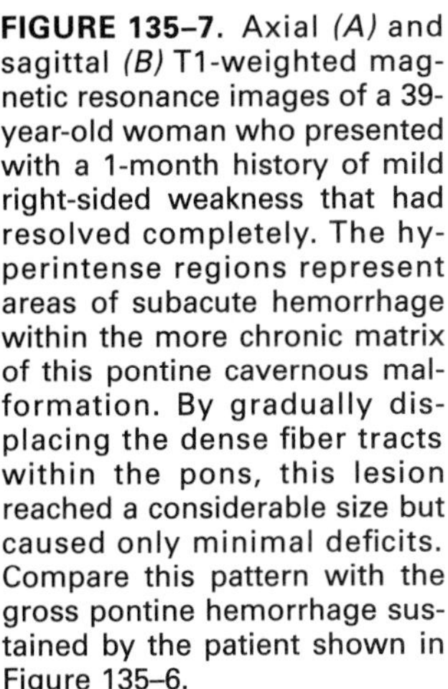

FIGURE 135–7. Axial *(A)* and sagittal *(B)* T1-weighted magnetic resonance images of a 39-year-old woman who presented with a 1-month history of mild right-sided weakness that had resolved completely. The hyperintense regions represent areas of subacute hemorrhage within the more chronic matrix of this pontine cavernous malformation. By gradually displacing the dense fiber tracts within the pons, this lesion reached a considerable size but caused only minimal deficits. Compare this pattern with the gross pontine hemorrhage sustained by the patient shown in Figure 135–6.

TABLE 135–2 ■ **Natural History of Cavernous Malformations**

AUTHOR, YEAR	RATE OF SYMPTOMATIC HEMORRHAGE	COMMENTS
Del Curling et al,[17] 1991	0.1% per lesion/year	Retrospective study based on patients' historical recall of hemorrhagic events. Assumed all lesions were present from birth
Robinson et al,[16] 1991	0.7% per lesion/year	Prospective study
Zabramski et al,[20] 1994	1.2% per lesion/year	Prospective magnetic resonance imaging study of patients with familial form of this disease. Overall rate of hemorrhage was 2.1% per lesion/year, but only 60% of episodes were symptomatic
Kondziolka et al,[38] 1995	1.3%/year (retrospective) 2.6%/year (prospective) 0.6%/year (incidental) 4.5%/year (symptomatic)	Found that rate of hemorrhage was significantly lower in patients presenting with incidental lesions compared with those with a previous history of symptomatic hemorrhage
Aiba et al,[39] 1995	0%/year (incidental) 0.4%/year (seizures) 22.3%/year (gross hemorrhage)	Prospective study. Found rate of hemorrhage was related to presentation: low in those presenting with seizures or incidental lesions; high after gross hemorrhage into the surrounding brain
Porter et al,[28] 1997	4.2%/year	Based on retrospective review from time of first symptomatic hemorrhage. Rate is remarkably similar to that reported for symptomatic lesions by Kondziolka et al[38]

the most common presentation for hemorrhage into supratentorial lesions; hemorrhage into brainstem and spinal cord cavernous malformations produces the sudden onset of focal deficits. Spontaneous improvement is common in this latter group and can result in a confusing clinical picture (e.g., diagnosis of multiple sclerosis) unless patients are evaluated with MRI.

The natural history of cavernous malformations is related to their presentation (Table 135–2). Incidental lesions and lesions discovered during the evaluation of nonspecific symptoms, such as headache, have a low risk of symptomatic hemorrhage—in the range of 0.1% to 0.6% per year. The risk of rebleeding is higher in patients with a history of previously symptomatic hemorrhage and varies with location and type of hemorrhage. The recurrent hemorrhage rate approaches 25% per year in patients with gross extralesional hemorrhage. Patients with gross hemorrhage into brainstem lesions are at the greatest risk of disability and death secondary to recurrent hemorrhage.

REFERENCES

1. Otten P, Pizzolato GP, Rilliet B, et al: A propos de 131 cas d'angiomes caverneux (cavernomes) du S.N.C. reperes par l'analyse retrospective de 24,535 autopsies [131 cases of cavernous angioma (cavernomas) of the CNS discovered by retrospective analysis of 24,535 autopsies]. Neurochirurgie 35:82–131, 1989.
2. McCormick WF: Pathology of vascular malformations of the brain. In Wilson CB, Stein BM (eds): Intracranial Arteriovenous Malformations. Baltimore, Williams & Wilkins, 1984, pp 44–63.
3. Sarwar M, McCormick WF: Intracerebral venous angioma: Case report and review. Arch Neurol 35:323–325, 1978.
4. Russell DS, Rubenstein LJ: Pathology of Tumors of the Nervous System, 5th ed. Baltimore, Williams & Wilkins, 1989.
5. Zabramski JM, Henn JS, Coons S: Pathology of cerebral vascular malformations. Neurosurg Clin N Am 10:395–410, 1999.
6. McCormick WF: The pathology of vascular ("arteriovenous") malformations. J Neurosurg 24:807–816, 1966.
7. Giombini S, Morello G: Cavernous angiomas of the brain: Account of fourteen personal cases and review of the literature. Acta Neurochir (Wien) 40:61–82, 1978.
8. Laberge-Le Couteulx S, Jung HH, Labauge P, et al: Truncating mutations in CCM1, encoding KRIT1, cause hereditary cavernous angiomas. Nat Genet 23:189–193, 1999.
9. Sahoo T, Johnson EW, Thomas JW, et al: Mutations in the gene encoding KRIT1, a Krev-1/rap1a binding protein, cause cerebral cavernous malformations (CCM1). Hum Mol Genet 8:2325–2333, 1999.
10. Voigt K, Yasargil MG: Cerebral cavernous haemangiomas or cavernomas: Incidence, pathology, localization, diagnosis, clinical features and treatment: Review of the literature and report of an unusual case. Neurochirurgia (Stuttg) 19:59–68, 1976.
11. Rigamonti D, Drayer BP, Johnson PC, et al: The MRI appearance of cavernous malformations (angiomas). J Neurosurg 67:518–524, 1987.
12. Gomori JM, Grossman RI, Goldberg HI, et al: Occult cerebral vascular malformations: High-field MR imaging. Radiology 158: 707–713, 1986.
13. Lemme-Plaghos L, Kucharczyk W, Brant-Zawadzki M, et al: MRI of angiographically occult vascular malformations. AJR Am J Roentgenol 146:1223–1228, 1986.
14. New PF, Ojemann RG, Davis KR, et al: MR and CT of occult vascular malformations of the brain. AJR Am J Roentgenol 147: 985–993, 1986.
15. Schorner W, Bradac GB, Treisch J, et al: Magnetic resonance imaging (MRI) in the diagnosis of cerebral arteriovenous angiomas. Neuroradiology 28:313–318, 1986.
16. Robinson JR, Awad IA, Little JR: Natural history of the cavernous angioma. J Neurosurg 75:709–714, 1991.
17. Del Curling O Jr, Kelly DL Jr, Elster AD, et al: An analysis of the natural history of cavernous angiomas. J Neurosurg 75:702–708, 1991.
18. Hayman LA, Evans RA, Ferrell RE, et al: Familial cavernous angiomas: Natural history and genetic study over a 5-year period. Am J Med Genet 11:147–160, 1982.
19. Rigamonti D, Hadley, MN, Drayer BP, et al: Cerebral cavernous malformations: Incidence and familial occurrence. N Engl J Med 319:343–347, 1988.
20. Zabramski JM, Wascher TM, Spetzler RF, et al: The natural history of familial cavernous malformations: Results of an ongoing study. J Neurosurg 80:422–432, 1994.
21. Labauge P, Laberge S, Brunereau L, et al: Hereditary cerebral cavernous angiomas: Clinical and genetic features in 57 French families. Societe Francaise de Neurochirurgie. Lancet 352:1892–1897, 1998.
22. Alvarez-Sabin J, Montalban J, Tintore M, et al: Pure sensory stroke due to midbrain haemorrhage [letter]. J Neurol Neurosurg Psychiatry 54:843, 1991.
23. Willmore LJ, Sypert GW, Munson JB: Recurrent seizures induced by cortical iron injection: A model of posttraumatic epilepsy. Ann Neurol 4:329–336, 1978.
24. Chusid JB, Kopelott LM: Epileptogenic effects of pure metals implanted in motor cortex of monkeys. J Appl Physiol 17:697–700, 1962.
25. Zimmerman RS, Spetzler RF, Lee KS, et al: Cavernous malformations of the brain stem. J Neurosurg 75:32–39, 1991.
26. Fritschi JA, Reulen HJ, Spetzler RF, et al: Cavernous malformations of the brain stem: A review of 139 cases. Acta Neurochir (Wien) 130:35–46, 1994.
27. Weil SM, Tew JM Jr: Surgical management of brain stem vascular malformations. Acta Neurochir (Wien) 105:14–23, 1990.
28. Porter PJ, Willinsky RA, Harper W, et al: Cerebral cavernous malformations: Natural history and prognosis after clinical deterioration with or without hemorrhage. J Neurosurg 87:190–197, 1997.
29. Brunken M, Sagehorn S, Leppien A, et al: De novo formation of a cavernoma in association with a preformed venous malformation during immunosuppressive treatment [German]. Zentralbl Neurochir 60:81–85, 1999.
30. Maraire JN, Abdulrauf SI, Berger S, et al: De novo development of a cavernous malformation of the spinal cord following spinal axis radiation: Case report. J Neurosurg 1999; 90:234-238, 1999.
31. Rosahl SK, Vorkapic P, Eghbal R, et al: Ossified and de novo cavernous malformations in the same patient. Clin Neurol Neurosurg 100:138–143, 1998.
32. Larson JJ, Ball WS, Bove KE, et al: Formation of intracerebral cavernous malformations after radiation treatment for central nervous system neoplasia in children. J Neurosurg 88:51–56, 1998.
33. Houtteville JP: Brain cavernoma: A dynamic lesion. Surg Neurol 48:610–614, 1997.
34. Detwiler PW, Porter RW, Zabramski JM, et al: De novo formation of a central nervous system cavernous malformation: Implications for predicting risk of hemorrhage: Case report and review of the literature. J Neurosurg 87:629–632, 1997.
35. Pozzati E, Giangaspero F, Marliani F, et al: Occult cerebrovascular malformations after irradiation. Neurosurgery 39:677–684, 1996.
36. Tekkok IH, Ventureyra EC: De novo familial cavernous malformation presenting with hemorrhage 12.5 years after the initial hemorrhagic ictus: Natural history of an infantile form. Pediatr Neurosurg 25:151–155, 1996.
37. Pozzati E, Acciarri N, Tognetti F, et al: Growth, subsequent bleeding, and de novo appearance of cerebral cavernous angiomas. Neurosurgery 38:662–670, 1996.
38. Kondziolka D, Lunsford LD, Kestle JR: The natural history of cerebral cavernous malformations. J Neurosurg 83:820–824, 1995.
39. Aiba T, Tanaka R, Koike T, et al: Natural history of intracranial cavernous malformations. J Neurosurg 83:56–59, 1995.
40. Jain KK, Robertson E: Recurrence of an excised cavernous hemangioma in the opposite cerebral hemisphere: Case report. J Neurosurg 33:453–456, 1970.
41. Wakai S, Ueda Y, Inoh S, et al: Angiographically occult angiomas: A report of thirteen cases with analysis of the cases documented in the literature. Neurosurgery 17:549–556, 1985.

CHAPTER **136**

The Genetics of Cerebral Cavernous Malformations

ERIC W. JOHNSON ■ DOUGLAS A. MARCHUK ■ JOSEPH M. ZABRAMSKI

Since first being described in the mid- to late 1800s, cerebral cavernous malformations (CCMs) have been of sporadic interest to the scientific and medical community. CCMs represent 5% to 15% of all cerebral vascular malformations. Two large retrospective reviews of more than 22,000 magnetic resonance imaging (MRI) studies yielded an incidence rate of 0.4% to 0.5% for cavernous malformations in the general population.[1, 2] This finding is almost identical to the incidence rates reported by McCormick[3] and Otten and colleagues[4] in postmortem studies of more than 30,000 cases.

CCMs occur in two forms. In the *sporadic* form, patients usually have one or two lesions and no family history of neurological disease. The *familial* form is characterized by multiple lesions and a strong family history of seizures. The presence of three or more lesions is almost pathognomonic for the familial form of the disease. Given that more than 40% of patients with the familial form of CCMs are asymptomatic, the autosomal dominant segregation pattern can be masked, particularly in smaller families.[5, 6] With careful history and MRI screening, 50% of sporadic cases at the authors' institution are found to be familial.

With the advent of MRI and recognition that many cases of CCMs have a familial component, the genetic basis of this disease became a subject of increasing research interest. This chapter examines the genetic details of the familial form of CCMs and the implications of these findings for the pathogenesis of this disease.

HISTORICAL BACKGROUND

Although the familial form of CCMs has the highest incidence among Hispanics, it has been described in almost every ethnic group that has been studied. The first suggestion that CCMs might be a hereditary disorder appeared in the German medical literature in 1928.[7] Sporadic reports of the familial occurrence of CCMs followed in the literature, but studies were hampered by the lack of a reliable diagnostic tool for identifying affected individuals.[8–10]

In 1982, Hayman and coworkers[11] published convincing evidence that the familial form of CCMs was inherited as an autosomal dominant disorder. The authors prospectively screened 43 members of a single large family with computed tomography (CT) and found lesions consistent with CCMs in 15. The results of the Hayman study emphasized the variable clinical penetrance of this disorder as well as the limitations of CT for detecting affected individuals.[11] Biochemical and red blood cell immunologic genetic linkage studies of 36 members of the family were performed, but no linkage could be established.

By the mid-1980s, the MRI characteristics of CCMs were well established, making it possible to diagnose accurately and screen patients for the familial form of this disease.[12–15] In February 1988, Mason and coworkers[16] presented a Hispanic family in whom 10 of 22 family members exhibited clinical signs and symptoms of CCMs. Five additional family members were found to have asymptomatic lesions, accentuating the need to screen all members of a CCM family, not just those with symptoms. This study was the first to present evidence that Hispanic families have a predisposition for the familial form of CCMs. In August 1988, Rigamonti and coworkers[6] showed the prevalence of CCMs in an additional five Hispanic families, confirming the presence of a connection between CCMs and Hispanics. With MRI, this group showed the fairly high prevalence of asymptomatic CCMs in the Hispanic population and subsequently in the general population. Many groups since have confirmed this observation.[2, 5, 17–19]

In 1994, collaborators at the Center for Medical Genetics in Marshfield, Wisconsin, and at the Barrow Neurological Institute in Phoenix, Arizona, linked the gene for familial CCMs, designated *CCM1*, to chromosome 7q (7q11-q22) in a large Hispanic family.[20, 21] Subsequent work by these investigators and others led to the identification of the mutated gene responsible for *CCM1*.[22, 23] Before this discussion is pursued further, key concepts involved in the genetic analysis of a disease are introduced.

LINKAGE ANALYSIS

In genetic studies, linkage analysis often is the first step in identifying the location of a genetic mutation responsible for a disease. This process of localization depends on three factors, as follows:

1. Multiple, short, repeated sequences along the genome can be used as *genetic markers* to identify particular segments of each chromosome, the so-called short tandem repeat polymorphic (STRP) markers.
2. Crossovers occur during gametogenesis: Genetic material is exchanged between two strands of complementary DNA (recombination) during the duplication and segregation of alleles for sexual reproduction.
3. The rate of crossover, or genetic recombination, is related directly to the distance between the marker and disease gene.

In linkage analysis, the investigator measures the frequency with which the disease gene and markers are inherited together, that is, how tightly they are linked. When the marker and disease gene are located immediately adjacent to each other, the frequency of recombination approaches 0. As the genetic distance increases, the frequency of recombination increases, approaching 0.5 when the marker and disease gene are on separate chromosomes. With sophisticated software, it is possible to calculate an odds ratio for linkage to a particular marker. In the genetic literature, the results of linkage analysis studies are reported as $\log_{10}$ of the odds (LOD score) for and against linkage to a particular marker. An LOD score of 3, odds of 1000 to 1, is considered positive evidence of linkage and is equivalent to a significance level of 0.05; an LOD score of 4, or 10,000 to 1, is equivalent to a significance level of 0.01.

CEREBRAL CAVERNOUS MALFORMATION GENETICS

Linkage analysis studies measure the linkage between phenotype (evidence of disease) and genetic markers. In many disease processes, the identification of affected individuals can be difficult because of variable penetrance. In patients with familial CCMs, only about 60% of affected individuals have symptoms.[5] If 40% of affected individuals are misclassified, linkage analysis never successfully localizes the gene responsible for the disease. Such was the case in 1982, when Hayman and colleagues[11] attempted linkage analysis using CT as the screening tool. The introduction of MRI made it possible to identify affected and unaffected individuals accurately.

Combining linkage analysis with MRI screening in several large Hispanic families with CCMs allowed accurate localization of the *CCM1* gene.[20, 21] In 1995, Dubovsky and associates[21] published findings linking the *CCM1* gene to a 33 million base-pair interval (33 cM) on the long arm of chromosome 7 (7q). Later that same year, Johnson and coworkers[24] significantly narrowed the area of interest for the *CCM1* gene. Their report first suggested that Hispanic families with *CCM1* shared a common ancestor in the not too distant past. The authors found that the affected members of these families had a common haplotype. This finding suggested that most of the affected individuals were descendants of one individual (the founder). This founding haplotype was present in most Hispanic families with *CCM1* but was absent in sporadic Hispanic cases. Variations in this familial Hispanic haplotype were considered evidence of ancestral crossover events and were used to help refine the *CCM1* interval. Using the shared haplotype information along with analysis of crossovers in affected individuals from the Hispanic and the white families, the region likely to contain the *CCM1* gene was reduced to a 2- to 4-cM segment of 7q between markers D7S2410 and D7S689.[24]

In an effort to facilitate the search for the *CCM1* gene, the CCM Consortium was established in early 1995 to coordinate the efforts of the numerous laboratories working to map and clone the *CCM1* gene. The Consortium included the genetics laboratories at Barrow Neurological Institute, the Marshfield Center for Medical Genetics, the University of Minnesota, Duke University, and the Green and Bogowski laboratories at the National Institutes of Health. The individual laboratories represented strengths in family collection and clinical assessment, genotyping, vascular genetics, mutation analysis, chromosome 7 physical mapping, and informatics. This type of approach should be a model for future gene-mapping efforts. This approach ensures maximum collaboration, reduces the demands on patients by eliminating *competition* for affected families, and helps to expedite the often tedious effort needed to find mutations.

After Dubovsky and coworkers[21] published the initial linkage data, other groups rapidly confirmed linkage of *CCM1* to the same region of 7q. Gunel and colleagues[25] found linkage in two CCM families. Analysis localized the gene to a 7-cM region of chromosome 7q, confirming the validity of the previously published *CCM1* critical interval. Marchuk and associates[26] showed linkage for *CCM1* in two additional families—one of Italian-American origin and one of Hispanic and Mexican-American origin. The linkage was to a slightly broader, overlapping 41-cM segment of 7q. Gil-Nagel and colleagues[27] showed linkage to a 15-cM segment in this same region in a large white kindred.

In 1996, Gunel and associates[28] used linkage dysequilibrium analysis in 14 Hispanic kindreds to narrow the area of interest on the *CCM1* gene to a 2- to 3-cM region on either side of the STRP marker D7S558. Results from these 14 apparently unrelated families indicated a high probability (better than 10,000 to 1) that the affected members were all descendants of one individual.

Within these initial studies were reports of many families, specifically non-Hispanic families, with either weak or no clear linkage to the *CCM1* locus on chromosome 7p. In 1998, Craig and coworkers[29] reported linkage analyses in 20 white families that showed evidence for two new loci. *CCM2* was also on chromosome 7 but on its short arm (7p15-p13), and *CCM3* was on the long arm of chromosome 3 at q25.2-q27. Analysis indicated that in the CCM population, 40% of families linked to *CCM1*, 20% linked to *CCM2*, and 40% linked

TABLE 136–1 ■ **Primers for Polymerase Chain Reaction Amplification and Sequencing of *KRIT1* Exons**

EXON SIZE	FORWARD PRIMER (SENSE)*	REVERSE PRIMER (ANTISENSE)*	PRODUCT SIZE
1	TCACTTTATTCCAGCTTTATTCC	AAAACGTCTTTTAAATCAGAGC	260
2	TGACAAAGCTCTTAATGGGT	GACTACAATGCATACAAATTGC	261
3	AAACAATTTTTACAGTCCTGTTG	AGAACAGTCTTGAAAAGAAGGA	280
4	CATTTCAGATGATCTTTTTAGG	TGTCATTACTTGTTATTCACTGCT	286
5	ATTGGATGACATTTTCCCTT	AGCCATCTAATCGTCTTTCC	281
6	AGCACATGAAGTTGAAGGAA	CCCAAAAAGGAATAATGAGG	292
7	GAAGTGCAGACAGTTTAATACAAA	CTCAACAGATTTTGTGCATTT	293
8	GCTTTTTCTTTTCCCATATT	TAGCACAAGACCATGCATAA	283
9	CGTTACTGAAAGCCATTTGT	CAGGACTATAAATTTAATCTACCTCTG	281
10	CAATGGTACATTTTCCTTTCA	AGGTTGGTACTGTTGTTTTAACT	329
11	CTGAACTATTATATTTAGAGCAGACA	CACAATAGTTTATGAAGTCCAAA	261
12	CCCAATGTCATGAATTTCC	GCTCGGCCAAAAGTAATA	233

*All primers read 5′ to 3′. Only forward primers were used for direct sequencing of the exons.
Adapted from Sahoo T, Johnson EW, Thomas JW, et al: Mutations in the gene encoding *KRIT1,* a Krev-1/rap1a binding protein, cause cerebral cavernous malformations *(CCM1).* Hum Mol Genet 8:2325–2333, 1999.

to *CCM3.* Initial evidence indicated variable penetrance of symptomatic disease for the three loci—about 88% for *CCM1,* 100% for *CCM2,* and 63% for *CCM3.* These differences could not be explained by differences in gender or age.

Laberge and coworkers[30] in France analyzed 36 non-Hispanic European CCM families using STRP markers from the *CCM1, CCM2,* and *CCM3* loci. An initial analysis of these non-Hispanic families showed that 65% linked to *CCM1.* In contrast to the Hispanic families with *CCM1,* there was no evidence of a shared haplotype to suggest a common ancestor for this population.

CCM1 GENE

The most exciting development in the genetics of CCMs has been the discovery by two independent groups of investigators that mutations in the *KRIT1* gene are responsible for *CCM1.*[22, 23] *KRIT1* encodes a novel Krev-1/rap1a binding protein[31] and is divided into 10 exons extending more than 37.7 kb of chromosome 7 genomic DNA (Table 136–1).[23, 31]

Few known genes fall within the *CCM1* critical interval. By virtue of its location, the *KRIT1* gene was a priority candidate for study after it was mapped to the *CCM1* interval.[31] The positional cloning-based search for the *CCM1* gene was facilitated by the availability of the complete genomic sequence for this region. The sequence provided access to novel STRP markers for refined haplotype construction and detailed information about known genes in the interval. It also allowed the use of gene-prediction programs to identify putative exons for mutation screening.

In total, 19 distinct *KRIT1* mutations were found among the 35 *CCM1* kindreds reported to date (Tables 136–2 and 136–3). In the Hispanic (Mexican-American) families (Table 136–2), most *CCM1* alleles consisted of the identical 742C>T (Q248X) *KRIT1* mutation. This mutation was present in 16 of the 19 Hispanic families of Mexican-American descent.[23] Other Mexican-American and non-Hispanic white *CCM1* kindreds harbor other *KRIT1* mutations.[22, 23]

TABLE 136–2 ■ ***KRIT1* Mutations in *CCM1* Families**

FAMILY NO.	MUTATION	PREDICTED EFFECT
Hispanic		
10, 11, 13, 14, 15, 16, 123, 128, 152, 200, 300, 500, 600, 800, 900, 1100	742C>T	Premature termination
12	1314delT	Frameshift in codon 438
400	1089delA	Frameshift in codon 363
1200	990T>A	Premature termination
White		
1	IVS4+1G>A	Splice site alteration
2	IVS8-2A>G	Splice site alteration
20	1089delA	Frameshift in codon 363
55	281C>G	Premature termination

Adapted from Sahoo T, Johnson EW, Thomas JW, et al: Mutations in the gene encoding *KRIT1,* a Krev-1/rap1a binding protein, cause cerebral cavernous malformations *(CCM1).* Hum Mol Genet 8:2325–2333, 1999.

TABLE 136–3 ■ ***KRIT1* Mutations in White *CCM1* Families**

FAMILY NO.	MUTATION	PREDICTED EFFECT
5	1348del(84bp)	Splice site alteration
6	1342delA	Premature termination
10	1283C>T	Premature termination
11	1430A>G	Splice site alteration
18	247insC	Frameshift/premature termination
19	261G>A	Premature termination
25	436delA	Premature termination
27	633delT	Premature termination
35	1012del(26bp)	Premature termination
41	615G>A	Premature termination
42	681delGAAT	Premature termination
58	1271insC	Frameshift/premature termination

Adapted from Laberge-le Couteulx S, Jung HH, Labauge P, et al: Truncating mutations in *CCM1,* encoding *KRIT1,* cause hereditary cavernous angiomas. Nat Genet 23:189–193, 1999.

Analysis of the genetic haplotype data for the Mexican-American families reveals a correlation between the *KRIT1* mutations and the common disease haplotype.[23] All 16 families with the 742C>T mutation share the common disease haplotype over the interval that includes *KRIT1* and extends to involve additional markers for variable distances in both directions. These data confirm that the families with the *CCM1* chromosome descended from a single common ancestor.

Further analysis of the haplotype data for the Hispanic families with unique *KRIT1* mutations reveals that they share a much smaller portion of the disease haplotype that does not extend beyond the region immediately surrounding *KRIT1*. Families 12, 400, and 1200 harbor unique *KRIT1* mutations and are not related to one another or the other 16 Hispanic families in Table 136–2. Failure to recognize that some of the markers used for determining whether families shared the common disease haplotype were relatively frequent in the Mexican-American population and had important implications.

The initial screening strategy for finding the *CCM1* gene was to concentrate efforts on families of Mexican-American descent with the purpose of mapping ancestral crossover events as a means of narrowing the region of interest. Although this approach was sound, the assumption that all Hispanic families were related to a common ancestor ultimately proved to be incorrect. The inappropriate inclusion of putative recombination events in families 12 and 1200 to define the region of interest erroneously diverted the initial candidate gene search approximately 0.5 cM telomeric of *KRIT1*.

There is no evidence for a common disease haplotype in non-Hispanic white families.[24, 30] Distinct *KRIT1* mutations were found in each of the 16 white *CCM1* families (see Tables 136–2 and 136–3). Sahoo and colleagues[23] noted the same mutation in two apparently unrelated families (see Table 136–2): family 20, a white kindred, and family 400, a Mexican-American kindred. The mutation consists of the loss of a single A in a run of six As, which may explain its independent origin.

The *CCM1* mutations identified to date fall into one of three classes: frameshift, premature chain termination, and splice site mutations. They all predict truncated CCM1 proteins that likely severely disrupt the normal assembly or function of *KRIT1*. No missense mutations have been identified.

KRIT1 FUNCTION

The function of the KRIT1-encoded protein and its role in angiogenesis are areas of ongoing research. Initially, KRIT1 was isolated as a binding protein associated with Krev-1/rap1a.[31] Krev-1/rap1a has the ability to revert partially the transformed phenotype of Kirsten sarcoma virus–transformed cells. It is also a member of the Ras family of guanosine triphosphatases (GTPases) with tumor-suppressing activity for the Ras oncogenes.[32–35] Identical protein residues in Krev-1/rap1a and Ras are responsible for interaction with effectors, indicating that these two proteins mediate opposing effects through common downstream messengers such as Raf-1, B-Raf, and Ral-GDS.[35–41] The homology between the Krev-1/rap1a protein and Ras, its ability to interact with most of the cellular effectors of Ras, and its ability to revert the oncogenic effect of Ras in vivo suggest that Krev-1/rap1a behaves as a tumor suppressor in the cell. The finding that Krev-1/rap1a can bind tightly a number of Ras effectors, including the Ras GTPase-activating protein (Ras-GAP), and act as a competitive inhibitor of Ras-GAP interaction supports this hypothesis.

The predicted protein sequence of *KRIT1* provides some insight into its role. The 529–amino acid sequence has a predicted molecular weight of 60.8 kd, reflecting the presence of a large number of aromatic residues, particularly tyrosines.[31] The KRIT1 protein sequence has many regions that are predicted to be hydrophobic, including a single transmembrane domain at amino acids 339 through 359. Interaction with Krev1/rap1a is specific to the carboxy-terminal end of the KRIT1 protein; a short deletion (amino acids 483 through 529) results in an almost total loss of interaction.[31]

The amino-terminal end of *KRIT1* (amino acids 83 through 215) contains three ankyrin repeats.[23] Ankyrin repeats are interactive domains that mediate association with other cellular partners. Multiple classes of proteins possess ankyrin repeats, but they are extremely abundant in cytoskeletal and membrane-attached proteins. In conjunction with the hydrophobic character and predicted transmembrane domain for *KRIT1* and the known localization of Krev-1/rap1a to endosomal compartments,[42, 43] the presence of multiple ankyrin repeats suggests that *KRIT1* is associated with intracellular membranes.

The expression profiles of *KRIT1* and Krev-1/rap1a provide few hints about its role in vascular development. Krev-1/rap1a is expressed in a variety of tissues, including the small blood vessels of many organs.[44] Northern blot analysis of *KRIT1* showed weak expression in the blood vessels of heart, muscle, and brain but not in other tissues.[31]

The localization of *KRIT1* to 7q21-22 is particularly interesting because chromosomal alterations in 7q22 have been implicated in a variety of cancers, including myeloid disorders and uterine leiomyomata.[45–53] Although the role of Krev-1/rap1a has not been investigated in these classes of malignancies, a characteristic feature of chromosome 7 monosomy and 7q22 deletions is their occurrence as secondary events after hyperactivation of Ras or mutation of the Ras-GAP protein neurofibromatosis 1 (*NF-1*) gene.[48, 54–56] Insofar as Krev-1/rap1a appears to function as a regulator of Ras activity, deletion of *KRIT1*, a potential positive regulator of Krev-1/rap1a activity, may provide an indirect mechanism to enhance Ras-dependent tumor growth.

CONCLUSION

A working model for the *CCM1* mutations would be that CCMs are benign vascular tumors that develop as a result of an alteration in important growth control pathways involving the regulation of Krev-1/rap1a by the *KRIT1* protein. In support of this hypothesis, the Krev-1/rap1a pathway is known to be altered in tuberous sclerosis type 2 (TSC2), an autosomal dominant condition characterized by benign neurocutaneous tumors. TSC2, similar to CCM, often is associated with seizure activity. The TSC2 gene product, tuberin, functions as a tumor-suppressor protein by acting as a GTPase-activating protein for Krev-1/rap1a.[57, 58] Somatic inactivation or loss of heterozygosity of the wild-type tuberin allele in TSC2-associated tumors leads to unregulated growth.[58, 59]

The focal nature of CCMs suggests that these vascular tumors may develop secondary to loss of the wild-type *KRIT1* allele in the developing cerebral vasculature. A two-hit model, with a central tumor-suppressor function of *KRIT1*, would be similar to the mechanism of tuberin inactivation in TSC2-associated tumors. Alternatively, the cause of vascular lesions may relate to a mechanical or environmental trigger in the cerebral vasculature, coupled with the underlying genetic defect in *KRIT1*. Whatever the exact mechanism, the data point to a role for the *KRIT1* and Krev-1/rap1a pathway in the pathogenesis of CCMs and potentially in that of other cerebrovascular disorders.

Recent analysis of genomic sequence encompassing the region containing *KRIT1* in both human and mouse using exon/gene prediction programs identified a number of putative exons upstream of the previously described and published "first" exon.[60 61] These potential exons show homology to a series of overlapping ESTs present in the mouse and human EST databases that are contiguous with and extend upstream of the 5′ end of the *KRIT1* cDNA sequence. RT-PCR and 5′ RACE experiments confirm the existence of four additional coding exons, resulting in 207 additional amino acids upstream of the originally described translational start site. We have identified a novel frameshift mutation in one of the newly identified exons of *KRIT1* in a *CCM1* family. These data extend and establish the authentic *KTRI1* amino acid sequence and suggest that the additional *KRIT1* exons may harbor mutations in other *CCM1* families that have yet to show a *KRIT1* mutation.[61]

REFERENCES

1. Del Curling O Jr, Kelly DL Jr, Elster AD, et al: An analysis of the natural history of cavernous angiomas. J Neurosurg 75:702–708, 1991.
2. Robinson JR, Awad IA, Little JR: Natural history of the cavernous angioma. J Neurosurg 75:709–714, 1991.
3. McCormick WF: Pathology of vascular malformations of the brain. In Wilson CB, Stein BM (eds): Intracranial Arteriovenous Malformations. Baltimore, Williams & Wilkins, 1984, pp 44–63.
4. Otten P, Pizzolato GP, Rilliet B, et al: 131 cases of cavernous angioma (cavernomas) of the CNS, discovered by retrospective analysis of 24,535 autopsies [in French]. Neurochirurgie 35:82–83, 128–131, 1989.
5. Zabramski JM, Wascher TM, Spetzler RF, et al: The natural history of familial cavernous malformations: Results of an ongoing study. J Neurosurg 80:422–432, 1994.
6. Rigamonti D, Hadley MN, Drayer BP, et al: Cerebral cavernous malformations: Incidence and familial occurrence. N Engl J Med 319:343–347, 1988.
7. Kufs H: Uber heredofamiliare angiomatose des gehirns und der retina, ihre beziehungen zueinander und zur angiomatose der haut. Zentralbl Neurol Psychiat 113:651–686, 1928.
8. Clark JV: Familial occurrence of cavernous angiomata of the brain. J Neurol Neurosurg Psychiatry 33:871–876, 1970.
9. Michael JC, Levin PM: Multiple telangiectases of the brain: A discussion of hereditary factors in their development. Arch Neurol Psychiatry 36:514–529, 1936.
10. Bicknell JM, Carlow TJ, Kornfeld M, et al: Familial cavernous angiomas. Arch Neurol 35:746–749, 1978.
11. Hayman LA, Evans RA, Ferrell RE, et al: Familial cavernous angiomas: Natural history and genetic study over a 5-year period. Am J Med Genet 11:147–160, 1982.
12. Rigamonti D, Drayer BP, Johnson PC, et al: The MRI appearance of cavernous malformations (angiomas). J Neurosurg 67:518–524, 1987.
13. Gomori JM, Grossman RI, Goldberg HI, et al: Occult cerebral vascular malformations: High-field MR imaging. Radiology 158: 707–713, 1986.
14. Lemme-Plaghos L, Kucharczyk W, Brant-Zawadzki M, et al: MRI of angiographically occult vascular malformations. AJR Am J Roentgenol 146:1223–1228, 1986.
15. Schorner W, Bradac GB, Treisch J, et al: Magnetic resonance imaging (MRI) in the diagnosis of cerebral arteriovenous angiomas. Neuroradiology 28:313–318, 1986.
16. Mason I, Aase JM, Orrison WW, et al: Familial cavernous angiomas of the brain in an Hispanic family. Neurology 38:324–326, 1988.
17. Requena I, Arias M, Lopez-Ibor L, et al: Cavernomas of the central nervous system: Clinical and neuroimaging manifestations in 47 patients. J Neurol Neurosurg Psychiatry 54:590–594, 1991.
18. Dobyns WB, Michels VV, Groover RV, et al: Familial cavernous malformations of the central nervous system and retina. Ann Neurol 21:578–583, 1987.
19. Allard JC, Hochberg FH, Franklin PD, et al: Magnetic resonance imaging in a family with hereditary cerebral arteriovenous malformations. Arch Neurol 46:184–187, 1989.
20. Kurth JH, Dubovsky J, Zabramski JM, et al: Genetic linkage of the familial cavernous malformation (CM) gene to chromosome 7q. Am J Med Genet 55(suppl):A15, 1994.
21. Dubovsky J, Zabramski JM, Kurth J, et al: A gene responsible for cavernous malformations of the brain maps to chromosome 7q. Hum Mol Genet 4:453–458, 1995.
22. Laberge-le Couteulx S, Jung HH, Labauge P, et al: Truncating mutations in CCM1, encoding KRIT1, cause hereditary cavernous angiomas. Nat Genet 23:189–193, 1999.
23. Sahoo T, Johnson EW, Thomas JW, et al: Mutations in the gene encoding KRIT1, a Krev-1/rap1a binding protein, cause cerebral cavernous malformations (CCM1). Hum Mol Genet 8:2325–2333, 1999.
24. Johnson EW, Iyer LM, Rich SS, et al: Refined localization of the cerebral cavernous malformation gene (CCM1) to a 4-cM interval of chromosome 7q contained in a well-defined YAC contig. Genome Res 5:368–380, 1995.
25. Gunel M, Awad IA, Anson J, et al: Mapping a gene causing cerebral cavernous malformation to 7q11.2-q21. Proc Natl Acad Sci U S A 92:6620–6624, 1995.
26. Marchuk DA, Gallione CJ, Morrison LA, et al: A locus for cerebral cavernous malformations maps to chromosome 7q in two families. Genomics 28:311–314, 1995.
27. Gil-Nagel A, Dubovsky J, Wilcox KJ, et al: Familial cerebral cavernous angioma: A gene localized to a 15-cM interval on chromosome 7q [published erratum appears in Ann Neurol 1996 Sep;40(3):480]. Ann Neurol 39:807–810, 1996.
28. Gunel M, Awad IA, Finberg K, et al: A founder mutation as a cause of cerebral cavernous malformation in Hispanic Americans. N Engl J Med 334:946–951, 1996.
29. Craig HD, Gunel M, Cepeda O, et al: Multilocus linkage identifies two new loci for a mendelian form of stroke, cerebral cavernous malformation, at 7p15-13 and 3q25.2-27. Hum Mol Genet 7: 1851–1858, 1998.
30. Laberge S, Labauge P, Marechal E, et al: Genetic heterogeneity

and absence of founder effect in a series of 36 French cerebral cavernous angiomas families. Eur J Hum Genet 7:499–504, 1999.
31. Serebriiskii I, Estojak J, Sonoda G, et al: Association of Krev-1/rap1a with Krit1, a novel ankyrin repeat-containing protein encoded by a gene mapping to 7q21-22. Oncogene 15:1043–1049, 1997.
32. Kitayama H, Sugimoto Y, Matsuzaki T, et al: A ras-related gene with transformation suppressor activity. Cell 56:77–84, 1989.
33. Frech M, John J, Pizon V, et al: Inhibition of GTPase activating protein stimulation of Ras-p21 GTPase by the Krev-1 gene product. Science 249:169–171, 1990.
34. Zhang K, Papageorge AG, Martin P, et al: Heterogeneous amino acids in Ras and Rap1A specifying sensitivity to GAP proteins. Science 254:1630–1634, 1991.
35. Zhang K, Noda M, Vass WC, et al: Identification of small clusters of divergent amino acids that mediate the opposing effects of ras and Krev-1. Science 249:162–165, 1990.
36. Hu CD, Kariya K, Tamada M, et al: Cysteine-rich region of Raf-1 interacts with activator domain of post-translationally modified Ha-Ras. J Biol Chem 270:30274–30277, 1995.
37. Marshall MS, Davis LJ, Keys RD, et al: Identification of amino acid residues required for Ras p21 target activation. Mol Cell Biol 11:3997–4004, 1991.
38. Maruta H, Holden J, Sizeland A, et al: The residues of Ras and Rap proteins that determine their GAP specificities. J Biol Chem 266:11661–11668, 1991.
39. Herrmann C, Horn G, Spaargaren M, et al: Differential interaction of the ras family GTP-binding proteins H-Ras, Rap1A, and R-Ras with the putative effector molecules Raf kinase and Ral-guanine nucleotide exchange factor. J Biol Chem 271:6794–6800, 1996.
40. Urano T, Emkey R, Feig LA: Ral-GTPases mediate a distinct downstream signaling pathway from Ras that facilitates cellular transformation. EMBO J 15:810–816, 1996.
41. Hu CD, Kariya K, Okada T, et al: Effect of phosphorylation on activities of Rap1A to interact with Raf-1 and to suppress Ras-dependent Raf-1 activation. J Biol Chem 274:48–51, 1999.
42. Beranger F, Goud B, Tavitian A, et al: Association of the Ras-antagonistic Rap1/Krev-1 proteins with the Golgi complex. Proc Natl Acad Sci U S A 88:1606–1610, 1991.
43. Pizon V, Desjardins M, Bucci C, et al: Association of Rap1a and Rap1b proteins with late endocytic/phagocytic compartments and Rap2a with the Golgi complex. J Cell Sci 107(pt 6):1661–1670, 1994.
44. Wienecke R, Maize JC Jr, Reed JA, et al: Expression of the TSC2 product tuberin and its target Rap1 in normal human tissues. Am J Pathol 150:43–50, 1997.
45. Pedersen-Bjergaard J, Vindelov L, Philip P, et al: Varying involvement of peripheral granulocytes in the clonal abnormal-7 in bone marrow cells in preleukemia secondary to treatment of other malignant tumors: Cytogenetic results compared with results of flow cytometric DNA analysis and neutrophil chemotaxis. Blood 60:172–179, 1982.
46. Kere J, Ruutu T, Davies KA, et al: Chromosome 7 long arm deletion in myeloid disorders: A narrow breakpoint region in 7q22 defined by molecular mapping. Blood 73:230–234, 1989.
47. Kere J, Ruutu T, Lahtinen R, et al: Molecular characterization of chromosome 7 long arm deletions in myeloid disorders. Blood 70:1349–1353, 1987.
48. Luna-Fineman S, Shannon KM, Lange BJ: Childhood monosomy 7: Epidemiology, biology, and mechanistic implications. Blood 85:1985–1999, 1995.
49. Ogata T, Ayusawa D, Namba M, et al: Chromosome 7 suppresses indefinite division of nontumorigenic immortalized human fibroblast cell lines KMST-6 and SUSM-1. Mol Cell Biol 13:6036–6043, 1993.
50. Pedersen-Bjergaard J, Philip P, Larsen SO, et al: Chromosome aberrations and prognostic factors in therapy-related myelodysplasia and acute nonlymphocytic leukemia. Blood 76:1083–1091, 1990.
51. Sargent MS, Weremowicz S, Rein MS, et al: Translocations in 7q22 define a critical region in uterine leiomyomata. Cancer Genet Cytogenet 77:65–68, 1994.
52. Weiss K, Stass S, Williams D, et al: Childhood monosomy 7 syndrome: Clinical and in vitro studies. Leukemia 1:97–104, 1987.
53. Yamada T, Shippey CA, Martineau M, et al: Demonstration of acquired hemizygosity and clonality in acute lymphoblastic leukemia with chromosome 7 abnormalities using hypervariable DNA probes. Genes Chromosomes Cancer 2:88–93, 1990.
54. Ballester R, Marchuk D, Boguski M, et al: The NF1 locus encodes a protein functionally related to mammalian GAP and yeast IRA proteins. Cell 63:851–859, 1990.
55. Martin GA, Viskochil D, Bollag G, et al: The GAP-related domain of the neurofibromatosis type 1 gene product interacts with ras p21. Cell 63:843–849, 1990.
56. Viskochil D, Buchberg AM, Xu G, et al: Deletions and a translocation interrupt a cloned gene at the neurofibromatosis type 1 locus. Cell 62:187–192, 1990.
57. Wienecke R, Konig A, DeClue JE: Identification of tuberin, the tuberous sclerosis-2 product: Tuberin possesses specific Rap1-GAP activity. J Biol Chem 270:16409–16414, 1995.
58. Soucek T, Pusch O, Wienecke R, et al: Role of the tuberous sclerosis gene-2 product in cell cycle control: Loss of the tuberous sclerosis gene-2 induces quiescent cells to enter S phase. J Biol Chem 272:29301–29308, 1997.
59. Maheshwar MM, Cheadle JP, Jones AC, et al: The GAP-related domain of tuberin, the product of the TSC2 gene, is a target for missense mutations in tuberous sclerosis. Hum Mol Genet 6:1991–1996, 1997.
60. Zhang J, Clatterbuck RE, Rigamonti D, Dietz HC: Cloning of the murine *Krit1* cDNA reveals novel mammalian 5′ coding exons. Genomics 70:392–395, 2000.
61. Sahoo T, Goenaga-Diaz E, Serebriiskii IG, et al: Computational and experimental analyses reveal previously undetected coding exons of the *Krit1* (*CCM1*) gene. Genomics 71:123–126, 2001.

CHAPTER 137

Surgical Management of Supratentorial Cavernous Malformations

Kenneth P. Vives ■ Murat Gunel ■ Issam A. Awad

Therapeutic decisions about supratentorial cavernous malformations (CMs) are dictated by the range of clinical manifestations of these lesions. Patients may suffer from overt hemorrhage, or lesions may expand by microhemorrhage and cavern proliferation, causing symptomatic mass effect. They may also disrupt brain function through seizure activity thought to be mediated by iron deposition and gliosis of surrounding brain parenchyma.[1-3] Thus, the goal of intervention may be to prevent hemorrhage, decrease mass effect, or eliminate or reduce seizure activity.

These potential benefits must be weighed against the risks of treatment in individual patients. Overall, several common clinical scenarios are encountered (Table 137–1). These include asymptomatic or incidentally discovered lesions in association with nonspecific symptoms, those presenting after a first seizure or with well-controlled epilepsy, cases associated with longstanding or intractable epilepsy, and cases in which lesional hemorrhage or expansion causes focal neurological deficits or apoplectic clinical presentation. The indications and objectives of management are different in each of these scenarios and are influenced by other factors such as the patient's age and sex, lesion location, and multiplicity of lesions. Other special considerations may arise with lesions associated with a venous malformation or with dural-based lesions.

The definition of the term *hemorrhage* in association with CMs merits discussion. The inherent pathophysiology of CMs is that of repeated microhemorrhage. On histopathology, lesional hemorrhage is a hallmark sine qua non of every CM. It is reflected by the reticulated signal on magnetic resonance imaging (MRI) and by the typical "ring" of low-intensity signal from hemosiderin deposition in perilesional parenchyma. Lesions may exhibit intracavernous or intercavernous hemorrhagic expansion or repeated microhemorrhages in association with cavern proliferation. Gross hemorrhage beyond the boundaries of the lesion may cause focal mass effect or, less commonly, apoplectic clinical deterioration from large intracerebral hematomas or from subarachnoid or intraventricular extension. The clinical manifestations of hemorrhage are clearly related to its volume and location. The term *symptomatic hemorrhage* therefore includes a spectrum of clinical manifestations. Clinically relevant hemorrhages may represent chronic "ooze" associated with proliferative lesion expansion, acute intralesional bleeding, and more overt or gross hemorrhage beyond lesion boundaries. The latter may be apoplectic.

TABLE 137–1 ■ **Typical Clinical Scenarios Associated with Supratentorial Cavernous Malformations**

Asymptomatic or incidentally discovered solitary lesions
New-onset seizures or well-controlled epilepsy
Intractable epilepsy
Clinically significant hemorrhagic events
Mass effect without evidence of overt hemorrhage
Multiple or familial cavernous malformations

MANAGEMENT OPTIONS AND EXPECTED OUTCOMES

Expectant and Medical Management

Expectant management of CMs consists of MRI follow-up performed at regular intervals, with the aim of detecting lesion expansion or hemorrhage. It is often advised when patients have minimal or no associated symptoms and when the CM is deep or inaccessible. Patients are counseled about the symptoms of hemorrhage and to seek medical attention should they arise. They are cautioned that the use of anticoagulants may predispose to more serious sequelae should bleeding occur. Further, female patients of childbearing age are warned of the possible increased risk of lesion proliferation during pregnancy. Patients with familial CMs are counseled regarding the autosomal dominant inheritance of the disease, including incomplete penetrance and the genesis of de novo lesions. There is no evidence that limitations on exercise alter the clinical behavior of CMs, although intralesional pressures have been shown to increase with Valsalva's maneuvers.[4] Hence, it may be judicious to refrain from intense strenuous activities.

Medical management is essentially limited to treatment of an associated seizure disorder. A supratentorial CM is associated with an estimated 2.4%/year cumulative risk of new seizures.[5] Reports of the outcome of surgical resection of solitary CMs in association with a history of epilepsy reveal that 75% to 88% of patients become seizure free.[6–8] Risk factors for continued seizures include female sex, incomplete resection, greater number of preoperative seizures, and greater severity and duration of preoperative seizures.[6, 8] Lesion location in a particular lobe of the brain is not associated with persistent postoperative seizures.[6] Excision of a solitary supratentorial CM provides the best chance of seizure control and a high likelihood of a seizure-free outcome off anticonvulsant medications. No pharmacotherapy is available to reduce or stabilize lesions.

Radiotherapy and Stereotactic Radiosurgery

There is no evidence that conventional external beam radiotherapy favorably alters the natural history of CMs. In fact, there is concern that radiation may promote the genesis of de novo lesions.[9–14]

Stereotactic radiosurgery has been associated with high rates of focal neurological deficits, and there is no convincing evidence that it substantially reduces the hemorrhage rate.[15–20] Kondziolka and colleagues[21] treated 47 patients with stereotactic radiosurgery and compared pre- and post-treatment hemorrhage rates. Their patients were not typical of most surgical series, as there was a preponderance of brainstem or deep-seated lesions. They demonstrated a significant decrease in the hemorrhage rate to 8.8% in the first 2 years after treatment, and a further decrease to 1.1% in the following 4 years. After the procedure, however, 26% of patients experienced a neurological exacerbation, which correlated with hyperintense change in T2-weighted signals; deficits were permanent in 4%. Another study confirmed these findings,[19] revealing a high complication rate and no significant difference between the post-treatment hemorrhage rate and the reported natural history of hemorrhage from CM. Both series confirmed a decrease in hemorrhage rate over time—from 2 to 4 years after treatment. But this reduced hemorrhage rate is not comparable to the zero rebleed rate after complete lesion excision. These results and the high complication rate make radiosurgical treatment less favorable for patients with surgically accessible lesions. For patients with deep-seated and truly inaccessible lesions, radiosurgery may be considered.[21, 22] Current radiosurgical protocols advocate reduced treatment dosimetry (not exceeding 15 Gy at the lesion border) in an effort to minimize radiation-induced morbidity.[21]

Surgical Resection

Surgical resection of accessible supratentorial lesions is associated with low rates of morbidity and mortality. Repeat hemorrhages in patients with completely resected lesions have not been reported, except in patients with multiple lesions. Surgical resections for deep-seated lesions are associated with higher rates of morbidity.[23–26] As with brainstem lesions, most neurological setbacks resolve several weeks or months after surgery. The management strategy differs slightly, based on the exact location of these lesions. Thalamic or capsular lesions may be managed similarly to brainstem lesions. Surgical intervention may be warranted when the CM presents itself to a pial or ependymal surface, whereas more conservative management is considered for deep lesions that are not approachable through an accessible surgical corridor. Pineal region malformations often present with symptoms of mass effect, necessitating decompression.

MANAGEMENT STRATEGIES

Asymptomatic or Incidentally Discovered Solitary Cavernous Malformations

Lesions may be discovered incidentally in the course of imaging studies for nonspecific or unrelated symptoms (Fig. 137–1). Headaches may reflect occult bleeding or are likely incidental to the lesion. Patients with no history of clinical hemorrhage have an annual bleed rate of 0.39% to 0.6%.[27–31] This rate is lower than that associated with arteriovenous malformations. A first hemorrhage from a CM is rarely life threatening but may result in significant morbidity from which the patient may or may not fully recover. Before intervention is considered solely on the basis of preventing hemorrhage, the host-related factors that may affect hemorrhage risk or its consequences must be examined. One factor is patient age, with a greater actuarial risk for younger patients based on cumulative annualized lifetime risk. Another factor is sex. Several studies have suggested a possible increased risk of hemorrhage in females,[5, 30] especially during pregnancy,[9, 28, 32] but other studies have not substantiated this increased risk.[29, 31]

Lesional location is also a factor that must be considered. Supratentorial lesions constitute approximately 75% to 88% of lesions and have a lower risk of clinically significant hemorrhage compared with infratentorial lesions.[9, 32, 33] A hemorrhage may have worse consequences in some locations than in others. Lesions in or near the rolandic regions, speech areas, calcarine cortex, internal capsule, or thalamus may exhibit overt symptoms after minor bleeding. Other lesions in more polar lobar locations may expand significantly or exhibit extralesional hemorrhage with little or no overt clinical sequelae. More gradual effects on memory or integrative brain function are rarely identified by the patient or clinician.

The risk-benefit considerations of intervention for patients with lesions located in critical areas are also different. Although the consequences of hemorrhage are more serious, the surgical approach is also associated with greater risk. Hence, the threshold for surgical intervention in more eloquent locations is higher, although the potential benefit of lesion excision is also

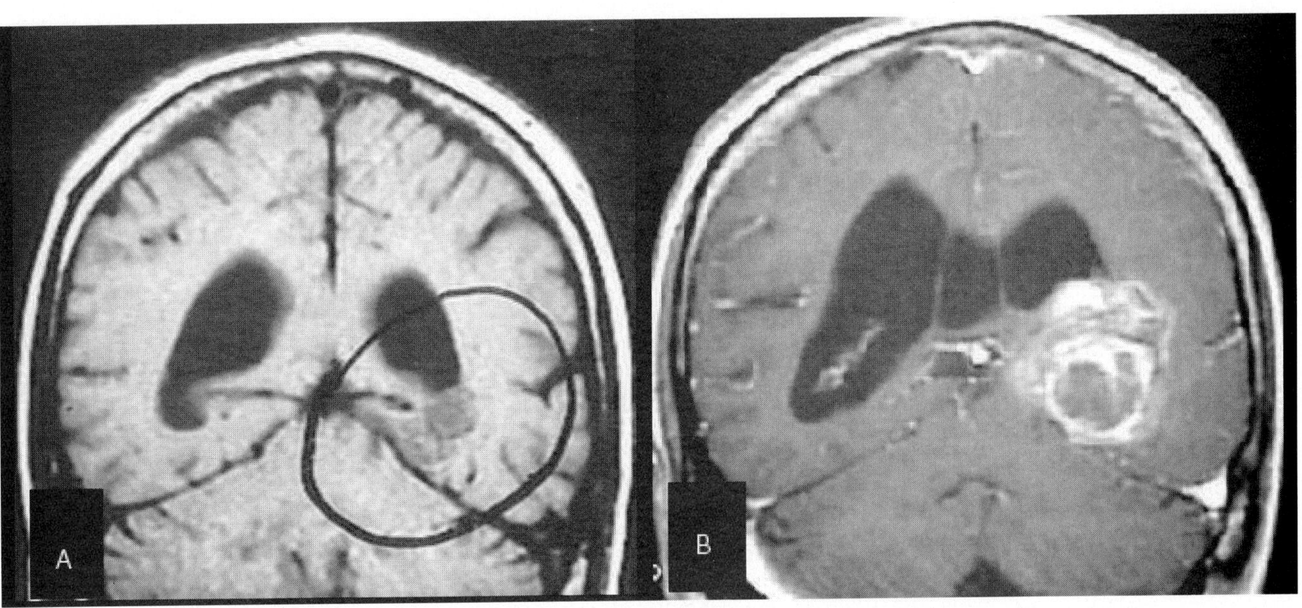

FIGURE 137–1. This elderly patient was originally followed expectantly for a left medial occipitotemporal cavernous malformation associated with headaches and no other specific symptoms. *A*, Original magnetic resonance imaging (MRI) scan reveals a 2-cm lesion without evidence of recent hemorrhage. *B*, At follow-up the lesion had grown through intralesional hemorrhage. Gadolinium-enhanced coronal MRI scan shows a septated heterogeneous lesion in the medial occipitotemporal area, inferior to the atrium of the lateral ventricle, with hydrocephalus. This patient was treated with a ventriculoperitoneal shunt and lesion excision via the inferior temporal sulcus.

greater. The psychological burden of knowing that he or she has a lesion that, without warning, may hemorrhage and substantially affect the patient's neurological status, employment, and family life needs to be considered. Severe headache or a slight physiologic change can frequently cause patients anxiety, necessitating frequent clinical evaluation and imaging studies.

Modern surgical series reveal that a solitary superficial CM can be resected with few complications and no deaths beyond the standard risks of anesthesia. Thus, we offer young, asymptomatic patients the option of resection of solitary accessible lesions, even if they are located in areas of critical cortical function. For asymptomatic lesions that are more difficult to access without substantial risk, the threshold for intervention is higher. Younger patients are presented with the option of accepting a higher surgical risk up front to ensure protection from serious hemorrhage at an unpredictable time in the future, with potentially devastating consequences. Alternatively, patients can be managed expectantly, with follow-up MRI scans annually or sooner if symptoms arise. Patients are counseled to be prepared to consider lesion excision if the CM grows or bleeds.

Overt Hemorrhage

Patients with a history of overt symptomatic hemorrhage may have an annual risk of recurrent hemorrhage as high as 4.5%/year,[30–32] approximately four times the annual bleed rate for patients without a history of hemorrhage. Other studies, however, failed to find an association between history of hemorrhage and subsequent bleeds.[5] There is evidence that hemorrhages can cluster over time.[30, 31, 34] Patients with symptomatic hemorrhages (Fig. 137–2) may present with an array of manifestations, depending on the lesion's location: headaches, focal neurological deficits, seizures, and, rarely, herniation and coma. The indications for urgent operative intervention in these patients are usually based on the continued rate of neurological decline and the evident or anticipated consequences of mass effect from the hematoma. Thus, the goal of intervention is not only to prevent a rehemorrhage but also to decompress neural tissue and relieve mass effect.

Some patients present with intracerebral hemorrhage of unknown cause (Fig. 137–3), and a CM may be discovered during emergent decompression of the hematoma. As long as the lesion is resected completely at surgery and its removal is verified by delayed postoperative MRI, no further intervention is warranted. In patients suspected of harboring a CM but without evidence of one during initial imaging of an intracerebral hematoma, the need for operative intervention is multifactorial. Some patients may have definitive indications for urgent craniotomy for decompression, as delineated earlier. In patients without evidence of continued decline or problems with intracranial pressure, two strategies may be considered. The first consists of elective exploration soon after the clinical event. The second is expectant management until other diagnostic modalities offer a clearer picture of the possible underlying cause. Early elective exploration in otherwise healthy patients offers the possible benefit of a briefer stay in the intensive care unit and in the hospi-

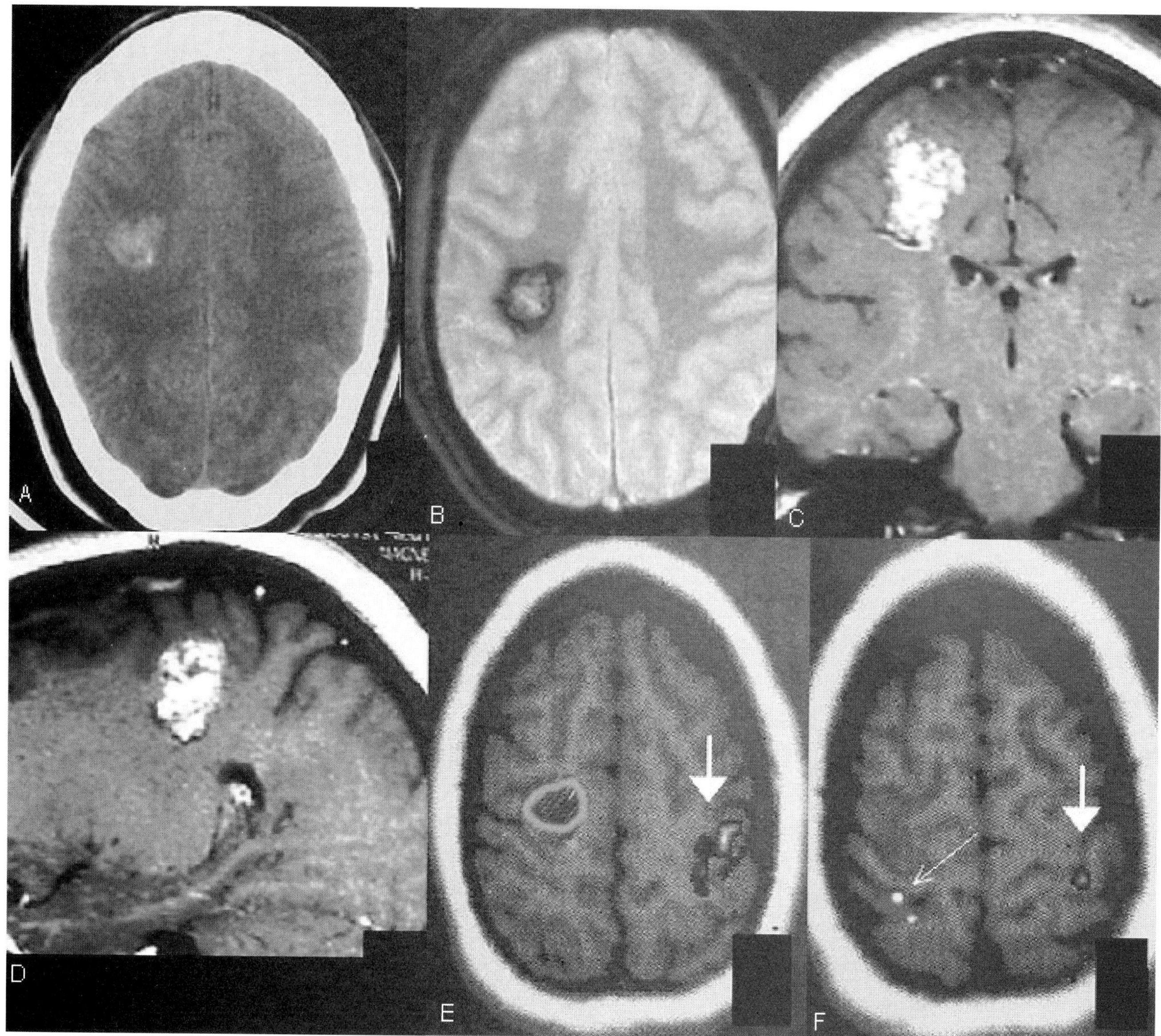

FIGURE 137–2. Patient with a lobar cavernous malformation (CM) with an acute intralesional hemorrhage. *A*, Noncontrast computed tomographic scan reveals a right frontal CM with evidence of acute hemorrhage. *B–D*, Axial proton-density, coronal T2-weighted, and sagittal T1-weighted magnetic resonance imaging (MRI) scans reveal the location of the CM at the gray-white junction, extending into the centrum semiovale adjacent to the rolandic area. Functional MRI was performed to delineate the relationship of the lesion to functional brain areas. The lesion is outlined in gray. *E*, The right motor hand area contralateral to the lesion is shown *(large arrow)*. *F*, The left motor hand area *(small arrow)* is shown to be one full gyrus posterior to the lesion. A frameless stereotactic craniotomy was performed to remove the lesion. Access was obtained through the superior frontal sulcus. Postoperatively, the patient experienced a temporary hemiparesis that rapidly resolved.

tal, because many of these patients require close observation after a hemorrhage to monitor for the consequences of delayed edema and mass effect. This need would be eliminated if the hematoma were evacuated at the time of exploration. In addition, early diagnosis may avoid the need for further treatment or follow-up. Expectant management can be offered to patients with risk factors that make craniotomy more hazardous, such as advanced age or significant cardiac disease, or to patients with an expressed desire to avoid surgery. Follow-up imaging is performed after 2 and 6 weeks, or at a time when the hematoma will have resorbed enough so that any underlying pathology will be evident. In view of the risks of rebleeding, prompt intervention must be considered as soon as a suspected CM becomes apparent.

Mass Effect or Focal Neurological Deficits

Patients may exhibit a neurological deficit due to the compression of critical areas of brain function. The indications for surgery are to decompress neural tissue

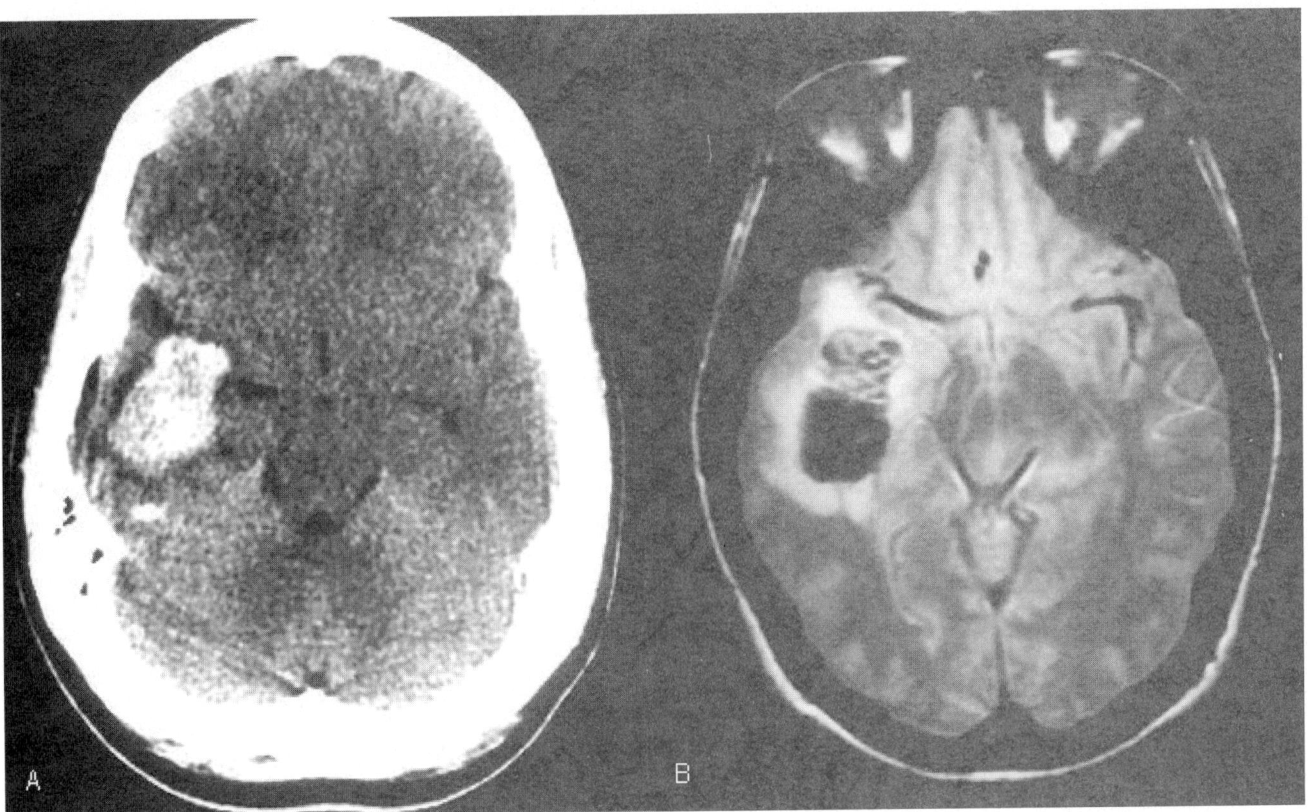

FIGURE 137–3. Patient presenting with an acute intracerebral hematoma from an underlying cavernous malformation (CM). *A*, Noncontrast computed tomographic scan demonstrates an acute right temporal hematoma with mild mass effect. *B*, Proton-density magnetic resonance imaging scan reveals an area just anterior to the hematoma cavity with hemosiderin and signal characteristics of a CM.

and prevent further deterioration from additional hemorrhages or lesion expansion. The rate of neurological decline and the location of the lesion need to be considered carefully in these patients. Intralesional hemorrhage and occasionally perilesional edema may cause acute neurological signs. In certain areas, such as the optic chiasm, the threshold for ischemia may be reached with microscopic growth of a lesion, resulting in rapid functional decline. Obviously, these patients require urgent decompression and resection to prevent further loss of function and to enhance any chance of recovering function.

For patients with slower rates of decline or fixed focal deficits, the rationale of management is similar to that for patients who present with asymptomatic lesions. Patients with surgically accessible lesions should be recommended for resection, and patients with deep lesions should be counseled about the risks and benefits of surgery, weighed against the option of continued expectant management, as discussed earlier. A threshold of neurological decline is often reached when patients and clinicians agree that the risks of surgery for deeper or less accessible lesions are justified.

New-Onset Seizures

A new-onset seizure occurs in patients with known CMs at an estimated rate of 2.4%/patient-year, cumulative over time.[5] Overall, approximately 4.3% to 11% of patients develop new seizures during 1 to 5 years of follow-up.[5, 29, 31] A seizure may reflect recent lesion hemorrhage. In other instances, there may be no indication of recent bleeding or change in lesion size. If seizures can be controlled easily with medications, the indications for surgery in these patients are similar to those for patients with asymptomatic CMs. One must also consider the need for seizure medications, their side effects, and, for many, the need to monitor serum blood levels. Some of these patients may become seizure free over time; others will become intractable to medications and may require evaluation for lesion resection to help control their seizures. Patients often consider the option of excision of a solitary CM to prevent seizure intractability or to enable the discontinuation of anticonvulsant medication.[6]

Long-Standing or Intractable Epilepsy

A seizure disorder is associated with 23% to 51% of CMs.[31, 35] The rate of recurrent seizures in this population is 5.5%/patient-year.[5] In general, patients with CMs who present with the primary complaint of intractable seizures and no clear history of major hemorrhagic events should undergo an abbreviated version of the standard workup for patients with intractable epilepsy. This evaluation may include interictal and ictal scalp electroencephalographic monitoring with video recording of seizure symptoms, interictal and ictal single photon emission computed tomography imaging or 18-fluoro-2-deoxyglucose positron emission tomography imaging, and neuropsychological examination. Patients whose data are concordant with the lesion location by MRI may benefit from functional imaging or Wada testing to delineate critical areas of highly functional brain in relation to the lesion. The specific surgical strategy in such cases is somewhat controversial. Options include lesionectomy alone; lesionectomy plus resection of adjacent abnormal tissue identified by vision, by texture, or by imaging; and lesionectomy plus resection of adjacent or even remote cortex that has been identified by electrophysiologic study as an area of epileptogenicity. These other areas are usually identified as either zones of ictal onset (as identified by ictal monitoring) or areas of abnormal interictal activity (identified by interictal monitoring or intraoperative electrocorticography).

The CMs themselves do not harbor neural tissue and thus cannot generate seizures. There must be a volume of adjacent tissue from which the seizures arise. Theoretically, if the process by which this tissue became epileptogenic is reversible, removal of the lesion alone could render a cure. Conversely, if this tissue has been damaged irreversibly, lesionectomy alone will not affect the epileptogenic process. Surgical manipulation and postoperative changes also may enhance or inhibit epileptogenicity. There is probably some critical volume of tissue that, if resected or disconnected, would render the patient seizure free. It may consist of tissue adjacent to the lesion, or it may be remote, as in cases of so-called dual pathology. The exact means of identifying this tissue (by visual or pathologic inspection, by ictal onset, or by electrocorticography) continues to be an area of controversy and debate.

Other Lesions Mimicking Cavernous Malformations

The MRI appearance of a CM is characteristic but not totally specific. Neoplastic lesions may closely mimic the appearance of a CM (Fig. 137–4), most notably hemorrhagic metastases (i.e., melanoma) and some gliomas associated with calcification or hemorrhage (i.e., oligodendroglioma, pleomorphic xanthoastrocytoma). Overt hemorrhage may totally obscure typical MRI features of any underlying pathology, and the MRI appearance of subacute hematoma may closely resemble that of a CM. An occult or angiographically overt arteriovenous malformation may be confused with a CM—the former in the setting of negative angiography,

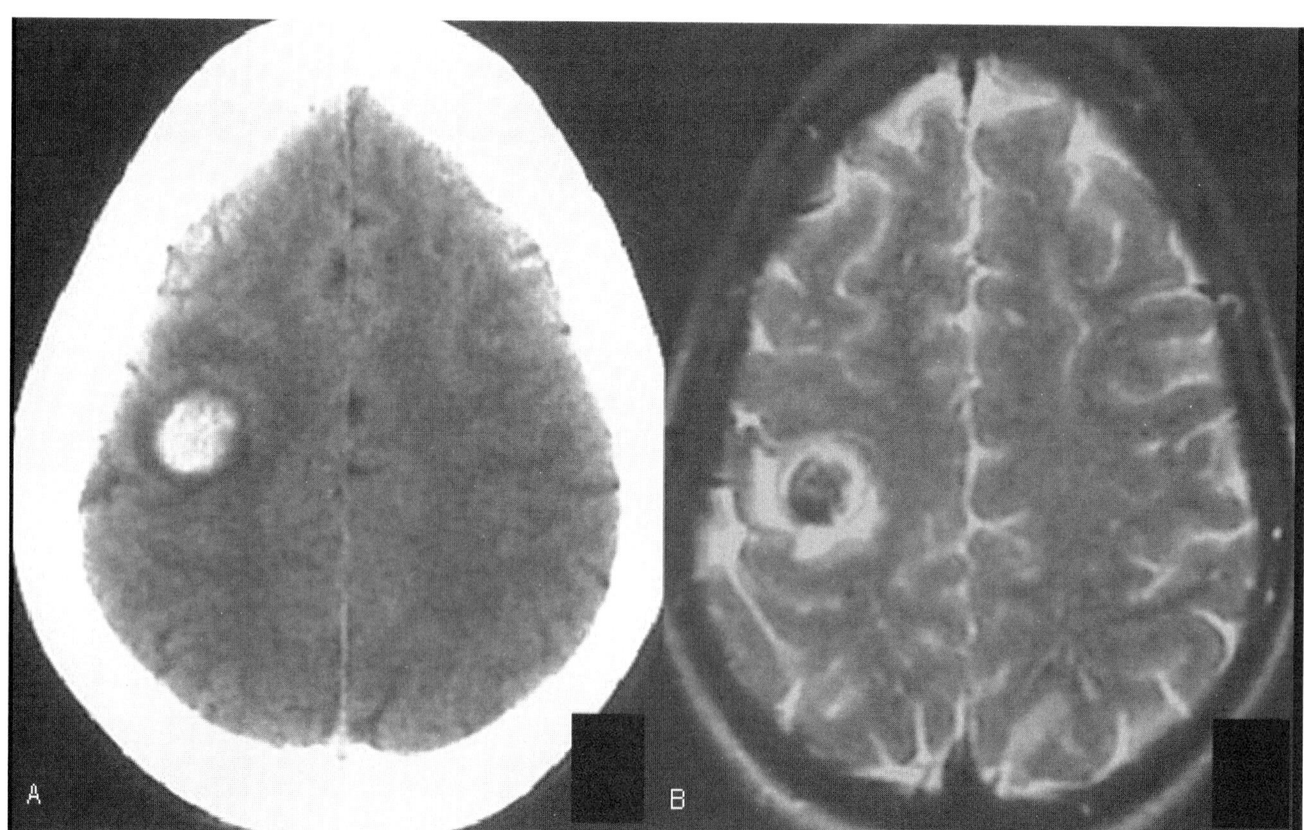

FIGURE 137–4. Patient with a right rolandic lesion mimicking a cavernous malformation. *A*, Axial noncontrast computed tomographic scan reveals a sharply demarcated right frontal hemorrhage with a small amount of adjacent edema. *B*, Axial T2-weighted magnetic resonance imaging scan reveals a heterogeneous hypointense lesion in the right frontal lobe at the gray-white junction, with mild mass effect and adjacent edema. At the time of stereotactic craniotomy, a hemorrhagic tumor was encountered and resected completely. Pathology revealed a pleomorphic xanthoastrocytoma.

and the latter because a draining vein is mistaken for a venous anomaly associated with the CM (Fig. 137–5).

The presence of multiple lesions may be suggestive of CM, although multifocal metastases can mimic this picture. Hereditary hemorrhagic telangiectasia (Osler-Weber-Rendu disease) is also associated with multifocal vascular malformations, although these lesions are overt on angiography and have a distinct appearance on MRI scans. A careful history and systemic medical evaluation often uncover evidence in support of these diseases. In other instances, close follow-up of the lesions is required, with a low threshold for biopsy of atypical or expanding lesions.

SURGICAL MANAGEMENT

Preoperative Planning

Preoperative imaging studies for patients undergoing craniotomy for hemispheric CMs should include MRI scans with both T1- and T2-weighted images in three planes. In addition, gadolinium-enhanced MRI should be performed in at least one plane. This modality can help elucidate venous malformations or other regional venous dysmorphisms that can occur in association with mixed CMs and venous malformations. Fluid-attenuated inversion recovery images may help delineate the boundaries of lesions abutting a pial or ependymal surface. Patients who harbor lesions in areas of critical brain function may benefit from functional imaging to identify a surgical corridor that minimizes the risk of incurring a neurological deficit (see Figs. 137–2*C* and *D*). The preoperative mapping of critical areas, such as primary motor or sensory areas for the hand or foot, in relation to the lesion allows better planning of the craniotomy. This information may be supplemented by intraoperative mapping for precise guidance of a sulcal approach or corticectomy. The coregistration with images acquired for intracranial navigation systems (frameless stereotaxy) may assist in the intraoperative localization of these areas.

Frame-based or frameless stereotactic devices are frequently used to minimize the size and invasiveness of a craniotomy and especially to guide transsulcal approaches to subcortical lesions or CMs in rolandic areas. For more superficial polar lesions, we frequently use dot-localizing computed tomography.[36] Either the night before or the morning of surgery, the awake patient is brought to the computed tomographic scanner, and a localizing grid is secured to the patient's head. A localizing marker is placed over the lesion, using computed tomographic guidance. Hence, the craniotomy can be centered precisely without added intraoperative time. Cortical insonation by B-mode ultrasonography may help reveal subcortical locations at surgery.

Surgical Technique

Surgical strategies are modified based on the location of the lesion, the presence or absence of an associated venous malformation, or a coexistent overt hematoma. After a craniotomy flap has been created and the dura opened, the lesion itself is localized. If the lesion reaches the surface of the brain, it may appear as a purple-blue mulberry-like structure surrounded by an area of hemosiderosis. Otherwise, intraoperative ultrasonography or stereotaxy is used to localize subcortical lesions, especially smaller CMs. In patients with an apparent hematoma on neuroimaging, access into the hematoma cavity provides an initial plane of dissection.

Intraoperative cortical mapping may help identify areas of critical function to be avoided during the resection. Preoperative functional imaging can also be referenced and may be more helpful if coregistered with stereotactic images for precise delineation of the areas of function (see Figs. 137–2*D* and *E*). Owing to the possible presence of associated venous malformations, the cortical venous drainage pattern should be inspected before resection. When addressing the CM itself, a gliotic pseudocapsule typically allows a dissection plane. The lesion is often shrunk by bipolar coagulation or by emptying larger blood-filled caverns. The surrounding gliotic plane is then used to resect the lesion en bloc. Working circumferentially around the lesion, the gliotic plane is identified, and a cotton patty is placed to preserve the plane of dissection. In this manner, the lesion is dissected circumferentially from all sides until it is free. It is then removed and sent for histopathologic examination.

After the lesion's removal, the resection bed should be carefully inspected under magnification for small satellite lesions,[37] which should be coagulated or resected. If the lesion was located well away from areas of critical function, surrounding hemosiderin-stained brain may be resected because of its possible epileptogenicity. This is considered more imperative in patients with a history of seizures, even if they are well controlled on medications, to enhance the patient's chances of successfully withdrawing from pharmacotherapy. After careful hemostasis, the cavity can be lined with a procoagulant material, and a routine closure can be performed.

Associated Venous Malformations

On preoperative imaging, approximately 24% of patients with CMs may have obvious venous malformations in proximity to the CM (Fig. 137–6).[38] Other CMs may be associated with abnormal adjacent venous structures. An area of regional venous dysmorphism often surrounds the lesion. A venous malformation itself may be the sole source of venous drainage for the area of surrounding brain. Resection of the venous malformation may cause hemorrhagic cortical venous infarction. For this reason, every effort is made to preserve these associated venous malformations at the time the CM is resected. Venous malformations are extremely common in the general population; however, their close proximity to CMs when the two coexist has led to speculation regarding their etiologic relationship.[4, 39–42] There is the possibility of postoperative for-

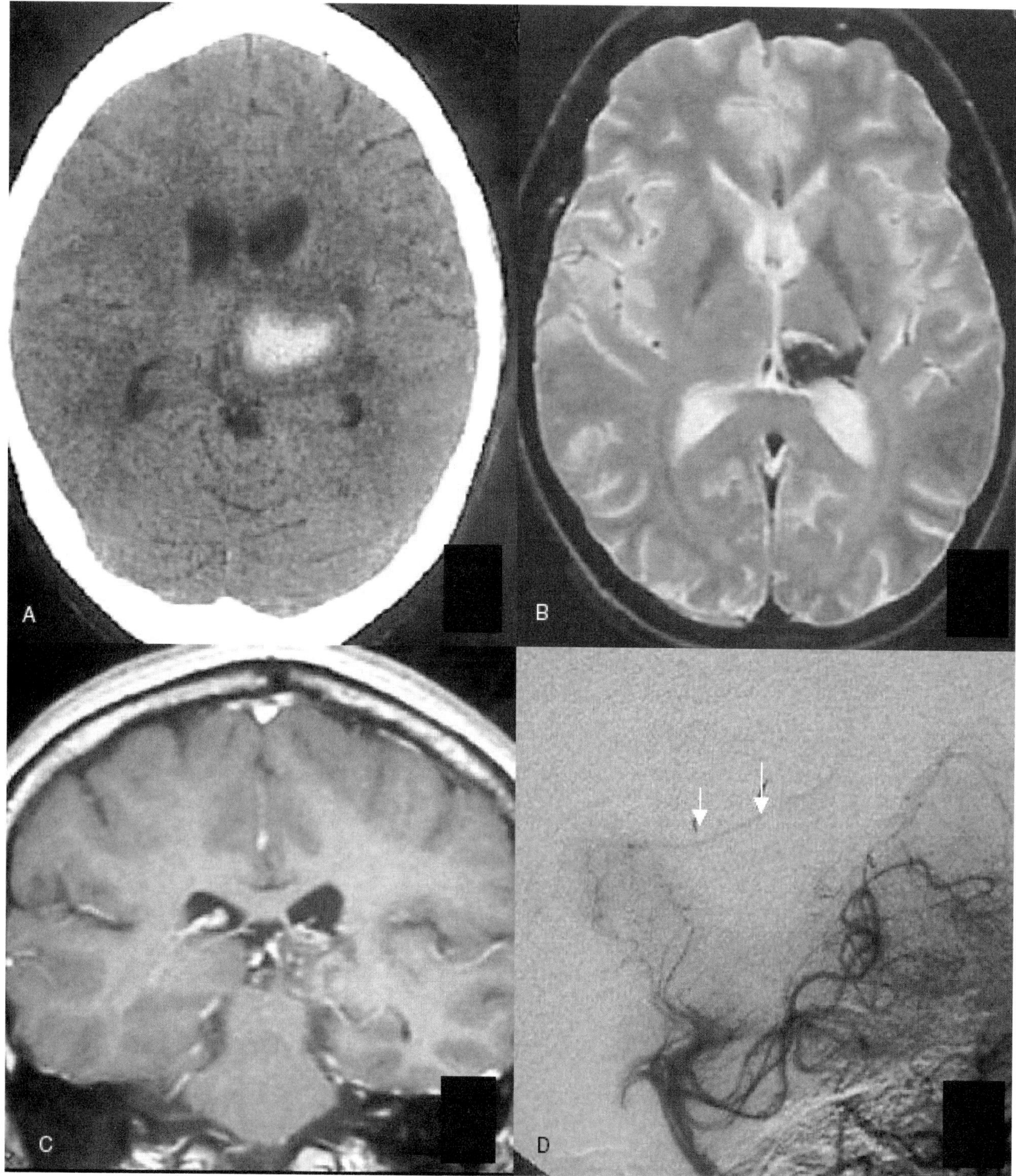

FIGURE 137–5. Patient with a lesion suspicious for a cavernous malformation in the right posterior thalamus. *A*, Noncontrast computed tomographic scan reveals a hemorrhagic lesion in the left pulvinar. *B*, T2-weighted magnetic resonance imaging (MRI) scan reveals a heterogeneous lesion with a small area of hyperintensity anteriorly. *C*, Coronal T2-weighted MRI scan shows a mixed lesion in close proximity to the deep venous system. *D*, Vertebral artery angiogram demonstrates an early filling vein draining posteriorly *(arrows)*. An arteriovenous malformation was found at craniotomy.

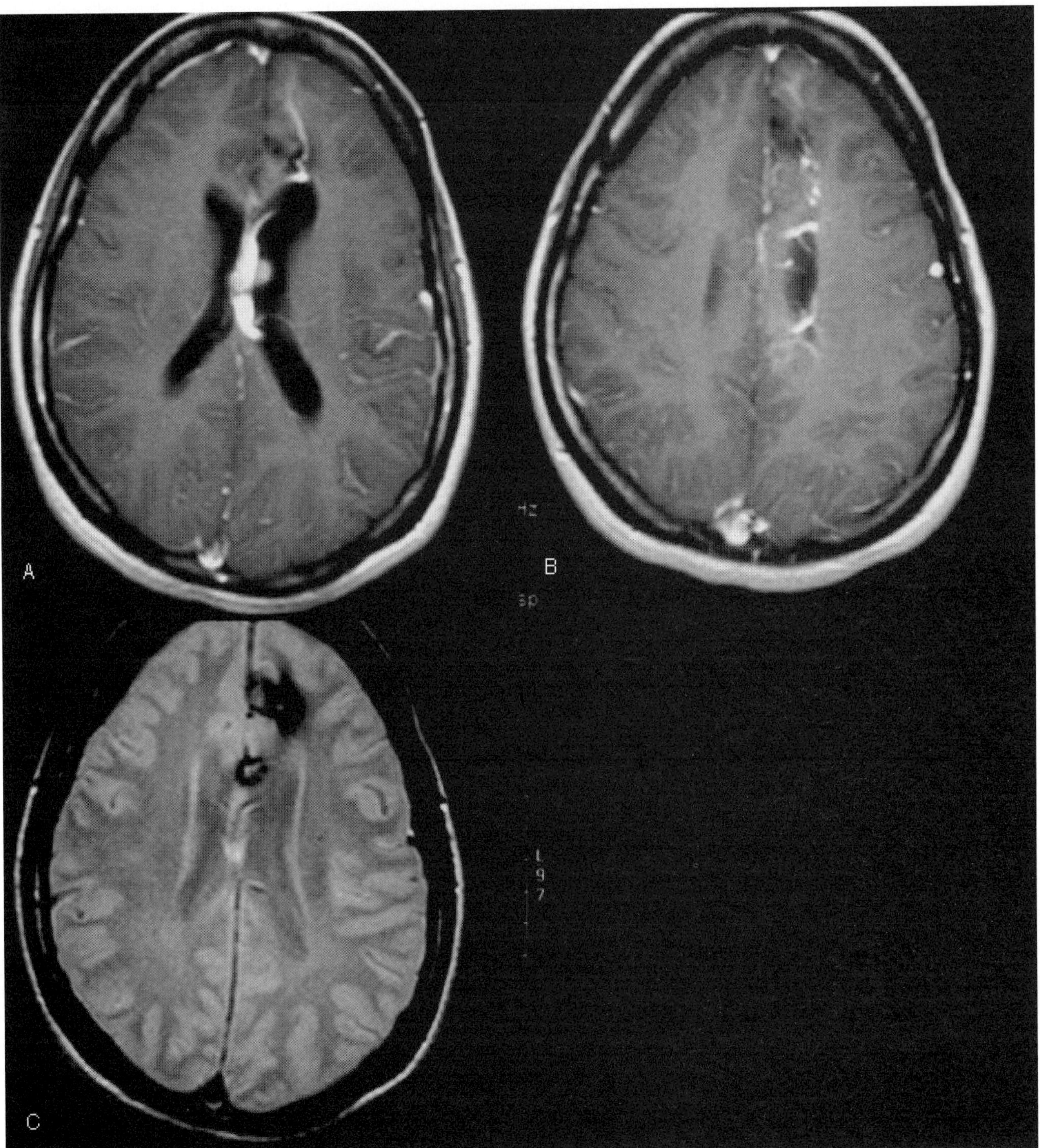

FIGURE 137–6. Patient with a medial frontal cavernous malformation (CM) with associated venous malformations. Axial gadolinium-enhanced magnetic resonance imaging (MRI) scans reveal two venous malformations—one in the left frontopolar region *(A)* inferior to the lesion, and another posterior to the lesion *(B)* draining into the internal cerebral veins. Proton-density MRI scan *(C)* shows a typical rim of low-intensity signal characteristic of CMs. A possible satellite lesion is visible posteromedially.

mation of de novo CMs in association with venous malformations. We recommend follow-up surveillance of these patients with serial imaging, despite successful excision of the CM component of the lesion.

Patients with Intractable Epilepsy

When a CM is excised with the primary aim of controlling intractable seizures, the preoperative evaluation should verify that the area of the CM is, in fact, the source of seizure activity. In cases of a solitary CM, clinical seizure semiology (preictal, ictal, and postictal symptoms and signs), electroencephalographic lateralization or localization of interictal or ictal-onset epileptiform activity, and functional or neuropsychological tests are analyzed for concordant information localized to the region of the CM. For patients with concordant data, the resection is performed in the usual fashion as described earlier. Although iron deposition in the surrounding brain is thought to be the etiologic factor in seizure genesis,[1–3, 43] the data on the relationship between resection of surrounding hemosiderosis at the time of CM resection and postoperative seizure control are equivocal.[8] In general, we recommend resection of the surrounding area of hemosiderosis when this is possible without causing postoperative deficits.

It is possible that an area of independent ictal genesis exists in some patients harboring a CM.[44–47] Theoretically, in patients with a prolonged history of seizures with a focal extrahippocampal onset, the seizures may propagate to the hippocampus and cause excitotoxic damage. This damage may result in a distinct focus in the mesial temporal lobe or other areas that can independently generate seizures. In most instances, the relative contribution of each substrate of the dual pathology (CM versus mesial temporal lobe sclerosis) to the seizure disorder remains speculative. When a patient has clear evidence of hippocampal sclerosis (by atrophy on MRI, neuropsychological testing, and functional imaging) in association with a temporal lobe CM, resection of both structures can be undertaken simultaneously. When this relationship is less clear and ictal monitoring indicates that at least some of the seizures originate in the area of the CM, a lesionectomy alone should be performed, especially in the absence of convincing evidence of hippocampal dysfunction (i.e., normal neuropsychological testing and functional imaging).

When preoperative evaluation reveals evidence of epileptogenicity remote from the CM or in the common scenario of multiple CMs (see later), a detailed epilepsy evaluation with invasive electrodes is recommended to delineate the epileptogenic zone precisely. A solitary CM or the largest lesion is not always the cause of an intractable seizure disorder.

Capsular and Thalamic Cavernous Malformations

As stated earlier, the surgical resection of capsular and thalamic CMs is associated with greater morbidity rates than those reported for more superficial hemispheric lesions. These patients typically present with more severe preoperative neurological deficits. Our

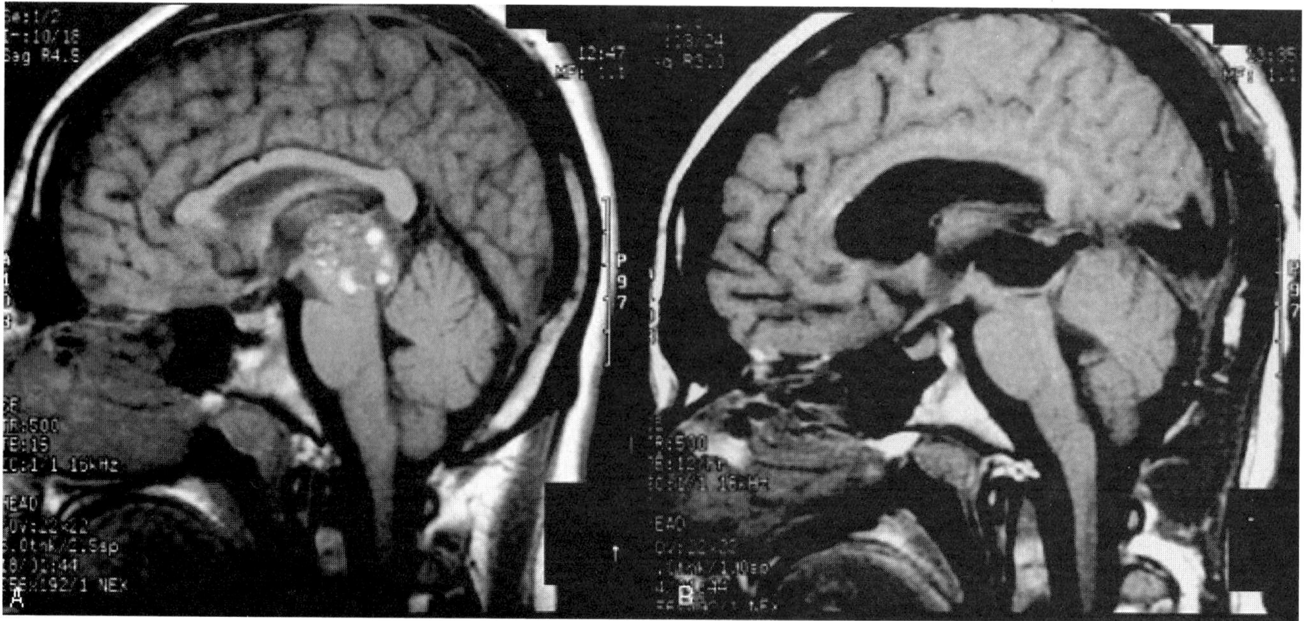

FIGURE 137–7. A 15-year-old boy with a posterior thalamic-mesencephalic cavernous malformation presented with acute headache, hemiparesis, hemisensory loss, and hemianopsia. *A*, Preoperative sagittal T1-weighted magnetic resonance imaging (MRI) scan reveals a large heterogeneous mass in the posterior thalamus, extending to the posterior pial surface of the pulvinar. In this case, a suboccipital transtentorial approach was used to visualize the lesion and the adjacent venous structures. *B*, Postoperative T1-weighted MRI scan confirms total excision.

management strategy is to resect only those lesions that reach a ventricular or pial surface. Surgical approaches are chosen by the surface presentation of the lesion (Figs. 137–7 and 137–8). More anterior lesions can be approached via a transcallosal route. Lateral thalamic lesions can be approached via a transcortical route through the superior parietal lobule, whereas medial posterior lesions can be resected via a posterior

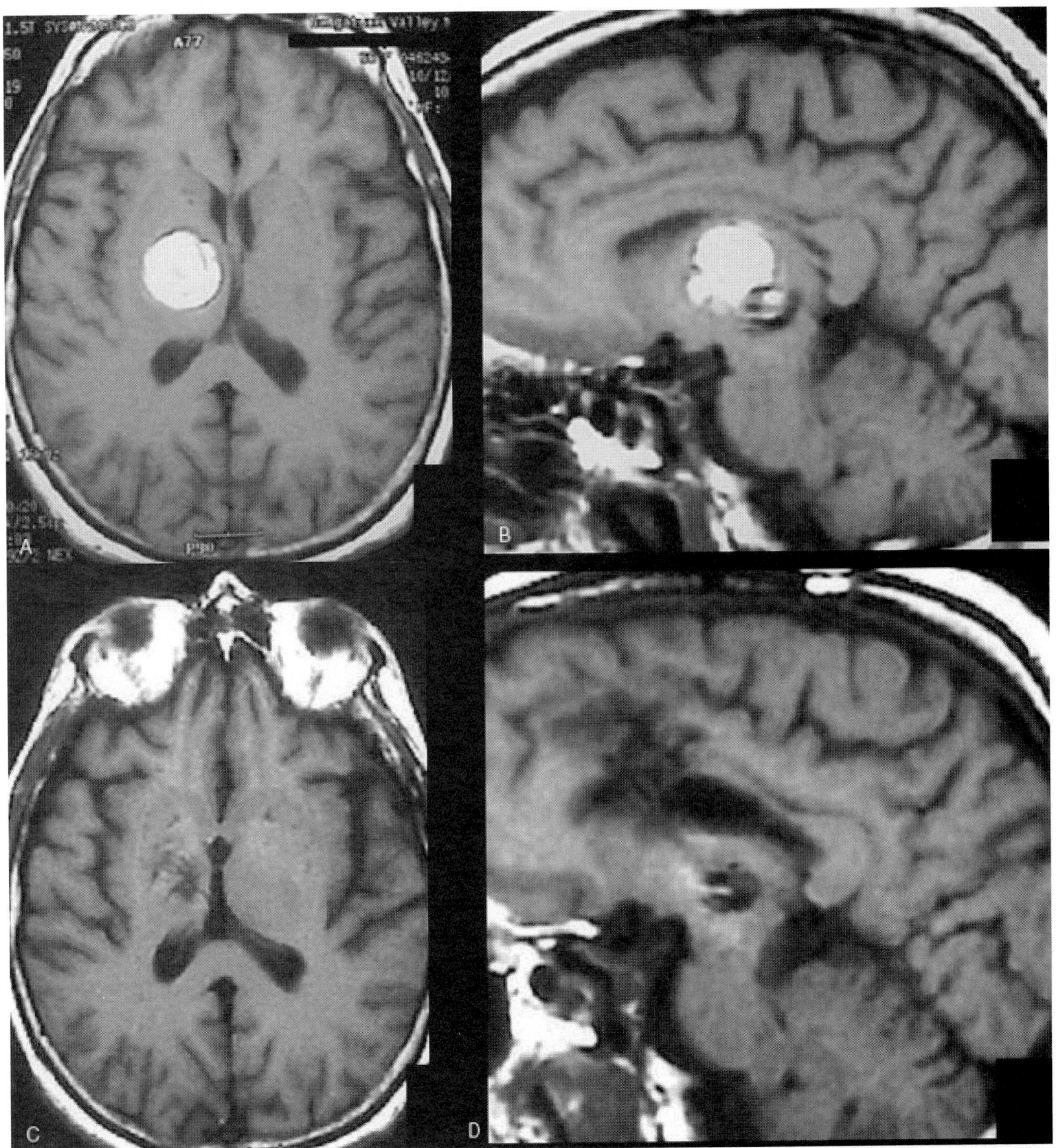

FIGURE 137–8. Patient with a midthalamic cavernous malformation (CM) presenting with repetitive hemorrhages. Axial *(A)* and sagittal *(B)* T1-weighted magnetic resonance imaging (MRI) scans show the CM located in the anterior right thalamus. On the sagittal MRI scan, the lesion can be seen approximating the third ventricular ependymal surface of the thalamus. The CM was approached via an interhemispheric transcallosal route. Postoperative axial *(C)* and sagittal *(D)* T1-weighted MRI scans confirm total removal of the lesion. The patient recovered completely, without a hint of residual hemiparesis 2 months after surgery.

interhemispheric approach. We have found frameless stereotaxy especially useful for guiding surgical approaches in these cases. These lesions are best removed by internal decompression when possible and careful blunt dissection with conservative use of electrocauterization.

Optic Pathway Cavernous Malformations

CMs within the optic apparatus are rarely encountered, and few cases of their surgical resection have been reported.[48, 49] These patients may present with acute, subacute, or progressive visual disturbances. As described by Maitland and coworkers,[50] "chiasmal apoplexy" may occur with the abrupt onset of headache, a sudden change in visual acuity, and visual field changes. Clinical presentation and computed tomographic scans may mimic subarachnoid hemorrhage from an anterior communicating artery aneurysm. Negative angiography and characteristic MRI scans usually establish the diagnosis. The rehemorrhage rate for lesions in this area may be as high as 25%.[48] Patients with sudden changes in vision or rapidly progressive deficits need an urgent craniotomy. These lesions can be approached via pterional or subfrontal lamina terminalis–type routes.

Other CMs may compromise vision by involvement of the lateral geniculate body; the geniculocalcarine projections in the temporal, parietal, or occipital lobe; or the calcarine cortex. Lesion resection is typically associated with some degree of recovery of visual field compromise.

Pineal Cavernous Malformations

A review by Slavin and colleagues[51] revealed only 12 case reports of pineal region CMs in the literature. These lesions account for less than 1% of CMs of the central nervous system. These patients may present with signs of increased intracranial pressure, ocular symptoms from compression of the tectal plate, and other neurological or neuroendocrine abnormalities from compression of adjacent structures. For patients with ventriculomegaly, external ventricular drainage or shunt placement may be considered. Interhemispheric transsplenial, suboccipital transtentorial, and supracerebellar infratentorial surgical approaches can be used successfully, depending on the exact location and extent of the lesion (Fig. 137–9).

Multiple Lesions

Typically, treatment in patients harboring multiple CMs is aimed at addressing the symptomatic lesion. Often, it is obvious that one particular lesion has hemorrhaged or is much larger, or its location is consistent with the patient's clinical symptoms or signs. Surgery is planned to address the symptomatic lesion and pos-

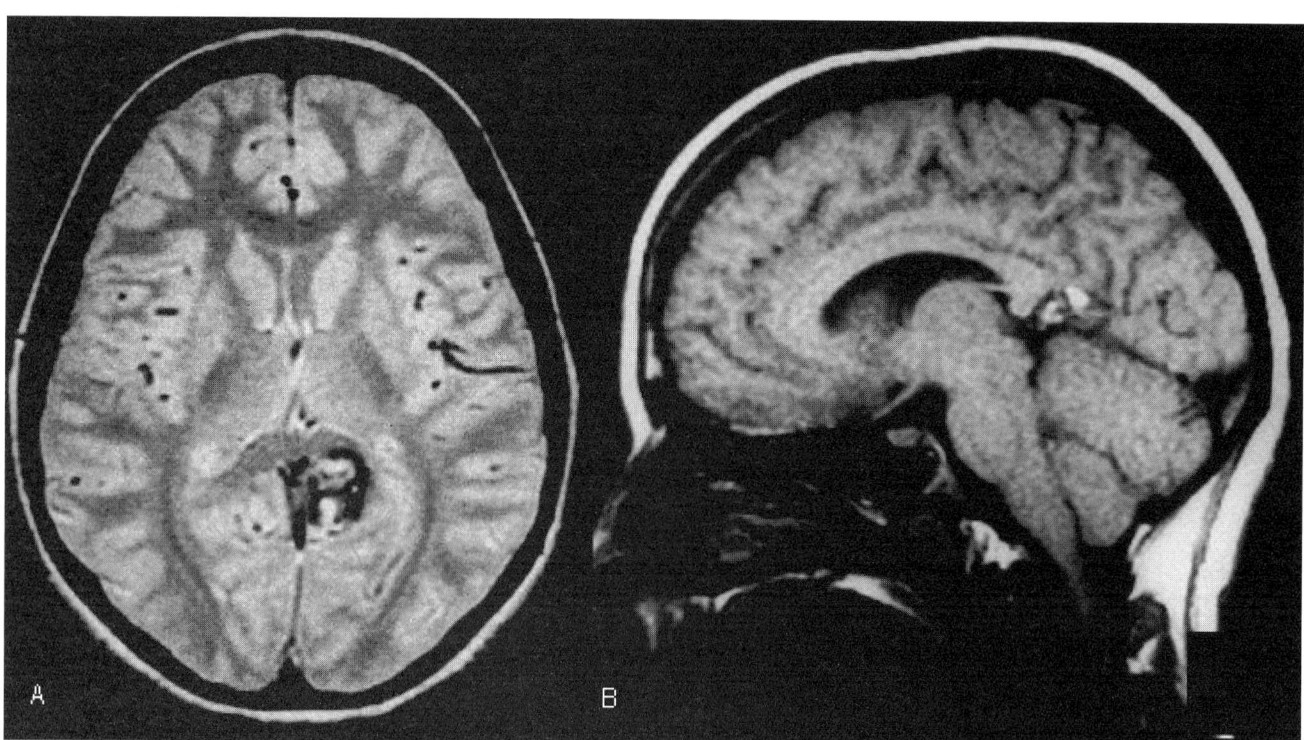

FIGURE 137–9. Patient with a right pineal region–medial occipital cavernous malformation presenting with headaches and hemianopsia. Axial proton-density magnetic resonance imaging (MRI) scan *(A)* and sagittal T1-weighted MRI scan *(B)* show the lesion medial to the atrium in the medial occipital lobe, reaching the interhemispheric pial surface posterior to the splenium of the corpus callosum. An occipital interhemispheric approach was used for total removal of the lesion. The patient's visual field deficit partially resolved.

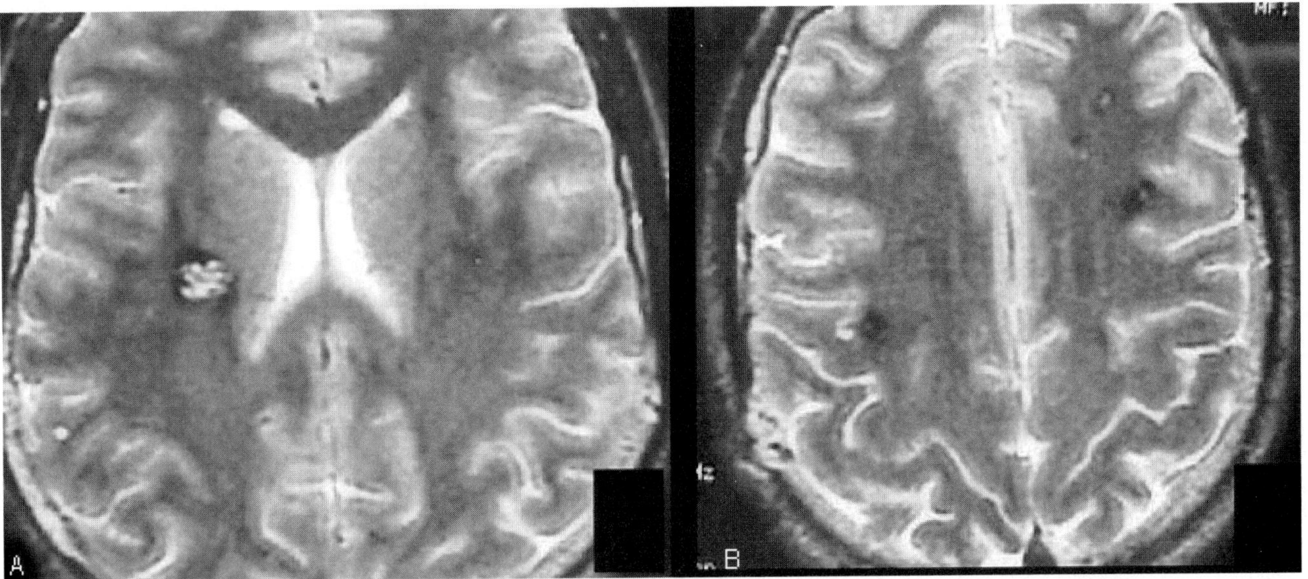

FIGURE 137–10. Hispanic man presenting with multiple cavernous malformations (CMs), the largest of which is in the right frontal area at the gray-white junction. Axial T2-weighted magnetic resonance imaging scans reveal four separate areas of hypointensity consistent with CMs. *A*, One lesion is inferior in the right superior aspect of the posterior limb of the internal capsule. *B*, A second lesion is in the right prerolandic gyrus, and the remaining two lesions are in the left anterior frontal lobe.

sibly any nearby lesions if they can be resected through the same craniotomy without placing the patient at significant added risk.

A distinct problem arises in patients who harbor multiple CMs and epilepsy (Fig. 137–10). It may be difficult to pinpoint a specific lesion as being responsible for the generation of seizures. In some cases, concordance of ictal scalp electroencephalography, neuropsychological examination, and lesion location with seizure semiology may point to a specific lesion. In other cases, intracranial monitoring may be necessary to delineate the specific epileptogenic lesion. Mostly in the setting of multiple CMs, an occult associated vascular lesion may be responsible for the seizures, while more overt lesions are, in fact, incidental to the epilepsy.

In general, the threshold of surgical intervention is higher for patients with multiple CMs, with close expectant follow-up and consideration of excision of growing or symptomatic lesions. Patients with familial CMs are at risk for the formation of de novo CMs.[9, 29, 52–54] It has been suggested that most patients with multiple CMs may have a genetically inherited form of the disease with variable clinical penetrance.[55, 56]

Dural-Based Cavernous Malformations

These lesions have identical histopathology to the typical CMs of the brain, but several features set them apart clinically. Most dural-based CMs are found in the middle fossa, followed by the cerebellopontine angle, the tentorium, and the convexities. These lesions most frequently present with headache. Those in the cavernous sinus region may cause ocular signs, visual field deficits, hormonal imbalances, and other cranial nerve palsies.[57, 58] On imaging, these lesions may be mistaken for meningiomas. On MRI, they typically do not have a reticulated core or the rim of signal hypointensity invariably seen with intraparenchymal CMs. Dural-based lesions enhance strongly and homogeneously with gadolinium.[58–60] Compared with their intraparenchymal counterparts, these lesions rarely manifest with hemorrhage.[59] Specifically, dural-based CMs in the middle cranial fossa may have substantial vascularity and tend to bleed profusely on attempted excision. In these cases, it may be advantageous to perform preoperative angiography with embolization[61] or possibly external radiation or stereotactic radiosurgery to reduce vascularity before proceeding to excision.[62, 63] Resection of lesions in the middle cranial fossa may be associated with a morbidity rate as high as 38%,[58] whereas supratentorial lesions outside the middle fossa can usually be resected without permanent sequelae.[59]

REFERENCES

1. Willmore LJ, Triggs WJ, Gray JD: The role of iron-induced hippocampal peroxidation in acute epileptogenesis. Brain Res 382: 422–426, 1986.
2. Shiota A, Hiramatsu M, Mori A: Amino acid neurotransmitters in iron-induced epileptic foci of rats. Res Commun Chem Pathol Pharmacol 66:123–133, 1989.
3. Moriwaki A, Hattori Y, Nishida N, et al: Electrocorticographic characterization of chronic iron-induced epilepsy in rats. Neurosci Lett 110:72–76, 1990.
4. Little JR, Awad IA, Jones SC, et al: Vascular pressures and cortical blood flow in cavernous angioma of the brain. J Neurosurg 73: 555–559, 1990.
5. Moriarity JL, Wetzel M, Clatterbuck RE, et al: The natural history of cavernous malformations: A prospective study of 68 patients. Neurosurgery 44:1166–1171, 1999.
6. Cohen DS, Zubay GP, Goodman RR: Seizure outcome after lesionectomy for cavernous malformations. J Neurosurg 83:237–242, 1995.

7. Casazza M, Broggi G, Franzini A, et al: Supratentorial cavernous angiomas and epileptic seizures: Preoperative course and postoperative outcome. Neurosurgery 39:26–32, 1996.
8. Zevgaridis D, van Velthoven V, Ebeling U, et al: Seizure control following surgery in supratentorial cavernous malformations: A retrospective study in 77 patients. Acta Neurochir (Wien) 138: 672–677, 1996.
9. Pozzati E, Acciarri N, Tognetti F, et al: Growth, subsequent bleeding, and de novo appearance of cerebral cavernous angiomas. Neurosurgery 38:662–669, 1996.
10. Novelli PM, Reigel DH, Langham Gleason P, et al: Multiple cavernous angiomas after high-dose whole-brain radiation therapy. Pediatr Neurosurg 26:322–325, 1997.
11. Alexander MJ, DeSalles AA, Tomiyasu U: Multiple radiation-induced intracranial lesions after treatment for pituitary adenoma: Case report. J Neurosurg 88:111–115, 1998.
12. Larson JJ, Ball WS, Bove KE, et al: Formation of intracerebral cavernous malformations after radiation treatment for central nervous system neoplasia in children. J Neurosurg 88:51–56, 1998.
13. Maeder P, Gudinchet F, Meuli R, et al: Development of a cavernous malformation of the brain. AJNR Am J Neuroradiol 19: 1141–1143, 1998.
14. Maraire JN, Abdulrauf SI, Berger S, et al: De novo development of a cavernous malformation of the spinal cord following spinal axis radiation: Case report. J Neurosurg 90(Suppl):234–238, 1999.
15. Coffey RJ, Lunsford LD, Bissonette D, et al: Stereotactic gamma radiosurgery for intracranial vascular malformations and tumors: Report of the initial North American experience in 331 patients. Stereotact Funct Neurosurg 54:535–540, 1990.
16. Lunsford LD, Kondziolka D, Bissonette DJ, et al: Stereotactic radiosurgery of brain vascular malformations. Neurosurg Clin N Am 3:79–98, 1992.
17. Lunsford LD, Kondziolka D, Flickinger JC: Stereotactic radiosurgery: Current spectrum and results. Clin Neurosurg 38:405–444, 1992.
18. Amin-Hanjani S, Ogilvy CS, Candia GJ, et al: Stereotactic radiosurgery for cavernous malformations: Kjellberg's experience with proton beam therapy in 98 cases at the Harvard cyclotron. Neurosurgery 42:1229–1236, 1998.
19. Karlsson B, Kihlstrom L, Lindquist C, et al: Radiosurgery for cavernous malformations. J Neurosurg 88:293–297, 1998.
20. Yoon PH, Kim DI, Jeon P, et al: Cerebral cavernous malformations: Serial magnetic resonance imaging findings in patients with and without gamma knife surgery. Neurol Med Chir (Tokyo) 38(Suppl):255–261, 1998.
21. Kondziolka D, Lunsford LD, Flickinger JC, et al: Reduction of hemorrhage risk after stereotactic radiosurgery for cavernous malformations. J Neurosurg 83:825–831, 1995.
22. Maesawa S, Kondziolka D, Lunsford LD: Stereotactic radiosurgery for management of deep brain cavernous malformations. Neurosurg Clin N Am 10:503–511, 1999.
23. Voigt K, Yasargil MG: Cerebral cavernous haemangiomas or cavernomas: Incidence, pathology, localization, diagnosis, clinical features and treatment. Review of the literature and report of an unusual case. Neurochirurgia (Stuttg) 19:59–68, 1976.
24. Simard JM, Garcia-Bengochea F, Ballinger WE Jr, et al: Cavernous angioma: A review of 126 collected and 12 new clinical cases. Neurosurgery 18:162–172, 1986.
25. Vaquero J, Salazar J, Martinez R, et al: Cavernomas of the central nervous system: Clinical syndromes, CT scan diagnosis, and prognosis after surgical treatment in 25 cases. Acta Neurochir (Wien) 85:29–33, 1987.
26. Bertalanffy H, Gilsbach JM, Eggert HR, et al: Microsurgery of deep-seated cavernous angiomas: Report of 26 cases. Acta Neurochir (Wien) 108:91–99, 1991.
27. Del Curling O Jr, Kelly DL Jr, Elster AD, et al: An analysis of the natural history of cavernous angiomas. J Neurosurg 75:702–708, 1991.
28. Robinson JR, Awad IA, Little JR: Natural history of the cavernous angioma. J Neurosurg 75:709–714, 1991.
29. Zabramski JM, Wascher TM, Spetzler RF, et al: The natural history of familial cavernous malformations: Results of an ongoing study. J Neurosurg 80:422–432, 1994.
30. Aiba T, Tanaka R, Koike T, et al: Natural history of intracranial cavernous malformations. J Neurosurg 83:56–59, 1995.
31. Kondziolka D, Lunsford LD, Kestle JR: The natural history of cerebral cavernous malformations. J Neurosurg 83:820–824, 1995.
32. Robinson JR Jr, Awad IA, Magdinec M, et al: Factors predisposing to clinical disability in patients with cavernous malformations of the brain. Neurosurgery 32:730–735, 1993.
33. Porter PJ, Willinsky RA, Harper W, et al: Cerebral cavernous malformations: Natural history and prognosis after clinical deterioration with or without hemorrhage. J Neurosurg 87:190–197, 1997.
34. Tung H, Giannotta SL, Chandrasoma PT, et al: Recurrent intraparenchymal hemorrhages from angiographically occult vascular malformations. J Neurosurg 73:174–180, 1990.
35. Requena I, Arias M, Lopez-Ibor L, et al: Cavernomas of the central nervous system: Clinical and neuroimaging manifestations in 47 patients. J Neurol Neurosurg Psychiatry 54:590–594, 1991.
36. Hirschberg H: Localization of brain tumors with a simple scalp-mounted fiducial device: Technical note. J Neurosurg 70:280–281, 1989.
37. Jellinger K: Vascular malformations of the central nervous system: A morphological overview. Neurosurg Rev 9:177–216, 1986.
38. Abdulrauf SI, Kaynar MY, Awad IA: A comparison of the clinical profile of cavernous malformations with and without associated venous malformations. Neurosurgery 44:41–46, 1999.
39. Rigamonti D, Spetzler RF, Medina M, et al: Cerebral venous malformations. J Neurosurg 73:560–564, 1990.
40. Awad IA, Robinson JR: Cavernous malformations and epilepsy. In Awad IA, Barrow DL (eds): Cavernous Malformations. Park Ridge, Ill, American Association of Neurological Surgeons, 1993, pp 49–64.
41. Wilms G, Bleus E, Demaerel P, et al: Simultaneous occurrence of developmental venous anomalies and cavernous angiomas. AJNR Am J Neuroradiol 15:1247–1254, 1994.
42. McLaughlin MR, Kondziolka D, Flickinger JC, et al: The prospective natural history of cerebral venous malformations. Neurosurgery 43:195–200, 1998.
43. Kraemer DL, Awad IA: Vascular malformations and epilepsy: Clinical considerations and basic mechanisms. Epilepsia 35(Suppl 6):S30–S43, 1994.
44. Cascino GD, Jack CRJ, Parisi JE, et al: Operative strategy in patients with MRI-identified dual pathology and temporal lobe epilepsy. Epilepsy Res 14:175–182, 1993.
45. Dodick DW, Cascino GD, Meyer FB: Vascular malformations and intractable epilepsy: Outcome after surgical treatment. Mayo Clin Proc 69:741–745, 1994.
46. Cendes F, Cook MJ, Watson C, et al: Frequency and characteristics of dual pathology in patients with lesional epilepsy. Neurology 45:2058–2064, 1995.
47. Li LM, Cendes F, Watson C, et al: Surgical treatment of patients with single and dual pathology: Relevance of lesion and of hippocampal atrophy to seizure outcome. Neurology 48:437–444, 1997.
48. Shibuya M, Baskaya MK, Saito K, et al: Cavernous malformations of the optic chiasma. Acta Neurochir (Wien) 136:29–36, 1995.
49. Arrue P, Thorn-Kany M, Vally P, et al: Cavernous hemangioma of the intracranial optic pathways: CT and MRI. J Comput Assist Tomogr 23:357–361, 1999.
50. Maitland CG, Abiko S, Hoyt WF, et al: Chiasmal apoplexy: Report of four cases. J Neurosurg 56:118–122, 1982.
51. Slavin KV, Dujovny M, McDonald LW, et al: Pineal region: Rare location of a cavernous haemangioma. Neurol Res 16:133–136, 1994.
52. Tekkok IH, Ventureyra EC: De novo familial cavernous malformation presenting with hemorrhage 12.5 years after the initial hemorrhagic ictus: Natural history of an infantile form. Pediatr Neurosurg 25:151–155, 1996.
53. Detwiler PW, Porter RW, Zabramski JM, et al: De novo formation of a central nervous system cavernous malformation: Implications for predicting risk of hemorrhage. Case report and review of the literature. J Neurosurg 87:629–632, 1997.
54. Houtteville JP: Brain cavernoma: A dynamic lesion. Surg Neurol 48:610–614, 1997.

55. Gunel M, Awad IA, Finberg K, et al: A founder mutation as a cause of cerebral cavernous malformation in Hispanic Americans. N Engl J Med 334:946–951, 1996.
56. Labauge P, Laberge S, Brunereau L, et al: Hereditary cerebral cavernous angiomas: Clinical and genetic features in 57 French families. Societe Francaise de Neurochirurgie. Lancet 352:1892–1897, 1998.
57. Kawai K, Fukui M, Tanaka A, et al: Extracerebral cavernous hemangioma of the middle fossa. Surg Neurol 9:19–25, 1978.
58. Momoshima S, Shiga H, Yuasa Y, et al: MR findings in extracerebral cavernous angiomas of the middle cranial fossa: Report of two cases and review of the literature. AJNR Am J Neuroradiol 12:756–760, 1991.
59. Lewis AI, Tew JM Jr, Payner TD, et al: Dural cavernous angiomas outside the middle cranial fossa: A report of two cases. Neurosurgery 35:498–504, 1994.
60. Vogler R, Castillo M: Dural cavernous angioma: MR features. AJNR Am J Neuroradiol 16:773–775, 1995.
61. Namba S: Extracerebral cavernous hemangioma of the middle cranial fossa. Surg Neurol 19:379–388, 1983.
62. Shibata S, Mori K: Effect of radiation therapy on extracerebral cavernous hemangioma in the middle fossa: Report of three cases. J Neurosurg 67:919–922, 1987.
63. Rigamonti D, Pappas CT, Spetzler RF, et al: Extracerebral cavernous angiomas of the middle fossa. Neurosurgery 27:306–310, 1990.

CHAPTER **138**

Infratentorial Cavernous Malformations

RANDALL W. PORTER ■ PAUL W. DETWILER ■ ROBERT F. SPETZLER

Despite advances in surgical techniques and frameless stereotaxy, surgery on the brainstem remains one of the most technically challenging operations.[1] The first reference to the brainstem was made in the Middle Ages, probably by Albertus Magnus, who proposed that the midbrain was the origin of the imagination.[1] Later, during the Renaissance, Vesalius provided a more detailed account of the midbrain, corpora quadrigemina, pineal gland, and superior and inferior cerebellar peduncles.[2]

In 1830, Sir Charles Bell said of his brainstem drawings (as reported by Jeffersen), "He who makes himself master of this plate can have no difficulty in comprehending the whole nervous system."[3] Although his statement may have been an ambitious oversimplification, it is still true that the brainstem is one of the most dangerous and intimidating areas of the human body on which to operate. In 1890, Braun reported the first successful operation on a cerebellar abscess.[4] At the turn of the 19th century, however, operations on the cerebellum were associated with mortality rates that exceeded 50%.

In the first half of the 20th century, brainstem surgery was guided by ventriculography. In 1912, Frazier reported a posterior fossa approach used to section the eighth cranial nerve for the treatment of Ménière's disease.[5] Not until the discovery of computed tomography were major strides in imaging the brainstem made. Current techniques include detailed preoperative visualization with magnetic resonance imaging (MRI), intraoperative frameless stereotactic guidance, monitoring of brainstem auditory evoked responses (BAERs), and skull base approaches that enable safe and extensive exposure of the entire brainstem.

In the realm of intrinsic brainstem lesions, brainstem cavernous malformations are ideal lesions to resect. They are histologically benign and contain no neural tissue. If removed completely, they are one of the few curable brainstem tumors. The successful and safe resection of these lesions, however, did not become routine until skull base and frameless stereotactic techniques were developed. In 1851, Virchow reported the first case of a brainstem hemangioma, and more than a century later, Russell coined the term *cryptic vascular malformation* to classify these lesions as distinct entities.[6] In 1953, Teilmann reviewed the 46 cases of vascular malformations of the pons that had been reported in the literature up to that time.[7] During the next half-century, numerous authors resected these lesions, with good results.[8–28]

NATURAL HISTORY

Cavernous malformations account for 5% to 13% of the vascular lesions occurring in the central nervous system.[29–31] They affect 0.4% to 0.9% of the population and are composed of thin endothelial layers of large capillaries without intervening brain parenchyma.[9, 32–34] They have a propensity to hemorrhage and rehemorrhage. Cavernous malformations can grow through red cell diapedesis and form membranes similar to subdural hematomas. Of all central nervous system cavernomas, 9% to 35% are found in the brainstem.[10, 35, 36]

With the advent of MRI and more sophisticated techniques, cavernous malformations have been diagnosed with increasing frequency. Their radiographic appearance is pathognomonic.[37] In the hyperacute period, hemorrhage is isointense with brain tissue on T1-weighted images with a short TR (repetition time) and hypointense on T2-weighted images with a long TR/TE (echo delay). Subacute hematomas (3 weeks to several months old) have a classic salt-and-pepper appearance. They are characterized by a hyperintense center (methemoglobin) on both T1-weighted (Fig. 138–1) and T2-weighted images and a hypointense surrounding rim of hemosiderin, especially on the latter images. Gradient-echo images in particular can be used to screen for small occult lesions (Fig. 138–2).[38]

In our experience, cavernous malformations are always associated with venous anomalies. The latter may manifest as classic venous malformations with the characteristic caput medusae appearance or as smaller, radiographically occult anomalies seen only at surgery. In fact, venous anomalies likely play a role in the genesis and recurrence of cavernomas.

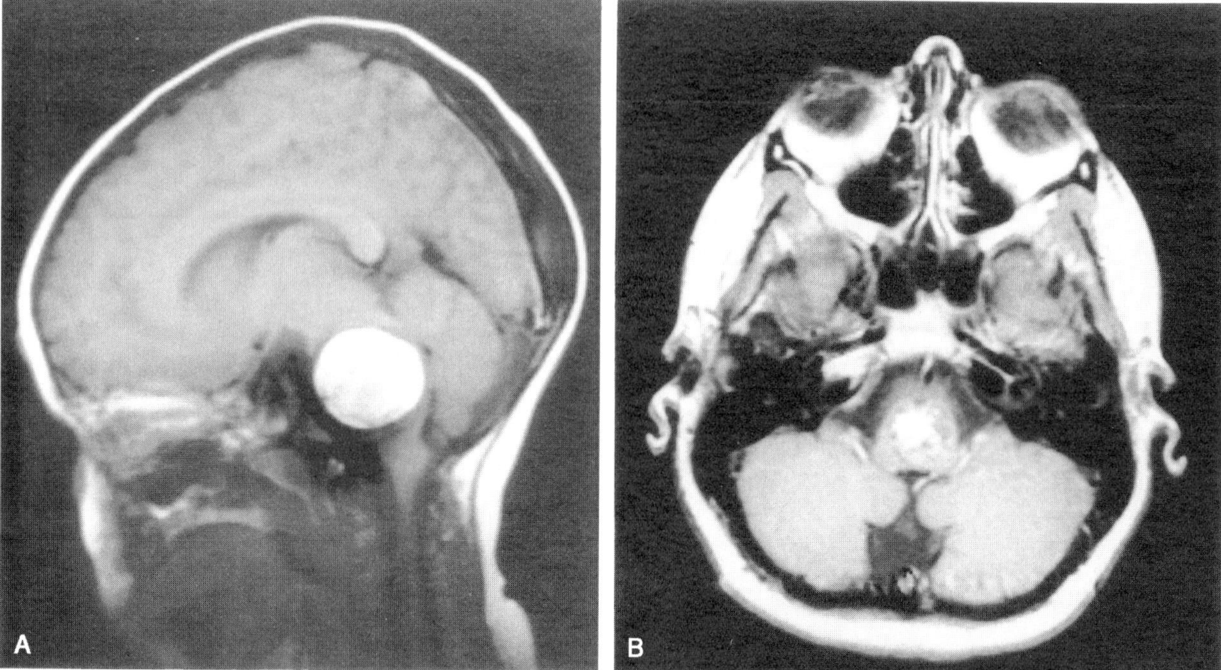

FIGURE 138–1. *A*, Sagittal T1-weighted magnetic resonance imaging (MRI) scan reveals a massive hemorrhage within the substance of the pons with a homogeneous hyperintense signal compatible with subacute blood products. *B*, Axial T1-weighted MRI scan from a 16-year-old girl with heterogeneous blood products from hemorrhages of different ages within the cavernous malformation of the medulla.

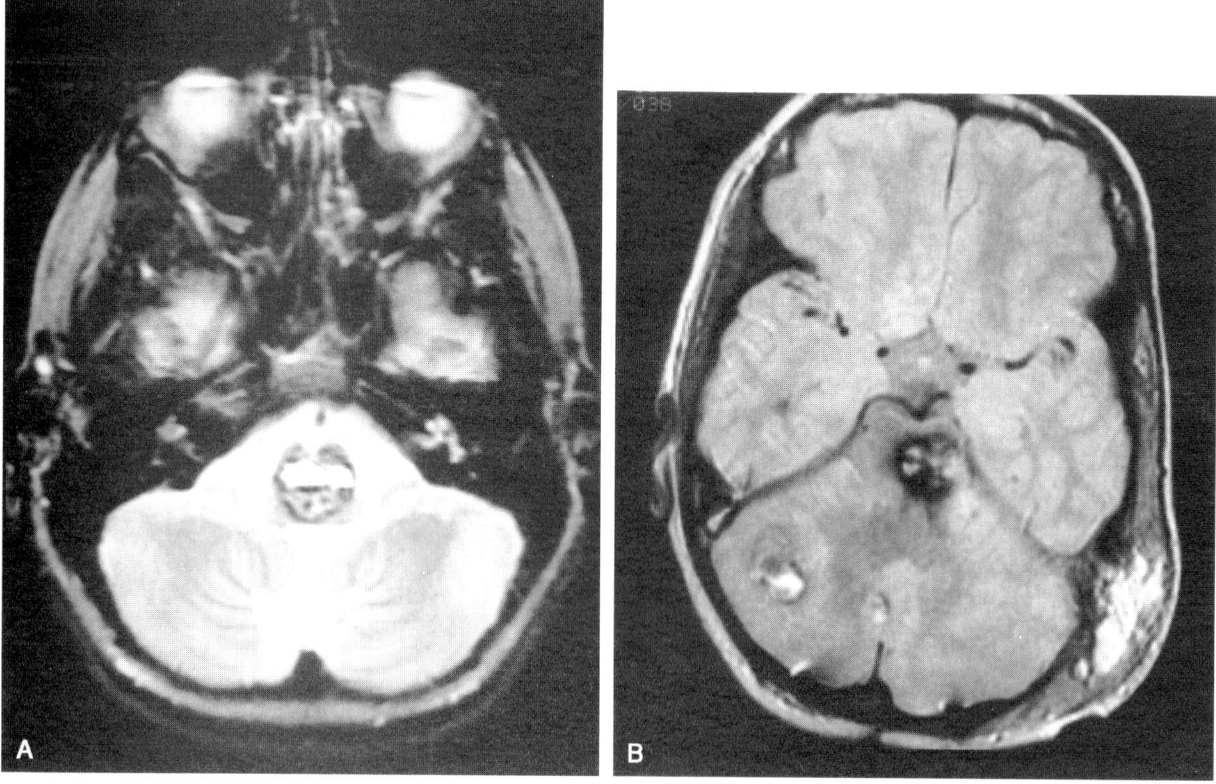

FIGURE 138–2. *A*, T2-weighted magnetic resonance imaging scan reveals various intensities of blood products with layers of fluid within the center of the medulla, consistent with new and old hemorrhage. *B*, Gradient-echo sequencing reveals multiple cavernous malformations with hypointense rims of surrounding hemosiderin.

TABLE 138–1 ■ **Surgical Series of Cavernous Malformations of the Brainstem**

AUTHOR	NO. OF PATIENTS	
	Total	Surgically Treated
Porter et al, 1999[28]	100	86
Sathi et al, 1996[25]	50	23
Zimmerman et al, 1991[18]	24	16
Fahlbusch et al, 1990[16]	20	10
Bertalanffy et al, 1991[14]	15	13
Fritschi et al, 1994[35]	15	9
Amin-Hanjani et al, 1998[27]	14	14

Modified from Porter RW, Detwiler PW, Spetzler RF, et al: Cavernous malformations of the brainstem: Experience with 100 patients. J Neurosurg 90:50–58, 1999.

Few large clinical series of brainstem cavernous malformations exist, and fewer than 300 cases have been reported (Table 138–1).[14, 18, 25, 27, 28, 35] Thus, their natural history remains poorly defined. Brainstem cavernous malformations may be found incidentally, or they can manifest with severe neurological deficits.[35] Although histologically benign, brainstem cavernous malformations can cause devastating neurological consequences or death. The most common symptoms, however, include multiple neurological deficits, depending on the presence of an expanding hemorrhage or the lesion's location. Constitutional symptoms such as headache, nausea, and vomiting are also common. Hemorrhage usually causes the acute onset of symptoms, but slowly expansile lesions may cause neurological deficits to worsen gradually. Clinically, these patients may appear to have brainstem stroke, tumor, or infection. Alternatively, the waxing and waning of the symptoms can mimic multiple sclerosis.

Kondziolka and coworkers[36] reported prospective hemorrhage and rehemorrhage rates of 2.4% and 5% per year, respectively. In our institutional retrospective review, hemorrhage and rehemorrhage rates were 5% and 30%, respectively.[28] The timing of a subsequent hemorrhage, however, is impossible to predict. The interval between hemorrhages has ranged from hours to 17 years.[28] With each hemorrhage, symptoms tend to worsen and then improve, but less so after each incident. After one hemorrhage, the likelihood of a subsequent hemorrhage is substantially higher than in patients with silent lesions.[12, 20, 35, 36] Further, the lesion's location appears to affect the risk of symptomatic hemorrhage; the hemorrhage rate of infratentorial lesions may be 30 times that of lesions in the supratentorial compartment.[39]

The risk of hemorrhage is affected by how *hemorrhage* is defined. We define a hemorrhagic episode as a clinical history of an apoplectic episode or evidence of subacute or acute blood production on computed tomography or MRI. The characteristic hypointense ring seen on T2-weighted MRI, however, is due to hemosiderin and does not, in our opinion, define an acute hemorrhagic episode.

SURGICAL INDICATIONS

Lesions are considered appropriate for surgical resection if they reach the pial surface, hemorrhage repeatedly with progressive neurological deficits, manifest with acute hemorrhage outside the lesion capsule, or cause significant mass effect from large intralesional hemorrhages (Table 138–2). Typically, we resect only clearly exophytic lesions in this location. In the floor of the fourth ventricle, we recommend avoiding a myelotomy through even the thinnest amount of tissue. The thickness of the rim is best ascertained on T1-weighted MRI (Fig. 138–3). Lesions that clearly reach the pial surface on T1-weighted imaging can be considered for resection.

Patients should not be considered for surgical therapy if they have severe concomitant medical problems or if they have had a single hemorrhagic episode from a lesion that does not reach the pial surface. In our experience, these patients can be followed conservatively until they suffer at least one more hemorrhage. This rule is especially true if even the thinnest rim of tissue in the floor of the fourth ventricle must be traversed. If patients develop fixed deficits after another hemorrhage, surgery should be offered as a treatment option. Conservative therapy, however, is still a reasonable option if the symptoms resolve completely. Such lesions usually rehemorrhage, especially in young patients, and then often reach the pial surface. Once patients have experienced several hemorrhages, they may be more willing to accept the inherent risks associated with brainstem surgery.

To facilitate the removal of acute hemorrhage, we typically wait 3 to 5 days for a hematoma to liquefy. If the patient is deteriorating rapidly, however, the brainstem may need to be decompressed in an emergent fashion. Acute hematomas tend to be tenacious and to require more manipulation of the surrounding parenchyma than do more subacute, yet liquefied, clots.

Unlike most other surgical and medical diseases, children do not always endure surgery on brainstem cavernous malformations better than adults. In our series, 3 of 11 children had worse outcomes than adults.[28] Given the small number of cases, however, the significance of this outcome is difficult to determine. Pediatric lesions are considered for resection only after multiple episodes of hemorrhage.

TABLE 138–2 ■ **Surgical Indications for Brainstem Cavernous Malformations**

Exophytic lesions (reaching the pial surface)
Rapid or progressive neurological deterioration
Hemorrhage outside lesion capsule
Significant mass effect
Multiple debilitating hemorrhages

Adapted from Porter RW, Detwiler PW, Spetzler RF: Surgical technique for resection of cavernous malformations of the brain stem. Operative Techn. Neurosurg 3:124–130, 2000.

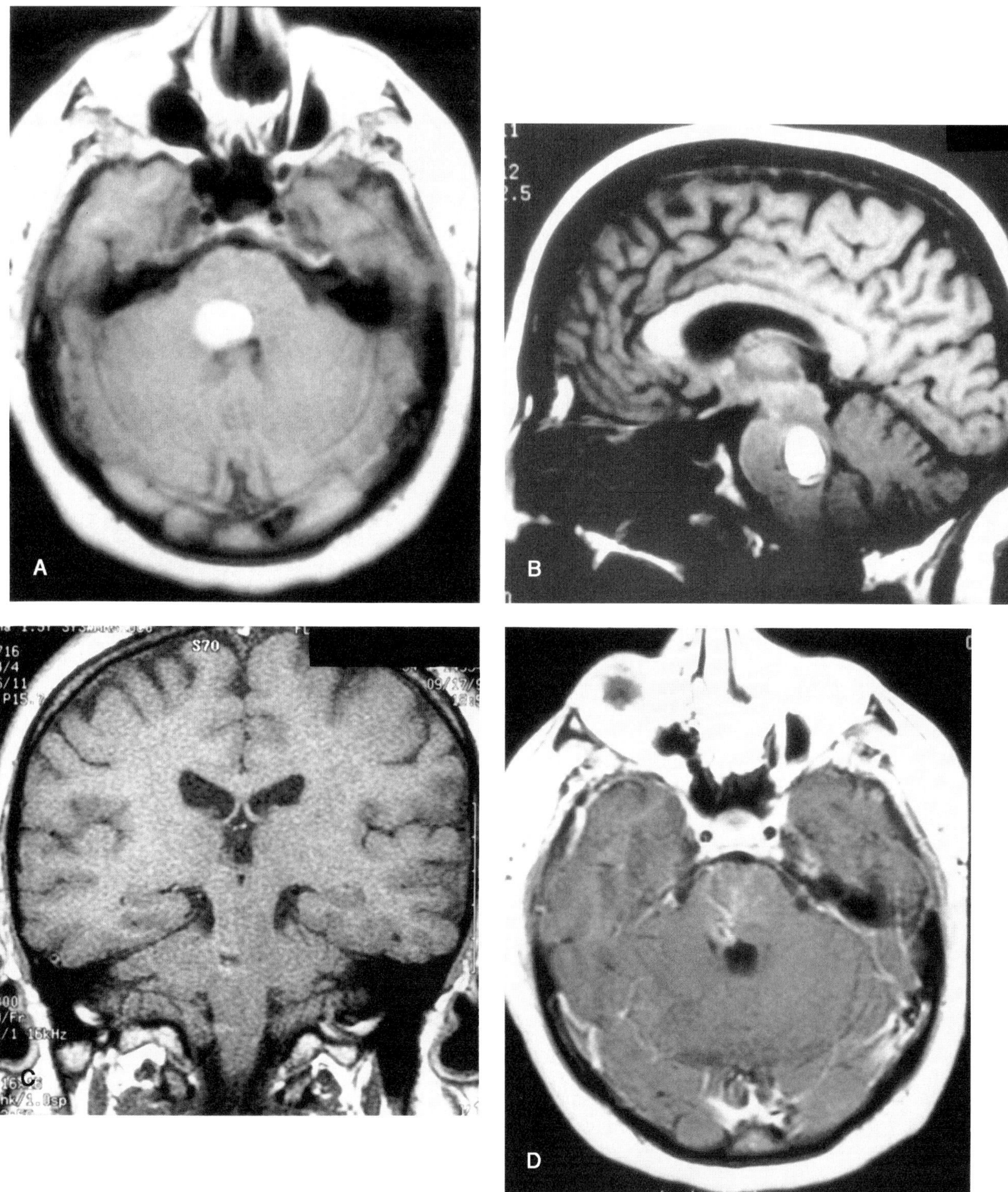

FIGURE 138–3. A 32-year-old Hispanic woman presented with left body numbness, dysmetria, and ataxia. Axial *(A)* and sagittal *(B)* T1-weighted magnetic resonance imaging (MRI) scans revealed a cavernoma of the pons that reached the surface of the floor of the fourth ventricle. The lesion was resected through a suboccipital approach. Coronal *(C)* and axial *(D)* MRI scans 2 years later reveal no recurrence and preservation of the venous anomaly. (From Porter RW, Detwiler PW, Spetzler RF: Surgical technique for resection of cavernous malformations of the brain stem. Operative Techn Neurosurg 3:124–130, 2000.)

OPERATIVE PROCEDURE

Preoperative Considerations

The goals of surgery are to minimize the amount of normal brainstem tissue traversed while completely excising the lesion and to preserve an associated venous anomaly or malformation. If a large venous malformation is occluded, venous infarction may result.[40]

Once the decision to operate has been made, obtaining preoperative consent can be as important as surgical technique. Patients should be educated that their deficits are likely to worsen after surgery but then typically improve over time. They should be told that the surgical experience is similar to having another hemorrhage. They should also be warned that a tracheostomy or feeding tube may be necessary on a short-term basis and that a moderate course of rehabilitation will likely be necessary. Such information eases patients' anxiety and provides them with realistic expectations about the process.

To determine the best surgical approach, we use the "two-point method."[41] One point is placed in the center of the lesion, and a second is placed where the lesion most closely reaches the pial surface. The two points are connected, and the resultant straight line through the least eloquent tissue dictates the most appropriate surgical approach (Fig. 138–4). Preoperative permanent neurological deficits, such as seventh or eighth cranial nerve palsies, can also influence the choice of approach. Such deficits, for example, may make a translabyrinthine or transcochlear approach more attractive.

Preoperative and intraoperative MRI with frameless stereotactic guidance is an invaluable tool. We use the Elekta View scope (Medtronics, Minneapolis, MN), a frameless stereotactic system that tracks the surgeon's focal point with respect to the lesion's location and operative trajectory.

Intraoperative Monitoring

Intraoperative monitoring during brainstem surgery is a valuable adjunct to help minimize complications. At our institution, somatosensory evoked potentials (SEPs), compressed spectral analysis or electroencepha-

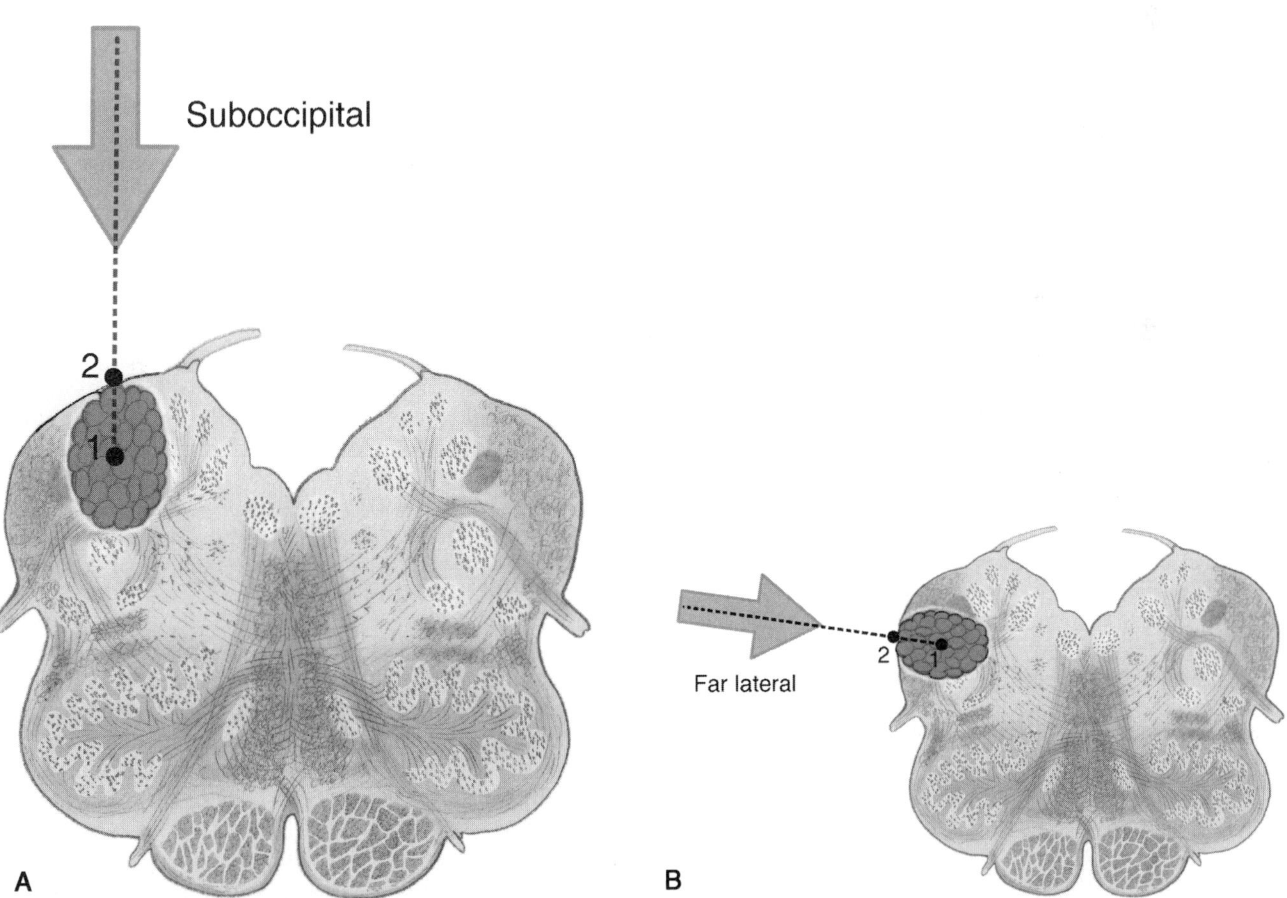

FIGURE 138–4. Artist's rendition of the "two-point" method applied to medullary cavernous malformations in similar locations. The first point is placed in the center of the lesion (1), and the second is placed at the point where the lesion comes closest to the surface (2). A line connecting the two points determines the optimal approach. These two lesions require different surgical approaches, the suboccipital *(A)* and the far-lateral *(B)*, because the points where they reach the surface are different. (From Porter RW, Detwiler PW, Spetzler RF: Surgical technique for resection of cavernous malformations of the brain stem. Operative Techn Neurosurg 3:124–130, 2000.)

lography, and BAERs are monitored routinely. These monitoring techniques should be applied *before* and *after* positioning, because excessive flexion or rotation of the neck can cause disastrous outcomes such as vascular compression, brachial plexopathy, spinal cord injury in the presence of spondylosis, or excessive venous pressure.

Although these techniques provide continual feedback, postoperative neurological deficits are not always preceded by a change in the recorded waveforms, and false negatives can occur.[42] Consequently, the pathway being monitored must be relevant to the operation. Baseline recordings are useful so that a change can be evaluated as a relative rather than an absolute change. The surgeon can then make adjustments accordingly.

BAERs are central signals as they relate to the cochlear nucleus and can be monitored during surgery on an intrinsic pontine lesion. Intraoperative changes in wave latencies suggest an interruption in the auditory pathways. BAERs, however, reflect only the auditory pathways; they do not reflect global brainstem function. Thus, damage to motor or other cranial nerve nuclei can go undetected. When the floor of the fourth ventricle is involved, the facial colliculus can be stimulated to localize it accurately and to minimize the chance of embarrassing the function of the seventh or eighth cranial nerve.[43–46] Disciplined and meticulous surgical technique is the best means of avoiding postoperative deficits.[47]

Surgical Technique

If intrinsic lesions fail to reach the pial surface, normal brainstem tissue will be violated during surgery. In this case, an opening is made using hemosiderin staining or a bulge in the brainstem as a guide. In addition, the two-point method must be applied in conjunction with frameless stereotactic guidance. In contrast, exophytic lesions are readily apparent, assuming the correct surgical approach was chosen. Lesions usually have the characteristic "mulberry" appearance with a thin layer of arachnoid (Fig. 138–5).

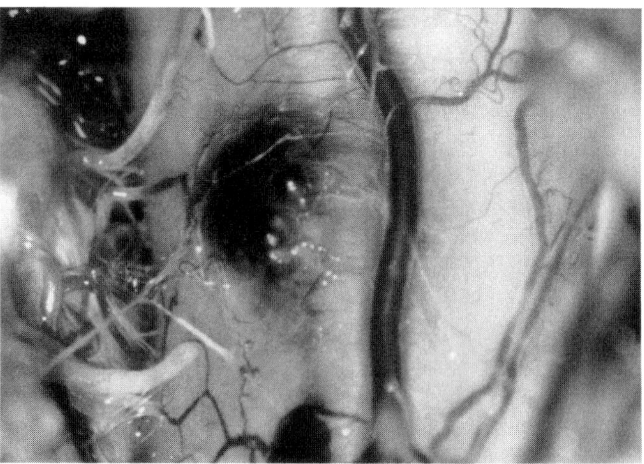

FIGURE 138–5. Exophytic cavernoma of the medulla with the classic "mulberry" appearance. A concomitant associated venous malformation is present to the right of the lesion. (From Porter RW, Detwiler PW, Spetzler RF: Surgical technique for resection of cavernous malformations of the brain stem. Operative Techn Neurosurg 3:124–130, 2000.)

The lesion can be entered with bipolar cauterization. Acute, subacute, and chronic blood products can be suctioned. The capillary network or hemangiomatous portion can then be gently dissected with microdissectors while the surrounding parenchyma is preserved. Microscissors may be necessary to detach the lesion from surrounding tissue. During dissection, the surgeon should be mindful of the ubiquitous venous anomaly (Fig. 138–6). If a large, associated venous malformation is entered and coagulated, venous infarction and a devastating outcome can result.[28] Smaller venous tributaries, however, can usually be coagulated and transected with impunity. If the surgeon is unsure of their significance, associated veins within the resection cavity should be preserved.

Because of the small size of the opening made in the brainstem to access the lesion, it can be very difficult to determine whether the cavernoma has been completely resected, given the depth and darkness of the cavity. Again, the use of frameless stereotaxy with a state-of-the-art microscope is essential to maximize the chance of complete removal. Despite the availability of these contemporary techniques, however, the surgeon cannot always be certain that the lesion has been resected completely without causing damage to surrounding structures. Thus, it is preferable to err on the side of caution, performing a conservative curettage and assessing the resection with postoperative MRI. It is always better to stage a procedure rather than risk the patient's neurological function.

Postoperative Management

Typically, patients are left intubated for 24 hours after surgery. They are extubated only after they demonstrate a good cough and gag reflex in the intensive care unit. Evaluation of postoperative swallowing is recommended in patients whose function could be at risk owing to the lesion's location. Short-term (months) tracheostomy or feeding tubes should be placed when these functions appear to be less than optimal. This need should not be interpreted as a treatment failure, because few patients require these adjuncts on a long-term basis.[28] If patients are warned of the potential need preoperatively, they tend to accept these procedures more readily after surgery.

If the patient is stable, MRI is usually obtained on postoperative day 1 to assess for the presence of residual lesion and to serve as a baseline for comparing future studies. Hemosiderin staining makes assessing the extent of resection difficult. Consequently, follow-up imaging should be obtained annually for the first few years to monitor for progression or recurrence.

Despite postoperative MRI scans consistent with a radiographic cure, recurrence rates can be as high as 5%,[28] and the physician should always be suspicious of residual lesions. However, venous malformations associated with hemosiderin staining can mimic cavernomas. Further, even patients who have had "com-

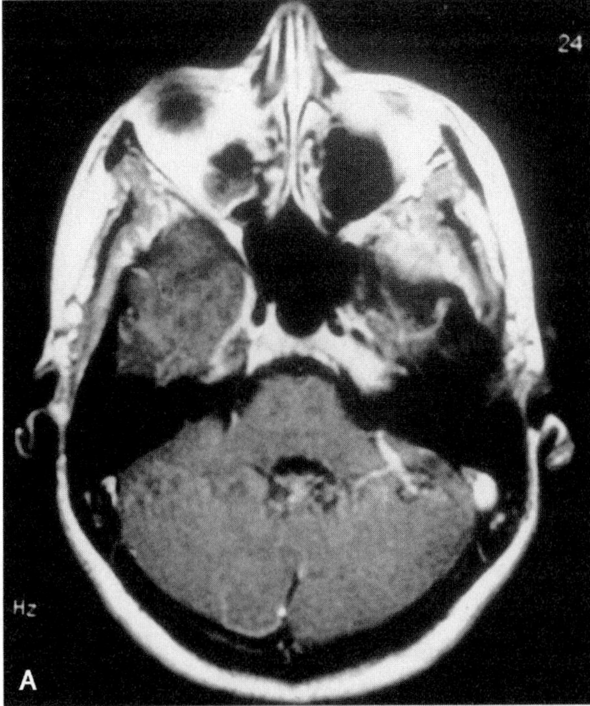

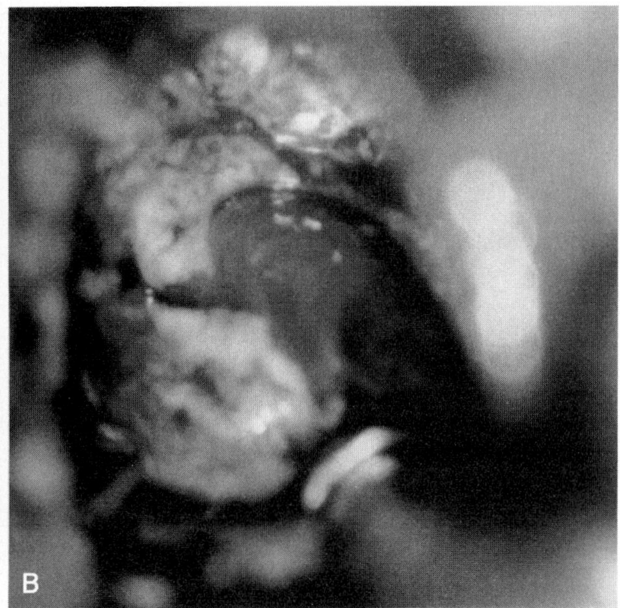

FIGURE 138–6. A 24-year-old woman presented with nystagmus, ataxia, and oscillopsia. Magnetic resonance imaging scan *(A)* and intraoperative photograph *(B)* show the associated venous malformation. (From Porter RW, Detwiler PW, Spetzler RF: Surgical technique for resection of cavernous malformations of the brain stem. Operative Techn Neurosurg 3:124–130, 2000.)

plete" resections can develop a recurrence years later.[28] This trend may reflect the presence of an unrecognized residual lesion at surgery or a de novo lesion that developed as a result of an associated venous anomaly. A careful, annual clinical and radiographic follow-up should be instituted for all patients. Symptomatic patients may need to be evaluated more frequently. If patients are symptom free and the MRI scan is negative, the follow-up intervals can be increased at the surgeon's discretion.

SURGICAL APPROACHES

The suboccipital, orbitozygomatic, retrosigmoid, far-lateral, and infratentorial-supracerebellar approaches are reviewed here. The petrosal approaches are reviewed elsewhere in this textbook. Overall, such approaches provide access to the pons, with anterior access increasing as more bone is removed. The subtemporal approach is rarely used alone; it is usually combined with the orbitozygomatic osteotomy to access the lateral midbrain. The combined approach, also reviewed elsewhere in this text, provides access to lesions of the midbrain and pontomesencephalic junction that extend above and below the tentorium (Fig. 138–7). This latter approach is being used with less frequency at our institution.

Suboccipital Approach

In this approach, the patient is placed prone on chest rolls or a laminectomy frame, and the neck is flexed to open the space between the foramen magnum and C1. After a strip shave, a midline skin incision is made extending from approximately C3 to the inion. The fascia is opened, producing a Y-shaped cuff with its base attached to the inion. This technique helps identify the avascular midline plane between the semispinalis capitis, trapezius, and splenius capitis muscles and provides a watertight fascial closure at the end of the procedure. The posterior cervical musculature is elevated from the suboccipital bone using subperiosteal dissection and retracted laterally with fishhooks (Fig. 138–8). A suboccipital craniotomy is fashioned using the Midas Rex drill (Medtronics, Midas Rex, Fort Worth, TX) with a B1 bit and footplate. A bur hole can be made over the cerebellar hemisphere. Alternatively, the footplate can be placed under the foramen magnum. The dura is opened in a Y-shaped fashion, with its base along the torcular (Fig. 138–9). Using the suboccipital approach, the surgeon can reach the posterior cervicomedullary junction inferiorly, the midline floor of the fourth ventricle, and the medial aspect of the middle cerebellar peduncle. Lesions of the posterior midbrain can also be accessed by splitting the superior cerebellar vermis or superior medullary velum or by the supracerebellar-infratentorial approach.

If a lesion is to be approached through the floor of the fourth ventricle, the location of cranial nerve nuclei becomes relevant. In 1993, Kyoshima and coauthors[44] described "safe entry zones" above and below the facial colliculus. Bogucki and colleagues[48] later modified the zones to access intrapontine lesions. The *infrafacial* zone has a line 2 mm lateral to the median sulcus on its

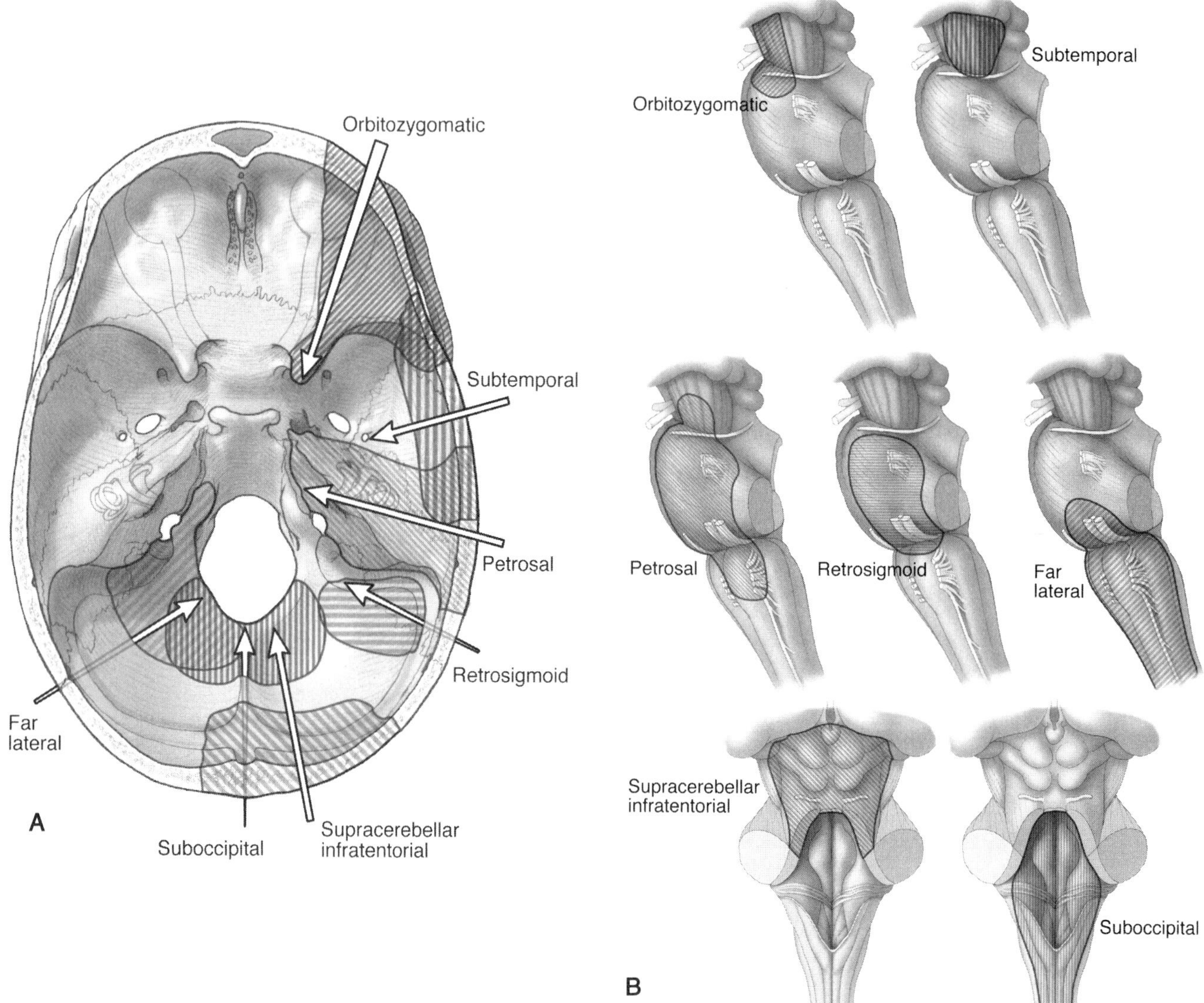

FIGURE 138–7. *A*, Axial illustration of the skull base depicting the extent of bone removal required by each approach. *B*, Lateral and posterior views of the brainstem showing the various skull base approaches used to access the corresponding shaded areas of the brainstem. (From Porter RW, Detwiler PW, Spetzler RF: Surgical approaches to the brain stem. Operative Techn Neurosurg 3: 114–123, 2000.)

medial border, the hypoglossal triangle on its inferior border, the facial colliculus on its superior border, and the vestibular area laterally. The *suprafacial* zone has the following boundaries: laterally, the superior cerebellar peduncle; medially, a vertical line 2 mm lateral to the median sulcus; superiorly, the frenulum veli; and inferiorly, the facial colliculus.[48] Tumors, however, can distort normal anatomy, obscuring these landmarks. In such cases, the facial colliculus can be stimulated directly while the facial nerve is monitored.

At the end of the case, the dura and fascia are closed in layers, and the bone flap is replaced. Fibrin glue can be used on the dural suture line and bone cement in the craniotomy defect to minimize the chance of a cerebrospinal fluid (CSF) leak. It is useful to release the head holder during fascial and muscle closure, because significant spasms can occur, precluding adequate reapproximation of the suboccipital musculature to the occiput.

Orbitozygomatic Approach

The orbitozygomatic approach is used to access the anterior and lateral midbrain, interpeduncular region, rostral pons, pontomesencephalic junction, and caudal to mid–third ventricle.[49–51] In 1986, Hakuba and associates[50] first described this approach for lesions of the parasellar region, interpeduncular fossa, medial sphenoid wing, Meckel's cave, and basilar tip. The main advantage is that it permits downward retraction of the globe of the eye to gain an upward and oblique view of the interpeduncular fossa and third ventricle. The technique, as performed at our institution, has been detailed elsewhere[51] and is reviewed here briefly.

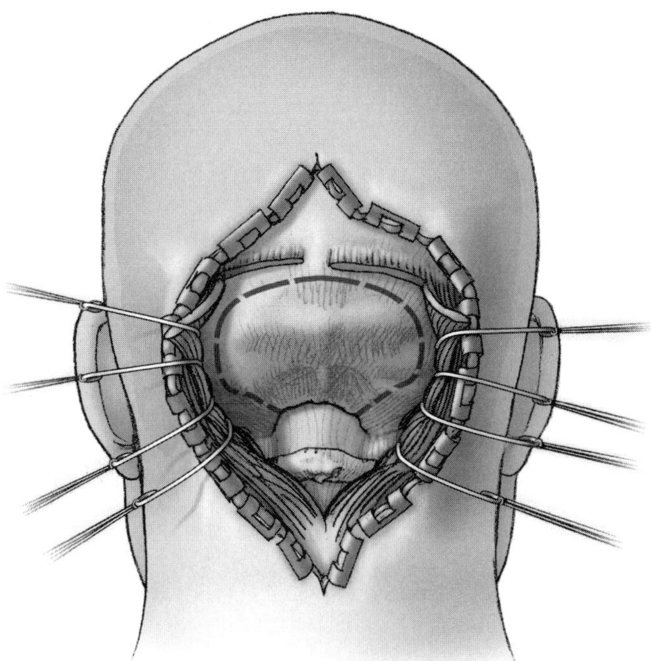

FIGURE 138–8. Extent of the craniotomy required for the suboccipital approach. Fishhooks, rather than traditional retractors, are used for muscle retraction to bring the surgeon's hands closer to the operative field. (From Porter RW, Detwiler PW, Spetzler RF: Surgical approaches to the brain stem. Operative Techn Neurosurg 3:114–123, 2000.)

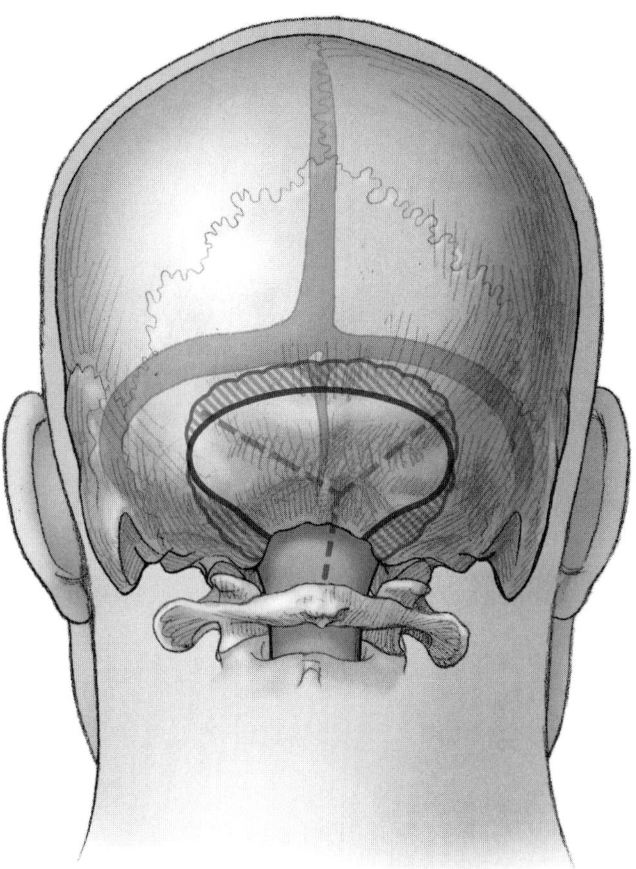

FIGURE 138–9. The dura is opened using a Y-shaped configuration. The inferior limb of the incision is just off the midline to avoid the occipital sinus and to ensure that it is crossed only once. (From Porter RW, Detwiler PW, Spetzler RF: Surgical approaches to the brain stem. Operative Techn Neurosurg 3:114–123, 2000.)

The patient is positioned supine with the head rotated 30 to 60 degrees. Less rotation provides access to lesions of the posterior fossa. Slight extension of the neck, so that the malar eminence is the most superior point of the operative field, causes the frontal lobe to fall away from the anterior cranial fossa.[49] The scalp incision extends from the root of the zygoma, 1 cm anterior to the tragus, to the midline or medial contralateral line. Alternatively, a bicoronal skin incision can be used.[50] A vascularized pericranial flap should be preserved during the opening for use at the end of the procedure to isolate the exenterated frontal sinus should it be violated during the osteotomy. The temporalis fascia is incised along the posterior border of the skin incision and extended anteriorly just below the superior temporal line.

A dissection plane is then developed between the temporalis fascia and muscle, below the second fat pad. Next, the frontozygomatic and temporal zygomatic processes and superior orbital rim are exposed by elevating the temporalis fascia off the respective bony surfaces with a periosteal elevator. The periorbita is freed from within the orbit with a curet, and thin Telfa (Johnson & Johnson, Raynham, MA) strips are left in place to protect the periorbita. The elevator should not be passed too deeply toward the cone of the orbit, because the optic nerve can be damaged. After the temporalis muscle is elevated and retracted from the squamous temporal bone, a standard pterional craniotomy is performed, followed by the orbitozygomatic osteotomy. Peripheral tack-up holes are drilled around the craniotomy, and sutures are placed. The temporalis muscle is again released and placed over the craniectomy defect in preparation for the orbitozygomatic osteotomy.

An oscillating saw is used to make six osteotomies (Fig. 138–10). The first osteotomy is made at the base of the zygoma by placing the saw on the zygomatic root just above the temporalis muscle. The blade is oriented anteriorly, medially, and obliquely. It must not be placed too deep, to avoid violating the capsule of the temporomandibular joint. The second cut begins just anterior and inferior to the temporal process of the zygomatic bone and proceeds laterally to medially while directed slightly inferiorly. It stops in the midportion of the malar eminence at the zygomaticofacial foramen, which is connected with the third cut. This latter cut extends from the inferior orbital fissure within the orbit through the orbital surface of the temporal bone, connecting the second cut at an apex. The inferior orbital fissure can first be identified with a No. 4 Penfield dissector, after which the tip of the saw can be placed. An inverted V is thus created on the malar eminence; the left and right links are the second and third cuts, respectively. The fourth cut extends through

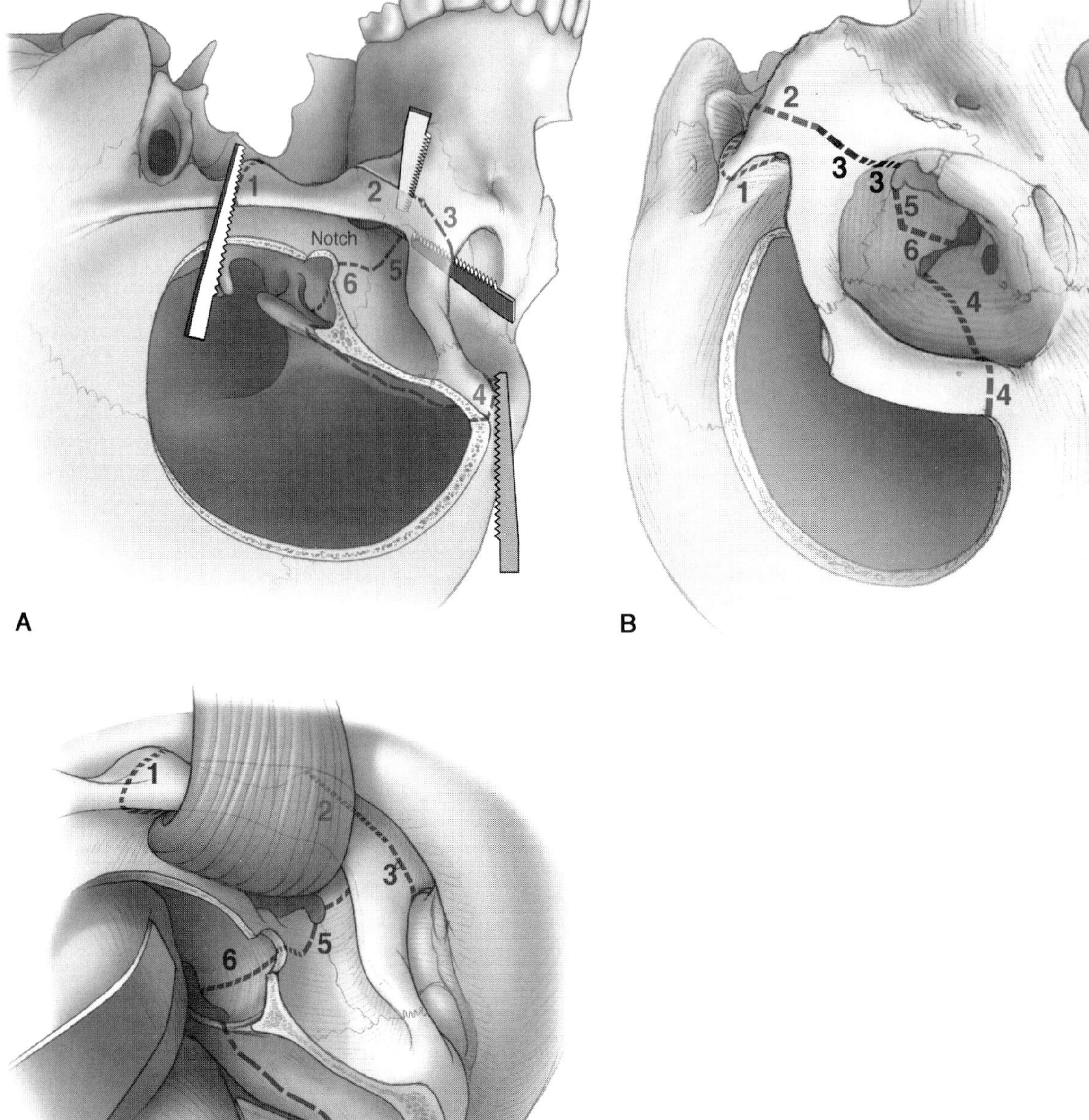

FIGURE 138–10. *A*, Lateral view of the osteotomies required for an orbitozygomatic approach. An anterior subtemporal notch can be made to facilitate a connection between the fifth and sixth cuts. *B*, Intraorbital perspective shows the osteotomies required. *C*, The fourth, fifth, and sixth osteotomies are depicted. A residual bony island can be left after the last cut is made and removed with a rongeur. (From Porter RW, Detwiler PW, Spetzler RF: Surgical approaches to the brain stem. Operative Techn Neurosurg 3:114–123, 2000.)

the orbital surface of the frontal bone posteriorly toward the superior orbital fissure. If more medial access is required, the supraorbital nerve can be mobilized from its foramen using an osteotome. If the foramen is high above the orbital rim, the nerve can be sacrificed, but forehead numbness will result. The fifth cut is made from outside the lateral orbital wall. It extends posteriorly from the inferior orbital fissure across the greater wing of the sphenoid bone and through the posterior orbit. The final (sixth) cut extends from the fifth cut to the superior orbital fissure. Alternatively, it can connect the fourth and fifth cuts just proximal to the superior orbital fissure. A rongeur can be used to remove the residual bony island of the greater wing of the sphenoid until the dural fold of the superior orbital fissure is identified.

To ensure precise reapproximation at closure, cranial fixation plate holes can be drilled before the osteotomy is removed. Typically, 1.5-mm or smaller cranial fixation plates are used. The dural opening extends from the medial superior orbital margin to the temporal tip in a semilunar fashion. It is tacked anteroinferiorly, which permits downward retraction of the globe. Tacking sutures are placed deep toward the orbital apex and anchored around the secure fishhooks. The operative microscope is then brought into the field, and a trans-sylvian or subtemporal approach is undertaken in an atraumatic fashion. The uncus can be retracted posteriorly, allowing access to Liliquest's membrane and the interpeduncular fossa. The working distance to lesions in the parasellar region and the interpeduncular fossa is about 3 cm shorter with an orbitozygomatic approach than with a standard frontotemporal approach.[50] A more upward and oblique view of the sylvian fissure, third ventricle, and upper brainstem can be achieved (Fig. 138–11), with less retraction on the temporal and frontal lobes.[50] We have used fast-absorbing Vicryl sutures (Ethicon, Johnson & Johnson Professionals, Inc., Somerville, NJ) in a running fashion to close the skin. This white suture does not require removal and simply disintegrates in about 2 weeks.

Patients should be forewarned of significant postoperative periorbital edema and diplopia, which usually resolves within a week. They should begin jaw exercises on postoperative day 1 to avoid restricted range of motion at the temporomandibular joint due to scarring of the temporomandibular ligament and joint capsule. Complications can include temporary or permanent paresis of the frontalis muscle, temporary orbital swelling, enophthalmos of an entrapped globe, cranial neuropathy, and CSF leakage. Cosmetic results are usually good or excellent. Atrophy of the temporalis muscle can be minimized by using monopolar cauterization judiciously and by reapproximating the superior aspect of the temporalis muscle to a small muscle cuff of fascia left along the superior temporal line.

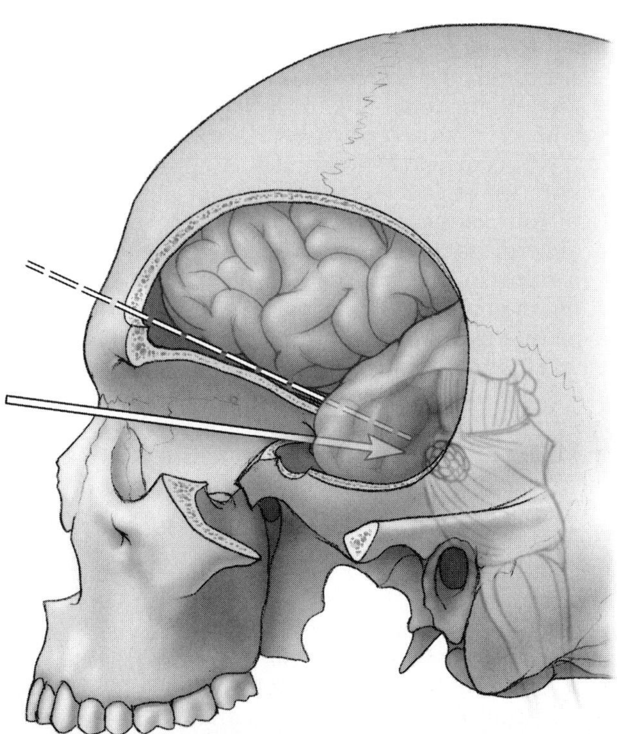

FIGURE 138–11. A flatter view to the brainstem can be achieved after the orbital roof is removed and the globe is retracted inferiorly. (From Porter RW, Detwiler PW, Spetzler RF: Surgical approaches to the brain stem. Operative Techn Neurosurg 3:114–123, 2000.)

Retrosigmoid Approach

The retrosigmoid approach offers access to the posterolateral pons, lateral middle cerebellar peduncle, superior lateral medulla, and cerebellopontine angle. The patient can be positioned lateral, prone, or supine with a sandbag beneath the ipsilateral shoulder. In the supine position, the head is turned flat, parallel with the floor, and the neck is flexed such that a finger can be placed between the mandible and clavicle. Excessive rotation or flexion during positioning can cause neurovascular compromise, especially in patients with extracranial carotid disease or degenerative cervical spondylosis. Baseline SEPs should therefore be recorded before and after positioning. If the SEPs change, the patient should be repositioned. Alternatively, the patient can be placed prone or in the lateral decubitus position.

The skin incision starts above the auricle and curves behind the ear inferiorly, 4 to 6 cm behind the mastoid and 6 to 8 cm behind the external auditory canal. Inferiorly, it extends just below the mastoid tip into the sternocleidomastoid muscle. Subperiosteal elevation of the muscle should reveal the digastric groove. If the incision is placed too far anteriorly, the scalp, muscle, and bone obscure visualization of the cerebellopontine angle.

The sinuses can be identified with frameless stereotactic guidance. Surgical judgment should always prevail, because the surgeon should be familiar with surface skull landmarks that approximate the locations of the major sinuses. The asterion is an unreliable external landmark for the transverse-sigmoid junction, but a line drawn from the root of the zygoma to the inion (the superior nuchal line) is a good approximation of the transverse sinus.[52] Typically, the transverse-sigmoid junction is avoided by placing the bur hole below this line or 2 cm below the asterion, two thirds of it behind and one third of it in front of the occipitomastoid suture.[53]

After the bur hole is completed, a craniotomy behind the sigmoid sinus and below the transverse sinuses can be fashioned (Fig. 138–12). The bone up to the transverse and sigmoid sinuses can be rongeured to expose their edges. Alternatively, the mastoid air cells can be drilled directly to expose the sigmoid and transverse sinuses, and then the craniotomy can be performed. A line connecting the junction of the squamosal and parietomastoid sutures to the tip of the mastoid process approximates the course of the descending portion of the sigmoid sinus.[52] The bone over

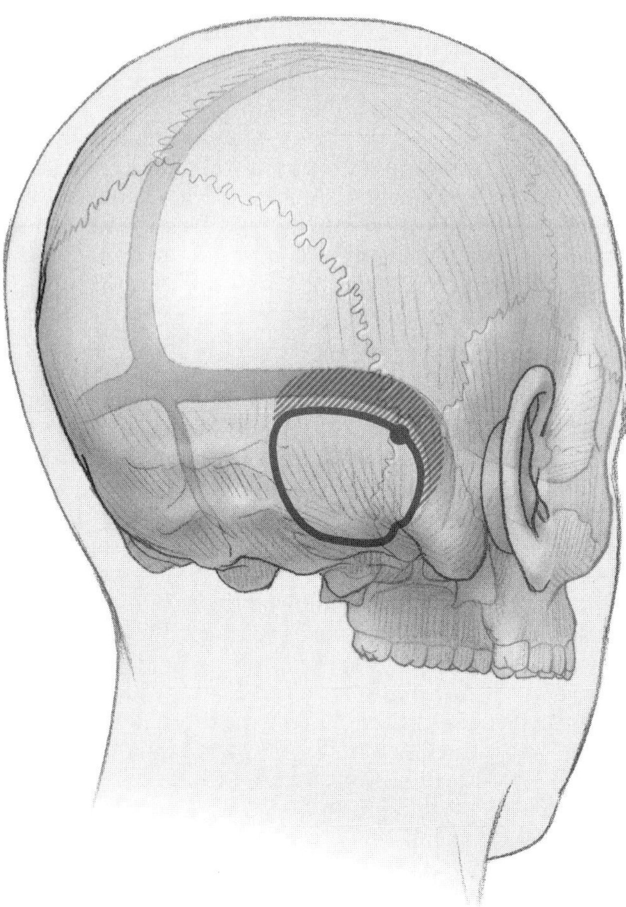

FIGURE 138–12. In the retrosigmoid approach, a bur hole is made at the transverse-sigmoid junction, and the craniotomy is made posterior and inferior to the bur hole. (From Porter RW, Detwiler PW, Spetzler RF: Surgical approaches to the brain stem. Operative Techn Neurosurg 3:114–123, 2000.)

the sigmoid and transverse sinuses can be drilled, first with a cutting bur and then with a diamond bur, leaving a thin shell of inner cortical bone. The remaining thin shell of bone can be removed safely with a Penfield dissector or curet. If the sinus is entered during drilling, Gelfoam (Upjohn, Kalamazoo, MI) or Nu-Knit gauze (Johnson & Johnson, Arlington, TX) should be laid on top of the hole, but not inserted into it, followed by a cottonoid. Mastoid air cells violated during the exposure should be obliterated with bone wax to avoid CSF leakage.

To relax the cerebellum, some surgeons prefer to place a lumbar drain before surgery to release CSF while the dura is opened. Alternatively, a small linear incision, angled in the direction of the jugular bulbar, can be made over the cerebellar hemisphere. Strips of Telfa sponge (Kendall, Mansfield, MA) are placed on top of the hemisphere, and CSF is released after the arachnoid over the cerebellomedullary cistern is opened. Once the dura is opened, CSF must be released quickly, because the cerebellum can "swell," depending on the size of the lesion. After the cerebellum is relaxed, the dural opening is completed in a curvilinear fashion with its base on the transverse-sigmoid junction. For even better exposure, a slit is cut toward the transverse-sigmoid junction. The dura is then tacked up anteriorly in the form of two or three triangles.

Intradurally, the junction of the tentorium and petrous bone at the superior and lateral extents of the dural opening should be visualized.[54] Cranial nerves IV through XI can be identified (Fig. 138–13). If necessary, the petrosal vein can be resected with impunity. Lesions of the lateral pons, lateral cerebellar hemisphere, and pontomedullary junction can be resected through this approach.

The dura is closed primarily or with a dural patch graft. Fibrin glue should be applied to the suture line to prevent CSF leakage, and bone substitute can be used to replace the craniectomized bone. If a patient develops a CSF leak, a lumbar drain is placed for 3 days. If the leak has stopped at that point, the drain is removed. If the CSF leak persists, a lumboperitoneal shunt should be considered, or the patient should be returned to surgery for reclosure and rewaxing of the air cells. More recently, we have successfully applied Tisseal (Baxter Healthcare, Glendale, CA) fibrin glue to the internal auditory canal to treat CSF leaks.

Far-Lateral Approach

The far-lateral or transcondylar approach has several modifications and variations. It basically involves a partial condylectomy, with or without resection of the lateral mass of C1. It allows the surgeon to achieve an anterolateral trajectory to the brainstem, and it eliminates the need to traverse contaminated mucosal structures through the transoral or transfacial route. Thus, the risk of meningitis, CSF leakage, or both can be minimized. First described by Heros[55] and later modified by Spetzler and Grahm,[56] this approach provides access to lesions of the vertebrobasilar junction, inferolateral pons, anterolateral medulla, and upper cervical spinal cord. Its potential disadvantages include craniocervical instability,[57] vertebral artery injury, wound infection, meningitis, or lower cranial nerve deficits.

Various positions, including the modified park-bench, sitting, lateral decubitus, supine with the head rotated, and lateral or half-lateral decubitus, have been used with this approach. At our institution, we prefer a modified park-bench position in which the operating table is extended 10 to 20 cm by placing a rigid plastic board under the mattress (Fig. 138–14). The dependent arm is cradled in a padded sling between the table edge and the Mayfield head holder (Codman, Inc., Raynham, MA).

The clivus is brought perpendicular to the floor by performing four maneuvers on the neck: (1) flexion in the anteroposterior plane until the chin is one fingerbreadth from the clavicle, (2) rotation 45 degrees contralateral to the side of the lesion, (3) lateral flexion 30 degrees down toward the opposite shoulder (also the floor), and (4) slight distraction, increasing the interval between the foramen magnum and C1 so that the surgeon can look down the axis of the brainstem and

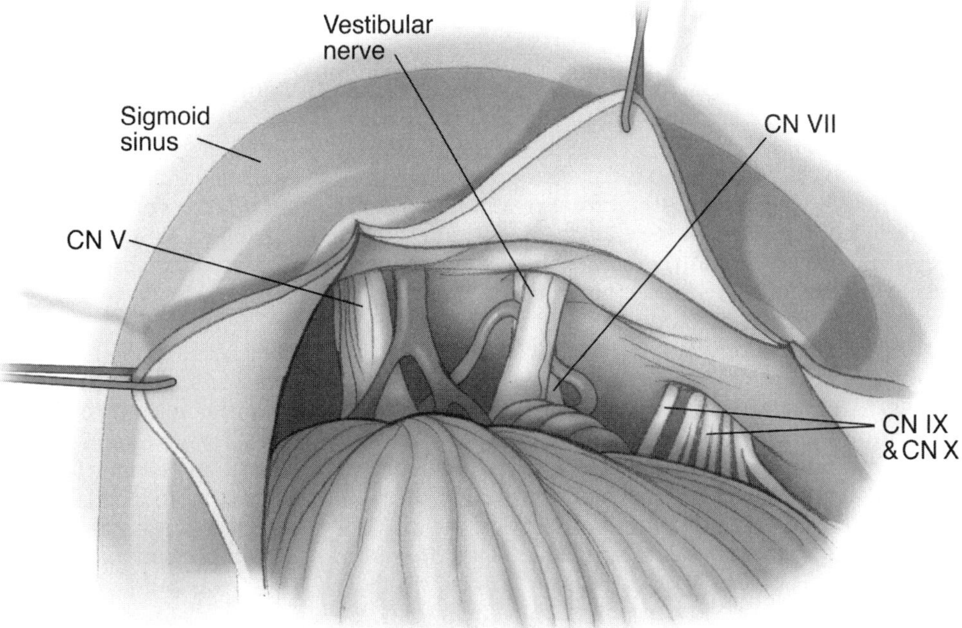

FIGURE 138–13. The structures of the cerebellopontine angle are revealed after the dura is opened during a retrosigmoid approach. CN, cranial nerve. (From Porter RW, Detwiler PW, Spetzler RF: Surgical approaches to the brain stem. Operative Techn Neurosurg 3: 114–123, 2000.)

work between the horizontally oriented cranial nerves. The ipsilateral shoulder should also be retracted inferiorly with cloth tape to allow greater freedom of movement with the microscope (see Fig. 138–14). SEPs should be monitored before and after positioning to avoid a stretch injury to the brachial plexus. The patient should be taped securely to the bed to permit frequent and extreme rotation.

The skin incision begins in the midline at C2 or C3 and proceeds superiorly, curving anteriorly and laterally to the mastoid tip. Monopolar cauterization is used to develop a plane below the superficial muscle fascia. A small muscle cuff is cut and left attached to the superior nuchal line for reapproximation of the fascia and muscles at the end of the procedure. The midline dissection is carried down the avascular ligamentum nuchae, and the muscle flap is reflected inferolaterally with fishhooks and a Leyla bar (Aesculap, San Francisco, CA). Muscle is then stripped off the laminae of C1 and C2 with a Penfield dissector or gauze sponge.

The posterior arch of C1 is removed with a Kerrison rongeur or the drill. The lateral aspect of the ipsilateral C1 posterior arch is further removed with a rongeur to the lateral aspect of the dura. The extradural vertebral artery, which lies on top of the sulcus arteriosus, can be followed into the foramen transversarium with a Woodson or dental instrument. The venous plexus surrounding the artery can be the source of profuse bleeding, which can be controlled with Nu-Knit gauze and bipolar coagulation. The foramen transversarium can

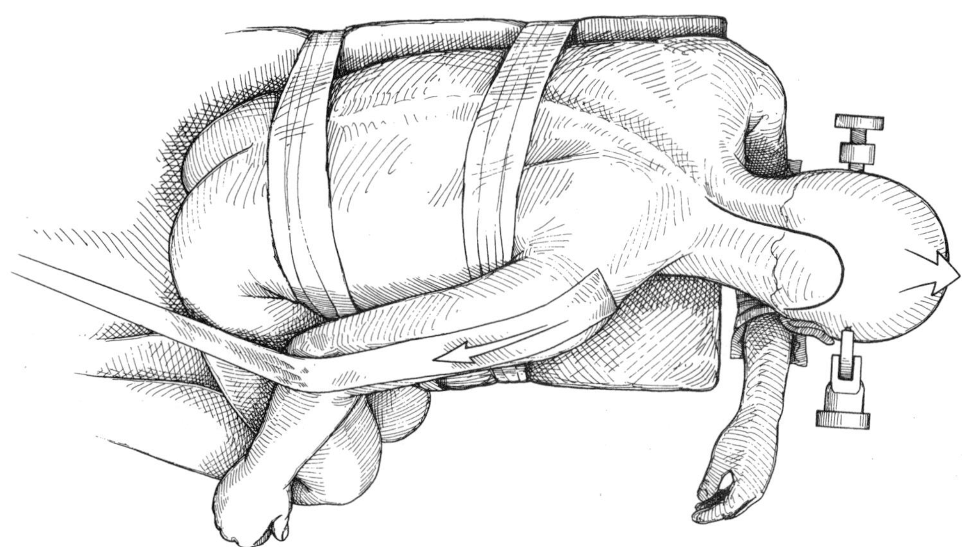

FIGURE 138–14. Patient position and skin incision for the far-lateral approach. A lateral decubitus position is used, with the contralateral arm cradled beyond the edge of the bed. The head is distracted rostrally, and the ipsilateral shoulder is pulled caudally to increase visualization of the clivus. An inverted hockey-stock incision is used. (Courtesy of Barrow Neurological Institute, Phoenix, AZ.)

be unroofed by sliding the footplate of a Kerrison punch into it (Fig. 138–15). Alternatively, a diamond bur can be used to skeletonize the vertebral artery. The C2 nerve root between C1 and C2 should be preserved to avoid occipital numbness. The occipitoatlantal membrane is dissected off the foramen magnum with a curved curet to prepare for the craniotomy.

A lateral suboccipital craniotomy extends from the midline down to the foramen magnum and laterally to the retromastoid region (Fig. 138–16). If the preoperative MRI reveals considerable mass effect, the craniotomy should extend across both cerebellar hemispheres so that the cerebellum has room to swell after the dura is opened. This also allows easier access to the cisterna magna. The lateral foramen magnum is drilled laterally to include the posteromedial one third to one half of the occipital condyle. This maneuver can be performed safely by drilling within the center of the condyle (with a diamond bur) and leaving a thin eggshell of bone that can be removed with rongeurs. The operating microscope provides superior lighting during the drilling process. The condylar emissary vein, when entered, should be expected to produce heavy venous bleeding, but it can be controlled with bone wax, paddies, and Nu-Knit. Visualization of this vein indicates sufficient anterior bony removal. The hypoglossal canal, which should not be seen during the exposure, is situated anterior and medial to the anterior third of the condyle.

The foramen transversarium can be unroofed with a rongeur or diamond bur, and the vertebral artery can be mobilized. The vertebral artery can be retracted medially, and the lateral mass of C1 can also be drilled (Figs. 138–17 and 138–18). The two limbs of the C-shaped dural opening are placed over the upper cervical cord and cerebellum, respectively (Fig. 138–19), to allow a greater anterolateral exposure. The dura is tacked laterally with suture. Initially, the arachnoid is left intact to prevent extradural blood from contaminating the subarachnoid space. Once extradural bleeding is controlled, the arachnoid is opened and tacked to the dural edge with hemoclips.

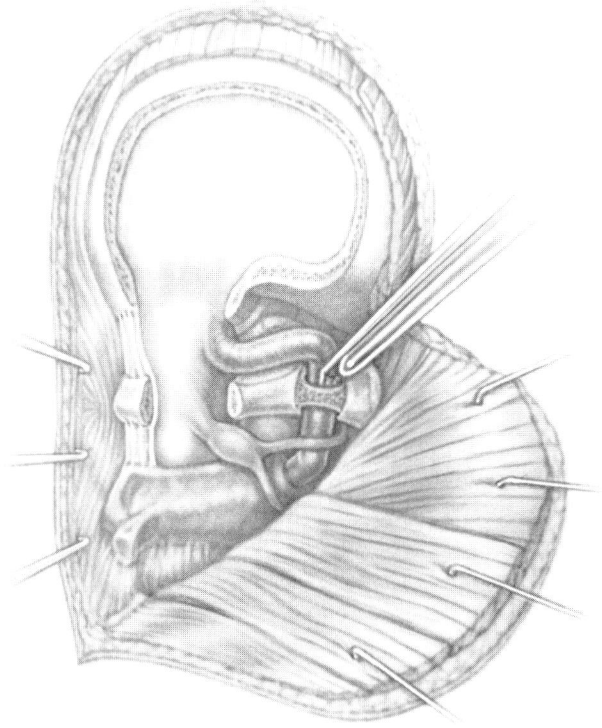

FIGURE 138–15. A Kerrison punch is placed in the foramen transversarium to unroof the vertebral artery. (Courtesy of Barrow Neurological Institute, Phoenix, AZ.)

The medulla, upper cervical cord, and lower cranial nerves can now be visualized. Structures that can be accessed include the cerebellar tonsils; C1 and C2 rootlets; cerebellum; lower pons; cranial nerves IX, X, XI, and XII; vertebral arteries; and ipsilateral posterior inferior cerebellar artery (Fig. 138–20). An extended far-lateral approach, which combines a far-lateral and retrosigmoid approach, provides access to the lower pons and pontomedullary junction in addition to the exposure achieved with the far-lateral approach.

Supracerebellar-Infratentorial Approach

In 1936, Dandy first described a supratentorial parafalcine approach to the pineal-tectal region.[58] He used the semisitting position and in some cases sectioned the corpus callosum, probably damaging the deep galenic venous system with resultant cerebral edema. He lacked the benefit of the operating microscope, MRI, frameless stereotaxy, and advanced neuroanesthetic techniques. Thus, not surprisingly, complication rates were high. As techniques evolved, it became apparent that the infratentorial route would more safely access the same area by dissecting below the galenic venous system.

This approach was initially described by Krause[59] and later popularized by Stein.[60] The supracerebellar-infratentorial approach permits exposure of malformations involving the midline tectal and pineal regions. Positioning is the same as for the suboccipital approach, but the angle of the tentorium must be considered. In the ideal position, the tentorium is perpendicular to the floor. This positioning can be checked preoperatively with frameless stereotactic guidance. The craniotomy should extend above and below the transverse sinus to expose the transverse sinus–torcular junction (Fig. 138–21). This craniotomy permits greater retraction of the tentorium superiorly compared with a pure suboccipital craniotomy. It can be performed safely by placing a single bur hole lateral to the superior sagittal sinus using the equivalent of the Midas Rex (Medtronic Midas Rex, Fort Worth, TX) footplate and drill bit. Before the sinus is crossed, the surgeon should reverse the footplate and irrigate through the craniotomy line to confirm that the plate is extradural.

The dura is opened in an inverted V shape with the base on the edge of the transverse sinuses. Bridging veins from the superior aspect of the cerebellum that drain into the transverse sinus are coagulated and divided to permit downward retraction of the cerebellum. If these veins are not coagulated early in the

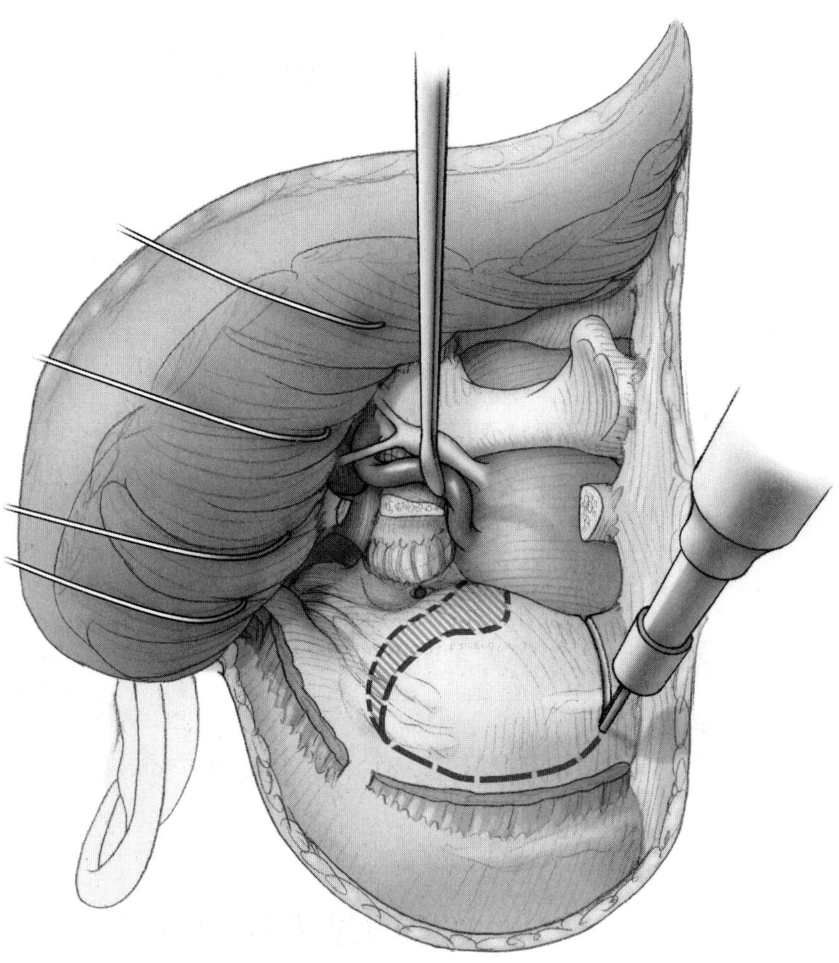

FIGURE 138–16. The craniotomy used for the far-lateral approach extends from the foramen magnum to the retromastoid area to the midline. The vertebral artery can be protected with a Penfield dissector. (From Porter RW, Detwiler PW, Spetzler RF: Surgical approaches to the brain stem. Operative Techn Neurosurg 3:114–123, 2000.)

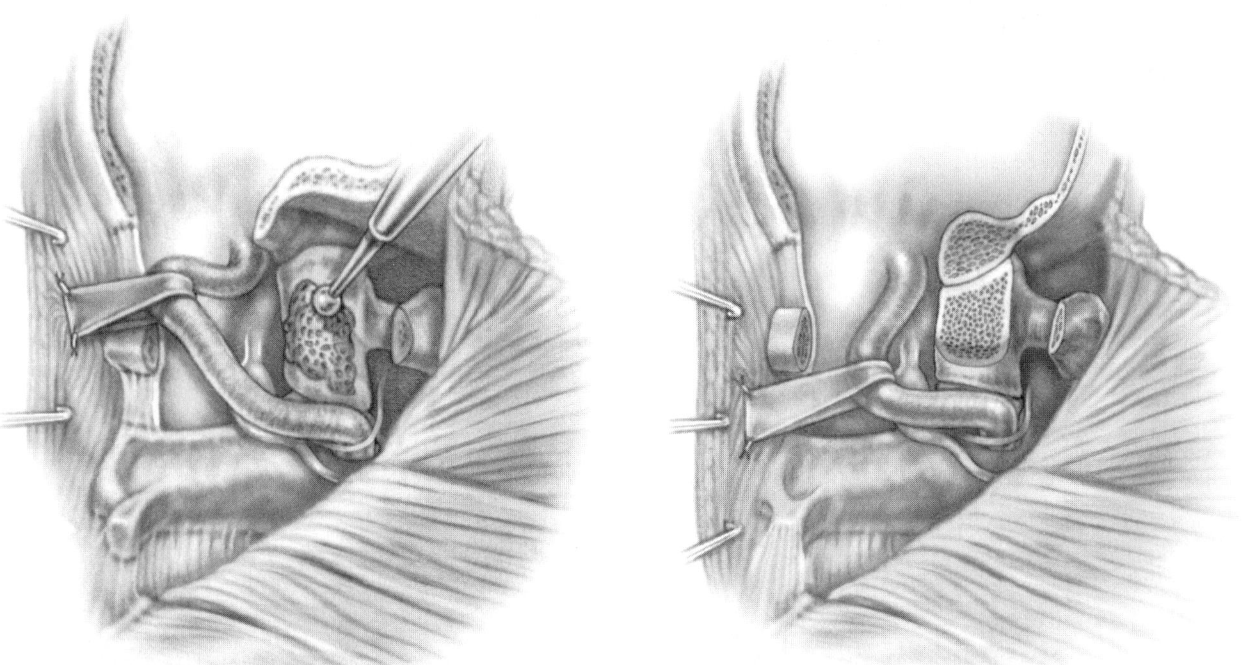

FIGURE 138–17. A diamond bur is used to drill the lateral mass of C1 while the vertebral artery is retracted medially. (Courtesy of Barrow Neurological Institute, Phoenix, AZ.)

FIGURE 138–18. Extent of bony removal after a far-lateral craniotomy with transposition of the vertebral artery. (Courtesy of Barrow Neurological Institute, Phoenix, AZ.)

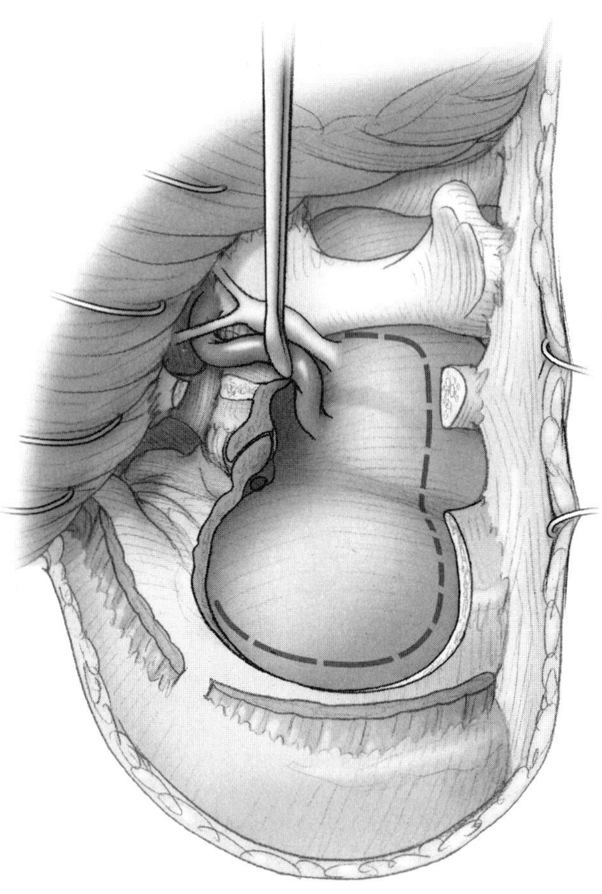

FIGURE 138–19. A C-shaped dural opening extending from the upper cervical spine to the lateral cerebellum allows a more lateral-anterior trajectory to the brainstem. (From Porter RW, Detwiler PW, Spetzler RF: Surgical approaches to the brain stem. Operative Techn Neurosurg 3:114–123, 2000.)

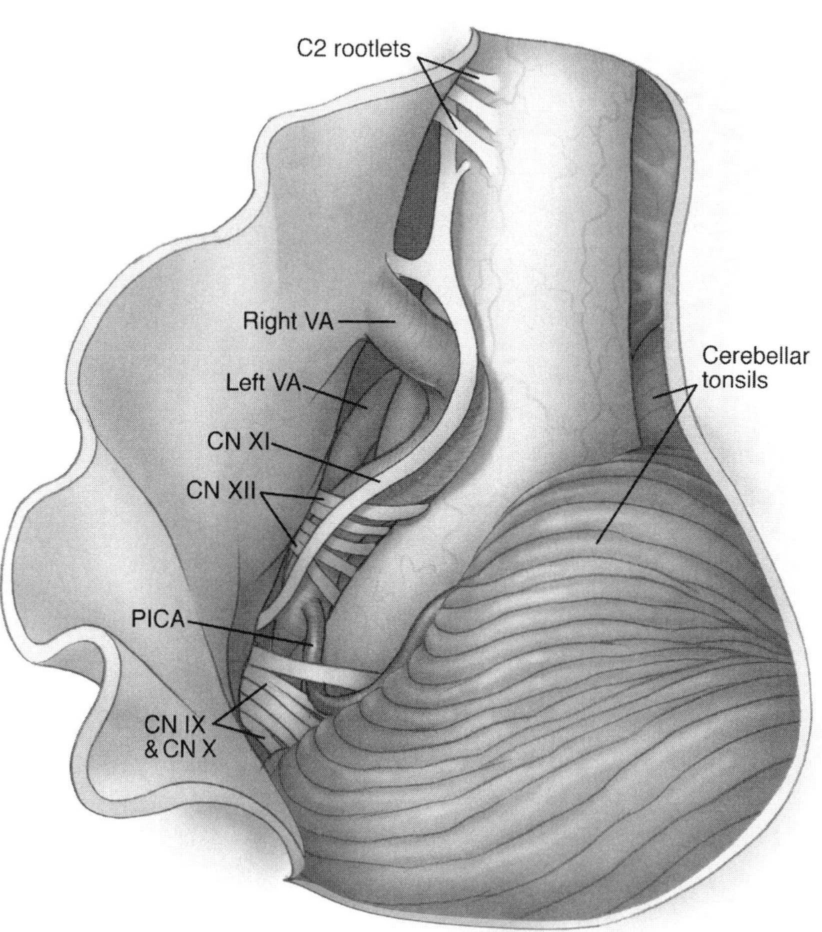

FIGURE 138–20. Illustration of the intradural exposure achieved by the far-lateral approach. The cervicomedullary junction to the pons can be visualized. CN, cranial nerve; PICA, posterior inferior cerebellar artery. (From Porter RW, Detwiler PW, Spetzler RF: Surgical approaches to the brain stem. Operative Techn Neurosurg 3:114–130, 2000.)

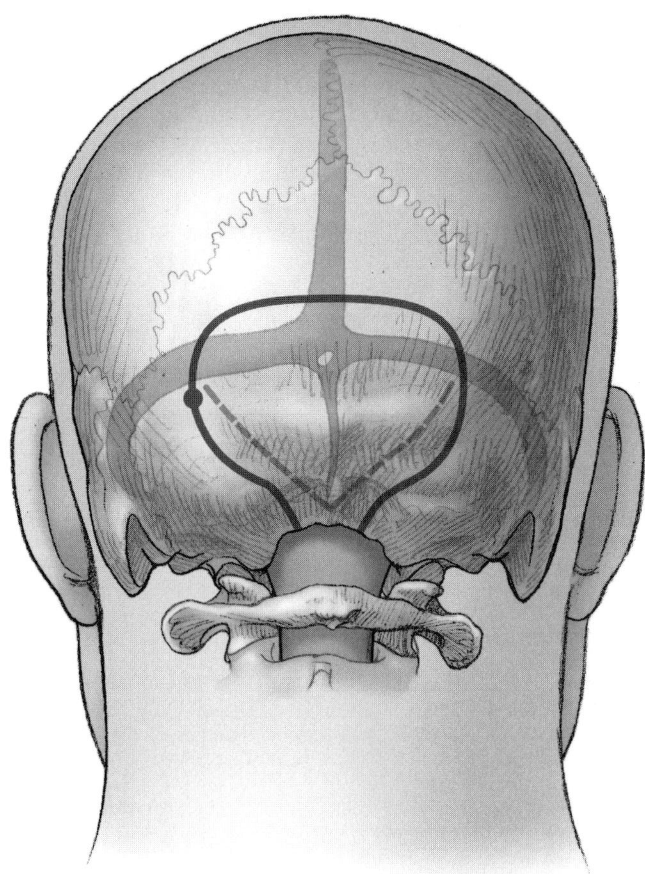

FIGURE 138–21. The craniotomy for the supracerebellar-infratentorial approach extends across all three sinuses, allowing the dura to retract the tentorium superiorly without obstructing bone over the torcular. (From Porter RW, Detwiler PW, Spetzler RF: Surgical approaches to the brain stem. Operative Techn Neurosurg 3:114–123, 2000.)

procedure, severe venous bleeding can occur during retraction. They must be coagulated as close to the surface of the cerebellum as possible to leave a pedicle on the surface of the tentorium. If they are avulsed at the interface of the tentorium, coagulation is not only futile but may enlarge the hole in the sinus and cause disastrous bleeding. If this occurs, a piece of Nu-Knit larger than the defect should be patched over the hole. A paddy is then placed over the hemostatic agent and can be held in place with a retractor during the remainder of the procedure. At the end of the procedure, the retractor is removed, and the Nu-Knit will adhere to the venous opening.

During the approach to the deep galenic system, the arachnoid is often thick and should be divided over the veins as close to the cerebellum as possible. Care must be taken to identify the vein of Galen, internal cerebral veins, basal veins of Rosenthal, occipital veins, pineal veins, and precentral cerebellar vein. If possible, the last should be preserved; if not, it can usually be coagulated and divided with impunity. Further exposure can be achieved by incising the tentorium 1 cm lateral to the straight sinus. The upper vermis can also be resected to explore the lower posterior midbrain and anterior medullary velum.

The cavernoma is dissected with the usual set of instruments. Long bipolar coagulation devices and microdissectors, including down-biting, up-biting, and straight microdissectors, should be used. Long suction instruments, ultrasonic aspirators, pituitary rongeurs, and tumor forceps are also useful. The resection bed should be inspected for residual lesion and venous anomalies. The dura should be closed in a watertight fashion with a dural patch and fibrin glue, if necessary.

This approach restricts maneuvers to below the deep galenic system and avoids traversing brain tissue. No normal tissue is violated if the lesion is ventral to the velum interposition and deep venous system.[61] The limitations of the approach are defined by the superolateral extension of lesions above the tentorium, which can be difficult to reach from an infratentorial exposure.

Paramedian[33] and lateral (retrosigmoid) supracerebellar-infratentorial[62, 63] approaches have also been described. The former is performed through a paramedian craniotomy 2 to 3 cm off midline and provides direct access to the cerebellomesencephalic fissure, inferior colliculus, fourth cranial nerve, and superior cerebellar peduncle.[64] The latter approach is through a retrosigmoid-infratentorial craniotomy and provides access to lesions of the lateral quadrigeminal plate, superior cerebellar peduncles, and trigeminal nerves.[62, 63]

PATIENT OUTCOMES

Between 1984 and 1998,[28] 100 patients (mean age, 37 years; range, 3 to 64 years) with brainstem cavernous malformations were evaluated at Barrow Neurological Institute. Asian patients accounted for 1%; Hispanic, 21%; and white, 78%. Fourteen percent of the patients had a family history of cavernous malformations. Of these lesions, 39% were in the pons, 16% in the midbrain, 16% in the medulla, 15% in the pontomesencephalic junction, 10% in the pontomedullary junction, and 1% in the midbrain-thalamic region. Two percent of the lesions involved more than two levels.

Typically, the lesion's location influenced the clinical presentation. Most patients had multiple neurological signs, which included (in order of frequency) cranial nerve deficits, sensory complaints (i.e., numbness, burning, or paresthesia), paresis or plegia, ataxia or gait disturbance, dysmetria, speech difficulties, and decreased level of consciousness or coma. Patients also presented with multiple symptoms: headache, vertigo or dizziness, nausea or vomiting, trigeminal neuropathy, hiccups, seizures (without convexity lesions), respiratory distress, hydrocephalus, neck pain, syncope, and tremor. Three percent of the cavernous malformations of the brainstem were found incidentally.

Eighty-six patients underwent surgical resection of their lesions. The following approaches were used: suboccipital (30%), far-lateral (19%), orbitozygomatic (13%), supracerebellar-infratentorial (9%), retrosigmoid (8%), retrolabyrinthine (6%), subtemporal (5%), combined (3.5%), pterional (2%), translabyrinthine (2%), transcochlear (1%), and occipital interhemispheric (1%). All 86 patients who underwent surgery had a venous anomaly intimately associated with the cavernous malformation.

Twelve percent of all surgical patients had neurological deficits at their follow-up examination. New permanent cranial nerve deficits occurred in 7%, increased weakness in 2%, and brachial plexopathy related to the modified park-bench position in 1%. Ten percent of the patients required short-term tracheostomy or feeding tubes, but only 2% required these adjuncts on a long-term basis.

The mean and median follow-up periods were 35 months and 24 months, respectively (range, 1 month to 14 years). Ninety-six percent of the patients were available for follow-up. Eighty-seven percent of the surgical patients were the same or better, 9% were worse, and 3.5% had died. In the nonsurgical group, 58% were the same or better, 32% were worse, and 8% had died.

As with other skull base and brainstem approaches, complication rates were not inconsequential. Temporary or permanent complications occurred in 35% of our cases; permanent complications were present in 12% at late follow-up. These complications included new neurological deficits, brachial plexopathy, meningitis, long-term tracheostomy or feeding tube, recurrence, sinus tear, CSF leak, wound infection, meningitis, pneumonia, and pulmonary embolus.

Outcomes were evaluated using the Glasgow Outcome Scale (GOS) score and compared with baseline values. The mean preoperative GOS score for all surgical patients at presentation was 4.4 (range, 2 to 5). Preoperative GOS scores for the operated group were as follows: GOS 5, 49%; GOS 4, 42%; GOS 3, 8%; GOS 2, 1%; and GOS 1, 0%. At a mean follow-up of 35 months, the mean GOS score was 4.53 (range, 1 to 5). Postoperative GOS scores were as follows: GOS 5, 73%; GOS 4, 17%; GOS 3, 6%; and GOS 2, 1%. Three patients (3%) died—one from a venous infarction, and two from cardiopulmonary arrest. Since this series was reported,[28] we have reviewed an additional 100 cases. Conservative management was recommended for slightly less than half these patients.

CONCLUSION

To achieve optimal results when performing surgery on the brainstem, surgeons must be familiar with all the available options, the involved anatomy, and the natural history of the disease. There is no replacement for in-depth study, skull base laboratory dissections, and experience. Conservative therapy is appropriate for patients with brainstem cavernous malformations that are asymptomatic and for those who have had a single nondevastating hemorrhage. Patients who suffer repeated hemorrhages or progressive neurological deficits should be considered for surgical resection, especially if the lesion abuts a pial surface. The two-point method can be used to help choose the appropriate skull base approach. When surgery is performed on cavernous malformations of the brainstem, associated venous anomalies should be expected, and their major tributaries should be preserved. Early postoperative MRI can be used as a baseline and to determine the degree of lesion resection. Meticulous radiographic and clinical follow-up are necessary to monitor for residual or recurrent disease. Complications can occur, and extensive informed consent should be obtained.

REFERENCES

1. Morcos JJ, Haines SJ: History of brain stem surgery. Neurosurg Clin N Am 4:357–365, 1993.
2. Vesalius A: De Humani Corpis Fabrica. Joporiui, 1943.
3. Jeffersen SG: The reticular formation and clinical neurology. In Jeffersen SG (ed): Reticular Formation of the Brain. Boston, Little Brown, 1958, pp 729–738.
4. Braun E: Case of Schwartze. Die Erfolge der Trepanation bei dem otitis chen Hirnabscess. Arch Onrenheilk 29:161–200, 1890.
5. Frazier CH: Intracranial division of the auditory nerve for persistent aural vertigo. Surg Gynecol Obstet 13:524–529, 1912.
6. Russell DS, Falconer MA, Beck DJK, et al: The pathology of spontaneous intracranial hemorrhage. Proc R Soc Med 47:689–704, 1954.
7. Teilmann K: Hemangiomas of the pons. Arch Neurol Psychiatry 69:208–223, 1953.
8. Giombini S, Morello G: Cavernous angiomas of the brain: Account of fourteen personal cases and review of the literature. Acta Neurochir (Wien) 40:61–82, 1978.
9. Del Curling O Jr, Kelly DL Jr, Elster AD, et al: An analysis of the natural history of cavernous angiomas. J Neurosurg 75:702–708, 1991.
10. Simard JM, Garcia-Bengochea F, Ballinger WE Jr, et al: Cavernous angioma: A review of 126 collected and 12 new clinical cases. Neurosurgery 18:162–172, 1986.
11. Abe M, Kjellberg RN, Adams RD: Clinical presentations of vascular malformations of the brain stem: Comparison of angiographically positive and negative types. J Neurol Neurosurg Psychiatry 52:167–175, 1989.
12. Sakai N, Yamada H, Tanigawara T, et al: Surgical treatment of cavernous angioma involving the brainstem and review of the literature. Acta Neurochir (Wien) 113:138–143, 1991.
13. Zabramski JM, Kawaguchi S, Spetzler RF: Management of brainstem cavernous malformations. Contemp Neurosurg 16:1–6, 1994.
14. Bertalanffy H, Gilsbach JM, Eggert H-R, et al: Microsurgery of deep-seated cavernous angiomas: Report of 26 cases. Acta Neurochir (Wien) 108:91–99, 1991.
15. Isaman F, Conesa G: Cavernous angiomas of the brain stem. Neurosurg Clin N Am 4:507–518, 1993.
16. Fahlbusch R, Strauss C, Huk W, et al: Surgical removal of pontomesencephalic cavernous hemangiomas. Neurosurgery 26:449–457, 1990.
17. Weil S, Tew JM Jr, Steiner L: Comparison of radiosurgery and microsurgery for treatment of cavernous malformations of the brain stem [abstract]. J Neurosurg 72:336A, 1990.
18. Zimmerman RS, Spetzler RF, Lee KS, et al: Cavernous malformations of the brain stem. J Neurosurg 75:32–39, 1991.
19. Lewis AI, Tew JM Jr: Management of thalamic–basal ganglia and brain-stem vascular malformations. Clin Neurosurg 41:83–111, 1994.
20. Aiba T, Tanaka R, Koike T, et al: Natural history of intracranial cavernous malformations. J Neurosurg 83:56–59, 1995.
21. Konovalov AN, Spallone A, Makhmudov UB, et al: Surgical management of hematomas of the brain stem. J Neurosurg 73: 181–186, 1990.
22. Tung H, Giannotta SL, Chandrasoma PT, et al: Recurrent intraparenchymal hemorrhages from angiographically occult vascular malformations. J Neurosurg 73:174–180, 1990.
23. Becker DH, Townsend JJ, Kramer RA, et al: Occult cerebrovascular malformations: A series of 18 histologically verified cases with negative angiography. Brain 102:249–287, 1979.

24. Crawford JV, Russell DS: Cryptic arteriovenous and venous hamartomas of the brain. J Neurol Neurosurg Psychiatry 19:1–11, 1956.
25. Sathi S, Lewis AI, Tew JM Jr: The natural history of the brainstem cavernous malformations [abstract]. Program for Joint Section on Cerebrovascular Surgery, AANS and CNS, Jan 23, 1996, San Antonio, TX.
26. Wascher TM, Spetzler RF: Cavernous malformations of the brain stem. In Carter LP, Spetzler RF (eds): Neurovascular Surgery. New York, McGraw-Hill, 1995, pp 541–555.
27. Amin-Hanjani S, Ogilvy CS, Ojemann RG, et al: Risks of surgical management for cavernous malformations of the nervous system. Neurosurgery 42:1220–1228, 1998.
28. Porter RW, Detwiler PW, Lawton MT, et al: Cavernous malformation of the brain stem: Experience with 100 patients. J Neurosurg 90:50–58, 1999.
29. Jellinger K: The morphology of centrally-situated angiomas. In Pia HW, Gleave JRW, Grote E, et al (eds): Cerebral Angiomas: Advances in Diagnosis and Therapy. New York, Springer-Verlag, 1975, pp 9–20.
30. McCormick WF, Hardman JM, Boulter TR: Vascular malformation ("angiomas") of the brain, with special reference to those occurring in the posterior fossa. J Neurosurg 28:241–251, 1968.
31. Sarwar M, McCormick WF: Intracerebral venous angioma: Case report and review. Arch Neurol 35:323–325, 1978.
32. McCormick WF: The pathology of vascular ("arteriovenous") malformations. J Neurosurg 24:807–816, 1966.
33. Sage MR, Brophy BP, Sweeney C, et al: Cavernous haemangiomas (angiomas) of the brain: Clinically significant lesions. Australas Radiol 37:147–155, 1993.
34. Robinson JR, Awad IA, Little JR: Natural history of the cavernous angioma. J Neurosurg 75:709–714, 1991.
35. Fritschi JA, Reulen H-J, Spetzler RF, et al: Cavernous malformations of the brain stem: A review of 139 cases. Acta Neurochir (Wien) 130:35–46, 1994.
36. Kondziolka D, Lunsford LD, Kestle JRW: The natural history of cerebral cavernous malformations. J Neurosurg 83:820–824, 1995.
37. Maraire JN, Awad IA: Intracranial cavernous malformations: Lesion behavior and management strategies. Neurosurgery 37:591–605, 1995.
38. Sigal R, Krief O, Houtteville JP, et al: Occult cerebrovascular malformations: Follow-up with MR imaging. Radiology 176:815–819, 1990.
39. Porter PJ, Willinsky RA, Harper W, et al: Cerebral cavernous malformations: Natural history and prognosis after clinical deterioration with or without hemorrhage. J Neurosurg 87:190–197, 1997.
40. Senegor M, Dohrmann GJ, Wollmann RL: Venous angiomas of the posterior fossa should be considered as anomalous venous drainage. Surg Neurol 19:26–32, 1983.
41. Brown AP, Thompson BG, Spetzler RF: The two-point method: Evaluating brain stem lesions. BNI Q 12:20–24, 1996.
42. Ginsburg HH, Shetter AG, Raudzens PA: Postoperative paraplegia with preserved intraoperative somatosensory evoked potentials: Case report. J Neurosurg 63:296–300, 1985.
43. Katsuta T, Morioka T, Fujii K, et al: Physiological localization of the facial colliculus during direct surgery on an intrinsic brain stem lesion. Neurosurgery 32:861–863, 1993.
44. Kyoshima K, Kobayashi S, Gibo H, et al: A study of safe entry zones via the floor of the fourth ventricle for brain-stem lesions: Report of three cases. J Neurosurg 78:987–993, 1993.
45. Strauss C, Fahlbusch R: Anatomical aspects for surgery within the floor of the IVth ventricle. Zentralbl Neurochir 58:7–12, 1997.
46. Morota N, Deletis V, Lee M, et al: Functional anatomic relationship between brain stem tumors and cranial motor nuclei. Neurosurgery 39:787–794, 1996.
47. Virchow R: Über die Erweiterung klëinerer Gefäsfe. Arch Pathol Anat 3:425–462, 1851.
48. Bogucki J, Gielecki J, Czernicki Z: The anatomical aspects of a surgical approach through the floor of the fourth ventricle. Acta Neurochir (Wien) 139:1014–1019, 1997.
49. Fujitsu K, Kuwabara T: Zygomatic approach for lesions in the interpeduncular cistern. J Neurosurg 62:340–343, 1985.
50. Hakuba A, Liu S, Nishimura S: The orbitozygomatic infratemporal approach: A new surgical technique. Surg Neurol 26:271–276, 1986.
51. Zabramski JM, Kiris T, Sankhla SK, et al: Orbitozygomatic craniotomy: Technical note. J Neurosurg 89:336–341, 1998.
52. Day JD, Kellogg JX, Tschabitscher M, et al: Surface and superficial surgical anatomy of the posterolateral cranial base: Significance for surgical planning and approach. Neurosurgery 38:1079–1084, 1996.
53. Rhoton AL Jr: Comments on Day et al: Surface and superficial surgical anatomy of the posterolateral cranial base: Significance for surgical planning and approach. Neurosurgery 38:1083–1084, 1996.
54. Spetzler RF, Daspit CP, Pappas CTE: The combined supra- and infratentorial approach for lesions of the petrous and clival regions: Experience with 46 cases. J Neurosurg 76:588–599, 1992.
55. Heros RC: Lateral suboccipital approach for vertebral and vertebrobasilar artery lesions. J Neurosurg 64:559–562, 1986.
56. Spetzler RF, Grahm TW: The far-lateral approach to the inferior clivus and the upper cervical region: Technical note. BNI Q 6: 35–38, 1990.
57. Vishteh AG, Crawford NR, Melton MS, et al: Stability of the craniovertebral junction after unilateral occipital condyle resection: A biomechanical study. J Neurosurg 90:91–98, 1999.
58. Dandy WE: Operative experience in cases of pineal tumor. Arch Surg 33:19–46, 1936.
59. Krause F: Operative Freilengung der Vierhagel nebst Beobachtungen über Hir and bekompression. Zentralb Chir 53:2817–2819, 1926.
60. Stein BM: The infratentorial supracerebellar approach to pineal lesions. J Neurosurg 35:197–202, 1971.
61. Stein BM: Surgical approach to the pineal tumors. In Wilkins RH, Rengachary SS (eds): Neurosurgery Update I. Diagnosis, Operative Technique and Neuro-Oncology. New York, McGraw-Hill, 1990, pp 389–398.
62. Laborde G, Gilsbach JM, Harders A, et al: Experience with the infratentorial supracerebellar approach in lesions of the quadrigeminal region, posterior third ventricle, culmen cerebelli, and cerebellar peduncle. Acta Neurochir (Wien) 114:135–138, 1992.
63. Pendl G, Vorkapic P, Koniyama M: Microsurgery of midbrain lesions. Neurosurgery 26:641–648, 1990.
64. Ogata N, Yonekawa Y: Paramedian supracerebellar approach to the upper brain stem and peduncular lesions. Neurosurgery 40: 101–105, 1997.

CHAPTER 139

Cavernous Carotid Fistulas

SANJAY GHOSH ■ DONALD LARSEN ■ J. DIAZ DAY

Carotid cavernous fistula originally was termed *pulsatile exophthalmos* based on the symptoms produced by this vascular disorder. The first recorded treatment of pulsatile exophthalmos was by Travers in 1809.[1] Travers found that compression of the ipsilateral carotid artery caused the orbital bruit to stop and the exophthalmos to decrease. Without using anesthesia, Travers ligated the patient's common carotid artery, which resulted in complete resolution of the patient's symptoms, as shown in the engraving from Travers' original article (Fig. 139-1).

Despite successfully treating this condition, Travers mistakenly theorized that pulsatile exophthalmos was due to a problem in the orbit. The intracranial origin of pulsatile exophthalmos was not realized until 1823. During an autopsy on a patient who had this condition, Guthrie observed an ophthalmic artery aneurysm. Soon after in France, Baron performed an autopsy on a patient who also had pulsatile exophthalmos. He found the patient to have an abnormal communication between the cavernous sinus and the internal carotid artery (ICA). These investigators were the first to establish the fact that pulsating exophthalmos was due to pathology within the cranial vault, such as an aneurysm or carotid artery fenestration, rather than pathology of the orbit.

These clinical and pathologic observations shaped the early treatment paradigms for pulsatile exophthalmos. Direct digital compression of the ipsilateral common carotid artery was used as a first-line treatment for pulsatile exophthalmos. In the early 1900s, some clinicians achieved carotid compression by placing a wooden frame around the neck and placing a compressive rubber stopper into the carotid artery (Fig. 139-2). This method of digital or mechanical compression was effective in 37% of cases reported on in 1907 by de Schweinitz and Holloway.[1] This mechanical compression technique was used to ascertain whether the patients could tolerate occlusion of the vessel without suffering an ischemic event.

In the early 1900s, ligation of the common carotid artery was used as the next treatment option if simple carotid compression was not effective. Of 84 patients treated in this manner by de Schweinitz and Holloway, 68% initially were cured with 7% mortality. During the same era of the early 1900s, some surgeons elected to ligate only the ICA. This ligation resulted in relief of pulsatile exophthalmos in 87% of patients with 8% mortality. Common carotid artery and ICA ligation successfully treated pulsatile exophthalmos in most cases, albeit with a relatively high mortality.

In 1935, Dandy[2] introduced a new treatment for cases of pulsatile exophthalmos that were refractory to carotid ligation. Dandy correctly surmised that carotid artery ligation resulted in clot formation and thrombosis of the fistula. He believed that treatment failure was due to retrograde flow through the circle of Willis, above the site of ligature. Consequently, in patients who failed cervical carotid ligation, Dandy performed a craniotomy and clipped the ICA just proximal to the posterior communicating artery. According to Dandy, this technique effectively isolated the aneurysm or arterial tear from the remainder of the cerebral circulation.

MICROSURGERY

A combination of carotid compression, cervical carotid ligation, and Dandy's intracranial carotid clipping was the standard of treatment for many years. Despite being effective in many cases, these techniques had an unacceptably high mortality. Although the early series reported 7% to 8% mortality, Stern and colleagues,[3] in 1967, reported a 26% mortality rate among patients treated using a combination of cervical and intracranial carotid artery ligation. Some cavernous carotid fistulas persisted despite ligation of the cervical carotid artery and ICA. These factors led Parkinson[4] to devise direct surgical approaches to the cavernous sinus to allow obliteration of the fistula, while preserving the patency of the carotid artery.

In 1974, Parkinson and associates[5] described an anatomic corridor to the cavernous sinus bound by the trochlear and oculomotor nerves above and the first division of the trigeminal nerve below. This region of the cavernous sinus was exposed through an intradural, subtemporal approach. Incision of the dura at this point provided direct access to the intracavernous portion of the carotid artery, while averting injury to the cranial nerves. This region also is referred to as the lateral triangle of the cavernous sinus. Parkinson used the access of the lateral triangle to allow direct repair of carotid cavernous fistulas or direct packing of the cavernous sinus with obliteration of the venous channels. These procedures initially were performed under cardiac arrest to minimize blood loss with opening of the cavernous sinus and carotid artery. Parkinson obliterated many cavernous carotid fistulas successfully, while preserving the patency of the carotid artery.

The modern techniques of skull base surgery further refined Parkinson's triangular corridor to cavernous carotid fistulas. Parkinson's original approach required significant direct temporal lobe retraction and sacrifice of the temporal bridging veins. Parkinson's exposure provided access to only one triangle of the eight triangles of the cavernous sinus, and it initially required cardiac bypass to minimize blood loss.[4, 5] The extradural temporopolar approach to the cavernous sinus allows complete exposure of the cavernous sinus, while preserving the anterior venous drainage of the temporal lobe. This exposure also minimizes direct retraction of the brain. Day and Fukushima[6] reported on the use of the extradural temporopolar approach combined with an intradural approach to obliterate dural cavernous carotid fistulas. Their exposure provided direct access to Parkinson's triangle and the seven other triangles of the cavernous sinus. Through these eight corridors, Day and Fukushima[6] successfully obliterated dural cavernous carotid fistulas, while preserving the cranial nerves in almost 90% of cases. Modern microsurgical techniques have made it possible to obliterate cavernous carotid fistulas safely. Despite such significant technical advances, microsurgery has been supplanted by endovascular neurosurgery as the primary treatment modality for cavernous carotid fistulas. Today, most cavernous carotid fistulas are managed by endovascular techniques.

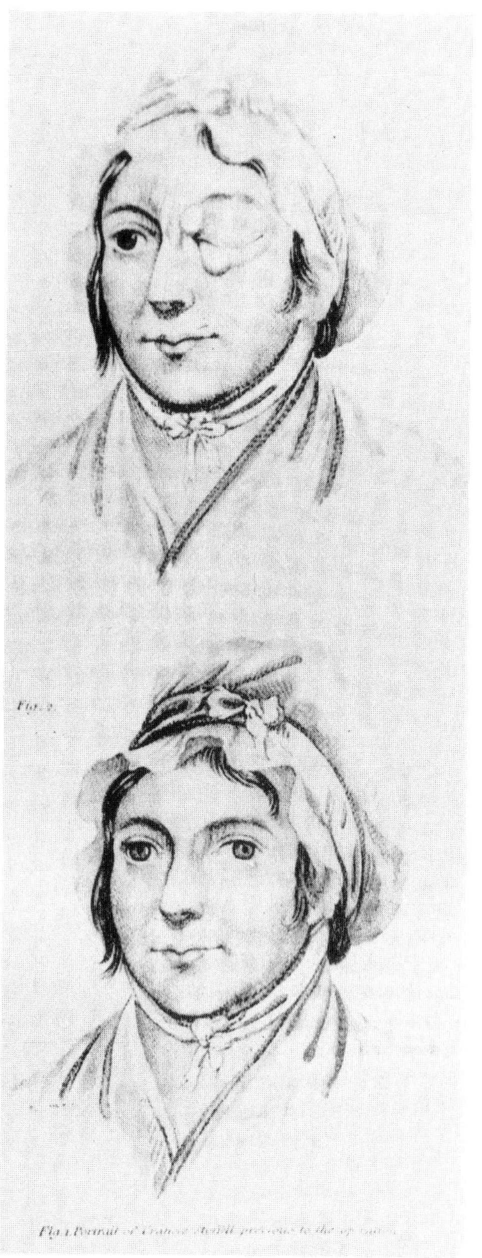

FIGURE 139–1. Illustration from Locke's article[1] shows exophthalmos secondary to carotid cavernous sinus fistula formation.

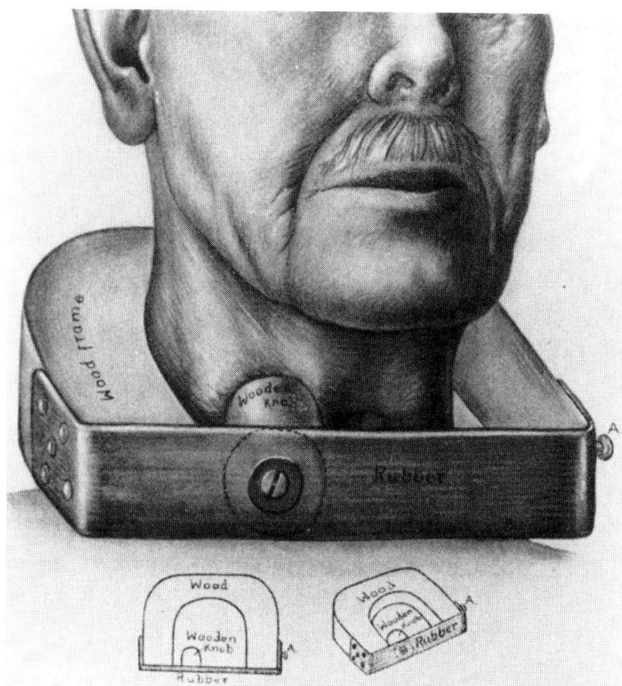

FIGURE 139–2. Device used in early 20th century for manual carotid artery compression for the treatment of carotid cavernous fistulas.

ENDOVASCULAR NEUROSURGERY

Modern endovascular treatment of carotid cavernous fistulas may be successful individually through the venous system or through the arterial supply or may require a combination of the approaches. The venous approach is achieved through either the superior orbital vein or the petrosal sinuses. Peterson and colleagues[7] described one of the earliest attempts to treat carotid cavernous fistulas by the superior orbital vein. Peterson and colleagues[7] reported placement of a copper wire through a dilated superior ophthalmic vein and thrombosis of the fistula by passing current through the wire. This initial attempt was complicated by spasm and thrombosis of the ipsilateral carotid artery. Hosobuchi[8] later reported successful electrothrombosis of carotid cavernous fistulas using a similar technique, while preserving the patency of the carotid artery.

Carotid cavernous fistulas also may be approached posteriorly through the petrosal sinuses. Debrun and coworkers[9, 10] provided one of the earliest descriptions of transvenous embolization of carotid cavernous fistulas, accessed through the inferior petrosal sinus. These clinicians obliterated the fistulas by deploying a detachable balloon into the cavernous sinus. Today, transvenous embolization is preferred with fibered platinum microcoils rather than balloons because they can be delivered through smaller catheters and have an inherent thrombogenicity, which promotes thrombosis of the cavernous sinus and closes the fistula.[11]

Arterial endovascular treatment of carotid cavernous fistulas may involve the following either as a single treatment or in combination: direct detachable balloon embolization of the fistulous connection, intracavernous or proximal internal carotid vessel occlusion, transarterial packing of the cavernous sinus, or embolization of feeding vessels with various materials. Endovascular intracavernous carotid artery occlusion first was described by Serbinenko in 1970.[12] Serbinenko devised a catheter with an inflatable balloon that floated to the intracavernous carotid artery. Access was obtained by direct carotid puncture. When the balloon was in position, Serbinenko filled the balloon with a mixture of silicon polymer and tantalum powder to occlude the parent vessel permanently and treat the carotid cavernous fistula. When the balloon was inflated, the catheter was cut and allowed to float within the arterial system proximal to the balloon. Serbinenko later developed a detachable latex balloon catheter that could be deployed safely to treat carotid cavernous fistulas. In the United States, Hieshima developed a silicone detachable balloon with a self-sealing valve that still is employed to date.[12]

In the interest of preserving the ICA, these pioneering neurosurgeons began to place the detachable balloons into the cavernous sinus with the hope of avoiding compromise of the carotid artery lumen. This procedure entails placement of a catheter by the Seldinger technique through the femoral artery to the affected ICA. The catheter is steered through the hole in the carotid artery until the balloon lies within the cavernous sinus. The balloon is inflated and detached within the cavernous sinus. The balloon then occludes the fistula by blocking the abnormal connection between the artery and the cavernous sinus.

Debrun and coworkers[9] reported one of the earliest series using this technique. They preserved the patency of the ICA in 59% of cases of traumatic carotid cavernous fistulas treated using this technique. The transarterial balloon occlusion technique is most effective when the carotid cavernous fistula is due to an isolated tear within the carotid artery itself. When the fistula is composed of multiple feeding vessels from either the ICA or external carotid artery, it is necessary to employ more sophisticated means. Carotid cavernous fistulas with multiple feeding vessels often require selective catheterization of the feeding vessels and injection of an occlusive polymer, such as polyvinyl alcohol.[13]

Today, the management of carotid cavernous fistulas is primarily with endovascular techniques. Microsurgical treatment using skull base approaches is reserved for carotid cavernous fistulas that cannot be treated by endovascular means. The optimal treatment of a carotid cavernous fistula can be determined by analyzing the exact anatomic substrate of the fistula itself. The classification scheme proposed by Barrow and associates[13] is an excellent means to categorize carotid cavernous fistulas and predict which treatment strategy would be most effective.

CLASSIFICATION AND CAUSE

Carotid cavernous fistulas are classified best by the precise anatomic substrate of the lesion based on digital subtraction angiography. Barrow and associates[13] established a simple yet elegant scheme to categorize these fistulas based on angiographic criteria. Type A fistulas are direct shunts between the ICA and the cavernous sinus. These fistulas are most commonly the result of significant blunt cranial trauma from motor vehicle accidents, fights, and falls.[14] Direct carotid cavernous fistulas also may arise from penetrating cranial trauma from a knife or projectile.[15, 16] Such direct fistulas may be iatrogenic from perforation of the carotid artery during various procedures, including Fogarty catheter placement during carotid endarterectomy, transsphenoidal craniotomy, percutaneous radiofrequency ablation of the trigeminal nerve, and nasopharyngeal surgery. Type A fistulas also may arise from rupture of an intracavernous carotid artery aneurysm. These direct lesions rarely may occur spontaneously, without any antecedent trauma or surgical manipulation.[10] Direct fistulas also may occur in disorders characterized by abnormalities in collagen deposition and the media of the arterial wall, such as Ehlers-Danlos syndrome, fibromuscular dysplasia, pseudoxanthoma elasticum, and cavernous ICA aneurysms.[11, 17–22] Type A fistulas are high-flow lesions and tend not to resolve spontaneously.[10]

The remaining three categories of carotid cavernous fistulas are distinct from type A lesions. Types B, C, and D carotid cavernous fistulas are dural arteriovenous malformations rather than frank disruptions in the vessel wall. These three fistulas are distinct based on the source of the feeding arteries to the dural arteriovenous malformation. Type B dural shunts consist of feeding vessels from the intracavernous carotid artery. Type C fistulas consist of feeding vessels from only the external carotid artery to the cavernous sinus. Type D lesions have feeding vessels from the ICA and external carotid artery. Types B, C, and D lesions may be either high flow or low flow. They may occur spontaneously or as a result of minor trauma. The precise cause of dural arteriovenous fistulas is unknown and the subject of considerable speculation. These lesions are more likely to undergo spontaneous thrombosis than type A fistulas.

The decision to treat a carotid cavernous fistula is based on the patient's symptoms and whether the angiographic appearance of the fistula shows high-risk features for intracranial hemorrhage.[23]

SYMPTOMS AND PATHOPHYSIOLOGY

Carotid cavernous fistulas produce a constellation of symptoms that arise from abnormally elevated pressure within the cavernous sinus. This elevation in intracavernous pressure is transmitted anteriorly to the orbital veins or posteriorly to the inferior petrosal sinus. The elevation of venous pressure in the orbit gives rise to chemosis, exophthalmos, and bruit. Vinuela and associates[24] observed proptosis or exophthalmos among 90% of patients with spontaneous carotid cavernous fistulas. Of their patients, 90% had significant chemosis. Orbital bruits that were noticed by the patients occurred less frequently in 25% of cases. These patients also may develop swelling of the eyelids, which may produce considerable cosmetic deformity with time (see Fig. 139-1).

Diplopia is a common symptom among patients with carotid cavernous fistulas. Double vision may arise by several distinct mechanisms. The first is by cranial nerve dysfunction resulting from arterialized pressure within the cavernous sinus and resultant ischemia of the vasa nervosum. In the case of aneurysms, the cranial nerves may be compressed directly by the arterial dilatation. The abducent nerve is the most frequently affected in patients with type A fistulas; this is due to the proximity of the sixth nerve to the carotid artery within the cavernous sinus.[14] The second mechanism of diplopia in carotid cavernous fistula is mechanical restriction of the extraocular muscles. The restriction of muscle function is due to vascular engorgement of the muscles from elevated venous pressure. Such myopathy may produce diplopia that does not fit the pattern of a single cranial nerve palsy.

One of the most serious consequences of carotid cavernous fistulas is visual loss. In the early series of de Schweinitz and Holloway of 1908, 89% of patients had visual loss.[25] Sattler, in 1920, observed functional blindness in half of his patients.[25] These early series show that untreated or incompletely treated carotid cavernous fistulas often result in significant visual loss. The cause of visual loss in these patients is due to three mechanisms that all compromise perfusion of the retina. The first is by retinal ischemia. This occurs when the low resistance and high flow of the fistula preferentially shunts blood away from the ophthalmic artery. The blood flow to the retina is put in jeopardy and may result in frank visual loss. The second mechanism is by marked elevation of the intraorbital venous pressure. Such an elevation in venous pressure reduces the arteriovenous gradient within the retina and compromises retinal perfusion.[25] The third mechanism that contributes to visual loss is elevation of intraocular pressure. The vascular engorgement that yields extraocular muscle dysfunction and proptosis also produces a rise in intraocular pressure. This rise in intraocular pressure further compromises the effective perfusion of the retina and may lead to visual loss. The extent and progression of visual loss is paramount in determining the need for endovascular or surgical treatment of carotid cavernous fistulas. Patients with these lesions must have their vision monitored. Management decisions are shaped by the stability or instability of the patient's vision and related symptoms.

Epistaxis and intracranial hemorrhage are not well-recognized complications of carotid cavernous fistulas. In 1920, Sattler's literature review of 322 cases of carotid cavernous fistulas revealed 5 fatal cases of epistaxis and 3 intracerebral hematomas.[26] These hemorrhagic complications also have been described in contemporary case reports.[27–29] Goto and colleagues[28] observed fatal hemorrhage in 4 of 148 patients who had type A carotid cavernous fistulas. D'Angelo and coworkers[27] postulated the reason for intracerebral hemorrhage in some patients with carotid cavernous fistulas. At the time of angiography, they observed large, dilated, tortuous cerebral veins in the presence of carotid cavernous fistulas. These dilated veins were arterialized at the time of craniotomy. D'Angelo and coworkers[27] theorized that this abnormal high pressure and flow through the venous system is susceptible to rupture and the formation of intracerebral or subarachnoid hemorrhage. The work of Sattler and Goto suggested that 3% of all carotid cavernous fistulas present with intracerebral hemorrhage. Although the precise actuarial risk remains to be determined, the issue of intracerebral hemorrhage must be considered when planning the management of these lesions.

Halbach and colleagues[23] identified other angiographic and clinical criteria to help recognize high-risk carotid cavernous fistulas. Angiographic features that were associated with increased morbidity and mortality included the presence of a pseudoaneurysm, large varix of the cavernous sinus, thrombosis of venous outflow pathways distant from the fistula, and venous drainage to cortical veins. In their series of 155 patients with carotid cavernous fistulas, 21 patients had a varix of the cavernous sinus. Three of these 21 patients went on to have subarachnoid hemorrhage, which proved universally fatal.

In addition to angiographic findings, Halbach and colleagues[23] identified clinical signs and symptoms that characterize a high-risk carotid cavernous fistula. These signs and symptoms include increased intracranial pressure, rapidly progressing proptosis, diminished visual acuity, hemorrhage, and transient ischemic attacks. The work of these authors suggests that the presence of any of these findings should prompt treatment of the offending fistulas.

TREATMENT

The treatment options for carotid cavernous fistulas include manual carotid and jugular compression, endovascular treatment, and microsurgery. Conservative treatment with digital compression of the ipsilateral carotid artery and jugular vein is effective for some indirect carotid cavernous fistulas. In 1924, Locke[1] found manual compression of the ipsilateral carotid artery to be effective in 26% of cases (see Fig. 139-2). More recently, Halbach and colleagues[30] successfully treated 30% of patients with indirect carotid cavernous fistulas with manual compression alone. Halbach and colleagues[30] instructed patients to compress their own carotid artery with the contralateral hand for 10 seconds several times an hour. This compression was performed with the patients sitting or laying down. The contralateral hand was used to perform the compression. This was done so that should ischemia and weakness develop, the compressing hand would fall away from the neck. Before initiation of treatment, these patients were monitored for the development of symptomatic bradycardia with carotid compression. The patients were warned to cease carotid and jugular compression immediately if they developed any symptoms of cerebral ischemia, such as weakness, sensory changes, or altered mental status. With this technique of intermittent manual compression, thrombosis of the indirect carotid cavernous fistula was achieved within 4 to 6 weeks in 30% of all cases.[30]

One relative contraindication for carotid-jugular compression in the treatment of indirect fistulas is significant cortical venous drainage.[30] Patients with carotid cavernous fistulas that drain posteriorly through the petrosal sinuses and the cortical venous system are at significant risk of intracerebral hemorrhage.[27] Compression of the internal jugular vein in theory could elevate cerebral venous pressure and result in venous infarction or hemorrhage.

Patients with types B, C, or D carotid cavernous fistulas with mild symptoms, absence of cortical venous drainage, no evidence of significant carotid artery atherosclerosis, and stable vision may undergo a trial of manual carotid and jugular compression. If patients develop progression of visual loss or other symptoms while undergoing a conservative trial, they should have interventional treatment. Although compression is effective 30% of the time for indirect carotid cavernous fistulas, these conservative measures are not effective for type A or direct carotid cavernous fistulas. Type A fistulas are a direct tear within the carotid artery and, as a result, are high pressure. Consequently, they are much less likely to undergo spontaneous thrombosis than indirect fistulas. Goto and associates[28] reported on 148 patients with type A or direct carotid cavernous fistulas. Of 148 patients, 4 (2.7%) died from hemorrhage before therapy could be implemented. Only 3% of these patients had spontaneous resolution of type A fistulas without intervention. Patients with type A carotid cavernous fistulas must be advised that fatal hemorrhage is almost as likely as spontaneous resolution of these lesions. Consequently, a more aggressive therapeutic approach for these lesions is warranted.

Endovascular Neurosurgery

The decision to treat a carotid cavernous fistula involves an analysis of many factors related to cause, symptoms and clinical course, angiographic features, and the patient's medical condition. Many patients who have fistulas associated with trauma may have other organ system injuries requiring more immediate attention. Elderly patients with minimal symptoms and low-risk indirect fistulas may opt for no treatment at all. Certain situations demand urgent treatment, such as rapid visual decline, increased intracranial pressure, and evidence of cortical venous drainage.[23, 27] Formal ophthalmologic evaluation of visual acuity and intraocular pressure can be extremely valuable in the decision to intervene. The goal of treatment, treatment strategy, and assessment of risks and benefits must be defined clearly before endovascular procedures for carotid cavernous fistula.

Balloon Embolization

Transarterial deployment of detachable balloons is the treatment of choice for direct carotid cavernous fistulas. We prefer detachable silicone balloons mounted on microcathers designed for intracranial endovascular procedures. Ideally the balloon is flow directed into the rent between the cavernous ICA and the cavernous sinus. The balloon is inflated with an iso-osmolar contrast agent within the cavernous sinus, blocking all arterial flow without compromising the ICA lumen. The balloon is detached in this position after arteriography confirms closure of the fistula and preservation of the intracranial ICA flow, effectively curing the carotid cavernous fistula. Occasionally nondetachable silicone balloons are positioned adjacent to the detachable balloon to assist in deployment or within the ICA to reduce flow before deployment.

Successful balloon embolization is not always possible. The carotid injury or the cavernous sinus may not be of the appropriate size to accept proper placement or stable positioning of the balloon. Bone fragments or foreign bodies may puncture the balloon. These patients may require transvenous approaches or parent artery sacrifice to obliterate the fistula.

Parent artery sacrifice should be performed only after other treatment modalities have been exhausted. If ICA occlusion is required, test occlusion should be performed before permanent sacrifice, unless there is evidence that the patient otherwise would tolerate ICA occlusion. In the situation of complete ipsilateral steal into the fistula (no intracranial filling) with adequate cross-filling and collateral supply to the brain, the patient is likely to tolerate ICA occlusion.

Advantages of endovascular treatment include the ability to perform the procedure under local anesthesia with continuous neurological evaluation, reduction of blood loss compared with craniotomy and elimination of many other risk factors associated with open procedures, immediate angiographic assessment of changing hemodynamics during treatment, and initiation of treatment immediately after diagnosis (may be important in acute visual decline). Disadvantages include thromboembolic and ischemic events secondary to intravascular devices and manipulation; development of a pseudoaneurysm at the site of the fistula with delayed balloon deflation or migration; and alteration of hemodynamics resulting in acute orbital engorgement or cortical venous enlargement, possibly resulting in visual compromise or intracranial swelling or hemorrhage.

Coil Embolization

If balloon occlusion of a direct carotid cavernous fistula is not technically possible, arterial or venous microcoil placement may be required. Transarterial fibered platinum microcoil placement generally is not performed because of the risk of ICA entry with possible occlusive or thromboembolic consequences. Electrolytically detachable platinum alloy fibered Guglielmi Detachable Coils (GDC) (Target Therapeutics) are available for transarterial embolization of carotid cavernous fistulas. Deployment of these coils is more precise than pushable coils and may reduce the risk of nontarget embolization should inadvertent deployment in the parent artery occur.

Transvenous coil occlusion of carotid cavernous fistula drainage is a much more common treatment. In general, a microcatheter is used to cannulate the cavernous sinus through the inferior petrosal sinus. If this access cannot be gained successfully, facial vein, periorbital vein, or superior orbital approaches may be employed. These are usually possible from a transfemoral route; however, cutdown or direct stick may be necessary depending on the patient's anatomy. If the arterial opening into the cavernous sinus is large, occasionally a transarterial temporary balloon or permanent stent may be required to prevent coil embolization into the parent ICA during transvenous coil packing.

Careful analysis of the anatomy of the carotid cavernous fistula is required when the cavernous sinus has been accessed by way of the microcatheter before the deployment of any coils. The standard drainage of the cavernous sinus is through the inferior petrosal sinus. In the setting of a carotid cavernous fistula, arterialized blood often flows through the superior ophthalmic vein and cortical veins. These veins have been recruited to handle the excess flow into the cavernous sinus. Premature or inadvertent closure of the inferior petrosal sinus could pressurize these veins acutely and cause an acute rise in intraocular, intraorbital, or intracranial pressure. Consequently, visual damage or intracerebral hemorrhage may occur.

When the superior orbital vein is engorged, transvenous coiling usually begins in this vessel, gradually working back through the cavernous sinus toward the inferior petrosal sinus. Cortical venous drainage must be occluded before occluding the inferior petrosal sinus. Packing of the site of the fistula within the cavernous sinus is usually curative.

Other Embolic Agents

Although balloon embolization generally is reserved for arterial embolization of direct carotid cavernous fistulas, other agents are available for the treatment of these lesions. Indirect carotid cavernous fistulas previously have been described as lesions that often have complex arterial supply. It is rare to cure these lesions with transarterial embolization alone. Embolization with polyvinyl alcohol particles alone usually results in delayed recanalization of the fistula. It is also rare to be able to embolize the entire fistula transarterially because the fistulas frequently are supplied by myriad residual branches that are too small to catheterize subselectively. The role of particle embolization of these lesions is to slow down temporarily the arterial flow to the fistula, while performing transvenous coil embolization of the cavernous sinus. One must be aware, however, that the blood supply to cranial nerves III to XII can arise from the branches supplying the fistula, and embolization of these vessels may result in cranial nerve dysfunction.

Microsurgery

Endovascular neurosurgery is usually successful in treating direct carotid cavernous fistulas. For type A fistulas, Debrun and colleagues[10] found transarterial detachable balloon occlusion to be successful in 97% of cases. The remaining 3% of patients required direct surgical exposure of the cavernous carotid artery to repair the fistula. Similar to type A fistulas, most indirect or types B, C, and D fistulas resolve with either conservative treatment or embolization therapy.[9, 10, 13] Some fistulas may be difficult to manage with endovascular treatment alone.[6, 10] In early series, Debrun and colleagues[10] found embolization to be effective in only 46% of patients with type D fistulas. The remaining 54% of patients required adjuvant microsurgery or lived with persistent fistulas. Significant technical advances in endovascular neurosurgery have improved significantly the efficacy of embolization; however, fistulas that cannot be managed by endovascular means require direct microsurgical treatment.[6, 10, 31, 32]

Day and Fukushima[6] described the microsurgical management of type D fistulas that failed endovascular therapy. All nine of their patients had progression of symptoms and persistence of fistulas despite endovascular therapy. The residual feeding vessel in every case was the meningohypophyseal trunk (Figs. 139-3 and 139-4). These patients were managed with a combined intradural and extradural frontotemporal approach to the cavernous sinus.[14, 15] All nine fistulas were obliterated successfully using this technique.

Most carotid cavernous fistulas are treated successfully with endovascular techniques. Patients with persistent fistulas and progression of symptoms despite endovascular therapy must have microsurgical ablation of the fistulas. Modern skull base surgery has made it possible to expose and negotiate the cavernous sinus safely, while preserving the cranial nerves, carotid artery, critical venous pathways, and brain.[4–6, 31, 33] Exposure of the entire cavernous sinus is achieved best by using a combined intradural and extradural frontotemporal approach.[6, 31, 33]

Surgical Technique of Frontotemporal Approach to the Cavernous Sinus

The frontotemporal approach to the cavernous sinus is initiated after satisfactory induction of general anesthe-

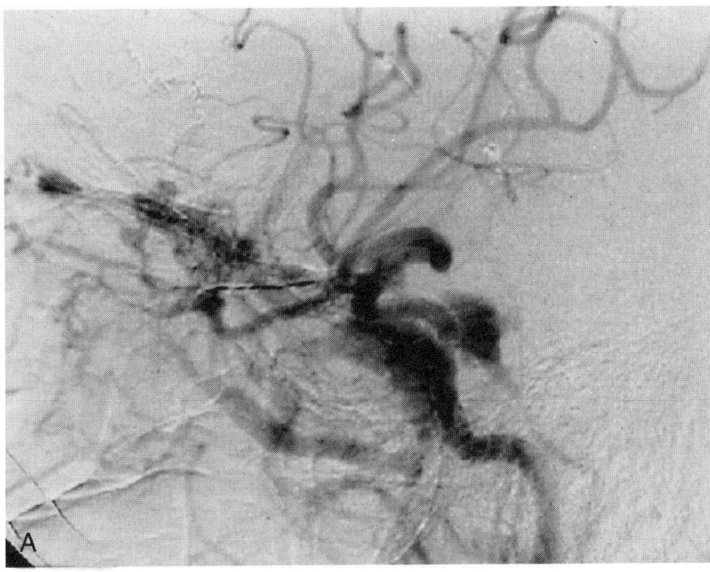

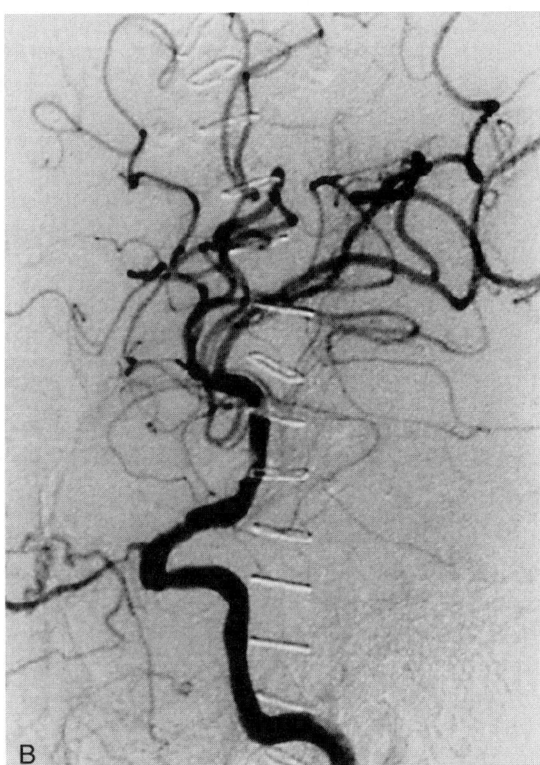

FIGURE 139–3. *A,* Angiogram of a 67-year-old patient after coil embolization by way of the transvenous approach who had continued deterioration of vision. *B,* Postoperative angiogram shows occlusion of the fistula.

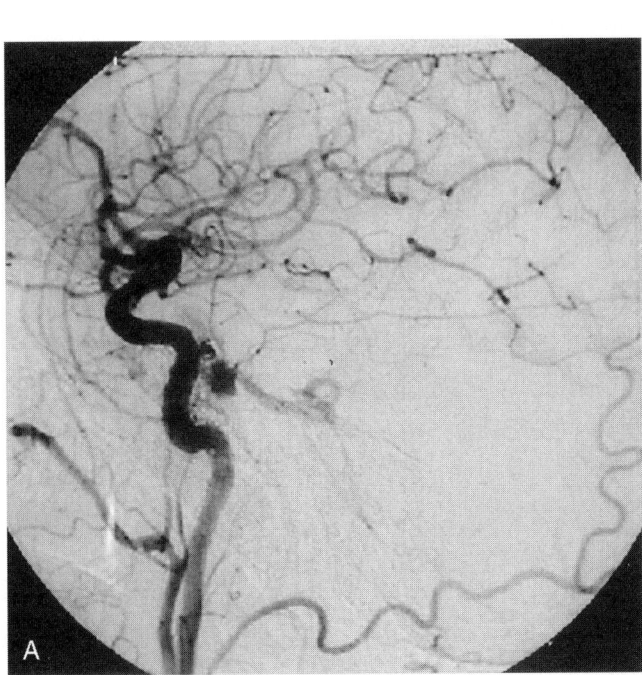

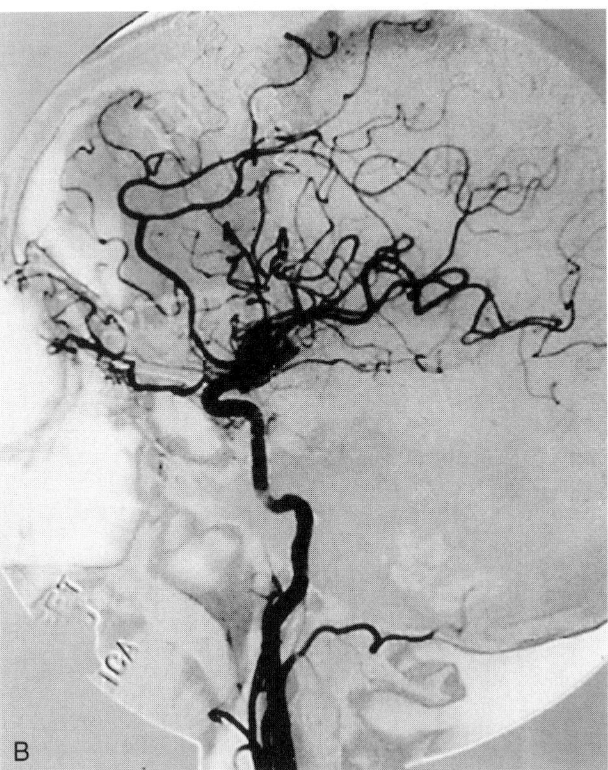

FIGURE 139–4. *A,* Cerebral angiogram after transvenous partial embolization of a carotid cavernous fistula in a 42-year-old woman. Her vision continued to deteriorate with increased intraocular pressures, and she had elevated cerebral venous pressure secondary to continued filling of a petrosal vein. *B,* Postoperative angiogram shows complete occlusion by direct microsurgery.

sia. The head is placed in three-pin fixation and rotated approximately 45 degrees. A routine pterional-type scalp incision is made. The temporalis muscle is incised and elevated with the periosteum using a retrograde dissection technique.[34] Monopolar cauterization of the muscle is limited to prevent future atrophy of the muscle. The musculocutaneous flap is elevated anteriorly to the orbital rim. A frontotemporal craniotomy is cut one third above and two thirds below the superior temporal line. The dura is elevated away from the frontal and temporal cranial base. The sphenoid ridge is flattened medially to the meningo-orbital artery.

Next, the pertinent cranial nerves are skeletonized using a high-speed drill. The optic canal is unroofed. This leads to the anterior clinoid process, on the lateral border of the optic nerve. The anterior clinoid is removed, while paying close attention to the optic nerve on the medial border, the oculomotor nerve on the lateral border, and the carotid artery along the inferior border. The superior orbital fissure, foramen rotundum, and foramen ovale are unroofed to expose 5 to 8 mm of the respective dural sleeves. The middle meningeal artery is identified at the foramen spinosum and ligated. When the bony work is complete, the dura propria over the temporal lobe is separated from the outer cavernous membrane. Bleeding may come from small openings in the cavernous sinus, and this is controlled with the gentle packing of Surgicel. The dura propria is elevated to the incisural edge and petrous ridge. Up to this point, the posterolateral, posteromedial, anteromedial, anterolateral, and far lateral cavernous triangles are exposed (triangles 1, 5, 6, 7, and 8 of Fig. 139-5).

Medially the dura is opened in an L-shaped manner that goes from the optic nerve sheath across the sylvian fissure and along the tuberculum sella. The fibrous dural ring around the carotid artery is opened. This provides exposure of the medial, superior, and lateral cavernous triangles (triangles 2, 3, and 4, Fig. 139-5).

The effective obliteration of the carotid cavernous fistula relies on packing a sufficient amount of oxidized cellulose in the correct position within each triangular corridor. This packing results in compression of the abnormal vascular channels, while preserving the adjacent cranial nerves. Overpacking in any direction can lead to carotid occlusion or cranial nerve palsy. Consequently, it is important to understand the precise anatomic substrate of each triangular corridor of entry into the cavernous sinus.

The anteromedial triangle (triangle 1, Fig. 139-5) is an epidural space that contains the subclinoidal segment of the carotid artery.[35, 36] This area is bordered by the lateral border of the intracanalicular optic nerve, the medial wall of the superior orbital fissure dura, and the dural ring surrounding the carotid artery as it enters the subarachnoid space. This segment of the

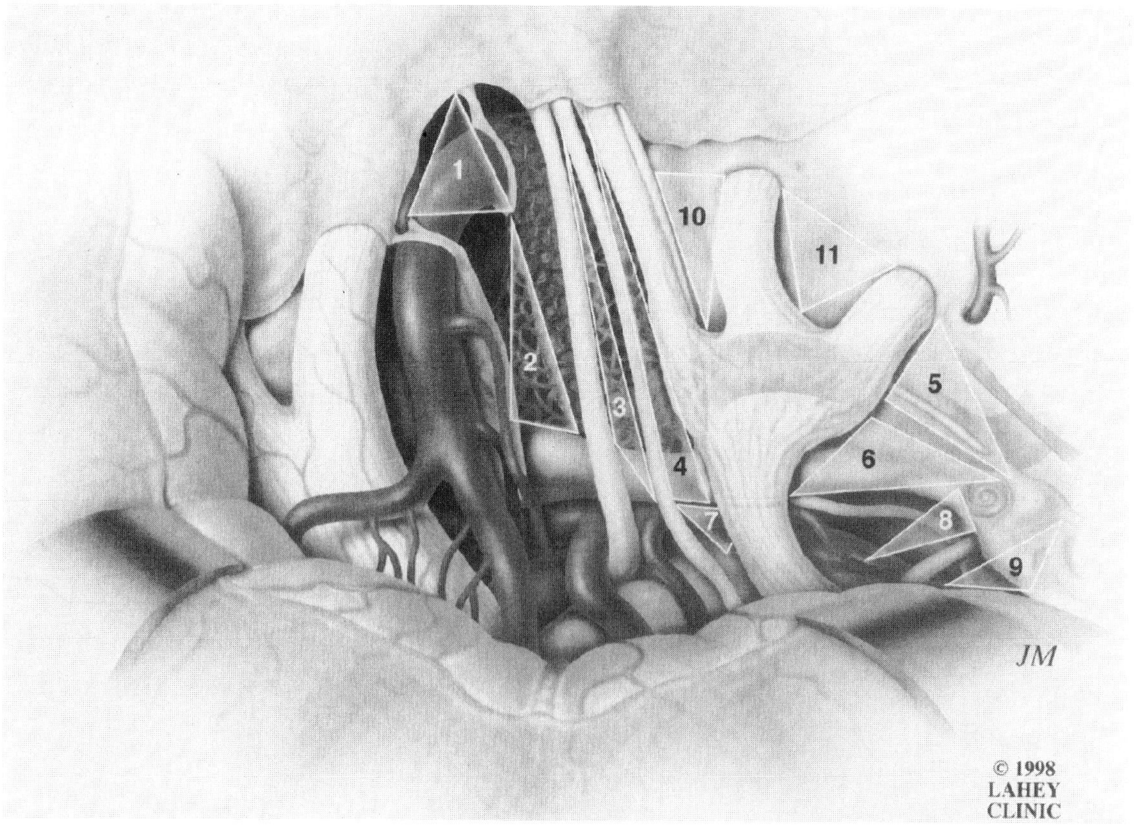

FIGURE 139–5. Geometric organization of the entry corridors to the cavernous sinus. 1, anteromedial triangle; 2, medial triangle; 3, superior triangle; 4, lateral triangle (Parkinson's); 5, posterolateral triangle (Glasscock's); 6, posteromedial triangle (Kawase's); 7, posteroinferior triangle; 8, premeatal triangle; 9, postmeatal triangle; 10, anterolateral triangle; 11, far lateral triangle.

carotid artery often is surrounded by a venous plexus, which communicates with the cavernous sinus. In treating carotid cavernous fistulas, this segment must be packed. Heavy packing of the oxidized cellulose in this triangle potentially may occlude the carotid artery.

The medial triangle (triangle 2, Fig. 139-5) is bound by the oculomotor nerve as it enters the cavernous sinus, the posterior clinoid process, and the subclinoidal carotid artery. Packing of embolic material in the lateral and anterior direction carries risk to the carotid artery and occulomotor nerve. The posterior and inferior portion of this triangle leads to the basilar venous plexus of the clivus and the inferior petrosal sinus. A large amount of material may be packed in this direction without harm.

The superior triangle (triangle 3, Fig. 139-5) is bound by the oculomotor and trochlear nerves. The posterior margin of this triangle is the porus oculomotorius and porus trochlearis, which are the dural penetration of these cranial nerves into the cavernous sinus. The superior triangle often provides access to the origin of the meningohypophyseal trunk. Occlusion of this vessel may be achieved through this space. Packing of embolic material may be performed in the posterior and medial directions. This packing augments occlusion of communications with the basilar venous plexus and inferior petrosal sinus. Excessive packing anteriorly and laterally can risk the cavernous carotid artery and the oculomotor and trochlear nerves.

The lateral or Parkinson's triangle (triangle 4, Fig. 139-5) is the anatomic corridor originally used by Parkinson to access the cavernous carotid artery.[4, 5] This corridor is bound superiorly by the trochlear nerve and inferiorly by the ophthalmic division of the trigeminal nerve (V1). Packing in the anterior and lateral directions poses a risk to the sixth nerve, V1, and the carotid artery. Posterior packing also risks the abducent nerve. Medial packing is a safe means of occluding the communication to the inferior petrosal sinus. This triangle often is used to expose type A fistulas that have failed endovascular treatment.

The posterolateral triangle, also known as Glasscock's triangle (triangle 5, Fig. 139-5), is the location of the horizontal intrapetrous carotid artery. This triangle is bound by the posterior rim of foramen ovale, the mandibular division of the trigeminal nerve, the middle meningeal artery, and the cochlear apex. This triangle may need to be opened for proximal control of the intracavernous carotid artery and to occlude fistulous connections to the pterygoid venous plexus.

The posteromedial triangle, which is also known as Kawase's triangle (triangle 6, Fig. 139-5), is an island of bone in the petrous apex.[37, 38] This triangle is bound by the porus trigeminus, cochlea, and posterior border of V3. Removal of bone in this region provides access to the posterior cavernous sinus region. This provides access to fistulous connections to the superior petrosal sinus, inferior petrosal sinus, and petrosal veins.

The anterolateral triangle (triangle 7, Fig. 139-5) is the area between the ophthalmic and maxillary divisions of the trigeminal nerves. This corridor is important in the treatment of carotid cavernous fistulas. The superior ophthalmic vein typically communicates with the cavernous sinus in this area. Packing toward the orbit may be performed with impunity; however, aggressive posterior packing may occlude the carotid artery or injure the abducent nerve.

The far-lateral triangle (triangle 8, Fig. 139-5) is a space bound by the second and third divisions of the trigeminal nerve (V2 and V3). This area commonly contains the sphenoid emissary vein, which provides a pathway from the cavernous sinus to the pterygoid plexus. Packing toward the base of this triangle to occlude the sphenoid emissary vein is performed safely. Posterior packing within this triangle must be performed with care because it may occlude the carotid artery as it crosses the foramen lacerum.

In the direct, microsurgical management of type D carotid cavernous fistulas, all of the cavernous triangles are opened and packed. The type D fistulas are diffuse lesions and generally require full exposure of the cavernous sinus for successful obliteration. The surgical approach may be tailored, however, based on the results of the postembolization angiogram. If the sole feeding vessel is the meningohypophyseal trunk, selective opening of the superior or lateral triangle may be performed.

This technique has been applied successfully in the management of type D carotid cavernous fistulas.[6] Day and Fukushima[6] reported on their experience with nine patients using the combined extradural and intradural frontotemporal approach to the cavernous sinus. In all nine cases, complete resolution of the carotid cavernous fistula was achieved, as documented by postoperative angiography. Cranial nerve palsies were minimized by adhering to the triangular corridors that are bound by the cranial nerves. Only one patient had persistent diplopia from cranial nerve palsy after surgery (11%). By packing between the cranial nerves, within the triangles, permanent injury to the cranial nerves is limited or avoided. Many of the patients had temporary diplopia that resolved by 3 months after surgery. In this series, the patency of the carotid artery was preserved in seven of nine cases, or 78% of the time. Of the two patients with compromised carotid arteries, one had transient hemiparesis that subsequently resolved. The other patient had postoperative occlusion of the carotid artery and developed a persistent hemiparesis. This situation results in an 11% incidence of stroke using this technique. Vision was preserved at the preoperative level or improved in all patients. Overall the combined extradural and intradural frontotemporal approach to the cavernous sinus is a relatively safe and effective means to deal with persistent type D carotid cavernous fistulas. With a detailed knowledge of the triangular corridors to the cavernous sinus, cranial nerves may be preserved in almost 90% of cases, and stroke may be averted with the same frequency.

Radiosurgery

Some centers have investigated the use of stereotactic radiosurgery in the treatment of carotid cavernous fistulas.[39–42] Ionizing radiation has been used for other intracranial vascular malformations.[43–49] Radiation presumably leads to vessel occlusion by invoking blood vessel intimal hyperplasia.[39, 40] Barcia-Salorio and colleagues[39, 40] reported on 25 patients with carotid cavernous fistulas. They treated 22 patients with indirect or types B, C, or D fistulas with stereotactic radiosurgery alone. They also presented three patients with type A fistulas that were refractory to carotid artery trapping.

Radiosurgery was performed by this group by placement of a stereotactic frame followed by a localizing angiogram. The patients then received 30 to 40 Gy to the lesion using a cobalt radiation source. Of the patients with indirect fistulas, 20 of 22 closed in a mean period of 7.5 months after radiosurgery, as documented by angiography. Symptoms improved a mean 2.37 months after radiosurgery. Of the three patients with trapped type A fistulas, one patient had resolution of symptoms 6 months after radiosurgery, and the other two had no relief with radiosurgery. This study shows successful treatment of indirect carotid cavernous fistulas using stereotactic guidance and an external cobalt source of radiation. The system that Barcia-Salorio and colleagues employed had 35 fixed portals to focus the radiation.[50]

Many centers in the United States now use the Leksell gamma knife system to deliver cobalt radiation. This system uses 201 fixed portals to focus the ionizing radiation on a single point within the stereotactic head frame. Pollock and coworkers[42] reported on 20 patients with indirect carotid cavernous fistulas who were treated with the Leksell gamma knife system. In this small group of 20 patients, 7 were treated with radiosurgery alone, and 13 received radiation after endovascular therapy. The patients were treated with a median of 3 isocenters and a range of 1 to 10 isocenters. Treatment planning was performed to have the lesion conform to the 50% isodose curve. The median dosage to the 50% isodose line was 20 Gy. With a mean follow-up of 36 months after radiosurgery, 19 patients had improvement of clinical symptoms. This improvement proved temporary in 3 patients, who required further transvenous or transarterial embolization 4 to 12 months after radiosurgery. Follow-up angiography was performed on 15 of the patients, of whom 13 showed complete obliteration of the carotid cavernous fistulas.[42]

These data show that radiosurgery may be effective in treating some indirect carotid cavernous fistulas; however, this technique has several important limitations. First, it takes a mean of 7.5 months for radiosurgery to exact an effect on the lesion.[39–41, 51] Radiosurgery is an inappropriate treatment choice for patients who have progressive visual loss, neurological deficit, or high-risk cortical venous drainage. Second, the permanence of radiotherapy in the management of carotid cavernous fistulas is unclear. Pollock and coworkers[42] observed a 15% recurrence (3 of 20 patients) among patients treated with radiosurgery. The symptoms recurred 4 to 12 months after radiosurgery, necessitating further endovascular treatment. More long-term data are necessary to ascertain the true actuarial control rate of radiosurgery. Third, radiosurgery does not seem to have any role in the management of direct or type A carotid cavernous fistulas. Debrun and associates[9] estimated that many type A carotid cavernous fistulas consist of single holes within the arterial wall that are 2 to 6 mm in diameter. The work of Barcia-Salorio suggested that radiation is not effective in obliterating such a large defect in the arterial wall.[39–41, 51] Consequently, radiosurgery does not seem to be a reasonable option for type A carotid cavernous fistulas.

A fourth major consideration in the use of radiosurgery for carotid cavernous fistulas is the long-term effects of radiation. In contrast to patients with metastatic malignancies, patients with carotid cavernous fistulas have normal life expectancies. Consequently the possibility of long-term neurovascular complications or malignancy cannot be overlooked.[52–55] Brada and associates[53] analyzed patients who had partial resection of pituitary adenomas and adjuvant radiation therapy. They observed a 1.3% cumulative risk of developing malignancy 10 years after radiation treatment and a 1.9% cumulative risk at 20 years.[7] These radiation-induced sarcomas tend to occur in a delayed manner. Chang and coworkers[54] observed sarcomas 4 to 15 years after cranial irradiation. When radiation-induced sarcomas occur, they are often fatal. Chang and coworkers[54] observed 86% fatality (six of seven patients) among patients with radiation-induced sarcomas, with a median survival of 19 months.

A presumed benefit of stereotactic radiosurgery is that radiation delivery to adjacent tissue is minimized through the use of many overlapping beams or portals. In the case of the Leksell gamma unit, it is 201 fixed channels.[56] Despite this fact, case reports have emerged that describe the development of fatal malignancies in patients who were treated with stereotactic radiosurgery for other benign conditions, such as vestibular schwannoma and meningioma.[57–59] These patients developed fatal malignancies on average 5 to 6 years after radiation treatment.[58] Radiation-induced sarcoma is an infrequent but potentially fatal complication of radiation therapy that must be considered when treating patients with benign diseases. Although early data show some promise, the precise role of radiosurgery in the management of indirect carotid cavernous fistulas remains to be determined.

SUMMARY

Endovascular neurosurgery has emerged as the primary treatment modality for direct and indirect carotid cavernous fistulas. When endovascular techniques are not successful, direct exposure of the cavernous sinus using the techniques of modern skull base microsurgery is necessary. The use of stereotactic radiosurgery as an adjunct to endovascular neurosurgery has shown some promise in preliminary clinical studies.

REFERENCES

1. Locke CE: Intracranial arteriovenous aneurysm or pulsating exophthalmos. Ann Surg 80:1–24, 1924.

2. Dandy W: The treatment of carotid cavernous arteriovenous aneurysms. Ann Surg 102:916–926, 1935.
3. Stern WE, Brown J, Alksne J: The surgical challenge of carotid cavernous fistula: The critical role of intracranial circulatory dynamics. J Neurosurg 27:298–308, 1967.
4. Parkinson D: A surgical approach to the cavernous portion of the internal carotid artery: Anatomical studies and case report. J Neurosurg 23:474–483, 1965.
5. Parkinson D, Downs AR, Whytehead LL, Syslak WB: Carotid cavernous fistula: Direct repair with preservation of carotid. Surgery 76:882–889, 1974.
6. Day JD, Fukushima T: Direct microsurgery of dural arteriovenous malformation type carotid-cavernous sinus fistulas: Indications, technique, and results. Neurosurgery 41:1119–1124, discussion 1124–1126, 1997.
7. Peterson E, Valberg J, Whittingham D: Electrically induced thrombosis of the cavernous sinus in the treatment of carotid cavernous fistula. Excerpta Med Int Congr Series 193:105, 1969.
8. Hosobuchi Y: Electrothrombosis of carotid-cavernous fistula. J Neurosurg 42:76–85, 1975.
9. Debrun G, Lacour P, Vinuela F, et al: Treatment of 54 traumatic carotid-cavernous fistulas. J Neurosurg 55:678–692, 1981.
10. Debrun GM, Vinuela F, Fox AJ, et al: Indications for treatment and classification of 132 carotid-cavernous fistulas. Neurosurgery 22:285–289, 1988.
11. Halbach VV, Higashida RT, Barnwell SL, et al: Transarterial platinum coil embolization of carotid-cavernous fistulas. AJNR Am J Neuroradiol 12:429–433, 1991.
12. Teitelbaum GP, Larsen DW, Zelman V, et al: A tribute to Dr. Fedor A. Serbinenko, founder of endovascular neurosurgery. Neurosurgery 46:462–469, discussion 469–470, 2000.
13. Barrow DL, Spector RH, Braun IF, et al: Classification and treatment of spontaneous carotid-cavernous sinus fistulas. J Neurosurg 62:248–256, 1985.
14. Kupersmith MJ, Berenstein A, Flamm E, Ransohoff J: Neuroophthalmologic abnormalities and intravascular therapy of traumatic carotid cavernous fistulas. Ophthalmology 93:906–912, 1986.
15. Bullock R, van Dellen JR: Acute carotid-cavernous fistula with retained knife blade after transorbital stab wound. Surg Neurol 24:555–558, 1985.
16. Kieck CF, de Villiers JC: Vascular lesions due to transcranial stab wounds. J Neurosurg 60:42–46, 1984.
17. Debrun GM, Aletich VA, Miller NR, DeKeiser RJ: Three cases of spontaneous direct carotid cavernous fistulas associated with Ehlers-Danlos syndrome type IV. Surg Neurol 46:247–252, 1996.
18. Farley MK, Clark RD, Fallor MK, et al: Spontaneous carotid-cavernous fistula and the Ehlers-Danlos syndromes. Ophthalmology 90:1337–1342, 1983.
19. Graf CJ: Spontaneous carotid-cavernous fistula: Ehlers-Danlos syndrome and related conditions. Arch Neurol 13:662–672, 1965.
20. Hollister D: Heritable disorders of connective tissue: Ehlers-Danlos syndrome. Pediatr Clin North Am 25:575–591, 1978.
21. Kanner AA, Maimon S, Rappaport ZH: Treatment of spontaneous carotid-cavernous fistula in Ehlers-Danlos syndrome by transvenous occlusion with Guglielmi detachable coils: Case report and review of the literature. J Neurosurg 93:689–692, 2000.
22. Schievink WI, Piepgras DG, Earnest FT, Gordon H: Spontaneous carotid-cavernous fistulae in Ehlers-Danlos syndrome Type IV: Case report. J Neurosurg 74:991–998, 1991.
23. Halbach VV, Hieshima GB, Higashida RT, Reicher M: Carotid cavernous fistulae: Indications for urgent treatment. AJR Am J Roentgenol 149:587–593, 1987.
24. Vinuela F, Fox AJ, Debrun GM, et al: Spontaneous carotid-cavernous fistulas: Clinical, radiological, and therapeutic considerations: Experience with 20 cases. J Neurosurg 60:976–984, 1984.
25. Sanders M, Hoyt W: Hypoxic ocular sequelae of carotid-cavernous fistulae. Br J Ophthalmol 53:82–97, 1969.
26. Miller N, Newman N (eds): Walsh and Hoyt's Clinical Neuro-Ophthalmology, 5th ed. Baltimore, Williams & Wilkins, 1998, pp 2165–2207.
27. d'Angelo VA, Monte V, Scialfa G, et al: Intracerebral venous hemorrhage in "high-risk" carotid-cavernous fistula. Surg Neurol 30:387–390, 1988.
28. Goto K, Hieshima GB, Higashida RT, et al: Treatment of direct carotid cavernous sinus fistulae: Various therapeutic approaches and results in 148 cases. Acta Radiol 369(Suppl):576–579, 1986.
29. Mullan S: Treatment of carotid-cavernous fistulas by cavernous sinus occlusion. J Neurosurg 50:131–144, 1979.
30. Halbach VV, Higashida RT, Hieshima GB, et al: Dural fistulas involving the cavernous sinus: Results of treatment in 30 patients. Radiology 163:437–442, 1987.
31. Day JD, Giannotta SL, Fukushima T: Extradural temporopolar approach to lesions of the upper basilar artery and infrachiasmatic region. J Neurosurg 81:230–235, 1994.
32. Tu YK, Liu HM, Hu SC: Direct surgery of carotid cavernous fistulae and dural arteriovenous malformations of the cavernous sinus. Neurosurgery 41:798–805, discussion 805–806, 1997.
33. Day JD, Fukushima T, Giannotta SL: Cranial base approaches to posterior circulation aneurysms. J Neurosurg 87:544–554, 1997.
34. Oikawa S, Mizuno M, Muraoka S, Kobayashi S: Retrograde dissection of the temporalis muscle preventing muscle atrophy for pterional craniotomy: Technical note. J Neurosurg 84:297–299, 1996.
35. Dolenc V: Direct microsurgical repair of intracavernous vascular lesions. J Neurosurg 58:824–831, 1983.
36. Dolenc VV: A combined epi- and subdural direct approach to carotid-ophthalmic artery aneurysms. J Neurosurg 62:667–672, 1985.
37. Kawase T, Shiobara R, Toya S: Anterior transpetrosal-transtentorial approach for sphenopetroclival meningiomas: Surgical method and results in 10 patients. Neurosurgery 28:869–875, discussion 875–876, 1991.
38. Kawase T, Toya S, Shiobara R, Mine T: Transpetrosal approach for aneurysms of the lower basilar artery. J Neurosurg 63:857–861, 1985.
39. Barcia-Salorio JL, Soler F, Barcia JA, Hernandez G: Radiosurgery of carotid-cavernous fistulae. Acta Neurochir 62(Suppl):10–12, 1994.
40. Barcia-Salorio JL, Soler F, Barcia JA, Hernandez G: Stereotactic radiosurgery for the treatment of low-flow carotid-cavernous fistulae: Results in a series of 25 cases. Stereotact Funct Neurosurg 63:266–270, 1994.
41. Barcia-Salorio JL, Soler F, Hernandez G, Barcia JA: Radiosurgical treatment of low flow carotid-cavernous fistulae. Acta Neurochir 52(Suppl):93–95, 1991.
42. Pollock BE, Nichols DA, Garrity JA, et al: Stereotactic radiosurgery and particulate embolization for cavernous sinus dural arteriovenous fistulae. Neurosurgery 45:459–466, discussion 466–467, 1999.
43. Kurita H, Kawamoto S, Sasaki T, et al: Results of radiosurgery for brain stem arteriovenous malformations. J Neurol Neurosurg Psychiatry 68:563–570, 2000; see comments.
44. Maesawa S, Flickinger JC, Kondziolka D, Lunsford LD: Repeated radiosurgery for incompletely obliterated arteriovenous malformations. J Neurosurg 92:961–970, 2000.
45. Massager N, Regis J, Kondziolka D, et al: Gamma knife radiosurgery for brainstem arteriovenous malformations: Preliminary results. J Neurosurg 93(Suppl 3):102–103, 2000.
46. Massoud TF, Hademenos GJ, De Salles AA, Solberg TD: Experimental radiosurgery simulations using a theoretical model of cerebral arteriovenous malformations. Stroke 31:2466–2477, 2000; in process citation.
47. Payne BR, Prasad D, Steiner M, et al: Gamma surgery for vein of Galen malformations. J Neurosurg 93:229–236, 2000.
48. Richling B, Killer M: Endovascular management of patients with cerebral arteriovenous malformations. Neurosurg Clin N Am 11: 123–145, 2000.
49. Schlienger M, Atlan D, Lefkopoulos D, et al: Linac radiosurgery for cerebral arteriovenous malformations: Results in 169 patients. Int J Radiat Oncol Biol Phys 46:1135–1142, 2000.
50. Yu C: Principles of stereotactic radiosurgery. In Petrovich Z, Brady LW, Apuzzo ML, et al (eds): Combined Modality Therapy of Central Nervous System Tumors. New York, Springer, 2000, pp 81–107.
51. Barcia-Salorio JL, Barcia JA, Soler F, et al: Stereotactic radiotherapy plus radiosurgical boost in the treatment of large cerebral arteriovenous malformations. Acta Neurochir 58(Suppl):98–100, 1993.
52. Arlen M, Higinbotham NL, Huvos AG, et al: Radiation-induced sarcoma of bone. Cancer 28:1087–1099, 1971.
53. Brada M, Ford D, Ashley S, et al: Risk of second brain tumour

after conservative surgery and radiotherapy for pituitary adenoma. BMJ 304:1343–1346, 1992.
54. Chang SM, Barker FG 2nd, Larson DA, et al: Sarcomas subsequent to cranial irradiation. Neurosurgery 36:685–690, 1995.
55. Ducatman BS, Scheithauer BW: Postirradiation neurofibrosarcoma. Cancer 51:1028–1033, 1983.
56. Leksell L: Stereotactic radiosurgery. J Neurol Neurosurg Psychiatry 46:797–803, 1983.
57. Comey CH, McLaughlin MR, Jho HD, et al: Death from a malignant cerebellopontine angle triton tumor despite stereotactic radiosurgery: Case report. J Neurosurg 89:653–658, 1998; see comments.
58. Fagan P, Chang P, Turner J: Triton tumor letter to the editor. J Neurosurg 90:987–989, 1999.
59. Thomsen J, Mirz F, Wetke R, et al: Intracranial sarcoma in a patient with neurofibromatosis type 2 treated with gamma knife radiosurgery for vestibular schwannoma. Am J Otol 21:364–370, 2000.

PART XI SPINAL ARTERIOVENOUS MALFORMATIONS

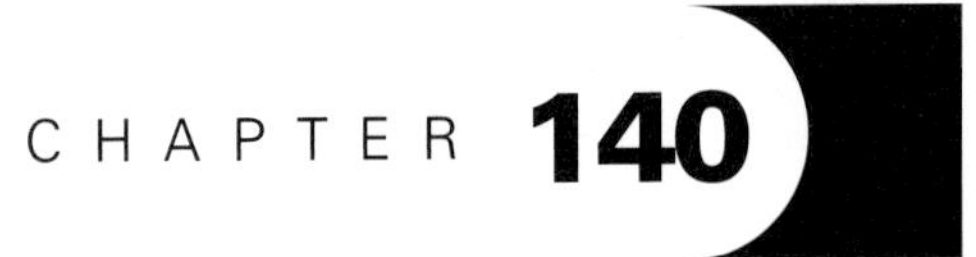

Classification of Spinal Cord Vascular Lesions

HOWARD A. RIINA ■ PAUL W. DETWILER ■ RANDALL W. PORTER ■ ROBERT F. SPETZLER

This chapter presents a modified classification system for spinal cord vascular lesions based on the senior author's (RFS) experience with their treatment. Three major types of lesions are introduced (Table 140–1): neoplastic, aneurysmal, and arteriovenous (AV). Neoplasms are subclassified as hemangioblastomas and cavernous malformations; spinal aneurysmal lesions are apparent. The AV lesions are subclassified as AV fistulas and AV malformations (AVMs). Fistulas are subdivided into extradural and intradural lesions, with intradural lesions further characterized as dorsal or ventral. AVMs are divided into extradural-intradural, intramedullary, and conus malformations. As with any classification system, the goal of this one is to provide a common language for communication to help improve diagnosis and treatment.

TABLE 140–1 ■ **Modified Classification System for Spinal Cord Vascular Malfunctions**

Neoplastic Vascular Lesions
- Hemangioblastomas
- Cavernous malformations

Spinal Aneurysms

Arteriovenous Lesions
- Arteriovenous fistulas
  - Extradural
  - Intradural
    - Dorsal (subtypes A and B)
    - Ventral (subtypes A, B, and C)
- Arteriovenous malformations
  - Extradural-intradural
  - Intramedullary
    - Compact
    - Diffuse
  - Conus

NEOPLASTIC VASCULAR LESIONS

Both hemangioblastomas and cavernous malformations occur sporadically and in a familial pattern and are also known to appear and grow spontaneously.[1]

Hemangioblastomas

Hemangioblastomas are composed of three cell types: endothelial cell–associated pericytes, lipid-laden stromal cells, and endothelial cells.[2] As familial lesions, they occur in the setting of von Hippel-Lindau disease. Erythropoietin production by tumor cells can result in polycythemia. Hemangioblastomas are usually intramedullary, abutting the leptomeninges (Fig. 140–1; see color section in this volume), but they have been observed in other locations, including within the cerebellum and along nerve roots.[3] The cerebellum is the most common site. Despite their varied locations throughout the neuraxis (intracranial and intraspinal), these lesions are histopathologically similar. They can be highly vascular and pose the same difficulties for resection as do AVMs. As in the cerebellum, hemangioblastomas can be associated with a non-neoplastic cystic cavity, which, in the spinal cord, may mimic a syrinx (Fig. 140–2; see color section in this volume).[4]

Cavernous Malformations

In this classification system, cavernous malformations are regarded as neoplastic because their behavior paral-

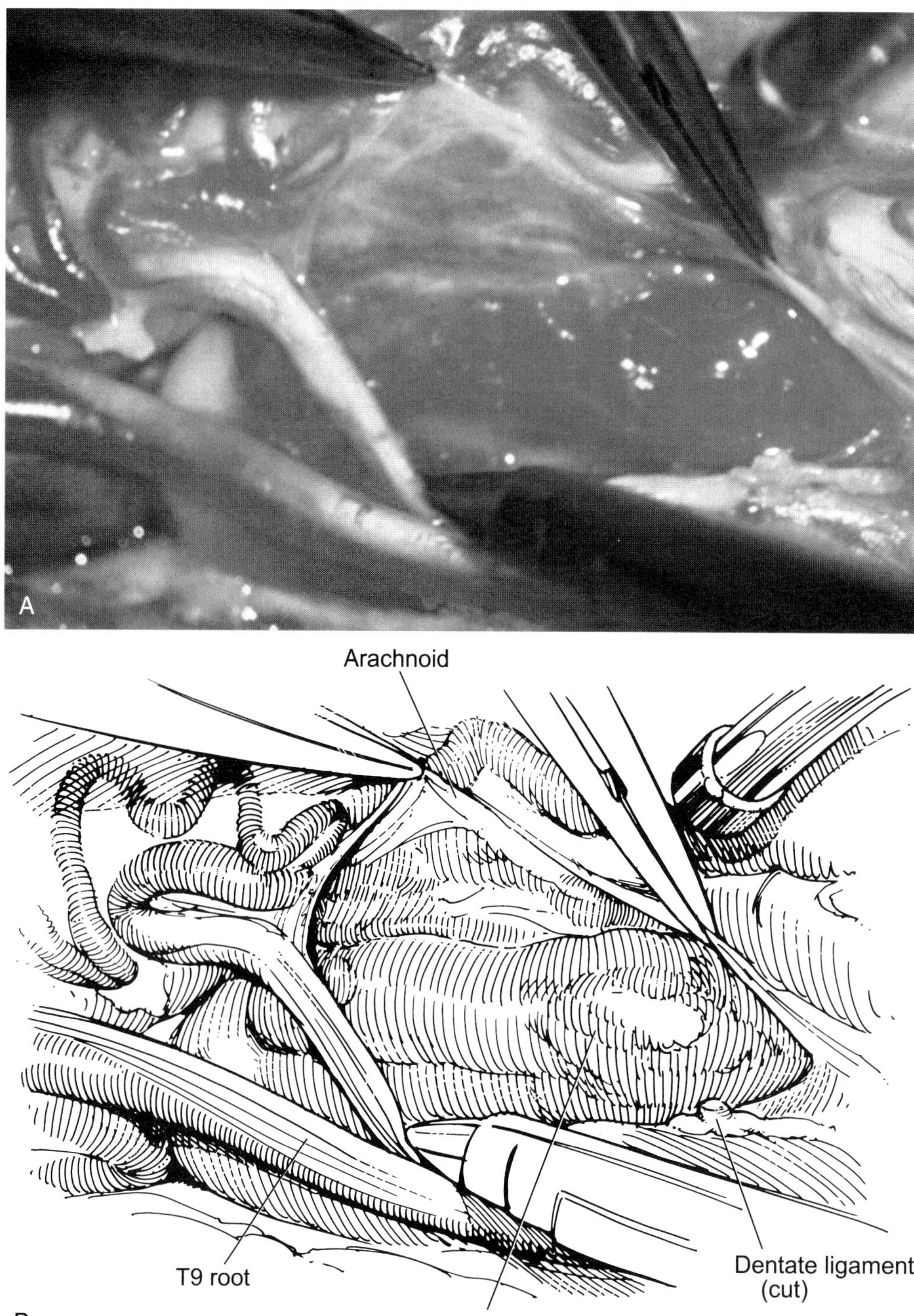

FIGURE 140–1. Intramedullary T9 hemangioblastoma situated arteriorly. The dentate ligament is cut (see color section in this volume). *A,* Intraoperative photograph. *B,* Corresponding illustration. (From Spetzler RF, Koos WT, Richling B, Lang J: Color Atlas of Microneurosurgery, vol 3, 2nd ed. Stuttgart, Germany, Georg Thieme Verlag, 1999.)

lels that of a neoplastic lesion. They are associated with a known and identifiable chromosomal abnormality and occur sporadically as well as in a familial pattern (particularly among Mexican Americans).[5] They can appear and grow spontaneously.[6] These angiographically occult lesions are composed of sinusoidal vascular channels lined with endothelium, surrounded by a hemosiderin-stained gliotic rim of tissue (Fig. 140–3; see color section in this volume).[7] Calcification is frequently observed. Cavernous malformations always occur in conjunction with a developmental venous anomaly.[8] They have been observed in the cerebrum,

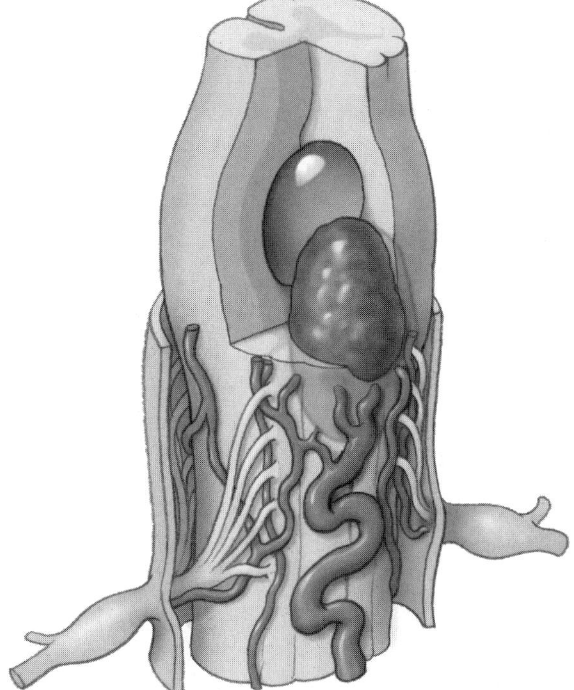

FIGURE 140–2. Cystic hemangioblastoma of the spinal cord (see color section in this volume). (Courtesy of Barrow Neurological Institute, Phoenix, AZ.)

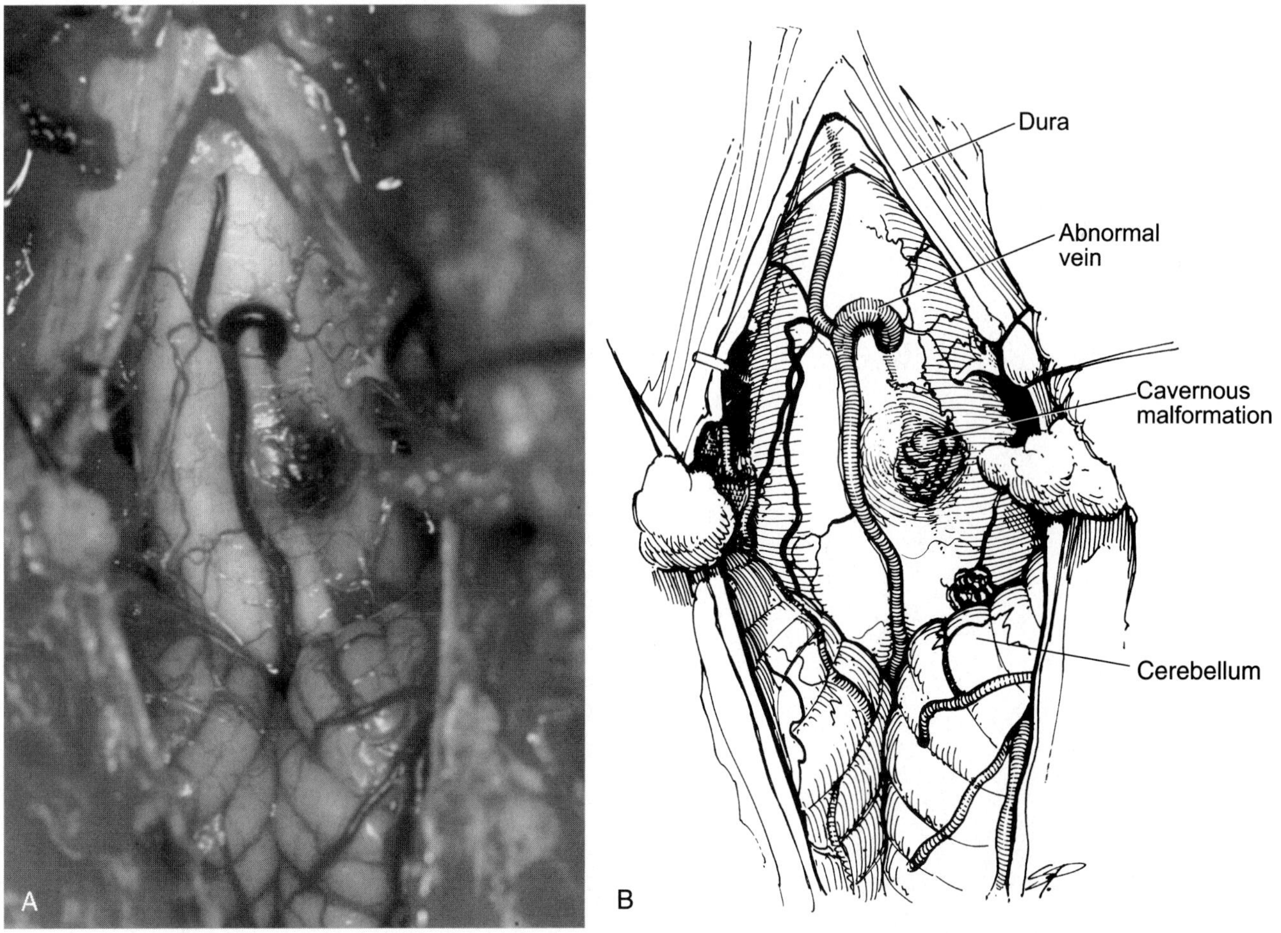

FIGURE 140–3. Intraoperative photograph *(A)* and corresponding illustration *(B)* of a spinal cavernous malformation and associated venous anomaly (see color section in this volume). The cerebellum is at the bottom of the photograph. (From Spetzler RF, Koos WT, Richling B, Lang J: Color Atlas of Microneurosurgery, vol 3, 2nd ed. Stuttgart, Germany, Georg Thieme Verlag, 1999.)

brainstem, cerebellum, and spinal cord. When a cavernous malformation is resected, the integrity of this venous anomaly must be preserved, despite its aberrant nature, because it serves as normal venous drainage to the surrounding tissue. Injury to or disturbance of this venous structure can result in catastrophic venous infarction.

SPINAL CORD ANEURYSMS

Arterial aneurysms involving the spinal vasculature are rare. They are usually found as flow-related lesions in conjunction with spinal cord AVMs.[9, 10] Like intracranial aneurysms, they are believed to develop from intimal defects subjected to abnormal shear forces related to blood flow (Fig. 140–4). Treatment of aneurysms involving the spinal cord vasculature is complex. For aneurysms associated with AVMs, it has been argued that treatment or partial treatment of the AVM, with the resulting alteration in blood flow, may cause the aneurysm to regress. Whenever possible, the primary treatment of a spinal aneurysm is sacrifice of the parent radicular vessel. This is obviously impossible when the anterior spinal artery or its main supply is involved. In such cases, no treatment, flow modification, or direct exclusion from the circulation should be considered. We have seen two spinal aneurysmal lesions, both of which manifested after subarachnoid hemorrhage. One lesion involved the artery of Adamkiewicz and hence was in direct line with the blood supply to the anterior spinal artery. This lesion was wrapped. The second lesion involved the radicular vessel with no contribution to the anterior spinal artery; it was treated by occluding the radicular vessel in question.

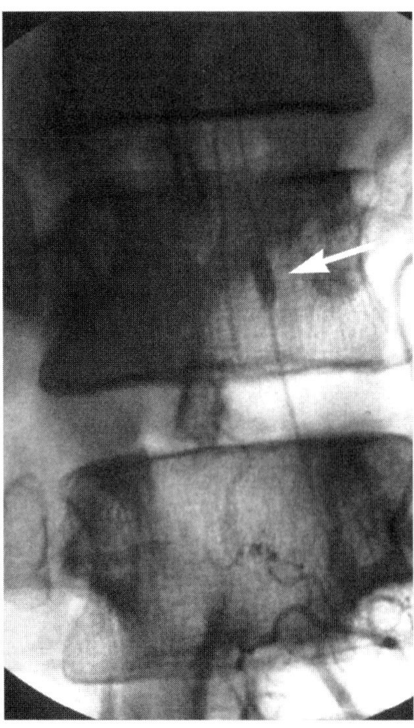

FIGURE 140–4. Spinal artery aneurysm arising from the artery of Adamkiewicz *(arrow).* (From Vishteh AG, Brown A, Spetzler, RF: Aneurysm of the intradural artery of Adamkiewicz treated with muslin wrapping: Technical case report. Neurosurgery 40: 207–209, 1997. With permission from Lippincott Williams & Wilkins.)

ARTERIOVENOUS FISTULAS AND ARTERIOVENOUS MALFORMATIONS OF THE SPINAL CORD

Extradural Arteriovenous Fistulas

Extradural AV fistulas usually become symptomatic with progressive myelopathy related to spinal cord compression, venous congestion, or arterial steal.[11, 12] Initially, they are often diagnosed with magnetic resonance imaging (MRI) of the spinal cord; however, the diagnostic gold standard remains spinal angiography. Fistulas represent a direct connection between an extradural artery and vein (Fig. 140–5; see color section in this volume). They are high-flow lesions that create an engorged epidural venous complex, which subsequently compresses the spinal cord by mass effect. The high venous pressure generated in the epidural venous system prevents venous outflow from the spinal cord parenchyma, leading to venous hypertension. This dilated epidural venous complex also serves as an arterial sink that generates vascular steal. These fistulas are usually accessible and can be treated effectively with endovascular techniques. Today, open surgical intervention is rarely required.

Intradural Arteriovenous Fistulas

Dorsal Intradural Arteriovenous Fistulas. These lesions, also known as type I spinal AVMs, are the most common spinal vascular malformation. They usually become symptomatic with progressive myelopathy caused by venous hypertension (Fig. 140–6; see color section in this volume).[13] Occasionally, they present with hemorrhage.[14] Diagnostic evaluation usually begins with MRI of the spinal cord, followed by spinal angiography. Spinal angiography demonstrates a slow-flow lesion supplied by a dorsal radicular vessel. When only a single feeding vessel is encountered, the lesion is considered a type A fistula; when more than one feeding vessel is involved, it is referred to as a type B or multiple dorsal intradural fistula.[15]

Dorsal intradural AV fistulas most often occur in the thoracic spine. Classically, the involved artery or arteries enter the dura at the dural root sleeve, where the fistula is formed. The result is arterialization of the spinal venous vasculature, which, along with venous outflow obstruction, generates venous hypertension and subsequent myelopathy. Patients have progressive neurological symptoms that can be arrested only by eliminating the fistulous component.[16]

These lesions are best treated surgically. Endovascular surgery is often too proximal, leading to recurrence;

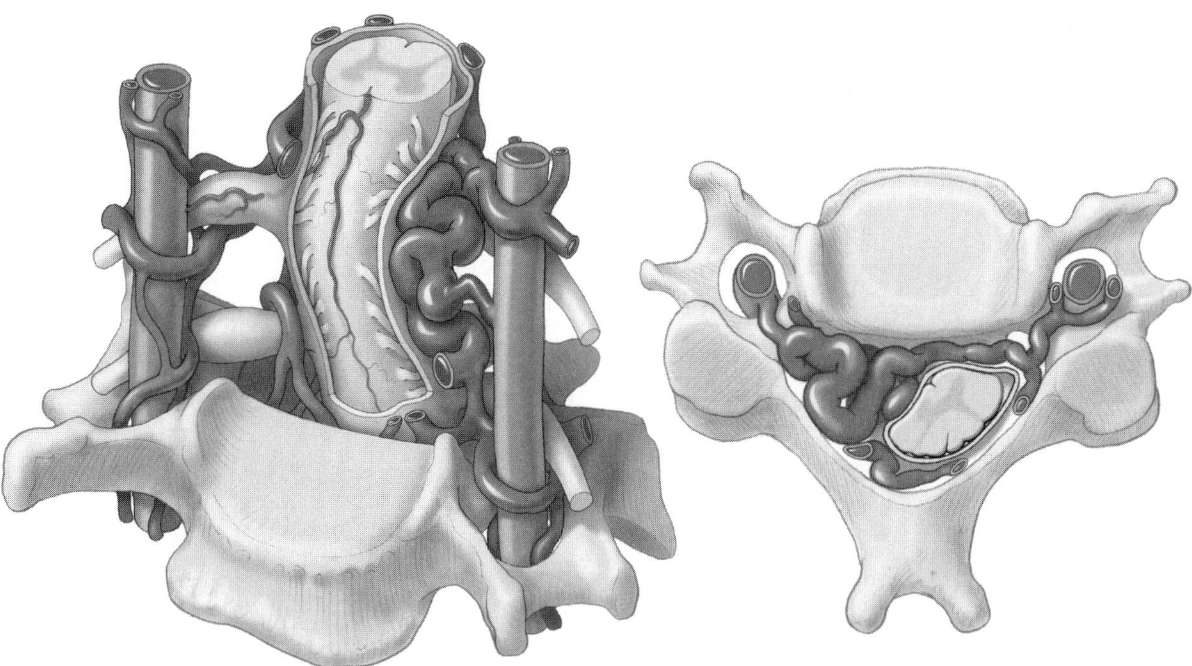

FIGURE 140–5. Extradural arteriovenous fistula (see color section in this volume). (From Spetzler RF, Detwiler PW, Riina HA, Porter RW: Modified classification of spinal cord vascular lesions. J Neurosurg [Spine 2] 96:145–156, 2002.)

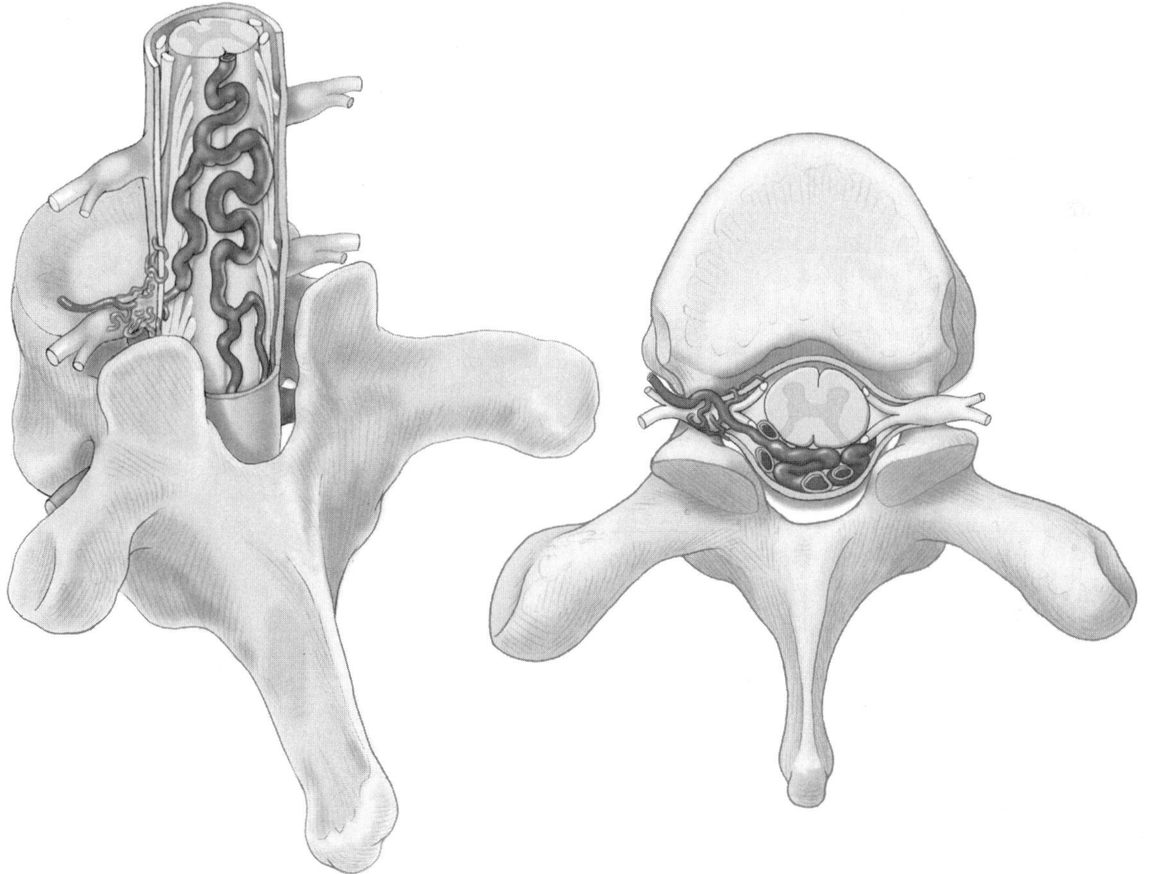

FIGURE 140–6. Dorsal intradural arteriovenous fistula (see color section in this volume). (From Spetzler RF, Detwiler PW, Riina HA, Porter RW: Modified classification of spinal cord vascular lesions. J Neurosurg [Spine 2] 96:145–156, 2002.)

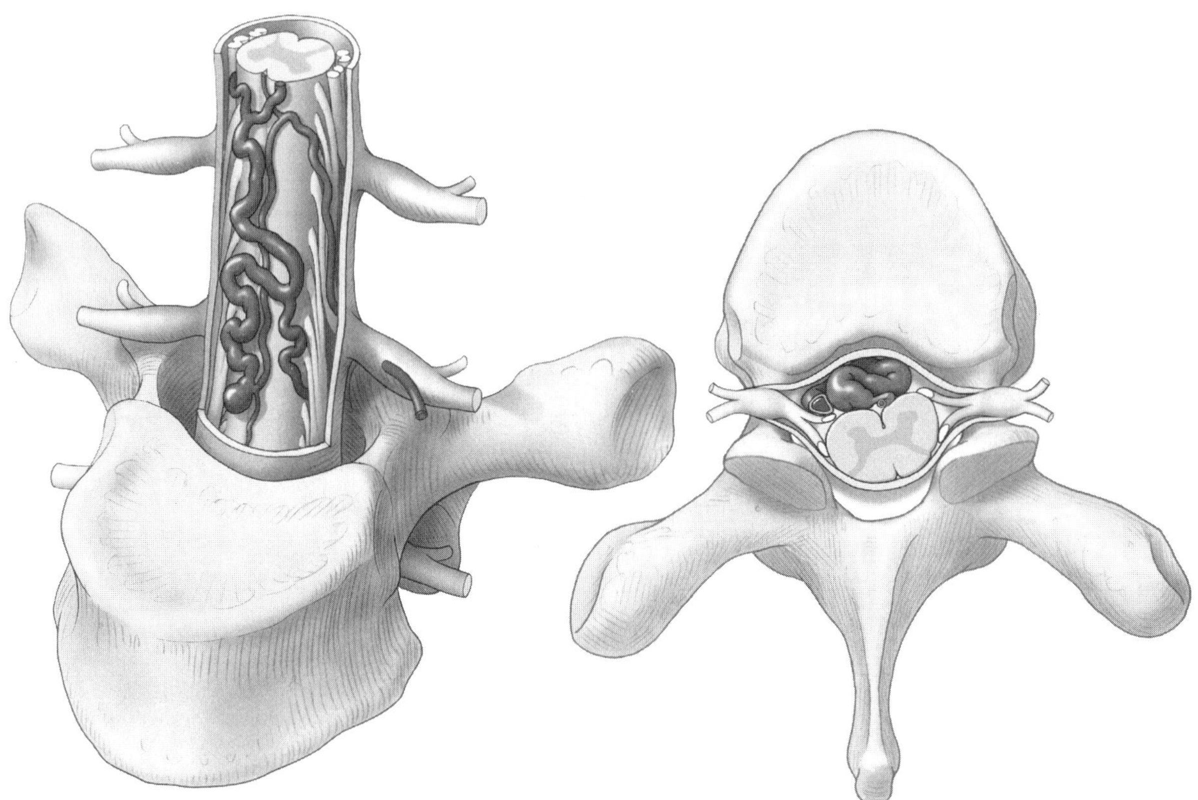

FIGURE 140–7. Ventral intradural arteriovenous fistula (see color section in this volume). (From Spetzler RF, Detwiler PW, Riina HA, Porter RW: Modified classification of spinal cord vascular lesions. J Neurosurg [Spine 2] 96:145–156, 2002.)

when it is too distal, venous hypertension can be aggravated. At surgery, an intradural fistulous connection is identified and interrupted, thereby curing the lesion. We have never seen an extradural component to these well-described lesions, nor have we seen the changes in the epidural venous plexus that would be expected if the fistula had an extradural component. Prominent epidural vessels encountered represent dural recruitment to the fistula.

Ventral Intradural Arteriovenous Fistulas. In the old nomenclature, the ventral intradural AV fistulas first described by Merland and coworkers[17] are the type IV malformations categorized by Heros and colleagues.[18] We have preserved Merland's subclassification: A denotes a small, B denotes a medium, and C denotes a large fistula (Fig. 140–7; see color section in this volume).[15]

Ventral intradural AV fistulas are midline lesions. Their blood supply is from the anterior spinal artery, and the fistulous component connects to the dilated and engorged venous system (Fig. 140–8; see color section in this volume).[19] They are high-flow lesions when characterized by spinal angiography.

Symptoms are often related to hemorrhage, compression, or venous hypertension. Patients with ventral intradural AV fistulas can present with progressive myelopathy related to compression from either a venous aneurysm or venous congestion. We have also

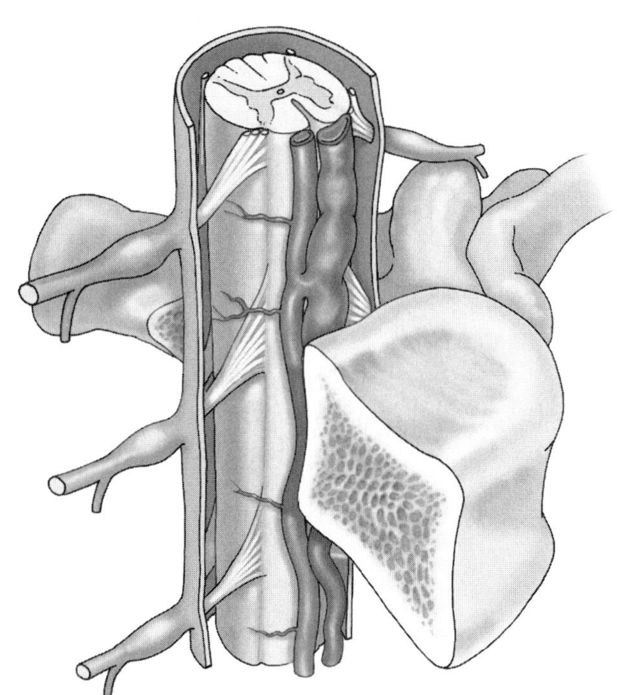

FIGURE 140–8. Ventral intradural arteriovenous fistula with connection to a dilated, engorged venous system (see color section in this volume). (Courtesy of Barrow Neurological Institute, Phoenix, AZ.)

seen patients present with subarachnoid hemorrhage. Patients usually undergo MRI of the spine before spinal angiography. Besides the high flow, spinal angiography usually shows a feeder originating from the anterior spinal artery.

Type A fistulas have the smallest shunt and slowest blood flow and therefore less venous hypertension and compression related to venous aneurysmal dilatation than the other types. Type B fistulas have somewhat larger shunts and higher blood flow and therefore are associated with a greater degree of venous hypertension. Type C fistulas have large shunts, very high flow, and significant degrees of venous hypertension. In these patients, venous congestion can cause significant compression and contribute to myelopathy. As the size of the shunt and velocity of the blood flow increase, the symptoms related to vascular steal and venous hypertension become more prominent. A significant number of these lesions can be treated endovascularly, but if this is unsuccessful, they can be treated surgically for direct fistula interruption.

Extradural-Intradural Arteriovenous Malformations

In the older nomenclature, extradural-intradural AVMs are known as juvenile AVMs, metameric AVMs, or type III AVMs.[20, 21] As their name implies, these complex lesions have both extra- and intradural components (Fig. 140–9; see color section in this volume). The malformation can include part of the vertebral body, be involved extradurally, and have significant intradural and intramedullary components. Patients often present with pain and progressive myelopathy related to compression and arterial steal.[20] Hemorrhage can occur as well. Patients usually undergo MRI, followed by spinal angiography. Spinal angiography reveals a high-flow lesion with multiple feeders that involve all layers of the spinal cord, as well as the surrounding vertebral bodies and musculature. We have had the most success using a multidisciplinary treatment approach that combines endovascular therapies with surgical resection. These lesions can be highly complex and difficult to cure.

Intramedullary Arteriovenous Malformations

Intramedullary AVMs, also known as type II AVMs, glomus-type AVMs, classic AVMs, angioma arteriovenosum, and angioma racemosum arteriovenous, are the spinal vascular malformations that most closely resemble intracranial cerebral AVMs (Fig. 140–10; see color section in this volume).[22, 23] They often present with acute myelopathy; however, patients with long-standing lesions often have progressive myelopathy. Pain is frequently associated with these lesions. Symptoms can be related to compression, arterial steal, and sometimes hemorrhage.[24] Patients undergo MRI of the spine, followed by spinal angiography. Spinal angiography often reveals multiple feeding vessels from the anterior and posterior spinal arteries to these high-flow lesions. We further subdivide these lesions based on the architecture of the nidus, which can be either diffuse or compact (Figs. 140–11 and 140–12; see color section in this volume). The type of nidus has implica-

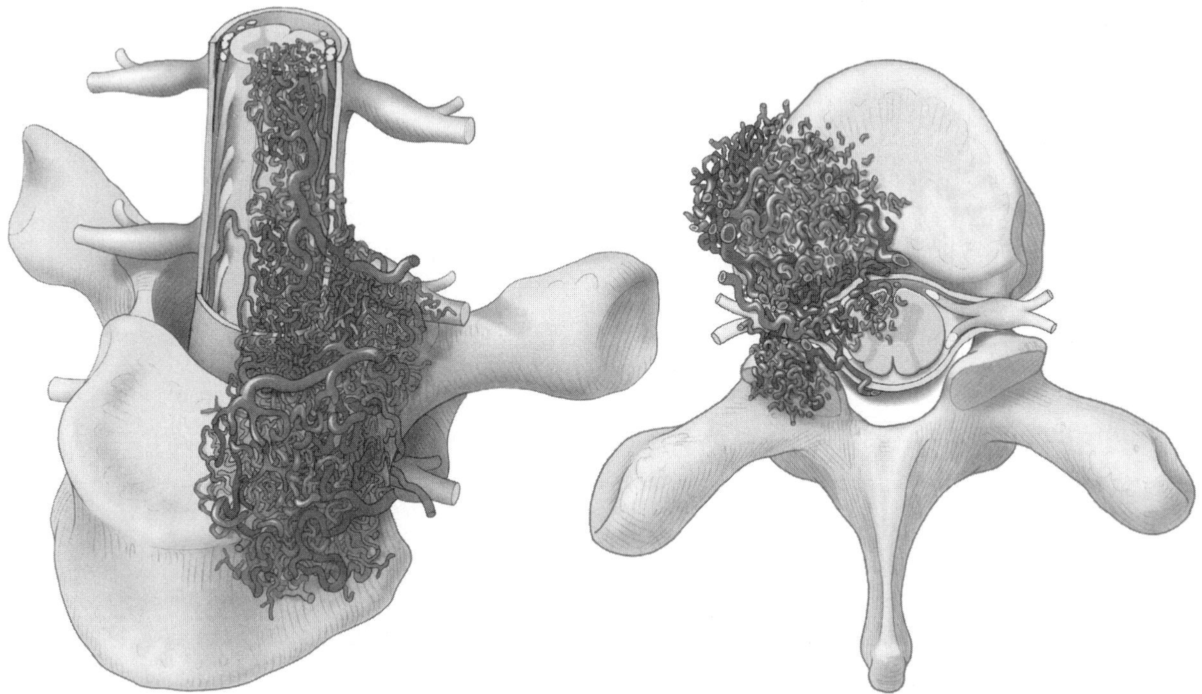

FIGURE 140–9. Complex extradural-intradural spinal arteriovenous malformation (see color section in this volume). (From Spetzler RF, Detwiler PW, Riina HA, Porter RW: Modified classification of spinal cord vascular lesions. J Neurosurg [Spine 2] 96:145–156, 2002.)

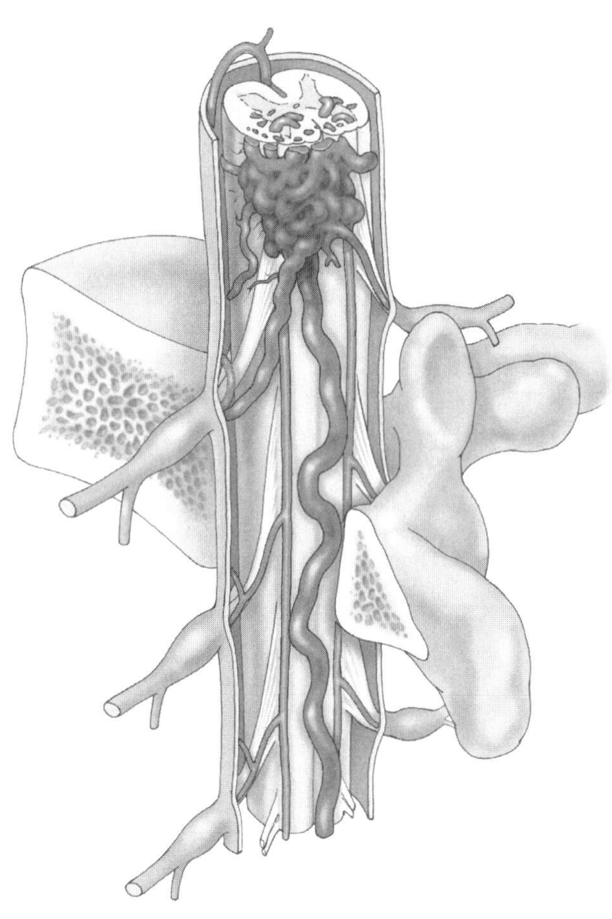

FIGURE 140–10. Intramedullary arteriovenous malformation (see color section in this volume). (Courtesy of Barrow Neurological Institute, Phoenix, AZ.)

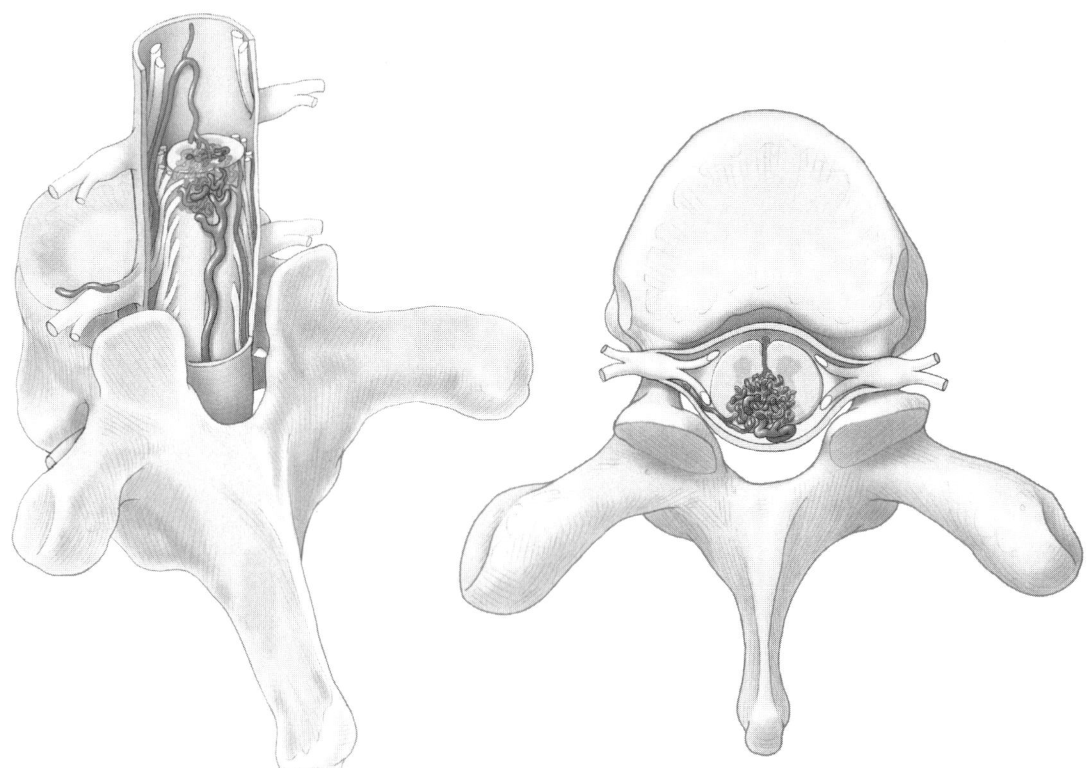

FIGURE 140–11. Intramedullary arteriovenous malformation with a compact nidus (see color section in this volume). (From Spetzler RF, Detwiler PW, Riina HA, Porter RW: Modified classification of spinal cord vascular lesions. J Neurosurg [Spine 2] 96:145–156, 2002.)

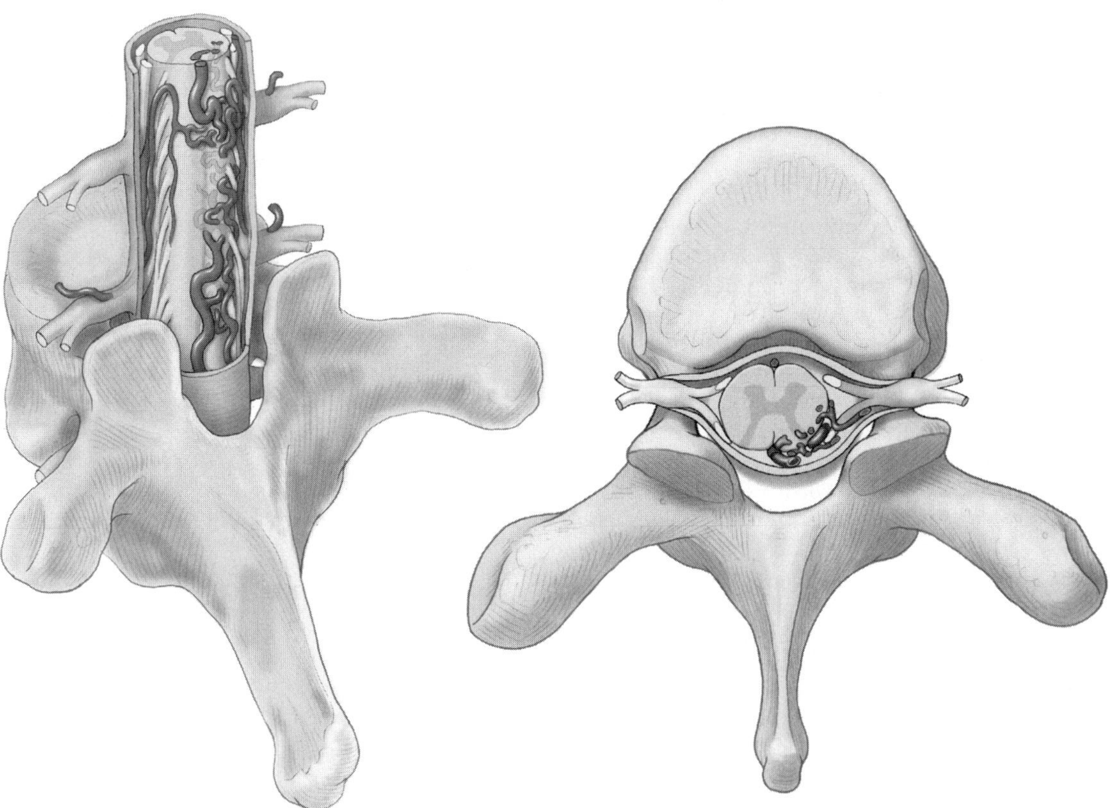

FIGURE 140–12. Intramedullary arteriovenous malformation with a diffuse nidus (see color section in this volume). (From Spetzler RF, Detwiler PW, Riina HA, Porter RW: Modified classification of spinal cord vascular lesions. J Neurosurg [Spine 2] 96:145–156, 2002.)

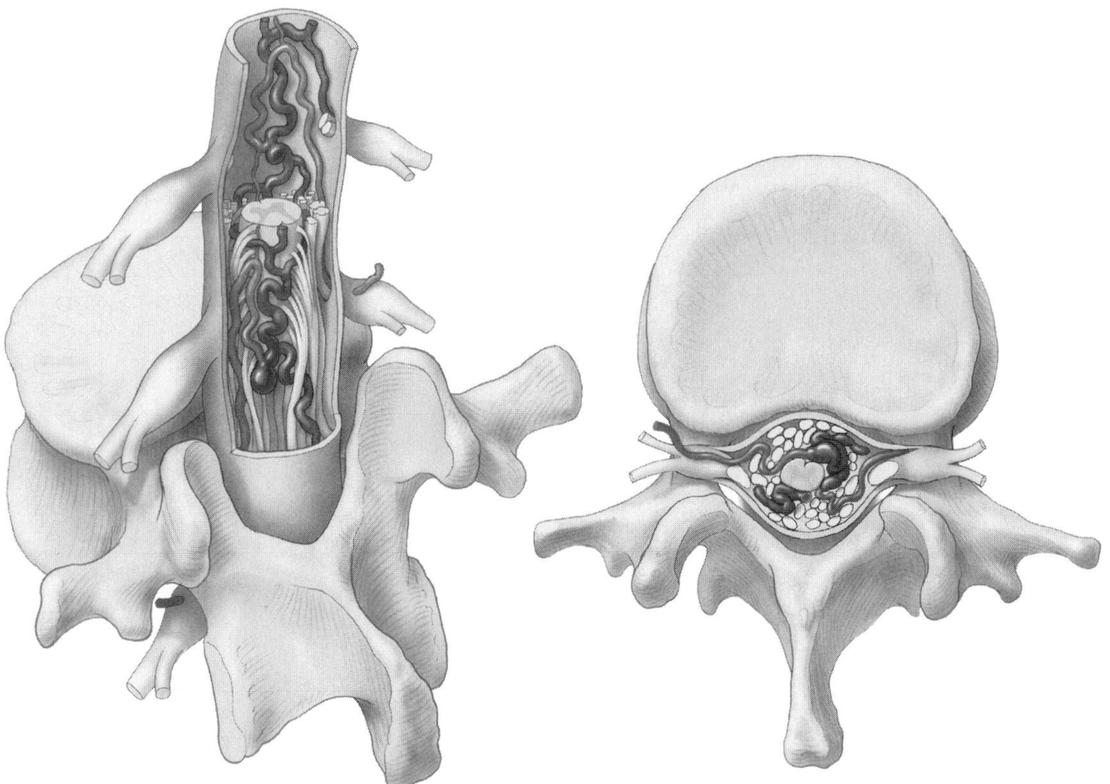

FIGURE 140–13. Conus arteriovenous malformation (see color section in this volume). (From Spetzler RF, Detwiler PW, Riina HA, Porter RW: Modified classification of spinal cord vascular lesions. J Neurosurg [Spine 2] 96:145–156, 2002.)

tions for resectability. If the basic tenets of AVM surgery are followed, lesions with a compact nidus are often amenable to surgical resection, whereas diffuse lesions are more difficult to resect.

Conus Arteriovenous Malformations

Conus AVMs are location specific and have features of both AV fistulas and AVMs of the spinal cord but are distinct to the conus and cauda equina (Fig. 140–13; see color section in this volume). They can be both peri- and intramedullary, often with a diffuse border. Patients become symptomatic with progressive myeloradiculopathy and occasional subarachnoid hemorrhage. Symptoms are related to venous hypertension, venous compression, and hemorrhage. Patients undergo spinal MRI followed by spinal angiography, which demonstrates multiple arterial feeders, usually more than one nidus, and a pattern of complex venous drainage. Because of their unique angioarchitecture, complete resection of conus AVMs is difficult to achieve. A combination of endovascular and surgical approaches has led to a high rate of obliteration. Intraoperative angiography is helpful in the management of these complex lesions.

REFERENCES

1. Anson JA, Spetzler RF: Surgical resection of intramedullary spinal cord cavernous malformations. J Neurosurg 78:446–451, 1993.
2. Guidetti B, Fortuna A: Surgical treatment of intramedullary hemangioblastoma of the spinal cord: Report of six cases. J Neurosurg 60:530–541, 1984.
3. Browne TR, Adams RD, Roberson GH: Hemangioblastoma of the spinal cord: Review and report of five cases. Arch Neurol 33: 435–441, 1976.
4. Enomoto H, Shibata T, Ito A, et al: Multiple hemangioblastomas accompanied by syringomyelia in the cerebellum and the spinal cord. Surg Neurol 22:197–203, 1984.
5. Rigamonti D, Hadley MN, Drayer BP, et al: Cerebral cavernous malformations: Incidence and familial occurrence. N Engl J Med 319:343–347, 1988.
6. Cosgrove GR, Bertrand G, Fontaine S, et al: Cavernous angiomas of the spinal cord. J Neurosurg 68:31–36, 1988.
7. McCormick PC, Michelsen WJ, Post KD, et al: Cavernous malformations of the spinal cord. Neurosurgery 23:459–463, 1988.
8. Vishteh AG, Sankhla S, Anson JA, et al: Surgical resection of intramedullary spinal cord cavernous malformations: Delayed complications, long-term outcomes, and association with cryptic venous malformations. Neurosurgery 41:1094–1101, 1997.
9. Vishteh AG, Brown AP, Spetzler RF: Aneurysm of the intradural artery of Adamkiewicz treated with muslin wrapping: Technical case report. Neurosurgery 40:207–209, 1997.
10. El Mahdi MA, Rudwan MA, Khaffaji SM, et al: A giant spinal aneurysm with cord and root compression. J Neurol Neurosurg Psychiatry 52:532–535, 1989.
11. Heier LA, Lee BCP: A dural spinal arteriovenous malformation with epidural venous drainage: A case report. AJNR Am J Neuroradiol 8:561–563, 1987.
12. Arnaud O, Bille F, Pouget J, et al: Epidural arteriovenous fistula with perimedullary venous drainage: Case report. Neuroradiology 36:490–491, 1994.
13. Bederson JB, Spetzler RF: Pathophysiology of type I spinal dural arteriovenous malformations. BNI Q 12:23–32, 1996.
14. Aminoff MJ, Barnard RO, Logue V: The pathophysiology of spinal vascular malformations. J Neurol Sci 23:255–263, 1974.
15. Anson JA, Spetzler RF: Classification of spinal arteriovenous malformations and implications for treatment. BNI Q 8:2–8, 1992.
16. Aminoff MJ, Logue V: Clinical features of spinal vascular malformations. Brain 97:197–210, 1974.
17. Merland JJ, Riche MC, Chiras J: Intraspinal extramedullary arteriovenous fistulae draining into the medullary veins [French]. J Neuroradiol 7:271–320, 1980.
18. Heros RC, Debrun GM, Ojemann RG, et al: Direct spinal arteriovenous fistula: A new type of spinal AVM. Case report. J Neurosurg 64:134–139, 1986.
19. Barrow DL, Colohan ART, Dawson R: Intradural perimedullary arteriovenous fistulas (type IV spinal cord arteriovenous malformations). J Neurosurg 81:221–229, 1994.
20. Spetzler RF, Zabramski JM, Flom RA: Management of juvenile spinal AVMs by embolization and operative excision: Case report. J Neurosurg 70:628–632, 1989.
21. Rudy DC, Woodside JR: Familial juvenile type III spinal cord arteriovenous malformation: Urodynamic findings. J Urol 130: 946–947, 1983.
22. Cogen P, Stein BM: Spinal cord arteriovenous malformations with significant intramedullary components. J Neurosurg 59:471–478, 1983.
23. Connolly ES Jr, Zubay GP, McCormick PC, et al: The posterior approach to a series of glomus (type II) intramedullary spinal cord arteriovenous malformations. Neurosurgery 42:774–786, 1998.
24. Djindjian M, Djindjian R, Hurth M, et al: Steal phenomena in spinal arteriovenous malformations [French]. J Neuroradiol 5: 187–201, 1978.

CHAPTER 141

Endovascular Treatment of Spinal Cord Arteriovenous Malformations

GAVIN W. BRITZ ■ JOSEPH ESKRIDGE

Vascular lesions of the spinal cord are a heterogeneous group of conditions that result from either congenital or acquired abnormalities of the spinal vasculature. The pathology, natural history, and treatment of these conditions are variable. Although these conditions were first recognized in the late 19th century, recent advancements in magnetic resonance imaging (MRI), superselective angiography, and endovascular therapy have contributed significantly to a better understanding and treatment of spinal vascular malformations. Angiographic diagnosis and endovascular treatment were initially reported by Djindjian and colleagues[1, 2] in France and by Doppman and associates[3, 4] in the United States as an alternative to the surgical ligation of feeding arteries. Since then, this approach has been accepted as the first line of treatment in many cases.[5–7]

The literature on spinal vascular malformations contains a great deal of confusing nomenclature. Therefore, an understanding of the classification of these lesions is important, because treatment and outcome differ depending on the type of lesion.

CLASSIFICATION

The classification of vascular lesions of the spinal cord has undergone an evolutionary process, based on our understanding of the clinicopathologic and then the radiologic features of these lesions.[8] Early classification schemes were based on pathologic specimens from autopsies and the operating room. Modern classification systems are based primarily on the nidus concept or, less often, on the type of artery involved, as identified by selective angiography.[8]

More recently, two important classification schemes have been described. The first was reported by Berenstein and Lasjaunias[9] in 1992 and then adapted by Niimi and Berenstein[10] in 1999 (Table 141–1). This classification divides lesions into fistulas or arteriovenous malformations (AVMs) that are found either within the cord itself (spinal cord vascular lesions) or in the surrounding dura or paraspinal regions. In addition, spinal cord telangiectasias and cavernous malformations are considered separately.

The second, and probably more widely accepted, classification was described by Anson and Spetzler[11] in 1992. They divided these lesions into four types, I to IV (Table 141–2). Type I consists of an arteriovenous fistula (AVF) located between a dural branch of the spinal ramus of a radicular artery and an intradural medullary vein. Type II is an AVM with a compact nidus located within the spinal cord. Type III is an extensive AVM often extending into the vertebral body and the surrounding paraspinal tissues. Type IV is an intradural AVF located just outside the spinal cord substance (perimedullary). Lesions similar to Type IV lesions had been divided into three subtypes by Gueguen and coworkers[12] in 1987. Type A is a simple perimedullary fistula fed by a single arterial branch, type B is an intermediate-sized fistula with multiple dilated arterial feeders, and type C is a large perimedullary fistula with multiple giant perimedullary arterial feeders.

Recently, Spetzler and colleagues[13] proposed a new

TABLE 141–1 ■ **Classification of Spinal and Spinal Cord Vascular Lesions**

- Spinal vascular lesions
  - Spinal dural arteriovenous fistulas
    - Isolated
    - Multiple
  - Spinal extradural and paraspinal arteriovenous fistulas
    - Isolated
    - Associated with systemic dysplasia (e.g., von Recklinghausen's disease)
- Spinal cord vascular lesions
  - Spinal cord vascular malformations
    - Isolated
      - Arteriovenous malformations
      - Arteriovenous fistulas
    - Multiple
      - Metameric (Cobb syndrome and other associations)
      - Nonmetameric (Rendu-Osler-Weber, Klippel-Trénaunay, and other syndromes)
- Spinal cord telangiectasias
- Cavernous vascular malformations (cavernomas)

From Niimi Y, Berenstein A: Endovascular treatment of spinal vascular malformations. Neurosurg Clin N Am 10:47–71, 1999.

TABLE 141–2 ■ Classification of Spinal Arteriovenous Malformations

TYPE	DESCRIPTION
I	Arteriovenous fistula located between a dural branch of the spinal ramus of a radicular artery and an intradural medullary vein
II	Intramedullary glomus malformation with a compact nidus within the substance of the spinal cord
III	Extensive arteriovenous malformation often extending into the vertebral body and paraspinal tissues
IV	Intradural perimedullary arteriovenous fistula
IV = A	Simple perimedullary fistula fed by a single arterial branch
IV = B	Intermediate-sized fistula with multiple dilated arterial feeders
IV = C	Large perimedullary fistula with multiple giant arterial feeders

From Anson JA, Spetzler RF: Classification of spinal arteriovenous malformations and implications for treatment. BNI Q 8:2–8, 1992.

classification that represents an evolution from these earlier systems (Table 141–3). Lesions are divided into three broad categories: neoplasms, aneurysms, and arteriovenous lesions. Neoplastic vascular lesions include hemangioblastomas and cavernous malformations. Spinal cord arteriovenous lesions are divided into AVFs and AVMs. AVFs are then subdivided into those that are extradural and those that are intradural, with intradural lesions categorized as either dorsal or ventral. AVMs are subdivided into extradural-intradural and intradural malformations. Intradural lesions are further subdivided into intramedullary, intramedullary-extramedullary, and those found in the conus medullaris.

The remainder of this chapter focuses on endovascular therapy of AVMs, because combining a discussion of neoplastic vascular lesions with one of vascular malformations is questionable.[14] To avoid confusing nomenclature, we use the most recent classification described by Spetzler and colleagues[13] to assimilate the available data on the endovascular treatment of spinal cord AVMs.

TABLE 141–3 ■ Classification of Spinal Cord Vascular Malformations

- Neoplastic vascular lesions
  - Hemangioblastomas
  - Cavernous malformations
- Spinal aneurysms
- Arteriovenous lesions
  - Artervenous fistulas
    - Extradural
    - Intradural
      - Ventral
        - Small shunt
        - Medium shunt
        - Large shunt
      - Dorsal
        - Single feeder
        - Multiple feeder
  - Arteriovenous malformations
    - Extradural-intradural
    - Intradural
    - Conus medullaris

From Spetzler RF, Detwiler PW, Riina H, Porter RW: Modified classification of spinal cord vascular lesions. J Neurosurg (Spine) 96:145–156, 2002.

EVALUATION OF SPINAL CORD ARTERIOVENOUS MALFORMATIONS

Magnetic Resonance Imaging

Spinal angiography is invasive and has associated risks and should therefore be reserved for patients who are likely to have spinal vascular malformations and for those who require endovascular therapy. This is particularly true since the advent of MRI, which is currently the best modality for noninvasive evaluation. At present, computed tomography and myelography are rarely needed and have limited value in the evaluation of spinal vascular malformations. Characteristic MRI features of spinal vascular malformations include the demonstration of signal voids secondary to dilated arteries or veins, which can be within or on the surface of the spinal cord. In addition, MRI is useful in evaluating associated findings such as spinal cord edema, hematomyelia, thrombosis, cavitation, atrophy, and venous drainage.[10, 15, 16]

Advances in MRI technology have improved the diagnosis and localization of spinal vascular malformations. Postcontrast magnetic resonance angiography (MRA) complements standard spinal MRI by improving the detection and display of normal and abnormal intradural vessels, primarily veins. The detection of abnormal veins facilitates the diagnosis of spinal vascular malformations and vascular tumors. The most useful application has been in the demonstration of the medullary vein into which the fistula drains, thus allowing noninvasive identification of the spinal level of the fistula.[17] Saraf-Lavi and associates[18] performed a study using contrast-enhanced MRA to determine its sensitivity, specificity, and ability to predict the vertebral level in patients with spinal dural AVFs. Twenty patients with surgically proven dural AVFs (diagnosed with radiographic digital subtraction angiography) and 11 control patients who had normal digital subtraction angiography findings underwent routine MRI plus three-dimensional contrast-enhanced MRA of the spine. Images were reviewed in two stages (stage 1, MRI only; stage 2, MRI plus MRA) by three neuroradiologists who were blinded to the final diagnoses. The sensitivity, specificity, and accuracy of the three reviewers in detecting the presence of fistulas ranged from 85% to 90%, 82% to 100%, and 87% to 90%, respectively, for stage 1, compared with 80% to 100%, 82%, and 82% to 94%, respectively, for stage 2. For each reviewer, there was no significant difference between the values for stages 1 and 2; however, among the reviewers, one of the more experienced neuroradiologists had a significantly greater sensitivity than a less experienced neuroradiologist for stage 2. On average, the percentage of true positive results for which the correct fistula level was predicted increased from 15% for stage 1 to

50% for stage 2, and the correct level plus or minus one level was predicted in 73% of cases for stage 2.

MRA is also particularly useful in evaluating spinal vascular malformations after treatment. Mascalchi and coworkers[19] recently examined 34 patients with spinal vascular malformations (30 dural AVFs, 2 perimedullary AVFs, and 2 intramedullary AVMs) using MRA and MRI before and after endovascular or surgical treatment. MRA showed residual flow in perimedullary vessels in seven patients with dural fistulas after embolization with liquid adhesive. In all seven, treatment failure was confirmed with arteriography. Long-lasting disappearance of flow in perimedullary vessels was demonstrated with MRA in 22 patients with dural fistulas. MRI demonstrated normalization of spinal cord volume in 16 of 22 patients and signal intensity on T2-weighted images in 3 patients. Disappearance of cord enhancement was observed in 5 of 21 patients, and disappearance of perimedullary enhanced vessels was demonstrated in 6 of 13 patients. In one additional patient with a dural fistula treated with embolization, early post-treatment MRA showed disappearance of flow in perimedullary vessels, which reappeared at follow-up and was consistent with reopening of a small residual fistula. Post-treatment MRA demonstrated transient reduction of flow in the nidus in two patients with intramedullary malformations treated with embolization. Permanent disappearance of flow in the perimedullary vessel was seen after endovascular treatment in two patients with perimedullary fistulas. Therefore, it appears that MRA is more sensitive than MRI in depicting residual or recurrent flow in peri- or intramedullary vessels, which indicates patency of the vascular malformation.[19]

Angiography

Angiography remains the gold standard in the evaluation of spinal vascular malformations. It confirms the diagnosis and determines the feasibility for either surgical or endovascular treatment. Preferably, spinal angiography is performed with the patient under general anesthesia and with controlled respiration to avoid motion artifact caused by breathing. This increases the resolution of images, which is important in making the correct diagnosis and avoiding complications such as missing a small spinal cord artery, which can lead to disastrous results during embolization. For a patient under general anesthesia, breathing motion can be controlled by temporarily stopping the ventilator during an actual angiographic run.

The goal of the angiographic evaluation is to demonstrate the angioarchitecture of the pathology and the normal spinal cord blood supply above and below the lesion. This includes demonstrating the anterior and posterior spinal arteries. The majority of this information can be obtained by straight anteroposterior views. Occasionally, lateral and oblique views are required to localize the lesion to the intradural space. For cervical lesions, bilateral vertebral arteries, ascending and deep cervical arteries, and supreme intercostal arteries need to be evaluated. Occasionally, for larger lesions in the cervical region, the occipital and ascending pharyngeal arteries may provide an indirect supply.[6, 9, 10] It is also important that the evaluation be continued until the blood supply for the normal spinal cord is demonstrated. For thoracic and upper lumber lesions, bilateral intercostal arteries and lumbar arteries are studied until the entire blood supply to the lesion and the normal spinal cord above and below the lesion is demonstrated. If spinal cord arteries are not seen on the lumbar artery angiogram, lateral and median sacral arteries should be studied, because the spinal cord artery can be derived from them via the filum terminale.[20, 21]

The basic technique of spinal angiography is the same for all diseases involving the spinal cord. A high-volume injection is not necessary; however, prolonged filming (>30 seconds) is mandatory in spinal dural AVFs, which reflects their slow-flow nature.

If a spinal dural AVF is not discovered despite bilateral angiography from the supreme intercostal artery to the internal iliac artery, the external carotid arteries and the vertebral arteries should be studied to rule out an intracranial pial or dural AVM draining to the spinal cord.

ENDOVASCULAR TREATMENT

The goal of endovascular treatment of spinal vascular malformations is the obliteration of either the fistula in AVFs or the abnormal vessels in AVMs. Endovascular therapy of spinal vascular malformations should be performed with the patient under general anesthesia, as described earlier for spinal angiography using controlled respiration. Many different catheters are available for cannulation of the required vessels, which include the vertebral arteries, ascending and deep cervical arteries, supreme intercostal arteries, intercostal arteries, lumbar arteries, and lateral and median sacral arteries.

Once the pathology is identified, selective and superselective catheterization can be performed into the feeding pedicle with a microcatheter, which in most cases is used with a guide wire. The development of hydrophilic coatings for both microcatheters and micro–guide wires has improved the ability to reach the distal lesion supplied by a small feeder. The value of performing superselective catheterization is that it allows occlusion of the fistula or AVM nidus without compromising supply to the normal spinal cord by going beyond the branch that supplies the cord. Further, it provides direct access to the pathology; proximal occlusion without reaching the pathology has no long-lasting effect and makes further treatment difficult.

Some authors have described the use of physiologic monitoring with somatosensory evoked potentials (SEPs) and motor evoked potentials (MEPs) during embolization.[5, 10, 22, 23] In these situations, a continuous infusion of propofol and fentanyl is used rather than halogenated agents or muscle relaxants.[24, 25] This allows the detection of abnormal spinal cord function that may be related to the embolization; if an abnormality is detected, the physician can either abandon the procedure or change the position of the catheter. Because the changes picked up by physiologic monitoring may occur in a delayed fashion after the insult, chemical provocative testing can be performed under SEP and MEP monitoring.[26] The chemical provocative test is performed by injecting 50 to 75 mg of amobarbital sodium (Amytal Sodium) followed by 20 to 40 mg of lidocaine (Xylocaine).[10] Amobarbital is used to test the functional changes of neurons, and lidocaine is used to test axonal function. If a decrease in the amplitude (of 50%) or increase in the latency (>10%) of SEPs or the disappearance of MEPs is induced by the chemical provocative test, embolization from this catheter position is aborted. Recovery of SEPs and MEPs to the baseline usually occurs within 5 to 10 minutes. Further superselective catheterization of the same pedicle or another pedicle is performed after searching for a safer catheter position.

After embolization, the patient should be admitted to a neurosurgical intensive care unit and continuously monitored for neurological changes. Corticosteroids are frequently used to minimize spinal cord swelling in patients with spinal cord AVMs; those with AVFs often do not require steroids. In patients with large AVFs or when there is significant preexisting venous congestion, heparinization should be considered to prevent progressive venous thrombosis and worsening of the patient's neurological condition.

Different embolic agents are available to treat spinal cord vascular malformations, and there are different opinions regarding the best embolic agent. The choices include particulate agents such as polyvinyl alcohol (PVA) and microspheres, glues, and a variety of coils.[27–29] The advantage of PVA is its ease of use; however, the occlusive effect tends to be temporary, and PVA use is frequently associated with recanalization.[9, 10, 27, 28] Liquid adhesive, such as *N*-butyl cyanoacrylate (NBCA), is currently the best agent in terms of a long-lasting effect; however, it is cumbersome to use and requires that the microcatheter be advanced up to the nidus or fistula. Coil embolization is often used only for large fistulas and aneurysms.

ARTERIOVENOUS LESIONS

Spinal cord arteriovenous lesions have been divided into AVFs and AVMs, and each is discussed separately (see Table 141–3).

Arteriovenous Fistulas

EXTRADURAL ARTERIOVENOUS FISTULAS

Spetzler and colleagues[13] described these lesions as fistulas secondary to a direct connection between an extradural artery and vein that leads to the development of a high-flow fistula and engorgement of the epidural venous system. The location of the fistula may be epidural or between the two layers of the dura mater. The epidural venous engorgement is due to the exclusive drainage to the epidural vein.[5, 30–32] In some cases, however, drainage into both the intradural and epidural veins has been reported.[33, 34] The patient can present with myelopathy,[35, 36] radiculopathy,[36–38] subarachnoid hemorrhage,[37] and, rarely, a spontaneous epidural hematoma.[39] Myelopathy can be caused by venous hypertension and congestion of the spinal cord or by mass effect by the dilated epidural vein. Radiculopathy is most likely caused by mass effect, but disturbance of venous drainage of the nerve root may be a contributing factor. Subarachnoid hemorrhage occurs in those that have intradural venous drainage. Symptoms can rarely be attributed to the shunting of large quantities of arterial blood into the venous system or to steal of blood flow from the spinal cord.[13] Extradural AVFs are treated almost exclusively by endovascular procedures and only rarely require open surgery.[10, 13] Endovascular treatment involves embolization of the arterial feeder.

INTRADURAL ARTERIOVENOUS FISTULAS

Intradural AVFs are the most controversial lesions in terms of origin, pathophysiology, and treatment. Using Spetzler and colleagues'[13] classification, intradural dorsal and intradural ventral lesions are considered distinct entities.

Intradural Dorsal Arteriovenous Fistulas (Type 1; SCAVMs) (Fig. 141–1)

Intradural dorsal AVFs are the most common type of spinal AVF. They are also known as type I malformations,[11, 13] spinal dural AVFs,[9, 10] long dorsal AVFs,[40] angioma racemosum[41] dorsal extramedullary AVFs, and angioma venosum racemosum.[41–43] They usually present after age 40 years. In a report by Berenstein and Lasjaunias[5, 9] of 172 cases, 85% of the patients were men, and their mean age at the time of diagnosis was 55 years. In a recent report by Eskandar and coworkers,[44] the records and angiograms of all patients with spinal dural AVFs treated at Massachusetts General Hospital over a 6-year period (1992 to 1998) were reviewed. A total of 26 patients with spinal dural AVFs were treated, which included 22 men and 4 women with a mean age of 65 years (range, 39 to 79 years). Lesions were located in the following areas: 5 in the foramen magnum or the cervical region, 13 in the thoracic, 5 in the lumbar, and 3 in the sacral.[44] The predominance in the thoracic region is consistent with reports by other authors.[5, 9, 13, 45]

Clinically, patients usually present with a progressive myelopathy. It is also common for patients to have a history of pain in the back or legs. By the time of diagnosis, most patients also have bladder or bowel and sexual dysfunction. The mode of progression of the myelopathy is variable; it can be continuous, step-ladder type, or waxing and waning with gradual progression. Symptoms can be aggravated by activities causing increased intra-abdominal pressure, such as bending or straining. Approximately 10% to 20% of patients experience acute exacerbation of myelopathy with or without pain but without hemorrhage. The

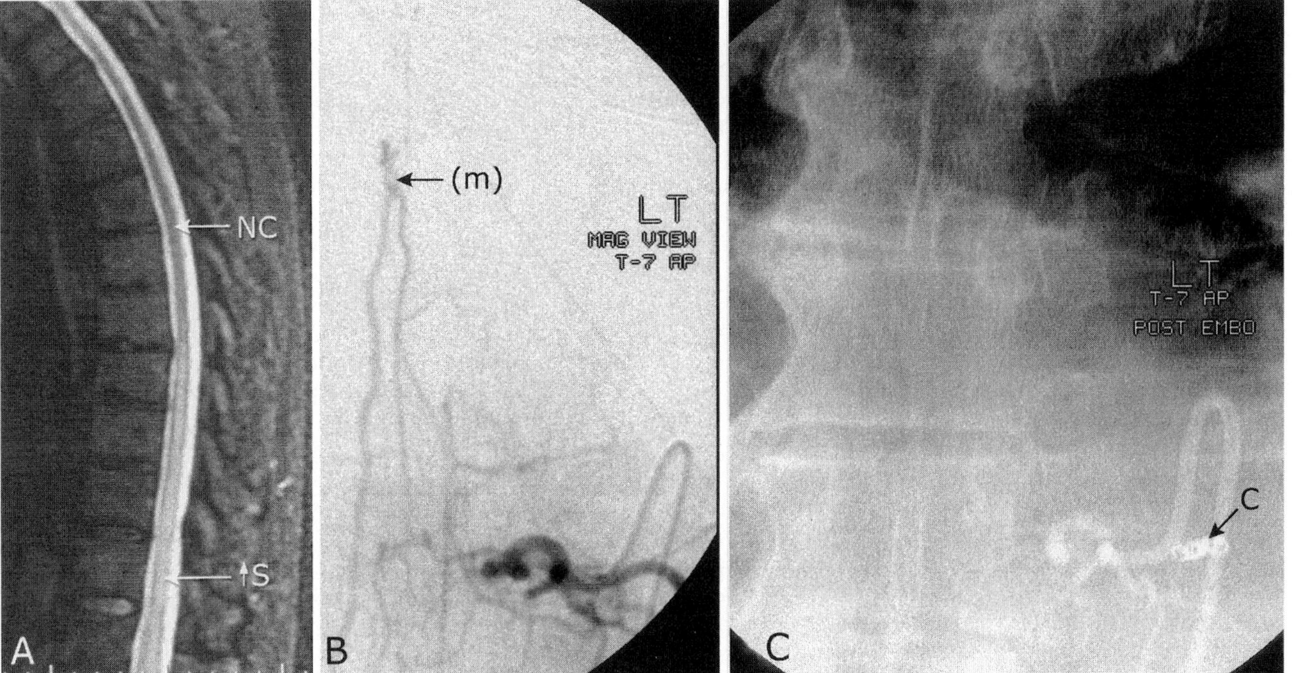

FIGURE 141–1. A patient presented with progressive myelopathy and a diagnosis of spinal dural arteriovenous fistula was made after MRI and spinal angiography were performed. *A*,This saggital T2-weighted MRI demonstrates increased signal in the conus and thoracic spinal cord (*S*), with normal spinal cord signal (*NC*) noted above. *B*, This spinal angiogram demonstrates a dural fistula that is feeding off of the left T7 radicular pedicle with nidus located at approximately the T5 level in midline and with a slow draining vein in the midline to approximately the T10 level. The anterior spinal artery was noted to arise off of the left T9 pedicle. Embolization was then performed. *C*, This image, taken after embolization, shows no flow in the dural AV fistula, with coils noted (*C*). Embolization consisted of placing the microcatheter in the proximal portion of the intercostal artery where two 3 × 2 coils were deployed to block subsequent preferential flow of glue through the intercostal artery and rather directed into the dural AV fistula.

cause of this acute exacerbation is probably acute decompensation of the already damaged drainage of the spinal cord as a result of thrombosis or other additional hemodynamic changes.[5, 9, 10] Aminoff and Logue[46] detailed the clinical prognosis of these lesions in 60 cases. In seven patients who presented with acute-onset symptoms, there was no further progression. In the remaining 53 patients, symptoms progressed gradually, and 5 of these patients suffered acute neurological events. Within 3 years of the onset of functional lower extremity impairment, half the patients had become severely disabled. These outcomes led to the present dogma that progressive neurological deterioration can be halted only by eliminating the fistula.[13] This is supported by Niimi and coauthors'[47] 1997 report on a series of 49 patients with severe neurological deficits at the time of treatment. Although all the patients improved significantly after treatment, those treated within 7 days after acute exacerbation had better outcomes than those treated later.

The primary pathophysiology of intradural dorsal AVFs is venous hypertension. In rare cases, patients may experience clinical deterioration secondary to hemorrhage.[48, 49] Spinal dural AVFs are located within the dura covering a spinal nerve root arterializing the coronal venous plexus. They are usually supplied by a dural branch of the dorsospinal artery and drained by a single radicular vein, which then drains into intradural perimedullary veins.[5, 33, 50, 51] The radicular vein penetrates the dura away from the nerve root in 40% of cases.[10] This disposition of the draining vein enables a bimetameric supply to the spinal dural AVF, which occurred in eight of the cases (16%) reported by Niimi and Berenstein.[10] These lesions have been divided into two subtypes: type A, with a single feeding artery, and type B, with multiple feeding arteries.[11]

Intraoperative inspection of the dorsal nerve roots reveals a vascularized pedicle or pedicles, which feed the AVF in the subarachnoid space. The presence of an AVF in the dural root sleeve has been repeatedly verified histologically, but no extradural arteriovenous abnormality exists; otherwise, engorgement of the epidural venous plexus would be expected. Although there are numerous extradural and dural vessels, they compromise the dural recruitment process to feed the intradural fistula. If the fistula were extradural or within the dura, the drainage would empty into the rich vascular epidural or dural venous system instead of into the high-resistance coronal venous plexus. When more than one feeding vessel is present (type B), they form a single intradural fistula, providing further support for the intradural location of the AVF.[13] Measurements of epidural venous pressure, which is the same as central venous pressure, support this contention.[13] The development of spinal dural AVFs causes venous hypertension, which leads to hypoperfusion of the spinal cord. This is demonstrated on angiogram by the slow-flow shunt, with delayed clearance of contrast from the draining perimedullary veins and prolonged circulation time in the anterior spinal artery (ASA).[10] The venous drainage is usually cranial on the posterior surface of the spinal cord. It has been postulated that venous drainage on the anterior surface of the spinal cord or in the caudal direction indicates a more severely compromised spinal cord venous drainage and correlates with severity of the clinical symptoms.[5, 10]

Treatment is indicated in most, if not all, patients with spinal dural AVFs to at least stop the progression of myelopathy. Elderly patients with a long history of complete paraplegia may not be candidates for treatment, however, because they are unlikely to obtain functional recovery by occlusion of the fistula. Spinal dural AVFs can be treated by embolization, surgery, or both. Institutions with a surgical bias cite the high rates of recurrence and progressive myelopathy associated with embolization.[52–54] In addition, in surgical series, the reported morbidity rate is extremely low and the success rate is high.[13, 55–57] Spinal dural AVFs that have arterial feeders arising from the same pedicle as the spinal cord artery should be treated by surgery.[47] Institutions that favor embolization as the treatment of choice cite its less invasive nature compared with surgery, the ability to perform embolization in the same sitting as diagnostic angiography, the possibility of early rehabilitation (started the day after embolization), and the ability to perform surgery if embolization fails.[10]

No long-term follow-up data are available to support either contention. However, a recent report by Eskandar and coworkers[44] on their experience with endovascular and surgical therapy for spinal dural AVFs provided much insight.[44] As stated earlier, those authors reviewed the records and angiograms of 26 patients with spinal dural AVFs treated from 1992 to 1998. During this period, the intention was to treat all patients with embolization initially and to reserve surgery for those in whom endovascular treatment failed or in whom the pretreatment evaluation suggested that endovascular therapy would be ineffective or unsafe. Of the 26 patients, 23 (88%) underwent embolization and 3 (12%) underwent surgery as the primary mode of treatment. Of the 23 patients in whom embolization was performed or attempted, 9 (39%) ultimately required surgery. All patients were stabilized or improved following definitive treatment, as assessed by Aminoff-Logue scores. The authors concluded that endovascular therapy can be successful as an initial treatment for the majority of patients; however, there is a 39% failure rate, which is not observed following surgical therapy.

Techniques for catheterization and embolization are similar to those used for other spinal vascular abnormalities, except that a flow-guided catheter may not be successful in these slow-flow lesions; therefore, a wire-assisted microcatheter is preferred. Provocative testing is not necessary.[10] Superselective angiography from the microcatheter should be performed before embolization, because a spinal cord artery may not be visualized owing to its slow flow on the angiogram done at the orifice of the segmental artery. With regard to the choice of embolic agent, NBCA provides a more permanent result, as PVA particles are known to recanalize. Coils and particles are occasionally used to protect normal territories before embolization of the direct feeder with NBCA. The goal of embolization is to penetrate a column of NBCA to the proximal portion of the draining vein through the fistula. Both underpenetration and overpenetration of NBCA should be avoided. Underpenetration causes proximal occlusion and recurrence of the AVF as a result of collateralization. Overpenetration and occlusion of perimedullary veins can cause aggravation of venous hypertension and the associated myelopathy. A control angiogram after embolization should be performed on the contralateral segmental artery at the same level as the feeding pedicle and on segmental arteries two levels above and below on both sides to rule out collateral circulation reconstituting the fistula. An angiogram of the ASA may show immediate improvement of the spinal cord circulation.[5, 10]

Intradural Ventral Arteriovenous Fistulas (Type IV; SCAVFs) (Fig. 141–2)

Heros and associates[58] introduced the term *type IV lesion* in 1986, and Gueguen and coworkers[12] divided ventral fistulas into three subtypes: 1, 2, and 3. Anson and Spetzler[11] reclassified the subtypes as IV-A, IV-B, and IV-C; in Spetzler and colleagues'[13] most recent classification, these subtypes have been maintained.[13] Type A, B, and C fistulas are progressively larger shunts, with the last characterized by a giant fistula and a markedly distended venous network. As the size and flow of the fistula increase, the signs and symptoms attributable to progressive vascular steal and spinal cord compression become more pronounced.[13]

In 1977, Djindjian and coworkers[59] described perimedullary or intradural ventral AVFs, which originate directly from the ASA and have a direct fistula to an enlarged venous network, with no intervening capillary system.[60, 61] Blood flow through the lesions is rapid and can produce flow-related aneurysms and venous hypertension.[13] They are more common in the pediatric population and in patients with Rendu-Osler-Weber syndrome; other syndromes known to be associated with them are neurofibromatosis and Klippel-Trénaunay and Parkes-Weber syndromes.[6, 62]

These fistulas can be treated with either surgical or endovascular intervention, but the patency of the ASA must be maintained.[58] Some authors believe that surgery should be performed for the majority of cases, and most reserve endovascular therapy for large fistulas or as an adjunct to surgery, because it is easier to maintain the integrity of the ASA with surgery.[60, 63–66] Endovascular therapy requires the delivery of PVA, NBCA, and coils to the fistula.

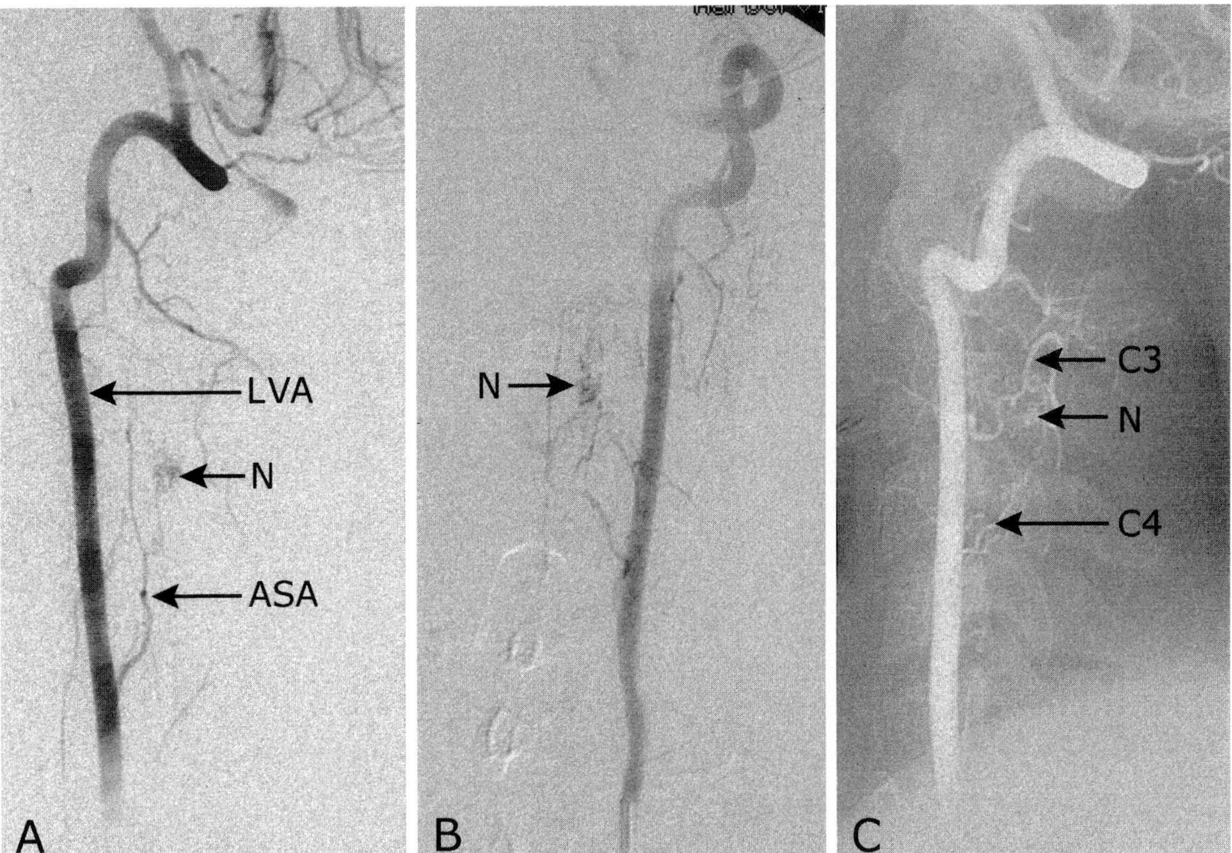

FIGURE 141–2. A patient presented with an acute cervical cord hemorrhage and the MRI suggested an associated vascular malformation. A spinal angiogram was then performed, which demonstrated an intermedullary arterial venous malformation at the C3 and C4 levels of the spinal cord supplied by anterior spinal artery and distal cervical branches of the right vertebral artery. *A*, *B*, left vertebral artery, lateral (*A*) and anteroposterior (*B*) views. A small arteriovenous malformation nidus (*N*) within the mid cervical cord is demonstrated at the C3 level. This is supplied by a small branch arising from the anterior spinal artery which is derived from a C6 branch from the left vertebral artery (*LVA*). The posterior spinal arteries are not visualized. *C*, Right vertebral artery. Lateral view again shows a small arteriovenous malformation nidus (*N*) within the spinal cord at the C3 level. This is supplied by right C3 and right C4 vertebral artery branches, with venous drainage along the posterior dural venous plexus. The anterior and posterior spinal arteries are not seen on the right-sided injections. Due to the small size of the branches supplying the malformation, the patient underwent surgical resection without any associated embolization.

Arteriovenous Malformations

Spinal cord AVMs are supplied by spinal cord arteries and drained by spinal cord veins. They are differentiated from AVFs by the presence of a nidus. Spinal cord AVMs can be located extradurally, intradurally, or both. Intradural AVMs can be found on the surface of the spinal cord or within the cord itself.

EXTRADURAL-INTRADURAL ARTERIOVENOUS MALFORMATIONS

Extradural-intradural AVMs are uncommon and have also been referred to as juvenile, metameric, or type III AVMs.[67–70] Metameric AVMs involving the skin, vertebrae, and spinal cord are part of the Cobb syndrome.[5] They respect no tissue boundaries and can be extensive. Complete surgical resection is often difficult without significant risk of neurological morbidity.[13] Owing to the extensive nature of these lesions, a multidisciplinary approach is required. Embolization is vital and often constitutes definitive management of these leions.[71] Embolization of multiple feeding arteries is required, with the delivery of PVA, NBCA, and coils, often in combination. Occasionally, this is followed by a staged resection.[13]

INTRADURAL ARTERIOVENOUS MALFORMATIONS (Type II, SCAVMs, Glomus Type) (Fig. 141–3)

Intramedullary AVMs are characterized by a nidus, similar to intracranial AVMs. These lesions were previously referred to as classic AVMs, glomus-type lesions, type II AVMs, angioma arteriovenosum, and angioma racemosum arteriovenous lesions.[11, 13, 43, 72–77] There is a slight male predominance, and they can occur at any level of the spinal cord; they are found in

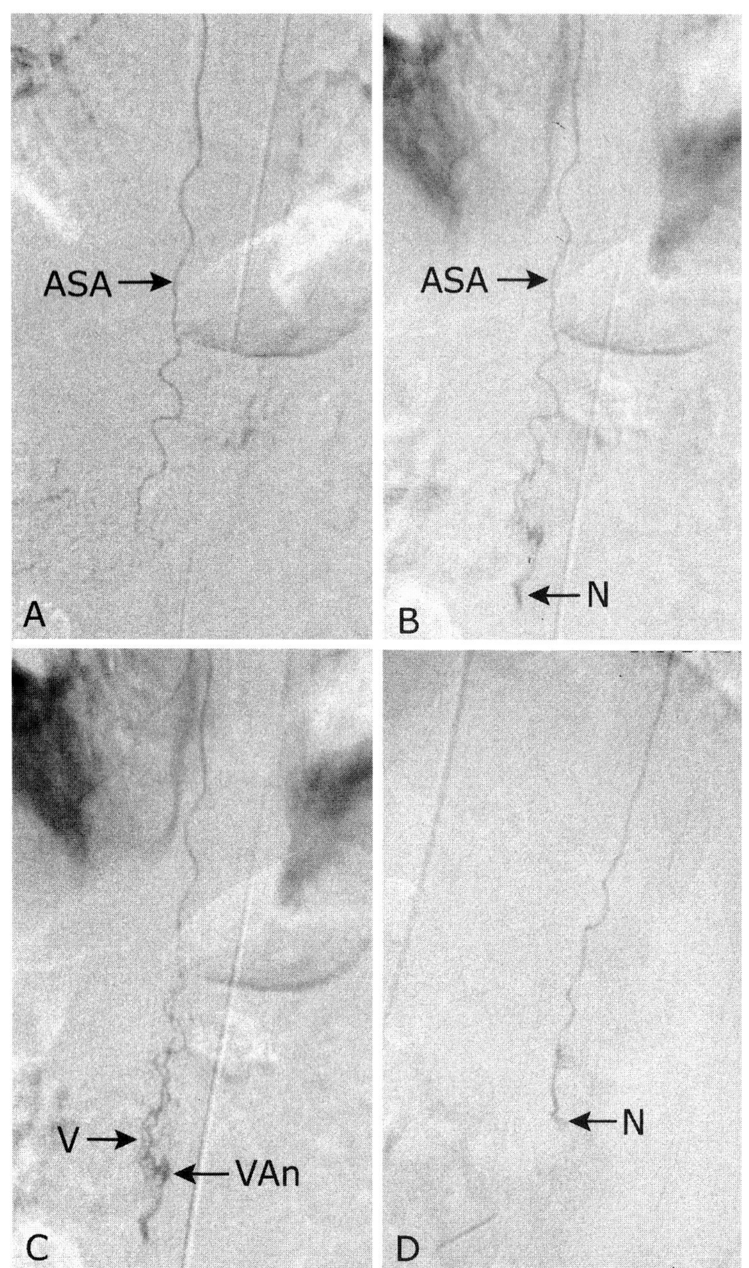

FIGURE 141–3. A patient presented with progressive myelopathy and his MRI was suspicious for a vascular malformation. He subsequently underwent a spinal angiogram, which demonstrated a small perimedullary arteriovenous fistula (Type IV, or ventral intradural arteriovenous fistula at the conus). *A*, Right T7 intercostal injection demonstrates a prominent anterior spinal artery (*ASA*) coursing downward to the L1 level. *B*, A small nidus (*N*) is noted on a longer imaging, with rapid filling of vein (*v*) on image *C* and a small venous aneurysm (*VAn*) is also noted. *D*, Lateral imaging demonstrates that the lesion lies ventral to the conus (*N*) and becomes important to differentiate between a perimedullary fistula and a conus AVM. No embolization was possible without endangering the integrity of the anterior spinal artery.

the cervical area in 30% of cases and in the thoracolumbar area in 70%, which is grossly proportional to the volume of the spinal cord in each segment.[5, 10, 45, 78]

In the majority of patients, symptoms occur before 16 years of age.[5] MRI has significantly improved the diagnosis after presentation, which usually consists of either subarachnoid hemorrhage or hematomyelia. Recurrent hemorrhage is more common than in cerebral malformations, and 40% of these AVMs rebleed within the first year after the initial hemorrhage.[5, 10] The hemorrhage is frequently associated with significant neurological deficits, and each ictus is associated with significant mortality of 10% to 20%.[10] Less frequently, a patient presents with acute or progressive neurological deterioration related to an ischemic cause, without evidence of hemorrhage. This is usually secondary to thrombosis of the draining veins and the resulting venous hypertension or mass effect from a dilated draining vein.[5, 7, 10] Some authors believe that a progressive myelopathy can occur secondary to vascular steal,[79] but others disagree.[10] Rarely, the diagnosis is made in patients with no neurological signs or symptoms, based on a workup for unrelated symptoms or associated metameric or skin lesions.

The poor prognosis of untreated spinal cord AVMs justifies aggressive intervention, especially in young patients, even if there are significant neurological deficits.[5, 10, 13] When neurological deficits exist because of recent hemorrhage, treatment is usually delayed to permit maximal recovery before the initiation of treatment.

The diagnosis can be made using MRI, but angiography is necessary to define the exact angioarchitecture of the lesion. This allows a clear understanding of the lesion, which is vital for planning and executing treatment. Spinal cord AVMs are supplied by multiple branches of the anterior and posterior spinal arteries and are characterized by high pressure, relatively low resistance, and high blood flow.[13] The nidus can be either compact or diffuse.[13] Aneurysms associated with spinal cord AVMs are common.[13, 80]

Some authors believe that surgical resection remains the mainstay of treatment.[73] In a recent series, complete resection was not possible in only 8% of cases.[13] Many other authors believe that embolization should be considered the treatment of choice,[10] and others have demonstrated that in select cases, embolization can be the definitive treatment.[81]

As described earlier, embolization should be performed with the patient under general anesthesia and with SEP and MEP monitoring. Chemical provocative testing should be considered, and superselective catheterization should be done to allow for occlusion of the nidus without compromising the blood supply to the normal spinal cord.

CONUS MEDULLARIS ARTERIOVENOUS MALFORMATIONS (Fig. 141–4)

Spetzler and colleagues[13] proposed that conus medullaris AVMs constitute a separate category of lesions characterized by multiple feeding arteries, multiple nidi, and complex venous drainage.[13] They have multiple direct arteriovenous shunts that derive their blood supply from the anterior and posterior spinal arteries

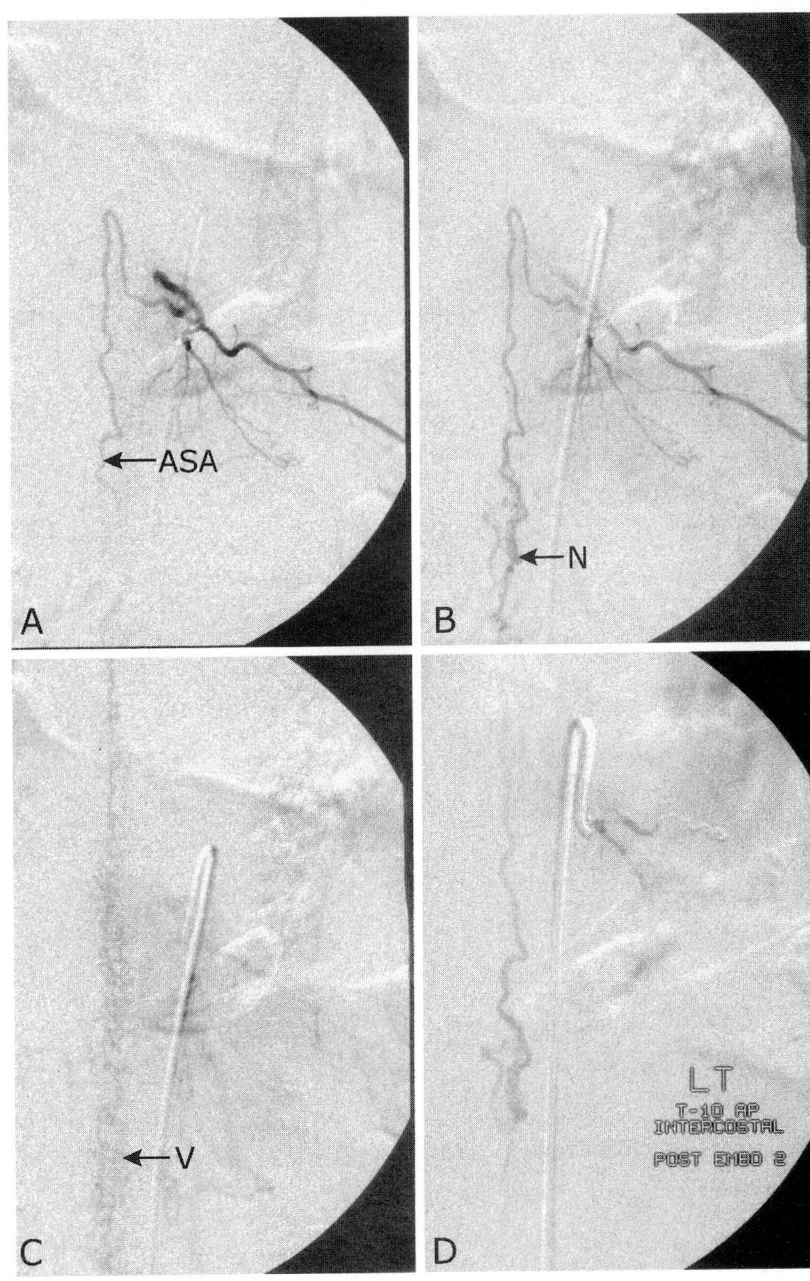

FIGURE 141–4. This patient presented with progressive myelopathy. Spinal angiography demonstrated a conus AVM supplied by the artery of Adamkiewicz off the left T10. Images *A*, *B*, and *C* demonstrate the artery of Adamkiewicz filling with abnormal filling of tortuous vessels. Arteries (*ASA*), veins (*v*), and the nidus (*N*) are also noted. As this lesion was within the substance of the conus and the patient did not want to take the risk of surgery, palliative embolization was performed. Palliative embolization has the goal of decreasing the arterial flow and therefore the associated venous hypertension. It is important to achieve this goal without creating stasis or occlusion of the ASA. Embolization was performed with the deployement of two 3 × 2 coils to improve flow dynamics for delivery of PVA particles. Then, 6 ml of 150- to 250-μ PVA particles suspended in 50 ml of nonionic contrast were then delivered under direct fluoroscopic visualization. This was followed by embolization of the anterior spinal artery using PVA 6-0 silk. *D*, Post embolization image which demonstrates delayed filling of the nidus. Patient reported an improvement in symptoms.

and have glomus-type nidi that are usually extramedullary and pial based, but they may also have an intramedullary component. They are always located in the conus medullaris and cauda equina but can extend along the entire filum terminale. These lesions can be treated with both surgery and embolization, and the experience of Spetzler and colleagues[13] is that this type of lesion is best treated using aggressive embolization and subsequent resection.

SPINAL CORD ANEURYSMS

Spinal cord aneurysms are most commonly associated with spinal cord AVMs.[5, 10] Treatment of these aneurysms is directed at both the aneurysm and the associated AVM. Embolization of the feeding artery is fundamental in treating both aspects of the condition. The principles of treatment are similar to those discussed earlier for spinal cord AVMs. Spetzler and colleagues[13] classify spinal cord aneurysms unrelated to AVMs as a separate entity. The pathophysiology of these aneurysms is related to blood flow and dissection.[82–84] Patients usually present with subarachnoid hemorrhage and sudden-onset low back pain. The aneurysm can involve the radicular arteries, the artery of Adamkiewicz, and the ASA.[82–84] Treatment is usually surgical.

REFERENCES

1. Djindjian R, Dumesnil M, Faure C, et al: Etude angio-graphique d'un angiome intra-rachidien. Rev Neurol 106:278, 1962.
2. Djindjian R, Houdart R, COphignon J, et al: Premiers essais d'embolisation par voie Mmorale dans un cas dlangiome medullaire et dans un cas d'angiome ali-ment~ par la carotide exteme. Rev Neurol 125:119, 1971.
3. Doppman J, Di Chiro G: Subtraction-angiography of spinal cord vascular malformations: Report of a case. J Neurosurg 23:140, 1965.
4. Doppman J, Di Chiro G, Ommaya A: Percutaneous embolization of spinal cord arteriovenous malformations. J Neurosurg 34: 48, 1971.
5. Berenstein A, Lasjaunias P: Spine and spinal cord vascular lesions. In Endovascular Treatment of Spine and Spinal Cord Lesions, vol 5. Berlin, Springer-Verlag, 1992, p l.
6. Berenstein A, Choi I, Neophytides A, et al: Endovascular treatment of spinal cord arteriovenous malformations (SCAVMs). AJNR Am J Neuroradiol 10:898, 1999.
7. Rodesch G, Pongpech H, Alvarez H, et al: Spinal cord arteriovenous malformations in a pediatric population: Children below 15 years of age. The place of endovascular management. Intervent Neuroradiol 1:29, 1995.
8. Marsh WR: Vascular lesions of the spinal cord: History and classification. Neurosurg Clin N Am 10:1–8, 1999.
9. Berenstein A, Lasjaunias P: Spine and spinal cord vascular lesions. In Endovascular Treatment of Spine and Spinal Cord Lesions, vol 5. Berlin, Springer-Verlag, 1992, p 2.
10. Niimi Y, Berenstein A: Endovascular treatment of spinal vascular malformations. Neurosurg Clin N Am 10:47–71, 1999.
11. Anson JA, Spetzler RF: Classification of spinal arteriovenous malformations and implications for treatment. BNI Q 8:2–8, 1992.
12. Gueguen B, Merland JJ, Riche MC: Vascular malformations of the spinal cord: Intrathecal perimedullary arteriovenous fistulas fed by medullary arteries. Neurology 37:969–979, 1987.
13. Spetzler RF, Detwiler PW, Riina H, Porter RW: Modified classification of spinal cord vascular lesions. J Neurosurg (Spine) 96: 145–156, 2002.
14. Barrow DL: Spinal cord vascular lesions. J Neurosurg (Spine) 96: 143–144, 2002.
15. Dormont D, Gelbert F, Assouline E, et al: MR imaging of spinal cord arteriovenous malformations at 0.5 T: Study of 34 cases. AJNR Am J Neuroradiol 9:833, 1988.
16. Minami S, Sagoh T, Nishimura K, et al: Spinal arteriovenous malformation: MR imaging. Radiology 169:109, 1988.
17. Bowen BC, Pattany PM: MR angiography of the spine. Magn Reson Imaging Clin N Am 6:165–178, 1998.
18. Saraf-Lavi E, Bowen BC, Quencer RM, et al: Detection of spinal dural arteriovenous fistulae with MR imaging and contrast-enhanced MR angiography. AJNR Am J Neuroradiol 23:858–867, 2002.
19. Mascalchi M, Ferrito G, Quilici N, et al: Spinal vascular malformations: MR angiography after treatment. Radiology 219:346–353, 2001.
20. Schaat TJ, Salzman KL, Stevens EA: Sacral origin of a spinal dural arteriovenous fistula: Case report and review. Spine 27: 893–897, 2002.
21. Akiyama H, Katayama S, Tanaka K, Korosue K: [Multiple spinal arteriovenous fistulas occurring at conus medullaris and dura of the sacral region: A case report.] No Shinkei Geka 29:1177–1181, 2001.
22. Berenstein A, Young Y, Ransohoff T, et al: Somatosensory evoked potentials during spinal angiography and therapeutic transvascular embolization. J Neurosurg 60:777, 1984.
23. Linden D, Berlit P: Spinal arteriovenous malformations: Clinical and neurophysiological findings. J Neurol 243:9, 1996.
24. Kothbauer K, Deletis V, Epstein F: Intraoperative spinal cord monitoring for intramedullary surgery: An essential adjunct. Pediatr Neurosurg 26:247, 1997.
25. KothbauerK, Pryor J, Berenstein A, et al: Motor evoked potentials predicting early recovery from paraparesis after embolization of a spinal dural arteriovenous fistula. Intervent Neuroradiol 4: 81, 1998.
26. Doppman J, Girton M, Oldfield E: Spinal Wada test. Radiology 161:319, 1986.
27. Scialfa G, Scotti G, Biondi A, De Grandi C: Embolization of vascular malformations of the spinal cord. J Neurosurg Sci 29: 1–9, 1985.
28. Phadke RV, Venkatesh SK, Kumar S, et al: Embolization of cranial/spinal tumours and vascular malformations with hydrogel microspheres: An experience of 69 cases. Acta Radiol 43:15–20, 2002.
29. Radek A, Maciejczak A, Zajgner J, et al: [Embolization of AVMs of thoracic spinal cord with histoacryl glue.] Neurol Neurochir Pol 30:333–345, 1996.
30. Heier LA, Lee BCP: A dural spinal arteriovenous malformation with epidural venous drainage: A case report. AJNR Am J Neuroradiol 8:561–563, 1987.
31. Pirouzmand F, Wallace M, Willinsky R: Spinal epidural arteriovenous fistula with intramedullary reflux. J Neurosurg 87:633, 1997.
32. Tanaka K, Waga S, Kojima T, et al: Spinal dural arteriovenous malformation: Report of an unusual case. Neurosurgery 24:915, 1989.
33. Afshar T, Doppman J, Oldfield E: Surgical interruption of intradural draining vein as curative treatment of spinal dural arteriovenous fistulas. J Neurosurg 82:196, 1995.
34. Arnaud O, Bille F, Pouget J: Epidural arteriovenous fistula with perimedullary venous drainage: Case report. Neuroradiology 36: 490–491, 1994.
35. Bradac G, Simon R, Schramm J: Cervical epidural AVM: Report of a case of uncommon location. Neuroradiology 14:97, 1977.
36. Willinsky R, TerBrugge K, Montanera W, et al: Spinal epidural arteriovenous fistulas: Arterial and venous approaches to embolization. AJNR Am J Neuroradiol 14:812, 1993.
37. Cahan L, Higashida R, Halbach V, et al: Variants of radiculomeningeal vascular malformations of the spine. J Neurosurg 66:333, 1987.
38. Han S, Love M, Simeone F: Diagnosis and treatment of a lumbar extradural arteriovenous malformation. AJNR Am J Neuoradiol 8:1129, 1987.
39. Miyagi Y, Miyazono M, Kamikaseda K: Spinal epidural vascular malformation presenting in association with a spontaneously resolved acute epidural hematoma: Case report. J Neurosurg 88: 909–911, 1998.
40. Malis LI: Microsurgery for spinal cord arteriovenous malformations. Clin Neurosurg 26:543–555, 1979.

41. Krayenbühl H, Yasargil MG, McClintock HG: Treatment of spinal cord vascular malformations by surgical excision. J Neurosurg 30:427–435, 1969.
42. Newman MJD: Racemose angioma of the spinal cord. Q J Med 109:97–108, 1959.
43. Wyburn-Mason R: The Vascular Abnormalities and Tumours of the Spinal Cord and Its Membranes. London, H Klimptom, 1943, p 196.
44. Eskandar EN, Borges LF, Budzik RF Jr, et al: Spinal dural arteriovenous fistulas: Experience with endovascular and surgical therapy. J Neurosurg. 96(2 Suppl):162–167, 2002.
45. Rosenblum B, Oldfield H, Doppman J, et al: Spinal arteriovenous malformations: A comparison of dural arteriovenous fistulas and intradural AVMs in 81 patients. J Neurosurg 67:795, 1987.
46. Aminoff MJ, Logue V: The prognosis of patients with spinal vascular malformations. Brain 97:211–218, 1974.
47. Niimi Y, Berenstein A, Setton A, et al: Embolization of spinal dural arteriovenous fistulae: Results and follow-up. Neurosurgery 40:675, 1997.
48. Aminoff MJ, Barnard RO, Logue V: The pathophysiology of spinal vascular malformations. J Neurol Sci 23:255–263, 1974.
49. Bederson JB, Spetzler RF: Pathophysiology of type I spinal dural arteriovenous malformations. BNI Q 12:23–32, 1996.
50. Lougue V: Angiomas of the spinal cord: Review of the pathogenesis, clinical features, and results of surgery. J Neurol Neurosurg Psychiatry 42:1, 1979.
51. Merland T, Riche M, Chiras J: Les fistules arterio-veineuses intracanalaires, extra-medullaires a drainage veineux medullaire. J Neuroradiol 7:271, 1980.
52. Hall WA, Oldfield EH, Doppman JL: Recanalization of spinal arteriovenous malformations following embolization. J Neurosurg 70:714–720, 1989.
53. Morgan MK, Marsh WR: Management of spinal dural arteriovenous malformations. J Neurosurg 70:832–836, 1989.
54. Nichols DA, Rufenacht DA, Jack CR Jr: Embolization of spinal dural arteriovenous fistula with polyvinyl alcohol particles: Experience in 14 patients. AJNR Am J Neuroradiol 13:933–940, 1992.
55. Huffmann BC, Gilsbach JM, Thron A: Spinal dural arteriovenous fistulas: A plea for neurosurgical treatment. Acta Neurochir (Wien) 135:44–51, 1995.
56. Lee TT, Gromelski EB, Bowen BC: Diagnostic and surgical management of spinal dural arteriovenous fistulas. Neurosurgery 43: 242–247, 1998.
57. Symon L, Kuyama H, Kendall B: Dural arteriovenous malformations of the spine: Clinical features and surgical results in 55 cases. J Neurosurg 60:238–247, 1984.
58. Heros RC, Debrun GM, Ojemann RG: Direct spinal arteriovenous fistula: A new type of spinal AVM: Case report. J Neurosurg 64: 134–139, 1986.
59. Djindjian M, Djindjian R, Rey A: Intradural extramedullary spinal arterio-venous malformations fed by the anterior spinal artery. Surg Neurol 8:85–93, 1977.
60. Barrow DL, Colohan ART, Dawson R: Intradural perimedullary arteriovenous fistulas (type IV spinal cord arteriovenous malformations). J Neurosurg 81:221–229, 1994.
61. Benhaiem-Sigaux N, Zerah M, Gherardi R: A retromedullary arteriovenous fistula associated with the Klippel-Trenaunay-Weber syndrome: A clinicopathologic study. Acta Neuropathol (Berl) 66:318–324, 1985.
62. Riche M, Modenesi-Freitas J, Djindjian M, et al: Arteriovenous malformations (AVM) of the spinal cord in children. Neuroradiology 22:171, 1982.
63. Glasser R, Masson R, Mickle JP: Embolization of a dural arteriovenous fistula of the ventral cervical spinal canal in a nine-year-old boy. Neurosurgery 33:1089–1094, 1993.
64. Halbach VV, Higashida RT, Dowd CF: Treatment of giant intradural (perimedullary) arteriovenous fistulas. Neurosurgery 33: 972–980, 1993.
65. Riché MC, Melki JP, Merland JJ: Embolization of spinal cord vascular malformations via the anterior spinal artery. AJNR Am J Neuroradiol 4:378–381, 1983.
66. Sure U, Wakat JP, Gatscher S, et al: Spinal type IV arteriovenous malformations (perimedullary fistulas) in children. Childs Nerv Syst 16:508–515, 2000.
67. Kerber CW, Cromwell LD, Sheptak PE: Intraarterial cyanoacrylate: An adjunct in the treatment of spinal/paraspinal arteriovenous malformations. AJR Am J Roentgenol 103:99–103, 1978.
68. Rudy DC, Woodside JR: Familial juvenile type III spinal cord arteriovenous malformation: Urodynamic findings. J Urol 130: 946–947, 1983.
69. Singhal AB, Drago S, Sheth SG: Ruptured type III cervical spinal cord arteriovenous malformation as a cause of acute quadriparesis. J Assoc Physicians India 43:565–566, 1995.
70. Spetzler RF, Zabramski JM, Flom RA: Management of juvenile spinal AVMs by embolization and operative excision: Case report. J Neurosurg 70:628–632, 1989.
71. Bao YH, Ling F: Classification and therapeutic modalities of spinal vascular malformations in 80 patients. Neurosurgery 40: 75–81, 1997.
72. Cogen P, Stein BM: Spinal cord arteriovenous malformations with significant intramedullary components. J Neurosurg 59:471–478, 1983.
73. Connolly ES Jr, Zubay GP, McCormick PC: The posterior approach to a series of glomus (type II) intramedullary spinal cord arteriovenous malformations. Neurosurgery 42:774–786, 1998.
74. Ommaya AK, Di Chiro G, Doppman JL: Ligation of arterial supply in the treatment of spinal cord arteriovenous malformations. J Neurosurg 30:679–692, 1969.
75. Owen MP, Brown RH, Spetzler RF: Excision of intramedullary arteriovenous malformation using intraoperative spinal cord monitoring. Surg Neurol 12:271–276, 1979.
76. Raynor RB, Weiner R: Transthoracic approach to an intramedullary vascular malformation of the thoracic spinal cord. Neurosurgery 10:631–634, 1982.
77. Yasargil MG, DeLong WB, Guarnaschelli JJ: Complete microsurgical excision of cervical extramedullary and intramedullary vascular malformations. Surg Neurol 4:211–224, 1975.
78. Djindjian R: Clinical symptomatology and natural history of arteriovenous malformations of the spinal cord: A study of the clinical aspects and prognosis, based on 150 cases. In Pia H, Djindjian R (eds): Spinal Angiomas: Advances in Diagnosis and Therapy. Berlin, Springer, 1978, pp 75–81.
79. Djindjian M, Djindjian R, Hurth M: [Steal phenomena in spinal arteriovenous malformations.] J Neuroradiol 5:187–201, 1978.
80. Biondi A, Merland JJ, Hodes JE: Aneurysms of spinal arteries associated with intramedullary arteriovenous malformations. I. Angiographic and clinical aspects. AJNR Am J Neuroradiol 13: 913–922, 1992.
81. Ausman JI, Gold LH, Tadavarthy SM: Intraparenchymal embolization for obliteration of an intramedullary AVM of the spinal cord: Technical note. J Neurosurg 47:119–125, 1977.
82. El Mahdi MA, Rudwan MA, Khaffaji SM: A giant spinal aneurysm with cord and root compression. J Neurol Neurosurg Psychiatry 52:532–535, 1989.
83. Smith BS, Penka CF, Erickson LS: Subarachnoid hemorrhage due to anterior spinal artery aneurysm. Neurosurgery 18:217–219, 1986.
84. Vishteh AG, Brown AP, Spetzler RF: Aneurysm of the intradural artery of Adamkiewicz treated with muslin wrapping: Technical case report. Neurosurgery 40:207–209, 1997.

CHAPTER **142**

Spinal Arteriovenous Malformations

B. GREGORY THOMPSON ■ EDWARD H. OLDFIELD

Patients with spinal arteriovenous malformations (AVMs) may have an insidious, subacute, or acute onset of symptoms, depending on the type of AVM and the mechanism of cord injury. Before recommending treatment, one must consider the expected clinical course based on the natural history of the type of vascular abnormality and the potential risks and benefits of the proposed treatment. However, knowledge of the natural history of spinal vascular abnormalities is incomplete. As with other rare disorders for which therapy is attempted, the natural history is known only from retrospective studies, and additional factors mitigate the usefulness of previous studies. Most information on the natural history of spinal AVMs was acquired when they were all considered to be congenital AVMs of the spinal cord. In the past 2 decades, there have been significant advances in the understanding and treatment of spinal AVMs. Fundamental observations have been made regarding their true anatomy and pathophysiology, which in turn have enabled more effective and safer treatment. It is now generally recognized that the spinal vascular abnormalities are not a single entity but comprise several biologically distinct forms. Based on an understanding of the epidemiology, anatomy, pathophysiology, mechanism of origin, clinical presentation, and prognosis, four major types of spinal vascular abnormalities are now recognized: dural arteriovenous fistulas (AVFs), AVMs of the spinal cord, perimedullary (pial) AVFs, and cavernous angiomas (Table 142–1).[1, 2]

Although the mode of clinical presentation suggests a specific pathophysiologic process, which implies the particular type and location of an AVM, a definite diagnosis requires a methodical imaging evaluation. Before embarking on treatment, the clinician must consider (1) the type of vascular abnormality affecting the patient, (2) the likely clinical course based on the natural history of that type of lesion in relation to the age and overall medical condition of the patient, (3) the specific vascular anatomy of the lesion and its relationship to the vessels supplying the spinal cord (Fig. 142–1), and (4) the relative risks and benefits of the proposed treatment.

TABLE 142–1 ■ **Classification of Spinal Vascular Abnormalities Based on Distinct Biologic Features**

Dural arteriovenous fistulas (AVFs)
Intradural arteriovenous malformations (AVMs)
Spinal cord AVMs
Juvenile AVMs
Glomus AVMs
Perimedullary AVFs
Cavernous angiomas

Adapted from Oldfield E, Doppman J: Spinal arteriovenous malformations. Clin Neurosurg 34:161–183, 1988.

HISTORY AND CLASSIFICATION

Elsberg performed the first successful operation for a spinal AVM in 1914.[3] Before surgery his patient was densely paraparetic and bedridden and had sensory loss below the T9 dermatomal level. Operative exploration revealed an abnormal posterior "dilated spinal vein" that entered the spinal dura adjacent to the dural penetration of the posterior root of the ninth thoracic spinal nerve. Elsberg excised 2 cm of the abnormal vessel as it penetrated the spinal dura. Postoperatively the patient improved dramatically, with complete neurological recovery by 3 months after surgery.[3, 4]

The classification of spinal AVMs has evolved with, and been limited by, the technology available to study them. The earliest analyses of spinal AVMs were based solely on postmortem histopathologic examinations. In 1925, Sargent reviewed the 21 previously reported cases of spinal AVM and concluded that 19 of them were "venous angiomas."[5] In his 1943 review of 110 cases, Wyburn-Mason classified spinal cord vascular malformations into two histologic groups, arteriovenous angiomas and purely venous angiomas, the latter accounting for approximately two thirds of all cases.[6] The venous angioma type was described as a mass of distended, blue pial vessels on the surface of the spinal cord. For consistency with Virchow's original classification of vascular anomalies, Wyburn-Mason called this type "angioma racemosum venosum." Thus, these early classifications suggested that a majority of spinal AVMs were venous lesions on the surface of the cord.[1]

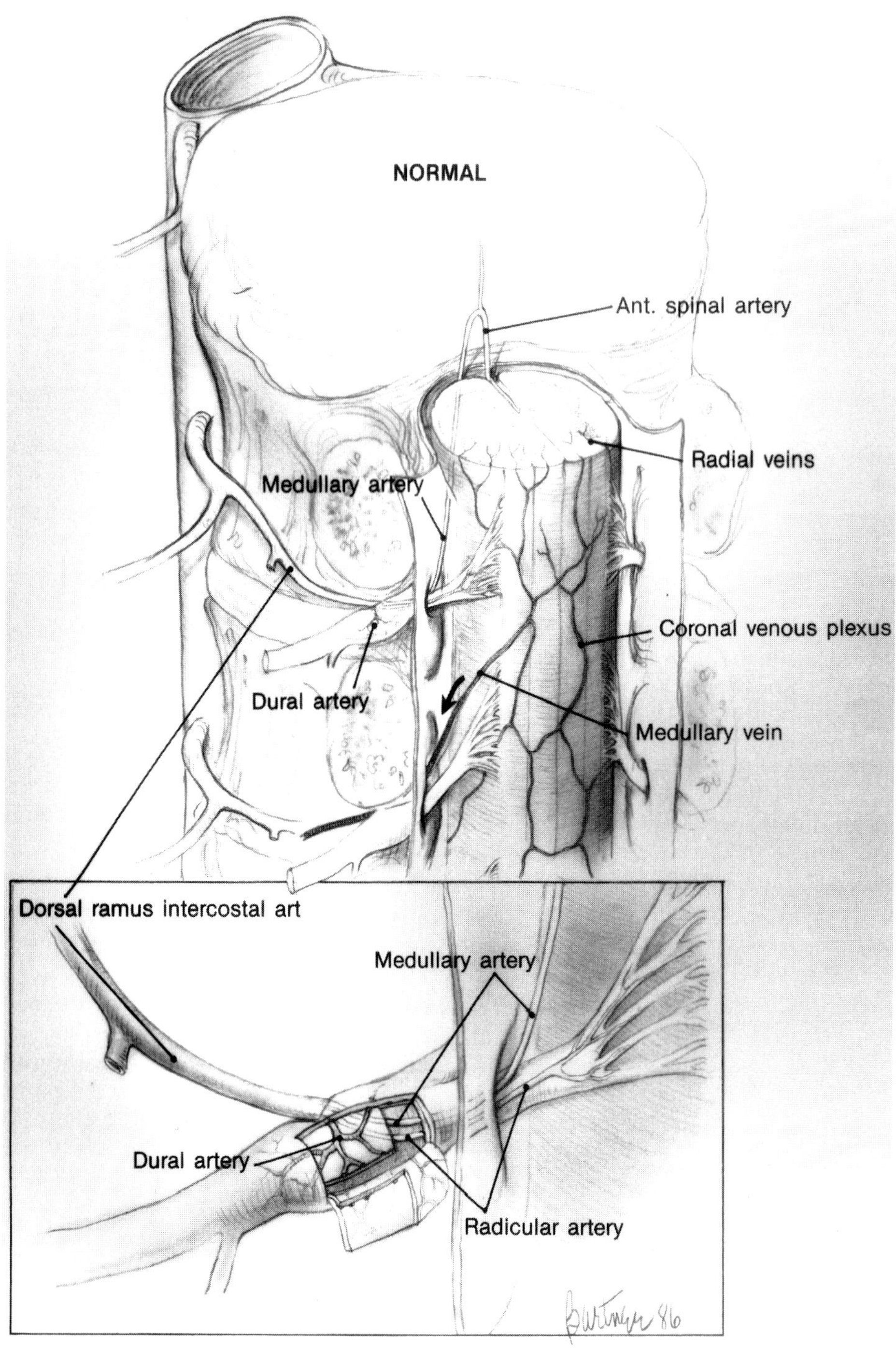

FIGURE 142–1. Normal spinal vascular anatomy. At each segmental level, the spinal ramus of each intercostal artery (or its equivalent at the cervical and lumbar levels) divides, after entering the intervertebral foramen and penetrating the outer surface of the dura, into radicular arteries, which supply the anterior or posterior nerve roots, and a dural artery, which provides arterial blood to the spinal dura and the nerve root sleeve. At some levels, the intervertebral portion of the spinal ramus of the intercostal artery also is the origin of a medullary artery, which penetrates the dura adjacent to the nerve root ganglion, ascends, and joins the anterior or a posterior spinal artery to supply the spinal cord. The spinal cord is drained by radial veins, which carry the blood to the surface to the coronal venous plexus, a plexiform network of interconnecting veins in the pia, or to sulcal veins. These are drained by medullary veins that pierce the dura adjacent to the dural penetration of the nerve roots to carry the blood to the extradural veins. (Drawing by Howard Bartner, NIH; from Oldfield E, Doppman J: Spinal arteriovenous malformations. Clin Neurosurg 34:161–183, 1988.)

The introduction of spinal aortography and then selective spinal arteriography by Doppman and Djindjian and their coworkers in the 1960s allowed clinicians to confirm the presence of spinal AVMs and to define their anatomy in living patients for the first time. Demonstration of the radiographic anatomy of spinal AVMs in vivo resulted in a more precise arteriographic classification of these lesions based on their vascular anatomy and pattern of blood flow, rather than on postmortem pathology.[7–11] Hence, spinal AVMs were classified radiographically into three categories.[7, 8] Type I, the "single coiled vessel type," constituted 80% to 85% of all spinal AVMs. Type II, or "glomus," and type III, or "juvenile," AVMs accounted for 15% to 20% of all lesions. Although investigators were able to demonstrate the site of the AVF only in type II and III lesions, in all three types the nidus was thought to be within the spinal cord.[1]

The juvenile- and glomus-type malformations, although accounting for a minority of all spinal AVMs, were initially described more accurately than the single coiled vessel type. Arteriographically, they were composed of a discrete nidus in the substance of the spinal cord and had at least one medullary artery that supplied blood to the spinal cord as well as to the AVM. The juvenile type was considered analogous to cerebral AVMs. It occurred primarily in children and young adults, had multiple large feeding vessels supplying a large AVM, had rapid shunting of blood flow, and was often associated with a spinal bruit. The glomus type also had a distinctive radiographic appearance. Typically, a single feeding artery supplied a small nidus of delicate vessels occupying a short segment of spinal cord.

The single coiled vessel lesion, the most common of the three types, was described as a single, continuous, tightly coiled vessel on the surface of the spinal cord. Blood flow through this lesion was generally slow, often requiring nearly 20 seconds for clearance of contrast material. These spinal AVMs were usually supplied by one or two feeding vessels that were thought to supply the AVM but not the spinal cord. In contrast to the juvenile and glomus types, in this type the nidus of the arteriovenous shunt was not identified. The arteriographic classification was adopted by surgeons, who theorized, but were never able to demonstrate, that the nidus of the AVM was located in multiple penetrating parenchymal vessels between the dorsolateral arterial plexus and the single coiled vessel on the cord surface. This theory, concomitant with the advent of microneurosurgery in the 1960s, led to surgical stripping of the engorged, thin-walled vessels from the surface of the cord as the preferred treatment.[12, 13]

In 1977, Kendall and Logue identified AVFs in the

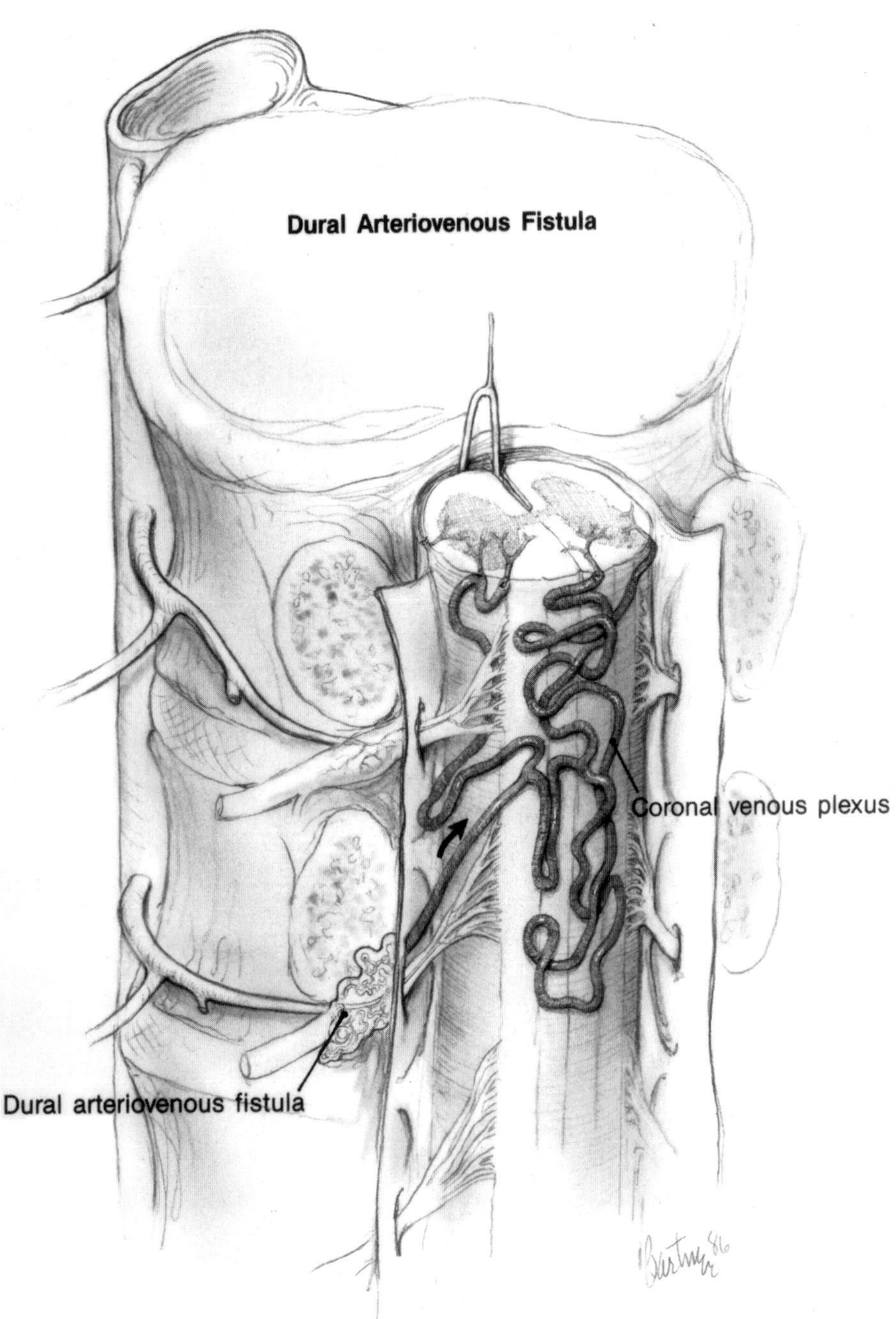

FIGURE 142–2. Vascular anatomy of dural arteriovenous fistula (AVF). Dural AVFs are supplied by a dural artery and drained by a medullary vein, which carries the arterialized blood retrograde to the normal direction of venous drainage to the coronal venous plexus, which becomes elongated, tortuous, and dilated by the reception of arterial blood. Because of the valveless nature of the intradural venous system, the increased venous pressure within the coronal venous plexus is transmitted to the spinal cord and causes venous congestion and myelopathy. (Drawing by Howard Bartner, NIH; from Oldfield E, Doppman J: Spinal arteriovenous malformations. Clin Neurosurg 34:161–183, 1988.)

dural sleeve of spinal nerve roots in nine patients who had radiographic findings otherwise completely consistent with the single coiled vessel type of spinal AVM.[14] After simple surgical excision of the dural AVF, the patients improved. Hence, lesions that were previously considered pial venous angiomas or single coiled vessel AVMs by earlier classifications were now recognized to be dural AVFs in the spinal nerve root sleeve and adjacent spinal dura. The typical single coiled vessel morphology of these lesions is now acknowledged to be the result of chronic metamorphosis of the vessels of the coronal venous plexus by the arterialization of normal pial veins into dilated, serpentine, thin-walled vessels on the surface of the spinal cord.

Two additional advances in the understanding and classification of spinal AVMs have occurred in the past 25 years. First was the recognition by Djindjian and colleagues in 1977 that some intradural lesions that were previously considered AVMs of the spinal cord are actually simple AVFs in the pia (perimedullary AVFs).[15] Second was the recognition of an additional important category of vascular lesion that was previously thought to be extremely rare, because there was no diagnostic study that could reveal it before the introduction of computed tomographic scanning. This lesion is the cavernous angioma (also called cavernous malformation), which has a predisposition to hemorrhage repeatedly. Its true incidence has become evident only since the introduction of magnetic resonance imaging (MRI).

With the recognition that former type I AVMs were actually dural AVFs, the identification of perimedullary AVFs, the recognition of the clinical importance of cavernous angiomas, and the increased understanding of the pathophysiology underlying the natural history and clinical presentation of the different types of spinal AVMs, it has become clear that each major type is a distinct biologic entity (Figs. 142–2 to 142–7). Thus, a

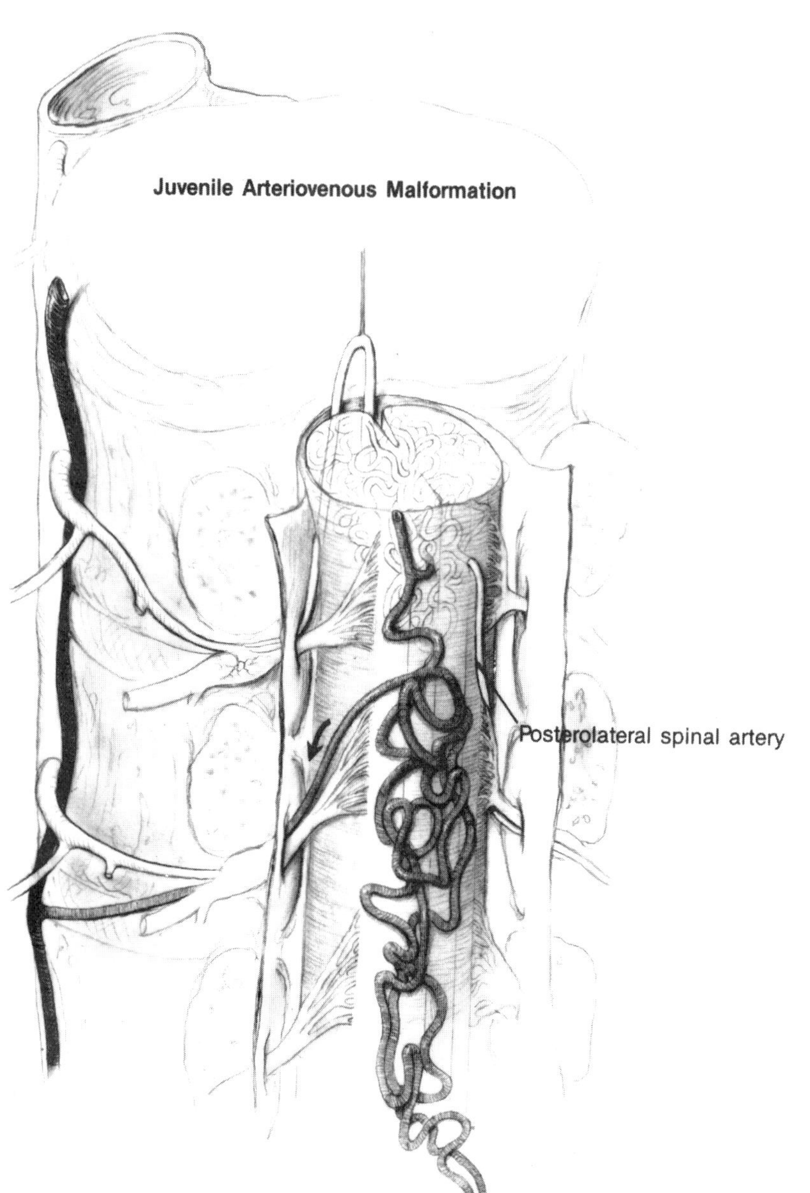

FIGURE 142–3. Vascular anatomy of the juvenile type of intramedullary arteriovenous malformation (AVM). Juvenile-type intramedullary AVMs are fed by enlarged medullary arteries via dilated anterior and posterior spinal arteries. The nidus of the AVM is often extensive, filling the spinal canal, and commonly contains neural tissue within the interstices of the vessels of the AVM. (Drawing by Howard Bartner, NIH; from Oldfield E, Doppman J: Spinal arteriovenous malformations. Clin Neurosurg 34: 161–183, 1988.)

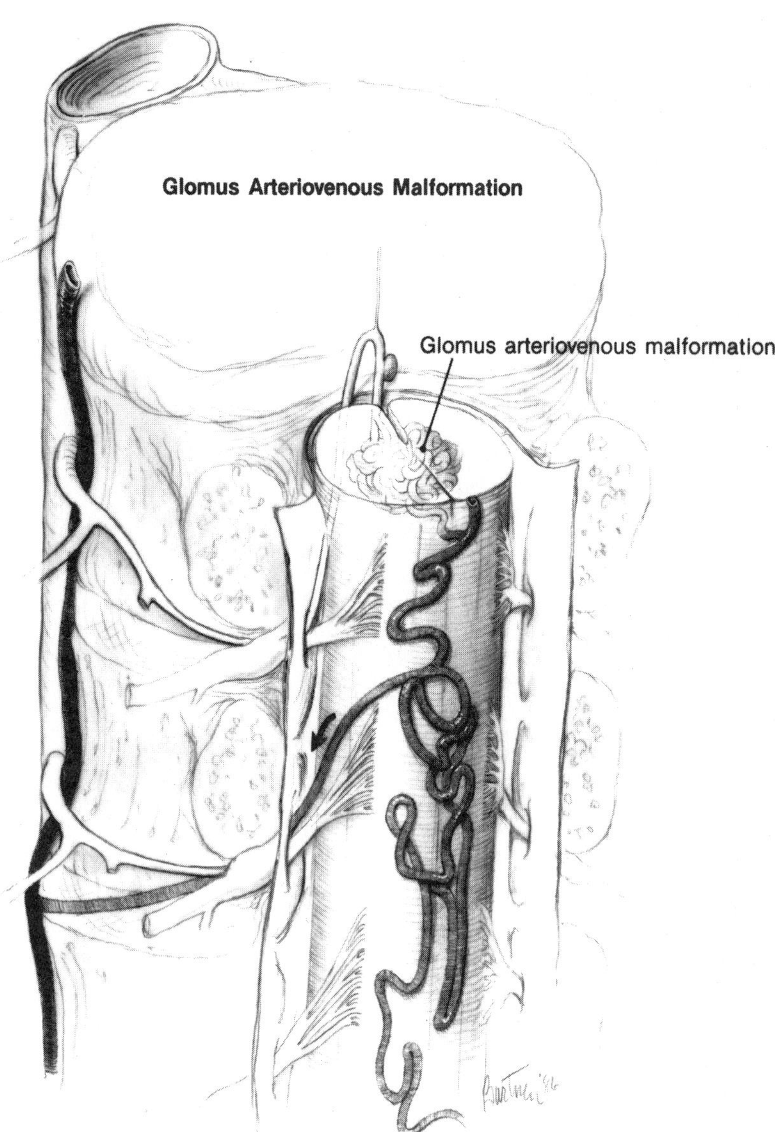

FIGURE 142–4. Vascular anatomy of the glomus type of intramedullary arteriovenous malformation (AVM). The nidus of glomus-type intramedullary AVMs is a tightly packed congerie of blood vessels confined to a short segment of the spinal cord. These AVMs, commonly found in the anterior half of the spinal cord, are usually supplied by the anterior spinal artery. (Drawing by Howard Bartner, NIH; from Oldfield E, Doppman J: Spinal arteriovenous malformations. Clin Neurosurg 34:161–183, 1988.)

reclassification of spinal AVMs was necessary to provide terminology that accurately described the lesion and allowed logical categorization based on biologically distinct categories rather than on the use of old terms and categorization schemes that were based on a mistaken understanding of the true nature of the lesions, used abstract terms (e.g., type I spinal AVM) rather than comprehensible and clearly descriptive terms for the various lesions, and permitted different authors to use the same term in substantially different ways.[7, 8] Hence, three main types of spinal vascular malformations with definite biologic differences (e.g., anatomy, pathogenesis, pathophysiology, epidemiology, clinical features) are now recognized: dural AVFs, intradural vascular malformations (which include AVMs of the spinal cord and intradural AVFs), and cavernous angiomas of the spinal cord (see Table 142–1 and Fig. 142–7). In dural AVFs, the arteriovenous nidus is embedded in the dura, usually in the spinal nerve root sleeve and contiguous dura (see Fig. 142–2). In the intradural vascular malformations, the arteriovenous shunt is either buried in the substance of the spinal cord (AVMs; see Figs. 142–3 and 142–4) or in the pia or subarachnoid space (perimedullary AVFs; see Fig. 142–5). Cavernous angiomas (see Fig. 142–6), which are not demonstrated by spinal arteriography but have highly characteristic MRI findings, are rarely mistaken for the other types of spinal vascular abnormalities.

VASCULAR ANATOMY AND PATHOGENESIS

Normal Vascular Anatomy of Spinal Cord and Dura

The clinical diagnosis of the various subtypes of spinal AVMs and the correct interpretation of diagnostic studies require an understanding of the spinal vascular anatomy. Hence, knowledge of the normal spinal vascular anatomy is necessary to fully appreciate the blood supply, arteriographic features, and pathophysiology

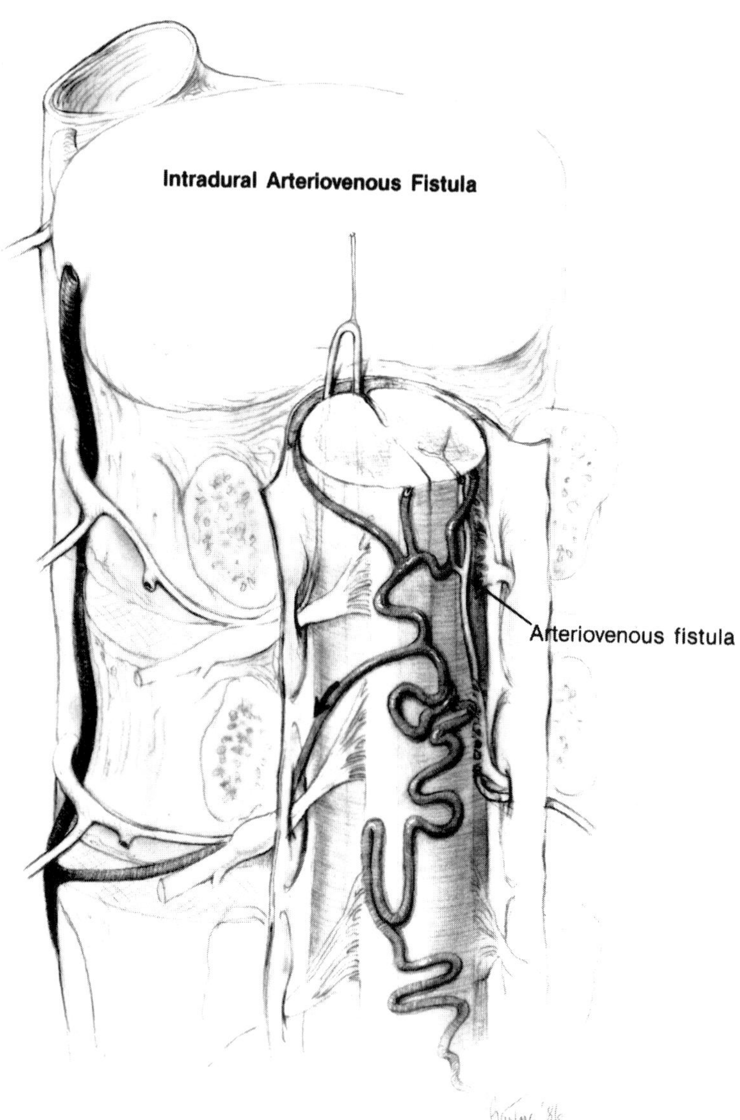

FIGURE 142–5. Vascular anatomy of a perimedullary (pial) arteriovenous fistula (AVF). Medullary arteries provide the arterial supply, in this instance, via a posterior spinal artery. Most intradural AVFs occur in the lower thoracic or lumbar area and are supplied by the anterior spinal artery. Large perimedullary AVFs often have associated venous varices at the junction of the arterial and venous elements in which the portion of the vein just distal to the arteriovenous shunt is dilated. Many of these lesions are not as simple as the one illustrated here. They can have more than one simple fistula in the same region of the pia, and, at surgery, the tortuosity and dilatation of the venous drainage often obscure the site of the AVF beneath a nest of blood vessels. (Drawing by Howard Bartner, NIH; from Oldfield E, Doppman J: Spinal arteriovenous malformations. Clin Neurosurg 34:161–183, 1988.)

underlying cord injury in each type of spinal vascular malformation.

ARTERIAL ANATOMY

The spinal cord is supplied by two arterial networks, the anterior and posterior arterial systems (see Fig. 142–1). The anterior plexus is derived from the anterior spinal artery, which extends along the entire length of the spinal cord in the anterior median fissure and is the origin of sulcal arteries, which leave the anterior spinal artery at a 90-degree angle to perfuse the anterior two thirds of the spinal cord. The anterior horns, corticospinal tracts, and spinothalamic tracts are perfused by this anterior spinal arterial distribution. The posterior system is a network of plexiform collaterals between two posterolateral arteries. It supplies the posterior third of the spinal cord, including a portion of the corticospinal tracts and the entire dorsal column.[8–10, 16–18] Both the anterior and the posterior arterial systems are supplied by medullary arteries.

During the first 6 months of gestation, paired bilateral medullary arteries supply anterior and posterolateral arteries at each segmental level of the spinal cord. By the third trimester, however, most medullary arteries have regressed, and, in adults, only 6 to 10 remain to supply the spinal cord.[16] Medullary arteries in the cervical region are derived from the vertebral arteries and branches of the thyrocervical trunk. Medullary arteries in the thoracic and lumbar regions arise from a branch of the segmental vessels from the aorta and iliac arteries, specifically the intervertebral segment of the spinal ramus of the posterior segmental (intercostal) arteries (see Fig. 142–1).

The largest and most important of these 6 to 10 medullary arteries is the arteria radicularis anterior magna, or the artery of Adamkiewicz. It serves as the major blood supply to the mid- and lower thoracic and lumbar segments of the spinal cord and typically originates on the left side between T8 and L2; however, it may arise from T3 to L4 and may be on either side.[19] The upper thoracic portion of the spinal cord, above

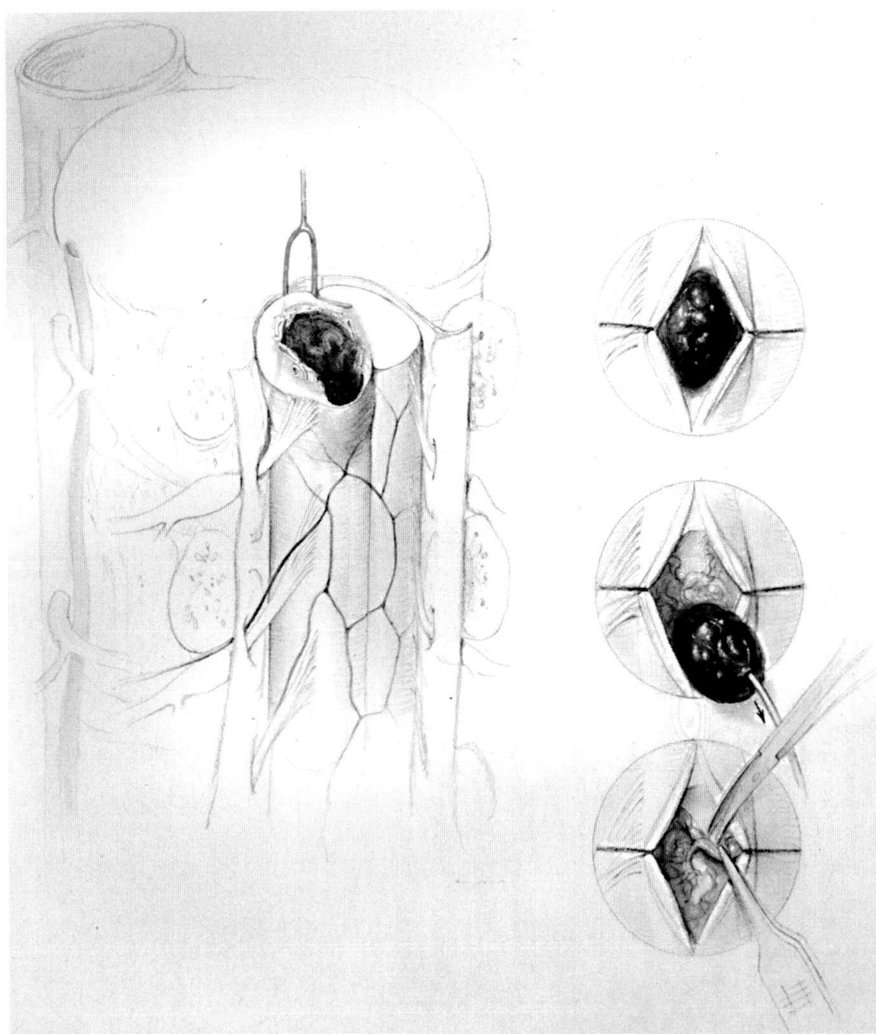

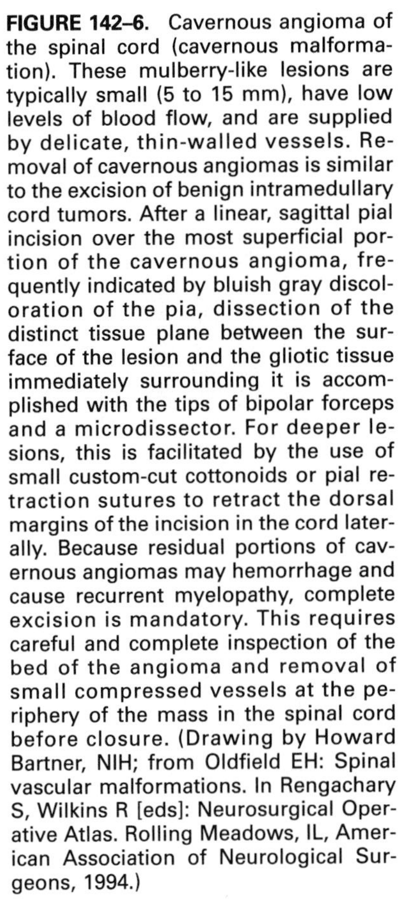

FIGURE 142–6. Cavernous angioma of the spinal cord (cavernous malformation). These mulberry-like lesions are typically small (5 to 15 mm), have low levels of blood flow, and are supplied by delicate, thin-walled vessels. Removal of cavernous angiomas is similar to the excision of benign intramedullary cord tumors. After a linear, sagittal pial incision over the most superficial portion of the cavernous angioma, frequently indicated by bluish gray discoloration of the pia, dissection of the distinct tissue plane between the surface of the lesion and the gliotic tissue immediately surrounding it is accomplished with the tips of bipolar forceps and a microdissector. For deeper lesions, this is facilitated by the use of small custom-cut cottonoids or pial retraction sutures to retract the dorsal margins of the incision in the cord laterally. Because residual portions of cavernous angiomas may hemorrhage and cause recurrent myelopathy, complete excision is mandatory. This requires careful and complete inspection of the bed of the angioma and removal of small compressed vessels at the periphery of the mass in the spinal cord before closure. (Drawing by Howard Bartner, NIH; from Oldfield EH: Spinal vascular malformations. In Rengachary S, Wilkins R [eds]: Neurosurgical Operative Atlas. Rolling Meadows, IL, American Association of Neurological Surgeons, 1994.)

the region perfused by the artery of Adamkiewicz and below the relatively well-collateralized cervical region, is a "watershed" or arterial border zone. It is particularly susceptible to hemodynamic ischemia and is the site of watershed infarcts of the spinal cord induced by severe hypotension.

In addition to the medullary arteries, which supply only the spinal cord, there are two other important terminal branches of the intervertebral artery (the posterior spinal ramus of each segmental artery), as well as the radicular arteries (which supply the nerve roots) and the dural arteries (which supply the dural root sleeves and spinal dura). These arteries persist at each segmental level into adulthood (see Fig. 142–1).

VENOUS ANATOMY

The spinal cord venous system, like the arterial system, is composed of two radially arranged vascular networks (see Fig. 142–1). The sulcal veins in the anterior median fissure and the radial veins in the dorsal and anterolateral portions of the spinal cord drain to the coronal venous plexus on the cord surface.[20] This pial venous plexus is drained by medullary veins to the epidural venous plexus. The medullary veins—which, like the medullary arteries, are not present at each segmental level but arise sporadically along the long axis of the spinal cord—cross the subarachnoid space and penetrate the dura adjacent to the dural penetration of the nerve roots.[20] Venous structures within the intrathecal space lack valves, but functional valves at the level of the dural penetration of the medullary veins prevent retrograde venous flow from the epidural (Batson's) plexus to the intradural space.[17, 20] In the region of the cervicomedullary junction, the venous system of the brainstem and the spinal cord freely communicate.

Vascular Anatomy of Spinal Vascular Abnormalities

DURAL ARTERIOVENOUS FISTULAS

Figures 142–2 and 142–8 illustrate the typical pathologic and arteriographic anatomy of spinal dural AVFs. The AVF, a low-flow shunt in the dural sleeve of a spinal nerve root, is supplied by the dural branch of the intervertebral artery. A medullary vein, the sole

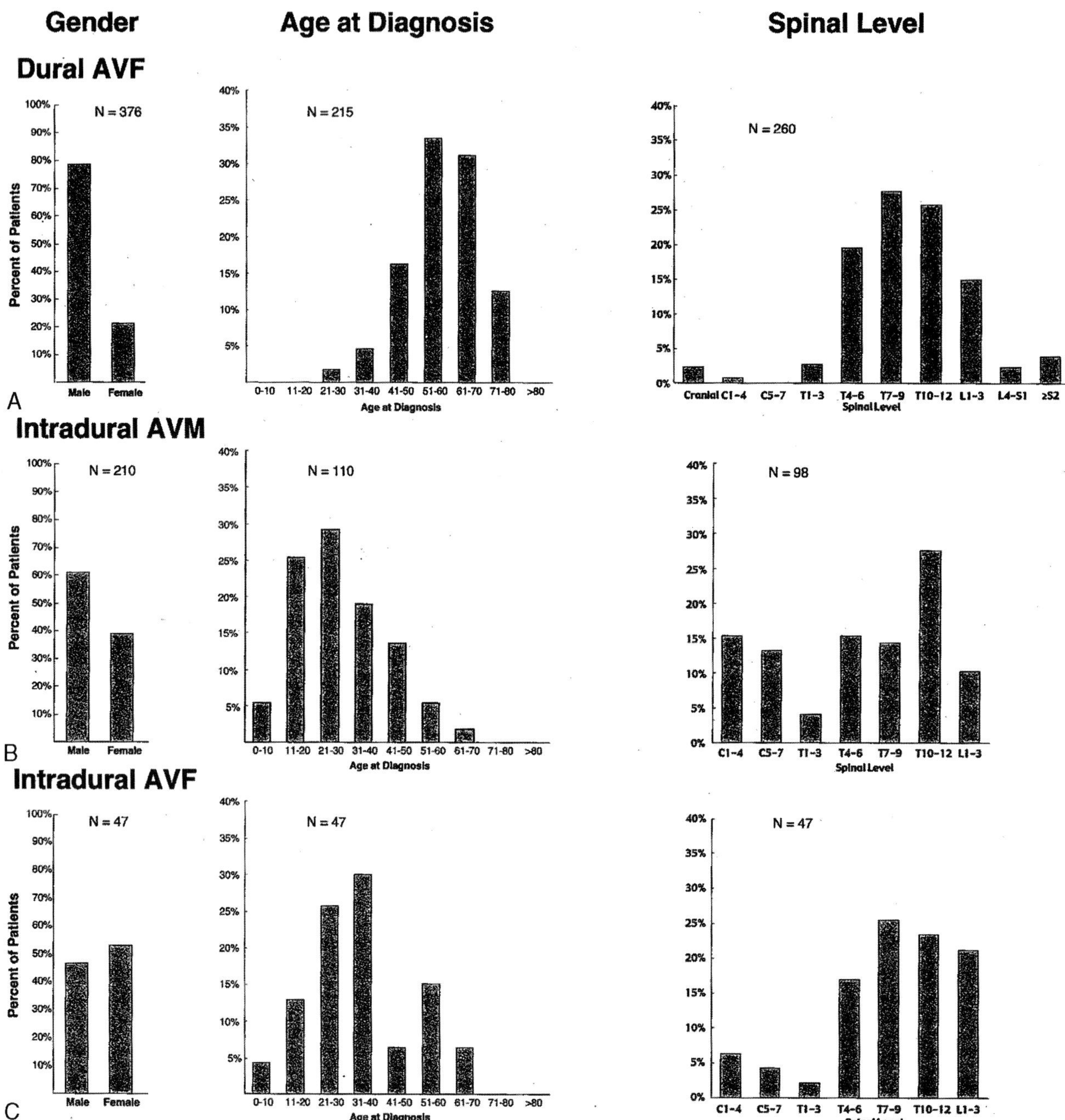

FIGURE 142–7. Distribution of patients with spinal dural arteriovenous fistulas (AVFs) *(A)*, intradural spinal arteriovenous malformations (AVMs) (*B*; most reports include AVMs and AVFs), and perimedullary AVFs *(C)* by gender, age at diagnosis, and level of AVF along the long axis of the spine. The distinct differences in the distribution of patients with these three types of spinal vascular abnormalities indicate that they are biologically discrete disorders and support the general classification depicted in Table 142–1. (Compiled from data from the following references: dural AVFs—gender,[22, 23, 40, 49, 86, 97–99, 102, 139–143] age,[22, 23, 40, 97, 139, 140] and level[14, 22, 23, 40, 49, 86, 98, 102, 139–143]; intradural AVMs—gender,[23, 46, 56, 142, 143] and age and level[23, 56, 142, 143]; intradural AVFs—gender, age, and level.[15, 25, 59, 60, 142] From Oldfield EH, et al: submitted for publication.)

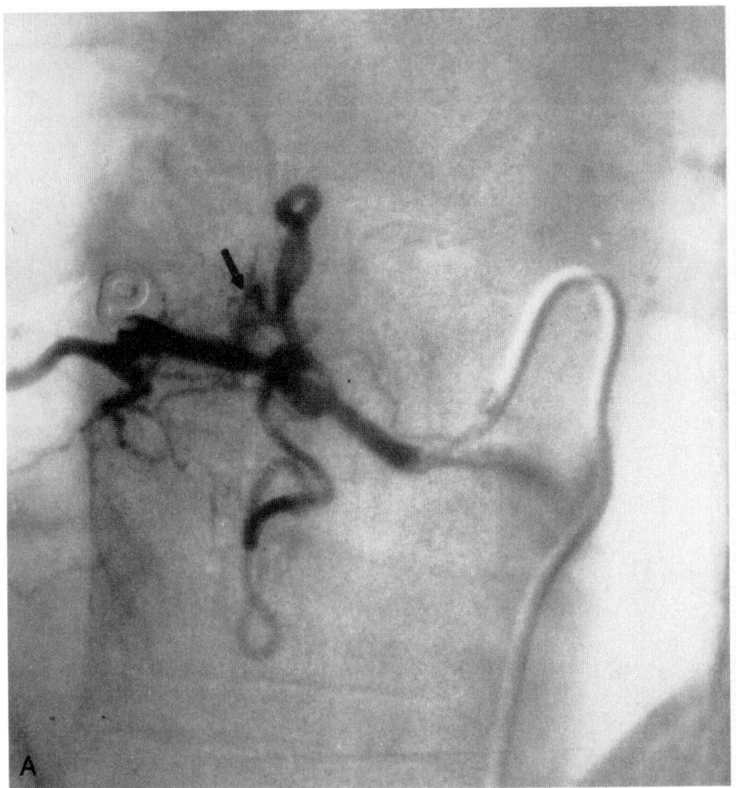

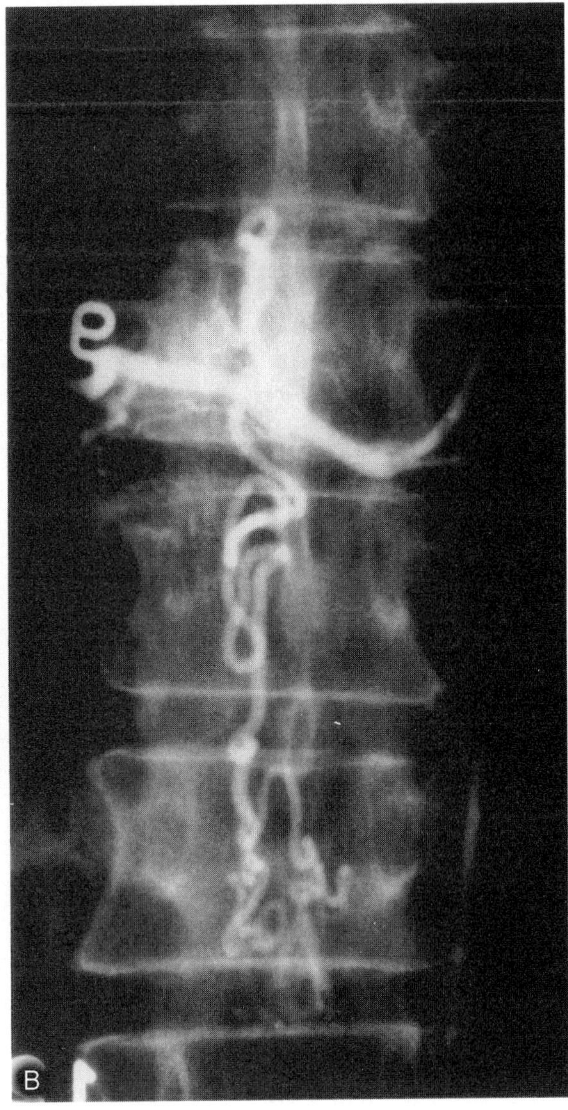

FIGURE 142–8. Selective spinal arteriogram of a spinal dural arteriovenous fistula (AVF) embedded in the root sleeve of the ninth thoracic nerve root and the adjacent spinal dura in a 56-year-old man with progressive myelopathy. With spinal dural AVFs, the nidus of the fistula is typically in the intervertebral foramen *(A, arrow)* and the lateral aspect of the spinal canal and drains into the dilated, tortuous intradural veins on the cord surface, covering several levels of the spinal cord *(B)*. Unlike the AVF seen here, in which the initial venous drainage is caudal, most dural AVFs drain in a predominantly rostral direction. (From Oldfield EH, DiChiro G, Quindlen EA: Successful treatment of a group of spinal cord arteriovenous malformations by interruption of dural fistula. J Neurosurg 59:1019–1030, 1983.)

venous outflow from the dural AVF, carries the shunted arterial blood retrograde to the normal direction of venous flow to the coronal venous plexus.[4] Microarteriography of specimens in which the spinal dural AVF was excised en bloc demonstrates that the nidus in the dura is in the dural root sleeve and the adjacent spinal dura and that it is a simple network of a small number of separate vessels that converge into the medullary vein just beneath the inner layer of dura (Fig. 142–9).[21]

The absence of other routes of regional venous drainage,[22, 23] which would normally be provided by medullary veins, to carry excess blood flow from the coronal venous plexus through the dura and into the extradural venous system, results in rostral flow of the arterialized blood in the coronal venous plexus, reaching the cranial venous system in most patients. The diversion of blood under high pressure by the arterialized medullary vein from the dural AVF and into the coronal venous plexus, combined with the absence of normal pathways for venous drainage, results in dilatation, elongation, and tortuosity of the vessels of the coronal venous plexus. Moreover, because the intrathecal venous system is valveless, the radial and sulcal veins transmit the high pressure directly to the spinal cord, producing venous congestion, venous hypertension, reduced arterial perfusion pressure, ischemia, and myelopathy (see further on).

INTRADURAL ARTERIOVENOUS MALFORMATIONS

The nidus of intradural AVMs (Figs. 142–10, and 142–11; see also Figs. 142–3 and 142–4) is embedded within the spinal cord or partially intra- and extramedullary. Intradural AVMs are more uniformly distributed along the length of the spinal cord than are dural AVFs or perimedullary AVFs (see Fig. 142–7). They are usually supplied by one or more enlarged medullary arteries that supply the spinal cord as well.

Juvenile Type. The anatomic features of juvenile-type intradural AVMs are represented in Figures 142–3 and 142–10. These lesions are fed by multiple enlarged

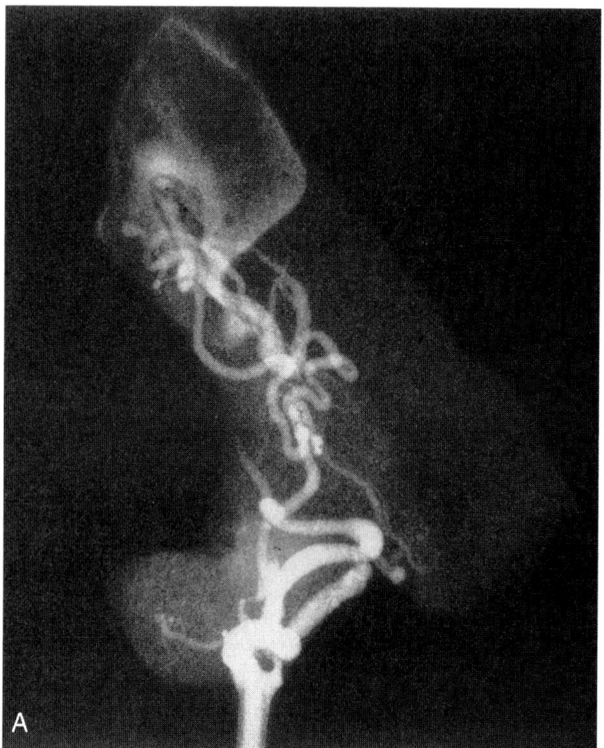

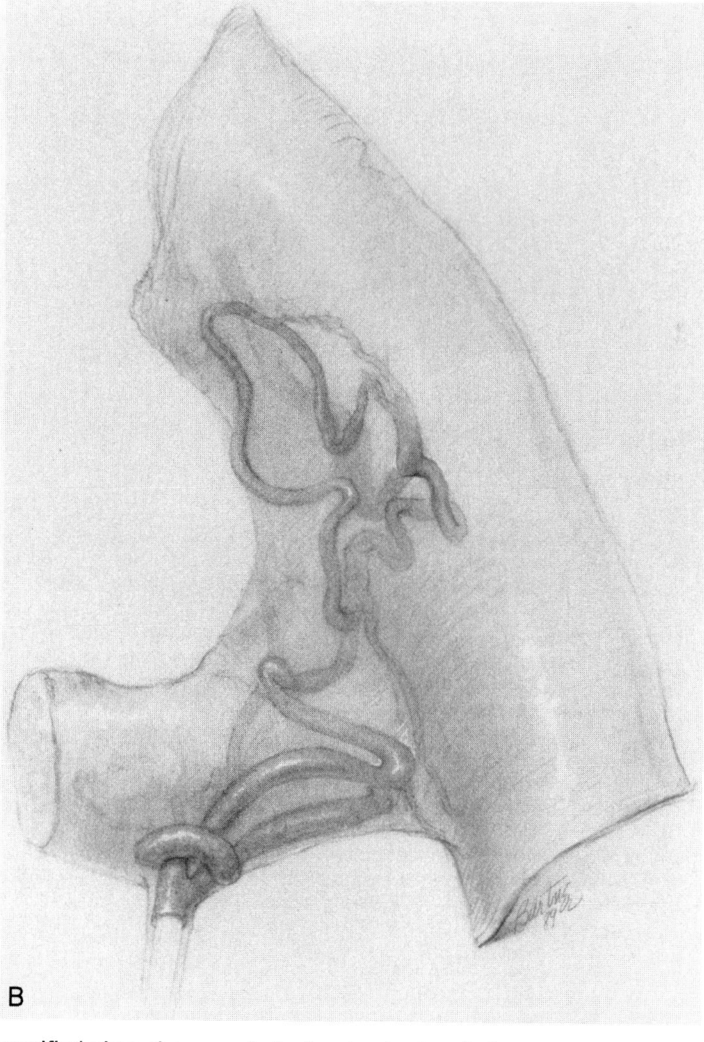

FIGURE 142–9. Microarteriogram. *A*, In this magnified view, the cannula in the dural artery is just visible at the lower end of the photograph. The shadow of the dural nerve root sleeve can be seen just above it. At the upper end, a stellate flare represents spillage of contrast agent from the cut end of the medullary vein. *B*, An artist's sketch of the microarteriogram highlights the sinuous path taken by the primary vascular loops from which the shunt is constructed. The dural artery splits immediately into two loops, which coalesce in the dura at the axilla of the root and then split in the dura again into two arterial loops on the root's shoulder. When the two vessels rejoin (midportion of the image), they penetrate the dura to join the medullary vein. Note the absence of any true glomus of capillaries, indicating that these lesions are arteriovenous fistulas, not arteriovenous malformations. (*B*, Drawn by Howard Bartner, NIH; from McCutcheon IE, Doppman JL, Oldfield EH: Microvascular anatomy of dural arteriovenous abnormalities of the spine: A microangiographic study. J Neurosurg 84: 215–220, 1996.)

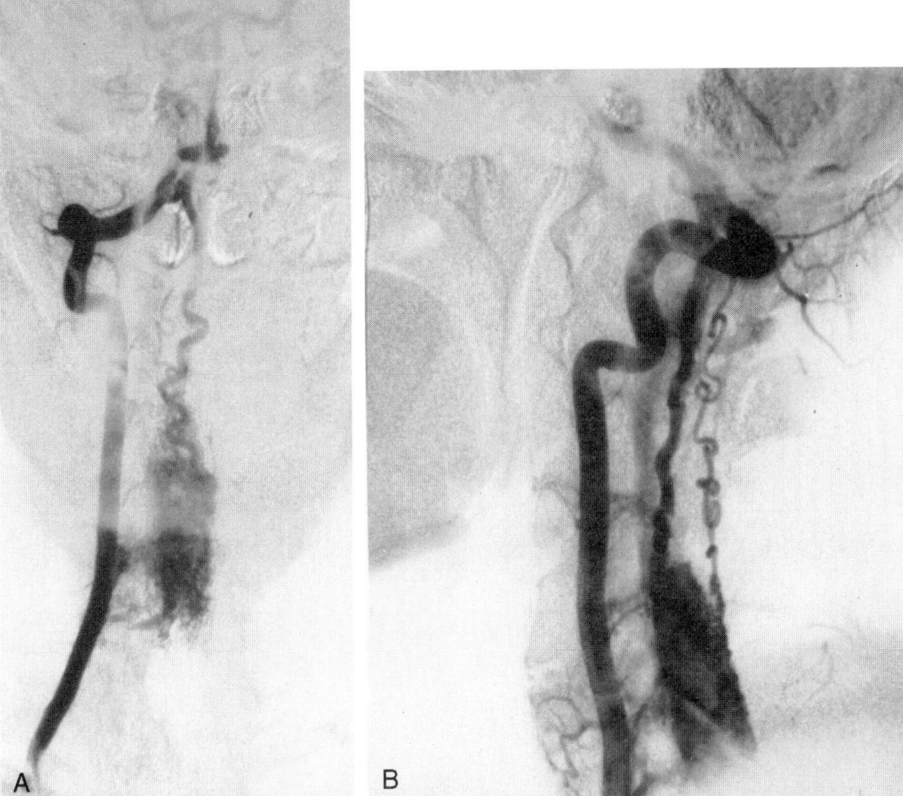

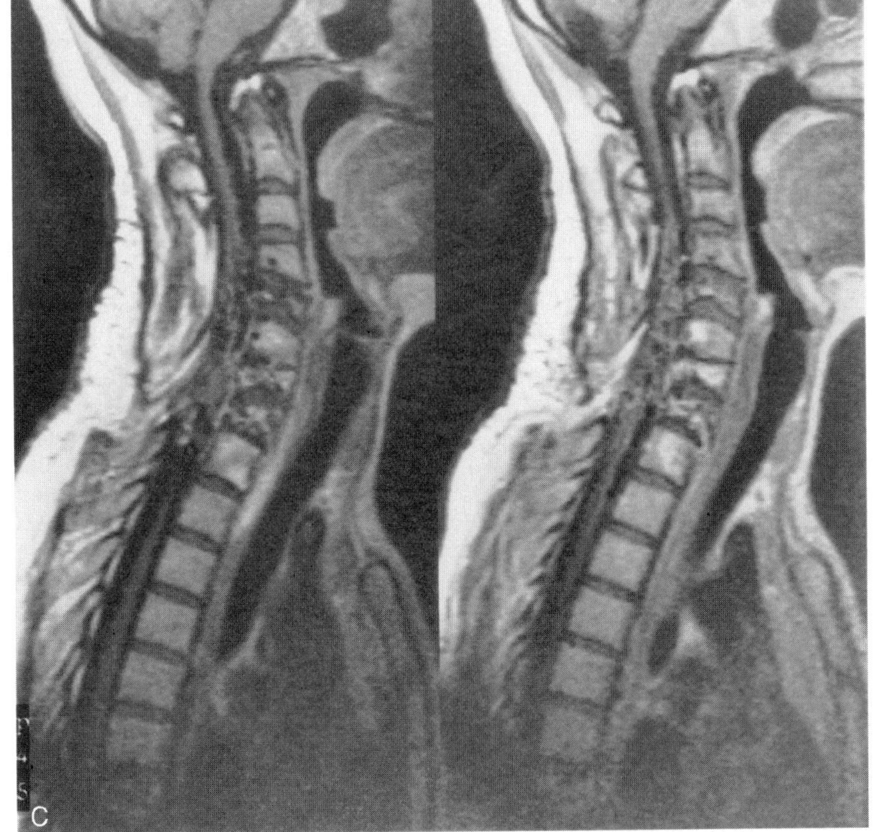

FIGURE 142–10. Juvenile-type intramedullary arteriovenous malformation (AVM) of the cervical and thoracic segments of the spine in a 26-year-old deaf and mute woman with progressive quadriparesis that was eliminating her ability to communicate by signing. Right vertebral arteriography, anteroposterior *(A)* and lateral *(B)* views, demonstrates the superior aspect of a large intramedullary AVM that extends from C4 to T2. The nidus of the AVM fills the spinal canal from front to back and from side to side. On sagittal T1-weighted magnetic resonance imaging scan *(C)*, the signal void from the AVM clearly involves not only the cross-sectional area of the spinal cord but also the anterior and posterior elements of the spine and paraspinous soft tissue, a distribution that was confirmed by additional arteriography. (From Thompson B, Oldfield E: Spinal vascular malformations. In Carter L, Spetzler R, Hamilton M [eds]: Neurovascular Surgery. New York, McGraw-Hill, 1994, pp 1167–1195.)

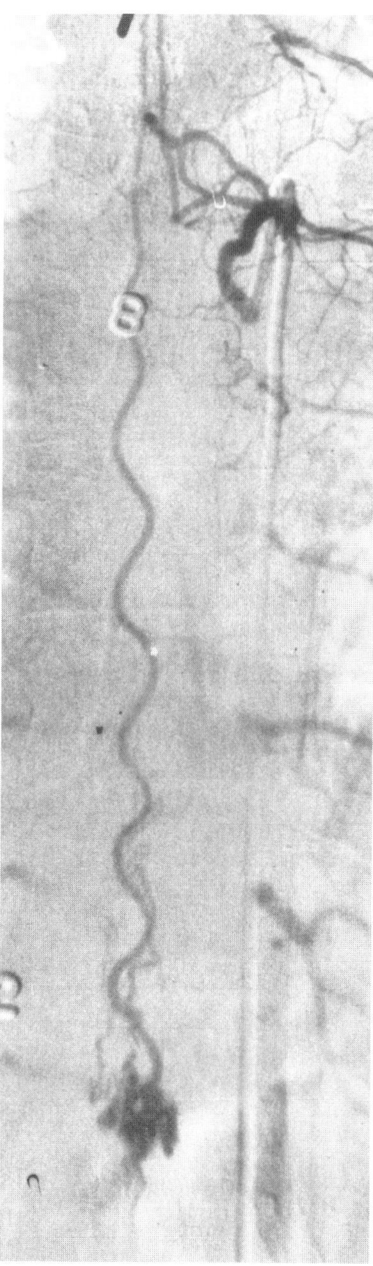

FIGURE 142–11. Selective spinal cord arteriogram demonstrating a glomus-type intramedullary arteriovenous malformation (AVM) supplied by the anterior spinal artery via the artery of Adamkiewicz. (From Oldfield EH, DiChiro G, Quindlen EA: Successful treatment of a group of spinal cord arteriovenous malformations by interruption of dural fistula. J Neurosurg 59:1019–1030, 1983.)

medullary arteries, via anterior and posterolateral spinal arteries, and may have a voluminous arteriovenous nidus that completely fills the thecal sac. The nidus typically has neural tissue within its interstices. Juvenile AVMs frequently involve the vertebral column and the paraspinous soft tissues (metameric form; see Fig. 142–10). Unlike dural AVFs, these are high-flow AVMs; a spinal bruit may indicate their presence.

Glomus Type. The nidus in the glomus subtype of intradural AVMs is a compact tangle of blood vessels that is confined to a short segment of cord (see Figs. 142–4 and 142–11). These lesions typically lie in the anterior half of the spinal cord and are supplied by one or two medullary arteries via the anterior spinal artery.

PERIMEDULLARY ARTERIOVENOUS FISTULAS

The anatomic derangement in intradural AVFs is depicted in Figures 142–5 and 142–12. In these lesions, a direct pial fistulous communication lies between an intradural spinal artery and the coronal venous plexus. The absence of intervening small vessels (i.e., a glomus) at the AVF defines the lesion. The fistula may arise from the anterior or posterolateral spinal arteries but is more commonly supplied by the anterior spinal artery.[15, 24–26] Intradural AVFs are often associated with a venous varix at the arterial-to-venous transition.

CAVERNOUS ANGIOMAS

Considering that cavernous angiomas are usually angiographically occult, it is not surprising that the spinal cord vascular anatomy is not altered by them (see Fig. 142–6). These mulberry-like lesions are typically small (5 to 15 mm), have a low level of blood flow, and are supplied by delicate thin-walled vessels. A rim of hemosiderin and gliosis, the product of previous small hemorrhages, typically surrounds these well-demarcated lesions. Cavernous malformations may occur in association with cerebral cavernous malformations and may occur at more than one level of the spinal cord when they are associated with familial multiple cavernous angiomatosis,[27, 28] which is now known to be an autosomal-dominant trait that maps to chromosome 7q.[29–35]

CAUSE, PATHOPHYSIOLOGY, CLINICAL PRESENTATION, AND NATURAL HISTORY

This section discusses the cause, pathophysiology, clinical presentation, and natural history of each type of vascular abnormality. Dural AVFs are the most common type, have similar pathophysiology of cord injury from patient to patient, and have a relatively stereotypic clinical course, permitting prediction of a patient's prognosis with reasonable accuracy. In contrast, the other types of AVMs are less common and have a more sporadic and less predictable clinical course, and the pathophysiology of cord injury varies from patient to patient (e.g., hemorrhage, venous congestion, vascular steal, aneurysm formation with cord compression). Cavernous angiomas, which have conspicuously different clinical and radiographic features and do not pose a problem of differential diagnosis, are considered last.

Dural Arteriovenous Fistulas

Spinal dural AVFs are distinguished from intradural AVMs by their cause, pathophysiology, incidence, age

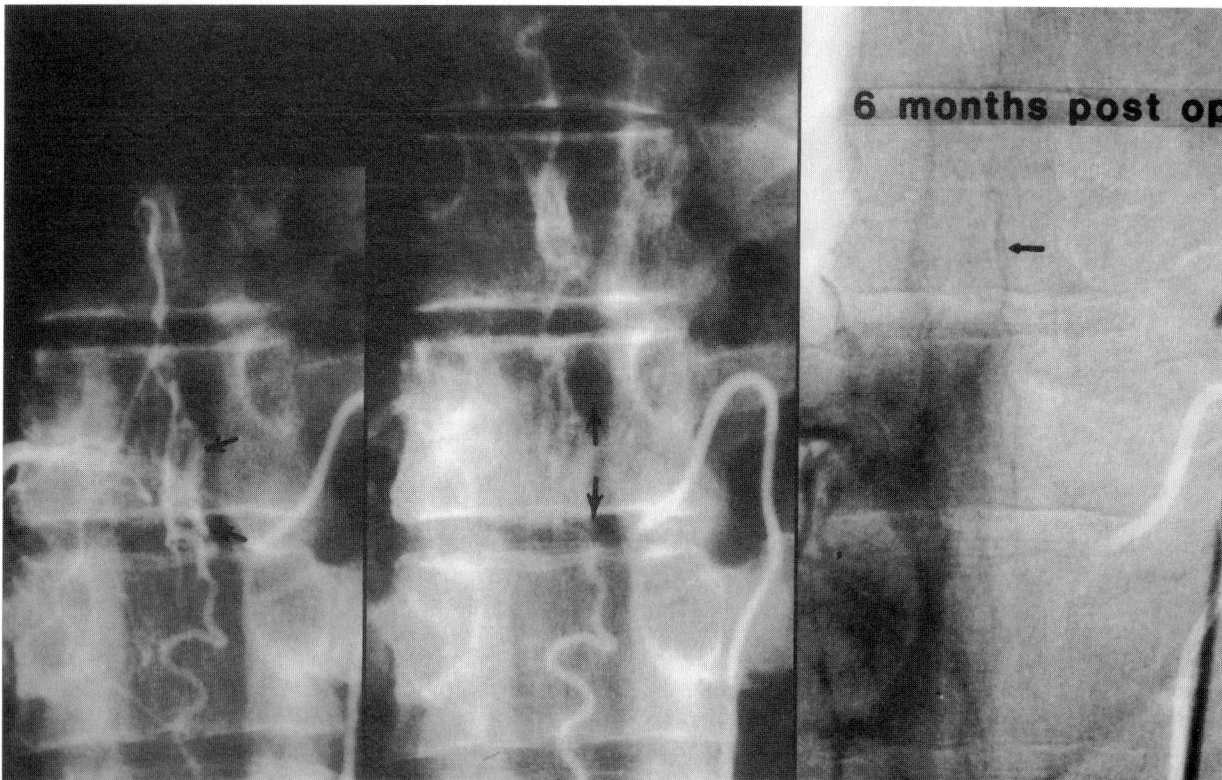

FIGURE 142–12. Posterolateral perimedullary arteriovenous fistula (AVF). *Left,* Selective spinal arteriography demonstrates that the nidus of this relatively small pial AVF is supplied by the descending limb of a posterior spinal artery, that there is more than one arteriovenous shunt, and that the arterial-to-venous shunting occurs at a moderate pace. The site of the nidus *(arrows)* is identified just proximal to the site of initial venous dilatation and by the site from which the venous flow diverges rostrally and caudally *(middle, arrows). Right,* The feeding vessel has returned to a more normal size 6 months after surgical excision and the absence of filling of the AVF.

at symptom onset, distribution along the spinal axis (see Fig. 142–7), and neurological presentation and progression (Table 142–2).[1, 23] These distinguishing characteristics are important, because effective treatment of these lesions requires early recognition and clinical differentiation from intradural spinal AVMs.

Although the exact mechanism underlying the origin of dural AVFs is unknown, the late onset of symptoms, lack of association with other vascular anomalies, strong predilection for the lower spinal segments, absence of medullary veins in these patients,[22, 23, 36] predominant occurrence in men, and occasional development of similar lesions by acquired means, such as traumatic paraspinal AVFs[37] and postoperative dural AVFs,[38] suggest that these lesions are acquired.[1, 23] The pathophysiology of the progressive myelopathy produced by these lesions is clear: dural AVFs are low-flow arteriovenous shunts that induce venous hypertension. By directly measuring the venous pressure in the coronal venous plexus at surgery in patients with spinal dural AVFs, Hassler and coworkers demonstrated that the venous pressure in the spinal cord averages 74% of the simultaneous mean systemic arterial pressure.[39] Therefore, by the time of treatment, these patients have venous hypertension severe enough to reduce spinal cord arterial perfusion pres-

TABLE 142–2 ■ **Comparison of Clinical Syndromes of Dural Arteriovenous Fistulas and Intradural Arteriovenous Malformations**

	DURAL AVF (N = 27)	INTRADURAL AVM* (N = 54)
Gender	Predominantly male	Male or female
Mean age (yr) at diagnosis	46	24
Onset of symptoms	Gradual (85%)	Acute (37%)
SAH	0	50%
First symptom	Paresis (44%)	SAH (32%)
Spinal bruit	0	6%
Exacerbation of symptoms by activity	70%	15%
Arms affected	0	11%

*Includes perimedullary AVFs.

AVF, arteriovenous fistula; AVM, arteriovenous malformation; SAH, subarachnoid hemorrhage. Adapted from Rosenblum B, Oldfield EH, Doppman JL, DiChiro G: Spinal arteriovenous malformations: A comparison of dural arteriovenous fistulas and intradural AVMs in 81 patients. J Neurosurg 67:795–802, 1987.

sure to less than 30% of normal (spinal cord perfusion pressure = mean arterial pressure − venous pressure), resulting in venous congestion, spinal cord ischemia, and progressive cord injury with clinical myelopathy. The clinical result of progressive cord injury from venous hypertension is an insidious but progressive decline in motor and sensory function, which is the mode of presentation in 85% to 95% of patients with dural AVFs.[23, 40] However, about 5% to 15% of patients with dural AVFs experience episodes of acute myelopathic exacerbation (Foix-Alajouanine syndrome).[41] The rapid worsening in such cases likely indicates profound venous congestion that, unless treated expeditiously to eliminate venous hypertension, will result in venous thrombosis and irreversible cord injury.[42] An even rarer presentation, and one that has been reported in only a few patients with dural AVFs, is acute hemorrhage.

For clinical diagnosis, it is important to remember that dural AVFs are distinguished from intradural AVMs by a number of clinical features (see Fig. 142–7 and Table 142–2).[23] Unlike intradural AVMs, dural AVFs have a strong male predilection (>80%) and present in the latter half of life (80% of patients have symptom onset after age 40).[23] Dural AVFs have a strong tendency to occur in the lower thoracic and lumbar regions.[23] In the National Institutes of Health (NIH) experience, 85% occurred below T6, and 100% below T3.[23] Consequently, patients with spinal dural AVFs are unlikely to have upper extremity involvement and typically present with an insidious onset of paraparesis or sphincter dysfunction. Low back or radicular pain often precedes the onset of a gradually progressive myelopathy. Patients with dural AVFs often report symptomatic worsening during physical exertion (neurogenic claudication) or with certain postural changes (see Table 142–2).[23]

There are no studies of the untreated natural history of patients with dural AVFs. The first report describing them was not published until 1977.[14] With that report, it became apparent that treatment was simple, safe, and effective. Thus, a prospective study of their natural history without treatment has not been possible and cannot be justified now or in the future. However, the natural history of dural AVFs can be deduced from studies performed before the recognition of their existence and from studies of the condition of patients at treatment.[43] This opportunity is based on their high prevalence among patients with spinal AVMs; their distinguishing epidemiologic and clinical features,[1, 23] which are distinct enough to permit their identification with reasonable accuracy in prior studies[44–47]; and the consistency of their clinical course. The information available to examine the natural history comes principally from a retrospective analysis performed by Aminoff and Logue and reported in 1974.[44, 45] Although their study began before the introduction of selective spinal arteriography, it clearly reveals the natural history of patients with dural AVFs. It was composed predominantly of adult males with thoracolumbar lesions (49 of the 60 patients were ≥41 years old, 43 of those 49 were males, and 55 of the 60 lesions [92%] were in the thoracic or lumbar spinal segments)[44] that had never hemorrhaged (90%), features that distinguish patients with dural AVFs from those with other types of spinal AVMs.[43] The course of the disease, as defined by their study, was one of progressive neurological decline and functional disability. Twenty percent of the 60 patients required crutches or were nonambulatory by 6 months after the onset of symptoms other than pain (Fig. 142–13). Fifty percent of the patients were severely disabled (confined to a wheelchair or bed) within 3 years of the onset of gait impairment, and 91% had restricted activity within 3 years of the onset of symptoms.[44, 45] Similarly, in their 1976 report, which included 23 patients with type I AVMs (now known to be dural AVFs), Tobin and Layton noted, "There seems to be a distinct natural history for patients who have the angiographic Type I arteriovenous malformation. These usually have a slowly progressive course, evolving over 2 to 3 years, leading to nearly complete paraplegia and bowel or bladder incontinence. Few of these patients seem to have other modes of presentation."[47]

In contrast to the gradual, slowly progressive decline in motor and sensory function over 2 to 3 years,[1, 14, 23, 40, 45, 47–49] about 15% of patients with dural AVFs have more rapid, subacute neurological worsening (Foix-Alajouanine syndrome). This deterioration is unpredictable and indicates severe venous congestion, which, unless treated immediately, will lead to venous thrombosis, infarction, and irreversible loss of neurological function.[41, 42]

Intradural Arteriovenous Malformations

Spinal cord AVMs, unlike dural AVFs, occur in males and females with nearly equal incidence (see Fig. 142–7). Further, intradural vascular malformations of the spinal cord have an earlier onset of symptoms, a higher incidence of association with other vascular anomalies, and a more uniform distribution along the spinal axis than do dural AVFs (see Fig. 142–7).[23] Collectively, these observations suggest that AVMs of the spinal cord are congenital lesions, most likely the result of inborn errors of vascular embryogenesis (Table 142–3). The embryologic insult likely occurs before day 18 of gestation, as the spinal cord vasculature is fully developed by that time.

Although current understanding of the pathophysiology of myelopathy in medullary AVMs (juvenile and glomus types) suggests that the mechanism may not be the same in all patients, the high flow rates associated with this type of spinal AVM underlie all the putative mechanisms. In contrast to patients with dural AVFs, an acute initial presentation with the sudden onset of back pain, suboccipital pain, and meningismus or sudden loss of consciousness occurs in many patients with AVMs of the spinal cord; subarachnoid or intramedullary hemorrhage occurs as the initial presentation in about 35% of patients, and by the time of diagnosis, about 50% of patients have had one or more hemorrhage (Tables 142–2 and 142–4).[23] The incidence of hemorrhage is even higher in children. In 38 children younger than 15 years with AVMs of the spinal cord

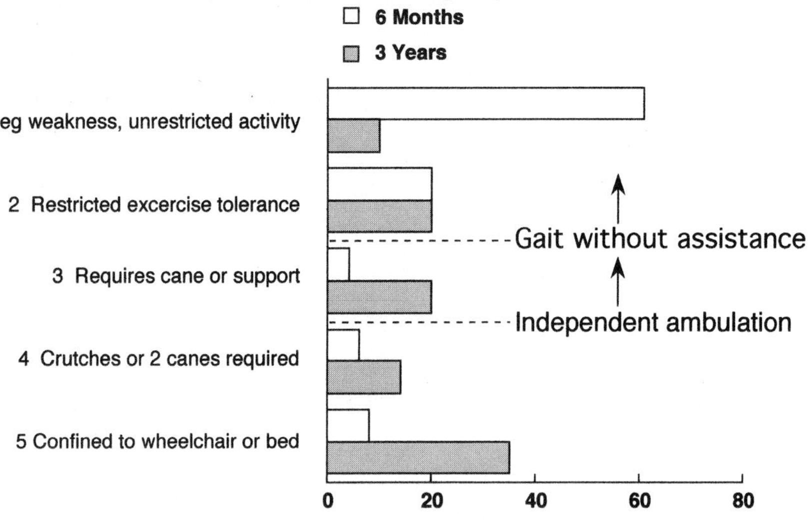

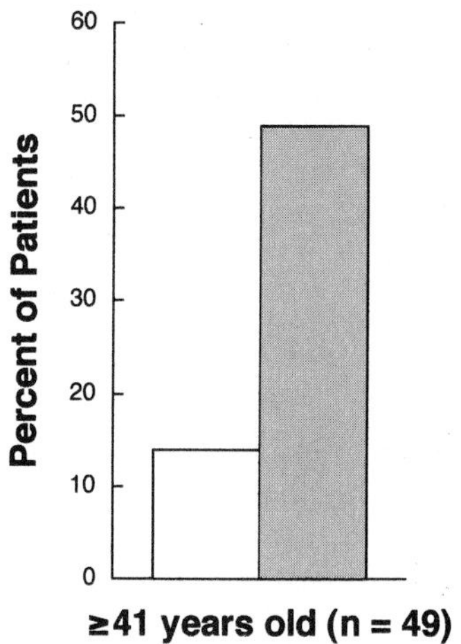

FIGURE 142–13. Degree of functional disability at 6 months and 3 years after the onset of symptoms in 49 patients aged 41 years or older reported by Aminoff and Logue.[45] Almost all these patients had spinal dural arteriovenous fistulas. Note that the greatest change in function between 6 months and 3 years is among patients with minimal neurological deficit who progressed to severe functional disability. By 3 years, half the patients were confined to wheelchairs or had to use crutches to ambulate. (From Oldfield E: Spinal vascular malformations. In Swash M [ed]: Outcomes in Neurological and Neurosurgical Disorders. Cambridge, UK, Cambridge University Press, 1998.)

reported by Riche and colleagues, 84% had an acute initial onset of symptoms, 59% of which were associated with sudden impairment of motor function.[50] The high incidence of associated arterial aneurysms and the 13% to 37% incidence of associated vascular abnormalities elsewhere in the central nervous system[23, 46, 51] may partially explain the high incidence of hemorrhage.

About half of all patients with intramedullary AVMs do not experience the acute deterioration that accompanies hemorrhage. The gradual loss of neurological function in these patients suggests a different mechanism of cord injury.[23] Several mechanisms of this progressive form of myelopathy have been proposed, including ischemia resulting from vascular steal,[52, 53] mechanical compression by aneurysm, and medullary venous congestion.[23] Because intradural AVMs are high-flow shunts, because the medullary arteries that supply the arteriovenous nidus of these lesions also routinely supply the spinal cord, and because visible, often enlarged, medullary veins provide venous drainage into the extradural venous system in most of these lesions,[23] a vascular steal phenomenon may be the most logical explanation in many patients with progressive loss of neurological function.

The natural history of intradural AVMs, similar to the pathophysiologic mechanism of cord injury, is incompletely defined and variable. Data on long-term disability without therapy are unavailable, as these lesions are usually treated when they are diagnosed. Many reports suggest that AVMs of the spinal cord cause recurrent hemorrhages or progressive neurological disability over the first few months or years after they are diagnosed (see Table 142–4). In the 90 patients with intradural AVMs of all types reported by Hurth and associates, 69% had acute episodes of stepwise

TABLE 142–3 ■ **Comparison of Acquired versus Congenital Vascular Malformations**

	ACQUIRED DURAL AVF	CONGENITAL AVM OF THE SPINAL CORD
Gender	Predominantly male	Male or female
Onset of symptoms	Later half adulthood	Child or young adult
Associated congenital malformation	Never	Occasionally
Distribution along spine	Lower half	Diffuse
Normal spinal venous pathways	Absent	Present

AVF, arteriovenous fistula; AVM, arteriovenous malformation. From Oldfield E, Doppman J: Spinal arteriovenous malformations. Clin Neurosurg 34:161–183, 1988.

TABLE 142–4 ■ **Presentation and Natural History of Intradural Arteriovenous Malformations**

		PRESENTATION		EVOLUTION		
AUTHOR/ YEAR*	**NO. OF PATIENTS**	**Age at Onset of Symptoms**	**Initial Symptoms**	**At Diagnosis or Treatment**	**Progressive Evolution**	**Associated with Deterioration**
Hurth et al, 1978[46]	90	86% <40 yr	SAH in 36%	SAH in 39%; SAH in 55% of patients <15 yr	Recurrent SAH (1 fatal) in 39% of patients with SAH; stepwise progression in 69%	SAH with "violent physical efforts," pregnancy, minor trauma
Riche et al, 1982[†50]	38	All <15 yr	Acute onset in 84%, associated with sudden motor impairment in 19 of the 32 patients (59%)	SAH in 55%	71% with successive acute attack(s); 17% with gradually progressing evolution	Exertion
Rosenblum et al, 1987	54	Mean, 27 yr	Acute onset in 50% of patients; SAH in 10 of 14 patients (71%) with glomus AVMs	At diagnosis, paresis in 93%, sensory loss in 74%, bladder dysfunction in 74%, hemorrhage in 52%; at treatment, 74% were moderately or severely disabled (cane, crutches, or wheelchair), only 26% had unaided ambulation		Posture (17%), activity (15%), pregnancy (6%), Valsalva (13%), injury (13%)
Biondi et al, 1990[54]	40	Mean, 20 yr	SAH in 58%	SAH in 68%; 75% moderately or severely disabled	31% had relapse with worsening between treatments during 6-yr (mean) follow-up	
Yasargil et al, 1984	41	76% <41 yr	SAH in 59%	SAH in 76%; 63% moderately or severely disabled	Stepwise progression in 40%	

*All series include patients with perimedullary arteriovenous fistulas, except Yasargil et al, which includes only patients with intramedullary AVMs, and Biondi et al, which includes only thoracic, intramedullary AVMs.

†Includes only patients <15 yr.

SAH, subarachnoid hemorrhage.

AVM, arteriovenous malformation;

From Oldfield, EH: Spinal vascular malformations. In Swash M (ed): Outcomes in Neurological and Neurosurgical Disorders. Cambridge University Press, 1998.

neurological progression, and 39% of the patients with previous hemorrhage had at least one additional hemorrhage (fatal in one patient).[46] Similarly, in the 38 patients with thoracic medullary AVMs treated by Biondi and colleagues with repeated, yearly embolization with particles of polyvinyl alcohol (PVA), 31% relapsed with neurological worsening between treatments (average of 6 years of treatment).[54] Pregnancy, vigorous exertion, and minor trauma may cause rapid progression of symptoms or be associated with an increased risk of hemorrhage (see Table 142–4).

Most authors characterize the prognosis of these patients as grave and consider the natural history sufficiently unpredictable and hazardous to justify the risks of treatment.[1, 23, 25, 46, 50, 54–56] However, it must be acknowledged that the natural history varies greatly among individual patients and that the prognosis in some of them is not always grim. Retrospective evaluation of Aminoff and Logue's series[43] indicates that in half the patients whose presentation was acute—a presentation more likely to be associated with intradural AVMs—there was no subsequent neurological progression.[44, 45] Similar observations were made by Tobin and Layton in their report on the natural history of patients with spinal AVMs, in which they reported a progressive course leading to paraplegia over 2 to 3 years in patients with features that now suggest dural AVFs, but "such a relationship was not as clear" for intradural AVMs.[47] Hurth and associates noted that 80% of the 17 untreated patients with AVMs in the cervical segments of the spinal cord were independent and capable of carrying out their jobs 5 years after diagnosis, and 5 patients who were untreated or incompletely treated were unchanged 15 years after diagnosis, demonstrating the "slow progression of disease . . . in a limited number of cases." Further, 60% of their 17 untreated patients with thoracic AVMs at 5 years, and 41% of 17 untreated or incompletely treated patients at 15 years, were "self-sufficient and relatively well."[46] The dilemma in making decisions for individual patients is that we have no reliable guidelines that permit us to identify these patients prospectively.

Thus, although the neurological prognosis is guarded for untreated adults with intradural AVMs, it may not be as dismal as it is for patients with dural AVFs. This must be considered when undertaking treatment of intradural AVMs, because, in some cases, attempts to permanently eliminate the AVM are associated with significant risk.

An exception to this are children with symptomatic AVMs of the spinal cord. In the retrospective assessment of 38 children younger than 15 years by Riche and colleagues, symptoms had a sudden onset in 84%; in 60% of these, there was sudden impairment of motor function, often associated with physical effort.[50] The sudden onset was commonly followed by a period of remission, but with successive attacks in 71% and subarachnoid hemorrhagse in 55%. Unlike in adults, a gradually progressive evolution of the syndrome occurred in only 17% of the 38 children.

Perimedullary Arteriovenous Fistulas

Perimedullary AVFs, which lie in the pia on the surface of the spinal cord, constitute about 10% to 20% of all spinal AVMs.[15, 23, 57] They are distributed equally between males and females, and most are associated with the onset of symptoms in the first half of adult life; the average age at diagnosis is older than that of patients with AVMs of the spinal cord but younger than that of patients with dural AVFs (see Fig. 142–7). However, they may also present in childhood, as early as 3 weeks of age.[58, 59] Their anatomic distribution along the spinal axis is bimodal, predominantly in the thoracolumbar region, particularly at the conus medullaris and, to a lesser extent, in the upper cervical region (see Fig. 142–7).[15, 23, 57, 59, 60]

The existence of these lesions in early childhood suggests a congenital mechanism of origin. However, they may present in late adulthood, and there are two reported cases in which a perimedullary AVF was acquired as a result of surgery. One arose in the conus medullaris in a 28-year-old 5 years after resection of a teratoma of the filum terminale.[25] In the other case, a 35-year-old presented with a perimedullary AVF in the conus medullaris 1 year after resection of an ependymoma at the same site.[59]

Clinical presentation is a slowly progressing myelopathy or radiculopathy, which occurs in about 80% of patients, or subarachnoid hemorrhage, which affects about 20% of patients.[23] For therapeutic purposes, Merland and colleagues categorized perimedullary AVFs into three distinct types (Table 142–5). Type I is a small, simple fistula supplied by a single feeder, usually the terminal portion of a thin anterior spinal artery, but in some instances a posterior spinal artery. The flow through the fistula is usually slow and ascending in the vessels of the coronal venous plexus, which are only slightly tortuous and dilated. Type II AVFs are supplied by one or two main arterial feeders via several distinct arterial pedicles that converge to form multiple discrete shunts and drain into a dilated and tortuous venous system with a relatively high flow rate (see Fig. 142–12). Type III AVFs, which account for the majority of the pial AVFs, are single giant AVFs with very high blood flow located in the cervical or lower thoracolumbar level. They are fed by several branches of the posterior or anterior spinal arteries, which are hugely dilated and converge into a single shunt draining into a giant venous ectasia (Fig. 142–14).[25, 57]

Initially, it appeared as though there were no distinctive clinical presentations among the various types of perimedullary AVFs, but, with more experience, it has become apparent that only type II and III AVFs hemorrhage or produce compression of the spinal cord by venous ectasia.[57] Despite this, most patients have grad-

TABLE 142–5 ■ **Categories of Perimedullary Arteriovenous Fistulas**

TYPE	AVF	ARTERIAL SUPPLY; SITE OF AVF	BLOOD FLOW; VENOUS DRAINAGE	PATHOPHYSIOLOGY OF MYELOPATHY	TREATMENT
I	Single small pial AVF	Single slender arterial feeder, usually ASA, into small AVF; anterior conus medullaris or proximal filum terminale	Low; slow ascending venous drainage via slightly dilated and tortuous pial veins	Venous hypertension	Surgery
II	Several discrete pial shunts; nidus size is small to medium	Several dilated arterial feeders, ASA or PSA, which converge to nidus in region of conus anterolaterally or posterolaterally	Moderate-high through fistula, but rostral venous drainage is slow via dilated and tortuous pial veins	Venous hypertension, hemorrhage	Surgery, embolization, or both
III	Single giant pial AVF	Multiple hugely dilated ASAs and PSAs, which converge into single large AVF; cervical, thoracic, or lumbar region	Rapid and high; drains rapidly, directly into large venous ectasia or varix and then laterally via greatly enlarged veins into epidural venous system	Hemorrhage, cord compression by varix	Embolic occlusion with latex balloon, surgery, or embolization and surgery

ASA, anterior spinal artery; AVF, arteriovenous fistula; PSA, posterior spinal artery.

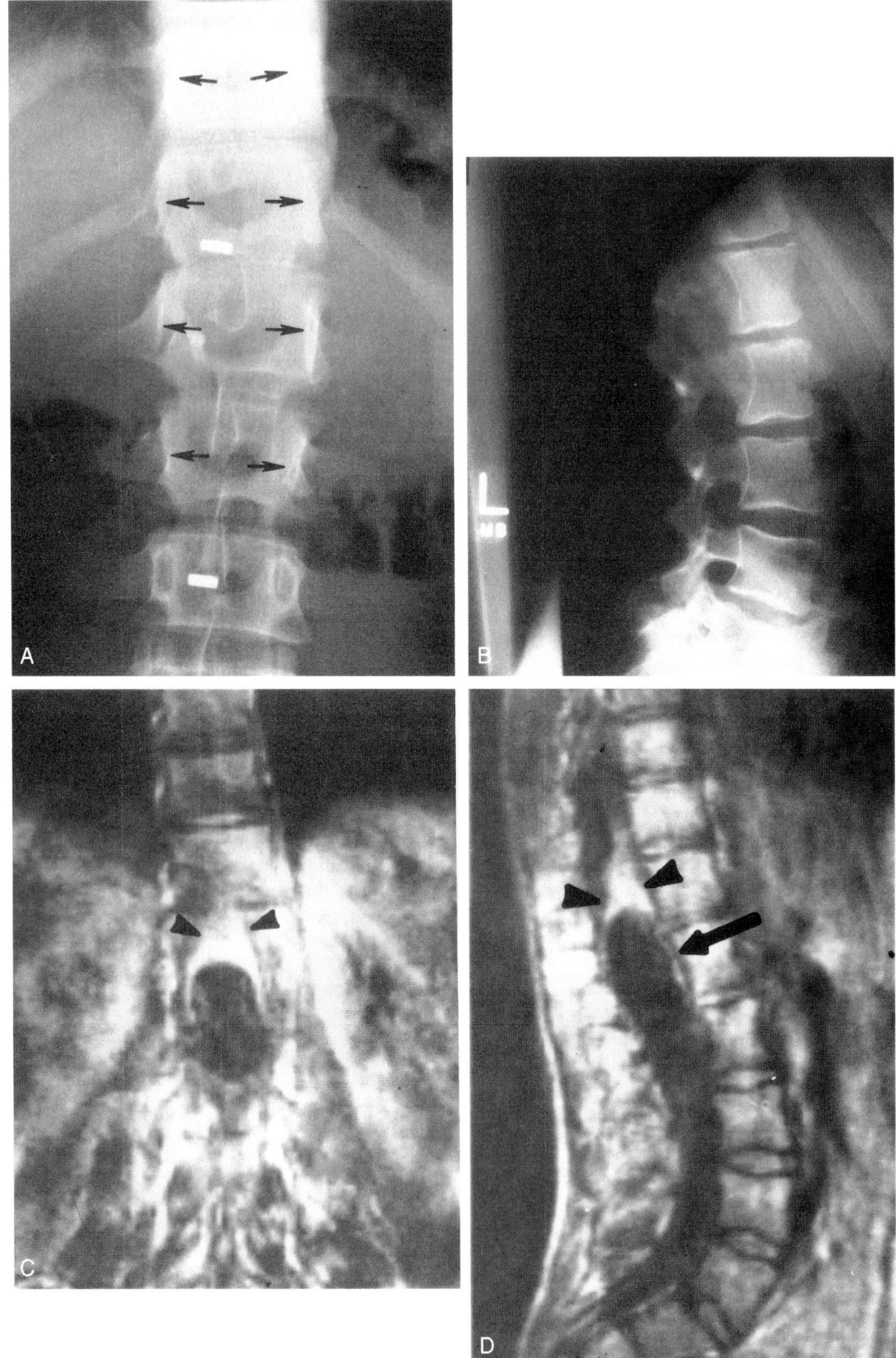

FIGURE 142–14. Fourteen-year-old boy with a congenital intradural arteriovenous fistula (AVF) associated with a massive intramedullary aneurysm-varix at the site of arterial-to-venous transition. Anteroposterior *(A)* and lateral *(B)* lumbothoracic spine radiographs reveal medial erosion of pedicles *(A, arrows)* and scalloping of the posterior aspect of several vertebrae *(B)*. Coronal *(C)* and sagittal *(D)* magnetic resonance imaging (MRI) scans (spin echo [SE] 500/40) show the spinal cord *(arrowheads)* splayed around a large intramedullary aneurysm (signal void; *D, arrow)*.

Illustration continued on following page

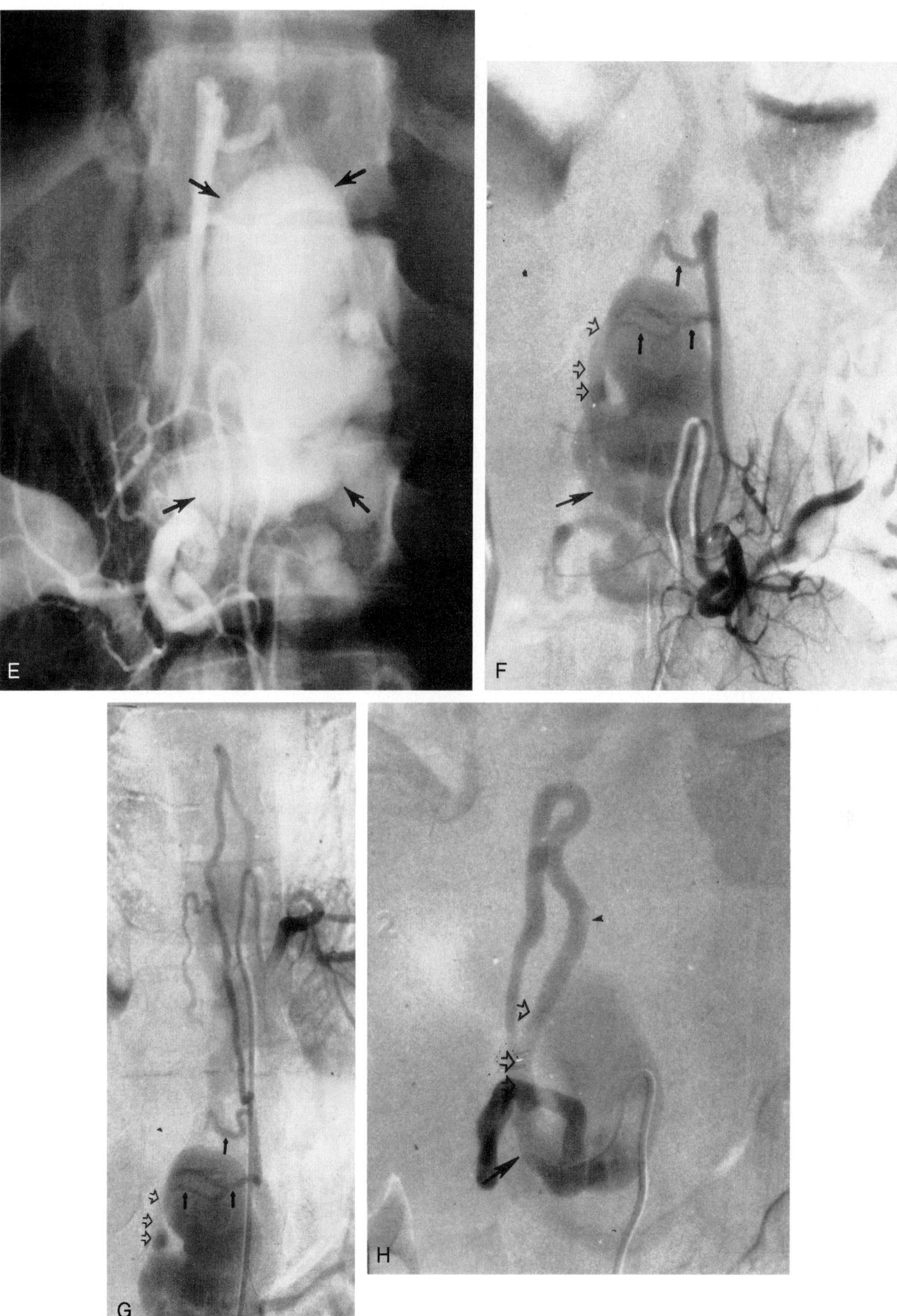

FIGURE 142–14. *Continued.* Selective spinal arteriography *(E–H)* reveals a huge varix *(E, arrows)* expanding the spinal canal in association with an AVF *(F and H, arrows)*. The fistula was supplied by several vessels that converged to form a simple AVF *(F and H, arrows)* via a common trunk *(F–H, open arrows)*.

Illustration continued on following page

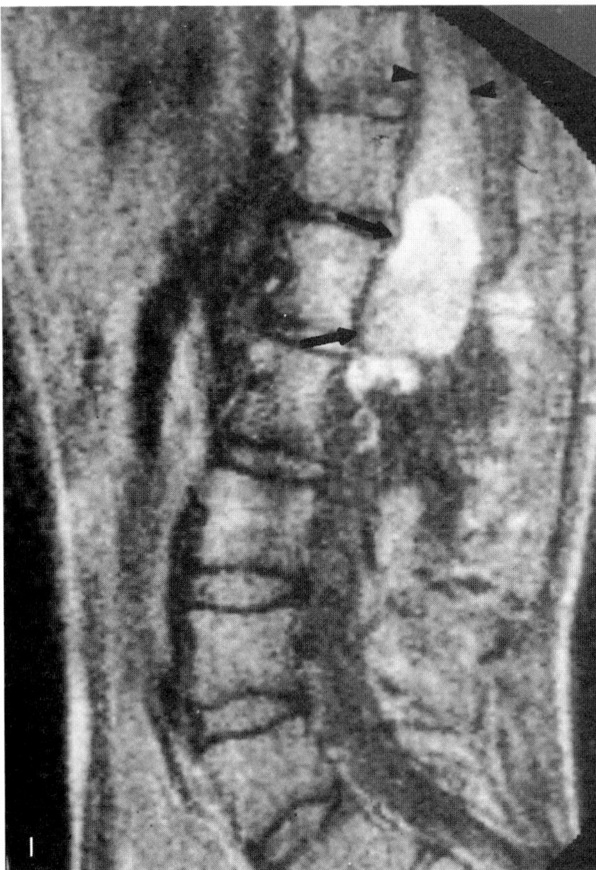

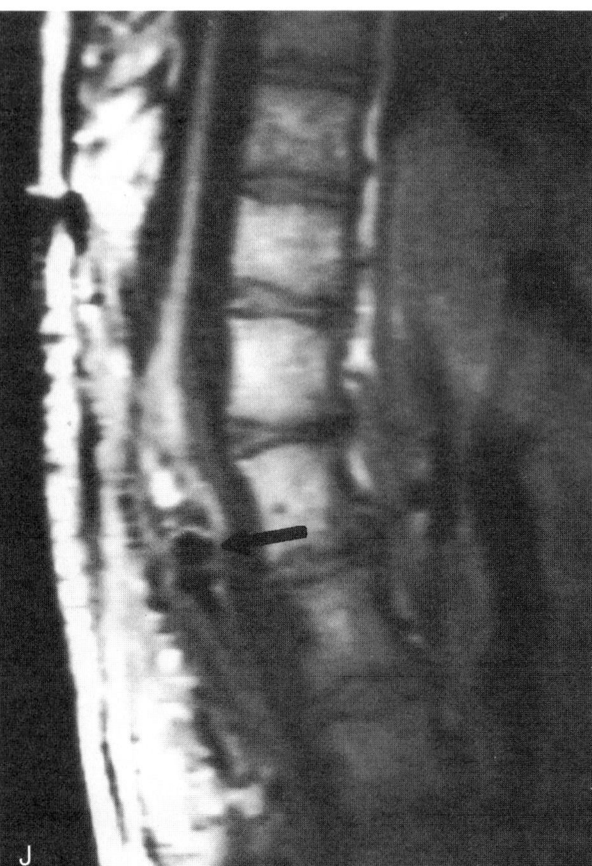

FIGURE 142–14. *Continued.* One week after interruption of the AVF, the MRI scan (SE 500/40) showed a high signal in the aneurysm *(I, arrows)*, indicating thrombosis (*arrowheads* show the spinal cord). On the MRI scan 18 months later *(J)*, the thrombosed aneurysm has shrunk to a small focus with a persistent descending vein *(arrow)*. Dilatation of the subarachnoid space and the atrophic spinal cord can be seen above the site of the varix. (From Doppman JL, DiChiro G, Dwyer AJ, et al: Magnetic resonance imaging of spinal arteriovenous malformations. J Neurosurg 66:830–834, 1987.)

ually progressive neurological loss[23, 57] that is similar to the progression associated with the venous hypertension underlying the myelopathy of spinal dural AVFs. Barrow and colleagues directly quantified venous hypertension in the venous drainage of two patients with spinal dural AVFs and progressive myelopathy and related the venous pressures with the clinical and MRI findings.[59] This mechanism probably accounts for the myelopathy in most patients with type I AVFs, as they do not hemorrhage, they are not associated with venous ectasia and cord compression, and the rate of transit from the arterial to the venous system is much too slow to produce vascular steal. However, because type II and III AVFs are always supplied by an artery that also supplies the spinal cord, it is likely that vascular steal accounts for the myelopathy in at least some of these patients with rapid shunting of blood and generous venous drainage pathways on arteriography.

Retrospective studies of the clinical history before treatment provide the only information on the natural history of this type of AVM. They suggest a relentless progression from myelopathy to paraplegia within 5 to 7 years of the onset of symptoms in patients presenting with myelopathy without hemorrhage, and there is a high incidence of repeated hemorrhage in patients presenting with hemorrhage.[15, 23, 25, 57, 59]

Cavernous Angiomas

Cavernous angiomas, also known as cavernous malformations, cavernous hemangiomas, and cavernomas, are distributed along the entire length of the neuraxis and represent 5% to 12% of all spinal vascular abnormalities.[29, 61] They are distributed proportional to the volume of nervous tissue, so many more arise in the brain than in the spinal cord.[62] Cavernous angiomas in the spinal cord are histologically identical to those in brain. They typically occur as an intramedullary mass but may present as an epidural lesion.

Studies have identified a familial variant of the disease (familial multiple cavernous angiomatosis) with multiple cavernomas and autosomal-dominant transmission.[27, 28, 63–68] Genetic studies on patients from affected families have localized the genetic abnormality to chromosome 7q.[30–35, 68–74] Although cavernomas are associated with familial transmission, they do not necessarily arise early in life. They have been documented to arise de novo (with and without a family history) in the brain and spinal cord as new lesions in patients with prior negative computed tomography and MRI scans and after irradiation of the cranial and spinal axes in adults and children.[75–78]

Although cavernous angiomas are low-flow lesions, the pathogenesis of myelopathy is usually via hematomyelia. Symptomatic lesions have a hemosiderin ring on MRI and a hemosiderin-stained gliotic capsule at surgery, suggesting repeated small hemorrhages (Fig. 142–15). Small lesions may remain clinically silent throughout life, only to be discovered at postmortem examination. Symptomatic cavernous angiomas tend to present in early adulthood through middle age (third to sixth decades).[62]

The clinical presentation varies greatly among patients, but there are four common patterns: discrete acute episodic progression over months or years, slowly progressive decline of neurological function over months or years, acute onset and rapid progression, and slowly progressive loss of function after an acute onset of mild neurological symptoms.[79] Cavernomas in the spinal cord, like those in the brainstem, are more commonly symptomatic than are those in the cerebral hemispheres. The available information on symptomatic lesions indicates a tendency toward further neurological impairment associated with repeated small hemorrhages.[79]

DIAGNOSTIC IMAGING

Although dural AVFs are distinguished clinically from intradural AVMs by age at onset of symptoms, distribution along the spinal axis, and neurological presentation,[23] the specific diagnosis must be confirmed with imaging studies. Clinical features are useful only insofar as they guide the clinician through the proper diagnostic tests toward an accurate diagnosis and appropriate treatment. The imaging evaluation ultimately determines the proper intervention, because effective management is predicated on establishing the precise type of vascular abnormality and the specific anatomy of the lesion.

The radiographic evaluation of spinal AVMs has two components: screening studies, generally used for the initial evaluation of patients with progressive radiculomyelopathies, and vascular imaging studies for diagnostic confirmation and anatomic definition.

Screening Studies

As a group, spinal AVMs are only one of myriad causes of progressive radiculomyelopathy. The clinical differential diagnosis includes cervical spondylosis, amyotrophic lateral sclerosis, intervertebral disk disease, neoplasia, syringomyelia, multiple sclerosis, and infection. There is no single pathognomonic sign or symptom specifically indicative of spinal AVMs. Plain films of the spine and MRI are used to guide the choice of further investigations.

Initial screening examinations with plain films of the spine are usually helpful only to rule out other causes of radiculomyelopathy, such as spondylosis, vertebral tumor, or fracture. Occasionally, high-flow AVMs cause increased interpedicular distance at the level of the AVM (see Fig. 142–14), but there are no specific findings for spinal AVMs on plain films.

MAGNETIC RESONANCE IMAGING

Owing to its lower risk and its capacity for multiplanar imaging, MRI has replaced myelography as the initial diagnostic procedure in patients with myelopathy. With spinal AVMs, MRI abnormalities may be produced by abnormal vessels in the subarachnoid space, by the nidus of an intramedullary AVM in the spinal cord, or by changes in the spinal cord produced by venous congestion, myelomalacia, infarction, or hemorrhage.[80–85] MRI is noninvasive and often provides the initial diagnosis of an AVM; it may also distinguish intramedullary AVMs from perimedullary AVFs and dural AVFs. Ideally, MRI should be performed with a 1.5-tesla machine using a spinal coil.

Patients with spinal vascular malformations, except those with cavernous angiomas, often demonstrate a serpentine pattern of low signal in the subarachnoid space on T1- and T2-weighted MRI scans. This pattern of signal void is due to flow in dilated, tortuous vessels of the arterialized coronal venous plexus. These arterialized pial veins may focally indent the cord surface and produce a scalloped appearance on sagittal T1-weighted images (Fig. 142–16*B* and *C*). The abnormal signal produced by the enlarged coronal venous plexus is frequently most prominent in the posterior pia and subarachnoid space.

Dural Arteriovenous Fistulas. Patients with dural AVFs demonstrate a wide range of MRI findings.[81, 82] T1- and T2-weighted images, when abnormal, reveal an area of focal cord expansion, most commonly affecting the conus; there is a central area of low or high signal on T1-weighted images and increased signal intensity on T2-weighted images in the thoracolumbar segments of a cord swollen from venous congestion (see Fig. 142–16*A* and *B*). In the large study of Gilbertson and coworkers, increased T2 signal in the cord was the most common finding, and it occurred in all patients.[86] Studies obtained immediately after intravenous gadolinium-DTPA reveal enhancement of the vessels of the coronal venous plexus (see Fig. 142–16C) and may produce enhancement of the most severely involved segments of the spinal cord; delayed imaging after gadolinium (40 to 45 minutes) may reveal an increase in the extent of enhancement to involve the entire enlarged lower portion of the spinal cord (Fig. 142–17).[85] Whether gadolinium enhancement of the spinal cord indicates edema, venous congestion, or loss of integrity of the blood-brain barrier associated with ischemic injury remains to be determined. Although the sensitivity of T2 signal changes is high, T2 signal abnormality and enhancement of the spinal cord on T1-weighted images are nonspecific features, and some patients do not have visible contrast enhancement of the congested vessels of the coronal venous plexus

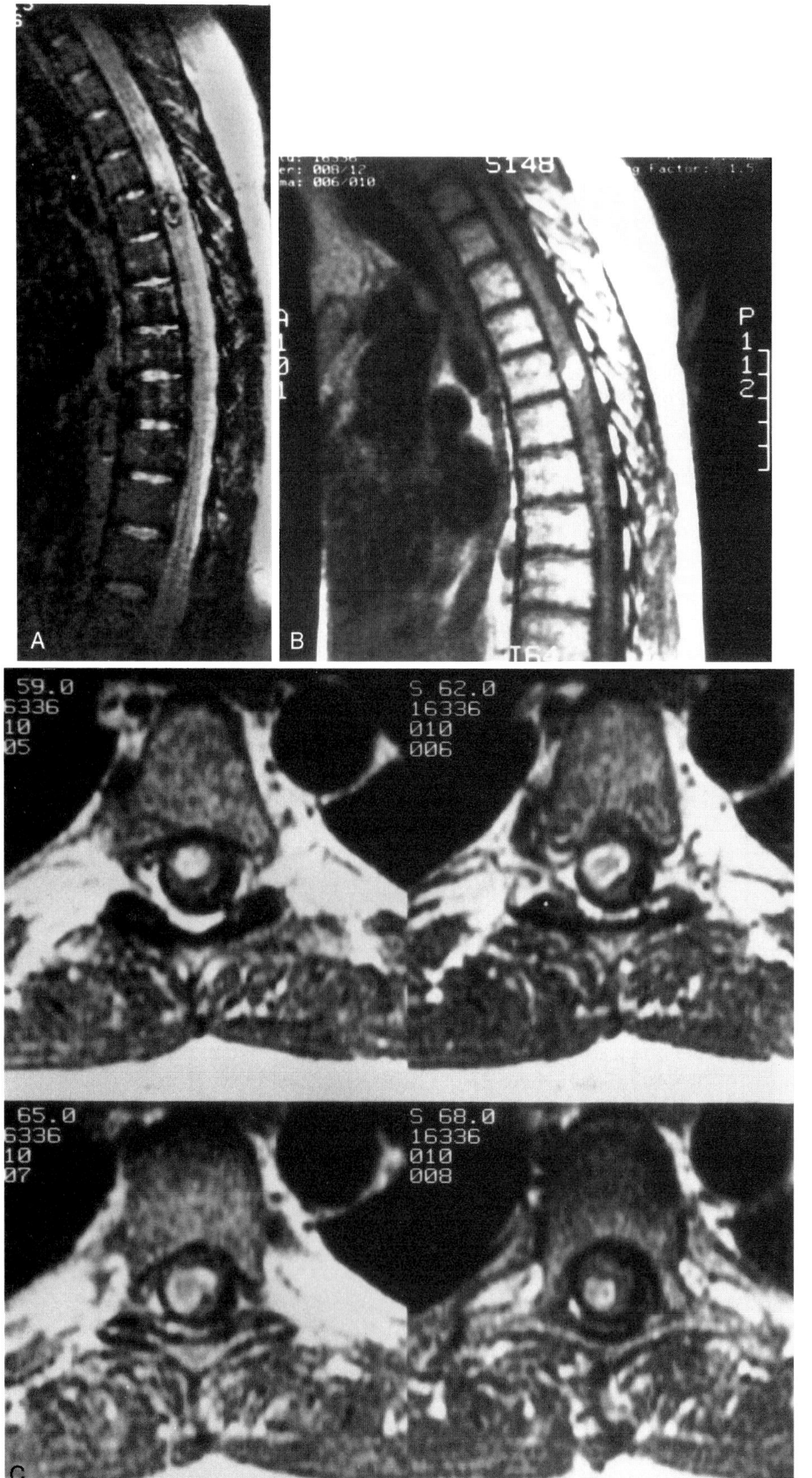

FIGURE 142–15. Magnetic resonance imaging (MRI) appearance of a typical cavernous angioma of the spinal cord. T1- and T2-weighted MRI scans of the angioma, which are similar to those of cavernous malformations in the brain, typically demonstrate a well-delineated spherical or oblong intramedullary lesion of mixed signal—predominantly low signal surrounding scattered areas of increased signal on T2-weighted images. The MRI findings depend on the age of the blood products. This angioma, in the midthoracic portion of the spinal cord, is shown on T2-weighted (TR 2000, TE 40) sagittal *(A)*, T1-weighted (TR 500, TE 20) sagittal *(B)*, and T1-weighted (TR 650, TE 25) axial *(C)* MRI scans. It was associated with chronic paraparesis that was progressing in a stuttering, subacute manner. The high signal on T1-weighted images *(B* and *C)* is consistent with methemoglobin accumulation in the subacute intramedullary hematoma, which was confirmed at surgery. (From Oldfield EH: Spinal vascular malformations. In Rengachary S, Wilkins R, [eds]: Neurosurgical Operative Atlas. Rolling Meadows, IL, American Association of Neurological Surgeons, 1994.)

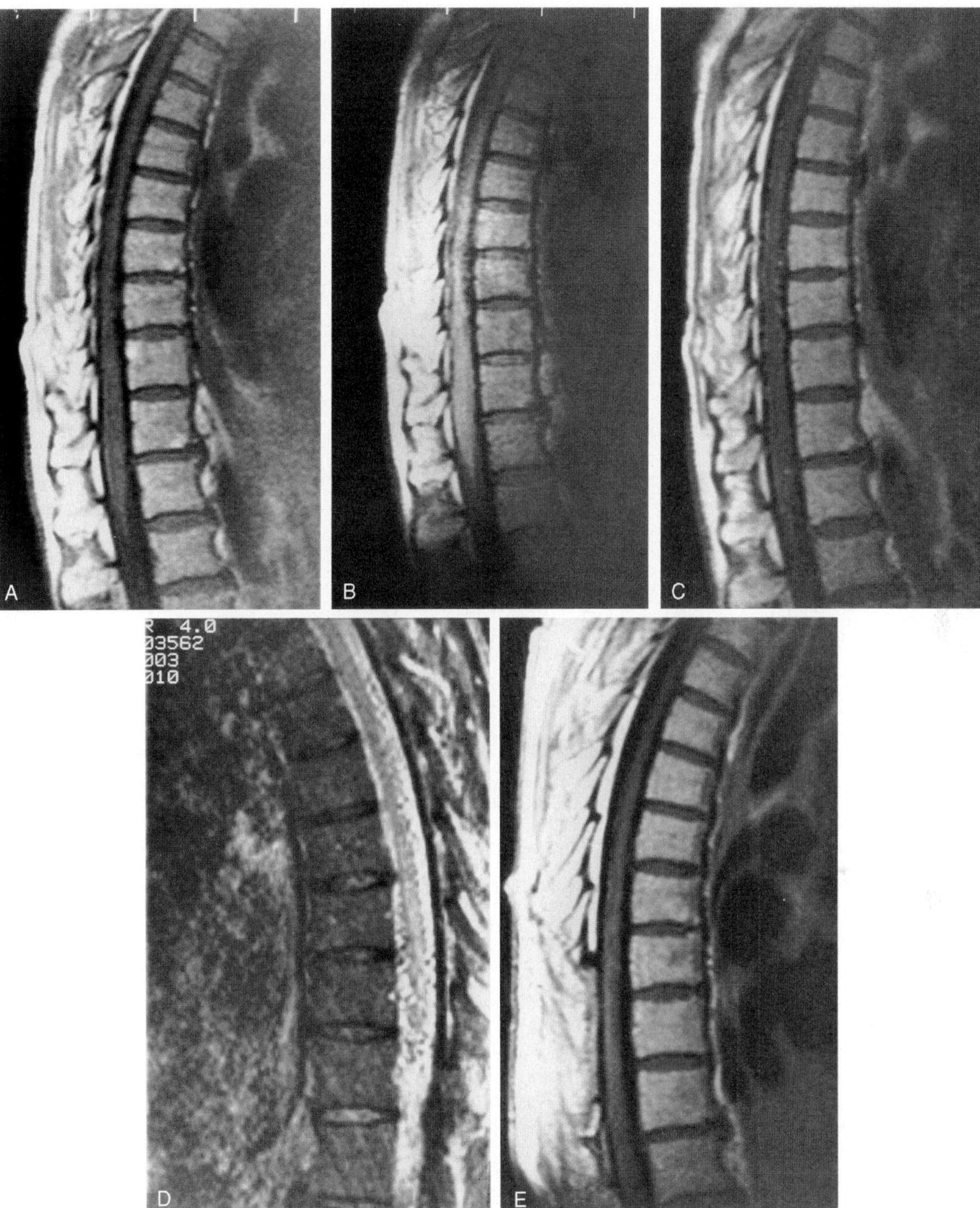

FIGURE 142–16. Sagittal spinal magnetic resonance imaging (MRI) scans of a 66-year-old man with a spinal dural arteriovenous fistula (AVF) at T9-10. Before contrast injection, T1-weighted (TE 400, TR 16) images reveal an area of focal cord expansion affecting the conus *(A)* and an increased signal intensity with T2-weighted (TR 2000, TE 20) proton density imaging (*B)* in the thoracolumbar segments of a cord swollen from venous congestion. Immediately after injection of gadolinium-DTPA *(C)*, T1-weighted images (TR 400, TE 16) reveal enhancement of the vessels of the coronal venous plexus (compare the same MRI technique without enhancement in *A*). T2-weighted imaging techniques that show cerebrospinal fluid brightly often prominently depict the abnormal vessels on the surface of the cord *(D)* and in the cerebrospinal fluid. As seen on T1-weighted (TR 417, TE 16) MRI performed after gadolinium-DTPA injection 8 months after excison of the spinal dural AVF *(E)*, elimination of the fistula resulted in resolution of the swollen appearance of the spinal cord and disappearance of the abnormal enhancing vessels on the cord surface. (From Thompson B, Oldfield E: Spinal vascular malformations. In Carter L, Spetzler R, Hamilton M [eds]: Neurovascular Surgery. New York, McGraw-Hill, 1994, pp 1167–1195.)

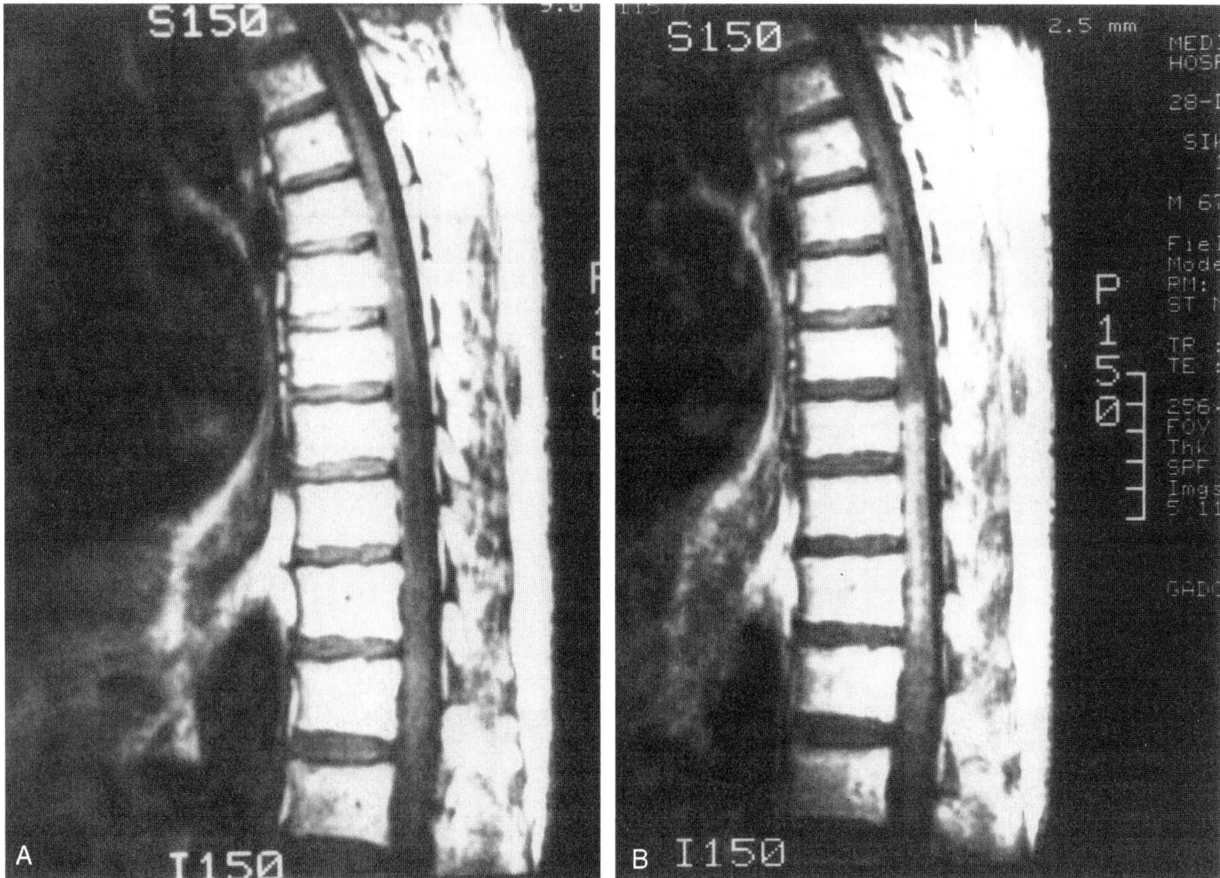

FIGURE 142–17. T1-weighted magnetic resonance imaging (MRI) scan of a patient with severe paraparesis from a thoracic dural arteriovenous fistula (AVF). *A*, Note the nonspecific widening of the midthoracic portion of the cord and the low signal before administration of gadolinium. *B*, Images after intravenous gadolinium show nonspecific enhancement of the central region of the spinal cord most severely affected. Note that the MRI findings in this patient do not establish the diagnosis of a spinal dural AVF or even suggest the presence of an arteriovenous malformation. MRI may be normal or only nonspecifically abnormal in patients with spinal dural AVFs. (From Thompson B, Oldfield E: Spinal vascular malformations. In Carter L, Spetzler R, Hamilton M [eds]: Neurovascular Surgery. New York, McGraw-Hill, 1994, pp 1167–1195.)

(see Fig. 142–17). It has recently been suggested that a peripheral hypointensity on T2-weighted images of the spinal cord is a consistent and specific diagnostic feature of venous congestion associated with dural AVFs.[87]

Surgical elimination of the spinal dural AVF results in diminishment of the swollen appearance of the spinal cord, induces resolution of the abnormal T2 hyperintensity in the spinal cord, and eliminates enhancement of the abnormal vessels of the coronal venous plexus over the weeks or months after surgery (see Fig. 142–16).[88, 89]

Intradural Arteriovenous Malformations and Arteriovenous Fistulas. At the site of intramedullary AVMs, T1-weighted images usually demonstrate a focal signal flow void comprising multiple channels with a serpentine pattern in an area of local expansion of the spinal cord (Fig. 142–18).[81, 84] The position of the nidus in the axial plane of the cord is established with sagittal and axial images, sometimes permitting the exact intramedullary position of an AVM to be recognized, and occasionally distinguishing perimedullary AVFs from intramedullary AVMs that are partially intra- and extramedullary (see Fig. 142–18*A* and *B*).[81, 84] Subacute hemorrhage is seen as increased signal on T1-weighted studies. An aneurysm or a venous varix associated with an AVM or an AVF, respectively, is recognized as a globular-shaped region of flow void (see Fig. 142–14*C* and *D*).[80, 81, 90] Occlusion of the nidus with emboli or thrombosis of a varix after interruption of an AVF can be confirmed by loss of the signal flow void on T1 images.[81]

Although MRI may suggest a spinal vascular malformation and the need for further spinal arteriographic evaluation, if MRI is performed only without contrast, the images may either be normal or show nonspecific changes in patients with dural AVFs (see Fig. 142–17). Because dural AVFs are the most common type of spinal vascular malformation and the type most amenable to treatment, patients with unexplained progressive myelopathy or radiculopathy and a normal unenhanced MRI study require additional diagnostic evaluation with MRI with contrast.

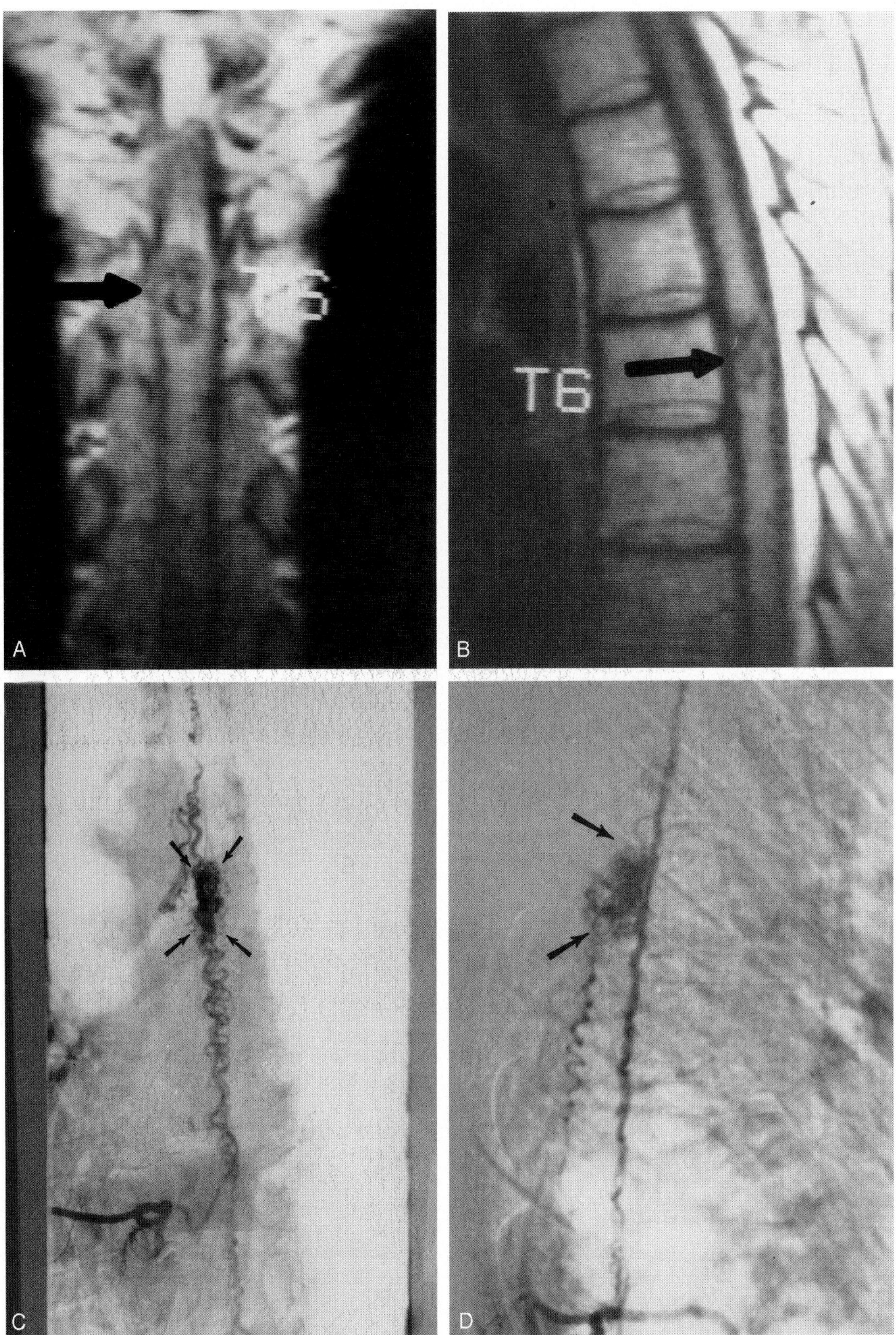

FIGURE 142–18. *A and B,* Magnetic resonance imaging (MRI) scans of an intramedullary arteriovenous malformation (AVM). Because of the rapid flow within the vessels of intramedullary AVMs, they have areas of flow void on MRI. *A,* Coronal T2-weighted (1000/75) MRI scan reveals an intramedullary nidus *(arrow)* at the T6 vertebral level. *B,* Sagittal T1-weighted (SE 600/25) MRI scan shows the nidus *(arrow)* more clearly. At selective spinal arteriography, the anteroposterior *(C)* and lateral *(D)* views in the early venous phase confirm the intramedullary location of the nidus *(arrows).* (From Doppman J, DiChiro G, Dwyer A, et al: Magnetic resonance imaging of spinal cord arteriovenous malformations. J Neurosurg 66:830–834, 1987.)

Cavernous Angiomas. The results of arteriography and myelography are usually normal, so MRI is the most important diagnostic test to detect cavernous angiomas.[29, 61] MRI typically demonstrates a well-delineated, predominantly low-signal spherical or oblong intramedullary lesion with scattered heterogeneous areas of increased signal (see Fig. 142–15). The decreased signal is due to hemosiderin deposition along the periphery of and within the malformation. However, the absence of a true "flow void" signal is consistent with these low-flow lesions. On T2-weighted images, this mix of signal intensity produces the familiar "target" configuration that is typical of cavernous malformations (see Fig. 142–15*A*).

Exceptions to the foregoing description do occur. The MRI appearance can vary, depending on the age of small foci of hemorrhage at distinct sites in the cavernous angioma. These variations include increased T2 signal in the spinal cord surrounding the lesion (from myelomalacia or edema), areas of acute hemorrhage that are isointense or hypointense on T1-weighted images and hypointense on T2-weighted images, T1 hyperintensity and T2 hypointensity at foci of hemorrhage between a few days and 2 weeks old, and evolution from hyperintensity to hypointensity on T1- and T2-weighted studies as the blood products liquefy and are broken down over the following weeks and months. Enhancement with gadolinium-DTPA varies from patient to patient.

MYELOGRAPHY

It is important to remember that myelography is a sensitive diagnostic screening test for spinal AVMs. A technically acceptable myelogram reliably demonstrates abnormal vascularity as serpentine filling voids in the subarachnoid space in all types of spinal vascular abnormalities (Fig. 142–19), except cavernous angiomas. Therefore, in a patient with equivocal findings on MRI, myelography that fails to demonstrate abnormal vessels in the subarachnoid space obviates the need for spinal arteriography. However, once the diagnosis of spinal AVM has been confirmed with MRI or myelography, spinal arteriography is necessary to establish the type of spinal AVM, define the precise anatomic location of the nidus of the AVM, and identify the arterial supply to the AVM and to the spinal cord.

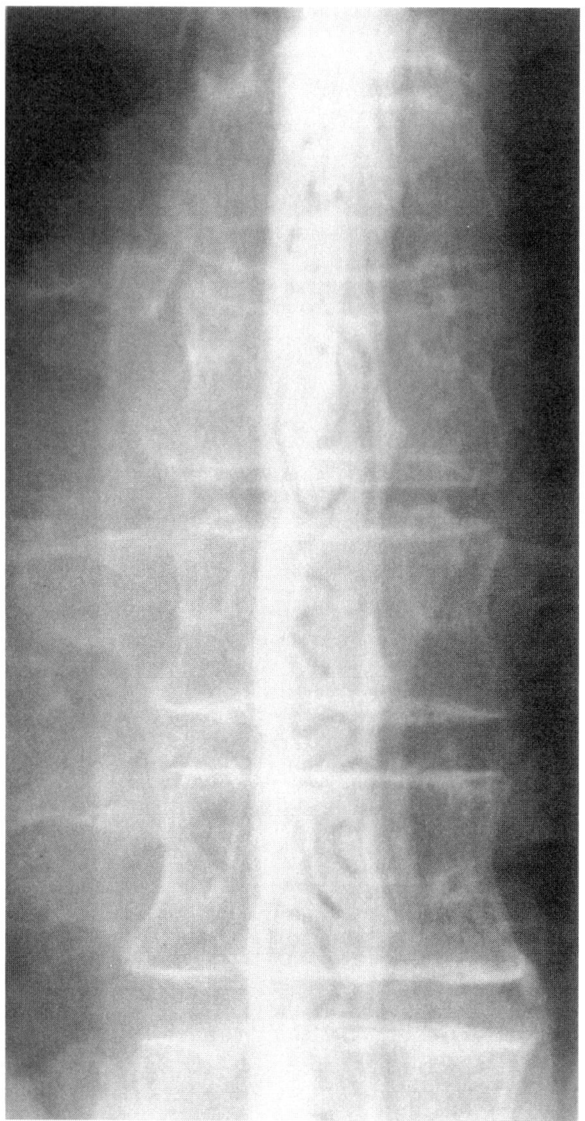

FIGURE 142–19. Myelogram of a patient with a spinal dural arteriovenous fistula. The dilated coronal venous plexus is evident on the dorsal surface of the spinal cord. (From Muraszko KM, Oldfield EH: Vascular malformations of the spinal cord and dura. Neurosurg Clin N Am 1:631–652, 1990.)

Selective Spinal Arteriography

Because successful treatment of spinal AVMs requires detailed understanding of the regional vascular anatomy, spinal arteriography is indispensable. It provides precise anatomic information about four items that are crucial to the surgeon or interventional neuroradiologist: the type of AVM, the exact location and anatomic configuration of the nidus of the AVM, the identification of the feeding vessels to the AVM, and the regional vascular anatomy of the spinal cord. Table 142–6 summarizes the major features distinguishing the dural AVFs from intradural AVMs of the spinal cord and perimedullary AVFs.

Dural Arteriovenous Fistulas. Selective spinal arteriography of dural AVFs demonstrates intrathecal drainage of the fistula, via an arterialized medullary vein, into the dilated, tortuous veins of the coronal venous plexus (see Fig. 142–8); in most patients, this occurs predominantly along the posterior surface of the spinal cord. In some patients, it also discloses the nidus of the AVF in the intervertebral foramen and lateral aspect of the spinal canal (see Fig. 142–8*A*). A prolonged view of the venous phase after selective injection of the artery feeding the AVF fully defines the abnormal venous anatomy, as these low-flow lesions often require 15 seconds or more for the contrast material to dissipate.

Intracranial dural AVFs that drain inferiorly into the spinal venous system and cause myelopathy can mimic spinal dural AVFs clinically and on MRI and myelo-

TABLE 142-6 ■ **Radiographic Features Distinguishing Dural and Intradural Malformations**

	DURAL AVM (*N* = 27)	INTRADURAL AVM* (*N* = 54)
Site of nidus	Lateral canal 100%	Within cord 80% Ventral cord surface 11% Dorsal cord surface 9%
Level of spine	Lower half	Diffuse
Rapid flow	0	80%
Associated spinal aneurysm	0	44%
Common supply of AVM and medullary artery	15%	100%
Route of venous drainage	Rostral 100% Caudal 4%	Rostral 81% Caudal 72%

*Includes perimedullary AVFs.

AVF, arteriovenous fistula; AVM, arteriovenous malformation. Adapted from Rosenblum B, Oldfield EH, Doppman JL, DiChiro G: Spinal arteriovenous malformations: A comparison of dural arteriovenous fistulas and intradural AVMs in 81 patients. J Neurosurg 67:795–802, 1987.

graphic studies (Fig. 142–20).[91–93] The AVF in these patients is located in the dura of the posterior fossa convexity or the tentorium and is supplied by branches of the internal or external carotid arteries. Myelopathy occurs when the arterialized venous drainage has access to the valveless spinal venous system. Hence, if a patient with myelopathy has MRI or myelographic findings of a dilated, tortuous coronal venous plexus but normal spinal arteriography, he or she should undergo carotid arteriography to search for a dural AVF of the tentorium or posterior fossa. Similarly, because sacral dural AVFs with intrathecal medullary venous drainage and consequent myelopathy may be supplied by branches of the iliac arteries,[94, 95] it is important for the arteriogram to include selective injection of all arteries potentially supplying the sacral dura if selective spinal arteriography is negative.

Intradural Arteriovenous Malformations. Selective spinal arteriography of glomus-type AVMs typically demonstrates a dense mass of blood vessels confined to a short segment of spinal cord. These lesions may be supplied solely by the anterior spinal artery (see Fig. 142–11) or by the anterior and posterior spinal arteries.

Juvenile-type spinal AVMs have multiple feeding vessels and occupy a larger volume of spinal cord. The nidus is usually large and contains spinal cord tissue within its interstices. In the metameric form, paraspinous soft tissues may also be involved (see Fig. 142–10).

Direct AVFs in the pia may be perfused by the anterior or posterior spinal arteries. These are on the cord surface or, rarely, on the filum terminale. The most common type, type III, is often associated with extensive venous enlargement and variceal formation. For the smaller, type I AVFs, the exact site of the fistula can often be determined as the point at which the feeding artery abruptly dilates, as it joins the venous drainage (see Fig. 142–12). Angiomyelotomography is useful to detect small perimedullary AVFs (type I), to distinguish them from AVMs of the spinal cord, and to enhance the precision of the definition of the vascular anatomy of the AVF before treatment.[15, 25, 57]

TREATMENT AND OUTCOME

The ideal treatment for spinal AVMs is one that permanently obliterates the nidus of the AVM without compromising spinal cord blood supply or damaging the spinal cord. Whether this can be safely accomplished and by which means depend largely on the type of spinal AVM and the technical constraints imposed by its anatomy.

Dural Arteriovenous Fistulas

SURGERY

The goal of treatment of spinal dural AVFs is permanent elimination of venous congestion of the spinal cord. This goal, which may be accomplished through excision, obliteration or occlusion of the nidus, or interruption of venous drainage from the fistula between the dura and the dilated coronal venous plexus, has not always been the objective of treatment. When spinal arteriography was first introduced in the 1960s, the AVF was not identified in the spinal dura but was thought to reside in the arterialized pial veins of the coronal venous plexus. Consequently, these dilated, tortuous, arterialized coronal veins were mistaken for the nidus of the AVM and became the target of microneurosurgical operations designed to "strip" the cord of the purported pial nidus.[13, 55, 96, 97] Unfortunately, this treatment often exacerbated, rather than eliminated, the venous congestion. Further, these stripping procedures involved an extensive multilevel laminectomy, a tedious and unnecessary pial dissection, and a higher risk of morbidity to the patient. Moreover, the veins being excised were the normal veins of the coronal plexus that had been altered in appearance by the reception of blood under high pressure and flow.[4] Recognition of the actual location of the dural AVF implied that effective treatment of most spinal vascular malformations should be directed at the dural nidus of the fistula. Simple interruption of the AVF produces permanent resolution of venous congestion and improvement of myelopathy in many patients.[1, 14, 23, 40, 49, 93, 98–100]

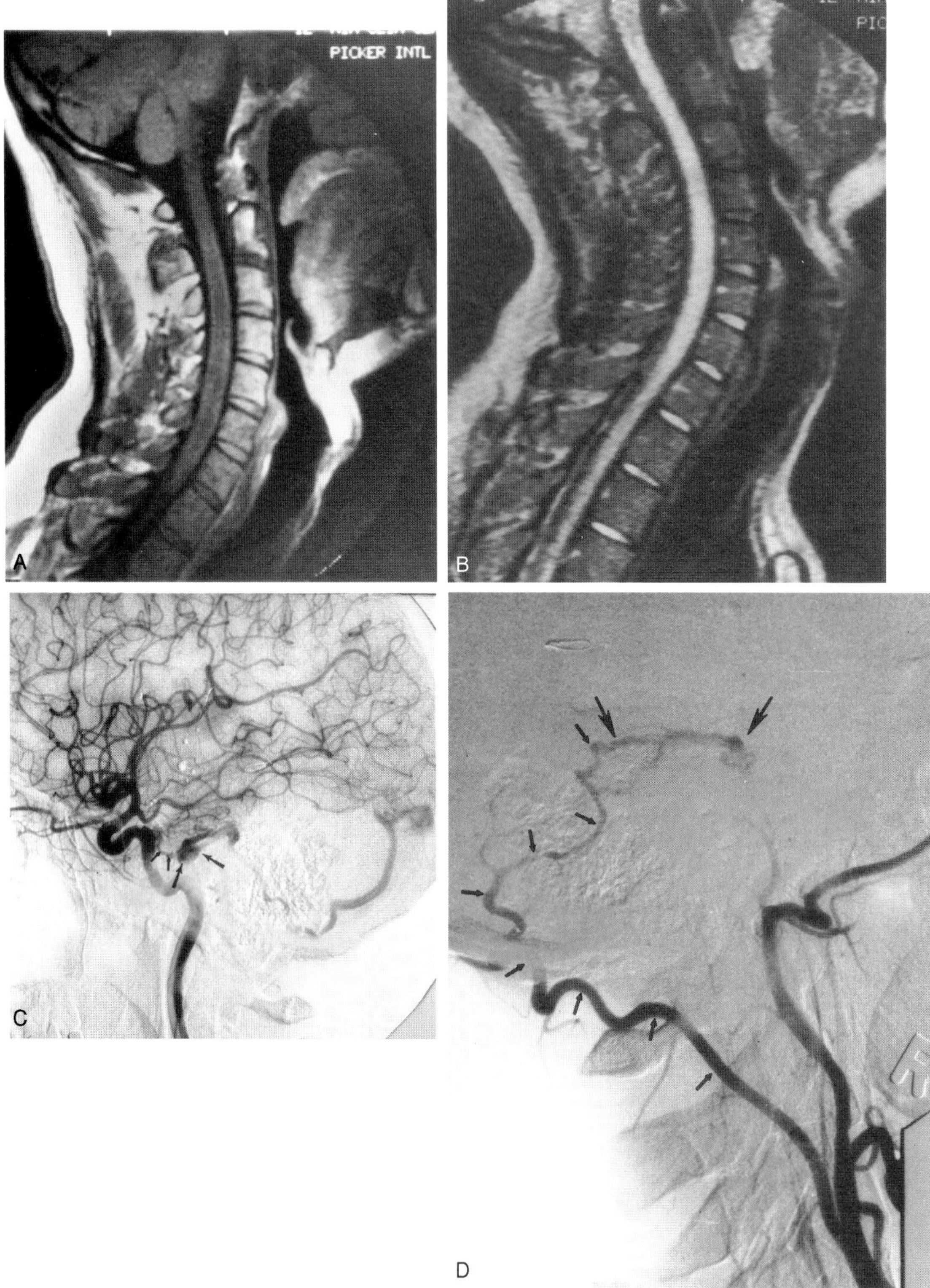

FIGURE 142–20. Forty-one-year-old man with progressive quadriparesis, beginning in the lower extremities, from spinal medullary venous drainage of an intracranial dural arteriovenous fistula (AVF) of the tentorium at the petrous apex. T1-weighted (TE 550, TR 22) magnetic resonance imaging (MRI) scan *(A)* reveals expansion of the cord and abnormal cord signal from C2 to T1. T2-weighted (TE 2000, TR 80) MRI scan *(B)* discloses a high signal in an expanded cord from C1 to T1. Note the absence of abnormal signal void in the subarachnoid vessels on MRI. Carotid arteriography demonstrates an intracranial dural AVF *(C and D, large arrows)* supplied by the tentorial branch of the right internal carotid artery *(C, small arrows)* and by the occipital branch of the right external carotid artery *(D, small arrows)*.

Illustration continued on following page

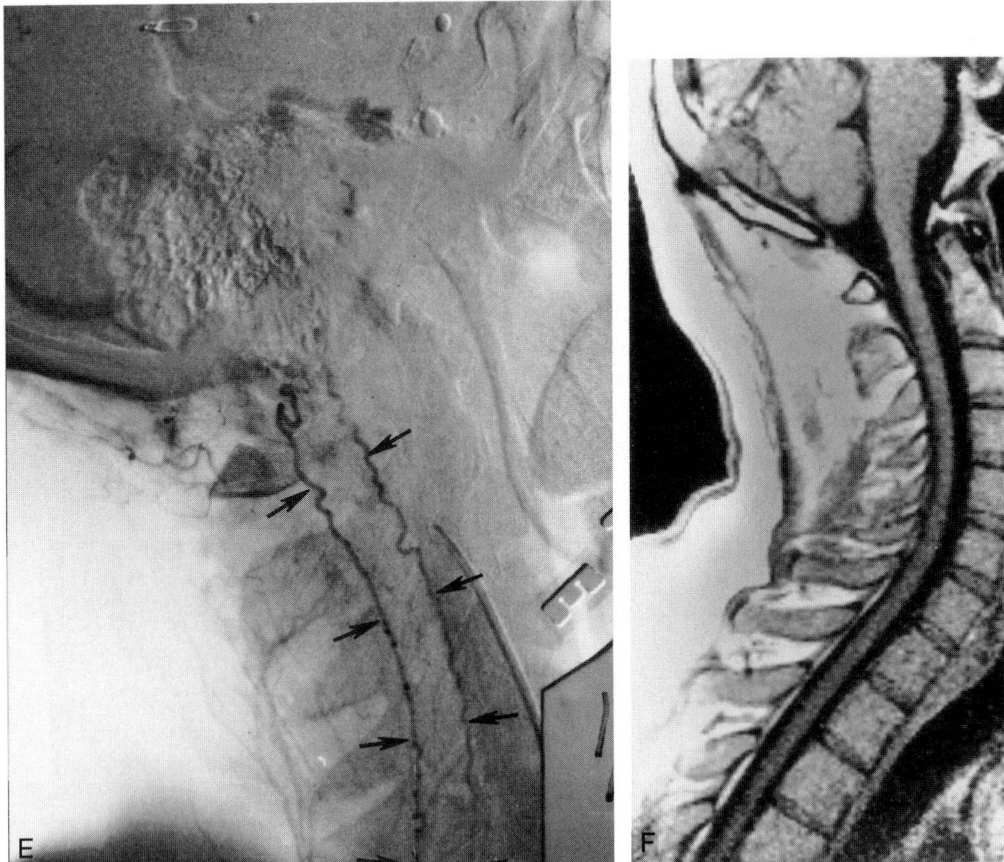

FIGURE 142–20. *Continued.* The blood enters the petrosal vein and empties into the anterior and posterior spinal veins *(E, arrows)* after internal carotid artery and external carotid artery *(E)* injection. There is prolonged spinal venous drainage *(E)*. Sagittal T1-weighted (TR 417, TE 16) MRI 4 years after interruption of the AVF *(F)* reveals return of the normal signal intensity and remission of the expanded spinal cord. (From Wrobel C, Oldfield E, DiChiro G, et al: Myelopathy due to intracranial dural arteriovenous fistulas draining intrathecally into spinal medullary veins: Report of three cases. J Neurosurg 69:934, 1988.)

Operative treatment of dural AVFs begins with a laminectomy one level above and one level below the level of the dural nidus and the intramedullary vein that drains the fistula. After a midline dural opening, the arterialized medullary vein is identified. This vessel almost always penetrates the dura at the site of the dural penetration of the posterior nerve rootlets (Figs. 142–2 and 142–21). To confirm that the vessel to be interrupted is the medullary vein draining the dural AVF and not a medullary artery, its configuration is compared with the anatomy disclosed in the venous phase of the preoperative arteriogram, and it is followed as it crosses the subarachnoid space and joins the abnormal-appearing coronal venous plexus (Figs. 142–21 and 142–22). Following its identification and confirmation, the arterialized medullary vein is coagulated with bipolar forceps over 4 to 6 mm and sharply divided as it penetrates the inner layer of dura, between the dura and the engorged coronal venous plexus. Interruption of the medullary vein usually produces a visible change in venous turgor, and after a few minutes, the color of the arterialized coronal venous plexus may change from red to blue. However, it should be noted that interruption of the medullary vein usually does *not* produce an immediate or dramatic change in venous color (perhaps because of shunting of blood through a spinal cord capillary bed that is maximally dilated to supply the cord in the face of severely diminished perfusion pressure).

Special Circumstances. In the experience at the NIH, the only patient with persistence of a spinal dural AVF after surgical interruption of the vein draining it intradurally was one with extradural *and* intradural venous drainage of the fistula, a setting in which the flow through the dural AVF remained patent.[100] In this rare circumstance, the dural fistula should be excised or obliterated with bipolar cautery, but only if the segmental intercostal artery feeding the dural fistula is not also the origin of a medullary artery supplying the spinal cord.[100] Because the artery of Adamkiewicz also arises from this region, it is particularly important to note that 5% to 15% of dural AVFs are supplied from intercostal arteries that also supply the spinal cord via a medullary artery (Fig. 142–23).[23, 101] When the same segmental vessel (intercostal artery or one of its equivalents) supplies the AVF and the spinal cord,[101] simple intradural interruption of the arterialized medullary

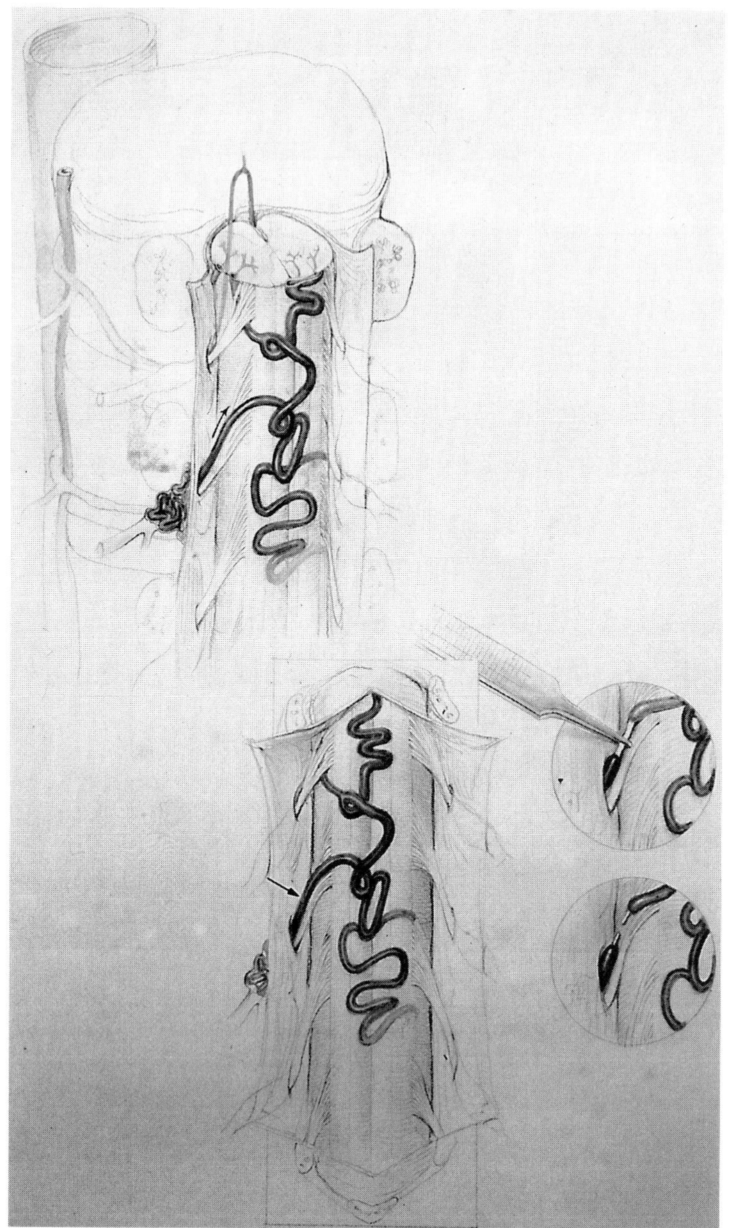

FIGURE 142–21. Most dural arteriovenous fistulas (AVFs) can be permanently obliterated by identifying the site of intradural penetration of the arterialized vein draining the dural AVF (almost always next to the dural penetration of the nerve root), coagulating a segment of it with bipolar forceps, and sharply dividing it. (Drawing by Howard Bartner, NIH; from Oldfield EH: Spinal vascular malformations. In Rengachary S, Wilkins R, [eds]: Neurosurgical Operative Atlas. Rolling Meadows, IL, American Association of Neurological Surgeons, 1994.

vein alone is the treatment of choice, as it provides lasting obliteration of the fistula and is the only treatment that does not risk arterial occlusion and cord infarction (see Fig. 142–23).[1, 93, 100]

Outcome. Operative treatment of dural AVFs is safe and consistently interrupts the progression of neurological deficits.[1, 4, 14, 23, 40, 49] When the series from the National Hospital for Nervous Disease[40] and the NIH[23] are combined (total of 76 patients), 37 of the 49 severely disabled (Aminoff and Logue grades 3 to 5) patients (76%) had improved gait after surgery (Fig. 142–24). Further, 26 of 27 patients (96%) with disability but unaided locomotion retained independent ambulation, and 17 of the 27 (63%) improved. Of the 76 patients, 70 (92%) either stabilized or improved. Improvement in control of micturition and independent ambulation is achieved in most patients after surgery.[23, 40] Patients with more advanced preoperative disability are likely to be stabilized but are less likely to improve after surgery.[4, 14, 23, 40, 43, 49] These observations have been confirmed in more recent reports.[98, 99] One retrospective study of 25 patients found a tendency toward moderate, but definite, functional decline several years after treatment.[102] This occurred more commonly in patients with a more prolonged clinical course before treatment and in patients with more severe neurological deficits at treatment. Thus, this functional decline may represent the additive effects of age on the original neurological damage.

In summary, neurological outcome is closely related to the preoperative neurological function of the patient (see Fig. 142–24). Patients who are diagnosed and treated early, before progression of myelopathy and neurological impairment, retain their pretreatment neurological function or improve. Finally, because simple

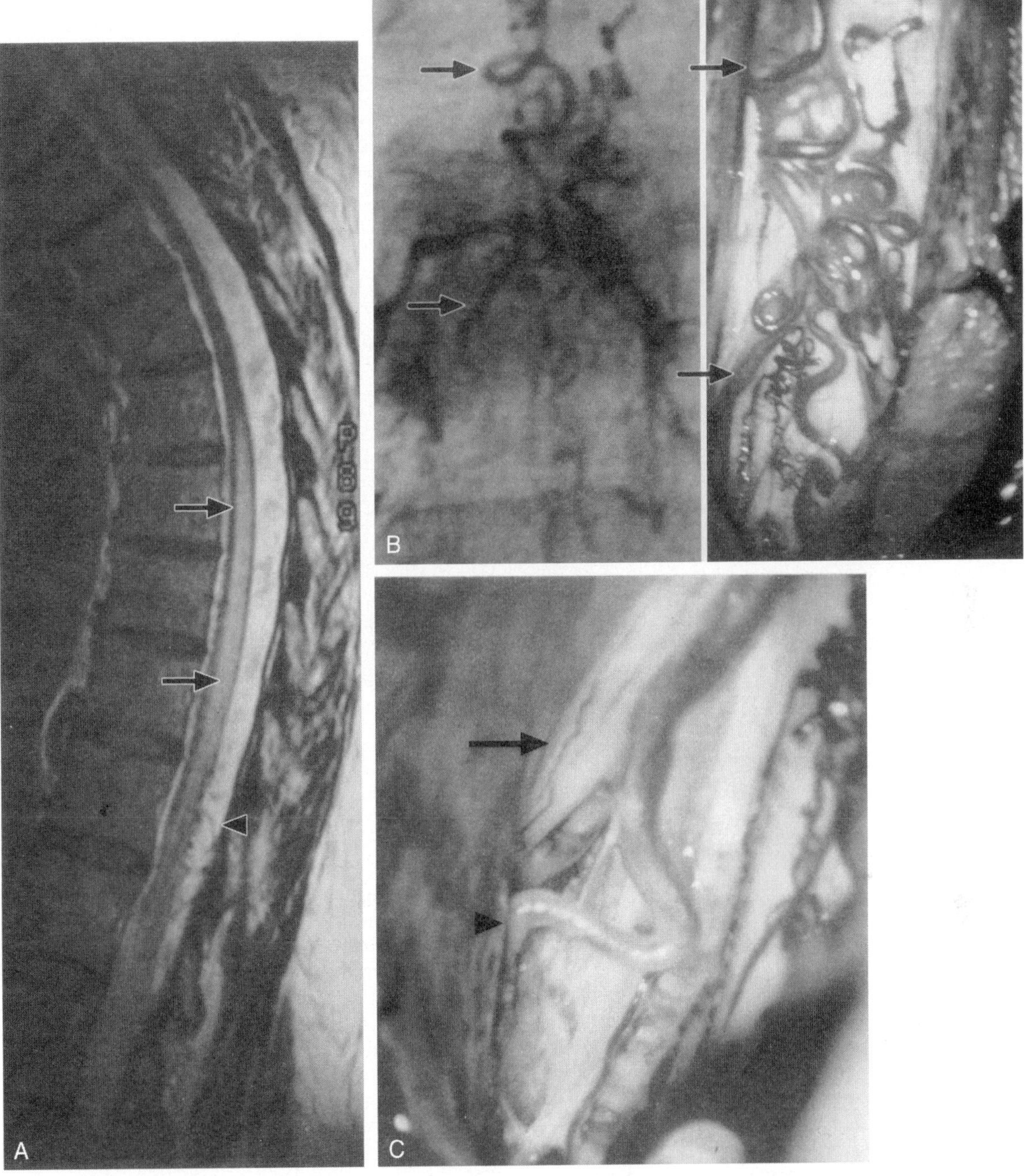

FIGURE 142–22. A 67-year-old woman with a 6-month history of progressive gait disturbance, lower extremity claudication, and bladder dysfunction. *A*, T2-weighted noncontrast sagittal magnetic resonance imaging (MRI) scan of the thoracic spine. There is abnormal bright signal *(arrows)* within the substance of the thoracic cord, with accompanying expansion of the spinal cord. Serpentine flow voids *(arrowhead)* can be seen dorsal to the spinal cord. *B*, Preoperative arteriogram and intraoperative view. An anteroposterior spinal arteriogram (left; seen from the surgeon's view) demonstrates filling of the spinal dural arteriovenous fistula (AVF) and the pattern of the vessels of the coronal venous plexus. Note the congruency of the vascular pattern compared to an intraoperative view (right) of the dorsal surface of the spinal cord at the same level. By studying the vascular pattern of the arteriogram, correlation with the intradural vessels (*top arrows*) is possible, which allows ready identification of the intradural draining vein *(bottom arrows)*. *C*, Intradural draining vein (medullary vein). This magnified view demonstrates the relationship of the intradural draining vein of the AVF *(arrowhead)* to the dural penetration of the nerve root *(arrow)*. The fistula is effectively treated with coagulation and division of this vessel. (From Watson JC, Oldfield EH: The surgical management of spinal dural vascular malformations. Neurosurg Clinic N Am 10:73–87, 1999.)

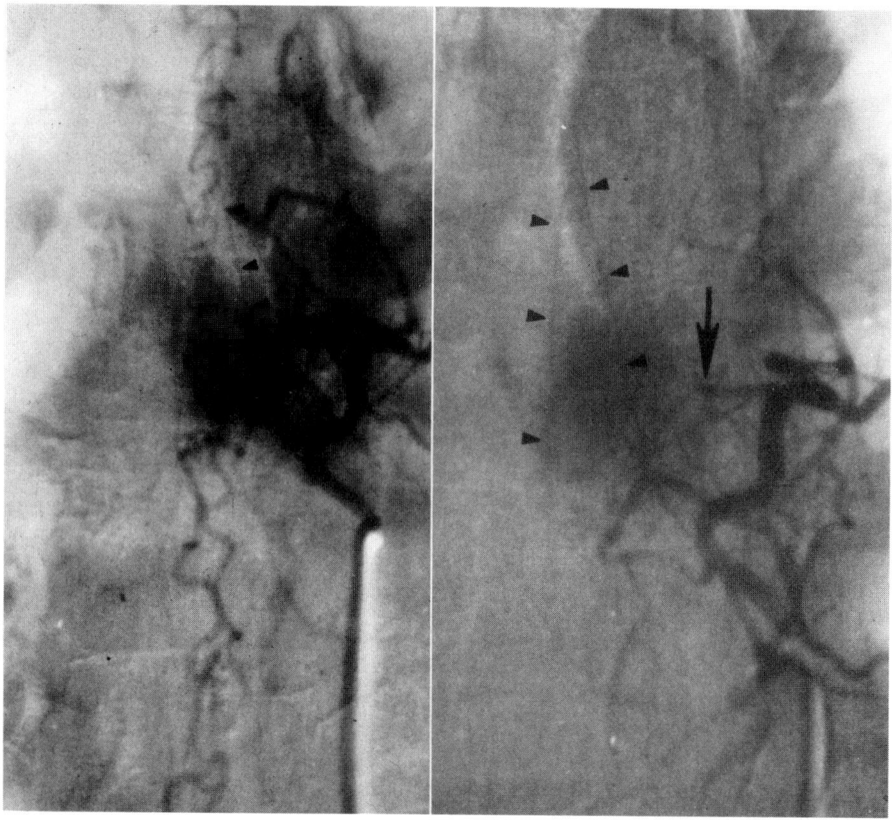

FIGURE 142–23. Selective spinal arteriogram in a 36-year-old man with a spinal dural arteriovenous fistula (AVF) at the seventh thoracic nerve root. *Left,* The left seventh thoracic intercostal artery provides a common origin of the arterial supply to the dural AVF (just caudal and to the patient's left of the *lower arrowhead)* and to the artery of Adamkiewicz *(arrowheads). Right,* Following surgical interruption of the medullary vein draining the dural AVF intradurally, the dural fistula no longer opacifies. The *large arrow* designates the abrupt termination of the vessel previously supplying the AVF. (From Oldfield E, Doppman J: Spinal arteriovenous malformations. Clin Neurosurg 34: 161–183, 1988.)

interruption of the venous drainage of a spinal dural AVF provides lasting occlusion of the fistula,[100] as it does for cranial dural AVFs,[103] this has been used to support the concept that the venous approach to the treatment of certain dural AVFs can be used successfully alone.[103, 104]

EMBOLIZATION

Although dural AVFs can be treated by transarterial embolization, the durability of embolic occlusion and neurological improvement has been problematic. Additionally, embolization cannot be safely used in patients with common arterial supply to the dural AVF and the spinal cord (see Fig. 142–23).[1, 23, 101]

With particulate embolization, symptomatic improvement is usually only transient, as the embolized dural AVF recanalizes, and recurrent myelopathy follows.[97, 105] Embolization with liquid polymerizing agents (isobutyl-2-cyanoacrylate [IBC]) is used at some centers as primary treatment of patients with spinal dural AVFs. It has been argued that embolization with liquid agents will pass distally into the feeding artery, reach the nidus of the dural AVF and the vein draining it, and provide permanent obliteration of the fistula. However, it is generally accepted that embolic occlusion with these agents does not provide complete or permanent occlusion of other types of central nervous system AVFs and AVMs.[106] Further, although minimal clinical or arteriographic follow-up has been performed in patients with spinal dural AVFs occluded with liquid agents, the incidence of recanalization is high, as is the frequency with which patients require additional therapy later.[98, 99, 107] Merland and colleagues noted persistent flow through the dural AVF requiring immediate surgery in 14 of 45 patients embolized with IBC.[108] Niimi and associates examined the outcome of 47 patients in whom embolic therapy was used for spinal dural AVFs.[109] In 8 of the 47 (17%), the inadequacy of therapy was recognized immediately (partial embolization), because the acrylic did not reach the fistula or an anterior or posterior spinal artery arose at the same level. Two of these eight patients were followed for less than 1 month, but five of the six patients followed for more than 1 month required additional treatment. Of the remaining 39 patients, 4 were followed for less than 1 month (one of whom had recanalized already), and 35 were followed for at least 1 month, 18 of whom (51%) had recurrence. Overall, 26 of the 43 patients (60%) who were followed for at least 1 month either had inadequate therapy at the outset (eight patients) or had a known recurrence of the AVF. Many of the patients who had not yet recanalized had been followed for less than 1 year,[109] an interval known to be inadequate for establishing the permanency of occlusion.[106]

As summarized earlier, regardless of the therapy used, most patients who have neurological deficits at treatment have some degree of residual deficit. Because of the risk of incomplete therapy, or therapy that is transient, the patient has the anxiety of not knowing whether the residual neurological impairment is the result of partial treatment or of recanalization of the AVF, which might be treatable. It also requires frequent

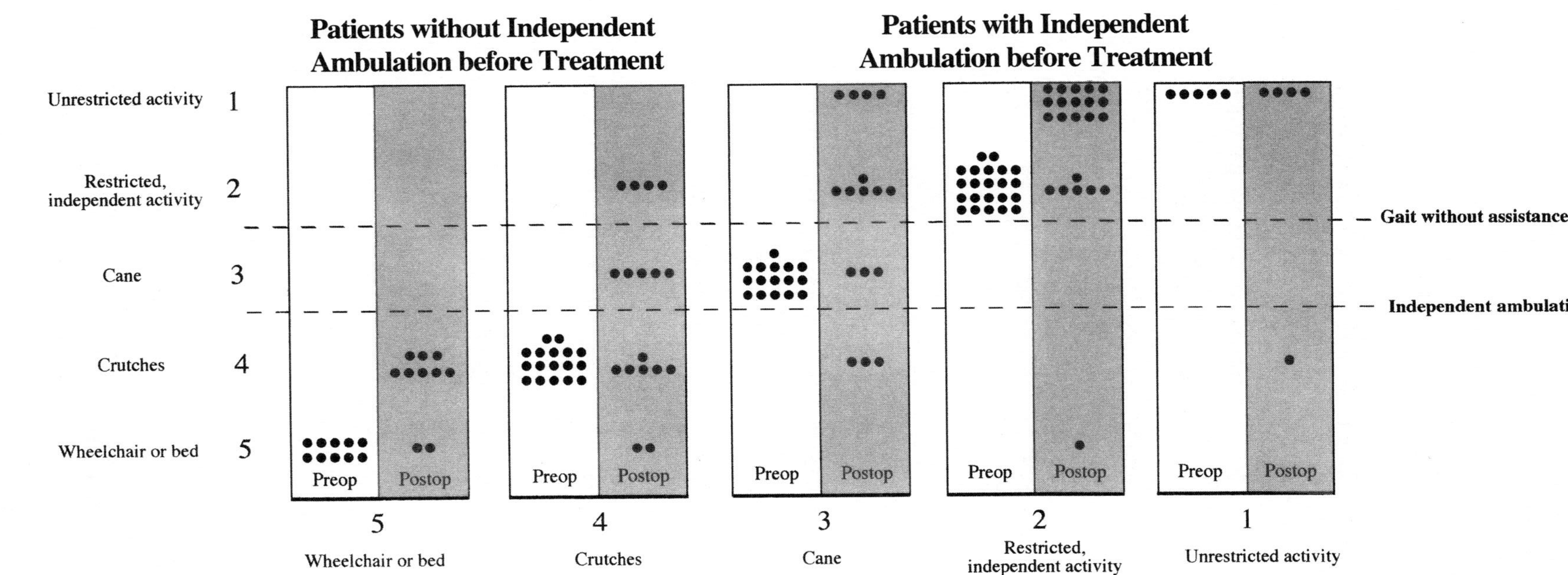

FIGURE 142–24. Relationship of preoperative functional state and postoperative outcome in patients with dural arteriovenous fistulas (AVFs). The outcome after surgery is directly related to the patient's neurological status preoperatively. Generally, patients who walk independently before treatment do so after treatment. Note, however, that most patients were not treated until they had already acquired severe functional disability. Early diagnosis and therapy offer the best outcome. (Adapted from Muraszko KM, Oldfield EH: Vascular malformations of the spinal cord and dura. Neurosurg Clin N Am 1:631–652, 1990. Data from Rosenblum B, Oldfield EH, Doppman JL: Pathogenesis of spinal arteriovenous malformations. J Neurosurg 67:795–802, 1987; Symon L, Kuyama H, Kendall B: Dural arteriovenous malformations of the spine: Clinical features and surgical results in 55 cases. J Neurosurg 60:238–247, 1984.)

radiologic reassessment to establish if recurrence has occurred.

Finally, hemorrhage[110] and delayed paraplegia[22, 56] after embolization of spinal dural AVFs with IBC have been reported. This suggests either propagation of venous thrombosis into the coronal venous plexus or passage of embolic material through the AVF and into the coronal venous plexus, exacerbating venous hypertension and leading to hemorrhage or venous infarction.

Perhaps the most appropriate use of embolization is in the treatment of patients with Foix-Alajouanine syndrome and incipient venous thrombosis and spinal cord infarction. A patient with an untreated dural AVF and rapid symptomatic progression has perilously high venous hypertension and is at risk for venous thrombosis and irreversible cord injury. Transarterial embolization of the fistula in these patients provides immediate reduction in venous congestion until definitive surgical treatment can be performed.[42]

Thus, treatment limited to simple interruption of the vein draining the AVF intradurally is optimal in most patients, as it eliminates venous hypertension without risk to the normal vessels that supply the spinal cord and provides lasting and curative treatment.

Intradural Vascular Malformations

The ideal therapy for intradural vascular malformations is one that completely and permanently obliterates the AVM while preserving the blood supply to the spinal cord. However, the feasibility of this goal and how it can best be accomplished (with surgery alone, embolization alone, or surgery after embolization) depend on the type, size, location, and blood supply of the vascular malformation. In vascular malformations with certain adverse risk factors (large size, location in the thoracic or lumbar segments of the spinal cord, involvement of the ventral half of the spinal cord, complex blood supply associated with extension anterior to the ventral cord surface, and multiple feeding vessels from the anterior spinal artery), preservation of neurological function and avoidance of iatrogenic disability may mandate less than definitive treatment, regardless of the therapeutic approach.

SURGERY

A number of general principles apply to the surgical management of all intradural AVMs.[13, 55, 56, 111–113] Surgery should be attempted only after careful consideration of the vascular anatomy of the lesion and the adjacent spinal cord as depicted by selective spinal arteriography. After acute subarachnoid or intraparenchymal hemorrhage, surgery is best delayed to permit clot lysis and absorption. Preoperative embolization with particulate material or occlusion of giant feeders with balloon occlusion reduces the blood flow and tension in the AVM or AVF. Because it commonly leaves small particles in feeding vessels to a greater extent than in venous drainage vessels (EHO, personal observations), preoperative particulate embolization can also assist the surgeon in defining the feeding arteries during surgery. The operating microscope and appropriate microsurgical instrumentation are mandatory. Operative exposure must extend at least one level above and one level below the nidus of the AVM. The dura should be opened in the midline, and the arachnoid is preserved to avoid laceration of any delicate, distended, or adherent vessels underlying the dural opening. The use of small (2 to 3 mm × 10 to 15 mm) rectangular cotton pledgets or stay sutures secured to the pia-arachnoid facilitates retraction and exposure provided by myelotomy for intramedullary vascular malformations. Painstaking hemostasis is crucial to maintain optimal visualization of the nidus of the AVM. The vascular anatomy defined on the preoperative angiogram must be carefully correlated to that seen intraoperatively to identify and confirm the major feeding and draining vessels and to plan the sequence of steps for excision.

Intraoperative ultrasonography with a directional flow probe or intraoperative arteriography[114, 115] may be helpful to localize the intramedullary nidus and to distinguish afferent from efferent vessels. Bipolar cautery, used judiciously, can reduce the size and turgor of the AVM. Continuous bipolar irrigation maintains optimal visualization and prevents adherence to friable vessels. Large feeding vessels may require ligatures or clips, but metallic clips are generally avoided so as not to interfere with the results of postoperative imaging. Generally, one major draining vein is preserved until the last arterial feeders have been taken. Intraoperative arteriography can be used to detect residual AVM that is still patent,[114, 115] but it may not detect small portions of thrombosed nidus that recanalize later. Hemostasis is completely reassessed before closure. The dura is closed in watertight fashion.

For certain ventral AVMs or AVFs, Martin and coworkers[116] and Markert and colleagues[117] described exposure of the ventrolateral quadrant of the spinal cord through an extended posterolateral approach that can be used in the cervical and thoracic regions. This technique includes a midline skin incision with a transverse extension at the level of the lesion, unilateral division and retraction of the paraspinous muscles, laminectomy and unilateral removal of facets and pedicles, dural incision over the dorsal root entry zone, multilevel division of the ipsilateral dentate ligaments, and elevation and rotation of the spinal cord with dentate traction stitches. This technique provides exposure of the ventral root entry zone, the ipsilateral half of the ventral surface of the spinal cord, and the anterior spinal artery, although the surface of the spinal cord beyond the anterior spinal artery is not seen well.

Intramedullary Arteriovenous Malformations. Circumferential dissection is carried out along the gliotic plane between the intramedullary AVM and the adjacent neural tissue (Fig. 142–25). To facilitate dissection of the deeper portions of the AVM, the dorsal portion of the spinal cord is gently retracted laterally with small cottonoids or fine pial sutures attached to the dura laterally. Although the outcome of operative treat-

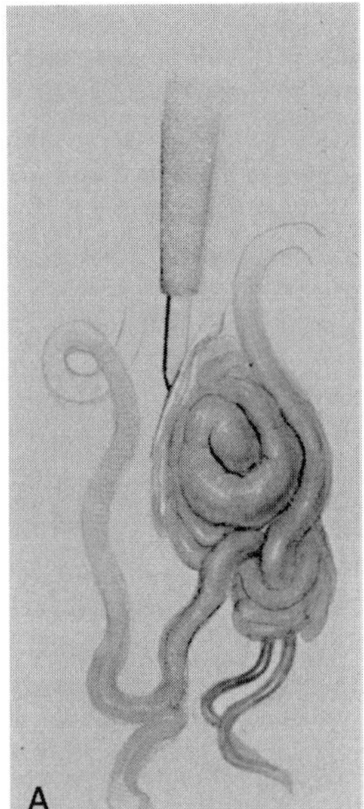

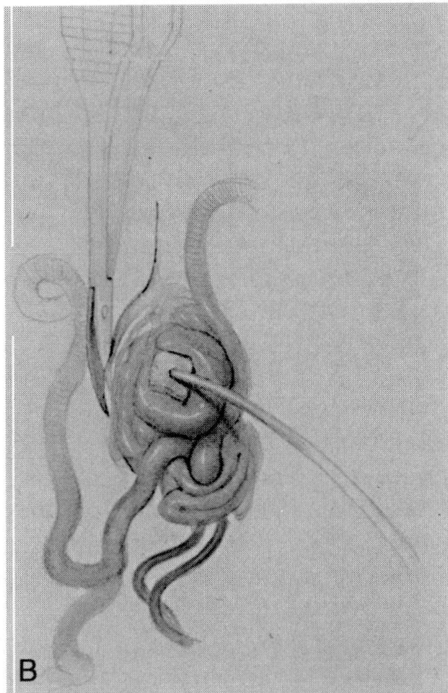

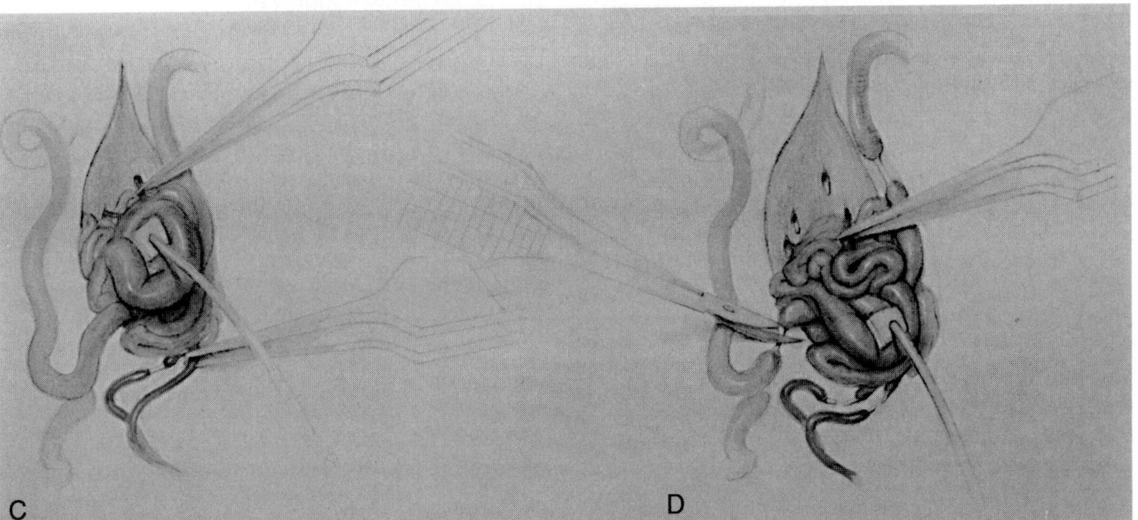

FIGURE 142–25. *A and B,* After separating the arachnoid from the arteriovenous malformation (AVM), a diamond knife is used to incise the pia at the edge of the nidus. To obtain the exposure neccesary for excision of the deep portion of the AVM, the pial incision is extended a few millimeters rostrally and caudally, usually in the midline. *C and D,* The superficial feeding vessels are interrupted sharply after they have been coagulated with bipolar cautery. Gentle retraction with a microsucker, with the tip of a small cottonoid and the suction on low setting; dissection with the tips of the bipolar forceps in the gliotic plane between the malformation and the spinal cord; and elevation of the malformation while working from one pole upward or downward to expose, coagulate, and interrupt the vessels entering and leaving the malformation ventrally result in dissection of the nidus of the malformation from the surrounding spinal cord. Small custom-cut cottonoids and, if necessary, pial traction sutures are used to maintain adequate separation of the spinal cord from the nidus of the AVM for dissection. As the margins of the malformation are dissected, bipolar coagulation is used to gradually shrink the AVM and render it less susceptible to rupture during manipulation. Progressive shrinking of the AVM by coagulation also reduces turgidity in the nidus as the dissection proceeds. Generally, at least one of the major draining veins is preserved patent until dissection around the periphery of the malformation has been completed and all feeding vessels have been occluded. However, when the AVM is occluded by presurgical embolization, this may not be necessary. (Drawing by Howard Bartner, NIH; from Oldfield EH: Spinal vascular malformations. In Rengachary S, Wilkins R [eds]: Neurosurgical Operative Atlas. Rolling Meadows, IL, American Association of Neurological Surgeons, 1994.)

ment of spinal intramedullary AVMs is, in general, less satisfactory than the results of treatment of dural AVFs, there are several characteristics of glomus-type intramedullary AVMs that often render them technically less problematic than juvenile-type lesions. Unlike juvenile-type AVMs, glomus lesions are generally compact, lack intertwined neural elements, and usually have a single arterial feeding vessel.[23] In addition, the cervical region has a more abundant collateral system than do the thoracolumbar cord segments, permitting total surgical excision of certain cervical intramedullary lesions.[13, 23, 55, 56, 118, 119] However, if a relatively large lesion is situated entirely intraparenchymally in the anterior half of the spinal cord, complete excision may yield unacceptable neurological deficits. Operative intervention may be inadvisable in this circumstance.

Owing to their relative infrequency, no adequate long-term study has been done to compare surgical and embolic treatment for intramedullary AVMs in the cervical region. However, intramedullary AVMs in the thoracic and lumbar regions pose a substantially greater operative risk because of their more tenuous collateral blood supply. Ventral intramedullary lesions in these segments are usually treated with repeated arteriographic embolization (see later).[54]

Because they are voluminous, high-flow lesions that usually contain neural tissue within the interstices of the component vessels of the AVM and derive their arterial supply from multiple medullary arteries that also supply the spinal cord, most juvenile-type intramedullary AVMs are considered inoperable. For patients with progressive myelopathy or hemorrhage, embolization is usually recommended (see later).[54] An exception is a dorsally located lesion that is partly intramedullary and partly extramedullary.[13, 55, 56, 112, 119, 120] Presurgical or intraoperative embolization permits an easier and safer excision and may improve the chances of total excision of these lesions.[119, 121–123]

Outcome. Reports of the results of surgery for intamedullary AVMs are all influenced by selection bias. Although the results of surgery have been reported for small series of patients, many have been isolated cases, and none of the surgical series indicated the population of patients from which the surgical patients were selected. Clearly, patients were selected to undergo surgery because of the likelihood of a successful and safe excision, rather than submitting all patients with AVMs to surgical therapy.

Further, the natural history of intramedullary AVMs is variable (see earlier), and the arteriographic outcome of surgery is known only for 3 years after surgery (Table 142–7). Early postoperative arteriography revealed persistent AVM in as many as 40% of patients treated surgically during the 1960s and 1970s.[23] At 3 years after surgery, about 30% to 50% of patients are improved, 30% to 50% remain unchanged, and 10% to 20% are worse. However, there are limited data on the incidence of persistent AVM, even as early as 3 years, and no long-term data exist on the incidence of clinical relapse or progression because of incomplete surgical excision. Moreover, there are no studies of delayed arteriographic follow-up more than 1 year after surgical treatment of intradural AVMs. The short-term clinical results (3-year follow-up) of surgery clearly indicate superior results in patients who receive treatment before serious neurological deficits arise (Fig. 142–26). However, this must be balanced against the knowledge that some patients have an innocuous clinical course for many years without any treatment (see earlier, and personal observations of EHO).

EMBOLIZATION

Embolic occlusion of spinal AVMs developed as a natural extension of the introduction and refinement of

TABLE 142–7 ■ **Results of Treatment of Intradural Arteriovenous Malformations**

			POSTOPERATIVE ARTERIOGRAPHY		FUNCTIONAL STATUS AFTER TREATMENT			
AUTHOR/ YEAR	NO. OF PATIENTS	LEVEL OF NIDUS	Immediate (Persistent AVM)	Delayed (Persistent Recurrent AVM)	Follow-up (mean, yr)	Improved (%)	Unchanged (%)	Worse (%)
Surgery								
Rosenblum et al, 1987*	43	17% cervical, 83% thoracolumbar	32 (41%)	0	3	33	51	14
Yasargil et al, 1984†	41	46% cervical, 54% thoracolumbar	0	0	3	48	32	20
Conolly et al, 1998†	15	20% cervical, 80% thoracolumbar	15 (7%)	10 (30%)‡	3.8	40	53	7
Embolization								
Biondi et al, 1990†	35	100% thoracic		35 (100%)	6	63	26	11

*Includes patients with perimedullary AVFs.
†Includes only intramedullary AVMs.
‡Only 2 of 10 patients studied >1 yr after surgery.
From Oldfield EH: Spinal vascular informations. In Swash M (ed): Outcomes in Neurological and Neurosurgical Disorders. Cambridge, UK, Cambridge University Press, 1998.

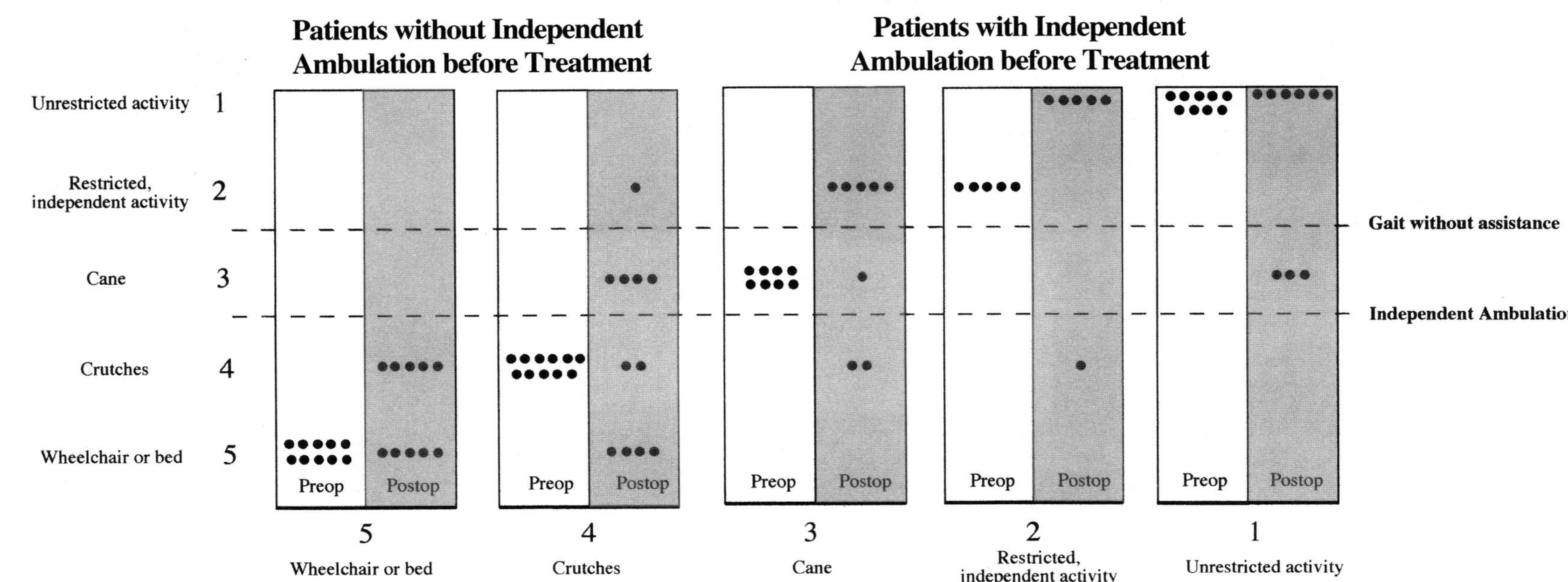

FIGURE 142–26. Relationship of preoperative functional state and postoperative outcome in patients with intramedullary arteriovenous malformations. As in patients with dural arteriovenous fistulas (AVFs), the outcome after surgery is directly related to the patient's neurological status preoperatively. Generally, patients who walked independently before treatment do so after treatment. Note, however, that many patients were not treated until they had already acquired severe functional disability. As in patients with dural AVFs (see Fig. 142–24), early diagnosis and therapy offer the best outcome for patients in both groups. (From Muraszko KM, Oldfield EH: Vascular malformations of the spinal cord and dura. Neurosurg Clin N Am 1:631–652, 1990. Data from Rosenblum B, Oldfield EH, Doppman JL: Pathogenesis of spinal arteriovenous malformations. J Neurosurg 67:795–802, 1987.)

selective spinal arteriography.[9, 122, 124] With certain intradural AVMs, embolization is used alone. Because the incidence of recanalization after embolic occlusion is quite high,[105, 125] embolization may be used before surgery for lesions that can be excised with acceptable risk. The nidus of an intramedullary AVM, as occurs in hemangioblastomas,[80] is often composed of several independent vascular compartments with varying degrees of overlapping common supply. Embolization, including the use of liquid embolizing materials such as the polymerizing acrylics, rarely permanently occludes the entire nidus of the AVM. For this reason, some clinicians who once advocated the routine use of glue for embolizing intradural spinal AVMs no longer do so because of the low incidence of lasting occlusion and the incidence of complications associated with it.[51, 54]

Consideration of embolization requires careful assessment of the anatomy of the blood supply, including the size of the vessels supplying the AVM, and the level of the lesion. For success, one must occlude the nidus of the AVM but not obstruct a vessel supplying the AVM and the spinal cord proximal or distal to the nidus. Because the feeding artery is often a medullary artery or the anterior spinal artery, occlusion may immediately interrupt the blood supply to the spinal cord, especially in lesions below the upper thoracic level. Cervical AVMs are safer to embolize because of the presence of greater collateral sources of blood supply in that region.

Arteriography is used frequently during progressive embolic occlusion for assessment purposes. Selection of the catheter depends on how close the tip of the catheter must be to the nidus of the AVM for selective occlusion of the AVM while preserving the blood supply of the spinal cord and on whether particulate or liquid embolic material is used.

Although several particulate materials have been used to occlude spinal AVMs, including Gelfoam, PVA sponge microparticles, silk threads, and clot, the most commonly used particulate is PVA in the 150- to 250-μm diameter range. Selection of the size of the particles is based on the desire to have them pass freely through the conducting vessels, the medullary arteries, the anterior or posterior spinal artery, and the enlarged sulcal vessels to the AVM, without occluding the normal sulcal vessels. Because the diameter of the normal anterior spinal artery is 340 to 1100 μm and the diameter of the normal sulcal ateries is 60 to 72 μm, PVA of 150- to 250-μm diameter should pass through the anterior spinal artery, not enter the normal sulcal arteries, and pass into the enlarged sulcal arteries supplying the AVM.[126, 127] When the vessel providing the most direct route to the AVM is particularly difficult to engage with a catheter, such as feeding arteries from the cervical segment of the vertebral artery, the particles can be embolized in a flow-directed manner toward the nidus via temporary or permanent balloon occlusion of the artery just distal to the origin of the feeding vessel. With particulate embolization, progressive occlusion of the malformation is carefully monitored with repeated arteriographic examination, and the embolization is terminated when the lesion is almost completely occluded (in situ PVA continues to cause clot to form and propagate after completion of the procedure) or when there is retrograde reflux of the contrast medium proximal to the catheter tip, indicating that flow-directed targeting of the nidus will no longer occur. Liquid materials (e.g., IBC), which are less embolic, require placement of the catheter tip at the edge of the nidus of the AVM and injection of a small amount of the polymer.

The most common side effect of complete embolic occlusion of spinal AVMs is new neurological deficits that arise 24 to 48 hours after embolization. These deficits may be related to propagation of venous thrombosis in the enlarged coronal venous plexus, which is sluggishly carrying only the venous drainage of the spinal cord. To avoid this complication, patients are routinely anticoagulated with heparin for 48 to 60 hours after the procedure. Repeat arteriography is obtained 7 to 10 days later, with additional embolization as needed and at intervals of 1 to 2 years, or when neurological symptoms or signs recur.

Even though embolization of spinal AVMs with PVA does not provide lasting elimination of flow through the AVM, it plays an important role in the current management of patients with intradural AVMs. Presurgical particulate embolization makes surgery easier, and when used as the only therapy, it reduces the risk of hemorrhage (which could cause quadriplegia or death), mollifies the severity of spasticity in some patients, and, most important, delays neurological progression in most patients. The results obtained by Biondi and colleagues—who advocate routine yearly arteriography and embolization with PVA (Ivalon) particles, regardless of symptoms—suggest that serial endovascular embolization with PVA provides safe and successful management of most patients with AVMs in the thoracic region of the spinal cord.[54] Their long-term follow-up (mean, 6 years) of 35 patients showed that although no patients had complete, permanent obliteration of the AVM (most patients had a <50% reduction in AVM size), nearly two thirds were clinically improved at the end of the study. One of us (EHO) has several patients with thoracic or lumbar ventral intramedullary AVMs that receive their blood supply from the anterior spinal artery whose neurological status has been stabilized for several years by repetitive particulate embolic occlusion when symptoms recur.

As with surgery of intradural AVMs, the best results with embolization are obtained in patients without major neurological deficits before treatment.[11, 23, 51, 54, 110, 122, 125–127] Selective catheterization and embolization are associated with risks of occlusion of the anterior spinal artery and paraplegia or quadriplegia; perforation of an intradural vessel with the catheter and subarachnoid or intramedullary hemorrhage[125]; and passage of the emboli through the AVM into the venous system, causing hemorrhage or venous infarction,[110] or into the distal vessels of the parent artery, such as the basilar artery when using the vertebral artery to reach the AVM.

SUMMARY OF TREATMENT SELECTION FOR INTRAMEDULLARY MALFORMATIONS

As a result of rapidly and simultaneously evolving classification schemes, diagnostic techniques, surgical instrumentation, catheter sophistication, and other factors, the results of contemporary surgery, alone or after embolization, for intradural AVMs are unknown. The information on surgery is limited to series that began 2 to 3 decades ago. The three surgical and single embolization series included in Table 142–7 are the only published series of more than 10 patients that permit tabulation of the data. Further, for individual patients, there appear to be prominent selection biases for the use of surgery, embolization, or combined treatment in all series, surgical or embolization, large or small. For instance, although most intradural AVMs are in the thoracic or thoracolumbar segments of the spinal cord, with few exceptions,[55] the published reports emphasizing surgical success focus on patients with cervical lesions,[56, 111, 119] which arise in segments of the spinal cord with the greatest collateral blood supply. Further, there is a conspicuous bias for surgery for lesions in the dorsal half of the spinal cord, exemplified by the tendency to provide surgical therapy for "long dorsal AVMs" before they were recognized to be the products of dural AVFs. Dorsal intramedullary AVMs are less likely to receive their blood supply from the anterior spinal artery and are associated with less surgical risk than are ventral lesions.[112] The tendency to avoid subjecting patients in good condition to a therapeutic procedure that risks leaving them paraplegic results in a longer delay from diagnosis to surgical treatment with more difficult AVMs. In the NIH series, the average duration from the onset of symptoms to treatment was 2.7 years for dural AVFs, compared with 4.2 years for intradural AVMs, and patients with intradural AVMs were more likely to have worse functional grades at treatment than were patients with dural AVFs.[23]

Some of the factors that underlie bias in the selection of surgical or embolic therapy may act in opposite ways at different centers. Some centers reserve the surgery-only option for patients who cannot be treated effectively with embolization, whereas others select the more accessible, "safer" lesions (smaller, well-defined AVMs; direct AVFs; cervical AVMs; dorsal lesions) for surgery. In addition, there are nuances in the manner of reporting outcomes that must be acknowledged. Patients who are treated when they are paraplegic or quadriplegic are rarely made worse as a result of therapy. Thus, those who treat patients earlier can easily have a greater percentage of patients who are worse after treatment than before, despite superior long-term preservation of neurological function.

Many of the outcome data from early reports do not reflect significant advances in diagnostic techniques, current knowledge of the various subtypes of AVMs, details of anatomy that can now be obtained before treatment with MRI and the rapid-sequence imaging available with intra-arterial digital techniques, the advantages of more selective arteriography, or the significant advances in the equipment and techniques of interventional radiology and surgery. Further, certain lesions are treated more effectively with surgery, and certain others are treated best with embolization. Still others are more effectively treated by combining preoperative particulate embolization with surgery afterward. Thus, direct comparisons of surgical and embolic therapy cannot be reliably made and, in the modern era of treatment, may not be very meaningful.

In most patients with intradural spinal AVMs, treatment should be recommended when the diagnosis is established. When arteriography reveals that an intradural AVM or AVF can be *completely excised with limited risk*, because of its permanence, surgery alone or surgery after embolization should be considered. When lesions are identified, by arteriography or during surgery, as having unacceptable risks associated with complete excision, embolization should be considered.

Perimedullary Arteriovenous Fistulas

With intradural AVFs, the goal of treatment is precise interruption of the abnormal communication between the artery and vein. Elimination of the extramedullary fistulous connection of perimedullary AVFs may be achieved by surgery[15, 24–26, 51] or embolization.[15, 25, 128] For treatment purposes, these lesions have been divided by Merland and associates into three groups based on the caliber, length, and number of vessels supplying and draining the fistula (see Table 142–5): small fistulas in the conus or filum terminale supplied by a long, thin anterior spinal artery (type I); larger fistulas in the pia posterolaterally or anterolaterally composed of several discrete shunts and fed by enlarged anterior or posterior spinal arteries (type II; see Fig. 142–12); and the most common type, single giant fistulas supplied by several enormously enlarged anterior and posterior spinal arteries (type III; see Figs. 142–14 and 142–27).[25, 51] In AVFs is which a long, small-caliber anterior spinal artery is the sole feeding vessel (type I perimedullary AVFs), embolization usually is not safe, and surgical intervention is generally safer and effective.[24–26, 90] With type II lesions, embolization may be useful to reduce blood flow through the AVF in preparation for surgery, but it is usually not curative when used alone, perhaps because of the multiplicity of the constituents of the AVF.[57] Thus, surgical intervention is generally accepted as the treatment of choice for posterior or posterolateral perimedullary AVFs (Figs. 142–12 and 142–28) or when embolization is inherently dangerous.[25, 57, 59, 60] Surgical interruption of AVFs supplied by the anterior spinal artery on the ventral surface of the cord in the midline has been successfully performed via a transvertebral approach[24] and by posterolateral approaches with rotation of the spinal cord.[26, 116, 117] Patients with the giant simple fistulas (type III AVF) can be treated with selective occlusion by detachable balloons (which permits a trial occlusion before disengagement), occlusion with a coil, interruption with surgery (see Fig. 142–14), or a combination of embolic and surgical approaches (see Fig. 142–27).[25, 51] In perimedullary AVFs, as in the other forms of AVMs, better results are obtained in patients who re-

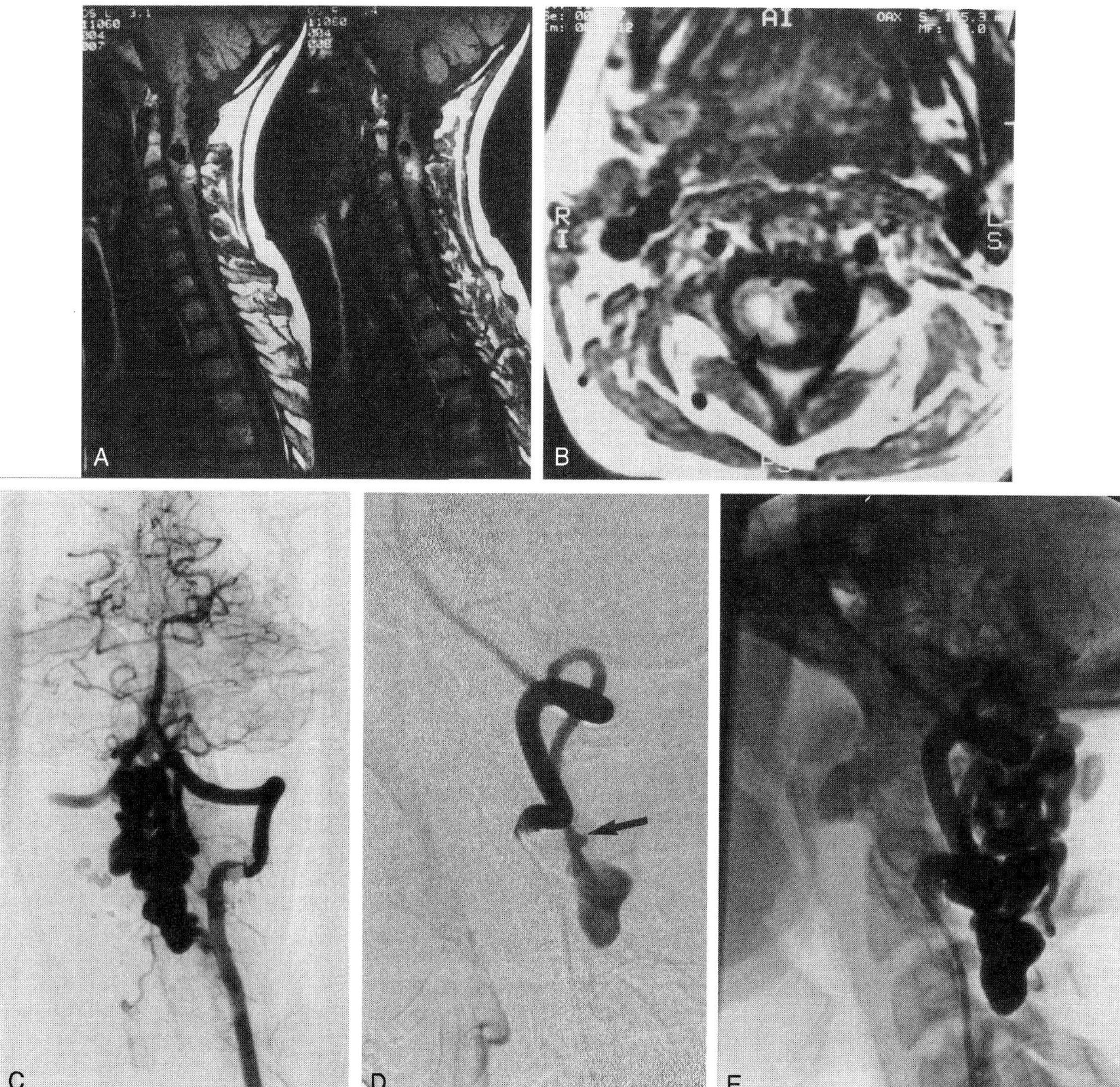

FIGURE 142–27. T1-weighted sagittal and axial magnetic resonance imaging (MRI) scans *(A and B)*, performed without contrast; selective left vertebral arteriography using standard "cut films" (*C*, anteroposterior view); and rapid-sequence (10 frames/second) digital imaging (*D and E*, lateral view) of a direct arteriovenous fistula (AVF) in the pia in the upper cervical segments (C2 and C3) of the spinal cord in a 17-year-old girl who had nearly normal neurological function despite having had four prior hemorrhages, including a "stroke" at age 7 years. She had the abrupt onset of severe headache, stiff neck, and weakness and numbness of the left upper and lower extremities 11 days before admission. With MRI *(A and B)*, the patent (low intramedullary and extramedullary signal) and thrombosed (high intramedullary signal, *arrows*) portions of a large, multinodular intramedullary varix and the extensive collection of abnormal vessels in the upper cervical subarachnoid space and cisterna magna are apparent. With routine selective arteriography *(C)*, it appears to be an arteriovenous malformation of the spinal cord with extensive blood flow. Flow through the lesion was so fast that only rapid-sequence digital imaging *(D)* could clearly demonstrate that it was an AVF, as well as the presence of a small aneurysm *(arrow)* just proximal to the AVF and the large varix at the site of the fistula. Multiple feeding vessels converged at the site of the AVF, which was at the upper margin of the large intramedullary aneurysm *(D)*. Note that in the next frame in the series *(E)*, performed just 100 msec after *D*, the coiled, dilated, arterialized veins conceal the site of the fistula and obscure visualization of the aneurysm. To reduce blood flow through the fistula, a coil was positioned in the distal portion of the principal feeding artery, a posterior spinal artery, at the level of the small aneurysm *(D)* the day before the fistula and the large aneurysm were excised.

Illustration continued on following page

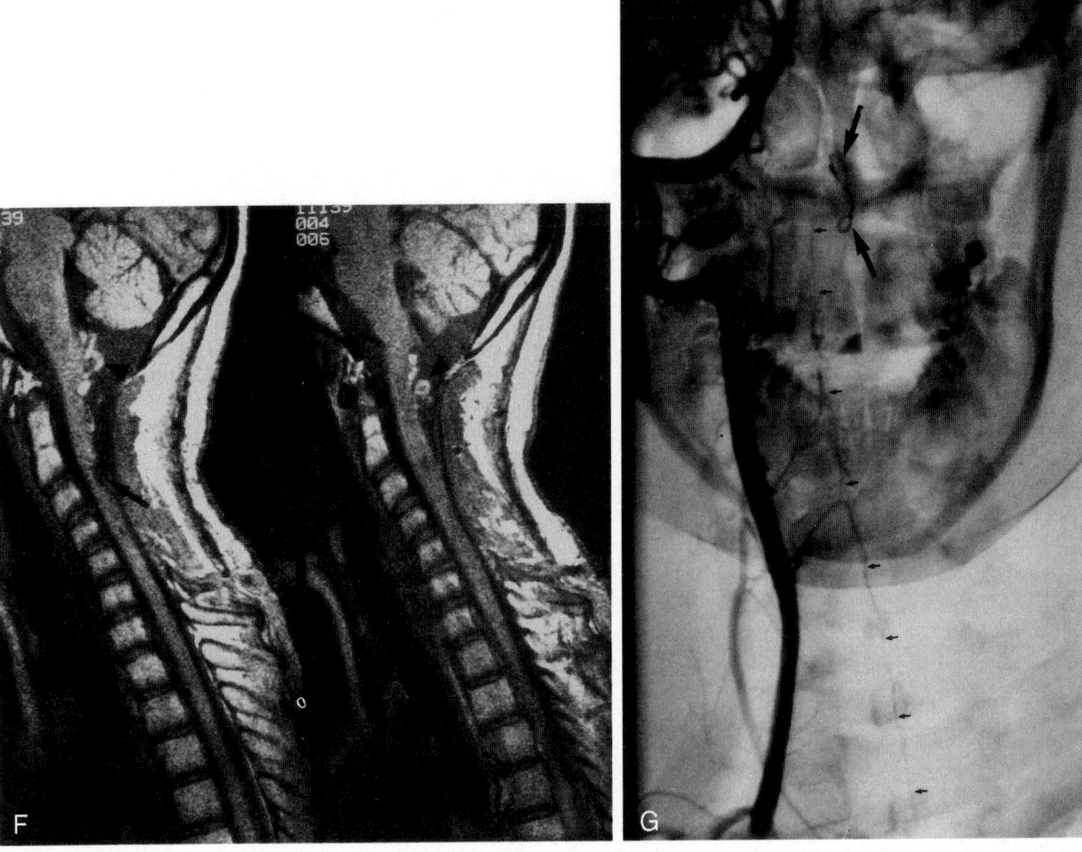

FIGURE 142–27. *Continued.* After surgery, sagittal T1-weighted MRI *(F)* revealed no abnormal signal void at the site of the previous aneurysms *(arrow)* and thrombosis of some of the abnormal veins *(arrowheads).* Arteriography *(G)* confirmed patency of the anterior spinal artery *(small arrowheads).* The *arrows* in *G* indicate the coil placed in the principal feeding vessel, a posterior spinal artery originating from the left vertebral artery, via catheterization with a 3F Tracker catheter. (From Oldfield EH: Spinal vascular malformations. In Rengachary S, Wilkins R, [eds]: Neurosurgical Operative Atlas. Rolling Meadows, IL, American Association of Neurological Surgeons, 1994.)

ceive early diagnosis and interruption before they have serious neurological deficits.[23, 25, 57, 60]

Cavernous Angiomas

Most cavernous angiomas of the spinal cord are diagnosed after they cause myelopathy by a cycle of repeated small hemorrhages and gliosis. The usual considerations for surgery of intraparenchymal cord lesions must be considered. Lesions lying in the dorsal half of the cord, which are immediately accessible with a limited myelotomy over the most superficial aspect of the lesion (frequently indicated by bluish gray discoloration of the pia; see Fig. 142–6), require less manipulation of the spinal cord for exposure, are associated with less risk of additional neurological injury during surgery, and have a more favorable prognosis for improvement after removal than do the ventral lesions. Techniques for removing cavernous angiomas are similar to those for excising benign intramedullary spinal cord tumors, with the exception that at some sites the margin of the cavernoma may be more adherent to the contiguous spinal cord than is common in benign tumors. Because residual portions of cavernous angiomas, left in situ during surgery, tend to rehemorrhage and cause recurrent myelopathy,[129, 130] complete excision is mandatory and requires careful inspection of the bed of the angioma in the spinal cord before closure.[29, 79, 130–132]

With cavernous angiomas, the outcome after surgery, as with dural and intradural spinal AVMs, depends greatly on the patient's neurological function before surgery.[29, 79, 129–131, 133–137] Fifteen percent to 25% of patients with spinal cord cavernous angiomas have an increased deficit immediately after surgery. However, these generally resolve with time, leaving most patients with improvement or stabilization of their neurological deficits. Thus, the early and long-term outcome of surgical excision of cavernomas of the spinal cord is one of improvement or stabilization.[129, 130, 135]

Unlike in patients with significant or progressing neurological deficits, excision of asymptomatic spinal cord cavernous malformations is controversial, primarily because information on their natural history is in-

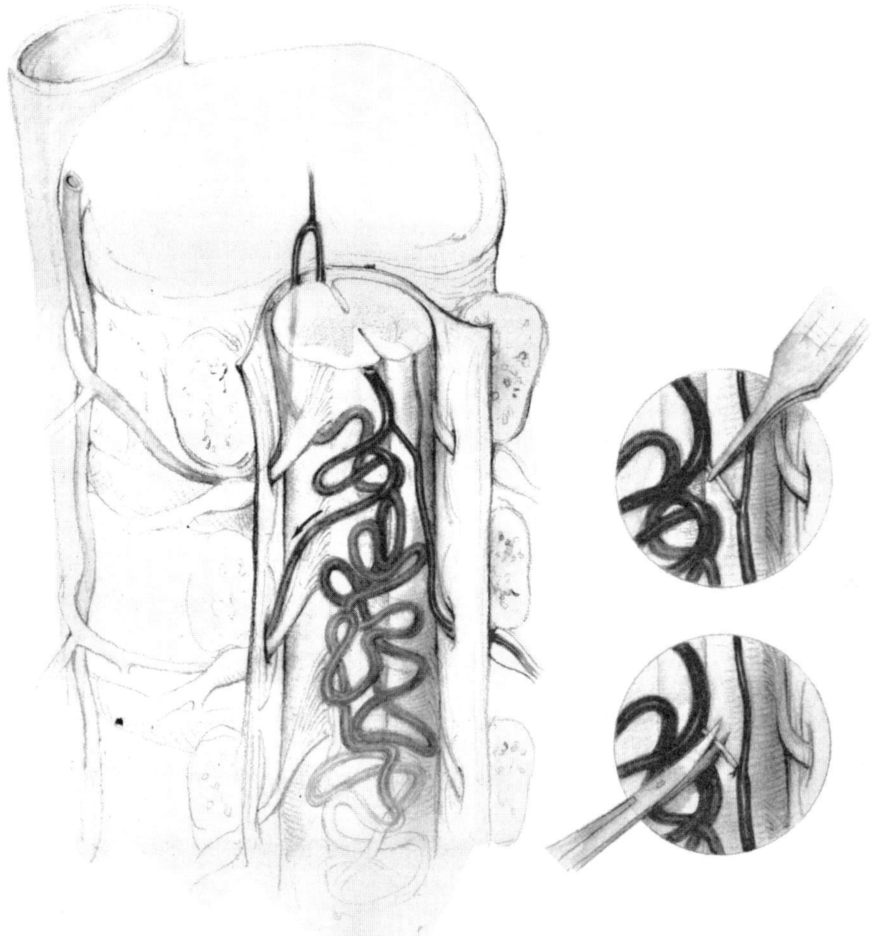

FIGURE 142–28. Intradural arteriovenous fistula (AVF) in the pia (perimedullary AVF). Medullary arteries provide the arterial supply, in this instance via a posterior spinal artery. Note the dilatation of the vein just distal to the arteriovenous shunt. The site of arterial-to-venous transition is identified, and after bipolar coagulation of a 4- to 6-mm segment of the distal portion of the artery to the AVF, the arteriovenous shunt is interrupted on the distal portion of the arterial side of the fistula, beyond the last arterial branch to the spinal cord. In some instances, a small clip or ligature is required, but most feeders can be managed by bipolar coagulation and sharp interruption alone. Many of these lesions are not as simple as the one illustrated here. These lesions can have more than one simple fistula in the same region of the pia, and the tortuosity and dilatation of the venous drainage often obscure the site of the AVF beneath a nest of blood vessels. (Drawing by Howard Bartner, NIH; from Oldfield EH: Spinal vascular malformations. In Rengachary S, Wilkins R [eds]: Neurosurgical Operative Atlas. Rolling Meadows, IL, American Association of Neurological Surgeons 1994.)

complete. Some cavernous angiomas remain asymptomatic and undetected or are detected incidentally, such as during spinal screening in a patient with a symptom-producing cavernous angioma of the brain. One recent clinicoradiographic study of the natural history of familial, mostly cerebral, cavernous malformations reported a 6.5% annual rate of symptomatic (re)hemorrhage,[138] but it is unclear whether these data can be extrapolated to the treatment of asymptomatic cavernous malformations of the spinal cord. Therefore, recommendations for treatment must consider the patient's symptoms, evidence of progression, and projected risks of surgery. Until more information is available, there is no compelling argument for treatment of asymptomtic cavernous angiomas of the spinal cord.

SUMMARY

The increased understanding of the epidemiology, pathophysiology, and anatomy of vascular lesions affecting the spinal cord over the past 2 decades permits them to be categorized based on distinctive biologic features. Current techniques of diagnosis and treatment permit early detection, precise anatomic definition, and successful treatment of most patients with spinal vascular malformations. Although MRI is increasingly useful, myelography is also a sensitive screening test for spinal AVMS in patients with a typical clinical syndrome and ambiguous findings on MRI. Selective spinal arteriography is required for categorization of the AVM, anatomic definition of the vascular supply of the AVM and spinal cord in the region of the AVM, and optimal treatment.

Successful management of spinal AVMs and avoidance of neurological impairment are highly dependent on the type of lesion and the timing of treatment. The dural AVF is the most common type of spinal AVM and the most amenable to treatment. Venous congestion, the cause of myelopathy in these lesions, is effectively treated by interruption of the medullary vein as it enters the subarachnoid space, between the dural nidus and the coronal venous plexus. Embolization of an untreated dural AVF in an acutely deteriorating patient stabilizes the deficit and provides adequate time for definitive surgical treatment.

Definitive treatment of intradural AVMS of the spinal cord is more difficult than that for dural AVFs. Intradural spinal AVMs impair cord function by hemorrhage, venous congestion, compression by aneurysm or varix, and ischemia secondary to vascular steal. Patients with inoperable thoracic or lumbar intramedullary AVMs can often be successfully managed with serial endovascular particulate embolization. Although no definitive studies are available, certain cervical intramedullary lesions can best be treated surgically if they are small and have a pial presentation. Most perimedullary AVFs can be effectively treated with surgical interruption, embolic occlusion, or embolization combined with surgery. Most symptom-producing cavernous malformations of the spinal cord can be easily diagnosed with MRI and treated safely and effectively by surgical excision.

The outcome after treatment of dural AVFs, intradural AVMs of the spinal cord, perimedullary AVFs, and cavernous angiomas depends not only on the type and location of the lesion but also on the patient's preoperative neurological function. Patients who are ambulatory before treatment are usually ambulatory after treatment. Optimal outcome depends on early diagnosis and intervention.

REFERENCES

1. Oldfield E, Doppman J: Spinal arteriovenous malformations. Clin Neurosurg 34:161–183, 1988.
2. Oldfield EH: Spinal arteriovenous malformations. In Wilkins RH, Rengachary SS (eds): Neurosurgery Update II. New York, McGraw-Hill, 1991, pp 186–196.
3. Elsberg C: Diagnosis and Treatment of Surgical Diseases of Spinal Cord and Its Membranes. Philadelphia, Saunders, 1916.
4. Oldfield EH, DiChiro G, Quindlen EA: Successful treatment of a group of spinal cord arteriovenous malformations by interruption of dural fistula. J Neurosurg 59:1019–1030, 1983.
5. Sargent P: Hemangioma of the pia mater causing compression paraplegia. Brain 48:259–267, 1925.
6. Wyburn-Mason R: The Vascular Abnormalities and Tumors of the Spinal Cord and Its Membranes. London, H. Klimpton, 1943.
7. Baker HL, Love JG, Layton DD: Angiographic and surgical aspects of spinal vascular anomalies. Radiology 88:1078–1085, 1967.
8. DiChiro G, Doppman J, Ommaya A: Selective arteriography of arteriovenous aneurysms of spinal cord. Radiology 88:1067–1077, 1967.
9. Doppman J, DiChiro G, Ommaya A: Selective Arteriography of the Spinal Cord. St. Louis, Warren H. Green, 1969.
10. Doppman J: The nidus concept of spinal cord arteriovenous fistulas: A surgical recommendation based upon angiographic observations. Br J Radiol 44:758–763, 1971.
11. Newton T, Adams J: Angiographic demonstration and nonsurgical embolization of spinal cord angioma. Radiology 91:873, 1968.
12. Krayenbuhl H, Yasargil M, McClintock H: Treatment of spinal cord vascular malformations by surgical excision. J Neurosurg 30:427–435, 1969.
13. Malis L: Microsurgery for spinal cord arteriovenous malformations. Clin Neurosurg 26:543–555, 1979.
14. Kendall B, Logue V: Spinal epidural angiomatous malformations draining into intrathecal veins. Neuroradiology 3:181–189, 1977.
15. Djindjian M, Djindjian R, Rey A, et al: Intradural extramedullary spinal arteriovenous malformations fed by the anterior spinal artery. Surg Neurol 8:85–93, 1977.
16. Gillilan L: The arterial blood supply to the human spinal cord. J Comp Neurol 110:75, 1958.
17. Suh T, Alexander L: Vascular system of the human spinal cord. Arch Neurol Psychiatry 41:659–677, 1939.
18. Turnbull I: Microvasculature of the human spinal cord. J Neurosurg 35:141–147, 1971.
19. Taveras J, Wood E: Diagnostic neuroradiolgy. In Taveras J, Wood E (eds): Baltimore, Williams & Wilkins, 1976, pp 1180–1181.
20. Gillilan L: Veins of the spinal cord: Anatomic details; suggested clinical applications. Neurology 20:860–868, 1970.
21. McCutcheon IE, Doppman JL, Oldfield EH: Microvascular anatomy of dural arteriovenous abnormalities of the spine: A microangiographic study. J Neurosurg 84:215–220, 1996.
22. Merland J, Riche M, Chiras J: Intraspinal extramedullary arteriovenous fistulae draining into the medullary veins. J Neuroradiol 7:271–320, 1980.
23. Rosenblum B, Oldfield E, Doppman J, DiChiro G: Spinal arteriovenous malformations: A comparison of dural arteriovenous fistulas and intradural AVMs in 81 patients. J Neurosurg 67: 795–802, 1987.
24. Heros R, Debrun G, Ojemann R, et al: Direct spinal arteriovenous fistula: A new type of spinal AVM: Case report. J Neurosurg 64:134, 1986.
25. Gueguen B, Merland J, Riche M, Rey A: Vascular malformations of the spinal cord: Intrathecal perimedullary arteriovenous fistulas fed by medullary arteries. Neurology 37:969–979, 1987.
26. Aminoff M, Gutin P, Norman D: Unusual type of spinal arteriovenous malformation. Neurosurgery 22:589–591, 1988.
27. Rigamonti D, Hadley M, Drayer B, et al: Cerebral cavernous malformations: Incidence and familial occurrence. N Engl J Med 319:343–347, 1988.
28. Bicknell J, Carlow T, Kornfeld M: Familial cavernous angiomas. Arch Neurol 35:746, 1978.
29. Cosgrove G, Bertrand G, Fontaine S, et al: Cavernous angiomas of the spinal cord. J Neurosurg 68:31–34, 1988.
30. Craig HD, Gunel M, Cepeda O, et al: Multilocus linkage identifies two new loci for a mendelian form of stroke, cerebral cavernous malformation, at 7p15-13 and 3q25.2-27. Hum Mol Genet 7:1851–1858, 1998.
31. Gunel M, Awad IA, Anson J, Lifton RP: Mapping a gene causing cerebral cavernous malformation to 7q11.2-q21. Proc Natl Acad Sci U S A 92:6620–6624, 1995.
32. Gunel M, Awad IA, Finberg K, et al: Genetic heterogeneity of inherited cerebral cavernous malformation. Neurosurgery 38: 1265–1271, 1996.
33. Gunel M, Awad IA, Finberg K, et al: A founder mutation as a cause of cerebral cavernous malformation in Hispanic Americans. N Engl J Med 334:946–951, 1996.
34. Dubovsky J, Zabramski JM, Kurth J, et al: A gene responsible for cavernous malformations of the brain maps to chromosome 7q. Hum Mol Genet 4:453–458, 1995.
35. Polymeropoulos MH, Hurko O, Hsu F, et al: Linkage of the locus for cerebral cavernous hemangiomas to human chromosome 7q in four families of Mexican-American descent. Neurology 48:752–757, 1997.
36. Brunereau L, Gobin YP, Meder JF, et al: Intracranial dural arteriovenous fistulas with spinal venous drainage: Relation between clinical presentation and angiographic findings. AJNR Am J Neuroradiol 17:1549–1554, 1996.
37. Weingrad DN, Doppman JL, Chreitien PB, DiChiro G: Paraplegia due to posttraumatic pelvic arteriovenous fistula treated by surgery and embolization. J Neurosurg 50:805–810, 1979.
38. Yoshino O, Matsui H, Hirano N, Tsuji H: Acquired dural arteriovenous malformation of the lumbar spine: Case report. Neurosurgery 42:1387–1389, 1998.
39. Hassler W, Thron A, Grote E: Hemodynamics of spinal dural arteriovenous fistulas: An intraoperative study. J Neurosurg 70: 360, 1989.
40. Symon L, Kuyama H, Kendall B: Dural arteriovenous malformations of the spine: Clinical features and surgical results in 55 cases. J Neurosurg 60:238–247, 1984.
41. Foix C, Alajouanine T: La melite necrotique subaique. Rev Neurol 2:1, 1926.
42. Criscuolo G, Oldfield E, Doppman J: Reversible acute and subacute myelopathy in patient with dural arteriovenous fistulas: Foix-Alajouanine syndrome reconsidered. J Neurosurg 70:354, 1989.
43. Oldfield E: Spinal vascular malformations. In Swash M (ed): Outcomes in Neurological and Neurosurgical Disorders. Cambridge, UK, Cambridge University Press, 1998.
44. Aminoff M, Logue V: Clinical features of spinal vascular malformations. Brain 97:197–210, 1974.
45. Aminoff M, Logue V: The prognosis of patients with spinal vascular malformations. Brain 97:211–218, 1974.

46. Hurth M, Houdart R, Djindjian R, et al: Arteriovenous malformations of the spinal cord: Clinical, anatomical and therapeutic considerations—a series of 150 cases. Progr Neurol Surg 9: 238–266, 1978.
47. Tobin W, Layton D: The diagnosis and natural history of spinal cord arteriovenous malformations. Mayo Clin Proc 51:637–646, 1976.
48. Aminoff M, Barnard R, Logue V: The pathophysiology of spinal vascular malformations. J Neurol Sci 23:255–263, 1974.
49. Logue V: Angiomas of the spinal cord: Review of the pathogenesis, clinical features, and results of surgery. J Neurol Neurosurg Psychiatry 42:1–11, 1979.
50. Riche M, Modensesi-Freitas J, Djindjian M, Merland J: Arteriovenous malformations (AVM) of the spinal cord in children: A review of 38 cases. Neuroradiology 22:171–180, 1982.
51. Riche M, Melki J, Merland J: Embolization of spinal cord vascular malformations via the anterior spinal artery. AJNR Am J Neuroradiol 4:378–381, 1983.
52. Djindjian M, Djindjian R, Hurth M, et al: Steal phenomenon in spinal arteriovenous malformations. J Neuroradiol 5:187, 1978.
53. Bandyopadhyay S, Sheth RD: Acute spinal cord infarction: Vascular steal in arteriovenous malformation. J Child Neurol 14: 685–687, 1999.
54. Biondi A, Merland JJ, Reizine D, et al: Embolization with particles in thoracic intramedullary arteriovenous malformations: Long-term angiographic and clinical results. Radiology 177:651–658, 1990.
55. Cogen P, Stein B: Spinal cord arteriovenous malformations with significant intramedullary components. J Neurosurg 59:471–478, 1983.
56. Yasargil M, Symon L, Teddy P: Arteriovenous malformations of the spinal cord. In Symon L (ed): Advances and Technical Standards in Neurosurgery, vol 11. Vienna, Springer-Verlag, 1984, pp 61–102.
57. Mourier KL, Gobin YP, George B, et al: Intradural perimedullary arteriovenous fistulae: Results of surgical and endovascular treatment in a series of 35 cases. Neurosurgery 32:885–891, 1993.
58. Sure U, Wakat J, Gatscher S, et al: Spinal type IV arteriovenous malformations (perimedullary fistulas) in children. Childs Nerv Syst 16:508–515, 2000.
59. Barrow DL, Colohan AR, Dawson R: Intradural perimedullary arteriovenous fistulas (type IV spinal cord arteriovenous malformations). J Neurosurg 81:221–229, 1994.
60. Hida K, Iwasaki Y, Goto K, et al: Results of the surgical treatment of perimedullary arteriovenous fistulas with special reference to embolization. J Neurosurg 90:198–205, 1999.
61. Simard J, Garcia-Bengochea F, Ballinger W, et al: Cavernous angioma: A review of 126 collected and 12 new clinical cases. Neurosurgery 18:162, 1986.
62. Voight K, Yasargil M: Cerebral cavernous hemangiomas or cavernomas: Incidence, pathology, localization, diagnosis, clinical features and treatment. Review of the literature and report of an unusual case. Neurochirurgica (Stuttg) 19:59, 1976.
63. Brunereau L, Labauge P, Tournier-Lasserve E, et al: Familial form of intracranial cavernous angioma: MR imaging findings in 51 families. French Society of Neurosurgery. Radiology 214: 209–216, 2000.
64. Hayman LA, Evans RA, Ferrell RE, et al: Familial cavernous angiomas: Natural history and genetic study over a 5-year period. Am J Med Genet 11:147–160, 1982.
65. Labauge P, Laberge S, Brunereau L, et al: Hereditary cerebral cavernous angiomas: Clinical and genetic features in 57 French families. Societe Francaise de Neurochirurgie. Lancet 352:1892–1897, 1998.
66. Passarin MG, Salviati A, Gambina G, et al: Familial cavernous hemangioma with atypical neuroimaging. Ital J Neurol Sci 17: 295–300, 1996.
67. Siegel AM: Familial cavernous angioma: An unknown, known disease [editorial; comment]. Acta Neurol Scand 98:369–371, 1998.
68. Siegel AM, Andermann E, Badhwar A, et al: Anticipation in familial cavernous angioma: A study of 52 families from International Familial Cavernous Angioma Study. IFCAS Group [letter]. Lancet 352:1676–1677, 1998.
69. Gil-Nagel A, Dubovsky J, Wilcox KJ, et al: Familial cerebral cavernous angioma: A gene localized to a 15-cM interval on chromosome 7q. Ann Neurol 39:807–810, 1996; erratum in Ann Neurol 40:480, 1996.
70. Johnson EW, Iyer LM, Rich SS, et al: Refined localization of the cerebral cavernous malformation gene (CCM1) to a 4-cM interval of chromosome 7q contained in a well-defined YAC contig. Genome Res 5:368–380, 1995.
71. Laberge S, Labauge P, Marechal E, et al: Genetic heterogeneity and absence of founder effect in a series of 36 French cerebral cavernous angiomas families. Eur J Hum Genet 7:499–504, 1999.
72. Notelet L, Chapon F, Khoury S, et al: Familial cavernous malformations in a large French kindred: Mapping of the gene to the CCM1 locus on chromosome 7q. J Neurol Neurosurg Psychiatry 63:40–45, 1997.
73. Siegel AM, Andermann F, Badhwar A, et al: Anticipation in familial cavernous angioma: Ascertainment bias or genetic cause. Acta Neurol Scand 98:372–376, 1998; see comments.
74. Zhang J, Clatterbuck RE, Rigamonti D, Dietz HC: Mutations in KRIT1 in familial cerebral cavernous malformations. Neurosurgery 46:1272–1277, discussion 1277–1279, 2000.
75. Maraire JN, Abdulrauf SI, Berger S, et al: De novo development of a cavernous malformation of the spinal cord following spinal axis radiation: Case report. J Neurosurg 90:234–238, 1999.
76. Massa-Micon B, Luparello V, Bergui M, Pagni CA: De novo cavernoma case report and review of literature. Surg Neurol 53: 484–487, 2000.
77. Larson H, Ball W, Bove K, et al: Formation of intracerebral cavernous malformations after radiation treatment for central nervous system neoplasia in children. J Neurosurg 88:51–56, 1998.
78. Novelli P, Reigel D, Gleatson P, Yunis E: Multiple cavernous angiomas after high-dose whole-brain radiation therapy. Pediatr Neurosurg 26:322–325, 1997.
79. Ogilvy C, Louis D, Ojemann R: Intramedullary cavernous angiomas of the spinal cord: Clinical presentation, pathological features, and surgical management. Neurosurgery 31:219–230, 1992.
80. DiChiro G, Doppman J, Dwyer A, et al: Tumors and arteriovenous malformations of the spinal cord: Assessment using MR. Radiology 156:689–697, 1985.
81. Doppman J, DiChiro G, Dwyer A, et al: Magnetic resonance imaging of spinal cord arteriovenous malformations. J Neurosurg 66:830–834, 1987.
82. Masaryk T, Ross J, Modic M, et al: Radiculomeningeal vascular malformations of the spine: MR imaging. Radiology 164:845–849, 1987.
83. Minami S, Sagoh T, Nishimura K, et al: Spinal arteriovenous malformations: MR imaging. Radiology 169:109–115, 1988.
84. Dormont D, Gelbert F, Assouline E, et al: MR imaging of spinal arteriovenous malformations at 0.5 T: Study of 34 cases. AJNR Am J Neuroradiol 9:833–838, 1988.
85. Terwey B, Becker H, Thron A, Vahldiek G: Gadolinium-DTPA enhanced MR imaging of spinal dural arteriovenous fistulas. J Comput Assist Tomogr 13:30–37, 1989.
86. Gilbertson JR, Miller GM, Goldman MS, Marsh WR: Spinal dural arteriovenous fistulas: MR and myelographic findings. AJNR Am J Neuroradiol 16:2049–2057, 1995.
87. Hurst RW, Grossman RI: Peripheral spinal cord hypointensity on T2-weighted MR images: A reliable imaging sign of venous hypertensive myelopathy. AJNR Am J Neuroradiol 21:781–786, 2000; see comments.
88. Willinsky RA, terBrugge K, Montanera W, et al: Posttreatment MR findings in spinal dural arteriovenous malformations. AJNR Am J Neuroradiol 16:2063–2071, 1995.
89. Horikoshi T, Hida K, Iwasaki Y, et al: Chronological changes in MRI findings of spinal dural arteriovenous fistula. Surg Neurol 53:243–249, 2000.
90. Mourier KL, Gelbert F, Rey A, et al: Spinal dural arteriovenous malformations with perimedullary drainage: Indications and results of surgery in 30 cases. Acta Neurochir (Wien) 100:136–141, 1989.
91. Woimant F, Merland J, Riche M, et al: Syndrome bulbo-medullaire en rapport avec une fistule arterio-venueuse meningee

dusinus lateral a drainage veineux medullaire. Rev Neurol 138: 559–566, 1982.

92. Wrobel CJ, Oldfield EH, DiChiro G, et al: Myelopathy due to intracranial dural arteriovenous fistulas draining intrathecally into spinal medullary veins: Report of three cases. J Neurosurg 69:934–939, 1988.
93. Thompson B, Oldfield E: Spinal vascular malformations. In Carter L, Spetzler R, Hamilton M (eds): Neurovascular Surgery. New York, McGraw-Hill, 1994, pp 1167–1195.
94. Stein SC, Ommaya A, Doppman JL, DiChiro G: Arteriovenous malformation of the cauda equina with arterial supply from branches of the internal iliac arteries. J Neurosurg 36:649–651, 1972.
95. Larsen DW, Halbach VV, Teitelbaum GP, et al: Spinal dural arteriovenous fistulas supplied by branches of the internal iliac arteries. Surg Neurol 43:35–40, discussion 40–41, 1995.
96. Leussenhop A, De La Cruz T: The surgical excision of spinal intradural vascular malformations. J Neurosurg 330:552, 1969.
97. Morgan MK, Marsh WR: Management of spinal dural arteriovenous malformations. J Neurosurg 70:832–836, 1989.
98. Behrens S, Thron A: Long-term follow-up and outcome in patients treated for spinal dural arteriovenous fistula. J Neurol 246:181–185, 1999.
99. Westphal M, Koch C: Management of spinal dural arteriovenous fistulae using an interdisciplinary neuroradiological/neurosurgical approach: Experience with 47 cases. Neurosurgery 45: 451–457, discussion 457–458, 1999.
100. Afshar JK, Doppman JL, Oldfield EH: Surgical interruption of intradural draining vein as curative treatment of spinal dural arteriovenous fistulas. J Neurosurg 82:196–200, 1995; see comments.
101. Doppman J, DiChiro G, Oldfield E: Origin of spinal arteriovenous malformation and normal cord vasculature from a common segmental artery: Angiographic and therapeutic considerations. Radiology 154:687–689, 1985.
102. Tacconi L, Lopez Izquierdo BC, Symon L: Outcome and prognostic factors in the surgical treatment of spinal dural arteriovenous fistulas: A long-term study. Br J Neurosurg 11:298–305, 1997.
103. Thompson BG, Doppman JL, Oldfield EH: Treatment of cranial dural arteriovenous fistulae by interruption of leptomeningeal venous drainage. J Neurosurg 80:617–623, 1994.
104. Mullan S: Reflections upon the nature and management of intracranial and intraspinal vascular malformations and fistulae. J Neurosurg 80:606–616, 1994.
105. Hall W, Oldfield E, Doppman J: Recanalization of spinal cord arteriovenous malformations following embolization. J Neurosurg 70:714, 1989.
106. Gruber A, Mazal P, Bavinski G, et al: Repermeation of partially embolized cerebral arteriovenous malformations: A clinical, radiologic, and histologic study. AJNR Am J Neuroradiol 17: 1323–1331, 1996.
107. Birchall D, Hughes DG, West CG: Recanalisation of spinal dural arteriovenous fistula after successful embolisation. J Neurol Neurosurg Psychiatry 68:792–793, 2000.
108. Merland J, Assouline E, Rufenacht D, et al: Dural spinal arteriovenous fistulae draining into medullary veins: Clinical and radiological results of treatment (embolization and surgery) in 56 cases. In XIIIth Congress of the European Society of Neuroradiology. Amsterdam, Elsevier, 1985.
109. Niimi Y, Berenstein A, Setton A, Neophytides A: Embolization of spinal dural arteriovenous fistulae: Results and follow-up. Neurosurgery 40:675–682, discussion 682–683, 1997.
110. Djindjian R: Embolization of angiomas of the spinal cord. Surg Neurol 4:411–420, 1975.
111. Yasargil M, DeLong W, Guarnaschelli J: Complete microsurgical excision of cervical extramedullary and intramedullary vascular malformations. Surg Neurol 4:211–224, 1975.
112. Connolly ES Jr, Zubay GP, McCormick PC, Stein BM: The posterior approach to a series of glomus (type II) intramedullary spinal cord arteriovenous malformations. Neurosurgery 42:774–785, discussion 785–786, 1998.
113. Oldfield EH: Technique.
114. Schievink WI, Vishteh AG, McDougall CG, Spetzler RF: Intraoperative spinal angiography. J Neurosurg 90:48–51, 1999.
115. Barrow DL, Boyer KL, Joseph GJ: Intraoperative angiography in the management of neurovascular disorders. Neurosurgery 30:153–159, 1992; see comments.
116. Martin NA, Khanna RK, Batzdorf U: Posterolateral cervical or thoracic approach with spinal cord rotation for vascular malformations or tumors of the ventrolateral spinal cord. J Neurosurg 83:254–261, 1995; see comments.
117. Markert JM, Chandler WF, Deveikis JP, Ross DA: Use of the extreme lateral approach in the surgical treatment of an intradural ventral cervical spinal cord vascular malformation: Technical case report. Neurosurgery 38:412–415, 1996.
118. Touho H, Karasawa J, Shishido H, et al: Successful excision of a juvenile-type spinal arteriovenous malformation following intraoperative embolization: Case report. J Neurosurg 75:647–651, 1991.
119. Spetzler RF, Zabramski JM, Flom RA: Management of juvenile spinal AVMs by embolization and operative excision: Case report. J Neurosurg 70:628–632, 1989.
120. Houdart R, Djindjian R, Hurth M, Rey A: Treatment of angiomas of the spinal cord. Surg Neurol 2:186–194, 1974.
121. Ausman J, Gold L, Tadavarthy S, et al: Intraparenchymal embolization for obliteration of an intramedullary AVM of the spinal cord. J Neurosurg 47:119–125, 1977.
122. Doppman J, DiChiro G, Ommaya A: Percutaneous embolisation of spinal cord arteriovenous malformations. J Neurosurg 34: 48–55, 1971.
123. Latchaw R, Harris R, Chou S, et al: Combined embolization and operation in the treatment of cervical arteriovenous malformations. Neurosurgery 6:131–137, 1980.
124. Doppman J, DiChiro G, Ommaya A: Obliteration of spinal-cord arteriovenous malformations by percutaneous embolisation. Lancet 1:477, 1968.
125. Touho H, Karasawa J, Ohnishi H, et al: Superselective embolization of spinal arteriovenous malformations using the Tracker catheter. Surg Neurol 38:85–94, 1992.
126. Horton J, Latchaw R, Gold L, et al: Embolisation of intramedullary arteriovenous malformations of the spinal cord. AJNR Am J Neuroradiol 7:113–118, 1986.
127. Theron J, Cosgrove R, Melanson D, Ethier R: Spinal arteriovenous malformations: Advances in therapeutic embolization. Radiology 158:163–169, 1986.
128. Riche M, Scialfa G, Gueguen B, Merland J: Giant extramedullary arteriovenous fistulas supplied by the anterior spinal artery: Treatment by detachable balloons. AJNR Am J Neuroradiol 4: 391–394, 1983.
129. Amin-Hanjani S, Ogilvy CS, Ojemann R, Crowell RM: Risks of surgical management for cavernous malformations of the nervous system. Neurosurgery 42:1220–1228, 1998.
130. Vishteh A, Sankhla S, Anson J, et al: Surgical resection of intramedullary spinal cord cavernous malformations: Delayed complications, long-term outcomes, and associated cryptic venous malformations. Neurosurgery 41:1094–1101, 1997.
131. Anson JA, Spetzler RF: Surgical resection of intramedullary spinal cord cavernous malformations. J Neurosurg 78:446–451, 1993.
132. Tyndel F, Bilboa J, Hudson A, Colapinto E: Hemangioma calcificans of the spinal cord. Can J Neurol Sci 12:321–322, 1985.
133. McCormick P, Michelsen W, Post K, et al: Cavernous malformations of the spinal cord. Neurosurgery 23:459–463, 1988.
134. Cantore G, Delfini R, Cervoni L, et al: Intramedullary cavernous angiomas of the spinal cord: Report of six cases. Surg Neurol 43:448–452, 1995.
135. Cristante L, Herrmann H: Radical excision of intramedullary cavernous angiomas. Neurosurgery 43:424–431, 1998.
136. Padovani R, Acciarri N, Giulioni M, et al: Cavernous angiomas of the spinal district: Surgical treatment of 11 patients. Eur Spine J 6:298–303, 1997.
137. Harrison MJ, Eisenberg MB, Ullman JS, et al: Symptomatic cavernous malformations affecting the spine and spinal cord. Neurosurgery 37:195–204, discussion 204–205, 1995.
138. Zabramski JM, Wascher TM, Spetzler RF, et al: The natural history of familial cavernous malformations: Results of an ongoing study. J Neurosurg 80:422–432, 1994.
139. Ushikoshi S, Hida K, Kikuchi Y, et al: Functional prognosis after treatment of spinal dural arteriovenous fistulas. Neurol Med Chir (Tokyo) 39:206–212, discussion 212–213, 1999.

140. Lee TT, Gromelski EB, Bowen BC, Green BA: Diagnostic and surgical management of spinal dural arteriovenous fistulas. Neurosurgery 43:242–246, discussion 246–247, 1998.
141. Benhaiem N, Porrier J, Hurth M: Arteriovenous fistula of the meninges draining into the spinal veins: A histological study of 28 cases. Acta Neuropathol (Berl) 62:103–111, 1983.
142. Lundqvist C, Berthelsen B, Sullivan M, et al: Spinal arteriovenous malformations: Neurological aspects and results of embolization. Acta Neurol Scand 82:51–58, 1990.
143. Koenig E, Thron A, Schrader V, Dichgans J: Spinal arteriovenous malformations and fistulae: Clinical, neuroradiological and neurophysiological findings. J Neurol 236:260–266, 1989.

PART XII PREGNANCY AND TREATMENT OF VASCULAR DISEASE

CHAPTER 143

Pregnancy and Treatment of Vascular Disease

MARK R. HARRIGAN ■ B. GREGORY THOMPSON

Cerebrovascular disorders during pregnancy and the puerperium are infrequent but can be devastating to the mother and the fetus. Approximately 0.67% of all women of childbearing age give birth each year.[1] The precise incidence of cerebrovascular disease during pregnancy is uncertain. Estimates range from 0.3 to 9 per 100,000 deliveries[2–4]; the wide variability of these estimates is likely due to differing referral patterns and the low incidence of cerebrovascular disease in the childbearing age group in general.[5] Of maternal deaths, however, 12% to 80% are due to cerebrovascular disease.[6–8] Cerebrovascular disease during pregnancy results in higher maternal and fetal mortality and morbidity rates than in nonpregnant women of the same age.[8–10]

Cerebrovascular disorders affecting pregnant women most commonly include aneurysmal subarachnoid hemorrhage, angiomatous intracerebral hemorrhage, and ischemic stroke secondary to arterial occlusion or intracranial venous thrombosis. Other vascular disorders associated with pregnancy include oncotic aneurysms and intracerebral hemorrhage secondary to metastatic choriocarcinoma, cavernous-carotid fistulas, and pituitary apoplexy.

Physiologic changes during pregnancy, maternal and fetal needs, and disorders unique to pregnancy all present special problems to neurosurgeons managing pregnant patients with a cerebrovascular disorder. The diagnosis and management of cerebrovascular disease during pregnancy have changed dramatically. New imaging technologies, better understanding of the physiology of pregnancy, and advances in cerebrovascular surgery have enabled neurosurgeons to meet better the needs of pregnant patients.

PHYSIOLOGIC CHANGES DURING PREGNANCY

A wide variety of hemodynamic, cardiovascular, and hormonal changes that occur during pregnancy may increase the risk of intracranial vascular events and significantly affect neurosurgical management. Plasma volume increases 40% to 50% by term, and total blood volume increases 25% to 40%.[11] There are relative reductions in hemoglobin and hematocrit levels (physiologic anemia of pregnancy) because erythrocyte volume increases only about 20%.[11] These reductions are minimized with folic acid and iron supplementation; a normal minimum hematocrit level for pregnancy is 35%, and normal hemoglobin levels are 11 to 12 g/dL.[11]

Heart rate and stroke volume, the components of cardiac output, increase 29% and 18%, producing a 60% increase in cardiac output.[5, 11–13] This increase occurs during the first two trimesters of gestation, then cardiac output remains constant until term.[12, 14] An estrogen-induced reduction in uterine and systemic vascular resistance occurs to provide adequate blood flow to the uterus.[11] Arterial blood pressure may decrease 10% because the increase in cardiac output does not match the decrease in peripheral resistance.[12] Arterial pressure increases at term, and cardiac output increases by an additional 20% during uterine contractions.[5] In the third trimester, significant compression of the aorta and inferior vena cava by the gravid uterus can occur in the supine position and cause changes in blood pressure and distribution of blood flow.[7]

Uterine blood flow increases throughout pregnancy and accounts for 10% of cardiac output at term. Uterine blood flow varies directly with maternal blood pressure, placing the fetus at risk of hypoperfusion during maternal hypotension.[15] Umbilical blood vessels are sensitive to pH and constrict in response to maternal hyperventilation, which can place the fetus at risk of hypoperfusion.[16]

During pregnancy, a respiratory alkalosis occurs to balance a metabolic acidosis. Alveolar minute ventilation increases 50% to 70% because of a 40% rise in tidal volume and a 15% increase in respiratory rate.[11]

Arterial carbon dioxide tension ($Pa{CO_2}$) is reduced to about 32 mm Hg, whereas blood pH remains normal.

Regional cerebral blood flow, as measured by single-photon emission computed tomography (SPECT), increases from 7 to 19 weeks of gestation, ranging from an increase of 9.1% in the frontal lobes to 16.7% in the cerebellum.[17] The hemodynamic stress of labor may alter cerebral blood flow temporarily. During a Valsalva maneuver, blood flow through the internal carotid artery decreases 21%.[18]

Hemodynamic and hormonal changes in pregnancy lead to alterations in blood vessel wall structure, and these changes in turn may influence the behavior of vascular lesions.[5, 8, 19, 20] Progesterone, estrogen, and prostacyclins are believed to have direct effects on vascular smooth muscle, leading to generalized vasodilation in the uterus, kidneys, and skin.[12] Intimal hyperplasia of arteries and veins has been observed as well as thickening, reticular fragmentation, and loss of normal elastic corrugation of the vessel media.[12]

Many alterations in coagulation factor concentrations and blood viscosity occur during pregnancy. Thrombin formation[21]; tissue plasminogen inhibition[22]; and serum concentrations of fibrinogen[21, 23, 24] and clotting factors VII, VIII, IX, and X increase.[25–27] Fibrinolytic activity,[22, 24] tissue-type plasminogen activator,[22] and protein S[28, 29] are reduced. Platelets become more aggregable in the second and third trimesters and the puerperium.[21, 30] Although blood viscosity decreases as a result of enlargement of the plasma volume and a decrease in the hematocrit level, the combined effect of these changes is a hypercoagulable state during pregnancy and 3 weeks postpartum.[31]

PHARMACOLOGIC CONSIDERATIONS

The physiologic changes of pregnancy alter the pharmacokinetics of most drugs. Drug absorption, metabolism, clearance, protein binding, and volume of distribution all are in a state of flux throughout pregnancy. Many drugs commonly used in neurosurgery can affect the fetus adversely.[8]

Anticonvulsants

Seizure prophylaxis is necessary in many patients with cerebrovascular disorders, and control of preexisting seizure disorders is particularly important in patients with unruptured aneurysms and arteriovenous malformations (AVMs). Seizures first begin during pregnancy in 13% of all women with epilepsy,[32, 33] and pregnant women with epilepsy constitute 0.5% of all pregnancies,[34] underscoring the importance of anticonvulsants in some patients during pregnancy.

All of the commonly used anticonvulsants are established human teratogens. The greatest teratogenic risk is in the first trimester. Congenital malformations occur in 4% to 5% of the children of epileptics, a rate almost twice that of the general population.[35, 36] This high incidence is likely to be due, at least in part, to anticonvulsants. The risk of seizures, with associated maternal and fetal hypoxia and acidosis, justifies the use of anticonvulsants in pregnant patients at risk, however.[5, 8, 36–38]

Phenytoin administration can lead to the fetal hydantoin syndrome, which includes intrauterine growth retardation, microcephaly, mental retardation, and limb defects.[39] Phenobarbital and primidone are associated with craniofacial abnormalities, retarded skeletal development, limb abnormalities, and psychomotor delay.[40, 41] Carbamazepine is associated with fingernail hypoplasia, developmental delay, craniofacial abnormalities, cardiac defects,[42] and spina bifida.[43] Valproic acid is associated with fetal distress; neural tube defects; and the fetal valproate syndrome, which includes brachycephaly, mental retardation, and cardiovascular and genitourinary abnormalities.[44, 45] Benzodiazepines have a relatively low rate of teratogenicity in animal studies, but human studies have shown some association with craniofacial anomalies.[40]

Although the overall teratogenic potential of any one anticonvulsant is not substantially different from that of any other,[8, 36, 37] there is marginal evidence that carbamazepine is the most favorable.[46] Although phenytoin, phenobarbital, and valproic acid are classified by the U.S. Food and Drug Administration as Category D drugs (risk in pregnancy is definite but may be acceptable), carbamazepine is classified as a Category C drug (risk in pregnancy is unknown).[47] The maternal risk of drug-induced agranulocytosis or aplastic anemia, coupled with the fact that carbamazepine can be administered orally only, reduces the advantages of carbamazepine over the other commonly used anticonvulsants.[5]

Several general guidelines exist to minimize the risk of complications from anticonvulsant therapy. First, anticonvulsants should be limited to patients at significant risk of developing a seizure disorder. Second, physiologic changes of pregnancy alter the pharmacokinetics of all commonly used anticonvulsants in many ways, necessitating use of the lowest possible dose and frequent monitoring (at least monthly) of serum anticonvulsant levels. Drug metabolism gradually returns to normal during the puerperium, indicating that anticonvulsant levels should be monitored for at least 1 month postpartum.[8] Third, vitamin K and folate supplementation are recommended during pregnancy to oppose anticonvulsant interaction with folic acid and phytomenadione (vitamin K) metabolism, which can increase the risk of neural tube defects and early neonatal bleeding.[34] Anticonvulsant monotherapy is preferred over polytherapy when possible.[48] The newer anticonvulsants are not recommended in pregnancy and require further research to prove their safety in humans.[34, 38] With proper management, 95% of pregnancies in women taking anticonvulsants have favorable outcomes.[34, 49]

Anticoagulants

Short-term anticoagulation is needed for management of acute ischemic stroke, venous sinus thrombosis, deep venous thrombosis, and some neurovascular procedures. Long-term anticoagulation is necessary for pregnant patients at risk of embolic stroke, such as women with artificial heart valves. Anticoagulation during pregnancy is associated with significant risk, but measures can be taken to minimize the risk and to provide a normal outcome in approximately two thirds of cases.[50–52]

Heparin does not cross the placental barrier.[51, 53] No known congenital abnormalities are associated with heparin use during pregnancy,[40] and fetal hemorrhage is not a risk.[40] Heparin anticoagulation is associated with the same maternal risks in pregnant patients as in nonpregnant patients,[40] however, including maternal hemorrhage, thrombocytopenia,[54] anaphylaxis, fat necrosis, and alopecia.[53] Osteoporosis also is a risk; 36% of women who received heparin during pregnancy had decreased bone density after delivery.[55] Maternal hemorrhage is the most common and significant risk, occurring in about 10% of pregnant patients taking heparin, and it is associated with a 2% mortality rate.[51–53] Stillbirth has been reported in one eighth of cases and prematurity in one fifth.[50]

Coumarin derivatives cross the placental barrier and are established teratogens. Reports of the incidence of congenital anomalies in the children of pregnant patients treated with coumarin are 30%.[50, 52, 53] The most common fetal effect of coumarin is the fetal warfarin syndrome, consisting of facial abnormalities, scoliosis, low birth weight, hypoplasia of the digits or extremities, and developmental retardation.[40] Fetal warfarin syndrome results from coumarin exposure during the first trimester, specifically from the sixth to the ninth week of gestation.[50, 52, 53] Spontaneous abortion is a significant risk associated with coumarin treatment during the first trimester.[56] Abnormalities associated with coumarin exposure during the second and third trimesters are less common and include central nervous system and ocular developmental anomalies, mental retardation, spasticity, seizure disorders, deafness, scoliosis, and growth retardation.[50–52, 57] Prematurity, stillbirth, and fetal hemorrhage also are reported in pregnant women taking coumarin.[58, 59]

The choice of anticoagulant for use during pregnancy depends on the stage of pregnancy. Use of heparin during the first trimester has resulted in good outcomes with respect to the fetal warfarin syndrome in most cases.[52, 57, 60] Most authors recommend substitution of coumarin during the second and third trimesters, given the relative safety of this drug after the first trimester.[40] Use of heparin during the final month of pregnancy allows rapid control of coagulation parameters during delivery. Alternatively, subcutaneous injection of low-molecular-weight heparin can be used safely throughout pregnancy and has a lower incidence of associated osteoporosis than unfractionated heparin.[61] Coagulation parameters must be monitored frequently, particularly in the final months of pregnancy, when higher doses of anticoagulants may be required to oppose the physiologic hypercoagulable state that occurs toward term.[52] The patient should be kept fully appraised of the risks and benefits of anticoagulation during pregnancy.[40]

Antiplatelet Agents

Antiplatelet agents are useful in patients with or at risk of ischemic stroke. Low doses of aspirin (60 to 150 mg) in the second and third trimesters were safe in a large clinical trial of the drug for the prevention of preeclampsia.[62] The safety of aspirin in the first trimester or of higher doses is unknown.[63] No teratogenic effects of ticlopidine have been reported in animal studies, but human studies have not been done.[64] Ticlopidine is recommended for patients who are unable to tolerate aspirin or if symptoms recur while patients are on aspirin.[64]

Mannitol

The osmotic diuretic mannitol is effective in treating elevated intracranial pressure. Mannitol crosses the placenta, however, and can increase fetal plasma osmolarity.[65] The potential for fetal dehydration led early authors to recommend against the use of mannitol in pregnant patients.[7] Fetal outcome data are limited, however,[40] and mannitol has been used without apparent adverse sequelae.[66] Consequently, more recent recommendations have favored the limited use of mannitol in cases of life-threatening elevated intracranial pressure.[65, 67]

Nimodipine

The calcium channel blocker nimodipine improves outcomes in patients with aneurysmal subarachnoid hemorrhage. Although there is some experimental evidence that nimodipine is associated with congenital malformations and intrauterine growth retardation,[68, 69] no adequate human studies have evaluated the risk of taking this drug during pregnancy.[40] Several authors recommend that nimodipine be offered to all patients in Hunt and Hess grades I to II after subarachnoid hemorrhage, with appropriate discussion of the possible risks and benefits with the mother, if possible.[31, 40] The blood pressure of pregnant patients treated with nimodipine should be monitored closely to avoid hypotension.[5] Postpartum patients on nimodipine should be advised against breast-feeding because the drug is highly concentrated in breast milk.[68, 69]

Antihypertensives

Hypertension occurs in one third of all pregnancies and usually is associated with preeclampsia or eclampsia.[5] Sustained or paroxysmal hypertension in pregnant patients with cerebrovascular disease is a substantial risk factor for further complications and should be treated. Antihypertensives should be used with caution, however. Uterine blood flow varies directly with maternal blood pressure, and any intervention that lowers maternal blood pressure can lower fetal blood flow to dangerous levels.[8] Maternal hypotension to less than 100 mm Hg systolic can produce uterine hypoperfusion and fetal bradycardia.[15] Prolonged maternal hypotension in animal models produces behavioral changes in the offspring that closely resemble cerebral palsy.[15]

Sodium nitroprusside has been used successfully in pregnant patients undergoing aneurysm surgery[66, 70]; however, fetal toxicity has been shown in animal studies.[71] The National High Blood Pressure Education Working Group recommended methyldopa for nonsevere hypertension during pregnancy and hydralazine for severe hypertension (diastolic blood pressure >104 mm Hg).[72]

Antifibrinolytic Agents

Antifibrinolytic therapy with ε-aminocaproic acid or tranexamic acid has been used in patients with subarachnoid hemorrhage to inhibit lysis of the clot within the aneurysm to prevent rebleeding. This approach is attractive in pregnant patients with subarachnoid hemorrhage, who have a higher incidence of rebleeding than nonpregnant patients. These agents are associated with an increased risk of thrombotic side effects, however, and are not recommended for use in pregnant patients.[5, 65]

OPERATIVE CONSIDERATIONS

Alterations in pulmonary mechanics have important implications in anesthetic management. Increased alveolar minute ventilation results in faster anesthetic induction, a 25% to 40% decrease in the minimal anesthetic concentration, and an increase in the risk of toxicity of inhalational anesthetics.[11] Also, physiologic hyperventilation of pregnancy results in a typical $Pa{CO_2}$ of 32 mm Hg, with a normal pH. Similar to the cerebral vasculature, the umbilical vessels are sensitive to pH and are responsive to hyperventilation. These factors should be considered when hyperventilation is used intraoperatively or to manage elevated intracranial pressure.

During any operation on a pregnant woman, the fetal heart rate should be monitored continuously with an abdominal Doppler transducer.[73] Tachycardia and loss of normal beat-to-beat variability are early signs of fetal distress. Fetal bradycardia is an indication of more severe maternal hypotension and uterine hypoperfusion.[66]

The supine position is used often for craniotomy. In more than 90% of pregnant women at term, however, the inferior vena cava is obstructed completely by the uterus when the women lie supine.[74] The obstruction can produce maternal and fetal hypotension, which can be eliminated by placing patients in a lateral decubitus position for the operation.[5] Moderate hypothermia can provide cerebral protection during vascular surgery and appears to be well tolerated by mother and fetus.[38, 75–77] Induced hypotension can be useful during craniotomy for vascular lesions.[66, 70, 78] Caution must be used during maneuvers to reduce maternal blood pressure because uterine perfusion is not autoregulated and may be reduced during maternal hypotension. Isoflurane anesthesia can be used to induce hypotension[5, 79] and is not associated with a significant reduction in uterine blood flow.[80] Although some animal studies have indicated that sodium nitroprusside crosses the placenta and leads to cyanide accumulation in the fetus,[71] the drug has been used successfully during aneurysm surgery.[66, 70]

DIAGNOSTIC EVALUATION

All neurologic imaging modalities are available for evaluation of pregnant patients and should be used when indicated. Head computed tomography (CT) is the initial diagnostic procedure of choice for pregnant patients suspected of having an intracranial hemorrhagic or ischemic stroke. Four-vessel cerebral angiography is useful to identify suspected vascular lesions. The diagnostic yield of angiography in aneurysmal subarachnoid hemorrhage during pregnancy is reported to be superior to that of the general population.[5, 81–83]

Head CT and cerebral angiography can be performed safely during pregnancy. Current recommendations for radiation exposure of the fetus include a maximum dose of 0.5 rem (roentgen-equivalent-man).[84] By shielding the uterus with a lead apron, the maximum dose to the fetus during a head CT is less than 0.05 rem and less than 0.1 rem during cerebral angiography.[40] Iodinated contrast agents are physiologically inert and pose little risk to the fetus.[85] Adequate hydration should be provided during the administration of iodinated contrast material to avoid fetal dehydration.[8]

No experimental or human data indicate that magnetic resonance imaging (MRI) is unsafe for pregnant women or the fetus.[40] Long-term data on fetal outcome are lacking, however, and the teratogenic potential of gadopentetate dimeglumine has not been assessed in humans.[8] Most authors recommend caution in using MRI in pregnant patients, particularly during the first trimester.[86] Informed consent should be obtained before MRI is used.[40]

ANEURYSMS AND SUBARACHNOID HEMORRHAGE

The incidence of spontaneous subarachnoid hemorrhage during pregnancy ranges from 0.01% to 0.05% of all pregnancies.[5, 8, 87] Dias and Sekhar[8] found the mean age for pregnant patients with aneurysmal hemorrhage to be 29.4 years, and the mean gestational age to be 30.5 weeks. The overall mortality rate is 35%, which is comparable to that of the nonpregnant population.[8] The risk of hemorrhage increases with advancing gestational age, peaking at 30 to 34 weeks.[8] The effect of parity on subarachnoid hemorrhage is unclear. Although Robinson and colleagues[77] found that multiparous women have an increased incidence of ruptured cerebral aneurysms, others have reported that the incidence is higher in primigravidas.[7, 8] Rehemorrhage during the pregnancy occurs in 33% to 50% of cases and is associated with a maternal mortality rate of 70%.[5, 8, 20, 82, 88]

Clinical Features

As with subarachnoid hemorrhage in the general population, trauma is the most common cause of subarachnoid hemorrhage in pregnant patients.[5] Likewise, the clinical features of aneurysmal subarachnoid hemorrhage in pregnant patients are similar to those of nonpregnant patients.[8] "The worst headache of my life" is the most common presenting complaint. A history of a sentinel headache may be present in 50% of cases.[89] Other clinical manifestations include a brief loss of consciousness, meningismus, nausea and vomiting, focal neurologic deficits, seizures, and depressed mental status. Hypertension has been implicated as a causative factor in subarachnoid hemorrhage during pregnancy, occurring in 29% of patients with antepartum aneurysmal hemorrhage and in 67% of patients with postpartum aneurysmal hemorrhage.[8]

Diagnosis

Subarachnoid hemorrhage can be identified on CT in more than 90% of cases.[81] Lumbar puncture should be performed when clinical suspicion of subarachnoid hemorrhage is high. When the diagnosis is confirmed by CT or lumbar puncture, a four-vessel angiogram should be obtained promptly. Three-dimensional CT angiography can be useful to identify the vascular lesion and surrounding brain and skull base structures and to permit better planning of the operative approach.

Preeclampsia and eclampsia are more common than subarachnoid hemorrhage in pregnant women. These disorders can manifest with features similar to those of spontaneous subarachnoid hemorrhage and are the principal diagnoses from which aneurysmal subarachnoid hemorrhage should be distinguished. Preeclampsia is defined as the presence of hypertension in pregnant patients accompanied by proteinuria, edema, or both. Preeclampsia typically occurs after the 24th week of pregnancy and usually in primiparas. Severe preeclampsia can include a sharp increase in blood pressure, hyperreflexia, neurologic changes, and visual disturbances. Eclampsia is defined as the occurrence of seizures in a preeclamptic patient not attributable to other causes. Laboratory findings characteristic of preeclampsia and eclampsia can be found in aneurysmal subarachnoid hemorrhage; albuminuria is present in 20% to 30% of pregnant patients with aneurysmal subarachnoid hemorrhage.[8] The opening pressure at the time of lumbar puncture can be elevated after an eclamptic seizure and after rupture of a cerebral aneurysm.[7] Radiologic studies, such as head CT, can help differentiate eclamptic disorders from aneurysmal subarachnoid hemorrhage. Eclampsia can cause intracranial hemorrhage. Of patients with fatal eclampsia, 40% exhibit subarachnoid hemorrhage or intraparenchymal hemorrhage on autopsy,[90, 91] although the incidence in nonfatal cases is unknown.[8] Typical CT findings in eclampsia are multiple subcortical petechial hemorrhages or a single, large intracerebral hematoma.[8] On T2-weighted MRI, small areas of increased signal intensity in the deep or subcortical white matter are present in 50% of women with eclampsia.[92]

Apart from eclamptic disorders, aneurysmal subarachnoid hemorrhage during pregnancy must be distinguished from a ruptured AVM, the next most common cause of intracranial hemorrhage during pregnancy. In a review of 154 cases of intracranial hemorrhage during pregnancy, Dias and Sekhar[8] found aneurysms to be the cause in 77% of patients and AVMs in 23%. Other causes of spontaneous subarachnoid hemorrhage during pregnancy include disseminated intravascular coagulopathy,[93] sickle cell anemia,[93] anticoagulation therapy,[94] cocaine abuse,[95] metastatic choriocarcinoma,[96] Moyamoya disease,[97] and spinal vascular anomalies.[5]

Neurosurgical Management

When aneurysmal subarachnoid hemorrhage has been diagnosed, treatment begins with medical stabilization of the patient. Placement of an arterial catheter permits continuous monitoring of blood pressure and treatment of hypertension and hypotension. Maternal hypotension should be avoided because the fetus is passively dependent on maternal blood pressure for adequate perfusion and vulnerable to maternal hypotension. As in nonpregnant patients with subarachnoid hemorrhage, seizure prophylaxis and treatment with nimodipine in anticipation of vasospasm are important. Continuous fetal heart rate monitoring is essential. Adequate analgesia, sedation, and antiemetics should be provided.

The risk of recurrent bleeding during the remainder of pregnancy for patients with an untreated aneurysm is 33% to 50%[82, 91] with a maternal mortality rate of 50% to 68%.[20, 82, 88] In an analysis of 118 pregnant patients with aneurysmal subarachnoid hemorrhage, Dias and Sekhar[8] found that surgical treatment of a ruptured aneurysm was associated with significantly lower maternal and fetal mortality rates than conservative treatment. These findings have led to the recommendation that the decision to operate after subarachnoid hemorrhage during pregnancy should be based on neurosurgical criteria, and the method of delivery should be based on obstetric considerations.[8] Obstetric issues should take priority over neurosurgical concerns during active labor (which can be precipitated by the hemorrhage), eclampsia, or fetal distress. Delivery should be performed promptly by cesarean section, followed as soon as possible by neurosurgical treatment.[5, 98]

The standard treatment of a ruptured aneurysm in any patient is to exclude it from the circulation. Craniotomy with clip ligation of the aneurysm usually is effective, and endovascular techniques have permitted treatment of patients with high-grade subarachnoid hemorrhage who are not suitable candidates for craniotomy. Moderate hypothermia[38, 75–77] and, rarely, induced hypotension[66, 70] can be useful adjuncts during surgery.

Approximately 30% of nonpregnant patients develop symptomatic vasospasm after subarachnoid hemorrhage. The incidence of vasospasm in pregnant patients is unknown.[5] Some authors suggest, however, that the hemodynamic changes that occur during pregnancy, such as physiologic hemodilution and volume expansion, protect the patient from ischemic injury caused by cerebral vasospasm.[81] Options for treatment of symptomatic vasospasm in the general population include hyperdynamic therapy, with intravascular volume expansion and vasopressors, and angioplasty. No information is available in the literature to provide guidelines for the use of these methods in pregnant patients.[5]

Obstetric Management

Early authors recommended delivery by cesarean section after treatment of a ruptured aneurysm to minimize the hemodynamic stresses of labor and delivery. The risk of bleeding during vaginal delivery is not significantly different from that during cesarean section,[77] however, and many reports have indicated that mortality rates after vaginal delivery or cesarean section are not significantly different for pregnant patients with vascular disorders.[7, 8, 19, 99] Neither vaginal delivery nor cesarean section seems to offer a significant advantage for patients with subarachnoid hemorrhage. The method of delivery in most situations should be selected according to obstetric rather than neurosurgical criteria. The safety of oxytocic agents, such as oxytocin, in patients with intracranial vascular lesions is unclear because these agents can cause maternal hypertension. Careful use of these agents, with vigilant attention to blood pressure control, appears to be tolerated, however.[5, 78, 100, 101]

Patients should be followed before, during, and after neurosurgical procedures with continuous fetal monitoring. If persistent fetal distress appears and is not reversed by changes in oxygenation, positioning, or blood pressure, emergent cesarean delivery should be performed. If labor begins and delivery becomes imminent during craniotomy, the intracranial procedure should be suspended, the bone flap temporarily replaced if possible, and the child delivered vaginally or by cesarean section according to obstetric indications. The intracranial procedure should be resumed after delivery. Obstetric methods to minimize bleeding during vaginal delivery include caudal or epidural anesthesia, shortening of the second stage of labor, and low forceps delivery. A neonatologist or a pediatric intensivist should be available for care of the anesthetized infant.[8, 77] Cesarean delivery can be used for fetal salvage when the mother is moribund and in the third trimester.[102]

Outcomes

In most series, maternal mortality rates from subarachnoid hemorrhage range from 30% to 50%[7, 8] but have been reported as high as 83%.[103] Dias and Sekhar[8] found the overall maternal mortality rate from aneurysmal subarachnoid hemorrhage to be 35%, which is similar to that of the nonpregnant population. The fetal mortality rate was 17%. The maternal mortality rate after subarachnoid hemorrhage varies directly with clinical (Hunt and Hess) grade, reaching a peak at Hunt and Hess grade V.[8] The maternal mortality rate in patients undergoing antepartum surgery for the ruptured aneurysm (11%) was significantly lower than for patients not undergoing surgery (63%).[8] The fetal mortality rate was significantly better after surgery (5%) compared with patients not undergoing surgery (27%).[8]

Unruptured Aneurysms

The overall risk of subarachnoid hemorrhage in patients in the general population harboring an intracranial aneurysm is 1% to 2% per year.[104, 105] The risk of aneurysmal subarachnoid hemorrhage in pregnant patients has not been established firmly, but most reports agree that pregnancy does confer an increased risk of rupture five times that of nonpregnant women in the same age group.[5, 106] The incidence of rupture increases with advancing maternal age[5, 77, 106] and as gestation progresses.[5] These observations, combined with the substantial risk of subarachnoid hemorrhage to the mother and the fetus, argue in favor of treating an incidentally discovered aneurysm before patients become pregnant.

ARTERIOVENOUS MALFORMATIONS AND ANGIOMATOUS HEMORRHAGE

Rupture of an AVM is a relatively common cause of intracranial hemorrhage during pregnancy. Although AVMs account for about 35% of intracranial hemorrhages in the general population, they are the cause of 21% to 48% of hemorrhages during pregnancy and the puerperium.[5, 8, 19, 83] These reports of a heightened proportion of angiomatous hemorrhage among pregnant women may reflect referral patterns as well as features of the general population in the reproductive age group. Pregnancy does not appear to confer an increased risk of hemorrhage in pregnant women harboring an AVM, however.[107–109] In a review of 540 pregnancies in women with AVMs referred for proton-beam therapy, Horton and coworkers[109] found a 35% risk of hemorrhage, which is not significantly different from that of the general population. Dias and Sekhar[8] found the mean age for patients with angiomatous hemorrhage to be 26.7 years and the mean gestational age to be 30 weeks.

Clinical Features

As in the general population, hemorrhage is the most common initial manifestation of an AVM, occurring in about 87% of pregnant patients.[83] The initial condition of pregnant patients with this diagnosis is worse than that of the general population. About 57% of pregnant patients are either stuporous or comatose at presentation.[8] Seizures, headache, mass effect, and ischemic symptoms resulting from steal phenomena are other possible presenting features of AVMs. Hypertension is present in 17% of pregnant patients with angiomatous hemorrhage.[8]

Diagnosis

The workup of pregnant patients with an intracranial hemorrhage suspected of having an AVM is similar to the workup of pregnant patients with aneurysmal subarachnoid hemorrhage. CT, angiography, MRI, and three-dimensional CT angiography are useful for diagnosis and operative planning. Intracranial hemorrhage resulting from a ruptured AVM must be differentiated from many other causes of hemorrhage associated with pregnancy, such as eclampsia, aneurysmal subarachnoid hemorrhage, metastatic choriocarcinoma, pituitary apoplexy, sinus thrombosis, and hemorrhagic transformation of an ischemic stroke.

Neurosurgical Management

The medical management of pregnant patients with a ruptured AVM is identical to the management of patients with aneurysmal subarachnoid hemorrhage. Hemodynamic stabilization, strict control of seizure activity, and continuous fetal heart rate monitoring are important. In contrast to aneurysmal subarachnoid hemorrhage, the benefit of surgical treatment of the intracranial lesion is less clear. The incidence of rehemorrhage from an AVM is higher in pregnant patients than in the general population. Although 3% to 6% of nonpregnant patients rehemorrhage within the first year after an initial hemorrhage, about 25% of pregnant patients rehemorrhage during the same pregnancy.[5, 38, 83] Surgery does prevent rehemorrhage; however, the benefit of surgery to outcome is not proven. In an analysis of 32 pregnant patients with angiomatous hemorrhage, Dias and Sekhar[8] did not find a significant advantage for surgical management compared with nonsurgical management in terms of maternal or fetal mortality rates. Despite this finding, most authors recommend that the decision to operate on patients with angiomatous hemorrhage during pregnancy should be based on neurosurgical rather than obstetric criteria.[8, 19, 38] Craniotomy and evacuation of the hematoma with resection of the AVM offer the greatest and most immediate protection against rehemorrhage. Hypothermia can be used to provide cerebral protection during the procedure.[38, 75] Treatment alternatives, such as radiosurgery and endovascular embolization, do not reduce the risk of rehemorrhage as quickly and may increase the chance of hemorrhage initially.[5]

Obstetric Management

Obstetric guidelines for the management of angiomatous hemorrhage are similar to recommendations for the care of patients with aneurysmal subarachnoid hemorrhage and are not reiterated here. Dias and Sekhar[8] did not find a significant advantage for either cesarean or vaginal delivery. The choice of delivery method should be based on obstetric rather than neurosurgical criteria.[38]

Outcomes

Maternal and fetal mortality rates from angiomatous hemorrhage are significant. Dias and Sekhar[8] found the overall maternal mortality rate to be 28% and the fetal mortality rate to be 14%. The maternal mortality rate compares unfavorably with that of the general population, which is about 10% for a ruptured AVM.

Unruptured Arteriovenous Malformations

Although pregnancy does not appear to increase the risk of hemorrhage from an AVM, the significant mortality rate associated with rupture during pregnancy justifies treatment of known AVMs in women of reproductive age before pregnancy. Also, because AVMs are associated significantly with seizure disorders, particularly in younger patients, ablation of an AVM may help reduce the chance of patients having a seizure disorder during pregnancy and avert the risks that accompany epilepsy and anticonvulsant use during pregnancy. Whether an AVM is treated by surgical resection, embolization, or radiosurgery, pregnancy should be deferred until treatment is completed.[109, 110]

CEREBRAL ISCHEMIA AND STROKE

Estimates of the incidence of cerebral infarction among pregnant women vary widely, ranging from 0.004% to 0.2% of all deliveries.[4] Most reports indicate that pregnancy increases the risk of ischemic stroke in women of reproductive age, but the magnitude of the risk is unclear. Estimates of relative risk of ischemic stroke during pregnancy extend from 1.16%[10] to 13%.[111]

Arterial Occlusion

Arterial embolism or thrombosis accounts for 60% to 80% of cases of ischemic stroke during pregnancy.[111] Stroke secondary to arterial occlusion tends to occur during the second and third trimesters of pregnancy and during the first week after delivery.[111] This gestational pattern corresponds to the appearance of the hypercoagulable state in the latter stages of pregnancy and the puerperium. The causes of arterial occlusion are listed in Table 143–1.

All patients suspected of having an ischemic stroke should undergo a thorough radiologic and laboratory investigation. CT is a good initial study to exclude hemorrhagic stroke and can identify some cases of ischemic stroke, depending on the region of the brain affected and the length of time since arterial occlusion. MRI has greater sensitivity and resolution than CT. Angiography can be useful, particularly when intra-arterial thrombolytic treatment is anticipated. Helpful initial laboratory investigations include a complete blood count, electrolytes, erythrocyte sedimentation rate, coagulation studies, and urinalysis. When a cardiac source is suspected, a chest radiograph, an electrocardiogram, and an echocardiogram should be obtained. Transesophageal echocardiography is superior

TABLE 143–1 ■ **Causes of Cerebral Ischemia or Stroke During Pregnancy and the Puerperium**

ARTERIAL OCCLUSION	VENOUS OCCLUSION
Cardiac	Hypercoagulable state
Infective endocarditis	Trauma
Rheumatic heart disease	Infection
Mitral valve prolapse	Polycythemia vera
Atrial fibrillation	Leukemia
Prosthetic heart valves	Dehydration
Atrial myxoma	Sickle cell anemia
Paradoxical embolism	Behçet's disease
Peripartum cardiomyopathy	Air embolism
Noncardiac	
Atherosclerosis	
Takayasu's disease	
Hypertension	
Antiphospholipid antibodies	
Air embolism	
Fat embolism	
Amniotic fluid embolism	
Illicit drug use	
Eclampsia	
Cerebral vasospasm	
Disseminated intravascular coagulation	
Sickle cell disease	
Thrombotic thrombocytopenic purpura	
Systemic lupus erythematosus	
Vasculitis	
Postpartum cerebral vasospasm	

to transthoracic echocardiography and is safe for pregnant patients.[112] Carotid duplex and magnetic resonance angiography are noninvasive techniques to investigate extracranial carotid disease.

Potential interventions for arterial occlusion in pregnant women include antiplatelet agents and anticoagulation; these medications were discussed in detail previously. Appropriate medical care, including intravenous hydration, antibiotics, and treatment of seizure disorders, is important when indicated.

Venous Thrombosis

Intracranial venous thrombosis occurs with an estimated incidence of 1 in 2500 to 1 in 10,000 deliveries[113] and accounts for 20% to 40% of cases of ischemic stroke during pregnancy.[111] This disorder tends to occur in multiparous women, 3 days to 4 weeks after childbirth, with most cases occurring in the second or third week postpartum.[9, 111, 113–115] Intracranial venous thrombosis during pregnancy is less common.[113, 116–118] Most cases are idiopathic,[118] although many systemic conditions can predispose toward intracranial venous thrombosis (see Table 143–1).

More than 70% of cases involve occlusion of multiple venous sinuses or cerebral veins.[119] Cortical veins are involved more commonly than deep cerebral and cerebellar veins.[118] Headache is the most common presenting symptom.[120] Other common clinical features are nausea and vomiting, seizures, focal neurologic deficits, fever, and altered mental status.[118]

Diagnosis of intracranial venous thrombosis is based on clinical findings and radiologic studies. CT, MRI, and angiography are useful. Investigation into possible predisposing factors with tests such as coagulation studies is important. When the diagnosis is confirmed, management begins with adequate hydration and treatment of elevated intracranial pressure, hydrocephalus, and seizures.[118] Treatment options for intracranial venous thrombosis include high doses of heparin (1000 IU/hour to start; activated partial thromboplastin time >1.5 to 2 times control) and endovascular fibrinolysis followed by heparinization and surgical thrombectomy.[118] Einhaupl and colleagues[121] found that patients receiving intravenous heparin for intracranial venous thrombosis had significantly better neurologic outcomes and mortality rates compared with patients receiving placebo treatment. Underlying predisposing disorders, such as sinusitis, also must be treated.[118]

Mortality rates for intracranial venous thrombosis of 33% have been reported[9]; however, neurologic outcomes for survivors usually are good.[118] Srinivasan[9] found that 59% of patients recovered without significant neurologic disability.

OTHER VASCULAR PROBLEMS ASSOCIATED WITH PREGNANCY

Metastatic Choriocarcinoma

Metastatic choriocarcinoma is a rare cause of intracerebral hemorrhage and oncotic intracranial aneurysms. Choriocarcinoma is a form of gestational trophoblastic neoplasia and is the most malignant tumor associated with pregnancy,[96] occurring in about 1 in 20,000 pregnancies.[122] The mechanism of metastasis is hematogenous and is based on the ability of normal chorionic tissue to penetrate the uterine wall in search of blood vessels to nourish the fetus. In the cerebral vasculature, trophoblasts infiltrate the vessels just as they would in the uterus. Damaged vessels may thrombose, form an embolus, or weaken the vessel wall and form an aneurysm or varicosity.[96, 123] Metastatic choriocarcinoma to the brain has a high rate of spontaneous hemorrhage, second only to metastatic melanoma[96]; at autopsy, most metastatic brain lesions are found to be hemorrhagic.[124] Intracranial hemorrhage is the mode of presentation in two thirds of cerebral metastases.[125]

Intracranial hemorrhage secondary to metastatic choriocarcinoma may be intracerebral, subdural, or subarachnoid[126]; however, it is uncommon for a patient to harbor multiple intracranial vascular disorders.[126, 127] Intracerebral hemorrhage can be located at any site in the brain where metastases have occurred. Oncotic aneurysms usually develop at distal sites in the distribution of the middle cerebral artery.[127, 128] The aneurysms can be single or multiple, large or small, and smooth or irregular.[129] Typically, aneurysms are fusiform.[130] Intracranial hemorrhage is treated by craniotomy and clot evacuation. Oncotic aneurysms should be clipped or excised[96, 126, 129] because they have a tendency to rehemorrhage[131] or to cause thrombosis of the distal artery.[132] A combination of radiation and multiagent chemotherapy is recommended for patients with choriocarcinoma brain metastases; these patients have an overall survival rate of 18%.[133]

Postpartum Cerebral Vasospasm

Cerebral vasospasm is a rare complication of pregnancy and usually occurs during the postpartum period and for 3 weeks after delivery. The cause is not understood, but evidence indicates that postpartum vasospasm is a variant of eclampsia.[134] Clinical features include severe headache, fluctuating neurologic deficits, and stroke.[135] Hyperdynamic therapy combined with nimodipine may be effective treatment for this disorder.[134]

Carotid-Cavernous Fistula

The spontaneous formation of a carotid-cavernous fistula rarely is associated with pregnancy and the puerperium.[136–138] Hemodynamic changes, combined with alterations in the blood vessel wall concomitant with pregnancy, may predispose to this lesion. The most common presenting symptom is unilateral frontal headache, often accompanied by ipsilateral conjunctival injection and visual symptoms.[65] This lesion tends to occur during the second half of pregnancy or the puerperium.[65] The fistulas resolve spontaneously in 60% of cases,[136] although successful treatment by embolization of the carotid artery has been reported.[137]

Pituitary Apoplexy

Severe shock around the time of delivery can lead to pituitary infarction and postpartum hypopituitarism (Sheehan's syndrome). Stimulation of prolactin-secreting cells in the adenohypophysis during pregnancy causes enlargement of the pituitary, putting it at risk of ischemia should severe hypotension occur. Infarction occurs in the region of the hypophyseal artery and rarely involves the neurohypophysis.[65] Treatment consists of hormone replacement therapy.

REFERENCES

1. Guyer B, Strobino DM, Ventura SJ, et al: Annual summary of vital statistics—1994. Pediatrics 96:1029–1039, 1995.
2. Sachs BP, Brown DA, Driscoll SG, et al: Maternal mortality in Massachusetts: Trends and prevention. N Engl J Med 31: 667–672, 1987.
3. Sharshar T, Lamy C, Mas JL: Incidence and causes of strokes associated with pregnancy and puerperium: A study in public hospitals of Ile de France. Stroke in Pregnancy Study Group. Stroke 26:930–936, 1995.
4. Wiebers DO, Whisnant JP: The incidence of stroke among pregnant women in Rochester, Minn, 1955 through 1979. JAMA 254: 3055–3057, 1985.
5. Sawin P: Spontaneous subarachnoid hemorrhage in pregnancy and the puerperium. In Loftus C (ed): Neurosurgical Aspects of Pregnancy. Park Ridge, IL, American Association of Neurological Surgeons, 1996, pp 85–99.
6. Gibbs CE: Maternal death due to stroke. Am J Obstet Gynecol 119:69–75, 1974.
7. Barrett JM, van Hooydonk JE, Boehm FH: Pregnancy-related rupture of arterial aneurysms. Obstet Gynecol Surv 37:557–566, 1982.
8. Dias MS, Sekhar LN: Intracranial hemorrhage from aneurysms and arteriovenous malformations during pregnancy and the puerperium. Neurosurgery 27:855–866, 1990.
9. Srinivasan K: Cerebral venous and arterial thrombosis in pregnancy and puerperium: A study of 135 patients. Angiology 34: 731–746, 1983.
10. Sandmire HH: Maternal mortality in Wisconsin: Cerebral vascular accident. Wisc Med J 88:23–24, 1989.
11. Pedersen H, Finster M: Anesthetic risk in the pregnant surgical patient. Anesthesiology 51:439–451, 1979.
12. Swift D: Changes in cardiovascular and cerebrovascular function during pregnancy. In Loftus C (ed): Neurosurgical Aspects of Pregnancy. Park Ridge, IL, American Association of Neurological Surgeons, 1996, pp 39–43.
13. Mabie WC, DiSessa TG, Crocker LG, et al: A longitudinal study of cardiac output in normal human pregnancy. Am J Obstet Gynecol 170:849–856, 1994.
14. Hunter S, Robson SC: Adaptation of the maternal heart in pregnancy. Br Heart J 68:540–543, 1992.
15. Rosen M: Cerebrovascular lesions and tumors in the pregnant patient. In Newfield P, Cottrell J (eds): Handbook of Neuroanesthesia: Clinical and Physiologic Essentials. Boston, Little, Brown, 1983, pp 227–244.
16. Meschia G: Placental respiratory gas exchange and fetal oxygenation. In Creasy R, Resnick R (eds): Maternal-Fetal Medicine: Principles and Practice. Philadelphia, WB Saunders, 1984, pp 274–285.
17. Ikeda T, Ikenoue T, Mori N, et al: Effect of early pregnancy on maternal regional cerebral blood flow. Am J Obstet Gynecol 168:1303–1308, 1993.
18. Greenfield JC Jr, Rembert JC, Tindall GT: Transient changes in cerebral vascular resistance during the Valsalva maneuver in man. Stroke 15:76–79, 1984.
19. Amias AG: Cerebral vascular disease in pregnancy: I. Haemorrhage. J Obstet Gynaecol Br Commonw 77:100–120, 1970.
20. Daane TA, Tandy RW: Rupture of congenital intracranial aneurysm in pregnancy. Obstet Gynecol 15:305–314, 1960.
21. Pinto S, Abbate R, Rostagno C, et al: Increased thrombin generation in normal pregnancy. Acta Eur Fertil 19:263–267, 1988.
22. Wright JG, Cooper P, Astedt B, et al: Fibrinolysis during normal human pregnancy: Complex inter-relationships between plasma levels of tissue plasminogen activator and inhibitors and the euglobulin clot lysis time. Br J Haematol 69:253–258, 1988.
23. Fletcher AP, Alkjaersig NK, Burstein R: The influence of pregnancy upon blood coagulation and plasma fibrinolytic enzyme function. Am J Obstet Gynecol 134:743–751, 1979.
24. Bonnar J, McNicol GP, Douglas AS: Fibrinolytic enzyme system and pregnancy. BMJ 3:387–389, 1969.
25. Chan SY, Chan PH, Ho PC, et al: Factor VIII-related antigen levels in normal pregnancy and puerperium. Eur J Obstet Gynecol Reprod Biol 19:199–204, 1985.
26. Nilsson IM, Kullander S: Coagulation and fibrinolytic studies during pregnancy. Acta Obstet Gynecol Scand 46:273–285, 1967.
27. Whitfield LR, Lele AS, Levy G: Effect of pregnancy on the relationship between concentration and anticoagulant action of heparin. Clin Pharmacol Ther 34:23–28, 1983.
28. de Boer K, ten Cate JW, Sturk A, et al: Enhanced thrombin generation in normal and hypertensive pregnancy. Am J Obstet Gynecol 160:95–100, 1989.
29. Malm J, Laurell M, Dahlback B: Changes in the plasma levels of vitamin K-dependent proteins C and S and of C4b-binding protein during pregnancy and oral contraception. Br J Haematol 68:437–443, 1988.
30. Lewis PJ, Boylan P, Friedman LA, et al: Prostacyclin in pregnancy. BMJ 280:1581–1582, 1980.
31. Stern B: Cerebrovascular disease and pregnancy. In Goldstein P, Stern B (eds): Neurological Disorders of Pregnancy, 2nd ed. Mt Kisco, NY, Futura, 1992, pp 51–84.
32. Knight AH, Rhind EG: Epilepsy and pregnancy: A study of 153 pregnancies in 59 patients. Epilepsia 16:99–110, 1975.
33. Krumholz A: Epilepsy and pregnancy. In Goldstein P (ed): Neurological Disorders of Pregnancy. New York, Futura, 1986, pp 65–88.
34. Nulman I, Laslo D, Koren G: Treatment of epilepsy in pregnancy. Drugs 57:535–544, 1999.

35. Bjerkedal T, Bahna SL: The course and outcome of pregnancy in women with epilepsy. Acta Obstet Gynecol Scand 52:245–248, 1973.
36. American Academy of Pediatrics Committee on Drugs: Anticonvulsants and pregnancy. Pediatrics 63:331–333, 1979.
37. Montouris GD, Fenichel GM, McLain LW Jr: The pregnant epileptic: A review and recommendations. Arch Neurol 36:601–603, 1979.
38. Sadasivan B, Malik GM, Lee C, et al: Vascular malformations and pregnancy. Surg Neurol 33:305–313, 1990.
39. Hanson JW, Smith DW: The fetal hydantoin syndrome. J Pediatr 87:424–428, 1975.
40. Piper J: Fetal toxicity of common neurosurgical drugs. In Loftus C (ed): Neurosurgical Aspects of Pregnancy. Park Ridge, IL, American Association of Neurological Surgeons, 1996, pp 1–20.
41. Seip M: Growth retardation, dysmorphic facies and minor malformations following massive exposure to phenobarbital in utero. Acta Paediatr Scand 65:617–621, 1976.
42. Jones KL, Lacro RV, Johnson KA, et al: Pattern of malformations in the children of women treated with carbamazepine during pregnancy. N Engl J Med 320:1661–1666, 1989.
43. Rosa FW: Spina bifida in infants of women treated with carbamazepine during pregnancy. N Engl J Med 324:674–677, 1991.
44. Tein I, MacGregor DL: Possible valproate teratogenicity. Arch Neurol 42:291–293, 1985.
45. Bailey CJ, Pool RW, Poskitt EM, et al: Valproic acid and fetal abnormality. BMJ 286:190, 1983.
46. Saunders M: Epilepsy in women of childbearing age. BMJ 299: 581, 1989.
47. Fed Reg 44:37, 434–437, 467, 1980.
48. Morrell MJ: Guidelines for the care of women with epilepsy. Neurology 51(5 suppl 4):S21-27, 1998.
49. Sabers A, a'Rogvi-Hansen B, Dam M, et al: Pregnancy and epilepsy: A retrospective study of 151 pregnancies. Acta Neurol Scand 97:164–170, 1998.
50. Hall JG, Pauli RM, Wilson KM: Maternal and fetal sequelae of anticoagulation during pregnancy. Am J Med 68:122–140, 1980.
51. Bonnar J: Venous thromboembolism and pregnancy. Clin Obstet Gynaecol 8:455–473, 1981.
52. Iturbe-Alessio I, Fonseca MC, Mutchinik O, et al: Risks of anticoagulant therapy in pregnant women with artificial heart valves. N Engl J Med 315:1390–1393, 1986.
53. Angel J, Knuppel R, Hoffman M, et al: Anticoagulant use in pregnancy. In Petrie R (ed): Perinatal Pharmacology. Oradell, NJ, Medical Economics Books, 1989, pp 95–108.
54. Calhoun BC, Hesser J: Heparin-associated antibody with pregnancy: Discussion of two cases. Am J Obstet Gynecol 156: 964–966, 1987.
55. Barbour L, Kick SD, Steiner JF, et al: A prospective study of heparin-induced osteoporosis in pregnancy using bone densitometry. Am J Obstet Gynecol 170:862–869, 1994.
56. Sareli P, England MJ, Berk MR, et al: Maternal and fetal sequelae of anticoagulation during pregnancy in patients with mechanical heart valve prostheses. Am J Cardiol 63:1462–1465, 1989.
57. Shaul WL, Hall JG: Multiple congenital anomalies associated with oral anticoagulants. Am J Obstet Gynecol 127:191–198, 1977.
58. Lecuru F, Desnos M, Taurelle R: Anticoagulant therapy in pregnancy: Report of 54 cases. Acta Obstet Gynecol Scand 75:217–221, 1996.
59. Astedt B: Antenatal drugs affecting vitamin K status of the fetus and the newborn. Semin Thromb Hemost 21:364–370, 1995.
60. Oakley C: Valve prostheses and pregnancy. Br Heart J 58:303–305, 1987.
61. Sanson BJ, Lensing AW, Prins MH, et al: Safety of low-molecular-weight heparin in pregnancy: A systematic review. Thromb Haemost 81:668–672, 1999.
62. CLASP (Collaborative Low-Dose Aspirin Study in Pregnancy) Collaborative Group: CLASP: A randomized trial of low-dose aspirin for the prevention and treatment of pre-eclampsia among 9364 pregnant women. Lancet 343:619–629, 1994.
63. Ginsberg JS, Hirsh J: Use of antithrombotic agents during pregnancy. Chest 102(4 suppl):385S–390S, 1992.
64. Davis P, Jacoby M, Adams H: Cerebral embolism in pregnant women. In Loftus C (ed): Neurosurgical Aspects of Pregnancy. Park Ridge, IL, American Association of Neurological Surgeons, 1996, pp 135–146.
65. Donaldson J: Neurology of Pregnancy, 2nd ed. London, WB Saunders, 1989.
66. Willoughby JS: Sodium nitroprusside, pregnancy and multiple intracranial aneurysms. Anaesth Intensive Care 12:358–360, 1984.
67. Briggs G, Freeman R, Yaffe S: Drugs in Pregnancy and Lactation: A Reference Guide to Fetal and Neonatal Risk, 5th ed. Baltimore, Williams & Wilkins, 1998, p 646.
68. McEvoy G, Litvak K, Welsh O, et al: AHFS Drug Information 94. Bethesda, MD, American Society of Hospital Pharmacists, 1994, pp 1182–1187.
69. Nimotop Packaging Insert. Bayer Corporation, West Haven, Conn, 2001.
70. Rigg D, McDonagh A: Use of sodium nitroprusside for deliberate hypotension during pregnancy. Br J Anaesth 53:985–987, 1981.
71. Penning D: Fetal effects of anesthesia. In Loftus C (ed): Neurosurgical Aspects of Pregnancy. Park Ridge, IL, American Association of Neurological Surgeons, 1996, pp 29–38.
72. National High Blood Pressure Education Program Working Group: Report on high blood pressure in pregnancy. Am J Obstet Gynecol 163:1691–1712, 1990.
73. van Buul BJ, Nijhuis JG, Slappendel R, et al: General anesthesia for surgical repair of intracranial aneurysm in pregnancy: Effects on fetal heart rate. Am J Perinatol 10:183–186, 1993.
74. Nau H, Rating D, Koch S, et al: Valproic acid and its metabolites: Placental transfer, neonatal pharmacokinetics, transfer via mother's milk, and clinical status in neonates of epileptic mothers. J Pharmacol Exp Ther 219:768–777, 1981.
75. Matsuki A, Oyama T: Operation under hypothermia in a pregnant woman with an intracranial arteriovenous malformation. Can Anaesth Soc J 19:184–191, 1972.
76. Hehre F: Hypothermia for operations during pregnancy. Anesth Analg 44:424–428, 1965.
77. Robinson JL, Hall CJ, Sedzimir CB: Subarachnoid hemorrhage in pregnancy. J Neurosurg 36:27–33, 1972.
78. Minielly R, Yuzpe AA, Drake CG: Subarachnoid hemorrhage secondary to ruptured cerebral aneurysm in pregnancy. Obstet Gynecol 53:64–70, 1978.
79. Newman B, Lam AM: Induced hypotension for clipping of a cerebral aneurysm during pregnancy: A case report and brief review. Anesth Analg 65:675–678, 1986.
80. Palahniuk RJ, Shnider SM: Maternal and fetal cardiovascular acid-base changes during halothane and isoflurane anesthesia in the pregnant ewe. Anesthesiology 41:462–472, 1974.
81. Giannotta SL, Daniels J, Goide SH, et al: Ruptured intracranial aneurysms during pregnancy: A report of four cases. J Reprod Med 31:139–147, 1986.
82. Pool JL: Treatment of intracranial aneurysms during pregnancy. JAMA 192:209–214, 1965.
83. Robinson JL, Hall CS, Sedzimir CB: Arteriovenous malformations, aneurysms, and pregnancy. J Neurosurg 41:63–70, 1974.
84. National Council on Radiation Protection and Measurements: Recommendations on Limits for Exposure to Ionizing Radiation (NCRP Report No. 91). Bethesda, Md, National Council on Radiation Protection, 1987.
85. Dalessio D: Neurologic diseases. In Burrow G, Ferris T (eds): Medical Complications During Pregnancy, 2nd ed. Philadelphia, WB Saunders, 1982, pp 435–447.
86. National Institutes of Health Consensus Conference: Magnetic resonance imaging. JAMA 259:2132–2138, 1988.
87. Maymon R, Fejgin M: Intracranial hemorrhage during pregnancy and puerperium. Obstet Gynecol Surv 45:157–159, 1990.
88. Cannell D, Botterell E: Subarachnoid hemorrhage and pregnancy. Am J Obstet Gynecol 72:844–855, 1956.
89. Verweij RD, Wijdicks EF, Gijn JV: Warning headache in aneurysmal subarachnoid hemorrhage: A case-control study. Arch Neurol 45:1019–1020, 1988.
90. Donnelly J, Locke F: Causes of death in 533 fatal cases of toxemia of pregnancy. Am J Obstet Gynecol 68:184–190, 1954.
91. Schwartz J: Pregnancy complicated by subarachnoid hemorrhage. Am J Obstet Gynecol 62:539–547, 1951.
92. Digre K, Varner M, Crawford S, et al: Magnetic resonance

imaging (MRI) in severe pre-eclampsia and eclampsia. Neurology 37(suppl 1):95, 1987.
93. Barno A, Freeman DW: Maternal deaths due to spontaneous subarachnoid hemorrhage. Am J Obstet Gynecol 125:384–392, 1976.
94. Hirsh J, Cade JF, Gallus AS: Anticoagulants in pregnancy: A review of indications and complications. Am Heart J 83:301–305, 1972.
95. Henderson CE, Torbey M: Rupture of intracranial aneurysm associated with cocaine use during pregnancy. Am J Perinatol 5:142–143, 1988.
96. Salcman M: Choriocarcinoma in pregnancy. In Loftus C (ed): Neurosurgical Aspects of Pregnancy. Park Ridge, IL, American Association of Neurological Surgeons, 1996, pp 147–155.
97. Enomoto H, Goto H: Moyamoya disease presenting as intracerebral hemorrhage during pregnancy: Case report and review of the literature. Neurosurgery 20:33–35, 1987.
98. Lennon RL, Sundt TM Jr, Gronert GA: Combined cesarean section and clipping of intracerebral aneurysm. Anesthesiology 60:240–242, 1984.
99. Pedowitz P, Perrell A: Aneurysms complicated by pregnancy: II. Aneurysms of the cerebral vessels. Am J Obstet Gynecol 73: 736–749, 1957.
100. Laidler JA, Jackson IJ, Redfern N: The management of caesarean section in a patient with an intracranial arteriovenous malformation. Anaesthesia 44:490–491, 1989.
101. Tuttleman RM, Gleicher N: Central nervous system hemorrhage complicating pregnancy. Obstet Gynecol 58:651–657, 1981.
102. Heikkinen JE, Rinne RI, Alahuhta SM, et al: Life support for 10 weeks with successful fetal outcome after fatal maternal brain hemorrhage. BMJ 290:1237–1238, 1985.
103. Miller HJ, Hinkley CM: Berry aneurysms in pregnancy: A 10 year report. South Med J 63:279–285, 1970.
104. Juvela S, Porras M, Heiskanen O: Natural history of unruptured intracranial aneurysms: A long-term follow-up study. J Neurosurg 79:174–182, 1993.
105. Jane JA, Kassell NF, Torner JC, et al: The natural history of aneurysms and arteriovenous malformations. J Neurosurg 62: 321–323, 1985.
106. Wiebers D: Subarachnoid hemorrhage in pregnancy. Semin Neurol 8:226–229, 1988.
107. Parkinson D, Bachers G: Arteriovenous malformations: Summary of 100 consecutive supratentorial cases. J Neurosurg 53: 285–299, 1980.
108. Itoyama Y, Uemura S, Ushio Y, et al: Natural course of unoperated intracranial arteriovenous malformations: Study of 50 cases. J Neurosurg 71:805–809, 1989.
109. Horton JC, Chambers WA, Lyons SL, et al: Pregnancy and the risk of hemorrhage from cerebral arteriovenous malformations. Neurosurgery 27:867–872, 1990.
110. Kjellberg RN, Hanamura T, Davis KR, et al: Bragg-peak proton-beam therapy for arteriovenous malformations of the brain. N Engl J Med 309:269–274, 1983.
111. Wiebers DO: Ischemic cerebrovascular complications of pregnancy. Arch Neurol 42:1106–1113, 1985.
112. Stoddard MF, Longaker RA, Vuocolo LM, et al: Transesophageal echocardiography in the pregnant patient. Am Heart J 124: 785–787, 1992.
113. Bansal BC, Gupta RR, Prakash C: Stroke during pregnancy and puerperium in young females below the age of 40 years as a result of cerebral venous/venous sinus thrombosis. Jpn Heart J 21:171–183, 1980.
114. Estanol B, Rodriguez A, Conte G, et al: Intracranial venous thrombosis in young women. Stroke 10:680–684, 1979.
115. Imai WK, Everhart FR Jr, Sanders JM Jr: Cerebral venous sinus thrombosis: Report of a case and review of the literature. Pediatrics 70:965–970, 1982.
116. Fehr PE: Sagittal sinus thrombosis in early pregnancy. Obstet Gynecol 59(suppl):7S–9S, 1982.
117. Lavin PJ, Bone I, Lamb JT, et al: Intracranial venous thrombosis in the first trimester of pregnancy. J Neurol Neurosurg Psychiatry 41:726–729, 1978.
118. Hamilton M, Ziai W, Hull R, et al: Venous thrombotic disorders in pregnancy. In Loftus C (ed): Neurosurgical Aspects of Pregnancy. Park Ridge, IL, American Association of Neurological Surgeons, 1996, pp 101–134.
119. Bousser MG, Chiras J, Bories J, et al: Cerebral venous thrombosis—a review of 38 cases. Stroke 16:199–213, 1985.
120. Galan HL, McDowell AB, Johnson PR, et al: Puerperal cerebral venous thrombosis associated with decreased free protein S: A case report. J Reprod Med 40:859–862, 1995.
121. Einhaupl KM, Villringer A, Meister W, et al: Heparin treatment in sinus venous thrombosis [published erratum appears in Lancet 1991; 338(8772):958]. Lancet 338:597–600, 1991.
122. Buckley JD: The epidemiology of molar pregnancy and choriocarcinoma. Clin Obstet Gynecol 27:153–159, 1984.
123. Vaughn HG Jr, Howard RG: Intracranial hemorrhage due to metastatic chorionepithelioma. Neurology 12:771–777, 1962.
124. Kobayashi T, Kida Y, Yoshida J, et al: Brain metastasis of choriocarcinoma. Surg Neurol 17:395–403, 1982.
125. Ishizuka T, Tomoda Y, Kaseki S, et al: Intracranial metastases of choriocarcinoma: A clinicopathologic study. Cancer 52:1896–1903, 1983.
126. Weir B, McDonald N, Mielke R: Intracranial vascular complications of choriocarcinoma. Neurosurgery 2:138–142, 1978.
127. Siegle JM, Caputy AJ, Manz H, et al: Multiple oncotic intracranial aneurysms and cardiac metastasis from choriocarcinoma: Case report and review of the literature. Neurosurgery 20:39–42, 1987.
128. Giannakopoulos G, Nair S, Snider C, et al: Implications for the pathogenesis of aneurysm formation: Metastatic choriocarcinoma with spontaneous splenic rupture: Case report and a review. Surg Neurol 38:236–240, 1992.
129. Momma F, Beck H, Miyamoto T, et al: Intracranial aneurysm due to metastatic choriocarcinoma. Surg Neurol 25:74–76, 1986.
130. Pullar M, Blumbergs PC, Phillips GE, et al: Neoplastic cerebral aneurysm from metastatic gestational choriocarcinoma. Neurosurgery 63:644–647, 1985.
131. Stilip T, Bucy P, Brewer J: Cure of metastatic choriocarcinoma of the brain. JAMA 221:276–279, 1972.
132. Nakahara T, Nonaka N, Kinoshita K, et al: Subarachnoid hemorrhage and aneurysmal change of cerebral arteries due to metastases of chorioepithelioma [Japanese]. No Shinkei Geka 3:777–782, 1975.
133. Bakri YN, Pedersen P, Nassar M: Normal pregnancy after curative multiagent chemotherapy for choriocarcinoma with brain metastases. Acta Obstet Gynecol Scand 70:611–613, 1991.
134. Akins PT, Levy KJ, Cross AH, et al: Postpartum cerebral vasospasm treated with hypervolemic therapy. Am J Obstet Gynecol 175:1386–1388, 1996.
135. Geraghty JJ, Hoch DB, Robert ME, et al: Fatal puerperal cerebral vasospasm and stroke in a young woman. Neurology 41:1145–1147, 1991.
136. Lin TK, Chang CN, Wai YY: Spontaneous intracerebral hematoma from an occult carotid-cavernous fistula during pregnancy and puerperium: Case report. J Neurosurg 76:714–717, 1992.
137. Raskind R, Johnson N, Hance D: Carotid cavernous fistula in pregnancy. Angiology 28:671–676, 1977.
138. Toya S, Shiobara R, Izumi J, et al: Spontaneous carotid-cavernous fistula during pregnancy or in the postpartum stage: Report of two cases. J Neurosurg 54:252–256, 1981.

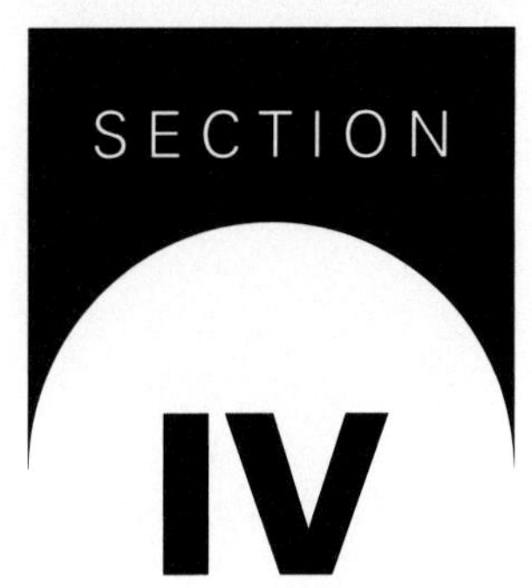

Epilepsy

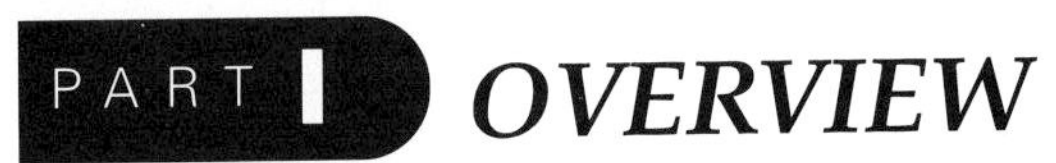

CHAPTER 144

General and Historical Considerations of Epilepsy Surgery

ELDAD HADAR ■ JÜRGEN LÜDERS

The objective of resective epilepsy surgery is the complete resection of the *epileptogenic zone,* which is the area of cortex indispensable for the generation of clinical seizures. Modern epileptologists use a variety of diagnostic tools, such as analysis of seizure semiology, electrophysiologic recordings, functional testing, and neuroimaging techniques, to define the location and boundaries of the epileptogenic zone. These diagnostic methods define different cortical zones (symptomatogenic zone, irritative zone, ictal onset zone, functional deficit zone, and the epileptogenic lesion), all of which are a more or less precise index of the location and extent of the epileptogenic zone. The ability to define precisely the epileptogenic zone is essentially a function of the sensitivities and specificities of the diagnostic methods. These modern techniques not only permit definition of the location of all the areas mentioned, but also have significantly increased the ability to define precisely the boundaries of these areas. A historical review of epilepsy surgery shows that initially epileptologists were able only to define the symptomatogenic zone and had to use this isolated information to deduce the most likely location and extent of the epileptogenic zone. Progressive introduction of new diagnostic techniques allowed epileptologists then to start to define some of the other zones listed previously. Further refinement of these techniques and the introduction of new techniques permit the definition of each zone with an unprecedented degree of accuracy; this in turn made definition of the epileptogenic zone progressively more precise.

This chapter gives an overview of the five zones used to define the epileptogenic zone. We describe the history of epilepsy surgery in terms of the development of the different diagnostic techniques necessary to define these five zones—*era of the symptomatogenic zone, era of the irritative and seizure onset zones, era of the epileptogenic lesion,* and *era of the functional deficit zone.* As tests capable of describing a new cortical zone have been developed, they usually have been added to the diagnostic armamentarium with the intent to provide supplementary, not redundant, information. In some cases, however, the development of new, more sensitive or specific methodologies to define a given zone has led to the abandonment of older techniques. A typical example is the development of high-resolution magnetic resonance imaging (MRI) technology. High-resolution MRI almost completely has replaced computed tomography (CT) scans in the presurgical evaluation.

DESCRIPTION OF CORTICAL ZONES

Symptomatogenic Zone

The symptomatogenic zone is the area of cortex that, when activated by an epileptiform discharge, reproduces the initial ictal symptoms. The zone is defined by careful analysis of the ictal symptoms that can be done with a thorough seizure history and analysis of ictal video recordings. The precision with which the epileptologist can define the location and extent of the symptomatogenic zone depends on the specific ictal symptoms. A highly localized somatosensory aura, such as paresthesias of one or two fingers at the beginning of the seizure, clearly localizes the symptomatogenic zone to the corresponding primary sensory area. In contrast, a poorly defined body sensation has little localizing or lateralizing value. There are many other ictal signs or symptoms whose localizing and lateralizing value falls in between these two extremes.

There may be no overlap between the symptomatogenic zone and the epileptogenic zone. The best method with which to define the symptomatogenic zones of the brain is direct cortical electrical stimulation, which produces conditions closely resembling activation of the cortex by an epileptiform discharge. Electrical stimulation reveals that most of the human cortex is symptomatically *silent*, strongly suggesting that its activation by an epileptiform discharge would not produce any symptoms unless there is spreading of the electrical activity to adjacent eloquent cortex. The presence of ictal symptoms may be caused by generation of the seizure from a zone of eloquent cortex. More frequently, however, ictal symptoms are produced by spreading of the discharge from an epileptogenic zone located in a symptomatically silent area to a distant area of eloquent cortex that is outside the epileptogenic zone.

Electrical stimulation studies have shown that symptoms can be elicited from eloquent cortex only if the stimulus parameters are *strong* enough. The stimulus has to have appropriate frequency, the individual stimuli have to be of sufficient duration and intensity, and the duration of the stimulus train has to be adequate. We would not expect any symptoms from an epileptiform discharge unless it fulfills these criteria. This explains the frequent observation that an epileptiform discharge is recorded from a symptomatogenic zone without producing the corresponding symptoms. All the limitations previously outlined have to be considered when trying to define the epileptogenic zone by a careful analysis of ictal symptoms.

Irritative Zone

The irritative zone is the area of cortical tissue that generates interictal electrographic spikes. These spikes can be considered as *miniseizures*. If they are of sufficient *strength* and are generated within an eloquent cortical area, spikes can give rise to clinical symptoms. A typical example is localized myoclonic jerks that can be seen in patients with spikes in the primary motor cortex. Not all spikes give rise to afterdischarges, however. In general, isolated, independent spikes do not generate any clinical symptoms regardless of whether they are located in silent or eloquent cortex. To produce symptoms, the spikes have to give rise to runs of epileptiform discharges that have sufficient strength to induce symptoms when they invade a symptomatogenic zone. This explains why the seizure onset zone, discussed next, is usually a subset of the irritative zone.

Seizure Onset Zone

The seizure onset zone is the area of cortex from which clinical seizures are generated. Similar to the irritative zone, it is localized most commonly by either scalp or invasive electroencephalography (EEG) techniques. In contrast to the irritative zone, the location of the seizure onset zone also can be determined by ictal single-photon emission computed tomography (SPECT) and more recently by functional MRI. This section first discusses the limitations of EEG as a technique to evaluate the ictal onset zone. We then analyze if the same limitations apply to ictal SPECT or functional MRI, and we compare these techniques with EEG.

The seizure onset zone is usually the portion of the irritative zone that generates spikes capable of producing afterdischarges. These repetitive spikes frequently have enough strength to produce clinical ictal symptoms when they are generated in or spread to eloquent cortex. In general, afterdischarges also have a tendency to spread into adjacent cortex. It has been thought that precise definition of the seizure onset zone should provide an accurate definition of the epileptogenic zone. There are two problems, however, that greatly limit the ability of the seizure onset zone to act as a marker of the epileptogenic zone.

The first problem is that there is no methodology that permits precise definition of the seizure onset zone. Scalp electrodes give an excellent overview of the electrical activity of the brain and frequently suggest the side and approximate location of the seizure onset. Using these electrodes, the epileptologist can obtain broad coverage of the brain surface. Scalp EEG has relatively low sensitivity for the detection of the seizure onset, however, because the surface electrodes are located at a relatively great distance from the cortex and are separated from the brain by a series of barriers that interfere significantly with the transmission of the electrical signals. The afterdischarge generated locally at the seizure onset zone usually is too small to be detected by scalp electrodes. These electrodes are capable of detecting a seizure discharge only after it has extended considerably and has activated a relatively large area of cortex. Invasive cortical surface electrodes record activity from an extremely limited region of the brain. By eliminating distance and insulating barriers, each electrode records the cortical area covered by only that electrode. Invasive electrodes are inherently sensitive for the detection of afterdischarges but are able to define the seizure origin accurately only if they directly cover the seizure onset zone. Because of the difficulties in obtaining broad cortical coverage, it is unusual that invasive electrodes are actually located over the entire seizure onset zone. Instead the invasive recording typically is limited to a zone near the exact seizure onset zone or covers only a portion of this zone. On the rare occasion when the epileptologist may be able to define the precise location of the seizure onset zone by EEG, it is exceptional that this technology also allows definition of the borders of the epileptogenic zone.

The second problem to consider is that the actual seizure onset zone may not correspond with the epileptogenic zone (cortical area from which clinical seizures may arise). The epileptogenic zone may be more or less extensive than the seizure onset zone (Figs. 144–1 and 144–2). When the epileptogenic zone is smaller than the seizure onset zone, partial resection of the seizure onset zone may lead to seizure freedom because the remaining seizure onset zone has been weakened sufficiently, rendering it incapable of generating further seizures. Conversely, when the epileptogenic zone is greater than the seizure onset zone, even total resection of the seizure onset zone would not result in seizure freedom. This phenomenon occurs when a patient has seizure onset zones of different thresholds within a single epileptogenic zone. The seizure onset

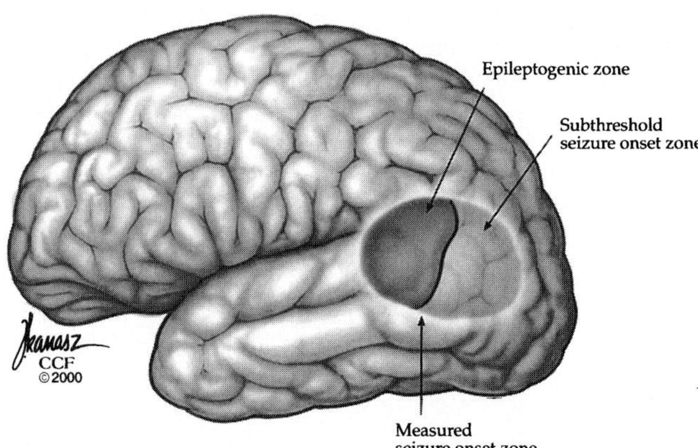

FIGURE 144–1. The seizure onset zone as measured by a variety of techniques is larger than the epileptogenic zone. Resection of the epileptogenic zone alone is sufficient to eliminate clinically evident seizures. The remaining portion of the seizure onset zone electrographically exhibits epileptiform activity but at a level below the threshold for the clinical manifestation of seizures.

zone of lowest threshold generates all the usual seizures and is the only one that can be measured directly. When this zone has been resected, however, another seizure onset zone of higher threshold may become clinically evident. There is no way to predict, even with the most modern technology, if additional, higher-threshold seizure onset zones exist. The cortical area of interest now becomes a *potential epileptogenic zone* containing one or more seizure onset zones. There are almost insurmountable practical barriers that make the actual seizure onset zone an imprecise index of the epileptogenic zone.

How do newer tests such as ictal SPECT and functional MRI that are designed to measure the seizure onset zone compare with scalp and invasive EEG? SPECT and functional MRI measure local changes in cerebral blood flow (a relative increase of ictal blood flow with respect to the interictal state). This increase of blood flow is a direct autoregulatory response to the hyperactivity of neurons during epileptogenic activation. Given that these changes are seen in regions of neuronal excitation, we would expect that SPECT and functional MRI would have the same theoretical limitations as EEG. Similar to EEG, neither SPECT nor functional MRI can identify a *potential epileptogenic zone* if it has not reached its threshold of activation. Regarding the sensitivities of these tests for detecting the seizure onset zone, numerous studies show a higher rate of false localization with either ictal SPECT or functional MRI than that shown with scalp EEG.[1–4] Invasive EEG always detects the seizure onset, often long before the initiation of clinical symptoms, indicating that, with regard to sensitivity, it is still the gold standard in mapping the seizure onset zone. The advantage of these imaging studies for localization is that they evaluate noninvasively all areas of the brain with the same degree of accuracy, including deeper regions of gray matter that are inaccessible to monitoring by scalp EEG. Although EEG and ictal SPECT are used to evaluate the same parameter, both techniques have significant problems regarding sensitivity. The two techniques do not provide identical information and should be considered to provide complementary data. The use of functional MRI to evaluate the seizure onset zone requires that the patient have a seizure while being scanned. This limitation makes functional MRI a practical test only in patients with frequent seizures.

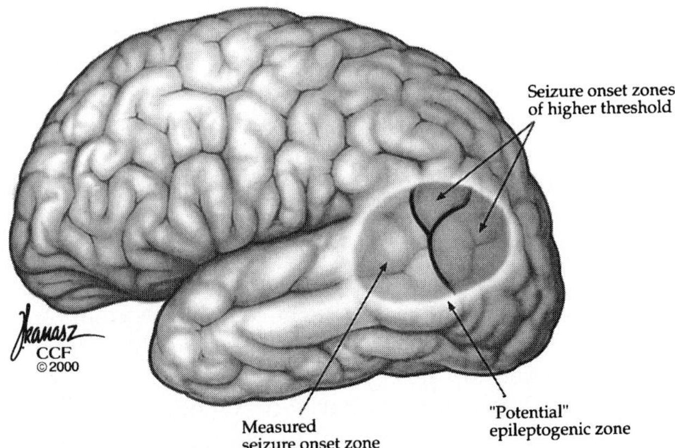

FIGURE 144–2. The measured seizure onset zone is smaller than the epileptogenic zone when adjacent seizure onset zones of higher threshold exist. Before surgical resection, only the measured seizure onset zone is believed to be responsible for generating clinical seizure activity. When this zone is resected, the adjacent seizure onset zones may become clinically evident. The true epileptogenic zone encompasses all of the seizure onset zones.

Epileptogenic Lesion

The epileptogenic lesion is a radiographic lesion that is the cause of the epileptic seizures. The best way to define this today is by high-resolution MRI. Not all lesions seen in a patient with epileptic seizures are epileptogenic, however. Some radiographic lesions may be unrelated to the clinical seizures. For this reason, when a lesion is seen on the MRI study, other methods still need to be used to verify (usually by video/EEG monitoring) that the radiographic lesion is responsible for the patient's seizures. A related problem is the definition of epileptogenicity in cases with dual or multiple pathology. Additional testing is necessary to define which of the lesions is epileptogenic. In cases in which two or more lesions are placed in close spatial proximity, the problem of attributing epileptogenicity to one lesion or another frequently can be resolved only with the use of invasive EEG technology.

The problem of the relationship of the epileptogenic zone with the epileptogenic lesion is similar to its relationship with the seizure onset zone discussed earlier. It has been thought that complete resection of the radiographic epileptogenic lesion is necessary to obtain seizure freedom. This is not always true, however, as evidenced by cases in which only partial lesion resection was possible (because of its location in eloquent cortex) with resultant complete seizure freedom. This situation implies that the remainder of the radiographic lesion either was never epileptogenic or was dependent on the resected tissue to elicit seizures. A more common clinical scenario occurs when seizures persist despite complete resection of the lesion visible on MRI. This is frequently the case in patients with cortical dysplasia or post-traumatic epilepsy. There are two possible explanations for this phenomenon. Many lesions are not intrinsically epileptogenic but induce seizures by generating reactions in the surrounding brain tissue with which they are in contact. Some of these lesions may induce microchanges in the brain tissue located at a significant distance from the epileptogenic lesion. These microchanges are epileptogenic, and in these cases selective resection of the MRI-visible epileptogenic lesion frequently is not sufficient to abolish all the seizures. Another explanation addresses the sensitivity of MRI in detecting the complete lesion. Brain tissue adjacent to a radiographic lesion may consist of lesional tissue of a lesser pathologic severity. This tissue, although potentially epileptogenic, may remain invisible on MRI. This is frequently the situation with cortical dysplasia, in which only the "tip of the iceberg" is visible on MRI. Failure to resect these MRI-invisible lesions can lead to persistence of seizures after seizure surgery. This is the most likely explanation for the relatively high frequency of surgical failure in patients with neocortical dysplasia.

There is no direct method to determine if an additional epileptogenic zone that is invisible on MRI surrounds any given epileptogenic lesion. The only way the epileptologist can try to predict the presence of a perilesional epileptogenic rim is by understanding the nature of the MRI-visible lesion. Well-delineated brain tumors and cavernous angiomas tend to produce epileptogenicity only in the MRI-visible lesion; lesionectomy usually is successful in these cases. As mentioned previously, cases with cortical dysplasia or post-traumatic epilepsy typically require more extensive resections for a successful outcome.

Area of Functional Deficit

The area of functional deficit is the area of cortex that is functionally abnormal in the interictal period. This dysfunction may be a direct result of the destructive effect of the lesion or may be functionally mediated (i.e., abnormal neuronal transmission that may affect brain function locally or at a considerable distance from the epileptogenic tissue). A variety of methods can be used to measure the functional deficit zone. Neurologic examination, neuropsychological testing, positron emission tomography (PET) scan, and interictal SPECT are some examples.

The relationship between these different tests and the location of the epileptogenic zone is complex and difficult to define even in individual cases. This difficulty is related to the fact that these tests measure parameters such as global brain function (general neurological examination) or brain physiology (local glucose metabolism or blood perfusion) but no factors more directly related to epileptogenesis. Some of these changes may be the result of a nonepileptogenic lesion or may occur at considerable distance from the primary seizure focus. The value of presurgically defining the functional deficit zone is relatively limited compared with the measurement of zones more directly related to the seizures. A typical example is seen in patients with pure mesial temporal sclerosis. PET studies often reveal extensive hypometabolic regions outside the mesial temporal structures. The epileptogenic zone usually is limited to the mesial temporal region, and seizure freedom often is achieved with resection of this tissue alone. Another example is seen in patients with extensive nonepileptogenic lesions in addition to a more limited epileptogenic lesion. Both types of lesions may produce a widespread functional deficit zone as defined by neurological testing, neuropsychological testing, PET, and interictal SPECT.

Despite all these limitations, good correlation of the functional deficit zone with the other zones defined previously provides additional supportive information regarding the location of the epileptogenic zone. Clear discrepancies between the results obtained in the tests used to define the different cortical zones make accurate definition of the epileptogenic zone difficult and frequently are a reason to request more sensitive, specific tests, such as invasive monitoring.

Epileptogenic Zone

The epileptogenic zone is the area of cortex that is required to generate epileptic seizures. This area may include an actual epileptogenic zone, which is the cortical area generating seizures before surgery (see earlier; equivalent to or smaller than the actual seizure onset zone), and a *potential epileptogenic zone*, which is an area of cortex that may generate seizures after the presurgical seizure onset zone has been resected. No diagnostic modality currently is available that can be used to measure directly the entire epileptogenic zone. This is because we cannot exclude the possible existence of a potential epileptogenic zone, which would become clinically apparent only postoperatively. The epileptogenic zone is a theoretical concept. If the patient is seizure-free after surgery, we conclude that the epileptogenic zone must have been included in the surgical resection.

Because the epileptogenic zone cannot be measured directly, its location must be inferred indirectly by defining the other zones discussed previously. When all of these data are concordant, the determination is easy. These cases are rare. In most cases, there is some degree of discrepancy between the five different zones. Attempts should be made to find a plausible explanation for these discrepancies, taking into consideration the basic principles outlined earlier. It is difficult to define the epileptogenic zone accurately when no adequate explanation for the discrepant location or extent of the different zones is found. In these cases, surgery should be deferred, while more precise testing, such as invasive video/EEG, is performed. As discussed earlier, however, invasive recordings are limited by their extent of cortical coverage. They should be used only in cases in which there is a clear hypothesis regarding the location of seizure onset and in which a specific question must be answered (e.g., from which lesion the seizure discharge originates in a patient with dual pathology or in patients with bilateral mesial temporal sclerosis).

Future Tests

There is a definite need to develop additional tests that can define the epileptogenic zone more directly. It is likely that these developments will be in functional neuroimaging. All widely available functional neuroimaging techniques (mainly PET and interictal SPECT) measure only nonspecific brain physiology, such as regional metabolism or blood flow. Further developments may make it possible to image directly the distribution of neurotransmitters involved in the pathogenesis of epilepsy. This imaging may allow us not only to define different types of epileptogenic lesions based on neurotransmitter and receptor physiology, but also to give a measurement of potential epileptogenic zones that currently are undetectable preoperatively. Refinements of the currently available diagnostic techniques may increase the accuracy with which epileptologists define the different zones, giving epileptologists some additional power even if they do not solve some of the essential theoretical limitations discussed before.

HISTORY OF EPILEPSY SURGERY

As previously stated, the objective of resective epilepsy surgery is the complete resection of the epileptogenic zone. This principle has remained constant since the origins of epilepsy surgery in the late 1870s. The means by which the epileptogenic zone is defined has undergone an evolution during this time, however, that parallels the evolution of technologic advances in neurodiagnostic testing. With the development and implementation of new testing modalities, new theories of defining the epileptogenic zone and new preoperative workups have evolved. The history of epilepsy surgery can be recounted by tracing the different theories of localizing the epileptogenic zone (Fig. 144–3).

Era of the Symptomatogenic Zone (1879–1935)

When the surgical treatment of epilepsy began, the location of the epileptogenic zone was determined almost exclusively by trying to locate the symptomatogenic zone. The concept that the symptomatogenic zone is a good estimate of the location of the epileptogenic zone was a by-product of the pioneering 19th

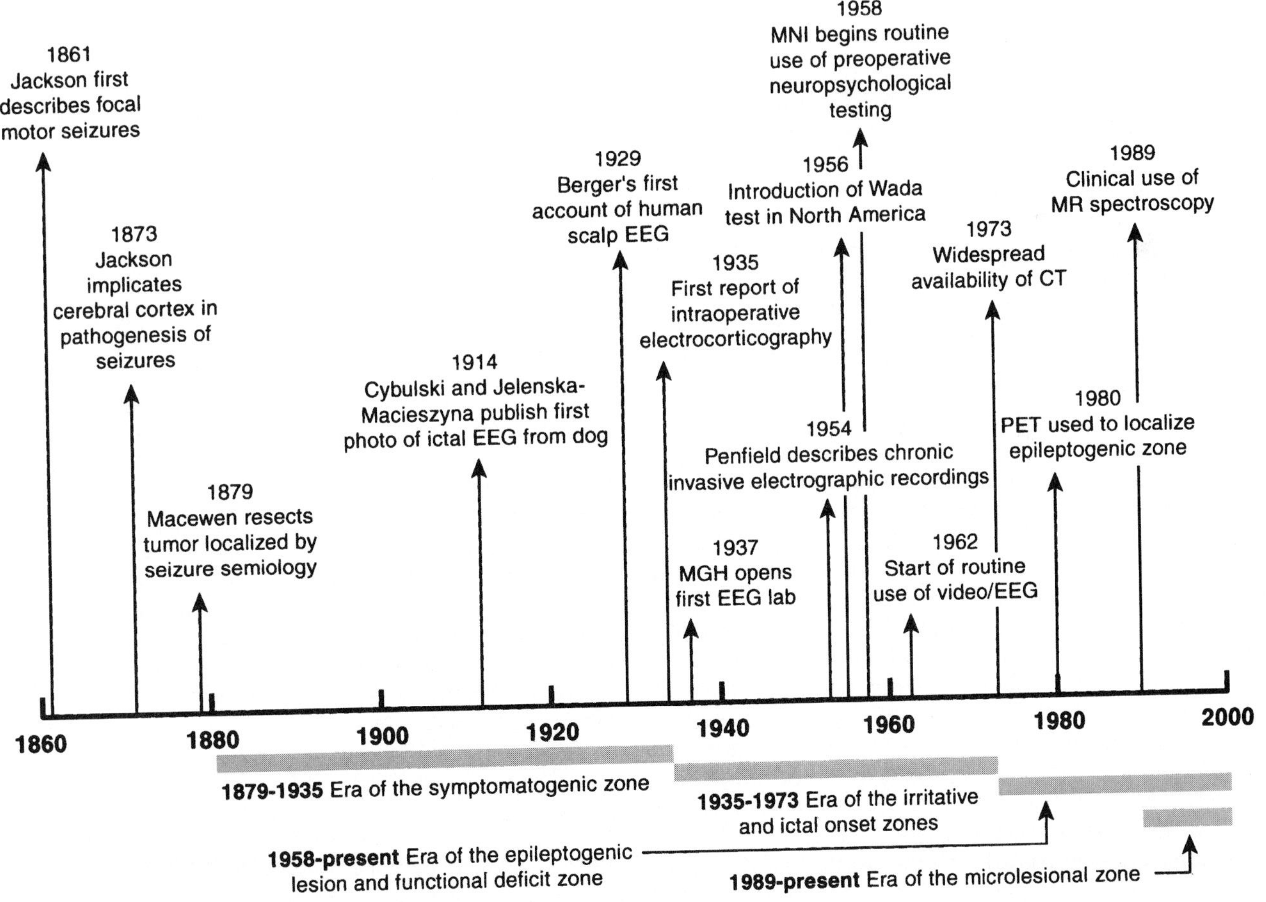

FIGURE 144–3. Timeline shows the history of epilepsy surgery. The major eras of thought pertaining to the localization of the epileptogenic zone are indicated at the bottom of the diagram. The vertical arrows indicate significant events that defined these eras.

century works of Jackson in clinical epilepsy. At that time, Jackson started to use ictal symptoms for cerebral localization in patients with partial epilepsies. Jackson's theories of epileptogenesis still prevail today and formulate the basis of our clinical understanding of epilepsy.

Before the work of Jackson and his pioneering theories of epileptogenesis, many theories had been proposed. By the early 19th century, the old ideas of seizures being caused by demonic possession had given way to the understanding of epilepsy as a physical illness. In 1836, Hall[5] published a theory of reflex action and applied it to epileptogenesis. Hall's animal experiments showed that motor reflexes were mediated through the spinal cord or the medulla oblongata. Hall proposed that epileptic seizures were caused by irritations of the afferent limb of the reflex arc. He asserted that disorders of dental, gastric, or intestinal origin could produce such irritation and lead to seizures. Hall[5] had difficulty explaining the loss of consciousness but believed this phenomenon was secondary to venous congestion from contraction of the neck musculature during a seizure. Hall's hypothesis was supported by Brown-Séquard,[6] who also believed that epilepsy is initiated by peripheral irritation and that the site of epileptogenesis is the medulla. Brown-Séquard differed from Hall in that he believed the loss of consciousness to be due to a reflex vasospasm causing cerebral ischemia.[7]

John Hughlings Jackson was born in Yorkshire, in April 1835. He trained at York Hospital Medical School from 1850 to 1855. In 1855–1856, Jackson studied in London at St. Bartholomew's Hospital with Paget. Jackson then returned to York, where he worked as House Physician at the York Dispensary for 3 years. In 1859, Jackson returned to London, where Hutchinson arranged for Jackson a position as Lecturer in Pathology, Morbid Anatomy, and Histology at The London Hospital Medical School. During the next several years, Jackson wrote and contributed many articles to the *Medical Times and Gazette*. In 1862, Jackson was appointed Assistant Physician at the National Hospital for the Relief and Cure of the Paralysed and Epileptic (now the National Hospital for Neurology and Neurosurgery), Queen Square, London, and full physician in 1867.[8–10]

Jackson first started writing about epilepsy in 1861, when he joined the staff of the *Medical Times and Gazette* as a medical correspondent and published an article entitled "Syphilitic Affections of the Nervous System."[11] In this article, Jackson[11] discussed seizures that are incomplete, unilateral *epileptiform convulsions* without loss of consciousness. His wife, having previously suffered a cerebral thrombosis, suffered from the same type of focal motor seizures, which became known as jacksonian epilepsy.[12] Jackson held to the popular view of the 1860s that the corpus striatum was the highest point in the motor tract, and he initially believed the pathology of focal motor epilepsy to be located in the basal ganglia.[7, 13] In 1863, however, Jackson began to recognize that the hemispheres frequently were involved in the generation of motor seizures. He wrote that the "autopsies of patients who have died after syphilitic epilepsy appear to show, the cause is obvious organic disease on the side of the brain, opposite to the side of the body convulsed, frequently on the surface of the hemisphere."[14] From 1863 to 1870, Jackson provided additional evidence that led him to recognize the role of the cerebral cortex in motor function and in epilepsy.

Jackson based his theories of cerebral localization and epileptogenesis on clinical observations and autopsy studies. He never carried out animal experiments to prove his conclusions.[15] In 1870, experimental studies by Fritsch and Hitzig provided experimental proof that electrical stimulation of the dog's frontal cortex could cause movement in the body on the opposite side. Hitzig[16] later stated that these experiments confirmed physiologically "that which Hughlings Jackson had concluded from clinical fact." Ferrier[17] confirmed these studies in London through electrical stimulation and ablation studies in animals. In 1873, Ferrier[17] stated, "The proximate causes of the different epilepsies, are as Hughlings Jackson supposes, 'discharging lesions' of the different centers in the cerebral hemispheres." By 1873, Jackson[18] had made his conclusive definition of epilepsy, which still stands today: "epilepsy is the name for occasional, sudden, excessive, rapid and local discharges of grey matter."

The belief that the epileptogenic zone could be localized based solely on symptoms paved the way for epilepsy surgery. The work of Jackson, Ferrier, Horsley, and Gowers was taking place at a time when a new trend in neuroscience recognized that certain somatic functions were attributable to specific locations in the brain. This trend led to concepts of cortical localization in epilepsy that revolutionized the way in which neuroscientists examined this disease process. In 1879, using such localization principles, Macewen,[19] a neurosurgeon working in Glasgow, correctly determined the location of a patient's frontal meningioma and resected the lesion. The patient survived and was cured of his seizures. In 1884, Bennet, with the help of Jackson, had in his care a patient who had seizures of increasing frequency involving the left side, leading to loss of consciousness and generalized seizures. Based primarily on this clinical observation, Bennet and Jackson localized the presumed lesion, and on November 25, 1884, Godlee found and resected a tumor from this site.[20, 21] During the next several years, Horsley,[22] working with Jackson and Ferrier, performed several operations for the treatment of epilepsy basing the localization of the resected tissue on symptoms. Until the introduction of EEG by Berger, localization in epilepsy surgery was based primarily on determination of the symptomatogenic zone.

Era of the Irritative and Ictal Onset Zones (1935–1973)

With the discovery of EEG as a tool to record interictal and ictal cortical activity, epileptologists soon realized that now they had a technique available that, together with the description of the ictal seizure symptoms, would allow them to define the epileptogenic zone with more precision. The first published report of electrical brain waves and sensory evoked potentials occurred in 1875, when Caton published his work on animal experiments in the *British Medical Journal*.[23, 24] Caton, working with the brains of monkeys and rabbits, showed a relationship between variation in electrical current and movement of the animal's head and neck. When recording the cortical region believed to be that for eyelids, Caton[24] showed that light to the opposite retina caused a change in brain waves. Beck later showed spontaneous electrical activity in the brains of dogs and rabbits in 1890.[23, 25] The first experimentally induced seizures recorded by EEG occurred in Russia in 1912 by Kaufmann,[26] a former student of Pavlov. Kaufmann showed abnormal brain waves in dogs after craniotomies were performed and tonic-clonic seizures were induced, but he did not have the equipment to photograph his data.[27] In 1914, Cybulski and Jelenska-Macieszyna[28] published the first photograph of an ictal EEG. The seizure was induced with electrical stimulation of the dog's cerebral cortex.[27, 28] The greatest advance in EEG came in 1929, when Berger[29] published his first work on scalp recordings of human EEG.[23]

Hans Berger was born on May 21, 1873, in Franconia. Berger first studied mathematics in Berlin, then changed his career and studied medicine in Würzburg, Berlin, Munich, Jena, and Kiel. Berger received his degree in Jena and began his work there at the Friedrich Schiller University Hospital. He became Chair and Director of the hospital in 1919.[30]

Berger was aware of Caton and Beck's work and unsuccessfully tried to study the electrical activity in the brain of animals from 1902 through 1910.[27] His research was interrupted during World War I, when he worked as an army neuropsychiatrist. When Berger returned to Jena, he was appointed chair of the Department of Neuropsychiatry, and his research resumed in 1920. Berger's first successful reading of scalp electrical activity occurred in 1924, when he recorded from the scalp of a patient who had a cranial defect secondary to a previous therapeutic trephination. Berger eventually developed EEG to record human brain activity from the scalp. His findings were published in the *Archiv für Psychiatrie und Nervenkrankheiten*.[29] Berger[31] mentioned his findings on interictal EEG activity as early as 1933. His work at first was met with skepticism; however, his findings finally were confirmed by Adrian and Matthews in 1934[32] and soon thereafter by Jasper and Carmichael in 1935.[33]

EEG quickly became clinically relevant. Fischer and Lowenbach[34] were the first to show epileptiform spikes in 1934.[23] Jasper[35] and Gibbs and colleagues[36] described the interictal spike as the hallmark of epilepsy in 1936. Schwab established the first clinic in the United States to perform EEG and to charge for its services in 1937 at the Massachusetts General Hospital.[27, 37] Penfield, who founded the Montreal Neurological Institute (MNI) in 1934, quickly recognized the great potential of EEG to define the epileptogenic zone better. Penfield convinced Jasper to join him in Montreal, and in January 1939 the MNI opened its laboratory of EEG and neurophysiology, the first of its kind to be dedicated to selecting epilepsy patients for surgery and providing the techniques for intraoperative recordings.[38, 39] Penfield and Erickson's book *Epilepsy and Cerebral Localization* contains a chapter by Jasper entitled "Electroencephalography."[40] This is one of the first reviews on the application of EEG to epilepsy and epilepsy surgery. This new technology allowed localization of seizures that occurred outside of eloquent cortical areas, such as the temporal lobes. In 1951, Bailey and Gibbs[41] reported on a series of 25 patients who had undergone temporal lobectomy based solely on EEG criteria. Their results were encouraging and helped to establish EEG as the primary modality of seizure localization in the workup of patients for surgical resection.[12]

In 1935, Foerster and Altenburger[42] published the first report of intraoperative electrocorticography (ECoG), which is the direct measurement of electrical activity from the human cerebral cortex during surgery (Fig. 144–4). Many others, including reports by Schwartz and Kerr in 1940[44] and Scarff and Rahm in 1941,[43] quickly followed. ECoG made it possible to measure brain electrical activity with much greater precision than scalp EEG by positioning the electrodes directly on the cortical surface. This eliminated the nearly 10-fold attenuation the electrical signal suffers when recorded through the skull and the scalp, which are media of high electrical resistance. From the beginning, ECoG has been used as a method to define the irritative zone (region of interictal spikes) with more

Electrocorticography

Tumor

Periphery of Tumor

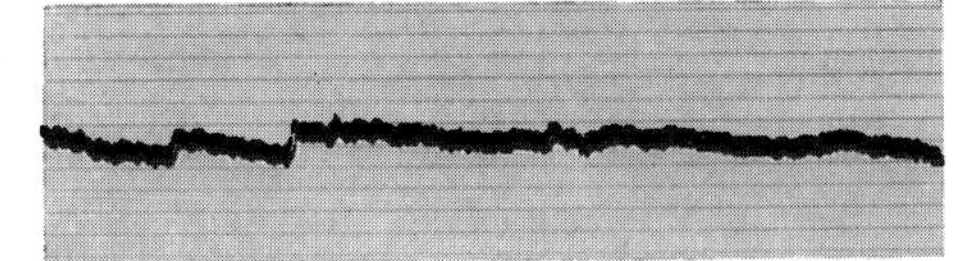

Healthy Cortex

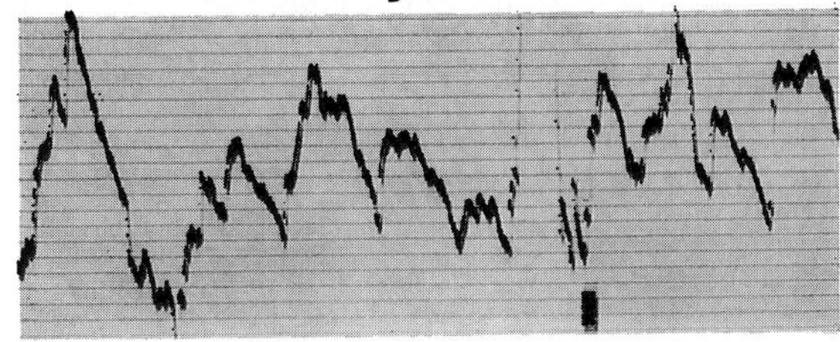

FIGURE 144–4. Tracing of the first intraoperative human electrocorticogram. (From Foerster FM, Altenburger H: Elektrobiologische vorgange an der menslichen Himrinde. Dtsch Z Nervenkr 135:277–288, 1935.)

precision during surgery. The logical assumption at that time was that total resection of the irritative zone was essential to achieve seizure freedom. By the early 1950s, ECoG was considered an indispensable tool in any epilepsy surgery program. Researchers soon realized, however, that successful outcomes also occurred in patients in whom complete resection of the irritative zone was not possible for a variety of reasons. This led to the eventual abandonment of ECoG in the late 1950s in some centers.[45–47] Falconer's[48] decision to perform standard temporal lobectomies for patients with temporal lobe epilepsy was linked closely to the observation that precise definition of the irritative zone by ECoG apparently did not affect the surgical outcome in these patients. Others, such as those at the Montreal Neurological Institute, also recognized the limitations of ECoG but continue its use today because of their belief that definition of the irritative zone still may play some role in the definition of the epileptogenic zone. Although ECoG is an extremely sensitive technique to define the irritative zone, initial enthusiasm faded as researchers realized the limitations of the irritative zone, even if accurately defined by ECoG, in determining the limits of the epileptogenic zone. Today in most centers, the impact that ECoG has on the final surgical decision is minimal, and many epilepsy surgery centers have abandoned its use.

The relatively poor technical quality of scalp EEG recordings obtained at the initial stages of clinical EEG explains the early attempts that researchers made to record electrical activity directly from the brain surface. Initially, recordings were obtained only during surgery (ECoG). ECoG was helpful in defining the irritative zone, but definition of the seizure onset zone remained elusive. Invasive recordings using chronically implanted electrodes were designed because investigators wanted to take advantage of the power of direct cortical recordings to define better the ictal onset zone. In 1954, long before the introduction of the CT scan into clinical practice in 1973 and the beginning of the era of the epileptogenic lesion, Penfield and Jasper[49] started using chronically implanted epidural strips of wires in an attempt to increase the sensitivity of EEG to define the seizure onset zone. This work soon was followed by the report of Ajmone-Marsan and Van Buren in 1958.[50] By the 1960s, Bancaud and Talairach[51–54] had developed and popularized the use of depth electrodes. These investigators used multicontact shaft electrodes that were implanted deep into brain parenchyma to reach mesial cortical structures and deep gray matter. The *stereoencephalography* of the French School soon had a major impact on epilepsy surgery centers. In essentially all European epilepsy centers, evaluation with depth electrodes using the technique developed by Talairach and Bancaud (or a slight modification of it) was required for surgical candidates before any surgical procedure was considered. Soon, depth electrodes were introduced in North America and became part of the standard evaluation of epilepsy surgery candidates.[55] Chronic invasive EEG recordings, which were introduced before the beginning of the epileptogenic lesion era, still play an important role today in more advanced epilepsy surgery centers.[56]

Parallel with the development of progressively more sophisticated techniques to define the irritative and ictal onset zones, epileptologists refined the precision to determine the symptomatogenic zone by developing recording techniques that allowed careful analysis of ictal symptoms and their correlation with the simultaneously recorded EEG. In 1938, attempts were made to combine EEG with video monitoring. At the 96th meeting of the American Psychiatric Association, Schwab showed moving pictures taken from two separate cameras simultaneously, one of the patient and the other of the EEG tracing.[27] In 1949, Hunter and Jasper[57] published their method of simultaneously recording the EEG tracing and the patient using a single camera. With the advent of the television in the 1950s, recording became easier. Goldensohn[58] started using a closed-circuit television system in 1962. This development was the start of the video/EEG technology that has been the essential diagnostic tool in presurgical evaluation of surgical candidates. With the introduction of new methods to define new cortical zones of completely different pathophysiologic significance, technologic advances have increased the ability to define better previously recognized cortical zones.

Era of the Epileptogenic Lesion and Functional Deficit Zone (1958–Present)

In 1973, the CT scan became available as a clinical tool.[59–63] Initially, CT had little impact on epilepsy surgery, in which major structural lesions already had been detected by the tools available at that time (clinical history, neurologic examination, interictal EEG, cerebrospinal analysis, and in some cases angiography or pneumoencephalography). It soon was discovered, however, that CT scans could detect some lesions that were clinically silent. Eventually, CT became a standard tool in most epilepsy centers. Patients who were candidates for epilepsy surgery were scanned to ensure that prominent lesions were not missed.

The real impact of anatomic neuroimaging on presurgical evaluation of patients undergoing epilepsy surgery came with the development of MRI. MRI studies first were performed on humans in the late 1970s.[12,64] By the early 1980s, MRI became routinely available for clinical use, and its role in evaluating epilepsy patients was becoming recognized.[65,66] With the introduction of high-resolution MRI in the mid-1980s, it had become well established that this imaging modality is more sensitive than CT in detecting lesions that cause seizure disorders.[67–71]

The history of the development of anatomic imaging is linked closely in time with the development of functional neuroimaging techniques that permit the evaluation of the functional deficit zone in patients who are candidates for epilepsy surgery. Some evaluation of the functional deficit zone was already possible, however, before the introduction of neuroimaging. This evaluation began with the work of Gall who, more than any other scientist, put the concept of cortical localization into use in the early 19th century.[13] By the mid-19th century, the standard neurological examination was understood well enough to allow localization of functional deficits if they were severe and affected some of the highly eloquent areas of the brain, such as the primary afferent and efferent areas (e.g., hemiparesis, cortical sensory deficits, visual field defects). Such deficits typically affect only a few surgical candidates whose lesions do not involve eloquent cortical areas. In patients undergoing surgery in the late 19th century, this technique already had some influence on the decision regarding the location of the epileptogenic zone.

The second category of testing that helped in defining the functional deficit zone in patients with epilepsy was neuropsychological testing. With the availability at the MNI of large numbers of patients who had undergone anterior temporal resection, Milner[72–74] attributed specialized functions to the left and right temporal lobes. By the late 1950s, this work led to systematic presurgical and postsurgical neuropsychological testing for all epilepsy surgery candidates. Milner's group also was the first to apply this test modality for localization of the epileptogenic zone.[75] By the early 1970s, extensive neuropsychological testing was considered an essential part of the workup for epilepsy surgery.[76–79] Three objectives of obtaining such data historically have been (1) establishment of baseline function for comparison with future test results, (2) lateralization and localization of the seizure focus, and (3) prediction of postoperative cognitive outcome.[80] With the development of other, more powerful tests to evaluate cortical areas of functional deficit, however, the role of neuropsychological testing in the presurgical evaluation changed. Epileptologists now seldom rely on the results of neuropsychological testing to lateralize or localize the epileptogenic zone. In modern epileptology, neuropsychology influences the decision regarding the location of the epileptogenic zone only if it shows markedly discrepant findings with other test results. A typical example is a striking verbal memory deficit in a right-handed patient with radiographic and electrographic evidence of right mesial temporal sclerosis and no other confounding factors that could explain dominance switching. Neuropsychological testing remains, however, an indispensable tool for prognosis of postsurgical neuropsychological deficits and for defining the potential for postsurgical neuropsychological rehabilitation. The intracarotid amobarbital procedure, or *Wada test*, which first was described in 1949 by Wada,[81] was used initially to lateralize only language function. The Wada test was introduced in North America in 1956 at the MNI.[82] In 1959, use of the Wada test was expanded to lateralize memory function in an attempt to identify areas of functional deficit and to predict postsurgical outcome.[83, 84] In modern neuropsychology, the Wada test is used mainly to lateralize eloquent cortex with regard to language and memory and is used only secondarily as a supplementary method to determine the localization of the epileptogenic zone. Use of the Wada test varies among institutions, with some centers testing all epilepsy surgery candidates and others selecting only a subset of these patients.

From the beginning of epilepsy surgery, decisions regarding the location of the epileptogenic zone were influenced by tests whose goal was to define functional deficit areas. It was the development of modern functional neuroimaging techniques in the late 1970s, however, that ushered in the functional deficit era. These developments centered on the field of nuclear medicine imaging. The two types of isotopic emission tomographic studies developed and refined during this time were PET and SPECT.

Brownell and Sweet recognized the potential of positron emission detection in imaging as early as 1953. The first positron scanner was developed at the Massachusetts General Hospital in 1970, but its clinical utility became manifest only with the technologic advances made in instrumentation, cyclotrons, and computational support.[85] In 1980, Kuhl and associates[86] published the first report of the use of PET to aid in the cortical localization of seizures. Kuhl and Engel[86–88] then showed that areas of interictal cortical hypometabolism imaged by fluorodeoxyglucose (FDG) PET in patients with temporal lobe epilepsy correlated extremely well with the presumed lateralization of the epileptogenic zone as defined by depth EEG (the gold standard at the time). Later the value of FDG PET in the lateralization and localization of extratemporal epilepsies was shown by many investigators.[89–91]

Parallel to the development of PET as a technique to define cortical areas of functional deficit, SPECT was introduced. Kuhl and Edwards[92] first introduced the concept of SPECT imaging in the early 1960s. The technique seldom was used until the 1970s, when technologic developments, especially in digital computers, allowed widespread clinical utility. The use of SPECT in the workup of epilepsy patients initially was introduced as an alternative, more affordable technique than PET to measure regional blood flow changes (usually a good reflection of regional metabolic changes). Many reports appeared suggesting that interictal SPECT alterations closely parallel the changes seen by PET technology.[93–96] More detailed studies revealed, however, that interictal SPECT was significantly less sensitive and specific than PET.[97–99] Although SPECT technology has its place in the workup of epilepsy surgery candidates, interictal SPECT alone seldom is used to evaluate functional deficit zones. PET studies, using a variety of other ligands such as flumazenil, currently are being evaluated in an attempt to find a methodology that may identify more precisely the area of functional deficit or give a more specific measurement of epileptogenicity.

FUTURE OF EPILEPSY SURGERY

More recent technologic developments not only have made available new techniques that triggered the *epileptogenic lesion/functional deficit zone era* of epilepsy surgery, but also have provided other modern techniques that permit better definition of most of the more classic cortical zones. With regard to the symptomatogenic zone, the advances since the 1980s have led to a better understanding of the location of different symptomatogenic zones and their relationships with the location of the epileptogenic zone. Definition of the location of the symptomatogenic zones was achieved mainly by detailed cortical stimulation studies in an extrasurgical setting.[100, 101]

With regard to the irritative/ictal onset zone, some significant advances were made. Analog EEG has been replaced almost completely by digital technology that greatly facilitates the review of the massive amount of EEG data collected during an EEG/video evaluation.[102–104] This technology has removed significant constraints of EEG data collection. Now the technologist needs to be concerned only with collecting an artifact-free record with good notation. If the interpreter is dissatisfied with the montage, it can be reformatted easily to a new montage. Changing variables, such as chart speed, gain, and filters, is simple and can enhance the interpretation of individual electrographic events.[102] Digital technology allows for automatic spike and seizure detection, computer-based surface mapping of EEG voltages, and source localization of EEG generators.[105]

The evolution of magnetoencephalography (MEG) has provided additional data for definition of the irritative zone. The development of MEG began in the 1960s with the work of Cohen,[106] a physicist at the Massachusetts Institute of Technology. During the next 2 decades, interest in this modality grew with the publication of several important papers from researchers at New York University.[107–111] In 1982, researchers at the University of California, Los Angeles, first described the use of MEG to localize epileptiform discharges in human subjects, leading to the first clinical consideration for this technique.[112] Today, MEG is used in epilepsy workups for two primary tasks: (1) localization of the seizure focus and (2) functional mapping of normal cortical areas.[113]

MEG recordings are based on the detection of small magnetic fluxes generated from intraneuronal electrical currents. A typical MEG device uses an array with 80 channels to record spikes over both hemispheres. Using anatomic or surface references, the MEG recordings can be coregistered with MRI images and displayed as a composite. This fusion of structural and functional data is termed *magnetic source imaging*.

How does MEG compare with EEG in the workup of epilepsy surgery candidates? In contrast to EEG, MEG measures magnetic fluxes, which are not attenuated by barriers such as dura, bone, and scalp, leading to minimal signal loss and distortion. These anatomic barriers insulate and distort the electrical signals detected by EEG in unpredictable ways, especially in the presence of previous traumatic and surgical defects.[114, 115] Such distortion makes coregistration of EEG sampling arrays with structural images inaccurate. This gives MEG a theoretical advantage in localization over EEG, which has been shown in experimental comparisons between these two techniques.[115–120] The strength of the measured magnetic flux decreases as a function of the cube of the distance from the source. This makes sampling of deep-seated foci difficult. The measurement of magnetic fluxes from the cortical surface depends on the orientation of the measured neuronal population to the detector. As a result of this fact, MEG devices are capable of sampling only neurons that are oriented parallel to the scalp (i.e., neurons that line the sulci). Neurons that are contained in the gyral surfaces are oriented perpendicular to the scalp and cannot be sampled by MEG.[121] EEG and MEG appear to provide complementary data in the workup of epilepsy surgery candidates.

With regard to the seizure onset zone, ictal SPECT has been refined into a routine part of the workup of surgical candidates in many epilepsy centers. As previously stated, interictal SPECT alone has shown little utility in the workup of epilepsy surgery candidates. In contrast to the interictal state, in which areas of decreased cortical blood flow and metabolism are measured, the ictal state is characterized by increases in both of these measurements in the region of the seizure focus. Horsley[122] first described this in 1892 when he observed hyperemic cortical changes during a patient's intraoperative seizure. Although SPECT shows regional blood flow, PET measures regional cerebral metabolic activity and has provided more clinically useful information in interictal studies. The use of PET for ictal studies has several logistic challenges given the need for tracer injection before the seizure. The use of SPECT to show ictal hyperperfusion first was described in 1983[123] and since has been refined in multiple studies.[124, 125] Characteristic and diagnostic patterns of blood flow in the postictal period have been shown to aid in seizure localization in patients with temporal lobe epilepsy[98, 126–128] and extratemporal epilepsy.[129, 130]

It is likely that with the development of new neuroimaging methods, the most important advances in the presurgical evaluation of patients with intractable epilepsy will be the availability of more precise markers of microscopic lesional zones. Such methods would allow epileptologists to map directly the actual and *potential* epileptogenic zones. Magnetic resonance spectroscopy is a noninvasive technique that can be used to measure selected chemical components of the brain tissue (e.g., the ratio between *N*-acetylaspartate and choline/creatine).[131–133] Abnormal magnetic resonance spectroscopy findings suggest some degree of brain tissue pathology even if no lesion is shown with standard anatomic imaging techniques (e.g., high-resolution MRI, fluid-attenuated inversion recovery [FLAIR]). Future advances in neuroimaging techniques will allow epileptologists to image various neurotransmitters directly and permit direct visualization of the actual and the potential epileptogenic zones. Various types and degrees of pathologic change affect these zones, and it is likely that modern neuroimaging techniques will permit classification of the epileptogenic zones according to such variables (e.g., alteration of neurotransmitters, dysfunction of ion channels, alteration of structural cellular proteins). We believe that direct visualization of these *microscopic* cellular alterations will mark the beginning of the *era of the microlesional zone*. The precise understanding of the pathophysiology of the epileptogenic zone that will accompany the identification of these microlesional zones also should lead to a more rational approach to epilepsy surgery and, it is hoped, to better surgical outcomes.

REFERENCES

1. Jackson GD, et al: Functional magnetic resonance imaging of focal seizures. Neurology 44:850–856, 1994.
2. Lee BI, et al: Single photon emission computed tomography-EEG relations in temporal lobe epilepsy. Neurology 49:981–991, 1997.
3. Detre JA, et al: Localization of subclinical ictal activity by functional magnetic resonance imaging: Correlation with invasive monitoring. Ann Neurol 38:618–624, 1995.
4. Warach S, et al: Hyperperfusion of ictal seizure focus demonstrated by MR perfusion imaging. AJNR Am J Neuroradiol 15: 965–968, 1994.
5. Hall M: Lectures on the Nervous System and Its Diseases. London, Sherwood, Gilbert & Piper, 1836.
6. Brown-Sequard CE: Course of Lectures on the Physiology and Pathology of the Nervous System. Philadelphia, Lippincott & Co, 1860.
7. Eadie MJ: XIXth century pre-Jacksonian concepts of epileptogenesis. Clin Exp Neurol 29:26–31, 1992.
8. Critchley M, Critchley EA: John Hughlings Jackson: Father of English Neurology. New York, Oxford University Press, 1998.
9. Swash M: John Hughlings-Jackson: a sesquicentennial tribute. J Neurol Neurosurg Psychiatry 49:981–985, 1986.
10. Tyler KL: Hughlings Jackson: The early development of his ideas on epilepsy. J Hist Med Allied Sci 39:55–64, 1984.
11. Jackson JH: Syphilitic affections of the nervous system. Medical Times and Gazette, 1861.
12. Kuzniecky RI, Jackson GD: Magnetic Resonance in Epilepsy. New York, Raven Press, 1995.
13. Finger S: Origins of Neuroscience. New York, Oxford University Press, 1994.
14. Jackson JH: Convulsive spasms of the right hand and arm preceding epileptic seizures. Medical Times and Gazette 1:110–111, 1863.
15. Reynolds EH: Hughlings Jackson: A Yorkshireman's contribution to epilepsy. Arch Neurol 45:675–678, 1988.
16. Hitzig E: Hughlings Jackson and the cortical motor centres in the light of physiological research. Brain 23:545–581, 1900.
17. Ferrier D: Experimental researches in cerebral physiology and pathology. Rep West Riding Lunatic Asylum 3:30–96, 1873.
18. Jackson JH: On the anatomical, physiological, and pathological investigation of epilepsies. Rep West Riding Lunatic Asylum 3: 315–339, 1873.
19. Macewen W: Tumor of the dura mater removed during life in a person affected with epilepsy. Glasgow Med J 12:210, 1879.
20. Green JR: The beginnings of cerebral localization and neurological surgery. BNI Quarterly 1:12–28, 1985.
21. Bennet AH, Godlee RJ: Excision of a tumour from the brain. Lancet 1:1090–1091, 1884.
22. Horsley V: Ten consecutive cases of operations upon the brain and cranial cavity to illustrate the details and safety of the method employed. BMJ 863–865, 1887.
23. Swartz BE, Goldensohn ES: Timeline of the history of EEG and associated fields. Electroencephalogr Clin Neurophysiol 106: 173–176, 1998.
24. Caton R: The electric currents of the brain. BMJ 2:278, 1875.
25. Brazier MAB: A History of the Electrical Activity of the Brain: The First Half-Century. London, Pitman, 1961.
26. Kaufmann PY: Electrical phenomena in cerebral cortex [in Russian]. Obz Psikhiatr Nev Eksper 7–8:403, 1912.
27. Goldensohn ES, Porter RJ, Schwartzkroin PA: The American Epilepsy Society: An historic perspective on 50 years of advances in research. Epilepsia 38:124–150, 1997.
28. Cybulski N, Jelenska-Macieszyna X: Action currents of the cerebral cortex [in Polish]. Bull Acad Sci Cracov B:776–781, 1914.
29. Berger H: Uber das Electrenkephalogramm des Menschen. Arch Psychiatr Nervenkr 87:527–570, 1929.
30. Wiedemann HR: Hans Berger (1873–1941). Eur J Pediatr 153: 705, 1994.
31. Berger H: Uber das Electrenkephalogramm des Menschen. Arch Psychiatr Nervenkr 100:301–320, 1933.
32. Adrian ED, Matthews BHC: The Berger rhythm: Potential changes from the occipital lobes in man. Brain 57:355–385, 1934.
33. Jasper HH, Carmichael L: Electrical potentials from the intact human brain. Science 81:51–53, 1935.
34. Fischer MH, Lowenbach H: Aktionsstrome des Zentralnervensystems unter der Einwikung von Krampfgiften: I. Miteilung Strychnin und Pikrotoxin. Arch Exp Pathol Pharmakol 174: 357–382, 1934.
35. Jasper HH: Localized analyses of the function of the human brain by the electro-encephalogram. Arch Neurol Psychiatry 36: 1131–1134, 1936.
36. Gibbs FA, Lennox WG, Gibbs EL: The electroencephalogram in diagnosis and in localization of epileptic seizures. Arch Neurol Psychiatry 36:1225–1235, 1936.
37. Brazier MAB: The EEG Journal loses one of its founders. Electroencephalogr Clin Neurophysiol 33:i–ii, 1972.
38. Feindel W: Toward a surgical cure for epilepsy: The work of Wilder Penfield and his school at the Montreal Neurological Institute. In Engel J (ed): Surgical Treatment of the Epilepsies. Philadelphia, Lippincott-Raven, 1996, pp 1–9.
39. Jasper HH: History of the early development of electroencephalography and clinical neurophysiology at the Montreal Neurological Institute: The first 25 years 1939–1964. Can J Neurol Sci 18(4 Suppl):533–548, 1991.
40. Jasper HH: Electroencephalography. In Penfield W, Erickson TC (eds): Epilepsy and Cerebral Localization. Springfield, IL, Charles C Thomas, 1941, pp 380–454.
41. Bailey P, Gibbs FA: The surgical treatment of psychomotor epilepsy. JAMA 145:365–370, 1951.
42. Foerster FM, Altenburger H: Elektrobiologische Vorgange an der menslichen Hirnrinde. Dtsch Z Nervenkr 135:277–288, 1935.
43. Scarff JE, Rahm WE: The human electro-corticogram: A report of spontaneous electrical potentials obtained from the exposed human brain. J Neurophysiol 4:418–426, 1941.
44. Schwartz HG, Kerr AS: Electrical activity of the exposed human brain: Description of technique and report of cases. Arch Neurol Psychiatr 43:457–559, 1940.
45. Walker AE, Lichtenstein S, Marshall C: A critical analysis of electrocorticography in temporal lobe epilepsy. Arch Neurol 2: 172–182, 1960.
46. Falconer MA: Discussion. In Baldwin M, Bailey P (eds): Temporal Lobe Epilepsy. Springfield, IL, Charles C Thomas, 1958, pp 483–499.
47. David M, Dell MB: Considerations on "temporal lobe" epilepsy and its surgical treatment. In Lorentz de Haas AM (ed): Lectures on Epilepsy. Amsterdam, Elsevier, 1958, pp 1–28.
48. Falconer MA: Discussion on the surgery of temporal lobe epilepsy: Surgical and pathological aspects. Proc R Soc Med 46: 971–974, 1953.
49. Penfield W, Jasper H: Epilepsy and the Functional Anatomy of the Human Brain. Boston, Little, Brown, 1954.
50. Ajmone-Marsan C, VanBuren JM: Epileptiform activity in cortical and subcortical structures in the temporal lobe of man. In Baldwin M, Bailey P (eds): Temporal Lobe Epilepsy. Springfield, IL, Charles C Thomas, 1958, pp 78–108.
51. Bancaud J, et al: La stereo-electroencephalographie dans l'epilepsie: Informations neurophysiopathologiques appotees par l'investigation functionelle stereotaxique. Paris, Masson, 1965.
52. Talairach J, David M, Tournoux P: L'exploration chirugicale stereotaxique du lobe temporale dans l'epilepsie temporale. Paris, Masson et Cie, 1958.
53. Talairach J, Bancaud J: Stereotactic approach to epilepsy. Prog Neurol Surg 5:297–354, 1973.
54. Talairach J, Bancaud J: Stereotaxic exploration and therapy in epilepsy. In Vinken PJ, Bruyn CS (eds): The Epilepsies: Handbook of Clinical Neurology. Amsterdam, Elsevier, 1974, pp 758–782.
55. Crandall PH, Walter RD, Rand RW: Clinical applications of studies on stereotactically implanted electrodes in temporal lobe epilepsy. J Neurosurg 20:827–840, 1963.

56. Blatt DR, Roper SN, Friedman WA: Invasive monitoring of limbic epilepsy using stereotactic depth and subdural strip electrodes: Surgical technique. Surg Neurol 48:74–79, 1997.
57. Hunter J, Jasper H: A method of simultaneous analysis of seizures and EEG on film. Electroencephalogr Clin Neurophysiol 1:113, 1949.
58. Goldensohn ES: Simultaneous recording of EEG and clinical seizures using kinescope. Electroencephalogr Clin Neurophysiol 21:623, 1966.
59. Ambrose J: Computerized transverse axial scanning (tomography): 2. Clinical application. Br J Radiol 46:1023–1047, 1973.
60. Ambrose J, Hounsfield G: Computerized transverse axial tomography. Br J Radiol 46:148–149, 1973.
61. Ambrose JA: Computerized transverse axial tomography. Br J Radiol 46:401, 1973.
62. Ambrose JA: The usefulness of computerized transverse axial scanning in problems arising from cerebral haemorrhage, infarction or oedema. Br J Radiol 46:736, 1973.
63. Hounsfield GN: Computerized transverse axial scanning (tomography): 1. Description of system. Br J Radiol 46:1016–1022, 1973.
64. Gadian DG: Nuclear Magnetic Resonance and Its Applications to Living Systems. New York, Oxford University Press, 1982.
65. Oldendorf WH: The use and promise of nuclear magnetic resonance imaging in epilepsy. Epilepsia 25(Suppl 2):S105–117, 1984.
66. Sostman HD, et al: Preliminary observations on magnetic resonance imaging in refractory epilepsy. Magn Reson Imaging 2: 301–306, 1984.
67. Heinz ER, et al: Efficacy of MR vs CT in epilepsy. AJR Am J Roentgenol 152:347–352, 1989.
68. Laster DW, et al: Chronic seizure disorders: Contribution of MR imaging when CT is normal. AJNR Am J Neuroradiol 6: 177–180, 1985.
69. Latack JT, et al: Patients with partial seizures: Evaluation by MR, CT, and PET imaging. Radiology 159:159–163, 1986.
70. Ormson MJ, et al: Cryptic structural lesions in refractory partial epilepsy: MR imaging and CT studies. Radiology 160:215–219, 1986.
71. Schorner W, Meencke HJ, Felix R: Temporal-lobe epilepsy: Comparison of CT and MR imaging. AJR Am J Roentgenol 149: 1231–1239, 1987.
72. Milner B, Penfield W: The effect of hippocampal lesions on recent memory. Trans Am Neurol Assoc 80:42–48, 1955.
73. Milner B: Psychological defects produced by temporal-lobe excision. Res Publ Assoc Nerv Ment Dis 36:244–257, 1958.
74. Milner B: Interhemispheric differences in the localization of psychological processes in man. Br Med Bull 27:272–277, 1971.
75. Milner B: Psychological aspects of focal epilepsy and its neurosurgical management. Adv Neurol 8:299–321, 1975.
76. Lezak MD: Neuropsychological Assessment, 2nd ed. New York, Oxford University Press, 1983.
77. Rausch R, Babb TL: Hippocampal neuron loss and memory scores before and after temporal lobe surgery for epilepsy. Arch Neurol 50:812–817, 1993.
78. Sass KJ, et al: Verbal memory impairment correlates with hippocampal pyramidal cell density. Neurology 40:1694–1697, 1990.
79. Trenerry MR, et al: MRI hippocampal volumes and memory function before and after temporal lobectomy. Neurology 43: 1800–1805, 1993.
80. Chelune G: Using neuropsychological data to forecast postsurgical cognitive outcome. In Luders HO (ed): Epilepsy Surgery. New York, Raven Press, 1992, pp 477–485.
81. Wada J: A new method for the determination of the side of cerebral speech dominance: A preliminary report on the intracarotid injection of sodium amytal in man. Igaku Seibutsugaku 14:221–222, 1949.
82. Wada J, Rasmussen T: Intracarotid injection of sodium amytal for the lateralization of cerebral speech dominance: Experimental and clinical observations. J Neurosurg 17:266–282, 1960.
83. Milner B, Branch C, Rasmussen T: Study of short-term memory after intracarotid injection of sodium amytal. Trans Am Neurol Assoc 87:224–226, 1962.
84. Blume WT, et al: Intracarotid amobarbital test of language and memory before temporal lobectomy for seizure control. Neurology 23:812–819, 1973.
85. Early PJ: Positron emission tomography (PET). In Early PJ, Sodee D (eds): Principles and Practice of Nuclear Medicine. St. Louis, Mosby, 1995, p 314.
86. Kuhl DE, et al: Epileptic patterns of local cerebral metabolism and perfusion in humans determined by emission computed tomography of 18FDG and 13NH3. Ann Neurol 8:348–360, 1980.
87. Engel J Jr, et al: Comparative localization of epileptic foci in partial epilepsy by PCT and EEG. Ann Neurol 12:529–537, 1982.
88. Engel J Jr, et al: Interictal cerebral glucose metabolism in partial epilepsy and its relation to EEG changes. Ann Neurol 12:510–517, 1982.
89. Swartz BE, et al: Neuroimaging in patients with seizures of probable frontal lobe origin. Epilepsia 30:547–558, 1989.
90. Theodore WH, et al: Complex partial seizures: Cerebral structure and cerebral function. Epilepsia 27:576–582, 1986.
91. Henry TR, et al: Interictal cerebral metabolism in partial epilepsies of neocortical origin. Epilepsy Res 10:174–182, 1991.
92. Kuhl DE, Edwards RQ: Image separation radioisotope scanning. Radiology 80:653, 1963.
93. Ryding E, et al: SPECT measurements with 99mTc-HM-PAO in focal epilepsy. J Cereb Blood Flow Metab 8:S95–100, 1988.
94. Podreka I, et al: Initial experience with technetium-99m HM-PAO brain SPECT. J Nucl Med 28:1657–1666, 1987.
95. Biersack HJ, et al: 99mTc-labelled hexamethylpropyleneamine oxime photon emission scans in epilepsy [letter]. Lancet 2:1436–1437, 1985.
96. Biersack HJ, et al: HM-PAO brain SPECT and epilepsy. Nucl Med Commun 8:513–518, 1987.
97. Lee BI, et al: HIPDM-SPECT in patients with medically intractable complex partial seizures: Ictal study. Arch Neurol 45:397–402, 1988.
98. Rowe CC, et al: Visual and quantitative analysis of interictal SPECT with technetium-99m-HMPAO in temporal lobe epilepsy. J Nucl Med 32:1688–1694, 1991.
99. Stefan H, et al: Functional and morphological abnormalities in temporal lobe epilepsy: A comparison of interictal and ictal EEG, CT, MRI, SPECT and PET. J Neurol 234:377–384, 1987.
100. Lüders HO (ed): Epileptic Seizures: Pathophysiology and Clinical Semiology. Philadelphia, Churchill Livingstone, 2000.
101. Feindel W: Brain stimulation combined with electrocorticography in the surgery of epilepsy: Historical highlights. Electroencephalogr Clin Neurophysiol 48(Suppl):1–8, 1998.
102. Swartz BE: The advantages of digital over analog recording techniques. Electroencephalogr Clin Neurophysiol 106:113–117, 1998.
103. Gotman J: The use of computers in analysis and display of EEG and evoked potentials. In Daly DD, Pedley TA (eds): Current Practice of Clinical Electroencephalography. New York, Raven Press, 1990, pp 51–84.
104. Blum DE: Computer-based electroencephalography: Technical basics, basis for new applications, and potential pitfalls. Electroencephalogr Clin Neurophysiol 106:118–126, 1998.
105. Duffy FH, Burchfiel JL, Lombroso CT: Brain electrical activity mapping (BEAM): A method for extending the clinical utility of EEG and evoked potential data. Ann Neurol 5:309–321, 1979.
106. Cohen D: Magnetoencephalography: Evidence of magnetic fields produced by alpha-rhythm currents. Science 161:784–786, 1968.
107. Okada YC, Williamson SJ, Kaufman L: Magnetic field of the human sensorimotor cortex. Int J Neurosci 17:33–38, 1982.
108. Williamson SJ, Kaufman L: Analysis of neuromagnetic signals. In Gevins A, Remond A (eds): Handbook of Electroencephalography and Clinical Neurophysiology. Amsterdam, Elsevier, 1987, pp 405–448.
109. Kaufman L, Williamson SJ: Magnetic location of cortical activity. Ann N Y Acad Sci 388:197–213, 1982.
110. Kaufman L, Williamson SJ: The neuromagnetic field. In Cracco RQ, Bodis-Wolner I (eds): Evoked Potentials: Frontiers of Clinical Science. New York, Alan R. Liss, 1986, pp 85–98.
111. Brenner D, Williamson SJ, Kaufman L: Visually evoked magnetic fields of the human brain. Science 190:480–482, 1975.
112. Barth DS, et al: Neuromagnetic localization of epileptiform spike activity in the human brain. Science 218:891–894, 1982.
113. Rowley HA, Roberts TP: Functional localization by magnetoencephalography. Neuroimaging Clin N Am 5:695–710, 1995.

114. Cuffin BN: Effects of local variations in skull and scalp thickness on EEG's and MEG's. IEEE Trans Biomed Eng 40:42–48, 1993.
115. Williamson SJ, et al: Advantages and limitations of magnetic source imaging. Brain Topogr 4:169–180, 1991.
116. Hari R, et al: MEG versus EEG localization test [letter]. Ann Neurol 30:222–224, 1991.
117. Williamson SJ: MEG versus EEG localization test [letter]. Ann Neurol 30:222–224, 1991.
118. Balish M, et al: Localization of implanted dipoles by magnetoencephalography. Neurology 41:1072–1076, 1991.
119. Cohen D, et al: MEG versus EEG localization test using implanted sources in the human brain. Ann Neurol 28:811–817, 1990.
120. Rose DF, et al: Magnetoencephalographic localization of subdural dipoles in a patient with temporal lobe epilepsy. Epilepsia 32:635–641, 1991.
121. Hari R, Kaukoranta E: Neuromagnetic studies of somatosensory system: Principles and examples. Prog Neurobiol 24:233–256, 1985.
122. Horsley V: An address on the origin and seat of epileptic disturbance. BMJ 1:693–696, 1892.
123. Uren RF, et al: Single-photon emission computed tomography: A method of measuring cerebral blood flow in three dimensions (preliminary results of studies in patients with epilepsy and stroke). Med J Aust 1:411–413, 1983.
124. Newton MR, et al: Postictal switch in blood flow distribution and temporal lobe seizures. J Neurol Neurosurg Psychiatry 55: 891–894, 1992.
125. Stefan H, et al: Regional cerebral blood flow during focal seizures of temporal and frontocentral onset. Ann Neurol 27:162–166, 1990.
126. Rowe CC, et al: Postictal SPET in epilepsy [letter]. Lancet 1: 389–390, 1989.
127. Rowe CC, et al: Localization of epileptic foci with postictal single photon emission computed tomography. Ann Neurol 26: 660–668, 1989.
128. Rowe CC, et al: Patterns of postictal cerebral blood flow in temporal lobe epilepsy: Qualitative and quantitative analysis. Neurology 41:1096–1103, 1991.
129. Brinkmann BH, et al: Quantitative and clinical analysis of SPECT image registration for epilepsy studies. J Nucl Med 40: 1098–1105, 1999.
130. O'Brien TJ, et al: The practical utility of performing peri-ictal SPECT in the evaluation of children with partial epilepsy. Pediatr Neurol 19:15–22, 1998.
131. Petroff OA, et al: High-field proton magnetic resonance spectroscopy of human cerebrum obtained during surgery for epilepsy. Neurology 39:1197–1202, 1989.
132. Urenjak J, et al: Specific expression of N-acetylaspartate in neurons, oligodendrocyte-type-2 astrocyte progenitors, and immature oligodendrocytes in vitro. J Neurochem 59:55–61, 1992.
133. Urenjak J, et al: Proton nuclear magnetic resonance spectroscopy unambiguously identifies different neural cell types. J Neurosci 13:981–989, 1993.

CHAPTER **145**

Basic Science of Post-traumatic Epilepsy

RAIMONDO D'AMBROSIO

The past decades of neuroscience research have brought to light a tight parallelism between the basic mechanisms of brain function and those of epilepsy. Indeed, every process contributing to the regulation of neuronal function may potentially be involved in epilepsy. Given the great number of cellular features that are already known to be involved in the regulation of neuronal excitability, and because epileptiform activity may be the ultimate consequence of even a slight change in the activity of a single type of ion channel, no feature of the brain should be disregarded a priori. With so many potential causes for altered neuronal excitability, it is not surprising that there are equally numerous causes for epilepsy. Epilepsy, in fact, is not a single disease. Although abnormal neuronal activity is present in all its manifestations, epilepsy is a neurological disorder that encompasses several syndromes with a broad spectrum of symptoms arising from a large number of known and unknown disorders of brain function. Epileptic syndromes are broadly classified as symptomatic or idiopathic. When epilepsy is not associated with brain lesions or abnormalities other than the seizures themselves, it is termed idiopathic. In symptomatic epilepsy, seizures are the result of an identifiable lesion of the brain. Clinical manifestations may be equally diverse, ranging from momentary behavioral arrest to tonic-clonic convulsions. The diversity of causes and clinical manifestations of the various epilepsies has important implications for the development of therapeutic strategies. Because there are many potential causes of seizure precipitation, it is unlikely that drugs targeting only a few of these mechanisms will ever result in complete control of seizures. Antiepileptic drugs targeting only the final common step of seizure precipitation, neuronal bursting and synchronization, are unlikely to fully control all forms of seizures or, especially, to prevent the onset of the seizures themselves, that is, be antiepileptogenic. In fact, the significant number of patients that have poorly controlled seizures suggests that many seizuregenic mechanisms are not targeted by any of the current available antiepileptic drugs.

This chapter focuses on one form of symptomatic epilepsy, the post-traumatic, and to stimulate the search for a better treatment, I discuss certain basic mechanisms that are thought to be involved in its development and maintenance. The presented proepileptic mechanisms may be classified as being either synaptic or nonsynaptic. Synaptic mechanisms of epilepsies are those that depend on synaptic and intrinsic neuronal function. Nonsynaptic mechanisms of epilepsies are those that lead to seizure generation or epileptogenesis through changes in extracellular space function and homeostasis.

SYNAPTIC MECHANISMS OF POST-TRAUMATIC EPILEPSY

Selective Vulnerability of Hilar Neurons

One of the hypothesized synaptic mechanisms is selective hippocampal neuronal loss. This hypothesis was first put forward by Lowenstein and colleagues[1] in 1992. Consistent with the neuronal loss and hippocampal sclerosis observed after traumatic brain injury (TBI) in humans, a single event of fluid percussion injury (FPI), a clinically relevant model of TBI,[2] caused hilar neuron loss in the rat. The resulting hippocampal damage was accompanied by hyperexcitability of the dentate gyrus, as demonstrated by in vivo stimulation of the perforant pathway (Fig. 145–1), and was shown to be associated with spatial memory impairment.[3] Lyeth and colleages[4] showed that midline FPI also caused spatial learning deficits in rats. Because hilar neurons have an overall inhibitory effect on the dentate gyrus, the original work by Lowenstein and colleagues offered for the first time an explanation of the neurobiologic substrate of post-traumatic impairment in cognitive function and seizures: post-traumatic disinhibition due to hilar neuron loss. At the time, most reports considered these neurological deficits a consequence of diffuse axonal damage,[5] vascular abnormalities,[6] or changes in neurochemical transmission.[4] Because the hippocampus is known to have an important role in certain aspects of memory,[7] the discovery that even moderate injury crucially affects

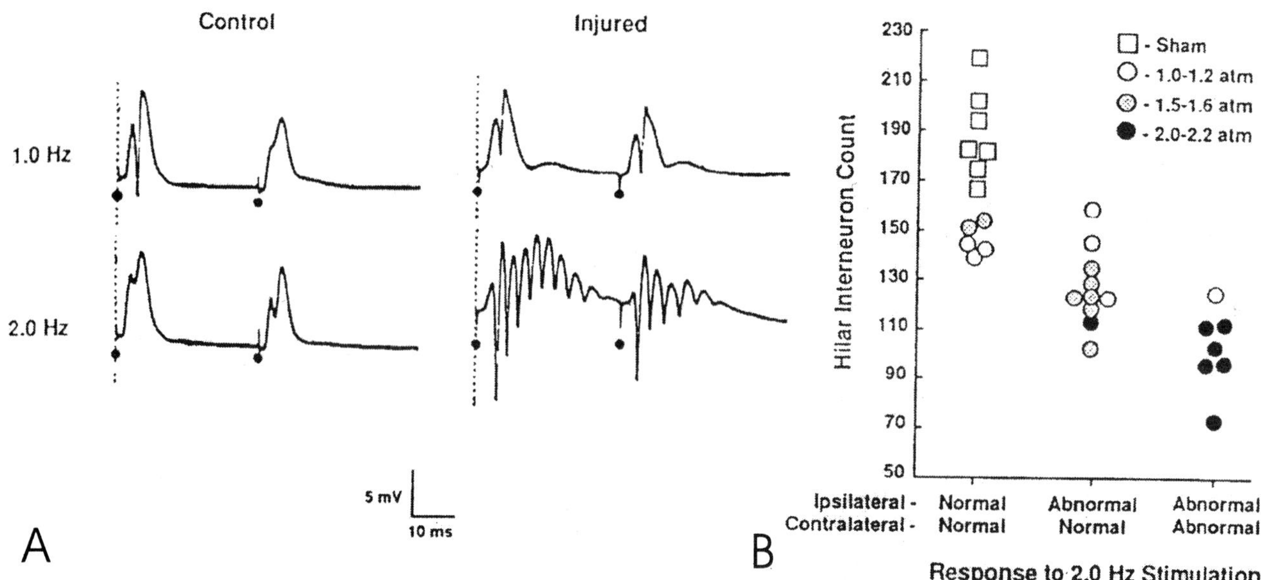

FIGURE 145–1. Hippocampal frequency-dependent hyperexcitability following traumatic brain injury. *A,* Responses in a control animal *(left)* and an animal with a 1.5-atm injury *(right)* to paired pulses with a 40-millisecond interval at 1 and 2 Hz. Notice the loss of inhibition at 2 Hz in the injured hippocampus, evidenced by the appearance of large, multiple dentate granule population spikes. *Solid circles* indicate the stimulus artifact. *B,* Relationship between the electrophysiology and the hilar neuron count and injury severity. The electrophysiologic results for each animal were categorized as normal bilaterally, abnormal ipsilateral to injury, or abnormal bilaterally. (From Lowenstein DH, Thomas MJ, Smith DH, McIntosh TK: Selective vulnerability of dentate hilar neurons following traumatic brain injury: A potential mechanistic link between head trauma and disorders of the hippocampus. J Neurosci 12:4846–4853, 1992.)

both the survival of hippocampal hilar neurons and the excitability of the dentate gyrus was important. While the observed loss of hilar neurons may be seizuregenic per se, the disparity between the acute loss of hilar neurons and the delayed onset of chronic seizures casts doubt on their causal linkage. If hilar inhibition of dentate gyrus is lost immediately after trauma, which is certainly a pro-seizuregenic factor, why does a silent period always occur between the initiating insult and chronic seizures? Recent studies have identified additional factors that could account for the delayed onset of seizures.

It was first shown that the rat hippocampus is hyperexcitable 1 week after FPI.[1] This observation was later extended to demonstrate changes in hippocampal structure and excitability at chronic times.[8, 9] These observations were confirmed using another model of closed head injury, the cortical impact injury.[10] The work of both groups suggests that recovery of inhibition, due to the time-dependent sprouting of post-traumatic mossy fibers, which results in a secondary increase in excitatory drive to target inhibitory interneurons in the hilus, occurs at chronic time points. These observations have been taken to suggest that progressive reactive synaptogenesis, and not disinhibition, is the likely cause of the frequency-dependent dentate gyrus hyperexcitability. Although this remains a possibility, surviving inhibitory cells or new replacement cells may have altered physiology and may not be exerting a full-fledged inhibitory control at all frequencies despite being reinnervated by sprouting mossy fibers.

Post-traumatic Sprouting

The role of reactive synaptogenesis ("sprouting") in the generation of chronic seizures remains controversial. This process has been thought to be associated with recovery of function after brain damage, since it has been shown that newly generated synapses are functional after mechanical[10, 11] and chemical injury.[12–14] Mossy fiber sprouting is a typical pathologic feature in humans and animals with temporal lobe seizures. Studies have suggested that chronic axonal sprouting and synaptic reorganization play a role in human post-traumatic epilepsy.[15–19] This line of thinking originates from the observations that granule cells receive aberrant excitatory innervation from sprouted mossy fibers[12, 20] and from the notion that fine regulation of excitatory drive has a crucial role in neuronal synchronization and seizure precipitation.[21]

Because of methodological pitfalls, it is unknown whether sprouting is necessary for the first seizures to appear or whether it is a consequence of their appearance. The protein synthesis inhibitor cycloheximide was found to block mossy fiber sprouting but not to prevent either the onset of seizures or the frequency of spontaneous seizures following status epilepticus.[22, 23] This line of evidence suggests that sprouting is not required for epileptogenesis to occur, but it does not address the issue of whether such invasive interventions with cycloheximide, while interfering with the sprouting process, are seizuregenic by other mechanisms. A later study[24] has examined whether sprouting of hippocampal mossy fibers is present at the time of appearance of the first spontaneous seizures in the rat and is critical for the occurrence of spontaneous epileptic seizures. Epilepsy was induced by electrical stimulation of the lateral nucleus of the amygdala until the rats developed status epilepticus. Rats were then monitored until they developed a second, spontaneous seizure and for 11 days thereafter. Sprouting density was measured by Timm staining, while neuronal damage was assessed in the hilus using thionine staining. Sprouting correlated with the neuronal damage and not with the time of onset of chronic seizures. In addition, animals that did not develop seizures also had sprouting. Such observations suggest that, although mossy fiber sprouting is present in all animals with spontaneous seizures, its presence is not necessary for their occurrence. Sprouting is also observed under pseudophysiologic conditions: sprouting of mossy fibers and of Schaffer collaterals can be induced experimentally by long-term potentiation (LTP), a paradigm of synaptic memory.[25, 26] Sprouting may represent an increase in excitatory drive that, as discussed below, may or may not be proseizuregenic, depending on many factors, including the neuronal type targeted, and changes in excitability of the postsynaptic neurons. Thus, sprouting may be secondary to the epileptogenic processes, rather than causal.

Post-traumatic Changes in Synaptic Transduction

Excess activation of ionotropic glutamatergic receptor channels, classified as *N*-methyl-D-aspartate (NMDA) or non-NMDA receptors, results in the flux of Na^+, K^+, and Ca^{2+} and in neuronal injury and death.[27, 28] Therefore, toxicity due to excess excitation (i.e., excitotoxicity) has been suggested to be a contributing factor in the pathology of TBI. This hypothesis is supported by observation that glutamate is neurotoxic in vitro[29] and that extracellular glutamate levels are elevated acutely after TBI in vivo.[30, 31] These observations have prompted the use of glutamate receptor antagonists in the treatment of TBI. These antagonists have been found to be neuroprotective in different models of TBI.[32] In addition to the possibility that trauma-induced elevation in extracellular glutamate may excessively activate glutamatergic receptor channels, there is recent evidence that TBI affects the activity of the glutamatergic channels themselves. Mechanical deformation of cells in an in vitro model of stretch injury[33] acutely altered the properties of the NMDA receptor channel so that Mg^{2+} could not block it in a voltage-dependent manner.[34] Such loss in Mg^{2+}-mediated blockade resulted in elevated intracellular Ca^{2+} levels when cells were challenged with exogenous NMDA.[34] It has also been shown that stretch injury directly alters α-amino-3-hydroxy-5-methyl-4-isoxazolepropionate (AMPA) receptor channels, causing an acute enhancement of AMPA-mediated current due to the loss of AMPA-dependent desensitization[35] (Fig. 145–2). The acute post-traumatic increase in NMDA and AMPA receptor–mediated synaptic drive would be expected to exacerbate the glutamatergic excitation after traumatic head injury. Given these post-traumatic changes in glutamatergic ion channel receptor activity and the central role these receptors play in neuronal excitability and synaptic plasticity, one would predict that the post-traumatic brain might suffer from overexcitation, and therefore excitotoxicity, but also from altered synaptic plasticity. Such changes may, in turn, affect neural computation, memory formation, and network excitability. It is therefore not surprising that memory and cognitive impairments are the most common neurological disorders after TBI.

Miyazaki and colleagues[36] observed a persistent sup-

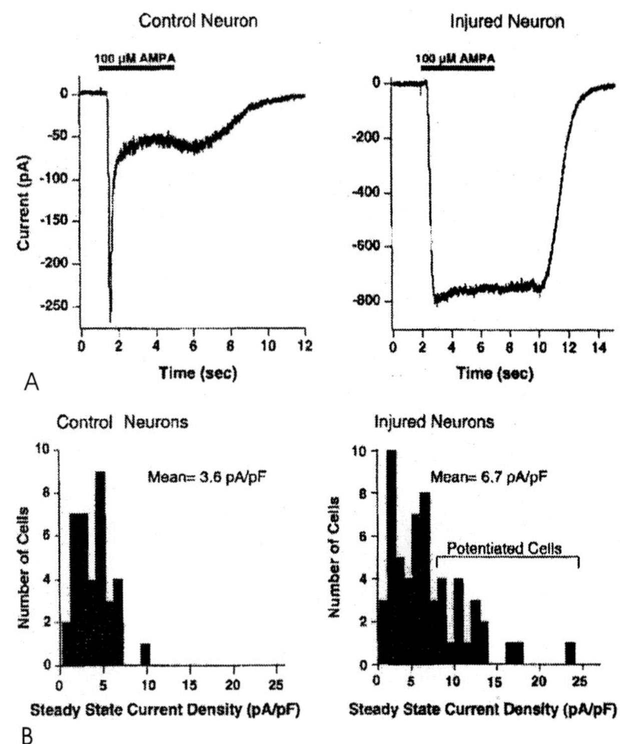

FIGURE 145–2. Mechanical injury potentiates AMPA receptor–elicited whole-cell currents. *A*, Representative patch-clamp recordings were made of whole-cell currents elicited by the application of 100 μM AMPA *(bars)* to an uninjured neuron *(left)* and a stretch-injured neuron *(right)*. Cells were voltage clamped at −40 mV. The uninjured neuron displayed desensitizing and steady-state current components. In contrast, the injured neuron displayed increased current amplitude and apparent loss of desensitization. *B*, A subpopulation of injured neurons exhibit altered AMPA channel function in response to mechanical stretch injury in culture. Whole-cell currents were normalized by cell capacitance and expressed as current densities. Amplitude histograms show AMPA-elicited, whole-cell, steady-state current densities in uninjured neurons *(left)* and stretch-injured neurons *(right)*. (From Goforth PB, Ellis EF, Satin LS: Enhancement of AMPA-mediated current after traumatic injury in cortical neurons. J Neurosci 19:7367–7374, 1999.)

pression of hippocampal LTP after TBI. They investigated changes in in vivo synaptic responses (i.e., population postsynaptic potentials) of CA1 pyramidal cells of the rat hippocampus to stimulation of the Schaffer collateral/commissural pathways 2 to 3 hours after lateral FPI. The changes observed after injury included a decrease in population spike threshold but not excitatory postsynaptic potential (EPSP) thresholds, decreases in the maximal amplitudes of both population spikes and EPSPs, and the suppression of LTP. In 1995, Reeves and colleagues[37] described changes in hippocampal LTP and cellular excitability 2, 7, and 15 days after midline FPI. They found that a significant LTP of the population EPSP slope could be induced only in controls, and no recovery to control levels was observed for any postinjury time point. Since LTP is thought to reflect cellular processes involved in memory formation, the observed post-traumatic suppression of LTP offers an electrophysiologic correlate of enduring memory deficits in humans after TBI.

To further delineate the cellular basis of TBI-mediated disruption of mechanisms implicated in memory, D'Ambrosio and colleagues[38] used it in vitro hippocampal slices obtained 2 days following midline FPI to study LTP and long-term depression (LTD), a form of synaptic plasticity complementary to LTP and similarly dependent on NMDA glutamate receptors (Fig. 145–3). These experiments revealed a loss of LTP in post-FPI slices similar to that reported by Miyazaki and colleagues.[36]

The persistence of impaired synaptic potentiation in vitro supports the concept that FPI causes a long-lasting synaptic modification that precludes further potentiation. However, the synaptic machinery appeared not to be impaired, because LTD could be equally induced in control and FPI slices. Therefore, the most likely candidate for post-traumatic impairment of LTP appears to be LTP itself. In fact, previously fully potentiated pathways cannot endure successive LTP. According to this hypothesis, the large and sudden increase in extracellular K^+ and glutamate, observed immediately after injury, would account for a nonspecific and pathologic potentiation of hippocampal synapses. This hypothesis is supported by previous work demonstrating transient elevation of extracellular K^+ can induce LTP because it causes nonspecific glutamate release and neuronal depolarization.[39] The post-traumatic pathologic LTP, by persisting at chronic time points after the insult, could shift the overall synaptic drive toward a nonspecific excitation, facilitating the precipitation of seizures in a manner similar to that hypothesized for sprouting.

Kindling as a Synaptic Epileptogenic Mechanism after Traumatic Brain Injury

In 1967, Graham Goddard[40] observed that the seizure threshold was progressively lowered by repetitive stimulation. He found that seizures could be induced in rats by applying a series of subliminal electrical brain stimulations. The concept of kindling was born. This model of epileptogenesis has been widely used to study epileptogenesis because it was recognized that seizures themselves could facilitate the onset of later seizures. In addition, it was found that some of the pathologic features commonly found in human epileptic brain are reproduced in the kindled brain (cellular and molecular changes and sprouting). However, the model is limited because it can only model a mechanism of secondary epileptogenesis in an already abnormal brain. In addition, it was shown by Wada that experimental kindling in animals is more easily obtained in animals that are lower in the phylogenetic scale.[40a]

The occurrence of epilepsy after TBI depends on the type and severity of the injury.[41] Seizures that occur acutely after injury do not predict the development of epilepsy. The progressive sickening of the post-traumatic brain toward the development of a chronic epileptic condition ("epileptogenesis") has been the subject of much research since it provides a theoretical window in which to intervene to prevent subsequent seizures. Unfortunately, all attempts to block the onset of post-traumatic epilepsy have failed. All clinical trials conducted to date have shown that classic antiepileptic drugs, although effective in treating acute post-traumatic seizures, are ineffective as prophylactic treatment,[42] and therefore that antiepileptic drugs are not necessarily antiepileptogenic. Classic antiepileptic drugs (e.g., phenytoin, phenobarbital, carbamazepine) were found to hinder epileptogenicity caused by kindling.[43, 44] Recent work has shed light on the epileptogenic processes initiated by trauma. Graber and Prince[45] hypothesized that epileptogenesis after cortical injury depended on processes initiated and/or maintained by neuronal firing and therefore might be prevented by blocking the voltage-operated sodium channels during the latent period. These investigators used a rat model of cortical injury consisting in islands of neocortex isolated by undercuts from the surrounding gray matter, with pial vasculature left intact. This model is very different from the human post-traumatic condition, lacking its unique focal and diffuse mechanical and hemorrhage component, and may complicate the interpretation of the data. Nonetheless, cortical hyperexcitability developed within the neocortical island after a latent period of 1 to 2 weeks and persisted many months after the insults. If epileptogenesis after injury depends on neuronal firing during the latent period, it should be prevented by suppressing neuronal electrical activity. The investigators chronically applied tetrodotoxin (TTX), a potent sodium channel blocker, embedded in a noninflammatory polymer, over the island of cortex. Two weeks later, neocortical slices were obtained and studied electrophysiologically. They found that TTX was effective in preventing epileptogenesis only when applied within 11 or more days after injury, demonstrating the existence of an epileptogenic period.

These data suggest that the latent period is relatively short. The acute changes that promote neuronal discharge and synaptic drive may ultimately be epileptogenic by kindling. This interpretation could account for the observation of several proseizuregenic mechanisms

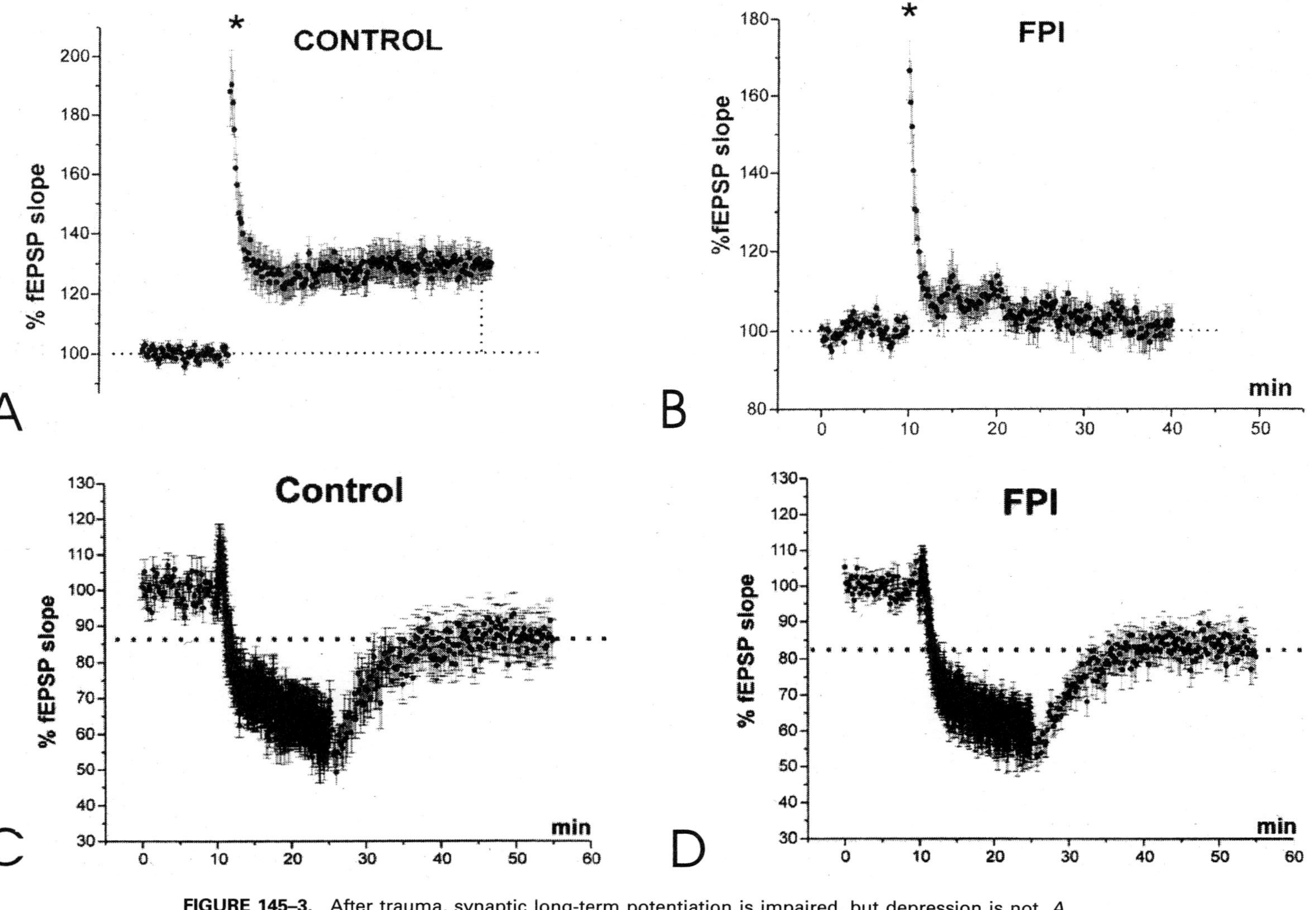

FIGURE 145–3. After trauma, synaptic long-term potentiation is impaired, but depression is not. *A,* Long-term potentiation (LTP) in control slices was elicited by a tetanic stimulation consisting of two 1-second trains of pulses at 100 Hz *(asterisks).* LTP evaluated at 30 minutes from induction was 30% ± 4%. *B,* After identical tetanic stimulation paradigms, no statistically significant LTP could be induced in slices obtained from fluid percussion injury (FPI) rats (1% ± 3%; control versus FPI, $P <$ .001). In contrast to LTP, long-term depression can be induced after FPI. In control slices, LTD was induced by 15 minutes of orthodromic stimulation at 1 Hz. *D,* A similar pattern of LTD induction and maintenance was observed in slices obtained from FPI animals. (Adapted from D'Ambrosio R, Maris DO, Grady MS, et al: Selective loss of hippocampal long-term potentiation, but not depression, following fluid percussion injury. Brain Res 786:64–79, 1998.)

acutely after trauma, and chronic seizures after a silent period, the time needed for kindling. This hypothesis is attractive on the basis of esthetic considerations, but it is difficult to justify in view of the clinical data available. The problem is that classic antiepileptic drugs may control seizures after TBI but fail to prevent the development of post-traumatic epilepsy.[42] If classic antiepileptic drugs prevent seizure-induced kindling but not the development of post-traumatic epilepsy, something epileptogenic other than kindling must occur during the "latent" period.

NONSYNAPTIC MECHANISMS OF POST-TRAUMATIC EPILEPSY

There has been relatively little research investigating pathophysiological changes in brain microenvironment homeostasis after TBI. Alterations in the microenvironment can result in neuronal hyperexcitability, synchronization, and ultimately in epilepsy.[46] Glial cells play a crucial role in the regulation of the brain environment, and the role of astrocytes in brain ion homeostasis and regulation of extracellular neurotransmitters is well documented. In particular, neuronal excitability and function crucially depend on proper regulation of intracellular and extracellular ions (particularly K^+) and of neurotransmitters (particularly glutamate and γ-aminobutyric acid [GABA]). Therefore, post-traumatic changes in glial cell physiology are central to the issue of nonsynaptic mechanisms of post-traumatic epilepsy.

Extracellular Potassium Ion Homeostasis under Physiologic Conditions and after Traumatic Brain Injury

During neuronal activity, extruded K^+ accumulates in the extracellular space. Because the extracellular concentration of potassium ions ($[K^+]_o$) is much smaller than its intracellular concentrations, even a modest increase in $[K^+]_o$ results in a significant dissipation of the K^+ gradient across the cell membrane. Since neuronal excitability, neuronal resting membrane potential, and inhibitory postsynaptic potentials all depend in a critical manner on the K^+ gradient, $[K^+]_o$ must be finely and effectively regulated. K^+ cannot be metabolized to other inactive substances, and its exchange between brain tissue and the bloodstream is negligible under normal conditions.[47] Thus, K^+ can only be redistributed. $[K^+]_o$ is regulated by cellular mechanisms that have different properties. There are three major cellular mechanisms involved in brain K^+ homeostasis (Fig. 145–4).

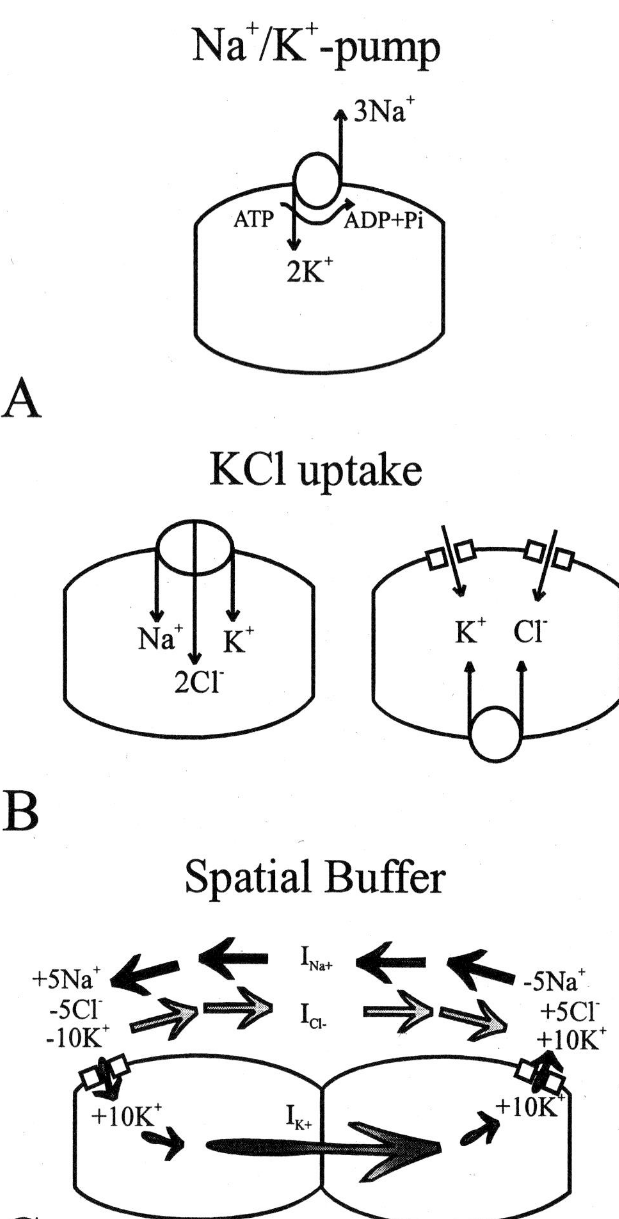

FIGURE 145–4. Schematics of the basic mechanisms of extracellular K^+ homeostasis after traumatic brain injury. *A,* The Na^+-K^+ pump is the housekeeper for all cellular ionic gradients. It requires ATP to extrude intracellular Na^+ and take up extracellular K^+ in neurons and glial cells. *B,* KCl uptake can occur in neurons and glial cells by passive shuffling of K^+ and Cl^-, with or without Na^+, through a membrane transporter or by pairing K^+ and Cl^- ionic currents through membrane ion channels. *C,* The spatial buffer mechanism of extracellular K^+ removal is a prerogative of glial cells. Extracellular K^+ is shunted from extracellular sites of accumulation to distal sites as an ionic current of K^+ conducted through glial cells. The intraglial K^+ current is closed extracellularly by currents carried by Na^+ and Cl^-.

UPTAKE OF POTASSIUM IONS BY THE SODIUM-POTASSIUM PUMP

The Na^+-K^+ pump is the housekeeper of ion gradients across cell membranes since it sets the main gradients for Na^+ and K^+ that are then used by ion channels, cotransporters and exchangers for their activity. The Na^+-K^+ pump hydrolyzes ATP to pump Na^+ out of the cell in exchange for K^+. The pump's activity[48] is modulated by $[Na^+]_{in}$ and $[K^+]_o$, and thus detects accumulation of extracellular K^+ and intracellular Na^+. Ouabain, by blocking the Na^+-K^+ pump, causes extracellular K^+ accumulation and seizures.[49] Post-traumatic decrease in tissue ATP content has been recently described.[50, 51] Thus, reduction of tissue Na^+-K^+ pump activity is expected[52, 53] and contributes to the post-traumatic impairment of extracellular K^+ homeostasis.[54–56]

NET UPTAKE OF POTASSIUM CHLORIDE

The accumulation of KCl into glia has been reported in several studies in acutely isolated slices of neocortex[57, 58] and hippocampus[59] and in cultured astrocytes[60, 61] or oligodendrocytes.[62] Ballanyi and coworkers[57] demonstrated the presence of KCl uptake in guinea-pig olfactory cortex slices by direct measure of $[Cl^-]_{in}$ with ion-selective microelectrodes. Coles and coworkers[63] showed the same phenomenon in the bee retina. Different routes are available for chloride to enter and leave the cells.

SPATIAL BUFFER

The spatial buffer mechanism provides for the redistribution of K^+ away from sites of extracellular local accumulation. Under resting conditions, glial membrane potential (E_K) is close to glial E_K. Neuronal activity locally increases $[K^+]_o$, which causes local glial E_K to shift to a more positive value. Thus, glial membrane potential becomes transiently more negative than the E_K, creating a gradient for inward K^+ currents. K^+ enters the glial cell through membrane K^+ channels, generating a local membrane depolarization. This local membrane depolarization propagates electrotonically to the rest of the glial cell membrane and to other glial cells coupled via gap junctions. When such a depolarizing electrotonic potential reaches spatially distal glial membranes facing normal $[K^+]_o$, an outward current of K^+ is generated that allows an equivalent amount of K^+ to leave the cell.[64–66]

Glial cells can perform spatial buffering because of their unique membrane properties. They extend over considerable distance and show extensive cell-to-cell coupling through gap junctions. This electrical coupling, although not required for the spatial buffer to work, facilitates the shunting of K^+ current to distal sites, thus reducing the depolarization of the glial membrane facing the focal increase of K^+ and preserving the electrochemical gradient for K^+ influx. It has been calculated that glial membrane K^+ conductance enables extracellular K^+ to be cleared more effectively than if there were simply a larger extracellular space, due to the establishment of an electrochemical K^+ gradient.[67] Indeed, a decrease in glial membrane K^+ conductance leads to the impairment of extracellular K^+ regulation.[54, 67] Spatial buffer has been directly demonstrated in a variety of tissue preparations: in acutely dissociated cells,[68–72] in the retina,[73] in brain slices,[74] and in the rest of the central nervous system.[65, 67, 75–77] Several studies[54, 55, 57,] have shown that blockade of glial inwardly rectifying K^+ channels results in impairment of extracellular K^+ regulation.

Relevant to the efficiency of active extracellular homeostasis in the post-traumatic brain, a significant drop in cerebral ATP has been observed following trauma. A decrease in cellular ATP has been demonstrated after lateral cortical impact in the mouse.[51] Using an in vitro model of stretch injury, it was also shown that cultured astrocytes are the most sensitive cell type in the rat brain.[33, 53] Neurons and astrocytes undergo a drop in intracellular ATP when exposed to

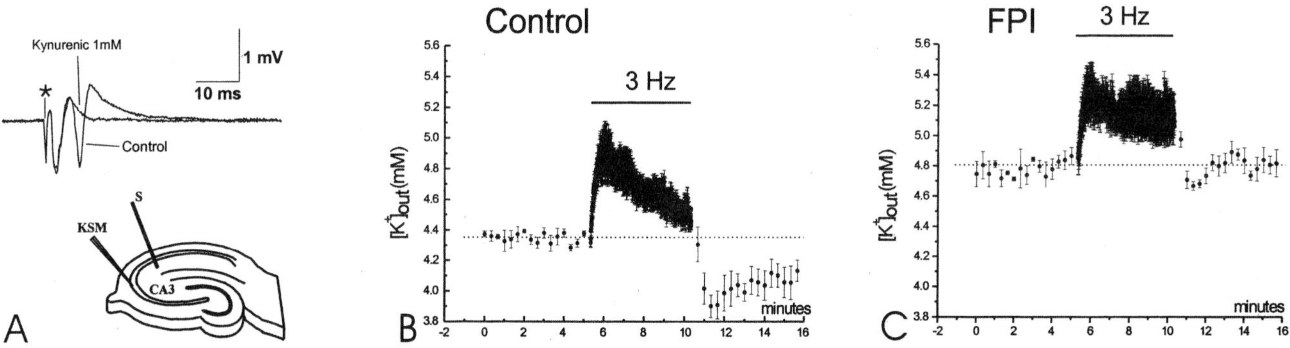

FIGURE 145–5. Abnormal accumulation of extracellular potassium during controlled neuronal firing in the post-traumatic brain. *A,* Field electrode and K^+-selective microelectrodes were placed in CA3 stratum pyramidale. The stimulating electrode was placed in CA2 stratum radiatum. Baseline values were obtained at 0.05 Hz of stimulation. Bath application of kynurenic acid (1 mM) and ZD-7288 (10 μM) abolished recurrent spikes and afterdischarge and maintained constant neuronal activation, as assessed by the amplitude of the antidromic spike per pulse of stimulation. *B,* In control slices, 3-Hz antidromic stimulation induced the rise of the extracellular potassium concentration ($[K^+]_o$) that peaked and then recovered toward the baseline. In the next 5 minutes of 0.05-Hz stimulation, $[K^+]_o$ markedly undershot baseline values and then recovered toward baseline. *C,* In slices obtained after fluid percussion injury, 3-Hz stimulation induced the rise of $[K^+]_o$ that did not recover during the high-frequency stimulation protocol and did not undershoot after its termination. The abnormal K^+ accumulation cannot be ascribed to altered neuronal firing but is the result of impaired K^+ homeostasis. (From D'Ambrosio R, Maris DO, Grady MS, et al: Impaired K(+) homeostasis and altered electrophysiological properties of post-traumatic hippocampal glia. J Neurosci 19:8152–8162, 1999.)

moderate stretch injury. Neurons recover within 24 hours, but astrocytes recover more slowly or do not recover at all, depending on the degree of the injury. When exposed to mild stretch injury, neurons and endothelial cells are the most resistant.[50, 53, 78] Rat whole-brain homogenates have a 50% reduction in ATP content after mild FPI.[50] This post-traumatic drop in cellular ATP was found to cause failure of the Na^+-K^+ pump in neurons in culture after stretch injury[53] and in situ after FPI.[52] It should be noted that neuronal membrane depolarization, directly caused by a decrease in Na^+-K^+ pump activity, may be per se pro-seizuregenic, as suggested in the rat hilus after FPI.[52] In addition, the data on impaired post-traumatic tissue energetics suggest that ion homeostasis is likely to be impaired after TBI.

Using microdialysis, Katayama and colleagues[30] showed that TBI caused an acute elevation of extracellular K^+ in the brain. This elevation was transient and, depending on the degree of injury, recovered toward baseline within an hour.[30] However, given the low spatial-temporal resolution inherent in the microdialysis technique, others have approached the issue of $[K^+]_o$ in the post-traumatic brain using K^+-selective microelectrodes. By taking advantage of the FPI,[2] a clinically relevant in vivo model of TBI, combined with the study of acutely isolated hippocampal slices, D'Ambrosio and colleagues demonstrated an impairment of extracellular K^+ homeostasis 2 days after moderate midline FPI.[54] Post-FPI slices exhibited elevated baseline $[K^+]_o$ and altered neuronal activity–induced extracellular K^+ accumulation; the latter did not appear to be caused by enhanced K^+ release from neurons (Fig. 145–5).

Extracellular K^+ homeostasis depends on dedicated cellular mechanisms whose activity may be affected following trauma. Recent experiments have shown that extracellular K^+ regulation, mediated by the neuronal and glial Na^+-K^+ pump, is likely to be impaired after FPI.[54–56] In addition to the overall activity of the Na^+-K^+ pump in neurons and glia, other post-traumatic changes in glial electrophysiology were found to result in impaired extracellular K^+ homeostasis. After FPI in the rat, complex and inward rectifier cell membranes exhibited a loss of inwardly rectifying K^+ currents (Fig. 145–6). The inward rectifier K^+ current is known to be an efficient passive mechanism for buffering extracellular K^+ and contributes to K^+ influx into glia in situ.[57, 79] In addition to loss of inward K^+ currents, complex cells had a dramatic loss of transient outward currents; because this current is activated by depolarizations, it could contribute to the maintenance of the membrane potential after changes in extracellular K^+ and thus be involved in K^+ homeostasis (Fig. 145–7). The finding that post-traumatic reactive glia have decreased membrane conductance to K^+ is consistent with previous reports by others showing loss of inward K^+ currents in reactive glia from human epileptic foci[80] and in an in vitro model of injury-induced reactive gliosis.[81]

The observation of post-traumatic changes of glial K^+ conductance has led us to conclude that post-traumatic glia have impaired passive uptake of K^+ through ion channels. This hypothesis was first put forward more than 30 years ago by Pollen and Trachtenberg,[82] who hypothesized a critical role for reactive glia in post-traumatic epilepsy through impairment of K^+ homeostasis. However, without proper control of neuronal excitability, in vivo experiments were unable to prove that reactive glia impaired extracellular K^+ homeostasis,[83–85] and the central role of glia malfunction could not be accurately determined. We addressed this issue by taking advantage of a combination of K^+-selective microelectrodes and pharmacologic manipulations allowed by the hippocampal slice preparation.[54, 55]

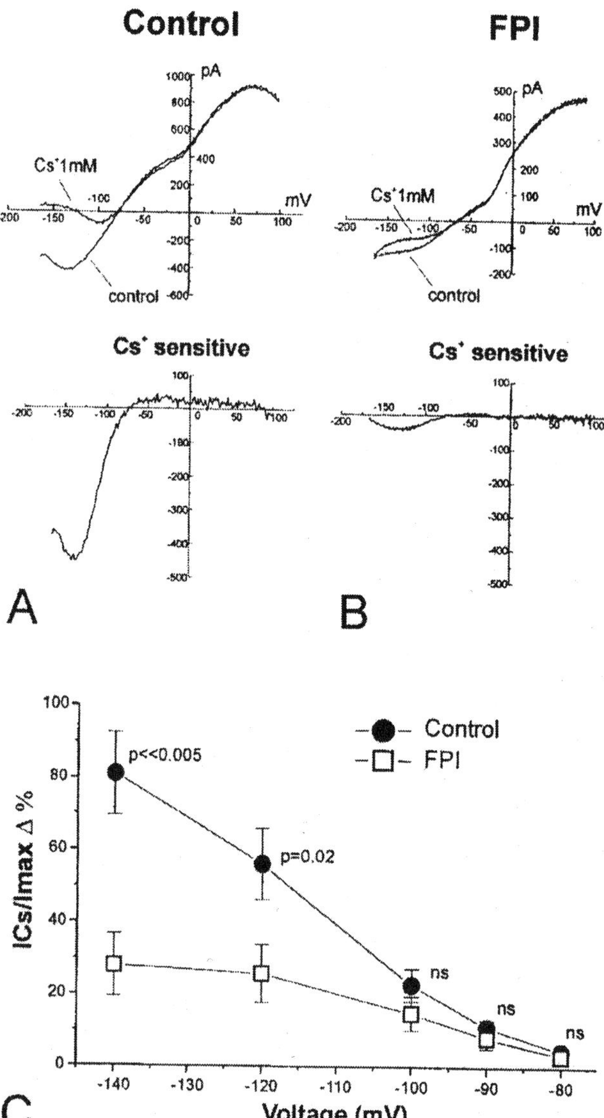

FIGURE 145–6. Post-traumatic glia have altered membrane K^+ current expression. *A*, Complex glial cells lose inward K^+ currents after midline fluid percussion injury (FPI). Complex cells in control hippocampal slices exhibited a large Cs^+-sensitive component. *B*, In contrast, complex cells in post-FPI hippocampal slices displayed decreased Cs^+ sensitivity 2 days after injury. *C*, The percentages of Cs^+-sensitive currents (I_{Cs}) for complex cells in normal and in post-FPI hippocampus are shown. (From D'Ambrosio R, Maris DO, Grady MS, et al: Impaired K(+) homeostasis and altered electrophysiological properties of post-traumatic hippocampal glia. J Neurosci 19:8152–8162, 1999.)

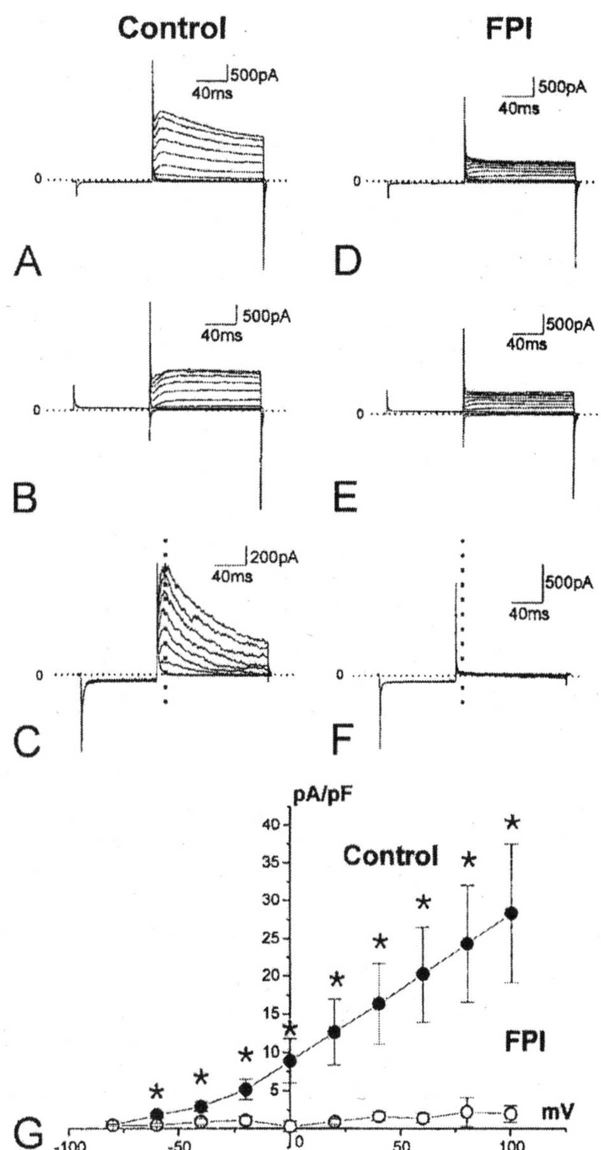

FIGURE 145–7. Complex glial cells lose K^+ transient outward currents after midline fluid percussion injury (FPI). *A* and *D,* Complex cells are endowed with depolarization-induced transient outward currents that can be induced by voltage commands consisting of a conditioning steps to −80 mV, followed by depolarization in 10-mV increments. *B* and *E,* When the conditioning step was set at −40 mV, the transient outward current was inactivated, and only a delayed rectifier current was observed. *C* and *F,* Transient outward current computed as the difference between protocols in *A* and *B*. Post-FPI complex cells showed a dramatic loss of the transient outward current, and no current is detectable as a difference. *G,* Relationship between the peak evoked current density in normal and post-FPI complex cells. *Asterisks* represent statistical significance at $P < .02$. (From D'Ambrosio R, Maris DO, Grady MS, et al: Impaired K(+) homeostasis and altered electrophysiological properties of post-traumatic hippocampal glia. J Neurosci 19:8152–8162, 1999.)

Consequences of Extracellular Potassium Accumulation

Previous work has demonstrated the sensitivity of in situ neurons to elevated extracellular K^+ and has led to acceptance of the high-K^+ model of epileptiform activity.[86–90] It is well known that moderate elevation in $[K^+]_o$ results in epileptiform bursts in hippocampal slices,[91] although the specific mechanisms underlying this phenomenon are still debated. $[K^+]_o$ could induce epileptiform activity by reducing the amplitude of the inhibitory postsynaptic potentials mediated by $GABA_A$ receptors or could synchronize pyramidal neuronal firing by increasing the phasic inhibition of inhibitory interneurons. More recently an alternative explanation has been put forward. The excitability of a cortical network is determined by neuronal connectivity and by the firing properties of the individual neurons. Most of these neurons are *regular spiking cells*—that is, they generate a single spike in response to a brief current injection or fire an accommodating train of action potentials on stimulation just above threshold. Other neurons are *bursters*—that is, they generate a cluster of several spikes riding a shoulder of slow membrane depolarization. Such cell types are not uniformly distributed in the neocortex and hippocampus, but rather in specific regions such as layer V of the neocortex or the CA3 subregion of the hippocampus. It was shown by Jensen and colleagues[90] that the levels of extracellular K^+ affect the burstiness of cortical neurons. These investigators demonstrated that, rather than falling into two distinct categories (i.e., regular spiking and bursters), the firing patterns of pyramidal neurons constitute a continuum that extends from nonbursters to bursters. Furthermore, the relative position of each neuron within this burstiness scale is flexible and depends on $[K^+]_o$ (Fig. 145–8). It has been shown that elevated K^+ is sufficient for interictal discharge to appear in brain slices.[89] In addition, it has been shown that the increase in $[K^+]_o$ is important in the transition from interictal to ictal state.[89, 92] Lastly, it is worth noticing that a nonsynaptic mechanism such as post-traumatic accumulation of extracellular K^+ or glutamate, by acting on neuronal targets, could increase synaptic strength and neuronal activity.

Glutamate Homeostasis after Traumatic Injury

Normal levels of extracellular glutamate, a primary excitatory neurotransmitter, are finely regulated by rapid uptake into neuronal and glial cells by specialized transporters. Increased extracellular levels of glutamate have been observed in the neocortex acutely after TBI, the causes of which are not fully understood and may depend on either increased release or decreased reuptake from neurons or glia. Nonspecific glutamate release from mechanically injured cells and excess synaptic activity occurs acutely after injury.[30] An acute, nonspecific increase in extracellular glutamate may be directly responsible for chronic seizures by triggering slow-activating proepileptogenic mechanisms. Indeed, it is known that excess glutamatergic activation participates in secondary neuronal damage after TBI. However, chronically impaired glutamate homeostasis could have a major impact on neuronal excitability after TBI.

Recent evidence suggests that the glial glutamate

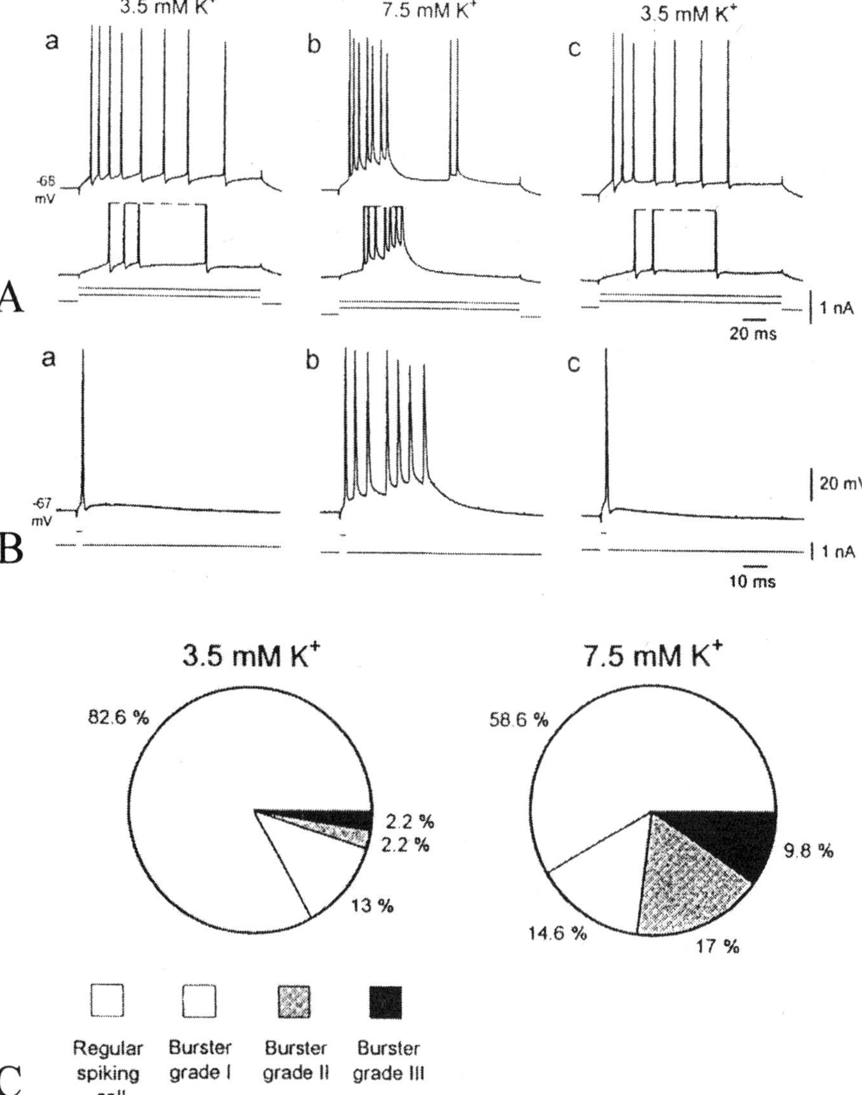

FIGURE 145–8. Reversible conversion of a regular spiking pyramidal cell into a grade II burster by raising the extracellular potassium ion concentration ($[K^+]_o$). The resting potential was maintained at −68 mV in high $[K^+]_o$ by steady injection of a negative current, as indicated in the current traces. *A,* At normal $[K^+]_o$ (3.5 mM), prolonged depolarizing pulses elicited accommodating trains of independent action potentials (a). Raising $[K^+]_o$ to 7.5 mM converted the firing pattern to burst mode (b). This effect promptly reversed on washing with standard saline (c). *B,* In normal $[K^+]_o$, the neuron fired only a solitary spike when briefly depolarized. Raising $[K^+]_o$ reversibly transformed this response into a burst (b and c). *C,* distribution of different firing patterns of CA1 pyramidal cells in normal and high $[K^+]_o$. Cell populations in 3.5 and 7.5 mM $[K^+]_o$ were classified as four distinct groups: irregular spiking cells and grade I, grade II, and grade III bursters. Notice that the increase in the fraction of bursters in high $[K^+]_o$ is mostly caused by the appearance of bursters of grade II and III. (Adapted from Jensen M, Azouz R, Yaari Y: Variant firing patterns in rat hippocampal pyramidal cells modulated by extracellular potassium. J Neurophysiol 71:831–839, 1994.)

transporter protein GLT-1, found mainly in the neocortex and hippocampus, has a key role in the regulation of baseline glutamate levels. Rao and colleagues[93] showed for the first time that the post-traumatic brain exhibits decreased expression of GLT-1 at chronic time points after controlled cortical impact. This work was confirmed in a ferrous chloride model of post-traumatic epilepsy,[94] in which decreased cortical levels of astrocytic GLT-1 protein were found.[95] In addition, it has been shown that antisense knockdown of GLT-1 exacerbates hippocampal neuronal damage after TBI.[96] The possibility that the post-traumatic brain suffers from decreased glial uptake of extracellular glutamate is very interesting.

CONCLUSIONS

Numerous synaptic and nonsynaptic substrates of post-traumatic hyperexcitability have been found, and it could be argued that we have a pretty good understanding of why the brain is hyperexcitable immediately after TBI. However, much work still needs to be done to elucidate the specific epileptogenic mechanisms that occur during the silent period that follows a single event of TBI and that precedes the onset of post-traumatic chronic seizures. Such work would benefit from the development of models of post-traumatic epilepsy that better reproduce the features of the human post-traumatic condition.

ACKNOWLEDGMENTS

I gratefully acknowledge the past support of the Epilepsy Foundation of America and the current support of the National Institute of Neurological Disorders and Stroke (NS 40823).

REFERENCES

1. Lowenstein DH, Thomas MJ, Smith DH, McIntosh TK: Selective vulnerability of dentate hilar neurons following traumatic brain

injury: A potential mechanistic link between head trauma and disorders of the hippocampus. J Neurosci 12:4846–4853, 1992.
2. Dixon CE, Lyeth BG, Povlishock JT, et al: A fluid percussion model of experimental brain injury in the rat. J Neurosurg 67: 110–119, 1987.
3. Smith D, Okiyama K, Thomas M, et al: Evaluation of memory dysfunction following experimental brain injury using the Morris water maze. J Neurotrauma 8:259–269, 1991.
4. Lyeth B, Jenkins L, Dixon R, et al: Prolonged memory impairment in the absence of hippocampal cell death following traumatic brain injury in the rat. Brain Res 526:249–258, 1990.
5. Povlishock J, Becker D, Cheng C, Vaughan G: Axonal change in minor head injury. J Neuropathol Exp Neurol 42:225–242, 1983.
6. Lewelt W, Jenkins L, Miller J: Autoregulation of cerebral blood flow after experimental fluid percussion injury of the brain. J Neurosurg 53:500–511, 1980.
7. Amaral D: Memory: Anatomical organization of candidate brain regions. In Mountcastle V, Plum F, Geiger S (eds): Handbook of Physiology: The Nervous System, vol V. Higher Functions of the Brain, part I. Bethesda, MD, American Physiology Society, 1987, pp 211–294.
8. Coulter DA, Rafiq A, Shumate M, et al: Brain injury-induced enhanced limbic epileptogenesis: Anatomical and physiological parallels to an animal model of temporal lobe epilepsy. Epilepsy Res 26:81–91, 1996.
9. Santhakumar V, Ratzliff AD, Jeng J, et al: Long-term hyperexcitability in the hippocampus after experimental head trauma. Ann Neurol 50:708–717, 2001.
10. Golarai G, Greenwood AC, Feeney DM, Connor JA: Physiological and structural evidence for hippocampal involvement in persistent seizure susceptibility after traumatic brain injury. J Neurosci 21:8523–8537, 2001.
11. McKinney RA, Debanne D, Gahwiler BH, Thompson SM: Lesion-induced axonal sprouting and hyperexcitability in the hippocampus in vitro: Implications for the genesis of posttraumatic epilepsy. Nat Med 3:990–996, 1997.
12. Tauck DL, Nadler JV: Evidence of functional mossy fiber sprouting in hippocampal formation of kainic acid-treated rats. J Neurosci 5:1016–1022, 1985.
13. Scharfman HE, Goodman JH, Sollas AL: Granule-like neurons at the hilar/CA3 border after status epilepticus and their synchrony with area CA3 pyramidal cells: Functional implications of seizure-induced neurogenesis. J Neurosci 20:6144–6158, 2000.
14. Scharfman HE, Smith KL, Goodman JH, Sollas AL: Survival of dentate hilar mossy cells after pilocarpine-induced seizures and their synchronized burst discharges with area CA3 pyramidal cells. Neuroscience 104:741–759, 2001.
15. Scheff S, Benardo I, Cotman C: Progressive brain damage accelerates axon sprouting in the adult rat. Science 197:795–797, 1977.
16. Buzsaki G, Ponomareff GL, Bayardo F, et al: Neuronal activity in the subcortically denervated hippocampus: A chronic model for epilepsy. Neuroscience 28:527–538, 1989.
17. Sutula T, Cascino G, Cavazos J, et al: Mossy fiber synaptic reorganization in the epileptic human temporal lobe. Ann Neurol 26: 321–330, 1989.
18. Ben-Ari Y, Represa A: Brief seizure episodes induce long-term potentiation and mossy fibre sprouting in the hippocampus. Trends Neurosci 13:312–318, 1990.
19. Dudek FE, Obenaus A, Schweitzer JS, Wuarin JP: Functional significance of hippocampal plasticity in epileptic brain: Electrophysiological changes of the dentate granule cells associated with mossy fiber sprouting. Hippocampus 4:259–265, 1994.
20. Cotman CW, Nadler JV: Reactive synaptogenesis in the hippocampus. In Cotman CW (ed): Neuronal Plasticity. New York, Raven Press, 1978, pp 227–271.
21. Traub RD, Miles R: Neuronal Networks of the Hippocampus. New York, Cambridge University Press, 1991.
22. Longo BM, Mello L: Blockade of pilocarpine- or kainate-induced mossy fiber sprouting by cycloheximide does not prevent subsequent epileptogenesis in rats. Neurosci Lett 226:163–166, 1997.
23. Longo BM, Mello L: Supragranular mossy fiber sprouting is not necessary for spontaneous seizures in the intrahippocampal kainate model of epilepsy in the rat. Epilepsy Res 32:172–182, 1998.
24. Nissinen J, Lukasiuk K, Pitkanen A: Is mossy fiber sprouting present at the time of the first spontaneous seizures in rat experimental temporal lobe epilepsy? Hippocampus 11:299–310, 2001.
25. Bliss TV, Lomo T: Long-lasting potentiation of synaptic transmission in the dentate area of the anaesthetized rabbit following stimulation of the perforant path. J Physiol 232:331–356, 1973.
26. Adams B, Lee M, Fahnestock M, Racine RJ: Long-term potentiation trains induce mossy fiber sprouting. Brain Res 775:193–197, 1997.
27. Rothman SM, Olney JW: Glutamate and the pathophysiology of hypoxic-ischemic brain damage. Ann Neurol 19:105–111, 1986.
28. Choi DW: Ionic dependence of glutamate neurotoxicity. J Neurosci 7:369–379, 1987.
29. Choi DW: Glutamate neurotoxicity in cortical cell culture is calcium dependent. Neurosci Lett 58:293–297, 1985.
30. Katayama Y, Becker DP, Tamura T, Hovda DA: Massive increases in extracellular potassium and the indiscriminate release of glutamate following concussive brain injury. J Neurosurg 73:889–900, 1990.
31. Nilsson P, Hillered L, Ponten U, Ungerstedt U: Changes in cortical extracellular levels of energy-related metabolites and amino acids following concussive brain injury in rats. J Cereb Blood Flow Metab 10:631–637, 1990.
32. McIntosh TK, Juhler M, Wieloch T: Novel pharmacologic strategies in the treatment of experimental traumatic brain injury: 1998. J Neurotrauma 15:731–769, 1998.
33. Ellis EF, McKinney JS, Willoughby KA, et al: A new model for rapid stretch-induced injury of cells in culture: Characterization of the model using astrocytes. *J Neurotrauma* 12:325–339, 1995.
34. Zhang L, Rzigalinski BA, Ellis EF, Satin LS: Reduction of voltage-dependent Mg^{2+} blockade of NMDA current in mechanically injured neurons. Science 274:1921–1923, 1996.
35. Goforth PB, Ellis EF, Satin LS: Enhancement of AMPA-mediated current after traumatic injury in cortical neurons. J Neurosci 19: 7367–7374, 1999.
36. Miyazaki S, Katayama Y, Lyeth BG, et al: Enduring suppression of hippocampal long-term potentiation following traumatic brain injury in rat. Brain Res 585:335–339, 1992.
37. Reeves TM, Lyeth BG, Povlishock JT: Long-term potentiation deficits and excitability changes following traumatic brain injury. Exp Brain Res 106:248–256, 1995.
38. D'Ambrosio R, Maris DO, Grady MS, et al: Selective loss of hippocampal long-term potentiation, but not depression, following fluid percussion injury. Brain Res 786:64–79, 1998.
39. Fleck MW, Palmer AM, Barrionuevo G: Potassium-induced long-term potentiation in rat hippocampal slices. Brain Res 580:100–105, 1992.
40. Goddard GV: Development of epileptic seizures through brain stimulation at low intensity. Nature 214:1020–1021, 1967.
40a. Wada JA: The clinical relevance of kindling: Species, brain sites and brain susceptibility. In Livington KE, Hornykiewicz H (eds): Limbic Mechanisms: The Continuing Evolution of the Limbic System Concept. New York, Plenum Press, 1978, pp 369–388.
41. Annegers JF, Grabow JD, Groover RV, et al: Seizures after head trauma: A population study. Neurology 30:683–689, 1980.
42. Temkin NR, Jarell AD, Andereson GD: Antiepileptogenic agents. How close are we? Drugs 61:1045–1055, 2001.
43. Wada JA, Sato M, Wake A, et al: Prophylactic effects of phenytoin, phenobarbital, and carbamazepine examined in kindling cat preparations. Arch Neurol 33:426–434, 1976.
44. Silver JM, Shin C, Mcnamara JO: Antiepileptogenic effects of conventional anticonvulsant in the kindling model of epilepsy. Ann Neurol 29:356–363, 1991.
45. Graber KD, Prince DA: Tetrodotoxin prevents posttraumatic epileptogenesis in the rats. Ann Neurol 46:234–242, 1999.
46. Schwartzkroin PA, Baraban SC, Hochman DW: Osmolarity, ionic flux, and changes in brain excitability. Epilepsy Res 32:275–285, 1998.
47. Mutsuga N, Schuette WH, Lewis DV: The contribution of local blood flow to the rapid clearance of potassium from the cortical extracellular space. Brain Res 116:431–436, 1976.
48. Thomas RC: Membrane current and intracellular sodium changes in a snail neurone during extrusion of injected sodium. J Physiol 201:459–514, 1969.
49. Pedley TA, Zuckermann EC, Glaser GH: Epileptogenic effects of localized ventricular perfusion of ouabain on dorsal hippocampus. Exp Neurol 25:207–219, 1969.

50. Ahmed SM, Rzigalinski BA, Willoughby KA, et al: Stretch-induced injury alters mitochondrial membrane potential and cellular ATP in cultured astrocytes and neurons. J Neurochem 74: 1951–1960, 2000.
51. Mautes AE, Thome D, Steudel WI, et al: Changes in regional energy metabolism after closed head injury in the rat. J Mol Neurosci 16:33–39, 2001.
52. Ross ST, Soltesz I: Selective depolarization of interneurons in the early posttraumatic dentate gyrus: Involvement of the Na(+)/K(+)-ATPase. J Neurophysiol 83:2916–2930, 2000.
53. Tavalin SJ, Ellis EF, Satin LS: Mechanical perturbation of cultured cortical neurons reveals a stretch-induced delayed depolarization. J Neurophysiol 74:2767–2773, 1995.
54. D'Ambrosio R, Maris DO, Grady MS, et al: Impaired K(+) homeostasis and altered electrophysiological properties of posttraumatic hippocampal glia. J Neurosci 19:8152–8162, 1999.
55. D'Ambrosio R, Gordon DS, Winn HR: Differential role of KIR channel and Na(+)/K(+)-pump in the regulation of extracellular K(+) in rat hippocampus. J Neurophysiol 87:87–102, 2002.
56. D'Ambrosio R, Gordon D: Chronic impairment of extracellular K+ homeostasis following traumatic brain injury in the rat. Paper presented at the American Epilepsy Society Meeting, 2002, Seattle, WA.
57. Ballanyi K, Grafe P, Bruggencate G: Ion activities and potassium uptake mechanisms of glial cells in guinea-pig olfactory cortex slices. J Physiol 382:159–174, 1987.
58. Ballanyi K: Functional role of ion transporters and neurotransmitter receptors in glia. In Vernadakis A, Roots B (eds): Neuron-Glia Interrelations during Phylogeny. II. Plasticity and Regeneration. Totowa, NJ, Humana Press, 1995, pp 197–219.
59. Mac Vicar BA, Tse FWY, Crichton SA, Kettenmann H: GABA-activated Cl^- channels in astrocytes of hippocampal slices. J Neurosci 9:3577–3583, 1989.
60. Walz W, Hinks EC: Carrier-mediated KCl accumulation accompanied by water movements is involved in the control of physiological K^+ levels by astrocytes. Brain Res 343:44–51, 1985.
61. Rose CR, Ransom BR: Intracellular sodium homeostasis in rat hippocampal astrocytes. J Physiol (Lond) 491:292–305, 1996.
62. Hoppe D, Kettenmann H: Carrier-mediated Cl^- transport in cultured mouse oligodendrocytes. J Neurosci Res 23:467–475, 1989.
63. Coles JA, Schneider-Picard G: Increase in glial intracellular K^+ in drone retina caused by photostimulation but not mediated by an increase in extracellular K^+. Glia 2:213–222, 1989.
64. Gardner-Medwin AR: A new framework for assessment of potassium-buffering mechanisms. Ann N Y Acad Sci 481:287–302, 1986.
65. Kettenmann H, Ransom BR (eds): Neuroglia. New York, Oxford University Press, 1995.
66. Orkand RK: Glial-interstitial fluid exchange. Ann N Y Acad Sci 481:269–272, 1986.
67. Gardner-Medwin AR, Coles JA: Dispersal of potassium through glia [abstract 1507]. Proc Int Union Physiol Sci 14:427, 1980.
68. Newman EA: Regional specialization of retinal glial cell membrane. Nature 309:155–157, 1984.
69. Newman EA, Frambach DA, Odette LL: Control of extracellular potassium levels by retinal glial cell K^+ siphoning. Science 225: 1174–1175, 1984.
70. Brew H, Attwell D: Is the potassium channel distribution in glial cells optimal for spatial buffering of potassium? Biophys J 48: 843–847, 1985.
71. Nilius B, Reichenbach A: Efficient K^+ buffering by mammalian retinal glial cells is due to cooperation of specialized ion channels. Pflugers Arch 411:654–660, 1988.
72. Karwoski CJ, Lu HK, Newman EA: Spatial buffering of light-evoked potassium increases by retinal Muller (glial) cells. Science 244:578–580, 1989.
73. Oakley B, Katz BJ, Xu Z, Zheng J: Spatial buffering of extracellular potassium by Muller (glial) cells in the toad retina. Exp Eye Res 55:539–550, 1992.
74. Holthoff K, Witte OW: Directed spatial potassium redistribution in rat neocortex. Glia 29:288–292, 2000.
75. Orkand RK, Nicholls JG, Kuffler SW: Effect of nerve impulses on the membrane potential of glial cells in the CNS of amphybia. J Neurophysiol 29:788–806, 1966.
76. Gardner-Medwin AR: Analysis of potassium dynamics in mammalian brain tissue. J Physiol (Lond) 335:393–426, 1983.
77. Walz W: Role of astrocytes in the clearance of excess extracellular potassium. Neurochem Int 36:291–300, 2000.
78. McKinney JS, Willoughby KA, Liang S, Ellis EF: Stretch-induced injury of cultured neuronal, glial, and endothelial cells: Effect of polyethylene glycol-conjugated superoxide dismutase. Stroke 27: 934–940, 1996.
79. D'Ambrosio R, Wenzel J, Schwartzkroin PA, et al: Functional specialization and topographic segregation of hippocampal astrocytes. J Neurosci 18:4425–4438, 1998.
80. Bordey A, Sontheimer H: Properties of human glial cells associated with epileptic seizure foci. Epilepsy Res 32:286–303, 1998.
81. MacFarlane SN, Sontheimer H: Electrophysiological changes that accompany reactive gliosis in vitro. J Neurosci 17:7316–7329, 1997.
82. Pollen DA, Trachtenberg MC: Neuroglia: Gliosis and focal epilepsy. Science 167:1252–1253, 1970.
83. Glötzner FL : Membrane properties of neuroglia in epileptogenic gliosis. Brain Res 55:159–171, 1973.
84. Pedley TA, Fisher RS, Prince D: Focal gliosis and potassium movement in mammalian cortex. Exp Neurol 50:346–361, 1976.
85. Lewis DV, Mutsuga N, Schuette WH, Van Buren J: Potassium clearance and reactive gliosis in alumina gel lesion. Epilepsia 18: 499–506, 1977.
86. Meltzer SJ: On the toxicology of potassium chlorate, with a demonstration of the effects of intracerebral injections. Am J Physiol 3:ix, 1899.
87. Feldberg W, Sherwood SL: Effects of calcium and potassium injected into the cerebral ventricles of the cat. J Physiol (Lond) 139:408–416, 1957.
88. Zuckermann EC, Glaser GH: Hippocampal epileptic activity induced by localized ventricular perfusion with high-potassium cerebrospinal fluid. Exp Neurol 20:87–110, 1968.
89. Traynelis SF, Dingledine R: Potassium-induced spontaneous electrographic seizures in the rat hippocampal slice. J Neurophysiol 59:259–276, 1988.
90. Jensen M, Azouz R, Yaari Y: Variant firing patterns in rat hippocampal pyramidal cells modulated by extracellular potassium. J Neurophysiol 71:831–839, 1994.
91. Rutecki PA, Lebeda FJ, Johnston D: Epileptiform activity induced by changes in extracellular potassium in hippocampus. J Neurophysiol 54:1363–1374, 1985.
92. Dichter MA, Herman CJ, Selzer M: Silent cells during interictal discharges and seizures in hippocampal penicillin foci. Evidence for the role of extracellular K^+ in the transition from the interictal state to seizures. Brain Res 48:173–183, 1972.
93. Rao VLR, Baskaya MK, Dogan A, et al: Traumatic brain injury down-regulates glial glutamate transporter (GLT-1 and GLAST) proteins in rat brain. J Neurochem 70:2020–2027, 1998.
94. Willmore LJ, Sypert GW, Munson JB: Recurrent seizures induced by cortical iron injection: A model of posttraumatic epilepsy. Ann Neurol 4:329–336, 1978.
95. Samuelsson C, Kumlien E, Flink R, et al: Decreased cortical levels of astrocytic glutamate transport protein GLT-1 in a rat model of posttraumatic epilepsy. Neurosci Lett 289:185–188, 2000.
96. Rao VL, Dogan A, Bowen KK, et al: Antisense knockdown of the glial glutamate transporter GLT-1 exacerbates hippocampal neuronal damage following traumatic injury to rat brain. Eur J Neurosci 13:119–128, 2001.

RECOMMENDED READINGS

For more in-depth readings on the basic mechanisms of the epilepsies, I recommend (in chronological order):

Schwartzkroin PA: Epilepsy: Models, Mechanisms, and Concepts. Cambridge, Cambridge University Press, 1993.

Degado-Escueta AV, Wilson WA, Olsen RW, Porter RJ: Jasper's Basic Mechanisms of the Epilepsies, 3rd ed. Philadelphia, Lippincott-Williams&Wilkins, 1999.

Engel JR, Pedley TA: Epilepsy: A Comprehensive Textbook. Philadelphia, Lippincott-Raven 1997.

CHAPTER 146

Approaches to the Diagnosis and Classification of Epilepsy

MARK D. HOLMES ■ JOHN W. MILLER

HISTORICAL PERSPECTIVE

Epilepsy is a condition with recurrent seizures and is one of the most common neurological conditions.[1] Hippocrates proposed that seizures are the result of abnormal brain function nearly 2400 years ago. He believed that the "sacred disease" was the result of abnormal "brain consistency" and rejected the idea that the gods cause seizures. Galen, in AD 175, described epilepsy as either idiopathic or symptomatic. Until the mid-19th century, physicians advocated an enormous number of useless remedies to remove the putative causes of seizures.[2] In the mid and latter half of the 19th century, Calmeil, Delasiauve, and Hughlings Jackson made the crucial differentiation between generalized and partial seizures. Jackson began to localize different types of seizures to particular brain regions.[3]

The first significant therapeutic advance in epilepsy management was Locock's observation of the effectiveness of bromides in women with catamenial seizures in 1857. In 1912, Hauptman discovered that phenobarbital was a useful antiseizure medication, and currently, this drug is the most commonly used treatment for epilepsy worldwide. The first antiepileptic drug discovered by systematic screening of compounds against experimental seizures in laboratory animals was phenytoin, which was identified by Merritt and Putnam in 1938.[2] This approach has been used to discover more than 36 antiepileptic agents since the 1950s.[4]

The first diagnostic test for diagnosing and characterizing seizures, the electroencephalogram (EEG), was developed by Berger in 1929.[5] Further technologic advances include the development in the 1970s and 1980s of synchronized EEG-audiovisual recording methods to characterize and correlate clinical seizure phenomena with ictal EEG changes,[6] customized neuropsychological testing batteries,[7] and several sophisticated neuroimaging techniques.[8] High-resolution magnetic resonance imaging (MRI), magnetic resonance spectroscopy, positron emission tomography, and single-photon emission computed tomography (SPECT) are imaging tools used to localize and identify the anatomic substrate of seizures. Developments in molecular biology and genetics have led to further understanding of the pathophysiology of epilepsy.[9]

In the modern era of antiepileptic drug development and technologic progress, epileptologists recognized the practical need to characterize accurately seizure type and epilepsy syndrome. A common language to describe ictal phenomena proved essential for communication between clinicians, providing direction to basic and clinical research, and optimal patient care. By the 1990s, the approach to medical management and surgical therapy for refractory epilepsy became based on an understanding of which seizure types, associated with recognized syndromes, are most amenable to specific modes of treatment. The first response to the need for a common language was formalized by the International League Against Epilepsy (ILAE), which published a classification of epileptic seizures in the 1960s. This scheme, with a revision issued in 1981, divided seizures into partial and generalized categories and is the most commonly used classification.[10] The ILAE classification of seizure types addressed neither the cause nor the anatomic origin of seizures, however, and in 1985 and 1989, the ILAE, in an effort to correct these shortcomings, developed a classification of the *epilepsies* and *epileptic syndromes*.[11] The new scheme maintained the fundamental dichotomy between *localization-related* and *generalized* epilepsies, and subdivided these further into *symptomatic*, *cryptogenic*, and *idiopathic* forms. Further refinements in the classification of seizure types and epilepsy syndromes are likely as the neurobiology of human epilepsy is understood better.

DEFINITIONS OF SEIZURE AND EPILEPSY

A *seizure* is the clinical manifestation of excessive, synchronous, abnormal firing of large populations of neurons that can result from many different causes. Seizures usually are self-limited. The word *epilepsy* is derived from the Greek verb *epilamvanein* ("to be seized," "to be taken hold of," "to be attacked"). Epilepsy is not a specific disease, but rather a broad spectrum of neurological conditions whose hallmark is that of recurring, unprovoked seizures. Cause, genetic and environmental substrates, associated neurological deficits, personality and psychosocial development, cognitive abilities, seizure types, sites of ictal onset, and responses to medical management may vary enormously, resulting in marked differences in the quality of life and disability experienced by persons with epilepsy.

Seizures are remarkably common, with the lifetime risk of suffering one or more seizures being greater than 9% by age 80.[12] The ages of highest incidence are infancy and early childhood and old age. At any given time, at least 1% of the population is under treatment for epilepsy.

TABLE 146–1 ■ **Risk Ratio for Epilepsy for Specific Prenatal and Perinatal Adverse Events***

Mental retardation and cerebral palsy	50.0
Cerebral palsy	12.0
Mental retardation	9.0
Neonatal hypoxia	5.1
Maternal hemorrhage	3.6
Neonatal seizures	3.0
Small for gestational age	2.6
Perinatal problems	1.8
Prematurity	1.4
Low birth weight	1.4
Obstetric problems	1.1
Delivery problems	1.1
Toxemia	1.0
Baseline	1.0

*Ratio of >1 indicates increased risk.
Data from Hauser W: Incidence and prevalence. In Engel J Jr, Pedley T (eds): Epilepsy: A Comprehensive Textbook. Philadelphia, Lippincott-Raven, 1998.

PATHOPHYSIOLOGY AND CAUSES

The epilepsies, although a heterogeneous group of disorders, have as a common feature a tendency for hyperexcitability to develop in one or more regions of the central nervous system (CNS).[13] Experimental models suggest that this tendency is the result of several different mechanisms. Neuronal excitability may be altered by changes in voltage-gated and transmitter-gated ion channels. When permanent changes in excitatory synapses or in local recurrent excitatory circuitry occur, seizures may result. Similarly, focal reductions in inhibitory neurotransmission may lead to hyperexcitability. Many neuromodulators and second messengers have been implicated in seizure expression as well as for overall susceptibility to epileptogenesis. Alterations in gene expression may relate to neuronal activation, injury, and seizures. The architecture and physiology of the neocortex, limbic system, thalamus, basal ganglia, and brainstem and the interconnectedness of these structures play important roles in seizure type and propagation. Developmental aberrations in cerebral cortex (under genetic control in many cases) and changes in cellular plasticity of neurons with age or in response to injury appear to be important factors in epileptogenesis.[13]

Risk factors for epilepsy are age dependent. For epilepsy beginning in childhood, head injury, CNS infection, mental retardation, and cerebral palsy are associated. Table 146–1 outlines the risk ratio for epilepsy for specific adverse events in early childhood.[12] Febrile seizures, although for the most part a benign condition, may be a risk factor for afebrile seizures in a few cases. Epidemiologic evidence suggests that there may be select groups of patients with febrile seizures who develop mesial temporal sclerosis and temporal lobe epilepsy or other epilepsy syndromes.[14]

For adults, several established risk factors are known. Severe head injury, particularly with penetrating wounds, poses the greatest risk. Minor head trauma, with only brief loss of consciousness and without skull fracture, or intracerebral injury does not carry a significant risk of subsequent epilepsy. Other important factors include CNS infection, CNS neoplasm, and cerebrovascular disease. Potential risk factors for epilepsy include multiple sclerosis, Alzheimer's disease, left ventricular hypertrophy, risk factors for embolic stroke, use of alcohol and illicit drugs, and acute symptomatic seizures. Table 146–2 relates the risk ratio for epilepsy with specific factors.[12]

With the advent of molecular biologic techniques, the role of genetic factors in the cause of neurological diseases, including the epilepsies, has become increasingly understood. Many clearly identified genetic disorders that may have epilepsy as part of the clinical spectrum are known. The genetic role in specific epilepsy syndromes may be complicated, however, and

TABLE 146–2 ■ **Risk Ratio for Epilepsy for Specific Risk Factors***

Military head injury	580.0
Severe civilian head injury	29.0
Cerebrovascular disease	20.0
Encephalitis	16.0
Alzheimer's disease	10.0
Hypertension/left ventricular hypertrophy	7.3
Moderate civilian head injury	4.0
Multiple sclerosis	4.0
Bacterial meningitis	4.0
Depression	3.7
Alcohol abuse	3.0
Heroin usage	3.0
Embolic risk factors	2.3
Aseptic meningitis	2.0
Mild civilian head injury	1.5
Tricyclic antidepressant drug usage	1.5
Electroconvulsive shock therapy	1.5
Neuroleptic drug usage	1.3
Hypertension	1.3
No risk	1.0
Treated left ventricular hypertrophy	0.7
Marijuana usage	0.4

*Ratio of >1 indicates increased risk.
Data from Hauser W: Incidence and prevalence. In Engel J Jr, Pedley T (eds): Epilepsy: A Comprehensive Textbook. Philadelphia, Lippincott-Raven, 1998.

TABLE 146–3 ■ **Genetics and Epilepsy**

I. Generalized epilepsies
  A. Simple inheritance
    1. Benign familial neonatal convulsions
    2. Progressive myoclonus epilepsies
  B. Complex inheritance
    1. Idiopathic generalized epilepsies
      a. Juvenile myoclonic epilepsy
      b. Other idiopathic generalized syndromes
    2. Myoclonic-astatic epilepsy
II. Localization-related epilepsies
  A. Simple inheritance
    1. Benign familial infantile convulsions
    2. Autosomal dominant nocturnal frontal lobe epilepsy
    3. Familial temporal lobe epilepsy
    4. Other single-gene syndromes
  B. Complex inheritance
    1. Idiopathic syndromes
    2. Cryptogenic/symptomatic syndromes

From European Epilepsy Academy Teaching Course: Genetics and Epilepsy. Epilepsia 40(suppl 3):1–40, 1999.

TABLE 146–4 ■ **Classification of Epileptic Seizures**

I. Partial seizures
  A. Simple partial
  B. Complex partial
    1. Impairment of consciousness at onset
    2. Simple partial onset progressing to complex partial
  C. Partial seizures evolving to generalized tonic-clonic convulsions
    1. Simple partial evolving to generalized tonic-clonic convulsions
    2. Complex evolving to generalized tonic-clonic convulsions, including those with simple partial onset
II. Generalized seizures
  A. Absence
  B. Myoclonic
  C. Tonic
  D. Clonic
  E. Atonic
  F. Tonic-clonic
III. Unclassified

From Commission on Classification and Terminology, International League Against Epilepsy: Proposal for revised clinical and electroencephalographic classification of epileptic seizures. Epilepsia 22:489–501, 1981.

for generalized and localization-related epilepsies, the inheritance may be simple or complex. Genetic causation may range from the only, or major, causative factor in some syndromes to a less significant factor in others. For some epilepsies (particularly symptomatic localization-related), acquired, *classic* risk factors may interact with the genetic to result in the clinical syndrome. Table 146–3 summarizes epilepsy syndromes that are known to have at least in part a genetic basis.[9]

CLASSIFICATION OF SEIZURES

Most epileptic seizures can be characterized as partial or generalized.[10] Partial seizures, based on EEG data, are assumed to arise from focal brain regions with variable spread to adjacent or distant brain areas. Generalized seizures appear to begin bilaterally from both hemispheres based on EEG findings and the clinical seizure. Under the ILAE classification scheme (Table 146–4), the partial seizures are subdivided further into simple or complex partial forms, depending on whether consciousness is impaired. The generalized seizures are subdivided into six subtypes depending on clinical manifestations.

Simple partial seizures are partial seizures without impairment of consciousness and may have motor, somatosensory, autonomic, or psychic symptoms. Consciousness is responsiveness to the external environment. Complex partial seizures may begin as simple partial seizures and progress to impairment of consciousness, often with accompanying automatisms. Complex partial attacks also may begin with consciousness impaired at the outset, and automatisms may or may not be present. Simple and complex partial seizures may evolve into secondarily generalized tonic-clonic seizures, if ictal activity spreads extensively to deep areas of the brain.

Generalized seizures may or may not have demonstrable impairment of consciousness. Absence seizures have a sudden onset with interruption of ongoing activity. The attack ends abruptly as well, usually after several seconds. Other associated features may include variable impairment of consciousness and, with prolonged absences, automatic behavior, or mild tonic, clonic, or atonic components. The generalized tonic-clonic seizure (convulsion) is the most frequently encountered of the generalized seizures. Consciousness is lost at the outset and accompanied by sustained contractions of the muscles (*tonic phase*), followed after a variable period by repetitive muscle contractions (*clonic phase*). A generalized clonic seizure is a convulsion that lacks the tonic phase, whereas a tonic seizure is characterized by sudden loss of consciousness with rigid contraction of extremity or axial musculature. Myoclonic (*jerk*) seizures consist of brief, sudden, shocklike muscle contractions that may be bilateral and widespread or may affect only individual muscle groups. An astatic seizure is accompanied by sudden loss or change of muscle tone, with loss of posture, and variable impairment of consciousness.

The ILAE classification of seizure types includes a category of *unclassified epileptic seizures*, to accommodate ictal phenomena that cannot be characterized further because of incomplete data. An addendum to the classification references the various forms of prolonged or repeated epileptic seizures, including status epilepticus.

CLASSIFICATION OF THE EPILEPSIES

The epileptic syndromes can be categorized two ways: (1) by cause—idiopathic, symptomatic, or cryptogenic—or (2) by anatomy, with the component seizures of the syndrome originating focally (localization-related) or synchronously from both sides (generalized).[11] The causes of idiopathic syndromes are not known, but genetic or hereditary causes are possible. Symptomatic epilepsy syndromes are considered to be the result of known or suspected disorders of the CNS. The term *cryptogenic* means that the cause of the disorder is hidden; cryptogenic epilepsies are presumed to be symptomatic. It is likely that localization-related and generalized epilepsy syndromes that now are considered to be cryptogenic in the future will be categorized differently, when more specific causes, including genetic, are established. Table 146–5 outlines the ILAE classification of the epilepsies and epileptic syndromes.

The ILAE classification of the epilepsies includes the recognition that some syndromes, primarily because of insufficient data, cannot be categorized at present as either localization-related or generalized. A category for syndromes that are situation-related is included in the scheme, such as febrile seizures, isolated seizures or status epilepticus, and seizures that occur in association with acute systemic illnesses (e.g., metabolic or toxic disorders). An appendix to the classification includes a listing of symptomatic generalized syndromes that have known, specific causes.

TABLE 146–5 ■ **Classification of Epilepsies and Epileptic Syndromes**

- I. Localization-related
  - A. Idiopathic (with age-related onset)
    1. Benign childhood epilepsy with centrotemporal spikes
    2. Childhood epilepsy with occipital paroxysms
    3. Primary reading epilepsy
  - B. Symptomatic
    1. Chronic progressive epilepsia partialis continua of childhood
  - C. Cryptogenic
    1. Temporal lobe epilepsies
    2. Frontal lobe epilepsies
    3. Parietal lobe epilepsies
    4. Occipital lobe epilepsies
    5. Bilobar and multilobar epilepsies
- II. Generalized
  - A. Idiopathic (with age-related onset)
    1. Benign neonatal familial convulsions
    2. Benign neonatal convulsions
    3. Benign myoclonic epilepsy in infancy
    4. Childhood absence epilepsy
    5. Juvenile absence epilepsy
    6. Juvenile myoclonic epilepsy
    7. Other idiopathic generalized epilepsy syndromes not defined
    8. Epilepsies with seizures precipitated by specific modes of activation
  - B. Cryptogenic or symptomatic (in order of age)
    1. West syndrome
    2. Lennox-Gastaut syndrome
    3. Epilepsy with myoclonic-astatic seizures
    4. Epilepsy with myoclonic absence
  - C. Symptomatic
    1. Early myoclonic encephalopathy
    2. Early infantile epileptic encephalopathy with burst-suppression
    3. Other symptomatic generalized epilepsies not defined above
    4. Specific syndromes
- III. Epilepsies and syndromes undetermined as to whether focal or generalized
- IV. Special syndromes
  - A. Situation-related
    1. Febrile seizures
    2. Isolated seizures or isolated status epilepticus
    3. Acute symptomatic seizures (e.g., secondary to metabolic or toxic factors)

From Commission on Classification and Terminology, International League Against Epilepsy: Proposal for revised classification of epilepsies and epileptic syndromes. Epilepsia 30:389–399, 1989.

SEIZURES COMMONLY ENCOUNTERED IN NEUROSURGICAL PRACTICE

Acute Symptomatic Seizures

Acute symptomatic seizures occur in the setting of illness or trauma that affects the CNS.[15] Such seizures, not regarded as epilepsy, occur within the first week of an insult. They may be partial or generalized, usually secondarily generalized, in nature, depending on the nature of the underlying condition. In general, acute symptomatic seizures may increase the risk for epilepsy by a factor of at least 3. In adults with moderate or severe head injury, acute symptomatic seizures are associated with a ninefold increased risk of recurring seizures. One half of all military casualties with penetrating brain injuries and early seizures develop epilepsy. The risk of unprovoked late seizures is increased threefold to fourfold when acute symptomatic seizures occur in the setting of postoperative surgery for vascular or ventricular disease, cerebrovascular disease, viral encephalitis, and bacterial meningitis.[16]

Status Epilepticus

Status epilepticus is characterized by repetitive or prolonged seizures. It is operationally defined as two or more seizures without full recovery between seizures or as a continuous seizure lasting 30 minutes or more, although it is evident that prolonged convulsive seizures are serious and require urgent medical intervention well before 30 minutes. Status epilepticus may manifest as generalized convulsive status, or it may assume nonconvulsive forms that include complex partial, simple partial, absence, or myoclonic status. The generalized convulsive form of status epilepticus is a medical emergency, with the potential for severe systemic or neuronal injury. Mortality from status epilepticus ranges from 8% to 32%, with adults at greater risk of death than children.[17] The most common identifiable causes of status epilepticus in pediatric patients (<16 years old) are CNS infections, antiepileptic medication changes, metabolic derangements, and congenital anomalies. In adults, cerebrovascular disease, antiepileptic medication changes, anoxic brain injury, substance abuse, and metabolic disturbances account for the major recognized causes.[18]

Secondary Epilepsy

The secondary epilepsies occur as a result of acquired disorders of the brain. In neurosurgical practice, the most commonly encountered seizures are those that occur in the setting of symptomatic or cryptogenic localization-related epilepsies. Such seizures may be the result of traumatic or surgical brain injury, neoplasm, or mesial temporal sclerosis, among other causes, and manifest as simple or complex partial attacks, with or without secondarily generalized tonic-clonic convulsions.

Medically Refractory Epilepsies

Despite the optimal use of antiepileptic medications, at least 25% of patients with epilepsy do not have complete control of seizures. Of these medically refractory individuals, a significant number of adults and children may benefit from resective neurosurgery. Most have a localization-related syndrome, with causes that reflect the known acquired risk factors for epilepsy. The most frequently evaluated epilepsy syndrome is refractory temporal lobe epilepsy, often the result of mesial temporal sclerosis. Some localization-related syndromes that may be wholly or in part genetic in origin, including conditions such as focal cortical dysplasia or tuberous sclerosis, may be amenable to surgical therapy in some cases.

DIAGNOSIS OF SEIZURES

Neurological History and Examination

Epileptic seizures must be distinguished from other causes of transient involuntary behavior or disturbance of neurological function, including syncope, migraine, transient ischemic attacks, movement disorders, parasomnias, and psychogenic spells. The most important means to establish the diagnosis is the moment-to-moment description of the episode. This description includes typical precipitants, warnings, subjective and externally visible manifestations of the event, and the patient's postictal state. Although only the patient can describe subjective sensations and feelings during auras and simple partial seizures, witnesses to the episodes usually are better able to describe involuntary movements and the patient's level of responsiveness and consciousness. With complex partial or generalized tonic-clonic seizures, it should be determined whether the patient also has simple partial seizures preceding the seizures or at other times. The examiner should inquire whether there is a history of childhood seizures, family history of seizures, past severe head trauma, risk factors for neoplasm or cerebrovascular disease, or a history of any other neurological condition. A careful neurological examination should be performed. A focal deficit could be due to an underlying structural process or could be a transient postictal deficit from a recent partial seizure. The general physical examination should look for clues of underlying cause, such as evidence of cardiac, cerebrovascular, or neoplastic disease.

The manifestations of seizures are so diverse as to defy a useful, comprehensive operational clinical definition and are much more varied than other neurological spells. Seizures most often are brief, stereotyped, discrete episodes; however, most patients with recurring seizures can group their episodes into a small number of types. Although straightforward generalized tonic-clonic seizures in acute settings may be recognized easily, for less commonplace forms of clinical spells, evaluation by a neurologist with clinical experience in the diverse manifestations of seizures is the cornerstone of diagnosis, with laboratory testing being used primarily to investigate the cause. Only occasionally is long-term video EEG recording of clinical spells necessary to clarify the diagnosis. This is especially the case when there is a suspicion of psychogenic episodes (*pseudoseizures*) mimicking epileptic seizures.

Laboratory Evaluation and Electroencephalogram

Patients with new onset of seizures should have an MRI study or a contrast-enhanced CT scan to look for structural causes. Basic screening hematologic and metabolic studies should include determination of sodium and magnesium and, in some cases, thyroid function tests. Prolactin levels have been used to distinguish between epileptic seizures and nonepileptic spells. Levels are elevated after 80% of generalized tonic-clonic seizures, 75% of complex partial seizures of temporal origin, but only 12.5% of frontal lobe complex partial seizures.[20] A significantly elevated prolactin level is evidence that a patient's spells are epileptic seizures; a normal prolactin level by itself is not proof that spells are not seizures.

The routine EEG is a particularly useful and inexpensive means of confirming the diagnosis of seizures and classifying them. Focal interictal epileptiform (Fig. 146–1) activity consists of brief electrical discharges that may occur on the EEG of patients with epilepsy at times when seizures are not occurring. These abnormalities consist of spikes (shorter than 70 msec), sharp waves (70 to 200 msec), or generalized spike-and-wave complexes and may be seen in about 50% of initial EEGs on epileptic patients and in 90% after multiple tracings.[21] Interictal epileptiform abnormalities have a high correlation with clinical evidence of seizures, and if seizures are not present, they nevertheless may be associated with structural brain disease.[22, 23] Such ab-

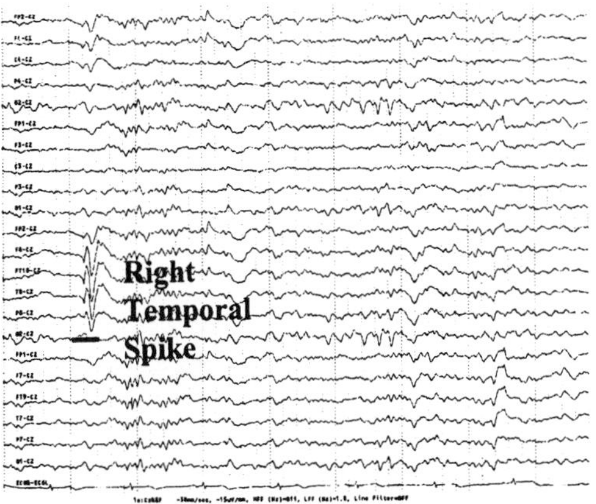

FIGURE 146–1. Interictal spike.

normalities are rare in normal patients.[24] The association between an interictal abnormality and a possible seizure disorder depends on its location and characteristics. Seizures are seen with 90% of children with temporal spikes, 75% of children with frontal spikes, and less than 54% of children with central and occipital spikes.[25] With multifocal spikes (three independent foci with at least one on each hemisphere), there is a 76% chance of seizures.[26] The most common epileptiform finding in patients with generalized seizures is generalized spike or multispike and slow wave activity, which often is activated by hyperventilation, photic stimulation, or sleep.

Periodic lateralized epileptiform discharges are spike or sharp waves that repeat in a nearly periodic fashion, every 1 to 3 seconds.[27] These usually are associated with the acute medically resistant focal or secondarily generalized seizures[27] and impaired consciousness. Most patients have an acute or subacute neurological illness, such as cerebral infarction, often watershed infarction from hypotensive and hypoxic episodes.[28, 29] Other causes include tumors, infection, trauma, intracerebral and subarachnoid hemorrhages, and subdural hematomas.[28, 29] Interictal epileptiform abnormalities are a reliable indicator of a potential seizure focus because they result from a characteristic neurophysiologic event, the paroxysmal depolarizing shift.[30, 31] The paroxysmal depolarizing shift is generated by thousands of neurons simultaneously undergoing large depolarization with superimposed action potentials, with synaptic events and intrinsic cellular currents participating. EEG spikes and sharp waves are due to the slow depolarizing currents of this phenomenon. An increase in depolarizing events and a loss of inhibitory mechanisms can lead to persistence and propagation of the discharge as a seizure.

The actual ictal EEG manifestations of partial seizures (Fig. 146–2) are nearly as varied as their clinical manifestations. The focal electrographic changes consist of attenuation of background rhythms, incrementing spikes or sharp waves, sinusoidal rhythms, and low-amplitude beta frequency activity and often display progressive evolution and change in morphology, amplitude, and frequency. This change may not be seen on the scalp EEG if an insufficient region of the cortex is involved, as with simple partial seizures or epilepsia partialis continua.

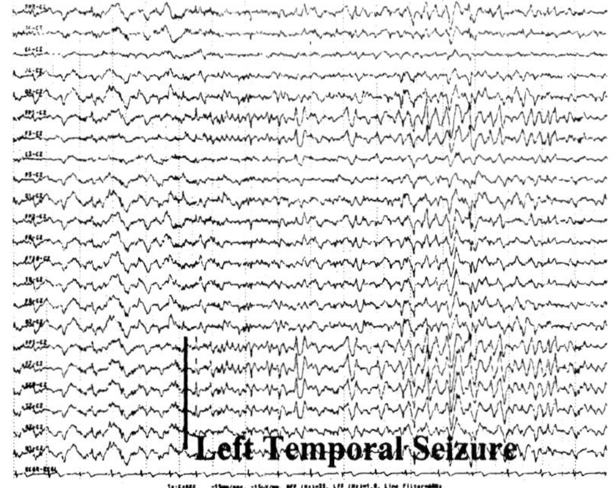

FIGURE 146–2. Partial seizure.

If psychogenic spells (*nonepileptic seizures*) are suspected or if neurosurgical treatment is being considered, the most useful procedure is an extended EEG with videotaping of behavior to capture typical spells. The EEG with videotaping determines if the spells are epileptic seizures and if their initial classification was correct. Ambulatory cassette EEG is not adequate to document pseudoseizures because of the lack of videotaping to characterize behavior and correlate it with the EEG and because of technical shortcomings of unmonitored recordings.

DIFFERENTIAL DIAGNOSIS OF SEIZURES

Physiologic Nonepileptic Seizures

The term *nonepileptic seizures* refers to events that in fact are not seizures. Physiologic causes of episodes that may mimic or be mistaken for seizures include transient ischemic attacks, syncope, vertigo of peripheral origin, transient global amnesia, parasomnias, and episodic movement disorders.

Neurocardiogenic syncope is distinguished from seizures by its typical prodrome, brief duration, and rapid return to normal consciousness. Occasionally, one or two myoclonic jerks may occur with the onset, but otherwise patients are limp and unresponsive during the event.

Parasomnias are age related, often dramatic behavioral events occurring during sleep. They generally are benign and are not associated with other medical disorders. Parasomnias associated with arousal include confusional arousals, somnambulism (sleep walking), and parvor nocturnus (sleep terrors). Sleep-wake transition disorders include rhythmic movement disorders, sleep starts, somniloquy (sleep talking), and nocturnal leg cramps. Parasomnias occurring in rapid-eye-movement (REM) sleep include nightmares, sleep paralysis, sleep-related priaprism, sleep-related sinus arrest, and REM sleep behavior disorder. The only common parasomnia in adults is REM sleep behavior disorder, which consists of semipurposeful movements during REM sleep—the acting out of dreams.

Transient global amnesia consists of episodes of isolated memory dysfunction with inability to form new memories, and variable retrograde amnesia without other neurological deficits. Although occasionally complex partial seizures may present with a history of amnesic periods without witnessed loss of responsiveness, transient global amnesia is distinguished by its typical duration of 5 to 6 hours and the fact that it seldom recurs.[32]

Episodic movement disorders are an infrequent differential diagnosis for seizures. Paroxysmal kinesogenic choreoathetosis consists of brief, movement-induced limb dystonia. It is not associated with EEG changes and is considered a movement disorder, rather than epileptic, although it responds to antiepileptic medication.

Nonphysiologic Nonepileptic Seizures

The manifestations of nonphysiologic nonepileptic seizures are diverse but most often are distinguished from epileptic seizures because they usually do not have a stereotyped evolution of behavior and may be prolonged. These seizures are diagnosed by the congruence of evidence of associated psychopathology on history or neuropsychological testing, with behavior manifestations that are inconsistent or atypical for epileptic seizures, and a lack of EEG changes during the episodes. Many simple partial seizures and some brief complex partial seizures may not have detectable ictal changes on scalp EEG recording, however. Long-term video EEG monitoring generally is required for the conclusive documentation of nonepileptic seizures. About 10% of patients with nonepileptic seizures also have evidence of concomitant epileptic seizures, but in these patients, usually one or the other type of episode is the active problem.

SUMMARY AND CONCLUSIONS

Epileptic seizures are common neurological events with diverse causes. Most patients with suspected seizures can be diagnosed correctly by a careful interview of the patient and witnesses. A simple routine or awake/sleep EEG is an inexpensive means of confirming the diagnosis and classifying the seizures correctly. Diagnostic tests, including standard blood tests and, in most cases, a neuroimaging study, are needed to look for the cause. Correct classification of seizure type and epilepsy syndrome is needed for correct treatment and determination of prognosis. Long-term video EEG monitoring should be used for patients with frequent spells that are resistant to treatment to confirm the diagnosis and, in some cases, to determine if the patient is a candidate for neurosurgical treatment.

REFERENCES

1. Temkin O: The Falling Sickness, 2nd ed. Baltimore, Johns Hopkins Press, 1971.
2. Scott D: The History of Epileptic Therapy: Account of How Medication Was Discovered. Pearl River, NY, Parthenon Publishing Group, 1993.
3. Taylor J (ed): Selected Writings of John Hughlings Jackson. New York, Basic Books, 1958.
4. Levy R, Mattson R, Meldrum B (eds): Antiepileptic Drugs, 4th ed. New York, Raven Press, 1995.
5. Berger H: On the electroencephalogram in man. Arch Psychiatr Neurol 100:301–320, 1933.
6. Goldensohn E: Simultaneous recording of EEG and clinical seizures using kinescope. Electroencephalogr Clin Neurophysiol 21: 623, 1966.
7. Dodrill C, Matthews C: The role of neuropsychology in the assessment and treatment of persons with epilepsy. Am Psychol 47:1139–1142, 1992.
8. Duncan J, Johannessen S (eds): The use of neuroimaging techniques in the diagnosis and treatment of epilepsy. Epilepsia 38(suppl 10):1–65, 1997.
9. European Epilepsy Academy Teaching Course: Genetics and epilepsy. Epilepsia 40(suppl 3):1–40, 1999.
10. Commission on Classification and Terminology, International League Against Epilepsy: Proposal for revised clinical and electroencephalographic classification of epileptic seizures. Epilepsia 22:489–501, 1981.
11. Commission on Classification and Terminology, International League Against Epilepsy: Proposal for revised classification of epilepsies and epileptic syndromes. Epilepsia 30:389–399, 1989.
12. Hauser W: Incidence and prevalence. In Engel J Jr, Pedley T (eds): Epilepsy: A Comprehensive Textbook. Philadelphia, Lippincott-Raven, 1998.
13. Delgado-Escueta A, Wilson W, Olsen R, Porter R (eds): Basic Mechanisms of the Epilepsies, 3rd ed. Philadelphia, Lippincott Williams & Wilkins, 1999.
14. Bruton C: The Neuropathology of Temporal Lobe Epilepsy. New York, Oxford University Press, 1988.
15. Annegers J, Hauser W, Lee J, Rocca W: Acute symptomatic seizures in Rochester, Minnesota. Epilepsia 36:327–333, 1995.
16. Hesdorffer D, Verity C: Risk factors. In Engel J Jr, Pedley T (eds): Epilepsy: A Comprehensive Textbook. Philadelphia, Lippincott-Raven, 1998.
17. Towne A, Pellock J, Ko D, DeLorenzo R: Determinants of mortality in status epilepticus: A retrospective study of 292 adult patients. Epilepsia 35:27–34, 1995.
18. DeLorenzo R, Towne A, Pellock J, Ko D: Status epilepticus in children, adults, and the elderly. Epilepsia 33(suppl 4):15–25, 1992.
19. Engel J Jr: Surgery for seizures. N Engl J Med 334:647–652, 1996.
20. Meierkord H, Shorvon S, Lightman S, Trimble M: Comparison of the effects of frontal and temporal lobe partial seizures on prolactin levels. Arch Neurol 49:225–230, 1992.
21. Salinsky M, Kanter R, Dasheiff RM: Effectiveness of multiple EEGs in supporting the diagnosis of epilepsy: An operational curve. Epilepsia 28:331–334, 1987.
22. Ajmone-Marsan C, Zivin LS: Factors related to the occurrence of typical paroxysmal abnormalities in the EEG records of epileptic patients. Epilepsia 11:361–381, 1970.
23. Daly DD: Use of the EEG for diagnosis and evaluation of epileptic seizures and nonepileptic episodic disorders. In Klass DW, Daly DD (eds): Current Practice of Clinical Electroencephalography. New York, Raven Press, 1979.
24. Eeg-Olofsson O, Petersen I, Sellden U: The development of the electroencephalogram in normal children from the age of 1 through 15 years: Paroxysmal activity. Neuropaediatrie 4:375, 1971.
25. Kellaway P: The incidence, significance and natural history of spike foci in children. In Henry CE (ed): Current Clinical Neurophysiology: Update on EEG and Evoked Potentials. Amsterdam, Elsevier/North Holland, 1980, pp 151–175.
26. Blume WT: Clinical and electroencephalographic correlates of the multiple independent spike foci pattern in children. Ann Neurol 4:541, 1978.
27. Chatrian GE, Shah CM, Leffman H: The significance of periodic lateralized epileptiform discharges in EEG: An electrographic, clinical, and pathological study. Electroencephalogr Clin Neurophysiol 17:177, 1964.
28. Dauben RD, Adams AH: Periodic lateralized epileptiform discharges in EEG: A review with special attention to etiology and recurrence. Clin Electroencephalogr 8:116, 1974.
29. Porecha HP, Reilly E: Clinical correlations of periodic lateralized epileptiform discharges. Clin Electroencephalogr 8:191, 1977.
30. Benardo LS, Pedley TA: Basic mechanisms of epileptic seizures. Cleve Clin Q 51:195, 1984.
31. Dichter MA, Ayala GF: Cellular mechanisms of epilepsy: A status report. Science 237:157, 1987.
32. Miller JW, Petersen RL, Metter EJ, et al: Transient global amnesia: Clinical characteristics and prognosis. Neurology 37:733–737, 1987.

CHAPTER **147**

Antiepileptic Medications: Principles of Clinical Use

BLAISE F. D. BOURGEOIS

Several new antiepileptic drugs have been introduced, and there now is a relatively large number of drugs to choose from when treating a newly diagnosed or uncontrolled patient with seizures. Although the newer drugs have not solved the problem of intractable epilepsy, they offer a welcome addition to the therapeutic armamentarium of epilepsy because each one has advantages with regard to efficacy, safety, pharmacokinetics, or interactions. The established, or older, drugs remain the drugs of first choice for most seizure types because most physicians treating epilepsy still are more familiar with the established drugs and have concerns about long-term safety of the newer drugs. As a group, most newer antiepileptic drugs offer the main advantages of relative safety, or favorable pharmacokinetics and interaction profiles, or the absence of the need for blood level or other routine laboratory monitoring.

This chapter presents a systematic review of the clinical pharmacology of each of the main established antiepileptic drugs and of the newer antiepileptic drugs, including pharmacokinetics, interactions, dosage, efficacy profile, and safety profile. The pharmacokinetic properties as well as doses and therapeutic ranges of the antiepileptic drugs to be discussed are summarized in Table 147–1. Principles of drug treatment of epilepsy are discussed, such as the decision to initiate long-term prophylactic drug treatment, the sequence of drug choices for various seizure types or syndromes (Table 147–2), initiation and monitoring of antiepileptic therapy, and discontinuation of treatment.

CLINICAL PHARMACOLOGY OF ANTIEPILEPTIC DRUGS

Phenytoin

Phenytoin (PHT) is one of the most widely used antiepileptic drugs. In addition to its good efficacy against convulsive seizures and decades of experience with its safety profile, PHT can be loaded rapidly without need to titrate the dose slowly. This property is particularly valuable in neurosurgical practice. The volume of distribution of PHT is about 0.75 L/kg (see Table 147–1). A dose of 7.5 mg/kg given intravenously raises the level by 10 mg/L. PHT elimination is unique among antiepileptic drugs because it is saturable at therapeutic concentrations.[1] This saturable elimination has been shown in all age groups.[2, 3] Saturable elimination results in a nonlinear relationship between maintenance dose and steady-state concentrations. Especially in the upper therapeutic range, small dosage increases can cause relatively large increases in levels. PHT does not have an elimination half-life because the time for the level to decrease by 50% becomes longer at higher levels. Steady-state levels are reached only 2 to 3 weeks after a patient has been on a stable maintenance dose. To achieve average levels of about 15 mg/L, adult patients must usually take 5 to 6 mg/kg/day, which corresponds to 350 to 450 mg/day. The common dose of 300 mg/day results in levels of 10 mg/L or less in most adult patients. PHT is a potent enzyme inducer and lowers the level of many other drugs. This affects other antiepileptic drugs, such as carbamazepine, valproate, felbamate, lamotrigine, topiramate, and tiagabine, as well as many other drugs, including warfarin (Coumadin), oral contraceptives, and cyclosporine. PHT is highly protein bound and is displaced from serum proteins by valproate. This displacement increases the free fraction of PHT and makes total serum levels unreliable.

The spectrum of activity of PHT includes partial seizures (simple or complex without or with secondary generalization), generalized convulsive seizures, status epilepticus,[4] and neonatal seizures.[5] Intravenous administrations of PHT can cause bradyarrhythmia and hypotension as well as skin necrosis.[6] This local irritation in particular can be avoided by using the prodrug phosphenytoin instead of PHT for intravenous administration. The total dose in PHT equivalents is the same for phosphenytoin as for PHT, but the rate of administration of phosphenytoin is up to 150 mg/minute (or 3 mg/kg/minute) instead of 50 mg/minute (or 1 mg/kg/minute) for PHT.

The dose-related central nervous system side effects of PHT are nystagmus, ataxia, and lethargy. PHT can

TABLE 147–1 ■ **Pharmacokinetic Parameters of Antiepileptic Drugs**

	F (%)	T_{max} (hr)	Vd (L/kg)	PROT. BIND. (%)	$T_{1/2}$ (hr)	T_{ss} (days)	THER. RANGE mg/L		DOSE mg/kg/day
							mg/L	μmol/L	
Carbamazepine	75–85	4–12	0.8–2	75	20–50* 5–20*	20–30*	3–12	12–50	10–30
Felbamate	>90	2–6	0.75	25	14–23	4	—	—	40–80
Gabapentin	30–60	2–3	0.85	0	5–9	2	—	—	30–40
Lamotrigine	>90	1–3	1.0	55	15–60	3–1	—	—	1–15
Oxcarbazepine (10-OH-carbamazepine)	>90	—	—	45	10–15	2	8–20	30–80	15–30
Phenobarbital	>90	0.54	0.55	45	65–110	15–20	10–30	4–130	2–5
Phenytoin	>90	2–12	0.75	90	10–60†	15–20	3–20	12–80	5–10
Primidone	>90	2–4	0.75	<10	8–15	—	—	—	10–20
Tiagabine	>90	1–2	1.4	96	2–9	1–2	—	—	0.1–1
Topiramate	>80	1–4	0.65	15	12–30	3–5	—	—	5–10
Valproate	>90	1–8‡	0.16	70–93†	5–15	2	50–100	50–700	15–30

*Steady-state values for half-life and serum levels are reached only after complete autoinduction.
†Concentration dependent.
‡Absorption of enteric-coated tablets is delayed.
F, bioavailability; T_{max}, time interval between ingestion and maximal serum concentration; Vd, volume or distribution, Prot. Bind., protein binding, fracture bound to serum proteins; $T_{1/2}$, elimination half-time; T_{ss}, steady-state time; Ther. Range, therapeutic range of serum concentration.

cause various forms of hypersensitivity reactions[7] as well as a hypersensitivity syndrome.[8] Other acute reactions to PHT include movement disorders. Chronic or delayed adverse effects include gingival hyperplasia, hirsutism, peripheral neuropathy, and bone demineralization secondary to reduced vitamin D levels.

Carbamazepine

Among neurologists, carbamazepine (CBZ) is the most commonly used drug of first choice against partial and secondarily generalized seizures. The elimination kinetics of CBZ are linear.[9] The characteristic feature of CBZ elimination is the autoinduction of its metabolism.[10] This autoinduction results in an increase of the CBZ clearance during the first weeks of treatment, unless the patient already is taking another enzyme-inducing drug, such as PHT, phenobarbital, or primidone. Accordingly the elimination half-life of CBZ decreases from about 36 hours to 10 to 20 hours (see Table 147–1).[11] The practical consequence is that the dose of CBZ must be increased progressively during the first 3 to 4 weeks of treatment from 100 to 200 mg/day to 600 to 800 mg/day. Further dosage increases can be made as needed and as tolerated. Because of the relatively short half-life after induction, the regular CBZ preparations are best given three times a day. Slow-release preparations, such as Tegretol-XR and Carbatrol, are given every 12 hours. CBZ is involved in many pharmacokinetic interactions. Similar to phenytoin, it is an enzyme inducer (see earlier). Other enzyme-inducing drugs, such as PHT, phenobarbital, and primidone, accelerate CBZ metabolism to a degree that exceeds CBZ autoinduction.

CBZ is effective against partial seizures without or with secondary generalization as well as against generalized tonic-clonic seizures. A double-blind controlled comparison has shown that, against partial and secondarily generalized seizures, PHT, CBZ, phenobarbital, and primidone are about equally effective in terms of seizure.[12] There is no parenteral preparation for CBZ, and it is not used in the treatment of status epilepticus or of neonatal seizures. In terms of adverse effects, CBZ benefits from many years of patient exposure. Dose-related central nervous system toxicity is the most common side effect. This toxicity may subside with time, can be minimized by careful titration, and is related closely to the CBZ serum levels.[13] Other side effects include neuropenia and rare, severe blood dyscrasias,[14] hyponatremia, movement disorders, allergic rashes, and hypersensitivity syndrome.

Valproate

Valproate (VPA) is unique because of its broad spectrum of activity against various seizure types. The absorption from enteric-coated VPA tablets can be delayed by several hours, but once it begins, it is rapid. Other oral preparations have a rapid and early absorption except for enteric-coated sprinkles, which have an intermediate absorption pattern. In serum, VPA is highly bound to proteins and tends to displace other drugs, such as PHT. The elimination half-life of VPA varies as a function of comedication. In adults, the half-life is 13 to 16 hours in the absence of inducing drugs[15] and 9 hours in induced patients.[16] In addition to displacement from serum proteins, VPA is involved in two types of pharmacokinetic interactions: Its metabolism is accelerated by inducing drugs such as PHT, CBZ, phenobarbital, and primidone, and VPA itself can prolong the elimination (and raise the levels) of other drugs, such as phenobarbital, ethosuximide, lamotrigine, and felbamate. The initial target dose of VPA is 15 mg/kg/day and can be attained within a few days. Higher doses of 60 mg/kg/day or more may be necessary in certain patients, especially those taking inducing drugs.

VPA has a broad spectrum of activity. In addition to

TABLE 147-2 ■ **Place of Newer Antiepileptic Drugs in the Treatment Sequence of Seizures and Epileptic Syndromes in Children**

Partial Seizures with or without Secondary Generalization	
First choice	Carbamazepine, phenytoin
Second choice	Gabapentin, lamotrigine, topiramate, valproate
Third choice	Tiagabine, phenobarbital, primidone
Consider	Benzodiazepine, acetazolamide, vigabatrin, felbamate
Generalized Tonic-Clonic Seizures	
First choice	Valproate, carbamazepine, phenytoin
Second choice	Topiramate, lamotrigine
Third choice	Phenobarbital, primidone
Absence Seizures	
Before age 10 years	
First choice	Ethosuximide, valproate
Second choice	Lamotrigine
Consider	Methsuximide, acetazolamide, benzodiazepine, topiramate
After age 10 years	
First choice	Valproate
Second choice	Lamotrigine
Third choice	Ethosuximide, methsuximide, acetazolamide, benzodiazepine, topiramate
Juvenile Myoclonic Epilepsy	
First choice	Valproate
Second choice	Lamotrigine, clonazepam, topiramate
Third choice	Phenobarbital, primidone, carbamazepine, phenytoin
Consider	Felbamate
Lennox-Gastaut and Related Syndromes	
First choice	Valproate
Second choice	Topiramate, lamotrigine
Third choice	Ketogenic diet, felbamate, benzodiazepine, phenobarbital
Consider	Ethosuximide, methsuximide, ACTH or steroids, pyridoxine, vigabatrin
Infantile Spasms	
First choice	ACTH, vigabatrin
Second choice	Valproate
Third choice	Topiramate, lamotrigine, tiagabine, benzodiazepine
Consider	Pyridoxine, felbamate
Benign Epilepsy with Centrotemporal Spikes	
First choice	Gabapentin, valproate
Second choice	Carbamazepine, phenytoin
Third choice	Phenobarbital, primidone, benzodiazepine
Consider	Lamotrigine, topiramate

ACTH, adrenocorticotropic hormone.

being about as effective as CBZ against partial seizures,[17] VPA is highly effective against absence seizures, generalized tonic-clonic seizures, and myoclonic seizures. It is the drug of first choice in patients with primary (idiopathic) generalized epilepsies. It is useful in the treatment of infantile spasms[18] and the Lennox-Gastaut syndrome. VPA has several side effects, affecting different systems and of variable severity. Mild side effects include transient hair loss and dose-related tremor. VPA is not sedative, but drowsiness and lethargy may appear in some patients at levels around 100 mg/L as well as idiosyncratic stuporous states at therapeutic levels.[19] Gastrointestinal upset is less common with enteric-coated tablets. Fatal hepatotoxicity[20] and pancreatitis[21] are the most serious complications of VPA treatment. Thrombocytopenia, in conjunction with other VPA-mediated disturbances of hemostasis, such as impaired platelet function, fibrinogen depletion, and coagulation factor deficiencies,[22] may cause excessive bleeding. The common practice of withdrawing VPA before elective surgery is recommended, although reports have found no objective evidence of excessive operative bleeding in patients maintained on VPA.[23, 24] In women of childbearing age, concerns associated with VPA treatment include not only the increased risk of neural tube defects in the fetus, but also an increased risk of polycystic ovaries and metabolic and endocrine disturbances.[25]

Phenobarbital and Primidone

The use of phenobarbital (PB) and primidone (PRM) for the treatment of seizures has declined steadily because of their central nervous system side effects and the availability of an increasing number of alternatives. PB and PRM produce more sedative and behavioral side effects than most other antiepileptic drugs, but they have relatively little systemic toxicity. PB has excellent pharmacokinetic properties, can be administered intravenously and intramuscularly, is effective in status epilepticus, and is inexpensive. The volume of distribution of PB is 0.55 L/kg. The elimination half-life of PB averages 80 to 100 hours in adults and newborns and is shorter in infants and children. Maintenance doses range from 2 to 5 mg/kg/day. Although treatment with PRM results in the accumulation of significant levels of PB, PRM has independent pharmacologic activity and probably is not just a prodrug. PRM itself has a much shorter half-life than PB. Daily dosage requirements of PRM are about five times higher than those of PB. As an enzyme inducer, PB causes pharmacokinetic interactions that are shared by other enzyme-inducing drugs and by PRM because of the derived PB. Other enzyme-inducing drugs, in particular PHT,[26] accelerate the conversion of PRM to PB, increasing the PB-to-PRM serum level ratio.

PB and PRM are as effective against partial and secondarily generalized seizures as CBZ and PHT but were found to be associated with more treatment failures because of mostly early central nervous system side effects.[12] PB can be used in the treatment of status epilepticus and neonatal seizures as well as for the prophylaxis of febrile seizures. In addition to the well-known sedative and behavioral side effects, PB and PRM can cause allergic reactions. Use over many years may be associated with connective tissue disorders, such as Dupuytren's contracture and frozen shoulder.

Felbamate

Because of potentially serious side effects, felbamate (FBM) currently is used only in special circumstances. Its pharmacokinetic parameters are summarized in Table 147–1. FBM is involved in multiple pharmacokinetic interactions. Levels of FBM are decreased by enzyme-inducing drugs. FBM raises levels of PHT and VPA. The recommended initial dose of FBM is 1200 mg/day (15 mg/kg/day) during the first week. This dose can be doubled at the beginning of the second week and tripled at the beginning of the third week. It is prudent to reduce the dose of other antiepileptic drugs by about one third when FBM is introduced. In double-blind studies, FBM was shown to be effective against partial onset seizures[27, 28] as well as in the treatment of Lennox-Gastaut syndrome.[29] Uncontrolled reports have suggested efficacy of FBM against absence seizures, juvenile myoclonic epilepsy, and infantile spasms.

The main common side effects of FBM have been nausea and vomiting, anorexia, weight loss, somnolence, and insomnia. Within 1 year after its marketing, it became evident that FBM was associated with a relatively high incidence of potentially fatal aplastic anemia[30] and hepatic necrosis.[31] Currently the main indication for FBM is as a drug of third choice in the treatment of the Lennox-Gastaut syndrome and against focal onset seizures.

Gabapentin

Gabapentin (GBP) differs from previously used antiepileptic drugs by the fact that it is eliminated entirely by the kidneys. As a consequence, it has no pharmacokinetic interactions. GBP absorption is saturable, and the daily dose should be administered three or four times a day, especially at high doses.[32] Initial target doses of GBP are about 1800 mg/day (30 mg/kg/day). Doses above 3600 mg/day (60 to 100 mg/kg/day) often are well tolerated and may be necessary to achieve the maximal benefit.

GBP has been shown in double-blind trials to be effective against focal onset seizures.[33] More recently, GBP was found to be superior to placebo in a double-blind study in patients with benign epilepsy of childhood with centrotemporal spikes (rolandic epilepsy).[34] Serious side effects of GBP appear to be exceedingly rare.[35]

Lamotrigine

Among the newer antiepileptic drugs, lamotrigine (LTG) is unique in its relatively broad spectrum of activity. LTG has a relatively long half-life (see Table 147–1) and can be administered two times a day. The pharmacokinetic interactions of LTG are the marked reduction of its levels by enzyme-inducing drugs and the marked elevation of its levels by VPA.[36] As a consequence of these interactions, dosage requirements for LTG vary from patient to patient. Patients taking VPA should receive 25 mg/day or less (0.2 mg/kg/day) during the first 2 weeks of treatment. Patients taking enzyme-inducing drugs without VPA may be started on higher doses. A slow titration with dosage increases at intervals of 2 weeks is important because it seems to reduce the risk of potentially severe rash associated with LTG.[37] Against focal onset seizures, LTG appears to be as effective as CBZ and PHT.[38, 39] LTG also has been found to be effective in the treatment of Lennox-Gastaut syndrome,[40] absence seizures, generalized tonic-clonic seizures, juvenile myoclonic epilepsy, and infantile spasms.

Topiramate

The pharmacokinetic parameters of topiramate (TPM) are summarized in Table 147–1. TPM can be administered two times a day in most cases. The main pharmacokinetic interaction involving TPM consists of an approximately twofold increase in its clearance by enzyme-inducing antiepileptic drugs.[41] To reduce the incidence of early side effects, the dose of TPM needs to be titrated slowly. The initial dosage should be 25 to 50 mg/day (0.5 to 1.0 mg/kg/day) with weekly increases by the same amount, aiming for an initial target dose of 200 to 400 mg/day (5 to 6 mg/kg/day). The efficacy of TPM was found to be relatively high against focal onset seizures in an analysis comparing trials of several newer antiepileptic drugs.[42] TPM was found to be effective in double-blind studies of patients with generalized tonic-clonic seizures[43] and in patients with Lennox-Gastaut syndrome.[44] The most common side effects of TPM include somnolence, impaired concentration, confusion, and abnormal thinking. Other side effects include anorexia, weight loss, and nephrolithiasis.

Tiagabine

Among the newer antiepileptic drugs, tiagabine (TGB) is the one for which there is the least amount of clinical experience. TGB has a short half-life (see Table 147–1), which becomes shorter in the presence of enzyme-inducing drugs. There are no other pharmacokinetic interactions. When TGB is introduced, the dose should be titrated slowly with weekly increments.

So far, the known clinical efficacy of TGB is limited to partial onset seizures without or with secondary generalization.[45] TGB does not appear to have severe or potentially life-threatening side effects. The main side effects include dizziness, tremor, difficulty with concentration, nervousness, and emotional lability.[45]

PRINCIPLES OF TREATMENT

Decision to Initiate Antiepileptic Drug Therapy

After a first seizure, the decision to treat or not to treat is based not only on the risk of seizure recurrence alone, but also on the potential risks associated with seizure recurrence and the potential risks associated with chronic antiepileptic therapy. There is good overall agreement that routine treatment after a first unprovoked seizure is not indicated in all cases. The decision has to be individualized, taking into account all the available information on a given patient as well as the patient's own preference. Certain factors have been associated with an increased risk of seizure recurrence, such as a remote symptomatic seizure, a focal onset seizure, a history of prior acute symptomatic seizures, epileptiform abnormalities on electroencephalography (EEG), a first seizure presenting as status epilepticus, and a first seizure followed by Todd's paralysis. Inversely, factors associated with a lower risk of seizure recurrence include an idiopathic generalized tonic-clonic seizure and the absence of epileptiform abnormalities on EEG. As a group, adults tend to have a higher risk of seizure recurrence after a first seizure and are more likely to be treated after a first seizure.

Antiepileptic Drug Selection by Seizure Type or Epilepsy Syndrome

When a decision to treat has been made, the first step is to determine the drug of first choice for the patient. The choice of an antiepileptic drug is based first on the seizure type or on the epileptic syndrome. Among the drugs available for a particular seizure type or syndrome, the choice is based mainly on the adverse effect profile, taking into consideration the patient's age and gender as well preference. The place of any antiepileptic in the treatment sequence of epilepsy is not established firmly and not strictly scientifically determined. This is because, especially for the newer drugs, there have been no head-to-head comparisons of their efficacy against any given seizure type or epilepsy syndrome. With this concept in mind, Table 147–2 assigns places to antiepileptic drugs in the treatment sequence of seizures. The listing of drugs as second and third choices applies only to patients whose seizures could not be controlled with a drug of first choice.

Basic Principles of Antiepileptic Drug Use

When the drug of first choice has been selected in an untreated patient, this drug almost always is used in monotherapy. An initial target dose is achieved, either rapidly or during several weeks, depending on the drug. Further dosage increases are dictated more by seizure control and side effects than by drug levels. The simple rule that the optimal drug dose is "as much as necessary, as little as possible" too often is disregarded. If the seizures do not come under control initially, the conclusion that the drug has failed should not be reached unless the maximal tolerated dose has been reached. The maximal tolerated dose, or subtoxic dose, is just below the dose at which dose-related side effects have appeared. Invariably, children, especially infants, have higher drug clearances and require significantly higher doses in milligrams per kilograms per day to achieve the same drug levels. Inversely, elderly patients often require lower doses, not only because they have lower clearances, but also because they may be more sensitive to the side effects.

If the first drug fails to control the seizures at the maximal tolerated dose, a second drug is selected. When a therapeutic dose or level of the second drug has been reached, the first drug should be tapered. It is exceptional for a drug combination to provide better seizure control than adequate monotherapy with either one of the two drugs alone. If drug levels are available, they should be used judiciously, with the understanding that the therapeutic range provided by the laboratory is a rough guideline and never should replace clinical observation and judgment. While monitoring a patient on antiepileptic drug therapy, it should be kept in mind that physicians invariably underestimate patients' lack of compliance with drug intake. Besides judiciously used drug levels, only a few antiepileptic drugs require periodic monitoring of laboratory values: complete blood count with CBZ therapy and complete blood count and liver function tests with VPA and FBM therapy. Discussing side effects of the medications and asking patients to report possible symptoms of adverse events is more important than laboratory monitoring.

Discontinuation of Antiepileptic Drug Therapy

Similar to the initiation of therapy, discontinuation is based on a risk versus benefit analysis. Factors shown to increase the risk of seizure recurrence after stopping antiepileptic therapy include a known remote cause, seizure onset after the age of 12 years, a family history of epilepsy in patients with idiopathic epilepsy, focal or generalized slowing on EEG before discontinuation, a history of atypical febrile seizures, and an IQ of less than 50. The 2-year recurrence risk after drug discontinuation may vary from about 10% in patients with none of these risk factors to about 80% in patients with remote symptomatic seizures and three risk factors. Contrary to widespread belief, seizure control almost always can be re-established with medication if seizures recur after discontinuation. In general, the decision to discontinue an antiepileptic drug is made after 2 years without seizures. Because there is usually no urgency, the drug should be tapered slowly during a period of at least 3 months. In patients who have become seizure-free after epilepsy surgery, it is a common practice to reduce the number of antiepileptic drugs after 1 year and to discontinue all drugs after 2 years.[46]

REFERENCES

1. Arnold K, Gerber N: The rate of decline of diphenylhydantoin in human plasma. Clin Pharmacol Ther 11:121–134, 1969.
2. Dodson WE: The nonlinear kinetics of phenytoin in children. Neurology 32:42–48, 1982.
3. Bourgeois BFD, Dodson WE: Phenytoin elimination in newborns. Neurology 33:173–178, 1983.
4. Cloyd J, Gumnit R, McLain W: Status epilepticus: The role of intravenous phenytoin. JAMA 244:1479–1481, 1980.
5. Painter MJ, Pippinger C, Wasterlain C, et al: Phenobarbital and phenytoin in neonatal seizures: Metabolism and tissue distribution. Neurology 31:1107–1112, 1981.
6. O'Brien T, Cascino G, So E, Hanna D: Incidence and clinical consequence of the purple glove syndrome in patients receiving intravenous phenytoin. Neurology 51:1034–1039, 1998.
7. Haruda F: Phenytoin hypersensitivity: 38 cases. Neurology 29: 1480–1485, 1979.

8. Schlienger R, Shear N: Antiepileptic drug hypersensitivity syndrome. Epilepsia 39(Suppl 7):S3–7, 1998.
9. Perucca E, Bittencourt P, Richens A: Effect of dose increments on serum carbamazepine concentration in epileptic patients. Clin Pharmacokinet 5:576–582, 1980.
10. Bertilsson L, Bengt H, Gunnel T, et al: Autoinduction of carbamazepine metabolism in children examined by a stable isotope technique. Clin Pharmacol Ther 27:83–88, 1980.
11. Eichelbaum M, Ekbom K, Bertilsson L, et al: Plasma kinetics of carbamazepine and its epoxide metabolite in man after single and multiple doses. Clin Pharmacol 8:337–341, 1975.
12. Mattson RH, Cramer JA, Collins JF, et al: Comparison of carbamazepine, phenobarbital, phenytoin and primidone in partial and secondarily generalized tonic-clonic seizures. N Eng J Med 313:145–151, 1985.
13. Hoppener R, Kuyer A, Meijer J, Hulsman J: Correlation between daily fluctuations of carbamazepine serum levels and intermittent side effects. Epilepsia 21:341–350, 1980.
14. Tohen M, Castillo J, Baldessarini R, et al: Blood dyscrasias with carbamazepine and valproate: A pharmacoepidemiological study of 2,228 patients at risk. Am J Psychiatry 152:413–418, 1995.
15. Gugler R, Schell A, Eichelbaum M, et al: Disposition of valproic acid in man. Eur J Clin Pharmacol 12:125–132, 1977.
16. Perucca E, Gatti G, Frigo GM, et al: Disposition of sodium valproate in epileptic patients. Br J Clin Pharmacol 5:495–499, 1978.
17. Mattson RH, Cramer JA, Collins JF, Department of VA Epilepsy Cooperative Study No. 264 Group: A comparison of valproate with carbamazepine for the treatment of complex partial seizures and secondarily generalized tonic-clonic seizures in adults. N Engl J Med 327:765–771, 1992.
18. Bachman DS: Use of valproic acid in treatment of infantile spasms. Arch Neurol 39:49–52, 1982.
19. Marescaux C, Warter JM, Micheletti G, et al: Stuporous episodes during treatment with sodium valproate: Report of seven cases. Epilepsia 23:297–305, 1982.
20. Bryant A, Dreifuss FE: Valproic acid hepatic fatalities: III. U.S. experience since 1986. Neurology 46:465–469, 1996.
21. Asconapé JJ, Penry JK, Dreifuss FE, et al: Valproate-associated pancreatitis. Epilepsia 34:177–183, 1993.
22. Gidal B, Spencer N, Maly M, et al: Valproate-mediated disturbances of hemostasis: Relationship to dose and plasma concentration. Neurology 44:1418–1422, 1994.
23. Ward MM, Barbaro NM, Laxer KD, Rampil IJ: Preoperative valproate administration does not increase blood loss during temporal lobectomy. Epilepsia 37:98–101, 1996.
24. Anderson GD, Lin YX, Berge C, Ojemann G: Absence of bleeding complications in patients undergoing cortical surgery while receiving valproate treatment. J Neurosurg 87:252–256, 1997.
25. Isojarvi JI, Laatikainen TJ, Knip M, et al: Obesity and endocrine disorders in women taking valproate for epilepsy. Ann Neurol 39:579–584, 1996.
26. Cloyd JC, Miller KW, Leppik IE: Primidone kinetics: Effects of concurrent drugs and duration of therapy. Clin Pharmacol Ther 29:402–407, 1981.
27. Bourgeois BFD: Pharmacokinetics and pharmacodynamics in clinical practice. In Wyllie E (ed): The Treatment of Epilepsy: Principles and Practice. Philadelphia, Lea & Febiger, 1993, pp 726–734.
28. Faught E, Sachdeo RC, Remler MP, et al: Felbamate monotherapy for partial-onset seizures: An active-control trial. Neurology 43: 688–692, 1993.
29. The Felbamate Study Group in Lennox-Gastaut Syndrome: Efficacy of felbamate in childhood epileptic encephalopathy (Lennox-Gastaut syndrome). N Engl J Med 328:29–33, 1993.
30. Kaufman D, Kelly J, Anderson T, et al: Evaluation of case reports of aplastic anemia among patients treated with felbamate. Epilepsia 38:1265–1269, 1997.
31. O'Neil M, Perdun C, Wilson M, et al: Felbamate-associated fatal acute hepatic necrosis. Neurology 46:1457–1459, 1996.
32. Gidal B, DeCerce J, Bockbrader H, et al: Gabapentin bioavailability: Effect of dose and frequency of administration in adult patients with epilepsy. Epilepsy Res 31:91–99, 1998.
33. Leiderman D: Gabapentin as add-on therapy for refractory partial epilepsy: Results of five placebo-controlled trials. Epilepsia 35:S74–S76, 1994.
34. Bourgeois B, Brown L, Pellock J, et al: Gabapentin (neurontin) monotherapy in children with benign childhood epilepsy with centrotemporal spikes (BECTS): A 36-week, double-blind, placebo-controlled study. Epilepsia 39:163, 1998.
35. McLean M, Morrell M, Willmore L, et al: Safety and tolerability of gabapentin as adjunctive therapy in a large, multicenter study. Epilepsia 40:965–972, 1998.
36. Vauzelle-Kervroedan F, Rey E, Cieuta C, et al: Influence of concurrent antiepileptic medication on the pharmacokinetics of lamotrigine as add-on therapy in epileptic children. Br J Clin Pharmacol 41:325–330, 1996.
37. Guberman A, Besag F, Brodie M, et al: Lamotrigine-associated rash: Risk/benefit considerations in adults and children. Epilepsia 40:985–996, 1998.
38. Brodie M, Richens A, Yuen A: Double-blind comparison of lamotrigine and carbamazepine in newly diagnosed epilepsy. Lancet 345:476–479, 1995.
39. Steiner T, Dellaportas C, Findley L, et al: Lamotrigine monotherapy in newly diagnosed untreated epilepsy: A double-blind comparison with phenytoin. Epilepsia 40:601–607, 1999.
40. Motte J, Trevathan E, Arvidsson JF, et al: Lamotrigine for generalized seizures associated with the Lennox-Gastaut syndrome. N Engl J Med 337:1807–1812, 1997.
41. Bourgeois B: Drug interaction profile of topiramate. In: International League Against Epilepsy. Philadelphia, Lippincott-Raven, 1996.
42. Marson A, Kadir Z, Chadwick D: New antiepileptic drugs: A systematic review of their efficacy and tolerability. BMJ 313: 1169–1174, 1996.
43. Biton V, Montouris G, Ritter F, et al: A randomized, placebo-controlled study of topiramate in primary generalized tonic-clonic seizures. Neurology 52:1330–1337, 1999.
44. Sachdeo R, Glauser T, Ritter F, et al: A double-blind, randomized trial of topiramate in Lennox-Gastaut syndrome. Neurology 52: 1882–1887, 1999.
45. Uthman B, Rowan A, Ahmann P, et al: Tiagabine for complex partial seizures: A randomized, add-on, dose-response trial. Arch Neurol 55:56–62, 1998.
46. Andermann F, Bourgeois BF, Leppik IE, et al: Postoperative pharmacotherapy and discontinuation of antiepileptic drugs. In Engel J (ed): Surgical Treatment of the Epilepsies. New York, Raven Press, 1993, pp 679–684.

PART II PREOPERATIVE EVALUATION FOR EPILEPSY SURGERY

CHAPTER 148

Single-Photon Emission Computed Tomography and Positron Emission Tomography

DAVID H. LEWIS

Nuclear medicine uses internally administered radioactivity for the diagnosis and treatment of disease. Functional neuroimaging with nuclear medicine comprises brain metabolic, perfusion, and neuroreceptor three-dimensional scanning with positron emission tomography (PET) and single-photon emission computed tomography (SPECT). Other nuclear medicine applications for central nervous system imaging in two dimensions include cerebrospinal fluid studies for either leak or communicating, normotensive hydrocephalus; evaluation of cerebrospinal fluid diversionary shunts; and cerebral perfusion scans for the assessment of brain death. This chapter chiefly covers the applications of SPECT and PET. In contrast to anatomic techniques such as conventional computed tomography (CT) and magnetic resonance imaging (MRI), these nuclear medicine methods image and measure the physiology and pathophysiology in tissue, which often can be the earliest and most sensitive manifestation of disease.

PET is an exceptional tool for the study of brain function with scientific rigor and quantitative accuracy. SPECT, used clinically and in research, is the most available, cost-effective, and widespread nuclear medicine technique. Both techniques image and measure radioactivity in the brain emitted by specific radiopharmaceuticals, which are localized within the central nervous system. The distribution of this radioactivity from an intravenous injection reflects many pertinent states in health and disease, depending on the radiopharmaceutical employed. PET imaging of the brain uptake of fluorine-18 fluorodeoxyglucose (FDG) is used to evaluate regional brain glucose metabolism in disorders such as neoplasia and epilepsy. Oxygen-15 water studies with PET are used to map brain perfusion and function with stimulus testing that is performed while the patient or subject is in the tomograph. Gaseous oxygen-15 studies are used to measure oxygen extraction fraction (OEF), which is an important parameter in occlusive cerebrovascular disease. SPECT imaging with technetium (Tc)-99m hexamethylpropyleneamine oxime (HMPAO, exametazime) or Tc-99m ethyl cysteinate dimer (bicisate) is used to evaluate regional cerebral perfusion in dementia, epilepsy, and cerebrovascular disorders.[1,2] These SPECT cerebral perfusion radiopharmaceuticals also can be used in stimulus testing of brain function, which can be done outside of the scanner because these radiopharmaceuticals have a longer half-life (6 hours) than PET compounds and are fixed in the brain early after injection with a temporal resolution of less than 1 minute for activation paradigms.

Other compounds used for imaging in PET and SPECT include radiotracers to image γ-aminobutyric acid (GABA)-A receptors (C-11 flumazenil, I-123 iomazenil), opiate receptors (C-11 carfentanil), dopaminergic system (F-18 fluorodopa, C-11 raclopride, C-11 risperidol, I-123 IBZM, I-123 beta-CIT, I-123 IBF), and brain metabolism of amino acids and DNA synthesis in tumors (C-11 methionine, C-11 thymidine) and imaging of tissue hypoxia (F-18 fluoromisonidazole, I-123 IAZA). These radiopharmaceuticals have been used solely in investigational studies in brain disorders.

The physical principle behind PET is that the radiopharmaceutical decays by positron emission. The positron undergoes an annihilation reaction with an electron after a brief transit in tissue, which is based on the energy of the positron. As the annihilation reaction converts the mass of the positron and electron into energy based on $E = mc^2$, two 511-keV photons are emitted in opposite directions and are intercepted by scintillation detectors, which emit light pulses in response. Coincidence circuitry in the camera determines whether the two gamma rays are in coincidence and accepted data or are rejected as scatter and random events. To a great extent, only the photons depicting the location of the decaying radioactivity in the body are collected. Transmission imaging also is performed in PET, to correct for photon attenuation in the body. Scatter corrections are applied to improve accuracy and image quality. Because of the short half-life of the PET radiopharmaceuticals, with the exception of F-18, which has a half-life of 2 hours, almost all injections of tracers such as C-11, O-15, and N-13 must be performed in the tomograph and images acquired immediately. For quantitative accuracy, arterial blood sampling and metabolite analysis are performed to derive numeric physiologic parameters in tissue.

In SPECT, injections rarely are performed in the scanner, and imaging is much more flexible. I-123 or Tc-99m radiopharmaceuticals can be injected and scanned several hours later. The Tc-99m radiopharmaceuticals that depict regional cerebral perfusion are fixed in the brain shortly after injection, and these tracers can be injected during seizure ictus, with balloon occlusion testing; or with intravenous acetazolamide cerebrovascular reserve testing; then the scan can be performed at a later time. The Tc-99m tracers decay by isomeric transition and emit a single monoenergetic gamma ray of 140 keV with each decay of Tc-99m to Tc-99. These gamma rays also interact with the scintillation detector to create the images, which are reconstructed into volumetric three-dimensional data. For the brain with intact skull, attenuation compensation is achieved in SPECT by way of a software correction of activity based on uniform attenuating media and an attenuation factor. Transmission imaging can be employed but has not been performed routinely because most manufacturers have not incorporated transmission attenuation correction in the devices that are commercially available. I-123 compounds, such as I-123 iofetamine (blood flow), I-123 HIPDM (blood flow), and I-123 iomazenil (GABA-A) are not commercially available in the United States but are used investigationally.

EPILEPSY

Interictal PET in epilepsy has been used for seizure focus lateralization for years. Sites of interictal hypometabolism are identified with FDG PET in approximately 70% of patients with temporal lobe epilepsy and about 60% of patients with frontal lobe–onset seizures. Specificity of FDG PET is excellent with less than 5% false localizations of the seizure focus compared with depth electrodes.[3]

Work with C-11 flumazenil PET has shown efficacy in describing the integrity of GABA-A receptors in partial epilepsy. C-11 flumazenil PET has been shown to match closely hippocampal sclerosis in temporal lobe epilepsy compared with resected tissue cell counts and in vitro quantitative autoradiography.[4] In addition, compared with FDG PET, C-11 flumazenil shows the pathologic focus in a more circumscribed fashion[5] because F-18 FDG PET measures metabolism at the focus and surrounding tissue, which may reflect a large area of diaschisis, whereas C-11 flumazenil PET images the benzodiazepine receptor integrity. C-11 flumazenil PET also has been shown to have efficacy in neocortical epilepsy.[6]

Other investigations into receptor imaging with PET in partial epilepsy have found increased μ and δ opiate receptors in temporal lobe epilepsy.[7] Increasingly, these studies of receptor imaging in epilepsy are being evaluated not only in terms of patient management, but also in shedding light on the neurobiology of epilepsy, which could lead to discovery of new drugs. PET also is being used investigationally in an array of disorders to evaluate receptor integrity and function in movement disorders, psychiatry, and chemical dependence and drug addiction.

In the clinical diagnosis and management of complex partial epilepsy, SPECT used with ictal injections of radiopharmaceutical has proved to be the ideal imaging method for the lateralization and localization of seizure onset (Fig. 148–1; see color section in this volume). Ictal SPECT is characterized by focal hyperperfusion in the epileptogenic zone. In a direct comparison with interictal FDG PET with ictal SPECT in temporal lobe epilepsy, Ho and colleagues[8] showed 89% sensitivity for localization with certainty with ictal SPECT; the figure for PET was 63%. SPECT also performed better in the situation of negative MRI findings. In this study, false lateralization was rare with SPECT, as opposed to the experience of Lee and associates.[9] It is clear from these studies, however, that correlation of timing of injections with electroencephalographic and clinical data is crucial for the use of this technique because it is not an entirely independent test for confirmation of seizure onset. One must take into account practical issues, such as length of seizure and transit time for an intravenous administration of radiotracer to go from antecubital vein to brain and be highly extracted on the first pass. A dose that is administered 10 seconds before the termination of a seizure may reach an immediately postictal brain. Postictal SPECT also has been shown to have a sensitivity of approximately 70% (similar to interictal PET in temporal lobe epilepsy), and timing and comparison of injections with electroencephalographic data are crucial.[10] The postictal SPECT in temporal lobe epilepsy shows a large zone of hypoperfusion in the hemisphere of onset. Interictal SPECT has less sensitivity for seizure focus localization. Devous and colleagues[11] reported in a meta-analysis of brain perfusion SPECT in epilepsy that the interictal sensitivity is about 50% for unilateral hypoperfusion. Most investigators now agree, however, and it has been shown by Spanaki and colleagues[12] that ictal/interictal quantitative difference analysis provides for the best

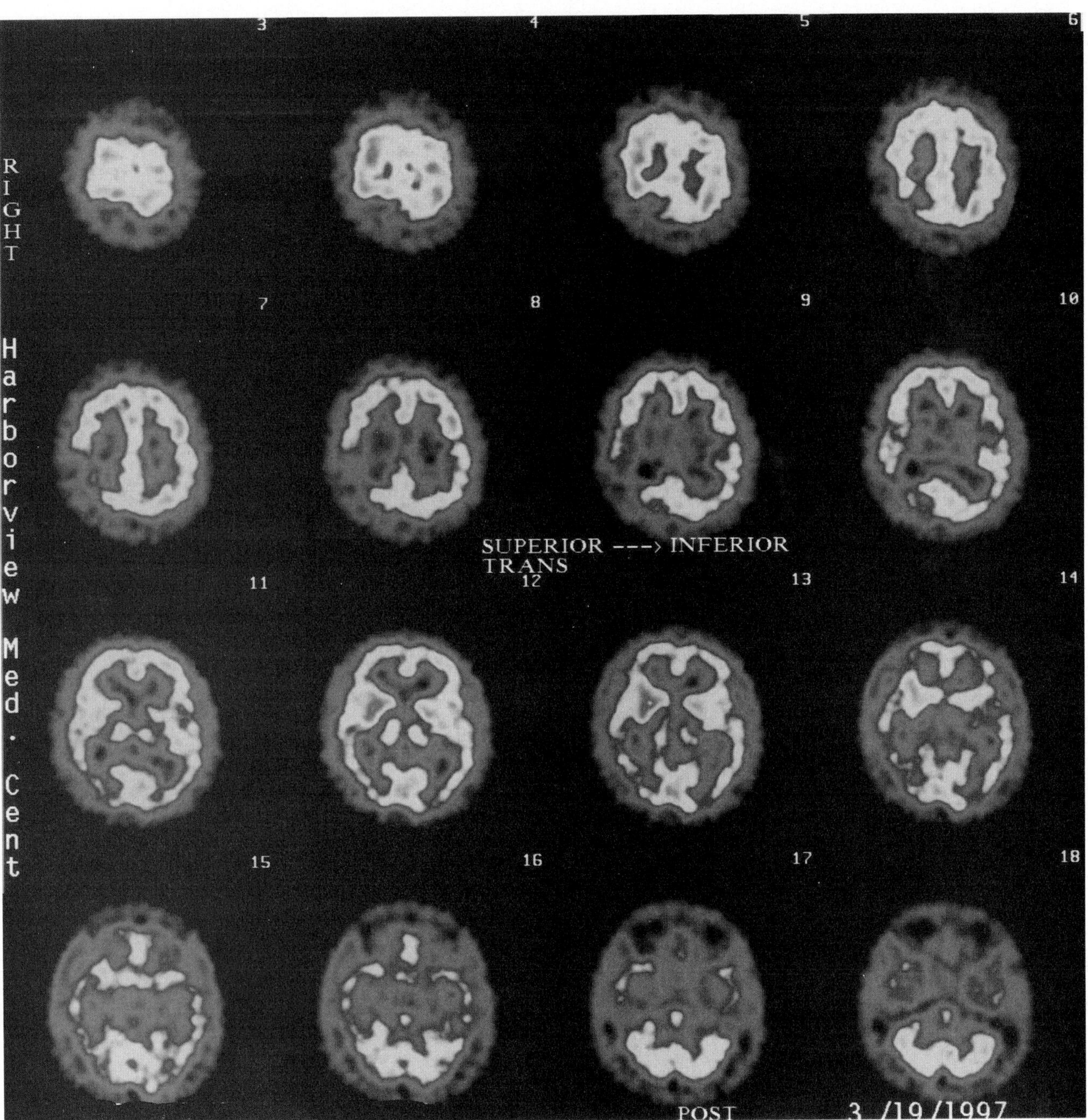

FIGURE 148–1. Transverse axial view of ictal injection of technetium-99m ethyl cysteinate dimer for regional cerebral perfusion in epilepsy. This patient had intractable epilepsy despite previous surgical resection in the right parietal cortex. Ictal image shows hyperperfusion *(red zone)* in the right insular cortex. After resection of this area, the patient was seizure-free (see color section in this volume).

and most reliable seizure focus localization for nuclear medicine studies in complex partial epilepsy. It is crucial to review timing of injections; after image acquisition, it is essential that coregistration software be used to align the SPECT images (to MRI also if possible) and to perform the subtraction analysis. There are commercial and research computer hardware and software packages that now enable any nuclear medicine laboratory to perform this work.

SPECT brain imaging may be applied to the study of neuroreceptors. In the study of complex partial epilepsy, I-123 iomazenil has been used to evaluate GABA-A receptors in the central nervous system. This radiopharmaceutical is available in Europe and Japan but has not been approved for use in the United States for clinical studies. It has been well characterized as a high-affinity ligand for the GABA-A receptor.[13] Results of a European multicenter study showed improved diagnostic value of I-123 iomazenil SPECT scans compared with interictal regional cerebral blood flow SPECT scans in epilepsy.[14] Similar to PET studies with C-11 flumazenil, the I-123 iomazenil SPECT studies show more circumscribed lesions compared with PET F-18 FDG studies.[15]

CEREBROVASCULAR DISEASE

The manifestations of cerebrovascular disease include acute stroke (ischemic and hemorrhagic), transient ischemic attacks (TIA) of either embolic or hemodynamic origin, and cerebral vasospasm as a consequence of subarachnoid hemorrhage. The application of PET in the acute evaluation of stroke is technologically and economically challenging given that the longest lived tracer (F-18) has a half-life of 2 hours, and the uptake phase of F-18 FDG is about 30 minutes. SPECT is much more available and easier, given the ubiquitous generator production of Tc-99m and the ready availability of perfusion tracers in kit formulations. In TIA as manifested by hemodynamic failure, PET studies showed patients with increased OEF (stage II hemodynamic failure) ipsilateral to carotid occlusion are at increased risk for subsequent ipsilateral stroke compared with patients without increased OEF (P = .005).[16] Patients who have increased OEF but who do not have follow-up clinical manifestations of stroke have evidence of interval reduction of OEF on subsequent PET.[17] This reduction in OEF over time is due to improvement in collateral blood flow. Functional studies of blood flow and oxygen metabolism using PET may have prognostic significance and merit revisitation of the external carotid/internal carotid bypass question in affected individuals with chronic cerebral hypoperfusion.[18]

SPECT imaging of cerebral perfusion has been the most applicable nuclear medicine test for imaging stroke shortly after ictus, TIA, and cerebral vasospasm–induced hypoperfusion after subarachnoid hemorrhage. The radiopharmaceuticals used for this imaging in the United States are Tc-99m HMPAO and Tc-99m ethyl cysteinate dimer. The widespread availability of SPECT camera systems and ready availability of the radiopharmaceuticals lead to practical usage of these techniques. There are no contraindications to the use of these radiopharmaceuticals or camera systems in patients with neurological emergencies.

In regard to prognosis after completed stroke, Alexandrov and colleagues[19] evaluated 458 patients with Tc-99m HMPAO SPECT. The results of their analysis of a simple visual interpretation scheme showed that SPECT readings had additional prognostic value independent of the Canadian Neurologic Scale. The diagnostic impact of SPECT was in the first 72 hours, when the focal low perfusion abnormality compared with the focal absence of perfusion on the images was able to improve the predictive value of the Canadian Neurologic Scale score for outcome.

In smaller studies performed during the first 48 hours and within 6 hours of stroke, SPECT with Tc-99m HMPAO and Tc-99m ethyl cysteinate dimer have high sensitivity and specificity for cortical infarction and can allow distinction of transient ischemia from infarction by semiquantitative regional activity thresholds.[20–22] Regional cerebral blood flow images and ratios from region-of-interest analysis can aid in diagnosis and prediction of outcome.

Options in acute stroke for acute therapy may include thrombolysis or decompressive craniectomy for malignant middle cerebral artery infarction. Ueda and colleagues[23] explored SPECT Tc-99m HMPAO imaging in 30 patients who had complete recanalization from intra-arterial thrombolysis within 12 hours of ictus.[23] They concluded that patients with semiquantitative analysis of SPECT showing greater than 55% of cerebellar flow in the affected vascular territory may be salvageable even beyond 6 hours; showing between 55% and 35% uptake may be salvageable with early treatment (<5 hours); and showing less than 35% uptake predicted hemorrhagic transformation within the critical time window. Fatal ischemic brain edema also can be predicted by early SPECT showing a complete deficit in an entire middle cerebral artery territory.[24] Perhaps decompressive craniectomy early after ictus in patients with malignant middle cerebral artery may prevent herniation and death. Further studies are necessary to investigate the merits of this aggressive approach to middle cerebral artery stroke.

In chronic cerebrovascular disease with clear evidence of hemodynamic-type TIA, cerebrovascular reserve can be studied with SPECT using acetazolamide and, in sulfa-allergic patients, carbon dioxide inhalation. Acetazolamide and carbon dioxide induce cerebrovascular arterial and arteriolar dilatation, which may result in an increase in cerebral blood flow by a factor of 30% to 50% above baseline and resting flow in normal vascular beds, but not in patients with hemodynamically significant cerebrovascular disease.[25, 26] Studies using xenon-133 for cerebral blood flow measurements with cerebral vasodilatory stress using acetazolamide showed promising results for improved outcome after external carotid/internal carotid bypass.[27] These cerebrovascular "stress" tests also can be performed with the Tc-99m-labeled tracers with high-quality imaging results in patients with cerebrovascular disease (Fig. 148–2; see color section in this volume).[28]

Hemorrhagic stroke requires computed tomographic scan for diagnosis. Most of these strokes are due to subarachnoid hemorrhage from aneurysmal rupture. Early aneurysm surgical clipping or obliteration by other means attempts to reduce the risk of rebleeding, which is the most lethal event in the ensuing period. When the aneurysm is addressed, SPECT and transcranial Doppler (TCD) are used as complementary tests to evaluate for cerebral vasospasm and the effect of this phenomenon on cerebral perfusion. SPECT is performed after the aneurysm has been obliterated and serves as a baseline for vasospasm, which usually occurs 4 to 12 days after the hemorrhage. TCD also is performed at baseline, then usually at daily intervals. If TCD shows progressively increasing vasospasm as a result of elevated erythrocyte velocities or the patient manifests new signs or symptoms compatible with vasospasm,[29] SPECT is repeated to evaluate for interval change in regional cerebral perfusion. One caveat: If

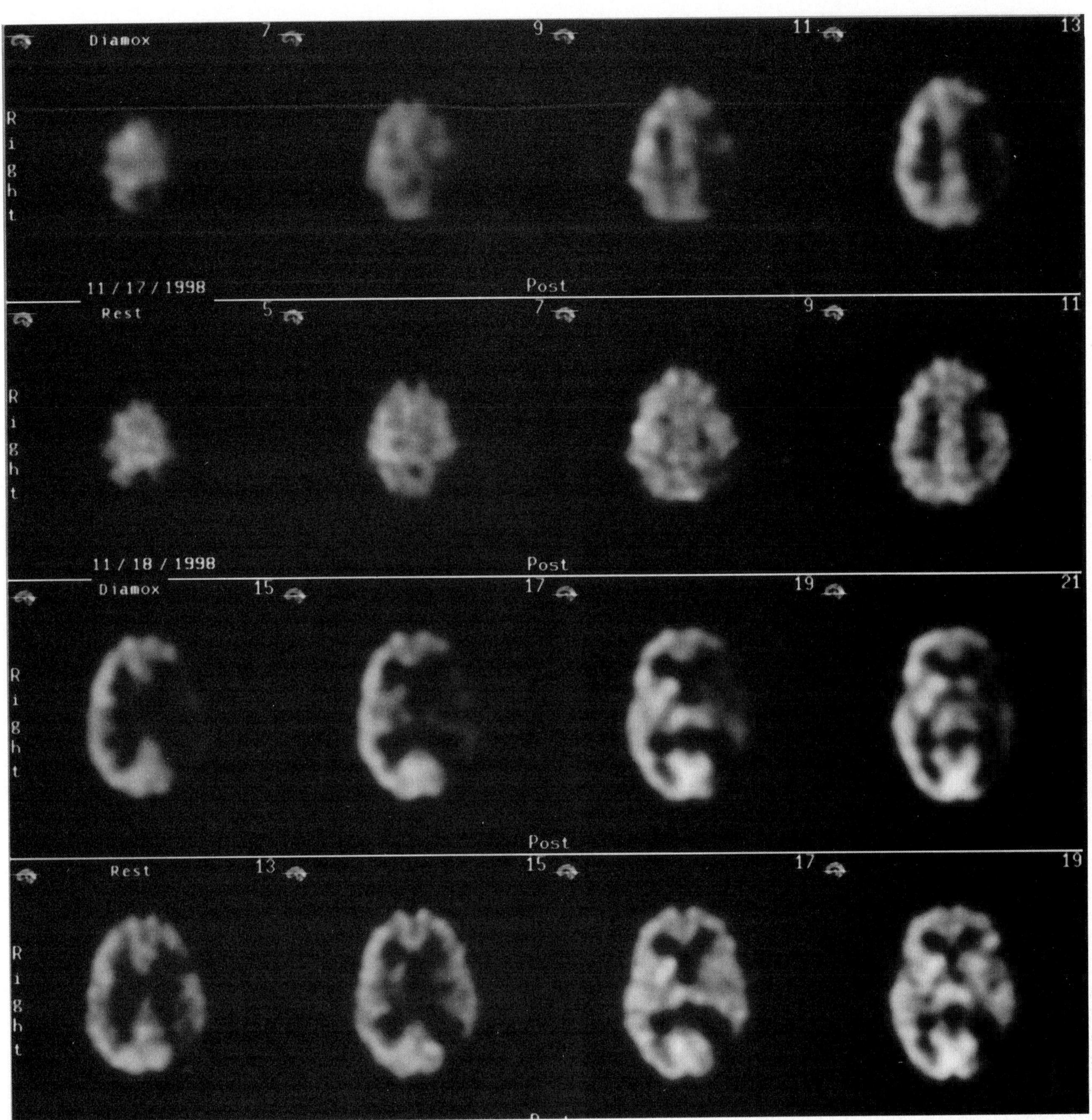

FIGURE 148–2. Transverse axial view of cerebral perfusion SPECT with technetium-99m ethyl cysteinate dimer with acetazolamide challenge *(rows 1 and 3)* and at rest. Images show severe lack of vasodilatory reserve in the left hemisphere with residual fixed defects in the watershed zones (see color section in this volume).

the phenomenon is truly global and balanced with all vessels affected equally, a semiquantitative or qualitative method such as SPECT may not detect this global change. Other methods such as xenon CT or xenon-133 SPECT can detect global changes because they are quantitative and yield flow results in mL/100 g/min.

SPECT and TCD are complementary in the noninvasive evaluation of cerebral vasospasm after subarachnoid hemorrhage.[30] TCD gauges vascular narrowing by measurement of erythrocyte flow velocities in the proximal vessels and branches of the circle of Willis. SPECT evaluates the tissue perfusion, which may be intact in the setting of intact autoregulation or collateral blood flow despite vasospasm on TCD. When SPECT shows a new decrement in perfusion despite proper medical therapy for vasospasm, this technique can indicate that a patient may need more aggressive treatment with endovascular therapy, such as balloon angioplasty or intra-arterial papaverine administration, or more aggressive hemodynamic therapy.[31, 32]

SPECT and TCD have been used to investigate the effect of endovascular therapy in cerebral vasospasm

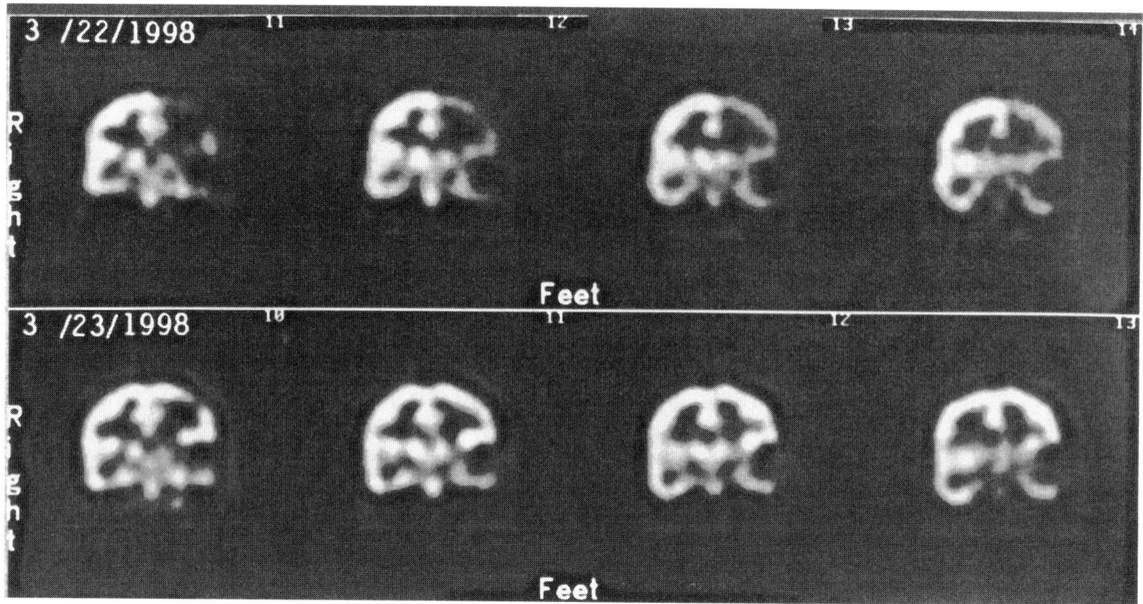

FIGURE 148–3. Coronal axial view of technetium-99m ethyl cysteinate dimer cerebral perfusion SPECT images before *(top)* and after *(bottom)* left middle cerebral artery balloon angioplasty for severe left middle cerebral artery vasospasm after subarachnoid hemorrhage. Images show significant improvement in perfusion to the left hemisphere (see color section in this volume).

(Fig. 148–3; see color section in this volume). Using these techniques, Elliott and colleagues[33] showed that balloon angioplasty is a more effective treatment of cerebral hypoperfusion secondary to vasospasm compared with papaverine. In distal vessel vasospasm that TCD may not detect but SPECT documents, intra-arterial papaverine is safe and can be effective.[34]

SPECT can be used with temporary balloon occlusion tests to evaluate cerebrovascular reserve in the setting of anticipated surgical sacrifice of the internal carotid artery. Tc-99m-labeled perfusion radiopharmaceutical is administered by peripheral venous injection, while the balloon is inflated in the angiographic suite. The SPECT scan is performed after the occlusion test is completed. This is in contrast to xenon CT, which would require the balloon to be inflated during CT xenon imaging. Inadequate reserve can be shown on the SPECT study compared with a baseline, resting examination. One caveat: If hypotension occurs in the operating room, this is not mimicked in the balloon occlusion test, and reserve may be affected significantly by a drop in blood pressure that would go unpredicted by the preoperative study. The results of this SPECT study of hemodynamic reserve may cause alteration in the surgical planning.[35]

SPECT can be used to describe the intra-arterial delivery of amobarbital to the brain for presurgical evaluation of memory and language function in one hemisphere. The Tc-99m-labeled tracer is coadministered with the intra-arterial amobarbital. SPECT is performed after the test is completed. Jeffery and colleagues[36] showed that in 18 of 25 patients, amobarbital was not delivered to the mesial temporal cortex by absence of uptake of tracer in that area on the scan.

ONCOLOGY

SPECT and PET have been used in the diagnosis and evaluation of response to treatment of tumors of the brain. SPECT with thallium-201 has been used in evaluation of recurrent gliomas[37] and in human immunodeficiency virus disease, in which the differential diagnosis of a brain lesion includes inflammatory and infectious processes versus lymphoma. Lymphoma largely has increased uptake of thallium-201, whereas the infectious and inflammatory processes usually do not show uptake of thallium-201.[38]

PET, with higher resolution and use of F-18 FDG, has an advantage over thallium-201, which requires breakdown of the blood-brain barrier for entry of the cationic radionuclide into the tumor. F-18 FDG normally traverses the blood-brain barrier and localizes in neurons. One of the problems with PET F-18 FDG is distinguishing uptake in normal brain from that of uptake in the glioma. For this reason, coregistration techniques of CT or MRI or both to PET are essential. After surgery, there is no enhanced uptake of FDG because of the surgery or use of glucocorticoids; early PET can assess for residual tumor or early recurrence, as long as coregistration to anatomic imaging is used with rigor and attention to detail.[39]

Imaging of cellular proliferation in brain tumors can be achieved by using C-11 thymidine and PET (Fig. 148–4). Kinetic and metabolite analyses of the data from PET and arterial blood sampling can estimate the flux of thymidine incorporation into DNA.[40] Using these data about the rate of DNA synthesis, perhaps new experimental therapies can be assessed in their ability to interfere with cellular proliferation with in vivo imaging.

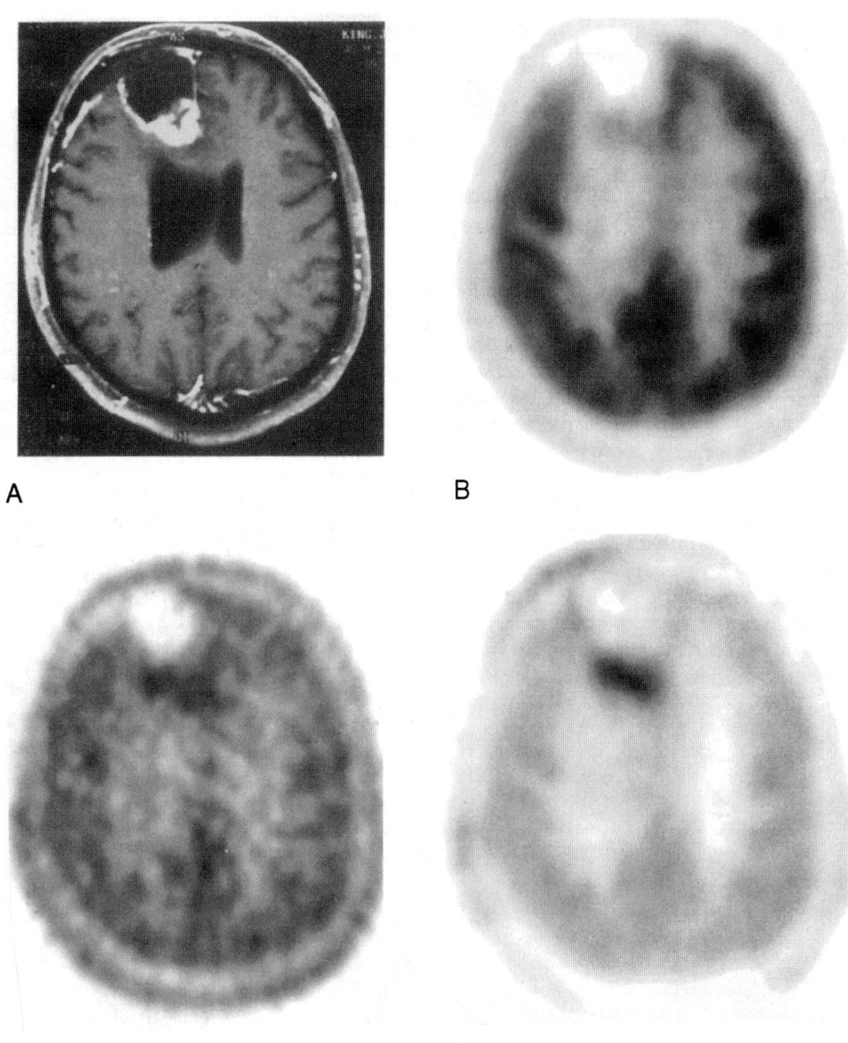

FIGURE 148–4. Images of a patient with recurrent right frontal glioma. *A,* Contrast-enhanced magnetic resonance imaging. *B,* Fluorine-18 fluorodeoxyglucose. *C,* Summed 20- to 60-minute thymidine image. *D,* Thymidine flux constant image using compartmental model and mixture analysis. Note the focus of increased thymidine flux in the posterior aspect of the tumor resection cavity. (From Eary JF, Mankoff DA, Spence AM, et al: 2-[C-11]Thymidine imaging of malignant brain tumors. Cancer Res 56:615–621, 1999; reprinted with permission from Cancer Research.)

TRAUMA

X-ray CT is the most important imaging tool in the evaluation of acute head trauma. Many studies in acute head trauma have reported that SPECT imaging of cerebral blood flow early after traumatic brain injury shows more cerebral lesions than head CT.[41–43] Also, in minor head trauma, if the SPECT is normal, the outcome is uniformly good.[44] If vascular injury or compromise is associated with blunt or penetrating traumatic brain injury, SPECT may indicate the severity of the vascular insult on brain perfusion. Also, in the follow-up of patients after mild head injury, it has been shown that SPECT is more sensitive than MRI or CT, and the abnormalities in perfusion were common in patients with persistent postconcussive syndrome.[45]

PET is impractical to employ in patients with acute traumatic brain injury; however, results similar to the previous discussion in regard to SPECT have been found with PET F-18 FDG scans in patients with a history of mild traumatic brain injury. Abnormalities have been found that help to explain the behavioral and cognitive deficits shown by such patients.[46]

Finally, although not using SPECT or PET techniques, portable cerebral blood flow scanning with single-photon emitting brain perfusion radiopharmaceuticals allows for the timely and important corroboration of the clinical impression of brain death in patients with traumatic brain injury or other brain insults. The scan is rapid to perform and often can be done portably if a gamma camera in the institution is a mobile unit. The results represent a robust standard for brain death corroboration when they show total cessation of the blood flow to the cerebrum and hindbrain.[47, 48]

REFERENCES

1. Assessment of brain SPECT: Report of the Therapeutics and Technology Assessment Subcommittee of the American Academy of Neurology. Neurology 46:278–285, 1996.
2. Masdeu JC, Brass LM, Holman BL, Kushner MJ: Brain single-photon emission computed tomography. Neurology 44:1970–1977, 1994.
3. Devinsky O, Pacia S: Epilepsy surgery. Neurol Clin 11:951–971, 1993.
4. Burdette DE, Sakurai SY, Henry TR, et al: Temporal lobe central benzodiazepine binding in unilateral mesial temporal lobe epilepsy. Neurology 45:934–941, 1995.

5. Szelies B, Weber-Luxenburger G, Pawlik G, et al: MRI-guided flumazenil- and FDG-PET in temporal lobe epilepsy. Neuroimage 3:109–118, 1996.
6. Richardson MP, Koepp MJ, Brooks DJ, Duncan JS: C-11-flumazenil PET in neocortical epilepsy. Neurology 51:485–492, 1998.
7. Frost JJ, Mayber HS, Fisher RS: Mu-opiate receptors measured by positron emission tomography are increased in temporal lobe epilepsy. Ann Neurol 23:231–237, 1988.
8. Ho SS, Berkovic SF, Berlangieri SU, et al: Comparison of ictal SPECT and interictal PET in the presurgical evaluation of temporal lobe epilepsy. Ann Neurol 347:738–745, 1995.
9. Lee BI, Lee JD, Kim JY, et al: Single photon emission computed tomography-EEG relations in temporal lobe epilepsy. Neurology 49:981–991, 1997.
10. Rowe CC, Berkovi SF, Sia STB, et al: Localization of epileptic foci with postictal single photon emission computed tomography. Ann Neurol 26:660–668, 1989.
11. Devous MD Sr, Thisted RA, Morgan GF, et al: SPECT brain imaging in epilepsy: A meta-analysis. J Nucl Med 39:285–293, 1998.
12. Spanaki MV, Spencer SS, Corsi M, et al: Sensitivity and specificity of quantitative difference SPECT analysis in seizure localization. J Nucl Med 40:730–736, 1999.
13. Beer HF, Blauenstein PA, Hasler PH, et al: In vitro and in vivo evaluation of iodine-123-Ro 16-0154: A new imaging agent for SPECT investigations of benzodiazepine receptors. J Nucl Med 31:1007–1014, 1990.
14. Schubiger PA, Hasler PH, Beer-Wohlfahrt H, et al: Evaluation of multicentre study with iomazenil—a benzodiazepine receptor ligand. Nucl Med Commun 12:569–582, 1991.
15. Tanaka F, Yonekura Y, Ikeda A, et al: Presurgical identification of epileptic foci with iodine-123 iomazenil SPET: Comparison with brain perfusion SPET and FDG PET. Eur J Nucl Med 24: 27–34, 1997.
16. Derdeyn CP, Yundt KD, Videen TO, et al: Increased oxygen extraction fraction is associated with prior ischemic events in patients with carotid occlusion. Stroke 29:754–758, 1998.
17. Derdeyn CP, Videen TO, Fritsch SM, et al: Compensatory mechanisms for chronic cerebral hypoperfusion in patients with carotid occlusion. Stroke 30:1019–1024, 1999.
18. Klijn CJ, Kapelle LJ, Tulleken CA, Van Gijn J: Symptomatic carotid artery occlusion: A reappraisal of hemodynamic factors. Stroke 28:2084–2093, 1997.
19. Alexandrov AV, Black SE, Ehrlich LE, et al: Simple visual analysis of brain perfusion on HMPAO SPECT predicts early outcome in acute stroke. Stroke 27:1537–1542, 1996.
20. Baird AE, Austin MC, McKay WJ, Donnan GA: Sensitivity and specificity of Tc-99m HMPAO SPECT cerebral perfusion measurements during the first 48 hours for the localization of cerebral infarction. Stroke 28:976–980, 1997.
21. Shimosegawa E, Hatazawa J, Inugami A, et al: Cerebral infarction within 6 hours of onset: Prediction of completed infarction with technetium-99m-HMPAO SPECT. J Nucl Med 35:1097–1103, 1994.
22. Berrouschot J, Barthel H, Hesse S, et al: Differentiation between transient ischemic attack and ischemic stroke within the first six hours after onset of symptoms by using Tc-99m ECD-SPECT. J Cerebral Blood Flow Metab 18:921–929, 1998.
23. Ueda T, Sakaki S, Yuh WTC, et al: Outcome in acute stroke with successful intra-arterial thrombolysis and predictive value of initial single-photon emission-computed tomography. J Cerebral Blood Flow Metab 19:99–108, 1999.
24. Berrouschot J, Barthel H, von Kummer R, et al: Technetium-99m-ethyl-cysteinate-dimer single-photon emission CT can predict fatal ischemic brain edema. Stroke 29:2556–2562, 1998.
25. Bonte FJ, Devous MD Sr, Reisch JS: The effect of acetazolamide on regional cerebral blood flow in normal human subjects as measured by single photon emission computed tomography. Invest Radiol 23:564–568, 1988.
26. Bonte FJ, Devous MD Sr, Ajmani AK, et al: The effect of acetazolamide on regional cerebral blood flow in patients with Alzheimer's disease or stroke as measured by single-photon emission computed tomography. Invest Radiol 24:99–103, 1989.
27. Schmiedek P, Piepgras A, Leinsinger G, et al: Improvement of cerebrovascular reserve capacity by EC-IC arterial bypass surgery in patients with ICA oclusion and hemodynamic cerebral ischemia. J Neurosurg 81:236–244, 1994.
28. Ramsay SC, Yeates MG, Lord RS, et al: Use of technetium-99m-HMPAO to demonstrate changes in flow reserve following carotid endarterectomy. J Nucl Med 32:1382–1386, 1991.
29. Davis SM, Andrews JT, Lichtenstein M, et al: Correlations between cerebral arterial velocities, blood flow, and delayed ischemia after subarachnoid hemorrhage. Stroke 23:492–497, 1992.
30. Lewis DH, Hsu S, Eskridge J, et al: Brain SPECT and transcranial Doppler ultrasound in vasospasm-induced delayed cerebral ischemia after subarachnoid hemorrhage. J Stroke Cerebrovasc Dis 2:12–21, 1992.
31. Lewis DH, Eskridge JM, Newell DW, et al: Brain SPECT and the effect of cerebral angioplasty in delayed ischemia due to vasospasm. J Nucl Med 33:1789–1796, 1992.
32. Lewis DH, Eskridge JM, McAuliffe W, et al: Effect of intra-arterial papaverine on cerebral blood flow in vasospasm after subarachnoid hemorrhage: A study using single-photon emission computed tomography. J Stroke Cerebrovasc Dis 5:24–28, 1995.
33. Elliott JP, Newell DW, Lam DJ, et al: Comparison of balloon angioplasty and papaverine infusion for the treatment of vasospasm following aneurysmal subarachnoid hemorrhage. J Neurosurg 88:277–284, 1998.
34. Lewis DH, Newell DW, Winn HR: Delayed ischemia due to cerebral vasospasm occult to transcranial Doppler: An important role for cerebral perfusion SPECT. Clin Nucl Med 22:238–240, 1997.
35. Eckard DA, Purdy PD, Bonte FJ: Temporary occlusion of the carotid artery combined with brain blood flow imaging as a test to predict tolerance to permanent carotid sacrifice. AJNR Am J Neuroradiol 13:1565–1569, 1992.
36. Jeffery PJ, Monsein LH, Szabo Z, et al: Mapping the distribution of amobarbital sodium in the intra-carotid Wada test by use of Tc-99m HMPAO with SPECT. Radiology 178:847–850, 1991.
37. Carvalho PA, Schwartz RB, Alexander E III, et al: Detection of recurrent gliomas with quantitative thallium-201/technetium-99m HMPAO single-photon emission computerized tomography. J Neurosurg 77:565–570, 1992.
38. Lorberboym M, Estok L, Machac J, et al: Rapid differential diagnosis of cerebral toxoplasmosis and primary central nervous system lymphoma by thallium-201 SPECT. J Nucl Med 37:1150–1154, 1996.
39. Glantz MJ, Hoffman JM, Coleman RE, et al: Identification of early recurrence of primary central nervous system tumors by F-18-fluorodeoxyglucose positron emisssion tomography. Ann Neurol 29:347–355, 1991.
40. Eary JF, Mankoff DA, Spence AM, et al: 2-(C-11)Thymidine imaging of malignant brain tumors. Cancer Res 59:615–621, 1999.
41. Abdel-Dayem HM, Sadek SA, Kouris K, et al: Changes in cerebral perfusion after acute head injury: Comparison of CT with Tc-99m HMPAO SPECT. Radiology 165:221–226, 1987.
42. Roper SN, Mena I, King WA, et al: An analysis of cerebral blood flow in acute closed head injury using technetium-99m-HMPAO SPECT and computed tomography. J Nucl Med 32:684–687, 1991.
43. Masdeu J, Van Heertum RL, Kleinman A, et al: Early single-photon emission computed tomography in mild head trauma. J Neuroimaging 4:177, 1994.
44. Jacobs A, Put E, Ingels M, Bossuyt A: Prospective evaluation of technetium-99m HMPAO SPECT in mild and moderate traumatic brain injury. J Nucl Med 35:942–947, 1994.
45. Kant R, Smith-Seemiller L, Isaac G, Duffy J: Tc-HMPAO SPECT in persistent post-concussion syndrome after mild head injury: Comparison with MRI/CT. Brain Inj 11:115–124, 1997.
46. Gross H, Kling A, Henry G, et al: Local cerebral glucose metabolism in patients with long-term behavioral and cognitive deficits following mild TBI. J Neuropyschiatry Clin Neurosci 8:324–334, 1996.
47. Reid RH, Gulenchyn KY, Ballinger JR: Clinical use of technetium-99m HM-PAO for determination of brain death. J Nucl Med 30: 1621–1626, 1989.
48. Idea RJ, Lewis DH: Trauma cases of Harborview Medical Center: Timely diagnosis of brain death in an emergency trauma center. AJR Am J Roentgenol 163:927–928, 1994.

CHAPTER **149**

Preoperative Evaluation for Epilepsy Surgery: Computed Tomography and Magnetic Resonance Imaging

RICHARD A. BRONEN

Neuroimaging has changed dramatically the preoperative evaluation and management for epilepsy surgery. Of the various neuroimaging modalities, magnetic resonance imaging (MRI) has had the greatest impact on classification and understanding of epilepsy syndromes by "shifting emphasis from the electroclinical diagnosis to brain substrate or structural abnormalities from which the electrical and clinical features of epilepsy syndrome originate."[1] This chapter reviews the role of computed tomography (CT), MRI, and magnetic resonance spectroscopy (MRS) before and after epilepsy.

COMPUTED TOMOGRAPHY SCANNING AND EPILEPSY SURGERY

The primary role of structural neuroimaging is to locate and define anatomic epileptogenic lesions; CT was the first cross-sectional neuroimaging technique to do this and had a major impact on epilepsy evaluation from the 1970s through the 1980s. CT scanning can detect neoplastic, vascular, and atrophic abnormalities, especially if the lesions are large, extratemporal, or calcified. CT may yield better results than MRI in certain conditions, such as the following: (1) in identifying *tram-track* calcification of the cortex associated with Sturge-Weber syndrome (Fig. 149-1), (2) in identifying calcification associated with cysticercosis, and (3) in identifying calcification of subependymal tubers in tuberous sclerosis.

Compared with MRI, CT offers several advantages: CT scanners are more widely available, images are interpreted easily, and the examination can be performed rapidly. CT imaging continues to be better than MRI for detection of calcification and acute hemorrhage. Disadvantages include poor image quality through the temporal fossa because of beam hardening artifact (an unfortunate location because most partial seizures originate from this region), lack of multiplanar imaging, radiation exposure, and increased risk of contrast reaction compared with MRI contrast material. A new generation of multislice slip-ring CT scanners is available, however, that can reconstruct instantly in multiple planes and eliminate much of the bone artifact that occurs with imaging the middle cranial fossa.

CT often is the first imaging study performed in patients presenting to emergency departments with new onset seizures. CT in particular is the first imaging study for elderly patients, in whom an acute hemorrhage or infarct may be the precipitating factor. CT imaging of chronic epilepsy patients has been abandoned at epilepsy centers, however, because of the marked superiority of MRI for evaluating intractable epilepsy.[2–12]

A series of investigations that compared preoperative MRI with CT scanning for patients undergoing resective surgery for medically refractory epilepsy confirmed the clear advantages of MRI.[11–13] In a study of 117 patients with correlative histology, sensitivities for detecting *positive pathology* were 95% by MRI and 32% by CT (Fig. 149-2), and specificities were 87% by MRI and 93% by CT; positive pathology was defined as lesions or hippocampal sclerosis at histopathology, whereas negative pathology was defined as either normal tissue or gliosis.[11] MRI detected an abnormality at the *surgical site* in 86% compared with 28% for CT (Fig. 149-3). MRI predicted the pathologic substrate in 88% versus 35% for CT. The probability of a positive CT scan in a patient with a negative MRI study was 0% (although CT detected calcification in 15%), whereas the probability of a positive MRI study in a patient with a negative CT scan was 80%. Multiple findings were observed in 3% of CT scans and 17% of MRI studies.[11]

In terms of postoperative seizure outcomes, the epileptogenic zone was detected in 95% of cases by MRI versus 30% by CT in 80 patients who were seizure-free postoperatively.[12] The positive predictive value of MRI for good seizure outcome was 80% compared with 77% with CT (i.e., if imaging was positive, how likely will a patient have a good outcome). The negative predictive

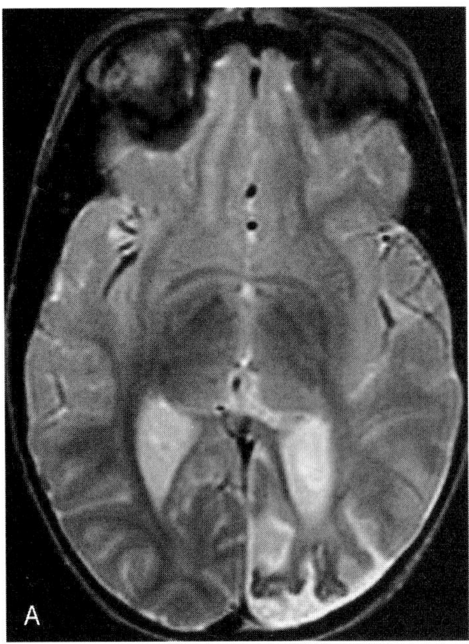

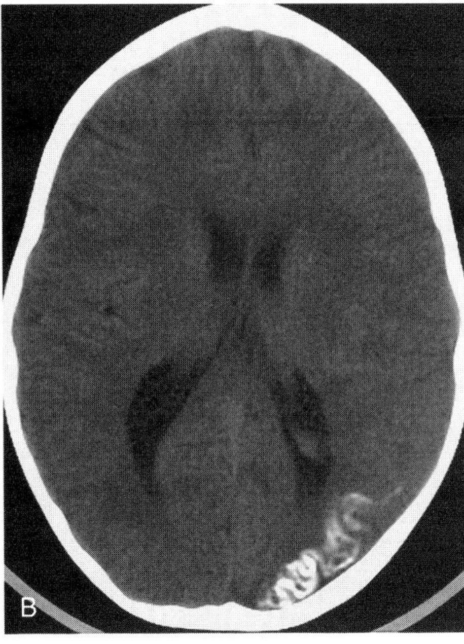

FIGURE 149–1. Utility of computed tomography (CT). *A,* Axial T2-weighted magnetic resonance image shows left occipital lobe volume loss. On careful inspection, there is an adjacent subtle hypointense cortical rim, consistent with hemosiderin or calcification. *B,* Axial nonenhanced CT scan through the same region shows cortical calcification indicative of Sturge-Weber syndrome.

value of MRI was 71% and CT was 28% (i.e., if imaging was normal, how likely will a patient have a poor outcome). Because of a decreased need for intracranial electroencephalography (EEG) monitoring with MRI compared with CT, a substantial cost savings was found by replacing CT with MRI evaluations.[13]

Based on these and other studies, it is concluded that CT has no role in the presurgical diagnostic evaluation of the patient with medically refractory epilepsy, despite its advantage for detection of calcification. A single imaging abnormality on CT or MRI in a patient with intractable epilepsy is a good predictor of successful postoperative seizure outcome, but MRI is more sensitive than CT for detecting the epileptogenic zone. MRI is a much better predictor of a poor postoperative seizure outcome when the imaging study is normal. These results show unequivocally that MRI is superior to CT for detecting an epileptogenic focus, predicting

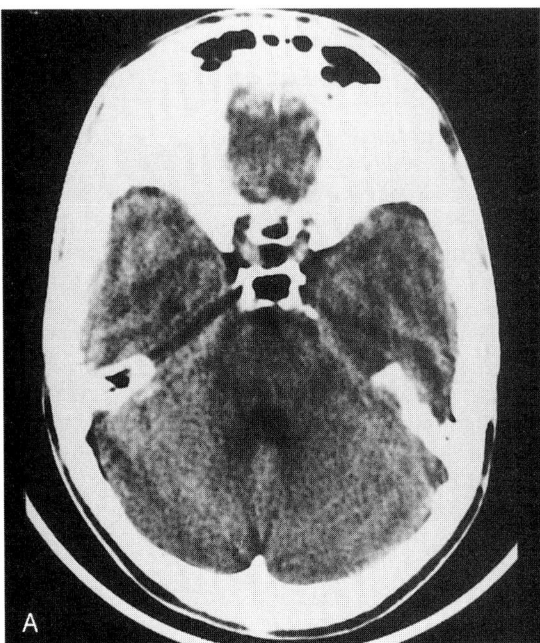

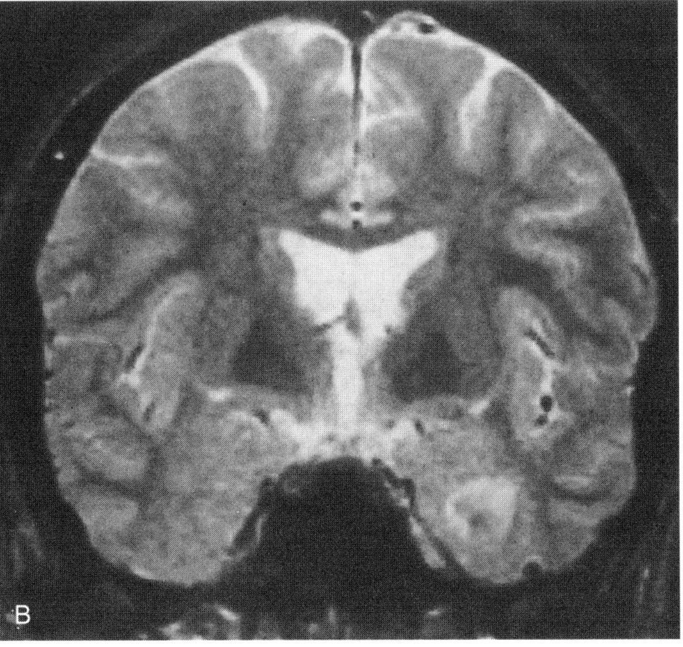

FIGURE 149–2. Utility of magnetic resonance imaging. *A,* Axial computed tomography (CT) scan is normal. *B,* Coronal T2-weighted magnetic resonance image easily detects the left temporal lobe tumor, a glioma. Beam-hardening artifact was partially responsible for inability to visualize this tumor by CT. (From Bronen RA, Fulbright RK, Spencer DD, et al: Refractory epilepsy: Comparison of MR imaging, CT, and histopathologic findings in 117 patients. Radiology 201:97–105, 1996.)

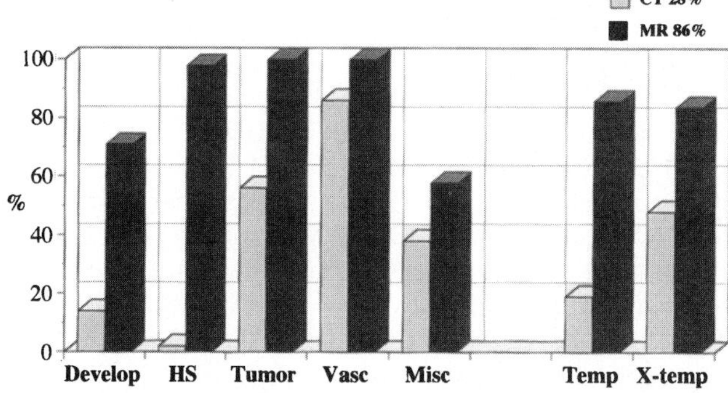

FIGURE 149–3. Sensitivity for detecting epileptogenic abnormalities by computed tomography and magnetic resonance imaging as compared with histopathology in 117 cases.[11] Develop, developmental anomalies; HS, hippocampal sclerosis; Vasc, vascular lesions; Misc, miscellaneous; Temp, temporal lobe abnormalities; X-temp, extratemporal lesions.

seizure outcome after surgery, and decreasing health costs associated with preoperative evaluation of intractable epilepsy requiring surgical amelioration.[11–13]

MAGNETIC RESONANCE IMAGING AND EPILEPSY SURGERY

The primary role of MRI is to locate and define anatomic epileptogenic lesions. The sensitivity for detecting epileptogenic anomalies depends on the type of population studied. Although the yield is much lower in patients with new onset seizures as opposed to patients with medically intractable epilepsy, MRI is still important. In a group of 263 patients with first-seizure presentation studied by King and colleagues,[14] 38 (14%) epileptogenic abnormalities were detected with MRI, including 17 tumors. Of the subgroup classified as generalized seizures ($n = 50$), only one patient presented with an imaging abnormality—an occipital lobe tumor. This patient subsequently was reclassified as having partial seizures with secondary generalization. Based on these findings, the authors recommended that MRI be performed in all seizure patients except patients with idiopathic generalized epilepsies and benign rolandic epilepsy.

In patients with intractable epilepsy, sensitivity for identifying epileptogenic abnormalities with MRI varies depending on the characteristics of the group studied (e.g., children versus adults) and on the underlying substrate (e.g., neoplasms versus cortical dysgenesis) (see Fig. 149-3). In one series of patients with intractable epilepsy, MRI had an overall sensitivity of 86% compared with surgical findings.[11] For temporal lobe epilepsy, MRI sensitivity (compared with pathologic findings) is 75% to 100% for hippocampal sclerosis and greater than 95% for neoplasms and vascular malformations.[15–26] Specificity for detecting an epileptogenic focus by MRI is about 70% to 85% for hippocampal sclerosis and greater than 90% for focal abnormalities, such as tumors. It is crucial to correlate clinical and electrical data with the static anatomic findings on MRI to avoid surgery resulting from false-positive findings (Fig. 149-4).[27] The sensitivity for detecting abnormalities on MRI in children undergoing epilepsy surgery has been reported as greater than 75%.[28–31] There is decreased sensitivity for detection of cortical dysgenesis (also known as malformations of cortical development or *cortical dysplasia*) because these abnormalities may be subtle or microscopic and beyond the resolution of conventional MRI.

In addition to its role in detection of epileptogenic abnormalities, MRI is useful in several different capacities in preparation for epilepsy surgery. MRI can depict the relationship between an epileptic abnormality and functionally important tissue (such as motor or lan-

FIGURE 149–4. *A,* Axial T2-weighted magnetic resonance image shows a lesion *(arrow)* with a central hyperintense complex component, surrounded by a hypointense (hemosiderin) rim. This is consistent with a hemorrhagic vascular malformation, most likely a cavernous hemangioma. In most seizure cases, this lesion would be the source of seizures. *B,* Because of discongruent preoperative localization, the patient underwent intracranial electroencephalography monitoring, and a contralateral focus was localized to the supplementary motor region and resected, as shown by computed tomography. Cavernous hemangiomas may calcify *(arrow* in *B).*

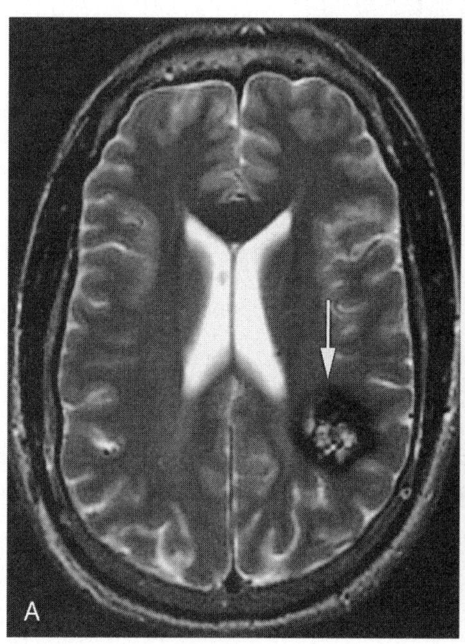

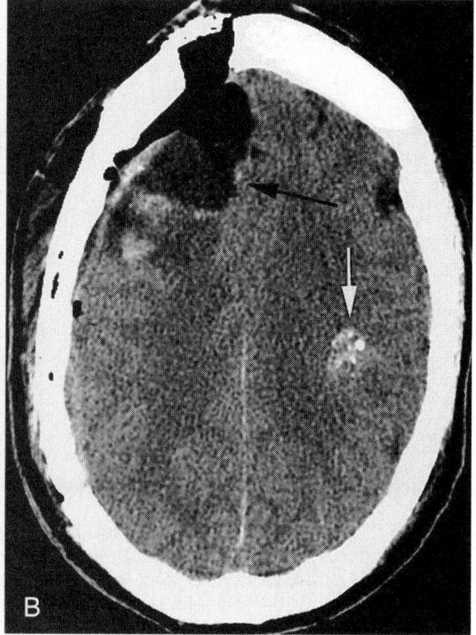

guage cortex), especially when combined with functional MRI. Coregistration of positron emission tomography (PET) and single-photon emission computed tomography (SPECT) images with MRI facilitates anatomic localization of PET and SPECT findings.[32]

MRI findings may influence whether the patient is a candidate for surgery, the type of surgery, the need for invasive EEG evaluation, and the prognosis for postoperative seizure control. Concordance of noninvasive tests with the MRI findings may preclude the need for invasive EEG testing.[33] MRI is useful in planning the placement of invasive electrodes, such as the surgical placement of subdural or depth electrodes. Because MRI of intracranial electrodes can be performed safely,[34] verification of the exact anatomic distribution of contacts is possible, allowing the region of surgery to be determined precisely (Fig. 149-5). Postoperatively, MRI may identify reasons for surgical failures, such as inadequate tissue resection, and it can monitor recurrence of tumors during follow-up examinations.

Several studies have shown that MRI findings can predict postoperative seizure outcome. A *successful seizure outcome* after temporal lobectomy is achieved in 70% to 95% of temporal lobe epilepsy patients who have MRI evidence of hippocampal sclerosis compared with only 40% to 55% in whom the MRI is normal.[12, 26, 35–37] In a study of 135 patients by Berkovic and coworkers,[37] a *seizure-free* state (for ≥2 years) was found to be dependent on substrate identified by MRI—a seizure-free state was obtained in 80% with focal lesions (i.e., tumors or cavernous malformations) compared with 62% with MRI findings of hippocampal sclerosis and 36% with normal MRI studies.

The advent of MRI has resulted in a dramatic change in the intracranial EEG algorithm for epilepsy surgery.

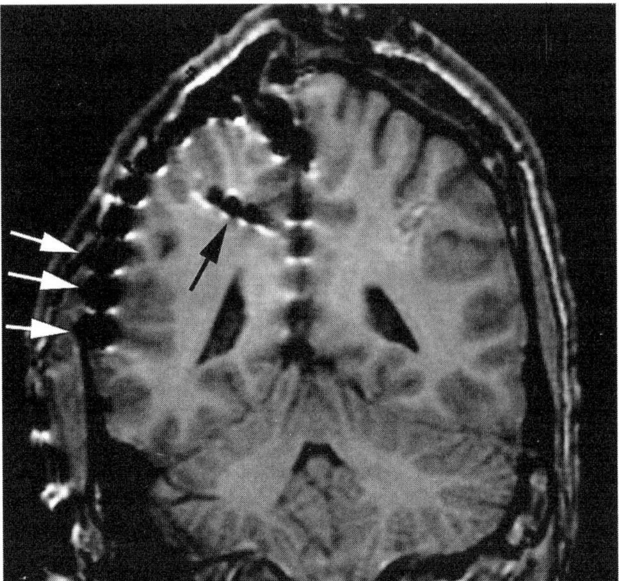

FIGURE 149–5. Magnetic resonance imaging performed with subdural *(white arrows)* and depth *(black arrow)* electrodes in place. Each arrow points to an electrode contact (or rather the magnetic susceptibility artifact created by the contact) on this coronal T1-weighted image.

Previously, all surgical patients had invasive EEG electrode placement, a procedure associated with a 2% to 5% complication rate, several weeks of hospitalization, and costs of $50,000.[38, 39] The paradigm for preoperative localization has shifted from emphasis on electrical data to neuroimaging findings. If MRI reveals a lesion or hippocampal sclerosis, the Yale Surgery Program does not use invasive EEG if MRI and scalp EEG are concordant, as long as other studies are not discordant (i.e., PET or SPECT).[33] Invasive EEG is indicated when MRI and scalp EEG are discordant, when there is more than one MRI abnormality, when MRI shows a large atrophic region or a developmental abnormality, and when MRI or other evidence indicates that mapping of brain function is indicated.

Magnetic Resonance Imaging of Pathologic Substrates

Substrate groups can be defined by common features such as histopathology and anatomy, mechanism of seizure generation, surgical treatment, and outcome. One such classification system, proposed by Spencer,[40] divides epilepsy into five substrates: (1) hippocampal sclerosis; (2) neoplasms; (3) vascular malformations; (4) developmental anomalies; and (5) miscellaneous, composed mostly of substrates associated with gliosis. MRI has a sensitivity of 88% for predicting the correct substrate category in subjects with intractable epilepsy.[11]

HIPPOCAMPAL SCLEROSIS (MESIAL TEMPORAL SCLEROSIS)

Familiarity with the normal anatomy of the hippocampus is essential for correct interpretation of hippocampal imaging abnormalities.[41–47] The hippocampus is a curved structure situated on the medial aspect of the temporal lobe (Fig. 149-6). Three regions of hippocampus can be defined, based on morphology and relationship to the brainstem—the *hippocampal head, body,* and *tail.* The head is located at the anterior aspect of the brainstem. The hippocampal head can be identified by digitations that resemble toes of the feet and also is referred to as the *pes hippocampus.* The body is a cylindrically shaped structure situated adjacent to the brainstem. The tail narrows rapidly as it sweeps upward behind the brainstem. In cross-section, the hippocampus is a complex functional unit composed of two interlocking U-shaped gray matter structures, the *cornu ammonis* and the *dentate gyrus* (Fig. 149-7). The *alveus, fimbria,* and *fornix* are white matter tracts that connect the hippocampus to subcortical structures, such as the hypothalamus, thalamus, and septal nuclei. The white matter of alveus converges medially to form the fimbria, which in turn forms the fornix. Structures adjacent to the hippocampus include the subiculum and white matter of the *parahippocampal gyrus* inferiorly; the *ambient cistern* medially, which separates the hippocampus from the brainstem; the *choriodal fissure* and *temporal horn* superiorly; and the *temporal horn* laterally.

MRI of the amygdala and hippocampus is per-

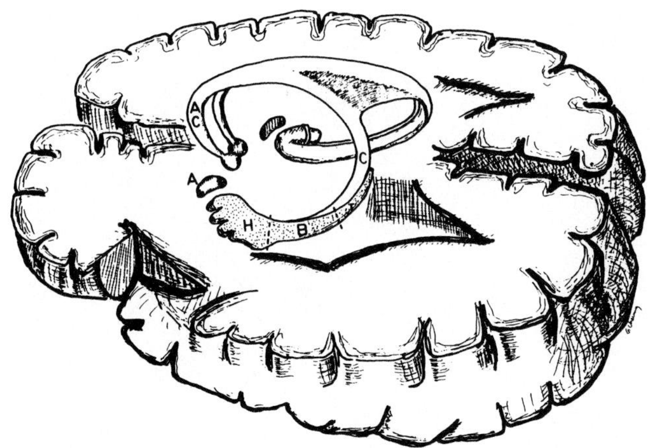

FIGURE 149–6. Diagram of hippocampus and fornix viewed from above. The amygdala (A) is anterior-superior to the hippocampal head (H), the digitated anterior bulbous portion of hippocampus. The hippocampus is uniform along its body (B), then narrows posterior at its tail (T). The main efferent pathway is the fornix. C, crus of fornix; AC, anterior columns of fornix. (From Bronen RA, Cheung G: Relationship of hippocampal and amygdala to coronal MRI landmarks. Magn Reson Imaging 9:449–457, 1991.)

formed best in the coronal plane, perpendicular to the long axis of the hippocampus (Fig. 149-8). The amygdala and hippocampus are isointense to gray matter on all pulse sequences. The hippocampus may be slightly hyperintense to gray matter on fluid-attenuated inversion recovery (FLAIR) sequences, however, because of inadequate suppression of water. The best landmark for separating amygdala from hippocampus is the anterior temporal horn, known as the *uncal recess*. The amygdala is always superior to the temporal horn. When there is a paucity of cerebrospinal fluid within the uncal recess of the temporal horn, the alveus (i.e., the white matter along the superior aspect of the hippocampal head) can be used to delineate the borders of these structures. The amygdala-hippocampal junction occurs at the level of the suprasellar cistern and basilar artery bifurcation. The hippocampal head can be recognized by its digitations and bulbous appearance. The hippocampal body appears as an oval gray matter structure, capped by the white matter of the alveus and fimbria. The internal architecture of the hippocampus may be visualized with high-resolution studies, using fast spin echo or inversion recovery techniques (see Figs. 149-7 and 149-8*D*). The hippocampal tail narrows markedly as it ascends around the brainstem. Many centers use the crus of the fornix to delineate the posterior boundary of the hippocampus for quantitative studies.[42–45, 47–49]

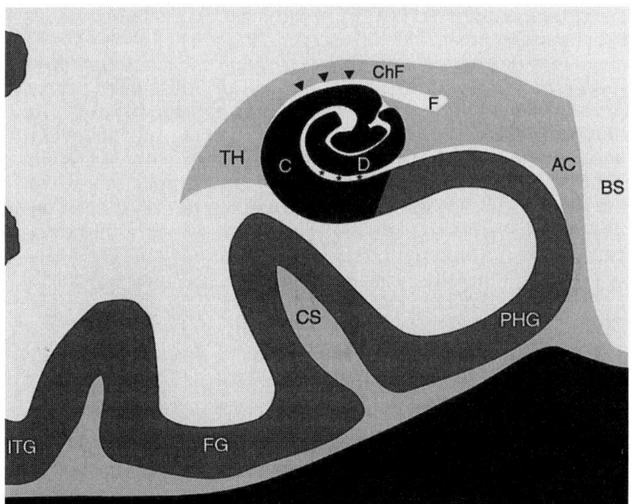

FIGURE 149–7. Diagram of a coronal slice through the medial temporal lobe. The hippocampus is composed of 2 U-shaped lamina of gray matter, the cornu ammonis (C) and dentate gyrus (D). Between them is the white matter of the molecular layer (*). The hippocampus is bordered by the alveus *(arrowheads)*, choroid fissure (ChF), and temporal horn (TH) superiorly. The alveus converges medially to form the fimbria (F), which in turn is a component of the fornix. The ambient cistern (AC) and brainstem (BS) are situated medially. Inferior to the hippocampus is the parahippocampal white matter and gyrus (PHG). The temporal horn (TH) borders the hippocampus on its lateral aspect. CS, collateral sulcus; FG, fusiform gyrus or lateral occipital-temporal gyrus; ITG, inferior temporal gyrus. (From Bronen RA: Epilepsy: The role of MR imaging. AJR Am J Roentgenol 159:1165–1174, 1992.)

The principal MRI features of hippocampal sclerosis are hippocampal atrophy and hyperintense signal changes on long TR (or T2-weighted) images (Figs. 149-9 through 149-12).[7, 15–19, 21, 23–26, 50, 51] These findings occur in approximately 80% to 95% of patients with surgically proven hippocampal sclerosis. T2-relaxometry is abnormal in 70% of hippocampal sclerosis.[20] T2-relaxometry refers to performing a quantitative measurement of T2 signal of the hippocampus (i.e., quantitation of the hyperintensity on T2-weighted images). This measurement usually is performed as a multiecho single slice sequence through the hippocampal body at the level of the mid brainstem. Although most reports have concentrated on patients with intractable temporal lobe epilepsy, MRI findings of hippocampal sclerosis also can be found in subjects that are medically well controlled.[52]

A variety of neuroimaging techniques have shown that abnormalities are not confined strictly to the hippocampus in patients with hippocampal sclerosis. There is widespread dysfunction of the temporal lobe, as indicated by findings on MRI, MRS, SPECT, and PET.[1, 53] Other MRI findings associated with hippocampal sclerosis include the following ipsilateral changes: loss of the hippocampal internal architecture (disappearance of molecular layers), loss of hippocampal head digitations, temporal horn dilation, temporal lobe atrophy, atrophy of the parahippocampal gyral white matter between the hippocampus and collateral sulcus (sometimes referred to as *collateral white matter*), hyperintensity in the anterior temporal lobe white matter, and changes associated with wallerian degeneration of hippocampal efferent pathways—atrophy of fornix and mammillary bodies.[50, 54–58]

How does qualitative visual inspection compare with quantitative analysis of hippocampal volume? The current consensus is that quantitative methods marginally increase sensitivity over visual analysis and are not needed for routine clinical evaluation.[15, 59, 60] One

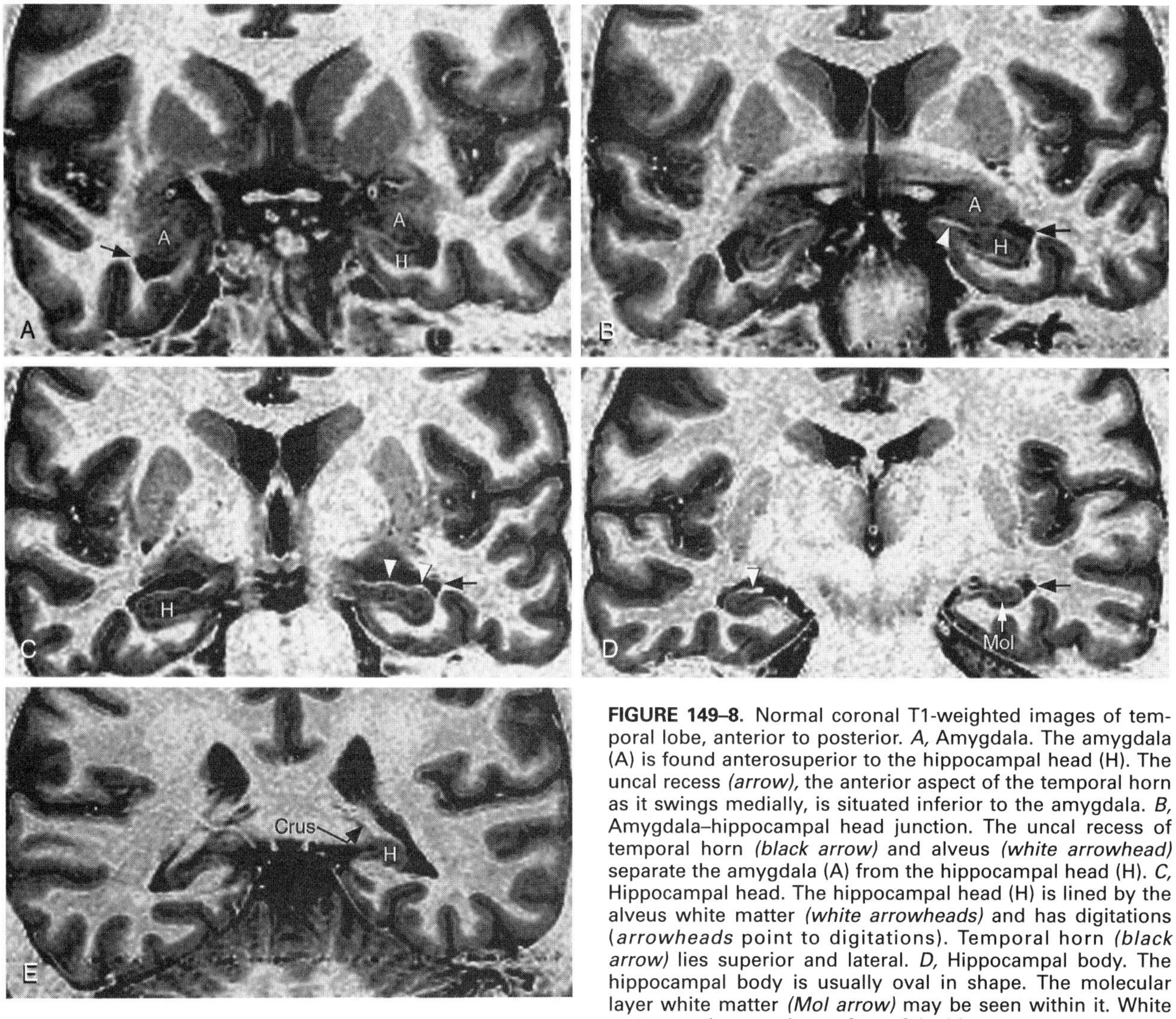

FIGURE 149–8. Normal coronal T1-weighted images of temporal lobe, anterior to posterior. *A,* Amygdala. The amygdala (A) is found anterosuperior to the hippocampal head (H). The uncal recess *(arrow),* the anterior aspect of the temporal horn as it swings medially, is situated inferior to the amygdala. *B,* Amygdala–hippocampal head junction. The uncal recess of temporal horn *(black arrow)* and alveus *(white arrowhead)* separate the amygdala (A) from the hippocampal head (H). *C,* Hippocampal head. The hippocampal head (H) is lined by the alveus white matter *(white arrowheads)* and has digitations (*arrowheads* point to digitations). Temporal horn *(black arrow)* lies superior and lateral. *D,* Hippocampal body. The hippocampal body is usually oval in shape. The molecular layer white matter *(Mol arrow)* may be seen within it. White matter on the superior surface of the hippocampus represents the alveus and fimbria *(arrowhead).* Temporal horn is lateral and superior *(black arrow). E,* Hippocampal tail. The hippocampal tail (H) is found posterior to the brainstem. Crus, crus of fornix. (Magnetic resonance images are inverted photographically; sequence is inversion recovery.)

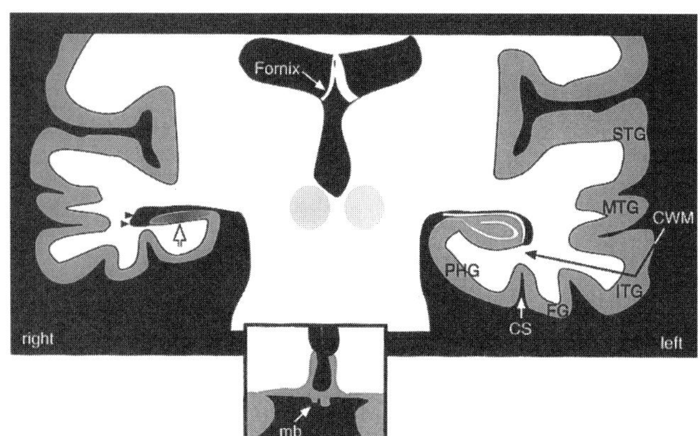

FIGURE 149–9. Diagram of right hippocampal sclerosis on a coronal T1-weighted image. The right hippocampus *(outlined arrow)* is small and hypointense—it would be hyperintense or bright on a T2-weighted image. The internal architecture (i.e., molecular layer) of the hippocampus is lost on the right. Secondary magnetic resonance imaging findings of hippocampal sclerosis include ipsilateral temporal horn dilation *(arrowheads)* and ipsilateral atrophy of the temporal lobe, collateral white matter (CWM), fornix, and mammillary body (mb). STG, superior temporal gyrus; MTG, middle temporal gyrus; ITG, inferior temporal gyrus; FG, fusiform gyrus; CS, collateral sulcus; PHG, parahippocampal gyrus. (From Bronen RA: MR imaging of mesial temporal sclerosis: How much is enough? AJNR Am J Neuroradiol 19: 15–17, 1998.)

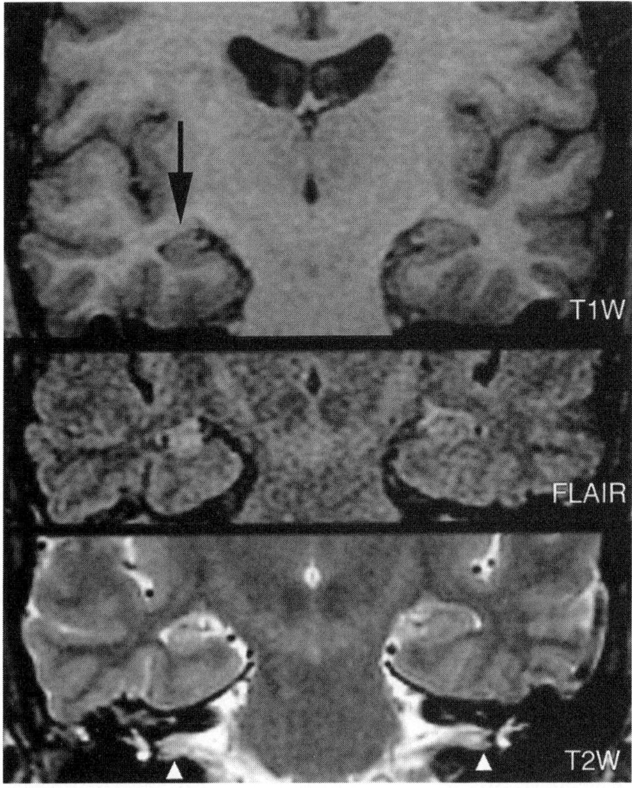

FIGURE 149–10. Right hippocampal sclerosis, composite magnetic resonance images. The right hippocampus *(arrow)* is slightly smaller than the left and is slightly hyperintense on fluid-attenuated inversion recovery (FLAIR) and T2-weighted images. The ipsilateral fornix and temporal lobes are slightly smaller. There is no head rotation to account for, as indicated by the symmetry of the internal auditory canals *(arrowheads* on T2-weighted image).

report found no difference between these techniques.[61] Hippocampal atrophy is identified in 80% to 90% by simple visual inspection, whereas quantitative methods routinely achieve sensitivities of 90% to 95%. Detection of unilateral atrophy by simple visual inspection is accurate when there is greater than 15% loss of volume quantitatively.[62] Quantitative methods for volume and T2-relaxometry may be useful, however, for detecting bilateral hippocampal abnormalities; mild bilateral hippocampal atrophy without signal changes is difficult to detect visually. About 10% to 20% of patients with hippocampal atrophy have atrophy bilaterally. Bilateral hippocampal atrophy is frequent in patients with temporal lobe developmental malformations.[63] Several series confirmed that surgical success is predicted by removal of the EEG-identified seizure onset area, not the more atrophic hippocampus in subjects with bilateral hippocampal atrophy.[64, 65]

Many centers use quantitative hippocampal volume measurements for clinical purposes. Quantitative measurements are especially important for research, however, allowing one to test a hypothesis that relates structure to clinical and pathologic measures.[59] The disadvantages of volumetrics include operator time, the need for dedicated personnel and dedicated workstation and software, and the inconvenience of accumulating a true representative sample of control subjects. MRI hippocampal volume has been correlated with hippocampal cell loss, memory indices, childhood febrile seizures, and successful postoperative outcome.[35, 37, 51, 66–68] Many studies have correlated hippocampal atrophy with duration of epilepsy.[69–72] One study by Tasch and associates[72] found MRI evidence that persistent seizures by themselves are responsible for ongoing neuronal dysfunction and loss in patients with temporal lobe epilepsy. Generalized seizures appear to cause progressive brain dysfunction—frequent generalized seizures were correlated with bilateral temporal lobe metabolic dysfunction by MRS and ipsilateral atrophy by MRI volumetry. These findings suggest early intervention for seizure control is indicated to prevent further and progressive brain injury.[73]

MRI has provided invaluable information for understanding the cause of hippocampal sclerosis. Some evidence suggests that hippocampal sclerosis is an acquired entity, whereas other evidence suggests it is a developmental anomaly. Hippocampal sclerosis may represent a common end point for a group of heterogeneous disorders. Several lines of evidence indicate an acquired cause. Time-dependent changes of the hippocampus have occurred after prolonged seizures or prolonged febrile seizures: The hippocampus initially becomes enlarged and hyperintense, then later atrophies.[74, 75] A quantitative MRI study of three monozygous twin pairs in which the index twin had temporal lobe epilepsy and hippocampal sclerosis found no indication of hippocampal sclerosis in the unaffected twin.[76] Animal models have shown that intense limbic

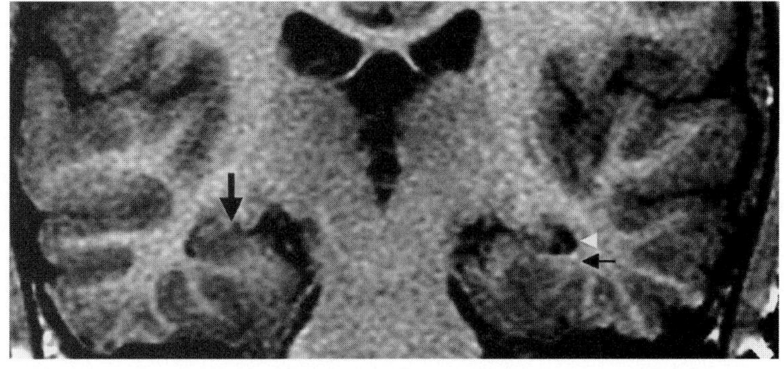

FIGURE 149–11. Left hippocampal sclerosis, coronal T1-weighted image through hippocampal body. Compare the normal right hippocampus *(large arrow)* with the atrophic left hippocampus. The left hippocampus was hyperintense on long TR images (not shown). Secondary signs of hippocampal sclerosis include temporal horn dilation *(arrowhead),* collateral white matter atrophy *(small arrow),* and temporal lobe atrophy. The loss of the white matter inferior to the left hippocampus makes it difficult to distinguish hippocampus from neocortical gray matter. The diagnosis was surgically proven hippocampal sclerosis.

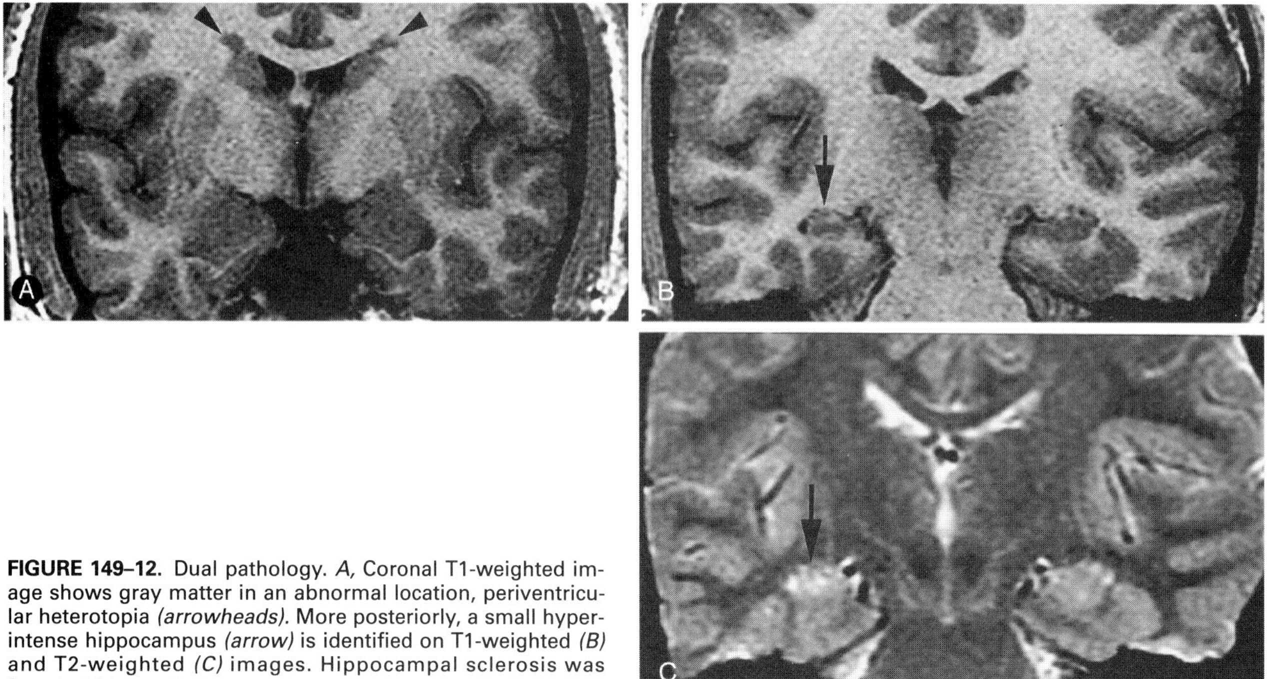

FIGURE 149–12. Dual pathology. *A,* Coronal T1-weighted image shows gray matter in an abnormal location, periventricular heterotopia *(arrowheads).* More posteriorly, a small hyperintense hippocampus *(arrow)* is identified on T1-weighted *(B)* and T2-weighted *(C)* images. Hippocampal sclerosis was found at histopathology.

seizures result in a pattern of hippocampal damage similar to hippocampal sclerosis.[77]

Other evidence suggests that hippocampal atrophy is a developmental abnormality. Hippocampal sclerosis is associated with a second abnormality in 15% of cases (dual pathology), which frequently is a developmental anomaly.[78] A study of two families with febrile convulsions found left hippocampal atrophy in 19 of 23 family members; only 2 had epilepsy, and 6 of 10 without febrile convulsions also had left hippocampal sclerosis.[79] Several investigators found widespread cerebral changes associated with a subgroup of hippocampal sclerosis, suggesting a developmental anomaly.[80, 81] Patients with widespread MRI changes have poorer postoperative seizure outcomes.

Focal atrophy of the amygdala has been associated with temporal lobe epilepsy. Compared with patients with hippocampal atrophy, patients with amygdala atrophy have a more prolonged postictal confusion state, a lower incidence of early febrile convulsions, older age at epilepsy onset, lower frequency of secondary generalized tonic-clonic seizures, and lesser memory dysfunction.[82] T2 relaxometry and FLAIR techniques are useful for detecting abnormalities of the amygdala that are not visualized with routine MRI sequences.[83]

In surgical epilepsy patients with focal extrahippocampal imaging abnormalities, 15% also have hippocampal sclerosis.[78] This combination of hippocampal sclerosis with an extrahippocampal abnormality is referred to as *dual pathology* (Fig. 149-12). After identifying a possible epileptogenic anomaly, it is still important to continue to scrutinize the rest of the MRI scan for additional abnormalities. The most frequent abnormalities associated with hippocampal sclerosis are cortical dysgenesis. Patients with dual pathology have a poorer postoperative seizure outcome, unless both abnormalities are resected.[80, 84]

At Yale, the algorithm for the surgical evaluation and management of hippocampal sclerosis has been driven by the MRI findings (Fig. 149-13). In a patient

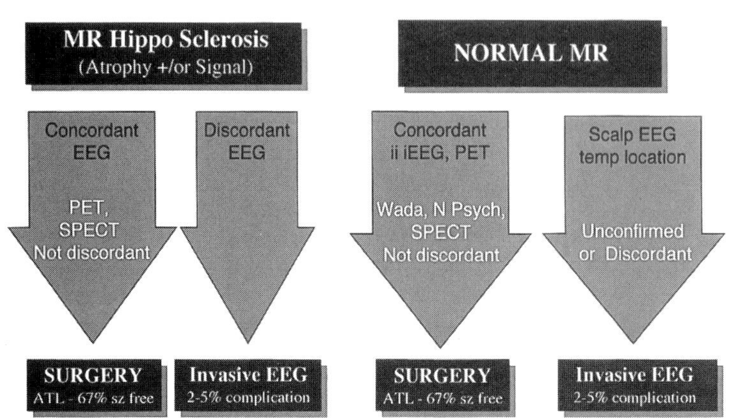

FIGURE 149–13. Surgical algorithm for temporal lobe epilepsy based on magnetic resonance imaging findings of hippocampal sclerosis. Hippo sclerosis, hippocampal sclerosis; EEG, scalp electroencephalography unless otherwise specified; ii iEEG, interictal and ictal scalp EEG; Wada, intracarotid artery amobarbital injection for lateralizing speech and memory; N Pysch, neuropsychological testing and assessment; ATL, anterior temporal lobectomy; sz free, seizure-free postoperatively.

with temporal lobe epilepsy, if the MRI suggests hippocampal sclerosis and the scalp EEG findings are concordant, a temporal lobectomy is performed without prior invasive EEG, provided that there are no other discordant tests.[33] Approximately 67% of patients enjoy a sustained (≥2 years) seizure-free state after surgery, and most of the rest have improved seizure control.[85] If MRI and scalp EEG localization is discordant, the patient must undergo an invasive EEG evaluation to determine if he or she is a candidate for surgery and to establish the resection site.[33] If MRI is normal, ictal EEG, interictal EEG, and PET all must be concordant before temporal lobectomy can be performed. This latter condition occurs infrequently in our experience, and most surgical candidates with normal MRI scans undergo invasive EEG before surgery.

NEOPLASTIC AND VASCULAR LESIONS

MRI has almost 100% sensitivity for depicting epileptic neoplastic and vascular lesions.[22] These lesions have many features in common, with most occurring in the temporal lobe (68%) adjacent to or in the cerebral cortex (85%). Some lesions may be present for decades. The chronicity and peripheral location can result in calvarial erosion (in a third of cases) (Fig. 149-14). Although most of these lesions are associated with mass effect, more than a third have no mass effect. For neoplasms, it is difficult to predict the histologic type based on MRI features.[86] Some tumors, such as gangliogliomas and dysembryoplastic neuroepithelial tumors, frequently are associated with chronic intractable seizures. Vascular lesions often have characteristic MRI findings allowing differentiation from other abnormalities in most cases. Cavernous hemangiomas have a central region of hyperintensity caused by chronic blood products, which is surrounded by a rim of signal void (owing to hemosiderin) (see Fig. 149-4).[87] Thrombosed arteriovenous malformations, also known as *occult vascular malformations*, may have an identical appearance.[88] High-flow vascular malformations present as curvilinear signal voids on MRI.[86] Venous angiomas, also known as *venous malformations*, appear to have no relationship to seizure generation, although there is evidence for an association of venous angiomas with cavernous malformations.[89]

DEVELOPMENTAL ANOMALIES

Developmental disorders are a more significant cause of seizures than commonly was appreciated until MRI became available—about 2% in pre-MRI surgical series compared with 4% to 25% in adult MRI series and 10% to 50% in pediatric MRI series.[90–94] Many anomalies are linked to genetic abnormalities. Surgery for cortical dysgenesis is not straightforward, even when a distinct imaging abnormality is visualized, for several reasons: Imaging findings may be diffuse, bilateral, or both, and the epileptogenic zone does not necessarily correspond to the MRI finding. Although many of these anomalies are highly epileptogenic, the region of seizure generation may be separate or more widespread than the anatomic lesion.[93, 95–98] Because of this discordance, surgical candidates with malformations of cortical development often merit an intracranial electrode study.[33, 99] Cortical dysgenesis in the temporal lobe often is accompanied by hippocampal or amygdala atrophy (dual pathology in 87%), and this atrophy often is bilateral.[63]

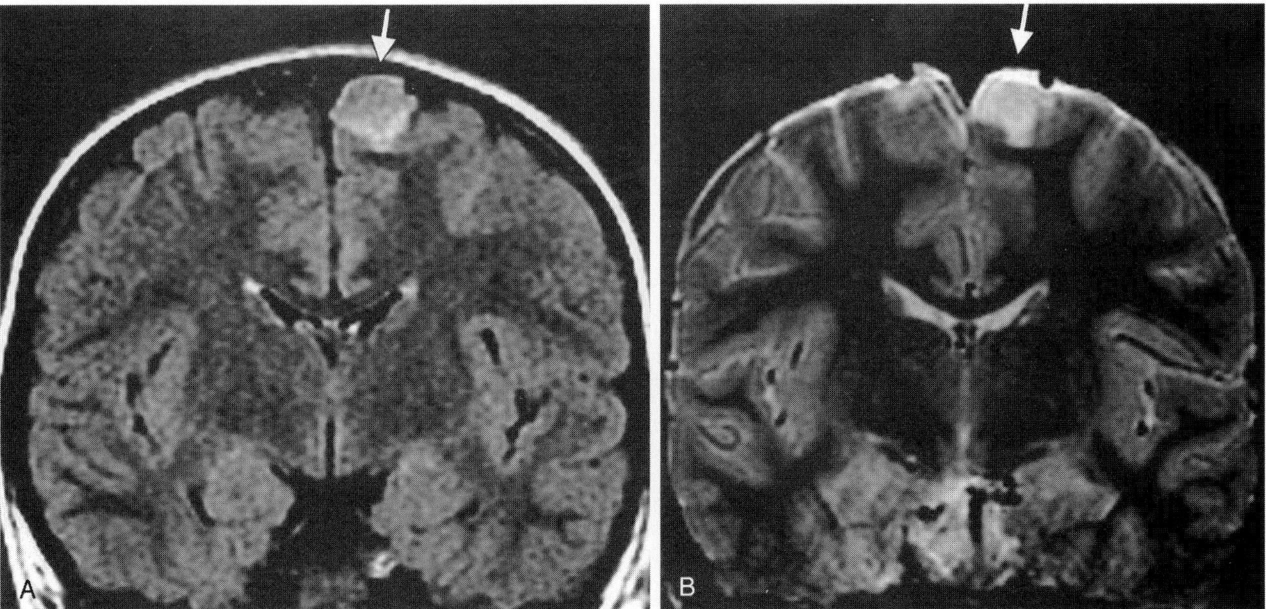

FIGURE 149–14. Tumors causing epilepsy usually are near or in the cortex. Although this tumor *(arrow)* appears extra-axial on the proton density–weighted image *(A)*, the T2-weighted image *(B)* defines its true involvement in the cortex. It is difficult to predict histology based on magnetic resonance imaging. This proven dysembryoplastic neuroepithelial tumor often is found in the cortex and may have a multiloculated appearance, in contrast to this case.

Malformations of cortical development can be classified into four categories, based on (1) abnormal cell proliferation, (2) abnormal migration, (3) abnormal cortical organization, and (4) none of the above (miscellaneous group).[100]

Abnormal cell proliferation can be due to either neuronal or glial proliferation. *Abnormal glial proliferation* consists of developmental tumors, such as dysembryoplastic neuroepithelial tumor, ganglioglioma, and gangliocytoma. These anomalies usually are found in or adjacent to the cortex and appear as focal lesions on MRI, often with a cystic component (see Fig. 149-14). *Abnormal neuronal proliferation* is typified by the balloon cell proliferative disorders—tuberous sclerosis, balloon cell focal cortical dysplasia of Taylor (or cortical dysplasia type II), and hemimegalencephaly. Balloon cells are giant progenitor cells with characteristics of neurons and glia. Balloon cell focal cortical dysplasia of Taylor and tuberous sclerosis have similar imaging characteristics.[101] Cortical lesions are hyperintense on T2-weighted images, often are associated with cortical thickening, and have radial bands extending to the ventricle. In contrast to tuberous sclerosis, balloon cell focal cortical dysplasia of Taylor is not associated with other cortical tubers, subependymal tubers, or characteristic cutaneous or systemic manifestations. Because balloon cell focal cortical dysplasia is hyperintense on T2-weighted images, it often is misinterpreted as a tumor. In contrast to neoplasms, balloon cell dysplasia frequently is associated with cortical thickening, homogeneous subcortical white matter hyperintensity, and radial bands extending to the ventricle (Fig. 149-15). This distinction may be crucial for surgical management.[101] Imaging findings of hemimegalencephaly include enlargement of one (or portions of) hemisphere and ipsilateral enlargement of the lateral ventricle, hyperintensity of the white matter, heterotopia, and cortical thickening (Fig. 149-16).

Abnormal neuronal migration includes the agyria-pachygyria spectrum (encompassing lissencephaly and subcortical band heterotopia) and heterotopic gray matter. These disorders often have a genetic cause and may be sex-linked. Although findings may be subtle, it is important to detect imaging abnormalities because resective surgical strategies and results are poor.[102] Heterotopia nodules (i.e., gray matter located in an abnor-

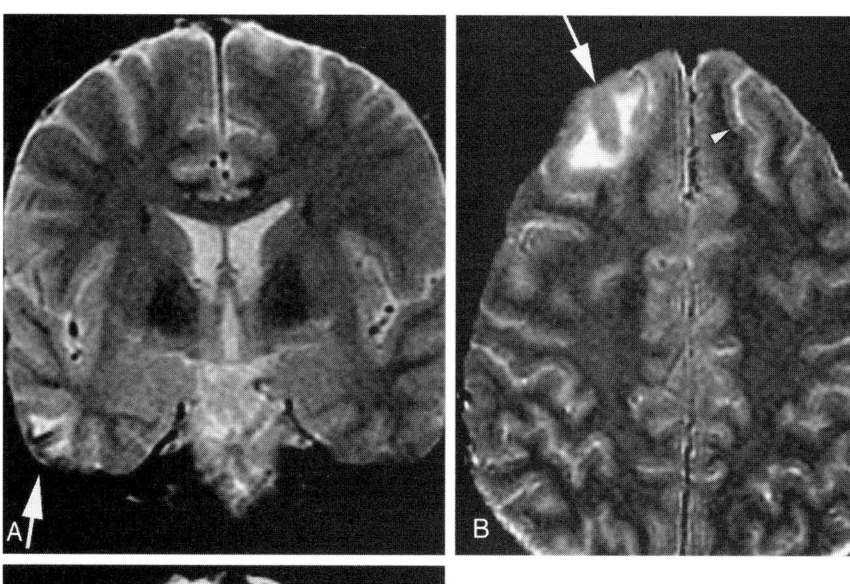

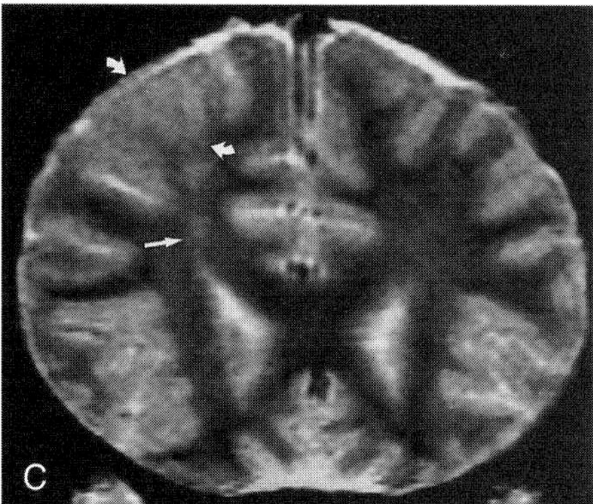

FIGURE 149–15. Tumor versus dysgenesis. *A* and *B*, The lesion on the coronal T2-weighted image in *A* has a similar appearance to that on the axial T2-weighted image in *B*. Both images have subcortical white matter hyperintensity *(arrows)*. The low-grade glioma in *A* is not associated with cortical thickening, however. The balloon cell focal cortical dysplasia of Taylor in *B* and the coronal T2-weighted image in *C* are associated with cortical thickening (in *B*, compare thickened cortex adjacent to *arrow* to normal cortex adjacent to *arrowhead;* in *C*, thickened cortex is found between *curved arrows*). The dysplasia is associated with a radial band (*arrow* in *C*) extending from ventricle to lesion. (From Bronen RA, Vives K, Kim JH, et al: MR of focal cortical dysplasia of Taylor, balloon cell subtype: Differentiation from low-grade tumors. AJNR Am J Neuroradiol 18:1141–1151, 1997.)

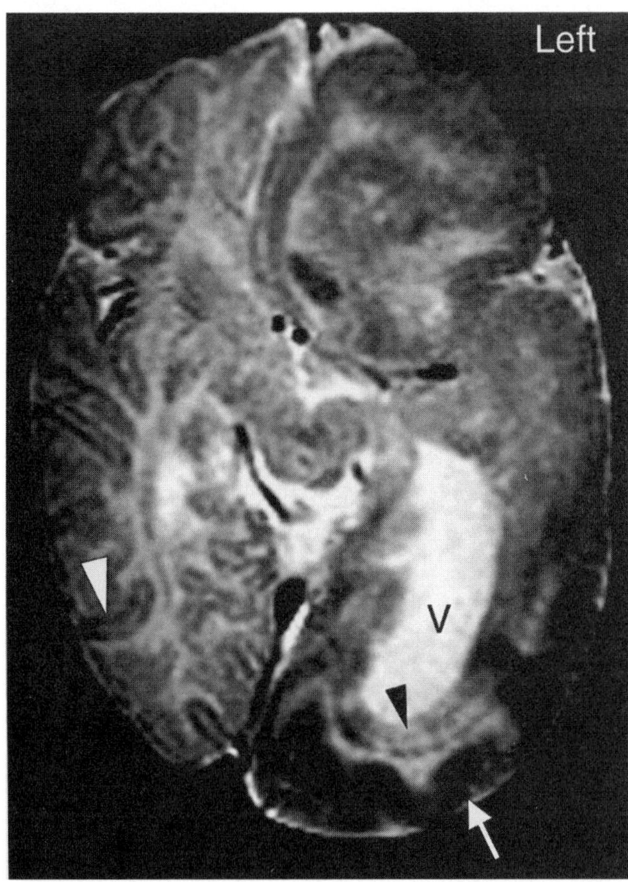

FIGURE 149–16. Hemimegalencephaly, axial T2-weighted image. The left hemisphere is markedly enlarged and dysplastic. The ipsilateral lateral ventricle (V) is enlarged. Heterotopic gray matter bands *(black arrowhead)* can be seen. The cortex is markedly thickened *(white arrow)*, especially when compared with normal cortex *(white arrowhead)*.

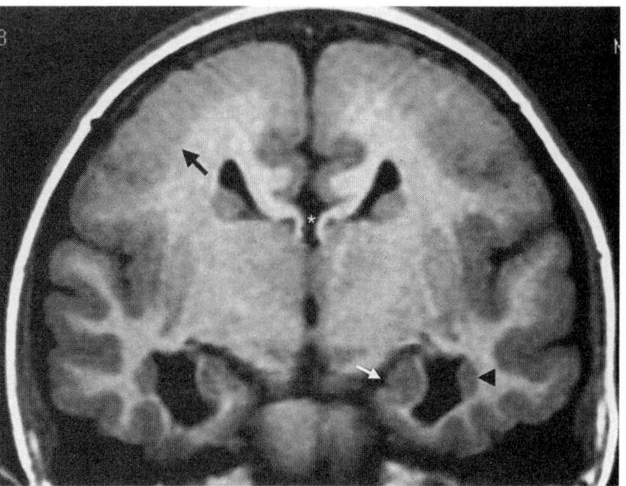

FIGURE 149–17. Pachygyria and heterotopia. Coronal T1-weighted image illustrates findings of pachygyria—a paucity of sulci in the frontal lobes bilaterally, associated with diffuse cortical thickening and indistinctness of the gray–white matter junction *(black arrow)*. Contrast this with the normal cortex in the temporal lobes. There is associated bilateral periventricular heterotopia *(black arrowhead)*. Agenesis of corpus callosum (*) and bilaterally unfolded vertical hippocampi *(white arrow)* also are present.

mal location) have been found to be associated with malformations in the overlying cortical plate and abnormal connectivity.[103] Heterotopia often presents on MRI as abnormal gray matter located in the periventricular regions bilaterally, especially posteriorly (Fig. 149-17; see also Fig. 149-12). This may be part of the X-linked dominant syndrome of periventricular nodular heterotopia (also known as *subependymal heterotopia*).[104] The classic lissencephaly associated with the *LIS1* gene anomaly has imaging findings of cortical thickening associated with smooth gyri (agyria) or a paucity of gyri (pachygyria) or a combination of both (see Fig. 149-17). X-linked lissencephaly (associated with a defect in the *DCX/XLIS* gene) presents as lissencephaly in males and with a double cortex or subcortical band heterotopia in females.[105–108]

Abnormal cortical organization includes polymicrogyria, schizencephaly, and non–balloon cell focal cortical dysplasia of Taylor. Most entities in this category are associated with cortical thickening, blurring of the gray–white matter junction, a cerebrospinal fluid cleft, or sulcal morphologic changes on MRI. Polymicrogyria commonly affects the sylvian fissure region, as with the congenital bilateral perisylvian syndrome. These patients have seizures, congenital pseudobulbar paresis, developmental delay, and bilateral opercular abnormalities consisting of polymicrogyria lining the sylvian fissure. On MRI, thickened opercular cortex and abnormal sylvian morphology are apparent (Fig. 149-18).[109] Schizencephaly usually is lined by polymicrogyria and is defined as a cerebrospinal fluid cleft extending from pia to ependyma. Focal cortical dysplasia of Taylor without balloon cells is not well described by imaging

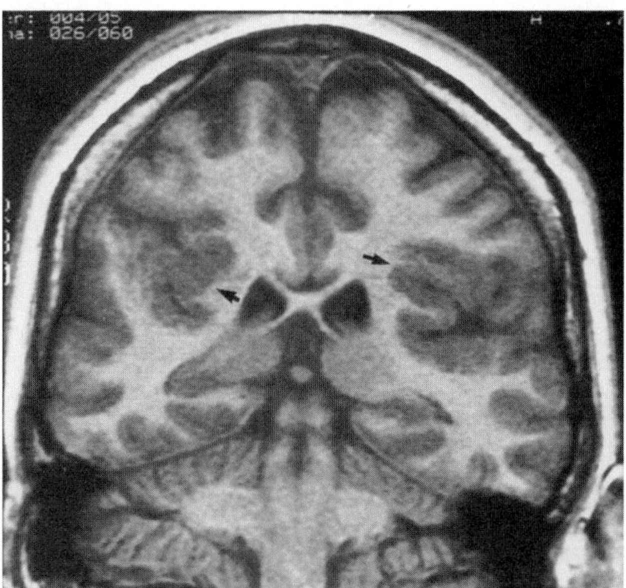

FIGURE 149–18. Congenital bilateral perisylvian syndrome. The gray matter lining the sylvian fissure bilaterally is abnormal in configuration and thickness *(arrows)* on this coronal T1-weighted image. This usually is due to polymicrogyria.

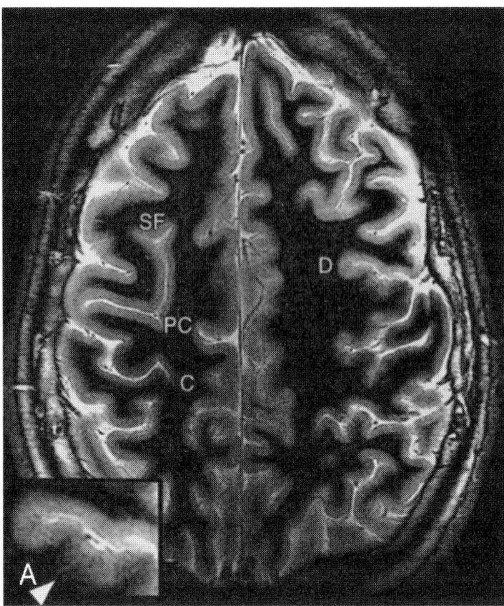

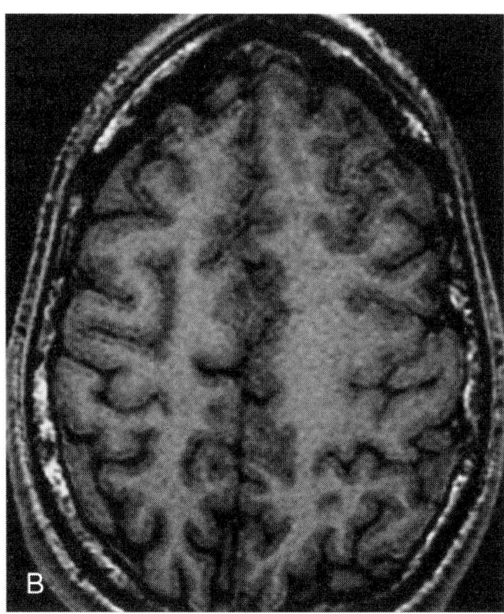

FIGURE 149–19. Presumed non–balloon cell focal cortical dysplasia. *A,* Axial inversion recovery sequence produced within a phased-array coil. The normal pattern of superior frontal (SF), precentral (PC), and central (C) sulci is disrupted on the left side. The high-quality image obtained with the phased-array coils allows one to discern abnormalities of the cortical gray matter. The insert of a dysplastic (D) gyrus shows irregularity of cortical thickness *(arrowhead). B,* Axial spoiled gradient recalled echo (SPGR) image obtained with a conventional head coil also shows the sulcal morphologic changes, but there is no clear abnormality of the cortical gray matter.

but appears to have cortical thickening, sulcal morphologic changes, and blurring of the gray–white matter junction without hyperintensity on T2-weighted imaging (Fig. 149-19).[110] Findings may be subtle, and specialized imaging strategies are necessary, including the use of thin section and high-resolution imaging.

The *miscellaneous dysgenesis category* includes hypothalamic hamartomas. These lesions have intrinsic epileptogenesis.[111] On MRI, these lesions usually are isointense to gray matter on all sequences, although they occasionally may be slightly hyperintense on T2-weighted imaging. Hypothalamic hamartomas can be classified into two categories based on their MRI appearance.[112] The parahypothalamic type is defined as a hamartoma attached to the floor of the third ventricle or tuber cinereum hamartoma—these are associated with precocious puberty but not seizures. The intrahypothalamic type is defined as a hamartoma involved or enveloped by the hypothalamus with distortion of the third ventricle by the lesion (Fig. 149-20). This

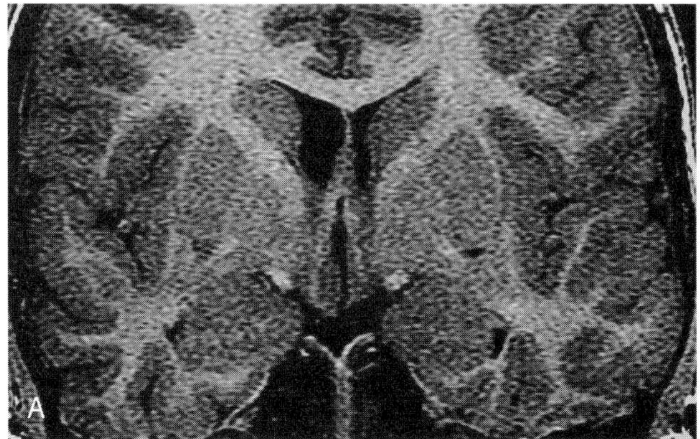

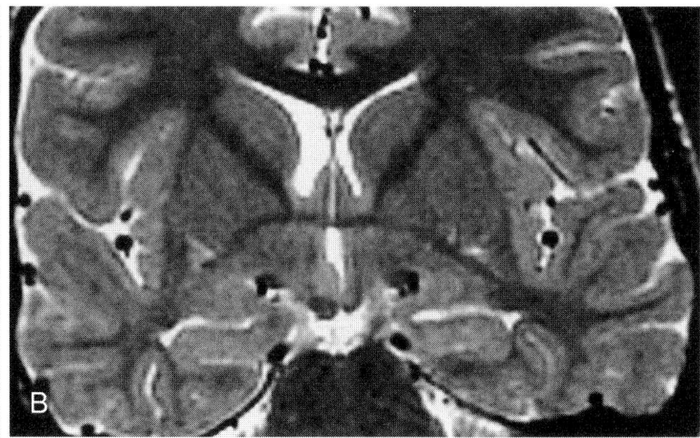

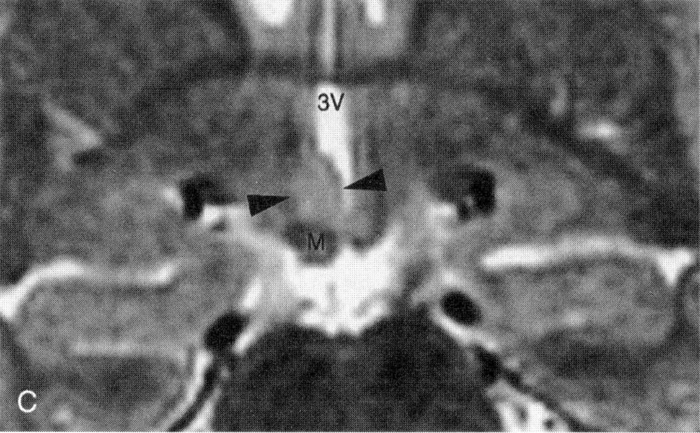

FIGURE 149–20. Hypothalamic hamartoma. This patient underwent several magnetic resonance imaging studies for a presumed right medial frontal seizure focus, before the seizure source was found. There is a subtle abnormality of the right hypothalamus on coronal T1-weighted *(A)* and T2-weighted *(B)* images. *C,* Magnification of *B* shows a hypothalamic mass *(arrowheads)* isointense to gray matter, bulging into the third ventricle (3V) and displacing the mammillary body (M) inferiorly—imaging findings consistent with hypothalamic hamartoma.

type usually is associated with medically intractable seizures and may be associated with precocious puberty.[112]

GLIOSIS AND MISCELLANEOUS ABNORMALITIES

A diffuse group of abnormalities that usually is associated with gliosis includes inflammatory and atrophic abnormalities. Large atrophic entities, such as those associated with infantile hemiplegia, Sturge-Weber syndrome, or end-stage Rasmussen's encephalitis, are easy to visualize with neuroimaging techniques.[86] A subset of patients undergoing surgery for temporal lobe epilepsy has hippocampal gliosis without neuronal loss by histopathology. In this condition, sometimes referred to as *paradoxical medial temporal lobe epilepsy,* MRI usually is normal, and postoperative outcome is poor.[24, 40]

Transient MRI signal changes have been associated with status epilepticus, a prolonged ictus, or multiple persistent seizures occurring just before imaging.[113–118] There usually is hyperintense signal change on long TR images, and this may be associated with abnormal contrast enhancement. This can be problematic if there are multifocal seizures, but surgical intervention is based on a single focus identified by imaging that turns out to be transient (Fig. 149-21). In some cases, prolonged focal seizures or a prolonged focal febrile seizure can result in hippocampal injury with signal changes and hippocampal enlargement in the acute setting (thought to be due to edema) followed by atrophy and hyperintensity on T2-weighted images.[74, 75] Status epilepticus can result in decreased diffusion on diffusion-weighted imaging.[119]

Incidental Findings

Many findings detected with MRI appear to have no relationship to epileptogenicity and are incidental, including venous angiomas, arachnoid cysts, and choroidal fissure cysts.[89, 120] Choroidal fissure cysts are isointense with cerebrospinal fluid and do not enhance with contrast material. The high-resolution coronal imaging used for seizure imaging has led to detection of several developmental variants. A large unilateral perivascular (Virchow-Robin) space situated either inferior to the basal ganglia or in the extreme and external capsules could be confused with a hyperintense tumor or pathologic lesion on high-resolution T2-weighted images.[121] The hippocampal sulcus remnant should not be mistaken for tumors or hippocampal sclerosis (Fig. 149-22). This normal variant is isointense to cerebrospinal fluid on all pulse sequences, is usually 1 to 2 mm in

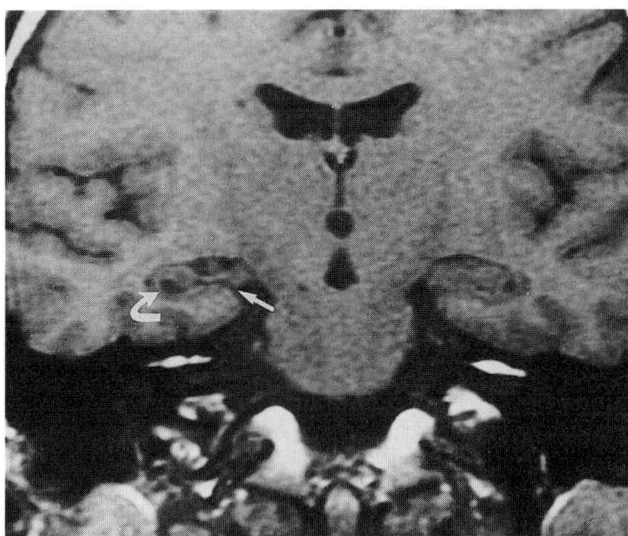

FIGURE 149–22. Coronal T1-weighted image of hippocampal sulcal remnant. When the medial aspect of the hippocampal sulcus *(straight white arrow)* does not obliterate in utero, a residual cavity—the hippocampal sulcal remnant *(curved white arrow)*—may persist, as it does bilaterally in this subject. In contrast to a pathologic lesion of the hippocampus, the remnant is isointense to cerebrospinal fluid on all pulse sequences and is contiguous with the hippocampal sulcus. (From Bronen RA, Cheung G: MRI of the normal hippocampus. Magn Reson Imaging 9:497–500, 1991.)

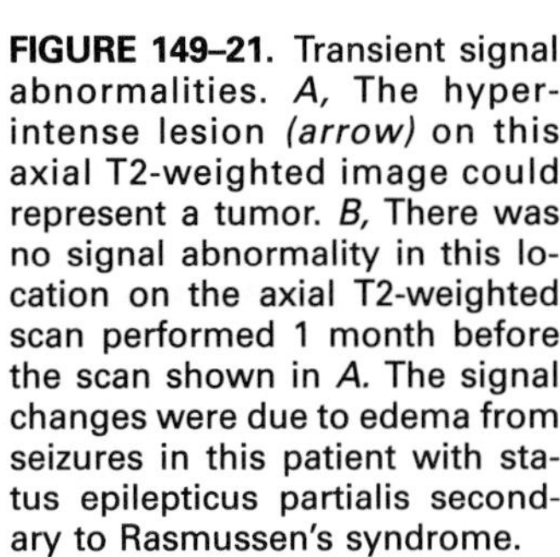

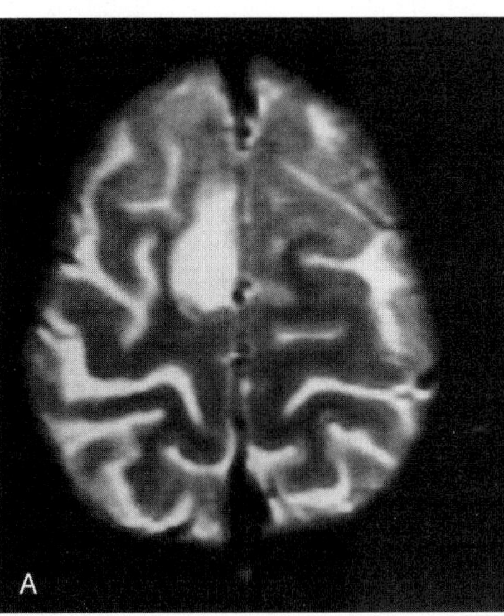

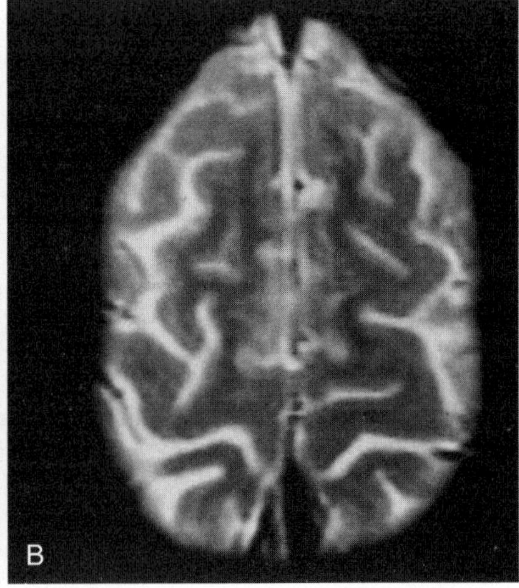

FIGURE 149–21. Transient signal abnormalities. *A,* The hyperintense lesion *(arrow)* on this axial T2-weighted image could represent a tumor. *B,* There was no signal abnormality in this location on the axial T2-weighted scan performed 1 month before the scan shown in *A.* The signal changes were due to edema from seizures in this patient with status epilepticus partialis secondary to Rasmussen's syndrome.

diameter, is situated between the dentate gyrus and cornu ammonis, and occurs in 10% to 20% of subjects.[44, 122, 123] It develops when the hippocampal sulcus does not involute normally medially in utero, resulting in a residual cystic cavity within the hippocampus that appears hyperintense on T2-weighted images.

Magnetic Resonance Imaging Techniques and Interpretation

Because of the subtle nature of many epileptogenic abnormalities and the need to image hippocampal changes, most centers use a dedicated protocol for MRI of seizure patients. Although protocols vary, high-resolution, three-dimensional–volume imaging is used for evaluating developmental abnormalities and quantifying the hippocampus and other regions. For assessing hippocampal and amygdala volumes, most authors use criteria established by Watson and coworkers[47] for defining anatomic boundaries. Coronal imaging, using three-dimensional volumes, high-resolution fast spin echo, or inversion recovery sequences, is important for evaluating hippocampal size and internal architecture.[23, 49, 124–126] T2-weighted images are important for assessing hippocampal signal changes and for evaluating the rest of the brain for focal abnormalities. The FLAIR sequence provides T2-weighted contrast with suppression of high signal intensity of cerebrospinal fluid. Jack and associates[23] found that FLAIR imaging was superior to T2-weighted imaging for hippocampal sclerosis. Wieshmann and colleagues[127] found FLAIR sequences to be particularly useful for identifying neocortical lesions (occasionally showing lesions when other sequences were normal), but not helpful for mild hippocampal sclerosis or heterotopia. Jackson[1] uses a stepwise approach in his evaluation of the epilepsy patient: If the initial MRI study is normal, he uses progressively more sophisticated techniques, (e.g., quantitation of volume and signal intensities and spectroscopy) to discover focal brain dysfunction. Contrast enhancement is not useful for routine MRI of seizure patients and is not helpful for diagnosing hippocampal sclerosis.[128–130] In selected cases of patients with focal lesions (suggestive of neoplastic or vascular diseases) or hemiatrophy (possibly representing Sturge-Weber syndrome), a contrast-enhanced MRI scan may yield additional information. A systematic approach for evaluating MRI scans is crucial for correct interpretation, realizing that imaging findings are only a component of the entire patient evaluation (Fig. 149-23).[131]

Routine MRI, quantitative volumes, quantitative T2 values, and MRS have well-established clinical and research uses. High-resolution MRI can be obtained by using a high field strength magnet or phase array surface coils—and they can detect previously unseen developmental abnormalities (see Fig. 149-19).[132] The value of performing ictal functional MRI or diffusion-weighted imaging for routine clinical cases is unknown because there is limited experience.[133] Functional MRI has evolved into a crucial component of the presurgical evaluation for mapping motor, language, and other crucial functions and is discussed in another section.[134]

H ippocampal size & signal
I AC & atrium (√ & correct for head rotation)
P eriventricular heterotopia
P eripheral
  Sulcal morphology abn
  Atrophy
  Gray matter thickening
  Encephalocele
O bvious lesion

FIGURE 149–23. HIPPO SAGE—mnemonic for using a systematic approach for interpretation of magnetic resonance images from a seizure patient. One must take into account head rotation, by assessing internal auditory canal (IAC) and lateral ventricular atria symmetry, when evaluating the hippocampus. Epileptogenic lesions that are easy to miss include periventricular heterotopia and subtle abnormalities at the periphery of the brain. The obvious lesion should be assessed last. Abn = abnormality.

MAGNETIC RESONANCE SPECTROSCOPY

MRS is a noninvasive means of investigating cerebral chemistry. MRS can be performed with either proton (^{1}H) or phosphorus (^{31}P) spectra and is evaluated with a single voxel or with many voxels simultaneously (multivoxel MRS is referred to as *chemical-shift imaging* or magnetic resonance spectroscopic imaging). ^{31}P MRS can show energy depletion and metabolic dysfunction, as evidenced by increased inorganic phosphate, reduced phosphomonoesters, and increased pH. Although a paucity of clinical data exists, ^{31}P MRS can lateralize temporal lobe epilepsy in 65% to 75% of cases.[135] In contrast to ^{1}H MRS, ^{31}P MRS cannot be performed on routine MRI systems, ^{31}P MRS uses much larger voxel sizes, and signal-to-noise ratio is decreased markedly.

Proton MRS can be performed on most clinical high field strength MRI systems using single voxel methods. Chemical-shift imaging technology is available on some clinical systems as well. Chemical-shift imaging has the advantage of better brain coverage and smaller voxel sizes, but it is more difficult to perform and prone to artifacts. Proton MRS can estimate concentrations of *N*-acetyl-aspartate (NAA), creatine (Cr), and choline-containing compounds (CHO). NAA is located primarily within neurons, and a decreased NAA/Cr or NAA/(Cr + CHO) ratio signifies neuronal loss and dysfunction.

Decreased NAA ratios can lateralize temporal lobe

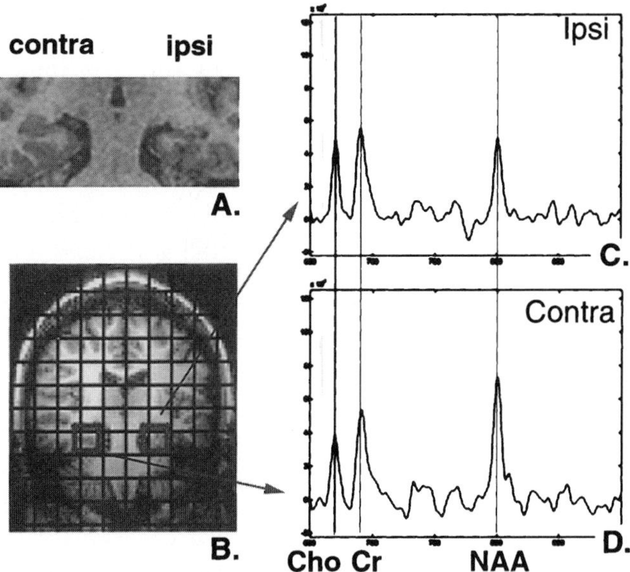

FIGURE 149–24. [1]H spectroscopy of temporal lobe epilepsy. *A,* Coronal T1-weighted image shows left hippocampal atrophy (ipsi) consistent with hippocampal sclerosis. *B,* Spectroscopic imaging yields spectra from multivoxels with spectra from ipsilateral abnormal hippocampus (ipsi) shown in *C* and the normal contralateral one (contra) in *D.* Compare the height of the peaks of NAA to Cr. The NAA/Cr ratio is decreased ipsilaterally. NAA, *N*-acetyl aspartate; Cr, creatine; Cho, choline. (Images courtesy of Hoby Hetherton and Edward Novotny.)

epilepsy in 65% to 96%, with bilateral changes occurring in 35% to 45% of patients.[135–137] In temporal lobe epilepsy patients with normal MRI studies, decreased NAA ratios can provide lateralizing information in at least 20% of cases (Fig. 149-24).[138, 139] Ipsilateral NAA concentrations cannot predict postoperative outcome for mesial temporal lobe epilepsy.[140, 141] Decreased NAA/Cr ratio in the nonoperated contralateral temporal lobe (i.e., bilateral temporal lobe dysfunction by MRS) was associated with surgical failure, however. MRS in extratemporal lobe epilepsy appears to be less accurate.

^{1}H MRS findings associated with cortical dysgenesis have been mixed, in part because of the variety of dysgenetic abnormalities evaluated.[142–144] Decreased NAA/Cr ratio has been found with focal cortical dysplasia. Some groups found NAA changes with heterotopia or polymicrogyria, whereas others did not. There may be metabolic abnormalities contralateral to the dysgenetic abnormality. Increases in γ-aminobutyric acid (GABA) and other amino acids have been found associated with cortical dysgenesis and tuberous sclerosis. No relationship has been found so far, however, between metabolic dysfunction and either seizure frequency or EEG findings.

Proton MRS can be used to estimate the cerebral concentrations of several neurotransmitters—GABA, glutamate, and glutamine.[145–150] This may become useful for characterizing neurometabolic abnormalities associated with various epilepsy syndromes, then studying the effects of different antiepileptic drugs and surgical treatments on neurotransmitter levels. In the future, cerebral transmitter levels rather than antiepileptic drug blood levels may be used to determine the correct dose of drug (Fig. 149-25).[151] Accurate determination of GABA, glutamate, and glutamine is technically much more difficult than determining NAA/Cr levels, however.

IMAGING AFTER SURGICAL PROCEDURES

Several groups have studied imaging findings after surgical procedures in epilepsy patients. After depth

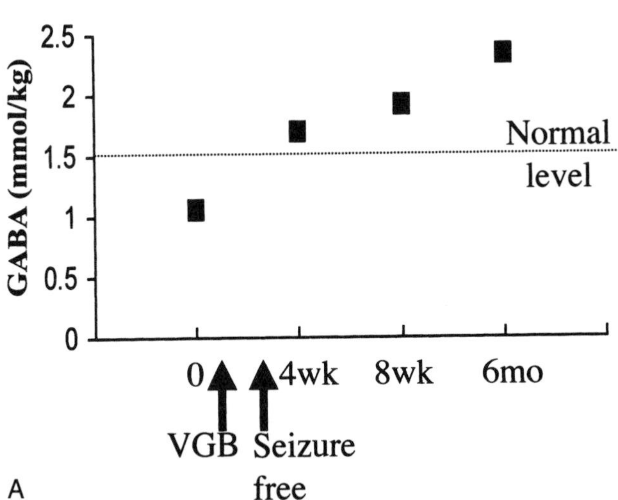

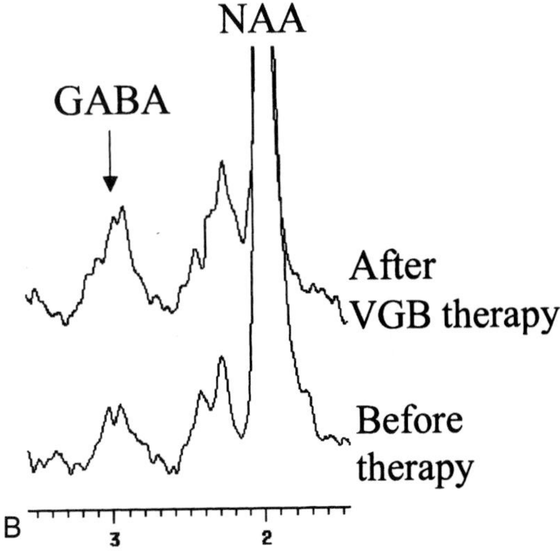

FIGURE 149–25. Brain neurotransmitter levels and drug effects can be assessed with ^{1}H spectroscopy using special techniques. *A,* Cerebral μ-aminobutyric acid (GABA) levels in a 2-year-old with seizures were subnormal. After changing from valproate to vigabatrin (VGB), GABA levels increased, and the seizures stopped. *B,* Spectra before and after vigabatrin therapy—compare the height of the GABA peaks. (From Novotny EJ, Hyder F, Shevell M, et al: GABA changes with vigabatrin in the developing human brain. Epilepsia 40:462–466, 1999.)

electrode placement, signal abnormalities were found in 43% of the tracts, consisting of punctate hyperintensities on T2-weighted images in most cases.[152] MRI with electrodes in place can be performed to determine contact positions (see Fig. 149-5). For evaluating corpus callosotomy subjects, thin sagittal T1-weighted images are optimal.[153] In children undergoing hemispherectomy surgery, early complications (e.g., epidural collections, parenchymal hemorrhage, infection, and early hydrocephalus) are visualized equally well with CT or MRI. MRI is the preferred method for detecting more chronic complications, such as septations or hemosiderin deposition leading to siderosis.[154]

In patients with temporal lobectomy, knowledge of the evolution of contrast enhancement patterns on postoperative CT or MRI brain images can help in differentiating benign from neoplastic changes.[155, 156] In the first 5 days, a thin linear enhancement pattern occurs on MRI at the surgical margin. From 1 week to 1 month after surgery, this pattern evolves into a thick linear or nodular (i.e., tumor-like) enhancement pattern (Fig. 149-26). Dural enhancement occurs uniformly after surgery and can persist for years. After temporal lobectomy, extra-axial fluid can be visualized during the first month after surgery, but disappears by 2 months. Intracranial air can be detected in 89% of MRI studies obtained during the first 4 days but was absent after day 5.[156] After temporal lobectomy, the choroid plexus enlarges and sags into the resection site along with the temporal lobe. During the first week after temporal lobectomy, an enlarged, markedly enhancing choroid plexus occurs in most cases and may mimic neoplastic enhancement.[157]

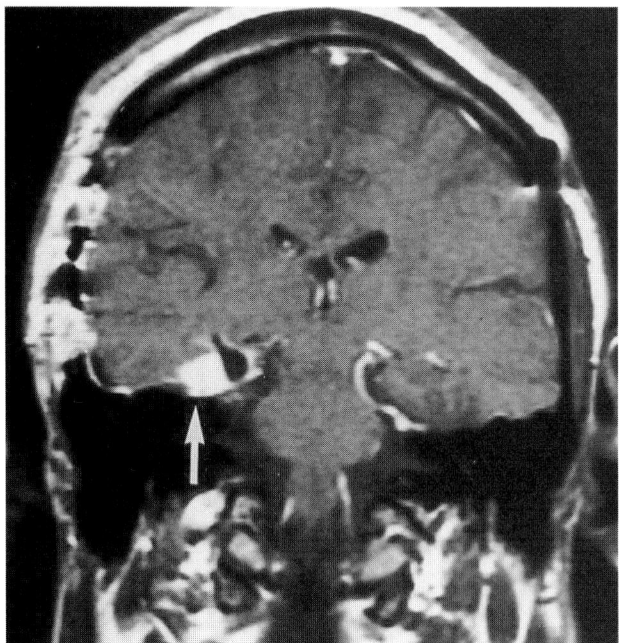

FIGURE 149–26. Postoperative contrast-enhanced coronal image. Three weeks after temporal lobectomy for hippocampal sclerosis, there is marked nodular-like enhancement of the brain parenchyma at the surgical margin *(arrow)*, which could be confused with tumor in a different circumstance. (From Sato N, Bronen RA, Sze G, et al: Postoperative changes in the brain: MR imaging findings in patients without neoplasms. Radiology 204: 839–846, 1997.)

Several groups have developed methods for evaluating the amount of postoperative volume resection, in an effort to assess this parameter with postoperative seizure outcome, different surgical techniques, and neuropsychological function.[158] Although overall volume resected does not correlate with seizure outcome, successful seizure outcome can be correlated with specific regions of resection, such as the extent of mesiobasal resection.[159–161]

REFERENCES

1. Jackson GD: Visual analysis in mesial temporal sclerosis. In Cascino GD, Jack CR Jr (eds): Neuroimaging in Epilepsy: Principles and Practice. Newton, MA, Butterworth-Heinemann, 1996, pp 73–110.
2. Laster DW, Penry JK, Ball DR, et al: Chronic seizure disorders: Contribution of MR imaging when CT is normal. AJNR Am J Neuroradiol 6:177–180, 1985.
3. Latack JT, Abou-Khalil BW, Siegel GJ, et al: Patients with partial seizures: Evaluation by MR, CT, and PET imaging. Radiology 159:159–163, 1986.
4. Lesser RP, Modic MT, Weinstein MA, et al: Magnetic resonance imaging (1.5 Tesla) in patients with intractable focal seizures. Arch Neurol 43:367–371, 1986.
5. Ormson MJ, Kispert DB, Sharbrough FW, et al: Cryptic structural lesions in refractory partial epilepsy: MR imaging and CT studies. Radiology 160:215–219, 1986.
6. Sperling MR, Wilson G, Engel JJ, et al: Magnetic resonance imaging in intractable partial epilepsy: Correlative studies. Ann Neurol 20:57–62, 1986.
7. Kuzniecky R, de la Sayette V, Ethier R, et al: Magnetic resonance imaging in temporal lobe epilepsy: Pathological correlations. Ann Neurol 22:341–347, 1987.
8. Schörner W, Meencke HJ, Felix R: Temporal-lobe epilepsy: Comparison of CT and MR imaging. AJR Am J Roentgenol 149: 1231–1239, 1987.
9. Brooks BS, King DW, El Gammal T, et al: MR imaging in patients with intractable complex partial epileptic seizures. AJNR Am J Neuroradiol 11:93–99, 1990.
10. Theodore WH, Katz D, Kufta C, et al: Pathology of temporal lobe foci: Correlation with CT, MRI, and PET. Neurology 40: 797–803, 1990.
11. Bronen RA, Fulbright RK, Spencer DD, et al: Refractory epilepsy: Comparison of MR imaging, CT, and histopathologic findings in 117 patients. Radiology 201:97–105, 1996.
12. Bronen RA, Fulbright RF, Spencer SS, et al: Comparison of MR and CT imaging of refractory epilepsy: Correlation with postoperative seizure outcome in 109 patients. Int J Neuroradiol 3:140–146, 1997.
13. Bronen RA, Fulbright RF, Spencer SS, et al: Economic impact of replacing CT with MR imaging for refractory epilepsy. Magn Reson Imaging 15:857–862, 1997.
14. King MA, Newton MR, Jackson GD, et al: Epileptology of the first-seizure presentation: A clinical, electroencephalographic, and magnetic resonance imaging study of 300 consecutive patients. Lancet 352:1007–1011, 1998.
15. Jack CR Jr, Sharbrough FW, Twomey CK, et al: Temporal lobe seizures: Lateralization with MR volume measurements of the hippocampal formation. Radiology 175:423–429, 1990.
16. Ashtari M, Barr WB, Schaul N, et al: Three-dimensional fast low-angle shot imaging and computerized volume measurement of the hippocampus in patients with chronic epilepsy of the temporal lobe. AJNR Am J Neuroradiol 12:941–947, 1991.
17. Cook MJ, Fish DR, Shorvon SD, et al: Hippocampal volumetric and morphometric studies in frontal and temporal lobe epilepsy. Brain 115:1001–1015, 1992.
18. Cendes F, Andermann F, Gloor P, et al: MRI volumetric mea-

surement of amygdala and hippocampus in temporal lobe epilepsy. Neurology 43:719–725, 1993.
19. Spencer SS, McCarthy G, Spencer DD: Diagnosis of medial temporal lobe seizure onset: Relative specificity and sensitivity of quantitative MRI. Neurology 43:2117–2124, 1993.
20. Jackson GD, Connelly A, Duncan JS, et al: Detection of hippocampal pathology in intractable partial epilepsy: Increased sensitivity with quantitative magnetic resonance T2 relaxometry. Neurology 43:1793–1799, 1993.
21. Spencer SS: The relative contributions of MRI, SPECT, and PET imaging in epilepsy. Epilepsia 35(suppl 6):S72–S89, 1994.
22. Bronen RA, Fulbright RK, Spencer DD, et al: MR characteristics of neoplasms and vascular malformations associated with epilepsy. Magn Reson Imaging 13:1153–1162, 1995.
23. Jack CR Jr, Rydberg CH, Krecke KN, et al: Mesial temporal sclerosis: Diagnosis with fluid-attenuated inversion-recovery versus spin-echo MR imaging. Radiology 199:367–373, 1996.
24. Bronen RA, Fulbright RF, King D, et al: Qualitative MR imaging of refractory temporal lobe epilepsy requiring surgery: Correlation with pathology and seizure outcome after surgery. AJR Am J Roentgenol 169:875–882, 1997.
25. Jackson GD, Berkovic SF, Tress BM, et al: Hippocampal sclerosis can be reliably detected by magnetic resonance imaging. Neurology 40:1869–1875, 1990.
26. Lee DH, Gao FQ, Rogers JM, et al: MR in temporal lobe epilepsy: Analysis with pathologic confirmation. AJNR Am J Neuroradiol 19:19–27, 1998.
27. Holmes MD, Wilensky AJ, Ojemann GA, et al: Hippocampal or neocortical lesions on magnetic resonance imaging do not necessarily indicate site of ictal onsets in partial epilepsy. Ann Neurol 45:461–465, 1999.
28. Cascino GD, Jack CR Jr, Parisi JE, et al: MRI in the presurgical evaluation of patients with frontal lobe epilepsy and children with temporal lobe epilepsy: Pathologic correlation and prognostic importance. Epilepsy Res 11:51–59, 1992.
29. Grattan SJ, Harvey AS, Desmond PM, et al: Hippocampal sclerosis in children with intractable temporal lobe epilepsy: Detection with MR imaging. AJR Am J Roentgenol 161:1045–1048, 1993.
30. Kuzniecky R, Murro A, King D, et al: Magnetic resonance imaging in childhood intractable partial epilepsies: Pathologic correlations. Neurology 43:681–687, 1993.
31. Wyllie E, Comair YG, Kotagal P, et al: Epilepsy surgery in infants. Epilepsia 37:625–637, 1996.
32. Zubel IG, Spencer SS, Imam K, et al: Difference images calculated from ictal and interictal technetium-99m-HMPAO SPECT scans of epilepsy. J Nucl Med 36:684–689, 1995.
33. Spencer SS: Selection of candidate for invasive monitoring. In Cascino GD, Jack CR Jr (eds): Neuroimaging in Epilepsy: Principles and Practice. Newton, MA, Butterworth-Heinemann, 1996, pp 219–234.
34. Davis LM, Spencer DD, Spencer SS, et al: MR imaging of implanted depth and subdural electrodes: Is it safe? Epilepsy Res 35:95–98, 1999.
35. Jack CR Jr, Sharbrough FW, Cascino GD, et al: Magnetic resonance image-based hippocampal volumetry: Correlation with outcome after temporal lobectomy. Ann Neurol 31:138–146, 1992.
36. Garcia PA, Laxer KD, Barbaro NM, et al: Prognostic value of qualitative magnetic resonance imaging hippocampal abnormalities in patients undergoing temporal lobectomy for medically refractory seizures. Epilepsia 35:520–524, 1994.
37. Berkovic SF, McIntosh AM, Kalnins RM, et al: Preoperative MRI predicts outcome of temporal lobectomy: An actuarial analysis. Neurology 45:1358–1363, 1995.
38. Van Buren JM: Complications of surgical procedures in the diagnosis and treatment of epilepsy. In Engel JJ (ed): Surgical Treatment of the Epilepsies. New York, Raven Press, 1987, pp 465–475.
39. Behrens E, Schramm J, Zentner J, et al: Surgical and neurological complications in a series of 708 epilepsy surgery procedures. Neurosurgery 41:1–9, 1997.
40. Spencer DD: Classifying the epilepsies by substrate. Clin Neurosci 2:104–109, 1994.
41. Duvernoy HM: The Human Hippocampus: Functional Anatomy, Vascularization and Serial Sections with MRI, 2nd ed. Berlin, Springer-Verlag, 1998.
42. Naidich TP, Daniels DL, Haughton VM, et al: Hippocampal formation and related structures of the limbic lobe: Anatomic-MR correlation: Part 1. Surface features and coronal sections. Radiology 162:747–754, 1987.
43. Naidich TP, Daniels DL, Haughton VM, et al: Hippocampal formation and related structures of the limbic lobe: Anatomic-MR correlation: Part II. Sagittal sections. Radiology 162:755–761, 1987.
44. Bronen RA, Cheung G: MRI of the normal hippocampus. Magn Reson Imaging 9:497–500, 1991.
45. Bronen RA, Cheung G: Relationship of hippocampal and amygdala to coronal MRI landmarks. Magn Reson Imaging 9:449–457, 1991.
46. Bronen R, Cheung G: MRI of the temporal lobe: Normal variations with special reference toward epilepsy. Magn Reson Imaging 9:501–507, 1991.
47. Watson C, Andermann F, Gloor P, et al: Anatomic basis of amygdaloid and hippocampal volume measurement by magnetic resonance imaging. Neurology 42:1743–1750, 1992.
48. Bronen RA: Anatomy of the temporal lobe. In Spencer SS, Spencer DD (eds): Surgery for Epilepsy. Boston, Blackwell, 1991, pp 103–118.
49. Jackson GD, Berkovic SF, Duncan JS, et al: Optimizing the diagnosis of hippocampal sclerosis using MR imaging. AJNR Am J Neuroradiol 14:753–762, 1993.
50. Bronen RA, Cheung G, Charles JT, et al: Imaging findings in hippocampal sclerosis: Correlation with pathology. AJNR Am J Neuroradiol 12:933–940, 1991.
51. Lencz T, McCarthy G, Bronen RA, et al: Quantitative magnetic resonance imaging in temporal lobe epilepsy: Relationship to neuropathology and neuropsychological function. Ann Neurol 31:629–637, 1992.
52. Kim WJ, Park SC, Lee SJ, et al: The prognosis for control of seizures with medications in patients with MRI evidence for mesial temporal sclerosis. Epilepsia 40:290–293, 1999.
53. Duncan JS: Imaging and epilepsy. Brain 120:339–377, 1997.
54. Mamourian AC, Brown DB: Asymmetric mamillary bodies: MR identification. AJNR Am J Neuroradiol 14:1332–1335, 1993.
55. Baldwin GN, Tsuruda JS, Maravilla KR, et al: The fornix in patients with seizures caused by unilateral hippocampal sclerosis: Detection of unilateral volume loss on MR images. AJR Am J Roentgenol 162:1185–1189, 1994.
56. Bronen RA: MR imaging of mesial temporal sclerosis: How much is enough? AJNR Am J Neuroradiol 19:15–17, 1998.
57. Oppenheim C, Dormont D, Biondi A, et al: Loss of digitations of the hippocampal head on high-resolution fast spin-echo MR: A sign of mesial temporal sclerosis. AJNR Am J Neuroradiol 19:457–463, 1998.
58. Meiners LC, Witkamp TD, De Kort GAP, et al: Relevance of temporal lobe white matter changes in hippocampal sclerosis: Magnetic resonance imaging and histology. Invest Radiol 34: 38–45, 1999.
59. Jack CR: Epilepsy: Surgery and imaging. Radiology 189:635–646, 1993.
60. Bronen R, Anderson A, Spencer D: Quantitative MR for epilepsy: A clinical and research tool? AJNR Am J Neuroradiol 15: 1157–1160, 1994.
61. Cheon JE, Chang KH, Kim HD, et al: MR of hippocampal sclerosis: Comparison of qualitative and quantitative assessments. AJNR Am J Neuroradiol 19:465–468, 1998.
62. Van Paesschen W, Sisodiya S, Connelly A, et al: Quantitative hippocampal MRI and intractable temporal lobe epilepsy. Neurology 45:2233–2240, 1995.
63. Ho SS, Kuzniecky RI, Gilliam F, et al: Temporal lobe developmental malformations and epilepsy: Dual pathology and bilateral hippocampal abnormalities. Neurology 50:748–754, 1998.
64. King D, Spencer SS, McCarthy G, et al: Bilateral hippocampal atrophy in medial temporal lobe epilepsy. Epilepsia 36:905–910, 1995.
65. Fish DR, Spencer SS: Clinical correlations: MRI and EEG. Magn Reson Imaging 13:1113–1117, 1995.
66. Trenerry MR, Jack CR Jr, Sharbrough FW, et al: Quantitative MRI hippocampal volumes: Association with onset and dura-

tion of epilepsy, and febrile convulsions in temporal lobectomy patients. Epilepsy Res 15:247–252, 1993.
67. Trenerry MR, Jack CR Jr, Ivnik RJ, et al: MRI hippocampal volumes and memory function before and after temporal lobectomy. Neurology 43:1800–1805, 1993.
68. Jackson GD: Temporal lobe epilepsy. In Kuzniecky RI, Jackson GD (eds): Magnetic Resonance in Epilepsy. New York, Raven Press, 1995, pp 107–182.
69. Van Paesschen W, Connelly A, King MD, et al: The spectrum of hippocampal sclerosis: A quantitative magnetic resonance imaging study. Ann Neurol 41:41–51, 1997.
70. Salmenpera T, Kalviainen R, Partanen K, et al: Hippocampal damage caused by seizures in temporal lobe epilepsy. Lancet 351:35, 1998.
71. Kalviainen R, Salmenpera T, Partanen K, et al: Recurrent seizures may cause hippocampal damage in temporal lobe epilepsy. Neurology 50:1377–1382, 1998.
72. Tasch E, Cendes F, Li LM, et al: Neuroimaging evidence of progressive neuronal loss and dysfunction in temporal lobe epilepsy. Ann Neurol 45:568–576, 1999.
73. Sutula TP, Hermann B: Progression in mesial temporal lobe epilepsy. Ann Neurol 45:553–556, 1999.
74. Tien RD, Felsberg GJ: The hippocampus in status epilepticus: Demonstration of signal intensity and morphologic changes with sequential fast spin-echo MR imaging. Radiology 194:249–256, 1995.
75. Van Landingham KE, Heinz ER, Cavazos JE, et al: Magnetic resonance imaging evidence of hippocampal injury after prolonged focal febrile convulsions. Ann Neurol 43:413–426, 1998.
76. Jackson GD, McIntosh AM, Briellmann RS, et al: Hippocampal sclerosis studied in identical twins. Neurology 51:78–84, 1998.
77. Sutula TP, Cavazos JE, Woodard AR: Long-term structural and functional alterations induced in the hippocampus by kindling: Implications for memory dysfunction and the development of epilepsy. Hippocampus 4:254–258, 1994.
78. Cendes F, Cook MJ, Watson C, et al: Frequency and characteristics of dual pathology in patients with lesional epilepsy. Neurology 45:2058–2064, 1995.
79. Fernández G, Effenberger O, Vinz B, et al: Hippocampal malformation as a cause of familial febrile convulsions and subsequent hippocampal sclerosis. Neurology 50:909–917, 1998.
80. Sisodiya SM, Moran N, Free SL, et al: Correlation of widespread preoperative magnetic resonance imaging changes with unsuccessful surgery for hippocampal sclerosis. Ann Neurol 41:490–496, 1997.
81. Marsh L, Morrell MJ, Shear PK, et al: Cortical and hippocampal volume deficits in temporal lobe epilepsy. Epilepsia 38:576–587, 1997.
82. Guerreiro C, Cendes F, Li LM, et al: Clinical patterns of patients with temporal lobe epilepsy and pure amygdalar atrophy. Epilepsia 40:453–461, 1999.
83. Van Paesschen W, Connelly A, Johnson CL, et al: The amygdala and intractable temporal lobe epilepsy: A quantitative magnetic resonance imaging study [published erratum appears in Neurology 1997 Jun;48(6):1751]. Neurology 47:1021–1031, 1996.
84. Li LM, Cendes F, Andermann F, et al: Surgical outcome in patients with epilepsy and dual pathology. Brain 122:799–805, 1999.
85. Spencer SS: Long-term outcome after epilepsy surgery. Epilepsia 37:807–813, 1996.
86. Friedland RJ, Bronen RA: Magnetic resonance imaging of neoplastic, vascular and indeterminate substrates. In Cascino GD, Jack CR Jr (eds): Neuroimaging in Epilepsy: Principles and Practice. Newton, MA, Butterworth-Heinemann, 1996, pp 29–50.
87. Rigamonti D, Drayer BP, Johnson PC, et al: The MRI appearance of cavernous malformations (angiomas). J Neurosurg 67:518–524, 1987.
88. Rapacki TF, Brantley MJ, Furlow TJ, et al: Heterogeneity of cerebral cavernous hemangiomas diagnosed by MR imaging. J Comput Assist Tomogr 14:18–25, 1990.
89. Topper R, Jurgens E, Reul J, et al: Clinical significance of intracranial developmental venous anomalies. J Neurol Neurosurg Psychiatry 67:234–238, 1999.
90. Brodtkorb E, Nilsen G, Smevik O, et al: Epilepsy and anomalies of neuronal migration: MRI and clinical aspects. Acta Neurol Scand 86:24–32, 1992.
91. Jackson GD: New techniques in magnetic resonance and epilepsy. Epilepsia 1994.
92. Kuzniecky RI: Neuroimaging in pediatric epilepsy. Epilepsia 37: S10–S21, 1996.
93. Raymond AA, Fish DR, Sisodiya SM, et al: Abnormalities of gyration, heterotopias, tuberous sclerosis, focal cortical dysplasia, microdysgenesis, dysembryoplastic neuroepithelial tumour and dysgenesis of the archicortex in epilepsy: Clinical, EEG and neuroimaging features in 100 adult patients. Brain 118: 629–660, 1995.
94. Wyllie E, Comair YG, Kotagal P, et al: Seizure outcome after epilepsy surgery in children and adolescents. Ann Neurol 44: 740–748, 1998.
95. Sisodiya SM, Free SL, Stevens JM, et al: Widespread cerebral structural changes in patients with cortical dysgenesis and epilepsy. Brain 118:1039–1050, 1995.
96. Palmini A, Gambardella A, Andermann F, et al: Operative strategies for patients with cortical dysplastic lesions and intractable epilepsy. Epilepsia 1994.
97. Richardson MP, Koepp MJ, Brooks DJ, et al: Cerebral activation in malformations of cortical development. Brain 121:1295–1304, 1998.
98. Jacobs KM, Gutnick MJ, Prince DA: Hyperexcitability in a model of cortical maldevelopment. Cereb Cortex 6:514–523, 1996.
99. Kuzniecky RI: Magnetic resonance imaging in cerebral developmental malformations and epilepsy. In Cascino GD, Jack CR Jr (eds): Neuroimaging in Epilepsy: Principles and Practice. Newton, MA, Butterworth-Heinemann, 1996, pp 51–63.
100. Barkovich AJ, Kuzniecky RI, Dobyns WB, et al: A classification scheme for malformations of cortical development. Neuropediatrics 27:59–63, 1996.
101. Bronen RA, Vives K, Kim JH, et al: MR of focal cortical dysplasia of Taylor, balloon cell subtype: Differentiation from low grade tumors. AJNR Am J Neuroradiol 18:1141–1151, 1997.
102. Dubeau F, Tampieri D, Lee N, et al: Periventricular and subcortical nodular heterotopia: A study of 33 patients. Brain 118: 1273–1287, 1995.
103. Hannan AJ, Servotte S, Katsnelson A, et al: Characterization of nodular neuronal heterotopia in children. Brain 122:219–238, 1999.
104. Huttenlocher PR, Taravath S, Mojtahedi S: Periventricular heterotopia and epilepsy. Neurology 44:51–55, 1994.
105. Reiner O, Carrozzo R, Shen Y, et al: Isolation of a Miller-Dieker lissencephaly gene containing G protein beta-subunit-like repeats. Nature 364:717–721, 1993.
106. Dobyns WB, Reiner O, Carrozzo R, et al: Lissencephaly: A human brain malformation associated with deletion of the LIS1 gene located at chromosome 17p13. JAMA 270:2838–2842, 1993.
107. Pilz DT, Matsumoto N, Minnerath S, et al: LIS1 and XLIS (DCX) mutations cause most classical lissencephaly, but different patterns of malformation. Hum Mol Genet 7:2029–2037, 1998.
108. Gleeson JG, Minnerath SR, Fox JW, et al: Characterization of mutations in the gene double cortin in patients with double cortex syndrome. Ann Neurol 45:146–153, 1999.
109. Kuzniecky R, Andermann F, Guerrini R: Congenital bilateral perisylvian syndrome: Study of 31 patients. The CBPS Multicenter Collaborative Study. Lancet 341:608–612, 1993.
110. Chan S, Chin SS, Nordli DR, et al: Prospective magnetic resonance imaging identification of focal cortical dysplasia, including the non-balloon cell subtype. Ann Neurol 44:749–757, 1998.
111. Kuzniecky R, Guthrie B, Mountz J, et al: Intrinsic epileptogenesis of hypothalamic hamartomas in gelastic epilepsy. Ann Neurol 42:60–67, 1997.
112. Arita K, Ikawa F, Kurisu K, et al: The relationship between magnetic resonance imaging findings and clinical manifestations of hypothalamic hamartoma. J Neurosurg 91:212–220, 1999.
113. Jayakumar PN, Taly AB, Mohan PK: Transient computerised tomographic (CT) abnormalities following partial seizures. Acta Neurol Scand 72:26–29, 1985.
114. Kramer RE, Luders H, Lesser RP, et al: Transient focal abnormalities of neuroimaging studies during focal status epilepticus. Epilepsia 28:528–532, 1987.
115. Riela AR, Sires BP, Penry JK: Transient magnetic resonance

imaging abnormalities during partial status epilepticus. J Child Neurol 6:143–145, 1991.
116. Horowitz SW, Merchut M, Fine M, et al: Complex partial seizure-induced transient MR enhancement. J Comput Assist Tomogr 16:814–816, 1992.
117. Chan S, Chin SS, Kartha K, et al: Reversible signal abnormalities in the hippocampus and neocortex after prolonged seizures. AJNR Am J Neuroradiol 17:1725–1731, 1996.
118. Meierkord H, Wieshmann U, Niehaus L, et al: Structural consequences of status epilepticus demonstrated with serial magnetic resonance imaging. Acta Neurol Scand 96:127–132, 1997.
119. Zhong J, Petroff O, Prichard J, et al: Changes in water diffusion and relaxation properties of rat cerebrum during status epilepticus. Magn Reson Med 30:241–246, 1993.
120. Arroyo S, Santamaria J: What is the relationship between arachnoid cysts and seizure foci? Epilepsia 38:1098–1102, 1997.
121. Song CJ, Kim JH, Kier EL, et al: MR and histology of subinsular T2-weighted bright spots: Virchow-Robbin spaces of the extreme capsule and insula cortex. Radiology (in press).
122. Sasaki M, Sone M, Ehara S, et al: Hippocampal sulcus remnant: Potential cause of change in signal intensity in the hippocampus. Radiology 188:743–746, 1993.
123. Kier EL, Kim JH, Fulbright RK, et al: Embryology of the human fetal hippocampus: MR imaging, anatomy, and histology. AJNR Am J Neuroradiol 18:525–532, 1997.
124. Tien RD, Felsberg GJ, Castro C, et al: Complex partial seizures and mesial temporal sclerosis: Evaluation with fast spin-echo MR imaging. Radiology 189:835–842, 1993.
125. Jack CR Jr, Krecke KN, Luetmer PH, et al: Diagnosis of mesial temporal sclerosis with conventional versus fast spin-echo MR imaging. Radiology 192:123–127, 1994.
126. Jackson GD: The diagnosis of hippocampal sclerosis: Other techniques. Magn Reson Imaging 13:1081–1093, 1995.
127. Wieshmann UC, Free SL, Everitt AD, et al: Magnetic resonance imaging in epilepsy with a fast FLAIR sequence. J Neurol Neurosurg Psychiatry 61:357–361, 1996.
128. Cascino GD, Hirschorn KA, Jack CR, et al: Gadolinium-DTPA-enhanced magnetic resonance imaging in intractable partial epilepsy. Neurology 39:1115–1118, 1989.
129. Elster AD, Mirza W: MR imaging in chronic partial epilepsy: Role of contrast enhancement. AJNR Am J Neuroradiol 12: 165–170, 1991.
130. Bronen RA: Is there any role for gadopentetate dimeglumine administration when searching for mesial temporal sclerosis in patients with seizures? AJR Am J Roentgenol 164:503, 1995.
131. Bronen RA, Fulbright RK, Kim JH, et al: A systematic approach for interpreting MR images of the seizure patient. AJR Am J Roentgenol 169:241–247, 1997.
132. Grant PE, Barkovich AJ, Wald LL, et al: High-resolution surface-coil MR of cortical lesions in medically refractory epilepsy: A prospective study. AJNR Am J Neuroradiol 18:291–301, 1997.
133. Hugg JW, Butterworth EJ, Kuzniecky RI: Diffusion mapping applied to mesial temporal lobe epilepsy: Preliminary observations. Neurology 53:173–176, 1999.
134. Jack CR Jr, Lee CC, Riederer SJ: Functional magnetic resonance imaging. In Cascino GD, Jack CR Jr (eds): Neuroimaging in Epilepsy: Principles and Practice. Newton, MA, Butterworth-Heinemann, 1996, pp 151–164.
135. Kuzniecky R: Magnetic resonance spectroscopy in focal epilepsy: P-31 and H-1 spectroscopy. Rev Neurol 155:495–498, 1999.
136. Garcia PA, Laxer KD, Ng T: Application of spectroscopic imaging in epilepsy. Magn Reson Imaging 13:1181–1185, 1995.
137. Kuzniecky R, Hugg JW, Hetherington H, et al: Relative utility of H-1 spectroscopic imaging and hippocampal volumetry in the lateralization of mesial temporal lobe epilepsy. Neurology 51:66–71, 1998.
138. Connelly A, Van Paesschen W, Porter DA, et al: Proton magnetic resonance spectroscopy in MRI-negative temporal lobe epilepsy. Neurology 51:61–66, 1998.
139. Woermann FG, McLean MA, Bartlett PA, et al: Short echo time single-voxel H-1 magnetic resonance spectroscopy in magnetic resonance imaging negative temporal lobe epilepsy: Different biochemical profile compared with hippocampal sclerosis. Ann Neurol 45:369–376, 1999.
140. Duc CO, Trabesinger AH, Weber OM, et al: Quantitative H-1 MRS in the evaluation of mesial temporal lobe epilepsy in vivo. Magn Reson Imaging 16:969–979, 1998.
141. Kuzniecky R, Hugg J, Hetherington H, et al: Predictive value of H-1 MRSI for outcome in temporal lobectomy. Neurology 53: 694–698, 1999.
142. Kuzniecky R, Hetherington H, Pan J, et al: Proton spectroscopic imaging at 4.1 tesla in patients with malformations of cortical development and epilepsy. Neurology 48:1018–1024, 1997.
143. Simone IL, Federico F, Tortorella C, et al: Metabolic changes in neuronal migration disorders: Evaluation by combined MRI and proton MRS. Epilepsia 40:872–879, 1999.
144. Aasly J, Silfvenius H, Aas TC, et al: Proton magnetic resonance spectroscopy of brain biopsies from patients with intractable epilepsy. Epilepsy Res 35:211–217, 1999.
145. Rothman DL, Petroff OA, Behar KL, et al: Localized 1H NMR measurements of gamma-aminobutyric acid in human brain in vivo. PNAS 90:5662–5666, 1993.
146. Petroff OA, Rothman DL, Behar KL, et al: Human brain GABA levels rise rapidly after initiation of vigabatrin therapy. Neurology 47:1567–1571, 1996.
147. Petroff OA, Rothman DL, Behar KL, et al: Low brain GABA level is associated with poor seizure control. Ann Neurol 40: 908–911, 1996.
148. Petroff OA, Hyder F, Mattson RH, et al: Topiramate increases brain GABA, homocarnosine, and pyrrolidinone in patients with epilepsy. Neurology 52:473–478, 1999.
149. Petroff OAC, Hyder F, Collins T, et al: Acute effects of vigabatrin on brain GABA and homocarnosine in patients with complex partial seizures. Epilepsia 40:958–964, 1999.
150. Petroff OAC, Rothman DL, Behar KL, et al: Effects of valproate and other antiepileptic drugs on brain glutamate, glutamine, and GABA in patients with refractory complex partial seizures. Seizure 8:120–127, 1999.
151. Novotny EJ, Hyder F, Shevell M, et al: GABA changes with vigabatrin in the developing human brain. Epilepsia 40:462–466, 1999.
152. Merriam MA, Bronen RA, Spencer DD, et al: MR findings after depth electrode implantation for medically refractory epilepsy. AJNR Am J Neuroradiol 14:1343–1346, 1993.
153. Harris RD, Roberts DW, Cromwell LD: MR imaging of corpus callosotomy. AJNR Am J Neuroradiol 10:677–680, 1989.
154. Dietrich RB, el Saden S, Chugani HT, et al: Resective surgery for intractable epilepsy in children: Radiologic evaluation. AJNR Am J Neuroradiol 12:1149–1158, 1991.
155. Laohaprasit V, Silbergeld DL, Ojemann GA, et al: Postoperative CT contrast enhancement following lobectomy for epilepsy. J Neurosurg 73:392–395, 1990.
156. Sato N, Bronen RA, Sze G, et al: Postoperative changes in the brain: MR imaging findings in patients without neoplasms. Radiology 204:839–846, 1997.
157. Saluja S, Sato N, Kawamura Y, et al: Choroid plexus changes after temporal lobectomy. AJNR Am J Neurol (submitted).
158. Moran NF, Lemieux L, Maudgil D, et al: Analysis of temporal lobe resections in MR images. Epilepsia 40:1077–1084, 1999.
159. Jack CR Jr, Sharbrough FW, Marsh WR: Use of MR imaging for quantitative evaluation of resection for temporal lobe epilepsy. Radiology 169:463–468, 1988.
160. Siegel AM, Wieser HG, Wichmann W, et al: Relationships between MR-imaged total amount of tissue removed, resection scores of specific mediobasal limbic subcompartments and clinical outcome following selective amygdalohippocampectomy. Epilepsy Res 6:56–65, 1990.
161. Nayel MH, Awad IA, Luders H: Extent of mesiobasal resection determines outcome after temporal lobectomy for intractable complex partial seizures. Neurosurgery 29:55–60, 1991.
162. Bronen RA: Epilepsy: The role of MR imaging. AJR Am J Roentgenol 159:1165–1174, 1992.

The Intracarotid Amobarbital Procedure or Wada Test

CARL B. DODRILL

HISTORICAL PERSPECTIVE

In 1949, Wada[1] reported that a unilateral intracarotid injection of sodium amobarbital produced sharply diminished functioning of the ipsilateral hemisphere without interruption of vital functions and without intolerable side effects. The potential value of the procedure for neurosurgery was recognized, for it was clear that the procedure could help to determine the lateralization of speech functions in patients who were to undergo surgical procedures in eloquent cortex. By 1954, Wada had completed intracarotid amobarbital studies successfully in 80 humans.[2] Branch and colleagues[3] soon thereafter reported on the safe application of the procedure to 123 patients, and the procedure was established. Although the method often has been called the *Wada test* after its founder, the term *intracarotid amobarbital procedure* (IAP) is technically more adequate, and it is used throughout this chapter.

The original use of the IAP was to determine the lateralization of speech functions, and this remains its best established use. A second use for the IAP, proposed by Milner and coworkers,[4] was to avoid the severe anterograde amnesia that can result with bilateral mesial temporal structures becoming dysfunctional after surgery.[5,6] Reasoning that the IAP might be a useful method of evaluating memory, Milner and coworkers[4] reported on memory studies in 50 patients undergoing the IAP. Using a simple memory testing paradigm, these investigators found memory dysfunction in 12 of the 50 patients, but always after injection of the hemisphere contralateral to the known seizure focus. Surgery on the focus never produced postoperative amnesia, and it was concluded that the IAP was an appropriate method for assessing the risk of postoperative amnesia in patients undergoing temporal lobectomy in which a portion of the mesial temporal lobes might be removed. The assessment of memory became a part of the IAP in nearly every case in which it is undertaken.

Since the 1960s, several additional uses have been proposed for the IAP. These uses include reaffirming the laterality of an epileptic focus,[7–10] predicting postoperative seizure control,[7,11,12] identifying the likely extent of hippocampal sclerosis,[13–15] and distinguishing between lateral neocortical and mesial temporal lobe epilepsy.[16] The IAP has potential to provide valuable information in these contexts,[17] but these applications are not discussed further because the focus of this chapter is on the more general uses of the IAP—to evaluate speech and memory.

UNDERLYING ASSUMPTIONS

Two basic conceptualizations have emerged about how the IAP operates and what is being tested with it. Historically the theory has been that the hemisphere perfused with amobarbital is nonfunctional, and so testing taking place at that time must be evaluating the functioning of the other hemisphere. This simple understanding of how the IAP works is in significant error because only a portion of any hemisphere is perfused by the standard dose of amobarbital delivered through the distribution of the internal carotid artery. It is no doubt true that a significant portion of that hemisphere continues to be operative.

A second basic conceptualization about the IAP is that it provides an estimate of the postoperative changes that may occur if surgery is done on the same side as the injection. This conceptualization makes no assumptions about the side opposite the injection or its functioning. This second viewpoint is most likely to be of assistance to the neurosurgeon, and this is the viewpoint that is adopted here. The pros and cons of these viewpoints in the context of predicting memory loss after surgery have been discussed in some detail.[18] The distinction between the two basic points of view is most important, and it leads to different conclusions about how the IAP operates.

BASIC TERMINOLOGY

One particularly troublesome problem in terminology that has resulted in confusion in this field has been the failure to distinguish between *speech* and *language*. *Speech* refers to the power or ability to talk, whereas *language* refers to the communication of thoughts and feelings and the meanings behind vocal utterances. The terms are quite different, but in the scientific literature they commonly are not distinguished. The result has been substantial confusion with definite consequences for neurosurgery. Neurosurgeons need to know which cortical areas are responsible for the production of speech because it is these areas that, if disturbed at the time of surgery, may result in dysphasia or language-related deficits. By focusing on the areas responsible for the production of speech, the IAP can be of great value in accurately lateralizing those areas for the neurosurgeon. The fact that areas in both cerebral hemispheres are related to various aspects of language, although of interest, is of less value to the neurosurgeon because many of those areas, even if removed surgically, do not produce dysphasia after surgery. Using the IAP to find the areas responsible for the production of speech rather than language is discussed in this chapter.

Also of value is the distinction between *typical* and *atypical* speech lateralization. *Typical speech* refers to the power or ability to talk being associated with only the left hemisphere. This is the usual circumstance for most patients. *Atypical speech* refers to speech associated with the right cerebral hemisphere alone or with both cerebral hemispheres. *Bilaterally represented speech* refers to having some essential speech functions on the left and other essential speech functions on the right. Except for rare circumstances, these speech functions are not duplicative, and surgery on either side can result in postoperative dysphasia in bilateral speech cases. In these cases, the IAP results on either side independently provide evidence for disruption of speech on that side.

GENERAL INTRACAROTID AMOBARBITAL PROCEDURE

The IAP varies in how it is executed in centers around the world.[17] The features common to all IAPs are few, but they include the introduction of amobarbital into a portion of the arterial system of one cerebral hemisphere and some type of testing of the impact of the barbiturate on cognitive functioning. Beyond this simple statement of procedure, little can be offered that is applicable universally across all centers performing the procedure. Nevertheless, to undertake the procedure systematically, decisions must be made about several variables, the most important of which are now discussed.

Patients to Whom the Procedure Is Applied

Most commonly, the IAP is applied to patients for whom elective surgery is being planned that probably or possibly will involve eloquent cortex—cortex that involves memory or the production of speech. Patients typically included are patients for whom left temporal or frontal resections are being planned and persons who are not strictly right-handed. These patient groups represent the minimum to which the IAP should be applied.

Although the guidelines presented in the previous paragraph are reasonable and generally accepted, it is better to determine the patient groups to whom the test should be applied based on actually determined atypical speech. Consequently, I reviewed the 836 cases with uncomplicated results on whom I had done IAPs during a 26-year period (1974 to 1999). Most of these patients had epilepsy and were being considered for cortical resection surgery, but some had arteriovenous malformations or tumors rather than epilepsy as their primary problem. All patients were classified as *left speech*, *right speech*, or *bilateral speech* based on the IAP, and this was done in the same way during the 26-year period. The results for the entire sample are presented in Table 150–1 along with results for handedness groups and groups based on side of surgery.

Perhaps the most remarkable finding in Table 150–1 is that atypical (right, bilateral) speech in this neurological sample is common. It is seen most commonly in left-handed patients having surgery on the left (55.8%); and in right-handed patients with surgery on the right, it appears in 3.6% of the cases. In interpreting these figures, one should bear in mind the population being sampled, which includes 233 people with onsets of neurological problems in the first 5 years of life. It is evident that the incidence of atypical speech is more common than has been thought, and this argues for using the IAP more broadly than often has been the case. Although it has not been possible to check the accuracy of the IAP with respect to speech lateralization in every case by cortical mapping, in many cases we have done mapping at this institution and we have followed up patients after surgery. In only one case did the IAP fail to find speech where it was discovered at

TABLE 150–1 ■ **Incidence of Left, Right, and Bilateral Speech in 836 Cases with Valid Wada Tests***

GROUP	LEFT (%)	RIGHT (%)	BILATERAL (%)
All patients (n = 836)	85.4	7.9	6.7
Handedness (n = 803)			
Right (n = 648)	92.8	2.3	4.9
Left (n = 155)	54.2	31.0	14.8
Side of surgery (n = 784)			
Right (n = 335)	93.1	3.6	3.3
Left (n = 449)	80.2	10.7	9.1
Handedness plus side of surgery (n = 766)			
Surgery on right (n = 329)			
Right-handed (n = 278)	96.4	1.4	2.2
Left-handed (n = 51)	76.5	15.7	7.8
Surgery on left (n = 437)			
Right-handed (n = 342)	90.1	2.9	7.0
Left-handed (n = 95)	44.2	37.9	17.9

*Conducted during a 26-year period at the University of Washington, Seattle.

surgery, and this is the only error in speech lateralization that we have been able to associate with the IAP in 26 years. Done properly, the IAP is an accurate procedure that can be relied on by neurosurgeons to prevent postsurgical language-related problems.

Sides Tested and the Order of Testing

Previously, there has been discussion about whether it is necessary to perfuse both cerebral hemispheres. There is now a reasonably good consensus, however, that all necessary information is *not* obtained from a single injection. Bilateral speech cases never can be identified with unilateral injections, and a comparison of the performances of the two hemispheres is never possible unless both are injected. Certainty of conclusions is increased greatly by perfusing both cerebral hemispheres. For these and other reasons, at least 84% of centers using the IAP "always to almost always" perfuse both hemispheres with each test.[17] We routinely do this in Seattle, the only exception being when one cerebral hemisphere is small or damaged so badly and epileptic that there is an increased probability of a convulsion if the one good hemisphere is perfused. In that case, the bad hemisphere only would be perfused.

There are advantages in perfusing the side of surgical interest first. In the experience at this institution, occasionally it was possible to do only a single injection for a variety of reasons, including the patient having a seizure, equipment failure, loss of cooperation of the patient, emergent need to use the angiographic facility, and problems with drug carryover.[19] All of these are reasons to do the side of surgical interest first.

Dosing and Administration of Amobarbital

No other aspect is more important for the successful completion of an IAP than the correct dosing and delivery of the amobarbital. Many guidelines are offered to assist the reader in planning these studies. There is a substantial degree of variability from one patient to the next in terms of the ideal amount of drug, however, and a portion of this variability is not predictable. More drug or less drug than is ideal may be given on occasion.

An overall guideline for dosing is that only as much drug need be used as is necessary to obtain the required information. If fairly coarse cognitive measures are used, more drug is needed; if more sensitive cognitive tests are available, less drug is needed. The doses recommended here are less than the doses commonly found in the literature. With an adequately sensitive cognitive test, there is no need for more drug, and by using less, important side effects are minimized, including confusion, lethargy, reduced cooperation, and *wet-dog shakes*, mimicking chills and fever but not involving a temperature change. When dosing is done correctly with minimal drug, it routinely is possible to do both sides in the same session, and the problems associated with carryover from one injection to the next[19] are largely sidestepped.

The injections done on each side typically involve a three-way stopcock with the drug injected during a 4- to 6-second period and with an immediate chasing through with saline. Thirty minutes between the amobarbital injections clears most but not all of the drug.

Guidelines for dosing are summarized in Table 150–2. For adults, there is a small but worthwhile difference in dosage requirements depending on gender. On average, men's brains are approximately 13% heavier than women's brains,[20, 21] and practical experience has shown that if one gives the same dose to men and women, there is a tendency to overdose women unnecessarily (or underdose men). In my experience with sensitive cognitive measures, 100 mg of amobarbital for women and 112.5 mg for men is sufficient. Although small, the difference in dose between the genders is worthwhile.

Other alterations in dose are indicated in Table 150–2. An underlying principle is that the dose should be altered when a condition is present that is likely to affect the patient's response to the drug. There needs to be an adequate impact of the drug on the tests being used, but an excessive impact is not desirable because it is more difficult for the patient and the examiner. If the first injection for a patient has proved to be more

TABLE 150–2 ■ **Guidelines for Amobarbital Dosing***

VARIABLE/GROUP	DOSE/ADJUSTMENT
Adults (age 16 and older)	
Gender	
Men	Use 112.5 mg
Women	Use 100 mg
Cognitive/neuropsychological limitations	
Moderate impairment (IQ 60–75)	Reduce dose by 12.5 mg
Severe impairment (IQ <60)	Reduce dose by 25 mg
Major behavioral/psychiatric problems likely to affect cooperation	Reduce dose by 12.5 mg
Presence of AVM or vascular anomalies likely to pool the amobarbital	Increase dose by 25–50 mg based on size of anomaly
Weight of patient	Make no alteration regardless of weight
Baseline barbiturate/other medications	Make no alteration regardless of medications
Children (age 5–15)	
Age (yr)	
5–8	Use 62.5 mg
9–12	Use 75 mg
13–15	Use 87.5 mg
Cognitive/neuropsychological limitations	Use dose in age grouping based on mental age†
Major behavioral/psychiatric problems	Consider reducing dose by 12.5 mg if age 9 or older
Gender	Make no alterations regardless of gender

*These are suggested doses that require alteration from one case to the next. It is assumed that each 50 mg of amobarbital is mixed with 1 mL of saline. Expect considerable fluctuation from one patient to the next.

†For example, if age = 12 and IQ = 50, mental age = 6; use 62.5 mg.

than required, one routinely would consider reducing the drug for the second injection by 12.5 to 25 mg on occasion. If the first injection was so light that an adequate measure of behavioral change was not obtained, a second injection can be done on that side within a few minutes with more drug. A third injection is possible on the other side, routinely without difficulty.

The anterior hippocampus is not perfused adequately by the distribution of the middle cerebral artery, and it has been suggested that a selective approach through the posterior cerebral artery should be used. This approach has been used at times,[22, 23] but the risks involved are unacceptably high, and the approach has all but been abandoned. Also, although the anterior hippocampus is not perfused directly by the amobarbital delivered by means of the internal carotid artery, its functioning clearly is affected. This has been shown through studies of depth electrodes during the IAP[24, 25] and by the use of single-photon emission computed tomography (SPECT).[26, 27] There is no need for posterior artery studies to evaluate the functioning of the hippocampus.

Selective Injections

A considerable degree of variation from one patient to the next exists in terms of the areas perfused by the amobarbital. One may wish to plan restricted resections, and in cases in which these resections are in areas adjacent to eloquent cortex, a selective or superselective injection of amobarbital may provide important guidance for the surgery. Although these studies are accomplished only infrequently and are outside the main focus of this chapter, a detailed treatment of this topic is available.[28]

Electroencephalography Recordings

The best survey of the practices of epilepsy programs shows that 69% use simultaneous electroencephalography (EEG) during the IAP to help confirm drug effect.[17] One quarter of the centers seldom or never use EEG. EEG is not used routinely during the IAP at this institution. I do not believe that EEG is worth the effort, inconvenience, and expense involved. There is some question as to the accuracy of EEG, especially in identifying amobarbital cross-perfusion.[29] The electrodes may be perceived as a barrier by the radiologist, and the presence of an EEG machine may congest further an already crowded room.

PSYCHOLOGICAL TESTING PROCEDURES

A variety of psychological testing procedures are used to evaluate speech and memory at different centers.[17] Because each center tends to use its own protocol, comparability is limited. Because of this, I began using other protocols in addition to my own to compare among more than one testing procedure. This effort has proved to be profitable in permitting the comparison of more than one method of memory assessment.[30]

A principal consideration in selecting test materials for the IAP is the limited time in which testing can be accomplished. This is especially the case on the side associated with speech, in which a speech blockage and prominent aphasia can make testing especially difficult for a time, after which much of the drug effect may have dissipated, and the time for valid testing often is reduced markedly. Testing before this time often is fraught with difficulties because the patient can give little response, and it is often impossible to determine if the materials have been registered adequately by the patient for memory testing. Efforts to deal with this problem have met with limited success, and this is perhaps the most important technical problem yet to be solved with the IAP.

Combining speech and memory testing in an efficient paradigm is to great advantage in view of the limited testing time. One way to do this is what is done here at the University of Washington in Seattle, where speech and memory are evaluated simultaneously in a repetitive three-part procedure. First, the patient is asked to name a solid object in the form of a complete sentence by saying, "This is a . . . ," then naming the object. By having the patient say "This is a . . . ," a larger sample of speech is obtained, and it is easier to evaluate a potential speech blockage. Second, a distractor task is inserted to make memory testing possible, and this consists of having the patient read a short sentence printed on a card. Third, the patient is asked to recall the object shown before the card. This procedure increases reliability and potentially validity by making several trials per minute routinely possible. It permits the calculation of error rates, and it is simpler than most protocols, which have several unrelated tasks that must be undertaken sequentially, most of which provide ancillary rather than core information. The only additional task that is accomplished with this procedure is the periodic checking of grip strength. This procedure evaluates recall rather than recognition memory (recall memory is the type of memory problem most commonly reported after epilepsy surgery), and it does so when the drug is present rather than at a later point. The materials used for this procedure are shown in Figure 150–1 (see color section in this volume).

Although the procedure just described is appealing by its simplicity and its ability to produce easily interpreted data, it is not the procedure used most commonly. The most common procedure is to have the patient perform various language-related tasks to evaluate speech and language and to expose the patient to 5 to 10 stimuli of various types for which recognition memory is evaluated after the procedure is over and the patient has returned to baseline functioning. It is a mistake to assume that this paradigm is superior to the one described previously in predicting memory loss after surgery. Actually, the opposite is true.[30]

Accuracy of Speech Lateralization

There is no doubt that with reasonable care, the IAP can identify the hemispheres associated with speech

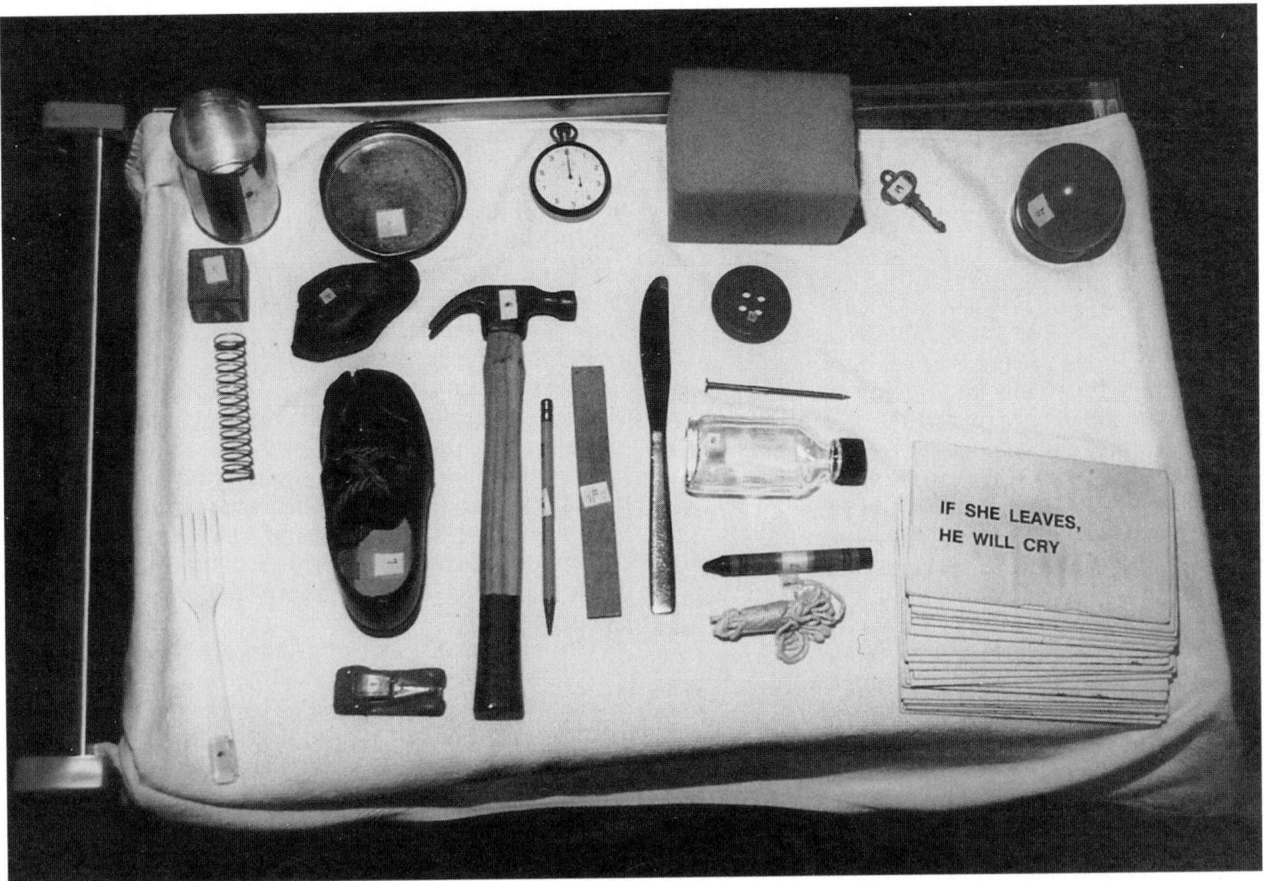

FIGURE 150–1. Psychological test materials used in the Seattle form of the intracarotid amobarbital procedure. (See color section in this volume.)

functions with great accuracy. In my experience, in 890 studies done in 869 patients, the IAP has been incorrect in the lateralization of speech in only one case in which a patient proved to have bilateral speech, when the IAP found speech on the right side only. Our experience is similar to that of other centers, which rarely report any inaccuracy in connection with speech lateralization.

Some authors have attempted to describe lateralization of linguistic functions on a continuum rather than as left, right, or bilateral.[31, 32] In cases in which this has been attempted, the authors routinely evaluate various aspects of language functions rather than speech. There is no question that some linguistic functions are located in various parts of the brain, and these are worthy of study. Surgery in most of these areas does not produce aphasia, however. Rather, surgery in the area related to the production of speech produces these problems, and this is the information the neurosurgeon needs for planning surgery.

Accuracy of Memory Assessment

Perhaps no other topic has attracted greater interest than the degree to which the IAP can presage memory losses after surgery. Originally the focus was on the prevention of global amnestic losses, and the IAP has been successful in this area.[33, 34] Although such a use of the IAP can be considered established, a more broadly applicable task for IAP memory testing has arisen. This is the common need to warn of troublesome mild to moderate verbal memory losses after surgery. This task has proved to be much more difficult, and few articles showing the usefulness of the IAP in this context are found and none before 1991.[34]

Since 1991, six data-based articles have been published on using IAP memory measures to predict mild to moderate memory changes after surgery. The first of these[35] failed to show statistically significant predictive power of the IAP, but in the other five cases,[30, 36–39] the IAP was shown to be able to predict memory changes after surgery to some degree. Although in each case the prediction was imperfect, the best predictions appeared in cases when a multivariate procedure was used that considered not only the IAP results, but also other variables that had shown predictive capabilities, such as age at onset of seizures (late onset predicts memory loss[40]), age at surgery (later surgery predicts loss[40, 41]), hippocampal sclerosis (lack of hippocampal sclerosis on surgery side predicts loss[42]), and preoperative verbal memory level (good verbal memory level predicts loss[43]). Within this context, the IAP is likely to be found to be of moderate value in predicting memory loss after surgery.

COMPLICATIONS DURING THE INTRACAROTID AMOBARBITAL PROCEDURE AND INTERPRETATION OF OUTCOME

Cerebral angiograms are associated with a low rate of complications, including strokes and severe vasospasm. Although patients undergoing the IAP typically are younger rather than older, the complication rate must be considered in calculating the risks versus benefits of the IAP. In one series[44] of 447 IAPs, the complication rate was 0.96%, whereas in the series of 836 patients reported in Table 150–1, the complication rate was 0.45%. In six of the eight patients reported as experiencing complications in these two series, symptoms resolved within 24 hours so that in only two cases (0.16%) were there persisting symptoms. In view of the fact that the possibility of finding atypical speech is at least 3.6% (see Table 150–1), the benefits appear to be many times greater than the risks, especially because persisting aphasia can arise from lobectomy.

Sedation and behavioral complications are much more common than neurological sequelae with the IAP as well as more troublesome.[45, 46] These difficulties can include confusion and combative behavior necessitating restraint for some minutes. At the extreme, personnel can be struck by a patient, and although this has happened to me only once in 900 studies, it reflects a volatile situation that renders little information and represents a safety issue for all concerned. From personal experience, it is possible to minimize this problem by doing the following: (1) establishing significant rapport with each patient, including showing significant interest in each patient personally and taking the time to show that interest; (2) getting an objective appraisal of the patient's abilities and their responses to stressful situations (I typically am able to do this through a full-day neuropsychological evaluation before doing the IAP; the patient's responses to the stressful tests give a good idea of likely responses with the IAP and how to handle that patient); and (3) selecting the correct drug dosage (see Table 150–2). Our average amobarbital dose among 749 adults was 106 mg, which is substantially less than the 125 mg used by Blum and colleagues[45] and far less than the 160 mg used by Lee and associates[46] when these investigators reported sedation and behavioral complications. These difficulties are most likely to occur in persons with diminished intelligence, substantial neuropsychological impairment, and psychiatric disturbances, groups for whom the dose must be reduced. Although it is not possible to eliminate this behavior in every case, by following the recommendations in Table 150–2 in addition to establishing rapport and knowing patients well, most adverse behavioral reactions can be avoided, while still obtaining valid studies.

ALTERNATE PROCEDURES AND THE FUTURE OF THE INTRACAROTID AMOBARBITAL PROCEDURE

Many procedures other than the IAP have been used in an effort to lateralize speech and to assess memory with techniques having a lower risk than the IAP, including standard magnetic resonance imaging (MRI),[14, 47] functional MRI,[48–52] SPECT,[53, 54] positron emission tomography,[55] magnetic source imaging,[56] transcranial magnetic stimulation,[57] and Doppler sonography.[58] Each technique has some promise for replicating findings from the IAP for speech, memory, or both. In no instance, however, has enough work been done on a method that a confident statement can be made about the ability of the method to replicate the IAP. Although functional MRI appears to be the most promising approach, it is not clear that it currently is capable of making the finer distinctions in speech lateralization (e.g., right speech versus bilateral speech).

One matter of great importance in essentially all of the studies of these alternate techniques is that all pertain to complex aspects of language or memory or both rather than to the production of speech. Despite the allure of these studies that evaluate complex cognitive functions, the neurosurgeon must continue to be concerned about identifying sites of speech production because it is the removal of any of these areas, rather than any area pertaining to *language*, that reliably produces persisting postoperative language-related problems. These studies of language produce findings related to both cerebral hemispheres in most patients, but it is safe to remove some of these areas at surgery without risk of postoperative deficit. At present, it appears that only the IAP reliably can make this distinction preoperatively.

The future of the IAP hinges on the ability of alternative procedures to identify reliably areas in which surgery carries a risk of producing persisting language-related deficits. If an alternative procedure can be found that carries fewer risks, it is likely to replace the IAP in time. Until this is the case, the IAP will continue to be done in centers throughout the world.

REFERENCES

1. Wada J: [A new method for the determination of the side of cerebral speech dominance: A preliminary report on the intracarotid injection of Sodium Amytal in man.] Igaku Seibutsugaku 14:221–222, 1949.
2. Wada J, Rasmussen T: Intracarotid injection of sodium amytal for the lateralization of cerebral speech dominance: Experimental and clinical observations. J Neurosurg 17:266–282, 1960.
3. Branch C, Milner B, Rasmussen T: Intracarotid Sodium Amytal for the lateralization of cerebral speech dominance. J Neurosurg 21:399–405, 1964.
4. Milner B, Branch C, Rasmussen T: Study of short-term memory after intracarotid injection of Sodium Amytal. Trans Am Neurol Assoc 87:224–226, 1962.
5. Scoville WF, Milner B: Loss of recent memory after bilateral hippocampal lesions. J Neurol Neurosurg Psychiatry 20:11–21, 1957.
6. Penfield W, Milner B: Memory deficits produced by bilateral

lesions in the hippocampal zone. AMA Arch Neurol Psych 79: 475–497, 1958.
7. Perrine K, Westerveld M, Sass KJ, et al: Wada memory disparities predict seizure laterality and postoperative seizure control. Epilepsia 36:851–856, 1995.
8. Rausch R, Babb TL, Engel J, Crandall PH: Memory following intracarotid amobarbital injection contralateral to hippocampal damage. Arch Neurol 46:783–788, 1989.
9. Rosenbaum T, Laxer K, Stanulis R, et al: Localization of temporal lobe seizure foci by Wada testing. In Wolf P, Dam M, Janz D, Dreifuss FE (eds): Advances in Epileptology, vol 16. New York, Raven Press, 1987, pp 319–321.
10. Swearer JM, Kane KJ, Phillips CA, et al: Predictive value of the intracarotid amobarbital test in bihemispheric seizure onset. Neurology 52:409–411, 1999.
11. Loring DW, Meador KJ, Lee GP, et al: Wada memory performance predicts seizure outcome following anterior temporal lobectomy. Neurology 44:2322–2324, 1994.
12. Sperling MR, Saykin AJ, Glosser G, et al: Predictors of outcome after anterior temporal lobectomy: The intracarotid amobarbital test. Neurology 44:2325–2330, 1994.
13. Davies KG, Hermann BP, Foley KT: Relation between intracarotid amobarbital memory asymmetry scores and hippocampal sclerosis in patients undergoing anterior temporal lobe resections. Epilepsia 37:522–525, 1996.
14. Loring DW, Murro AM, Meador KJ, et al: Wada memory testing and hippocampal volume measurements in the evaluation for temporal lobectomy. Neurology 43:1789–1793, 1993.
15. Sass KJ, Lencz T, Westerveld M, et al: The neural substrate of memory impairment demonstrated by the intracarotid amobarbital procedure. Arch Neurol 48:48–52, 1991.
16. Hamberger MJ, Walczak TS, Goodman RR: Intracarotid amobarbital procedure memory performance and age at first risk for seizures distinguish between lateral neocortical and mesial temporal lobe epilepsy. Epilepsia 37:1088–1092, 1996.
17. Rausch R, Silfvenius H, Wieser H-G, et al: Intraarterial amobarbital procedures. In Engel J (ed): Surgical Treatment of the Epilepsies, 2nd ed. New York, Raven Press, 1993, pp 341–357.
18. Chelune G: Hippocampal adequacy versus functional reserve: Predicting memory functions following temporal lobectomy. Arch Clin Neuropsychol 10:413–432, 1995.
19. Grote CL, Wierenga BA, Smith MC, et al: Wada difference a day makes: Interpretive cautions regarding same-day injections. Neurology 52:1577–1582, 1999.
20. Passingham RE: Brain size and intelligence in man. Brain Behav Evol 16:253–270, 1979.
21. Wittelson SF: The brain connection: The corpus callosum is larger in left-handers. Science 229:665–668, 1985.
22. Jack CR, Nichols DA, Sharbrough FW, et al: Selective posterior cerebral artery Amytal test for evaluating memory function before surgery for temporal lobe seizure. Neuroradiology 168:787–793, 1988.
23. Morton N, Polkey CE, Cox T, Morris RG: Episodic memory dysfunction during Sodium Amytal testing of epileptic patients in relation to posterior cerebral artery perfusion. J Clin Exp Neuropsychol 18:24–37, 1996.
24. Gotman J, Bouwer MS, Jones-Gotman M: Intracranial EEG study of brain structures affected by internal carotid injection of amobarbital. Neurology 42:2136–2142, 1992.
25. Adachi N, Onuma T, Suzuki I, et al: Intracarotid amobarbital injection produces hippocampal EEG changes in patients with temporal lobe epilepsy. Epilepsy Res 15:75–78, 1993.
26. Urbach H, Kurthen M, Klemm E, et al: Amobarbital effects on the posterior hippocampus during the intracarotid amobarbital test. Neurology 52:1596–1602, 1999.
27. Kim BG, Lee SK, Woo Nam H, et al: Evaluation of functional changes in the medial temporal region during intracarotid amobarbital procedure by use of SPECT. Epilepsia 40:424–429, 1999.
28. Wieser H-G, Muller S, Schiess R, et al: The anterior and posterior selective temporal lobe amobarbital tests: Angiographic, clinical, electroencephalographic, PET, SPECT findings, and memory performance. Brain Cogn 33:71–97, 1997.
29. Hong SB, Kim K, Seo DW, et al: Contralateral EEG slowing and amobarbital distribution in Wada test: An intracarotid SPECT study. Epilepsia 41:207–212, 2000.
30. Dodrill CB, Ojemann GA: An exploratory comparison of three methods of memory assessment with the intracarotid amobarbital procedure. Brain Cogn 33:210–223, 1997.
31. Benbadis SR, Dinner DS, Chelune GJ, et al: Objective criteria for reporting language dominance by intracarotid amobarbital procedure. J Clin Exp Neuropsychol 17:682–690, 1995.
32. Loring DW, Meador KJ, Lee GP, et al: Cerebral language lateralization: Evidence from intracarotid amobarbital testing. Neuropsychologia 28:831–838, 1990.
33. Loring DW, Hermann BP, Meador KJ, et al: Amnesia after unilateral temporal lobectomy: A case report. Epilepsia 35:757–763, 1994.
34. Rausch R, Langfitt JT: Memory evaluation during the intracarotid sodium amobarbital procedure. In Luders H (ed): Epilepsy Surgery. New York, Raven Press, 1991, pp 507–514.
35. Wyllie E, Haugle R, Awad I, et al: Intracarotid amobarbital procedure: I. Prediction of decreased modality-specific memory scores after temporal lobectomy. Epilepsia 32:857–864, 1991.
36. Loring DW, Meador KJ, Lee GP, et al: Wada memory asymmetries predict verbal memory decline after anterior temporal lobectomy. Neurology 45:1329–1333, 1995.
37. Chelune GJ: Hippocampal adequacy versus functional reserve: Predicting memory functions following temporal lobectomy. Arch Clin Neuropsychol 10:413–432, 1995.
38. Kneebone AC, Chelune GJ, Dinner DS, et al: Intracarotid amobarbital procedure as a predictor of material-specific memory change after anterior temporal lobectomy. Epilepsia 36:857–865, 1995.
39. Jokeit H, Ebner A, Holthausen H, et al: Individual prediction of change in delayed recall of prose passages after left-sided anterior temporal lobectomy. Neurology 49:481–487, 1997.
40. Hermann BP, Seidenberg M, Haltiner A, Wyler AR: Relationship of age at onset, chronologic age, and adequacy of preoperative performance to verbal memory change after anterior temporal lobectomy. Epilepsia 36:137–145, 1995.
41. Helstaedter C, Elger CE: Functional plasticity after left anterior temporal lobectomy: Reconstitution and compensation of verbal memory functions. Epilepsia 39:399–406, 1998.
42. Seidenberg M, Hermann B, Wyler AR, et al: Neuropsychological outcome following anterior temporal lobectomy in patients with and without the syndrome of mesial temporal lobe epilepsy. Neuropsychology 12:303–316, 1998.
43. Chelune GJ, Naugle RI, Luders H, Awad IA: Prediction of cognitive change as a function of preoperative ability status among temporal lobectomy patients seen at 6-month follow-up. Neurology 41:399–404, 1991.
44. Macken MP, Morris HM: Complications of the Wada test: A review of Cleveland Clinic experience. Epilepsia 40(suppl 7): 84, 1999.
45. Blum D, Bortz JJ, Ehsan T: Factors affecting degree of sedation after intracarotid Amytal injection. J Epilepsy 10:42–46, 1997.
46. Lee GP, Loring DW, Meador, KJ, et al: Severe behavioral complications following intracarotid sodium amobarbital injection: Implications for hemispheric asymmetry of emotion. Neurology 38: 1233–1236, 1988.
47. Charles PD, Abou-Khalil R, Abou-Khalil B, et al: MRI asymmetries and language dominance. Neurology 44:2050–2054, 1994.
48. Benson RR, FitzGerald BSEE, LeSueur LL, et al: Language dominance determined by whole brain functional MRI in patients with brain lesions. Neurology 52:798–809, 1999.
49. Binder JR, Swanson SJ, Hammeke TA, et al: Determination of language dominance using function MRI: A comparison with the Wada test. Neurology 46:978–984, 1996.
50. Gaillard WD, Hertz-Pannier L, Mott SH, et al: Functional anatomy of cognitive development: fMRI of verbal fluency in children and adults. Neurology 54:180–185, 2000.
51. Loring DW, Meador KJ, Allison JD, Wright JC: Relationship between motor and language activation using fMRI. Neurology 54:981–983, 2000.
52. Pujol J, Deus J, Losilla JM, Capdevila A: Cerebral lateralization of language in normal left-handed people studied by functional MRI. Neurology 52:1038–1043, 1999.
53. McMackin D, Dubeau F, Jones-Gotman M, et al: Assessment of the functional effect of the intracarotid sodium amobarbital procedure using co-registered MRI/HMPAO-SPECT and SEEG. Brain Cogn 33:50–70, 1997.

54. McMackin D, Jones-Gotman M, Dubeau F, et al: Regional cerebral blood flow and language dominance: SPECT during intracarotid amobarbital testing. Neurology 50:943–950, 1998.
55. Salanova V, Morris III HH, Rehm P, et al: Comparison of the intracarotid amobarbital procedure and interictal cerebral 18-fluorodeoxyglucose positron emission tomography scans in refractory temporal lobe epilepsy. Epilepsia 33:635–638, 1992.
56. Breier JI, Simos PG, Zouridakis G, et al: Language dominance determined by magnetic source imaging. Neurology 53:938–945, 1999.
57. Jennum P, Friberg L, Fuglsang-Frederiksen A, Dam M: Speech localization using repetitive transcranial magnetic stimulation. Neurology 44:269–273, 1994.
58. Rihs F, Sturzenegger M, Gutbrod K, et al: Determination of language dominance: Wada test confirms transcranial Doppler sonography. Neurology 52:1591–1596, 1999.

CHAPTER **151**

Functional Magnetic Resonance Imaging in Epilepsy Surgery

THOMAS A. HAMMEKE ■ WADE M. MUELLER ■ SARA J. SWANSON ■ JEFFREY R. BINDER

Brain surgery is an effective treatment for individuals with medically intractable focal epilepsy.[1–5] The best seizure control occurs when a single seizure focus can be identified and the maximal excision of epileptogenic tissue is accomplished.[6] Seizure control must be weighed against functional loss. Thus, determination of the appropriateness of surgery requires identification of the seizure focus as well as evaluation of the surgical risks. Functional brain mapping techniques can contribute to this process in several ways. First, by determining the location of important brain functions, mapping techniques can help predict the risk of postoperative language, memory, sensory, and motor deficits and enable adjustments in the surgical procedure to minimize such deficits. Second, asymmetries in interictal blood flow and temporal lobe functional activation can identify diseased brain tissue in which seizures are thought to originate. Third, techniques for detecting ictal discharges or hemodynamic or metabolic changes can be used to directly localize the origin of seizures.

Traditional techniques for presurgical functional mapping include the intracarotid amobarbital, or Wada, test[7, 8]; subdural grid stimulation mapping[9, 10]; intraoperative stimulation mapping[10–12]; and metabolic and functional neuroimaging techniques such as single photon emission computed tomography (SPECT) and positron emission tomography (PET).[13, 14] These methods, though useful, are relatively invasive (Wada, subdural grids, intraoperative stimulation mapping), costly, or not widely available (PET). Despite the use of these techniques, measurable language or memory decline after dominant hemisphere temporal lobe surgery for epilepsy occurs at a rate of 40% to 60%.[15–19] Methods for locating epileptogenic foci continue to improve, yet uncertainty about localization in individual patients continues to be a major problem affecting surgical eligibility and outcome.[20–25] A significant proportion of patients require invasive or semi-invasive recording techniques, adding to the economic cost and to the risk of a surgical approach.[11, 24, 26]

Functional magnetic resonance imaging (fMRI) is a noninvasive technique for detecting localized, event-related changes in MRI signal.[27–29] These changes are due to regional increases in blood flow that accompany neural activation and lead to paradoxically increased blood oxygenation in local vascular beds.[30] Because oxygenated blood is less paramagnetic than deoxygenated blood,[31] the increase in blood oxygenation results in locally increased field homogeneity, less intravoxel dephasing of proton spins, and increased MRI signal,[32] which is often referred to as blood oxygenation level–dependent (BOLD) signal.[33] The relationship between axonal and synaptic activity and fMRI signal was recently measured directly using an animal model[34]; however, the precise coupling of neural activity and hemodynamic response is not fully understood.[35, 36]

The fMRI technique possesses a number of important and inherent capabilities. First, and most important, the technique is safe, requiring no invasive procedures or radiation exposure. The safety of fMRI allows activation protocols to be thoroughly tested in normal volunteers before clinical use; enables the collection of large data sets in individual patients, with resultant enhancement of statistical power; and permits studies to be repeated, if necessary, without additional risk. Second, the relatively small size of fMRI voxels (typically 2 to 4 mm) results in excellent spatial resolution. Functional data can be registered with higher-resolution structural images acquired at the same brain locations in the same session, permitting functional loci to be identified more precisely with specific anatomic loci. Third, a large number of activation procedures can be performed in each subject during a single session, enabling localization of a wide variety of cognitive processes and systems. Fourth, fMRI can be implemented on the MRI scanners already in place at most medical facilities.

This chapter reviews the methodologic issues pertinent to the use of this technology in epilepsy. It then examines the progress to date on the use of fMRI to lateralize and localize language, memory, and sensorimotor functions in epilepsy patients and to assist in the localization of the seizure focus. For a broader review of the specific techniques used in fMRI, the reader is referred elsewhere.[28, 37, 38]

GENERAL METHODOLOGIC ISSUES

The exponential growth of brain mapping publications using fMRI technology proves its value in demonstrating relationships between brain structure and function.[39] There is a growing trend toward the use of presurgical functional maps to assist in assessing the feasibility of surgical resection, for surgical planning, and to select patients for invasive functional mapping procedures.[40] However, the true clinical value of the technology will ultimately be determined by the ability of individual activation protocols to accomplish their stated purpose. To be of clinical value, an activation protocol needs to be reliable (e.g., repeatable from one test to another), sensitive to the function of interest, and specific to the predictions being made. The clinical applicability of fMRI will also depend on the proportion of patients able to undergo the procedure, the rate of adverse reactions, and the rate of technical failure. These characteristics will ultimately determine how widespread the use of fMRI becomes and, therefore, its ultimate impact on patient management.

Reliability

Because fMRI techniques are safe, they lend themselves to study of test-test reliability. In one such investigation, Binder and colleagues[41] found that repetition of a language activation protocol (described later) within an fMRI session showed a strong correlation of the language lateralization profiles between the two activation runs ($r = 0.89$), demonstrating that such language activation protocols can be highly reliable. Little information is available to date on the reliability of activation profiles across imaging sessions. Preliminary studies imply that when sources of variance between sessions are controlled, activation maps from motor and cognitive tasks can be highly reliable.[42]

Sensitivity

For functional maps to be useful in planning brain surgery, it is important to know whether all areas crucial for cognitive functions have been successfully detected. More simply, are "inactive" areas in functional maps necessarily safe to remove? Critical to the sensitivity of an imaging protocol is careful design of the activation and control tasks. Most functional neuroimaging studies use some variation of the "task subtraction" method. In this approach, brain activity in response to an experimental task is measured after subtraction of activity during a control task or "rest" period. The difference between the two states is assumed to represent the substrate specific to the function of interest. When studying complex cognitive functions in which one component operation or a focused set of operations is of experimental interest, the control task is designed to include all the components of the target task except the component of interest. An example is the design used by Binder and colleagues,[43] based on tasks introduced by Démonet and associates.[44] In this study of cerebral dominance and localization patterns, language function was defined as the combined processing of speech sounds and word meaning. The experimental task involved hearing animal names and responding to those names in a way that met semantic criteria (found in the United States and used by humans). The control task involved listening to tone sequences and responding to those sequences that contained two high (750 Hz) tones. The hypothesized component operations involved in these two tasks are illustrated in Table 151–1. Subtraction of the shared attentional, working memory, early auditory processing, and response components was intended to delineate those brain regions specific to linguistic operations involved in making a semantic decision.

Although the logic of the task subtraction method seems straightforward, misleading results can and often do occur. The validity of the task subtraction method depends on an assumption that the subjects are doing only what is asked of them, an assumption that is often unjustified. For example, subjects may engage in processing that is "unsolicited," that is, not required to perform the task. This may take the form of "automatic" processing of familiar sensory stimuli (e.g., activation of semantic circuitry when exposed to stimuli that are speechlike), episodic memory encoding, processing that is entirely unrelated to the task (e.g., thinking about something during "rest" periods), or continued processing of activation-related stimuli during the rest or control condition.

These types of unsolicited processing have been demonstrated to occur and can have significant effects on activation-control subtractions.[45–47] For example, when studying the distribution of language functions with a word generation task, it is common to use word repetition or reading as the control task. This activation-control task contrast typically produces activation in the inferior regions of the left frontal lobe[48–51] but little activation in temporal and temporal-parietal regions, which have also been associated with language functions through lesion studies.[52–55] However, when language processing tasks are contrasted with a control task using nonlinguistic stimuli, areas of activation are more widely distributed throughout the hemisphere, including parietal and temporal regions.[44, 56, 57]

TABLE 151–1 ■ **Hypothesized Functional Components in the Semantic Decision Task versus a Tone Discrimination Task**

FUNCTIONAL COMPONENT	TONE DISCRIMINATION	SEMANTIC DECISION
Semantic processing		+
Phonetic processing		+
Attention, working memory	+	+
Auditory processing	+	+
Motor response	+	+

Related to unwanted activation from automatic processing is activation from unsolicited, self-initiated cognitive operations (e.g., thinking) that may be occurring during the so-called "resting" state or during states in which attentional demands from an assigned task are minimal. Examples of such control tasks include conditions with no overt stimulation, passive stimulation, or visual fixation, as well as tasks in which performance requirements are so brief or trivial as to leave the subject with considerable time for task-unrelated processing. Subjects may be very "active" during such states, engaging in processes that involve linguistic or semantic representations, as illustrated in a study by Binder and colleagues.[45] In this study, a number of left hemisphere brain regions, including the angular gyrus, posterior cingulate gyrus, medial frontal lobe, and parts of the medial temporal lobe, showed no activation from a language task when "rest" was used as a baseline but did show activation when contrasted with a perceptual discrimination task. Thus, the use of "rest" or simple word stimuli in control conditions for language activation studies may obscure activation from the language tasks, thereby producing an inaccurate picture of language zones from the activation-control subtraction. Similar problems in protocol sensitivity have been demonstrated to occur in studies of episodic memory.[47] Development of memory control tasks is difficult because episodic memory, or the memory for events embedded in time and place, occurs automatically. Thus, the problem in studies involving language or memory is not designing a task that turns a process on but rather designing a task that turns it off.

Specificity

Also important to the use of functional maps in surgical planning is determining whether "active" areas observed during cognitive tasks are necessarily crucial for these cognitive functions. If so, then anesthetization (as in the Wada test) or surgical excision of these areas would be expected to produce deficits that can be predicted from fMRI data. If these correlations are reliable, fMRI could be substituted for the more invasive Wada test and might be useful for planning optimal surgical resection boundaries. Conversely, there may be activated regions observed by fMRI that play an ancillary rather than a crucial role or carry out processes that are not relevant to cognitive outcome. In this case, planning surgical resection to spare these areas would be inappropriate and could lead to suboptimal seizure control.

Interpretation of Individual Variation

Although it is tempting to interpret differences in activation maps between subjects as evidence of differences in brain organization or pathology, other sources of variance need to be considered first. Magnetic field inhomogeneities and subject movement are common sources of interpretive error. Subject movement can create signal changes that are sometimes indistinguishable from task-related signals. Because task-related fMRI signals are in part related to the "duty cycle" of the task, intersubject differences may be due to differences in time "on task." Other factors that may account for intersubject variability include attention and effort, emotional state, task strategy, age, handedness, sex, educational level, extent of brain pathology, medications, and prescan diet (e.g., blood glucose and caffeine levels). Techniques for minimizing variability of activation include the use of (1) strategies to optimize homogeneity in the magnetic field, (2) head restraint systems, (3) postscan image registration to minimize the effects of gross motion, (4) behavioral performance matching across subjects by adjusting task difficulty on the basis of accuracy or processing time, (5) tasks and training techniques that minimize variation in processing strategy, and (6) functional indexes that are relatively unaffected by the overall level or extent of activation (e.g., ratio measures that compare relative degrees of brain activation in different regions of the same subject).

Practical Matters

Not all patients with epilepsy are suitable candidates for fMRI studies. In addition to the usual safety requirements for studies in high magnetic fields, body weight (obesity) and shape (macrocephaly, short neck, large girth) may prevent a patient from entering the bore of the magnet or prevent the patient from viewing visual stimuli. Claustrophobic reactions may prevent an individual's study or attainment of acceptable data. Most fMRI studies require the subject to remain relatively motionless for 1 to 2 hours, a feat that is impossible for some. Many patients may not be able to understand or comply with the instructions for the activation protocol. In our own investigations, we have found that individuals whose IQ is less than 80 often have difficulty performing our language and memory activation protocols due to an inability to discriminate between tones used during the control task, limited semantic knowledge, or slowed mental processing speed.

The effects of systemic illnesses and medications on BOLD signal properties have not been well investigated. Hematocrit has a positive linear relationship to the BOLD response.[58] Caffeine is a cerebral vasoconstrictor that causes a decrease in resting BOLD signal but does not suppress the hemodynamic response from task activation, thereby producing an enhanced task-activated BOLD contrast.[59] Cocaine and methylphenidate were shown to have no significant effect on BOLD signal in two studies,[60, 61] but *d*-amphetamine was found to increase the number of voxels activated by simple auditory and motor tasks.[62] Alcohol was found in one study to reduce BOLD signal by about 33%.[63] Sell and colleagues[64] demonstrated a reduction in the number of significantly activated voxels during a visual activation paradigm after intravenous heroin injection. Ratio measures of activation that compare different regions of brain might be less affected by such reductions in gain; however, spurious or less reliable ratios might be generated when the absolute number of activated voxels in regions of interest is low.[65] The effects of antiepileptic medications on BOLD contrast have not been systematically studied to date.

IMAGING LANGUAGE LATERALIZATION AND LOCALIZATION

Clinically apparent deficits in language, typically dysnomia, occur in 8% to 14% of patients after dominant anterior temporal lobectomy (ATL),[66, 67] and measurable naming deficits occur in up to 40% to 60% of such patients when tested with sensitive regression-based techniques.[15, 16, 18] Thus, determination of cerebral dominance and localization of language functions within the dominant hemisphere are important for minimizing postoperative language morbidity in epilepsy surgery.

Many research groups have reported left-lateralized fMRI responses during a variety of language tasks.[43, 68–76] Asymmetry in hemispheric activation can be identified in individuals (as opposed to group studies) with fMRI, making it useful for individual case management. Preliminary results also suggest a high level of agreement between fMRI and Wada tests on measures of language dominance.[72, 77–86] Other studies have examined the relationship between fMRI language activation foci and language areas identified by intraoperative stimulation mapping, with encouraging results in small groups of patients.[87–90] There is reason to believe that fMRI may be more sensitive than PET in detecting language zones.[76] Whole-brain imaging is now widely available, making it possible to perform comprehensive studies of the distribution of language functions. Overall, these findings indicate that a variety of different fMRI language protocols used in a variety of settings can establish cerebral dominance.

The more commonly used language activation protocols have involved word generation to letters, categories, or verbs; determination of rhymes from text; word or sentence reading; simple auditory or reading comprehension; and semantic decisions to auditory or written stimuli. Although activation during these protocols is typically asymmetrical, all give rise to bilateral activation to some degree. Also, although there is some overlap in the activation maps obtained from the different protocols, there is also considerable variability in the activation patterns seen.[71, 91–94] This may be related as much to the different types of control conditions used by different investigators as to the actual activation brought about by the language task used (as discussed earlier). In general, protocols using word generation tasks and phonologic decisions (e.g., rhyme detection) tend to activate inferior frontal and midfrontal regions, with inconsistent activation of temporal and parietal lobes. Protocols requiring semantic decisions tend to show more consistent activation of temporal and parietal cortices in addition to the dominant frontal lobe.[69, 71] It is useful to note that none of the language activation protocols used in these studies reliably activates the anterior temporal lobe,[85, 95] the most common site of epilepsy surgery.

One language activation protocol that has been investigated thoroughly is the semantic decision paradigm.[43, 45, 95–97] Cognitive systems thought to be preferentially activated by the semantic task include phonologic input, word form, and semantic access networks. This protocol has been applied to more than 160 normal subjects and has been contrasted with various passive and active control states.[45, 95, 98, 99] These studies have consistently demonstrated strong left-lateralization of the semantic task activation, which can be seen in individual patients (see Figure 151–1 for examples of left, mixed, and right dominant activations). Commonly activated regions include the left prefrontal cortex (inferior frontal, rostral and caudal middle frontal, and superior frontal gyri; anterior cingulate gyrus), left angular gyrus, anterior superior temporal sulcus, left middle and posterior inferior temporal gyri, left fusiform and parahippocampal gyri, left anterior hippocampus, left posterior cingulate gyrus, and left thalamus. This pattern was highly reproducible across randomly selected groups of right- and left-handed healthy adults.[95, 98, 99]

Binder and colleagues studied the lateralization patterns produced during this task paradigm using a normalized language laterality index (LI), reflecting the interhemispheric difference between active voxel counts in left (L) and right (R) homologous regions of interest: $LI = (L - R)/(L + R)$. This index ranges from -1 (all active voxels in the right hemisphere) to $+1$ (all active voxels in the left hemisphere). The characteristics of this variable and the biologic factors that influence it were studied in two large series of normal subjects.[65, 99] The first study involved 100 right-handed control subjects (52 men). LIs in this group ranged from strong left dominance ($LI = 0.97$) to roughly symmetrical representation ($LI = -0.05$), with a group median LI of 0.66. Using a dominance classification scheme based on previous Wada studies, 94% of subjects were left dominant, 6% were symmetrical, and none had right dominance. Although a slight age effect (i.e., greater symmetry of language representation) was found ($r = -0.23$, $P < 0.05$), no sex differences were observed using voxel-wise or region-of-interest comparisons between men and women.[98]

In a second study, 50 non–right-handed (left-handed and ambidextrous) normal subjects (26 women) were scanned using the same semantic decision protocol.[99] Atypical (symmetrical or right-lateralized) language dominance was much more frequent in this group, with 14% showing symmetrical activation and 8% showing right dominance. A quantitative index of handedness computed from the Edinburgh Inventory[100] was positively correlated with language LI ($P < 0.05$). Subjects with a family history of left-handedness were less strongly lateralized for language than were those without left-handed relatives (mean = 0.32 versus 0.51, $P < 0.05$), providing functional imaging evidence of a genetic basis for language lateralization.

Language Lateralization in Patients with Epilepsy

The semantic decision protocol was used in a group of 50 right-handed patients with epilepsy to determine

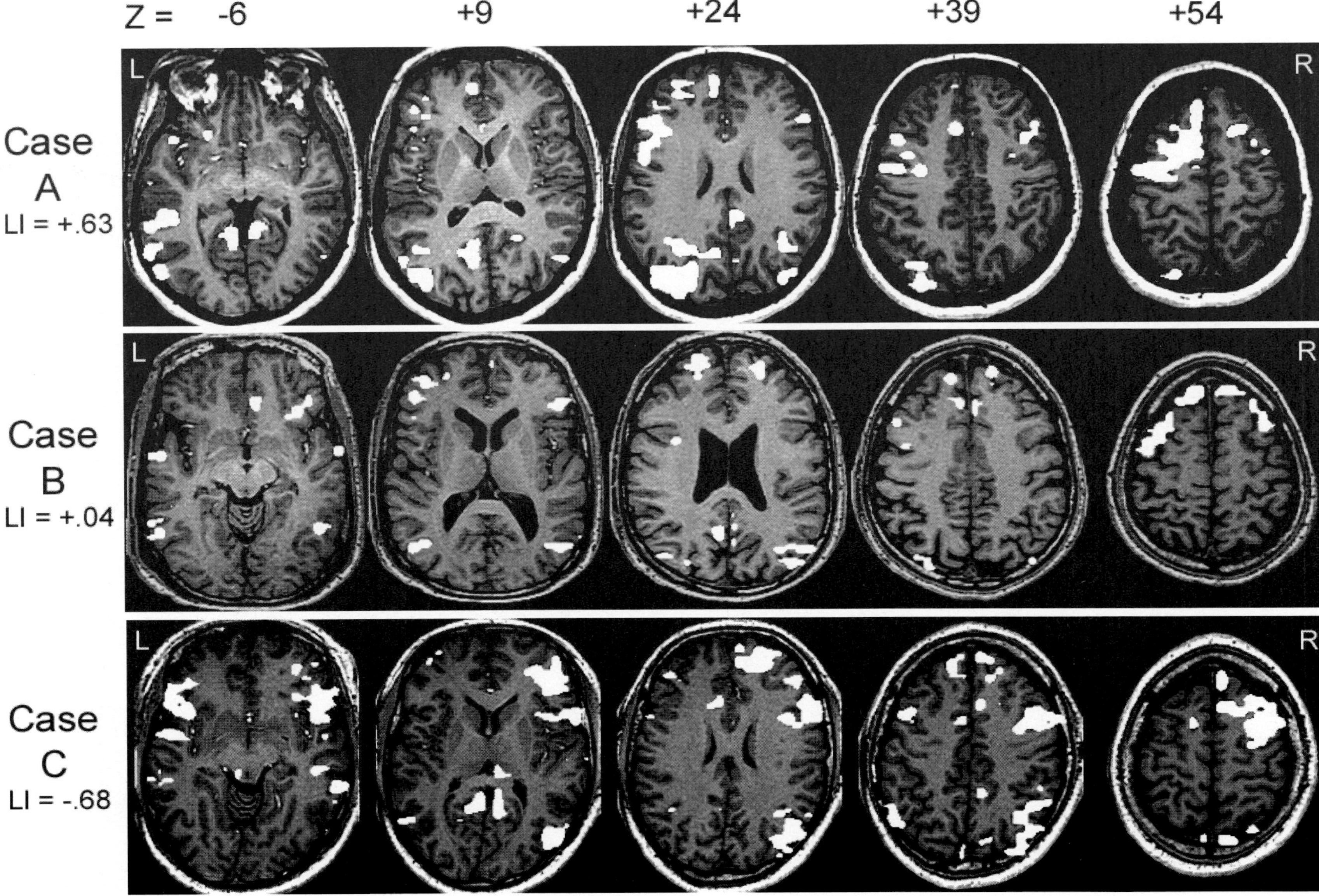

FIGURE 151–1. Case examples of lateralization of language functions with functional magnetic resonance imaging using activation from a semantic decision task contrasted with that from a tone discrimination task. Axial images at five levels of Z are provided after image registration in Talairach[191] coordinates. Areas of activation (represented in white) exceed the statistical threshold of $P < 0.01$ and a cluster size threshold of 300 μL. The lateralization index (LI) is calculated by tabulating the number of task-activated voxels in each cerebral hemisphere, such that LI = (left − right)/(left + right). Case A shows strong left hemisphere lateralization. Case B shows activation that is approximately equally distributed between the hemispheres. Case C shows strong right hemisphere lateralization.

whether lateralization is altered in any systematic way relative to normal right-handed controls.[65] Compared with the control group, epilepsy patients had a significantly higher incidence of atypical language lateralization—22% of patients with epilepsy versus 6% of control subjects ($P < 0.01$). Atypical lateralization increased in those with a younger age at onset of epilepsy ($r = 0.50$, $P < 0.001$). These results are in agreement with previous Wada studies showing similar relationships, further validating the fMRI lateralization measure. They also emphasize the importance of measuring language lateralization before surgery, particularly in patients with long-standing epilepsy. In a study of 61 patients with right-sided and 66 patients with left-sided seizures, Swanson and coworkers[101] found that fMRI language lateralization was shifted more to the right hemisphere in patients with left-sided seizures that began before 6 years of age ($r = 0.36$, $P < 0.001$). This reorganization of language to the right was found to be correlated with poorer preoperative naming abilities.

Comparisons with Wada Language Testing

Across a variety of different activation protocols and Wada procedures, preliminary results suggest a high level of agreement between fMRI and Wada tests on measures of language.[72, 77–86] Most of these studies had relatively small sample sizes (7 to 13 patients) and relatively few crossed-dominant individuals. Binder and colleagues published the largest series to date and attempted to study the statistical relationship between language dominance determined from the semantic decision protocol and a quantified index of language laterality from Wada testing. In the first series of 22 consecutive patients with epilepsy, fMRI LI was found to be highly correlated with language asymmetry determined by the Wada test ($r = 0.96$).[80] In a subsequent analysis, dominance classification by Wada and the fMRI semantic decision protocol was concordant in 48 of 49 (98%) consecutive patients with valid examinations.[41]

Prediction of Postoperative Language Morbidity

More important than concordance with Wada testing is whether fMRI language protocols can predict language decline after ATL surgery. The only specific study of this issue to date is encouraging. Sabsevitz and coworkers[102] measured the relationship between semantic decision fMRI LIs and the change between pre- and postoperative scores on the Boston Naming Test. Included were 55 patients about equally distributed between right and left ATL. ATL was performed by a neurosurgeon without benefit of fMRI language maps. As expected, greater activation in the left temporal region of interest (ROI) relative to the right ROI correlated significantly with postoperative naming decline ($r = -0.54$, $P = 0.02$).

Surgical Planning with Functional Magnetic Resonance Imaging Language Maps

It remains to be established whether fMRI language activation maps will allow more precise planning of surgical resections. At least three significant problems complicate progress in this area: (1) inconsistencies in language maps produced by different activation protocols; (2) the failure to find an activation protocol that reliably activates the anterior temporal lobe, where the majority of epilepsy surgeries are performed[71, 85, 95]; and (3) an inadequate understanding of the specificity of fMRI activation.

As indicated earlier, the different fMRI language activation protocols have produced markedly different patterns of activation.[71, 81, 85, 91–94, 103] Although minor variance in activation profiles is plausible, due to different demands on separate subcomponents of language function by different activation tasks, this does not account for the full range of variance in these studies. Rather, these findings suggest that activation maps are strongly dependent on the specific contrast between the language and control tasks used in the activation protocol (discussed earlier). Also, none of these language protocols is associated with robust anterior temporal lobe activation. Because the dominant anterior temporal lobe is known to contribute to language processing,[57, 104–110] and because left ATL can result in language decline,[15, 16, 18, 111–114] it follows that these protocols are not detecting crucial language areas. Clearly, further language activation task development is necessary.

In addition, it may be necessary to incorporate multiple activation protocols before a complete picture of language zones in an individual can be discerned.[71] For example, rare patients show a dissociation on the Wada test between performance on language tasks emphasizing speech output (repetition, counting) and those emphasizing comprehension, suggesting that in these cases the capacity for speech production resides in one hemisphere and speech comprehension in the other.[12, 115] In the few cases encountered in our studies, fMRI findings using the semantic decision–tone contrast were more closely aligned with the comprehension component of the Wada test.[116]

It is conceivable that some regions activated during language tasks may play a minor, supportive role rather than a critical role in language, and resection of these active foci may not produce clinically relevant or persistent deficits. Systematic studies of such specificity for surgical planning have yet to be done.

IMAGING MEDIAL TEMPORAL (MEMORY) ACTIVATION

Equally important in the presurgical evaluation of temporal lobe epilepsy (TLE) is the study of long-term episodic memory systems. Functional imaging of long-term memory systems is potentially useful in two ways. First, the identification of functionally hypoactive temporal lobe memory areas may have predictive value for the localization of seizure foci in TLE. Second, maps of temporal lobe activation associated with long-term memory encoding tasks may help predict the risk of postoperative memory encoding deficits from temporal lobectomy and could assist in planning optimal surgical excision boundaries that spare functional tissue.

Human lesion studies suggest that the medial temporal lobe (MTL) is critical for creating a stable representation of explicit events in long-term memory.[117, 118] Current models propose that the MTL coordinates unimodal and multimodal association cortex activity during perception, comprehension, and response to a stimulus event (or "episode"). Coordination of activity in these systems creates a linkage among the salient stimulus elements (including the environment or context in which the stimulus occurs), stored knowledge (e.g., semantic or spatial information) associated with these elements, and behavioral responses by the subject to the stimulus, creating a unitary representation of the episode for later retrieval from long-term memory.[119–121] However, attempts to use functional imaging to capture the processes in the MTL related to the formation of new memories have lagged behind the functional imaging of other cognitive operations.

Several factors might explain the relatively low success rate in previous attempts to detect activation in the MTL. The hippocampal formation in the MTL is relatively small in comparison to the volume elements (voxels) used in functional imaging, particularly those used in PET. Within-voxel averaging of signals from active and inactive structures may thus impair detection of hippocampal activity when larger voxels are used. In fMRI, loss of signal commonly occurs near air-tissue interfaces due to macroscopic field inhomogeneities. A brain region that is often affected by this phenomenon is the ventral-medial temporal pole, including, in some cases, parts of the amygdala and anterior entorhinal cortex,[122] thus obscuring detection of BOLD responses in these regions. Finally, the "control" state used in subtraction analyses is probably critical, in that detection of MTL activation is difficult if MTL activity continues to occur during the control condition.[47] Some evidence suggests that MTL encoding processes continue beyond the duration of the stimulus or event.[119, 123] Baseline signal levels in the MTL may thus vary, depending on the encoding demands of prior stimuli, the elapsed time since stimulus presentation, and concurrent task demands imposed during the baseline condition.

Bilateral posterior MTL (primarily posterior parahippocampus) activation during the encoding of spatial and verbal episodes has been demonstrated in numerous human fMRI studies.[47, 124–132] Many of these experiments involved a comparison between the encoding of novel and repeating environmental scenes. This task presumably involves the encoding of both the spatial configuration of the scene and a verbal configuration involving semantic associations of components of the scene. These results suggest that the posterior MTL plays a role in encoding novel scenes, with the magnitude of activation related to the strength of encoding, as measured by success on later recognition testing.[124, 125, 132] Consistent with this finding, Detre and associates[133] found that activation of posterior MTL regions can be used to predict memory lateralization in TLE. These investigators used an environmental-scene encoding task in which subjects were asked to memorize each stimulus. In the baseline condition, subjects passively viewed a repeating nonsense stimulus (a spatially scrambled picture). Asymmetry of activation in the posterior MTL was then used to calculate a memory lateralization score. Lateralization scores on fMRI corresponded closely with memory lateralization indexes calculated from the memory portion of the Wada test.

Cognitive factors that modulate MTL activity are not fully understood. A clue suggested by activation in this region during semantic language tasks is that the anterior MTL may be sensitive to the relational properties of an encoded episode.[128, 134–136] Meaningful stimuli, such as words and pictures, that can be tied to a larger semantic or spatial context may engage the anterior MTL by eliciting widespread activation of stored knowledge in polymodal association areas.[128, 134–138] In contrast, stimuli that are relatively meaningless should not elicit such relational processing. We tested this idea by comparing visual encoding tasks that differed in terms of either stimulus novelty or meaningfulness.[139] During two task contrasts, 34 normal, right-handed subjects were scanned. In the novelty contrast, encoding of novel scenes was compared with encoding of repeating scenes, similar to several previous studies.[126, 130, 140] For both conditions, the task was to decide whether the pictures represented indoor or outdoor scenes. In the relational processing contrast, encoding of novel pictures was compared with encoding of novel, incoherent (spatially scrambled) images. The task with the scrambled images was to decide whether the left and right halves of the image matched. The novelty contrast produced activation primarily in the posterior parahippocampus bilaterally, replicating prior studies. The relational contrast produced activation bilaterally in the anterior MTL, particularly in the anterior hippocampus (see Figure 151–2 for an example of hippocampal activation with this protocol).[139]

As a first step in validating this "scene encoding" protocol in epilepsy patients, we compared MTL functional LIs based on this protocol with LIs derived from Wada memory testing and with asymmetry scores derived from hippocampal volumetric measurement.[141] Functional MRI LIs were calculated for several MTL ROIs, including the anterior hippocampus, posterior hippocampus, anterior parahippocampus–fusiform gyrus, posterior parahippocampus–fusiform gyrus, and anterior temporal lobe (defined as all temporal lobe tissue anterior to a coronal plane through the posterior margin of the interpeduncular cistern), and for various combinations of these ROIs. Each ROI was derived by manually tracing the ROI in 30 to 40 individual brains and then averaging the tracings to create a probabilistic map of the ROI in stereotaxic space. Wada LIs and hippocampal asymmetry indexes were calculated by

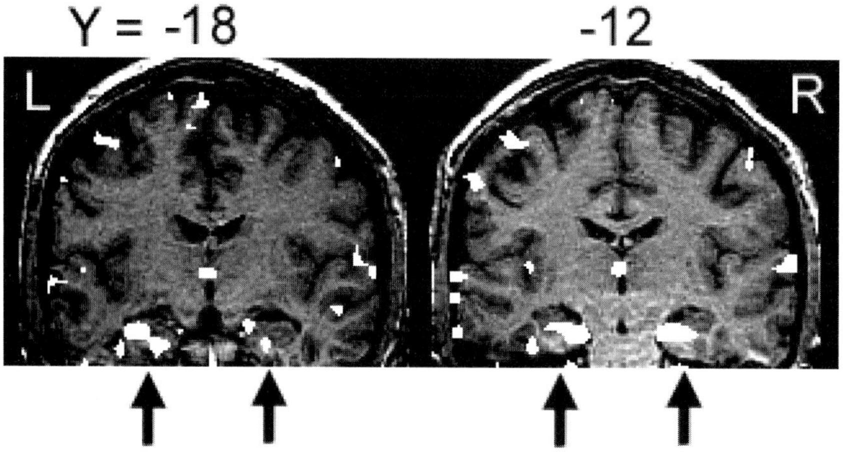

FIGURE 151–2. An example of hippocampal activation from blood oxygen level–dependent (BOLD) functional magnetic resonance imaging using signal increase from a scene encoding task contrasted with that from a perceptual discrimination task in a patient with right temporal lobe epilepsy. Coronal images in two planes of Y dimension are provided after image registration in Talairach[191] coordinates. Areas of activation (represented in white) exceed the statistical threshold of $P < 0.01$ and a cluster size threshold of 200 μL. Note that although hippocampal activation is bilateral, it is asymmetrical, with less activation occurring on the side of the seizure focus.

methods similar to those used by others.[7, 142] In a study of 55 patients diagnosed with probable TLE who had valid Wada memory testing, the Wada memory LI was modestly correlated with the anterior hippocampus fMRI LI ($r = 0.43$, $P = 0.001$) and less so with the posterior hippocampus LI ($r = 0.26$, $P = 0.058$). Hippocampal volume asymmetry indexes were correlated with the anterior hippocampus fMRI LI ($r = 0.46$, $P = 0.004$), the posterior hippocampus LI ($r = 0.33$, $P = 0.04$), and the combined anterior and posterior hippocampus LI ($r = 0.49$, $P = 0.002$), but not with LIs based on other ROIs. These data provide preliminary evidence for the validity of using scene encoding fMRI as an index of MTL functional asymmetry. More important, they demonstrate that functional activation in the hippocampus proper, and particularly in the anterior hippocampus, is much more closely linked to functional and anatomic asymmetries associated with TLE than is functional activation in nonhippocampal MTL regions, in agreement with a recent PET study.[143]

Another major aim of preoperative functional mapping in TLE is to estimate the risk of postoperative memory decline from left ATL surgery. Although a number of research groups are actively working on this issue, to date, there are limited data on fMRI as a predictor of memory outcome. One study found that memory activation asymmetries in an amygdalohippocampal ROI from preoperative fMRI correlated with postoperative changes in recognition memory performance.[144]

LATERALIZING THE SEIZURE FOCUS IN TEMPORAL LOBE EPILEPSY

More important than concordance with Wada testing or structural MRI is whether fMRI can be used to predict the side of seizure focus. Preliminary studies have focused on asymmetry of activation in the MTL, with the assumption that the side of decreased activation represents the epileptic temporal lobe. In a series of eight patients, Killgore and colleagues[145] found that activation asymmetry during a visual memory task predicted 1-year postoperative seizure control as well as the asymmetry in Wada memory scores. Wada and fMRI data were found to provide complementary information that collectively enhanced prediction accuracy. Jokeit and colleagues[127] studied 30 epileptic patients (16 left and 14 right TLE) and 17 healthy controls with a mental navigation task that required retrieval of knowledge about places that were familiar to the individuals. Although they found no systematic interhemispheric differences in MTL activation in their control subjects, interhemispheric differences correctly classified the side of seizures in 90% of those with epilepsy, yielding a sensitivity of 0.93 and a specificity of 0.88.

Binder and colleagues presented a larger series using their visual scene memory protocol and also found that prediction of side of seizure focus was comparable to Wada memory testing.[146, 147] Of 49 patients with probable TLE based on ictal video-electroencephalogram, Wada testing, and structural MRI, supplemented when necessary by invasive electroencephalogram, 24 were considered to have left TLE and 25 right TLE. Activation asymmetry was significantly more right-lateralized in the left TLE group than in the right TLE group for the anterior hippocampus ($P = 0.004$) but not for the posterior hippocampus or parahippocampus. Functional MRI correctly predicted the side of seizure focus in 73% of the patients. These results were similar to Wada memory testing, which also produced significantly more right-lateralized asymmetry scores in the left TLE group and correctly classified 81% of the patients. Thus, the predictive power of fMRI appears to be comparable to that of Wada memory testing, but it depends on the specific brain region in which activation asymmetry is assessed.

ICTAL LOCALIZATION OF SEIZURES

The technical ability to simultaneously record electrophysiologic activity and BOLD signal has made it possible to localize more directly the focus of seizure onset or the regions of abnormal discharge.[148, 149] Several investigators have been successful in using BOLD contrast to localize the origin of abnormal discharges.[150–156]

These investigators found evidence of increased perfusion during the intervals of abnormal electrical discharges. The initiation of an fMRI scan can be triggered by the first signs of abnormal discharge and then compared with an image obtained in the absence of epileptiform discharges.[156] Alternatively, a predefined ictal pattern on electroencephalogram can be used to trigger the scanner.[153] Bookheimer[157] described a patient with reflex epilepsy in whom seizures occurred with eye closure, an ideal circumstance for fMRI study. BOLD signal can also be used to identify the subcortical circuitry associated with the ictal events, thereby facilitating an understanding of the semiology of the seizure.[151] This strategy of localizing the source and distribution of abnormal discharges is not limited to patients who have frank seizures in the MRI scanner; it can also be used to detect subclinical neuroelectrical events.[150, 155, 156]

It remains to be seen how useful fMRI may be for this application in intractable epilepsy. Abnormal electrical discharges need to occur on a relatively frequent basis, either spontaneously or through elicitation by drugs or external stimulation, in order to make this method practical. The ideal patient is one with simple motor or sensory seizures, or one with complex partial seizures with minimal movement, in whom abnormal discharges occur frequently or can be readily precipitated. Imaging several events aids in the precision of localization. Ideally, ictal activity should be verified by electroencephalogram recordings acquired concurrently with fMRI. An additional interpretive problem regarding seizure origin arises when there are multiple areas of cortical activation, a situation that requires further refinement of image processing methods to optimize temporal resolution of the signal. It is also important to discriminate movement artifacts from BOLD signal contrast.[158] Patients who have secondary generalization from partial seizures would likely be excluded from study owing to movement artifacts.

IMAGING SENSORY AND MOTOR FUNCTIONS

Robust BOLD signal, often of a magnitude of 3% to 4% change on a 1.5-tesla system, can be easily achieved in sensory and motor cortices, making it relatively easy to determine boundaries of functional tissue in these cortical regions.[72, 159–163] A number of activation protocols are now available that enable one to study the functional integrity of the retinotopic organization of the visual cortex,[164–166] tonotopic organization of auditory cortices,[167, 168] and somatotopic organization in somatosensory and motor cortices.[169–172]

The sensorimotor homunculus can be easily identified with toe wiggling, finger tapping, and tongue movements. Simple somatosensory stimulation might include brushing the surface of the skin, passive joint position changes, or air puffs. In general, the more complex the stimulus or movement, and the more attentional systems engaged by it, the more distributed the activation becomes. It is possible to stimulate multiple sensory and motor systems simultaneously if specificity of activation is not an issue.[72] The magnitude of the BOLD signal in primary sensory and motor areas is roughly linearly related to the speed at which stimuli must be processed or movement occurs.[27, 173–176] Activation can be identified in dysplastic tissue,[154, 177–179] in edematous tissue,[162, 180] and within ischemic zones.[181] Functional tissue is typically distorted and displaced by mass lesions.[160, 162, 163, 178, 180] The accuracy of these functional maps has been studied with transcranial magnetic stimulation,[182, 183] intraoperative cortical stimulation,[72, 160, 162, 171, 178, 182, 184–187] and PET,[188] and the congruence between procedures is typically within 3 to 5 mm. Other recent studies have advised caution about precise reliance on fMRI maps owing to image distortion, which is common in echoplanar imaging.[189, 190]

Still, a fundamental question for predicting postoperative morbidity is whether all activation seen in fMRI is critical to performing the function in question. In our own experience, surgical disconnection of tissue that shows preoperative fMRI task activation does not always result in postoperative deficit. Additional research is necessary before these relationships are better understood. Functional MRI certainly has the potential to help us understand the nature of functional tissue. For example, Beauchamp and colleagues[181] demonstrated that tissue in the occipital lobe of a stroke patient with visual field and color vision deficits that appeared to be damaged in clinical scans apparently retained functional capacity when visual stimuli were presented during fMRI. Thus, fMRI not only offers the ability to define the boundaries of functional tissue in presurgical populations; it also may assist in identifying tissue that can participate in the recovery of function.

CONCLUSION

There is reason to be excited about the application of fMRI to the evaluation of patients for epilepsy surgery. The technology has evolved rapidly and offers a generally safe and reliable means of brain mapping, with excellent repeatability and spatial resolution. Activation protocols have been developed that reliably establish cerebral dominance for language and memory functions, creating the possibility of an alternative to the Wada examination in the presurgical workup of intractable epilepsy (although preliminary data suggest that these two procedures may provide complementary information). Information derived from fMRI protocols shows excellent promise for predicting the outcome of seizure surgery, in terms of both seizure control and morbidity. Considerable progress has also been made in localizing cognitive, sensory, and motor functions and in detecting seizures with fMRI.

Still, there is reason to be cautious about the clinical application of fMRI. As with any new diagnostic test, sources of error in interpretation need to be understood before the test is implemented clinically. Procedures for determining when a study is technically valid need to be developed, likely requiring close attention to movement, motivation, and task compliance. Because the sensitivity and specificity of the technology are highly protocol specific, each activation protocol will have to be studied in some detail to learn its predictive characteristics before clinical implementation. Using fMRI procedures to predict low-frequency events (e.g., aphasia or amnesia following temporal lobectomy) will require a large normative population to accurately estimate risk. Last, sources of error in overlaying echoplanar functional maps on anatomic maps will need to be overcome before precise estimation of functional boundaries can be used to tailor surgical resections.

REFERENCES

1. Engel J Jr, Van Ness PC, Rasmussen TB, Ojemann LM: Outcome with respect to epileptic seizures. In Engel J Jr (ed): Surgical Treatment of the Epilepsies. New York, Raven Press, 1993, pp 609–621.
2. Vickrey BG, Hays RD, Hermann BP, et al: Outcomes with respect to quality of life. In Engel J Jr (ed): Surgical Treatment of the Epilepsies. New York, Raven Press, 1993, pp 623–635.
3. Sperling MR, O'Connor MJ, Saykin AJ, et al: Temporal lobectomy for refractory epilepsy. JAMA 276:470–475, 1996.
4. Salanova V, Markand O, Worth R: Longitudinal follow-up in 145 patients with medically refractory temporal lobe epilepsy treated surgically between 1984 and 1995. Epilepsia 40:1417–1423, 1999.
5. Wiebe S, Blume WT, Girvin JP, et al: A randomized, controlled trial of surgery for temporal-lobe epilepsy. N Engl J Med 345: 311–318, 2001.
6. Luders H, Lesser RP, Dinner DS, et al: Commentary: Chronic intracranial recording and stimulation with subdural electrodes. In Engel J Jr (ed): Surgical Treatment of the Epilepsies. New York, Raven Press, 1993, pp 297–321.
7. Loring DW, Meador KJ, Lee GP, King DW: Amobarbital Effects and Lateralized Brain Function: The Wada Test. New York, Springer-Verlag, 1992.
8. Wada J, Rasmussen TB: Intracarotid injection of sodium amytal for the lateralization of cerebral speech dominance. J Neurosurg 17:266–282, 1960.
9. Arroyo S, Lesser RP, Awad IA, et al: Subdural and epidural grids and strips. In Engel J Jr (ed): Surgical Treatment of the Epilepsies. New York, Raven Press, 1993, pp 377–386.
10. Lesser RP, Luders H, Klem G, et al: Extraoperative cortical functional localization in patients with epilepsy. J Clin Neurophysiol 4:27–53, 1987.
11. Benbadis S, Wyllie E, Bingaman WE: Intracranial electroencephalography and localization studies. In Wyllie E (ed): The Treatment of Epilepsy: Principles and Practice. Philadelphia, Lippincott Williams & Wilkins, 2001, pp 1067–1075.
12. Ojemann G, Ojemann J, Lettich E, Berger M: Cortical language localization in left, dominant hemisphere: An electrical stimulation mapping investigation in 117 patients. J Neurosurg 71: 316–326, 1989.
13. Gaillard WD: Metabolic and functional neuroimaging. In Wyllie E (ed): The Treatment of Epilepsy: Principles and Practice. Philadelphia, Lippincott Williams & Wilkins, 2001, pp 1053–1056.
14. Pardo FS, Aronen HJ, Kennedy D, et al: Functional cerebral imaging in the evaluation and radiotherapeutic treatment planning of patients with malignant glioma. Int J Radiat Oncol Biol Phys 30:663–669, 1994.
15. Bell BD, Davies KG, Hermann BP, Walters G: Confrontation naming after anterior temporal lobectomy is related to age of acquisition of the object names. Neuropsychologia 38:83–92, 2000.
16. Brown SP, Swanson SJ, Sabsevitz DS, et al: Assessing language outcome after temporal lobectomy using regression-based change norms. J Int Neuropsychol Soc 8:270, 2002.
17. Chelune CJ, Naugle RI, Luders H, Sediak J: Individual change after epilepsy surgery: Practice effects and base-rate information. Neuropsychology 7:41–52, 1993.
18. Davies KG, Bell BD, Bush AJ, et al: Naming decline after left anterior temporal lobectomy correlates with pathological status of resected hippocampus. Epilepsia 39:407–419, 1998.
19. Martin RC, Sawrie SM, Roth DL, et al: Individual memory change after anterior temporal lobectomy: A base rate analysis using regression-based outcome methodology. Epilepsia 39: 1075–1082, 1998.
20. Berkovic SF, McIntosh AM, Kalnins RM, et al: Preoperative MRI predicts outcome of temporal lobectomy: An actuarial analysis. Neurology 45:1358–1363, 1995.
21. Dodrill CB, Wilkus RJ, Ojemann GA, et al: Multidisciplinary prediction of seizure relief from cortical resection surgery. Ann Neurol 20:2–12, 1986.
22. So N, Gloor P, Quesney LF, et al: Depth electrode investigations in patients with bitemporal epileptiform abnormalities. Ann Neurol 25:423–431, 1989.
23. Spencer SS: Depth electroencephalography in selection of refractory epilepsy for surgery. Ann Neurol 9:207–214, 1981.
24. Spencer SS, Soares JC: Depth electrodes. In Engel J Jr (ed): Surgical Treatment of the Epilepsies. New York, Raven Press, 1993, pp 359–376.
25. Spencer SS: Selection of candidates for temporal resection. In Wyllie E (ed): The Treatment of Epilepsy: Principles and Practice. Philadelphia, Lippincott Williams & Wilkins, 2001, pp 1031–1041.
26. Pilcher WH, Rusyniak WG: Complications of epilepsy surgery. Neurosurg Clin N Am 4:311–325, 1993.
27. Kwong KK, Belliveau JW, Chesler DA, et al: Dynamic magnetic resonance imaging of human brain activity during primary sensory stimulation. Proc Natl Acad Sci U S A 89:5675–5679, 1992.
28. Moonen CTW, Bandettini PA: Functional MRI. New York, Springer-Verlag, 1999.
29. Ogawa S, Tank DW, Menon R, et al: Intrinsic signal changes accompanying sensory stimulation: Functional brain mapping with magnetic resonance imaging. Proc Natl Acad Sci U S A 89:5951–5955, 1992.
30. Fox PT, Raichle ME: Focal physiological uncoupling of cerebral blood flow and oxidative metabolism during somatosensory stimuluation in human subjects. Proc Natl Acad Sci U S A 83: 1140–1144, 1986.
31. Thulborn KR, Waterton JC, Matthews PM, Radda GK: Oxygenation dependence of the transverse relaxation time of water protons in whole blood at high field. Biochim Biophys Acta 714: 265–270, 1982.
32. Ogawa S, Lee TM, Kay AR, Tank DW: Brain magnetic resonance imaging with contrast dependent on blood oxygenation. Proc Natl Acad Sci U S A 87:9868–9872, 1990.
33. Bandettini PA, Wong EC, Hinks RS, et al: Time course EPI of human brain function during task activation. Magn Reson Med 25:390–397, 1992.
34. Logothetis NK, Pauls J, Augath M, et al: Neurophysiological investigation of the basis of the fMRI signal. Nature 412:150–157, 2001.
35. Arthurs OJ, Boniface S: How well do we understand the neural origins of the fMRI BOLD signal? Trends Neurosci 25:27–31, 2002.
36. Heeger DJ, Ress D: What does fMRI tell us about neuronal activity? Nat Rev Neurosci 3:142–151, 2002.
37. D'Esposito M: Functional neuroimaging of cognition. Semin Neurol 20:487–498, 2000.
38. Nadeau SE, Crosson B: A guide to the functional imaging of cognitive processes. Neuropsychiatry Neuropsychol Behav Neurol 8:143–162, 1995.
39. Cabeza R, Nyberg L: Imaging cognition II: An empirical review of 275 PET and fMRI studies. J Cogn Neurosci 12:1–47, 2000.
40. Lee CC, Ward HA, Sharbrough FW, et al: Assessment of functional MR imaging in neurosurgical planning. AJNR Am J Neuroradiol 20:1511–1519, 1999.
41. Binder JR, Hammeke TA, Possing ET, et al: Reliability and validity of language dominance assessment with functional MRI. Neurology 56(Suppl):A158, 2001.
42. Noll DC, Genovese CR, Nystrom LE, et al: Estimating test-retest reliability in functional MR imaging. II. Application to motor and cognitive activation studies. Magn Reson Med 38:508–517, 1997.
43. Binder JR, Rao SM, Hammeke TA, et al: Lateralized human brain language systems demonstrated by task subtraction functional magnetic resonance imaging. Arch Neurol 52:593–601, 1995.
44. Démonet JF, Chollet F, Ramsay S, et al: The anatomy of phono-

logical and semantic processing in normal subjects. Brain 115(Pt 6):1753–1768, 1992.
45. Binder JR, Frost JA, Hammeke TA, et al: Conceptual processing during the conscious resting state: A functional MRI study. J Cogn Neurosci 11:80–95, 1999.
46. Price CJ, Wise RJ, Frackowiak RS: Demonstrating the implicit processing of visually presented words and pseudowords. Cereb Cortex 6:62–70, 1996.
47. Stark CE, Squire LR: When zero is not zero: The problem of ambiguous baseline conditions in fMRI. Proc Natl Acad Sci U S A 98:12760–12766, 2001.
48. Buckner RL, Raichle ME, Petersen SE: Dissociation of human prefrontal cortical areas across different speech production tasks and gender groups. J Neurophysiol 74:2163–2173, 1995.
49. Petersen SE, Fox PT, Posner MI, et al: Positron emission tomographic studies of the cortical anatomy of single-word processing. Nature 331:585–589, 1988.
50. Raichle ME, Fiez JA, Videen TO, et al: Practice-related changes in human brain functional anatomy during nonmotor learning. Cereb Cortex 4:8–26, 1994.
51. Buckner RL, Petersen SE, Ojemann JG, et al: Functional anatomical studies of explicit and implicit memory retrieval tasks. J Neurosci 15(Pt 1):12–29, 1995.
52. Damasio AR: Aphasia. N Engl J Med 326:531–539, 1992.
53. Geschwind N: Disconnexion syndromes in animals and man. Brain 88:237–294, 1965.
54. Luria AR: Higher Cortical Functions in Man. New York, Basic Books, 1966.
55. Damasio H, Damasio AR: Lesion Analysis in Neuropsychology. Oxford, Oxford University Press, 1989.
56. Binder JR: Neuroanatomy of language processing studied with functional MRI. Clin Neurosci 4:87–94, 1997.
57. Damasio H, Grabowski TJ, Tranel D, et al: A neural basis for lexical retrieval. Nature 380:499–505, 1996.
58. Levin JM, Frederick BB, Ross MH, et al: Influence of baseline hematocrit and hemodilution on BOLD fMRI activation. Magn Reson Imaging 19:1055–1062, 2001.
59. Mulderink TA, Gitelman DR, Mesulam MM, Parrish TB: On the use of caffeine as a contrast booster for BOLD fMRI studies. Neuroimage 15:37–44, 2002.
60. Gollub RL, Breiter HC, Kantor H, et al: Cocaine decreases cortical cerebral blood flow but does not obscure regional activation in functional magnetic resonance imaging in human subjects. J Cereb Blood Flow Metab 18:724–734, 1998.
61. Rao SM, Salmeron BJ, Durgerian S, et al: Effects of methylphenidate on functional MRI blood-oxygen-level-dependent contrast. Am J Psychiatry 157:1697–1699, 2000.
62. Uftring SJ, Wachtel SR, Chu D, et al: An fMRI study of the effect of amphetamine on brain activity. Neuropsychopharmacology 25:925–935, 2001.
63. Levin JM, Ross MH, Mendelson JH, et al: Reduction in BOLD fMRI response to primary visual stimulation following alcohol ingestion. Psychiatry Res 82:135–146, 1998.
64. Sell LA, Simmons A, Lemmens GM, et al: Functional magnetic resonance imaging of the acute effect of intravenous heroin administration on visual activation in long-term heroin addicts: Results from a feasibility study. Drug Alcohol Depend 49:55–60, 1997.
65. Springer JA, Binder JR, Hammeke TA, et al: Language dominance in neurologically normal and epilepsy subjects: A functional MRI study. Brain 122(Pt 11):2033–2046, 1999.
66. Ojemann GA: Mapping of neuropsychological language parameters at surgery. Int Anesthesiol Clin 24:115–131, 1986.
67. Swanson SJ, Lisk LM, Morris GL, et al: Language function following temporal lobectomy with functional mapping. Epilepsia 35(Suppl 8):103, 1994.
68. Bavelier G, Corkin S, Jezzard P, et al: Sentence reading: A functional MRI study at 4 tesla. J Cogn Neurosci 9:664–686, 1997.
69. Billingsley RL, McAndrews MP, Crawley AP, Mikulis DJ: Functional MRI of phonological and semantic processing in temporal lobe epilepsy. Brain 124(Pt 6):1218–1227, 2001.
70. Chee MW, O'Craven KM, Bergida R, et al: Auditory and visual word processing studied with fMRI. Hum Brain Map 7:15–28, 1999.
71. Gaillard WD, Bookheimer SY, Cohen M: The use of fMRI in neocortical epilepsy. Adv Neurol 84:391–404, 2000.
72. Hirsch J, Ruge MI, Kim KH, et al: An integrated functional magnetic resonance imaging procedure for preoperative mapping of cortical areas associated with tactile, motor, language, and visual functions. Neurosurgery 47:711–721, 2000.
73. Poldrack RA, Wagner AD, Prull MW, et al: Functional specialization for semantic and phonological processing in the left inferior prefrontal cortex. Neuroimage 10:15–35, 1999.
74. Pujol J, Deus J, Losilla JM, Capdevila A: Cerebral lateralization of language in normal left-handed people studied by functional MRI. Neurology 52:1038–1043, 1999.
75. Shaywitz BA, Shaywitz SE, Pugh KR, et al: Sex differences in the functional organization of the brain for language. Nature 373:607–609, 1995.
76. Xiong J, Rao S, Gao JH, et al: Evaluation of hemispheric dominance for language using functional MRI: A comparison with positron emission tomography. Hum Brain Map 6:42–58, 1998.
77. Bahn MM, Lin W, Silbergeld DL, et al: Localization of language cortices by functional MR imaging compared with intracarotid amobarbital hemispheric sedation. AJR Am J Roentgenol 169: 575–579, 1997.
78. Bazin B, Cohen L, Lehericy S, et al: Study of hemispheric lateralization of language regions by functional MRI: Validation with the Wada test. Rev Neurol (Paris) 156:145–148, 2000.
79. Benson RR, FitzGerald DB, LeSueur LL, et al: Language dominance determined by whole brain functional MRI in patients with brain lesions. Neurology 52:798–809, 1999.
80. Binder JR, Swanson SJ, Hammeke TA, et al: Determination of language dominance using functional MRI: A comparison with the Wada test. Neurology 46:978–984, 1996.
81. Carpentier A, Pugh KR, Westerveld M, et al: Functional MRI of language processing: Dependence on input modality and temporal lobe epilepsy. Epilepsia 42:1241–1254, 2001.
82. Desmond JE, Sum JM, Wagner AD, et al: Functional MRI measurement of language lateralization in Wada-tested patients. Brain 118:1411–1419, 1995.
83. Gao X, Jiang C, Lu C, Shen T: Determination of the dominant language hemisphere by functional MRI in patients with temporal lobe epilepsy. Chin Med J 114:711–713, 2001.
84. Hertz-Pannier L, Gaillard WD, Mott SH, et al: Noninvasive assessment of language dominance in children and adolescents with functional MRI: A preliminary study. Neurology 48:1003–1012, 1997.
85. Lehericy S, Cohen L, Bazin B, et al: Functional MR evaluation of temporal and frontal language dominance compared with the Wada test. Neurology 54:1625–1633, 2000.
86. Yetkin FZ, Swanson S, Fischer M, et al: Functional MR of frontal lobe activation: Comparison with Wada language results. AJNR Am J Neuroradiol 19:1095–1098, 1998.
87. FitzGerald DB, Cosgrove GR, Ronner S, et al: Location of language in the cortex: A comparison between functional MR imaging and electrocortical stimulation. AJNR Am J Neuroradiol 18:1529–1539, 1997.
88. Ruge MI, Victor J, Hosain S, et al: Concordance between functional magnetic resonance imaging and intraoperative language mapping. Stereotact Funct Neurosurg 72:95–102, 1999.
89. Stapleton SR, Kiriakopoulos E, Mikulis D, et al: Combined utility of functional MRI, cortical mapping, and frameless stereotaxy in the resection of lesions in eloquent areas of brain in children. Pediatr Neurosurg 26:68–82, 1997.
90. Yetkin FZ, Mueller WM, Hammeke TA, et al: Functional magnetic resonance imaging mapping of the sensorimotor cortex with tactile stimulation. Neurosurgery 36:921–925, 1995.
91. Binder JR, Achten E, Constable RT, et al: Functional MRI in epilepsy. Epilepsia 43(Suppl 1):51–63, 2002.
92. Bookheimer SY, Dapretto M, Karmarkar U: Functional MRI in children with epilepsy. Dev Neurosci 21:191–199, 1999.
93. Detre JA, Floyd TF: Functional MRI and its applications to the clinical neurosciences. Neuroscientist 7:64–79, 2001.
94. Hammeke TA, Bellgowan PS, Binder JR: fMRI: Methodology—cognitive function mapping. Adv Neurol 83: 221–233, 2000.
95. Binder JR, Frost JA, Hammeke TA, et al: Human brain language areas identified by functional magnetic resonance imaging. J Neurosci 17:353–362, 1997.
96. Binder JR, Robinson C, Frost JA, et al: Localization of linguistic

and non-linguistic speech-processing systems using functional MRI (FMRI). Neurology 45:371, 1995.
97. Binder JR, Frost JA, Hammeke TA, et al: Function of the left planum temporale in auditory and linguistic processing. Brain 119:1239–1247, 1996.
98. Frost JA, Binder JR, Springer JA, et al: Language processing is strongly left lateralized in both sexes: Evidence from functional MRI. Brain 122(Pt 2):199–208, 1999.
99. Szaflarski J, Binder JR, Possing ET, et al: Language lateralization in left-handed and ambidextrous people: fMRI data. Neurology 59:238–244, 2002.
100. Oldfield RC: The assessment and analysis of handedness: The Edinburgh Inventory. Neuropsychologia 9:97–113, 1971.
101. Swanson SJ, Binder JR, Possing ET, et al: FMRI language laterality during a semantic task: Age of onset and side of seizure focus effects. J Int Neuropsychol Soc 8:222, 2002.
102. Sabsevitz DS, Swanson SJ, Hammeke TA, et al: Predicting naming deficits following left anterior temporal lobectomy using fMRI. J Int Neuropsychol Soc 8:317, 2002.
103. Lurito JT, Dzemidzic M: Determination of cerebral hemisphere language dominance with functional magnetic resonance imaging. Neuroimaging Clin N Am 11:355–363, 2001.
104. Cannestra AF, Bookheimer SY, Pouratian N, et al: Temporal and topographical characterization of language cortices using intraoperative optical intrinsic signals. Neuroimage 12:41–54, 2000.
105. Grabowski TJ, Damasio H, Tranel D, et al: A role for left temporal pole in the retrieval of words for unique entities. Hum Brain Map 13:199–212, 2001.
106. Hamberger MJ, Goodman RR, Perrine K, Tamny T: Anatomic dissociation of auditory and visual naming in the lateral temporal cortex. Neurology 56:56–61, 2001.
107. Mazoyer BM, Tzourio N, Frak V, et al: The cortical representation of language. J Cogn Neurosci 5:467–479, 1993.
108. Price CJ, Wise RJ, Warburton EA, et al: Hearing and saying: The functional neuro-anatomy of auditory word processing. Brain 119(Pt 3):919–931, 1996.
109. Price CJ, Moore CJ, Humphreys GW, Wise RJS: Segregating semantic from phonological processes during reading. J Cogn Neurosci 9:727–733, 1997.
110. Scott SK, Blank CC, Rosen S, Wise RJ: Identification of a pathway for intelligible speech in the left temporal lobe. Brain 123(Pt 12):2400–2406, 2000.
111. Chelune CJ: Using neuropsychological data to forecast postsurgical cognitive outcome. In Luders H (ed): Epilepsy Surgery. New York, Raven Press, 1991, pp 477–485.
112. Hermann BP, Wyler AR, Somes G, Clement L: Dysnomia after left anterior temporal lobectomy without functional mapping: Frequency and correlates. Neurosurgery 35:52–56, 1994.
113. Langfitt JT, Rausch R: Word-finding deficits persist after left anterotemporal lobectomy. Arch Neurol 53:72–76, 1996.
114. Strauss E, Semenza C, Hunter M, et al: Left anterior lobectomy and category-specific naming. Brain Cogn 43:403–406, 2000.
115. Risse GL, Gates JR, Fangman MC: A reconsideration of bilateral language representation based on the intracarotid amobarbital procedure. Brain Cogn 33:118–132, 1997.
116. Swanson SJ, Binder JR, Hammeke TA, et al: The relationship between Wada and fMRI language scores in patients with interhemispheric dissociation of language skills. Epilepsia 39:245, 1998.
117. Cohen JD, Perlstein WM, Braver TS, et al: Temporal dynamics of brain activation during a working memory task. Nature 386: 604–607, 1997.
118. Sass KJ, Spencer DD, Kim JH, et al: Verbal memory impairment correlates with hippocampal pyramidal cell density. Neurology 40:1694–1697, 1990.
119. Alvarez P, Squire LR: Memory consolidation and the medial temporal lobe: A simple network model. Proc Natl Acad Sci U S A 91:7041–7045, 1994.
120. McClelland JL, McNaughton BL, O'Reilly RC: Why there are complementary learning systems in the hippocampus and neocortex: Insights from the success and failures of connectivist models of learning and memory. Psychol Rev 102:409–457, 1995.
121. McClelland JL, Goddard NH: Considerations arising from a complementary learning systems perspective on hippocampus and neocortex. Hippocampus 6:654–665, 1996.
122. Binder J, Price C: Functional imaging of language. In Cabeza R, Kingstone A (eds): Handbook of Functional Neuroimaging of Cognition. Cambridge, MA: MIT Press, 2001, pp 187–251.
123. Kim JJ, Fanselow MS: Modality-specific retrograde amnesia of fear. Science 256:675–677, 1992.
124. Constable RT, Carpentier A, Pugh K, et al: Investigation of the human hippocampal formation using a randomized event-related paradigm and Z-shimmed functional MRI. Neuroimage 12:55–62, 2000.
125. Fernandez G, Weyerts H, Schrader-Bolsche M, et al: Successful verbal encoding into episodic memory engages the posterior hippocampus: A parametrically analyzed functional magnetic resonance imaging study. J Neurosci 18:1841–1847, 1998.
126. Gabrieli JDE, Brewer JB, Desmond JE, Glover GH: Separate neural bases of two fundamental memory processes in the human medial temporal lobe. Science 276:264–266, 1997.
127. Jokeit H, Okujava M, Woermann FG: Memory fMRI lateralizes temporal lobe epilepsy. Neurology 57:1786–1793, 2001.
128. Martin A: Automatic activation of the medial temporal lobe during encoding: Lateralized influences of meaning and novelty. Hippocampus 9:62–70, 1999.
129. Rombouts SA, Barkhof F, Witter MP, et al: Anterior medial temporal lobe activation during attempted retrieval of encoded visuospatial scenes: An event-related fMRI study. Neuroimage 14(1 Pt 1):67–76, 2001.
130. Stern CE, Corkin S, Gonzalez RG, et al: The hippocampal formation participates in novel picture encoding: Evidence from functional magnetic resonance imaging. Proc Natl Acad Sci U S A 93:8660–8665, 1996.
131. Stern CE, Sherman SJ, Kirchhoff BA, Hasselmo ME: Medial temporal and prefrontal contributions to working memory tasks with novel and familiar stimuli. Hippocampus 11:337–346, 2001.
132. Wagner AD, Schacter DL, Rotte M, et al: Building memories: Remembering and forgetting of verbal experiences as predicted by brain activity. Science 281:1188–1191, 1998.
133. Detre JA, Maccotta L, King D, et al: Functional MRI lateralization of memory in temporal lobe epilepsy. Neurology 50:926–932, 1998.
134. Cohen NJ, Eichenbaum H: Memory, Amnesia, and the Hippocampal System. Cambridge, MA: MIT Press, 1993.
135. Henke K, Weber B, Kneifel S, et al: Human hippocampus associates information in memory. Proc Natl Acad Sci U S A 96: 5884–5889, 1999.
136. Schacter DL, Curran T, Reiman EM, et al: Medial temporal lobe activation during episodic encoding and retrieval: A PET study. Hippocampus 9:575–581, 1999.
137. Craik FIM, Lockhart RS: Levels of processing: A framework for memory research. J Verb Learn Verb Behav 11:671–684, 1972.
138. Squire LR, Butters N: Neuropsychology of Memory, 2nd ed. New York, Guilford Press, 1992.
139. Bellgowan PS, Binder JR, Possing ET, et al: Comparison tasks dissociate anterior and posterior hippocampal activation during novel scene encoding. J Cogn Neurosci 11(Suppl 11):20, 1999.
140. Tulving E, Markowitsch HJ, Craik FIM, et al: Novelty and familiarity activations in PET studies of memory encoding and retrieval. Cereb Cortex 6:71–79, 1996.
141. Swanson SJ, Sabsevitz DS, Spanaki MV, et al: Functional magnetic resonance imaging (fMRI) hippocampal activation asymmetry correlates with hippocampal volume and Wada memory asymmetries in epilepsy surgery candidates. Epilepsia 42:79, 2001.
142. Jack CR Jr, Theodore WH, Cook M, McCarthy G: MRI-based hippocampal volumetrics: Data acquisition, normal ranges, and optimal protocol. Magn Reson Imaging 13:1057–1064, 1995.
143. Hong SB, Roh SY, Kim SE, Seo DW: Correlation of temporal lobe glucose metabolism with the Wada memory test. Epilepsia 41:1554–1559, 2000.
144. Casasanto DJ, Glosser G, Killgore WDS, et al: Presurgical fMRI predicts memory outcome following anterior temporal lobectomy. J Int Neuropsychol Soc 7:183, 2001.
145. Killgore WD, Glosser G, Casasanto DJ, et al: Functional MRI and the Wada test provide complementary information for predicting post-operative seizure control. Seizure 8:450–455, 1999.
146. Binder JR, Bellgowan PSF, Swanson SJ, et al: FMRI activation asymmetry predicts side of seizure focus in temporal lobe epilepsy. Neuroimage 11:S155, 2000.

147. Spanaki MV, Binder JR, Swanson SJ, et al: Prediction of seizure focus lateralization using functional MRI in temporal lobe. Neurology 56(Suppl 3):A389–A390, 2001.
148. Ives JR, Warach S, Schmitt F, et al: Monitoring the patient's EEG during echo planar MRI. Electroencephalogr Clin Neurophysiol 87:417–420, 1993.
149. Lemieux L, Allen PJ, Franconi F, et al: Recording of EEG during fMRI experiments: Patient safety. Magn Reson Med 38:943–952, 1997.
150. Detre JA, Sirven JI, Alsop DC, et al: Localization of subclinical ictal activity by functional magnetic resonance imaging: Correlation with invasive monitoring. Ann Neurol 38:618–624, 1995.
151. Detre JA, Alsop DC, Aguirre GK, Sperling MR: Coupling of cortical and thalamic ictal activity in human partial epilepsy: Demonstration by functional magnetic resonance imaging. Epilepsia 37:657–661, 1996.
152. Jackson GD, Connelly A, Cross JH, et al: Functional magnetic resonance imaging of focal seizures. Neurology 44:850–856, 1994.
153. Lazeyras F, Blanke O, Perrig S, et al: EEG-triggered functional MRI in patients with pharmacoresistant epilepsy. J Magn Reson Imaging 12:177–185, 2000.
154. Schwartz TH, Resor SR Jr, De La PR, Goodman RR: Functional magnetic resonance imaging localization of ictal onset to a dysplastic cleft with simultaneous sensorimotor mapping: Intraoperative electrophysiological confirmation and postoperative follow-up: Technical note. Neurosurgery 43:639–644, 1998.
155. Symms MR, Allen PJ, Woermann FG, et al: Reproducible localization of interictal epileptiform discharges using EEG-triggered fMRI. Phys Med Biol 44:N161–N168, 1999.
156. Warach S, Ives JR, Schlaug G, et al: EEG-triggered echo-planar functional MRI in epilepsy. Neurology 47:89–93, 1996.
157. Bookheimer SY: Functional MRI applications in clinical epilepsy. Neuroimage 4(3 Pt 3):S139–S146, 1996.
158. Hill RA, Chiappa KH, Huang-Hellinger F, Jenkins BG: EEG during MR imaging: Differentiation of movement artifact from paroxysmal cortical activity. Neurology 45:1942–1943, 1995.
159. Atlas SW, Howard RS, Maldjian J, et al: Functional magnetic resonance imaging of regional brain activity in patients with intracerebral gliomas: Findings and implications for clinical management. Neurosurgery 38:329–338, 1996.
160. Achten E, Jackson GD, Cameron JA, et al: Presurgical evaluation of the motor hand area with functional MR imaging in patients with tumors and dysplastic lesions. Radiology 210:529–538, 1999.
161. Lee CC, Jack CR Jr, Riederer SJ: Use of functional magnetic resonance imaging. Neurosurg Clin N Am 7:665–683, 1996.
162. Mueller WM, Yetkin FZ, Hammeke TA, et al: Functional magnetic resonance imaging mapping of the motor cortex in patients with cerebral tumors. Neurosurgery 39:515–520, 1996.
163. Pujol J, Conesa G, Deus J, et al: Clinical application of functional magnetic resonance imaging in presurgical identification of the central sulcus. J Neurosurg 88:863–869, 1998.
164. DeYoe EA, Carman GJ, Bandettini P, et al: Mapping striate and extrastriate visual areas in human cerebral cortex. Proc Natl Acad Sci U S A 93:2382–2386, 1996.
165. Engel S, Zhang X, Wandell B: Colour tuning in human visual cortex measured with functional magnetic resonance imaging. Nature 388:68–71, 1997.
166. Miki A, Liu GT, Modestino EJ, et al: Functional magnetic resonance imaging of the visual system. Curr Opin Ophthalmol 12: 423–431, 2001.
167. Melcher JR, Talavage TM, Harms MR: Functional MRI of the auditory system. In Moonen CTW, Bandettini PA (eds): Functional MRI. New York, Springer, 1999, pp 393–406.
168. Strainer JC, Ulmer JL, Yetkin FZ, et al: Functional MR of the primary auditory cortex: An analysis of pure tone activation and tone discrimination. AJNR Am J Neuroradiol 18:601–610, 1997.
169. Hallett M, Sadato N, Honda M, et al: Functional MRI of the sensorimotor system. In Moonen CTW, Bandettini PA (eds): Functional MRI. New York, Springer, 1999, pp 381–391.
170. Maldjian JA, Gottschalk A, Patel RS, et al: The sensory somatotopic map of the human hand demonstrated at 4 tesla. Neuroimage 10:55–62, 1999.
171. Puce A, Constable RT, Luby ML, et al: Functional magnetic resonance imaging of sensory and motor cortex: Comparison with electrophysiological localization. J Neurosurg 83:262–270, 1995.
172. Rao SM, Binder JR, Hammeke TA, et al: Somatotopic mapping of the human primary motor cortex with functional magnetic resonance imaging. Neurology 45:919–924, 1995.
173. Binder JR, Rao SM, Hammeke TA, et al: Effects of stimulus rate on signal response during functional magnetic resonance imaging of auditory cortex. Brain Res Cogn Brain Res 2:31–38, 1994.
174. Dai TH, Liu JZ, Sahgal V, et al: Relationship between muscle output and functional MRI–measured brain activation. Exp Brain Res 140:290–300, 2001.
175. Dhankhar A, Wexler BE, Fulbright RK, et al: Functional magnetic resonance imaging assessment of the human brain auditory cortex response to increasing word presentation rates. J Neurophysiol 77:476–483, 1997.
176. Rao SM, Bandettini PA, Binder JR, et al: Relationship between finger movement rate and functional magnetic resonance signal change in human primary motor cortex. J Cereb Blood Flow Metab 16:1250–1254, 1996.
177. Pinard J, Feydy A, Carlier R, et al: Functional MRI in double cortex: Functionality of heterotopia. Neurology 54:1531–1533, 2000.
178. Schlosser MJ, McCarthy G, Fulbright RK, et al: Cerebral vascular malformations adjacent to sensorimotor and visual cortex: Functional magnetic resonance imaging studies before and after therapeutic intervention. Stroke 28:1130–1137, 1997.
179. Spreer J, Dietz M, Raab P, et al: Functional MRI of language-related activation in left frontal schizencephaly. J Comput Assist Tomogr 24:732–734, 2000.
180. Jack CR, Lee CC, Ward SJ, Riederer SJ: The role of functional MRI in planning perirolandic surgery. In Moonen CTW, Bandettini PA (eds): Functional MRI. New York, Springer, 1999, pp 539–550.
181. Beauchamp MS, Haxby JV, Rosen AC, DeYoe EA: A functional MRI case study of acquired cerebral dyschromatopsia. Neuropsychologia 38:1170–1179, 2000.
182. Krings T, Foltys H, Reinges MH, et al: Navigated transcranial magnetic stimulation for presurgical planning—correlation with functional MRI. Minim Invasive Neurosurg 44:234–239, 2001.
183. Macdonell RA, Jackson GD, Curatolo JM, et al: Motor cortex localization using functional MRI and transcranial magnetic stimulation. Neurology 53:1462–1467, 1999.
184. Chapman PH, Buchbinder BR, Cosgrove GR, Jiang HJ: Functional magnetic resonance imaging for cortical mapping in pediatric neurosurgery. Pediatr Neurosurg 23:122–126, 1995.
185. Jack CR Jr, Twomey CK, Zinsmeister AR, et al: Sensory motor cortex: Correlation of presurgical mapping with function MR imaging and invasive cortical mapping. Radiology 190:85–92, 1994.
186. Schlosser MJ, Luby M, Spencer DD, et al: Comparative localization of auditory comprehension by using functional magnetic resonance imaging and cortical stimulation. J Neurosurg 91: 626–635, 1999.
187. Yousry TA, Schmid UD, Jassoy AG, et al: Topography of the cortical motor hand area: Prospective study with functional MR imaging and direct motor mapping at surgery. Radiology 195: 23–29, 1995.
188. Krings T, Schreckenberger M, Rohde V, et al: Metabolic and electrophysiological validation of functional MRI. J Neurol Neurosurg Psychiatry 71:762–771, 2001.
189. Kober H, Nimsky C, Moller M, et al: Correlation of sensorimotor activation with functional magnetic resonance imaging and magnetoencephalography in presurgical functional imaging: A spatial analysis. Neuroimage 14:1214–1228, 2001.
190. Roux FE, Boulanouar K, Ibarrola D, et al: Importance and limitations of the validation of functional MRI of motor function and language using preoperative cortical stimulation. J Neuroradiol 26(1 Suppl):S82–S88, 1999.
191. Talairach J, Tournoux P: Co-planar Stereotaxic Atlas of the Human Brain: 3D Proportional System: An Approach to Cerebral Imaging. New York, Georg Thieme, 1988.

CHAPTER **152**

Identification of Candidates for Epilepsy Surgery

G. REES COSGROVE ■ ANDREW J. COLE

In most patients with epilepsy, seizures can be well controlled with appropriate medication. Current estimates indicate, however, that 20% to 30% of patients with epilepsy are refractory to all forms of medical therapy.[1] These medically intractable patients are candidates for surgical treatment in an attempt to achieve better seizure control. Another group of patients who might benefit are patients whose seizures may be relatively well controlled but who have certain characteristic presentations or lesions that strongly suggest surgical intervention might be curative. Overall, the most important determinant of a successful surgical outcome is the identification and selection of patients for surgery. This process requires detailed presurgical evaluation to characterize seizure type, frequency, site of onset, psychosocial functioning, and degree of disability to select the most appropriate treatment from a variety of surgical options. This type of evaluation is carried out best at a multidisciplinary center experienced in the investigation and treatment of epilepsy. This chapter identifies the clinical, electrophysiologic, and radiographic characteristics that make certain patients good candidates for surgery. The essential elements of the presurgical evaluation that allow for appropriate selection of patients for surgical intervention are outlined.

DEFINITIONS

There are many types of seizures and different forms of epilepsy. A *seizure* is a paroxysmal, self-limited change in behavior associated with excessive electrical discharge from the central nervous system. *Epilepsy* is a condition of recurrent seizures. *Medical intractability* is a condition of recurrent seizures despite optimal treatment under the direction of an experienced neurologist during a 2- to 3-year period.[2, 3]

IDENTIFICATION OF SURGICAL CANDIDATES

Whether the patient's seizures are suspected of being focal or generalized, it generally is agreed that only patients with continued seizures intractable to optimal medical management are considered for surgery. Much discussion has occurred regarding an acceptable definition of medical intractability.

Operationally, if a patient's seizures remain uncontrolled after 2 years of working with an experienced neurologist, the epilepsy reasonably can be considered medically intractable. Although the continued development of new antiepileptic drugs may force modification of this definition in the future, the introduction of many new drugs since the mid-1990s already has complicated the task of determining medical intractability. In general, for patients with partial seizures, we begin with a trial of phenytoin or carbamazepine followed by a trial of valproic acid. If these first-line major anticonvulsants do not provide adequate seizure control, successive trials of adjunctive agents, such as lamotrigine, topiramate, tiagabine, gabapentin, levtiracetan or zonisamide, may be considered. Occasional success with one of these added agents should lead to an attempt at monotherapy with the successful drug. Because of the number of agents available, trials of every agent in every combination are impractical; a reasonable number of trials should be conducted systematically and expeditiously. Particular attention should focus on side effects and adverse events because an inability to tolerate an effective agent must be considered a medical failure. Patients rarely show a sustained benefit from added drugs if they fail trials of the primary first-line agents. Except in special situations, there is no clear role for long-term treatment with barbiturates when less toxic and equally effective alternatives exist.

Another group of patients with epilepsy exists that might be considered for surgical treatment even if they do not have severe medically intractable seizures. These patients may have seizures that are relatively well controlled on medications but are symptomatic because of a cortical lesion, such as a low-grade glioma or cavernous angioma. Many patients with lesional epilepsy have an excellent chance of becoming seizure-free with surgical intervention, especially patients with small, focal, but highly epileptogenic lesions. Engel[4] coined the term *surgically curable epilepsy* for these patients and considered them ideal surgical candidates that might not have to meet strict criteria of medical intractability before surgery is considered.

The incidence of lesional epilepsy has been estimated to represent 20% to 30% of cases with intractable seizures and appears to be increasing owing to the widespread availability of magnetic resonance imaging (MRI).[5] Many patients with a first seizure undergo an MRI scan, and a *symptomatic lesion* is discovered. In these cases, therapeutic strategies typically are directed against the specific pathology, and seizure control rarely is a problem. In other cases, patients with seizure disorders of long duration eventually may undergo neuroimaging that detects a causative lesion and become excellent candidates for more detailed evaluation. After the determination that a patient is medically intractable and has a form of epilepsy that may be amenable to surgical treatment, the final decision regarding the selection of that patient for surgery depends in large part on the results of a detailed and comprehensive presurgical evaluation.

PRESURGICAL EVALUATION

The goal of epilepsy surgery is to identify an abnormal area of cortex from which the seizures originate and remove it without causing any significant functional impairment. The primary components of the presurgical evaluation include a detailed clinical history and physical examination, advanced neuroimaging, video/EEG monitoring, neuropsychological testing, and assessment of psychosocial functioning (Table 152–1). The major surgical questions one hopes to answer with this evaluation are the following: (1) Are the seizures focal or generalized? (2) If focal, are they temporal or extratemporal in origin? (3) Is there a lesion associated with the seizures? (4) If surgery is undertaken, what functional deficits, if any, might be anticipated?

TABLE 152–1 ■ **Presurgical Evaluation**

Phase I: Noninvasive
Clinical examination
Neuroimaging
MRI
PET
SPECT (ictal)
Electrophysiologic
Routine EEG
24-hour intensive video/EEG monitoring
Ambulatory
Inpatient
Neuropsychological testing
Psychosocial evaluation
Phase II: Invasive
Electrophysiologic
24-hour intensive video/EEG monitoring
Epidural electrodes
Subdural electrodes
Intracerebral electrodes
Neuropsychological testing
Intracarotid amobarbital test

MRI, magnetic resonance imaging; PET, positron emission tomography; SPECT, single-photon emission computed tomography; EEG, electroencephalography.

Clinical Features

The presurgical evaluation of a patient with medically intractable epilepsy begins with a complete history and physical examination. One attempts to classify the different kinds of seizures as well as the frequency, severity, and duration of each type. The clinical semiology of these events can yield important localizing information to the experienced clinician.

Complex partial seizures of temporal lobe origin typically are preceded by an aura. Most commonly, patients describe an abdominal sensation and nausea, usually unpleasant, that characteristically rises up into the chest and throat. Less frequently, patients describe experiential phenomena, such as déjà vu; jamais vu; depersonalization; olfactory, gustatory, or auditory hallucinations; or visual disturbances such as micropsia or macropsia. Sometimes a witness may report that the patient must have a warning because he or she routinely takes protective action before a seizure even though he or she may be amnestic for the event. Ictal behavior is variable but commonly includes a blank stare; oral-alimentary automatisms, such as salivation, lip smacking, or swallowing; and variable appendicular automatisms, such as finger tapping or picking at clothes. Early speech arrest suggests dominant hemisphere involvement, as does prolonged postictal dysphasia. By contrast, ictal speech supports the hypothesis of nondominant hemispheric seizure onset.[6]

Frontal seizures often begin without any warning. They are frequently nocturnal and may be brief. Orbitofrontal attacks may be clinically indistinguishable from seizures of anterior temporal lobe origin. Ictal behavior can be bizarre, including complex, rhythmic, and sometimes violent automatisms that frequently are bilateral and often involve the lower extremities. Shouted verbal outbursts are common, occasionally with blasphemous content. These ictal automatisms or manifestations sometimes are mistaken for pseudoseizures because of their histrionic appearance. Supplementary motor attacks may begin with stereotyped tonic motor activity characterized by head version toward the contralateral side with elevation of the ipsilateral arm and extension of the contralateral arm into the so-called fencer's position. Frequently the postictal period after any frontal lobe seizure is brief or nonexistent.[7]

Seizures of parietal origin may be preceded by somatosensory auras, but a vague, poorly described sensation of dizziness may be a more common early feature. Consciousness often is well preserved perhaps because of the relative paucity of projections to limbic or contralateral structures. Ictal behavior is highly variable and often is dependent on pathways of propagation.[8]

Occipital attacks frequently begin with positive visual phenomena. In general, these phenomena are primary, bright, usually uncolored images perceived in the contralateral visual hemifield without definable or recognizable forms. Well-formed complex visual hallucinations are more likely to occur in association with temporal attacks. Rich occipitotemporal projections result in frequent progression from restricted occipital discharges to events that also involve temporal structures.[9]

Ictal semiology is rich and varied. The diligent physician may be rewarded with extraordinary insight into the localization of epileptic foci and their relationship to cortical function. It is crucial to interview a reliable witness along with the patient because most individuals are unable to provide an accurate first-hand account of their own ictal behavior. At times, the clinical features of the seizure are so distinct that they may localize the seizure onset clearly to a specific region of the cortex. Simple partial seizures with episodes of speech arrest but no loss of awareness imply onset in the dominant frontal operculum. Similarly, the localizing value of a seizure in a patient with focal tonic contraction and elevation of the right arm and hand is extremely compelling and implicates either the left rolandic cortex or supplementary motor regions.

It is important to determine the age of onset, response to treatment, and familial tendency toward seizures. The pregnancy and delivery history is helpful in assessing congenital or early acquired abnormalities. Other medical history of significance includes a history of febrile seizures, head injury, or intracranial infection. The adequacy of medication trials must be assessed to ensure that the patient is truly refractory to medical therapy.

On examination, the clinician looks for obvious asymmetries of development compatible with an early structural central nervous system lesion and focal neurological or cognitive abnormalities suggestive of acquired disease. In most patients, however, the neurological examination is completely normal.

Neuroimaging

Modern neuroimaging is crucial to surgical decision making. In the past, skull radiographs, ventriculograms, pneumoencephalography, and computed tomography (CT) scans showed indirect evidence of cerebral pathology in the form of focal or diffuse atrophy or space-occupying lesions. MRI has replaced CT as the imaging study of choice to evaluate patients with epilepsy. MRI is an extremely sensitive tool that can detect abnormalities of the brain with exceptional anatomic detail. MRI is especially sensitive for detecting focal atrophy (e.g., hippocampal atrophy), indolent gliomas, cortical dysplasias, cerebral gliosis, and small structural lesions of the neocortex.[5] MRI can show associated features of mass effect, focal atrophy, or calvarial molding. Occasionally, MRI can identify obvious dual pathology, such as distinct hippocampal atrophy associated with a neocortical temporal lesion. New high-resolution MRI using phased array surface coils can reveal previously undetectable lesions because of improved spatial resolution.[10] Subtle abnormalities, such as cortical dysplasia, can be visualized using these techniques, allowing for a more focused presurgical evaluation in the region of anatomic abnormality (Fig. 152–1).

Functional imaging visualizes alterations in cerebral metabolism or perfusion using positron emission tomography (PET) and single-photon emission computed tomography (SPECT). These studies reveal epileptic areas as hypometabolic between seizures and hypermetabolic during seizures (Fig. 152–2).[11, 12] Although they lack the spatial resolution of MRI, PET and SPECT can play an important role in the localization of abnormal cortex. Ictal SPECT studies can be obtained if an appropriate radioisotope is injected within seconds of a seizure onset. The isotope is concentrated in the region of seizure onset, and imaging studies can be obtained several hours after injection to show the area of ictal onset. These studies have been useful in many patients with occult epileptic foci.[13]

Advances in functional MRI can provide important information regarding the localization of eloquent cortex adjacent to lesions or planned resection lines. The

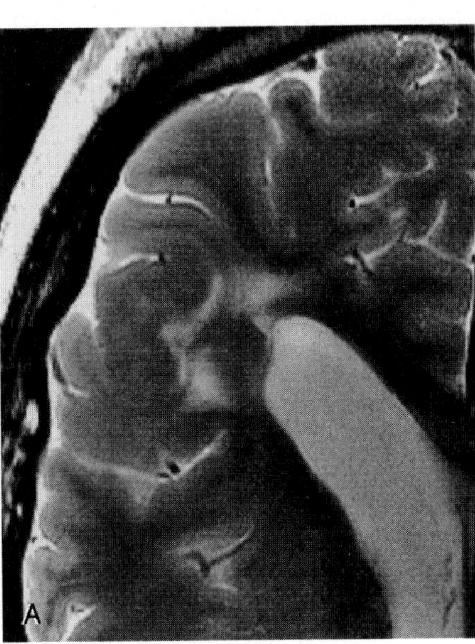

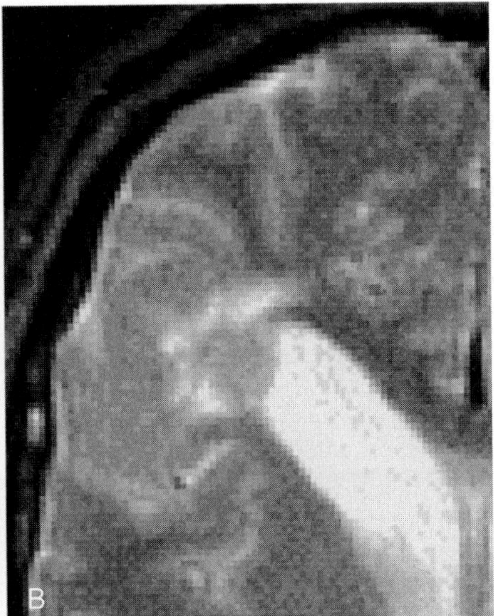

FIGURE 152–1. High-resolution phased array magnetic resonance image of a patient with intractable right frontal lobe epilepsy. Standard T2-weighted images *(B)* show subcortical periventricular lesion, but the extent of the focal cortical dysplasia is much more evident on the high-resolution images *(A)*. Note the clarity of the cortical ribbon and the improved gray–white matter junction definition.

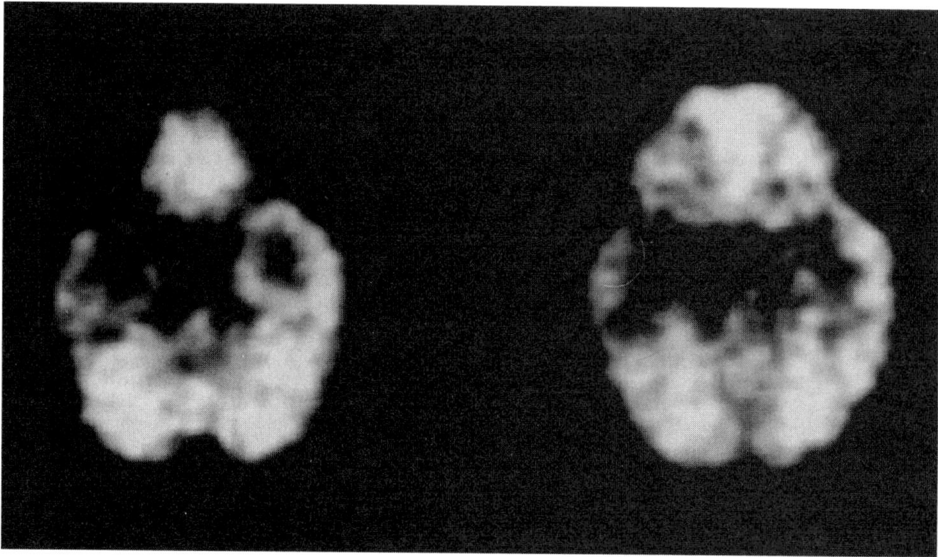

FIGURE 152–2. Interictal 18-fluorodeoxyglucose positron emission tomography scan (axial slices) in a patient with intractable complex partial seizures. Note the decreased metabolic activity throughout the right temporal lobe but most prominently in the mesial structures.

newest method of localizing cortical function is with functional MRI. This powerful neuroimaging technique can create an anatomic and functional model of a patient's brain.[14] Rapid echoplanar imaging performed while the patient engages in a specific task (i.e., fist clenching, tongue movement, verb generation) detects small changes in signal intensity related to changes in cerebral blood flow.[15] Intensive computerized image processing can define the areas of cortex activated by the specific task. Concurrent three-dimensional rendering of cerebral topography, cortical veins, and related pathology gives an unprecedented display of crucial relational anatomy. By combining detailed anatomic information with precise physiologic information, functional MRI is capable of creating a structural and functional model of an individual's brain (Fig. 152–3). In the future, magnetic resonance spectroscopy may provide distinct neurochemical information on mass lesions

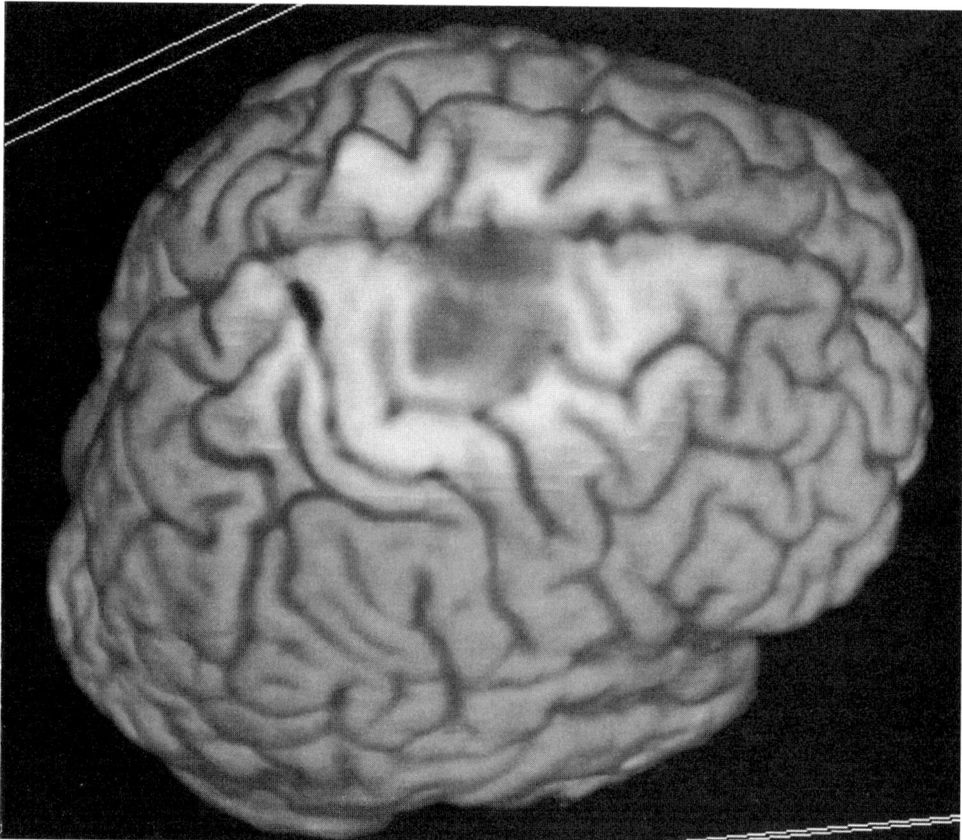

FIGURE 152–3. Functional magnetic resonance image superimposed on a three-dimensional surface rendering of a patient with focal motor seizures of the left hand. This image shows a low-grade glioma in the right superior frontal gyrus immediately anterior to the rolandic somatomotor area for hand function. Area of cortical activation during a left finger-tapping task is identified in red. (See color section in this volume.)

that might correlate with specific histopathology. Given these advances, it is likely that MRI will play an increasing role in the presurgical evaluation of epilepsy patients.

Other noninvasive cerebral mapping techniques that have evolved to localize functionally important cortical areas are magnetoencephalography and activated PET.[16, 17] Both techniques can localize certain cortical functions noninvasively but require dedicated units that are not widely available.

Electroencephalography

Electroencephalography (EEG) is the cornerstone of the presurgical evaluation. Analysis of unselected EEG activity between events (*interictal*) or of specific activity during events (*ictal*) can provide evidence of focal electrical dysfunction. Although certain interictal EEG abnormalities (spike and slow wave complexes) can be of localizing value, in general it is considered extremely important to record the EEG and the patient's behavior during the spontaneous occurrence of the patient's habitual events. Video/EEG monitoring can record the EEG continuously during a 24-hour period, which allows for careful inspection of the record during any symptomatic event. Sophisticated computer hardware and software enable automatic detection of spontaneous interictal epileptiform transients and electrographic seizures that otherwise might have gone unrecognized.[18] The EEG activity at the beginning of the seizure before spread to adjacent areas is most important in terms of localization, and if a specific cortical area is involved consistently at the onset, that area is likely to be the site of seizure origin. Patients often are hospitalized with reduction in antiseizure medications and may be recorded for 7 to 14 days to capture three to five of their habitual seizures.

Consistent and convincing interictal EEG evidence of epileptiform activity originating in one specific cortical region may provide adequate localizing information in some selected cases. In a patient with intractable complex partial seizures and a low-grade glioma in the mesial temporal lobe, consistent interictal epileptiform activity on scalp EEG from the same temporal lobe would make the patient a reasonable candidate for surgery even without ictal EEG recordings.

Neuropsychological Testing

Detailed neuropsychological testing is performed to reveal specific focal or multifocal cognitive deficits that might be correlated with the neuroimaging and EEG. This testing not only may help in localizing an abnormal area of the brain, but also serves as a comparison for postsurgical evaluation. An intracarotid amobarbital test may be performed as a prelude to surgery in selected patients to lateralize language and memory function to help avoid neurocognitive deficits.[19]

Psychosocial Assessment

Psychosocial evaluation is important to assess current level of functioning and to ensure that realistic goals and attitudes are engendered in the patient and the family before surgery.

DIAGNOSTIC SURGICAL OPTIONS

When a primary epileptogenic region or seizure focus is suspected but remains obscure despite appropriate neuroimaging and scalp (*noninvasive*) video/EEG recordings, some form of implanted (*invasive*) electrodes may be indicated. Intracranial electrodes can be placed in areas not readily sampled by routine surface electrodes and can give more precise EEG information because of their proximity to discharging areas of the brain and the lack of movement and muscle artifact on the recordings. These electrodes have the disadvantages, however, of sampling from a relatively small area of cerebrum surrounding the contact points and the fact that they are accompanied by a surgical risk.[20] Placement of intracranial electrodes should be undertaken only after appropriate noninvasive monitoring has been completed so that a hypothesis of seizure onset has been formulated and a clear goal of the investigation has been defined. The diagnostic surgical options of implanted electrodes include epidural, subdural, and intracerebral or depth electrodes.

Epidural Electrodes

Epidural electrodes are used infrequently and generally only for lateralization and approximate localization of seizure onset.[21] These electrodes are placed through tiny openings in the skull with the electrode contact resting on the dura to provide a high-amplitude EEG signal without muscle or movement artifact. Because they do not penetrate the dura, the risk of infection is minor. These electrodes can record only from the lateral convexity of the cerebral hemispheres and are limited in their spatial resolution.

Subdural Electrodes

Subdural electrodes are placed on the surface of the brain in the form of rectangular grids or linear strips with flat metal contact points mounted in flexible plastic. The grids require a craniotomy for placement and are limited to unilateral application. The strip electrodes can be placed through bur holes over the lateral convexity or under the frontal or temporal lobes.[22] It is difficult to place the electrodes in the interhemispheric fissure to record from parasagittal regions because of technical risks associated with large cortical bridging veins. The major advantage of subdural electrodes is that they do not penetrate cerebral tissue and can record from a relatively wide area of the cortical surface. Subdural electrodes can be used for extraoperative cortical stimulation to map out specific areas of cortical function. Subdural electrodes cannot record directly from the deep cerebral structures (i.e., amygdala, hippocampus, and cingulum), which are characteristically involved in many medically refractory partial epilepsies. They also have a small risk (approximately 4%) of intracranial infection and hemorrhage.[23]

Intracerebral Depth Electrodes

Intracerebral depth electrodes can be placed stereotactically into deep cerebral structures with the aid of CT, MRI, and angiography. Most centers use flexible electrodes with multiple contact points that are placed through small holes in the skull and secured with some form of cranial fixation. Electrodes usually are targeted toward the amygdala, hippocampus, orbitofrontal, and cingulate regions and may be inserted through a lateral or vertex approach. Using a lateral approach, stereotactic cerebral angiography must be used to avoid major blood vessels during placement of the depth electrodes. Depth electrodes may be used in combination with scalp or subdural electrodes for more extensive coverage. Depth electrode investigation generally is indicated for patients with bitemporal, bifrontal, or frontal temporal seizures and can localize a focal area of seizure onset not possible with scalp recordings.[24] The major complications of depth electrodes include hemorrhage and infection with mortality and morbidity rates between 1% and 4%.[23] The intracranial monitoring incurs greater risk than resective surgery itself and is considerably more expensive than a noninvasive evaluation, thus should be used only when necessary. With modern neuroimaging, the use of invasive intracranial monitoring has declined from about 40% to 50% of patients in most centers to 10% to 20%.

SURGICAL DECISION MAKING

If the information obtained during the noninvasive presurgical evaluation consistently points toward a single area of the brain as being the site of seizure onset, the patient may be taken directly to surgery for resection of that area. If neuroimaging shows a well-characterized lesion (i.e., unilateral hippocampal atrophy, cavernous angioma, focal cortical dysplasia) and is supported by the clinical features of the seizures, surgery may be reasonable without the general requirement for ictal EEG data. If the data gathered from the clinical examination, imaging studies, and noninvasive EEG evaluation are conflicting or disparities arise in the presumed localization of the seizure, invasive intracranial monitoring is warranted. This is especially true in the extratemporal epilepsies, in which EEG localization is notoriously difficult. If a localized area of seizure onset is confirmed, these patients too can undergo resective surgery.

CONCLUSIONS

The success or failure of the surgical treatment of epilepsy depends in large part on the proper identification and selection of patients. Advances in neuroimaging and long-term EEG monitoring have enabled a greater accuracy in the localization of the seizure focus with overall surgical results better than those previously obtained. It is hoped that continued improvements in the selection process and the presurgical evaluation will improve the results of surgical intervention in the future.

REFERENCES

1. Robb P: Focal epilepsy: The problem, prevalence, and contributing factors. Adv Neurol 8:11-22, 1975.
2. Commission on Classification and Terminology of the International League Against Epilepsy: Proposal for revised clinical and electro-graphic classification of epileptic seizures. Epilepsia 26: 258–268, 1985.
3. Commission on Classification and Terminology of the International League Against Epilepsy: Proposal for classification of epilepsies and epileptic syndromes. Epilepsia 26:268–278, 1985.
4. Engel J: Surgery for seizures. N Engl J Med 334:647–652, 1996.
5. Lessor R, Modic M, Weinstein M, et al: MRI in patients with intractable epilepsy. Arch Neurol 43:367–371, 1986.
6. Palmini A, Gloor P: The localizing value of auras in partial seizures. Neurology 42:801–808, 1992.
7. Geier S, Bancaud J, Talairach J, et al: The seizures of frontal lobe epilepsy. Neurology 27:951–958, 1975.
8. Williamson PD, Boon A, Thadani VM, et al: Parietal lobe epilepsy: Diagnostic considerations and results of surgery. Ann Neurol 31:193–201, 1992.
9. Ludwig B, Ajmone Marson C: Clinical ictal patterns in epileptic patients with occipital electroencephalographic foci. Neurology 25:463–471, 1975.
10. Grant PE, Barkovich AJ, Wald LL, et al: High-resolution surface-coil MR of cortical lesions in medically refractory epilepsy: A prospective study. AJNR Am J Neuroradiol 18:291–301, 1997.
11. Engel J, Kuhl N, Phelps M, Crandall P: Comparative localization of epileptic foci in partial epilepsy by PET and EEG. Ann Neurol 12:529–537, 1982.
12. Lee B, Marklan O, Siddiqui A, et al: Single photon emission computed tomography (SPECT) brain imaging, intractable complex partial seizures. Neurology 36:1471–1477, 1986.
13. Marks DA, Katz A, Hoffer P, et al: Localization of extratemporal epileptic foci during ictal single photon emission computed tomography. Ann Neurol 31:250–255, 1992.
14. Cosgrove GR, Buchbinder BR, Jiang H: Functional magnetic resonance imaging for intracranial navigation. Neurosurg Clin North Am 7:313–322, 1996.
15. Belliveau JW, Kennedy DN, McKinstry RC, et al: Functional mapping of the human visual cortex by magnetic resonance imaging. Science 254:716–719, 1991.
16. Nakasato N, Levesque M, Barth DS, et al: Comparisons of MEG, EEG and ECoG source localization in neocortical partial epilepsy in humans. Electroencephalogr Clin Neurophysiol 92:171–178, 1992.
17. Fox PT, Burton H, Raichle M: Mapping human somatosensory cortex with positron emission tomography. J Neurosurg 67:34–43, 1987.
18. Quesney LF, Gloor P (eds): Localization of epileptic foci: long-term monitoring in epilepsy. Electroencephalogr Clin Neurophysiol 37(suppl):S165–S200, 1985.
19. Wada J, Rasmussen T: Intracarotid injection of sodium amobarbital for the lateralization of speech dominance: Experimental and clinical observations. J Neurosurg 17:226–282, 1960.
20. Gloor P: Neuronal generators, the problem of localization and volume conductor theory in electroencephalography. J Clin Neurophysiol 2:327–354, 1985.
21. Barnett GH, Burgess RC, Awad IA, et al: Epidural peg electrodes for the presurgical evaluation of intractable epilepsy. Neurosurgery 27:113–115, 1990.
22. Wyler AR, Ojemann GA, Lettich E, Ward AA: Subdural strip electrodes for localizing epileptogenic foci. J Neurosurg 60:1195–1200, 1984.
23. Van Buren JM: Complications of surgical procedures in the diagnosis and treatment of epilepsy. In Engel J Jr (ed): Surgical Treatment of the Epilepsies. New York, Raven Press, 1987, pp 465–475.
24. Spencer S: Depth electroencephalography in selection of refractory epilepsy for surgery. Ann Neurol 9:207–214, 1981.

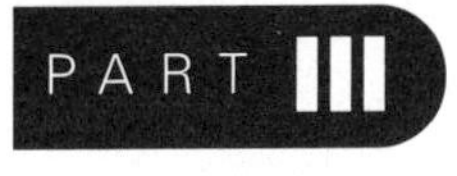

INTRAOPERATIVE MAPPING AND MONITORING FOR CORTICAL RESECTIONS

CHAPTER **153**

Motor, Sensory, and Language Mapping and Monitoring for Cortical Resections

JAMES SCHUSTER ■ DANIEL L. SILBERGELD

Electrical stimulation of human cortex was first reported in 1874 by Bartholow.[1] It was subsequently used to identify sensory and motor cortex,[2, 3] and, since the landmark work of Penfield and Rasmussen,[4] cortical mapping using both stimulating and recording techniques has become an integral part of the neurosurgical armamentarium. Refinements of functional mapping techniques[5–8] have reduced operative morbidity and led to a better understanding of cortical organization and function. Identification of functional cortex, including rolandic cortex and speech cortex, enables the surgeon to avoid these areas when formulating a surgical strategy. Mapping can also be used to guide resections in areas of "secondary" function, including the insula,[9] face motor cortex,[10] and supplementary motor areas (SMAs).[11] In addition to preserving cerebral function during surgery, these techniques allow surgeons to more extensively resect lesions or epileptic regions in the brain with increased safety.[12] Additionally, advances in functional imaging, including functional magnetic resonance imaging (fMRI), positron emission tomography, and frameless stereotactic navigational systems, have contributed to our understanding of cerebral functional topography and are being used to guide surgical resections. However, it must be emphasized that functional imaging identifies *involved* cortex, not necessarily cortex *essential* for function, which is better identified by cortical stimulation mapping.

PATIENT SELECTION

Somatosensory evoked potential (SSEP) and cortical stimulation mapping of motor cortex can be performed in patients under either general or local anesthesia; however, intraoperative language mapping and cortical stimulation mapping of sensory cortex require an awake, cooperative patient. Although there is no specific age cutoff, awake mapping in children younger than 10 years old can be difficult. Also, awake procedures in patients with psychiatric problems or developmental delay should be avoided. Obesity and pulmonary problems, including airway difficulties such as sleep apnea, are relative contraindications for awake procedures. If an awake procedure is not feasible and language mapping is necessary, a subdural or epidural electrode grid can be used for extraoperative functional mapping and seizure monitoring. This requires an additional operative procedure, but it is sometimes unavoidable.

PREOPERATIVE LOCALIZATION

Scalp and Skull Localization

Several methods have been described for localizing cortical structures (i.e., sylvian fissure, central sulcus) based on external skull landmarks. The sylvian fissure can be approximated by following a line connecting the lateral canthus and a point three fourths the distance along the line from the nasion to the inion (Fig. 153–1).[13] The angular gyrus is generally positioned just above the pinna, but there is well recognized individual variability.[7] Alternatively, the angular artery is located approximately 6 cm above the external auditory meatus.

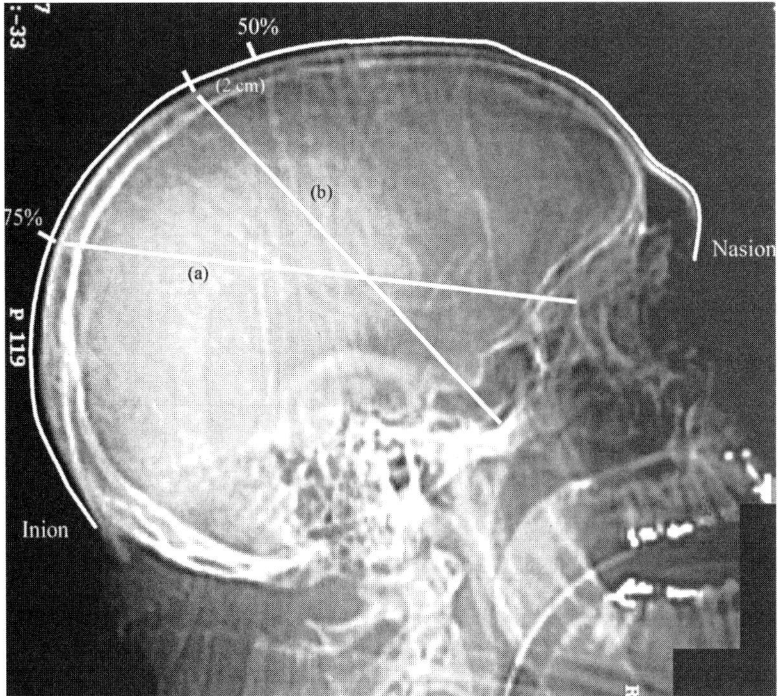

FIGURE 153–1. Landmarks used to localize sylvian fissure *(A)* and central sulcus *(B)*.

There are several methods for locating rolandic cortex. In general, the motor strip is located 4 to 5.4 cm behind the coronal suture,[14] with the superior aspect lying approximately on a perpendicular line drawn from the external auditory meatus to the midline. The central sulcus can be approximated by a line connecting a point 2 cm posterior to the midposition of an arch connecting the nasion to the inion and a point 5 cm straight up from the external auditory meatus[15] or to the midzygomatic point (see Fig. 153–1).[13] Other methods of localizing the central sulcus and sylvian fissure by external landmarks involve the construction of Taylor-Haughton lines.[16]

Imaging

Berger and colleagues showed that axial T2-weighted MRI consistently localized the central sulcus, whereas parasagittal and far lateral sagittal images readily identified rolandic (sensorimotor) cortex as a functional unit, based on the marginal ramus of the cingulate sulcus and insula, respectively.[17]

Functional MRI has shown utility in localizing rolandic cortex. However, the precision can be variable, with up to a 20-mm discrepancy with electrical stimulation mapping.[18] Mueller and coworkers were able to show a correlation between preoperative localization of rolandic cortex and intraoperative mapping, although motor and sensory localization overlapped on fMRI.[19, 20] They also showed that these techniques can be successfully applied in patients with tumors,[19] but other data suggest that tumors may alter regional activation and therefore the accuracy of fMRI.[21] Finally, Fox and associates advocated using strong vibrotactile stimuli to localize somatosensory cortex using positron emission tomography.[22]

The amobarbital (Amytal) Wada test has long been the gold standard for determining language dominance and evaluating lateralizing memory function.[23] However, it is an invasive procedure with all the inherent risks of cerebral angiography. Additionally, the results can be difficult to interpret when there is significant intracranial vascular shunting, as with arteriovenous malformations.

Positron emission tomography and fMRI have been used extensively for the localization of language. Functional MRI has been shown to be equivalent to Wada testing for determining the hemisphere of language dominance.[24, 25] However, Benson and colleagues[26] demonstrated that with fMRI, localization of object naming is considerably less reliable than that of verb generation. The identification of specific language sites within the dominant hemisphere is also less precise. Localization of number counting in the frontal sites has disagreed with electrical stimulation mapping by up to 20 mm.[18] Bookheimer and coworkers,[27] using positron emission tomography, showed that object naming activated predominantly the inferior temporal and frontal regions, with no activation of lateral temporal cortex—an area that routinely produces naming errors with direct electrical stimulation mapping.[7] Applying a battery of tests and combining the images may improve the ability to localize language,[27, 28] but it is unclear if imaging techniques are precise enough in localizing essential language to be used for planning surgical resections. The reliability of functional imaging for evaluating lateralized memory function continues to be evaluated.[29–31]

ANESTHESIA

When SSEP monitoring is performed under general anesthesia, halogenated anesthetic agents should be avoided, because they may increase the latency of cortical SSEPs.[32] High-dose barbiturate or propofol anesthesia may lead to burst suppression activity and is therefore contraindicated. Nitrous oxide combined with thiopental sodium (Pentothal) or low-dose propofol is an excellent general anesthetic for these studies.[32, 33] Obviously, with rolandic cortex mapping, muscle relaxants are avoided. Additionally, higher stimulation currents are generally required when the patient is under general anesthesia.

Awake language mapping is carried out using intravenous propofol. Pin fixation of the skull is well tolerated with local anesthetic injection but is not required. When pin fixation is not used, a skull clamp is attached to the bone edge to serve as a fixation point for self-retaining retractors, a support for the electrocorticography harness, and a means of controlling the head as the patient awakens from anesthesia. Urinary catheters are generally placed preoperatively, but male patients can use a urine bottle intraoperatively without difficulty. Airway issues are of prime concern, and some have advocated using a temporary laryngeal mask for the initial portion of the procedure when the patient is asleep. In addition to propofol, a generous local regional block (1% lidocaine, 0.25% bupivacaine [Marcaine], 1:200,000 epinephrine) is required for the scalp and bone work, including the dura near the middle meningeal artery at the skull base. There is significant individual variability with regard to the metabolism of propofol and thus to patient awakening after its discontinuation. Finally, to protect the brain, the dura is not opened until the patient is completely awake and cooperative.

INTRAOPERATIVE SEIZURES

With stimulation mapping, the potential exists for inducing seizures and subsequent brain swelling. It is therefore imperative to ensure adequate anticonvulsant levels perioperatively. Measures for terminating intraoperative seizures include the administration of short-acting benzodiazepines, cold irrigation solution applied to the cortex,[34] and deeper levels of general anesthetic in intubated patients.

INTRAOPERATIVE LOCALIZATION

Topography

Even with the availability of intraoperative navigational devices, a basic understanding of the topographic organization of the central sulcus is essential. Numerous detailed descriptions of brain sulci are available.[35–37] Duvernoy and Cabanis offer the following description: "The central sulcus can be identified at the vertex of the hemisphere, where it causes a significant notch curving backwards, and visible on the medial surface. From this point of origin, the cental sulcus courses inferiorly and obliquely following a sinuous course: the upper and lower parts anteriorly convex (superior and inferior genu) and the middle anteriorly concave. The lower end of the sulcus is separated from the lateral fissure by the subcentral gyrus."[36]

Localization of Somatosensory Cortex Using Somatosensory Evoked Potentials

SSEP mapping provides a quick, reliable means of identifying the primary somatosensory gyrus (and therefore rolandic localization) in both adult and pediatric populations. SSEPs can be performed under general anesthesia or in awake patients. SSEP mapping has an advantage over stimulation mapping, in that seizures cannot be evoked because the cortex itself is not stimulated.[38]

Techniques for intraoperative SSEP mapping are similar to those used for routine diagnostic studies. Usually, a peripheral nerve such as the median nerve at the wrist is stimulated, because its robust signal can be recorded at the cortical surface. Other nerves such as the tibial nerve can also be used.[38] Stimulation is performed at a rate of 2 to 5 Hz, with a 0.1- to 0.3-msec pulse duration. The current is adjusted to produce a minimal (not painful) twitch so that muscle activity can just be visualized. Mechanical and thermal stimulation can be used as well.[39] The stimulus generates a signal that is transmitted via the spinothalamic pathways to the medial lemniscus, then to the thalamus, and finally to the contralateral somatosensory cortex. Compared with scalp recordings, SSEP recordings made from the cortical surface have much higher voltages (10 to 100 mV). Recording typically uses a low-frequency cutoff of 1 Hz, a high-frequency filter of 3000 Hz, and an analysis time of 100 msec. Usually, trials of 100 to 200 stimuli are needed to elicit well-defined responses from somatosensory cortex.[38] Cortical responses have a number of different components designated by their positive (P) or negative (N) polarity with respect to the reference electrode. The number following the P or N represents the typical latency (in milliseconds) of the peaks. For instance, following median nerve stimulation, the contralateral somatosensory gyrus shows an initial N20 component, followed by a P25 component.

Two types of recording montages are used. The first is a *referential montage* in which each of the recording electrodes is referenced to an electrode that is out of the field of interest and usually off the cortical surface. The second type is a *bipolar montage*, in which each electrode is referenced to an adjacent electrode. When using a referential montage, somatosensory cortex is located beneath the electrode from which the waveform with the highest amplitude is recorded. In contrast, when using a bipolar montage, one looks for phase reversal across the somatosensory gyrus (Fig. 153–2). Following craniotomy and durotomy, an array of electrodes is placed in the axial (transverse) plane on the cortical surface. An eight-contact electrode strip

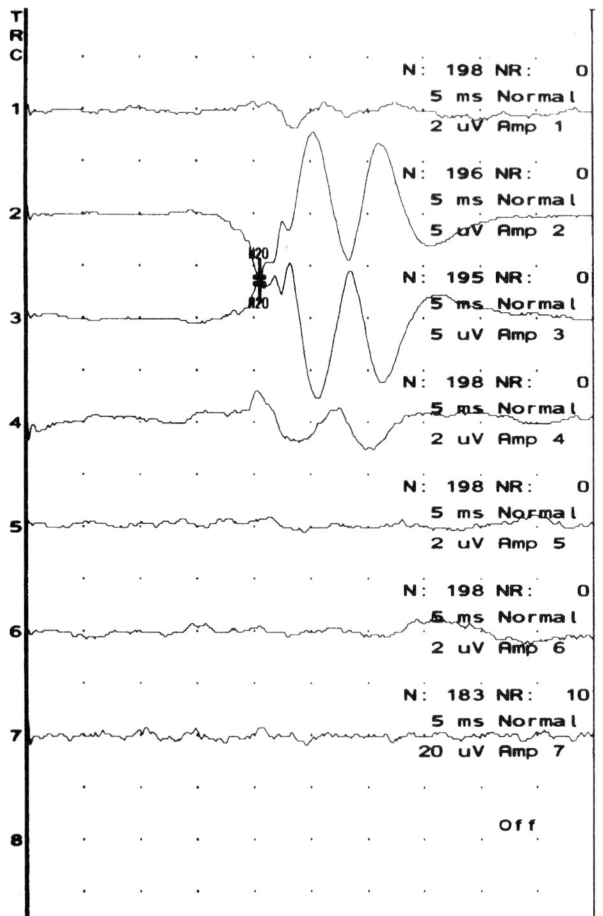

FIGURE 153–2. Somatosensory cortex localization by the identification of phase reversal (leads 2 and 3) using an eight-contact strip electrode and a bipolar recording montage.

(1 cm center-to-center spacing) is adequate. The electrode contacts should extend over areas of the brain anterior and posterior to the presumed somatosensory gyrus (4 cm above the sylvian fissure for the median nerve; at the vertex or just past it for the tibial nerve).

Electrodes may be placed on the dura (especially helpful in reoperation and postmeningitis cases, when the dura is adherent to the underlying cortex)[40] as well as directly on the cortical surface. If the craniotomy does not expose rolandic cortex, an electrode strip can be slid beneath the edge of the craniotomy to reach distant cortical regions.[41] A series of recordings is then made from the cortical surface by moving the electrode to different areas to verify localization of somatosensory cortex.

Cortical Stimulation Motor and Sensory Mapping

Functional localization by cortical stimulation mapping has been performed for more than 40 years.[8] Although this technique is reliable, it is often difficult to elicit responses in children or in adults who are under general anesthesia. Stimulation mapping of somatosensory cortex requires an awake patient, but motor cortex can be stimulated with the patient under general anesthesia. During cortical stimulation, it is important to bear in mind that repetitive stimulation at or near the same site, or with higher currents, can elicit local or generalized seizure activity. Therefore, the patient must have adequate serum anticonvulsant levels preoperatively, and a short-acting intravenous anticonvulsant (e.g., midazolam [Versed], lorazepam [Ativan]) should be readily available to the anesthesiologist in the event that seizures are elicited.

A constant-current, biphasic square wave, 60-Hz, bipolar stimulator (Ojemann Stimulator, Radionics Sales Corp.; 5mm between electrodes) set at 2 to 10 mA is used to elicit movement, sensation, or both in the awake patient.[12] Higher current settings may be necessary in younger children, in patients under general anesthesia, or when stimulating through the dura.[40] In children younger than 5 years of age, motor response to electrical stimulation can be difficult to elicit, requiring longer pulses at higher currents.[42] It is best to start at lower current settings (2 mA in an awake patient under local anesthetic, 4 mA in a patient under general anesthesia) and gradually increase the current (2-mA increments) until sensation or movement is elicited; this avoids eliciting seizure activity. Additionally, maximal stimulation efficiency requires stimulation of the cortex nearest to the central sulcus. Rarely, motor cortex stimulation blocks instead of elicits motor movement.[43]

Using this technique, the entire sensory and motor homunculi can be mapped. The technique can also be used to identify descending subcortical motor fibers when resections extend below the cortical surface, such as during SMA resections and insular resections. When performing subcortical motor mapping, the current needed to elicit movement is the same as or lower than the current needed at the cortical surface. When the resection is very close to functional cortex, it is helpful to periodically repeat the stimulation mapping procedure (the average current penetration is approximately 2 to 3 mm) to verify that cortical and subcortical functional regions are not damaged.

INTRAOPERATIVE MAPPING OF LANGUAGE CORTEX

When performing resections in the dominant hemisphere, preservation of language function is of paramount importance, as permanent language deficits can be one of the most disabling and distressing surgical complications for patients and their families. Because there is significant individual variability with regard to the number and location of essential language sites, standard anatomic resections do not always spare language function. Although resections in or near functional brain can be made safer by localizing important brain functions, the surgeon must be aware of a number of pitfalls to avoid producing functional deficits. The techniques currently available for mapping language function, including methodology, rationale, and pitfalls, are discussed here.

In contrast to mapping rolandic cortex, language cortex mapping depends on electrical blockade of cortical function rather than elicitation of function.[7] The techniques for awake craniotomy have been described elsewhere.[12, 33] Most patients, even children as young as 10 years, have little difficulty with the procedure, especially when propofol anesthesia[33] is used during placement of the field block, cranial opening, the majority of the resection, and closure.

It is first necessary to determine the after-discharge threshold so that depolarization is not propagated to nearby cortex, which may elicit local seizure phenomena or give false-negative or false-positive results. Therefore, electrocorticography must be performed during stimulation. A U-shaped electrode holder attached to the skull at the edge of the craniotomy (Grass model CE1) is used to place carbon-tipped electrodes over the exposed cortical surface, spaced approximately 10 to 20 mm apart (Fig. 153–3). Alternatively, strip electrodes can be placed at the edges of the exposed cortex. Bipolar stimulation is then used, starting with a current of 2 mA. The current is gradually increased (0.5- to 1-mA increments) with successive stimulations until the after-discharge threshold is determined. The current used for language mapping is then set to 0.5 to 1 mA below the after-discharge threshold. The duration of stimulation for setting after-discharges is the same as the duration of each slide presentation. A shorter duration of stimulation permits a higher current level to be used and shortens the mapping procedure.

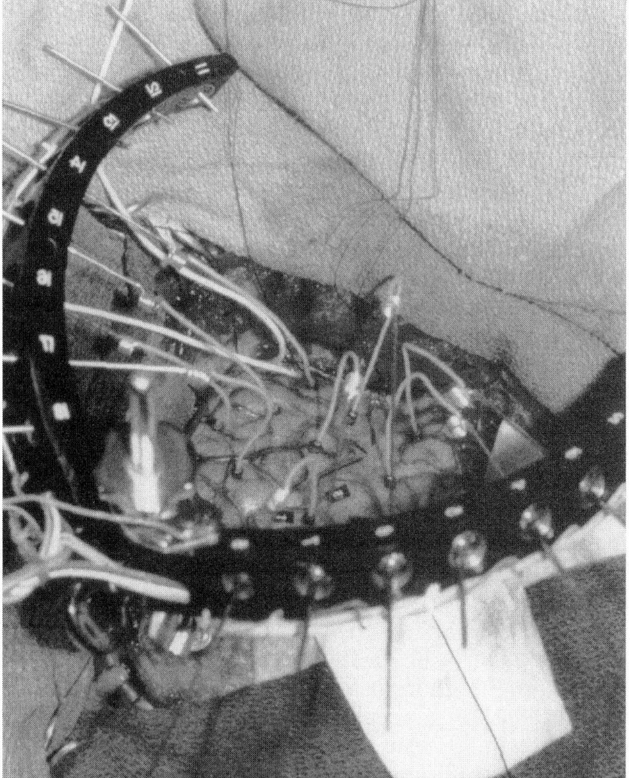

FIGURE 153–3. U-shaped electrode holder, which is attached to the skull at the edge of the craniotomy and used to position the carbon-tipped electrodes over the exposed cortical surface.

Fifteen to twenty perisylvian sites are selected and marked with small (5 by 5 mm) numbered tags before mapping (Fig. 153–4). Sites for stimulation mapping are randomly selected to cover all exposed cortex, including areas where essential language is likely to be located and those near or overlying the site of resection. The patient is shown images of simple objects using a computer or slide projector. A new image is shown every 2 to 4 seconds (depending on the patient's verbal ability). Cortical stimulation is applied before the presentation of each image and is continued until there is a correct response or the next image is presented. Each preselected site is stimulated three to four times, though never twice in succession. Sites where stimulation produces consistent speech arrest or anomia are considered essential to language function. It has been demonstrated that resections within 10 mm of essential language cortex will lead to transient postoperative speech difficulties.[7] Any injury to essential language areas will lead to permanent difficulties. When the resection is within 2 cm of the identified language area, it is best to have the patient continue naming objects during the part of the resection that is close to the identified language site. The resection should proceed slowly and be halted if naming errors occur. Haglund and colleagues determined that if resections near eloquent language cortex avoid resection within 10 to 20 mm along a continuous gyrus, a postoperative language deficit is unlikely.[44, 45]

As stated previously, it is important to remember that the topography of essential language varies from individual to individual.[7] Furthermore, patients who are adept in more than one language have separate essential language areas for each language. Standard anatomic temporal lobe resections (e.g., measured resections, resections anterior to the central sulcus, resections anterior to the vein of Labbé) do not always spare essential language areas. Ojemann and coworkers[7] found that subjects typically have two language areas—one in the posterior inferior frontal gyrus, and one in the posterior temporal lobe. However, individuals display a wide variety of language topography, and some have three or more sites identified. Furthermore, the specific language task performed by the patient may lead to the identification of different language sites.[46] Finally, when mapping motor speech, the surgeon must first identify face motor cortex. When stimulated, this area can evoke blockage of speech and therefore may be incorrectly identified as the motor speech area.

The basal language area[47] can probably be resected with relative impunity, indicating that although this site is involved in language function, it is not essential. Electrical stimulation of this area produced total global receptive and expressive aphasia, but resection produced no long-lasting language changes.[47]

As with the other types of mapping described earlier, language mapping can be performed through the

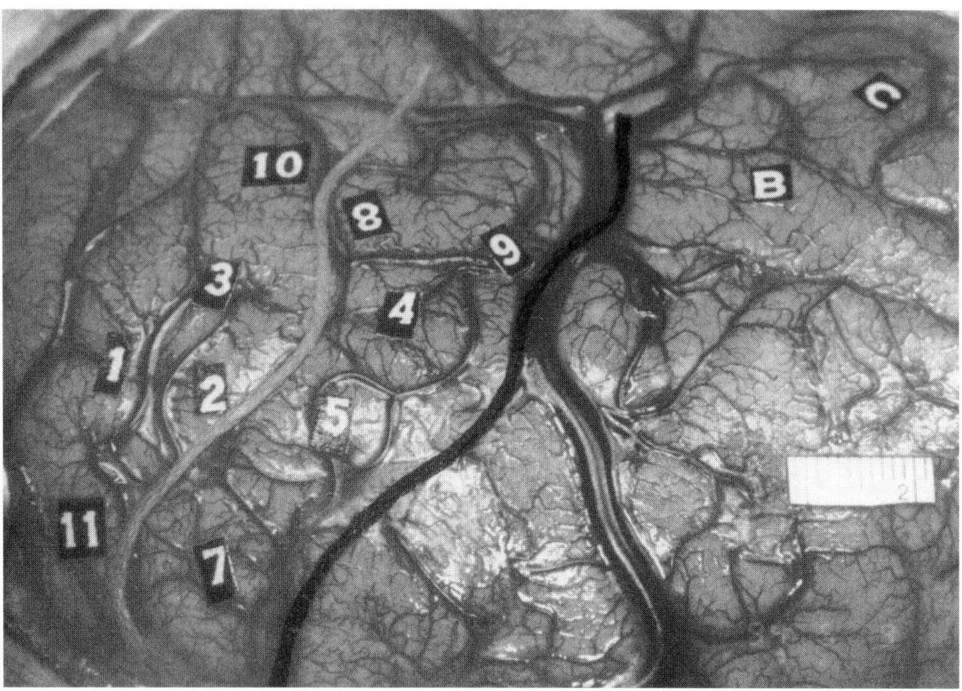

FIGURE 153–4. Number and letter arrangement used for mapping reference points. (The contrasting colored sutures are used to mark the sulcal boundaries.)

dura or directly on the cortical surface.[40] When the surgeon wishes to stimulate unexposed cortex, this can be accomplished by sliding a strip electrode beneath the edge of the bone flap and then using a device that attaches to the electrode lead wire connection, which permits direct bipolar stimulation (Fig. 153–5).[41]

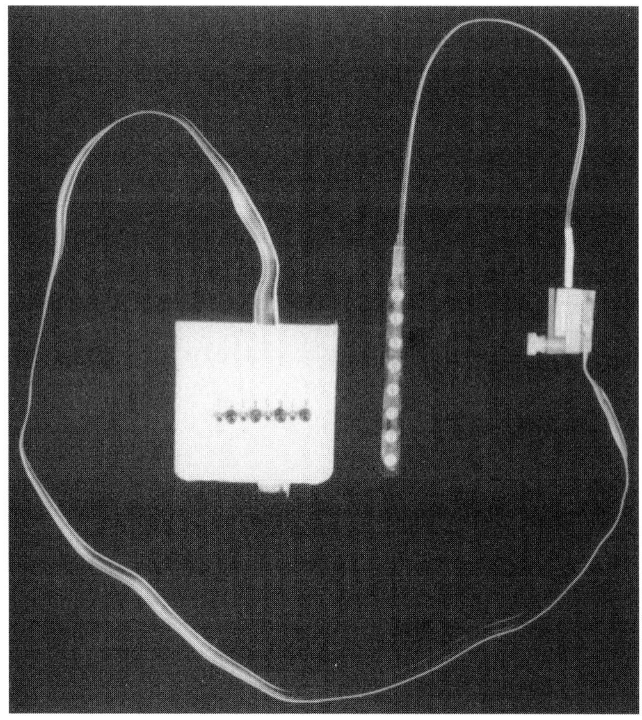

FIGURE 153–5. Strip electrode used for stimulating unexposed cortex.

EXTRAOPERATIVE MAPPING OF LANGUAGE CORTEX

As stated previously, if an awake procedure is not feasible (e.g., in a young child) and language mapping is necessary, a subdural or epidural electrode grid can be used for extraoperative functional mapping and seizure monitoring. Although the procedure is generally well tolerated, it carries the infection risk of chronically implanted hardware, and antibiotic coverage for the duration of the implantation is routinely used. Other shortcomings include less precise spatial resolution (a 1-cm interval between electrode contacts, versus 5-mm separation with stimulation probes), a fixed electrode orientation, and pain that is occasionally associated with awake extraoperative stimulation.

SPECIAL CONSIDERATIONS

Face Motor Cortex

Intrinsic tumors involving the nondominant face motor cortex can be safely removed using brain mapping techniques to localize inferior rolandic cortex and avoid resection of the hand motor cortex and descending subcortical motor pathways. Permanent disability is prevented because of the bilateral representation of face motor function at the neocortical level. However, owing to language localization in cortical zones contiguous with the dominant hemisphere face motor cortex, there is a significant risk of permanent postoperative dysarthria. Therefore, dominant face motor cortex resections should be performed with continual concomitant language testing.[10]

Supplementary Motor Area

Fried and associates[48] performed stimulation of the SMA with subdural electrode grids placed on the medial surface of the cerebral hemispheres in 13 patients with intractable epilepsy undergoing evaluation for surgical treatment. They demonstrated somatotopic organization, with the lower extremities represented posteriorly, the head and face anteriorly, and the upper extremities between these two regions. Anterior to the supplementary motor representation of the face, vocalization and speech arrest or slowing of speech were evoked. With intraoperative cortical and subcortical mapping to identify primary motor cortex and descending motor fibers, large tumor resections of the dominant hemisphere SMA can be performed safely; however, they may be accompanied by a dramatic but reversible syndrome of transient speech and motor deficits termed the SMA syndrome.[11] These deficits are related to one of the SMA's putative functions—namely, motor initiation, including speech function. If cortical and subcortical motor pathways stimulate at the end of the case, the postoperative deficits will most likely improve.

Insula

Surgery for intra-axial insulo-opercular lesions in the dominant hemisphere carries a risk of speech and motor deficits. Frequent intraoperative stimulation mapping is helpful for safe resection.[9, 49, 50]

Arcuate Fasciculus

Classic teaching and the evaluation of patients with strokes have suggested that damage to the arcuate fasciculus (a white matter tract in the inferior portion of the superior longitudinal fasciculus, superior to the insula and extreme capsule, connecting temporal and frontal language zones) causes impaired speech repetition. Shuren and coworkers[51] and Santiago and colleagues[52] reported cases in which the accepted anatomic location of the arcuate fasciculus was clearly resected without causing a deficit in language function, suggesting that, at least in these patients, the arcuate fasciculus was not necessary for speech repetition in the classic sense. Resections in this region can be carried out while the patient continues naming objects if the surgeon is concerned about proximity to essential speech cortex.

Resecting Language Cortex in Children

Duchowney and associates[53] found that in their patients who underwent cortical mapping for epilepsy, lesions acquired before the age of 5 years may cause language to relocate to the opposite hemisphere, but only when language cortex is destroyed. Several other studies demonstrated recovery of language by its relocation to the other hemisphere after postnatal dominant hemisphere insults. This process was inversely related to age, as the youngest children showed the best recovery.[54–57]

Tumors and Vascular Malformations in Functional Cortex

It was once widely believed that intrinsic tumors could be resected safely if the tumor removal stayed within the confines of the grossly abnormal tissue. Several retrospective studies[58, 59] have called this premise into doubt, because functioning motor, sensory, and language tissue can be located within grossly obvious tumor or in the surrounding infiltrated brain. This is clearly demonstrated by large asymptomatic brainstem or thalamic tumors that cannot be surgically removed without incurring disabling deficits.

PITFALLS OF CORTICAL MAPPING

Although cortical mapping is an important tool, potential pitfalls must be recognized if it is to be used safely and effectively. These pitfalls can be separated into two main categories: inability to identify functional cortex, and injury to functional cortex once it has been identified.

In young patients, stimulation motor mapping is often not possible. SSEPs must be used to localize rolandic cortex. Under general anesthesia, SSEPs and motor cortex localization may prove difficult. Nitrous oxide and narcotic anesthesia is best for such mapping.

Inability to identify functional cortex does not prove that one is not in functional cortex. It may indicate a problem with mapping, not that resection is necessarily safe. During localization of speech cortex, electrocorticography must be used to determine the after-discharge threshold. This ensures that no local seizures are elicited by stimulation. There are often more than two essential speech areas.[7] Therefore, the entire region to be resected should be mapped (i.e., mapping should not be stopped simply because two speech area have been identified). For speech cortex, the patient should continue naming objects during resection of abutting cortex or white matter. Vascular injury in the neighborhood of functional cortex must be avoided. Superficial lesional distortion of cortex does not indicate that underlying white matter has (or has not) been displaced. Ascending or descending fibers may not travel perpendicular to the gyral crown.

CONCLUSIONS

Despite recent advocacy of aggressive, "radical" surgical resections for intrinsic brain tumors of all grades, and the increasing number of cortical resections and disconnections being performed for epilepsy, it is imperative to minimize the patient's risk of functional deficit. Resections near functional cortex can be made safer with the mapping techniques described. However, any resection in or near functional cortex carries a clear risk of postoperative functional deficits. As stated by Penfield in 1954: "Throughout the analysis of every case, the clinician should be, first and foremost, a wise physician and an understanding friend to the patient. He should weigh for him the chances of success by surgery and balance this against the best that conservative treatment can promise. He must see the whole problem in the perspective of the patient's own outlook upon life."[8]

REFERENCES

1. Bartholow R: Experimental investigations into function of the human brain. Am J Med Sci 67:305–313, 1874.
2. Foerster O: The cerebral cortex of man. Lancet 109:309–312, 1931.
3. Cushing H: A note upon the faradic stimulation of the postcentral gyrus in conscious patients. Brain 32:44–54, 1909.
4. Penfield W, Rasmussen T: The Cerebral Cortex of Man: A Clinical Study of Localization and Function. New York, Macmillan, 1950.
5. Kelley DL, Goldring S, O'Leary JL: Average evoked somatosensory responses from exposed cortex of man. Arch Neurol 13: 1–13, 1965.
6. Ojemann GA: Cortical organization of language. J Neurosci 11: 2281–2287, 1991.
7. Ojemann G, Ojemann J, Lettich E, et al: Cortical language localization in left, dominant hemisphere: An electrical stimulation mapping investigation in 117 patients. J Neurosurg 71:316–326, 1989.
8. Penfield W, Jasper H: Epilepsy and the Functional Anatomy of the Human Brain. Boston, Little, Brown, 1954.
9. Zentner J, Meyer B, Stangl A, et al: Intrinsic tumors of the insula: A prospective surgical study of 30 patients. J Neurosurg 85: 263–271, 1996; see comments.
10. LeRoux PD, Berger MS, Haglund MM, et al: Resection of intrinsic tumors from nondominant face motor cortex using stimulation mapping: Report of two cases. Surg Neurol 36:44–48, 1991.
11. Rostomily RC, Berger MS, Ojemann GA, et al: Postoperative deficits and functional recovery following removal of tumors involving the dominant hemisphere supplementary motor area. J Neurosurg 75:62–68, 1991.
12. Silbergeld DL, Ojemann GA: The tailored temporal lobectomy. Neurosurg Clin N Am 4:273–281, 1993.
13. Keen WW: Surgery of the Head: Surgery, Its Principles and Practices. Philadelphia, WB Saunders, 1908.
14. Kido DK, LeMay M, Levinson AW, et al: Computed tomographic localization of the precentral gyrus. Radiology 135:373–377, 1980.
15. Anderson JE: Grant's Atlas of Anatomy. Baltimore, Williams & Wilkins, 1978.
16. Willis WD, Grossman RG: The Brain and Its Environment, 3rd ed. St. Louis, CV Mosby, 1981.
17. Berger MS, Cohen WA, Ojemann GA: Correlation of motor cortex brain mapping data with magnetic resonance imaging. J Neurosurg 72:383–387, 1990; see comments.
18. Yetkin FZ, Mueller WM, Morris GL, et al: Functional MR activation correlated with intraoperative cortical mapping. AJNR Am J Neuroradiol 18:1311–1315, 1997.
19. Mueller WM, Yetkin FZ, Hammeke TA, et al: Functional magnetic resonance imaging mapping of the motor cortex in patients with cerebral tumors. Neurosurgery 39:515–520, discussion 520–521, 1996.
20. Mueller WM, Yetkin FZ, Haughton VM: Functional magnetic resonance imaging of the somatosensory cortex. Neurosurg Clin N Am 8:373–381, 1997.
21. Ojemann JG, Neil JM, MacLeod AM, et al: Increased functional vascular response in the region of a glioma. J Cereb Blood Flow Metab 18:148–153, 1998.
22. Fox PT, Burton H, Raichle ME: Mapping human somatosensory cortex with positron emission tomography. J Neurosurg 67:34–43, 1987.
23. Wada J, Rasmussen T: Intracranial injection of Amytal for the lateralization of cerebral speech dominance. J Neurosurg 17:266–282, 1960.
24. Bahn MM, Lin W, Silbergeld DL, et al: Localization of language cortices by functional MR imaging compared with intracarotid amobarbital hemispheric sedation. AJR Am J Roentgenol 169: 575–579, 1997.
25. Yetkin FZ, Swanson S, Fischer M, et al: Functional MR of frontal lobe activation: Comparison with Wada language results. AJNR Am J Neuroradiol 19:1095–1098, 1998.
26. Benson RR, FitzGerald DB, LeSueur LL, et al: Language dominance determined by whole brain functional MRI in patients with brain lesions. Neurology 52:798–809, 1999.
27. Bookheimer SY, Zeffiro TA, Blaxton T, et al: A direct comparison of PET activation and electrocortical stimulation mapping for language localization. Neurology 48:1056–1065, 1997.
28. FitzGerald DB, Cosgrove GR, Ronner S, et al: Location of language in the cortex: A comparison between functional MR imaging and electrocortical stimulation. AJNR Am J Neuroradiol 18:1529–1539, 1997.
29. Theodore WH: Positron emission tomography and single photon emission computed tomography. Curr Opin Neurol 9:89–92, 1996.
30. Bly BM, Kosslyn SM: Functional anatomy of object recognition in humans: Evidence from positron emission tomography and functional magnetic resonance imaging. Curr Opin Neurol 10: 5–9, 1997.
31. Tulving E, Habib R, Nyberg L, et al: Positron emission tomography correlations in and beyond medial temporal lobes. Hippocampus 9:71–82, 1999.
32. Gordon E: The neurophysiology of anaesthesia. In Stockard JJ, Bickford RG (eds): A Basis and Practice of Neuroanaesthesia. Amsterdam, Excerpta Medica, 1975, pp 3–46.
33. Silbergeld DL, Mueller WM, Colley PS, et al: Use of propofol (Diprivan) for awake craniotomies: Technical note. Surg Neurol 38:271–272, 1992.
34. Sartorius CJ, Berger MS: Rapid termination of intraoperative stimulation-evoked seizures with application of cold Ringer's lactate to the cortex: Technical note. J Neurosurg 88:349–351, 1998.
35. Abernathy CD, Kubik S, Ono M: Atlas of the Cerebral Sulci. New York, Thieme Medical Publishers, 1990.
36. Duvernoy HM, Cabanis EA: The Human Brain: Surface, Three-Dimensional Sectional Anatomy with MRI, and Vascularization. New York, Springer Verlag, 1992.
37. Symington J: The central fissure of the cerebrum. J Anat Physiol 47:321–339, 1913.
38. Silbergeld DL, Miller JW: Intraoperative cerebral mapping and monitoring. Contemp Neurosurg 18:1–6, 1996.
39. Snyder AZ: Steady-state vibration evoked potentials: Descriptions of technique and characterization of responses. Electroencephalogr Clin Neurophysiol 84:257–268, 1992.
40. Silbergeld DL: Intraoperative transdural functional mapping: Technical note. J Neurosurg 80:756–758, 1994.
41. Silbergeld DL: A new device for cortical stimulation mapping of surgically unexposed cortex: Technical note. J Neurosurg 79: 612–614, 1993.
42. Jayakar P, Alvarez LA, Duchowny MS, et al: A safe and effective paradigm to functionally map the cortex in childhood. J Clin Neurophysiol 9:288–293, 1992.
43. Luders HO, Lesser RP, Dinner DS, et al: A negative motor response elicited by electrical stimulation of the human frontal cortex. Adv Neurol 57:149–157, 1992.
44. Ojemann GA: Brain organization for language from the perspective of electrical stimulation mapping. Behav Brain Sci 2:189–230, 1983.
45. Haglund MM, Berger MS, Shamseldin M, et al: Cortical localization of temporal lobe language sites in patients with gliomas. Neurosurgery 34:567–576, 1994.
46. Schwartz TH, Ojemann GA, Haglund MM, et al: Cerebral lateralization of neuronal activity during naming, reading and line-matching. Brain Res Cogn Brain Res 4:263–273, 1996.
47. Luders H, Lesser RP, Hahn J, et al: Basal temporal language area. Brain 114(Pt 2):743–754, 1991.
48. Fried I, Katz A, McCarthy G, et al: Functional organization of human supplementary motor cortex studied by electrical stimulation. J Neurosci 11):3656–3666, 1991.
49. Kumabe T, Nakasato N, Suzuki K, et al: Two-staged resection of a left frontal astrocytoma involving the operculum and insula using intraoperative neurophysiological monitoring—case report. Neurol Med Chir (Tokyo) 38:503–507, 1998.
50. Ture U, Yasargil DC, Al-Mefty O, et al: Topographic anatomy of the insular region. J Neurosurg 90:720–733, 1999.

51. Shuren JE, Schefft BK, Yeh HS, et al: Repetition and the arcuate fasciculus. J Neurol 242:596–598, 1995.
52. Santiago P, Ojemann GA, Silbergeld DL: Surgical disruption of the arcuate fasciculus does not result in aphasia. 1998, p. 250.
53. Duchowny M, Jayakar P, Harvey AS, et al: Language cortex representation: Effects of developmental versus acquired pathology. Ann Neurol 40:31–38, 1996.
54. Cummings JL, Benson DF, Walsh MJ, et al: Left-to-right transfer of language dominance: A case study. Neurology 29:1547–1550, 1979.
55. Rasmussen T, Milner B: The role of early left-brain injury in determining lateralization of cerebral speech functions. Ann N Y Acad Sci 299:355–369, 1977.
56. Vargha-Khadem F, O'Gorman AM, Watters GV: Aphasia and handedness in relation to hemispheric side, age at injury and severity of cerebral lesion during childhood. Brain 108(Pt 3): 677–696, 1985.
57. Woods BT, Carey S: Language deficits after apparent clinical recovery from childhood aphasia. Ann Neurol 6:405–409, 1979.
58. Skirboll SS, Ojemann GA, Berger MS, et al: Functional cortex and subcortical white matter located within gliomas. Neurosurgery 38:678–684, discussion 684–685, 1996.
59. Ojemann JG, Miller JW, Silbergeld DL: Preserved function in brain invaded by tumor. Neurosurgery 39:253–258, discussion 258–259, 1996.

CHAPTER 154

Monitoring and Mapping of Vision in the Neurosurgical Patient

KATHLEEN R. TOZER ■ STEPHEN L. SKIRBOLL ■ H. RICHARD WINN

Mapping brain function and monitoring the nervous system before and during neurosurgical procedures is an important tool in the management of the neurosurgical patient. Methods for brain monitoring and mapping include brainstem auditory evoked potential and cranial nerve monitoring, as well as intraoperative cortical mapping to localize somatosensory, motor, or language function. Increasingly, noninvasive localization of function using methods such as functional magnetic resonance imaging (fMRI), positron-emission tomography (PET), and magnetoencephalography (MEG) are supplementing more traditional mapping techniques. These techniques, along with standard structural imaging, are allowing neurosurgical intervention for resection of lesions, including epileptogenic foci, which have been considered unresectable in the past.[1, 2]

Unlike motor, sensory, and language function, the visual system has been a less well established target for physiologic monitoring and mapping. Although the anatomic pathway underlying transmission of visual information from the retina to the occipital cortex is well characterized, the visual system has been refractory to intraoperative monitoring. Much experimental data on mapping cortical visual function exist, but intraoperative mapping of visual cortical function is undertaken significantly less frequently than mapping of other brain functions. This chapter reviews the anatomic visual pathway and addresses work related to preoperative mapping of visual function and to intraoperative monitoring of the optic nerve and visual cortex.

ANATOMY

The visual system is one of the most studied and well defined neuroanatomic circuits.[3, 4] Light enters the pupil and strikes the retina on the nasal or temporal hemifield. As depicted in Figure 154–1, information from the right visual field strikes the temporal hemifield of the left retina and the nasal hemifield of the right retina. Information from the left visual field strikes the right retinal temporal hemifield and the left retinal nasal hemifield. From there, the information from the right or left retina travels through the optic nerve to the optic chiasm, where visual information from the right visual field is separated from the left visual field and subsequently travels to the contralateral occipital cortex through the thalamus. An ordered representation of the retina, from medial to lateral and superior to inferior aspects, is retained.

At the optic chiasm, nerve fibers from the nasal half of the retina cross to join the temporal fibers from the contralateral retina. When the fibers from the contralateral nasal retina join the temporal fibers, they initially loop anteriorly for a short distance in contralateral optic nerve before traveling together caudally in the optic tract toward the thalamus. A lesion in the optic nerve close to the chiasm can affect the visual field of the ipsilateral eye and the contralateral temporal visual field. From the chiasm, the optic tracts sweep back around the rostral midbrain to the lateral geniculate body (LGB) of the thalamus.

The first relay in the visual pathway is at the LGB, a small nucleus of the thalamus ventral to the pulvinar. Crossed and uncrossed fibers remain segregated and terminate in six alternating layers. Layers II, III, and V receive fibers from the ipsilateral temporal retina. Layers I, IV, and VI receive fibers from the contralateral nasal retina. Layers I and II are the magnocellular layers, containing large neurons that rapidly carry information encoding changes in the visual image. Layers III through VI are parvocellular layers and are composed of many smaller neurons that encode color and detailed spatial and form information. These layers retain the anatomic organization of the retinal fibers, with the superior retina (i.e., inferior visual field) projecting to the medial LGB and the inferior retina (i.e., superior visual field) projecting to the lateral LGB. The macula projects to the posterior LGB.

The neurons of the LGB give rise to the optic radiations, also called the geniculocalcarine tract. This tract traverses the internal capsule, passes around the lateral ventricle, and terminates in the visual cortex. A bundle of the optic tract courses forward over the temporal horn of the lateral ventricle, forming Meyer's loop.

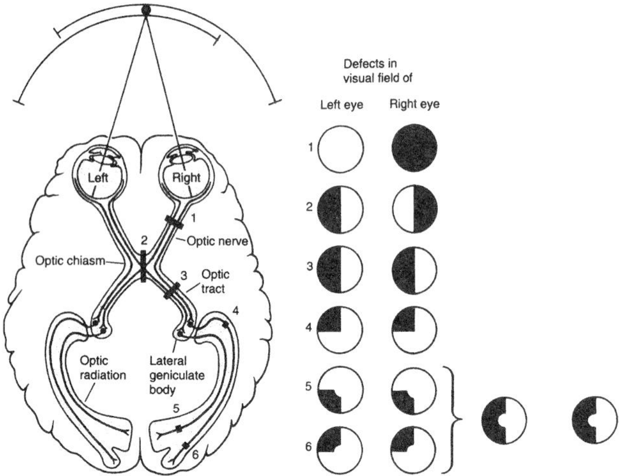

FIGURE 154–1. Schematic representation of the visual pathway with sample lesions and corresponding visual field defects. An optic nerve lesion (1) results in monocular blindness. Transection of the chiasm (2) causes loss of bilateral nasal fibers and a corresponding bitemporal defect. An optic tract lesion (3) results in contralateral hemianopsia. Meyer's loop lesion (4) results in contralateral superior quadrantanopsia. Superior and inferior calcarine sulcus lesions (5, 6) result in contralateral inferior and superior quadrantanopsia, respectively. Notice that the macula is spared because of the separation of the macular representation. (Adapted from Mason C, Kandel ER: Central visual pathways. In Kandel ER, Schwartz JH, Jessell TM [eds]: Principles of Neural Science, 3rd ed. East Norwalk, CT, Appleton & Lange, 1991.)

These fibers carry information from the contralateral superior visual field. The remainder of the tract, carrying contralateral inferior visual field fibers, takes a more direct route around the ventricle. The optic tract terminates in the primary visual cortex of the occipital lobe.

The primary visual cortex, like the rest of the visual system, retains a precise anatomic organization along the banks of the calcarine sulcus in the medial occipital lobe. Fibers carrying information from the superior visual field synapse on neurons along the inferior bank of the calcarine sulcus. Fibers representing the inferior visual fields synapse along the superior bank of the calcarine sulcus. The macula is responsible for the central 10 degrees of the visual field, and its fibers terminate on the posterior one third of the visual cortex. Between 50% and 60% of the posterior striate cortex represents the macula. In contrast, the anterior two thirds of the visual cortex receives representation of the nonmacular visual field.[5] Visual association cortex lies anterior, superior, and inferior to the primary visual cortex.

The precise segregation and anatomic correlation of visual information from the retina to the occipital lobe allows for localization of pathology based on clinical visual field deficits, as summarized in Figure 154–1. Lesions in the optic nerve cause unilateral blindness (see Fig. 154–1 [1]). Retrochiasmatic lesions of the optic tract affect the contralateral visual field (see Fig. 154–1 [3]). Selective lesions of Meyer's loop (see Fig. 154–1 [4]) affect the contralateral superior visual field, and lesions of distinct portions of the calcarine cortex affect distinct areas of the visual field (see Fig. 154–1 [5, 6]). Traditional visual field testing can be used to define visual field deficits, which can then be correlated with pathology evident on standard computed tomography and MRI.

The location and pathology of surgical lesions affecting the visual system vary. They may include lesions compressing the optic nerve or chiasm that arise from adjacent structures. Examples include sellar and parasellar lesions such as pituitary adenomas and craniopharyngiomas. The optic tract may be compromised by intrinsic or metastatic brain tumors, abscesses, and by vascular lesions such as arteriovenous malformations (AVMs). Such lesions may also affect the occipital lobe and invade or displace the striate cortex. Extra-axial lesions such as meningiomas may compress the visual pathway anywhere from the optic apparatus to the visual cortex. Epileptic foci may be immediately adjacent to or within the visual pathway. The utility of mapping and monitoring visual function depends on the nature and location of the particular lesion. Modalities such as visual evoked potential (VEP) monitoring, fMRI, PET, MEG, and direct cortical stimulation can be used alone or in combination to plan the optimal treatment for patients with lesions affecting the visual system.

INTRAOPERATIVE VISUAL MONITORING

Intraoperative monitoring of visual function has been widely reported and has had mixed success. The primary means of visual monitoring has been with VEPs. Unlike monitoring somatosensory evoked potentials or brainstem auditory evoked potentials, VEPs are less well established as a reliable means of physiologic monitoring. Some groups have had reasonable success, however, using a variety of stimulation protocols and outcome measurements. Although the difficulties with VEP monitoring are multifactorial, they are perhaps not insurmountable.

VEPs are often used in the diagnosis of neurological diseases. VEPs are best at assessing macular and optic nerve function. They also can provide information about chiasmatic defects but are not useful for assessing cortical function. A patient with cortical blindness can have normal VEPs if the anterior visual apparatus is intact.[6] Conversely, VEPs can be undetectable with a compromised optic nerve, even if some function is retained.

VEPs are measured by providing a visual stimulus and recording an electrical response through scalp electrodes. The typical stimulus in an awake patient is a shifting black and white checkerboard pattern that reverses colors at a defined frequency (i.e., pattern reversal stimulus). A second type of stimulus is a flashing light. The pattern reversal stimulated VEPs tend to be larger and more reproducible. Changes in total luminescence, pattern size, contrast, focus, pupillary size, and physiologic factors, among other things, can affect the VEP waveform.

A typical VEP response to a pattern reversal stimulus consists of a positive deflection with a latency of 100 msec flanked by negative deflections at 70 and 145 msec (Fig. 154–2). A second positive deflection may follow. These responses are called P100, N70, and N145. Alternatively, the first and second positive deflections may be called P1 and P2, and the first two negative deflections may be called N1 and N2. The latency and amplitude of the waveform are two values that can be compared for monitoring. Response latencies between eyes can be variable in normal individuals. Latency differences of greater than 10 msec between eyes suggest pathology. An absent P100 response or a P100 response with a latency longer than the 95th to 99th percentile is abnormal. The N70 peak can also exhibit normal variability. For operative monitoring, waveform stability is more important than obtaining a robust stereotypic waveform.

Intraoperative VEP recording is complicated by several factors.[17] The operating room can be a difficult environment in which to record signals because of background noise. Anesthesia can affect VEPs dramatically through general depression of cortical function; changes in blood pressure, ventilation and oxygenation status; pupillary size; and anesthetic drugs. The anesthetized patient cannot focus on a visual stimulus. A reliable property of the VEP response must be chosen to monitor.

Anesthesia must be undertaken carefully to minimize the affects of anesthetic drugs and physiologic factors on VEPs. In one study of surgical patients without visual problems who were undergoing noncranial surgery, VEPs were monitored under intravenous anesthesia.[7] A similar regimen to that used for other physiologic monitoring, such as somatosensory evoked potentials, was used. After induction of anesthesia, P100 latency increased, and waveform amplitude decreased. In some cases, recognizable VEPs disappeared completely.[2] If surgical decisions are to be made based on VEP monitoring, the other variables must be minimized, so that changes in VEPs reflect compromise of the visual circuit rather than other factors.

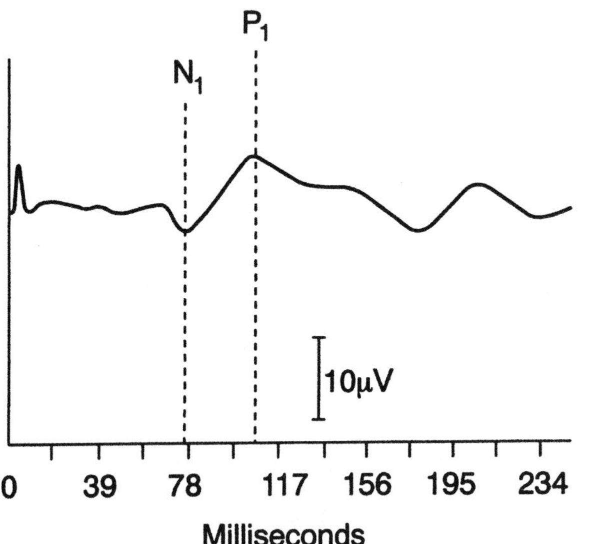

FIGURE 154–2. Representative visual evoked potential in response to a phase-reversal stimulus. Labeled are the N70 (N1) and P100 (P1) deflections, at approximately 70 and 100 msec, respectively. The N2 and P2 deflections are present but unlabeled. (From Jones NS: Visual evoked potentials in endoscopic and anterior skull base surgery: A review. J Laryngol Otol 3: 515, 1997.)

Choosing a proper visual stimulus protocol is also important for recording VEPs. Because anesthetized patients cannot focus on a visual stimulus such as a checkerboard pattern, flashes of light are most commonly used. Some methods used include special goggles that provide flashing light from light-emitting diodes (LEDs) through closed eyelids. Depending on the type of surgery, the goggles may interfere with surgical positioning. A contact lens photostimulator has also been used to deliver a flashing light stimulus. Eyelid sutures may be required to hold the contact lenses in place. Regardless of the stimulus method, pupillary size affects the amplitude and latency of the response. Any medication that changes the pupillary size, such as mydriatics or narcotics, affects the VEPs.

The appropriate aspect of the VEP waveform must be chosen to monitor. For example, the peak latency or the waveform amplitude of any of the characteristic deflections may be followed. Most often, the P100 latency is followed, as is the maximum amplitude between the negative and positive deflections. VEPs and other evoked potentials are monitored by an electrophysiologist. Any change in the waveform must be communicated to the surgeon and anesthesiologist.

VEP monitoring has been used in a variety of surgical procedures. Any procedure in which the orbital contents are at risk could benefit from optic nerve monitoring. Orbital decompression, optic nerve decompression, or endoscopic sinus surgery are some examples. VEP monitoring may also prove useful in monitoring visual function during complex spine procedures, during which visual function may be unexpectedly lost. The underlying pathophysiology is unclear, but some have advocated using VEPs in these procedures.

In one series using VEP monitoring during orbital surgery for dysthyroid eye disease, orbital tumors, or orbital trauma, VEP changes of a defined temporal profile correlated with intraoperative compromise of the visual system and postoperative deficits.[8] VEP waveform amplitudes in response to a flashing light stimulus through contact lenses were monitored. Diminishment of VEPs correlated with direct pressure on the optic nerve or displacement of the globe, as well as with hypotension, halothane or isoflurane use, or displacement of the contact lens stimulator. On releasing pressure on the optic apparatus, VEPs usually returned to baseline within 3 minutes. If the VEPs were absent for more than 4 minutes, the patient was more likely to have postoperative deficits. Using 4 minutes as the critical period allows some false-positive results. False-negative results, which are clinically more significant, did not occur in this series. Monitoring also slightly lengthened operating room time, because changes in VEPs resulted in a search for the cause, whether it was related to surgery or other factors.

Other reports have shown changes in flash-simulated VEPs have no correlation with postoperative visual acuity.[18] However, VEPs can be a guide to when surgical manipulation should cease, at least temporarily, to allow for recovery. Persistent prolongation may predict transient postoperative changes.[9]

VEPs have also been used to monitor the anterior visual pathway during operations involving the sellar and parasellar regions. Several series have used VEP monitoring during transsphenoidal resections of pituitary tumors. One study[10] of 22 patients with pituitary macroadenomas found that VEP monitoring improved postoperative visual fields but not postoperative visual acuity. Decreased P100 latency correlated with this improvement in visual fields. A second study[11] reported immediate improvement in waveform latency and amplitude after optic chiasm decompression, which correlated with postoperative visual improvement. One way VEPs may improve postoperative function is to allow a more radical resection to be performed.

VEPs have been reported in a variety of other procedures, including craniofacial surgery,[12] resections of sellar meningiomas and cysts,[13] and during treatment of AVMs.[13] In one case, VEPs changed during selective embolization of the distal branches of the posterior cerebral artery supplying an AVM. The VEPs recovered with repositioning of the vascular catheter. In a second case, VEPs improved when the draining vein of an occipital AVM was clipped, and visual function was preserved postoperatively. Although many instances of monitoring optic pathways with VEPs are reported, they are still not routinely used for surgical monitoring.

The origin of VEPs has been studied in patients with implanted subdural electrodes undergoing long-term invasive electrocorticography for seizure localization. VEPs have been recorded directly from the cortex during presentation of visual stimuli. The VEP amplitude recorded directly at the cortex is 10-fold higher than at the scalp, but the latencies are similar.[14] In normal occipital lobes, VEPs map to the mesial occipital lobe, superior calcarine fissure, occipital pole, lingual gyrus, and lateral occipital lobe in a temporal pattern.[14, 15] There appear to be multiple generators. VEP responses evoked by stimulation of one visual hemifield arise from the contralateral occipital lobe.[16]

VEPs measured by scalp electrodes are the result of multiple generators from both hemispheres. This probably contributes to the variability and relative lack of specificity of VEP changes.

In summary, VEPs have been studied extensively for monitoring of visual pathways for preoperative assessment, and to a lesser degree, VEPs have been used intraoperatively. Results during surgery have been decidedly mixed, and the technique is not widely used. Although VEP stability is improved by monitoring directly at the occipital cortex with subdural electrodes, it would be hard to justify the additional risk of implanting electrodes in patients with anterior visual pathway pathology. However, if noninvasive VEPs could be perfected, they could provide a powerful means of monitoring the optic nerve and chiasm during a variety of orbital and anterior skull base procedures.

PREOPERATIVE VISION MAPPING

Preoperative vision mapping uses noninvasive methods such functional MRI, ^{15}O-PET, and MEG to localize visual function to specific brain regions. Stimuli used to provoke functional responses vary. Some studies use red or white flashing lights to the entire visual field by means of an external light source[19] or through specialized goggles.[20, 21] Visual stimulation is usually flashed at 8 to 10 Hz. Other studies use LED arrays on goggles to stimulate particular visual regions.[22] More complex visual stimuli are also used. A pattern reversal protocol calls for a black and white checkerboard pattern that reverses the colors of the squares at a defined rate.[23, 24]

Functional Magnetic Resonance Imaging

Functional MRI is thought to detect physiologic activation of the brain by differential tissue oxygenation.[25, 26] When a specific region of cortex is activated, regional cerebral blood flow increases, resulting in relative hyperoxemia. As the level of oxyhemoglobin rises, the relative concentration of deoxyhemoglobin falls in the capillaries, venules, and draining veins of the activated cortex. Deoxyhemoglobin is paramagnetic, whereas oxyhemoglobin is not. Gradient-echo, T2-weighted images can detect the difference between concentrations of oxyhemoglobin and deoxyhemoglobin in the hyperoxemic cortex compared with the resting cortex.[25, 26] This method of detecting brain activation based on deoxyhemoglobin concentration is called blood oxygen level–dependent (BOLD) contrast MRI. Some controversy exists, however, regarding the exact nature of signal elicited during fMRI mapping.

There are some inherent advantages and disadvantages to fMRI imaging. No additional contrast need be given when using the BOLD protocol, unlike, for example, imaging with PET. Initial fMRI studies used stronger magnets, often 4.0 Tesla,[22] which are only available at a few centers. Subsequent studies, however, found the use of 1.5-T magnets, the strength used for standard MRI imaging, to be sufficient.[19–21, 23, 24] Functional MRI can be performed during the same sitting as a standard MRI, and the images can be superimposed on anatomic MR images. Spatial resolution may be on the order of anatomic MRI, at 1 mm, and temporal resolution on the order of 3 to 5 seconds.[20]

Disadvantages include the need for patient perseverance and cooperation. MR studies can take time, and any additional time needed to obtain functional images may not be tolerated.[14, 16] Patients must keep their heads still to obtain accurate images. The data must be analyzed appropriately with specialized software. One study[21] found that the detection of functional activation depended on the analysis threshold chosen, with a caveat against operator-dependent activation patterns. MRI studies are expensive, but much of the hardware needed to perform fMRI is already in place, and the additional risks to patients of this procedure are small.

Functional MRI has been used as a scientific tool to map visual areas in experimental animals and in normal human volunteers. Several studies have considered fMRI images of patients with neurosurgical diseases. The aims of these studies have been multiple. Many studies focus primarily on motor, sensory, or language mapping, but a few studies also include visual cortex mapping. These have included patients with a variety of lesions, including tumors, epileptic foci, and vascular malformations.

In one study,[21] three patients with AVMs were studied with fMRI. Although the focus was primarily on motor and speech mapping, the visual cortex was also mapped. The stimulus was provided by goggles containing an array of LEDs, arranged to provide a stimulus to a particular visual hemifield. In these cases, the visual data were not reported to have changed surgical management, unlike the speech and motor data.

Another group[20] studied four patients using fMRI and other modalities to study motor, language, and in two patients, vision localization. The two patients in whom vision was mapped had intractable seizures. One patient had a temporal occipital cyst with a temporal focus for her seizures. The other patient had no clearly defined seizure focus but had visual auras preceding his seizures. In the first patient, fMRI showed functional visual cortex medial to the cyst wall (Fig. 154–3*B*). This was corroborated by the PET data and by intraoperative stimulation. Identification of this functional cortex altered surgical management. The second patient had bilateral visual cortex activation. This did not change surgical management, which involved electrode implantation.

A third study[19] reported using fMRI mapping for 12 patients with space-occupying lesions posterior to the

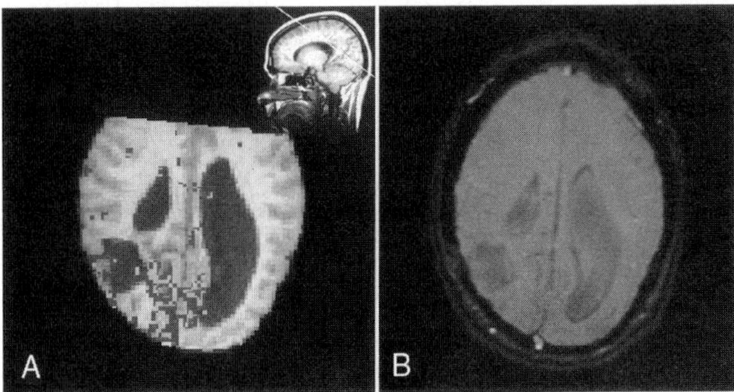

FIGURE 154–3. Positron-emission tomography (PET) *(A)* and functional magnetic resonance imaging (fMRI) *(B)* of a patient with a temporo-occipital cyst and visual activation medial to the cyst. *A*, ^{15}O-water PET is superimposed on a T1-weighted image. Dark pixels represent activation after visual stimulation. *B*, The fMRI of the same plane of the section is superimposed on a T2-weighted image. Pixels represent activation. (Adapted from Fried I, Nenov VI, Ojemann SG, Woods RP: Functional MR and PET imaging of rolandic and visual cortices for neurosurgical planning. J Neurosurg 83:854–861, 1995.)

optic chiasm. Some lesions involved the occipital lobe, whereas others affected the optic radiations or lateral geniculate nucleus, leaving the occipital lobe parenchyma grossly intact. The pathologic diagnosis included intrinsic tumors, metastases, and one abscess. Traditional visual field mapping was also performed. In all cases, the unaffected hemisphere was compared with the affected hemisphere. Unaffected hemispheres revealed activation along the calcarine fissure, as seen in healthy volunteers. In affected hemispheres, activation was diminished or absent, regardless of whether the visual cortex was directly involved in the lesion or deafferented by a lesion involving anterior visual structures.

Visual field evaluation correlated with alterations of visual cortical activation. For example, in 7 of 7 patients with hemianopsia, contralateral visual cortex activation was diminished. A patient with a central homonymous scotoma demonstrated absent activation of the contralateral occipital pole and intact anterior activation.[19]

In another study,[23] fMRI activation was compared between surgical patients with tumors, epilepsy, or cerebrovascular malformations and healthy volunteers. This group examined localization of motor cortex, sensory cortex, Broca's region, and in six patients, visual cortex. Patients viewed a pattern reversal stimulus projected onto a screen by a mirror mounted on the head coil. Activity was found by fMRI in the visual cortex of all of the healthy volunteers and in 6 of 6 patients with lesions in this area. This signal was in the calcarine sulcus or inferior occipital gyrus. Homonymous visual field defects were consistent with fMRI cortical maps compared with activity in the unaffected hemisphere.

Masouka and coworkers[24] reported fMRI studies of 10 patients with occipital epilepsy, 3 of whom had a structural abnormality (e.g., atrophy, hamartoma, heterotopia). A pattern reversal stimulus was used with full and half fields on a screen. Normal patients showed variability in the size and symmetry of functional activation patterns. Functional MRI activation patterns were graded as symmetrical or markedly asymmetrical to allow for normal variability. When comparing activation patterns in patients with occipital lobe epilepsy with unaffected patients, more epilepsy patients were rated abnormal. All four epilepsy patients with symmetrical activation patterns did not activate in either hemisphere. Epilepsy patients with asymmetric maps tended to have concordant abnormal activation and side of ictal electroencephalography (EEG).

Roux and colleagues[21] examined 11 patients with tumors and visual field defects, including quadranopsia, homonymous, and bitemporal hemianopsia. Twelve unaffected patients were used as a comparison. Formal visual field testing was performed, as well as fMRI using a photic stimulus. Tumors were intrinsic gliomas or meningiomas, except for one hypophyseal adenoma. In four patients with tumor removed from calcarine cortex but involving optic radiations or the trigone, no visual cortex activation was seen, consistent with a deafferentation effect. Functional MR activation did occur in infiltrated parenchyma adjacent to the tumor, but no activation was identified within the main portion of the tumor. Using an intraoperative frameless stereotactic device and image guidance with correlated fMRI and anatomic MRI data, this group spared brain with functional activation. None of the patients in this series experienced worsened postoperative visual deficits. One patient with a hypophyseal adenoma and bitemporal hemianopsia had no activation of contralateral visual cortex preoperatively with unilateral stimulation, as expected if the nasal fibers are compromised. A second fMRI was obtained after a transsphenoidal resection, revealing a return of bilateral cortical activation after unilateral visual stimulation.

In summary, fMRI is a useful technique to identify visual cortex in normal and some pathologic conditions. Its use in motor, language, and somatosensory mapping is widespread. It is noninvasive and involves little additional risk to the patient. The physiologic basis of fMRI is still being studied, and its usefulness in certain diseases (e.g., AVMs) is unclear. An absence of detection of functional tissue by fMRI does not necessarily ensure that no viable functional tissue is present.[21] Despite this, as fMRI is increasingly used for neurosurgical mapping, its utility in delineating visual cortex should concomitantly improve.

Positron-Emission Tomography

PET is another technique that can be used to detect functional activation of cortical regions. Like fMRI, it has been used extensively for the experimental study of the functional anatomy of human and nonhuman brains. Clinical application of PET to detect functional regions in brains with pathologic processes is less well reported than fMRI use. Use of PET to study the visual system in neurosurgical diseases is even less commonly reported, but like fMRI, PET is a potentially powerful mapping tool for the visual system.

[^{15}O]-water PET noninvasively localizes cortical activation based on changes in cerebral blood flow.[20, 27] It does not detect white matter tracts. A special positron scanner is required that is often available only at specialized centers. Briefly, a visual stimulus similar to those described previously is given. At a defined time interval, a dose of radioactively labeled water ($H_2{}^{15}O$) is injected intravenously. The PET scanner then detects the distribution of the tracer in the cerebral blood flow. Increased flow results in a relative increase in concentration of the radiolabeled tracer and is a reflection of neuronal activation. Images obtained after a stimulus are compared with baseline images. In this way, changes in cerebral activation based on increased cerebral blood flow are detected. The PET scan can then be coregistered with an anatomic MR scan.[20, 27] The temporal resolution of PET imaging is approximately 50 seconds, the time it takes for the tracer to clear. The spatial resolution is improved by coregistering the images with an MR scan.

Two groups of investigators[20, 27] have used PET to evaluate visual function. Both groups were primarily studying motor and language mapping. Each reported one case of visual mapping with [^{15}O]-water PET, the first a patient with an occipital tumor,[27] and the second with a temporo-occipital cyst and seizures.[20] In both cases, the PET data were coregistered with an MR scan. In both cases, the functional data were taken into consideration when planning surgical resections. In the second case, PET data and fMRI data were concordant (see Fig. 154–3). A subdural grid had been implanted over the affected visual cortex.

The latter case is of particular interest because visual function was identified in the cortex medial to the temporo-occipital cyst by PET and fMRI. On stimulation of the subdural electrodes over the affected cortex, the patient reported flashes of light in the contralateral visual field. The resection was tailored to spare this cortex as much as possible. Postoperatively, the patient experienced a contralateral upper quadrant visual defect. In this case, the use of functional imaging and cortical stimulation may have spared the patient greater postoperative deficits.

In summary, to the limited extent that PET has been used to map visual cortex, it appears to provide a valid assay of visual function. The difference, if any, between visual functional information gleaned from PET or fMRI remains to be elucidated. The main disadvantage of PET is the need for a special and costly scanner that is only now becoming more widely available. Scanning with fMRI can be performed on a conventional scanner, which is readily accessible. For both methods, however, specialized expertise is still required.

Magnetoencephalography

MEG is a third noninvasive means of imaging cortical function and has been used to map visual cortex.[28–30] The theory behind MEG relies on the small magnetic fields that are induced by neuronal electrical currents. Physics dictates that these magnetic fields are orthogonal to the current flow. Neurons within the sulci elicit electrical currents tangential to the scalp (Fig. 154–4). These currents induce radial magnetic fields. The neurons along the gyral surface produce radial neuronal currents, resulting in magnetic field potentials tangential to the scalp. Neurons within a sulcus thus produce maximally detectable magnetic field changes.[29] These magnetic fields are relatively undistorted by overlying tissue. In contrast, the electrical potentials detected by EEG are summed responses of radial and tangential currents, which are then impeded by the overlying meninges, bone, and scalp.

The small magnetic fields are detected by a magnetometer to produce a map. A magnetometer is a large, commercially available device that requires a magnetically shielded room. Fiducial markers are used to register the patient's head. Magnetic fields are compared with and without stimulating vision. Visual stimuli used are similar to those described previously. The location and strength of stimulus-induced neuronal currents can be recorded. The resulting functional map can be coregistered with an MRI scan. This is referred to as magnetic source imaging (MSI).[28] Temporal resolution of MEG is on the order of milliseconds. Spatial

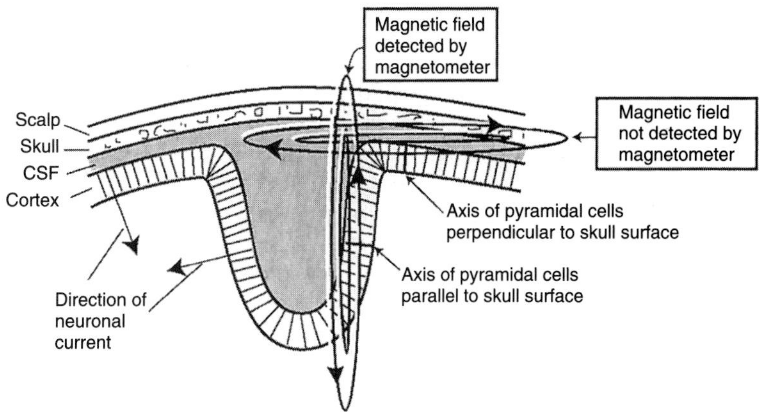

FIGURE 154–4. Schematic representation of magnetic fields induced by neuronal electrical currents. Notice that only neurons within the sulci elicit electric fields tangential to the surface, producing magnetic fields perpendicular to the surface and optimally detectable by the magnetometer. (Adapted from Alberstone CD, Skirboll SL, Benzel EC, et al: Magnetic source imaging and brain surgery: Presurgical and intraoperative planning in 26 patients. J Neurosurg 92:79–90, 2000.)

resolution is improved by coregistration with an MRI scan.

Advantages to this system include direct, noninvasive monitoring of neuronal activity in response to a stimulus. Temporal resolution is very good. The biggest disadvantage of MEG is the need for a magnetometer, which is expensive and not widely available. Although neuronal currents on the surface are detectable, deeper functional activation is not.

Visual cortical function has been mapped with MEG. One group[28] reported neuronal activation in the visual cortex peaking at latencies of 90 to 160 msec after stimulation. Activated cortex is contralateral to the stimulated visual hemifield. In one example, vision was mapped to cortex medial to a parieto-occipital AVM (Fig. 154–5). A second group reported MEG and MSI localization of the visual cortex in six patients with lesions, including gliomas, meningiomas, and one metastasis each in the peritrigonal, parieto-occipital, and temporal regions.[29] In one patient with an occipital meningioma and homonymous hemianopsia, MSI was used to localize visual cortex inferior to the mass. Based on this information, a parieto-occipital approach was planned rather than an occipital approach. Functional visual cortex was avoided, and postoperatively, the patient's vision remained unchanged.

In summary, functional MRI, PET, and MEG have all been used successfully to map visual function. The most widely reported modality for preoperative mapping is fMRI, but all three methods have advantages and disadvantages. All primarily map visual cortex rather than deeper white matter tracks. MEG maps neuronal activity directly and provides the best temporal resolution. Spatial resolution is improved by coregistration with MRI. MEG, however, uses the most specialized equipment and requires technical expertise. PET and fMRI have excellent spatial resolution and are more widely available. Both, however, indirectly map neuronal activation by relying on cerebral blood flow to detect functional cortex. All three methods can provide valuable information for operative planning and can potentially improve neurosurgical outcomes.

INTRAOPERATIVE MAPPING OF THE VISUAL CORTEX

Operative visual mapping encompasses three methods to detect functional visual cortex: implanted subdural electrodes, direct intraoperative stimulation, and VEPs. Functional mapping by means of cortical and subcortical stimulation is widely reported for somatosensory, motor, and language function.[1, 2] Subdural electrodes typically are used to monitor patients long term, using electrocorticography to isolate seizure foci. Somatosensory and language functions are also mapped between operations using these electrodes. Intraoperative cortical stimulation is used for motor, somatosensory, and language mapping, often during an awake craniotomy. Cortical stimulation has also been used to map functional visual cortex.

Stimulation of the visual cortex results in a variety of visual sensations. In early work toward developing a visual prosthesis for the blind, investigators reported

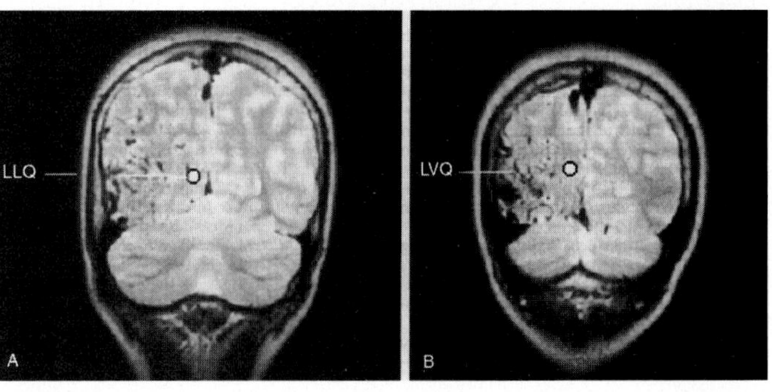

FIGURE 154–5. Magnetic source image of a parieto-occipital arteriovenous malformation (AVM). The magnetoencephalographic activation map was elicited by a visual stimulus coregistered with fast spin-echo, coronal magnetic resonance image and shows visual activation in cortex medial to the AVM. (Adapted from Rowley HA, Roberts TP: Functional localization by magnetoencephalography. Neuroimaging Clin N Am 5:695–710, 1995.)

the production of phosphenes on stimulating the occipital cortex.[30] Phosphenes are typically sensations of small, white flickers of light seen in the visual field contralateral to the site of stimulation. Subsequently, a variety of visual responses, including color, motion, and shapes have been reported in response to cortical stimulation.[31] For intraoperative mapping, the presence or absence of visual sensations is often sufficient for determining involvement of the stimulated cortex.

The first method of mapping visual cortex uses implanted subdural electrodes. The electrodes can be used to record responses or stimulate responses. The electrodes are implanted during an initial operation, often for long-term electrocorticography, to localize a seizure focus. Visual cortex can be mapped by evoking visual phenomena while stimulating through the subdural electrodes. This has been reported extensively for mapping normal anatomic localization of the human visual system.[31] Conversely, on presentation of a visual stimulus, the evoked responses over occipital cortex can be recorded to map activation.[32] Responses are greatest over the visual cortex and diminish at adjacent electrodes, enabling reasonable spatial resolution.[14]

The second method involves directly stimulating the occipital lobe in the operating room. This must be done as an awake craniotomy to allow the patient to report visual sensations. A craniotomy is performed under local anesthesia with monitored sedation. After exposure of the occipital cortex, an electrical stimulator providing a train of pulses is used to systematically probe the region of interest. Five such cases of mapping primary visual cortex were reported by Danks and colleagues.[33] In this study, the visual results were not separated from somatosensory, motor, or language mapping. In 96% of these cases, postoperative function was the same or better than preoperative function. Resection was done to within 0.5 cm from primary somatosensory cortex, including visual cortex.

Visual cortex mapping can also be undertaken under general anesthesia using VEPs. VEPs can be recorded directly at the visual cortex. This has been reported in one series of two patients with occipital epilepsy with implanted subdural grids for long-term monitoring.[32] VEPs were recorded preoperatively in both patients in response to flashing light and pattern reversal stimuli. Responses to photic driving were also recorded. VEP and photic responses colocalized to the same cortical region, a site distinct from the ictal focus. At the time of the epilepsy resection, intraoperative photic responses were recorded continuously under general anesthesia from the subdural electrodes. Recording continued during resection of the occipital seizure focus. Postoperatively, both patients had preserved central vision, although one of the two had a slight enlargement of her peripheral deficit.

CONCLUSIONS

Visual mapping and monitoring are still under development. Unlike motor, somatosensory, and language functions, intraoperative mapping of visual function is infrequently reported. The literature primarily consists of case reports and small series, often as an aside included in a report on a group of patients mapped for other modalities. The techniques for mapping visual function are available, and as the technology evolves, use will increase. Intraoperative visual monitoring, however, remains problematic. VEPs are not easily maintained in the operating room, nor are changes easily analyzed. With improvements in technology, however, intraoperative monitoring and mapping of vision could improve functional outcome, allow more radical treatment of intracranial pathology affecting vision, and become a powerful tool in neurosurgery.

REFERENCES

1. Skirboll SL, Ojemann GA, Berger MS, et al: Functional cortex and subcortical white matter located within gliomas. Neurosurgery 38:678–685, 1996.
2. Berger MS, Ojemann GA: Techniques of functional localization during removal of tumors involving the cerebral hemispheres. In Loftusc TV (ed): Intraoperative Monitoring Techniques in Neurosurgery. New York, McGraw-Hill, 1994, pp 113–127.
3. Mason C, Kandel ER: Central visual pathways. In Kandel ER, Schwartz JH, Jessell TM (eds): Principles of Neural Science, 3rd ed. East Norwalk, CT, Appleton & Lange, 1991.
4. Hubel DH, Wiesel TN: Brain mechanisms of vision. Sci Am 241: 150–162, 1979.
5. Holmes D, Lister WT: Disturbances of vision of cerebral lesions with special reference to cortical representation of the macula. Brain 39:34–73, 1916.
6. Celesia G: Visual evoked potentials in clinical neurology. In Aminoff M (ed): Electrodiagnosis in Clinical Neurology, 4th ed. Philadelphia, Churchill Livingstone, 1999.
7. Wiedemayer H, Fauser B, Armbruster W, et al: Visual evoked potentials for intraoperative neurophysiologic monitoring using total intravenous anesthesia. J Neurosurg Anesth 15:19–24, 2003.
8. Harding GF, Bland JD, Smith VH: Visual evoked potential monitoring of optic nerve function during surgery. J Neurol Neurosurg Psychiatry 53:890–895, 1990.
9. Jones NS: Visual evoked potentials in endoscopic and anterior skull base surgery: A review. J Laryngol Otol 3:513–516, 1997.
10. Chacko AG, Babu KS, Chandy MJ: Value of visual evoked potential monitoring during trans-sphenoidal pituitary surgery. Br J Neurosurg 10:275–278, 1996.
11. Feinsod M, Selhorst JB, Hoyt WF, Wilson CB: Monitoring optic nerve function during craniotomy. J Neurosurg 44:29–31, 1976.
12. Handel N, Law J, Hoehn R, Kirsch W: Monitoring visual evoked response during craniofacial surgery. Ann Plast Surg 2:257–8, 1979.
13. John ER, Chabot RJ, Prichep LS, et al: Real-time intraoperative monitoring during neurosurgical and neuroradiological procedures. J Clin Neurophysiol 6:125–158, 1989.
14. Noachtar S, Hashimoto T, Luders H: Pattern visual evoked potentials recorded from human occipital cortex with chronic subdural electrodes. Electroencephalogr Clin Neurophysiol 88:435–446, 1993.
15. Arroyo S, Lesser RT, Poon W, et al: Neuronal generators of visual evoked potentials in humans: Visual processing in the human cortex. Epilepsia 38:600–610, 1997.
16. Hoeppner TJ, Bergen D, Morrell F: Hemispheric asymmetry of visual evoked potentials in patients with well-defined occipital lesions. Electroencephalogr Clin Neurophysiol 57:310–319, 1984.
17. Grundy BL: Monitoring of sensory evoked potentials during neurosurgical operations: Methods and applications. Neurosurgery 11:556–575, 1982.
18. Silva ICE, Wang AD, Symon L: The application of flash visual evoked potentials during operations on the anterior visual pathways. Neurol Res 7:11–16, 1985.
19. Kollias SS, Landau K, Khan N, et al: Functional evaluation using magnetic resonance imaging of the visual cortex in patients with retrochiasmatic lesions. J Neurosurg 89:780–790, 1998.

20. Fried I, Nenov VI, Ojemann SG, Woods RP: Functional MR and PET imaging of rolandic and visual cortices for neurosurgical planning. J Neurosurg 83:854–861, 1995.
21. Roux FE, Ibarrola D, Lotterie JA, et al: Perimetric visual field and functional MRI correlation: Implications for image-guided surgery in occipital brain tumours. J Neurol Neurosurg Psychiatry 71:505–514, 2001.
22. Latchaw RE, Hu X, Ugurbil K, et al: Functional magnetic resonance imaging as management tool for cerebral arteriovenous malformations. Neurosurgery 37:619–625, 1995.
23. Hirsch J, Ruge MI, Kim KH, et al: An integrated functional magnetic resonance imaging procedure for preoperative mapping of cortical areas associated with tactile, motor, language, and visual functions. Neurosurgery 47:711–721, 2000.
24. Masuoka LK, Anderson AW, Gore JC, et al: Functional magnetic resonance imaging identifies abnormal visual cortical function in patients with occipital lobe epilepsy. Epilepsia 40:1248–1253, 1999.
25. Ogawa S, Lee TM, Kay AR, Tank DW: Brain magnetic resonance imaging with contrast dependent on blood oxygenation. Proc Natl Acad Sci U S A 87:9868–9872, 1990.
26. Ogawa S, Tank DW, Menon R, et al: Intrinsic signal changes with sensory stimulation: Functional brain mapping with magnetic resonance imaging. Proc Natl Acad Sci U S A 89:5951–5955, 1992.
27. Vinas FC, Zamorano L, Mueller RA, et al: [^{15}O]-water PET and intraoperative brain mapping: A comparison in the localization of eloquent cortex. Neurol Res 19:601–608, 1997.
28. Rowley HA, Roberts TP: Functional localization by magnetoencephalography. Neuroimaging Clin N Am 5:695–710, 1995.
29. Alberstone CD, Skirboll SL, Benzel EC, et al: Magnetic source imaging and brain surgery: Presurgical and intraoperative planning in 26 patients. J Neurosurg 92:79–90, 2000.
30. Brindley GS, Lewin WS: The sensations produced by electrical stimulation of the visual cortex. J Physiol 196:479–493, 1968.
31. Lee HW, Hong SB, Seo DW, et al: Mapping of functional organization in human visual cortex. Neurology 54:849–854, 2000.
32. Curatolo JM, MacDonell RAL, Berkovic SF, Fabinyi GCA: Intraoperative monitoring to preserve central visual fields during occipital corticectomy for epilepsy. J Clin Neurosci 7:234–237, 2000.
33. Danks RA, Aglio LS, Gugino LD, Black PM: Craniotomy under local anesthesia and monitored conscious sedation for the resection of tumors involving eloquent cortex. J Neurooncol 49:131–139, 2000.

CHAPTER 155

Intracranial Monitoring

KENNETH P. VIVES ■ SUNGHOON LEE ■ KEVIN MCCARTHY
DENNIS D. SPENCER

RATIONALE

Intracranial monitoring is one of an increasing number of tools available to neurosurgeons for the investigation of brain physiology and pathophysiology. The investigative process for neurological diseases always begins with the patient's history and a physical examination, which provide clues about the current state of brain function and dysfunction. For periodic disorders, such as epilepsy, examination of the patient during the ictus and immediately after can provide further information about the areas of the brain involved. Neuroimaging with modalities such as computed tomography and magnetic resonance imaging (MRI) can further elucidate anatomic details of pathology and its relation to surrounding brain structures. Taken one step further, functional MRI can, in some patients, visualize areas of brain related to specific functions. Although these techniques are promising, the number of specific brain functions that can be mapped is limited. In many cases in which long-standing pathology exists and plasticity has allowed the relocation of function—perhaps in a more diffuse pattern—this type of imaging may not reveal the precise areas involved. Further, the tasks that patients have to perform may be demanding, especially while confined in the MRI gantry. Such problems may be magnified in children and the neurologically impaired. Other imaging modalities, such as single photon emission computed tomography, can identify areas with abnormal blood flow, and positron emission tomography and magnetic resonance spectroscopy can identify areas of abnormal metabolism. These studies are somewhat lacking in anatomic resolution but can be enhanced by coregistration with anatomic MRI.

Scalp electroencephalograms (EEGs) may provide clues to the regional localization of electrophysiologic disturbance; however, the anatomic resolution provided by such studies is inadequate to delineate the relationship of involved and uninvolved structures and allow safe operative intervention. The thick layers of skin and skull protect the fragile structures of the central nervous system, but they hinder electrophysiologic localization within the brain.

Thus, despite technical advances in functional and metabolic imaging and more sophisticated analysis of interictal abnormal electrophysiology using dipole modeling or magnetoencephalography, there are only two ways that the surgeon can be assured of localizing the epileptogenic substrate. The first is indirect, involving the use of MRI to identify anatomic abnormalities that are known to be highly epileptogenic, such as hippocampal atrophy in the setting of medial temporal lobe epilepsy or low-grade tumors. The second is using electrodes to directly record from suspected areas of brain. The goal of such studies is twofold: to elucidate areas of brain pathology (i.e., epileptogenicity), and to localize brain functions in order to assess the potential risks and benefits of further intervention. Although the remainder of this chapter focuses primarily on intracranial monitoring for epilepsy, the use of these devices for extraoperative brain mapping is also addressed.

HISTORY

The contributions of Otto von Guericke and later Ewald von Kleist and Pieter van Musschenbroek of Leyden in the late 1600s and early 1700s provided scientists with the means to generate and discharge static electricity. Although abundant hypotheses existed regarding the possible role of electricity in nerve conduction and muscle conduction, Luigi Galvani was among the earliest scientists to demonstrate the role of, as he termed it, "animal electricity" in his experiments with frog leg preparations. Using both electrostatic machines and static electricity generated from storms, he demonstrated contraction of the muscle in response to the discharge of electricity and published these results in 1791. Galvani believed that these contractions resulted from the discharge of electricity from within the preparation; fortunately, not all agreed. Volta argued that extrinsic electricity was responsible, having been conducted into the tissue, possibly through the nerves. In the early 1800s, Hans Christian Oersted and J. S. C. Schweigger developed devices to measure small amounts of electricity (galvanometers). The development of such sensitive instruments allowed Richard Caton to record "feeble currents of the brain" directly from the cerebral cortex of animals in 1875.[1] Fifty-four years later, Hans Berger is credited with being the first to describe the human EEG. His initial measurements were performed on patients with skull defects or trephine holes and later on intact patients. In 1931, he recorded spike-wave activity from the brain of a person with epilepsy. Similarly, in 1935, Frederic and Erna Gibbs recorded comparable spike-wave patterns with a frequency of 3 Hz from the scalp of a woman suffering from petit mal seizures. In 1939, Sachs, Schwartz, and Kerr first recorded such activity directly from the surface of the human brain. Victor Horseley had been using direct cortical stimulation to guide resections for epilepsy, but it was Wilder Penfield and Herbert H. Jasper who began recording abnormal electrical activity directly from the surface of the brain at the time of such surgery. The first use of stereotactic depth electrodes for the treatment of intractable seizures dates to 1950, when E. A. Spiegel and H. T. Wycis recorded from and subsequently lesioned the lateral thalamus in an attempt to relieve seizures. These and other early studies emphasized the use of interictal recordings to guide resections. Talairach and Bancaud[2] realized the limited ability of interictal activity to delineate the areas of paroxysmal ictal discharge, and with this influence, American neurosurgeon Paul H. Crandall began chronic monitoring for the recording of spontaneous seizures in 1973.

INDICATIONS

Epilepsy

Patients being evaluated for intractable epilepsy undergo a fairly standard workup, with some variability from center to center. Tertiary care centers, where patients with intractable seizures are referred for surgical evaluation, initially screen patients for appropriateness. In general, patients with focal epilepsy that manifests as one consistent seizure type are likely to have an anatomic substrate for their symptomatic seizures. A second group of patients likely to benefit from surgery consists of those with multiple seizure types but with one type that is more frequent or more disabling. Last are those patients with suspected diffuse or bihemispheric seizures that cause drop attacks upon generalization. These patients may be candidates for monitoring before consideration of corpus callostomy.

At Yale, we believe that the ictal onset best defines the volume of tissue that, when resected, will render the patient seizure free. The primary goal of intracranial monitoring for resections for epilepsy is to define this volume. It is worthwhile to note that not all institutions use these data in the same way. Some believe that interictal activity should play a major role in defining the resection and may use intraoperative interictal recordings to define the limits of resection.

In a typical phased epilepsy surgery evaluation, patients undergo a detailed history-taking and physical examination, followed by MRI and outpatient EEG. This is usually followed by inpatient continuous audiovisual EEG to further document interictal EEG patterns and to capture detailed semiologic data, along with ictal EEG patterns. During this time, patients may undergo interictal and ictal single photon emission computed tomography and interictal positron emission tomography. Neuropsychological examination may take place at this time as well. At the end of this period of monitoring, all the data are examined in detail to assess whether a specific area is responsible for the seizures. A decision tree is presented in Figures 155–1 and 155–2. Each part of the preoperative data set has its own characteristics that must be weighed in making the decision as to concordance. Some data, by their very nature, point to only broad areas of brain dysfunction, whereas others may be very specific. Other pieces of data, such as the ictal scalp EEG, may be regional at best and confer more weight to an MRI structural abnormality, or the ictal EEG may indicate multifocality or generalization or be characterized only by muscle artifact.

Concordance of these data with an MRI abnormality is necessary to proceed to operation without further monitoring. Several scenarios are likely. An initial determination can be made whether the patient has a lesion present on MRI. Patients with lesions can then be divided based on whether their other data are concordant or nonconcordant (see Figs. 155–1 and 155–2). In general, patients with abnormal MRIs and concordant data are good candidates for resection. In those with normal MRIs, intracranial monitoring is necessary to delineate the areas of brain to be resected. The study may be designed as a focused study to cover the areas of brain identified by the initial data set as being potentially epileptogenic. In general, if the patient has one predominant seizure type, an ictal EEG may point to a particular area for invasive study. Some patients may have multiple areas of ictal onset but a common spread pattern, thus generating a single seizure type. Other patients may have a single area of ictal generation with a variable spread pattern, which manifests as multiple seizure types. Seizure onset in particular areas of the brain may be prone to rapid spread, making the ictal EEG appear bilateral or diffuse.

These and many other factors need to be considered before deciding that a patient is or is not a candidate for further investigation. For example, a patient may have an ictal EEG that specifies one hemisphere, semiology on audiovisual EEG that is consistently lobar (hemifield flashing lights from one occipital lobe), single photon emission computed tomography and positron emission tomography scans confirming regionally abnormal blood flow and metabolism, and neuropsychological testing that is abnormal but nonspecific. An

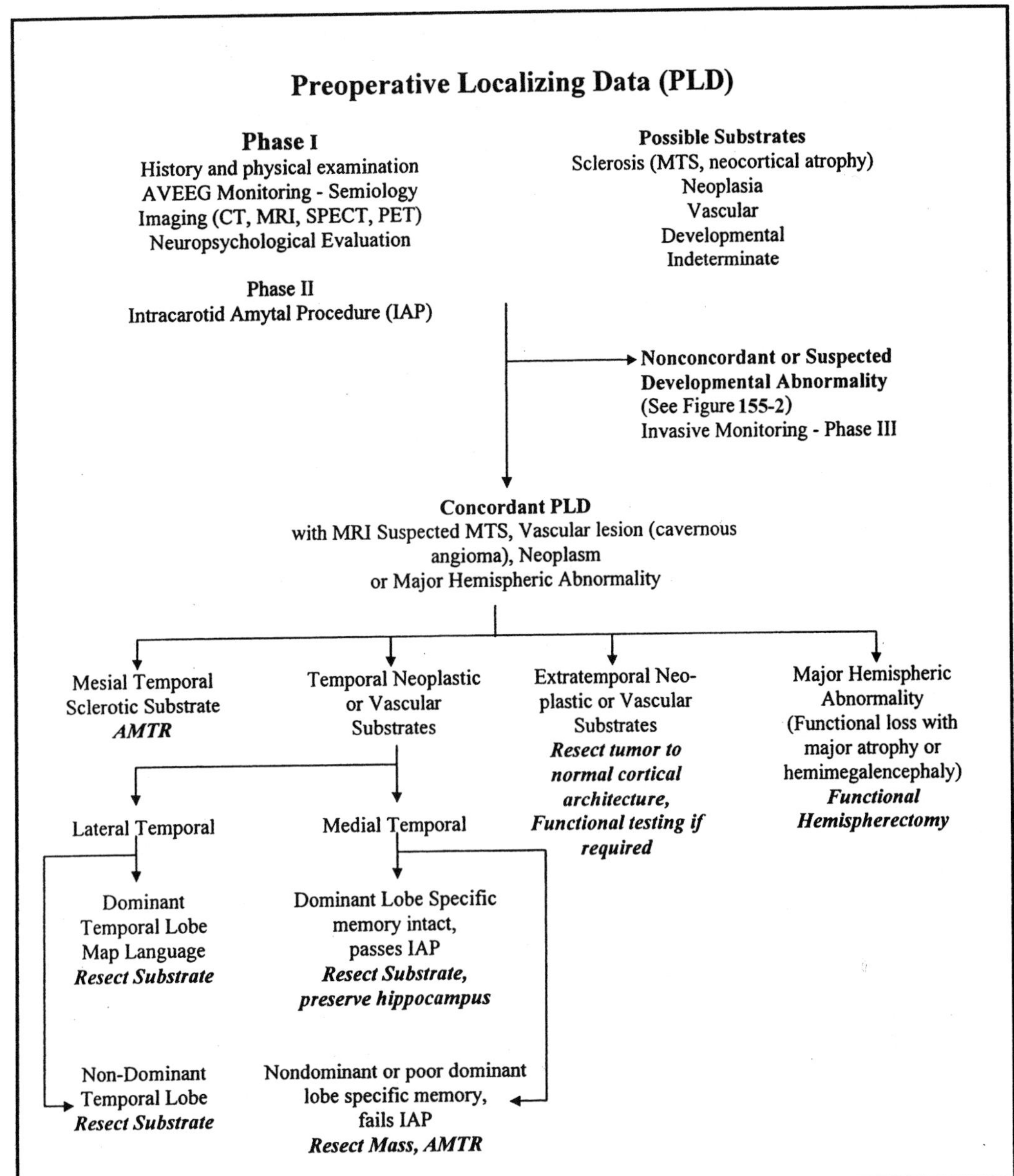

FIGURE 155–1. Part one of a decision-making tree for the evaluation of patients with intractable epilepsy.

invasive study should be designed to cover the posterior aspect of the hemisphere in question.

The other set of patients consists of those with evidence of a tumor, vascular malformation, or hippocampal sclerosis on MRI. Typically, these patients, in whom the other data are concordant, proceed to surgery without intracranial monitoring. Exceptions are patients with evidence of brain developmental disorders on neuroimaging. These patients may have more diffuse brain abnormalities, and at our center, the threshold for invasive monitoring in these cases is low. In many cases in which a lesion is present and the other data are concordant, further study is warranted to ensure that the lesion is or is not responsible for the seizures. In other cases, patients may have multiple lesions, but all the data point to one particular lesion as being responsible for the seizures. Unless there are pressing reasons to address one of the other lesions (e.g., a patient with multiple cavernous malformations, one of which is larger and has evidence of hemorrhage, but the data point to a smaller lesion without evidence of hemorrhage), many of these patients can proceed directly to surgery.

A special case involves patients with lesions and evidence of hippocampal sclerosis. There is speculation in the literature about the relationship of these entities.[3–6] It is possible that an extrahippocampal lesion may cause seizures that spread through the hippocampus. Over time, this spread pattern could damage the hippocampus through excitotoxicity, rendering it an independent source of seizures. At our institution, in general, patients with temporal lobe lesions and evidence of hippocampal atrophy and dysfunction (temporal lobe–specific poor memory) in whom the other data are concordant for the temporal lobe undergo a combined resection of the lesion and the hippocampus.

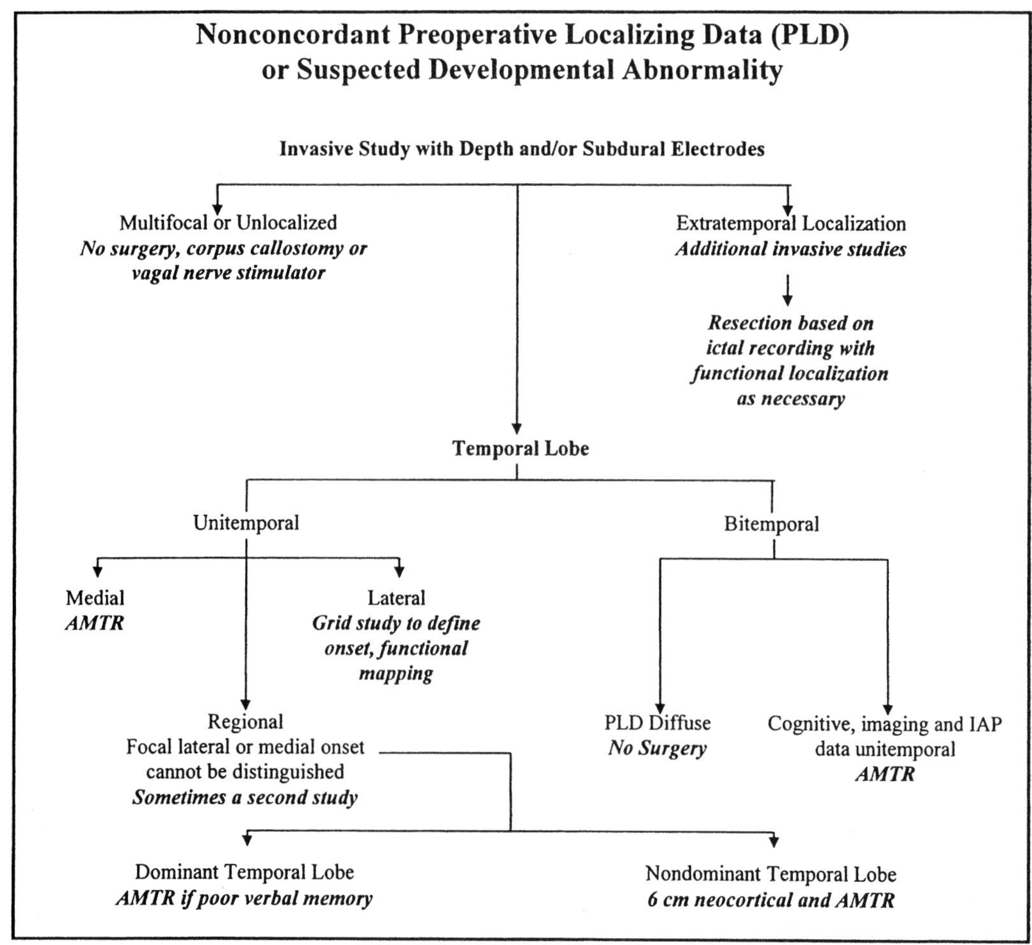

FIGURE 155–2. Part two of a decision-making tree for the evaluation of patients with epilepsy.

The more medial the lesion, the more likely we are to assume true dual pathology and resect both. Patients without evidence of hippocampal dysfunction on neuropsychological studies and intracarotid amobarbital (Amytal) testing usually undergo lesionectomy without hippocampectomy, regardless of the volume of the hippocampus, although a small portion of these patients may need further resection.

Brain Mapping

A separate indication for intracranial monitoring for patients without epilepsy is for extraoperative brain mapping. The goal is typically to map the areas of appreciable function in relation to a lesion (1) to provide data about the risks of surgical resection so that the clinician and patient can make a decision about the appropriateness of surgery and (2) to allow surgical planning to minimize those risks. In some instances, intraoperative monitoring may be the most efficient way to address these issues. The mapping of simple motor modalities can be accomplished at surgery through direct cortical stimulation. Similarly, sensory mapping can be performed via somatosensory evoked potentials. Intraoperative language mapping requires an awake patient who can participate at the time of surgery and demonstrate reversible deficits during cortical stimulation. Testing of higher cognitive function may be difficult during surgery owing to the complexity of the tasks that must be performed. Beyond these straightforward tests, particular patients and particular types of mapping may make extraoperative mapping more desirable.

Some patients, such as children and adults who are unable to cooperate, may be unable to participate in an awake craniotomy. The claustrophobic nature of the drapes, even if they are transparent, can be overwhelming. No matter how good the anesthesia, the discomfort from the craniotomy may also be a hindrance. Even preoperative language testing in children may be difficult, because the patient is required to focus on the tests for a substantial period; the same can be said of neurologically impaired adults. Other brain modalities may be difficult to map intraoperatively. For example, a professional in the field of personal relations who has a lesion in the posterior fusiform gyrus near the facial recognition area may not desire a resection if he or she could be substantially impaired. Mapping this area requires multiple visual stimuli that would be difficult to accomplish intraoperatively.

HARDWARE

A variety of electrodes is available for use in electrophysiologic monitoring. A combination of depth electrodes and subdural strip or grid electrodes is routinely used in most situations. In certain situations in which the plane between the dura and brain surface is scarred and safe dissection is impossible, epidural peg electrodes can be used. Some centers supplement scalp studies or intracranial studies with foramen ovale or sphenoidal electrodes. The construction, surgical technique, and use of each are discussed here.

Depth Electrodes

Depth electrodes are typically constructed with one or more contacts on a thin shaft with a blunt tip to minimize traumatic brain and vascular injury. Both rigid and flexible types exist. For insertion, the flexible electrodes are made rigid through a stylet that is fixed adjacent to the electrode or placed down the center and removed after insertion. An added advantage is that these electrodes can be tunneled subcutaneously, reducing the risk of infection. The contacts themselves are usually made of platinum or platinum-iridium construction and spaced from 3 to 10 mm apart. For multicontact electrodes, individual insulated wires run up the inner cannula of the hollow electrode and present to contacts that can be connected to a ribbon cable. Electrodes with multiple contacts can be used to record along the longitudinal dimension of a structure, such as the hippocampus (Fig. 155–3), or they may allow the simultaneous recording of a deep structure and the cortical surface through which the electrode was inserted (Fig. 155–4).

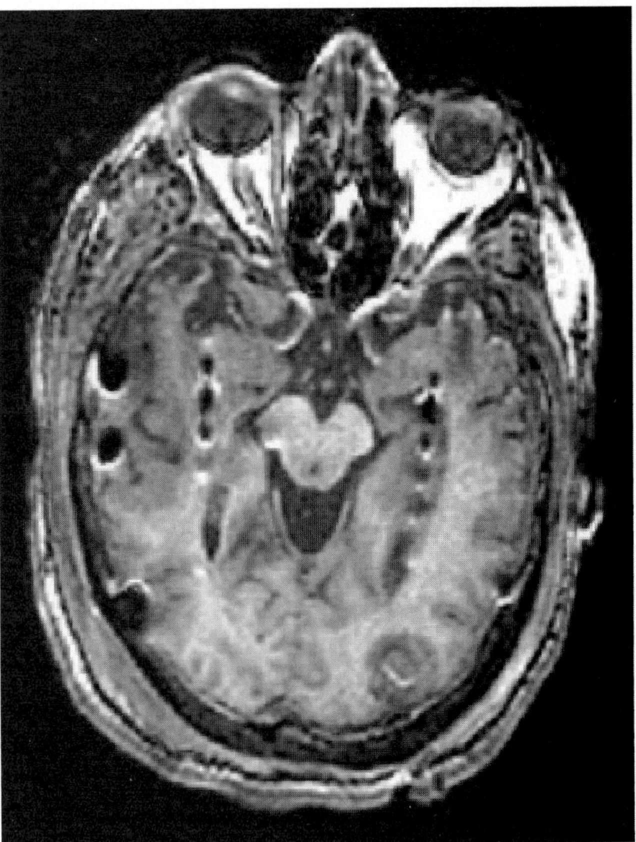

FIGURE 155–3. Postoperative axial, T1-weighted magnetic resonance imaging scan illustrating the placement of bilateral, longitudinal hippocampal depth electrodes from the occipital approach. This allows sampling of electrophysiologic data along the length of the hippocampus. Subdural strips provide lateral neocortical coverage.

Subdural Electrodes—Strips and Grids

Subdural strips are typically constructed from a flexible material that conforms to the surface anatomy of the brain. Usually they have multiple contacts in one or more columns to allow simultaneous recording from different areas of the cortex. In general, two types are used: one that consists of a thin shaft or reed with multiple contacts (similar to the depth electrodes), and one in which multiple disks are embedded in a thin sheet of Silastic. We find the second type to be more useful because of the enhanced ability to direct the electrodes to specific sites from a remote bur hole. The larger contact surface and the Silastic coating make cortical stimulation possible without dural pain. The wires then exit together in a hollow Silastic tube and present to contacts that can be connected to a ribbon cable (Fig. 155–5). The contacts are constructed of stainless steel or platinum.

Most grids are similarly constructed, but they have columns of multiple contacts for a wider area of coverage (Fig. 155–6; see also Fig. 155–5). These terminate in multiple thin, hollow tubes with contacts for connecting to ribbon cables. One special type is an L-shaped grid for recording from the medial surface of the hemisphere (Fig. 155–7). Once again, the contacts may be made of platinum or stainless steel. The platinum construction allows for safe postoperative MRI (see Fig. 155–6).[7]

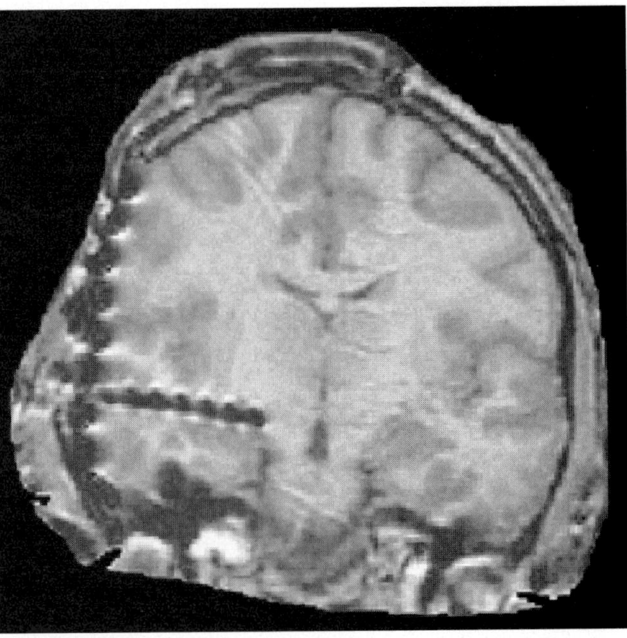

FIGURE 155–4. Postoperative coronal, T1-weighted magnetic resonance imaging scan illustrating the simultaneous placement of an orthogonal depth electrode and a right frontotemporal grid.

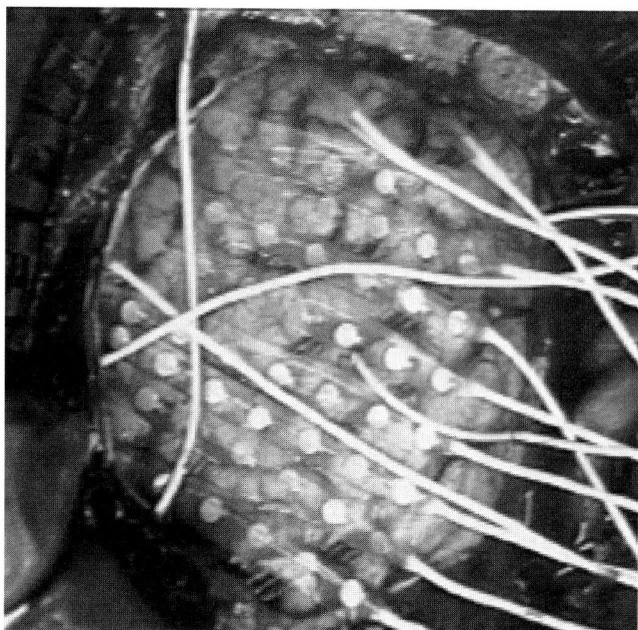

FIGURE 155–5. Intraoperative photograph illustrating simultaneous grid, strip, and depth electrode placement. This grid was fenestrated between columns to allow the placement of the depth electrode and to achieve better conformance with the brain surface.

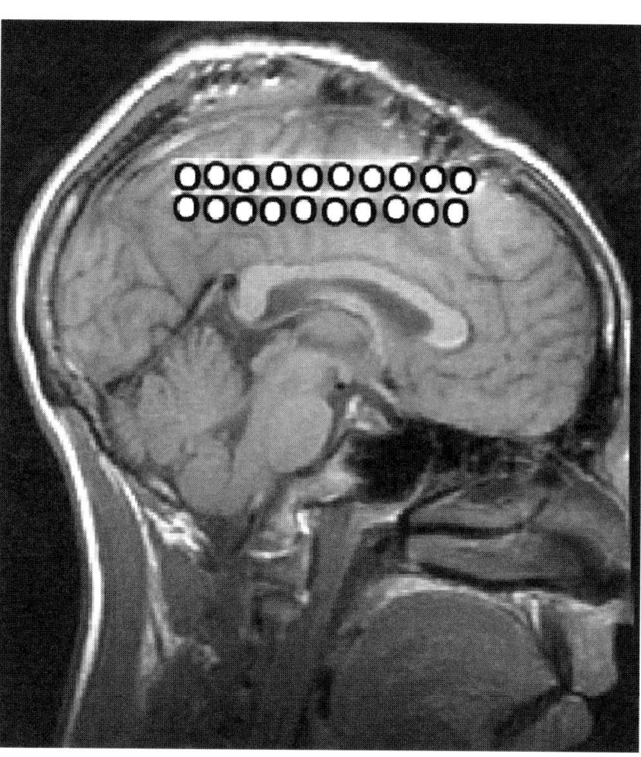

FIGURE 155–7. Postoperative sagittal magnetic resonance imaging scan illustrating the use of an L-shaped medial interhemispheric grid for a patient with seizures suspected of arising in the supplementary motor area.

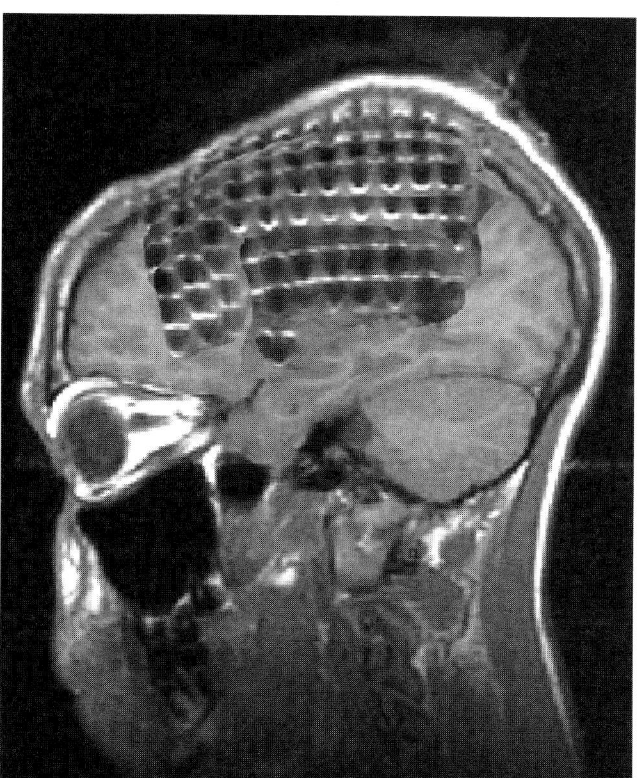

FIGURE 155–6. Postoperative magnetic resonance imaging scan illustrating grid placement. This is a composite image created by collapsing multiple sagittal images to allow the simultaneous viewing of electrodes in different planes.

Epidural Peg Electrodes

The recording of electrical activity from the placement of electrodes in the epidural space traces its history to Penfield and Jasper, who used epidural ball electrodes in a few difficult cases.[8] In comparison to scalp EEGs, epidural recordings have the advantage of providing an improved signal-to-noise ratio. This effect is created by reducing the volume conduction and amplitude attenuation and by eliminating the myogenic and kinesiogenic artifacts inherent to scalp EEG recordings.[9] Epidural recording has also been considered an alternative to subdural and intraparenchymal monitoring because of its semi-invasive nature and the presumed advantage of fewer infectious and hemorrhagic complications.

Epidural electrode designs have included ball electrodes,[8] screws,[9] and pegs.[10] Epidural screws and peg electrodes are widely applied in some epilepsy surgery centers. The screw is usually made of titanium, with a tapered shaft to prevent overpenetration.[9] Screw length varies to allow for stable placement and to accommodate the varying thicknesses of scalp and calvaria. The screw head is hexagonal to allow easy placement and removal of the electrodes with a wrench. Right-angled EEG monitoring leads can be placed in the screw head.[9] Epidural peg electrodes are composed of mushroom-shaped Silastic elastomer, and the stalk tapers from a diameter of 4.7 mm to a diameter of 0.5 mm. At the base of the stalk, either stainless steel or platinum tips are used to conduct the electrical current. The tips are continuous with Teflon-coated steel wire that is tunneled through the peg, exiting through the cap. Strip arrays of epidural electrodes have also been described.[11]

Foramen Ovale and Sphenoidal Electrodes

Foramen ovale electrodes were first developed in 1985 as a semi-invasive EEG alternative to intracerebral depth electrodes in the evaluation of mesial temporal lobe epilepsy.[12] These electrodes generally consist of helical, wound, Teflon-coated silver wires that end in multicontact poles.[13] The construct is mounted on a thin stainless steel wire. The mechanical properties conferred to this construct allow appropriate flexibility to avoid puncturing of the pia-arachnoid layer. The external diameter allows easy passage through a specially constructed 18-gauge introducer cannula.[12]

Sphenoidal electrodes are used by many epilepsy centers as an adjunct to standard scalp EEG electrodes for the evaluation of temporal lobe epilepsy. These electrodes, in conjunction with scalp EEGs, can help determine whether the focus of the seizure is in the medial or lateral aspect of the temporal lobe. Sphenoidal electrodes were originally rigid, allowing for only short-term monitoring, but they have evolved to a flexible design. Teflon-coated single or multiple wires have silver or stainless steel tips, are flexible, and may be applied for EEG recordings for up to 3 weeks.[14]

Recording Equipment

Following implantation, the leads are connected to an isolation box to prevent any inadvertent current from entering the patient. Impedances are checked with a small current in the vicinity of 10 nA.[15] The isolation box is then connected to a multichannel amplifier and a recording system. Typically, systems with at least 64 channel capabilities are used; however, more extensive studies necessitate more channels. An initial montage with sampling from the contacts of each implanted device is used. Information gained as the study continues usually dictates changes in the montage to focus on the relevant areas. Simultaneous video recordings provide the information necessary to correlate semiology with electrophysiologic data.

DESIGN OF STUDIES

Epilepsy Studies

In general terms, the preoperative localizing data dictate the areas to be studied. Localizing data from the seizure semiology, scalp ictal EEGs, neuroimaging, and neuropsychological data are combined to establish which areas are suspected of being involved in seizure generation. Several typical scenarios are typically encountered. Patients with lesions and discordant data typically require grid coverage over the lesion, as well as strip and depth electrode coverage of areas as indicated by the other preoperative data. Patients with developmental abnormalities require special consideration. In contrast to most other lesions, these malformative lesions may be inherently capable of seizure generation. Subdural grid coverage may not identify the seizure source if it is located deep in a malformed area of gray matter; depth electrode coverage of the lesion itself may be required. Other less accessible lesions may also be suitable for depth electrodes, such as the medial hemisphere or insula (see Fig. 155–4). Patients with multiple lesions typically require coverage over the most likely responsible lesions, as well as other potential epileptogenic regions demonstrated on preoperative studies. In patients with suspected bilateral medial temporal lobe seizures, bilateral hippocampal depth electrode studies are used in combination with limited bilateral temporal lobe strip coverage (see Fig. 155–3).

Patients without lesions but with concordant preoperative data undergo a focused study of the suspected area of brain, as well as sampling of other areas. For patients with discordant preoperative data and negative MRIs, a broad study is designed, using any localizing data to direct the study. Many times, despite the paucity of imaging abnormalities and conflicting data, an invasive study may be useful. Usually, patients arrive at this stage because seizure semiology is reproducible and may be distinct enough to define an area of seizure generation. This semiologic information can at least be used to help construct the study.

Two important facts must be kept in mind when designing and interpreting such studies. First, one cannot cover all possible epileptogenic locations with electrodes, and caution must be taken when interpreting electrical activity at the edge of grids or the end of strips. A source just beyond the area of coverage may appear to originate from these edge contacts. A clear voltage reversal between two adjacent electrodes is much better evidence of localization. Second, grids and strips record only from the surface of the brain. Gray matter in the sulci is also sampled from the surface, with similar problems to scalp EEG recordings.

Brain Mapping Studies

Typically, these focused studies cover the areas of the lesion, as well as adjacent functional brain. In most locations, a subdural grid is well suited to such studies. In other cases, regional venous anatomy may dictate the use of custom-cut grids or subdural strips to avoid sacrificing a critical vein. For example, with lesions in the posterior fusiform gyrus, the location of the vein of Labbé may make grid placement difficult.

OPERATIVE CONSIDERATIONS

Preoperative Evaluation

Patients undergoing intracranial monitoring require routine preoperative management similar to that of any other patient undergoing craniotomy. Coagulation studies and particularly a bleeding time are necessary to screen for occult disorders of hemostasis. Many patients who require intracranial monitoring have also undergone intracarotid Amytal testing, so the arterial and particularly the venous phase of the angiogram can be reviewed preoperatively to identify areas where the venous anatomy may limit the ability to place electrodes. For patients who have not undergone an angiogram and in whom the preoperative plan for electrodes requires defining the vascular anatomy, such as interhemispheric studies or studies around the vein of Labbé, a preoperative magnetic resonance venogram may be helpful. In patients who have seizures at particular times of the month, such as catamenial epilepsy, the study should be timed so that the monitoring precedes that period by several days. In general, epilepsy patients need to be carefully counseled about the possibility of lengthy studies that require them to be confined to a single room for, in rare instances, weeks at a time. The electrodes and head dressing can be heavy and difficult to tolerate for some patients. Particularly with grid placement, we have found that the operation itself may cause a period of decreased seizure activity that may prolong studies.

Placement of subdural strips or grids often requires the use of mild hyperventilation and mannitol administration to provide adequate brain relaxation, thus necessitating general anesthesia. Depth electrodes may be inserted under local anesthesia with sedation; however, it is rare that such studies are performed without the simultaneous use of subdural strips.

Depth Electrodes

The insertion of depth electrodes is a stereotactic procedure, using either fixed frame or frameless devices. Identifying vascular structures using anatomic MRI is most useful when coregistered with magnetic resonance angiography and venography. The planned trajectory can be reviewed so as to avoid these structures en route to the target. In contrast to biopsies, multiple contacts along the electrode trajectory need to be optimally positioned to obtain the maximal amount of information.

Following prepping and draping, the area of skin through which the electrode is to be inserted is identified with stereotaxy. Usually, a small, vertical, linear incision is used in the parasagittal occipital bone for longitudinal hippocampal placement (see Fig. 155–3). Incisions for orthogonal temporal, frontal, or parietal study vary with location, but thoughtful consideration should be given to the design of the skin incision so that it can be incorporated into a larger incision at the time of future resection. In patients with very thick bone, the trajectory of the depth electrode needs to be taken into account when creating the bur hole so as to avoid having the trajectory blocked by the bone edge. Following bur hole placement, the dura is coagulated and opened. If necessary, the entry point is replanned to avoid surface vessels. The electrode is then measured to ensure placement at the appropriate depth. Following the coagulation and incision of the pia-arachnoid, the electrode is inserted with the proper X-Y-Z coordinates, feeling for areas of resistance as the electrode is passed. If unexpected resistance is met, the stereotaxy system is checked, the MRI trajectory is reviewed, and passage is reattempted. The stylet is then removed, and the electrode is tunneled under the skin using a cannula and trocar. A purse-string 4–0 nylon suture is placed at the site of exit from the skin and tied down; then two separate 3–0 nylon sutures

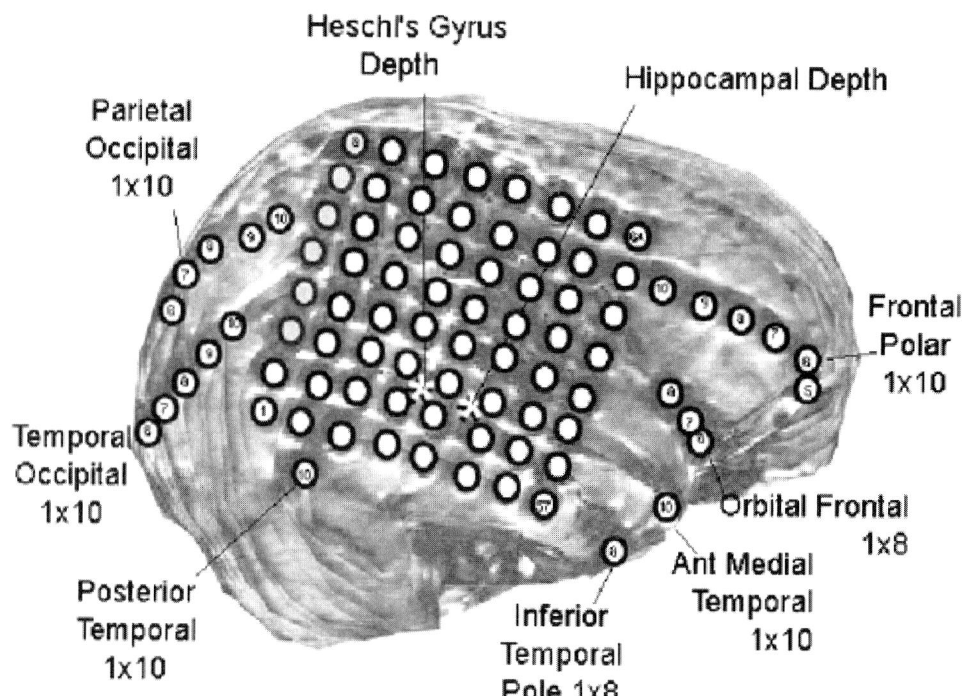

FIGURE 155–8. Composite image from postoperative magnetic resonance imaging scans illustrating the combined placement of multiple subdural strips, a subdural grid, and two depth electrodes.

are used to secure the electrode to the skin. The ends of these electrodes are typically marked so that they can be identified postoperatively with the head dressing on. Following placement, the location of the electrode, along with its identifying mark, is recorded in the patient's chart. Gelfoam is then placed in the bur hole, and the skin is closed. In many instances, a depth electrode must be placed orthogonally through a grid that has been placed (see Fig. 155–4). In these cases, a small hole needs to be created in the grid to place the electrode. The electrode is sutured to the grid and tunneled out through the base of the flap.

When turning a large craniotomy flap, such as that needed for subdural grids, the brain may shift a number of millimeters. This shift occurs primarily at the cortical surface, not at the more medial structures such as the hippocampus, thus making the preoperative stereotaxy valid for the placement of depth electrodes (Fig. 155–8). Regardless, it is preferable to place the depth electrodes before cortical settling.

Over the past several years, we have been using frameless magnetic resonance stereotaxy (Acciss OMI) almost exclusively for the insertion of depth electrodes (Fig. 155–9). This system allows stereotactic placement when multiple targets are planned in one hemisphere during grid placements. The absence of a frame prevents interference with the craniotomy and obviates the need to reset the X-Y-Z coordinates for each trajectory.

Subdural Strips

Before prepping, the skin incision should be marked. Localization can be performed with simple craniometric measurement in accompaniment with MRI, or stereotaxy can be used as an aid. Once again, the possible

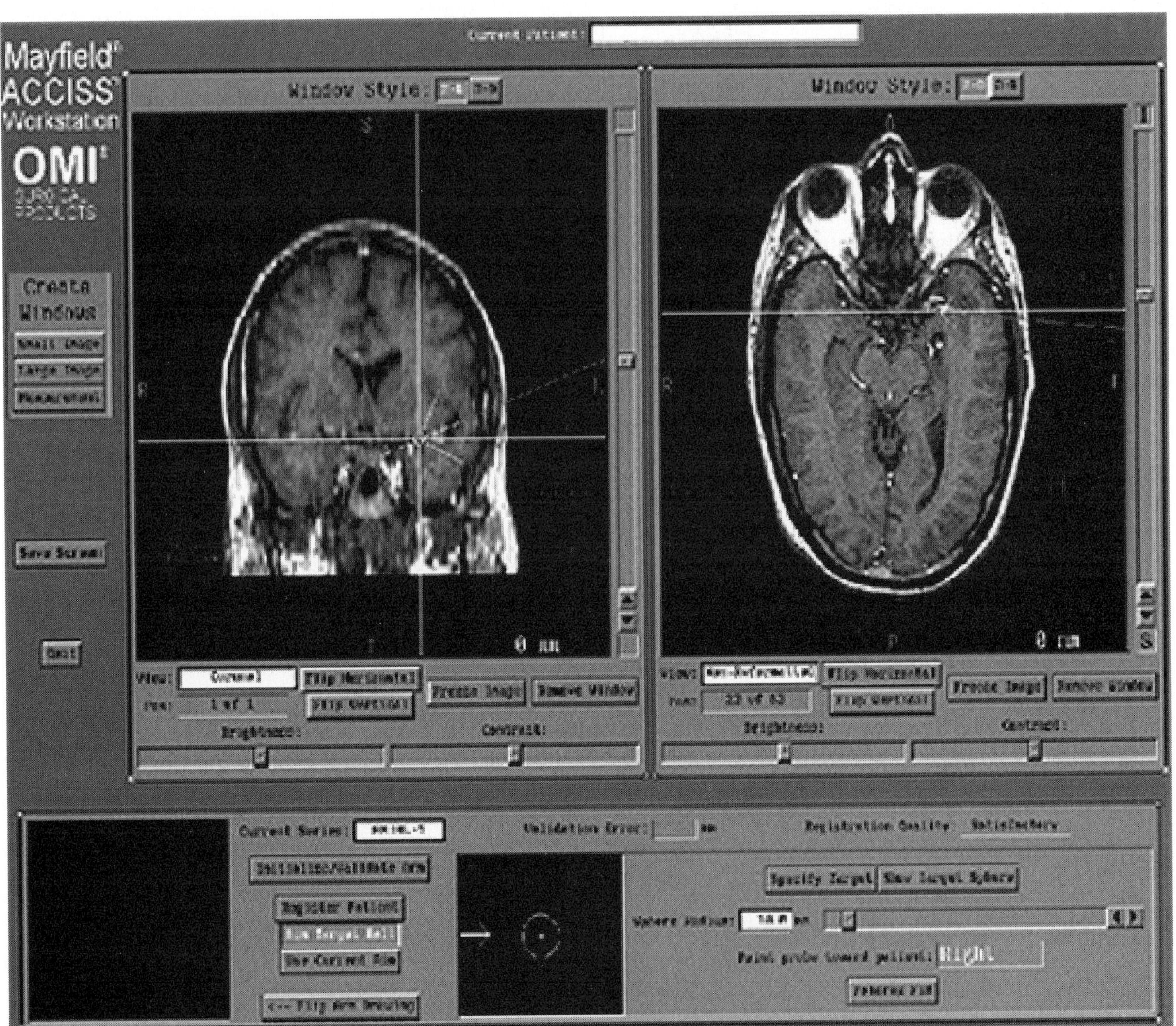

FIGURE 155–9. Screen capture of frameless stereotaxy software for the insertion of an orthogonal amygdala depth electrode.

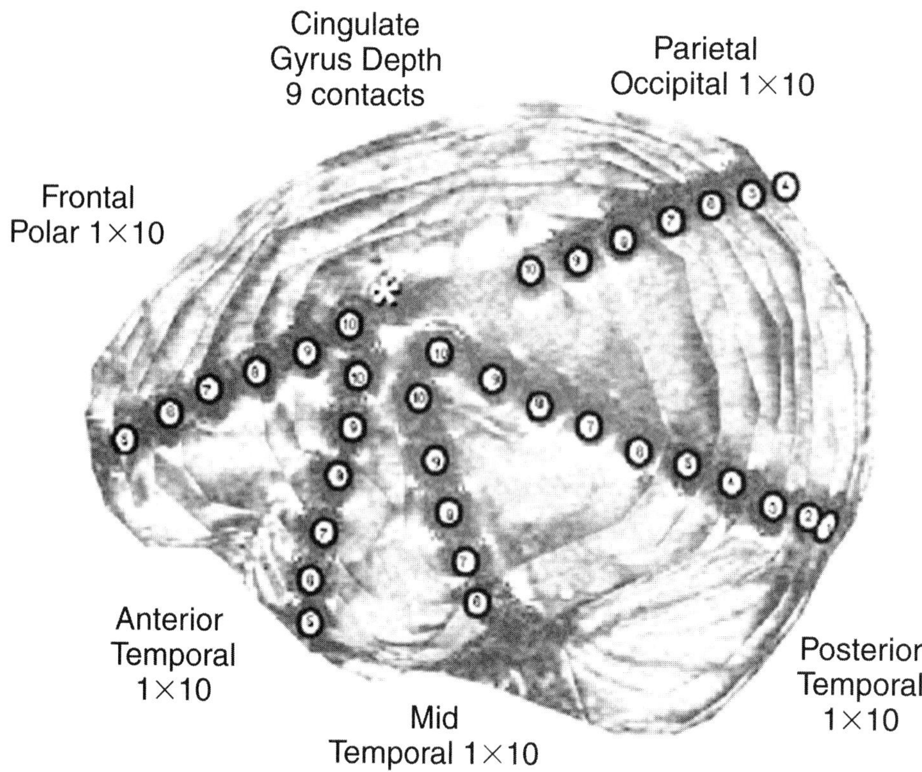

FIGURE 155–10. Composite image from postoperative magnetic resonance imaging scans illustrating the type of placement that can be achieved through a low frontal trough corresponding to the typical upper limb of a craniotomy for an anteromedial temporal resection.

need to incorporate incisions into a future larger incision for resection should be considered. For example, for patients undergoing temporal lobe strip studies in whom an anteromedial temporal lobe resection may be required, we typically make the skin incision for the subdural strip insertion in the same location as the upper limb of the temporal lobe craniotomy incision (Fig. 155–10). Following skin incision, a bony trough is created in the anteroposterior direction by making multiple bur holes and connecting them with a cutting bur. After bony removal, the dura is coagulated and opened. The strips are inserted with a pair of forceps, directing them toward the desired target using a steady stream of irrigation under the strip. This irrigation helps the strip slide smoothly over the surface of the brain and prevents trauma. If any resistance is felt, the strip is removed and reinserted. These areas of resistance may represent bridging cortical veins and thus should be avoided to prevent hemorrhage under the bone, which the surgeon has no access to through the same craniotomy. Finding the correct trajectory and depth of insertion for a given cortical location requires both patience and experience. Following insertion, the intended position is recorded in the patient's chart, and the electrode is tunneled through the skin. A purse-string suture is placed around the site of exit, and the electrode is secured with a separate skin suture. Gelfoam is placed over the dural incision, and the skin is closed.

Subdural Grids

Placement of large subdural grids requires a craniotomy flap of the same approximate size as the grid (see Figs. 155–5 and 155–6). Once again, the skin flap should be designed so that, if necessary, it can be incorporated into an incision for resection. The skin is incised in a U-shaped fashion and reflected, leaving the periosteum intact. A periosteal graft is then harvested for use in dural closure following grid placement. The bone flap is removed, and the bone is cleaned thoroughly and sent to the bone bank for the duration of the study. Alternatively, an incision in the abdomen can be made and the bone inserted subcutaneously for safekeeping until the time of replacement, or it can be left in the craniotomy site but not secured tightly to the skull. Following hemostasis, the dura is opened, removed in a circumferential fashion, and stored until closure. This denervates the dura and decreases postoperative headache. A digital photograph of the brain is then taken. The grid is placed on the brain in the appropriate position, and the multiple leads are tunneled subcutaneously and brought out through the base of the skin flap, if possible. Purse-string sutures are placed around each exit site, and each electrode is secured to the skin with a separate suture. An additional photograph is then taken with the grid, strips, and depth electrodes in place. These photographs often reveal gyral anatomy and electrode placement that cannot be obtained even with three-dimensional reconstructed MRI scans. The dura is then closed using the previously harvested periosteal and dural grafts. An epidural drain is placed and tunneled through a distant separate stab incision. A "sleeper stitch" is placed around the drain exit site and wrapped around the drain. This is used to secure the skin when the drain is removed the following morning. The skin is then closed in two layers.

Epidural Peg Electrodes

The surgical placement of epidural peg or screw electrodes can be done with the patient under general or local anesthesia. The patient's head is placed in a favorable position for exposure of the desired brain area for electrographic examination, and multiple skin incisions of approximately 1.5 cm are made for the placement of epidural peg electrodes. For the placement of epidural screw electrodes, only 0.5-cm stab incisions are required. Small twist-drill bur holes are made. When placing epidural screws, the electrodes are hand tightened and then secured with a wrench. When placing epidural peg electrodes, appropriate stalk-length electrodes are selected and placed securely with a wrench until the cap of the peg can be covered by the edges of the galea, and the electrode wires are tunneled through the subcutaneous space. Usually, the placement of epidural strips and grids requires a craniotomy.

Foramen Ovale and Sphenoidal Electrodes

Härtel's landmarks[16] are used to insert foramen ovale and sphenoidal electrodes. The introductory cannula is inserted 3 cm lateral to the oral commissure and passed to the foramen ovale using Kirschner's technique[17] under fluoroscopic guidance. The cannula is guided along a line formed by the intersection of two orthogonal planes. The first plane is defined by the insertion point and the point on the lower eyelid corresponding to the medial border of the pupil. The second plane is defined by the insertion point and the point 5 cm anterior to the external auditory meatus. Cerebrospinal fluid return is visualized with the removal of the inner cannula. The electrode is then placed through the cannula, usually without resistance, until its expected placement in the cistern. The cannula is then withdrawn, and the electrodes are fixed to the skin with gauze and adhesive tape. The removal of foramen ovale electrodes does not require anesthesia. Transient spasm or dysesthesias may be elicited during the withdrawal of electrodes in the ipsilateral teeth.

Sphenoidal electrode placement is performed percutaneously under the zygomatic arch, to rest near the foramen ovale. The electrodes are directed toward the midportion of the foramen ovale. Following insertion, the electrodes are taped securely to the skin and attached to a standard EEG jack.

POSTOPERATIVE CARE

The head is wrapped in a bulky head dressing with a chin strap and the electrodes exiting from one or two sites. This type of dressing is necessary to prevent dislodgment of the electrodes during seizures and to contain any minor cerebrospinal fluid leaks. Patients who undergo grid placement are usually placed on a three-day tapering course of methylprednisolone (Solu-Medrol). An MRI is obtained the following morning to localize the electrodes. Before sending the patient for an MRI, care is taken to ensure that none of the electrodes forms a loop. The signal artifact from the contacts themselves prevents computed tomographic scans from delineating postoperative complications.[7] In addition, the superior resolution of MRI provides anatomic detail that is not possible to obtain with computed tomographic scanning. We typically perform interictal single photon emission computed tomography at this time for later subtraction from an ictal injection.

Complications include depth electrodes associated with small intraparenchymal hematomas (2%), subdural electrodes mistakenly placed intraparenchymally (4%),[18] and depth electrodes in the wrong position (2%).[19]

After MRI, the patient is taken to the epilepsy unit and connected to the monitoring equipment. The exiting electrodes and their connections must be tethered to the dressing. Wyler and colleagues[20] found no difference in rates of meningitis in patients receiving continuous antibiotics after subdural strip placement versus those receiving only perioperative coverage; thus, our patients are routinely placed on a 24-hour course of antibiotics and then receive no antibiotics during the remainder of the study unless other indications arise. Cerebrospinal fluid leaks may occur in up to 19% of patients,[21] so the head dressing is checked twice daily for evidence of leakage. A wet dressing is changed using sterile technique, and the source of the leak is sought and sutured. Patients commonly experience low-grade fever and headache following the procedure. These fevers do not correlate with intracranial infection,[21] but care should be taken to evaluate patients with prolonged fever. Headache is especially troublesome after grid placement, and patients may require narcotics for 36 to 48 hours.

At the end of monitoring, the patient is returned to the operating room. Probes and strips can be removed with gentle, steady traction without reopening the incision. Patients who have undergone grid placement are intubated and placed in pins, and the exiting leads from any grids and strips are tied in a bundle with an umbilical tape that extends below the sterile field. Following sterile preparation, the sutures are removed, and the head is reprepped. The patient is draped, and the incision is reopened. The leads are cut intradurally and then removed from the sterile field by pulling on the umbilical tape outside the field. The dura is reopened, and the grid is removed. Neocortical resections are performed at this time using the acquired ictal data and functional mapping from grid stimulation. If ictal onset is localized to the medial temporal lobe, the electrodes are removed, and the patient is brought back for a standard anteromedial temporal lobe resection in approximately 4 to 6 weeks. This avoids retraction of the mildly edematous brain caused by the electrode study. Following any planned resection of tissue, the dura is closed, and the banked bone flap is reinserted and secured.

OUTCOME WITH INTRACRANIAL MONITORING

The outcome of resection for patients undergoing intracranial monitoring for epilepsy is linked to the selected population that undergoes such monitoring and the interpretation of data from such studies. We have outlined the general criteria used to select these patients for study, but the process is dynamic and changes over time. Patients with the best outcomes from surgical resection are those with hippocampal sclerosis or circumscribed lesions and concordant data. The majority of these patients do not require monitoring. Patients selected for invasive study are less likely to have excellent outcomes, owing to the nonconcordance of their preoperative data or to the nonlesional extratemporal location.

Approximately 64% to 94% of patients are found to have sufficient localizing information to proceed to resection after intracranial study.[19, 22–24] Thus, many more patients can be offered resection, compared with patients evaluated with scalp EEGs only.[25] An increasing percentage of patients monitored are those with extratemporal epilepsy, because MRI identifies most lesions and hippocampal atrophy.

Following resection, 28% to 64% of patients are seizure free.[19, 22] The range is so wide because series from different centers have substantially varied patient populations, experience, and indications for intracranial monitoring. In 21 patients with seizures localizing to the temporal lobe, Cascino and coworkers[26] found that only 9 of 21 patients were seizure free after resection. The largest number of patients with inferior outcomes had normal MRI scans (without hippocampal atrophy), along with three patients who had hypothalamic masses and were thought to have gelastic seizures.

The role of epidural peg and screw electrodes has not been fully defined in the presurgical evaluation of epilepsy patients. The main advantages are their relative ease of placement and the likely decreased rates of major complications associated with subdural and intraparenchymal monitoring. Although the signal-to-noise ratio is significantly improved when epidural monitoring is compared with scalp EEG, it provides a lower density of coverage than does subdural or intraparenchymal monitoring and does not allow for the definition of functional anatomy. These issues regarding the density of coverage may be overcome in part by the placement of epidural grid electrodes, which requires a craniotomy.

Surgical outcome following the preoperative use of epidural arrays was reported by Goldring and Gregorie,[11] who reviewed 100 cases in which epidural electrode arrays were used to define the epileptic focus. Sixty-four percent of the epileptic children and 62% of the epileptic adults had "good" outcomes. Nevertheless, questions remain about the accuracy with which epidural electrodes define the seizure focus and whether surgical outcomes based on their results are comparable to those of resections based on more invasive monitoring.

The efficacy of foramen ovale electrodes in identifying the mesiolimbic temporal lobe as the epileptogenic substrate has been examined on a limited basis. Wieser and Siegel[12] reported favorable outcomes in candidates for amygdalohippocampectomy who were studied preoperatively with foramen ovale electrodes; similar outcomes were reported in that group (64% seizure free) and in the group studied with stereoelectroencephalography (59% seizure free).

The advantages of formen ovale electrodes are their semi-invasiveness, relative ease of placement, and elimination of the increased risk associated with the placement of depth electrodes and subdural grids and strips.[27] They may also be more cost-effective.[28] One drawback involves the interpretation of the information generated without the appropriate context of having accurate electrographic information from other alternative epileptogenic sites. The most serious drawback may be the possibility of falsely localizing the seizure focus to the mesial temporal lobe and missing the real epileptogenic focus, which may be in the neocortical temporal lobe or in an extratemporal location. Some centers with extensive experience with this technique emphasize the need to closely examine the ictal seizure discharge pattern and the clinical seizure semiology, as well as the scalp EEG, when interpreting the results recorded from formen ovale electrodes.[12] In light of the significant theoretical disadvantage of false localization, foramen ovale electrodes have not been used at our institution. We favor the techniques of intracranial depth electrodes and subdural grids and strips, which remain the gold standard in this field. Rather than replacing invasive monitoring, foramen ovale electrodes may have a more rational place as an adjunct, perhaps in the selection of patients for further invasive electrographic localization.

Early studies comparing sphenoidal electrodes to scalp EEG electrodes revealed that in patients suspected of having mesial temporal lobe epilepsy, the spike amplitude was largest in sphenoidal electrodes. It was believed that the proximity of these electrodes to the basal medial aspect of the temporal lobe increased their sensitivity for detecting mesial temporal discharges.[29] This notion of sphenoidal spikes' specificity for mesial temporal discharges has been questioned, however; Marks and coworkers[30] found that the large sphenoidal spikes may be associated with extratemporal and extrahippocampal foci. The localizing value and the specificity of sphenoidal electrodes remain unclearly defined. We recommend that when sphenoidal recordings are being used to guide surgical resection, they be interpreted in the context of corroborative evidence from invasive EEGs and other presurgical diagnostic methods.

SUMMARY

The use of intracranial monitoring to delineate brain function and dysfunction is largely dependent on the investigator's use of preoperative data to define a specific question that can be answered through the design and implementation of a study. Specific thought must be given not only to which areas are to be studied but also to which areas are to be omitted from the study. The recording and analysis of electrophysiologic data and data gained through stimulation studies can be used to determine the area of resection for epilepsy surgery, the anatomic relationship of a lesion to functional brain areas, or both. Electrophysiologic data constitute only a small amount of information that can be gained through such studies. A whole range of biosensors that, in the future, may detect changes in neurotransmitter levels, electrolyte disturbances, or metabolism can be envisioned to arm the neurosurgeon with more detailed information to allow safer, more successful resections.

REFERENCES

1. Brazier MAB: A History of the Electrical Activity of the Brain: The First Half-Century. New York, Macmillan, 1961.
2. Talairach J, Bancaud J: Lesion, "irritative" zone and epileptogenic focus. Confin Neurol 27:91–94, 1966.
3. Cascino GD, Jack CR, Parisi JE, et al: MRI-detected hippocampal formation atrophy in temporal lobe lesional epilepsy: Identification of dual pathology. Ann Neurol 32:245, 1992.
4. Cascino GD, Jack CRJ, Parisi JE, et al: Operative strategy in patients with MRI-identified dual pathology and temporal lobe epilepsy. Epilepsy Res 14:175–182, 1993.
5. Cendes F, Cook MJ, Watson C, et al: Frequency and characteristics of dual pathology in patients with lesional epilepsy. Neurology 45:2058–2064, 1995.
6. Li LM, Cendes F, Watson C, et al: Surgical treatment of patients with single and dual pathology: Relevance of lesion and of hippocampal atrophy to seizure outcome. Neurology 48:437–444, 1997.
7. Silberbusch MA, Rothman MI, Bergey GK, et al: Subdural grid implantation for intracranial EEG recording: CT and MR appearance. AJNR Am J Neuroradiol 19:1089–1093, 1998.
8. Penfield W, Jasper HH: Epilepsy and the Functional Anatomy of the Human Brain, 1st ed. Boston, Little, Brown, 1954.
9. Ross DA, Henry TR, Dickinson LD: A percutaneous epidural screw electrode for intracranial electroencephalogram recordings. Neurosurgery 33:332–334, 1993.
10. Barnett GH, Burgess RC, Awad IA, et al: Epidural peg electrodes for the presurgical evaluation of intractable epilepsy. Neurosurgery 27:113–115, 1990.
11. Goldring S, Gregorie EM: Surgical management of epilepsy using epidural recordings to localize the seizure focus: Review of 100 cases. J Neurosurg 60:457–466, 1984.
12. Wieser HG, Siegel AM: Analysis of foramen ovale electrode-recorded seizures and correlation with outcome following amygdalohippocampectomy. Epilepsia 32:838–850, 1991.
13. Wieser HG, Elger CE, Stodieck SR: The "foramen ovale electrode": A new recording method for the preoperative evaluation of patients suffering from mesio-basal temporal lobe epilepsy. Electroencephalogr Clin Neurophysiol 61:314–322, 1985.
14. Wilkus RJ, Thompson PM: Sphenoidal electrode positions and basal EEG during long term monitoring. Epilepsia 26:137–142, 1985.
15. Spencer SS: Intracranial recording. In Spencer SS, Spencer DD (eds): Surgery for Epilepsy. Boston, Blackwell Scientific, 1991, pp 54–65.
16. Härtel F: Über die intracranielle Injektionbehandlung der Trigeminusneuralgie. Med Klin 10:582–584, 1914.
17. Kirschner M: Zur Elektrokoagulation des Ganglion Gasseri. Zentralbl Chir 47:2841–2843, 1932.
18. Ross DA, Brunberg JA, Drury I, et al: Intracerebral depth electrode monitoring in partial epilepsy: The morbidity and efficacy of placement using magnetic resonance image–guided stereotactic surgery. Neurosurgery 39:327–333, 1996.
19. Rosenbaum TJ, Laxer KD, Vessely M, et al: Subdural electrodes for seizure focus localization. Neurosurgery 19:73–81, 1986.
20. Wyler AR, Walker G, Somes G: The morbidity of long-term seizure monitoring using subdural strip electrodes. J Neurosurg 74:734–737, 1991.
21. Swartz BE, Rich JR, Dwan PS, et al: The safety and efficacy of chronically implanted subdural electrodes: A prospective study. Surg Neurol 46:87–93, 1996.
22. Wyler AR, Ojemann GA, Lettich E, et al: Subdural strip electrodes for localizing epileptogenic foci. J Neurosurg 60:1195–1200, 1984.
23. Spencer SS, Spencer DD, Williamson PD, et al: Combined depth and subdural electrode investigation in uncontrolled epilepsy. Neurology 40:74–79, 1990.
24. Behrens E, Zentner J, van Roost D, et al: Subdural and depth electrodes in the presurgical evaluation of epilepsy. Acta Neurochir (Wien) 128:84–87, 1994.
25. Spencer SS: Depth electroencephalography in selection of refractory epilepsy for surgery. Ann Neurol 9:207–214, 1981.
26. Cascino GD, Trenerry MR, Sharbrough FW, et al: Depth electrode studies in temporal lobe epilepsy: Relation to quantitative magnetic resonance imaging and operative outcome. Epilepsia 36:230–235, 1995.
27. Awad IA, Assirati JA Jr, Burgess R, et al: A new class of electrodes of "intermediate invasiveness": Preliminary experience with epidural pegs and foramen ovale electrodes in the mapping of seizure foci. Neurol Res 13:177–183, 1991.
28. Carter DA, Lassiter AT, Brown JA: Cost-efficient localization of seizures of mesiotemporal onset with foramen-ovale electrodes. Neurol Res 20:153–160, 1998.
29. Pacia SV, Ebersole JS: Intracranial EEG substrates of scalp ictal patterns from temporal lobe foci. Epilepsia 38:642–654, 1997.
30. Marks DA, Katz A, Booke J, et al: Comparison and correlation of surface and sphenoidal electrodes with simultaneous intracranial recording: An interictal study. Electroencephalogr Clin Neurophysiol 82:23–29, 1992.

CHAPTER 156

Epilepsy Surgery: Outcome and Complications

WEBSTER H. PILCHER

The past 15 years have witnessed a dramatic expansion of epilepsy monitoring and surgery as a neuroscience subspecialty.[1, 2] The proliferation of multidisciplinary epilepsy centers has increased our capacity to provide comprehensive evaluations of patients with intractable epilepsy (Fig. 156–1), leading to greater numbers of patients being offered surgical treatment (Fig. 156–2).

In addition to traditional diagnostic and surgical procedures, contemporary surgical approaches include selective amygdalohippocampectomy (SAH), multiple subpial transection (MST), keyhole deafferentation hemispherotomies, radiosurgery, and neuroaugmentative approaches, including deep brain stimulation (DBS) and vagal nerve stimulation (Fig. 156–3).

Advances in our understanding of intractable epilepsies have facilitated a discrete taxonomy of surgically remediable syndromes (Fig. 156–4).[1] Each syndrome and each new treatment approach engenders a new data set with regard to seizure outcome, complications (i.e., surgical, neurological, neuropsychological, and psychobehavioral), health outcomes expressed in terms of alterations in quality of life, and cost-effectiveness of alternative therapeutic interventions.

EPIDEMIOLOGY AND LIFETIME COST OF INTRACTABLE EPILEPSY

Epilepsy is a common disorder, afflicting 1.3% or 2 million Americans, with 1 in 10 having at least one seizure over the course of a lifetime.[3] In 1990, 300,000 Americans experienced a new-onset seizure, with 147,000 diagnosed as epileptic.[4] Eight percent or 21,000 were projected to experience frequent, intractable seizures, and this small group accounts for the preponderant burden of unemployment and epilepsy-related deaths. Estimates of the lifetime cost of intractable epilepsy incorporate *direct cost* (i.e., medical care cost) and *indirect cost* (i.e., lost earnings). This small group of intractable epileptics accounted for 40% of the projected direct cost and 72% of the projected indirect cost of all epileptics diagnosed in 1990, totaling more than 3 billion dollars for this small cohort, or $147,000 per patient. Beyond these estimates, the burden of epilepsy incorporates additional, unmeasurable indirect costs that include the cost of pain, suffering, and reduction in the quality of life of epileptic patients and their caretakers.[4]

ADVANCES IN OUTCOME ASSESSMENT OF EPILEPSY SURGERY

The historical gold standard of outcome assessment after epilepsy surgery has been provided by studies of seizure reduction after surgery. The syndrome of intractable epilepsy, however, embraces comorbidities beyond frequent, intractable seizures, which include psychosocial, psychiatric, and neuropsychological impairments and medication toxicity and excess mortality rates (Fig. 156–5).[5, 6] Contemporary studies also emphasize health outcomes commensurate with the World Health Organization (WHO) definition of health as "a state of complete physical, mental, and social well-being."[3, 5]

During the past decade, epilepsy-specific, health-related quality of life (HRQOL) instruments have been developed to assess the impact of epilepsy surgery on health and quality of life of patients with intractable epilepsy. These instruments incorporate generic measures of health status previously validated in studies of health outcomes in other disease states and epilepsy-specific measures of health status that are more sensitive to the cognitive, memory, and role limitation issues implicit in the disease of intractable epilepsy (Fig. 156–6).[5, 7] A clear relationship has been documented between psychosocial status and quality of seizure control in medically managed epileptics.[8] Similarly, in postoperative patients, seizure-free patients score more favorably than patients having auras or recurrent seizures on a variety of measures.[9] Elimination of seizures postoperatively also improves the HRQOL of epilepsy patients compared with patients with other diseases, including heart disease, hypertension, and diabetes.[10] A Canadian prospective, randomized, controlled trial of epilepsy surgery versus best medical management

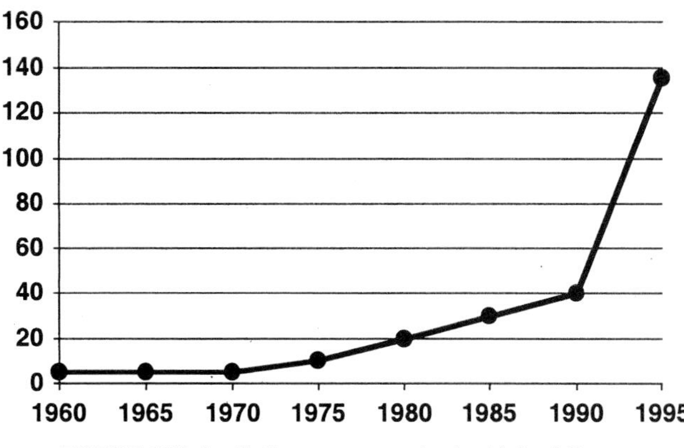

FIGURE 156–1. Epilepsy centers in the United States.

Procedure	Before 1986 ❖	1986-90 ◆
ATLX	2336	4862
SAH	----	568
Neocortical Resection	825	1073
Lesionectomy	----	440

❖ 39 Centers
◆ 107 Centers

FIGURE 156–2. Worldwide surgical procedures for temporal lobe epilepsy.

SURGICAL APPROACHES	
Resective Surgery	Temporal Lobe Resections ("standard," anteromedial selective amygdalohippocampectomy); Extratemporal Resections; Lesional Resections, Anatomic or Functional Hemispherectomy
Radiosurgery	Mesial Temporal Lobe Epilepsy; Hypothalamic Hamartomas with Gelastic Seizures
Disconnection Surgery	Corpus Callosotomy; Keyhole Hemispherotomies; Multiple Subpial Transections
Neuroaugmentative Surgery	Vagal Nerve Stimulator (VNS); Deep Brain Stimulation (DBS)
Diagnostic Surgery	Depth Electrodes; Subdural Strip Electrodes; Subdural Grid Electrodes

FIGURE 156–3. Surgical approaches for epilepsy.

Temporal Lobe Epilepsy (TLE)	Idiopathic; Mesial Temporal Sclerosis/MTLE; Lesional (Tumor, Vascular Malformation, Developmental, Ischemic, Traumatic)
Extratemporal Epilepsy	Idiopathic; Lesional (Tumor, Vascular Malformation, Developmental, Ischemic; Traumatic)
Catastrophic Epilepsy	Lesional; (Hemimegalencephaly, Diffuse Cortical Dysplasias, Sturge-Weber, Rasmussen's, Porencephalic Cysts)
Secondarily Generalized Epilepsies	Lennox-Gastaut

FIGURE 156–4. Surgically remediable syndromes.

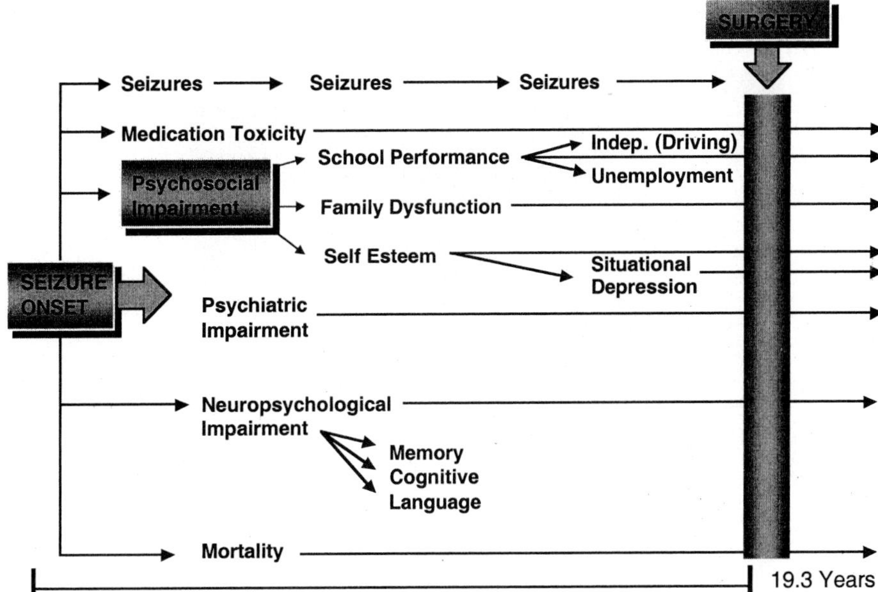

FIGURE 156–5. Temporal lobe epilepsy as a chronic illness.

in 80 patients documented improved seizure outcomes and HRQOL in operated patients.[2]

Advances in epidemiologic and "health outcomes" investigations have facilitated cost-effectiveness studies of epilepsy surgery. Cost-effectiveness studies incorporate established patient preferences for being in certain health states, along with cost estimates of each health state, to assess the cost-effectiveness of surgical intervention. *Health states* are typically quantified on a scale of 0 to 1. For example, preference-based values for epilepsy-related health states include a healthy, disease-free patient (1.0), a patient with intractable complex partial seizures (0.62), and a postoperative, seizure-free patient (0.8911). This approach permits calculation of *quality-adjusted life-years* (QALYs) by multiplying expected postoperative survival in years by the appropriate quality-adjustment factor (from 0 to 1) that reflects the outcome state.[11, 12] The number of QALYs added to a patient's life by successful epilepsy surgery can be estimated (Fig. 156–7), and when combined with the cost of therapy, it can be expressed as the cost (in dollars) of providing an incremental QALY to the life of a patient with intractable epilepsy. The cost-effectiveness of surgical intervention can then be expressed in various ways, providing a measure of the cost-effectiveness of epilepsy surgery, which can be compared with other, unrelated health care interventions.

TEMPORAL LOBE RESECTIONS

Surgically Remediable Syndromes

The prototypical syndrome of mesial temporal lobe epilepsy incorporates a history of an early insult in infancy or childhood,[13, 14] hippocampal sclerosis and atrophy on magnetic resonance imaging (MRI),[15] an abnormal creatine-to-NAA (Cr/NAA) ratio on magnetic resonance spectroscopy (MRS),[16] temporal hypometabolism on interictal positron emission tomography (PET),[17, 18] and a characteristic pattern of hyperperfusion and hypoperfusion on ictal single photon emission computed tomography (SPECT).[13] Electroencephalographic studies reveal an anteromedial epileptogenic zone, and Wada testing reveals appropriate memory deficits.[19] Histopathologic study of resected hippocampi reveals loss of principal hippocampal neurons, synaptic reorganization, sprouting of mossy fibers, and enhanced expression of glutamate receptors.[20, 21]

Generic (Rand SF-36)	• Emotional well being • Role limitations due to: Emotional Problems Physical Problems • Energy/Fatigue • Social Function • Pain • Physical Function • Health Perceptions
Epilepsy Specific	• Cognitive Functions • Role Limitations Due to Memory Problems

FIGURE 156–6. The Epilepsy Surgery Inventory (ESI-55) is a health-related quality of life measure for epilepsy.

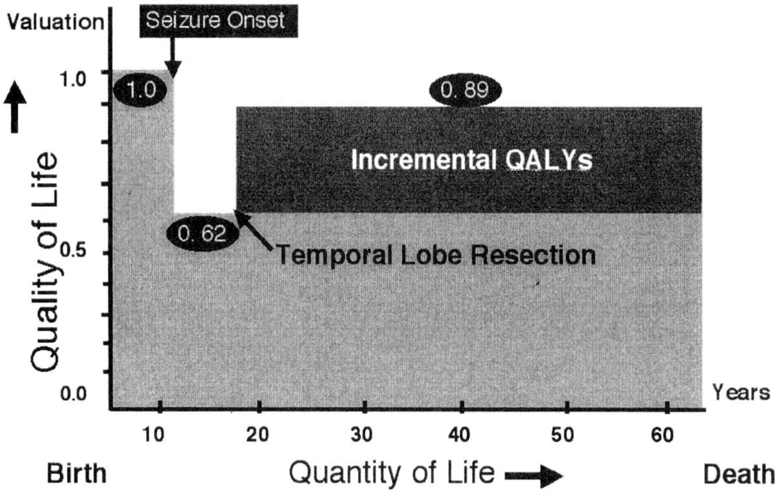

FIGURE 156–7. Estimated number of quality-adjusted life years (QALYs) added to a patient's life after successful epilepsy surgery.

A smaller population of patients with *cryptogenic* TLE have normal MRI scans preoperatively.[14] Patients with *lesional* TLE present with temporal lobe neoplasms, vascular malformations, disorders of cortical development, or traumatic or ischemic insults within the temporal lobe. These lesions may variably involve mesial temporal lobe structures or may be associated with hippocampal sclerosis (i.e., dual pathology),[22] leading to distinct surgical approaches and outcomes

Surgical Approaches for Mesial Temporal Lobe Epilepsy

The traditional en bloc temporal lobectomy incorporated a 5- to 6-cm lateral resection along with a portion of the amygdala and anterior hippocampus.[23, 24] More centers now employ a focused anteromedial resection in which a restricted resection of middle and inferior temporal gyrus is combined with thorough hippocampal removal.[25–27] The trans-sylvian SAH permits exclusive resection of medial structures.[28, 29] Awake surgery with intraoperative electrocorticography and functional brain mapping permits tailored resection of lateral and medial structures.[30, 31]

SEIZURE OUTCOMES

Classification Schemes

Studies have demonstrated that HRQOL and psychosocial measures may not improve significantly with as much as a 70% reduction of seizure frequency postoperatively.[32] In recognition of the benefits derived when seizure freedom or near–seizure freedom is achieved postoperatively, contemporary seizure outcome classification schemes emphasize patterns of seizure reduction that are likely to affect quality of life.[33–35] The Engel classification scheme (Fig. 156–8) provides four categories of seizure outcome: I, seizure free; II, rare seizures (i.e., two to three per year); III, worthwhile improvement (>90% reduction); and IV, no worthwhile improvement (<90% reduction).[34]

Improvement in Seizure Outcomes

Early investigations of temporal lobe resections during an era in which the lateral resection was emphasized documented seizure-free outcomes of 27% to 44% in long-term follow-up assessments.[36–40] Engel compared worldwide outcomes of earlier (1949 to 1984) and more recent (1986 to 1990) eras and documented superior outcomes in contemporary series (Fig. 156–9).[1, 33] This improvement was thought to result from improved methods of patient selection and convergence of surgical resection approaches to emphasize medial resections.

Seizure Outcomes Over Time

The protean expressions of seizure outcomes after surgical intervention have become a subject of considerable interest in long-term studies of postoperative patients. These studies have revealed that, for many individual patients, seizure control is not static but may fluctuate over time.

Sperling and colleagues[35] studied 89 patients with TLE who underwent anterior temporal lobe resections between 1986 and 1990 and were followed postopera-

I. Free of Disabling Seizures
- Auras
- ≥ 2 yr Sz Free
- GTC with Drug Withdrawal

II. Rare Disabling Seizures (≤ 2 yr)
- ≥ 2 yr
- Nocturnal Seizures Only

III. Worthwhile Improvement
- ≥ 2 yr

IV. No Worthwhile Improvement (≤ 90%)

FIGURE 156–8. Engel outcome classification.

Procedure	PTs.	Sz. Free (2 Yr)	>90%	<90%
PALM DESERT 1986: 39 CENTERS (1949-84)				
ATLX	2336	55.5%	27.7%	16.8%
PALM DESERT 1992: 107 CENTERS (1986-90)				
ATLX	3579	67.9%	24.0%	8.1%
AHX	413	68.8%	22.3%	9.0%
Lx	293	66.6%	21.5%	11.9%

FIGURE 156–9. Worldwide outcomes after anterior temporal lobe resection for seizure.

tively for 5 years. The percentage of patients in class I (i.e., seizure free over the past year) remained constant at 70% over the follow-up period. Only 55% of patients were seizure free over the entire 5-year period after surgery. Of the patients who experienced postoperative seizures, 55% had the first seizure by 6 months postoperatively, and 93% had the first seizure by 2 years postoperatively (Fig. 156–10). Patients who were seizure free over the first 2 years after surgery were likely to remain seizure free thereafter.

In a 5-year outcome study of 148 operated TLE patients, 44.6% were completely seizure free since surgery at the 4.8-year follow-up, with 62% seizure free over the past year.[41] In another 5-year follow-up study of 135 patients, 62% of patients with mesial temporal sclerosis (MTS) were seizure free for the last 2 years of the study, whereas only 50% were seizure free for the entire 5-year period.[42]

Acute, Postoperative Seizures and Late Improvement

Seizures occurring in the immediate postoperative period were traditionally disregarded because early seizures after stroke and head injury were not reliably predictive of late seizure outcome.[33] In early studies, Rasmussen and others[43–45] described a "running down" phenomenon in 15% to 20% of patients, in which early postoperative seizures dissipated over time, with subsequent improved control. In a contemporary study, running down was reported in only 5% of TLE patients and occurred more frequently in patients with preoperative unilateral epileptiform discharges.[46] Other studies suggest that seizures occurring in the first postoperative week may portend a less favorable outcome in adult[47, 48] and pediatric patients.[49]

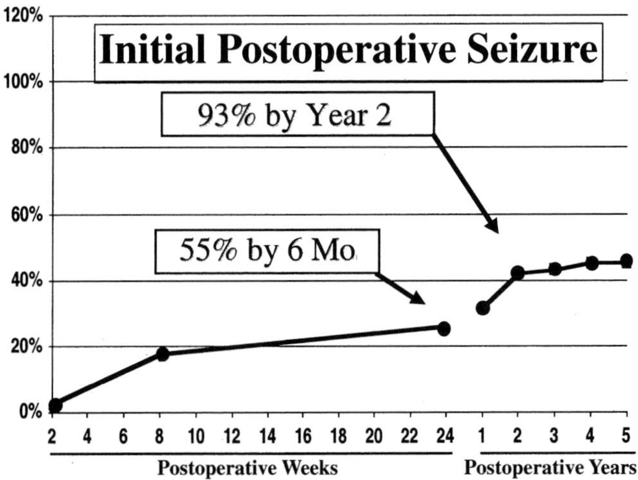

FIGURE 156–10. Percentage of patients who had initial postoperative seizures after anterior temporal lobe resection.

Surgical versus Best Medical Management

A 5-year follow-up study compared seizure outcomes of 148 operated and 94 unoperated TLE patients.[41] Seizure freedom during the final year of follow-up was achieved in 62% of operated and 7.5% of nonoperated patients. Complete seizure freedom over the entire study period was achieved in 44.6% of operated and 4.3% of nonoperated patients. None of the nonoperated patients and 8.8% of the operated patients were antiepileptic drug (AED) free at follow-up. Other adult studies have documented AED freedom in 21%[50] and 35%[51] of patients at 1- and 2-year follow-up evaluations, respectively. Pediatric studies have documented 30% to 44% AED-free rates at 2 years[51, 52] and 30%, 35%, and 60% AED-free rates at 2, 5, and 10 years postoperatively, respectively.[53]

The only prospective, randomized, controlled study of surgical versus best medical management for TLE compared the outcome of surgery in 40 medically managed patients with 40 surgically managed patients.[2] At the 1-year follow-up assessment, 58% of the surgically treated and only 8% of the medically treated patients were seizure free.

Pathologic Substrate of Mesial Temporal Lobe Epilepsy

The pathologic features of hippocampal sclerosis (i.e., MTS) incorporate the loss of principal neurons (i.e., atrophy), glial proliferation (i.e., gliosis), and sprouting of dentate granule cells.[54, 55] When hippocampal principal neuron loss exceeds 50%, hippocampal atrophy is visible on MRI,[54] and gliosis manifests as high signal intensity on flare and T2-weighted images. Some degree of hippocampal sclerosis occurs contralateral to the side of resection, and it may be undetected by standard MRI assessment. In 5% to 10% of cases, overt, bilateral MTS is visible on MRI.[56]

Imaging, Neuropsychological, Electrographic, and Clinical Features

The presence of unilateral MTS, side-specific neuropsychological deficits, and ipsilateral electrographic abnormalities constitutes a favorable substrate for surgical intervention. Good outcomes were achieved in 91% of patients with MRI-defined unilateral MTS, in 62% with bilateral MTS, and in only 50% of patients without MTS.[57] A subset of bilateral MTS patients may have unilateral onsets as defined by depth electrode recordings of ictal onset, and in one study, four of five patients were rendered seizure free at 2-year follow-up.[56] PET hypometabolism highly correlates with MRI and histologically confirmed hippocampal atrophy.[58, 59] In a 1-year postoperative follow-up study, 83% of patients with restricted mesial temporal lobe hypometabolism on PET were seizure free, whereas only 38% of patients with normal PET scans or evidence of multilobar hypometabolism were seizure free.[18] In a 5-year outcome assessment of 135 operated patients, 80% of patients with foreign tissue lesions, 62% of patients with MTS, and 36% of patients with normal hippocampi were seizure free for the 2 years preceding the completion of the study.[42] Multivariate analyses may improve prediction of outcome.[60] When patients presented with MTS, a known cause of epilepsy, and absence of generalized seizures, 93% experienced a satisfactory outcome. Satisfactory outcomes were achieved in 78% to 83% when two of these features were present, in 53% to 61% when one was present, and in 29% when none was present.[61] Corroborative evidence of lateralized hippocampal dysfunction provided by a lateralized memory deficit on the intracarotid Amytal test (i.e., Wada Test) is independently predictive of seizure-free outcome.[19, 62]

Interictal[52, 63] and ictal[60, 64, 65] electroencephalograms provide independent evidence for the side of seizure onset. In a comparative study, concordance of MRI and interictal electroencephalographic findings was most closely associated with favorable surgical outcome in patients with nonlesional TLE.[66] A 5-year follow-up study demonstrated that 26 (92.9%) of 28 patients with a consistent, unilateral, anterior-midtemporal epileptiform focus without discordant findings in other studies had at least 75% reduction in seizures and that 61% of these patients were seizure free 5 years postoperatively.[63]

In a review of 126 articles on temporal lobe resection published between 1991 and 2001, the median seizure-free rate was 70%, and of 63 factors analyzed, good outcome was associated with preoperative MTS, anterior temporal localization of interictal epileptiform activity, absence of preoperative generalized seizures, and absence of seizures in the first postoperative week.[67] Age at seizure onset, preoperative seizure frequency, and extent of lateral resection had no association with outcome.

Age at the time of surgery (>45 years old) may be related to seizure outcome, with some studies suggesting less favorable outcomes[68] and others suggesting that advanced age does not predispose to a less favorable outcome.[69, 70]

Extent of Cortical and Hippocampal Resection

In early studies, lateral resection alone often yielded disappointing results with regard to seizure freedom.[71] Two studies, one of which was a randomized, prospective trial, suggested that the extent of lateral resection does not correlate with seizure outcome.[72, 73] Feindel and Rasmussen[74] reported that 53 of 100 patients were seizure free after a standard lateral resection was combined with a complete amygdalectomy and minimal hippocampal resection. The favorable outcomes after SAH,[34, 75] the effectiveness of removal of residual posterior hippocampus in reoperative surgery[76, 77] and the identification of posterior hippocampal onsets in depth electrode studies[25] all suggest that a thorough hippocampal resection may be essential to optimize seizure outcome. In contrast to earlier reports that the extent of mesial resection had no association with seizure outcome, two studies addressed this issue effectively.[67] The first study of 94 TLE patients, for whom postoperative MRI was employed to confirm the extent of the medial resection, revealed a correlation of the extent of the mesiobasal resection with seizure outcome, regardless of the extent of lateral resection.[78] In a separate, randomized, prospective, longitudinal, blinded study, 70 patients with unilateral ictal onsets determined by intracranial recordings underwent temporal lobe resections, which were randomized to partial or total hippocampectomy.[27] At 1- and 2-year follow-up, the group with complete hippocampectomy experienced superior seizure outcomes (69% versus 38% seizure free at 1 year) without increased neuropsychological or neurological morbidity.

Impact of the Surgical Approach

Although rare patients may harbor epileptogenic zones exclusively in the lateral temporal neocortex,[79] most candidates for nonlesional temporal lobe resection express the syndrome of mesial temporal lobe epilepsy for which resection of mesial structures is now emphasized.[13] A long-term follow-up study of 50 patients managed with lateral resection alone revealed that 44% were seizure free at follow-up.[80] In Engel's compilation of seizure outcomes from 107 centers worldwide, seizure outcomes were similar between centers and surgical approaches, provided that mesial structures were adequately resected.[1] In single-center studies, SAH and standard resections produced similar results.[57] In the SAH series of Wieser and colleagues,[75] a cohort of 22 (73%) of 30 TLE patients with depth electrodes confirmed that those with hippocampal onsets were seizure free postoperatively. These results after SAH compare favorably with those of studies of patients with histologically confirmed MTS undergoing standard anteromesial resections, in which 67% were seizure free at the 5-year follow-up assessment.[81]

A single-center study documented the seizure outcomes of 321 patients undergoing various temporal lobe resections between 1989 and 1997.[82] This series incorporated 96 standard anterior temporal resections, 84 restricted lateral and generous mesial resections, and 91 SAH procedures. A significant percentage underwent preoperative invasive diagnostic procedures. The notable finding was the absence of significant differences in seizure outcomes for the three operative cohorts in which different resection strategies were employed.

Stereotactic Radiosurgery

An initial report of gamma knife radiosurgical treatment of 25 patients with intractable mesial temporal lobe epilepsy found that 13 of 16 patients seizure free at 24 months, with 2 of 16 improved.[83] Two patients were immediately seizure free. A dose of 20 to 25 Gy at the 50% isodose line was employed with a target volume of 6500 to 7500 mm^3. The median interval to seizure cessation was 10.5 months. Minimal side effects were reported, including headache, nausea, and vomiting, which resolved with steroids.

Intraoperative Electrocorticography

Despite its long history, the contribution of electrocorticography to improved seizure outcomes remains ill defined and controversial. Early studies of "tailored" resections suggested that electrocorticography had some predictive value, particularly if spikes were entirely absent before resection or abundant after resection.[45, 84, 85] Study[31] findings support the use of electrocorticography to tailor the hippocampal resection and to optimize seizure outcomes while preserving some of the hippocampus. In two studies conducted at different centers of standard, nontailored anteromesial resections with maximal hippocampectomy and using electrocorticography before and after resection, the electrocorticographic findings did not correlate with outcome.[86, 87] Other studies provide support for a rather limited value of electrocorticography in contemporary temporal lobe surgery.[72, 88, 89] In patients with intractable epilepsy and temporal or extratemporal tumors resected only to normal tissue margins, the extramarginal spike distribution did not correlate with outcome.[90] Although electrocorticographic recordings in selected, infrequent cases may permit tailoring of resection to improve seizure outcome, the association of electrocorticographic spikes with outcome across populations of TLE patients is not well defined.[67]

NEUROPSYCHOLOGICAL OUTCOMES

Neuropsychological assessment provides information that is useful in the selection of candidates for surgical intervention and as a tool to predict and assess adverse outcomes of surgery. Of particular concern are losses of memory function, including global amnesia and material-specific memory deficits affecting short-term verbal and visual spatial memory. Potential cognitive losses and adverse psychosocial and psychiatric outcomes are also considered.

Cognitive Outcome

Intellectual function is generally preserved in adults[35] and children[91] after temporal lobe resection, and when seizure control is achieved, improvement in some measures have been reported. In the Graduate Hospital series of 89 consecutive patients undergoing dominant[42] and nondominant[47] resections, measures of verbal IQ were unchanged postoperatively, and improvements in performance IQ and full-scale IQ were realized.[35] In part, these improvements were considered attributable to the practice effect. Other centers have reported similar findings, including improvement of verbal IQ after nondominant resections and of performance IQ after dominant resections.[92–95]

Global Memory Deficits

Although uncommon, global memory deficits after temporal lobe resection are among the most disabling of the complications of epilepsy surgery. Milner[96] described two patients with global amnesia in an early Montreal Neurological Institute series of 90 dominant temporal resections. These patients exhibited a syndrome of profound anterograde memory loss with preservation of cognitive performance, personality, early memory, and technical skills.[97, 98] Other early reports described global amnesia after unilateral resection in the dominant or nondominant hemispheres.[94, 98, 99] Evidence that hippocampal rather than lateral neocortical removal is critical to the production of global amnesia is provided by a report of a patient undergoing a staged resection in whom global amnesia occurred only after the hippocampus was removed[96] and by reports of global amnesia after SAH.[100] Contemporary series report rare postoperative global memory deficits, with a frequency of 1%,[94, 101–103] whereas a less profound postoperative "severe amnesia" may be more common.[104]

Intracarotid Amytal Procedure: The Wada Test

The Wada test was originally developed to determine hemispheric lateralization of language function,[105] but was subsequently adapted by Milner and colleagues[106] to provide a measure of the risk to memory function postoperatively. The Wada test has been employed to identify patients at risk for global memory loss,[107] and such losses are uncommon because the Wada test was universally adopted. Reports of favorable memory outcome in patients who failed the Wada test preoperatively (i.e., false positives) have called into question the reliability of this procedure in some patients.[108] The

Wada test has also been useful in identifying lateralized temporal lobe dysfunction and as a predictor of seizure laterality,[109, 110] and more recently, it has been used to predict material-specific memory losses (particularly verbal memory losses) after surgery.[62, 111] Complications of the Wada test include the complications of transfemoral carotid angiography, including thromboembolism and stroke (0.5% to 1.0%), allergic contrast reactions (1 in 40,000), and local complications of femoral puncture.[103] Rare deaths have been reported.[107] In the future, functional MRI memory assessments may augment or supplant this procedure.[112]

Material-Specific Memory Deficits

Reported material-specific memory deficits include losses of short-term verbal and nonverbal memory postoperatively. In particular, short-term verbal memory losses are common after dominant temporal lobe resections, with significant decrements in verbal memory reported in 25% to 50% of operated patients.[113] Verbal memory losses may accompany nondominant resections, although at a much lower frequency.[113] Nonverbal memory deficits are less commonly identified, even after nondominant resections,[114] and some investigators report that these losses may be obscured by practice effects.[113] In the Graduate Hospital series, evidence of significant short-term verbal memory loss was identified in many patients after dominant temporal lobe resections, with a trend toward improvement after nondominant temporal lobe resections.[35] In a series of 321 TLE patients undergoing a variety of surgical approaches to nonlesional and lesional TLE over 10 years, verbal memory declined in 34%, improved in 19%, and remained stable in 46%.[82] Preoperatively, weak performance on measures of verbal memory, young age at surgery, and operations on the right (nondominant) side were associated with stability or improvement in verbal memory. Short-term nonverbal memory measures exhibited similar rates of improvement and deterioration. Preoperatively, weak nonverbal memory and left-sided (dominant) operations were associated with improvement, whereas better performance preoperatively and older age were associated with deterioration.[82]

The high frequency with which verbal memory impairment occurs after dominant temporal lobe surgery has stimulated interest in predicting which patients are at risk for postoperative deficits. Studies have documented significantly greater risk for verbal memory loss in two categories of patients: those with intact memory function and a normal hippocampus ipsilateral to the seizure focus (i.e., functional adequacy hypothesis) and those with ipsilateral hippocampal atrophy but impaired memory function contralateral to the seizure focus to be resected (i.e., functional reserve hypothesis).[115] Patients with left TLE and a reversed Wada memory asymmetry score (i.e., best memory performance by the epileptogenic, left temporal lobe, with poor right temporal lobe performance) have a greater risk for memory morbidity after left-sided resection and poorer seizure outcome postoperatively.[116] Patients with dominant hippocampal atrophy who undergo contralateral, nondominant resections are also at risk for verbal memory deficits.[117] Preoperative MRI studies of hippocampal volumes and left hippocampal MRS profiles (Cr/NAA) also help predict the risk to verbal memory performance after surgery.[16]

In one study, a multivariate risk factor model for predicting postoperative verbal memory decline was developed in which five risk factors were independently associated with outcome: dominant hemisphere resection, MRI findings other than exclusively ipsilateral MTS, intact preoperative delayed recall verbal memory, relatively poorer preoperative immediate recall verbal memory, and intact ipsilateral memory performance on the Wada test.[118] Using this model, individual patients can be apprised of the risk to their verbal memory function after surgery.

Standard Anterior Temporal Lobe Resection versus Selective Amygdalohippocampectomy: Memory Outcome

For patients thought to be at risk for global or material-specific memory deficits postoperatively, various management strategies have been proposed to reduce the losses, including memory mapping in the temporal neocortex[119] with restriction of neocortical resection, SAH, or simple denial of surgery to these patients. With reports of global amnesia occurring in patients undergoing SAH,[100] attention turned to the possible advantage of selective mesial resection from the standpoint of preservation of material-specific memory, especially short-term verbal memory function. Although some early outcome studies in small series of patients suggested a possible advantage of SAH versus standard anterior temporal lobe resection from the standpoint of postoperative memory outcome,[50, 120] others produced conflicting results.[121]

Report of a large study population of 140 patients undergoing right (74 patients) or left (66 patients) SAH revealed declines in verbal learning and memory in 32% of the right-sided and 51% of the left-sided resections.[122] This study did not support the concept that SAH patients experience less memory loss than patients undergoing standard resections. The left SAH patients were particularly at risk when preoperative testing revealed intact verbal memory function, late onset of epilepsy, and the absence of MTS on MRI. Collateral damage to adjacent temporolateral tissue during the trans-sylvian dissection may augment losses engendered by hippocampal resection.[122, 123] The role of deafferentation of temporal circuitry during resection of parahippocampal gyrus, amygdala, and hippocampus also needs to be considered and is supported by PET evidence of worsening hypometabolism of the remaining temporal lobe neocortex after SAH.[124]

Postoperative Language Dysfunction

After dominant temporal lobe resections, a syndrome of transitory postoperative dysnomia or aphasia is observed in as many as 30% of operated patients, and it gradually disappears over a few weeks.[125] This occurs even when resections are guided by intraoperative or extraoperative language mapping.[126, 127] The cause of this transitory phenomenon is unclear, but it is more common when resections are carried to within 1 to 2 cm of essential language sites as determined by mapping procedures.[119, 128] Other causes may include resection of inferior temporal lobe inessential language sites,[129] brain retraction with associated neuroparalytic edema,[130, 131] and deafferentation of white matter pathways. Some investigators have suggested that such word finding deficits represent an acute postoperative exacerbation of preoperative deficits common in patients with TLE and that resolution normally occurs within 1 year.[132]

Although some investigations of naming have not revealed enduring deficits at 6 and 18 months postoperatively,[126, 133, 134] others[125, 135, 136] have suggested that significant, persistent word-finding difficulties occur commonly after standard or anteromesial temporal lobe resections. Such deficits have been associated with early risk factors for the development of seizures[135] and with the pathologic state of the resected hippocampus.[137] In one study, a subset of 7% of patients undergoing standard dominant resections exhibited persistent postoperative dysnomia.[136]

These findings, along with Ojemann's description of enduring language deficits after resections within 1 to 2 cm of identified language sites,[138] have stimulated interest in the value of intraoperative mapping and in tailoring of lateral neocortical resection. Ojemann suggested that up to 17% of patients undergoing left temporal resections 4.0 to 4.5 cm from the temporal tip (i.e., standard temporal lobe resection) without mapping would experience postoperative deficits.[139] Some centers employ cortical resections restricted to 3 cm of the middle and inferior gyrus without mapping and have reported minimal postoperative language deficits.[25] With the general trend toward such restricted lateral cortical resections in the temporal lobe, language mapping is less commonly employed. The possibility that even such restricted resections may engender deficits not seen in patients undergoing mapping has not been studied.

Persistent, severe dysphasia has been reported in 1% to 2% of patients undergoing dominant temporal resections, even with language mapping.[77, 94, 140, 141] Such adverse postoperative outcomes occur as a result of resection of essential language cortex or are caused by manipulation of or thrombosis of middle cerebral or anterior choroidal arteries.[142]

NEUROBEHAVIORAL AND PSYCHOSOCIAL OUTCOMES

Psychiatric Outcome

Psychiatric morbidity in patients with epilepsy ranges from 15% to 50% in various studies.[143, 144] There is a high prevalence of psychopathology, including depression, in candidates for temporal lobe resection preoperatively and postoperatively.[145, 146] One study reported postoperative improvement or resolution of longstanding depressive symptoms in 47% of patients undergoing temporal lobe resections, suggesting that preoperative depression is not a contraindication to surgery.[147] In this same study, depression occurred de novo in 10% of operated patients. Improvement in depression postoperatively is more reliable in patients who are rendered seizure free.[148, 149] Preoperative prediction of the risk for chronic depressive symptoms postoperatively may be possible using measures of emotional adjustment, such as the Washington Psychosocial Seizure Inventory.[149]

The early postoperative period is characterized by the dynamic expression of various psychopathologic conditions, and in one study, one half of the patients with no psychopathology preoperatively had developed symptoms of anxiety, depression, and emotional lability 6 weeks after surgery.[150] Other reports have documented new psychiatric problems in 31% of patients and resolution of psychiatric diagnoses in 15% of patients in the 6 months after surgery.[145] In one extraordinary study, 10% of 121 operated TLE patients required postoperative psychiatric hospitalization, particularly those with bilateral spike discharges preoperatively.[151] The de novo appearance of hypomania requiring psychiatric hospitalization[152] and postoperative psychogenic seizures, particularly in female patients undergoing right temporal lobe surgery,[145, 153] as well as neurotic or psychotic symptoms in 9 of 100 operated cases,[154] fortify the mandate for comprehensive psychosocial and psychiatric assessments preoperatively and postoperatively. In the context of a thorough preoperative evaluation, a history of psychotic symptoms does not represent an absolute contraindication to surgical intervention, although exacerbation of symptoms may occur postoperatively.

Psychosocial Outcome

The syndrome of intractable TLE embraces comorbidities beyond the encumbrance of frequent, intractable seizures, including psyochosocial, psychiatric, and neuropsychological impairments; medication toxicities; and excess mortality rates. These impairments develop as the result of frequent, disabling seizures during critical stages of personal development and may not resolve immediately after surgery (see Fig. 156–5).

Patients are aware of epilepsy-associated disabilities and hope for their resolution after surgery. In a study of 69 preoperative patients, their aims for epilepsy surgery beyond seizure freedom included desire for work, ability to drive, independence, socializing, and freedom from antiepileptic medications.[6] The psychosocial outcomes of successful surgery were assessed in a 5-year follow-up study of long-term changes in life performance of 61 surgically managed and 23 medically managed, temporal lobe epileptics.[155] In this study, 68% of the surgery group exhibited improved psychosocial status compared with 5% of the medically managed group. Individuals who had surgery were more likely to be driving, working full time, living independently, and financially independent. Remaining seizure free was not a prerequisite for improvement in psychosocial measures in this study, although other investigations have documented diminished psychosocial adjustment in patients with recurrent seizures.[156]

Health-Related Quality of Life

Contemporary outcome studies incorporate measures of health outcomes in which the patient's perspective becomes an integral aspect of the assessment.[157] To facilitate HRQOL studies of epilepsy surgery patients, assessment tools such as the Epilepsy Surgery Inventory (ESI-55)[7] have been developed and validated for use in this population. This instrument incorporates a "generic core" adapted from the RAND 36-Item Health Survey, along with 12 epilepsy-specific items addressing domains of cognitive function, role limitations due to memory problems, and health perceptions.[9] Vickrey and coworkers[7] documented improved HRQOL in postoperative, seizure-free patients compared with patients with persistent auras and with persistent seizures. In another study of 2-year postoperative patients, seizure-free patients and those with 90% reduction experienced significant improvement in HRQOL.[51] Compared with the health status of patients with other chronic diseases, postoperative patients with persistent seizures scored less well than patients with heart disease, hypertension, or diabetes. When patients were seizure free postoperatively, they scored better than patients with these illnesses.[10]

Other instruments developed to assess HRQOL have included the Quality of Life in Epilepsy-89 (QOLIE-89)[158] and a shorter version, the QOLIE-10.[157] In a study of 37 nonsurgical and 53 surgical patients evaluated preoperatively and at 1 and 2 years postoperatively, significant improvement on 10 of the 17 scales of QOLIE-89 was identified for patients who were entirely seizure free, with more improvement at the 2-year follow-up than at the 1-year follow-up evaluation. Notably, patients with persistent auras were not significantly improved compared with patients with persistent seizures.[159] At the 1-year follow-up assessment, in a randomized, prospective, controlled trial of surgical therapy versus best medical management for TLE, the surgical group scored better on the QOLIE-89[64, 74] and in measures of school or job performance (56% or 39%).[2]

Cost-Effectiveness of Surgical Treatment

Wiebe and colleagues[12] used decision-analysis modeling and an intention-to-treat approach to compare medical with surgical treatment of intractable TLE in a Canadian population of 200 patients treated surgically or medically for 35 years. In their model, surgery required a larger initial expenditure. By 8 years postoperatively, however, the cost savings engendered by the 57 seizure-free patients made surgery less expensive across the entire cohort of surgical patients. Surgical therapy was more cost-effective than medical management in this population.

In a decision-analysis model of surgical versus best medical management of intractable TLE, using Rochester, New York, cost data, Langfitt[11] addressed the relative cost-effectiveness of opposing treatments. Intrinsic to this investigation was the expression of the cost-effectiveness of treatment as a *marginal cost-effectiveness ratio* (MCER), which represents the dollar cost per QALY added to treated patients' lives postoperatively. Each postoperative outcome state was assigned a quality adjustment on the basis of ESI-55 scores achieved by 42 patients undergoing evaluation for surgery. With a state of total health adjusted to 1.0, patients with intractable seizures preoperatively were adjusted to 0.62, and postoperative states were adjusted as follows: no seizures (0.89), auras only (0.80), and recurrent complex partial seizures (0.72). In this model, a patient rendered seizure free after surgery would improve from 0.62 to 0.89 on the adjustment scale, and if the

Treatment	MCER's (1995 US $/QALY)
◆ Lifetime TB screening 20 y.o. BM vs. None	324,537
◆ MRI vs. CT in dx. of dementia	146,400
◆ Stenting vs. balloon angioplasty (symptomatic single-vessel CAD)	29,893
◆ Asymptomatic intracranial aneurysm repair	28,441
◆ Early AAA repair vs. watchful waiting	20,454
◆ ATLX vs. medical management for MIE	15,581
◆ Estrogen in severely osteoporotic women to prevent hip fx vs. none	5,827

FIGURE 156–11. The marginal cost-effectiveness ratio (MCER) for treatment.

patient lived for 40 years in this state of health, the patient would accrue an additional 10 QALYs. The calculated MCER was $15,581/QALY, which compares quite favorably with the cost of other health care interventions (Fig. 156–11). In another American study, a cost-effectiveness ratio of $27,200 per QALY was determined.[160]

OUTCOMES AND COMPLICATIONS OF DIAGNOSTIC AND SURGICAL PROCEDURES

Epilepsy surgery is safe and effective. Nevertheless, invasive diagnostic procedures and definitive surgical interventions do carry some risk, which must be considered when recommending surgical intervention to patients with intractable seizures.

Diagnostic Procedures

DEPTH ELECTRODES

In the past, intracerebral depth electrodes were employed routinely in the preoperative evaluation of most patients for temporal lobe resection.[161] In contemporary practice, improved imaging and surface electroencephalographic monitoring methods have reduced the need for invasive recordings in many cases. Depth electrodes are particularly sensitive to localized discharges emanating from deep structures such as the amygdala and hippocampus and require brain penetration to reach the areas of interest. This requirement of brain penetration carries a risk of infection (1% to 4%) and intracerebral hemorrhage that has been observed in 3% of patients after parasagittal placements and in 1% after lateral placements.[103] In one early series, 2 of 163 patients died, one from posterior cerebral artery laceration and another after laceration of a parasagittal bridging vein.[162] Studies using contemporary stereotactic methods have reported fewer adverse outcomes. A study reported minor complications in none of 18 patients[163] and in 5 of 115 patients without any permanent neurological deficits.[164] Bilateral intrahippocampal depth electrodes may be associated with verbal memory decline postoperatively.[122]

SUBDURAL STRIP ELECTRODES

Subdural strip electrodes were popularized[165] as an alternative to depth electrode implantation. Although strip electrodes cannot directly sample activity from deep structures, they do not require brain penetration while providing extensive coverage of neocortical areas. In an extensive series of 350 patients, two cases of meningitis, one brain abscess associated with hemiparesis, and three superficial wound infections were reported.[165] In a prospective study of 55 patients undergoing implantation of subdural electrodes, unexpected adverse effects included fever higher than 102°F (5%), migraine (5%), and temporalis muscle fibrosis (5%). In a multicenter study of 131 patients undergoing strip implantation, only five minor complications, including three small hematomas not requiring evacuation, were identified.[166]

SUBDURAL GRID ELECTRODES

Subdural grid electrodes are used to sample electrographic data from wide expanses of neocortex and to map eloquent brain regions through electrical stimulation methods. Because they require a craniotomy for placement and because numerous electrode cables must exit the cranium through cutaneous puncture, infections constitute the most common complication of these procedures. Infection rates of 22% were identified in an early Cleveland Clinic series, which declined to 7% when cables were tunneled to exit percutaneously.[127] A contemporary series of 49 patients undergoing grid implantation reported a 4% infection rate, subdural hematoma formation requiring emergency evacuation in 8%, and brain swelling in 2%.[167] Other series reported subdural hematoma formation in 8% and increased intracranial pressure requiring premature removal of the grid.[103] Careful tunneling of cables, perioperative antibiotic management, avoidance of injury to or compression of bridging veins, and judicious use of Decadron and mannitol have been recommended.[103]

Resective Temporal Lobe Surgery

In a review[103] of the accumulated worldwide experience with temporal lobe resective surgery before 1993, significant, impairing complications were uncommon but included death,[38, 94, 163, 168–170]; infection[94, 103, 130]; hemiparesis due to manipulation or thrombosis of the middle cerebral artery or anterior choroidal vasculature or to direct brainstem injury or resection[169, 171–174]; visual field deficits due to resection of Meyer's loop fibers in the roof of the temporal horn[175, 176] or hemianopsia[141, 177, 178] due to excessive tissue resection or to infarction; postoperative hematoma formation[38, 94, 168]; and rare cranial nerve III[169, 172] and cranial nerve VII[179] palsies. In one review,[103] there was a trend in the direction of reduced mortality and morbidity over time in large, single-center series and in a worldwide survey of 2282 operations performed from 1928 through 1973.[38]

In a contemporary, single-center study of temporal lobe surgery in 456 consecutive patients, 28 complications were reported (8.5%), including no mortalities, meningitis (1.5%), subdural hematoma (0.6%), deep vein thrombosis (1.2%), and neurological complications (5%), nine (2.7%) of which resulted in permanent morbidity.[82] In another single-center study of 215 patients undergoing temporal lobe surgery between 1984 and 1999, complications included mild hemiparesis,[2] hemianopsia,[1] transient cranial nerve palsies,[7] and transient language difficulties.[8, 180] In a multicenter study in Sweden, the complications of 449 operated patients at six centers were reviewed.[166] In 247 temporal lobe resections, one death occurred; the 62-year-old woman had experienced a postoperative hematoma. Hemiparesis occurred in five patients, once after a neocortical resection and four times after resections involving the hippocampus. These complications were thought to be caused by anterior choroidal artery infarction and manipulation of "perforating vessels." Other complications included hemianopsia (0.4%) and cranial nerve injury (0.9%). Age correlated with the severity of complications in the overall series, with only one of four major complications occurring in patients younger than 35 years. "Manipulation hemiplegia," originally described by Penfield[174] as caused by manipulation of middle cerebral artery and anterior choroidal artery vessels in the sylvian fissure causing hemiparesis, was thought to be more likely in older patients with atherosclerosis and hypertension and constituted the major complications of temporal lobe surgery in the group older than 35 years. In a Norwegian epilepsy surgery series,[181, 182] "large" complications occurred in 1 of 64 patients younger than 19 years and in 7 of 61 adult patients, confirming a greater risk for postoperative complications among older patients. This association was bolstered by an American study of 215 operations performed between 1983 and 1999 in which permanent complications occurred in 3 of 215 patients and occurred only in patients 30 years old or older.[180]

Reports of unusual complications after temporal lobe resection include four cases of cerebellar hemorrhage thought to be associated with postoperative epidural suction drains[183] and diplopia associated with transient trochlear nerve palsy in 3 of 22 patients.[184]

The annual death rate attributable to epilepsy, which reflects accidents, suicide, and sudden, unexpected death due to epilepsy (SUDEP), is higher in patients with chronic epilepsy than in the general population. Studies of the impact of postoperative seizure freedom have revealed that successful temporal lobe surgery lowers but does not normalize the overall mortality associated with chronic epilepsy.[185] In the Graduate Hospital series,[35] all late mortalities (4 of 89), including three SUDEPs and one suicide, occurred in patients with recurrent seizures. In another study of 215 patients undergoing temporal lobe surgery between 1984 and 1999, late mortalities were studied and occurred in 2% (3 of 148) of seizure-free patients and 11.9% (8 of 67) of patients with recurrent seizures.[180] Deaths occurred during seizures,[3] SUD,[3] suicide,[2] accidents,[2] and as a result of malignancy.[1] The preponderance of late mortalities occurred in the group of patients with recurrent seizures. No cases of SUDEP occurred in the seizure-free group.

Extratemporal Resective Surgery

EXTRATEMPORAL EPILEPSIES AND PROCEDURES

The protean clinical manifestations of the extratemporal epilepsies result from the varied pathogenetic features of these disorders and the eloquent brain regions that are affected by seizures arising in the broad expanse of the frontal, parietal, and occipital lobes. Patients with extratemporal epilepsies present for surgery less commonly (35%) than those with TLEs (65%).[1] Epileptogenic regions are often large and ill defined, mandating larger resections. Lesions of various types predominate in this group. Surgical approaches include lobar and multilobar, central, and tailored resections; topectomy; and multiple subpial transactions. As a result of the proximity to eloquent brain regions and the often ill-defined epileptogenic zone in extratemporal disorders, intraoperative and extraoperative brain mapping procedures are used more commonly than in temporal lobe surgery. Extratemporal resections are often combined with callosotomy or multiple subpial transactions to improve efficacy. In a series of 2177 patients over 51 years at the Montreal Neurological Institute, resective operations included temporal (56%), frontal (18%), central or rolandic (7%), parietal (6%), and occipital (1%) multilobar resections and hemispherectomy (11%).[103, 186]

SEIZURE OUTCOMES

The outcome of extratemporal resections has historically been less favorable than for temporal lobe surgery, with approximately 45% patients becoming seizure free in a worldwide compilation (1986 through 1990) after surgery.[1] Contemporary reports suggest improved outcomes as a result of improved imaging, patient selection, mapping, and surgical methods. In a representative study of 60 patients with extratemporal epilepsy,[187] structural abnormalities were present in 50 (83%). Resection locations were frontal,[36] parietal,[7] and occipital.[13] Extraoperative mapping with grids and strips was performed in 5%, and the remainder underwent intraoperative electrocorticographic mapping. At the 4-year follow-up evaluation, 61% of patients with focal lesions were seizure free, compared with 20% of patients without histopathologic abnormalities. In a series of 39 patients undergoing frontal lobe resections, with adjunctive MST and callosotomy when appropriate, 72% were judged to be Engel class I or II postoperatively.[188] In another study of 25 patients undergoing frontal surgery, 24 underwent intracranial monitoring, and 80% were Engel class I or II postoperatively (64% were seizure free).[189] In this series, patients without lesions had better outcomes than those with lesions. In a review of frontal lobe epilepsies (1987 through 1994) treated in 68 resections, 72% of lesional and 40% of nonlesional patients had excellent outcomes (i.e., Engel class I or II), with seizure-free rates of 44% and 24%, respectively.[190] In a report of seizure outcomes for 37 patients with intractable frontal tumoral epilepsy in whom tumor resection only was attempted independent of electrocorticographic data, 67% of patients had Engel class I or II outcomes, and 35% were seizure free.[191]

COMPLICATIONS OF RESECTION

Complications of extratemporal resections include complications of invasive monitoring with grids, surgical complications of resection or MST, and neurological sequelae of intentional resection of or inadvertent injury to regions of eloquent cortex. Complications in a study of 60 extratemporal procedures included three wound infections and three neurological deficits (i.e., hemiparesis in two and aphasia in one), which slowly resolved.[187] In frontal lobe resections, Broca's area within the posterior 2.5 cm of the opercular, inferior frontal gyrus is usually spared,[187] and language sites identified by stimulation mapping techniques within the middle frontal gyrus may contribute, if resected, to transient or long-standing expressive aphasias.[139] Resection of the supplementary motor cortex may engender a striking syndrome of postoperative mutism, contralateral neglect, or hemiparesis and diminished spontaneous movement, which usually resolves spontaneously over weeks.[192, 193]

The cognitive effects of frontal resections are usually well tolerated.[194] Preservation of draining veins and arterial supply to the central area are key considerations.[103] Partial resection of the nondominant face motor cortex is usually well tolerated, but complete removal may produce long-standing perioral weakness.[76, 195, 196] The superior resection margin should stay 2 to 3 mm below the lowest elicited thumb response. Rasmussen describes successful removal of the dominant face motor cortex, provided that vascular supply to the central area is meticulously preserved.[195, 196] Resection of the hand motor area produces a permanent deficit of fine motor control, and resection of the hand sensory area also produces significant functional impairment.[103] Resection of the leg motor cortex produces an initial flaccid paralysis of the contralateral leg, followed by gradual partial recovery of ambulatory capacity over months.[195, 196] Large parietal resections behind Rolandic cortex can be accomplished with a low rate of hemiparesis (0.5%).[195] When resections are extended into the parietal operculum, visual field defects may occur if resections are carried deep into the white matter.[169, 196] A nondominant parietal syndrome appears in some patients after large parietal resections, and in the dominant hemisphere, Wernicke's area must be respected. In the occipital lobe, complete resection produces the expected contralateral hemianopsia, and excision to within 2 cm of Wernicke's area may elicit a dyslexia.[196]

Lesional Epilepsy

TEMPORAL LOBE EPILEPSY

Lesions of various types are identified in 15% to 30% of patients with intractable temporal lobe epilepsy.[197, 198] These lesions may be neoplastic (e.g., astrocytoma, ganglioglioma, pleomorphic xanthoastrocytoma, DNET), vascular (e.g., cavernous hemangioma, arteriovenous malformation, angioma), dysgenetic (e.g., microdysgenesis, focal or diffuse dysplasia, Sturge-Weber, tuberous sclerosis), traumatic, or ischemic. In a review of 167 patients with temporal or extratemporal lesions, 15% (particularly those with neuronal migration disorders) presented with hippocampal sclerosis, or *dual pathology*.[22] In further investigations of dual pathology, significant hippocampal neuron loss was identified in cases of lesions located adjacent to the hippocampus and in patients with a history of "early injury."[199, 200]

In patients with temporal lesions and intractable epilepsy, studies of lesional resection alone, without resection of mesial structures (i.e., *lesionectomy*) produced disappointing results, with 22%,[201] 19%,[202] and 43%,[203] rendered seizure free in small series. In cases of laterally located lesions, seizure outcome is improved when complete lesion resection is achieved.[78] When lesional removal is performed along with a standard mesial resection, seizure outcomes were improved, with 85%,[203] 91%,[204] and 92%[205] rendered seizure free in various series. Other investigators have recommended gross total resection of the lesion along with an additional 5 to 10 mm of adjacent epileptogenic tissue (i.e., *lesionectomy plus*) and sparing of mesial structures in the case of lateral lesions without dual pathology (i.e., normal hippocampus), and they have reported favorable seizure outcomes with this approach.[82, 207] In patients with temporal lobe lesions and dual pathology, resection of the mesial structures along with the lesion has been recommended.[208]

The value of electrocorticography in guiding decisions regarding extent of extralesional tissue resection is controversial[209] and has been addressed in reports of patients with TLE and various tumors[72, 127, 202, 205] or arteriovenous malformations,[204] suggesting an advantage conferred by resection of epileptogenic tissue, including mesial structures, along with lesional resection. Despite a possible advantage from the standpoint of seizure control, hippocampal resection in lesional cases may engender in selected patients significant neuropsychological morbidity, particularly in dominant resections when evidence of hippocampal sclerosis is absent on MRI. When the hippocampus is not invaded by tumor, the lesionectomy plus approach may confer less morbidity in dominant resections while maintaining favorable seizure outcomes.[207] Excision of the presumed epileptogenic region without lesional resection yields poor results.[209]

EXTRATEMPORAL LESIONAL EPILEPSY

Lesional resection alone has provided favorable results in extratemporal sites, with 9 (64%) of 14 seizure free[201] and 17 (94%) of 18 seizure free[210] in representative series. In a meta-analysis of the available literature that addressed lesional epilepsy in all sites, 44% of patients were seizure free after simple excision, and 67% were seizure free after "seizure surgery."[211] Lesionectomy with removal of hemosiderin-stained brain produced seizure freedom in 73% of patients with occult vascular malformations.[212]

Cortical dysplasias are associated with a unique pattern of intrinsic epileptogenicity, and intraoperative electrocorticography is thought by some investigators to provide useful information to guide resection and ensure optimal seizure outcome.[213, 214] In a large series of patients undergoing surgery for focal epilepsy due to cortical dysplasias, 49% were seizure free, with 58% of those undergoing complete resection seizure free and 27% of those with incomplete resection seizure free.[215] Another report suggested universal seizure freedom in 16 of 16 patients with Taylor's balloon cell–type cortical dysplasia after complete lesionectomy without electrocorticography.[216] Other neuronal migration abnormalities, such as double cortex, do not benefit from resective surgery.[217]

Subcortical Lesional Epilepsy

HYPOTHALAMIC HAMARTOMAS

Intrahypothalamic hypothalamic hamartomas may be associated with intractable partial, gelastic and generalized seizures,[218] and retardation and behavioral disorders, whereas precocious puberty predominates in the "parahypothalamic" subset.[219] Although several reports document the successful surgical removal of these lesions through transcallosal or modified subfrontal approaches[220] and relief of seizures, such intrahypothalamic surgery raises concern regarding complications of the approach to (i.e., transcallosal) direct intrahypothalamic resection of these lesions. Reports of successful treatment of hypothalamic hamartomas with improvement in seizures in many patients and minimal complications suggest an attractive alternative to open surgery.[221–224] In a multicenter study of 10 patients undergoing gamma knife treatment in seven centers, 4 patients were seizure free, 1 had rare nocturnal seizures, 1 had rare partial seizures, and 2 were improved.[222] Minimal side effects were reported.

CEREBELLAR SEIZURES

The classic teaching that epileptic seizures do not arise from the cerebellar cortex has been challenged by several reports of focal motor seizures with secondary generalization arising in the cerebellum.[225, 226] Investigations have used video-electroencephalographic monitoring and intraoperative recordings to confirm that a cerebellar ganglioglioma can engender interictal and ictal discharges and that removal of this lesion can lead to resolution of these events.[225, 226] A review of the available literature revealed seizure freedom in five of eight patients after resection of cerebellar lesions, including five gangliogliomas, two hamartomas, and one astrocytoma. Seizures with semiology similar to "cerebellar seizures" have been reported in association with hamartomas of the floor of the fourth ventricle, along with resolution after resection of these lesions.[227]

Disconnection Surgery

MULTIPLE SUBPIAL TRANSECTIONS

MST was developed by Morrell and colleagues[228] to permit the treatment of partial epilepsies that reside exclusively or partially within eloquent cortical regions. In a review of the Rush-Presbyterian experience with 100 patients, the seizure outcomes were stratified according to MST performed alone (32 patients) or in conjunction with cortical resection (68 patients). Class I and II outcomes were achieved, respectively, using MST alone in 38% and 25% of patients with partial seizures, in 58% and 13% using MST alone in patients with Landau-Kleffner syndrome, and in 49% and 10% in conjunction with resection procedures. In a report[229] from Bonn of 20 MST procedures performed without resection, less favorable outcomes were documented. Postoperatively, patients were categorized as follows: class I (1 patient), class II (1), class III (7), and class IV (11). A review[230] of the Yale experience with 12 patients undergoing MST with or without resection also revealed less favorable outcomes, including Engel class II (1 patient), class III (2), and class IV (9) results. A study[231] of long-term outcome reported a late increase in seizure frequency in 19% of patients treated with MST with or without resection. A meta-analysis of aggregate international experience with 211 patients at six centers revealed 53 undergoing MST alone and 158 undergoing MST plus resection.[232] *Excellent outcome,* defined as more than 95% seizure reduction, was achieved with MST plus resection in 68% of patients with complex partial seizures and with MST alone in 62% of patients with complex partial seizures.

As increasing numbers of patients were offered this procedure and experience with MST accumulated, the neurological deficits originating from operated eloquent cortex have become a topic of considerable interest. In the Rush-Presbyterian review of 100 patients, MST in Broca's area (23 patients) was associated with reduction in verbal fluency but preservation of spoken and written language abilities.[228] Fifty percent of the patients with Landau-Kleffner syndrome recovered age-appropriate speech, with 30% requiring speech therapy. In 41 of 45 patients undergoing MST in Wernicke's area, receptive function, including comprehension of spoken and written words, remained intact. One patient suffered a deep hemorrhage, worsening the speech deficit. In 44 transections in the hand motor cortex, strength was preserved, and activities of daily living could be performed with the affected hand. In seven transections in the leg area, which were described as technically difficult, two patients suffered footdrop due to subcortical venous hemorrhage. After 56 transections within the postcentral gyrus, persistent sensory loss was demonstrated in only one patient. Overall neurological complications were observed in 17%, with permanent deficits identified in 7%. No deaths occurred. In the Bonn series of 20 isolated MST procedures, there were seven neurological complications, all of which were resolved after several weeks, and four cases of "surgical complications." Two cases of "remarkable" intraoperative brain swelling and edema were described, with a large intracerebral hematoma discovered in one patient.[229] One subdural hygroma and one infected bone flap also occurred in this series. In a pediatric series, 25 patients underwent MST, with outcomes of class I or II (10 patients), class III (12), and class IV (3).[233] No mortalities or significant morbidities occurred.

CORPUS CALLOSOTOMY

The procedure of subtotal or staged, total corpus callosotomy has been recommended less frequently since the widespread introduction of the vagal nerve stimulator. Nevertheless, an abundant literature attests to the utility of this procedure as palliative treatment in patients with multiple or poorly lateralized (and unresectable) epileptogenic foci, secondarily generalized tonic-clonic seizures, and injurious drop attacks due to tonic or atonic seizures with resultant falls and injury.[234–237] Early studies revealed increased focal seizures in 25% of patients undergoing callosotomy.[236] In 70% of patients, elimination or more than 80% reduction of seizures has been reported.[235, 236, 238]

In a series of 23 patients with intractable, generalized seizures, 17 underwent partial division and 6 underwent total division of the corpus callosum. Forty-one percent of patients were completely free or nearly free of the seizure types targeted for treatment, and 45% experienced a more than 50% reduction in seizure frequency.[239] Four developed simple partial motor seizures postoperatively. Retarded patients experienced poorer outcomes. Fifty-seven percent of patients experienced a transient disconnection syndrome that resolved. One patient experienced a clinically silent, right, frontal infarction related to venous thrombosis. The average hospital stay was 7.7 days.

Callosotomy is particularly effective for drop attacks, and in a study[240] of 52 patients with drop attacks (i.e., tonic or atonic seizures), 42 (81%) of 52 patients were completely relieved of drop attacks, with better results occurring in patients with total callosal section. Two adult patients exhibited a marked disconnection syndrome, which gradually remitted, and 14 patients experienced transient akinetic states, which resolved in several weeks. No deaths and one epidural hematoma were observed. In another study[241] of 20 patients followed for 3 years, 50% exhibited a marked improvement in quality of life, and 50% had relief of more than one half of their seizures. In a cohort of 17 patients, 9 patients experienced more than 80% reduction in targeted seizures, and overall, 88% of parents reported satisfaction with the surgical outcome, citing improved alertness and responsiveness.[242]

A rich literature is available to document the surgical and functional complications attributable to corpus callosotomy, with significantly more complications occurring in earlier series.[103, 205] Complications consist of acute disconnection syndromes, which are more common with total callosotomy, and the rare split brain syndrome. Subtotal (70% to 80%) callosotomy has been recommended as an initial procedure to minimize this complication. Surgical complications related to obtaining access to the interhemispheric fissure include venous compromise with hemorrhage and infarction. With current microsurgical approaches, patient selection, and perioperative management, callosotomy is a safe procedure that is somewhat underused.

Neuroaugmentative Surgery

LEFT VAGUS NERVE STIMULATION

Since U.S. Food and Drug Administration approval of left vagus nerve stimulation (VNS) for the palliative treatment of patients older than 12 years of age with intractable partial seizures was obtained in 1997, more than 16,000 patients have undergone the implantation of a vagus nerve stimulator over the left vagus nerve.[243, 244] In prospective clinical trials, median partial seizure reduction of 34% after 3 months and 45% at 12 months were achieved in patient groups younger than and older than 50 years old. Twenty percent of patients at 12 months had seizure reductions of 75% or more, exhibiting the phenomenon of improved seizure control over time.[243, 244] At 3 months, generalized seizures were reduced by 46%. Improvements in mood[245] have been reported, with worsening of figural memory when the VNS is on during memory tasks[246] but with no change in cognitive functions.[246] In patients with more than 50% improvement in seizure frequency, quality of life measures were improved.[247, 248] Reported side effects include voice alteration, hoarseness, throat or neck pain, headache, cough, and dyspnea, which are most evident during stimulation.[249] Adverse events in adults over the 12 years that the VNS has been used include infection requiring antibiotics or device removal and transient paralysis of the left vocal cord with hoarseness and aspiration.[250] An extraordinary report of self-inflicted vocal cord paralysis in two developmentally disabled patients by manipulation and rotation of the pulse generator within the subclavicular pocket mandates that patients be observed for device manipulation.[251] In a review of adverse events in 24 children implanted with the VNS, 15 events occurred in 11 patients. These complications included lead fractures, wound erythema, requested removal of the device, abscess, malfunction, gastrostomy, recurrent psychosis, and diminished speech volume.[249] Removal of electrodes from the vagus nerve can be difficult, and a report of resolution of a deep wound infection with antibiotics alone suggests that this may not always be necessary.[252] No increase in sudden, unexpected, unexplained death with the VNS was identified when implanted patients were compared with appropriate cohort populations.[253]

DEEP BRAIN STIMULATION

In the past, brain stimulation in the cerebellum; anterior, centromedian, and ventralis intermedius thalamic nuclei; and the caudate nucleus has been attempted for the modulation of cortical excitability.[254, 255] Electrical stimulation of the hippocampus has also been tried in an attempt to block temporal lobe seizures.[256] In an initial report of patients with DBS in the subthalamic nucleus, daytime seizures were reduced by more than 80%.[254]

Hemispherectomy and Hemispherotomy

The catastrophic epilepsies, in which panhemispheric syndromes are associated with intractable seizures, include Rasmussen's encephalitis, developmental syndromes (i.e., hemimeganencephaly, tuberous sclerosis, hamartomas, Sturge-Weber syndrome), and congenital hemiplegia or porencephaly.[257]

RESECTIVE PROCEDURES

Although the original surgical approach of anatomic, complete, en bloc hemispherectomy with sparing of the basal ganglia, hypothalamus, and diencephalon[76, 195, 258] was successful from the standpoint of seizure control, the immediate and delayed complications were daunting.[103] In particular, these procedures created a large area of denuded, unsupported subcortical tissue and significant volumes of intracranial dead space, which led to repeated microhemorrhages and subdural membrane formation, referred to as *superficial cerebral hemosiderosis*. Many years after surgery (36 years in one report), hydrocephalus,[259] increased intracranial pressure, neurological demise, or even death[260] complicated the postoperative course in as many as 38% of patients.[261]

An alternative approach of *hemispheric decortication* in a large pediatric series of 52 cases,[257] in which a lobe-by-lobe removal was accomplished, was associated with favorable seizure outcome (26 of 48 patients were seizure free) and a reduced rate of delayed complications. Nevertheless, three patients died in the perioperative period, and intraoperative blood loss and coagulopathy complicated the clinical course, particularly in children without brain atrophy or with hemimegalencephaly. Another alternative of *cerebral hemicorticectomy,* in which the entire cortical surface is degloved to the level of the white matter, was associated with 8 of 11 patients who were seizure free postoperatively, one case of hydrocephalus, and no deaths or delayed complications.[262]

FUNCTIONAL HEMISPHERECTOMY

Postoperative complications were significantly reduced with the introduction by Rasmussen of the technique of modified or *functional hemispherectomy,* in which a generous central and temporal resection is juxtaposed with deafferentation of the frontal and occipital lobes.[76, 196] With deafferentation rather than removal of the frontal and occipital lobes, the volume of intracranial dead space is reduced, and in a 7.3-year follow-up study of 14 patients, no hemosiderosis or hydrocephalus occurred, and 10 of 14 patients were seizure free.

During the past decade, the approach of hemispheric deafferentation as a preferred alternative to resection has been advanced by several investigators, all of whom performed increasingly limited resections in concert with hemispheric deafferentation. Villemure and Mascott[263] introduced the *peri-insular hemispherotomy,* in which a smaller craniotomy and a much reduced peri-insular (i.e., opercular frontal, parietal, and temporal) resection are combined with deafferentation of the frontal, parietal, occipital, and temporal lobes. In addition to a favorable seizure outcome (i.e., 9 of 11 patients were seizure free, and 1 of 11 improved 95%), reduced operative time and perioperative and delayed complications were documented.

The *trans-sylvian keyhole functional hemispherectomy* advanced by Schramm and colleagues[264, 265] represents a true minimalist approach to hemispheric deafferentation. A linear scalp incision and a 4 × 4 cm craniotomy provide the limited exposure required for a trans-sylvian approach to the circular sulcus, through which access to the entire ventricular system is gained. Transventricular hemispheric deafferentation and amygdalohippocampectomy are performed, with significantly reduced blood loss and a mean operating time of 3.6 hours, contrasting with the 6.3 hours needed for a Rasmussen-type functional hemispherectomy. For 20 patients, 88% were seizure free, and seizures improved for 6%. This approach is facilitated in patients with hemispheric atrophy and not recommended for hemimegalencephaly. In a modification of this technique, Shimizu and Taketoshi[266] described 34 patients undergoing a transopercular hemispherotomy, after which 67% of patients were seizure free.

REFERENCES

1. Engel J: Surgery for seizures. N Engl J Med 334:647–652, 1996.
2. Wiebe A, Blume W, Girvin, J, et al: A randomized, controlled trial of surgery for temporal-lobe epilepsy. N Engl J Med 345: 311–318, 2001.
3. Rowland LP, et al: National Institutes of Health Consensus Development Conference Statement: Surgery for Epilepsy, March 19–21, 1990, .
4. Begley CE, Annegers JF, Lairson DR, et al: Cost of epilepsy in the United States: A model based on incidence and prognosis. Epilepsia 35:1230–1243, 1994.
5. Devinsky O, Vickrey BG, Cramer JA, et al: Development of the Quality of Life in Epilepsy Inventory. Epilepsia 36:1089–1104, 1995.
6. Taylor DC, McMackin D, Staunton H, et al: Patients' aims for epilepsy surgery: Desires beyond seizure freedom. Epilepsia 42: 629–633, 2001.
7. Vickrey BG, Hays RD, Graber J, et al: A health-related quality of life instrument for patients evaluated for epilepsy surgery. Med Care 30:299–319, 1992.
8. Jacoby A, Baker G, Steen N, et al: The clinical course of epilepsy and its psychosocial correlates: Findings from a U.K. community study. Epilepsia 37:148–161, 1996.
9. Vickrey BG: A procedure for developing a quality of life measure for epilepsy surgery patients. Epilepsia 34 (Suppl 4):S22–S27, 1993.
10. Vickrey BG, Hays RD, Rausch R, et al: Quality of life of epilepsy surgery patients as compared with outpatients with hypertension, diabetes, heart disease and/or depressive symptoms. Epilepsia 35:597–607, 1994.
11. Langfitt JT: Cost-effectiveness of anterotemporal lobectomy for medically intractable complex partial epilepsy. Epilepsia 38:154–163, 1997.
12. Wiebe S, Gafni A, Blume WT, et al: An economic evaluation of surgery for temporal lobe epilepsy. J Epilepsy 8:227–235, 1995.
13. Engel J: Epilepsy surgery. Curr Opin Neurol 7:140–147, 1994.
14. Wieser H, Engel J, Williamson P, et al: Surgically remediable temporal lobe syndromes. In Engel J Jr (ed): Surgical Treatment of the Epilepsies, 2nd ed. New York, Raven Press, 1993, pp 49–63.
15. Jack CR, Sharbrough FW, Twomey CK, et al: Temporal lobe seizures: Lateralization with MR volume measurements of the hippocampal formation. Radiology 175:423–429, 1990.
16. Sawrie SM, Martin RC, Knowlton R, et al: Relationships among hippocampal voltmetry, proton magnetic resonance spectroscopy and verbal memory in temporal lobe epilepsy. Epilepsia 42:1403–1407, 2001.
17. Salanova V, Markand O, Worth R: Focal functional deficits in temporal lobe epilepsy of PET scans and the intracarotid amobarbital procedure: Comparison of patients with unitemporal epilepsy with those requiring intracranial recordings. Epilepsia 42:198–203, 2001.
18. Manno EM, Sperling MR, Ding X, et al: Predictors of outcome

after anterior temporal lobectomy: Positron emission tomography. Neurology 44:2331–2336, 1994.
19. Sperling MR, Saykin AJ, Glosser G, et al: Predictors of outcome after anterior temporal lobectomy: The intracarotid amobarbital test. Neurology 44:2325–2330, 1994.
20. Nakasato N, Levesque MF, Babb TL: Seizure outcome following standard temporal lobectomy: Correlation with hippocampal neuron loss and extrahippocampal pathology. J Neurosurg 77: 194–200, 1992.
21. Lynd-Balta E, Pilcher WH, Joseph SA: Distribution of AMPA receptor subunits in the hippocampal formation of temporal lobe epilepsy patients. Neuroscience 72:15–29, 1996.
22. Cendes F, Andermann F, Gloor P, et al: Atrophy of mesial structures in patients with temporal lobe epilepsy: Cause or consequence of repeated seizures? Ann Neurol 34:795–801, 1993.
23. Walker AE: Surgery for epilepsy. In Magnus O, Lorentz de Hass AM (eds): Handbook of Clinical Neurology. 15. The Epilepsies. Amsterdam, North Holland, 1974, pp 739–757.
24. Crandall PH: Standard *en bloc* anterior temporal lobectomy. In Spencer SS, Spencer DD (eds): Surgery for Epilepsy. Boston, Blackwell Science, 1991.
25. Spencer DD, Spencer SS, Mattson RH, et al: Access to the posterior temporal lobe structures in the surgical treatment of temporal lobe epilepsy. Neurosurgery 15:667–671, 1984.
26. Spencer DD, Inserni J: Temporal lobectomy. In Luders H (ed): Epilepsy Surgery. New York, Raven Press, 1992, pp 533–545.
27. Wyler AR, Hermann BP, Somes G: Extent of medial temporal resection on outcome from anterior temporal lobectomy: A randomized prospective study. Neurosurgery 37:982–991, 1995.
28. Wieser HG, Yasargil G: Selective amygdalo-hippocampectomy as a surgical treatment of mediobasal limbic epilepsy. Surg Neurol 17:445–457, 1984.
29. Yasargil MG, Teddy P, Roth P: Selective amygdalohippocampectomy: Operative anatomy and surgical technique. Adv Tech Stand Neurosurg 12:93–123, 1985.
30. Ojemann GA: Intraoperative tailoring of temporal lobe resections. In Engel J Jr (ed): Surgical Treatment of the Epilepsies, 2nd ed. New York, Raven Press, 1993, pp 481–488.
31. McKhann GM II, Schoenfeld-McNeill JS, Born DE, et al: Intraoperative hippocampal electrocorticography to predict the extent of hippocampal resection in temporal lobe epilepsy surgery. J Neurosurg 93:44–52, 2000.
32. Hermann BP, Wyler AR, Ackerman B, et al: Short-term psychological outcome of anterior temporal lobectomy. J Neurosurg 71:327–334, 1989.
33. Engel J Jr: Outcome with respect to epileptic seizures. In Engel J Jr (ed): Surgical Treatment of the Epilepsies. New York, Raven Press, 1987, pp 553–571.
34. Engel J Jr, Van Ness PC, Rasmussen TB, et al: Outcome with respect to epileptic seizures. In Engel J Jr (ed): Surgical Treatment of the Epilepsies, 2nd ed. New York, Raven Press, 1993, pp 609–621.
35. Sperling M, O'Connor M, Saykin A, et al: Temporal lobectomy for refractory epilepsy. JAMA 276:470–475, 1996.
36. Penfield W, Flanigan H: Surgical therapy of temporal lobe seizures. Arch Neurol Psychiatry 64:491–500, 1950.
37. Bailey P: Surgical treatment of psychomotor epilepsy: Five year followup. South Med J 54:299–301, 1961.
38. Jensen I: Temporal lobe surgery around the world. Acta Neurol Scand 52:354–373, 1975.
40. Rasmussen TB: Surgical treatment of the complex partial seizures: Results, lessons and problems. Epilepsia 24(Suppl 1): 65–76, 1983.
41. Bien CG, Kurthen M, Baron K, et al: Long-term seizure outcome and antiepileptic drug treatment in surgically treated temporal lobe epilepsy patients: A controlled study. Epilepsia 42:1416–1421, 2001.
42. Berkovic SF, McIntosh AM, Kalnins RM, et al: Preoperative MRI predicts outcome of temporal lobectomy. Neurology 45: 1358–1363, 1995.
43. Bladin PF: Post-temporal lobectomy seizures. Clin Exp Neurol 24:77–83, 1987.
44. Rasmussen T: Cortical resection for medically refractory focal epilepsy: Results, lessons and questions. In Rasmussen T, Marino R (eds): Functional Neurosurgery. New York, Raven Press, 1979, pp 253–269.
45. Salanova V, Andermann F, Rasmussen T, et al: The running down phenomena in temporal lobe epilepsy. Brain 119:989–996, 1996.
46. Ficker DM, So EL, Mosewich RK, et al: Improvement and deterioration of seizure control during the postsurgical course of epilepsy surgery patients. Epilepsia 40:62–67, 1999.
47. Garcia PA, Barbaro NM, Laxer KD: The prognostic value of postoperative seizures following epilepsy surgery. Neurology 41:1511–1512, 1991.
48. Luders H, Murphy D, Awad I, et al: Quantitative analysis of seizure frequency 1 week and 6, 12 and 24 months after surgery of epilepsy. Epilepsia 35:1174–1178, 1994.
49. Park K, Buchhalter J, McClelland R, et al: Frequency and significance of acute postoperative seizures following epilepsy surgery in children and adolescents. Epilepsia 43:874–881, 2002.
50. Wieser HG: Selective amygdalo-hippocampectomy for temporal lobe epilepsy. Epilepsia 29(Suppl 2):S100–S113, 1988.
51. McLachlan RS, Rose KJ, Derry PA, et al: Health-related quality of life and seizure control in temporal lobe epilepsy. Ann Neurol 41:482–489, 1997.
52. Gilliam F, Wyllie E, Kashden J, et al: Epilepsy surgery outcome: Comprehensive assessment in children. Neurology 48:1368–1374, 1997.
53. Mathern GW, Giza CC, Yudovin S, et al: Postoperative seizure control and antiepileptic drug use in pediatric epilepsy surgery patients: The UCLA experience, 1986–1997. Epilepsia 40:1740–1749, 1999.
54. De Lanerolle NC, Kim JH, Brines ML: Cellular and molecular alterations in partial epilepsy. Clin Neurosci 2:64–81, 1994.
55. Babb TL, Kupfer WR, Pretorius JK, et al: Synaptic reorganization by mossy fibers in human epileptic fascia dentate. Neuroscience 42:351–363, 1991.
56. King D, Spencer SS, McCarthy G, et al: Bilateral hippocampal atrophy in medial temporal lobe epilepsy. Epilepsia 36:905–910, 1995.
57. Arruda F, Cendes F, Andermann F, et al: Mesial atrophy and outcome after amygdalohippocampectomy or temporal lobe removal. Ann Neurol 40:446–450, 1996.
58. Semah F, Baulac M, Hasboun D, et al: Is interictal temporal hypometabolism related to mesial temporal sclerosis? A positron emission tomography/magnetic resonance imaging confrontation. Epilepsia 36:447–456, 1995.
59. Engel J Jr, Brown WJ, Kuhl DE, et al: Pathological findings underlying focal temporal lobe hypometabolism in partial epilepsy. Ann Neurol 12:518–528, 1982.
60. Spencer SS, McCarthy G, Spencer DD: Diagnosis of medial temporal lobe seizure onset: Relative specificity and sensitivity of quantitative MRI. Neurology 43:2117–2124, 1993.
61. Spencer SS: Long term outcome after epilepsy surgery. Epilepsia 37:807–813, 1996.
62. Loring DW, Meador KJ, Lee GP, et al: Wada memory asymmetries predict verbal memory decline after anterior temporal lobectomy. Neurology 45:1329–1333, 1995.
63. Holmes MD, Dodrill CB, Ojemann LM, et al: Five-year outcome after epilepsy surgery in nonmonitored and monitored surgical candidates. Epilepsia 37:748–752, 1996.
64. Risinger M, Engel J, Van Ness P, et al: Ictal localization of temporal lobe seizures with scalp/sphenoidal recordings. Neurology 39:1288–1293, 1989.
65. Murro A, Park Y, King D, et al: Seizure localization in temporal lobe epilepsy: A comparison of scalp-sphenoidal and volumetric MRI. Neurology 43:2531–2533, 1993.
66. Gilliam F, Bowling S, Bilir E, et al: Association of combined MRI, interictal EEG and ictal EEG results with outcome and pathology after temporal lobectomy. Epilepsia 38:1315–1320, 1997.
67. McIntosh AM, Wilson SJ: Seizure outcome after temporal lobectomy: Current research practice and findings. Epilepsia 42:1288–1307, 2001.
68. Sirven JI, Malamut BL: Temporal lobectomy outcome in older versus younger adults. Neurology 54:2166–2170, 2000.
69. Boling W, Andermann F, Reutens D, et al: Surgery for temporal lobe epilepsy in older patients. J Neurosurg 95:242–248, 2001.
70. McLachlan RS, Chovaz CJ, Blume WT, et al: Temporal lobectomy for intractable epilepsy in patients over age 45 years. Neurology 42:662–665, 1992.

71. Penfield W, Jasper H: Epilepsy and the functional anatomy of the human brain. Boston, Little, Brown, 1954, pp 739–817.
72. Cascino GD, Trenerry MR, Jack CR Jr, et al: Electrocorticography and temporal lobe epilepsy: Relationship to quantitative MRI and operative outcome. Epilepsia 36:692–696, 1995.
73. Hermann B, Davies K, Foley K, et al: Visual confrontation naming outcome after standard left anterior temporal lobectomy with sparing versus resection of the superior temporal gyrus: A randomized prospective clinical trial. Epilepsia 40: 1070–1076, 1999.
74. Feindel A, Rasmussen T: Temporal lobectomy with amygdalectomy and minimal hippocampal resection: Review of 100 cases. Can J Neurol Sci 18:603–605, 1991.
75. Wieser HG, Siegel G, Yasargil G: The Zurich Amygdalohippocampectomy series: A cohort up-date. Acta Neurochir Suppl 50: 122–127, 1990.
76. Rasmussen T: Surgery for epilepsy arising in regions other than the temporal and frontal lobes. In Advances in Neurology, vol 8. Neurosurgical Management of the Epilepsies, vol 8. New York, Raven Press, 1975, pp 207–226.
77. Rasmussen T: Surgical treatment of patients with complex partial seizures. In Penry JK, Daly DD (eds): Advances in Neurology, vol 11. New York, Raven Press, 1975, pp 415–449.
78. Nayel MH, Awad IA, Luders H: Extent of mesiobasal resection determines outcome after temporal lobectomy for intractable complex partial seizures. Neurosurgery 29:55–61, 1991.
79. Walczak T: Neocortical temporal lobe epilepsy: Characterizing the syndrome. Epilepsia 36:633–635, 1995.
80. Keogan M, McMackin D, Peng S, et al: Temporal neocorticectomy in management of intractable epilepsy: Long term outcome and predictive factors. Epilepsia 33:852–861, 1989.
81. Hennessy MJ, Elwes RD, Rabe-Hesketh S, et al: Prognostic factors in the surgical treatment of medically intractable epilepsy associated with mesial temporal sclerosis. Acta Neurol Scand 103:344–350, 2001.
82. Clusmann H, Schramm J, Kral T, et al: Prognostic factors and outcome after different types of resection for temporal lobe epilepsy. J Neurosurg 97:1131–1141, 2002.
83. Regis J, Bartonomei F, Rey M, et al: Gamma knife surgery for mesial temporal lobe epilepsy. J Neurosurg 93:141–146, 2000.
84. Fiol ME, Gates JR, Torres F, et al: The prognostic value of residual spikes in the postexcision electrocorticogram after temporal lobectomy. Neurology 41:512–516, 1991.
85. McBride MC, Binnie CD, Janota I, et al: Predictive value of intraoperative electrocorticograms in resective epilepsy surgery. Ann Neurol 30:526–532, 1991.
86. Schwartz TH, Bazil CW, Walczak TS, et al: The predictive value of intraoperative electrocorticography in resections for limbic epilepsy associated with mesial temporal sclerosis. Neurosurgery 40:302–311, 1997.
87. Tran TA, Spencer SS, Marks D, et al: Significance of spikes recorded on electrocorticography in nonlesional medial temporal lobe epilepsy. Ann Neurol 38:763–770, 1995.
88. Kanazawa O, Blume WT, Girvin JP: Significance of spikes at temporal lobe electrocorticography. Epilepsia 37:50–55, 1996.
89. Tuunainen A, Nousiainen U, Mervaala E, et al: Postoperative EEG and electrocorticography: Relation to clinical outcome in patients with temporal lobe surgery. Epilepsia 35:1165–1173, 1994.
90. Tran TA, Spencer SS, Javidan M, et al: Significance of spikes recorded on intraoperative electrocorticography in patients with brain tumor and epilepsy. Epilepsia 38:1132–1139, 1997.
91. Westerveld M, Sass K, Chelune GJ, et al: Temporal lobectomy in children: Cognitive outcome. J Neurosurg 92:24–30, 2000.
92. Milner B: Visual recognition and recall after right temporal lobe excision in man. Neuropsychologia 6:191–209, 1968.
93. Milner B: Psychological aspects of focal epilepsy and its neurosurgical management. Adv Neurol 8:299–321, 1975.
94. Olivier A: Risk and benefit in the surgery of epilepsy: Complications and positive results on seizure tendency and intellectual function. Acta Neurol Scand S78:114–120, 1988.
95. Rausch R, Crandall P: Psychological status related to surgical control of temporal lobe seizures. Epilepsia 23:191–201, 1982.
96. Milner B: Psychological defects produced by temporal lobe excision. Res Publ Assoc Res Nerv Ment Dis 36:244–257, 1958.
97. Scoville WB, Milner B: Loss of recent memory after bilateral hippocampal lesions: 1957. J Neuropsychiatry Clin Neurosci 12: 103–113, 2000.
98. Dimsdale H, Logue V, Piercy M: A case of persisting impairment of recent memory following right temporal lobectomy. Neuropsychologia 1:287–298, 1964.
99. Walker E: Recent memory loss in unilateral temporal lesions. Arch Neurol Psychiatry 78:543–552, 1957.
100. Rausch R. Psychological evaluation. In Engel J Jr (ed): Surgical Treatment of the Epilepsies. New York, Raven Press, 1987, pp 181–95.
101. King D, Flanigan H, Gallagher B, et al: Temporal lobectomy for partial complex seizures: Evaluation, results and 1 year follow up. Neurology 36:334–339, 1986.
102. Walczak T, Radtke R, McNamara J, et al: Anterior temporal lobectomy for complex partial seizures: Evaluation, results and long-term follow up in 100 cases. Neurology 40:413–418, 1990.
103. Pilcher WH, Ojemann GA: Presurgical evaluation and epilepsy surgery. In Apuzzo MLJ (ed): Brain Surgery: Complication Avoidance and Management. New York, Churchill Livingstone, 1993.
104. McClone J, Black SE: Criterion-based validity of an intracarotid amobarbital recognition-memory protocol. Epilepsia 40:430–438, 1999.
105. Wada J, Rasmussen T: Intracarotid injection of sodium amytal for the lateralization of cerebral speech dominance: Experimental and clinical observations. J Neurosurg 17:266–282, 1960.
106. Milner B, Branch C, Rasmussen T: Study of short-term memory after intracarotid injection of sodium amytal. Trans Am Neurol Assoc 87:224–226, 1962.
107. Jones-Gotman MJ: Commentary: Psychological evaluation; testing hippocampal function. In Engel J Jr (ed): Surgical Treatment of the Epilepsies. New York, Raven Press, 1987, pp 203–211.
108. Kubu CS, Girvin JP, McLachlan RS, et al: Does the intracarotid amobarbital procedure predict global amnesia after temporal lobectomy? Epilepsia 41:1321–1329, 2000.
109. Wyllie E, Naugle R, Chelune G, et al: Intracarotid amobarbital procedure. II. Lateralizing value in evaluation for temporal lobectomy. Epilepsia 32:865–869, 1991.
110. Perrine K, Westerveld M, Sass KJ, et al: Wada memory disparities predict seizure laterality and postoperative seizure control. Epilepsia 36:851–856, 1995.
111. Sabsevitz DS, Swanson SJ, Morris GL, et al: Memory outcome after left anterior temporal lobectomy in patients with expected and reversed Wada memory asymmetry scores. Epilepsia 42: 1408–1415, 2001.
112. Golby AJ, Poldrack RA, Illes J, et al: Memory lateralization in medial temporal lobe epilepsy assessed by functional MRI. Epilepsia 43:855–863, 2002.
113. Martin RC, Sawrie SM, Roth, DL, et al: Individual memory change after anterior temporal lobectomy: A base rate analysis using regression-based outcome methodology. Epilepsia 39: 1075–1082, 1998.
114. Trenerry MR: Neuropsychologic assessment in surgical treatment of epilepsy. Mayo Clin Proc 71:1196–1200, 1996.
115. Chelune GJ: Hippocampal adequacy versus functional reserve: Predicting memory functions following temporal lobectomy. Arch Clin Neuropsychol 10:413–432, 1995.
116. Davies KG, Hermann BP, Foley KT: Relation between intracarotid amobarbital memory asymmetry scores and hippocampal sclerosis in patients undergoing anterior temporal lobe resections. Epilepsia 37:522–525, 1996.
117. Trenerry MR, Jack CR, Ivnik RJ, et al: MRI hippocampal volumes and memory function before and after temporal lobectomy. Neurology 43:1800–1805, 1993.
118. Stroup E, Langfitt J, Berg M, et al: Predicting verbal memory decline following anterior temporal lobectomy. Neurology 2003 (in press).
119. Ojemann GA, Dodrill CS: Intraoperative techniques for reducing language and memory deficits with left temporal lobectomy. In Advances in Epileptology, vol 16. New York, Raven Press, 1987, pp 327–330.
120. Pauli E, Pickel S, Schulemann H, et al: Neuropsychologic findings depending on the type of the resection in temporal lobe epilepsy. Adv Neurol 81:373–7, 1999.

121. Goldstein LH, Polkey CE: Short-term cognitive changes after unilateral temporal lobectomy or unilateral amygdalo-hippocampectomy for the relief of temporal lobe epilepsy. J Neurol Neurosurg Psychiatry 56:135–140, 1993.
122. Gleissner U, Helmstaedter C, Schramm J, et al: Memory outcome after selective amygdalohippocampectomy: A study in 140 patients with temporal lobe epilepsy. Epilepsia 43:87–95, 2002.
123. Van Roost D, Clusmann H, Urbach H et al. Transcortical keyhole approach versus transsylvian approach for selective amygdalohippocampectomy: Which procedure is better? Acta Neurochir 142:1191, 2000.
124. Dupont S, Croize A, Semah F, et al: Is amygdalohippocampectomy really selective in medial temporal lobe epilepsy? A study using positron emission tomography with (18) fluorodeoxyglucose. Epilepsia 42:731–740, 2001.
125. Langfitt JT, Rausch R: Word-finding deficits persist after left anterotemporal lobectomy. Arch Neurol 53:72–76, 1996.
126. Stafiniak P, Saykin AJ, Sperling MR, et al: Acute naming deficits following dominant temporal lobectomy: Prediction by age at first risk for seizures. Neurology 40:1509–1512, 1990.
127. Wyllie E, Luders H, Morris H, et al: Clinical outcome after complete or partial cortical resection for intractable epilepsy. Neurology 37:1634–1641, 1987.
128. Ojemann G: Surgical therapy for medically intractable epilepsy. J Neurosurg 66:489–499, 1987.
129. Luders H, Lesser R, Dinner D et al. Language deficits elicited by electrical stimulation of the fusiform gyrus. In Engel J Jr (ed): Fundamental mechanisms of human brain function. New York, Raven Press, 1987, pp 83–90.
130. Penfield W: Pitfalls and success in surgical treatment of focal epilepsy. Br Med J xx:669–672, 1958.
131. Penfield W, Milner B: Memory deficit produced by bilateral lesions in the hippocampal zone. Arch Neurol Psychiatry 79: 475–497, 1958.
132. Chelune GJ: Using neuropsychological data to predict postsurgical cognitive outcome. In Luders HO (ed): Epilepsy Surgery. New York, Raven Press, 1992, pp 477–486.
133. Davies KG, Maxwell RE, Beniak TE, et al: Language function after temporal lobectomy without stimulation mapping of cortical function. Epilepsia 36:130–136, 1995.
134. Hermann BP, Wyler AR, Somes G: Language function following anterior temporal lobectomy. J Neurosurg 74:560–566, 1991.
135. Saykin AJ, Stafiniak P, Robinson LJ, et al: Language before and after temporal lobectomy: Specificity of acute changes and relation to early risk factors. Epilepsia 36:1071–1077, 1995.
136. Hermann BP, Wyler AR, Somes G: Dysnomia after left anterior temporal lobectomy without functional mapping: Frequency and correlates. Neurosurgery 35:52–57, 1994.
137. Davies KG, Bell BD: Naming decline after left anterior temporal lobectomy correlates with pathological status of resected hippocampus. Epilepsia 39:407–419, 1998.
138. Ojemann G: Brain organization of language from the perspective of electrical stimulation mapping. Behav Brain Sci 6:189–230, 1983.
139. Ojemann G, Ojemann J, Lettich E, et al: Cortical language localization in left dominant hemisphere. J Neurosurg 71:316–326, 1989.
140. Rasmussen T: Cortical resection in the treatment of focal epilepsy. Adv Neurol 8:139–154, 1975.
141. Katz A, Awad I, Kong A, et al: Extent of resection in temporal lobectomy for epilepsy. II. Memory changes and neurologic complications. Epilepsia 30:763–771, 1989.
142. Helgason C, Bergen D, Bleck T, et al: Infarction after surgery for focal epilepsy: Manipulation hemiplegia revisited. Epilepsia 28:340–345, 1987.
143. Fenwick P.: Psychiatric assessment and temporal lobectomy. Acta Neurol Scand S78:96–101, 1988.
144. Fenwick PB, Blumer D, Caplan R, et al: Presurgical psychiatric assessment. In Engel J Jr (ed): Surgical Treatment of the Epilepsies, 2nd ed. New York, Raven Press, 1993, pp 273–90.
145. Glosser G, Zwil AS, Glosser DS, et al: Psychiatric aspects of temporal lobe epilepsy before and after anterior temporal lobectomy. J Neurol Neurosurg Psychiatry 68:53–58, 2000.
146. Matsuura M: Indication for anterior temporal lobectomy in patients with temporal lobe epilepsy and psychopathology. Epilepsia 41:39–42, 2000.
147. Altshuler L, Rausch R, Delrahim S, et al: Temporal lobe epilepsy, temporal lobectomy and major depression. J Neuropsychiatry Clin Neurosci 11:436–443, 1999.
148. Herman BP, Wyler AR: Depression, locus of control and the effects of epilepsy surgery. Epilepsia 30:332–338, 1989.
149. Derry P, Rose K, McLachlan RS: Moderators of the effect of preoperative emotional adjustment on postoperative depression after surgery for temporal lobe epilepsy. Epilepsia 41:177–185, 2000.
150. Ring HA, Moriarty J: A prospective study of the early postsurgical psychiatric associations of epilepsy surgery. J Neurol Neurosurg Psychiatry 64:601–604, 1998.
151. Anhoury S, Brown RJ, Krishnamoorthy ES, et al: Psychiatric outcome after temporal lobectomy: A predictive study. Epilepsia 41:1608–1615, 2000.
152. Kanemoto K: Hypomania after temporal lobectomy: A sequel to the increased excitability of the residual temporal lobe? J Neurol Neurosurg Psychiatry 59:448–454, 1995.
153. Montenegro MA, Guerreiro MM.: *De novo* psychogenic seizures after epilepsy surgery: A case report. Arq Neuropsiquiatr 58: 535–537, 2000.
154. Mayanagi Y, Watanabe E: Psychiatric and neuropsychological problems in epilepsy surgery: Analysis of 100 cases that underwent surgery. Epilepsia 42:19–23, 2001.
155. Jones JE, Berven NL, Ramirez L, et al: Long-term psychosocial outcomes of anterior temporal lobectomy. Epilepsia 43:896–903, 2002.
156. Wheelock I, Peterson C, Buchtel HA: Presurgery expectations, postsurgery satisfaction and psychosocial adjustment after epilepsy surgery. Epilepsia 39:487–494, 1998.
157. Cramer JA, Perrine K, Devinsky O, et al: Development and cross-cultural translations of a 31-item quality of life in epilepsy inventory. Epilepsia 39:81–88, 1998.
158. Devinsky O, Perrine K, Hirsch J, et al: Relation of cortical language distribution and cognitive function in surgical epilepsy patients. Epilepsia 41:400–404, 2000.
159. Markand O, Salanova V: Health-related quality of life outcome in medically refractory epilepsy treated with anterior temporal lobectomy. Epilepsia 41:749–759, 2000.
160. King JT, Sperling MR: A cost-effectiveness analysis of anterior temporal lobectomy for intractable temporal lobe epilepsy. J Neurosurg 87:20–28, 1997.
161. Diehl B, Luders HO: Temporal lobe epilepsy: When are invasive recordings needed? Epilepsia 41(Suppl 3):S61–S74, 2000.
162. Engel J Jr, Crandall PH, Rausch R: The partial epilepsies. In Rosenberg RN (ed): The Clinical Neurosciences, vol 2. New York, Churchill Livingstone, 1983, p 1249.
163. Blatt DR, Roper SM: Invasive monitoring of limbic epilepsy using stereotactic depth and subdural strip electrodes: Surgical technique. Surg Neurol 48:74–79, 1997.
164. Fernandez GA, Hufnagel A: Safety of intrahippocampal depth electrodes for presurgical evaluation of patients with intractable epilepsy. Epilepsia 38:922–929, 1997.
165. Wyler AR, Ojemann GA, Lettich E, et al: Subdural strip electrodes for localizing epileptogenic foci. J Neurosurg 60:1195–1200, 1984.
166. Rydenhag B, Silander HC: Complications of epilepsy surgery after 654 procedures in Sweden, September 1990–1995: A multicenter study based on the Swedish National Epilepsy Surgery Register. Neurosurgery 49:51–57, 2001.
167. Lee WS, Lee JK: Complications and results of subdural grid electrode implantation in epilepsy surgery. Surg Neurol 54: 346–351, 2000.
168. Rasmussen T: The role of surgery in the treatment of focal epilepsy. Clin Neurosurg 16:288–314, 1968.
169. Van Buren JM: Complications of surgical procedures in the diagnosis and treatment of epilepsy. In Engel J Jr (ed): Surgical Treatment of the Epilepsies. New York, Raven Press, 1987, pp 465–475.
170. Ojemann G: Temporal lobectomy tailored to electrocorticography and functional mapping. In Spences S, Spencer D (eds): Surgery for Epilepsy. New York, Blackwell Science, 1991, pp 137–145.

171. Silfvenius H, Gloor P, Rasmussen T: Evaluation of insular ablation in surgical treatment of temporal lobe epilepsy. Epilepsia 5:307–320, 1964.
172. Crandall PH: Postoperative management and criteria for evaluation. In Purpura DP, Penry JK, Walter RD (eds): Advances in Neurology, vol 8. Neurosurgical Management of the Epilepsies. New York, Raven Press, 1975, pp 265–279.
173. Ojemann GA: Neurosurgical management of epilepsy: A personal perspective in 1983. Appl Neurophysiol 46:11–18, 1985.
174. Penfield W, Lende R, Rasmussen T: Manipulation hemiplegia. J Neurosurg 18:760–776, 1961.
175. Babb T, Wilson CL, Crandall P: Asymmetry and ventral course of the human geniculostriate pathway as determined by hippocampal visual evoked potentials and subsequent visual field defects after temporal lobectomy. Exp Brain Res 47:317–328, 1982.
176. Falconer M, Wilson J: Visual field changes following anterior temporal lobectomy: Their significance in relation to Myer's loop of the optic radiation. Brain 81:1–14, 1958.
177. Marino R, Rasmussen T: Visual field changes after temporal lobectomy in man. Neurology 18:825–835, 1968.
178. Van Buren JM, Baldwin M: The architecture of the optic radiation in the temporal lobe of man. Brain 81:15–40, 1958.
179. Anderson J, Awad I, Hahn J: Delayed facial nerve palsy after temporal lobectomy for epilepsy: Report of four cases and discussion of possible mechanisms. Neurosurgery 28:453–456, 1991.
180. Salanova V, Markand O, Worth R: Temporal lobe epilepsy surgery: Outcome, complications and late mortality rate in 215 patients. Epilepsia 43:170–174, 2002.
181. Guldvog B, Loyning Y, Hauglie-Hanssen E, et al: Surgical treatment for partial epilepsy among Norwegian adults. Epilepsia 35:540–553, 1994.
182. Guldvog B, Loyning Y, Hauglie-Hanssen E, et al: Surgical treatment for partial epilepsy among Norwegian children and adolescents. Epilepsia 35:554–565, 1994.
183. Toczek MT, Morrell MJ, Silverberg GA: Cerebellar hemorrhage complicating temporal lobectomy. J Neurosurg 85:718–722, 1996.
184. Jacobson DM, Warner JJ, Ruggles KH: Transient trochlear nerve palsy following anterior temporal lobectomy for epilepsy. Neurology 45:1465–1468, 1995.
185. Hennessy MJ, Langan Y: A study of mortality after temporal lobe epilepsy surgery. Neurology 53:1276–83, 1999.
186. Olivier A: Extratemporal resections in the surgical treatment of epilepsy. In Spencer SS, Spencer DD (eds): Surgery for Epilepsy. Boston, Blackwell Scientific Publications, 1991.
187. Zentner J, Hufnagel A, Ostertun B, et al: Surgical treatment of extratemporal epilepsy: Clinical, radiologic and histopathologic findings in 60 patients. Epilepsia 37:1072–1080, 1996.
188. Shimizu H, Maehara T: Neuronal disconnection for the surgical treatment of pediatric epilepsy. Epilepsia 41:28–30, 2000.
189. Jobst BC, Siefel AM, Thadani VM, et al: Intractable seizures of frontal lobe origin: Clinical characteristics, localizing signs and results of surgery. Epilepsia 41:1139–1152, 2000.
190. Mosewich RK, So EL, O'Brien TJ, et al: Factors predictive of the outcome of frontal lobe epilepsy surgery. Epilepsia 41:843–849, 2000.
191. Zaatreh MM, Spencer DD, Thompson JL, et al: Frontal lobe tumoral epilepsy: Clinical, neurophysiologic features and predictors of surgical outcome. Epilepsia 43:727–733, 2002.
192. Zentner J, Hufnagel A, Pechstein U, et al: Functional results after resective procedures involving the supplementary motor area. J Neurosurg 85:542–549, 1996.
193. Fontaine D, Capelle L, Duffau H: Somatotopy of the supplementary motor area: Evidence from correlation of the extent of surgical resection with the clinical patterns of deficit. Neurosurgery 50:297–305, 2002.
194. Milner B: Visually guided maze learning in man: Effects of bilateral hippocampal, bilateral frontal and unilateral cerebral lesions. Neuropsychologia 3:317–338, 1965.
195. Rasmussen T: Surgery of frontal lobe epilepsy. In Purpura DP, Penry JK, Walter RD (eds): Advances in Neurology, vol 8. New York, Raven Press, 1975, pp 197–205.
196. Rasmussen T. Commentary: Extratemporal cortical excisions and hemispherectomy. In Engel J Jr (ed): Surgical Treatment of the Epilepsies. New York, Raven Press, 1987, pp 417–424.
197. Babb TL, Brown WJ: Pathological findings in epilepsy. In Engel J Jr (ed): Surgical Treatment of the Epilepsies. New York, Raven Press, 1987, pp 511–540.
198. Spencer DD, Spencer SS, Mattson RH, et al: Temporal lobe masses in patients with intractable partial epilepsy. Neurology 34:432–436, 1984.
199. Fried I, Kim J, Spencer D: Hippocampal pathology in patients with intractable seizures and temporal lobe masses. J Neurosurg 76:735–740, 1992.
200. Mathern GW, Babb TL, Pretorius JK, et al: The pathophysiologic relationships between lesion pathology, intracranial ictal EEG onsets, and hippocampal neuron losses in temporal lobe epilepsy. Epilepsy Res 21:133–147, 1995.
201. Cascino GD, Kelly PJ, Sharbrough F, et al: Long-term follow-up of stereotactic lesionectomy in partial epilepsy: Predictive factors and electroencephalographic results. Epilepsia 33:639–644, 1992.
202. Jooma R, Yeh H, Privitera M, et al: Lesionectomy versus electrophysiologically guided resection for temporal lobe tumors manifesting with complex partial seizures. J Neurosurg 83:231–236, 1995.
203. Moore J, Cascino G, Trenerry M, et al: A comparative study of lesionectomy versus corticectomy in patients with temporal lobe lesional epilepsy. J Epilepsy 6:239–242, 1999.
204. Yeh HS, Kashwagi S, Tew J, et al: Surgical management of epilepsy associated with cerebral arteriovenous malformations. J Neurosurgery 72:216–223, 1990.
205. Pilcher WH, Silbergeld DL, Berger MS, et al: Intraoperative electrocorticography during tumor resection: Impact on seizure outcome in patients with gangliogliomas. J Neurosurg 78:891–902, 1993.
206. Pilcher W, Roberts, D, Flanigin F: Complications of Epilepsy Surgery. In Engel J Jr (ed): Surgical Treatment of the Epilepsies, 2nd ed. New York, Raven Press, 1993, pp 565–581.
207. Schramm J, Kral T: Surgical treatment for neocortical temporal lobe epilepsy: Clinical and surgical aspects and seizure outcome. J Neurosurg 94:33–42, 2001.
208. Cascino GD, Jack CR, Parisi JE, et al: Operative strategy in patients with MRI-identified dual pathology and temporal lobe epilepsy. Epilepsy Res 14:175–182, 1993.
209. Fried I, Cascino G: Lesional surgery. In Engel J Jr (ed): Surgical Treatment of the Epilepsies, 2nd ed. New York, Raven Press, 1993, pp 501–509.
210. Awad I, Rosenfeld J, Ahl J, et al: Intractable epilepsy and structural lesions of the brain: Mapping, resection strategies and seizure outcome. Epilepsia 32:179–186, 1991.
211. Weber J, Silbergeld D, Winn HR: Surgical resection of epileptogenic cortex associated with structural lesions. Neurosurg Clin N Am 4:327–336, 1993.
212. Kraemer DL, Griebel ML, Lee N, et al: Surgical outcome in patients with epilepsy with occult vascular malformations treated with lesionectomy. Epilepsia 39:600–607, 1998.
213. Palmini A, Gambardella A, Andermann F, et al: Intrinsic epileptogenicity of human dysplastic cortex as suggested by corticography and surgical results. Ann Neurol 37:476–487, 1995.
214. Hong S, Kang K, Seo D, et al: Surgical treatment of intractable epilepsy accompanying cortical dysplasia. J Neurosurg 93:766–773, 2000.
215. Edwards J, Wyllie E, Ruggeri P, et al: Seizure outcome after surgery for epilepsy due to malformation of cortical development. Neurology 55:1110–1114, 2000.
216. Urbach H, Scheffler B, Heinrichsmeier, et al: Focal cortical dysplasia of Taylor's balloon cell type: A clinicopathological entity with characteristic neuroimaging and histopathological features and favorable postsurgical outcome. Epilepsia 43:33–40, 2002.
217. Bernasconi A, Martinez V, Rosa-Neto P, et al: Surgical resection for intractable epilepsy in "double cortex" syndrome yields inadequate results. Epilepsia 42:1124–1129, 2001.
218. Kuzniecky R, Guthrie B: Intrinsic epileptogenesis of hypothalamic hamartomas in gelastic epilepsy. Ann Neurol 42:60–67, 1997.
219. Arita K, Ikawa F: The relationship between magnetic resonance imaging findings and clinical manifestations of hypothalamic hamartoma. J Neurosurg 91:212–220, 1999.
220. Rosenfeld JV, Harvey AS: Transcallosal resection of hypothala-

mic hamartomas, with control of seizures, in children with gelastic epilepsy. Neurosurgery 48:108–118, 2001.
221. Unger F, Schrottiner O, Haselberger K, et al: Gamma knife radiosurgery for hypothalamic hamartomas in patients with medically intractable epilepsy and precocious puberty. J Neurosurg 92:726–731, 2000.
222. Regis J, Fabrice B, de Toffol B, et al: Gamma knife surgery for epilepsy related to hypothalamic hamartomas. Neurosurgery 47:1343–1352, 2000.
223. Parrent AG: Stereotactic radiofrequency ablation for the treatment of gelastic seizures associated with hypothalamic hamartoma: Case report. J Neurosurg 91:881–884, 1999.
224. Dunoyer C, Ragheb J, Resnick T, et al: The use of stereotactic radiosurgery to treat intractable childhood partial epilepsy. Epilepsia 43:292–300, 2002.
225. Mesiwala AH, Kuratani JD, Avellino AM, et al: Focal motor seizures with secondary generalization arising in the cerebellum. J Neurosurg 97:190–196, 2002.
226. Chae JH, Kim SK, Wang KC, et al: Hemifacial seizure of cerebellar ganglioglioma origin: Seizure control by tumor resection. Epilepsia 42:1204–1207, 2001.
227. Delalande O, Rodriguez D, Chiron C, et al: Successful surgical relief of seizures associated with hamartoma of the floor of the fourth ventricle in children: Report of two cases. Neurosurgery 49:726–731, 2001.
228. Smith MC: Multiple subpial transections in patients with extratemporal epilepsy. Epilepsia 39(Suppl 4):S81–S89, 1998.
229. Schramm J, Aliashkevich A, Grunwald T: Multiple subpial transactions: Outcome and complications in 20 patients who did not undergo resection. J Neurosurg 97:39–47, 2002.
230. Mulligan LP, Spencer DD, Spencer SS: Multiple subpial transactions: The Yale experience. Epilepsia 42:226–229, 2001.
231. Orbach D, Romanelli P, Devinsky O, et al: Late seizure recurrence after multiple subpial transactions. Epilepsia 42:1130–1133, 2001.
232. Spencer SS, Schramm J, Wyler A, et al: Multiple subpial transection for intractable partial epilepsy: An international meta-analysis. Epilepsia 43:141–145, 2002.
233. Shimizu H, Maehara T: Neuronal disconnection for the surgical treatment of pediatric epilepsy. Epilepsia 41:28–30, 2000.
234. Purves SJ: Selection of patients for corpus callosum section. In Spencer SS, Spencer DD (eds): Surgery for Epilepsy. Boston, Blackwell Scientific Publications, 1991, p 69.
235. Spencer SS: Corpus callosum section and other disconnection procedures for medically intractable epilepsy. Epilepsia 29(Suppl 2):S85–S99, 1988.
236. Spencer SS, Spencer DD, Williamson PD, et al: Corpus callosotomy for epilepsy. I. Seizure effects. Neurology 38:19–24, 1988.
237. Wilson DH, Reeves A, Gazzaniga M, et al: Cerebral commisurotomy for control of intractable seizures. Neurology 27:708–715, 1977.
238. Purves SJ, Wada JA, Woodhurst WB, et al: Results of anterior corpus callosum section in 24 patients with medically intractable seizures. Neurology 38:1194–1201, 1988.
239. Sorenson JM, Wheless JW, Baumgartner JE, et al: Corpus callosotomy for medically intractable seizures. Pediatr Neurosurg 27:260–267, 1997.
240. Maehara T, Shimizu H: Surgical outcome of corpus callosotomy in patients with drop attacks. Epilepsia 42:67–71, 2001.
241. Andersen B, Rogvi-Hansen B, Kruse-Larsen C, et al: Corpus callosotomy: Seizure and psychosocial outcome, a 39 month follow-up of 20 patients. Epilepsy Res 23:77–85, 1996.
242. Gilliam F, Wyllie E, Kotagal P, et al: Parental assessment of functional outcome after corpus callosotomy. Epilepsia 37:753–757, 1996.
243. Schachter SC, Wheless JW: The evolving place of vagus nerve stimulation therapy. Neurology 59(Suppl 4):S1–S2, 2002.
244. Schachter SC: Vagus nerve stimulation therapy summary: Five years after FDA approval. Neurology 59(Suppl 4):S15–S20, 2002.
245. Elger G, Hoppe C, Falkai P, et al: Vagus nerve stimulation is associated with mood improvements in epilepsy patients. Epilepsy Res 42:203–210, 2000.
246. Helmstaedter C, Hope C, Elger CE: Memory alterations during acute high intensity vagus nerve stimulation. Epilepsy Res 47: 37–42, 2001.
247. Dodrill CB, Morris GL: Effects of vagal nerve stimulation on cognition and quality of life in epilepsy. Epilepsy Behav 2: 46–53, 2001.
248. Morrow JI, Bingham E, Crain JJ, et al: Vagal nerve stimulation in patients with refractory epilepsy: Effect on seizure frequency, severity and quality of life. Seizure 9:442–445, 2000.
249. Murphy JV: Left vagal nerve stimulation in children with medically refractory epilepsy. J Pediatr 134:563–566, 1999.
250. Ben-Menachem E, Hellstrom K, Verstappen D: Analysis of direct hospital costs before and 18 months after treatment with vagus nerve stimulation therapy in 43 patients. Neurology 50(Suppl 4):S44–S47, 2002.
251. Kalkanis JG, Krisha P, Espinose JA, et al: Self-inflicted vocal cord paralysis in patients with vagus nerve stimulators. J Neurosurg 96:949–951, 2002.
252. Ortler M, Luef G, Kofler A, et al: Deep wound infection after vagus nerve stimulator implantation: Treatment without removal of the device. Epilepsia 42:133–135, 2001.
253. Annegers JF, Coan SP, Hauser WA, et al: Epilepsy, vagal nerve stimulation by the NCP system, mortality and sudden, unexpected, unexplained death. Epilepsia 39:206–212, 1998.
254. Benabid AL, Minotti L, Koudsie A, et al: Antiepileptic effect of high-frequency stimulation of the subthalamic nucleus (corpus luysi) in a case of medically intractable epilepsy caused by focal dysplasia: A 30 month follow-up: Technical case report. Neurosurgery 50:1385–1392, 2002.
255. Velasco F, Velasco M, Velasco AL, et al: Electrical stimulation of the centromedian thalamic nucleus in control of seizures: Long-term studies. Epilepsia 36:63–71, 1995.
256. Velasco M, Velasco F, Velasco AL, et al: Subacute electrical stimulation of the hippocampus blocks intractable temporal lobe seizures and paroxysmal EEG activities. Epilepsia 41:158–169, 2000.
257. Carson B, Javedan S, Freeman J, et al: Hemispherectomy: A hemidecortication approach and review of 52 cases. J Neurosurg 84:903–911, 1996.
258. Krynauw R: Infantile hemiplegia treated by removing one cerebral hemisphere. J Neurol Neurosurg Psychiatry 13:243–267, 1950.
259. Kalkanis S, Blumenfeld H, Sherman JC, et al: Delayed complications thirty-six years after hemispherectomy: A case report. Epilepsia 37:758–762, 1996.
260. White H: Cerebral hemispherectomy in the treatment of infantile hemiplegia. Confin Neurol 21:1, 1961.
261. Wilson P: Cerebral hemispherectomy for infantile hemiplegia. Brain 93:147–180, 1970.
262. Winston, K: Cerebral hemicorticectomy for epilepsy. J Neurosurg 77:889–895, 1992.
263. Villemure JG, Mascott CR: Peri-insular hemispherotomy: Surgical principles and anatomy. Neurosurgery 37:975–981, 1995.
264. Schramm J, Behrens E, Entzian W: Hemispherical deafferentation: An alternative to functional hemispherectomy. Neurosurgery 36:509–516, 1995.
265. Schramm J, Kral T, Clusmann H: Transsylvian keyhole functional hemispherectomy. Neurosurgery 49:891–901, 2001.
266. Shimizu H, Taketoshi M: Modification of peri-insular hemispherotomy and surgical results. Neurosurgery 47:367–373, 2000.

CHAPTER **157**

Surgery for Extratemporal Lobe Epilepsy

JAMES W. LEIPHART ■ ITZHAK FRIED

One of the most significant developments in epilepsy surgery has been the recognition of surgically remediable syndromes of epilepsy.[1] Foremost among these has been the syndrome of mesial temporal lobe epilepsy characterized by distinct patterns of semiology, electroencephalographic signature, imaging correlates, and histopathology.[2] The hallmark of this syndrome is hippocampal sclerosis, which underlies a hyperexcitable, recurrent, and pharmacologically resistant pattern of electrical activity. From the surgeon's standpoint, the significance of this syndrome is the feasibility of a uniform surgical approach to the disease, which previously was regarded as a spectrum of electrical abnormalities but now is recognized as a uniform entity.

In contrast, extratemporal epilepsy presents a complex challenge for the surgeon. Because there is no analog to the distinct pathology found in mesial temporal lobe epilepsy, there is no uniform resection plan for extratemporal epilepsy. The surgeon has to deal with a spectrum of resection plans, seeking an ablation that is (1) sufficient and necessary to achieve seizure control and (2) functionally feasible (i.e., it should incur a neurological consequence acceptable to the patient). This resection zone may be characterized by one or more of the following features: (1) concordance with the seizure semiology, (2) a focal abnormality on electroencephalography (EEG) or magnetoencephalography (MEG) or both, (3) a focal abnormality on magnetic resonance imaging (MRI), (4) a focal metabolic abnormality, and (5) concordance with neurocognitive impairment. The existence of a focal MRI abnormality is probably the most important feature in the surgical approach to extratemporal epilepsy. The presence of a focal abnormality immediately classifies a case as extratemporal *lesional* epilepsy. It usually means a better surgical prognosis. Much of the challenge in surgery for extratemporal epilepsy is in the so-called nonlesional cases. In these cases, the resection cannot rely on a MRI abnormality, although pathologic studies of the resected tissue may reveal a lesion not detected by MRI preoperatively. The resection relies on EEG (scalp or intracranial) and alternative imaging techniques, such as positron emission tomography (PET), MEG, single-photon emission computed tomography (SPECT), and magnetic resonance spectroscopy (MRS).

As mesial temporal lobe epilepsy has become better defined as a clinicopathologic entity with a standard surgical approach,[2, 3] extratemporal lobe epilepsy syndromes and their surgical treatments have become more distinct in comparison. The semiologies of extratemporal neocortical epilepsy are less well characterized, even when localization is to a single lobe (frontal, temporal, or parietal). Extratemporal lobe epilepsies also tend to spread rapidly, making localization based on their clinical characteristics difficult. In some cases, especially in the frontal lobes, seizures cross to the contralateral side quickly, making lateralization difficult as well.

Temporal lobe epilepsy has proved especially amenable to surgical intervention because of the functional feasibility of resection in the anterior and anteromedial part of the temporal lobe. Careful neurocognitive, Wada, and functional imaging testing and electrical stimulation mapping in selected cases can minimize the possibility of language or memory impairment. Frequently the surgical resection can be tailored to the temporal tip and sclerotic hippocampus, limiting the potential for cognitive deficit. Extratemporal lobe epilepsies frequently involve regions that have motor, sensory, language, or other critical cognitive functions. This potential for impairment has largely precluded the development of routine, stereotyped surgical techniques or approaches, making each operative intervention a tailored resection.

In contrast to temporal lobe epilepsy, which frequently has the consistent underlying pathology of hippocampal sclerosis, extratemporal lobe epilepsies have a wide variety of underlying pathologies ranging from tumors and other space-occupying lesions to developmental abnormalities to trauma. As might be expected, each different underlying pathologic substrate may be associated with a different expected surgical outcome for seizure control. In addition, there is a subset of cases of extratemporal epilepsy for which no structural substrate is found either in preoperative imaging or in tissue histopathology.

Technologic advances have provided modern alternatives to resective surgery for medically intractable epilepsy, but none has supplanted surgical resection in efficacy. These alternatives include stimulation methods, such as vagal nerve stimulation or deep brain stimulation. The rate of significant seizure control with vagal nerve stimulation is approximately 30% to 50%.[4] Deep brain stimulation for severe intractable epilepsy is still largely experimental, and even more recent protocols using stimulation of subthalamic nucleus or anterior thalamus have achieved only a modest rate of success.[5, 6] Technologic advances also have made resective surgery safer from mortality and morbidity standpoints. Advances in neurosurgical techniques and neuroanesthesia have made operative mortality a rare occurrence. Advances in functional imaging and stimulation brain mapping and intraoperative image guidance help minimize the chance of neurological deficit. These considerations require that the surgical team have a good understanding of the different extratemporal seizure syndromes and the surgical risks and seizure control rates for each, so that a discussion among the surgical team members and with the patient can lead to an optimal decision-making process.

This chapter discusses various important aspects of extratemporal lobe epilepsy surgery, including the characteristics, risks, and outcomes of the epilepsies localized to each individual extratemporal lobe and the various pathologies underlying the extratemporal lobe epilepsies, with their differences in postoperative seizure control outcomes. Also described are the preoperative and intraoperative techniques used to (1) localize the seizure focus for resection and (2) establish the limitations of the resective area to avoid neurological deficit, with emphasis on more recent advances that have the potential to facilitate greatly the safety and efficacy of resective surgery for extratemporal lobe epilepsy.

LOBAR DISTRIBUTION OF EXTRATEMPORAL LOBE EPILEPSY

The distribution of lobes involved in various reported surgical series of extratemporal epilepsy may be skewed by the relative risk of ablative surgery in each lobe considered and may not represent the natural distribution of seizures in the general population of all patients with epilepsy. The surgical series are particularly instructive, however, because they provide a view of cases in which relatively good localization has been achieved. The confidence in localization increases with invasive subdural or depth electrode monitoring, intraoperative stimulation-induced replication of the seizure characteristics, and verification of seizure control postoperatively. Any or all of these criteria can be applied to the classification of surgical epilepsy patients but not nonsurgical patients.

Much of the early understanding of the surgical treatment of extratemporal lobe epilepsies comes from the work of Penfield and Rasmussen at the Montreal Neurological Institute.[7–12] In their epilepsy surgery series, these authors excluded patients with tumors as being a distinct class in terms of natural histories, surgical approaches, and outcomes.[8] They classified the precentral and postcentral gyri together as a separate entity, the central region, owing to their combined involvement in sensorimotor functions and their unique function compared with the functions of the other lobes.[11, 13] In one surgical series, 56% of patients had seizure onset in the temporal lobe; 18%, in the frontal lobe; 7%, in the central region; 6%, in the parietal lobe; 1%, in the occipital lobe; and 11%, in multiple lobes.[12] Other epilepsy surgery series found similar lobar proportions with 45% to 64% frontal, 7% to 13% parietal, 2% to 23% occipital, and 23% to 44% multiple lobe seizure onset zones.[14–17]

In surgical series, pediatric epilepsy patients typically have a higher incidence of extratemporal lobe than temporal lobe epilepsy, and the reverse is true for adult epilepsy patients.[10, 18–21] A review of the University of California Los Angeles (UCLA) experience with pediatric lobar and multilobar resective surgery for epilepsy from 1986 to 2000 revealed 35% temporal lobe, 12% frontal lobe, 3% parietal lobe, 4% occipital lobe, and 47% multilobe patients.[22] In the epilepsy surgery series by Eriksson and colleagues,[15] pediatric and adult patients were analyzed separately. Of the adult resections, 76% were temporal lobe, whereas only 25% were temporal lobe in the children. The extratemporal lobe epilepsy surgeries at Miami Children's Hospital included 62% frontal, 15% parietal and occipital, and 23% multiple lobes.[20]

Parietal lobe epilepsy and occipital lobe epilepsy are rare in surgical series, a finding reported by several authors.[23, 24] This rare incidence may be due to the relative resistance of these regions of the brain to the development of seizures, the difficulty identifying these seizures because of the ambiguity of symptoms referable to seizures from these areas, or the higher chance of permanent postoperative neurological deficit. The data also illustrate one of the characteristics of extratemporal lobe epilepsy that make it more refractory to surgical therapy than temporal lobe epilepsy—the higher incidence of widespread pathology involving more than one lobe.

FRONTAL LOBE EPILEPSY

The frontal lobe is the largest lobe of the brain, encompassing several distinct anatomic-functional units, including the primary motor region; supplementary motor areas; language areas in the dominant frontal operculum; the frontal eye fields; part of the cingulate gyrus; a component of the limbic system; the orbitofrontal and ventromedial regions, which play a major role in the regulation of emotions; and the dorsolateral frontal region, which has major cognitive function, especially working memory. The regions responsible for clearly observable motor functions, the primary and supplementary motor areas, were the earliest to be classified anatomically[25, 26] and were the earliest targets for surgical therapy of epilepsy.[27–30] The clinical syndromes of primary and secondary motor cortex seizures are fairly well agreed on. Characterization of primary motor cortex seizures essentially has remained unaltered since the investigations of Penfield and Jasper,[31] consisting of focal clonic jerks without loss of consciousness if generalization does not occur. Supplementary motor cortex seizure morphology has been described by Ajmone-Marsan and Ralston[32] and has been characterized by more complex motor semiology, including combined movements of extremities and head version.

Seizures in other regions of the frontal lobe have shown significant variability, resulting in difficulty in characterizing classic frontal lobe epilepsy syndromes.[33] Based on characterization of seizures in patients with depth electrode recording, Bancaud and Talairach[34] offered classification of frontal lobe epilepsies to (1) inferior frontal gyrus seizures in either dominant or nondominant hemispheres with speech arrest, tonic or tonic-clonic contractions at the ipsilateral angle of the mouth, swallowing, salivation, gustatory hallucinations, vegetative signs, respiratory deficits, and possibly simple motor manifestations; (2) medial intermediate frontal seizures originating in the mesial frontal lobe, anterior to the supplementary motor cortex, superior to the cingulate gyrus, and posterior to the polar region with frontal-type absence or complex motor seizures; (3) dorsolateral intermediate frontal seizures with contralateral deviation of the eyes followed by aversion of the head; (4) anterior cingulate gyrus seizures with intense fright, expressions of fear, and aggressive verbalizations and acts; (5) frontopolar seizures with dissociation from the environment, fixed eyes, immobility, flexion and turning of the head, falling, and tonic-clonic generalization; (6) orbitofrontal seizures with either olfactory illusions and hallucinations or vegetative symptoms, including cardiovascular, respiratory, or digestive system involvement; (7) operculoinsular suprasylvian seizures with a variety of symptoms, including somatomotor involvement of the face and upper and lower limbs, disorders of verbal expression, contralateral oculocephalic deviation, dissociation from the environment, and postictal speech deficits. These syndromes are not universally accepted, with some authors expressing skepticism concerning the feasibility of anatomic localization from seizure semiology.[35]

Localization of a single resectable focus in frontal lobe epilepsy is typically difficult because of the propensity for extensive epileptic zones with multiple pathways allowing for rapid ictal spread within the frontal lobe and to other lobes and the contralateral side.[36] Even a determination of lateralization can be difficult.[37] In the absence of a distinct focal structural lesion, localization of frontal lobe epilepsy foci almost always requires intracranial ictal recording, either with subdural electrodes[36] or depth electrodes.[34] The findings from these evaluations, combined with the variety of anatomic imaging modalities available, are the basis on which surgical resection plans are made.

Because of the difficulty in localization of the seizure focus, it is not surprising that seizure reduction outcomes of surgery for frontal lobe epilepsy are modest compared with surgical outcomes for temporal lobe seizures. An additional factor may be the increased restraint in cortical resection resulting from the relative involvement of critical functions in the frontal lobe.[38, 39] Generous resections of the frontal lobe for epilepsy have been described, including total frontal lobectomy on the nondominant side and resection of the lateral sensorimotor cortex to nearly 3 cm above the sylvian fissure.[9, 12, 40] Any transient deficit from loss of a frontal eye field or the supplementary motor cortex is likely to resolve eventually. Special care is taken, however, to preserve speech areas in the frontal operculum of the dominant hemisphere, a region in which incurred deficits are likely to remain permanent. Care is taken in resecting primary motor cortex, especially in the hand region or in the dominant hemisphere face region, because fine motor movement could be permanently affected.[27, 41, 42] Functional MRI can be helpful in delineating these motor areas preoperatively.[43]

In Rasmussen's series[11] of surgical resections for frontal lobe epilepsy, only 26% of the patients became seizure-free, and 30% had marked reduction in seizure tendency. In considering central resections alone, better results were reported, with 60% seizure-free and 30% with marked reduction in seizure frequency, but this was after reoperation for some patients.[9] For frontal lobe resections in children, Rasmussen[11] reported dismal rates of seizure control, with only 9% seizure-free and 20% with a significant reduction in seizures. Other authors reported variable seizure control rates after frontal resections for seizures, with seizure-free rates of 28%,[15] 50%,[16] and 57%[44] and significant reduction in seizures in 31%[16] and 7%[44] depending on the series. The frontal epilepsy syndromes remain relatively resistant to surgical intervention.

■ CLINICAL CASE 1

A 29-year-old woman presented for surgical evaluation for complex partial seizures dating back to 8 years of age, when she was diagnosed with Sturge-Weber syndrome. Her seizures were characterized by unresponsiveness, a blank stare, eyelid flutter, and rubbing her fingers together or rubbing her arms. These seizures typically would last 10 to 40 seconds; she had 15 to 25 seizures per month with occasional generalization. Her seizures had proved resistant to multiple pharmacologic agents. Her interictal EEG showed generalized frontotemporal slowing, right greater than left; right, frontally predominant polyspike and wave discharges; and isolated right temporal spike discharges. During EEG video telemetry, the patient's seizures were characterized by wide-eyed staring, lifting of both arms above the head, rubbing the face, and moving the pillow and covers. EEG recorded during these episodes suggested frontal lobe seizures with the possibility of right frontal onset, but because of rapid propagation to the left frontal lobe, the possibility of bilateral or left frontal onset could not be ruled out. MRI and an angiogram during intracarotid sodium amobarbital testing showed a right frontal venous angioma (Fig. 157-1*A*). The intracarotid sodium amobarbital test indicated that the left hemisphere was dominant for language. MEG results were consistent with widespread right anterior frontal and

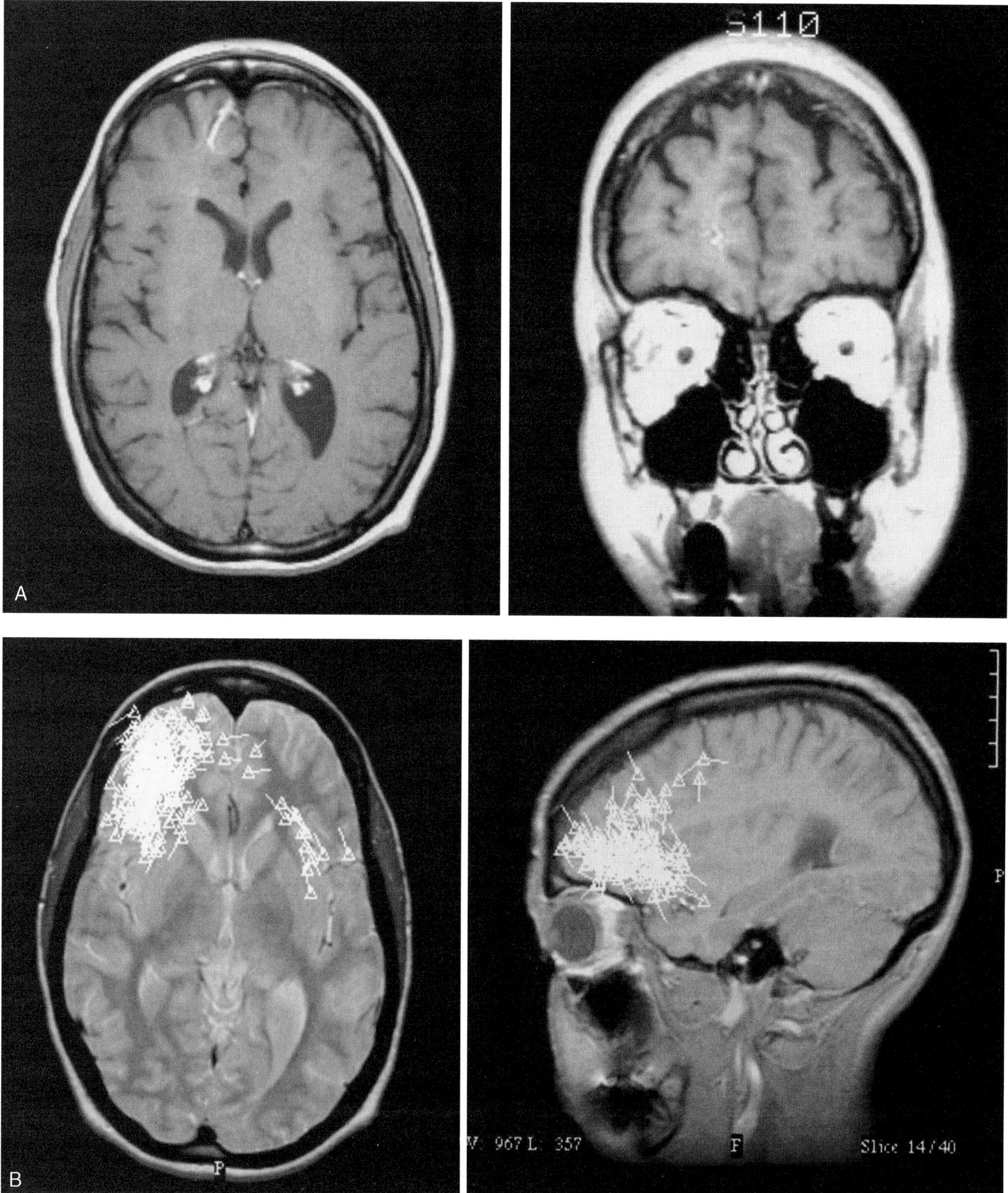

FIGURE 157-1. Clinical case 1. *A,* Preoperative magnetic resonance imaging (MRI) shows right frontal venous angioma in the region consistent with electroencephalographic localization of the seizure focus. *B,* Magnetoencephalogram superimposed on MRI shows epileptiform spikes localized to the frontopolar region, consistent with the area of the venous angioma seen on MRI in *A.*

Illustration continued on following page

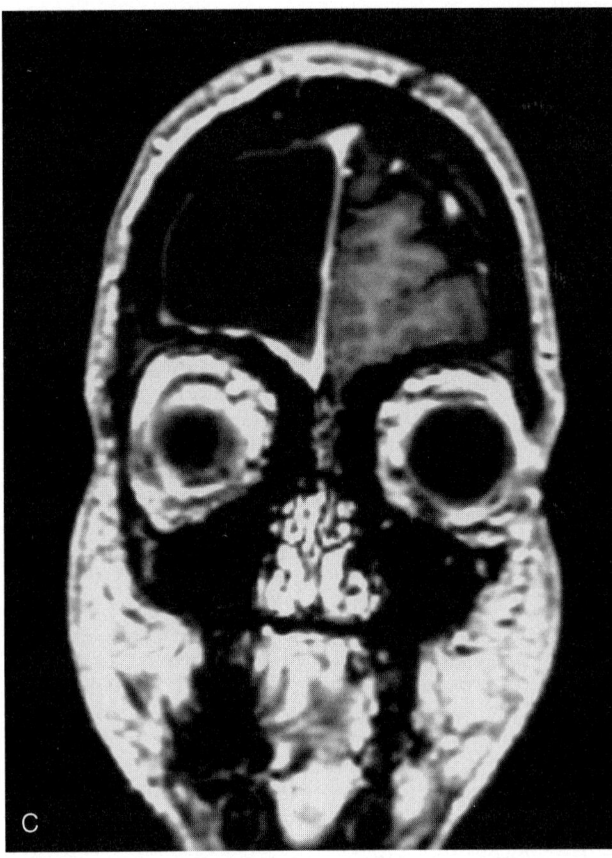

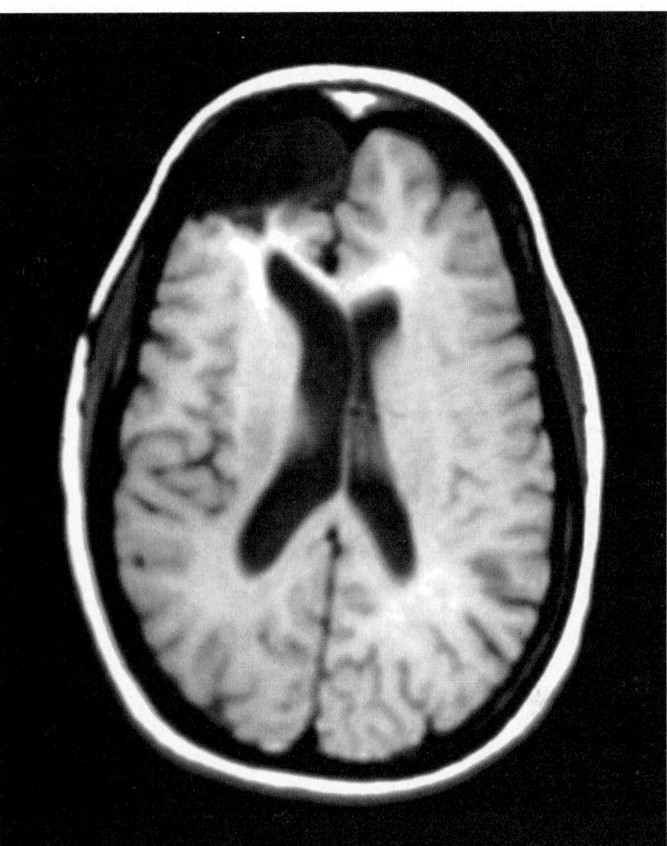

FIGURE 157-1. *Continued. C,* Postoperative MRI shows resection of the frontopolar region, including the venous angioma seen in *A.*

orbitofrontal activity, but with some activity in the left frontal region (see Fig. 157-1*B*).

Based on the MEG findings, subdural grid and strip electrodes were surgically placed over the right frontal region extending over the mesial and lateral frontal and the orbitofrontal regions. Ictal recordings from these electrodes showed onset in the anterior right frontal lobe. Electrocorticography at the time of resective surgery showed spiking activity at the anterior, mesial, and lateral extents of the craniotomy in the right frontal lobe. The tissue surrounding the venous angioma was resected en bloc, consisting mostly of the middle frontal gyrus with some additional cortical tissue at the frontal pole (see Fig. 157-1*C*). The resection included the anterior mesial frontal region. Somatosensory evoked potential mapping indicated a margin of safety between the posterior border of the resection and the rolandic cortex. Postresection electrocorticography showed no residual spiking activity, so the resection was carried no further. The pathology reading for the resected tissue was cortical dysplasia. Postoperatively the patient was seizure-free and remained so at 5-year follow-up.

This case of frontal polar involvement shows the usefulness of integrating several different modalities of evaluation, including semiology, EEG, MRI, MEG, subdural electrodes, and electrocorticography, when there is ambiguity concerning the seizure focus. Even if no single test is definitive, if all tests suggest the same region as the seizure focus, resective surgery is likely to be successful. This case also shows that a lesion seen on MRI cannot stand alone in the planning of resection for epilepsy because anatomic findings, such as the lesion identified preoperatively as venous angioma, may not be responsible for generation of the seizures; in this case, a large area of cortical dysplasia was resected after the MEG-guided grid study delineated the origin of the seizures.

PARIETAL LOBE EPILEPSY

Parietal lobe epilepsy is relatively rare in series of epilepsy surgeries, perhaps due to an innate seizure resistance of the region or the reluctance of surgeons to resect tissue in this area. Seizures originating in the parietal area have not received as much investigation as frontal lobe or temporal lobe seizure syndromes. Parietal lobe seizures typically are characterized by somatosensory auras[45, 46] and pain, paresthesia, vertigo, head and eye deviation, complex visual hallucinations, sensations of body movements, and actual complex movements of the extremities.[47–49] Outside of the primary sensory cortex, there is a paucity of reported clinical and electrophysiologic correlates of seizure activity.[47] Combined with a tendency for seizures to spread quickly to other regions of the brain,[46] this paucity makes characterization and localization of the seizure focus difficult based on semiology and scalp EEG. Similar to frontal lobe epilepsy, focal lesions on MRI or other imaging modalities are paramount in selecting the appropriate surgical resection site.

Tailored resections of the parietal lobe usually do not include the primary somatosensory cortex because of the importance of this cortex in the production of skilled movement, as described by Penfield and Erickson.[50] Similar to primary motor cortex, it has been suggested that primary sensory cortex can be resected nearly 3 cm above the sylvian fissure in nondominant and dominant hemispheres without significant deficit as long as tongue, thumb, and lip areas are identified and preserved.[40] Any resection of the parietal lobe in the dominant hemisphere should remain above the intraparietal sulcus to prevent any damage to the receptive language center.[40] In general, resections in the parietal dominant hemisphere should take into consideration the high probability of language deficits in the vicinity of the sylvian fissure and more superiorly in regions such as the angular gyrus. In general, resections in the dominant parietal lobe should be carried out only after electrical stimulation mapping. Preoperative functional MRI can be useful to provide a general idea of language representation in the region but cannot be relied on with respect to final surgical decision making. With significant resection of the parietal lobe, a contralateral inferior quadrantanopsia should be expected.[40] The nondominant parietal lobe mediates important visuospatial functions. Large resections in this lobe cannot be undertaken without severe impairment in spatial cognition. We have used focal resections in the nondominant parietal lobe when invasive monitoring showed a fairly circumscribed epileptogenic region (see Clinical Case 2) but resorted to multiple subpial transactions when large nondominant parietal territory was involved (see Clinical Case 4).

Surgical seizure control outcomes after parietal resections are reportedly slightly better than outcomes seen after frontal lobe resections. In the series on parietal lobe resections for epilepsy from Rasmussen's group, 45.5% of patients were seizure-free or had only auras persisting postoperatively, and 40.5% had worthwhile improvement in seizures.[8] In other series, the seizure-free rates after parietal lobe resection for seizure foci were 50%,[15] 57%,[16] 90%,[23] and 100% (three patients),[44] and the rates of significant seizure improvement were 29%[16] and 10%.[23]

■ CLINICAL CASE 2

An 18-year-old right-handed man with seizures since the age of 6 was admitted for presurgical evaluation. His seizures were characterized by an aura of impending doom. Initially, his seizures consisted of 20 seconds of staring, but later the semiology changed to staring and dystonic posturing in a sitting position with outstretched arms lasting 20 seconds, occasionally followed by left face and arm twitching with drooling. Postictally after the longer seizures, he had left-hand weakness and dysarthric speech. On average, he had more than one seizure per day. The patient was placed on several different antiepileptic medications and had a vagal nerve stimulator placed without alleviating the seizures. Video EEG monitoring showed rare right temporal spike and wave complexes with seizure activity originating in the right temporal region. MRI was unremarkable, but PET showed right inferior parietal hypometabolism (Fig. 157-2*A*). MEG showed dipoles in the right posterior temporal and inferior parietal regions (see Fig. 157-2*B*). These tests suggested possible temporal and parietal lobe involvement; accordingly, subdural electrodes were surgically placed to cover the frontotemporoparietal region, with strips covering the basal temporal lobe, anterior frontal lobe, posterior parietal region, and superior frontoparietal junction. These subdural electrodes localized the region of seizure onset to the right temporoparietal cortex, including the supramarginal gyrus and posterior superior temporal gyrus. The region of ictal onset corresponded well to the region of interictal abnormalities, although smaller. For resective surgery, intraoperative evoked potentials and electrical stimulation mapping were used to define the rolandic cortex. Intraoperative electrocorticography confirmed localization of the epileptogenic region to the temporoparietal junction and was similar to the interictal localization obtained by the long-term recordings with the subdural grid. Resection included the area surrounding the posterior edge of the sylvian fissure on the parietal and the temporal sides. Subpial transections were performed at the anterior border of the resection cavity, where interictal abnormalities were observed close to the somatosensory cortex. Postresection electrocorticography showed slowing but no residual spikes. Pathology examination of the resected tissue revealed no histologic abnormalities. The patient has remained seizure-free for more than 1 year, although longer follow-up is required to assess the success of surgery.

This case shows the combined used of various modalities to plan surgery. Scalp EEG, MEG, and SPECT were useful in directing the placement of invasive electrodes. The resection included the entire ictal onset zone but not the entire zone of interictal abnormalities, which was larger. Multiple subpial transection was used to address the remaining region of interictal abnormalities, close to the rolandic cortex, and to avoid a large resection in the nondominant parietal lobe.

OCCIPITAL LOBE EPILEPSY

Occipital lobe epilepsy is also rare. Clinically, occipital lobe epilepsy is characterized most often by visual auras.[7,24,51] These visual auras are elementary in nature, being described as lights, spots, or simple shapes that can be flashing or moving. Formed visual hallucinations are more suggestive of temporal lobe epilepsy, either primary or from spread of an occipital lobe seizure. Another clinical feature of occipital lobe epilepsy is episodic blindness,[7,51–53] which can involve half of the visual field or the entire visual field. Other signs observed with occipital seizures include blinking and tonic or clonic eye deviation.[7,51] Occipital lobe seizures can spread rapidly to the temporal lobe, making the localization of their onset difficult and occasionally leading to relatively ineffective temporal lobectomy.[51]

Resective surgery for occipital lobe epilepsy almost certainly is going to lead to some degree of visual deficit,[40] and this procedure must be considered carefully by the patient and the surgical team. It would be a tragedy for a patient to undertake surgical intervention for seizure control in anticipation of regaining a driver's license simply to have the license denied be-

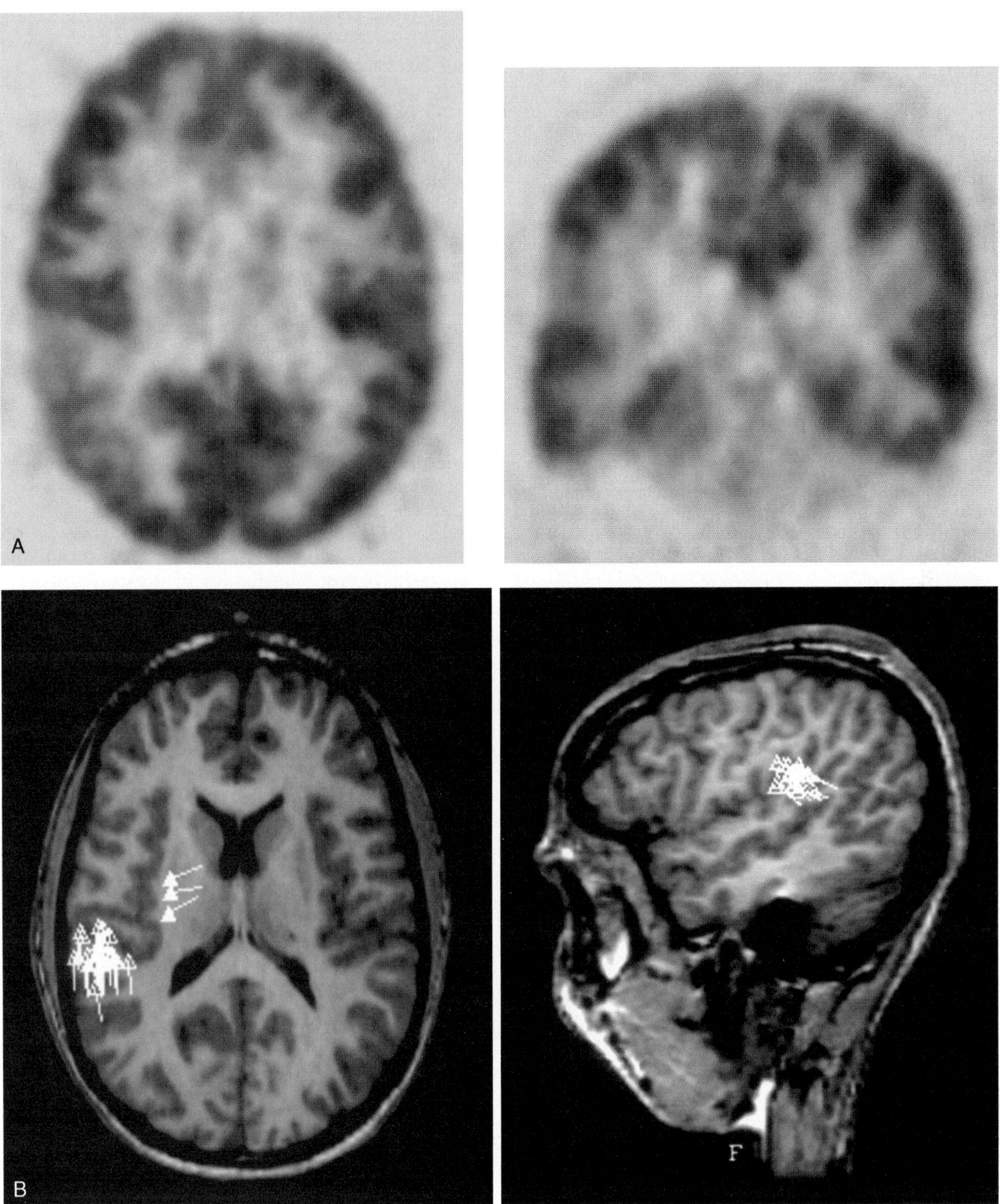

FIGURE 157-2. Clinical case 2. *A,* Positron emission tomography (PET) shows a region of hypometabolism in the right lateral parietal lobe. *B,* Magnetoencephalogram superimposed on magnetic resonance imaging shows spiking activity focused in the right parietal lobe, consistent with the findings of PET in *A.*

cause of a dense hemianopsia. Many of these patients have preoperative visual field deficits, however, especially if there is a mass underlying the seizure disorder, and there is a risk in not controlling the seizures because permanent blindness has been described after recurrent, uncontrolled occipital seizures.[54] Given the frequent spread of occipital lobe seizures to the temporal lobe, resections sometimes are designed to include some portion of the temporal lobe.[7, 14, 51]

Postoperative seizure control outcome for occipital

lobe epilepsy patients varied significantly among series. In one series, only 20% were seizure-free, but 60% were significantly improved.[44] Other series reported better results, with seizure-free rates of 46%,[7] 47%,[24] 50%,[15] and 62%[16] and significant reduction of seizures in 12%,[24] 22%,[7] and 38%.[16] Generally, these were slightly better rates of seizure control compared with the frontal lobe epilepsy resections. Similar to frontal lobe resective surgery for epilepsy, the seizure control outcomes for occipital lobe epilepsy may suffer because of a more conservative approach in the extent of cortical resection.

■ CLINICAL CASE 3

A 38-year-old man who has had seizures since the age of 13 initially had generalized tonic-clonic seizures that would occur at night, but 5 years before surgery, he began having seizures during the day in which he would become disoriented, experience vertigo and partial loss of awareness, and turn his head and eyes to the right. The generalized tonic-clonic seizures began with lifting of the right arm and lasted for 0.5 to 2 minutes. He typically had 5 to 10 focal seizures per day and 1 to 2 generalized seizures per month. On video EEG monitoring, the seizures appeared to begin in the left occipital region but almost instantly spread to the left parasagittal area. On MEG, he had dipoles not only in the mesial part of the left occipital lobe, but also in bilateral central parietal areas (Fig. 157-3*A*). MRI and SPECT were unremarkable, and PET showed no regions of focal hypometabolism. Neuropsychological testing indicated nondominant hemisphere involvement. Intracranial depth electrodes were stereotactically placed in the right occipital, right parietal, right parahippocampal gyrus, right supplementary motor, left occipital, left posterior parietal, left parietal, left parahippocampal gyrus, and left supplementary motor areas (see Fig. 157-3*B*). Seizure evaluation with these electrodes indicated a left frontal onset for the seizures. The depth electrodes were removed, and at a later time, frontal subdural grid and strip electrodes were placed through bilateral frontal craniotomies with extensive sampling of the left mesial frontal region. A left mesial frontal focus was delineated, and this region was resected with electrocorticography guidance and somatosensory evoked potential and stimulation mapping of motor cortex. The pathology was consistent with a cavernous hemangioma, a lesion that was not seen on any of the preoperative imaging studies. The patient is currently nearly 3 years seizure-free after surgery.

This case shows the complexity involved in localizing an extratemporal seizure focus and illustrates how easily noninvasive tests can point to an incorrect seizure focus. In such cases, depth electrodes are used to identify a broad region of onset. When the region has been identified, extensive sampling can be achieved by focused subdural electrode arrays, which are used to identify the discrete epileptogenic region and map the region by electrical stimulation. In this case, depth electrodes in the parietal and occipital lobes and frontal subdural electrodes were essential in localizing the seizure focus to the frontal lobe, rather than to the posterior target suggested by noninvasive monitoring.

MULTILOBAR RESECTIONS

Extratemporal lobe epilepsy may involve more than one lobe, particularly in pediatric patients,[22] and multilobar resections that involve two or three lobes may be necessary. The more common multilobar resection patterns are frontal-temporal,[14] frontal-parietal, and temporal-occipital.[22] These resections are designed around preserving regions of important function, such as motor-sensoryf cortex and language areas. When the epileptogenic region is extensive enough to involve entirely or almost entirely the cortex of one cerebral hemisphere, removal or disconnection of the whole hemisphere may be in order.[55, 56] The original procedure to accomplish this was hemispherectomy, in which the entire hemisphere neocortex was resected. Functional hemispherectomy and hemispherotomy procedures were developed in an attempt to leave intact some of the brain tissue for structural purposes to alleviate the issues of cerebral shift and large subdural hygromas. These procedures were designed to remove only the amount of tissue necessary to disconnect the hemisphere's neocortex completely from the other parts of the brain. The larger resections more commonly are reserved for pediatric patients, who have the best opportunity for regaining neurological function over time. In the series by Eriksson and coworkers[15] that compared pediatric and adult epilepsy surgeries, there were eight hemispherectomies in the pediatric group and none in the adult group. The procedure has been used in adult patients with hemispheric atrophy and fixed unilateral motor deficit. Given the inevitable minimum neurological deficit of decreased fine motor control and the higher risk of surgical complications than other epilepsy surgeries (16% in one series[17]), these procedures should be considered only for severe epilepsy syndromes with full comprehension of the risks by the family and only by a surgeon who is experienced in this specific type of surgery.

OTHER SURGICAL TECHNIQUES

Direct resection is not the only surgical procedure available to treat intractable extratemporal lobe epilepsies. In general, the other surgical methods can be classified as disconnection procedures and stimulation procedures.

Disconnection Procedures

MULTIPLE SUBPIAL TRANSECTION

Multiple subpial transection involves inserting a specially designed instrument through the pia at one side of a gyrus and transecting the cortical ribbon of that gyrus subpially to the other side of the gyrus. Subpial transections traditionally are performed approximately every 5 to 10 mm along the length of each gyrus within a region of epileptogenicity. These transections are thought to divide the fibers connecting adjacent regions of the cortex, while leaving the projection fibers in and out of the region intact. This procedure has shown some efficacy in eliminating or reducing seizures without compromising the function of the cortical region. Subpial transections typically are used in regions of

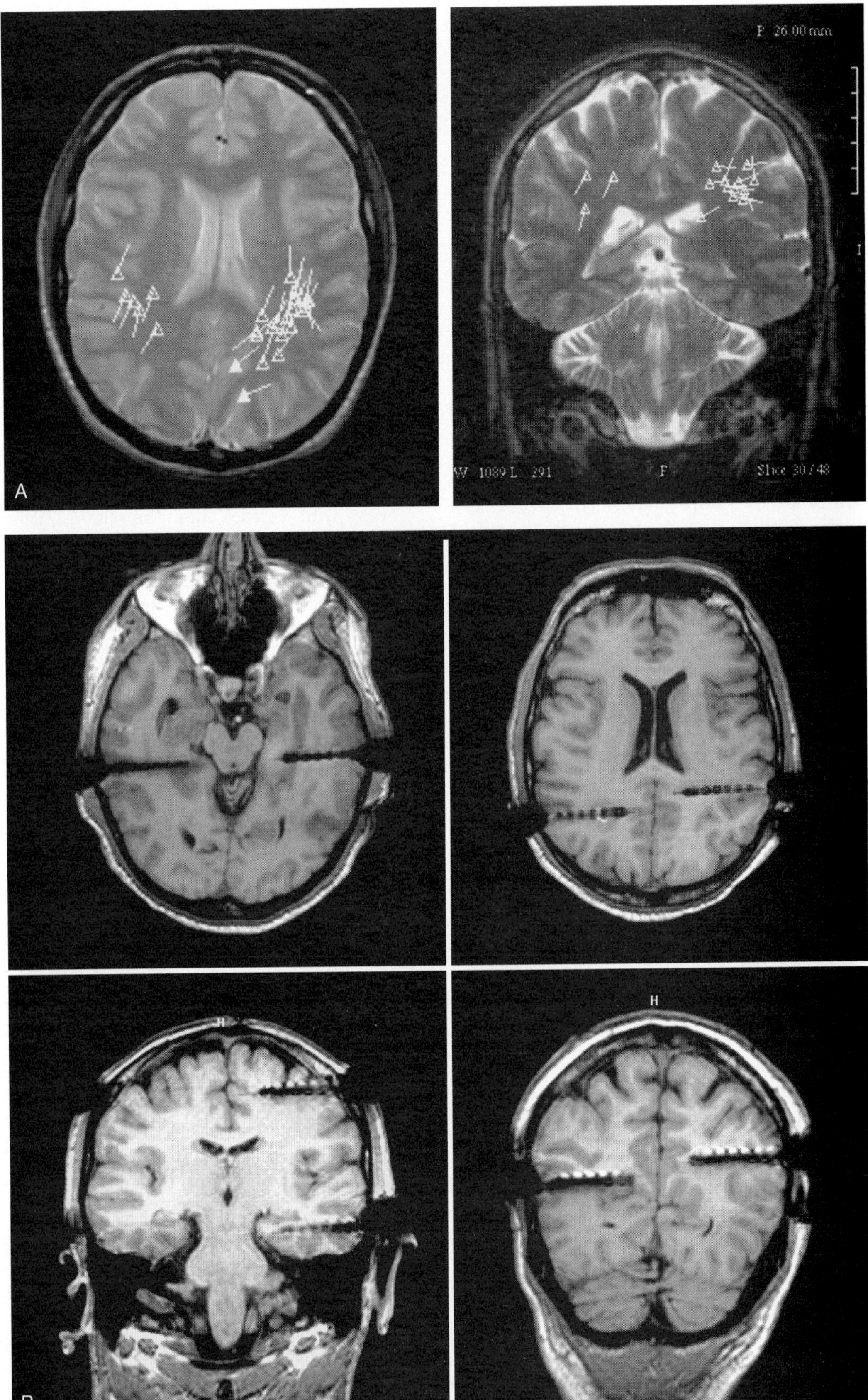

FIGURE 157-3. Clinical case 3. *A,* Magnetoencephalogram superimposed on magnetic resonance imaging (MRI) shows bilateral parietal spikes, more on the left than the right. *B,* MRI shows placement of depth electrodes. (MRI artifact exaggerates the size of the electrodes, which have a diameter of 1.3 mm.)

cortex with critical functions (see Clinical Case 4) and can be performed in combination with tissue resection techniques.[57–59]

CORPUS CALLOSUM SECTION (CORPUS CALLOSOTOMY)

In corpus callosotomy, a portion of the corpus callosum, usually the anterior two thirds, is divided in an attempt to eliminate most connections from one cerebral hemisphere to the other, in this way curtailing sudden generalization by preventing spread of seizures from one side of the brain to the other. Corpus callosotomy is indicated in cases of drop attacks in which the seizures spread throughout the brain so quickly as to cause a complete flaccid paralysis and falling, posing considerable risk of serious injury. These patients are severely affected by the resulting repeated head traumas. Corpus callosotomy does not eliminate the seizures but is designed to change the character of the seizures to eliminate the drop attacks. This is not considered first-line surgical therapy for the treatment of seizures, but rather a rare procedure for a specific indication. In some cases of nonlesional frontal lobe epilepsy, anterior corpus callosum section has been used in combination with a frontal resection to improve seizure outcome.[60] Vagal nerve stimulation has replaced corpus callosum section in some cases as the first-line surgical therapy for severe generalized atonic seizures.

HEMISPHEROTOMY

Hemispherotomy is essentially a disconnection procedure designed to replace radical or functional hemispherectomy procedures. Rather than resection of part or all of the affected hemisphere, the procedure aims at disconnecting it from subcortical structures and from the contralateral hemisphere. Several variants of the procedure have been described.[61–64]

Stimulation Procedures

Implantable stimulation devices have added to the surgical options to treat medically intractable epilepsy. The vagal nerve stimulator has been commercially available for years. This device is 30% to 50% effective in providing at least 50% reduction in seizures for patients with medically intractable seizures who are not surgical candidates.[4, 65] These devices are especially important in the treatment of extratemporal lobe epilepsy because the foci are more likely to be located in areas not amenable to surgical resection. Various deep brain stimulator targets have been investigated as potential targets for the treatment of medically intractable epilepsy. The use of deep brain stimulation in the centromedian and anterior nuclei of the thalamus[6, 66, 67] and in the subthalamic nucleus[68, 69] has shown modest efficacy in control of medically intractable epilepsy. Techniques are being developed using seizure-identifying algorithms to predict seizures and prevent them with triggered stimulation.[70, 71] These various stimulation techniques under development would provide more options for patients with extratemporal lobe epilepsy who are not candidates for surgical resection.

■ CLINICAL CASE 4

A 36-year-old man had his first seizure at the age of 32. Seizures typically were characterized by visual hallucinations of the number 103 followed by loss of awareness and the behaviors of cheering and clapping, then postictal confusion and sleepiness. He was having approximately two to three seizures per week, only one third of which began with a visual aura. The seizures had proved resistant to pharmacotherapy with four different medications in various combinations. Interictal scalp EEG showed right parietal spike and slow wave activity, and video EEG monitoring captured three complex partial seizures that localized to the right central parietal region and one rapidly secondarily generalized seizure in which his head turned to the left before generalization. MRI was normal, but PET showed mild right temporal hypometabolism. MEG showed clusters of spike activity over the posterior temporal and parietal regions of the right hemisphere (Fig. 157-4*A*). The patient had subdural grid electrodes surgically placed through a right temporal/parietal/occipital craniotomy (see Fig. 157-4*B*). Activity recorded from these subdural electrodes showed diffuse onset of the seizures from the right parietal and temporal regions. After extraoperative monitoring, the patient returned to the operating room for surgical treatment of the epilepsy. Stimulation motor mapping and electrocorticography were performed. A biopsy specimen was taken from a region well behind rolandic cortex, showing no abnormality on pathology analysis. Multiple subpial transections were carried out guided by electrocorticography during surgery and the information obtained from the subdural grids before the operation. Multiple subpial transections were used because the seizure focus overlapped regions of rolandic cortex and extensive regions of the nondominant parietal lobe.

Electrocorticography was much improved after the multiple subpial transections, but residual spikes remained, so further subpial transections were performed. The final electrocorticography was improved further. The patient's postoperative course was unremarkable, and in a 4-year follow-up period, he remained seizure-free. This case shows the potential efficacy of subpial transections in alleviating seizures located in cortex that is not amenable to wide surgical resection.

FIGURE 157-4. Clinical case 4. *A,* Magnetoencephalogram superimposed on magnetic resonance imaging (MRI) shows spikes primarily localized to the right lateral parietal and posterior temporal lobes but with some spikes in the left parietal lobe. LD1, LD2, and LD5 denote dipoles related to the somatosensory representation of the left-hand digits. *B,* Three-dimensional reconstruction of MRI shows approximate location of the subdural electrodes over the right parietal, occipital, and temporal lobes.

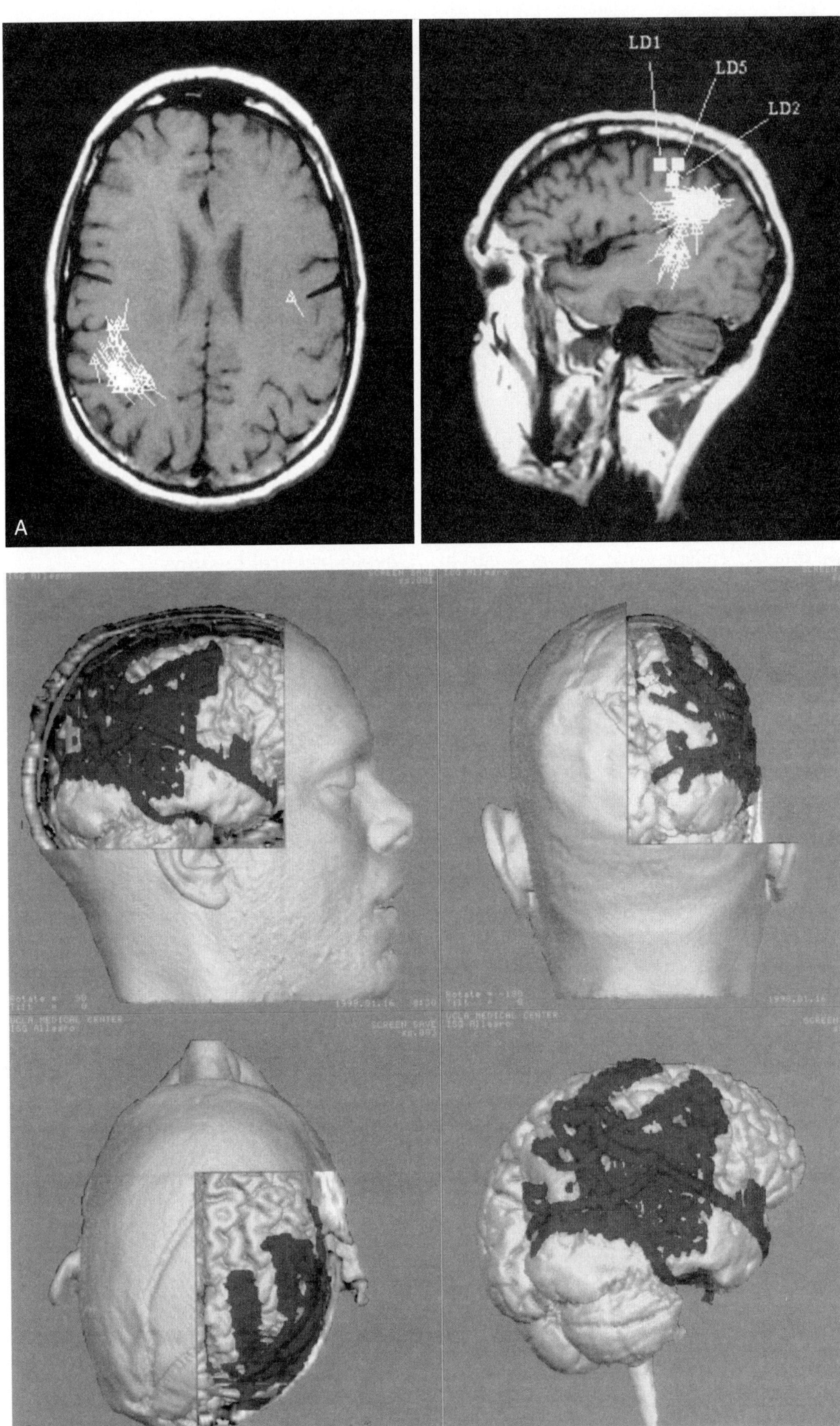
LD1
LD5
LD2
A
B

PATHOLOGIC SUBSTRATES

The pathologic substrates underlying extratemporal lobe epilepsy syndromes are important in planning surgery and seem to have an impact on the seizure control outcomes of patients. Focal abnormalities, such as tumors, vascular lesions, and some cortical abnormalities, may have relatively distinct borders that are differentiated more easily from normal brain tissue intraoperatively. This differentiation facilitates identification of the epileptogenic substrate and complete removal of the entire abnormality. Analysis of several extratemporal lobe epilepsy surgery series showed various categories of epileptogenic pathologies.[7–11, 14–16, 22–24, 44, 46, 51, 72]

Neoplastic Lesions

Neoplasms frequently underly epileptic foci. These tumors can be low-grade astrocytomas, oligodendrogliomas, gangliogliomas, dysembryoplastic neuroepithelial tumors, and others. They may involve the limbic system,[73] but also are seen commonly in extratemporal locations. In general, epileptogenic tumors occur in young people, are slow growing, and involve the cortical gray matter. These tumors can be addressed best with an extended lesionectomy in an effort to remove the tumor and its margins in the surrounding brain. As long as the entire lesion with margins is removed, the outcome after resection of neoplasms is good, with seizure-free rates around 80%,[16, 24] although lower success rates have been reported also.[44] In the UCLA pediatric series, patients with tumors had the best seizure control outcomes.[22] Surgical outcome depends on the extent of resection. Partial resections of neoplasms usually yield poor seizure outcome, and best results are achieved with reresection of the lesion and surrounding margins. It is controversial whether resection of additional contiguous tissue based on electrocorticography is beneficial.[74, 75]

Vascular Lesions

The two vascular lesions classically associated with seizures are arteriovenous malformations and cavernous hemangiomas. The detection of cavernous hemangiomas representing seizure foci has been increasing since the development and refinement of MRI in the preoperative evaluation for epilepsy surgery. Venous angiomas also have been found in patients with epilepsy, but they usually are not considered to be the cause of the seizures. Some associated underlying developmental abnormality may be the culprit, as is illustrated in Clinical Case 1. The other vascular abnormality listed in some surgical epilepsy series is seen in Sturge-Weber syndrome, a pathology more commonly seen in pediatric patients. Zentner and associates[16] found that non-neoplastic focal lesions, including arteriovenous malformations and cavernous hemangiomas, had seizure-free rates of 52%. Seizure outcomes after removal of cavernous angiomas appear to be comparable to outcomes after resections of neoplasms. We believe that removal of the margins of this lesion is important in achieving good seizure outcome.

Gliotic Lesions

Gliotic lesions, including traumatic, ischemic, and postinflammatory pathologies, are predominant in older surgical series that span several decades of operative experience. This is especially true of series predating the use of computed tomography (CT) or MRI. Many of these lesions are related to perinatal or birth trauma or anoxia. Improvements in obstetric care have contributed to the relatively small incidence of these pathologies in modern epilepsy surgery series. Gliotic lesions remain a significant cause of epilepsy, however, especially in the pediatric population. This category includes infectious and inflammatory lesions, some of which have resolved, leaving behind gliotic scar tissue, and others, such as Rasmussen's encephalitis, that are slow and indolent, progressing until the entire hemisphere is involved. Seizures resulting from gliotic lesions can be difficult to control surgically.[44]

Developmental Lesions

Abnormalities of neuronal migration and development are recognized increasingly as a cause of intractable epilepsy. With modern neuroimaging, some of these lesions can be identified and treated surgically. The most common developmental abnormality underlying seizures is cortical dysplasia. Other common developmental abnormalities include polymicrogyria and other cortical gyral malformations. Tuberous sclerosis and heterotopias also have been reported as lesions underlying epilepsy. Developmental lesions are seen more commonly in pediatric epilepsy patients and may involve extensive regions of cortex, sometimes involving more than one lobe. Seizure-free rates of 36% to 50% have been reported after resection of developmental lesions.[24, 44] Of this group, best seizure control outcome has been achieved with resection of focal cortical dysplasia.[22, 24]

Normal Tissue

In general, surgical resections that yield tissue with no histopathologic abnormalities are a minority. In many cases, the changes are minimal and nonspecific but still are described as gliosis. The significance of this diagnosis is unclear. It also may be the case that surgeons are less inclined to operate on normal-appearing substrates. Typically, nonlesional extratemporal epilepsy surgeries have yielded a seizure-free rate ranging from 0% to 20%.[16, 24, 44]

EVALUATIVE TECHNIQUES IN EXTRATEMPORAL LOBE EPILEPSY

Preoperative Evaluation

Because extratemporal lobe epileptic foci in general are difficult to localize by semiology or scalp EEG, other ancillary techniques are required to obtain a concordant assessment of the localization of the seizure focus for resection, particularly in the absence of a distinct structural abnormality on MRI. In many cases, invasive monitoring with intracranial electrodes is required. As part of the presurgical workup, three questions need to be answered: (1) Is there a structural substrate for the disease? (2) Are there physiologic markers for the zone that needs to be removed? (3) Are there functional constraints to removal of the epileptogenic focus?

VIDEO ELECTROENCEPHALOGRAPHY MONITORING

Modern imaging modalities provide information essential for preoperative epilepsy surgery evaluation. The role of video and scalp EEG monitoring has changed concurrently with the development of more advanced imaging techniques. It has a vital but different role as one of several tools used to localize the resection area. Together, several testing modalities make up the clinical picture. In the presence of a distinct lesion, it is still important to establish the relationship between the lesion and seizure onset. In some cases, lesions may not be related to seizures, and in rare cases presumed epilepsy patients with space-occupying lesions were found to have nonepileptic seizures (i.e., pseudoseizures). EEG monitoring is especially important in cases with multiple structural lesions, such as tuberous sclerosis or familial multiple cavernous angiomas, in which each of the lesions could be the causative substrate underlying the epileptic syndrome. In some epilepsy patients, there is no focal abnormality on imaging studies, and video EEG monitoring remains the primary modality in localization of the epileptic focus. In many of these cases, invasive monitoring is necessary for precise localization.

INVASIVE ELECTRODE MONITORING

Invasive monitoring with surgically implanted electrodes is frequently necessary for more accurate localization of the epileptic focus than can be provided by scalp EEG, especially with extratemporal lobe epilepsy. Depth electrodes have several contacts along their length and are surgically placed in specific locations within the brain parenchyma using frame-based or frameless stereotactic guidance. Depth electrodes allow for the investigation of mesial, basal, and deep structures. They are especially helpful in the evaluation of mesial temporal lobe epilepsy syndromes or in cases in which patterns of spread from extratemporal focus may involve the mesial temporal lobe rapidly. Examples are distinguishing mesial temporal lobe epilepsy from orbitofrontal epilepsy or mesial temporal lobe epilepsy from occipital lobe epilepsy. Orbitofrontal and occipital seizures often rapidly spread to the temporal lobe. Depth electrode recording can be useful in lateralizing frontal lobe epilepsy, when contralateral spread is fast.

Subdural or epidural grid and strip electrodes are surgically placed in direct apposition to the cortex, either through bur holes or by craniotomy. Grid electrodes are especially useful in extratemporal lobe epilepsy because they provide sampling of the cortical activity over the cerebral convexities, and they make possible recording from more extensive territories. The main advantage of subdural grids is that they enable detailed sampling of a cortical region, along with functional mapping using electrical stimulation. This coverage can be essential in defining the anatomic extent of more diffuse epileptic foci that are seen frequently in extratemporal lobe epilepsy.

Invasive monitoring also can be performed in the epidural space using grid or peg electrodes. Epidural peg electrodes are surgically placed in small holes drilled into the skull such that they rest against the dura mater. They do not provide the same level of sensitivity or accuracy as depth and subdural electrodes, but they are useful in situations of significant subdural scarring in patients who have had prior surgery or trauma.

IMAGING

The most important imaging modality in preoperative planning for extratemporal epilepsy surgery is MRI.[76,77] Advances in anatomic definition provided by modern MRI have contributed immensely to the identification of epileptic foci. Localized, well-circumscribed lesions on MRI, whether contrast enhancing or signal abnormalities on the T2-weighted or fluid-attenuated inversion recovery (FLAIR) images, make clear the target of resection and signify a greater possibility of postoperative seizure control. FLAIR imaging can be particularly useful and should be part of the routine epilepsy MRI protocol.[78,79] More diffuse lesions have a poorer prognosis for postoperative seizure control, and the absence of a lesion on MRI denotes the worst prognosis for seizure control with surgery. Three-dimensional reconstructions of CT and magnetic resonance angiography images now can be fused with three-dimensional reconstructions of MRI in the frameless stereotactic system for more accurate representation of the vascular structures in relation to cortical anatomy. Careful three-dimensional reconstructions of the cortical surface can reveal surface abnormalities associated with developmental lesions. Imaging of the brain with invasive monitors in place also can be fused with the preoperative MRI to provide exact localization and verification of electrode placement.

Three imaging modalities have proved especially useful in the physiologic localization of the epileptogenic regions in extratemporal lobe epilepsy. The first of these is fluorine-18 fluorodeoxyglucose PET, which identifies areas of cortex of abnormal metabolic activity. Interictally epileptogenic zones tend to be hypometabolic relative to normal cortex, and ictally the region involved with the seizure may be hypermetabolic. PET has proved most useful in the workup of mesial temporal lobe epilepsy, but it also can help delineate extratemporal epileptic foci and verify the likely epileptogenicity of structural lesions seen on MRI. The second, more recently developed imaging modality is SPECT.

In SPECT scanning, a trace amount of radioisotope is injected intravenously, and areas of increased blood flow are revealed. When used in the ictal state and compared with the interictal state, it may show a significant seizure focus where increased neuronal activity results in increased blood flow.[80, 81] This technique has proved especially useful in tandem with coregistration to MRI.[82–84]

MEG registered to MRI (magnetic source imaging)[85] also has proved to be an effective tool for epilepsy surgery, especially in extratemporal epilepsy. MEG uses superconducting quantum interference device magnetometers to detect the magnetic fields associated with intraneuronal electrical currents. The magnetic field, which can indicate the epileptic focus, is not attenuated or distorted by the overlying skull and scalp, increasing accuracy of localization. MEG dipoles are registered to the MRI image using fiducials, allowing for structural localization in three dimensions. These images have proved useful in precise localization of extratemporal lobe epileptic foci (see Clinical Case 1).[86]

Another MRI modality showing promise in the localization of extratemporal seizure foci is magnetic resonance spectroscopy (MRS),[87, 88] which shows the relative distributions of various chemicals in selected areas of the brain. MRS has been explored extensively in mesial temporal lobe epilepsy, but also has been used in studies of extratemporal lobe epilepsy. Extratemporal epileptic foci have shown increased pH, decreased phosphomonoesters,[89] decreased *N*-acetyl aspartate (NAA), and decreased NAA-to-creatine and NAA-to-choline ratios.[87, 90, 91] MRS provides another view of the epileptogenic area and with further development may enjoy wider use by clinicians.

Functional MRI is a relatively new imaging technology that provides information on specific activation of cortical processing zones during motor, sensory, and cognitive functions. This modality holds promise as a preoperative tool to define the relationship of cortical functional anatomy and the epileptogenic zone.[43] Functional MRI is useful in the delineation of functional cortical anatomy for frontal lobe epilepsy resections, especially for motor areas. Although the clinical utility of functional MRI activation outside rolandic cortex is controversial,[77] it provides a noninvasive preliminary to intraoperative mapping, avoiding craniotomy in cases in which the deficits would be unacceptable. It also is useful in determining hemispheric language dominance and it correlates well with results obtained by the Wada test.[92] In addition to its role in defining functional cortical zones, functional MRI is developing as a tool to localize interictal epileptiform discharges. Simultaneous EEG recording and event-related functional MRI allows the linking of epileptiform activity with local brain hemodynamic changes.[93, 94]

NEUROPSYCHOLOGICAL TESTING

Careful neuropsychological testing can provide information concerning the impact of the epileptic focus on regional neurological function.[95] This testing can be especially important in frontal lobe epilepsy because specific abnormalities can manifest on testing, even though routine neurological examination appears normal. Frontal lobe epilepsy patients with either preoperative or postoperative deficits have difficulty with mental flexibility, planning, and fluency (verbal fluency from the left frontal lobe and nonverbal fluency from the right frontal lobe). Parietal lobe deficits are uncommon except in patients with extensive parietal lesions. Distortion in copying of a complex figure representing distortion in conceptualization of spatial representation can be associated with parietal lobe lesions, right more than left, and somatosensory tests sometimes show differences in these patients. Occipital lobe lesions may be manifested by visual field deficits, and if these are significant, they may interfere with cognitive visual tests. Lateral occipital defects have profound cognitive effects on visual cognitive tasks only if they are bilateral, although unilateral occipitotemporal lesions may be accompanied by material-specific neurocognitive deficits depending on the hemisphere involved.

The other important preoperative neuropsychological test commonly employed is the intracarotid amobarbital procedure or Wada test.[96, 97] The patient's language and memory functions are tested during an injection of a barbiturate into one cerebral hemisphere to block function on that side, and the test sometimes is repeated with injection on the other side. The memory component of the test usually is required in temporal lobe epilepsy in which mesial temporal resection is considered. For extratemporal epilepsy, the memory part of the Wada test is less important. Establishing the side of language dominance is crucial, however, in planning frontal lobe and parietal lobe epilepsy surgery. Developments in functional MRI hold promise in using this noninvasive modality to determine language hemispheric dominance,[98] potentially obviating the need for the more invasive amobarbital procedure, which requires angiography and amobarbital administration.

Intraoperative Evaluation

INTRAOPERATIVE MAPPING

It is often necessary to evaluate localization of functions such as language and movement in patients who are undergoing extratemporal lobe resections for seizures. Preoperative functional MRI is useful in providing a general impression of these functional regions in relation to the proposed site of resection. Functional MRI currently is still under development, however, and so most surgeons perform the gold standard intraoperative electrical stimulation mapping for proposed resections near regions of motor, sensory, or language cortex. In patients for whom EEG monitoring using grid electrodes is indicated for localization focus, extraoperative mapping is performed on the ward.

For intraoperative language or sensory mapping, the patient needs to be fully conscious and able to cooperate. For motor mapping, patient cooperation is not required, and the procedure can be carried out under general, albeit light and nonparalytic anesthesia. When patient cooperation is required, the operation is performed under local anesthesia with intravenous sedation during periods of the procedure when the patient's cooperation is not required. Agents such as propofol have improved greatly the ability to carry out such procedures with reasonable patient comfort. An alternative method, which we often use, is asleep-awake-asleep anesthesia,[99] in which the procedure is started with general anesthesia and intubation, enabling the routine neurosurgical craniotomy protocol including cranial fixation and image-guided surgery. Only at the stage of the procedure when mapping is required is the patient allowed to emerge from general anesthesia and subsequently is extubated, leaving a small guide through the vocal cords. After mapping, the patient can be reintubated and fully anesthetized. Electrical stimulation mapping or patient testing can be carried out throughout the resection if the resection is close to functional processing zones.

INTRAOPERATIVE ELECTROCORTICOGRAPHY

Extratemporal lobe epilepsy surgeries require extensive preoperative testing to localize and define the seizure focus as discussed previously. Even with this significant preoperative workup, it is frequently necessary to perform intraoperative electrocorticography to define the seizure focus further and plan the extent of resection. To perform electrocorticography, grid electrodes of various sizes and configurations or individual electrodes are placed directly on the exposed cerebral cortex over suspected regions of epileptogenesis, and electrical activity is recorded. Anesthesia is lightened as much as possible during electrocorticography so as not to suppress epileptic activity. Spike activity usually is taken as an indication of an epileptogenic zone, but sometimes severe slowing of activity is considered also. After tissue resection, electrocorticography can be performed around the borders of the resection cavity to verify the elimination of pathologic electrical activity.

Another electrophysiologic technique used intraoperatively is evoked potential sensorimotor mapping, which can be performed with the patient under general anesthesia. To perform evoked potential sensorimotor mapping, a small electrical current stimulates the median nerve at the hand, and somatosensory evoked potentials are recorded from the cortical surface over suspected rolandic cortex. Phase reversal of the N20 median nerve somatosensory-evoked potential from one strip electrode lead to the next defines the central sulcus, with the precentral motor area anterior and the postcentral sensory area posterior. This process indirectly identifies the motor cortex and does not provide the detailed map offered by electrical stimulation mapping.

FRAMELESS STEREOTAXY

The use of frameless stereotactic equipment in neurosurgery has become widespread in all areas, including epilepsy surgery,[100] and it is especially useful in extratemporal lobe epilepsy surgery. As discussed previously, extratemporal lobe epilepsy has a better prognosis for postoperative seizure control if a structural lesion can be identified on imaging as the seizure focus. This improved prognosis depends on the ability to resect the lesion completely at the time of surgery. Complete resection can be especially difficult for the pathologic lesions underlying extratemporal lobe epilepsy because they frequently appear similar to normal brain tissue and do not have distinct borders. Frameless stereotactic systems can guide the surgeon directly to the lesion and help determine the borders of the lesion based on the imaging.

Frameless stereotaxy is also useful in cases of nonlesional extratemporal lobe epilepsy. Many of the evaluation modalities described previously, such as MEG and SPECT, can be combined with the three-dimensional images to help guide the surgery. CT or MRI images with invasive electrodes in place can be fused with preoperative MRI images to help localize the epileptogenic tissue more accurately during surgery.[101] Functional MRI can be added to suggest functional regions that may require extensive stimulation mapping. The use of frameless stereotaxy in extratemporal lobe epilepsy holds considerable promise in improving the safety and efficacy of surgery.

NEW MODALITIES IN DEVELOPMENT

Novel intraoperative techniques are being developed that should prove useful in extratemporal lobe epilepsy surgery. One of these is interventional MRI, which has been used in epilepsy surgery, mainly for temporal lobe epilepsy,[102, 103] although it is applicable to extratemporal lobe epilepsy as well. This technology has undergone considerable improvement in adjustment to the operating room environment. In its application to epilepsy surgery, it is especially useful because it enables the use of various sequences intraoperatively, including FLAIR sequences, which are sensitive to the subtle tissue changes seen sometimes in epileptogenic lesions. With larger resections, especially those involving multiple lobes, brain shift poses difficulties for traditional image-guided navigation. Interventional MRI allows for intraoperative evaluation of the extent of resection without confounds of brain shift.

Intraoperative optical imaging of intrinsic signals (iOIS) is another technique under development that should prove useful during surgical resection of extratemporal epileptic foci. The equipment is attached to the microscope and allows for detection of cortical regions that are active during specific activities, such as hand movement and language. Intraoperative studies using this technique suggest that iOIS provides more detailed information about cortical function than stimulation mapping,[104] and functions localized by iOIS seem to correspond to functional MRI localization.[105] Animal studies indicate that this process holds promise for localizing seizure foci intraoperatively.[106]

CONCLUSION

Extratemporal lobe epilepsies present a unique challenge to the neurosurgeon because of the frequent lack of obvious underlying pathology and the presence of diffuse and variable underlying pathologies frequently involving cortical regions with critical neurological functions. The key to successful extratemporal lobe epilepsy surgery is the use of the specific preoperative and intraoperative technologies available to define a region where resection is necessary and sufficient to achieve seizure control with minimal neurological sequelae. Localizing a focal lesion responsible for the seizures is associated with the best seizure control outcome if the entire lesion can be resected. Nonlesional extratemporal lobe epilepsies have a more modest prognosis for postoperative seizure control and usually require the use of more modalities, including invasive electrodes, in planning the resection. Preoperative functional scans, intraoperative mapping techniques, and subpial transections when indicated minimize the risk of neurological deficit associated with resection. With the appropriate tools and careful multimodality evaluation at every stage, extratemporal lobe epilepsy surgery provides a reasonable chance of complete seizure control.

REFERENCES

1. Duchowny MS, Harvey AS, Sperling MR, et al: Indications and criteria for surgical intervention. In Engel J Jr, Pedley TA (eds): Epilepsy: A Comprehensive Textbook. Philadelphia, Lippincott-Raven, 1997, pp 1677–1685.
2. Engel J Jr: Introduction to temporal lobe epilepsy. Epilepsy Res 26:141–150, 1996.
3. Fried I: Anatomic temporal lobe resections for temporal lobe epilepsy. Neurosurg Clin N Am 4:233–242, 1993.
4. Binnie CD: Vagus nerve stimulation for epilepsy: A review. Seizure 9:161–169, 2000.
5. Loddenkemper T, Pan A, Neme S, et al: Deep brain stimulation in epilepsy. J Clin Neurophysiol 18:514–532, 2001.
6. Fisher RS, Uematsu S, Krauss GL, et al: Placebo-controlled pilot study of centromedian thalamic stimulation in treatment of intractable seizures. Epilepsia 33:841–851, 1992.
7. Salanova V, Andermann F, Olivier A, et al: Occipital lobe epilepsy: Electroclinical manifestations, electrocorticography, cortical stimulation and outcome in 42 patients treated between 1930 and 1991: Surgery of occipital lobe epilepsy. Brain 115(Pt 6): 1655–1680, 1992.
8. Salanova V, Andermann F, Rasmussen T, et al: Parietal lobe epilepsy: Clinical manifestations and outcome in 82 patients treated surgically between 1929 and 1988. Brain 118(Pt 3):607–627, 1995.
9. Lehman R, Andermann F, Olivier A, et al: Seizures with onset in the sensorimotor face area: Clinical patterns and results of surgical treatment in 20 patients. Epilepsia 35:1117–1124, 1994.
10. Fish DR, Smith SJ, Quesney LF, et al: Surgical treatment of children with medically intractable frontal or temporal lobe epilepsy: Results and highlights of 40 years' experience. Epilepsia 34:244–247, 1993.
11. Rasmussen T: Tailoring of cortical excisions for frontal lobe epilepsy. Can J Neurol Sci 18(4 Suppl):606–610, 1991.
12. Rasmussen T: Surgery for central, parietal and occipital epilepsy. Can J Neurol Sci 18(4 Suppl):611–616, 1991.
13. Rasmussen T: Surgery for epilepsy arising in regions other than the temporal and frontal lobes. Adv Neurol 8:207–226, 1975.
14. Holmes MD, Kutsy RL, Ojemann GA, et al: Interictal, unifocal spikes in refractory extratemporal epilepsy predict ictal origin and postsurgical outcome. Clin Neurophysiol 111:1802–1808, 2000.
15. Eriksson S, Malmgren K, Rydenhag B, et al: Surgical treatment of epilepsy—clinical, radiological and histopathological findings in 139 children and adults. Acta Neurol Scand 99:8–15, 1999.
16. Zentner J, Hufnagel A, Ostertun B, et al: Surgical treatment of extratemporal epilepsy: Clinical, radiologic, and histopathologic findings in 60 patients. Epilepsia 37:1072–1080, 1996.
17. Behrens E, Schramm J, Zentner J, et al: Surgical and neurological complications in a series of 708 epilepsy surgery procedures. Neurosurgery 41:1–9, discussion 9–10, 1997.
18. Duchowny MS, Resnick TJ, Alvarez LA, et al: Focal resection for malignant partial seizures in infancy. Neurology 40:980–984, 1990.
19. Wyllie E, Comair YG, Kotagal P, et al: Epilepsy surgery in infants. Epilepsia 37:625–637, 1996.
20. Prats AR, Morrison G, Wolf AL: Focal cortical resections for the treatment of extratemporal epilepsy in children. Neurosurg Clin N Am 6:533–540, 1995.
21. Duchowny M, Levin B, Jayakar P, et al: Temporal lobectomy in early childhood. Epilepsia 33:298–303, 1992.
22. Leiphart JW, Peacock WJ, Mathern GW: Lobar and multilobar resections for medically intractable pediatric epilepsy. Pediatr Neurosurg 34:311–318, 2001.
23. Cascino GD, Hulihan JF, Sharbrough FW, et al: Parietal lobe lesional epilepsy: Electroclinical correlation and operative outcome. Epilepsia 34:522–527, 1993.
24. Aykut-Bingol C, Bronen RA, Kim JH, et al: Surgical outcome in occipital lobe epilepsy: Implications for pathophysiology. Ann Neurol 44:60–69, 1998.
25. Jackson JH: On the anatomical and physiological localization in the brain. Lancet 1:84–85, 1873.
26. Horsley V: The motor cortex of the brain and the mechanism of the will. BMJ 1:111–115, 1885.
27. Horsley V: Ten consecutive cases of operation upon the brain and cranial cavity to illustrate the details and safety of the method employed. BMJ 1:863–865, 1887.
28. Horsley V: The Linacre lecture on the so-called motor area of the brain. BMJ 2:125–137, 1909.
29. Keen WW: Three successful cases of cerebral surgery. Am J Med Sci 96:330–365, 1888.
30. Lloyd HJ, Deaver JB: A case of focal epilepsy successfully treated by trephining and excision of the motor cortex. Am J Med Sci 96:471–481, 1888.
31. Penfield W, Jasper H: Epilepsy and the Functional Anatomy of the Brain. Boston, Little, Brown, 1954.
32. Ajmone-Marsan C, Ralston BL: The Epileptic Seizure: Its Functional Morphology and Diagnosis Significance: A Clinical-Electrographic Analysis of Metrazol Induced Attacks. Springfield, IL, Charles C Thomas, 1957.
33. Chauvel P, Trottier S, Vignal JP, et al: Somatomotor seizures of frontal lobe origin. Adv Neurol 57:185–232, 1992.
34. Bancaud J, Talairach J: Clinical semiology of frontal lobe seizures. Adv Neurol 57:3–58, 1992.
35. Williamson PD, Engel J Jr, Munari C: Anatomic classification of localization-related epilepsies. In Engel J Jr, Pedley TA (eds): Epilepsy: A Comprehensive Textbook. Philadelphia, Lippincott-Raven, 1997, pp 2405–2416.
36. Toczek MT, Morrell MJ, Risinger MW, et al: Intracranial ictal recordings in mesial frontal lobe epilepsy. J Clin Neurophysiol 14:499–506, 1997.
37. Bleasel A, Kotagal P, Kankirawatana P, et al: Lateralizing value and semiology of ictal limb posturing and version in temporal lobe and extratemporal epilepsy. Epilepsia 38:168–174, 1997.
38. Salanova V, Quesney LF, Rasmussen T, et al: Reevaluation of surgical failures and the role of reoperation in 39 patients with frontal lobe epilepsy. Epilepsia 35:70–80, 1994.
39. Williamson PD, Mattson RH, Spencer SS, et al: Complex partial seizures of frontal lobe origin: Problems with diagnosis and management. Epilepsia 24:516, 1983.
40. Olivier A, Awad IA: Extratemporal resections. In Engel J Jr (ed): Surgical Treatment of the Epilepsies, 2nd ed. New York, Raven Press, 1993, pp 489–500.
41. Penfield W, Jasper H: Epilepsy and the Functional Anatomy of the Human Brain. Boston, Little, Brown, 1954.
42. Penfield W, Rasmussen T: A clinical study of localization of function. In: The Cerebral Cortex of Man. New York, MacMillan, 1950, pp 184–186.
43. Gaillard WD, Bookheimer SY, Cohen M: The use of fMRI in neocortical epilepsy. Adv Neurol 84:391–404, 2000.
44. Adler J, Erba G, Winston KR, et al: Results of surgery for

extratemporal partial epilepsy that began in childhood. Arch Neurol 48:133–140, 1991.
45. Ajmone-Marsan C, Goldhammer L: Clinical patterns and electrographic data in cases of partial seizures of frontal-central-parietal origin. In Brazier MAB (ed): Epilepsy, Its Phenomena in Man. New York, Academic Press, 1973, pp 235–258.
46. Williamson PD, Boon PA, Thadani VM, et al: Parietal lobe epilepsy: Diagnostic considerations and results of surgery. Ann Neurol 31:193–201, 1992.
47. Niedermeyer E: Special types of epilepsy according to the site of focus. In Niedermeyer E (ed): Compendium of the Epilepsies. Springfield, IL, Charles C Thomas, 1974, pp 106–144.
48. Foerster O, Penfield W: The structural basis of traumatic epilepsy and results of radical operation. Brain 53:99–119, 1930.
49. Penfield W, Gage L: Cerebral localization of epileptic manifestations. Arch Neurol Psychiatry 30:709–727, 1933.
50. Penfield W, Erickson TC: Epilepsy and Cerebral Localization. Baltimore, Charles C Thomas, 1941.
51. Williamson PD, Thadani VM, Darcey TM, et al: Occipital lobe epilepsy: Clinical characteristics, seizure spread patterns, and results of surgery. Ann Neurol 31:3–13, 1992.
52. Huott AD, Madison DS, Niedermeyer E: Occipital lobe epilepsy: A clinical and electroencephalographic study. Eur Neurol 11: 325–339, 1974.
53. Olivier A, Gloor P, Andermann F, et al: Occipitotemporal epilepsy studied with stereotaxically implanted depth electrodes and successfully treated by temporal resection. Ann Neurol 11: 428–432, 1982.
54. Aldrich MS, Vanderzant CW, Alessi AG, et al: Ictal cortical blindness with permanent visual loss. Epilepsia 30:116–120, 1989.
55. Schramm J: Hemispherectomy techniques. Neurosurg Clin N Am 13:113–134, 2002.
56. Vining EP, Freeman JM, Pillas DJ, et al: Why would you remove half a brain? The outcome of 58 children after hemispherectomy: The Johns Hopkins experience: 1968 to 1996. Pediatrics 100(2 Pt 1):163–171, 1997.
57. Wyler AR, Wilkus RJ, Rostad SW, et al: Multiple subpial transections for partial seizures in sensorimotor cortex. Neurosurgery 37:1122–1127, discussion 1127–1128, 1995.
58. Wyler AR: Multiple subpial transections in neocortical epilepsy: Part II. Adv Neurol 84:635–642, 2000.
59. Mulligan LP, Spencer DD, Spencer SS: Multiple subpial transections: The Yale experience. Epilepsia 42:226–229, 2001.
60. Laskowitz DT, Sperling MR, French JA, et al: The syndrome of frontal lobe epilepsy: Characteristics and surgical management. Neurology 45:780–787, 1995.
61. Villemure JG, Vernet O, Delalande O: Hemispheric disconnection: Callosotomy and hemispherotomy. Adv Tech Stand Neurosurg 26:25–78, 2000.
62. Villemure JG, Mascott CR: Peri-insular hemispherotomy: Surgical principles and anatomy. Neurosurgery 37:975–981, 1995.
63. Schramm J, Behrens E, Entzian W: Hemispherical deafferentation: An alternative to functional hemispherectomy. Neurosurgery 36:509–515, discussion 515–516, 1995.
64. Delalande O, Pinard JM, Basdevant C, et al: Hemispherotomy: A new procedure for central disconnection. Epilepsia 33(Suppl 3):99–100, 1992.
65. McLachlan RS: Vagus nerve stimulation for intractable epilepsy: A review. J Clin Neurophysiol 14:358–368, 1997.
66. Velasco M, Velasco F, Velasco AL, et al: Acute and chronic electrical stimulation of the centromedian thalamic nucleus: Modulation of reticulo-cortical systems and predictor factors for generalized seizure control. Arch Med Res 31:304–315, 2000.
67. Velasco F, Velasco M, Velasco AL, et al: Electrical stimulation of the centromedian thalamic nucleus in control of seizures: Long-term studies. Epilepsia 36:63–71, 1995.
68. Benabid AL, Koudsie A, Benazzouz A, et al: Deep brain stimulation of the corpus luysi (subthalamic nucleus) and other targets in Parkinson's disease: Extension to new indications such as dystonia and epilepsy. J Neurol 248(Suppl 3):III37–III47, 2001.
69. Benabid AL, Minotti L, Koudsie A, et al: Antiepileptic effect of high-frequency stimulation of the subthalamic nucleus (corpus luysi) in a case of medically intractable epilepsy caused by focal dysplasia: A 30-month follow-up: Technical case report. Neurosurgery 50:1385–1392, 2002.
70. Jerger KK, Netoff TI, Francis JT, et al: Early seizure detection. J Clin Neurophysiol 18:259–268, 2001.
71. Gluckman BJ, Nguyen H, Weinstein SL, et al: Adaptive electric field control of epileptic seizures. J Neurosci 21:590–600, 2001.
72. Jobst BC, Siegel AM, Thadani VM, et al: Intractable seizures of frontal lobe origin: Clinical characteristics, localizing signs, and results of surgery. Epilepsia 41:1139–1152, 2000.
73. Fried I, Kim JH, Spencer DD: Limbic and neocortical gliomas associated with intractable seizures: A distinct clinicopathological group. Neurosurgery 34:815–823, discussion 823–824, 1994.
74. Fried I: Management of low-grade gliomas: Results of resections without electrocorticography. Clin Neurosurg 42:453–463, 1995.
75. Berger MS, Ghatan S, Haglund MM, et al: Low-grade gliomas associated with intractable epilepsy: Seizure outcome utilizing electrocorticography during tumor resection. J Neurosurg 79: 62–69, 1993.
76. Fried I: Magnetic resonance imaging and epilepsy: Neurosurgical decision making. Magn Reson Imaging 13:1163–1170, 1995.
77. Fried I: Functional neuroimaging in presurgical localization of essential cortical processing zones. Adv Neurol 83:297–303, 2000.
78. Wieshmann UC, Free SL, Everitt AD, et al: Magnetic resonance imaging in epilepsy with a fast FLAIR sequence. J Neurol Neurosurg Psychiatry 61:357–361, 1996.
79. Riederer SJ, Jack CR, Grimm RC, et al: New technical developments in magnetic resonance imaging of epilepsy. Magn Reson Imaging 13:1095–1098, 1995.
80. Harvey AS, Hopkins IJ, Bowe JM, et al: Frontal lobe epilepsy: Clinical seizure characteristics and localization with ictal 99mTc-HMPAO SPECT. Neurology 43:1966–1980, 1993.
81. Ho SS, Berkovic SF, Newton MR, et al: Parietal lobe epilepsy: Clinical features and seizure localization by ictal SPECT. Neurology 44:2277–2284, 1994.
82. O'Brien TJ, So EL, Mullan BP, et al: Subtraction ictal SPECT co-registered to MRI improves clinical usefulness of SPECT in localizing the surgical seizure focus. Neurology 50:445–454, 1998.
83. O'Brien TJ, So EL, Mullan BP, et al: Subtraction SPECT co-registered to MRI improves postictal SPECT localization of seizure foci. Neurology 52:137–146, 1999.
84. O'Brien TJ, So EL, Mullan BP, et al: Subtraction peri-ictal SPECT is predictive of extratemporal epilepsy surgery outcome. Neurology 55:1668–1677, 2000.
85. Wheless JW, Willmore LJ, Breier JI, et al: A comparison of magnetoencephalography, MRI, and V-EEG in patients evaluated for epilepsy surgery. Epilepsia 40:931–941, 1999.
86. Ebersole JS, Squires KC, Eliashiv SD, et al: Applications of magnetic source imaging in evaluation of candidates for epilepsy surgery. Neuroimaging Clin N Am 5:267–288, 1995.
87. Lundbom N, Gaily E, Vuori K, et al: Proton spectroscopic imaging shows abnormalities in glial and neuronal cell pools in frontal lobe epilepsy. Epilepsia 42:1507–1514, 2001.
88. Laxer KD: Magnetic resonance spectroscopy in neocortical epilepsies. Adv Neurol 84:405–414, 2000.
89. Garcia PA, Laxer KD, van der Grond J, et al: Phosphorus magnetic resonance spectroscopic imaging in patients with frontal lobe epilepsy. Ann Neurol 35:217–221, 1994.
90. Garcia PA, Laxer KD, van der Grond J, et al: Proton magnetic resonance spectroscopic imaging in patients with frontal lobe epilepsy. Ann Neurol 37:279–281, 1995.
91. Stanley JA, Cendes F, Dubeau F, et al: Proton magnetic resonance spectroscopic imaging in patients with extratemporal epilepsy. Epilepsia 39:267–273, 1998.
92. Andelman F, Neufeld M, Reider-Groswasser I, et al: [Presurgical neuropsychological assessment in epilepsy: The Wada test]. Harefuah 138:440–444, 519, 2000.
93. Lemieux L, Krakow K, Fish DR: Comparison of spike-triggered functional MRI BOLD activation and EEG dipole model localization. Neuroimage 14:1097–1104, 2001.
94. Krakow K, Woermann FG, Symms MR, et al: EEG-triggered functional MRI of interictal epileptiform activity in patients with partial seizures. Brain 122:1679–1688, 1999.
95. Jones-Gotman M: Clinical neuropsychology and neocortical epilepsies. Adv Neurol 84:457–462, 2000.
96. Wada J, Rasmussen T: Intracarotid injection of sodium amytal

for the lateralization of cerebral speech dominance: Experimental and clinical observations. J Neurosurg 17:266–282, 1960.
97. Rausch R, Silfvenius H, Wieser H-G, et al: Intraarterial amobarbital procedures. In Engel J Jr (ed): Surgical Treatment of the Epilepsies, 2nd ed. New York, Raven Press, 1993, pp 341–357.
98. Ramsey NF, Sommer IE, Rutten GJ, et al: Combined analysis of language tasks in fMRI improves assessment of hemispheric dominance for language functions in individual subjects. Neuroimage 13:719–733, 2001.
99. Huncke K, Van de Wiele B, Fried I, et al: The asleep-awake-asleep anesthetic technique for intraoperative language mapping. Neurosurgery 42:1312–1316, discussion 1316–1317, 1998.
100. Eisner W, Burtscher J, Bale R, et al: Use of neuronavigation and electrophysiology in surgery of subcortically located lesions in the sensorimotor strip. J Neurol Neurosurg Psychiatry 72: 378–381, 2002.
101. Schulze-Bonhage AH, Huppertz HJ, Comeau RM, et al: Visualization of subdural strip and grid electrodes using curvilinear reformatting of 3D MR imaging data sets. AJNR Am J Neuroradiol 23:400–403, 2002.
102. Kaibara T, Myles ST, Lee MA, et al: Optimizing epilepsy surgery with intraoperative MR imaging. Epilepsia 43:425–429, 2002.
103. Schwartz TH, Marks D, Pak J, et al: Standardization of amygdalohippocampectomy with intraoperative magnetic resonance imaging: Preliminary experience. Epilepsia 43:430–436, 2002.
104. Cannestra AF, Bookheimer SY, Pouratian N, et al: Temporal and topographical characterization of language cortices using intraoperative optical intrinsic signals. Neuroimage 12:41–54, 2000.
105. Cannestra AF, Pouratian N, Bookheimer SY, et al: Temporal spatial differences observed by functional MRI and human intraoperative optical imaging. Cereb Cortex 11:773–782, 2001.
106. Chen JW, O'Farrell AM, Toga AW: Optical intrinsic signal imaging in a rodent seizure model. Neurology 55:312–315, 2000.

CHAPTER 158

Standard Temporal Lobectomy and Transsylvian Amygdalohippocampectomy

ROBERT E. MAXWELL ■ RAMACHANDRA TUMMALA

From the large experience accumulated over the past half century a consensus has developed that temporal lobectomy is an effective means of treating medically refractory partial-complex epilepsy of temporal lobe origin. Controversy still exists regarding the timing of surgery and the relative merits of different operative approaches and techniques.

The electroencephalogram obtained by scalp or invasive recording is used to identify and localize interictal and ictal discharges. This is then correlated with pathologic changes identified within the temporal lobe by magnetic resonance imaging (MRI) and in complex cases by evidence of metabolic derangements detected with positron emission tomography (PET).[1] Neuropsychometric cognitive testing with assessment of language and memory lateralization completes the presurgical evaluation and guides the final decisions regarding surgical approach and extent of resection. The final common denominator determining the choice of temporal lobe surgery is the clear and indisputable convergence of data confirming the presence of unilateral temporal lobe epilepsy.

Most neurosurgeons working with epileptologists rely on a relatively standard medial resection that includes the anterior 1.5 to 2.5 cm of hippocampus, the dentate gyrus, a portion of the parahippocampus, and the uncus, including the uncal portion of the amygdala. The extent of lateral temporal resection varies according to electrodiagnostic data, evidence regarding side of language dominance, MRI evidence of neocortical abnormalities, and, to some extent, the experience and preference of the epilepsy neurosurgeon. Tailored resections based on invasive monitoring are selectively performed in cases where interictal and ictal recording and functional mapping are deemed necessary to ensure adequate and/or safe resection margins.

An alternative surgical approach for patients with both the pathology and the seizure onset limited to the mesiobasal structures of the temporal lobe is selective amygdalohippocampectomy. This approach was first proposed by Niemeyer in 1958 using a transcortical incision through the middle temporal gyrus.[2] Interest in selective medial temporal resection was later rekindled by the favorable results of the transsylvian approach to amygdalohippocampectomy described by Wieser and Yasargil.[3] Other neurosurgeons have subsequently described alternative approaches to selective amygdalohippocampectomy. Olivier described an approach through the anterior-superior temporal gyrus.[4] Rougier and colleagues proposed an approach through the superior temporal sulcus.[5] Hori and associates described a subtemporal approach.[6]

STANDARD ANTERIOR TEMPORAL LOBECTOMY

The standard anterior temporal lobectomy involves resection of the anterior 4.5 cm of the middle and inferior temporal gyri, although some neurosurgeons may include the inferior portion of the superior temporal gyrus. This approach allows for visualization and subsequent en bloc resection of the medial temporal structures.

The patient is placed in a supine position with the head turned to the opposite side using skull fixation with pins. The ipsilateral shoulder is placed on a roll to lessen torsion on the neck and any compromise of venous return from the head. The head is slightly extended and the vertex tilted slightly toward the floor.

A question mark–shaped incision is made starting at the superior border of the zygomatic arch just in front of the tragus. The incision extends posteriorly just above the auricle and then superiorly and anteriorly to the hairline. This incision spares the temporalis branch of the facial nerve to the frontalis muscle and can also be fashioned to spare the main stem of the superficial temporal artery.[7]

The scalp and temporalis muscles are elevated subperiosteally by sharp dissection as a single flap and reflected forward. Better access to the anterior temporal fossa is ultimately afforded if the temporalis muscle is mobilized off the zygomatic arch for a distance of at least 2 cm. The temporalis muscle and scalp are retracted anteriorly.

A free bone flap offers the optimum exposure in the middle cranial fossa. Trephination of the skull is performed with a craniotome at sufficiently close intervals that the dura mater can be separated from the inner table of the skull before turning the bone flap with a high-speed air drill. Extra care in separating the dura mater from the inner table of the skull lessens the risk of tearing the dura mater and possibly lacerating the underlying cortex and cortical vessels prematurely. This is particularly important if electrocorticography or placement of a subdural grid electrode array or temporal strips is being considered for invasive monitoring. Before the dura mater is opened, the skull and free bone flap may be prepared for subsequent closure by drilling holes for tack-up sutures. Thorough hemostasis is also best achieved at this time by waxing the bony diploë and tamponading any epidural venous bleeding. The temporal bone is inspected for any opening of the mastoid air cells, which are carefully packed and sealed to prevent communication with the middle fossa, thereby lessening the risk of a cerebrospinal fluid fistula and possible meningitis.

The branches of the middle meningeal artery are next coagulated at any sites where they cross the durotomy, which is planned at least 0.5 cm from the skull margin to allow for easy closure of the dura mater. The dural flap can be fashioned in a number of ways, but reflecting the flap anteriorly over the sphenoid wing and temporalis muscle best preserves the vascularity and viability of the dural flap. During the procedure, the dura mater is protected and kept moist to avoid shrinkage and the need for duraplasty at the time of closure.

The sylvian fissure is next carefully identified by observing the location of the sphenoid ridge separating the frontal lobe from the anterior temporal lobe. The middle cerebral veins may vary in location relative to the sylvian fissure and are not as dependable a landmark as the sphenoid ridge.

It is at this stage of the operation when divergent approaches to temporal lobe epilepsy surgery occur, depending on the perceived nature and location of the pathologic process and the preference of the neurosurgeon and epileptologist. Those favoring a tailored temporal lobectomy guided by electrodiagnostic mapping will proceed with electrocorticography at this juncture. The anterior medial temporal resection varies from the standard anterior temporal lobectomy primarily by limiting the amount of lateral neocortical temporal lobe tissue excised during exposure of the medial temporal lobe structures.

Conventional wisdom and cortical mapping studies strongly suggest that the anterior 4.5 cm of even the dominant temporal lobe usually can be resected without significant compromise of neurological function, particularly if the superior temporal gyrus is spared. A small "pie in the sky" sliver of contralateral superior quadrant visual field deficit may be elicited on careful examination after interruption of the most anterior fibers in the geniculocalcarine loop around the tip of the inferior horn of the lateral ventricle. This deficit, if present, is not clinically significant. A standard anterior temporal lobectomy is, therefore, generally defined as one safely confined to the anterior 4.5 cm of the temporal lobe sparing all or part of the superior temporal gyrus.

The temporal lobe dissection is initiated by bipolar coagulation of the pia mater and pial vessels along the superior temporal gyrus or sulcus and then at a right angle across the middle and inferior temporal gyri at the posterior limit of the planned resection. The pia mater is sectioned and subpial dissection of the underlying cortex and white matter carried out by aspiration, with care being taken to identify, bipolar coagulate, and divide any penetrating blood vessels.

Patients suffering epilepsy may have small, atrophic, or maldeveloped temporal lobes with subtle variations in expected anatomy. The pia-arachnoid plane between the limen insulae and the temporal lobe must be recognized and respected during the subpial dissection to avoid injury to the candelabra branches of the M2 segment of the middle cerebral artery. The neurosurgeon can best appreciate variations in anatomic relationships by studying coronal MR images and thereby avoid carrying the neocortical part of the resection medial to the inferior circular sulcus of the insula.

The primary line of dissection is then continued in an inferomedial direction across the white matter on a plane that if continued would pass lateral to the tentorial edge of the incisura.[8] On entering the inferior horn of the lateral ventricle, the choroid plexus is protected and ventricular soilage avoided by gently placing a thin cottonoid strip in the opening of the ventricle. The lateral temporal lobe dissection is then continued by deviating the dissection plane vertically toward the floor of the middle fossa so the plane transects the lateral entorhinal portion of the parahippocampal gyrus just medial to the rhinal sulcus anteriorly and the collateral sulcus more posterior. The subpial transection along the floor of the middle fossa is completed by coagulating and sectioning the pia-arachnoid. Care is taken during this maneuver to avoid heat transfer to the floor of the middle fossa dura mater because this could result in injury to the trigeminal nerve if the dura mater is thin or absent, as is sometimes the case.

Before attempting to lift or deliver the lateral temporal lobe from the middle fossa, the surgeon examines the temporal pole and undersurface of the temporal lobe for bridging veins, which are then bipolar coagulated and divided adjacent to the brain before delivering the lateral temporal lobe en bloc. Preserving venous drainage until the lateral temporal lobe resection is nearly completed avoids unnecessary venous stasis and engorgement and lessens edema and venous bleeding during the procedure.

Magnification facilitates resection of the mesiotemporal lobe structures, including en bloc removal of the hippocampus and delivery of the uncus with the temporal portion of the amygdala and parahippocampal gyrus from the incisura. The operating microscope offers several advantages over surgical loupes. These include superior optics, better lighting, variable magnification and focal length, an observer arm, and the opportunity for television monitoring and recording.

The extent of mesiotemporal resection necessary to provide optimum control of partial-complex seizures of temporal lobe origin is controversial and data are inconclusive. The neural structures generally included under the rubric of mesiotemporal lobe are the hippocampus, fimbria, dentate gyrus, temporal amygdala, uncus, and parahippocampal gyrus.

The previously described lateral anterior temporal lobectomy exposes the inferior horn of the lateral ventricle and in effect disconnects the hippocampus on its lateral side. En bloc resection of the hippocampus involves opening the choroidal fissure by developing the plane between the choroid plexus and the dorsal surface of the hippocampus at the taenia fimbria. The choroid plexus is thereby left attached to the ependyma and pia mater on the undersurface of the thalamus via the taenia thalami. It is helpful for purposes of orientation to recognize that the inferior choroidal point marking the anterior limit of the choroid plexus in the inferior horn of the lateral ventricle correlates with where the pes of the hippocampus merges with the head of the hippocampus as it angles anteroinferomedially, forming the medial surface of the inferior horn of the lateral ventricle.

From this stage of the operation on, the surgeon has several technical options for consideration depending on the extent of the mesiotemporal structures to be removed; the need or desirability for obtaining tissue en bloc to study architectural detail or to perform cell counts or histochemical studies; and the considerations dictated by the pathologic substrate, whether mesiotemporal sclerosis, neoplasia, tissue herniation, or adhesive arachnoiditis along the inferomedial surface of the uncus and parahippocampal gyrus. Partial hippocampectomy can almost always be done safely en bloc. Sometimes, depending on the factors already noted, it is prudent to consider subpial resection of at least portions of the uncus and parahippocampal gyrus when they are adhesed to the arachnoid membrane within the ambien cistern with the contiguous anterior choroidal and posterior cerebral arteries and the trochlear and oculomotor nerves.

After the hippocampus is exposed along the medial surface of the inferior horn of the lateral ventricle, the inferior choroidal point is identified, and the choroidal fissure is opened, en bloc resection of the hippocampus can proceed by first dissecting through the uncal recess anterior to the head of the hippocampus where it angles inferomedially. This line of dissection is carried medial through the amygdala and semilunar gyrus to a point on the apex of the uncus just posterior to the rhinal sulcus. A modest amount of subpial resection at this point exposes the arachnoid membrane and the underlying oculomotor nerve and posterior cerebral artery. The dissection is not carried superior to the plane of the inferior choroidal point so as not to encroach on the globus pallidus where it merges with the amygdalar complex. As the dissection proceeds posteriorly, small hippocampal arteries are encountered as they pass from the anterior choroidal and posterior cerebral arteries through the hippocampal sulcus. These vessels are carefully coagulated and divided immediately adjacent to the brain to avoid injury or traction to a vascular loop of the anterior choroidal artery supplying the internal capsule.

The posterior extent of the hippocampectomy is completed by disconnecting the body and parahippocampal tissue down to the floor of the middle fossa and the tentorium. It is rarely necessary to include the tail of the hippocampus. A standard, nontailored resection usually includes 2.5 cm of the hippocampus, although resection can be extended into the tail of the hippocampus. Some epilepsy centers use intraoperative electrocorticography during this stage of the resection to detect residual interictal spikes and thereby tailor the posterior extent of the mesial resection in an attempt to eliminate the last vestige of potentially epileptogenic tissue.

With completion of the resection, the surgeon can see the contents of the ambien cistern unless the arachnoid membrane is thick or cloudy from preexisting inflammation. The edge of the tentorium cerebri is seen with the oculomotor nerve passing beneath its edge. The trochlear nerve is usually not seen unless looked for just under the edge of the tentorium. The visualized vascular anatomy is somewhat variable but can include the internal carotid artery, the posterior cerebral artery, the posterior communicating artery, the superior cerebellar artery, and the anterior choroidal artery. The basal vein of Rosenthal is often seen. The midbrain is recognized just beyond or deep to the posterior cerebral artery. The arachnoid plane separating the medial temporal structures from the neural and vascular contents of the ambien cistern must be recognized and preserved to avoid neurological complications. The recognition of this anatomy may be more difficult when there has been previous surgery or severe arachnoiditis in this region.

SELECTIVE AMYGDALOHIPPOCAMPECTOMY

History and Indications

The importance of the mesiobasal limbic structures in temporal lobe epilepsy is well established. In contrast, seizures of temporal neocortical origin are relatively uncommon. Hughlings Jackson was the first to demonstrate a mesiotemporal lesion as a cause of psychomotor epilepsy.[9] Extensive neurophysiologic work has revealed the roles of the uncus, hippocampus, amygdala, dentate gyrus, parahippocampal gyrus, entorhinal cortex, and piriform area in the origin and spread of temporal lobe seizures. Thus, the mesiobasal temporal structures represent the predominant anatomic, functional, pathologic, and consequently the surgical substrate of partial complex epilepsy of temporal lobe origin. Stereotactic depth recordings have helped determine that the amygdala and hippocampus are the most important relays in the limbic system. Temporal lobe epilepsy surgery may be successful because of the deafferentation of the hippocampus from entorhinal input or because of the collective removal of these structures.[3]

Anterior temporal lobectomy remains an appropriate surgical treatment for mesiobasal lobe epilepsy. In recent years, however, there has been a trend toward reducing the extent of neocortical resection and limiting the resection of temporal lobe tissue to the mesiobasal limbic structures. This relatively new strategy has been facilitated by the introduction of the operating microscope and microneurosurgical techniques.

As outlined at the beginning of this chapter, five different surgical approaches, all of which are transventricular, have been described for selective amygdalohippocampectomy. The transsylvian approach, although perhaps more technically challenging, deserves review because of the success reported for this approach, although the follow up was limited. Olivier, who departed from his initially reported transcortical approach through the superior temporal gyrus, has more reported success with the transcortical route through the middle temporal gyrus as a modification of Niemeyer's original technique.[4]

All patients evaluated for selective amygdalohippocampectomy in the Zurich series had medically refractory partial-complex epilepsy localized to a unilateral mesiobasal temporal area involving the amygdala and hippocampus.[10] The goal of selective amygdalohippocampectomy is to remove the uncal portion of the amygdala, the anterior portion of the hippocampus, and a portion of the parahippocampal gyrus with its entorhinal cortex. Evaluation with MRI, including volumetric studies, has encouraged clinical investigators to classify temporal lobe epilepsy based on the presence of unilateral atrophy, bilateral atrophy, or no atrophy of the mesiobasal limbic structures. Patients with unilateral atrophy appear to have shown the best seizure control postoperatively.[11–13] Selective amygdalohippocampectomy offers an acceptable alternative to temporal lobectomy only in patients with a well-defined, localized seizure onset in the mesiobasal temporal region.

Surgical Technique

The transsylvian selective amygdalohippocampectomy can be performed through an elliptical craniotomy centered over the frontal sphenotemporal region. The craniotomy can be smaller than that used for a standard temporal lobectomy. The posterior ridge of the lesser wing of the sphenoid bone and the posterolateral orbital rim are drilled down to the level of the anterior clinoid process. A semicircular dural flap is turned and reflected over the sphenoid ridge. Tack-up sutures are placed through the dural edges to lessen epidural oozing, and the dural flap is covered with moistened sponges to prevent desiccation and facilitate dural closure.

Under the operating microscope, the frontolateral orbital aspect of the frontal lobe is gently retracted to expose the carotid and chiasmatic cisterns. The carotid cistern is then entered by opening the arachnoid between the optic nerve and the internal carotid artery. The release of cerebrospinal fluid during this maneuver relaxes the brain. Additional relaxation can be achieved by opening the arachnoid lateral to the internal carotid artery and first segment of the anterior cerebral artery.

A thorough knowledge of the microvascular anatomy in the region of the sylvian fissure is essential when using the transsylvian approach.[14] The lateral branches of the internal carotid artery (including the posterior communicating artery) and the perforating uncal arteries are identified along with the oculomotor nerve. The proximal sylvian fissure is opened by dividing the arachnoid membrane by sharp dissection. Dissection usually is facilitated by proceeding along the frontal lobe side of the middle cerebral vein complex. In those cases where many branches of the middle cerebral vein obstruct a medial approach, a lateral dissection can be performed along the medial surface of the superior temporal gyrus. As the dissection proceeds deeper into the sylvian fissure, longer fine-tipped instrumentation is necessary. The completed transsylvian dissection extends from the internal carotid artery for a distance of 2 cm distal to the middle cerebral artery bifurcation. This exposes the proximal M2 segment of the middle cerebral artery and the anterior third of the insula. On completion of this portion of the exposure, branches of the M1 segment of the middle cerebral artery including the temporal polar, anterior temporal, and posterior temporal arteries and the lenticulostriate arteries are visualized.

A 1.5-cm incision is then made through the anterior temporal stem at the level of the middle cerebral artery bifurcation lateral to the inferior trunk of the M2 segment of the middle cerebral artery. The inferior circular sulcus of the insula is entered inferiorly through the temporal stem at the level of or just posterior to the limen insulae. This approach leads to the temporal horn of the lateral ventricle, which is then opened by means of a gentle spreading action with fine-tipped forceps. Care is taken not to aspirate the choroid plexus. This provides exposure of the lateral, superior, and posterior portions of the amygdala, which is identified by its hazelnut brown color. Resection of basal, lateral, and cortical nuclei of the amygdala by aspiration and sharp dissection then proceeds in the medial and superior inferior directions toward the optic tract. The lateral boundary of the removal of amygdalar tissue is the rhinal sulcus. Subependymal veins draining the amygdala course along the medial ventricular wall. Traction injury to these veins may result in significant bleeding. The medial structures in the amygdala, including the medial and central nuclei, are preserved.

The temporal horn of the lateral ventricle is unroofed for a distance of 2.5 to 3 cm from its tip. The operating microscope is angled in a more posteroinferior direction, exposing the choroid plexus and the hippocampus. The choroid plexus is protected with a thin, moistened, cotton pad, and the tela choroidea is revealed at the choroidal fissure. The anterior choroidal artery, the hippocampal vein, and branches of the basal vein of Rosenthal may sometimes be visualized through the tela choroidea. This thin membrane is opened with fine microdissectors to expose the taenia fimbria and the lateral peduncle of the midbrain.

The small uncal and hippocampal branches of the anterior choroidal artery may be coagulated and divided, but all other branches must be preserved. Opening the choroidal fissure along the taenia fimbria exposes the subiculum within the lateral wing of the transverse fissure. The underlying hippocampal arteries usually originating from the P2 or P3 segments of the posterior cerebral artery are coagulated and divided.

The hippocampus and parahippocampal gyrus can then be transected adjacent to the ascending area of the fimbria and hippocampal tail at the level of the posterior rim of the cerebral peduncle. The transection follows inferolaterally in the direction of the collateral sulcus and tentorial edge. The dissection along the collateral sulcus is semicircular within the temporal horn and extends to the tentorial edge. Small arterial branches entering the parahippocampal gyrus can be coagulated and divided within the collateral sulcus. This allows lateral reflection of the dissected mesiotemporal structure and exposure of hippocampal veins that can now be divided. On completion of their dissection, the uncus, amygdala, hippocampus, and parahippocampal gyrus can be removed en bloc. After irrigation and thorough hemostasis the wound is ready for closure.

The en bloc resection of the anterior portion of the hippocampus and parahippocampal gyrus by this approach may in some cases prove to be complex and tedious. An alternative, piecemeal aspiration and removal of the mesiobasal temporal structures can be performed. The entry point through the roof of the temporal horn as approached through the inferior circular sulcus of the insula is less than 1 cm from the lateral geniculate body of the thalamus. Furthermore, no clear-cut demarcation exists between the lateral geniculate body and the temporal horn. There is, therefore, the potential for injury to the thalamus with this approach. There is also no clear demarcation between the globus pallidus and amygdala. The transsylvian route also disrupts the uncinate fasciculus and the anterior commissure. The resection of the mesiobasal temporal epileptic region is, therefore, performed in conjunction with interruption of the main seizure propagation pathways.

The transcortical selective amygdalohippocampectomy as originally described by Niemeyer and later modified and advocated by others offers the advantage of relatively fewer vascular tissue planes for the surgeon to work through and the option of greater exposure of the medial basal structures when necessary. MRI-based frameless stereotactic systems and interventional MR operating suites may assist with localization and orientation.

The position of the amygdala and hippocampus is established, and a stereotactic reference may be used to assist the extent of exposure and resection by means of these techniques. The temporal horn is approximately 3 cm deep to the surface of the middle temporal gyrus. A subpial dissection along the inferior margin of the superior temporal sulcus will lead the surgeon in the direction of the temporal horn. On entering the ventricle, several landmarks guide the hippocampal resection. The lateral ventricular sulcus lying between the hippocampus and the collateral eminence is first identified. By retracting the choroid plexus posterosuperiorly, the choroid fissure and the apex of the uncus can be seen. The temporal horn is then unroofed sufficiently to identify the tail of the hippocampus.

The medial temporal resection then proceeds with a subpial resection of the parahippocampal gyrus along its anteroposterior axis. The posterior cerebral artery lies on the other side of the pia along the medial border of this gyrus. Anterior dissection to the parahippocampal gyrus leads to the anterior uncus. Once the parahippocampal gyrus is empty, the hippocampus is rotated laterally, transected at the junction of the body and tail, and lifted to reveal the hippocampal sulcus. The fimbria is then resected and followed into the apex of the uncus. The anterior portion of the uncus is resected subpially to avoid injury to the third nerve or cerebral peduncle. The posterior limit of the hippocampal resection is the lateral mesencephalic sulcus between the cerebral peduncle and tectum. Resection of the amygdala can be performed once the entorhinal sulcus is identified. The entire temporal amygdala is located within the boundaries of the uncus.

COMPLICATIONS OF TEMPORAL LOBE SURGERY FOR EPILEPSY

The morbidity and mortality from temporal lobe surgery for epilepsy have decreased with improvements in patient selection, preoperative evaluation, operative technique, and postoperative care. Comparative data are still inadequate to compare the advantages of more tailored resections such as selective amygdalohippocampectomy to standard temporal lobectomy because of smaller patient cohorts, limited follow-up data, and variations in patient selection.

The mortality from temporal lobe surgery is less than 1%, and in more recent series from epilepsy centers no deaths have occurred after several hundred consecutive surgeries.[15] The epilepsy surgery population is young and usually otherwise healthy. The age-adjusted death rate for epileptics is three times that of the nonepileptic population. The risk of mortality is, therefore, not considered a contraindication to surgery in epilepsy centers with an extensive experience with temporal lobectomy.

Morbidity after temporal lobe surgery for epilepsy varies according to a number of factors, which include extent and location of the resection, age and condition of the patient, and the experience of the surgeon. The patient and family need to be informed about transient side effects that occur after standard temporal lobectomy. Examples include a dysnomia following resections in the lateral temporal lobe that may last a few days and then completely resolve. Another common side effect is a small opposite superior quadrantic visual field deficit that most likely would go unnoticed by the patients if not brought to attention during testing of confrontation visual fields. This subclinical deficit is the result of aspirating white matter around the superolateral aspect of the inferior horn 4.0 to 5.0 cm back from the temporal pole and thereby disrupting the most anterior portion of the geniculocalcarine tract. A transient diplopia or blurred vision that clears on covering one eye sometimes occurs as a side effect of manipulating the oculomotor nerve as the uncus and the parahippocampal gyrus are delivered from the incisura. These symptoms may last for as short a time as a few hours or may persist up to 2 to 3 months before resolving.

Another very serious potential, but fortunately rare, complication of temporal lobectomy is that of direct trauma to the cerebral peduncle or midbrain. This complication is a result of the arachnoidal plane between the medial temporal lobe and the structures of the ambien cistern being violated. This complication is more likely to occur in the presence of a neoplasm or vascular malformation or in the presence of significant scar or severe arachnoiditis associated with previous infection, surgery, or hemorrhage in this region. In cases where these anatomic problems are anticipated, either a conservative approach or reliance on modern imaging technology such as intraoperative MRI or frameless stereotaxy for localization may offer significant advantages.

The morbidity and mortality from anterior temporal lobe surgery for epilepsy have decreased with improvements in patient selection, preoperative evaluation, operative technique, and postoperative care. Comparative data are still inadequate to compare the advantages of more tailored resections to standard temporal lobectomy because of smaller patient cohorts, limited follow-up data, and variations in patient selection.

The most significant and potentially disabling complications of temporal lobectomy are the result of infarction of tissue supplied by branches of the middle cerebral artery, anterior choroidal artery, posterior choroidal artery, and posterior communicating artery. Transient hemiparesis is reported to occur in up to 5% of patients undergoing temporal lobe surgery.[16] Permanent, disabling hemiparesis or hemiplegia is reported to occur in 2% to 3% of patients undergoing temporal lobectomy.[16, 17]

There are several sites where vascular injury resulting in hemiparesis can occur during standard temporal lobectomy. These include the candelabra branches of the middle cerebral artery coursing over the surface of the insula; the choroid plexus in the inferior horn of the lateral ventricle; the middle cerebral artery branches looping through the superior temporal gyrus; and the anterior choroidal, posterior choroidal, and posterior cerebral arteries and perforating branches coursing through or adjacent to the choroidal fissure. The volume of vascular ischemic tissue injury may be small but result in significant weakness, as in the case of injury to a branch of the anterior choroidal artery supplying the genu or posterior limb of the internal capsule. Larger infarcts may involve the diencephalon, retrolenticular structures posterior to the internal capsule, deep white matter, and cortex, resulting not only in hemiparesis but also in visual field deficits and dysphasia when the dominant hemisphere is involved.

Certain anatomic and pathologic substrates are more vulnerable to vascular injury and complications resulting from surgical trauma. Patients suffering previous severe trauma, temporal lobe surgery, or meningitis often have severe gliosis, dense arachnoidal adhesions, and atrophy that distorts tissue planes and normal anatomy. In some cases, scarring is so severe that usual subpial dissection techniques are not applicable and ultrasonic fractionation and sharp dissection are necessary to deliver pathologic tissue. Densely gliotic tissue and scarring increase the chance for traction injury to vessels within the incisura and hippocampal sulcus as the hippocampus, parahippocampal gyrus, and uncus are being exposed and delivered from the region of the incisura. The arachnoidal plane separating the medial temporal lobe structures from the cerebral peduncle may be obliterated in patients with previous meningitis or trauma, and extra attentiveness may be necessary in select cases to recognize and avoid crossing this plane.

A symptomatic minor "pie in the sky" visual field deficit detectable on formal testing is relatively common, particularly during the first few days after temporal lobectomy before tissue edema subsides. This finding is the result of anatomic or functional disturbance of the most anterior fibers of the geniculocalcarine optic radiation in the roof of the inferior horn of the lateral ventricle. The superolateral wall of the inferior horn is opened to expose the hippocampus. Experience has suggested that superior quadrantic visual field deficits can be lessened by limiting the extent of the ventricular opening.[18, 19] Hemianoptic visual field deficits usually result from vascular injury during resection of the medial temporal structures and are usually accompanied by hemiparesis when they occur.

Transient diplopia after temporal lobectomy is usually secondary to traction on the ipsilateral oculomotor nerve during delivery of the uncus and parahippocampal tissue. On rare occasions the trochlear nerve may be injured where it passes adjacent to the hiatus of the incisura beneath the tentorium cerebelli. Rare instances of transdural injury to the trigeminal or even facial nerve have also occurred during temporal lobectomy. The latter complications are avoided by not coagulating or traumatizing the dura mater along the anterior plane of the petrous ridge or along the floor of the middle fossa.

Transient and persistent language deficits may occur after temporal lobectomy in the dominant hemisphere. Preoperative neuropsychometric testing and amobarbital (Amytal Sodium) (Wada) testing may influence the surgical approach and extent of resection. Many epilepsy centers use cortical mapping to help tailor the resection in an effort to avoid dysphasia, but even with this precaution the incidence of transient language deficits exceeds 25%.[17, 20] Dysnomia resolving over several days coincides with the time course of evolving and resolving brain edema within and adjacent to language cortex in the posterior and basal temporal lobe.[21]

Persistent language deficits occur after infarctions in the distribution of the anterior choroidal or middle cerebral arteries in the dominant hemisphere.[22, 23] In the absence of vascular complications, the trend toward smaller neocortical resections and tailored resections in the dominant temporal lobe has resulted in a modest reduction in the incidence of postoperative dysnomia as determined by a multilingual aphasia battery administered 6 months after surgery.[24] Patients with good seizure control suffering from postoperative dysnomia generally show marked improvement by the 1-year anniversary of their surgery.[20]

Headache is the most common patient complaint after temporal lobectomy. This varies considerably from patient to patient, considering the relatively standard nature of the procedure. Higher functioning patients tend to suffer and complain more and longer about pain during their convalescence. Factors contributing to headache include incision and closure of the temporalis muscle and fascia, aseptic meningitis secondary to blood products in the cerebrospinal fluid, and muscular and scalp pain associated with prolonged skeletal fixation with the neck turned and somewhat extended.

Postoperative epidural and subdural hematomas are rarely a problem after temporal lobectomy. The internal decompression of the middle fossa and incisura reduces the opportunity for modest masses and tissue shifts to compromise the brainstem. Significant postoperative infections producing septic meningitis, subdural abscess, or bone flap infection are uncommon.[15]

OUTCOMES OF TEMPORAL LOBE RESECTION FOR EPILEPSY

Temporal lobe limbic resection is the most frequently applied surgical procedure for intractable epilepsy, and multiple technical approaches have been described. Thus far, no prospective randomized studies have been reported evaluating the overall outcome of temporal lobe surgery for epilepsy, including seizure control, the neuropsychological outcome of surgery, and the impact on quality of life from the surgery.

In 1950, Penfield and Flanigin reviewed 68 temporal lobe resections carried out between 1939 and 1949 and reported relief of seizures in 50% of the patients.[25] Since that time, thousands of additional patients undergoing temporal lobe resective surgery for epilepsy have been reported.[26, 27] Thirty-two reports from 29 centers using methods of outcomes meta-analysis show an aggregate seizure-free rate of 67.6% when all mesial temporal resections, from the most conservative to the most radical, are included.[28] The data compiled to date indicate that prior to 1985 approximately 56% of patients undergoing temporal lobe surgery for partial complex epilepsy achieved complete control of their seizures and another 28% had notable improvement. Since the mid 1980s, close to 70% of patients with temporal lobe seizures have complete control after limbic resections whether by anterior temporal lobectomy or amygdalohippocampectomy and fewer than 10% of patients show no improvement after surgery. Furthermore, more centers are performing epilepsy surgery as selection criteria are better defined, operative risks have lessened with improved technology, and the benefits of limbic resection when compared with the natural history of the disease have been recognized.

Only a few studies of the extent of hippocampal resection have been reported.[29–33] The only randomized prospective controlled study was that of Wyler and colleagues in which patients underwent anterior mediotemporal resections with either a standard radical hippocampectomy to the level of the superior caliculus or a more limited hippocampectomy to the anterior edge of the superior peduncle. They reported that the total hippocampectomy group had a 69% seizure-free outcome compared with 38% for the partial hippocampectomy group.[33]

Extensive experience with cortical stimulation mapping of language areas within the temporal lobe has found that stimulation eliciting dysnomia and other language distortions occurs in variable locations on the temporal surface of the dominant hemisphere. Resection of these areas is thought to result in permanent fluent language deficits. These areas are rarely located more anteriorly than 4.5 cm from the temporal pole on the middle temporal gyrus and more anteriorly than 3 cm on the superior temporal gyrus.[34] Several studies have shown no demonstrable declines in language function in patients after anterior mesial temporal resections.[33, 35–37]

There is a strong correlation between the risk of verbal memory loss after dominant temporal resection and the degree of mesial temporal sclerosis. The absence of hippocampal sclerosis is a strong risk factor for the development of verbal memory loss, whereas patients with hippocampal sclerosis show no deterioration in memory after dominant temporal lobectomy.[35, 38, 39]

There is considerable anecdotal information to suggest that temporal lobectomy and its modifications are of benefit in improving quality of life, particularly when seizures are completely controlled and the amount of anticonvulsant medication can be reduced or eliminated.[40] Documentation to date has not been sufficient, however, to assess accurately and quantify the overall and precise effect of limbic resections on quality of life.

Surgery, even when resulting in complete seizure control, has not been documented to improve employment status.[41] Perhaps carefully controlled studies evaluating the impact of early, compared with late, surgical intervention after the onset of partial complex epilepsy of temporal lobe origin will provide answers regarding the effectiveness of surgery on work and school performance, employability, degree of independence, and interpersonal relationships.

It is also recognized that poor patient selection and complications may impact adversely the quality of life when new deficits are superimposed on preexisting conditions.

CONCLUSION

Evidence suggests that seizure control after limbic resections is predicated on the identification and resection of a pathologic substrate consistent with the seizure semiology. Patients with focal structural lesions in the temporal lobe or with MRI-documented evidence of mesial temporal sclerosis with electrodiagnostic correlation have better seizure control after surgery than patients with multifocal or diffuse localization or nonspecific pathology.

Optimum results after temporal lobe surgery are observed in the presence of mesial temporal sclerosis when accompanied by a history of early febrile seizures and neuropsychometric evidence of memory deficits on the ipsilateral side. An electrodiagnostic pattern predictive of a good seizure outcome would be one with ictal onset in the anterior medial temporal lobe and, ideally, no or limited propagation and slowing in the contralateral temporal lobe.

Neurosurgeons have had success achieving control of partial complex seizures of medial temporal lobe origin both by means of a more or less standard anterior temporal lobectomy and by more selective approaches such as transsylvian or transcortical amygdalohippocampectomy. Experience has shown, however, that success in achieving seizure control depends on the neurosurgeon removing the critical volume of epileptogenic tissue responsible for the seizures with information often inadequate to know with 100% confidence what that volume of tissue is and precisely where its limits are located or defined.

Evidence strongly suggests that the best opportunity for achieving complete seizure control is offered by surgical approaches permitting adequate removal of the uncal portion of the amygdala, the anterior 2 to 3 cm of the hippocampus, and the adjacent anterior temporal cortex, including the parahippocampal gyrus that is rapidly recruited as the seizure spreads. To the extent the neurosurgeon is confident this goal is achieved by the approach selected, then that approach is appropriate, providing it can be done efficiently with an acceptable risk of complications and morbidity.

Selective amygdalohippocampectomy has the intuitive appeal of offering seizure control by means of a more limited exposure with less brain tissue removal. These theoretical advantages, however, are tempered by a number of considerations that the neurosurgeon analyzes when planning a surgical approach.

First of all, what is the pathologic and anatomic substrate the patient presents that will influence the likely success of a given approach and, particularly, what is likely to be the volume of tissue necessary to remove that will achieve complete seizure control. Long-term follow-up data have been limited to validate that selective and more limited tissue resection is as effective in seizure control as standard temporal lobectomy, and the reports on selective amygdalohippocampectomy have been from relatively few centers.

Adequate removal of the uncus with the temporal portion of the amygdala, the majority of the hippocampus, and the parahippocampal gyrus may prove difficult on occasion for even a skilled and experienced surgeon familiar with the intricacies and variations in the anatomy offered by the transsylvian approach. Marked gliosis, arachnoiditis, and variations in anatomy may limit exposure and compromise the adequacy of tissue removal. The removal of anterolateral temporal neocortex and subcortical white matter ensures not only adequate exposure for removal of the critical mass of medial temporal lobe tissue but also more complete disconnection of these areas from pathways for rapid generalization. Furthermore, not only is additional tissue from the lateral temporal lobe available for pathologic assessment, but the exposure of the amygdalohippocampal complex provided by lateral anterior temporal lobectomy also permits a more satisfactory en bloc presentation of medial temporal tissues to the pathologist.

It is important for the epilepsy surgeon to evaluate his or her experience combined with the evidence provided by preoperative evaluation of the neuropsychometric studies, electrodiagnostic testing, neuroimaging, and assessment of the patient's perspective toward incomplete seizure control and possible surgical side effects and complications before deciding on a selective, or more standard, approach to temporal lobe resection for epilepsy.

REFERENCES

1. Latock J, Abou-Khalil V, Siegal G, et al: Patients with partial seizures: evaluation by MR, CT, and PET imaging. Radiology 159:159–163, 1986.
2. Niemeyer P: The transventricular amygdalohippocampectomy in temporal lobe epilepsy. In Baldwin M, Baily P (eds): Temporal Lobe Epilepsy. Springfield, Ill, Charles C Thomas, 1958, pp 461–482.
3. Wieser H, Yasargil G: Selective amygdalohippocampectomy as a surgical treatment of mesiobasal limbic epilepsy. Surg Neurol 17: 445–457, 1982.
4. Olivier A: Transcortical selective amygdalohippocampectomy in temporal lobe epilepsy. Can J Neurol Sci 27(Suppl 1):68–76, 2000.
5. Rougier A, Saint-Hilaire J, Loiseau P, et al: Evaluation and surgical treatment of the epilepsies. Neurochirugie 38:3–112, 1992.
6. Hori T, Tabuchi S, Kurosaki M, et al: Subtemporal amygdalohippocampectomy for treating medically intractable temporal lobe epilepsy. Neurosurgery 33:50–56, 1993.
7. Maxwell R: Cerebral lobectomies. In Apuzzo M (ed): Brain Surgery Complication Avoidance and Management. New York, Churchill Livingstone, 1993, p 448, Figure 16–63.
8. Maxwell R: Cerebral lobectomies. In Apuzzo M (ed): Brain Surgery Complication Avoidance and Management. New York, Churchill Livingstone, 1993, p 451, Figure 16–66A.
9. Jackson J, Colman W: Case of epilepsy with tasting movements and "dreamy state" with very small patch of softening in the left uncinate gyrus. Brain 21:580–590, 1898.
10. Yasargil M, Wieser H, Valavanis A, et al: Surgery and results of selective amygdala-hippocampectomy in one hundred patients with nonlesional limbic epilepsy. Neurosurg Clin North Am 4: 243–261, 1993.
11. Kitchen N, Thomas D, Thompson P, et al: Open stereotactic amygdalohippocampectomy—clinical, psychometric, and MRI follow-up. Acta Neurochir (Wien) 123:33–38, 1993.
12. Wieser H, Siegel A, Yasargil G: The Zurich amygdalo-hippocampectomy series: A short up-date. Acta Neurochir Suppl (Wien) 50:122–127, 1990.
13. Renowden S, Matkovic Z, Adams C, et al: Selective amygdalohippocampectomy for hippocampal sclerosis: Postoperative MR appearance. Am J Neuroradiol 16:1855–1861, 1995.
14. Yasargil G, Teddy P, Roth P: Selective amygdalo-hippocampec-

tomy: Operative anatomy and surgical technique. In Symon L, Brihaye J, Guidetti B, et al (eds): Advances and Technical Standards in Neurosurgery. Vienna, Springer, 1985, pp 93–123.
15. Olivier A: Risk and benefit in the surgery of epilepsy: Complications and positive results on seizure tendency and intellectual function. Acta Neurol Scand Suppl 117:114–120, 1988.
16. Van Buren J: Complications of surgical procedures in the diagnosis and treatment of epilepsy. In Engel J (ed): Surgical Treatment of the Epilepsies. New York, Raven, 1987, pp 465–475.
17. Wyllie E, Luders H, Morris H, et al: Clinical outcome after complete or partial cortical resection for intractable epilepsy. Neurology 37:1634–1641, 1987.
18. Marino R, Rasmussen T: Visual field changes after temporal lobectomy in man. Neurology 18:825–835, 1968.
19. Van Buren J, Baldwin M: The architecture of the optic radiation in the temporal lobe of man. Brain 81:15–40, 1958.
20. Stafiniak P, Saykin A, Sperling M, et al: Acute naming deficits following dominant temporal lobectomy: Prediction by age at first risk for seizures. Neurology 40:1509–1512, 1990.
21. Ojemann G: Surgical therapy for medically intractable epilepsy. J Neurosurg 66:489–499, 1987.
22. Helgason C, Caplan L, Goodwin J, et al: Anterior choroidal artery-territory infarction. Arch Neurol 43:681–686, 1986.
23. Helgason C, Bergen D, Bleck T, et al: Infarction after surgery for focal epilepsy: Manipulation hemiplegia revisited. Epilepsia 28: 340–345, 1987.
24. Hermann B, Wyler A: Comparative results of temporal lobectomy under local or general anesthesia: Language outcome. J Epilepsy 1:127–134, 1988.
25. Penfield W, Flanigin H: Surgical therapy of temporal lobe seizures. Arch Neurol Psychiatry 64:491–500, 1950.
26. Jensen I: Temporal lobe surgery around the world. Acta Neurol Scand 52:354–373, 1975.
27. Engel J Jr, Van Ness P, Rasmussen T, et al: Outcome with respect to epileptic seizures. In Engel J Jr (ed): Surgical Treatment of the Epilepsies, 2nd ed. New York, Raven Press, 1993, pp 609–621.
28. Kim R, Spencer D: Surgery for mesial temporal sclerosis. In Schmidek H, Sweet W (eds): Operative Neurosurgical Techniques. Philadelphia, WB Saunders, 2000, pp 1436–1444.
29. Awad I, Katz A, Hahn J, et al: Extent of resection in temporal lobectomy for epilepsy: Part I. Interobserver analysis and correlation with seizure outcome. Epilepsia 30:756–762, 1989.
30. Jooma R, Yeh H, Privitera M, et al: Seizure control and extent of mesial temporal resection. Acta Neurochir (Wien) 133:44–49, 1995.
31. Kanner A, Kaydanova Y, de Toledo-Morrell L, et al: Tailored anterior temporal lobectomy: Relation between extent of resection of mesial structures and postsurgical seizure outcome. Arch Neurol 52:173–178, 1995.
32. Nayel M, Awad I, Luders H: Extent of mesiobasal resection determines outcome after temporal lobectomy for intractable complex partial seizures. Neurosurgery 29:55–60, 1991.
33. Wyler A, Hermann B, Somes G: Extent of medial temporal resection on outcome from anterior temporal lobectomy: A randomized prospective study. Neurosurgery 37:982–990, 1995.
34. Ojemann G, Ojemann J, Lettich E, et al: Cortical language localization in left, dominant hemisphere. J Neurosurg 71:316–326, 1989.
35. Hermann B, Wyler A, Somes G: Language function following anterior temporal lobectomy. J Neurosurg 74:560–566, 1991.
36. Katz A, Awad I, Kong A, et al: Extent of resection in temporal lobectomy for epilepsy. Part II. Memory changes and neurologic complications. Epilepsia 30:763–771, 1989.
37. Wolf R, Ivnik R, Hirschorn K, et al: Neurocognitive efficiency following left temporal lobectomy: Standard versus limited resection. J Neurosurg 79:76–83, 1993.
38. Hermann B, Wyler A: Effects of anterior temporal lobectomy on language function: A controlled study. Ann Neurol 23:585–588, 1988.
39. Loring D, Lee G, Meador K, et al: Hippocampal contribution to verbal recent memory following dominant-hemisphere temporal lobectomy. J Clin Exp Neuropsychol 13:575–586, 1991.
40. Rausch R, Crandall P: Psychological status related to surgical control of temporal lobe seizures. Epilepsia 23:191–202, 1982.
41. Bladin P: Psychosocial difficulties and outcome after temporal lobectomy. Epilepsia 33:898–907, 1992.

CHAPTER **159**

Tailored Resections for Epilepsy

ANDREW N. MILES ■ GEORGE A. OJEMANN

Surgery for epilepsy has two main aims. The primary objective is removal of the epileptogenic zone, defined as the total area of brain that is necessary and sufficient to generate seizures and that must be removed to abolish seizures.[1] However, the second aim is to achieve the primary objective without producing new neurological or cognitive deficits. Tailored resections for epilepsy use data derived from electrocorticography (ECoG) in an attempt to identify the epileptogenic zone and data derived from functional mapping to identify eloquent cortex. Such data may be derived intra- or extraoperatively and may place varying amounts of emphasis on interictal or ictal recordings.

The earliest resections for epilepsy, beginning with Horsley's[2] initial experience in 1886 and including the series of Krause[3] and Foerster,[4, 5] were tailored to include gross lesions and portions of cortex with functions reflected in the initial symptoms of the patient's ictal semiology. Most of those resections were in rolandic cortex, as that was one of the few areas of brain where the ictal semiology provided accurate functional localization. The classic form of the tailored resection for epilepsy appeared with the development of electroencephalography (EEG) in the 1930s. In medically refractory patients, scalp EEG identified interictal epileptiform abnormalities localized in other brain areas, particularly the temporal lobe. Resections in the temporal lobe were tailored to the location of interictal epileptiform abnormalities recorded on intraoperative ECoG. Resections were also tailored to avoid "eloquent" areas in the individual patient, as identified by electrical stimulation mapping, initially of motor and sensory cortex, and later of language.[6] This technique was especially well developed at the Montreal Neurological Institute in the 1940s and 1950s, with an extensive experience reported by Penfield and Jasper.[7]

A separate school of tailored resections emphasized ictal recordings through intracranial electrodes. As initially developed by Talairach and associates,[8] recordings were obtained through acute and chronic depth electrodes placed at potential sites of seizure onset suggested by the patient's ictal semiology. More recently, these ictal recordings have been obtained through chronic subdural grid and strip electrodes,[9] as well as chronic depth electrodes.[10–12] In addition, there has been increased interest in using the techniques developed for tailored epilepsy surgery to resect intracerebral neoplastic lesions, based on the premise that the epileptogenic zone lies in adjacent macroscopically normal brain.[13, 14]

The recognition that many patients with medically refractory temporal lobe epilepsy (TLE) had pathologic abnormalities in mesial temporal structures, especially the hippocampus,[15] provided the basis for developing anatomically standardized operations for TLE that emphasize the resection of specific anatomic structures, rather than tailoring the resection to the pathophysiologic abnormalities present on ECoG in an individual patient. The original anatomically standardized resection for medically refractory TLE was the en bloc anterior temporal lobectomy first developed by Falconer.[16] This has been modified by varying the extent of medial temporal and lateral neocortical resection, with the aim of reducing the risk of postoperative cognitive deficits.[17] The extent of temporal neocortical resection in standardized operations was further modified with the development of the transcortical transventricular amygdalohippocampectomy by Niemeyer[18] and the trans-sylvian amygdalohippocampectomy by Wieser and Yasargil.[19]

TEMPORAL LOBE EPILEPSY OF MESIAL TEMPORAL ORIGIN

The pioneering neurosurgeons who first removed the temporal lobe for epilepsy based on EEG and ECoG findings included Penfield,[20] working with the neurophysiologist Jasper,[21] and Bailey and Gibbs.[22] With the advent of the anatomically standardized en bloc resection[16] and its subsequent modifications, numerous authors have advocated either tailored or anatomically standardized procedures for mesial TLE. However, no randomized, controlled trials comparing the two approaches exist, and published series using one or the other approach report similar outcomes. The use of tailored resections for medically refractory mesial TLE therefore remains controversial.

Anatomically standardized resections for medically refractory mesial TLE are based on the premise that resection of structural pathology identified on imaging studies will include the epileptogenic zone. They also assume that the location of eloquent areas, such as language cortex, is sufficiently uniform that they can be avoided by conforming to the anatomic landmarks defining the standardized resection. Tailored resections for mesial TLE, in contrast, emphasize the importance of a patient's individual pathophysiology by altering the degree of resection based on the location of interictal epileptiform discharges and the location of eloquent cortex as determined by functional mapping. Tailored resections are based on the premise that there is considerable individual variability in the extent and location of both the epileptogenic zone and eloquent cortex and that this variability can be identified using interictal epileptiform discharge data from ECoG and functional mapping.

There are two major areas of controversy in the use of tailored resections for medically refractory mesial TLE that derive from the aims of epilepsy surgery stated in the first paragraph: removal of the epileptogenic zone without producing neurological or cognitive deficits. The first point of contention is the use of interictal epileptiform discharges on intraoperative ECoG to identify the epileptogenic zone. Although there is general agreement that identification of the ictal onset zone using chronic extraoperative ECoG is not required if seizure semiology, interictal or ictal scalp EEG, and magnetic resonance imaging (MRI) data are concordant,[23] it is controversial whether interictal intraoperative ECoG adds any information that more accurately identifies the epileptogenic zone and allows the extent of resection to be tailored to this information. The second point of contention is the use of functional mapping techniques to identify temporal lobe cortex essential for language and memory, with the aim of tailoring the resection to minimize the risk of disturbing this eloquent cortex.

In tailoring a temporal lobe resection to a patient's individual pathophysiology, the surgeon aims to use data from the preresection ECoG to guide the extent of resection and data from the postresection ECoG to assess the adequacy of resection in terms of the likelihood of a good seizure outcome. However, the literature examining the relationship between pre- and postresection ECoG and seizure outcome is contradictory. Early reports suggested a better outcome when all spike foci identified on preresection interictal ECoG were resected. Jasper and coworkers[21] documented a good seizure outcome in 59% of patients with complete excision of cortex producing interictal spikes, compared with only 37% of patients with partial excision. More recently, Binnie and colleagues[24] also demonstrated that preresection ECoG findings were predictive of outcome. They found that the presence of maximal epileptiform spikes in extratemporal regions on preresection ECoG was associated with a good seizure outcome in only 30% of cases, compared with a good outcome in 71% of cases when the region of maximal epileptiform discharges was within the temporal lobe. When patients with extratemporal discharges were excluded, the presence of maximal discharges in posterior temporal regions was associated with a worse seizure outcome; only 47% of such patients had good seizure outcomes, compared with 76% of patients without maximal posterior temporal discharges. It is unknown whether tailoring the resection to include maximal discharges in posterior temporal regions would have improved seizure outcome, because these surgeons perform only anatomically standardized en bloc resections. Other reports examining preresection ECoG findings as a predictor of seizure outcome have not found a correlation between features such as location of maximal spike amplitude or spike frequency and outcome.[25–28] This is consistent with an earlier report demonstrating that the area of cortex defined by the presence of interictal spikes on ECoG or EEG, defined as the irritative zone,[1] often markedly exceeds the area of cortex that must be excised to achieve a satisfactory outcome.[29]

Reports examining postresection ECoG findings as a predictor of seizure outcome are also conflicting, with the majority failing to find a correlation between the presence of residual spikes on interictal ECoG and seizure outcome.[24, 27–37] Others have suggested that the presence of interictal epileptiform discharges on postresection ECoG portends a poor seizure outcome.[21, 38–41] Bengzon and associates[38] reported that 72% of patients with a poor seizure outcome and 36% of patients with a good seizure outcome had persistent epileptiform abnormalities on postresection ECoG. Similarly, Fiol and colleagues[39] found that the presence of spontaneous residual ECoG spikes was significantly associated with a less favorable prognosis; only 47% of patients with residual spikes were seizure free, compared with 72% without.

In almost all published reports, the intraoperative ECoG is analyzed by visual inspection to determine features that are assumed to correlate with the presumed epileptogenic zone, such as location of maximal spike frequency or amplitude. It has been suggested, however, that computer analysis of the ECoG may facilitate identification of the epileptogenic zone.[37] Alarcon and coworkers[42] hypothesized that regions where the earliest interictal spikes are found, which they defined as "leading regions," are located in the epileptogenic zone. They proposed that these leading regions behave as pacemakers for interictal spike activity in surrounding or even relatively remote cortex and that sites where secondary propagated activity occurs (equivalent to Luders's irritative zone)[1] have less epileptogenic potential and do not need to be excised. However, because the latency between interictal spikes recorded at different sites is usually less than 200 msec,[43] which is too short to be easily detected by visual assessment of the ECoG, computer analysis of digital ECoG recordings is required. Alarcon's group developed a computer algorithm that identifies the latency between spikes in all channels where the spike is detected. This algorithm has been evaluated retrospectively on 42 patients from their series who underwent anatomically standardized temporal lobectomies for medically refractory seizures.[24, 42] Using the algorithm to identify leading regions revealed a significant relationship between surgical removal of leading regions and seizure outcome. Eighty-six percent of patients with a good outcome (Engel class I and II)[44] had all leading regions excised, and 83% of patients with a poor outcome (Engel class III and IV) had at least one leading region remaining. Based on these results, the authors calculated that if they had tailored their resections to the location of leading regions instead of performing standardized resections, and if they had been able to remove all identified leading regions, the proportion of good outcomes in their series would have increased from 71% to 95%. These results are currently being evaluated both retrospectively and prospectively in a larger series of patients.[24]

An additional confounding issue when attempting to interpret the literature on intraoperative ECoG is that the majority of reports have focused on recordings obtained from subtemporal and lateral temporal neocortex to guide the extent of temporal neocortical resection, rather than direct hippocampal recordings to guide the extent of mesial resection. It has been suggested that an optimal seizure outcome depends on an extensive hippocampal resection.[17, 45] This belief is based on reports demonstrating that patients with less complete hippocampal resections had worse seizure outcomes,[45–47] and that the majority of patients with recurrent seizures after temporal resection had residual mesial temporal structures on MRI, the subsequent resection of which was associated with a good seizure outcome.[48, 49] However, several authors who used direct intraoperative interictal ECoG recordings from the hippocampus as a guide to the extent of resection have challenged the view that a maximal hippocampal resection is necessary for a good seizure outcome.[50–55] Jooma and coworkers[51] used direct intraoperative recordings from the hippocampus to guide the extent of mesial resection and analyzed their results retrospectively in 70 patients. They found no difference in seizure outcome between patients who underwent very limited mesial resection (corticoamygdalectomy) owing to the presence of spiking restricted to the amygdala region and those who underwent, in addition, varying degrees of hippocampal resection based on the extent of interictal hippocampal spiking on ECoG. Reviewing the Montreal experience, Rasmussen and Feindel found no significant difference in seizure outcome in patients undergoing corticoamygdalectomy versus the additional resection of at least 50% of the hippocampus.[50, 54] More recently, McKhann and associates[53] reported on the University of Washington experience. Similar to Jooma's group,[51] they found no correlation between the extent of hippocampal resection and seizure outcome, provided there were no spikes on postresection hippocampal ECoG recordings. There was, however, a significant correlation between the presence of spikes on postresection hippocampal ECoG and seizure outcome. Only 29% of patients who had postresection spikes in the hippocampus were seizure free, compared with 73% with no hippocampal spikes. These results suggest that intraoperative hippocampal ECoG recordings can be used to tailor the extent of hippocampal resection without compromising seizure outcome. Although the University of Washington experience has been that the presence of spikes on postresection hippocampal recordings is associated with a poor seizure outcome and that intraoperative hippocampal recordings can be used to tailor the mesial resection to the patient's individual pathophysiology (limiting the extent of hippocampal resection according to the location of hippocampal spikes without compromising seizure outcome), the overall seizure outcome is no different from that reported with standardized anatomic resections with maximal hippocampal resection.

If there is conflicting evidence that tailored temporal lobe resections are associated with better seizure outcomes than standardized anatomic resections, what evidence is there to support tailored resections based on the second goal of epilepsy surgery: avoidance of neurological or cognitive deficits? In TLE surgery, the functionally essential areas that must be avoided are those for language and memory, particularly material-specific memory (verbal memory in dominant temporal lobes, and visuospatial memory in nondominant temporal lobes). Cortical stimulation mapping of language suggests significant individual variability in location of dominant hemisphere perisylvian sites essential for language.[56–60] In an electrical stimulation mapping investigation of 117 patients undergoing dominant temporal lobe resections, Ojemann and colleagues[58] demonstrated stimulation-evoked naming errors within 3 to 4 cm of the temporal pole along the middle temporal gyrus in 5% of cases, and along the superior temporal gyrus in 14% of cases. These sites are within the boundaries of an anatomically standardized temporal lobe resection. Similar individual variability and location of language-essential sites within the boundaries of a standard dominant temporal lobe resection have been found by others.[61] The utility of cortical stimulation language mapping as a technique to minimize the risk of language deficits following dominant hemisphere resections has been demonstrated by Ojemann and coworkers.[62, 63] In their series, no patient with a resection margin greater than 1 cm away from a language site identified by intraoperative cortical stimulation–evoked naming errors had permanent language deficits postoperatively. In contrast, all patients with resections less than 0.7 cm away from such sites had postoperative language deficits persisting for 1 to 4 weeks; in 43% of patients, the deficits were permanent.[62] A number of risk factors for atypical language-essential sites, particularly anteriorly in the dominant temporal lobe, potentially within the boundaries of a standardized dominant temporal lobe resection, have been identified. These include early age of seizure onset, low preoperative verbal IQ score, left-handedness, right hemisphere memory dominance, and absence of early risk factors for subsequent development of epilepsy.[58, 61, 64–67]

A relationship between temporal lobe resections and memory deficits was first established by Penfield, Scoville, and Milner in the 1950s.[68, 69] They observed that bilateral removal of the uncus, amygdala, and anterior hippocampus was associated with persistent global impairment of recent memory. Subsequently, Milner[70] demonstrated memory deficits that were material specific according to the side of temporal lobe resection (dominant, verbal and nondominant, visuospatial), with the severity of these deficits being related to the extent of unilateral hippocampal removal. More recent reports have documented substantial verbal memory deficits after dominant anterior temporal lobectomies.[71–76]

A number of reports have suggested that larger hippocampal resections are associated with greater deficits in verbal memory following dominant resections and in visuospatial memory following nondominant resections.[70, 71, 77–82] Some reports, however, have not found any correlation between memory outcome and extent of hippocampal resection.[45, 83, 84] In one of these,[45] total hippocampectomy was associated with greater decline in postoperative verbal memory performance than was partial hippocampal removal, although the results did not achieve statistical significance.

A number of variables have been identified that are associated with an increased risk of verbal memory decline following dominant temporal lobe resection. These include high preoperative verbal memory scores, absence of ipsilateral hippocampal atrophy on MRI, absence of ipsilateral hippocampal sclerosis on pathologic analysis of the operative specimen, results of the preoperative intracarotid amobarbital procedure, late age of seizure onset, and male sex.[75, 85–95] The decision to limit the extent of mesial resection with the aim of reducing the risk of postoperative memory deficits is most often based on the presence of such preoperative factors, because there is no reliable way to test hippocampal memory functions intraoperatively. However, a technique to temporarily inactivate the hippocampus during awake craniotomies for temporal lobe resection using topically applied cold water has been reported.[96, 97] The authors described 12 patients who failed preoperative ipsilateral intracarotid amobarbital procedures, suggesting that the contralateral temporal lobe would not sustain memory postoperatively. Intraoperative ipsilateral hippocampal cooling suggested contralateral memory function in 11 of the 12, and none of the 11 developed postoperative memory disturbance.[96]

Evidence from cortical stimulation mapping of verbal memory in the dominant temporal lobe suggests that, in addition to the role played by the hippocampus, the lateral temporal neocortex has a significant role in the mediation of verbal memory, particularly in input and storage aspects.[98–101] Ojemann and Dodrill[99, 100] have shown that there is considerable variability in the exact lateral temporal location of sites related to memory, with a significant minority of sites being identified within the boundaries of lateral resection in anatomically standardized operations.[99, 100, 102] There are thus two variables that must be considered when tailoring the extent of temporal lobe resection to minimize the risk of postoperative memory deficits: extent of medial hippocampal resection, and extent of lateral temporal neocortex resection. In contrast to hippocampal memory function, lateral temporal neocortical memory function can be tested using standard techniques of cortical stimulation during an awake craniotomy. Using a previously described technique for intraoperative mapping of language and verbal memory by direct cortical stimulation in an awake patient,[102] Ojemann and Dodrill[99, 100] demonstrated a significant correlation between postoperative verbal memory scores and extent of lateral temporal lobe resection. The presence of intraoperative stimulation-evoked memory errors within the anterior temporal resection, or within 2 cm of its margin, identified 90% of cases with postoperative memory deficits. The absence of errors identified 70% of cases without such deficits.[100]

The tailoring of resections for mesial TLE based on the location of interictal epileptiform discharges recorded on intraoperative ECoG and the location of eloquent cortex determined by functional mapping of language and verbal memory remains controversial. At the University of Washington, we perform intraoperative ECoG from the lateral and basal surfaces of the temporal lobe before resection of the lateral temporal neocortex. Although the majority of patients undergoing resection for TLE at this institution have predominant interictal epileptiform discharges on intraoperative ECoG arising from the medial basal portion of the temporal lobe, a significant minority of patients have interictal discharges maximal from both basal and lateral temporal surfaces.[103] In these cases, the extent of lateral resection is tailored to the location of interictal discharges on the lateral temporal surface, reflecting our contention that, at least in some patients, the lateral temporal neocortex contributes to the temporal lobe epileptic process, and localized lateral temporal interictal discharges are an indicator of this contribution. This is supported by previous published data from the University of Washington.[104–107] In an experimental primate model of chronic epilepsy, excision of the area of interictal epileptiform activity was required to control seizures.[105] Clinically, localized interictal epileptiform discharges on scalp EEG have been identified as a predictor of a good seizure outcome.[104, 106, 107]

Following resection of the lateral temporal neocortex, intraoperative ECoG is performed directly from the hippocampus. The extent of hippocampal resection is tailored to the extent of interictal epileptiform discharges recorded from the hippocampus. The University of Washington experience is that the hippocampus can be spared without sacrificing seizure control, provided the hippocampal resection includes all ECoG-identified electrophysiologically abnormal tissue.[53] This provides further support for the role of localized interictal epileptiform discharges as an indicator of the epileptogenic zone. Although this approach has not been associated with better seizure outcomes than those reported by other groups, preserving electrophysiologically normal hippocampus, particularly if it is also radiologically or histologically normal, may reduce the risk of postoperative memory loss. There is some evidence that sparing the hippocampus can prevent postoperative memory decline, particularly in those who are most at risk.[79, 108] Analysis of our results also demonstrates that the extent of dominant temporal medial resection is directly proportional to the postoperative decline in measures of verbal memory, particularly in patients with a normal hippocampus or mild mesial temporal sclerosis on histologic analysis of the operative specimen or a normal hippocampus on preoperative MRI.

In addition to being tailored to a patient's individual pathophysiology, resections in the dominant temporal lobe are tailored to the location of eloquent cortex as identified by functional mapping in an awake patient. It is an ongoing controversy whether excluding sites found to be essential for language and memory by direct cortical stimulation, particularly in patients with identified risk factors, reduces the risk of postoperative deficits. The University of Washington experience has been that avoiding sites with stimulation-evoked changes in memory and naming reduces the risk of a postoperative decline in measures of memory and language.[63, 100] However, other epilepsy surgery units have not found a difference in postoperative memory and language function in patients undergoing anatomically standardized versus tailored temporal lobe resections.[78, 84, 109–111]

NONLESIONAL NEOCORTICAL TEMPORAL AND EXTRATEMPORAL EPILEPSY

In the setting of nonlesional neocortical temporal and extratemporal epilepsy, there are no anatomically standardized resections, and current imaging technologies such as MRI do not identify a lesion. Resections must therefore be tailored to the patient's individual pathophysiology in some way. Controversy arises in these cases over the specific technique used to tailor the resection to include the epileptogenic zone. Resections for nonlesional neocortical epilepsy may be based on information derived from acute intraoperative or chronic extraoperative ECoG. This reflects differing views on whether regions with interictal epileptiform discharges on intraoperative ECoG or ictal onset zones on extraoperative ECoG more accurately identify the epileptogenic zone.

Although it might seem intuitive that the ictal onset zone localized with chronic extraoperative ECoG is most likely to identify the epileptogenic zone, this is not necessarily the case. The reported results of resective surgery directed specifically at sites of ictal onset are no different from those of resective surgery directed at sites of interictal activity,[103, 112] suggesting that neither location completely identifies the epileptogenic zone. There is also evidence from experimental animal models of epilepsy of the value of interictal epileptiform discharges in identifying the epileptogenic zone.[105, 113] In these models, interictal and ictal epileptiform activity occurs at the same sites,[113] or excision of the interictal epileptiform activity is also required to control seizures.[105] In the clinical setting, the presence of unilateral focal interictal epileptiform discharges on scalp EEG has been identified as a predictor of good seizure outcome.[106, 114–117] There is some suggestion that, at least in the setting of nonlesional neocortical temporal and extratemporal epilepsy, the combined area identified by the presence of both interictal and ictal epileptiform activity may localize the epileptogenic area more precisely.[33, 118–122] Using chronic extraoperative ECoG to identify both the ictal onset zone and sites with interictal epileptiform discharges in 13 patients, Bautista and associates[118] demonstrated that all patients with interictal activity beyond the resection margins had poor seizure outcomes, even though the ictal onset zone was identified and resected. All patients with nonlesional epilepsy who had resection of both the ictal onset zone and sites with interictal activity had good seizure outcomes. Similar results have been obtained by others.[33, 120]

Resections for nonlesional neocortical epilepsy must also be tailored to avoid functionally eloquent cortex such as that related to motor, sensory, language, and memory functions, which may be in close proximity to the ictal onset zone. In the temporal lobe, this area is often outside the boundaries of what are deemed to be "safe" lateral resections according to the criteria for standardized temporal lobe resections. Extratemporally, the planned area of resection may be in close proximity to or within motor, sensory, and language cortex. In resections for neocortical epilepsy, therefore, the need for functional mapping is less controversial and more of a necessity. Eloquent cortex can be identified using either intraoperative direct brain stimulation techniques or extraoperative stimulation by means of implanted subdural electrodes. The technique used depends in part on the surgeon's philosophy about the relative value of interictal versus ictal recordings as a guide to the extent of resection. Other issues also play a role in the decision. Extraoperative techniques permit mapping over a prolonged time or over several separate sessions, allowing precise mapping and restimulation to confirm questionable results. Extraoperative techniques are required for patients who are unlikely to tolerate an awake craniotomy for intraoperative mapping, such as young children. Potential disadvantages of extraoperative techniques include the necessity of two separate craniotomies and the morbidity associated with chronic subdural electrode implantation. However, several studies have demonstrated the safety and low morbidity associated with extraoperative techniques.[123–126] Extraoperative mapping techniques also substantially increase the cost of the presurgical evaluation, and they are probably less precise than intraoperative techniques.[103] For example, intraoperative mapping often demonstrates essential language sites in areas of cortex 1 cm in extent with sharp boundaries,[58] whereas extraoperative mapping usually shows less focal localization.[127] However, the potential effects of this difference in terms of the relative risk of damaging eloquent cortex are unknown, given that no randomized trial of extraoperative versus intraoperative techniques has compared outcomes in terms of incidence of neurological deficits or, for that matter, seizure-free outcomes.

EPILEPSY ASSOCIATED WITH STRUCTURAL LESIONS

Surgical resection of structural lesions can involve resection of the lesion alone (lesionectomy) or resection of the lesion and epileptogenic cortex (seizure surgery). A tailored resection may be performed in either case, with the resection tailored to avoid eloquent cortex in the former and to excise epileptogenic cortex and avoid eloquent cortex in the latter. Tailoring a resection to avoid eloquent cortex is the less controversial of these two concepts. A number of reports demonstrate that lesions within or adjacent to eloquent cortex can be safely resected using either intraoperative direct brain stimulation techniques or extraoperative stimulation by means of implanted subdural electrodes to identify functional cortex and minimize the risk of postoperative functional deficit.[62, 128–133] Once again, the technique chosen to identify eloquent cortex depends in part on the surgeon's philosophy with regard to two controversial issues: First, is seizure surgery for structural lesions—that is, the resection of lesion and epileptogenic cortex—associated with better seizure outcomes than lesionectomy alone? Second, if so, should the epileptogenic cortex be identified by the location of interictal epileptiform discharges found during acute intraoperative ECoG, by the location of the ictal onset zone found during chronic extraoperative ECoG via implanted subdural electrodes, or by both?

Several studies have compared lesionectomy and seizure surgery in terms of seizure outcome in an attempt to answer the first question, with contradictory results.[13, 134–141] All these studies have a number of problems, such as inadequate follow-up, marked heterogeneity in type of lesion included, and lack of randomization, that make it difficult to draw overall conclusions. The relative merit of lesionectomy versus seizure surgery is likely to depend on a number of factors, such as the nature and location of the lesion, the preoperative duration of seizures, and the initial response to medical therapy. Weber and coworkers[142] performed a meta-analysis of the available literature evaluating seizure outcome following lesionectomy or seizure surgery and separated the results according to the nature of the structural lesion. They found that at 2-year follow-up, the percentage of patients with persistent seizures following lesionectomy ranged from 1.4 to 4 times that following seizure surgery, depending on the nature of the lesion. Low-grade astrocytomas, gangliogliomas, and vascular malformations were most successfully treated with seizure surgery, and high-grade gliomas were associated with a high proportion of continuing seizures, irrespective of the type of surgery.

Other factors have been shown to influence the likelihood of continuing or recurrent seizures following surgery for structural lesions. Several reports have demonstrated that, irrespective of the nature of the lesion, patients with fewer seizures before presentation, shorter preoperative seizure history, or seizures that readily responded to antiepileptic medications are more likely to be seizure free following lesionectomy alone.[139, 140, 143–147] Concordance of preoperative data—that is, ictal semiology and interictal and ictal EEG all consistent with lesion location on imaging—has also been associated with good seizure outcomes following lesionectomy.[148–151] Lesion location may influence seizure outcome. Lesionectomy for structural lesions in the temporal lobe may be more likely associated with persistent or recurrent seizures than is seizure surgery with resection of mesial temporal structures in addition to extratemporal lesionectomy.[138, 151, 152] Extent of resection of gliomas has been associated with seizure outcome.[13, 134] Awad and colleagues[13] demonstrated that macroscopically complete resection was associated with postoperative seizure control in 93% of their cases. However, when macroscopically complete resection was not possible, incomplete resection of the tumor but complete resection of the seizure focus identified with interictal or ictal scalp EEG and chronically implanted subdural electrodes was associated with seizure control in 83% of cases.

The relative merits of interictal versus ictal recordings in identifying the epileptogenic zone in patients with structural lesions and medically refractory epilepsy are also controversial. Several studies attempted to address the relative value of one technique or the other, although no randomized, controlled comparisons are available.[13, 14, 118, 139, 153–155] Awad and colleagues[13] demonstrated that resecting the ictal onset zone identified by chronic subdural electrodes in patients with incompletely resected gliomas was associated with markedly greater seizure control rates than incomplete resection of both tumor and ictal onset zone. Others demonstrated that improved seizure outcomes are associated with the absence of interictal epileptiform activity outside the resection margins on intraoperative preresection or postresection ECoG.[139, 154, 155]

TECHNICAL ASPECTS OF TAILORED RESECTION AT THE UNIVERSITY OF WASHINGTON

Resections tailored to the location of interictal epileptiform discharges on ECoG and eloquent cortex identified by electrical stimulation mapping can be conducted with the patient under general anesthesia, except that there is no intraoperative technique for individually localizing language or memory in that setting. However, because general anesthesia interferes with the accuracy of both techniques to some extent, ideally, they are used in awake patients. The advent of propofol intravenous anesthesia has made awake craniotomy much easier for both the patient and the surgeon.[156] The only demand now made on patients is that they hold still for 1 to 2 hours while awake. Thus, the technique can be used in children aged 12 years or older and in most adolescents and adults. It can also be safely used in the presence of an intracranial mass, although the brain will be slightly tighter than is usually observed with modem endotracheal anesthesia, and it may be necessary to be slightly more aggressive with the use of intravenous osmotic agents in that setting compared with general anesthesia. Although propofol alters the ECoG when it is administered, those effects rapidly clear when it is discontinued.

We now use only the lateral position with propofol. In that position, we have had no difficulties maintaining an airway, whereas some problems have occurred in patients in the supine position. The patient is positioned while awake, with particular attention to comfort. The head rests on a foam ring, and skeletal fixation is not used. Propofol anesthesia is then induced intravenously. Once the patient is asleep, a local anesthetic field block is placed, using a mixture of equal volumes of 0.5% lidocaine and 0.25% bupivacaine, both with 1:200,000 epinephrine. Propofol is not a particularly good analgesic, so a patient under propofol anesthesia often shows some reaction to the placement of this block. The block is performed by first making injections slowly through a needle, initially 30 gauge, at sites near the major scalp nerves and then completing the block around the entire area of the planned incision. Use of small amounts of intravenous fentanyl is of value in reducing the patient's response to placement of the block. If the incision is to extend to the root of the zygoma, the temporalis muscle is also infiltrated. The scalp incision and craniotomy then proceed in the usual manner. Once the dura is exposed, dural pain sensation is blocked by intradural injection of small quantities of local anesthetic around the middle meningeal artery, using the 30-gauge needle. A clamp is placed on the skull at the edge of the craniotomy, not only to provide a place to attach ECoG recording equipment but also to provide a handle to control the head if the patient becomes restless.

At this point, all pain-sensitive structures have been blocked with local anesthetic, and the bone removal is completed with the patient asleep. The lateral surface of the brain is insensitive to pain or touch. We usually wake the patient before opening the dura, unless that opening is expected to be very tedious, such as when extensive pial-dural adhesions are anticipated. The patient is usually conversant within 5 to 15 minutes of stopping the propofol. At that time, the patient is reminded that he or she is in the operating room and should not move his or her head without first asking. The longest period before waking in our experience has been 45 minutes. The patient usually wakens abruptly, which is a major advantage of propofol, and there is commonly no period of confusion. Very rarely, a patient may have seizures when awake. Short-acting benzodiazepines or barbiturates may be needed to control them, but use of these drugs interferes with subsequent recording and stimulation.

The standard technique for individually identifying functionally important areas is electrical stimulation mapping. The topic of functional mapping is covered in another chapter. However, pertinent aspects of the technique used at the University of Washington are discussed here. Several technical factors are important to successful stimulation mapping:

1. Mapping is difficult beyond the edges of the craniotomy. The exposure should thus be generous and include likely locations of functionally important areas.
2. Sites where language is located must be identified, because only then does the absence of language changes indicate cortex that can be resected with a low risk of aphasia. This also requires that the exposure include likely sites for language.
3. The stimulating current must be sufficient to alter function in cortex, but not so great as to evoke a seizure.
4. The patient must make few errors on the language measure in the absence of stimulation. Only a few samples of stimulation effect at any one site can be obtained. If there are many errors in the absence of stimulation, errors during stimulation may be random events and not related to stimulation effects at that site. We regularly obtain three samples of stimulation effect at each site. For errors on all samples to have less than a 5% probability of being random events, the error rate in the absence of stimulation must not exceed 20%. Thus, stimulation mapping is of limited value in severely aphasic patients. Patients with mild aphasia may not be able to name with a low enough control error rate, but they may be able to read single words or can be continuously engaged in conversation during stimulation, although neither technique is as satisfactory as naming for localizing language.

The only parameters of stimulation varied at the University of Washington are the current level and train duration. All stimulations use 60-Hz trains of biphasic pulses, each phase 1 msec in duration, delivered from a constant current stimulator across 1-mm stainless steel bipolar ball electrodes placed 5 mm apart. Most other contemporary stimulation techniques use shorter pulses, often 0.3 msec for each phase, and some use 30-Hz frequency but are otherwise similar. Levels of electrical charge that produce histologic changes in tissue have been extensively studied in animals.[157] Histologic examination of stimulation sites in resected human cortex has not shown any changes in our patients (unpublished data). Moreover, patients' performance in the absence of stimulation does not deteriorate after repeated stimulations. These findings indicate that stimulation at the indicated parameters does not permanently alter cortex.

After the patient is wakened and the dura opened, ECoG recording is performed. As the patient recovers from the propofol anesthesia, a typical burst-suppression ECoG pattern is seen, which changes to a continuous recording once the patient is awake. An additional advantage of propofol, in our view, is in recording the interictal ECoG in the small number of patients who have interictal epileptiform activity predominantly during sleep. It is our impression that rapidly waking and then resedating these patients with propofol allows the identification of interictal discharges during this period that would not be seen during recording with the patient fully awake. The goal of the ECoG recording is to delineate the full extent of interictal spikes. To this end, subdural strip electrodes are placed over cortical areas not immediately under the craniotomy, such as basal temporal cortex, orbital frontal surface, or medial face of a hemisphere. Recordings are obtained from the lateral surface through carbon ball electrodes. We use referential ECoG recordings to a linked neck reference. Ten to 15 minutes of continuous ECoG recording is observed before the next phase of the procedure.

At the completion of this recording, sensorimotor cortex is first identified. We use stimulus trains beginning at 2 mÅ, asking the patient for any evoked sensory responses, while an assistant looks for any overt movements. Current is increased at 1-mÅ intervals until responses are obtained. The site of each positive response is identified with a sterile numbered ticket. Motor cortex can also be identified with stimulation of the patient under general anesthesia, so long as the patient is not paralyzed. However, patient responses under general anesthesia are much less focal, no sensory information is available, and tongue movements are difficult to identify. Recording of somatosensory evoked responses is an alternative technique for identifying sensory cortex while the patient is under general anesthesia, but in patients who are awake, that procedure requires more time and provides less information than stimulation mapping.

Following identification of the rolandic cortex, sterile numbered tickets are placed across the remaining cortex that is to be mapped for language sites (Fig. 159–1). The choice of language measure to use with stimulation mapping is somewhat controversial. Penfield used object naming, which has an advantage as a screening measure for language function because all perisylvian aphasic syndromes include deficits in naming. This is the language measure most often used at the University of Washington.[58] However, others have used reading measures as a screening test.[9, 158]

Before commencing naming tasks, the afterdischarge threshold is established for the area of cortex that will undergo language mapping. A small current, commonly 2 mÅ between pulse peaks, is applied for 4 seconds to cortex adjacent to an ECoG electrode. In the case of temporal exposures, thresholds are first determined for more posterior electrodes. This stimulation is repeated at increasing currents until afterdischarges are evoked, the patient reports a response, or an arbitrary upper limit on current is reached, usually 10 mÅ between pulse peaks for direct cortical stimulation. The current is then reduced 1 mÅ below the afterdischarge threshold, and the threshold at the next most anterior electrode is determined. After all electrodes have been sampled, which takes 5 to 10 minutes, a current is selected for mapping that is at the lowest threshold for afterdischarge. The main reason for establishing the afterdischarge threshold is to avoid evoking a seizure. In addition, using the maximal current that can be applied without inducing a seizure minimizes the risk that failure to elicit speech arrest or a speech error at a given cortical site is due to an inadequate stimulating current rather than that the stimulated cortical site is noneloquent for language.

The patient then begins the naming task. We use slide pictures of common objects to elicit naming, showing each slide at 4-second intervals on a slide projector. A 4-second stimulation train is applied to one of the sites identified by a numbered ticket at the appearance of the second or third slide. An assistant records the patient's responses and the number of the site stimulated. Another site is stimulated two or three slides later, until all sites have been sampled once. The process is then repeated in a different order two more times, so that stimulation effects on naming have been determined three times for each site. Sites with re-

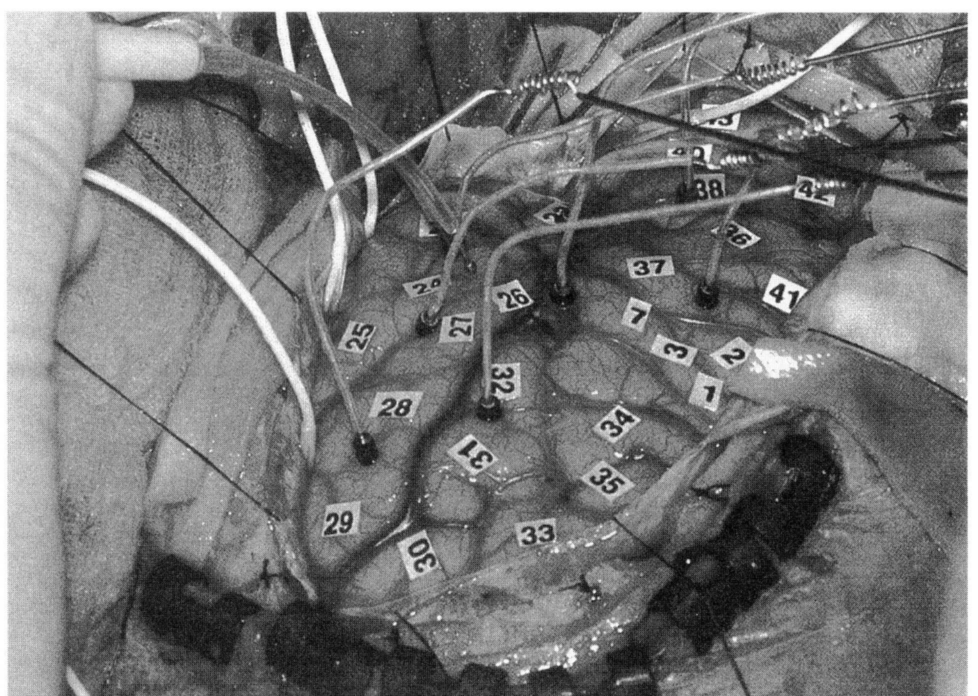

FIGURE 159–1. For language mapping, sterile numbered tickets are placed randomly across the cortex to be mapped. The awake patient then begins naming objects presented as slides on a projector screen. Every second or third slide, a cortical site adjacent to a numbered ticket is stimulated with the bipolar probe for 4 seconds while an assistant records the patient's response and the number of the site stimulated. This is repeated until each site has been stimulated at least three times.

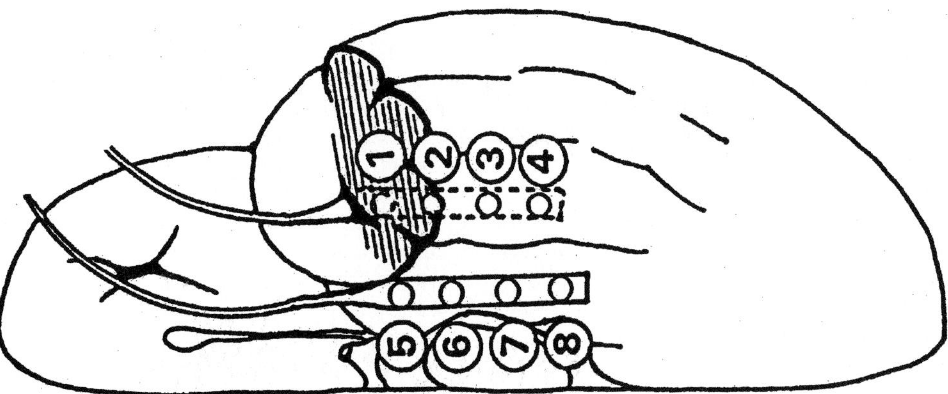

FIGURE 159–2. Following resection of the anterolateral temporal neocortex and opening of the ventricle, a four-contact strip electrode is placed directly on the hippocampus within the ventricle, and another is placed parallel to it on the parahippocampal gyrus, for intraoperative electrocorticography.

peated naming errors are considered essential for language. With this technique, stimulation effects on naming can be determined for 20 sites in about 20 minutes. Stimulation mapping with other language measures follows this same general plan, although the relation of applying the current to the behavioral measures may vary, especially when assessing memory. The senior author's protocol for assessing cortical stimulation effects on the input, storage, or retrieval phases of recent verbal memory has been published.[99]

The initial resection is designed to remove all tissue with interictal spikes identified during ECoG and any grossly evident lesion, unless the tissue is functionally important. The resection is usually undertaken after restarting propofol anesthesia, unless tissue very close to an area essential for language or motor functions is to be removed. In this case, that portion of the resection is performed while testing the patient's function, stopping the resection when the function begins to fail. If stopped at that point, any postoperative deficit is only transient. This technique is particularly important for the occasional patient in whom no language sites are identified during cortical stimulation in the region of the proposed resection. This may be because there is

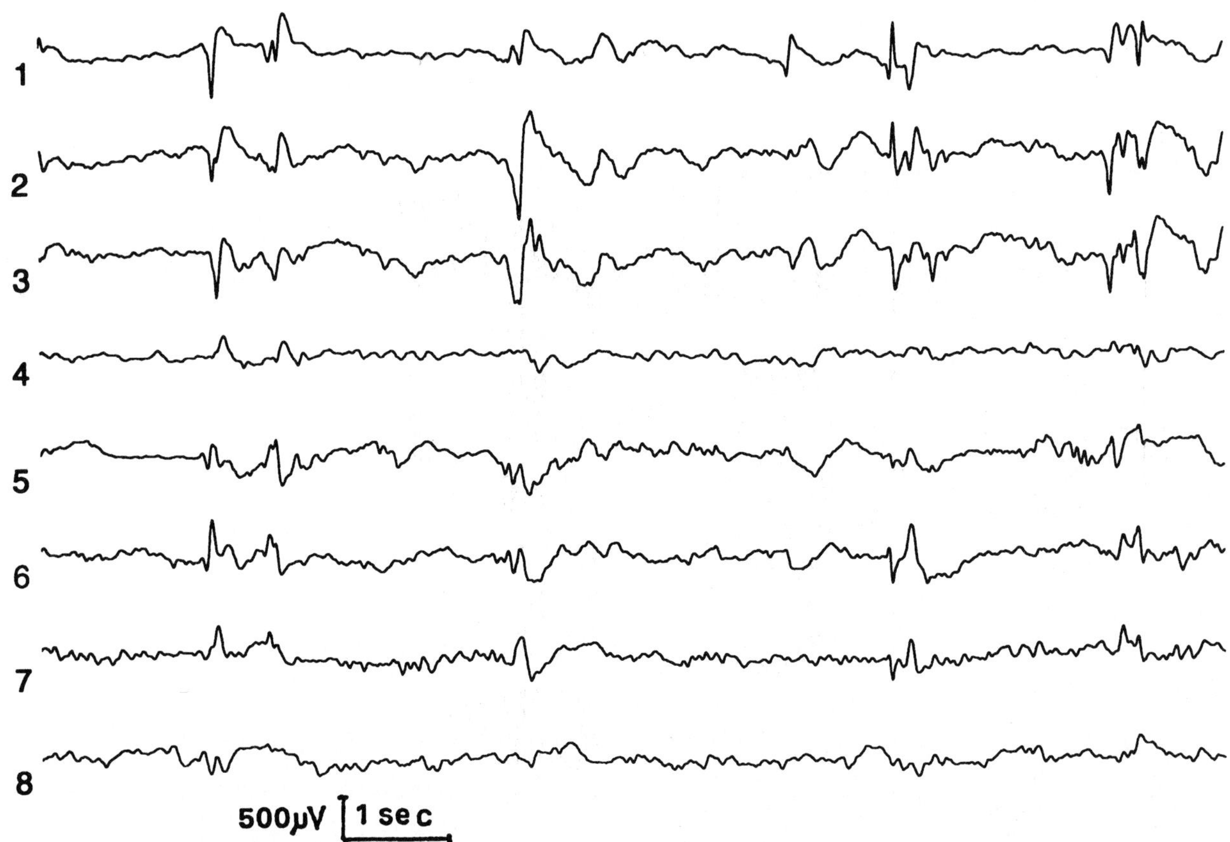

FIGURE 159–3. A typical intraoperative recording from the hippocampus (leads 1 to 4), and parahippocampal gyrus (leads 5 to 8). In this case, the hippocampus underlying contacts 1 to 3 would be resected, ending the hippocampal resection between contacts 3 and 4.

no eloquent cortex for language in the area stimulated. For example, in the senior author's series, naming sites were identified only in the frontal lobe in 17% and only in the temporoparietal lobe in 15% of patients, despite the classic model of language localization describing a frontal and temporoparietal site in all patients.[58] Alternatively, absence of language sites in the expected areas may reflect such low afterdischarge thresholds that the stimulating current is below that required to disrupt naming tasks. In this setting, the initial cortical resection is performed with the patient awake and performing naming tasks.

In temporal lobe resections, we repeat the ECoG recording after removing the lateral cortex and opening the ventricle, placing a four-contact subdural strip directly on the hippocampus and another one parallel to it on the parahippocampal gyrus (Fig. 159–2). Hippocampal surface interictal epileptiform spikes are typically positive, whereas those recorded from the parahippocampal gyrus are typically negative (Fig. 159–3). The location of interictal spikes on recordings from these electrodes is used to plan the extent of the medial temporal resection, unless concerns about memory necessitate a more limited hippocampal removal. Propofol is briefly turned off for this recording, restarted for the mesial resection, and then stopped again for a final ECoG recording after completion of the resection (Fig. 159–4). The presence of interictal spikes in some locations on this postresection ECoG, such as discharges in the insula, is not an indication for further resection. Following resection, interictal spikes sometimes appear at lateral cortical sites where they were previously absent. Whether this finding is an indication for further resection is still controversial, and we do not perform further resection in this setting. Propofol anesthesia is restarted for closure of the craniotomy.

CONCLUSION

Although the effectiveness of surgery for medically refractory epilepsy in carefully selected patients has been documented repeatedly, similarly good seizure outcomes have been demonstrated using several different techniques based on divergent views on the optimal method to identify Luders's putative epileptogenic zone. In addition, although avoiding neurological and cognitive morbidity is the goal of all resective epilepsy surgery, there are differing views on the variability of eloquent cortex, particularly for language and memory, and on the optimal functional mapping technique, either intraoperative or extraoperative. In the absence of any randomized, controlled trials with large numbers of matched cases, it is difficult to absolutely endorse any surgical philosophy for the management of medically refractory epilepsy.

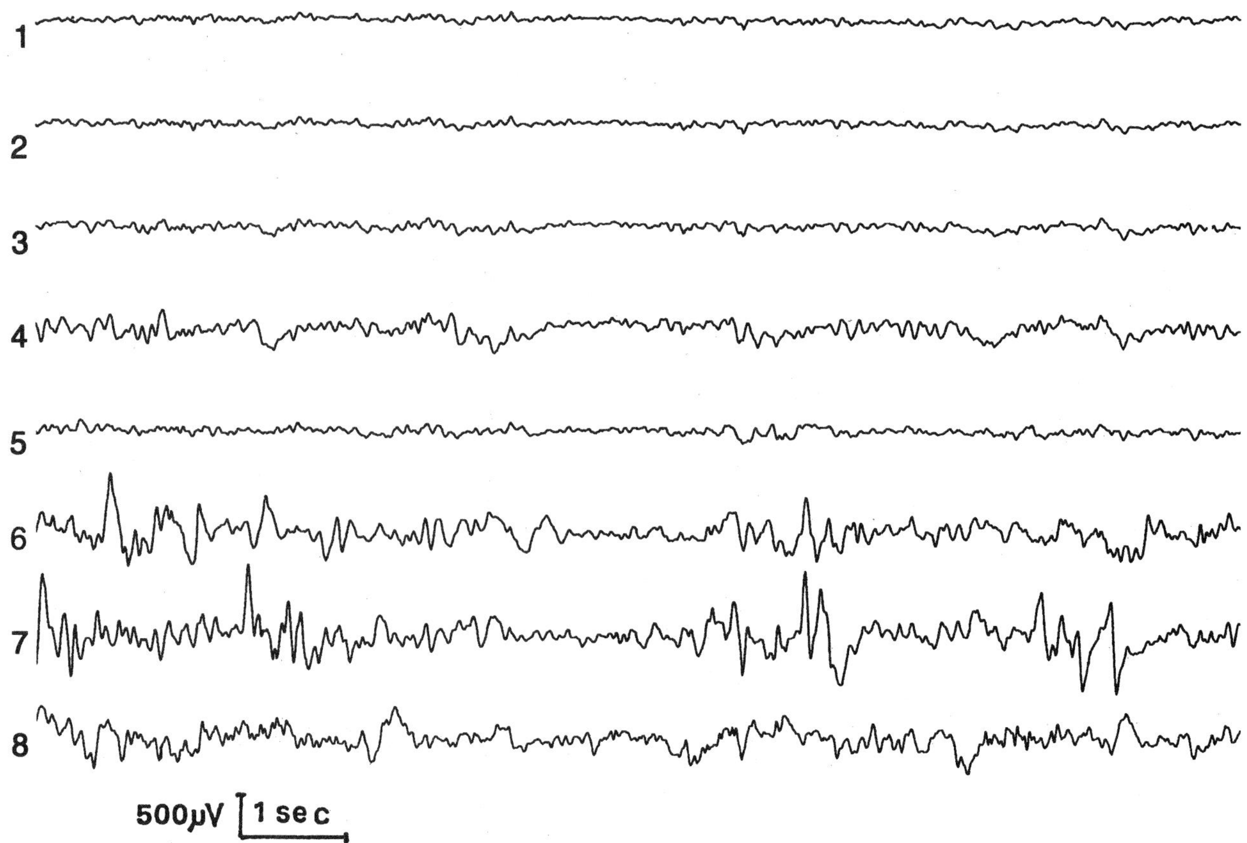

FIGURE 159–4. Following completion of the hippocampal resection, the two strip electrodes are repositioned in contact with residual hippocampus and parahippocampal gyrus, and electrocorticography is repeated. No further epileptiform discharges should be evident.

At the University of Washington, we tailor surgical resections for medically refractory epilepsy to the individual patient's pathophysiology and functional anatomy. In the setting of mesial TLE, intraoperative ECoG is performed before resection. In the majority of cases, no or few interictal discharges are identified from the lateral neocortex but are seen from the mesial basal region initially and then from the hippocampus when direct hippocampal recordings are performed after the lateral neocortical resection. In these cases, lateral resection is performed to allow access to the mesial structures. In all dominant temporal resections, language mapping is performed to identify eloquent language cortex and ensure that it is not located anteriorly within the proposed lateral resection. Memory mapping is also performed intraoperatively in selected patients considered to be at high risk for postoperative verbal memory decline based on the presence of preoperative risk factors such as high verbal memory scores, absence of ipsilateral hippocampal atrophy on MRI, results of the intracarotid amobarbital procedure, and late age of seizure onset. In the minority of cases found to have interictal discharges arising from both mesial basal and lateral temporal cortex, the lateral resection is tailored to include the lateral interictal discharges. Following the lateral resection, the extent of hippocampal resection is tailored to the location of interictal discharges recorded directly from the hippocampus.

In the setting of nonlesional neocortical epilepsy, invasive monitoring with subdural grids or strips is generally performed. The positioning of the grid for invasive recordings is determined from the seizure semiology and the location of ictal onset on scalp recordings. The subsequent resection is predominantly tailored to the ictal onset zone determined from the invasive recordings. However, areas of localized interictal epileptiform discharge are also resected if possible, based on our experience that exclusively unilateral, unifocal interictal epileptiform activity on scalp EEG is highly predictive of good seizure outcome.[107] The management of patients with structural lesions and epilepsy at our institution depends on the presence of risk factors associated with seizure recurrence following lesionectomy alone. If such factors are present, invasive monitoring and extraoperative functional mapping with subdural grids or strips are generally performed.

REFERENCES

1. Luders H, Awad I: Conceptual considerations. 51–62, 1992.
2. Horsley V: Brain surgery. BMJ 2:670–675, 1886.
3. Krause F: Die Operative Behandlung Der Epilepsie. Med Klin Berlin 5:1418–1422, 1909.
4. Foerster O: Zur Pathogenese Und Chirurgischen Behandlung Der Epilepsie. Zentralbl Chir 52:531–549, 1925.
5. Foerster O, Altenburger H: Elektrobiologische Vorgange an Der Menslichen Hirnrinde. Dtsch Z Nervenkr 135:277–288, 1935.
6. Penfield W, Roberts L: Speech and Brain Mechanisms. 1959.
7. Penfield W, Jasper H: Epilepsy and the Functional Anatomy of the Human Brain. 1954.
8. Talairach J, De Ajuriaguerra J, David M: Etudes Stereotaxiques Des Structures Encephaliques Profondes Chez L'Homme. Presse Med 60:605–609, 1952.
9. Luders H, Hahn J, Lesser RP, et al: Basal temporal subdural electrodes in the evaluation of patients with intractable epilepsy. Epilepsia 30:131–142, 1989.
10. Crandall PH, Walter RD, Rand RW: Clinical applications of studies on stereotactically implanted electrodes in temporal lobe epilepsy. J Neurosurg 20:827–840, 1963.
11. Lieb JP, Walsh GO, Babb TL, et al: A comparison of EEG seizure patterns recorded with surface and depth electrodes in patients with temporal lobe epilepsy. Epilepsia 17:137–160, 1976.
12. Spencer SS: Depth electroencephalography in selection of refractory epilepsy for surgery. Ann Neurol 9:207–214, 1981.
13. Awad IA, Rosenfeld J, Ahl J, et al: Intractable epilepsy and structural lesions of the brain: Mapping, resection strategies, and seizure outcome. Epilepsia 32:179–186, 1991.
14. Berger MS, Ghatan S, Haglund MM, et al: Low-grade gliomas associated with intractable epilepsy: Seizure outcome utilizing electrocorticography during tumor resection. J Neurosurg 79: 62–69, 1993.
15. Margerison JH, Corsellis JAN: Epilepsy in the temporal lobes. Brain 89:499–530, 1966.
16. Falconer MA: Discussion on the surgery of temporal lobe epilepsy. Proc R Soc Med 46:971–975, 1953.
17. Fried I: Anatomic temporal lobe resections for temporal lobe epilepsy. Neurosurg Clin N Am 4:233–242, 1993.
18. Niemeyer P: The transventricular amygdala-hippocampectomy in temporal lobe epilepsy. 461–482, 1958.
19. Wieser HG, Yasargil MG: Selective amygdalohippocampectomy as a surgical treatment of mesiobasal limbic epilepsy. Surg Neurol 17:445–457, 1982.
20. Penfield W, Flanigin HF: Surgical therapy of temporal lobe seizures. Arch Neurol Psychiatry 64:491–500, 1950.
21. Jasper H, Pertuisset B, Flanigin HF: EEG and cortical electrograms in patients with temporal lobe seizures. Arch Neurol Psychiatry 65:272–290, 1951.
22. Bailey P, Gibbs FA: The surgical treatment of psychomotor epilepsy. JAMA 145:365–370, 1951.
23. Diehl B, Luders HO: Temporal lobe epilepsy: When are invasive recordings needed? Epilepsia 41(Suppl 3):S61–S74, 2000.
24. Binnie CD, Alarcon G, Elwes RD, et al: Role of ECoG in "en bloc" temporal lobe resection: The Maudsley experience. Electroencephalogr Clin Neurophysiol Suppl 48:17–23, 1998.
25. Cascino GD, Trenerry MR, Jack CR Jr, et al: Electrocorticography and temporal lobe epilepsy: Relationship to quantitative MRI and operative outcome. Epilepsia 36:692–696, 1995.
26. McBride MC, Binnie CD, Janota I, Polkey CE: Predictive value of intraoperative electrocorticograms in resective epilepsy surgery. Ann Neurol 30:526–532, 1991.
27. Schwartz TH, Bazil CW, Walczak TS, et al: The predictive value of intraoperative electrocorticography in resections for limbic epilepsy associated with mesial temporal sclerosis. Neurosurgery 40:302–309, 1997.
28. Tran TA, Spencer SS, Marks D, et al: Significance of spikes recorded on electrocorticography in nonlesional medial temporal lobe epilepsy. Ann Neurol 38:763–770, 1995.
29. Engel J Jr, Driver MV, Falconer MA: Electrophysiological correlates of pathology and surgical results in temporal lobe epilepsy. Brain 98:129–156, 1975.
30. Kanazawa O, Blume WT, Girvin JP: Significance of spikes at temporal lobe electrocorticography. Epilepsia 37:50–55, 1996.
31. Rasmussen TB: Surgical treatment of complex partial seizures: Results, lessons, and problems. Epilepsia 24(Suppl 1):S65–S76, 1983.
32. Tuunainen A, Nousiainen U, Mervaala E, et al: Postoperative EEG and electrocorticography: Relation to clinical outcome in patients with temporal lobe surgery. Epilepsia 35:1165–1173, 1994.
33. Wyllie E, Luders H, Morris HH III, et al: Clinical outcome after complete or partial cortical resection for intractable epilepsy. Neurology 37:1634–1641, 1987.
34. Fenyes I, Zoltan I, Fenyes G: Temporal lobe epilepsies with deep seated epileptogenic foci. Arch Neurol 4:103–115, 1961.
35. Devinsky O, Canevini MP, Sato S, et al: Quantitative electrocorticography in patients undergoing temporal lobectomy. J Epilepsy 5:178–185, 1992.
36. Graf M, Niedermeyer E, Schiemann J, et al: Electrocorticogra-

phy: Information derived from intraoperative recordings during seizure surgery. Clin Electroencephalogr 15:83–91, 1984.
37. Chatrian GE, Tsai ML, Temkin NR, et al: Role of the ECoG in tailored temporal lobe resection: The University of Washington experience. Electroencephalogr Clin Neurophysiol Suppl 48:24–43, 1998.
38. Bengzon AR, Rasmussen T, Gloor P, et al: Prognostic factors in the surgical treatment of temporal lobe epileptics. Neurology 18:717–731, 1968.
39. Fiol ME, Gates JR, Torres F, Maxwell RE: The prognostic value of residual spikes in the postexcision electrocorticogram after temporal lobectomy. Neurology 41:512–516, 1991.
40. Stefan H, Quesney LF, Abou-Khalil B, Olivier A: Electrocorticography in temporal lobe epilepsy surgery. Acta Neurol Scand 83:65–72, 1991.
41. So N, Olivier A, Andermann F, et al: Results of surgical treatment in patients with bitemporal epileptiform abnormalities. Ann Neurol 25:432–439, 1989.
42. Alarcon G, Garcia Seoane JJ, Binnie CD, et al: Origin and propagation of interictal discharges in the acute electrocorticogram: Implications for pathophysiology and surgical treatment of temporal lobe epilepsy. Brain 120:2259–2282, 1997.
43. Alarcon G, Guy CN, Binnie CD, et al: Intracerebral propagation of interictal activity in partial epilepsy: Implications for source localisation. J Neurol Neurosurg Psychiatry 57:435–449, 1994.
44. Engel J Jr: Outcome with respect to epileptic seizures. 553–571, 1987.
45. Wyler AR, Hermann BP, Somes G: Extent of medial temporal resection on outcome from anterior temporal lobectomy: A randomized prospective study. Neurosurgery 37:982–990, 1995; see comments.
46. Nayel MH, Awad IA, Luders H: Extent of mesiobasal resection determines outcome after temporal lobectomy for intractable complex partial seizures. Neurosurgery 29:55–60, 1991.
47. Awad IA, Katz A, Hahn JF, et al: Extent of resection in temporal lobectomy for epilepsy. I. Interobserver analysis and correlation with seizure outcome. Epilepsia 30:756–762, 1989.
48. Awad IA, Nayel MH, Luders H: Second operation after the failure of previous resection for epilepsy. Neurosurgery 28:510–518, 1991.
49. Germano IM, Poulin N, Olivier A: Reoperation for recurrent temporal lobe epilepsy. J Neurosurg 81:31–36, 1994.
50. Feindel W, Rasmussen T: Temporal lobectomy with amygdalectomy and minimal hippocampal resection: Review of 100 cases. Can J Neurol Sci 18:603–605, 1991.
51. Jooma R, Yeh HS, Privitera MD, et al: Seizure control and extent of mesial temporal resection. Acta Neurochir (Wien) 133: 44–49, 1995.
52. Kanner AM, Kaydanova Y, Toledo-Morrell L, et al: Tailored anterior temporal lobectomy: Relation between extent of resection of mesial structures and postsurgical seizure outcome. Arch Neurol 52:173–178, 1995.
53. McKhann GM, Schoenfeld-McNeill J, Born DE, et al: Intraoperative hippocampal electrocorticography to predict the extent of hippocampal resection in temporal lobe epilepsy surgery. J Neurosurg 93:44–52, 2000.
54. Rasmussen T, Feindel W: Temporal lobectomy: Review of 100 cases with major hippocampectomy. Can J Neurol Sci 18:601–602, 1991.
55. Son EI, Howard MA, Ojemann GA, Lettich E: Comparing the extent of hippocampal removal to the outcome in terms of seizure control. Stereotact Funct Neurosurg 62:232–237, 1994.
56. Burnstine TH, Lesser RP, Hart J Jr, et al: Characterization of the basal temporal language area in patients with left temporal lobe epilepsy. Neurology 40:966–970, 1990.
57. Davies KG, Maxwell RE, Jennum P, et al: Language function following subdural grid-directed temporal lobectomy. Acta Neurol Scand 90:201–206, 1994.
58. Ojemann G, Ojemann J, Lettich E, Berger M: Cortical language localization in left, dominant hemisphere: An electrical stimulation mapping investigation in 117 patients. J Neurosurg 71: 316–326, 1989.
59. Ojemann GA, Whitaker HA: Language localization and variability. Brain Lang 6:239–260, 1978.
60. Ojemann GA: Individual variability in cortical localization of language. J Neurosurg 50:164–169, 1979.
61. Schwartz TH, Devinsky O, Doyle W, Perrine K: Preoperative predictors of anterior temporal language areas. J Neurosurg 89: 962–970, 1998.
62. Haglund MM, Berger MS, Shamseldin M, et al: Cortical localization of temporal lobe language sites in patients with gliomas. Neurosurgery 34:567–576, 1994.
63. Ojemann GA: Electrical stimulation and the neurobiology of language. Behav Brain Sci 6:221–230, 1983.
64. Devinsky O, Perrine K, Llinas R, et al: Anterior temporal language areas in patients with early onset of temporal lobe epilepsy. Ann Neurol 34:727–732, 1993.
65. Devinsky O, Perrine K, Hirsch J, et al: Relation of cortical language distribution and cognitive function in surgical epilepsy patients. Epilepsia 41:400–404, 2000.
66. Saykin AJ, Stafiniak P, Robinson LJ, et al: Language before and after temporal lobectomy: Specificity of acute changes and relation to early risk factors. Epilepsia 36:1071–1077, 1995.
67. Stafiniak P, Saykin AJ, Sperling MR, et al: Acute naming deficits following dominant temporal lobectomy: Prediction by age at 1st risk for seizures. Neurology 40:1509–1512, 1990.
68. Penfield W, Milner B: Memory deficit produced by bilateral lesions in the hippocampal zone. AMA Arch Neurol Psychiatry 79:475–497, 1958.
69. Scoville WB, Milner B: Loss of recent memory after bilateral hippocampal lesions: 1957 [classic article]. J Neuropsychiatry Clin Neurosci 12:103–113, 2000.
70. Milner B: Brain mechanisms suggested by studies of temporal lobes. 122–145, 1967.
71. Helmstaedter C, Elger CE: Cognitive consequences of two-thirds anterior temporal lobectomy on verbal memory in 144 patients: A three-month follow-up study. Epilepsia 37:171–180, 1996.
72. Hermann BP, Wyler AR, Bush AJ, Tabatabai FR: Differential effects of left and right anterior temporal lobectomy on verbal learning and memory performance. Epilepsia 33:289–297, 1992.
73. Ivnik RJ, Sharbrough FW, Laws ER Jr: Effects of anterior temporal lobectomy on cognitive function. J Clin Psychol 43:128–137, 1987.
74. Martin RC, Sawrie SM, Roth DL, et al: Individual memory change after anterior temporal lobectomy: A base rate analysis using regression-based outcome methodology. Epilepsia 39: 1075–1082, 1998.
75. Novelly RA, Augustine EA, Mattson RH, et al: Selective memory improvement and impairment in temporal lobectomy for epilepsy. Ann Neurol 15:64–67, 1984.
76. Powell GE, Polkey CE, McMillan T: The new Maudsley series of temporal lobectomy. I. Short-term cognitive effects. Br J Clin Psychol 24:109–124, 1985.
77. Baxendale SA, Thompson PJ, Kitchen ND: Postoperative hippocampal remnant shrinkage and memory decline: A dynamic process. Neurology 55:243–249, 2000.
78. Katz A, Awad IA, Kong AK, et al: Extent of resection in temporal lobectomy for epilepsy. II. Memory changes and neurologic complications. Epilepsia 30:763–771, 1989.
79. Kim HI, Olivier A, Jones-Gotman M, et al: Corticoamygdalectomy in memory-impaired patients. Stereotact Funct Neurosurg 58:162–167, 1992.
80. Milner B: Disorders of learning and memory after temporal lobe lesions in man. Clin Neurosurg 19:421–446, 1972.
81. Nunn JA, Polkey CE, Morris RG: Selective spatial memory impairment after right unilateral temporal lobectomy. Neuropsychologia 36:837–848, 1998.
82. Nunn JA, Graydon FJ, Polkey CE, Morris RG: Differential spatial memory impairment after right temporal lobectomy demonstrated using temporal titration. Brain 122:47–59, 1999.
83. Loring DW, Lee GP, Meador KJ, et al: Hippocampal contribution to verbal recent memory following dominant-hemisphere temporal lobectomy. J Clin Exp Neuropsychol 13:575–586, 1991.
84. Wolf RL, Ivnik RJ, Hirschorn KA, et al: Neurocognitive efficiency following left temporal lobectomy: Standard versus limited resection. J Neurosurg 79:76–83, 1993.
85. Baxendale SA, Van Paesschen W, Thompson PJ, et al: Hippocampal cell loss and gliosis: Relationship to preoperative and postoperative memory function. Neuropsychiatry Neuropsychol Behav Neurol 11:12–21, 1998.

86. Bell BD, Davies KG, Haltiner AM, Walters GL: Intracarotid amobarbital procedure and prediction of postoperative memory in patients with left temporal lobe epilepsy and hippocampal sclerosis. Epilepsia 41:992–997, 2000.
87. Bell BD, Davies KG: Anterior temporal lobectomy, hippocampal sclerosis, and memory: Recent neuropsychological findings. Neuropsychol Rev 8:25–41, 1998.
88. Davies KG, Bell BD, Bush AJ, et al: Naming decline after left anterior temporal lobectomy correlates with pathological status of resected hippocampus. Epilepsia 39:407–419, 1998.
89. Hermann BP, Wyler AR, Somes G, et al: Pathological status of the mesial temporal lobe predicts memory outcome from left anterior temporal lobectomy. Neurosurgery 31:652–656, 1992.
90. Kneebone AC, Chelune GJ, Dinner DS, et al: Intracarotid amobarbital procedure as a predictor of material-specific memory change after anterior temporal lobectomy. Epilepsia 36:857–865, 1995.
91. Sass KJ, Sass A, Westerveld M, et al: Specificity in the correlation of verbal memory and hippocampal neuron loss: Dissociation of memory, language, and verbal intellectual ability. J Clin Exp Neuropsychol 14:662–672, 1992.
92. Sass KJ, Westerveld M, Buchanan CP, et al: Degree of hippocampal neuron loss determines severity of verbal memory decrease after left anteromesiotemporal lobectomy. Epilepsia 35:1179–1186, 1994.
93. Seidenberg M, Hermann B, Wyler AR, et al: Neuropsychological outcome following anterior temporal lobectomy in patients with and without the syndrome of mesial temporal lobe epilepsy. Neuropsychology 12:303–316, 1998.
94. Trenerry MR, Jack CR Jr, Cascino GD, et al: Gender differences in post-temporal lobectomy verbal memory and relationships between MRI hippocampal volumes and preoperative verbal memory. Epilepsy Res 20:69–76, 1995.
95. Wyllie E, Naugle R, Awad I, et al: Intracarotid amobarbital procedure. I. Prediction of decreased modality-specific memory scores after temporal lobectomy. Epilepsia 32:857–864, 1991.
96. Lee GP, Loring DW, Smith JR, Flanigin HF: Intraoperative hippocampal cooling and Wada memory testing in the evaluation of amnesia risk following anterior temporal lobectomy. Arch Neurol 52:857–861, 1995.
97. Lee GP, Smith JR, Loring DW, Flanigin HF: Intraoperative thermal inactivation of the hippocampus in an effort to prevent global amnesia after temporal lobectomy. Epilepsia 36:892–898, 1995.
98. Helmstaedter C, Grunwald T, Lehnertz K, et al: Differential involvement of left temporolateral and temporomesial structures in verbal declarative learning and memory: Evidence from temporal lobe epilepsy. Brain Cogn 35:110–131, 1997.
99. Ojemann GA, Dodrill CB: Verbal memory deficits after left temporal lobectomy for epilepsy: Mechanism and intraoperative prediction. J Neurosurg 62:101–107, 1985.
100. Ojemann GA, Dodrill CB: Intraoperative techniques for reducing language and memory deficits with left temporal lobectomy. 327–330, 1987.
101. Perrine K, Devinsky O, Uysal S, et al: Left temporal neocortex mediation of verbal memory: Evidence from functional mapping with cortical stimulation. Neurology 44:1845–1850, 1994.
102. Ojemann GA: Organization of short-term verbal memory in language areas of human cortex: Evidence from electrical stimulation. Brain Lang 5:331–340, 1978.
103. Ojemann GA: Different approaches to resective epilepsy surgery: Standard and tailored. Epilepsy Res Suppl 5:169–174, 1992.
104. Dodrill CB, Wilkus RJ, Ojemann GA, et al: Multidisciplinary prediction of seizure relief from cortical resection surgery. Ann Neurol 20:2–12, 1986.
105. Harris AB: Absence of seizures or mirror foci in experimental epilepsy after excision of alumina and astrogliotic scar. Epilepsia 22:101–122, 1981.
106. Holmes MD, Dodrill CB, Wilensky AJ, et al: Unilateral focal preponderance of interictal epileptiform discharges as a predictor of seizure origin. Arch Neurol 53:228–232, 1996.
107. Holmes MD, Kutsy RL, Ojemann GA, et al: Interictal, unifocal spikes in refractory extratemporal epilepsy predict ictal origin and postsurgical outcome. Clin Neurophysiol 111:1802–1808, 2000.
108. Pauli E, Pickel S, Schulemann H, et al: Neuropsychologic findings depending on the type of the resection in temporal lobe epilepsy. Adv Neurol 81:371–377, 1999.
109. Davies KG, Maxwell RE, Beniak TE, et al: Language function after temporal lobectomy without stimulation mapping of cortical function. Epilepsia 36:130–136, 1995; see comments.
110. Hermann BP, Wyler AR, Somes G: Language function following anterior temporal lobectomy. J Neurosurg 74:560–566, 1991; see comments.
111. Hermann BP, Perrine K, Chelune GJ, et al: Visual confrontation naming following left anterior temporal lobectomy: A comparison of surgical approaches. Neuropsychology 13:3–9, 1999.
112. Ojemann G, Engel J Jr: Acute and chronic intracranial recording and stimulation. 263–289, 1987.
113. Luders H, Bustamanate L, Zablow L, et al: Quantitative studies of spike foci induced by minimal concentrations of penicillin. Electroencephalogr Clin Neurophysiol 48:80–89, 1980.
114. Cascino GD, Trenerry MR, So EL, et al: Routine EEG and temporal lobe epilepsy: Relation to long-term EEG monitoring, quantitative MRI, and operative outcome. Epilepsia 37:651–656, 1996.
115. Chee MW, Morris HH III, Antar MA, et al: Presurgical evaluation of temporal lobe epilepsy using interictal temporal spikes and positron emission tomography. Arch Neurol 50:45–48, 1993.
116. Gilliam F, Bowling S, Bilir E, et al: Association of combined MRI, interictal EEG, and ictal EEG results with outcome and pathology after temporal lobectomy. Epilepsia 38:1315–1320, 1997.
117. Schulz R, Luders HO, Hoppe M, et al: Interictal EEG and ictal scalp EEG propagation are highly predictive of surgical outcome in mesial temporal lobe epilepsy. Epilepsia 41:564–570, 2000.
118. Bautista RE, Cobbs MA, Spencer DD, Spencer SS: Prediction of surgical outcome by interictal epileptiform abnormalities during intracranial EEG monitoring in patients with extrahippocampal seizures. Epilepsia 40:880–890, 1999; see comments.
119. Hufnagel A, Elger CE, Pels H, et al: Prognostic significance of ictal and interictal epileptiform activity in temporal lobe epilepsy. Epilepsia 35:1146–1153, 1994.
120. Jennum P, Dhuna A, Davies K, et al: Outcome of resective surgery for intractable partial epilepsy guided by subdural electrode arrays. Acta Neurol Scand 87:434–437, 1993.
121. Wennberg R, Quesney F, Olivier A, Rasmussen T: Electrocorticography and outcome in frontal lobe epilepsy. Electroencephalogr Clin Neurophysiol 106:357–368, 1998.
122. Wennberg RA: Poor surgical outcome in patients with neocortical epilepsy is correlated with interictal epileptiform abnormalities outside the area of surgical resection [letter; comment]. Epilepsia 41:355–357, 2000.
123. Behrens E, Zentner J, Van Roost D, et al: Subdural and depth electrodes in the presurgical evaluation of epilepsy. Acta Neurochir (Wien) 128:84–87, 1994.
124. Swartz BE, Rich JR, Dwan PS, et al: The safety and efficacy of chronically implanted subdural electrodes: A prospective study. Surg Neurol 46:87–93, 1996.
125. Wiggins GC, Elisevich K, Smith BJ: Morbidity and infection in combined subdural grid and strip electrode investigation for intractable epilepsy. Epilepsy Res 37:73–80, 1999.
126. Wyler AR, Walker G, Somes G: The morbidity of long-term seizure monitoring using subdural strip electrodes. J Neurosurg 74:734–737, 1991; see comments.
127. Lesser R, Luders H, Dinner D, et al: The localisation of speech and writing functions in the frontal language area: Results of extraoperative cortical stimulation. Brain 107:275–291, 1984.
128. Berger MS, Kincaid J, Ojemann GA, Lettich E: Brain mapping techniques to maximize resection, safety, and seizure control in children with brain tumors. Neurosurgery 25:786–792, 1989.
129. Burchiel KJ, Clarke H, Ojemann GA, et al: Use of stimulation mapping and corticography in the excision of arteriovenous malformations in sensorimotor and language-related neocortex. Neurosurgery 24:322–327, 1989.
130. Devaux B, Chassoux F, Landre E, et al: Chronic intractable epilepsy associated with a tumor located in the central region: Functional mapping data and postoperative outcome. Stereotact Funct Neurosurg 69:229–238, 1997.
131. Gorecki JP, Smith RR, Wee AS: Excision of arteriovenous malfor-

mation in sensorimotor and language-related neocortex using stimulation mapping and corticography under local anesthesia. Stereotact Funct Neurosurg 58:89–, 1992.
132. Gregorie EM, Goldring S: Localization of function in the excision of lesions from the sensorimotor region. J Neurosurg 61: 1047–1054, 1984.
133. Son EI, Yi SD, Lee SW, et al: Surgery for seizure-related structural lesions of the brain with intraoperative acute recording (ECoG) and functional mapping. J Korean Med Sci 9:409–413, 1994.
134. Britton JW, Cascino GD, Sharbrough FW, Kelly PJ: Low-grade glial neoplasms and intractable partial epilepsy: Efficacy of surgical treatment. Epilepsia 35:1130–1135, 1994.
135. Casazza M, Avanzini G, Broggi G, et al: Epilepsy course in cerebral gangliogliomas: A study of 16 cases. Acta Neurochir Suppl (Wien) 46:17–20, 1989.
136. Goldring S, Rich KM, Picker S: Experience with gliomas in patients presenting with a chronic seizure disorder. Clin Neurosurg 33:15–42, 1986.
137. Goldring S, Gregorie EM: Experience with lesions that mimic gliomas in patients presenting with a chronic seizure disorder. Clin Neurosurg 33:43–70, 1986.
138. Jooma R, Yeh HS, Privitera MD, Gartner M: Lesionectomy versus electrophysiologically guided resection for temporal lobe tumors manifesting with complex partial seizures. J Neurosurg 83:231–236, 1995.
139. Rassi-Neto A, Ferraz FP, Campos CR, Braga FM: Patients with epileptic seizures and cerebral lesions who underwent lesionectomy restricted to or associated with the adjacent irritative area. Epilepsia 40:856–864, 1999.
140. Rossi GF, Pompucci A, Colicchio G, Scerrati M: Factors of surgical outcome in tumoural epilepsy. Acta Neurochir (Wien) 141: 819–824, 1999.
141. Spencer DD, Spencer SS, Mattson RH, Williamson PD: Intracerebral masses in patients with intractable partial epilepsy. Neurology 34:432–436, 1984.
142. Weber JP, Silbergeld DL, Winn HR: Surgical resection of epileptogenic cortex associated with structural lesions. Neurosurg Clin N Am 327–336, 1993.
143. Cappabianca P, Alfieri A, Maiuri F, et al: Supratentorial cavernous malformations and epilepsy: Seizure outcome after lesionectomy on a series of 35 patients. Clin Neurol Neurosurg 99: 179–183, 1997.
144. Cohen DS, Zubay GP, Goodman RR: Seizure outcome after lesionectomy for cavernous malformations. J Neurosurg 83:237–242, 1995.
145. Packer RJ, Sutton LN, Patel KM, et al: Seizure control following tumor surgery for childhood cortical low-grade gliomas. J Neurosurg 80:998–1003, 1994.
146. Yeh HS, Tew JM Jr, Gartner M: Seizure control after surgery on cerebral arteriovenous malformations. J Neurosurg 78:12–18, 1993.
147. Zevgaridis D, van Velthoven V, Ebeling U, Reulen HJ: Seizure control following surgery in supratentorial cavernous malformations: A retrospective study in 77 patients. Acta Neurochir (Wien) 138:672–677, 1996.
148. Casazza M, Broggi G, Franzini A, et al: Supratentorial cavernous angiomas and epileptic seizures: Preoperative course and postoperative outcome. Neurosurgery 39:26–32, 1996; see comments.
149. Casazza M, Avanzini G, Ciceri E, et al: Lesionectomy in epileptogenic temporal lobe lesions: Preoperative seizure course and postoperative outcome. Acta Neurochir Suppl (Wien) 68:64–69, 1997.
150. Kraemer DL, Griebel ML, Lee N, et al: Surgical outcome in patients with epilepsy with occult vascular malformations treated with lesionectomy. Epilepsia 39:600–607, 1998.
151. Lombardi D, Marsh R, de Tribolet N: Low grade glioma in intractable epilepsy: Lesionectomy versus epilepsy surgery. Acta Neurochir Suppl (Wien) 68:70–74, 1997.
152. Yeh HS, Kashiwagi S, Tew JM Jr, Berger TS: Surgical management of epilepsy associated with cerebral arteriovenous malformations. J Neurosurg 72:216–223, 1990.
153. Berger MS, Ghatan S, Geyer JR, et al: Seizure outcome in children with hemispheric tumors and associated intractable epilepsy: The role of tumor removal combined with seizure foci resection. Pediatr Neurosurg 17:185–191, 1991.
154. Tran TA, Spencer SS, Javidan M, et al: Significance of spikes recorded on intraoperative electrocorticography in patients with brain tumor and epilepsy. Epilepsia 38:1132–1139, 1997.
155. Wennberg R, Quesney LF, Lozano A, et al: Role of electrocorticography at surgery for lesion-related frontal lobe epilepsy. Can J Neurol Sci 26:33–39, 1999.
156. Silbergeld DL, Mueller WM, Colley PS, et al: Use of propofol (Diprivan) for awake craniotomies: Technical note. Surg Neurol 38:271–272, 1992.
157. Yuen TG, Agnew WF, Bullara LA, et al: Histological evaluation of neural damage from electrical stimulation: Considerations for the selection of parameters for clinical application. Neurosurgery 9:292–299, 1981.
158. Luders H, Lesser RP, Hahn J, et al: Basal temporal language area demonstrated by electrical stimulation. Neurology 36:505–510, 1986.

CHAPTER **160**

Topectomy: Uses and Indications

ATSUSHI UMEMURA ■ GORDON H. BALTUCH

Epilepsy remains one of the most common neurological disorders affecting adults and children. In most cases, seizures can be treated effectively with anticonvulsant medication. However, 5% to 10% of all new epilepsy patients ultimately become drug resistant.[1] These patients are considered to be medically intractable and should be considered for surgical treatment.

In the surgical treatment for epilepsy, there are two basic types of procedures: resection of epileptic focus and disconnection of electrical activity (Table 160–1). Resection is divided into hemispherectomy, lobectomy, and topectomy according to the area of the brain cut out. The term *topectomy* refers to resection of only the focal cerebral cortex identified as the source of seizures.

In general, resective procedures are much more effective at completely controlling seizures than disconnective procedures. The fundamental concept underlying a focal cortical resection is that the epileptic focus contains the epileptogenicity generating the patient's seizures. If this epileptogenic focus can be accurately identified and resected, the seizures will cease. The epileptogenicity is assumed to derive from neurons and their dendrites, but not axons.[2] Resection of only epileptogenic gray matter (i.e., cerebral cortex) rather than of white matter may be sufficient to suppress the seizures. Numerous pathologic studies have been performed on epileptogenic tissue removed from the human brain. The most characteristic and ubiquitous changes are the presence of gliosis, loss of neurons, and dendritic abnormalities.[3, 4]

The anterior temporal lobe and medial temporal structures are the most common part of the brain involved in epileptic foci, and resection of these structures is the most common type of epilepsy surgery. At the Montreal Neurological Institute, in a series covering the period from 1929 to 1980, the anatomic distribution of surgical resections in 2177 patients was as follows: temporal, 56%; frontal, 18%; central, 7%; parietal, 6%; occipital, 1%; and multilobar, 11%.[5] The term *topectomy* generally indicates resection of focal cerebral cortex from the frontal or parietal or the occipital lobes other than the temporal lobe. Generally, in the extratemporal resection, localization of the seizure origin is much more difficult, seizure outcome is less favorable, and there are higher risks of major morbidity than those in temporal resection.[6]

This chapter reviews the principles and methods of surgical localization and cortical resection in patients with extratemporal epilepsies.

TABLE 160–1 ■ **Surgical Treatment for Epilepsy**

Resection
Hemispherectomy: resection of cerebral hemisphere
Lobectomy: resection of one cerebral lobe
Topectomy: resection of focal cerebral cortex

Disconnection
Corpus callosotomy: disconnection of two hemispheres
Multiple subpial transection: disconnection of focal area of cerebral cortex

PATIENT SELECTION

As a general principle, surgical treatment for epilepsy should be considered when the seizure has not been controlled with adequate attempts of maximally tolerable doses of correct anticonvulsant medications; the seizure interferes with psychological and intellectual development, employment, or social performance; all potentially epileptogenic areas have matured, the seizure tendency (i.e., pattern and frequency) is stable, and there is no strong trend toward seizure reduction; and the patient is strongly motivated to cope with an exhaustive diagnostic regimen and a lengthy operative procedure under local anesthesia.[7–9] Chronic psychosis is a contraindication for surgical treatment, but epilepsy-related acute psychosis is not. Mental retardation is not a contraindication.[10, 11]

The length of time that patients have seizures before being referred for surgery has become shorter, and early intervention is recommended. For adults, the period was once 10 to 30 years, whereas adequate, but unsuccessful, antiepileptic drug therapy for 1 to 5 years may be sufficiently long enough for surgery to be considered today.[10]

Resective surgery should be considered only when

the seizure arises from a focal and not highly eloquent area of brain. Practically, this usually means that the focus is not in the speech or motor cortex. Multiple widespread or bilateral foci are usually contraindicated for resective surgery.

Clinical and electroencephalographic studies are necessary to confirm these criteria. Topectomy should be performed in noneloquent brain tissue. Multiple subpial transections may be indicated instead when eloquent brain is involved.

PRESURGICAL EVALUATION

The optimal resective surgery for epilepsy is to resect just enough neuronal tissue to eliminate seizures without causing additional unacceptable neurological or cognitive deficits. The purpose of presurgical evaluation in extratemporal cortical resection is determination of the volume of cortex involved in seizure initiation and propagation that must be removed. Surgery may be considered if this area is deemed to be resectable. As stated by Rasmussen,[12] epileptogenic lesions outside the temporal lobe are considerably more varied in extent and geographic configuration than the more common temporal lobe epileptogenic lesions. Several diagnostic tests are used for this purpose, but there is no consensus on how much information is needed before a particular surgical intervention can be recommended.[13]

The initial preoperative evaluation process includes careful examination of clinical seizure characteristics, ictal and interictal scalp electroencephalographic (EEG) findings, neuroimaging, and neuropsychological testing. The results of these tests should provide considerable lateralizing and localizing information. Usually, video-EEG monitoring is the gold standard of the evaluation. When noninvasive tests do not show the source of seizures clearly, an invasive test is considered. As for extratemporal nonlesional resection, localization of seizure focus is difficult, and invasive EEG studies are almost always required.[6]

Noninvasive Evaluation

SYMPTOMATIC LOCALIZATION

Some initial symptoms and signs have localizing value. A detailed history of the patient's behavior during the seizure includes a description of any aura, partial or generalized seizures, preservation or loss of consciousness, postictal dysphasia, or Todd's palsy. Although temporal lobe epilepsy is typically characterized by nonconvulsive seizures, extratemporal epilepsy more often generalizes.

In *frontal lobe seizures,* clinical localization of the seizure origin is extremely difficult because ictal behavioral manifestations in frontal lobe epilepsy largely result from seizure spread to neighboring or even more distant brain regions.[14] Rasmussen defined six types of onset:

1. Immediate loss of consciousness followed by generalized tonic-clonic convulsion
2. Loss of consciousness associated with initial head and eyes turning to the opposite side, followed by generalized convulsion, which suggests an origin in the anterior third of the frontal lobe
3. Initial turning of the head and eyes away from the side of the lesion with preserved consciousness and conscious contraversive attacks and then progressing to loss of consciousness and generalized convulsions, which suggests an origin in the convexity of the intermediate frontal region
4. Posturing movements of the body with tonic elevation of the contralateral arm, downward extension of the ipsilateral arm, and turning of the head away from the side of lesion, which suggests a discharging focus in the mesial aspect of the intermediate frontal region
5. A vague sensation in the head or in the body often followed by a brief arrest of activity, confused thinking, and staring, which is frequently followed by a generalized convulsive seizure
6. Seizure arising from the frontal lobe that may be associated with ictal or postictal automatisms, similar to those seen with temporal lobe epilepsy[15, 16]

In *central area seizures,* the attacks are somatomotor or somatosensory. In some patients, the attacks remain localized, but in most patients, a certain portion of the attacks progress to generalized convulsive seizures. Focal status epileptics and epilepsia partialis continua are particularly common.[16, 17]

In cases of *parietal lobe seizures,* most patients have attacks consisting of unilateral motor or sensory phenomena with additional features such as dizziness, cephalic sensation, contraversion, perceptual illusions, informed visual hallucinations, mental confusion, epigastric sensation, dysphasia, or automatism.[16, 17]

In *occipital lobe seizures,* visual symptomatology such as transient blindness or visual hallucinations usually characterized by flashes of lights, colored balls, and other geometric patterns have a strong relationship with seizure activity.[16]

Some initial seizure symptoms may not reflect the region of seizure origin, because many cortical regions, including most of the parietal lobe and the frontal-polar regions, are clinically silent in terms of seizure manifestations. In evaluating localization, it should be stressed that seizures originating in these regions may produce signs and symptoms only after spreading outside of the epileptogenic region.[18]

EXTRACRANIAL ELECTROENCEPHALOGRAPHY

The EEG assessment gives the most useful information on the location and size of the epileptogenic area. An interictal epileptiform abnormality consisting of spikes, spike and slow-wave complexes, sharp waves, and sharp- and slow-wave complexes repeated on several occasions may be significant.[19] Activation procedures such as medication withdrawal, hyperventilation, or drug-induced sleep may enhance abnormalities or even provoke a seizure.[7]

Long-term video-EEG monitoring is generally performed on an inpatient basis to correlate the seizure with appropriate electrical abnormalities and possibly to identify the seizure origin electrographically.[13] The specific clinical ictal symptoms can help greatly in some cases in which localization of the focus is problematic. The EEG pattern of seizure onset is most often rhythmic, fast, spikelike discharges, often building in amplitude.[9]

NEUROIMAGING

Magnetic resonance imaging (MRI) is the imaging modality of choice in patients with intractable partial epilepsy. Computed tomography (CT) is added to MRI because it demonstrates intracranial calcifications much better than MRI. MRI, especially three-dimensional volumetric studies, provides visualization of focal, dysplastic cortical lesions in many patients previously given a diagnosis of cryptogenic neocortical epilepsy.[13, 20] An MRI-identified epileptogenic lesion may indicate the cause of the seizure disorder. However, MRI-detected abnormalities should be highly correlated with the electrophysiologic findings before making a final determination about the origin of ictal onset.[21] MRI is extremely useful in the diagnosis of structural and developmental epileptogenic pathologies. Most have ischemic lesions or developmental lesions, specifically neuronal migration disorders.[22]

Structural lesions include ischemic infarctions (i.e., prenatal, perinatal, or postnatal), Sturge-Weber syndrome, and Rasmussen's encephalitis. For patients with Sturge-Weber syndrome, CT may provide diagnostic information of cerebral atrophy and intracranial calcifications. A progressive, unilateral cortical atrophy is demonstrated in Rasmussen's encephalitis. Among the developmental pathologies, unilateral megalencephaly is the most characteristic. The most common neuronal migration disorders are lissencephaly and diffuse pachygyria. A complete absence of gyri and sulci in lissencephaly and a few thick, wide gyri, separated by shallow sulci in diffuse pachygyria, are distinguished on MRI.[21]

Ictal-perfusion single photon–emission computed tomography (SPECT) may demonstrate increased blood flow at the site of seizure onset.[9, 23–25] The tracer isotope (usually technetium-99m hexamethyl-propyleneamineoxime [HMPAO]) is administered immediately after onset of seizure, and the scan may be obtained within several hours. There are some reports concerning localized hyperperfusion in ictal studies with frontal, parietal, or occipital epilepsies, but this technique is still used only in a few highly specialized epilepsy centers.[26, 27] Interictal SPECT has had limited value, occasionally showing locally reduced blood flow.[23]

Interictal positron-emission tomography (PET) with a tracer for glucose metabolism (i.e., ^{18}F-fluorodeoxyglucose) regularly demonstrates hypometabolism in the epileptic focus of temporal lobe epilepsy.[9, 28] However, PET is less reliable at identifying extratemporal, nonlesional foci.[19]

NEUROPSYCHOLOGICAL TESTING

Neuropsychological examinations contain a personality inventory and tests of memory, language function, and intelligence. These are useful in localization and lateralization of speech, memory, spatial, cognitive, and cerebral dominance functions. They also evaluate mental states such as mental retardation.[19, 29]

Invasive Evaluation

WADA TEST

Wada test (i.e., intracarotid Amytal test)[30] is performed to identify the dominant hemisphere for language function and the laterality of memory function. In the series from the Montreal Neurological Institute, 96% of right-handers had speech centers in the left cerebral hemisphere, and 4% had speech centers in the right hemisphere. In left-handed or ambidextrous individuals, 70% had speech areas on the left, 15% had speech areas on the right, and 15% had some representation of speech in each hemisphere. This test is necessary for all left-handed and ambidextrous patients and right-handed patients with some questionable evidence from psychological tests, x-ray films, electroencephalograms, or seizure patterns.[7] Unusual language lateralization is often seen in cases of the left hemisphere injury in early life or early onset of intractable epilepsy.[9]

INVASIVE ELECTROENCEPHALOGRAPHY

When an epileptogenic focus is not clearly lateralized (usually frontal lobe epilepsy) or localized after long-term scalp video–EEG monitoring, invasive EEG monitoring, which records information directly from the presumed epileptogenic region, is necessary for cortical resection. In extratemporal epilepsy, subdural strip electrodes are used primarily to lateralize an epileptogenic focus, and large subdural grids are used to define the limits of a focus that has already been lateralized but not sufficiently localized. It is important to cover as much as possible of the suspected area for accurate lateralization and localization.[19, 31–33]

Subdural strip electrodes are placed through a bur hole and passed blindly into the subdural space. Multiple electrodes may be inserted through one bur hole to cover wide regions of the brain. In patients with bifrontal discharges, strip electrodes are placed over the medial and lateral surfaces of the posterior frontal lobe from bur holes at the coronal suture, just off the midline.[9]

Subdural grid electrodes are placed with a craniotomy. These are used for determining the site of seizure onset over the convexity of one hemisphere and for extraoperative functional mapping (e.g., motor, sensory, speech functions) by stimulation of each electrode. Maximal removal area of an epileptogenic focus while preserving cortical function is determined by these evaluations.[5] In invasive EEG procedures, because the electrode leads are brought out through the scalp and the patient is monitored for a few weeks, the most common complication is infection, especially with a large subdural grid.[31]

SURGICAL PROCEDURE

General Principles

The extent of cortical resection is based on the results of the presurgical evaluation and of intraoperative recording and stimulation. However, resection of essential cortex, such as the language and precentral arm or leg motor cortex, should be absolutely avoided because producing a hemiparesis or aphasia is probably too severe a deficit to make the operation worthwhile for seizure control. Identification of language and motor cortex is particularly important in cortical resection.

Anatomically, the frontal Broca's speech area is identified in the opercular, inferior frontal gyrus (usually the posterior 2.5 cm of this gyrus). It is difficult to identify Wernicke's area strictly by anatomic criteria. The parietal speech area is identified 1 to 4 cm above the sylvian fissure and 2 to 4 cm behind the postcentral sulcus. The temporal speech areas usually extend posteriorly behind the level of the postcentral sulcus and 2 to 3 cm from the adjacent convolution above, behind Heschl's gyri, but the precise locations can vary. Language mapping is important in the cortical resection of a dominant hemisphere.[7, 8, 34]

Large frontal resections in the nondominant hemisphere can be carried out safely in front of the precentral gyrus. Identification of the precentral and postcentral gyrus is best accomplished by stimulation under local anesthesia.[5, 16] Resection of precentral arm or leg motor cortex is permitted only if significant contralateral paresis is already present.[9, 34] The lower precentral face area can be resected. This results in contralateral facial paresis, which subsequently improves but may leave some mild upper motoneuron facial weakness.[16]

Resection of the postcentral sensory arm or leg area causes profound proprioceptive deficit and is rarely indicated.[16, 34, 35] However, the lower 2.5 to 3 cm of the postcentral face area can be resected without significant deficit.[16] In the nondominant hemisphere, the entire parietal cortex posterior to the postcentral gyrus can be removed without a sensorimotor deficit.[16, 34, 36] Resection in the parietal operculum may produce contralateral lower quadrantic hemianopsia if resections are carried beyond the depths of the sulci into the white matter.[34, 35] In the dominant hemisphere, parietal lobe resections should be limited to the superior parietal lobule.[16]

Resection of occipital cortex may produce a disabling contralateral homonymous hemianopsia, and the seizures should be severe to warrant surgery. If vision is intact preoperatively, calcarine cortex and optic radiations are spared as much as possible. As essential cortex for reading is often more widespread than that for naming, excision within 2 cm of Wernicke's area may cause a persisting dyslexia.[34, 35]

Apart from functional anatomy, the vascular territory of each crucial artery or vein should be studied to assess the consequences of its occlusion during surgery. This approach is essential to minimize morbidity, especially for surgery of the motor and speech areas. Any ascending vein to the superior sagittal sinus draining from the central or postcentral sulci should be left intact to avoid significant morbidity.[5, 16]

Preoperative Care and Anesthesia

When preoperative EEG studies have localized the epileptogenic zone to a noneloquent cortical area, general anesthesia can be used.[16] However, when intraoperative electrocorticography is required, the use of drugs depressing cortical electrical activity, such as benzodiazepines and barbiturates, should be avoided for anesthesia. When functional mapping of motor, speech, and sensory areas is performed, the patient should be conscious and cooperative during the procedure. In this situation, local anesthesia with analgesic drugs (i.e., fentanyl and droperidol or propofol) should be used.[8, 37] Local anesthesia has the disadvantages of being more time consuming and of limiting the head position, and it cannot be used with uncooperative patients and young children. Constant supervision by a specially trained anesthesia team is essential.[5, 16]

Intraoperative Electrocorticography

The use of intraoperative electrocorticography is controversial. It is performed to further delineate the extent of epileptogenic zone. The primary epileptic neurons are found by interictal electrocorticographic spikes. Proponents of electrocorticography feel there is a clear relationship among the site of interictal discharges, the site of ictal onset, and the tissue that must be removed to control seizures. This hallmark is used to determine what part of brain should be resected.[5, 9, 38, 39] They feel that electrocorticography provides prognostic information by indicating the areas of residual discharges after cortical resection. Patients with no interictal discharges on postresection recordings are more likely to be seizure free than those with persistent discharges.[5, 38, 40] Other groups feel that electrocorticography offers no useful information.

Cortical Stimulation: Functional Mapping

The purpose of intraoperative cortical stimulation is to localize eloquent cortex such as motor cortex, sensory cortex, or language area in the dominant hemisphere. Functional mapping is necessary when cortical resections are carried out near the eloquent areas that should be spared. Identification of motor cortex is useful in any resection in posterior frontal or parietal lobes. Identification of language cortex is necessary in any dominant-hemisphere resection in perisylvian cortex and posterior superior frontal lobe.

The location of the central sulcus is determined with electrical stimulation of the precentral and postcentral gyri after preliminary identification. The suspected site of the motor and sensory cortex is stimulated and mapped with a motor response detected by the anesthetist or a sensory change reported by the patient.[9, 34, 38] In practice, the best way to identify the postcentral gyrus is to obtain sensory responses of the tongue area located at the bottom of the postcentral gyrus.[16, 41]

The frontal, parietal, and temporal language areas in the dominant hemisphere are stimulated while the patient carries out simple verbal tasks such as naming objects shown on picture cards. The language area is indicated if the patient says nothing (i.e., speech arrest) during stimulation or if the patient can talk but not name the object.[8, 9, 34, 38] However, a negative stimulation result does not always exclude the presence of speech function in the stimulated cortex. Because there is great variability in the exact localization of essential language areas, only intraoperative mapping can reliably determine the location of language centers.

Surgical Technique

Unlike temporal lobectomy, there are no anatomically standard operations for extratemporal cortical resection. Craniotomy is performed for resection of epileptic focus. The extent of the neocortical resection is determined according to the gross pathology and the result of electrocorticography and functional mapping. In general, areas with interictal discharges are resected. Essential motor and language areas should be preserved (preferably with a 2-cm or one-gyrus margin) regardless of involvement in the epileptic focus.[9] Special attention is given to the vascular supply of the area to be resected. The possible surgical and functional morbidity by occlusion of each artery and vein in the surgical field must be considered.[34] When the extent of the resection is determined, the area of excision is demarcated with a white thread and is parallel along the axis of a gyrus or perpendicular to two gyri across a sulcus. Because each of these factors differs among patients, the extent of the resection is tailored to each case.

A subpial dissection technique is used for cortical resection.[2, 5, 8, 9, 16, 34, 42, 43] This procedure was employed by Horsley in 1909 and has remained the basis of surgery of epilepsy. The pial surface is coagulated and incised in a relatively avascular area. The resection of a gyrus is then carried out in a subpial fashion. An ultrasonic aspirator at a low-suction and low-vibration setting is extremely useful for focal resections in a subpial plane. Meticulous, slow removal of epileptogenic gray matter is carried to the bottom of the sulcus without damaging vessels within the pia that may supply other nonresected tissue.

Hemostasis is achieved principally with topical agents such as Gelfoam or Surgicel and with minimal use of electrocautery. In topectomy, unnecessary resection of the underlying white matter is avoided to preserve the integrity of projection, association, and commissural fibers. Appropriate antiepileptic medication and dexamethasone are given after cortical resection.

Surgical Outcome

Extratemporal nonlesional resection is associated with much poorer seizure control and higher rates of major morbidity than lesional or temporal resection. Table 160–2 shows the seizure outcome reported by Engel and colleagues in 1993.[44] Extratemporal surgery results in 45% of patients who are seizure free and 35% who are improved.

In localized resective surgery, less than 5% of patients have some postoperative neurological deficit due to unintended vascular compromise or other accidental damage to essential neural tissue. However, most disturbances are transient and resolve within a period of months.[13]

TABLE 160–2 ■ **Outcome for Seizures**

OUTCOME	ATL (%)	ETR (%)
Seizure free	2429 (67.9)	363 (45.1)
Improved	860 (24.0)	283 (35.2)
Not improved	290 (8.1)	159 (19.8)
Total	3579 (100)	805 (100)

ATL, anterior temporal lobectomy; ETR, extratemporal resection.
From Engel J: Surgery for seizures. N Engl J Med 334: 647–652, 1996.

REFERENCES

1. Hauser WA: The natural history of drug-resistant epilepsy: Epidemiologic considerations. Epilepsy Res Suppl 5:25–28,1992.
2. Wyler AR: Focal cortical resections. In Wyler AR, Hermann BP (eds): The Surgical Management of Epilepsy. Boston, Butterworth-Heinemann, 1994, pp 129–138.
3. Schwartzkroin PA, Wyler AR: Mechanisms underlying epileptiform burst discharge. Ann Neurol 7:95–107, 1980.
4. Auer RN, Siesjo BK: Biological differences between ischemia, hypoglycemia, and epilepsy. Ann Neurol 24:699–707, 1988.
5. Olivier A, Awad IA: Extratemporal resections. In Engel J (ed): Surgical Treatment of the Epilepsies, 2nd ed. New York, Raven Press, 1993, pp 489–500.
6. Baltuch GH: Complex partial seizures: Surgical treatment. Curr Treat Options Neurol 1:353–357, 1999.
7. Hansebout RR: Surgery of epilepsy—current technique of cortical resection. In Schmidek HH, Sweet WH (eds): Operative Neurosurgical Techniques, Indications, Methods and Results, 2nd ed. Orlando, FL, Grune & Stratton, 1988, pp 1223–1234.
8. Marino R: Neurosurgical aspects of epilepsy in adults. In Youmans JR (ed): Neurological Surgery, 3rd ed. Philadelphia, WB Saunders, 1990, pp 4288–4326.
9. Ojemann GA: Surgical treatment of epilepsy. In Wilkins RH, Rengachary SS (eds): Neurosurgery, 2nd ed. New York, McGraw-Hill, 1996, pp 4173–4183.
10. Silfvenius H: Latest advances in epilepsy surgery. Acta Neurol Scand Suppl 162:11–16, 1995.
11. Engel J, Shewmon A: Who should be considered a surgical candidate? In Engel J (ed): Surgical Treatment of the Epilepsies, 2nd ed. New York, Raven Press, 1993, pp 23–34.
12. Rasmussen T: Commentary: Extratemporal cortical excisions and hemispherectomy. In Engel J (ed): Surgical Treatment of the Epilepsies. New York, Raven Press, 1987, pp 417–424.
13. Engel J: Surgery for seizures. N Engl J Med 334:647–652, 1996.
14. Quesney LF, Risinger MW, Shewmon A: Extracranial EEG evaluation. In Engel J (ed): Surgical Treatment of the Epilepsies, 2nd ed. New York, Raven Press, 1993, pp 173–195.
15. Rasmussen T: Surgery of frontal lobe epilepsy. In Purpura DP, Penry JK, Walter RD (eds): Advances in Neurology, vol 8. New York, Raven Press, 1975, pp 197–205.
16. Olivier A: Extratemporal cortical resections: Principles and methods. In Lüders H (ed): Epilepsy Surgery. New York, Raven Press, 1991, pp 559–568.
17. Rasmussen T: Surgery for epilepsy arising in regions other than

the temporal and frontal lobes. In Purpura DP, Penry JK, Walter RD (eds): Advances in neurology, vol 8. New York, Raven Press, 1975, pp 207–226.

18. Williamson PD, Ness PCV, Wieser HG, Quesney LF: Surgically remediable extratemporal syndrome. In Engel J (ed): Surgical Treatment of the Epilepsies, 2nd ed. New York, Raven Press, 1993, pp 65–76.
19. Wyler AR, Vossler DG: Surgical strategies for epilepsy. In Grossman RG, Loftus CM (eds): Principles of Neurosurgery, 2nd ed. Philadelphia, Lippincott-Raven Publishers, 1999, pp 737–755.
20. Barkovich AJ, Rowley HA, Andermann F: MR in partial epilepsy: Value of high-resolution volumetric techniques. AJNR Am J Neuroradiol 16:339–343, 1995.
21. Kuzniecky RI, Cascino GD, Palmini A, et al: Structural neuroimaging. In Engel J (ed): Surgical Treatment of the Epilepsies, 2nd ed. New York, Raven Press, 1993, pp 197–209.
22. Barkovich A, Chuang S, Norman D: MR of neuronal migration anomalies. AJNR Am J Neuroradiol 8:1009–1017, 1987.
23. Berkovic SF, Newton MR, Chiron C, Dulac O: Single photon emission tomography. In Engel J (ed): Surgical Treatment of the Epilepsies, 2nd ed. New York, Raven Press, 1993, pp 233–243.
24. Rowe CC, Berkovic SF, Sia STB, et al: Localization of epileptic foci with postictal single photon emission computed tomography. Ann Neurol 26:660–668, 1989.
25. Harvey AS, Hopkins IJ, Bowe JM, et al: Frontal lobe epilepsy: Clinical seizure characteristics and localization with ictal (99m)Tc-HMPAO SPECT. Neurology 43:1966–1980, 1993.
26. Lee BI, Markand ON, Wellman HN, et al: HIPDM single photon emission computed tomography brain imaging in partial onset secondarily generalized tonic-clonic seizures. Epilepsia 28:305–311, 1987.
27. Stefan H, Bauer J, Feistel H, et al: Regional cerebral blood flow during focal seizures of temporal and frontocentral onset. Ann Neurol 27:162–166, 1990.
28. Henry TR, Chugani HT, Abou-Khalil BW, et al: Positron emission tomography. In Engel J (ed): Surgical Treatment of the Epilepsies, 2nd ed. New York, Raven Press, 1993, pp 211–232.
29. Jones-Gotman M, Smith ML, Zatorre RJ: Neuropsychological testing for localizing and lateralizing the epileptogenic region. In Engel J (ed): Surgical Treatment of the Epilepsies, 2nd ed. New York, Raven Press, 1993, pp 245–261.
30. Wada J, Rasmussen T: Intracranial injection of Amytal for the localization of cerebral speech dominance. J Neurosurg 17:266–282, 1960.
31. Wyler AR: Diagnostic operative techniques in the treatment of epilepsy: Grids and strip electrodes. In Schmidek HH, Sweet WH (eds): Operative neurosurgical techniques, 3rd ed. Philadelphia, WB Saunders, 1995, pp 1265–1270.
32. Arroyo S, Lesser RP, Awad IA, et al: Subdural and epidural grids and strips. In Engel J (ed): Surgical Treatment of the Epilepsies, 2nd ed. New York, Raven Press, 1993, pp 377–386.
33. Wyler AR, Wilkus RJ, Blume WT: Strip electrodes. In Engel J (ed): Surgical Treatment of the Epilepsies, 2nd ed. New York, Raven Press, 1993, pp 387–397.
34. Pilcher WH, Ojemann GA: Presurgical evaluation and epilepsy surgery. In Apuzzo MLJ (ed): Brain Surgery: Complication Avoidance and Management. New York, Churchill Livingstone, 1993, pp 1525–1555.
35. Pilcher WH, Roberts DW, Flanigin HF, et al: Complications of epilepsy surgery. In Engel J (ed): Surgical Treatment of the Epilepsies, 2nd ed. New York, Raven Press, 1993, pp 565–581.
36. Corkin S, Milner B, Rasmussen T: Somatosensory thresholds: Contrasting effects of postcentral gyrus and posterior parietal-lobe excisions. Arch Neurol 23:41–58, 1970.
37. Ojemann GA: Awake operations with mapping in epilepsy. In Schmidek HH, Sweet WH (eds): Operative neurosurgical techniques, 3rd ed. Philadelphia, WB Saunders, 1995, pp 1317–1322.
38. Ojemann GA: Intraoperative electrocorticography and functional mapping. In Wyler AR, Hermann BP (eds): The Surgical Management of Epilepsy. Boston, Butterworth-Heinemann, 1994, pp 189–196.
39. Dodrill C, Wilkus R, Ojemann G, et al: Multidisciplinary prediction of seizure relief from cortical resection surgery. Ann Neurol 20:2–12, 1986.
40. Bengzon A, Rasmussen T, Gloor P, et al: Prognostic factors in the surgical treatment of temporal lobe epileptics. Neurology 18: 717–731, 1968.
41. Picard C, Olivier A: Sensory cortical tongue representation in man. J Neurosurg 59:781–789, 1983.
42. Penfield W, Jasper H: Epilepsy and the functional anatomy of the human brain. Boston, Little, Brown & Company, 1954.
43. Rasmussen T: Cortical resection in the treatment of focal epilepsy. In Purpura DP, Penry JK, Walter RD (eds): Advances in neurology, vol 8. New York, Raven Press, 1975, pp 139–154.
44. Engel J, Ness PCV, Rasmussen TB, Ojemann LM: Outcome with respect to epileptic seizures. In Engel J (ed): Surgical Treatment of the Epilepsies, 2nd ed. New York, Raven Press, 1993, pp 609–621.

CHAPTER **161**

Multiple Subpial Transection

RICHARD W. BYRNE ■ WALTER W. WHISLER

From the inception of epilepsy surgery, it has been clear that resective surgery for medically intractable seizure foci can be done in noneloquent areas with acceptably low rates of morbidity and with a reasonable chance for seizure control in carefully selected patients. Resection of seizure foci in eloquent cortex, however, results in unacceptable deficits. The surgical procedure of multiple subpial transection (MST) addresses this difficult problem by capitalizing on the difference between the vertical and horizontal organization of the brain.[1] The master organizational principle in the cerebral cortex is the functional vertical column, with its vertical orientation of incoming and outgoing fibers and blood supply.[2–4] At the same time, seizures spread horizontally through the gray matter. MST involves disconnecting the gray matter columns that lie in eloquent cortex. This technique can inhibit synchronization and spread of the seizure focus with minimal injury to the cortex. In this chapter we cover the history of the development of MST, patient selection, surgical indications, technique, results, pitfalls, and areas for further exploration.

HISTORY

In the 1930s two treatments emerged for patients with chronic epilepsy that brought hope for better seizure control. The anticonvulsant effects of phenytoin were discovered in 1938[5] and brought many patients with chronic epilepsy under control. At the same time, Wilder Penfield at the Montreal Neurological Institute expanded the use of surgical resection of seizure foci, primarily in the temporal lobe, for "psychomotor seizures."[6] News of Penfield's success spread, and in 1951, Percival Bailey and Fred Gibbs at the University of Illinois Neuropsychological Institute reported their results of temporal lobectomy for psychomotor seizures guided by electroencephalogram findings.[7] One class of patients that would not benefit from standard surgical therapy consisted of those with a seizure focus in eloquent cortex, because excision of this seizure focus would lead to unacceptable deficits.

Several discoveries in neuroscience in the 1950s and 1960s, along with his own work, led Frank Morrell to believe that a nonresective surgical therapy was possible. The first discovery, by Mountcastle,[2, 3] was that gray matter in the neocortex was organized in vertical functional columns with afferent and efferent connections perpendicular to the surface of the cortex. Although there are horizontal interconnections between neurons, experiments by Sperry and colleagues[8–10] demonstrated that if these horizontal connections are interrupted in the cat visual cortex, the function of that cortex is largely preserved. In these experiments, they placed mica plates into gray matter perpendicular to the cortical surface—thus severing the horizontal fibers in the cortex but preserving the vertical fibers. Visual testing showed a preservation of function. Experiments by Morrell demonstrated the role of these horizontal fibers in the synchronization and spread of an epileptic discharge.[11, 12] He found that in the monkey, he could inhibit the seizure focus but preserve the motor function when he transected through a penicillin-induced seizure focus in the motor cortex.[1] These findings led to a long-term collaboration in the surgical treatment of seizure foci in eloquent cortex between neurologist Morrell and neurosurgeon Walter Whisler, who had worked at the Illinois Neuropsychological Institute with Gibbs. As of 1999, Morrell and Whisler had treated more than 120 patients with MST at the Rush Epilepsy Center in Chicago, where they developed and perfected the technique. Since the report of their original series,[1] many other epilepsy centers have duplicated that success and reported their findings.[13–25]

PATIENT SELECTION

The great majority of surgical epilepsy cases can be treated with standard resective techniques such as temporal lobectomy with amygdalohippocampectomy and extratemporal resection in noneloquent cortex. Subpial transection is reserved for cases in which resection is not indicated or in which the seizure activity extends beyond the area of resection into eloquent cortex. The majority of these cases are dominant temporal lobe resections where MST is carried out on the posterior temporal lobe stump that contains residual seizure activity. By abolishing the capacity of the epileptogenic area to generate seizures, the surgical resection can be transformed from a failure into a palliative or curative procedure. MST has been used to treat patients with epileptogenic lesions of speech, motor, or primary sensory cortex.

MST can be used in the treatment of:

1. Epilepsia partialis continua
2. Focal sensory, somatosensory, or visual cortex seizures
3. Resection with evidence of epileptogenic activity in adjacent eloquent areas
4. Landau-Kleffner syndrome
5. Rasmussen's encephalitis[26]
6. Resection in noneloquent areas such as the nondominant posterior temporal lobe to avoid a homonymous hemianopia, or when the size of the resection would increase the operative risk

Landau-Kleffner syndrome (LKS) was described in 1957 by Landau and Kleffner[27] after they evaluated a group of children with acquired epileptic aphasia. After developing normally and acquiring the ability to speak and to understand speech, these children had progressive loss of speech function. No clear precipitating event or illness occurred to cause the loss, but they had infrequent clinical seizures and an electroencephalogram pattern of near-continuous slow spike and wave discharge in slow-wave sleep, primarily in the parasylvian area.

Although LKS is one of the "benign rolandic epilepsies" that remit after several years, the abnormal course of speech and behavioral development is anything but benign.[28, 29] The term *benign* is deceiving. Although the seizures and the slow spike and wave discharge of LKS usually resolve in the late teenage years, the chance for the development of language and intellectual skills has largely passed by then. If LKS is allowed to follow its course without intervention, these children have little chance for normal speech and behavior. Anticonvulsants are helpful in controlling the overt clinical seizures sometimes seen in LKS, but they do not reverse the continuous spike and wave discharge that bombards the speech areas, inhibiting speech function. In most cases, massive doses of steroids inhibit the slow spike and wave discharge and allow the return of speech function temporarily and sometimes quite dramatically. The problem with steroid treatment is that very large doses are needed for many years through the child's critical period of development. Serious, permanent side effects inevitably occur, which limits the effectiveness of steroid therapy.

If, after a thorough evaluation, a clear diagnosis of severe, medically intractable LKS is made and a clearly demarcated parasylvian focal seizure onset is demonstrated with monitoring, magnetoencephalography, and a methohexital suppression test, surgery is considered. If the focal onset is in an area of noneloquent cortex, standard resective surgery of the seizure focus is considered. If the seizure focus lies in parasylvian cortex in a probable speech area, MST is considered. Because these children are, by definition, aphasic, Wada testing and intraoperative mapping are not possible. Our surgical experience with LKS now numbers more than 20 cases. Long-term follow-up is available in 16 cases, with excellent results.[28, 30]

OPERATIVE PROCEDURE

If subdural grid recording and mapping have been done, general anesthesia with methohexital is used. Methohexital has been shown to induce epileptic activity, with some evidence that it preferentially induces the primary seizure focus.[31–33]

If intraoperative mapping is planned, lighter doses of methohexital are used, along with intravenous sedation and generous use of local anesthetic. Our choice for local anesthetic is a mixture of 1% lidocaine and 0.25% bupivacaine to block the occipital, temporal, and supraorbital nerves. Patients are positioned with the planned operative exposure superior in the field and the head in three-point fixation. A standard craniotomy with an exposure large enough to allow electrocorticography is done. Electrocorticography is performed using a grid and specially placed cylindrical electrodes as needed. In most cases in which MST is being considered, the seizure focus lies in both eloquent and noneloquent cortex. In these cases, surgical resection is performed in the noneloquent cortex to within 1.5 cm of eloquent cortex, as delineated by intraoperative or subdural grid stimulation mapping using standard techniques.[34, 35] If repeat electrocorticography does not show a significant resolution of the interictal activity and the primary residual focus lies within eloquent cortex, MST is performed on the crown of the involved gyri at 5-mm intervals through the gray matter. Transections are made in parallel rows in the direction perpendicular to the long axis of the gyrus (Fig. 161–1). If significant resolution of the seizure focus is noted on electrocorticography, no further transection is done. If no significant resolution is noted and a clearly focal area is active in spite of transection of the crown of the gyrus in that area, transection is sometimes carried out vertically into the gray matter within the depth of the sulcus. This is illustrated in a cadaver in Figure 161–2. This transection is performed along the same plane as the transection of the crown. If the primary seizure focus is truly in the MST area, these maneuvers will stop or significantly reduce the intraictal epileptic discharges. If they do not, it is possible that the preoperative evaluation and electrocorticography have not shown the primary seizure focus, which may be projecting from a distance.

In the less common scenario, the seizure focus is located entirely in eloquent cortex. In these cases, MST is the only surgical option. The procedure is done as described earlier, the only exception being that there is no cortical resection. This is commonly the case in LKS.

All the intraoperative decision making relies on electrocorticography and the preoperative evaluation. Evidence of a true focal-onset seizure focus with spread through the surrounding cortex must be differentiated from mere cortical "spiking," which is not appropriate for treatment with MST. This requires an experienced

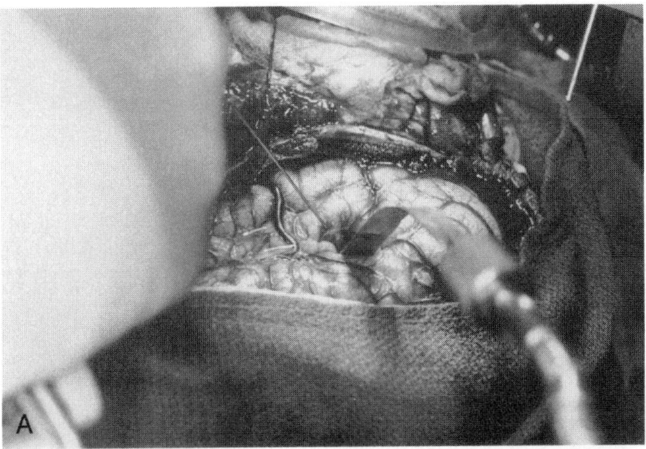

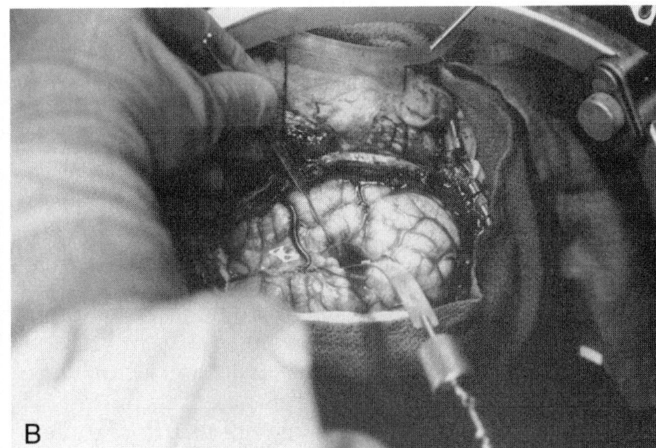

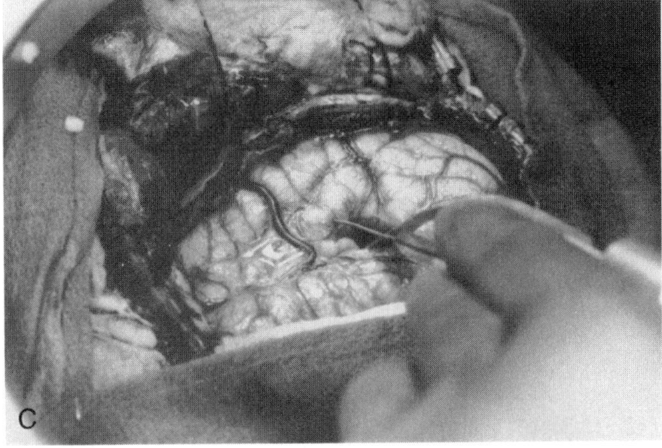

FIGURE 161–1. *A*, A 20-gauge needle is used to open a hole in the pia in an avascular area. *B*, The transection hook enters through the hole. *C*, The hook is advanced stepwise across the gyrus, with the tip of the hook visible beneath the pia. The transector is then withdrawn along the same path.

epileptologist familiar with the interpretation of electrocorticography.

TRANSECTIONS

Transections are performed with a specially designed fine, malleable wire that is bent into a 4-mm blunt hook at the tip (Fig. 161–3). The hook of the subpial transector (Whisler-Morrell Subpial Transector, Redman Neurotechnologists, Lake Zurich, IL) measures 4 mm in length because the average depth of gray matter in neocortex is 4 mm.[1] This hook is bent at an obtuse angle of 105 degrees relative to the main shaft of the wire. The wire is connected to a rectangular handle with the tip of the hook aligned with the flat sides of the handle. This is important because it prevents the hook from going into the cortex at any angle other than perpendicular. If the hook is advanced through the cortex at an angle off the perpendicular, extensive undercutting of the cortex will result, with corresponding deficits. The transection hook shank can be bent to any shape necessary for use in technically difficult locations. This is useful in the intrahemispheric motor and visual cortex, and in the posterior temporal lobe when the sylvian fissure is opened to allow access to the depths of the fissure.

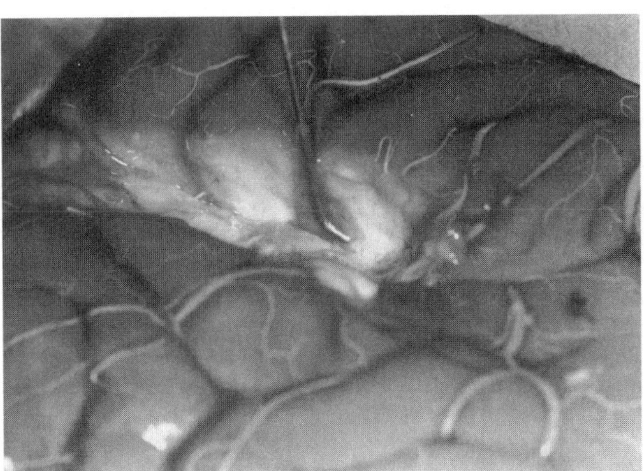

FIGURE 161–2. On a cadaver specimen in the coronal plane, the transector is seen advancing into the depth of a sulcus. The tip is reversed and pointed away from the sulcus to lessen the possibility of vessel injury.

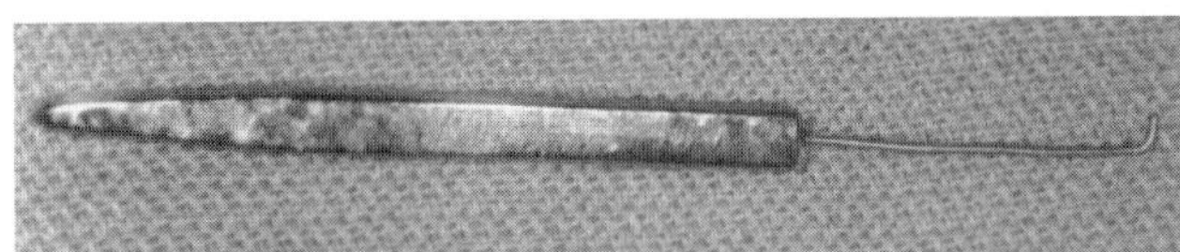

FIGURE 161–3. The transector has three parts. The rectangular handle is connected to a malleable wire with a 4-mm tip. The tip is angled at 105 degrees to prevent vessel snagging.

The area to be transected is carefully inspected. The gyral and microgyral patterns are noted. The course of the vascular supply and bypassing vessels is traced. After electrocorticography, transections are usually begun in the most dependent area, because subarachnoid bleeding may occur. If the transections were begun in a more superior area, the subarachnoid blood would quickly obscure the more dependent areas. If a large amount of subarachnoid blood accumulates, a small opening can be made in the pia to let the blood escape. Each transection is begun by opening a hole in an avascular area of the pia. This is done at the edge of a sulcus with a 20-gauge needle. As the transector hook enters the gray matter through this hole, it is important to keep the hook vertically oriented to avoid undercutting and to avoid advancing the tip too deep and thus injuring white matter. The hook is advanced in a stepwise fashion in a straight line across the crown of the gyrus in a direction perpendicular to the long axis of the gyrus. The hook is then withdrawn along the same path, with the tip of the hook visible just below the pia.[36–38] As the hook is withdrawn from the pial puncture hole, a small amount of blood sometimes escapes. This is easily controlled with a small piece of Gelfoam and gentle pressure. The next transection line is made parallel to and 5 mm from the first. Because the hook is 4 mm long, it can be used to estimate the distance to the next transection line. The transections are thus done along the gyrus in the area of the seizure focus. If enough subarachnoid bleeding occurs to obscure the gyrus, another area can be transected while waiting for the blood to clear. Using this technique and the Whisler-Morrell hook, we have never encountered bleeding that could not be controlled with gentle pressure.

Great care must be taken to note the course of the major blood vessels, particularly around the sylvian fissure and the intrahemispheric fissure. When a transection must be done in the depths of a sulcus or a fissure, the hook is inserted upside down, with the tip pointed away from the pial surface. This lessens the likelihood of snagging a vessel in the sulcus or fissure. The obtuse angle of the hook also helps lessen the likelihood of vessel snagging. In cases of parasylvian-onset epilepsy, it is often useful to open the sylvian fissure under the microscope in order to record from the depths of the fissure and to transect under direct vision (Fig. 161–4). There are cases in which transection at 5-mm intervals is not possible because of microgyral patterns or a large confluence of vessels, which may cover the area to be transected. After a few minutes, the subpial transection lines become visible; because of microscopic bleeding, they are maroon (Fig. 161–5).

PATHOLOGY

When MST is performed, acute pathologic changes are consistent with microscopic focal injury along the transection line (Fig. 161–6). On the transection line, hemorrhage, edema, and mild cell injury are seen. When the transection lines are done properly and are perpendicular to the gyral surface, the columns of cell bodies and their vertical afferent and efferent fibers are preserved. In the study by Pierre-Louis and colleagues,[39] the majority of transections were entirely in gray matter and were perpendicular to the gyral surface.

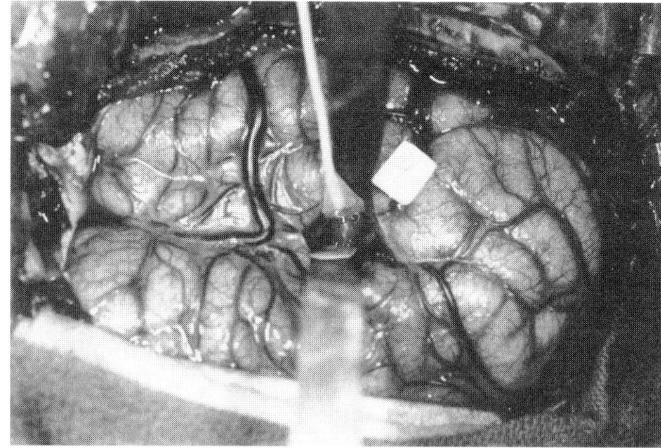

FIGURE 161–4. In cases of parasylvian-onset epilepsy, the sylvian fissure is opened under the microscope, recordings are made in the depths of the sulcus, and transections are made at the base of the sylvian fissure under direct vision.

RADIOLOGY AND FUNCTIONAL IMAGING

Acute changes from MST seen on computed tomography and magnetic resonance imaging include small subcortical hemorrhages and edema, with a loss of definition of the gray-white junction. On magnetic resonance imaging, the transections themselves can often be seen acutely. At 6 months, magnetic resonance im-

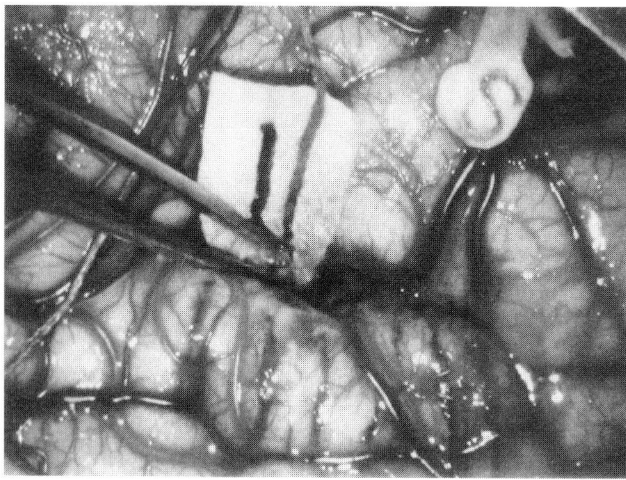

FIGURE 161–5. After transections are completed, fine lines can be seen beneath the pia at 5-mm intervals. Petechial bleeding is easily controlled with Gelfoam and gentle pressure.

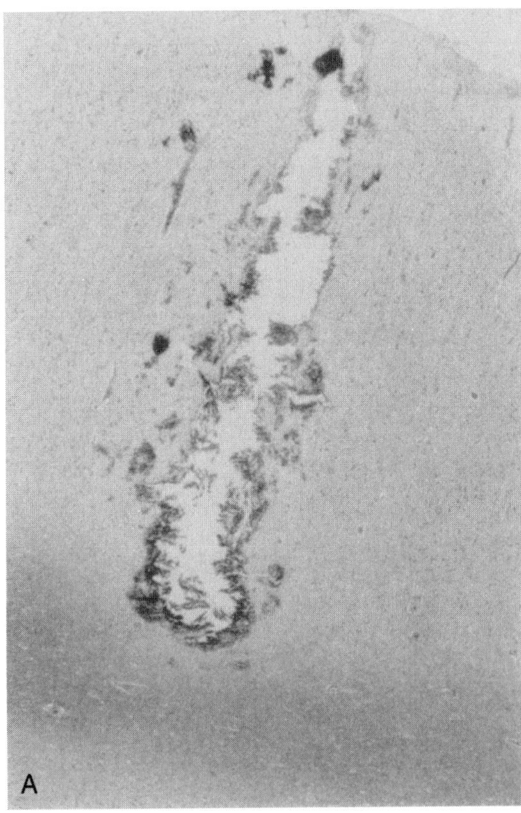

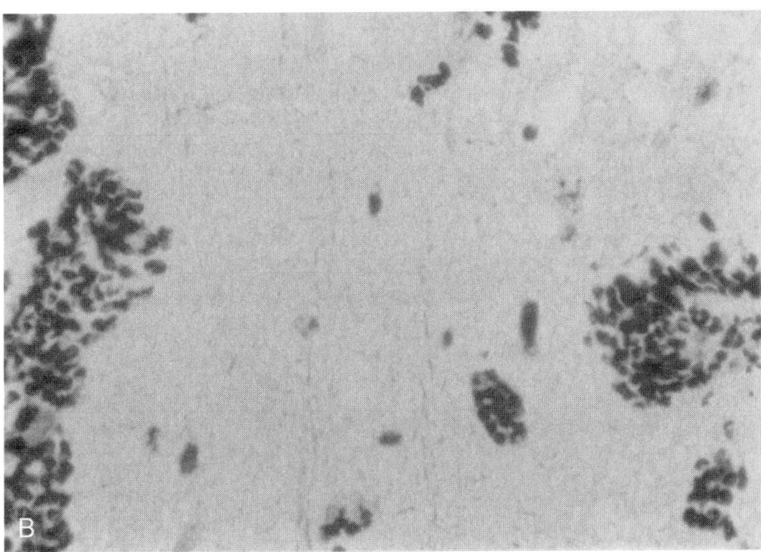

FIGURE 161–6. Pathology of multiple subpial transection is illustrated with hematoxylin-eosin staining. The transection shown reaches down to the white matter but remains within gray matter. Edema and mild inflammatory changes are noted on higher power. Intervening vertical cell columns are preserved.

aging shows clear, fine transections in the gray matter. If subcortical hemorrhage occurs, microcystic changes and focal gyral atrophy may be seen.

Hashizume and Tanaka[40] demonstrated the effects of MST on an experimental seizure focus. In a kainic acid rat seizure model, they found that MST suppressed the spread of seizure activity to the ipsilateral hemisphere and reduced the frequency of seizures but did not eliminate them. They tested glucose metabolism in the transected cortex and found that it was not altered, suggesting that function of the cortex was preserved.

COMPLICATIONS

In our series of more than 100 patients and in published series by others, there have been no deaths (Table 161–1). In the early postoperative period, most patients who have MST in eloquent cortex have subtle, transient deficits corresponding to the area transected. These deficits are most pronounced in the first week after surgery. As the edema and microhemorrhage resolve, most patients return to their baseline function within 2 to 4 weeks. In many patients undergoing careful, detailed examination, deficits in fine motor

TABLE 161–1 ■ **Postsurgical Outcome**

		SIGNIFICANT WORTHWHILE IMPROVEMENT		NO SIGNIFICANT IMPROVEMENT		NEUROLOGICAL COMPLICATIONS	
		Engel's Classification					
SURGICAL PROCEDURE	*n*	*Class I (%)*	*Class II (%)*	*Class III (%)*	*Class IV (%)*	**Transient (%)**	**Permanent (%)**
MST only, partial seizures	16	6 (37.5)	4 (25)	2 (12.5)	4 (25)	1 (6)	3 (19)
MST only, LKS	16	9 (57.7)	2 (12.5)	2 (12.5)	3 (18)	2 (12.5)	—
MST/resection	68	33 (48.5)	7 (10)	16 (23.5)	12 (18)	7 (10)	4 (6)
Total	100	48	13	20	19	10	7

LKS, Landau-Kleffner syndrome; MST, multiple subpial transection.

From Morrell F, Kanner A, Whisler W: Multiple subpial transection. In Stefan H, Andermann F (eds): Plasticity in Epilepsy. New York, Lippincott-Raven, 1998.

TABLE 161–2 ■ **Postsurgical Outcome after Multiple Subpial Transection (MST) at Epilepsy Centers**

		SIGNIFICANT IMPROVEMENT		NO WORTHWHILE IMPROVEMENT		NEUROLOGICAL COMPLICATIONS	
AUTHOR	***n***	**MST Only**	**MST/Resection**	**MST Only**	**MST/Resection**	***n***	**Type (*n*)**
Shimizu et al[20]	12	12	—	0	0	0	—
Devinsky et al[17]	3	0	0	0	0	2	Mild speech deficits (2)
Sawhney et al[18]	21	8	12	1	0	0	—
Lui et al*	50	32	—	18	—	0	—
Wyler et al[14]	6	6	—	0	—	1	Mild motor deficits (1)
Hufnagel et al[19]	22	4	15	2	1	7	Mild speech deficits (2) Mild motor deficits (3) Overt speech deficits (2)
Pacia et al[13]	21	3	18	0	1	9	Mild dysnomia (7) Moderate dysphasia (1) Loss of proprioception in hand (1)
Rush Epilepsy Center	100	25	56	7	12	17	Permanent (7) Transient (8) Sensorimotor (13)
Total (%)	235 (38.3)	90 (44.3)	104 (12)	28 (6)	14 (15.4)	36	

* In this study, it was not clear whether MST alone or MST and resection were performed.
From Morrell F, Kanner A, Whisler W: Multiple subpial transection. In Stefan H, Andermann F (eds): Plasticity in Epilepsy. New York, Lippincott-Raven, 1998.

control or speech can be detected, but in almost all cases, the patients do not notice these findings themselves.

In our series, there was a 5% incidence of permanent, disabling complications corresponding to the area transected. In two cases, motor deficits arose after retraction and transection of the intrahemispheric leg motor cortex. Two cases of postoperative dysphasia occurred after transection of speech areas. One case of hemiparesis occurred after a basal ganglia hemorrhage distant from the site of transection. There were eight cases of deficits corresponding to the area transected that lasted longer than the expected 2 to 4 weeks, but these eventually resolved over several months. One was a speech deficit, and seven were related to sensory or motor function. Seven other complications occurred that were clearly related to resection or craniotomy. A permanent visual field loss and a permanent sensory loss were clearly related to surgical resection. A transient sixth nerve palsy was related to temporal lobe resection. A single case of meningitis, orchitis, and phlebitis was related to the craniotomy and resolved with appropriate treatment. Our final permanent complication rate was 7%.

Complication rates similar to ours have been reported in other series (Table 161–2). A period of transient dysfunction has also been commonly noted. Higher complication rates can be expected if the interval of transection is narrowed to 4 mm or closer.[16] Although a perpendicular transection through cortex causes little damage to the surrounding neurons, as the pathologic studies indicate, it does cause some damage.[39, 41] As the interval is narrowed, one would expect a higher percentage of neurons in the cortex to be injured. This would also be expected if the depths of the sulci in the cortical area were transected. This maneuver is not routinely done at our center but is done routinely by some surgeons. And because there is a learning curve to this technique, higher complication rates can be expected with less experienced surgeons.

SEIZURE OUTCOME

To evaluate the effects of MST on seizure outcome, it is useful to look at MST in the following categories:

1. MST for focal-onset epilepsy where MST is the only procedure done.
2. MST for focal-onset epilepsy where a cortical resection of noneloquent cortex is also done. In these cases, the preoperative evaluation showed seizure activity in eloquent and noneloquent cortex, and the cortical resection had no significant effect on electrocorticography. MST was then done on adjacent eloquent cortex.
3. MST for LKS.

Seizure outcome after MST should be analyzed in this fashion because the cortical resection done in the majority of cases introduces a confounding variable: one cannot be certain whether the MST or the resection had the effect on seizure outcome. In these cases, one can be certain only that the MST had an effect on the electrocorticography. Also, many of these patients had previously been rejected for epilepsy surgery at other centers because of the location of their seizure focus. These patients have posterior-lateral dominant temporal lobe seizure foci or seizure foci around the central sulcus or in the primary visual cortex. The group that had MST as the only surgical intervention gives the clearest indication of the effect of MST on seizure outcome, because there are fewer confounding variables and the pathology is more uniform in this group. Seizure outcome in cases of LKS is a secondary issue. Control of overt clinical seizures is not the objective in this syndrome, because many patients do not have obvious seizures. The application of MST in LKS is done with the objective of eliminating the constant slow spike and wave discharge in the parasylvian cortex and allowing the return of speech function. In these cases, return of speech function is the primary measurable objective and must be measured against historical controls.

In 16 cases of MST alone for focal-onset seizures in eloquent cortex with at least 2 years of follow-up, 6 patients were made seizure free (see Table 161–1). An additional 6 patients had only rare seizures or had a 90% or greater seizure reduction. Four patients had no worthwhile benefit. Overall, 75% of patients in this category had a worthwhile Engel's class I to III seizure outcome. Long-term outcome analysis in this group is under way. All these patients would have been rejected for standard resective surgery, so their outcomes should be compared to best medical therapy. Other groups have reported similar results (see Table 161–2). In Wyler and coworkers' series of six patients with uniform pathology in sensorimotor cortex, all six had a significant reduction in their seizures.[32] There was only one mild motor deficit.

The next category of patients had a combination of MST and resection, which is the most common type of case in our series. We have found that it is rare for a seizure focus to lie entirely in eloquent cortex. A total of 82% of patients in this category were seizure free or had a significant reduction in their seizures (Engel's class I to III; see Table 161–1).

The last category of patients treated with MST is LKS patients. Of the 20 patients who had MST at the Rush Epilepsy Center, 16 patients have had more than 2 years of follow-up. In 9 of the 16 cases, transections in the involved parasylvian cortex resolved the continuous spike and wave discharge. In 11 cases, significant improvement in speech was noted on detailed speech evaluation at 2 years' follow-up. The best predictor of postoperative improvement was length of time from surgery.[42] In these cases, the speech outcome is compared to historical controls, because an age-matched control group is not available in this rare syndrome. Compared to published series demonstrating the natural history of LKS, the speech outcome of the surgical series is significantly improved.

CONCLUSIONS

Our initial experience with MST was reported in 1989.[1] In that group of the most intractable cases, 11 of 20 patients were seizure free after follow-up of at least 5 years. Subsequent cases in which MST was performed without resection proved the independent efficacy of the procedure. Since then, MST has proved helpful in cases of intractable epilepsy with foci in unresectable cortex. Similar results at other centers confirm its efficacy and safety if done properly on well-selected patients. The exact mechanism of action of MST is being delineated with functional testing. Other centers trying MST have added different techniques and new protocols.[13, 14, 16] As we learn more about MST and about the nature of epileptogenic cortex, the technique will be further refined and will likely result in improved outcomes in patients with unresectable seizure foci.

REFERENCES

1. Morrell F, Whisler WW, Bleck T: Multiple subpial transection: A new approach to the surgical treatment of focal epilepsy. J Neurosurg 70:231–239, 1989.
2. Mountcastle VB: Modality and topographic properties of single neurons of cat's somatic sensory cortex. J Neurophysiol 20:408–434, 1957.
3. Mountcastle VB: The columnar organization of the neocortex. Brain 120:701–722, 1957.
4. Asanuma H: Recent developments in the study of the columnar arrangement of neurons within the motor cortex. Physiol Rev 55: 143–156, 1975.
5. Merritt HH, Putnam TJ: Sodium diphenylhydantoinate in treatment of convulsive disorders. JAMA 111:1068–1073, 1938.
6. Feindel W: Development of surgical therapy of epilepsy at the Montreal Neurological Institute. Can J Neurol Sci 18:549–553, 1991.
7. Bailey P, Gibbs FA: The surgical treatment of psychomotor epilepsy. JAMA 145:365–370, 1951.
8. Sperry RW: Physiological plasticity and brain circuit theory. In Harlow HF, Woolsey CN (eds): Biological and Biochemical Bases of Behavior. Madison, University of Wisconsin Press, 1958, pp 33–37.
9. Sperry RW, Miner N: Pattern perception following insertion of mica plates into visual cortex. J Comp Physiol Psychol 48:463–469, 1955.
10. Sperry RW, Miner N, Myers RE: Visual pattern perception following subpial slicing and tantalum wire implantation in visual cortex. J Comp Physiol Psychol 48:50–58, 1955.
11. Morrell F: Microelectrode studies in chronic epileptic foci. Epilepsia 2:81–88, 1961.
12. Morrell F: Cellular pathophysiology of focal epilepsy. Epilepsia 10:495–505, 1969.
13. Pacia SV, Devinsky O, Perrine K, et al: Multiple subpial transections for intractable partial seizures: Seizure outcome. J Epilepsy 10:86–91, 1997.
14. Wyler AR, Wilkus RJ, Rotard SW, et al: Multiple subpial transection for partial seizures in sensorimotor cortex. Neurosurgery 37: 1122–1128, 1995.
15. Rougier A, Sundstrom L, Claverie B, et al: Multiple subpial transection: Report of 7 cases. Epilepsy Res 24:57–63, 1996.
16. Patil AA, Andrews RV, Torkelson R: Surgical treatment of intractable seizures with multilobar or bihemispheric seizure foci (MLBHSF). Surg Neurol 47:72–78, 1997.
17. Devinsky O, Perrine K, Vazquez B, et al: Multiple subpial transections in the language cortex. Brain 117:255–265, 1994.
18. Sawhney IMS, Robertson JA, Polkey CE, et al: Multiple subpial transection: A review of 21 cases. J Neurol Neurosurg Psychiatry 58:344–349, 1995.
19. Hufnagel A, Zenter J, Fernandez G, et al: Multiple subpial transection for control of epileptic seizures: Effectiveness and safety. Epilepsia 38:678–688, 1997.
20. Shimizu H, Suzuki I, Ishijima B, et al: Multiple subpial transection (MST) for the control of seizures that originated in unresectable cortical foci. Jpn J Psychiatr Neurol 45:354–356, 1991.
21. Honovar M, Janota I, Polkey CE: Rasmussen's encephalitis in surgery for epilepsy. Dev Med Child Neurol 34:1–4, 1992.
22. Zonghui L, Quanjun Z, Shiyue L, et al: Multiple subpial transection for treatment of intractable epilepsy. Chin Med J 108:539–541, 1995.
23. Tanake T, Yonemasu Y: Basic and clinical approaches for surgical

treatment of intractable epilepsies. Clin Neurol 34:1237–1239, 1994.
24. Neville BRG, Harkness WFJ, Cross JH: Surgical treatment of severe autistic regression in childhood epilepsy. Pediatr Neurol 16:137–140, 1997.
25. Patil AA, Andrews R, Torkelson R: Minimally invasive surgical approach for intractable seizures. Stereotact Funct Neurosurg 65: 86–89, 1995.
26. Morrell F, Whisler WW, Smith MC: Multiple subpial transection in Rasmussen's encephalitis. In Andermann F (ed): Chronic Encephalitis and Epilepsy: Rasmussen's Syndrome. Boston, Butterworth-Heinemann, 1991, pp 219–234.
27. Landau W, Kleffner F: Syndrome of acquired aphasia with convulsive disorder in children. Neurology 7:523–530, 1957.
28. Morrell F, Whisler WW, Smith MC, et al: Landau-Kleffner syndrome: Treatment with subpial intracortical transection. Brain 118:1529–1546, 1995.
29. Rintahaka PJ, Chugani HT, Sankar R: Landau-Kleffner syndrome with continuous spikes and waves during slow-wave sleep. J Child Neurol 10:127–133, 1995.
30. Morrell F, Kanner AM, Hoeppner TJ, et al: Multiple subpial transection for selected cases of Landau-Kleffner syndrome. In Tuxhorn I, Holthausen H, Boenigk HE (eds): Pediatric Epilepsy Syndromes and Their Surgical Treatment. London, John Libbey (in press).
31. Hufnagel A, Burr W, Elger CE, et al: Localization of the epileptic focus during methohexital-induced anesthesia. Epilepsia 33:271–284, 1992.
32. Wyler AR, Richey ET, Atkinson RA, et al: Methohexital activation of epileptogenic foci during acute electrocorticography. Epilepsia 28:490–494, 1987.
33. Hardiman O, Coughlan A, O'Moore B, et al: Interictal spike localization with methohexital: Preoperative activation and surgical follow-up. Epilepsia 28:335–339, 1987.
34. Lesser RP, Luders H, Klem G, et al: Extraoperative cortical functional localization in patients with epilepsy. J Clin Neurophysiol 4:27–53, 1987.
35. Ojemann G, Whitaker HA: Language localization and variability. Brain Lang 81:239–260, 1978.
36. Whisler WW: Multiple subpial transection. In Rengachary SS (ed): Neurosurgical Operative Atlas, Vol 6. Park Ridge, Ill, American Association of Neurological Surgeons, 1997, pp 125–129.
37. Morrell F, Kanner AM, Whisler WW: Multiple subpial transection. In Stefan H, Andermann F (eds): Plasticity in Epilepsy. New York, Lippincott-Raven, 1998.
38. Whisler WW: Multiple subpial transection. In Kaye A, Black P (eds): Operative Neurosurgery. United Kingdom, Churchill Livingstone, 1997.
39. Pierre-Louis SJC, Smith MC, Morrell F, et al: Anatomical effects of multiple subpial transection. Epilepsia 34:104(S), 1993.
40. Hashizume K, Tanaka T: Multiple subpial transection in kainic acid–induced focal cortical seizure. Epilepsy Res 32:389–399, 1998.
41. Kauffmann W, Kraus G, Uematsu S, et al: Treatment of epilepsy with multiple subpial transections: An acute histological analysis in human subjects. Epilepsia 37:342–352, 1996.
42. Grote CL, VanSlyke P, Hoeppner JA: Language outcome following multiple subpial transection for Landau-Kleffner syndrome. Brain 122(Pt 3):561–566, 1999.

CHAPTER **162**

Vagus Nerve Stimulation for Intractable Epilepsy

ARUN PAUL AMAR ■ MICHAEL L. LEVY ■ MICHAEL L. J. APUZZO

Vagus nerve stimulation (VNS) delivered via the implantable Neurocybernetic Prosthesis (NCP) from Cyberonics, Inc. (Houston, Tex) is emerging as a novel adjunct in the management of patients with medically refractory seizures. This device delivers intermittent electrical stimulation to the left cervical vagus nerve trunk, which secondarily transmits rostral impulses to exert widespread effects on neuronal excitability throughout the central nervous system. We have comprehensively reviewed the theoretical rationale, practical background, and clinical application of VNS in previous publications.[1–3] The operative procedure for implanting the NCP has also been presented in detail elsewhere.[4, 5]

ANATOMY AND PHYSIOLOGY OF THE VAGUS NERVE

Although the vagus nerve is generally regarded as an efferent projection that innervates the larynx and provides parasympathetic control of the heart, lungs, and gastrointestinal tract, the majority of its fibers are special visceral and general somatic afferents leading toward the brain.[1]

Several branches of the vagus nerve arise cephalad to the midcervical trunk, where the VNS electrodes are applied.[5] These include projections to the pharynx and carotid sinus, as well as superior and inferior cervical cardiac branches leading to the cardiac plexus. Both the right and left vagus nerves carry cardiac efferent fibers, but anatomic studies in dogs suggest that those on the right side preferentially supply the sinoatrial node of the heart, while those on the left side preferentially innervate the atrioventricular node. For this reason, the NCP system is generally inserted on the left side. Nevertheless, stimulation of the left vagus nerve may rarely cause bradycardia or asystole, even at approved settings.

As mentioned, the NCP is generally applied to the midcervical portion of the vagus nerve trunk, distal to the origin of the superior and inferior cervical cardiac branches; this may be another reason why the incidence of bradycardia is low.[5] Nonetheless, the diameter, appearance, and location of the cardiac branches may approximate those of the nerve trunk itself, and care must be taken to avoid mistaking the two. If the cardiac branches are stimulated directly, small currents as low as 0.8 mA may produce significant bradycardia.[5]

The midcervical portion of the vagus nerve is relatively free of branches.[5] The superior laryngeal nerve arises rostral to the carotid bifurcation before descending toward the larynx, and high currents applied to the midcervical nerve trunk may recruit these fibers, leading to tightness or pain in the pharynx or larynx. The recurrent laryngeal nerve travels with the main trunk and branches caudally at the level of the aortic arch before ascending in the tracheoesophageal groove. As a result, hoarseness is a common occurrence during periods of stimulation or after NCP implantation.

REGIONAL ANATOMY OF THE CAROTID SHEATH

In addition to branches of the vagus nerve trunk, several other nerves in the vicinity of the carotid sheath are at risk from the implantation procedure itself or from subsequent stimulation. The hypoglossal nerve arises cephalad to the midcervical region, making unilateral tongue weakness an infrequent complication of NCP implantation. The phrenic nerve lies deep to a fascial plane beneath the carotid sheath, and hemiparalysis of the diaphragm has been reported with stimulation at high output currents, though not as an operative complication.

The sympathetic trunk lies deep and medial to the common carotid artery. It gives off fibers that ascend with the internal carotid artery toward the intracranial contents. We are aware of one case of Horner's syndrome following insertion of the VNS device, due to either manipulation of the sympathetic plexus itself or traction on the sympathetic fibers around the internal carotid artery.

Weakness in the muscles of the lower face may result from injury to branches of the facial nerve, which ramify through the caudal aspect of the parotid gland. In general, hypoglossal and facial nerve injuries are more common sequelae of carotid endarterectomy incisions, which tend to be higher than those used for placement of the VNS device.

THEORETICAL BASIS OF VAGUS NERVE STIMULATION

As with many other anticonvulsant therapies, information about the neural mechanisms underlying VNS lags behind the appreciation of its clinical efficacy.[2] The exact means by which VNS modulates seizure activity and its locus of action have been reviewed elsewhere but remain uncertain.[1, 2] It was initially proposed that VNS works by recruiting afferent C fibers and A delta fibers within the nerve, but this contention has been challenged by observations that VNS retains its antiepileptic effects even after selective destruction of these small unmyelinated fibers by capsaicin treatment.

Vagal afferent fibers originate from receptors in the viscera and terminate in diffuse areas of the central nervous system, many of which are potential sites of epileptogenesis.[2] These include the cerebellum, diencephalon, amygdala, hippocampus, insular cortex, and multiple brainstem centers. Some of these projections relay through the nucleus tractus solitarius, whereas others form direct, monosynaptic connections with their targets. Although it remains unclear which of these pathways underlie the mechanism of VNS action, the locus coeruleus and raphe nucleus appear to be key intermediaries, because bilateral chemical lesions of these centers abolish the seizure-suppressing effects of VNS therapy in animal models.

These results imply that norepinephrine and serotonin, which are diffusely released by the locus coeruleus and raphe nucleus, respectively, may mediate the anticonvulsant actions of VNS.[2] Indeed, these two neurotransmitters are known to modulate the seizure threshold in some parts of the brain by inducing interneurons to release γ-aminobutyric acid (GABA), leading to widespread inhibition of neuronal excitability throughout the brain. However, the levels of GABA and serotonin metabolites in the cerebrospinal fluid of patients undergoing VNS appear to be inversely correlated with the efficacy of treatment, and the neurotransmitter systems that mediate the antiepileptic actions of VNS remain uncertain.

Recently, some animal studies suggested that VNS derives its mechanism of action from cardiac rate and conduction changes leading to transient cerebral ischemia, rather than direct effects on neurotransmitter release or neuronal membrane conductance. However, such experiments conflict with the majority of human studies, which report no significant effects on cardiac performance in response to VNS therapy. Although studies of cerebral blood flow using positron emission tomography have delineated some regions of decreased perfusion, such changes are presumed to reflect altered synaptic activities rather than global impairment of systemic hemodynamics. These studies' findings are inconsistent, and they suffer from many methodologic variations that may confound their results; however, they may help elucidate the mechanism of VNS action and eventually even predict the likelihood of a favorable outcome.[2]

CLINICAL UTILITY OF VAGUS NERVE STIMULATION

Clinical experience with VNS began in 1988 with the first human implant of the NCP system. Since then, more than 1000 patients have participated in seven clinical trials in 26 countries, and more than 3000 patient-years of data have accrued. These studies confirm the long-term safety, efficacy, feasibility, and tolerability of VNS, as well as the durability of the NCP. VNS was approved by the U.S. Food and Drug Administration in 1997, and in 1999, the Therapeutics and Technology Subcommittee of the American Association of Neurology declared VNS a "safe and effective" therapeutic modality, based on a preponderance of class I evidence.[6] Although VNS requires a large initial investment, owing to the price of the device itself as well as the cost of its surgical insertion, cost-benefit analysis suggests that the expense of VNS is recovered within 2 years of follow-up.[7]

A recent meta-analysis of 454 patients enrolled in one of five controlled clinical trials (two double-blind and three open-label studies) suggests that the response of individual patients to VNS varies widely.[4a] One percent to 2% of subjects enjoy complete seizure cessation, others derive no benefit, and the remainder experience intermediate results. Approximately 43% of patients achieve a 50% reduction in baseline seizure frequency. Although this figure is similar to the initial results of many new drug trials, VNS differs significantly, in that its efficacy is maintained during prolonged stimulation and, unlike treatment with chronic antiepileptic medication, overall seizure control actually improves with time. The median reduction in seizure frequency for the entire group was 35% at 1 year, 43% at 2 years, and 44% at 3 years.[4a] These results were obtained using a "last visit carried forward" analysis, which minimizes selection bias by extrapolating data from nonresponders who exit the trial and thus tends to underestimate the efficacy among responders. For patients persisting in the trial (declining N analysis), sustained efficacy is even greater. In general, long-term continuation rates are high, reflecting the unique profile of safety, efficacy, and tolerability that VNS provides.

Adverse effects are typically transient, mild, and limited to cycles of stimulation. Initially, patients may experience voice alteration (20% to 30%), paresthesias (10%), or cough (6%), but the incidence of these side effects diminishes greatly over time. Surgical complications are rare but include infection requiring explantation (~1%), vocal cord injury (<1%), and lower facial paresis (<1%). Physiologic perturbations are highly unusual, and device failure is also very uncommon.

VNS offers several advantages over pharmacotherapy and other surgical modalities.[1] These include the lack of significant toxicity or neuropsychological deficits, the potential for reversibility, the potential for guaranteed treatment compliance, sustained efficacy over time, global improvements in quality of life and cognitive function, and the absence of adverse drug interactions. The potential efficacy and favorable side effect profile of VNS argue for its continued application in the management of medically refractory epilepsy.

PATIENT SELECTION

Epilepsy affects up to 1% of the general population.[1] It is the most prevalent neurological condition affecting people of all ages and the second most common neurological disorder overall. Despite recent advances in our understanding of the molecular and cellular basis of epilepsy and the development of several new medications directed against these mechanisms, satisfactory seizure control remains elusive in 30% to 40% of patients. About half of these patients have partial-onset seizures, and in the United States alone, there are at least 300,000 people with medically refractory partial-onset seizures. Although there is disagreement about which of these patients should undergo cerebral surgery, it is estimated that only 30,000 to 100,000 patients are appropriate candidates for temporal lobectomy, focal cortical resection, callosotomy, hemispherectomy, subpial transection, and other extant procedures.

The selection criteria for insertion of the NCP system are still evolving and reflect current governmental standards, institutional biases, and general guidelines from prior clinical trials.[1, 2] Presently, the device is approved by the Food and Drug Administration only "as an adjunctive therapy in reducing the frequency of seizures in adults and adolescents over 12 years of age with partial onset seizures which are refractory to antiepileptic medications." However, good results have been obtained with off-label use in children as young as 3 years old and in patients with Lennox-Gastaut or other primarily generalized seizure syndromes.[4b] Preliminary experience with infantile spasms has been disappointing, however. Patients with both idiopathic epilepsy and seizures with a structural cause are considered appropriate candidates. Of note, VNS has been used successfully in patients in whom previous surgical procedures failed, confirming the potential efficacy of VNS in highly refractory patient populations.

The definition of medical intractability varies from center to center. Standards from previous studies commonly required a frequency of at least six seizures per month and a seizure-free interval of no longer than 2 to 3 weeks despite therapy with multiple medications.[1, 2] However, seizure frequency, seizure type, severity of attacks, drug toxicity, and overall impact on quality of life must all be considered before a patient is deemed refractory to pharmacotherapy. Adequate monitoring of patient compliance and sufficient trials of investigational drugs must also be assured.

As noted earlier, the response to VNS is highly variable, and previous clinical trials failed to characterize the demographic factors that predict a favorable outcome.[1, 2] Furthermore, VNS is rarely curative. Although reduction in seizure frequency can dramatically affect patients' quality of life, residual seizures may still preclude them from driving a car, maintaining employment, or performing other basic functions. Therefore, at present, we do not consider implantation of the NCP an alternative to conventional epilepsy surgeries that offer a higher likelihood of seizure cessation. We generally reserve VNS for patients in whom such operations are not indicated, including those whose seizure focus is bilateral, is not associated with a structural abnormality, or cannot be completely resected due to overlap with functional cortex. Patients should undergo an extensive diagnostic algorithm that may include video monitoring, brain imaging, invasive or scalp electroencephalography, and neuropsychological testing to ascertain their eligibility for temporal lobectomy, focal cortical resection, subpial transection, callosotomy, hemispherectomy, or other, more proven treatment strategies. A discussion of the efficacy, risks, and benefits of such procedures versus those of VNS should then ensue.

For obvious reasons, the NCP system cannot be inserted in patients who have undergone a prior left cervical vagotomy. Furthermore, the safety of VNS has not been tested in several conditions in which impairment of vagus nerve function might produce deleterious effects. Thus, relative contraindications include progressive neurological or systemic disease, pregnancy, cardiac arrhythmia, asthma, chronic obstructive pulmonary disease, active peptic ulcer disease, and insulin-dependent diabetes mellitus.[1]

NEUROCYBERNETIC PROSTHESIS COMPONENTS

Figure 162–1 provides a schematic representation of VNS therapy.[2] A pulse generator inserted in the subcutaneous tissues of the upper left chest delivers intermittent electrical stimulation to the cervical vagus nerve trunk via a bifurcated helical lead.

In addition to the implantable lead and pulse generator, the NCP system includes a number of peripheral components, such as a telemetry wand that interrogates and programs the pulse generator noninvasively. This programming wand is powered by two 9-V batteries and is interfaced with an IBM-compatible computer that runs a menu-based software package furnished by Cyberonics (Fig. 162–2). The system also includes a hand-held magnet that patients can carry with them to alter the character of stimulation delivered by the generator.

The NCP model 100 pulse generator is approximately the same size and shape as a cardiac pacemaker (Fig. 162–3). It contains an epoxy resin header with receptacles that accept the connector pins extending from the bifurcated lead. The generator is powered by a single lithium battery encased in a hermetically sealed titanium module. Under normal conditions, the generator has a projected battery life of approximately

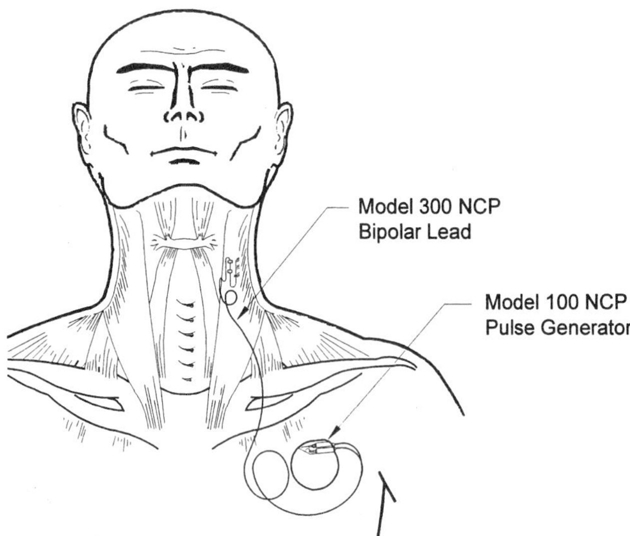

FIGURE 162–1. Schematic representation of vagus nerve stimulation therapy. A pulse generator inserted in the subcutaneous tissues of the upper left chest delivers intermittent electrical stimulation to the cervical vagus nerve trunk via a bifurcated helical lead. (Courtesy of Cyberonics, Inc., Houston, TX.)

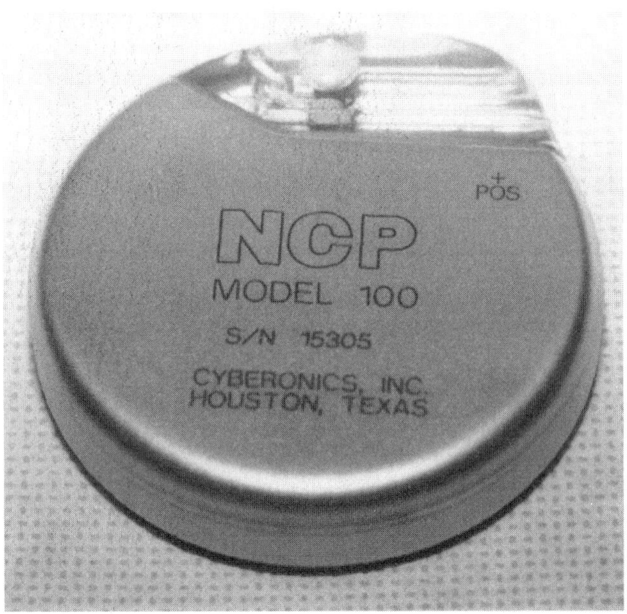

FIGURE 162–3. The Neurocybernetic Prosthesis model 100 pulse generator is approximately the same size and shape as a cardiac pacemaker.

4 to 6 years. Once it has expired, the generator can be replaced under local anesthesia during a simple outpatient procedure. A newer version of the pulse generator with an 8-year battery life (model 101) is currently available, and a third-generation model will soon be commercially available.

The generator contains an internal antenna that receives radiofrequency signals emitted from the telemetry wand and transfers them to a microprocessor that regulates the electrical output of the pulse generator. The generator delivers a charge-balanced waveform characterized by five programmable parameters: output current, signal frequency, pulse width, signal on-time, and signal off-time. These variables are titrated empirically in the outpatient setting, according to individual patient tolerance and seizure frequency. Altering the parameters of stimulation has various consequences on VNS efficacy, side effects, and battery life.

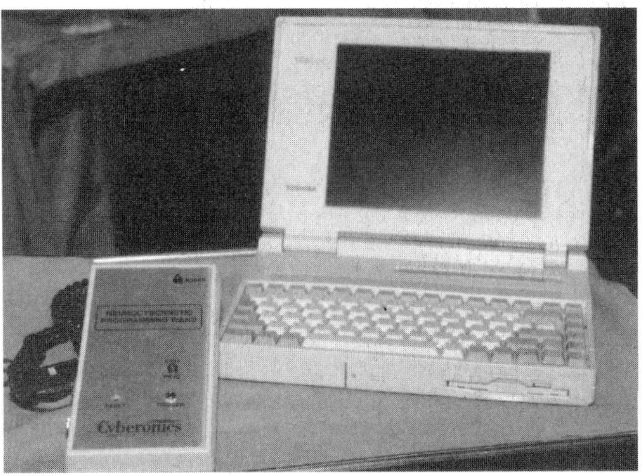

FIGURE 162–2. The Neurocybernetic Prosthesis telemetry wand interfaces with a laptop computer to permit noninvasive programming.

The generator has two accessories. One is a hairpin-shaped resistor that is used during preliminary electrodiagnostic testing before implantation to test the internal impedance of the generator. The other is a hexagonal torque wrench that is used to tighten the set screws that secure the lead connector pins to the epoxy resin header of the generator.

While the generator is still in its package, it can be interrogated by the telemetry wand. The generator must pass this system check before it is opened onto the sterile field. The failure rate of the generator is extremely low, but it is recommended that a backup generator be available in the operating room at all times.

The NCP model 300 bipolar lead is insulated by a silicone elastomer and can thus be safely implanted in patients with latex allergies. One end of the lead contains a pair of connector pins that insert directly into the generator; the opposite end contains an electrode array consisting of three discrete helical coils that wrap around the vagus nerve (Fig. 162–4). The middle and distal coils represent the positive and negative electrodes, respectively, and the most proximal one serves as an integral anchoring tether that prevents excessive force from being transmitted to the electrodes when the patient turns his or her neck. The leads come in two sizes, measured by the internal diameter of each helix. Although the majority of patients can be fitted with the 2-mm coil, it is desirable to have the 3-mm coil available in the operating room as well.

Each electrode helix contains three loops. Embedded inside the middle turn is a platinum ribbon coil that is welded to the lead wire. This shape permits the platinum ribbon to maintain optimal mechanical contact

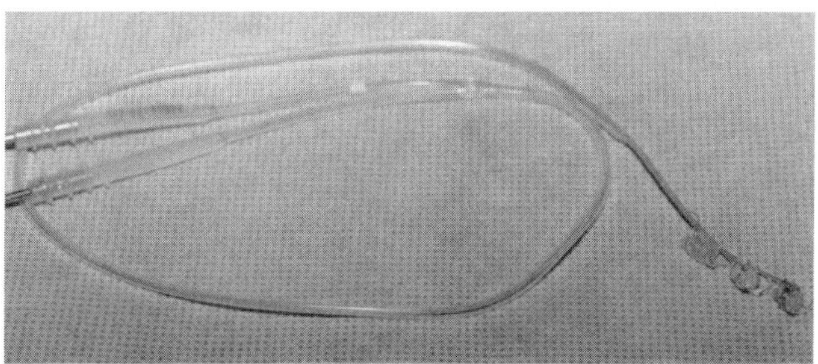

FIGURE 162–4. Neurocybernetic Prosthesis model 300 bipolar lead. One end of the lead contains a pair of connector pins that insert directly into the generator, and the opposite end contains an electrode array consisting of three discrete helical coils that wrap around the vagus nerve.

with the nerve. Suture tails extending from either end of the helix permit manipulation of the coils without injuring these platinum contacts. Damage to the vagus nerve itself is greatly reduced by the self-sizing, open helical design of the NCP electrode array, which permits body fluid interchange with the nerve. Thus, compared with cuff electrodes, mechanical trauma and ischemia to the nerve are minimized. The electrode is intended to fit snugly around the nerve while avoiding compression, thus allowing the electrode to move with the nerve and minimizing abrasion from relative movement of the nerve against the electrode.

The hand-held magnet performs several functions. When briefly passed across the chest pocket where the generator resides, it manually triggers a train of stimulation superimposed on the baseline output. Such on-demand stimulation can be initiated by the patient or a companion at the onset of an aura, in an effort to diminish or even abort an impending seizure. The parameters of this magnet-induced stimulation may differ from those of the prescheduled activation. Alternatively, if the device appears to be malfunctioning or if the patient wishes to terminate all stimulation for any other reason, the system can be indefinitely inactivated by applying the magnet over the generator site continuously. Finally, patients are instructed to test the device periodically by performing magnet-induced activation and verifying that stimulation occurs. Most patients can perceive the stimulation as a slight tingling sensation in the throat.

OPERATIVE PROCEDURE

General Considerations

The techniques and instruments required for placement of the NCP system are not arcane, and although the operation can be performed by anyone who is familiar with exposure of the carotid sheath, neurosurgeons are the ideal candidates because they maintain active roles in comprehensive epilepsy programs and participate in decisions about which patients should initiate VNS therapy.[4, 5]

The operation takes less than 2 hours and is typically performed with the patient under general anesthesia, thus minimizing the possibility that an intraoperative seizure might compromise the surgery.[4, 5] However, regional cervical blocks have also been used in awake patients. Although implantation can be performed as an outpatient procedure, it may be desirable to observe patients overnight for vocal cord dysfunction, dysphagia, respiratory compromise, or seizures induced by anesthesia, even though these complications are rare.

Prophylactic antibiotics are administered preoperatively and for 24 hours postoperatively.

Consideration must be given to the organization of the operating room to maximize the surgeon's access and minimize traffic within the area.[1, 4] Following endotracheal intubation, we rotate the table 90 degrees clockwise from the anesthesia setup, which lies alongside the patient's right foot. This permits the surgeon to stand at the patient's left and the assistant to stand at the patient's right. The scrub technician is positioned at the patient's head, affording ready access to each surgeon on either side. The electrophysiology staff remains behind the assistant's back but within reach of the scrub technician in order to conduct preimplant diagnostic testing once the generator has been placed within the sterile field.

The implantation procedure is conceptually straightforward.[4, 5] The first step involves creation of a chest pocket that accommodates the pulse generator. Next, through a separate incision, the carotid sheath is opened, the internal jugular vein mobilized, and the vagus nerve trunk isolated. The lead is tunneled within a subcutaneous tract between the two incisions. The helical electrodes are applied to the vagus nerve, and the lead connector pins are attached to the generator. After additional electrodiagnostic testing, the lead and generator are secured to adjacent tissue, and the wounds are closed in standard, multilayer fashion.

Many aspects of the operative technique have an impact on outcome and merit some prefatory discussion.[1, 4, 5] The importance of the surgeon's preoperative preparation cannot be overemphasized. Planning for placement of the VNS system requires a thorough anatomic understanding of the relevant neural, vascular, and muscular components of the anterior cervical triangle in order to minimize risk to the ansa cervicalis, recurrent laryngeal nerve, tributaries to the internal jugular vein, and other structures. By way of review, the vagus nerve lies in the carotid sheath wedged between the internal jugular vein and the carotid artery. The sternocleidomastoid muscle lies lateral and anterior to the sheath, and the sympathetic trunk lies deep and posterior. The recurrent laryngeal nerve, which supplies all muscles of the larynx except the cricothyroid, lies medially in the tracheoesophageal groove.

In addition to anatomic review, electrode model drills with practice devices supplied by the manufacturer help familiarize the surgeon with the technique and strategy of helix placement. Finally, before insertion of the first VNS system, team rehearsals should be conducted with all members of the surgical staff in the operating suite to review the room organization and reduce traffic in the area. These precautions may minimize the risk of hardware infection during the actual procedure.

Operative Technique

The patient is positioned supine with a shoulder roll beneath the scapulae to provide mild neck extension.[4, 5] This facilitates passage of the tunneling tool that connects the two incisions. The head is rotated 30 to 45 degrees toward the right, bringing the left sternocleidomastoid muscle into prominence.

Many options exist for placement of the skin incisions. Often, a 5-cm transverse chest incision is made approximately 8 cm below the clavicle, centered above the nipple. The underlying fat is dissected to the level of the pectoralis fascia, and a subcutaneous pocket is fashioned superiorly. Although others have suggested a deltopectoral incision with inferior dissection to create the pocket, we believe that the scar tissue formed beneath the pectoral incision helps prevent caudal migration of the generator. Recently, we have been using a lateral incision along the anterior fold of the axilla, which affords better cosmetic results, especially in women (Fig. 162–5).

Next, a 5-cm longitudinal incision is made along the anterior border of the sternocleidomastoid muscle, centered over its midpoint. Generally, this incision is a little lower than that for an endarterectomy. Alternatively, a transverse skin incision at C5-6, similar to the approach for an anterior cervical diskectomy, can be made (see Fig. 162–5). For an inexperienced surgeon, the longitudinal incision permits a wider exposure, which facilitates electrode placement through this aperture.

The platysma muscle is divided vertically, and the investing layer of deep cervical fascia is opened along the anterior border of the sternocleidomastoid, allowing it to be mobilized laterally. Following palpation of the carotid pulse, the neurovascular bundle is

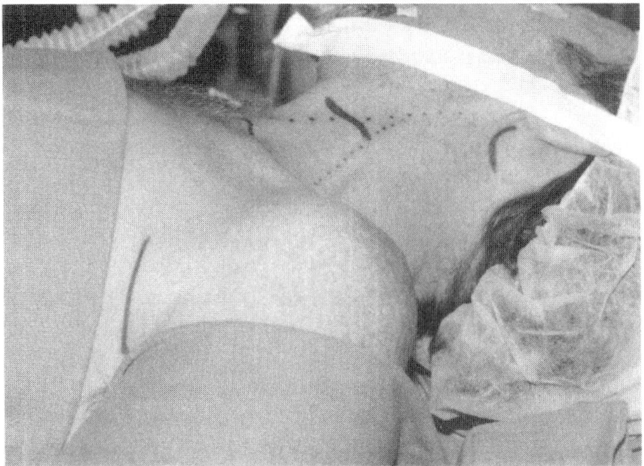

FIGURE 162–5. Proposed sites for the transverse incision of the neck and the anterior axillary incision of the chest. The positions of the anterior border of the sternocleidomastoid muscle, external jugular vein, clavicle, and mastoid tip have also been outlined for orientation.

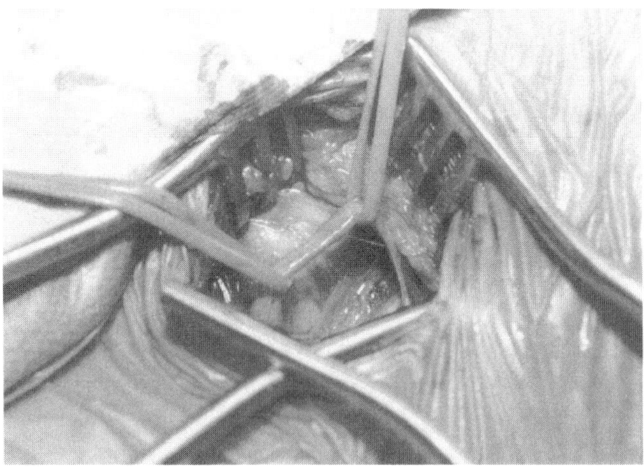

FIGURE 162–6. Isolation of the cervical vagus nerve trunk from other components of the neurovascular bundle. Dissection generally commences with retraction of the internal jugular vein using vessel loops. This technique minimizes injury to the nerve itself and the likelihood of postoperative complications.

identified and sharply incised to reveal its contents. Self-retaining retractors with blunt blades expedite this stage of the procedure. Care is taken to limit the exposure between the omohyoid muscle and the common facial vein complex, thus minimizing the potential risk to adjacent neurovascular structures.

Within the carotid sheath at the level of the thyroid cartilage, the vagus nerve is generally encountered deep and medial to the internal jugular vein, encased in firm areolar tissue lateral to the common carotid artery. There is great variability in the relative position of these structures, however, and the strategy by which the nerve is isolated from the remainder of the neurovascular bundle must take this individual diversity into account.

We attempt to minimize direct manipulation of the nerve itself. Instead, we prefer to mobilize the vessels away from the nerve. Dissection generally commences with isolation and retraction of the internal jugular vein using vessel loops (Fig. 162–6).

Next, the nerve trunk is identified and dissected with the aid of the operating microscope or surgical loupes. At least 3 to 4 cm of the nerve must be completely freed from its surrounding tissues. At this stage, we have found that inserting a blue background plastic sheet between the nerve and the underlying vessels greatly facilitates subsequent steps of the procedure. The technique of mobilizing the vessels away from the nerve usually preserves the vasa nervorum. This nuance may reduce the incidence of postoperative complications such as hoarseness.

A tunneling tool is then used to create a subcutaneous tract between the two incisions. The tool is directed from the cervical to pectoral sites, to minimize potential injury to the vascular structures of the neck.

Depending on the relative size of the exposed nerve, either a small or a large helical electrode is selected for insertion. The lead connector pins are passed through the tunnel and emerge from the chest incision, while the helical electrodes remain exposed in the cervical region. Before applying the electrodes, the lead wire should be directed parallel and lateral to the nerve, with the coils occupying the gap between them.

Each coil is applied by grasping the suture tail at either end and stretching the coil until its convolutions are eliminated. The central turn of this unfurled coil is applied either obliquely or perpendicularly across or beneath the vagus trunk and wrapped around the surface of the nerve. The coil is then redirected parallel to the nerve as the remainder of its loop is applied proximal and distal to this midpoint. The memory within the elongated coil causes it to reassume its helical configuration and conform to the nerve snugly. Either the positive or the negative terminal can be applied first, but the anchoring tether is generally applied last.

While all these maneuvers are taking place, additional electrodiagnostic testing of the generator is simultaneously carried out between the neurology team and the scrub technician. With the hairpin resistor inserted into the receptacles for the lead connector pins, the telemetry wand interrogates the device from within a sterile sheath to measure its internal impedance. Once the generator passes this preimplant diagnostic test, it is ready for insertion.

The lead connector pins are connected to the pulse generator and secured to their receptacles with set screws, using the hexagonal torque wrench. It is important to completely insert the hex wrench into its socket in the epoxy header in order to decompress the backpressure that builds up as the connector pins enter the receptacles. This step is essential for making good contact between the lead and the generator. If the connector pins fail to make such contact, the generator may attempt to overcome the resulting increased impedance by augmenting the output current, leading to intermittent symptoms of overstimulation.

Additional electrodiagnostic examination is performed to appraise the coupling of all connections and to verify the integrity of the overall system. Then a 1-minute lead test is performed at a frequency of 20 Hz with an output current of 1 mA and a pulse width of 500 msec. During this test stimulation, the patient's vital signs and electrocardiogram are monitored. Rarely, profound bradycardia results, necessitating the use of atropine. The incidence of this event is thought to be about 1 in 1000. If it occurs, attention should be directed to the lead to ensure that the electrodes encircle the vagus nerve trunk rather than one of its cardiac branches.[5] Following the test stimulation, the generator is restored to its inactive status until 1 to 2 weeks postoperatively. This waiting period allows for resolution of postoperative edema and proper fixation of the electrode to the nerve.

The redundant portion of the lead between the generator and electrode is secured to several areas of the cervical fascia with Silastic tie-downs. The objective is to form superficial and deep restraint configurations that help prevent excessive traction from being transmitted to the electrodes during repetitive neck motion. First, a U-shaped strain relief bend is made inferior to the anchoring tether, and the distal lead is secured to the fascia of the carotid sheath. Next, a strain relief loop is established by securing the lead to the superficial cervical fascia between the sternocleidomastoid and platysma muscles. Care is taken not to sew the lead directly to the muscle.

Finally, the generator is retracted into the subcutaneous pocket and secured to the pectoralis fascia with O-Prolene or similar nonabsorbable suture, using the suture hole contained within the epoxy resin header. Any excess lead is positioned in a separate pocket at the side of the generator. To prevent abrasion of the lead, however, it should not be placed behind the pulse generator. Wound closure then proceeds in standard multilayer fashion, using a subcuticular stitch for the skin. The cosmetic results are generally very good.

LEAD REMOVAL OR REVISION

In some circumstances, it may become necessary to remove or replace the electrodes that encircle the vagus nerve trunk. Although fibrosis and adhesions may develop in the vicinity of the vagus nerve, Espinosa and colleagues[8] demonstrated that the spiral electrodes can be safely removed from the nerve, even years after implantation.

COMPLICATION AVOIDANCE AND MANAGEMENT

In the meta-analysis mentioned earlier, the most commonly observed surgical complication was infection of either the generator site or the lead implantation site.[4a] The overall infection rate was 2.86%, but more than half of these patients were successfully treated with antibiotic therapy alone; only about 1.1% required explantation of the device.

Transient vocal cord paralysis is the second most common surgical complication of NCP implantation. The incidence of this event in the collective study experience was only 0.7%. However, because video stroboscopy and formal swallowing assessments are rarely performed after surgery, it is possible that more cases went undetected, and the true prevalence of vocal cord paresis is not known.[5] Fortunately, most reported cases resolve clinically.

Temporary lower facial hypesthesia or paralysis occurred in another 0.7% of patients in the meta-analysis.[4a] As stated earlier, excessively high surgical incisions could have been a cause.

To date, out of more than 5000 implantation procedures, only four cases of intraoperative bradycardia or asystole have been reported during the lead test, accounting for an incidence of less than 0.1%. Asconape and coworkers[9] analyzed the factors that potentially contribute to this event and the means of their prevention. As mentioned, the superior or inferior cervical cardiac branches might be mistaken for the vagus trunk itself, and correct positioning of the electrodes on the intended nerve must be verified. Proper placement of the skin incision, centered over the midcervical portion of the nerve, also helps avert this complication. Current spread to the cardiac nerves can be minimized by measures that insulate them from the midcervical trunk during the lead test, such as placement of a Silastic dam beneath the nerve trunk and removal of pooled blood or saline from the vicinity. Finally, the current should be ramped up in small increments during the lead test, starting with 0.25 mA.

As stated earlier, we prefer to mobilize the vascular structures away from the nerve trunk, thus minimizing direct manipulation of the nerve itself. We believe that this practice may improve the efficacy of subsequent stimulation and diminish the incidence of surgical complications such as hoarseness. Other precepts of good surgical technique, gained from experience and familiarity with the implantation procedure, also contribute to improved outcomes.

REFERENCES

1. Amar AP, Heck CN, Levy ML, et al: An institutional experience with cervical vagus nerve trunk stimulation for medically refractory epilepsy: Rationale, technique, and outcome. Neurosurgery 43:1265–1280, 1998.
2. Amar AP, Heck CN, DeGiorgio CM, et al: Experience with vagus nerve stimulation for intractable epilepsy: Some questions and answers. Neurol Med Chir (Tokyo) 39:489–495, 1999.
3. Amar AP, DeGiorgio CM, Tarver WB, et al: Long-term multicenter experience with vagus nerve stimulation for intractable partial seizures: Results of the XE5 trial. Stereotact Funct Neurosurg 73: 104–108, 1973.
4. Amar AP, Levy ML, Apuzzo MLJ: Vagus nerve stimulation for intractable epilepsy. In Rengechary S (ed): Neurosurgical Operative Atlas, vol 9. Rolling Meadows, IL. American Association of Neurological Surgeons, 2000, pp 179–188.

4a. Morris GL, Mueller WM: Vagus nerve stimulation study group E01-E05: Long-term treatment with vagus nerve stimulation in patients with refractory epilepsy. Neurology 53:1731–1735, 1999.

4b. Amar AP, Levy ML, McComb JG, Apuzzo MLJ: Vagus nerve stimulation for control of intractable seizures in childhood. Pediatr Neurosurg 34:218–223, 2001.

5. DeGiorgio CM, Amar AP, Apuzzo MLJ: Vagus nerve stimulation: Surgical anatomy, technique, and operative complications. In Schachter S, Schmidt D (eds): Vagal Nerve Stimulation. London, Dunitz, 2001, pp 31–50.
6. Fisher RS, Handforth A: Reassessment: Vagus nerve stimulation for epilepsy. Neurology 53:666–669, 1999.
7. Boon P, Vonck K, Vandekerckhove T, et al: Vagus nerve stimulation for medically refractory epilepsy: Efficacy and cost-benefit analysis. Acta Neurochir (Wien) 141:447–453, 1999.
8. Espinosa J, Aiello MT, Naritoku DK: Revision and removal of stimulating electrodes following long term therapy with the vagus nerve stimulator. Surg Neurol 51:659–664, 1999.
9. Asconape JJ, Moore DD, Zipes DP, et al: Bradycardia and asystole with the use of vagus nerve stimulation for the treatment of epilepsy: A rare complication of intraoperative device testing. Epilepsia 40:1452–1454, 1999.

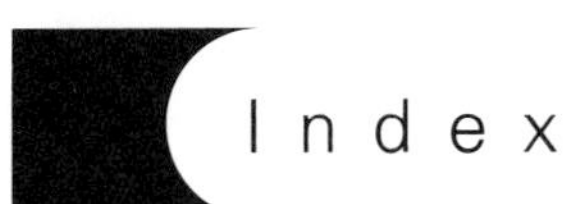

Index

Note: Page numbers followed by f indicate illustrations; those by a b, boxes; those by a t, tables.

ABC system, of cervical spine anterior screw-plate fixation, 4630t, 4635–4636, 4636f
ABCDEs, 5087–5088
Abdomen, trauma assessment of, 5089
Abducens nerve, 29, 316, 316f, 1899, 1974
  examination of, 266
    pediatric, 3173–3174
  injury to, in atlanto-occipital dislocation, 4929
  paresis of, 317, 318t, 320, 320f
Abortion, CNS transplantation tissue from, 2833, 2835
Abscess
  epidural. *See* Epidural abscess; Pyogenic infection, spinal.
  tuberculous, 1443
Absolute alcohol wash, for cerebral palsy, 3731
ABT-627, as angiogenesis antagonist, 779t
Abulia, 285
  in frontal lobe tumors, 830
Abuse, reporting obligations in, 411
Academic practice, legal issues regarding, 409–410
Accessory nerve, 1973–1974
Acetaminophen, for pain, 2959
Acetazolamide
  for brain edema, 802
  for elevated intracranial pressure, 1429
  for infantile posthemorrhagic hydrocephalus, 3411
Acetyl coenzyme A, synthesis of, 1483t
Acetylcholine, in action potential, 3814
Achilles tendonitis, vs. distal tibial nerve entrapment, 3936
Achondroplasia, 3362–3371
  apnea in, 3363–3364
  cervicomedullary compression in, 3364–3365
    decompression of, 3367–3368
      outcome of, 3369
    ventriculostomy for, 3367
  craniovertebral region, 3343, 3344f
  epidemiology of, 3362–3363
  genetics of, 3362–3363
  hydrocephalus in, 3365–3366, 3398
  intracranial pressure in, 3365–3366
  jugular bulb dehiscence in, 3364
  medical complications of, 3363–3364, 3363t
  neurologic complications of, 3363t
  neurologic vs. orthopedic aspects of, 3366
  psychosocial problems in, 3363
  reproduction in, 3363
  spinal stenosis in, 3365, 3366–3367
    decompression of, 3368–3369
      outcome of, 3369–3370
    recurrence of, 3370–3371, 3370f, 3371f
Acid-base metabolism, 123–126, 125f
Acidosis, cerebral, in head injury, 5050
Acoustic meatus, internal, 36f, 40f
Acoustic neuroma, 1147–1164. *See also* Brainstem, glioma of.
Acoustic neuroma *(Continued)*
  arterial involvement in, 1159, 1159t
  cerebellopontine angle
    anatomic distortions in, 1158–1159, 1158t
    auditory tests in, 335f–336f
    treatment of, 1163–1164, 1163f
  diagnosis of, 1149–1150, 1149f, 1152, 1153f
  facial nerve distortions in, 1158–1159, 1158t, 1159t
  features of, 1147, 1147f
  historical review of, 1147–1150, 1148f, 1149f
  in pregnancy, 872
  intracanalicular, 1162–1163, 1163f
  magnetic resonance imaging of, 1149, 1149f
  pathology of, 1152–1153, 1154f
  posterior fossa anatomic variations in, 1158–1159, 1158t
  radiosurgery for, 1154–1155, 4055–4056, 4059f
    complications in, 574
    linac, 4112
    vs. microsurgery, 1164, 4056, 4057t, 4058t
  surgery for, 1154–1158, 1158t
    complications of, 1161–1162
      avoidance of, 570–571
    cranial nerve preservation in, 1160–1161
    evolution of, 1150–1152
    facial nerve monitoring during, 1159–1160
    facial nerve paralysis after, 1161
    headache after, 1162
    middle fossa approach to, 1155
    morbidity in, 1161–1162
    mortality in, 1161
    neurophysiologic monitoring during, 1160
    outcome in, 1164
    posterior fossa intradural approach to, 925–926
    suboccipital approach to, 1156–1158, 1156f–1158f
    translabyrinthine approach to, 1148–1149, 1155–1156
  treatment of, 1147, 1150
    tumor size and, 1162–1164, 1163f
  venous involvement in, 1159, 1159t
  vs. facial nerve schwannoma, 1147, 1147f, 1148f
  vs. meningioma, 1153
  vs. peripheral schwannoma, 1153, 1154f
Acoustic radiation, 9
Acoustic reflex, hearing assessment with, 334, 335f–336f
Acquired immunodeficiency syndrome (AIDS)
  neuropathy in, 3841
  primary central nervous system lymphoma in, 1069–1070, 1071f
Acquired immunodeficiency syndrome (AIDS) *(Continued)*
  pyogenic spinal infections in, 4363–4364
    differential diagnosis of, 4371
    medical management of, 4379
  reporting obligations in, 411–412
  systemic lymphoma in, 1070, 1072
Acromegaly
  carpal tunnel syndrome in, 3890
  diagnosis of, in pregnancy, 868
  dopamine agonists for, 1193
  growth hormone excess and, 1189, 1190
  neuropathy in, 3843
  radiation therapy for, 1193, 4035–4036
  radiosurgery for, 4062
  recurrence of, 1193–1194
  somatostatin analogs for, 1192–1193
  surgery for, 1176
Actin, in axonal regeneration, 197
Actinomyces israelii, spinal infection with, 4295
Actinomycin, for Ewing's sarcoma, 4850
Actinomycosis, spinal, 4385
Action potential, 73
  calcium, 219, 220, 222–224
  conductance changes during, 220–221, 221f
  electrodiagnostic testing of, 3851–3852, 3851f
  generation of, 220–221, 221f
  glial, 221
  ion currents in, 219
  maintenance of, 224–225
  motor unit, polyphasic nature and, 3856–3857, 3856f
  muscle fiber, spontaneous, peripheral nervous system abnormalities with, 3856, 3856t
  neuronal, 3813, 3813f, 3814b
  repolarization of, 220, 224–225
  sodium, 220–222
Adamantinoma, pituitary, 1207
Adaptive development, 3170, 3170t
Adductor reflex testing, pediatric, 3180
Adenoassociated viruses
  as central nervous system gene therapy vector, 4166–4167
  as vectors, 818
Adenocarcinoma, paranasal sinus, 1312
Adenohypophysis, morphology of, 1171–1172
Adenoid cystic carcinoma, paranasal sinus, 1312, 1313f
Adenoma, pituitary. *See* Pituitary adenoma.
Adenosine
  for pain, 2966
  in cerebral autoregulation, 1475
  in cerebral blood flow–metabolism coupling, 1489
Adenosine triphosphate, 119–120
  after brain injury, 2455–2456
  generation of, 118–119, 119f
  in cerebral metabolism, 1479, 1482
  in focal cerebral ischemia, 134, 134f
  in neurons, 1486

Adenoviruses
as vectors, 818
cytopathic capability of, 822
in angiosuppressive gene therapy, 783
in herpes simplex virus thymidine kinase gene transfer, 820
Adherens junctions, in blood-brain barrier, 157
Adhesion molecules
in axon targeting, 201
in blood-brain barrier function, 12
in cerebral ischemia, 140–141, 141t
in malignant glioma, 760–763
T-cell–arresting, 682
Adhesions, lysis of, 2976
Adie's pupil, 322, 322f
Adrenal medulla, transplantation of, 2831
pain control by, 3141
stereotactic surgery in, 2661
Adrenalectomy, for Cushing's disease, 1199
α-Adrenergic agonists, for bladder outlet incontinence, 380–381
α-Adrenergic antagonists
for bladder outlet retention, 380
for bladder retention, 377
Adrenocorticotropic hormone, for multiple sclerosis, 1454t, 1455
Adrenoleukodystrophy
familial spastic paraplegia in, 4319
vs. multiple sclerosis, 1453
Advance directives, 414
Advanced Trauma Life Support, 555
Adventitious movements, examination of, 268
Age
blood-brain barrier in, 166–167
in aneurysm outcome, 1800
in aneurysm rupture, 1789
in arteriovenous malformation hemorrhage risk, 2192, 2192t
in bullet wounds, 5224–5225, 5224t
in cerebellar astrocytoma, 3655
in cerebrospinal fluid shunt infection, 3420
in intervertebral disk degeneration, 4395–4396
in intracerebral hemorrhage surgery, 1741–1742
in intracranial hematoma, 5072
in lumbar stenosis surgical complications, 4535
in mild head injury, 5067
in Parkinson's disease, 2735
in pediatric lumbar disk herniation, 3560
in supratentorial arteriovenous malformation surgery, 2232
AGM-1470 (TNP-470), for glioma invasion, 766
Agrin, in neuromuscular junction formation, 201
AIDS. *See* Acquired immunodeficiency syndrome (AIDS).
Air conduction testing, 331, 331f, 332f
Air embolism
ependymoma surgery and, 3628–3629
medulloblastoma surgery and, 3645
patient positioning and, 614–615
pediatric craniotomy and, 3190f, 3191
posterior fossa surgery and, 555
prone positioning and, 603
Airways
assessment of, 5087
management of
during pediatric surgery, 3188–3189, 3189t
Airways *(Continued)*
in cervical spine trauma, 4888
in craniofacial surgery, 3329
in traumatic brain injury, 5089, 5127–5128
obstruction of, in craniofacial trauma, 5246
Akathisia, 2730
Akinesia, 2673, 2730
subthalamic nucleus stimulation for, 2822
Akinetic mutism, 284, 285t
Alar ligaments, 3537, 4925, 4926f
disruption of, 3333
pediatric, rupture of, 3529
Albright's syndrome, skull in, 1401, 1402f
Alcohol, for spasticity, 2866t
Alcohol use
bone health and, 4234
in bullet wounds, 5225–5226
in mild head injury, 5067
neuropathy in, 3843
stroke risk in, 1616
vs. brain death, 398
Alendronate, for osteoporosis, 4233
Alexander's disease
astrocytes in, 111
glial fibrillary acidic protein in, 111
Alkaloids, 882
Alkylating agents
for malignant glioma, 975
pharmacology of, 880–882
O^6-Alkylguanine-DNA-alkyltransferase (AGT)
in DNA tumor cell repair, 878
inhibition of, 879
Allergies, medications, past medical history/pregnancy, last meal, events (AMPLE), 5088
Allodynia, 2926–2927, 3120t, 3821, 3831
Allograft, 2829t, 4617–4618
in cervical spine fusion, 4622, 4628f
in thoracic spine fusion, 4975–4978
Alopecia, headrests and, 610
Alpha fetoprotein
in germ cell tumors, 1014, 1014t
neural tube defect screening with, 3219
Alpha motoneuron, 2875, 2876, 2876f
excitatory polysynaptic pathways affecting, 2876, 2877f
hyperexcitability of, 2877
monosynaptic connection affecting, 2876
Alteplase, spontaneous intracerebral hemorrhage in, 1735
Altered mental status. *See* Consciousness, altered states (loss) of.
Alveus, 9, 2486, 2487f
Alzheimer's disease
apoptosis in, 2710
immune-inflammatory network in, 684
microglia in, 90
neuronal cell death in, 83
Parkinson's disease with, 2759
positron emission tomography of, 484–485, 484f, 485f, 2759
Amantadine, for multiple sclerosis, 1454t
Ambient cistern, 2486, 2487f
Ambient gyrus, 26, 26f
Ambulation, in cerebral palsy, 3725–3727, 3729–3730, 3733
after selective dorsal rhizotomy, 3743–3744
predictors of, 3739, 3743
Ameloblastoma, 1207
Amenorrhea-galactorrhea syndrome, prolactinoma and, 1185
American Society for Peripheral Nerve, 3798, 3799t
American Spinal Cord Association Classification, 242t
Amino acids
excitatory, in ischemic injury, 1516–1517, 1517f
transport of, across blood-brain barrier, 160–161, 160t, 161f
γ-Aminobutyric acid (GABA)
extracellular space and, 230
in vagus nerve stimulation, 2644
synthesis of, astrocytes in, 107
γ-Aminobutyric acid (GABA) agonists, for pain, 2964–2965
γ-Aminobutyric acid (GABA) receptors, 2699, 2700f
distribution of, 2689f
for baclofen, 2883, 2883f
in globus pallidus, 2688–2689, 2688f
in striatum, 2686–2687, 2686f
in subthalamic nucleus, 2690–2691
positron emission tomography of, 2476
single-photon emission computed tomography of, 2477–2478
ε-Aminocaproic acid, in pregnancy, 2424
Aminoglycosides
for Ménière's disease, 2906
for vertigo, 2906
ototoxicity from, 350
Amiodarone, pseudotumor cerebri from, 1424
Amitriptyline, for pain, 2960, 3838
Ammonia
astrocyte detoxification of, 104f–105f, 107
brain levels of, in hepatic coma, 295
Amnesia
after mild head injury, 5073
forniceal surgery and, 1259–1260
transient global, vs. seizure, 2466
Amniocentesis, neural tube defect screening with, 3219
Amobarbital, intracarotid injection of. *See* Intracarotid amobarbital procedure.
Amphetamines, spontaneous intracerebral hemorrhage with, 1735
Amphibians, spinal cord regeneration in, 4156
Amphotericin B, for spinal candidiasis, 4389
AMPLE (allergies, medications, past medical history/pregnancy, last meal, events), 5088
Amputation, pain syndromes after, spinal cord stimulation for, 3114
Amygdala, 10f, 12f
atrophy of, in temporal lobe epilepsy, 2490
extratemporal, 11
magnetic resonance imaging of, 2486–2487, 2488f
temporal, 11
Amygdalar vein, 1239
Amygdalohippocampectomy, transsylvian selective, 2607–2609
Amyloid, 83
microglia infiltration of, 90, 91f
Amyloidosis, in lumbar stenosis, 4527
Amyotrophic lateral sclerosis, 4319, 4320
peripheral neuropathy in, 3846–3847
weakness in, 272
Amyotrophy
diabetic, 3842–3843, 4511
differential diagnosis of, 4527
neuralgic, 3840–3841

Amytal test. *See* Intracarotid amobarbital procedure.
Anal reflex testing, 367
Analgesia
in intracranial pressure management, 5127, 5127t
nucleus caudalis ablation and, 3049
Analytic studies, 249–253
Anastomoses
circuminfundibular, 19
during brain embolization procedures, 859, 860t, 861f
Martin-Gruber, 3898
posterior inferior cerebellar artery–to–posterior inferior cerebellar artery, 2115
Riche-Cannieu, 3898
Anastomotic vein
inferior, 17
superior, 17
Anatomic gifts, legal issues regarding, 415–416
Ancrod, trials for, 1496–1497, 1497t
Androgen, in bone metabolism, 4232–4233
Androgen receptors, in meningioma, 1108
Anemia
congenital, macrocephaly in, 428
in extracranial head injury, 5057
in traumatic brain injury, 5122f, 5123–5124, 5136
iron-deficiency, pseudotumor cerebri in, 1425
microcytic, pseudotumor cerebri in, 1425
nonpernicious, neuronal degeneration in, 4321
prevention of, 1852
sickle cell
pediatric, spinal infections in, 3566
subarachnoid hemorrhage in, 1832
treatment of, 5136
Anencephaly, 81, 3215, 4256
Anesthesia, 3821
brainstem auditory evoked potentials in, 1508
cerebral physiology for, 1503–1504, 1504t
cerebral protection in, 1515–1523
deep hypothermic circulatory arrest in, 1528–1537. *See also* Circulatory arrest, deep hypothermic.
electroencephalography in, 1506–1507, 1506f
evaluation before, 547–558
cardiac risk in, 550
cardiovascular system in, 549–550
cerebral blood flow in, 551
cerebrovascular physiology in, 551–552
endocrine system in, 550
gastrointestinal system in, 550
hematologic system in, 550
history in, 548
in emergencies, 550
in epilepsy, 557
in head injury, 555–556, 556t
in intracranial tumors, 552
in neuroradiology, 557–558
in non-neurosurgical procedures, 558
in posterior fossa procedures, 554–555
in spinal surgery, 556–557, 557t
in vascular diseases, 552–554, 552t, 553t
intracranial pressure in, 551–552
laboratory studies in, 550–558
neurological system in, 548–549
physical examination in, 548
Anesthesia *(Continued)*
physical status in, 548, 548t
renal system in, 550
respiratory system in, 549
systemic assessment in, 548–550
Glasgow Coma Scale in, 1505, 1505t
in aneurysms, 1509–1511, 1509t
in anterior circulation aneurysms, 1871–1872
in arteriovenous malformations, 1511–1512
in cavernous malformations, 1512
in cerebrovascular disease, 1503–1512
in cordotomy, 3062
in craniotomy, 5149–5150
in deep hypothermic circulatory arrest, 1534–1535
in epilepsy surgery, 2621
in moyamoya, 1719
in occlusive cerebrovascular disease, 1508–1509
in posterior fossa arteriovenous malformations, 2260
in pregnancy, 873
in proximal internal carotid artery aneurysms, 1907
in spinal vascular surgery, 1512
in thoracic spine fracture, 4968
intracranial pressure and, 1504–1505
local, pediatric, 3190
neonatal, 3194
neurophysiologic monitoring in, 1505–1508, 1505t, 1506f, 1507f
pediatric, 3187–3196
airway management in, 3188–3189, 3189t
anticonvulsant therapy and, 3189, 3190f
cerebral edema prevention in, 3189–3190
emergence from, 3192–3193, 3193t
fasting before, 3187–3188, 3188t
fluid maintenance in, 3189, 3190t
head positioning for, 3192
induction of, 3188
maintenance of, 3189–3190, 3189t, 3190f, 3190t
monitoring of, 3190–3191, 3190f, 3191t
pharmacologic agents in, 3189, 3189t
positioning for, 3191–3192, 3192t
postoperative management in, 3193
prone positioning for, 3192, 3192f
thermal homeostasis in, 3191
vascular access in, 3190
venous air embolism in, 3190f, 3191
preemptive, 2927
prone positioning complications in, 603
somatosensory evoked potentials in, 1507–1508, 1507f
Anesthesia dolorosa, 2989t, 3120t
Anesthetics, 1508
local
for spasticity, 2865, 2866t
for trigeminal neuralgia, 2993
neural blockade with, 2970–2984. *See also* Neural blockade.
neurophysiologic monitoring effects of, 3191, 3191t
ophthalmic, for trigeminal neuralgia, 2993
Aneurysmal bone cyst
cervical spine, 4843, 4844f
imaging of, 529, 539f
pediatric, 3567–3568
Aneurysmal bone cyst *(Continued)*
skull, 1388–1389
pediatric, 3721
spinal, 4296t, 4297, 4354, 4354f, 4837, 4843, 4844f
pediatric, 3589, 3590f
Aneurysms. *See also* specific intracranial location, e.g., Cerebral artery, distal anterior, aneurysms of.
angiography of, 1806
anterior circulation, surgery for, 1868–1893
anatomy for, 1878–1879
anesthesia in, 1871–1872
angiography during, 1869, 1870f, 1871, 1872, 1873f, 1874f
arachnoid dissection in, 1878
blood pressure in, 1872
brain relaxation in, 1872
brain retraction in, 1878
clipping in, 1878–1879
computed tomography in, 1872
craniotomy in, 1872, 1875–1877, 1876f
dissection in, 1878
interhemispheric exposure in, 1879–1880
intradural procedure in, 1878–1880
medical considerations in, 1868–1869
monitoring during, 1872
operating microscope in, 1869
positioning for, 1869
preparation for, 1868–1872
stereotaxy in, 1871, 1871f
transsylvian exposure in, 1879
arterial bypass procedures for, 2107–2108. *See also* Arterial bypass.
arteriovenous malformations with, 1801, 1802f, 2152, 2164–2166, 2191, 2212, 2213f, 2214f, 2235, 2252, 2252f
embolization for, 2124–2125, 2124f, 2125f
hemorrhage risk with, 2191
microsurgery for, 2124–2125, 2124f, 2125f
radiosurgery for, 2125, 2125f
rupture of, 2187–2188
treatment of, 2123–2125
atherosclerotic, deep hypothermic circulatory arrest for, 1528–1529, 1529f
balloon occlusion of, 2057–2060, 2058f
carotid artery disease in, 1801
cerebral vasospasm in, 1841
circulatory arrest for, 1807
clipping of, 1822–1823, 2107–2108
historical aspects of, 1462, 1462f
dissecting, penetrating trauma and, 2132
embolization of, 2060–2062, 2061f
aneurysm size and, 2066–2067
balloon-remodeling technique in, 2062, 2062f
coil complications in, 2071, 2072
failure of, surgery after, 2122–2123, 2122f
histopathologic changes after, 2070–2071
hydrocephalus after, 2070
infection in, 2072
ischemia during, 2071
rupture during, 2071–2072
stent-coil technique in, 2063–2064, 2063f
surgery with, 2072–2074, 2073f
vasospasm after, 2069–2070
vs. surgery, 2066

Aneurysms *(Continued)*
endoscopy for, 1806
endovascular occlusion of, 1803–1806, 2057–2074, 2121. *See also* Guglielmi detachable coil embolization.
after bypass, 2115, 2117
after subarachnoid hemorrhage, 1804–1805
alternate techniques for, 1806–1807
balloon occlusion in, 2057–2060, 2058f
deconstructive approach to, 2057–2060
outcome factors in, 1804, 1804f, 1804t
reconstructive approach to, 2060–2064
residual aneurysm after, 1803–1804
safety of, 1803
vs. surgery, 1805–1806
familial, 1774–1776
epidemiology of, 1774, 1774t
evaluation of, 1775–1776, 1776t
gene mutations in, 1776
gene-environment interactions in, 1776
inheritance pattern in, 1774–1775
rupture of, 1775
screening for, 1775, 1775t
flow-related, arteriovenous malformation and, 2164–2165
fusiform, 1801
arterial bypass for, 2117–2118
basilar artery, 1593, 1594f
genetics of, 1769–1776
giant. *See* Giant aneurysms.
historical considerations in, 1461–1462, 1462f
Hunt and Hess grading of, 1509, 1509t
hunterian ligation for, 1806
hypothermia for, 1807
in alpha-antitrypsin deficiency, 1771–1772
in autosomal polycystic kidney disease, 1769–1770
in autosomal polycystic liver disease, 1770, 1776
in Marfan's syndrome, 1772
in neurofibromatosis type 1, 1772–1773
in pregnancy, 2424–2426
in pseudoxanthoma elasticum, 1773
in type IV Ehlers-Danlos syndrome, 1770–1771, 1771t
infectious, 2101–2105
clinical manifestations of, 2103
diagnosis of, 2103–2104
epidemiology of, 2101
imaging of, 2103–2104
microbiology of, 2102
natural history of, 2103
outcome of, 2105
pathophysiology of, 2102
treatment of, 2104–2105
intracranial hemorrhage in, 2121
intranidal, arteriovenous malformation and, 2165
magnetic resonance angiography of, 1591–1593, 1592f, 1593f
mass effect in, 2067
micro-, 1801–1802
multiple, treatment of, 2121–2122
mycotic, 1801, 2101
outcome in, 1800
parent artery occlusion for, 1806, 2057–2060, 2058f
partially thrombosed, deep hypothermic circulatory arrest for, 1529, 1529f
pediatric, 1801, 3448–3452
assessment of, 3450–3451, 3450f
development of, 3448

Aneurysms *(Continued)*
disorders associated with, 3449
distribution of, 3449–3450
human immunodeficiency virus infection with, 3449, 3449f
imaging of, 3451, 3451f
natural history of, 3450
ophthalmoplegia in, 3450f, 3451
pathology of, 3448–3449, 3448f, 3449f
trauma and, 3448–3449, 3448f, 3451f
treatment of, 3451–3452
posterior circulation, 1971–2002
anatomic distribution of, 1975–1976
angiography of, 1976–1977
clinical presentation of, 1976
diagnostic studies for, 1976–1977
endovascular treatment of, 2002
giant, 1975–1976
hypothermic circulatory arrest for, 2000, 2002
magnetic resonance imaging of, 1977
revascularization for, 1999–2000, 2000t, 2001f
rupture of, 1976
saccular, 1975
surgical approaches to, 1971–2002, 1971t, 1972f, 1972t, 1973t
anatomy in, 1973–1975, 1975f
basilar apex, 1977–1987
basilar trunk, 1987–1993
inner skull base, 1973t
outer cranial, 1972t
selection of, 1997, 1999
vertebral trunk, 1993–1997
vascular malformations in, 1976
posterior fossa arteriovenous malformations with, 2252, 2252f
pregnancy in, 1800–1801
revascularization for, 2107–2108
rupture of, 1509, 1796–1800
cerebral arterial wall changes after, 1845, 1846f
cerebral vasospasm from. *See* Vasospasm.
during angiography, 1819
hydrocephalus in, 1799
in arteriovenous malformation surgery, 2187–2188
intracerebral hemorrhage in, 1798–1799
intraventricular hemorrhage in, 1799
poor-grade, 1797, 1798f
rebleeding in, 1796
subarachnoid hemorrhage in, 553, 1813, 1815–1816, 1816f
surgery for
complications of, 1799–1800
timing of, 1796–1797
vasospasm in, 1799
saccular, 1591
in circle of Willis, 1592
in moyamoya, 1717–1718
spinal cord, 2356, 2356f, 2372, 4821
subarachnoid hemorrhage in. *See* Subarachnoid hemorrhage.
supratentorial arteriovenous malformation with, 2235
surgery for
decision making in, 1793–1807
failure of, coil embolization after, 2123, 2123f
ischemia prevention in, 1522
trapping techniques in, 1806–1807
transcranial Doppler ultrasonography of, 1548, 1549f

Aneurysms *(Continued)*
traumatic, 1801, 2131–2133, 5207–5208, 5207f–5210f, 5211
clinical presentation of, 2132
diagnosis of, 2132–2133
false, 2131
true, 2131
treatment of, 1509, 2121–2123
anesthesia in, 1509–1511, 1509t
deep hypothermic circulatory arrest in, 1529
vasospasm effects of, 1842
unruptured
embolization of, 2067
endovascular occlusion of, 1805
grading of, 1797, 1797f
natural history of, 1781, 1783–1787, 1783t, 1793, 1794t
outcome in, age and, 1800
prevalence of, 1782–1783
rupture of, 1793–1794, 1794t
age and, 1789
cigarette smoking and, 1790
confounding factors in, 1787–1790
gender and, 1790
growth and, 1788
hypertension and, 1789–1790
location in, 1787–1788
multiple aneurysms and, 1788
size in, 1787
symptomatic lesions and, 1788–1789
surgery for
efficacy of, 1794
outcome in, 1795, 1795f
patient selection in, 1795–1796, 1796f, 1796t
risk in, 1794–1795, 1794t, 1796t
Angina pectoris, spinal cord stimulation for, 3113
Angiofibroma, juvenile nasopharyngeal
angiography of, 1353–1354
clinical presentation of, 1351, 1351t
embolization of, 1354, 1354f
epidemiology of, 1351
histogenesis of, 1351
imaging of, 1352–1353, 1352f, 1353f
intracranial extension in, 1357
outcome in, 1357, 1358f
radiotherapy for, 1357–1358
staging of, 1353, 1354t
surgical approaches to, 1354–1357, 1355t
infratemporal fossa, 1357
lateral skull base, 1357
Le Fort I, 1356–1357, 1356f
transfacial, 1355–1356
transnasal, 1355
transpalatal, 1355
Angiogenesis, 719–720, 771–785
antagonists for, 776–783
angiogenic growth factors as, 778t, 780–781
endothelial cell inhibitors as, 777t, 778–780
integrin inhibitors as, 778t, 781
protease inhibitors as, 776–777, 777t
concepts of, 773, 774t, 775t
control of, 774t
evolution of, 773, 774t
historical perspective on, 771–774, 773f, 774f
in brain tumors, 771–785
in malignant phenotype, 771, 772f
inhibitors of, 773–774, 775t
discovery of, 772–773, 773f
mechanisms of, 782–783

Angiogenesis *(Continued)*
invasiveness and, 773
mediators of, 774t
regulation of, gene therapy for, 783, 821–822
research on, 783–784, 785
stimulators of, 773–774, 775t
discovery of, 772–773, 773f
Angiogenesis dependency, 774t
Angiogenesis factors, tumor, 773, 775t
Angiogenic drugs, discovery of, 774–775, 775f, 776f
Angiogenic growth factors
antagonists of, 778t, 780–781
in brain tumors, 731
Angiography
spinal, 506
vs. carotid duplex ultrasonography, 1566–1567
Angiolipoma, 3693
spinal, 4843
Angioma
arteriovenous, 2375
cavernous. *See* Cavernous malformations.
osseous, 1368
retinal, in von Hippel-Lindau disease, 1053
venous, 2375
Angioma arteriovenosum. *See* Spinal cord, arteriovenous malformations of.
Angioma racemosum. *See* Spinal cord, arteriovenous fistula of.
Angioma racemosum venosum, 2375
Angiomatosis, encephaloretinofacial, 2154–2155
Angionecrosis, after arteriovenous malformation embolization, 2226, 2227f
Angiopathy
cerebral amyloid, spontaneous intracerebral hemorrhage in, 1735, 1736f
diabetic, differential diagnosis of, 4527
Angioplasty
balloon
for carotid restenosis, 1666
for cerebral vasospasm, 1856–1857, 1857f, 1858f
of carotid artery, 1651–1658. *See also* Carotid angioplasty.
Angiosarcoma, 1142
scalp, 1414
Angiostatin, angiosuppressive therapy with, 779–780
Angiosuppressive therapy, 776–783
gene therapy in, 783
surrogate markers for, 783–784
vs. chemotherapy, 784–785, 784t
Angiozyme, angiosuppressive therapy with, 780
Angular gyrus, 4f, 5, 2531
Angular ramus, 4f
Anisocoria, 302, 322
Anisotropic diffusion imaging, 943, 944f
Ankle reflex testing, pediatric, 3180
Ankle-foot orthotic, for cerebral palsy, 3730
Ankylosing spondylitis, 4303, 4303t, 4304f, 4349, 4350f, 4459–4462, 4479, 4480
cause of, 4459–4460
clinical features of, 4460–4462, 4460t, 4461f
craniocervical junction, 4580
criteria for, 4466, 4466t
Ankylosing spondylitis *(Continued)*
diagnostic evaluation of, 4464–4466, 4465f
epidemiology of, 4459
extraspinal findings in, 4461–4462
features of, 4463t
fractures in, 4469–4470, 4470f
imaging of, 541, 544
juvenile-onset, 3567
nonsurgical treatment of, 4466–4467
outcomes of, 4470–4471
pathology of, 4460
radiography of, 4464–4465, 4465f
spine in, 4460–4461, 4460t, 4461f
surgery for, 4467–4469, 4468f, 4469f
complications of, 4469–4470, 4470f
indications for, 4463–4464
Ankylosis, cervical. *See* Cervical spondylotic myelopathy.
Annuloplasty, intradiskal electrothermal, 4791–4792, 4793f
Annulus fibrosus, 4327–4328
aging effects on, 4396
peripheral, 4185
tear of, magnetic resonance imaging of, 507f, 508
Anoxia, potassium increases in, 102
Antacids, in ependymoma surgery, 3630
Antecollis, 2896t
rotatory, 2893, 2894f, 2895
Anterior angle, 32
Anterior cingulate cortex, stimulation of, 3122
Anterior circulation aneurysms. *See* Aneurysms, anterior circulation.
Anterior column, trauma to, imaging of, 519
Anterior commissure, 8f, 14f
radiologic features of, 2769–2770
Anterior cord syndrome, 4310, 4311
Anterior fontanelle
delayed closure of, 431
small, 431
Anterior fossa, 422
encephalocele of, 3205–3211. *See also* Encephalocele, anterior.
weakness of, 426
Anterior horizontal ramus, 4f
Anterior horn cell disease, 272
Anterior iliac crest, bone graft harvest from, 4602–4605, 4602f–4604f
Anterior interosseous syndrome, 3925
Anterior longitudinal ligament, 4186
Anterior screw-plate fixation. *See* Cervical spine, anterior screw-plate fixation of.
Anterior spinal artery syndrome, 4311, 4890, 4890f
vs. thoracic disk herniation, 4492
Anterior Thoracolumbar Locking Plate system, 4684–4685, 4685f, 4719, 4721–4722, 4721f
Anterolateral margin, 32
Anterosuperior margin, 32
Antiapoptotic genes, 718–719
Antibiotics
for bullet wounds, 5230
for distal anterior cerebral artery aneurysm surgery, 1950
for infectious aneurysms, 2104–2105
for pyogenic spinal infection, 4379, 4381
bacteriologic diagnosis and, 4369
for shunt infection, 3423–3424
for traumatic cerebrospinal fluid fistula, 5270–5271
in shunt infection prevention, 3422
Antibiotics *(Continued)*
ototoxic, for Ménière's disease, 2906
prophylactic
after cervical laminoforaminotomy, 4416
after cervical laminoplasty, 4419
in craniofacial trauma, 5248
in traumatic brain injury, 5129
Antibody(ies)
effector function of, 680
movement of, 682–683
myelin-blocking, 4169
Anticholinergic drugs, for dystonia, 2796
Anticoagulants
for blunt cerebrovascular injury, 5217
for carotid artery injury, 1671
in carotid endarterectomy, 1633–1634
pregnancy effects on, 2422–2423
spontaneous intracerebral hemorrhage from, 1734–1735
Anticonvulsants
for chronic pain, 2959–2960
for dystonia, 2796
for trigeminal neuralgia, 2990, 2990t, 2996
intracranial pressure and, 189
neural tube defects from, 3218
pediatric, anesthesia in, 3189, 3190f
postoperative, in bullet wounds, 5240–5241
pregnancy effects on, 2422
prophylactic, in bullet wounds, 5230–5231
Antidepressants
for pain, 2966
for trigeminal neuralgia, 2990, 2991t
modulation sites for, 2954f
tricyclic
for failed back syndrome, 4337
for neuropathic pain, 3838
for pain, 2960, 2966
mechanisms of, 2964
side effects of, 2964
Antidiuretic hormone
after aneurysmal subarachnoid hemorrhage, 1829–1830
release of, after pituitary resection, 3679
Antiepileptic drugs, 2469–2473
clinical pharmacology of, 2469–2472
discontinuation of, 2473
epileptic syndrome and, 2471t, 2473
failure of, pediatric, 3760
for glial tumors, 870–871
for post-traumatic epilepsy, 2454
initiation of, 2472–2473
pharmacokinetics of, 2470t
principles of, 2473
seizure type and, 2471t, 2473
selection of, 2470t, 2473
Antifibrinolytic agents, pregnancy effects on, 2424
Antigen(s)
astrocytoma, 890
brain tumor, 677
cell surface, 676
immune response to, 679–680
presentation of
by microglial cells, 889–890
direct vs. indirect, 678
in central nervous system, 887, 889–890
MHC in, 677–679, 678f
to T cells, 887, 888f
processing of, 676
recognition of, 676–677

Antigen(s) *(Continued)*
re-presentation of, to migrant T cells, 682
tumor, 887, 889f
identification of, 674
vaccines using, 893
Antigen receptors, 675–677
Antigenic determinants, 675–676
Antigen-presenting cells, 678, 887, 889
dendritic cells as, 893
Antihypertensive agents
in traumatic brain injury, 5127, 5128t
intracranial pressure and, 187–188
pregnancy effects on, 2423–2424
Anti-ICAM-1 antibody, in ischemia protection, 1522
Anti-inflammatory agents
for chronic pain, 2959
modulation sites for, 2954f
Antinuclear antibodies, in rheumatoid arthritis, 4570
Antioccludin antibodies, 156
Antiplatelet agents, pregnancy effects on, 2423
Antisense oligonucleotides, for recurrent carotid stenosis, 1665
Antisiphon devices, in cerebrospinal fluid shunt, 3378–3379, 3378f
Antisocial behavior, in traumatic brain injury response, 5193t
Antispasmodics, 3788
for cerebral palsy, 3731, 3732
Antithrombotics, for cerebral venous thrombosis, 1726–1727
α_1-Antitrypsin deficiency, aneurysms in, 1771–1772
alpha$_1$-Antitrypsin gene, 1772
Antley-Bixler syndrome, 3164
Anxiety
after traumatic brain injury, 5296
depression with, anterior cingulotomy for, 2856–2857, 2857f
in chronic pain, 2966
Anxiolytics, for pain, 2966
Aortic arch, atherosclerosis of, magnetic resonance angiography of, 1590, 1591f
APC, 744
Apert's syndrome, 3318, 3320f
historical aspects of, 3164
surgery for
Le Fort III osteotomy in, 3326–3327
monoblock osteotomy in, 3327, 3328f
treatment of, 3321
Aphasia
after temporal lobe resection, 2572–2573
after traumatic brain injury, 5186
fluent, 264
middle carotid artery infarction and, 1614
nonfluent, 264
subcortical, stroke and, 1608
testing for, 264–265, 264t
Apical dental ligament, 4925, 4926f
Apnea
in achondroplasia, 3363–3364
in traumatic brain injury, 5128
Apnea test, 398, 398t
Apneustic breathing, in consciousness assessment, 283
Apo-2 ligand, in astrocytoma immunotherapy, 894
Apolipoprotein (apo A-I), in blood-brain barrier, 162
Apoplexy
historical aspects of, 1463
pituitary, 1175–1176, 1202–1203
Apoptosis, 82, 718–719
after central nervous system injury, 4155–4156
cell proliferation and, in tumor growth, 689
in Alzheimer's disease, 2710
in angiogenesis, 773, 774t
in immune response, 680
in ischemic injury, 1519, 1519f
in Parkinson's disease, 2710
in traumatic brain injury, 5030
invasion and, 774t
regulators of, 743
vs. necrosis, 130–132, 131f
Apractic syndromes, middle carotid artery infarction and, 1615
Aqueduct, 14f
Aqueduct of Sylvius, obstruction of
endoscopic third ventriculostomy for, 3393–3394
hydrocephalus from, 3391, 3392f
shunt failure in, 3393
treatment of, 3392–3393
Arachidonic acid
in blood-brain barrier function, 12
in ischemic injury, 1518
metabolism of, 1472–1473, 1472f
Arachnoid, 1099
dissection of, in anterior circulation aneurysm surgery, 1878
embryology of, 3289
Arachnoid cisterns, anatomy of, 1926–1927, 1927f, 1929
Arachnoid cyst, 3289–3299
along lateral cerebral convexity, 3295
clinical presentation of, 3290–3291
development of, 3289
distribution of, 3290, 3290t
imaging of, 541, 542f, 3291–3292, 3291f, 3292f
in sylvian fissure, 3292–3293, 3293f
infratentorial, 3298–3299
intrasellar, 3295, 3295f
pathology of, 3289–3290
posterior fossa, 3298, 3298f
quadrigeminal, 3297–3298, 3297f
radiologic features of, 839
retrochiasmatic, 3294f
shunt for, 3291
spinal cord, 4821
suprasellar, 3293–3295, 3294f, 3295f
supratentorial, 3292–3298
trauma and, 3289
treatment of, 3290–3291
Arachnoid granulations, 1100, 1100f
Arachnoid villi, 1100
occlusion of
hydrocephalus from, 3397–3398, 3397f, 3398f
treatment of, 3398
Arachnoiditis, imaging of, 541, 541f, 542f
Arcade of Struthers, 3902
Arcuate fasciculus, resection of, language assessment during, 2537
Arcuate ligament of Osborne, 3903
Area postrema, 33f
pediatric, ependymoma of, 3625, 3625t
L-Arginine, in cerebral blood flow regulation, 1470t, 1471
Arix, 55t
Arm
anterior interosseous nerve in, surgery on, 650–651, 651f
median nerve in, surgery on, 650, 650f, 651f
Arm *(Continued)*
pain in
dorsal rhizotomy for, 3041–3042
surgery for, 3026t
posterior interosseous nerve in, surgery on, 651
radial nerve in, surgery on, 651
Arrhythmias
after aneurysmal subarachnoid hemorrhage, 1828–1829
in thoracoscopy, 4769
thoracic endoscopic sympathectomy for, 3097
Arteria radicularis anterior magna, 2380
Arterial bypass, 2108–2118
aneurysm occlusion after, 2115, 2117
cervical-to-petrous, 1672f, 1673
collateral circulation and, 2107
complications of, 2117
distal vertebral artery–to–occipital artery, 1709
external carotid artery–to–distal vertebral artery, 1706, 1708f, 1709–1710, 1711f
extracranial carotid artery–to–middle cerebral artery saphenous vein interposition graft in, 2110–2111, 2111f, 2112f
extracranial carotid artery–to–posterior cerebral artery saphenous vein interposition graft in, 2111, 2113
extracranial-intracranial, vs. carotid artery sacrifice, 1892–1893
for aneurysms, 1807, 2107–2108
for fusiform aneurysms, 2117–2118
for giant aneurysms, 2117–2118
for skull base tumors, 2108
graft patency in, 2117
in hemodynamic failure, 1603–1604
ischemia prevention in, 1522
management after, 2117
middle cerebral artery, 1673–1674
monitoring during, 2109
occipital artery–to–posterior inferior cerebral artery graft in, 2113, 2115, 2115f, 2116f
outcome of, 2117–2118
patent artery and, 2107
patient selection in, 1807
pericallosal-to-pericallosal, 2115
petrous-to-supraclinoid, 1673f–1674f, 1674
petrous-to-supraclinoid carotid saphenous vein graft in, 2109, 2109f, 2110f
preoperative planning for, 2108
saphenous vein interposition graft in, 2110, 2111f, 2112f
superficial temporal artery–to–middle cerebral artery, 2113, 2113f, 2114f
superficial temporal artery–to–superior cerebellar artery, 2115
type I, 2109–2110, 2109f, 2110f
type II, 2110, 2111f, 2112f
types of, 2108–2115, 2109f
Arterial pressure
cerebrospinal fluid circulation and, 3387
in cerebral blood flow, 1504
Arterial reanastomosis, primary, 2115
Arterial reconstruction, 2115
historical considerations in, 1463
Arterial-capillary-venous hypertensive syndrome, in arteriovenous malformation, 2189, 2190f–2191f
Arteriosclerotic disease, carotid artery, preoperative evaluation for, 552–553, 552t

Arteriovascular malformations, 2137–2155, 2138t. *See also* specific type, e.g., Developmental venous anomalies.
Arteriovenous differentiation of oxygen ($AVDO_2$), 5048, 5048t
  autoregulation effects on, 5048, 5053, 5053t
Arteriovenous fistula
  dural, 2171–2173, 2377–2379
    arteriography of, 2400–2401, 2402f–2403f
    classification of, 2173, 2173t
    clinical features of, 2172–2173, 2386–2388
    definition of, 2171–2172
    distribution of, 2382f
    embolization for, 2127–2128, 2128f, 2406, 2408
    epidemiology of, 2172
    extradural-intradural venous drainage in, 2403–2404, 2406f
    functional disability in, 2388, 2389f
    headache in, 2172
    hemorrhage in, 2172–2173
    imaging of, 537, 538f
    location of, 2172, 2173
    magnetic resonance angiography of, 1593, 1596, 1596f
    magnetic resonance imaging of, 2395, 2398, 2398f
    nidus of, 2379, 2383, 2383f
    outcome in, 2404, 2406, 2407f
    pathogenesis of, 2171–2172
    prognosis for, 2173
    pulsatile tinnitus in, 2172
    radiosurgery for, 2128, 2128f
    surgery for, 2127–2128, 2401–2403, 2404f–2407f, 2406
    symptoms of, 2173
    synonyms for, 2171
    treatment of, 2126–2128
    vascular anatomy of, 2377f, 2381, 2383, 2384f, 2386, 2387f
    vs. intradural arteriovenous malformations, 2386–2387, 2387t, 2388, 2400, 2401t
  extracranial vertebral artery, 1694
  extradural, 2356, 2357f, 2366
  intradural
    dorsal, 2356, 2357f, 2358, 2366–2368, 2367f
    ventral, 2358, 2358f, 2359, 2368, 2369f
  perimedullary, 2378
    anatomy of, 2380f, 2386, 2387f
    clinical features of, 2391, 2392f–2394f, 2394
    embolization of, 2413, 2414f–2415f
    radiographic features of, 2401t
    surgery for, 2413, 2416f
    treatment of, 2413, 2414f–2416f, 2415
    types of, 2391, 2391t
  peripheral nerve involvement in, 3949
  spinal cord, 2366–2368
  traumatic, 5204
Arteriovenous malformations, 2147–2155, 2159–2167
  anesthesia in, 1511–1512
  aneurysms with. *See* Aneurysms, arteriovenous malformations with.
  angiography of, 2162
  anterior callosal, 2242, 2242f
  asymptomatic, 2161
  behavior of, 2164
  brainstem. *See* Brainstem, arteriovenous malformations of.

Arteriovenous malformations *(Continued)*
  capillary telangiectasia and, 2153
  caudate, 2246
  cavernous, 4319
  cavernous malformation and, 2154
  cerebellar, 2251
    arterial supply/venous outflow in, 2256–2257, 2257f, 2258f
    imaging of, 2254–2255, 2254f
    surgery for, 2260–2263, 2261f–2263f
  classification of, 2185–2187, 2186f, 2187t
  clinical presentation of, 2148–2149, 2149f, 2161–2163
    in pregnancy, 2426–2427
  conus medullaris, 2362, 2371–2372, 2371f
  definition of, 2159–2160
  developmental venous anomalies and, 2153–2154
  diagnosis of, in pregnancy, 2427
  dural, 2283–2290, 2343, 4318, 4318f
    classification of, 2284, 2286–2288, 2286f–2289f
    clinical manifestations of, 2283–2284
    etiology of, 2283
    imaging of, 2284, 2285f
    natural history of, 2283–2284
    superior sagittal sinus
      clinical manifestations of, 2284
      imaging of, 2287–2288, 2288f, 2289f
      treatment of, 2290
    transverse-sigmoid
      clinical manifestations of, 2284
      imaging of, 2286–2287, 2286f, 2287f
      treatment of, 2288–2290
    treatment of, 2288
      outcomes of, 2290
  embolization of, 2126, 2151–2152, 2223–2229
    catheters for, 2224–2225
    flow control in, 2225
    histopathologic findings after, 2226, 2226f, 2227f, 2228
    material for, 2225
    morphologic criteria for, 2223–2224
    nidus accessibility in, 2223–2224
    nidus hemodynamics in, 2224
    outcome of, 2228–2229
    repermeation after, 2226, 2226f
    results of, 2196–2198, 2197f
    risk in, 2225–2226
    size in, 2224
    visual evoked potentials during, 2544
  endovascular treatment of, 2205–2220
    anatomic factors in, 2211–2212
    aneurysms and, 2212, 2213f, 2214f
    angiography in, 2206, 2211, 2211f
    clinical factors in, 2205–2206
    combination, 2217–2218
    complications of, 2219f, 2220
    curative, 2212, 2215f, 2216f
    embolization techniques in, 2218
    morphologic factors in, 2206, 2211, 2211f
    outcome in, 2218, 2218t, 2220, 2220t
    palliative, 2212, 2216–2217
    patient selection in, 2205
    preoperative embolization in, 2217
    symptoms and, 2206, 2207f–2210f
  epidemiology of, 2147, 2160–2161
  extradural-intradural, 2359, 2359f
  functional decline in, 2192
  giant. *See* Giant arteriovenous malformations.
  headache in, 2163, 2206
  heavy-particle radiosurgery for, 3991–3992, 3992f

Arteriovenous malformations *(Continued)*
  hemorrhage in, 2121, 2161–2163, 2188, 2206, 2207f–2210f
    after radiosurgery, 4081–4082
    effects of, 2191–2192
    recurrent, 2163–2164
    risk for, 2191
      age in, 2192, 2192t
  historical aspects of, 1462–1463
  hypothalamic, 2243
  imaging of, 2138t, 2149–2150, 2150f, 2151f, 2160, 2164
  in extratemporal lobe epilepsy, 2598
  in pregnancy, 2166, 2426–2427
  insular, 2237–2238
  internal capsule, 2246
  intradural, 4318
    acquired vs. congenital, 2388, 2389t
    arteriography of, 2401
    clinical features of, 2388–2389
    glomus (type II), 2376–2377
      vascular anatomy of, 2379f, 2386
    historical aspects of, 2375–2379
    juvenile (type III), 2376–2377
      vascular anatomy of, 2378f, 2383, 2385f, 2386
    magnetic resonance imaging of, 2398, 2399f
    natural history of, 2388–2391, 2390t
    prognosis of, 2390–2391
    single coiled vessel (type I), 2376, 2377
    vascular anatomy of, 2383, 2384f–2387f, 2386
    vs. dural arteriovenous fistulas, 2386–2387, 2387t, 2388, 2400, 2401t
  intramedullary, 2359, 2360f, 2361f, 2362
    magnetic resonance imaging of, 2398, 2399f
    outcome in, 2410, 2410t, 2411f
    surgery, 2408, 2409f, 2410
  intraventricular, 2243, 2244f, 2245f, 2246
  magnetic resonance angiography of, 1593, 1595f
  magnetic resonance imaging of, 469–471, 470f
  medial temporal, 2239–2241, 2240f
  micro-, with parenchymal hematoma, 2215f
  microsurgery for, 2126
  mixed, 2152–2154
  morbidity in, 2163
  mortality in, 2163
  multimodality treatment for, 4084
  natural history of, 2138t, 2148–2149, 2149f, 2191–2192, 4080–4081
  neurological deficit in, 2163, 2206, 2210f
  neuropsychological assessment in, 388–389, 389t
  observation of, 2191–2192, 2192t
  outcome in, 2163–2164
    in pregnancy, 2427
  parasagittal, 2238–2239
  paratrigonal, 2240–2241, 2240f, 2241f
  parieto-occipital, magnetoencephalography of, 2547, 2547f
  pathogenesis of, 2159–2160
  pathology of, 2138t, 2148, 2148f
  pediatric, 2166–2167, 3452–3457
    aneurysm with, 3448
    assessment of, 3453–3454
    development of, 3452
    embolization of, 3455–3456
    hemorrhage in, 3453
    imaging of, 3454, 3454f, 3455f

Arteriovenous malformations *(Continued)*
natural history of, 3453
pathology of, 3452
radiosurgery for, 3456, 3457f
results in, 3456–3457
rupture of, 3452–3453
seizures in, 3454
subarachnoid hemorrhage in, 3447–3448
surgery on, 3195
treatment of, 3454–3455
positron emission tomography of, 1604
posterior callosal, 2242–2243, 2243f
posterior fossa, 2251–2265. *See also* Posterior fossa, arteriovenous malformations of.
preoperative evaluation in, 554
putamen, 2246
radiation therapy for
cure rates in, 2194, 2194t
delayed cure by, 2194–2195
hemorrhage after, 2194
mortality/morbidity risks with, 2199, 2199t
necrosis after, 2195–2196, 2195f, 2196t
results of, 2193–2196
seizure after, 2196
surgery with, 2198
vs. microsurgery, 2198–2199
radiosurgery for, 4073–4085
complications of, 4080–4084
dose selection in, 4076
failure of
reasons for, 4079–4080
salvage retreatment after, 4084
follow-up after, 4077–4078
head ring application in, 4074
patient selection for, 4073–4074
radiation delivery in, 4077
results of, 4079
stereotactic image acquisition in, 4074, 4075f
technique of, 4073–4078, 4075f–4077f
treatment planning in, 4074–4076, 4076f
scalp, 1414
seizures in, 2163, 2196, 2206
size of, 2162
Spetzler-Martin grading system for, 2185–2187, 2186f, 2187t
spinal, 2375–2417, 4315t, 4318–4319, 4318f
arteriography of, 2400–2401, 2401t, 2402f–2403f
causes of, 2386–2395
classification of, 2375–2379
clinical presentation of, 2386–2395
imaging of, 536–537, 2395–2401
magnetic resonance imaging of, 2395, 2397f
myelography of, 2400, 2400f
natural history of, 2386–2395
pathogenesis of, 2379–2386
pathophysiology of, 2386–2395
screening studies for, 2395–2400
treatment of, 2401–2416
vascular anatomy in, 2379–2386
spinal cord, 2363–2372. *See also* Spinal cord, arteriovenous malformations of.
staged-volume radiosurgery for, 2126
stereotactic radiosurgery for, 2126, 2151
embolization before, 2217–2218
subarachnoid hemorrhage in, 2149, 2149f
supratentorial, 2231–2248

Arteriovenous malformations *(Continued)*
anatomic classification of, 2237, 2238f
classification of, 2248
coexisting intracranial aneurysm with, 2235
convexity, 2237
diagnosis of, 2232, 2233f
embolization of, 2234–2235
grading of, 2234
identification of, 2236
microsurgery for, 2235–2237
pathogenesis of, 2231–2232
radiosurgery for, 2235
surgery for, 2232–2247
angiography during, 2246
apex dissection in, 2237
complications of, 2246–2247
cost-effectiveness of, 2234
craniotomy in, 2236
decision making in, 2248
deep arterial pedicle dissection in, 2237
follow-up after, 2246
hemostasis in, 2237
indications for, 2232, 2234
intensive care after, 2246
lesion-related factors in, 2232, 2234
nidus dissection in, 2236–2237
outcome of, 2247, 2247t
patient-related factors in, 2232
positioning for, 2236
preoperative measures for, 2236
superficial feeding arteries in, 2236
surgeon-related factors in, 2234
timing of, 2235–2236
venous drainage in, 2237
surgery for
aneurysm rupture during, 2187–2188
arterial-capillary-venous hypertensive syndrome in, 2189, 2190f–2191f
brain eloquence in, 2187
cerebral circulatory pressures in, 2188–2189, 2188f
complications of, 2187–2191
deep venous drainage in, 2187
edema during, 2188
hemorrhage during, 2187, 2188
hyperemia in, 2188
in pregnancy, 2427
neurological deficits after, 2192–2193, 2193f
perfusion pressure breakthrough in, 2188
results of, 2192–2193, 2193f, 2193t
risk in, 2150, 2151t
seizures after, 2189, 2191, 2193, 2193t
thrombosis in, 2189, 2189f
vasospasm in, 2189, 2191f
sylvian, 2237–2238, 2239f
syndromic, 2154–2155
synonyms for, 2159
temporal lobe, homonymous visual field defects in, 314f, 315
thalamic, 2246
third ventricular, 2242–2243
transcranial Doppler ultrasonography of, 1547–1548
transitional forms of, 2152–2154
treatment of, 2138t, 2150–2152, 2151t
clinical significance and, 2205
decision making in, 2185–2201
individualized, 2198–2199, 2199t
perioperative management in, 2200, 2200t
unruptured, in pregnancy, 2427

Arteriovenous malformations *(Continued)*
vasospasm in, 1841
venous drainage pattern of, 2162–2163
vermian, arterial supply/venous outflow in, 2256, 2256f
vision mapping in, functional magnetic resonance imaging for, 2545
vs. supratentorial cavernous malformation, 2311, 2312f
Artery(ies)
injury to
neurological deficit from, 935, 936f
transsphenoidal surgery and, 1182
occlusion of, in pregnancy, 2427–2428, 2428t
temporary occlusion of, 1520
Artery of Adamkiewicz, 2380, 4310–4311
Artery of Heubner, 28f
Arthritis
enteropathic, 4351
peripheral, in ankylosing spondylitis, 4461
psoriatic, 4350–4351, 4462, 4463t
reactive, 4462–4463, 4463t
rheumatoid, 4351
Arthrodesis, in spine stabilization surgery, 4339–4343, 4341f, 4342f
Arthropathy
enteropathic, 4463, 4463t
psoriatic, 4350–4351
craniocervical junction, 4580
Articular capsular ligament, 4925, 4926f
Ascending ramus, 4f
Ash, 53t
Ashworth Scale, 242t, 2864, 2864t
in cerebral palsy, 3725, 3726t, 3750, 3750t
in spasticity, 2880–2881, 2881t
Aspartate, in traumatic brain injury, 5025
Aspen collar, 4898f
Aspergillosis, spinal, 4387–4388
Aspergillus, infectious aneurysms from, 2102
Aspiration
bur hole, 1753
for intracerebral hemorrhage, 1753–1756, 1760t
mechanically assisted, 1754–1755
stereotactic, 1753–1754, 1756, 1760t
Aspirin
for carotid artery disease, 1617
in carotid endarterectomy, 1644
in pregnancy, 2423
spontaneous intracerebral hemorrhage from, 1735
Assistive devices, for cerebral palsy, 3730, 3732–3733
Asterion, 423f
Astroblastoma, 993–994, 994f
third ventricular, 1246
Astrocytes, 83–84, 97–112
after central nervous system injury, 4168
ammonia detoxification by, 104f–105f, 107
amyloid plaque infiltration by, 90, 91f
calcium ion waves in, 110
classification of, 86
clinical implications of, 110–112
connexins in, 101
contact spacing of, 99, 100f–101f
cortical, 97, 98f
end-feet of, 99, 100f–101f
ensheathing glia and, 4163
fibroblast growth factor receptor in, 728
fibrous, 86, 99, 100f–101f
functions of, 84f, 102–110

Astrocytes *(Continued)*
gap junction communication in, 227
glutamate in, 1485
synthesis of, 104f–105f, 106–107
transporters for, 102–103, 104f–105f, 106
glycogen in, 99, 101, 109, 111
glycogenesis in, 1485
gray matter, 85–86
identification of, 99
in axonal regeneration, 204–205
in blood-brain barrier regulation, 109–110
in brain endothelium function, 158
in brain injury recovery, 5031
in cerebral blood flow–metabolism coupling, 1489
in cerebral metabolism, 1486–1487
in genetic disease, 111
in glucose metabolism, 107, 108f
in ion homeostasis, 102, 103f, 104f
in nervous system regeneration, 4155
in neuronal metabolism, 107, 108f, 109
in D-serine synthesis, 107
in stroke, 111–112
ischemia tolerance of, 111
lineage of, 97–98, 98f
malignant progression in, 725
physiology of, 101–102
protoplasmic, 86, 99, 100f–101f
structure of, 98–99, 100f–101f, 101
subcortical, 97, 98f
types of, 83–84
white matter, 84–85
Astrocytoma, 4296t
anaplastic
brainstem, 985, 985f
chemotherapy for, 976
classification of, 662, 662t
diagnosis of, 972, 973f
epidemiology of, 969
gene alterations in, 751t
genetics of, 969–970
prognosis for, 977–978
radiation therapy for, 975, 4021–4022
radiologic features of, 844, 844f
seizures in, 828
surgery for, 974, 974f
vascular endothelial growth factor receptors in, 733
antigens to, 890
benign, radiologic features of, 845–847, 845f
bromodeoxyuridine marking of, 693
cerebellar. *See* Cerebellar astrocytoma.
cerebral
desmoplastic, of infancy, 991
superficial, 990
circumscribed, 663–664
classification of, 661–664, 661t
angiogenesis in, 772
cystic, 450, 451f
cytometric cell-cycle analysis of, 694–695
desmoplastic, pediatric, 663, 850
diffuse fibrillary, 661–663
DNA polymerase marking of, 694
fibrillary, 1246
fibroblast growth factor expression in, 727–728
gemistocytic, 661
gene alterations in, 751t
giant cell
radiologic features of, 844
subependymal, 991–992, 992f
classification of, 663

Astrocytoma *(Continued)*
foramen of Monro obstruction from, 3390, 3391f
third ventricular, 1246
glutamate transporters in, 106
grading of, 662t, 689–690
growth factors expressed by, 726t
imaging of, 525
immune system evasion by, 891
immunotherapy for
autoimmune disease in, 894
immunization site in, 893–894
tumor necrosis factor in, 894–895
incidence of, 950
juvenile pilocytic, 1246
Ki-67/MIB-1 marking of, 695–696
low-grade
histopathology of, 951–952, 951f
interstitial brachytherapy for, 4104
prognostic factors in, 965
radiologic features of, 844, 844f
lymphocytes in, 890
magnetic resonance imaging of, 450, 450f–453f, 452–453
magnetic resonance spectroscopy of, 452f, 453
male:female ratio in, 953
malignant, linac radiosurgery for, 4113–4114
MIB-1 labeling index for, 696, 697t, 698
molecular markers for, 696, 697t, 698
oligodendrocyte progenitor cells and, 92–93
pediatric, 3697
pathology of, 3700
surgery for, 3702
pilocytic, 986–988
classification of, 663
clinical presentation of, 986
gene alterations in, 751t
imaging of, 845–846, 845f, 986, 987f
juvenile
biopsy of, 3666
surgery for, 3667, 3667f
MIB-1 labeling index for, 699, 700t
natural history of, 986
optic pathway, pediatric, 3595
pathology of, 986–987
proliferation markers for, 699
treatment of, 987–988
pilomyxoid, 663
platelet-derived growth factor in, 730
proliferating cell nuclear antigen marking of, 693
protoplasmic, 661
radiologic features of, 835, 842–847, 843f–844f
spinal cord, 4040, 4302, 4302f, 4825–4826, 4825f, 4826f
radiation therapy for, 4042, 4043, 4043t
surgery for, 4043
treatment of, 4828–4829, 4831
third ventricular, 1246
^{3}H-thymidine marking of, 692
TP53 mutation in, 950
transforming growth factor-β in, 730–731
vascular endothelial growth factor in, 733
Astrogliogenesis, 97, 98f
Astrogliosis, 204
Ataxia
autosomal-dominant, 2738–2740
autosomal-recessive, 2738

Ataxia *(Continued)*
cerebellar
after medulloblastoma surgery, 1037
urologic disorders in, 373–374
episodic, 2739–2740
hereditary, 2740
ion channels in, 225t
nucleus caudalis DREZ ablation and, 3054, 3087–3088
pediatric, 3180
progressive, 4316t, 4320–4321
spinocerebellar, 2739
urologic disorders in, 373–374
with oculomotor apraxia, 2738
with vitamin E deficiency, 2738
Ataxia-telangiectasia, 2738
Ataxic breathing, in consciousness assessment, 282–283
Ataxic cerebral palsy, 3725
Atherosclerosis
aortic arch, magnetic resonance angiography of, 1590, 1591f
carotid artery, 1613–1618. *See also* Carotid artery, atherosclerosis of.
ischemic optic neuropathy in, 306
stenosis from, transcranial Doppler ultrasonography of, 1554
vertebral artery, 1694
magnetic resonance angiography of, 1590, 1591f
Atherothrombosis, 1495
Athetosis, in cerebral palsy, 3724, 3727
Athetotic movements, pediatric, assessment of, 3180
Atlantal ligament, transverse, 3331, 3537
Atlantis system, of cervical spine anterior screw-plate fixation, 4630t, 4633–4635, 4633f–4635f
Atlantoaxial joint, 3331
anatomy of, 4939
biomechanics of, 4187
complex fracture of, 4934, 4935, 4935f
fractures of, 4906, 4906f, 4907f
injury to, biomechanics of, 4188
instability of, 3333
in Down syndrome, 3337–3338, 3338f
in skeletal dysplasia, 3343
pediatric
anatomy of, 3537–3538
biomechanics of, 3537–3538, 3538f
fusion of, 3547, 3548f, 3549f
instrumentation with, 3547, 3549–3550, 3549f, 3550f
rotatory fixation of, 3537–3543
classification of, 3538–3540, 3539f–3541f
radiography of, 3538–3540, 3539f–3541f
treatment of, 3541, 3542f
systemic disorders affecting, 3542–3543
transarticular screw fixation of, 3547, 3549–3550, 3549f, 3550f
translational subluxation of, 3541–3542
subluxation of, rheumatoid arthritis and, 4571–4572, 4571f, 4573
surgery for, 4578, 4580f
Atlantoaxial motion segment, 3333
Atlanto-occipital dislocation, 4655, 4902–4903, 4925, 4928–4933
classification of, 4931, 4932f
clinical presentation of, 4928–4929
dens-bastion line in, 4929–4930, 4930f
evaluation of, 4929–4931
magnetic resonance imaging of, 4931, 4931f

Atlanto-occipital dislocation *(Continued)*
mechanism of, 4928
pediatric, 3528–3537
classification of, 3531
clinical presentation of, 3531–3532
hyperextension-distraction forces in, 3530
pathology of, 3529–3531, 3531f
radiography of, 3532–3536, 3532f–3537f
tectorial membrane in, 3531, 3531f
treatment of, 3536–3537
Powers ratio in, 4930–4931, 4930f
radiography of, 4929, 4929f
traction for, 4932–4933
treatment of, 4931–4933
Wackenheim's line in, 4929, 4930f
X-line method in, 4930f, 4931
Atlanto-occipital joint. *See also* Craniovertebral junction.
dissociation of, 518f, 519, 519f
embryology of, 3331–3332
fusion of. *See* Occipitocervical fusion.
pediatric
anatomy of, 3528–3529, 3530f
biomechanics of, 3528–3529
injury to, 3516
instrumentation fusion of, 3550–3552, 3551f–3553f
Atlanto-occipital ligament, 4925, 4926f
Atlas
assimilation of, 3339–3340, 3340f
bifid, 3338
diseases of, 4800t
vertebral formation in, 3332
Atlas fracture, 4903, 4903f, 4925, 4933–4935
burst, 501, 519
classification of, 4934, 4934f
clinical presentation of, 4933–4934
evaluation of, 4934
imaging of, 518f, 519, 519f
mechanism of, 4933
radiography of, 4934, 4935f
treatment of, 4935
Atracurium, 1508
Atrial natriuretic factor, after aneurysmal subarachnoid hemorrhage, 1829–1830
Atrial veins, 17, 1239
Atrium, 7f, 8, 8f, 12f, 13, 15f
Atrophy, denervation, 201
Attention, after traumatic brain injury, 5186–5187
Attorney-in-fact, 409
Atypical teratoid-rhabdoid tumors
cerebellar, 999
classification of, 669
Audiometry, pure-tone, 331–332, 331f, 332f
Auditory apparatus, in temporal bone fractures, 5276
Auditory brainstem evoked response
hearing assessment with, 334–335, 336f
in auditory neuropathy, 336–337
Auditory canal, schwannoma of, 459, 459f
Auditory evoked potential recordings
of auditory neuropathy, 335–337
with cochlear implants, 337
Auditory nerve, pediatric, examination of, 3175–3176
Auditory neuropathy, testing for, 335–337
Auditory system
dysfunction of, pediatric basilar skull fracture and, 3468
examination of, 267
function of
measures of, 330–338
Auditory system *(Continued)*
objective measures of, 333–338
subjective measures of, 330–333, 331f–333f
mechanical receptors for, 74, 74f
Auscultation, for bruits, 269
Autograft, 2829t, 4616–4617
for pyogenic spinal infection, 4376f–4379f
in cervical spine fusion, 4622
Autoimmune disease
immunotherapy and, 894
peripheral nerves in, 3816
Automated percutaneous lumbar diskectomy, 4776–4780
complications of, 4779
historical perspective on, 4776–4777
indications for, 4777–4778
results of, 4779
technique of, 4778–4779
Autonomic nervous system
bladder innervation by, 358, 358f
dysfunction of, in peripheral nerve injury, 3822
in lower urinary tract function, 359–360
in pain, 3820–3821
Autonomic neuropathy, diabetic, 3842
Autopsy, legal issues regarding, 416
Autoregulation
after traumatic brain injury, 5084
cerebral blood flow, 5048, 5053, 5053t
in traumatic brain injury, 5120
theories on, 5049–5050
failure of, 1601, 1601t
in head injury, 5051–5052, 5053f
metabolic, 5048, 5051–5052
of cerebral metabolism. *See* Cerebral autoregulation.
pressure, 5048–5049, 5049f, 5052
theories of, 5049–5050
viscosity, 5049, 5052, 5053t
Autosomal-dominant disorders, 273
Autosomal-recessive disorders, 273
Avulsion, in craniofacial trauma, 5249
Awake position, 597t, 600, 601f, 602f
Awakening, in deep hypothermic circulatory arrest, 1536
Axilla, median nerve entrapment at, 3924
Axillary nerve, palsy of, 3824, 3825f
Axis
anatomy of, 4939
biomechanics of, 4939
diseases of, 4800t
fractures of, 4903–4906, 4903f–4907f, 4904t, 4906t, 4925, 4939–4947
imaging of, 518f, 519, 519f
traumatic spondylolisthesis of, 520f, 521, 4945–4947, 4946t
Axolemma, in remyelination, 198
Axon(s)
collateral sprouting of, 3785
conduction velocity of, 86
degeneration of, 3961–3962, 3961f, 3962f
calcium in, 199
peripheral neuropathy from, 3835, 3836t
diffuse injury to, 5045–5046, 5046t, 5091, 5092f
disconnection pathways in, 5028, 5028f
in multiple sclerosis, 1451
in traumatic brain injury, 5045–5046, 5046t, 5105–5106, 5107f
magnetic resonance imaging of, 469, 5093, 5095f
Axon(s) *(Continued)*
pathophysiology of, 5105–5106, 5107f
pediatric, 3463
therapy in, 5028–5029, 5029t
growth of, 80–81
guidance of, 80–81
failure of, 82, 82f
in myelinated nerve fiber, 3958–3960, 3960f
in nociception, 2922, 2923
motor function and, 3831, 3833, 4157
myelination and, 86–87, 86f
peripheral nervous system, in central nervous system repair, 4161–4162
regeneration of, 87, 89f, 195, 196f, 3785, 5032
after central nervous system injury, 202–203
collaterals in, 200–201
distal nerve stump in, 198–199
growth cones in, 198
macrophages in, 206
neuromuscular junction in, 201
neurotrophic receptors in, 197–198
stimulation of, 202
targeting of, 200–201
time in, 198
repair of. *See* Central nervous system, repair of.
retraction of, 3785
retrograde degeneration in, 4156
structure of, 78
transection of
chromatolytic changes in, 3961
pathophysiology of, 3967, 3968f–3969f
Axon hillock, 72f, 73, 78
Axonotmesis
grading of, 3825t, 3826
needle electromyography of, 3860–3861
nerve conduction studies of, 3860
Axoplasm, 78
Axotomy
dorsal root ganglion neurons in, 3815, 3815f
neurotransmitters after, 197–198
traumatic brain injury and, 5028–5029, 5028f, 5029t
Azathioprine
for multiple sclerosis, 1454t, 1455
for sarcoidosis, 1439

B cells
antigen receptors on, 675–676, 677
antigen recognition by, 676, 680
in immune response, 675
movement of, 682–683
B7, in astrocytoma treatment, 893
Babinski sign, 268
pediatric, 3181
Back pain. *See also* Low back pain.
in Ewing's sarcoma, 4848
in lumbar disk disease, after surgery, 4517–4518, 4517f, 4518f
in osteoid osteoma, 4837
in pyogenic spinal infection, 4366
in spinal metastases, 4855, 4855f
Backboard, for cervical spine trauma, 4888
Baclofen
for bladder outlet retention, 380
for cerebral palsy, 3731, 3748–3749
for multiple sclerosis, 1454t
for pain, 2964–2965
for trigeminal neuralgia, 2990t, 2993
formulations of, 3748

Baclofen *(Continued)*
intrathecal
cerebrospinal fluid concentration of, 2883–2884, 2884f, 3749
complications of, 3753–3754
delivery systems for, 2886
distribution of, 2883–2884, 2884f
dosage of, 3750, 3751–3752
duration of action of, 3749
efficacy of, 2884–2885, 2885f, 2885t, 3752–3753, 3752t
for cerebral palsy, 3732, 3749–3756
for dystonia, 2748, 2748f, 2749t
for spasticity, 2750–2751, 2751t, 2866t, 2867, 2882–2887, 3788
GABA receptors and, 3748, 3749
kinetics of, 2883–2884, 2884f
mechanism of action of, 3748
patient selection for, 2886–2887, 2886t, 3750, 3751t, 3754–3755
pharmacokinetics of, 3749
physiologic effects of, 2883, 2883f
pump for, 3749–3754, 3749f, 3750f
response to, 3750
side effects of, 2885–2886, 3748–3749
tolerance to, 2885–2886
vs. dorsal rhizotomy, 3752–3753, 3752t
Bacteremia, pyogenic spinal infections in, 4364
Bacterial infection. *See also* specific infection.
myelitis from, 4312t, 4313
pyogenic. *See* Pyogenic infection.
Bacteriology, neoplastic disease treatment and, 711–712
Bacteroides, spinal infection from, 4365
Bad, 719
Bak, 719
Baker's cyst, 3934
Balance disturbance, after temporal bone fracture, 5281
Baldness, headrests and, 610
Ballism, 2720
Ballismus, 2676
Balloon angioplasty
for carotid restenosis, 1666
for cerebral vasospasm, 1856–1857, 1857f, 1858f
Balloon cells, proliferation of, 2492
Balloon compression, for trigeminal neuralgia, 3000–3002, 3001f
Balloon occlusion, of aneurysms, 2057–2060, 2058f
Baló's concentric sclerosis, 1452
Band of Giacomini, 27
Bands of Büngner, 3961, 3962f
Barbiturate coma
in bullet wounds, 5231
intracranial hypertension treatment by, 5133–5134
Barbiturates, 1508
after head injury, 5097
brain protection with, 5059
cerebral metabolic rate of oxygen and, 1532
in carotid endarterectomy, 1626–1627
in craniotomy, 5150
in hypothermic circulatory arrest, 1511
in ischemia protection, 1521
intracranial pressure and, 188–189
Barthel Index, 243t, 5288
Basal arteries, craniopharyngioma attached to, 3672, 3673f
Basal cell carcinoma
scalp, 1409–1410
Basal cell carcinoma *(Continued)*
skull, 1398, 1399f
staging of, 1410
Basal ganglia, 11
anatomy of, 2671, 2672f, 2683–2695, 2699, 2700f, 2730–2731
"anterior," 19
in dystonia, 2795–2796, 2796f
in micturition, 359
in movement disorders, 2699–2701, 2700f–2701f, 2702t, 2703, 2824–2825
in obsessive-compulsive disorders, 2854–2855
in psychiatric disorders, 2855
in urologic dysfunction, 373
input to, 2671–2672
intrinsic connections of, 2672–2673
motor thalamic nuclei inputs from, 2691, 2692f
organization of, 2683, 2684f
output projections of, 2673
synaptic connectivity of, 2683–2695, 2730–2731. *See also* specific structure, e.g., Striatum.
thalamic nuclei inputs to, 2693, 2694f
thalamocortical circuit and, 2699–2701, 2700f, 2702t, 2703
in Huntington's disease, 2718
venous drainage of, 1238
Basal vein, 10f, 15f, 35f, 36f
segments of, 23–24, 24f
Basement membrane, 3814
glioma spread through, 760
Basic fibroblast growth factor, 51
in angiogenesis, 719, 771, 773
in brain injury recovery, 5031–5032
in recurrent carotid artery stenosis, 1663
Basic helix-loop-helix structure, 51
Basigin gene, 158
Basilar apex
anatomy of, 1974–1975, 1975f
aneurysms of, 1975, 2025, 2041–2052
arteriovenous malformations with, 1976
coil embolization for, 2051–2052
complications in, 2051
endovascular treatment of, 2051–2052
extended orbitozygomatic approach to, 1982, 1985, 1985f
medial petrosectomy for, 1986–1987
orbitozygomatic-pterional approach to, 1982, 1983f–1984f
pterional approach to, 2049–2050
pterional-transsylvian approach to, 1978, 1978f–1981f, 1982
pure transsylvian approach to, 2042–2047, 2043f
clipping in, 2047
craniotomy in, 2043–2044, 2045f, 2046f
positioning in, 2043, 2044f
scalp incision in, 2043, 2045f
subarachnoid exposure in, 2044, 2046–2047
skull base approach to, 1985–1987, 1986f
subtemporal approach to, 1977–1978, 1977f, 2042, 2047–2049, 2047f, 2048f
surgery for, 2042–2051
anatomy in, 2041–2042
approaches to, 1977–1987, 2025
temporary occlusion for, 2050–2051
transclinoidal approach to, 1985
transclinoidal-extracavernous approach to, 1986, 1986f
Basilar apex *(Continued)*
transclinoidal-transcavernous approach to, 1985
treatment timing for, 2050
giant aneurysm of, deep hypothermic circulatory arrest for, 1529, 1530f
perforating arteries of, 1974–1975, 1975f
Basilar artery, 22f, 36f, 37, 38f
anatomy of, 1974, 2026
aneurysms of, 2025–2038
clinical presentation of, 2025–2026
combined petrosal approach to, 2030–2032, 2031f–2033f
combined supra-/infratentorial approach to, 1990–1991, 1990f
complications of, 2036–2038
embolization of, 2067–2068
extended retrolabyrinthine approach to, 1987f–1988f, 1988–1989
extradural temporopolar approach to, 2029–2030, 2030f, 2031f
extreme lateral inferior transtubercular approach to, 2034–2036, 2035f–2037f
middle fossa approach to, 1991, 1992f, 1993
results of, 2038
retrolabyrinthine transsigmoid approach to, 2032–2034, 2033f–2035f
subtemporal transtentorial approach to, 2026–2027, 2026f, 2027f
surgical approaches to, 1985, 1987–1993, 2026–2036
hypothermic circulatory arrest in, 2037
rupture during, 2037
transcochlear approach to, 1987f–1988f, 1989–1990
translabyrinthine approach to, 1987f–1988f, 1989
transoral approach to, 1993, 1993f
transpetrosal approach to, 1987–1990, 1987f–1988f, 1988t
transsylvian approach to, 2027–2029, 2028f, 2029f
blunt trauma to, 5212
fusiform aneurysms of, 1593, 1594f
intermittent insufficiency of, 1692
occlusion of, 5212
paramedian perforating branches of, rupture of, 1739
Basilar impression, 3340
congenital developmental, 3341–3343, 3343f
Basilar invagination, 3340–3341, 3341f
Ballismus, 2729
Bathrocephaly, 428–429
Batimastat (BB-94), for glioma invasion, 766
Battered child syndrome, evaluation of, 3499–3500, 3500f
Bax, 719
Bayliss effect, 1475
BB-94 (batimastat), for glioma invasion, 766
Bcl-2, 718, 743
cell protection by, 1519
in carotid body tumors, 1678
Bcl-x, 718
Bcl-xl, 718–719
Becquerel, 4007
Behavior management, in traumatic brain injury, 5294–5295
Behavioral disturbances, pediatric, neurorehabilitation of, 3789

Behavioral therapy, pain treatment with, 2966
  regression of benefit in, 2940–2941
Bell's cruciate paralysis, 4871, 4871f
Bence Jones protein, in multiple myeloma, 4854
BendMeister rod bender, 4659f, 4660
Benedikt's syndrome, 273
Benton Controlled Oral Word Association Test (COWAT), 5186
Benzel-Kesterson interspinous wiring modification, 4645, 4647f
Benzodiazepines, 1508
  for dystonia, 2796
  for pain, 2966
  in intracranial pressure management, 5127, 5127t
  in pregnancy, 2422
Beriberi, neuropathy in, 3844
Bernard-Horner syndrome, in nerve plexus injury, 3970
Bethanechol, for multiple sclerosis, 1455t
Biceps reflex testing, pediatric, 3180
Biglycan, 4230
Bilharziosis, spinal, 4390
Bing's sign, 268
Bioartificial materials, for central nervous system repair, 4163
Biochemical markers, for neoplastic meningitis, 1232
Biomechanics
  of atlantoaxial joint, 4187, 4188
  of axis, 4939
  of cervical spine, 4187–4190, 4193–4194, 4432
  of craniovertebral junction, 3333–3334
  of facet joints, 4185
  of internal spinal fixation, 4592–4596, 4593f, 4594f
  of intervertebral disk, 4185–4186
  of lumbar spine, 4191, 4714–4715
  of pediatric atlantoaxial joint, 3537–3538, 3538f
  of pediatric atlanto-occipital joint, 3528–3529
  of pediatric spinal injury, 3515–3516
  of spinal cord injury without radiographic abnormality, 3516
  of spine, 4181–4199, 4586, 4587f, 4588–4589
  of spondylolisthesis, 4543–4547
  of thoracic spine, 4190–4191, 4953–4954, 4953f–4955f
  of thoracic spine fixation, 4195–4198
  of thoracic spine fractures, 4192, 4195–4198
  of thoracic spine posterior procedures, 4694–4695
  of vertebrae, 4184–4185
Biopsy
  complications in, 573, 573t
  endoscopic, 3430
  in frameless stereotactic surgery, 945–946
  in pyogenic spinal infection, 4369, 4370f
  muscle, 3963–3964
  of pineal region tumors, 1014–1016, 1014f, 1014t
  of third ventricle tumors, 1248–1249
  peripheral nerve, 3837, 3838t, 3962–3963
  surgical navigation in, 945–946
Birbeck granules, in eosinophilic granuloma, 4843
Birth history, 3169–3170
Birth trauma, 3481–3486
Birth trauma *(Continued)*
  brachial plexus injury in, 3488–3495, Brachial plexus, obstretic injury to
  epidural hematoma in, 3483–3484, 3483f
  incidence of, 3481
  intracranial hemorrhage in, 3483–3485, 3483f–3486f
  posterior fossa subdural hematoma in, 3484–3485, 3485f, 3486f
  risk factors for, 3481
  scalp injury in, 3481–3482
  subdural hematoma in, 3484, 3484f
Bisphosphonates, in bone metabolism, 4233
Bisulfan, for ependymoma, 1048t
Bithermal caloric test, 344–345, 344f
Biventral lobule, 30f, 33f
Bladder
  anatomy of, 357–358, 357f, 358f
  autonomic receptors in, 358, 358f
  distention of, 364
  dysfunction of, in cerebral palsy, 3728, 3732, 3744–3745
  filling dysfunction of, 364–365, 365f
  neuromuscular function of, 363
  reflex contraction of, 377
  storage dysfunction of, 364–365, 365f
    treatment of, 378–379
  storage function of, 363
  voiding dysfunction of, 365
Bladder outlet resistance, 359
Bladder outlet retention, treatment of, 379–380
Blastocyst, development of, 4239, 4240f
Blastomycosis
  cranial destruction in, 430, 430f
  spinal, 4388f, 4389
Bleomycin, for craniopharyngioma, 1219, 3683–3684
Blepharospasm, 2729
Blindness
  in trigeminal schwannoma, 1345, 1345f
  monocular, 2541, 2542f
    optic nerve lesions, 2542, 2542f
  patient positioning and, 612–614
  prone positioning and, 603–604
Blink response, pediatric, 3173
Blood pressure. *See also* Arterial pressure.
  in cervical spine trauma, 4888, 4889
  in intracerebral hemorrhage, 1740
  in pregnancy, 2421
  in stroke, 1500–1501
  in trauma, 5090
Blood transfusion, 2829
Blood vessels, lumbar spine and, surgical anatomy of, 4706
Blood viscosity
  hypothermia effects on, 1532
  in head injury, 5058–5059
Blood-brain barrier, 153–170
  adherens junctions in, 157
  amino acid transport across, 160–161, 160t, 161f
  anatomic, 159
  capillaries of, 154
  cell biology of, 154–159, 155f
  contrast media penetration of, 164
  diseases affecting, 163–167
  disruption of, in chemotherapy, 879
  drug delivery across, 15–18, 16f
  endothelial cells forming, 153–154
  functional, 159
  gap junctions in, 157
  glucose transport across, 154, 159–160, 159f
Blood-brain barrier *(Continued)*
  GLUT-1 in, 158–159
  glutamate transport across, 161–162
  γ-glutamyltranspeptidase in, 158, 161
  immune cell passage through, 890
  in aging, 166–167
  in brain injury, 166
  in brain tumors, 164–165, 165t
  in cerebral edema, 165–166
  in cerebral ischemia, 166
  in cerebral metabolism, 1487
  in chemotherapy, 878
  in epilepsy, 166
  in experimental allergic encephalomyelitis, 164
  in hypertension, 166
  in immune response, 673
  in multidrug resistance, 162–163
  in multiple sclerosis, 164
  in radiation injury, 166
  in stress, 166
  inflammation effects on, 163–164
  ion transport across, 162
  ketone body transfer across, 1485
  lipoprotein transport across, 162
  macromolecular passage through, 154–155
  markers of, 157–159
  maturation of, 158
  microenvironmental influences on, 157–159
  morphology of, 154–155, 155f
  neurotransmitter transport in, 154, 161–162
  opening of
    chemotherapy delivery via, 153
    for brain edema, 802–803
  pediatric, 3462
  pericytes in, 153
  perivascular glia in, 153
  permeability of, 154, 155f
    cellular mechanisms of, 163
    disease effects on, 11–15
    lipophilicity and, 15, 16f
    to nucleosides, 158
    to nucleotides, 157–158
  physiology of, 791–792, 792f
  protective metabolic function of, 161
  receptor-mediated transport across, 163
  regulation of, astrocytes in, 109–110
  tight junctions in, 156–157, 159f
  transcellular endocytosis in, 159f
  transcellular lipophilic pathway in, 159f
  transcytosis through, 163
  transendothelial pathways of, drug delivery via, 159, 159f
  transport across, 156, 159–163, 159f
Blood–cerebrospinal fluid barrier, 791–792, 792f
Blood-tumor barrier, 17
Bmp4, 53t
Bobble-head doll syndrome, in suprasellar cysts, 3294
Bohlman triple-wire technique, 4645–4646, 4647f–4648f
Bone
  abnormalities of, head shape and, 3300
  anatomy of, 4227–4229, 4228f, 4613–4614
  biochemistry of, 4614–4615
  calcium in, 4231
  cancellous, 4227–4229, 4228f, 4613–4614
  cellular elements of, 4229, 4230f, 4614
  cortical, 4227, 4228f, 4613
  formation of, 4231–4233, 4231f, 4232t, 4613
    in spondyloarthropathies, 4460

Bone (Continued)
growth of
radiation-induced delay of, 4042
regulatory proteins in, 4614, 4614t
health of
alcohol and, 4234
body weight and, 4234–4235
caffeine and, 4234
exercise and, 4234
smoking and, 4233–4234
histology of, 4229–4231, 4230f
hypertrophy of, growth hormone excess and, 1189–1190
magnesium in, 4231
metabolic disease of, 4347–4349, 4348f
molecular biology of, 4614–4615
phosphorus in, 4231
repair of, 4614–4615
woven, 4614
Bone conduction testing, 331, 331f, 332f
Bone cyst, aneurysmal. *See* Aneurysmal bone cyst.
Bone grafts, 4615–4618
allograft, 2829t, 4606, 4617–4618
in cervical spine fusion, 4622, 4628f
autograft, 2829t, 4606–4607, 4616–4617
cervical spine fusion with, 4622
cancellous, 4616, 4619
ceramic, 4618
clinical applications of, 4606–4608, 4607f, 4608f
complications of, 4603–4606, 4603f, 4604f, 4606f
cortical, 4615–4616
incorporation of, 4619
demineralized bone matrix in, 4618
for pyogenic spinal infection, 4376–4378, 4379f
from anterior iliac crest, 4602–4605, 4602f–4604f
from posterior iliac crest, 4605–4606, 4606f
future of, 4608–4609, 4609t
harvesting of, 4601–4606, 4602f–4604f, 4606f
healing of
electromagnetic stimulation in, 4619
factors in, 4619–4620
physiology of, 4618–4619
historical perspective on, 4599
immunogenicity of, 4616t, 4617
in cervical spine fixation, 4420, 4423, 4423f, 4607–4608, 4607f, 4622, 4626–4627, 4626f, 4626t
with interspinous wiring, 4645–4646, 4647f
in cervical spine fusion, 4607–4608, 4607f
in craniofacial repair, 5252, 5256f
in occipitocervical fusion, 4666
in thoracolumbar fusion, 4608, 4608f
incorporation of
creeping substitution in, 4619
stages in, 4618–4619
osteogenic cells in, 4615, 4616t
properties of, 4615–4616, 4616t
recombinant human bone morphogenetic protein, 4618
spinal fusion principles and, 4599–4600
structural support by, 4615–4616, 4616t
substrates for, 4600–4601
types of, 4616–4618
Bone growth factors, 4608–4609, 4609t, 4614–4615
in posterior longitudinal ligament ossification, 4476
Bone marrow transplantation, for Ewing's sarcoma, 4850
Bone matrix, 4229–4231
demineralized, 4618
Bone metabolism, 4227–4236
anatomic considerations of, 4227–4229, 4228f
androgen in, 4232–4233
bisphosphonates in, 4233
calcitonin in, 4232
disorders of, 4235–4236
estrogen in, 4232
histologic considerations of, 4229–4231, 4230f
insulin in, 4233
parathyroid hormone in, 4231–4232
remodeling process in, 4231, 4231f
smoking and, 4233–4234
steroid hormones in, 4233
vitamin D in, 4232, 4232t
Bone morphogenetic proteins, 4609
in osteoinduction, 4615
in posterior longitudinal ligament ossification, 4476
interbody fusion with, for lumbar disk disease, 4792–4794, 4793f
Bone scan
for pyogenic spinal infection, 4368, 4369f
for spinal metastases, 4858
for spinal tumors, 4836
osteoid osteoma, 4837, 4838f
Bone sialoprotein, 4230
Bone softening syndromes, 3341–3343, 3343f
Bone tumors. *See* Osseous tumors.
Bony labyrinth, 327
Borderline personality, in traumatic brain injury response, 5193t
Bossing
biparietal, 428
frontal, 428
Botulinum toxin
for cerebral palsy, 3731–3732
for dystonia, 2796
for spasticity, 2866t, 3788
peripheral nerve effects of, 3816
Botulism, 270
Bowel function
in cerebral palsy, 3727, 3732
in neurourinary disorders, 366
Braces, for cerebral palsy, 3730
Brachial neuritis, 3840
Brachial neuropathy, 3840
Brachial plexitis, 3840
radiation-induced, vs. peripheral nerve tumors, 3876, 3878f
Brachial plexus
anatomy of, 647–648
avulsion of
delivery and, 3489–3490
dorsal root entry zone ablation for, 3046
magnetic resonance imaging of, 3885
pain after, 3046
in breast cancer, 3954
obstetric injury to, 3488–3495, 3969, 3975
causes of, 3976
classification of, 3976–3977, 3976t
clinical presentation of, 3489–3490
complications of, 3494
elbow function in, 3980t
electrodiagnosis of, 3974, 3978, 3978t, 3979t, 3980f
evaluation of, 3490–3491, 3491f
Brachial plexus (Continued)
hand function in, 3980t
historical aspects of, 3488
incidence of, 3975–3976
infraclavicular, 3970
localization of, 3861
medial rotation contracture in, 3981, 3982f
natural history of, 3977–3978
nerve root avulsion in, 3970, 3971f
operative findings in, 3978–3979
outcomes in, 3494–3495, 3494t
pathophysiology of, 3488–3489, 3489f
patterns of, 3490
posterior shoulder dislocation in, 3981, 3982f, 3983, 3983t, 3985
treatment of, 3984f–3986f, 3985–3987, 3986t
pseudomeningocele with, 3491, 3491f
range of motion in, 3981f
recovery from, 3489, 3489t
recording of, 3979, 3980f, 3980t, 3981, 3981f
risk factors for, 3489, 3976
rupture in, 3490
secondary reconstruction in, 3495
severity of, 3970
shoulder function in, 3980t
spinal nerve injury in, 3979, 3979t, 3980f
supraclavicular, 3970
surgery for, 3491–3494, 3492f, 3493f. *See also* Brachial plexus, surgery on.
treatment of, 3970, 3972–3973, 3972f–3974f
palsy of
antenatal development of, 3488–3489
obstetric. *See* Brachial plexus, obstetric injury to.
positioning and, 611–612
surgery on
electrodiagnostic monitoring during, 3868, 3869f, 3870, 3870f
exposures in, 648–650, 649f, 650f, 3491–3492, 3492f
grafting procedures in, 3493, 3493f
historical aspects of, 3488
infraclavicular approach to, 649–650, 650f
neuroma resection in, 3492–3493
neurotization in, 3493–3494
positioning for, 607–608, 648
supraclavicular approach to, 648–649, 649f
Brachial vein, 36f
Brachioradialis muscle, paralysis of, in radial nerve entrapment, 3928
Brachioradialis reflex testing, pediatric, 3180
Brachytherapy, 4007
for brain tumors, 4095–4107
follow-up after, 4101
interstitial, 4095–4096
for brain metastases, 4104, 4105t
for low-grade astrocytoma, 4104
for malignant glioma, 4101–4104, 4102t, 4103t
for skull base tumors, 4105
implantation technique in, 4098–4100, 4098t, 4099f, 4100f
patient selection for, 4097–4098
pediatric, 4105
radiobiology of, 4096–4097, 4096t
intracavitary, 4095–4096

Brachytherapy *(Continued)*
for craniopharyngioma, 4105–4106, 4106t
for cystic glioma, 4106–4107
implantation technique in, 4100–4101
patient selection for, 4098
radiobiology of, 4096–4097, 4096t
Bracing, complications of, 576
Bradykinesia
definition of, 2673, 2730
in Parkinson's disease, 2732
radiosurgical pallidotomy for, 4090–4091, 4090f, 4091f, 4091t
Bradykinin
blood-brain barrier permeability and, 17
release of, 2953, 2954f
Bragg peak effect, 4006
in stereotactic radiosurgery, 3990, 3992f
Brain
anatomy of, 3–40
nasoiniac line in, 630
antibody effect on, 683
antigen clearance from, 679–680
arteriovenous malformations in. *See under* Arteriovenous malformations.
as "immunoprivileged" site, 12
atrophy of, shaking-impact syndrome and, 3502f
blood barrier with. *See* Blood-brain barrier.
bullet wounds to, 5223–5241. *See also* Bullet wounds.
capillary endothelium of, 155–156
capillary telangiectasia of. *See* Capillary telangiectasia.
chemical composition of, pediatric, 3462
development of, oligodendrocyte progenitor cells in, 91–92, 92f
developmental venous anomalies of. *See* Developmental venous anomalies.
electrical failure of, 1468
endothelium of, 157
energy metabolism in
astrocyte regulation of, 86
positron emission tomography of, 488–489
field potentials in, 230–231
glucose metabolism in, 86, 117–118, 118f, 154, 1482–1484, 5047–5048
astrocytes in, 107, 108f
features of, 1483t
positron emission tomography of, 1601
stages of, 1484f
growth of, 3462
herniation in. *See* Herniation syndromes.
homeostasis of, 154
immune effectors in, 681–683
immune privilege of, 673, 680
immune regulation in, 683–685, 683f, 684f
immune response in, 673–685. *See also* Immune response; Inflammation.
in shaking-impact syndrome, 3501–3502, 3502f
infection of, after débridement, 5236
magnetic resonance imaging of, 439–473. *See also* Magnetic resonance imaging.
metabolism in. *See* Cerebral metabolism.
metastases to. *See* Brain metastases.
necrosis of, growing fracture and, 3469, 3469f
oligodendrocyte progenitor cells in, 92
pediatric, attributes of, 3462–3463

Brain *(Continued)*
physiology of, 1503–1504, 1504t, 1601
anesthesia and, 551–552
Po_2 of, in traumatic brain injury, 5118, 5119, 5119f
primary lymphoma of, in pregnancy, 872
protection of, in head injury, 5059
stereotactic biopsy of, complications of, 573, 573t
temperature of, in head injury, 5124, 5124f
transport-mediated drug accumulation in, 15–16
viscoelastic properties of, cerebrospinal fluid and, 3387, 3388f, 3389
Brain contusion, 5041–5042
Brain death, 285t, 393–403
angiography of, 399
blood flow measurements in, 399
brainstem auditory evoked potentials in, 400–401
brainstem reflex in, 397, 397t
causes of, 397–398
clinical determination of, 396–399, 396t–398t
confirmation of, 399–401, 400t
consultation about, 397, 397t
declaration of, 394–396, 395t
diagnosis of, 394
electroencephalography of, 400, 400t
family approach in, 403, 403t
imaging of, 400
pediatric, 401–403, 402t
radionuclide studies of, 399
somatosensory evoked potentials in, 401
transcranial Doppler ultrasonography of, 399–400, 1553–1554
transplantation and, 395, 395t, 403, 403t
Brain edema. *See* Cerebral edema.
Brain injury. *See also* Head injury; Stroke.
acquired, pediatric, neurorehabilitation of, 3788–3790
blood-brain barrier in, 166
diffuse, pediatric, 3462–3463
glutamate-induced, 111
hyperglycemia-mediated, 128–130
in hydrocephalus, 3408
metabolic effects of, in recovery, 3784
mild, pediatric, 3461–3469
skull fracture with, 3465–3470, 5042, 5042t
without skull fracture, 3461–3465, 5039–5043
assessment of, 3463–3464
computed tomography of, 3464
epidemiology of, 3461, 3461f
outcome of, 3465
pathophysiology of, 3463
treatment of, 3464–3465
organic, 5190
positron emission tomography of, 488–491, 490t
traumatic, 5103–5137
acceleration/deceleration in, 5085–5086, 5085f
anemia in, 5122f, 5123–5124, 5136
angular acceleration and, 5040, 5040f
apoptosis in, 5030
assessment of, 5288–5291
attention after, 5186–5187
autoregulation after, 5084
axonal damage in, 5084–5085
axotomy in, 5028–5029, 5028f, 5029t
Barthel Index in, 5288

Brain injury *(Continued)*
baseline values in, 5290
behavior management in, 5294–5295
biomechanical considerations in, 5085–5086, 5085f
brain temperature in, 5124, 5124f
brain tissue Po_2 in, 5118, 5119, 5119f
calcium homeostasis in, 5025–5027
calpain activation in, 5027
caspases in, 5030
cellular mechanisms in, 5084
cerebral blood flow in, 5109–5112, 5109t, 5110t
control of, 5145, 5147f
in treatment plans, 5120, 5121f
management of, 5125
monitoring of, 5115–5116, 5116f
transcranial Doppler flow velocity of, 5114–5115
cerebral ischemia in
monitoring of, 5113–5120, 5116f–5119f
treatment of, 5134–5135, 5135t
cerebral oxygen saturation in, near-infrared spectroscopy of, 5118–5119
cerebral perfusion pressure in, 5114
management of, 5124–5125, 5125f, 5126–5129, 5126t
clinical trials in, 5105
cognitive function after, 5185–5188
cognitive function before, 5188–5190
cognitive rehabilitation in, 5293–5294
coma data banks in, 5103, 5104t
comorbid medical complications of, 5197
concentration after, 5186–5187
contact loading in, 5085
cytokines in, 5029
diabetes insipidus in, 5131
diffuse axonal, 5045–5046, 5046t, 5105–5106, 5107f
drug treatment of, 5103
edema after, 5083–5084
emotional sequelae of, 5190–5194
epilepsy after. *See* Epilepsy, post-traumatic.
evaluation of, 5083–5098
examination of, 5089–5092, 5091f, 5092f
excitotoxic pathway antagonism for, 5026, 5026f
executive functioning after, 5187–5188
extracellular potassium homeostasis after, 2454–2456, 2454f–2457f
fever in, 5128, 5136
focal vs. diffuse, 5041–5046
classification of, 5041, 5041t
free fatty acids in, 5026
functional assessment of, 5288–5289, 5288t, 5289t, 5291
Functional Independence Measure in, 5288, 5289t
Galveston Orientation and Amnesia Test in, 5289
gene expression in, 5028
Glasgow Coma Scale in, 5088, 5088t, 5288, 5288t
glutamate homeostasis after, 2457–2458
glutamatergic receptor channels in, 2451–2452, 2451f
gunshot wounds and, 5085–5086
hematoma in, 5106, 5107f, 5108
hemodynamics in, 5096–5097

Brain injury *(Continued)*
hemorrhagic contusion in, 5107f, 5108
hippocampal long-term potentiation after, 2452, 2453f
hippocampus in, 2449, 2450f
history in, 5089
hydroxyl radical production in, 5084
hyperemia in, 5109t, 5110t, 5111
hyperglycemia in, 5131
hypernatremia in, 5131
hypocapnia in, 5120, 5122f, 5123
hyponatremia syndrome in, 5130–5131, 5130f
hypoperfusion in, 5109t, 5110–5111, 5110t
hypotension after, 5096
hypoxia in, 5122f, 5123, 5135–5136
inertial loading in, 5085
interpersonal sequelae of, 5181, 5182, 5182t, 5183f
intracranial hemorrhage after, 5083
intracranial hypertension in, 5109, 5111
management of, 5126–5129, 5131–5134, 5132t
monitoring of, 5113–5114
intracranial pressure in, treatment of, 5124, 5125, 5145, 5146f
intrapersonal sequelae of, 5181, 5182, 5182t, 5183f
invasive procedures in, 5097–5098
jugular venous oxygen saturation in
monitoring of, 5116–5118, 5116f–5118f
secondary ischemic insults and, 5120, 5122f, 5123–5124
laboratory tests in, 5098
language function after, 5185–5186
learning after, 5187
leukocytes in, 5029
major injury in, 5095–5096
mechanisms of, 5039–5040
medications in, 5097
memory after, 5187
mild
classification of, 5195, 5195t
differential diagnosis of, 5197–5198, 5198t
outcome evaluation in, 5196–5197
patient approach in, 5198–5199
rehabilitation of, 5295
mild sequelae to, 5194–5198
mitochondrial dysfunction in, 5027
Model Systems Program for, 5296
motivational capacity after, 5191–5192
neurocognitive assessment of, 5289–5290, 5290t
neurocognitive sequelae of, 5182–5190, 5183t
neurogenesis in, 5033
neurogenic sequelae of, 5197
neurological assessment in, 5089–5095. *See also* Neurological assessment.
neurological monitoring in, 5112–5124
neuronal death after, 5084–5085
neuropsychological evaluation in
constructivist approach in, 5182
discipline-specific vs. patient-oriented, 5181–5182
neuropsychological testing in, 5289–5291, 5290t
oxygen delivery after, 5084
oxygenation in, 5096
pathophysiology of, 5105–5106, 5107f, 5108–5112, 5109t, 5110t

Brain injury *(Continued)*
penetrating, 5085–5086
prehospital management of, 5086–5087
premorbid emotional functioning in, 5192–5194, 5193t
premorbid problems of, 5197, 5198t
primary, 5103, 5104f
classification of, 5107f, 5108
vs. secondary, 5039
primary survey in, 5087–5088, 5088t
primary vs. secondary, 5083, 5083f
prognosis of, 5290–5291
psychogenic sequelae of, 5197
psychomotor-visuomotor function after, 5188
radiography of, 5092–5093, 5093f–5095f
Rancho Los Amigos Levels of Cognitive Functioning Scale in, 5288–5289, 5289t
reactive oxygen species in, 5026–5027
recovery from, 5025–5033
cytokines in, 5031
growth factors in, 5031–5032
rehabilitation of, 5287–5296. *See also* Rehabilitation.
relearning in, 5191
resuscitation in, 5083–5098, 5088t
salt wasting in, 5130–5131, 5130f
secondary, 5039, 5083–5085, 5083f, 5085t, 5103, 5104f, 5108–5112
vs. primary, 5039
secondary gain in, 5197–5198, 5198t
secondary ischemic insults in, 5111, 5112, 5120–5124, 5122f
cerebral causes of, 5120, 5122f
systemic causes of, 5120, 5122f, 5123–5124
treatment of, 5135–5137, 5136f
secondary survey in, 5088–5089
seizures in, 5120, 5122f, 5128–5129, 5136–5137
self-awareness after, 5192
sensory perceptual function after, 5188
sequelae of, 5181–5199
severity of, 5290–5291
spontaneous recovery in, 5191
superoxide production in, 5084
surgery for
anesthesia for, 5149–5150
bleeding after, 5174, 5176
bur holes in, 5150, 5153, 5153f
complications of, 5174, 5176, 5176f–5178f, 5178
positioning for, 5149, 5149f
preparation for, 5146, 5148–5150, 5149f
swelling after, 5176, 5176f, 5177f
timing in, 5131
ventriculostomy in, 5097–5098, 5150, 5151f–5152f
swelling in, 5108–5109
syndrome of inappropriate antidiuretic hormone secretion in, 5130, 5130f
trauma team in, 5087
treatment of, 5124–5137, 5145–5178
acute, 5095–5098
airway management in, 5127–5128
anticonvulsants in, 5128–5129, 5129t
antihypertensives in, 5127, 5128t
approaches to, 5124–5126, 5125f, 5126f
conservative, 5145–5146, 5148f
fluid/electrolyte management in, 28f, 5130–5131

Brain injury *(Continued)*
gastric ulcer prophylaxis in, 5129
guidelines for, 5103–5105
head elevation in, 5126–5127
history of, 5103–5105, 5104t, 5105t
Lund therapy in, 5125, 5125f, 5126t
nutrition in, 5129–5130
prehospital, 5086–5087
prophylactic antibiotics in, 5129
sedation/analgesia in, 5127, 5127t
thromboembolism prophylaxis in, 5129
triage in, 5095–5096
vasodilatory cascade in, 5124, 5125f
vasospasm in, 1840–1841, 5111–5112
ventilation in, 5096
visuoconstructual abilities after, 5186
visuocoperceptual abilities after, 5186
visuospatial abilities after, 5186
weakness in, 5131–5132, 5132f
Brain laceration, 5042
Brain mapping, 2531–2537
in epilepsy, 2511
intracranial monitoring for, 2554
study design in, 2557
Brain metastases, 1077–1093
chemotherapy for, 1078, 1092–1093
corticosteroids for, 1078
epidemiology of, 1077–1078
incidence of, 1077, 4015
interstitial brachytherapy for, 4095, 4104, 4105t
magnetic resonance imaging of, 457, 457f, 458f
medical treatment of, 4015
melanoma and, stereotactic radiosurgery for, 1091–1092
primary tumor and, 1077–1078, 4015
radiation therapy for, 1078–1080, 1079f, 4015–4018
altered fractionation schemes for, 1079
complications of, 1080, 4024
dose-fractionation schemes for, 1078–1079
dose-response relationship in, 4016–4017
fractionation trials in, 4015–4016, 4016t
patient parameters in, 1078
prognostic factors in, survival and, 4017, 4017t
prophylactic, in small cell lung cancer, 1080
radiosensitizers in, 1080
repeat, 4018
sensitizer trials in, 4016, 4016t
stereotactic radiosurgery after, 1092
whole brain, 4017–4018, 4018t
radiosurgery for, 4065–4068, 4066t, 4067f, 4095
linac, 4114
recurrent
stereotactic radiosurgery for, 1092
surgical approaches to, 1085
renal cell carcinoma and, stereotactic radiosurgery for, 1091
stereotactic radiosurgery for, 1088–1092, 1089t
radiation therapy with, 1090–1091, 1091t
vs. surgery, 1089–1090
surgery for, 1080–1088
anatomy in, 1084, 1084f
approaches in, 1083, 1084–1085, 1086f
cerebellar, 1084, 1085, 1085f, 1086f
clinical assessment in, 1082–1083

Brain metastases *(Continued)*
histologic type in, 1082
intraventricular, 1085, 1086f
morbidity after, 1088
mortality in, 1085, 1087
outcome in, 1085, 1087–1088, 1087t
patient selection for, 1081–1083
prognostic factors in, 1081–1083
radiation therapy after, 1083, 1083f
radiography in, 1081–1082
supratentorial, 1084, 1084f
survival after, 1087t, 1088
tumor location in, 1081–1082
tumor number in, 1081
tumor size in, 1081
vs. radiosurgery, 4067–4068
treatment of, 1078–1093
Brain natriuretic peptide, after aneurysmal subarachnoid hemorrhage, 1830
Brain tumors
age in, 808
angiogenesis in, 771–785. *See also* Angiogenesis.
antigens of, 673, 677
blood-brain barrier in, 16–17, 153, 164–165, 165t
brachytherapy for, 4095–4107
cerebral vasospasm in, 1841
chemicals and, 811
chemotherapy for, 153, 660
classification of, 661–672
clinical manifestations of, 827–831
congenital conditions associated with, 811
considerations in, 659–660
demographics of, 808, 808t
diet and, 810
electrophysiologic abnormalities in, 230
embolization of, 857–862
agents for, 858–859, 858t
anastomoses during, 859, 860t, 861f
complications of, 859, 860t, 861f
efficacy of, 859, 862
provocative testing in, 859
technique of, 857–858
vascular risk during, 859, 860t
endovascular occlusion for, 862–864
cerebral blood flow evaluation in, 862–863
complications of, 863
predictive value of, 863–864
technique of, 862
environmental risk factors for, 809–811
epidemiology of, 807–809, 808t, 809t
extra-axial
radiologic features of, 835, 836–839
vs. intra-axial, 835
familial clustering of, 811
focal manifestations of, 829–831, 829t
functional magnetic resonance imaging of, 852–853, 853f
gender in, 808, 808t
gene alterations in, 750, 751t
gene therapy for, 817–822. *See also* Gene therapy.
gene transfer–mediated drug targeting for, 818–820, 818f–820f
geography of, 808
grading of, 689
growth factors in, 725–733. *See also* specific growth factor, e.g., Fibroblast growth factor.
headache in, 828
hereditary syndromes associated with, 811–813, 812t

Brain tumors *(Continued)*
herniation syndromes in, 826–827, 826f, 826t
histopathology of, 661–672
proliferation markers in, 689, 690f
imaging of, 659
immunology in, 887–895
immunotherapy for, 673, 891–895
effector function in, 681, 681f
immunization site in, 893–894
tumor necrosis factor-α in, 684–685
in multiple sclerosis, 1452
in pregnancy, 867–874
in twins, 811
industrial exposure and, 810
infection and, 810
intra-axial
radiologic features of, 835, 842–852
vs. extra-axial, 835
intracranial pressure in, 180, 552
intraparenchymal, 835, 840–841
invasion in, experimental models for, 763–765
Jacksonian seizures in, 829
Karnofsky performance scale in, 830, 830t
malignant
angiogenesis in, 771, 772f
radiation therapy for, 4015–4024
manifestations of, 827–829, 827t–829t
meningitis and, 1231–1234
mental changes in, 827–828, 827t
metabolism of, 487–488, 487f–490f
metals and, 811
micro, T cells in, 675, 675f
mortality rates in, 809
neurology of, 825–833
nonmetal elements and, 811
occupational exposure and, 810
of disordered embryogenesis, 3687–3693. *See also* specific type, e.g., Colloid cyst.
oncogenesis of, 659
papilledema in, 828–829
pathophysiology of, 825–827, 826f, 826t
pesticides and, 811
positron emission tomography of, 487–488, 487f–490f, 2480, 2481f
preoperative evaluation in, 552
proliferation markers for
mitotic activity as, 689–692
molecular, 692–696
tumor-specific data on, 696–705
race in, 808, 808t
radiation and, 809–810
radiation therapy for, 659–660, 3990
radiologic features of, 835–854
radiosurgery for, 659
seizures in, 828, 828t
single-photon emission computed tomography of, 2480
socioeconomic effects in, 808
spontaneous intracerebral hemorrhage in, 1735
subcortical, 943, 945f
surgery for, 899–907. *See also* Craniotomy.
advances in, 659
care after, 906–907
evaluation before, 899
frameless stereotaxy in, 901
imaging before, 899–901
incisions in, 902
intracranial pressure and, 900, 900f
navigation systems in, 941–947. *See also* Stereotactic surgery, frameless.

Brain tumors *(Continued)*
positioning for, 902
preparation for, 901–902
timing of, 900, 900f
tumor removal in, 905–906
symptoms of, 825–827, 826f, 826t
tobacco and, 810
trauma and, 810–811
treatment of, drug delivery in, 16–17
tumor suppressor genes in, 739–744
vs. multiple sclerosis, 1450t
Brain volume, intracranial pressure and, 187–189
Brain-derived neurotrophic factor
after peripheral nerve injury, 3967–3968
in central nervous system regeneration, 4155
in central nervous system repair, 4165
in central nervous system transplantation, 2843–2844
in Parkinson's disease, 2706
Brainstem, 29, 30f
ablative procedures on, 3045–3056
anaplastic astrocytoma of, 985, 985f
anterior, veins of, 34, 35f
arteriovenous malformations of, 2251, 2251f
arterial supply/venous outflow in, 2257
deep, 2257, 2264f, 2265, 2265f
superficial, 2257, 2263–2265, 2263f, 2264f
surgery for, 2263–2265, 2263f–2265f
cavernous malformations of, 2294–2295, 2295f, 2321–2338
hemorrhage risk in, 2323
natural history of, 2321, 2322f, 2323, 2323t
outcome in, 2337–2338
surgery for, 2326, 2326f, 2327f
approaches to, 2325, 2325f, 2327, 2328f
care after, 2326–2327
far-lateral approach to, 2332–2334, 2333f–2336f
indications for, 2323, 2323t, 2324f
monitoring during, 2325–2326
orbitozygomatic approach to, 2328–2331, 2330f, 2331f
retrosigmoid approach to, 2331–2332, 2332f, 2333f
suboccipital approach to, 2327–2328, 2329f
supracerebellar-infratentorial approach to, 2334, 2337, 2337f
surgical series of, 2323, 2323t
diseases of, 272
ependymoma of, surgical complications in, 3629
glioma of, 984–986
cervicomedullary, 984
classification of, 984
clinical presentation of, 984
diffuse, 984
pediatric, 3663–3664
exophytic, 984–985
pediatric, 3669
focal, 831, 984
pediatric, 3664
histopathology of, 984–985
imaging of, 984–985
immune enhancement in, 683–684
magnetic resonance imaging of, 450, 451f, 452
metastatic, pediatric, 3669

Brainstem *(Continued)*
natural history of, 984
outcomes in, 985–986, 3669
pathology of, 984–985, 985f
pediatric, 3663–3670
chemotherapy for, 3669, 3669t
classification of, 3663t
complications of, 3667–3668
differential diagnosis of, 3664
frequency of, 3663
historical aspects of, 3663
imaging of, 3664–3666, 3665f, 3666f
pathogenesis of, 3664
prognosis of, 3664–3665, 3665f
radiation therapy for, 3668–3669, 3668f, 3668t
surgery for, 3666–3667, 3667f
treatment of, 985–986
hemorrhage of, 1739–1740, 1739f
in consciousness, 278, 279f
in parkinsonism, 2675
injury to, transsphenoidal surgery and, 1182
lesions of
physical features of, 274
pupillary dilation in, 288, 288f
sensory loss in, 274, 274f
vertigo in, 352
medulloblastoma of, 1035f
meningioma of, vs. acoustic neuroma, 1150f
monitoring of, in ependymoma surgery, 3630–3631
opioid-sensitive areas of, 2954f
pain-relief procedures on, 3073–3081
pediatric, surgery on, 3194t
posterior circulation aneurysm and, 1976
Brainstem auditory evoked potentials
in altered consciousness, 297
in anesthesia, 1508
Brainstem reflexes, absence of, in brain death determination, 397, 397t
Breast cancer
brachial plexus involvement by, 3954
in pregnancy, 872
intramedullary metastases from, 526f
meningioma in, 1105
orbital metastasis in, 1376
skull metastases in, 1392, 1392f
Breathing
apneustic, 283
assessment of, 5087
in cervical spine trauma, 4888, 4889
ataxic, 282–283
in consciousness assessment, 282–283, 283f
Bromocriptine
during pregnancy, 1189
for acromegaly, 1193
for meningioma, 1110
for pituitary adenoma, 868–869
for prolactinoma, 1186–1187
Bromodeoxyuridine
as tumor proliferation marker, 692–693
in meningioma, 1103
Brown-Séquard syndrome, 272, 4397, 4872, 4889–4890, 4890f
after spinal hemangioma treatment, 4841
vs. thoracic disk herniation, 4492
Brucellosis, spinal, 4385–4386
Bruising, in battered child syndrome, 3499, 3499f
Bruits
auscultation for, 269
cervical, in stroke, 1622–1623
Bruns-Garland syndrome, 4511
BudR, in malignant glioma radiosensitization, 4020
Bulb, 9
Bulbocavernous reflex
monitoring of, in pediatric intramedullary tumors, 3712
testing of, 367, 367f
Bullet wounds, 5223–5241
adjunctive therapy for, 5230–5231
age in, 5224–5225, 5224t
alcohol use and, 5225–5226
angiography of, 5228–5229
bone fragments in, infection from, 5236
brain edema in, 5235
bullet caliber in, 5225
cerebrovascular injury in, 5203–5204
circumstances in, 5225
compressed cisterns in, 5230
computed tomography of, 5229–5230, 5229t
cortical contusions in, 5234
débridement for, complications of, 5236–5237, 5237t
demographics of, 5224–5226, 5224t
disseminated intravascular coagulation in, 5236
drug use and, 5225–5226
effects of, 5223–5224
energy transfer in, 5223
evaluation of, 5227–5228, 5228t
field resuscitation in, 5226
Glasgow Coma Score in, 5237–5240, 5237t, 5238t
hypotension effects in, 5226
hypoxia in, 5226
intracranial bleeding in, 5230
intracranial hematomas in, 5234–5235
level of consciousness in, 5227–5228, 5228t
mechanism of death in, 5223–5224
metal fragments in, infection from, 5236
missile fragmentation in, 5230
missile track in, 5223, 5229, 5229t
missile trajectory in, 5223
mortality in, 5230
hospital admission timing and, 5227
operation rate and, 5227
surgery and, 5232, 5232t, 5234, 5236t
motor release findings in, 5228
outcome in, 5237–5239, 5237t, 5238t
penetrating head injury from, 5085–5086
peripheral nerve injury in, 3827
pupillary findings in, 5228, 5228t
race in, 5224t, 5225
radiography of, 5228
reporting obligations in, 411
seizure after, 5240–5241
skull fracture from, 5223
suicide in, 5224t, 5225
surgery for, 5231–5234, 5232t, 5234t
mortality in, 5232, 5232t, 5234, 5236t
patient selection in, 5239–5240
thoracic spine, 4981
transventricular injury in, 5229–5230
vascular injury in, 5235–5236
ventricular injury in, 5236
wounds associated with, 5237
Bupivacaine
for spasticity, 2865, 2866t
intrathecal, 3141
peripheral nerve effects of, 3816
Bur holes
exploratory, 5150, 5153, 5153f
in anterior communicating artery aneurysm surgery, 1932–1933, 1932f
Bur holes *(Continued)*
in traumatic brain injury surgery, 5150, 5153, 5153f
Burns, nerve damage in, 3827
Burst fracture. *See* Fracture(s), burst.
Burst lobe, 5044
Bypass. *See also* Arterial bypass; Venous bypass.
cardiopulmonary, in deep hypothermic circulatory arrest, 1534
Bystander effect, 818

C1620A, 3362
C1620G, 3362
Cables
braided, 4592, 4592f
in occipitocervical fusion, 4660–4661, 4660f–4662f
in posterior subaxial cervical fixation, 4644–4650, 4645f–4649f
Cadherins, in malignant glioma, 763
Caffeine, bone health and, 4234
Cahill oblique facet wiring technique, 4646, 4648f
CAI, as angiogenesis antagonist, 779t
Calamus scriptorius, 34
Calbindin, substantia nigra pars compacta lesions and, 2706
Calcar avis, 8, 8f, 12f
Calcarine artery, 23
Calcarine cortex, lesions of, visual field defects from, 2542, 2542f
Calcarine sulcus, 3, 10f, 22f, 24f, 25, 26f
anterior, 25
posterior, 25
Calcarine vein
anterior, 28
posterior, 28
Calcification
in brain tumors, 836
in spinal chondrosarcoma, 4847
in spinal chordoma, 4848
Calcitonin
in bone metabolism, 4232
intrathecal, 3141
Calcitonin gene–related peptide
expression of, after axonal transection, 3967
for cerebral vasospasm, 1854
in axonal regeneration, 197
release of, 2953
Calcium
action potentials and, 219, 220, 222–224
astrocyte movement of, 110
homeostasis of, 122–123, 123f, 124f
in axonal degeneration, 199
in blood-brain permeability, 11
in bone, 4231
in cell death, 126–128
in cerebral blood flow–metabolism coupling, 1489–1490
in ischemic injury, 1517, 1518f
in traumatic brain injury, 5025–5027
metabolism of, ion homeostasis and, 120–123, 121f–124f
release of, in cerebral autoregulation, 1476
Calcium carbonate, in bone, 4614
Calcium channel blockers
for aneurysmal subarachnoid hemorrhage, 1852–1853, 1854f
for cerebral vasospasm, 1547
in ischemia protection, 1522
Calcium channels, 120, 121f, 220t

Calcium channels (Continued)
activation of, 3814
mutations in, 223–224
subunits of, 223, 3814
voltage-gated, 222–223, 223t
Calcium phosphate, in bone, 4614
Calcium pyrophosphate dehydrate deposition disease, at craniocervical junction, 4580–4581, 4583f
California Concussion Scale, 5195, 5196f
Callahan facet wiring technique, 4649, 4649f
Callosal sulcus, 3, 24f
Callosomarginal artery, 1925, 1946, 1946f
distal anterior cerebral artery aneurysm arising from, 1949f, 1950f
Caloric testing, 344–345, 344f
Calpain, in traumatic brain injury, 5027
Calvaria
basal cell carcinoma of, 1398, 1399f
fracture of, 425–427, 426f, 427f
in Chiari malformation type II, 3349–3350, 3350f
osteoma of, 1383
Paget's disease of, 1400
Canalithiasis, 2903
Canalization, occult spinal dysraphism and, 3258, 3258f
Cancer
gene therapy for, 712
incidence of, spinal metastases and, 4854
mutations in, 714
pain in
dorsal rhizotomy for, 3034, 3040, 3040t
dorsal root entry zone procedures for, 3045
ganglionectomy for, 3034, 3040, 3040t
intrathecal morphine for, 3133–3134, 3134f
midbrain tractotomy for, 3054
Candida albicans, infectious intracranial aneurysms from, 2102
Candidiasis, spinal, 4389–4390
Cannulation, in deep hypothermic circulatory arrest, 1534
Cantilever beam techniques, in internal spinal fixation, 4593–4596, 4595f
Capillary(ies), in blood-brain barrier, 154
Capillary hemangioma
in congenital lumbosacral lipoma, 3237
in occult spinal dysraphism, 3259, 3260f, 3261
vascular endothelial growth factor in, 733
Capillary malformations. *See* Capillary telangiectasia.
Capillary telangiectasia, 2137–2139
arteriovenous malformations and, 2153
cavernous malformations and, 2153
clinical presentation of, 2138t, 2139, 2176
definition of, 2175–2176
developmental venous anomalies and, 2152–2153
epidemiology of, 2137, 2176
focal deficit in, 2176
hemorrhage in, 2176
imaging of, 472, 2138t, 2139, 2175
natural history of, 2138t, 2139
pathogenesis of, 2175–2176
pathology of, 2137, 2138t, 2139
treatment of, 2138t, 2139
Capreomycin, for tuberculosis, 1441
Capsaicin, for trigeminal neuralgia, 2993
Capsular ligaments, 4187
Captopril, angiosuppressive therapy with, 782
Capusulotomy, anterior, for psychiatric disorders, 2859, 2859f
Caput medusae, in developmental venous anomalies, 2140, 2140f
Carbamazepine
for multiple sclerosis, 1454t
for neuropathic pain, 3839
for trigeminal neuralgia, 2990t, 2991–2992, 2996
in pregnancy, 2422
pharmacology of, 2470, 2470t
Carbolic acid, for cerebral palsy, 3731
Carbon dioxide
hypothermia effects on, 1532
in altered consciousness, 295
in traumatic brain injury, 5089–5090
Carbon dioxide reactivity
in cerebral blood flow regulation, 5050
in head injury, 5052–5053
in transcranial Doppler ultrasonography, 1544, 1544f, 1550
in traumatic brain injury, 5120, 5122f, 5123
Carbon monoxide, in cerebral blood flow regulation, 1472
Carboplatin
for ependymoma, 1048, 1048t
pharmacology of, 881–882
Carboxyamido-triazole, angiosuppressive therapy with, 782
Carcinoembryonic antigen, in meningioma, 1108
Carcinomatosis, spinal, imaging of, 527, 529, 529f
Cardiac output, in pregnancy, 2421
Cardiac risk index, for surgery, 550
Cardiomegaly, in vein of Galen malformations, 3435, 3435f
Cardiopulmonary bypass, in deep hypothermic circulatory arrest, 1534
Cardiovascular system
disorders of
in aneurysmal subarachnoid hemorrhage, 1828–1829
prone positioning and, 603
in spinal cord injury, 557, 4881
preoperative assessment of, 549–550
subarachnoid hemorrhage effects on, 553
Carmustine
for ependymoma, 1048t
for malignant glioma, 975–976
in malignant glioma radiosensitization, 4019–4020
pharmacology of, 880–881
Carotid angioplasty
saphenous vein graft in, 1627–1629, 1628f
stenting with, 1651–1658
complications of, 1657–1658
outcome of, 1657–1658
patient selection for, 1651, 1652f, 1653–1654, 1653f
restenosis after, 1657
technique of, 1654–1657, 1655f, 1656f
Carotid artery
aneurysms of, 1801
transsylvian exposure for, 1879
angiography of, vs. carotid duplex ultrasonography, 1566–1567
atherosclerosis of, 1613–1618
Chlamydia pneumoniae in, 1613
clinical manifestations of, 1614–1615, 1614t
history of, 1613
ischemic stroke in, 1614
Carotid artery (Continued)
magnetic resonance angiography of, 1588–1590, 1588f–1590f
pathology of, 1613–1614
plaque in, 1613–1614
preoperative evaluation for, 552–553, 552t
shear stress in, 1614
ulceration of, in stroke, 1624–1625, 1624f
bifurcation of
aneurysms of, 1889
lesions of, 1626
bruits of, 1615
cavernous connection with. *See* Cavernous carotid fistula.
cervical, diseases of, 1677–1687
common
atherosclerosis of, 1651
compression of, for carotid cavernous fistula formation, 2341, 2342f
middle vertebral artery transposition to, 1703, 1705f
proximal vertebral artery transposition to, 1700, 1701f, 1702f
dissection of, 276t
angioplasty for, 1654
magnetic resonance angiography of, 1590–1591, 1592f
transcranial Doppler ultrasonography of, 1552
external
aneurysms of, 1682–1684, 1683f, 1684f
in glomus jugulare tumors, 1299f, 1300
middle cerebral artery saphenous vein graft with, 2110–2111, 2111f, 2112f
posterior cerebral artery saphenous vein graft with, 2111, 2113
vertebral artery bypass with, 1706, 1708f, 1709–1710, 1711f
fibromuscular dysplasia of, 1681–1682, 1682f
in carotid endarterectomy, 1633, 1633f, 1634f
injury to, 1669–1675
blunt, 5204, 5204f, 5205
clinical manifestations of, 1669–1670
diagnosis of, 1670–1671
endovascular stents for, 1675, 5217–5218, 5218t
historical aspects of, 1669
medical treatment of, 1671
pathogenesis of, 1669
penetrating, 1670, 1670f, 5203–5204
surgery for, 1671–1675, 5217
outcomes in, 1674–1675
transsphenoidal surgery and, 569
internal, 15f, 18f, 19, 22f, 28f
anatomy of, 1924, 1924f
aneurysms of, 1683f, 1684, 1684f, 1919
balloon occlusion of, 2057–2058, 2058f
blunt trauma to, 5211–5212
cavernous segment of, 1895–1896, 1897f–1898f
aneurysms of, 1899–1900, 1901f, 1909
branches of, 1896
cavernous sinus and, fistula between. *See* Cavernous carotid fistula.
cervical
exposure of, 1907
middle cerebral artery bypass for, 1673–1674
petrous bypass for, 1672f, 1673

Carotid artery *(Continued)*
choroidal segment of, 19
clinoidal segment of, 1896, 1897f–1898f
aneurysms of
anterolateral variant of, 1901–1903, 1902f–1903f
clipping technique for, 1909, 1910f
imaging of, 1899
medial variant of, 1901–1903, 1902f–1903f
treatment of, 1903–1904
types of, 1901–1903, 1902f–1903f
communicating segment of, 19, 1916–1917
aneurysms of, 1917–1918, 1917t
dissecting aneurysm of, 1880, 1881f, 1882f
giant aneurysm of, 1870f
in anterior communicating artery aneurysm surgery, 1933
in skull base tumors, 2108
infundibulum of, 1920
intracavernous aneurysms of, surgery for, 1881–1882, 1884–1885, 1884f
ischemic injury to, 1614
lesions of, 1626
angioplasty for, 1653–1654
occlusion of, 1640–1641, 1641f, 1642–1643
ischemia risk in, 2107
ophthalmic segment of, 19, 1896, 1897f–1898f
aneurysms of, 1886–1887, 1888f
clinical presentation of, 1904, 1905f–1906f
clipping technique for, 1909, 1911f
dorsal variant, 1904
embolization of, 2068–2069
imaging of, 1899
treatment of, 1904, 1906
types of, 1904
branches of, 1896, 1898
petrous-to-supraclinoid bypass for, 1673f–1674f, 1674
precavernous, 1344
in trigeminal schwannoma, 1347, 1348f
proximal
aneurysms of, 1895
bony resection for, 1907, 1908f
circulatory arrest for, 1907, 1909
clipping technique for, 1909–1910, 1910f, 1911f
closure for, 1910
complications of, 1911–1912
dural sheaths in, 1895
giant, 1909–1910
postoperative care in, 1910–1911
surgery for, 1907–1912
bends in, 1896
pseudoaneurysms of, 1684, 1684f, 1880, 1883f
saccular aneurysms of, 1915–1920
imaging of, 1915
outcome in, 1920, 1920t
subarachnoid hemorrhage grading in, 1915–1916, 1916t
surgery for, 1915–1916, 1920
sacrifice of, vs. extracranial-intracranial bypass, 1892–1893
segments of, 1895–1896, 1897f–1898f
supraclinoid, aneurysms of, 1919–1920
temporary balloon occlusion of, single-photon emission computed tomography with, 2480

Carotid artery *(Continued)*
transcranial Doppler ultrasonography of, 1541, 1541f
traumatic aneurysms of, 5207, 5207f–5208f
intrapetrous, aneurysms of, 1880–1881, 1881f–1883f
middle, ischemic injury to, 1614–1615
occlusion of, 1554
petrous, 36f
radiation stenosis of, 1685–1687, 1686f
recurrent stenosis of, 1661–1667
angioplasty for, 1652f, 1653, 1653f
clinical presentation of, 1664
diagnosis of, 1664
etiology of, 1661–1662
histopathology of, 1663–1664, 1663f
incidence of, 1661, 1662t
pathogenesis of, 1662–1664
treatment of
medical, 1664–1665
surgical, 1665–1666, 1665f, 1666f
resection of, interposition graft in, 1665–1666, 1666f
shunt for, 1629–1630, 1629f
embolization from, 1643
spontaneous dissection of, 1684–1685, 1686f
stenosis of, 1622
after endarterectomy, 1644
endarterectomy for, 1621–1645. *See also* Carotid endarterectomy.
radiation-induced, 1654
stroke risk in, 1615
transient ischemic attacks in, 1623
superficial temporal–middle cerebral artery bypass for, 1674
thrombosis of, carotid endarterectomy and, 1643–1644
Carotid artery disease, 1613–1618. *See also* Atherosclerosis.
hemodynamic effects of, 1601–1602, 1602f
medical management of, 1616–1618
natural history of, 1615–1616
platelet antiaggregant therapy for, 1617–1618
risk factors for, 1616–1617
transient ischemic attacks and, 1613
ultrasonography of, 1565–1566, 1566f
Carotid body, 1677
anatomy of, 1677–1678
tumors of, 1677–1681
β-adrenergic blockade in, 1679
clinical presentation of, 1678
genetics of, 1678
growth of, 1679–1680
histology of, 1678, 1678f
imaging of, 1678–1679, 1679f, 1680f
metastatic, 1680
radiation therapy for, 1681
surgery for, 1680–1681
Carotid cave
anatomy of, 1885, 1885f
aneurysms of, 1885–1886, 1885f
Carotid cavernous fistula. *See* Cavernous carotid fistula.
Carotid cistern, 1926–1927, 1927f
Carotid endarterectomy, 1621–1645
anesthesia for, 1509
barbiturates in, 1626–1627
care after, 1639–1640
carotid artery shunt in, 1629–1630, 1629f
cerebral protection in, 1626–1627
clinical studies of, 1625–1626

Carotid endarterectomy *(Continued)*
closure in, 1637–1639, 1637f–1639f
complications of, 1643–1645
controversies in, 1626
effectiveness of, 1651
embolization in, 1643
for restenosis, 1662
for stenosis, 1661
historical background on, 1621–1622
in tandem lesions, 1626
intracerebral hemorrhage in, 1644–1645
myocardial infarction in, 1645
operating microscope in, 1630–1631, 1631f
patch angioplasty with, for recurrent stenosis, 1665–1666, 1665f, 1666f
patient selection for, 1651, 1652f, 1653, 1653f
restenosis after, 1657
saphenous vein grafts in, 1627–1629, 1628f
stroke risk and, 1615–1616
technique of, 1631–1637, 1631f–1636f
thrombosis in, 1643–1644
transcranial Doppler ultrasonography monitoring during, 1548–1550
Carotid sheath, nerves surrounding, 2643–2644
Carotid siphon, lesions of, 1626
Carotid thromboendarterectomy, 1640–1643, 1641f
Carotid-oculomotor membrane, 1895
Carpal joint, radial, innervation of, 3898
Carpal tunnel, anatomy of, 3889
Carpal tunnel syndrome, 3889–3894
causes of, 3877–3878, 3889–3890
diagnosis of, 3890–3891
electrophysiologic studies of, 3877, 3890–3891
magnetic resonance imaging of, 3878–3879
magnetic resonance neurography of, 3874f
median nerve demyelination in, 3853
median nerve entrapment in, 3923–3924
needle electromyography in, 3858
nerve conduction studies in, 3857–3858
presentation of, 3876–3877
treatment of, 3891
complications of, 3894
endoscopic release procedure in, 3893–3894, 3893f
open release procedure in, 3891–3893, 3892f
Carpenter's syndrome, 3320–3321
historical aspects of, 3164
Cart1, 53t
Cartilage-hair hypoplasia, atlantoaxial instability in, 3543
Case reports/series, 248–249
Case-control studies, 249
Caspar headholder, 4622, 4623f
Caspar system, of cervical spine anterior screw-plate fixation, 4630t, 4631–4632, 4631f
Caspases, in traumatic brain injury, 5030
Catatonia, vs. coma, 293
Catheters
complications of, 3140
epidural, infections from, 4384–4385
for arteriovenous malformation embolization, 2224–2225
for bladder outlet incontinence, 381
for intrathecal drug infusion, 3136–3138
for urinary retention, 377–378

Catheters (*Continued*)
ventricular
in cerebrospinal fluid shunt, 3379–3380, 3380f
obstruction of, 3382–3383
Cauda equina, 4989f
compression of
decompression for, 4998
in pyogenic spinal infection, 4364
in spinal stenosis, 4521
treatment of, 4374
recovery of, 4989–4990
sensory loss in, 272, 272f
Cauda equina syndrome, 4872
in lumbosacral spine tumors, 4041
lumbar diskectomy and, 580
Caudal agenesis, 4269–4270, 4269f
Caudal point, 38
Caudal regression syndrome, 4317
Caudate
arteriovenous malformation of, 2246
hematoma of, 1737
Caudate nucleus. *See* Nucleus caudalis.
Caudomedial artery, 39
Causalgia, 3831
definition of, 3094
pain in, 3820–3821
sympathectomy for, 3094
vicious cycle hypothesis of, 3094
Cavernoma. *See* Cavernous malformations.
Cavernous angioma. *See* Cavernous malformations.
Cavernous angiomatosis, familial multiple, 2394
Cavernous carotid fistula, 1771, 2341–2350, 5211
carotid-jugular compression for, 2345
classification of, 2343–2344
clinical presentation of, 5212, 5214
embolic agents for, 2346
embolization of
balloon, 2345–2346
coil, 2346
endovascular treatment of, 2342–2343, 2345
historical aspects of, 2341, 2342f
in pregnancy, 2429
in type IV Ehlers-Danlos syndrome, 1771
intracaverous internal carotid artery aneurysm and, 1882, 1884–1885
microsurgery for, 2341–2342, 2346, 2347f
radiosurgery for, 2349–2350
surgery for, 2346, 2348–2349, 2348f
symptoms of, 2344
treatment of, 2344–2350
Cavernous hemangioma. *See* Cavernous malformations.
Cavernous malformations, 1373, 2142–2147, 2167–2171, 2292–2298, 4315t
anesthesia in, 1512
arteriovenous malformations and, 2154
asymptomatic, 2169
behavior of, 2171
brainstem, 2294–2295, 2295f, 2321–2338. *See also* Brainstem, cavernous malformations of.
capillary telangiectasia and, 2153
capsular, 2314–2316
central skull base, 1268
cerebral
familial, 2299
CCM1 in, 2300–2301
genetic markers in, 2300

Cavernous malformations (*Continued*)
genetics of, 2299–2303
historical background for, 2299
Krev-1/rap1a pathway in, 2303
KRIT1 mutations in, 2301–2302, 2303
linkage analysis of, 2299–2300
magnetic resonance imaging of, 2300
sporadic, 2299
classification of, 2167–2168, 2167t
clinical presentation of, 2138t, 2144, 2169–2170, 2293–2295, 2293f–2297f
cryptic, 2167
definition of, 2167–2168
developmental venous anomalies and, 2153
dural-based, 2317
epidemiology of, 2142, 2168–2169, 2292–2293
extradural, 4821
familial, 2293, 2293f, 2295
focal deficit in, 2170
genetics of, 2168
hemorrhage in, 2169–2170, 2170t, 2293–2294, 2293f–2296f, 2295, 2296
morbidity and mortality of, 2170–2171
imaging of, 2138t, 2144–2145, 2145f, 2146f, 2167–2168
in extratemporal lobe epilepsy, 2598
incidence of, 2292, 2293t
infratentorial, 2321–2338. *See also* Brainstem, cavernous malformations of.
intradural, 4826, 4830f
magnetic resonance imaging of, 471, 471f, 2167–2168, 2167t, 2292, 2293f–2297f
natural history of, 2138t, 2144, 2295–2296, 2297f
neurological deficit in, 2294, 2295f
occult, 2167
optic pathway, 2316
outcome in, 2170–2171
pathology of, 2138t, 2142–2144, 2143f
pineal, 2316, 2316f
scalp, 1413–1414
seizure in, 2169, 2171, 2294, 2294f
spinal cord, 2353–2354, 2355f, 2356. *See also* Spinal cord, cavernous malformations of.
sporadic, 2293, 2295
supratentorial, 2305–2317
clinical scenarios associated with, 2305, 2305t
epilepsy in, 2310
expectant management of, 2305–2306
hemorrhage in, 2305, 2307–2308, 2308f, 2309f
incidental, 2306–2307, 2307f
intractable epilepsy with, 2314
lesions mimicking, 2310–2311, 2310f, 2312f
long-standing seizure in, 2310
mass effect in, 2309
medical management of, 2306
multiple, 2316–2317, 2317f
neurological deficits in, 2309
new-onset seizure in, 2309
radiotherapy for, 2306
stereotactic radiosurgery for, 2306
surgery for, 2306, 2311–2318
imaging before, 2311
venous malformations associated with, 2311, 2313f, 2314
vs. arteriovenous malformation, 2311, 2312f

Cavernous malformations (*Continued*)
synonyms for, 2167
thalamic, 2314–2316, 2314f, 2315f
third ventricular, 1247
treatment of, 2138t, 2146–2147
vascular anatomy of, 2386
Cavernous sinus, 1895
anatomy of, 918–919, 919f, 920f
frontotemporal surgical approach to, 2346, 2348–2349, 2348f
inferior, artery of, 1896
injury to, transsphenoidal surgery and, 1182
internal carotid artery and, fistula between. *See* Cavernous carotid fistula.
lateral triangle of, 2341–2342
meningioma of, 1118, 1118f, 1278
septic thrombosis of, 1421
triangles of, 2346, 2348–2349, 2348f
tumors of, 1265
Cavernous sinus syndrome, intracavernous internal carotid artery aneurysm and, 1881–1882
Cavitation
post-traumatic, 206
spinal cord, 4317
CCM1, 2142, 2168
KRIT1 mutations and, 2301–2302, 2301t
localization of, 2300–2301
CCM2, 2142, 2168
localization of, 2300–2301
CCM3, 2142, 2168
localization of, 2300–2301
CD4
in antigen recognition, 678
in multiple sclerosis, 1450
CD8, in antigen recognition, 678
CD40–CD40 ligand system, in antigen-presenting cell activation, 893
CDK4, 1411
CDKN2, 1411
CDKN2/p16/INK4a, 741
Celecoxib, for pain, 2959
Celiac plexus block, 2983–2984
fluoroscopy in, 2973, 2973f, 2974f
Cell(s)
calcium metabolism in, 122f
electrical measurements in, 216, 217f
electrical properties of, 215–216, 216f, 218–219, 219f
major histocompatibility complex expression in, 678
migration of, 681–683
proliferation of, in malignant phenotype, 771, 772f
Cell adhesion molecules
in central nervous system repair, 4156–4157, 4162
in malignant glioma, 760–761, 763
Cell cycle, 716–718, 717f
regulation of, tumor suppressor genes in, 741
Cell cycle analysis, cytometric, tumor proliferation marking by, 694–695
Cell cycle arrest pathways, in glioma, 717–718, 717f
Cell cycle modulators, in gene therapy, 820–821
Cell death, 82–83. *See also* Apoptosis.
apoptotic vs. necrotic, 130–132, 131f
calcium hypothesis of, 126
calcium-related, 126–128
excitotoxic hypothesis of, 126
genetic program for, 133

Cell death *(Continued)*
glutamate-related, 126–128
in global ischemia, 132–133
mitochondrial failure and, 132–133
pathways for, 133
programmed, 718–719
protein synthesis and, 132
Cell membrane, ion selectivity of, 219
Cell Saver system, 4968
Cell swelling, 228
Cell-cell signaling, 774t
Cellular signaling proteins, as tumor suppressor genes, 741–743
Central deafferentation syndromes, 3018t
Central herniation, 826, 826t, 5055t, 5056
rostral-caudal progression of, 292, 292f
Central lobule, 30f, 31f
Central nervous system
abnormal sensory feedback to, in parkinsonian tremor, 2774
antigen presentation in, 887, 889–890
B cells in, 683
congenital tumors of, 811
disorders of, blood-brain barrier in, 153
drug penetration of, 17–18
electrophysiology of, 215–232
hemangioblastoma of, 1053–1060. *See also* Hemangioblastoma.
immune-inflammatory network in, 673–685. *See also* Immune response; Inflammation.
in urinary tract function, 359–360, 359f, 360f
inflammation of, 135–136
neuroimmunology and, 4155
injury to, 202–206
apoptosis after, 4155–4156
astrocytes in, 86, 204–205
chronic responses to, 4156
gene expression after, 4154–4155
inflammation in, 205–206
neurons in, 202–203
oligodendrocytes in, 203–204
pediatric, 3463
recovery from, 5025–5033
response to, 202
retrograde neuronal changes after, 4156
secondary effects of, 206
sequelae to, 4154–4156
transneuronal degeneration after, 4156
vs. peripheral nervous system injury, 3968–3969
wallerian degeneration after, 4156
lymphocytes in, 890
malformations of, gene mutations and, 46t
metastases to
chemotherapy for, 17
classification of, 671–672
magnetic resonance imaging of, 457, 457f, 458f
peripheral nervous system and, 3809
physiology of, 216, 217f
primary lymphoma of. *See* Lymphoma, primary central nervous system.
regulation of, astrocytes in, 86
repair of, 4153–4169
after incomplete injury, 4157
bioartificial regeneration environments in, 4163
biologic methods in, 4158
developmental rationale for, 4156–4157
dorsal root entry zone in, 4161–4162

Central nervous system *(Continued)*
embryonic tissue transplantation in, 4158
ensheathing glia in, 4162–4163
evaluation of, 4158
evidence supporting, 4156–4157
extracellular matrix in, 4168
gene therapy in, 4166–4167
glial cellular transplantation in, 4161–4163
glial scarring in, 4167–4168
in chronic injury, 4169
in immature mammals, 4156
in nonmammalian species, 4156
inflammatory cell transplantation in, 4164
inhibition reduction in, 4168, 4169
intraspinal embryonic tissue transplantation in, 4159
intrinsic regenerative capacity in, 4164–4169
mammalian lower extremity function and, 4157
mechanisms of, 4153–4154
models for, 4157–4158
myelin inhibition of, 4168–4169
myelin repair in, 4164
peripheral nerve grafts in, 4161, 4162
physical methods in, 4164
Schwann cells in, 4162
strategies for, 4158–4169
trophic molecules in, 4164–4166
undifferentiated, renewable cells in, 4159–4161
vs. plasticity, 4154
replacement in, 4154
secondary lymphoma of, 1074
stimulation of, 3119
transplantation in, 2829–2847. *See also* Transplantation.
tuberculosis of, 1439–1443
tumors of
chemotherapy for, 877–878
classification of, 4023
cyst with, 671t
extra-axial
radiologic features of, 835, 836–839
vs. intra-axial, 835
functional magnetic resonance imaging of, 852–853, 853f
intra-axial
radiologic features of, 835, 842–852
vs. extra-axial, 835
intraparenchymal, radiologic features of, 835, 840–841
radiologic features of, 835–854
xanthogranuloma of, 1443–1444
Central spinal cord syndrome, 4397, 4890, 4890f
Central sulcus, 3, 4f, 24f
in craniometrics, 630–631
localization of, 2532, 2532f
magnetic resonance imaging of, 2532
of insula, 5, 6f
topography of, 2533
Centromedian-parafascicular nuclear complex, subthalamic nucleus projections from, 2690
Centrum semiovale, venous drainage of, 1238
Cephalocele, 3198
Cephalohematoma
calcified, pediatric, 3717, 3718f
linear skull fracture and, 3482
scalp injury and, 3482
skull, 1404

Cephalothin, in pediatric glioma surgery, 3598
Ceramic bone graft, 4618
c-ERB2, in medulloblastoma, 3641
Cerebellar artery
anterior inferior, 36f, 37–39, 40f, 1974, 2026
embolization of, 2258
in arteriovenous malformations, 2256–2257, 2257f
occlusion of, ischemia risk with, 2107
origin of, aneurysms arising at, 2025
saccular aneurysm of, 1975
basilar superior, 2026
inferior, aneurysms of, 2025
rupture of, 1787
posterior inferior, 36f, 37–39, 40f, 1973–1974
anastomosis of, 2115
aneurysms of, 1975
clinical significance of, 2007–2008
diagnosis of, 2013–2014
endovascular occlusion of, 2019, 2021
far lateral suboccipital approach to, 2015, 2017f
lateral/medial suboccipital approach to, 2018
midline suboccipital approach to, 2018–2019
outcome in, 2020–2021
preoperative evaluation for, 2014
presentation of, 2009, 2010t–2012t, 2013, 2013f
rupture of, 2009
subarachnoid hemorrhage in, 2013, 2013f
surgical complications of, 2019–2020
treatment indications for, 2007–2008, 2008f
embolization of, 2258
in arteriovenous malformations, 2256–2257, 2256f, 2257f
occlusion of, ischemia risk with, 2107
superficial temporal artery bypass to, 2115
superior, 36f, 38f, 39–40, 1974, 1975
aneurysms of, 1975
embolization of, 2258
in arteriovenous malformations, 2256–2257, 2256f, 2257f
trigeminal nerve compression by, 3013
trigeminal nerve and, 1344
Cerebellar astrocytoma
pediatric, 3655–3660
age in, 3655
clinical presentation of, 3655, 3656t
complications of, 3659, 3659t
fibrillary, 3657, 3657f, 3658
follow-up for, 3660
histology of, 3656–3658, 3657f
imaging of, 3655–3656, 3656f
location of, 3656
outcome in, 3659–3660
radiation therapy for, 3660
sex in, 3655
surgery for, 3658–3659
pilocytic, juvenile, 3656–3657, 3657f
Cerebellar ataxia
after medulloblastoma surgery, 1037
urologic disorders in, 373–374
Cerebellar fissure, precentral, 32
Cerebellar hemisphere
arteriovenous malformations of, 2251
arterial supply/venous outflow in, 2256–2257, 2257f, 2258f

Cerebellar hemisphere *(Continued)*
imaging of, 2254–2255, 2254f
surgery for, 2261–2262, 2262f
crossed diaschisis of, stroke and, 1607, 1608f
insulo-opercular lesions in, surgery for, stimulation mapping during, 2537
Cerebellar incisura
anterior, 32
posterior, 32, 33f, 34
Cerebellar invasion, in Chiari malformation type II, 3352, 3352f
Cerebellar peduncle
inferior, 33f
middle, 29, 31f, 33f, 36f
superior, 31f, 33f
Cerebellar tentorium
arachnoid cyst of, 3292–3299
cavernous malformations of, 2317. *See also* Brainstem, cavernous malformations of; Cavernous malformations, supratentorial.
in Chiari malformation type II, 3350–3351
meningioma of, 1114
Cerebellar tonsils
arteriovenous malformations of, surgery for, 2262–2263, 2263f
displacement of, in Chiari malformation type I, 3347–3348
herniation of, 826t, 827, 5055t, 5056, 5091, 5092f
bullet wounds and, 5224
in Chiari malformation type I, 3349, 3350f
Cerebellar vein, precentral, 15f, 36f
Cerebellar vermis, arteriovenous malformations of, surgery for, 2260–2261, 2261f
Cerebellomedullary fissure, vein of, 34
Cerebellomesencephalic fissure, 31f, 32
Cerebellopontine angle
acoustic neuroma of
anatomic distortions in, 1158–1159, 1158t
auditory tests in, 335f–336f
treatment of, 1163–1164, 1163f
arterial supply of, 40, 40f
cavernous malformation of, 2317
choroid plexus tumor of, surgery for, 3618, 3619
cyst of, 3298
epidermoid tumor of, 3690
retrosigmoid approach to, 927
facial nerve schwannoma of, 1147, 1147f
vs. acoustic neuroma, 1147, 1147f, 1148f
globular tumor of, 1147f
meningioma of, 838f, 1119, 1119f, 1120f
surgical complications in, 568
retrosigmoid approach to, 920, 921f
schwannoma of, magnetic resonance imaging of, 459, 460f
tumors of, 831
supine positioning for, 607
Cerebellopontine angle syndrome, in trigeminal schwannoma, 1345–1346
Cerebellopontine fissure, 30, 30f
vein of, 36f
Cerebellothalamic projection, 2692f, 2693
Cerebellum, 29–34, 31f, 33f
atypical teratoid-rhabdoid tumors of, 999
dysfunction of
motor loss in, 274
urologic disorders in, 373–374
Cerebellum *(Continued)*
dysplastic gangliocytoma of, 666
ganglioglioma of, in epilepsy, 2578
hemorrhage in, 1736, 1737t, 1738–1739, 1739f
in Chiari malformation type II, 3351–3352, 3352f
in micturition, 359
metastases to, surgical approaches to, 1084, 1085, 1085f, 1086f
motor thalamic nuclei inputs from, 2691, 2692f
neuroblastoma of, 3640
petrosal surface of, 30–32, 31f
veins of, 34
suboccipital surface of, 33–34
veins of, 34
tentorial surface of, 10f, 32–33, 33f
veins of, 34, 35f
tumors of, 831
Cerebral acidosis, in head injury, 5050
Cerebral amyloid angiopathy, spontaneous intracerebral hemorrhage in, 1735, 1736f
Cerebral artery
aneurysms of, deep hypothermic circulatory arrest for, 1528–1529, 1529f–1531f, 1531
anterior, 26f, 27
A2 segment of, perforators of, 1925
aneurysms of, 1871f, 1892, 1919, 1923
rupture of, 1787
embryology of, 1923
segments of, 1923–1925, 1924f
blunt trauma to, 5212
distal anterior
anatomy of, 1945–1947, 1946f, 1947f
aneurysms of, 1939, 1945–1956
clinical characteristics of, 1947–1948, 1948t
historical background on, 1945
imaging of, 1948–1949, 1949f, 1950f
interhemispheric exposure for, 1880
multiple, 1947, 1948t
outcomes in, 1942
presentation of, 1939–1940, 1940f
rupture of, 1947
sites for, 1946–1947
subarachnoid hemorrhage in, 1947
surgery for, 1939–1942, 1940f, 1949–1952, 1951f, 1953f, 1954f
adjuncts to, 1940f, 1941
craniotomy in, 1940f, 1941
dissection/clipping in, 1941–1942, 1941f
head position in, 1941
incision in, 1940f, 1941
interhemispheric dissection in, 1941
results of, 1952–1956, 1954t
traumatic, 1947–1948
anomalies of, 1946, 1947f
infarction of, 1952
fibrosis of, 1847–1848
middle, 22f
anatomy of, 1959–1960
aneurysms of, 1919, 1959–1969
angiography of, 1873f, 1874f
clinical presentation of, 1960
embolization for, 1969, 2069
epidemiology of, 1959
imaging of, 1960, 1961f
outcome in, 1965, 1967–1969
rupture of, 1787
superior temporal gyrus approach to, 1963, 1965
Cerebral artery *(Continued)*
surgery for, 1890–1891, 1960–1969
care after, 1965
superficial temporal artery in, 1965, 1967f, 1968f
timing of, 1960, 1962
transsylvian approaches to, 1879, 1962–1963, 1963f–1965f
bifurcation of, aneurysms of, 1965, 1967f
branches of, 1959–1960
diseases of, 1602
in moyamoya, 1717f
in sylvian arteriovenous malformation, 2237, 2239f
occlusion of, ischemia and, 133–134, 134f, 1520, 2107
segments of, 13–14
sphenoid (M1) segment of, 21, 1924f
stroke involvement of, positron emission tomography of, 1601, 1603f
superficial temporal artery bypass to, 2113, 2113f, 2114f
traumatic pseudoaneurysm of, 5208, 5209f–5210f
occlusion of, 5212
posterior, 10f, 15f, 18f, 19, 22f, 36f, 1974
ambient segment of, 2052
anatomy of, 2052
aneurysms of, 2041, 2042, 2052–2053
hypoplastic, 1976
saccular aneurysm of, 1975
segments of, 21, 2052
posterior inferior, 38f
proximal anterior, aneurysms of, surgery for, 1930–1936. *See also* Communicating artery, anterior, aneurysms of, surgery for.
temporary clipping of, 1528
transcranial Doppler ultrasonography of, 1541, 1541f–1543f
vasospasm effect on, 1844–1845, 1845f, 1846f
Cerebral atrophy, microcephaly in, 428
Cerebral autoregulation, 181–182, 182f, 1474–1479, 5048–5050, 5049f, 5053, 5053t
arteriovenous difference in oxygen in, 5053, 5053t
blood viscosity in, 5049, 5052
after head injury, 5052, 5053t
calcium release in, 1476
carbon dioxide reactivity in, 5050, 5052–5053, 5053t
cerebral blood volume in, 5053, 5053t
cerebral metabolism in, 5048, 5051–5052, 5053, 5053t
cerebral perfusion pressure in, 1474, 5048–5049, 5049f
after head injury, 5052
definition of, 1474
endothelium in, 1476
in traumatic brain injury, 5084, 5120
mechanisms of, 1475–1478, 1477f, 1477t
metabolic, 5048
in head injury, 5051–5052
myogenic hypothesis of, 1475
neurogenic hypothesis of, 1476, 1477
principles of, 1475, 1475f
theories of, 5049–5050
transcranial Doppler ultrasonography of, 1550–1552, 1551f, 1555
Cerebral autosomal dominant arteriopathy with subcortical infarcts and leukoencephalopathy, 82, 82f

Cerebral blood flow, 1467–1474
after traumatic brain injury, 5084
arterial pressure and, 1504
augmentation of, 1521
autoregulation of. *See* Cerebral autoregulation.
calculation of, xenon computed tomography in, 1569–1570, 1571f
cerebral blood volume and, 5050
cerebral perfusion pressure and, 1467
cerebrospinal fluid and, 3387, 3388f, 3389
cerebrovascular resistance and, 1467
concepts of, 1467–1469
evaluation of, in vessel occlusion procedures, 862–863
hemodynamics of, 1467–1468
hyperventilation and, 5123, 5132–5133
in head injury, 5051–5053, 5051f, 5051t, 5053t
in infantile posthemorrhagic hydrocephalus, 3408
in pregnancy, 2422
in stroke, 1606–1607
in subarachnoid hemorrhage, 1814–1815
in subdural hematoma, 5044, 5106
in traumatic brain injury, 5109–5112, 5109t, 5110t
in vasospasm, 5046
intracranial pressure and, 186–187
ischemia and, 5051
jugular venous oxygen saturation and, 5116–5118, 5117f, 5118f
management of, 5125, 5134–5135, 5135t, 5145, 5147f
mannitol effects on, 5052, 5053t
measurement of, 1478–1479, 1480t–1481t
xenon computed tomography in. *See* Xenon computed tomography.
monitoring of, 5115–5116, 5116f
Monro-Kellie doctrine in, 1469
neuronal dysfunction and, 5051, 5051f
$Paco_2$ effect on, 1477–1478, 1477f
Pao_2 effect on, 1478, 1478f
pediatric, 3462
physiology of, 180, 1504
positron emission tomography of, 488–489, 490t, 1601, 1603f
preoperative evaluation and, 551
regulation of, 1469–1474
carbon monoxide in, 1472
endothelins in, 1474
nitric oxide in, 1470–1472, 1470t, 1471f
oxygen-derived free radicals in, 1473–1474
vasoactive mediators in, 1469, 1469t
vs. cerebral autoregulation, 1474
rheologic concepts of, 1468
shear rate in, 1468
systemic hypertension effects on, 5127
thresholds for, 1468, 1469t, 1515, 1516f
transcranial Doppler ultrasonography of, in trauma, 1550, 5114–5115
viscosity of, 1468
Cerebral blood flow velocity, subarachnoid hemorrhage effect on, 1545–1547, 1546f
Cerebral blood flow–metabolism coupling, 1488–1490
adenosine in, 1489
astrocytes in, 1489
calcium in, 1489–1490
chemical mediators of, 1488–1489
hydrogen ions in, 1489
mediators of, 1488t
Cerebral blood flow–metabolism coupling *(Continued)*
nitric oxide in, 1490
perivascular nerves in, 1489
potassium channels in, 1489–1490
potassium ions in, 1488–1489
Cerebral blood volume
autoregulation effects on, 5053, 5053t
cerebral blood flow and, 5050
determination of, 5054–5055
in head injury, 5052
in subarachnoid hemorrhage, 1814–1815
in vasospasm, 5046
intracranial pressure and, 186–187, 1469, 5054–5055
magnetic resonance imaging of, 466, 466f, 467f
physiology of, 180
positron emission tomography of, 488–489, 490t, 1601
Cerebral convexity, cysts of, 3295
Cerebral cortex
in micturition, 359, 360f
injury to, urologic disorders from, 373
resection of. *See* Topectomy.
surgical complications of, 1258
topography of, 423, 423f
Cerebral edema, 791
after débridement, 5236
blood-brain barrier in, 165–166
classification of, 792–793, 792f–795f
cytotoxic, 13, 791, 792–793, 792f, 5084
definition of, 791
historical aspects of, 791
hydrostatic, 791
in brain tumors, 827
in bullet wounds, 5235
in traumatic brain injury, 5083–5084, 5108–5109
intact-barrier, 791
interstitial, 791, 793, 795f
intracranial pressure in, 180, 187–188
mediators of, 801
open-barrier, 791
osmotic, 791, 793
prevention of, in pediatric anesthesia, 3189–3190
surgery and, 566, 934–935, 934f, 5176, 5176f, 5177f
treatment of, 801–803
Lund therapy in, 5125, 5125f
tumor-associated, 793
blood supply in, 795, 796f
imaging of, 799, 800f
mechanisms of, 795, 796f, 797f
neuroradiographic characteristics of, 795, 798f, 799
tumor-host interactions and, 791–803
vascular permeability factor/vascular endothelial growth factor in, 793, 795, 801
vasogenic, 13, 791, 793, 793f, 794f, 5083–5084
resolution of, 799, 801
vs. brain swelling, 791
Cerebral hemispheres
cysts of, 3296, 3296f, 3297f
in consciousness, 279
information transfer between, transcallosal surgery and, 1259
lesions of, 274
tumors of, 830
pediatric, 3697–3703
chemotherapy for, 3702–3703
epidemiology of, 3697
Cerebral hemispheres *(Continued)*
imaging of, 3697–3700, 3698f–3701f
pathology of, 3700–3702
presentation of, 3697
prognosis of, 3703
radiation therapy for, 3702–3703
surgery for, 3702
Cerebral hypoperfusion, transient ischemic attacks from, 1624
Cerebral infarction, 1495
vasospasm and, blood velocities in, 1546
Cerebral ischemia
adhesion molecules in, 140–141, 141t
apoptosis vs. necrosis in, 130–132, 131f
blood-brain barrier in, 166
brain metabolism in, 117
calcium homeostasis in, 122–123, 123f, 124f
carotid endarterectomy and, transcranial Doppler ultrasonography of, 1550
cell death in, 126–128
chemokines in, 136–137, 137t, 140
complement system in, 142
cytokines in, 138–140
focal, 117, 133–135
global, 117, 132–133
head injury and, 5051, 5051f, 5051t
transcranial Doppler ultrasonography of, 1552
hydrogen ions in, 123–124, 126
hyperglycemia-mediated, 128–130
immunosuppressants in, 135
in cerebral palsy, 3736–3737, 3736f
in pregnancy, 2427–2428, 2428t
in vagus nerve stimulation, 2644
inflammation in
cell-protective effects of, 138
growth-promoting effects of, 138
mechanisms of, 137
mediators of, 135–143
triggers of, 138
inflammatory cells in, 136, 136t
magnetic resonance imaging of, 466–467, 468f, 469
monitoring of, in traumatic brain injury, 5113–5120, 5116f–5119f
monocytes in, 136, 137–138
neutrophils in, 136, 137–138, 141–142, 143f
nitric oxide inhibitors in, 135
pathophysiology of, hypothermic cerebral protection and, 1532
pH in, 124–126, 125f
reactive oxygen species inhibitors in, 135
spin trap nitrones in, 134–135, 134f
subdural hematoma and, 5044
treatment of, in traumatic brain injury, 5134–5135, 5135t
vasospasm and, 1839
Cerebral lymphoma. *See* Central nervous system, primary lymphoma of.
Cerebral metabolic rate of glucose (CMRG), 5048, 5048t, 5052
positron emission tomography of, 480, 482, 488–489, 490t
Cerebral metabolic rate of oxygen (CMRO), 1503, 5048, 5048t
in barbiturate coma, 5134
in head injury, 5050, 5051
in luxury perfusion, 5052
in seizures, 5120
in subarachnoid hemorrhage, 1814–1815
ischemia and, 5051
positron emission tomography of, 488–489, 490t, 1603f

Cerebral metabolism, 1479, 1482–1487
  acid-base metabolism in, 123–126, 125f
  adenosine triphosphate in, 119–120, 1479, 1482
    generation of, 118–119, 119f
  astrocytes in, 1486–1487
  autoregulation of. *See* Cerebral autoregulation.
  blood-brain barrier in, 1487
  calcium homeostasis in, 120–123, 121f–124f
  definition of, 1479
  glutamate in, 1485–1486, 1485f
  in head injury, 5050–5051
  indices of, 1479
  ketone bodies in, 1485
  mitochondria in, 117–120, 118f, 119f
  neurons in, 1486
  of glucose, 1482–1484, 1483t, 1484f
  of glycogen, 1484–1485
  pathways of, 1482–1486
  physiology of, 5047–5048, 5048t
  regional aberrations of, positron emission tomography of, 490–491, 491f
  resting, in Parkinson's disease, 2759
  structural elements in, 1486–1487
Cerebral oxygenation measurement
  brain tissue Po_2 in, 5118, 5119, 5119f
  in treatment plans, 5120, 5121f
  jugular venous oxygen saturation in, 5116–5118, 5116f–5118f
  near-infrared spectroscopy in, 5118–5119
Cerebral palsy, 3723
  adjunctive therapies in, 3733
  ambulation in, 3725–3727, 3729–3730, 3733
    predictors of, 3739, 3743
  assistive devices for, 3730
  ataxic, 3725
  birth weight and, 3723
  causes of, 3723
  classification of, 3723–3725
  clinical presentation of, 3725, 3726t, 3747
  cognitive function in, 3727, 3744
  complications of, 3727–3729
  definition of, 3723
  diagnosis of, 3725, 3726t
  differential diagnosis of, 3725
  dorsal rhizotomy for, 3747–3756. *See also* Selective dorsal rhizotomy.
  drug therapy for, 3730–3732, 3749–3756
  dystonia in, 2748
  epidemiology of, 3723
  extrapyramidal (dyskinetic), 3724–3725
  gait abnormalities in, 3729–3730, 3743–3744
  hypertonia in, 3754–3755
  intrathecal baclofen for, 3732, 3749–3756. *See also* Baclofen, intrathecal.
  movement disorders in, 3724–3727, 3726t, 3729–3730, 3747–3748
  oral baclofen for, 3748–3749
  orthotics for, 3730
  periventricular leukomalacia in, 3736, 3736f, 3737f
  prognosis for, 3725–3727
  pyramidal, 3723–3724
  recreational activities in, 3733
  rigidity in, 3724
  risk factors for, 3723
  selective dorsal rhizotomy for, 3736–3745. *See also* Selective dorsal rhizotomy.
  severity of, 3725, 3726t, 3750, 3750t
Cerebral palsy *(Continued)*
  spasticity in, 2751, 2751f, 3725–3727, 3729, 3730–3732, 3747–3748
    after dorsal rhizotomy, 3743
    deleterious effects of, 3737
    dorsal rhizotomy for, 3736–3745
    pathogenesis of, 3736–3737, 3736f, 3737f
    treatment of, 3754–3756
  speech problems in, 3727, 3730, 3732
  treatment of, 3754–3755
  with hemiplegia, 3724
Cerebral peduncles, 29, 3054
  lesions of, 273, 273f
    temporal lobectomy and, 2610
Cerebral perfusion pressure, 181–182, 551
  cerebral blood flow and, 1467
  hemodynamic impairment and, 1601, 1601t, 1602f
  in cerebral autoregulation, 1474, 5048–5049, 5049f, 5052
  in cerebral blood flow, 5134
  in head injury, 5058
  in increased intracranial pressure, 566, 1504
  in subdural hematoma, 5044
  in traumatic brain injury, 5084, 5096, 5114, 5124–5129, 5125f, 5126t
  mean arterial pressure and, 1467
  metabolic impairment and, 1601, 1601t, 1602f
  occlusive disease effects on, 1554
  pediatric, 3462
  positron emission tomography of, 489–490, 490t
  regulation of, 5048–5049
Cerebral vasospasm, 1839–1859. *See also* Vasospasm.
Cerebral veins
  anterior, 24f
  deep middle, 17, 24f
  internal, 14f, 15f, 35f, 1239
  obstruction of, pseudotumor cerebri from, 1420–1422, 1424t
  thrombosis of. *See* Cerebral venous thrombosis.
Cerebral venous thrombosis, 1723–1730
  angiography of, 1726, 1726f
  antithrombotics for, 1726–1727
  clinical presentation of, 1724
  computed tomography of, 1724, 1725f
  diagnosis of, 1724–1726, 1725f, 1726f
  endovascular thrombolytics for, 1727–1729, 1727t, 1728f, 1729f
  incidence of, 1724
  interventional neuroradiology for, 1727–1729, 1727t, 1728f, 1729f
  magnetic resonance angiography of, 1597, 1597f
  magnetic resonance imaging of, 1724–1726, 1725f, 1726f
  outcome in, 1729–1730
  pathogenesis of, 1723–1724
  surgery for, 1729
  thrombolytics for, 1727
  treatment of, 1726–1729
Cerebrospinal fluid
  absorption of, 179
  antigen transport of, 679
  chemotherapy via, 878
    in neoplastic meningitis, 1233–1234
  circulation of, historical aspects of, 3147–3151, 3148f
  composition of, 154, 178, 178t
  diversion of, 185–186
Cerebrospinal fluid *(Continued)*
    in lateral ventricle tumors, 1244
    in third ventricular tumors, 1251
    sites for, 3374, 3374t
  drainage of. *See also* Cerebrospinal fluid shunt.
    for infantile posthemorrhagic hydrocephalus, 3411, 3412f, 3413–3414
    in intracranial hypertension, 5133
    in intracranial pressure management, 5058
    in sagittal sinus pressure increases, 3400, 3401f
  dynamics of, 178–179, 179f, 3387, 3388f, 3389
  ex vacuo collections of, child abuse and, 3507
  formation of, 178, 179
  glioma dissemination via, 760
  hydraulic circuit of, 3387, 3388f
  in achondroplasia, 3365–3366
  in arachnoid cyst, 3289–3290
  in choroid plexus tumors, 3613
  in germ cell tumor surgery, 3608
  in intracranial pressure, 5054
  in neoplastic meningitis, 1231–1232
  in primary central nervous system lymphoma, 1069–1070
  in sarcoidosis, 1437
  in spinal cord stimulation, 3108
  in spinal metastases, 4856
  in subarachnoid hemorrhage, 1817–1818, 1818t
  leakage of, 276t. *See also* Cerebrospinal fluid fistula.
    acoustic neuroma surgery and, 570, 571
    craniofacial trauma and, 5247–5248
    frontal sinus repair and, 5252–5253
    glomus jugulare tumor surgery and, 1306–1307
    pediatric intramedullary tumor surgery and, 3713
    skull base surgery and, 571
    spinal surgery and, 574–576
    thoracic spine fracture and, 4982
    transsphenoidal surgery and, 1180
  nuclear medicine studies of, 2475
  obstruction of, 1505
    at aqueduct of Sylvius, 3391–3393, 3392f
    at basal cisterns, 3395, 3395f
    at foramen of Monro, 3389–3391, 3390f, 3391f
    at fourth ventricle outlet foramina, 3393–3394, 3394f, 3395f
    between spinal and cortical subarachnoid spaces, 3394–3397, 3395f
  pathways of, 3387, 3388f
  physiology of, 175, 178, 178t
  pressure differentials in, 3389
  resorption of, 1505
  source of, historical aspects of, 3151
  storage of, 179
  tension pneumocephalus and, 616
Cerebrospinal fluid fistula
  lumbar stenosis surgery and, 4462
  temporal bone fracture and, 5279–5280, 5280f
  traumatic, 5267–5272
    bedside tests for, 5269
    classification of, 5267
    clinical presentation of, 5268–5269

Cerebrospinal fluid fistula *(Continued)*
early, 5267
history in, 5268
identification of, 5269–5270
imaging of, 5269–5270
infection prophylaxis in, 5270–5271
laboratory tests for, 5269
late, 5267
meningitis in, 5268–5269
pathophysiology of, 5267–5268
physical examination of, 5268
pneumocephalus in, 5269
spontaneous, 5267
surgery for, 5271–5272
treatment of, 5270–5272
Cerebrospinal fluid pressure, in intracranial pressure, 5054
Cerebrospinal fluid shunt, 3374–3383
antisiphon devices in, 3378–3379, 3378f
catheters for, 3379–3380, 3380f
obstruction of, 3382–3383
design of, brain biomechanical models in, 3381–3382
differential pressure valves in, 3376–3377
externally adjustable differential pressure valves in, 3377
flow-regulated valves in, 3378, 3378f
for infantile posthemorrhagic hydrocephalus, 3412f, 3413, 3414
gravity-actuated valves in, 3379, 3379f
historical aspects of, 3374–3375, 3374t
horizontal-vertical valve in, 3379, 3379f
hydrodynamics of, 3375, 3375f, 3376f, 3380–3381
hydrostatic pressure in, 3375, 3376f
in vitro testing of, 3380–3381
infection of, 3419–3424
age and, 3420
evaluation of, 3420–3422, 3421f
organisms in, 3422–3423
outcome in, 3424
presentation of, 3420
prevention of, 3422
rate of, 3419
risk factors for, 3420
skin bacteria and, 3420
timing of, 3419–3420
treatment of, 3423–3424
obstruction of, clearance of, 3382–3383
pressure-flow curve for, 3375, 3375f
programmable valves in, 3377, 3377f
siphoning in, 3376, 3376f, 3377f
valves in, 3376–3379, 3381–3382
Cerebrovascular accidents. *See* Stroke.
Cerebrovascular disease
anesthesia for, 1503–1512
historical considerations in, 1461–1465
ischemic, preoperative evaluation for, 552–553, 552t
occlusive, anesthesia for, 1508–1509
positron emission tomography of, 1600–1609, 2478
single-photon emission computed tomography of, 2478–2480, 2479f, 2480f
transcranial Doppler ultrasonography in, 1554–1555
treatment of, 2121–2128
Cerebrovascular injury, traumatic, 5203–5219
aneurysm in, 5207–5208, 5207f–5210f, 5211
blunt (nonpenetrating), 5204–5207
angiography of, 5214–5215
Cerebrovascular injury *(Continued)*
anticoagulation for, 5217
clinical presentation of, 5211–5212
common pathway in, 5206
diagnosis of, 5214–5215
endovascular treatment for, 5217–5219, 5218f
grading of, 5216
imaging of, 5215
intimal disruption in, 5206
mechanisms of, 5206–5207
screening for, 5216
surgery for, 5216–5217
treatment of, 5216–5219, 5218f
clinical presentation of, 5211–5214
diagnosis of, 5214–5216
epidemiology of, 5203–5211
historical background on, 5203
mechanisms of, 5203–5211
penetrating, 5203–5204
clinical presentation of, 5211
diagnosis of, 5214
Cerebrovascular innervation, 1476–1477, 1477t
Cerebrovascular malformations, historical considerations in, 1462–1463
Cerebrovascular reactivity, in head injury, 5051–5053, 5053t
Cerebrovascular resistance, cerebral blood flow and, 1467
Cerebrovascular surgery, cytoprotective strategies for, 1520–1522
Cerebrum
anatomy of, 3–28
anterior segment of, 25–26
association fibers of, 6–7, 7f
basal surface of, 17–24
arterial relationships of, 19–23, 20f, 22f
neural relationships of, 17–19, 18f
venous relationships of, 23–24, 24f
lateral surface of, 3–17
arterial relationships in, 13–16
neural structures in, 3–13
venous relationships in, 16–17
lobes of, 16
medial surface of, 24–28
arterial relationships in, 27, 28f
neural relationships in, 24–27, 26f
venous relationships in, 28
posterior segment of, 26
sulci of, 3
Cervical artery, aneurysms of, surgery for, 1880–1881, 1881f–1883f
Cervical bruit, in stroke, 1622–1623
Cervical collar
complications from, 576
for spinal trauma, 4888, 4898f, 4899
Cervical disk disease, 4395–4404
after hyperextension-hyperflexion injury, 4919–4920
clinical presentation of, 4396–4397, 4410
herniation in, 4410
hyperextension-hyperflexion injury and, 4919
imaging of, 4397–4398
biodynamics and, 4410–4412, 4411f, 4412f
in spondylosis, 4447
magnetic resonance imaging of, 4411–4412, 4412f
nonoperative treatment of, 4398
pathology of, 4409–4410
pathophysiology of, 4395–4396
pediatric, 3560
imaging of, 3562
surgery for, 3563–3564
Cervical disk disease *(Continued)*
posterior approach to, 4409–4428
radiculopathy in, 271–272, 272t, 4396
surgery for, 4399–4404
Cervical diskectomy, 4439–4440, 4439f, 4440f, 4625–4626, 4625f, 4625t
Cervical facet joint
medial branch of, denervation of, 2977, 2980
pain referral patterns in, 2979f
Cervical nerve roots, inflammation of, 505f
Cervical orthoses, 3334, 4898–4899, 4898f, 4899f
for multiple myeloma, 4854
Cervical radiculopathy, magnetic resonance imaging of, 3882–3883, 3883f
Cervical spine
acceleration-deceleration injury to, 4915
anatomy of, 4431–4432
aneurysmal bone cyst of, 4843, 4844f
anterior approaches to, 4431–4443
complication avoidance in, 576–578
in trauma, 4901
anterior screw-plate fixation of, 4621–4637
ABC system of, 4630t, 4635–4636, 4636f
Atlantis system of, 4630t, 4633–4635, 4633f–4635f
bone grafting in, 4626, 4626f, 4626t
bone healing in, 4626–4627
Caspar system of, 4630t, 4631–4632, 4631f
closure in, 4629
Codman, 4630t, 4633, 4633f
complications of, 4636–4637
diskectomy in, 4625–4626, 4625f
follow-up to, 4629
fusion in, 4627–4629, 4628f
incision for, 4622–4623, 4623f
indications for, 4621–4622
midline orientation in, 4625, 4625t
Orion system of, 4630t, 4632–4633, 4632f
orthoses in, 4629
plate fixation in, 4626, 4626f, 4626t
positioning for, 4622, 4623f
preparation for, 4622
soft tissue dissection in, 4623–4624, 4624f
Synthes system of, 4630t, 4632, 4632f
systems for, 4629, 4630t, 4631–4636
vertebral column exposure in, 4623–4624, 4624f
anterior ventromedian approach to, complication avoidance in, 576–577
arterial supply of, 4310–4311
biomechanics of, 4187, 4432
facetectomy and, 4193–4194
in atlantoaxial injury, 4188
in burst fracture, 4189
in extension injury, 4190
in flexion-compression injury, 4189–4190
in lower injury, 4188–4189
in rotation injury, 4190
cantilever injury to, 4915
chordoma of, 4848
dislocation of
bilateral, 4909, 4909f
unilateral, 4908–4909
disorders of, ependymoma surgery and, 3630
extension of, in ankylosing spondylitis, 4460, 4461f

Cervical spine (*Continued*)
fractures of, 4896–4897
airway management in, 5246
computed tomography of, 502f
jumped facets in, 520f, 521
fusion of, 4440, 4626–4629, 4628f
biomechanics in, 4193–4194
bone grafts in, 4607–4608, 4607f
ganglionectomy in, 3035–3036, 3037f
hyperextension of, 4896, 4909
carotid artery injury in, 5204, 5204f
central cord syndrome in, 4890
hyperextension-hyperflexion injury to, 4915–4922
clinical presentation of, 4918–4919
historical aspects of, 4915
imaging of, 4920–4921
litigation in, 4920
mechanism of, 4915–4917
motor vehicle accidents and, 4915–4917
outcome in, 4922
pathology of, 4917–4918
prognosis of, 4919–4920
treatment of, 4921–4922
hyperflexion of, 4896
anterior cord syndrome in, 4890
bilateral facet dislocations from, 4909, 4909f
carotid artery injury in, 5204, 5204f
internal fixation of, 4596–4597, 4596f, 4597f, 4901–4902
anterior, 4440, 4442
biomechanics in, 4194
C1–2 transarticular, 4748–4751, 4751f
image-guided navigation for, 4748–4751, 4751f, 4752f
posterior, 4419–4424, 4422f, 4423f, 4639–4653
anesthesia for, 4643
articular mass screw-plate and screw-rod fixation in, 4650–4653, 4651f, 4652t
exposure for, 4643–4644
interlaminar clamps in, 4650, 4650f
monitoring during, 4643
patient positioning for, 4643
postoperative care after, 4653
wire and cable techniques in, 4644–4650, 4645f–4649f
Jefferson fracture of, 501f
ligamentous disease of, 4395–4404
clinical presentation of, 4396–4397
imaging of, 4397–4398
nonoperative treatment of, 4398
surgery for, 4399–4404
lower, anterior approach to, 635
metastases to, imaging of, 531, 531f
middle, anterior approach to, 635
multiple myeloma of, 4854
myelopathy of, 4397
surgery for, 4400–4404, 4402f–4404f
osteoid osteoma of, 4837, 4838f
pain in, 4396
surgery for, 4399
pediatric
flexion injury of, 3516
internal fixation of, 3546
posterior fusion of, 3546–3547
pseudosubluxation of, 3515
posterior approaches to, 4639–4653
complication avoidance in, 578–579
historical perspective on, 4639
in trauma, 4901–4902
indications for, 4639–4641, 4640t

Cervical spine (*Continued*)
instrumentation constructs for, 4641–4642, 4641t, 4642t
pyogenic infection of, surgery for, 4372f–4375f, 4374–4375
radiculopathy of, 4396–4397, 4399–4400, 4399f, 4400f
surgery for, 4399–4400, 4399f, 4400f
treatment of, 4412–4413, 4427
radiography of, 500–501, 500f, 501f
rheumatoid arthritis of, 4571, 4571f
radiologic features of, 4574, 4574f–4577f
rotation of, 3537–3538, 3538f
screw fixation of, complication avoidance in, 577–578
sprain of, 4915
stability of, 4897
restoration of, 4640, 4898–4902, 4898f, 4899f
strain of, 4915
subaxial, fracture of, 4934
surgical approaches to, 631–636
historical aspects of, 4395
posterior, 635–636
prone position in, 635–636
sitting position in, 636
traction for, in spinal cord injury, 4873–4874, 4875f, 4891–4892, 4892f
trauma to, 4149, 4307, 4885–4910
acute care of, 4887–4896, 4890f–4892f
biomechanics in, 4188–4189
child abuse and, 3507
classification of, 4896
epidemiology of, 4886–4887
historical considerations in, 4885–4886
imaging of, 517–519, 518f–520f, 521, 4892–4896
pediatric, 4887, 4910
stability restoration after, 4640, 4898–4902, 4898f, 4899f
treatment of
emergency room, 4889–4892, 4890f–4892f
prehospital, 4887–4889
surgical, 4899–4902
vertebral artery trauma in, 5205–5206
without radiographic abnormality, 4910
upper
anterior approach to, 632, 633f, 634–635, 634f
retropharyngeal prevascular approach to, 632, 634, 634f
retropharyngeal retrovascular approach to, 634–635
transoral approach to, 632
Cervical spondylosis
anterior approaches to, 4431–4443
complications of, 4443–4444, 4443f
historical perspective on, 4431
technique of, 4436–4439, 4437f, 4438f
diskectomy and corpectomy in, 4439–4440, 4439f–4441f
plating in, 4440, 4442
clinical manifestations of, 4433–4434
diagnosis of, 4434–4436, 4435f
pathophysiology of, 4432–4433
Cervical spondylotic myelopathy, 4397, 4447–4456
clinical presentation of, 4410, 4448–4449
natural history of, 4448
pathophysiology of, 4447–4448
radiography of, 4449–4450, 4450f
surgery for, 4400–4404, 4402f–4404f, 4450–4456

Cervical spondylotic myelopathy (*Continued*)
anesthesia for, 4414–4415
anterior approach to, 4451, 4452f
approaches to, 4450–4451
complications of, 4424–4427, 4424t, 4426f
indications for, 4413, 4414f, 4414t
laminectomy in, 4414t, 4416–4418, 4417f, 4418f, 4451–4452
posterior segmental instrumentation and, 4419–4424, 4422f, 4423f
laminoforaminotomy in, 4415–4416, 4415f, 4427
posterior spinal fusion and, 4416, 4416f, 4417f
laminoplasty in, 4418–4419, 4418f–4421f, 4425
outcome of, 4427–4428, 4452, 4453t–4454t, 4455–4456, 4455f
patient positioning for, 4414
patient selection for, 4450
posterior approach to, 4451–4452
preoperative evaluation for, 4414
treatment of, 4412–4428, 4413, 4450
vs. multiple sclerosis, 1455
Cervicomedullary compression
achondroplasia and, 3364–3365
decompression of, 3367–3368
outcome of, 3369
Down syndrome and, 3338
Cervicothoracic junction, surgical approaches to, 631–636. *See also* Cervical spine, surgical approaches to.
Cervicothoracic orthoses, 4899
Cesarean section, after ruptured aneurysm treatment, 2426
c-fos, traumatic brain injury and, 5028
Chamberlain's line, 423f, 424
Chance fracture, 521, 522f, 4967t
biomechanics in, 4192
Channelopathy, 225t
Charcot-Marie-Tooth disease, 3815–3816
neuropathy in, 3845
Chemical receptors, 74–75
Chemicals
brain tumors and, 811
neuropathy from, 3843–3844
parkinsonism from, 2716
Chemodectoma, skull, 1396–1397, 1397f
Chemokines
effector function of, 680
in cerebral ischemia, 136–137, 137t, 140
Chemonucleolysis, for lumbar disk disease, 4771–4776, 4774f
Chemoreceptors, 3809
Chemotherapy, 877–882. *See also* specific agent.
O^6-alkylguanine-DNA-alkyltransferase inhibition in, 879
antituberculous, 4387
approaches to, 879–880
blood-brain barrier in, 878
disruption of, 153, 879
blood-tumor barrier in, 878
central nervous system pharmacology in, 878–879
concentration of, at tumor site, 878–879
delivery of, 16–17
DNA repair in, 877–878
drug resistance in, 877–878
reversal of, 879
for brain metastases, 1078, 1092–1093
for brain tumors, 660
for brainstem glioma, pediatric, 3669, 3669t
for central nervous system metastases, 17

Chemotherapy *(Continued)*
for cerebral hemisphere tumors, pediatric, 3702–3703
for craniopharyngioma, 1219, 3683–3684
for ependymoma, 1048, 1048t
for esthesioneuroblastoma, 1335, 1337
for Ewing's sarcoma, 4850
for glial tumors, 871
for low-grade glioma, 964
for malignant glioma, 975–976
for medulloblastoma, 1005, 1038–1039
pediatric, 3647, 3648, 3649
for multiple myeloma, 4854
for neoplastic meningitis, 1233–1234
for paranasal sinus tumors, 1327, 1328f–1329f
for pineal region tumors, 1025
for primary central nervous system lymphoma, 1072, 1073t, 4023
high-dose, 879
interstitial, 880
intra-arterial, 879–880
intratumoral, 880
limitations of, 877–878
pharmacology of, 880–882
systemic administration of, 878
vs. angiosuppressive therapy, 784–785, 784t
Chest pain, hyperextension-hyperflexion injury and, 4918
Cheyne-Stokes respirations, in consciousness assessment, 282
Chiari malformation, 3347–3359
definition of, 3347, 3347t
fourth ventricle outlet foramina obstruction in, 3393
hindbrain herniation in, 3353–3354
historical aspects of, 3347
imaging of, 3355
in basilar invagination, 3340–3341
pathogenesis of, 3353–3354
surgery for, complications of, 3359
type 0, 3353, 3353f
type 1.5, 3353
type I, 3347t
asymptomatic, 3357f
findings in, 3347–3349, 3348f–3350f
imaging of, 533, 3355–3356
outcome in, 3469
signs/symptoms of, 3354–3355, 3354t
surgery for, 3356–3358, 3357f
symptomatic, 3357f
type II, 3215, 3217f, 3347t, 4270–4271, 4270f, 4271t
asymptomatic, 3358f
findings in, 3349–3352, 3350f–3352f
imaging of, 533, 534f, 3356
in myelomeningocele, 3215, 3216f, 3217f, 3223–3224
outcome in, 3469
surgery for, 3358–3359, 3358f
symptomatic, 3358f
type III, 3347t, 3352
type IV, 3347t, 3352
Chiasma
diffuse glioma of, pediatric, 3596, 3597
trauma to, 312f
Chiasmatic cistern, 1927f, 1929
Child abuse, 3499–3512
adjudicatory hearing in, 3509–3510
cerebrospinal fluid collection in, 3507
child protective services in, 3509
chronic extracerebral fluid collections in, 3505–3506, 3506f
shunts for, 3506–3507, 3507f

Child abuse *(Continued)*
civil proceedings in, 3509–3510, 3510t
criminal proceedings in, 3509–3510, 3510t
definition of, 3499
dispositional hearing in, 3510
evaluation of, 3499–3505
expert witness in, 3510–3511
head injury in, 3461, 3499
outcomes of, 3508
treatment of, 3505–3507
in older children, 3504–3505, 3504f
law enforcement agencies in, 3509
legal outcomes in, 3511–3512
mandated reporters for, 3508–3509
medicolegal considerations in, 3508–3512
physician reporting responsibilities in, 3508–3509
physician testimony in, 3510–3510
prevention of, 3512
social outcomes in, 3511–3512
spinal injury in, 3507–3508, 3508f
Child protective services, in child abuse, 3509
Children
achondroplasia in, 3362–3371
anesthesia in, 3187–3196
aneurysms in, 1801, 3448–3452
antiepileptic drugs for, 2471t
arachnoid cyst in, 3289–3299
arteriovenous malformations in, 2166–2167, 3447–3448, 3452–3457
atlantoaxial rotatory fixation in, 3537–3543
atlanto-occipital dislocation in, 3528–3537
brain death in, 401–403, 402t
brain of, 3462–3463
brain tumors in, of disordered embryogenesis, 3687–3693
brainstem glioma in, 3663–3670
cause of death in, 3461, 3461f
cerebellar astrocytoma in, 3655–3660
cerebral hemisphere tumors in, 3697–3703
cerebral palsy in, 3723–3733
cervical spine trauma in, 4887
without radiographic abnormality, 4910
Chiari malformations in, 3347–3359
choroid plexus tumors in, 3612–3620
craniofacial syndromes in, 3315–3329
craniopharyngioma in, 3671–3684
craniosynostosis in, 3300–3312
Dandy-Walker syndrome in, 3285–3287
developmental craniovertebral abnormalities in, 3331–3344
diskitis in, 4293, 4382
encephaloceles in, 3198–3211
eosinophilic granuloma in, 4843
ependymoma in, 3623–3634
epilepsy in, 3758–3765, 3769–3777
germ cell tumors in, 3603–3610
growing skull fractures in, 427, 427f
head injury in, 3473–3478
hydrocephalus in, 3387–3403
imaging in, 3196
interstitial brachytherapy for, 4105
intervertebral disk diseases in, 3559–3568
intradural extramedullary metastases in, 529
intraventricular hemorrhage in, 3463
language cortex resection in, 2537
lipomyelomeningocele in, 3229–3243

Children *(Continued)*
medulloblastoma in, 3639–3649
mild brain injury in, 3461–3469
skull fracture with, 3465–3470
without skull fracture, 3461–3465
myelocystocele in, 3224–3225, 3225f, 3280–3281, 3280f
myelomeningocele in, 3215–3224
neurological examination in, 3169–3186
neurorehabilitation in, 3783–3790
neurosurgery in, 3145–3164
occult spinal dysraphism in, 3257–3281
odontoid fractures in, 3333
optic pathway gliomas in, 3595–3599
orbital fracture in, 5261f, 5262f
perioperative concerns in, 3187–3188, 3187t, 3188t
primitive neuroectodermal tumors in. *See* Primitive neuroectodermal tumors.
pyogenic spinal infections in, 4381–4382
skull fracture in, 3465–3470, 5261f
skull of, 3462–3463
skull tumors in, 3717–3721
spinal cord tumors in, 3707–3714
spinal tumors in, 3587–3592
radiation therapy for, 4046–4047
spondylolisthesis in, 3571–3583
subarachnoid hemorrhage in, 1832
surgery on
evaluation before, 3187–3188, 3187t, 3188t
fasting before, 3187–3188, 3188t
in emergencies, 3193–3194, 3194t
management after, 3193
tethered spinal cord in, 3245–3254
vein of Galen malformations in, 3433–3444
withholding treatment from, 415
Chinese lettering, in Chiari malformation type II, 3351, 3351f
Chlamydia pneumoniae
in carotid atherosclerosis, 1613
multiple sclerosis from, 1449
Chlorambucil, for sarcoidosis, 1439
Chlorhexidine, in epidural catheter placement, 4385
Chloride, in neurons, 3812, 3812t
Chloride channels, 220t
in glioma, 230
Cholesteatoma, 3690
Cholesterol, in xanthogranuloma formation, 1444
Chondrification
failed, 4280–4281, 4281f
in vertebral column development, 4273–4274, 4274f
Chondroblastoma, 1365
Chondroitin sulfate, in central nervous system repair failure, 4168
Chondroitin sulfate proteoglycans
in axonal growth failure, 205
in malignant glioma, 762
Chondroma, 1364–1365
central skull base, 1267
skull, 1386–1388, 1388f
spinal, 4840, 4841f
Chondromyxoid fibroma, 1365
Chondrosarcoma, 1142, 1283–1292, 4296t, 4298–4299
central skull base, 1267
classic, 1284
clinical presentation of, 1284–1285
cranial, 1283–1292
dedifferentiated, 1284

Chondrosarcoma (Continued)
dural invasion in, 1285–1286
imaging of, 1285
mesenchymal, 1142, 1284
pathology of, 1284
radiation therapy for, 1290–1291
radiosurgery for, 1291, 4068
signs/symptoms of, 1284, 1284t
skull, 1390, 1390f
skull base, radiosurgery for, 4068
spinal, 4357, 4837, 4846–4848, 4847f, 4849f
from osteochondroma, 4840
imaging of, 532–533, 532f
surgery for, 1285–1290
approaches to, 1286–1290, 1286t
complications of, 1292, 1292t
extended subfrontal approach to, 1286–1287, 1286f
frontotemporal-orbitozygomatic approach in, 1287
lateral transcondylar approach in, 1288, 1289f
petrosal approach in, 1288–1290
preauricular subtemporal-infratemporal approach in, 1287–1288, 1288f, 1289f
results of, 1291–1292, 1291t, 1292t
subtemporal, transcavernous, transpetrous apex approach in, 1287
transpharyngeal-transpalatal approach in, 1287
vertebral column, radiation therapy for, 4049
Chordoid glioma, third ventricle, 664
Chordoma, 1283–1292, 4296t, 4298, 4299f
chondroid, 1283
clivus/craniovertebral junction, 4804–4808
imaging of, 4805, 4805f–4806f
pathology of, 4804–4805
presentation of, 4805
radiation therapy for, 4807
surgery for, 4805–4808, 4808f
dedifferentiated, 1283, 1284
dural invasion in, 1285–1286
imaging of, 1285
MIB-1 labeling index for, 704, 704t
pathology of, 1283–1284
physaliphorous cells in, 1283
proliferation markers for, 704, 704t
radiation therapy for, 1290–1291
radiosurgery for, 1291, 4068
signs/symptoms of, 1284, 1284t
skull, 1283–1292, 1390–1392, 1391f
skull base, 1267, 4799
interstitial brachytherapy for, 4105
radiosurgery for, 4068
spinal, 4357, 4357f, 4837
imaging of, 4848, 4849f
pediatric, 3567
surgery for, 1285–1290
approaches to, 1286–1290, 1286t
complications of, 1292, 1292t
extended subfrontal approach to, 1286–1287, 1286f
frontotemporal-orbitozygomatic approach to, 1287
lateral transcondylar approach to, 1288, 1289f
petrosal approach to, 1288–1290
preauricular subtemporal-infratemporal approach to, 1287–1288, 1288f, 1289f

Chordoma (Continued)
results of, 1290f, 1291–1292, 1291t, 1292t
subtemporal, transcavernous, transpetrous apex approach to, 1287
transpharyngeal-transpalatal approach to, 1287
vertebral column
radiation therapy for, 4048–4049
stereotactic radiosurgery for, 4049
Chorea, 2717–2720. *See also* specific condition, e.g., Huntington's disease.
benign hereditary, 2719, 2736
causes of, 2717t
clinical presentation of, 2747
definition of, 2676, 2729
disorders causing, 2736–2737
pediatric, 3179
sporadic, 2719
surgery for, 2747, 2747f
Sydenham's, 2736, 2762
obsessive-compulsive disorder in, 2854
systemic lupus erythematosus with, 2762
thalamic stimulation for, 2747, 2747f
vascular causes of, 2737
Choreoathetosis, 2729
Chorioallantoic membrane assay, in angiogenesis antagonist discovery, 775, 776f
Choriocarcinoma
classification of, 667t, 668
metastatic, in pregnancy, 2428–2429
pediatric, 3607–3608
Choroid plexus, 8f, 12f, 14f, 30–31, 31f, 32, 40f
arteriovenous malformation of, 2243, 2244f
carcinoma of, 3619
classification of, 665, 665t
diffuse villous hypertrophy of, 3613
papilloma of, 3612
classification of, 665, 665t
in pregnancy, 872
magnetic resonance imaging of, 453, 455f
metastatic, 3617
pathology of, 3614, 3616f
radiologic features of, 840
third ventricular, 1246
vs. carcinoma, 3614, 3617, 3617f
tumors of, 3612–3620
anatomic distribution of, 3612
clinical features of, 3612–3613
complications of, 3619–3620
diagnosis of, 3613–3614
differential diagnosis of, 3617
DNA sequences in, 3617
histopathologic classification of, 665, 665t
historical aspects of, 3612
hydrocephalus in, 3613
imaging of, 3613–3614, 3615f, 3616f
immunohistochemistry of, 3617
incidence of, 3612–3620
pathology of, 3614, 3616f, 3617, 3617f
pediatric, 3612–3620
prognosis of, 3619–3620
proliferation markers for, 701
surgery for, 3617–3619
xanthogranuloma of, 1444
Choroidal artery, 1240, 1240f
anterior, 21, 22f, 1918
aneurysms of, 1887, 1918–1919

Choroidal artery (Continued)
giant aneurysm of, 1870f
infarction of, 1615
lateral posterior, 22
medial posterior, 14f, 21–22, 22f
posterior, 22f
infarction of, 1615
Choroidal fissure, 10f, 11, 2486, 2487f
cyst of, 2495
Choroidal plexus, 13
Choroidal point, 12f, 37
inferior, 10f, 26
Choroidal vein, 17
Chromaffin cells, transplantation of, 2831
Chromolysis, after peripheral nerve axonal injury, 197
Chromosome 22, in meningioma, 1106–1107, 1106f, 1107f
Chymopapain
for lumbar disk disease, 4771–4776, 4774f
spontaneous intracerebral hemorrhage in, 1735
Cigarette smoking. *See* Tobacco.
Ciliary neurotrophic factor
after peripheral nerve injury, 3967, 3968
astrocytic release of, 4168
in central nervous system repair, 4160, 4165
Cingulate gyrus, 24f, 26f
Cingulate sulcus, 24f
Cingulotomy, 3030
anterior, for psychiatric disorders, 2856–2857, 2857f
Cingulum, 6–7
Ciprofloxacin, for tuberculosis, 1441
Circle of Willis, 1266
compensatory function of, in carotid occlusion, 1554
saccular aneurysms in, 1592
three-dimensional imaging of, 433, 434f
transcranial Doppler ultrasonography of, 1543f
Circular collimators, 4139, 4139f, 4140f
Circular sulcus, 5, 6f
Circulation, assessment of, 5087–5088
in cervical spine trauma, 4888
Circulatory arrest, deep hypothermic, 1528–1537. *See also* Deep hypothermic circulatory arrest.
Circumflex artery
long, 21
short, 21, 22f
Circuminfundibular anastomosis, 19
Cisplatin, 881
for paranasal sinus tumors, 1327
Citicoline
in ischemia protection, 1522
trials for, 1498
c-jun, in carotid body tumors, 1678
Claudication
neurogenic. *See* Neurogenic claudication.
vascular. *See* Vascular claudication.
Claustrum, 8f, 12f
Clawing, in ulnar nerve entrapment, 3925
Clay shoveler's fracture, 4909–4910
Clinical agreement, 240–241, 241t
Clinical target volume, 4011
Clinoid process
anatomy of, 1266
anterior, 15f, 1266, 1895, 1896f
removal of, 1907
dural anatomy of, 1895, 1897f–1898f
meningioma of, 1115–1116, 1116f, 1117f
neural anatomy of, 1897f–1898f, 1898

Clinoid process *(Continued)*
osseous anatomy of, 1895, 1896f
posterior, in basilar apex aneurysm approach, 1985
vascular anatomy of, 1895–1896, 1897f–1898f, 1898
Clipping, of aneurysms, 1822–1823, 2107–2108
historical aspects of, 1462, 1462f
Clivus
anatomy of, 1266
bipartite, 3338
chordoma of, 1391, 1391f, 4804–4808
imaging of, 4805, 4805f–4806f
pathology of, 4804–4805
presentation of, 4805
radiation therapy for, 4807
surgery for, 4805–4808, 4808f
diseases of, 4800t
in Chiari malformation type I, 3348
Clonazepam
for multiple sclerosis, 1454t
for trigeminal neuralgia, 2990t, 2993
Clonidine
for cerebral palsy, 3731
for pain, 2965
intrathecal, 3141
Clonus, testing of, 3181
Clopidogrel, for carotid artery disease, 1617–1618
Closed lip, 62f, 63
CM101, angiosuppressive therapy with, 783
CM101/ZDO101, as angiogenesis antagonist, 779t
c-myc
in carotid body tumors, 1678
in medulloblastoma, 3640–3641
Cnot, 53t
CNS. *See* Central nervous system.
Coagulation, in pregnancy, 2422
Coagulopathy
hypothermia-induced, 1533
in cerebral venous thrombosis, 1723
in deep hypothermic circulatory arrest, 1536
in mild head injury, 5074
renal failure with, 1747, 1752f, 1753
Coasting, 3843
Cobalamin deficiency, neuropathy from, 3844
Cocaine
spontaneous intracerebral hemorrhage in, 1735
subarachnoid hemorrhage from, 1832
Coccidioidomycosis, spinal, 4390
Cochlea, 327, 328f
in temporal bone fracture, 5281
innervation of, 329f
otoacoustic emissions from, 337–338
Cochlear implants
electrically evoked auditory potentials with, 337
indications for, 353–354, 354f
Cochlear nerve, 40f, 329f
pediatric, 3175–3176
preservation of, in acoustic neuroma surgery, 1160
Cochlear system, 327–330
Codman cervical spine anterior screw-plate fixation, 4630t, 4633, 4633f
Cogan's syndrome, endolymphatic hydrops in, 349–350
Cognitive function
after epilepsy surgery, 2571
Cognitive function *(Continued)*
assessment of, 5185–5188
ependymoma surgery and, 3630
in anterior communicating artery aneurysms, 1937
in cerebral palsy, 3727
after dorsal rhizotomy, 3731
premorbid estimate of, 5188–5190
rehabilitation of
in traumatic brain injury, 5293–5294
pediatric, 3789
Cohort studies, 249–250
Collagen
deficiency of, in carotid artery dissection, 1685
extracellular lattice of, in cerebral vasospasm, 1847–1848
in malignant glioma, 761
type I, 4229, 4614
type III, in Ehlers-Danlos syndrome type IV, 1771
Collateral eminence, 7f, 12f, 18f
Collateral ligament, medial, 3926
Collateral sulcus, 3, 12f, 18–19, 18f, 26f
Collateral trigone, 7f, 8, 8f, 12f
Collicular point, 21
Collimation, multileaf, 4139–4142, 4139f–4142f
Collimators
circular, 4139, 4139f, 4140f
in radiation therapy, 4012
Colloid cyst, 3687–3689
diagnosis of, 3688, 3689f
endoscopic removal of, 3430, 3430f
of anterior third ventricle, 3390
pathology of, 3687–3688
presentation of, 3688
surgery for, 3688–3689
third ventricular, 1245–1246
surgical approach to, 1251
xanthogranuloma from, 1444
Colpocephaly, in Chiari malformation type II, 3350
Coma, 284, 285t
awakening from, 3861–3862
barbiturate
in bullet wounds, 5231
intracranial hypertension treatment by, 5133–5134
brainstem auditory evoked potentials in, 401
in pregnancy, 295, 295t
intracranial hypertension in, 5109
prognosis of, 297–298, 297t, 298f
structural lesions and, 278f
vs. catatonia, 293
Coma data banks, in traumatic brain injury, 5103, 5104t
Coma dépassé, 394
Combretastatins, angiosuppressive therapy with, 779
Communicating artery
anterior, 22f, 27, 28f
anatomy of, 1924f, 1925
aneurysms of, 1923–1938
angiography of, 1892f
clinical presentation of, 1930, 1930f, 1931f
complications of, 1936–1937
interhemispheric exposure for, 1879–1880
lamina terminalis cistern origin of, 1927, 1927f
orientation of, 1928f–1929f
outcomes of, 1937–1938
Communicating artery *(Continued)*
radiography of, 1930, 1930f, 1931f
rupture of, 1787
surgery for, 1891–1892, 1930–1936
A1 segment exposure in, 1933–1934, 1933f
A1-A2 complex vessels in, 1934–1935, 1935f
adjuncts to, 1931
aneurysm neck dissection in, 1935–1936
approaches to, 1877, 1929–1930, 1929t
aspiration in, 1936
bur holes in, 1932–1933, 1932f
clipping in, 1936
craniotomy placement in, 1931–1932
dural opening in, 1932f, 1933
gyrus rectus resection in, 1934, 1934f
head position in, 1932
incision in, 1932, 1932f
internal carotid artery exposure in, 1933
optic nerve exposure in, 1933
papaverine in, 1936
sylvian fissure dissection in, 1933
temporalis muscle dissection in, 1932, 1932f
embryology of, 1923
microsurgical anatomy of, 1923–1929
perforators of, 1925
posterior, 19–20, 22f, 28f
anatomy of, 1916–1917
aneurysms of, 1917, 1917t
surgery for, 1887, 1889
treatment of, 1917–1918
Communication
in cerebral palsy, 3727, 3730, 3732
after dorsal rhizotomy, 3744
rehabilitation of, pediatric, 3789
Comparative genomic hybridization, 747, 748f
Compartment syndrome, nerve injury in, 3827
Complement system, in cerebral ischemia, 142
Complete sulcus, 18
Complex regional pain syndrome
diagnosis of, sympathetic nerve blocks in, 2981
nomenclature for, 3094
thoracic endoscopic sympathectomy for, 3101t
Complications
avoidance of, 561–582
intraoperative monitoring in, 562
patient positioning in, 561–563
catastrophic, 563–565
cranial fixation, 562–563
surgical risk factors and, 565–582
Compound muscle action potential
distal motor latency in, 3853
in brachial plexus surgery, 3868, 3869f
in median nerve tumor surgery, 3866, 3868, 3868f
lesion site and, 3854, 3854f
nerve assessment by, 3866
nerve conduction studies of, 3853–3855, 3854f
Compound nerve action potential
from surgical field, 3864
in peripheral nerve surgery monitoring, 3863

Compound nerve action potential (Continued)
- nerve assessment by, 3866
- within surgical field, 3864

Compression, peripheral nerve injury in, 3827–3828
Compression fracture. *See* Fracture(s), compression.
Compression sleeves, 4968
Compression therapy, for transverse-sigmoid dural arteriovenous malformation, 2288
Compton effect, in radiation therapy, 4006, 4006f
Computed tomography, 5019
- before epilepsy surgery, 2483–2485, 2484f, 2485f
- in surgical navigation, 946
- skull, 419, 432–433
- spinal, 501–503, 502f, 4145
- xenon. *See* Xenon computed tomography.

Computer, in image-guided spinal navigation, 4743–4756
Concentration
- after hyperextension-hyperflexion injury, 4919
- after traumatic brain injury, 5186–5187

Concentrative nucleoside transporters, 158
Concorde position, 597t, 604, 604f
Concussion, 5045
- labyrinthine, 5281
- pediatric, 3463
- temporal bone fracture and, 5281
- vestibular, 5281

Conditioning lesions, in central nervous system repair, 4164
Conduction, during action potential, 220–221, 221f
Conduction block, nerve conduction studies of, 3860
Conductor, 215
Confusion, in pregnancy, 295, 295t
Congenital anomalies
- cranial destruction in, 429–430
- spinal, imaging of, 533–536
- vertigo in, 2902

Congenital deformities, of axial skeleton, 4317–4318
Congenital lumbosacral lipoma. *See* Lipoma, congenital lumbosacral.
Congenital malformations. *See also* specific malformations.
- neural, 4256–4271, 4256t
- spinal, 4148, 4276–4281, 4276f–4281f, 4315t, 4316–4319, 4317f, 4318f

Congenital spondylolisthesis, 4541, 4542f
- pathogenesis of, 4543–4544
- treatment of, 4550–4551

Coning, 1504–1505
Connective tissue, in spasticity, 2879–2880
Connective tissue disorders, heritable, aneurysms with, 1769–1773, 1770t
Connexins, in astrocytes, 101
Conotoxin, peripheral nerve effects of, 3816
Conradi's syndrome, 3334
Consciousness
- after surgery, 906–907
- altered states (loss) of, 275, 283–286, 285t
  - brainstem auditory evoked potentials in, 297
  - causes of, 282, 282t
  - diagnosis of, 294t
  - differential diagnosis of, 277–298
  - electroencephalography in, 296–297, 296f
  - in injury severity estimation, 5195–5196
  - in mild head injury, 5073
  - intracranial pressure monitoring in, 295–296
  - mechanisms of, 277–278, 278f
  - respiratory failure in, 282–283, 283f
  - somatosensory evoked potentials in, 297
  - treatment of, 292–295
- assessment of, 281–292, 281t
  - Glasgow Coma Scale in, 286–287, 286t
  - in herniation syndromes, 290–292, 291t, 292f
  - in intracranial catastrophe, 289–292, 291t, 292f
  - ocular movement abnormalities in, 288–289
  - oculovestibular response testing in, 289, 290f, 290t
  - Pediatric Coma Scale in, 287–289, 288f
  - physical examination in, 282–283, 283f
  - pupillary response in, 287–288
- clouding of, 283
- definition of, 277, 393
- level of, in bullet wounds, 5227–5228, 5228t
- neuroanatomy of, 278–280, 279f
- neurophysiology of, 280–281, 280f
- self-awareness in, 283

Constipation, in cerebral palsy, 3727, 3732
Contact guidance, in peripheral nerve regeneration, 3804–3805
Contractures, in cerebral palsy, 3728, 3732
Contrast media, blood-brain barrier effects of, 164
Contusion(s)
- brain, 5041–5042
- cerebral, 5159, 5159f
  - evacuation of, 5159, 5160f–5161f, 5162
- hemorrhagic, in traumatic brain injury, 5107f, 5108
- in mild head injury, 5070, 5071t
- magnetic resonance imaging of, 469
- pediatric, 3463
- peripheral nerve injury from, 3827
- shaking-impact syndrome and, 3501, 3504f

Conus medullaris, 4989f
- arteriovenous malformations of, 2371–2372, 2371f
- ascent of, 4245, 4247f
- dysraphic anomalies of, 3247–3248
- lesions of, sensory loss in, 272, 272f
- lipoma of, 3229
- tethering of, by tight filum terminale, 3247

Conus medullaris syndrome, 4872
Conversion hysteria, pediatric, back pain in, 3568
Coordination, examination of, 267–268
- pediatric, 3179

Copper chelators, as angiogenesis antagonists, 778t, 781–782, 782f
Copper depletion, in angiogenesis, 775, 776f
Coprolalia, 2730
Copropraxia, 2730
Copula pyramidis, 31f
Copular point, 31f, 32, 37
Cordectomy, for spasticity, 2870
Cordotomy
- anatomy for, 3059–3061, 3060f
- complications of, 3068–3070
- for pain, 3059–3070
- historical aspects of, 2913–2914, 3059
- lateral spinothalamic tract in, 3060, 3060f
- open, 3067–3068
  - anterior, 3068, 3068f
  - posterior, 3067–3068, 3067f
- patient selection for, 3061
- percutaneous technique of, 3061–3067
  - anatomic localization in, 3062–3063, 3063f–3066f
  - anesthesia for, 3062
  - anterior, 3063, 3066f
  - bilateral, 3066–3067
  - care after, 3067
  - computed tomography–guided, 3063, 3064f, 3065f
  - dentate ligament in, 3063, 3066f
  - electrode system calibration in, 3061, 3062f
  - instrumentation in, 3061, 3062f
  - lesions in, 3065–3066
  - physiologic localization in, 3063, 3065
  - positioning for, 3062
  - preparation before, 3061–3062
  - x-ray–guided, 3063, 3066f
- results of, 3068–3070

Cornea, assessment of, 302, 304, 304f
Cornu ammonis, 2486, 2487f
Corona radiata, 7f
Coronal suture, 423f
Corpectomy
- cervical, anterior, 4439–4440, 4441f
- complications of, 577
- for pyogenic spinal infection, 4372f, 4374–4376, 4377f–4379f
- in cervical spine fixation, 4625–4626, 4628f
- thoracic, 4767, 4768f
  - anterior, 4974–4978, 4976f–4977f
  - vertebral reconstruction after, 4767, 4768f, 4769

Corpus callosotomy
- complications of, 1243–1244
- for extratemporal lobe epilepsy, 2596
- for third ventricle tumors, 1253–1254
- seizure outcome after, 2578–2579

Corpus callosum, 4f, 7f, 8f, 9, 24f, 1237, 1238f
- agenesis of, in Dandy-Walker syndrome, 3286
- anterior
  - arteriovenous malformation of, 2242, 2242f
  - damage to, 265
- genu of, 14f
- glioma spread through, 757, 759–760
- hematoma of, in distal anterior cerebral artery aneurysms, 1948
- lipoma of, 3693
- median artery of. *see* Cerebral artery, anterior.
- posterior
  - arteriovenous malformation of, 2242–2243, 2243f
  - damage to, 265
- rostrum of, 15f
- splenium of, 13
- surgical complications of, 1258–1259
- venous drainage of, 1238

Cortex
- abnormal organization of, 2493
- anterior cingulate, 2932–2933

Cortex *(Continued)*
area of functional deficit of, 2438
contusions of, bullet wounds and, 5234
developmental anomalies of, classification of, 2492
eloquent, seizure control in, 2635
epileptogenic lesions of, 2437–2438
surgical history of, 2442–2443
epileptogenic zone of, 2438–2439
function of, testing of, 264–265, 264f, 264t
functional deficit zone of, surgical history of, 2442–2443
insular, 2933
irritative zone of, 2436
surgical history of, 2440–2442, 2441f
mapping of, 2531–2538
patient selection in, 2531
motor, stimulation mapping of, 2534
neuronal development in, 79f
seizure onset zone of, 2436–2437, 2437f
sensory, 2931–2932
functional magnetic resonance imaging of, 2519
stimulation mapping of, 2534
patient selection in, 2531
somatosensory area of, 2932, 2933f
somatosensory evoked potential mapping of, 2533–2534, 2534f
spinothalamic tract and, 2927, 2930f
stimulation mapping of, seizures during, 2533
structure localization in, before surgery, 2531–2532, 2532f
symptomatogenic zone of, 2435–2436
surgical history of, 2439–2440
tumors of, resection of, 2537
vascular malformations in, resection of, 2537
zones of, 2435–2438
Cortical dysgenesis
magnetic resonance imaging of, 2491
magnetic resonance spectroscopy of, 2497
vs. tumor, 2492, 2492f
Cortical dysplasia
in epileptic resection, 2577–2578
in extratemporal lobe epilepsy, 2598
magnetic resonance imaging of, 2485
non–balloon cell focal, magnetic resonance imaging of, 2493–2494, 2494f
Corticobasal degeneration, 2715
positron emission tomography of, 2761–2762
vs. Parkinson's disease, 2735
Corticospinal tract
decussation of, 4871, 4871f
in lower urinary tract function, 362
Corticosteroids
epidural injections of, 2973–2976, 2975t. *See also* Epidural steroid injections.
for aneurysmal subarachnoid hemorrhage, 1822
for brain edema, 801–802, 5134
for brain metastases, 1078
for bullet wounds, 5230
for chronic inflammatory demyelinating polyradiculoneuropathy, 3840
for glial tumors, 870
for intracerebral hemorrhage, 1740
for medulloblastoma, 3644
for pain, 2959
for primary central nervous system lymphoma, 1072
Corticosteroids *(Continued)*
for primitive neuroectodermal tumors, 1003
for pseudotumor cerebri, 1429
for pyogenic spinal infection, 4376
for sarcoidosis, 1438–1439
for spinal cord compression, 4047
for spinal cord injury, 4874, 4876
for spinal metastases, 4858
for therapeutic injections, 2970
for traumatic brain injury, 5097
for tumor-associated edema, 13–14
intracranial pressure and, 188
osteoporosis from, 4235
pseudotumor cerebri from, 1423, 1425
Corticostriatal projection, functional organization of, 2683–2685
Corticosubthalamic projection, 2690
Corticotrophin-releasing hormone test, in Cushing's disease, 1196
Cortisol, measurement of, 1196
Costotransversectomy, 640
for thoracic disk herniation, 4981
vs. other techniques, 4758, 4758t
Costovertebral triangle, 4765–4766
Cotrel-Dubousset rod–multiple hook construct, in lumbar spine fixation, 4734, 4734f
Cotrel-Dubousset rod-screw plate
in occipitocervical fusion, 4661, 4663f
in thoracic spine fixation, 4969–4972, 4970f–4972f
Coumarin, in pregnancy, 2423
Court proceedings
in child abuse, 3509–3510, 3510t
in life-sustaining treatment refusal, 415
^{11}C-PK 11195, glial marking by, 1609
Cranial fixation, complications of, 562–563
Cranial nerves
examination of, 265–267
I. *See* Olfactory nerve.
II. *See* Optic nerve.
III. *See* Oculomotor nerve.
in acoustic neuroma, 1159, 1159t
in craniovertebral junction tumors, 4800
in skull base surgery, 1266
inferior petrosal sinus and, 1302, 1302f
injury to
after skull base surgery, 572
in atlanto-occipital dislocation, 4928–4929
IV. *See* Trochlear nerve.
IX. *See* Glossopharyngeal nerve.
monitoring of, in ependymoma surgery, 3630–3631
palsy of
glomus jugulare tumor embolization and, 1300–1301
glomus jugulare tumors and, 1305–1306
in basilar trunk aneurysms, 2037
in sarcoidosis, 1435–1436
pediatric basilar skull fracture and, 3467–3468
pediatric, examination of, 3173–3176
posterior circulation aneurysm and, 1976
preservation of, in acoustic neuroma surgery, 1160–1161
schwannoma of
magnetic resonance imaging of, 459–460, 460f
radiologic features of, 837
V. *See* Trigeminal nerve.
VI. *See* Abducens nerve.
VII. *See* Facial nerve.
Cranial nerves *(Continued)*
VIII. *See* Vestibular-auditory nerve.
X. *See* Vagus nerve.
XI. *See* Spinal accessory nerve.
XII. *See* Hypoglossal nerve.
Cranial neuralgia, 3018t
Cranial neuropathy, 318t
Cranial settling, 4571
Craniectomy, historical aspects of, 3159–3161, 3161f–3163f
Craniocervical junction
acquired abnormalities of, 4569–4583
metastases to, 4860
osseous relationships at, 519
rheumatoid arthritis of
radiologic features of, 4574, 4574f–4577f
surgical indications for, 4574–4575, 4578
treatment of, 4578–4580, 4579f–4581f
seronegative spondyloarthritis of, 4580–4581, 4582f, 4583f
Craniofacial anomalies
historical aspects of, 3155–3164
in utero compression and, 3301
Craniofacial resection, for paranasal sinus tumors, 1318–1320, 1320f–1322f
Craniofacial syndromes, 3315–3329. *See also* specific type, e.g., Crouzon's syndrome.
evaluation of, 3316–3317
fibroblast growth factor receptor mutations in, 3315–3316
functional matrix theory of, 3315
historical aspects of, 3315–3316, 3316f
hydrocephalus in, 3398–3399
radiography of, 3317, 3317f
surgery for, 3321–3329
complications of, 3328–3329
distraction osteogenesis in, 3327–3328
Le Fort III osteotomy in, 3326–3327
monoblock osteotomy in, 3327, 3328f
psychological considerations in, 3318
timing of, 3317–3318
Craniofacial trauma, 5245–5266
airway management in, 5246, 5246t, 5247f
avulsion flap in, 5249
central fractures in, 5251
combined central and lateral fractures in, 5251
comminuted fracture in, 5260f
ears in, 5251
eyelids in, 5251
facial nerve in, 5251
fractures in, 5251–5262
classification of, 5251
clinical examination of, 5252
radiography of, 5252
treatment of, 5252–5262
bone flap in, 5260f
bone graft in, 5252, 5256f
bone material for, 5258f–5259f
frontal sinus repair in, 5252–5253
galea-frontalis flap in, 5258f–5259f
historical approaches to, 5251–5252
priorities in, 5245–5246
sequence of, 5253, 5256, 5256f
surgical, 5252, 5253f–5256f
technical problems in, 5256–5257, 5257f–5263f, 5262
hemorrhage in, 5246–5247
infection in, 5248
laceration in, 5249
lateral fractures in, 5251

Craniofacial trauma *(Continued)*
lips in, 5251
multiple fractures in, 5245
nose in, 5251
occlusion in, 5248–5249
ocular injury in, 5247
panfacial injuries in, 5262–5266
parotid gland/duct in, 5251–5252
pathogenesis of, 5251
patterns of, 5251
regional considerations in, 5250–5251
rhinorrhea in, 5247–5248
soft tissue injury in, 5249–5251
tattoo in, 5249
tissue loss in, 5249–5250
Craniolacunia, in Chiari malformation type II, 3349–3350, 3350f
Craniometrics, 630
Craniopharyngeal fat tumor, 1207
Craniopharyngeal pouch tumor, 1207
Craniopharyngioma, 1207–1219
adamantinomatous, 1211, 1212f
brachytherapy for, 4095–4096, 4097
intracavitary, 4098, 4105–4106, 4106t
central skull base, 1267
chemotherapy for, 1219
classification of, 671, 1212–1213
clinical presentation of, 1210–1211
embryology of, 1207–1208
endocrine deficits in, 1210
epidemiology of, 1208
historical aspects of, 1207
imaging of, 1208–1210, 1209f, 1272f
MIB-1 labeling index for, 704, 705t
observation of, 1213
outcome in, adult vs. pediatric, 1218
papillary, 1211–1212, 1212f
pathology of, 1211–1212, 1211f, 1212f
pediatric, 3671–3684
chemotherapy for, 3683–3684
cysts in, 3675
aspiration of, 3679, 3680f
endocrine function in, 3675
historical aspects of, 3671
hydrocephalus in, 3675, 3676f
imaging of, 3674–3675, 3674f, 3675f
incidence of, 3672–3673, 3673f
intracystic irradiation in, 3683
pathology of, 3671–3672, 3672f, 3673f
pituitary stalk preservation in, 3679, 3679f
radiation therapy for, 3681–3683, 3681f–3683f
signs/symptoms of, 3673–3674
stereotactic radiosurgery for, 3682–3683
surgery for, 3675–3679, 3676f–3680f, 3676t
care after, 3679
results of, 3680–3681
proliferation markers for, 704
radiation therapy for, 1218–1219
recurrence of, 1217–1218
stereotactic radiosurgery for, 1219
surgery for, 1213–1218, 1214f
bifrontal basal interhemispheric approach to, 1215
pterional approach to, 1215
resection extent in, 1217
results of, 1216–1217
stereotactic cyst decompression in, 1216
subfrontal approach to, 1214–1215
superior approach to, 1216
temporal approach to, 1215

Craniopharyngioma *(Continued)*
transsphenoidal approach to, 1215–1216
third ventricular, 1247
treatment of, 1213–1219
visual disturbances from, 1210
Cranioplasty, 5174, 5175f
Craniosynostosis, 428, 428f. *See also* specific disorder, e.g., Crouzon's syndrome.
bilateral coronal, 3310–3311
historical aspects of, 3155–3164
lambdoid, 3310
metopic, 3309–3310, 3310f
multisuture, 3311
nonsyndromic, frequency of, 3315
outcome in, 3311–3312
patterns of, 3305t
physical disorders with, 3315
primary
chromosomal anomalies in, 3305
gene mapping in, 3305–3306
genetic factors in, 3305–3306
inheritance patterns in, 3305
primary nonsyndromic, 3304–3305
sagittal, 3306–3307, 3306f–3308f
computed tomography of, 3306, 3307f
radiography of, 3306, 3306f
surgery for, 3306–3307, 3307f, 3308f
secondary, 3311
surgery for
complications of, 3328–3329
distraction osteogenesis in, 3327–3328
historical aspects of, 3159–3162, 3161f–3163f, 3316
in neonates, 3194
Le Fort III osteotomy in, 3326–3327
monoblock osteotomy in, 3327, 3328f
syndromic
frequency of, 3315
historical aspects of, 3315–3316, 3316f
unilateral coronal
assessment of, 3308–3309, 3309f
surgery for, 3309
vs. microcephaly, historical aspects of, 3162
Craniotomy, 623–636
anterior parasagittal, 634, 634f
awake position for, 597t, 600, 601f, 602f
bifrontal, 5159, 5160f–5161f, 5162
bleeding control in, 1872, 1875, 5174, 5176
complications of, 932t
cosmetic considerations in, 1872
drills in, 1875
exposures in, 630–631, 631f
for anterior circulation aneurysms, 1872, 1875–1877, 1876f
for intracerebral hemorrhage, 1745–1746
frontal, 1877
frontosphenotemporal, 1932, 1932f
orbitozygomatic extension with, 632–633, 632f
frontotemporal, 902–903, 1978, 1978f–1981f
head positioning in, 630
hematoma after, 5176, 5177f, 5178f, 5179
historical aspects of, 623–624
in pure transsylvian approach, 2043–2044, 2045f, 2046f
in third ventricular tumors, 1249–1251, 1250f
lateral cerebellar, 904–905
lateral position for, 628, 629f
lateral suboccipital, far-lateral transcondylar extension with, 635–636, 636f

Craniotomy *(Continued)*
Mayfield skull fixation in, 624–625, 624f–626f, 627
midline cerebellar, 904
midline suboccipital, 634–635, 635f
minimal-access, 942, 943f
optimal-access, 942
parasagittal, 903–904
parietal-occipital, 903
patient positioning for, 627–630, 628f, 629f
posterior parasagittal, 634
prone position for, 628–630, 629f
pterional, 1875, 1978, 1978f–1981f
pterional-orbitozygomatic, 1875–1877, 1876f
standard, 632–636
subtemporal, 633, 633f
supine position for, 628, 628f
surgical navigation systems in, 942–945
critical brain tissue in, 942–943, 944f, 945f
for subcortical tumors, 943, 945f
resection control with, 943–945, 945t
techniques for, 631–632
Craniovertebral junction. *See also* Atlanto-occipital joint.
anatomy of, 3331
biomechanics of, 3333–3334
blood supply of, 3331
craniometric reference lines for, 424–425, 424f, 425f
developmental abnormalities of, 3331–3344
atlantoaxial subluxation in, 3333
atlas assimilation in, 3339–3340
basilar invagination in, 3340–3341
cervical orthoses for, 3334
classification of, 3334, 3334t
clinical presentation of, 3334–3335, 3335t
craniometry in, 3335, 3336f
epidemiology of, 3334
foramen magnum in, 3338, 3339f
imaging of, 3335–3336, 3336f
in Down syndrome, 3337–3338, 3338f
in Grisel's syndrome, 3337, 3337f
spina bifida in, 3333
treatment of, 3336–3337
types of, 3332–3333, 3337–3341
diseases of, 4655, 4800t
embryology of, 3331–3332, 4275–4276, 4275f
eosinophilic granuloma of, 4809
injury to, 4925
ligamentous anatomy of, 4925–4926, 4926f
lymphatic drainage of, 3331
neurenteric cyst of, 4813f, 4814
neurinoma of, 4813–4814
neurofibroma of, 4812–4813, 4812f
osteoid osteoma of, 4809
pediatric, anatomy of, 3528–3529, 3530f
plasmacytoma of, 4808–4809, 4810f
range of motion at, 4655
tumors of, 4799–4814, 4800t
clinical manifestations of, 4799–4801
electrophysiology of, 4801
extradural, 4804–4809
imaging of, 4801
intradural, 4809, 4811–4814
at C1–2, 4812–4814
surgical approaches to, 4801, 4802f, 4803t, 4804

C-reactive protein
in postoperative diskitis, 4383
in pyogenic spinal infections, 4366
Cremasteric reflex testing, pediatric, 3181
Cribriform-ethmoid junction, fracture of, rhinorrhea in, 5267–5268
Crimes, reporting obligations in, 411
Crista ampullaris, 339
Crista galli, 1266
Cross-clamping, hypoperfusion from, transcranial Doppler ultrasonography of, 1548–1549
Crossed extension stepping reflex, in cerebral palsy, 3725, 3726t
Crossed straight leg raising test, 4512, 4512f
Cross-sectional surveys, 249
Crouzon's syndrome, 3318, 3319f
historical aspects of, 3158f, 3162, 3164, 3164f
hydrocephalus in, 3398
surgery for
Le Fort III osteotomy in, 3326–3327
monoblock osteotomy in, 3327, 3328f
treatment of, 3321
Cruciate ligament, 4925, 4926f
in dens aplasia-hypoplasia, 3341
transverse, disruption of, 3333
Crus cerebri, 10f, 21, 29, 30f, 33f, 3073
Crush injury
prone positioning and, 603
spinal cord, without radiographic abnormality, 3523
Crutch palsy, 3928
Crying, in facial nerve testing, 3174
Cryorhizotomy, for spasticity, 2868–2870, 2868f
Cryptic vascular malformation, 2321
Cryptococcus neoformans, central nervous system infection with, 4295
Cubital tunnel, 3898, 3902
intraneural pressure in, 3901
Cubital tunnel syndrome
anterior transmuscular transposition for, 3912, 3913f
decompression for, 3909–3910
differential diagnosis of, 3903
elbow flexion test for, 3904, 3905f
evaluation of, 3906, 3906f–3908f, 3908
grading of, 3927
intramuscular transposition for, 3911–3912
medial epicondylectomy for, 3910–3911
nerve stimulators for, 3916, 3916f
neurolysis for, 3915–3916
recurrent, 3914–3915
secondary transmuscular transposition for, 3915
subcutaneous transposition for, 3911
submuscular transposition for, 3911
surgery for, 3909–3912, 3913f, 3927–3928
care after, 3916–3917, 3917f
results of, 3914, 3914t
ulnar nerve entrapment in, 3926–3928
Culmen, 30f
Cuneolingual gyrus, 26f
Cuneus, 24f, 25, 26f
Cupula, 329f, 339
Cupulolithiasis, 2903
temporal bone fracture and, 5281
Curare, peripheral nerve effects of, 3816
Currarino's triad, 4267–4269, 4269f
Cushing's disease, 1195–1199
adrenalectomy for, 1199
clinical features of, 1195
Cushing's disease *(Continued)*
corticotroph adenomas in, 1195
drugs for, 1199
imaging of, 1197
laboratory tests for, 1195–1197
Nelson's syndrome progression with, 1199
persistent, treatment of, 1198
radiation therapy for, 1198–1199, 4035
radiosurgery for, 4062–4063
surgery for, 1176, 1197–1198, 1198t
treatment of, 1197–1199
vs. adrenocorticotrophic hormone–producing lesions, 1196
vs. Cushing's syndrome, 1194
Cushing's response, 5090
Cushing's syndrome
causes of, 1194
cortisol levels in, 1196
differential diagnosis of, 1194–1195, 1194t
vs. Cushing's disease, 1194
Cushing's ulcer, ependymoma surgery and, 3630
Cutaneous nerve
lateral dorsal, 653
lateral femoral, entrapment of, 3933
medial antebrachial, 3899, 3899f
Cutaneous reflexes, examination of, 268–269
Cutting cones, 4614
Cyclo-oxygenase
in arachidonic acid metabolism, 1473
in ischemia, 127
inhibition of, anti-inflammatory effects of, 2959
Cyclophosphamide
for Ewing's sarcoma, 4850
for multifocal motor neuropathy, 3840
for multiple sclerosis, 1454t, 1455
for sarcoidosis, 1439
Cycloserine, for tuberculosis, 1441
Cyclosporine
for sarcoidosis, 1439
pseudotumor cerebri from, 1424
Cyclosporine A
for multifocal motor neuropathy, 3840
in central nervous system injury, 5027
Cyclotron, in positron emission tomography, 477–479, 478f
Cyproheptadine, for pituitary adenoma, 869
Cyst
aneurysmal bone. *See* Aneurysmal bone cyst.
arachnoid. *See* Arachnoid cyst.
Baker's, 3934
cerebellopontine angle, 3298
cerebral convexity, 3295
cerebral hemisphere, 3296, 3296f, 3297f
choroidal fissure, 2495
dermoid. *See* Dermoid cyst.
ependymal
histopathologic classification of, 664–665, 664t
vs. neurenteric cyst, 1229
epidermoid. *See* Epidermoid cyst.
ganglion, 3947t, 3948
decompressive surgery for, 4337
magnetic resonance imaging of, 3875–3876, 3877f
in central nervous system tumors, 671t
in pediatric craniopharyngioma, 3675, 3679, 3680f
intraspinal, pediatric, 3568
intraventricular, endoscopic management of, 3429
Cyst *(Continued)*
leptomeningeal, 1404–1405, 1405f, 3717
neurenteric, 1226–1229, 3272–3273, 4263–4266, 4263f–4267f, 4317
at C1–2, 4813f, 4814
at craniovertebral junction, 4813f, 4814
imaging of, 535, 536f, 1227f–1228f, 1228–1229
vs. ependymal cyst, 1229
of hemispheric fissure, 3296–3297, 3297f
pineal, 1012, 1012f
quadrigeminal, 3297–3298, 3297f
sella turcica, 3295, 3295f
suprasellar cistern, 3293–3295, 3294f, 3295f
sylvian fissure, 3292–3293, 3293f
synovial
imaging of, 512, 513f–514f
vs. lumbar disk disease, 4511, 4511f
third ventricular, 1247
ventricular, endoscopic management of, 3429
Cysticercosis, 4390
magnetic resonance imaging of, 463, 465f
Cystoplasty, reduction, 378
Cytarabine, for neoplastic meningitis, 1233
Cytogenetics, 747, 748f
Cytokine-induced neutrophil chemoattractant, in cerebral ischemia, 140
Cytokines
effector function of, 680
helper T cell–secreted, 678
in blood-brain barrier function, 12
in brain injury recovery, 5031
in central nervous system, 4155
in cerebral ischemia, 136, 137t, 138–140
in distal nerve stump, 200
in traumatic brain injury, 5029
inflammatory, for CNS injury, 205–206
pro-inflammatory, 682
Cytomegalovirus
in carotid atherosclerosis, 1613
polyradiculopathy from, 3841
Cytometry, cell-cycle analysis by, tumor proliferation marking by, 694–695
Cytopathic-oncolytic viruses, gene therapy with, 822
Cytoprotection, 1520–1522
Cytoskeleton, in cell death, 128
Cytostatics, for glioma invasion, 765–766

Dab1, 53t
Dactylitis, in spondyloarthropathy, 4460
Danazol, pseudotumor cerebri from, 1424
Dandy-Walker syndrome, 3285–3287
fourth ventricle outlet foramina obstruction in, 3393, 3394, 3394f
hydrocephalus in, 3285–3286, 3287f
imaging of, 3286f, 3287f
in posterior encephalocele, 3201f
Dandy-Walker variant, 3285
Dantrium, for spasticity, 2866t
Dantrolene
for cerebral palsy, 3731
for multiple sclerosis, 1454t
for spasticity, 2866t, 2867–2868, 3788
DCC/Netrin 1, 743
DCX, 53t
in lissencephaly, 61
Death
colloid cyst and, 3688
definition of, 393

Death *(Continued)*
determination of, 415
diagnosis of, 393–394
Débridement
for postoperative spinal infection, 4384
for pyogenic spinal infection, 4375–4376, 4376f, 4378
for spinal tuberculosis, 4387
of bullet wounds, 5236–5237, 5237t
Decompression
for cervical degenerative disease, 4409–4428
for cubital tunnel syndrome, 3909–3910
for degenerative spondylolisthesis, 3581–3583
for failed back syndrome, 4337–4339
for lumbar fracture, 5004–5005
for pyogenic spinal infection, 4374–4375, 4379
for spinal cord injury, 4878–4880
for spinal metastases, 4858–4862, 4860f–4863f
for spinal stenosis, 3368–3369
for spinal tuberculosis, 4387
for thoracic disk herniation, 4981
for thoracic spine fracture, 4972–4978, 4974f–4977f, 4980
for thoracolumbar scoliosis, 4562
for thoracolumbar spine fracture, 5000–5002, 5000t, 5001f, 5001t
microvascular, of trigeminal nerve, 3005–3014
neurovascular, for vertigo, 2909
of cauda equina compression, 4998
of cervicomedullary compression, 3367–3368
of spinal cord compression, 4998
of ulnar nerve entrapment, 3909–3910
of vertebral arteries, 1700, 1702, 1703, 1705f, 1709
stereotactic, for craniopharyngioma, 1216
thoracic spine
anterior, 4973–4978, 4974f–4977f
posterolateral, 4972–4973
transoral, for upper cervical spine, 4751–4752, 4752f
transthoracic, 4974, 4975–4978, 4975f
Decorin, 4230–4231
Deep brain stimulation, 3026–3027
chronic pain treatment with, 3119–3129, 3123
complications of, 3128–3129
electrode implantation in, 3125–3126
functional magnetic resonance imaging in, 3122
generator implantation in, 3126
head frame for, 3123
hemorrhage in, 3128, 3128t
historical aspects of, 3119–3120
mechanisms of, 3121–3122
microelectrode recording in, 3124
outcomes in, 3126–3128, 3127t, 3128t
paresthesia-producing targets in, 3121–3122, 3122t
patient selection in, 3120–3121, 3121t
periaqueductal gray targets in, 3121, 3121t, 3122, 3125, 3125f
periventricular gray targets in, 3121, 3121t, 3122, 3125
procedure in, 3126–3127
site selection in, 3121, 3121t, 3122t
stimulation trial in, 3126
target selection in, 3123, 3124
technique of, 3122–3126
Deep brain stimulation *(Continued)*
for Parkinson's disease, 2662, 2662f
movement disorder treatment with, 2803–2825. *See also* specific target, e.g., Globus pallidus, internal.
atlases in, 2808–2809
basal ganglia targeting in, 2804
clinical validation in, 2809
complications of, 2822–2824
computed tomography in, 2808
coordinates in, 2809, 2809f
costs of, 2825
electrode implantation in, 2810, 2811f, 2812–2813, 2812f
electrophysiologic studies in, 2813, 2814f–2816f, 2815–2817
generators in, 2817–2819, 2818f, 2824
indications for, 2819–2820
lesion targeting in, 2805–2810
magnetic resonance imaging in, 2804–2805, 2806f–2808f, 2807–2808
microadjustments in, 2815–2817
microrecording in, 2813, 2815, 2815f
parallel processing model and, 2819
patient selection in, 2819–2820
radiography in, 2804
results of, 2820–2822
side-effects of, 2824
software for, 2810
target localization in, 2819, 2824
ventriculography in, 2804, 2805–2807, 2805f
vs. ablation, 2824
vs. neural grafts, 2824
seizure outcome with, 2579
vs. thalamotomy, 2780
Deep hypothermic circulatory arrest, 1528–1537, 2108
cannulation sites in, 1534
cerebral ischemia pathophysiology and, 1532
complications in, 1536
for posterior circulation aneurysms, 2000, 2002
history of, 1528
in aneurysm treatment, 1511, 1528–1529, 1529f–1531f, 1531, 1807
indications for
anatomic factors in, 1528–1529, 1529f–1531f, 1531
patient-related factors in, 1531–1532, 1531t
medical evaluation before, 1533–1534
neuroanesthetic management in, 1534–1535
patient preparation for, 1534
results of, 1536–1537
surgical management in, 1535–1536
technical preparations before, 1533
techniques for, 1533–1536
Deep tendon reflexes
in peripheral neuropathy, 3833
testing of, 3824–3825
Deep venous thrombosis, 563–564
Degenerative disease
neuronal, 4315t–4316t, 4319–4321, 4320f
spinal, 4147–4148
cervical. *See* Cervical disk disease.
lumbar. *See* Lumbar disk disease.
thoracic. *See* Thoracic disk herniation.
vs. pyogenic infection, 4371
Degenerative spondylolisthesis
pathogenesis of, 4545–4546, 4545f, 4546f
treatment of, 4551–4553, 4552f
Dehydration, intracranial hypertension treatment by, 5133
Dejerine-Sottas disease, 536, 537f
Delirium, 286
after traumatic brain injury, 5296
Delivery
brachial plexus injury in, 3488–3495. *See also* Brachial plexus, obstetric injury to.
epidural hematoma in, 3483–3484, 3483f
in neoplastic disease, 873
intracranial hemorrhage in, 3483–3485, 3483f–3486f
intraparenchymal hemorrhage in, 3485
posterior fossa subdural hematoma in, 3484–3485, 3485f, 3486f
scalp injury in, 3481–3482
skull fracture in, 3482–3483, 3482f
subdural hematoma in, 3484, 3484f
traumatic. *See also* Birth trauma; Brachial plexus, obstetric injury to.
vertex, brachial plexus injury in, 3488, 3489f
Delta, 53t
Dementia, 285–286
colloid cyst and, 3688
Lewy body
apoptosis in, 2710
clinical features of, 2712
forms of, 2708–2709
neuritic Alzheimer's disease changes in, 2712
pathology of, 2712–2713
substantia nigra pars compacta in, 2706f
positron emission tomography of, 484–485
thalamic, strategic infarcts and, 1609
Demyelination, 3961, 3961f
imaging of, 541, 543f
in multiple sclerosis, 1450–1451
in sensory nerve action potential, 3853, 3853f
primary, 3962
radiation-induced, 854
secondary, 3962
segmental, 3962
urologic disorders in, 375
vertigo in, 2902
Dendrite(s), 72f, 73
antigen presentation by, 893
structure of, 77
Denervation
prolonged, 201
urologic disorders in, 375
Denervation hypersensitivity, in cerebral vasospasm, 1849
Dens
aplasia-hypoplasia of, 3341
fracture of. *See also* Odontoid fracture.
imaging of, 519, 519f
Dentate gyrus, 26f, 27, 2486, 2487f
Dentate ligament, 3060, 3060f
in cordotomy, 3063, 3066f
triangular processes of, 36f
Dentate tubercle, 31f
Dentatorubropallidoluysian atrophy, 2718–2719, 2740
Dentition, in craniofacial trauma, 5248–5249
2-Deoxyglucose, in positron emission tomography, 480, 481t, 482
Dependency
definition of, 3783–3784
in traumatic brain injury response, 5193t
Depolarization, 3813, 3813f
Depolarizing potentials, 228

Depression
in chronic pain, 2960, 2966
in epilepsy, 2573
in traumatic brain injury, 5193t, 5296
neurosurgery for, 2856
subcaudate tractotomy for, 2857–2858, 2858f
Depth-dose curves, in radiation therapy, 4008, 4008f
Dermal pit, in congenital lumbosacral lipoma, 3237
Dermal sinus, 4259–4260, 4259f
dorsal, 4316
Dermatomal somatosensory evoked potentials, intraoperative, 4216–4219, 4218t
Dermatomes
cervical, 271, 271f
lower limb, 271, 271f
radicular, 2922f
thoracic, 271, 271f
Dermatomyositis, 833
Dermoid cyst, 1224–1226, 3691–3692, 4259–4260
congenital, 4317
intraspinal, 3275f
orbital, 1374
pial, 3689
radiologic features of, 841, 841f
skull, 1385–1386
pediatric, 3718–3719, 3719f
Dermomyotome, formation of, 4272–4275
Descriptive cohort studies, 249
Descriptive studies, 247–249
Desipramine, for neuropathic pain, 3838
Desmoid tumors, 3946–3948, 3947f, 3947t
Desmoplastic infantile ganglioglioma, 850
Detrusor hyperreflexia, postural, 365, 365f
Detrusor instability, 366
Detrusor muscle, frontal cortex areas for, 359, 360f
Detrusor muscle receptors, 361–362, 362f
Developmental disorders, 52, 56–64
epilepsy from, magnetic resonance imaging of, 2491–2495, 2492f–2494f
Developmental history, 3170, 3170t
Developmental reflexes, testing of, 3181–3182
Developmental venous anomalies, 2139–2142, 2173–2175
arteriovenous malformations and, 2153–2154
capillary telangiectasia and, 2152–2153
cavernous malformations and, 2153, 2311, 2313f, 2314, 2321
clinical features of, 2138t, 2140, 2174–2175, 2174t
definition of, 2173–2174
epidemiology of, 2139, 2174
focal deficit in, 2175
headache in, 2175
hemorrhage in, 2174–2175
imaging of, 2138t, 2140–2141, 2140f, 2141f
in epilepsy, 2491
magnetic resonance imaging of, 471–472, 472f
morbidity and mortality of, 2175
natural history of, 2138t, 2140
pathogenesis of, 2173–2174
pathology of, 2138t, 2139–2140
seizure in, 2175
synonyms for, 2173
treatment of, 2138t, 2141–2142
with supratentorial cavernous malformation, 2311, 2313f, 2314
Devic's disease, 1452, 4314
Dexamethasone
for glial tumors, 870
for spinal cord compression, 4047
for spinal metastases, 4858
in pediatric glioma surgery, 3598
Dexamethasone suppression test, for hypercortisolemia, 1196
Diabetes insipidus
after craniopharyngioma surgery, 3679
after subarachnoid hemorrhage, 1830
germ cell tumors in, 3608
in traumatic brain injury, 5131
pineal region tumors and, 1013
transsphenoidal surgery and, 569
Diabetes mellitus
after pituitary surgery, 1191
in carpal tunnel syndrome, 3889–3890
lumbar spinal stenosis in, 4527
neural tube defect from, 3218–3219
posterior longitudinal ligament ossification in, 4475–4476
stroke risk in, 1616
Diabetic amyotrophy, 3842–3843, 4511
Diabetic neuropathy, 3842–3843
acute mono-, 3843
autonomic, 3842
proximal, 3842–3843
sensorimotor, 3842
sensory, 3842
tramadol for, 3838
Diagnostic tests, 250
accuracy of, 497–499, 498t, 499t
assessment of, 257–258
clinical decision rules in, 237–238
disease prevalence and, 236–237, 237t, 238t, 498–499, 498t, 499t
evaluation of, 497–499
impact of, 499
likelihood ratios in, 235, 237
patient outcome and, 499
predictive value of, 236, 238t, 497–498, 498t
probability in, 235–236, 235–238, 236f
properties of, 236–237, 236t–238t
receiver operator characteristic curve of, 499, 499f
sensitivity of, 236, 238t, 497, 498t
signs and symptoms and, 237, 238t
societal outcome and, 499
specificity of, 236, 238t, 497, 498t
statistics in, 235–238
technical capacity of, 497
Diaphragma sellae, meningioma of, 1117
Diaschisis, 3784
crossed cerebellar, stroke and, 1607, 1608f
thalamocortical, stroke and, 1608–1609
Diastatic suture, 427
Diastematomyelia, 3267, 3267f, 4317, 4317f
imaging of, 535
tethering point in, 3270, 3272, 3272f
Diazepam
before arteriovenous malformation radiosurgery, 4074
for bladder outlet retention, 380
for cerebral palsy, 3731
for multiple sclerosis, 1454t
for spasticity, 2866t, 2867, 3788
for vertigo, 2906
physiologic effects of, 2883, 2883f
Diaziquone, for neoplastic meningitis, 1233
Diencephalon
in Chiari malformation type II, 3351
opioid-sensitive areas of, 2954f
Diet, brain tumors and, 810
Diffuse intravascular coagulation, 564
Diffusion, in magnetic resonance imaging, 446–447
Digital nerve
dorsal, 653
entrapment of, 3936
Dimples
in occult spinal dysraphism, 3259, 3260f
in tethered spinal cord, 3249, 3249f
Diplegia, spastic, in cerebral palsy, 3724, 3725–3727, 3729, 3731–3732, 3747
Diplomyelia, 3267–3268, 3267f, 4317
Diplopia, 317
after midbrain tractotomy, 3056
binocular, 317
examination of, 266, 317
history of, 317
in cavernous carotid fistula, 2344
in olfactory groove meningioma, 1273, 1274f, 1275f
monocular, 317
symptomatic treatment of, 321
transient, temporal lobectomy and, 2610
Dipyridamole
for carotid artery disease, 1618
in carotid endarterectomy, 1644
Disability, 3783
assessment of, 5088, 5088t
Disability Rating Scale, 242t
Disconnection syndromes, testing for, 265
Disequilibrium, 347t
Diskectomy
cervical, 4439–4440, 4439f, 4440f, 4625–4626, 4625f, 4625t
complication avoidance in, 577
endoscopic, 3431
infection after, 4383
lumbar
complication avoidance in, 580–581
endoscopic, 4783–4788
percutaneous
automated, 4776–4780
laser-assisted, 4780–4783
spondylolisthesis after, 4543, 4546–4547
thoracoscopic, 4765–4769
indications for, 4765
micro technique in, 4766–4767, 4767f
Diskitis
after diskography, 4384
imaging of, 540, 540f
pain in, 4293
pediatric, 3566, 4382
examination of, 3561–3562
imaging of, 3562
postoperative, 4383
Diskogenic pain, 4328
Diskography, 506
in lumbar disk disease, 4513
infection after, 4384
Dislocation
atlanto-occipital, 4902–4903
axial skeleton, 4307t
cervical spine
bilateral, 4909, 4909f
unilateral, 4908–4909
hip, in cerebral palsy, 3728
thoracic spine, 4959–4960, 4960f, 4962–4964, 4962t, 4963f
surgery for, 4980–4981
treatment guidelines for, 4967t
vertebral, congenital, 4279–4280, 4280f
Disseminated intravascular coagulation, bullet wound and, 5236

Diuretics
  for brain edema, 802
  intracranial pressure and, 189
Dix-Hallpike maneuver, 275
Dizziness, 275
  causes of, 347t, 348
  mechanisms of, 347t, 348
Dkk1, 53t
Dlx1, 53t
DMBT1, 744
DNA
  construction of, 713
  fragmentation of, in cell death, 128
  radiation interactions with, 3999
DNA analysis, 747–752, 748f–751f
DNA polymerase, as tumor proliferation marker, 694
DNA repair genes, 739
Dolichocephaly, assessment of, 3301
Doll's eye, 289
^{18}F-Dopa, uptake of, positron emission tomography of, 2755–2757, 2756f, 2757f
L-Dopa, blood-brain barrier transport of, 161
Dopa decarboxylase, positron emission tomography of, 2755, 2756f
L-Dopa–carbidopa, for parkinsonian tremor, 2775
Dopamine
  in movement disorders, 2701, 2703
  in striatal output pathways, 2701–2702
Dopamine agonists
  for acromegaly, 1193
  for Parkinson's disease, 2733
Dopamine D_1 binding, positron emission tomography of, 2758
Dopamine receptors, 2699, 2700f
  in striatum, 2687, 2700
Dopamine-depleting drugs, for dystonia, 2796
Dopaminergic agents, for prolactinoma, 1186–1187
Dopaminergic neurons
  in akinetic-rigid Parkinson's disease, 2708
  substantia nigra pars compacta, in Parkinson's disease, 2704, 2706, 2706f
Dopaminergic system
  lesions of, embryonic tissue transplantation for, 4158
  positron emission tomography of, 482–483
Dopaminergic therapy
  dyskinesia from, 2677
  dystonia in, 2677
Doppler effect, 1540
Doppler shift, 1562, 1564f, 1565f
Doppler ultrasonography, transcranial. *See* Transcranial Doppler ultrasonography.
Doppler ultrasound, history of, 1540
Dormancy therapy, 773
Dorsal column postsynaptic system, 2930, 2932f
Dorsal column stimulation, for spasticity, 2866t
Dorsal horn
  neurochemical pathways in, 2953, 2955f
  sensory processing in, 2953, 2955
Dorsal midbrain syndrome, 322–323
Dorsal rhizotomy, 3028, 3033–3042
  complications of, 3039–3040
  evaluation before, 3035
Dorsal rhizotomy *(Continued)*
  for cancer pain, 3034, 3040, 3040t
  for cerebral palsy, 3736–3745. *See also* Selective dorsal rhizotomy.
  for spasticity, 2661, 2866t
  historical aspects of, 3033
  indications for, 3034–3035
  modifications of, 3039
  results of, 3040–3042, 3040t, 3041t
Dorsal root entry zone, in central nervous system repair, 4161–4162
Dorsal root entry zone procedures, 3028, 3045–3056
  care after, 3048, 3053
  complications of, 3048, 3053–3054
  for cancer pain, 3045
  for spasticity, 2870
  indications for, 3046
  management before, 3046–3047
  mechanism of, 3045
  microsurgical section in, 3047–3048
  nucleus caudalis, for facial pain, 3085–3090
  technique of, 3047
Dorsal root ganglion, 71, 72f, 2922
  aberrant course of, 2923, 2923f
  axotomy effects on, 3815, 3815f
  death of, in peripheral nerve injury, 197
  radiofrequency lesions of, 3037–3038
  regeneration of, in peripheral vs. central nervous system injury, 202
Dorsomedial nucleus, 3079
  lesions in, 3080
Dorsum sellae, 1266
Dose-escalation studies, 251
Dose-volume histogram, in radiation therapy, 4011, 4012f
Double cortex, 81, 81f
Double-cortin, 81
Down syndrome
  atlantoaxial instability in, 3543
  craniovertebral junction abnormalities in, 3334, 3337–3338, 3338f
Doxazosin, for bladder outlet retention, 380
Doxorubicin, for Ewing's sarcoma, 4850
Dracuncular infection, spinal, 4390
DREZ. *See* Dorsal root entry zone.
Drooling, in cerebral palsy, 3727, 3732
Drug abuse
  in bullet wounds, 5225–5226
  pyogenic spinal infections from, 4364, 4365, 4370–4371
  vs. brain death, 398
Drugs
  antiepileptic. *See* Antiepileptic drugs.
  chorea from, 2736
  delivery of
    across blood-brain barrier, 15–18, 16f
    through central nervous system, 17–18
    transcellular shuttles for, 153
  endocytosis of, 16
  evaluation of, 253–254
  for failed back syndrome, 4336–4337
  for recurrent carotid stenosis, 1664–1665
  gene transfer–mediated targeting of, 818–820, 818f–820f
  in spinal cord injury, 4874, 4876
  in vivo monitoring of, positron emission tomography in, 491
  intrathecal infusion of, 3133–3141
    alternative approaches to, 3141
    catheters in, 3136–3138
    complications of, 3140–3141
    equipment for, 3136–3140
Drugs *(Continued)*
    for cancer pain, 3133–3134, 3134f
    for neurogenic pain, 3135
    for pain, 3133–3141
    for severe chronic pain, 3134–3135, 3135f
    patient selection in, 3133–3135
    pump implantation for, 3138–3140, 3138f, 3139f
    pumps in, 3136–3138, 3137f
    studies on, 3133t
    surgical complications in, 3140
    tolerance in, 3134–3135, 3134f, 3140–3141
  neuropathy from, 3843–3844
  parkinsonism from, 2716
  Parkinson's disease from, 2735
  pregnancy effects on, 2422–2424
  resistance to, blood-brain barrier in, 15, 162–163
  spontaneous intracerebral hemorrhage with, 1735
Dsl1, 53t
Dumbbell tumors, 4817, 4818f
  treatment of, 4822–4823
Dura, 36f, 1099
  opening of, 1932f, 1933
Dural ring, 1895
Dural sinus, thrombosis of. *See* Cerebral venous thrombosis.
Duret's hemorrhage, of uncal herniation, 5091, 5092f
Durotomy, in lumbar disk disease, 4517
Dynorphin receptors, in striatum, 2687
Dysangiogenesis, hemorrhagic, 2143
Dysarthria
  in brain tumors, 829
  ventral intermedialis nucleus stimulation and, 2823
Dysdiadochokinesis, 3179
Dysembryoplastic neuroepithelial tumors, radiologic features of, 849–850, 850f
Dysesthesia, 3831
  after midbrain tractotomy, 3056
  facial, mesencephalotomy for, 3078
  vs. thoracic disk herniation, 4492
Dyskinesia
  deep brain stimulation for, 2820
  definition of, 2730
  drug-induced, 2677
  in cerebral palsy, 3725
  pallidotomy for, 2790, 4090–4091
  Parkinson's, positron emission tomography of, 2758
  subthalamic nucleus stimulation for, 2821
  tardive, 2730, 2762
Dysmetria
  nucleus caudalis DREZ ablation and, 3087–3088
  pediatric, 3179
Dysnomia
  temporal lobectomy and, 2610–2611
  transitory, after temporal lobe resection, 2572–2573
Dysostoses, odontoid process, 3343
Dysphasia, temporal lobectomy and, 2610
Dysphonia, spasmodic, 2729
Dystonia, 2677–2678, 2720–2721, 2737–2738
  action, 2677
  basal ganglia in, 2795–2796, 2796f
  cerebellar stimulation for, 2797
  classification of, 2795
  craniofacial, 2721
  deep brain stimulation for, 2798, 2820

Dystonia *(Continued)*
definition of, 2729
dopa-responsive, 2737, 2765
dorsal column stimulation for, 2797
focal, 2738
heredodegenerative, 2721
idiopathic torsion, positron emission tomography of, 2764–2765
in cerebral palsy, 3724, 3725, 3731–3732, 3747–3748, 3751t
intrathecal baclofen for, 2748, 2748f, 2749t
medical therapy for, 2796
nonkinesigenic, 2737
pallidotomy for, 2797–2798
parkinsonism and, 2678, 2721, 2737
vs. dopa-responsive dystonia, 2765
x-linked (Lubac), 2721
paroxysmal, 2737
paroxysmal kinesigenic, 2737
pediatric, assessment of, 3179–3180
peripheral denervation for, 2797
plus, 2737
primary, 2737, 2795
primary inherited, 2721
primary torsion, 2721
reciprocal innervation in, 2891
secondary, 2721, 2737, 2795
severity of, 3751t
spasmodic torticollis in, 2891
surgery for, 2748, 2796–2799
microelectrode recording in, 2798–2799
patient selection in, 2796–2797
thalamic stimulation for, 2821
thalamotomy for, 2797–2798
treatment of, 2737–2738
with myoclonus, 2721
Dystopia, orbital, 5257, 5262
in roof fracture, 5261f, 5262f
Dysuria, 365
DYT1, in primary dystonia, 2721
DYT5, 2737
DYT11, 2737

EAAC1, 103
EAAT4, 103
EAAT5, 103
Ear(s)
hair cell of, 74, 74f
in craniofacial trauma, 5251
Ebselen, for cerebral vasospasm, 1854
E-cadherin, in meningioma, 1103
Echinococcal infection, spinal, 4390
Eclampsia, 2425
Edema
brain. *See* Cerebral edema.
dependent, prone positioning and, 563
in arteriovenous malformation, 2188
in astrocytoma, 836
ischemic, 5055
neurotoxic, 5055
postoperative, 566
tumor-associated, 13
Edward's sleeves, in thoracic spine fixation, 4969f
EGFR
in glioblastoma, 950
in glioblastoma multiforme, 726
in glioma, 716
EGR2, 53t
Ehlers-Danlos syndrome type IV, 1770–1771, 1771t
intracranial aneurysms in, 1771

Eicosanoids
in blood-brain barrier function, 12
in cerebral blood flow regulation, 1472–1473, 1472f
in cerebral vasospasm, 1848–1849
Ejaculation
in neurogenic disorders, 366
retrograde, anterior lumbar approach and, 580
Elbow
brachial plexus obstetric palsy and, 3980t
ulnar nerve entrapment at, 3897–3917. *See also* Ulnar nerve, entrapment of, elbow-level.
ulnar nerve surgery and, 652
Electrical auditory brainstem response, with cochlear implants, 337
Electrical injury, peripheral nerve, 3828
Electrical stimulation, 3107–3116
deep brain. *See* Deep brain stimulation.
electrode computer adjustment in, 3115–3116, 3115f
electromyographic recording and, 4223–4224
for cerebral palsy, 3731
for chronic pain, 3107–3116
for failed back surgery syndrome, 3112–3113
for urinary retention, 378
implanted pulse generators for, 3110–3111, 3111f
mechanisms of, 3107–3108
peripheral nerve, 3112–3114
electrodes for, 3109–3110, 3110f
screening protocols for, 3111–3112
spinal cord, 3112–3114
complications of, 3115t
contraindications to, 3115t
electrodes for, 3108–3109, 3108f–3110f
for angina pectoris, 3113
for ischemic pain, 3113
for low back pain, 3113
for peripheral nerve injury, 3113
for reflex sympathetic dystrophy, 3113–3114
indications for, 3112–3114
outcomes of, 3114–3115, 3114f
vs. reoperation, 3112–3113
Electrocardiogram, subarachnoid hemorrhage effects on, 553–554
Electrocorticogram, in ischemia prevention, 1523f
Electrodes
computer adjustment for, in electrical stimulation, 3115–3116, 3115f
depth, 2555, 2555f, 2558–2559, 2558f, 2559f
epidural peg, 2556–2557
insertion of, 2561
for electrophysiologic studies, 2554–2557, 2555f, 2556f
foramen ovale, 2557, 2561
implantable
deep brain stimulation with, 2810, 2811f, 2812–2813, 2812f, 3125–3126
spinal cord stimulation with, 3108–3109, 3108f–3110f
in cordotomy, 3061, 3062f
in epilepsy, 2486, 2486f, 2529, 2530, 2535, 2599
in peripheral nerve surgery monitoring, 3863
in trigeminal neuralgia, 2997, 2998f

Electrodes *(Continued)*
intracranial monitoring with, 2554–2557, 2555f, 2556f
insertion of, 2558–2561, 2558f–2560f
percutaneous, peripheral nerve stimulation with, 3109–3110, 3110f
sphenoidal, 2557
subdural, 2555, 2556f, 2559–2560, 2560f
Electrodiagnostic studies. *See* Electromyography; Electrophysiologic studies; Nerve conduction studies.
Electroencephalography, 230–231
desynchronization of, 280
in altered consciousness, 296–297, 296f
in anesthesia, 1506–1507, 1506f
scalp, 2551
Electrolytes
in altered consciousness, 295
in anterior communicating artery aneurysms, 1937
in subarachnoid hemorrhage, 554, 1829–1830, 1830t
management of, in traumatic brain injury, 5130–5131, 5130f
Electromagnetic stimulation, in bone healing, 4619
Electromyography, 3851
fundamentals of, 3851–3852, 3851f
in selective dorsal rhizotomy, 3741–3742, 3741f, 3742t
indications for, 3851
intraoperative, 4219–4222, 4220t, 4221f, 4222f
needle, 3856–3857, 3856f, 3856t
interference pattern in, 3857
motor unit action potential size and, 3856–3857, 3856f
of carpal tunnel syndrome, 3858
of peripheral nerve trauma, 3860–3861
of radiculopathy, 3859
of ulnar neuropathy, 3858–3859
positive sharp waves in, 3856, 3856f
recruitment in, 3857
spontaneous muscle fiber action potentials in, 3856, 3856t
spontaneous free-running
in peripheral nerve surgery monitoring, 3863, 3865
of thenar muscles, 3866, 3867f
triggered
in median nerve tumor surgery, 3866, 3867f
in peripheral nerve surgery monitoring, 3862, 3864
Electronystagmography, 343–346, 344f, 346f
Electrophysiologic studies
electrodes for, 2554–2557, 2555f, 2556f
in neurosurgery, 230–232, 232t
in thoracic spine fracture, 4967–4968
intraoperative
historical review of, 4203–4204
medicolegal aspects of, 4224–4225
methodological overview of, 4204
nerve root involvement and, 4216–4222
of spinal cord and nerve roots, 4203–4225
space-occupying lesions and, 4222–4224
spinal cord function and, 4204–4215
tethered cords and, 4222–4224
of central nervous system, 215–232
physical principles of, 216, 217f
recording equipment for, 2557
terminology in, 216t

Electrothermal annuloplasty, intradiskal, 4791–4792, 4793f
Electrothrombosis, in Guglielmi detachable coil embolization, 2070
Embolic agents, 858–859, 858t
  for cavernous carotid fistula, 2346
Embolism
  ependymoma surgery and, 3628–3629
  extracranial vertebral artery, 1694–1695, 1697
  in Guglielmi detachable coil embolization, 2071
  in pregnancy, 2427–2428
  medulloblastoma surgery and, 3645
  patient positioning and, 614–615
  pediatric craniotomy and, 3190f, 3191
  posterior fossa surgery and, 555
  prone positioning and, 603
  pulmonary, 563–564
  transcranial Doppler ultrasonography of, 1544
  venous air, 563
    posterior fossa surgery and, 555
Embolization
  in carotid endarterectomy, 1643
  of aneurysms. *See* Aneurysms, embolization of.
  of arteriovenous malformations. *See* Arteriovenous malformations, embolization of.
  of brain tumors. *See* Brain tumors, embolization of.
  of cavernous carotid fistula, 2345–2346
  of cerebellar artery, 2258
  of dural arteriovenous fistula, 2127–2128, 2128f, 2406, 2408
  of glomus jugulare tumors, 1300–1301, 1307
  of intradural vascular malformations, 2410, 2412
  of juvenile nasopharyngeal angiofibroma, 1354, 1354f
  of perimedullary arteriovenous fistula, 2413, 2414f–2415f
  of posterior fossa arteriovenous malformations, 2257–2258
  of spinal aneurysmal bone cyst, 4843
  of spinal hemangioma, 4841, 4842f
  of spinal tumors, 4836
    metastatic, 4861, 4861f
  of vein of Galen malformations, 3443–3444, 3444f
  selective arterial, in vertebral artery trauma, 5218–5219
  transarterial, for transverse-sigmoid dural arteriovenous malformation, 2288–2289
  with Guglielmi detachable coil. *See* Guglielmi detachable coil embolization.
Embolus
  aberrant, in arteriovenous malformations, 2225
  intracranial, transcranial Doppler ultrasonography of, 1555
  postoperative, transcranial Doppler ultrasonography of, 1549–1550
Embryonal cancer, classification of, 667–669, 667t, 668t
Embryonic organizer, neuroectoderm induction by, 4253–4254
Embryonic tissue, transplantation of, for neurodegenerative lesions, 4158–4159
Embryonic vesicles, 46, 47f
EMD 121974, integrin blocking by, 781
Emergency surgery, preoperative evaluation for, 550
Emotional status
  after traumatic brain injury, 5190–5194
  assessment of, 5191
    neurosurgeon's role in, 5191–5194, 5193t
  premorbid, estimation of, 5192–5194, 5193t
EMX1, 53t
EMX2, 53t
En-1, 50, 53t
En-2, 50, 53t
Encephalitis
  limbic, 832–833
  pseudotumor cerebri in, 1425
  Rasmussen's, magnetic resonance imaging of, 2495, 2495f
Encephalitis lethargica, postencephalitic parkinsonism in, 2715
Encephalocele, 3198–3211
  anterior, 3205–3211
    basal, 3205–3206, 3206f
    classification of, 3205, 3206f
    diagnosis of, 3206–3207, 3207f, 3208f
    imaging of, 3207, 3208f
    pathogenesis of, 3199
    prognosis of, 3211
    sincipital, 3205–3206, 3206f
    surgery for, 3209–3211, 3210f
      timing of, 3207–3209
  atretic, 3201f, 3205, 3206f
  classification of, 3198, 3199t
  definition of, 3198, 3199f
  epidemiology of, 3198
  incidence of, 3198
  occipital, 3200
    findings with, 3201–3202
    imaging of, 3201f
  occipitocervical, 3200
  occult, 3205
  parietal, 3200
    findings with, 3202, 3202f, 3203f
    syndromes associated with, 3202
  pathogenesis of, 3198–3200
  posterior, 3200–3205
    findings with, 3201–3202, 3202f, 3203f
    imaging of, 3200, 3200f, 3201f
    outcome in, 3205
    prenatal diagnosis of, 3200, 3200f, 3201f
    surgery for, 3202–3205, 3204f, 3205f
  rudimentary, 3205
  surgery for, in neonates, 3194
Encephaloduroarteriomyosynangiosis, 1464
  for moyamoya, 1718
Encephalomyelitis, 832–833
  experimental allergic, blood-brain barrier in, 164
Encephalopathy, pugilistic, 2717
Enchondroma. *See* Chondroma.
End plates
  marrow changes in, magnetic resonance imaging of, 508, 508f
  pediatric, 3515
End points, surrogate vs. true, 238–239
Endarterectomy
  carotid artery. *See* Carotid endarterectomy.
  historical aspects of, 1463
Endocarditis
  infectious intracranial aneurysms from, 2101, 2103, 2104
  pyogenic spinal infections and, 4370
Endochondral ossification, 4613
Endocrine system
  disorders of
    in growth hormone–secreting pituitary adenoma, 1189–1190
    medulloblastoma surgery and, 3648
  in craniopharyngioma, 1210
  preoperative evaluation of, 550
Endocytosis
  in blood-brain barrier, 159f
  of drugs, 16
Endodermal sinus tumor, magnetic resonance imaging of, 3607f, 3608
End-of-life issues, legal, 414–416
Endogenous modulators, in angiogenesis, 775t
Endolymph, movement and, 341, 341f
Endolymphatic hydrops, vs. Ménière's disease, 349–350
Endolymphatic sac, surgery on, 2908
Endonasal septal pushover technique, 1178
Endoneurium, of peripheral nerves, 3958, 3959f
Endonucleases, in apoptosis, 1519
Endoscope
  fiberoptic, 3427, 3428f
  rigid, 3427, 3428f
  viewing systems for, 3427
Endoscopic diskectomy, lumbar, 4783–4788
  historical perspective on, 4783–4784
  indications for, 4784
  results of, 4785–4788
  technique of, 4784–4785, 4786f, 4787f
Endoscopy, 3427–3431
  applications of, 3428–3431
  complications of, 3431
  for intracerebral hemorrhage, 1755
  historical aspects of, 3427
  in pediatric hydrocephalus treatment, 3429–3430, 3429f
  in transsphenoidal approach, 1178
  irrigation during, 3427–3428
  membrane fenestration with, 3429–3430, 3429f
  microsurgery with, 3430
  of aneurysms, 1806
  of sympathetic nervous system, 3093
  of syringomyelia, 3430–3431
  of third ventricle tumors, 1249
  of urinary disorders, 368
  tumor biopsy with, 3430
  ventricular catheter positioning with, 3428, 3429f
Endostatin, angiosuppressive therapy with, 779
Endothelial barrier antigen, 157, 158
Endothelial cell inhibitors, as angiogenesis antagonist, 777t, 778–780
Endothelial cell migration assay, in angiogenesis antagonist discovery, 775, 776f
Endothelial cells
  activated, 725
  in blood-brain barrier, 109–110, 153–154
  in bystander effect, 818, 818f
  peripheral endothelium vs., 155–156
Endothelial factors, in cerebral blood flow autoregulation, 5049–5050
Endothelin(s), in cerebral blood flow regulation, 1474
Endothelin-1
  angiosuppressive therapy with, 782–783
  in blood-brain permeability, 11
  in cerebral vasospasm, 1849
Endothelium, in cerebral autoregulation, 1476

Endothelium-derived relaxing factor. *See* Nitric oxide.
Endothoracic fascia, 4674
Endotracheal tube, complications of, patient positioning and, 609–610
Endovascular occlusion
  for cerebral vasospasm, 1547
  for spinal aneurysmal bone cyst, 4843
  for spinal hemangioma, 4841, 4842f
  historical considerations in, 1464–1465
  of aneurysms, 1803–1806, 2057–2074, 2121. *See also* Aneurysms, embolization of; Aneurysms, endovascular occlusion of.
  of brain tumors, 862–864
Engle Class, 242t
Enkephalin receptors, in striatum, 2687
Enlimomab, in ischemia protection, 1522
Enophthalmos, orbital blow-out fracture and, 5257f
Entacapone, for Parkinson's disease, 2733
Enteric infection, after myelomeningocele repair, 3223
Enterocolitis, necrotizing, after myelomeningocele repair, 3223
Enterogenous cyst. *See* Neurenteric cyst.
Enteroviruses, myelitis from, 4311, 4312t
Enthesis, 4580
Enthesitis, in spondyloarthropathies, 4460
Enthesopathies, 4475–4487. *See also* Posterior longitudinal ligament, ossification of.
  anatomy and physiology in, 4479–4480
Environment control, 5088
Environmental awareness, after traumatic brain injury, 5192
Eosinophilic granuloma
  craniovertebral junction, 4809
  spinal, 4296t, 4297–4298, 4355, 4837, 4843, 4845f
    pediatric, 3567, 3591, 3592f
Ependyma, 97
Ependymal cells, 49, 83, 93
Ependymal cyst
  histopathologic classification of, 664–665, 664t
  vs. neurenteric cyst, 1229
Ependymoblastoma, 669
Ependymoma, 1043–1048, 4296t
  anaplastic, 664–665, 664t
  cause of, 1044
  chemotherapy for, 1048, 1048t
  classification of, 664–665, 664t, 1044–1045, 1045t
  diagnosis of, 1044–1046
  epidemiology of, 1044
  filum terminale, 4296t, 4300–4301
    treatment of, 4824
  fourth ventricle, 3624, 3625, 3626f, 3627
  gene alterations in, 751t
  imaging of, 525, 525f
  immunohistology of, 1046
  in pregnancy, 872
  light microscopy of, 1045–1046
  locations of, 1043
  magnetic resonance imaging of, 453, 454f, 1046
  metastatic, 527, 528f
  myxopapillary, 665, 701
  pediatric, 3623–3634, 3697
    chemotherapy for, 3631–3632, 3632f, 3703
    complications of, 3628–3631
    dissemination of, 3626
    epidemiology of, 3623
Ependymoma *(Continued)*
    genetic factors in, 3623
    grading of, 3624
    hydrocephalus in, 3626–3627
    imaging of, 3625–3626, 3625f, 3626f, 3626t, 3699
    neurophysiologic monitoring in, 3630–3631
    pathology of, 3623–3624, 3624f
    quality of life after, 3634
    radiation therapy for, 3631, 3631t
    recurrent, 3634
    signs/symptoms of, 3624–3625, 3625t
    surgery for, 3627–3628, 3628f
    survival in, 3632–3634, 3633f, 3633t
    treatment of, 3626–3628
  platelet-derived growth factor in, 730
  posterior fossa, 3624, 3630
  proliferation markers for, 700–701
  radiation therapy for, 1047–1048
  radiologic features of, 840
  rates of, 1044
  recurrence of, 1043
  resection of, 1043, 1047
  spinal cord, 4040, 4302, 4826, 4827f
    MIB-1 labeling index for, 701, 701t
    radiation therapy for, 4042, 4043, 4043t
    surgery for, 4043
    treatment of, 4828
  third ventricular, 1246
  treatment of, 1046–1048
  ultrastructure of, 1046
  variants of, 1045, 1045t
  ventricular, MIB-1 labeling index for, 700–701, 700t
Ephrins, 80
Epiblast, 47, 4239, 4240f, 4241
Epidemiology, 235–259. *See also* Diagnostic tests; Outcomes assessment.
  analytic studies in, 249–253
  case reports/series in, 248–249
  case-control studies in, 249
  cohort studies in, 249–250
  common biases in, 247, 248t
  cross-sectional surveys in, 249
  descriptive cohort studies in, 249
  descriptive studies in, 247–249
  diagnosis studies in, 250
  dose-escalation studies in, 251
  individual studies in, 248–249
  interventional studies in, 251–252
  medical literature assessment in, 257–259
  meta-analysis in, 252–253
  natural history studies in, 250–251
  observational studies in, 249–251
  population correlation studies in, 247–248
  randomized, controlled studies in, 251–252
  study designs in, 247–253, 247t
Epidermal growth factor, 726
  in central nervous system repair, 4160
Epidermal growth factor receptor
  in brain tumors, 726–727
  in gliomas, 715
Epidermoid cyst, 1207, 1223–1224, 3690–3691, 3690f, 3691f, 4259–4260
  cerebellopontine angle, retrosigmoid approach to, 927
  congenital, 4317
  imaging of, 1224, 1225f
  orbital, 1374
  pial, 3689
  radiologic features of, 838–839
Epidermoid cyst *(Continued)*
  skull, 1385–1386, 1386f
    pediatric, 3718–3719
  vs. trigeminal schwannoma, 1348
Epidural abscess. *See also* Pyogenic infection, spinal.
  clinical presentation of, 4366
  incidence of, 4363–4364
  magnetic resonance imaging of, 4379, 4380f
  myelitis in, 4313
  neurological deficit in, 4373–4374
  outcome of, 4381, 4382f
  pain in, 4291, 4293, 4293f
  pediatric, 3566
  postdiskography, 4384
  treatment of, 4378–4379, 4380f
Epidural catheters, infections from, 4384–4385
Epidural hematoma, 5042–5043
  after arterial bypass, 2117
  delivery and, 3483–3484, 3483f
  evacuation of, 5154, 5157, 5157f
  in mild head injury, 5070, 5071t
  in traumatic brain injury, 5083, 5106, 5107f
  magnetic resonance imaging of, 469
  pediatric, head injury and, 3475–3476, 3475f, 3476t, 3477
  postoperative, 936, 937f
  spinal cord compression in, 523, 524f
  treatment of, 5146
Epidural scar, postoperative, 580
Epidural space
  abscess of, pain from, 4291, 4293, 4293f
  infection of, imaging of, 540, 540f
Epidural steroid injections, 2974–2976
  approaches to, 2976
  contraindications to, 2974, 2975t
  fluoroscopy in, 2973–2974
  indications for, 2974, 2975t
  interlaminar, 2975
  limitations of, 2974, 2975t
  outcomes in, 2976
  rationale for, 2974
  transforaminal, 2975–2976
Epilepsy. *See also* Seizures.
  area of functional deficit in, 2438
  as chronic illness, 2565, 2567f
  blood-brain barrier in, 166
  brain mapping in, 2511, 2557
  cavernous malformations in, 2314
  cerebellar ganglioglioma in, 2578
  chemical-shift imaging of, 2496–2497, 2497f
  classification of, 2463–2464, 2464t
  clinical features of, 2526–2527
  cognitive outcome in, 2571
  corpus callosotomy for, 2578–2579
  cortical zones in, 2435–2439
    epileptogenic, 2438–2439
    irritative, 2436
    seizure onset, 2436–2437, 2437f
    symptomatogenic, 2435–2436
  cost of, 2565
  cryptogenic, 2461
  death rate in, 2576
  deep brain stimulation for, 2579
  definition of, 2461–2462, 2525
  developmental disorders and, magnetic resonance imaging of, 2491–2495, 2492f–2494f
  diagnosis of, 2461–2467
    complications of, 2575
    electrode-based, 2529–2530

Epilepsy *(Continued)*
disconnection surgery for, 2578–2579
drugs for. *See* Antiepileptic drugs.
dual pathology in, 2490, 2490f
dysgenesis in, magnetic resonance imaging of, 2494–2495, 2494f
electrode use in
complications of, 2575
magnetic resonance imaging during, 2486, 2486f
electroencephalography of, 2529
epidemiology of, 2565
epileptogenic cortex in, resection of, 2620
epileptogenic lesion in, 2437–2438
extratemporal lobe, 2587
alternative treatment of, 2588
corpus callosotomy for, 2596
developmental lesions in, 2598
distribution of, 2588
electrode monitoring of, 2599
evaluation of
before surgery, 2598–2600
during surgery, 2600–2601
gliotic lesions in, 2598
hemispherotomy for, 2596
localization of, 2587
magnetic resonance imaging of, 2587, 2599–2600
multiple subpial transection for, 2594, 2595f, 2596
neoplasms in, 2598
neuropsychological testing in, 2600
nonlesional neocortical, 2619
pathology of, 2587, 2598
positron emission tomography of, 486–487
surgery for, 2587–2602
challenges in, 2587–2588
complications of, 2576–2577
disconnection procedures in, 2594, 2595f, 2596
electrocorticography in, 2601
frameless stereotaxy in, 2601
imaging in, 2601
multilobar procedures in, 2594
seizure outcome after, 2576–2578
stimulation mapping in, 2600–2601
stimulation procedures in, 2596, 2596f–2597f
vascular lesions in, 2598
video electroencephalography monitoring of, 2599
frontal lobe, 2588–2589, 2590f–2591f, 2591
classification of, 2589
localization of, 2589
neuropsychological testing in, 2600
pediatric, 3770
functional hemispherectomy for, 2580
functional magnetic resonance imaging in, 2511–2520
drug effects on, 2513–2514
language lateralization and, 2514, 2515f, 2516
patient selection for, 2513
reliability of, 2512
sensitivity of, 2512–2513, 2512t
specificity of, 2513
variation in, 2513
generalized, 2461
genetic factors in, 2462–2463, 2463t
gliosis in, magnetic resonance imaging of, 2495
health-related quality of life in, 2565, 2567f, 2574

Epilepsy *(Continued)*
hemispherotomy for, 2580
hippocampal sclerosis in, 2490, 2490f
historical perspective on, 2461
hypothalamic hamartoma in, 2578
idiopathic, 2449, 2461
in cerebral palsy, 3728
in low-grade glioma, 953
in supratentorial cavernous malformation, 2310
incidence of, after aneurysmal subarachnoid hemorrhage, 1825–1826, 1826t
intracranial monitoring in
study design for, 2557
surgery after, 2561–2562
intractable, definition of, 3769
ion channels in, 225t
language dysfunction in, 2572–2573
language lateralization in, 2514, 2516
left vagus nerve stimulation for, 2579
lesionectomy in, 2620
localization-related, 2461
long-term memory systems in, functional magnetic resonance imaging of, 2516–2518
magnetic resonance imaging of, 2527–2528, 2527f, 2528f
incidental findings in, 2495–2496, 2495f
interpretation of, 2496, 2496f
magnetic resonance spectroscopy of, 2496–2497, 2497f
medial temporal activation in, functional magnetic resonance imaging of, 2516–2518
medically intractable, 2525
medically refractory, 2465
memory loss in, 2571–2572
multilobar, pediatric, 3771
multiple subpial transection for, 2635–2641. *See also* Multiple subpial transection.
neuroaugmentative surgery for, 2579
neuropsychological testing in, 2529
nonlesional neocortical, electrode monitoring in, 2625
occipital lobe, 2588–2589, 2592–2594, 2593f
pediatric, 3770–3771
panhemispheric syndromes with, 2579
parasylvian-onset, 2638, 2638f
parietal lobe, 2588, 2591–2592
pediatric, 3770
pathophysiology of, 2462–2463, 2462t, 2463t
pediatric
causes of, 3758
diagnosis of, 3771–3772
electrocorticography of, 3771
electroencephalography of, 3771
epidemiology of, 3769
focal nature of, 3760
imaging of, 3771
medically intractable, 3760
pathology of, 3775–3776, 3775t
positron emission tomography of, 3771
presentation of, 3770–3771
surgery for, 3773–3775
amobarbital test before, 3765
brain plasticity and, 3759
candidates for, 3759–3760
complications of, 3758–3759, 3777, 3777t

Epilepsy *(Continued)*
development after, 3759
evaluation before, 3758, 3760–3765
historical aspects of, 3772–3773
imaging before, 3763–3765, 3764f, 3765f
magnetic resonance imaging before, 3764, 3764f
magnetic resonance spectroscopy before, 3765
multifocal subpial transection in, 3775, 3776
neuropsychological assessment before, 3765
positron emission tomography before, 3764, 3765f
repeat, 3775
results of, 3776
seizures after, 3759
single-photon computed tomography before, 3764–3765
types of, 3758
video electroencephalogram monitoring before, 3760–3763, 3761f–3763f
surgery on, 3195
vs. adult epilepsy, 3770
positron emission tomography of, 485–487, 486t, 2476–2477, 2527, 2528f
post-traumatic, 2449–2458
extracellular potassium homeostasis in, 2454–2456, 2454f–2457f
glutamate homeostasis in, 2457–2458
hilar neuron loss in, 2449–2450, 2450f
mechanisms of, 2449–2454
nonsynaptic mechanisms of, 2454–2458
sodium-potassium pump in, 2454–2455
synaptic kindling mechanism in, 2451–2452, 2451f
synaptic transduction in, 2451–2452, 2451f
synaptogenesis in, 2450–2451
psychomotor, mesiotemporal lesion and, 2607
psychosocial assessment in, 2529
quality-adjusted life-years in, 2567, 2568f
radiosurgery for, 4093
seizure outcome after, 2570–2571
Rasmussen's encephalitis and, magnetic resonance imaging of, 2495, 2495f
risk factors for, 2462, 2462t
secondary, 2464–2465
seizure localization in
extracranial electroencephalography in, 2630–2631
functional magnetic resonance imaging in, 2518–2519
imaging in, 2631
intracarotid amobarbital test in, 2631
invasive electroencephalography in, 2631–2632
symptomatic, 2630
surgery for, 2525–2530. *See also* Topectomy.
anesthesia in, 2620–2621
approaches to, 2565, 2566f
candidate identification in, 2525–2526
computed tomography before, 2483–2485, 2484f, 2485f
decision making in, 2530
disconnection in, 2629, 2629t
electrical stimulation mapping in, 2621

Epilepsy *(Continued)*
electrocorticography in, 2621–2622, 2623f, 2624, 2624f
electrophysiologic recording methods in, 231, 232t
epileptogenic zone in, 2435
evaluation before, 2526–2529, 2526t
functional magnetic resonance imaging in, 2516
future of, 2443–2445
history of, 2439–2443, 2439f
imaging in, 2442–2443, 2497–2498, 2498f
in era of epileptogenic lesion, 2442–2443
in era of functional deficit zone, 2442–2443
in era of irritative/ictal onset zones, 2440–2442, 2441f, 2444
in era of microlesional zone, 2445
in era of seizure onset zone, 2444
in era of symptomatogenic zone, 2439–2440
in structural lesions, 2620
increases in, 2565, 2566f
intracranial monitoring evaluation in, 2552–2554, 2553f, 2554f
language decline after, functional magnetic resonance imaging of, 2516
language mapping in, 2622–2624, 2622f
magnetic resonance imaging before, 2483, 2484f–2496f, 2485–2496
magnetic resonance spectroscopy before, 2496–2497, 2497f
magnetic source imaging in, 2444
magnetoencephalography in, 2444
marginal cost-effectiveness ratio for, 2574–2575, 2574f
memory mapping in, 2625
neurobehavioral outcome after, 2573–2575
neuropsychological outcome after, 2571–2573
outcome after, 2565, 2567, 2567f, 2568f
positioning in, 2621
psychiatric outcome after, 2573
psychosocial outcome after, 2573–2574
resection in, 2629, 2629t
seizure outcome after, 2568–2571, 2568f, 2569f
assessment of, 2565, 2567f, 2568f
classification schemes for, 2568, 2568f
electrocorticography and, 2571
electrography and, 2570
imaging features and, 2570
magnetic resonance imaging of, 2486
surgical technique and, 2570–2571
surgical vs. medical treatment in, 2569
sensorimotor cortex identification in, 2622
single-photon emission computed tomography before, 2476–2477, 2477
sodium channels in, 222
stereotactic, 557
supplementary motor area in, cortical stimulation mapping of, 2537
tailored resections in, 2615–2625
symptomatic, 2449, 2461

Epilepsy *(Continued)*
temporal lobe
amygdala atrophy in, 2490
anterior lobectomy for, 2605–2607
complications of, 2610
outcome in, 2611
chemical-shift imaging of, 2497, 2497f
clinical features of, 2570
electrocorticography in, 2616–2617, 2618, 2625
electroencephalography of, 2570
hippocampal sclerosis in, 2569–2570
imaging of, 2567–2568, 2570
lesional, 2568
seizure outcome in, 2577
magnetic resonance imaging of, 486
magnetic resonance spectroscopy of, 486
magnetoencephalography of, 486
nonlesional neocortical, surgery for, 2619
paradoxical medial, magnetic resonance imaging of, 2495, 2495f
pediatric, 3770
positron emission tomography of, 485–486, 486t
single photon emission computed tomography of, 486
surgery for, 2568, 2615–2619
complications of, 2575, 2609–2611
historical aspects of, 2615
memory loss and, 2617–2618
outcomes of, 2611–2612
seizure outcome after, 2568, 2569f
transsylvian selective amygdalohippocampectomy for, 2607–2609
tumors and, magnetic resonance imaging of, 2491, 2491f
U. S. centers for, 2565, 2566f
vagus nerve stimulation for, 2643–2650. *See also* Vagus nerve, stimulation of.
vascular lesions and, 2491
vertigo in, 2902
Epilepsy Surgery Inventory, 2565, 2567f
Epileptic syndromes, 2461
classification of, 2463–2464, 2464t
surgery for, 2565, 2566f
Epileptogenesis
localization of, 2551
surgical history of, 2442–2443
trauma and, 2452
Epileptogenic tumors, 2598
Epileptogenic zone, 2438–2439
potential, 2437, 2438, 2444
resection of, 2435
Epiphysis, slipped, 3564–3565
Epistaxis, in cavernous carotid fistula, 2344
Epitopes, 676
recognition of, 677
spreading of, 676
Epitrochleoanconeus, in ulnar nerve compression, 3903
Epoxygenase, in arachidonic acid metabolism, 1473
Epstein-Barr virus
multiple sclerosis from, 1449
paranasal sinus tumors and, 1312
Equilibrative nucleoside transporters, 158
Equilibrium potential, for potassium, 3812
Erb's palsy, 3822–3823, 3822f
Erection, 366
Erythrocyte sedimentation rate
in postoperative diskitis, 4383
in pyogenic spinal infections, 4366
after antibiotic treatment, 4379, 4381

Erythropoietin, in hemangioblastoma, 1055
E-selectin, in cerebral ischemia, 140–141
Esthesioneuroblastoma, 1333–1341, 1395–1396, 1396f
grading of, 1333, 1334t
imaging of, 1333–1334, 1335f
of paranasal sinus, 1313, 1314t
outcome in, 1340–1341
pathology of, 1333, 1334f
physical examination of, 1333
radiation therapy for, 1334–1335, 1337
recurrence of, 1340, 1340t
staging of, 1333, 1335t
surgery for, 1337–1340, 1338f, 1339f
frontal sinus in, 1338, 1338f
pericranial flap in, 1336f–1337f, 1337
treatment of, 1334–1340
complications of, 1340
Estrogen
deficiency of, in prolactinoma, 1185
in bone metabolism, 4232
Estrogen receptors, in meningioma, 1107–1108
Estrogen replacement therapy, pseudotumor cerebri from, 1423
Ethambutol, for tuberculosis, 1441
Ethionamide, for tuberculosis, 1441
Ethmoid cells, in anterior skull base, 910, 912f
Ethmoidal neurovascular bundle, posterior, 1321f
Ethmoidal sinus
adenocarcinoma of, occupational exposure and, 1
tumors of, staging of, 1317, 1318t
Etidocaine, for spasticity, 2865, 2866t
Etidronate, for osteoporosis, 4233
Etomidate, 1508
in carotid endarterectomy, 1627
in craniotomy, 5150
in ischemia protection, 1521
Etoposide
for ependymoma, 1048t
pharmacology of, 882
European Organization for Research and Treatment of Cancer Quality of Life Questionnaire C30, 243t
Evidence-based practice, 254–257
cumulative evidence evaluation in, 255–256, 255t, 256t
future of, 256
medical literature assessment in, 254–255, 255f, 255t, 257–259
outcome assessment in, 256
self-education resources for, 255t
skills for, 254, 255t
Evoked potentials, in ischemia prevention, 1523f
Ewing's sarcoma, 1143, 4296t, 4299, 4300f
extraosseous, 3953
primitive neuroectodermal, 3953
skull, 1393–1394, 1394f
spinal, 4356–4357, 4837, 4848–4850
imaging of, 4848, 4850f
radiation therapy for, 4049
Excitotoxicity, in ischemic injury, 1517
Exclusion, in outcomes assessment, 245
Executive functioning, after traumatic brain injury, 5187–5188
Exercise, bone health and, 4234
Exogenous substances, pseudotumor cerebri from, 1422–1425, 1424t
Exophthalmos
carotid cavernous sinus fistula formation and, 2341, 2342f

Exophthalmos (Continued)
fibrous dysplasia and, 1366
in craniofacial repair, 5257
pulsatile, 2341
Expert witness, 413
in child abuse, 3510–3511
Exposure, assessment of, 5088
Extension injury
to cervical spine, 4890, 4896, 4909
to thoracic spine, 4961, 4962f
External auditory canal, in temporal bone fracture, 5276, 5278f, 5280, 5281
External ventricular drainage, for infantile posthemorrhagic hydrocephalus, 3412f, 3413
Extracellular matrix
in central nervous system repair, 4168
molecules of, in malignant glioma, 761–763
Extracellular matrix proteins, in distal nerve stump, 200
Extracellular space
astrocytes and, 101–102
homeostasis in
loss of, 230
maintenance of, 228, 229f, 230
potassium accumulation in, 228
size of, glial regulation of, 230
Extracerebral fluid collection, chronic, child abuse and, 3505–3506, 3506f
shunts for, 3506–3507, 3507f
Extracerebral space, enlargement of, child abuse and, 3505, 3506f
Extracranial carotid artery–to–middle cerebral artery saphenous vein interposition graft, 2110–2111, 2111f, 2112f
Extracranial carotid artery–to–posterior cerebral artery saphenous vein interposition graft, 2111, 2113
Extracranial radiosurgery, 4069, 4143
Extracranial-intracranial bypass, 2107
Extradural tumor, sensory signs of, 269–270, 270f
Extraocular muscles, 316
pediatric, examination of, 3174
Extremity(ies)
lower
abnormalities of, nerve damage and, 3833, 3833f
central nervous system repair and, 4157
digital nerve entrapment in, 3936
discrepancies between, in occult spinal dysraphism, 3262, 3264, 3264f
entrapment syndromes of, magnetic resonance imaging of, 3882, 3882f
pain in, 3026t
peripheral nerve disorders in, 3822
peripheral nerve entrapment in, 3933–3936
peripheral nerve surgery in, 652–655, 654f, 655f
weakness in, colloid cyst and, 3688
upper
anterior interosseous nerve in, surgery on, 650–651, 651f
functional deficits in, upper extremity nerve disorders and, 3823
in brachial plexus obstetric palsy, 3980t
in cervical spondylotic myelopathy, 4448, 4449
innervation of, 3898
Extremity(ies) (Continued)
ischemia of, thoracic endoscopic sympathectomy for, 4762
median nerve in
entrapment of, 3924
surgery on, 650, 650f, 651f
pain in
dorsal rhizotomy for, 3041–3042
hyperextension-hyperflexion injury and, 4918
surgery for, 3026t
peripheral nerve disorders in, 3822, 3822f
hand deficits in, 3863
peripheral nerve surgery in, 647–652, 649f–652f
positioning of, 647–652, 649f–652f
posterior interosseous nerve surgery in, 651
radial nerve surgery in, 651
radiculopathy of, 272t
Eye(s)
injury to, 5247
lymphoma of, 1068–1069
position of, inframedial bulge in, 5257f
Eye movements, 316–323
abnormalities of, 288–289
in sarcoidosis, 1436
compensatory, 340f
vestibulo-ocular reflex and, 341, 341f
disorders of, 317–321
examination of, 317, 317b
in benign positional nystagmus, 342–343, 343f
in coma, 293
in Glasgow Coma Scale, 286t, 287
in vestibular system testing, 346–347
midbrain in, 3054
pediatric, examination of, 3174
Eyelids, in craniofacial trauma, 5251

Face
numbness in, in trigeminal schwannoma, 1344f, 1345
somatotopic organization of, 3048–3049
three-dimensional imaging of, 433, 435f
trauma to. *See* Craniofacial trauma.
Facet joint(s)
aging effects on, 4396
arthropathy of, 2977–2978, 2979f
biomechanics of, 4185
cervical
dislocation of, 4908–4909, 4909f
laminectomy of, posterior cervical segmental instrumentation and, 4419–4424, 4422f, 4423f
medial branch of, denervation of, 2977, 2980
pain referral patterns in, 2979f
wiring of, 4646–4650, 4648f, 4649f
degeneration of, radiologic features of, 512, 513f
denervation procedures for, 2976–2981
ganglion cyst of, decompressive surgery for, 4337
innervation of, 2977, 2978f
lumbar, 4328
arthropathy of, 2977–2978, 2979f
injections into, 2977
intra-articular injections into, 2977
medial branch of, 2977, 2978f
denervation of, 2977, 2980
Facet joint(s) (Continued)
percutaneous radiofrequency rhizotomy of, 3038–3039
pain syndromes affecting, 4330
pediatric, 3515
posterior, in intervertebral disk degeneration, 4329
pyogenic infection of, 4381
thoracic, 4953
dislocation of, 4959–4960, 4962–4964, 4962t, 4963f
surgery for, 4980–4981
treatment guidelines for, 4967t
medial branch of, 2976, 2977f
denervation of, 2978–2980, 2980t
outcomes in, 2980–2981
pain referral patterns in, 2979f
Facetectomy, cervical
biomechanics in, 4193–4194
complications of, 4427
Facial colliculus, 33f
Facial nerve, 40f, 329f
dysfunction of
glomus jugulare tumors and, 1305, 1306
in acoustic neuroma, 1158–1159, 1158t, 1159t
vision examination in, 302, 304, 304f
examination of, 266–267
injury to
diagnosis of, 5282–5283
epidemiology of, 5282
grading scales for, 5275, 5276t
in craniofacial trauma, 5251
in sarcoidosis, 1435
pathophysiology of, 5282
skull base surgery and, 572
temporal bone fracture and, 5282–5284
treatment of, 5283–5284
vagus nerve stimulator implantation and, 2643–2644
monitoring of, during acoustic neuroma surgery, 1159–1160
paralysis of, acoustic neuroma surgery and, 570, 1161
pediatric
examination of, 3175
traumatic neuropathy of, 3468
preservation of, in acoustic neuroma surgery, 1160
schwannoma of, vs. acoustic neuroma, 1147, 1147f, 1148f
Facial pain
atypical, 2989t, 3018t
diagnostic clues in, 2988, 2989t
differential diagnosis of, 3018t
DREZ nucleus caudalis ablation for, 3085–3090
history of, 2987
in trigeminal schwannoma, 1344
Fahraeus-Lindqvist effect, 1468
Failed back syndrome
anatomy in, 4327–4328
classification of, 4330, 4330t
clinical evaluation of, 4332–4336
diskogenic pain treatment and, 4328
electrical stimulation for, 3112–3113
history of, 4332–4333
imaging of, 4333–4334, 4333f–4335f
inflammatory, 4331
mechanical instability, 4331
myofascial, 4330
neural compression, 4330–4331
neurodiagnostic testing of, 4334
neuropathic, 4331

Failed back syndrome *(Continued)*
pathology of, 4328–4329
physical examination of, 4332–4333
physiologic testing of, 4334
physiology of, 4327–4328
psychological, social, economic testing of, 4334, 4336
psychosocioeconomic, 4332
treatment of, 4336–4343
decompressive surgery in, 4337–4339
epidural fibrosis after, 4337
ganglionectomy in, 3042
neuropathic pain surgery in, 4343
pharmacologic, 4336–4337
psychosocioeconomic, 4338
rehabilitation in, 4336
stabilization-arthrodesis surgery in, 4339–4343, 4341f, 4342f
surgical, 4338–4343
types of, 4329–4332
False negative, 497
False positive, 497
Falx cerebri
in Chiari malformation type II, 3351, 3351f
meningioma of, 1112–1113
Familial cancer syndrome, 969
Familial polyposis, brain tumors in, 812t, 813
Family, in life-sustaining treatment refusal, 415
Family history, 263–264
Farnesyl transferase inhibitors, angiosuppressive therapy with, 780
Fas ligand, in astrocytoma development, 891
Fas/Apo1/CD95, 743
Fasciculations, 268
Fastigium, 31f
Fat, in Cushing's disease, 1195
Fatigue, in neuromuscular junction disorders, 270
Fatty acids, free, after traumatic brain injury, 5026
Fazio-Londe syndrome, 4319, 4320
FCMD, in lissencephaly, 61
Fecal incontinence, in cerebral palsy, 3727, 3732
Feeding problems, in cerebral palsy, 3727
Felbamate, pharmacology of, 2470t, 2471–2472
Femoral cutaneous nerve, lateral, entrapment of, 3933
Fertility, prolactinoma and, 1188–1189
Fetal tissue, in neurogenesis, 5033
Fetal tissue transplantation, 2830–2843, 4158
abortion in, 2833, 2833t
assessment before, 2832–2833, 2832t
chromaffin cells in, 2831
donation protocols in, 2833
donor age determination in, 2833, 2834f, 2834t, 2835
mesencephalic tissue in, 2831–2832
grafting procedures for, 2836–2837
preparation techniques for, 2835–2836, 2835f
patient selection in, 2832
postoperative care in, 2837–2838
results of, 2838–2839, 2840t, 2841, 2842t, 2843t
Fetus
central nervous system development in, 2833, 2834f
Parkinson's disease effects on, positron emission tomography of, 2757–2758, 2758f
Fever
in pediatric neurorehabilitation, 3787
in traumatic brain injury, 5124, 5124f, 5128, 5136
pain associated with, 4290–4295, 4291t
treatment of, 5136
FGFR3, in achondroplasia, 3362, 3363
Fibrillation potentials, 3856, 3856t
Fibrillin-1, 1772
Fibrinolysis, for intracerebral hemorrhage, 1753–1754
Fibrinolytic agents, spontaneous intracerebral hemorrhage with, 1735
Fibroblast growth factor
in axonal regeneration, 200
in brain tumors, 727–728
in central nervous system repair, 4160, 4162
in glioma, 716
Fibroblast growth factor receptor
in brain tumors, 728
in craniofacial syndromes, 3315–3316
Fibrolysis, subarachnoid blood clot, 1852
Fibroma, ossifying, 1367
Fibromuscular cushions, 2148
Fibromuscular dysplasia, carotid artery, 1681–1682, 1682f
Fibromyalgia, 4331
Fibromyositis, 4331
Fibromyxochondroma, 1365
Fibronectin, in malignant glioma, 761
Fibrosarcoma, 1142–1143, 1143f
skull, 1389–1390, 1390f
Fibrosis, cerebral arterial, in vasospasm, 1847–1848
Fibrous dysplasia, 1365–1367
monostotic, 3590–3591
orbital, 1374–1375
osteogenic sarcoma with, 1389, 1389f
radiologic aspects of, 1365–1366, 1365f
signs/symptoms of, 1366
skull, 1401–1402, 1402f, 1403f
pediatric, 3719, 3720f
spinal, pediatric, 3590–3591, 3591f
treatment of
indications for, 1366
surgical, 1366–1367, 1367f
Fibrovascular stroma, in bone graft incorporation, 4619
Fick equation, 5048
Field potentials, 230–231
Filum terminale
dysgenesis of, 3264–3266, 3265f, 3266f
dysraphic anomalies of, 3247–3248
ependymoma of, 4296t, 4300–4301, 4819
treatment of, 4824
hypertrophic, 3264, 3265f
lipoma of, 3229
split spinal cord from, 3248, 3248f
paraganglioma of, classification of, 666–667
thickened, 4266–4267
tight, 4316
development of, 3247
Fimbria, 9, 2486, 2487f
Finger-to-nose test, 3179
Fishes, spinal cord regeneration in, 4156
Fistula
arteriovenous. *See* Arteriovenous fistula.
cavernous carotid. *See* Cavernous carotid fistula.
cerebrospinal fluid. *See* Cerebrospinal fluid fistula.
perilymph
temporal bone fracture and, 5281–5282
Fistula *(Continued)*
tympanotomy for, 2907
vertigo in, 2903–2904
traumatic, 2132
Fixation, internal. *See* Internal fixation.
Flap(s), galea-frontalis, in craniofacial trauma, 5258f–5259f
Flexion injury
to cervical spine, 4890, 4896, 4909, 4909f
to thoracic spine, 4958–4959, 4959f, 4962, 4962t
Flexion-rotation injury, to thoracic spine, 4959–4960, 4960f, 4980–4981
Flexor carpi ulnaris, in ulnar nerve compression, 3903
Flexor superficialis muscle, median nerve entrapment at, 3924
Flexor synovialis, in carpal tunnel syndrome, 3890
Flexor-pronator aponeurosis, in ulnar nerve compression, 3903
FLNA, 53t
Flocculus, 30, 30f, 31, 31f, 34, 36f, 40f
peduncle of, 32, 33f
Floor plate, notochord and, in primary neurulation, 4254–4255
Flow cytometry, in tumor proliferation marking, 694–695
Fluid management
in traumatic brain injury, 5130–5131, 5130f
intracranial pressure and, 188
Fluid pressure injury
hippocampus effects of, 2449, 2450
synaptic modification from, 2452, 2453f
Fluid shifts, in deep hypothermic circulatory arrest, 1536
^{11}C-Flumazenil, neuronal marking by, 1609
Fluorescence in situ hybridization, 747, 748f
2-[^{18}F]Fluoro-2-deoxy-D-glucose (FDG), positron emission tomography with, 480, 481t, 482
in brain tumors, 487, 487f–489f
in Huntington's disease, 483, 484f
of regional hypermetabolism, 490, 491f
[^{18}F]6-Fluoro-L-dopa, in positron emission tomography, 482, 483f
^{18}F-Fluoromisonidazole, hypoxia marking by, 1609
Fluoroscopy, image-guided spinal navigation and, 4754–4755, 4755f
5-Fluorouracil, for paranasal sinus tumors, 1327
Foam cells, in xanthogranuloma formation, 1444
Folate
deficiency of, neural tube defects from, 3217–3218
supplemental, 3218, 3218t
Foley catheter, complications of, patient positioning and, 614
Folic acid
deficiency of, in occult spinal dysraphism, 3257–3258
recommended daily allowances for, 3218
supplemental, in pregnancy, 871
Folium, 34
Folstein Mini-Mental Status Testing, 242t
Fontan's space, 4674
Foot
abnormalities of, nerve damage and, 3833, 3833f
digital nerve entrapment in, 3936
Foot drop, nerve injury and, 3823

Football injuries, to cervical spine, 4887
Foramen caecum, inferior, 30f
Foramen magnum
erosion of, 431
in achondroplasia, 3364
in Chiari malformation type I, 3348
in craniovertebral junction developmental abnormalities, 3338, 3339f
meningioma of, 1121, 1122f, 1123, 1123f, 4809, 4811–4812, 4811f
tumors of, 4800–4801
Foramen magnum basilar angle, 425, 425f
Foramen of Luschka, 32
rhomboid lip of, 30–31, 31f
Foramen of Magendie, historical aspects of, 3150
Foramen of Monro, 4f, 7, 7f, 8f, 9, 10f, 14f, 15f
colloid cyst in, 3687
in third ventricular tumor surgery, 1255–1256
obstruction of
giant cell astrocytoma and, 3390, 3391f
hydrocephalus from, 3389–3391, 3390f, 3391f
shunt failure in, 3390–3391
treatment of, 3390
Foramen ovale
electrodes in, 2557, 2561
in thermal rhizotomy, 2999, 2999f
Forceps major, 8
Forearm
anterior interosseous nerve surgery in, 650–651, 651f
median nerve surgery in, 650–651, 650f, 651f
posterior interosseous nerve surgery in, 651, 652f
radial nerve surgery in, 651, 652f
ulnar nerve surgery in, 652
Foregut cyst. *See* Neurenteric cyst.
Foreign body
in upper airway obstruction, 5246
retained, in spinal surgery, 575
Foreign body giant cells, after arteriovenous malformation embolization, 2226, 2227f
Fornix, 7f, 8f, 10–11, 10f, 14f, 15f, 26f, 1237, 1238f, 2486, 2487f
crus of, 11
surgical complications of, 1259–1260
venous drainage of, 1238
Fourth ventricle, 29–32, 30f, 31f
cavernous malformations of, 2323
choroid plexus tumors of, 3618
dermoid tumor of, 3691
ependymoma of, pediatric, 3624, 3625, 3626f, 3627
floor of, 34
glioma of, pediatric, 3666, 3667
in Chiari malformation type II, 3350, 3351f
junctional part of, 34
outlet foramina of, obstruction of, 3393, 3394f
shunt failure in, 3394
treatment of, 3393–3394, 3395f
petrosal surface of, 30–32, 30f, 31f
roof of, 31, 31f
veins of, 35f
suboccipital surface of, 33–34
tentorial surface of, 32–33, 33f
tumors of, 831
Foxa2, 53t
Foxb1, 53t
Fractionated stereotactic radiotherapy, 4136, 4138, 4138f
linacs for, 4115
Fracture(s)
atlantoaxial, 4906, 4906f, 4907f
atlas, 4903, 4903f, 4925, 4933–4935. *See also* Atlas fracture.
axial, 4903–4906, 4903f–4907f, 4904t, 4906t, 4925, 4939–4947
imaging of, 518f, 519, 519f
pain in, 4306–4307, 4307t
burst
atlas, 501f, 519
cervical spine, 4896–4897, 4907, 4908f
biomechanics of, 4189
lumbar spine, 4993, 4995f
percutaneous screws/rods in, 5006, 5006f
treatment of, 4999
thoracic spine, 4955, 4956f, 4962, 4962t
biomechanics of, 4192
Denis type D, 4960f
stable vs. unstable, 4959, 4959f
surgery for, 4979–4980
treatment guidelines for, 4967t
thoracolumbar spine, 521, 522f, 4993, 4995f
treatment of, 4999
calvarial, 425–427, 426f, 427f
cervical spine, 4896–4897. *See also* Cervical spine, trauma to.
Chance, 521, 522f
clay shoveler's, 4910
complex atlantoaxial, 4934, 4935f
compression
cervical spine, 4907
metastases and, 531, 531f, 4855, 4856f
thoracic spine, 4955, 4956f, 4958, 4959f, 4961–4962, 4962t
surgery for, 4979
treatment guidelines for, 4967t
craniofacial, 5251–5262. *See also* Craniofacial trauma.
dens, 519, 519f
depressed. *See* Skull fracture, depressed.
flexion, thoracic spine, 4958–4959, 4959f
flexion-rotation, thoracic spine, 4959–4960, 4960f, 4980–4981
hangman's, 520, 520f, 4905–4906, 4905f, 4906f, 4906t, 4940f, 4945–4947, 4946t
humeral
radial nerve entrapment in, 3928
shaking-impact syndrome and, 3502f
Jefferson's, 501f, 519, 4903, 4903f, 4934, 4934f
limbus vertebral, in lumbar spinal stenosis, 4531
lumbar spine
classification of, 4992–4997, 4993t
flexion-distraction, 521, 522f
seat belt–type injury and, 4993, 4996f
surgery for, decompression/ instrumentation in, 5004–5005
occipital condyle, 4902, 4925
classification of, 4927, 4927f
clinical presentation of, 4926–4927
delivery and, 3483, 3483f
diagnosis of, 4927, 4927f
treatment of, 4927–4928
odontoid, 4934, 4939–4947. *See also* Odontoid fracture.
pelvic, lumbosacral plexus injury in, 3970
posterior arch, 4933
Fracture(s) *(Continued)*
rhinorrhea in, 5267–5268
sacral, 5011–5016. *See also* Sacral fracture.
sella turcica, cerebrospinal fluid fistula in, 5267
skull, 425–427, 426f, 427f, 5057. *See also* Skull fracture.
skull base, 427–428
cerebrospinal fluid fistula in, 5267
three-dimensional imaging of, 435f, 436
spinal
imaging of, 517–523
in ankylosing spondylitis, 4461, 4469–4470, 4470f
unstable, 4877–4878
subaxial, 4907–4908, 4908f, 4908t
teardrop, 4907–4908, 4908f
temporal bone, 5275–5284
thoracic spine, 4951–4982. *See also* Thoracic spine, fractures of.
thoracolumbar spine, 521, 521f, 522f, 4149, 4997–4998. *See also* Thoracolumbar spine fracture.
wedge compression, 521, 521f
lumbar spine, 4993, 4994f
treatment of, 4998–4999, 4999f
thoracic spine, 4952, 4958, 4959f
Fracture-dislocation, thoracolumbar spine, 4993, 4996–4997, 4997f
treatment of, 4999
Frankel/ASIA Impairment, 242t
Fraud, legal issues in, 413–414
Free radical scavengers, for brain edema, 802
Free radicals
after traumatic brain injury, 5084
in cerebral vasospasm, 1848
in ischemic injury, 1517–1518
radiation and, 3999
Freezing, 2730
Friedreich's ataxia, 4320–4321
Frontal bone
comminuted fracture of, 5260f
depressed fracture of, three-dimensional imaging of, 433, 433f
segmental fracture of, 435f
Frontal cortex, in psychiatric disorders, 2855
Frontal gyrus
inferior, 3, 4f
medial, 24f
middle, 3, 4f
superior, 3, 4f
Frontal horn, 4f, 7, 7f, 8f, 15f, 1237, 1238f
in Chiari malformation type II, 3350
tumors of
transcallosal approach to, 1241–1242
transcortical approach to, 1242
veins of, 17
Frontal lobe, 3–4, 4f
arteriovenous malformation of, 2243
basal surface of, 17
hemorrhage of, 1738, 1738f
in micturition, 359, 360, 360f
injury to, urologic disorders from, 373
orbital surface of, 17
resection of, complications of, 2577
seizures in, 2589
tumors of, 830
venous drainage of, 16, 23, 24f, 28
Frontal sinus
compound injury to, 5166
surgery for, 5166, 5168f–5169f, 5170

Frontal sinus *(Continued)*
fracture of, 425
bone material for, 5258f–5259f
rhinorrhea in, 5268
in esthesioneuroblastoma surgery, 1338, 1338f
repair of, 5252–5253
trauma to, 5259f
Frontal sulcus, superior, 4f
Frontal veins
inferior, 23
medial, 28
Fronto-orbital artery, 26f
Fronto-orbital vein, 24f
Frontopolar artery, 26f, 27
Frontosphenoid suture, 1321f
Frontosylvian vein, 16
Frontotemporal region, epidural hematoma of, 5043
Frozen back syndrome, 4329
Functional Independence Measure, 243t, 5288, 5289t
Functional magnetic resonance imaging, 448–449, 449f, 852–853, 853f
in vision mapping, 2544–2546, 2545f
Functional radiosurgery, 4087–4093, 4114–4116. *See also* Radiosurgery.
Fundus, pediatric, examination of, 3173
Fungal infection
axial spine, 4295
magnetic resonance imaging of, 463
mycotic aneurysm from, 2102
myelitis from, 4312t, 4313
spinal, 4387–4390, 4388f, 4389f
Furosemide
brain dehydration with, 1505
for pseudotumor cerebri, 1429
in distal anterior cerebral artery aneurysm surgery, 1950
Fusiform gyrus, 18f
Fusion
anterior lumbar interbody, 4717, 4718f
laparoscopic, 4788–4791, 4790f
Spine-Tech BAK device for, 4722, 4723f–4724f
atlantoaxial, pediatric, 3547, 3548f, 3549f
instrumentation with, 3547, 3549–3550, 3549f, 3550f
bone grafts in, 4613–4620. *See also* Bone grafts.
cervical spine, 4440, 4626–4629, 4628f
biomechanics in, 4193–4194
bone grafts in, 4607–4608, 4607f, 4622, 4628f
for degenerative spondylolisthesis, 4532–4533
for lumbar spinal stenosis, 4533–4534
for spondylolysis, 4554, 4554f
healing of, tobacco and, 4619–4620
interbody, with bone morphogenetic protein, 4792–4794, 4793f
occipitocervical, 4655–4668
of neural folds, 4250–4251
pediatric, unintentional extension of, 3552–3553
posterior
laminoforaminotomy with, 4416, 4416f, 4417f
of pediatric cervical spine, 3546–3547
posterior lumbar interbody, complication avoidance in, 581–582
premature, of sutures, 3304–3305, 3305t
principles of, 4599–4600
spondylolisthesis after, 4547, 4548f
thoracic spine, allograft in, 4975–4978

Fusion *(Continued)*
thoracolumbar spine, bone grafts in, 4608, 4608f
transthoracic, anterior, 4680–4683, 4681f, 4682f
decompression and, for burst fracture, 4980
F-wave, 3855, 3855f

G protein, in McCune-Albright syndrome, 3719
G protein–linked receptor molecules, 75
G_1 pathway, 717, 717f
G207 virus, cytopathic-oncolytic capability of, 822
G380R, in achondroplasia, 3362
GABAergic interneurons, migration of, 80
Gabapentin
for cerebral palsy, 3731
for multiple sclerosis, 1454t
for neuropathic pain, 2960, 3838
for pain, 2965
pharmacology of, 2470t, 2472
Gag response testing, pediatric, 3186
Gait. *See also* Ambulation.
abnormalities of
in brain tumors, 829–830
in cerebral palsy, 3729–3730
in Parkinson's disease, 2732
analysis of, 269, 3744
antalgic, 3180
ataxic, 3180. *See also* Ataxia.
determinants of, 3729
hemiplegic, 3180
pediatric, assessment of, 3180
spastic, 3180
Galactorrhea, in prolactinoma, 1185
Galveston Orientation and Amnesia Test, 5195, 5195t, 5289
Gamma knife radiosurgery, 4115, 4117–4121, 4118f–4121f, 4131–4132. *See also* Radiosurgery.
Gammopathy, monoclonal, 3841
Ganciclovir, in gene transfer, 819
Gangliocytoma
cerebellar dysplastic, 666
classification of, 666
Ganglioglioma, 981–984, 4302
clinical presentation of, 981
desmoplastic infantile, 991
in epilepsy, 2578
MIB-1 labeling index for, 702, 702t
natural history of, 981
outcome of, 983–984
pathology of, 982–983
pediatric, 3699–3700, 3700f, 3701f
intramedullary, 3709f
pathology of, 3701
surgery for, 3702
proliferation markers for, 702, 702t
radiography of, 981–982, 982f
radiologic features of, 846f, 847
treatment of, 983–984
Ganglion cyst, 3947t, 3948
decompressive surgery for, 4337
magnetic resonance imaging of, 3875–3876, 3877f
Ganglionectomy, 3028, 3033–3042
cervical, 3035–3036, 3037f
complications of, 3039–3040
dorsal root, 3035–3037
evaluation before, 3035
for cancer pain, 3034, 3040, 3040t
indications for, 3034–3035

Ganglionectomy *(Continued)*
lumbar, 3035–3037
modifications of, 3039
percutaneous radiofrequency, 3037–3038
results of, 3040–3042, 3040t, 3041t
thoracic, 3035, 3036f
Ganglioneuroblastoma, 1394
Ganglioneuroma, 1394
peripheral nerve involvement in, 3950
spinal cord, 4821
Gangliosides, in spinal cord injury, 4876
Gap junctions
electrical communication through, 226–227
in blood-brain barrier, 157
Gardner's syndrome, brain tumors in, 812t, 813
Gardner-Wells tongs, in cervical traction, 4891
Gasserian ganglion, 3048
trigeminal nerve and, 1344
Gastrocnemius muscle, 653
Gastrocytoma. *See* Neurenteric cyst.
Gastrointestinal tract
disorders of
after aneurysmal subarachnoid hemorrhage, 1831
in cerebral palsy, 3727
in pediatric neurorehabilitation, 3787
in spinal cord injury management, 4881
preoperative evaluation of, 550
Gastrulation, 47, 4240f, 4241, 4271–4272
disorders of, 4263–4266, 4263f–4267f, 4277
in cyst development, 1223, 1226
Gate control theory, of pain, 2915, 2953, 3107, 3119
Gaze
conjugate, examination of, 266
disturbances of, supranuclear abnormalities and, 3174
periodic alternating, 293
ping-pong, 293
Gaze test, of vestibular function, 345
Gbx2, 53t
Gender
in aneurysm rupture, 1790
in intracranial hematoma, 5072
in mild head injury, 5067
in pediatric lumbar disk herniation, 3560
Gene(s), 712–714
after central nervous system injury, 4154–4155
characterization of, 712
developmental families of, 51–52, 51t
expression of, 713–714
in mice, 714
traumatic brain injury and, 5028
homeotic, 51
in brain tumors, 750, 751t
in central nervous system malformations, 46t
manipulation of, 712
organizer, 51, 51t, 53t–55t
regulator, 51, 51t, 52, 53t–55t
transfer of, 817
positron emission tomography of, 492, 492f
transfection in, 713
viral vectors in, 713–714
Gene mapping, in primary craniosynostosis, 3305–3306
Gene therapy, 817–822
adenoviral vectors for, 818
angiosuppression with, 783

Gene therapy *(Continued)*
antiangiogenic, 821–822
cell cycle modulators in, 820–821
cytopathic-oncolytic viruses in, 822
for brain tumors, 818–822
for central nervous system repair, 4166–4167
for gliomas, 711–721
for lumbar disk disease, 4794–4795
for neoplastic meningitis, 1233
for recurrent carotid stenosis, 1665
immune modulation in, 821
in CNS transplantation, 2844–2845
retroviral vectors for, 817–818
suicide, 818–820, 818f–820f
transfer-mediated drug targeting in, 818–820, 818f–820f
tumor suppressor genes in, 820–821
vector systems for, 818
Generalization, 235
Generators, implantable
for deep brain stimulation, 2817–2819, 2818f, 2824, 3126
for electrical stimulation, 3110–3111, 3111f
Genetic factors
in achondroplasia, 3362–3363
in anaplastic astrocytoma, 969–970
in aneurysms, 1769–1776
in carotid body tumors, 1678
in cavernous malformations, 2168
in familial cerebral cavernous malformations, 2299–2303
in glioblastoma multiforme, 969–970
in hemangioblastoma, 1053–1054, 1054t
in hypochondroplasia, 3362
in malignant glioma, 969–970
in neurological disease, 263–264
in neurotraumatology, 5021
in posterior longitudinal ligament ossification, 4475, 4476–4477
in thanatophoric dysplasia, 3362
in von Hippel-Lindau disease, 1053–1054
Geniculate body, 10f, 12f
Geniculocalcarine tract, 2541–2542
Gentamicin, for Ménière's disease, 2906
Geranylgeranyl transferase inhibitors, angiosuppressive therapy with, 780
Germ cell tumors
classification of, 667–668, 667t, 3603, 3603t
congenital, 3604
mixed, 667–668, 667t
nongerminoma, 667–668, 3603
pediatric, 3604, 3607–3608, 3607f
chemotherapy for, 3610
location of, 3606
radiation therapy for, 3609–3610
surgery for, 3608
pediatric, 3603–3610
chemotherapy for, 3610
clinical presentation of, 3604, 3606
diagnosis of, 3606–3608
epidemiology of, 3604, 3605f
location of, 3604
radiation therapy for, 3608–3610
surgery for, 3608, 3609f
pure vs. mixed, 1015t
radiation therapy for, 4023–4024
radiologic features of, 839
treatment of, tumor type and, 3603–3604
tumorigenesis of, 3603, 3603f, 3604f
Germinal matrix
embryology of, 3405–3406, 3406f
subependymal, hemorrhage into, 3405, 3406f. *See also* Hydrocephalus, infantile posthemorrhagic.

Germinal matrix *(Continued)*
injury pattern in, 3407, 3407f
neuropathology from, 3407–3408
pathogenesis of, 3406f, 3407
severity of, 3408, 3408t
Germinoma
classification of, 667, 667t
pediatric
chemotherapy for, 3610
diagnosis of, 3606–3607, 3606f
magnetic resonance imaging of, 3605f
radiation therapy for, 3608–3609
surgery for, 3608
pure, pediatric, 3604, 3606
radiation therapy for, 4023–4024
radiologic features of, 839, 839f, 849
third ventricular, 1247
Giacomini's band, 26f
Giant aneurysms, 2079–2096
arterial bypass for, 2117–2118
clinical presentation of, 2081
deep hypothermic circulatory arrest for, 1529, 1530f, 1531, 1531f
diagnosis of, 2081, 2082f, 2083
distribution of, 2080t
embolization of, 2067
endovascular occlusion of, 1805, 2093, 2096, 2096f
epidemiology of, 2080
historical considerations in, 2079–2080, 2080t
incidence of, 2080
outcome in, 2079, 2080t
pathophysiology of, 2080–2081
surgery for, 1802–1803, 2089–2093
aneurysmectomy in, 2093, 2094f, 2095f
anterior circulation approach to, 2084, 2084f–2086f
bypass techniques in, 2091, 2092f, 2093, 2093f
clipping techniques in, 2090, 2090f
combined approach to, 2088–2089, 2089f
far-lateral approach to, 2087–2088, 2088f
interhemispheric approach to, 2087
occlusion techniques in, 2090–2091, 2091f–2095, 2093
orbitozygomatic approach to, 2087, 2087f
orbitozygomatic pterional approach to, 2084, 2084f–2086f
posterior circulation approach to, 2087–2089, 2087f–2089f
skull base approach to, 2083–2084, 2083f, 2083t
subtemporal approach to, 2089
transpetrosal approach to, 2087, 2088f
vascular control in, 2089–2090
treatment of, 2083–2096
Giant arteriovenous malformations, 2267–2280
embolization of, 2269–2270
hemodynamics of, 2268–2269
imaging of, 2269
location of, 2268
microsurgery for, 2270–2272
presentation of, 2267
stereotactic radiosurgery for, 2270
surgery for
angiography during, 2273
complications of, 2273, 2274f–2279f, 2275, 2280
contraindications to, 2268
evaluation before, 2269

Giant arteriovenous malformations *(Continued)*
hypothermia during, 2273
indications for, 2267–2268
monitoring during, 2272
multimodality treatment of, 2272
outcomes of, 2273
stereotaxis during, 2273
ultrasound during, 2273
treatment of, 2125–2126
Giant cell arteritis, anterior ischemic optic neuropathy in, 306, 307
Giant cell astrocytoma
radiologic features of, 844
subependymal, 991–992, 992f
classification of, 663
foramen of Monro obstruction from, 3390, 3391f
third ventricular, 1246
Giant cell tumors, 1367
in Paget's disease, 1400
skull, 1388
spinal, 4296t, 4297, 4355, 4355f, 4837, 4851f
imaging of, 4850, 4852f
pediatric, 3589
Gibbous deformity, in pyogenic spinal infection, 4366
Gigantism, growth hormone excess and, 1189
Gilford orthoses, 4899
Gilles de la Tourette syndrome, 2722
Glabella, loss of, in craniofacial trauma, 5262
Glasgow Coma Scale, 242t, 286–287, 286t, 5040–5041, 5041t
assessment with, 5103, 5104t
eye opening in, 287
in altered consciousness management, 293
in anesthesia, 1505, 1505t
in children, 3464
in head injury, 555–556, 556t, 5088, 5088t
in mild head injury, 5073
in neurological assessment, 5090
in neurotraumatology, 5018
in pediatric head injury, 3473, 3474, 3474t
in trauma assessment, 5088, 5088t
in traumatic brain injury, 5145–5146, 5288, 5288t
intracranial pressure monitoring and, 185
strengths and limits to, 5194–5196, 5195t, 5196f
Glasgow Coma Score
in bullet wounds, 5237–5240, 5237t, 5238t
intraoperative hypotension and, 1551–1552
Glasgow Outcome Scale, 242t, 5103, 5105t
in brainstem cavernous malformation outcome, 2338
GLAST, 103, 104f–105f, 230
Glatitramer acetate, for multiple sclerosis, 1454t, 1455
Glia
extracellular space size and, 230
gap junction communication in, 227
ion channels in, 219–226, 225, 226f
Glia-derived neurotrophic factor
after peripheral nerve injury, 3967, 3968
in nervous system regeneration, 4155
Glial action potentials, 221

Glial cell(s)
abnormal proliferation of, 2492
in central nervous system repair, 4162–4163
in potassium spatial buffering, 2455
potassium ion distribution by, 102, 104f
radical, 79f, 80, 84, 97, 98f
Glial cell line–derived growth factor
delivery of, positron emission tomography in, 492–493, 493f
in axonal regeneration, 199–200
Glial cell line–derived neurotrophic factor
in axonal regeneration, 200
in central nervous system transplantation, 2843–2844
Glial fibrillary acidic protein, 97
after central nervous system injury, 4168
in Alexander's disease, 111
in diffuse fibrillary astrocytoma, 661
in medulloblastoma, 3640, 3646
Glial membrane potential, in potassium redistribution, 2455
Glial scar, in axonal regeneration, 205
Glial tumors, 4296t
in pregnancy, 870–871, 870f
mixed, classification of, 665–667, 666t
oligodendrocyte progenitor cells and, 92–93
radiosurgery for, 4063–4065, 4064t
spinal cord, 4825
third ventricular, 1246
Glioblastoma
brachytherapy for, 4097
classification of, 662
contiguous spread of, 757
deep vein thrombosis risk in, 939
EGFR amplification in, 950
fibroblast growth factor receptor in, 728
gene alterations in, 751t
low copper diet in, 781
multifocal spread of, 758, 758f
mutations in, 715
platelet-derived growth factor receptor in, 730
vascular endothelial growth factor receptor in, 733
Glioblastoma multiforme
anaplastic, 969
bromodeoxyuridine marking of, 693
cytometric cell-cycle analysis of, 695
diagnosis of, 972, 973f
DNA polymerase marking of, 694
genetics of, 726, 969–970
histopathology of, 970–971, 971f
incidence of, 4018
interstitial brachytherapy for, 4097
Ki-67/MIB-1 marking of, 696
necrosis in, 843f–844f, 844
prognosis for, 977–978
proliferating cell nuclear antigen marking of, 694
radiation therapy for, 975
radiologic features of, 842, 842f
radiosurgery for, 4063–4065, 4064t
recurrent, treatment of, 976–977, 977f
seizures in, 828
third ventricular, 1246
^{3}H-thymidine marking of, 692
vascular endothelial growth factor in, 733
Glioblastosis cerebri, classification of, 662–663
Gliofibroma, 990
Gliogenesis, 97, 98f
Glioma, 981–994. *See also* specific type, e.g., Astrocytoma.
angionecrotic, 772
brain edema in, 795
brainstem. *See* Brainstem, glioma of.
bromodeoxyuridine marking of, 692–693
"butterfly," 970f
cell cycle arrest pathways in, 717–718
cellular biology of, 714–720
chordoid, third ventricle, 664
cystic, intracavitary brachytherapy for, 4106–4107
diffuse chiasmatic, pediatric, 3596, 3597
DNA polymerase marking of, 694
electrophysiologic abnormalities in, 230
endothelial proliferation in, 771–772
exophytic chiasmatic-hypothalamic, pediatric, 3596, 3597, 3598
gene therapy for, 711–721
incidence of, 808–809, 809t, 950
insulin-like growth factors in, 728–729
intramedullary, pediatric, 3708
low-grade, 950–966
chemotherapy for, 964
computer-assisted stereotactic resections of, 956
histopathology of, 951–953, 951f, 952f
magnetic resonance imaging of, 953, 954f
magnetic resonance spectroscopy of, 954, 955f
malignant transformation of, 954–956
misdiagnosis of, 955
outcome in, 965–966
preoperative characteristics of, 953–954, 954f, 955f
prognostic factors in, 964–965
radiation therapy for, 962–964, 963t
stereotactic biopsy of, 955–956
surgery for, 955–962
frameless navigation systems in, 956, 958f
imaging during, 956–957
magnetic source imaging in, 956, 957f
prognosis of, 957, 959, 959t–962t
sonographic navigation in, 956, 958f
stimulation mapping techniques in, 956, 956f
timing of, 955–956
type of, 956–957
magnetic resonance imaging of, 449–450, 450f–454f, 452–453
malignant, 757–766, 969–978, 4018
adhesion molecules in, 760–763
brachytherapy for, 757
cadherins in, 763
cell surface adhesion molecules in, 763
chemotherapy for, 975–976
collagen in, 761
computed tomography of, 758–759
contiguous spread of, 757
diagnosis of, 972, 973f
distant recurrence of, 757–758
epidemiology of, 969
extracellular matrix molecules in, 761–763
familial, 969–970
fibronectin in, 761
genetics of, 969–970
glycoproteins in, 762
glycosaminoglycan in, 762
grading of, 970–972, 970f–972f
histopathology of, 970–972, 970f–972f
hyaluronate receptors in, 763
Glioma *(Continued)*
immunoglobulin superfamily in, 763
integrins in, 763
interstitial brachytherapy for, 4101–4104, 4102t, 4103t
intraoperative mapping techniques for, 974, 974f
invasion in, 757–766
laminin in, 761
magnetic resonance imaging of, 758–759
multifocal, 758, 758f
neutron therapy for, 4020–4021
pediatric, chemotherapy for, 3703
prognosis for, 977–978
proteoglycans in, 762–763
radiation therapy for, 974–975
high-dose, 4019, 4019t
particle beam radiation in, 4020–4021
prognostic factors in, 4021, 4021t
radiosensitization of, 4019–4020
radiosurgery for, 758, 4063–4065, 4064t
recurrent, 4103–4104, 4103t
seizures in, 828
spread of
along basement membrane, 760, 760f
animal models of, 764–765
anti-invasion therapy for, 765–766
by cerebrospinal fluid, 760
clinical patterns of, 757–758
cytostatics for, 765–766
experimental models for, 763–765
mechanism of, 759–760, 760f
molecular basis of, 760
through white matter, 759–760
surgery for, 972–974, 974f
tenascin in, 761–762
thrombospondin in, 762
treatment of, 972–977
molecular biology of, 714–720
mutations in, 714–715
optic nerve, 309, 1373
focal manifestations of, 831
prechiasmatic, pediatric, 3596
optic pathway, pediatric, 3595–3599. *See also* Optic pathway glioma, pediatric.
proliferating cell nuclear antigen marking of, 693
proliferation markers for, 689–705, 690f, 690t
mitotic activity as, 689–692
molecular, 692–696
signal transduction in, 715–716, 716f
surgery for
complication avoidance in, 566–567, 566t, 567t
tumor removal in, 905
^{3}H-thymidine marking of, 692
treatment of
angiogenesis in, 720
cell cycle arrest pathways in, 717f, 718
invasion and, 720
molecular targets for, 720, 721f
programmed cell death in, 719
signal transduction in, 716, 716f
usual types of, 981–994
vascular endothelial growth factor in, 733
vascular endothelial growth factor receptors in, 733
ventricular, endoscopic treatment of, 3429, 3429f

Gliomatosis cerebri
  magnetic resonance imaging of, 452
  radiologic features of, 842, 842f
Gliosarcoma, 1141
  histopathology of, 970–971, 972f
Gliosis, 204
Gliotic lesions, in extratemporal lobe epilepsy, 2598
Globus pallidus, 10f, 11, 12f, 13, 2671, 2672, 2672f, 2673, 2730
  γ-aminobutyric acid receptors in, 2688–2689, 2688f
  external, 2683, 2731
    projections of, 2687, 2699
    stimulation of, 2819
    striatal projection to, 2700–2701
  glutamate receptors in, 2688–2689, 2688f
  in drug-induced dyskinesia, 2677
  in dystonia, 2678
  in Huntington's disease, 2676
  in parkinsonism, 2673–2674, 2674f
  in subthalamic nucleus lesions, 2676
  internal, 2683, 2731
    in basal ganglia–thalamocortical circuits, 2699, 2700f
    projections to tegmental pedunculopontine nucleus from, 2693, 2694f, 2695
    projections to thalamus from, 2691–2693, 2692f
    stimulation of, 2804, 2805f, 2817
      complications of, 2823
      electrophysiologic studies in, 2813, 2815
      results of, 2821
    subthalamic nucleus projection to, 2701
  lesions of, surgery for, 2675
  neurons of, 2688–2689, 2688f
  progressive atrophy of, 2719–2720
  stereotactic surgery on, in Parkinson's disease, 2659
Globus pallidus internalis, stereotactic surgery on, 2660
Glomus body, 8f
  distribution of, 1297
  tumors arising from, 1297
Glomus jugulare tumors, 1295–1308
  blood supply of, 1307
  classification of, 1297–1298, 1298t
  clinical presentation of, 1298
  diagnosis of, 1298
  embolization of, 1300–1301, 1300f, 1307
  epidemiology of, 1298
  extension routes of, 1297
  historical perspective on, 1295–1297
  jugular body location in, 1295
  laboratory studies for, 1300
  natural history of, 1298
  outcome in, 1308
  pathology of, 1297–1298, 1297f
  radiation therapy for, 1305
  radiologic features of, 1298–1300, 1299f
  skull, 1397, 1397f
  surgical approaches to, 1301–1305
    blood control during, 1307
    cerebrospinal fluid leak after, 1306–1307
    complications of, 1305–1308, 1306t
    cranial nerve deficit after, 1305–1306
    infection with, 1307
    infratemporal fossa, 1304–1305, 1305f
    jugular foramen anatomy in, 1301–1302, 1301f
    lateral skull base, 1302–1304, 1303f, 1304f
Glomus jugulare tumors *(Continued)*
    meningitis after, 1307
    modified lateral skull base, 1304, 1305f
    wound healing in, 1307
  treatment of, 1300–1305
Glomus jugularis, 1295
Glomus tissue, 1295
Glomus tumors
  classification of, 1297
  historical perspective on, 1295, 1296
  peripheral nerve involvement in, 3950
  radiation therapy for, 1297
  skull, 1396–1397, 1397f
  stereotactic radiosurgery for, 1297
Glossopharyngeal nerve, 1973–1974
  examination of, 267
    pediatric, 3176
Glossopharyngeal neuralgia, 2989t
GLT-1, 103, 104f–105f, 230
Glucocorticoid receptors, in meningioma, 1108
Glucocorticoids
  for ankylosing spondylitis, 4467
  for brain edema, 801–802
  in bone metabolism, 4233
Glucose, 123
  brain metabolism of, 86, 117–118, 118f, 154, 1482–1484, 1483t, 1484f, 5047–5048
    astrocytes in, 107, 108f, 1487
    features of, 1483t
    positron emission tomography of, 1601
    stages of, 1484f
  in ischemia protection, 1521
  transport of, across blood-brain barrier, 15, 159–160, 159f
GLUT-1
  in blood-brain barrier, 15, 158–159
  in brain glucose transport, 159–160
GLUT-3, in brain glucose transport, 160
Glutamate
  as nociceptive synaptic neurotransmitter, 2927
  extracellular space and, 230
  in brain injury, 111
  in cell death, 126–128
  in cerebral metabolism, 1485–1486, 1485f
  in immune control, 684
  in traumatic brain injury, 2457–2458, 5084
  neurotoxicity from, in ischemic injury, 1517
  release of, 2953
  synthesis of, 104f–105f, 106–107
  transporters for, 230
    across blood-brain barrier, 161–162, 161f
    in astrocytes, 102–103, 104f–105f, 106
  uptake of, 103, 104f–105f, 106
Glutamate antagonists, in ischemia protection, 1522
Glutamate receptors, 2699, 2700f
  distribution of, 2689f
  in globus pallidus, 2688–2689, 2688f
  in striatum, 2686, 2686f
  in subthalamic nucleus, 2690–2691
  in traumatic brain injury, 5025–5026, 5026f
Glutamate-glutamine cycle, 104f–105f, 106
Glutamatergic receptor channels, in traumatic brain injury, 2451–2452, 2451f
Glutamine
  synthesis of, in astrocytes, 1486–1487
Glutamine *(Continued)*
  transport of, across blood-brain barrier, 160–161
γ-Glutamyltranspeptidase (GGT), in blood-brain barrier, 158, 161
Gluteal cleft
  in occult spinal dysraphism, 3261, 3262f
  in tethered spinal cord, 3249, 3249f
Glycerol
  intracranial pressure and, 189
  rhizotomy with, for trigeminal neuralgia, 2999–3000
Glycine antagonist, trials for, 1498
Glycocalyx, in postoperative spinal infections, 4384
Glycogen
  cerebral metabolism of, 1484–1485
  in astrocytes, 99, 101, 109
Glycogenesis, 1484–1485
Glycolysis, 118, 123
  aerobic, 1482, 1483–1484, 1483t
  anaerobic, in ischemic injury, 1515, 1517, 1517f
  in head injury, 5050–5051
Glycoprotein
  in malignant glioma, 762
  myelin-associated, axonal regeneration and, 199
P-Glycoprotein
  in multidrug resistance, 162–163, 877
  in multidrug resistance reversal, 879
Glycosaminoglycan, in malignant glioma, 762
Goiter, pituitary adenoma and, 1200
GOK/STIM 1, 744
Goldenhar's syndrome, craniovertebral junction abnormalities in, 3334
Goldman equation, 218–219
Golgi apparatus, 78
Gonadal insufficiency, in craniopharyngioma, 1210
Good Samaritan laws, 408
Gorlin's syndrome, medulloblastoma in, 997, 3639
Grafts, 2829, 2829t
  anterior interbody, in thoracic spine, 4680–4681
  bone. *See* Bone grafts.
  central nervous system, 2829, 2829t
  complications of, in anterior cervical approaches, 577
  extracranial carotid artery–to–middle cerebral artery saphenous vein interposition, 2110–2111, 2111f, 2112f
  extracranial carotid artery–to–posterior cerebral artery saphenous vein interposition, 2111, 2113
  in brachial plexus surgery, 3493, 3493f
  in pediatric internal fixation, 3546
  interposition, in carotid artery resection, 1665–1666, 1666f
  mesencephalic tissue, 2836–2837
  nerve, historical aspects of, 3803
  neural, vs. deep brain stimulation, 2824
  occipital artery–to–posterior inferior cerebral artery, 2113, 2115, 2115f, 2116f
  patency of, 2117
  peripheral nerve
    historical aspects of, 3803
    in central nervous system repair, 4161, 4162
  petrous-to-supraclinoid carotid saphenous vein, 2109, 2109f, 2110f

Grafts *(Continued)*
saphenous vein interposition, 2109–2111, 2111f, 2112f, 2113
in carotid artery procedures, 1627–1629, 1628f
sural nerve, in brachial plexus surgery, 3492
vein
for middle vertebral artery, 1703, 1705f
for proximal vertebral artery, 1700, 1701f
Grandiosity, in traumatic brain injury response, 5193t
Granular cell tumor, 3947t, 3948
neurohypophysis, 671
Granulation tissue, in bone graft incorporation, 4619
Granule cells, migration of, 80
Granulocyte-macrophage colony-stimulating factor (GM-CSF), in tumor vaccines, 892–893
Granuloma
cholesterol, 1443
eosinophilic
skull, 1400
spinal, 4355, 4837, 4843, 4845f
Granulomatous disease
pain in, 4293–4295, 4294f
radiologic features of, 835
spinal, 4352
imaging of, 541, 543f
Graphesthesia, pediatric, 3184
Grasp response testing, 3182
Graves' disease, 323
Graves' ophthalmopathy, 1376–1377
Gray, 4007
Gray matter
astrocytes in, 85–86
organization of, 2635
spinal cord
in nociception, 2923–2926, 2924f, 2925f, 2953, 2955
laminae in, 2923–2924, 2924f, 2927
neurons in, 2924, 2924f
primary afferent neurons of, 2924–2926, 2925f
Great horizontal fissure, 33f, 34
vein of, 35f
Greenstick osteotomy, in cervical laminoplasty, 4419–4420, 4419f
Grisel's syndrome, craniovertebral junction abnormalities in, 3337, 3337f
Grob "Y" screw plate, 4667f
Gross tumor volume, 4011, 4011f
Growth cone, axonal, 80
Growth factor receptors
brain tumor–related, 725–726, 726t
in glioma, 715
Growth factors
bone, 4608–4609, 4609t, 4614–4615
in posterior longitudinal ligament ossification, 4476
brain tumor–related, 725–733. *See also* specific factor, e.g., Fibroblast growth factor.
types of, 725–726, 726t
in angiogenesis, 775t
in brain injury recovery, 5031–5032
in distal nerve stump, 200
in medulloblastoma, 1033
modulation of, 733, 733t
suppression mechanisms for, 732f–733f, 733
Growth hormone
after pituitary surgery, 1191–1192, 1192t
in growth hormone–secreting pituitary adenoma, 1190
pseudotumor cerebri from, 1424
Growth hormone–releasing hormone–producing tumor, 1190
Growth retardation, in cerebral palsy, 3727, 3748
Growth-associated protein 43
after traumatic brain injury, 5032
in axonal regeneration, 197
Growth-promoting gene products, in axonal regeneration, 197
Gsc, 53t
Guam, Parkinson-dementia complex of, 2716
Guanosine monophosphate, cyclic, in cerebral blood flow regulation, 1470t
Guanosine triphosphatase–activating protein, 1773
Guanylate cyclase, in cerebral blood flow regulation, 1470t
Guardians, 409
Guglielmi detachable coil embolization
aneurysm rupture in, 2071–2072
aneurysm size and, 2066–2067
angiographic follow-up in, 2065–2066, 2065f
balloon-remodeling technique with, 2062, 2062f
coil herniation in, 2071
coil unraveling in, 2072
components of, 2060–2061, 2061f
histopathologic changes after, 2070–2071
hydrocephalus after, 2069–2070
in mass effect, 2067
infection in, 2072
ischemia during, 2071
of basilar bifurcation aneurysms, 2067–2068
of cavernous carotid fistula, 2346
of internal carotid artery ophthalmic segment aneurysm, 2068–2069
of middle cerebral artery aneurysm, 1969, 2069
of unruptured aneurysms, 2067
outcome in, 2064–2066, 2065f
rebleeding after, 2069
stent-coil technique with, 2063–2064, 2063f
surgical approach combined with, 2072–2074, 2073f
technique of, 2061–2062
thromboembolic complications of, 2071
vasospasm after, 2069–2070
Guilford brace, pediatric, 3544
Guillain-Barré syndrome, 3839
demyelinating polyneuropathy in, 3853
human immunodeficiency virus infection and, 3841
pathology of, 3816
Guinea worm infection, spinal, 4390
Gulf War, blood-brain barrier effects of, 14
Gunshot wounds. *See* Bullet wounds.
Guyon's canal, ulnar nerve entrapment in, 3928
GV150526, trials for, 1498
Gyri, 60f, 61
Gyrus rectus, resection of, 1934, 1934f

Habenula, 1245
Habenular commissure, 14f
Hagen-Poiseuille equation, 1468
Hair cells, vestibular, 74, 74f, 339, 340–341, 340f
Hair follicle tumors, 1415
Hair tuft
in congenital lumbosacral lipoma, 3236–3237
in occult spinal dysraphism, 3261, 3261f
Hallervorden-Spatz disease, 2720
Hallpike maneuver, vestibular function and, 342, 343f, 345
Hallucinations, baclofen and, 2886
Halo vest, 3334, 4899, 4899f
complications of, 576
for craniovertebral junction anomalies, 3336
for multiple myeloma, 4854
for odontoid fractures, 4940–4941
pediatric
complications of, 3543–3544
infection in, 3544
pin loosening in, 3543–3544
Halstead-Reitan Neuropsychological Test Battery, 386
Hamartoma, 992–993
hypothalamic
in epilepsy, 2578
magnetic resonance imaging of, 2494–2495, 2494f
Hamstring muscles, in isthmic spondylolisthesis, 3573
Hand
functional deficits in, upper extremity nerve disorders and, 3823
in brachial plexus obstetric palsy, 3980t
innervation of, 3898
myelopathic, 4448, 4449
Handicap, definition of, 3783
Hand-Schüller-Christian disease, 3719
Hand-Schüller-Christian syndrome, 1400–1401
Hangman's fracture, 520, 520f, 4905–4906, 4905f, 4906f, 4906t, 4940f, 4945–4947, 4946t
Harm, studies about, 259
Harms cage, for pyogenic spinal infection, 4376f–4379f
Harrington rod system, 4597
for thoracic spine fracture, 4952, 4964, 4969, 4969f
Head
elevation of, intracranial pressure and, 187
extension of, 2892–2893, 2892f, 2893f, 2896t
flexion of, 2893, 2895, 2896t
lateral tilting of, 2892, 2892f, 2895, 2896t
movements of, 2896t
cartesian axes and, 2891
pain in, surgery for, 3025t
positioning of, in craniotomy, 630
rotation of, 2892, 2892f, 2893, 2895, 2896t
secondary survey of, in trauma, 5090
shape abnormalities of, assessment of, 3300
size of, body size and, 3462
skeletal fixation of
complication avoidance in, 562–563
complications of, 610
Head circumference curves, in external hydrocephalus, 3397, 3397f
Head frame, for deep brain stimulation, 3123
Head injury. *See also* Brain injury.
airway management in, 5246
atlanto-occipital dislocation in, 4928

Head injury *(Continued)*
birth trauma and, 3481–3486. *See also* Birth trauma.
blood-brain barrier in, 166
brain dysfunction following, 5051t
brain protection in, 5059
carbon dioxide reactivity in, 5052–5053
cerebral autoregulation in, 5051–5052, 5053f
cerebral blood flow disturbances in, 5051–5053, 5051f, 5051t, 5053t
cerebral blood volume in, 5052
cerebral hypotension in, 1551–1552
cerebral ischemia in, 1552, 5051, 5051f, 5051t
cerebral metabolic disturbances in, 5050–5051
cerebral perfusion pressure management in, 5058
cerebrovascular reactivity in, 5051–5053, 5053t
child abuse and, 3499
outcomes of, 3508
treatment of, 3505–3507
circulatory stages after, 5046–5047, 5047t
classification of, 5040–5041, 5041t
extracranial, 5056–5057
anemia in, 5057
arterial hypoxia in, 5056
hyperglycemia in, 5057
pyrexia in, 5056–5057
systemic hypotension in, 5056
intracranial hypertension in, 184
intracranial pressure in, 5053–5055, 5054f
intraventricular hemorrhage in, 5047
luxury perfusion (hyperemia) in, 5051–5052
magnetic resonance imaging of, 469
meningioma from, 1104–1105
mild, 5065–5079
age in, 5067, 5072
amnesia after, 5073
causes of, 5066–5067, 5067t, 5072
coagulopathy in, 5074
computed tomography of, 5065, 5066t, 5069–5070, 5074–5075, 5077t
definition of, 5065–5066, 5066t
epidemiology of, 5066
gender in, 5067, 5072
Glasgow Coma Scale in, 5067–5069, 5068t, 5073
headache, vomiting, nausea in, 5072
hematoma in, 5071
risk factors for, 5071–5075
intracranial abnormalities in, 5070
lesion type in, 5070, 5071t
loss of consciousness in, 5073
magnetic resonance imaging of, 5077–5078
mental status in, 5073
neurological deficits in, 5072
neurological deterioration in, 5071
neurological examination in, 5077t
outcomes in, 5075
positron emission tomography of, 5079
race in, 5072
radiography of, 5076, 5077t
risk factors in, 5071–5075
seizures in, 5073
single photon emission computed tomography of, 5078
skull fracture in, 5074
substance abuse in, 5067
surgery for, 5070–5071

Head injury *(Continued)*
treatment of, 5075–5076, 5076t, 5077t, 5078f
mortality from, 5039, 5039t
pediatric, 3473–3478
epidemiology of, 3473
epidural hematoma in, 3475–3476, 3475f, 3476t
evaluation of, 3474–3475, 3474t
Glasgow Coma Scale in, 3473, 3474, 3474t
hyperventilation in, 3474–3475
intraparenchymal hematoma in, 3476
mass lesions in, 3475–3476
moderate, 3476–3477
monitoring of, 3478
outcomes in, 3477–3478
pathophysiology of, 3473–3474
recovery from, 3478
subarachnoid hemorrhage in, 3476, 3477f
subdural hematoma in, 3475f, 3476
surgery for, 3195–3196
physical processes causing, 5040
preoperative evaluation in, 555–556, 556t
pressure autoregulation after, 5052
prognosis of, blood flow velocity in, 1552
secondary brain displacement in, 5055–5056, 5055t
severity scale for, 5041, 5041t
transcranial Doppler ultrasonography after, 1550–1552, 1551f
traumatic aneurysm in, 2131–2133
treatment of, 5057–5059
intracranial pressure management in, 5057–5058
viscosity autoregulation after, 5052, 5053t
Headache, 276
after acoustic neuroma surgery, 1162
causes of, 276t
hyperextension-hyperflexion injury and, 4918
in arteriovenous malformations, 2163, 2206
in brain tumors, 828
in carotid artery dissection, 1685
in colloid cyst, 3688
in dural arteriovenous fistula, 2172
in increased intracranial pressure, 183
in low-grade glioma, 953
in pseudotumor cerebri, 1419
in subarachnoid hemorrhage, 1815
in venous malformation, 2175
migraine, 276t
temporal lobectomy and, 2611
tension-type, 276t
Headrests, pressure necrosis from, 610
Health states, 2567
Healthcare fraud, legal issues in, 413–414
Health-related quality of life, in epilepsy, 2574
Health-related quality of life instruments, in epilepsy, 2565, 2567f
Hearing
physiology of, 328–330
preservation of, in acoustic neuroma surgery, 1160
Hearing assessment
acoustic reflex in, 334, 335f–336f
air conduction testing in, 331, 331f, 332f
auditory brainstem evoked response in, 334–335, 336f
bone conduction testing in, 331, 331f, 332f

Hearing assessment *(Continued)*
electrically evoked auditory potentials in, 337
immittance studies in, 333–334, 335f
in auditory neuropathy, 336–337
masking in, 331–332
objective measures in, 333–338
otoacoustic emission measures in, 337–338
pediatric, 3175–3176
pure-tone audiometry in, 331–332, 331f, 332f
speech audiometry in, 332–333, 333f
subjective measures in, 330–333, 331f–333f
tuning fork tests in, 330
tympanometry in, 333–334
Hearing loss
acoustic neuroma surgery and, 570
after midbrain tractotomy, 3056
conductive, in temporal bone fracture, 5280–5281
in brain tumors, 829
in cerebral palsy, 3728
in temporal bone fracture, 5280
in trigeminal schwannoma, 1345, 1345f
sensorineural, in temporal bone fracture, 5281
Heart, in infectious intracranial aneurysm, 2104
Heart disease
embolization in, 1495
in stroke, 1625
Heart failure, in vein of Galen malformations, 3434–3435, 3435f, 3441–3442
Heat injury, peripheral nerve, 3828
Heel-to-shin test, 3179
Helicotrema, 328
Hemangioblastoma, 1053–1060
angiography of, 1056, 1057f
capillary, 670–671, 671t
clinical presentation of, 1054–1055
conditions related to, 1058–1060
cystic, spinal cord, 2355f
diagnosis of, 1055–1056, 1055f–1057f
epidemiology of, 1053–1054, 1054t
gene alterations in, 751t
genetics of, 1053–1054, 1054t
imaging of, 525, 525f
in pregnancy, 872
intramedullary, 4302
magnetic resonance imaging of, 1055–1056, 1055f, 1056f
MIB-1 labeling index for, 703
pathology of, 1058, 1059f, 1060f
peripheral nerve involvement in, 3949–3950
polycythemia in, 1055
proliferation markers for, 703–704
radiation therapy for, 1058
radiologic features of, 850, 851f
spinal cord, 1054, 2353, 2354f, 2355f, 4825, 4826, 4828f
treatment of, 4828, 4831
sporadic, 1054
supratentorial, 1054–1055
surgery for, 1056–1058
treatment of, 1056–1058
Hemangioma, 4297
capillary
in congenital lumbosacral lipoma, 3237
in occult spinal dysraphism, 3259, 3260f, 3261

Hemangioma (Continued)
vascular endothelial growth factor in, 733
cavernous. See Cavernous malformations.
in tethered spinal cord, 3249, 3249f
peripheral nerve involvement in, 3949
scalp, 1413–1414
skull, 1384–1385
pediatric, 3720–3721
spinal, imaging of, 4841, 4842f
vertebral body, 4354–4355, 4355f, 4837, 4840–4843, 4842f
imaging of, 532
pediatric, 3589–3590
Hemangiopericytoma, 1133
meningeal, 1133–1138. See also Meningeal hemangiopericytoma.
MIB-1 labeling index for, 703, 704t
orbital, 1375
peripheral nerve involvement in, 3950
proliferation markers for, 703, 704t
radiation therapy for, 4023
radiologic features of, 841
Hematocrit
in head injury, 5058–5059
in pregnancy, 2421
Hematologic system, preoperative evaluation of, 550
Hematoma
after craniotomy, 5176, 5177f, 5178f, 5179
after skull base surgery, 571
bullet wounds and, 5230, 5234–5235
caudate, 1737
epidural. See Epidural hematoma.
in anterior cervical approaches, 577
in anticoagulant therapy, 1735
in bone graft incorporation, 4618–4619
in spontaneous intracerebral hemorrhage, 1737–1740, 1737f–1739f
in traumatic brain injury, 5106, 5107f, 5108
infratentorial
progression of, 1744
volume of, 1743
intracerebral, 5045, 5159, 5159f
evacuation of, 5159, 5160f–5161f, 5162
in traumatic brain injury, 5106, 5107f, 5108
postoperative, 936
under extradural hematoma, 5157
parenchymal, micro-arteriovenous malformation with, 2215f
pediatric, head injury and, 3475–3476, 3475f, 3476t
peripheral nerve involvement in, 3949
posterior fossa
diagnosis of, 5162, 5163f
evacuation of, 5162–5163, 5164f–5165f
postoperative, neurological deficit from, 935–936, 937f
prevention of, 565
subdural. See Subdural hematoma.
subgaleal, scalp injury and, 3481–3482
supratentorial
craniotomy for, 5153–5154, 5155f–5156f
progression of, treatment and, 1743–1744
sitting position and, 606
volume of, outcome and, 1742–1743, 1743f
temporal lobe, 1747, 1750f–1751f
evacuation of, 5146, 5148f
traumatic, 5042, 5042t
Hematoma (Continued)
traumatic brain injury and, 5083
volume of
postevacuation intracranial pressure and, 1755, 1756f
surgical effect of, 1742–1743, 1743f
Hematopoietic cells, 4614
Hemialexia, left, corpus callosum section and, 1244
Hemianopsia
homonymous, in posterior cerebral artery stroke, 5212, 5213f
stroke and, 1608
Hemiballismus, 2676, 2720
basal ganglia changes in, 2675f
pediatric, assessment of, 3179
Hemicord syndrome. See Brown-Séquard syndrome.
Hemilaminotomy, lumbar, complication avoidance in, 580
Hemimegalencephaly, magnetic resonance imaging of, 2492, 2492f, 2493f
Hemimetameric somitic shift, 4277–4278, 4277f
Hemimyelomeningocele, 3215
Hemineglect, middle carotid artery infarction and, 1615
Hemiparesis
atlanto-occipital dislocation and, 4928–4929
contralateral, in epidural hematoma, 5043
in subarachnoid hemorrhage, 1816
ipsilateral, 5091
temporal lobectomy and, 2610
Hemiplegia
spastic, in cerebral palsy, 3724, 3725–3727
temporal lobe resection and, 2576
Hemispherectomy
for epilepsy, 2579–2580
functional, 2580
seizure outcome with, 2580
trans-sylvian keyhole functional, 2580
Hemispheric decortication, for epilepsy, 2580
Hemispheric vein
inferior, 35f
superior, 36f
Hemispherotomy
for epilepsy, 2579–2580, 2596
peri-insular, 2580
Hemivertebra, 4277–4278, 4277f, 4281, 4281f
Hemodilution, in intracerebral hemorrhage, 1740
Hemodynamic failure, 1601–1604
clinical correlates in, 1603–1604
misery perfusion in, 1601–1602, 1602f
Hemodynamic steal, 1601
Hemodynamics
in pregnancy, 2422
transcranial Doppler ultrasonography of, 1554–1555
Hemoglobin
in head injury, 5058–5059
in pregnancy, 2421
Hemorrhage
after traumatic brain injury, 5083
angiomatous, in pregnancy, 2426–2427
arteriovenous malformations and, 2121, 2161–2163, 2188, 2191–2192, 2206, 2207f–2210f
after radiation therapy, 2194
after radiosurgery, 4081–4082
Hemorrhage (Continued)
after surgery, 2246–2247, 2273, 2274f–2279f, 2275, 2280
aneurysms and, 2165
risk for, 2191
age in, 2192, 2192t
brain surgery and, 5174, 5176
brainstem, 1739–1740, 1739f
cerebellar, 1736, 1737t, 1738–1739, 1739f
control of, 5087–5088
delivery and, 3483–3485, 3483f–3486f
diffuse intravascular coagulation in, 564
germinal matrix–intraventricular, 3405, 3406f. See also Hydrocephalus, infantile posthemorrhagic.
injury pattern in, 3407, 3407f
neuropathology from, 3407–3408
pathogenesis of, 3406f, 3407
severity of, 3408, 3408t
in aneurysms, 2121
in brainstem cavernous malformations, 2323
in bullet wounds, 5230, 5234–5235
in capillary telangiectasia, 2176
in cavernous carotid fistula, 2344
in cavernous malformations, 2169–2170, 2170t, 2293–2294, 2293f–2296f, 2295, 2296
in craniofacial trauma, 5246–5247
in deep brain stimulation, 3128, 3128t
in dural arteriovenous fistula, 2172–2173
in giant arteriovenous malformation, 2267
in malignant phenotype, 771, 772f
in moyamoya, 1716
in pallidotomy, 2790
in posterior fossa arteriovenous malformations, 2252
in spinal intradural arteriovenous malformations, 2388–2389
in supratentorial cavernous malformations, 2305, 2307–2308, 2308f, 2309f
in temporal bone fracture, 5280
in traumatic aneurysm dissection, 2133
in venous malformation, 2174–2175
in xanthogranuloma formation, 1444
into neurovascular sheath, 3975
into subependymal germinal matrix, 3405, 3406f
intracerebral. See Intracerebral hemorrhage.
intraparenchymal, delivery and, 3485
intraventricular, 5047
aneurysm rupture and, 1824
pediatric, 3463
lobar, 1738, 1738f
pontine, 1739–1740, 1739f
punctate, 5046
putaminal, 1737, 1737f, 1746, 1746f–1748f
recurrent, in arteriovenous malformation, 2163–2164
shaking-impact syndrome and, 3501, 3502f
spontaneous, spinal, 4310t, 4311
stereotactic surgery and, 2779
Strich, 5046
subarachnoid. See Subarachnoid hemorrhage.
thalamic, 1737–1738, 1738f
tissue plasminogen activator and, 1500
Hemorrhagic angiogenic proliferation, 2143
Hemorrhagic dysangiogenesis, 2143

Hemosiderosis
seizures from, 2314
superficial cerebral, 2580
Hemostasis
in cervical laminoforaminotomy, 4416
in cervical laminoplasty, 4419
in supratentorial arteriovenous malformation surgery, 2237
Hensen's node, 47, 4239, 4240f, 4241
Heparan sulfate proteoglycans, in malignant glioma, 762
Heparin
in carotid endarterectomy, 1633–1634
in cerebral venous thrombosis, 1726–1727
in deep venous thrombosis prevention, 564
in pregnancy, 2423
in recurrent carotid artery stenosis, 1662–1663
spontaneous intracerebral hemorrhage with, 1735
Hepatitis
neuropathy from, 3842
transmission of, by allograft bone, 4617
Hepatocyte growth factor–scatter factor, 773
Hepatolenticular degeneration, 2735
Hereditary motor and sensory neuropathy, imaging of, 536, 537f
Hereditary neuropathy, 3845–3846
with liability to pressure palsy, 3845–3846
Herniation syndromes, 290–292
central, 826, 826t, 5055t, 5056
rostral-caudal progression of, 292, 292f
definition of, 291
effects of, 293
in brain tumors, 826–827, 826f, 826t
intracranial pressure in, 183
posterior (tectal), 5055t, 5056
sites for, 5055, 5055t
subfalcine (cingulate), 5055, 5055t
tonsillar, 826t, 827, 5055t, 5056, 5091, 5092f
bullet wounds and, 5224
in Chiari malformation type I, 3349, 3350f
transtentorial, 826
treatment of, 827
types of, 291t
uncal, 826, 826t, 5055–5056, 5055t, 5091, 5091f
Duret's hemorrhage in, 5091, 5092f
Heroin
blood-brain barrier transport of, 15
spontaneous intracerebral hemorrhage from, 1735
Herpes simplex virus
as central nervous system gene therapy vector, 4166–4167
multiple sclerosis from, 1449
mutant, cytopathic-oncolytic capability of, 822
Herpes simplex virus thymidine kinase gene, vector transfer of, 818–820, 819f, 820f
Herpes zoster infection
myelitis in, 4312–4313
neuropathy from, 3841–3842
Herpesvirus B, myelitis from, 4311, 4312t
Herpesviruses
as vectors, 818
myelitis from, 4311, 4312t
Heschl's gyrus, 5, 6f, 14, 15f
HESX1, 53t
Heterotopia
magnetic resonance imaging of, 2493, 2493f
periventricular, 61
subcortical laminar, 61, 62f
Heterotopic nodules, 63, 63f
Heterotopic ossification, in brain injury rehabilitation, 5295
Heubner's artery, 22f
Hieron osteon, 5011
Hindbrain herniation
in Chiari malformation, 3353–3354
posterior fossa volume reduction and, 3340
Hip dislocation/subluxation, in cerebral palsy, 3728
after dorsal rhizotomy, 3744
Hippel-Lindau syndrome, 4302
Hippocampal sulcus, remnant of, magnetic resonance imaging of, 2495, 2495f
Hippocampal vein, 17
longitudinal, 24f
transverse, 1239
Hippocampectomy, 2607
Hippocampus, 7f, 8f, 9, 10f, 11, 12f, 15f, 18f, 26f
atrophy of, 2487, 2489
as developmental abnormality, 2490
gray matter structures of, 2486, 2487f
long-term potentiation in, after traumatic brain injury, 2452, 2453f
magnetic resonance imaging of, 2486–2487, 2488f
neuronal loss in, in post-traumatic epilepsy, 2449–2450, 2450f
regions of, 2486, 2487f
resection of, memory loss and, 2618
sclerosis of
magnetic resonance imaging of, 2486–2487, 2487f–2490f, 2489–2491
surgical algorithm for, 2490–2491, 2490f
Hippus, 288
Histamine, release of, 2953, 2954f
Histiocytoma, fibrous, 1143
orbital, 1375
Histiocytosis, Langerhans cell
pediatric, 3591
skull, 1400–1401, 1401f
pediatric, 3719–3720, 3720f
spinal, 4355, 4837, 4843, 4845f
pediatric, 3567
Histiocytosis X, pediatric, 3591
skull, 3719–3720, 3720f
History, 263–264
Histrionic personality, in traumatic brain injury response, 5193, 5193t
H-neu, 744
Hoarseness, 267
Hoffman reflex, 4410
Holoprosencephaly, 52, 56–57, 56f, 57f, 81
alobar, 56
middle interhemispheric variant of, 57
semilobar, 56–57
Homeoboxes, 51
Homeodomain, 48, 51
Homeostasis, extracellular, maintenance of, 228, 229f, 230
Homocystine, stroke risk in, 1617
Hook-rod construct
lumbar, 4733, 4733f
complication avoidance in, 582
multiple hooks in, 4734, 4734f
thoracic, 4969–4972, 4970f–4972f
Hooks
sublaminar, 4971–4972, 4972f
transverse, 4972, 4972f
Hormonal therapy, for meningioma, 1110–1111
Hormones, in pregnancy, 2422
Horner's syndrome, 322, 323f, 5212
avoidance of, in thoracic sympathectomy, 3099f, 3100f
stellate ganglion block and, 2982
thoracic endoscopic sympathectomy and, 3101
vagus nerve stimulator implantation and, 2643
vs. thoracic disk herniation, 4492
House/Brackman Scale for Facial Nerve, 242t
Hox, 52, 53t, 3332
H-reflex, 3855, 3855f
HT7 antigen, 158
β-Human chorionic gonadotropin, in germ cell tumors, 1014, 1014t
Human herpesvirus type 6, multiple sclerosis from, 1449
Human immunodeficiency virus (HIV)
in trauma, 5087
transmission of, by allograft bone, 4617
Human immunodeficiency virus (HIV) infection
in pediatric aneurysms, 3449, 3449f
myelitis from, 4311, 4312t, 4313
neuropathy from, 3841
tuberculosis in, spinal, 4386–4387
tuberculous spondylitis in, 4293–4294
Human immunodeficiency virus (HIV) testing, informed consent for, 409
Human leukocyte antigen (HLA) B27
in ankylosing spondylitis, 4459
in posterior longitudinal ligament ossification, 4476
Human T-cell lymphotropic virus type I
multiple sclerosis from, 1449
myelitis from, 4311, 4312t, 4313
Humerus
fracture of
radial nerve entrapment in, 3928
shaking-impact syndrome and, 3502f
supracondylar process of, median nerve entrapment by, 3924
Hunt & Hess, 242t
Hunt and Hess grade, 1509, 1509t
Hunter-Hurler syndrome, 4479
Huntington's disease, 2676–2677, 2717–2718, 2736
basal ganglia–thalamocortical circuit in, 2718
positron emission tomography of, 2762–2764, 2763f
substantia nigra pars compacta in, 2706f
Hyaluronate receptors, in malignant glioma, 763
Hyaluronic acid, in malignant glioma, 763
Hydatid disease, spinal, 4390
Hydrocephalus
after giant arteriovenous malformation surgery, 2280
after subarachnoid hemorrhage, 1823–1824, 1823t, 1824f
aneurysm rupture and, 1510, 1799
classification of, 3146–3147
historical aspects of, 3145–3153
in achondroplasia, 3365–3366
in Chiari malformation type II, 3350
in choroid plexus tumors, 3613
in Dandy-Walker syndrome, 3285–3286, 3287f

Hydrocephalus (Continued)
in epidermoid tumor, 3690
in germ cell tumors, 3608
in medulloblastoma, 3643–3644
in midbrain glioma, 3666
in pineal region tumors, 1014
in sarcoidosis, 1436, 1439
in spina bifida, 3222, 3223
in suprasellar cysts, 3294
in vein of Galen malformations, 3442, 3442f, 3443
infantile posthemorrhagic, 3405–3415
brain injury in, 3408
cerebral blood flow in, 3408
cerebrospinal fluid drainage in, 3411, 3412f, 3413–3414
clinical presentation of, 3408–3409
course of, 3409–3410
definition of, 3405
diagnosis of, 3408–3409
epidemiology of, 3405, 3405t
external ventricular drainage for, 3412f, 3413
germinal matrix–intraventricular hemorrhage and, 3407–3408, 3407f, 3408t
hypoxic-ischemic injury in, 3408
intraventricular fibrinolysis for, 3411
lumbar puncture for, 3411, 3412f, 3413
medical management of, 3410–3411
monitoring of, 3410f
observation for, 3410
outcome in, 3414–3415
pathophysiology of, 3405–3408, 3406f, 3407f, 3408t
prevention of, 3409, 3410f
treatment of, 3410–3414
ventricular access devices for, 3412f, 3413–3414
ventricular tap for, 3412f, 3413
ventriculoperitoneal shunt for, 3414
ventriculosubgaleal shunt for, 3412f, 3413
lateral ventricle tumors and, 1244
medical treatment of, historical aspects of, 3151
pediatric, 3387–3403
aqueduct of Sylvius obstruction and, 3391–3393, 3392f
arachnoid villi occlusion and, 3397–3398, 3397f, 3398f
biomechanical models of, 3381–3382
biventricular, 3390
brain injury in, 3408
cerebrospinal fluid obstruction site in, 3389
classification based on, 3389–3400
communicating, 3389
compartmentalized, 3429
external, 3397
head circumference curves in, 3397, 3397f
extraventricular obstructive, 3389
fetal management of, 3220
foramen of Monro obstruction and, 3389–3391, 3390f, 3391f
fourth ventricle outlet foramina obstruction and, 3393–3394, 3394f, 3395f
in achondroplasia, 3398
in craniopharyngioma, 3675, 3676f
in ependymoma, 3626–3627
in intramedullary tumors, 3708
intraventricular obstructive, 3389
monoventricular, 3391f

Hydrocephalus (Continued)
multiloculated, 3394
noncommunicating, 3389
pathophysiology of, 3387, 3388f, 3389
sagittal sinus pressure increases and, 3398–3399, 3399f
shunt failure in, 3399–3400, 3400f, 3401f
treatment of, 3399
shunt complications in, 3400–3402, 3402f
spinal-cortical subarachnoid space obstruction and, 3394–3397
trauma and, 3477
treatment of, endoscopy in, 3429–3430, 3429f
posterior circulation aneurysm and, 1976
shunt-dependent, aneurysm embolization and, 2070
shunts for. *See* Cerebrospinal fluid shunt.
surgery for, historical aspects of, 3151–3153, 3152f
treatment of
before surgery, 1036
in primitive neuroectodermal tumors, 1002–1003
unilateral, 3429
Hydrochloroquine, for sarcoidosis, 1439
Hydrogen
in cerebral blood flow–metabolism coupling, 1489
in cerebral ischemia, 123–124, 126
Hydrogen nucleus, in magnetic resonance imaging, 439
Hydromyelia, 4315t, 4317
Hydrostatic pressure, in cerebrospinal fluid shunt, 3375, 3376f
Hydrosyringomyelia, in spina bifida, 3216
Hydroxyl, 1473
Hyoscyamine, for multiple sclerosis, 1455t
Hyperactivity, in traumatic brain injury response, 5193t
Hyperalgesia, 3120t
nerve growth factor in, 2956
secondary, 2926–2927
Hypercholesterolemia, stroke risk in, 1616–1617
Hypercoagulable states, cerebral venous thrombosis from, 1723
Hypercortisolemia
adrenocorticotropic hormone–dependent, vs. adrenocorticotropic hormone–independent, 1196
diagnosis of, 1196
Hyperekplexia, 2730
Hyperemia
absolute, 5084
in arteriovenous malformation, 2188
in traumatic brain injury, 5084, 5109t, 5110t, 5111
intracranial hypertension and, 5111
intracranial pressure and, 186–187
luxury, head injury and, 5051–5052
relative, 5084
true, 490
Hyperesthesia, 3821, 3831
Hyperextension
cervical, 4896, 4909
carotid artery injury in, 5204, 5204f
central cord syndrome in, 4890
spinal cord injury without radiographic abnormality and, 3521, 3521f
thoracic, 4961, 4962f

Hyperextension-hyperflexion injury, cervical spine, 4915–4922. *See also* Cervical spine, hyperextension-hyperflexion injury to.
Hyperflexion
cervical, 4896
anterior cord syndrome in, 4890
bilateral facet dislocations from, 4909, 4909f
carotid artery injury in, 5204, 5204f
thoracic, 4958–4959, 4959f, 4962, 4962t
Hyperglycemia
in extracranial head injury, 5057
in traumatic brain injury, 5131
ischemic damage from, 128–130
pH and, 129–130
Hyperhidrosis, thoracic endoscopic sympathectomy for, 3097, 3100t, 3101, 4762
Hyperkinetic disorders, 2676
Hypernatremia, in traumatic brain injury, 5131
Hyperostosis
ankylosing, in lumbar spinal stenosis, 4527
cervical, in spondylosis, 4447
diffuse idiopathic skeletal, 4476, 4478f
in meningioma, 1102, 1103f, 1362, 1363f
Hyperostosis frontalis interna, 1402–1403, 1403f
Hyperpathia, 3120t
Hyperperfusion, 490
in arteriovenous malformations, 1604
postoperative, transcranial Doppler ultrasonography of, 1550
Hyperpolarization, 3813, 3813f
Hyperprolactinemia, in pituitary adenoma, 1174–1175
Hypertelorism, orbital
anterior fossa encephalocele with, 3207f
surgery for, 3322, 3324–3326, 3325f
Hypertension
anterior ischemic optic neuropathy in, 306f
carotid endarterectomy and, 1644
for cerebral vasospasm, 1855
for ischemic neurological deficits, 1840
in altered consciousness, 294–295
in aneurysm rupture, 1789–1790
in intracerebral hemorrhage, 1740
in ischemia protection, 1521
in pontine hemorrhage, 1739
in pregnancy, 2423–2424
intracranial. *See* Intracranial hypertension.
lobar hemorrhage from, 1738
stroke risk in, 1616
treatment of, in traumatic brain injury, 5127, 5128t
venous
hydrocephalus from, 3398–3400, 3399f, 3400f, 3442
in spinal cord arteriovenous fistulas, 2367, 2368, 2387–2388
Hyperthermia, brain death and, 398
Hyperthyroidism
chorea with, 2736–2737
pituitary adenoma and, 1200
secondary, surgery for, 1176
Hypertonia
muscle, 3178
pediatric, 3177–3178
spastic, 3178
Hyperventilation, 275
cerebral blood flow and, 5132–5133

Hyperventilation (Continued)
in pediatric head injury, 3474–3475
in traumatic brain injury, 5120, 5122f, 5123
intracranial pressure and, 187, 5058
Hypervolemia, for cerebral vasospasm, 1855
Hypoadrenalism, in pediatric craniopharyngioma, 3675
Hypocapnia
in traumatic brain injury, 5120, 5122f, 5123, 5135
intracranial pressure reduction by, 5057
treatment of, 5135
Hypochondroplasia, genetics of, 3362
Hypoesthesia, 3821
Hypoglossal nerve
dysfunction of, glomus jugulare tumors and, 1305
examination of, 267
pediatric, 3176
vagus nerve stimulator implantation and, 2643
Hypoglossal triangle, 33f
Hypogonadism, prolactinoma and, 1185
Hypokalemia, surgery and, 550
Hypometabolism
contralateral hemisphere, stroke and, 1607–1608
in stroke recovery, 1609
Hyponatremia, after subarachnoid hemorrhage, 1829–1830
Hyponatremia syndrome, in traumatic brain injury, 5130–5131, 5130f
Hypoparathyroidism, posterior longitudinal ligament ossification in, 4476
Hypophonia, subthalamic nucleus stimulation for, 2821
Hypophosphatemia, in altered consciousness, 295
Hypophyseal artery, superior, 19, 1896, 1898
aneurysm of, 1904
Hypophysectomy, 3030
Hypopituitarism
in pregnancy, 2429
transsphenoidal surgery and, 1182
Hypotension
in altered consciousness, 295
in bullet wounds, 5226
in cervical spine trauma, 4888, 4889
in head injury, 1551–1552
in pregnancy, 2423–2424
in trauma, 5090
in traumatic brain injury, 5096, 5120, 5122f
treatment of, 5135, 5136f
intraoperative, outcome in, 1551–1552
systemic, 1528
in extracranial head injury, 5056–5057
Hypothalamic sulcus, 14f
Hypothalamus, 13
after brain death, 398
arteriovenous malformation of, 2243
glioma of, pediatric, 3596
injury to, transsphenoidal surgery and, 569, 1181–1182
pituitary adenoma of, 1174
sarcoidosis of, 1436
stimulation of, 2854
Hypothermia
brain death and, 398
brain protection with, 5059
coma from, 294
Hypothermia (Continued)
in aneurysm treatment, 1807
in giant arteriovenous malformation surgery, 2273
in intracranial hypertension treatment, 5134
in ischemia protection, 1521, 1532
intracranial pressure and, 189
protective. See Deep hypothermic circulatory arrest.
side effects of, 1532–1533, 1533t
Hypothyroidism
in pediatric craniopharyngioma, 3675
neuropathy in, 3843
Hypotonia, pediatric, 3178
Hypovolemia, after aneurysmal subarachnoid hemorrhage, 1829
Hypoxia
in bullet wounds, 5226
in extracranial head injury, 5056–5057
in infantile posthemorrhagic hydrocephalus, 3408
in traumatic brain injury, 5122f, 5123, 5135–5136
myelination delay from, 64
pediatric tolerance for, 3462
radiomarkers for, 1609
treatment of, 5135–5136
Hysteria, conversion, pediatric, 3568

Idarubicin, for ependymoma, 1048t
Ifosfamide, for ependymoma, 1048, 1048t
Iliac crest, posterior, bone graft harvest from, 4605–4606, 4606f
IM862
angiosuppressive therapy with, 783
as angiogenesis antagonist, 779t
Image cytometry, in tumor proliferation marking, 694–695
Image-guided spinal navigation, 4743–4756
clinical applications of, 4747–4753
fluoroscopic, 4754–4755, 4755f
for anterior thoracolumbar surgery, 4752–4753, 4754f
for cervical spine screw fixation, 4748–4751, 4751f, 4752f
for pedicle fixation, 4747–4748, 4748f–4750f
for transoral surgery, 4751–4752, 4752f
pitfalls of, 4753–4754
principles of, 4743–4747, 4744f–4746f
Immobilization, after cervical spine trauma, 4887, 4888–4889
Immune modulation, of tumors, 821
Immune response, 674–675, 675f
adaptive, 674
antigenic determinants in, 675–676
blood-brain barrier in, 12
effector function in, 673, 680–681, 681f
for brain targets, 681–683
historical perspective on, 673–674
in central nervous system, 673–685
initiation of, 679–680
site-specific features of, 683–685, 683f, 684f
T cells in, 677–679, 678f
Immune system
astrocytoma evasion of, 891
in cerebral vasospasm, 1847
Immune-associated antitumor effect, in gene transfer, 818–819
Immune-inflammatory network, 675
in neurodegenerative disorders, 684
Immunoblastic sarcoma. See Central nervous system, primary lymphoma of.
Immunoblot, 753, 753f
Immunocompromise
primary central nervous system lymphoma in, 1067, 1069, 1070f
pyogenic spinal infections in, 4363–4364
differential diagnosis of, 4371
medical management of, 4379
outcome of, 4381
Immunogenicity, of bone grafts, 4616t, 4617
Immunoglobulin
for chronic inflammatory demyelinating polyradiculoneuropathy, 3840
for Guillain-Barré syndrome, 3839
Immunoglobulin G, blood-brain barrier transcytosis of, 163
Immunoglobulin superfamily, in malignant glioma, 763
Immunology, central nervous system inflammation and, 4155
Immunosuppressants, in focal cerebral ischemia, 135
Immunosuppression, tumor-induced, 681, 892
Immunotherapy
autoimmune disease and, 894
for brain tumors, 891–895
immunization site in, 893–894
Impairment, 3783
IN-1 antibody, in neuron regeneration, 204, 5032
Incidentaloma, 1170
Inclusion tumor, 3689–3690, 3689t
Incontinence
in cerebral palsy, 3727, 3728, 3732, 3744–3745
in multiple sclerosis, 1452
in occult spinal dysraphism, 3259, 3259f
urinary. See Urinary incontinence.
Index test, 497
Individual studies, 248–249
Indomethacin, pseudotumor cerebri from, 1424
Induction, 47–48, 48t
Industrial exposure, brain tumors and, 810
Infarction
choroidal artery, 1615
distal anterior cerebral artery, 1952
in stroke, 1622
magnetic resonance imaging of, 463–464, 465f, 466
middle carotid artery, 1615
periventricular hemorrhagic, 3407, 3407f
pons, 273
spinal cord, 4310–4311, 4310t
imaging of, 537, 539f
Infection. See also specific infection.
after skull base surgery, 572
after spinal surgery, 4383–4384, 4518–4519, 4982
brain tumors and, 810
extravascular, aneurysm from, 2101, 2102
in ankylosing spondylitis, 4459
in bullet wounds, 5236
in carotid atherosclerosis, 1613
in cerebral venous thrombosis, 1723
in cerebrospinal fluid shunt, 3419–3424. See also Cerebrospinal fluid shunt, infection of.
in craniofacial surgery, 3328–3329
in craniofacial trauma, 5248

Infection *(Continued)*
in Cushing's disease, 1195
in glomus jugulare tumor surgery, 1307
in pediatric neurorehabilitation, 3787
in traumatic cerebrospinal fluid fistula, 5270–5271
magnetic resonance imaging of, 461–463, 462f–464f
of cephalohematoma, 3482
of halo vest pins, 3544
pain associated with, 4290–4295, 4291t
peripheral neuropathy from, 3832t, 3841–3842
postoperative, 938, 938f
pulmonary, in spinal cord injury, 4881
spinal, imaging of, 537–544
Inferior fovea, 33f, 34
Inferior frontal sulcus, 3
Inferior occipitofrontal fasciculus, 6, 7f
Inferior vermis, 34
Inflammation, 674
after arteriovenous malformation embolization, 2226, 2227f
"bad" vs. "good," 206
blood-brain barrier effects of, 163–164
cell-protective effects of, 138
central nervous system, 135–136
injury and, 205–206
neuroimmunology and, 4155
cranial destruction in, 430, 430f
growth-promoting effects of, 138
in Alzheimer's disease, 90
in carotid atherosclerosis, 1614
in cerebral ischemia, 135–143. *See also* Cerebral ischemia, inflammation in.
in cerebral vasospasm, 1847
in ischemic injury, 1518–1519
in osteoid osteoma, 4837
in stroke, 142–143
in subarachnoid hemorrhage, 1831
innate, 674
mechanisms of, 137
mediators of, 135–143, 674, 2956
modulation of, 2953, 2954f
neurogenic, 2921
nociceptive primary afferent neurons in, 2921
of cervical nerve roots, 505f
orbital, 1376
peripheral nervous system, in regeneration, 4155
spinal, imaging of, 537–544
third ventricular, 1247
triggers of, 138
Inflammatory bowel disease, craniocervical junction disease and, 4580
Inflammatory cells
in cerebral ischemia, 136, 136t
transplantation of, for central nervous system repair, 4164
Inflammatory syndrome, low back pain in, 4331
Informed consent, 408
during pregnancy, 409
for human immunodeficiency virus testing, 409
for minors, 408–409
Infraclavicular plexus, neurogenic sarcoma of, 3953f
Infundibular arteries, 19
Infundibular recess, 14f
Inhalation agents, cerebral physiology and, 551
Initiative, in frontal lobe tumors, 830
Injection injury, peripheral nerve, 3828
INK4a-ARF, in glioma, 717, 717f, 718
Inner ear, anatomy of, 327, 328f, 329f
Inotropic agents, cerebral blood flow effects of, 5134–5135, 5135t
Inoue-Melnick virus, meningioma from, 1105
Insecurity, in traumatic brain injury response, 5193t
Instrumentation. *See also* specific type.
cervical spine, complication avoidance in, 577, 578, 579
for spinal internal fixation, 4589–4592
in pediatric atlantoaxial fusion, 3547, 3549–3550, 3549f, 3550f
spinal, infections after, 4383–4384, 4982
Insula, 5–6, 6f, 12f, 15f
anterior limiting sulcus of, 4f, 7f, 8f, 15f
arteriovenous malformation of, 2237–2238
Insular cleft, 5, 6f
Insulin, in bone metabolism, 4233
Insulin-like growth factor, 197
after peripheral nerve injury, 3968
in axonal regeneration, 200
in brain tumors, 728–729
Insulin-like growth factor receptors, in brain tumors, 728–729
Integrins
in malignant glioma, 763
inhibitors of, as angiogenesis antagonists, 778t, 781
Integument, in spinal cord injury management, 4881–4882
Intellectual function, in frontal lobe tumor, 830
Intelligence quotient (IQ)
after epilepsy surgery, 2571
after traumatic brain injury, 5185
before traumatic brain injury, 5189
Intensity-modulated radiotherapy, 4142–4143
Interbrachial sulcus, 32
Intercellular adhesion molecule 1
in cerebral ischemia, 140–141
in stroke, 142
Intercostal muscles, 4674
Intercostal neuralgia, dorsal rhizotomy for, 3041
Interferon
for neoplastic meningitis, 1233
in multiple sclerosis, 1450
Interferon-α, angiosuppressive therapy with, 780–781
Interferon-β, for multiple sclerosis, 1454t, 1455
Interferon-γ
in brainstem, 684, 684f
in MHC expression, 683, 683f
in recurrent carotid artery stenosis, 1663
Interferon-inducible protein, in cerebral ischemia, 140
Interhemispheric fissure, cysts of, 3296–3297, 3297f
Interlaminar clamps, 4650, 4650f
Interleukin(s), in cerebral ischemia, 136
Interleukin-1
in axonal regeneration, 199
in multiple sclerosis, 1450
in nervous system regeneration, 4155
in Schwann cell proliferation, 200
in traumatic brain injury, 5029
Interleukin-1α, in cerebral ischemia, 138–139
Interleukin-1β, in cerebral ischemia, 138–139
Interleukin-2
in brain tumors, 887
in multiple sclerosis, 1450
in neoplastic meningitis, 1233
Interleukin-6
in brain injury recovery, 5031
in cerebral ischemia, 139
in distal nerve stump, 200
Interleukin-7, in tumor vaccines, 892
Interleukin-8, in angiogenesis, 719
Interleukin-10, in cerebral ischemia, 139–140
Interleukin-12
in angiosuppressive therapy, 779t, 783
in multiple sclerosis, 1450
Intermedius nerve, 40f
Intermuscular septum, medial, in ulnar nerve compression, 3902
Internal auditory canal
structural relationships in, 329f, 339
surgical approaches to, 922–923
tumors of, 920, 922f
Internal capsule, 9, 10f
anterior limb of, 4f, 8f
arteriovenous malformation of, 2246
genu of, 1237, 1238f
stimulation of, 3119, 3125
venous drainage of, 1238
Internal fixation
cervical spine. *See* Cervical spine, internal fixation of.
for mandibular fractures, 5264–5265
in airway management, 5246, 5247f
lumbar spine. *See* Lumbar spine, internal fixation of.
pediatric, 3545–3546
bone graft in, 3546
cervical spine, 3546
for atlantoaxial rotatory injury, 3541, 3542f
nonunion in, 3546
spinal, 4145–4148, 4586–4597
biomechanics in, 4586, 4587f, 4588–4589, 4592–4596, 4593f, 4594f
cantilever beam techniques for, 4593–4596, 4595f
cervical, 4596–4597, 4596f, 4597f
distraction techniques for, 4592, 4593f
for metastases, 4858–4862, 4859t, 4860f, 4864f
goals of, 4586
hardware optimization in, 4596
image-guided navigation for, 4747–4751, 4748f–4752f
instrumentation for, 4589–4592
rods and plates for, 4591–4592
screws for, 4589–4591, 4590f, 4591f
tension band techniques for, 4592–4593, 4594f
thoracolumbar, 4597
three-point techniques for, 4592, 4594f
wires for, 4592, 4592f
thoracic spine, 4965
historical perspective on, 4952
posterior, 4969–4972, 4970f–4972f
for compression fracture, 4979
techniques of, 4695–4699, 4696f–4699f
principles of, 4967–4968
Internodal segment, 3810
Internodes, in peripheral nerve entrapment, 3922
Interosseous muscle, weakness of, 3925
Interosseous nerve
anterior, surgery on, 650–651, 651f

Interosseous nerve (*Continued*)
posterior
entrapment of, 3929–3930
surgery on, 651, 652f
Interpeduncular cistern, 1975
Interpeduncular fossa, 30f
Interpeduncular sulcus, 32, 33f
Interspinous ligament, 4187
Intertransverse ligaments, 4187
Interventional studies, 251–252
Intervertebral artery, 2381
Intervertebral disk
aging effects on, 4395–4396
biomechanics of, 4185–4186
bulging of, 508, 508f, 509f
degenerative disease of
annular tears in, 507f, 508
disk abnormalities in, 508–509, 508f–511f
end plate marrow changes in, 508, 508f
evaluation of, 507–508, 507f, 508f
pathology of, 4328–4329
radiological studies of, 507–516
herniation of, 508–509, 508f
complication avoidance in, 581
decompressive surgery for, 4337, 4981
extrusions in, 509, 511f
imaging of, 508–509, 4333f–4335f
in cervical spine. *See* Cervical disk disease.
in lumbar spinal stenosis, 4530–4531
in lumbar spine. *See* Lumbar disk disease.
in thoracic spine. *See* Thoracic disk herniation.
nerve root in, 271, 4330
olisthy with, 4532
pain in, 4328
protrusions in, 509, 510f
recurrent, 4330
lumbar, diseases of. *See* Lumbar disk disease.
pediatric, 3515
anatomy of, 3559–3560
calcified cervical, 3566–3567, 3566f
degeneration of, in isthmic spondylolisthesis, 3577–3578
development of, 3559–3560
diseases of, 3559–3568
clinical presentation of, 3560–3562
historical aspects of, 3559
pathophysiology of, 3560
herniation of
differential diagnosis of, 3564–3568, 3565t
outcomes in, 3564, 3564t
surgery for, 3563–3564
traumatic, 3564
treatment of, 3563
pseudobulge of, 512, 512f
recurrent, vs. scar, 515, 516f
retained fragment of
decompressive surgery for, 4337
reherniation of, 580
sequestered, 509, 4410
Intima, disruption of, in blunt cerebrovascular injury, 5204, 5206
Intracarotid amobarbital procedure, 2503–2508, 2571–2572
alternatives to, 2508
before pediatric epilepsy surgery, 3765
bilateral speech in, 2504, 2504t
cerebral hemispheres tested in, 2505
complications of, 2508
Intracarotid amobarbital procedure (*Continued*)
dosing in, 2505–2506, 2505t, 2508
electroencephalography in, 2506
historical perspective on, 2503
language center localization with, 2532
left speech in, 2504, 2504t
mechanism of, 2503
memory assessment accuracy in, 2506, 2507–2508
patient selection for, 2504–2505
posterior cerebral artery in, 2506
psychological tests in, 2506–2508, 2507f
right speech in, 2504, 2504t
seizure localization with, 2631
selective injections in, 2506
speech lateralization accuracy in, 2506–2507
terminology for, 2503–2504
vs. functional magnetic resonance imaging, 2516
Intracerebral hematoma, 5045
Intracerebral hemorrhage
aneurysm rupture and, 1798–1799
carotid endarterectomy and, 1644–1645
in pregnancy, 2166
in subarachnoid hemorrhage, 1825
spontaneous, 1733–1764
anticoagulant therapy and, 1734–1735
blood pressure control in, 1740
bur hole aspiration for, 1753
case studies about, 1746–1747, 1746f–1752f, 1753
causes of, 1734–1735, 1734t
cerebellar hemorrhage in, 1736, 1737t
cerebral amyloid angiopathy and, 1735, 1736f
craniotomy for, 1745–1746
definition of, 1733
diagnosis of, 1736–1737
drug use and, 1735
epidemiology of, 1734
fibrinolytic therapy for, 1753–1754
hematoma location in, 1737–1740, 1737f–1739f
historical review of, 1733–1734
imaging of, 1736–1737
intracranial pressure monitoring in, 1755–1756, 1756f
intracranial tumors and, 1735
mechanically assisted aspiration for, 1754–1755
neuroendoscopic techniques for, 1755
outcome of, 1756, 1757t, 1758, 1758f–1759f, 1760t, 1761, 1762t–1763t, 1764, 1764f
pathogenesis of, 1735–1736
pathology of, 1735–1736
stereotactic aspiration for, 1753–1754
surgery for, 1741–1756
age effects on, 1741–1742
hematoma volume effects on, 1742–1743, 1743f
progression and, 1743–1744
rationale for, 1741
techniques in, 1745–1747, 1746f–1752f, 1753–1756, 1756f
timing of, 1744–1745
treatment of, 1740–1741
medical vs. surgical, 1756–1764
Intracranial catastrophe, signs of, 289–292, 291t, 292f
Intracranial hypertension, 184, 1504
blood-brain barrier in, 166
hyperemia and, 5111
Intracranial hypertension (*Continued*)
in chronic extracerebral fluid collections, 3506
in traumatic brain injury, 5109, 5120, 5122f
monitoring of, 5113
complications of, 5113
indications for, 5114
normal values in, 5113–5114
treatment of, 187–188
barbiturate coma in, 5133–5134
cerebrospinal fluid drainage in, 5133
dehydration in, 5133
hyperventilation in, 5132–5133
in traumatic brain injury, 5126–5129, 5131–5134
osmotherapy in, 5133
pharmacologic paralysis in, 5131–5132, 5132f, 5132t
Intracranial monitoring, 2551–2562
brain mapping in, 2554, 2557
care after, 2561
considerations in, 2557–2561, 2558f–2560f
electrodes for, 2554–2557, 2555f, 2556f
insertion of, 2558–2561, 2558f–2560f
hardware for, 2554–2557, 2555f, 2556f
history of, 2551–2552
indications for, 2552–2554, 2553f, 2554f
outcome with, 2561–2562
preoperative evaluation in, 2557–2558
recording equipment for, 2557
study design in, 2557
Intracranial pressure, 176–177, 177f
after ventriculostomy, 3367
autoregulation of, 181–182, 182f
brain volume and, 187–189
cerebral blood volume and, 1469
definition of, 176–177, 177f
elevation of, 180
effects of, 181–183, 182f
postoperative, 566
symptoms of, 183
transcranial Doppler ultrasonography of, 1552–1553, 1553f
factors governing, 179f
in achondroplasia, 3365
in anesthesia, 1504–1505
in aneurysm rupture, 1510
in brain edema, 180
in brain tumors, 180
in craniopharyngioma, 1210
in head injury, 555, 5053–5055, 5054f
in herniation syndromes, 183
in intracerebral hemorrhage, 1740
in intracranial tumors, 552
in primary central nervous system lymphoma, 1069, 1069t
in pseudotumor cerebri, 1426, 1428–1429
in sitting position, 606
in subarachnoid hemorrhage, 180, 1813–1814, 1824–1825
in subdural hematoma, 5044, 5106
in surgery timing, 900, 900f
in traumatic brain injury, 5096
in tuberculosis, 1440
Lundberg's classification of, 184, 184f
management of, 185–190, 1429
analgesia in, 5127, 5127t
cerebral blood flow in, 186–187
cerebral blood volume reduction in, 186–187
cerebrospinal fluid diversion in, 185–186
drug therapy in, 187–189
external drainage in, 189

Intracranial pressure *(Continued)*
fluid resuscitation in, 188
head position in, 187, 5126–5127
hyperventilation in, 187
in head injury, 5057–5058
in traumatic brain injury, 5124, 5125, 5126–5129, 5145, 5146f
sedation in, 5127, 5127t
venous outflow resistance in, 5126–5127
mannitol effects on, in head injury, 5052, 5053t
masses and, 189
measurement of, 176, 176f, 185
ventriculostomy in, 5150, 5151f–5152f
monitoring of, 183–185, 184f
in altered consciousness, 295–296
in bullet wounds, 5231
in intracerebral hemorrhage, 1755–1756, 1756f
normal, 175–176, 176f
papilledema and, 305–306, 306f
physiology of, 175–190
predictive values and, 238t
preoperative evaluation and, 551–552
pressure-volume index in, 5054, 5054f
pressure-volume relationships and, 180–181, 181f
reduction of, 186t
refractory, 182
respiratory activity in, 176, 176f
steady-state dynamics of, 177–178
systemic hypertension effects on, 5127
Intracranial stenosis, 1543–1544
Intradiskal electrothermal annuloplasty, 4791–4792, 4793f
Intralaminar nucleus, in consciousness, 279
Intralimbic gyrus, 26f
Intraparenchymal hematoma
pediatric, head injury and, 3476
traumatic brain injury and, 5083
Intraparietal sulcus, 4, 4f
Intrathecal drug infusion, 3133–3141. *See also* Drugs, intrathecal infusion of.
Intraventricular hemorrhage, in pediatric arteriovenous malformations, 3447–3448
Intubation
complications of, patient positioning and, 609–610
neurological assessment and, 5090
pediatric, 3546
tracheal, in spinal cord injury, 557, 557t
Invasiveness
angiogenesis and, 773
malignant phenotype in, 771, 772f
Inverse steal response, in traumatic brain injury, 5123
Inverted radial reflex, 4410
Iododeoxyuridine, in malignant glioma radiosensitization, 4020
Ion(s)
distribution of, in resting membrane potential, 3812, 3812t
homeostasis of
astrocytes in, 102, 103f, 104f
calcium metabolism and, 120–123, 121f–124f
transport of, in blood-brain barrier, 162
Ion channel blockers
axonal conduction effects of, 2954f
for chronic pain, 2959–2960
Ion channels, 219–226, 220t
glial, 225, 226f
Ion channels *(Continued)*
in nociception, 2917–2918
neurological disorders and, 225t
selectivity of, 219–220
sodium, 220–222, 221f
Ion currents, 215
expression of, 226
resting membrane potential and, 218
Irinotecan, for ependymoma, 1048t
Iritis, in ankylosing spondylitis, 4461
Iron, in cavernous malformation, 2143, 2143f
Irradiation plexitis, vs. metastatic cancer, 3954
Ischemia. *See also* Stroke.
after arterial bypass, 2117
after giant arteriovenous malformation surgery, 2280
apoptosis in, 1519, 1519f
arachidonic acid metabolites in, 1518
calcium homeostasis in, 1517, 1518f
cerebral. *See* Cerebral ischemia.
cross-clamp, intraluminal shunt for, 1549
cyclo-oxygenase-2 in, 127
cytoprotective strategies for, 1520–1522
duration of
limitation of, 1520–1521
neurological injury and, 1495–1496, 1496f
reversibility and, 1516, 1517f
energy failure in, 1515, 1517, 1517f
excitotoxicity in, 1517
glutamate neurotoxicity in, 1517
Guglielmi detachable coil embolization and, 2071
hyperglycemia-mediated, 128–130
hyperventilation-induced, 187
in basilar trunk aneurysms, 2036–2037
in infantile posthemorrhagic hydrocephalus, 3408
in traumatic brain injury, 5111, 5112
inflammation in, 1518–1519
mechanisms of, 1519–1520, 1520f
medical treatment of, 1495–1501
pathophysiology of, 1515–1520
hypothermic protection and, 1532
in cerebral arteries, 1532
perfusion pressure effects on, 1504
peripheral nerve injury in, 3827–3828
potassium increases in, 102
prevention of
barbiturates in, 1521
blood flow augmentation in, 1521
cytoprotective agents in, 1521–1522
etomidate in, 1521
glucose limitation in, 1521
hypothermia in, 1521
limiting ischemia duration in, 1520–1521
propofol in, 1521
surgical protocol for, 1522–1523, 1523f
reactive oxygen species in, 1517–1518
secondary, traumatic brain injury and, 5111, 5112, 5120–5124, 5122f
cerebral causes of, 5120, 5122f
systemic causes of, 5120, 5122f, 5123–5124
treatment of, 5135–5137, 5136f
upper extremity, thoracic endoscopic sympathectomy for, 4762
vasospastic, 1850
vertebrobasilar, medical treatment of, 1696–1697
vessel occlusion procedures and, 864
Ischemia *(Continued)*
Ischemic core, 1605
Ischemic pain, peripheral vascular disease and, spinal cord stimulation for, 3113
Ischemic penumbra, 1496, 1516, 1601, 1601t
positron emission tomography of, 1605
Island of Reil, 5–6, 6f
Isoflurane, 1508
Isograft, 2829t
Isola spinal system, 4969, 4970f
Isoniazid, for tuberculosis, 1441, 4387
Isotopes, in brachytherapy, 4096, 4096t
Isthmic spondylolisthesis, 4541, 4542f
pathogenesis of, 4544
treatment of, 4551
pediatric, 4550–4551

Jackson table, 643
in thoracic spine fracture, 4968
Jacksonian seizures, in brain tumors, 829
Jackson-Weiss syndrome, 3164
Jacobson's nerve, in glomus jugular tumor classification, 1297
Japanese Orthopedic Association Scale, 243t
Jaw stretch reflex testing, pediatric, 3180
Jefferson's fracture, 501f, 519, 4903, 4903f, 4934, 4934f
Joint(s), nociceptors of, 2921
Joint capsule injury, 4917
Joint contractures, in cerebral palsy, 3728, 3732
Jugular body, 1295
Jugular bulb
dehiscence of, in achondroplasia, 3364
historical perspective on, 1295
tumors arising from, 1297
Jugular canal, enlargement of, 431
Jugular foramen, 36f
anatomy of, 1301–1302, 1301f
cervical-transmastoid approach to, 927–928, 928f
cranial nerves and, 1302, 1302f
intradural-extradural approach to, 927–928, 928f
meningioma of, 1120–1121, 1122f
Jugular vein, occlusion of, papilledema from, 1421–1422
Jugular venous oxygen saturation ($SjvO_2$), in traumatic brain injury
cerebral blood flow and, 5116–5118, 5117f, 5118f
secondary ischemic insults and, 5120, 5122f, 5123–5124
junB, traumatic brain injury and, 5028
Juvenile nasopharyngeal angiofibroma. *See* Angiofibroma, juvenile nasopharyngeal.

Kanamycin, for tuberculosis, 1441
Kaneda SR Anterior Spinal System, 4684, 4685f
implantation of, 4686–4689, 4687f
Kaposi's sarcoma, scalp, 1414
Karnofsky Performance Scale, 243t
in brain tumors, 830, 830t
in thoracic spine tumors, 4672
interstitial brachytherapy and, 4097
Katz Adjustment Scale, Revised, 5191
Kendrick extrication device, 4888
Kennedy's disease, 4319, 4320
Keratosis, scalp, 1409

Kernohan's notch phenomenon, 292
Ketamine, 1508
cerebral physiology and, 551
for pain, 2965
Ketoconazole, for pituitary adenoma, 869
Ketone bodies, blood-brain barrier transfer of, 1485
Ketoprofen, pseudotumor cerebri from, 1424
Ki-67, as tumor proliferation marker, 695–696
Kidney(s), preoperative evaluation of, 550
Kiloh-Nevin syndrome, 3925
Kinocilia, 341
Kjer's dominant optic atrophy, 313
Klaus height index, 424–425, 424f
Klippel-Feil syndrome
atlas assimilation in, 3339, 3340
imaging of, 536f
in Chiari malformation type I, 3348
Knobloch's syndrome, in parietal encephalocele, 3202
Knockout mice, 714
Knudson's two-hit hypothesis, 739–740, 740f
Kostuik-Harrington device, 4684
Krebs cycle, in glucose metabolism, 1482, 1483t, 1484
Krev-1/rap1a pathway, in familial cerebral cavernous malformations, 2303
KRIT1, mutations in, 2301–2302, 2301t
Krox-20, 51
Kyphoscoliosis
in pediatric intramedullary tumors, 3708
radiation-induced, 4042
Kyphosis, 4306
congenital, 4318
in spina bifida, 3223
pediatric, 3565–3566
fixation for, 3546–3547
pediatric intramedullary tumor surgery and, 3713
postoperative, after cervical laminectomy, 4425–4427, 4426f
thoracic, 4953, 4953f
in ankylosing spondylitis, 4460, 4461f

L1, in central nervous system repair, 4162
L1CAM, 53t
L2/HNK-1, in axon targeting, 201
Labyrinth, sound transmission in, 330
Labyrinthectomy, 2908
Labyrinthine fistula test, 342
Labyrinthitis
circumscribed, 351
serous, 351
suppurative, 351
vertigo in, 2903
Laceration
brain, 5041–5042
in craniofacial trauma, 5249
peripheral nerve injury in, 3827
Lacertus fibrosus muscle, median nerve entrapment at, 3924
Lactate, 123
astrocyte production of, 107, 108f, 109
Lactate-oxygen index, 5048
Lambdoid suture, 423f
Lambert-Eaton myasthenic syndrome
calcium channel mutations in, 223–224
clinical manifestations of, 833
ion channels in, 225t
pathology of, 3816
Lamina terminalis, 13, 14f
Lamina terminalis *(Continued)*
anterior communicating artery aneurysm origin in, 1927, 1927f
Laminectomy
cervical
complications of, 4424–4427, 4424t, 4426f
for degenerative disease, 4416–4418, 4417f, 4418f
with posterior segmental instrumentation, 4419–4424, 4422f, 4423f
indications for, 4414t
outcome of, 4427–4428
for metastases, 4858–4862, 4860f–4863f
lumbar
complication avoidance in, 581
infection after, 4383
olisthy after, 4532
regression of benefit in, 2940
spondylolisthesis after, 4543, 4544f
pathogenesis of, 4546–4547
thoracic, 4497, 4498f
biomechanics in, 4194–4195
complication avoidance in, 579
for bullet wounds, 4981
Laminin
in axonal regeneration, 200
in central nervous system repair, 4162
in malignant glioma, 761
Laminoforaminotomy, cervical, 4415–4416, 4415f, 4427
Laminoplasty, for cervical degenerative disease, 4418–4419, 4418f–4421f, 4425
Laminotomy, posterolateral decompression with, for thoracic fracture, 4973, 4974f
Lamotrigine, 2470t, 2472
Landau reflex, in cerebral palsy, 3725, 3726t
Landau-Kleffner syndrome, multiple subpial transection for, 2636
seizure outcome in, 2641
Langerhans cell histiocytosis
pediatric, 3591
skull, 1400–1401, 1401f
pediatric, 3719–3720, 3720f
spinal, 4355, 4837, 4843, 4845f
pediatric, 3567
Language
after traumatic brain injury, 5185–5186
callostomy effects on, 1244
delays in, cerebral palsy and, 3727, 3730, 3732
after dorsal rhizotomy, 3744
development of, 3170, 3170t
evaluation of, 264, 264f
single-photon emission computed tomography of, 2480
lateralization of, functional magnetic resonance imaging of, 2514, 2515f, 2516
temporal lobectomy effects on, 2610–2611
vs. speech, 2504
Language centers
imaging localization of, 2532
intracarotid amobarbital test for, 2532
resection of, in children, 2537
stimulation mapping of
anesthesia for, 2533
during face motor cortex resection, 2536
extraoperative, 2536
intraoperative, 2534–2536, 2535f, 2536f
Laparoscopic anterior interbody fusion
historical perspective on, 4788
indications for, 4788–4789
results of, 4789–4791
technique of, 4789, 4790f
Laparotomy, pain after, dorsal rhizotomy for, 3041
Laser, pulse-dye, for cerebral vasospasm, 1857
Laser-assisted percutaneous diskectomy, lumbar, 4780–4783
complications of, 4782, 4783
historical perspective on, 4780–4781
indications for, 4781
results of, 4782–4783
technique of, 4781–4782
Lateral angle, 32
Lateral femoral cutaneous nerve, entrapment of, 3933
Lateral mass plates, cervical, 4423–4424
Lateral medullary plate syndrome
mesencephalotomy for, 3077
sensory loss in, 273–274, 274f
Lateral parietotemporal line, 3
Lateral position, 597t, 598, 599f, 600
complication avoidance in, 562
for craniotomy, 628, 629f
Lateral recess, 31f, 32
artery of, 39
vein of, 35f
Lateral ventricle, 5, 7–11, 7f, 8f, 10f
anatomy of, 1237–1240, 1238f–1240f
arterial supply of, 1240, 1240f
atrium of, 1237, 1238f
tumors of, 1242–1243
body of, 1237, 1238f
tumors of, 1242
veins of, 17
choroid plexus tumors in, 3612
meningioma of, 1113
structures of, 1237–1238, 1238f
surgery on, venous ligation in, 1239–1240
tumors of, 1237–1245. *See also* specific site, e.g., Frontal horn.
benign, 1241
clinical presentation of, 1241
complications of, 1243–1245
malignant, 1241
outcome in, 1243–1245
primary, 1240
secondary, 1240–1241
surgical approaches to, 1241, 1242f
venous drainage of, 1238–1240, 1239f
xanthogranuloma of, 1443
Lateroanteocollis, 2894f, 2895
Laterocollis, 2892, 2892f, 2896t
rotatory, 2893, 2893f
Lateroretrocollis, 2894f, 2895
Latex allergy, in myelomeningocele, 3224
Lathyrism, familial spastic paraplegia in, 4319
Law enforcement, in child abuse, 3509
Le Fort fracture, complex, 5265–5266
Learning, after traumatic brain injury, 5187
Leber's hereditary optic neuropathy, 313
Leg(s)
discrepancies between, in occult spinal dysraphism, 3262, 3264, 3264f
pain in, surgery for, 3026t
Legal issues, 407–416
academic medical practice and, 409–410
confidentiality and, 411–412
end-of-life issues and, 414–416

Legal issues *(Continued)*
enforcement provisions in, 408
good Samaritan laws and, 408
in cervical hyperextension-hyperflexion injury, 4920
in child abuse, 3508–3512
informed consent and, 408
during pregnancy, 409
for human immunodeficiency virus testing, 409
for minors, 408–409
intraoperative electrophysiologic monitoring and, 4224–4225
medical malpractice and, 412–413
patient referrals and, 407
peer review committees and, 410–411
physician-patient privilege and, 411–412
records and, 411
reimbursement and, 413–414
reporting obligations and, 411–412
screening and, 407
stabilization and, 407
transfer and, 407–408
treatment obligations and, 408
Lemon sign, in Chiari malformation type II, 3349, 3350f
Lenticulostriate arteries, lateral, 21
Lentiform nucleus, 4f, 8f, 10f, 12f
Leprosy, neuropathy from, 3842
Leptin, blood-brain barrier transport of, 163
Leptomeningeal cyst, 3717
pediatric, 3707
Leptomeninges
lymphoma of, 1074
neoplasia of. *See* Meningitis, neoplastic.
Lesegue test, 4512, 4512f
Lethargy, 283
Letterer-Siwe disease, 1400, 3719
Leukemia
meningitis in, 1231–1234
Philadelphia chromosome in, 740
Leukocyte(s)
blood-borne, in inflammatory response, 674
homing of, 682
in cerebral ischemia, 136, 141–142, 143f
in traumatic brain injury, 5029
passive migration of, 681
Leukocyte inhibitory factor, in distal nerve stump, 200
Leukoencephalopathy, progressive multifocal, 832, 833
Leukotrienes
in blood-brain barrier permeability, 13
in cerebral vasospasm, 1848–1849
Leuprolide acetate, pseudotumor cerebri from, 1424
Levator scapulae, denervation of, 2897–2898
Levodopa, for Parkinson's disease, 2732–2733
Levonorgestrel, pseudotumor cerebri from, 1424
Lewy bodies, 2704
biologic significance of, 2709–2710
components of, 2709
detection of
α-synuclein staining in, 2709
ubiquitin staining in, 2709
in Parkinson's disease, 2708–2709
Lewy body dementia
apoptosis in, 2710
clinical features of, 2712
forms of, 2708–2709
Lewy body dementia *(Continued)*
neuritic Alzheimer's disease changes in, 2712
pathology of, 2712–2713
substantia nigra pars compacta in, 2706f
Lewy body disease, 2703–2713. *See also* Parkinson's disease.
diffuse, vs. Parkinson's disease, 2735
Parkinson's disease with, positron emission tomography of, 2759
α-synuclein in, 2703
Lhermitte's sign, 4397, 4410
Lhx2, 54t
Lhx9, 54t
Liability, attending physicians,' 410
Lidocaine
for spasticity, 2865, 2866t
peripheral nerve effects of, 3816
Life, definition of, 393
Life expectancy, 1781, 1782t
Life-sustaining treatment, 414
refusal of, 415
termination of, 414–415
Li-Fraumeni syndrome
brain tumors in, 812t, 813
malignant glioma in, 969
Ligament(s), spinal
biomechanics of, 4186–4187
injury to, imaging of, 523, 524f
Ligamentous laxity, in degenerative spondylolisthesis, 3580
Ligamentum flavum, 4186–4187
in spinal stenosis, 4521
ossification of, 4479
Ligamentum nuchae, 4925, 4926f
Light-headedness, presyncopal, 275, 347t
Likelihood ratio, 235, 237
Lim, 54t
LIM mineralization protein-1, 4609
Limbic system
antidepressant-sensitive areas of, 2954f
in pain perception, 2955–2956
in psychiatric disorders, 2854, 2855
leucotomy of, for psychiatric disorders, 2858–2859, 2858f
surgery on, 2854
Limen insulae, 4f, 5, 6f
Limiting sulcus, 5–6, 6f
Linac radiosurgery, 4111–4116, 4132–4133, 4132f. *See also* Radiosurgery.
dose planning for, 4134–4136, 4135f–4137f
for benign tumors, 4111–4112
for malignant tumors, 4112–4114
stereotactic imaging and localization in, 4133–4134
system requirements for, 4133, 4134f
Lindau's tumor, 1053
Linear accelerator–based radiosurgery. *See* Linac radiosurgery.
Lingual gyrus, 18f
Lipases, in arachidonic acid release, 1472–1473, 1472f
Lipid, peroxidation of, in cerebral vasospasm, 1848
Lipid membrane, transcellular passage through, 15
Lipofibrohamartoma, 3948–3949, 3949f
Lipolysis, ischemia and, 126–127
Lipoma, 3693, 3693f, 3948–3949, 3949f
congenital lumbosacral, 3229
anatomy of, 3230–3233, 3230f–3233f
caudal, 3230, 3230f, 3231–3232, 3232f
clinical presentation of, 3236–3238
complications in, 3242
Lipoma *(Continued)*
computed tomography of, 3239
dorsal, 3230–3231, 3230f
embryology of, 3233–3235, 3234f
in adults, 3238
magnetic resonance imaging of, 3238
neurological deficits in, 3237
orthopedic syndrome in, 3237
outcome in, 3242–3243
pathophysiology of, 3235–3236
radiography of, 3238
scoliosis in, 3238
somatosensory evoked potentials in, 3239
spinal cord retethering in, 3242
surgery for, 3239–3242, 3241f
transitional, 3230, 3230f, 3231
ultrasonography of, 3238
urodynamic studies in, 3239
urologic syndrome in, 3237–3238
conus medullaris, 3229
filum terminale, 3229
split spinal cord from, 3248, 3248f
intradural, 4316–4317
lumbosacral spine, occult spinal dysraphism in, 3229. *See also* Lipomyelomeningocele.
radiologic features of, 841
skull, 1389
spinal cord, 4260–4263, 4261f, 4262f, 4826, 4829f
Lipomeningomyelocystocele, 3226
Lipomyelocele, 3229, 4317
Lipomyelomeningocele, 3215, 3229–3243, 4317. *See also* Lipoma, congenital lumbosacral.
Lipophilicity, blood-brain barrier permeability and, 15, 16f
Lipoprotein, blood-brain barrier transport of, 162
Lipoxygenase, in arachidonic acid metabolism, 1473
Lips, in craniofacial trauma, 5251
Lis1, 54t, 61
Lissauer's tract, 2923, 2923f
Lissencephaly, 61, 61f
magnetic resonance imaging of, 2493
neuron migration failure and, 81
Lithium carbonate, pseudotumor cerebri from, 1422–1423
Lithotomy, peripheral nerve injuries in, 612
Liver, after subarachnoid hemorrhage, 1831
Lobectomy, anterior temporal, 2605–2607
complications of, 2610
outcome in, 2611
Locked-in syndrome, 273, 285, 285t
Locus ceruleus
in vagus nerve stimulation, 2644
stimulation of, 3122
Lomustine
for ependymoma, 1048t
for malignant glioma, 976
pharmacology of, 880–881
Long gyrus, anterior, of insula, 5, 6f
Long QT syndrome, ion channels in, 225t
Longitudinal ligament
anterior, 4186
posterior. *See* Posterior longitudinal ligament.
Longus colli muscle, rupture of, auto accidents and, 4917
Lordosis, 4306
congenital, 4318

Loss-of-heterozygosity analysis, 750, 750f
Low back, anatomy of, 4327–4328
Low back pain, 4147. *See also* Failed back syndrome.
causes of, 4327, 4329
hyperextension-hyperflexion injury and, 4918
in ankylosing spondylitis, 4349, 4350f, 4460–4461, 4460t
in enteropathic arthritis, 4351
in infection, 4351–4352, 4351f, 4352f
in inflammatory disorders, 4349–4351, 4350f
in metabolic bone disease, 4347–4349
in myofascial pain syndrome, 4351
in osteomalacia, 4347–4348
in osteoporosis, 4348–4349, 4348f
in Paget's disease, 4349
in pelvic disorders, 4359
in psoriatic arthropathy, 4350–4351
in Reiter's syndrome, 4350
in retroperitoneal disorders, 4359
in rheumatoid arthritis, 4351
in spondylolisthesis, 3572–3573
inflammatory syndrome in, 4331
mechanical (instability) syndrome in, 4331
myofascial syndrome in, 4330
neural compression syndrome in, 4330–4331
neuropathic syndrome in, 4331
pediatric
in intervertebral disk disease, 3559t
in spinal tumors, 3587
prevalence of, 4327
psychosocioeconomic syndrome in, 4332
radicular, 4328
rehabilitation for, 4330
spinal cord stimulation for, 3113
spinal origin of, 4329
classification of, 4330, 4330t
surgery for, 4337–4343
decision making in, 4329–4330
indications for, 4329
Low-birth-weight infants, cerebral palsy in, 3723, 3724t, 3736
Lubeluzole
in ischemia protection, 1522
tissue plasminogen activator with, 1498
Lüchenschädel, in Chiari malformation type II, 3349–3350, 3350f
Lumbago, 4330
Lumbar disk, 4327–4328
Lumbar disk disease, 4507–4519, 4704, 4731, 4737, 4771–4795
anatomic considerations in, 4507–4508, 4507f
anterior procedures for, 4788–4791
automated percutaneous diskectomy for, 4776–4780
bone morphogenetic protein for, interbody fusion with, 4792–4794, 4793f
chemonucleolysis for, 4771–4776
complications of, 4775
historical perspective on, 4771–4772
indications for, 4772
results of, 4775
technique of, 4773–4775, 4774f
clinical presentation of, 4510–4513, 4511f–4513f
computed tomography of, 4513, 4513f
degenerative, 4704
differential diagnosis of, 4510–4511, 4511f
Lumbar disk disease *(Continued)*
endoscopic diskectomy for, 4783–4788, 4786f, 4787f
far lateral herniation in, 4530
fusion in, 4531
outcome in, 4531
surgery for, 4530–4531
gene therapy for, 4794–4795
historical perspective on, 4507
imaging of, 4512–4513, 4513f
intradiskal electrothermal annuloplasty for, 4791–4792, 4793f
laparoscopic anterior interbody fusion for, 4788–4791, 4790f
laser-assisted percutaneous diskectomy for, 4780–4783
magnetic resonance imaging of, 4512–4513, 4513f
pathophysiology of, 4508–4510, 4508f–4510f
pediatric, 3560–3562
differential diagnosis of, 3561, 3564–3568, 3565t
epidemiology of, 3560
examination of, 3561–3562
history of, 3560–3561, 3561t
imaging of, 3562–3563, 3563f
outcome in, 3564, 3564t
pain in, 3560–3561
signs of, 3561t
surgery for, 3564
symptoms of, 3561t
pedicle fixation in, biomechanics in, 4198
physical examination in, 4511–4512, 4512f
posterior procedures for, 4771–4788
surgery for
complications of
intraoperative, 4517
postoperative, 4517–4519, 4517f, 4518f
indications for, 4513–4514
technique of, 4514–4517, 4515f, 4516f
symptoms of, 4510, 4511f
urologic disorders in, 375
Lumbar diskectomy
complication avoidance in, 580–581
endoscopic, 4783–4788, 4786f, 4787f
percutaneous
automated, 4776–4780
laser-assisted, 4780–4783
Lumbar facet joint, 4328
arthropathy of, 2977–2978, 2979f
injections into, 2977
intra-articular injections into, 2977
medial branch of, 2977, 2978f
denervation of, 2977, 2980
percutaneous radiofrequency rhizotomy of, 3038–3039
pain syndromes affecting, 4330
Lumbar puncture
for infantile posthemorrhagic hydrocephalus, 3411, 3412f, 3413
in spinal metastases, 4856
in subarachnoid hemorrhage, 1817–1818, 1818t
Lumbar spine
anatomy of, 4327–4328, 4705, 4705f
anterior interbody fusion of, 4340, 4717, 4718f
laparoscopic, 4788–4791, 4790f
anterior procedures on, 4701–4725
biomechanics of, 4714–4715
complication avoidance in, 579–580
Lumbar spine *(Continued)*
complications of, 4722, 4724
historical perspective on, 4701
indications for, 4701–4704
innovations in, 4724
surgical approaches in, 4707–4714, 4709f–4713f
arthrodesis-stabilization of, 4339–4343, 4341f, 4342f
biomechanics of, 4191
chordoma of, 4848, 4849f
diseases of, endoscopic treatment of, 3431
eosinophilic granuloma of, 3591, 3592f
extension of, 4328
flexion of, 4328
in ankylosing spondylitis, 4460, 4461f
flexion-compression injury to, 4191–4192
flexion-distraction fracture of, 521, 522f
fracture of
burst, 4993, 4995f
percutaneous screws/rods in, 5006, 5006f
treatment of, 4999
classification of, 4992–4997, 4993t
seat belt–type injury and, 4993, 4996f
surgery for, decompression/ instrumentation in, 5004–5005
wedge compression, 4993, 4994f
treatment of, 4998–4999, 4999f
fracture-dislocation of, 4993, 4996–4997, 4997f
treatment of, 4999
fusion of, complication avoidance in, 581–582
ganglionectomy in, 3035–3037
great vessels and, 4706
iatrogenic instability of, 4735–4736
infection of, 4704
pyogenic, 4376, 4378f
injury to, 4702–4704, 4731, 4732t, 4987–5006
anatomic influences in, 4991–4992
evaluation of, 4987–4991
Frankel classification of, 4988, 4988t
imaging of, 4990–4991, 4990f, 4991f
methylprednisolone in, 4988
motor index score in, 4988, 4988t
neurological examination in, 4988–4990, 4988t, 4989f
outcomes in, 5005–5006
posterior instrumentation for, 4734–4735
spinal examination in, 4988
treatment of, 4997
internal fixation of, 4342, 4342f, 4597, 4715–4717, 4716f–4718f
anterior, complications of, 4722, 4724
implantation techniques for, 4717–4722, 4719f–4721f, 4723f–4724f
posterior, 4731–4740, 4733–4734, 4733f–4735f
posterior rod-hook constructs in, 4733, 4733f
posterior rod–multiple hook constructs in, 4734, 4734f
posterior wire-rod constructs in, 4733–4734, 4734f
screw-plate constructs in, 4716–4717, 4717f
screw-rod constructs in, 4715–4716, 4716f
transpedicular screws in, 4734, 4735f
neuronal structures of, 4706–4707, 4708f

Lumbar spine (Continued)
olisthy of, 4531–4532
pediatric, osteoid osteoma of, 3588, 3588f
posterior interbody fusion of, 4340
posterior procedures on, 4731–4740
complication avoidance in, 580–581
indications for, 4731–4732
instrumentation for, 4733–4734, 4733f–4735f
outcomes of, 4734–4737
technical considerations in, 4737–4738
technique of, 4738–4740, 4738f, 4739f
radiography of, 501, 502f, 4732–4733
reoperation on, 4339
seat belt–type injury to, treatment of, 4999
segmental instability syndrome of, posterior fixation systems for, 4341–4342, 4342f
segmental stabilization of, 4341, 4341f
spinal cord injury without radiographic abnormality in, 3523
spondylolysis of, radiography of, 501, 502f
stenosis of, 4521–4536. *See also* Spinal stenosis, lumbar.
surgical approaches to, 4707–4714
anterior, 640–642
anterolateral, 640, 641f
endoscopic transperitoneal, 642
indications for, 4329
paramedian, 641, 642f, 643f
retroperitoneal, 4710, 4711f–4713f
posterior, 642–643
retroperitoneal, 4708
for disk disease, 4791
ventrolateral, 4708–4710, 4709f, 4710f
transperitoneal, 4710, 4712, 4714
tumors of, 4701–4702, 4732
vs. lumbar disk disease, 4510–4511
ventral musculature and, 4705–4706, 4706f, 4707f
visceral structures and, 4707
Lumbar sympathetic block, 2984
Lumbosacral plexopathy, idiopathic, 3841
Lumbosacral plexus injury, 3969
severity of, 3970
treatment of, 3973
Lumbosacral spine
congenital lipoma of, 3229. *See also* Lipoma, congenital lumbosacral.
lipoma of, occult spinal dysraphism in, 3229. *See also* Lipomyelomeningocele.
Lund therapy, 5125, 5125f, 5126t
Lung(s)
in traumatic brain injury, 5123
infections of, in spinal cord injury, 4881
rheumatoid arthritis involvement of, 4572–4573
Lung cancer
in pregnancy, 872
metastatic
to orbit, 1376
to skull, 1392
small cell, prophylactic radiation therapy for, 1080
Lupus glomerulonephritis, tuberculosis in, 1442f
Luque construct, lumbar, 4733–4734, 4734f
complication avoidance in, 582
Luxury perfusion, 490, 1601, 1603f
in head injury, 5051–5052
Lyme disease
myelitis in, 4313
neuropathy from, 3842
reporting obligations in, 411–412
vs. multiple sclerosis, 1453, 1453t
Lymphangioma, 3947t, 3948
skull, 1384–1385, 1385f
Lymphocytes
cytotoxic T, 678
immune specificity of, 679
in astrocytoma, 890
in central nervous system, 890
in immune response, 674–675, 675f
tumor-infiltrating, 887
Lymphoid tissue, secondary, in immune response initiation, 679
Lymphokine-activated killer cells, for brain tumors, 887
Lymphoma
angiotrophic, classification of, 670
cerebral, 1067–1074. *See also* Lymphoma, primary central nervous system.
leptomeningeal, 1074
meningitis in, 1231–1234
of skull, 1393, 1394f
primary central nervous system, 1067–1074
AIDS-associated, 1069–1070, 1071f
cerebrospinal fluid in, 1069–1070
chemotherapy for, 1072, 1073t, 4023
classification of, 670
clinical features of, 1068–1069, 1069t
diagnosis of, 1069–1070, 1070f, 1071f, 1072
epidemiology of, 1067, 1068t
in pregnancy, 872
incidence of, 809
magnetic resonance imaging of, 1069, 1070f, 1071f
neoplastic lymphoid cells in, 1068, 1069f
ocular manifestations of, 1068–1069
pathology of, 1067–1068, 1068f, 1069f
radiation therapy for, 1072, 1073t, 4022–4023
recurrent, 1073–1074
risk factors for, 1068t
surgery for, 1072–1073
symptoms of, 1069, 1069t
treatment of, 1072–1073
vs. secondary cerebral lymphoma, 1070
radiologic features of, 529, 529f, 835, 849, 849f
Lymphotoxin, in multiple sclerosis, 1450

Machado-Joseph disease, 2719
Macrocephaly, 428, 428f
vein of Galen malformation with, 2216f
Macroglia, lineage pathways for, 97–98, 98f
Macrophage inflammatory protein, in cerebral ischemia, 140
Macrophages
in axonal regeneration, 206
in central nervous system, 4155
in central nervous system repair, 4164
in cerebral ischemia, 136
in distal nerve stump, 199
in peripheral nervous system injury, 195
radiomarkers for, 1609
Macrosomia, in Dandy-Walker syndrome, 3286
Macula, 2542
Maffucci's syndrome, chondroma with, 1387, 4840
Mafosfamide, for neoplastic meningitis, 1233
Magnesium, in bone, 4231
Magnetic resonance angiography, 1575–1597
black blood, signal loss and, 1577, 1578f
clinical applications of, 1588–1597
contrast-enhanced, 1586–1588, 1587f
elliptical centric view order in, 1587
fluoroscopic triggering in, 1587
single-phase, 1587–1588
test bolus timing in, 1587
of carotid artery atherosclerosis, 1588–1590, 1588f–1590f
of extracranial circulation, 1588–1591
of intracranial circulation, 1591–1597
phase contrast, 1584–1586
bipolar gradient in, 1584–1585, 1585f
flow velocity quantification in, 1586
two-dimensional, 1586, 1586f
phase difference image in, 1585
techniques in, 1582–1588
time of flight, 1582–1584
three-dimensional, 1583–1584, 1584f, 1585f
magnetization transfer, 1584
MOTSA, 1584, 1584f
TONE pulse, 1584, 1585f
venetian blind artifact in, 1584
zero filling, 1584, 1585f
two-dimensional, 1583, 1583f
lipid suppression in, 1583, 1583f
Magnetic resonance imaging, 439–473
amplitude effects in, 1575–1579, 1576f–1579f, 1580
clinical, 449
diffusion in, 446–447
displacement artifact in, 1577–1578, 1579f, 1580
echo planar image in, 444, 446, 447f
entry-slice effect in, 1576, 1577f
fast spin echo, 444, 445f
flow compensation in, 1581–1582
flow effects in, 1575–1582
flow-related enhancement in, 1575, 1576f
functional, 448–449, 449f, 852–853, 853f
in vision mapping, 2544–2546, 2545f
gadolinium contrast, 443–444
ghosting artifacts in, 1581, 1582f
gradient echo, 444
gradient moment nulling in, 1581–1582
gradients in, 441, 441f
historical aspects of, 439
hydrogen nucleus in, 439
image contrast in, origin of, 441–443, 442f
image weighting in, 443, 443t
in surgical navigation systems, 943, 944f, 946
inconsistent phase in, 1581
in-flow effect in, 1575, 1576f
intravoxel phasing dispersion in, 1580–1581, 1581f
inversion recovery, 444, 446f
isochromat in, 1580, 1581f
magnets for, 439
magnitude effects in, 1575–1580, 1576f–1579f
nuclear spins in, 439–440, 440f
of peripheral nerve disorders, 3873–3886
perfusion in, 447
phase effects in, 1580–1582, 1580f–1582f

Magnetic resonance imaging *(Continued)*
physics of, 439–443
pulsatile flow in, 1581, 1582f
radiofrequency coil in, 440, 440f
relaxation rates in, 442, 442f
screening, 449
signal in
creation of, 439–440, 440f
detection of, 440, 440f, 441f
localization of, 441, 441f
skull, 432–433
spatial presaturation in, 1577
spectroscopy in, 447–448, 448f
spin echo, 443, 443f, 443t
signal loss with, 1576–1577, 1577f, 1578f
spinal, 503–505, 505f, 4145
T1 saturation in, 1575
tailored examination with, 449
TOF effects in, 1575–1579, 1576f–1579f, 1580
tridirectional flow compensation in, 1579f, 1580
voxel intensity in, 441–442
wash-in effect in, 1575, 1576f
Magnetic resonance neurography
for peripheral nerve disorders, 3873–3875, 3874f
spinal, 504, 505f
Magnetic resonance spectroscopy, spinal, 504–505
Magnetic resonance stereotaxy, frameless, depth electrode insertion with, 2559, 2559f
Magnetoencephalography, vision mapping with, 2546–2547, 2547f
Major histocompatibility complex (MHC)
detection of, 678
expression of, 678–679, 678f
in antigen re-presentation, 682
in antigen presentation, 887
in blood-brain barrier function, 12
in multiple sclerosis, 1450
peptide-, T-cell receptor recognition of, 676, 679
polymorphism in, 679
Major histocompatibility complex (MHC) restriction, 679
Malformation(s), neuronal development defects and, 81–82, 81f
Malignancy, 2989t
Malignant phenotype, switch to, 773, 774t
Malignant reticulosis. *See* Central nervous system, primary lymphoma of.
Malignant tumors of neural sheath origin, 3951, 3952t, 3953–3954, 3953f
Malignant tumors of nonneural sheath origin, 3954–3955, 3955f
Mamillary body, 14f
Mandated reporters, for child abuse, 3508–3509
Mandible
fracture of
airway management in, 5246
plate fixation for, 5264–5265
positioning of, in rigid fixation, 5265
Mannitol
administration of, blood-brain barrier in, 17
brain dehydration with, 1505
for pediatric cerebral edema, 3190
in distal anterior cerebral artery aneurysm surgery, 1950
in intracranial pressure management, 189, 5058, 5097
Mannitol *(Continued)*
in ischemia prevention, 1522
in pediatric glioma surgery, 3598
pregnancy effects on, 2423
Marfan's syndrome, aneurysms in, 1772
Marginal ramus, 24–25, 24f
Marimastat, angiosuppressive therapy with, 776–777
Martin-Gruber anastomosis, 3898
Mash1, 54t
Masking, in hearing assessment, 331–332
Massa intermedia, 13, 14f, 15f, 22f
in Chiari malformation type II, 3351
Matching, in outcomes assessment, 245
Math1, 54t
Math5, 54t
Matrix Gla protein, 4230
Matrix metalloproteinase
for glioma invasion, 766
in multiple sclerosis, 1450
Maxilla
dentition of, 5249
fracture of, sagittal, 5265
Maxillary sinus tumors, staging of, 1317, 1318t
Mayfield skull fixation, 624–625, 624f–626f, 627, 4657, 4657f
in thoracic spine fracture, 4968
McCune-Albright syndrome, 3590, 3719
skull in, 1401, 1402f
McGill Pain Questionnaire, 243t
McGregor's line, 423f, 424
McRae's line, 424f, 425
MDR1, 162
MDR2, 162
Mean arterial pressure, cerebral perfusion pressure and, 1467
Measurement, 238–244
choice of, 241, 244
clinical agreement in, 240–241, 241t
instruments for, 241, 242t–243t
reliability in, 239–240
responsiveness in, 239, 240
surrogate vs. true end points in, 238–239
techniques of, 239–241
validity in, 239
MECA-32, 158
Mechanical (instability) pain syndrome, 4331
arthrodesis-stabilization of, 4340
Mechanoreceptors, 73–74, 74f, 3809
Meckel-Gruber syndrome, in parietal encephalocele, 3202
Meckel's cave, meningioma of, 1278
Meckel's ganglion blockade, 2982
Medial antebrachial cutaneous nerve, 3899, 3899f
Medial lemniscus, 3074–3075, 3079
stimulation of, 3122, 3125
Medial longitudinal fasciculus
in consciousness, 289
pediatric, examination of, 3174
Median eminence, 33f, 34
Median fissure, 29
anterior, 30f
Median nerve
anatomy of, 3889, 3924
conduction studies of, 3857–3858
demyelination of, 3853
entrapment of
above wrist, 3924–3925
at wrist, 3889, 3923–3924. *See also* Carpal tunnel syndrome.
by supracondylar process, 3924
in upper forearm, 3924–3925
Median nerve *(Continued)*
somatosensory evoked potentials of, in coma prognostication, 3861
surgical approaches to
exposure for, 650–651, 650f, 651f
positioning for, 608, 650
tumors of, electrodiagnostic testing for, 3866, 3866f–3868f, 3868
Median sulcus, 33f
Medicaid, legal issues in, 413
Medical literature, critical assessment of, 257–259
Medical malpractice, 412
expert witness in, 413
lawsuit in, 412
physician's role in, 412–413
Medical records
confidentiality of, 411
of minors, 411
Medical Research Council Grading System, 243t
Medicare, legal issues in, 407, 413
Medicare-Medicaid antikickback statute, 413–414
Medicine, academic practice of, legal issues regarding, 409–410
Medulla, 29
glioma of, pediatric, 3667
lateral, lesions of, 273–274, 274f
Medullary artery, 2380–2381
Medullary stria, 33f
Medullary vein, 35f, 2381, 2383, 2384f
Medullary velum
inferior, 31f, 32, 33f, 35f
superior, 31f, 33f
Medulloblastoma, 1031–1040
anaplastic, 3640
biologic indicators in, 1006, 1006t
chemotherapy for, 1005, 1038–1039
classification of, 668–669, 1031, 1032t, 1034, 1036t
clinical presentation of, 1033
complications of, 1004
definition of, 997, 998
desmoplastic, 668, 998, 999f, 1032
epidemiology of, 1031, 1032t
gene alterations in, 751t
histogenesis of, 1032–1033
hydrocephalus in, treatment of, 1002–1003
imaging of, 1033–1034, 1034f–1036f
in pregnancy, 872
large cell, 668, 3640
metastases in, 1002, 1003f, 1034
molecular biology of, 1033
neurotrophins in, 729
outcome in, 1004–1007
pathology of, 998–999, 1031–1032, 1032f
pediatric, 3639–3649
chemotherapy for, 3647–3648, 3702
complications of, 3648–3649
differential diagnosis of, 3640
epidemiology of, 3639
extent of, 3646
genetic abnormalities in, 3640–3641
growth factors in, 3640–3641
hydrocephalus in, 3643–3644
imaging of, 3641–3643, 3641f–3643f
metastatic, 3642
pathology of, 3639–3641
prognosis of, 3646
radiation therapy for, 3646–3647
complications of, 3648
recurrence of, 3649
shunts in, 3643–3644

Medulloblastoma (Continued)
staging of, 3646
surgery for, 3643–3645
complications of, 3645–3646
platelet-derived growth factor in, 730
platelet-derived growth factor receptor in, 730
radiation therapy for, 1005–1006, 1038
radiography of, 1000, 1001f, 1002, 1003f
radiologic features of, 847, 849
recurrent, 1006–1007, 1039
signs/symptoms of, 1000
staging of, 1034–1036, 1036t, 1037t
surgery for, 1036–1038
surveillance of, 1039, 1039t
terminology for, 1031
treatment of, 1036–1039
algorithm for, 1040, 1040f
complications of, 1037–1038
sequelae of, 1039–1040
vs. primitive neuroectodermal tumors, 1032
Medulloblastoma cerebelli, 1031
Medulloepithelioma, 669
Megalencephaly, benign familial, head circumference curves in, 3397, 3397f
Meige's syndrome, 2721
Meissner's corpuscle, 74, 74f, 3809, 3810f
Melanocytic nevus, scalp, 1410–1411
Melanoma
brain metastases in, 1078
stereotactic radiosurgery for, 1091–1092
epidemiology of, 1411
in pregnancy, 872
radiologic features of, 852
scalp, 1411–1413, 1412f
staging of, 1411–1412
treatment of, 1412–1413, 1412f
Melanoma antigen-encoding (MAGE) gene, 890
Melanosis, neurocutaneous, brain tumors in, 812t, 813
Melatonin, in pineal parenchymal cell tumors, 1014
Membrane potential, of astrocytes, 101
Membrane-associated guanylate kinase homologue (MAGUK) proteins, 156
Membranous labyrinth, 327
Memory
evaluation of, 264, 264f, 265
single-photon emission computed tomography in, 2480
intracarotid amobarbital testing of, 2506, 2507–2508
Memory loss
anterior temporal lobe resection and, vs. amygdalohippocampectomy, 2572
forniceal surgery and, 1259–1260
global, after epilepsy surgery, 2571
hyperextension-hyperflexion injury and, 4919
intracarotid amobarbital procedure for, 2571–2572
material-specific, after epilepsy surgery, 2572
temporal lobe resections and, 2617–2618
third ventricular tumor surgery and, 1258
traumatic brain injury and, 2451, 2452, 2453f, 5187
MEN1, 744
Ménière's disease
endolymphatic sac procedures for, 2908
treatment of, 2906
vertigo in, 349–350, 2902, 2903f
Meningeal artery, posterior, 37
Meningeal hemangiopericytoma, 1133–1138
classification of, 670
clinical findings in, 1134
imaging of, 1134, 1135f, 1136f
incidence of, 1134
metastatic, 1137, 1137t
molecular biology of, 1133–1134
pathology of, 1133, 1134f
prognosis of, 1137–1138
recurrent, 1136–1137, 1137t
survival in, 1137, 1137t
treatment of, 1134, 1136, 1137f
Meninges
arterial supply of, 1108, 1109t
embryology of, 1099–1100, 1100f
in Chiari malformation type I, 3349
in Chiari malformation type II, 3350–3351
tumors of, classification of, 669–670, 669t, 1100t
Meningioangiomatosis, 670
Meningioma, 1099–1127, 1362–1364, 1363f, 3949, 4296t
anaplastic, 1102, 1102f
angioblastic, 1133
angiography of, 1108, 1109t
anterior skull base, 910, 910f, 1364
atypical, 1102, 1102f
brain edema in, 795, 796f, 797f
brainstem, vs. acoustic neuroma, 1150f
cavernous sinus, 1118, 1118f
surgical approach to, 1278
central skull base, 1265, 1267
cerebellopontine angle, 1119, 1119f, 1120f
classification of, 669–670, 669t
clinical behavior of, 1103
clinoidal, 1115–1116, 1116f, 1117f
clival, 1120, 1120f
convexity, 1111, 1111f
cranial thickening from, 429, 429f
diaphragma sellae, 1117
distribution of, 1101–1102
dural, surgery for, 905
epidemiology of, 1104
etiology of, 1104–1106
extraneuraxial, 1103–1104
falcine, 1112–1113
fibroblastic, 1101, 1101f
foramen magnum, 1121, 1122f, 1123, 1123f, 4809, 4811–4812, 4811f
genetic aspects of, 751t, 1106–1107, 1106f, 1107f
global, bone invasion in, 1364, 1364f
grading of, 1101t, 1109, 1109t, 1110t
hemangiopericytic, 1102
historical background on, 1099
hormonal therapy for, 1110–1111
hyperostosing "en plaque," 1362–1363, 1363f, 1364
hyperostosis in, 1102, 1103f
imaging of, 526, 526f
immunohistochemistry of, 1102, 1103, 1103f
in breast cancer, 1105
in pregnancy, 871–872, 872f
incidence of, 809
insulin-like growth factors in, 728–729
interstitial brachytherapy for, 4105
intraosseous, 1103–1104
intraventricular, 1113
jugular foramen, 1120–1121, 1122f
magnetic resonance imaging of, 453, 455, 456f
Meningioma (Continued)
malignant, 1138
radiation therapy for, 4023
malignant potential of, 1103
meningothelial, 1101, 1101f
metastases in, 1104
MIB-1 labeling index for, 702–703, 703t
multiple, 1103
nonsurgical treatment of, 1110–1111
olfactory groove, 1114–1115, 1115f, 1265
imaging of, 1268, 1270f–1275f, 1273, 1275
surgical approach to, 1276
results of, 1279t, 1280
optic nerve, 309, 1118–1119
optic nerve sheath, 1372
orbital, 1118–1119, 1372
parasagittal, 1111–1112, 1112f, 1113f
clinical presentation of, 1268, 1268f, 1269f
surgical approach to, 1276, 1277f, 1278
results of, 1278, 1279t, 1280
pathology of, 1100–1104, 1100t, 1101f–1103f
periorbital, 1372
petroclival, 1119–1120, 1120f, 1121f
platelet-derived growth factor in, 730
posterior fossa, 1119–1120, 1119f–1121f
proliferation markers for, 702–703, 703t
radiation therapy for, 1110
radiation-induced, 1105, 1105f
radiologic features of, 835, 836, 837f, 838f, 1108–1109, 1109t
radiosurgery for, 4056, 4059, 4060t, 4061f, 4062f
linac, 4111–4112
receptors in, 1107–1108
recurrent, 568, 1109–1110
seizures and, 568, 568t
skull, 1397–1398, 1398f, 1399f
skull base
radiosurgical complications in, 574
surgical approaches to, 1123–1127
sphenoid petroclival, 1120, 1120f
sphenoid planum, 1364
sphenoid wing, 1115, 1372
spinal cord, 4300, 4819, 4819f
treatment of, 4823–4824
stereotactic radiation therapy for, outcome in, 4030
superior sagittal sinus, 1265
surgery for, 1109–1110, 1111–1123
complication avoidance in, 567–568, 568t
posterior fossa intradural approach to, 925–927, 926f
tentorial, 1114
third ventricular, 1246
transitional, 1101, 1101f
trauma and, 1104–1105
tuberculum sellae, 1116–1118, 1117f
surgical approach to, 1276
variants of, 1102
vascular endothelial growth factor in, 733
vascular supply to, 860t
venous thrombosis in, 1105–1106
viruses and, 1105
vs. acoustic neuroma, 1153
vs. fibrosarcoma, 1143
vs. trigeminal schwannoma, 1347–1348
Meningioma en plaque, 1100
Meningitis
acoustic neuroma surgery and, 571
after myelomeningocele repair, 3223

Meningitis (Continued)
aseptic
ependymoma surgery and, 3629–3630
in epidermoid tumor, 3690
medulloblastoma surgery and, 3645
bacterial, magnetic resonance imaging of, 461–463, 463f
glomus jugulare tumor surgery and, 1307
in dermal sinus tracts, 3274
in pyogenic spinal infection, 4371, 4371f
in sarcoidosis, 1436
in traumatic cerebrospinal fluid fistula, 5268–5271
neoplastic, 1231–1234
chemotherapy for, 1233–1234
clinical presentation of, 1231
imaging of, 1232
incidence of, 1231
laboratory findings in, 1231–1232
pathology of, 1232
radiotherapy for, 1233
staging of, 1232–1233
surgery for, 1233
treatment of, 1233–1234
pseudotumor cerebri in, 1425
transsphenoidal surgery and, 1182
tuberculous, 1440
magnetic resonance imaging of, 463, 464f
viral, magnetic resonance imaging of, 461, 462f
Meningocele, 4259
anterior, 3278–3280, 3279f, 3280f
definition of, 3215
posterior, 3276, 3276f–3278f, 3278
spina bifida aperta with, 4316
Meningocele manqué, 3280
mesencephalic, 3205
Meningothelial cells, tumors of, 1142t
Menstrual cycle, in prolactinoma, 1185
Mental retardation
familial, with brain tumors, 811
in cerebral palsy, 3727
neuron migration failure and, 81
Mental status
in brain tumors, 827–828, 827t
in mild head injury, 5073
Mental status examination, pediatric, 3171–3172
Mepitiostane, for meningioma, 1110
Meralgia paresthetica, 3933–3934
Merkel cells, 74, 74f
Merkel receptor, 3809, 3810f
Merlin, in meningioma, 1107
Mesencephalic nucleus, 3048
Mesencephalic sulcus, lateral, 10f, 32–33, 33f
Mesencephalic syndrome, 322–323
Mesencephalic tissue grafts, 2836–2837
Mesencephalic vein, lateral, 36f
Mesencephalon
anatomy of, 3073–3075, 3074f
in Chiari malformation type II, 3351
Mesencephalotomy, 3073–3079
historical development of, 3075–3077, 3076f
indications for, 3077–3078, 3077f
results of, 3078–3079
stimulation studies in, 3076–3077, 3076f
technique of, 3078
Mesenchymal tumors, 1142t
Meta-analysis, 252–253
Metabolic disorders, osseous, 4235–4236, 4308–4309, 4347–4349, 4348f. See also Bone metabolism.
Metabolism, reduction of, in ischemia protection, 1521
Metabolites, vasoactive, in cerebral blood flow autoregulation, 5049–5050
Metals, brain tumors and, 811
Metastases
brain. See Brain metastases.
central nervous system, radiologic features of, 851–852, 852f
from spinal osteosarcoma, 4845
hemorrhagic
radiologic features of, 851–852
vs. supratentorial cavernous malformation, 2311
in pregnancy, 872
intradural extramedullary, imaging of, 527, 528f, 529
paranasal sinuses, 1313, 1315f
radiologic features of, 835
scalp, 1416
skull, 1392–1395, 1392f–1395f
spinal. See Spinal metastases.
surgery for, tumor removal in, 905
vs. irradiation plexitis, 3954
vs. trigeminal schwannoma, 1347
Metencephalon, in Chiari malformation type II, 3351–3352, 3352f
Methotrexate
for multiple sclerosis, 1454t, 1455
for neoplastic meningitis, 1233
for primary central nervous system lymphoma, 1072
for sarcoidosis, 1439
Methylmethacrylate, vertebral reconstruction with, 4767, 4768f, 4769
Methylprednisolone
for cerebral vasospasm, 1854
for cervical spine trauma, 4890–4891
for glial tumors, 870
for multiple sclerosis, 1454t
for spinal cord injury, 4988
in cervical spine fixation, 4622
in CNS inflammation, 206
in occipitocervical fusion, 4657
Metopic suture, 431–432
Mexiletine, for neuropathic pain, 3838
Meyerding classification, of spondylolisthesis, 3572, 3572f
Meyer's loop, 9, 2541
lesions of, visual field defects from, 2542, 2542f
mGluR2 receptor, in striatum, 2686, 2686f
MHC. See Major histocompatibility complex (MHC).
Miami-J collar, 4898f
MIB-1 labeling index, 695–696
for astrocytoma, 696, 697t, 698
for chordoma, 704, 704t
for craniopharyngioma, 704, 705t
for ependymomas, 700–701, 700t, 701t
for ganglioglioma, 702, 702t
for hemangioblastoma, 703
for hemangiopericytoma, 703, 704t
for meningioma, 702–703, 703t
for neurocytoma, 701–702, 702t
for oligodendroglioma, 699, 699t
for pilocytic astrocytoma, 699, 700t
for pleomorphic xanthoastrocytoma, 700
for schwannoma, 704
Mice
knockout, 714
transgenic, 714
Microarrays, 753–754, 754f
Microcephaly, 428
Microglia, 83
Microglia (Continued)
after central nervous system injury, 4168
amyloid plaque infiltration by, 90, 91f
distribution of, 87, 89f
function of, 87–88, 90f, 91f
in blood-brain barrier, 153
radiomarkers for, 1609
ramified, 88
"reactive," 88, 90, 90f
sources for, stem cells as, 93, 94f
turnover of, 90–91
Microglial cells
antigen presentation by, 889–890
in axonal regeneration, 206
Microgliomatosis. See Central nervous system, primary lymphoma of.
Microsurgery, endoscopic, 3430
Microtubule-associated protein 1B, after traumatic brain injury, 5032
Micturition, 363
frontal lobes in, 359, 360f
intravesical pressure in, 365
neuromuscular function of, 363
parasympathetic nervous system arcs in, 361–362, 362f
pontine center for, 359, 359f
reflex, 365
sensation of, 365
suprapontine centers in, 360–361
supraspinal arcs in, 360–361
sympathetic nervous system arcs in, 361, 361f
urgency of, 364–365
Midazolam, pediatric, 3188
Midbrain, 14f, 15f, 29
anatomy of, 3054
compression of, pineal region tumors and, 1013
glioma of, pediatric, 3666, 3666f
hemorrhage of, 5091, 5092f
in Chiari malformation type II, 3351
syndromes affecting, 272–273
tegmentum of, 10f
tractotomy of, 3045, 3054–3056
complications of, 3055–3056
electrical stimulation in, 3055, 3055t
evaluation before, 3055
indications for, 3054–3055
Midbrain syndrome, dorsal, 322–323
Middle ear, glomus jugulare tumor of, 1297, 1299f
Middle fossa, 422–423
anterior approaches to, 919, 919f
cavernous malformation of, 2317
enlargement of, 431
erosion of, 431
extradural approach to, 921–923, 923f
fracture of, rhinorrhea in, 5268
intradural approach to, 920, 920f, 923–924
trigeminal schwannoma of, 1346, 1349
weakness of, 426
Mifepristone, for meningioma, 1110
Migraine, 276t
familial hemiplegic, ion channels in, 225t
vertigo in, 352, 2901–2902
Millard-Gubler syndrome, 273, 273f
Miller-Fisher syndrome, 3839
Millon Clinical Multi-Axial Inventory, 5192
Minerva jacket, 4899, 4899f
complications of, 3544
Minimally conscious state, 284
Minimally responsive state, 284
Mini-mental Status Examination, 264, 264f
Miniseizures, 2436

Minnesota Multiphasic Personality Inventory-2, 5192
Minocycline, pseudotumor cerebri from, 1424
Minors
informed consent for, 408–409
medical care decisions by, 411
medical records of, 411
Miosis, 288
Misery perfusion, 489, 1601, 1602f
Misonidazole, in malignant glioma radiosensitization, 4019–4020
Missile injury. *See also* Bullet wounds.
peripheral nerve, 3827
traumatic aneurysms from, 2131
Mitochondria
dysfunction of, 274
after traumatic brain injury, 5027
in cell death, 132–133
in brain metabolism, 117–120, 118f, 119f
Mitochondrial permeability transition megapore, 5027
Mitogens, 48
Mitosis, tumor grading with, 689–692
frequency in, 691–692
molecular marker correlation with, 692
presence vs. absence in, 691
Mitoxantrone, for multiple sclerosis, 1454t, 1455
Mixed channels, 220t
MK 801, in intracerebral hemorrhage, 1741
Mnr2, 54t
Modeling, in outcomes assessment, 245
Modified Ashworth scale, in cerebral palsy, 3725, 3726t
Molecular markers
mitotic activity correlation with, 692
proliferation, 692–696
Molecular medicine, positron emission tomography in, 491–493, 492f, 493f
Monoclonal antibodies, for neoplastic meningitis, 1233
Monoclonal gammopathy, 3841
Monocytes, in cerebral ischemia, 136, 137–138
Mononeuritis, 271
Mononeuritis multiplex, 3834, 3834t
Mononeuropathy
diabetic, 3843
physical features of, 270–271
Mononeuropathy multiplex, 271, 3834, 3834t
Monro-Kellie doctrine, 178, 1469
MOPP therapy, for ependymoma, 1048, 1048t
Morcellation technique, historical aspects of, 3161, 3163f
Morning stiffness, pain with, 4302–4303, 4303t, 4304f
Moro reflex
in cerebral palsy, 3725, 3726t
testing of, 3181–3182
Morphine
intrathecal
complications of, 3140
for cancer pain, 3133–3134
pump for, regression of benefit in, 2941
tolerance to, 3134, 3134f, 3140–3141
transport of, across blood-brain barrier, 15
Morquio's syndrome
atlantoaxial instability in, 3543
craniovertebral junction abnormalities in, 3334
spinal stenosis in, 4479–4480
Morton's neuroma, 3936
Motion segment, 4181, 4182f
instability of, 4331
Motivation, after traumatic brain injury, 5191–5192
Motoneuron(s), 75, 3811f
combined upper/lower degenerative diseases of, 4320–4321, 4320f
degeneration of, 4315t
disorders of, symptoms of, 3833
hyperexcitability of, 2877–2878, 2878f
injury sensitivity of, 3967
lower, degenerative diseases of, 4319–4320
spinal vs. cranial, survival of, 195
upper, degenerative diseases of, 4319
Motoneuron disease, in cervical spondylotic myelopathy, 4448–4449
Motor axons, degeneration of, compound muscle action potential in, 3854, 3854f
Motor cortex
corticosubthalamic projection from, 2690
functional magnetic resonance imaging of, 2519
language mapping and, 2536
seizures in, 2589
somatosensory evoked potential mapping of, 2531
stimulation mapping of, patient selection in, 2531, 2534
stimulation of, 2819, 3027
Motor disturbances
in frontal lobe tumors, 830
in peripheral nerve disorders, 3821–3822, 3821f
Motor end plate, 3814
Motor evoked potentials
in pediatric intramedullary tumors, 3711–3712, 3712f
intraoperative, 4211–4215, 4212t, 4213f, 4213t, 4215f, 4216f
Motor examination, 267–268
in peripheral nerve disorders, 3822–3823, 3823f
pediatric, 3176–3180
Motor nerve fibers, efferent endings of, 3809
Motor nerve terminal, 3811f
transmission at, 3813–3814
Motor nerves, measurement of, 3803
Motor nucleus, periurethral striated muscle and, 360, 360f
Motor reflexes
in Glasgow Coma Scale, 286t, 287
vestibular system in, 340
Motor system, functional magnetic resonance imaging of, 2519
Motor thalamic nuclei
basal ganglia inputs to, 2691, 2692f
cerebellar inputs to, 2691, 2692f
nomenclature of, 2691, 2691t
Motor thalamus, 2691–2693
Motor unit action potential, polyphasic nature and, 3856–3857, 3856f
Motor units, recruitment of, 3857
Motor vehicle accidents
atlanto-occipital dislocation in, 4928
atlas fracture in, 4933
hyperextension-hyperflexion cervical spine injury, 4915–4917
Movement
control of, 2875–2876, 2876f
vestibular system and, 340–341, 340f, 341f
Movement disorders, 2729–2740. *See also* Parkinsonism; Parkinson's disease.
akinetic-rigid, 2699, 2699t, 2703–2717
atactic, 2699, 2699t
basal ganglia in, 2671–2673, 2672f, 2699–2701, 2700f–2701f, 2702t, 2703, 2824–2825
classification of, 2699, 2699t, 2703, 2703t
deep brain stimulation for. *See* Deep brain stimulation, movement disorder treatment with.
definitions in, 2729–2730
dopamine effects in, 2701, 2703
episodic, vs. seizure, 2466–2467
history in, 2745
hyperkinetic, 2717–2722
basal ganglia–thalamocortical circuit in, 2701f
pathophysiology of, 2676
hyperkinetic-rigid, 2699, 2699t
hypokinetic, basal ganglia–thalamocortical circuit in, 2701f
in cerebral palsy, 3724–3727, 3726t, 3729–3730, 3747–3748
neuroglial inclusions in, 2702t, 2703
neuropathology of, 2699–2722
pediatric, examination for, 3179–3180
physical examination in, 2745–2746
positron emission tomography of, 482–485, 2755–2765
radiotracers in, 2755, 2756t
surgery for, 2671–2678, 2803
ablation vs. stimulation in, 2752
contraindications to, 2752
electrophysiologic recording methods in, 231, 232t
evaluation scales for, 2752t
patient selection in, 2745–2752
terminology in, 2729–2730
types of, 2676–2678
Moyamoya, 1715–1721
angiography of, 1716
cerebral blood flow in, 1717
clinical presentation of, 1716
computed tomography of, 1717
diagnosis of, 1716–1718
differential diagnosis of, 1717
electroencephalography of, 1717
epidemiology of, 1715
etiology of, 1715
magnetic resonance imaging of, 1716
medical treatment of, 1718
pathogenesis of, 1715
pathology of, 1716
pediatric, surgery on, 3195
positron emission tomography of, 1602
pregnancy in, 1720
saccular aneurysms with, 1717–1718
surgery for, 1718–1720, 1719f
treatment of, 1718–1720
Mucocele
orbital, 1375
skull, 1404
Mucopolysaccharidosis
odontoid process involvement in, 3344
spinal stenosis in, 4479–4480
Mucormycosis, spinal, 4389f
Multialkylator, for ependymoma, 1048t
Multidrug resistance–associated protein, 162
Multifocal motor neuropathy, 3840
Multileaf collimation, 4139–4142, 4139f–4142f

Multiple endocrine neoplasia type 1 (MEN-1) syndrome, pituitary tumors in, 1170
Multiple familial polyposis. *See* Turcot's syndrome.
Multiple myeloma, 4296t, 4298
 magnetic resonance imaging of, 532, 4852–4854, 4853f
 skull, 1392–1393, 1393f
 spinal, 1393, 1393f, 4356, 4356f, 4850, 4852–4854, 4853f
 vs. plasmacytoma, 4808–4809
Multiple organ syndrome, polyneuropathy in, 5132
Multiple sclerosis, 1449–1456
 benign, 1451–1452
 blood-brain barrier in, 164
 clinical presentation of, 1451–1452
 course of, 1451–1452
 demyelinative myelitis in, 4314, 4314f
 diagnosis of, 1452–1453
 differential diagnosis of, 1453, 1453t, 1455
 epidemiology of, 1449
 genetic basis of, 1449
 hyperacute, 1452
 imaging of, 541, 543f, 1452–1453
 immunopathogenesis of, 1449–1450
 Marburg variant, 1452
 pathology of, 1450–1451
 primary progressive, 1451
 prognosis of, 1452
 relapsing-remitting, 1451
 treatment of, 1454t–1455t, 1455–1456
 vertigo in, 352, 2902
 vs. brain tumor, 1450t
Multiple subpial transection, 2635–2641
 anesthesia in, 2636
 complications of, 2640, 2640t
 electrocorticography in, 2636
 historical aspects of, 2635
 outcomes of, 2639–2640, 2639t
 pathology of, 2638, 2639f
 patient selection for, 2635–2636
 principle of, 2635
 seizure outcome after, 2578, 2640–2641
 transections in, 2636, 2637f, 2638, 2638f
 transector for, 2637, 2637f
Multiple system atrophy, 2703
 akinetic-rigid form, 2708
 cytoplasmic inclusions in, 2713–2714
 neurodegeneration in, clinical subtypes and, 2713–2714
 pathogenesis of, 2714
 positron emission tomography of, 2761
 striatal neurons in, 2708
 substantia nigra pars compacta in, 2706f
 α-synuclein in, 2703
 vs. Parkinson's disease, 2735
Muscimol, in intracerebral hemorrhage, 1740–1741
Muscle(s)
 agonist, 2891
 antagonist, 2891
 asymmetry of, 3822, 3823f
 biopsy of, 3963–3964
  needle, 3964
  open, 3964
 disorders of, weakness in, 270
 nociceptors of, 2921
 progressive atrophy of, in lower motor neuron degenerative disease, 4319
 stretch of. *See* Stretch reflex.
 synergistic, 2891
Muscle(s) *(Continued)*
 testing of, in peripheral nerve disorders, 3822–3823, 3823f
 ventral lumbar, 4705–4706, 4706f, 4707f
Muscle bulk, pediatric, assessment of, 3178
Muscle fiber action potential, spontaneous, peripheral nervous system abnormalities with, 3856, 3856t
Muscle fibers
 complex repetitive discharges from, 3856
 in spasticity, 2879–2880
Muscle lengthening, for cerebral palsy, 3732
Muscle relaxants, 1508
 cerebrovascular effects of, in traumatic brain injury, 5131–5132, 5132t
 for failed back syndrome, 4337
 for tracheal intubation, 557
 in craniotomy, 5150
Muscle spindle, 2875–2876, 2876f, 3809, 3810f
Muscle strength, pediatric, assessment of, 3178–3179, 3178t
Muscle tone, pediatric, examination of, 3177–3178
Musculocutaneous nerve, entrapment of, 3933
Mutagenesis, 818
Mutism
 after medulloblastoma surgery, 1038
 akinetic, in frontal lobe tumors, 830
 ependymoma surgery and, 3629
 medulloblastoma surgery and, 1004, 3645–3646
 transcallosal surgery and, 1258–1259
Myasthenia gravis
 ion channels in, 225t
 ocular, 323
 pathology of, 3816
 physical features of, 270
Myasthenic syndrome, 270
Mycobacterium tuberculosis, 1440
 infectious aneurysms from, 2102
Mycoplasma pneumoniae, myelitis from, 4313
Mydriasis, pharmacologic, 322
Myelencephalon, in Chiari malformation type II, 3352
Myelin, 86–87, 86f
 central nervous system repair inhibition by, 4168–4169
 in axonal regeneration, 204
 repair of, cellular transplantation in, 4164
Myelin internode, 86, 86f, 87, 88f
Myelin sheath, 3810, 3811f
Myelin-associated glycoprotein, inhibitory activity of, 4169
Myelination, 63t, 64, 64t, 86–87, 86f
 pediatric, 3462
Myelin-blocking antibodies, 4169
Myelitis
 acute necrotizing, 4314
 bacterial, 4312t, 4313
 demyelinative, in multiple sclerosis, 4314, 4314f
 epidural abscess in, 4313
 fungal, 4312t, 4313
 noninfectious inflammatory, 4313–4314, 4314f
 parasitic, 4312t, 4313
 postinfectious, 4313–4314
 postvaccinal, 4313–4314
 transverse, in multiple sclerosis, 1452
 viral, 4311–4313, 4312t
Myelocele, spina bifida aperta with, 4316
Myelocystocele, 3224–3225, 3225f, 3280–3281, 3280f, 4316
 anatomy in, 3225
 epidemiology of, 3225
 etiology of, 3226
 history of, 3225
 outcome of, 3226
 pathogenesis of, 3225–3226
 prenatal diagnosis of, 3226
 terminal, 3215, 4267, 4268f
 treatment of, 3226
Myelodysplasia, 3245
Myelography
 computed tomography, of pyogenic spinal infection, 4368, 4369f
 spinal, 505–506
Myeloma globulin, in multiple myeloma, 4854
Myelomeningocele, 4256–4259, 4258f, 4259f
 anatomy in, 3215–3216
 Chiari malformation type II in, 3215, 3216f, 3217f, 3223–3224, 3351
 chromosomal abnormalities in, 3219
 differential diagnosis of, 3219
 epidemiology of, 3217
 etiology of, 3217–3219, 3218t
 examples of, 3215, 3216f
 historical aspects of, 3155, 3157f
 history of, 3216
 hydrocephalus in, 3216
 latex allergy in, 3224
 orthopedic consultation in, 3224
 pathogenesis of, 3217
 pediatric, 3215–3224
 perinatal management of, 3220–3223, 3222f
 prenatal counseling for, 3219–3220
 prenatal diagnosis of, 3219
 prognosis of, 3219–3220
 sibling risk in, 3220
 spina bifida aperta with, 4316
 surgery for, 3221–3223, 3222f
  complications of, 3223–3224
  in neonates, 3194, 3194f
 terminology for, 3215
Myelopathy
 cervical, 4397
  in rheumatoid arthritis, 4573
 in cervical spondylosis. *See* Cervical spondylotic myelopathy.
 in perimedullary arteriovenous fistula, 2394
 progressive
  in conus medullaris arteriovenous malformations, 2371f
  in dural arteriovenous fistula, 2366–2367, 2367f
  in intradural arteriovenous malformations, 2370, 2370f
 sensory patterns in, 272
 spinal cord, radiation therapy and, 4046
Myelotomy, 3029
 for spasticity, 2866t, 2870
Myerson's sign, 269
Myoblastoma, 3947t, 3948
Myocardial infarction, carotid endarterectomy and, 1645
Myocardial ischemia
 in subarachnoid hemorrhage, 1869
 surgery and, 549–550
Myocardium, hypothermia effects on, 1533
Myoclonus, 2722, 2738, 2751
 clinical manifestations of, 833
 definition of, 2729

Myoclonus (Continued)
dystonia with, 2721
pediatric, assessment of, 3179–3180
segmental, 2722
Myoclonus-dystonia, 2737
Myofascial pain syndrome
in cerebral palsy, 3728
low back pain in, 4330, 4351
Myopathy
critical illness, 5131–5132, 5132f
in sarcoidosis, 1436
ion channel disorders in, 225t
weakness in, 270
Myosin light chain kinase, in cerebral vasospasm, 1848
Myositis ossificans, 3947, 3947f, 3947t
Myotonia
ion channels in, 225t
pediatric, 3178
sodium channel, 225t
Myotonia congenita, ion channels in, 225t
Myxedema coma, treatment of, 293–294
Myxochondroma, 1365

N450K, in achondroplasia, 3362
Na-K-ATPase
in blood-brain barrier ion transport, 162
in neuronal potassium uptake, 228, 230
Nalidixic acid, pseudotumor cerebri from, 1423
Narcotics
for failed back syndrome, 4336
in craniotomy, 5150
in intracranial pressure management, 5127, 5127t
Nasal bone, in craniofacial trauma, 5262
Nasal cavity, complications in, transsphenoidal surgery and, 569, 1182–1183
Nasoiniac line, 630–631, 631f
Nasopharynx
juvenile angiofibroma of, 1351–1359. *See also* Angiofibroma, juvenile nasopharyngeal.
squamous cell carcinoma of, 1398, 1399f
National Adult Reading Test, 5189
National Institutes of Health Stroke Scale, 242t, 1498, 1499t
Natriuresis, after subarachnoid hemorrhage, 1829–1830
Natural history studies, 250–251
assessment of, 258
Nausea, 275
Neck
pain in
dorsal rhizotomy for, 3041–3042
hyperextension-hyperflexion injury and, 4918
surgery for, 3025t
penetrating injuries to, 1670
trauma assessment of, 5088–5089
zones of, 1670, 1670f
Necrosis, 82–83
impending, 1601, 1601t
in astrocytoma, 835–836
in glioblastoma multiforme, 843f–844f, 844
in malignant phenotype, 771, 772f
radiation, in arteriovenous malformation, 2195–2196, 2195f, 2196t
vs. apoptosis, 130–132, 131f
Necrotizing enterocolitis, after myelomeningocele repair, 3223
Neglect, reporting obligations in, 411
Nelson's syndrome, 1199–1200
Neonates
emergency surgery on, 3193–3194, 3194t
vein of Galen malformation in, 3435, 3435f
Neoplasia, cranial destruction in, 430
Neoplastic meningitis, 1231–1234
Neovascularization, angiogenic-induced, 821–822
Nernst equation, 218, 3812
Nerve cell body, 72f, 73, 77–78
Nerve conduction, 86–87, 86f
Nerve conduction studies, 3851–3857
fundamentals of, 3851–3852, 3851f
F-wave in, 3855, 3855f
H-reflex in, 3855, 3855f
in carpal tunnel syndrome, 3857–3858
in peripheral nerve trauma, 3860, 3861
in radiculopathy, 3859
in ulnar neuropathy, 3858–3859
indications for, 3851
late responses in, 3855, 3855f
of compound muscle action potential, 3853–3855, 3854f
of sensory nerve action potential, 3852–3853, 3852f, 3853f
repetitive stimulation in, 3855–3856
Nerve fibers
myelinated, 3958–3960, 3960f
unmyelinated, 3960, 3960f
Nerve grafts, historical aspects of, 3803
Nerve growth factor, 195, 3805
after peripheral nerve injury, 3967
brain-derived, 197, 200
development and, 3975
in brain injury recovery, 5031
in central nervous system repair, 4165–4166
in distal nerve stump, 200
in inflammation, 2956
in nervous system regeneration, 4155
neurotropic function of, 4165
Nerve of Henle, 3898
Nerve of Kuntz, sectioning of, 3099f, 3100
Nerve plexus injury, 3969–3973
diagnosis of, 3970
severity of, 3970, 3971f
treatment of, 3970, 3972–3973, 3972f–3974f
Nerve roots
avulsion of, 3970, 3971f
pain in, 3821
cervical, inflammation of, 505f
disease involvement of, 271–272, 271f, 272f
in cervical laminoforaminotomy, 4416
intraoperative electrophysiologic monitoring of, 4203–4204, 4216–4222
paresis of, after cervical laminectomy, 4425
selective injection of, 2975–2976
Nerve sheath tumor, 3941, 4296t, 4300, 4301f
benign, 3942–3946, 3943f–3945f, 3946t
surgical results for, 3945–3946, 3945f, 3946t
pediatric, 3714, 3714f
spinal cord, 4040, 4817–4818, 4818f
treatment of, 4822–4824
Nerve stump, distal
cellular responses in, 199–200
cytokines in, 200
extracellular matrix proteins in, 200
growth factors in, 200
Nerve stump (Continued)
neurotrophic factors in, 200
pathway specificity in, 200–201
prolonged denervation of, 201
regeneration in, 198–199
Nervous system
pattern formation in, 78, 79f
redundancy in, 3785
vicarious functioning in, 3785
Nervous system injury, functional recovery after, 3784–3786
Neural blockade, 2970–2984
complications of, 2972
diagnostic, 2970, 2971t
fluoroscopy in, 2972–2974, 2973f, 2974f
limitations of, 2970–2972
risks of, 2972
standards for, 2972
therapeutic, 2970
training for, 2972
Neural cell transplantation, 93, 94f
Neural compression syndrome
decompressive surgery for, 4337
low back pain in, 4330–4331
reoperation for, 4339
Neural crest
fate of, 4255
formation of, 4243
Neural folds, fusion of, 4250–4251
Neural foramina, stenosis of, 515
osteophytes and, 509, 512f
Neural induction, 47
primary, 78
Neural placode, 3215, 3216f
Neural plate
bending of, 4248–4250, 4249f
shaping of, 4246, 4248, 4248f
Neural tube
formation of, 4243, 4244f
patterning of, 51, 51t
regionalization of, 50–51
segmentation of, 48, 48t, 50–51
Neural tube defect, 4256–4259, 4258f, 4259f. *See also* Myelomeningocele.
alpha fetoprotein screening for, 3219
anticonvulsants and, 3218
definition of, 3215
diabetes mellitus and, 3218–3219
folate deficiency and, 3217–3218
obesity and, 3219
open, folic acid deficiency and, 3257
risk factors for, 3218t
Neuralgia
cranial, 3018t
postherpetic, 2989t, 3842
dorsal rhizotomy for, 3041
mesencephalotomy for, 3077–3078
vs. trigeminal neuralgia, 2988
trigeminal. *See* Trigeminal neuralgia.
Neurapraxia
grading of, 3825–3826, 3825t
needle electromyography of, 3860–3861
nerve conduction studies of, 3860
Neuraxis, rostrocaudal and metameric specification of, 4255–4256
Neurectomy, 3028
for trigeminal neuralgia, 3003
Neuregulins, in brain tumors, 727
Neurenteric cyst, 1226–1229, 3272–3273, 4263–4266, 4263f–4267f, 4317
at C1–2, 4813f, 4814
at craniovertebral junction, 4813f, 4814
imaging of, 535, 536f, 1227f–1228f, 1228–1229
vs. ependymal cyst, 1229

Neurilemmoma, scalp, 1414–1415
Neurinoma
at C1–2, 4813–4814
cranial nerve, retrosigmoid approach to, 927, 927f
trigeminal nerve. *See* Trigeminal neurinoma.
vs. trigeminal schwannoma, 1347
Neuritic tangle, 83
Neuritis
optic, 308–309, 308f
in multiple sclerosis, 1452
vestibular, 350
uncompensated, 2903
vertigo in, 2902–2903
Neuro D, 54t
Neuroacanthocytosis, 2719, 2736
Neuroaxonal dystrophy, 2720
Neurobehavioral Rating Scale, 5191
Neurobiology, restorative, 4153. *See also* Central nervous system, repair of.
Neuroblastoma, 3953–3954
cerebellar, 3640
cerebral, 669
definition of, 998
insulin-like growth factors in, 729
olfactory, 1395–1396, 1396f
orbital metastasis in, 1376
skull, 1394–1395, 1395f
Neuroblasts
disorders of, 58, 61, 61f–63f
migration of, 58–59, 59f, 60f, 61
proliferation of, 57–58, 58f
Neurocan, in central nervous system repair failure, 4168
Neurochemicals, in immune control, 684
Neurocutaneous melanosis, brain tumors in, 812t, 813
Neurocysticercosis, third ventricle in, 1247
Neurocytoma, 4302
classification of, 666
proliferation markers for, 701–702, 702t
radiologic features of, 841, 841f
third ventricular, 1246
Neurodegenerative disease, 82–83
embryonic tissue transplantation for, 4158–4159
inflammatory mediators in, 674
Neurodevelopmental treatment, for cerebral palsy, 3731
Neurodysgenesis, 424
Neuroectoderm
induction of, by embryonic organizer, 4253–4254
prospective, localization of, 4241, 4241f
Neuroectodermal tumors, supratentorial primitive, 669
Neuroembryology, 45–64
embryonic vesicles in, 46, 47f
terminal period in, 46
Neuroendocrine carcinoma, paranasal sinus, 1312–1313
chemoradiation therapy for, 1327, 1328f–1329f
Neuroendoscopy, 3427–3431. *See also* Endoscopy.
Neuroepithelial cells, 49
Neuroepithelial cyst. *See* Neurenteric cyst.
Neuroepithelial stem cells, 98, 98f
Neuroepithelial tumors
desmoplastic, 990–991
dysembryoplastic, 666
pediatric
imaging of, 3699, 3699f
Neuroepithelial tumors *(Continued)*
pathology of, 3701–3702
surgery for, 3702
proliferation markers for, 701
Neurofibroma, 3941, 3944, 3944f, 4296t
at C1–2, 4812–4813, 4812f
diffuse, 1374
imaging of, 526–527, 527f
magnetic resonance imaging of, 3875–3876, 3876f
orbital, 1373–1374
plexiform, 527f, 1373–1374
scalp, 1414–1415
spinal cord, treatment of, 4822–4823
surgery for, 3944–3945, 3944f, 3945f
results of, 3945f, 3946, 3946t
Neurofibromatosis, 4817
genetic basis of, 742
malignant glioma in, 969
malignant tumors of neural sheath origin in, 3951
neurofibroma with, surgical results for, 3946, 3946t
schwannoma in, 3941, 3942f
Neurofibromatosis type 1
aneurysms in, 1772–1773
brain tumors in, 812, 812t
brainstem glioma in, 3664
Neurofibromatosis type 2, brain tumors in, 812, 812t
Neurofibromin, 742, 1773
Neurofilaments, 78
Neurogenesis, 57–58, 58f, 78, 79f, 80
disorders of, 58
in traumatic brain injury, 5033
Neurogenic claudication, 4305
in spinal stenosis, 4521
vs. vascular claudication, 4527
Neurogenic pain, intrathecal drugs for, 3135
Neurogenic shock, 4872
Neuroglia, 83–94. *See also* Glia.
Neuroglial inclusions, in movement disorders, 2702t, 2703
Neurohypophysis, granular cell tumor of, 671
Neurokinin, inflammation mediation by, 2956
Neuroleptics, for trigeminal neuralgia, 2990–2991
Neurological assessment
blood pressure management in, 5090
brainstem in, 5091–5092
carbon dioxide levels in, 5089–5090
Cushing response in, 5090
examination in, 5089–5092, 5091f, 5092f
Glasgow Coma Scale in, 5090
herniation syndromes in, 5091, 5091f
history in, 5089
in skull fracture, 5093, 5094f
in thoracic spine fracture, 4968
in traumatic brain injury, 5089–5095
intubation and, 5090
pupillary examination in, 5090–5091
radiographic evaluation in, 5092–5093, 5093f–5095f
reflexes in, 5091
Neurological deficit, 4309–4321
acute paresis/paralysis in, 4310–4311, 4310t
after arteriovenous malformation surgery, 2192–2193, 2193f
after cervical laminectomy, 4424–4425
after surgery, 907
after thoracic spine fracture, 4982
Neurological deficit *(Continued)*
callostomy and, 1244
chronic, progressive, 4314–4321, 4315t–4316t
classification of, in rheumatoid arthritis, 4575, 4578, 4578t
delayed ischemic, 1839
after cerebral vasospasm, 1545
blood flow velocities and, 1547
diagnostic studies for, 4309–4310
evaluation of, 4309
in arteriovenous malformations, 2163, 2206, 2210f
in cavernous malformations, 2294, 2295f
in congenital lumbosacral lipoma, 3237
in congenital malformations, 4316–4319, 4317f, 4318f
in epidural abscess, 4373–4374, 4381
in sacral fractures, 5014
in supratentorial cavernous malformation, 2309
location of, 4309
parent carotid artery occlusion and, 2060
postoperative hematoma and, 935–936, 937f
reversibility of, ischemia duration and, 1516, 1517f
spinal cord growth and, 3236
spinal cord infarction and, 4310–4311
spontaneous spinal hemorrhage and, 4311
subacute, progressive, 4311–4314, 4312t, 4314f
surgery and, 932f, 933
vascular events in, 4310–4311, 4310t
Neurological disease
causes of, 274–275
ion channel disorders in, 225t
localization of, 269–274
nerve root involvement in, 271–272, 271f, 272f
Neurological examination, 264–265, 264f, 264t
pediatric, 3169–3186
adaptive development in, 3170, 3170t
birth history in, 3169–3170
chief complaint in, 3169
cranial nerve examination in, 3173–3176
developmental history in, 3170, 3170t
developmental reflexes in, 3181–3182
family history in, 3170–3171
history in, 3169–3171
in neonates, 3184–3185
in older infants, 3185–3186
in young children, 3185–3186
in young infants, 3184–3185
language development in, 3170, 3170t
mental status examination in, 3171–3172
motor examination in, 3176–3180
physical examination in, 3171–3184
reflex testing in, 3180–3181
somatosensory examination in, 3182–3184
speech assessment in, 3176
preoperative, 548–549
Neurological history, 263–264
Neurological signs
internuclear, 270
segmental, 269–270, 270f
supranuclear, 270
suprasegmental, 269–270, 270f
Neurological status
assessment of, 5088, 5088t

Neurological status (Continued)
monitoring of, in traumatic brain injury, 5112–5113
Neurology, behavioral, 385
Neurolysis, 2978–2981
radiofrequency, for spasticity, 2866t
Neurolytics, for cerebral palsy, 3731–3732
Neuroma
grading of, 3825t, 3826
painful, 3821
resection of, in brachial plexus surgery, 3492–3493
sodium channel disorders and, 3815, 3815f
Neuromeres, 50
Neuromonitoring, of peripheral nerves, 3862–3866
Neuromuscular blockade, in traumatic brain injury, 5131–5132, 5132t
Neuromuscular junction, 3809, 3811f, 3814
chemical synaptic transmission at, 227
disorders of, physical characteristics of, 270
in axon regeneration, 201
Neuromyelitis optica, 4314
Neuromyopathy, carcinomatous, 3954
Neuron(s), 71–83
action potential conduction in, 3813, 3814b
action potential generation in, 3813, 3813f
as equivalent circuit, 3814b, 3814f
axonal growth mode of, 198
axotomized, survival of, 197
central nervous system injury effects on, 4154
death of, 82–83
definition of, 71, 72f
degeneration of, after central nervous system injury, 4156
depression of, in consciousness levels, 279–280
development of, 78, 79f, 80–81
defects during, 81–82, 81f
effector, 75
energy metabolism in, astrocytes in, 107, 108f, 109
excitability of, 228, 230
function of, 71–73, 72f
in cerebral metabolism, 1486
in spinal cord gray matter, 2924–2926, 2924f, 2925f
injury to, free radicals in, 1473
injury-induced death of, 3967
ion channels in, 219–226
ion currents in, 226
lumbar spine, 4706–4707, 4708f
maturation of, 80–81
failure of, 82
migration of, 80
abnormalities of, 2492–2493
failures of, 81–82, 81f
neuropeptide expression in, injury and, 3967–3968, 3968f–3969f
organization of, 75
pattern formation in, 78, 79f
failure of, 81
proliferation of, 97
abnormalities of, 2492
radiomarkers for, 1609
regeneration of, 5032
after central nervous system injury, 202–203
replacement of, 4159
resting membrane potential in, 3812, 3812t
Neuron(s) (Continued)
retrograde changes in, after central nervous system injury, 4156
saltatory conduction in, 3813
sensory, 73–75, 74f
sodium action potentials in, 221
sources for, stem cells as, 93, 94f
staining methods for, 75–77, 76f
structure of, 71, 72f, 75–78, 76f
survival of, after peripheral nerve injury, 195, 197–202
visualization of, 75–77, 76f
Neuronal action potential, 3813, 3813f, 3814b
Neuronal degenerative disease, 4315t–4316t, 4319–4321, 4320f
subacute combined/combined system disease, of nonpernicious anemia type, 4321
Neuronal tumors, histopathologic classification of, 665–667, 666t
Neuronopathy, subacute sensory, 832
Neuro-ophthalmology, 301–323
Neuro-otology, 327–354
Neuropathic pain, 2956–2957, 3024, 3120, 3831
deep brain stimulation for, 3127–3128, 3127t, 3128t
surgery for, 4343
trigeminal, 3018t
Neuropathy
compressive, 3900, 3901f, 3902f
critical illness, 5131–5132, 5132f
entrapment, 3820, 3900
magnetic resonance imaging of, 3876–3883
multiple, 3900
facial, brain embolization procedures and, 859
hypertrophic, localized, 3950–3951
multifocal motor, 3840
toxic, 3832t, 3843–3844
traumatic, pediatric, 3468, 3468f
urologic disorders in, 375
Neuropeptides
after axotomy, 197–198
after neural injury, 3967
Neuroplasty, 2976
Neuroprotection
cytoprotective strategies for, 1520–1522
in intracerebral hemorrhage, 1740–1741
intraoperative, 1515–1523
trials for, 1498
Neuropsychological assessment, 385–391
abbreviated tests in, 388
brain-sensitive tests in, 387
case studies of, 388–391, 389t, 390t
general tests in, 388
in arteriovenous malformation, 388–389, 389t
in intractable seizures, 390–391, 390t
in traumatic brain injury, 5289–5290, 5290t
rationale for, 385–386
referral for, 386–387, 386t
tests for, 387–388, 388t, 5183–5185
normative values in, 5184–5185
reliability in, 5184
standardization in, 5183
validity in, 5184
Neuropsychology, 385–391, 5020
clinical, 385
cognitive domains of, 5183t
experimental, 385
historical perspective on, 385
Neuroreceptors, single-photon emission computed tomography of, 2477–2478
Neurorehabilitation, 3783–3790
definition of, 3783
functional recovery in, 3784–3786
pediatric, 3783, 3786–3787
behavioral, 3789
brain injury and, 3788–3790
cognitive, 3789
communication, 3789
seizure, 3789–3790
spasticity and, 3787–3788
Neurosarcoidosis, 1435. See also Sarcoidosis.
Neurosecretory cells, 75
Neurosurgeon, in emotional status evaluation, 5191–5194, 5193t
Neurosurgery
cellular and molecular, 4153. See also Central nervous system, repair of.
electrophysiologic methods in, 231–232, 232t
functional
definition of, 2653–2654
history of, 2653–2664
origins of, 2654–2655, 2654f
stereotactic and functional, 2664
Neurosyphilis, myelitis in, 4313
Neurothelin, 158
Neurotmesis
grading of, 3825t, 3826
needle electromyography of, 3860–3861
nerve conduction studies of, 3860
Neurotomy
alcohol, 3018–3019, 3019f
for trigeminal neuralgia, 3018–3020
surgical, 3019–3020, 3020f
Neurotoxicity, methamphetamine-induced, positron emission tomography of, 492–493, 493f
Neurotransmitters
after axotomy, 197–198
blood-brain barrier transport and, 154, 161–162
cerebral concentrations of, magnetic resonance spectroscopy of, 2497, 2497f
in cerebral autoregulation, 1476–1477
inflammatory mediators as, 674
release of, nociceptor stimulation and, 2953, 2954f
Neurotraumatology, 5018–5021
clinical advances in, 5018–5019
computed tomography introduction and, 5019
experimental models in, 5020
genetic factors in, 5021
historical aspects of, 5017–5021, 5018t
monitoring in, 5020–5021
neuropsychology in, 5020
Traumatic Coma Data Bank and, 5019
Neurotrophic factor receptors
after axotomy, 197–198
in brain tumors, 729
Neurotrophic factors
ciliary, 195, 200
glial cell line–derived, 197
in brain tumors, 729
in central nervous system transplantation, 2843–2844
in distal nerve stump, 200
release of, after axonal injury, 195, 197
Neurotrophin(s)
apoptosis reduction by, 4156
in axonal regeneration, 203

Neurotrophin(s) *(Continued)*
in brain tumors, 729
in central nervous system repair, 4164–4166
Neurotrophin-4/5, 195, 197, 200
Neurotropism, in peripheral nerve regeneration, 3804–3805
Neurourology, 357–381
Neurulation, 48–50, 49f, 49t
congenital lumbosacral lipoma and, 3233–3234
failure of, terminology for, 3215
molecular control of, 4251–4256, 4252f
occult spinal dysraphism and, 3258, 3258f
primary, 50, 4243, 4244f
mechanisms of, 4245–4251, 4248f, 4249f
specification of notochord and floor plate in, 4254–4255
secondary, 50, 4243–4245, 4245f, 4246f
disorders of, 4266–4269, 4268f, 4269f
Neutron therapy, 4008
Neutrophils, in cerebral ischemia, 136, 137–138, 141–142, 143f
Nevoid basal cell carcinoma, medulloblastoma in, 997, 3639
Nevoid basal cell carcinoma syndrome
brain tumors in, 812–813, 812t
genetic basis of, 742–743
medulloblastoma in, 1033
Nevus, melanocytic, scalp, 1410–1411
Nevus sebaceous of Jadassohn, 1415
Newborns, withholding treatment from, 415
NF-1, 742
NF-2, 744, 1044
in meningioma, 1106, 1107
NG-2, in central nervous system repair inhibition, 4168
Ngn1, 54t
NG-nitro-L-arginine methyl ester (L-NAME), in cerebral blood flow autoregulation, 5049
Nicaraven, for cerebral vasospasm, 1854
Nigrostriatal circuit, 2700
Nigrothalamic projection, 2691, 2692f, 2693
Nimodipine
for subarachnoid hemorrhage, 1852–1853, 1854f
for vasospasm, 1840
pregnancy effects on, 2423
Nissl substance, 78
Nitric oxide, 1473
endothelin-1 and, 1474
in blood-brain barrier regulation, 11, 162
in cell death, 128
in cerebral blood flow regulation, 1470–1472, 1470t, 1471f, 5049
in cerebral blood flow–metabolism coupling, 1490
in cerebral vasospasm, 1849
in ischemic injury, 1517–1518
in multiple sclerosis, 1450
inhibitors of, in focal cerebral ischemia, 135
Nitric oxide synthase
in cerebral blood flow regulation, 1470, 1470t, 1471
in free radical production, 1473
Nitric oxide synthase inhibitors, in ischemia protection, 1522
Nitrogen, metabolism of, after subarachnoid hemorrhage, 1831
Nitrogen mustard, ototoxicity from, 350–351
Nitrosourea, 880–881
Nizofenone, for cerebral vasospasm, 1854
Nkx2–1, 54t
Nkx2–2, 54t
Nkx6–1, 54t
Nkx6–2, 54t
N-methyl-D-aspartate antagonists
for pain, 2965–2966
intrathecal, 3141
N-methyl-D-aspartate receptors
in cerebral blood flow autoregulation, 5049
in neuropathic pain, 2957
in traumatic brain injury, 2451–2452, 2451f, 5025, 5026f
Nocardia asteroides
infectious intracranial aneurysms from, 2102
spinal infections from, 4385
Nociception
anterior cingulate cortex in, 2932–2933
ascending pathways in, 2927–2931
dorsal column postsynaptic system in, 2930, 2932f
in gray matter, 2953, 2955
insular cortex in, 2933
pathways of, 2928f
propriospinal multisynaptic ascending system in, 2930
somatosensory cortices in, 2932, 2933f
spinomesencephalic tract in, 2930, 2931f
spinoreticular tract in, 2930, 2931f
spinothalamic tract in, 2927, 2928f–2930f, 2930
transduction mechanisms in, 2917–2919
trigeminal brainstem nuclear complex in, 2930–2931, 2933f
Nociceptive fibers, 2917, 2918t
stimulus response of, 2917, 2918f
Nociceptive primary afferent neurons, 2917, 2918t
activation of, 2919–2920, 2953, 2954f
amino acids of, 2926–2927
axons of, 2922
chemosensitive, 2919, 2919f
heat sensitive, 2918–2919
in inflammation, 2921
mechanosensitive, 2919
neuropeptides of, 2926–2927
sensitization of, 2920–2921, 2920f
stimulus response of, 2917, 2918f
synaptic neurotransmitters of, 2926–2927
tissue innervation by, 2921f, 2922–2923, 2922f
Nociceptors, 3809
activation of, 2919–2920
chemosensitive, 2921
heat sensitive, 2918–2919, 2921
in spinal cord gray matter, 2923–2926, 2924f, 2925f
joint, 2921
mechanical, 2919
mechano-heat, 2921
muscle, 2921
polymodal C fiber, 2921
sensitization of, 2920–2921, 2920f
superficial, 2921
visceral, 2921–2922
Nocutria, 365
Node of Ranvier, 3810, 3950
Nog, 54t
NOGO, in axonal regeneration, 204
Nogo, neuron regeneration and, 5032
Nogo A, 4168
Non-Friedreich's ataxia, 4320–4321
Non-Hodgkin's lymphoma. *See also* Lymphoma.
in primary central nervous system lymphoma, 1068
skull, 1393, 1394f
Nonmetal elements, brain tumors and, 811
Nonnnerve sheath tumors, 3946–3951, 3947t
Nonsteroidal anti-inflammatory drugs
for ankylosing spondylitis, 4466–4467
for cervical disk disease, 4398, 4412, 4414
for failed back syndrome, 4336
for pain, 2959
North American blastomycosis, spinal, 4388f, 4389
North American Spine Society Questionnaire, 243t
Northern blot analysis, 752, 752f
Nortriptyline, for neuropathic pain, 3838
Nose
in craniofacial trauma, 5251
in transsphenoidal surgery, 1177–1178
Notch, 48
Notch, 54t
Notochord, 47, 4241–4243, 4242f
chordomas from, 4848
formation of, 4241–4243, 4242f
specification of, in primary neurulation, 4254–4255
Nottingham Health Profile, 243t
Nuclear magnetic resonance, 439
Nuclei ventrales posteriores thalami, 2927
stereotactic surgery on, in Parkinson's disease, 2659
Nucleolar organizing regions, as tumor proliferation markers, 695
Nucleosides
blood-brain barrier permeability to, 158
transporters of, 158
Nucleotides, blood-brain barrier permeability to, 157–158
Nucleus accumbens, 2683
Nucleus amygdalae, 9
Nucleus caudalis, 7f, 8, 8f, 10f, 13, 15f, 1237, 1238f, 2683
anatomy of, 3085
coagulation of, 3053
DREZ ablation of, 3045
care after, 3053
complications of, 3053–3054, 3087–3088
evaluation before, 3049, 3051
for facial pain, 3085–3090
historical aspects of, 3086
impedance recording in, 3087
indications for, 3049, 3050t–3051t
outcome in, 3049, 3052t, 3088, 3090
patient selection for, 3086
somatosensory evoked potentials in, 3087, 3089f
technique of, 3051–3052, 3086–3087, 3087f–3089f
fetal mesencephalic grafting in, 2836–2837
in nociception, 3045
stimulation of, 3119
Nucleus dentatus, 33, 33f
Nucleus interpolaris, 3085
Nucleus oralis, 3085
Nucleus pulposus, 4327–4328
degeneration of, 4328–4329
herniated, 4304–4305
Nucleus raphe magnus
in vagus nerve stimulation, 2644
stimulation of, 3122

Nucleus reticularis gigantocellularis, stimulation of, 3122
Nucleus reticularis thalami, in selective attention, 280
Nucleus ventralis anterior thalami, 2691, 2691t
stereotactic surgery on, in Parkinson's disease, 2659
Nucleus ventralis intermedius thalami
destruction of, for tremor, 2803
in radiosurgical thalamotomy, 4087, 4088, 4088f
stereotactic surgery on, in Parkinson's disease, 2659–2660
stimulation of, 2804, 2805f, 2815–2816
complications of, 2823
coordinates for, 2809–2810, 2810t
electrophysiologic studies in, 2813
results of, 2820–2821
Nucleus ventralis lateral thalami, 2691, 2691t
Nucleus ventrocaudalis parvicellularis, 3079
Nucleus ventroposterolateral stimulation, 3119
Nucleus ventroposteromedial stimulation, 3119
Nuclues ventralis posteromedial thalami, 2929f
Numb, 54t
Numbness, 3831
distribution of, in length-dependent peripheral neuropathy, 3833, 3833f
Nutrition
deficiency of, neuropathy from, 3844
in pediatric neurorehabilitation, 3786
in traumatic brain injury, 5129–5130
Nystagmus
after medulloblastoma surgery, 1037
benign paroxysmal positional, 342, 343f
congenital, 3174
gaze-evoked, 3174
in vestibular testing, 2905
jerk, 3174
pediatric, 3174–3175
spontaneous, 342
statis positional, 342
vestibular, 342, 3174

Obesity
in pseudotumor cerebri, 1429
neural tube defect from, 3219
surgery and, 549
Obex, 33f
Observational studies, 249–251
Obsessive-compulsive disorder
anterior capsulotomy for, 2859, 2859f
anterior cingulotomy for, 2857
cortical-striatal-thalamic circuits in, 2854
frontal-striatal-pallidal-thalamic circuits in, 2855
limbic leucotomy for, 2858
magnetic resonance imaging of, 2855
neurosurgery for, 2856
subcaudate tractotomy for, 2857–2858, 2858f
Tourette's syndrome and, 2854–2855
Obtundation, 283–284
Occipital artery
distal vertebral artery bypass to, 1709
posterior inferior cerebral artery bypass with, 2113, 2115, 2115f, 2116f
Occipital bone, osteodiastasis of, 3483, 3483f
Occipital condyle fracture, 4902, 4925
classification of, 4927, 4927f
clinical presentation of, 4926–4927
delivery and, 3483, 3483f
diagnosis of, 4927, 4927f
treatment of, 4927–4928
vertical, 3483, 3483f
Occipital horn, 8, 8f, 9, 1237, 1238f
Occipital lobe, 5, 18f, 26f
hemorrhage of, 1738
lesions of, homonymous visual field defects from, 315, 315f–316f
seizures in, 2592–2594, 2593f
stimulation of, visual cortex mapping by, 2548
tumors of, 831
venous drainage of, 17, 23, 28
visual cortex of, 2542, 2542f
Occipital nerve
in carotid endarterectomy, 1632
injury to
acoustic neuroma surgery and, 1162
ataxia from, 2980
Occipital neuralgia
dorsal rhizotomy for, 3040–3041, 3041t
ganglionectomy for, 3040–3041, 3041t
Occipital ramus, anterior, 4f
Occipital sulcus, lateral, 5
Occipital vein, internal, 28
Occipitoatlantoaxial joint
lymphatic drainage of, 3331
rotational abnormality of, in Grisel's syndrome, 3337, 3337f
Occipitobasilar vein, 23
Occipitocervical dislocation, 4902–4903
Occipitocervical fusion, 4655–4668
after trauma, 4901
bone grafts in, 4666
complications of, 4668
Cotrel-Dubousset rod-screw plate in, 4661, 4663f
fixation plates in, 4666, 4667f
follow-up to, 4666–4668
for odontoid infection, 4373f–4375f, 4375
hardware failure in, 4655, 4656f
iliac crest wiring in, 4661, 4662f
imaging during, 4658
indications for, 4656
instrumentation in, 4658–4666
lateral mass screws in, 4665–4666, 4666f, 4667f
levels included in, 4656
metal implants for, 4661, 4663f
orthoses in, 4666–4668
pars interarticularis screws in, 4662, 4664–4665, 4664f, 4665f
positioning for, 4657–4658, 4657f
preparation before, 4656–4657
rod bender for, 4659f, 4660
screw-based techniques for, 4661–4662, 4664f
skin incision in, 4658, 4658f
soft tissue dissection in, 4658, 4658f
sublaminar cable placement in, 4660–4661, 4660f–4662f
suboccipital cable placement in, 4660–4661, 4660f
transarticular screws in, 4662, 4664–4665, 4664f, 4665f
Vicryl suture in, 4660, 4661f
wiring techniques for, 4659f–4663f, 4660–4661
Occipitomastoid suture, 423f
Occipitotemporal gyrus, 18f
Occipitotemporal sulcus, 18, 18f
Occludin, 156
Occlusion, in craniofacial trauma, 5248–5249
Occult spinal dysraphism, 3257–3281. *See also* Spinal dysraphism, occult.
Occupational hazards
brain tumors and, 810
paranasal sinus tumors from, 1311, 1311t
Occupational therapy, in cerebral palsy, 3730–3731
Octreotide
for acromegaly, 1192–1193
for pituitary adenoma, 869
Ocular movements. *See* Eye movements.
Ocular myoclonus, 293
Oculocephalic reflex
in consciousness assessment, 289
in pediatric assessment, 3174
Oculomotor nerve, 10f, 15f, 18f, 22f, 36f, 316, 316f, 1898–1899, 1975
aberrant regeneration of, 321
complete palsy of, 321
examination of, 266
pediatric, 3173, 3174
palsy of, 272–273, 273f
paresis of, 319t, 320
parietal/incomplete paresis of, 321, 321f
posterior communicating artery aneurysms and, 1887
Oculomotor nuclei, 3074
Oculosympathetic paresis, 322, 323f
Oculovestibular response testing, in conscious assessment, 289, 290f, 290t
Odontoid fracture, 3341, 4903–4904, 4904f, 4904t, 4934, 4939–4947
atlanto-occipital dislocation in, 4928
classification of, 4904f, 4904t, 4939, 4940f, 4940t
internal fixation of, 4596
pediatric, 3333
screw fixation of, 3550
type I, 4903, 4904f, 4904t, 4939
type II, 4903–4904, 4904f, 4904t, 4939–4943
anterior screw fixation of, 4943
nonsurgical treatment of, 4940–4942
nonunion of, 4941, 4941t, 4942f
surgery for, 4942–4943
type III, 4904, 4904f, 4904t, 4943
anterior screw fixation of, 4943, 4944f–4946f, 4945
Odontoid process
anomalies of, 3341–3344, 3342f–3344f
blood supply to, 3331
in mucopolysaccharidosis, 3344
pyogenic infection of, 4373f–4375f, 4375
retroflexion of, in Chiari malformation type I, 3348, 3348f
rheumatoid arthritis of, 4571–4572, 4571f
skeletal dysplasia of, 3343–3344
vertical migration of, 4571
vertical penetration of, in rheumatoid arthritis, 4571, 4572f
OEIS (omphalocele, bladder exstrophy, imperforate anus, spinal defect) complex, 3226
Ofloxacin, for tuberculosis, 1441
Ohm's law, 216, 218, 1467, 3814b, 3814f
Oil-water partition coefficient, of blood-brain barrier, 15, 16f
Olfactory ensheathing cells
in axonal regeneration, 203
in central nervous system repair, 4162–4163
Olfactory epithelium, 1312

Olfactory groove
anatomy of, 1266
meningioma of, 910, 910f, 1114–1115, 1115f, 1265
diagnosis of, 1268, 1270f–1275f, 1273, 1275
imaging of, 1268, 1270f–1275f, 1273, 1275
surgical approach to, 1276
results of, 1279t, 1280
Olfactory nerve, examination of, 265
pediatric, 3173
Olfactory neuroblastoma, 1312–1313, 1395–1396, 1396f
immunocytologic differentiation of, 1313t, 1314f
Olfactory striae, 18f
Olfactory tract, 10f, 14f, 15f, 18f, 22f, 24f, 28f
dissection of, in aneurysm surgery, 1879
Olfactory vein, 24f
Oligemia, 1601, 1601t
Oligoastrocytoma
anaplastic, 664
cytometric cell-cycle analysis of, 695
mixed, 664
chemotherapy for, 976
proliferation markers for, 698–699
Oligodendroblast, 98
Oligodendrocyte(s), 83, 86–87, 86f
in axonal regeneration, 203–204
Oligodendrocyte progenitor cells, 83, 91–93
distribution of, 87, 89f
function of, 91
glial neoplasms and, 92–93
in brain development, 91–92, 92f
Oligodendroglioma, 4302
anaplastic, 664
radiation therapy for, 4022
classification of, 664
cytometric cell-cycle analysis of, 695
DNA polymerase marking of, 694
gene alterations in, 751t
grading of, mitotic activity in, 690
incidence of, 950
low-grade, histopathology of, 952–953, 952f
magnetic resonance imaging of, 453, 454f
male:female ratio in, 953
malignant
chemotherapy for, 976
histopathology of, 943–944, 972f
prognosis for, 978
radiation therapy for, 975
MIB-1 labeling index for, 699, 699t
mixed, 953
oligodendrocyte progenitor cells and, 92–93
pediatric, 3697
chemotherapy for, 3703
imaging of, 3698f, 3699
pathology of, 3700
platelet-derived growth factor in, 730
prognostic factors in, 965
proliferation markers for, 698–699
radiologic features of, 847, 847f
seizures in, 828
TP53 mutation in, 950–951
Olisthy
after laminectomy, 4532
disk herniation with, 4532
lumbar spine, 4531–4532
surgery for, 4532
unstable, fusion for, 4532–4533
Ollier's disease, chondroma with, 1387, 4840
Omohyoid muscle, in carotid endarterectomy, 1632
Oncogenes, in angiogenesis, 775t
Oncogenesis, 659
Onion whorl disease, 3950–3951
Onuf's nucleus, in urinary tract function, 360
Open lip, 62f, 63
Opercular cleft, 5, 6f
Opercule rolandique, 3
Operculoinsular compartment, 5
Ophthalmic artery, 19, 1896
aneurysms of, 1904
surgery for, 1886–1887, 1888f
Ophthalmopathy, Graves,' 1376–1377
Ophthalmoplegia
in pediatric aneurysms, 3450f, 3451
orbital tumors and, 1371
Ophthalmoscopy, 265
Opioid receptors
in epilepsy, 2476
sites for, 2955, 2955f, 2960–2961
Opioids, 1508
antinociceptive effects of, 2960
endogenous, in deep brain stimulation, 3122
for nonmalignant pain, 2961
for pain, 2960–2964
for trigeminal neuralgia, 2991
modulation sites for, 2954f
patient-physician contract for, 2962, 2962f–2963f
physical dependence on, 2961–2962
responsiveness of, 2961
side effects of, 2961
sites of action of, 2960–2961
tolerance to, 2961
Opsoclonus, 293, 833, 2722, 3174–3175
Optic canals, tuberculum sellae meningioma in, 1117, 1117f
Optic chiasm, 10f, 24f, 2541
chiasmatic cistern and, 1927f, 1929
compression of, 313f
lesions of, 313–314, 313f, 314f
lesions posterior to, vision mapping in, 2545
radiation vasculitis of, 314f
Optic disk
anterior ischemic neuropathy of, 306–308, 307f
bow-tie atrophy of, 309, 312f
drusen of, 309, 311f, 312f
edema of
causes of, 304t
differential diagnosis of, 304t, 305
in pseudotumor cerebri, 1426, 1427f
pallor of, 309, 312
Optic nerve, 10f, 14f, 15f, 1321f, 2541
anatomy of, 305, 305f
chiasmatic cistern and, 1927f, 1929
congenitally anomalous, 309, 312f
disorders of, 304t, 305
examination of, 265–266
pediatric, 3173
glioma of, 309, 831, 1373
prechiasmatic, pediatric, 3596
granulomatous disorders of, 309
in anterior communicating artery aneurysm surgery, 1933
lesions of, monocular blindness from, 2542, 2542f
lymphoproliferative disorders of, 309
meningioma of, 309, 1118–1119
Optic nerve *(Continued)*
traumatic neuropathy of, pediatric, 3468, 3468f
Optic nerve sheath
fenestration of, for pseudotumor cerebri, 1430
meningioma of, 1372
Optic neuritis, 308–309, 308f
in multiple sclerosis, 1452
Optic neuropathy
anterior ischemic, 306–308, 307f
compressive, 309, 310f, 323
hereditary, 312–313
infiltrative, 309, 311f
nutritional, 312
toxic, 312
traumatic, 313
Optic pathway
cavernous malformation of, 2316
pilocytic astrocytoma of, pediatric, 3595
Optic pathway glioma, pediatric, 3595–3599
chemotherapy for, 3598–3599
clinical presentation of, 3595–3596
outcome in, 3599
pathology of, 3595
radiation therapy for, 3598
surgery for, 3597–3598
treatment of, 3597–3599
Optic radiation, 8f, 9–10, 2541–2542
Optic recess, 14f
Optic tract, 10f, 12f, 18f, 24f
retrochiasmatic lesions of, 2542, 2542f
Oral cavity, surgical approaches through, complication avoidance in, 576
Oral contraceptives
in cerebral venous thrombosis, 1723–1724
in pseudotumor cerebri, 1423
Orbit
blow-out fracture of, enophthalmos from, 5257f
dermoid cyst of, 1374
distraction osteogenesis for, 3327–3328
epidermoid cyst of, 1374
exenteration of, in anterior skull base surgery, 913–914, 914f, 915f
fibrous dysplasia of, 1374–1375
fibrous histiocytoma of, 1375
fracture of, pediatric, 5261f
hemangiopericytoma of, 1375
hypertelorism of
anterior fossa encephalocele with, 3207f
surgery for, 3322, 3324–3326, 3325f
in Tolosa-Hunt syndrome, 1376
meningioma of, 1118–1119, 1372
metastases to, 1375–1376
mucocele of, 1375
neurofibroma of, 1373
nonspecific inflammation of, 1376
osteoma of, 1374
peripheral nerve tumors of, 1373–1374
pseudotumor of, 1376–1377
reconstruction of, in craniofacial trauma, 5257f
rhabdomyosarcoma of, 1375
schwannoma of, 1374
surgery on, visual evoked potentials during, 2543–2544
tumors of, 1371–1381
clinical presentation of, 1371
imaging of, 1371–1372
surgery for, 1377–1381
anteromedial orbitotomy in, 1380–1381, 1380f

Orbit (Continued)
approaches in, 1377–1378
fronto-temporo-orbital approach in, 1377f, 1378–1379
lateral microsurgical approach in, 1379–1380, 1379f
pterional approach in, 1379, 1379f
timing in, 1378
treatment of, 1372
Orbital dystopia, 5257, 5262
in roof fracture, 5261f, 5262f
Orbital fissure, superior, 1895, 1896f
Orbital gyrus, 17–18, 18f
Orbital roof
fracture of
depressed, 435f
displaced, 5262f
dystopia in, 5261f, 5262f
pediatric, 5261f
operative injury to, 5257
reconstruction of, 5261f
Orbital sulcus, 17
Orbital wall, blow-in fracture of, 5258f
Orbitectomy, for paranasal sinus tumors, 1322–1323, 1323f
Orbitofrontal artery, 27
Orbitopathy, dysthyroid, 1376–1377
Orbitotomy, anteromedial, for tumors, 1380–1381, 1380f
Organ of Corti, 328, 328f, 329f
Orion system, of cervical spine anterior screw-plate fixation, 4630t, 4632–4633, 4632f
Orthoses
cervical, 3334, 4898–4899, 4898f, 4899f
external
pediatric, complications of, 3543–3544, 3545f
vs. surgery, for spinal cord injury, 4876–4880
in occipitocervical fusion, 4666–4668
lumbar, in mechanical pain diagnosis, 4331
Orthotics, for cerebral palsy, 3730
Os odontoideum, 3333, 3341, 3342f
dystopic, 3341, 3341f
orthotopic, 3341
Oscillopsia, 275
vertigo in, 2904
Osler-Weber-Rendu disease, capillary telangiectasia with, 2176
Osmolarity, in altered consciousness, 295
Osmotherapy
for brain edema, 802
intracranial hypertension treatment by, 5133
Osseous tumors, 1361–1368
anterior basal skull reconstruction in, 1362
classification of, 1361
clinical presentation of, 1361
radiologic study of, 1361–1362
surgery for, 1362
types of, 1362–1368. *See also* specific tumor, e.g., Meningioma.
Ossification
cranial disorders of, 431–432
endochondral, 4613
failed, 4280–4281, 4281f
in vertebral column development, 4274–4275, 4274f
posterior longitudinal ligament, 4475–4487
Ossification centers, in skull formation, 3301
Ossifying fibroma, 1367
Osteitis deformans. *See* Paget's disease.
Osteoblastoma, 1367–1368, 1368f
pediatric, 3567
skull, 1384
pediatric, 3721
spinal, 4295, 4296t, 4297, 4353–4354, 4354f, 4837, 4839–4840, 4839f
pediatric, 3588–3589
vs. osteoid osteoma, 4809
Osteoblasts, 4614
Osteocalcin, 4230
Osteochondral dysplasia, odontoid process, 3343
Osteochondroma, 3947–3948, 3947t
skull, 1386–1388, 1388f
spinal, 4295, 4296t, 4354, 4840, 4841f
Osteoclastoma, 4355, 4355f
skull, 1388
Osteoclasts, 4614
Osteoconduction, in bone grafts, 4615, 4616t
Osteodiastasis, occipital, 3483, 3483f
Osteofibroma, 4809
Osteogenesis imperfecta, 3342, 3343f
Osteogenic cells, in bone grafts, 4615, 4616t
Osteogenic precursor cells, 4614
Osteogenic sarcoma, skull, 1389, 1389f
Osteoid, giant, 4809
Osteoid osteoma
cranial thickening from, 429, 429f
craniovertebral junction, 4809
pediatric, 3567
skull, 1384
spinal, 4295, 4296t, 4297, 4353, 4837, 4838f
pediatric, 3588, 3588f
vs. osteoblastoma, 4809
Osteoinduction
bone morphogenetic proteins and, 4615
of bone grafts, 4615, 4616t
Osteolysis, odontoid process, 3343
Osteoma, 1367, 1367f
orbital, 1374
skull, 1383–1384, 1384f
pediatric, 3721
Osteomalacia, 4235–4236, 4309, 4347–4348
Osteomyelitis
chronic recurrent multicentric, pediatric, 3566
spinal, 4351–4352, 4731–4732
antibiotics for, 4379, 4381
Candida, 4389–4390
imaging of, 537, 539–540, 540f
vertebral, pain in, 4290–4291, 4292f
vs. vertebral body neoplasms, 540–541
Osteomyxochondroma, 1365
Osteonectin, 4230
Osteophyte(s)
cervical, 4398
formation of
aging in, 4396
disk degeneration and, 4329
spinal, radiologic features of, 509, 512f
Osteophytic bars, cervical, in spondylosis, 4447
Osteopontin, 4230
Osteoporosis, 4235, 4308–4309, 4348–4349, 4348f
bisphosphonates in, 4233
in Cushing's disease, 1195
in prolactinoma, 1185
steroid-induced, 4235
Osteoporosis circumscripta cranii, 1400, 1400f
Osteosarcoma, spinal, 4356, 4837, 4845–4846, 4846f
radiation therapy for, 4049
Osteotomy
greenstick, in cervical laminoplasty, 4419–4420, 4419f
Le Fort III, in craniofacial syndromes, 3326–3327
monobloc, in craniofacial syndromes, 3327, 3328f
Oswestry Low Back Pain Disability Questionnaire, 243t
Otitis media, serous, glomus jugulare tumor surgery and, 1308
Otoacoustic emission testing, 337–338
of auditory neuropathy, 335–337
Otolith organs, 339, 339f
Otolithic crisis of Tumarkin, 349
Otoliths, 339
Otorhinorrhea, 5268
Otorrhea, 5267
Ototoxicity, drug-induced, 350–351
Otx1, 54t
Otx2, 50, 54t
Outcomes assessment, 244–247
alpha/beta error and power in, 245–246
bias in, 244
confidence intervals in, 246
confounding variables in, 244–245
exclusion in, 245
in evidence-based practice, 256
matching in, 245
modeling in, 245
multiple tests in, 246
randomization in, 245
standardization in, 245
statistical analysis in, 245–247
stratification in, 245
survival analysis in, 246–247
univariate vs. multivariate techniques in, 246
Overachievers, in traumatic brain injury response, 5193t
Overbite, 5249
Overjet, 5249
Oxcarbazepine, for trigeminal neuralgia, 2990t, 2993
Oxidative phosphorylation, in glucose metabolism, 1482, 1483t, 1484
Oxybutynin chloride, for multiple sclerosis, 1455t
Oxygen
cerebral metabolism of, 5047–5048
barbiturates and, 1532
positron emission tomography of, 1601
hypothermia effects on, 1532
Oxygen delivery, after traumatic brain injury, 5084
Oxygen extraction fraction, positron emission tomography of, 488–489, 490t, 1601
Oxygen-derived free radicals, in cerebral blood flow regulation, 1473–1474
Oxytocin, pseudotumor cerebri from, 1424

p14, in tumors, 718
p16, 1411
in gliomas, 715
in tumors, 718
p19/ARF, 743
p19/p14, in gliomas, 715
p21/WAF1/Cip1, 741
p27/Kip1, 741

p53, 717, 717f, 743
immune response to, 677
in angiogenesis, 774
in astrocytoma development, 890
in cell cycle control, 821
in gliomas, 715
in tumors, 676
p73, 743–744
Pachygyria, 61
magnetic resonance imaging of, 2493, 2493f
Pacinian corpuscle, 74, 74f, 3809, 3810f
$Paco_2$
cerebral blood flow effect of, 551, 1477–1478, 1477f, 1504
in subarachnoid hemorrhage, 1815
Padgett stages, 46
Paget's disease, 4235, 4309, 4349
skull, 1399–1400, 1400f
skull contour abnormalities in, 428, 428f
Pain
acute, 2956
vs. chronic pain, 3023–3024
acute localized, 4306–4309, 4307t, 4308f
benign, 3024
brainstem procedures for, 3073–3081. *See also* specific technique, e.g., Mesencephalotomy.
central, 2956, 2957, 3120, 3120t
cervical, surgery for, 4399
chronic, 2956
approach to, 2937–2949
behavioral therapy for, 2966
central sensitization in, 2957
centrally acting drugs for, 2960–2966
characteristics of, 3120, 3120t
compensation in, 2940, 2940t, 2945
deep brain stimulation for, 3026–3027, 3119–3129. *See also* Deep brain stimulation.
definition of, 2956
depression in, 2960, 2966
disability in, 2945
electrical stimulation for, 3107–3116. *See also* Electrical stimulation.
employment and, 2945
environmental mechanisms of, 2957–2959
frustrations in, 2949
intrathecal morphine for, 3134–3135, 3135f
liability in, 2940, 2940t
mechanisms of, 2956–2959
medical treatment of, 2953–2966
principles of, 2959
modulation sites for, 2953, 2954f, 2955–2956, 2955f
outcome expectations in, 2938–2940, 2940t
patient approach in, 2946–2948, 2946t, 2947f
peripherally acting drugs for, 2959–2960
physical therapy for, 2966
psychological aspects of, 2945–2946, 2957–2959, 2966
regression of benefit in, 2940–2941
somatization in, 2958
surgery for, 2938
aftercare planning for, 2947–2948
expectations for, 2948–2949
failure of, 2943–2944, 2949
limitations of, 2941–2943
patient goals in, 2947
patient's needs in, 2944–2945
Pain *(Continued)*
regression of benefit in, 2946
satisfaction in, 2948
surgeon's needs in, 2944
surgeon's role in, 2943–2944
vs. acute pain, 3023–3024
whiplash injury and, 4921
cingulotomy for, 3030
classification of, 3023–3024
cordotomy for, 3028–3029, 3059–3070. *See also* Cordotomy.
deafferentation, 3821
dorsal rhizotomy and, 3039
ganglionectomy and, 3039
definitions of, 2956
diskogenic, 4328, 4399
dorsal rhizotomy for, 3028. *See also* Dorsal rhizotomy.
dorsal root entry zone lesioning for, 3028
facial
atypical, 2989t
diagnostic clues in, 2988, 2989t
history of, 2987
fever/weight loss associated with, 4290–4295, 4291t
ganglionectomy for, 3028. *See also* Ganglionectomy.
gate control theory of, 2915, 2953, 3107, 3119
head, surgery for, 3025t
historical aspects of, 2913–2915, 4289
hypophysectomy for, 3030
imaging for, 4290
in axial skeletal infections, 4290–4295, 4291t
in cerebral palsy, 3728
in cervical disk degeneration, 4396
in Chiari malformation type I, 3354–3355
in Chiari malformation type II, 3355, 3355t
in lumbar disk disease, after surgery, 4517–4518, 4517f, 4518f
in morning stiffness, 4302–4303, 4303t, 4304f
in pediatric lumbar disk herniation, 3560–3561
in peripheral nerve damage, 3820–3821
in pyogenic spinal infection, 4366
intraspinal opioids for, 2915
intrathecal drug infusion for, 3133–3141. *See also* Drugs, intrathecal infusion of.
intrathecal morphine for, 3140
laboratory studies for, 4289–4290
malignant, 3024
mechanical, 4303–4306, 4305t, 4306f
motor cortex stimulation for, 3027
myelotomy for, 3029
neck
hyperextension-hyperflexion injury and, 4918
surgery for, 3025t
neural blockade for, 2970–2984. *See also* Neural blockade and specific nerve block.
neuraxial drug infusion for, 3027
neurectomy for, 3028
neurogenic, 3120t
intrathecal drugs for, 3135
neurological deficit and, 4309–4321
neuromatrix theory of, 2957, 2958f
neuropathic, 2956–2957, 3024, 3120, 3831
deep brain stimulation for, 3127–3128, 3127t, 3128t
Pain *(Continued)*
surgery for, 4343
trigeminal, 3018t
nociceptive, 2956, 3024, 3120
deep brain stimulation for, 3126–3127
nonpharmacological adjuvants for, 3024
peripheral mechanisms in, 2956
peripheral nerve stimulation for, 3026
physiologic anatomy of, 2917–2934
psychogenic, 2956
radicular, 4328
mechanical cause of, 4304
radiculopathic, 4329
sensation of, spinothalamic tract in, 2927
spinal cord stimulation for, 3026
spinal disorders presenting with, 4289–4309
stimulation therapies for, 3026–3027
surgery for, 3023–3030
ablative, 3027–3030
augmentative, 3025–3027, 3025t, 3026t
electrophysiologic recording methods in, 231, 232t
historical aspects of, 2913, 2914t
in treatment scheme, 3024
patient selection in, 3025
procedures in, 3025–3030, 3025t
sympathectomy for, 3028, 3093–3102. *See also* Sympathectomy.
sympathetic-independent, 3094
sympathetic-mediated, 3094
diagnosis of, 3095
differentiation of, 3095
laboratory studies for, 3095
paravertebral sympathetic block for, 3096
pathophysiology of, 3094–3095
thoracic endoscopic sympathectomy for, 3096–3097
terminology for, 3120, 3120t
thalamic, 3120
thalamotomy for, 3030
tissue transplantation techniques for, 3141
transmission of, 2953, 2954f
treatment of, progression in, 3024
tumor-related, 4835
from Ewing's sarcoma, 4848
from osteoid osteoma, 4837
in recumbency/nighttime, 4295, 4296t, 4297–4298
in spinal metastases, 4855, 4855f
Pain sensation testing, pediatric, 3182–3183
Palatal fracture, sagittal, 5265–5266
PAL-E, 158
Pallidoluysian atrophy, 2719
Pallidonigral degeneration, 2719
Pallidonigroluysian degeneration, 2719
Pallidonigroluysian neuroaxonal dystrophy, 2720
Pallidothalamic projection, 2692f, 2693
Pallidotomy, 2733, 2759, 2785–2792
cerebral activation effects of, 2760
complications in, 573, 574t
complications of, 2788, 2790, 2790t
evaluation before, 2786–2787
increased use of, 2785, 2785f
indications for, 2786
lesion making in, 2787–2788
mapping in, 2787, 2788f, 2789f
outcome in, 2790–2791, 2791f, 2791t
radiosurgical, 4090–4091, 4090f, 4091f, 4091t
technique of, 2787–2788
vs. subthalamic nucleus stimulation, 2824

Palmar grasp, in cerebral palsy, 3725, 3726t
Palsy, pressure, patient positioning and, 610–612, 612t
Pan plexus, injury to, 3821f
Pancoast's syndrome, intralaminar thalamotomy for, 3077
Pancreas, carcinoma of, thoracic endoscopic sympathectomy for, 4762–4763
Pancreatitis, chronic, celiac plexus block for, 2983
Pancuronium, 1508
Panfacial injury, 5262–5266, 5264f
  treatment of, 5265–5266
Pannus, rheumatoid, 4570
PaO_2, in cerebral blood flow regulation, 551, 1478, 1478f
Papaverine
  for cerebral vasospasm, 1854, 1856, 1856f, 1857
  in anterior communicating artery aneurysm surgery, 1936
Papez circuit, limbic system and, 2854
Papilledema, 305–306, 306f
  in brain tumors, 828–829
  in increased intracranial pressure, 183
  in pseudotumor cerebri, 1419, 1420f–1423f
Papilloma, choroid plexus. *See* Choroid plexus, papilloma of.
Paracentral lobule, 25
Paracentral ramus, 24, 24f
Parachute response testing, 3182
Paraganglia, tumors of, 1678
Paraganglioma
  filum terminale, 666–667
  skull, 1396–1397, 1397f
  spinal cord, 4821
  vascular supply to, 860t
Parahippocampal gyrus, 12f, 15f, 18f, 25, 26f, 2486, 2487f
Paralysis
  acute, 4310–4311, 4310t
  anesthesia positioning and, 611
  pediatric intramedullary tumor surgery and, 3713
  pharmacologic, in traumatic brain injury, 5131–5132, 5132t
  succinylcholine and, 270
Paramedian fissure, 29
Paramedian nuclei, 33f
Paranasal sinus(es)
  adenocarcinoma of, 910, 911f, 1312
  adenoid cystic carcinoma of, 1312, 1313f
  injury to, 425, 426f
  metastases to, 1313, 1315f
  neuroendocrine carcinoma of, 1312–1313
    chemoradiation therapy for, 1327, 1328f–1329f
  osteoma of, 1383, 1384f
  squamous cell carcinoma of, 1312
  transitional (schneiderian) carcinoma of, 1312
Paranasal sinus tumors, 1311–1330
  adjuvant therapy for, 1326–1327
  chemotherapy for, 1327, 1328f–1329f
  classification of, 1317, 1318t
  computed tomography of, 1316f, 1317
  diagnosis of, 1315–1317
  epidemiology of, 1311–1312
  Epstein-Barr virus and, 1312
  extension of, 1315–1316
  histologic distribution of, 1313–1315, 1315t
Paranasal sinus tumors *(Continued)*
  magnetic resonance imaging of, 1317, 1317f, 1318f
  occupational hazards and, 1311, 1311t
  outcome in, 1327
  pathogenesis of, 1311–1312
  pathology of, 1312–1315, 1313f–1315f, 1313t–1315t
  radiation therapy for, 1327, 1328f–1329f
  rhinoscopy of, 1315, 1316f
  surgery for, 1318–1326
    complications of, 1326, 1326t
    craniofacial resection in, 1318–1320, 1320f–1322f
    lateral approaches to, 1323f–1325f, 1324–1326
    orbitectomy in, 1322–1323, 1323f
  treatment of, 1317–1318, 1318t, 1319f
Paraneoplastic cerebellar degeneration, 832
Paraneoplastic disorders, 832–833
Paraneoplastic syndrome
  neuropathy in, 3845
  vertigo in, 2902
Paraolfactory gyrus, 25
Paraolfactory sulcus, 25
Paraplegia
  from spinal metastases, 4859
  hereditary spastic, 4319
  patient positioning and, 615–616
Paraproteinemia
  in multiple myeloma, 4854
  in plasmacytoma, 4850, 4852
Parasagittal region, meningioma of
  diagnosis of, 1268, 1268f, 1269f
  surgical approach to, 1276, 1277f, 1278
    results of, 1278, 1279t, 1280
Parasagittal sinus, surgical complications of, 1258
Parasellar region
  anatomy of, 1266
  surgery on, visual evoked potentials during, 2544
  surgical anatomy of, 918–919, 919f, 920f
  tumors of, frontotemporal approach to, 918–919, 919f
Parasitic infection
  myelitis from, 4312t, 4313
  spinal, 4390
Parasomina, vs. seizure, 2466
Parasympathetic nervous system, in lower urinary tract function, 361–362, 362f
Parasympathomimetic agents, for bladder retention, 377
Paraterminal gyrus, 24f, 25
Parathyroid hormone, in bone metabolism, 4231–4232
Paravermian fissure, 34
Parenchymal tumors, cranial
  morbidity/mortality rates for, 566t
  surgical complications in, 566–567, 566t, 567t
Paresis
  acute, 4310–4311, 4310t
  nerve root, after cervical laminectomy, 4425
Paresthesia, 3831
  hyperextension-hyperflexion injury and, 4918
Parietal lobe, 4–5, 26f
  hemorrhage of, 1738
  inferior, 5
  seizures in, 2591–2592
  superior, 4
  tumors of, 830–831
  venous drainage of, 17, 28
Parietal lobule, superior, 4f
Parietal veins, 17
Parietooccipital artery, 23
Parietooccipital sulcus, 3, 10f, 22f, 24f, 26f
Parinaud's syndrome, 322–323, 1013
  examination in, 3174
PARK2, in familial Parkinson's disease, 2711
Parkinson-dementia complex of Guam, 2716
Parkinsonism, 2703
  causes of, 2703, 2703t
  definition of, 2703, 2731
  drug-related, 2716
  dystonia with, 2678, 2721
  experimental, positron emission tomography in, 492, 492f
  pathophysiology of, 2673–2676, 2674f, 2675f
  postencephalitic, 2715–2716
    substantia nigra pars compacta in, 2706f
  secondary, 2716–2717
  signs of, modified testing for, 268
  toxic, 2716
  vascular, 2716
Parkinson's disease, 2704–2712, 2706f, 2731–2735
  activation studies in, 2759–2760
  age of onset in, 2732
  akinetic-rigid type, 2707–2708
  apoptosis in, 2710
  bradykinesia in, 2732
  brain-derived neurotrophic factor in, 2706
  causes of, 2732
  clinical presentation of, 2830
  CNS transplantation for, 2830–2847. *See also* Fetal tissue transplantation.
  cognitive impairment in, Lewy bodies and, 2709
  deep brain stimulation for, 2733–2734, 2820
  dementia with, Lewy bodies in, 2712–2713
  diagnosis of, 2704, 2732t, 2746–2747
  differential diagnosis of, 2734–2735, 2746–2747
  dopamine transporter in, 2706
  dopaminergic system in, 2704, 2706, 2706f
    lesion type and, 2707–2708
  drug-induced, 2735
  dyskinesias in, 2733
  extranigral systems in, 2708
  familial, 2711–2712
  family history of, 2732
  fetal function in, positron emission tomography of, 2757–2758, 2758f
  fetal tissue transplantation for, 2830–2843. *See also* Fetal tissue transplantation.
  gait abnormalities in, 2732
  gene therapy for, 817
  idiopathic, 2704–2712
  incidence of, 2704, 2704t
  juvenile, 2710–2711, 2732
  lesion pattern in, 2707–2708
  Lewy bodies in, 2704, 2708–2709
  medical therapy for, 2732–2733
  misdiagnosis in, 2704, 2705t
  motor functions in, pallidotomy effects on, 2791t
  neuron degeneration in, 2710, 2711f
  neuronal cell death in, 2708–2709

Parkinson's disease *(Continued)*
oxidative stress in, 2706–2707
pallidotomy for, 2733, 2759, 2785–2792. *See also* Pallidotomy.
pathology of, 2704, 2706, 2706f
pathophysiology of, 2785–2792
positron emission tomography of, 482–483, 483f, 2755–2759, 2756f–2758f
postural instability in, 2732
preclinical, positron emission tomography of, 2756–2757
presynaptic dopaminergic system in, positron emission tomography of, 2755–2756, 2756f, 2757f
progression of, positron emission tomography of, 2757
radiosurgical pallidotomy for, 4090–4091, 4090f, 4091f, 4091t
rating scales for, 2746, 2746t
resting brain metabolism in, positron emission tomography of, 2759
rigidity in, 2732
secondary, 2704
staging of, 2746, 2747t
stereotactic surgery for, 2659, 2661, 2734, 2734t
substantia nigra pars compacta in, 2704, 2706, 2706f
subthalamic nucleus stimulation for, 2803–2804
positron emission tomography of, 2760
quality of life after, 2822
subthalamotomy for, 2733
surgery for, 2733–2734, 2734t, 2747
α-synuclein in, 2703, 2708
thalamic stimulation for, 2820–2821
tremor in, 2732, 2750, 2774–2776
central oscillator hypothesis of, 2774
dopaminergic function and, 2760
mechanisms of, 2774–2775
peripheral nerve hypothesis of, 2774
positron emission tomography of, 2760
thalamotomy for, 2775–2776
radiosurgical, 4087–4090, 4087t, 4088f, 4089f
tremor-dominant type, 2708
urologic disorders in, 373
vascular, 2735
Parotid duct, in craniofacial trauma, 5251–5252
Parotid gland, in craniofacial trauma, 5251–5252
Paroxysmal disorders, 275
Pars nervosa, 1301
Pars opercularis, 3, 4f, 5, 6f
Pars orbitalis, 3, 4f, 5, 6f
Pars triangularis, 3–4, 4f, 5, 6f
Pars venosa, 1301
Parsonage-Turner syndrome, 3840
Patellar reflex testing, pediatric, 3180
Patient approach, 4289–4321
Patient confidentiality
exceptions to, 411–412
to medical records, 411
Patient positioning, 595–616
air embolism in, 614–615
awake, 600, 601f, 602f
blindness in, 612–614
complications of, 603–604, 609–616
avoidance of, 561–562
Concorde, 597t, 604, 604f
for anterior transthoracic decompression, 4974–4975, 4976f
Patient positioning *(Continued)*
for craniotomy, 627–630, 628f, 629f
for peripheral nerve exposure, 607–609
for pineal region procedures, 1016–1017, 1017f
for posterior cervical stabilization, 4643
for thoracic spine fixation, 4971
for transsphenoidal procedures, 609
head fixation complications in, 562–563, 610
historical background on, 595–596
intubation complications in, 609–610
lateral, 597t, 598, 599f, 600
for craniotomy, 628, 629f
operating room considerations in, 609
paraplegia from, 615–616
pediatric, 609
peripheral nerve injuries in, 610–612, 612t
pressure palsies in, 610–612, 612t
prone, 600, 602–604, 602f
for craniotomy, 628–630, 629f
in posterior cervical approach, 636
quadriplegia from, 615
sitting, 597t, 604, 605f, 606–607
in posterior cervical approach, 636
tension pneumocephalus in, 616
supine, 596–598, 597t, 598f
for cerebellopontine angle tumors, 607
for craniotomy, 628, 628f
three-quarter, 597t, 607, 608f
urinary complications of, 614
Patient referrals, legal issues regarding, 407
Patient transfer, legal issues regarding, 407–408
Patterning, 51, 51t
Pavlov ratio, 4410, 4411f
PAX, 3332
in medulloblastoma, 3641
Pax, 52
Pax2, 50, 54t
Pax3, 54t
Pax5, 55t
Pax6, 55t
Payment, in academic practice, 409–410
Peacock system, for intensity-modulated radiotherapy, 4142
Pediatric Coma Scale, 287–289, 288f
Pedicle(s), thoracic, 4693–4694, 4765, 4971–4972, 4972f
biomechanics of fixation and, 4195–4198
sublaminar hooks and, 4971–4972, 4972f
Pedicle artery, aneurysm of, arteriovenous malformation and, 2165–2166
Pedicle erosion, in spinal metastases, 4855, 4855t, 4856f
Pedicle fixation
image-guided spinal navigation for, 4747–4748, 4748f–4750f
lumbar, 4738, 4740
Peduncular segment, anterior, 24f
Peduncular vein, 24f, 35f
Pedunculopontine nucleus, 2731
stimulation of, 2819
Peer review committees, legal issues affecting, 410–411
Pelvic plexus, 361
Pelvic tilt, from osteoid osteoma, 4837
Pelvis
disorders of, low back pain in, 4359
fracture of, lumbosacral plexus injury in, 3970
sacral fractures and, 5011
trauma assessment of, 5089
Pemoline, for multiple sclerosis, 1454t
Penicillamine
angiosuppressive therapy with, 780
in angiogenesis, 775, 776f
Penicillin, pseudotumor cerebri from, 1423
Pentoxifylline, for sarcoidosis, 1439
Peptide-MHC complex, T-cell receptor recognition of, 676, 679
Peptostreptococcus, spinal infection from, 4365
Perceptual function, examination of, 264, 264f, 265
Percutaneous lumbar diskectomy
automated, 4776–4780
laser-assisted, 4780–4783
Percutaneous transluminal angioplasty
for carotid restenosis, 1666
for cerebral vasospasm, 1856–1857, 1857f, 1858f
Perforated substance
anterior, 10f, 17, 18f, 19, 24f
posterior, 14f, 18f
Perforating arteries, anterior, 21, 22f
Perfusion
in magnetic resonance imaging, 447
luxury, 490, 1601, 1603f
in head injury, 5051–5052
misery, 489, 1601, 1602f
Perfusion pressure
in arteriovenous malformation, 2188
ischemia and, 1504
Perfusion pressure breakthrough
after supratentorial arteriovenous malformation surgery, 2247
in giant arteriovenous malformation, 2224–2225
Perfusion reserve, 1601
Periaqueductal gray stimulation, 3119–3122, 3121t, 3125, 3125f
Periaxonal space, 3959
Pericallosal artery, 14f, 27, 1946
anatomy of, 1924, 1924f, 1925
bypass procedures with, 2115
Pericallosal veins, posterior, 28
Pericytes, in blood-brain barrier, 12, 153
Perilymph fistula
temporal bone fracture and, 5281
tympanotomy for, 2907
vertigo in, 2903–2904
Perineum
pain in, dorsal rhizotomy/ganglionectomy for, 3042
trauma assessment of, 5089
Perineuroma, 3950
Periosteum, 4614
Peripheral endothelial cells, vs. brain, 155–156
Peripheral nerve endings, 3809, 3810f, 3811f
Peripheral nerve fibers, 3809
conduction velocity in, 3809, 3810t
myelinated, 3809
unmyelinated, 3809
Peripheral nerves
anatomy of, 647–648, 3809–3810, 3810f, 3811f
areas innervated by, 2922f
assessment of, neuromonitoring in, 3865–3866
autoimmune disorders of, 3816
barrier system of, 3960–3961
biopsy of, 3962–3963
blood supply to, 3899
chemical interference in, 3816
components of, staining techniques for, 3959t

Peripheral nerves (*Continued*)
compression of
discrimination testing in, 3803–3804, 3804f
histopathology of, 3900, 3901f, 3902f
connective tissue compartment of, 3958, 3959f
demyelinating diseases of, 3815–3816
disorders of
axonal degeneration/regeneration in, 3961–3962, 3961f, 3962f
magnetic resonance imaging of, 3873–3886
magnetic resonance neurography of, 3873–3875, 3874f
muscle signal changes in, magnetic resonance imaging of, 3884, 3884f
pathology of, 3814–3816, 3961–3962, 3961f, 3962f
physical features of, 270–271, 271f
vascular pathologic changes in, 3962
dissection of, neuromonitoring of, 3865
division of, 3967
electrodiagnostic evaluation of, 3851–3870
endoneurium of, 3958, 3959f
entrapment of, 3921–3936. *See also* specific type, e.g., Median nerve, entrapment of.
electrophysiologic tests of, 3922
internode in, 3922
ischemia in, 3922
lower extremity, 3933–3936
magnetic resonance imaging of, 3922–3923
mechanical deformation in, 3922
pathophysiology of, 3921–3922
signs/symptoms of, 3922
surgery for, 3923
treatment of, 3796–3797
types of, 3923–3936
upper extremity, 3923–3933
genetic diseases of, 3815–3816
grafting for, historical aspects of, 3803
injection into, 3974–3975
injury to
autonomic dysfunction in, 3822
axonotmetic, 3795, 3796f, 3884
treatment of, 3796
vs. neurotmetic, 3885, 3885t, 3886f
classification of, 3899, 3900f
compression and, 3827–3828
contusion and, 3827
electrical, 3828
electrodiagnostic testing in, 3860–3861
vs. magnetic resonance imaging, 3885, 3885t
electromyography of, 3973–3974
emergency room evaluation of, 3819–3820
evaluation of, 3795–3797
fifth-degree, 3899
first-degree, 3899
fourth-degree, 3899
functional recovery after, 201–202
grading of, 3825–3826, 3825t
clinical, 3796–3797, 3797t
pathologic, 3795–3796, 3796f
gunshot wounds and, 3827
history of, 3820–3822
iatrogenic, 3828–3829, 3974–3975
imaging of, 3974
in upper extremity, 3822, 3822f
injection, 3828
ischemia and, 3827–3828

Peripheral nerves (*Continued*)
laceration and, 3827
location of, 3861
magnetic resonance imaging of, 3883–3885, 3884f, 3885t, 3886f
electrodiagnostic testing and, 3885, 3885t
mechanism of, 3795, 3826–3829
motor deficit in, 3821–3822, 3821f
motor testing in, 3822–3823, 3823f
needle electromyography of, 3860–3861
nerve conduction studies of, 3860
neurapraxic, 3795, 3796f, 3884
magnetic resonance imaging of, 3884, 3885
treatment of, 3796
neurotmetic, 3795, 3796f, 3884
surgery for, 3796
pain in, 3820–3821
pathology of, 3815, 3815f
patient approach in, 3819–3829
patient positioning and, 610–612, 612t
peripheral nerve stimulation for, 3114
physical examination of, 3822–3825, 3822t
reflex testing in, 3824–3825
regeneration after, 3967–3968, 3968f–3969f
second-degree, 3899
sensory evaluation in, 3824, 3825f
sensory loss in, 3821, 3821f
sensory nerve action potential in, 3974
sixth-degree, 3899–3900, 3900f
somatosensory evoked potential in, 3974
spinal cord stimulation for, 3113
stretch and, 3827
thermal, 3828
third-degree, 3899
traction and, 3827
treatment of, 3967–3987
localization of, 3865
manipulation of, 3865
multiple compression of, 3900
myelin sheath of, 3810, 3811f
myelinated nerve fiber in, 3958–3960, 3960f
neuromonitoring of, 3862–3866
neurovascular sheath of, hemorrhage into, 3975
physiology of, 3809–3816
reconnection of, historical aspects of, 3800–3801, 3802f
regeneration of
historical aspects of, 3804–3805
reticular vs. neuron theories of, 3799–3800, 3799f, 3800f
repair of, epineurial vs. perineurial sutures in, historical aspects of, 3801, 3803
sensory fibers in, classification of, 2918t
stimulation of, 3026
electrodes for, 3109–3110, 3110f
implanted pulse generators for, 3110–3111, 3111f
indications for, 3112–3114
structure of, 3958–3961, 3959f, 3959t, 3960f
surgery on, 647–655
as subspecialty, 3805–3806, 3805f, 3806t
compound nerve action potentials in, 3863
electromyography during, 3862, 3864

Peripheral nerves (*Continued*)
exposure for, 648–650, 649f, 650f
historical aspects of, 3798–3806
neuromonitoring during, 3862–3866
patient positioning for, 607–609, 648
somatosensory evoked potentials during, 3862, 3863–3864
tethered, magnetic resonance imaging of, 3883
transmission in, 3812–3814
tumors of. *See also* specific type.
diagnosis of, 3941–3942, 3942f
magnetic resonance imaging of, 3875–3876, 3875f–3878f, 3941, 3942f
orbital, 1373–1374
surgery for, 3955
treatment of, 3941–3955
vs. lumbar disk disease, 4511
vs. radiation-induced plexitis, magnetic resonance imaging in, 3876, 3878f
unmyelinated nerve fiber in, 3960, 3960f
wallerian degeneration of, 3815
Peripheral nervous system
central nervous system and, 3809
inflammation of, in regeneration, 4155
injury to, 195–202
gene expression after, 4154–4155
neuronal survival after, 195, 197
axonal degeneration in, 199
axonal regeneration in, 198–201
growth-promoting gene products in, 197
neuromuscular junction in, 201
neuropeptides in, 197–198
neurotransmitters in, 197–198
prolonged degeneration in, 201
response to, 195, 196f
urologic disorders in, 375
vs. central nervous system injury, 3968–3969
neuronal cell migration in, 80
Peripheral neuropathy, 3831–3847
acquired vs. inherited, 3836, 3837t
alcoholic, 3843
ancillary tests for, 3837, 3838t
axonal, 3835, 3836t
biopsy in, 3837, 3838t, 3962–3963
chemicals and, 3843–3844
deficit distribution in, 3834t
demyelinating, 3835, 3835t
diabetic, 3842–3843
differential diagnosis of, 4527
diagnosis of, 3834–3837
disorders associated with, 3836–3837, 3837t
drugs and, 3843–3844
electromyography for, 3835, 3836t, 3837
endocrine, 3832t, 3842–3843
hereditary, 3832t, 3836, 3837t, 3845–3846
history in, 271
idiopathic, 3832t, 3846
immune-mediated, 3832t, 3839–3841
in amyotrophic lateral sclerosis, 3846–3847
in renal disease, 3846
in sarcoidosis, 1436
infectious, 3832t, 3841–3842
inflammatory, 3832t, 3839–3841
length-dependent, 3835, 3836t
numbness in, 3833, 3833f
lesion localization in, 3834, 3834t
tests for, 3835, 3836t
mechanism of, 3832t

Peripheral neuropathy *(Continued)*
  motor, 3831, 3832t, 3833, 3833f, 3834–3835, 3834t, 3835t
  neoplastic, 3832t, 3844–3845
  nerve conduction studies for, 3835, 3836t, 3837
  neuropathic pain in, 3838
  nutritional, 3832t, 3844
  onset of, 3835–3836, 3836t
  sensory, 3831, 3832t, 3834–3835, 3834t, 3835t
  symptoms/signs of, 3831, 3832t, 3833–3834, 3833f
  time course of, 3835–3836, 3836t
  toxic, 3832t
  treatment of, 3837–3839
  types of, 3832t
  vascular, 3832t, 3844
  vesicogenic retention in, 376
  vs. neurosurgical conditions, 3832t
Peripheral vascular disease, ischemic pain with, spinal cord stimulation for, 3113
Peripheral vascular surgery, sympathetic nerve blocks in, 2982
Periurethral muscle, frontal cortex areas for, 359, 360f
Periurethral striated muscle receptors, proprioceptive pathways from, 362, 363f
Perivascular nerves, in cerebral blood flow–metabolism coupling, 1489
Perivascular sarcoma. *See* Central nervous system, primary lymphoma of.
Perivascular space
  cell migration from, 682
  immune regulation in, 683
Periventricular gray stimulation, chronic pain treatment with, 3121, 3121t, 3122, 3125
Periventricular leukomalacia, in cerebral palsy, 3736, 3736f, 3737f
Permanent unconscious condition, 414
Permanent vegetative state, 393
Peroneal nerve
  common, 652–653
    entrapment of, 3935
  deep, 653
    entrapment of, 3935
  entrapment of, 3882, 3882f, 3934–3935
  palsy of, 4511
    magnetic resonance imaging of, 3884, 3884f
    recovery of, 3821, 3821f
  superficial branch of, entrapment of, 3935
  surgery on, 654, 654f, 655f
    magnetic resonance imaging after, 3886f
Peroneus longus muscle, 653
Persistent vegetative state, 284, 285t
Personality
  in brain tumors, 828
  in frontal lobe tumors, 830
  vulnerable preinjury, 5193, 5193t
Personhood, 393
Pes cavus, nerve damage and, 3833, 3833f
Pesticides, brain tumors and, 811
Petriellidium boydii, infectious intracranial aneurysms from, 2102
Petroclival region
  anatomy of, 1266
  anterior approaches to, 923
Petrosal fissure, 30, 30f
Petrosal nerve, 1344
Petrosal sinus
  inferior, 36f
    cranial nerves and, 1302, 1302f
    in Cushing's disease diagnosis, 1197
  superior, 31f, 36f
Petrosal vein, 1344
  superior, 34, 35f, 36f
Petrous apex
  cholesterol granuloma of, 1443
  erosion of, 431
Petrous bone
  anterior approaches to, 919–920, 919f–921f
  tympanic portion of, erosion of, 431
Petrous-to-supraclinoid bypass, 1673f–1674f, 1674
Pfeiffer's syndrome, 3318–3319, 3320f
  historical aspects of, 3164
  hydrocephalus in, 3399
  surgery for
    Le Fort III osteotomy in, 3326–3327
    monoblock osteotomy in, 3327, 3328f
  treatment of, 3321
pH
  hyperglycemia and, 129–130
  in brain death determination, 398
  in cerebral ischemia, 124–126, 125f
Phagocytes, effector function of, 680
Phalen test, 3825
Phantom limb, spinal cord stimulation for, 3114
Pharyngeal artery, ascending, in glomus jugulare tumor, 1300
Pharyngovertebral vein, 3331
Pharynx, rheumatoid arthritis involvement of, 4573
Phencyclidine, spontaneous intracerebral hemorrhage in, 1735
Phenobarbital
  in pregnancy, 2422
  pharmacology of, 2470t, 2471
Phenol
  for cerebral palsy, 3731
  for spasticity, 2865, 2866t, 2867
Phenoxybenzamine, for multiple sclerosis, 1455t
Phenylbutazone, for ankylosing spondylitis, 4466
Phenylpropanolamine
  for bladder outlet incontinence, 380–381
  spontaneous intracerebral hemorrhage in, 1735
Phenytoin
  for neuropathic pain, 3839
  for trigeminal neuralgia, 2990t, 2992
  in ischemia prevention, 1522
  in pediatric glioma surgery, 3598
  in pregnancy, 2422
  in seizure prophylaxis, 566
  pharmacology of, 2469–2470, 2470t
  posttraumatic seizure prevention with, 5097
  pseudotumor cerebri from, 1424
Pheochromocytoma, in von Hippel-Lindau disease, 1060
Philadelphia chromosome, in leukemia, 740
Philadelphia collar, 4898f, 4899
Phosphatidylinositol-3-kinase, in glioma, 715–716
Phosphocan, in central nervous system repair failure, 4168
Phosphofructokinase, in glucose metabolism, 1482
Phosphorus, in bone, 4231
Photoreceptor(s), 71, 72f
Phrenic nerve, vagus nerve stimulator implantation and, 2643
Physaliphorous cells, in chordoma, 1283
Physiatrist, 5287
Physical examination
  ancillary parts of, 269
  auscultation in, 269
  motor, 267–268
  neurological, 264–265, 264f, 264t
  of cranial nerves, 265–267
  of reflexes, 268–269
  of skin, 269
  of station and gait, 269
  sensory, 268
Physical receptors, 75
Physical status, awareness of, after traumatic brain injury, 5192
Physical therapy, in cerebral palsy, 3731
Physician reporting responsibilities, in child abuse, 3508–3509
Physician-patient privilege, 411–412
Pia mater, 1099
  arteriovenous fistula of. *See* Arteriovenous fistula, perimedullary.
Pick's disease, substantia nigra pars compacta in, 2706f
Pilocytic astrocytoma. *See* Astrocytoma, pilocytic.
Pilomatricoma, scalp, 1415
Pineal body, 1245
Pineal cell tumors, 839
Pineal gland, 13, 14f, 15f, 3692
  anatomy of, 818f, 1011
  cavernous malformation of, 2316, 2316f
  cyst of, 1012, 1012f
  germinoma of, pediatric, 3606
Pineal parenchymal tumors
  of intermediate differentiation, 667
  proliferation markers for, 705
Pineal recess, 14f
Pineal tumors, 1011–1026
  adjuvant therapy for, 1024–1025
  biologic markers for, 1014, 1014t
  chemotherapy for, 1025
  clinical features of, 1012–1014
  deep venous system and, 1013, 1013f
  diagnosis of, 1013–1014, 1013f
  focal manifestations of, 831
  germ cell, 3604
  histopathologic classification of, 667, 667t
  hydrocephalus in, management of, 1014
  nongerminoma germ cell, pediatric, 3606
  pathology of, 818f, 1011–1012
  radiation therapy for, 1024–1025
  radiologic features of, 839–840, 839f
  radiosurgery for, 1025, 4069
  stereotactic procedures for, 1015–1024
    approaches in, 1016
    care after, 1023
    complications of, 1023
    infratentorial-supracerebellar approach in, 1017, 1018f–1019f, 1020–1021
    occipital-transtentorial approach in, 1022, 1022f
    outcome of, 1023–1024, 1023t, 1024f
    patient positioning in
      lateral, 1017, 1017f
      prone, 1017, 1017f
      sitting, 1016–1017, 1017f
    transcallosal-interhemispheric approach in, 1021–1021, 1021f

Pineal tumors *(Continued)*
transcortical-transventricular approach in, 1022
workup after, 1024, 1024f
surgery for, 1015–1024
symptoms of, 1012–1013
tissue diagnosis in
biopsy vs. open resection for, 1014–1015, 1014f, 1014t
endoscopic biopsy for, 1016
treatment of, 1014–1015, 1015f, 1015t
Pinealoblastoma, 997–998. *See also* Primitive neuroectodermal tumors, supratentorial.
Pinealocytes, 1012
Pinealoma, 1012
Pineoblastoma, 998
classification of, 667, 667t, 669
radiologic features of, 839
Pineocytoma
classification of, 667, 667t
radiologic features of, 839
Ping-pong gaze, 293
Pins and needles, 3831
Piriformis syndrome, 4330, 4511
magnetic resonance imaging of, 3881–3882, 3881f
Pituitary adenoma
central skull base, 1267
classification of, 1172–1174, 1173t
clinical manifestations of, 1174–1175
compressive effects of, 1174
corticotroph, 1170, 1194–1200. *See also* Cushing's disease; Cushing's syndrome; Nelson's syndrome.
adrenocorticotropic hormone secretion in, 1194
diagnosis of, 868, 1175, 1273
functional, fractionated radiation therapy for, 4035–4036
functional classification of, 1172, 1173t
gonadotroph, 1170–1171
growth hormone–secreting (somatotroph), 1170, 1189–1194
clinical features of, 1189–1190
growth hormone levels in, 1190
medical treatment of, 1192–1193
radiation therapy for, 1193
recurrence of, 1193–1194, 1194t
remission of, 1191–1192, 1192t
surgery for, 1190–1192, 1192t
histopathology of, 1172
hormonal studies in, 868, 1175
hyperprolactinemia in, 1174–1175
hypothalamus compromise in, 1174
imaging classification of, 1173
imaging of, 1175
in pregnancy, 867–870, 869f
incidence of, 809, 1170
lactotroph. *See* Prolactinoma.
magnetic resonance imaging of, 455, 457, 457f, 868, 869f
mass effects in, 1176
nonfunctional, fractionated radiation therapy for, 4034–4035, 4034t, 4035f
null cell, 1200–1201
pathologic classification of, 1172–1173, 1173t
prolactin-producing, 1184–1189. *See also* Prolactinoma.
pterional approach to, 1183–1184
radiologic features of, 839–840
radiosurgery for, 4059, 4061–4063, 4062f, 4063t
sites of, cell type and, 1170
Pituitary adenoma *(Continued)*
surgery for, 1175–1184
approaches to, 1176–1177, 1176t
contraindications to, 1176
evaluation before, 1176
indications for, 1175–1176
third ventricular extension of, 1247
thyrotroph, 1170, 1200
transcranial approach to, 1183–1184
transsphenoidal approach to, 1177–1183
care after, 1180–1181
complications of, 1181–1183, 1181t
endonasal approaches in, 1177–1178
endonasal septal pushover technique in, 1178
endoscopy in, 1178
positioning for, 1177
reconstruction in, 1180
recurrence after, 1184t
remission after, 1184t
repeat, 1183
sphenoid sinus entry in, 1177–1179
sphenoidotomy in, 1179
sublabial approach in, 1178–1179
tumor removal in, 1179–1180
treatment of, 868–870, 1175
visual loss in, 1174
World Health Organization classification of, 1173–1174
Pituitary apoplexy, 1175–1176, 1202–1203
in pituitary adenoma, 868
Pituitary fossa, 422
transsphenoidal approaches to, supine positioning for, 609
Pituitary gland
adamantinoma of, 1207
adenoma of. *See* Pituitary adenoma.
anterior, morphology of, 1170
anterior insufficiency of, transsphenoidal surgery and, 569
arterial supply of, 19
carcinoma of, 1201–1202
metastases in, 1202
compression of, 1174
hormones secreted by, in tumor diagnosis, 1175
hypersecretion by, 1174
infarction of, in pregnancy, 2429
insufficiency of, 1174
macroadenoma of, magnetic resonance imaging of, 457, 457f
sarcoidosis of, 1436
tumors of. *See* Pituitary tumors.
Pituitary stalk, 14f
preservation of, in pediatric craniopharyngioma surgery, 3679, 3679f
Pituitary tumors, 1169–1203. *See also* Pituitary adenoma.
clinically nonfunctioning, 1200–1201
epidemiology of, 1170
focal manifestations of, 831
hormone secretion by, 1169
in multiple endocrine neoplasia type 1, 1170
in women, 1170
pathology of, 1170–1174
radiation therapy for, 4033–4036
dose selection in, 4033–4034
side effects of, 4036
stereotactic, 4030
technique of, 2661f, 4033
three-field arrangement in, 2661f, 4033
surgery for, history of, 1169–1170
Pitx, 55t
Pitx2, 51
Plagiocephaly
anterior
assessment of, 3301, 3301f, 3302f
deformational, 3301, 3301f
differential diagnosis of, 3301, 3302t
synostotic, 3301, 3302f
posterior
assessment of, 3302–3304, 3302f–3304f
deformational, 3303–3304, 3303t, 3304f
differential diagnosis of, 3303t
Planning target volume, 4011
Plantar fasciitis, vs. distal tibial nerve entrapment, 3936
Plantar nerve, 653
Planum polare, 5, 6f
Planum sphenoidale
anatomy of, 1266
meningioma of, 910, 910f
Planum temporale, 5, 6f
Plaque, in multiple sclerosis, 1451
Plasmacytoma
craniovertebral junction, 4808–4809, 4810f
solitary, 4296t, 4298
spinal, 4355–4356, 4837, 4850–4852
multiple myeloma from, 4854
vs. multiple myeloma, 4808–4809
Plasmapheresis
for chronic inflammatory demyelinating polyradiculoneuropathy, 3840
for Guillain-Barré syndrome, 3839
Plasticity
in nervous system injury recovery, 3785
in pediatric epilepsy surgery, 3759
pediatric, 3462
vs. regeneration, 4154
Platelet antiaggregant therapy, for carotid artery disease, 1617–1618
Platelet glycoprotein IIB-IIIa, for carotid artery disease, 1618
Platelet-derived growth factor, 729–730
in axonal regeneration, 200
in bone, 4614, 4615
in gliomas, 715
in recurrent carotid artery stenosis, 1663
Platelet-derived growth factor receptors, in brain tumors, 730
Plates
internal spinal fixation with, 4591–4592, 4901, 4902
anterior cervical, 4440, 4442
anterior thoracolumbar, 4684–4685, 4685f, 4719, 4721–4722, 4721f
in metastases, 4862, 4864f
posterior cervical, 4423–4424
mandible fracture fixation with, 5264–5265
occipitocervical fusion with, 4666, 4667f
Platinums, 881–882
Platybasia, 424, 3340
Pleomorphic xanthoastrocytoma, 988–990. *See also* Xanthoastrocytoma, pleomorphic.
Plexitis, radiation-induced
vs. metastatic cancer, 3954
vs. peripheral nerve tumors, magnetic resonance imaging in, 3876, 3878f
Pli de passage, 3, 4f
Plial vessels, molecular characterization of, 157
PMP22, 3845
Pneumocephalus
after skull base surgery, 571–572
esthesioneuroblastoma surgery and, 1340

Pneumocephalus (*Continued*)
in traumatic cerebrospinal fluid fistula, 5269
traumatic, 425, 426f
Pneumonia, in subarachnoid hemorrhage, 1827
Pneumonitis, complement-mediated, hypothermia and, 1533
PNU-145156E, angiosuppressive therapy with, 779t, 783
Po_2, in cerebral blood flow, 1504
Poiseuille's equation, 5048
Poliomyelitis, weakness in, 272
Poliovirus infection, myelitis from, 4311–4312
Polyadenosine diphosphate-ribose polymerase, in traumatic brain injury, 5027
Polycationic proteins, blood-brain barrier transcytosis of, 163
Polycystic kidney disease, autosomal, intracranial aneurysms in, 1769–1770
Polycystic liver disease, autosomal dominant, intracranial aneurysms in, 1770, 1776
Polycythemia, in hemangioblastoma, 1055
Polyglutamine repeat disorders, 2703t
Polymerase chain reaction, 712–713, 750–752, 750f, 751f
reverse transcription, 752, 753f
Polymicrogyria, 61
magnetic resonance imaging of, 2493, 2493f
Polymorphonuclear cells, in cerebral ischemia, 136
Polymyositis, clinical manifestations of, 833
Polyneuropathy, 3833
diabetic, 3842
sensory loss in, 271, 271f
Polyradiculoneuropathy, chronic inflammatory demyelinating, 3839–3840
Polyradiculopathy, cytomegalovirus, 3841
Polysialylated neural cell adhesion molecule, after traumatic brain injury, 5032
Pons, 29
cavernous malformations of, 2324f
glioma of, pediatric, 3663, 3667
hemorrhage of, 1739–1740, 1739f
in Chiari malformation type II, 3352
infarctions of, 273
syndromes affecting, 273, 273f
Pontine micturition center, 359, 359f, 360
Pontine sulcus, lateral, 30f
Pontine vein, transverse, 35f
Pontomedullary artery, 1974
Pontomedullary sulcus, 29, 39
Pontomesencephalic sulcus, 30f
Pontomesencephalic vein, anterior, 35f
Pontotrigeminal vein, 36f
Population correlation studies, 247–248
Portland Adaptability Inventory, 5191
Positional test, of vestibular function, 345
Positive supporting response, in cerebral palsy, 3725, 3726t
Positron emission tomography, 477–493, 1600–1609, 2475
biologic disease processes assessed by, 482
brain imaging in, 479–480, 479f
camera in, 479–480
clinical applications of, 485–491
cyclotron procedures in, 477–479, 478f

Positron emission tomography (*Continued*)
full width at half maximum in, 480
image reconstruction in, 480
in cerebrovascular disease, 1600–1609
in molecular medicine, 491–493, 492f, 493f
in oncology, 2480, 2481f
in vivo drug monitoring with, 491
of Alzheimer's disease, 484–485, 484f, 485f
of arteriovenous malformations, 1604
of brain injury, 488–491, 490t
of brain tumors, 487–488, 487f–490f
of cerebrovascular disease, 2478
of dementia, 484–485
of epilepsy, 485–487, 486t, 2476–2477
of extratemporal lobe epilepsy, 486–487
of hemodynamic failure, 1601–1604, 1602f, 1603f
of hemodynamic reserve, 1601–1602
of Huntington's disease, 483–484, 484f
of misery perfusion, 1601–1602, 1602f
of movement disorders, 482–485
of neurological dysfunction, 482–485
of Parkinson's disease, 482–483, 483f
of stroke, 1604–1607
of temporal lobe epilepsy, 485–486, 486t
of trauma, 2481
parametric images in, 480
physiologic variables in, 1600, 1600f, 1600t
principles of, 477–482, 2475–2476
radiochemical procedures in, 477–479, 478f, 478t
radiolabeled compounds for, 480, 481t
radiopharmaceuticals in, 2475
sensitivity of, 479
spatial resolution in, 479, 479f
techniques of, 1600–1601
tracer kinetic models in, 480, 481f
tracers in, 1600–1601
vision mapping with, 2546
Postcentral gyrus, 4f, 5, 6f, 24f
Postcentral sulcus, 4, 4f
Postclival fissure, 31f, 33f
Postconcussional disorder, 5197
Posterior arch, fracture of, 4933, 4934, 4934f
Posterior commissure, 12f, 14f, 15f
radiologic localization of, 2769–2770
Posterior fossa, 423
acoustic neuroma of
anatomic variations in, 1158–1159, 1158t
vascular involvement in, 1159, 1159t
anatomy of, 28–40
arachnoid cyst of, 3298, 3298f
arteries of, 36f, 37–40, 38f, 40f
arteriovenous malformations of, 2251–2265
aneurysms with, 2252, 2252f
classification of, 2256–2257, 2256f–2258f
clinical presentation of, 2251–2253, 2252f
fourth ventricle and, 2255, 2255f
hematoma of, evacuation of, 2253, 2253f, 2254, 2254f, 2255
hemorrhage in, 2252
imaging of, 2253–2255, 2254f, 2255f
preoperative embolization of, 2257–2258
prevalence of, 2251
seizure in, 2252–2253
stereotactic radiosurgery for, 2258–2259

Posterior fossa (*Continued*)
surgery for, 2259–2260, 2259f
patient selection in, 2253, 2253f
bullet wounds to, 5236
choroid plexus tumors of, 3612, 3613
surgery for, 3618
embryology of, 3332
encephalocele of, 3200–3205. *See also* Encephalocele, posterior.
ependymoma of, pediatric, 3624, 3630
epidermoid tumor of, 3691
epidural hematoma of, 5043, 5154
extradural approach to, 920, 921f, 924–925, 924f, 925f
height of, 424–425, 424f
hematoma of
diagnosis of, 5162, 5163f
evacuation of, 5162–5163, 5164f–5165f
in Chiari malformation type I, 3348, 3356
intradural approach to, 925–928
medulloblastoma of, 3641f
pediatric, 3639
chemotherapy for, 3702
meningioma of, 1119–1120, 1119f–1121f
presigmoid-subtemporal approach to, 924–925, 925f
primitive neuroectodermal tumors of. *See* Medulloblastoma.
retrosigmoid suprameatal approach to, 926, 926f
subdural hematoma of, delivery and, 3484–3485, 3485f, 3486f
surgery on, evaluation before, 554–555
three-dimensional imaging of, 435f
trauma to, magnetic resonance imaging of, 469
tumors of
pediatric, surgery for, 3194–3195, 3194t
vertigo in, 353
veins of, 34–35, 35f, 36f, 37
petrosal group of, 35
posterior (tentorial) group of, 37
superior (galenic) group of, 35, 37
weakness and, 426
Posterior fossa syndrome, medulloblastoma resection and, 1004
Posterior inferior cerebellar artery–to–posterior inferior cerebellar artery anastomosis, 2115
Posterior longitudinal ligament, 4186
ossification of, 4475–4487
anatomy and physiology in, 4477–4479, 4478f
clinical presentation of, 4480–4481
diagnosis of, 4481, 4482f–4484f
in lumbar stenosis, 4526–4527
natural history of, 4481
pathogenesis of, 4475–4477
pathology of, 4480
surgery for
procedure selection in, 4481–4485
techniques of, 4485–4486
treatment of, 4481
complications of, 4486
results of, 4486–4487, 4487f
rupture of, in spinal cord injury without radiographic abnormality, 3521, 3521f
Posterolateral fissure, 30, 30f
Postganglionic fibers, 2981
Postherpetic neuralgia, 2989t, 3842
dorsal rhizotomy for, 3041
mesencephalotomy for, 3077–3078
vs. trigeminal neuralgia, 2988

Postolivary sulcus, 29
Postoperative hyperperfusion syndrome, carotid endarterectomy and, transcranial Doppler ultrasonography of, 1550
Postpolio syndrome, 4319–4320
Post–subarachnoid hemorrhage vasculopathy. *See* Vasospasm.
Postsynaptic cell, 72f, 73
Postsynaptic potential
  excitatory, 227–228, 228t
  inhibitory, 227–228, 228t
Post-traumatic amnesia, in injury severity estimation, 5195–5196
Post-traumatic stress disorder, in traumatic brain injury response, 5193, 5193t
Postural instability, in Parkinson's disease, 2732
Posture
  frog-leg, 3177
  in ankylosing spondylitis, 4460, 4461f
  pediatric, examination of, 3177
Potassium
  astrocyte uptake of, 101, 102, 103f
  equilibrium potential for, 3812
  extracellular
    after fluid pressure injury, 2456, 2456f, 2457f
    after traumatic brain injury, 2454–2456, 2454f–2457f
    in epileptiform activity, 2457, 2458f
  in astrocytes, 1486
  in cerebral blood flow–metabolism coupling, 1488–1489
  in electrical synaptic transmission, 227
  in extracellular homeostasis, 228, 229f, 230
  in neuron excitability, 228, 230
  in neurons, 3812, 3812t
  resting membrane potential and, 218–219, 219f
Potassium channels, 220t, 224–225
  glial, 225
  in cerebral blood flow–metabolism coupling, 1489–1490
Potassium chloride, in glial cells, 2455
Potassium spatial buffering, 102, 104f, 228, 229f, 1486, 2455–2456, 2455f–2457f
Pou1f1, 54t
Precentral gyrus, 4f, 5, 6f, 24f
Precentral sulcus, 3, 4f
Precuneus, 24f, 25, 26f
Precursor cells
  astrocyte, 98, 98f
  glia-restricted, 98, 98f
  neuroepithelial, 4159–4160
  neuron-restricted, 98
Prednisone
  for multiple sclerosis, 1454t
  for optic neuritis, 309
  for sarcoidosis, 1439
Preeclampsia, 2425
Prefrontal cortex, dorsolateral, in motor control, 2759
Pregabalin, for pain, 2965
Preganglionic fibers, 2981
Pregnancy
  acoustic neuroma in, 872
  anesthesia in, 873
  aneurysms in, 2424–2426
  angiomatous hemorrhage in, 2426–2427
  anticoagulants in, 2422–2423
  anticonvulsants in, 2422
  antifibrinolytic agents in, 2424
  antihypertensives in, 2423–2424
Pregnancy *(Continued)*
  antiplatelet agents in, 2423
  arterial occlusion in, 2427–2428, 2428t
  arteriovenous malformations in, 2166, 2426–2427
  brain tumors in, 867–874
  breast cancer in, 872
  carotid-cavernous fistula in, 2429
  carpal tunnel syndrome in, 3890
  cerebral hemorrhage in, 2166
  cerebral ischemia in, 2427–2428, 2428t
  cerebral vasospasm after, 2429
  cerebrovascular disorders during, 2421–2429
  choroid plexus papilloma in, 872
  coma in, 295, 295t
  confusion in, 295, 295t
  craniotomy in, anesthesia for, 873
  drug effects of, 2422–2424
  ependymoma in, 872
  folic acid supplementation in, 871
  glial tumors in, 870–871, 870f
  growth hormone–secreting adenoma in, 869
  hemangioblastoma in, 872
  imaging during, 2424
  informed consent during, 409
  intracranial aneurysm in, 1800–1801
  lung cancer in, 872
  mannitol in, 2423
  medulloblastoma in, 872
  melanoma in, 872
  meningioma in, 871–872, 872f
  metastases in, 872
  metastatic choriocarcinoma in, 2428–2429
  moyamoya in, 1720
  nimodipine in, 2423
  physiologic changes during, 2421–2422
  pituitary adenoma in, 867–870, 869f
  pituitary apoplexy in, 2429
  primary brain lymphoma in, 872
  prolactinoma in, 1188–1189
  pseudotumor cerebri in, 872–873, 1430
  stroke in, 2427–2428, 2428t
  subarachnoid hemorrhage in, 2424–2426
  surgery during, 2424
  venous thrombosis in, 2428
Premamillary artery, 20
Premature infants
  cerebral palsy and, 3723, 3724t, 3736
  germinal matrix–intraventricular hemorrhage in. *See* Hydrocephalus, infantile posthemorrhagic.
  subgroups of, 3405, 3405t
Premotor cortex, lateral, 2759
Preolivary sulcus, 29, 30f, 37
Prepyramidal fissure, 33f
Prepyriform cortex, 26f
Pressor agents, cerebral blood flow effects of, 5134–5135, 5135t
Pressure, 176
Pressure palsy, patient positioning and, 610–612, 612t
Pressure reactivity index, 182, 182f
Pressure-volume curve, 177, 177f, 182, 182f
Pressure-volume index, 177, 177f, 182, 182f
  in intracranial compliance, 1504
  in intracranial pressure, 5054, 5054f
Presynaptic cell, 72–73, 72f
Presynaptic terminal, 78
Prevalence, 236–237, 237t
Primary fissure, 31f, 35f
Primidone
  in pregnancy, 2422
  pharmacology of, 2470t, 2471
Primitive neuroectodermal tumors, 997–1007, 3639
  biologic indicators in, 1006, 1006t
  complications of, 1004
  craniospinal irradiation in, 1005
  grading of, 1004, 1004t
  histopathologic classification of, 668–669, 668t
  history of, 997
  hydrocephalus management in, 1002–1003
  incidence of, 997–998
  insulin-like growth factors in, 729
  magnetic resonance imaging of, 461, 461f
  neurotrophins in, 729
  outcome in, 1004–1007, 1006t
  pathology of, 998–999, 998f–1000f
  pediatric, 3697
    pathology of, 3700
  posterior fossa. *See* Medulloblastoma.
  radiation therapy for, 4023
  radiography of, 1000, 1001f–1003f, 1002
  radiologic features of, 847, 848f, 849
  signs/symptoms of, 1000
  supratentorial, 997–998, 1031
    imaging of, 1002f
    outcome in, 1006
    pediatric, 3699, 3700f
      chemotherapy for, 3702
  terminology for, 997, 1031
  treatment of, 1002–1004
  tumor factors in, survival and, 1006, 1006t
  vs. medulloblastoma, 1032
Primitive node, 47
Primitive reflexes, in cerebral palsy, 3725, 3726t
Primitive streak, 47
  development of, 4239, 4240f
  regression of, 4241, 4242f
Prinomastat, angiosuppressive therapy with, 777
Proapoptotic genes, 719
Proatlas, segmentation abnormality of, 3338
Probability
  in diagnosis, 235–238
  post-test, 235–236, 236f
  pretest, 235–236, 236f
Procarbazine, 881
  for malignant glioma, 976
Progenitor cells
  in central nervous system repair, 4159, 4160, 4161
  transplantation of, 93, 94f
    in neural regeneration, 5033
Progesterone receptors, in meningioma, 1108
Progressive pallidum atrophy, 2719–2720
Progressive supranuclear palsy
  neurodegeneration in, 2714–2715
    histologic features of, 2714
  positron emission tomography of, 2761, 2762f
  striatal neurons in, 2708
  substantia nigra pars compacta in, 2706f
  vs. Parkinson's disease, 2735
Prolactin
  after pituitary surgery, 1191
  in growth hormone–secreting pituitary adenoma, 1190
  in meningioma, 1108
  in pituitary adenoma, 1174–1175
  in prolactinoma, 1185–1186

Prolactinoma, 1170
  clinical presentation of, 1185
  in pregnancy, 1188–1189
  laboratory studies for, 1185–1186
  macro-, 1185
    surgery for, 1188
  medical treatment of, 1186–1187
    in pregnancy, 1189
  micro-, 1185
    surgery for, 1187–1188
  radiation therapy for, 4036
  radiosurgery for, 4063
  surgery for, 1187–1189
    in pregnancy, 1189
    indications for, 1187, 1187t
    recurrence after, 1188
  tumor progression in, 1185
Proliferating cell nuclear antigen
  as tumor proliferation marker, 693–694
  in glioblastoma, 4097
  in meningioma, 1103, 1103f
Pronator syndrome, median nerve compression in, 3924–3925
Pronator teres muscle, median nerve entrapment at, 3924
Prone position, 597t, 600, 602–604, 602f
  complication avoidance in, 561–562
  dependent edema in, 563
  for craniotomy, 628–630, 629f
  in posterior cervical approach, 635–636
  orbital complications from, 576
Propionibacterium
  pyogenic spinal infections from, 4365
  shunt infection by, 3422–3423
Propofol, 1508
  cerebral physiology and, 551
  in craniotomy, 5149–5150
  in epilepsy surgery, 2621
  in ischemia protection, 1521
Proprioception
  pediatric, testing of, 3183–3184
  sensory nerve fibers in, 3809
Propriospinal multisynaptic ascending system, 2930
Proptosis, orbital tumors and, 1371
Prosencephalic vein, median, 3434
Prostaglandins
  in cerebral vasospasm, 1848–1849
  synthesis of, 2959
Prostate, transurethral resection of, for bladder outlet retention, 380
Prostatism, nocturia with, 365
Protease inhibitors, as angiogenesis antagonist, 776–777, 777t
Proteases
  in angiogenesis, 775t
  in apoptosis, 1519
  in axonal degeneration, 199
Protein
  as tumor antigens, 677
  phosphorylation of, in cell death, 127
  regulatory, in bone growth, 4614, 4614t
  synthesis of, in cell death, 132
Protein analysis, 752–753, 753f
Protein C, in cerebral venous thrombosis, 1723
Protein kinase C system, in cerebral vasospasm, 1848
Protein truncation test, 753
Proteoglycans
  in axonal growth failure, 205
  in bone, 4230
  in malignant glioma, 762–763
Proton radiosurgery, 4123–4129
  evolving technology in, 4129
  historical perspective on, 4123
  physical principles of, 4123–4127, 4124f–4126f
  technique of, 4128–4129
  treatment principles for, 4127–4128, 4128f
  vs. linac radiosurgery, 4115–4116
Proto-oncogenes, 739
Protuberance, 29
Prourokinase, trials of, 1496
Psammoma bodies, 1101, 1101f
P-selectin, in cerebral ischemia, 140–141
Pseudallescheria boydii, infectious intracranial aneurysms from, 2102
Pseudarthrosis
  after scoliosis surgery, 4566
  complication avoidance in, 577
Pseudoaneurysms
  displacement artifact and, 1579f
  internal carotid artery, 1880, 1883f
  peripheral nerve involvement in, 3949
  traumatic, 2131, 5208, 5209f–5210f
    after débridement, 5237
Pseudobulbar palsy, medulloblastoma surgery and, 3645–3646
Pseudochondroplasia, atlantoaxial instability in, 3543
Pseudocoma, 293
Pseudoephedrine
  for bladder outlet incontinence, 380–381
  spontaneous intracerebral hemorrhage in, 1735
Pseudomeningocele
  brachial plexus injury with, 3491, 3491f
  cerebellar astrocytoma surgery and, 3659
  ependymoma surgery and, 3630
  postoperative, 564–565
  spinal surgery and, 574–576
Pseudomonas
  infectious aneurysms from, 2102
  pyogenic spinal infections from, 4365, 4379f
Pseudoparkinsonism, arteriosclerotic, 2716
Pseudopod, in craniopharyngioma, 3672, 3672f
Pseudospondylolisthesis, 3580
Pseudotumor, orbital, 1376
Pseudotumor cerebri, 1419–1430
  causes of, 1419–1426
  cerebral venous drainage obstruction and, 1420–1422, 1424t
  clinical manifestations of, 1419, 1420f–1423f
  complications of, 1426
  conversion from hydrocephalus to, 3400, 3400f
  diagnosis of, 1426, 1427f, 1428
  endocrine dysfunction and, 1422, 1424t
  epidemiology of, 1419
  exogenous substances and, 1422–1425, 1424t
  familial, 1426
  headache in, 1419
  imaging of, 1426, 1427f
  in pregnancy, 872–873
  lumbar puncture in, 1426
  metabolic dysfunction and, 1422, 1424t
  optic disk in, 1426, 1427f
  papilledema in, 1419, 1420f–1423f
  pathophysiology of, 1426
  systemic illness and, 1425–1426, 1425t
Pseudotumor cerebri *(Continued)*
  treatment of, 1429–1430
    during pregnancy, 1430
  venous hypertension and, 3398
Pseudoxanthoma elasticum, intracranial aneurysms in, 1773
Psuedopuberty, precocious, 1013
Psychiatric disorders
  after traumatic brain injury, 5296
  anterior capsulotomy for, 2859, 2859f
  anterior cingulotomy for, 2856–2857, 2857f
  in epilepsy, 2573
  in failed back syndrome, 4337
  limbic leucotomy for, 2858–2859, 2858f
  neurosurgery for, 2853–2861
    anatomic basis for, 2854–2855
    approaches to, 2856–2861
    evaluation before, 2861
    historical perspective on, 2853–2854
    indications for, 2859–2860
    outcome in, 2860–2861
    patient selection in, 2855–2856
    repeat procedures in, 2860
  subcaudate tractotomy for, 2857–2858, 2858f
Psychological disturbances
  after glomus jugulare tumor surgery, 1308
  traumatic brain injury and, 5190–5191
  vs. multiple sclerosis, 1455
Psychological measurement, 385
Psychomotor function, after traumatic brain injury, 5188
Psychosocial problems, in achondroplasia, 3363
Psychosocioeconomic syndrome, low back pain in, 4332
Psychosurgery, 2853
  politics of, 2660–2661
Ptc, 54t
PTCH/SMOH/SHH, 742–743
PTEN, in glioma, 716
PTEN/MMAC1/TEP1, 742
Pterion, 423–424, 423f
Ptosis, examination of, 266
Pudendal nerve, in lower urinary tract function, 362, 362f, 363f
Pulmonary edema
  in subarachnoid hemorrhage, 1826–1827, 1869
  neurogenic, 1869
Pulmonary embolism, 563–564
Pulse repetition frequency, 1540
Pulvinar, thalamic, 10f, 11
Pumps, implantable
  complications of, 3140
  for intrathecal baclofen, 3749–3752, 3749f, 3750f, 3753–3754
  for intrathecal drug infusion, 3136–3140, 3137f–3139f
Pupil(s), 321–322, 322f, 323f
  abnormally large, 322, 322f
  abnormally small, 322, 323f
  dilation of, in brainstem lesions, 288, 288f
  examination of, 266
  football, 288
  in bullet wounds, 5228, 5228t
  near-light dissociation of, 322
  oval, 288
  size of, 322
Pupillary defect, relative afferent, 302, 304b

Pupillary response
examination of, 265
in Pediatric Coma Scale, 287–288, 288f
pediatric, 3173
Pupillary sparing, relative, in oculomotor neuropathy, 321
Purkinje cell, 71, 72f
Pursuit tests, of vestibular function, 345–346, 346f
Putamen, 7f, 12f, 2683
arteriovenous malformation of, 2246
fetal mesencephalic grafting in, 2836
hemorrhage of, 1737, 1737f, 1746, 1746f–1748f
Pyogenic infection, spinal, 4147, 4363–4382. *See also* specific infection.
clinical presentation of, 4365–4366
computed tomography of, 4366–4367, 4367f
conditions associated with, 4370–4371, 4371f
diagnosis of, 4366–4371, 4367f–4371f
differential diagnosis of, 4371–4372
epidemiology of, 4363–4364
epidural, pain in, 4291, 4293, 4293f
extraspinal manifestations of, 4371, 4371f
laboratory findings in, 4366
low back pain in, 4351–4352, 4351f, 4352f
magnetic resonance imaging of, 4367–4368, 4368f, 4370f, 4379, 4380f
medical management of, 4379, 4381
microbiology of, 4365
diagnostic, 4368–4369, 4370f
myelography of, 4368, 4369f
outcome of, 4381, 4382f
pain in, 4290–4291, 4292f
pathogenesis of, 4364–4365, 4365f
pediatric, 4381–4382
radiography of, 4366–4368, 4367f–4370f
surgery for, 4372–4376, 4372f–4378f
treatment of, 4372–4381, 4372f–4380f
Pyramid, 30f, 34
Pyramidal tract, in lower urinary tract function, 362
Pyrazinamide, for tuberculosis, 1441, 4387
Pyrexia, in extracranial head injury, 5056–5057
Pyridostigmine, blood-brain barrier transport of, 14
Pyridoxine deficiency, neuropathy from, 3844
Pyrimidines, halogenated, in malignant glioma radiosensitization, 4020
Pyruvate, in glucose metabolism, 1482, 1483, 1484f

Quadrangular lobule, 30f, 31f
Quadrantanopsia, 2542f
Quadrigeminal cistern, cyst of, 3297–3298, 3297f
Quadrigeminal plate, 36f, 3073
Quadrigeminal point, 21
Quadriplegia
atlanto-occipital dislocation and, 4928–4929
midcervical, posterior fossa surgery and, 555
sitting position and, 615
spastic, in cerebral palsy, 3724, 3725–3727, 3729, 3731–3732, 3747–3748
Quality-adjusted life-years, in epilepsy, 2567, 2568f

R248C, in achondroplasia, 3362–3363
Rabies virus, myelitis from, 4311, 4312t
Race
in bullet wounds, 5224t, 5225
in intracranial hematoma, 5072
Rad, 4007
Radial glial cells, 61
Radial glial fibers
disruption of, 63, 63f
in neuroblast migration, 58, 59f
Radial nerve
entrapment of, 3928–3930
above elbow, 3929
superficial sensory branch of, entrapment of, 3930
Radial tunnel syndrome, 3928
magnetic resonance imaging of, 3882, 3882f
Radial veins, 2381
Radiation
absorbed dose of, 4006–4007
biologic effects of, 4006, 4006f, 4007
brain tumors and, 809–810
carotid artery stenosis from, 1685–1687, 1686f
direct action of, 3999, 4006
DNA interactions with, 3999
effects of, 853–854
high linear energy transfer beams in, 4006, 4006f
in spinal fusion healing, 4620
indirect action of, 4006
ionizing, 3999
meningioma from, 1105, 1105f
myelopathy from, familial spastic paraplegia in, 4319
photon beam, 4007
units of, 4007
water interactions with, 3999
Radiation injury
blood-brain barrier in, 166
in arteriovenous malformation radiosurgery, 4082–4083
Radiation necrosis, after arteriovenous malformation radiation therapy, 2195–2196, 2195f, 2196t
Radiation survival curve, radiosensitizer effect on, 4001, 4003f
Radiation therapy, 3989–3990, 4005–4012. *See also* Brachytherapy.
additive quality of, 4001
automation in, 4012
buildup region in, 4001, 4002f
clinical target volume in, 4011
complications of, 4024
Compton effect in, 4006, 4006f
conformal, 4002–4003
depth-dose analysis in, 4008
depth-dose curves in, 4008, 4008f
differential cell repair in, 4000
dose in, 4000
dose-volume histogram in, 4011, 4012f
external beam, 4007–4008
falloff region in, 4001, 4002f
for benign skull base tumors, 4027–4030
for brain metastases, 4015–4018
for brain tumors, 659–660
for malignant brain tumors, 4015–4024
for pituitary tumors, 4033–4036
for spinal cord tumors, 4042–4047
Radiation therapy *(Continued)*
fractionated, 3999–4001, 4000f
gross tumor volume in, 4011, 4011f
heavy particle, 4008
historical aspects of, 3989–3990
hyperfractionation in, 4001
intensity-modulated, 4012, 4142–4143
interactions in, 4005–4006, 4006f
isocenter in, 4000
linear accelerators in, 4007–4008, 4007f, 4008f
multileaf collimators in, 4012
pair production in, 4005–4006
photoelectric effect in, 4005
physics of, 4005
planning target volume in, 4011
prior, radiosurgical dose prescription effect of, 4054
radiobiology in, 3999–4003
side effects of, 4036
simulation in, 4000, 4010, 4010f
stereotactic. *See also* Radiosurgery.
beam delivery systems for, 4138–4139
fractionated, 4136, 4138, 4138f
linacs for, 4115
radiobiology of, 4002–4003
target volume definitions in, 4011, 4011f
treatment planning in, 4008–4009, 4009f
computers in, 4010
contouring in, 4010
imaging in, 4009–4010, 4010f
three-dimensional, 4010–4011, 4011f
triangulation in, 4000
types of, 4007–4008, 4007f, 4008f
vs. stereotactic radiosurgery, 4012
Radical glial, 84
Radicular artery, 2381
spinal nerve root and, 3033–3034
Radiculopathy
cervical, 4396–4397
surgery for, 4399–4400, 4399f, 4400f
treatment of, 4412–4413, 4427
diabetic, 3843
electrodiagnostic studies of, 3859
in spinal stenosis, 4521
lower extremity, 4328
lumbar, 4329
upper extremity, signs/symptoms of, 272t
Radiobiology, 3999–4003
Radiography
skull, 419–422, 420f–422f
spinal, 500–501, 500f, 501f, 4145–4146
Radioisotopes, positron-emitting, 477–479, 478f, 478t
Radiolabeled compounds, in positron emission tomography, 480, 481t
Radiologic features, of central nervous system tumors, 835–854
Radionuclide imaging
of pyogenic spinal infection, 4368, 4369f
of spinal metastases, 4858
of spinal tumors, 4836
osteoid osteoma, 4837, 4838f
Radiosurgery, 4053–4069, 4131. *See also under* Stereotactic.
adjuvant, 4053
circular collimators in, 4139, 4139f, 4140f
complications from, 2280
dose planning for, 4054, 4076, 4134–4136, 4135f–4137f
extracranial, 4069, 4143
for arteriovenous malformations, 4073–4085
for brain metastases, 4065–4068, 4066t, 4067f, 4095, 4114

Radiosurgery *(Continued)*
for brain tumors, 659
for epilepsy, 4093
for malignant astrocytomas, 4113–4114
for malignant gliomas, 4063–4065, 4064t
for meningioma, 4056, 4059, 4060t, 4061f, 4062f, 4111–4112
for pineal region tumors, 4069
for pituitary tumors, 4059, 4061–4063, 4062f, 4063t
for skull base chondrosarcoma, 4068
for skull base chordoma, 4068
for trigeminal neuralgia, 3002–3003, 4091–4092, 4092t, 4093f
for tumors, 4053–4069. *See also* specific tumor.
for vestibular schwannomas, 4055–4056, 4057t, 4058t, 4059f, 4112
functional, 4087–4093, 4114–4116
future of, 4069
γ knife, 4115, 4117–4121, 4118f–4121f, 4131–4132
basic unit design for, 4117, 4118f
dose prescription in, 4119–4121
technique of, 4117–4118, 4119f
technology of, 4117
treatment planning in, 4118–4119, 4120f, 4121f
vs. linac radiosurgery, 4115
imaging for, 4053–4054
in pallidotomy, 4090–4091, 4090f, 4091f, 4091t
in thalamotomy, 2773–2774, 4087–4090, 4087t, 4088f, 4089f
linac, 4111–4116, 4132–4136, 4132f–4137f
multileaf collimation in, 4139–4142, 4139f–4142f
primary, 4053
proton, 4115–4116, 4123–4129
evolving technology in, 4129
historical perspective on, 4123
physical principles of, 4123–4127, 4124f–4126f
technique of, 4128–4129
treatment principles for, 4127–4128, 4128f
spinal, 4069
techniques for, 4054–4055, 4115–4116
Ramisectomy, posterior, 2897
Ramus, posterior primary, 4328
Rancho Los Amigos Levels of Cognitive Functioning Scale, 242t, 5288–5289, 5289t
Randomization, in outcomes assessment, 245
Randomized, controlled studies, 251–252
Ranklin Disability Scale, 242t
ras oncogene, in angiogenesis, 780
Rasmussen's encephalitis, magnetic resonance imaging of, 2495, 2495f
Raynaud's disease, thoracic endoscopic sympathectomy for, 4762
Raynaud's syndrome, thoracic endoscopic sympathectomy for, 3097
Rb pathway, in glioma, 717
Rb1, 741
Reactive nitrogen species, in cell death, 128
Reactive oxygen species
in cell death, 127–128
in ischemic injury, 1517–1518
in traumatic brain injury, 5026–5027
inhibitors of, 135
Receiver operator characteristic curve, 499, 499f
Receptor-mediated transport, across blood-brain barrier, 163
Recombinant human bone morphogenetic protein, 4618
Recreational activities, in cerebral palsy, 3733
Rectus gyrus, 10f, 17, 18f, 24f
Recurrent artery of Heubner, 27
anatomy of, 1925–1926, 1926f
Recurrent nerve of Luschka, 4328
Red reflex, 304, 304b
Reference test, 497, 498t
Reflex sympathetic dystrophy, 3094
spinal cord stimulation for, 3113–3114
thoracic endoscopic sympathectomy for, 4762
Reflexes
examination of, 268–269
in older infant, 3185
pediatric, 3180–3182
in cerebral palsy, 3725, 3726t, 3748
in cervical spondylotic myelopathy, 4410, 4449
Regeneration, 2829
vs. plasticity, 4154
Rehabilitation. *See also* Neurorehabilitation.
after traumatic brain injury, 5287–5296
assessment in, 5288–5291, 5288t–5290t
community-based model for, 5293
complications during, 5295–5296
historical aspects of, 5287–5288
medical model for, 5292–5293
for failed back syndrome, 4336
regression of benefit in, 2941
Reil's furrowed band, 31f, 33f
Reimbursement, legal aspects of, 413–414
Reinnervation, preferential motor, 201
Reissner's membrane, 328, 328f
Reiter's syndrome, 4350, 4463t
Relative luxury perfusion, 490
Reliability, 239–240
RELN, 55t, 61
Remains, disposition of, 416
Remak cell, 3960
Remyelination, 198, 3962
Renal artery, fibromuscular dysplasia of, 1681
Renal cell carcinoma
brain metastases in, stereotactic radiosurgery for, 1091
clear cell
in von Hippel-Lindau disease, 1053, 1059
metastatic, vs. hemangioblastoma, 1058
Renal disease, neuropathy in, 3846
Renal failure
coagulopathy with, 1747, 1752f, 1753
in encephalopathy, 295
patient positioning and, 614
postoperative, hypothermia and, 1533
Rendu-Osler-Weber syndrome, 2154
Renshaw cells, 2877
Reperfusion injury, 1495, 1517
Reporting obligations, 411–412
Reproduction
in achondroplasia, 3363
in Cushing's disease, 1195
Respiration, paralysis of, bullet wounds and, 5224
Respiratory failure, in altered consciousness, 282–283, 283f
Respiratory insufficiency
in cervical spine trauma, 4888, 4889
pseudotumor cerebri in, 1425
Respiratory mucosa, 1312
Respiratory system
disorders of
in aneurysmal subarachnoid hemorrhage, 1826–1828
in cerebral palsy, 3727–3728
in pregnancy, 2421–2422
in spinal cord injury management, 4880–4881
lateral spinothalamic tract and, 3060–3061
preoperative assessment of, 549
subarachnoid hemorrhage effects on, 554
Responsiveness, 239, 240
Resting energy expenditure, in traumatic brain injury, 5129–5130
Resting membrane potential, 216, 216f, 218
maintenance of, 219, 219f
neuronal, 3812, 3812t
potassium and, 218–219, 219f
Restriction fragment length polymorphisms, 749–750, 749f, 750f
Resuscitation, failure of, 394
Reticular formation, in consciousness, 278–279, 279f, 280
Reticulospinal tract, in lower urinary tract function, 362
Reticulum cell sarcoma. *See* Central nervous system, primary lymphoma of.
Retina, 2541
angioma of, in von Hippel-Lindau disease, 1053
Retinal-pigmented epithelial cells, central nervous system transplantation for, 2841
Retinoblastoma, 998
classification of, 669
hereditary, 739–740, 740f
mutations in, 739–740, 740f
spontaneous, 740, 740f
trilateral, 741
Retinoic acid, 52
Retrocollis, 2896t
inferior, 2893, 2893f
rotatory, 2893, 2893f
superior, 2892–2893, 2892f
Retroperitoneal space disorders
intraoperative, in lumbar disk disease, 4517
low back pain in, 4359
Retrotonsillar vein, inferior, 35f
Retroviruses
as vectors, 817–818
in CNS transplantation, 2845–2846, 2845t
in herpes simplex virus thymidine kinase gene transfer, 819–820
Revascularization. *See also* Arterial bypass; Venous bypass.
historical considerations in, 1463–1464
in aneurysm treatment, 2107–2108
in bone grafts, 4619
in moyamoya, 1718–1720, 1719f
in posterior circulation aneurysms, 1999–2000, 2000t, 2001f
Reverse transcription polymerase chain reaction, 752, 753f
Rhabdomyosarcoma, 1142
orbital, 1375
Rheology, 1468
Rheumatic disorders, spinal, 4303, 4303t
vs. lumbar disk disease, 4511
Rheumatoid arthritis, 4302–4303, 4303t, 4351, 4569–4580
atlantoaxial subluxation in, 4573

Rheumatoid arthritis *(Continued)*
cervical myelopathy in, 4573
clinical presentation of, 4573
craniocervical junction
radiologic features of, 4574, 4574f–4577f
surgical indications for, 4574–4575, 4578
treatment of, 4578–4580, 4579f–4581f
criteria for, 4570t
extra-articular manifestations of, 4572–4573
genetic susceptibility to, 4570
immunologic features of, 4569–4570, 4570t
in carpal tunnel syndrome, 3889–3890
juvenile
atlantoaxial instability in, 3543
craniocervical junction, 4580
neurological deficit in, 4575, 4578, 4578t
neurological signs in, 4573
paresthesia in, 4573
spinal involvement in, 4570–4572, 4571f, 4572f
treatment of, 4573
Rheumatoid basilar invagination, 4571
Rheumatoid factors, 4569–4570, 4570t
Rheumatoid translation, 4571
Rhinal sulcus, 18f, 19
Rhinorrhea, 5267
in craniofacial trauma, 5247–5248
pediatric basilar skull fracture and, 3467
transsphenoidal surgery and, 569–570, 1182
Rhizotomy
dorsal, 3028, 3033–3042. *See also* Dorsal rhizotomy.
extradural, 3037, 3038f
for spasticity, 2869–2870
glycerol, for trigeminal neuralgia, 2999–3000
intradural, 3037
partial sensory, for trigeminal neuralgia, 3017–3018
thermal, for trigeminal neuralgia, 2997–2999, 2998f, 2999f
Rhombomeres, 50
Rib(s)
heads of, 4765
thoracic spine motion and, 4953–4954
Riche-Cannieu anastomoses, 3898
Rifampin, for tuberculosis, 1441, 4387
Right to die, 414
Rigidity, 3178
decerebrate, 2863, 3178
definition of, 2673
in Parkinson's disease, 2732
nuchal, 3178
plastic, 3178
radiosurgical pallidotomy for, 4090–4091, 4090f, 4091f, 4091t
subthalamic nucleus stimulation for, 2822
Rinne test, 330
pediatric, 3175
RMP-7, blood-brain barrier permeability and, 17
RN33B cell line, in central nervous system repair, 4161
RNA analysis, 752, 752f, 753f
Rod-hook constructs, lumbar spine fixation with, 4733, 4733f
Rod–multiple hook constructs, lumbar spine fixation with, 4734, 4734f
Rods
for internal spine fixation, 4591–4592, 4952, 4969, 4969f
percutaneous, lumbar burst fracture fixation with, 5006, 5006f
Rod-screw constructs, lumbar spine fixation with, 4715–4716, 4716f
Rod-wire constructs, lumbar spine fixation with, 4733–4734, 4734f
Rogers interspinous wiring method, 4644–4645, 4644f
Rolandic cortex
functional magnetic resonance imaging of, 2532
imaging localization of, 2532
mapping of, anesthesia for, 2533
Rood technique, for cerebral palsy, 3731
Rostral sulcus, 25
Rotational testing, of vestibular function, 346, 347f
Rotatory fixation, atlantoaxial, pediatric, 3537–3543
classification of, 3538–3540, 3539f–3541f
radiography of, 3538–3540, 3539f–3541f
treatment of, 3541, 3542f
Round window, in sound transmission, 328f, 329
Roy-Camille occipitocervical plate, 4667f
Ruffini's corpuscle, 3809, 3810f
Ruffini's endings, 74, 74f

Saccade test, of vestibular function, 345
Saccular macula, 339, 339f
Saccule, 339, 339f
Sacral agenesis, imaging of, 535–536
Sacral fracture, 5011–5016
classification of, 5011–5013, 5012f–5014f
clinical presentation of, 5013–5014
imaging of, 5014–5015
indirect trauma in, 5012
neurological deficit in, 5014
pathophysiology of, 5011–5013, 5012f–5014f
treatment of, 5015–5016
zone I, 5012, 5012f, 5013f
zone II, 5013, 5013f
zone III, 5013, 5014f
Sacred bone, 5011
Sacrococcygeal region, development of, 4276
Sacrum
anatomy of, 5011
chordoma of, 4848
Ewing's sarcoma of, 4850f
extradural rhizotomy in, 3037, 3038f
giant cell tumor of, 4850, 4851–4852
lesions of
erectile dysfunction in, 366
micturition disorders in, 365
osteosarcoma of, 4846f
Saethre-Chotzen syndrome, 3319–3320
Sagittal balance, in cervical degenerative disease, 4410–4411, 4411f
Sagittal index, in thoracic fracture, 4967, 4968t
Sagittal sinus
inferior, 28
meningioma of, 1111–1112, 1112f, 1113f
superior, 28
dural arteriovenous malformation of, 2284
imaging of, 2287–2288, 2288f, 2289f
treatment of, 2290
Sagittal sinus *(Continued)*
meningioma of, 1265
surgical approach to, 1276
obstruction of, 1421
venous drainage of, 1266
surgical complications of, 1258
Sagittal suture, arteriovenous malformation of, 2238–2239
Salicylates, for trigeminal neuralgia, 2994
Salt wasting
after subarachnoid hemorrhage, 1830, 1830t
in traumatic brain injury, 5130–5131, 5130f
vs. syndrome of inappropriate secretion of antidiuretic hormone, 1830
Saltatory conduction, 87, 3813
S-antigen, in pineal parenchymal cell tumors, 1014
Saphenous nerve, entrapment of, 3934
Saphenous vein
bypass with, for giant/fusiform aneurysms, 2118
carotid angioplasty graft with, 1627–1629, 1628f
interposition grafts with, 2109–2111, 2111f, 2112f, 2113
Sarcoglioma, 1143
Sarcoidosis, 1435–1439
clinical presentation of, 1435–1436
diagnosis of, 1436–1438, 1437f, 1438f
hypothalamic, 1436
imaging of, 1437–1438, 1437f, 1438f
pathophysiology of, 1435
pituitary, 1436
pseudotumor cerebri in, 1425
radiologic features of, 841
spinal cord, 1436
treatment of, 1438–1439
vs. multiple sclerosis, 1453, 1453t
Sarcoma, 1141
circumscribed, cerebellar, 1143
meningeal, 1141–1146
classification of, 1141, 1142t
clinical significance of, 1141–1142
pathogenesis of, 1142–1143, 1143f
pathology of, 1142–1143, 1143f
mesenchymal
cause of, 1143
imaging of, 1144–1145, 1144f, 1145f
presentation of, 1144, 1144f
treatment of, 1145–1146
monstrocellular, 1143
neurogenic, 3951, 3952t, 3953–3954, 3953f
nonneurogenic, 3953
osteogenic, 4296t, 4299
skull, 1389, 1389f
soft tissue, scalp, 1413
Sarcomatosis, meningeal, 1141, 1143
Saxitoxin, peripheral nerve effects of, 3816
Scala media, 327, 328, 328f, 329f
Scala tympani, 327, 328f, 329f
Scala vestibuli, 327, 328, 328f, 329f
Scalp
angiosarcoma of, 1414
arteriovenous malformation of, 1414
basal cell carcinoma of, 1409–1410
hemangioma of, 1413–1414
in cortical structure localization, 2531–2532
injury to, 5057
delivery and, 3481–3482
Kaposi's sarcoma of, 1414
keratosis of, 1409
melanocytic nevus of, 1410–1411

Scalp *(Continued)*
melanoma of, 1411–1413, 1412f
metastases to, 1416
nervous tissue layer of, tumors of, 1414–1415
neurofibroma of, 1414–1415
pressure necrosis of, headrests and, 610
reconstructive procedures on, 1414f–1417f, 1416–1417
schwannoma of, 1414–1415
skin appendages of, 1415
skin tissue layer of, tumors of, 1409–1413
soft tissue layer of, tumors of, 1413
squamous cell carcinoma of, 1410
tumors of, 1409–1417
vascular tissue layer of, tumors of, 1413–1414
Scar, imaging of, 515, 516f
Scheie's syndrome, 4479
Scheuermann's disease, pediatric, 3565
Scheuermann's kyphosis, examination of, 3561
Schistosomiasis, spinal, 4390
Schizencephaly, 62f, 63
magnetic resonance imaging of, 2493
Schmorl's node, anterior, 3564–3565
Schober's flexion test, in ankylosing spondylitis, 4464
School records, in premorbid cognitive functioning estimate, 5189–5190
Schwabach's test, 330
Schwann cells, 87, 88f, 89f
in axonal regeneration, 199–200
in central nervous system repair, 4162
in demyelination/remyelination, 3962
in distal nerve stump, 199
in myelinated nerve fiber, 3959–3960
in peripheral nervous system injury, 195
in remyelination, 198
in trigeminal nerve, 1343–1344
transfected, in central nervous system gene therapy, 4167
Schwannoma, 3941–3943, 4296t
cerebellopontine angle, magnetic resonance imaging of, 459, 460f
computed tomography of, 526
cranial nerve, magnetic resonance imaging of, 459–460, 460f
facial nerve, vs. acoustic neuroma, 1147
gene alterations in, 751t
magnetic resonance imaging of, 457, 459–460, 459f, 460f, 526–527, 527f, 3875–3876, 3941, 3942f
orbital, 1374
pediatric, 3714, 3714f
proliferation markers for, 704
radiologic features of, 835, 836–837, 838f
scalp, 1414–1415
spinal cord, 4817–4818, 4818f
treatment of, 4822–4823
surgery for, 3943–3944, 3943f
results of, 3945–3946, 3946t
trigeminal, 924f, 1343–1349
clinical presentation of, 1344–1346, 1344f, 1345f
differential diagnosis of, 1347–1348
epidemiology of, 1343
outcome in, 1349
pathology of, 1343
radiologic evaluation of, 1346–1347, 1346f–1348f
radiosurgery for, 4068–4069
stereotactic radiosurgery for, 1349
surgery for, 1349
Schwannoma *(Continued)*
vestibular, 838f, 1152
magnetic resonance imaging of, 459, 459f
radiosurgery for, 4055–4056, 4057t, 4058t, 4059f
linac, 4112
stereotactic radiation therapy for, outcome in, 4030
Sciatic nerve
anatomy of, 652–653
entrapment of, 3934
surgery on
exposure for, 653–654, 654f
positioning for, 608–609, 653
Sciatica, 4330
cause of, 4328
predictive values and, 238t
Scintigraphy. *See* Radionuclide imaging.
SCIWORA. *See* Spinal cord injury without radiographic abnormality.
Scleroderma, sympathetic nerve blocks for, 2981
Sclerosis
amyotrophic lateral, 4319, 4320
peripheral neuropathy in, 3846–3847
weakness in, 272
primary lateral, 4319
Sclerotomes
failed fusion of, 4280–4281, 4281f
formation of, 4272–4275
occipital, 3332
anomalies of, 3333
Scoliosis, 4306
congenital, 4318
degenerative, 4533
in cerebral palsy, 3728–3729
in Chiari malformation type I, 3348, 3348f
pediatric intramedullary tumor surgery and, 3713
thoracolumbar, 4557–4567, 4558f
classification of, 4558–4559, 4559t
demographics of, 4557
evaluation of, 4559–4561, 4560f, 4561f
medical treatment of, 4561–4562
natural history of, 4557
surgery for, 4562–4564, 4564f, 4565f
care after, 4566–4567
results of, 4564–4566, 4564t, 4565t
symptoms of, 4557–4558
tumor-related, 4835, 4837
with occult spinal dysraphism, 3262, 3262f, 3263f
Scott's syndrome, atlantoaxial instability in, 3543
Screening, legal issues regarding, 407
Screw fixation
cervical spine
complication avoidance in, 577, 578, 579
image-guided navigation for, 4748–4751, 4751f, 4752f
lumbar spine
complication avoidance in, 582
transpedicular, 4734, 4735f, 4740
of pediatric odontoid fracture, 3550
transarticular, of pediatric atlantoaxial joint, 3547, 3549–3550, 3549f, 3550f
Screw-plate fixation
cervical spine, 4424, 4650, 4651f
anterior, 4621–4637
lumbar spine, 4716–4717, 4717f
Screw-rod fixation
cervical spine, posterior, 4650, 4652t
Screw-rod fixation *(Continued)*
lumbar spine, 4715–4716, 4716f
of spinal stenosis, 4534–4535
Screws
bending strength of, 4589, 4590f
cancellous, 4590
cannulated, 4591
constrained, 4591
cortical, 4590
in odontoid fracture fixation, 3550, 4943, 4944f–4946f, 4945
lag, 4590
lateral mass, in occipitocervical fusion, 4665–4666, 4666f, 4667f
nonself-tapping, 4590, 4590f
pars interarticularis, in occipitocervical fusion, 4662, 4664–4665, 4664f, 4665f
percutaneous, lumbar burst fracture fixation with, 5006, 5006f
plate/rod and, 4591, 4591f
pullout strength of, 4590
self-tapping, 4590, 4590f
spinal fixation with, 4589–4591, 4590f, 4591f, 4901–4902
transarticular, in occipitocervical fusion, 4662, 4664–4665, 4664f, 4665f
Seat belt injury
to cervical spine, 4887
to thoracic spine, 4960–4961, 4961f, 4962, 4962t
Secondary fissure, 34
Sedatives
intracranial pressure management with, 5058, 5127, 5127t
pediatric, preoperative, 3188
Segmentation anomalies, spinal, 4279, 4279f
imaging of, 535, 536f
Seizures, 275, 2461–2462. *See also* Epilepsy.
acute symptomatic, 2464
after arteriovenous malformation radiation therapy, 2196
after arteriovenous malformation surgery, 2189, 2191, 2193, 2193t
after giant arteriovenous malformation surgery, 2280
after supratentorial arteriovenous malformation surgery, 2247
astatic, 2463
baclofen and, 2886
blood-brain barrier in, 166
bullet wounds and, 5240–5241
classification of, 2463, 2463t
complex partial, of temporal lobe origin, 2526
definition of, 2461–2462, 2525
diagnosis of, 2465–2466, 2465f, 2466f
differential diagnosis of, 2466–2467
drugs for. *See* Antiepileptic drugs.
during cortical stimulation mapping, 2533
electroencephalography of, 2465–2466, 2465f, 2466f
frontal, 2526
generalized, 2463
generalized clonic, 2463
ictal localization of, functional magnetic resonance imaging in, 2518–2519
in arteriovenous malformations, 2163, 2164, 2206
in brain tumors, 828, 828t
in cavernous malformations, 2169, 2171, 2294, 2294f
in cerebral palsy, 3728
in low-grade glioma, 953

Seizures *(Continued)*
in mild head injury, 5073
in pediatric aneurysms, 3451
in pediatric arteriovenous malformations, 3454
in pediatric cerebral hemisphere tumors, 3697, 3698f
in posterior fossa arteriovenous malformations, 2252–2253
in sarcoidosis, 1436
in subarachnoid hemorrhage, 1825–1826, 1826t
in traumatic brain injury, 5120, 5122f, 5128–5129, 5136–5137
in tuberculosis, 1440
in venous malformation, 2175
intractable, neuropsychological assessment in, 390–391, 390t
laboratory evaluation of, 2465
lateral ventricle tumor resection and, 1243
lateralization of, functional magnetic resonance imaging in, 2518
localization of
extracranial electroencephalography in, 2630–2631
imaging in, 2631
intracarotid amobarbital test in, 2631
invasive electroencephalography in, 2631–2632
symptomatic, 2630
magnetic resonance imaging of, 472–473, 473f
meningioma and, 568, 568t
mini-, 2436
motor cortex, 2589
myoclonic, 2463
neurological examination of, 2465
neurological history in, 2465
new-onset, in supratentorial cavernous malformation, 2309
nonepileptic, 2466
nonphysiologic nonepileptic, 2467
of parietal origin, 2526
onset of, single-photon emission computed tomography of, 2476
partial, 2463, 2466, 2466f
pediatric brain injury and, 3464
physiologic nonepileptic, 2466–2467
postoperative, 565–566, 937–938
post-traumatic, pediatric, neurorehabilitation of, 3789–3790
psychogenic spells in, 2466
treatment of, 5128–5129, 5136–5137
unclassified epileptic, 2463
vision mapping in, imaging for, 2545, 2545f
Selective dorsal rhizotomy
complications of, 3742–3743
contraindications to, 3738–3739, 3738t
dorsal root sectioning in, 3741–3742, 3741f
dorsal root separation/identification in, 3740–3741, 3741f
electromyography in, 3741–3742, 3741f, 3742t
for cerebral palsy, 3736–3745
indications for, 3737–3738, 3737t, 3738t
laminectomy in, 3740
patient selection for, 3737–3738, 3737t, 3738t
postoperative course in, 3742–3743
preoperative evaluation for, 3739
results of, 3743–3744
technique of, 3739–3745
vs. intrathecal baclofen, 3752–3753, 3752t
Selective serotonin reuptake inhibitors, for pain, 2964, 2966
Selegiline, for Parkinson's disease, 2733
Self-awareness, after traumatic brain injury, 5192
Sella turcica
cyst of, 3295, 3295f
erosion of, 430–431
fracture of, cerebrospinal fluid fistula in, 5267
small, 430
unusual configurations of, 430–431
Sellar region
anatomy of, 1266
arachnoid cyst above, 3293–3295, 3294f, 3295f
arachnoid cyst in, 3295, 3295f
epidermoid tumor of, 3690
in transsphenoidal surgery, 1178, 1179
lesions of
differential diagnosis of, 1171, 1171t
radiologic features of, 839–840
surgery on, visual evoked potentials during, 2544
tumors of, classification of, 671
Semicircular canals, 338, 338f, 340f
mechanical receptors in, 74
vestibulo-ocular reflex and, 341, 341f
Semicircular ducts, 339
Semilunar gyrus, 25–26, 26f
Semilunar lobule
inferior, 30f, 33f
superior, 30f, 31f
Sensation
after traumatic brain injury, 5188
disturbances of, in brain tumors, 829
evaluation of, 268, 3824, 3825f
loss of, in peripheral nerve damage, 3821, 3821f
pediatric, testing of, 3184
Sensitivity, 236
Sensorimotor polyneuropathy, diabetic, 3842
Sensory cortex, 2931–2932
functional magnetic resonance imaging of, 2519
stimulation mapping of, 2534
patient selection in, 2531
Sensory nerve action potential
in demyelination, 3853, 3853f
nerve conduction studies of, 3852–3853, 3852f, 3853f
supramaximal stimulation in, 3852
temporal dispersion in, 3852
Sensory nerve fibers, 3809
Sensory nerves, measurement of, 3803–3804
Sensory neurons, injury sensitivity of, 3967
Sensory polyneuropathy, diabetic, 3842
Sensory receptors, 3810f
Sensory system
functional magnetic resonance imaging of, 2519
pediatric, examination of, 3182–3185
Sepsis
after myelomeningocele repair, 3223
polyneuropathy in, 5132
Septal vein, 17
anterior, 8f, 15f
Septum pellucidum, 7f, 12f
venous drainage of, 1238
Sequential Compression Sleeves, 4968
D-Serine, synthesis of, astrocytes in, 107
Serotonin
in vagus nerve stimulation, 2644
release of, 2953, 2954f
Sevoflurane, cerebral physiology and, 551
Sex, in cerebellar astrocytoma, 3655
Sexual dysfunction, in neurogenic urinary disorders, 366
Sexually transmitted diseases, reporting obligations in, 411–412
SF-36 Health Survey, 2872
Shaken baby syndrome, 3500–3501
Shaking-impact syndrome, 3500–3504
brain appearance in, 3501–3502
child abuse evaluation team in, 3501
contusion in, 3501, 3504f
differential diagnosis of, 3503–3504
intracranial hemorrhage in, 3501, 3502f
mechanism of, 3501, 3504
physical examination of, 3501
skeletal survey in, 3502–3503
spinal cord injury in, 3521, 3522f
subdural hematoma in, 3501, 3503f, 3504f
timing of, 3504
Shark tooth deformity, in Chiari malformation type II, 3350
Sharp waves, positive, 3856, 3856t
Shear injury, to thoracic spine, 4960, 4960f, 4963f
Sheehan's syndrome, 2429
SHH, 55t
Shh, 52
Shock
neurogenic, 4872
spinal, 4872–4873, 4888
Short Form Health Survey, 243t
Short gyrus, of insula, 5, 6f
Shoulder
medial rotation contracture of, brachial plexus obstetric injury and, 3981, 3982f
pain in, surgery for, 3026t
posterior dislocation of, brachial plexus obstetric injury and, 3981, 3982f, 3983
anterior approach to, 3984f–3986f, 3985–3987, 3986t
classification of, 3983, 3983t
diagnosis of, 3983, 3985
subscapularis recession for, 3985
Shoulder-girdle syndrome, 3840
Shrapnel injury, traumatic aneurysm from, 2132
Shunts
complications of, 3399–3400, 3400f
failure of
in aqueduct of Sylvius obstruction, 3393
in basal cistern obstruction, 3396–3397
in foramen of Monro obstruction, 3390–3391
in fourth ventricle outlet foramina obstruction, 3394
in sagittal sinus pressure increases, 3399–3400, 3400f, 3401f
predictive values and, 238t
for chronic extracerebral fluid collections, 3506–3507, 3507f
in medulloblastoma surgery, 3644
intraluminal, during carotid endarterectomy, 1548–1549
pediatric, complications of, 3400–3402, 3402f
Shy-Drager syndrome, neurodegeneration in, 2713

Sialoprotein, bone, 4230
Sibson's fascia, 4674
Sickle cell anemia
  pediatric, spinal infections in, 3566
  subarachnoid hemorrhage in, 1832
Sickness Impact Profile, 243t, 2872
Sigmoid sinus
  glomus jugulare tumor of, 1299, 1299f
  jugular foramen and, 1302
  thrombosis of, magnetic resonance angiography of, 1597, 1597f
  transverse, dural arteriovenous malformation of, 2284
    imaging of, 2286–2287, 2286f, 2287f
    treatment of, 2288–2290
Signal transduction
  in early neural development, 4251–4252, 4252f
  in glioma, 715–716, 716f
Signal transduction enzymes, in angiogenesis, 775t
Simple lobule, 30f, 31f
Single-photon emission computed tomography, 2475
  in oncology, 2480, 2481f
  of cerebrovascular disease, 2478–2480, 2479f, 2480f
  of epilepsy, 2476–2477, 2477
  of trauma, 2481
  physical principle of, 2476
  radiopharmaceuticals in, 2475
Sinonasal undifferentiated carcinoma, 1312, 1313
Sinus pericranii, 1403–1404
Sinus tracts
  dermal
    congenital, 3274–3276, 3275f, 3276f
    in occult spinal dysraphism, 3260f–3262f, 3261
  lumbar, in tethered spinal cord, 3249, 3250f
Sinuses, cerebrospinal fluid leakage at, 5267
Sinuvertebral nerve, 4328
Sitting position, 597t
  in posterior cervical approach, 636
  tension pneumocephalus in, 616
SIX3, 55t
Skeletal dysplasia
  craniovertebral junction abnormalities in, 3334
  odontoid process, 3343–3344
Skeletal fixation, head, complications of, 610
Skeleton, axial
  benign tumors of, 4295, 4296t, 4297–4298
  congenital deformities of, 4317–4318
  deformities of, 4315t
  dislocations of, 4307t
  fractures of, 4307t
  inflammatory disorders of, 4303t
  malignant tumors of, 4296t, 4298–4299, 4299f
Skin
  anomalies of, in congenital lumbosacral lipoma, 3236–3237
  examination of, 269
  flora of, in cerebrospinal fluid shunt infection, 3420
  in occult spinal dysraphism, 3259, 3260f–3262f, 3261
  sensory receptors in, 3810f
Skin appendages, scalp, 1415
Skull
  anatomy of, 1266–1267

Skull *(Continued)*
  aneurysmal bone cyst of, 1388–1389
    pediatric, 3721
  basal cell carcinoma of, 1398, 1399f
  bone neoplasms of, pediatric, 3720–3721
  calcifications within, 432
  cephalohematoma of, 1404
  chondroma of, 1386–1388, 1388f
  chondrosarcoma of, 1390, 1390f
  chordoma of, 1390–1392, 1391f
  computed tomography of, 419, 432–433
  congenital lesions of, 3718–3720
  contents of, 1504
  contour abnormalities of, 428–429, 428f
  convolutional markings on, 432
  density abnormalities of, 429, 429f
  depressed fracture of, 426–427, 426f, 427f
    delivery and, 3482, 3482f
  dermoid cyst of, 1385–1386
    pediatric, 3718–3719
  destruction of, 429–431, 430f
  ependymoma of, pediatric, 3623
  epidermoid tumors of, 1385–1386, 1386f, 3690–3691
    pediatric, 3718–3719
  erosion of, 429–431, 430f
  Ewing's sarcoma of, 1393–1394, 1394f
  fibrosarcoma of, 1389–1390, 1390f
  fibrous dysplasia of, 1401–1402, 1402f, 1403f
    pediatric, 3719, 3720f
  fractures of. *See* Skull fracture.
  giant cell tumors of, 1388
  hemangioma of, 1384–1385
    pediatric, 3720–3721
  imaging of, 432–433
  in Chiari malformation type II, 3349–3350, 3350f
  in cortical structure localization, 2531–2532
  in sinus pericranii, 1403–1404
  Langerhans cell histiocytosis of, 1400–1401, 1401f
  leptomeningeal cyst of, 1404–1405, 1405f
  lipoma of, 1389
  lymphangioma of, 1384–1385, 1385f
  magnetic resonance imaging of, 432–433
  maldevelopment of, functional matrix theory of, 3315
  meningioma of, 1397–1398, 1398f, 1399f
  metastases to, 1392–1395, 1392f–1395f
  molding of, vs. primary synostosis, 3301–3304
  mucocele of, 1404
  multiple myeloma of, 1392–1393, 1393f
  neuroblastoma of, 1394–1395, 1395f
  non-Hodgkin's lymphoma of, 1393, 1394f
  ossification disorders of, 431–432
  osteoblastoma of, 1384
    pediatric, 3721
  osteoclastoma of, 1388
  osteogenic sarcoma of, 1389, 1389f
  osteoid osteoma of, 1384
  osteoma of, 1383–1384, 1384f
    pediatric, 3721
  Paget's disease of, 1399–1400, 1400f
  paraganglioma of, 1396–1397, 1397f
  pediatric, 3462–3463
  radiography of, 419–422
    anatomy in, from lateral view, 422–423, 423f
    anteroposterior technique in, 419, 420f, 421
    basal technique in, 422, 422f

Skull *(Continued)*
    lateral technique in, 419, 420f
    posteroanterior technique in, 421
    Towne's anteroposterior technique in, 421, 421f
    Towne's posteroanterior technique in, 422
  radiologic features of, 419–436
  size abnormalities of, 428, 428f
  squamous cell carcinoma of, 1398, 1399f
  surgery on
    landmarks for, 423–424, 423f
    risk factors in, 565–574
  teratoma of, 1386, 1387f
  thickness abnormalities of, 429, 429f
  thinness abnormalities of, 429
  three-dimensional imaging of, 433, 433f–435f, 436
  trauma to, 425–428
    pediatric, 3717–3718, 3718f
  tumors of. *See* Skull tumors.
  vascular channels in, 423
  vascular markings on, 432
Skull base, 1266–1267
  adenocarcinoma of, 910, 911f
  anatomy of, 1266–1267
  anterior
    meningioma of, 910, 910f, 1364
    tumors of, 910, 911f, 913
  basilar invagination of, 424
  central
    bony structures of, 1266
    cavernous hemangioma of, 1268
    chondroma of, 1267
    chondrosarcoma of, 1267
    chordoma of, 1267
    craniopharyngioma of, 1267
    meningioma of, 1265, 1267
      surgical approach to, 1276, 1278
    neural structures of, 1266–1267
    pituitary adenoma of, 1267
    trigeminal neurinoma of, 1267
    tumors of, 1265–1266
      magnetic resonance imaging of, 920–921, 922f, 923f
      pathology of, 1267–1268
      surgical results in, 1280, 1280t
    vascular structures of, 1266
  cerebrospinal fluid leakage at, 5267
  chondroma of, 1364–1365, 1386, 1388f
  chondrosarcoma of, 1283–1292, 1284. *See also* Chondrosarcoma.
  chordoma of, 1283–1292, 4799. *See also* Chordoma.
  distraction osteogenesis for, 3327–3328
  embryology of, 3331–3332
  exposure of, in basilar apex aneurysm approach, 1985–1987, 1986f
  fibrous dysplasia of, 910, 911f
  fracture of, 427–428
    cerebrospinal fluid fistula in, 5267
    three-dimensional imaging of, 435f, 436
  lateral
    in sinonasal tumor exposure, 1324–1326, 1324f, 1325f
    jugular foramen and, 1302
  malformations of, in Chiari malformation type I, 3348
  meningioma of
    cranio-orbital zygomatic approach to, 1123–1124, 1124f
    operative closure for, 1127
    petrosal approaches to, 1125–1126, 1126f

Skull base *(Continued)*
radiosurgery for, complications in, 574
surgical approaches to, 1123–1127
transcondylar approach to, 1126–1127, 1127f
zygomatic extended middle fossa approach to, 1124–1125, 1124f, 1125f
metastatic carcinoma of, 1368
posterior, tumors of, magnetic resonance imaging of, 920–921, 922f, 923f
surgery on, complication avoidance in, 571–573
traumatic aneurysm in, 5207–5208
endovascular therapy for, 2133
tumors of. *See* Skull base tumors.
vascular injury in, magnetic resonance imaging of, 469
Skull base surgery, 909–928
anterior, 910–918
anatomy for, 910–911, 912f
combined approaches in, 916, 918
extracranial approach in, 913
orbital exenteration with, 913–914, 914f, 915f
intracranial approach in, 914–916, 916f, 917f
principles of, 911, 913
transfrontal extradural approach in, 915, 916f
transfrontal intradural approach in, 915–916, 917f
goals of, 909–910
historical aspects of, 909
lateral, 1302–1304, 1303f, 1304f
middle, 918–928
extradural approach to, 919, 919f
transpetrosal approaches in, 921–928
modified lateral, 1304, 1305f
posterior, 918–928
transpetrosal approaches in, 921–928
Skull base tumors, 1265–1281
clinical presentation of, 1268–1275
diagnosis of, 1268–1275
imaging of, 1268–1275
interstitial brachytherapy for, 4105
observation for, 4027
pathology of, 1267–1268
radiation therapy for, 4027, 4028f
revascularization for, 2108, 2109f
stereotactic radiation therapy for, 4029–4030, 4030f
stereotactic radiosurgery for, 4029
surgery for, 1275–1280, 4027–4029
three-dimensional imaging of, 433, 434f
Skull caliper traction, pediatric, complications of, 3543
Skull fracture, 425–427, 426f, 427f, 5057
aneurysm in, 2132
assessment of, 5093, 5094f
basal, 427–428
bullet wounds and, 5223
cephalohematoma with, 3482
delivery and, 3482–3483, 3482f
depressed, 426–427, 426f, 427f, 433, 433f, 435f, 5166, 5166f
epidural hematoma in, 5154
in mild head injury, 5070, 5071t
over venous sinus, 5170, 5171f
surgery for, 5166, 5167f
growing, 427, 427f, 1404–1405, 1405f, 3468–3470, 3469f, 3717–3718, 3718f
in mild head injury, 5074
intracranial hematoma and, 5042, 5042t
leptomeningeal cyst in, 1404–1405, 1405f
Skull fracture *(Continued)*
pediatric, 3465–3469, 5261f
basilar, 3467–3468, 3468f
comminuted, 3466–3467
complex, 3466–3467
compound, 3467
cosmetic repair in, 3466, 3467f
depressed, 3465–3466, 3466f, 3467f
"greenstick," 3466, 3466f
linear, 3465, 3465f
mild brain injury with, 3465–3470
subgaleal hematoma in, 3465, 3466f
ping-pong, 3147, 3466, 3466f
rhinorrhea in, 5267–5268
segmental, 435f
Skull tumors, 1265–1281, 1383–1405, 1384t
benign, 1383–1389
by direct extension, 1395–1399, 1396f–1399f
clinical presentation of, 1268–1275
diagnosis of, 1268–1275
embryonic, 1385–1386, 1386f, 1387f
imaging of, 1268–1275
malignant, 1389–1392, 1389f–1391f
pathology of, 1267–1268
pediatric, 3717–3721
epidemiology of, 3717
imaging of, 3717
primary, 1383–1392
secondary, 1392–1399
surgery for, 1275–1280
Smiling, in facial nerve testing, 3174
SMN, 55t
Smoking. *See* Tobacco.
SNCA, in familial Parkinson's disease, 2711
Snellen acuity chart, 301, 302f
SNX-111, intrathecal, 3141
Social awareness, after traumatic brain injury, 5192
Sodium, in neurons, 3812, 3812t
Sodium action potential, 219, 220–222, 3813, 3813f
Sodium channel myotonia, 225t
Sodium channels, 220t
after sensory neuron transection, 3815, 3815f
alpha subunits of, 222
beta subunits of, 222
gating of, 221
glial, 225, 226f
structure of, 221–222
tetrodotoxin blockage of, 221
Sodium nitroprusside
for cerebral vasospasm, 1857
in pregnancy, 2424
Sodium valproate, for trigeminal neuralgia, 2990t, 2993
Sodium-potassium pump, in post-traumatic epilepsy, 2454–2455
Soft tissue hypertrophy, growth hormone excess and, 1189–1190
Soft tissue injury
cervical spine, 4917
thoracic spine, 4981
Soft tissue sarcoma, scalp, 1413
Solitary fibrous tumor, 670
Solitary plasmacytoma, spinal, 4355–4356, 4850–4852
Somatoform disorders, in traumatic brain injury response, 5193, 5193t
Somatosensory cortex, 2932, 2933f
Somatosensory evoked potential mapping
anesthesia in, 2533
of somatosensory cortex, 2533–2534, 2534f
Somatosensory evoked potentials
dermatomal, intraoperative, 4216–4219, 4218t
during nucleus caudalis ablation, 3051–3052
in altered consciousness, 297
in anesthesia, 1507–1508, 1507f
in brachial plexus surgery, 3868, 3869f, 3870f
in distal nerve stimulation, 3864
in median nerve surgery, 3866, 3866f
in nerve root stimulation, 3864
in nucleus caudalis DREZ ablation, 3087, 3089f
in peripheral nerve surgery, 3862, 3863–3864
in radiculopathy, 3859
intraoperative, 4204–4211, 4205t, 4206f, 4206t, 4209f–4211f
median nerve, in coma prognostication, 3861
nerve assessment by, 3865–3866
Somatosensory gyrus, somatosensory evoked potential mapping of, 2533–2534, 2534f
Somatostatin, intrathecal, 3141
Somatostatin analogs, for acromegaly, 1192–1193
Somatostatin receptors, in meningioma, 1108
Somites, formation of, 4271–4272
Somitic columns, malalignment of, 4277–4278, 4277f
Somnolence, after midbrain tractotomy, 3056
Songer sublaminar cables, in thoracic spine fixation, 4969f
Sonic hedgehog, 81
in encephalocele, 3200
Sound waves, properties of, 1561, 1561f
Southern blotting, 748–750, 748f–750f
Space-occupying lesions, 276t
in sarcoidosis, 1436
intraoperative electrophysiologic monitoring of, 4222–4224
SPARC, in meningioma, 1103
Spasmodic torticollis, 2891–2899. *See also* Torticollis, spasmodic.
Spasticity, 2875
ablative surgery for, 2863–2872
abnormal descending control in, 2878–2879
active movement tests for, 2881–2882
alpha motoneuron in, 2875
anterior rhizotomy for, 2870
Ashworth scale for, 2880–2881, 2881t, 3725, 3726t, 3750, 3750t
cerebral palsy and, 2751, 2751f, 3725–3727, 3729, 3730–3732, 3747–3748
after dorsal rhizotomy, 3743
deleterious effects of, 3737
dorsal rhizotomy for, 3736–3745. *See also* Selective dorsal rhizotomy.
intrathecal baclofen for, 3748–3756. *See also* Baclofen, intrathecal.
pathogenesis of, 3736–3737, 3736f, 3737f
treatment of, 3754–3756
chemical neurolysis for, 2865, 2866t, 2867
clinical evaluation of, 2880–2881, 2880f, 2881t
cordectomy for, 2870
cryorhizotomy for, 2868–2870, 2868f

Spasticity *(Continued)*
deep tendon reflexes in, 2880, 2880f
definition of, 2875
dorsal root entry zone procedure for, 2870
drop test for, 2881, 2881f
evaluation of, 3739
flexor reflex in, disinhibition of, 2878–2879
hemifacial, surgery for, 2751–2752
historical aspects of, 2863–2864
in brain injury rehabilitation, 5295
intrathecal baclofen for, 2750–2751, 2751t, 2875, 2882–2887. *See also* Baclofen, intrathecal.
measurement of, 2880–2882
muscle fiber changes in, 2879–2880
muscle spindle in, 2875–2876, 2876f
muscle stretch reflex in, 2876–2878, 2876f–2878f, 2879t
myelotomy for, 2870
passive quantifiable tests of, 2881, 2881f
pathology of, 2863f
pediatric, management of, 3787–3788
pharmacologic treatment of, 2865, 2866t, 2867–2868
physiologic basis of, 2875–2880
posterior rhizotomy for, 2869–2870
pyramidal function in, 2879
selective dorsal rhizotomy for, 2750–2751, 2751f
soft tissue changes in, 2879–2880
spinal changes in, 2879
spinal cord surgery for, 2868–2870
stretch reflex in, disinhibition of, 2878
surgery for, 2661
treatment of, 2882–2887
outcome measures for, 2864–2865, 2864t
voluntary movement interference in, 2882
weakness in, in craniovertebral junction tumors, 4800
Spatial buffering, 102, 104f, 228, 229f, 230, 1486, 2455–2456, 2455f–2457f
Specificity, 236
Spectroscopy, in magnetic resonance imaging, 447–448, 448f
Speech
bilaterally represented, 2504
lateralization of, intracarotid amobarbital testing of, 2506–2507
pediatric, assessment of, 3176
typical vs. atypical, 2504
vs. language, 2504
Speech audiometry, in hearing assessment, 332–333, 333f
Speech impairment
after dorsal rhizotomy, 3744
in brain tumors, 829
in cerebral palsy, 3727, 3730, 3732
transcallosal surgery and, 1258
Speech recognition threshold, in hearing assessment, 332–333, 333f
Spemann organizer, 48
Sphenoid bone
drilling through, 1932–1933, 1932f
electrodes in, 2557, 2561
hyperostosing meningioma of, 1362–1363
meningioma of, 1398f
surgery across, complication avoidance in, 568–570, 568t
Sphenoid compartment, 4f, 5
Sphenoid planum, meningioma of, 1364, 1364f
Sphenoid sinus
in anterior skull base, 910, 912f
in transsphenoidal surgery, 1177–1178
Sphenoid wing
erosion of, 431
lesser, 4f
sinus of, 17
meningioma of, 1115, 1372
Sphenoidotomy, in transsphenoidal surgery, 1179
Sphenopalatine artery, bleeding from, 569
Sphenopalatine ganglion block, 2982
Sphenoparietal sinus, 17, 423
Sphincter, urethral
smooth muscle, 359, 359f
striated muscle, 359
Spin trap nitrones, in focal cerebral ischemia, 134–135, 134f
Spina bifida, 81. *See also* Myelomeningocele.
clinic for, 3224
combined, 4263–4266, 4263f–4267f
definition of, 3215
fetal management of, 3220
historical aspects of, 3154–3155, 3154f–3157f
history of, 3216
hydrocephalus with, 3222, 3223
kyphosis in, 3223
latex allergy in, 3224
renal management in, 3221
Spina bifida aperta, 533, 3215, 4316
Spina bifida cystica, 533, 3215
Spina bifida manifesta, 533
Spina bifida occulta, 3215. *See also* Spinal cord, tethered.
historical aspects of, 3245–3246
Spinal accessory nerve, examination of, 267
pediatric, 3176
Spinal artery
anterior, 36f, 1973, 2380
posterior, 37, 1973
Spinal columns
combined disorders of, 4320f, 4321
force vectors through, 4586, 4587f
stability via, 4586, 4587f, 4896–4897, 4954–4955, 4955f
Spinal cord, 4508
anatomy of, for cordotomy, 3059–3061, 3060f
aneurysms of, 2356, 2356f, 2372, 4821
arachnoid cyst of, 4821
arterial networks of, 2380–2381
arteriovenous fistula of, 2366–2368
dorsal intradural, 2356, 2357f, 2358
extradural, 2356, 2357f, 2366
extradural-intradural, 2359, 2359f
intradural
dorsal, 2366–2368, 2367f
ventral, 2368, 2369f
arteriovenous malformations of, 2363–2372
angiography of, 2365
classification of, 2363–2364, 2363t, 2364t
conus, 2362
electrophysiologic testing in, 2365–2366
endovascular treatment of, 2365–2366
extradural-intradural, 2369
intradural, 2369–2371, 2370f
intramedullary, 2359, 2360f, 2361f, 2362
magnetic resonance angiography of, 2365
Spinal cord *(Continued)*
magnetic resonance imaging of, 2364–2365
vs. multiple sclerosis, 1455
astrocytoma of, 4040, 4302, 4302f, 4825–4826, 4825f, 4826f
radiation therapy for, 4042, 4043, 4043t
surgery for, 4043
treatment of, 4828–4829, 4831
at thoracolumbar junction, 4989f
blood supply to, dorsal rhizotomy/ganglionectomy and, 3040
cavernous malformations of, 2353–2354, 2355f, 2356, 2379, 2381f, 4319
clinical features of, 2394–2395, 2396f
extradural, 4821
familial, 2394–2395
imaging of, 537, 539f, 2400
intradural, 4826, 4830f
treatment of, 2415–2416
cavitation of, 4315t
chronic, progressive neuronal degeneration of, 4314t–4315t, 4316
chronic ischemia of, 4314, 4315t–4316t, 4316
compression of, 4314, 4316
decompression for, 4998
in cervical spondylotic myelopathy, 4447–4448
in pyogenic spinal infection, 4364
metastases and, 4047
treatment of, 4374
diseases of
sensory loss in, 272, 273f
urologic disorders in, 374–375
electrical stimulation of, 3112–3114. *See also* Electrical stimulation.
embryology of, 4239–4282
ependymoma of, 4040, 4826, 4827f, 4828
radiation therapy for, 4042, 4043, 4043t
surgery for, 4043
extradural disease of, 4819–4821
extramedullary tumors of, 4296t
fetal development of, 4239–4282
field potentials in, 230–231
formation of, 3258–3259, 3258f
ganglioneuroma of, 4821
glial tumors of, 4825
glioma of, radiation therapy for, 4043
gray matter of, 3045–3046
in nociception, 2953, 2955
laminae in, 2923–2924, 2924f
projections of, 2927
neurons in, 2924, 2924f
nociception in, 2923–2926, 2924f, 2925f
primary afferent neurons of, 2924–2926, 2925f
hemangioblastoma of, 1054, 2353, 2354f, 2355f, 4825, 4826, 4828, 4828f
hypoperfusion of, in arteriovenous fistula, 2367
in cervical spondylotic myelopathy, 4447, 4449–4450, 4450f
in Chiari malformation type I, 3349, 3349f
in Chiari malformation type II, 3351
in lower urinary tract function, 359–360, 360f
in spasticity, 2879
infarction of, 4310–4311, 4310t
imaging of, 537, 539f
inflammation of, 4821
intraoperative electrophysiologic monitoring of, 4203–4225

Spinal cord (Continued)
- lipoma of, 4260–4263, 4261f, 4262f, 4826, 4829f
- meningioma of, 4819, 4819f
  - treatment of, 4823–4824
- metastatic cancer of, 4047–4048
- myelopathy of, radiation therapy and, 4046
- nerve sheath tumor of, 4040
  - treatment of, 4822–4824
- neurofibroma of, 4817–4818
  - treatment of, 4822–4823
- paraganglioma of, 4821
- pediatric, elasticity of, 3519
- retethering of, after congenital lumbosacral lipoma surgery, 3242
- sacral, diseases of, urologic disorders in, 374
- sarcoidosis of, 1436
- schwannoma of, 4817–4818, 4818f
  - treatment of, 4822–4823
- split, 3267–3272, 3267f–3273f, 4263–4266, 4263f–4267f, 4315t
  - embryogenesis of, 3268, 3271f
  - filum lipoma and, 3248, 3248f
  - treatment of, 3270, 3272, 3272f, 3273f
- sugar coating of, 527, 529f
- suprasacral, diseases of, urologic disorders in, 374
- tethered, 3245–3254, 3257
  - by lipoma, 3229. *See also* Lipomyelomeningocele.
  - clinical presentation of, 3249–3250, 3249f, 3250f
  - cutaneous stigmata in, 3249, 3249f, 3250f
  - diagnosis of, 3250–3251, 3250f, 3251f
  - embryology of, 3247–3248
  - historical aspects of, 3245–3246
  - imaging of, 533, 535f
  - in congenital lumbosacral lipoma, 3235–3236
  - intraoperative electrophysiologic monitoring of, 4222–4224
  - magnetic resonance imaging of, 3251, 3252f
  - outcome in, 3253–3254, 3253f
  - pathology of, 3247–3248, 3248f
  - pathophysiology of, 3248–3249
  - pediatric, 3565
  - radiography of, 3250–3251, 3250f
  - surgery for, 3251–3253, 3252f, 3253f
  - tight filum terminale and, 3247, 3248
  - ultrasonography of, 3251, 3251f
- vascular anatomy of, 2379–2381
- vascular lesions of
  - classification of, 2353–2362, 2353t, 2363–2364, 2363t, 2364t
  - neoplastic, 2353–2354, 2354f, 2355f, 2356
- venous system of, 2381
- ventral intradural arteriovenous fistula of, 2358–2359, 2358f

Spinal cord injury, 4146–4149, 4307–4308, 4308f, 4869–4882
- acute central cervical, 4871–4872
- Brown-Séquard syndrome and, 4872, 4889–4890, 4890f
- cervical traction for, 4873–4874, 4875f
- complete vs. incomplete, 4870
- completeness of, 4869–4871, 4870f
- corticosteroids in, 4874, 4876
- cruciate paralysis in, 4871, 4871f
- dorsal root entry zone ablation for, 3046, 3047

Spinal cord injury (Continued)
- drugs for, 4874, 4876
- endotracheal intubation and, 610
- epidemiology of, 4869
- etiology of, 4869
- gangliosides in, 4876
- imaging of, 523, 524f, 4876, 4877f, 4878f
- in cervical disk disease, 4397
- in intradural arteriovenous malformations, 2389–2390
- incidence of, 4869
- level of, 4869–4871, 4870f
- pediatric, 3515–3553
- penetrating, treatment of, 4880
- prevention of, 4869
- prognosis of, 4873
- research on, 4882
- spinal shock in, 4872–4873
- syndromes of, 4871–4873, 4889–4890, 4890f
- tracheal intubation in, 557, 557t
- treatment of, 4876–4882
  - decompression in, 4878–4880
  - emergency room, 4873–4876
  - in intensive care unit, 4880–4882
  - prehospital, 4873
  - surgery vs. external orthosis in, 4876–4880
- unstable fracture in, 4877–4878
- without radiographic abnormality. *See* Spinal cord injury without radiographic abnormality.

Spinal cord injury without radiographic abnormality, 3515, 3518–3526, 4910
- age in, 3516, 3519–3520, 3519f, 3520f
- biomechanics of, 3516
- cervical site of, 3519–3520, 3520f
- chemical blood state in, 3522, 3522t
- definition of, 3515, 3518
- delayed neurological deterioration in, 3520
- extraneural abnormalities in, 3521–3522, 3521f, 3522f
- hyperextension in, 3521, 3521f
- incidence of, 3519, 3519f
- magnetic resonance imaging of, 3520–3523, 3521f–3524f, 3522t
- mechanisms of, 3519
- neural abnormalities in, 3522–3523, 3522t, 3523f, 3524f
- occult vs. overt instability in, 3520
- outcome in, 3526, 3526f
- posterior longitudinal ligament rupture in, 3521, 3521f
- severity of, 3519, 3519f
- tectorial membrane hemorrhage in, 3521, 3522f
- thoracolumbar, 3523
- treatment of, 3523–3525, 3525f

Spinal cord stimulation, 3026
- complications of, 3115t
- contraindications to, 3115t
- for angina pectoris, 3113
- for failed back surgery syndrome, 3112–3113
- for ischemic pain, 3113
- for low back pain, 3113
- for peripheral nerve injury, 3113
- for reflex sympathetic dystrophy, 3113–3114
- implantable electrodes for, 3108–3109, 3108f–3110f
- implantable pulse generators for, 3110–3111, 3111f
- indications for, 3112–3114

Spinal cord stimulation (Continued)
- mechanism of, 3107–3108
- outcomes of, 3114–3115, 3114f
- regression of benefit in, 2941
- screening protocols for, 3111–3112
- vs. reoperation, 3112–3113

Spinal cord syndrome, anterior, 4872, 4890, 4890f

Spinal cord tumors, 4039, 4817–4832
- clinical presentation of, 4041
- epidemiology of, 4039
- extradural, 4040–4041
  - clinical features of, 4821
  - imaging of, 4821–4822
  - treatment of, 4822–4824
    - pediatric, 3714
- extramedullary, 4299–4301, 4301f, 4817–4824
  - etiology of, 4817–4821
  - incidence of, 4817–4821, 4817t
- imaging of, 4041
- inclusion, 4819–4821
- intradural
  - clinical features of, 4826–4827
  - imaging of, 4827–4828
  - treatment of, 4828–4832
- intradural extramedullary, 4040
  - pediatric, 3707–3714
    - epidemiology of, 3707
    - treatment of, 3714
  - radiation therapy for, 4045–4046
- intramedullary, 4039–4040, 4296t, 4301–4302, 4302f, 4824–4832
  - etiology of, 4825–4826, 4825f–4830f
  - incidence of, 4825–4826
  - pediatric, 3707–3714
    - characteristics of, 3707, 3707t
    - clinical presentation of, 3708, 3708t
    - epidemiology of, 3707, 3707t
    - histology of, 3707, 3708t
    - imaging of, 3708, 3709f, 3710, 3710f
    - laser for, 3710–3711
    - motor evoked potentials in, 3711–3712, 3712f
    - neurophysiologic monitoring in, 3711–3712, 3712f
    - outcome in, 3713
    - radiation therapy for, 3713–3714
    - surgery for, 3710–3711
      - complications of, 3713
    - ultrasonic aspiration of, 3710
  - radiation therapy for, 4045, 4045t
- metastatic, 4039, 4040–4041
- natural history of, 4039
- pain in, 4041
- pathology of, 4039
- prognosis of, 4041–4042
- radiation therapy for, 4042–4047
  - myelopathy after, 4046
  - pediatric effects of, 4046–4047
  - results of, 4044–4046, 4045t
  - sequelae of, 4046–4047
  - techniques of, 4044
- recumbency/nighttime pain associated with, 4295

Spinal dysraphism, 4316
- definition of, 3215, 3257
- historical aspects of, 3153–3155, 3154f, 3155f
- imaging of, 533, 534f
- occult, 3257–3281, 4315t, 4316–4317, 4317f. *See also* specific condition, e.g., Filum terminale, dysgenesis of.
  - clinical presentation of, 3259–3264, 3259t

Spinal dysraphism *(Continued)*
cutaneous lesions in, 3259, 3260f–3262f, 3261
definition of, 3257, 3258t
embryogenesis of, 3258–3259, 3258f
epidemiology of, 3257–3258
incontinence in, 3259, 3259f
lumbosacral lipoma and, 3229. *See also* Lipomyelomeningocele.
orthopedic manifestations of, 3261–3262, 3262f–3264f, 3263t, 3264
pediatric, 3565
scoliosis with, 3262, 3262f, 3263f
urologic anomalies in, 3264
open, 4315t, 4316
pediatric, surgery for, 3196
urologic disorders in, 374–375
Spinal internal fixation, 4586–4597. *See also* Internal fixation, spinal.
Spinal metastases, 4296t, 4298, 4357–4358, 4358f, 4836, 4854–4863
bone integrity in, 4861
classification of, 4854, 4854t
extent of involvement in, 4860–4861
imaging of, 525–526, 526f, 529, 531–532, 531f, 532f, 4855–4858, 4855f–4858f, 4855t
incidence of, 4854
lumbar, 4701–4702
management of, 4858–4862, 4859t, 4860f–4864f
patient debility in, 4861
prognosis for, 4862–4863, 4864t
signs/symptoms of, 4855, 4855f
spinal level of, 4860, 4860f–4861f
tumor location in, 4860
Spinal motion
in cervical spondylosis development, 4396
thoracic, 4954, 4954f
Spinal motion segment
elastic zone of, 4589
failure of, 4589
force vectors through, 4586, 4587f
internal fixation and, 4586
neutral zone of, 4589
range of motion of, 4588–4589, 4588f
Spinal muscular atrophy, in lower motor neuron degenerative disease, 4319–4320
Spinal nerve
avulsion of, repair of, 3970, 3972
branches of, 3033, 3034f
fibers of, 2921f, 2922
Spinal nerve root, 2923, 2923f
anatomy of, 3033–3034, 3034f
axon types of, 2921f, 2923
tumors of, imaging of, 526–527, 527f
Spinal nerve root sleeve, dural arteriovenous fistula of, 2377–2378
Spinal nucleus, anatomy of, 3085
Spinal reconstruction, for metastases, 4860, 4862f, 4863f
Spinal shock, 4872–4873, 4888
Spinal stability, 4145–4149, 4181–4182
clinical evaluation of, 4184
continuum concept of, microtrauma and, 4183–4184, 4184f
two- and three-column concepts of, 4182–4183, 4182f, 4183f, 4896–4897, 4954–4955, 4955f
Spinal stenosis. *See also* Posterior longitudinal ligament, ossification of.
Spinal stenosis *(Continued)*
achondroplasia and, decompression of, 3368–3369
outcome of, 3369–3370
acquired, 512, 514, 515f
cervical, with lumbar stenosis, 4526
imaging of, 512, 514–515, 515f, 516f
in achondroplasia, 3366–3367
in cervical spondylotic myelopathy, 4449
in mucopolysaccharidosis, 4479–4480
lateral recess, 514–515, 516f, 4521
lumbar, 4521–4536, 4737
acquired, 4521
amyloidosis with, 4527
anatomy of, 4521
ankylosing hyperostosis with, 4527
cervical/thoracic stenosis with, 4526
computed tomography of, 4522, 4523, 4523f–4526f, 4525
congenital, 4521
decompressive surgery for, 4337, 4338–4339
degenerative scoliosis with, 4533
degenerative spondylolisthesis with, 4531–4533
diagnosis of, 4522–4525
differential diagnosis of, 4526–4527
disk herniation in, surgery for, 4530–4531
electromyography of, 4525–4526
expansive laminaplasty for, 4530
fusion for, 4533–4534
anterior, 4535
pedicle screw-rod fixation in, 4534–4535
isthmic spondylolisthesis with, 4533
laminectomy for, 4527–4529
laminotomy for, 4529–4530
limbus vertebral fracture in, 4531
magnetic resonance imaging of, 4522–4523, 4522f, 4523f
nonsurgical treatment of, 4527
pathophysiology of, 4521
posterior longitudinal ligament ossification with, 4526–4527
second operations for, 4529
signs of, 4522
somatosensory evoked potentials in, 4525–4526
subluxation in, 512
surgery for, 4527–4530
complications of, 4535–4536
outcome of, 4535
symptoms of, 4521–4522
trumpet laminectomy for, 4530
yellow ligament ossification with, 4526–4527
pain in, 4305
pediatric, 3565
recurrent, in achondroplasia, 3370–3371, 3370f, 3371f
subarticular, 4521
thoracic, with lumbar stenosis, 4526
Spinal surgery, 631–643. *See also under* specific region, e.g., Cervical spine, surgical approaches to.
bone grafts in, 4613–4620. *See also* Bone grafts.
cerebrospinal fluid leak in, 574–575
challenges in, 4149
complication avoidance in, 574–582
evaluation before, 556–557, 557t
historical aspects of, 631
image-guided navigational systems for, 4743–4756
Spinal surgery *(Continued)*
imaging during, 575
pseudomeningocele in, 574–575
stereotactic, 576
Spinal tap, dermoids from, 3275f
Spinal tracts
in lower urinary tract function, 362–363, 363f
nucleus of, 3048
Spine
actinomycosis of, 4385
aneurysmal bone cyst of, 4354, 4354f
imaging of, 4843, 4844f
pediatric, 3589, 3590f
angiography of, 506
angiolipoma of, 4843
arteriovenous malformations of, 2375–2417. *See also* Arteriovenous malformations, spinal.
aspergillosis of, 4387–4388
atlantoaxial. *See* Atlantoaxial joint.
biomechanics of, 4181–4199, 4586, 4587f, 4588–4589
anatomic substructures in, 4184–4187
functional, 4187–4192
future studies of, 4198–4199
in spondylolisthesis, 4543–4547
motion segment in, 4181, 4182f
research techniques for, 4192–4193
treatment and, 4192–4198
blastomycosis of, 4388f, 4389
brucellosis of, 4385–4386
candidiasis of, 4389–4390
cervical. *See* Cervical spine.
chondroma of, 4840
chondrosarcoma of, 4357, 4837, 4846–4848
from osteochondroma, 4840
imaging of, 532–533, 532f, 4847, 4847f
chordoma of, 4357, 4357f, 4848, 4849f
pediatric, 3567
coccidioidomycosis of, 4390
computed tomography of, 501–503, 502f, 4145
congenital malformations of, 4148, 4276–4281, 4276f–4281f, 4315t, 4316–4319, 4317f, 4318f
imaging of, 533–536
cyst of, pediatric, 3568
deformities of
after selective dorsal rhizotomy, 3742–3743
pediatric intramedullary tumor surgery and, 3713
degenerative disease of, 4147–4148
osteophytes in, 509, 512f
radiologic features of, 507–516
vs. pyogenic infection, 4371
diskography of, 506
dislocation fracture of, 521, 523, 523f
disorders of
classification of, 4289, 4290f
pain in, 4289–4309
endoscopic procedures on, 3430–3431
eosinophilic granuloma of, 4296t, 4297–4298, 4355, 4837, 4843, 4845f
pediatric, 3567, 3591, 3592f
epidural abscess of. *See* Epidural abscess.
Ewing's sarcoma of, 4356–4357, 4837, 4848–4850, 4850f
radiation therapy for, 4049
fibrous dysplasia of, pediatric, 3590–3591, 3591f
formation of, 3258–3259, 3258f

Spine (Continued)
fractures of
imaging of, 517–523
in ankylosing spondylitis, 4461, 4469–4470, 4470f
unstable, 4877–4878
giant cell tumor of, 4355, 4355f, 4850, 4851–4852
pediatric, 3589
granulomatous disease of, 4352
imaging of, 541, 543f
in Chiari malformation type I, 3348, 3348f
in Chiari malformation type II, 3350
infection of, 4147, 4363–4390. *See also* Pyogenic infection, spinal and specific infection.
after epidural catheter placement, 4384–4385
iatrogenic, 4382–4385
imaging of, 537–544
postdiskography, 4384
postoperative, 4383–4384
inflammation of
imaging of, 537–544
pediatric, 3566–3567, 3566f
injury to, 4307–4308, 4308f
pediatric, 3564. *See also* specific injury.
age in, 3517–3518, 3517t, 3518t
biomechanics of, 3515–3516
causes of, 3516, 3516t
child abuse and, 3507–3508, 3508f
classification of, 3515
epidemiology of, 3516–3517, 3516t
outcome in, 3518
patterns of, 3517
predictions in, 3516
site of, 3517–3518, 3518t
treatment of, 3518
radiologic features of, 517–524
instantaneous axis of rotation of, 4587f, 4588
internal fixation of. *See* Internal fixation, spinal.
intradural arteriovenous malformations of. *See* Arteriovenous malformations, intradural.
intradural vascular malformations of, 2379
embolization for, 2410, 2412
outcome in, 2410, 2410t, 2411f
surgery for, 2408, 2409f, 2410
treatment of, 2408, 2413
Langerhans cell histiocytosis of, pediatric, 3567
ligaments of, 4186–4187
injury to, imaging of, 523, 524f
lumbar. *See* Lumbar spine.
magnetic resonance imaging of, 503–505, 505f, 4145
metastases to. *See* Spinal metastases.
mucormycosis of, 4389f
multiple myeloma of, 1393, 1393f, 4356, 4356f, 4850, 4852–4854, 4853f
myelography of, 505–506
neutral axis of, 4588
nocardiosis of, 4385
osteoblastoma of, 4353–4354, 4354f, 4839, 4839f
pediatric, 3588–3589
osteochondroma of, 4354, 4840, 4841, 4841f
osteoid osteoma of, 4353, 4837, 4838f
pediatric, 3588, 3588f
osteosarcoma of, 4356, 4845–4846, 4846f

Spine (Continued)
parasitic infections of, 4390
pediatric
flexion injury to, 3527, 3527f, 3529f
fusion of, unintentional extension of, 3552–3553
ligamentous instability in, 3526–3528, 3527f–3529f
mass lesions of, 3567–3568
stabilization of, complications of, 3543–3553
structural lesions of, 3564–3566
physiologic loading of, 4589
plasmacytoma of, 4355–4356, 4850–4852
multiple myeloma from, 4854
postoperative changes to, imaging of, 515–516, 516f
radiography of, 500–501, 500f, 501f, 4145–4146
radiologic features of, 497–544
evaluation of, 497–499, 498t, 499f, 499t
modalities for, 500–506
radiosurgery of, 4069
rheumatoid arthritis of, 4570–4572, 4571f, 4572f
sarcoid of, imaging of, 541, 544f
segmentation anomalies of, 4279, 4279f
imaging of, 535, 536f
spontaneous hemorrhage in, 4310t, 4311
thoracic. *See* Thoracic spine.
thoracoscopy of. *See* Thoracoscopy.
three-column model of, 4992, 4992f
tomography of, 505
tuberculosis of, 4386–4387
tumors of, 4148, 4352–4359, 4835–4864
angiography of, 4836
benign, 4353–4355, 4354f, 4355f, 4836
bony, 4837
cartilaginous, 4836–4837, 4840, 4841f
computed tomography of, 4836
embolization of, 4836
extradural, 529, 529f–532f, 531–533
extramedullary intradural, 4358–4359
imaging of, 525–533
intradural extramedullary, 526–527, 526f–529f, 529
intramedullary, 525–526, 525f, 526f, 4358
laboratory studies in, 4836
malignant, 4355–4358, 4836, 4845–4850, 4846f–4852f
metastatic, 4357–4358, 4358f, 4836, 4854–4863
osteogenic, 4837–4840, 4838f, 4839f
pediatric, 3567–3568, 3587–3592
primary, 4353–4357, 4354f–4357f, 4836–4837, 4836t
radiologic assessment of, 4835–4836
signs/symptoms of, 4835
vascular, 4837, 4840–4843, 4842f
ultrasonography of, 506
vascular anatomy of, 2375, 2376f
vascular malformations of, 4318–4319, 4318f
classification of, 2375–2376, 2375t
imaging of, 536–537, 538f, 539f
vascular surgery on, anesthesia for, 1512
Spine-Tech BAK interbody fusion device, 4722, 4723f–4724f
Spinomesencephalic tract, 2930, 2931f
Spinoreticular tract, 2930, 2931f
Spinothalamic tract, 2927, 2928f–2930f, 2930
ablative procedures in, 3045
anatomy of, 3075
in lower urinary tract function, 363

Spinothalamic tract (Continued)
lateral
descending respiratory pathway in, 3060–3061
in cordotomy, 3060–3061, 3060f
section of, historical aspects of, 3075
within midbrain, 3054
Spinous process, thoracic
fracture of, 4978–4979
osteochondroma of, 4840, 4841
Splanchnic nerve block, 2983–2984
Splint, molded body, 3544, 3545f
Spondylitis
in spondyloarthropathies, 4460
infectious, 3566
pediatric, 3566
tuberculous, 3566
pain in, 4293–4295, 4294f
Spondyloarthropathy, 4349–4351, 4350f, 4459–4471
classification of, 4462, 4462t
comparison of, 4463t
imaging of, 541, 544
seronegative, craniocervical junction, 4580–4581, 4582f, 4583f
undifferentiated, 4459, 4463
Spondylodesis, ventral derotation, 4684
Spondylodiskitis, 4461
postoperative, 4383
Spondylodiskopathy, 4461
Spondyloepiphyseal dysplasia
atlantoaxial instability in, 3543
odontoid process, 3343–3344
Spondylolisthesis, 3565, 3571–3584, 4305–4306, 4541–4554
biomechanics of, pathogenesis and, 4543–4547
classification of, 3571–3572
clinical findings in, 4541, 4543
congenital, 4541, 4542f
pathogenesis of, 4543–4544
treatment of, 4550–4551
definition of, 3571
degenerative, 509, 3580–3583, 4541, 4543f
after posterior lumbar instrumentation, 4736–4737
decompression for, 3581–3583
intact neural arch with
fusion for, 4532–4533
lumbar stenosis in, 4531–4533
olisthy in, 4531–4532
intertransverse process arthrodesis for, 3581–3583, 3582f, 3583f
natural history of, 3580
pathogenesis of, 4545–4546, 4545f, 4546f
surgical outcome in, 3582–3583, 3583f
treatment of, 3580–3581, 4551–4553, 4552f
differential diagnosis of, 3573
dysplastic, 3573, 3573f
epidemiology of, 3571, 3571f, 3572f
examination of, 3561
isthmic, 3574–3580, 4541, 4542f, 4543f
diagnosis of, 3575
disk degeneration in, 3577–3578
elongated pars interarticularis in, 3574, 3574f, 3577, 3577f
incidence of, 3574–3575
pathogenesis of, 4544
progression of, 3575
tight hamstrings in, 3573
treatment of, 3575–3578, 3577f, 3579f, 4551
in children, 4550–4551
types of, 3574

Spondylolisthesis *(Continued)*
  lysis with, fusion for, 4533
  measurement of, 3572, 3572f
  Meyerding classification of, 3572, 3572f
  pathologic, 3574, 3574f, 4541, 4546
  postlaminectomy, 3574, 3574f
  postsurgical, 4543, 4544f
    pathogenesis of, 4546–4547, 4548f
    treatment of, 4553–4554
  presentation of, 3572–3573
  radiologic features of, 509, 512, 513f, 4541–4543, 4542f–4544f, 4547–4549, 4549f, 4550f
  traumatic, 3573–3574
    axis, 520f, 521, 4905–4906, 4905f, 4906f, 4906t, 4945–4947, 4946t
    pathogenesis of, 4546
  treatment of, 4550–4554
Spondylolysis, 4305–4306, 4306f
  fusion techniques for, 4554, 4554f
  pediatric, 3565
    examination of, 3561
  postsurgical, treatment of, 4553–4554
  radiologic features of, 509, 512, 513f
Spondylolysis acquisita, 4543
Spondylometaphyseal dysplasia, atlantoaxial instability in, 3543
Spondylosis
  cervical, 4395–4397. *See also* Cervical spondylotic myelopathy.
    anterior approaches to, 4431–4443
  lumbar, radiography of, 501, 502f
Spondylosis deformans, 509
Spongioblastoma cerebelli, 3639
Spontaneity, in frontal lobe tumors, 830
Sports injuries, to cervical spine, 4889. *See also* Cervical spine, trauma to.
Squalamine, angiosuppressive therapy with, 779
Squamosal suture, 423f
Squamous cell carcinoma
  nasopharyngeal, 1398, 1399f
  paranasal sinus, 1312
  scalp, 1410
  staging of, 1410
Stab wounds, traumatic aneurysms from, 2131
Stabilization
  for spinal metastases, 4858–4862, 4859t, 4860f, 4864f
  legal issues regarding, 407
Stalk section effect, in pituitary adenoma, 1174–1175
Standardization, in outcomes assessment, 245
Staphylococcus aureus
  infectious intracranial aneurysms from, 2102
  pyogenic spinal infections from, 4365, 4376f
  shunt infection from, 3422
Staphylococcus epidermidis
  pyogenic spinal infections from, 4365
  shunt infection from, 3422
Star clusters, in developmental venous anomalies, 2140, 2140f
Starling's equation, in brain edema, 793
Station, examination of, 269
Statistics
  in diagnosis, 235–238
  in outcomes assessment, 245–247
Status epilepticus, 2464
Steele-Richardson-Olszewski syndrome, positron emission tomography of, 2761
Stellate ganglion block, 2982–2983
Stem cells
  characteristics of, 4159
  embryonic, differentiation of, 4160
  in central nervous system repair, 4160
  in central nervous system transplantation, 2841, 2843
  with neural capability, 93, 94f
Stenosis, intracranial, transcranial Doppler ultrasonography of, 1554
Stents, carotid angioplasty with, 1651–1658. *See also* Carotid angioplasty.
Stepping reflex, in cerebral palsy, 3725, 3726t
Stereocilia, 341
Stereopsis, 317
Stereotactic radiation therapy
  beam delivery systems for, 4138–4139
  fractionated, 4136, 4138, 4138f
    linacs for, 4115
Stereotactic radiosurgery, 3990–3995
  Bragg peak effect in, 3990, 3992f
  for arteriovenous malformations, 2126, 2151, 2217–2218
  for brain metastases, 1088–1092, 1089t, 1091t
  for cavernous malformations, 2306
  for chordoma, 4049
  for craniopharyngioma, 1219, 3682–3683
  for giant arteriovenous malformations, 2270
  for glomus tumors, 1297
  for posterior fossa arteriovenous malformations, 2258–2259
  for skull base tumors, 4029
  for trigeminal neuralgia, 3006, 3020–3021
  for trigeminal schwannoma, 1349
  frameless image-guided, 3994–3995, 3995f
  γ knife, 2660, 3992, 3993f, 4012
  heavy-particle, 3990–3992, 3991f, 3992f
  historical aspects of, 3990–3995
  history of, 2660
  in thalamotomy, 2773–2774, 4087–4090, 4087t, 4088f, 4089f
  linear accelerator, 2660, 3992, 3994, 3994f
  radiation beams in, 4012
  radiobiology of, 4001–4002, 4002f
  vs. radiation therapy, 4012
Stereotactic surgery, 2769–2774. *See also* Radiosurgery; Stereotactic radiosurgery.
  complications of, 573–574, 573t, 574t, 2779
  for adrenal medulla transplantation, 2661
  for epilepsy, 557
  for trigeminal neuralgia, 3020–3021
  frame-based, 2658–2659, 2658f
  frameless, 901, 2663f, 2664
    brain movement in, 942
    display in, 942
    economics of, 946–947
    head movement in, 942
    historical aspects of, 941
    imaging in, 941
    in biopsy, 945–946
    in craniotomy, 942–945, 943f–945f, 945t
    intraoperative imaging in, 946
    multimodality imaging in, 946
    pointing devices in, 941
    registration in, 941
  functional, historical aspects of, 2659–2660
Stereotactic surgery *(Continued)*
  historical aspects of, in pain surgery, 2914–2915
  history of, 2655–2657, 2656f, 2657f
  image-based, 2662–2664
  macrostimulation localization in, 2771, 2773
  medical therapy effects on, 2660
  microelectrode localization in, 2770–2771, 2770f–2772f
  physiologic localization in, 2770–2771, 2770f–2772f
  radiofrequency, 2773
  radiologic localization in, 2769–2770
  radiosurgery, 2773–2774
  semi-microelectrode localization in, 2771, 2773
  technologic innovation in, 2657–2659, 2658f
  volumetric guidance in, 2664
Sternocleidomastoid muscle
  denervation of, 2898
  pediatric, evaluation of, 3176
  rupture of, auto accidents and, 4917
Sterno-occipital mandibular immobilization brace, 4899
Stiff-man syndrome, 2886
Stimulation, supramaximal, 3852
Strabismus, pediatric, examination of, 3174
Straight leg raising test, 4512, 4512f
Straight sinus, 10f, 15f
Stratification, in outcomes assessment, 245
Streptococcus
  infectious intracranial aneurysms from, 2102
  pyogenic spinal infections from, 4365
Streptokinase, thrombolytics for, 1727
Streptomycin
  for Ménière's disease, 2906
  for tuberculosis, 1441
Stress, blood-brain barrier in, 166
Stretch, peripheral nerve injury from, 3827
Stretch reflex, 2876–2878, 2876f–2878f
  alpha motoneuron hyperexcitability in, 2877
  excitatory polysynaptic pathways in, 2876, 2877f
  γ motoneuron hyperexcitability in, 2877–2878, 2878f
  group II endings in, 2877
  inhibition in, 2878
  mechanisms in, 2878, 2879t
  monosynaptic connections in, 2876
  pediatric, 3180
  reciprocal inhibition in, 2876–2877
  recurrent inhibition in, 2877
Stretch-activated cation channels, in cerebral autoregulation, 1475–1476
Striae medullaris thalami, 13, 14f
Striatal interneurons, synaptic innervation of, 2689
Striate artery, medial, 1925–1926, 1926f
Striatofugal projections
  direct, 2687–2689, 2688f, 2689f, 2700
  indirect, 2687–2689, 2688f, 2689f, 2700–2701
Striatonigral degeneration, positron emission tomography of, 2761
Striatum, 11, 2671, 2672f, 2683, 2730–2731. *See also* specific projection, e.g., Corticostriatal projection.
  afferents to, 2683–2687
  γ-aminobutyric acid neurons in, 2684–2685
  γ-aminobutyric acid receptors in, 2686–2687, 2686f

Striatum (Continued)
aspiny neurons in, 2684–2685
cortical neurons in, 2685
dopaminergic denervation of, in akinetic-rigid Parkinson's disease, 2708
dopaminergic neurons in, 2687
dynorphin receptors in, 2687
enkephalin receptors in, 2687
glutamate receptors in, 2686, 2686f
hereditary necrosis of, 2719
in basal ganglia–thalamocortical circuits, 2699, 2700f
intralaminar thalamic nuclei in, 2685
lesions of, dystonia in, 2677
medium spiny neurons of, 2730–2731
substance P receptors in, 2687
Striola, 341
Striothalamic sulcus, 8, 8f, 10f
Stroke
behavioral recovery from, cortical hypometabolism in, 1609
cardiac disease in, 1625
carotid atherosclerosis and
plaque ulceration in, 1624–1625, 1624f
symptoms of, 1614–1615, 1614t
cervical bruit in, 1622–1623
contralateral cerebral effects of, 1607–1608
crossed cerebellar diaschisis in, 1607, 1608f
embolic
blunt vertebral artery injury and, 5212, 5213f
transcranial Doppler ultrasonography of, 1549–1550
epidemiology of, 1622
evaluation of, 1498, 1499t
glomus jugulare tumor embolization and, 1300
hemianopia from, 1608
hemorrhagic
single-photon emission computed tomography of, 2478–2479
transcranial Doppler ultrasonography of, 2478–2479
venous occlusion procedures and, 935, 935f
historical considerations in, 1463
in traumatic aneurysm dissection, 2133
incidence of, 1651
infarction and, 1622
inflammation in, 142–143
ipsilateral effects from, 1609
magnetic resonance imaging of, 463–464, 465f–468f, 466–467, 469
management of, 1500–1501
medical treatment of, 1495–1501
metabolic effects of, 1607–1609, 1608f
middle cerebral artery in, positron emission tomography of, 1603f
pathophysiology of, 1495–1496, 1495f, 1622–1626
astrocytes in, 111–112
characteristics of, 1622–1626
platelet antiaggregant therapy for, 1617–1618
positron emission tomography of, 1604–1607
clinical correlates in, 1606
irreversibly damaged tissue in, 1605
ischemic core in, 1605
ischemic penumbra in, 1605, 1606
spontaneous hyperperfusion in, 1606
therapy and, 1606–1607
Stroke (Continued)
risk factors for, 1615–1617
single photon emission computed tomography of, 1606, 2478
subcortical effects of, 1608–1609
surgery for, 1501
thalamocortical diaschisis from, 1608–1609
thrombolytic therapy for, 1496–1498, 1497t
tissue plasminogen activator for, 1498, 1499t, 1500, 1500t
transcranial Doppler ultrasonography in, 1554–1555
transient ischemic attacks and, 1624
vessel occlusion procedures and, 863
Stump pain, spinal cord stimulation for, 3114
Stupor, 284
Sturge-Weber syndrome
brain tumors in, 812t, 813
in extratemporal lobe epilepsy, 2598
Styloid process, 36f
SU5416, angiosuppressive therapy with, 780
SU6668, angiosuppressive therapy with, 780
Subarachnoid hemorrhage, 276t
aneurysmal, 1771, 1774, 1774t, 1813–1833
admitting orders for, 1821, 1821t
blood pressure management in, 1822
cardiovascular complications in, 1828–1829
catheter-based angiography of, 1818–1820
causes of, 1813, 1814t
cerebral blood flow in, 1814–1815
cerebral blood volume in, 1814–1815
cerebral metabolic rate for oxygen in, 1814–1815
cerebral vasospasm from. See Vasospasm.
clinical grading of, 1820, 1820t
cocaine use and, 1832
complications of, 1822–1826
computed tomography of, 1816–1817, 1816f, 1817f
delayed-onset neurological worsening after, 1849, 1849t
diabetes insipidus in, 1830, 1830t
diagnosis of, 1816–1820
evaluation of, 1815–1820
fluid/electrolyte disturbances in, 1829–1830, 1830t
gastrointestinal complications of, 1831
general care for, 1820–1822
grading of, 1816–1817, 1817f
headache in, 1815
hydrocephalus after, 1823–1824, 1823t, 1824f
in distal anterior cerebral artery aneurysms, 1947
in giant aneurysm, 2081
in middle cerebral artery aneurysms, 1960, 1962
in posterior inferior cerebellar artery aneurysm, 2009, 2013, 2013f, 2014
in pregnancy, 2424–2426
in sickle cell anemia, 1832
in vertebral artery aneurysm, 2009, 2013, 2013f, 2014
in vertebrobasilar junction aneurysm, 2009, 2013, 2014
incidence of, 1813
intracerebral hemorrhage in, 1825
intracranial pressure response to, 1813–1814, 1824–1825
intraventricular hemorrhage in, 1824
lumbar puncture in, 1817–1818, 1818t
magnetic resonance imaging of, 1818
medical complications of, 1826–1831, 1827t, 1868–1869
neurological complications of, 1827t, 1831, 1831t
outcome in, 1832, 1833t
$Paco_2$ in, 1815
pathophysiology of, 1813–1815
pediatric, 1832
rebleeding of, 1822–1823
respiratory complications of, 1826–1828
risk for
aneurysm growth and, 1788
in unruptured aneurysm, 1793–1794, 1794t
rupture in, 1509, 1510, 1815–1816
salt wasting in, 1830, 1830t
seizures in, 1825–1826, 1826t
signs/symptoms of, 1815–1816
syndrome of inappropriate secretion of antidiuretic hormone in, 1829–1830, 1830t
treatment of, 1820–1822, 2121–2122
venous thromboembolism in, 1828
blood clot management in, 1852, 1853f
blunt vertebral artery injury and, 5212
bullet wounds and, 5230
cardiovascular changes in, 553
cerebral arterial wall changes after, 1844–1845, 1845f
constrictive angiopathy of. See Vasospasm.
electrocardiographic changes after, 553–554
electrolyte disturbances and, 554
endovascular occlusion after, 1804–1805
grading of, 1915–1916, 1916t
hypovolemia after, prevention of, 1852
in arteriovenous malformations, 2149, 2149f
in pediatric arteriovenous malformations, 3447–3448
incidence of, 1783–1784
intracranial pressure in, 180
neurological grading of, 553, 553t
outcome of
age in, 1800
in pregnancy, 2426
pediatric, 3463, 3476, 3477f
perimesencephalic, 1842
preoperative evaluation for, 553–554
respiratory system effects of, 554
surgery for
complications after, 1799–1800
in pregnancy, 2425–2426
timing of, 1796–1797
traumatic
cerebral vasospasm after, 1552, 5046–5047, 5047t
external hydrocephalus in, 3397
vasospasm from, 1841, 1841f, 1846, 1847f
animal models of, 1844
cerebral blood flow velocity in, 1545–1547, 1546f
risk for, 1840
transcranial Doppler ultrasonography of, 1545–1547, 1545t, 1546f, 1547f
vitreous hemorrhage in, 1816

Subarachnoid space
blood clots in, 1845
formation of, cerebrospinal fluid alterations in, 3289
historical aspects of, 3149, 3149f
in anterior circulation aneurysm surgery, 1878
metastatic medulloblastoma of, 3642
pediatric, 3462
spinal to cortical obstruction in, hydrocephalus from, 3394–3397
Subaxial dislocations, 4908–4910, 4908t, 4909f
Subaxial fractures, 4907–4908, 4908f, 4908t
Subcallosal area, 25
Subcaudate tractotomy, for psychiatric disorders, 2857–2858, 2858f
Subcentral gyrus, 3
Subclavian steal syndrome, of extracranial vertebral artery, 1694, 1694f
Subcortical tumors, 831
Subdural hematoma, 5043–5045
acute, 5043–5044
after arterial bypass, 2117
chronic, 5044–5045, 5170, 5172, 5172f, 5173f
bur hole drainage of, 5173
child abuse and, 3505
cranioplasty for, 5174, 5175f
craniotomy for, 5174
shunting for, 5174
spontaneous regression of, 5172–5173
surgery for, 5172
twist drill drainage of, 5173–5174
classification of, 5043, 5043t
contusion/laceration and, 5044
delivery and, 3484, 3484f
evacuation of, 5158–5159, 5159f
imaging of, 5093, 5093f
magnetic resonance imaging of, 469
mild head injury and, 5070, 5071t
pediatric, head injury and, 3475f, 3476, 3477
posterior fossa, delivery and, 3484–3485, 3485f, 3486f
postoperative, 936, 937f
presentation of, 5157–5158, 5157f, 5158f
shaking-impact syndrome and, 3501, 3503f, 3504, 3504f
traumatic brain injury and, 5083, 5106, 5107f
treatment of, 5146, 5148f
Subdural space, fluid collections in, patient positioning and, 616
Subependymal germinal matrix hemorrhage, 3405, 3406f. *See also* Hydrocephalus, infantile posthemorrhagic.
injury pattern in, 3407, 3407f
neuropathology from, 3407–3408
pathogenesis of, 3406f, 3407
severity of, 3408, 3408t
Subependymoma
classification of, 665
radiologic features of, 840–841
third ventricular, 1246
Subfrontal gyrus, 1926, 1926f
Subfrontal sulcus, 1926, 1926f
Sublaminar cables, in thoracic spine fixation, 4969f
Subluxation
atlantoaxial, in rheumatoid arthritis, 4571–4572, 4571f, 4573
hip, in cerebral palsy, 3728
Subparietal sulcus, 25
Subpial transection, for extratemporal lobe epilepsy, 2594, 2595f, 2596
Substance abuse, in mild head injury, 5067
Substance P
after axonal transection, 3967
as nociceptive synaptic neurotransmitter, 2927
in immune control, 684
inflammation mediation by, 2956
release of, 2953, 2954f
Substance P receptors, in striatum, 2687
Substantia gelatinosa, 2924–2925, 3045–3046
in pain transmission, 2953
Substantia nigra, 10f, 11, 29, 2683, 2730
Substantia nigra pars compacta, 2671, 2731
cell degeneration in, 2710
dopaminergic neurons of, 2683
in Parkinson's disease, 2704, 2706, 2706f
dopaminergic projections of, 2699
in akinetic-rigid Parkinson's disease, 2707–2708
in basal ganglia–thalamocortical circuits, 2699, 2700f
striatal projection to, 2700
Substantia nigra pars reticularis, 2671, 2672, 2672f, 2673, 2731
γ-aminobutyric acid neurons in, 2683
in parkinsonism, 2674, 2674f
lesions of, surgery for, 2675
projections to tegmental pedunculopontine nucleus from, 2693, 2694f, 2695
projections to thalamus from, 2691–2693, 2692f
stimulation of, 2819
subthalamic nucleus projection to, 2701
Subthalamic nucleus, 11, 2671, 2672f, 2673, 2730, 2731
γ-aminobutyric acid receptors in, 2690–2691
deep brain stimulation of, 2662
glutamate receptors in, 2690–2691
glutamatergic projections to, 2690
in parkinsonism, 2674, 2674f
lesions of, 2676
surgery for, 2675
pallidal projections to, 2700–2701
projections of, 2699
stereotactic surgery on, 2660
stimulation of, 2803–2804, 2805f, 2817
complications of, 2823
coordinates for, 2809, 2810t
electrophysiologic studies in, 2815, 2816f
results of, 2821–2822
Subventricular zone, 79f, 80, 97–98
Succinylcholine, 1508
Sucking reflex testing, 3174, 3182
Sudden infant death syndrome, posterior plagiocephaly in, 3302
Sudeck's sign, 3538
Suicide, in bullet wounds, 5224t, 5225
Sulcal veins, 2381
Sulci, 60f, 61
cerebral, 3
Sulcus limitans, 33f
Sulfasalazine, for ankylosing spondylitis, 4467
Superficial reflex testing, pediatric, 3181
Superficial temporal artery–to–middle cerebral artery bypass, 2113, 2113f, 2114f
Superficial temporal artery–to–superior cerebellar artery bypass, 2115
Superior colliculus, 15f
brachium of, 10f
Superior fovea, 33f
Superior longitudinal fasciculus, 6, 7f
Superior sulcus, 3
Superolateral recess, 31f, 32, 33f
Superoxide, 1473
Superoxide dismutases, in traumatic brain injury, 5026
Supinator muscle, posterior interosseous nerve entrapment and, 3928
Supine position, 596–598, 597t, 598f
complication avoidance in, 561
for cerebellopontine angle tumors, 607
for craniotomy, 628, 628f
Supplementary motor area, cortical stimulation mapping of, 2537
Supracondylar process, median nerve entrapment by, 3924
Supraculminate vein, 36f
Supramarginal gyrus, 4f, 5, 6f
Supraolivary fossette, 29, 30f
Suprapineal recess, 14f
Suprapontine centers, in micturition, 360–361
Suprascapular nerve, entrapment of, 3932–3933
Suprascapular notch, entrapment neuropathy at, 3932
Suprasellar cistern, cysts of, 3293–3295, 3294f, 3295f
Suprasellar region
germ cell tumors of, 3604
germinoma of, pediatric, 3606
tumors of, 831
Supraspinous ligament, 4187
Supratentorium, surgery on, seizures after, 565
Sural nerve, 653
biopsy of, 3963
entrapment of, 3934
graft with, in brachial plexus surgery, 3492
Suramin, angiosuppressive therapy with, 775, 776f, 781
Surgery
evaluation before, 547–558
nerve damage in, 3975
non-neurological, in neurological patient, 558
risk factors in, 565–582
Surgical complications, 931–939
avoidance of, 932–939
frameless stereotaxis in, 933f, 934
retractor placement in, 934–935, 934f
brain edema as, 934–935, 934f
classification of, 888t, 931–932
deep vein thrombosis as, 939
definition of, 931
hematoma in, 935–936, 937f
infection as, 938, 938f
neurological, 933–937
partial resection and, 935, 935f
patient selection and, 932–939
regional, 937–938, 938f
seizure as, 937–938
surgical approach and, 932f, 933
systemic, 938–939
vascular injury in, 935, 935f, 936f
Surgical navigation, 941–947
brain movement in, 942
display in, 942
economics of, 946–947
head movement in, 942
historical aspects of, 941

Surgical navigation *(Continued)*
imaging in, 941
in biopsy, 945–946
in craniotomy, 942–945, 943f–945f, 945t
intraoperative imaging in, 946
multimodality imaging in, 946
pointing devices in, 941
registration in, 941
Sutures
anomalies of
head shape and, 3300
historical aspects of, 3158, 3158f, 3159f
coronal, 423f
diastatic, 427
lambdoid, 423f
metopic, 431–432
occipitomastoid, 423f
ossification of, 3301
premature fusion of, 3304–3305, 3305t
prominent, in infants, 431–432
squamosal, 423f
Swimmer's projection, in cervical spine radiography, 4894
Sylvian cistern, in aneurysm surgery, 1879
Sylvian fissure, 5–6, 6f
anatomy of, 2608
arachnoid cyst of, 3292–3293, 3293f
arteriovenous malformation of, 2237–2238, 2239f
dissection of, 1933
in craniometrics, 630–631
localization of, 2531, 2532f
posterior ramus of, 4, 4f
Sylvian fissure stem, 4f
Sylvian point, 14, 16
Sylvian triangle, 16
Sylvian vein, superficial, 17
Sympathectomy, 3028, 3093–3102
approaches to, 3096
historical aspects of, 3093–3094
lumbar endoscopic, 3102, 3102f
nomenclature in, 3094
patient selection for, 3095–3096
thoracic endoscopic, 3096–3102, 4762–4765
anatomic orientation for, 4763–4764, 4764f
care after, 3100
closure in, 4764
complications of, 3101–3102, 4765
dissection in, 3099–3100, 3099f
goals of, 4763
indications for, 3096–3097, 4762–4763, 4762t
instruments for, 3098–3099
intrathoracic anatomy in, 3098f, 3099
outcome in, 3100–3101, 3100t, 3101t, 4765
ports for, 3099
positioning for, 3097f, 3098, 3098f, 4763, 4763f
transection in, 4764, 4764f
unilateral vs. bilateral, 3095t
Sympathetic block, paravertebral, in sympathetic-mediated pain, 3096
Sympathetic dystrophy, 3094
Sympathetic fiber bundles, 1899
Sympathetic nerve trunk, vagus nerve stimulator implantation and, 2643
Sympathetic nervous system
afferent fibers of, 2981
anatomy of, 2981
blockade procedures in, 2981–2984
efferent fibers of, 2981
endoscopy of, 3093
Sympathetic nervous system *(Continued)*
in lower urinary tract function, 361, 361f
indications for, 2981–2982
Synapses, 71–73, 72f
ensheathment of, 86
in brain metabolism, 86
transduction in, in post-traumatic epilepsy, 2451–2452, 2451f
Synaptic terminal, 72f, 73
Synaptic transmission, 226–228
chemical, 227–228
electrical, 226–227
Synaptogenesis
in post-traumatic epilepsy, 2450–2451
reactive, 3785
Synchondrosis, neural central, 3332
Syncope, 275
neurocardiogenic, vs. seizure, 2466
Syndrome of inappropriate antidiuretic hormone secretion (SIADH)
after aneurysmal subarachnoid hemorrhage, 1829–1830, 1830t
in traumatic brain injury, 5130, 5130f
vs. salt wasting, 1830
Synostosis
bilateral coronal, surgery for, 3321
after age three, 3322
before age one, 3321–3322, 3322f, 3323f
coronal, deformational anterior plagiocephaly and, 3301f
primary, vs. skull molding, 3301–3304
sagittal, growth restriction in, 3315, 3316f
unilambdoid, vs. deformational plagiocephaly, 3302, 3302f, 3303f, 3303t
Synovial cyst
imaging of, 512, 513f–514f
vs. lumbar disk disease, 4511, 4511f
Synovitis, in spondyloarthropathies, 4460
Synthes system, of cervical spine anterior screw-plate fixation, 4630t, 4632, 4632f
α-Synuclein, 2703
in Lewy bodies detection, 2709
Synucleopathies, 2703–2714, 2703t
Syphilis
congenital, endolymphatic hydrops in, 350
myelitis in, 4313
Syringocele, 3226
Syringohydromyelia
imaging of, 533, 535f, 3356
in Chiari malformation type II, 3351
Syringomyelia, 4315t, 4317
cerebrospinal fluid obstruction and, 3393
embryonic tissue transplantation for, 4159
endoscopy in, 3430–3431
post-traumatic, 4308
terminal, 3273–3274, 3273f
Syringomyelocele, 3226
Syrinx (syringes), in Chiari malformation type I, 3349, 3349f
Systemic lupus erythematosus
chorea with, 2736
pseudotumor syndrome in, 1425
Systolic blood pressure, in bullet wounds, 5226

T cell receptor
diversity of, 890
peptide-MHC recognition by, 676
T cells
active extravasation by, 682
antigen presentation to, in brain tumor therapy, 887, 888f
antigen receptors on, 675–676, 677
antigen recognition by, 680
arrest of, 682
effector functions of, 680
helper, 678
in immune response initiation, 679
in multiple sclerosis, 1450
in immune response, 675, 675f
in multiple sclerosis, 1450
in perivascular space, 683
MHC class II–restricted, 678, 679
MHC class I–restricted, 678
migrant, antigen presentation to, 682
secreted factors of, 680
selective adhesion of, 682
Tactile sensibility, pediatric, 3183
Taenia thalami, 12–13
Tamoxifen, for meningioma, 1110
Tamsulosin, for bladder outlet retention, 380
Tapetum, 7f, 8f, 9
Tardy ulnar palsy, 3897, 3926
Tarlov cysts, 4511
Tarsal tunnel, 653
tibial nerve surgery at, 655, 655f
Tarsal tunnel syndrome, 3935–3936
Tattoo, accidental, in craniofacial trauma, 5249
Tauopathy, 2703, 2703t, 2714–2716
Taylor-Haughton lines, 631, 631f
Teardrop fractures, 4907–4908, 4908f
Technology, evaluation of, 253–254
Tectal beaking, in Chiari malformation type II, 3351
Tectal vein, 36f
Tectorial membrane, 4925–4926, 4926f
hemorrhage in, spinal cord injury without radiographic abnormality and, 3521, 3522f
pediatric, in atlanto-occipital dislocation, 3529, 3531, 3531f
Tectum, 29, 3054
Tegmental pedunculopontine nucleus
nigral projections to, 2693, 2694f, 2695
pallidal projections to, 2693, 2694f, 2695
Tegmentum, 29, 3054, 3074
Tela choroidea, 13, 31f, 33f, 35f, 36f
Telangiectasia
capillary. *See* Capillary telangiectasia.
radiation-induced, 854
Telencephalon, in Chiari malformation type II, 3351, 3351f
Telovelar junction, 33f
Temozolomide, 882
Temperature
in cerebral blood flow, 1504
instability of, in deep hypothermic circulatory arrest, 1536
pediatric, testing of, 3183
Temporal arteritis, 276t
Temporal artery
inferior, 22–23, 22f
superficial
bypass with, for moyamoya, 1719, 1719f, 1720f
in middle cerebral artery aneurysm, 1965, 1967f
middle cerebral artery bypass with, 1674, 2113, 2113f, 2114f
superior cerebellar artery bypass with, 2115

Temporal bone
erosion of, 431
fracture of, 5275–5284
assessment of, 5275–5276, 5276t
auditory function in, 5276
cerebrospinal fluid fistula in, 5279–5280, 5280f
classification of, 5276–5279, 5278f
clinical examination of, 5275
complications of, 5279–5284
facial nerve injury in, 5275, 5276t, 5282–5284
hearing loss in, 5280–5281
hemorrhage in, 5280
longitudinal, 5276, 5278f
mixed pattern, 5278
oblique, 5278
otic-sparing, 5279
prevention of, 5279
radiography of, 5275–5276, 5277f
resuscitation in, 5275
rhinorrhea in, 5268
transverse, 5276–5278, 5278f
vestibular function in, 5276
glomus jugulare tumor of, 1297, 1299f
jugular foramen and, 1302
meningioma of, 1398f
Temporal gyrus, 18f
inferior, 5, 18, 18f
middle, 4f, 5
superior, 4f, 5
venous drainage of, 17
Temporal horn, 7f, 8f, 9, 1237, 1238f, 2486, 2487f
enlargement of, subarachnoid hemorrhage and, 1816
tumors of, 1243
venous drainage of, 1239
Temporal lobe, 5, 12f, 18f
anterior, resection of, 2605–2607
amygdalohippocampectomy vs., memory loss in, 2572
complications of, 2610
outcomes in, 2568, 2569f, 2611
arteriovenous malformation of, homonymous visual field defects in, 314f, 315
basal surface of, 18–19
epidural hematoma in, 5154
hematoma in, 1747, 1750f–1751f
hemorrhage of, 1738
in hippocampal sclerosis, 2487
medial
arteriovenous malformation of, 2239–2241, 2240f, 2243, 2245f
memory areas of, functional magnetic resonance imaging of, 2516–2518
mesial portion of, 25
resection of
for epilepsy, 2567–2568
memory deficits after, 2571
tumors of, 830
venous drainage of, 17, 23, 28
Temporal pole, 10f
Temporal sulcus, 18f
inferior, 3, 5
superior, 4f, 5
Temporal veins, inferior, 23
Temporalis muscle, dissection of, 1932
Temporary artery, inferior, 22f
Temporobasal vein, 23, 24f
Temporomandibular joint
dislocation of, skull base surgery and, 572–573
pain in, hyperextension-hyperflexion injury and, 4918–4919
Temporo-occipital line, 3
Temporosylvian vein, 17, 24f
Tenascin
in axonal growth failure, 205
in central nervous system repair inhibition, 4168
in malignant glioma, 761–762
Tenascin C, in axonal regeneration, 200
Tendon reflexes
deep
in peripheral neuropathy, 3833
testing of, 367, 3824–3825
examination of, 268
Tendon transfers/lengthening, for cerebral palsy, 3732
Tennis elbow, resistant, 3928
Tenorium, 15f
Tenotomy, for spasticity, 2866t
Tension band techniques, for spinal internal fixation, 4592–4593, 4594f
Tension pneumocephalus, patient positioning and, 616
Tentorial sinus, 24f, 35f
lateral, 17
Teratocarcinoma cell line, in central nervous system repair, 4161
Teratoma, 3689, 3692–3693, 3692f
atypical, 3692
classification of, 667–668, 667t
pediatric
diagnosis of, 3607, 3607f
surgery for, 3608
skull, 1386, 1387f
with malignant transformation, 668
Terazosin, for bladder outlet retention, 380
Terminal condition, 414
Testimony, in child abuse, 3510
Tetanus prophylaxis, in bullet wounds, 5230
Tethered spinal cord. *See* Spinal cord, tethered.
Tetracaine, peripheral nerve effects of, 3816
Tetracycline, pseudotumor cerebri from, 1423–1424
Tetraplegia, 4870–4871
Tetrodotoxin
in epileptogenesis prevention, 2452
peripheral nerve effects of, 3816
Thalamic nucleus, basal ganglia inputs to, 2693, 2694f
Thalamic radiation, 9
Thalamic sensory relay nucleus, stimulation of, 3119, 3122, 3125, 3126
Thalamic syndrome, mesencephalotomy for, 3077
Thalamic veins
deep, 17
superficial, 17
Thalamocaudate vein, 1238–1239
Thalamocortical circuit, basal ganglia and, 2699–2701, 2703
Thalamogeniculate artery, 22f
Thalamoperforating artery
anterior, 20
posterior, 21, 22f
Thalamostriatal projection, 2685–2686
Thalamostriate vein, 8f, 15f, 1238
Thalamotomy, 3030, 3079–3081
complications of, 573, 2779–2780
for cerebellar tremor, 2779
for dystonia, 2797–2798
for essential tremor, 2776–2777, 2777f, 2777t
functional deficits after, 2779–2780
Thalamotomy *(Continued)*
historical development of, 3080
indications for, 3077, 3077f, 3080
stereotactic technique in, 2769–2774
macrostimulation localization in, 2771, 2773
microelectrode localization in, 2770–2771, 2770f–2772f
physiologic localization in, 2770–2771, 2770f–2772f
radiofrequency, 2773
radiologic localization in, 2769–2770
radiosurgical, 2773–2774, 4087–4090, 4087t, 4088f, 4089f
semi-microelectrode localization in, 2771, 2773
technique of, 3080–3081
tremor treatment with, 2769–2780
indications for, 2775
results of, 2775–2776
vs. thalamic deep brain stimulation, 2780
Thalamus, 7f, 8f, 10f, 11, 13, 15f, 26f, 1237, 1238f
anatomy of, 3079
arteriovenous malformation of, 2246
as central oscillator, 2774
cavernous malformation of, 2314–2316, 2314f, 2315f
glioma of, pediatric, 3663
hemorrhage of, 1737–1738, 1738f
in consciousness, 278–279
lateral geniculate body of, 2541
neurons of, 2774
nuclei of, electrophysiologic properties of, 2770–2771, 2770f–2772f
posterior ventral medial nucleus in, 2929f
stereotactic surgery on, in Parkinson's disease, 2659
stimulation of, 2661, 3119, 3122, 3125, 3126. *See also* Deep brain stimulation.
complications of, 2823
results of, 2820–2821
venous drainage of, 1238
ventral anterior nucleus of, 2691, 2691t
stereotactic surgery on, in Parkinson's disease, 2659
ventral lateral nucleus of, 2691, 2691t
ventral nuclear group in. *See also* Nucleus ventralis.
surgical lesions of, 2769
ventral posterior nucleus of, 2927
stereotactic surgery on, in Parkinson's disease, 2659
ventral posteromedial nucleus of, 2929f
Thalidomide
angiosuppressive therapy with, 780
for glioma invasion, 766
for sarcoidosis, 1439
Thanatophoric dysplasia, genetics of, 3362
Thenar muscle
atrophy of, in carpal tunnel syndrome, 3890
needle electromyography of, 3858
Therapy, studies about, 258–259
Thermal injury, peripheral nerve, 3828
Thermoreceptors, 3809
Thiamine deficiency, neuropathy from, 3844
Thiopental
cerebral physiology and, 551
in ischemia prevention, 1522

Thiotepa
for ependymoma, 1048t
for neoplastic meningitis, 1233
Third ventricle, 8f, 15f
anatomy of, 1245, 1245f, 1254, 1255f
arteriovenous malformation of, 2242–2243
astroblastoma of, 1246
astrocytoma of, 1246
cavernous malformations of, 1247
chordoid glioma of, 664
choroid plexus tumors in, 3612–3613
colloid cyst of, 1245–1246, 3390
endoscopic removal of, 3430, 3430f
surgical approach to, 1251
craniopharyngioma of, 1247
cystic lesions of, 1247
ependymoma of, 1246
fibrillary astrocytoma of, 1246
floor of, 19
germinoma of, 1247
glial tumors of, 1246
glioblastoma multiforme of, 1246
inflammation of, 1247
interpeduncular region of, 19
juvenile pilocytic astrocytoma of, 1246
meningioma of, 1246
metastatic neoplasms of, 1247
neural structures of, 1245, 1245f
neurocysticercosis involvement of, 1247
neurocytoma of, 1246
pituitary adenoma extension into, 1174, 1247
roof of, 13, 14f
subependymal giant cell astrocytoma of, 1246
subependymoma of, 1246
tumors of, 1245–1260
callostomy for, 1253–1254
cerebrospinal fluid diversion in, 1251
clinical presentation of, 1247
craniotomy for, 1249–1251, 1250f, 1252–1253
endoscopy of, 1249
interforniceal approach to, 1256–1257
mass excision in, 1257
operative closure for, 1257
outcome in, 1257–1260
pathology of, 1245–1247
stereotactic biopsy of, 1248–1249
surgical approaches to, 1247–1251, 1248f
complications of, 1257–1260
transcallosal approach to, 1249, 1250, 1251–1254
glucocorticoids for, 1252
imaging in, 1251–1252
positioning for, 1252
ventriculostomy for, 1252
transchoroidal trans–velum interpositum approach to, 1256
transcortical approach to, 1249
transforaminal approach to, 1255–1256
vascular structures of, 1245, 1245f
xanthogranuloma of, 1443
Thixotropy, 1468
Thoracic disk herniation, 4491–4503, 4981
clinical presentation of, 4491–4492, 4492t
differential diagnosis of, 4492
epidemiology of, 4491
historical perspective on, 4491
imaging of, 4492–4495, 4492f–4495f
after myelography, 4493, 4493f, 4494f
magnetic resonance imaging of, 4493–4495, 4494f, 4495f
Thoracic disk herniation *(Continued)*
pediatric, 3560
radiography of, 4492–4493
surgery for, 4495–4497, 4496f, 4496t, 4497f
anterior approaches in, 4497–4499, 4498f
complications of, 4502–4503, 4503t
lateral approaches in, 4499–4500
posterior approaches in, 4497, 4498f
results of, 4500–4502, 4502t
technique of, 4500, 4501f–4502f
Thoracic endoscopic sympathectomy, 3096–3102, 4762–4765. *See also* Sympathectomy, thoracic endoscopic.
Thoracic facet joint, 4953
dislocation of, 4959–4960, 4962–4964, 4962t, 4963f
surgery for, 4980–4981
treatment guidelines for, 4967t
medial branch of, 2977, 2978f
denervation of, 2977, 2980
pain referral patterns in, 2979f
Thoracic outlet
anatomy of, 3930–3931
peripheral nerve entrapment in, 3930
syndromes of, 3931–3932
surgery for, 3932
Thoracic outlet syndrome(s), 3880–3881, 3931–3932
magnetic resonance imaging of, 3880f, 3881
surgery for, 3932
Thoracic region, ganglionectomy in, 3035, 3036f
Thoracic spine
anatomy of, 4693–4694, 4765–4766, 4766f
aneurysmal bone cyst of, 4843
anterior procedures on, 4671–4690
biomechanics in, 4683–4684
complications of, 4690
fusion in, 4680–4683, 4681f, 4682f
historical background of, 4671
implantation principles for, 4685–4686, 4686f
Kaneda device and, 4686–4689, 4687f
ZPlate II system and, 4689–4690, 4689f
indications for, 4671–4673
instrumentation constructs for, 4684–4685, 4685f
lateral extracavitary approach in, 4676–4678, 4676–4678f
retropleural, 4678–4680, 4678f–4680f
surgical anatomy and, 4673–4675, 4674f, 4675f
T3–T4, 4675–4676
transpleural, 4680
biomechanics of, 4190–4191, 4953–4954, 4953f–4955f
anterior instrumentation and, 4683–4684
in burst fracture, 4192
in chance fracture, 4192
in flexion-compression injury, 4190–4191
laminectomy and, 4194–4195
long-segment instrumentation and, 4195
pedicle fixation and
in degenerative disease, 4198
in trauma, 4195–4198
posterior instrumentation and, 4694–4695
universal instrumentation and, 4195
Thoracic spine *(Continued)*
corpectomy of, 4767, 4768f
vertebral reconstruction after, 4767, 4768f, 4769
decompression of
anterior, 4973–4978, 4974f–4977f
posterolateral, 4972–4973
degenerative disease of, 4673
dislocation fracture of, 521, 523, 523f
dislocation of, 4959–4960, 4960f, 4962–4964, 4962t, 4963f
surgery for, 4980–4981
treatment guidelines for, 4967t
extension injury to, 4961, 4962f
flexion injury to, 4958–4959, 4959f
flexion-distraction injury to, 4960–4961, 4961f
treatment guidelines for, 4967
flexion-rotation injury to, 4959–4960, 4960f, 4980–4981
fractures of, 4149, 4951–4982
anatomic factors in, 4672–4673, 4953–4954
biomechanics in, 4192, 4195–4198
classification of, 4955–4957, 4956t, 4957f, 4961–4964, 4962t, 4963f
surgery and, 4965–4967, 4966f, 4967t, 4968t
complications of, 4981–4982
computed tomography of, 4955, 4956f
distribution of, 4954, 4955f
epidemiology of, 4952–4953, 4953f
historical perspective on, 4951–4952
instability and, 4954–4957, 4955f–4959f, 4956t
bracing of, 4967, 4968t
intraoperative ultrasonography of, 4978, 4978f
magnetic resonance imaging of, 4953f
mechanisms of, 4957–4961, 4959f–4962f
minor, 4978–4979
treatment of
initial, 4964
surgical, 4965–4978
vs. nonsurgical, 4964–4965
hemangioma of, 4842f
hyperextension of, 4961, 4962f
hyperflexion of, 4958–4959, 4959f, 4962, 4962t
infection of, 4673
injury to, child abuse and, 3508, 3508f
internal fixation of, 4597, 4965
historical perspective on, 4952
posterior
devices in, 4969–4972, 4969f–4972f
for compression fracture, 4979
techniques in, 4695–4699, 4696f–4699f
principles of, 4967–4968
multiple myeloma of, 4853f
plasmacytoma of, 4850
posterior procedures on, 4693–4699
anatomic considerations in, 4693–4694
biomechanics in, 4694–4695
techniques of, 4695–4699, 4696f–4699f
pyogenic infection of, 4375–4376, 4376f, 4377f
radiography of, 501
shear injury to, 4960, 4960f, 4963f
soft tissue injury to, 4981
spinal cord injury without radiographic abnormality of, 3523
surgery on, 636–640
anterior approach to, 637–639

Thoracic spine (Continued)
complication avoidance in, 579
posterior approach to, 640
posterolateral approach to, 639–640
posterolateral extracavitary approach to, 640
techniques for, 4758, 4758t
transpleural-retroperitoneal approach to, 637, 638f
sympathectomy of, endoscopic, 4762–4765. *See also* Sympathectomy, thoracic endoscopic.
thoracoscopy of. *See* Thoracoscopy.
tumors of, 4671–4672
Thoracic sympathetic block, 2983
Thoracolumbar scoliosis, 4557–4567, 4558f. *See also* Scoliosis, thoracolumbar.
Thoracolumbar spine
anterior
image-guided navigation of, 4752–4753, 4754f
locking plate system for, 4719, 4721–4722, 4721f
anterior segmental stabilization of, 4564–4565, 4565f
biomechanics of, 4190–4191
degenerative disease of, pedicle fixation in, biomechanics in, 4198
fracture-dislocation of, 4993, 4996–4997, 4997f
treatment of, 4999
fusion of, bone grafts in, 4608, 4608f
injury to, 4987–5006
anatomic influences in, 4991
evaluation of, 4987–4991
Frankel classification of, 4988, 4988t
fulcrum in, 4987, 4988f
imaging of, 4990–4991, 4990f, 4991f
methylprednisolone in, 4988
motor index score in, 4988, 4988t
neurological examination in, 4988–4990, 4988t, 4989f
outcomes in, 5005–5006
spinal examination in, 4988
treatment of, 4997
instability of, 4992
posterior segmental stabilization of, 4562–4563, 4564f
seat belt–type injury to, 4999
Thoracolumbar spine fracture, 4149, 4997–4998
burst, 4993, 4995f
treatment of, 4999
classification of, 4992–4997, 4993t
cord/nerve root syndromes in, 4927, 4989f
imaging of, 521, 521f, 522f
seat belt–type injury and, 4993, 4996f
surgery for
anterior instrumentation in, 5004
deformity correction in, 5004
neural decompression with, 5000–5002, 5000t, 5001f, 5001t
posterior instrumentation in, 5002, 5003f, 5004
treatment of, 4997–4998
wedge compression, 4993, 4994f
treatment of, 4998–4999, 4999f
Thoracoplasty, for scoliosis, 4566
Thoracoscopy, 639, 4757–4769
complications of, 4769
considerations in, 4759
contraindications to, 4758
diskectomy via, 4765–4769
indications for, 4765
micro technique in, 4766–4767, 4767f
Thoracoscopy (Continued)
education for, 4758–4759
for thoracic disk herniation, 4497–4499, 4498f
hemostasis during, 4759–4760
historical overview of, 4757
imaging with, 4759
indications for, 4757–4758, 4758t
instruments with, 4759
operating room setup for, 4760, 4760f
portal insertion in, 4760–4762, 4761f
spinal exposure in, 4762
vs. other techniques, 4757–4758, 4758t
wound closure in, 4762
Thoracotomy, 637
pain after, dorsal rhizotomy for, 3041
retropleural, 638–639, 639f, 4678–4680, 4678f–4680f
transpleural, 4680
vs. other techniques, 4758, 4758t
Three-quarter position, 597t, 607, 608f
Thrombocytopenic purpura, pseudotumor cerebri in, 1425–1426
Thromboembolism
giant aneurysm and, 2081
in subarachnoid hemorrhage, 1828
prevention of, in spinal cord injury, 4882
prophylaxis against, in traumatic brain injury, 5129
Thrombogenesis, 1495
Thrombolysis
mechanism of, 1496
of subarachnoid blood clot, 1852, 1853f
trials of, 1496–1498, 1497t
Thrombolytics, endovascular, for cerebral venous thrombosis, 1727–1729, 1727t, 1728f, 1729f
Thrombophlebitis, in deep hypothermic circulatory arrest, 1536
Thrombosis
arterial, in pregnancy, 2427–2428, 2428t
cerebral venous. *See* Cerebral venous thrombosis.
in arteriovenous malformation, 2188–2189, 2189f
in cavernous malformation, 2143, 2143f
in dural arteriovenous fistula, 2171
in Guglielmi detachable coil embolization, 2070, 2071
in meningioma, 1105–1106
intra-aneurysmal, parent artery occlusion and, 2059–2060
venous, 563–564
after giant arteriovenous malformation surgery, 2280
in pregnancy, 2428, 2428t
postoperative, 939
Thrombospondin, in malignant glioma, 762
Thromboxane A
in cerebral vasospasm, 1849
synthesis of, 2959
Thrombus
in recurrent carotid artery stenosis, 1662
vertebrobasilar, 1697
^{3}H-Thymidine, as tumor proliferation marker, 692
Thyroid artery, in carotid endarterectomy, 1632–1633
Thyroid gland, metastatic carcinoma of, to skull, 1392, 1392f
Thyroid-stimulating hormone, in pituitary adenoma, 1200
Tiagabine, 2470t, 2472
Tibial nerve, 653
Tibial nerve (Continued)
distal, entrapment of, 3935–3936
surgery on
at tarsal tunnel, 655, 655f
in leg, 654–655
positioning for, 608–609
Tibialis anterior muscle, 653
Tibialis posterior muscle, 653
Tic douloureux. *See* Trigeminal neuralgia.
Tickle, in pediatric sensory testing, 3183
Ticlopidine
for carotid artery disease, 1617
in pregnancy, 2423
Tics, 2721–2722
definition of, 2729–2730
pediatric, assessment of, 3179
Tight junctions
actin-myosin interaction in, 156
between endothelial cells, 155–156
electrical resistance of, 156–157
in blood-brain barrier, 156, 159f, 792
paracellular pathways of, 15
proteins associated with, 156
Tinel's sign, 3825, 3925
in ulnar nerve entrapment, 3903–3904
Tingling, 3831
Tinnitus
in dural arteriovenous fistula, 2172
in dural arteriovenous malformation, 2283, 2284
Tirilazad mesylate, for cerebral vasospasm, 1853–1854
Tissue plasminogen activator
criteria for, 1498, 1499t, 1500
dosage in, 1500, 1500t
for intracerebral hemorrhage, 1753
for intraventricular hemorrhage, 1824
for stroke, 1495
hemorrhagic complications of, 1500, 1735
lubeluzole with, 1498
protocol for, 1500t
subarachnoid blood clot fibrolysis with, 1852
thrombolytics for, 1727
trials for, 1496, 1497t
Titanium cage, in transthoracic decompression, 4974, 4975–4978, 4975f
Tizanidine
for cerebral palsy, 3731
for multiple sclerosis, 1454t
for spasticity, 2866t, 2868
TNP-470, angiosuppressive therapy with, 778–779
Toad64, 55t
Tobacco
bone health and, 4233–4234
brain tumors and, 810
in aneurysm rupture, 1790
in carotid artery stenosis, 1661
in familial intracranial aneurysms, 1776
in spinal fusion healing, 4619–4620
in stroke risk, 1616
surgery and, 549
Tocopherol deficiency, neuropathy from, 3844
Tolcapone, for Parkinson's disease, 2733
Tolosa-Hunt syndrome, orbit in, 1376
Tomography, spinal, 505
Tong traction, for cervical spine trauma, 4891–4892, 4892f, 4900
Tongue, pediatric, evaluation of, 3176
Tonic labyrinthine reflex, in cerebral palsy, 3725, 3726t

Tonic neck reflex
in cerebral palsy, 3725, 3726t
testing of, 3182
Tonsillar herniation, 826t, 827, 5055t, 5056, 5091, 5092f
in Chiari malformation type I, 3349, 3350f
Tonsils, 31f, 32
superior pole of, 33f
Topectomy, 2629–2633
anesthesia for, 2632
cortical stimulation during, 2632–2633
electrocorticography during, 2632
evaluation before, 2630–2632
outcome in, 2633, 2633t
patient selection for, 2629–2630
principles of, 2632
technique of, 2633
Topiramate, 2470t, 2472
Topoisomerase inhibitors, 882
Torcular Herophili
meningioma of, 1276
venous drainage of, 1266
Torticollis, 2729
atlas assimilation in, 3340
clinical forms of, 2891–2893, 2892f–2894f, 2895, 2896t
craniovertebral junction abnormalities in, 3334
rotatory, 2892, 2892f, 2896t
spasmodic, 2891–2899
electromyography of, 2895
physiopathology of, 2891
selective peripheral denervation for, 2897–2898
indications for, 2895
results of, 2898–2899, 2898t, 2899t
surgical techniques for, 7–8, 2896t
tumor-related, 4835
Touch, testing of, pediatric, 3183
Touch receptors, 73–74, 74f
Tourette's syndrome, obsessive-compulsive disorder in, 2854–2855
Toxins
neuropathy from, 3832t, 3843–3844
parkinsonism from, 2716
peripheral nerve effects of, 3816
Tp53
in cell cycle control, 820–821
in gliomas, 950–951
in malignant glioma, 969–970
Trace elements, in angiogenesis, 775t
Traction
cervical, 4891–4892, 4892f, 4900
peripheral nerve injury from, 3827
Traction response, testing of, 3182
Tractotomy, midbrain. *See* Midbrain, tractotomy of.
TRAIL, in astrocytoma immunotherapy, 894
Tramadol
for diabetic neuropathy, 3838
for failed back syndrome, 4336
for pain, 2964
Tranexamic acid, in pregnancy, 2424
Transcranial Doppler ultrasonography, 1540–1555
diagnosis with, 1543–1544, 1544f
during carotid endarterectomy, 1548–1550
examination techniques in, 1541–1543, 1541f–1543f, 1542t
flow velocity recording in, 1543–1544
historical aspects of, 1540–1541, 1542t
neurosurgical applications of, 1545–1554
Transcranial Doppler ultrasonography *(Continued)*
of aneurysms, 1548, 1549f
of arteriovenous malformation, 1547–1548
of brain death, 1553–1554
of cerebral vasospasm, 1545–1546, 1545t, 1850–1851
of cerebrovascular disease, 1554–1555
of emboli, 1544
of head injury, 1550–1552, 1551f
of increased intracranial pressure, 1552–1553, 1553f
of stroke, 1554–1555
of subarachnoid hemorrhage, 1545–1546, 1545t
predictive value of, 1547, 1548f
principles of, 1541–1544, 1544f
Transcription factors, 51, 743–744, 4252–4253
Transferrin
in cerebrospinal fluid fistula, 5269
transcytosis of, through blood-brain barrier, 163
Transforming growth factor, in stroke, 142
Transforming growth factor-α, in brain tumors, 726
Transforming growth factor-β
in astrocytoma treatment, 891, 892
in bone, 4609, 4614–4615
in brain tumors, 730–731
in cerebral ischemia, 140
Transfusion reaction, 564
Transgenic mice, 714
Transient ischemic attacks, 1623–1624, 1624f
carotid artery disease and, 1613, 1614–1615, 1614t
definition of, 1495–1496
in moyamoya, 1716
magnetic resonance angiography of, 1576f
positron emission tomography of, 2478
presentation of, 1624
single-photon emission computed tomography of, 2478
stroke in, 1624
thromboembolism and, 1623–1624, 1624f
Transitional (schneiderian) carcinoma, paranasal sinus, 1312
Transplantation, 2829, 2829t
central nervous system, 2829–2847, 2829t
adrenal medulla tissue in, 2831
brain death and, 395–396, 395t, 403, 403t
disease pathophysiology in, 2844
gene therapy trials in, 2844–2845
historical aspects of, 2829
intracerebral, 2843
neural cells in, 93, 94f
neurotrophic factors in, 2843–2844
Parkinson's disease treatment with, 2830–2843. *See also* Fetal tissue transplantation.
porcine xenografts for, 2841
retinal-pigmented epithelial cells for, 2841
retroviral vectors in, 2845–2846, 2845t
stem cells for, 2841, 2843
terminology for, 2829, 2830t
tissue sources for, 2841–2843
embryonic tissue, 4158, 4159
fetal tissue. *See* Fetal tissue transplantation.
glial cellular, 4161–4163
Transplantation *(Continued)*
inflammatory cell, 4164
Transtentorial herniation, 826
Transverse crest, 40f
Transverse ligament, in atlas fracture, 4933, 4934, 4935
Transverse sinus, thrombosis of, 1421
magnetic resonance angiography of, 1597, 1597f
Trapezius muscle, pediatric, 3176
Trapidil, for meningioma, 1110
Trauma
aneurysms from. *See* Aneurysms, traumatic.
brain tumors and, 810–811
cellular basis of, 5025–5033
cerebral venous thrombosis from, 1723
cerebrovascular. *See* Cerebrovascular injury, traumatic.
cranial destruction in, 430
craniofacial. *See* Craniofacial trauma.
death due to, central nervous system injury and, 5095
in pediatric lumbar disk herniation, 3560
magnetic resonance imaging of, 469
open, peripheral nerve injury in, 3820
pediatric, surgery for, 3195–3196
peripheral nerve injury in, evaluation of, 3819–3820
positron emission tomography of, 2481
recovery from, 5025–5033
resuscitation for, 5087–5089
primary survey in, 5087–5088, 5088t
secondary survey in, 5088–5089
single-photon emission computed tomography of, 2481
spinal, 4148–4149, 4307–4308, 4308f
cervical, 4885–4910
lumbar, 4702–4704, 4731, 4732t
thoracic, 4951–4982
spondylolisthesis from, 3573–3574
to brain. *See* Brain injury, traumatic.
Trauma team, 5087
Traumatic Coma Data Bank, 5019, 5103
Traumatic far-out syndrome, 5012
Traumatic spondylolisthesis, 4546
Treatment, legal obligations for, 408
Tremor
action, 2729
cerebellar, 2778–2779
classification of, 2750
definition of, 2729
differential diagnosis of, 2750t
environmental exposure and, 2750
essential, 2731, 2750, 2776–2778
deep brain stimulation for, 2820
mechanism of, 2772f, 2776
thalamotomy for, 2776–2777, 2777f, 2777t
results of, 2777–2778
ventral intermedius nucleus stimulation for, 2821
in Parkinson's disease, 2732
intention, 2750
kinetic, 2750
parkinsonian. *See* Parkinson's disease, tremor in.
pediatric, assessment of, 3179–3180
resting, 2729, 2750
senile, 2750
subthalamic nucleus stimulation for, 2822
surgery for, 2748, 2750, 2803
thalamotomy for, 2769–2780
vs. thalamic deep brain stimulation, 2780

Tremor *(Continued)*
ventral intermedius nucleus stimulation for, 2820–2821
Triage, 5095–5096
Tricarboxylic acid (TCA) cycle, glutamate in, 104f–105f, 106
Triceps reflex testing, pediatric, 3180
Trichogenic tumors, scalp, 1415
Tricyclic antidepressants
for failed back syndrome, 4337
for pain, 2960, 2966
mechanisms of, 2964
side effects of, 2964
Trigeminal brainstem nuclear complex, 2930–2931, 2933f
Trigeminal nerve, 29, 1975
anatomy of, 1343–1344, 2996–2997, 3048
descending tractotomy of, 3052–3053
disorders of, eye examination in, 302, 304, 304f
divisions of, cutaneous distribution of, 2926, 2927f
examination of, 266
first division of, 1899
glycerol rhizotomy of, 2999–3000
in sarcoidosis, 1436
injury to, acoustic neuroma surgery and, 570–571
microvascular decompression of, 3003, 3005–3014
care after, 3013–3014
complications of, 3013, 3014t
historical aspects of, 3005
neurophysiology before, 3007
outcome of, 3010–3013, 3011t, 3012f
patient history for, 3006
patient selection for, 3005–3006
physical examination for, 3006–3007, 3007t
technique of, 3007–3010, 3008f–3010f
vascular findings in, 3013, 3013t
nucleotomy of, 3053
pediatric, examination of, 3175
schwannoma of. *See* Schwannoma, trigeminal.
somatosensory evoked potentials of, during nucleus caudalis ablation, 3051
stereotactic tractotomy of, 3081
thermal rhizotomy of, 2997–2999, 2998f, 2999f
tractotomy of, 3085–3086
complications of, 3086
vessels compressing, 3013, 3013t
Trigeminal neuralgia, 2987
atypical, 2988
cause of, 2987–2988, 2997
diagnosis of, 2987–2988, 2996
differential diagnosis of, 2988, 2988t
distribution of, 3007, 3007t
epidemiology of, 2988
glycerol rhizotomy for, 3006
historical aspects of, 2913, 3005
medical treatment of, 2989–2994, 2989f
anticonvulsants in, 2990, 2990t, 2996
antidepressants in, 2990, 2991t
approach to, 2994
drugs in, 2991–2994
mechanism of, 2991
neuroleptics in, 2990–2991
opioids in, 2991
microvascular decompression for, 3005–3014. *See also* Trigeminal nerve, microvascular decompression of.
patient history for, 2987
Trigeminal neuralgia *(Continued)*
percutaneous treatment of, 2997–3003
balloon compression in, 3000–3002, 3001f
glycerol rhizotomy in, 2999–3000
microvascular decompression in, numbness and, 3003
peripheral neurectomy in, 3003
thermal rhizotomy in, 2997–2999, 2998f, 2999f
radiofrequency gasserian lesions of, 3006
radiosurgery for, 3002–3003, 4091–4092, 4092t, 4093f
stereotactic radiosurgery for, 3006, 3020–3021
surgery for
alternative treatments in, 3017–3021, 3018t
neurotomy procedures in, 3018–3020, 3019f, 3020f
partial sensory rhizotomy in, 3017–3018
surgical procedures for, 3006
Trigeminal neurinoma, central skull base, 1267
Trigeminal neuropathic pain, 2989t
Trigeminal nucleus, 2926, 2926f, 3085
Trigeminal point, 38
Trigone, 1237, 1238f
arteriovenous malformation of, 2240–2241, 2240f, 2241f
tumors of, 1242–1243
Trihexyphenidyl, for dystonia, 2796
Triple wire technique
in laminoforaminotomy, with posterior spinal fusion, 4416, 4416f, 4417f
in posterior cervical fusion, 4645–4646, 4647f–4648f
Triple-H therapy, for cerebral vasospasm, 1547
Trisomy 13, myelomeningocele with, 3219
Trisomy 18, myelomeningocele with, 3219
Trisomy 21
atlantoaxial instability in, 3543
craniovertebral junction abnormalities in, 3334, 3337–3338, 3338f
Triton tumor, 3953
Trochlear nerve, 36f, 316, 316f, 1344, 1899, 1975
examination of, 266
pediatric, 3173, 3174
palsy of, 319f, 320, 320f
True negative, 497
True positive, 497
Trunk pain, surgery for, 3026t
Tryosine hydroxylase, in akinetic-rigid Parkinson's disease, 2707
T-saw, in chordoma en bloc excision, 4848
TSC1, 55t, 744
TSC2, 742
TSRH universal spine instrumentation system, 4969, 4970f
Tuber, 34
Tuber cinereum, 14f
Tuberculoma, central nervous system, 1440–1441, 1442f
treatment of, 1443
Tuberculosis, 1439–1443
clinical presentation of, 1440
diagnosis of, 1440–1441, 1442f
pathogenesis of, 1440
pediatric, spondylitis in, 3566
reporting obligations in, 411–412
spinal, 4386–4387
pain in, 4293–4295, 4294f
treatment of, 1441, 1443
Tuberculum sellae
anatomy of, 1266
meningioma of, 1116–1118, 1117f
surgical approach to, 1276
Tuberous sclerosis
brain tumors in, 811–812, 812t
foramen of Monro giant cell astrocytoma in, 3391f
malignant glioma in, 969
subependymal giant cell astrocytoma in, 991–992, 992f
Tubulin, in axonal regeneration, 197
Tumor(s)
angiogenesis-dependent growth of, 773
axial skeleton
benign, 4295, 4296t, 4297–4298
malignant, 4296t, 4298–4299, 4299f
recumbency/nighttime pain associated with, 4295, 4296t, 4297–4298
endoscopic biopsy of, 3430
growth of, control of, 774t
inclusion, 3689–3690
classification of, 3689t
neuropathy from, 3844–3845
radiosurgery for, 4053–4069
removal of, 905–906
surgery for, in neonates, 3194–3195, 3194t
vs. lumbar spinal stenosis, 4527
Tumor antigens, 887, 889f
identification of, 674
vaccines using, 893
Tumor cells
as vaccines, 892–893
invasion by, 720
Tumor dormancy, 774t
Tumor markers, for pineal region tumors, 1014, 1014t
Tumor necrosis factor, in astrocytoma immunotherapy, 894–895
Tumor necrosis factor-α
in brain injury recovery, 5031
in cerebral ischemia, 139
in immunotherapy, 684–685
in multiple sclerosis, 1450
in stroke, 142
in traumatic brain injury, 5029
Tumor suppressor genes, 739–744
apoptosis regulators as, 743
as cell cycle regulators, 741
candidate, 741–744, 742f
cellular signaling proteins as, 741–743
evidence for, 739
identification of, 740–741
in brain tumors, 739–744
in gene therapy, 820–821
transcriptional regulators as, 743–744
Tumor-associated edema, 13
Tumor-brain barrier, in chemotherapy, 878
Tuning fork tests, 330
Tunnel of Corti, 328, 328f
Turcot's syndrome
brain tumors in, 812t, 813
malignant glioma in, 969
medulloblastoma in, 997, 3639
Twining projection, in cervical spine radiography, 4894
Twining's line, 423, 423f, 424–425, 424f
Twins, brain tumors in, 811
Twist, 55t
Tympanic membrane
in sound transmission, 328f, 329
in temporal bone fracture, 5280, 5281
Tympanometry, 333–334

Tympanum, transformer mechanism of, 329–330
Tyrosine kinase receptors, in glioma, 715

U74006F, for cerebral vasospasm, 1848
Ulcer(s)
ependymoma surgery and, 3630
mucosal, after aneurysmal subarachnoid hemorrhage, 1831
stress, in traumatic brain injury, 5129
Ulnar artery, innervation of, 3898
Ulnar nerve
anatomy of, 3897–3898, 3925
anomalous motor connections of, 3898
at elbow, 3900–3901
autonomous zones of, 3824
blood supply to, 3898–3899
entrapment of, 3925–3928
elbow-level, 3897–3917, 3926–3928
anterior transmuscular transposition for, 3912, 3913f
causes of, 3879, 3901–3903, 3902f
decompression of, 3909–3910
diagnosis of, 3879, 3903–3905, 3904f, 3905f, 3905t
electrodiagnosis of, 3905–3906
evaluation of, 3906, 3906f–3908f, 3908
flexion-pressure test for, 3904, 3905f
grading of, 3927
historical aspects of, 3897
intramuscular transposition for, 3911–3912
magnetic resonance imaging of, 3879f, 3880
medial epicondylectomy for, 3910–3911
nerve stimulators for, 3916, 3916f
neurolysis for, 3915–3916
pain evaluation in, 3906, 3906f–3908f, 3908
physical examination for, 3903, 3904f
points of, 3902, 3902f
recurrent, 3914–3915
results in, 3914, 3914t
secondary transmuscular transposition for, 3915
staging of, 3905t
subcutaneous transposition for, 3911
submuscular transposition for, 3911
surgery for, 3909–3912, 3913f, 3927–3928
medial antebrachial cutaneous nerve injury in, 3899
Tinel's sign in, 3903–3904
treatment of, 3879–3880, 3908–3909, 3909f
space-occupying lesions and, 3903
wrist-level, 3925–3926, 3928
hypermobility of, at elbow, 3903
injury to
positioning and, 612
surgery and, 3903
pseudoneuroma of, plexus formation and, 3903
sensory distribution of, 3898
subluxation of, 3903
surgery on, 652
historical aspects of, 3897, 3898t
Ulnar neuritis, post-traumatic, 3897
Ulnar neuropathy, elbow-level, 3822
needle electromyography of, 3859
nerve conduction studies of, 3858–3859
Ultrasonography, 1561–1567
A-mode, 1562, 1562f
B-mode, 1561–1562, 1563f
boundary separation in, 1565
diagnosis with, 1565–1567, 1566f
Doppler shift in, 1562, 1564f, 1565f
duplex
carotid artery, vs. angiography, 1566–1567
spectral analysis in, 1562–1565, 1564f, 1565f
intraoperative, 1567
in transthoracic decompression, 4978, 4978f
physics of, 1561–1565
sound wave properties in, 1561, 1561f
spinal, 506
transcranial Doppler. *See* Transcranial Doppler ultrasonography.
Uncal herniation, 826, 826t, 1504
Uncal notch, 25, 26f
Uncal recess, 11, 12f
Uncinate fasciculus, 6, 7f
Uncinate gyrus, 26f
Uncinate processes, pediatric, 3515
Unconsciousness, 282, 282t
Uncus, 4f, 12f, 15f, 18f, 22f, 24f, 25
Uniform Anatomical Gift Act, 415–416
Uniform Determination of Death Act, 394
Uniform Parkinson's Disease Rating Scale, 242t, 268
Universal segmental fixation systems
for thoracic spine fractures, 4969–4972, 4970f–4972f
thoracic spine biomechanics and, 4195
Urea, intracranial pressure and, 189
Urethra, 358
Urethral sphincter
mechanisms of, 358f, 359
pharmacologic relaxation of, 380
smooth muscle, 359, 359f
spinal cord control of, 360, 360f
striated muscle, 359
Urinary frequency, 365, 365f
Urinary incontinence
in cerebral palsy, 3728, 3732, 3744–3745
intrinsic sphincteric dysfunction and, 366
neurological disorders and, 365–366
of nonresistance, 366
outlet-based, 380–381
overflow, 366
paradoxical, 366
sphincteric mechanisms in, 358f, 359
stress, 366
total, 366
treatment of, 378–379
behavioral, 378
minimally invasive, 379
pharmacologic, 378–379
surgical, 379
urge, 359, 366
Urinary retention
neurogenic outlet dysfunction and, treatment of, 379–380
reduction cystoplasty for, 378
treatment of, 376–378, 377t
behavioral methods for, 376–377
minimally invasive, 377–378
pharmacologic, 377
reflex contractions in, 377
surgical, 378
Urinary tract, 357–381
anatomy of, 357–363
central nervous system centers for, 359–360, 359f, 360f
Urinary tract *(Continued)*
in spinal cord injury management, 4881
lower
functional arcs of, 360–363
neuroanatomy of, 359
neuromuscular function of, 363
neurophysiology of, 359
parasympathetic nervous system in, 361–362, 362f
pudendal system arcs in, 362, 362f, 363f
spinal tracts in, 362–363, 363f
supraspinal arcs of, 360–361
sympathetic nervous system in, 361, 361f
neurological disorders of
associated conditions in, 366–367
basal ganglia lesions and, 373
bedside urodynamic tests for, 370
bowel habits in, 366
cerebellar lesions and, 373–374
cerebral cortex lesions and, 373
classification of, 363–364
demyelinating lesions and, 375
denervation and, 375
electromyography in, 371–372, 372f
endoscopy for, 368
evaluation of, 364–373
filling cystometry in, 368–369, 369f
filling dysfunction symptoms in, 364–365, 365f
history of, 364–367
incontinence in, 365–366
laboratory tests for, 367–368
lumbar disk disease and, 375
neuropathy and, 375
peripheral lesions and, 375
physical examination of, 367, 367f
radiologic studies for, 368
reflex testing in, 367, 367f
sacral lesions and, 374
sexual dysfunction in, 366
spinal dysraphism and, 374–375
spinal lesions and, 374–375
storage dysfunction symptoms in, 364–365, 365f
suprasacral lesions and, 374
supraspinal lesions and, 373–374
treatment of, 375–381, 377t
urethral pressure profiles in, 370–371, 372f
urodynamic studies in, 368–373
uroflowmetry in, 370, 371f
videourodynamics in, 373
voiding cystometry in, 369–370, 370f
voiding dysfunction symptoms in, 365
neurophysiology of, 357–363
Urine storage, 363
Urine volume, postvoid residual, in urologic disorders, 367
Urokinase
for cerebral venous thrombosis, 1727, 1727t
for intracerebral hemorrhage, 1753
thrombolytics for, 1727
Uterine blood flow, in pregnancy, 2421
Utricle, 339, 339f
Utricular macula, 339, 339f
Uvula, 31f, 33f, 34

Vaccines
tumor cells as, 892–893
using tumor antigens, 893
Vaccinia virus, as vector, 818

Vagal triangle, 33f
Vagus nerve, 1973–1974
anatomy of, 2643
examination of, 267
pediatric, 3176
palsy of, glomus jugulare tumors and, 1306
stimulation of
adverse effects of, 2644
clinical experience with, 2644
components for, 2645–2647, 2646f, 2647f
device implantation for, 2647–2649, 2648f
complications of, 2649–2650
mechanism of, 2644
patient selection for, 2645
seizure outcome with, 2579
vs. other therapies, 2644–2645
Validity, 239
Valproate, 2470–2471, 2470t
Valproic acid, in pregnancy, 2422
Valves, cerebrospinal fluid shunt, 3376–3379, 3377f–3379f, 3381–3382
VanGilder's modified Klaus height index line, 424f, 425
Vanilloid receptor type 1, in heat transduction, 2918–2919
Varices, in supratentorial arteriovenous malformation, 2231
Vasa nervorum, 3899
Vascular accidents, vertigo in, 352
Vascular anomalies, pediatric, 3195
Vascular claudication, vs. neurogenic claudication, 4527
Vascular disease
cranial destruction in, 430
magnetic resonance imaging of, 466–467, 468f, 469
preoperative evaluation for, 552–554, 552t, 553t
Vascular endothelial growth factor
angiogenic growth factors and, 780
in angiogenesis, 719, 731, 771, 773
in angiosuppressive gene therapy, 783
in arteriovenous malformations, 3452
in astrocytes, 110
in brain tumors, 731, 733
Vascular endothelial growth factor receptors, in brain tumors, 733
Vascular lesions
spinal cord, classification of, 2363–2364, 2363t, 2364t
transsphenoidal surgery and, 1182
Vascular malformations
capillary telangiectasia with, 2176
classification of, 2159, 2160t
intradural, arteriovenous shunt in, 2379
magnetic resonance angiography of, 1593, 1595f, 1596, 1596f
magnetic resonance imaging of, 469–472, 470f–472f
natural history of, 2159–2176
occult, in epilepsy, 2491
spinal
imaging of, 536–537, 538f, 539f
intradural, 2379
syndromic, 2154–2155
Vascular permeability factor/vascular endothelial growth factor (VPF/VEGF), in brain edema, 793, 795, 801
Vascular phenotype, switch to, 773, 774t
Vasculitic neuropathy, 3844
Vasculitis
anterior ischemic optic neuropathy in, 306
Vasculitis *(Continued)*
peripheral nerve involvement in, 3962
radiation, chiasmatic, 314f
thoracic endoscopic sympathectomy for, 3097
vs. multiple sclerosis, 1453, 1453t
Vasculopathy, post–subarachnoid hemorrhage. *See* Vasospasm.
Vasoactive agents, in blood-brain permeability, 11
Vasoactive intestinal peptide, after axonal transection, 3967
Vasoconstriction
in cerebral vasospasm, 1848
intracranial pressure reduction by, 5057–5058
Vasogenic edema, in malignant phenotype, 771, 772f
Vasomotor reactivity, transcranial Doppler ultrasonography of, 1554–1555
Vasomotor reserve, transcranial Doppler ultrasonography of, 1554, 1555
Vasospasm, 1839–1859
aneurysm rupture and, 1799
aneurysm treatment and, 1842
angiographic, 1839, 1839f
arterial wall changes in, 1844–1845, 1845f, 1846f
arteriovenous malformations and, 1841
calcium channel blockers for, 1852–1853, 1854f
cerebral blood volume in, 5046
clinical, 1839
computed tomography angiography of, 1851, 1851f
definition of, 1839
diagnosis of, 1850
eicosanoids in, 1848–1849
endothelin in, 1849
endovascular reversal of, 1855–1856
epidemiology of, 1841–1842, 1841f, 1842t
etiology of, 1845
experimental models of, 1842, 1843t, 1844
extracellular collagen lattice contraction in, 1847–1848
fluid management in, 1852
historical perspective on, 1840
hyperdynamic therapy for, 1855
hypertension for, 1855
hypervolemia for, 1855
immune system in, 1847
in aneurysms, 1841
in arteriovenous malformation, 1841
in arteriovenous malformation resection, 2189, 2191f
in brain tumors, 1841
in pediatric aneurysms, 3451
in pregnancy, 2425–2426
in traumatic brain injury, 5109t, 5110t, 5111–5112, 5137
incidence of, 1841, 1841f
inflammation in, 1847
intra-aortic balloon counterpulsation for, 1855
magnetic resonance imaging of, 1851
neurogenic factors in, 1849
nitric oxide in, 1849
papaverine for, 1856, 1856f, 1857
pathogenesis of, 1846–1849, 1846t, 1847f
pathology of, 1844–1845, 1845f, 1846f
percutaneous transluminal balloon angioplasty for, 1856–1857, 1857f, 1858f
perimesencephalic subarachnoid hemorrhage and, 1842
Vasospasm *(Continued)*
pharmacologic prevention of, 1853–1854
postpartum, 2429
post-traumatic, 1840–1841
transcranial Doppler ultrasonography of, 1552
prevention of, 1852–1855, 1853f, 1854f, 1854t
approach to, 1857, 1859, 1859f
proliferative mechanisms in, 1847
reversal of, 1855–1859, 1855t
risk factors for, 1841–1842, 1842t
signs/symptoms of, 1849–1850
single-photon emission computed tomography of, 1851, 2478
structural theories of, 1847–1848
subarachnoid blood clot management in, 1852, 1853f
subarachnoid hemorrhage and, 1841, 1841f, 1842
single-photon emission computed tomography of, 2479–2480
transcranial Doppler ultrasonography of, 1545–1547, 1545t, 1546f, 1547f, 2479–2480
traumatic, 5046–5047, 5047t
symptomatic, 1839
transcranial Doppler ultrasonography of, 1850–1851
traumatic subarachnoid hemorrhage and, 5046–5047, 5047t
treatment of, 1855–1859, 1855t
approach to, 1857, 1859, 1859f
vessel effects of, 1547
triple-H therapy for, 1855
vasoconstriction in, 1848
xenon-enhanced computed tomography of, 1851
VATER association, lipomatous filum terminale in, 3264
Vectors, for central nervous system gene therapy, 4166
Vegetative state
permanent, 393
persistent, 284, 285t
Vein(s), occlusion of, hemorrhagic stroke from, 935, 935f
Vein grafts, for middle vertebral artery, 1703, 1705f
Vein of Galen, 14f, 15f, 24f, 34, 36f, 1239
anatomy of, 3433–3434, 3434f
malformations of, 3433–3444
angiographic classification of, 3436–3437, 3436f, 3437f
arteriovenous shunt in, 3434–3435
choroidal, 3436
classification of, 3434
clinical classification of, 3435, 3435f
diagnosis of, 3437–3438
embryology of, 3434
historical aspects of, 3433–3434
hydrocephalus in, 3442, 3442f, 3443
imaging of, 3437–3438, 3438f, 3439f
natural history of, 3438, 3440f, 3441, 3441f
outcomes in, 3444
parenchymal injury in, 3440f, 3441
partially treated, 3438, 3440f, 3441
pathophysiology of, 3434–3435
thrombosis of, 3441, 3441f
transtorcular embolization of, 3443–3444, 3444f
treatment of, 3441–3444, 3442f, 3444f
with macrocephaly, 2216f
Vein of Labbé, 17, 24f

Vein of Trolard, 17
Velum interpositum, 13
Vena cava, superior, occlusion of, 3398f
Veno-occlusive disease, cerebral, magnetic resonance angiography of, 1596–1597, 1597f
Venous air embolism, 563
  posterior fossa surgery and, 555
Venous angioma. *See* Developmental venous anomalies.
Venous bypass
  of distal vertebral artery, 1708f, 1709
  of proximal vertebral artery, 1700, 1701f
  saphenous vein, for giant/fusiform aneurysms, 2118
Venous malformations. *See* Developmental venous anomalies.
Venous occlusion, in pregnancy, 2428t
Venous outflow resistance, in intracranial pressure management, 5126–5127
Venous sinuses
  depressed skull fracture over, 5170, 5171f
  laceration of, 5211
  meningioma of, 567–568
  occlusion of, 5214
  trauma to, diagnosis of, 5215–5216
Ventilation
  in spinal cord injury, 557
  in traumatic brain injury, 5128
Ventral derotation spondylodesis, 4684
Ventricle(s)
  asymmetrical, after shunts, 3400, 3401f
  bullet wounds to, 5229–5230, 5236
  catheters in, 3379–3380, 3380f
    endoscopic positioning of, 3428, 3429f
    obstruction of, 3382–3383
  cysts of, endoscopic management of, 3429
  fibrinolysis in, for infantile posthemorrhagic hydrocephalus, 3411
  fourth. *See* Fourth ventricle.
  glioma of, endoscopic treatment of, 3429, 3429f
  hemorrhage into, 5047
    aneurysm rupture and, 1799
    from germinal matrix, 3405, 3406f. *See also* Hydrocephalus, infantile posthemorrhagic.
      injury pattern in, 3407, 3407f
      neuropathology from, 3407–3408
      pathogenesis of, 3406f, 3407
      severity of, 3408, 3408t
    pediatric, 3463
  hemorrhagic infarction of, 3407, 3407f
  in Chiari malformation type I, 3348
  in Chiari malformation type II, 3350
  lateral. *See* Lateral ventricle.
  meningioma of, 1113
  surgery effects on, 549
  third. *See* Third ventricle.
  tumors of, 1237–1261
Ventricular access devices, for infantile posthemorrhagic hydrocephalus, 3412f, 3413–3414
Ventricular cavity, 19
Ventricular shunts. *See* Shunts.
Ventricular tap, for infantile posthemorrhagic hydrocephalus, 3412f, 3413
Ventricular vein, 17
  inferior, 24f, 1239
Ventricular zone, 79f, 80, 97
Ventriculitis
  foramen of Monro obstruction from, 3390
  imaging of, 3421, 3421f
Ventriculocranial ratio, in aneurysmal subarachnoid hemorrhage, 1823–1824, 1823t, 1824f
Ventriculography, anterior/posterior commissure localization with, 2770
Ventriculostomy, 5150, 5151f–5152f
  endoscopic, 3429–3430
    for aqueduct of Sylvius obstruction, 3393–3394
  in achondroplasia, 3367
  in brain relaxation, 1872
  in germ cell tumors, 3608
  in traumatic brain injury surgery, 5150, 5151f–5152f
VentroFix system, 4684, 4685f, 4718–4719, 4719f, 4720f
Verbal Fluency Test, 5186
Verbal response, in Glasgow Coma Scale, 286t, 287
Vermian vein, 35f
Vermohemispheric fissure, 34
Verocay bodies, 3942
Vertebra(e)
  anomalies of, in occult spinal dysraphism, 3262, 3263f
  biomechanics of, 4184–4185
  cervical, 4432
  compression fracture of, metastases and, 531, 531f
  compression of, cervical spine injury and, 4917
  congenital dislocation of, 4279–4280, 4280f
  disordered alignment of, 4279–4280, 4280f
  disordered formation of, 4278–4279, 4278f
  disordered segmentation of, 4279, 4279f
  limbus, pediatric, 3564–3565
  limbus fracture of, in lumbar spinal stenosis, 4531
  malignancies of, pediatric, 3567
  metastases to, imaging of, 531, 531f
  occipital, 3333, 3338, 3339f
  osteomyelitis of, pain in, 4290–4291, 4292f
  thoracic, reconstruction of, 4767, 4768f, 4769
Vertebra plana, 4809
  in eosinophilic granuloma, 4843, 4845f
Vertebral artery, 36f, 37
  anatomy of, 1973–1974
  aneurysms of
    clinical significance of, 2007–2008
    diagnosis of, 2013–2014
    endovascular occlusion of, 2019, 2020–2021
    presentation of, 2009, 2010t–2012t, 2013, 2013f
    rupture of, 2008
    subarachnoid hemorrhage in, 2013, 2013f
    surgery for, 2014–2019, 2015f
      complications of, 2019–2020
      evaluation before, 2014
      far lateral suboccipital approach in, 2015, 2017f
      outcome of, 2020
      transfacial transclival approach in, 2015–2016, 2016f, 2017f
    treatment indications in, 2008–2009
Vertebral artery *(Continued)*
  atherosclerosis of, magnetic resonance angiography of, 1590, 1591f
  cervical, 4310–4311
  dissecting aneurysms of
    rupture of, 2008
    surgery for, 2019, 2019f
  dissection of, magnetic resonance angiography of, 1590–1591, 1592f
  distal, 1693, 1693f
    approaches to, 1706, 1707f, 1712t
    decompression of, 1709
    diseases of, surgery for, 1706, 1707f, 1708f, 1709–1710, 1710f, 1711f
    external carotid artery bypass to, 1706, 1708f, 1709–1710, 1711f
    occipital bypass to, 1709
    reconstruction of, 1706, 1708f, 1709
    stenosis of, 1709, 1710f
    vein bypass from, 1708f, 1709
  extracranial
    anatomy of, 1692–1693, 1693f
    arteriovenous fistula of, 1694
    atherosclerosis of, 1694
    compression of, 1694
    critical stenosis of, 1693
    diseases of, 1691–1712
      angiography of, 1691
      audiometry for, 1695
      brain imaging of, 1695–1696
      causes of, 1693–1694, 1694f
      cerebral angiography of, 1696
      diagnosis of, 1695–1696
      embolic causes in, 1694–1695, 1697
      endovascular treatment of, 1697, 1698f
      hemodynamic evaluation in, 1696
      history of, 1695
      laboratory tests for, 1695
      medical treatment of, 1696–1697, 1711
      outcome in, 1711–1712, 1712t
      pathophysiology of, 1693–1695
      physical examination of, 1695
      reconstruction procedures for, 1691–1692
      surgery for, 1697–1711
      symptoms of, 1692, 1692t
      vestibular tests for, 1695
    penetrating injury to, 1692
    spontaneous dissections of, 1694
    subclavian steal syndrome of, 1694, 1694f
    trauma to, 1694
  fusiform aneurysms of, surgery for, 2019, 2019f
  middle, 1693, 1693f
    approaches to, 1703, 1704f, 1712t
    decompression of, 1703, 1705f
    diseases of, surgery for, 1702–1703, 1704f–1706f
    endarterectomy for, 1703, 1705f
    transposition of, to common carotid artery, 1703, 1705f
    vein grafts for, 1703, 1705f
  occlusion of, 2107
  positional obstruction of, transcranial Doppler ultrasonography of, 1555
  proximal, 1692–1693, 1693f
    approaches to, 1697–1698, 1699f, 1712t
    decompression of, 1700, 1702
    diseases of, surgery for, 1697–1698, 1699f, 1700, 1701f, 1702, 1702f
    subclavian-vertebral endarterectomy of, 1700, 1701f

Vertebral artery *(Continued)*
transposition of, to common carotid artery, 1700, 1701f, 1702f
vein grafts for, 1700, 1701f
trauma to
blunt, 5205–5206, 5206f, 5212, 5213f
penetrating, 5203, 5204
selective arterial embolization for, 5218–5219
surgery for, 5217
traumatic aneurysm of, 5207, 5207f–5208f
Vertebral body
biomechanics of, 4185
chondrosarcoma of, 4846
eosinophilic granuloma of, 4843
hemangioma of, 4354–4355, 4355f, 4837, 4840–4843, 4842f
imaging of, 532
pediatric, 3589–3590
metastases to, 4047, 4861
neoplasms of, vs. osteomyelitis, 540–541
osteophytes of, 509, 512f
pediatric, 3515
thoracic, 4953, 4953f, 4958, 4959f
burst fracture of, 4962, 4980
wedge compression fracture through, 4952, 4958, 4959f
wedge compression fracture through, 521, 521f
Vertebral centrum
aplasia of, 4281, 4281f
hypoplasia of, 4281, 4281f
Vertebral column
cervical, 4623f, 4624f
development of
abnormal, 4276–4281, 4276f–4281f
normal, 4271–4276, 4273f–4275f
trauma to, 4148–4149
pediatric, 3515–3553
tumors of, pediatric, 3587–3592
Vertebral trunk aneurysms, surgical approaches to, 1993–1997
extended far-lateral, 1995, 1996f, 1997
far-lateral, 1994–1995, 1996f
far-lateral combined supra-/infratentorial, 1997, 1998f–1999f
midline suboccipital, 1993–1994, 1994f
Vertebrectomy
complication avoidance in, 577, 580
for giant cell tumor, 4850
thoracic, 4975–4978
thoracoscopic, 4765–4769
Vertebrobasilar insufficiency
positron emission tomography of, 1602
symptoms of, 1692, 1692t
vertigo in, 352–353, 1692
Vertebrobasilar ischemia
dizziness in, 2901
medical treatment of, 1696–1697
Vertebrobasilar junction aneurysms
clinical significance of, 2007–2008
diagnosis of, 2013–2014
endovascular occlusion of, 2019
outcome of, 2020–2021
presentation of, 2009, 2010t–2012t, 2013
rupture of, 2008, 2009, 2013
surgery for, 2014–2019, 2015f
complications of, 2019–2020
evaluation before, 2014
far-lateral suboccipital approach in, 2015, 2017f
outcome of, 2020
Vertebrobasilar junction aneurysms *(Continued)*
subtemporal-presigmoid transtentorial approach in, 2016, 2018, 2018f
transfacial transclival approach in, 2015–2016, 2016f, 2017f
treatment indications in, 2008–2009
Vertigo, 275, 2901–2909
aminoglycosides for, 2906
audiometry in, 2904
benign paroxysmal positional, 275, 348–349, 2903
surgery for, 2907–2908
temporal bone fracture and, 5281
vestibular rehabilitation for, 2906–2907
causes of, 347t
central, 347–348, 348t, 351–353, 2901–2902
clinical features of, 2904
congenital anomalies and, 2902
definition of, 347
demyelination and, 2902
diagnosis of, 2904–2905
differential diagnosis of, 347–353
electronystagmography in, 2905
epilepsy and, 2902
episodic, temporal bone fracture and, 5281
imaging for, 2905
labyrinthitis and, 2903
medical treatment of, 2905–2906
Ménière's disease and, 349–350, 2902, 2903f
migraine and, 2901–2902
neurovascular decompression for, 2909
oscillopsia and, 2904
paraneoplastic syndrome and, 2902
perilymph fistula and, 2903–2904
peripheral, 347–351, 348t, 2902–2904
post-traumatic, 350
rotational chair testing in, 2905
surgery for, 2907–2909, 2909f
temporal bone fracture and, 5281
vertebrobasilar insufficiency and, 1692
vertebrobasilar ischemia and, 2901–2902
vestibular nerve section for, 2909, 2909f
vestibular neuritis and, 2902–2903
vestibular rehabilitation for, 2906–2907
vestibular suppressants for, 2905–2906
vestibular system in, 341–342
vestibular testing in, 2905
Vesicointestinal fissure, 3226
Vestibular apparatus, in temporal bone fracture, 5276, 5281–5282
Vestibular area, 33f, 34
Vestibular disorders
central, 2901–2902
classification of, 2901–2904
peripheral, vertigo in, 2902–2904
surgery for, 2907
Vestibular end-organs, innervation of, 329f
Vestibular examination, 267, 2905
pediatric, 3176
Vestibular labyrinth
bony, 338, 338f
membranous, 338–339, 339f, 340f
Vestibular nerve, 329f, 339
inferior, 40f
pediatric, examination of, 3175–3176
section of, 2909, 2909f
superior, 40f
Vestibular neurectomy, 353
Vestibular neuritis, 350
uncompensated, 2903
vertigo in, 2902–2903
Vestibular schwannoma
magnetic resonance imaging of, 459, 459f
radiosurgery for, 4055–4056, 4057t, 4058t, 4059f
linac, 4112
stereotactic radiation therapy for, 4030
Vestibular suppressants, for vertigo, 2905–2906
Vestibular system, 338–342
anatomy of, 338–339, 338f, 339f
blood supply of, 339
function of
bithermal caloric test of, 344–345, 344f
electronystagmography of, 343–346, 344f, 346f
gaze test of, 345
Hallpike maneuver and, 342, 343f, 345
in pediatric basilar skull fracture, 3468
labyrinthine fistula test of, 342
objective measurement of, 343–347
positional tests of, 342–343, 343f, 345
pursuit tests of, 345–346, 346f
rotation tests of, 346, 347f
saccade test of, 345
tests of, 342–347
visual-vestibular interaction and, 346–347
hair cells in, 339, 340–341, 340f
in motor reflexes, 340
in vertigo, 341–342
mechanical receptors for, 74
nystagmus and, 342
peripheral, 340–341, 340f, 341f
physiology of, 340–342, 340f, 341f
supranuclear connections in, 339
Vestibular-auditory nerve, examination of, 267
Vestibule, 338
Vestibulocochlear labyrinth
bony, 327
membranous, 327
sound transmission in, 330
Vestibulo-ocular reflex, 346–347
semicircular canals and, 341, 341f
VHL, 743
Vibration testing, pediatric, 3183
Video electroencephalogram monitoring, for pediatric epilepsy, 3760–3763, 3761f–3763f
Vincristine, 882
for ependymoma, 1048, 1048t
for Ewing's sarcoma, 4850
for malignant glioma, 976
Virchow-Robin space, magnetic resonance imaging of, 2495
Viruses
adeno-
as vectors, 818, 4166–4167
cytopathic capability of, 822
in angiosuppressive gene therapy, 783
in herpes simplex virus thymidine kinase gene transfer, 820
as gene therapy vectors, 4166–4167
cytopathic-oncolytic, 822
meningioma from, 1105
multiple sclerosis from, 1449
neuropathy from, 3841–3842
Viscera
lumbar spine and, 4707
nociceptors of, 2921–2922
Vision
afferent aspects of, 301–315

Vision *(Continued)*
disorders of, history of, 301
examination of, 301–302, 302b, 302f–304f, 304–305, 304b
fibrous dysplasia effects on, 1366
Vision loss
in cavernous carotid fistula, 2344
in cerebral palsy, 3728
in olfactory groove meningioma, 1269, 1272f, 1273, 1273f
in optic pathway cavernous malformations, 2314
in orbital tumors, 1371
in pituitary adenoma, 1174
in transsphenoidal surgery, 1182
patient positioning and, 612–614
Vision mapping, 2544–2548
before surgery, 2544–2547, 2545f, 2547f
during surgery, 2547–2548
functional magnetic resonance imaging in, 2544–2546, 2545f
magnetoencephalography in, 2546–2547, 2547f
positron emission tomography in, 2546
visual evoked potential in, 2548
Visual acuity, examination of, 265, 301, 302f
pediatric, 3173
Visual Analogue Scale, 243t
Visual apparatus, in brain tumors, 829
Visual association cortex, 2542
Visual auras, in occipital lobe epilepsy, 2592
Visual cortex, 2542, 2542f
Visual disturbances, 347t
craniopharyngioma and, 1210
Visual evoked potentials, during surgery, 2542–2544, 2543f
Visual field defects
checkerboard, 315
homonymous
occipital lobe lesion and, 315, 315f–316f
temporal lobe lesion and, 314f, 315
temporal lobectomy and, 2610
Visual fields
confrontation testing of, 301, 302b, 303f
examination of, 265, 301–302
pediatric, 3173
left, 2541, 2542f
right, 2541, 2542f
Visual system
afferent
anatomy of, 305, 305f
disorders of, 305–315
anatomy of, 2541–2542, 2542f
efferent, 316–323
anatomy of, 316–317, 316f
disorders of, 317–321
lesions of, 314, 2542
monitoring of, during surgery, 2542–2544, 2543f
retrochiasmal lesions of, 314–315, 314f–316f
Visual-vestibulo-ocular reflex, 346–347
Visuoconstructual abilities, after traumatic brain injury, 5186
Visuomotor function, after traumatic brain injury, 5188
Visuoperceptual abilities, after traumatic brain injury, 5186
Visuospatial abilities, after traumatic brain injury, 5186
Vital signs, pediatric, 3191t
Vitamin A, pseudotumor cerebri from, 1424–1425
Vitamin B deficiency
combined neuronal degeneration/ system disease from, 4321
neuropathy from, 3844
Vitamin D
for osteomalacia, 4236
in bone metabolism, 4232
Vitamin E, for Parkinson's disease, 2733
Vitamin E deficiency
ataxia with, 2738
neuropathy from, 3844
Vitreous hemorrhage, in subarachnoid hemorrhage, 1816
Voiding dysfunction, 365
Vojta technique, for cerebral palsy, 3731
Vomiting, in increased intracranial pressure, 183
Von Economo's encephalitis, obsessive-compulsive disorder in, 2854
Von Hippel-Lindau disease
brain tumors in, 812t, 813
capillary hemangioblastoma in, 671
clear cell renal cell carcinoma in, 1059
genetics of, 1053–1054
hemangioblastoma with, 1053–1054, 1054t
lesions associated with, 1053, 1054t
pheochromocytoma in, 1060
screening for, 1060
Von Hippel-Lindau protein, 1053–1054
Von Hippel's tumor, 1053

Wada test. *See* Intracarotid amobarbital procedure.
Waldeyer's cells, 2924
Waldeyer's sheath, 358
Walker-Warburg syndrome, in parietal encephalocele, 3202
Walking, in cerebral palsy, 3725–3727, 3729–3730, 3733
after selective dorsal rhizotomy, 3743–3744
predictors of, 3739, 3743
Wallenberg's syndrome, 5212
Wallerian degeneration, 3815, 3961
after central nervous system injury, 199, 4156
Warfarin
for carotid artery disease, 1618
putaminal hemorrhage of, 1746, 1748f
Weakness
in critically ill, 5131–5132, 5132f
in neuromuscular junction disorders, 270
in polyneuropathy, 271, 271f
lower motor neuron type, 269
upper motor neuron type vs., 269
spastic, in craniovertebral junction tumors, 4800
Weber's syndrome, 273
Weber's test, 330
Wechsler Adult Intelligence Scale, 242t
after traumatic brain injury, 5185
WeeFIM, 243t
Weight loss
bone health and, 4234–4235
for pseudotumor cerebri, 1429
pain associated with, 4290–4295, 4291t
Welcker's basal angle, 425, 425f
Wellesley wedge, for spinal metastases, 4864f
Werdnig-Hoffman syndrome, 4319
Wernicke-Korsakoff syndrome, 3844
Western blot analysis, 753, 753f
Whiplash, 4915
Whiplash shake syndrome, external hydrocephalus in, 3397, 3397f
Whitaker Grade, 243t
White matter
astrocytes of, 84–85
collateral, in hippocampal sclerosis, 2487
demyelination of, in multiple sclerosis, 1450–1451
glioma spread through, 760
water content of, 3462
Whitehill interspinous wiring modification, 4645, 4646f
Wilson's disease, 2735–2736
[^{11}C]WIN 35,428
Parkinson's disease detection with, 482–483
Windshield wiper eyes, 293
Winking owl sign, in spinal metastases, 4855, 4855t, 4856f
Wire-rod construct, posterior, lumbar, 4733–4734, 4734f
Wires
in occipitocervical fusion, 4659f–4663f, 4660–4661
internal spinal fixation with, 4592, 4592f
cervical spine, 4644–4650, 4645f–4649f
in metastases, 4860, 4860f, 4862, 4864f
with laminectomy, for cervical degenerative disease, 4420–4423, 4422f, 4423f
with laminoforaminotomy, 4416, 4416f, 4417f
sublaminar, complication avoidance in, 582
Wnt, 52
Wnt1, 50, 55t
Wnt3, 55t
Wnt7, 55t
Wnt8, 55t
Wnt8c, 48
Wohlfart-Kugelberg-Welander disease, 4319
Women
carotid artery stenosis in, 1661–1662
pituitary tumors in, 1170
World Federation of Neurological Surgeons Grading Scale, 242t
Wounds, complications of, 564–565
after spinal surgery, 4383–4384
Wyburn-Mason syndrome, 2154–2155

Xanthoastrocytoma, pleomorphic, 988–990
classification of, 663
clinical presentation of, 988
natural history of, 988
outcome of, 990
pathology of, 988–990, 989f
pediatric, 3700, 3701f
pathology of, 3702
proliferation markers for, 700
radiography of, 988
radiologic features of, 844
treatment of, 990
Xanthogranuloma, 1443–1444
cystic, 1444
Xanthoma, 1443
Xenografts, 2829t
as brain tumor invasion model, 764–765

Xenografts *(Continued)*
in central nervous system transplantation, 2841
Xenon computed tomography, 1569–1573
cerebral blood flow calculation with, 1569–1570, 1571f
impact of, 1570, 1572
methodology of, 1569
validation of, 1572–1573, 1573f
X-linked disorders, 273

Yale orthosis, 4899
Yellow ligament, ossification of, in lumbar stenosis, 4526–4527
Yolk sac tumor, 667–668, 667t

Zellweger's syndrome, neuron migration failure and, 81
Zic1, 55t
Zidovudine, blood-brain barrier transport of, 162–163
Zielke ventral derotation spondylodesis, 4684
Zinc finger, 51
Zonula occludens-1 (ZO-1), 156
ZPlate II system, 4686, 4686f
implantation of, 4689–4690, 4689f
Zygapophyseal joint, injury to, 4917
Zygomatic arch, displaced, 5265